AAOS

40th Anniversary
ORANGE BOOK SERIES

Seventh Edition

Nancy Caroline's
Emergency
Care in the Streets

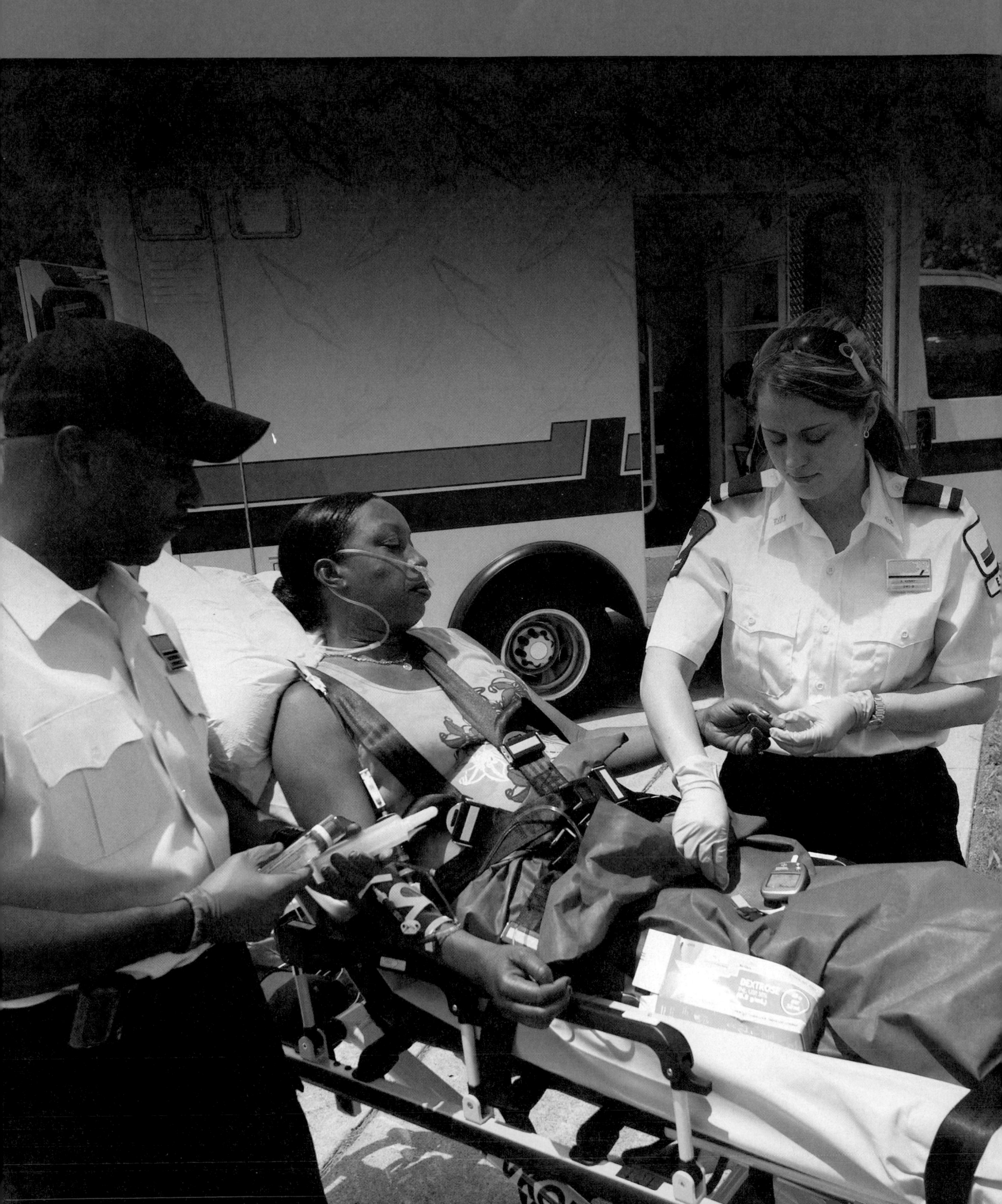

Nancy Caroline's

Emergency
Care in the Streets

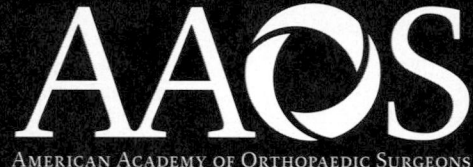

AMERICAN ACADEMY OF ORTHOPAEDIC SURGEONS

Series Editor:

Andrew N. Pollak, MD, FAAOS

Lead Editors:

Bob Elling, MPA, EMT-P

Mike Smith, BS, MICP

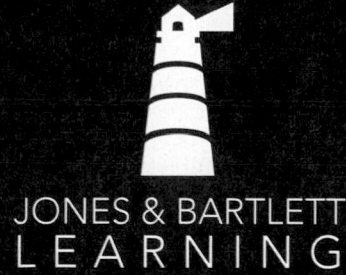

JONES & BARTLETT
LEARNING

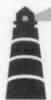

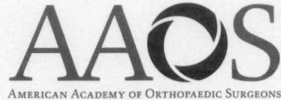

AMERICAN ACADEMY OF ORTHOPAEDIC SURGEONS

World Headquarters
Jones & Bartlett Learning
5 Wall Street
Burlington, MA 01803
978-443-5000
info@jblearning.com
www.jblearning.com

Jones & Bartlett Learning books and products are available through most bookstores and online booksellers. To contact Jones & Bartlett Learning directly, call 800-832-0034, fax 978-443-8000, or visit our website, www.jblearning.com.

Substantial discounts on bulk quantities of Jones & Bartlett Learning publications are available to corporations, professional associations, and other qualified organizations. For details and specific discount information, contact the special sales department at Jones & Bartlett Learning via the above contact information or send an email to specialsales@jblearning.com.

Production Credits:

Chairman, Board of Directors: Clayton Jones
Chief Executive Officer: Ty Field
President: James Homer
SVP, Editor-in-Chief: Michael Johnson
SVP, Chief Technology Officer: Dean Fossella
SVP, Chief Marketing Officer: Alison M. Pendergast
VP, Manufacturing and Inventory Control: Therese Connell
VP, Design and Production: Anne Spencer
Executive Publisher: Kimberly Brophy
Vice President of Sales, Public Safety Group: Matthew Maniscalco
Director of Sales, Public Safety Group: Patricia Einstein
Executive Acquisitions Editor—EMS: Christine Emerton
Managing Editor: Carol B. Guerrero
Editor: Amanda J. Green

Senior Editorial Assistant: Amber Hodge
Editorial Assistant: Carly Lavoie
Production Manager: Jenny L. Corriveau
Production Editor: Jessica deMartin
Associate Production Editor: Nora Menzi
Text Design: Anne Spencer
Cover Design: Kristin E. Parker
Rights and Permissions Manager: Katherine Crighton
Photo Research Supervisor: Anna Genoese
Composition: diacriTech
Cover Image: © Glen E. Ellman
Printing and Binding: Courier Companies
Cover Printing: Courier Companies

The procedures and protocols in this book are based on the most current recommendations of responsible medical sources. The American Academy of Orthopaedic Surgeons and the publisher, however, make no guarantee as to, and assume no responsibility for, the correctness, sufficiency, or completeness of such information or recommendations. Other or additional safety measures may be required under particular circumstances.

This textbook is intended solely as a guide to the appropriate procedures to be employed when rendering emergency care to the sick and injured. It is not intended as a statement of the standards of care required in any particular situation, because circumstances and the patient's physical condition can vary widely from one emergency to another. Nor is it intended that this textbook shall in any way advise emergency personnel concerning legal authority to perform the activities or procedures discussed. Such local determination should be made only with the aid of legal counsel.

Notice: The patients described in "You are the Medic" and "Assessment in Action," throughout this text, are fictitious.

Additional illustrations and photographic credits appear on pages 1479–1480, which constitutes a continuation of the copyright page.

Some images in this book feature models. These models do not necessarily endorse, represent, or participate in the activities represented in the images.

To order this product, use ISBN: 978-1-4496-4586-1

Library of Congress Cataloging-in-Publication Data
Caroline, Nancy L.
    Nancy Caroline's emergency care in the streets. —7th ed. / American Academy of Orthopaedic Surgeons.
        p. ; cm.
    Emergency care in the streets
    Includes index.
    ISBN-13: 978-1-4496-0922-1 (hardcover)
    ISBN-10: 1-4496-0922-8 (hardcover)
    1. Medical emergencies. 2. Emergency medical technicians. I. American Academy of Orthopaedic Surgeons. II. Title. III. Title: Emergency care in the streets.
    [DNLM: 1. Emergency Treatment. 2. Emergency Medical Services. 3. Emergency Medical Technicians. WB 105]
    RC86.7.C38 2012
    616.02'5—dc23
                                    2011017160
6048
Printed in the United States of America
15 14 13 12 11   10 9 8 7 6 5 4 3 2 1

Brief Contents

Contents

Skill Drills

Resources

Instructor Resources

Instructor's ToolKit DVD

ISBN: 978-1-4496-3609-8

The DVD includes:

- PowerPoint presentations with embedded video and animations
- Lecture outlines
- Teaching tips, enhancements, support materials, and preparation guidance
- Student activities and assignments
- Image and table bank
- Skill sheets
- Answers to end-of-chapter student questions

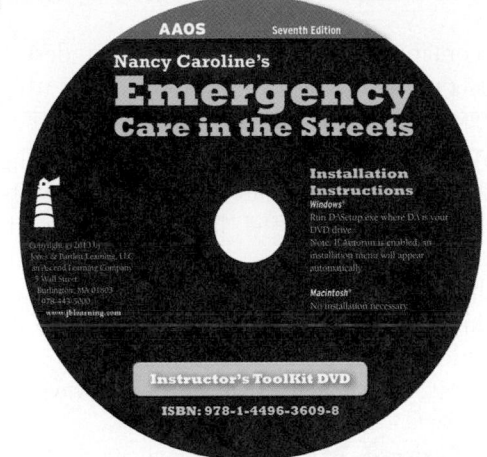

Instructor's TestBank CD

ISBN: 978-1-4496-3688-3

This powerful evaluation tool allows educators to gauge student competency through both general knowledge and critical-thinking questions. Each scenario-based, multiple-choice question is page-referenced to *Nancy Caroline's Emergency Care in the Streets, Seventh Edition*. Educators can originate tailor-made tests quickly and easily by selecting, editing, and printing a test along with an answer key.

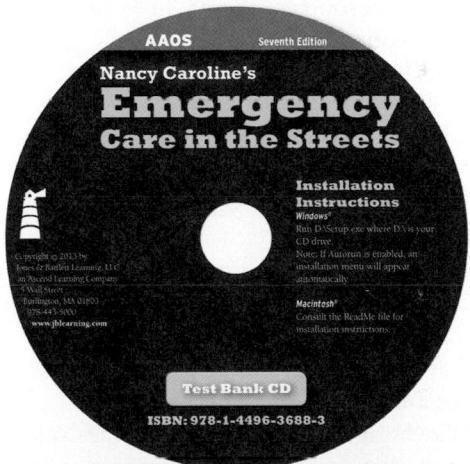

Student Resources

Student Workbook

ISBN: 978-1-4496-0924-5

This resource is designed to encourage critical-thinking and aid comprehension of the course material through a variety of activities:

- Realistic and engaging case studies
- ECG interpretation exercises
- "What would you do?" scenarios
- Skill drill activities
- Anatomy labeling exercises
- Medical vocabulary building exercises
- Complete the Patient Care Report

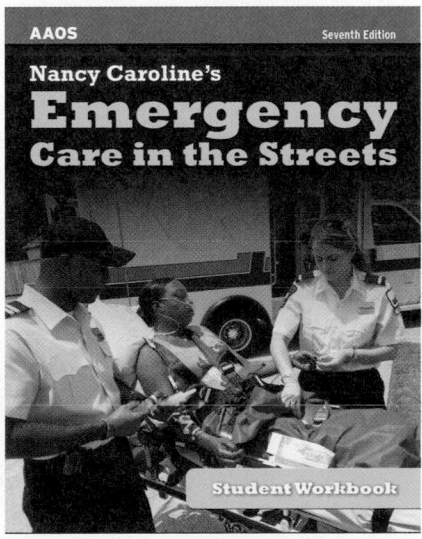

Digital Curriculum Solution Packages

Digital Curriculum Solution Packages allow educators to offer their students cutting-edge digital resources based on world-class medical content. The innovative, multifaceted online tools facilitate absolute understanding—how the human body works, how to apply the patient assessment process, how to be a confident, effective paramedic. This total comprehension and command of the content is the key to success on certification exams and in the field.

Gold standard content joins sound instructional design in a user-friendly online interface to give students a truly interactive, engaging learning experience with:

- **eBook/eWorkbook**: With the content of the *Seventh Edition* at the students' fingertips, students can take notes, listen to 9-1-1 calls, and watch animations and skill videos. Students can then reinforce their general knowledge, hone their critical-thinking skills, and perfect their psychomotor skills in the eWorkbook. The results are recorded in the integrated learning management system, *Navigate Course Manager*.
- **Navigate Course Manager**: Navigate is your complete online classroom environment. In addition to unlocking the resources offered in your package of choice, it is your tool for managing assignments, automatic grading, and classroom discussion.
- **Web Tools**: Unlock additional interactive and mobile educational resources such as a complete audio book, chapter pretests, interactive skill drills, and skill evaluation sheets.
- **Navigate TestPrep**: This dynamic tool is designed to help prepare students for state or national certification examinations by providing practice examinations and simulated certification examinations using case-based questions and detailed rationales.
- **Interactive Lectures**: Take the lectures out of the classroom! Covering the entire scope of the *National EMS Education Standards*, these interactive lectures provide anytime, anywhere access for students to an innovative educational environment.

Available packages include:

Advantage Package Print Edition:
ISBN: 978-1-4496-3817-1

- Printed Textbook
- Printed Student Workbook
- Navigate Course Manager
- Web Tools, including an Audio Book

Advantage Package Digital Edition:
ISBN: 978-1-4496-3818-4

- eBook/eWorkbook
- Navigate Course Manager
- Web Tools, including an Audio Book

Preferred Package:
ISBN: 978-1-4496-3821-4

- Printed Textbook
- Printed Student Workbook (optional)
- eBook/eWorkbook
- Navigate Course Manager
- Web Tools, including an Audio Book
- Navigate TestPrep

Premier Package:
ISBN: 978-1-4496-3822-1

- Printed Textbook
- Printed Student Workbook (optional)
- eBook/eWorkbook
- Navigate Course Manager
- Web Tools, including an Audio Book
- Navigate TestPrep
- Interactive Lectures

www.Paramedic.EMSzone.com
ISBN: 978-1-4496-3778-1

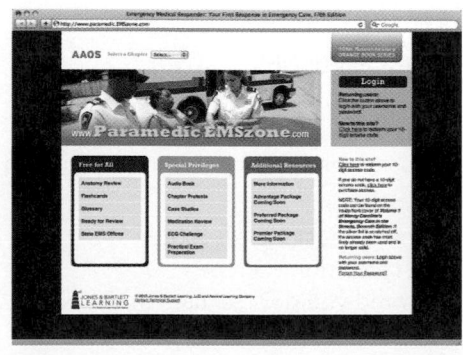

www.Paramedic.EMSzone.com is specifically designed to complement *Nancy Caroline's Emergency Care in the Streets, Seventh Edition.*

This engaging companion website provides a wealth of resources that are free and available to all, including:

- Anatomy Review
- Flashcards
- Glossary
- Ready for Review

The code printed on the front inside cover of this textbook provides students with special user privileges to:

- Audio Book
- Case Studies
- Chapter Pretests
- Practical Exam Preparation Tools
- Much More

Acknowledgments

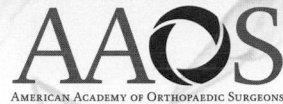 The American Academy of Orthopaedic Surgeons would like to acknowledge the editors, authors, and reviewers of *Nancy Caroline's Emergency Care in the Streets, Seventh Edition.*

Series Editor

Andrew N. Pollak, MD, FAAOS
Professor of Orthopaedics, Head, Division of Orthopaedic Traumatology, University of Maryland School of Medicine
Associate Director of Trauma, R Adams Cowley Shock Trauma Center, University of Maryland Medical Center
Medical Director, Baltimore County Fire Department
Baltimore, Maryland

Lead Editors

Bob Elling, MPA, EMT-P
Albany Medical Center—Clinical Instructor
Colonie EMS Department
Times Union Center EMS
Whiteface Mountain Medical Services
Colonie, New York

Mike Smith, BS, MICP
Program Chair, Lead Instructor, Emergency Medical and Health Services
Tacoma Community College
Tacoma, Washington

Authors

Chapter 1: Don Kimlicka, NREMT-P, CCEMT-P
Director/Field Paramedic
Clintonville Area Ambulance Service
Clintonville, Wisconsin
Field Paramedic
Great Divide Ambulance Service
Cable, Wisconsin

Chapter 1: David Ellis, BS, CCEMT-P, FP-C, CMTE
Program Manager
EagleMed, LLC
Greenville, South Carolina

Chapter 2: Don Kimlicka, NREMT-P, CCEMT-P
Director/Field Paramedic
Clintonville Area Ambulance Service
Clintonville, Wisconsin
Field Paramedic
Great Divide Ambulance Service
Cable, Wisconsin

Chapter 3: Elizabeth M. Wertz Evans, RN, BSN, MPM, FACMPE, CPHQ, CPHIMS, EMT-P, PHRN
Executive Director
Oncology Nursing Society
Pittsburgh, Pennsylvania

Chapter 4: Alan J. Azzara, Esq, EMT-P
EMS Legal and Compliance Consultant
Westport Island, Maine

Chapter 5: Randy E. Price, BS, NREMT-P
Training Manager
Piedmont Medical Center EMS
Rockhill, South Carolina

Chapter 6: Bryan Ware, EMT-P
Chief of EMS
Beulah, Colorado

Chapter 7: Nicholas J. Montelauro, AAS, NREMT-P, FP-C, NCEE
Trans-Care Ambulance
Terre Haute, Indiana

Chapter 8: Hugh Skerker
Troy, New York

Chapter 8: Bob Elling, MPA, EMT-P
Albany Medical Center—Clinical Instructor
Colonie EMS Department
Times Union Center EMS
Whiteface Mountain Medical Services
Colonie, New York

■ Authors continued

Chapter 9: Howard E. Huth, III, BA, EMT-P, CIC
Director
SUNY Cobleskill Paramedic Program
Cobleskill, New York
Paramedic Supervisor
Albany County Sheriff's Office EMS Unit
Voorheesville, New York

Chapter 10: Andrew Bartkus, RN, MSN, JD, CEN, CCRN, CFRN, NREMT-P, FP-C
Lifeguard Air Emergency Services
Albuquerque, New Mexico

Chapter 11: Keith Widmeier, NREMT-P, CCEMT-P, BS
Wayne County EMS
Monticello, Kentucky

Chapter 12: Michael D. Hummel, NREMT-P, I/C
Lead ALS Instructor/Clinical Coordinator
East Bay Medical Educators
Bristol, Rhode Island

Chapter 13: Alan W. Heckman, MSPAS, PA-C, NREMT-P, NCEE
Department of Emergency Medicine
Lehigh Valley Health Network
Allentown, Pennsylvania

Chapter 13: Mike Smith, BS, MICP
Program Chair, Lead Instructor, Emergency Medical and Health Services
Tacoma Community College
Tacoma, Washington

Chapter 14: Mike Smith, BS, MICP
Program Chair, Lead Instructor, Emergency Medical and Health Services
Tacoma Community College
Tacoma, Washington

Chapter 15: Stephen J. Rahm, NREMT-P
EMS Specialist/Faculty
Department of Emergency Health Sciences
University of Texas Health Science Center at San Antonio
San Antonio, Texas

Chapter 16: Charles D. Bortle, EdD, RRT, NREMT-P
Director, Center for Clinical Competency
Albert Einstein Medical Center
Philadelphia, Pennsylvania

Chapter 17: Scott J. Corcoran, BS, EMT-P
Erie Community College
Orchard Park, New York

Chapter 17: Christopher Touzeau, MS, RN, NREMT-P
Montgomery County Fire and Rescue
Rockville, Maryland

Chapter 18: Charles Sowerbrower, MEd, NREMT-P, CCP-C
Sinclair Community College
Dayton, Ohio

Chapter 19: William N. Martin, NREMT-P, CCT-P, CIC
North Country Life Flight
Saranac Lake, New York

Chapter 19: Bob Elling, MPA, EMT-P
Albany Medical Center—Clinical Instructor
Colonie EMS Department
Times Union Center EMS
Whiteface Mountain Medical Services
Colonie, New York

Chapter 19: Randy E. Price, BS, NREMT-P
Training Manager
Piedmont Medical Center EMS
Rockhill, South Carolina

Chapter 20: Charles Sowerbrower, MEd, NREMT-P, CCP-C
Sinclair Community College
Dayton, Ohio

Chapter 21: George E. Perry, EdD, NREMT-P
Vice President of Instruction
Blue Ridge Community and Technical College
Martinsburg, West Virginia

Chapter 22: Carol Gupton, BS, NREMT-P
Emergency Provider Instruction
Omaha, Nebraska

Chapter 23: Leaugeay C. Barnes, MS, CCEMT-P, NREMT-P
Oklahoma City Community College
Oklahoma City, Oklahoma

Chapter 24: David Ellis, BS, CCEMT-P, FP-C, CMTE
Program Manager
EagleMed LLC
Greenville, South Carolina

Chapter 25: Ann Bellows, RN, NREMTP, EdD
Outreach Education Opportunities
Las Cruces, New Mexico

Authors continued

Chapter 26: Katherine West, BSN, MSEd, CIC
Infection Control Consultant
Infection Control/Emerging Concepts, Inc.
Manassas, Virginia

Chapter 27: Mike Smith, BS, MICP
Program Chair, Lead Instructor, Emergency Medical and
Health Services
Tacoma Community College
Tacoma, Washington

Chapter 28: Chris Stratford, MS, BSN, RN, EMT
University of Utah, Center for Emergency Programs
Salt Lake City, Utah

Contributors

Andrew Bartkus, RN, MSN, JD, CEN, CCRN, CFRN, NREMT-P, FP-C
Lifeguard Air Emergency Services
Albuquerque, New Mexico

Rhonda J. Beck, NREMT-P
EMT/Paramedic Instructor
Darton College
Albany, Georgia
Crisp Regional EMS
Cordele, Georgia

Anthony Caliguire, Lieutenant REMT-P
Scotia Fire Department
Scotia, New York
Paramedic Instructor Coordinator
Hudson Valley Community College Paramedic Program
Troy, New York

Julie Chase, BS, NCEE, NREMT-P, FP-C
Virginia Airborne Search and Rescue Squad
Berryville, Virginia

Patty Maher, MPA, EMTP
Professor/Assistant Chair—EMS
Daytona State College
Daytona Beach, Florida

Jeanine Newton-Riner, EdD(s), MHSA, RRT, EMT-P
Operations Manager
CoastalEMS
Savannah, Georgia

Reviewers

James "Bud" Adams, AAS, NREMT-P
College of Southern Nevada
Las Vegas, Nevada

Sean M. Ahlers, MS, NREMT-P
Emergency Training Associates
Fargo, North Dakota

William Allen
National College of Technical
Instruction
Natick, Massachusetts

Linda V. Anderson, RN, BSN
Santa Rosa Junior College
Windsor, California

Deborah Baert
Kishwaukee Community Hospital
Genoa, Illinois

Blance Keith Bankston, NREMT-P
EMS Coordinator
LSU Fire and Emergency Training
Institute
Baton Rouge, Louisiana

Robin E. Bishop, BA, MICP, CHS III, MEP, DOIC
Crafton Hills College
Yucaipa, California

Tim Bobbitt, EMT, Paramedic
St. Charles County Ambulance
District
Florissant, Missouri

Barbara Booton, NREMT-P, EMS IC
Emergency Education
Brookings, South Dakota

Terry Brandt, NREMT-P
Montana State University—Great Falls
Great Falls, Montana

Lynn Browne-Wagner, MSN, RN
EMS Program Director
Northland Pioneer College
Holbrook, Arizona

Aaron R. Byington, MA, NREMT-P
Captain, Layton City Fire
Layton, Utah

Anthony Caliguire, REMT-P
Paramedic Instructor Coordinator
Hudson Valley Community College
Troy, New York

Wesley Carter, AAS, NREMT-P
Lenoir Community College
Kinston, North Carolina

Reviewers continued

Matthew G. Cassavechia, EMT-P
Director, Emergency Medical Services
Western Connecticut Health Care
Network
Danbury, Connecticut

Chris Chadwick, EMT-P
Training Officer
Shreveport Fire Academy
Shreveport, Louisiana

Brian Chamberlin, BS, FF/EMT-P
Atlantic Partners EMS/Kennebec
Valley Community College
Winslow, Maine

Russ Christiansen, NREMT-P,
CCEMTP
Paramedic Technology Program
Director
Casper College
Casper, Wyoming

Scott Cook, BAS, CCEMT-P
Southern Maine Community College
South Portland, Maine

Michael Crabtree, EMT-P/LI
McLean County Area EMS System
Bloomington, Illinois

Rocky E. Cramer, BS, MICT
Instructor/Coordinator
Paramedic Director
Flint Hills Technical College
Emporia, Kansas

Mike Cronin, EMT-P
EMS Coordinator/Paramedic Instructor
Mount Vernon Fire Department
Mount Vernon, Ohio

Rich Dandridge, BA, EMT-P
Training Officer
Warren County Ambulance District
Warrenton, Missouri

Tom Duffee, BA, EMT-B
EMS Program Coordinator
Clark State Community College
Springfield, Ohio

Dietrich Easter
UpState EMS Council/Jennings
Medcare
Easley, South Carolina

William Faust, MPA, NREMT-P
Gaston College
Gastonia, North Carolina

Patrick Flaherty, BS, NREMT-P
Sandy Springs Fire Rescue
Sandy Springs, Georgia

Mark Forgues, MEd, EMT-P
Massachusetts Institute of Technology
Cambridge, Massachusetts

Scott Frasard, PhD, EMT-P
Cardinal Health
Albuquerque, New Mexico

Robert Galligher, NREMTP
Supervisor/Education Coordinator
Vital Link EMS
Batesville, Arkansas

Leroy M. Garcia Jr, MAOM-L,
NREMT-P
Pueblo Community College
Pueblo, Colorado

David Glendenning, EMT-P
Field Training Officer
New Hanover Regional EMS
Cape Fear Community College
Wilmington, North Carolina

Doug Goodwin, AS, NREMT-P
Cleveland Community College
Shelby, North Carolina

Grant Goold, EdD
American River College
Sacramento, California

Karen Beasley Grabenstein,
NREMT-P, CICP
Training Officer
Bulloch County EMS
Statesboro, Georgia

Gary Green, EMT-P, EMS-I
Assistant Chief-EMS
Madison Township Fire Department
Newark,Ohio
Instructor
Mid-East Career and Technology
Center
Zanesville, Ohio

Jeffrey R. Grunow, MSN, NREMT-P
Associate Professor—Chair
Emergency Care & Rescue
Department
Weber State University
Ogden, Utah

Marisa Hanson, CCP/LP
Clinical Coordinator, MedStar EMS
Fort Worth, Texas

William E. Hathaway, BS, CC/
NREMT-P, VEMS I/C
Executive Director
Bennington Rescue Squad, Inc.
Bennington, Vermont

Gregg L. Heller, AS, CCEMT-P,
NREMT-P
Paramedic Program Coordinator
Ada County Paramedics
Boise, Idaho

Joel Henderson, AAS, NREMT-P,
CCEMTP
Program Director of EMS
Montana State University Great Falls
Great Falls, Montana

Lynn Henley, NREMT-P I/C
Director of Education & QA
AHA TC Coordinator
AAA Ambulance Service
Hattiesburg, Mississippi

Thomas R. Herron Jr, AAS,
NREMT-P
EMS Coordinator
Cape Fear Community College
Wilmington, North Carolina

Jeremy R. Hill, NREMT-P,
CCEMT-P, Level II Paramedic
Instructor, AAS
Lenoir Community College
Kinston, North Carolina

Mark Hollinger, RN, MICN, EMT
Educator and Consultant,
Department of Emergency Medicine,
Los Angeles County/USC Medical
Center
Senior Instructor, Los Angeles
County College of Nursing and
Allied Health
Los Angeles, California

Mark A. Huckaby, NREMT-P
EMS Coordinator, Grant Medical
Center LifeLink
Columbus, Ohio

Reviewers continued

James B. Huettenmueller, BS Ed, NREMTP
EMS Program Clinical Coordinador
Tulsa Tech
Tulsa, Oklahoma

Derek Hunt, NR/CCEMT-P, PNCCT, FP-C
ShandsCair
Shands at the University of Florida
Gainesville, Florida

Charlene Jansen, BS, MM, EMT-P
Mineral Area College
Park Hills, Missouri

Chad E. Jarvis, CCEMT-P
Rockingham Community College
Wentworth, North Carolina

Brian E. Johns, CCEMT-P, I/C
Lifestar EMS/Tri-State EMS Educators
West Ossipee, New Hampshire

Jay Johns, NREMTP, BSEd
EMS Educator, Memorial Hospital
Paramedic Program
EMS Educator, Southwestern Illinois
College EMS Program
Belleville, Illinois
Paramedic, Washington County
Ambulance
Nashville, Illinois

Janelle Johnson
Paramedic/Instructor
Metropolitan Emergency Medical
Service
Little Rock, Arkansas

Sue A. Kartman, CCEMT-P
EMS Instructor/Coordinator
WITC (Wisconsin Indianhead
Technical College)
MATC Madison
Madison, Wisconsin

Michael Keller, BS, NREMT-P
Gaston College, Department for EMS
Education
Gastonia, North Carolina

Timothy M. Kimble, NREMT-P
EMS Lieutenant
Fauquier County Department of Fire
Rescue & Emergency Management
Warrenton, Virginia

Karla Kimlicka, PTA, EMT-B
EMT-Basic
Great Divide Ambulance Service
Cable, Wisconsin

David J. Kleiman, NREMT-P, CCEMT-P
Paramedic Instructor
Chattahoochee Technical
College – North Metro Campus
Acworth, Georgia

Amy Krueger, NREMT-P
Jerome County Paramedics
Twin Falls, Idaho

Steven C. LeCroy, Sr, MA, NREMTP, CRTT
St. Petersburg College
St. Petersburg, Florida

Mary Levy, EMS RN
Clark County Unified Paramedic
Program
Las Vegas, Nevada

Scott Lindberg, NREMT-P
Faculty EMS Instructor
Hennepin Technical College
Eden Prairie, Minnesota

Kristina A. Long, NREMT-P, BAS
Program Director, Paramedicine
Flathead Valley Community College
Kalispell, Montana

Patty Maher, MPA, EMTP
Daytona State College
Daytona Beach, Florida

Norman D. "Chip" Mainville
New England Emergency Medical
Training
Harrisville, Rhode Island

Connie J. Mattera, MS, RN, EMT-P
EMS Administrative Director
Northwest Community EMS System
Arlington Heights, Illinois

James McCarragher, RN, MSN, NREMT-B, New Hampshire EMS Instructor/Coordinator
Cornish Rescue Squad
Cornish, New Hampshire

Timothy L. McCawley, AAS, NREMT-P
Bennett Fire Protection District # 7
Bennett, Colorado

Lynette McCullough, MCH, NREMT-P
EMS Program Director
Southern Crescent Technical College
Griffin, Georgia

Jeffrey J. McGovern, NREMT-P, CCEMT-P, EMS-I
APLS Program Coordinator
Lead Paramedic Instructor
New Haven Sponsor Hospital
Program
New Haven, Connecticut

Richard Meadows, EMT-P, RN, CCRN, BA, NCEE
Kanawha County Emergency Ambulance Authority Paramedic Program
Charleston, West Virginia

Dean C. Meenach, RN, BSN, CEN, CCRN, CPEN, EMT-P
Director of EMS Education
Mineral Area College
Park Hills, Missouri

Antoinette Melton-Tharrett, NREMT-P, Level III Kentucky Paramedic Instructor
Air-Evac Lifeteam
Albany, Kentucky

Lawrence "Lars" Mester, NREMT-P, EMT-T
Lakes Region General Hospital
Laconia, New Hampshire

Nicholas J. Montelauro, AAS, NREMT-P, FP-C, NCEE
Trans-Care Ambulance
Terre Haute, Indiana

William Montrie, AAS, EMT-P
Academic Program Chair – EMM/
FST, Owens Community College
Toledo, Ohio
Captain-Paramedic, Springfield
Township Fire Department
Holland, Ohio

Patrick M. Mroczek, EMT-P
Ret Field Chief, Chgo Fire Dept
Didactic Coordinator,
Malcolm X College
Chicago, Illinois

Angel J. Nater, MS, EMT-P
Seminole State College
Sanford, Florida

Reviewers continued

Gregory S. Neiman, BA, NREMT-P, CEMA (VA)
Virginia Office of EMS
Glen Allen, Virginia

Brad Newbury, AAS/NREMT-P I/C
Director
National Medical Education &
Training Center
West Bridgewater, Massachusetts

SGT Earl K. Newman III, NREMT-P, CCEMTP, Flight Medic
Rhode Island Army National Guard
Quonset Air National Guard Base
North Kingstown, Rhode Island

B. Jeanine Newton-Riner, EdD(s), MHSA, RRT, EMT-P
CoastalEMS
Savannah, Georgia

Laurie Oelslager, EdD, NREMT-P
South Central College
North Mankato, Minnesota

Mary Anne Pace, MPH, EMT
Education Program Manager
Ada County Paramedics
Boise, Idaho

Erica Marie Paredes, EMT, MBA, Clinical Specialist
Snowy River EMS Productions LLC
Phoenix, Arizona

Chad A. Parlier, AAS, NREMTP, CCEMTP
Davidson County CommunityCollege
Lexington, North Carolina

Christopher Patrello, BS, EMT-P I/C
Livingston County EMS
Howell, Michigan

Allen O. Patterson, BS, NREMT-P, LP, CCP, EMSC
National College of Technical
Instruction—Livermore
Livermore, California

Corey S. Pittman, NREMT-P, CCEMT-P, AASc-EMS, I/C
Mayland Community College
Spruce Pine, North Carolina

Kerry Sousa Pomelow, Paramedic, Education Coordinator
Maine EMS
Canaan, Maine

Lionel Powell, EMT-P
Crestview Medical Group
Salt Lake City, Utah

M. E. (Eddie) Pyle, RN, Paramedic
LSU Fire and Emergency Training
Institute
Baton Rouge, Louisiana

Sean C. Ralston, BS, NREMT-P, CCEMT-P
Regional EMS Coordinator
Maniilaq EMS
Kotzebue, Alaska

Mark J. Reed, EMT-Paramedic, NREMT-P
Emergency Medical Services Instructor, Portland Community College
Lieutenant/Paramedic, Retired,
Columbia River Fire & Rescue
Portland, Oregon

Louis Robinson, MS, NREMT-P
Kanawha Valley Community and
Technical College
Institute, West Virginia

Anthony Rowley, EMT-P
All State Career School
Lansdowne, Pennsylvania

Joseph J. Rubino, EMT-P, I/C
Course Coordinator, Instructor
Denton Township EMS Education
Prudenville, Michigan

Jennifer Russell, Paramedic
Bellingham, Washington

Ian T.T. Santee, MICT, MPA
Kapiolani Community College
Honolulu, Hawaii

Chris Schultz, MHA, NREMT-P, CMTE
Hennepin Technical College
Eden Prairie, Minnesota

Richard Shok, BSN, RN, EMS-I
Owner and Director
Code One Medical Solutions, LLC
Code One Training Solutions, LLC
East Hartford, Connecticut

Gursarn Singh, BS
EMS Director
University of Arkansas at Monticello
College of Technology, McGehee
McGehee, Arkansas

Alonzo W. Smith, BA, NREMT-P
Richland County Emergency Services
Department
Columbia, South Carolina

Shadrach Smith, BS Bio, Paramedic
Program Director and Lead
Instructor, Paramedic Advantage
Orange, California

George B. Snyder, BCJ, NREMT-P, CHEP, EMS-I/T
Director and Lead Instructor/EMS
Coordinator, The Institute for
Prehospital Care – Trumbull
Memorial Hospital
Warren, Ohio
Fire Chief, Burghill Vernon Fire
Department
Kinsman, Ohio

David Tauber, NREMT-P, CCEMT-P, FP-C, NCEE
Education Director, New Haven
Sponsor Hospital Program
New, Haven Connecticut
Executive Director, Advanced Life
Support Institute
Conway, New Hampshire

James A. Temple, BA, NREMT-P, CCP
EMS Coordinator EICC
Eastern Iowa Community Colleges
Davenport, Iowa

Elizabeth A. Tomyl, EMT-P
National College of Technical
Instruction
Natick, Massachusetts

Wayne D. Turner, EMT-P, EMSI
Cincinnati State Technical and
Community College
Cincinnati, Ohio

Eric Victorin, MBA, EMT-B (I)
The Valley Hospital Emergency
Medical Services
Ridgewood, New Jersey

Reviewers continued

Susan Vigh, MEd, BSRRT, NREMTP, EMSI
Polaris Career Center and Auburn Career Center
Middleburg Heights, Ohio

Carl Voskamp, LicP
Victoria College
Victoria, Texas

Michael L. Wallace, MPA, EMT-P, CCEMT-P
Central Jackson County Fire Protection District
Blue Springs, Missouri

Mark Warth, NREMT-P
EMS Training Coordinator
North Suburban Medical Center
Thornton, Colorado

Eric A. Wellman, BS, NREMT-P, CCEMTP
Southern Maine Community College
South Portland, Maine

Michael Wells, NREMT-P, CCEMT-P, CCP-C, BBA
Emergency Training Solutions
Mount Carmel, Tennessee

Richard C. Wilkinson, II, NRP, ALEM
Priority Medical Training
Harvest, Alabama

Monroe Yancie, AAS, EMTP
Primary Paramedic Instructor
IHM Academy of EMS
St. Louis, Missouri

David A. Young, BS, NREMT-P
Coordinator/Instructor EMS Programs
Western Piedmont Community College
Morganton, North Carolina

 ## Photoshoot Acknowledgements

We would like to thank the following people and institutions for their collaboration on the photoshoots for this project. Their assistance was greatly appreciated.

Medical Advisor: Anthony Caliguire, Lieutenant REMT-P
Scotia Fire Department
Scotia, New York
Paramedic Instructor Coordinator
Hudson Valley Community College
Paramedic Program
Troy, New York

Medical Advisor: Guy Peifer, EMT-P
Director of Paramedic Education
Borough of Manhattan Community College
City University of New York
New York, New York

Medical Advisor: Keith Widmeier, NREMT-P, CCEMT-P, BS
Wayne County EMS
Monticello, Kentucky

Baltimore City Fire Department
Baltimore, Maryland

Karly Biddison
Glen Arm, Maryland

Damian L. Briscoe
Baltimore, Maryland

Christopher Franklin
Sykesville, Maryland

Travis Frazier
Baltimore, Maryland

Anthony Goldman
Baltimore, Maryland

Neil Holmes
Baltimore, Maryland

John R. Morris, IV
West Grove, Pennsylvania

Michael Norris
Baltimore, Maryland

Sarah Sette
Baltimore, Maryland

Ashley Slack
Elkridge, Maryland

Brian Slack
Maryland Institute of Emergency Medical Services Systems
Baltimore, Maryland

Larry Smith
Laurel, Maryland

Tina M. Stoltz
Preston, Maryland

Ronn Wade
Director, Anatomical Services Division
University of Maryland School of Medicine
Director, State Anatomy Board
Maryland Department of Health and Mental Hygiene
Baltimore, Maryland

Kyle Walcott
Baltimore, Maryland

A. Michael Walker, II, NREMT, CHSS, TCC
Kenova Fire-Rescue
Kenova, West Virginia

Juan Wilson
Baltimore, Maryland

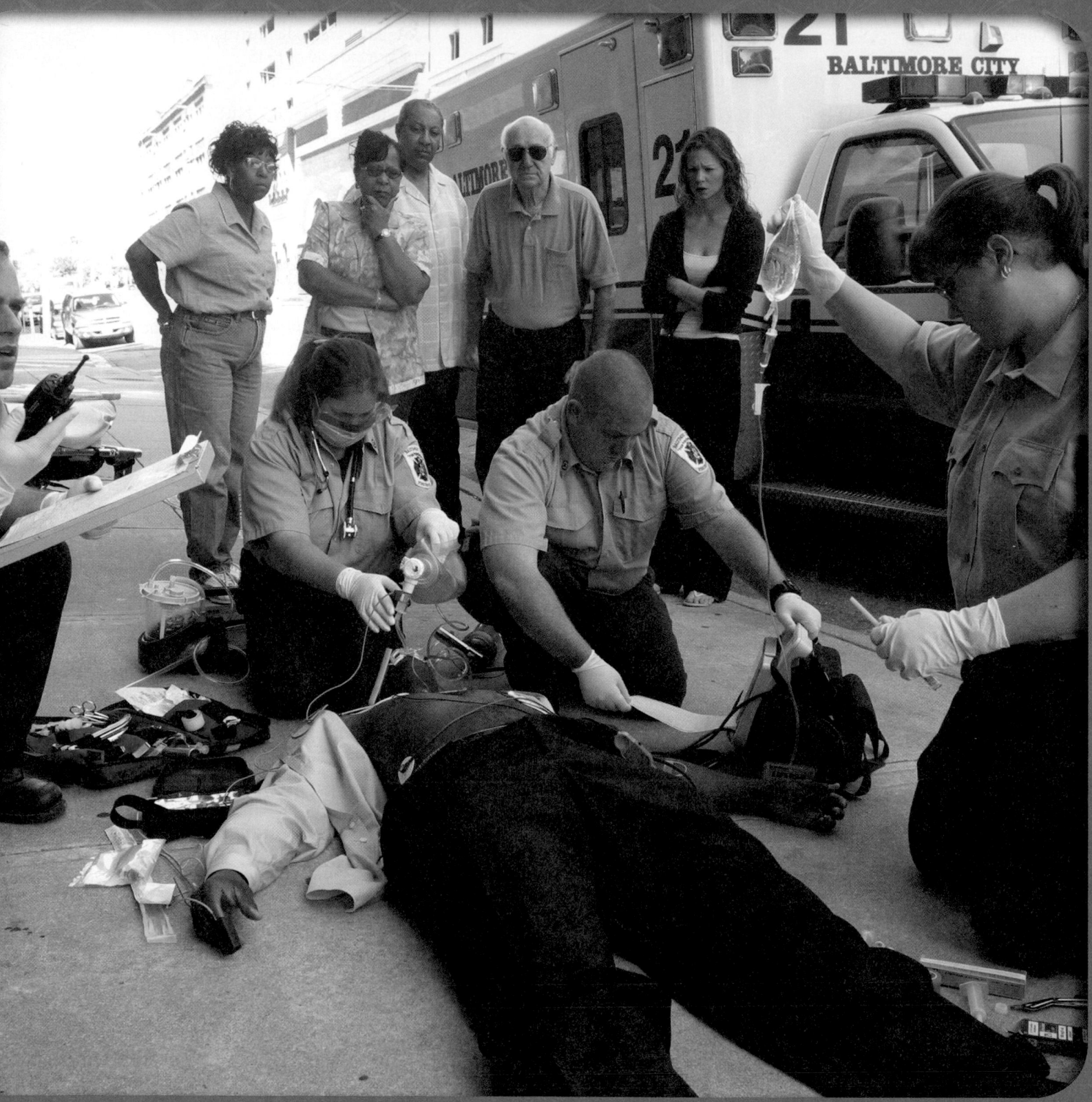

EMS Systems

National EMS Education Standard Competencies

Preparatory

Integrates comprehensive knowledge of the EMS system, safety/well-being of the paramedic, and medical/legal and ethical issues which is intended to improve the health of EMS personnel, patients, and the community.

Emergency Medical Services (EMS) Systems

- EMS systems (p 5)
- History of EMS (pp 5-6)
- Roles/responsibilities/professionalism of EMS personnel (pp 15-19)
- Quality improvement (pp 19-21)
- Patient safety (p 18)

Research

- Impact of research on emergency medical responder (EMR) care (p 21)
- Data collection (pp 22-23)
- Evidence-based decision making (p 25)
- Research principles to interpret literature and advocate evidence-based practice (pp 24-25)

Knowledge Objectives

1. List key developments in the history of EMS. (pp 5-8)
2. List the five main types of services that provide emergency care. (p 10)
3. Discuss the processes of licensure and certification. (pp 8-9)
4. Define reciprocity and explain its relevance to the practice of emergency care. (pp 9-10)
5. Discuss the role of the National Scope of Practice and the *National EMS Education Standards* as they relate to the levels of EMS education. (pp 10-12)
6. Discuss the critical points, required components, and system elements of EMS. (p 7)

7. Describe the levels of EMS education in terms of skill sets needed for each of the following: EMR, EMT, AEMT, and paramedic. (pp 11-12)
8. Describe various types of transports the paramedic may perform, including transports to specialty centers and interfacility transports. (p 13)
9. Discuss the paramedic's role in working with other health care providers and public safety agencies. (pp 13-14)
10. Discuss initial paramedic education and the importance of continuing education. (pp 12-13)
11. Describe the attributes that a paramedic is expected to possess. (pp 15-17)
12. Describe the roles and responsibilities of the paramedic. (pp 17-19)
13. Discuss issues relating to the appropriate method of transport, as well as non-transport situations. (pp 13, 18)
14. Describe how medical direction of an EMS system works and the paramedic's role in the process. (p 19)
15. Characterize the EMS system's role in prevention and public education in the community. (pp 16, 18-19, 23)
16. Discuss the purpose of the EMS continuous quality improvement (CQI) process. (pp 19-21)
17. Discuss examples of how errors can be prevented when providing EMS care. (p 21)
18. Discuss the importance of medical research and its role in refining EMS practices. (pp 21-22)
19. Define peer-reviewed literature and describe how this relates to a practicing paramedic. (p 24)
20. List and define types of research and subtypes within each category. (pp 22-23)
21. Discuss ethical considerations relating to conducting medical research. (pp 23-24)
22. Discuss evidence-based medicine and how to incorporate this concept into everyday paramedic practice. (p 25)

Skills Objectives

There are no skills objectives for this chapter.

Introduction

The <u>emergency medical services (EMS)</u> system continues to evolve. In the early days, a responder was called to a location for people who were ill or injured and simply transported them rapidly to a medical facility; this was often called "scoop and swoop" or "load and go." Because of the awareness of our communities and findings in research, society's expectations of an emergency medical provider have changed significantly. As a paramedic, you will encounter many different situations. Some will involve caring for very basic needs such as lending an ear to a person who needs a listener. Other situations will involve you assessing and treating any number of life-threatening conditions **Figure 1**. The public's perception of you will often be compared

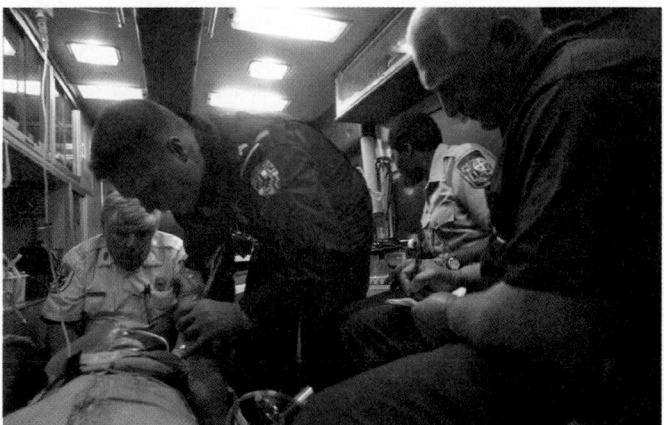

Figure 1 Today's prehospital care professionals are highly trained to provide a wide variety of medical services to the public.

with what is seen on television and read in published articles; it will also be based on your treatment of their loved ones. As you move forward in your education and career, you must always be ready for change because EMS continually evolves. Continued education is a must; what you learn today may not be the same expectation tomorrow. Remember to treat all people you encounter with respect and dignity. These people may be in the worst situation they have ever been exposed to in their lives.

EMS System Development

The History of EMS

Far back in history, you can find information that relates to the development of organized emergency medical services. The first recorded use of an ambulance was by the military during the Siege of Malaga in 1485. This was strictly a transport and no medical care was provided. During the 1800s, EMS started to make some headway with the following key developments:

- 1800s–Napoleon designated a vehicle and attendant to care for injuries on the battlefield
- 1860–The first recorded use of a medic/ambulance combination in the United States
- 1865–The first civilian ambulance came out of the Commercial Hospital in Cincinnati, Ohio
- 1869–The first ambulance service was started out of Bellevue Hospital in New York, New York
- 1899–The first operated automobile-type ambulance came out of Michael Reese Hospital in Chicago

The 1900s continued to see the evolution of EMS with minor changes occurring between World Wars I and II. In this time frame, a major shift occurred; because of a lack of manpower resulting from the wars, many hospital-based ambulance

YOU are the Medic   PART 1

At 1618 you are dispatched to the 300 block of Hunt Road for a crash involving a single vehicle and a motorcycle; you advise the dispatcher that you are en route. Three minutes later as you are nearing the crash scene, you notice a car sitting diagonally across the road and a motorcycle lying on its side about 20′ farther up from the car. You note fluid running from underneath the car and no one is inside the vehicle. A crowd of bystanders is gathered at a driveway and a man is holding a motorcycle helmet. You think this may be the rider until the man steps to the side of the crowd and you see someone lying supine on the ground. You also note two women who are trying to talk to a girl who appears to be in her late teens or early twenties; she is screaming hysterically. No other public safety agencies have arrived on scene.

As you exit the ambulance and approach the scene, you see that there is damage to the right front fender and the passenger door of the car. The man holding the helmet turns and calls to you to hurry. He tells you that he was driving the car and that he is fine, but that the motorcycle rider is "hurt bad."

1. What is your first action as you are approaching the scene and conducting a scene size-up?

2. What role does the EMS system play in this call?

services were shut down. Some key developments before 1950 included the following:

- 1926–Phoenix Fire Department adds service similar to present-day EMS
- 1928–Julien Stanley Wise launched the first rescue squad out of Roanoke, Virginia called Roanoke Life Saving Crew
- 1940s–Because of a shortage of medical personnel, the role of EMS was turned over to fire and police departments. Unfortunately, there were no minimum training standards set. Also, the role of providing emergency care was not always immediately accepted or welcomed.

The 20th Century and Modern Technology

After World War II and into the 1950s and 1960s, EMS began to make major strides forward. During the 1950s and the Korean War, military medical researchers recognized that bringing the hospital closer to the field might give patients a better chance of surviving. Helicopters were first used in 1951 during the Korean War. They brought patients to Mobile Army Surgical Hospitals (M*A*S*H units), which helped thousands of soldiers and civilians survive Figure 2 . In 1956, mouth-to-mouth resuscitation was developed by Drs Elan and Safar. The first portable defibrillator was developed by Johns Hopkins Hospital around this same time.

In the late 1950s and early 1960s, however, the focus moved back to bringing the hospital to the patient in some European countries. **Mobile intensive care units (MICUs)** were developed and staffed by specially trained physicians. This concept quickly spread to the United States, but US physicians were in short supply, and physicians who were interested had minimal expertise in the prehospital area. Some physicians then asked "Can a person who is not a physician be trained to perform advanced medical skills?" The answer was "Yes."

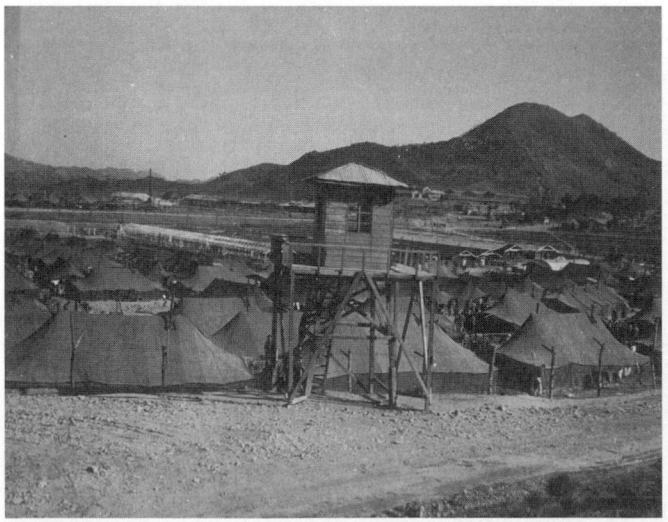

Figure 2 Temporary hospitals, such as this one in use during the Korean War, were set up to provide more rapid care for the injured.

In 1965 the National Academy of Science and the National Research Council released "The White Paper" or "Accidental Death and Disability: The Neglected Disease of Modern Society." Some of the findings in this white paper include the following:

- A lack of uniform laws and standards
- Ambulances and equipment were of poor quality
- Lack of communication between EMS and hospitals
- Lack of personnel training
- Hospitals only had part-time staff
- More people died in motor vehicle accidents than in the Vietnam war

From these findings, the white paper outlined 10 critical points for a functioning system. From these points the National Highway Safety Act was instituted in 1966. In this act the US Department of Transportation (US DOT) was created to provide authority and financial support for the development of basic and advanced life support programs. In 1968, the Task Force of the Committee of EMS drafted basic training standards, and 9-1-1 was created. Table 1 lists the critical points, required components, and system elements of EMS that ultimately developed as a result of publication of The White Paper.

In 1969, a year after basic training standards were developed, Dr Eugene Nagel, then of Miami, Florida, began training fire fighters from the Miami Fire Department with advanced emergency skills, thus creating the first true paramedic program Figure 3 . Dr Nagel took the use of advanced emergency treatment one step further. He developed a telemetry system that enabled fire fighters to transmit a patient's electrocardiogram to physicians at Jackson Memorial Hospital and to receive radio instructions from the physicians regarding what measures to take. Dr Nagel is often called the "Father of Paramedicine." Additionally in 1969, standards for ambulance design and equipment were published.

During the 1970s, advancements continued, helicopters became more available, and the National Registry of Emergency Medical Technicians (NREMT) began. The first EMT textbook, *Emergency Care and Transportation of the Sick and Injured*, was published by the American Academy of Orthopaedic Surgeons (AAOS) in 1971. In that same year, the AAOS began training EMTs nationwide through a national workshop. The first television-based program focused on EMS, *Emergency*, started a very successful 8-year run. In 1973 the Emergency Medical Services System Act defined 15 required components of an EMS system, listed in Table 1, with emphasis on regional development and trauma care. The act provided a structure and uniformity to the EMS system that came out of pioneering programs in Miami, Seattle, and Pittsburgh, and the Illinois Trauma System (Dr David Boyd). In 1974, after a federal report disclosed that less than half of ambulance personnel completed sufficient training, guidelines were published for the development and implementation of EMS systems. In 1975, the American Medical Association recognized emergency medicine as its own specialty branch of medicine. Many cities set up individual advanced EMS training, and regions added their own spin to what they thought was the essential standard of care, but it was not until 1977 that the first National Standard Curriculum for

Table 1 Critical Points, Required Components, and System Elements of EMS

Year	Source	Item
1966	The White Paper	Critical points for a functioning EMS system: 1. Develop collaborative strategies to identify and address community health and safety issues 2. Align the financial incentives of EMS and other health care providers and payers 3. Participate in community-based prevention efforts 4. Develop and pursue a national EMS research agenda 5. Pass EMS legislation in each state to support innovation and integration 6. Allocate adequate resources for medical direction 7. Develop information systems that link EMS across its continuum 8. Determine the costs and benefits of EMS to the community 9. Ensure nationwide availability of 9-1-1 as the emergency telephone number 10. Ensure that all calls for emergency help are automatically accompanied by location-identifying information
1973	The Emergency Medical Services Act	Required components of an EMS system: 1. Integration of health services 2. EMS research 3. Legislation and regulation 4. System finance 5. Human resources 6. Medical direction 7. Education and training systems 8. Public access and education 9. Prevention 10. Transportation 11. Communication systems 12. Clinical care facilities 13. Patient information and education systems 14. Mutual aid agreements 15. Evaluation
1980s/1990s	The National Highway Traffic and Safety Administration	EMS system elements: 1. Regulation and policy 2. Resource management 3. Human resources and training 4. Transportation 5. Facilities 6. Communication 7. Public information and education 8. Medical direction 9. Trauma systems 10. Evaluation

paramedics was developed by the US DOT. This first paramedic curriculum was based on the work of Dr Nancy Caroline.

Through the 1980s and 1990s, changes continued in EMS and the number of trained personnel grew. The National Highway Traffic Safety Administration (NHTSA) developed 10 system elements, listed in Table 1, in an effort to sustain EMS systems. Unfortunately federal funding and staff were reduced, and the responsibility for EMS was transferred to the states. Although it was made clear that the federal funding being provided was just "seed money" and that long-term local funding strategies needed to be developed, many states apparently believed that the federal dollars would not go away. Unfortunately, they did and to this day funding is still a major roadblock for local governments as well as states.

Several other major legislative initiatives also came about in this time frame, such as the EMS for Children (EMS-C) program

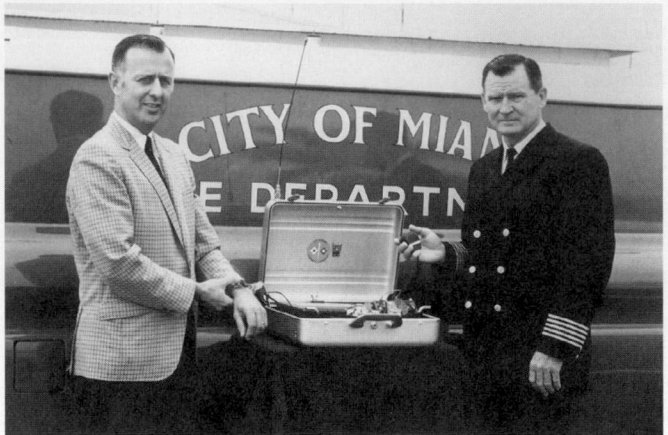

Figure 3 Dr Eugene Nagel, widely considered the father of paramedicine, provided much-needed leadership to the developing field of EMS training. Here he is shown (at left) in 1967 with Chief Larry Kenney of the Miami Fire Department, with the first telemetry package to be used by paramedics.

grant funding that was implemented in 1984. In 1986 an amendment was made to the Public Safety Officers Benefit Act in which families of Fire and EMS providers were compensated if the provider was killed in the line of duty. As progress continued into the 1990s, **trauma systems** started making headway. Some of these secondary programs received federal funding, but in present day are struggling to prove necessity and maintain the funding. Their expertise is vital to further advancement in EMS, but some of the suggested advancements are held back because of lack of funding.

■ Licensure, Certification, and Registration

On completing initial paramedic education, you will be eligible to take your state's certification examination. A **certification** examination is used to ensure that all health care providers have at least the same basic level of knowledge and skill. Once you have passed this examination, you will be eligible to apply for state licensure. **Licensure** is how states control who is allowed to practice as a health care provider. Different states refer to the authority granted to you to function as a paramedic as licensure, certification, or credentialing. For the purposes of this text, *licensure* will be used. Performing functions as a paramedic prior to licensure is unlawful, or to be more specific, considered practicing medicine without a license unless directly supervised by a paramedic program internship preceptor as a part of your training program.

Although holding a license shows that you have successfully completed initial education and met the requirements to achieve such a license, it does not mean that you can perform as a paramedic without or outside the supervision of your service's physician medical director. Agencies (state, local, and national) still require that paramedics receive **medical direction** (both online and off-line). The concept and principles of medical control will be discussed later in the chapter.

YOU *are the Medic*   PART 2

As you form your general impression of the patient, you observe that he is a young man who appears to be unresponsive. He is not wearing any protective clothing and some of the bystanders tell you that they took his helmet off "so he could breathe." You note that the patient is breathing, but his breaths are very shallow and he has some minor bleeding from an obvious fracture of his left lower leg. Before you reach the patient, the hysterical girl runs to you and begs you to hurry up and do something because her "boyfriend is dying!" She does not think you are moving fast enough. The two women try again to console her, but she is frantic. You ascertain that she was standing in the driveway while the boyfriend pulled away on his motorcycle, and that she was not involved in the crash.

Recording Time: 1 Minute	
Appearance	Pale, unmoving, obvious fracture of left lower leg
Level of consciousness	Unresponsive
Airway	Clear
Breathing	Rapid and shallow, possibly asymmetrical
Circulation	Rapid and weak radial pulses

3. What aspects of professionalism must be employed in this situation?

4. Aside from those noted in the previous question, what other roles and responsibilities are vital in your status as a health care professional?

Words of Wisdom

Nancy Lee Caroline was born in a Boston suburb to Leo and Zelda Caroline in 1944. Nancy had a strong social conscience and devoted her life to medicine, teaching, and her patients—and she had a superb sense of humor. She has often been rightly called the Mother of Paramedics because of her dedication to paramedic education. She died of multiple myeloma at age 58 in 2002.

Nancy's medical career began at the young age of 15 in the pathology laboratory of the famous Benjamin Castleman, MD, at Massachusetts General Hospital, where she conducted medical research long before she entered college. Nancy majored in linguistics at Radcliffe College, and received her MD from Case Western Reserve University in 1977. Thereafter she took a fellowship in Critical Care Medicine at the University of Pittsburgh. It was here that she began her groundbreaking work in paramedicine.

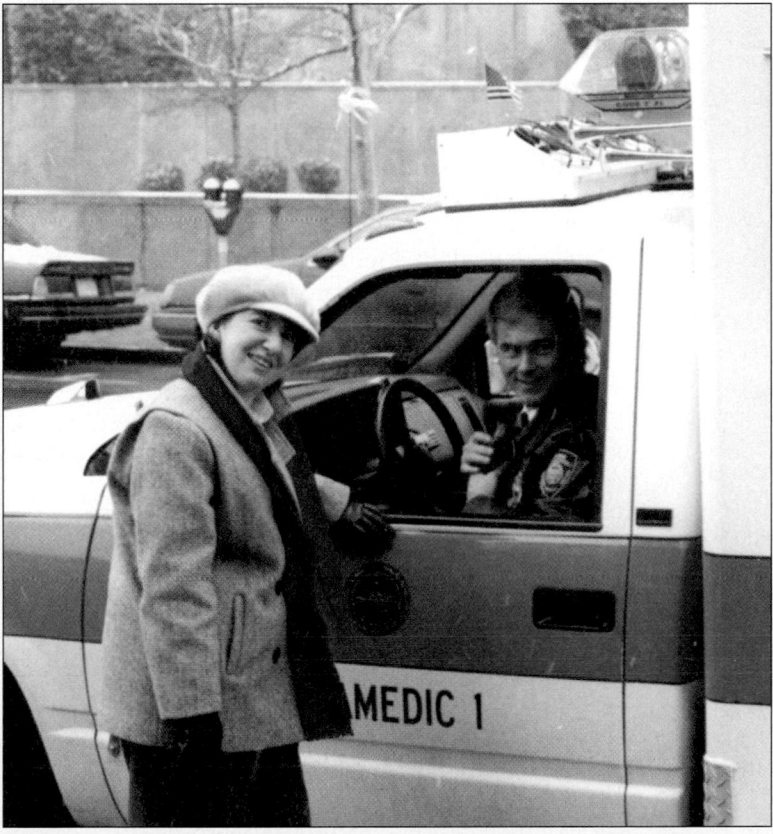

Around that time, the late Peter Safar, MD, was overseeing a US Department of Transportation grant to create a curriculum for paramedics. Dr. Safar offered Nancy an opportunity, as medical director of Freedom House Enterprises Ambulance Service, to train paramedics chosen from a group of African-American men who did not have a chance to complete their high school educations. Nancy was extremely successful—so successful that she was asked to write a curriculum for paramedic training, a curriculum that was published as the first edition of the textbook you are reading—*Emergency Care in the Streets*.

The list of Nancy's other accomplishments is long. She served as the first medical director of Israel's Red Cross society, where in addition to training the first Israeli paramedics, she took extensive Hebrew lessons (it was a point of pride for her to develop a knowledge of the languages in whatever country she was working). After her tenure there ended in 1981, Nancy relocated to Nairobi, Kenya, to become Senior Medical Officer of the African Medical and Research Foundation (AMREF), the foundation that oversees the famous Flying Doctor service. When she became aware of the devastating famine that overtook Ethiopia in the early 1980s, Nancy became a consultant for the League of Red Cross Societies, writing a handbook on basic life support and running classes on first aid for African nations. Nancy worked with the Ethiopian Orthodox Church to provide better nourishment and health care to children in over 600 orphanages. In addition, Nancy served as director of medical programs for the American Joint Distribution Committee in Addis Ababa.

Returning to Israel in 1987, she served as medical consultant for the Center for Educational Technology and for AMREF, developing training materials in emergency medicine and writing correspondence courses for rural health workers in Africa. She also served as an adjunct professor at the University of Pittsburgh's medical school, and, while volunteering in the Department of Oncology in Tel Hashomer, Nancy collaborated with Alexander Waller, MD, on the *Handbook of Palliative Care in Cancer*.

Nancy settled in Metulla, Israel. She realized there was a need for special care in north Israel for people with advanced cancer. In 1995, she founded the Hospice of the Upper Galilee (HUG). In 2002, she married geneticist and molecular biologist Lazarus Astrachan.

Nancy left the world too soon, but unquestionably left the world a better place. Despite all her accomplishments, the compliment that meant the most to her was to be called the Mother of Paramedics. Nancy was, no doubt, the best mother paramedics could have.

Finally, you may be required to be registered as well as licensed. **Registration** means that records of your education, state or local licensure, and recertification will be held by a recognized board of registration.

Additionally, some states require that paramedic graduates come from an accredited paramedic program. The Committee on Accreditation of Educational Programs for the EMS Professions (CoAEMSP) is the only accrediting agency for paramedic programs. The mission of the CoAEMSP is to continuously improve the quality of EMS education through accreditation and recognition services for the full range of EMS professions. Because of changes with the National Scope of Practice and the need to expand the professional image of EMS, the number of accredited paramedic education programs will grow significantly over the next few years.

■ Reciprocity

Be aware that each state has different licensing or certification requirements and procedures regardless of whether they follow the National Scope of Practice model. Granting certification to a provider from another state or agency is known as reciprocity. More than 40 states recognize National Registry certification as part of their reciprocity process. For reciprocity to be granted to an individual EMT or paramedic, most states will require you to hold current state certification and to be in good standing as well as having National Registry certification. Several states will require you to challenge their requirements; in other words, you may be required to go through that state's written and/or practical evaluations prior to reciprocity being granted. Others may request your education transcript and continuing education hours. You may be required to provide information for a background check. Because you will be an integral part of the health care system, most states want to be certain you do not have previous issues that could call into question your integrity or professionalism. Finally, some states will require a fee to process your reciprocity application and provide a license.

The EMS System

The modern-day EMS system is a complex network of coordinated services providing various levels of care to a community. These services work in unison to meet both the growing and standing needs of the citizens in the community in which they reside. As a paramedic, you are part of this network; therefore, you must stay active in your community to be able to meet the ever-changing needs. There are a variety of service types in present-day EMS, including the following:

- Fire-based
- Third service (municipalities)
- Private (both for profit and nonprofit)
- Hospital-based
- Hybrid or other

The EMS network begins with citizen involvement in the complex EMS system. The public in most cases does not understand EMS and only knows what is seen in newspapers, television, and movies. They need to be taught how to recognize what is an emergency and what is not, how to activate the EMS system, and how basic care can be provided before EMS arrives. Remember that the public usually does not have medical training or knowledge and a simple cut may be an emergency in their eyes.

When you are called to a "sick person" at 2 AM who only has a common cold and cannot sleep, you must avoid becoming angry at the patient, your career, or your EMS system. Instead, use this time to educate the public by offering sympathy and insight on cold treatment, and perhaps tactfully discuss why a cold is not an emergency. You will often respond to nonemergency calls. Factors that play a role in determining the outcome or likelihood of your patient's survival include the following:

- Bystander care
- Dispatch (including prearrival directions)
- Response (both mode and distance)
- Prehospital care provided (level of EMS-trained personnel)

Words of Wisdom

A patient may only experience once what a paramedic may experience hundreds of times. Understand the patient's anxiety.

- Transportation (ground ambulances, critical care units, air transport)
- Emergency department care (on-duty trained emergency physicians and staff)
- Definitive care (including trauma, pediatric, and neurologic specialists)
- Rehabilitation

When the public activates the EMS system, their first contact is usually a dispatcher. Requirements for dispatcher training vary greatly from state to state, and oftentimes dispatchers have to cover police and fire communications as well. Dispatchers must interpret the stressed caller's needs to determine if it is an emergency by extracting appropriate information, and then decide what resources need to be sent. Scene findings do not always exactly reflect the information received by dispatch and relayed to you. You must remember that dispatch is only able to provide information from what is told to them; never under- or overestimate that information. Despite this, you, as a paramedic, will be required to develop a care plan, decide on the appropriate transport method, and determine the appropriate receiving facility.

Being active in your community will keep you on top of the best local resources and enable you to answer questions regarding your patient care plan. You will ask yourself, "Does the receiving facility have the resources needed for this patient?" If the answer is no, the next question is, "Is there an appropriate facility within a reasonable distance?" And of course, you must remember that in some regions competent adult patients may be able to request the facility to which they are transported.

Special Populations

EMS systems must be capable of handling many different situations including obstetric, pediatric, and geriatric emergencies. Proper procedures, drug dosages, and even assessment techniques are often different in children, adults, and older people.

Levels of Education

Licensure of EMS personnel is a state function, subject to the laws and regulations of the state in which the EMS provider practices. For this reason, there is some variation from state to state in the scope of practice and in education and relicensure requirements. The following information explains how the system is supposed to work from the federal level to the local level.

At the federal level, NHTSA brought in experts from around the country to create the National EMS Scope of Practice Model. This document provides overarching guidelines as to what skills each level of EMS provider should be able to accomplish. The next step is the state level. Because licensure is a state function, laws are enacted to regulate how EMS providers will operate and are then executed by the state-level EMS administrative offices, which control licensure. Finally, the local medical director decides the day-to-day limits of EMS personnel. For example, the medications that will be carried on an ambulance or where patients are transported are the day-to-day operational concerns in which the medical director will have direct input.

The national guidelines are intended to create more consistent delivery of EMS across the country. The only way a medical director can allow a paramedic to perform a skill is if the state has already approved performance of that skill. The medical director can limit the scope of practice but cannot expand it beyond state law. Expanding the scope of practice requires state approval.

In 2009 the National Standard Curricula for all levels of EMS providers were revised to a new format and renamed the *National EMS Education Standards*. In the United States, NHTSA is the federal administrative source for these standards and related documents. The *National EMS Education Standards* for the four levels of EMS providers can be downloaded from the NHTSA's website at http://www.ems.gov. In addition, the NREMT is a nongovernmental agency that provides a national standard for testing and certification throughout the United States. Many states use the National Registry testing process for licensing their EMS providers and grant licensing reciprocity to NREMT-certified EMS personnel. It is important to remember, however, that EMS is regulated entirely by the state in which you are licensed.

The Dispatcher

The dispatcher plays a key role in an EMS call. He or she must receive and enter all information on the call, interpret the information, and in turn, relay it to the appropriate resources **Figure 4** . In some locations the dispatcher may be trained as an emergency medical dispatcher (EMD), which charges this person with the added task of giving simple prearrival instructions (ie, CPR, bleeding control) to a caller in hopes that this care may benefit the patient until EMS personnel are on scene.

Emergency Medical Responder

This level was known most recently as the "first responder." Not all states have this as a certification and/or licensing level, and for those states that do, there can be considerable variability in requirements and allowed skills. In the generic use of the term, an emergency medical responder (EMR) is usually a person trained in CPR and/or first aid. As a paramedic, one of your jobs will be to familiarize yourself with the level of training of the EMRs in your system.

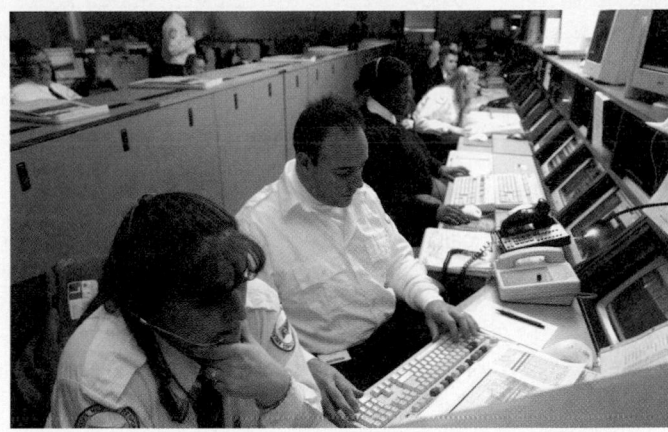

Figure 4 The dispatcher coordinates the entire rescue effort. He or she interprets a caller's information and then sends appropriate personnel and resources to the scene.

From an EMS point of view, an EMR has completed a course that covers the *National EMS Education Standards* for the EMR level. This training will help the EMR to be able to recognize the seriousness of a patient's condition, administer appropriate basic care, and relay information to the paramedic. EMRs are an essential level of provider to the EMS system, especially in rural areas **Figure 5** .

EMT

Recently changed from being called the EMT-Basic (EMT-B), the EMT is the backbone and primary provider level in many EMS systems. This is also the level of certification required before being able to enter a paramedic education program. Much lifesaving care is provided at this level.

In some states EMTs may be trained in advanced airway intervention, limited medication administration, and intravenous

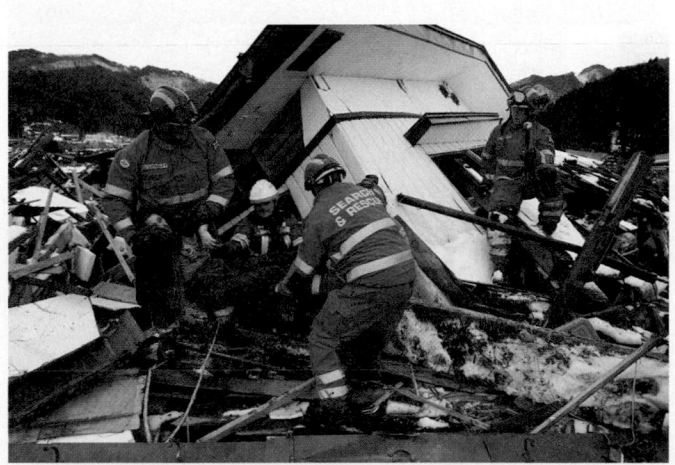

Figure 5 The emergency medical responder is critical for providing the initial emergency patient care, particularly when medical personnel must travel long distances to a scene.

(IV) fluid therapy; however, EMTs with this expanded scope of practice are not recognized at a different certification level per the *National EMS Education Standards*. In EMS, there are more providers trained and certified at the EMT level than at any other level **Figure 6** .

Advanced EMT

The level formerly called EMT-Intermediate (EMT-I) has gone through numerous changes over the years. It was initially developed in 1985 and was known as the EMT-I 85 level. The skill level for the EMT-I saw a significant change in 1999, when a major revision of the 1985 curriculum took place. More recently, changes made within the National Scope of Practice have eliminated the intermediate level, and it has been replaced with the Advanced EMT (AEMT) level. AEMTs are trained in more advanced pathophysiology, as well as some advanced procedures such as establishing IV access, administering IV fluids, performing blood glucose monitoring, and performing some advanced airway management.

Controversies

Some argue that in an urban setting all that is needed are AEMTs rather than paramedics, whereas others argue that AEMTs perform ALS skills without having adequate academic preparation and should be phased out. The jury is still out on whether this particular level of training will become an attractive option for jurisdictions and EMS providers.

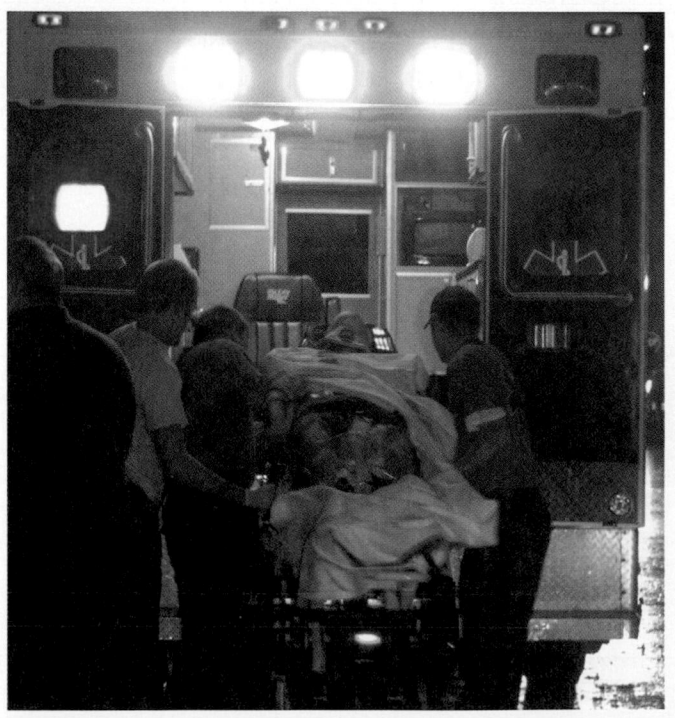

Figure 6 EMTs constitute the majority of EMS providers.

Paramedic

Currently paramedic is the highest EMS skill level at which you can be either certified or licensed at the national level. In 1998, the US DOT paramedic curriculum underwent major revisions and the level of training and skills increased greatly. In 2009 when the *National EMS Education Standards* were completed, the skills allowed at the paramedic level changed to some extent. Starting in 2013, to test through NREMT, a paramedic student must have attended an accredited institution. States that do not employ NREMT as their testing mechanism may not require that institutions be accredited. Although you may hold a license or certification independently, states still require paramedics to function directly under the guidance of a licensed physician and to be affiliated with a paramedic-level service.

Paramedic Education

Initial Education

Education may vary from state to state, but for the most part all states base their paramedic education programs on the *National EMS Education Standards* for the paramedic. As mentioned, significant changes were made to these standards, formerly called curricula, in 2009. A major recommendation was the inclusion of a college-level anatomy and physiology course as part of a training program. The *National EMS Education Standards* outline the minimum of what a paramedic must know to practice. States require varying hours of education, but the national average falls between 1,000 and 1,500 hours of combined classroom, clinical, and field education. Some leaders want to structure education so that the paramedic designation is achieved through an associate or bachelor's degree accredited program. A distinct benefit of this is that it can give paramedics credits that could be used in achieving higher-level college degrees.

Words of Wisdom

The number of calls you go on is not the deciding factor on how much more education you need.

Continuing Education

Most states require that paramedics show proof of hours spent in continuing education or refresher programs. Such programs keep you up-to-date on new research findings, new techniques, and skills, and help prevent degradation of skills used less frequently **Figure 7** . Continuing education can also showcase current issues in your state that impact you and your system's ability to provide quality emergency medical care. Continuing education can be enjoyable, and it should be. Whenever possible, you should attend conferences and seminars, ideally with some of them being out of your region and/or state, which helps broaden your knowledge base. It is certainly worth attending conferences that may not be designed for paramedics, such as those targeted

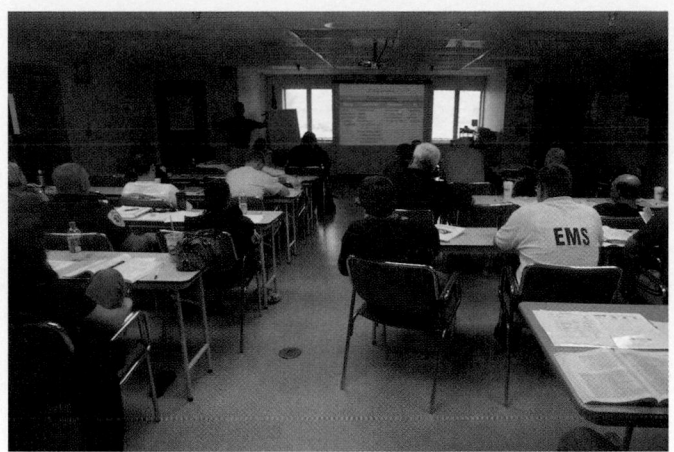

Figure 7 Continuing education can keep you up-to-date on technologic improvements that are continually made available to paramedics.

at nurses or physicians. Keep up with reading EMS journals. With the advancement of technology, Internet-based continuing education resources have expanded greatly; however, be sure that these programs meet your state or national requirements.

Get everyone on your service involved in postrun critiques—they can be beneficial in identifying problem areas in your practice. Postrun critiques are considered to be a form of continuing education in some states.

No matter what requirements are mandated by a state licensing agency, responsibility for continuing medical education ultimately rests with each individual paramedic. You know which areas of your knowledge have diminished and which skills require additional refresher efforts. You are the only person who will have to live with the questions and doubts that inevitably arise after something goes wrong in the field. Continuing medical education is a way to help make sure that things do not go wrong. A statement that should be remembered throughout a paramedic's career is: "Along with the privilege of being a paramedic comes a responsibility to continually educate and train oneself. You would expect no less from someone responding to you or your family." –Dr. Rob Puls, DC, CCEMT-P

Additional Types of Transports

Transport to Specialty Centers

In addition to hospital emergency departments, many EMS systems include specialty centers that focus on specific types of care (such as trauma, burns, poisoning, or psychiatric conditions) or specific types of patients (for example, children). Specialty centers require in-house staffs of surgeons and other specialists; other facilities must page operating teams, surgeons, or other specialists from outside the hospital. Typically, only a few hospitals in a region are designated as specialty centers. Transport time to a specialty center may be slightly longer than the time to an emergency department, but patients will receive definitive

care more quickly at a specialty center. You must know the location of the centers in your area and when, according to your protocol, you must transport the patient directly to one. Sometimes, air medical transport will be necessary. Local, regional, and state protocols will guide your decision in these instances.

Interfacility Transports

Many EMS services provide interfacility transportation for non-ambulatory patients or patients with acute and chronic medical conditions requiring medical monitoring. This transportation may include transferring patients to and from hospitals, skilled nursing facilities, board and care homes, or even their home residence.

During ambulance transportation, the health and well-being of the patient is your responsibility. You should obtain the patient's medical history, chief complaint, and latest vital signs and provide ongoing patient assessment. In certain circumstances, depending on local protocols, a nurse, physician, respiratory therapist, or medical team will accompany the patient, especially when the patient requires care that extends beyond the scope of practice of paramedics.

Working With Other Professionals

Working With Hospital Staff

You should become familiar with the hospital by observing hospital equipment and how it is used, the functions of staff members, and the policies and procedures in all emergency areas of the hospital. You will also learn about advances in emergency care and how to interact with hospital personnel. This experience will help you to understand how your care influences a patient's recovery and will emphasize the importance and benefits of proper prehospital care. It will also show you the consequences of delay, inadequate care, or poor judgment.

Physicians are not likely to be in the field with you to provide personal, on-the-spot instructions. However, you may consult with appropriate medical staff by using the radio through established medical control procedures. A physician or nurse may serve as an instructor for medical subjects in your education program. Through these experiences, you will become more comfortable using medical terms, interpreting patient signs and symptoms, and developing patient management skills. The best patient care occurs when all emergency care providers have close rapport. This rapport allows you and hospital staff the opportunity to discuss mutual problems and to benefit from each other's experiences.

Working With Public Safety Agencies

Some public safety personnel have EMS training. As a paramedic, you must become familiar with all the roles and responsibilities of these workers. Personnel from certain agencies are better prepared than you are to perform certain functions. For example, employees of a utility company are better equipped to control downed power lines than are you or your partner. Law enforcement personnel are better able to handle violent scenes and traffic control, while you and your partner are better able to provide emergency medical care Figure 8 . If you work together and recognize that each person has special training and a job to do at the scene, effective scene and patient management will result. Remember that the best, most efficient patient care is achieved through cooperation among agencies.

Continuity of Care

In addition to responding to EMS calls, taking care of the patient, transporting, and returning to service, EMS providers have responsibilities to the community. The community has expectations of EMS providers and, as health care providers and public servants, you must project confidence to the community you serve.

If you are working in the public sector rather than private sector, you should encourage people in the community to become involved in your service to some level. Present-day medicine focuses on prevention—getting involved in community efforts

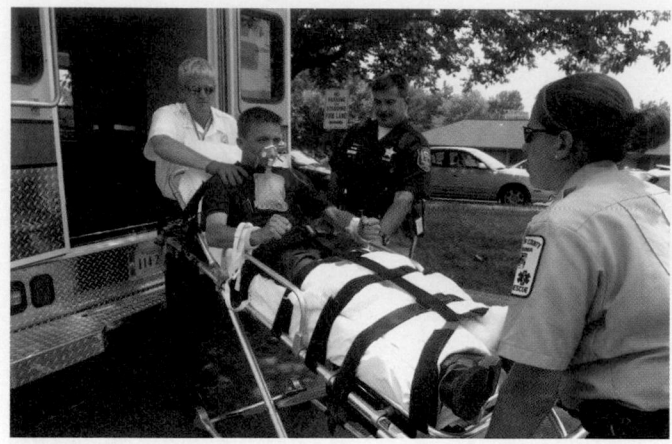

Figure 8 You will work with law enforcement personnel when dealing with violent patients.

YOU are the Medic   PART 3

A quick assessment reveals that the patient is unresponsive and the only visible injury is the patient's leg. You note damage to the left side of the helmet and ask the man holding it to place it on the passenger seat of your ambulance. While your partner is gathering immobilization equipment, fire department personnel arrive and you ask one of the fire fighters to talk with the girlfriend and find out as much information about the patient as possible.

Further assessment reveals very diminished breath sounds on the left side and distended neck veins. His radial pulses are weakening and increasing in rate. Your partner inserts an oral airway and begins ventilating the patient with a bag-mask device and 100% oxygen while the fire fighters assist you in packaging the patient on the long backboard. His left leg is secured to his right leg and bleeding is controlled with direct pressure and a dressing. He is loaded into the ambulance and you quickly obtain vital signs while the fire fighter who was talking to the girlfriend tells you that the patient is 22 years old, has no medical history, and takes no medications. The girlfriend does not think he is allergic to anything. He has a blood glucose level of 102 mg/dL and you note hyperresonance to percussion on the left side of his chest. The cardiac monitor shows a sinus tachycardia without ectopy.

Your partner tells you that it is becoming difficult to ventilate the patient. On the basis of your findings, you recognize that the patient has a pneumothorax that is developing tension. The only definitive treatment is a needle thoracostomy. Even though you have had training for performing this procedure, your standing orders do not allow it. A fire fighter takes over ventilations from your partner.

Recording Time: 6 Minutes	
Respirations	Assisting ventilations at 12 breaths/min
Pulse	138 beats/min, weak radials
Skin	Pale, cool, diaphoretic
Blood pressure	96/54 mm Hg
Oxygen saturation (Spo$_2$)	92% with ventilations by bag-mask device and 100% oxygen
Pupils	Equal but sluggish to react

5. Even though you do not have standing orders to perform a needle thoracostomy, you know this is what the patient needs. How will you handle this situation?

6. How will you make the determination of how and where to transport this patient?

is your opportunity to use your medical expertise for the people you serve. To start, take a look at your community and the type of calls you have most frequently. From this you can develop a variety of prevention strategies or activities within your community to reduce those types of calls. For example, perhaps your community has many calls relating to accidental falls. There are training programs available to help identify possible causes of falls. You can visit homes in your community to offer suggestions for prevention.

As a new paramedic, you are considered part of the health care and emergency services community. You will work side by side with other professional groups. For example, you will integrate your work with other medical professionals, law enforcement, emergency management and disaster services, home health groups, such as hospice, and of course emergency responders. It is vital that you understand your role as well as the roles of those with whom you interact to ensure that calls run as smoothly as possible. You must also be prepared for any number of situations, and establish expectations for each role.

Words of Wisdom

The best paramedics will continually refresh their basic life support skills as well as advanced life support skills.

National EMS Group Involvement

Many national and state organizations exist, and many invite paramedic membership. These organizations have an impact on the future direction of EMS, so it is very important for you to identify and become involved in them. You will also have access to many valuable resources to help you develop yourself and your service area and to improve your problem-solving skills. One of the common goals of many national and state organizations is to promote uniformity of EMS standards and practices. Some of these organizations are listed in Table 2.

Table 2 National EMS Organizations

- National Highway Traffic Safety Administration (NHTSA)
- National Association of Emergency Medical Service Physicians (NAEMSP)
- National Association of State EMS Officials (NAEMSO)
- National Association of EMS Educators (NAEMSE)
- National Registry of EMTs (NREMT)
- National Association of EMTs (NAEMT)
- Emergency Medical Services for Children (EMS-C)
- American College of Emergency Physicians (ACEP)
- American Ambulance Association (AAA)
- International Association of Flight and Critical Care Paramedics (IAFCCP)

Professionalism

During your paramedic education, you learn a vast amount of information designed to make you a **health care professional**, practicing at the paramedic level. A **profession** is a field of endeavor that requires a specialized set of knowledge, skills, and expertise, often gained after lengthy education.

A health care professional has the following attributes:

- Conforms to the same standards of other health care professions
- Provides quality patient care
- Instills pride in the profession
- Strives continuously for high standards
- Earns respect from others in the profession
- Meets high societal expectations of the profession whether on or off duty

As a paramedic, you must meet standards, competencies, and continuing education requirements. The paramedic profession has expected standards and performance parameters as well as a code of ethics. Collectively, these are the standards by which you will be measured as a paramedic.

It is imperative that you remember you are in a highly visible role in your community Figure 9. Professional image and behavior must be a top priority whether you are in uniform, on duty, or off duty in street clothes. You are a representative of the agency, city, county, district, or state you work in. It is said that people will make an initial judgment of you within the first 10 seconds of meeting you, even if you say nothing. As a paramedic, you will meet new people as an everyday part of your career. To provide the best possible care, you must instill confidence, plus establish and maintain credibility. As you walk into a situation, never forget that a significant part of your job is to continually show that you are concerned for the well-being of your patients and their families. Your appearance is also of utmost importance—it has more impact than you may think.

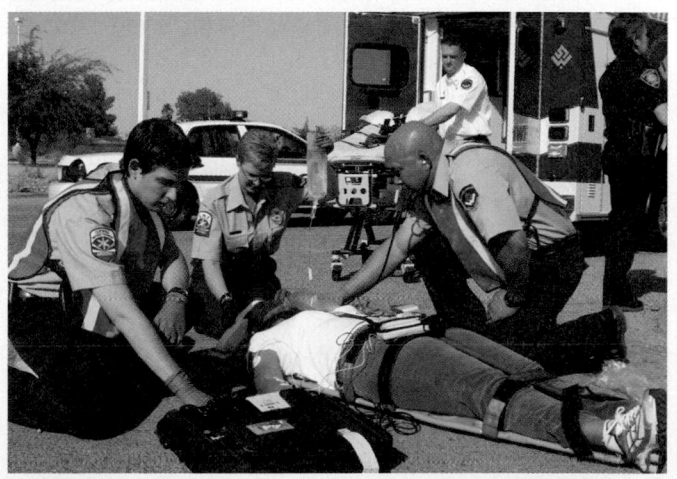

Figure 9 Adopting a professional attitude and appearance is a critical part of working with the public and earning their trust.

It is not appropriate to arrive at a call in dirty clothes, with dirty hands, and smelling offensively. You must look and act like a professional at all times.

You are an integral part of the entire health care system; therefore, you must present a professional image and treat others in the profession with the respect you would want to be treated with. It is inappropriate to argue with other health care providers or hospital staff, but there is an appropriate circumstance to have professional discussions regarding patient care. Remember that you are a patient advocate and it is appropriate for you to raise patient care issues professionally at appropriate times and locations. There may be occasions where differences of opinion exist; these are best addressed by contacting a supervisor. Such conversations may identify instances when other branches of health care do not follow the same practices as EMS, due to different expectations or requirements.

Other attributes of professionalism as a paramedic include the following:

- **Integrity.** The single most important attribute. Be open, honest, and truthful with your patients.
- **Empathy.** Show your patients, their families, and other health care professionals that you identified and understand their feelings. It is okay to show emotions to some extent.
- **Self-motivation.** You should have an internal drive for excellence, which is often a driving force to ensure that you always behave in a professional manner. You will need to continuously educate yourself, accept negative or constructive feedback, and perform with minimal supervision.
- **Confidence.** To instill confidence in your patients and colleagues, you must show that you are confident in your abilities and skills. Continually strive to be the best paramedic you can, for example, attend educational sessions and perform self critiques. These measures are only a few of the items available that will build confidence, thus helping you to run your calls smoothly and effectively.
- **Communications.** You must be able to express and exchange your ideas, thoughts, and findings with other professional colleagues. Make conscious reminders to yourself when interacting with patients and their families to listen well and speak directly, without using confusing medical terms. Clear, professional written documentation is also important. Record keeping and reporting is a responsibility of all EMS providers.
- **Teamwork and respect.** Teamwork is required in EMS. On every call, everyone must work together to achieve a common goal—to provide the best possible prehospital care to ensure the overall well-being of your patient. Most often in the field, the paramedic is the team leader. A team leader will not undermine his or her team regardless of his or her level, but instead will help guide and support the team, remaining flexible and open for change at any moment and communicating at an appropriate place and time with other members of the team to resolve problems. You must always be as respectful of others as you would expect them to be with you.
- **Patient advocacy.** You must always act in the best interest of the patient while respecting his or her wishes and beliefs, regardless of your own. This includes patients with special needs or those with different lifestyles, values, and cultures from your own. Never allow your personal feelings about a patient to have an impact on the care you provide. Respect those you serve. While you need to communicate to do your job, be sure that you maintain a high level of confidentiality. Whatever details you have to communicate about your patient, ensure that communication about the patient does not occur in front of anyone who is not on your team, this will be discussed in greater detail in the chapter, *Medical, Legal, and Ethical Issues*. When you talk to members of your team, do so quietly and with appropriate respect. Your role as a patient advocate means you should always be on the lookout for spousal abuse, child abuse or neglect, and elder abuse or neglect. Make sure you communicate your findings to the appropriate authorities.
- **Injury prevention.** A paramedic is in the unique position of seeing the patient's surroundings prior to transport. If you can spot a potential hazard (such as a loose rug at the top of the stairs), use your diplomatic skills and talk about your findings to the patient or a family member. Get involved with training programs such as those on the topics of fall prevention or child passenger safety. You may prevent a potential injury. Discuss the importance of using bike helmets, safety belts, and child car seats whenever you can. It is another way of preventing injuries.
- **Careful delivery of service.** A paramedic must deliver the highest quality patient care. Pay careful attention to detail and continuously evaluate and reevaluate your performance. Use other medical professionals as resources, not adversaries. Follow policies, protocols, and procedures as well as the orders of your superiors.
- **Time management.** Time management is an important skill in any profession. Using your time wisely, for example by prioritizing your patient's needs, keeping your ambulance always ready to go, and ensuring that you document each emergency call as soon as it has concluded, is a component of professional delivery of service.
- **Administration.** Part of the paramedic's role is administrative. In addition to documenting each call thoroughly and

professionally, you may be asked to take on special projects or station duties. As you advance in your career, you may also play a role in working with other agencies and forging partnerships with other public safety resources.

As the health care industry gains a better understanding of a paramedic's skills and abilities, more health care locations are using paramedic services within their organizations. For example, many hospitals now incorporate paramedics in their emergency departments and clinics. Physician offices also are identifying the benefits of using paramedic services within their organizations. With the recent advent of the emerging forms of influenza, some clinics and local public health departments used paramedics to administer vaccines, while in other locations paramedics help serve as home health nurses. Also, you will perform special types of transports beyond your standard 9-1-1 emergency calls. Your service may provide transfers between health care locations; these may include specialty services such as critical care, neonatal, or high-risk obstetric transfers. The expertise that a paramedic acquires is a very important part of the entire emergency medical environment; offer your abilities in all ways possible.

Roles and Responsibilities

So what does it actually mean to be a paramedic? What are my roles? What am I responsible for? These are questions that you should ask yourself throughout your career. The EMS system continues to grow and mature, and with those changes will come new roles and additional responsibilities. Some of the primary responsibilities are shown in **Figure 10** and include the following:

- **Preparation.** Be prepared physically, mentally, and emotionally. Keep up your knowledge and skill abilities. Be sure you have the appropriate equipment for your call and that it is in good working order.

Words of Wisdom

For safety, avoid wearing long necklaces, dangling earrings, or other jewelry that could interfere with your work.

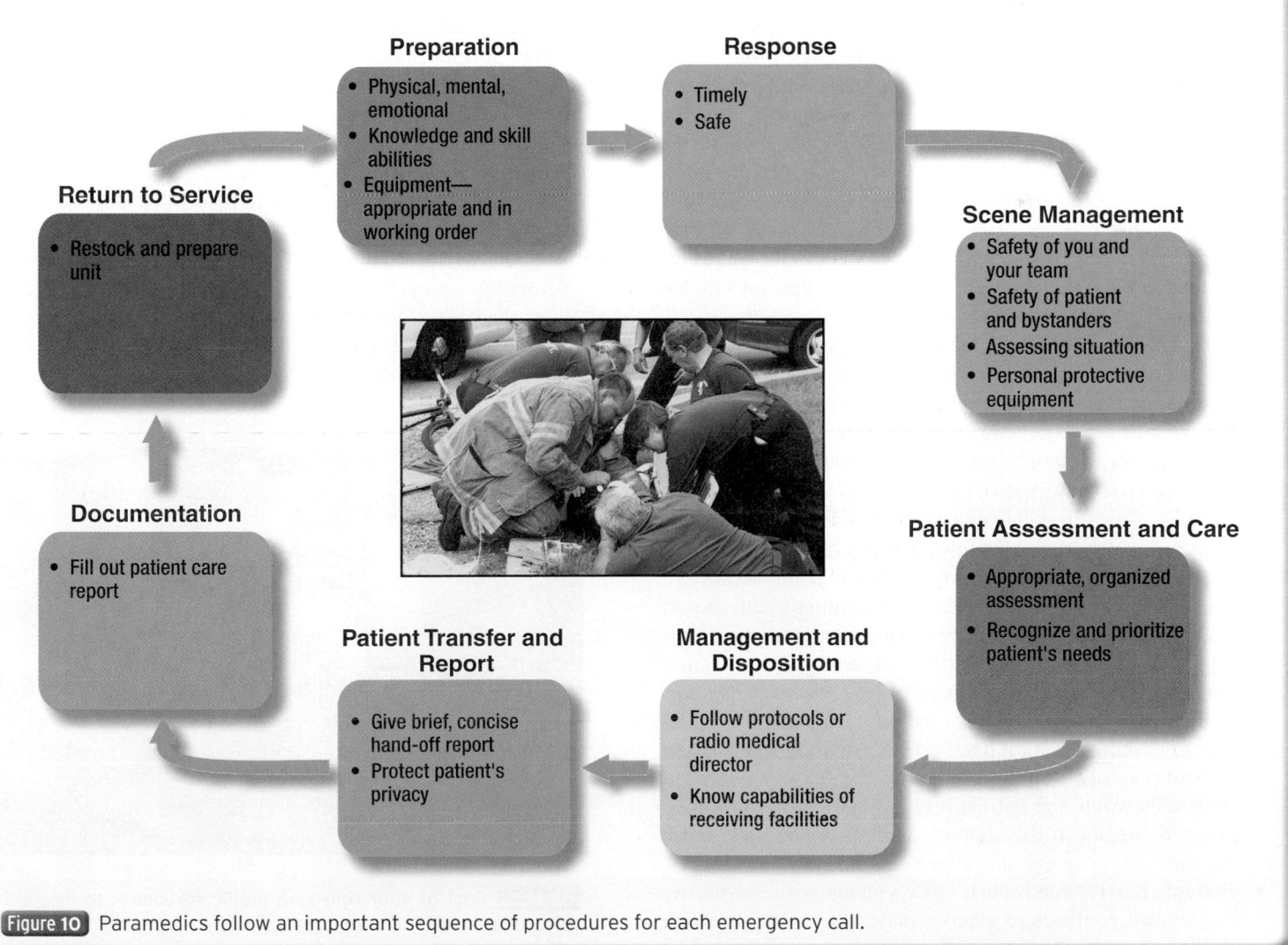

Preparation
- Physical, mental, emotional
- Knowledge and skill abilities
- Equipment— appropriate and in working order

Response
- Timely
- Safe

Scene Management
- Safety of you and your team
- Safety of patient and bystanders
- Assessing situation
- Personal protective equipment

Patient Assessment and Care
- Appropriate, organized assessment
- Recognize and prioritize patient's needs

Management and Disposition
- Follow protocols or radio medical director
- Know capabilities of receiving facilities

Patient Transfer and Report
- Give brief, concise hand-off report
- Protect patient's privacy

Documentation
- Fill out patient care report

Return to Service
- Restock and prepare unit

Figure 10 Paramedics follow an important sequence of procedures for each emergency call.

- **Response.** Responding to the event in a timely, safe manner is very important. High speed—running "hot" without due regard to the safety of yourself, your partner, your patient, and persons on the highway (even if they should get out of your way but do not)—is not acceptable.

- **Scene management.** Ensuring your own safety and the safety of your team is the first priority. You must also ensure the patient's safety and the safety of any bystanders. Part of your preparation before you reach the scene should include considering all possibilities from dispatch information. Once at the scene and assessing the situation, the nature of the call may give valuable information. Scene safety includes but is not limited to the use of personal protective equipment such as gloves, masks, or goggles. The paramedic often sets the example for safety to the members of the EMS team.

- **Patient assessment and care.** An appropriate organized assessment based on the principles you will learn in this textbook should be performed on all patients. You need to recognize and prioritize the patient's needs on the basis of the injuries he or she has sustained or the illness that most urgently needs treatment.

- **Management and disposition.** You must follow medical guidelines or protocols approved by your medical director and possibly your state. Sometimes, however, when you are in the field, you will discover that the protocols or guidelines might not cover the situation you are in. This is the time to make radio contact with your medical director and use critical thinking skills. Having a good working relationship with your medical director is critical. You are the eyes, ears, and touch of the medical director. Situations that require a protocol or guideline variance or a decision outside of your scope of practice need to be communicated with your medical director. If you are unable to make contact, you must weigh your decisions closely before any intervention and communicate to your medical director as soon as possible. Although most calls will require transport to an emergency department, you must also be aware of other transport and destination decisions. For example, a patient with carbon monoxide poisoning may need to be transported to a hospital with a hyperbaric chamber—would you know where it is and how to access it? Your local receiving facilities may not keep you apprised of their capabilities; therefore, it is your responsibility to know your area's local health care abilities. You should know which facilities have specialty cardiac programs, and which are capable of handling trauma or pediatric emergencies. Know the capabilities of all receiving facilities with which you may interact before a call; this will assist you in making the right decision or providing information to your patient and his or her family. You may also be faced with calls where the patient refuses your care; this will be covered further in the chapter, *Medical, Legal, and Ethical Issues*.

- **Patient transfer and report.** Once you arrive at the receiving facility, continue to act as a patient advocate and give the appropriate facility staff a brief, concise hand-off report. Once again, use discretion so that you protect your patient's privacy.

- **Documentation.** After you transfer the patient, it is extremely important that a patient care report be filled out, preferably immediately. The report serves as a legal record of what you did in the field. Physicians must document their care of patients—so must you. Guidelines for documentation will be covered in the chapter, *Documentation*.

- **Return to service.** Every person on the EMS team is responsible for restocking and preparing the unit as quickly as possible for the next call. Failure to do so can bring about serious legal consequences if another call comes in and the unit is not fully restocked and ready to respond.

Words of Wisdom

One of your responsibilities as an EMS professional is to provide emotional support. Remember that calming and reassuring the patient, the family, and other responders can go a long way in making you an effective paramedic.

You are looked upon as a health care professional, so take advantage of this role. Educate the public about what you do and its importance. Get involved with prevention, community, and leadership activities whenever possible **Figure 11**. Never miss an opportunity to teach the community about prevention of injury and illness. Explain to people how to appropriately use your services. For those areas where trained EMS staff are few and far between, use your abilities to promote programs that get the public involved in CPR training, one of the major determinants of whether or not a person in cardiac arrest will live or die.

In some regions, paramedics have other health care responsibilities such as working in clinics, free-standing emergency facilities, and hospitals. Home visits by paramedics under direct medical control are being considered. In recent years with the

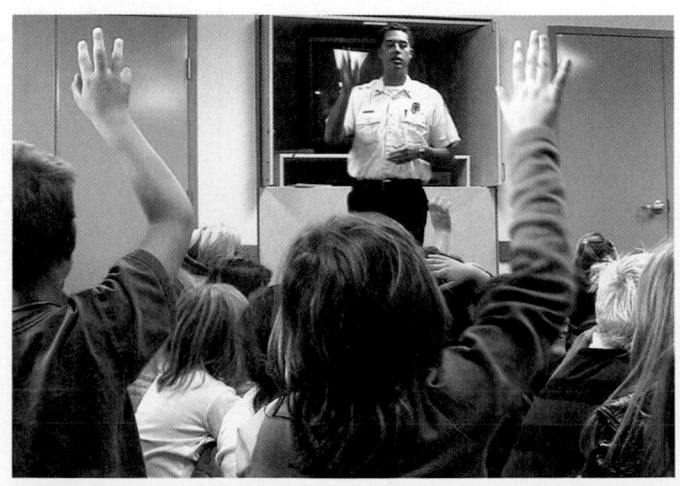

Figure 11 Part of your role as a public servant is to interact with and educate the public.

rise in influenza and possible pandemic issues, paramedics are being used to evaluate people at home and provide some immunization and medication administration.

Providers at all levels of EMS need to be advocates for prehospital health care, which often means setting out a well-thought-out campaign for EMS. Research your community, look at the strengths and weaknesses of the system, and develop plans for initiatives to improve the system. Many people lack an understanding of the role of EMS and do not recognize how vital EMS is until a loved one is unexpectedly taken ill. By involving yourself in your communities, you can both educate and advocate. It is up to all EMS personnel to educate the media and public. You must strive to stay at the top of your profession. Continue your education and become a mentor for new EMS professionals.

Words of Wisdom

In some cases you may encounter a physician on scene. If the physician is familiar with EMS protocols or happens to be your medical director, it can be a great help. But you may be caught between what the physician on the scene wants and the protocols that your medical director has given your service. Remember that you work with your physician medical director and you must adhere to the local protocols and standing orders.

You must remain calm and composed should the physician on the scene demand medical control of the situation.

Politely explain that all your actions must be in accordance with your EMS medical director's protocols. Point out that you can only transfer care of the patient to an onsite physician if that physician is now taking full responsibility for the patient and he or she will be present during transport, riding with the patient in your ambulance to the emergency department, as well as signing for any orders given.

Documentation and Communication

Documentation of equipment repairs and checks is nearly as important as documenting patient care.

■ Medical Direction

One of the distinctions in the differences among levels of EMS education is that the paramedic carries out advanced cardiology and pharmacologic skills. Paramedics do not have independent authority to act. Physicians who are educated about the levels and the extent of the education of EMS personnel play a vital role in running a service. The role of an EMS medical director may include the following:

- Educating and training personnel.
- Participating in the recommendation or selection of new personnel.
- Participating in or recommending equipment.
- Developing clinical protocols or guidelines in cooperation with other EMS personnel who are considered experts in the field.
- Developing and assisting in a quality improvement program.
- Providing input into patient care.
- Interfacing between EMS systems and other health care agencies.
- Serving as an EMS advocate to the community.
- Serving as the "medical conscience" of the EMS system.

The medical director also provides online and off-line medical control. **Online medical control** is medical direction given in real time to an EMS service or provider (either by radio or by electronic communication). **Off-line medical control** is medical direction given through a set of protocols, policies, and/or standards. The benefit to online medical control is that it provides immediate and specific patient care resources, allows telemetry transmission, allows for continuous quality improvement, and can render on-scene assistance. Off-line medical control allows for

the development of protocols or guidelines, standing orders, procedures, and training. A **protocol** or guideline is a treatment plan for a specific illness or injury. A **standing order** is a type of protocol or guideline that is a written document signed by the EMS system's medical director that outlines specific directions, permissions, and sometimes prohibitions regarding patient care that is rendered prior to contacting medical control (for example, defibrillation). Protocols or guidelines are usually developed in conjunction with national standards. For example, EMS personnel use the American Heart Association advanced cardiac life support algorithms as a protocol for cardiac patients (discussed in detail in the chapter, *Cardiovascular Emergencies*). Protocols also dictate what type of equipment and supplies are approved and needed as well as minimum expectations of personnel. The medical director also plays a role after the ambulance run. Medical directors help with patient care report review or even personally perform such reviews to ensure continuous quality improvement.

■ Improving System Quality

Making a good thing better should always be part of your paramedic career. A tool often used to continually evaluate your care is called **continuous quality improvement (CQI)**. **Quality control** is another process that evaluates problems and finds solutions. CQI is a process of assessing current practices and looking for ways to create ongoing improvement, thus reducing the chance of a problem arising in the first place. When properly developed and followed, a CQI program can help you and your service.

The process of CQI is dynamic, and your EMS system should develop a structure before a CQI assessment program is launched. A good CQI process should include the following:

- Identify any departmental or system-wide issues.
- Identify specific items that need to be measured.
- Conduct an in-depth review of the issue(s).
- Evaluate the issue(s) and develop a list of remedies.

- Develop an action plan for correction of issue(s).
- Enforce a plan of action, including time frames.
- Reexamine the issue.
- Identify and promote excellence found in patient care during the evaluation.
- Identify modifications that may be needed to protocols and standing orders.
- Identify situations that are currently not addressed by protocols and standing orders.

Although it may not be feasible, all ambulance runs should be reviewed. First and foremost the focus of CQI needs to be on improving patient care. Often providers show hesitation to use the CQI process because of fear of being ridiculed or reprimanded. To avoid this, it is important to use your CQI process not as a punitive tool, but as a constructive tool for continuous improvement.

Some services will choose to perform quality control as peer review **Figure 12** . Peer review can be a good learning experience if the people doing the reviewing have proper and consistent guidelines to follow and keep an open mind. No matter how good your education, you will still make mistakes and miss things from time to time. When a peer reviewer finds things you can improve, you should look at it as an educational tool. In an ideal system, the members of the peer review team rotate on and off, meaning that at some point you will also serve as a reviewer. Caution: never use this process as a tool to demean or belittle a

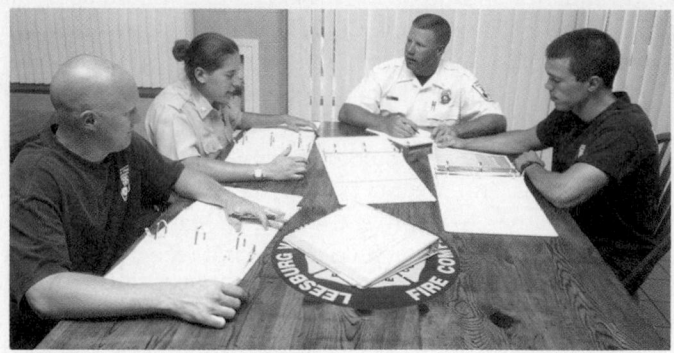

Figure 12 Peer reviews should be seen as a constructive part of paramedic practice.

fellow paramedic. Nor should you discuss your findings with anyone who is not identified as part of the review process. Be professional.

A comprehensive CQI program can help to prevent problems from arising by evaluating day-to-day operations and identifying possible stress points in these operations. These may include the following:

- Medical direction issues
- Education
- Communications

YOU are the Medic   PART 4

Due to the urgency of the situation, you tell your partner to get en route to the Mayfield Trauma Center that is 9 miles away. It is 1628. You call medical control and give a thorough description of the mechanism of injury, signs and symptoms, presentation, and vital signs and request orders to perform a needle thoracostomy en route. The physician tells you to go ahead with the procedure and to advise him of any changes.

As soon as you complete the procedure, the fire fighter tells you that there is less resistance as he ventilates the patient. You note that chest rise is almost symmetrical and his blood pressure and pulses improve. He is still unresponsive.

You arrive at the trauma center at 1638. You give your report to the receiving facility and complete your documentation while your partner cleans and restocks the ambulance. You save a copy of the report for your supervisor to add to a study being done on the benefits of prehospital needle thoracostomy. Ten minutes later you are in service and headed to another call.

Recording Time: 13 Minutes	
Respirations	12 breaths/min assisted with bag-mask ventilations
Pulse	118 beats/min
Skin	Pale, slightly diaphoretic
Blood pressure	104/62 mm Hg
Oxygen saturation (Spo$_2$)	98% on oxygen via bag-mask device
Pupils	Equal but sluggish to react

7. This situation is a good example of how EMS research may help future patients through evidence-based practice. Explain.

8. How is retrospective research beneficial for educating EMS personnel?

- Prehospital treatment
- Transportation issues
- Financial issues
- Receiving facility review
- Dispatch
- Public information and education
- Disaster planning
- Mutual aid

A function of the evaluation process for ensuring quality control is to determine ways to eliminate human error. To cut down on the potential for errors, ensure adequate lighting when handling medications and keep interruptions to a minimum. Keeping medications in a specific location and in their original packaging can also reduce the potential for errors.

High-risk activities include handing patients off. You must deal with the issues not only of the physical transfer of the patient from your stretcher, but also communication with the next caregiver in line. Providing a written copy of your assessment and treatment along with the verbal report helps to ensure coordinated care. It is imperative that you give a report of your care of the patient and any changes that may have occurred since you took over care. States often require that documentation be left with the patient. Other safety issues revolve around advanced airway management, medication administration, and safe transport (such as avoiding ambulance crashes and providing proper immobilization) of patients who may have potential traumatic injuries.

It is important that you strive to eliminate errors as much as possible. Understanding the circumstances of the errors helps to minimize them. There are three main sources of errors. They can occur as a result of a rules-based failure, a knowledge-based failure, or a skills-based failure (or any combination of these). For example, does a paramedic have the legal right to administer the particular medication needed by the patient? If not, a rules-based failure has occurred if a paramedic assists with the administration. Does a paramedic know all of the pertinent information about the medication being delivered? If not, a breakdown at this point, such as the administration of the wrong medication, would be referred to as a knowledge-based failure. Finally, is the equipment operating and being used properly? If not, a skills-based error has occurred. Any error can come from multiple sources.

Agencies need to have clear protocols, which are detailed plans that describe how certain patient issues, such as chest pain or shortness of breath, are to be managed. These protocols need to be understood by all paramedics within the service.

The environment can be part of the reason for errors. Are there ways to limit distractions? Can paramedics find what they need in a timely manner? Sometimes the solution is as easy as ensuring flashlights are available on all ambulances. Make sure all drugs and equipment are properly labeled and organized.

When you are about to perform a skill, ask yourself, "Why am I doing this?" Considering the reason for your actions allows you time to reflect and make a more informed decision. If you have considered what to do and cannot come up with a solution, ask for help. Talk with your partner, contact medical control, or call your EMS supervisor.

Another way for you to help limit medical errors is to use "cheat sheets." Have a copy of your protocol book with you. Emergency physicians have many reference materials available to them. Physicians recognize they cannot memorize everything, so referencing a book or a reliable Internet resource helps ensure the use of accurate information.

Preventing errors requires being conscientious of protocols and not allowing interruptions while providing patient care. Use downtime to refresh the skills you use less often. Use decision-making aids, such as algorithms, and reflect on what has been done as an informal critique for future improvement of your performance. Finally, after a troublesome call, sit down and talk. Talk with your partner and/or your supervisor. Discussing the events that just happened provides an excellent avenue for learning. Your discussions can help lead to changes in protocol, changes in how equipment is stocked, or even the purchase of new equipment.

■ EMS Research

As medicine has increasingly been drawn toward **evidence-based practice**, so has the EMS system. Although EMS systems have been used for more than 30 years, there is little or no evidence that the care that has been provided to patients is optimal. Patient care protocols should be based on scientific findings. A leading role in this effort to link scientific findings to patient care has been taken by the Department of Transportation National EMS Research Agenda, which is developing processes and setting goals for the optimization of prehospital emergency care. This research can force a dramatic departure from the standardized, non-evidence-based method of operation historically used in EMS. For example, recent studies have shown that a "hands only" CPR technique by bystanders improves outcomes in victims of sudden cardiac arrest. Previously, the treatment protocol dictated care for airway and breathing first for all patients and then care for circulation (the ABCs). Research has shown, however, that to provide the best outcome for patients in cardiac arrest, circulation should be addressed first, followed by care for airway and breathing (CAB). Similar studies are planned or in progress to either change or reaffirm the provided standards of care in prehospital medicine.

It is important to ensure that research is performed by properly educated researchers, typically persons who have a PhD or MD degree and an interest in EMS research. Both the National Registry of EMTs and the Robert Wood Johnson Foundation operate EMS-related research fellowships to aid in the development of EMS-focused researchers.

An increase in the number of higher learning education centers (colleges and universities) that provide an EMS track for students is a tremendous benefit to the EMS system. This allows the student to enter the EMS field not only trained as a paramedic, but also holding a bachelor's degree. Although the EMS field is currently primarily composed of providers who hold a license or certification, paramedic students who have bachelor's degrees will further enhance the profession within the medical community. Higher learning institutions also produce high-quality research, which then feeds back into the educational system and practice.

The Research Process

The first step in conducting research is to identify the specific problem, procedure, or question to be investigated. In general, a research topic usually arises when a certain practice is questioned. For example, the efficacy of endotracheal intubation and rapid sequence intubation in the field has been a popular research topic. Even if the topic has been researched before, this does not mean it cannot be revisited. Sometimes research findings can be flawed and a new process may identify flaws or enhance previous research findings. Once the question is determined, a **research agenda** is developed. This agenda specifies the questions to be answered and the precise methods in which the data will be gathered. Although numerous additional questions may arise from results during the study, the researcher must adhere to the research agenda and answer only the question at hand. Other items of interest encountered during the course of the research may themselves become topics of research in a separate study.

Once a qualified researcher has decided on a specific question to be answered, the next step is to determine the **research domain** in which the study should be conducted. A research domain is the area of research (clinical, systems, or education). A clinical domain, for example, would include stroke research involving clinical trials that would lead to improved patient care. A systems domain in EMS research would focus on operations, such as the effects of 24-hour shifts on patient care. An education domain would focus on how programs are taught, such as a study of the components that make up high-performing paramedic programs.

EMS research may be performed by EMS providers, but it is usually performed by persons with a master's degree or doctorate who are studying a particular branch of medicine or science. EMS research may be performed within a **research consortium**; this is a group of agencies working together to study a particular topic. Paramedics may be involved in collaborative research by gathering data. You may be part of a study to determine how much oxygen should be given to patients with shortness of breath, or you could be involved in a study to track the time it takes to transport serious trauma patients to the emergency department. Your job will be to ensure that you accurately gather and report data about the patients you encounter who fit within the study's parameters. The information gathered will then be analyzed by the researcher(s) to answer the question at hand. The results could then be shared with the rest of the EMS and scientific community to improve patient care practices. Evidence-based medical practice is based on such research.

Funding

When a research project begins, it is advisable for the researchers to use an **institutional review board (IRB)**. An institutional review board involves a group or institution that reviews the research. The requirements for review, which make research eligible for federal funding, were devised in 1966 by the US Public Health Service.

All research requires funding. In particular, large clinical trials or systems research can carry a significant fiscal cost. This cost is funded through a variety of sources, such as local or federal government, nonprofit foundation grants, and industry or corporate funding. To qualify for a federal or public grant, the study must first go through a rigorous evaluation process to ensure that it will answer a question within the domain covered by the grant. The methods and results are then subject to stipulations placed on them by the grantor. Similarly, nonprofit organizations or foundations will fund research into their specific areas of interest, and will typically have some control over the methods used. Corporate support can be in the form of a grant to a nonprofit research organization, or more commonly as a chartered research project to validate a product manufactured by the corporation, such as a new medication or medical equipment.

Any type of support given to a researcher is considered funding, including free lab space, travel, or assistants to help with the research. To prevent the appearance of bias or potential conflicts of interest, researchers need to disclose all sources of funding and support and maintain total transparency with regard to their research methods.

Types of Research

There are different types of research. The type of research that will yield the best results may depend on the research topic and what the researcher wishes to learn. Types include quantitative and qualitative.

Qualitative research focuses on questions within a context of surrounding events and concurrent processes and attempts to build a more complete, holistic picture. In other words, qualitative research takes into account the real-world factors that may have influenced the results of a study and may attempt to interpret the results to account for these factors. Oftentimes, qualitative research is used when specific answers cannot be identified in quantitative research. Qualitative research often involves the interpretation of previously published data by the researcher and making a statement of the findings. Qualitative methods investigate the why and how of decision making, not just what, where, and when. It is difficult to evaluate qualitative studies using set guidelines. Rather, each study must have a set of parameters specific to the question. Most medical research falls into the qualitative category.

Quantitative research is based on numeric data. Types of quantitative research include the following:

- **Experimental research.** A scientific approach to research in which a researcher controls, manipulates, and then measures one or more variables to ascertain how manipulating the variables affects the subjects. Experimental research is concerned with cause-and-effect relationships.
- **Nonexperimental research.** Descriptive research that does not involve experimentation using patients and manipulating variables to reach a conclusion. For example, a study

on the effectiveness of different levels of pain management would be unethical to conduct on humans; therefore, data would be gathered through interviewing patients and watching vital sign parameters.

- **Survey research.** In this type of research, conclusions are based on survey results. To be valid, researchers must identify what is being measured and determine the appropriate sample size. Additionally, the sample population must reflect the composition of the population being researched. For example, if a study of the incidence of cancer were conducted in an area that had a particularly high incidence of cancer, the results of that study would not be indicative of the whole country.

Retrospective research uses available data, for example, from medical records or patient care reports. Research may involve examining those records to determine the types of calls that required transport and areas in which the department can improve, such as in response and transport times. This information is then used to develop educational sessions for EMS personnel or can be used to plan public education and public prevention strategies. It may be necessary for the researcher to collaborate with a hospital or group of hospitals in gathering the necessary patient outcome information. In order to comply with federal laws such as the Healthcare Insurance Portability and Accountability Act (HIPAA), patient identification information may have to be deleted from records prior to the change of hands between agencies.

Many large retrospective studies collect and analyze data from widespread, sometimes nationwide, patient databases. Such databases link EMS, hospitals, and even posthospitalization providers into the system and allow for a broad, total picture of the patient population in question. Nationwide databases for cardiac arrest patients, patients requiring extracorporeal membrane oxygenation, and trauma registries exist within the United States. Nationwide databases are typically overseen by a centralized agency, for example, within the federal government; data are usually collected by state or local governments to populate the databases. The same techniques of data collection and analysis can be used at the local level for smaller research projects; data from various hospitals and EMS agencies can be entered into a centralized database that can then be used to study specific patient populations. For accurate research results, however, there must be clear-cut guidelines for data entry so that comparisons of data can be made.

In addition to retrospective research, other types of research include prospective research, cohort research, and case studies. **Prospective research** studies gather information as events occur in real time. A **cohort research** examines patterns of change, a sequence of events, or trends over time within a certain population or "cohort" of study subjects. Inversely, a **case study** method is the investigation and documentation of a single case over a period of time.

Additionally, these categories can be subgrouped as cross-sectional or longitudinal. The **cross-sectional design** collects all data at one point in time, essentially serving as a "snapshot" of events and information. The **longitudinal design** collects information at various set time intervals. Therefore, a prospective study must have, by design, a longitudinal data-gathering method, whereas retrospective, cohort, or case study research can utilize either a cross-sectional or longitudinal data collection technique.

Finally, a **literature review** is a form of research in which the existing literature is reviewed, and the researcher analyzes the collection of research to draw a conclusion.

Research Methods

A beginning step in conducting research is to identify the group or groups of people necessary for the research. Once the group(s) is identified, it may be refined further, such as limiting the research to people in a specific age bracket, with a certain medical condition, or of a specific gender. As an example, a researcher may wish to study women between the ages of 30 and 40 who have diabetes. Once the list of eligible subjects is identified, researchers randomly choose who will be part of the research. There are many different ways to achieve this. A list of subjects or groups can be computer-generated (**systematic sampling**) or time frame parameters can be set (**alternative time sampling**). Finally, the least preferred method is when subjects are manually assigned to a specific researcher (**convenience sampling**), rather than being randomly assigned. Even in the best cases, **sampling errors** can occur. For example, a study may fail to include all of the needed subjects, or there may be people in the study who meet criteria but still are not the best representation.

Parameters should be identified in research. Parameters outline the type of people who are appropriate for the study. Another tool to consider is **blinding**, in which subjects are not told the specifics of the project. There are single-, double-, and triple-blinded studies where one, two, or all parties are blinded, respectively. When participants of the research project are advised of all aspects of the project, it is known as an **unblinded study**.

As research continues, data will be acquired. The gathered statistics can be either in a **descriptive** or **inferential** format. In a descriptive format, observations are made, but no attempts are made to alter or change an event. In an inferential format, a hypothesis is used to prove one finding over another. Descriptive statistics can also be performed in either a qualitative or quantitative style. The quantitative approach covers additional variables, such as the mean, median, and mode. For example, in a study on diabetes in women who are between 30 and 40 years old, the mean age of study participants equals the average age of the subjects, the median age is the midpoint age of the subjects, and the mode is the most frequent age of the subjects. Finally, standard deviation outlines how much the scores in each set differ from the mean.

Ethical Considerations

As in many aspects of a profession, there are **ethical** items to consider when conducting research. One entity that monitors whether a study is conducted ethically is the study's IRB, whose primary purpose is to ensure the protection of study participants and to ensure appropriate conduct. Researchers must ensure that the risks will not outweigh the benefits. They must acquire consent from all subject(s) and be certain their rights and welfare are adequately protected. Any potential conflicts of interest to the study should be identified. For example, if a person is involved in a similar study, or is employed by the person or company performing the study, this would be considered a conflict of interest. Subjects must be allowed to participate voluntarily without being coerced. Subjects must also be informed of all potential risks that may occur and be allowed to withdraw from the research at any time Figure 13. At a minimum, the subjects should be advised they are protected by the Office of Human Research Protection. This office offers materials to those involved in research. The Food and Drug Administration also offers guidance for researchers on a variety of topic areas. To ensure the research is not flawed, the potential of subject withdrawal or any other possible variable that may affect the outcome should be identified before the study begins.

Patients who are potential participants in a clinical domain research trial must be informed about the study protocols prior to participating in the study. For example, a pharmaceutical corporation may have introduced a new clot-busting medication. To validate the effectiveness of the medication, patients are entered into a trial, in which they will either receive the new medication, a more well-studied medication, or perhaps a placebo. The patient would have to be informed of the potential effects of the study and sign a waiver to be entered into the program. In some cases a treatment that is being studied may be administered in emergency situations under waiver of informed consent; it is assumed that the patient would want the treatment to be given because of its lifesaving effects.

■ Evaluating Medical Research

Paramedics must know how to evaluate what is true medical research and what is a printed personal preference. When evaluating a research article, you must look for certain criteria in order to determine the quality of the research. Table 3 provides

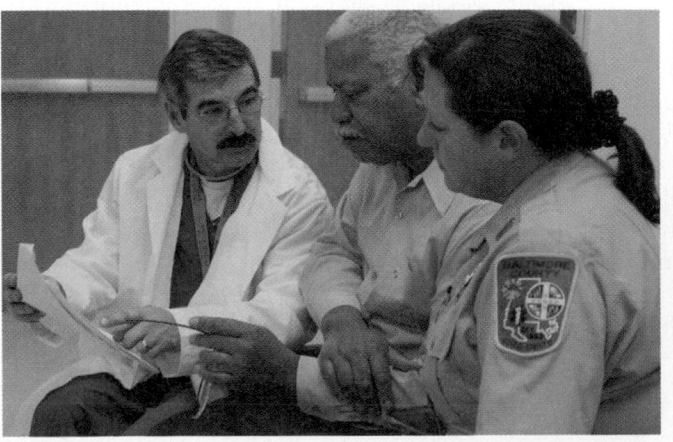

Figure 13 Any person who participates in a research study should be well informed of the study's goals as well as the potential risks and any potential benefits associated with participation.

Table 3 Fifteen Questions to Answer When Evaluating and Interpreting Research
1. Was the research peer reviewed?
2. What was the research hypothesis?
3. Was the study approved by an institutional review board and conducted ethically?
4. What was the population being studied?
5. What were the inclusion and exclusion criteria?
6. What method was used to acquire a sample of patients?
7. How many groups were the patients divided into?
8. How were the patients assigned to the groups?
9. What type of data was gathered?
10. Did the study have enough patients involved?
11. Are there any confounding variables unaccounted for?
12. Were the data analyzed correctly?
13. Is your conclusion logically based from the data?
14. Will it apply in local EMS systems?
15. Were the patients similar to those in your local EMS system?

15 questions to answer when evaluating and interpreting research. For example, does the article contain references to other research, or not? Is there input from expert peers? Does the article discuss previous research? When you review research, you must read every part, including the indexes.

The type of journal in which the research is published is also an important part of determining quality and validity. One method of ensuring quality and validity is through the **peer review** process. Many medical journals accept research studies from a wide variety of sources. Prior to publication, these studies are sent to subject matter experts (the author's "peers") for review of the content and research methods. The research and its conclusions are then accepted, revised, or rejected based on the findings of the peer review. This method allows for a greater checks-and-balances in ensuring quality of the research methods and validity of research conclusions. Many EMS and medical peer-reviewed journals are available in print.

Additionally, the widespread proliferation of medical information on the Internet has resulted in specific Internet sites becoming valid tools for accessing research. Sources range from a wide source such as Google Scholar, to more medically specific sources such as Medscape and PubMed, which contain a substantial number of published articles from various journals and publications. When you are reviewing the research available on a particular topic, this is a useful tool for finding peer-reviewed research.

As discussed, a research study must follow a structured process. It will define exactly what it is intended to be measured, the population affected, and the goal of the research. A good research article will have adequate data; for example, 5,000 people were identified and followed over a 5-year period, with data available from all persons involved. With any research topic, there are limitations as to what can be measured and how accurately. If in reviewing a research article, you find that some people backed out, died, or were omitted for any reason not originally anticipated or outlined, then the research will most likely be flawed.

Evidence-Based Practice

Evidence-based practice is becoming an integral part of functioning as an EMS provider. Patient care should be focused on the procedures that have proven useful in improving patient outcomes. There is a limited amount of prehospital EMS research relative to other areas of medical research; however, as EMS research continues, evidence-based practice will have a correspondingly greater role in EMS. High-quality patient care should focus on procedures useful in improving patient outcomes through sound research. It is important for EMS providers to stay up-to-date on the latest advances in health care. Every 3 to 5 years, the American Heart Association unveils a revised set of guidelines based on large amounts of evidence. The American Heart Association provides an excellent example of evidence-based medical decision making in progress. To learn more about the consensus on the science of resuscitation, refer to the website for the organization ILCOR, which is the International Liaison Committee on Resuscitation. These changes occur because more information is known. One word of caution: When reading new research results, make sure you understand what the results mean. Ask questions, and conduct some of your own research. Conclusions that seem too good to be true are usually not true.

To link medical research and evidence to patient care, you must ensure that the quality of the evidence is sufficient to justify changing patient care protocols. To ensure quality evidence, researchers have developed a generally accepted system for rating the quality of a study from I to IV, with Level I being considered the highest quality of evidence.

Level I evidence stems from research consisting of multiple studies on a widespread, large sample size. Additionally, the study must have randomization. The study does not just utilize the one procedure in question, but also uses other techniques as a basis of comparison of how results vary. If the new technique or medication used results in a significant positive effect or outcome when weighed against other methods, it is considered a high-quality study.

Level II evidence results from a single, randomly controlled trial, from multiple trials with small sample sizes, or from multiple large, randomly controlled studies that resulted in a moderate effect on patient outcome.

Level III evidence is divided into A, B, and C categories. A IIIA study is from a well-designed trial without randomization. IIIB studies consist of evidence from causal comparison and case or cohort studies. (Causal comparative studies investigate cause/effect relationships.) IIIC studies have evidence gathered from single experiments.

Level IV evidence, which is considered the lowest level, consists of reviews of descriptive studies or expert opinion or uncontrolled studies.

Quality EMS research has many benefits for the future. In all health care fields, research determines the effectiveness of treatment—what works and what does not work. Because funding for EMS continues to be a problem, it is important that EMS prove that what it does makes a difference. Proper research achieves this when it is outcome based, which means the topic generates thoughts on improving the overall patient outcome. Research can help identify which procedures, medications, and treatments work and which do not. Once a study is released and your medical director has decided to follow its recommendations, your service should measure the results of these new practices in your CQI program. These can be as simple as changing jump kit design to allow for a faster door-to-drug administration time for cardiac patients, to adding thousands of dollars of equipment to provide therapeutic hypothermia. These combined research efforts eventually will lead to a higher professional image to the community of the services that you provide.

YOU *are the Medic*   SUMMARY

1. What is your first action as you are approaching the scene and conducting a scene size-up?

As you are approaching the scene you should look not only for hazards, but also for the need for any additional resources. Radio the dispatcher to send the fire department for spilled fluids and additional help. Request law enforcement personnel for traffic control and/or crowd control. Are there any other hazards requiring specialized care such as downed power lines or hazardous materials? Do a quick visual inspection to determine the mechanism of injury. How many patients do you see? Call for additional units as soon as possible to minimize scene time and the length of time it will take for all patients to reach definitive care.

2. What role does the EMS system play in this call?

The EMS network begins with citizen involvement. The public must recognize a need and be aware of how to access the EMS system in your community. Once the EMS system has been activated, a dispatcher receives the information and processes or interprets the information, making the determination of whether this is an actual emergency, and then dispatches appropriate units. The dispatcher may be trained as an emergency medical dispatcher, and may give prearrival instructions to the caller to provide care until EMS is on scene.

As a paramedic, when you arrive on scene you will have to determine what is happening at the scene and develop a plan of care for the patient or patients. This includes deciding on the appropriate transport method and receiving facility. For this reason you must be aware of the best local resources that will meet the needs of the patient.

3. What aspects of professionalism must be employed in this situation?

As a health care professional you must provide care appropriate for your level of certification and do so in a manner that instills confidence in your patient as well as others on scene. You are in a highly visible role and are judged on your level of professionalism. You are a representative of your agency and as you enter a situation, you must continually show that you are truly concerned with the well-being of your patient and his or her family. Your appearance is also an important part of your professionalism. Remember that this is the first impression the public has of you and you want it to be a positive one.

In this situation, you must employ integrity as well as empathy when dealing with the patient's girlfriend. She is scared and upset, as most people are when faced with a traumatic situation. Communicating with her should not take precedence over patient care, but a kind word can make all the difference in instilling confidence in your ability. You should also be aware that she is possibly a valuable source of information for patient history because the patient is unable to speak for himself. If you deem the situation serious enough that the patient needs your immediate care, you may ask a partner or another responder to gather this information from her. You must work as a team with your partner and, in this case, the fire fighters to assess, package, and treat this patient. You could ask one of the fire fighters to talk with the

girlfriend and let her know that you are doing everything possible to help the patient and also to advise her of which hospital you are transporting him to. You should act as an advocate for this patient because he is unable to speak for himself and advise the hospital of any information received from the girlfriend on scene.

4. Aside from those noted in the previous question, what other roles and responsibilities are vital in your status as a health care professional?

Educating the public is a large part of your responsibility as a paramedic. You should involve yourself in prevention, community, and leadership activities whenever possible. The public should know how to appropriately use your services, and promotion of public involvement in activities such as CPR training are vital in areas where EMS resources are limited. These actions can be a major determinant in whether a patient lives or dies.

Some paramedics may work in clinics, emergency departments, and hospitals, and providers of all EMS levels need to be advocates for prehospital health care. Continue your education, become a mentor for new EMS professionals, and evaluate EMS research to stay well informed on the efficacy of EMS practices.

5. Even though you do not have standing orders to perform a needle thoracostomy, you know this is what the patient needs. How will you handle this situation?

If protocols do not cover the situation you are in, you must radio medical control for orders. It is imperative that you have a good working relationship with your medical director and the physicians at the hospitals where you frequently transport patients. You are the eyes and ears on the scene and as such, you must provide a clear picture of the circumstances for medical control when requesting orders for actions that fall outside of standing orders. Explain the situation, including all findings as well as pertinent negatives and vital signs, to the answering physician and provide the reason you are requesting this order. Include your estimated time of arrival in your report. This may play a major role in the determination to allow you to perform the requested procedure. Once the order is given, repeat it back to the physician. Perform the procedure, and then contact medical control with an update including current vital signs and the patient's response to treatment.

6. How will you make the determination of how and where to transport this patient?

Appropriate transport and destination decisions are often made through cooperation with other medical professionals. The patient's injuries and presentation should dictate whether he is taken to the closest facility (ie, cardiac arrest) or to a more appropriate location that may be farther away (ie, a trauma center in the case of this patient).

The patient in this scenario has an altered mental status and respiratory compromise, making this an emergency transport. If definitive care is a great distance, air transport may be a better option. He should be transported to a trauma center as opposed

YOU *are the Medic* | SUMMARY, *continued*

to a small local facility. The patient potentially needs surgical intervention, and transporting him to any facility other than a trauma center will only delay definitive care and increase the risk of morbidity or mortality.

7. This situation is a good example of how EMS research may help future patients through evidence-based practice. Explain.

Through evidence-based practice, patient care is focused on the procedures that have proven useful in improving patient outcomes—needle thoracostomy in this instance. Documentation of procedures that have benefited patients helps provide research that may lead to protocols or standing orders for patients with the same presentation in the future. High-quality patient care should focus on procedures useful in improving patient outcomes through sound research. Paramedics must stay up-to-date on the latest advances in health care. Organizations such as the American Heart Association are constantly updating their guidelines based on large amounts of evidence. Your entire career will be one of learning, and your experiences in patient care may help shape the future through research.

8. How is retrospective research beneficial for educating EMS personnel?

Retrospective research uses currently available information. Continuous quality improvement (CQI) is a form of retrospective research; examining patient care records can help determine opportunities for improvement and provides information to generate educational sessions for EMS personnel. It can also be used to plan public education and public prevention strategies. A comprehensive CQI program can help to prevent problems from arising by evaluating day-to-day operations and identifying possible stress points in these operations. It can also provide the basis for EMS research through evidence-based practice. The EMS industry is forced to not only prove through the scientific method that its practices are correct, but also that these practices are optimized for the greatest effect. The goal is to constantly strive to provide the best possible care for every patient. Through research, those ideas and practices that are proven obsolete are removed and new proven skills and procedures are introduced and taught.

EMS Patient Care Report (PCR)

Date: 04-20-11	**Incident No.:** 0457832	**Nature of Call:** MVC		**Location:** 300 block of Hunt Road	
Dispatched: 1618	**En Route:** 1618	**At Scene:** 1621	**Transport:** 1628	**At Hospital:** 1638	**In Service:** 1648

Patient Information

Age: 22 **Sex:** M **Weight (in kg [lb]):** 78 kg (172 lb)	**Allergies:** None known **Medications:** None **Past Medical History:** None **Chief Complaint:** AMS, possible pneumothorax, open fx of L lower leg

Vital Signs

Time: 1627	**BP:** 96/54	**Pulse:** 138	**Respirations:** 12	**Spo$_2$:** 92% on O$_2$ via bag-mask
Time: 1634	**BP:** 104/62	**Pulse:** 118	**Respirations:** 12	**Spo$_2$:** 98% on O$_2$ via bag-mask
Time:	**BP:**	**Pulse:**	**Respirations:**	**Spo$_2$:**

EMS Treatment
(circle all that apply)

Oxygen @ __15__ L/min via (circle one): NC NRM **Bag-mask device**	**Assisted Ventilation**	**Airway Adjunct:** Oral	CPR
Defibrillation	**Bleeding Control**	**Bandaging**	**Splinting**	**Other:** Cardiac monitor

Narrative

22-year-old man involved in an MVC—motorcycle rider who hit car, with AMS, possible pneumothorax, and open fx of L lower leg with minor bleeding. Helmet removed by bystanders prior to EMS arrival. On arrival pt supine on ground unresponsive, pupils equal but sluggish to react, presents with very diminished breath sounds on the left, hyperresonance to percussion, JVD, cardiac monitor showing sinus tach without ectopy, glucose 102 mg/dL. Skin pale, cool, diaphoretic. Inserted oropharyngeal airway, assisted ventilations with bag-mask, splinted L leg to R leg—bleeding controlled with direct pressure and bandaging, fully c-spine immobilized on long backboard with c-collar and blocks. Ventilations becoming increasingly difficult. Obtained orders from medical control for needle thoracostomy. After performing, neck veins are flat, Spo$_2$ increased to 98%, radial pulses stronger and increase in BP, easier to ventilate, no change in mental status. Transported to Mayfield Trauma Center without incident. **End of report**

Prep Kit

- World Wars I and II saw the development of ambulance corps to rapidly care for and remove injured soldiers from the battlefields.

- During the Korean and Vietnam Wars, wounded soldiers could be saved by using helicopters to rapidly remove them from the battlefields to a medical unit.

- In 1966 the National Academy of Science and the National Research Council released a "White Paper" outlining 10 critical points.
  - From these points the National Highway Safety Act was instituted in 1966.
  - The US Department of Transportation was also created.

- Paramedics are required to be licensed. This may also be called certification or credentialing. Performing functions as a paramedic prior to licensure is unlawful.

- The standards for prehospital emergency care and the people who provide it are governed by the laws in each state and are typically regulated by a state office of EMS.

- There are four levels of training: emergency medical responder, emergency medical technician, advanced emergency medical technician, and paramedic. At the paramedic level, personnel may perform invasive procedures under the direction of medical control.

- Paramedics may be involved in a variety of types of transports, including transports to specialty centers that focus on specific types of care of specific populations. They may also perform interfacility transports.

- Paramedics work with other health care providers and other public safety agencies. Becoming familiar with the roles and responsibilities of these parties will be beneficial when on EMS calls.

- Continuing education programs expose paramedics to new research findings and refresh their skills and knowledge.

- Each EMS system has a physician medical director who authorizes the providers in the service to provide medical care in the field. Medical control is off-line (indirect) or online (direct).

- The paramedic profession contains expected standards and performance parameters as well as a code of ethics.

- Professional attributes that a paramedic is expected to have include integrity, empathy, self-motivation, confidence, communication skills, teamwork, respect, patient advocacy, injury prevention efforts, careful delivery of service, time management skills, and administrative skills.

- Some of the primary paramedic responsibilities include preparation, response, scene management, patient assessment and care, management and disposition, patient transfer and report, documentation, and return to service.

- Quality control and continuous quality improvement are tools paramedics use to evaluate the care they provide to patients.

- Research helps bring together the findings of many professionals involved in EMS and brings forth a consensus of what EMS personnel should or should not do. Types of research include quantitative and qualitative research.

- There are many ethical considerations in conducting medical research. Researchers must obtain consent from all subjects, fully inform them of the research parameters, and ensure that the rights and welfare of subjects are protected.
- Paramedics must know how to evaluate medical research. Become familiar with criteria for determining the quality of the research, including how to recognize peer-reviewed literature, and how to use the Internet for finding quality research articles.
- Evidence-based practice is becoming an integral part of functioning as an EMS provider. Engage in reviewing medical literature as it becomes available, and make efforts to stay on top of changing guidelines related to your practice of paramedicine.

■ Vital Vocabulary

alternative time sampling Time parameters that are set during a research project.

blinding The method of not giving the specifics of a project to the people participating in a research or study.

case study A type of research in which a single case is investigated and documented over a period of time.

certification A process in which a person, an institution, or a program is evaluated and recognized as meeting certain predetermined standards to provide safe and ethical care.

cohort research A type of research that examines patterns of change, a sequence of events, or trends over time within a certain population of study subjects.

continuous quality improvement (CQI) A system of internal and external reviews and audits of all aspects of an EMS system.

convenience sampling A type of research in which subjects are manually assigned to a specific person or crew, rather than being randomly assigned; the least-preferred component of research.

cross-sectional design A data collection method in which all data at one point in time is collected, essentially serving as a "snapshot" of events and information.

descriptive A research format in which an observation of an event is made, but without attempts to alter or change it.

emergency medical services (EMS) A health care system designed to bring immediate on-scene care to those in need along with transport to a definitive medical care facility.

ethical A behavior expected by a person or group following a set of rules.

evidence-based practice The use of practices that have been proven to be effective in improving patient outcomes.

health care professional A person who follows specific professional attributes that are outlined in this profession.

inferential A research format that uses a hypothesis to prove one finding from another.

institutional review board (IRB) A group or institution that follows a set of requirements for review that were devised by the US Public Health Service.

licensure The process whereby a state allows qualified people to perform a regulated act.

literature review A form of research in which the existing literature is reviewed, and the researcher analyzes the collection of research to draw a conclusion.

longitudinal design A data collection method in which information is collected at various set time intervals, and not just at one time.

medical direction Direction given to an EMS service or provider by a physician.

mobile intensive care units (MICUs) An early title given to an ambulance-style unit.

off-line medical control Medical direction given through a set of protocols, policies, and/or standards.

online medical control Medical direction given in real time to an EMS service or provider.

parameters Outlined measures that may be difficult to obtain in a research project.

peer review The process used by medical magazines, journals, and other publications to ensure quality and validity of an article before publishing it, and which involves sending the article to subject matter experts for review of the content and research methods.

profession A specialized set of knowledge, skills, and/or expertise.

prospective research A type of research that gathers information as events occur in real time.

protocol A treatment plan developed for a specific illness or injury.

qualitative A type of descriptive statistic in research that does not use numeric information.

quality control The responsibility of the medical director to ensure that the appropriate medical care standards are met by EMS personnel on each call.

quantitative A type of measurement in research that uses a mean, median, and mode.

reciprocity The process of granting licensure or certification to a provider from another state or agency.

registration Providing information to an entity that stores it in some form of record book. In the context of EMS, records of your education, state or local licensure, and recertification are held by a recognized board.

research agenda The specific question(s) that a study aims to answer, and the precise methods in which the data will be gathered.

research consortium A group of agencies working together to study a particular topic.

research domain The area (clinical, systems, or education) that will be impacted by a study.

retrospective research Research performed from current available information.

sampling errors Expected errors that occur in the sampling phase of research.

standing order A type of protocol that is a written document signed by the EMS system's medical director that outlines specific directions, permissions, and sometimes prohibitions regarding patient care that is rendered prior to contacting medical control.

systematic sampling A computer-generated list of subjects or groups for research.

trauma systems The collaboration of prehospital and in-hospital medicine that focuses on optimizing the use of resources and assets of each with a primary goal of reducing the mortality and morbidity of trauma patients.

unblinded study A type of study in which the subjects are advised of all aspects of the study.

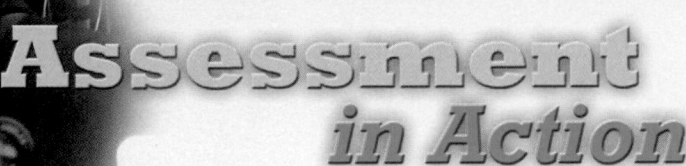

Assessment in Action

While on shift you and your partner are dispatched to a call for a 57-year-old man having chest pain. On arrival his wife tells you that he has an extensive cardiac history and hands you a bag full of medications. The patient is pale, diaphoretic, and clutching his chest. He says the pain is on the left side of his chest and radiating up into his jaw and down his left arm. He has not experienced relief from the nitroglycerin he took prior to your arrival.

During the primary assessment you notice that he is breathing at 22 breaths/min with adequate tidal volume and his oxygen saturation is 97% on room air. His radial pulse is rapid and irregular. He tells you that his pain is a "10" on a 1-10 scale. He is placed on the stretcher in a position of comfort and quickly loaded into the ambulance for further evaluation, treatment, and transport.

1. Which paramedic-level skill is needed for assessing this patient?
   A. IV therapy
   B. Oxygen administration
   C. Cardiac monitoring
   D. Administration of nitroglycerin

2. You recently read a study about the benefits of a prehospital infusion of potassium, insulin, and glucose for chest pain patients who meet certain criteria to provide fuel for dying cardiac cells. How could you implement the findings of this study into your paramedic care?
   A. Approach your supervisor to discuss the study.
   B. Perform a 12-lead ECG and administer an insulin injection to this patient.
   C. Call your medical director to discuss the study.
   D. All of the above

3. Once you have completed your paramedic course, you decide to work in another state. This may be accomplished through:
   A. reciprocity.
   B. certification.
   C. registration.
   D. licensure.

4. Paramedics are required to receive a set amount of continuing education based on the state in which they practice. How can continuing education credit be obtained?
   A. By attending conferences and seminars
   B. By reading EMS journals
   C. Through Internet-based continuing education providers
   D. All of the above

5. As a licensed paramedic you may be called on to perform advanced cardiology and pharmacologic skills that otherwise are only performed by physicians or other advanced practitioners. What gives the paramedic the authority to act?
   A. A medical director
   B. Protocols
   C. Standing orders
   D. Reciprocity

Additional Questions

6. While you are caring for a patient at the scene of an accident, a man steps forward and tells you that he is a physician and that he wants to assist in taking care of your patient. You do not recognize him, but he shows you physician credentials. How should you handle this situation?

7. Explain the purpose of EMS research and how to determine if a research article is high quality.

Workforce Safety and Wellness

National EMS Education Standard Competencies

Preparatory

Integrates comprehensive knowledge of the EMS system, safety/well-being of the paramedic, and medical/legal and ethical issues which is intended to improve the health of EMS personnel, patients, and the community.

Workforce Safety and Wellness

- Provider safety and well-being (pp 33-38)
- Standard safety precautions (p 48)
- Personal protective equipment (pp 48-50)
- Stress management (pp 39-43)
  - Dealing with death and dying (pp 43-45)
- Prevention of response-related injuries (pp 47-52)
- Prevention of work-related injuries (pp 36-37)
- Lifting and moving patients (pp 36-37)
- Disease transmission (pp 47-48)
- Wellness principles (pp 33-38)

Medicine

Integrates assessment findings with principles of epidemiology and pathophysiology to formulate a field impression and implement a comprehensive treatment/disposition plan for a patient with a medical complaint.

Infectious Diseases

Awareness of

- A patient who may have an infectious disease (pp 47-50)
- How to decontaminate equipment after treating a patient (chapter on *Transport Operations*)

Assessment and management of

- A patient who may have an infectious disease (chapter on *Infectious Diseases*)
- How to decontaminate the ambulance and equipment after treating a patient (chapter on *Transport Operations*)
- A patient who may be infected with a bloodborne pathogen (chapter on *Infectious Diseases*)
  - Human immunodeficiency virus (HIV) (chapter on *Infectious Diseases*)
  - Hepatitis B (chapter on *Infectious Diseases*)
- Antibiotic-resistant infections (chapter on *Infectious Diseases*)
- Current infectious diseases prevalent in the community (chapter on *Infectious Diseases*)

Anatomy, physiology, epidemiology, pathophysiology, psychosocial impact, presentations, prognosis, and management of

- HIV-related disease (chapter on *Infectious Diseases*)
- Hepatitis (chapter on *Infectious Diseases*)
- Pneumonia (chapter on *Infectious Diseases*)
- Meningococcal meningitis (chapter on *Infectious Diseases*)
- Tuberculosis (chapter on *Infectious Diseases*)
- Tetanus (chapter on *Infectious Diseases*)
- Viral diseases (chapter on *Infectious Diseases*)
- Sexually transmitted disease (chapter on *Infectious Diseases*)
- Gastroenteritis (chapter on *Infectious Diseases*)
- Fungal infections (chapter on *Infectious Diseases*)
- Rabies (chapter on *Infectious Diseases*)
- Scabies and lice (chapter on *Infectious Diseases*)
- Lyme disease (chapter on *Infectious Diseases*)
- Rocky Mountain Spotted Fever (chapter on *Infectious Diseases*)
- Antibiotic-resistant infections (chapter on *Infectious Diseases*)

Knowledge Objectives

1. State the steps that contribute to wellness and their importance in managing stress. (pp 33-38)
2. Understand the physiologic, physical, and psychological responses to stress. (pp 39-43)
3. Describe reactions to expect from critically ill and injured patients and how you can effectively work with patients exhibiting a range of behaviors. (pp 40-41)
4. Discuss techniques for working at particularly stressful situations, such as multiple-casualty scenes or the death of a child. (pp 42-46)
5. Describe posttraumatic stress disorder (PTSD) and steps that can be taken, including critical incident stress management, to decrease the likelihood that PTSD will develop. (p 46)
6. Describe issues concerning care of the dying patient, death, and the grieving process of family members. (pp 43-46)
7. Define "infectious disease" and "communicable disease." (p 47)
8. List various routes of disease transmission. (p 47)
9. Understand the standard precautions that are used to prevent infection when treating patients. (p 48)
10. Describe the steps to take for personal protection from airborne and bloodborne pathogens. (pp 48-50)
11. Explain postexposure management when exposed to patient blood or body fluids, including completing a postexposure report. (p 50)
12. Discuss the importance of ambulance cleaning and disinfection. (pp 49-50)
13. Describe the steps necessary to determine scene safety and to prevent work-related injuries at the scene. (pp 50-52)
14. List the various types of protective clothing you may need to wear to protect yourself from a variety of hazards. (p 50)
15. Discuss the different types of protective clothing worn to prevent injury. (pp 48-50)
16. Recognize the possibility of violent situations and the steps to take to deal with them. (pp 50-52)

Skills Objectives

1. Demonstrate the necessary steps to take to manage a potential exposure situation. (p 50)

Introduction

As a member of the EMS community, you are dedicated to providing prehospital emergency care and transport for the sick and injured, making your job gratifying, but also very demanding. Many skills are needed to deliver care, but some of the most important ones now stressed in current EMS education are those involving scene safety or safety in general. With the existence of scene hazards, environmental and human-made threats, and infectious diseases, scene safety remains crucial. Equally important are principles of how to take care of yourself—principles of wellness. The unique demands of EMS can be minimal or extreme. Oftentimes EMS providers do not get enough sleep or do not have enough time to eat or eat properly. Although there are many times on the job that you will not be able to get the proper sleep and nutrition you need, there is time outside of the job to take care of yourself. Simply put, if you have not prepared yourself, you may not be able to adequately serve your patients.

Present-day EMS continues to add more and more demands; therefore, being ready and able is more important than ever. As you begin your career, you may be assigned to a veteran paramedic who will serve as a mentor. The veteran may have been trained before wellness and safety training were given such high importance. Regardless of whom you will work with, this chapter is designed to highlight current suggestions for wellness and how to keep yourself ready for any emergency. Maintaining your health from the beginning will hopefully ensure a long, healthy, and satisfying career when you become that veteran in 20 to 30 years.

Components of Well-Being

Wellness was first defined in 1654 as the quality or state of being in good health, especially as an actively sought goal. A focus on wellness is indeed an important component of any EMS training program because it will enable providers to have a long, rewarding career in patient care.

Wellness is often considered to have three components: physical, mental, and emotional. Some believe that a fourth component, spiritual, is also essential.

Physical Well-Being

In health care, it is known that if providers are physically in shape, they are less likely to become injured and, if they do become injured, they may heal better. Muscle strength, flexibility, cardiac endurance, emotional equilibrium, posture (both sitting and standing), state of hydration, the foods you eat, and the amount of sleep you get all have an effect on your quality of life. Each of these factors may directly impact your chances of avoiding injury on the job. Also, you may be better able to deal with the mental stress associated with work in EMS. The American Heart Association's Simple 7 includes seven factors that have been found to improve heart health Figure 1, a major component of physical well-being. These factors include: get active, control cholesterol, eat better, manage blood pressure, lose weight, reduce blood sugar, and stop smoking. Taking these steps can improve mental well-being as well.

Nutrition

Present-day EMS has access to much more information regarding current guidelines about proper nutrition. In fact, as with anything in EMS, nutritional information is changing daily. Research often points out the consequences of poor nutrition—cardiac illness, type 2 diabetes, obesity, and a variety of medical conditions may result. However, many EMS services still require providers to work 24-hour shifts, oftentimes without meal or rest breaks. These on-the-job situations clearly challenge EMS providers who are trying to live a healthy lifestyle.

Today's education on nutrition suggests eating foods from the four main food groups (fruits and vegetables, meats, grains, and dairy products) in prescribed amounts. Research has shown that each person's requirements are different; therefore, nutritional requirements should be designed for individual needs. For example, a moderately active woman age 19 to

YOU *are the Medic*   **PART 1**

You are in a briefing at the office when a call comes in at 0712 for a possible cardiac arrest at 984 Solomon Street. You are en route 1 minute later. The traffic is very heavy at this time and you are becoming more and more agitated as you try to navigate through it. The frustration builds as you think about the work involved in running a code. You have not been sleeping well and were hoping for a slow morning to squeeze a nap in, but lately it seems as if you are repeating a never-ending cycle. You are not getting enough sleep, you are too tired to work out in the gym so your weight seems to be creeping up, and you eat too much junk food instead of regular meals simply because it is easier when you are on shift.

1. Your declining physical well-being is affecting your attitude and, in turn, your job. What can you do to change this?
2. Why is it so important to find ways to enhance your mental, emotional, and spiritual well-being?

Get Active

Why Get Active?

We all know that exercise is good for us, but nearly 70% of Americans do not get the physical activity they need. Living an active life is one of the most rewarding gifts you can give yourself and those you love. Simply put, daily physical activity increases your length and quality of life. If you get at least 30 minutes of moderate physical activity each day (like brisk walking), five times per week, you can almost guarantee yourself a healthier and more satisfying life while lowering your risks for heart disease, stroke and diabetes. Parents, your children need 60 minutes a day–every day–so when you get active, you're also modeling healthy living for the next generation.

The Price of Inactivity

If you exercise less than 150 minutes per week, you need to increase your activity level. Regular moderate intensity physical activity helps keep your heart in good condition. When you are inactive, you burn fewer calories, you are at higher risk for cholesterol problems, blood sugar and blood pressure problems, and your weight is often harder to manage. If that's not enough, physically active people nearly always report better moods, less stress, more energy and a better outlook on life.

What Can I Do To Get Active?

- Make the time
Nearly all of us feel time-crunched and over-scheduled. And although anyone can fall into a busyness trap, only you can make your health a priority over life's other demands. Even our nation's President sets aside time to exercise. It can be done and only you can say 'no' to interruptions and 'yes' to your good health!

- Start with walking
Walking is one of the best ways to get started. It's easy, it's social, it requires no special equipment, and it works! Just walk fast enough to get your heart rate up. Most of us can expect to cover 2 miles or more in a thirty minute block of time. If thirty minutes seems like an impossible goal, start with less. Some physical activity is always better than none! You can chart your progress as you work your way toward your goals.

To increase physical activity in your lifestyle try:

1. Parking farther away from your destination.
2. Taking short, brisk walks throughout the workday, in 10-minute chunks of time. After dinner, bring your dog along for a walk around the neighborhood.
3. Organizing school activities around physical activity.
4. Riding your bike or walking to work.

Figure 1 The American Heart Association's Simple 7 includes seven factors that have been found to improve heart health.

- **Oils.** Know your fats; make most fat sources from fish, nuts, and vegetable oils. Limit solid fats, like butter, stick margarine, shortening, and lard **Figure 3**.

Finally, it is a good idea to check the amount of sodium in canned and prepared foods, and choose those with lower amounts.

So, what do you think would be the best way for you to sustain your energy while on the job? Although it may be difficult because you really do not know what your shift will entail, preplan your meals. Keep yourself hydrated with bottled water, avoid soft drinks, and minimize your intake of caffeine. Carry numerous small snacks (like raisins, nuts, and fruits) that you can eat slowly and take with you to eat on the way back from a call. It is best to avoid fast food or high-fat foods because, although they may curb your hunger pains, in the long run they will not offer much to sustain your energy level.

Weight Control

EMS fieldwork calls on you to act quickly and accurately. Each day you must observe, assess, access, cope with, and control chaotic situations; therefore, staying fit is an important component for all

30 requires around 2,000 calories per day. This same calorie level is also suggested for sedentary men older than 50 years. The US Department of Agriculture (USDA) 2010 Dietary Guidelines focus on types of foods. The MyPlate icon shows relative portion sizes of the five food groups **Figure 2** :

- **Fruits.** Eat a variety of fruits; choose fresh, frozen, canned, or dried fruit. Go easy on fruit juices. Read labels; corn syrup should be avoided altogether. Look for products that have no sugar added.
- **Vegetables.** Vary the vegetables you eat; eat more dark green vegetables and orange vegetables, as well as dried beans and peas. Half of your plate should be fruits and vegetables.
- **Grains.** Make half your grains whole. Whole grains are healthier because they contain important nutrients that reduce the risk of disease. They also contain more protein and more fiber. Consume 3 ounces of whole grain bread, cereal, crackers, rice, or pasta every day. Look for the word "whole" before the grain name on the list of ingredients.
- **Meat and beans.** Go lean on protein; choose low-fat or lean meats and poultry. Bake, broil, or grill. Vary your choices with more fish, beans, peas, nuts, and seeds.
- **Dairy.** Eat calcium-rich foods, choosing low-fat or fat-free items. Choose fat-free or lowfat (1%) milk. If you cannot consume milk, choose lactose-free products or other calcium sources.

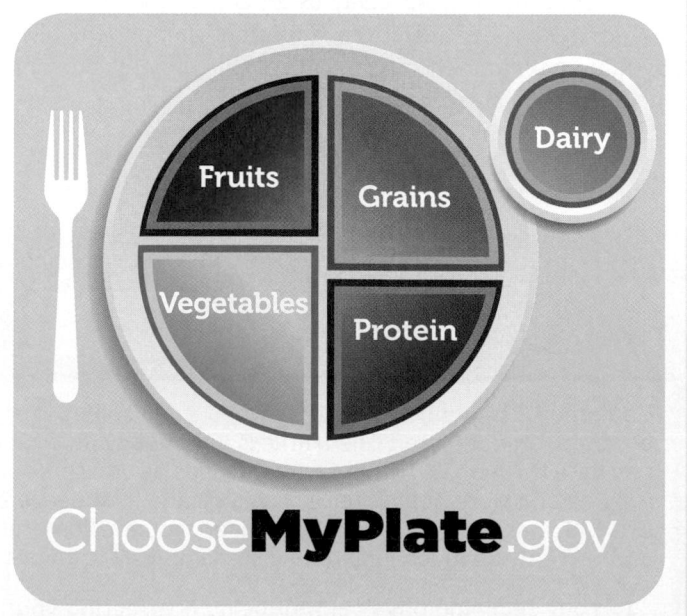

Figure 2 The USDA's MyPlate icon emphasizes healthy portions of vegetables, fruits, grains, proteins, and dairy.

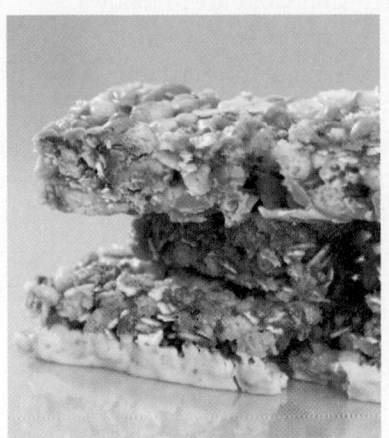

Figure 3 Health bars, smoothies, and energy drinks provide a quick, healthy alternative to fast foods.

people who work in the areas of public service. Oftentimes patterns you developed in your youth are harder to modify later in life, but it is never too late to make changes.

The USDA's 2010 Dietary Guidelines encourage lowering calorie intake, increasing physical activity, and making wiser food choices. The Guidelines discourage crash-dieting and instead recommend "eating fewer calories while increasing physical activity [as] the keys to controlling body weight." Diets are generally not as effective as making healthy food choices. It is also wise to eat less; the typical American consumes too many calories, which is ultimately stored as fat. Finally, the American Heart Association recommends that salt intake be minimized too.

However, gradual weight reduction is the key and it requires you to plan. Rather than taking coffee breaks, it is suggested that you take a walk or perform other forms of activity. If you must eat out, consider sharing a meal with your partner, eat oatmeal or cold cereal for breakfast, a salad with minimal or no dressing and half a sandwich for lunch, and a sensible dinner that consists of baked or broiled foods.

Exercise

Regular exercise has shown links to overall body weight, nutritional status, and hydration, and has been shown to improve sleep, mental capacity, ability to cope with stress, sex life, and overall long-term health. The exercise program for you depends on your personal preferences and goals. It should be something you enjoy and should be targeted at maintaining, or improving, three areas: your cardiovascular endurance, your flexibility, and your physical strength. If you are just beginning a program, it is recommended that you consult with your personal care physician.

In general, it is recommended that adults engage in at least 30 minutes of moderate to vigorous physical activity every day to help build optimal cardiovascular endurance. Working in a busy unit, you probably feel that you get that workout on every run, but activity on an EMS call does not meet the level of moderate to vigorous activity that raises your heart rate for the needed 30 minutes per day. To stay in good physical condition, you need to find a healthy balance between full-out physical activity (when you are "running hot") and no activity at all **Figure 4**. Present-day EMS services may provide their employees with workout equipment to use on each shift.

Depending on your level of health, there is a target heart rate you should try to achieve and attempt to reach every time you exercise; however, this should not be the goal if you are just beginning an exercise program. In that case, you should gradually increase your target heart rate. To find your target heart rate, calculate the following:

1. Identify your resting heart rate.
2. Take 220 and subtract your age in years. This total is your estimated maximum heart rate (not target range).
3. Take your maximum heart rate minus your resting heart rate. Depending on your level of health, multiply that figure by 60% to 80% (which means 0.6 to 0.8).
4. Add this figure to your resting heart rate.

Words of Wisdom

Tips for healthy eating include:
- Avoid oversized portions.
- Focus on fruits and vegetables.
- Vary the types of foods you eat. For example, choose alternate seafood, meat, and beans as your protein sources.
- Drink water instead of soda or other sugary drinks.
- Read food labels closely. Choose foods with lower calories, and lower amounts of fat, sugar, and sodium.

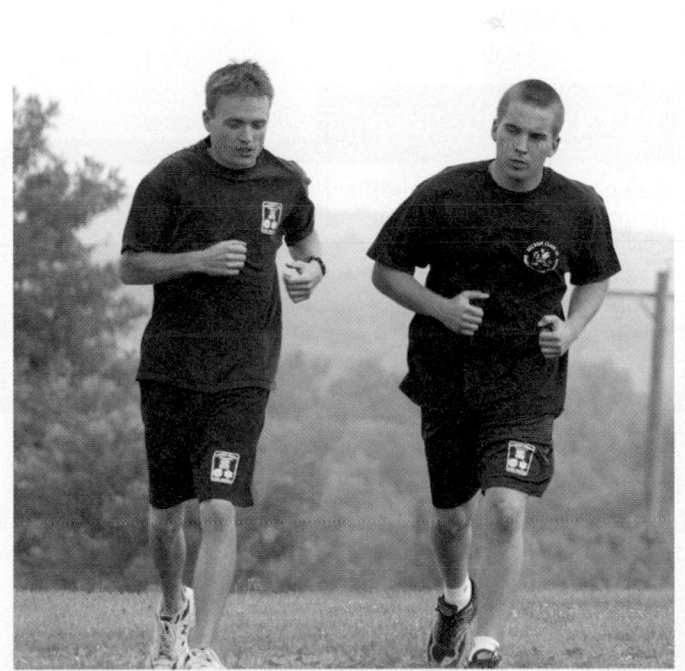

Figure 4 Regular exercise—apart from the work you do on calls—should be part of your daily or weekly routine.

For example, a 40-year-old man has a resting heart rate of 70 beats/min. Calculations would be as follows:

1. **Resting heart rate.**

   70 beats/min

2. **Maximum heart rate.**

   $220 - 40 = 180$ beats/min

3. **Maximum heart rate minus resting heart rate multiplied by 60% to 80% (we will use 70%, or 0.7).**

   $180 - 70 = 110 \times 0.7 = 77$

4. **Target heart rate.**

   $77 + 70 = 147$ beats/min

Smoking

Daily in your career you see the effects of smoking; therefore, if you do not smoke, do not start. You must also understand that everyone responds differently to smoke and some of your patients may be highly sensitive. If you smoke right before a call, the smell on your uniform may be enough to cause serious effects in an already sick patient.

If you are a smoker who is trying to quit, first understand that smoking is truly an addiction and quitting may not be easy. Talk to your primary care physician. There are a variety of programs that help to reduce a smoker's psychological dependency. These programs may include instructions, audiotapes, medications, and counseling to provide ongoing support. Other options that have been known to help some people are psychotherapy, hypnotism, and acupuncture.

Words of Wisdom

Being a paramedic in the field is physically and mentally demanding. Following simple guidelines for nutrition, exercise, and mental health will greatly enhance and prolong your career. Recruiting others you work with to join a health maintenance plan that includes these elements will foster teamwork as well as help maintain a balance between your career and your health.

Circadian Rhythms and Shift Work

EMS imposes schedules on paramedics that conflict with the body's circadian rhythms, or natural timing system. These rhythms are controlled by special areas of the brain, called the suprachiasmatic nuclei, which govern a person's "internal clock." Ignoring your circadian rhythms can cause you to experience consistent difficulty with sleep, higher thought functions, physical coordination, and even social functions. Try to determine what your natural rhythms are and design a schedule that is best for you. Research on circadian rhythms is only beginning to appear in medical journals, suggesting that someday a person might be able to alter his or her internal clock.

Some tips for dealing with shift work are as follows:

- Avoid caffeine.
- Eat healthy meals and try to eat at the same times every day.
- Keep a regular sleep schedule.

The most important point for all paramedics is: do not overlook the need for rest, whatever your rhythms. Current research and literature have shown that inadequate sleep has the same effect on the body and mind as being intoxicated. In this state, you would not want to be operating an emergency vehicle or administering medications.

Periodic Health Risk Assessments

Besides sleep, diet, exercise, hydration, and all the other things that make up a healthy lifestyle, you need to understand that hereditary factors may also have an effect on your overall health. Consider researching your immediate family's health history. Alzheimer disease, chemical addiction, cancer, cardiac illness, hypertension, migraine, mental illness, and stroke all feature prominent hereditary factors. The most common of all heredity health risk factors are heart disease and cancer.

Share this information with your personal physician. Work with him or her to set up a schedule for health assessments, building them into your routine physical checkups. Your physician should be your ally in screening for these diseases and in assessing your lifestyle as well as your heredity.

Body Mechanics

As a paramedic you will be required to lift and move a variety of patients. Some patients are small and light, whereas others may be significantly obese. There are a number of habits you can develop to prepare yourself to lift most weight ranges. They include the following actions:

- **Minimize the number of total body lifts you have to perform.** When patients need to be lifted, be prepared and plan the lift. In many cases, patients do not need to be lifted to a cot or any other location. For example, a patient with an arm laceration can stand and turn and sit on the cot or walk to the ambulance. Evaluate every situation to identify the easiest and safest way to lift or move a patient
- **Coordinate every lift prior to performing the lift.** Advise your patients regarding what they may experience during the lift so they do not panic. Once the lift is planned, use clear communication to execute it, such as "on the count of three, lift." Be sure that you plan and clarify with everyone, in advance, whether the lift will occur on three, or after you say "three."
- **Minimize the total amount of weight you have to lift.** If you have extra people around, ask for assistance. If possible, remove any unneeded equipment from the cot.
- **Never lift with your back.** Anyone who has spent a few years in EMS has made the mistake of lifting with his or her back. That can be a career-ender, unless you are lucky. To protect your back, follow these precautions **Figure 5**:
  - Always keep your back in a straight, upright position and lift without twisting.
  - When lifting, spread your legs about 15″ apart (shoulder width) and place your feet so that your center of gravity is properly balanced.

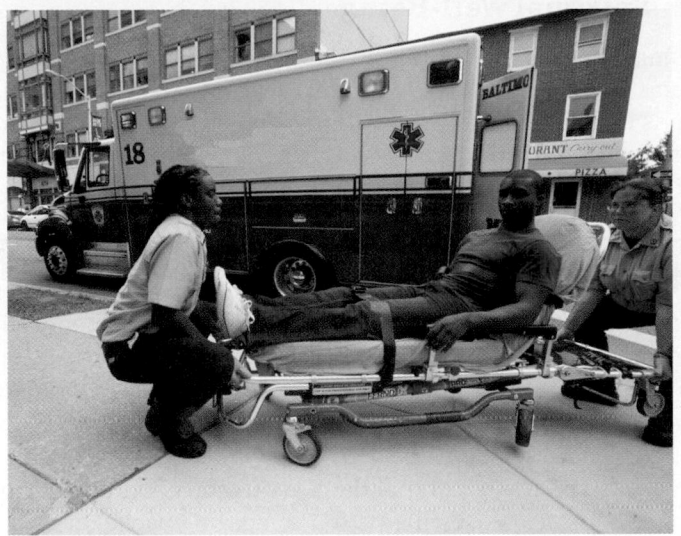

Figure 5 If your body is properly aligned when you lift, the line of force exerted against the spine occurs in an essentially straight line down the vertebrae. In this way, the vertebrae support the lift.

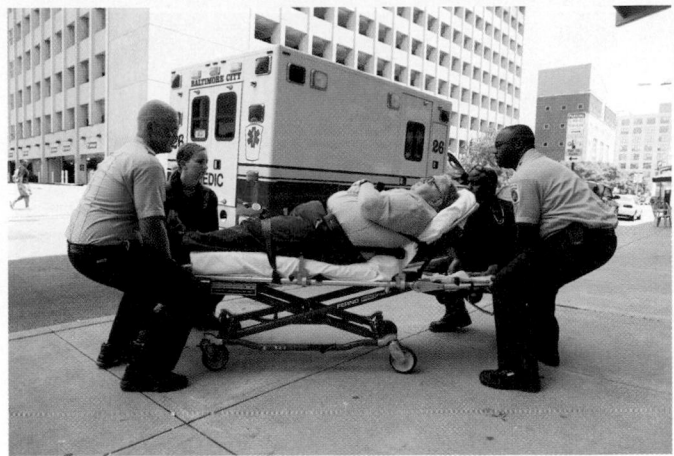

Figure 6 Never hesitate to ask for help from your coworkers, or to provide it when you are asked.

- Hold your back upright as you bring your upper body down by bending your legs.
- Lift by raising your upper body and arms and by straightening your legs until you are standing.
- Always lift with your legs, not with your back!
- Also, remember to breathe while lifting; do not hold your breath.

■ **Do not carry what you can put on wheels.** Position the ambulance, and the cot, as close to the patient as you can. Stair chairs have tracks to make going down stairs easier and safer.

■ **Ask for help.** Any time you need to move a patient who cannot or should not walk, consider the possibility of asking an extra person to help you **Figure 6**.

Mental Well-Being

As a paramedic you are not only exposed to diseases and injuries, you are also exposed and vulnerable to stress, especially when addressing the immediate needs of others. When a person is subjected to stress, the fight-or-flight system is activated. Preparing yourself on how you react when this system activates is crucial. For example, a physical conditioning regimen is a form of positive stress that allows a person to become more fit and better able to handle physical stress when it occurs. But when a person is unconditioned or if stress is overwhelming, the person cannot adapt as well when the fight-or-flight system kicks in. The fight-or-flight system creates physiologic responses to a profound stressor, including increased sympathetic tone, which results in dilation of the pupils, increased heart rate, dilation of the bronchi, mobilization of glucose, shunting of blood away from the gastrointestinal tract and cerebrum, and increased blood flow to the skeletal muscles. These actions help you deal with the situation immediately, relying on preplanning and gut instinct as your main resources, but to maintain your mental well-being for the long term, you need to be able to balance these situations by using appropriate coping skills.

A paramedic needs to be in control of his or her emotions. Is there a way paramedics can control their reactions? Absolutely. Remember, the most important thing you can do to control your behavior is to plan for it. There are many resources available to help you prepare. A simple thought to remember is that a professional is someone who can remain calm and think clearly when everything else is in disarray.

Emotional Well-Being

Professional caregivers have a natural interest in helping people. The key to remaining healthy in a lifelong practice of EMS is to make a deliberate effort to create a healthy balance between life at work and life away from work. Although many providers become very involved and dedicated to their work, it is important for you to separate yourself from your career from time to time and place focus on your personal life and family. All too frequently EMS providers and their families succumb unnecessarily to the effects of their career because they have not made that separation.

Every day EMS practitioners pour a large amount of energy into EMS, and while this is admirable, these providers need to be able to deal with the stress that they are exposed to on the job. A common stressor that you will be taught about is how to deal with patient disability and death. As a new provider you may feel that you can save or have a positive effect on every patient, but reality dictates that a patient's death, for example, is not your fault; some patients will not have a positive outcome regardless of what you do.

Good health care providers are strong, sensitive people **Figure 7**. However, these traits are also intertwined with normal emotional reactions to stressors of the job; therefore, EMS providers need to develop strategies for coping with stress. If you are approached by a coworker or leader who has noticed a negative change in your behavior, keep an open mind regarding

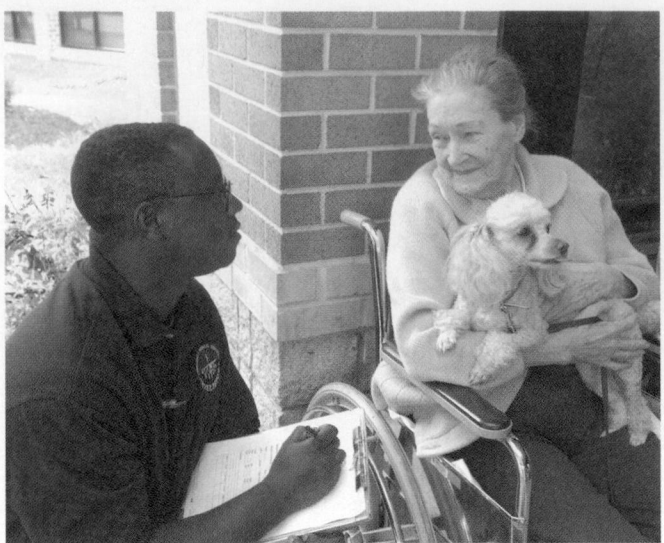

Figure 7 One thing that draws people to work as a paramedic is the pleasure of interacting closely with people.

what they see. If you note a change in your partner or other coworker, do not ignore it. You need to put aside any discomfort you may have about expressing your observations or fear of their reaction because the action you are taking may be the first step in moving someone away from disaster and back to emotional and physical well-being.

Spiritual Well-Being

Human spirituality is an unseen dimension of human experience. Some people address it with formal religion. Medical care supports the dignity and value of life and the sacredness of individuals. Your respect for the beliefs of patients or families will help in providing effective patient care.

Stress

Any event that causes us to react either physically, emotionally, or mentally is considered <u>stress</u>. Stress events may be pleasant, unpleasant, mild, or intense. Hans Selye, MD, PhD, considered the "father of stress theory," has defined biologic stress as the "nonspecific response of the body to any demand made upon it."

So, stress is a reaction of the body to any agent or situation (<u>stressor</u>) that requires the person to adapt. Adaptation of one sort or another is necessary for meeting the demands of everyday life. By itself, then, stress is neither a good thing nor a bad

Words of Wisdom

Some people may believe that showing emotion is a sign of weakness, and may not show the emotions you see in others in a similar situation. Everyone reacts differently to stressful events. Do not assume that people are not affected by stress because they do not react in the usual ways.

YOU are the Medic   PART 2

You arrive on scene 7 minutes later to realize you have been to this residence before, and you remember that this patient is a 23-year-old man with a history of leukemia whose condition has deteriorated rapidly during the past few weeks. Your heart drops as you remember the times that you have transported him and the conversations that you had. You remember thinking how you should appreciate how lucky you are to be healthy and have a good job. This courageous young man has always had something positive to say and a way of making everyone around him feel better. You immediately feel guilty for the way you have felt this morning—obviously your complaints come nowhere near the magnitude of this family's problems.

His mother ushers you into the house and tells you that he was feeling ill yesterday and would not eat last night. She just came in to check on him and found him not breathing.

Recording Time: 0 Minutes	
Appearance	Pale, cyanotic, appears lifeless
Level of consciousness	Unresponsive
Airway	Open and clear
Breathing	Apneic
Circulation	Pulseless
Skin	Cold to touch

3. The patient has been apneic for an undetermined amount of time. What is your next action?

4. On the basis of your previous interactions with the patient, what stage of the grieving process had he reached?

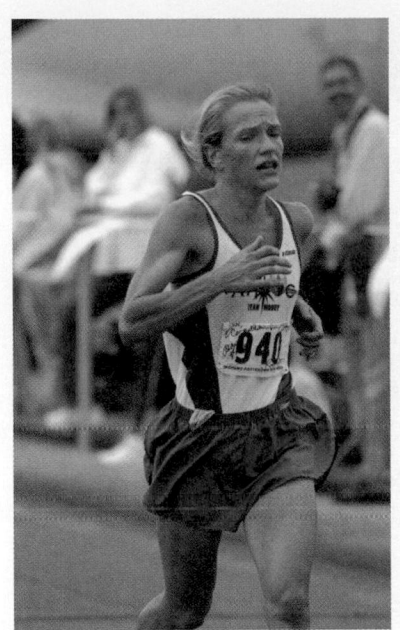

Figure 8 Some types of stress, called eustress, are positive and help push us to greater achievements.

thing; nor should stress be avoided. Selye classified stress into two categories: eustress (positive stress), the kind of stress that motivates a person to achieve; and distress (negative stress), the stress that a person finds overwhelming and debilitating **Figure 8**.

■ What Triggers Stress

A stress response often begins with events that are perceived as threatening or demanding, but the specific events that trigger the reaction vary enormously from person to person. The following factors trigger stress in most people:

- Loss of a loved one (death of a spouse or family member or going through a divorce) or of a valued possession
- Personal injury or illness
- Major life event (starting or finishing school, marriage, pregnancy, or having children leave home)
- Job-related stress (conflicts with others, excessive responsibility, the possibility of losing your job, or changing a job)

During the past three decades there have been a number of studies on the psychological stress levels in paramedics. The studies that seek to evaluate stress levels and compare them usually examine life-change units, or LCUs. These LCUs were originally described in the Life Chart Theory by Adolph Meyer and further explored by researchers Thomas Holmes and Richard Rahe. The researchers used the "Social Readjustment Rating Scale" that ranks 43 stress-producing events in a person's life and provides a weighted score for each event **Table 1**. The authors predicted that a score above 150 LCU could be associated with disease and illness (eg, heart attacks).

To deal effectively with stress, each person needs to make a personal appraisal of the stress triggers in his or her life and take action to minimize their effects.

■ The Physiology of Acute Stress

One of the fundamental models for stress evolved from studies of how humans responded to threats. It was observed that when a person perceived an event as threatening, a standard series of physiologic reactions was triggered, whatever the threat (this is why Selye referred to stress as a nonspecific response).

Typically, these physiologic reactions prepare us for fight-or-flight syndrome by activating the sympathetic nervous system (discussed further in the chapter on *Anatomy and Physiology*). For most people, the fight-or-flight response is a very useful and adaptive mechanism, mobilizing the person to either defend (fight) or to run away (flight) in the face of possible danger. In the modern world, however, the automatic fight-or-flight response to stressful circumstances is probably not as useful as it was in an earlier stage of evolution. Most of the stressors that people face today are not best solved by fighting or running away; instead, stress may be chronic, placing our bodies in a continuous, unrelieved state of alert, and may lead to chronic exhaustion and ill health.

Reactions to stress can be categorized as acute, delayed, or cumulative. Acute stress reactions occur during a stressful situation. The paramedic feels nervous and excited, and his or her ability to focus increases. If the stress of the situation becomes too great, a paramedic may experience emotional and physical reactions to stress.

Delayed stress reactions manifest after the stressful event. During the crisis, the paramedic is able to focus and function, but afterwards, he or she may be left with nervous, excited energy that continues to build. A paramedic may wish to learn certain stress management techniques to improve his or her chance of effectively managing stress when it occurs.

Cumulative stress reactions occur when a paramedic is exposed to prolonged or excessive stress. After the stressful event is over, he or she may be unable to shake off the effects. Inevitably, another stressful situation occurs. Each time, the paramedic finds it harder and harder to recover and becomes more and more exhausted.

Cumulative stress can have physical symptoms such as fatigue, changes in appetite, gastrointestinal problems, or headaches. Stress may cause insomnia or hypersomnia, irritability, inability to concentrate, and hyperactivity or underactivity. In addition, stress may manifest itself in psychological reactions such as fear, dull or nonresponsive behavior, depression, oversensitivity, anger, irritability, frustration, isolation, inability to concentrate, alcohol or drug abuse, and loss of interest in work or sexual activity. Often, today's fast-paced lifestyles compound these effects by not allowing a person to rest and recover after periods of stress. Prolonged or excessive stress has been proven to be a strong contributor to heart disease, hypertension, cancer, alcoholism, and depression.

■ How People React to Stressful Situations

Anyone—the patient, the family, bystanders, or health care professionals—who confronts critical illness or injury responds in some way to the stresses of each emergency.

Words of Wisdom

Learn to look for signs of stress in your coworkers and patients. Early discovery can often prevent the situation from worsening.

Table 1 Social Readjustment Rating Scale

Rank	Life Event	LCU	Rank	Life Event	LCU
1	Death of a spouse	100	23	Son or daughter leaving home	29
2	Divorce	73	24	Trouble with in-laws	29
3	Marital separation	65	25	Outstanding personal achievement	28
4	Jail term	63	26	Spouse begins or stops work	26
5	Death of close family member	63	27	Begin or end school	26
6	Personal injury or illness	53	28	Change in living conditions	25
7	Marriage	50	29	Revision of personal habits	24
8	Fired at work	47	30	Trouble with boss	23
9	Marital reconciliation	45	31	Change in work hours or conditions	20
10	Retirement	45	32	Change in residence	20
11	Change in health of family member	44	33	Change in schools	20
12	Pregnancy	40	34	Change in recreation	19
13	Sexual dysfunction	39	35	Change in church activities	19
14	Gain of new family member	39	36	Change in social activities	19
15	Business readjustment	39	37	Mortgage or loan of less than $10,000	17
16	Change in financial status	38	38	Change in sleeping habits	16
17	Death of close friend	37	39	Change in number of family get-togethers	15
18	Change to different line of work	36	40	Change in eating habits	13
19	Change in number of arguments with spouse	35	41	Vacation	13
20	Mortgage over $100,000	31	42	Christmas	12
21	Foreclosure of mortgage or loan	30	43	Minor violation of the law	11
22	Change in responsibilities at work	29			

Check off those events that currently apply to your life and add up the corresponding points. A score below 150 is thought to be within the range of normal stress. A score between 150 and 199 suggests a mild life crisis; between 200 and 299 points suggests a moderate life crisis; above 300 points is indicative of a major life crisis. (Reprinted with permission of the publisher from "The Social Readjustment Rating Scale" by T. H. Holmes and R. Rahe, *Journal of Psychosomatic Research*, vol. II, pp. 213-218. Copyright 1967 by Elsevier Science, Inc.)

Responses of Patients to Illness and Injury

Patients' responses to emergencies are determined by their personal methods of adapting to stress. It will help you as a paramedic to recognize certain common patterns of coping. A common response by the general public to stressors is anxiety. Some people will exhibit their anxiety by denying it; others become irritable or angry. Several common reactions, but in no particular order, include the following:

- **Fear.** Patients in these situations have realistic fears, such as fear of pain, disability, or death (or fear of their economic effects).
- **Anxiety.** Patients may experience diffuse anxiety, often stemming from a feeling of helplessness or a loss of control. People whose self-esteem depends on being active, independent, and aggressive are particularly vulnerable to anxiety when they become ill or injured.
- **Depression.** Depression is a natural response to loss. The patient who has had a stroke, for example, may have lost the ability to move an arm or leg on one side of the body and even the ability to speak, but can understand everything you say and do.
- **Anger.** Anger is one of the most difficult problems for many caregivers to deal with Figure 9 . A provider's natural tendency may be to think, "I am trying to save this person's life, and he is taking it out on me." It is crucial to remember that people often respond to discomfort or limitation of function through anger. Professional caregivers must realize that in certain circumstances a patient's anger may stem from fear and discomfort, and is not directed at them.
- **Confusion.** Confusion is especially common among older patients, in whom illness or injury may precipitate

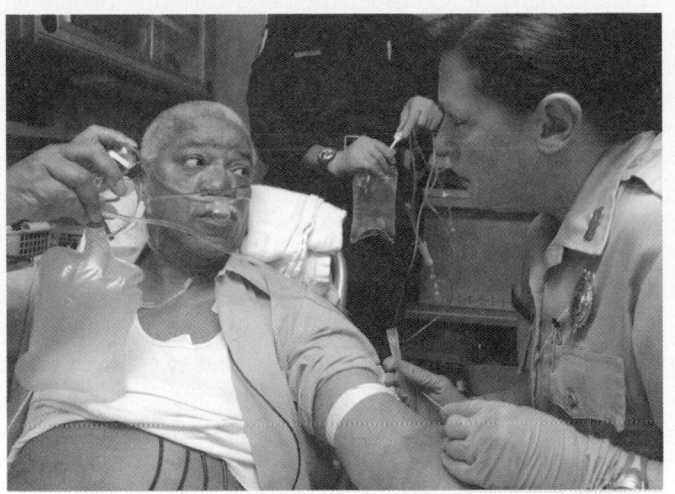

Figure 9 The sudden loss of control a patient feels when being treated during an emergency can lead to surprising and sometimes extreme reactions.

disorientation. Confusion is furthered by the presence of unfamiliar people and equipment, which may seem overwhelming. If a patient appears confused, it is very important to explain carefully at the outset who you are and what you plan to do

In addition to experiencing the reactions just described, some people may show one or more of the following psychologic **defense mechanisms**:

- **Denial**. Patients often ignore or diminish the seriousness of the situation. Some patients may dismiss all symptoms with words such as "only" or "a little." You may have to seek out others for reliable information in these cases.
- **Regression**. Regression is a return to an earlier age level of behavior or emotional adjustment. Children often exhibit this when under stress because of the fear of "getting in trouble." Adults also may revert to childish behaviors when under stress.
- **Projection**. Projection is attributing your own (sometimes unacceptable) feelings, motives, desires, or behavior to others. Patients who express vehement indignation or anger can unconsciously be denying their own "bad" behavior by attributing it to other people.
- **Displacement**. Displacement occurs when someone redirects an emotion from the original cause of the emotion (like a cardiac problem) to a more immediate substitute (like a paramedic). Displacement is often the operative mechanism when patients express anger at the paramedic, but in reality, patients are angry at someone else—themselves, a family member, fate, or just the situation.

As noted, most of the psychological stress responses are not under your patients' conscious control. Injured patients who respond with anger toward the paramedic often have no perspective on their unpleasant behavior. The reaction is automatic for the stressed patient.

Often, reactions to illness or injury are rooted in the patient's culture. Society today is multicultural, and some cultures may openly exhibit their anxieties in what might be termed inappropriate behavior in another culture. It is important for you to respect the culture of your patient.

Many Americans place great emphasis on making eye contact, having a firm handshake, and respecting personal space. Some patients may not make eye contact because their culture believes that lowered eyes shows deference to your authority and uniform. When making physical contact, obtain permission, if possible, beforehand. Learn the cultural differences of the populations you serve **Figure 10**.

Responses of Family, Friends, and Bystanders

Bystanders and family members may exhibit responses that are similar to those exhibited by patients. Family members may be anxious, panicky, or—especially if they are struggling with guilt—angry. Consciously or unconsciously, they may feel guilty for what has happened; they may believe, deep down, that if they had kept a closer eye on an injured child, for instance, he or she would not have run out into the street.

Paramedics must recognize that the patient's family and friends have concerns too and that their behavior, however unpleasant, arises from distress. Remain calm, and reassure them that at all times you are working under the physician's guidance in the best interests of the patient. You are entering a situation in which everyone is under stress, and there is no guarantee that people are going to behave appropriately.

In a situation involving multiple casualties, such as a train derailment, building collapse, or natural disaster (such as a tornado, flood, or earthquake), both victims and bystanders may react by becoming dazed, disorganized, or overwhelmed. The American Psychiatric Association has identified five categories of reactions in such circumstances. In general, people with these reactions should be removed from the scene, but not left

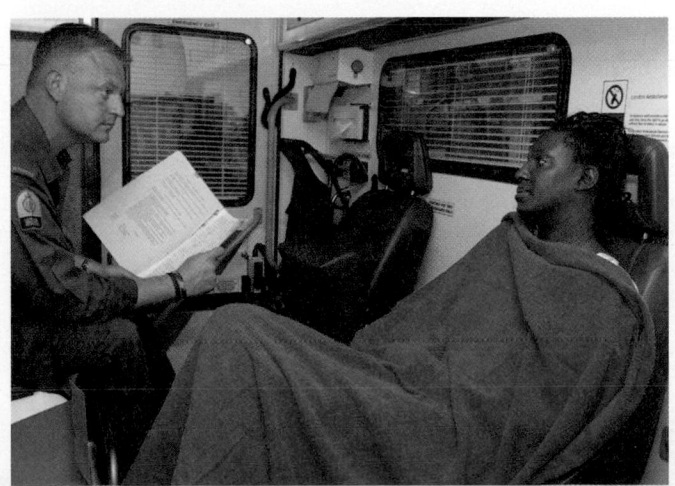

Figure 10 Particularly when serving people whose backgrounds are different from your own, you must always maintain an open, nonjudgmental attitude.

alone—find someone who is capable of handling them. The five categories are as follows:

- **Anxiety.** Reactions to such incidents are signs of extreme anxiety, which include sweating, trembling, weakness, nausea, and sometimes vomiting. People experiencing this response can recover fully within a few minutes and provide useful assistance if properly directed. EMS personnel are not immune to this type of reaction.
- **Blind panic.** A more worrisome reaction is blind panic, in which a person's judgment seems to disappear entirely. Blind panic is particularly dangerous because it is "catchy," and it may precipitate mass panic among others present.
- **Depression.** Depression is seen in the people who sit or stand in a numbed, dazed state. Depressed bystanders need to be brought back to reality as soon as possible.
- **Overreaction.** People who overreact tend to talk compulsively, joke inappropriately, become overly active, and race from one task to another without accomplishing anything useful.
- **Conversion hysteria.** In conversion hysteria, the patient subconsciously converts anxiety into a bodily dysfunction; he or she may be unable to see or hear or may become paralyzed in an extremity.

More details on how to cope with bystanders are found in the chapter on *Incident Management and Multiple-Casualty Incidents*, where multiple-casualty incidents are discussed.

Responses of the Paramedic

Paramedics are not immune to the stresses of emergency situations, and it is to be expected that you will sometimes experience a multitude of feelings, not all of them pleasant. These feelings are all perfectly natural, but it is preferable to keep control of them during an emergency. An attitude of outward calm and confidence on your part will do much to relieve the anxieties of others at the scene—and that too is part of a paramedic's therapeutic role.

One reaction that is common among health care professionals is a feeling of irritation at the patient who does not appear

to be particularly ill. Consider the possibility that people who call 9-1-1 with seemingly minor complaints are not calling for something minor at all—like a woman who called 9-1-1 because she could not get to sleep. Her problem was that it was her first night back home after the funeral of her husband. She was scared to death of her first night alone in the house and she did not know who to call.

Coping With Your Own Stress

Some early warning signs of your own stress include heart palpitations, rapid breathing, chest tightness, and sweating. Learn to feel yourself entering your fight-or-flight mode. You may notice rapid breathing and breathlessness, unnecessary shouting, and perhaps the use of curse words that you would not normally use. Often these signs are identified by others and alerted to you; do not become offended because this is the time for you to take appropriate action. There are many ways to prepare for or handle stress. The following are some management techniques available:

1. **Controlled breathing.** Take deep breaths in through the nose and out through the mouth. Controlled deep breathing may flood the body and brain with oxygen just prior to activation of the fight-or-flight system and may help prevent it from engaging.
2. **Progressive relaxation.** Progressive relaxation is a strategy in which you tighten and then relax specific muscle groups to initiate muscle relaxation throughout the body. This may be performed before, during, or after a call.
3. **Professional assistance.** Even the best paramedic may not be able to handle the continuous onslaught of stressful events. Seek out professional services such as employee assistance programs (EAP) or critical incident stress management (CISM) services described later in this chapter **Figure 11**.

Other coping strategies include focusing on the immediate situation while on duty. Remind yourself, "I will do my very best, but what I can do may not be enough."

Avoid excessive amounts of stimulants such as caffeine or the urge to use alcohol, cigarettes, or sleeping

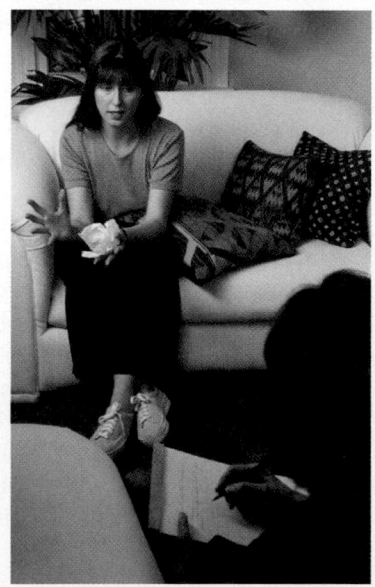

Figure 11 Consulting with a professional counselor or therapist can be an important part of dealing with stress and maintaining your emotional well-being.

aids after a stressful event. Attempt to get enough rest. Exercise vigorously and regularly. Identify things that make you laugh and find compatible partners at work.

Burnout

Why should EMS providers start worrying now about something that may (or may not) happen? Burnout needs to be considered now—at the earliest stage of paramedic training—because now is the time for you to start developing attitudes and habits that will help prevent burnout.

The dictionary defines **burnout** as the exhaustion of physical or emotional strength. Burnout, in fact, may be a consequence of chronic, unrelieved stress. The paramedic's job, by its very nature, is full of potential stresses. But burnout does not occur solely because of stress. There are more subtle stresses associated with interpersonal relations, pay, prestige, fringe benefits, and other issues. These complaints and stresses are, no doubt, legitimate. Burnout develops because of the way a person reacts to stress.

One person's eustress may be another's distress Figure 12 . The reason is that distress is a learned reaction, based on the way a person perceives and interprets the world around him or her. In other words, distress is nearly always the result of what a person believes. Here are some beliefs that are common among EMS personnel:

- I have to be perfect all the time.
- My safety depends on being able to anticipate every possible danger.
- I am totally responsible for what happens to patients; if they die, it is wholly my fault.
- If there is something I do not know, people will think less of me.
- A good paramedic never makes mistakes.

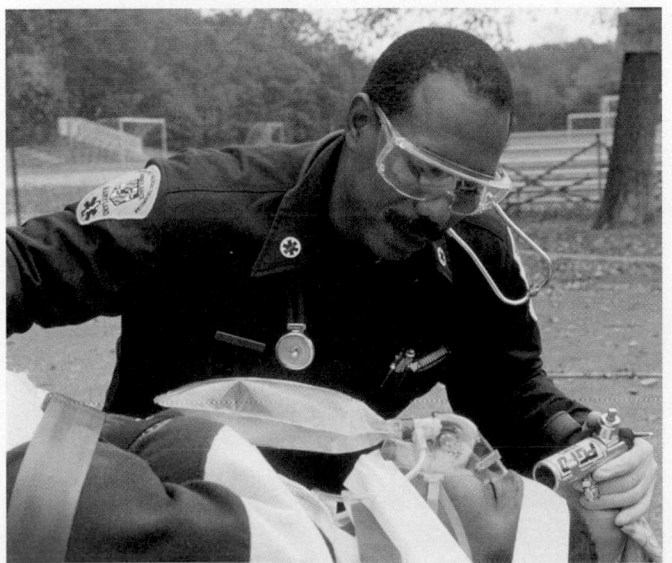

Figure 12 Dealing with stress as a paramedic requires the ability to emotionally distance yourself from the situation, and accepting the limits of what you can personally do.

These are all false beliefs and can lead to burnout. Prevention and relief of stress among EMS personnel begin with the recognition that such beliefs are unrealistic and invalid.

Like many of the conditions you will study in this textbook, burnout is a type of illness and it has signs and symptoms. The signs and symptoms may be trivial at first, but when ignored the illness grows in nature until it debilitates the paramedic. Symptoms of impending burnout include the following:

- Chronic fatigue and irritability
- Cynical, negative attitudes
- Lack of desire to report to work
- Emotional instability (crying easily, flying off the handle without provocation, laughing inappropriately)
- Changes in sleep patterns (insomnia or sleeping more than usual), and waking without feeling refreshed
- Feelings of being overwhelmed or being helpless or hopeless
- Loss of interest in hobbies
- Decreased ability to concentrate
- Declining health—having frequent colds, stomach upsets, and muscle aches and pains (especially headaches or backaches)
- Constant tightness in your muscles
- Overeating, smoking, or abusing drugs or alcohol

Some paramedics have been in the field for 20 years and show no signs of burnout, reporting to work every day with the same enthusiasm they did as rookies. What is their secret? In general, the paramedics who do not experience burnout are those who have learned to respect and value themselves. That is not as easy as it sounds. Practically speaking, what does it mean to respect and value yourself? How can you translate that attitude into concrete action? Some of the steps you can take to protect yourself from burnout are summarized in Table 2 .

Coping With Death and Dying

We all deal with death. What do you say to people who know they are dying? What do you say to a bereaved parent or spouse? How do you deal with your own feelings when a patient has died while under your care? These are all questions you need to be able to answer for yourself eventually, and it may take a lifetime to sort them out.

Death in the Western hemisphere is generally regarded as a traumatic experience, something to be feared and postponed as long as possible. Think about it— the paramedic's or average person's only experience with death is through death of another. As a paramedic, you will be there when people are born and you will be there when many of them die. Every one of these encounters is an honor—a most private moment in someone's life, to which you and a small number of your coworkers are invited. Why an honor? Because, in some cultures, these moments are a holy time, and regardless of culture, it is likely one of the most important moments in a person's life. Many patients will exhibit great dignity with their passing, and may show you how to die well someday.

Table 2   Nancy's Guidelines for Preventing Burnout

1. Paramedic heal thyself! Take care of your own health.
   - Get enough rest.
   - Eat a balanced diet.
   - Get regular physical exercise–at least 30 minutes of aerobic activity (walking, running, or swimming) three to four times a week.
   - Do not abuse your body. Smoking, overindulgence in alcohol, taking recreational drugs, or self-prescribing any other drugs are all forms of self-abuse.

2. Give yourself some "me" time every day. Some of the most stress-resistant paramedics are those who have learned the techniques of meditation and can thereby escape now and then to a quiet place within themselves. Try different methods of meditation or relaxation and see which one works best for you.

3. Learn how to relax Figure 13 .
   - Take time for hobbies.
   - Engage in social activities with people not involved in EMS.
   - Leave your job behind when your shift is over.

4. Do not make unreasonable demands on yourself.
   - Forget the idea that you have to be perfect. No one is perfect. If you do the best job you can, that is good enough.
   - You do not have to be right all the time. Accept the fact that now and then you will make a mistake–and that the world will not come to an end on account of it.

5. Do not make unreasonable demands on others.

6. Stay in touch with your feelings.
   - Find someone you can talk to. Share the stress.
   - Cry when you need to. There is no shame in being sad sometimes.

7. Learn techniques for shedding stress while on duty. Do not let stress accumulate.

8. Debrief after tough calls.

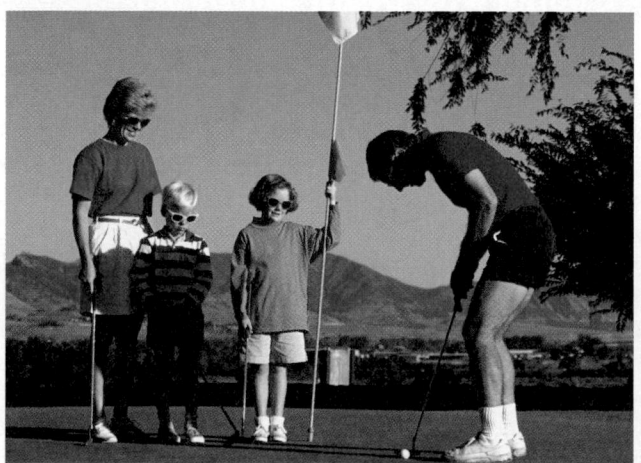

Figure 13 One of the best ways of dealing with the stress of working as a paramedic is to invest in relationships and activities outside of work that are meaningful to you.

As a paramedic, remember you will have the opportunity to help a great many people, but few will be successful resuscitations, no matter how long your career. What follows here are some general guidelines and techniques for dealing with the dying, their families, and your own stress.

■ Stages of the Grieving Process

In her classic study, *On Death and Dying*, Elisabeth Kübler-Ross, MD, defined five stages through which grieving people—usually the dying, but sometimes their survivors—often proceed Figure 14 . Each of these stages in some way helps the dying or their family members adapt to their own reality. It helps to be aware of these stages, and to consider the behavior of dying patients or their families in the context of the grieving process. Be aware that all people do not follow the stages in order and that you may arrive after a certain stage has already passed.

- **Stage 1: Denial.** It has already been discussed that denial is a mechanism by which people attempt to ignore a problem or pretend it does not exist. Denial is a way of buffering bad news until the person can mobilize the resources to deal with that news more effectively.
- **Stage 2: Anger.** When people can no longer deny the reality of a situation, anger over the loss replaces denial. They may ask, "Why me?" and displace their anger randomly to those around them. As mentioned earlier, such anger may be very difficult for health care personnel to deal with.
- **Stage 3: Bargaining.** When anger does not change the painful reality of a situation, people may resort to bargaining, that is, trying to make some sort of deal in hopes of postponing the inevitable ("If I can just live long enough to see my daughter's wedding, then I'll die in peace.").
- **Stage 4: Depression.** When bargaining fails to change the reality of a loss and people must come to terms with dying, there is suddenly an enormous sense of loss. They may become very quiet. They may want permission to express

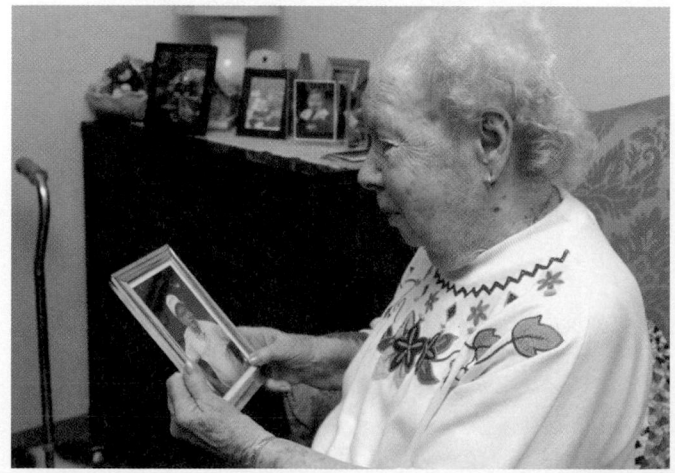

Figure 14 People usually go through a lengthy process of grieving before fully accepting the death of a loved one.

their sorrow—in words, in tears, or in what Kübler-Ross calls "the silence that goes beyond words." Acknowledge their loss and sadness, and if they act like they want to cry, offer some tissues or a towel. If they seem to want a hug, offer it. If they seem to just want to be quiet by themselves, do what you can to accommodate that as well.

- **Stage 5: Acceptance.** In the final stage of grief, people who are dying prepare to disengage from the world around them. They shed their fears and most of their other feelings as well and begin to loosen the ties that bind them to the living. When the dying enter this acceptance stage, it is often the family that is in need of the most help. Although families may know of an upcoming death, when that time actually comes, their emotions and reactions may change completely.

Dealing With the Dying Patient

People who are dying generally know, at the very least, that their situation is serious; they may, in fact, be well aware that they are dying and may want to talk about it. Some health care professionals are reluctant to discuss death with patients, so they try to maintain an attitude of reassurance by saying "everything will be alright." Perhaps the most important thing you can do for dying patients is to let them know that you understand and will talk about it if they wish. You do not need to come right out and ask, "Do you want to talk about dying?" You can simply say "If there is anything worrying you, I would be glad to listen."

Let patients talk as much as they wish 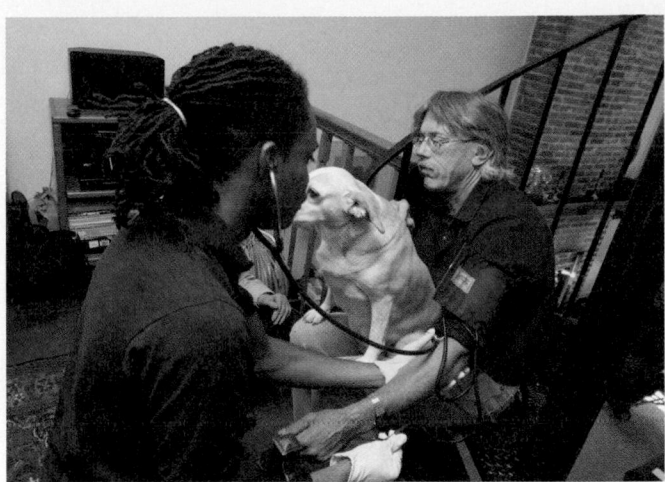. Make some physical contact. Hold their hand, put a hand on their shoulder, or make some other unmistakable gesture of empathy.

What if patients come straight out and ask you, "Am I going to die?" An answer should acknowledge the seriousness of their condition without taking away all hope. For example, you might say, "You seem to have had a severe heart attack. The situation is serious, but we will give you the best care available."

Dying patients also need to feel that they still have some control over their life. When people lose all control over their life, they may lose a large measure of their dignity and self-respect. As much as possible, explain to them what you are doing and allow them to participate in the treatment. Ask them if there is anyone they would like you to contact or if they have any special instructions they want conveyed to someone. If they

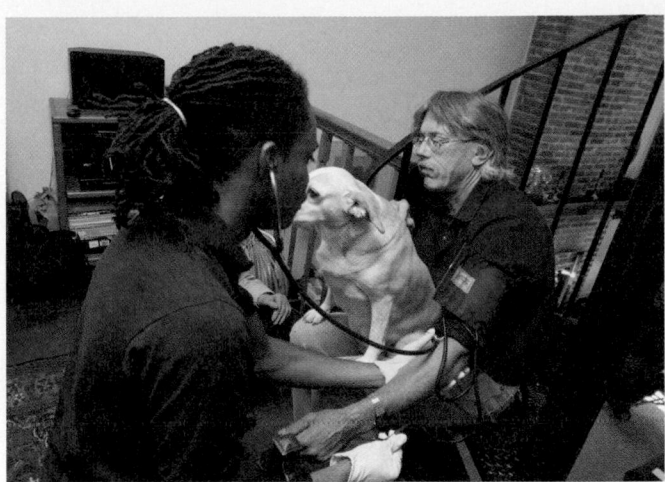

Figure 15 Be aware that each patient will have different ways of dealing with his or her immediate situation. Some may be relieved to talk openly about how they feel, while others may have a greater sense of privacy or stoicism.

do ask you to convey a message, write it down word-for-word as they state it to you. Also, know that experience tells us that people who know they are going to die will often look you in the eye and say, "I think I am going to die." Regardless, you should always provide the best care you can.

Dealing With a Grieving Family

Suppose you are called to the scene where a child has been run over by a truck. You can see at a glance that the child is dead. Two police officers are with the child's mother, who is crying hysterically.

The fact that there is nothing you can do for the child does not mean that the call is over. There is another "patient" at the scene—the child's mother—and the call is not over until you have done all you can for her **Figure 16**.

What kinds of things can you do for a grieving family? How can you help them begin the process of dealing with their loss? Here are a few guidelines:

- Do not try to hide the body of the deceased from the family, even if the body has been badly mutilated. People who are prevented from seeing the body of a loved one may

YOU are the Medic   PART 3

Your partner attaches the cardiac monitor to the patient and you note asystole in two leads. As you were lifting his shirt for your partner to attach the electrodes, you also noticed some lividity. Family members are starting to arrive. The patient's mother is becoming hysterical and is asking you to do something. She tells you that he cannot be dead, that she asked God to give him just a few more months. Your partner steps outside to call the dispatcher, law enforcement, and the coroner, and leaves you to talk with the family.

5. How will you explain the situation to the family, and what is your responsibility to them?

6. Which stage of grieving is seen in the patient's mother?

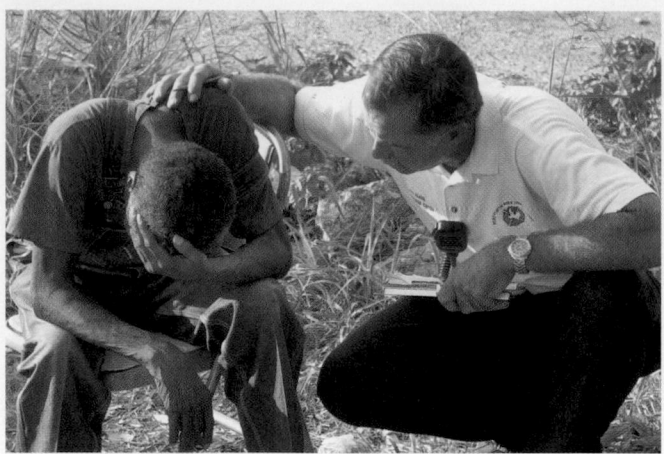

Figure 16 While on the scene, one of your responsibilities is to help family members through the initial period after the death of a loved one.

later have enormous difficulty working through their grief because they may not be able to get beyond their denial.

- For similar reasons, do not use euphemisms for death, such as "expired" or "passed away." The family needs to hear the word "dead."
- Do not be in a hurry to clear away all your resuscitation equipment. Let the family see the equipment before you start tidying up and packing away your gear, so that they will know that everything possible was done.
- Give the family some time with their loved one, especially when the victim is a child. If the death occurred in a public place, move the deceased into the ambulance and let the family say goodbye in their own way.
- Try to arrange for further support. This may be a neighbor, friend, or an offer to call the family's clergy.
- Accept the family's right to experience a variety of feelings—guilt, shock, denial, or anger.

Dealing With a Grieving Child

You need to be particularly sensitive to the emotional needs of children and how they differ depending on their age group. Children up to 3 years of age will be aware that something has happened and people are sad. Children 3 to 6 years of age believe that death is temporary and may continually ask when the person will return. The family should emphasize to the child that he or she was not responsible for the death and also that it is OK to cry when you are sad.

Children 6 to 9 years of age may mask their feelings in an effort to not look babyish. Family members should discuss the normal feelings of grieving with the child. Also, they should not hesitate to cry in front of the child.

Children 9 to 12 years of age may want to know details surrounding the incident. Family members should encourage the sharing of feelings and memories to facilitate the grieving process.

After the Call Is Over

Many calls can be real shockers. In those cases, everyone involved in the call is likely to experience some intense feelings. If these feelings stay bottled up, there may be all types of problems later. Therefore, every ambulance service needs to develop routine procedures for debriefing after any call that involved the death of a patient. All those who participated in the call need a chance to sit down together, in an atmosphere of confidentiality, and air their feelings about what happened.

Most calls should not disrupt your normal life functions. But, depending on a number of variables, some especially traumatic calls can preoccupy even well-adjusted providers for weeks or even months afterward. This is called **posttraumatic stress disorder (PTSD)**. By definition, a **critical incident** is one that overwhelms the ability of an EMS worker or an EMS system to cope with the experience, either at the scene or later.

Most paramedics never experience PTSD, but it can occur. Let your superiors know if you or a coworker is experiencing one or more signs of PTSD:

- You have trouble getting an incident out of your thoughts.
- You keep having flashbacks of an incident.
- You have nightmares or other sleep disturbances after an incident.
- Your appetite is not the same after an incident.
- After an incident, you laugh or cry for no good reason.
- You find yourself withdrawing from coworkers and family members after an incident.

Critical incident stress management (CISM) is a resource available for emergency personnel who have been involved in particularly traumatic calls or incidents. CISM is a process that was developed to address acute stress situations and potentially decrease the likelihood that PTSD will develop after such an incident. Although public safety organizations have used CISM for more than 20 years, there is no evidence that it is effective, or that its effects are not actually harmful. The following are suggested events where some sort of debriefing or management may be considered:

- Serious injury or death of a fellow worker in the line of duty
- Suicide of a fellow worker
- Multiple-casualty incidents, such as an airliner crash or train wreck
- Serious injury or death of a child
- Intense media attention to an incident

It is impossible to predict how any given person will react, but people should be offered opportunities to debrief. It should never be forced on them.

Many EMS systems have CISM teams to provide support after a traumatic call—but sometimes even during the incident itself. The intervention may take the form of a brief (usually about 30 minutes) defusing session right after the call, in which all who were involved in the incident are offered an opportunity to express their feelings about what happened. A formal debriefing is usually coordinated by one or more professional

Controversies

There are definitely two sides of the fence on the effectiveness of CISM. Psychology professionals and EMS professionals alike have debated this issue for some time. Be open-minded about the experience and then draw your own conclusion.

counselors 24 to 72 hours after an incident, when it becomes clear that the incident has had a serious impact and is causing persistent symptoms among the crew.

■ Disease Transmission

As a paramedic, you will be called on to treat and transport patients with a variety of communicable or infectious diseases. An **infectious disease** is a medical condition caused by the growth and spread of small, harmful organisms within the body. A **communicable disease** is a disease that can be spread from one person or species to another. The chapter on *Infectious Diseases*, covers care of patients with infectious diseases and protection from specific diseases in greater depth, while this chapter covers general protection of the paramedic against such diseases.

Immunizations, protective techniques, and simple handwashing can dramatically minimize the health care provider's risk of **infection**. When these protective measures are used, the risk of the health care provider contracting a serious communicable disease is negligible. Proper cleaning and disinfecting of the ambulance and equipment will help to prevent transfer of illnesses to other patients.

Along with personal protection, it is necessary to inform other health care workers who may come in contact with the patient of the potential risk. Discretion is imperative when communicating with other providers. Sensitive patient history should not be given out over the radio during your patient report. However, during your transfer of care, provide a complete patient history for the receiving facility. Also include all patient history in your written documentation.

Many people confuse the terms *infectious* and *contagious*. In fact, all contagious diseases are infectious, but only some infectious diseases are contagious. For example, pneumonia caused by pneumococcus bacteria is an infectious process, but it is not contagious. In other words, it will not be transmitted from one person to another. However, other infectious agents, such as the hepatitis B virus, are contagious because they can be transmitted from one person to another.

While all infections result from an invasion of body spaces and tissues by germs, different germs use different means of attack. These means are known as the mechanisms of transmission. **Transmission** is the way an infectious agent is spread. There are several ways infectious diseases can be transmitted, consisting of contact (direct or indirect), airborne, foodborne, and vector-borne (transmitted through insects or parasitic worms) transmission.

Contact transmission is the movement of an organism from one person to another through physical touch. There are two types of contact transmission: direct and indirect. **Direct contact** occurs when an organism is moved from one person to another through touching without any intermediary. **Bloodborne pathogens** are microorganisms that are present in human blood and can cause disease in humans if blood containing the pathogen enters the paramedic's bloodstream. Another example of direct contact is sexual transmission. Patients who are infected with the human immunodeficiency virus (HIV) can transfer the virus to their partners during sex.

Indirect contact involves the spread of infection between the patient with an infection to another person through an inanimate object. The object that transmits the infection is called a fomite. Needlesticks are an example of the spread of infection through indirect contact. In this case, the virus moves from the patient to the needle to the health care provider. This route of transmission was common many years ago before the advent of safety equipment such as needleless IV systems.

Airborne transmission involves spreading an infectious agent through mechanisms such as droplets or dust. The common cold is moved from person to person by coughing and sneezing. Because of airborne transmission, it is unsanitary to use your hands to cover a cough or sneeze because the organism travels onto your hands. Using a tissue when coughing or sneezing is better for controlling the spread of organisms, but you then have a piece of paper full of organisms. One of the best techniques to avoid contaminating your hands is to cough or sneeze into your arm/sleeve. Because you do not touch objects with your inner arms, the risk of moving the organism to an object or person is reduced. The organisms are trapped in the fabric and will eventually die.

■ Protecting Yourself

Much has changed in EMS since its inception. The use of personal protective equipment (PPE) was not common in the early years. It was a status symbol when you showed how much blood and dirt you were coated with. Surgeons in the 1800s took similar pride in their messy operating aprons, but they were transmitting infectious diseases. Present day EMS is changing continuously and new suggestions for protection are showing up frequently.

Thanks to the research and reporting done by the Centers for Disease Control and Prevention (CDC), EMS providers are now more aware that biohazards are an integral part of their profession and can have long-term effects on the health care worker if certain precautions are not adhered to. The CDC developed a set of **universal precautions** for health care workers to use in treating patients. EMS follows **standard precautions** rather than relying on universal precautions. Standard precautions differ from universal precautions in that they are designed to approach all body fluids as being potentially infectious.

In observing universal precautions only, you are assuming that only blood and certain body fluids pose only a risk for infectious diseases. Table 3 summarizes the CDC recommendations.

▇ Immunizations

As a paramedic, you are at risk for acquiring an infectious or communicable disease. Using basic protective measures can minimize the risk.

Prevention begins by maintaining your personal health. EMS personnel should receive annual health examinations. A history of all your childhood infectious diseases should be recorded and kept on file. Childhood infectious diseases include chickenpox, mumps, measles, rubella, and whooping cough. If you have not had one of these diseases, you must be immunized.

The CDC and the Occupational Safety and Health Administration (OSHA) have developed requirements for protection from bloodborne pathogens such as the hepatitis B virus. An immunization program should be in place in your EMS system. Immunizations should be kept up-to-date and recorded in your file. Recommended immunizations include the following:

- Tetanus-diphtheria boosters (every 10 years)
- Measles, mumps, rubella (MMR) vaccine
- Influenza vaccine (yearly)
- Hepatitis B vaccine
- Varicella (chickenpox) vaccine or having chickenpox

Table 3 Standard Precautions for the Care of All Patients in All Health Care Settings, Centers for Disease Control and Prevention 2007

Component	Recommendation
Hand hygiene	<ul><li>After touching blood, body fluids, secretions, excretions, or contaminated items</li><li>Immediately after removing gloves</li><li>Between patient contacts</li></ul>
Personal Protective Equipment	
Gloves	<ul><li>For touching blood, body fluids, secretions, excretions, or contaminated items</li><li>For touching mucous membranes and nonintact skin</li></ul>
Gown	<ul><li>During procedures and patient care activities when contact of the health care provider's clothing/exposed skin to blood, body fluids, secretions, excretions, or contaminated items is anticipated</li></ul>
Mask, eye protection, face shield	<ul><li>During procedures and patient care activities likely to generate splashes or sprays of blood, body fluids, secretions, or excretions. Examples include suctioning or endotracheal intubation</li></ul>
HEPA respirator	<ul><li>When working with a patient with tuberculosis</li></ul>
Patient Care Environment	
Soiled patient care equipment	<ul><li>Handle in a manner that prevents transfer of microorganisms to others and to the environment</li><li>Wear gloves if visibly contaminated</li><li>Hand hygiene</li></ul>
Environmental controls	<ul><li>Have procedures for the routine care, cleaning, and disinfection of environmental surfaces</li><li>Special attention to frequently touched surfaces within the ambulance (handrails, seats, cabinets, doors)</li><li>Have patients with tuberculosis wear a surgical mask</li></ul>
Textiles and laundry	<ul><li>Handle in a manner that prevents transfer of microorganisms to others and to the environment</li></ul>
Needles and other sharp objects	<ul><li>Do not recap, bend, break, or hand-manipulate used needles</li><li>Use safety features when available (needleless IV systems)</li><li>Place sharps in puncture-resistant containers</li></ul>
Special Circumstances	
Patient resuscitation	<ul><li>Use mouthpiece, resuscitation bag, or other ventilation devices to prevent contact with mouth and oral secretions</li></ul>
Respiratory hygiene/cough etiquette	<ul><li>Instruct symptomatic patients to cover mouth/nose when sneezing or coughing</li><li>Use tissues and dispose in no-touch receptacle</li><li>Perform hand hygiene after touching tissues</li><li>Place surgical mask on patient/provider</li><li>If mask cannot be used, maintain special separation distance (> 3′) if possible</li></ul>

You should also have a skin test for tuberculosis before you begin working as a paramedic. The purpose of the test is to identify anyone who has been exposed to tuberculosis in the past. Testing should be repeated every year. It is important to know that testing positive for a tuberculosis skin test does not mean that you have the disease; it indicates that you have been exposed. Additional follow-up will be needed to determine whether the disease is active. Other vaccines being investigated include pertussis (whooping cough) and *Staphylococcus aureus*. These vaccines are not currently recommended, but may be soon.

If you know that you will be transporting a patient who has a communicable disease, you have a definite advantage. This is when your health record will be valuable. If you have already had the disease or been vaccinated, you are not at risk. However, you will not always know whether a patient has a communicable disease. Therefore, you should always follow standard precautions if there is the possibility of exposure to blood or other body fluids.

Personal Protective Equipment and Practices

At a minimum, each ambulance should be equipped with certain PPE, not just because it is the law under OSHA, but because it is an important part of safety for yourself. At a minimum, you should have access to gloves, facial protection (masks and eyewear), gowns, and N95 respirators. The following paragraphs explain the importance of using infection control practices.

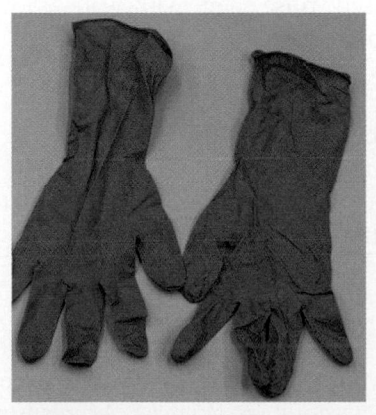

Figure 17 Nitrile gloves should be used on every EMS call.

Words of Wisdom

If you do not have access to soap and water, carry waterless hand cleaner wipes in your ambulance and use them instead. Isopropyl alcohol, the active ingredient they contain, is a very effective bactericide.

Whatever else you do, wash your hands.

Wear Gloves

Gloves are absolutely essential on any EMS call, and some patient encounters warrant more than one set of gloves for a caregiver, depending on the procedure, the patient's history, and the environment Figure 17. Anytime you intubate or start an IV line, consider following that with a new set of gloves before loading the patient and jumping aboard the ambulance. Be sure to take off your gloves before you drive.

Wash Your Hands

Get used to washing your hands before and after using the bathroom, before ingesting anything by mouth, before getting into your personal car, and before and after any physical contact between you and a patient or an instrument. Also wash your hands after you remove your gloves.

When you do wash your hands, wash them vigorously with antibacterial soap for at least 30 seconds before rinsing with clean water. Wash your hands, routinely and often. Turn that into a habit. Habits are reliable, even when you are stressed.

Use Lotion

Because of the need for frequent handwashing, your hands will begin cracking because the natural oils are also washed off your skin. Use hand lotion several times a day both on and off duty. Your skin is a very effective barrier to pathogens, as long as it has not been breached by the drying effects of frequent washing.

Use Eye Protection

Many seasoned paramedics make it their standard practice to wear anti-splash eyewear throughout any patient contact. That is a good idea. It is an absolute necessity during suctioning or intubation procedures. In fact, during intubation, a face shield may offer better protection.

Consider Wearing a Mask

Whether you or your patient is sick, wear a mask—to protect you, your patients, and your coworkers, from additional infections during a weakened state. If you are sick, stay at home; this is the best prevention.

Protect Your Body

Masks and gowns are appropriate whenever you care for a patient who is extremely messy or bloody Figure 18. A 30-gallon trash bag can be used as a two-armed glove to slide a patient from a couch or bed onto an ambulance cot if the patient is covered with feces, urine, or blood. Once the patient has been moved, you can simply turn the bag inside-out, squeeze the air out of it, tie a knot in its open end, and place it in a hazardous materials bag.

Incontinence barriers should be laid out on a surface when the patient is leaking any type of fluid or has skin lesions.

N95 or N100 Respirators

Read some of the recent statistics by the CDC regarding tuberculosis (TB) and you will realize that this is one of the most common diseases contracted. The CDC and world public health associations estimate that 1.7 billion people are affected with TB worldwide, with 3 million deaths a year. The chance of getting the TB bacillus makes it that much more important to wear the N95 or N100 respirator Figure 19 and not just a simple surgical mask.

Clean Your Ambulance and Equipment

Sanitize your patient compartment surfaces frequently, but especially the ambulance cot, the bench seat, the grab rails,

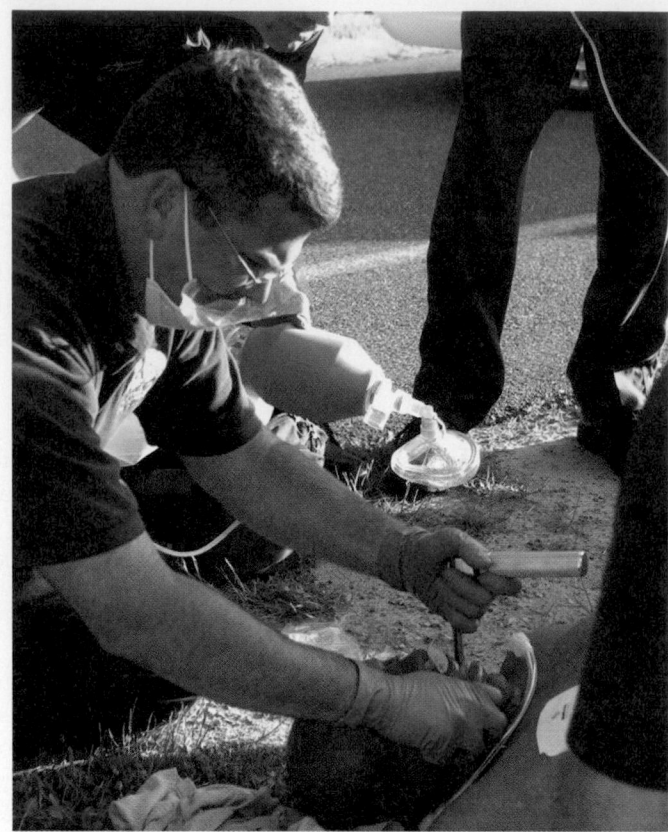

Figure 18 Paramedics always need to protect themselves from contact with any type of body fluids.

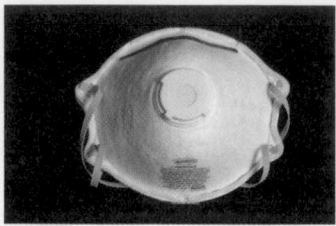

Figure 19 Specially designed respirator masks, such as the N95 or N100 respirator, protect against infection from tuberculosis bacteria.

Properly Dispose of Sharps

Disposal containers (large for the ambulance and small for carry-in gear) for sharps, such as needles and blades, are essential to protect crews against needle sticks or cuts **Figure 20** .

Consider Wearing Turnout Gear

Turnout gear can be bulky, expensive, and uncomfortable. It is not as protective against bullets or knives as are self-protective avoidance strategies, but it can protect the wearer from many kinds of chest and abdominal trauma such as those that occur during extrications and in emergency vehicle crashes.

Management of an Exposure

In the event that you have been exposed to a patient's blood or body fluids, follow your local EMS guidelines. Generally, any EMS provider who has been exposed should do the following:

- Turn care over to another EMS provider.
- Wash the affected area immediately with soap and water.
- If your eyes were exposed, rinse them with water for at least 20 minutes as soon as possible.
- Follow your department's infection control plan.
- Comply with all reporting requirements.
- Get a medical evaluation.
- Obtain proper immunization boosters.
- Document the incident, including the actions taken to reduce chances of infection.

Hostile Situations

In the past, EMS providers were expected to handle situations involving hostile patients without assistance. A position statement by the National Association of EMS Physicians in December 2003 outlined for the first time an official endorsement of the rights to safety not only of patients but also of their field caregivers. Most modern jurisdictions ask their EMS providers to stand back until police have defused the situation.

But EMS providers are also exposed to other kinds of hostile situations. If the element of hostility is known or can be anticipated in advance, EMS crews and their responders should never be allowed to arrive on scene first. Discipline yourself

the deck and deck hardware, and the interior and exterior areas around the door handles. These surfaces should be cleaned daily and after every call. Remove the cot mounts at least once a week to get rid of the dried blood and vomit that tend to accumulate there. Clean this area more often if you have had messy calls. Sanitize the phones and microphones as a matter of routine—especially the ones in the patient compartment, which you may have handled while wearing contaminated gloves.

Sanitize or replace your pen often. You typically handle it several times during every call, with your gloves on. Then, you handle it after the call, after you have washed your hands. Likewise, sanitize your stethoscope with alcohol or disinfectant wipes after every call.

Any piece of equipment that is intended for single use should be discarded in an appropriate hazardous materials bag. For any reusable piece of equipment that has had direct contact with the patient or patient's bodily fluids, use a commercial disinfecting agent for decontamination. Bleach diluted in water (1:10) can also be used as a disinfecting agent. Disinfecting kills many of the microorganisms on the surface of your equipment.

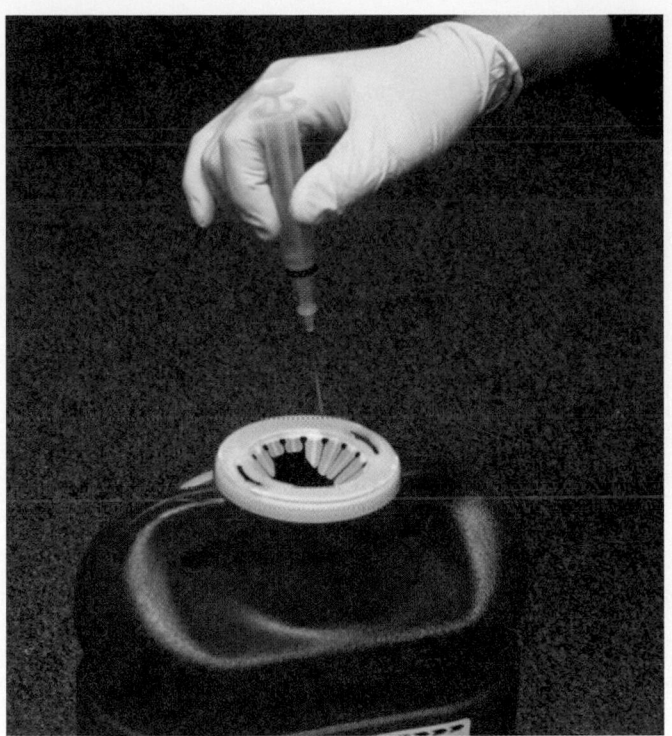

Figure 20 Any needles or blades must be disposed of in a sharps container.

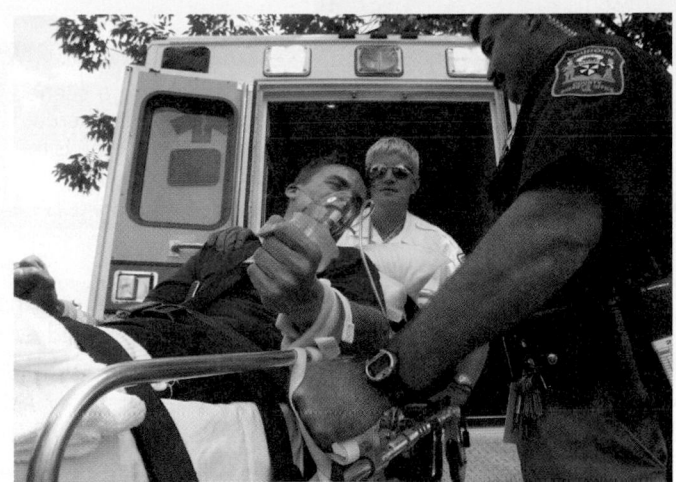

Figure 21 Do not hesitate to call for law enforcement if anyone's safety is in question.

to scrutinize all information that comes to you from others, and keep yourself on "yellow alert" any time you are on duty. Specifically, beware any call dispatched as a fight, stabbing, shooting, domestic disturbance, "person down," or "unknown medical aid." Every one of these calls is suspicious and warrants an initial response by police **Figure 21**. In addition, you should have the prerogative to ask for a police response to any call that your intuition suggests could be violent.

Do not be afraid of being less than a good caregiver if you ask for police to go in first. You will not be able to treat your patient if you are hurt.

Once you are in contact with a hostile patient, try hard to listen a lot more than you talk, and do not argue or ridicule.

Concentrate on de-escalating the patient's emotions. Many hostile patients who started out unwilling to go to the hospital became willing because of a crew member's patience, tactful reasoning, and reassurance.

Remember that anytime you are on someone else's turf, they have a clear advantage. You can expect them to know everything about their environment while you know nothing (including locations of weapons). Volatile patients in their home environment are much more dangerous there than anywhere else—especially in poor lighting.

Words of Wisdom

Some of the most dangerous calls are those that were not considered dangerous. The most worrisome calls are those with limited or vague information. If someone refuses to give information to a dispatcher, then law enforcement should respond to the scene first or with you to ascertain safety.

YOU *are the Medic*   PART 4

You hold his mom and tell her and the family that he has been down too long, that there is nothing that can be done. You explain that he has no cardiac activity and blood has started to pool in the dependent areas of his body. She is hysterical and begs you to do something. You calmly explain that it is too late and ask if you can call someone such as a pastor or priest. You also ask if he was a patient of hospice. She tells you that they did not think it was time for that. Her 19-year-old nephew steps in and accuses you of not knowing your job. He is becoming increasingly hostile. You know that law enforcement personnel are en route, but it may be a few minutes before they arrive.

7. How should you deal with a hostile bystander?

8. How will you deal with your own feelings and stress relating to this call?

Words of Wisdom

If you are the first unit arriving on the scene, do a scene assessment and notify other responding units of any actual or potential hazards that may be present. Your first job is to ensure the safety of the EMS crew—including yourself.

Finally, show empathy and understanding on the scene, and you will develop the trust of your patients. Knowledge of diverse cultures plays a major role in effective communication. The more you know about the people you serve, the more likely you will know their customs and expectations. You must also be diligent in your pursuit of treating all patients with respect and dignity, putting your personal prejudices aside.

■ Traffic Scenes

Regardless of where you are, motor vehicles move at high speeds, may carry hazardous substances, and may crash into one another in locations that are dangerous for you and all involved. It is important to stay aware of your surroundings, even the familiar ones that you see day in and day out.

Like any scene, your approach to traffic scenes always begins with your familiarity with the response area as to your best routing. This is critical information, because it also alerts those who might be available to help you with traffic control, air support, hazardous materials, terrain issues, and potential destinations.

Traffic may be only one of the many hazards at the scene of a motor vehicle crash **Figure 22**. For example, parking a hot,

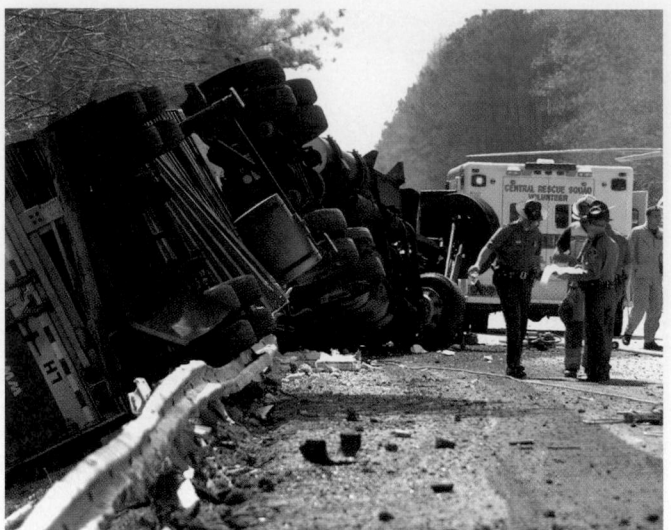

Figure 22 At a busy crash scene, it is important to place your vehicle in a safe, visible location, and to minimize the risk of any additional incidents.

running unit over dry grass may initiate a grass or vehicle fire. Remember that your primary concern at any scene is safety; safety for yourself as well as for those around you. Identify as many hazards as possible while you drive up and before leaving your unit.

Begin making physical observations a mile or so before you approach the scene. Watch the traffic, pay attention to the wind direction, look for smoke, and begin planning for evolving darkness and for weather-related issues. As you get closer, note the kinds of vehicles and obstacles involved. If traffic is not yet handled, determine the flow of traffic and how to control it initially.

How big an incident do you have, both in size and scope? Are you dealing with commercial carriers of industrial products? What resources will you need immediately? What is the topography? Where will fluids drain naturally? Where do you eventually want to park? What will your working space be? These are all important considerations.

Words of Wisdom

Safely operating emergency vehicles is an important part of any EMS provider's job. Principles of properly and safely operating an emergency vehicle include judicious use of lights and siren, proceeding cautiously through intersections, always remaining calm, and never assuming that other drivers will yield. These and other principles are covered in greater detail in the chapter on *Transport Operations*.

Lights and siren driving does not authorize a provider to ignore "due regard" or to drive at excessive speeds. Remember that ambulances do not handle as well as cars, they require significantly more time to stop, and control can be lost with far less maneuvering. Most states have specific rules or statutes on use of lights and siren.

Words of Wisdom

Scene safety should start early, with actions such as wearing a seat belt. As you and your partner prepare to respond to the scene, make sure you fasten your seat belts and shoulder harnesses before you move the ambulance.

YOU *are the Medic*   SUMMARY

1. Your declining physical well-being is affecting your attitude and, in turn, your job. What can you do to change this?

By staying in good physical shape, you are less likely to be injured on the job and you will be more capable of dealing with the mental stress that is also an integral part of being a paramedic. Making sure that you are well hydrated and getting proper nutrition are also important steps to take. Cardiac problems, type 2 diabetes, obesity, and possibly even Alzheimer disease are all consequences of poor nutrition.

Maintaining a healthy lifestyle can be difficult for EMS providers who work 24-hours shifts with no scheduled breaks. You should plan meals in advance and account for the possibility that you may not be near a microwave or refrigerator. Carry food in an insulated container and make choices that require minimal preparation. Follow the USDA MyPlate for recommendations. Also carry bottled water and snacks with you like raisins, nuts, and fruits. If you cannot exercise on duty, plan activities on the days you are off and make conscious decisions about your food choices.

Whereas exercise is important for weight management, it is also necessary for coping with stress. Regular vigorous exercise has been shown to improve your sleep, sex life, mental capacity, and overall long-term health. You should choose an activity that you enjoy because that will make you more likely to stick with it. Your exercise regimen should be targeted at maintaining or improving your cardiovascular endurance, your flexibility, and your physical strength. Try to engage in at least 30 minutes of moderate to vigorous physical activity most days of the week, and if you are a smoker, now is the time to stop!

It is also important to keep a regular sleep schedule, even though this is virtually impossible when working shift work. Get as much sleep as possible as time permits, avoid caffeine, and eat healthy meals—preferably at the same times every day. This will allow you to function at peak capacity even during stressful times.

2. Why is it so important to find ways to enhance your mental, emotional, and spiritual well-being?

Mild stress may be a good thing because it can enhance your mental acuity; however, overwhelming stress can push you into the fight-or-flight syndrome. Whereas the effects help you deal with the situation at hand, it can lead to crushing physical and mental strain if you do not learn appropriate coping skills. The physiologic response that occurs does so at the expense of your higher mental faculties. Your speech becomes clumsy, you forfeit depth perception and visual acuity, you lose fine motor control, and you may experience the jitters. You need to be able to think clearly and react properly. This can only be accomplished if your mental well-being is held in check. Employing techniques for coping before they are needed will help guide you when the situation arises.

To maintain your emotional health, you need a balance between your life at work and life away from work. Your entire life should not revolve around EMS. Doing your best job is a good boost for your self-esteem, but should not be all-encompassing. Maintain your skills and education and accept the fact that patients die. This is not something that you can control unless you are directly responsible for that death through your negligence. Otherwise, focus on the positive and allow the misfortunes of others to remind you of how fortunate you are. Being sensitive is part of what makes you a good caregiver; however, do not wear your feelings on your sleeve. Strive to do your best and remember that you are valuable and what you do does make a difference.

You may not be a member of an organized religious group, but if you are, you may find comfort in these beliefs. Medical care supports the dignity and value of life, and the sacredness of individuals. You must respect the beliefs of your patients, their families, and your coworkers. Respecting patients' beliefs will help you in managing effective patient care, and having a rich sense of your own spirituality will help to keep your life in good perspective.

3. The patient has been apneic for an undetermined amount of time. What is your next action?

The first step is to ensure that the patient cannot be resuscitated. Attach the cardiac monitor and check for asystole in two leads. If there is electrical activity, then you should proceed with cardiopulmonary resuscitation and follow local and ACLS protocols for the presenting rhythm. If the patient presents with asystole, or if there are other signs of obvious death, then you should refrain from disturbing the body and tell the family that it is past the time for anything to be done.

You should also notify the dispatcher, who will call law enforcement personnel and the coroner. In instances where the patient has an extended illness and there are no signs of foul play, an autopsy may not be required. In such cases, the funeral home may be notified to pick up the body at the home. If the patient's physician refuses to sign the death certificate without an autopsy, the body will be transported to a morgue. Law enforcement personnel should also be called any time there is a death. What may look to be a natural cause may turn out to be a criminal case. In most areas it is also standard for law enforcement personnel to write a report even for instances of obvious natural causes—such as an elderly person with a long history of cancer, etc.

4. On the basis of your previous interactions with the patient, what stage of the grieving process had he reached?

The patient had appeared to be prepared for the inevitable and had reached the acceptance stage. It can be difficult to interact with patients who are dealing with dying. They know it is inevitable, and everything is not going to be OK. However, it is generally better for them if they can talk about it. Family members may want to keep the patient's spirits up, as well as their own, and may find discussing death to be taboo. Offer to listen, and then be prepared to do so. It is also acceptable to offer a kind touch such as holding their hand, or putting a comforting hand on their shoulder. This should be dictated by what feels comfortable to the patient. Allowing the patient to participate in his or her care may also help them feel as if they still have some control over their life. Ask if there is anything you can do for them and if they ask you to give a message to someone, make sure to write it down so as not to forget.

YOU are the Medic   SUMMARY, continued

5. How will you explain the situation to the family, and what is your responsibility to them?

Telling the family that they have lost someone is never easy. Be direct. Do not "sugarcoat" the situation and do not use euphemisms for death. It is important to use the word "dead" or "died" to help the family move past their denial. Allow the family to see the body if they choose unless there is a potential crime scene. Give the family some time with the patient to allow them the chance to say goodbye. Try to arrange for further support as needed. Call a neighbor, religious person, or other family members to come over.

Probably the hardest part is to remind yourself not to take things personally if the family becomes upset with you. They may experience guilt, shock, denial, or anger, and you have to recognize that these are coping mechanisms that are not directed at you. Treat them with respect and empathy and allow them to work through their grief while offering to assist with whatever they may need.

6. Which stage of grieving is seen in the patient's mother?

She appears to be in two stages. She is still in denial, but is also trying to bargain. She understands that her son has an illness, but is still hopeful that the problem can be fixed. Her son's death, however, is reality, and she may move rapidly into the depression stage.

The loss of a child is a traumatic experience, no matter what the child's age. The "patient" you can help in this situation is the mother. Ask her what you can do to help. Suggest support groups that may be offered through the local hospital or other agencies. Each situation is different and should be handled based on the needs of the bereaved.

7. How should you deal with a hostile bystander?

The first step is to make sure that you remove yourself from a dangerous situation and request law enforcement personnel if they are not already en route. Removing yourself does not mean that you are abandoning your patient. You cannot provide care if you are injured. You would not normally go into a dangerous situation until law enforcement personnel have the scene secured. Use your intuition to help predict when a problem is developing. Intuition is the ability to process small details almost outside of your awareness. Once you are in contact with a hostile person, you should listen without arguing. Concentrate on de-escalating his or her emotions. An upset person does not listen or reason well. It is important to build a rapport with the person. This is based on empathy and understanding. While you do not want to say, "I know how you feel," it is important to stress, "I can only imagine how I might feel in your situation." Remember to put aside any personal prejudices and do your best to be understanding and accepting.

8. How will you deal with your own feelings and stress relating to this call?

You must understand that you cannot save every patient. You need to frequently remind yourself, "I will do my very best, but what I can do to help may not be enough." Dealing with stress is part of being a paramedic. When the situation involves a child, coworker, or family member, it can be much more difficult to handle.

This call could be particularly stressful because of your frame of mind en route to the call and your sudden change of emotions when you arrived on scene. Although death can be stressful, this situation could very easily be a trigger for acute stress. Talking with your partner should be the first step and possibly all that is needed. However, if you find yourself becoming more irritable, losing sleep, drinking more, or any other signs that indicate you are not coping well, it is imperative that you seek professional assistance. Most calls should not disrupt your normal daily functions, but if you find yourself preoccupied for weeks or months afterwards, you may be experiencing posttraumatic stress disorder. Report any concerns to your supervisor immediately and follow departmental policies for seeking help.

EMS Patient Care Report (PCR)

Date: 01-12-11	Incident No.: 1101034	Nature of Call: Possible cardiac arrest		Location: 984 Solomon Street	
Dispatched: 0712	En Route: 0713	At Scene: 0720	Transport:	At Hospital:	In Service: 0755

Patient Information	
Age: 23 Sex: M Weight (in kg [lb]): 70 kg (154 lb)	Allergies: No known drug allergies Medications: See list Past Medical History: Leukemia Chief Complaint: Cardiac arrest

Vital Signs				
Time: 0721	BP: 0	Pulse: 0	Respirations: 0	Spo$_2$:
Time:	BP:	Pulse:	Respirations:	Spo$_2$:
Time:	BP:	Pulse:	Respirations:	Spo$_2$:

YOU *are the Medic*   SUMMARY, *continued*

EMS Treatment (circle all that apply)			
Oxygen @ _____ L/min via (circle one): NC NRM Bag-mask device	Assisted Ventilation	Airway Adjunct:	CPR
Defibrillation	Bleeding Control	Bandaging	Splinting	**Other:** Cardiac monitor

Narrative
Dispatched to a possible cardiac arrest. Arrived on scene to find a 23-year-old man lying supine in bed apneic and pulseless. Mother states that pt refused to eat last pm and she found him "not breathing" just prior to calling EMS. Pt cold to touch, no obvious signs of injury, presents with dependent lividity. Cardiac monitor shows asystole in two leads. Pt has hx of leukemia and mother states "he has been getting worse over the past month." He was not a hospice pt. Mother also stated that he was not "feeling well" last pm. Advised dispatch to notify law enforcement and coroner of death. Stayed on scene with pt and family until turned over to coroner. **End of report**

Prep Kit

- Paramedics need to know how to ensure their own well-being.

- Wellness has at least four dimensions: physical, mental, emotional, and spiritual. It is important to keep all four dimensions healthy and balanced.

- The American Heart Association's Simple 7 are seven factors that have been found to improve heart health: get active, control cholesterol, eat better, manage blood pressure, lose weight, reduce blood sugar, and stop smoking.

- Nutrition plays a key role in maintaining day-to-day energy and maintaining a healthy body for life.

- Practice proper lifting techniques to protect your body and lengthen your career.
  - Minimize the number of total body lifts you have to perform.
  - Coordinate every lift in advance.
  - Minimize the total amount of weight you have to lift.
  - Never lift with your back.
  - Do not carry what you can put on wheels.
  - Ask for help anytime.

- Stress reactions can be acute, delayed, or cumulative. Post-traumatic stress disorder is a syndrome with onset following a traumatic, usually life-threatening event. Critical incident stress management is a process developed to address acute stress situations. Paramedics may also seek help through an employee assistance program.

- Learn how to effectively control stress so that it does not affect your wellness. Take appropriate action. Initial management techniques include the following:
  - Controlled breathing
  - Professional assistance
  - Progressive relaxation

- A patient's reaction to stress may include fear, anxiety, depression, anger, confusion, denial, regression, projection, and displacement.

- Health care professionals are not immune to the stresses of emergency situations and experience a multitude of feelings, not all of them pleasant.

- Burnout is a consequence of chronic, unrelieved stress.

- As a paramedic, you will be present when a lot of people are born and you will be there when a lot of people die.

- The patient who is dying may be aware of that fact and may want to talk about it. Be prepared to listen and provide empathy.

- A communicable disease is any disease that can be spread from person to person or animal to person. Infectious diseases can be transmitted by contact (direct or indirect), or they are airborne, foodborne, or vector-borne.

- Even if you are exposed to an infectious disease, your risk of becoming ill is small. Whether or not an acute infection occurs depends on several factors, including the amount and type of infectious organism and your resistance to that infection.

- You can take several steps to protect yourself against exposure to infectious diseases, including remaining up-to-date with recommended vaccinations, following standard precautions at all times, and handling all needles and other sharp objects with great care.

- Because it is often impossible to tell which patients have infectious diseases, you should avoid direct contact with the blood and body fluids of all patients.

- Standard precautions are protective measures designed to prevent health care workers from coming into contact with germs carried by patients. One extremely effective step is properly washing your hands. You must also use the proper personal protective equipment for the situation, including gloves, gowns, eye protection, masks, and possibly other specialized equipment.

- Infection control should be an important part of your daily routine. Be sure to follow the proper steps when dealing with potential exposure situations. You should know what to do if you are exposed to an airborne or bloodborne disease.

- Cleaning your ambulance and equipment is part of protecting yourself and your patients. Decontamination of equipment and supplies that have been potentially exposed to body substances requires a different cleansing routine than just soap and water; sterilization may be required.

- Keep yourself on alert while you are on duty. Do not be afraid to ask for the police to enter a scene first.

- During your career, you will be exposed to many hazards. Some situations will be life-threatening. In these cases you should be properly protected, or you must avoid the situation altogether.

- Scene hazards include traffic hazards, unstable vehicles, potential exposure to hazardous materials, electricity, and fire. Your safety is the most important consideration. Never approach a scene without first observing it from a safe distance.

- The most dangerous calls are your everyday ones because you become comfortable with them and may let down your guard.

- Your primary concern at any scene is safety—safety for yourself as well as those around you.

- Safe emergency vehicle operation is crucial to the safety of the paramedic, crew, and patient.

Vital Vocabulary

acute stress reaction Reaction to stress that occurs during a stressful situation.

airborne transmission The spread of an organism in aerosol form.

blind panic A fear reaction in which a person's judgment seems to disappear entirely; it is particularly dangerous because it may precipitate mass panic among others.

bloodborne pathogens Pathogenic microorganisms that are present in human blood and can cause disease in humans; include, but are not limited to, hepatitis B virus and human immunodeficiency virus.

burnout The exhaustion of physical or emotional strength.

communicable disease Any disease that can be spread from person to person or from animal to person.

conversion hysteria A reaction in which a person subconsciously transforms his or her anxiety into a bodily dysfunction; the person may be unable to see or hear or may become partially paralyzed.

critical incident An event that overwhelms the ability to cope with the experience, either at the scene or later.

critical incident stress management (CISM) A process that confronts responses to critical incidents and defuses them.

cumulative stress reaction Prolonged or excessive stress.

defense mechanisms Psychological ways to relieve stress; they are usually automatic or subconscious. Defense mechanisms include denial, regression, projection, and displacement.

delayed stress reaction Reaction to stress that occurs after a stressful situation.

denial An early response to a serious medical emergency, in which the severity of the emergency is diminished or minimized. Denial is the first coping mechanism for people who believe they are going to die.

direct contact Exposure to or transmission of a communicable disease from one person to another by physical contact.

displacement Redirection of an emotion from yourself to another person.

fight-or-flight syndrome A physiologic response to a profound stressor that helps a person deal with the situation at hand; features increased sympathetic tone and results in dilation of the pupils, increased heart rate, dilation of the bronchi, mobilization of glucose, shunting of blood away from the gastrointestinal tract and cerebrum, and increased blood flow to the skeletal muscles.

indirect contact Exposure or transmission of disease from one person to another by contact with a contaminated object.

infection The invasion of a host or host tissues by organisms such as bacteria, viruses, or parasites, with or without signs or symptoms of disease.

infection control Procedures to reduce transmission of infection among patients and health care personnel.

infectious disease A disease that is caused by infection or one that is capable of being transmitted with or without direct contact.

posttraumatic stress disorder (PTSD) A delayed stress reaction to a previous incident, often the result of one or more unresolved issues concerning the incident.

projection Blaming unacceptable feelings, motives, or desires on others.

regression A return to more childish behavior while under stress.

standard precautions Protective measures that have traditionally been developed by the CDC for use in dealing with objects, blood, body fluids, or other potential exposure risks of communicable disease.

stress A nonspecific response of the body to any demand made on it.

stressor Any agent or situation that causes stress.

transmission The way in which an infectious agent is spread: contact, airborne, by vehicles (for example, food or needles), or by vectors.

universal precautions Protective measures that have traditionally been developed by the CDC for use in dealing with objects, blood, body fluids, or other potential exposure risks of communicable disease.

Assessment in Action

I t is near dark and you are dispatched to the scene of a single-vehicle crash. On arrival at the scene you see a small pickup truck at the bottom of a ravine. A fire fighter on scene tells you there is one person inside and no signs of life have been observed. After picking your way through the debris down the treacherous embankment, you note that you can barely see the young man in the driver's seat. The fire fighter also states that it will take an extended period of time to extricate the patient.

The patient is not breathing and you cannot feel a carotid pulse. He also has brain matter exposed from a depressed skull fracture and blood is draining from his ear on the side you can see. You have no access to the rest of his body because the crumpled metal of the vehicle is encompassing him, so CPR is not an option. You contact medical control and are told not to attempt to resuscitate the patient.

1. While viewing the wreckage at the bottom of the ravine, it is natural for you to be bombarded with adrenaline and rush into an unsafe situation in an attempt to help the patient. It is critical that you remain calm in emergency situations. This requires controlling the fight-or-flight mechanism. All of the following are methods of coping with stress EXCEPT:
   A. controlled breathing.
   B. reframing.
   C. increased caffeine consumption.
   D. progressive relaxation.

2. If it were possible to untangle this patient from the vehicle, he would then have to be carried back up a significant grade to reach the ambulance. To reduce your exposure to damage when lifting your maximum weight, which of the following expresses the proper technique for lifting?
   A. Always lift with your back.
   B. Keep feet and knees together for proper balance.
   C. Place all equipment on the stretcher so you will only have to make one lift.
   D. Keep your back in a straight, upright position and lift without twisting.

3. You realize that you are extremely agitated and that your pulse rate is elevated. You also note an overwhelming sense of helplessness. Your patient that you were supposed to save is beyond your help. This, along with the other issues that have been building for weeks, can lead to what condition that is a consequence of chronic, unrelieved stress?
   A. Conversion hysteria
   B. Distress
   C. Burnout
   D. Anxiety

4. Very traumatic calls, such as this one, can preoccupy even well-adjusted providers for weeks or even months afterward. This is known as:
   A. a critical incident.
   B. posttraumatic stress disorder (PTSD).
   C. burnout.
   D. denial.

5. Motor vehicle crashes such as this have the potential for exposure to body fluids because of open injuries caused by broken glass and jagged metal. What personal protective equipment should be used for this situation?
   A. Gloves
   B. Mask
   C. N95 respirator
   D. Turnout gear

6. The death of the patient, along with the lack of ability to help, can trigger a stress response for you and it is natural to subconsciously attempt to relieve it. Regression and projection are types of:
   A. denial.
   B. defense mechanisms.
   C. displacement.
   D. reframing.

7. Situations such as this require that you be physically fit and well to access the patient. Along with the components of a healthy lifestyle, you should be aware of hereditary factors. The most common of all health risk factors are cancer and:
   A. heart disease.
   B. Alzheimer disease.
   C. chemical addiction.
   D. hypertension.

8. One definition of _____ is the "nonspecific response of the body to any demand made on it."
A. adaptation.
B. stress.
C. eustress.
D. distress.

Additional Questions

9. Traffic may be only one of the many hazards at the scene of a motor vehicle crash. What type of problems might you encounter en route to and after arrival at the scene?

10. When responding to a multiple-casualty incident, both victims and bystanders may react by becoming dazed, disorganized, or overwhelmed. What reactions in this circumstance may present a problem requiring that these persons be removed from the scene?

Public Health

National EMS Education Standard Competencies

Public Health

Applies fundamental knowledge of principles of public health and epidemiology including public health emergencies, health promotion, and illness and injury prevention.

Knowledge Objectives

1. Define public health and explain the goal of the public health field. (p 61)
2. List the major public health laws, regulations, and guidelines in place in the United States, and list the purpose of each. (pp 65-66)
3. Explain the paramedic's role in promoting public health, both in terms of illness and injury. (p 66)
4. Define primary prevention and secondary prevention, and give examples of each. (p 67)
5. Explain why EMS providers are in a unique position to promote public health. (pp 67-68)
6. Discuss the detrimental effects of injuries as related to public health. (pp 61-62)
7. Define intentional injuries and unintentional injuries. (pp 72-73)
8. Discuss the principles of injury prevention, including education, enforcement, engineering/environment, and economic incentives. (pp 68-69)
9. Discuss the concept of injury surveillance and how it relates to EMS. (pp 70-71)
10. List ways a paramedic can promote injury prevention in his or her community. (pp 71-72)
11. Discuss pediatric injuries and risk factors for them. (pp 73-74)
12. Describe the steps involved in organizing a community prevention program. (p 74)
13. Define and explain the relevance of a teachable moment in EMS. (pp 77-78)

Skills Objectives

There are no skills objectives for this chapter.

Introduction

Several years ago, San Diego paramedic Paul Maxwell went on a call for a possible drowning. A 2-year-old boy had wandered away from a day care facility and fallen into a neighbor's backyard pool. Despite everyone's best efforts, he could not be resuscitated. The mother was inconsolable and her cries haunted the paramedic.

Maxwell wondered how such tragedies could be prevented—if he could help it, he never wanted to go on another call like that again. Doing a little investigation, and looking up incidents on his EMS system's database, he discovered a pattern of increased drownings in his region. Maxwell made the decision to get involved. In cooperation with his EMS agency, he contacted other groups in his community with an interest in child safety. Using his system's data and motivated by his firsthand knowledge of the suffering that such a death inflicts, Maxwell began a coordinated and successful effort to reduce backyard pool drownings in his community, through both legislation and education. Although the reduction in drownings was incentive enough for Maxwell, he was recognized with a special award by the state of California.

This scenario demonstrates the important role in injury or illness prevention that an EMS provider can have. This chapter discusses injury and illness prevention as they relate to public health, and defines the EMS provider's role in promoting public health in his or her community.

Role of Public Health

According to the American Public Health Association (APHA), **public health** is defined as "the practice of preventing disease and promoting good health within groups of people" (2011). For a very long time, the health care system in the United States has concentrated on treating illness and injuries as opposed to their prevention. Health and wellness have only recently become more of a focus due to skyrocketing costs, the incidence of chronic disease, and health care reform.

Injuries as Public Health Threats

According to the National Center for Injury Prevention and Control, part of the Centers for Disease Control and Prevention (CDC), injuries are "the intentional or unintentional damage to the person resulting from acute exposure to thermal, mechanical, electrical, or chemical energy or from the absence of such essentials as heat or oxygen" (2011). Historically, injuries were not grouped together. Instead, they were reported under distinct umbrellas, which made it difficult to let the lay population see just how widespread injuries truly are Figure 1 . Grouping injuries as a common health problem makes it possible to consider the breadth and depth of the problem. It has enabled public health officials and other care providers to call attention to important problems and target more effective interventions.

Intentional injuries, such as assaults or suicide, are included in the definition of injury. EMS can often play a supporting role here too, but can usually have a greater impact in preventing **unintentional injuries**.

To many health experts, injury is the largest public health problem facing the country today. The following data were collected by the National Center for Health Statistics in 2007 (the latest available year for figures) Figure 2 :

- There were a total of 81.4 million injury-related visits to physician offices, emergency departments, and outpatient clinics.
- In total, 182,479 people died as a result of injury, or 60.5 deaths per 100,000 people.
- Of those, 42,031 were from motor vehicle crashes, 40,059 were from poisonings, and 31,224 were from firearms. (These numbers combine intentional and unintentional incidents. For example, while 31,224 deaths resulted from firearms, 613 of those were accidental.)
- Of those, 123,706 died of unintentional injuries and 58,340 died of intentional injuries (34,598 suicides and 18,361 homicides; and 5,381 deaths were undetermined).

YOU are the Medic   PART 1

On a sunny day you and your partner are dispatched at 1420 to the area of Hwy 232 and Needle Road for a motor vehicle crash. You have just admitted a patient to the emergency department, and it takes a few minutes to clean and prepare the ambulance for another run. The location of the call is outside of the city limits, so travel time will be extended, although traffic is generally not heavy at this time of day.

While you are en route, the dispatcher informs you that there are two patients and possibly an ejection. Because you suspect the injuries may be serious, you request that another unit be dispatched. You are familiar with this stretch of roadway; there have been multiple collisions in the same location. There is a sharp curve in the road just before a long, straight stretch. It is not unusual for a driver to lose control and end up in a ditch.

1. What is the proper response for this call?
2. What are the injury risks in this situation?

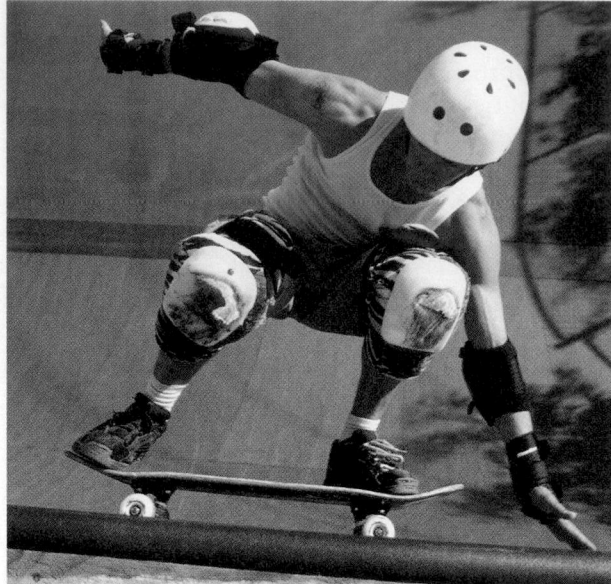 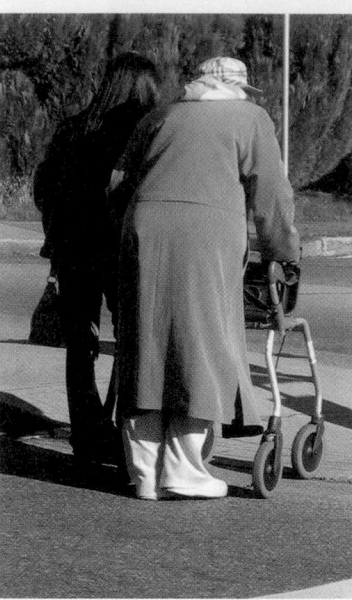

Figure 1 Injuries affect people of all age groups and physical abilities. For each potential injury, there are appropriate preventive measures that can and should be taken.

Total Deaths from Injury
182,479

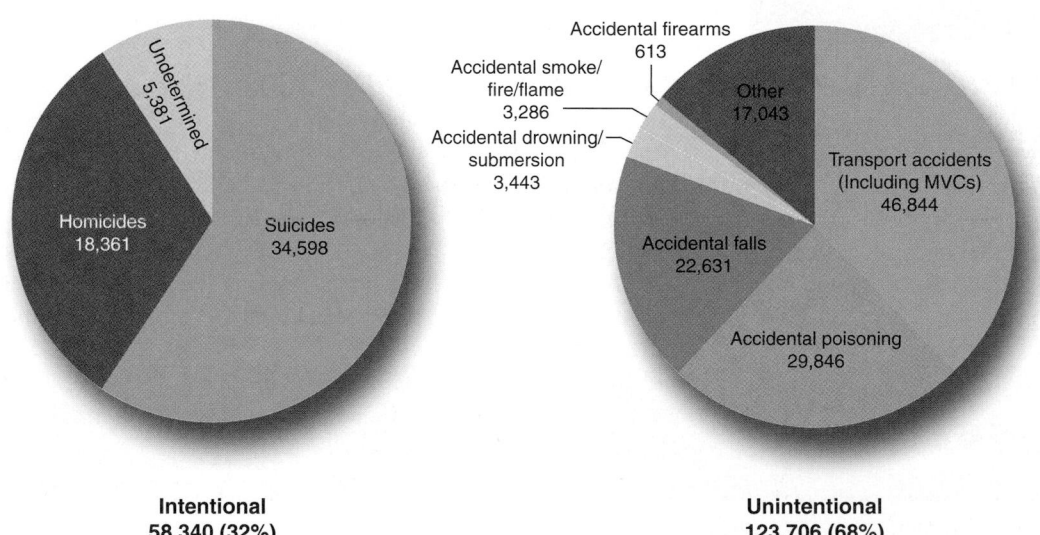

Intentional
58,340 (32%)

Unintentional
123,706 (68%)

Figure 2 The vast majority of injuries that occur are unintentional—particularly incidents related to driving.

Table 1 shows the top 10 causes of death in the United States in 2007. This information is extremely important in understanding the impact that injury has on different age groups. From ages 1 to 44 years, unintentional injuries are the leading killer. For all ages combined, unintentional injuries are the fifth leading killer behind heart disease, cancer, cerebrovascular events (stroke), and the effects of bronchitis, emphysema, and asthma.

How much do these injuries cost society, above and beyond the tremendous personal suffering? It is estimated that injuries requiring medical treatment cost $406 billion, with $80.2 billion for medical care and $326 billion for lost productivity (Centers for Disease Control and Prevention, 2007). Researchers are using this latter factor to measure the cost to society: **years of potential life lost**. It works like this: Assume a productive work life until age 65, and deduct the year of death from that age. Thus, an 18-year-old who dies in a car crash has lost 47 years of potential productive work life, while someone who dies of a stroke at age 63 years has lost 2 years. Because injuries are a leading cause of death in the young, it quickly adds up **Figure 3**. This method allows a comparison of the years of productive work life lost, disease by disease. This method can measure how many years of usefulness to society a child killed by an unintentional injury could have had, comparing those years with those of an older person who for example, had a myocardial infarction. The value of the comparison is to teach members of your community that the prevention of a childhood death is of great importance to the community. **Figure 4** compares years of potential productive work life lost by injury with other causes of death.

It is easier to measure death rates than to measure nonfatal (**morbidity**) injury rates because visits to clinics, emergency departments, physicians' offices, and other places for treatment are scattered in a number of agencies and professional groups.

The remainder was attributed to 412 from legal intervention (killed by law enforcement personnel) and 21 from war.

- Approximately 16,375 children between 12 and 19 years of age died in the United States. Of that number, almost 50% were unintentional, with one third of those due to car crashes.
- Teens died at the rate of 49.5 deaths per 100,000 people from 1999 to 2006.

Source: Centers for Disease Control and Prevention, 2010.

Table 1 Top 10 Causes of Death in 2007

1. Heart disease
2. Cancer
3. Stroke
4. Chronic, lower respiratory disease
5. Unintentional injuries
6. Alzheimer disease
7. Diabetes
8. Influenza and pneumonia
9. Kidney disease
10. Septicemia

Source: National Center for Health Statistics/National Vital Statistics Reports, 2007, United States.

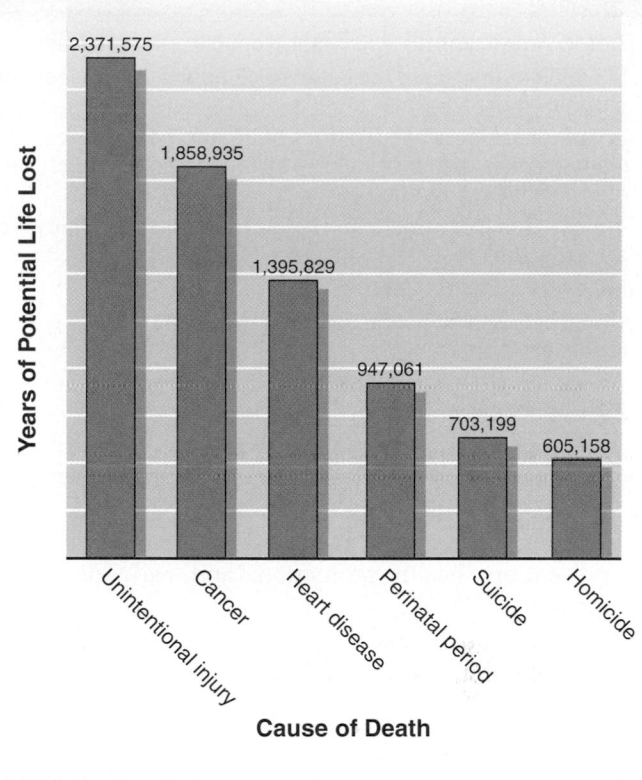

Cause of Death

Figure 4 Years of potential life lost categorized by cause of death.

Source: National Center for Injury Prevention and Control, 2007, United States.

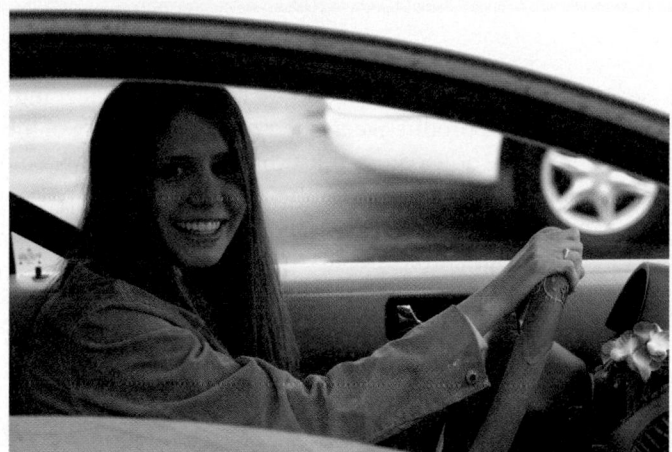

Figure 3 The regular use of a seat belt can have a dramatic effect on the number of years of potential life lost—particularly in younger age groups.

Illness and Disease as Public Health Threats

Illness and disease also represent significant threats to public health in the United States. Annual deaths for 7 out of 10 Americans are from chronic diseases, with cancer, heart disease, and stroke causing more than 50% of them. In 2005, almost 1 of every 2 adults, or 133 million Americans, had at least one chronic illness (Centers for Disease Control and Prevention, 2010). Causes include excessive alcohol intake, poor nutrition, tobacco use, and lack of physical activity Table 2.

In 2007, asthma, a common chronic illness, was the primary diagnosis for many children and adults presenting to the emergency department. The statistics are as follows:

- 121 visits per 10,000 children younger than age 5 years
- 59 visits per 10,000 people between 5 and 64 years of age
- 25 visits per 10,000 people age 65 and over (Niska, Bhuiya, & Xu, 2010)

In April of 2009, the H1N1 influenza virus was first detected in a 10-year-old patient in California. As an outbreak unfolded, the Centers for Disease Control (CDC) declared a US Public Health Emergency for H1N1 influenza, which eventually became a global pandemic as identified by the World Health Organization (WHO) in June of 2009. In September of that year, the Food and Drug Administration approved four vaccines for children and adults to try to prevent the disease. Through vaccination and ongoing communication from the CDC, prevention efforts targeted those people most susceptible to acquiring the illness, resulting in an expiration of the emergency in June of 2010 (Centers for Disease Control and Prevention, 2010).

Other health threats include contamination of the water supply, contamination of seafood (for example from oil leaks), radiation leaks, lack of sanitary conditions after natural disasters, and increased incidence of cancer after major incidents.

Public Health Efforts

The APHA recommends three major reforms to increase the attention given to wellness and prevention of illness and injury. We must:

1. Provide consistent, robust policy leadership that advocates for and funds multifaceted approaches to prevention and wellness.
2. Strengthen the ability of the public health system to facilitate and, as appropriate, provide community-based

Table 2 Chronic Diseases in the US

- 7 of 10 Americans die each year from chronic diseases
- 133 million Americans, or 1 of every 2 adults, had at least one chronic illness
- In Americans between the ages of 20 and 74, diabetes is the leading cause of kidney failure, blindness, and amputations of the lower extremities
- Almost 19 million Americans have limitations of activity from arthritis, the most common cause of disability
- 1 of every 3 adults is obese
- 1 in 5 children and young adults between the ages of 6 and 19 is obese
- One or more daily activities are limited in approximately 25% of people with chronic illnesses

Source: Centers for Disease Control and Prevention, 2010, United States.

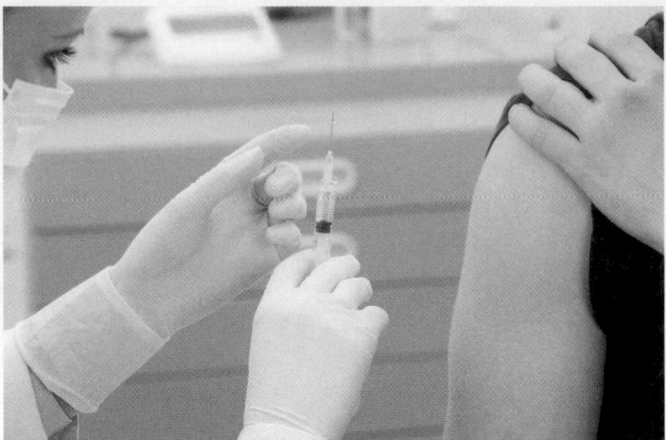

Figure 5 Vaccination programs allow the general public to receive flu vaccinations, helping to reduce the overall incidence of the flu.

prevention, health promotion, and early detection of disease.

3. Assume that all Americans have access to recommended clinical preventive services.

Public health efforts aim to have an impact on people within an entire city, community, state, or country. For example, a vaccination program conducted by a local health department may provide flu vaccines to children and adults in its community **Figure 5**. Through these efforts, people stay well during flu season, use health care resources less, continue going to school, and remain productive in their jobs. The quality of life is improved for the whole community, the economy is more stable with its workforce intact, and health care costs are lowered.

Preventing adverse health outcomes has been one of the goals of public health professionals. For example, aggressive education campaigns to promote the benefits of disease screening,

YOU are the Medic   PART 2

You arrive on scene 15 minutes later to find a single vehicle angled down into a ditch at the side of the road. The second unit is only a minute or two behind you. You can see a woman sitting in the driver's seat with a volunteer fire fighter holding cervical-spine control, and another woman is standing at the driver's window holding a crying infant who has blood on his face. A law enforcement officer is directing traffic. The scene appears safe as you approach. The woman holding the infant tells you that she was not involved in the crash but witnessed the infant in the car seat being thrown from the vehicle during the crash. She states that she took the infant out of the thrown car seat. The driver is crying, says she is fine, and tells you, "Just take care of my baby!" The driver was wearing her seat belt and her only complaint is ankle pain. You wait for the second unit to arrive to care for the mother.

You turn your attention to the crying infant, an 8-month-old boy, and immediately note that he has an approximate 1" laceration to the right side of his forehead with bleeding controlled and a large hematoma surrounding it. He also has slight angulation to his left forearm.

Recording Time: 0 Minutes	
Appearance	Agitated, normal skin color
Level of consciousness	Appropriate for age
Airway	Open and clear
Breathing	Rapid and gasping with crying
Circulation	Strong, rapid brachial pulse

3. What are the risk factors associated with the infant's injuries?

4. Is this a teachable moment?

injury prevention, and the importance of prenatal care have been successful. In adults, early detection of breast cancer, cervical cancer, and colorectal cancer have led to earlier treatment, better outcomes, and fewer deaths. The number of deaths from injury for children between 5 and 14 years of age dropped from 7.3 per 100,000 children in 2006 to 6.9 per 100,000 children in 2007. In 2008, preterm birth weights increased because there were more infants who had reached at least 37 weeks of gestation at birth. Adult smoking has decreased, and the age at which people begin to smoke is rising, both of which represent positive trends. These last accomplishments were made possible by efforts to decrease secondhand smoke by promoting smoke-free workplaces and passing laws that prohibit smoking in certain indoor facilities.

■ Public Health Laws, Regulations, and Guidelines

There are many rules, regulations, guidelines, and laws that govern public health. Some are federal while others are promulgated by individual states based on their specific circumstances and governmental hierarchy. A few examples are provided here Table 3.

The federal **Health Insurance Portability and Accountability Act (HIPAA)**, enacted in 1996, represented the first national standards established to protect the confidentiality of a patient's health information. The act outlines various conditions and situations in which a covered entity, in this instance the

Table 3 Public Health Laws, Regulations, and Guidelines to Improve Safety and Prevention

Law	Date	Description
Health Insurance Portability and Accountability Act (HIPAA)	Enacted in 1996	First national standards established to protect the confidentiality of a patient's health information
Various state laws regarding motorcycle helmets	As of April 2011	20 states and the District of Columbia legally require all riders to wear a helmet 27 states require some riders to wear a helmet 3 states (Illinois, Iowa, and New Hampshire) do not have a motorcycle helmet law
Various state laws regarding bicycle helmets	As of April 2011	No federal law States and localities began adopting laws in 1987; most apply to children younger than age 18 Some also cover skateboards, roller skates, in-line skates, and non-motorized scooters New Mexico first to include tricycle riders
Various state laws regarding automotive seat belts	As of April 2011	Most states have fines for not wearing a seat belt 21 states, the District of Columbia, and Puerto Rico make it a primary offense to not wear a seat belt; officer can stop the car and issue ticket New Hampshire has no seat belt law for adults
World Health Organization (WHO) Framework Convention on Tobacco Control (FCTC), regarding tobacco products	Established in 2005	International collaborative effort to reduce the demand and supply of tobacco
Family Smoking Prevention and Tobacco Control Act, Food and Drug Administration (FDA), regarding tobacco products	2009	Restrict the sale, distribution, and marketing of cigarettes and smokeless tobacco products to youth in the United States
State of New York regarding AEDs	2002	Law passed that requires at least one AED in each school and that at least one staff member is trained to use it Saved at least 54 lives in the past 6 years
State of Connecticut regarding AEDs	2009	Law that makes AEDs available in public schools; ensures that at least two staff members are trained to use them; prompted by the death of a 15-year-old student who died after collapsing during a run at school Companion bill reduces liability issues for AED users
Various state laws regarding tobacco products	As of April, 2011	Georgia, Idaho, New Hampshire, North Carolina, and Virginia have enacted smoking bans in particular places that do not fit other categories 11 states have no general statewide bans on smoking in nongovernment-owned spaces; require designation and warning signage for smoking and nonsmoking areas

EMS agency, is permitted to use and disclose **protected health information (PHI)**, the data that contain the patient's name, address, and other specific identifiers. HIPAA also addresses two other forms of data—a **limited data set** and data in which common identifiers are removed. A limited data set contains information necessary for public health and research, such as some geographic information, birth dates, and dates of treatment.

To address the issue of smoking, which is considered a serious public health hazard in the United States, multiple legislative efforts have occurred at the state, national, and international levels. In February 2010, the World Health Organization celebrated an important milestone in public health history with the 5-year anniversary of the first global public health treaty: Framework Convention on Tobacco Control (FCTC). Of 195 countries invited to participate, 168 have joined in this collaborative effort to reduce the demand and supply of tobacco. The treaty is helping its members by providing tools for governments to develop effective policies against the tobacco industry (WHO Framework Convention on Tobacco Control, 2010). The United States has not yet ratified this treaty; however, in June 2010, new regulations by the Food and Drug Administration (FDA) came into effect to restrict the sale and distribution and marketing of cigarettes and smokeless tobacco products to youth in the United States. Other laws have been enacted in many states to impose local smoking restrictions.

■ EMS Interface With Public Health

In November 2001, three organizations—the APHA, the National Association of EMS Physicians (NAEMSP), and the National Association of State EMS Directors—came together to create an agreement on the emergency medical and public health response to terrorism. Sponsored by the National Highway Traffic Safety Administration (NHTSA), these organizations met to discuss ways in which EMS and public health agencies could work more closely together to improve community health. They agreed to a set of principles that included leadership roles, the definition of EMS providers' roles, communication strategies, allocation of EMS resources, best practices, educational efforts, rural EMS systems, and the need for joint position statements, which outline how multiple organizations agree to certain standards.

Each year, the APHA designates September as National Preparedness Month to help people prepare for potential health emergencies. They sponsor the Get Ready campaign to help Americans, their families, and their communities prepare for hazards and disasters. Get Ready Day, one component of this campaign, is recognized on the third Tuesday of every September and provides tips to help people prepare for the following emergencies **Figure 6** :

- H1N1 safety
- Floods
- Heat waves
- Power outages
- Winter storms
- Earthquakes
- Emergencies at work

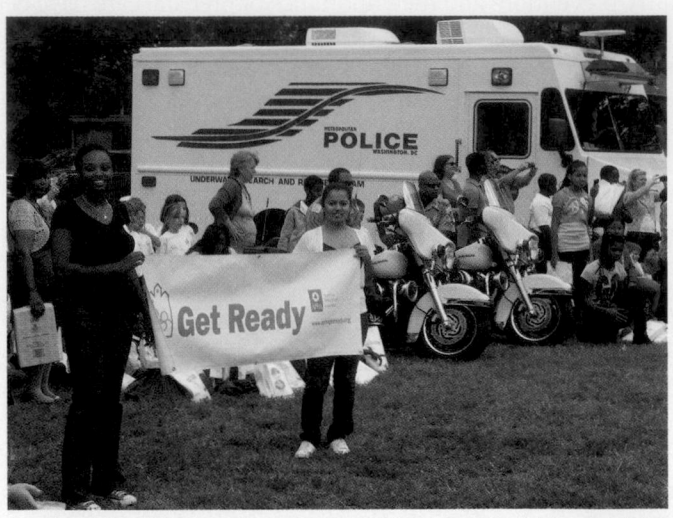

Figure 6 Get Ready Day, which occurs in September, is designated by the APHA as a way to prepare for potential health emergencies.

Activities such as Get Ready Day also represent opportunities for EMS personnel to be involved in public health initiatives. Programs can possibly be conducted year-round to create public awareness about safety and health issues. Bike safety and helmet workshops might occur in the spring to emphasize injury prevention. During the winter months in areas with snow, education can focus on safe driving, how and when to shovel snow, and what to do if a person cannot leave his or her home for a period of time due to weather conditions. Before and during flu season, EMS agencies might conduct a flu clinic in conjunction with their local hospital and primary care physician practices.

The Division of Emerging Infections and Surveillance Services at the CDC builds collaborative partnerships within the United States and abroad with the goal of detecting and responding to emerging infections. Their Epidemiology and Laboratory Capacity for Infectious Diseases program provides funding in all 50 states. Check with your state and local health departments to see what options exist for EMS participation.

■ Injury and Illness Prevention and EMS

More than a few paramedics have been motivated by their field experiences to work actively on prevention. Throughout the country, EMS providers are taking the lead or providing support in a wide variety of **interventions**—specific prevention measures or activities designed to increase positive health and safety outcomes **Figure 7** . From beginnings such as these, EMS has emerged as a strong advocate—and practitioner—of injury and illness prevention. EMS providers may participate in various injury prevention activities such as bike helmet rodeos, car seat checks, or swimming safety efforts at the local pool. Illness prevention initiatives such as flu inoculation programs or blood pressure monitoring are other ways for EMS providers to help identify the potential or lower the rate of chronic diseases in the community.

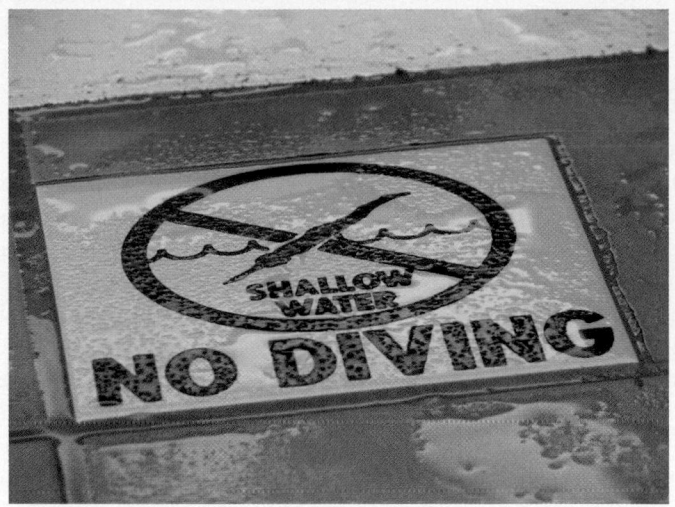

Figure 7 Many rules of public safety exist because of the persistent efforts of medical professionals and other involved citizens.

busy systems will find that time for prevention initiatives will be limited. However, there is a role for every EMS provider, at some level, in primary injury and illness prevention **Figure 8** . This includes, first and foremost, teaching others in the health care system and the public *why* you see an injury recurring at the same place or how an illness can be prevented.

The principles and techniques for illness prevention are not substantially different from those for injury prevention. For instance, the CDC sponsors the Healthy Communities Program to help communities and national networks direct more focus on the prevention of chronic diseases. They work with local and state health departments to support good health and decrease preventable risk factors at schools, health care sites, and work sites. Check with your local health department to see what programs might already exist and what opportunities are available for your EMS agency to start something new. If you discover a need for a prevention program—perhaps some of your elderly patients might not be getting their influenza or pneumococcal vaccines—apply the principles discussed in this section.

Common Roots

Injury prevention shares the common root of EMS—the historic National Academy of Sciences/National Research Council 1966 study, "Accidental Death and Disability: The Neglected Disease of Modern Society." The commission noted that just as EMS could help with trauma after an event, injury prevention initiatives could help before an accident happened.

Strengthening this link, the broader definition of injury prevention has always included EMS. **Primary prevention** is defined as keeping an injury from ever occurring. EMS traditionally has focused on **secondary prevention**, reducing the effects of an injury, disease, or other health problem that already exists.

In 1996 the *Consensus Statement on the EMS Role in Primary Injury Prevention* was published. Representing every imaginable EMS constituency, the authors of the statement made clear that primary injury prevention is an "essential" activity "that must be undertaken by the leaders, decision-makers, and providers of every EMS system."

As a paramedic, your priority is to respond to and treat illness and injury in your community. Providers in particularly

Why EMS Should Be Involved

Leaders in both EMS and the prevention field offer the following rationale:

- EMS providers are widely distributed in the population.
- EMS providers reflect the composition of the community they serve.
- In many rural communities, the EMT might be the most medically sophisticated person.

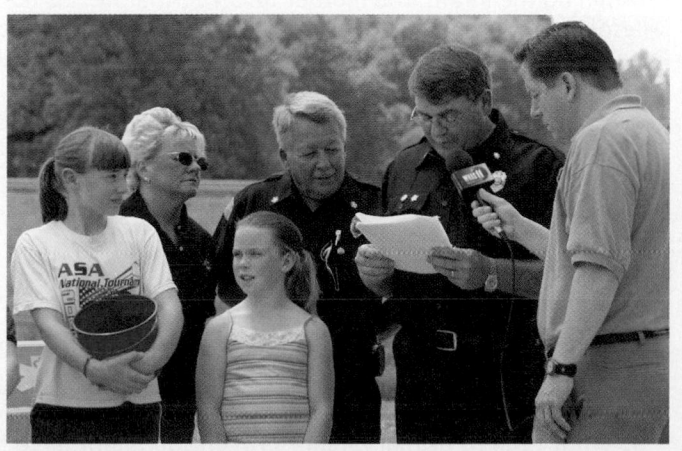

Figure 8 Embracing the full role of a paramedic means being involved in the concerns of your community.

- If properly coordinated, EMS would provide a formidable resource in the effort to reduce the overall injury burden.
- EMS providers are high-profile role models.
- EMS providers are perceived as champions of their patients.
- EMS providers are welcome in schools and other environments conducive to delivering the prevention message.
- Because they face the results of injuries and illness every day, EMS providers are perceived as authorities on prevention. (A paramedic talking to a city council about drowning prevention legislation, relating a true story about the suffering he or she witnessed, can be an extremely effective teacher.)

Special Populations

With a growing geriatric population, a good flu prevention program may be one of the keys to preventing an overload of the health care system. Evaluate all community options available to the older population in your area and bridge any gaps with programs to meet their needs and prevent illnesses related to the flu.

Principles of Injury and Illness Prevention

The 4 Es of Prevention

An injury risk or illness **risk** is a potentially hazardous situation in which the well-being of people can be harmed. Interventions need to combine *education* with three other types of interventions: *enforcement*, *engineering/environment*, and *economic incentives*. These are commonly referred to as the 4 Es of prevention **Figure 9**. The most effective prevention efforts reflect a combination of these interventions.

Education

Most paramedics know that people can behave in ways that cause them to become injured, ill, or put others at risk. Many people do not know and therefore cannot assess the risk of doing something—"I didn't know it was unsafe to put my baby's seat in the front passenger seat" or "I didn't think I needed a flu shot." Or people know the risk—"I won't wear seat belts, they are too uncomfortable" or "I don't believe in giving my baby all of those shots"—and disregard it anyway. Through education you can often inform people about potential dangers and then act to persuade them to change risky behavior. Show moms and dads how to use an infant car seat. Tell people about the horrors of being thrown from a vehicle. Relate general information about people you have treated who were at risk of death from the flu. Explain how pertussis, which was once nonexistent in the United States due to adequate vaccinations, is once again being seen in this country and why childhood immunizations are so important.

To be effective, messages need to be tailored to very specific groups and reinforced with meaningful rewards. Educational techniques that seem to be particularly promising include the use of contracts or participant commitment, incentives, behavioral feedback, and modeling.

However, despite your best efforts, even though some members of your community may know about a risk, their behavior will not necessarily change. A crucial advantage of any educational effort is that it can pave the way to legislative and environmental/technological changes.

YOU are the Medic   PART 3

You ask the woman holding the infant to hold his head still and try to keep his neck straight while your partner retrieves the immobilization equipment. The other ambulance has arrived on scene and is taking care of the mother. While you are examining the infant, the mother tells you that he has no significant medical history and takes no medications. He also has no allergies that she is aware of. No one is sure whether he lost consciousness. The woman holding the infant tells you that he was strapped into the car seat face down in the ditch crying when she got to him.

Recording Time: 3 Minutes	
Respirations	42 breaths/min
Pulse	138 beats/min
Skin	Pink, warm, and dry
Oxygen saturation (Spo₂)	99% on room air
Pupils	Equal and reactive to light

5. **What type of primary injury prevention might have helped this situation? Are there any automatic protections that would have worked?**

6. **Explain the Haddon matrix as it relates to your patient.**

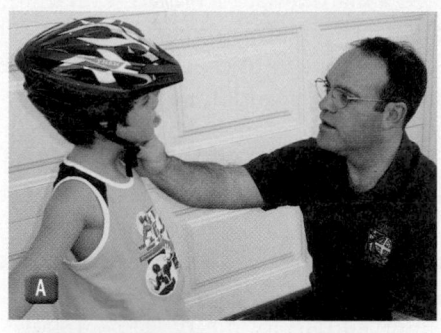
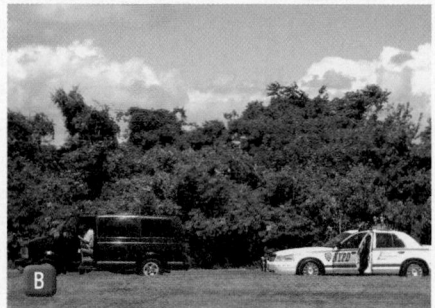
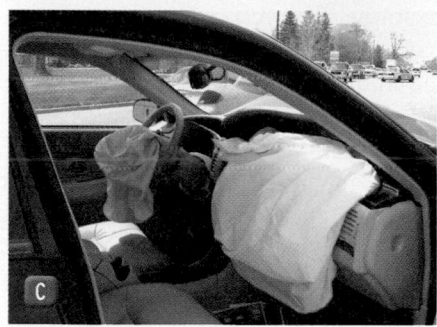
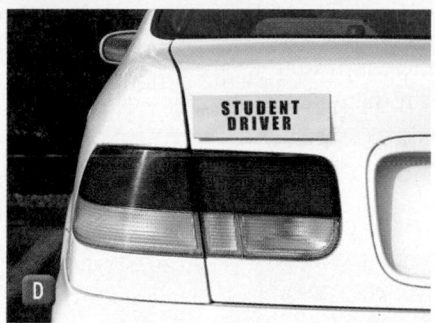

Figure 9   A. The 4 Es of prevention start with education. **B.** and **C.** Enforcement and engineering/environment contribute as well. **D.** Economic incentives, such as lower insurance rates for young drivers who have taken approved driver education programs or for adults who do not smoke, complete the picture.

Enforcement

Behavior can be forced to change by law (that is why it is called law enforcement). Legislation/regulation formulates rules that require people, manufacturers, and governments to comply with certain safety practices. Legislation is made by elected government bodies enacting laws that require safe practices. Regulations are made by bureaucracies or agencies that set policies and establish procedures that control the manufacture, sale, and/or use of products. Litigation sets policy when lawsuits are brought against manufacturers or distributors of dangerous products. For example, product liability litigation can encourage manufacturers to remove dangerous products from the market or make them safer. All these measures have been shown to be helpful in enforcement of safety regulations.

Engineering/Environment

Most EMS providers know spots where adding guardrails or smoothing out dangerous curves in a road could prevent crashes. Changing the design of products or spaces such as roads can offer automatic protection from injury, often without any conscious change of behavior by a person. These are called **passive interventions**.

For example, making child-resistant bottles is a passive intervention that reduces poisonings, and can be more effective than trying to keep the bottle out of a child's reach. Strategies to change the environment can include social, legal, political, and cultural approaches. Environmental modifications, which are often expensive, usually happen when the community's

awareness of the problem is raised, causing that community to accept responsibility for change.

Economic Incentives

Economic self-interest—saving money on health care costs or insurance rate reduction for careful drivers and nonsmokers—provides monetary incentives to reinforce safe behavior. The threat of lawsuits (and significant monetary damages) often causes manufacturers to improve the safety of consumer products—an economic loss that serves as an incentive to change behavior. Organizations also recognize the value of offering free or subsidized safety products (bike helmets, fire extinguishers, safety locks, smoking cessation kits, contraceptives) to encourage use.

The Value of Automatic Protections

Passive interventions—those that do not require a conscious decision to act—are often the most successful of all interventions. This approach is also referred to as automatic protection. Examples include the use of sprinkler systems in commercial buildings, air bags in automobiles, or the use of softer, yielding materials for playground surfaces. These measures provide 24-hour protection without requiring a conscious action or decision on the part of the user.

Consider the following injury prevention strategies, comparing education to automatic protection, in the case of head and chest injuries of drivers in motor vehicle crashes:

- **Option 1.** Educate people to buckle up every time they drive.
- **Option 2.** Require that car manufacturers install automatic seat belts and air bags.

The automatic protection offered by option 2 is more likely to reduce injuries because people do not have to do anything to protect themselves each time they are at risk. Again, however, a combination of approaches—education, enforcement, engineering/environmental modifications, and economic incentives—will result in the most effective strategy. Note that education is still an important aspect of the above examples. Motor vehicle passengers need to know that air bags do not replace the need for seat belts.

Models for Injury and Illness Prevention

A variety of visual models have been created to describe a health problem and how to approach it. The public health model identifies and seeks to control three factors: the host, the agent, and the environment. The public health model triumphed in the prevention and control of diseases such as malaria and polio, sometimes by attacking only two parts of the model. For example, to prevent malaria, you might develop a vaccine, spray pesticides to kill mosquitoes, and/or drain swamps to keep mosquitoes from breeding. These approaches target the host (people), the agent (mosquitoes), and the environment (swamps).

The public health model has been applied to a variety of injury problems. If you add the 4 Es of prevention, you can think through appropriate strategies for each part of the model (the host, the agent, and the environment). **Figure 10** sets out the three parts of the public health model using the example of bicycle-auto collisions.

The Haddon Matrix

William Haddon, Jr, MD, the National Highway Traffic Safety Administration's first director, had a mandate to find ways to prevent people from being killed and injured on the nation's

highways. Haddon created a matrix that identified several principles of injury prevention. The matrix proved so successful in helping researchers think about injuries, that it was named after Haddon: the **Haddon matrix**. Haddon added the factor of *time* to the previous models used to address the causes of injury. The host, agent, and environment are seen as factors that interact over time to cause injury. These factors correspond to three phases of the event: pre-event, event, and post-event. The matrix uses nine separate components to analyze the injury. The Haddon matrix encourages creative thinking in understanding the causes of and potential interventions for injury. **Table 4** shows a Haddon matrix for the example of bicycle-auto collisions.

Most EMS providers are trained to respond to the post-event—the period of time after an injury or illness has already occurred. The 9-1-1 call is received by the emergency medical dispatcher who sends a service unit to the scene. There, the team members administer emergency care, a form of secondary intervention that can change the outcome, severity, or result of the event.

You can use the Haddon matrix to trigger your fellow EMS providers and others in the community to think about and plan for strategies before the 9-1-1 call comes through. The pre-event phase can get everyone brainstorming about everything that can be done to prevent an injury from occurring. The event phase can get all people involved thinking about interventions to minimize an injury at the time of the event. The post-event phase can address ways to lessen the severity of the injury once it has occurred.

Injury prevention requires broad and innovative thinking to be most successful. The Haddon matrix helps you to think through which interventions can be effective at certain points in time. Addressing injury prevention within the context of a timeline—pre-event, event, and post-event—can expand your problem-solving capabilities beyond the answer of more education. Blaming the parent for lack of supervision or the driver for going too fast does not generate solutions to the problem of childhood injury. You can generate solutions with physical and measurable attributes using the Haddon matrix as a guide.

Injury and Illness Surveillance

Surveillance in injury and illness prevention does *not* mean watching over a criminal suspect! In prevention, it means watching over society by collecting and analyzing data. **Surveillance** is the ongoing, systematic collection, analysis, and interpretation of data essential to the planning, implementation,

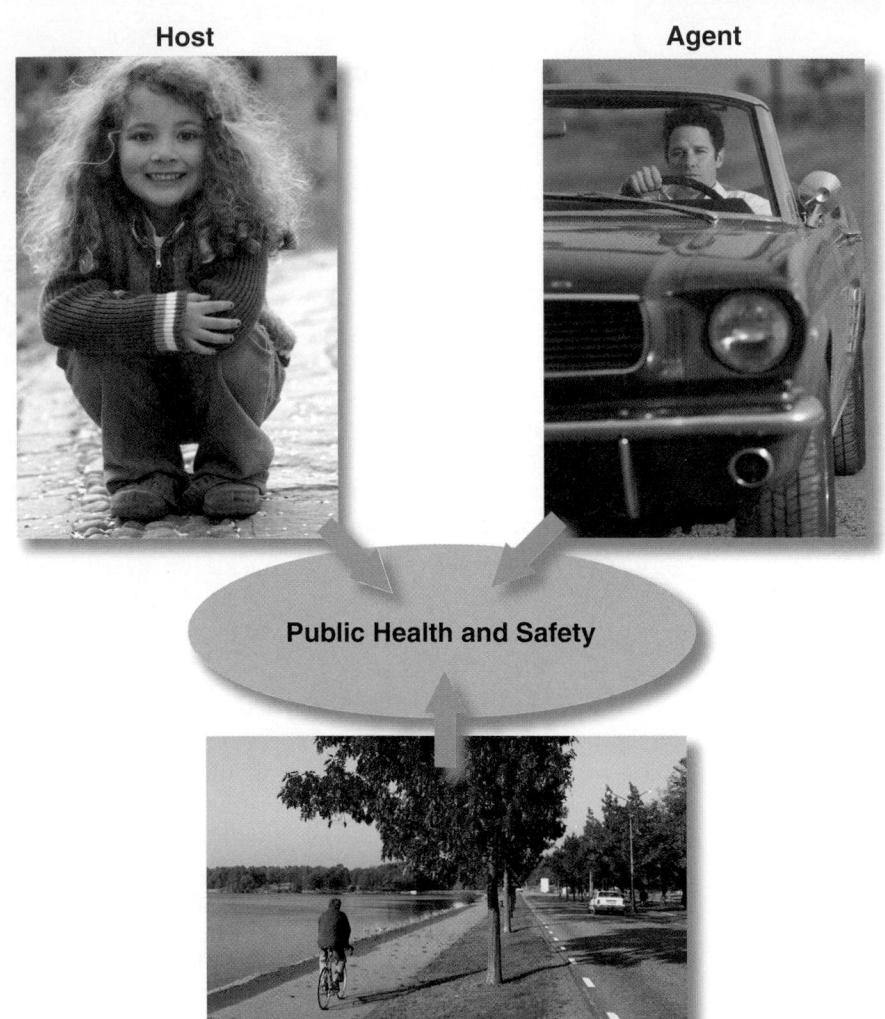

Host

Agent

Public Health and Safety

Environment

Figure 10 For bicycle-auto collisions, the public health model suggests the need to educate the child (host) and driver (agent) about safety, minimize the danger of serious injury through the required use of helmets, and perhaps create independent bike paths to separate children from traffic (environment).

Table 4   Childhood Motor Vehicle Occupant Injuries Using the Haddon Matrix

	Host (Human)	Agent (Car Seat/Vehicle)	Environment
Pre-Event	■ Wear seat belts and use car seats at all times. ■ Make sure babysitter, day care, and extended family members use car seat. ■ Drive defensively. ■ Reduce driving during high-risk times, such as rush hour, holiday weekends, or high-speed long distance travel.	■ Maintain up-to-date recall information on car seats. ■ Manufacture easy-to-use car seats. ■ Provide 3-point seat belts in rear seating positions. ■ Regulate good maintenance and safety features of vehicle.	■ Enforce seat belt and car seat laws. ■ Encourage safer roads with lower speeds, breakaway poles, and medians. ■ Encourage low-cost seat programs. ■ Conduct media and education campaigns about seat belts, car seats, drunk driving, and enforcement.
Event	■ Driver maintains control of vehicle. ■ Driver is belted. ■ Child is restrained.	■ Seat belts and correctly used car seats restrain and protect. ■ Vehicle design provides crash protection.	■ Breakaway signs and light poles are in place. ■ Guardrails and medians are in place.
Post-Event	■ Bystanders are trained in first response. ■ EMS personnel are expertly trained in treating pediatric injuries as well as car seat and seat belt extrications.	■ Ambulances are outfitted with up-to-date supplies and equipment designed for children.	■ Roadside call boxes are in place. ■ 9-1-1 and emergency medical dispatch systems are in place. ■ Adequate road shoulders for emergency use are in place. ■ There is quality EMS response and transport. ■ The patient is transported to a trauma center per protocol.

and evaluation of public health practice Figure 11 . These data are collected and then carefully disseminated to people or organizations that can use the data to effect change. The final link in the surveillance chain is the application of these data to interventions aimed at preventing injuries and illnesses.

A strong surveillance system is fundamental to creating an effective prevention program. To do the most good, you need to know who is being injured, where, and by what mechanism. For illness, you need to recognize the common illnesses and diseases within your own community. The news media may focus on a dramatic incident in which a dozen people are severely injured or closure of a school occurs due to a meningitis scare; but surveillance data might show that a commonplace, but less newsworthy injury (such as falls or flu among older people) is a greater threat to the community and more easily remedied.

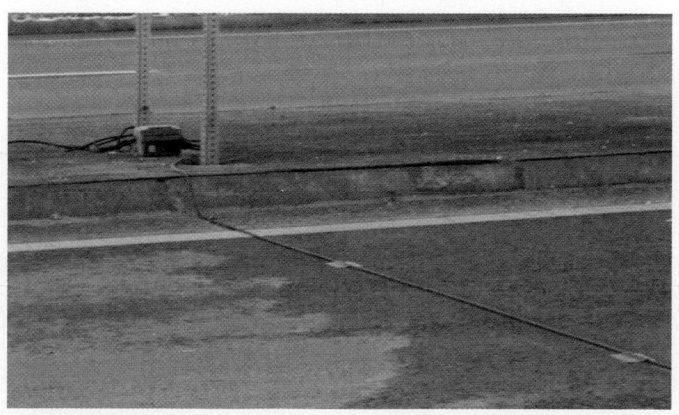

Figure 11   One type of surveillance that is familiar to anyone who drives is the use of technology that can tally the number of cars using a particular roadway.

Controversies

There is a theory that says if people keep falling off a mountain you should put a fence around the mountain to keep people from climbing it. Another theory says that you should tear down the mountain so that people can't fall off it. Yet another theory says that if you educate people on safe climbing you can prevent them from falling. Finally, there are some who believe an ambulance should be parked at the base of the mountain to save the people who keep falling. So goes the controversy of injury and potential interventions.

As part of the health system, paramedics need to triage their focus on prevention. Do not let the headlines be your guide.

■ Getting Started in Your Community

An abundance of problems faces every community. Each community requires the assessment of the problems that are impairing the health of the largest number of people. Otherwise, you may be overwhelmed with the enormity of the task.

There is a good chance that, eventually, you can roll up your sleeves and dig in to remedy even the problems that arise from the social conditions causing some illnesses and injuries. But it will give you and your community a good feeling to address a problem that will have the maximum impact on the community's well-being.

Documentation and Communication

Good documentation on prehospital care reports allows for more consistencies in data gathering, surveillance, and predictions of injury trends.

Recognizing Injury and Illness Patterns in Your Community

To be effective in prevention, you need to understand the patterns of injuries and illnesses that occur in your community and learn the characteristics of its population and environment and the types of risks that are present. Your regional or state EMS department or public health office will have the most data about injury and illness statistics and is a good starting place to gather information. Many states have this information on the Internet. There are a wide variety of other resources readily available online, including detailed information about specific problems, case studies, and expert assistance.

■ Intentional Injuries

Intentional injuries include suicides and suicide attempts, homicides, nonfatal batterings, violent assaults on women (including rapes and spousal abuse), and child and elder abuse.

Assaults are more likely to be fatal in the United States than in any other developed country **Figure 12**. In 2007 there were 18,361 homicides and 34,598 suicides. It is estimated there

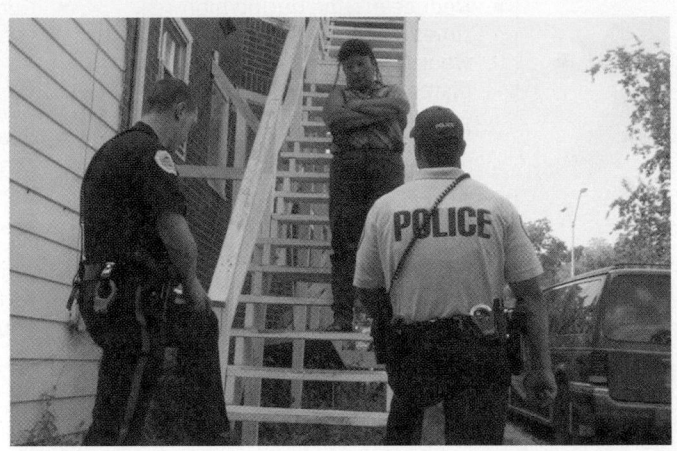

Figure 12 Intentional injuries include all cases of domestic and child abuse. As a citizen and medical professional, you are obligated to report all incidents of abuse or potentially abusive situations.

YOU are the Medic   PART 4

Your partner returns with a pediatric immobilization device and together you immobilize the infant. Once the infant is loaded into the ambulance, you gain IV access in his right antecubital fossa with a 24-gauge catheter and start an IV line of normal saline at a keep-vein-open rate. Even though he appears to be doing well, you decide to begin rapid transport to the closest trauma center because he has been ejected from a vehicle. You place him on oxygen via nasal cannula at 2 L/min and splint his left arm en route. You also clean and dress the wound on his head. He has relaxed and appears sleepy. You arrive at Midland Trauma Center at 1504. The pediatric trauma team is standing by for your report. Your partner restocks the truck while you transfer care and finish your PCR. You are back in service at 1511.

Recording Time: 10 Minutes	
Respirations	42 breaths/min
Pulse	126 beats/min
Skin	Pink, warm, and dry
Cardiac monitor	Sinus tachycardia without ectopy
Spo$_2$	100% on oxygen via nasal cannula @ 2 L/min
Pupils	Equal and reactive to light

7. What steps have you taken that would be considered secondary injury prevention?

8. How would you go about developing a prevention program to reduce this kind of injury in the future?

are nearly 7 million intentional injuries inflicted each year. Researchers are studying the causes of intentional violence in the United States. Certain factors emerge as numerically connected with intentional violence: being male, access to firearms, alcohol abuse, history of childhood abuse, mental illness, and poverty. These are all **risk factors**—characteristics that increase the chances of disease or injury.

It is often overwhelming to consider solutions when the challenges are linked to deeply rooted social ills. How can EMS personnel prevent intentional violence when it is clear that the scope of the problem is a wide one?

One way EMS providers have played important supporting roles in programs that seek to reduce suicide, domestic violence, and child abuse is by carefully reporting data and noting risk factors while on the scene. Also, EMS providers can be taught to identify injuries and risk factors associated with domestic violence or child abuse, and report them to the proper channels.

Remember, you are about to become a paramedic. What you do, your expectations of yourself, and your role will filter down to the other members of your crew. Being a conscientious observer will set an example.

Unintentional Injuries

Unintentional injuries have no premeditation; they are often called accidents. **Table 5** shows the top four causes of deaths from injury in 2007. Motor vehicle traffic incidents account for the most unintentional deaths (40%), followed by poisoning, firearms, and falls. Almost all motor vehicle deaths are classified as unintentional.

Words of Wisdom

Remember, you are also a member of "the public" so practice a safe lifestyle on and off the job. Wear seat belts, safety helmets, and appropriate high-visibility reflective vests when on the highway, and observe safety laws in everything you do.

Unintentional Injuries in Children

Many prevention programs have been strongly linked to children, for good reason. Each year 20 million children sustain an injury sufficiently severe to require medical attention, miss school, and/or require bed rest at a cost of $17 billion for medical treatment. Their developing bodies, including a larger head in proportion to the body, thinner skin, and a smaller airway, put them at higher risk of injury and of being more seriously affected by the injury than adults. Each year more than 14 million injured children require medical treatment **Figure 13**.

Grants, partners, and commercial sponsors support car seat inspections or donations of bike helmets for children because communities recognize that children are at risk. An additional reason to focus on children's issues is the "pass-along effect." Other family members benefit from the message too,

Table 5   Top 4 Causes of Death from Injury in 2007

1. Motor vehicle traffic incidents
2. Poisonings (of which 74.5% were unintentional)
3. Firearms (of which 55.6% were by suicide and 40.5% by homicide)
4. Falls

Source: The Centers for Disease Control and Prevention. National Center for Health Statistics/National Vital Statistics Reports, Deaths: Final Data for 2007, http://www.cdc.gov/nchs/data/nvsr/nvsr58/nvsr58_19.pdf. Accessed April 17, 2011.

such as when a third-grader insists that daddy buckle up too.

EMS for Children (EMSC) is a federal initiative that provides millions of dollars in funding to a wide variety of prevention and research programs. The National Safe Kids Campaign has more than 270 coalitions in all 50 states dedicated to reducing childhood injuries. Both have excellent websites, easily found by looking up their names in a search engine. They are good resources for generating ideas and gaining insight to what groups throughout the United States are doing.

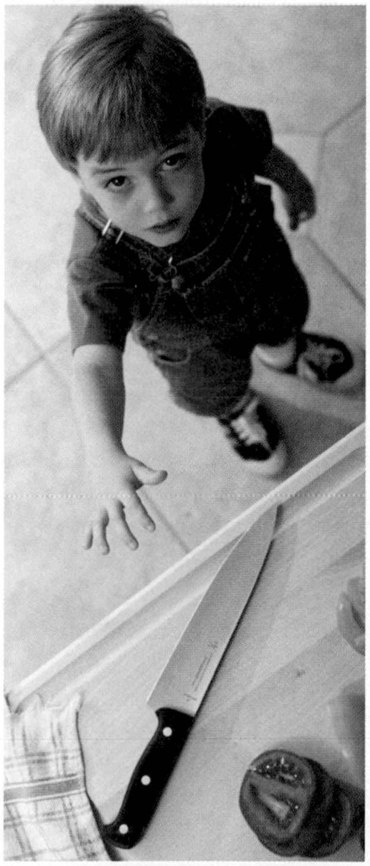

Risk Factors for Children

Children at greatest risk of injury are of lower socioeconomic status. The patterns of injury will differ from community to community, but just as the poorest children statistically are at risk of contracting a physiologic disease, they are also at risk of injury.

The CDC reports that home injuries of children occur most frequently where there is/are:

- Water, such as in the kitchen or bathroom, or a backyard swimming pool.
- Intense heat, such as in the kitchen or a backyard barbecue.

Figure 13 Children are at higher risk of sustaining serious injuries from an accident. Parents should always be aware of the potential dangers within reach of a child.

- Toxic agents, such as in the kitchen, bathroom, garage, or purse.
- High potential "energy," such as in stairwells or loaded firearms.

Many community members have a common belief that schools have become more violent and that intentional injuries are an increasing threat to students. Situations such as bullying and teen suicides are gaining more national attention. However, *unintentional* injuries—accidents—still represent a much greater threat to health.

School injuries occur most frequently during sports activities, industrial arts classes, and on playgrounds. Each year about 200,000 preschool and elementary children have injuries while playing on playgrounds. The cost of treating these children has been estimated to be around $1.2 billion. Severe injuries such as fractures, amputations, concussions, and dislocations occur in about 45% of the cases.

With the wide variety of injuries affecting children, how should you prioritize prevention efforts? Experts in public health suggest focusing on injuries that have high **mortality** (death) rates or hospitalization rates, that have a high long-term disability rate, or that have effective countermeasures. The highest priorities are assigned to those types of injuries that are common, severe, and readily preventable.

■ Illness Prevention

Traditionally, most efforts have focused on preventing injuries to adults and children. More attention is now being given to the prevention of illnesses and diseases, and EMS providers can play a major role in these initiatives. For example, there are five categories of behaviors that lead to an increased risk for poor health in adolescents:

- Tobacco use
- Alcohol and other drug use
- Sexual behaviors leading to sexually transmitted diseases (STDs) and unwanted pregnancies
- Unhealthy dietary behavior leading to obesity
- Physical inactivity leading to obesity (Centers for Disease Control and Prevention, 2010)

Paramedics and other EMS providers can organize or participate in programs that may possibly diminish these high-risk behaviors. In conjunction with the school nurse, consider conducting an assembly at a school to outline the availability of condoms and vaccines such as the one to prevent human papillomavirus (HPV), which is considered an STD and a cause of cervical cancer. This issue is a sensitive one yet requires direct prevention strategies to decrease the incidence of unwanted pregnancies and STDs. Check with your EMS manager before undertaking this initiative.

Something less controversial may be the issue of immunization against meningitis. This disease is very communicable, especially among teenagers who share water bottles, food, and engage in behaviors of close contact. Talk with the local pediatrician's office or the local pharmaceutical representative to see how you can participate in an awareness program to educate students and parents about vaccines to prevent this disease and where they can be obtained.

■ Community Organizing

Those in EMS who have created successful prevention programs give the following advice as you build your team and create an **implementation plan**:

- Identify a lead person to coordinate the effort.
- Build as broad a base of support as possible.
- Create a realistic time line for any project, keeping in mind that most must be ongoing to be effective.
- Gather data and facts that pinpoint who is being injured where, with what, and how frequently, or data on what types of diseases are most common in your community.
- Choose goals and objectives that are SMART—Simple, Measurable, Accurate, Reportable, and Trackable; build consensus in the community on the need for action.
- Make sure you understand the religious, ethnic, cultural, and language challenges that you may face in implementing an intervention.
- Do not reinvent the wheel—seek out others who have had success with similar interventions or who have expertise in public health.
- Anticipate opposition and expect some losses; turf battles are common but not inevitable.
- As you lobby to legislators, be brief in phone calls, visits, and testimony.
- Set up your program so that you can measure results and make changes as needed.
- Establish self-sustaining funding sources.
- Keep a sense of humor and persist—change does not happen overnight.

Words of Wisdom

For your first project, start small with realistic goals. Look for other communities that have best practices to share and learn from.

■ The Five Steps to Developing a Prevention Program

This step-by-step approach to establishing an injury prevention program, as advocated by the EMSC program, emphasizes the need to carefully establish goals and objectives, with measurable outcomes. (Although the following discusses childhood prevention programs, the methods can be applied to other age groups and their problems.)

1. **Conduct a Community Assessment** Bring people and groups together to assess what is already being accomplished in your region and to establish what resources (expertise, time, money) are potentially available. Make sure to invite people who represent the community at large, in all its

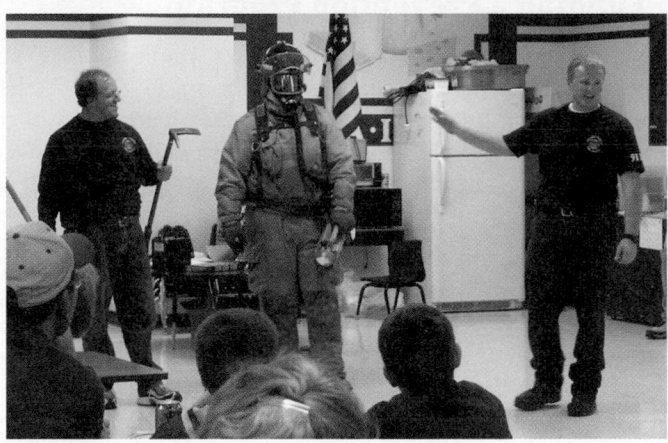

Figure 14 Fire prevention training is an example of ways in which public safety agencies engage in injury prevention activities.

diversity, including survivors of injuries or major illnesses and their families **Figure 14** . Recognize that there may be members who have had a loved one die as a result of a preventable injury or illness; these people can be powerful advocates. Potential partners include:

- EMS groups (private and public ground and air ambulance services, fire departments and fire fighter unions, volunteer services, rescue squads, lifeguards)
- Law enforcement (police departments and police officers, unions, sheriff's office, highway patrol, training academies)
- School groups (parent-teacher associations, student clubs, school boards, faculty)
- The media (management, editorial board members, staff reporters)
- Public health officials and health care providers (groups representing emergency physicians and nurses, pediatricians, managed care organizations, hospitals, clinics)
- Members of the business community (including those related to insurance, cars, sports, home improvements, safety equipment, local chambers of commerce)
- Religious organizations, civic groups, and service clubs (such as the Kiwanis and the Boy Scouts and Girl Scouts)
- Sports-related organizations (such as Little Leagues or YMCAs)
- Local chapters of nonprofit groups (such as SAFE KIDS Coalitions, Mothers Against Drunk Driving [MADD], the American Red Cross, the American Alzheimer's Association) **Figure 15**
- Local and national celebrities, community leaders, and elected officials

- Research groups (such as those at state universities, private colleges, community colleges)

2. **Define the Problem** On the basis of the community assessment and the data you have been able to gather, define the problem in specific quantifiable terms. For example, you should be able to answer the following questions for your community:

- What are the most frequent causes of fatal and nonfatal childhood injuries?
- What are the most frequent diseases and chronic illnesses in the community?
- What populations (by age, location, and other characteristics) are at highest risk of these injuries or illnesses? When and where are they occurring?
- Using the Haddon matrix, what other factors are associated with these causes?
- What, if anything, is already being done to prevent these injuries or illnesses?
- Is there an effective intervention available? What resources do you have in order to develop, implement, and evaluate different interventions?

3. **Set Goals and Objectives**

- **Goals** Make this a broad, general statement about the long-term changes the prevention initiatives are designed to make. (For example, a goal can be to decrease preventable injuries to children on the community's roadways.)
- **Objectives** Make these specific, time-limited, and quantifiable. There are two types: **process objectives** (1,000 child safety seats will be distributed to low income families within the next 18 months

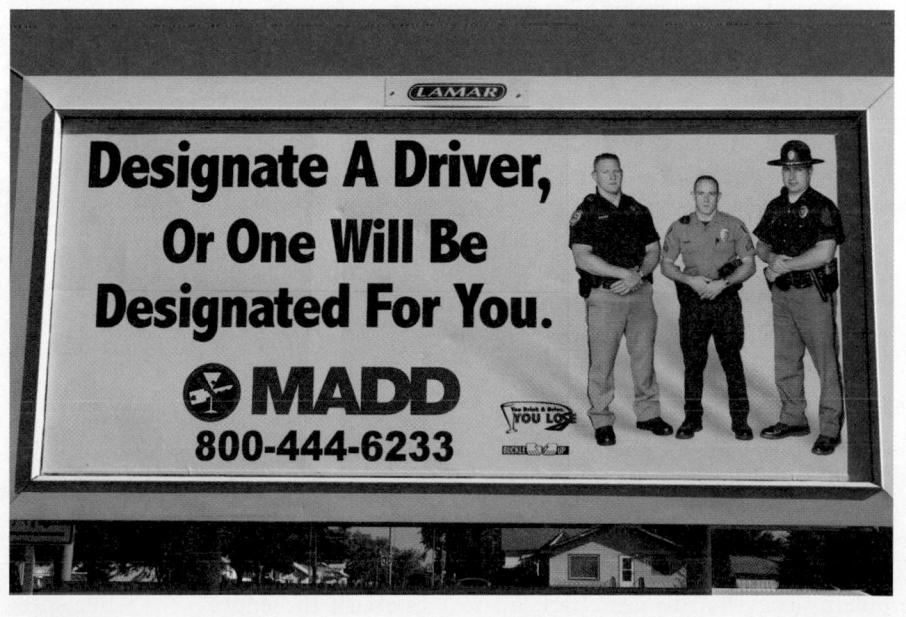

Figure 15 There are many organizations that can serve as potential partners in an injury prevention campaign.

or 500 elderly community members will receive the flu vaccine) and <u>outcome (impact) objectives</u> (the bicycle safety program will increase the rate of helmet use by children younger than 18 years from 30% to 50% within the next 18 months or the flu clinic will increase the number of flu vaccinations by 25% during the next year).

4. **Plan and Test Interventions** Interventions are the actions you take to accomplish your goals and objectives. Using the 4 Es of prevention and the Haddon matrix, brainstorm options. Consider the resources you have available to commit, and make sure you have thoroughly reviewed what others have already done. You may find communities have had success with similar interventions in similar populations. In that case, you can reliably duplicate their efforts as a process objective. (For example, other groups have shown that bike helmets reduce head injuries; you then need only to demonstrate increased usage of helmets in your targeted population.) Experienced prevention specialists also suggest that you be keenly aware of timing and cultural considerations as you plan your intervention. Getting a sample group together and testing the intervention before actually rolling out the entire program usually helps to improve your chances of success.

5. **Implement and Evaluate Interventions** To be credible, your intervention needs to be established so that the results can be measured quantitatively; that is, a formal <u>evaluation</u> will definitely tell you whether you met your goals and objectives. One EMS group knew from previous surveys that the seat belt usage rate in their community was well below the national average. They established an objective of improving seat belt usage in their community by 50%. Working with the department of public health in their state, they enacted a series of prevention programs. To measure the effectiveness of different interventions, they put volunteers at selected intersections around the city. They physically counted with a clicker every belted and nonbelted motorist who stopped in front of them. This is extremely important so that your experience can be shared with others. You want to spend your time and resources on efforts you can *show* make a difference. There is a science to planning, implementing, and evaluating an intervention. Seek out others who have knowledge and experience in this facet of injury or illness prevention; it will make for a better program.

Finally, be aware that many if not most interventions demand ongoing attention to be effective. Those EMS providers who had initial success in reducing backyard drownings saw the numbers go back up a few years after the initial burst of publicity and after enthusiasm for the interventions began to wane. Legislation to fence pools worked well but did not eliminate the problem. They had to gear back up to reestablish the educational interventions that had worked so well originally. Consider building long-term maintenance into any plan to continue the momentum of your program.

■ Funding a Prevention Program

Ideally, emergency services should have the resources and motivation to include primary prevention activities in their normal operating budget. As a relatively new expansion of the EMS mission, this likely will take time. But motivated services and people have found a variety of innovative ways to secure resources including:

- Partnering with the local media to create prevention messages, especially related to seasonal injuries or hazards.
- Seeking grants from regional, state, or national organizations, such as the EMSC program. (A good place to start is to contact your state EMS office about grant programs.)
- Seeking sponsorships from local nonprofit service organizations or commercial firms, including fire, EMS, Kiwanis organizations, and car dealerships.

Networking with other organizations interested in prevention often provides greater leverage in seeking grants or sponsorships. Perhaps the EMS provider donates the time of volunteers and is a credible voice in the community, whereas the partner provides organizational resources and knowledge about establishing a scientifically credible injury intervention.

■ How Every Provider Can Be Involved

Taking care of patients is the number one job of paramedics. Some will not have the time or inclination to get involved in every aspect of the primary injury and illness prevention measures discussed here. However, there are certain things paramedics can and should do, starting with preventing their own injuries and illnesses.

Primary prevention begins at home, so to speak, by taking care of yourself and at the same time presenting a role model for others in your service and for the community in general. Do you always wear seat belts, on and off duty? Do you smoke or excessively drink alcohol? Do you drive safely? Have you prepared yourself physically for the rigors of the job? Do you exercise on a regular basis? Do you practice safe lifting techniques? Have you taught your family and friends hands-only CPR? Do you always wear appropriate protective equipment? Do you always maintain scene safety? Do you get a flu shot each year? **Table 6** lists ways you can promote safety and health in your life and in the lives of others. Your employer will have policies regarding many of these safety issues, but it is up to you to implement them and to take seriously the risks you face every day on and off the job. Refer back to the chapter on *Workforce Safety and Wellness* to review the appropriate use of personal protective equipment and practices.

■ Responding to the Call

Perhaps the most ironic, if not most tragic, of all injuries are those caused when an ambulance collides with another vehicle while speeding to a scene, only to find out later the original call was not serious or even one requiring transport. Studies have shown that very few calls demand the use of siren and lights, and many departments now require all ambulances to stop at

Table 6 Tips for Promoting Safety and Health

- Teach children about safety measures, such as never inserting their fingers into a wall socket, avoiding the oven and stove, and avoiding the pool when adults are not present.
- Supervise children at all times.
- Once they are old enough to understand, teach children how to dial 9-1-1 and teach them when it is appropriate to do so.
- Program emergency phone numbers into your telephone. Include numbers for the local police department, fire department, and poison control. If your phone is not programmable, post these phone numbers in a nearby visible location such as on the refrigerator.
- Ensure that your home and its exterior are well lit and that surfaces are even.
- Ensure that all electrical cords are placed out of the flow of traffic.
- Avoid small rugs or runners that are not slip-resistant.
- Install and maintain smoke alarms.
- If your home uses gas heat, install and maintain carbon monoxide detectors.
- Use safety latches to prevent children opening drawers or cabinets that contain potentially dangerous substances, such as medicines or cleaning products.
- Install safety gates around stairs and swimming pools.
- Keep your hot water heater adjusted to less than 120°F to prevent burns.
- Teach hands-only CPR to your family and friends.

Adapted from: National Public Health Week April 4-10, 2011. American Public Health Association. http://www.nphw.org/nphw11/tips_home.htm. Accessed April 20, 2011.

every stop sign or red light *on every call*, and to maintain strict speed control. Prioritized dispatch systems using certified EMS dispatchers can provide sophisticated assessments of the need for different levels of response and can improve scene safety while reducing the need for unnecessary responses.

You can provide leadership within your own department for primary prevention by advocating policies or equipment that offer a safer environment or initiatives such as an EMS wellness program. At the same time, you can be a role model by how you personally approach the multitude of decisions you face each day regarding the risks of injury and diseases. It is impossible to be a credible advocate for prevention if you do not practice what you preach.

Education for EMS Providers

Every EMS provider should understand the fundamentals of prevention. This can easily be the focus of a continuing education program. Some states sponsor prevention workshops geared specifically to EMS providers. Contact your state EMS office to see if a workshop can be scheduled for your area, or contact your local public health office to see what training resources it might have available. There are also excellent self-paced courses and additional information available online.

The "Teachable Moment"

You are on the scene at the site of a crash between two vehicles. The injuries are not serious, and you notice one of the passengers was not wearing a seat belt. As you prepare him for transport, you look him in the eye and say, "You were very lucky this time … the other vehicle didn't hit you square. I've seen plenty of very bad injuries from crashes less serious than this. You really need to wear your seat belt *every* time you get in the car. It'll save your life."

You were involved in transporting a young student from the local high school who was later diagnosed with meningitis. You took this opportunity to learn more about meningitis, how it is transmitted, and what precautions you could take when treating future patients. Share this information with your colleagues, and distribute details about where meningitis vaccines are available.

Perhaps you are treating a patient on the second or third story of a house and notice children jumping off a couch or bed in front of an open window or screen. Explain to the family that it would be best to move the furniture in order to prevent a tragedy. In New York City, the law requiring bars/gates on windows of residences in high-rise buildings was revised after Eric Clapton's 5-year-old son, Conor, fell through an open window 53 stories to his death.

These were teachable moments. Educators tell us that there are times when people are more receptive to accepting advice than others. Near-misses like these make people realize their vulnerability and the true risk of their behavior—and the lesson is more likely to stick. The EMS provider is in the perfect position to articulate and reinforce this message. However, you must use good judgment and be sensitive to the situation **Figure 16**. Lecturing a parent immediately after a child has been seriously injured is not going to be effective. What makes a teachable moment?

- The injuries or illnesses are such that the parents, companions, or the patients themselves will be receptive to the message; you are aware of how ethnic and religious differences must temper the message.

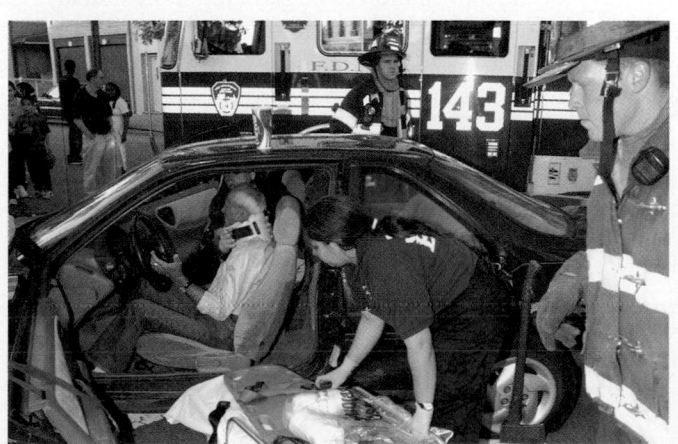

Figure 16 When injuries are not apparently serious, consider reinforcing the need for safety to prevent future injuries. Remind drivers and occupants of the importance of compliance with seat belt laws.

- The scene is conducive to delivering such a message in a nonthreatening, nonjudgmental way. You are not intruding inappropriately or causing embarrassment that could lead to the opposite reaction.
- There is a definitive prevention measure that could have helped, such as using a seat belt, getting a flu shot, correct installation of a car seat, stopping smoking, wearing a helmet, or keeping firearms locked and safe. Vague advice is less likely to have a lasting effect.

Words of Wisdom

The best teachable moments are those that convey positive reinforcement. If people are wearing seat belts properly and survive a crash with little or no injuries, tell them, "It's a good thing you had your seat belts on." You will notice smiles on their faces and they will likely remember your statement forever.

Collection/Analysis of Data and Research

In the opening paragraph of this chapter, it referred to data about backyard drownings. The importance of collecting data in measuring trends, validating interventions, assessing resources, and ultimately persuading others to act cannot be overestimated. For the EMS provider, this process starts with the prehospital care report. Standardized coding of incidents is required to collect useful data from far-flung sources. By accurately (and legibly) describing the details of the scene, the external mechanism of injury, the nature of the injury or illness, status of the patient's immunizations, and the use or absence of protective devices, EMS providers can supply important evidence of the scope of a problem and help in monitoring trends.

As a prevention advocate, assess your current prehospital care report to see if it can be modified to be a better tool. Are there ways for the information to be gathered more quickly? Can the information put into a computerized database be promptly updated, easily accessed, and searched? Are you able to use health information technology to record the data electronically?

Get involved in local, state, or national database systems. Often, much information is being gathered, but agencies are not consistent or timely in the process, are not sharing data, or do not have it on a common database. For the prevention field, the accurate and timely collection of data is critically important. In EMS, the goal is to put resources into those prevention interventions that can do the most good. This requires documenting injuries and illnesses and monitoring trends that can be tied to the effects of interventions.

Consider participating in local, regional, or national research projects. NHTSA and the Maternal and Child Health Bureau (MCHB) of the Health Resources Services Administration (HRSA) developed a National EMS Research Agenda as well as a National EMS Research Strategic Plan. The information you are collecting may be quite valuable to projects already in existence or those being considered. Talk with personnel from the local medical command center/hospital or university to see what might be available in your area.

Public health is a field that encompasses health promotion and disease prevention for groups of people. More attention is being given to health and wellness as opposed to simply treating injury and illness. Efforts such as vaccine programs, helmet safety education, and disease screening keep people well and decrease health care costs.

Prevention is something that everyone can do. Many veteran EMS providers have embraced a leadership role in primary prevention after witnessing too many episodes of needless suffering. These leaders recognize their unique role and use their positions to support interventions that make a difference. In their own lives and in their workplace, every EMS provider should be proactive in primary prevention, whether reducing the odds of a back injury by keeping fit, not smoking to reduce the potential for lung disease, using proper lifting techniques and protective gear, or taking advantage of a teachable moment with a patient.

Many extend this interest further, reaching out in their communities to become involved as leaders or supporters of a wide variety of prevention programs. They find personal satisfaction and professional fulfillment in the challenge of learning a new field, interacting with a new set of colleagues, and reducing the suffering of those they serve.

YOU *are the Medic*   SUMMARY

1. What is the proper response for this call?

As with any emergency call, it is imperative not to endanger yourself or others on the roadway while en route. Your dispatcher is the best resource for providing information. Wear your seat belts, stop at all red lights and stop signs, and drive with due regard for other drivers. In this scenario you will use lights and siren due to its urgency, but never assume that you are seen or heard and remember that you are *requesting* the right-of-way. Other considerations include weather, road construction, and the presence of school buses or children.

2. What are the injury risks in this situation?

An injury risk is a potentially hazardous situation that puts people in a position in which they may be harmed. Because there have been multiple crashes in this location, the environment may be a part of the problem. The negative bank of the curve contributes to the danger of the roadway, and this, combined with the potential for excessive speed, increases the likelihood of a crash. If an ejection occurs, lack of restraints is another injury risk. If a patient is under the influence of alcohol or other drugs, remember that the patient could become violent, and the scene may not be safe for you and your partner.

3. What are the risk factors associated with the infant's injuries?

First and foremost, the infant was ejected from the vehicle, which puts him at risk for significant injuries. Along with the visible injuries, the hematoma/laceration to his head and forearm fracture, you should maintain a high index of suspicion for occult injuries—those not readily seen. He was secured in a car seat, but it appears that the car seat was not properly secured in the vehicle. Because the seat was thrown from the vehicle, he had the potential to come into contact with the interior of the vehicle, a window or windshield, and any object outside the vehicle, including the ground. His extremities and head were extremely vulnerable to injury.

4. Is this a teachable moment?

No, this is not a teachable moment because of the potentially critical status of the infant. Teachable moments are points in time during which a person is receptive to accepting advice. At this time, giving advice to the mother is not going to be effective. She is concerned about the welfare of the child and she has injuries as well. The child also has the potential to be critically injured based on the mechanism of injury. In order to have a teachable moment, the injuries should be minor so that the person is receptive to the message. The scene must also be conducive to delivering the message in a nonthreatening, nonjudgmental way, and there has to have been a definitive prevention measure that could have helped—in this case, the car seat being properly secured in the vehicle.

5. What type of primary injury prevention might have helped this situation? Are there any automatic protections that would have worked?

Primary injury prevention is defined as keeping an injury from ever occurring. Prevention starts with recognition of potential problems or problem areas. Once these areas are identified, they can either be addressed through efforts such as environmental changes or providing safety equipment, or educating the public to avoid particular situations or to use appropriate safety devices properly.

Primary injury prevention may be addressed by changing speed limits, putting in guardrails, putting up stop signs or traffic lights, or modifying the existing roadway to straighten the curve. Educating the mother, and the general public, on the proper installation of a car seat would have prevented the infant from being ejected. A driver safety course for the mother is another form of primary injury prevention.

Automatic protections are more likely to reduce injuries because people do not have to take any steps to be protected each time they are at risk. The only automatic protections available in this instance are air bags. These would have benefited only the mother and work better in conjunction with proper seat belt use.

6. Explain the Haddon matrix as it relates to your patient.

The Haddon matrix was designed to identify several principles of injury prevention. Haddon surmised that the host (human), agent (car seat/vehicle), and environment are seen as factors that act over time to cause injury. These factors correspond to three phases of the event: pre-event, event, and post-event. By separating the causes of potential injuries, you are able to envision potential interventions.

As a paramedic, you normally respond after the injury has occurred (the post-event phase). By using the Haddon matrix you can plan strategies for the pre-event phase to prevent injuries from occurring. You can also think about the event phase and what interventions may minimize the actual injury, or the post-event phase and how to lessen the severity of the injury after it has occurred. You can decide which interventions can be effective at certain points in time. In this call you may view the event in the following manner:

- Pre-event:
    - Make sure a car seat is used and properly secured.
    - Drive defensively.
    - Car seat manufacturer must ensure that their products meet standards.
    - Vehicle should provide for easy installation.
    - Maintain vehicle in proper working order.
    - Enforce car seat laws.
    - Install guardrails, traffic lights, and stop signs.
    - Provide patrol in the area to enforce speed laws.
    - Offer education on the proper use of car seats.
- Event:
    - Child is properly restrained.
    - Driver maintains control of the vehicle.
    - Car seat is correctly used.
    - Vehicle design provides crash protection.
    - Guardrails, stop signs, traffic lights in place.

YOU are the Medic   SUMMARY, continued

- Post-event:
  - First responders are trained and available.
  - Paramedics are up-to-date with pediatric certifications.
  - Ambulance is stocked with pediatric supplies.
  - Enhanced 9-1-1 is available.
  - Road shoulder is sufficient for emergency use.
  - Trauma center is nearby.

7. What steps have you taken that would be considered secondary injury prevention?

Secondary injury prevention is aimed at reducing the effects of the injuries that have already occurred. The mechanism of injury indicates there is potential for spinal injuries. Asking the woman holding the infant to stabilize his head is the first step in secondary injury prevention. Immobilization of the infant in an appropriately sized device is the next step. Administering a low concentration of oxygen and gaining IV access with normal saline at a keep-vein-open rate are preventive measures in the event that the infant's status deteriorates. Monitoring the infant's vital signs, cardiac monitoring, and rapid transport are all required to ensure timely, appropriate treatment for the infant and to recognize any

changes in the infant's condition before you arrive at the trauma center.

8. How would you go about developing a prevention program to reduce this kind of injury in the future?

Conducting a community assessment to determine need is the first step for developing a prevention program. Researching call volume from this area would give you a starting point, along with pulling information from law enforcement and fire department calls from the same vicinity. Identify injury patterns and mechanisms of injury from the gathered data to formulate a definition of the problem. Set a goal for preventing crashes or injuries in this designated area and define objectives. Your objectives may be to offer workshops for car seat installation or to have guardrails installed. Plan and test your interventions. If there is a similar location where the crash rate has been high, research what was done there and if it was effective. Finally, implement and evaluate interventions. Put your plan into action and after a designated time frame, consider pulling the same data for the given time frame that you did in your original assessment to see whether there have been positive changes. On the basis of these results, you can then alter your goals and objectives to be more effective.

EMS Patient Care Report (PCR)

Date: 01-02-11	Incident No.: 1101234	Nature of Call: MVC	Location: Hwy 232 @ Needle Road		
Dispatched: 1420	En Route: 1422	At Scene: 1437	Transport: 1449	At Hospital: 1504	In Service: 1511

Patient Information

Age: 8 months Sex: M Weight (in kg [lb]): 10 kg (22 lb)	Allergies: No known drug allergies Medications: None Past Medical History: None Chief Complaint: Lac/hematoma to Ⓡ forehead, possible fx to Ⓛ forearm

Vital Signs

Time: 1440	BP:	Pulse: 138	Respirations: 42	Spo₂: 99% on room air
Time: 1447	BP:	Pulse: 126	Respirations: 42	Spo₂: 100% on O₂
Time:	BP:	Pulse:	Respirations:	Spo₂:

EMS Treatment
(circle all that apply)

Oxygen @ __2__ L/min via (circle one): (NC) NRM Bag-mask device	Assisted Ventilation	Airway Adjunct	CPR
Defibrillation	Bleeding Control	(Bandaging)	(Splinting) (Other:) Cardiac monitor

Narrative

Responded to a single-vehicle MVC where driver lost control. 8-month-old male secured in car seat was thrown from the vehicle and found face down in car seat in the ditch by bystander. Bystander stated car seat was not secured in vehicle. Pt removed from car seat by bystander prior to EMS arrival. On arrival, bystander was holding the infant, who was crying. Contacted dispatch to request additional unit to assess the mother. Pt presents with blood on face from approximate 1″ lac superior to right orbit with hematoma surrounding lac—bleeding controlled. Pt also presents with angulation to L forearm. Skin pink/warm/dry, PEARRL findings normal, unknown if there was any loss of consciousness. Had bystander support c-spine control while holding infant until immobilized with ped immobilization device. Vital signs normal for age, cardiac monitor showing sinus tach without ectopy. Gave O₂ via nasal cannula @ 2 L/min, 24-gauge IV Ⓡ antecubital fossa with normal saline at KVO rate, wound head dressed and bandaged, L forearm splinted. Rapid transport to Midland Trauma Center due to MOI. No changes en route. **End of report**

Prep Kit

Ready for Review

- Public health is a field that encompasses health promotion and disease prevention for groups of people. Public health-related issues can include disasters such as hurricanes and wildfires, or illness outbreaks such as the H1N1 flu outbreak.
- Federal, state, and international rules, regulations, guidelines and laws govern public health. Examples include HIPAA and a treaty initiated by the World Health Organization to reduce smoking.
- Every September is National Preparedness Month to help people prepare for potential health emergencies.
- Many paramedics have been motivated by their field experience to work actively on prevention.
- The 1966 National Academy of Sciences/National Research Council study, "Accidental Death and Disability: The Neglected Disease of Modern Society," noted that EMS could help with trauma after an event, and injury prevention could help prevent an accident before it happens.
- The 1996 Consensus Statement on the EMS Role in Primary Injury Prevention emphasized that primary injury prevention is an essential activity of EMS.
- EMS can play a supporting role in preventing intentional injuries and can have an even larger impact in preventing unintentional injuries.
- The years of potential life lost concept is another way to measure the cost of unintentional injury to society. It assumes that an average productive work life continues for 65 years. The age of death is deducted from 65, leaving the years of potential life lost.
- The 4 Es of prevention are:
  - Education
  - Enforcement
  - Engineering/environment
  - Economic incentives
- Automatic protections do not require a conscious decision to act and include air bags in automobiles.
- The Haddon matrix uses nine separate components to analyze injury. It encourages creative thinking in understanding the causes and potential interventions for injury.

- Surveillance is the ongoing systematic collection, analysis, and interpretation of data essential to the planning, implementation, and evaluation of public health practice.
- Paramedics need to triage their focus on prevention—do not let the headlines be your guide.
- The five steps to developing a prevention program are:
  - Conduct a community assessment.
  - Define the problem.
  - Set goals and objectives.
  - Plan and test interventions.
  - Implement and evaluate interventions.
- Primary prevention begins at home by taking care of yourself and presenting a role model for others in your service and in the community.
- The best teachable moments are those that convey positive reinforcement.
- The importance of collecting data in measuring trends, validating interventions, assessing resources, and ultimately persuading others to act cannot be overestimated.

Vital Vocabulary

<u>evaluation</u> Collection of the methods, skills, and activities necessary to determine whether a service or program is needed, likely to be used, conducted as planned, and actually helps people.

<u>Haddon matrix</u> A framework developed by William Haddon, Jr, MD, as a method to generate ideas about injury prevention that address the host, agent, and environment and their impact in the pre-event, event, and post-event phases of the injury process.

<u>Health Insurance Portability and Accountability Act (HIPAA)</u> The first national standards established to protect the confidentiality of a patient's health information.

<u>implementation plan</u> A strategy for carrying out an intervention; includes goals, objectives, activities, evaluation measures, resource assessment, and time line.

<u>intentional injuries</u> Injuries that are purposefully inflicted by a person on himself or herself or on another person; examples include suicide or attempted suicide, homicide, rape, assault, domestic abuse, elder abuse, and child abuse.

interventions In the context of prevention, specific measures or activities designed to meet a program objective; categories include education/behavior change, enforcement/legislation, engineering/technology, and economic incentives.

limited data set Information necessary for public health and research such as some geographic information, birth dates, and dates of treatment.

morbidity Number of nonfatally injured or disabled people; usually expressed as a rate, meaning the number of nonfatal injuries in a certain population in a given time period divided by the size of the population.

mortality Deaths caused by injury and disease; usually expressed as a rate, meaning the number of deaths in a certain population in a given time period divided by the size of the population.

outcome (impact) objectives State the intended effect of the program on participants or on the community in such terms as the participants' increased knowledge, changed behaviors or attitudes, or decreased injury rates.

passive interventions Something that offers automatic protection from injury or illness, often without requiring any conscious change of behavior by the person; child-resistant bottles and air bags are some examples.

primary prevention Keeping an injury or illness from occurring.

process objectives State how a program will be implemented, describing the service to be provided, the nature of the service, and to whom it will be directed.

protected health information (PHI) Data that contain the patient's name, address, and other specific identifiers.

public health An industry whose mission is to prevent disease and promote good health within groups of people.

risk A potentially hazardous situation that puts people in a position in which they could be harmed.

risk factors Characteristics of people, behaviors, or environments that increase the chances of disease or injury; some examples are alcohol use, poverty, smoking, or gender.

secondary prevention Reducing the effects of an injury or illness that has already happened.

surveillance The ongoing systematic collection, analysis, and interpretation of injury data essential to the planning, implementation, and evaluation of public health practice.

unintentional injuries Injuries that occur without intent to harm (commonly called accidents); some examples are motor vehicle crashes, poisonings, drownings, falls, and most burns.

years of potential life lost A way of measuring and comparing the overall impact of deaths resulting from different causes; calculated based on a fixed age minus the age at death.

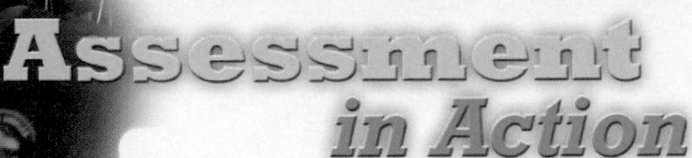

Assessment in Action

It is late afternoon and you have just attended a continuing education program on the importance of participating in injury prevention activities in your community. A sudden increase in the number of injuries involving children and elderly persons motivated your department to launch a campaign on injury awareness and prevention.

As you head back to the station you are dispatched to 875 Stanley Street for a possible burn. The dispatcher tells you that the caller is hysterical, repeating, "My baby is burned!" You respond that you are en route and approximately 5 minutes from the scene. On arrival you are met by a woman who is holding a 3-year-old boy. She tells you that her son pulled a pot of hot water off the stove down onto his arms. He has superficial thickness burns to both forearms and the back of his left hand. He has stopped crying and does not appear to be in a lot of distress.

1. During your class you have just learned that _____ are specific prevention measures or activities designed to increase positive health and safety outcomes.
   A. interventions
   B. passive interventions
   C. primary injury preventions
   D. secondary injury preventions

2. This incident was easily preventable by turning the pot handle inward on the stove to keep it out of the child's reach. This is known as:
   A. interventions.
   B. passive intervention.
   C. primary injury prevention.
   D. secondary injury prevention.

3. The child was curious and reached for the pot, pulling it down onto himself. This type of injury is:
   A. intentional.
   B. unintentional.
   C. passive.
   D. primary.

4. The _____ in this situation was the pot being turned so that it was in reach of the child.
   A. injury
   B. intervention
   C. incentive
   D. injury risk

5. As you are examining the child and dressing his injuries, you explain to his mother that it is important to have the handles of pots turned inward so that they are out of reach. This is known as a(n):
   A. teachable moment.
   B. evaluation.
   C. implementation plan.
   D. injury surveillance.

6. Even though most incidents such as this one that involve children are unintentional, there are those that are _____. This includes child abuse.
   A. preventable
   B. intentional
   C. teachable
   D. passive

7. It is important to educate the mother about how to make her home safe and prevent future injuries to her child. Interventions need to combine education with:
   A. enforcement, engineering/environment, and economic incentives.
   B. surveillance, goals, and objectives.
   C. implementation, evaluation, and data analysis.
   D. enforcement, process objectives, and passive interventions.

Additional Questions

8. Your department has discovered a need in your community for an injury prevention program. There has been a definite increase in call volume for falls and other unintentional injuries. Your supervisor has asked that you head up the program. How will you proceed?

9. Involvement in injury prevention is an important part of a paramedic's job. This should start with preventing your own injuries. How can this be achieved?

Medical, Legal, and Ethical Issues

National EMS Education Standard Competencies

Preparatory

Integrates comprehensive knowledge of the EMS system, safety/well-being of the paramedic, and medical/legal and ethical issues, which is intended to improve the health of EMS personnel, patients, and the community.

Medical/Legal and Ethics

- Consent/refusal of care (pp 96-97)
- Confidentiality (pp 86-87, 93-94)
- Advance directives (pp 105-106)
- Tort and criminal actions (pp 89-90)
- Evidence preservation (p 95)
- Statutory responsibilities (p 108)
- Mandatory reporting (pp 95-96)
- Health care regulation (pp 92-93, 94-95)
- Patient rights/advocacy (pp 103-105)
- End-of-life issues (pp 107-108)
- Ethical principles/moral obligations (pp 86-88)
- Ethical tests and decision making (pp 86-88, 97-99)

Knowledge Objectives

1. Differentiate between laws and ethics. (pp 86-91)
2. Describe medical ethics and discuss the implications for paramedics. (pp 86-88)
3. Discuss the legal system in the United States and how it affects paramedics. (pp 88-91)
4. Differentiate between civil and criminal law relevant to the paramedic. (pp 89-90)
5. Describe the process of a typical EMS lawsuit. (pp 90-91)
6. Discuss the legal and ethical accountability of paramedics. (pp 91-92)
7. Discuss legislation that affects the practice of paramedics. (p 92)
8. Differentiate between licensure and certification as they apply to the paramedic. (p 92)
9. Explain the importance and necessity of patient confidentiality and the standards for maintaining patient confidentiality that apply to the paramedic. (pp 93-94)

10. Discuss the legal and ethical issues surrounding patient transport. (pp 94-95)
11. Describe the actions that the paramedic should take to preserve evidence at a crime or crash scene. (p 95)
12. Explain the reporting requirements for special situations, including abuse, drug-related injuries, childbirth, suicide, and crime scenes. (pp 95-96)
13. Differentiate among expressed, informed, implied, and involuntary consent. (pp 96-97)
14. Describe the processes used by paramedics to determine consent or valid refusal, especially relative to the patient's decision-making capacity. (pp 97-99)
15. Identify the steps to take if a patient refuses care, and when to transport a patient against his or her will. (pp 97-99)
16. Identify methods for obtaining consent for minors, including exceptions for emancipated minors. (p 99)
17. Discuss the legal ramifications of patient restraint, both physical and chemical, for patient and practitioner safety. (pp 99-100)
18. Discuss the ethical implications of the allocation of resources and triage dilemmas. (p 100)
19. Describe the four elements that must be present in order to prove negligence: duty, breach of duty, proximate cause, and harm. (pp 100-103)
20. Discuss abandonment as it relates to the paramedic. (p 103)
21. Discuss patient rights, including autonomy, end-of-life decisions, and the moral and ethical implications of DNR orders and other advance directives. (pp 103-108)
22. Identify situations in which ceasing resuscitation efforts or not initiating resuscitation efforts would be appropriate for the paramedic in the field. (pp 106-107)
23. Discuss the responsibilities of the paramedic relative to resuscitation efforts for patients who are potential organ donors. (p 108)
24. Discuss common defenses to litigation, including contributory negligence. (pp 108-109)
25. List and describe forms of legal immunity that can apply to paramedics. (pp 108-109)
26. Discuss employment legislation regarding sexual harassment, discrimination, disabilities, FMLA, OSHA law, and other legislation that applies to paramedic practice. (pp 109-111)

Skills Objectives

There are no skills objectives for this chapter.

Introduction

All medical providers provide care under laws—like many human activities in a democracy. When you become a paramedic, you too will be governed by a set of laws affecting how you must treat patients. Ethics are principles, personal or societal, that determine what is right and wrong. One of the major differences between law and ethics is that laws have sanctions for violation that are enforceable **Figure 1**. Laws define our obligations and protect our rights and the rights of others. A paramedic responding to an emergency works within a framework of several types of laws that are set down by either (or both) the federal government or the state government:

- Motor vehicle laws for the operation of an emergency vehicle
- EMS legislation
- Medical licensing statutes and regulations
- Civil and criminal statutes about touching, treating, transporting, and possibly injuring another person
- Confidentiality laws such as the Health Insurance Portability and Accountability Act (HIPAA)

It is essential, therefore, that you have a basic understanding of laws and ethics applicable to prehospital emergency care. Failing to perform your job within the law can result in civil liability (malpractice suits against EMS providers are increasing) or even criminal liability. Practicing outside the law may also result in regulatory action within your state—a disciplinary hearing, for example—or action by your agency and medical director.

<u>Ethics</u> is the branch of philosophy that deals with the study and understanding of the distinction between right and wrong and the manner in which people apply concepts of right and wrong to their personal and professional lives. *Applied ethics* refers to the use of ethical values. In the past, the terms *ethics* and <u>*morality*</u> were sometimes distinguished from one another, but today, the two words are commonly used interchangeably and there is little, if any, meaningful difference between the two: a moral paramedic is an ethical paramedic.

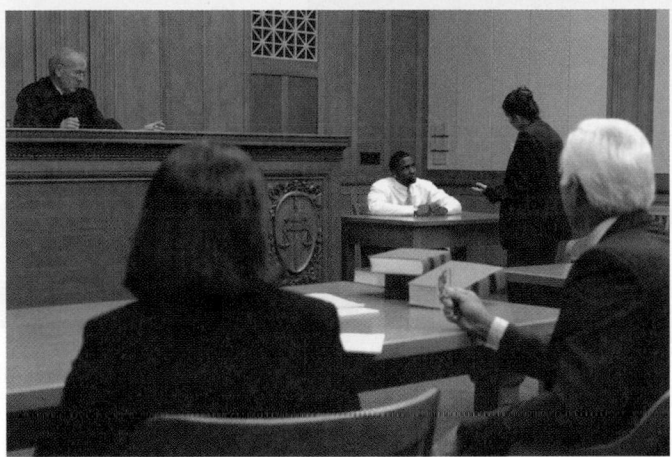

Figure 1 Unlike ethics, laws are enforceable rules that all citizens are obliged to follow. Paramedics are sometimes called into court to testify and provide evidence regarding cases under investigation or that are being litigated.

This chapter reviews important legal and ethical concepts affecting the paramedic. However, this text is only a framework to help your understanding of these issues. It cannot substitute for competent legal advice because many laws and legal obligations differ from state to state. Contact an attorney who specializes in the representation of medical professionals if you need legal advice related to your practice.

Words of Wisdom

Without question, your best legal protection is to provide a careful, detailed patient assessment and appropriate medical care, followed by complete and accurate documentation. Practice within your scope of practice and be respectful to patients and their property.

YOU *are the Medic* PART 1

You are eating breakfast at 0737 when you are dispatched to 487 Lenore Street for an unresponsive person. While you are en route, you and your partner discuss what could possibly be wrong with this patient—cardiac arrest, hypoglycemia, or stroke.

You arrive on scene at 0742 and are met at the ambulance by a woman who tells you that her 64-year-old mother is "acting strangely" this morning. She says that she would not respond to her at all and then she started "talking out of her head." She says her mother does not want to go to the hospital.

1. What type of consent is required to treat an unresponsive person?
2. What must you determine prior to allowing a patient to refuse care?

Words of Wisdom

Many state EMS offices have websites with information on laws that affect EMRs, EMTs, and paramedics. It is a good idea for you to review the laws of the state in which you are working.

■ Medical Ethics

It is important to understand the difference between your personal ethics and the ethics of your profession. Personal ethics are the product of your upbringing, family and community influences, your religious background, and your conscience. Professional ethics, on the other hand, arise out of the standards and practices of your profession, the Code of Professional Conduct, and in certain cases various state and federal laws such as HIPAA. Situations sometimes arise in which the personal ethical beliefs of a paramedic may come into conflict with the professional ethical standards. In almost every such case, the paramedic will be bound by professional ethics and must understand that personal ethics must be temporarily set aside.

As a paramedic, you must always be ethical in your practice and be aware of your own moral standards in your daily work. The interests of your patient must always take precedence over personal beliefs and standards Figure 2 .

Ethics related to the practice and delivery of health care is known as medical ethics (sometimes called bioethics). Your understanding of medical ethics must be formed as a part of, and consistent with, the general codes of the health care professional Figure 3 . Throughout history, there have been many published codes of ethics for health professionals. The Oath of Geneva, drafted by the World Medical Association in 1948, provides a good example; it is the oath taken by many medical students on

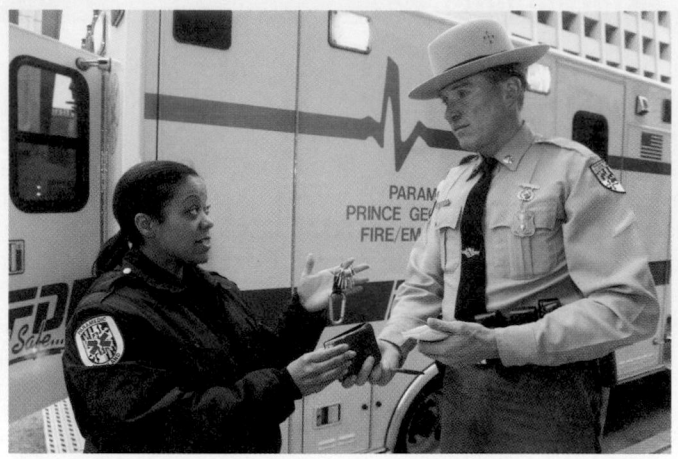

Figure 3 When people call 9-1-1, they trust you not only with providing proper medical care, but also with using sound ethical judgment—including the safeguarding of their personal possessions.

completion of their studies, at the time of being admitted to the medical profession:

"I solemnly pledge myself to consecrate my life to the service of humanity; I will give to my teachers the respect and gratitude which is their due; I will practice my profession with conscience and dignity; the health of my patient will be my first consideration; I will respect the secrets which are confided in me; I will maintain by all the means in my power the honor and noble traditions of the medical profession; my colleagues will be my brothers; I will not permit considerations of religion, nationality, race, party politics, or social standing to intervene between my duty and my patient; I will maintain the utmost respect for human life from the time of conception; even under threat, I will not make use of my medical knowledge contrary to the laws of humanity. I make these promises solemnly, freely and upon my honor."

Similar principles underlie the more detailed *Code of Ethics for Emergency Medical Technicians*, which was issued by the National Association of Emergency Medical Technicians in 1978 and is still in effect today:

"Professional status as an Emergency Medical Technician is maintained and enriched by the willingness of the individual practitioner to accept and fulfill obligations to society, other medical professionals, and the profession of Emergency Medical Technician. As an Emergency Medical Technician, I solemnly pledge myself to the following code of ethics:

- The fundamental responsibility of the Emergency Medical Technician is to conserve life, to alleviate suffering, and to promote health.
- The Emergency Medical Technician provides services based on human need, with respect for human dignity, unrestricted by considerations of nationality, race, creed, or status.

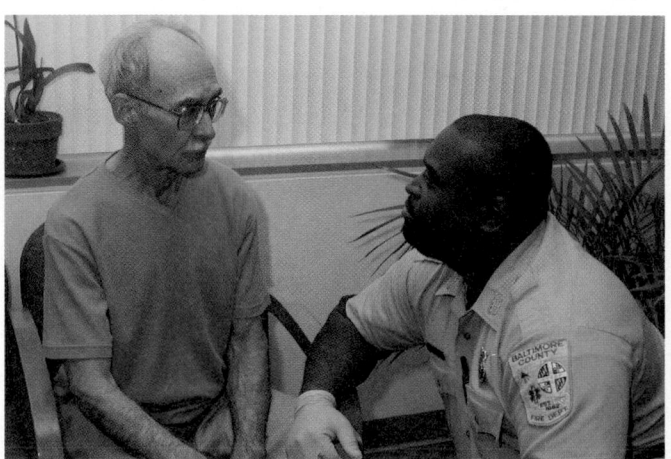

Figure 2 As a paramedic serving a diverse public, you will frequently work with people who have cultural backgrounds that are different from your own. Work to set aside your own personal beliefs when making decisions on the patient's behalf.

- The Emergency Medical Technician does not use professional knowledge and skill in any enterprise detrimental to the public good.
- The Emergency Medical Technician respects and holds in confidence all information of a confidential nature obtained in the course of professional work unless required by law to divulge such information.
- The Emergency Medical Technician as a citizen understands and upholds the laws and performs the duties of citizenship; as a professional person, the Emergency Medical Technician has a particular responsibility to work with other citizens and health professionals in promoting efforts to meet the health needs of the public.
- The Emergency Medical Technician maintains professional competence and demonstrates concern for the competence of other members of the medical profession.
- The Emergency Medical Technician assumes responsibility in defining and upholding standards of professional practice and education. The Emergency Medical Technician assumes responsibility for individual professional actions and judgment, both in dependent and independent emergency functions and knows and upholds the laws that affect the practice of the Emergency Medical Technician.
- The Emergency Medical Technician has the responsibility to participate in the study of and action on matters of legislation affecting Emergency Medical Technicians and emergency service to the public.
- The Emergency Medical Technician adheres to standards of personal ethics that reflect credit upon the profession.
- The Emergency Medical Technician may contribute to research in relation to a commercial product or service, but does not lend professional status to advertising, promotion, or sales.
- The Emergency Medical Technician, or groups of Emergency Medical Technicians, who advertise professional services, do so in conformity with the dignity of the profession.
- The Emergency Medical Technician has an obligation to protect the public by not delegating to a person less qualified any service which requires the professional competence of an Emergency Medical Technician.
- The Emergency Medical Technician works harmoniously with, and sustains confidence in, Emergency Medical Technician associates, the nurse, the physician, and other members of the health team.
- The Emergency Medical Technician refuses to participate in unethical procedures and assumes the responsibility to expose incompetence or unethical conduct in others to the appropriate authority.

In addition to the foregoing, your state may have its own code of ethics for EMS professionals and it is possible that the service or company you work for has its own set of policies, rules, or regulations that will provide guidance regarding ethical expectations of its employees. The ICARE program, developed by a group of EMS students and educators, incorporates many of the finest qualities of EMS professionals. ICARE (which

stands for integrity, compassion, accountability, respect, and empathy) is an excellent concept for all paramedics to remember and to incorporate into the care that they provide to their patients. All of the various codes and rules of right and wrong ultimately stem from a concern for the welfare of the patient, and it is a safe generalization that if you place the welfare of the patient ahead of all other considerations, you will rarely if ever commit an unethical act in medical care Figure 4.

It would be impossible to list all the ethical dilemmas potentially encountered in your work as a paramedic. Regardless of the ethical circumstances you may encounter, three basic ethical concepts, considered an inherent part of health care for centuries, should always be applied in making a decision. These ethical principles are: to do no harm, to act in good faith, and to act always in the patient's best interest.

The principle of *first, do no harm* (primum non nocere) essentially means that you should take all due care in ensuring that your patient receives the best possible care and that your actions do nothing to harm the patient. It requires you to take care in the way you assess, treat, and transport your patients so that you do nothing to exacerbate their medical condition or to cause an additional injury or medical problem.

The principles of acting in good faith and in the best interests of your patient go hand in hand. These principles are simply a reinforcement of your commitment to place the interests of the patient above all else and always to make decisions that are motivated by a clear desire to benefit your patient. You may at times make decisions on behalf of an unconscious or otherwise incompetent patient that the patient or a family member will later question. In such circumstances, you should be able to state confidently that the decision you made was motivated by your desire to benefit the patient.

Paramedics must be accountable for their actions at all times. How you handle teamwork, your personal attitude on the job, justice and respect for patient autonomy, and cultural

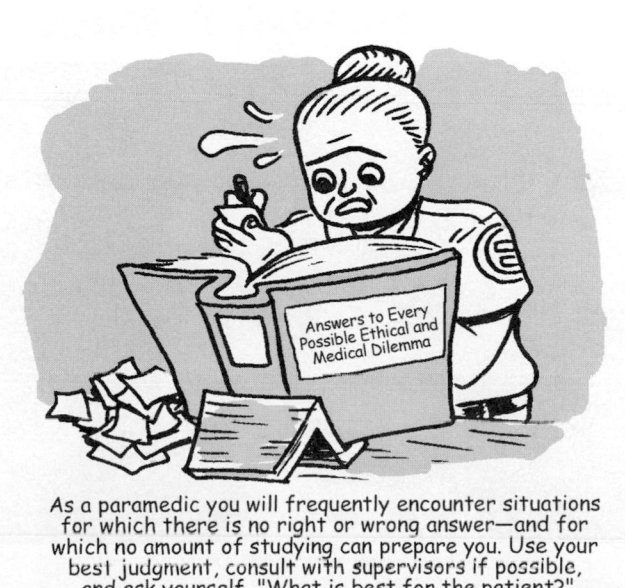

As a paramedic you will frequently encounter situations for which there is no right or wrong answer—and for which no amount of studying can prepare you. Use your best judgment, consult with supervisors if possible, and ask yourself, "What is best for the patient?"

Figure 4

or lifestyle diversity will ultimately shape your career. You must consider what type of a paramedic you want to become Figure 5 . It is helpful for you, as a new paramedic, to choose a mentor whose style and professionalism you wish to emulate.

Professional ethics are extremely important as EMS continues its pursuit of being recognized and funded in the same manner as the other medical professions. Immature, unprofessional behavior is unethical and has no place in this profession. Criminal acts, such as sexual misconduct, substance abuse, patient abuse, and harassment or stalking of coworkers, are both unethical and illegal. Off-duty misconduct can, and does, affect your reputation and may affect your employment as well. News stories that depict EMS personnel engaged in any immature or illegal activities serve to lessen the public's confidence in the services you provide. Inappropriate use of emergency vehicles, inappropriate visitors entertained at the station, and use of alcohol on duty are strictly forbidden.

You must always be respectful of patients and should never do anything to violate the trust that patients have in you as a professional. As a paramedic you are expected to honor the trust that has been bestowed on you as a member of the health care profession, to act ethically and professionally in every circumstance, and to avoid any misconduct that could call into question your ethics or integrity. Regrettably, there have been paramedics who have violated the ethical standards of their profession and have mistreated patients in a variety of ways. Such

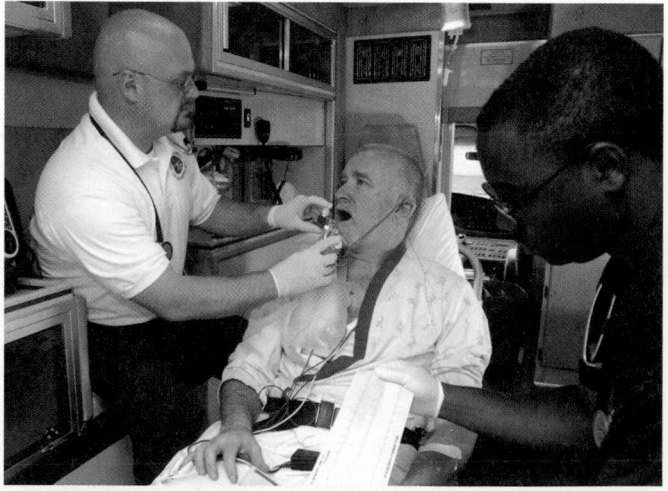

Figure 5 One of the best ways to hone your skills as a paramedic is to find a good mentor whose work ethic and attitude you admire.

misconduct has included discriminatory and abusive treatment, embellishing the patient assessment finding over the radio in an effort to obtain drug orders from the physician, and even sexual abuse. These violations of ethical standards have a negative impact on the profession itself, not just on those involved. Fortunately, these cases of misconduct are rare. The ethics of your profession require total commitment to acting in the best interest of your patient, and to otherwise conduct yourself in a professional and ethical manner at all times, meaning caring about your patients, coworkers, and the EMS system as a whole. Therefore, you should not overlook other EMS providers engaging in misbehavior. Misconduct should be promptly reported to the appropriate chain of command. Similarly, paramedics are obligated to report medical errors they make or witness to the medical director as soon as possible.

Paramedics who choose to become patient advocates, who participate in and actively seek out the best in training and professional development, and who put the good of the team above their own personal aspirations will ultimately succeed and be rewarded with a fulfilling career in EMS. Good ethics can be instilled by good mentors. People seem to perform best when they share themselves and work toward an end much greater than themselves. EMS is an evolving specialty, and the future of it lies in your hands.

Ethics and EMS Research

EMS practices have largely evolved like the rest of EMS—with "grass roots" effort and precious little research to confirm the effectiveness of the procedures used in the prehospital setting. Properly randomized, controlled studies in EMS are not common, but they are emerging. You must remember that the first principle of medical practice is to do no harm, and therefore must continue to seek further education about the effectiveness of EMS practice. Some of EMS care still relies on anecdotal experience that is unsupported by research. Some EMS procedures, however well-intentioned, prove not to be helpful to patients, and as a health care provider, you must act on those recommendations as well. Conducting EMS studies on critically ill or injured patients without their informed consent is a true ethical dilemma—many of the patients a paramedic sees in practice are critically ill or injured. These patients are usually unable to give consent, and their physical state is so compromised that even if they are conscious, they may not be able to absorb information to give informed consent. Continue to make yourself aware of how researchers are handling this issue and other ethical debates concerning patients in research.

The Legal System in the United States

Federal and state governments make, administer, and interpret laws that affect paramedics. Each level of government has three branches Figure 6 . The legislative branch, made up of elected officials (Congress at the federal level; state legislatures at the state level), actually makes the laws. The judicial branch (consisting of the court system) enforces and interprets laws and resolves disputes based on interpretation of laws.

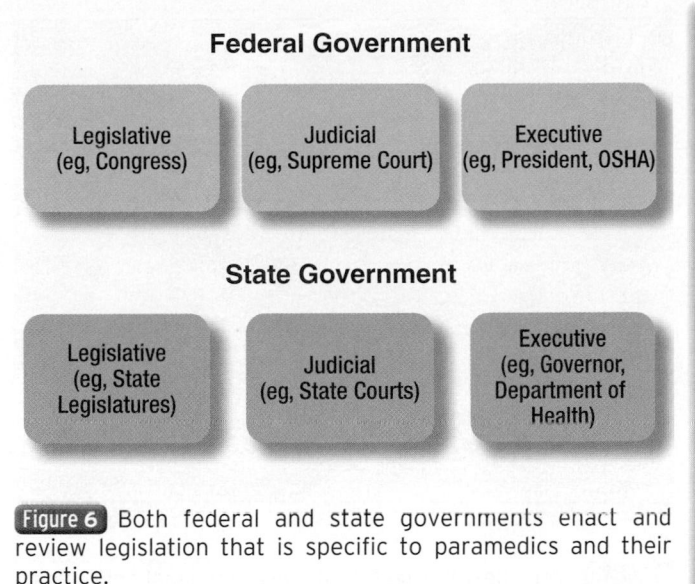

Federal Government

| Legislative (eg, Congress) | Judicial (eg, Supreme Court) | Executive (eg, President, OSHA) |

State Government

| Legislative (eg, State Legislatures) | Judicial (eg, State Courts) | Executive (eg, Governor, Department of Health) |

Figure 6 Both federal and state governments enact and review legislation that is specific to paramedics and their practice.

Courts have a number of levels, including trial courts and appellate courts. Although many people believe that all law comes from statutes passed by the legislative branch, this is not true. Court decisions, especially those issued by appellate courts, establish precedent and become the law of the state in which you live and practice as a paramedic. In most cases, these court decisions establish the standards of negligence that will apply if you are sued by a patient.

The third branch—the executive or administrative branch—reports to the president (in Washington, DC) or the governor (in your state capital) and is made up of various cabinets and agencies (the bureaucrats) that carry out and administer the laws. The agencies often use regulations to establish how things should be done. Agencies such as the Occupational Safety and Health Administration (OSHA) and the US Department of Transportation (DOT) at the federal level, and the Department of Health at the state level, are examples of parts of the administrative branch.

All states now have some type of legislation that sets out the framework for the EMS system. In addition, there may be administrative regulations that are set forth by state agencies or county governments that regulate the practice of paramedics. It is vital for you to know and understand the laws and administrative regulations that affect your practice in your home state.

■ Types of Law

Two kinds of law govern paramedics in court: civil law, under which a patient can sue you for a perceived injury, and criminal law, in which the state can prosecute you for breaking a legal statute. Malpractice suits are tried under civil law. Although some suits may be based on state statutes, most claims will arise out of principles of negligence established by prior court decisions. Many cases of medication misuse will be tried under criminal law.

A substantial part of civil law is concerned with establishing **liability**, or responsibility. When a person experiences an

injury and seeks redress for that injury, the judicial process must determine who was responsible. For example, a patient or (if the patient died) the survivor of a patient may be dissatisfied with the medical care the patient received. The patient or survivor may feel that inadequate care led to a bad outcome. People have a constitutional right to take legal action against the doctor, nurse, paramedic, or other involved parties. However, the person who is suing must prove that the medical providers he or she is suing caused harm by failing to provide medical care that met the accepted standards. A bad outcome alone does not necessarily mean the medical provider was negligent; the patient or survivor has to prove all of the elements of negligence before a lawsuit will be successful. A claim that contains all of the foregoing elements is sometimes referred to as an actionable cause.

A legal action of that sort is called a **civil suit**—that is, an action instituted by a private person or corporation (the **plaintiff**) against another private person or corporation (the **defendant**)—and the wrongful act that gives rise to a civil suit is called a **tort**. The law recognizes two classifications of torts: unintentional torts (commonly referred to as negligence) and intentional torts (those where there is an intent to cause harm). The objective of a civil suit is usually some sort of compensation (**damages**) for the injury the plaintiff sustained.

In medical liability cases, the plaintiff usually seeks monetary compensation for physical suffering, mental anguish, hospital and medical bills, and sometimes loss of earnings or earning capacity. In certain cases, the court may also award **punitive damages** if the misconduct of the EMS provider was intentional or constituted a reckless disregard for the safety of the public. To succeed in a civil suit, the plaintiff need only show that a preponderance of the believable evidence favors his or her position, and only 9 of the 12 jurors must agree.

Lawsuits against EMS providers most often result from emergency vehicle crashes. In the chapter *Public Health*, you learned about the importance of safe driving to your personal health and well-being. You should also be aware that safe driving is a key to preventing lawsuits. Vehicle crashes are all too common and cause expensive property damage as well as serious harm to patients, bystanders, and EMS providers **Figure 7**.

Other kinds of lawsuits against EMS providers are on the rise each year. Many of these lawsuits involve dispatch and transport issues, such as those involving a delayed transport response or patient deterioration after not being transported. Other lawsuits address the quality of the medical care provided by the EMS providers, especially paramedics.

Sometimes the same allegedly wrongful or harmful act that gave rise to a civil suit may also elicit criminal prosecution. A **criminal prosecution** is an action taken by the government against a person the prosecutors feel has violated criminal laws. In a criminal case, the government must prove guilt beyond all reasonable doubt to 12 jurors. If the government succeeds, the defendant can be fined or imprisoned or both.

The criminal laws most likely to apply to prehospital care include assault, battery, and false imprisonment or kidnapping. All of these are criminal actions resulting from complaints about a paramedic's behavior such as using improper restraining methods, making physical contact with a patient before asking

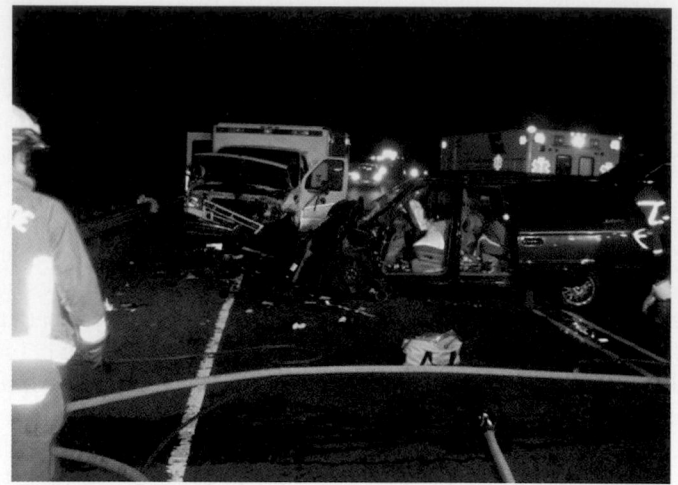

Figure 7 Many civil suits against paramedics arise from emergency vehicle collisions.

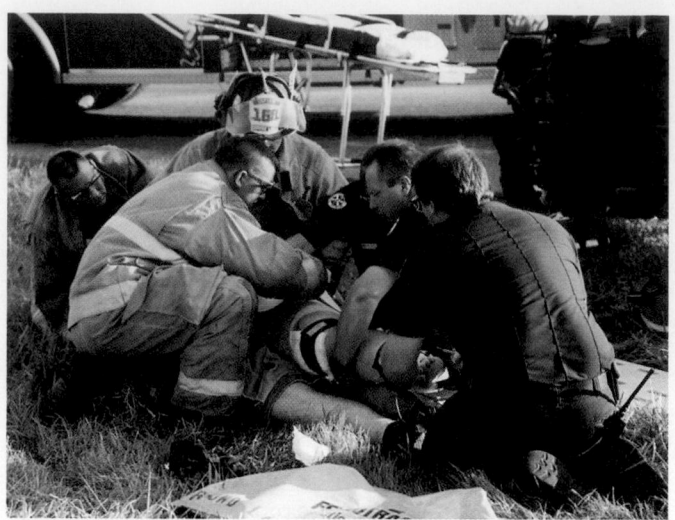

Figure 8 Your best prevention against any legal action is to keep the needs of your patient as your top priority.

a patient if you may touch him or her, or transporting a patient without his or her consent **Figure 8**. To prosecute a criminal charge of assault or battery, the prosecution generally needs to prove that there was intent to do harm. In a civil case, the plaintiff need only establish that the conduct took place without his or her consent. Criminal charges of false imprisonment or kidnapping are rarely filed against EMS providers. Civil suits alleging false imprisonment or kidnapping are much more common and usually arise out of circumstances in which the patient claims to have been transported or restrained against his or her will.

Whereas the vast majority of suits filed against EMS providers involve allegedly negligent or unintentional conduct, there are certain types of intentional tort claims that are occasionally filed. These include claims for assault, battery, defamation of character (libel and slander), and false imprisonment. **Assault** is said to occur when a person (the EMS provider) instills the fear of immediate bodily harm or breach of bodily security to another (the patient)—regardless of whether the threat of harm is actually carried out. **Battery** occurs when the defendant (the EMS provider) touches another person (the patient) without his or her consent. Here are rough working definitions of the difference: saying "I'm going to kick your teeth in" is assault; actually kicking the person's teeth in is battery. Just about any act of medical treatment performed without consent may be considered assault or battery or both, for such acts constitute a threat to the patient's bodily security ("Now I'm going to stick you with this needle…") and an unsanctioned contact with the patient's body.

False imprisonment occurs when a person is intentionally and unjustifiably detained against his or her will. In prehospital care, charges of false imprisonment may arise if a paramedic transports a patient without the patient's consent or uses restraints in a wrongful manner. In essence, your best protection against these charges is to obtain informed consent for almost everything you do. All medical care providers need

to get informed consent, but you will need some guidelines and tips (presented later in this chapter) that may not apply to most hospital-based personnel.

Paramedics may also be sued for **defamation**, which is intentionally making a false statement through written or verbal communication that injures a person's good name or reputation. **Libel** is making a false statement in the written form that injures a person's good name. When you write your patient care report, avoid using terms that may be considered insulting or offensive, such as "the patient appears to be drunk." Whatever your personal views, think about the way in which your run report would read in court. Do not let thoughtless comments become evidence against you.

Slander is verbally making a false statement that injures a person's good name. Once again, avoid using terms that could be considered offensive to the patient when you are passing along prehospital care information to emergency department personnel. Keep in mind always that your patient is most likely someone's son or daughter, husband or wife, brother or sister, or father or mother. How would you like information about members of your own family to be treated when information is relayed to the hospital?

Words of Wisdom

Being courteous, honest, and professional will prevent most patients from complaining or filing lawsuits.

The Legal Process

A civil suit begins when a dissatisfied patient contacts an attorney, who then files a document for a lawsuit (called a complaint) on behalf of the patient with a local court. The court where the action is first filed is generally referred to as the court of original jurisdiction. The complaint will contain the general allegations against the paramedic and the EMS system, but may not contain much specific information about what the patient thinks went wrong. The patient's attorney (or the attorney's staff) must hand deliver a copy of the complaint and a notice called a summons to all persons or agencies named in the lawsuit, notifying them of the complaint and the need to respond. From start to finish, a lawsuit may take several years. Because the lawsuit may not begin until several years after the paramedic sees the patient, good documentation is essential to defending a lawsuit.

In EMS, your attorney will usually be assigned to you by the insurance company that handles claims for your employer, whether the employer is a government or private agency. The response, or answer to the complaint, will be filed by your attorney. Once the complaint is filed and you (through your attorney) have answered, a period known as the discovery period begins. The discovery period can last anywhere from a few months to more than 2 years **Figure 9**. During the discovery period, the attorneys on both sides seek to find out as much about the case as possible. They will exchange written questions that must be answered by the parties under oath, exchange documents such as the patient's medical record, and take depositions (statements taken under oath). You should stay in touch with your attorney during this time and ask for a full explanation of everything that is happening. Your attorney will also prepare you for a deposition, instructing you where to go, what to wear, and how to respond to certain types of questions.

Attorneys may also file motions (requests for the court to take an action) and argue them before the judge. Your attorney will seek to have the lawsuit dismissed by filing motions. The plaintiff's attorney may ask the court to rule on certain portions of the claim by filing other motions. Either side may file motions asking the court to compel the other side to produce documents or information that is being withheld.

Most civil cases are resolved during a settlement process because it is expensive and time-consuming to take a case through trial. Settlement processes involve the parties and their attorneys in mediation, which is a conference set up to see if the parties can agree on a dollar amount that will resolve the case, or an arbitration, which is a mini-trial in which a single arbitrator or a panel of arbitrators will make a decision based on the evidence presented by both sides.

If the case does not resolve during the settlement process, it will proceed to trial. During a trial, the judge rules on what the law is and the jury decides what the facts are. Trial juries can be unpredictable; if they perceive that EMS has failed to meet community standards, large monetary damages can be rewarded. In most cases, the trial will be the final step in the judicial process, but the party that loses at trial always has the right to have the decision reviewed by an appellate court. Appeals are costly and time consuming, however, and only a small percentage of cases are ever appealed.

■ Legal Accountability of the Paramedic

■ The Paramedic and the Medical Director

The relationship between the paramedic and the medical director is complex and often not well understood. Ultimately, the paramedic has three lines of authority to answer to within the EMS system: the medical director, the licensing agency, and the employer. Although there is some overlap, it is important to keep these distinctions in mind. State EMS legislation usually requires that the paramedic perform advanced life-support procedures and skills only under the supervision of a physician. Legislation may also require the EMS system to have a medical director. Although the medical director is in a supervisory relationship with the paramedic, legally speaking, the paramedic is not the agent of the physician.

The acts of the paramedic, therefore, are not the actions of the physician, and the paramedic will be held accountable for his or her own actions. However, the medical director can be held legally accountable for failing to supervise the paramedic closely enough, or for failing to take action when the paramedic's performance is not up to standard. The medical director may restrict the paramedic's practice, or even withdraw supervision entirely from a paramedic if the medical director does not believe the paramedic is performing as he or she should. The medical director may also require certain remedial training if the paramedic is weak in some areas of practice. Although the medical director's remedial requirements may ultimately result in employment actions, medical directors are generally not held legally responsible for disciplinary actions taken by employers.

Many of the paramedic's activities require an order from a licensed physician. Orders may be given by radio or cell phone (online medical control) or instead may be defined by protocols,

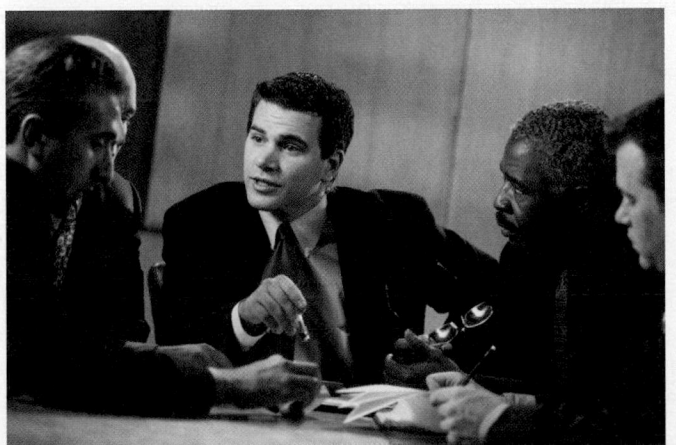

Figure 9 The process of a lawsuit can take years, and because of expenses associated with a trial, can result in out-of-court settlements.

Documentation and Communication

If you must deviate from your protocols because of unusual circumstances, consult with online medical control and make sure you document it well on your patient care report.

or standing orders (off-line medical control), but in any case, the paramedic is not at liberty to disregard or reverse a physician's order unless the paramedic truly believes that carrying out the order will harm the patient. That fact may give rise to difficult situations, such as instances in which paramedics find themselves at the scene of an emergency together with a physician who may not be knowledgeable in prehospital emergency care. Under those circumstances, the paramedics may feel that the orders of the on-scene physician are inappropriate. However, paramedics are on questionable legal ground if they choose to disregard a physician's orders, assuming the physician is licensed in that state and the order is appropriate. To avoid conflicts in such situations, it is best to ask the service medical director to develop protocols ahead of time defining the paramedic's relationship with the medical director of the service and with other physicians in the community, including bystander physicians. A physician is not required to ride to the hospital with EMS unless he or she has performed procedures above the level of the EMS providers or has otherwise assumed responsibility for patient care. Always be sure that the physician is licensed in your state, and document the physician's name and contact information, before allowing him or her to provide patient care. When conflicts do arise between paramedics and physician bystanders in the field, online medical control, not the paramedic, should resolve them.

■ EMS-Enabling Legislation

Most states now have what is called EMS-enabling legislation, defining how EMS is structured and designating responsibilities to government agencies. These laws also provide the state's framework for the paramedic's actual practice—what you are permitted to do in the field. For example, EMS legislation may define the need for a medical director, and may also define the scope of practice for the different levels of EMS personnel. You must be familiar with the EMS legislation in your state and any regulations that flow from those statutes.

■ Administrative Regulations

Administrative regulations—set forth by bureaucracies at the state and federal levels—affect and define the specific rules under which paramedics practice. For example, regulations may set out the precise skills and medications to be used by each level of EMS provider. Regulations—usually developed by either the state's Department of Health or the county agency responsible for regulating EMS practice—may further define the paramedic's role in emergency medical care of patients. Regulations may also define the requirements for licensure or certification, renewal requirements, continuing education requirements, and a list of behaviors that may subject paramedics to suspension or revocation of their license or certification.

If a paramedic provides less than adequate care, or fails to meet the requirements for recertification, the administrative agency may also take action against that paramedic's license. A license is not a right, but rather a privilege, granted by a government agency, allowing the paramedic to provide care to its citizens. Failure to abide by the regulations can have serious consequences.

Licensure and Certification

The terms licensure and certification are often confused because, in some states, paramedics are considered licensed but in others they are considered certified. Certification generally refers to a certain level of credentials based on hours of training and examination, and addresses criteria met for minimum competency. Certification may be granted by a governmental agency or by a private organization such as the American Heart Association or the American Red Cross. The fact that a paramedic has received certification from a private organization does not necessarily mean that he or she has authority to practice the skills included in that certification. Licensure refers to a carefully defined level of practice, usually granted by a government agency or local authority such as a state health department or county EMS authority. Often, these agencies themselves create and administer the licensing examinations. A license itself is a privilege granted by a government authority on certain conditions. The paramedic must comply with the government's requirements for professional behavior, continuing education, and licensure renewal, or risk losing that privilege. The rights and privileges conferred by licensing in one state may not be conferred in other states that certify, rather than license, paramedics.

Another concept that may be encountered by the paramedic is that of credentialing. Credentialing may be adopted by a specific EMS service as part of its employment requirements. For example, although you may be licensed as a paramedic by your state, the service for which you are seeking work may impose additional requirements as part of its eligibility standards. Typically, this may include things such as certification in CPR, trauma, or advanced cardiac life support (ACLS).

Discipline and Due Process

If a paramedic commits an infraction of the rules pertaining to licensure, the agency that granted the license may seek to restrict, suspend, or even revoke the privilege to practice.

When an administrative agency proposes a licensing action, the paramedic has a right to **due process**. Due process is a right to a fair procedure for the action the agency proposes to take. Due process has two components: notice and the opportunity to be heard. Notice means that the agency must notify the paramedic of the actions that allegedly constitute the infraction, usually by receipt of a certified letter containing a Notice of Contemplated Action. The letter informs the paramedic of the proposed action to be taken and the sections of the regulations the agency is alleging were violated. The letter also informs the paramedic of his or her right to a hearing and the procedure for requesting a hearing. The hearing provides an opportunity for the paramedic to tell his or her side of the story. If the licensing agency still believes licensure action is warranted after the hearing, it will send a Notice of Final Action. The paramedic may have appeal rights if a final licensure action is taken.

■ Medical Practice Act

In most states, physicians and other health care practitioners are enabled to function through the provisions of a **Medical Practice Act**. This act usually defines the minimum qualifications of those who may perform various health services, defines the skills that each type of practitioner is legally permitted to use, and establishes a means of licensure or certification for different categories of health care professionals. Requirements for relicensure or recertification based on continuing education and other factors may also be include in the Medical Practice Act. In some cases, Medical Practice Acts may require that a physician assume responsibility for competency of the paramedic through mandatory training, skill competency testing, and run review. You should become familiar with the terms of the Medical Practice Act in your state.

◼ Scope of Practice

The <u>scope of practice</u> for paramedics may be spelled out in their state's EMS legislation or regulations. The scope of practice is care that a paramedic is permitted to perform according to the state under its license or certification; however, a local medical director may not permit a paramedic to perform all of the skills or give all of the medications for which the paramedic is licensed or certified.

A paramedic carrying out procedures for which he or she is not authorized under the enabling legislation is practicing outside his or her scope of practice, which may be considered negligence or, in some states, even a criminal offense (considered practicing medicine without a license). The scope of practice should not be confused with the standard of care, which is what a reasonable paramedic in a similar situation would do. This is discussed later in this chapter.

◼ Health Insurance Portability and Accountability Act

The Health Insurance Portability and Accountability Act (<u>HIPAA</u>) provides stringent privacy requirements for patient information. The act was enacted in 1996 and provides for criminal sanctions as well as civil penalties for releasing a patient's private medical information in an unauthorized manner. Medical information can be disclosed only if it is necessary for a patient's treatment or for payment or medical/billing operations or when the release has been authorized in writing by the patient or a lawful patient representative. There are also several special situations that may require the release of patient information without the patient's authorization. These include legally mandated reporting (dog bites, gunshot wounds, child abuse), authorized data collection and research by public health agencies, authorized requests by law enforcement agencies, and information required to be disclosed pursuant to a valid subpoena. HIPAA requires each EMS agency to have a privacy officer responsible for ensuring that all protected health information (PHI) that the service deals with, in either written or electronic form, not be released in an unauthorized manner. This means you must be aware of where written patient information is at all times, and you cannot casually discuss a patient where you might be overheard—like in an elevator **Figure 10**. Use caution when you are giving reports or discussing patient information in other public places such as crash scenes or emergency department common

areas. Sharing patient stories with other paramedics may subject you to liability. Similarly, you must use caution when the media or the public is riding with your service to ensure that PHI is not disclosed without the patient's consent.

Some states also have laws pertaining to patient confidentiality; a breach of that confidentiality may allow patients to sue for unauthorized release of their medical information **Figure 11**.

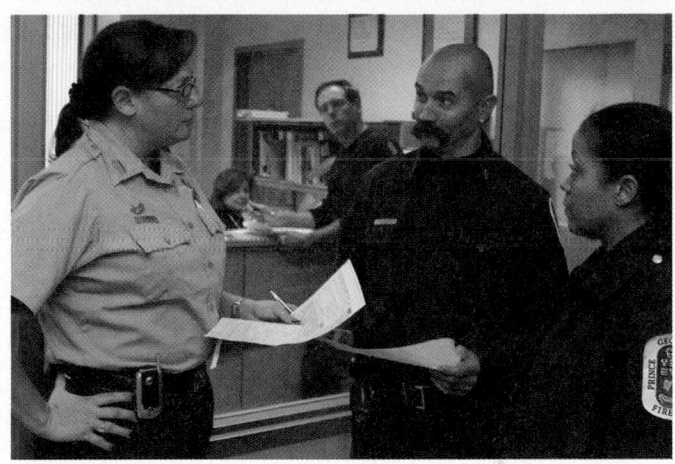

Figure 10 Remember that the HIPAA law guarantees a patient's confidentiality at all times. Be careful never to discuss a patient's condition in public.

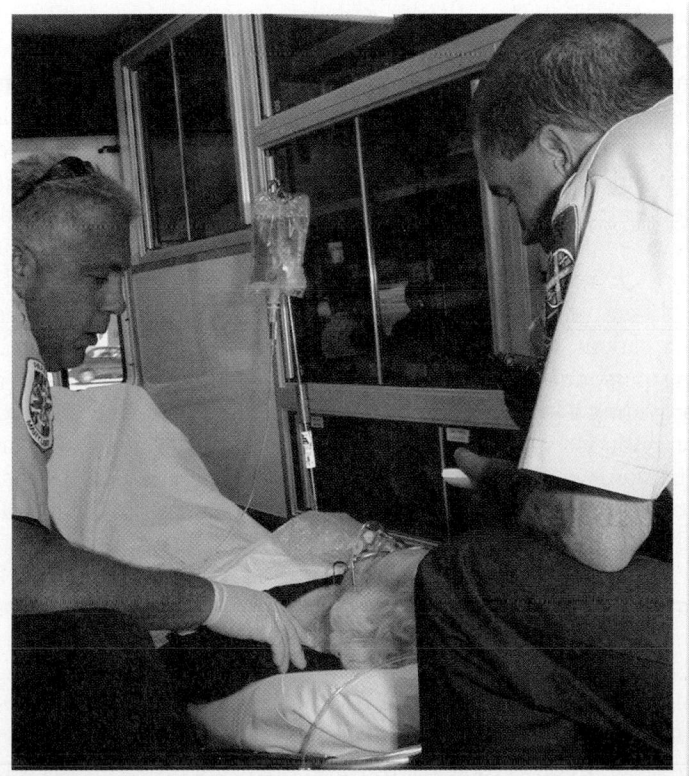

Figure 11 When you are communicating with a patient, be sensitive to his or her point of view, and the environment in which you choose to communicate.

Confidentiality is also a part of the Code of Ethics for Emergency Medical Technicians issued by the National Association of Emergency Medical Technicians (NAEMT). If your service receives a subpoena for a patient's PHI, be sure to notify legal counsel before releasing a patient's medical record to anyone.

HIPAA also requires you to provide patients with a copy of your service's privacy policies. Whereas this can often be difficult in an emergency setting, it is your obligation to do the best that you can to be in compliance with the law. Most services make up multipage leaflets that can be handed out to patients.

HIPAA also regulates the manner in which you and your service transmit PHI electronically. HIPAA security rules contain many provisions requiring various computer safeguards with which you must be familiar.

Your employer is required to provide you with HIPAA training at the time you are hired and then again on an annual basis.

Emergency Medical Treatment and Active Labor Act

The Emergency Medical Treatment and Active Labor Act (**EMTALA**) was enacted in 1986 to combat the practice of "patient dumping" and pays particular attention to the practice of sending women in labor to distant hospitals. Patient dumping occurs when a hospital emergency department denies medical screening or stabilizing treatment, or if it inappropriately transfers a person whose condition is not stable. Historically, most patient dumping occurred when a hospital discovered that the patient did not have health insurance or was otherwise unable to pay. In recent years, the term *economic triage* has been introduced. This term refers to the practice of making health care decisions based on the ability of the patient or the insurance carrier to provide payment for services. Whereas such considerations may have a place in certain aspects of the health care field, a paramedic or other emergency medical provider should never make a decision to treat or transport based on financial considerations, regardless of the current financial state of the EMS employer. The only consideration should be the needs of the patient; reimbursement issues should be addressed by billing personnel. Paramedics have occasionally been accused of providing a lower standard of care for indigent persons or those on public assistance; therefore, you should make sure that financial status never becomes a deciding factor in your practice. As a paramedic, you must always provide the highest possible quality of care to all patients regardless of their financial status.

As a paramedic, it is also important that you have a clear understanding of local protocols regarding the choice of hospitals to which you may transfer your patient. In some rural areas, there may be only one available hospital, but in other places there may be several options available. Some EMS systems simply require you to transfer the patient to the nearest hospital. In other systems, however, there are protocols that dictate that hospital selection be based on the specific needs of the patient. For example, some patients may require the services of a trauma center, a children's hospital, or a hospital with cardiac catheterization capabilities. Under some protocols, the choice of destination may be made by the paramedic alone, whereas in others the paramedic may be required to consult with medical control in making such decisions. It is important to become familiar with the protocols in your area of practice.

EMTALA can be enforced because it regulates hospitals that receive Medicare funding. EMTALA also issues severe fines for hospitals and doctors who violate its provisions. In addition, EMTALA further allows private persons to sue for violations of the act. Under most circumstances, neither an ambulance service nor a paramedic can be sued or charged with a violation under EMTALA. An ambulance service that is owned by a hospital, however, may be subject to a claim under EMTALA in certain cases.

EMTALA guarantees a medical screening examination, and treatment to stabilize any emergency medical conditions found, to any patient presenting to a hospital that has an emergency department **Figure 12**. It prohibits discrimination for any reason, including the ability to pay. Some urgent care centers may also be covered by EMTALA. Although EMTALA does not directly regulate paramedics, EMS is often the vehicle—both figuratively and literally—by which patient dumping takes place.

EMTALA also regulates patient transfers and applies to both the sending and receiving facilities. Paramedics should never transfer a patient who needs care that falls outside their scope of practice and they must feel comfortable that the patient is stable enough to transfer. A transferring hospital has an obligation to ensure that the transferring ambulance and crew are capable of meeting the needs of the patient during transfer and it should request an ambulance that is appropriately staffed and equipped. It would be a potential EMTALA violation if a hospital requested a BLS ambulance and crew to transport a patient with a serious cardiac condition who required cardiac monitoring and the administration of medication during the transport. Should a patient need a higher level of care, it is the responsibility of the transferring hospital to provide someone to ride along (a nurse, respiratory therapist, or even a physician). Paramedics should also make sure they have received all appropriate paperwork before leaving on a patient transfer, including all pertinent medical

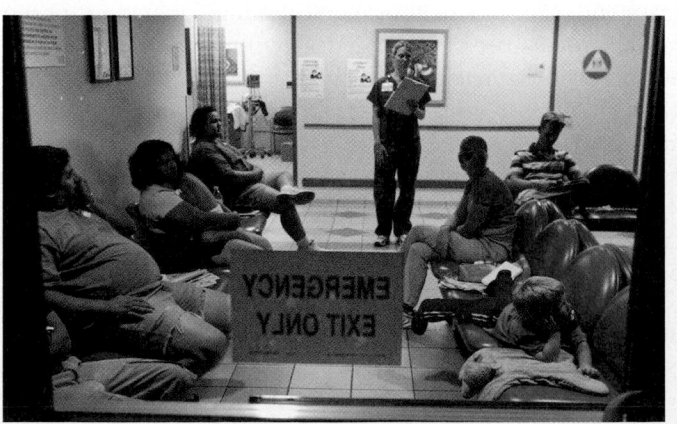

Figure 12 EMTALA legislation requires that every patient must receive emergency medical treatment—regardless of his or her ability to pay for medical treatment when it is received.

records, laboratory results, x-rays, and other documents. When you are arriving at the receiving hospital, that hospital should have a bed ready for the patient, after agreeing to accept the patient.

EMTALA issues are regulated by the Centers for Medicare and Medicaid Services (CMS) and carry severe monetary penalties—up to and including loss of Medicare funding—for hospitals that fail to comply. EMTALA has complex language that appears to be medical language but is actually legal language. For example, an *emergency medical condition* under EMTALA means what most paramedics would call an *acute situation*.

Emergency Vehicle Laws

Most states have specific statutes that define an emergency vehicle and what traffic should do when an emergency vehicle approaches. Although these laws vary somewhat from state to state, it is important to remember that these statutes still require emergency vehicles to be operated in a safe and prudent manner. Laws governing emergency vehicle operation do not authorize speeding, running red lights, or driving the vehicle in an unsafe manner, which can put the public at risk. Most state laws establish a higher standard for the emergency vehicle operator by making him or her responsible for operating the vehicle with due regard for the safety of all others. If a crash occurs, EMS providers will often be found at fault in civil cases brought against the drivers. Worse, if you are the driver, you might also be charged criminally for such situations. Although it is important for paramedics to know the laws of their state about emergency vehicle operation, it is also important to remember that the blue star of life on the side of your vehicle and the flashing red lights on top do not exempt you from defensive driving and common courtesy; you will be held responsible for your actions.

Transportation

Patients should be transported to the hospital of their choice when possible and reasonable; however, most EMS systems have protocols that direct paramedics to transport certain types of patients to particular hospitals. Examples of these patients include those who have experienced trauma, stroke, and cardiac events; homeless patients; mentally ill patients; and obese patients. The capability of each hospital to care for particular kinds of patients should guide the EMS system in developing transport protocols. Transportation of patients to a facility that does not have the ability to care for their particular illness or injury can result in liability for the paramedic.

Decisions made by paramedics not to transport patients at all have been the subject of litigation. A number of studies have demonstrated that paramedics should not be compelled to decide which patients need to be transported to the hospital for any health problems. The whole EMS system, including paramedics, does not have access to sophisticated diagnostic tools or radiography in the prehospital setting. Failure to transport a patient whose condition later deteriorates can bring about a lawsuit that is difficult to defend. Again, most EMS systems have protocols outlining when it is acceptable not to transport a patient, and many require consultation with online medical control.

Crime Scene and Emergency Scene Responsibilities

When you are handling a situation involving a death, or any potential crime scene, remember that it may take law enforcement officials some time to figure out whether the scene involved a suicide, homicide, or some other form of criminal activity. It is important for you to use extreme caution and not disturb or destroy potential evidence.

If the scene is a vehicle crash, do not move anything unless you have to—including broken glass, pieces of metal, or even a beer can. Leave dead bodies where they are until a coroner or medical examiner arrives to investigate.

If the incident scene is indoors, do not touch anything you do not have to touch, such as telephones or doorknobs, because of the risk of eliminating fingerprints. Carefully document any statements made by witnesses and get their contact information. Limit the number of EMS personnel who enter the scene because each person who enters the scene further contaminates what may later turn out to be a crime scene. If it is necessary to move furniture or other objects, be sure to notify law enforcement personnel that you have done so. Preserve any clothing that you remove from the patient, and make every attempt not to alter evidence on the clothing (eg, cutting through bullet or knife holes).

Remember that in rape cases the patient may carry vital pieces of evidence such as fiber, hair, sperm, or blood on his or her body—take care to protect this evidence.

If the scene involves a death, stay with the body until the police arrive, and protect the scene from contamination by bystanders, family members, media, or additional EMS personnel.

In most jurisdictions, a paramedic is not legally authorized to pronounce a patient dead. If you have any doubt about the possibility of saving the patient, initiate resuscitation and transport him or her to the hospital.

Special Populations

Be aware that at crime scenes the perpetrator may still be at or near the scene and could be a factor in when and how you care for your patient.

Mandatory Reporting

Each state has its own requirements regarding categories of cases that must be reported to the appropriate authorities. These cases include some of the most difficult ones a paramedic will see.

Virtually every state has laws requiring EMS providers to report suspected child and elder abuse. It is essential for you to be familiar with the reporting requirements of your own state. In most states, reporting laws also contain immunity provisions that protect the health care provider who files reports from legal liability, provided the report was not made with malicious intent. Failure to report is a crime and in many states has very serious implications. If your state requires you to report, complete the reporting yourself; do not pass along the information expecting someone else will make the report.

The obligation to report is most frequently applied to the following categories of cases:

- Neglect or abuse of children
- Neglect or abuse of older people
- Domestic violence
- Injury sustained during the commission of a felony, or specific injuries considered to be of suspicious origin (such as gunshot wounds or stab wounds)
- Drug-related injuries
- Childbirth occurring outside a licensed medical facility
- Rape
- Animal bites
- Certain communicable diseases

Because reporting requirements vary widely from state to state, learn the laws of your state and observe the reporting obligations that apply to you.

Special Populations

Do not forget to be observant and report any suspicious signs or symptoms to the proper authorities.

Coroner and Medical Examiner Cases

Every EMS system should have a list of procedures for cases that involve the coroner and medical examiner **Figure 13**. Although coroner laws vary somewhat from state to state, generally you should notify the police of all coroner cases, including the following situations:

- Obvious or suspected homicide
- Obvious or suspected suicide
- Any other violent or sudden, unexpected death
- Death of a prison inmate

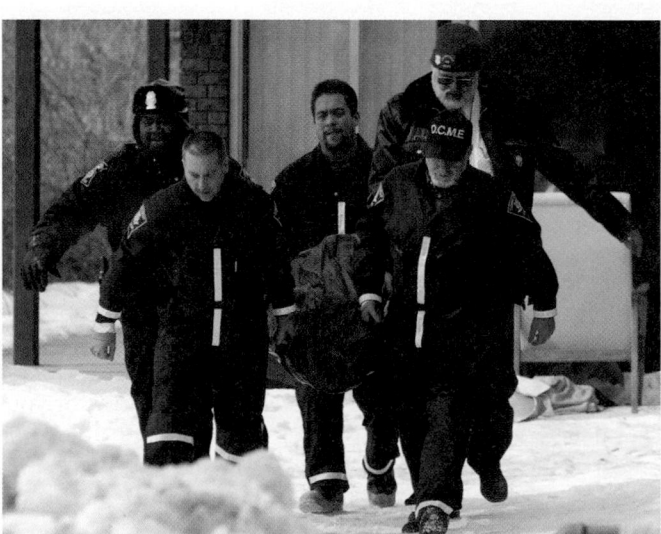

Figure 13 In any situation involving the death of a person, paramedics should contact the police or coroner with pertinent details depending on local protocols.

Paramedic—Patient Relationships

The most important premise affecting paramedics is one that does not appear in any of the statute books; it is the rule of doing what is best for the patient. Paramedics are trained in emergency medical care, not law. Every decision regarding patient care that you make, therefore, should be based on the standards of good medical care—not on the possible legal consequences. When you do what is best for the patient within your scope of practice, it is unlikely you will run afoul of the law—and in the event a lawsuit is initiated, your defense will be greatly enhanced if you have always kept the patient's best interest in mind.

Consent and Refusal

Prior to providing emergency medical care, you must obtain the **consent** of the patient. Any touching of a patient's body without consent may give rise to charges of assault and battery. The concept of consent refers to patients who are of legal age and who possess decision-making capacity, the capacity to make appropriate medical care decisions for themselves. Patients with decision-making capacity have the right to refuse all or part of the emergency medical care offered to them. You should be familiar with the two types of consent: informed consent and implied consent.

Informed consent must be obtained from every adult patient who has decision-making capacity. To obtain informed consent, use the following steps:

1. Describe the suspected problem to the patient.
2. Describe the treatment you would like to administer, and list potential risks associated with the proposed treatment.
3. Discuss any alternative types of treatment available.
4. Advise the patient regarding potential consequences of refusing treatment.

A number of things such as language barriers, emotional states, and mental abilities may impede you giving patients the information they need to make informed decisions. The key is to ensure that your patient understands what you are trying to do and grants you permission to treat. Whereas informed consent under emergency conditions may lack the formality seen in a hospital, you must document the patient's consent in your report to protect you against potential legal action.

Informed patient consent is routinely obtained verbally but may also be communicated through patient conduct, such as the patient rolling up a sleeve to allow you to take his or her blood pressure. **Expressed consent** is a type of informed consent that occurs when the patient does something, either by telling you or by taking some sort of action, that demonstrates he or she is giving you permission to provide care.

Implied consent is a form of consent assumed to be given by unconscious adults or by adults who are too ill or injured to consent verbally to emergency lifesaving treatment. In those cases, you assume that the patients would want care because of the severity of their condition, but the patients do not have decision-making capacity at the time that treatment is necessary.

Some EMS personnel incorrectly use the term <u>involuntary consent</u> to refer to situations in which a law enforcement officer or a legal guardian grants permission to treat someone who is under arrest (or otherwise in custody), incapacitated, a minor, or for other reasons. Involuntary consent is actually an oxymoron because consent can never be involuntary. Persons under arrest or in prison do not necessarily lose their right to be involved in medical treatment decisions. It is not uncommon for a law enforcement officer to direct EMS personnel to treat a person under arrest, but the paramedic should continue to follow informed consent guidelines. If a prisoner refuses treatment, medical control should be involved.

Decision-Making Capacity

Refusals, like consent, must be informed refusals, and all the same prerequisites apply. Patients must have decision-making capacity in order to be able to refuse care. <u>Decision-making capacity</u> is the ability of patients to understand the information you are providing to them, coupled with the ability to process that information and make a choice regarding medical care that is appropriate for them. You have a number of tools you can use to evaluate a patient's decision-making capacity, but the best one is your ability to talk to the patient to find out whether the patient understands what is happening to him or her. In addition, if pulse oximetry and blood glucose measurements are outside normal ranges, these readings can provide measurable information regarding your patient's ability to understand and communicate. Detailed documentation of decision-making capacity is important to include in your patient care report to show that the patient was able to understand your proposed plan of care.

If a conscious patient with decision-making capacity refuses to consent to treatment, that person may not be treated without a court order **Figure 14**. In such instances, you should consult with medical control for instructions. The most prudent approach is for you to inform the person in a calm and sympathetic manner of the possible consequences of refusing treatment. Keep in mind that many people who refuse medical treatment do so out of fear and emotional distress, and the patient's distress needs to be recognized and managed in an understanding way. It is not uncommon for patients to refuse treatment and transportation to the hospital because of a concern for the costs associated with the ambulance and hospital treatment. Addressing these concerns can be challenging for you and may require all of your "people skills."

It is not appropriate for you to consider the person who refuses treatment a "bad patient" and to behave in a hostile or

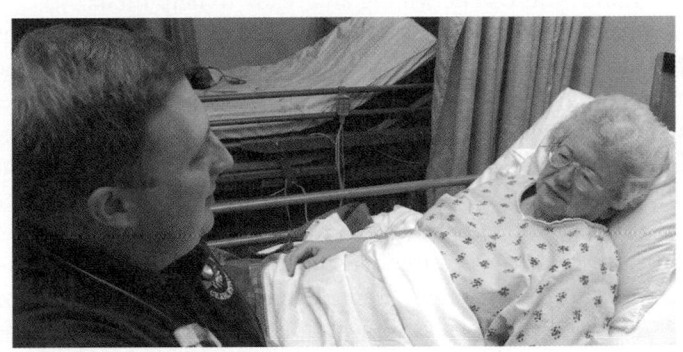

Figure 14 When a conscious patient with decision-making capacity makes a decision, you must respect that decision.

YOU are the Medic | PART 2 |

As you are led into the kitchen you see an older woman sitting at the kitchen table drinking coffee. She looks up as you walk in and starts to yell at her daughter. "I told you not to call them! I'm not going!" She is pale, frail-looking, and obviously very agitated. Her daughter tells you that her mother has had small strokes in the past as the result of a small brain tumor. She also tells you her mother does not have a do not resuscitate (DNR) order, but she does have an advance directive. She also takes medication for high blood pressure, hypothyroidism, and elevated cholesterol levels.

Recording Time: 0 Minutes	
Appearance	Pale, agitated
Level of consciousness	Appears alert
Airway	Open and clear
Breathing	Appears normal
Circulation	She is pale, but her nail beds are pink

3. What are the possible consequences of treating this patient without her consent?

4. On the basis of her history, what might be her problem?

aggressive manner toward him or her. Remember, you are at the scene to help the patient, so try to find out what is bothering the patient and why he or she is rejecting help, and always respect the patient's rights.

Consider that some patients refuse treatment as a way of denying that they have a problem—such as the middle-aged man with chest pain who refuses treatment in order to deny the possibility that he may be experiencing a heart attack. A sympathetic ear and a little reassurance on your part will often convert an unconvinced patient into someone you can help. Remember the phrase: "It never hurts to have these things checked out."

Having a patient speak with medical control by radio or telephone may be helpful at times. If the patient is still declining care after your explanation of the medical situation and the possible consequences of refusing treatment, there is not much further that you can do. However, even at that point, do not close any doors. Let patients know that, should they change their mind, you will be willing and ready to help them.

Maintain a courteous, sympathetic attitude. Let patients know that your chief concern is their well-being, and tell them that it is all right to change their mind. Urge patients to seek further medical evaluation from the physician of their choice. Help them make concrete plans for follow-up. Some patients will consent to transport but not consent to treatment; others may consent to treatment but refuse transport. If patients refuse transport, try to make sure that someone will be with them after you leave and always advise them to call back for help if needed.

As stated previously, your documentation of patient refusals is critically important should litigation arise in which the patient claims you committed abandonment. Document all findings of your assessment and mental status examination carefully, including the patient's history, the patient's stated reasons for refusing care, and all instructions and explanations given to the patient. Note how much time you spent attempting to provide care. The report should be signed by the patient and by an impartial observer (eg, a police officer, if available). The purpose of a witness/observer is to hear the exchange of the information, not just to sign a piece of paper with his or her name. Soliciting for signatures from others at the scene who may not have been paying attention to your conversation or the information exchanged with the patient may pose legal issues.

Prehospital refusal forms may look like the answer to documentation of a particularly difficult refusal problem you are encountering, but the forms must be backed up with action. Legally, you must have undertaken the process of attempting to obtain informed consent to treat the patient. Just because a patient has signed a refusal form does not mean that the patient has given you an informed refusal. You must have informed the patient of what you propose to do to care for him or her, and the potential risks of refusing that care, and provide that information in a manner he or she is capable of understanding.

It is often frustrating and difficult for the paramedic, like any other health care provider, to accept the fact that a patient may refuse all or part of care. However, it is important to respect a patient's rights, regardless of whether it is contrary to your beliefs or what you think you should be doing. Courts have upheld patient refusals when paramedics carefully documented a patient's decision-making capacity, and their explanation of the possible consequences of refusing care.

A problem sometimes arises in determining whether a person who refuses care or transport to a hospital has decision-making capacity. For example, you are called to help a patient who has had a seizure in a retail store. By the time you arrive, the seizure is over, and the patient is conscious. The patient says she is all right, and she refuses to go to the hospital. You smell alcohol on her breath. Does that patient possess the decision-making capacity to refuse treatment? To make that determination, you need to spend some time evaluating the patient. You should explain to her, "I cannot let you go until I have checked you over and until you talk to me enough to convince me that you are okay and that you understand your situation."

In general, any patient with an altered mental status or unstable vital signs probably cannot be considered able to refuse transport to the hospital. The paramedic must become proficient in quickly establishing whether a patient has decision-making capacity. The criteria for determining mental competence should be spelled out in detail in the protocols of every ambulance service. As a rule, such criteria will include the following:

- The patient is oriented to person, place, and day.
- The patient responds to questions appropriately.
- There is no significant mental impairment from alcohol, drugs, head injury, or other organic illness. (Ask family members, if present, whether the patient is behaving the way he or she normally does.) What constitutes significant mental impairment is a subjective judgment call.
- The patient demonstrates to you that he or she understands the nature of his or her condition and the risks of not going to the hospital for immediate care. This demonstration can take place only after the patient's condition and the risks of refusal have been thoroughly explained to the patient.
- The patient can describe a reasonable plan for follow-up care.
  - Oxygen saturation levels are within normal limits.
  - Blood glucose levels are within normal limits **Figure 15**.
  - The patient does not appear to have serious, distracting injuries that might impair rational decision making.

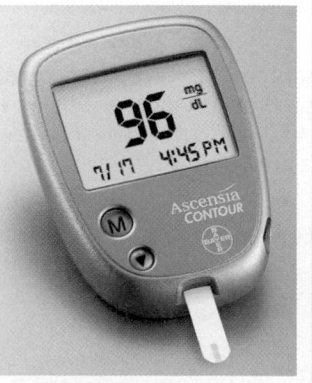

Figure 15 Remember that a patient's decision-making ability can be affected by the intake of alcohol or drugs, and by abnormal blood glucose or oxygen saturation levels.

When patients have a potentially life-threatening illness or injury and there is any doubt as to their decision-making capacity, it is always preferable to transport them to the hospital, even if it is against their will. The decision to allow a potentially impaired patient to refuse treatment is a medical decision, requiring judgment and experience. That decision is best made by a physician in the hospital, not by a paramedic on the street.

Some states have enacted emergency transportation statutes that permit EMS personnel to transport patients against their will under narrow circumstances. These statutes are designed to protect paramedics who make a good faith judgment that patients cannot make an informed decision because they do not have decision-making capacity. In 1993, New Mexico passed a law that permits transport without consent if the following criteria are met:

- There is online medical control.
- The provider is certified to at least the EMT level.
- The provider has made a good faith judgment.
- The patient is incapable of making an informed decision.
- The patient is reasonably likely to experience death or disability without medical intervention.

Psychiatric emergencies present particularly vexing problems of consent. When a person's life is not in danger, a police officer is generally the only person given the authority to restrain and transport that person against his or her will. An EMS system should not do so except at the express request of the police. Notably, neither a physician nor the patient's family may authorize such transport in most regions; they may authorize involuntary commitment, but their authority does not extend to the forcible transport of a patient against his or her will. Therefore, it is essential for every EMS service to establish protocols, based on local laws, for dealing with the mentally disturbed patient who refuses transport. In many instances, the participation of the police will be required, and the role of each agency involved should be clearly defined beforehand.

Controversies

The potential legal consequences of using reasonable force to bring a patient to the hospital (false imprisonment) are far less serious than the consequences—legal and medical—of a bad outcome (wrongful death or malpractice) if a patient in need of care is released at the scene. It is always preferable for you to err on the side of transporting a patient, but in all cases, consult with online medical control first.

■ Minors

Minors present special issues for the paramedic. Because minors have no legal status, they can neither refuse nor consent to medical care. In the case of children and adults who have legal guardians, consent must be obtained, if possible, from a parent or legal guardian of the patient. If the parent or guardian is not available, emergency treatment to sustain life may be undertaken without direct consent under the doctrine of implied consent. You should also be aware of the legal principle known as **in loco parentis**. This term literally means "in the place of the parent." This principle may apply in school, day care, or summer camp situations if a parent is unavailable. The school administrator or day care director may make treatment and transportation decisions on behalf of the minor.

A particularly difficult circumstance can arise if a parent or legal guardian refuses to grant consent to treat a minor who clearly requires lifesaving or limb-saving treatment. Although adults clearly have the right to refuse treatment for themselves, state laws generally do not permit a parent or guardian to deny treatment to a minor child. In fact, the failure of a parent to allow such treatment may constitute neglect. When confronted with such a circumstance, the paramedic should notify law enforcement and medical control. State law may permit the state to assume custody of the child for purposes of ensuring that necessary emergency treatment be provided.

Emancipated minors are under the legal age in a given state but can be treated as legal adults because of qualifying circumstances. Individual state law determines what circumstances qualify a minor as emancipated, although most states recognize any minor who has been emancipated by court order. Other states add criteria such as marriage, pregnancy, or active military service. Emancipated minors may be treated as adults when obtaining consent or refusal.

Special Populations

Although legislation varies in different areas, in most states, a pregnant teenager is "emancipated" during her pregnancy and can make all legal and medical decisions for herself and her unborn baby. However, the minute she delivers the baby, she once again assumes "minor" status, and her parents or legal guardians make all of her medical and legal decisions. She does, however, remain the legal guardian for her baby and can make all medical and legal decisions for her child (even though she cannot make them for herself).

Overall, obtaining consent for medical treatment may be one of the more difficult skills to acquire as a new paramedic; however, you will find that your expertise will build over time. A patient or even a child's guardian may not want you to assess and treat for a variety of reasons **Figure 16**. Therefore, keep in mind that as a patient advocate, you must anticipate potential problems for obtaining permission and be prepared to discuss the need for care.

Words of Wisdom

You should never tell patients that you are going to do a procedure. Instead, ask them if you can perform the procedure and explain to them why they need it.

■ Violent Patients and Restraints

The use of force by paramedics against patients has been the cause of numerous lawsuits in recent years. However, in the reality of today's EMS practice, you will encounter violent patients who must be restrained in order to protect the patients themselves and to protect those who are trying to care for them.

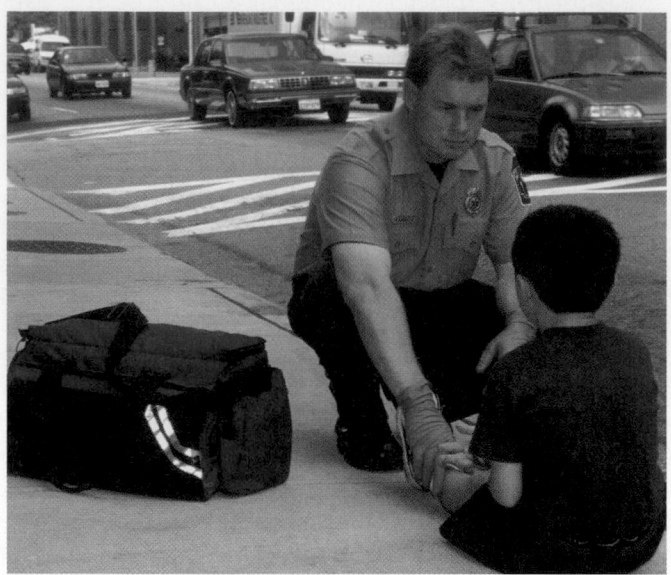

Figure 16 When you are dealing with a young child, explain to him or her the need for treatment, and consult his or her parent or guardian.

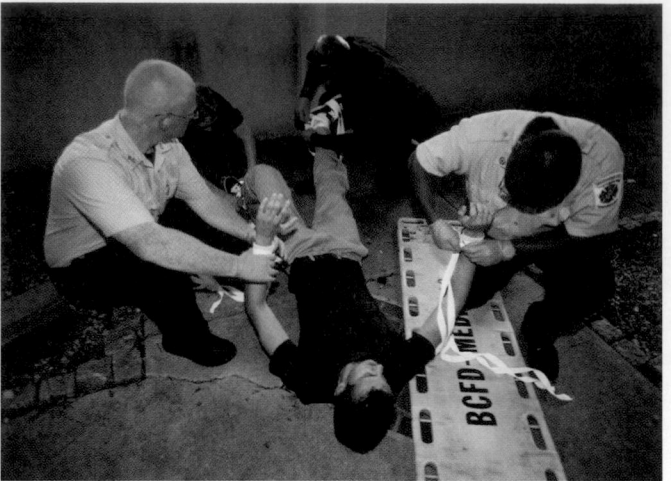

Figure 17 You should use restraint only when absolutely necessary to ensure your own safety and that of the patient. Remember that it will most likely take several strong people to fully restrain a patient.

Under the law, you can use force only in response to a patient's use of force against you. If you are attacked, you may defend yourself against the attack. However, the use of temporary disabling sprays, knives, or firearms are generally outside the scope of the paramedic's practice and are usually prohibited by the EMS agency. The amount of force that you are allowed to use under the law is either equal to or slightly greater than the force offered by the patient, and must be in response to the patient's actions. Violence against EMS providers is on the rise. For your own personal safety, do not enter a scene that is unsafe until law enforcement personnel can secure the scene and make it safe for you to enter.

In situations requiring patient restraint for medical reasons, it is important to understand that you may restrain patients only when the patients are a danger to themselves or to others **Figure 17**. Violence can be the result of hypoxia, hypoglycemia, mental illness, brain injury, drug abuse or overdose, alcohol, or a variety of other underlying medical and psychiatric causes. Specific medical protocols should cover what is considered appropriate in your EMS system for restraining patients, and should spell out what medications or devices are allowed for use in restraining patients. Many EMS systems now use medications (ie, chemical restraints), such as benzodiazepines or antipsychotics, to calm patients who are violent and need transportation to a hospital to discover the underlying medical or psychiatric cause of their outbursts.

■ Triage and Allocation of Resources

Resources of personnel and equipment most often become limited when an event occurs that creates a significant number of injured people. **Triage** is the process of establishing treatment priorities among the injured in order to best allocate the available resources to provide care to the most people. EMS services generally follow well-established triage protocols that have

been in use throughout the United States and other countries for many years. In some circumstances, the number of injured people requiring medical attention will exceed the number of medical personnel or equipment available to provide treatment. These situations, which may include natural disasters and terrorist acts, can present serious triage challenges to the paramedic.

Paramedics sometimes face ethical conflict regarding the allocation of limited resources during triage situations. For example, would you give special consideration to an injured person whom you knew personally? Would you be more likely to provide prompt care for an innocent incident victim while delaying care to the more seriously injured intoxicated driver who caused the incident? Would you be able to apply triage protocols objectively to a person who is abusive toward you? Could any bias you may have toward people of a certain race, religion, or nationality be set aside? These are among the ethical challenges that may confront you as a paramedic when performing triage. Triage requires you to be professional and ethical in every respect because decisions made during triage can affect life and death.

■ Negligence and Protection Against Negligence Claims

Unless there is some type of immunity, nothing can protect the paramedic from liability for gross **negligence**, a serious charge. Negligence occurs when a series of events happens:

1. The paramedic—or, in some cases, the EMS system—had a legal duty to the patient. For example, a paramedic hired to serve a community has a legal duty to the citizens of that community.
2. There was a breach of duty; that is, the person accused of negligence failed to act as another person with similar training would have acted under the same or similar

circumstances. Breach of duty may involve doing less than the person was trained to do (an error of omission; ie, a paramedic who fails to splint an injured extremity) or doing more than the person was trained to do (an error of commission; ie, a paramedic who sutures a laceration if doing so is not within the scope of practice).

3. The failure to act appropriately was the proximate cause (the first event in a chain of events) of the plaintiff's injury.
4. Harm resulted.

Paramedics and the EMS systems in which they work are protected from liability as long as they perform according to the standards for paramedics and EMS systems. Your best protection is to behave in all circumstances according to established procedures and standards set by national agencies, such as the guidelines for ambulance design and equipment from the National Highway Traffic Safety Administration (NHTSA). Although those standards are not law, they can be introduced as evidence in litigation and may affect the outcome of a lawsuit. It is therefore in your best interest to make sure that your vehicle is maintained in optimal condition and equipped according to prevailing standards.

Paramedics frequently ask if they should obtain their own insurance coverage despite the fact that they generally will be covered by the insurance provided by their employers. Although the insurance carried by your employer will generally cover you in any situation related to your employment, having additional insurance is often a good idea. Having your own liability policy will provide you with protection in several possible circumstances:

- If your employer's insurance carrier is required to pay out on a claim based on wrongdoing for which you are responsible, it is possible (though rare) that it will try to recover against you personally.
- If you are sued as a result of having provided off-duty emergency assistance.
- If you are an instructor teaching EMS-related classes outside the scope of your employment and are sued by a student or other party.

Insurance of this type is generally reasonably priced and may be a wise investment.

One aspect of negligence is whether there is "foreseeability." This concept implies that the injury, or harm, could have been predicted and therefore avoided if the proper precautions had been taken. For example, giving an incorrect dosage of a drug will foreseeably result in harm to a patient, just as running a red light while en route to a call may foreseeably result in a crash.

Negligence is commonly divided into three categories: malfeasance, misfeasance, and nonfeasance. **Malfeasance** occurs when a paramedic performs an act that he or she was never authorized to do, such as a medical intervention that is outside of the scope of practice. **Misfeasance** occurs when a paramedic performs an act that he or she is legally permitted to do but does so in an improper manner. For example, a paramedic administers a medication that is clearly within the scope of practice but accidentally calculates an incorrect dose. **Nonfeasance** occurs when the paramedic fails to perform an act that he or she is required or expected to perform. Failure to perform CPR when a patient goes into cardiac arrest would be an example of nonfeasance.

■ Elements of Negligence

Duty

Duty is prescribed by the law: it is what you, as an EMS provider, must do and how you must do it. Without question, your first duty as an EMS provider is to do no further harm to a patient.

The first element of negligence a patient must prove for a lawsuit to be successful is that of **duty**. The definitive *Black's Law Dictionary* defines duty relevant to medical negligence as "an obligation, to which law will give recognition and effect; to conform to a particular standard of conduct toward another." *Black's Law Dictionary* also states that if a person fails to perform according to that standard, "he becomes subject to liability to the person to whom the duty is owed for any injury sustained by that person of which the conduct is the legal cause."

Much confusion surrounds the concept of legal duty in EMS. For example, many paramedics think that they have a legal obligation to stop at roadside crashes simply because they are paramedics. However, in all but a few states, this is not the case. Although a paramedic may feel an ethical obligation to stop and assist, the law in most states does not require it. A paramedic is obligated to respond to calls when working a shift or while volunteering for a squad. Most services have a policy addressing the passing by another incident while en route to a call or en route to the hospital with a patient. The key is to make sure the appropriate personnel are dispatched if you cannot actually stop to render assistance due to the severity of the patient you are actually treating.

Another misconception is the idea that if you put a sticker that says "paramedic" on your vehicle, this somehow invokes a legal responsibility to stop at all emergencies. This is not true Figure 18 . However, the paramedic does have a legal duty to perform within the standard of care if a decision is made to stop and provide assistance. In addition, there is a further legal duty not to abandon the patient once treatment has begun. It is

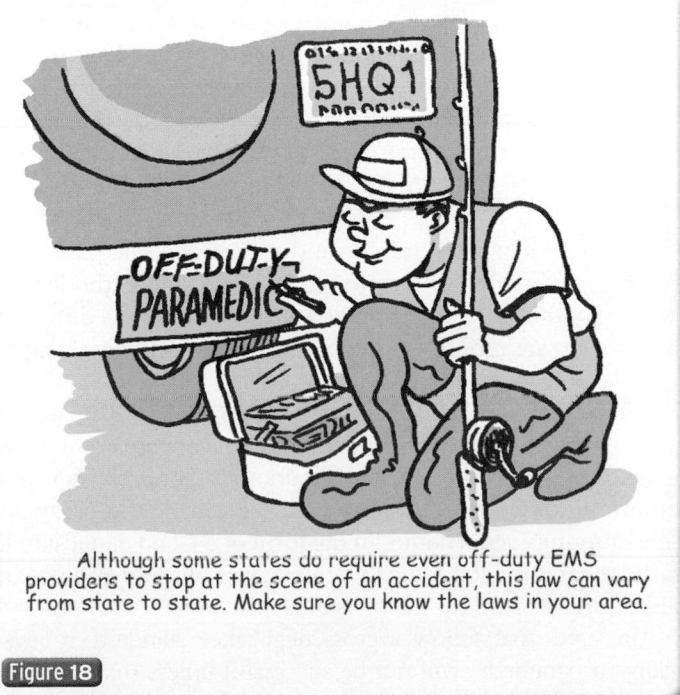

Although some states do require even off-duty EMS providers to stop at the scene of an accident, this law can vary from state to state. Make sure you know the laws in your area.

Figure 18

important to know what your legal obligations are when you are off duty. Find out what your state laws are, and educate your peers regarding these off-duty obligations.

The concept of duty extends to maintaining licensure or certification, attending continuing education courses, and maintaining your skills. Maintaining your health and psychological well-being so that you will be prepared for the rigors of prehospital patient care is essential. In addition, you have a duty to check your equipment at the beginning of each shift and ensure that all equipment is functioning properly. Finally, you have a duty to honor your patient's rights to privacy and their rights to refuse or limit the care you provide.

EMS agencies—and even entire EMS systems—can be held to a legal duty. EMS agencies have a duty to respond to calls for aid and to use mutual aid resources appropriately if call volume is too heavy to allow response within an appropriate time frame. Some EMS agencies may operate with contracts that specify legal duties, such as minimum response times.

Legal duty is a concept in the law that tells you what your standards of practice are. It is an unpredictable legal concept, often defined in the context of a case tried in a court of law. But the concept of legal duty is used by attorneys defending EMS providers. For example, in a lawsuit against an off-duty paramedic who stopped at a crash to render aid, the paramedic's attorney may attempt to show that the paramedic had no duty to the patient, but instead provided assistance he or she was not required by law to provide.

Remember, attorneys are often trained to work from the most general defense to the most specific elements of the case. Lack of legal duty is a general defense; however general it is, it may still be true.

Breach of Duty

The second element a patient must prove for a lawsuit to be successful is that the paramedic failed to perform within the **standard of care**. The standard of care is what a reasonable paramedic, in the same or similar situation, would have done. In a lawsuit, a jury will listen to the testimony of expert witnesses on both sides and ultimately decide whether the paramedic's care was reasonable or not. These expert witnesses will provide a number of sources on which to base their testimony about whether the paramedic's care was reasonable. Those sources will include their own training and experience; the paramedic's training, experience, and continuing education; textbooks; protocols; national standards; standard operating procedures; and the patient care report. Good documentation will go a long way to prove your high standards of care.

Some states differentiate between **ordinary negligence** and **gross negligence**. How high a standard of care a paramedic will be held to varies from one state to another. Some states provide immunity for all but the poorest care given by the paramedic. This immunity often comes in the form of a Good Samaritan law in those cases in which the paramedic was off duty and no compensation was paid for the assistance provided.

In states that follow a gross negligence standard, a lawsuit against a paramedic will not be successful unless that paramedic has seriously departed from the accepted standards. Actions

are grossly negligent if they are found to be willful or wanton (malicious) under the law. This is a difficult standard for a plaintiff to meet. Usually, either intentional conduct or recklessness is essential to a finding of willful or wanton conduct. For example, Ohio has defined willful and wanton misconduct as "the intent, purpose, or design to injure another" or "an intentional disregard of a clear duty or definite rule of conduct; a purpose not to discharge that duty; or the performance of wrongful acts with the knowledge of the likelihood of resulting injury." Other states have defined it as "reckless disregard," "utter indifference," or "conscious disregard" for the safety of others. If the paramedic can convince the jury that he or she acted in good faith, the paramedic will usually be acquitted (relieved from the charge) of gross negligence.

In other states, a plaintiff will only have to show ordinary negligence, which can be a failure to act or a simple mistake that causes harm to a patient. It is much easier for a plaintiff to prove negligence under the ordinary negligence standard.

In certain circumstances, a special theory of negligence known as **res ipsa loquitur** may apply even though the plaintiff is unable to demonstrate clearly the exact manner by which an injury occurred. *Res ipsa loquitur* means "the thing speaks for itself." Under this theory, you could be held liable upon a showing that the plaintiff was injured, that the instrumentality causing the injury was in your control, and that such injuries do not ordinarily occur unless there is negligence. For example, you and your partner are called to the home of a patient who lost consciousness as a result of an apparent drug overdose. While loading the patient into the ambulance, your partner slips, causing the stretcher to tip over; the patient strikes the ground and sustains a large laceration to his head. The patient later sues for negligence. Because the patient was unconscious at the time of the incident, he is unable to describe how the fall took place. Under the doctrine of *res ipsa loquitur*, the patient can prevail in his lawsuit by showing that he was under your care, that he sustained an injury, and that his injury would not have occurred unless there was negligence.

You should be aware of another type of negligence known as **negligence per se**. The principle of negligence per se is generally applied in those circumstances in which a paramedic inexcusably violates a statute. An example might be when a paramedic treats a patient even though his or her license is expired. A finding that a statute has been violated can sometimes lead to an automatic finding of negligence.

Proximate Cause

Even in cases in which the paramedic had a legal duty to the patient, and the paramedic breached the standard of care, a plaintiff must still link the act that fell below the standard of care directly to his or her injury by showing that the act (or failure to act) proximately caused the harm. *Black's Law Dictionary* defines **proximate cause** as "that which, in a natural and continuous sequence, unbroken by any intervening cause, produces injury, and without which the result would not have occurred." Simply stated, a plaintiff will have to prove that the paramedic's improper action, or failure to act, was the cause of the injury.

Failure to secure a patient on a backboard can be the proximate cause of severing the spinal cord. Proving that an act or a failure to act caused an injury is the most difficult part of a lawsuit to prove. For example, paramedics are treating a patient from a car crash who has a spinal cord injury and the paramedics drop the stretcher during patient care. The patient may try to show that his or her injury resulted from the dropped stretcher and not from the crash itself. Careful documentation of the patient's neurologic status at the time the paramedics first encounter the patient will be essential to their defense.

Harm

The final element plaintiffs must prove in a negligence lawsuit is that they were harmed. Although physical injury is usually part of any lawsuit for medical negligence, patients also may claim damages for emotional distress, loss of income, loss of enjoyment of life, loss of spousal consortium, loss of household services, and loss of future earning capacity. They will have to show that the paramedic's actions were proximate causes of each of these losses.

Abandonment

Abandonment is a form of negligence that involves the termination of care without the patient's consent. The term also implies that the patient had a continuing need for medical treatment and that the abrupt termination of treatment was the cause of subsequent injury or death. Therefore, once you have responded to an emergency, you may not leave a patient in need of medical treatment until another competent health care professional with an equal or higher level of training has taken responsibility for that patient's care. You must notify an appropriate health care professional of the patient's presence in the ED, and that you are transferring responsibility for care to that person.

It is also important that you complete a written report, which is often submitted electronically and frequently arrives after the call. It is important that the emergency department physician or nurse who is taking over care of your patient receive this report. The written report will permit the emergency department physician and staff to review what your findings were in the field, what medications you gave the patient, and what procedures you performed.

There are some situations that may not require transport but are not considered abandonment. EMS systems frequently receive calls for service for patients who may not really need treatment or transportation. A patient may have fallen and needs help getting up from the floor or may want your help administering his medication. Or, a patient who has a legitimate medical emergency, such as hypoglycemia, may feel fine after treatment and may not require transport to a hospital. Your local medical director should provide protocols for these situations. However, in general, it is a good idea to encourage transport.

In addition, some ambulance services, particularly in rural areas, may have a mix of providers of various levels of training and may not have a full staff of paramedics at all times. In those areas, even if a paramedic makes the initial response, the paramedic may not need to be part of the transport crew if the patient does not need advanced care. If in doubt, contact your medical control.

Many EMS systems provide a tiered response, with basic life support (BLS) providers reaching the patient quickly, followed by advanced life support (ALS) providers. If a BLS crew responds and makes an improper determination that a patient does not need ALS care, the system may be exposed to liability. Your service needs to work with every provider involved to set up protocols that provide guidance for the situations in which a BLS crew may cancel an incoming ALS crew.

■ Patient Autonomy

It is well established fact that patients have the right to direct their own care and to decide how they want their end-of-life medical care provided to them. This right, known as patient autonomy, has come to the forefront of medical ethics. In almost every case, except where the patient is a minor or lacks decision-making capacity, you must respect and honor the patient's right to make medical decisions, however irrational or unsound those decisions may appear.

Because medical technology has made the line between life and death more imprecise, a number of high-profile cases have brought the issue of patient autonomy to the forefront of the medical ethics debate in the past 20 years. Most recently, the Terri Schiavo case demonstrated that courts will ultimately support the right of a patient, or the patient's closest relative, to make end-of-life decisions **Figure 19**. Unfortunately Terri Schiavo did not leave written advance directives, which ultimately put the case in the hands of the courts (state and federal).

Patients' decisions may not be accepted by other members of the public or other members of the patient's family, but it is important for you to remember that our courts, including the United States Supreme Court, have clearly recognized the right of persons to make decisions about their own medical care, even if that decision will bring about the patient's death. Ethics has become the subject of many paramedic discussions because paramedics find themselves in the unique position of being accountable to more systems than the average health care provider in trying to respect the wishes of the patient **Figure 20**. The EMS system, your

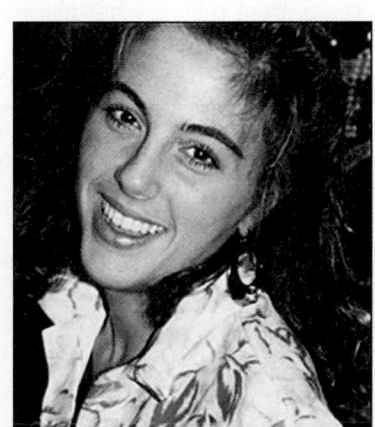

Figure 19 Because Terri Schiavo did not leave any directive about the type of care she wanted to receive, her case became a battleground between family members who held different viewpoints about care of the terminally ill.

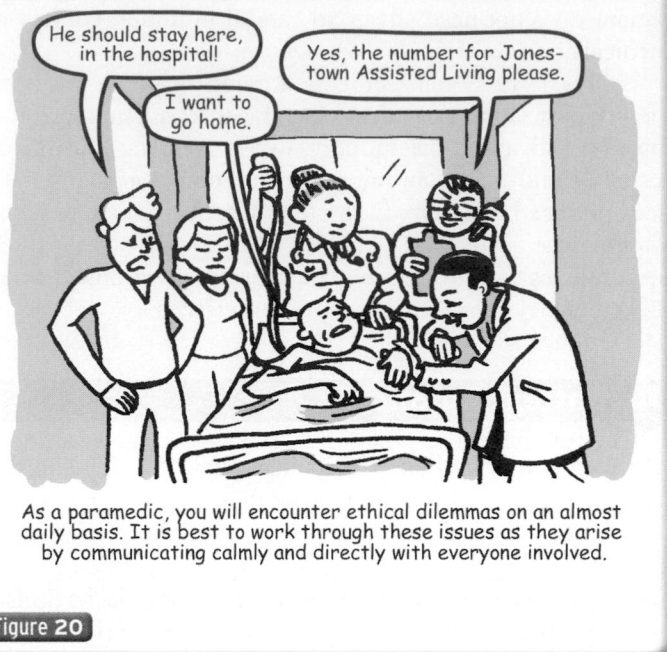

As a paramedic, you will encounter ethical dilemmas on an almost daily basis. It is best to work through these issues as they arise by communicating calmly and directly with everyone involved.

Figure 20

of the patient. These competing interests can create an ethical conflict that you will need to resolve through communication with all parties involved.

Occasionally, a physician will give an order that you feel is detrimental to the patient's best interests. It is important for you to immediately discuss with the physician why you feel that way. Remember, you are often in a better position to see what is going on with the patient, and a big part of your job is to communicate fully with the physician. A paramedic should never perform a procedure or administer a medication that he or she believes will be detrimental to the patient. For example, if a physician asks you to perform a procedure in which you are not trained or asks you to administer a medication in a dose that is well outside the range of your protocols, it is essential to obtain clarification from the physician and communicate your objections. You could discuss your current standing orders and offer a feasible alternative within your scope of practice, or you could request that the physician speak with your medical director. In all circumstances, act in the patient's best interest as his or her advocate.

A situation that is much more common is the necessity of treating patients against their wishes. This is generally permissible only in those situations in which the patient lacks decision-making capacity and consent is implied. If your patient is, for example, a man who does not want to admit he is having a myocardial

medical director, the EMS service for which you work, and your community's standard of care can compete with the wishes

YOU are the Medic   PART 3

The patient's daughter brings you a list of her mother's medications and you quickly review it—Coreg, Lisinopril, Synthroid, and Zocor. She also hands you a copy of the advance directive that states the patient wishes no heroic measures be taken if she is not breathing and does not have a pulse.

The patient tells you her name is Mary, but cannot tell you what day of the week it is or how old she is. She agrees to let you take her vital signs, but still says she will not go to the hospital. Measurement of her blood glucose level shows a reading of 138 mg/dL.

Her daughter tells you that her mother's symptoms have been going on for several days, but today she is worse. She keeps forgetting basic things and is now refusing to eat. She thinks her mother might be having "ministrokes" and her confusion is getting worse.

Recording Time: 4 Minutes	
Respirations	20 breaths/min, regular
Pulse	108 beats/min, strong radials
Skin	Cool and dry
Blood pressure	152/98 mm Hg
Oxygen saturation (Spo$_2$)	97% on room air
Pupils	Equal and reactive to light

5. Would it be considered abandonment if you left at this point?

6. Does her advance directive take precedence over her wishes?

infarction, you must use your best diplomatic negotiating skills, coupled with your medical knowledge, to persuade him to allow treatment and transport to the hospital **Figure 21**. These situations should be covered in protocols and discussed regularly and in detail with your medical director. Involve the patient's family, your supervisor, and medical control in obtaining the best care for your patient.

■ Advance Directives

An <u>advance directive</u> is usually a written document (but can also be an oral statement) that expresses the wants, needs, and desires of a patient in reference to his or her future medical care. Advance directives state what medical care the patient wants or does not want when the patient is unable to express his or her wishes. Living wills, do not resuscitate (DNR) orders, and organ donation orders are all advance directives.

Paramedics need to be aware that advance directives differ from state to state. In some states, a DNR order (also known as a resuscitation directive) may restrict any ALS care, whereas others provide for comfort care, including pain medications and oxygen therapy. In Colorado, a person designated as the medical durable power of attorney can revoke a resuscitation directive. However, in Montana, the patient or physician is the only one who can revoke a resuscitation directive. Because of these differences, you must know your own local and state protocols and regulations.

Whether EMS personnel are bound by advance directives is a function of state law—and such laws, like those that cover DNR orders, are usually strict, often limited to terminal patients in nursing homes or hospice care. Learning and following the laws of your state will provide a framework for decisions regarding advance directives.

Living Will and Health Care Power of Attorney

The <u>living will</u> and the <u>health care power of attorney</u> are types of advance directives in which a patient can express wishes regarding end-of-life medical care. These directives are sometimes called health care "durable" powers of attorney because they remain in effect once a patient loses decision-making capacity. The issue of dealing with powers of attorney can sometimes be confusing. First of all, you should be aware that there are various types of powers of attorney and not all of them authorize the designated agent to make decisions regarding health care. Elderly patients commonly execute powers of attorney that enable others to conduct financial affairs on their behalf and which have no effect on health care whatsoever. It is also possible that a power of attorney may have been executed outside the state in which the patient now resides and its effect within your state may be questionable. As a paramedic, you should ask to see the power of attorney and you should carefully review it to determine whether it authorizes the agent to make health care decisions. When you are in doubt, contact medical control for assistance.

Living wills generally require some kind of precondition to activate, such as a terminal illness or an irreversible coma. The living will should spell out exactly what kind of treatment a patient wishes to be given should he or she become incapacitated. A living will often contains a health care power of attorney, which designates another person (eg, a spouse, partner, adult sibling, or parent) to make health care decisions for the patient at any time the patient is unable to make those decisions. The person designated to make decisions does not have to be a relative, but may be someone close to the patient who understands his or her wishes. In those cases where the living will does not contain a health care power of attorney, its use in the field will be limited and once again, you should consult medical control.

The person who carries the health care power of attorney is often called the <u>surrogate decision maker</u> **Figure 22**. The surrogate decision maker is legally obligated to make decisions as the patient would want, and has presumably discussed these decisions with the patient. It is important to bear in mind that the surrogate decision maker has no authority until the patient

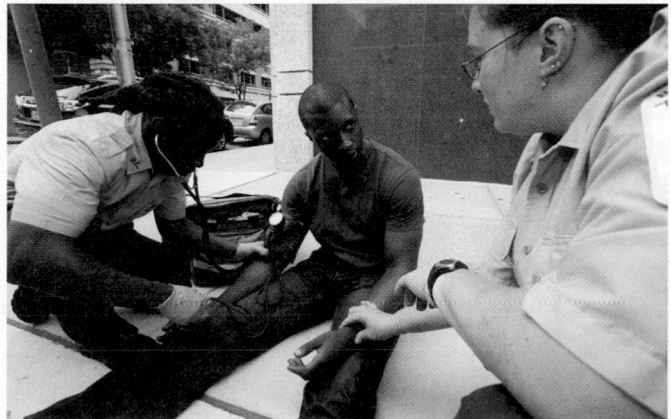

Figure 21 Remember that the decision to accept medical treatment is a difficult one. Give the patient time to think and to consider what feels right. Often, this is the first time the patient has had to face the reality of his or her medical condition.

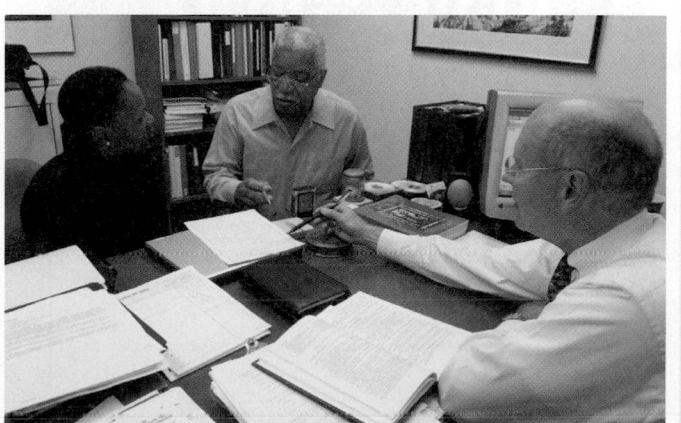

Figure 22 A surrogate decision maker (often a child or other close relative) is frequently designated when a person draws up a living will.

becomes incapable of making decisions. If you arrive on scene and find that a surrogate decision maker is attempting to make decisions that conflict with a competent patient's decisions, the patient's decisions are always the ones to be followed.

If you are unsure of the time of a cardiac arrest, begin care and immediately contact medical control to discuss termination of the resuscitative effort.

Words of Wisdom

Do not be confused: A living will is not the same as a DNR order. The living will allows for decisions to be made regarding DNR orders if a patient becomes incapacitated or unable to make his or her own decisions.

DNR Orders

A **do not resuscitate (DNR) order** (also referred to as *do not attempt resuscitation [DNAR]*) is an advance directive that describes which life-sustaining procedures, if any, should be performed if a patient's medical condition suddenly deteriorates. During the last 20 years, DNR orders were finally recognized in the prehospital setting **Figure 23**. EMS has now joined the medical community in recognizing that patients have the same rights to direct and refuse care outside the hospital that they do inside the hospital. Many states now have DNR forms specific to EMS, and most states have laws that govern the process of dying and what rights patients have to direct that process.

States have their own procedure for how to recognize a valid DNR order. Some states rely on a written physician order (which might not be available to the EMS provider), while others may require the patient to wear a bracelet or necklace. In some cases, such jewelry indicates that the patient has consented to the release of stored information, such as the patient's DNR status, to medical personnel **Figure 24**. In some states, DNR orders expire within a specified time frame and must be renewed to remain

valid, whereas others may have no expiration date. It may also be a requirement that the DNR order be executed within your state by a physician licensed to practice medicine within the state. You should be familiar with the documents used in your state and what you are expected to do if the documents are not available.

Although laws might differ from state to state, generally speaking, DNR orders must meet the following requirements to be valid:

- Clearly state the patient's medical problem(s)
- Signature of the patient or legal guardian
- Signature of one or more physicians
- In some states, DNR orders contain expiration dates, whereas in others, no expiration date is included. DNR orders with expiration dates must be dated in the preceding 12 months to be valid.

However, even in the presence of a DNR order, you are still obligated to provide supportive measures (oxygen, pain relief, and comfort) to a patient who is not in cardiac arrest, whenever possible. Each ambulance service, in consultation with its medical director and legal counsel, must develop a protocol to follow in these circumstances.

Withholding or Withdrawing Resuscitation

Current bioethical guidelines rely on the use of common sense and reasonable judgment in deciding when to stop CPR and resuscitation efforts, or to decline to initiate them at all. Numerous medical studies have shown that resuscitation of medical as well as trauma patients is sometimes futile at the onset or may become futile at some point. Futile resuscitation efforts—interventions that studies have shown do not benefit patients—are not medically or ethically indicated **Figure 25**.

Paramedics, especially those working in rural and wilderness situations, will need to consider the time it will take for a patient to reach definitive care at the hospital and the likelihood of survival. Occasionally you will hear a story about a patient who has recovered from what appeared to be a hopeless situation, providing motivation for you to attempt to save a patient under the most impossible circumstances. You must remember that rare survival cases should not be the guide to your decisions about

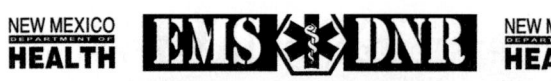

Figure 23 Do not resuscitate (DNR) orders can apply for a patient before he or she is taken to a hospital. Make sure you are familiar with the specific legalities of DNR orders in your area.

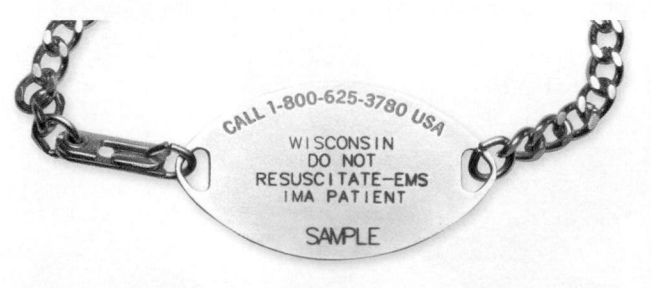

Figure 24 Medical identification bracelets can provide access to vital information about a patient, including important medical conditions and possible DNR orders. In the case of MedicAlert®, the EMS provider can obtain stored patient information from the MedicAlert Foundation.

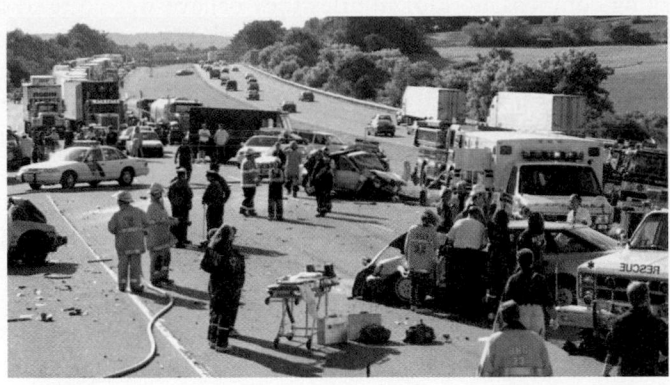

Figure 25 Although your instincts are always to try to sustain life at whatever cost, sometimes it is clear that resuscitation efforts will be futile, and should be withheld per local protocols.

resuscitation efforts, even though terminating lifesaving efforts in the field seems contrary to the instincts of health care providers.

Your focus should be to provide approximately 15 minutes of the best available method of resuscitation. If spontaneous circulation does not return within that time or no extenuating medical circumstances (eg, overdose, submersion, hypothermia) exist for the patient, termination of the resuscitation should be considered. Of course, written protocols should be followed.

Each state has different laws that may define the role of the paramedic in resuscitation issues. In some states, a paramedic may be able to "pronounce" death, while in other states only a medical investigator or physician may do so. State laws continue to govern your practice even if the patient is clinically deceased. Some of these laws include guidelines concerning situations in which even the most basic life support measures are inappropriate. For example, resuscitation should not be attempted on patients who are obviously dead (eg, livor/rigor mortis or putrefaction), or who have injuries incompatible with life (eg, decapitation). If resuscitation has already begun, cessation of these efforts in the field may be appropriate in cases of blunt trauma arrest, a prolonged rescue or response time, or other lengthy medical resuscitation efforts.

The decision to halt resuscitation is particularly difficult and emotional when you are caring for a pediatric patient. Studies have shown that paramedics feel particularly uncomfortable about terminating resuscitation in children. Paramedics and other medical professionals tend to be action-oriented people who feel that they must "do something" (as part of their moral code). However, in some situations, you can do more for the grieving family than for the child who has died. Ethically, you should be prepared to support the family, which can be the hardest part of the job.

Training, literature reviews, and open discussions about what actions are medically appropriate within EMS protocols should provide you guidance and ease concerns about difficult resuscitation situations. Continuing education regarding resuscitation issues may provide alternative viewpoints and a broader picture that allow you to make appropriate decisions in the field.

Acquire a thorough understanding of the basic consequences of typical EMS interventions. Ultimately, medical interventions and lifesaving attempts may prolong suffering or fail to return a patient to a meaningful life. When in doubt, do not hesitate to consult medical control. If communication is hindered because of terrain or wilderness conditions, your judgment will benefit from knowing about interventions and consequences of those interventions ahead of time.

End-of-Life Decisions

You will often deal with patients at the very end of their lives. These patients and their families should be treated with the utmost respect and empathy. You should never think: "Why did they bother to call 9-1-1 if they don't want us to do anything?" (This example represents the paramedic moral code getting in the way of the paramedic's medical ethics.) Instead, you must understand that the family of a dying patient, even one under hospice care, may not know how to check a pulse, and may not understand that difficult, agonal gasps may continue for hours before a patient actually dies. Furthermore, a loved one, despite knowing that death is near, will call for an ambulance, not knowing what else to do at the moment of death. Many people have never been with someone at the moment of death. If information and support is what they need, provide it—it is part of your job.

You should also remember to avoid imposing your own moral code on a patient whose value system may be different from your own. You will encounter dying patients with varied cultural beliefs; thus, you should be prepared to respect a patient's wishes even if the patient's lifestyle or religious beliefs differ greatly from your own.

You are likely to encounter confusing scenarios when the DNR paperwork may not be immediately available. It is permissible, if not obligatory, that you begin resuscitation efforts and then discontinue them (with agreement from online medical control) if and when the paperwork is confirmed. In other situations, the paperwork may be present, but family members may disagree with the DNR order and insist that you begin resuscitation. In these situations, avoid any hostile encounters while carrying out the patient's wishes to the best of your ability. Contact medical control in confusing situations involving resuscitation questions. The medical control physician can be a valuable resource in such circumstances.

Medical Orders for Life-Sustaining Treatment (MOLST)

An end-of-life document has emerged in recent years and is known as Medical Orders for Life-Sustaining Treatment (MOLST). Although similar to a DNR in many respects, the MOLST is more expansive. It is intended to be followed by all health care providers, not just EMS personnel. The DNR generally applies to patients who are in cardiac arrest whereas MOLST may apply to patients with impending pulmonary failure who are not in cardiac arrest. MOLST orders typically contain provisions that address the initiation of CPR, intubation, feeding tubes, the use of antibiotics, and **palliative care**. They apply only when the patient has lost decision-making capacity.

MOLST orders are not used in all states, and it is important that you check to see if your state has adopted such provisions.

Organ Donation

A major issue in medical ethics involves the potential for patients with mortal injuries to donate organs. Donor organs are badly needed within the medical system, with patients waiting years for a match.

Whether or not a patient should be kept alive for the sole purpose of organ donation is an issue that you should discuss with your medical director and local hospital system. The parameters for viable organs should be clearly spelled out within the individual EMS system. You should also understand the state law concerning organ donation: in many cases a patient must have witnessed informed consent, usually in writing.

In general, major organs such as the kidneys and liver are not appropriate for organ donation after prolonged hypotension or CPR. However, other tissue such as the corneas and skin may be valuable. Many states have programs that allow patients to agree to organ donation by making a notation on their driver's license **Figure 26** . If the patient's wishes regarding organ donation are not known, consent should be obtained from a family member before any arrangements are made to keep a patient alive solely for purposes of organ donation.

More resources that might be available to your system are workshops offered by organ transplant teams and EMS leaders as continuing education for paramedics in order to make you aware of the vital role of EMS in securing transplants.

■ Defenses to Litigation

Over the last 10 years, the media and public education have made the public more aware of what to expect from the local EMS system. If citizens perceive your response as delayed or your efforts as incompetent, they will often file lawsuits

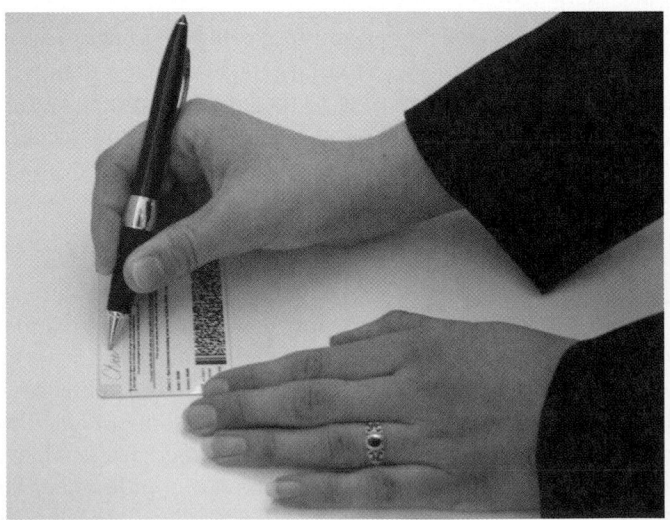

Figure 26 Most states have an organ donation form on the reverse side of the driver's license.

seeking compensation for injuries they believe were caused by inadequate EMS care. If you do not explain to your patients why you were delayed, or why a procedure is difficult, you leave yourself open to the consequences of unanswered questions that can lead a patient to seek legal action. In essence, your first defense to litigation is an open, informative, trust-based relationship with your patients. When this relationship is not possible or fails in its intent, and litigation occurs, several legal defenses may be used in the courtroom.

When a lawsuit is filed, the paramedic and the agency with which he or she is employed may implement one of two commonly used defenses: statute of limitations and contributory negligence. Every state has laws that limit the time within which a lawsuit may be filed. Such laws are called **statutes of limitations**. The time to file may be as short as 1 year in some states, whereas in other states the time may be as long as 5 or 6 years. A suit that is filed beyond these statutory periods can be dismissed as untimely. However, these statutory periods are typically extended for minors until the minor reaches the age of majority.

Another potential defense is known as **contributory negligence**. This will apply when the plaintiff has done something that contributes to his or her own injuries. For example, a paramedic encounters a patient with chest pain that appears to be cardiac in nature. Prior to administering nitroglycerin, the paramedic inquires about any recent use of erectile dysfunction medications. The patient denies the use of any such medication despite the fact that he used one of the medications several hours earlier. Shortly following the administration of nitroglycerin, the patient experiences a severe drop in blood pressure and almost dies as a result of the interaction between the nitroglycerin and erectile dysfunction medication. In the lawsuit that follows, the paramedic is able to assert the defense of contributory negligence because the patient failed to state that he had used the medication several hours earlier, and that usage clearly contributed to his adverse reaction to the nitroglycerin.

■ Good Samaritan Legislation

All but 13 states have some form of **Good Samaritan law** designed to provide **immunity** from liability to any member of the community who stops and helps at the scene of an emergency. Although the laws were initially passed to encourage the public to help at emergency scenes, many of these statutes also operate to provide some protection for EMS personnel who are off duty and assist at an emergency. The laws of most states limit the legal protection provided: the emergency care must be given free of charge (gratuitously). An EMT or paramedic providing emergency care while on duty is not, therefore, protected under Good Samaritan laws. As a general rule, if a paramedic has a legal duty to a patient, the Good Samaritan law will not protect him or her. Good Samaritan laws may help cover paramedics rendering assistance in another state, but they do not supersede the laws of the licensing agency in the paramedic's own state.

Most Good Samaritan laws also require that persons responding to an emergency do all that they can, within their knowledge, to support and sustain life and to prevent further injury. The paramedic is not expected to function as a physician;

but the paramedic is expected to deploy those skills that any other paramedic with similar training would use under the same or similar circumstances.

Courts have not been generous in applying the Good Samaritan law during routine EMS work. Courts have been applying the concept of immunity only during emergencies.

Governmental Immunity

An abiding principle of English law is that you cannot sue the queen (or king) because "the queen can do no wrong." In the United States, this concept, called sovereign immunity, has taken the form of legislation that identifies only limited types of lawsuits that can be filed against government agencies. Paramedics working for government agencies, such as a fire department, also have some governmental immunity for their actions. The immunity statutes may also set limited time frames in which lawsuits can be filed, and may limit the amount of money a plaintiff can recover.

Qualified Immunity

Governmental immunity does not cover civil rights violations, and attorneys have begun filing lawsuits against public sector paramedics for violating the civil rights of their patients. The most common complaint occurs when EMS personnel improperly restrain a violent patient or use excessive force to restrain a patient. Civil rights suits may also be filed when a paramedic's conduct deviates so far from the standard of care that a civil rights violation is said to occur.

Paramedics who work or volunteer for public agencies (such as fire departments), who are sued by patients alleging civil rights violations, may have another type of immunity called **qualified immunity**. Under this doctrine, the paramedic is held liable only when the plaintiff can show that the paramedic violated a clearly established law of which the paramedic should have known. This kind of immunity does not apply to tort cases.

Employment Law and the Paramedic

In addition to the legal issues that arise out of your role as a paramedic providing patient care, there are a number of important laws that affect your relationship with your employer. In fact, over the course of your career as a paramedic the chances of becoming involved in a legal issue regarding your employment are probably as great, if not greater, than your chances of being sued by a patient. The relationship between employer and employee involves an ever-increasing complexity of state and federal laws and regulations with which you should have a basic understanding.

Americans With Disabilities Act

The Americans With Disabilities Act (ADA) is a federal law that was adopted to protect qualified persons with disabilities from

YOU are the Medic   PART 4

You talk to Mary and explain to her that she needs to be evaluated. She starts to cry and tells you that, "they are just sending me to that hospital to die." You convince her that this is not true and that she needs to see a doctor so that she will feel better. She reluctantly agrees to go with you and says that she has a slight headache but otherwise feels fine. You perform a stroke assessment and see no signs of deficits.

At 0752, the patient is on a stretcher in the ambulance and you are en route to the hospital. You start a 20-gauge IV line in her left antecubital fossa and draw blood. You administer normal saline at a KVO rate. She will not tolerate a nasal cannula, so you just monitor her oxygen saturation level. The cardiac monitor shows a sinus tachycardia without ectopy.

You reassess her vital signs en route and transport her to Cedar's Medical Center. You arrive at the hospital at 0804. You give a report to the receiving nurse and are back in service at 0810.

Recording Time: 14 Minutes	
Respirations	18 breaths/min, regular
Pulse	102 beats/min, strong radials
Skin	Cool and dry
Blood pressure	162/94 mm Hg
Oxygen saturation (Spo$_2$)	98% on room air
Pupils	Equal and reactive to light

7. Had the patient continued to refuse treatment and transport, what options might you have exercised?

8. Under what type of consent was this patient treated?

being discriminated against in employment. The law generally applies to all employers with a minimum of 15 employees, but state laws providing similar protection may include employers with even fewer employees. The law applies to all aspects of employment including hiring, promotions, training, salary, benefits, and termination. A common misconception about the ADA is that it requires employers to hire disabled employees who may not be qualified for the job. This, of course, is not true. To be protected by the ADA, a person must meet the following two basic qualifications:

1. He or she must have a physical or mental disability that limits one or more major life activities such as hearing, seeing, walking, or speaking; and
2. He or she must possess the basic qualifications of the job and be able to perform the essential functions of the job adequately, with or without reasonable accommodations.

An employer may not inquire about an applicant's disability or require a medical examination until after a job offer has been made. If a disabled person would be able to perform the essential functions of the job using reasonable accommodations, the employer may be required to provide and pay for the cost of these accommodations. The law does not require an employer to provide accommodations that would result in an undue hardship to the employer or to other employees.

The ADA does not require an employer to give preference to a person with a disability. It simply requires that an employer make employment decisions based on reasons that are unrelated to the disability in which the applicant or employee is capable of performing the essential functions of the job.

Title VII of the Civil Rights Act

Title VII is the section of the Civil Rights Act that prohibits discrimination in employment based on race, color, religion, gender, or national origin. In addition, this section of the law provides protection against sexual harassment in the workplace. The antidiscrimination provisions of Title VII apply to all aspects of employment including recruiting, hiring, promotions, benefits, and termination. Like the ADA, Title VII applies only to businesses with more than 15 employees.

Today it is unusual for an employer to blatantly refuse to hire or promote someone based on race, gender, religion, color, or national origin. Successful claims of discrimination often involve the identification of a discriminatory hiring pattern that develops over time and that demonstrates that a particular class of persons, such as women or African Americans, are rarely hired or promoted and are vastly under-represented in the overall workforce.

Certain hiring practices violate Title VII even when these practices appear neutral. For example, what if an employer placed a classified ad seeking to hire paramedics and stated that one of the qualifications for the job was a minimum height of 5′ 9″? Although this qualification might seem neutral with respect to gender, it would have an obvious negative impact on the ability of women to be considered for the job because only a small percentage of women would meet the minimum height requirement. The burden would be on the employer to prove that it was necessary for a paramedic to be at least 5′ 9″ to

perform the functions of the job effectively. Clearly, the employer could not meet this burden.

Sexual Harassment

Sexual harassment litigation is one of the most common claims filed under Title VII, and it has seen its share of claims in EMS. There are two types of sexual harassment claims: (1) **quid pro quo** claims in which a person in authority attempts to exchange some work-related benefit such as a raise or promotion for sexual favors; and (2) **hostile environment** claims. These are claims in which the employer or an agent of the employer either creates or allows to continue an offensive practice related to sex that makes it uncomfortable or impossible for an employee to continue working. Most sexual harassment claims fall into the category of hostile environment. There is no precise definition in the law of the types of conduct that would constitute sexual harassment, but court decisions over the years have identified a number of circumstances that can be considered harassment. These include the following:

- Sexual jokes or comments
- Display of sexually offensive photographs or other material
- Unwelcome sexual advances
- Inappropriate and unwelcome touching or kissing
- Inappropriate inquiry into an employee's sex life

All employers have an obligation to prevent sexual harassment from occurring and to investigate any and all claims of sexual harassment promptly. As part of their obligation under the law, employers should provide training in sexual harassment for all newly hired employees and for all employees on an annual basis. As an employee, you should promptly report any conduct that you feel constitutes sexual harassment to your supervisor or to the organization's human resources department.

Additional Federal Laws Dealing With Discrimination

Several other federal laws prohibit various types of discrimination in the workplace. These include the following:

1. The *Pregnancy Discrimination Act* makes it illegal to discriminate in all areas of employment based on pregnancy, childbirth, or any medical condition related to pregnancy. This law was adopted in 1978 as an amendment to Title VII. Prior to the enactment of this law, it was not uncommon for employers to refuse to hire women who were pregnant or to terminate women once they became pregnant. The law also requires employers to provide health benefits and medical leave for pregnancy and childbirth equal to those provided for other medical conditions.
2. The *Equal Pay Act of 1963* makes it illegal to pay different rates of pay to men and women if they perform equal work in the same workplace. Executives and managers are generally exempt from the provisions of the law.
3. The *Age Discrimination in Employment Act of 1967* protects persons who are 40 years of age or older from discrimination in all aspects of employment based on age. The law applies to businesses with 15 or more employees.

State Laws

Many states have also passed laws that deal with discrimination in the workplace. For the most part, these laws address the same issues covered under federal law. In some cases, these laws provide more rights than the federal laws. For example, some state laws prohibit discrimination based on sexual orientation or marital status, neither of which is covered under federal law. Also, while under federal law many discrimination protections do not apply unless there are 15 or more employees, the laws of many states may apply when there are fewer employees. It is important to become familiar with the laws of your state.

Family Medical Leave Act

The Family and Medical Leave Act (FMLA) of 1993 is a federal law that grants eligible employees the right to take up to 12 weeks of unpaid leave per year under certain circumstances. To be eligible under the law, an employee must work for an employer with at least 50 employees and have worked for that employer for at least 12 months. Leave may be taken to deal with a medical condition of the employee or a family member or the birth or adoption of a child.

Some states have passed their own Family Leave Acts that may provide the employee with more rights than the federal law or which may apply to employers with fewer than 50 employees.

Occupational Safety and Health Administration

The Occupational Safety and Health Administration (OSHA) is the federal agency that regulates safety in the workplace. States may enforce regulations tighter than those set by OSHA but may not make regulations more lenient. All employers are covered either by OSHA or an OSHA-approved safety plan. Under the OSHA Act of 1970, all employers have several basic responsibilities including the following:

- To comply with all OSHA standards, rules, and regulations that are applicable to his or her business
- To provide all employees with a workplace that is free from hazards
- To warn employees of potential hazards
- To ensure that all employees are provided with appropriate safety equipment
- To establish and maintain a reporting system for all workplace injuries or illnesses
- To provide training for all employees

Health care employers have some additional responsibilities that are unique to their industry, including the following:

- Development of an exposure control plan to assist employees who may have been exposed to certain bloodborne pathogens
- Development of training programs for all newly hired employees as well as annual refresher training for all employees that address issues related to bloodborne pathogens
- Making the hepatitis B vaccine available at no charge to all employees
- Development of standards regarding the use of universal precautions

OSHA regulations and standards are often changing, and as a paramedic you should do your best to be as familiar as possible with these changes. In the EMS environment, thousands of EMS employees sustain injuries and illnesses each year. You share an obligation, along with your employer, to do all that you can to avoid injuries.

Ryan White Act

The Ryan White Act is a federal law that provides certain safeguards and protections for health care workers who are exposed or potentially exposed to certain designated diseases. The diseases that are covered have been established by the Centers for Disease Control and Prevention and include human immunodeficiency virus (HIV)/acquired immunodeficiency syndrome (AIDS), tuberculosis, hepatitis B, meningitis, diphtheria, hemorrhagic fevers, plague, and rabies.

The Act contains several important provisions, which include the following:

- Hospitals and emergency response employers are required to establish a notification system to be used when an exposure occurs.
- Employers must appoint a designated infection control officer to handle exposures and to assist all employees who may have been exposed.
- Access to the medical records of the patient who is the source of the exposure may be obtained to determine whether the patient has tested positively for, or is exhibiting signs and symptoms of a covered infectious disease.

Any paramedic who believes that he or she may have been exposed to an infectious disease should promptly notify his or her service's infection control officer.

National Labor Relations Act

Many paramedics are employed by EMS services that are unionized. This means that at some point the employees have elected to have a union represent them as their collective bargaining agent for purposes of negotiating issues such as compensation, benefits, and work conditions. The National Labor Relations Act, also known as the Wagner Act, is the primary law that establishes the rights of unions and union workers and regulates unfair labor practices by employers. Under this law, employees have a wide variety of rights with which they should become familiar. In addition to the provisions of the National Labor Relations Act, each state has its own set of laws that affect the rights of union members. In some states, "right to work laws" do not allow an employer or a union to require you to join a union as a condition to being hired or retained on the job. In other states, you may be required to join the union within a certain time period after you are hired.

YOU *are the Medic*   SUMMARY

1. What type of consent is required to treat an unresponsive person?

Any patients who are incapacitated and unable to make a decision for themselves are treated under implied consent. This applies to any patient who is too ill or injured to consent to emergency lifesaving treatment. It is assumed that the patient would want care because of the severity of his or her condition. Implied consent is also applied to minors or those adults who have guardians when there is a serious illness or injury and a parent or guardian is not present.

2. What must you determine prior to allowing a patient to refuse care?

You must first determine the patient's decision-making capacity. In order for a patient to refuse care, he or she must be able to understand the information given regarding their condition and care and be able to make a decision based on that information. As a general rule, a patient with an altered mental status or unstable vital signs probably cannot be considered able to refuse transport. To avoid potential legal action, you should follow the protocols for your service.

The first step in determining decision-making capacity is to talk to the patient. Is the patient oriented to person, place, and time? Does he or she respond appropriately to questions? Has there been any use of drugs or alcohol or has the patient possibly experienced some type of head trauma? Is there a history of any other organic illness such as dementia? A complete set of vital signs should be taken including blood glucose levels and oxygen saturation. If vital signs are within normal limits you should ensure that the patient understands the situation and if he or she is still refusing, the patient should be able to describe a plan for follow-up care to you. This may involve calling his or her personal physician or agreeing to go to the emergency department if symptoms worsen. Any patient who can demonstrate decision-making capacity has the right to refuse all or part of the care offered, but you should encourage the patient to be treated.

3. What are the possible consequences of treating this patient without her consent?

Treating a patient without his or her consent may be grounds for charges of assault, battery, and false imprisonment. Touching a patient without consent may result in charges of assault and battery. These charges may be the result of using improper restraining methods, not asking for permission prior to touching or making physical contact, or transporting a patient without his or her consent. However, the patient must be of legal age and demonstrate the ability to make informed decisions and refuse care.

Assault is defined as instilling fear of bodily harm or breach of bodily security to another person. You do not have to touch a patient to be charged with assault. Battery is the result of touching a person without permission. Almost any medical treatment performed without the patient's permission may be considered assault and/or battery. False imprisonment occurs when a person is intentionally and unjustifiably detained against his or her will.

This includes transport without consent or using restraints in a wrongful manner.

4. On the basis of her history, what might be her problem?

The patient has a history of transient ischemic attacks (TIAs), a brain tumor, hypothyroidism, hypertension, and hyperlipidemia. Any or all of these could be the problem or could be contributing factors. She is exhibiting symptoms similar to TIAs with the periods of unresponsiveness. However, because the confusion is lasting for more than 24 hours, there has to be another or an additional cause. The brain tumor could also be a major factor. It may be growing or pressing on certain areas of the brain that are causing the signs and symptoms of this patient. Hypertension may be a contributing factor for TIAs, or could exacerbate the brain tumor. Hypothyroidism causes a myriad of signs and symptoms, and taking too much or too little of her medication may result in the changes in mental status. Hyperlipidemia indicates that she already has an excess of cholesterol. If there are blockages in major vessels supplying the brain, hypoxia and an altered mental status may be the result.

5. Would it be considered abandonment if you left at this point?

Yes. The patient obviously has an altered mental status and abiding by her wishes not to be transported would be abandonment. Abandonment is the termination of care without the patient's consent. A patient with an altered mental status does not have decision-making capacity and cannot refuse. Abandonment is also a form of negligence. Once you respond to a call and make contact with a patient, you cannot legally release care of that patient unless the patient is competent to refuse care or you have turned care over to someone of equal or higher training.

You also should leave a copy of the patient care report with the person taking over care. This is a part of the patient's permanent record and provides a continuum of care. This may be difficult if you work for a busy service, but the patient care report is vital information for the physician and staff caring for the patient because it lists your patient findings, treatment, and response to treatment.

6. Does her advance directive take precedence over her wishes?

If she is capable of making informed decisions, then she can override the advance directive. In this situation, the patient is not in cardiac arrest so it is not an issue because her advance directive is specific to a cardiac arrest. An advance directive is a written document that expresses the wants, needs, and desires of a patient in reference to future health care. Do not resuscitate (DNR) orders specify that no treatment be performed at all; conversely, advance directives state specifically what the patient wants or does not want when he or she is unable to express his or her desires. For this patient, her advance directive is slightly different from a DNR because she wants no heroic measures taken; however, she does want basic life support. DNR orders, living wills, and organ donation orders are all advance directives.

YOU are the Medic — SUMMARY, continued

7. Had the patient continued to refuse treatment and transport, what options might you have exercised?

Having her daughter talk to her may have helped, but if all else fails then it becomes necessary to contact medical control for direction. She has proven to have an altered mental status and cannot refuse care because of her impaired decision-making capacity. Follow local protocols, and prior to contacting medical control, make sure you have all of the information concerning the patient—vital signs, blood glucose level, history, medications, and any findings—readily available.

Not only can medical control direct you in the proper handling of the patient, but having the patient speak directly to the physician on the phone may be enough to convince her that transport is necessary. Continue to be patient but firm in expressing to the patient why she needs to be transported for care.

8. Under what type of consent was this patient treated?

The patient was treated under informed consent as well as implied consent. She is confused about some things, which technically means that she can be treated under implied consent. The problem that she is experiencing may be the result of the brain tumor that she has or any of the other components of her history. It is possible that she is having TIAs and subsequently may have a stroke. These are potential life-threatening problems and she needs to be transported for further evaluation at the emergency department.

She was also treated under informed consent. She is not completely disoriented and understands most of what you are telling her. She agrees initially to allow you to take vital signs. She understands what you are about to do and gives you permission to do it. This is informed consent. She eventually consents and allows you to treat her as well as transport her to the closest, most appropriate facility.

EMS Patient Care Report (PCR)

Date: 02-02-11	Incident No.: 02110985	Nature of Call: Unresponsive person	Location: 487 Lenore Street		
Dispatched: 0737	En Route: 0738	At Scene: 0742	Transport: 0752	At Hospital: 0804	In Service: 0810

Patient Information

Age: 64	Allergies: Penicillin
Sex: F	Medications: Coreg, Synthroid, Zocor, Lisinopril
Weight (in kg [lb]): 69 kg (152 lb)	Past Medical History: HTN, brain tumor, TIAs, hyperlipidemia, hypothyroidism
	Chief Complaint: Slight headache, acting strangely, altered mental status

Vital Signs

Time: 0746	BP: 152/98	Pulse: 108	Respirations: 20	Spo_2: 97% on room air
Time: 0756	BP: 162/94	Pulse: 102	Respirations: 18	Spo_2: 98% on room air
Time:	BP:	Pulse:	Respirations:	Spo_2:

EMS Treatment
(circle all that apply)

Oxygen @ _____ L/min via (circle one): NC NRM Bag-mask device	Assisted Ventilation	Airway Adjunct:	CPR
Defibrillation	Bleeding Control	Bandaging	Splinting	(Other:) Cardiac monitor

Narrative

EMS responded to a possible unresponsive person to find a 64 y/o w/f complaining of "slight" headache and altered mental status. Pt alert, but confused, oriented to person, place, but not day. Daughter states that she has been this way for several days and has periods of not responding at all. Pt is ambulatory, no apparent distress noted, no neuro deficits. PEARRL, glucose is 138 mg/dL, heart monitor showing sinus tach without ectopy. Nothing else significant noted. Pt refused oxygen, but maintaining Spo_2 on room air within normal limits. 20-gauge IV L antecubital fossa with blood drawn for labs and NS at KVO. Transported to Cedar's Medical Center, no changes en route. **End of report**

Prep Kit

- Paramedics operate in a community that exposes them to professional liability and that requires them to have a solid understanding of law and ethics. Failing to perform their job as expected within the medical community, the legal community, and the regulations of the jurisdiction in which they function will expose them to civil and/or criminal liability.

- When personal ethics conflict with professional ethics, the paramedic usually will be bound by professional ethics and must temporarily set aside personal ethics.

- Three primary ethical principles for paramedics are to do no harm, act in good faith, and act in the patient's best interest.

- EMS research, while important, presents unique ethical dilemmas regarding informed patient consent. Staying aware of the issues and the latest research is the best way to promote the development of evidence-based practice for paramedics.

- The foundation of the legal system in the United States is the federal government. There are three branches of government: executive, judicial, and legislative.

- There are two types of law: civil and criminal.
  - Civil cases result in monetary damages.
  - Criminal cases result in incarceration of a person.

- Paramedics are particularly susceptible to charges of assault and battery. Assault is when you instill the fear of bodily harm in a person. Battery is when you (as a paramedic) unlawfully touch another person without his or her consent.

- False imprisonment can occur when a paramedic restrains a patient against his or her will. Protection against this charge can exist only if appropriate documentation and policy exist regarding the specific call.

- Defamation, slander, and libel present risks to paramedics when they make statements, either verbal or written, that injure a person's good name.

- Lawsuits follow a general process that starts with a complaint or notice of complaint, a response or answer by the defendant, discovery, settlement discussions, and trial process.

- Paramedics are subject to multiple legal jurisdictions, including state law, state regulations, local medical protocol, and departmental policy.

- Medical directors have a supervisory relationship over paramedics, but each paramedic is held personally responsible for his or her own actions.

- Your activities function as an extension of a series of medical directions from the medical director that are either online or off-line. These directives are binding on paramedics unless they believe that they will cause harm to the patient.

- State legislation enables paramedics to practice in every state. It is the responsibility of paramedics to understand the statutes of the state in which they practice.

- State jurisdictions issue paramedics either licenses or certificates. Paramedics must understand that the licensure or certification is a privilege extended by the governing authority that allows paramedics to practice within the enacting legislation.

- Paramedics have a right to due process, a fair procedure that includes appropriate legal notice of the action to be taken, and the opportunity to be heard before the licensing/certifying agency.

- State laws define scope of practice for the paramedic, which specifies the limits of practice allowed under the Medical Practice Act.

- HIPAA was enacted to protect patient information from unlawful and unnecessary dissemination.

- EMTALA is another federal law designed to prevent hospital emergency departments from turning patients away for any reason, including the ability to pay for care.

- Emergency vehicle operations must be performed in a manner that protects the public from further injury. No call can justify driving in a manner that endangers the public.

- Transportation to a certain medical facility should be determined by taking into account the patient's preference and the medical needs of the patient.

- Crime scenes present the intersection between EMS and law enforcement. Paramedics have an obligation to assist the law enforcement community in preservation of evidence and documentation of scenes or actions that may later be introduced on behalf of a criminal prosecution.

- Paramedics can be held legally responsible when they fail to report cases such as suspected abuse, domestic violence, gunshot/stab wounds, childbirth outside a medical facility, rape, infectious diseases, or animal bites.

- Suspected homicides, suicides, prison inmate deaths, and other violent or unexpected deaths should immediately be reported to local law enforcement personnel in order to allow a coroner or medical examiner to examine the body.

- All patients of sound mind have the legal right under the US Constitution to privacy, consent, and refusal. Paramedics cannot infringe on these inalienable rights unless they believe that patients are not of sound mind and pose a detriment to themselves or others.

- Patient refusals pose a large potential legal liability to paramedics. The only protection against a civil suit over a refusal will be the documentation at the time of the incident.
  - A refusal signature without narrative and evidence of a physical assessment is worthless.

- You must obtain informed consent from patients prior to any medical process, including examination.

- You must get expressed consent—action demonstrating permission to provide care—from patients before initiating treatment.

- Implied consent is said to exist when patients are unable to answer for themselves and paramedics deem that treatment is required.

- Determining the decision-making capacity of a patient can be tricky, but tools such as pulse oximetry and blood glucose measurements can provide factual documentation of patient awareness and ability to make clear decisions regarding his or her medical care. In any questionable circumstance, thorough documentation and consultation with medical control will provide the best protection against lawsuits.

- Minors pose challenges that local jurisdictions must address before a call occurs. In general, if the patient is a minor, the minor has neither the right to consent to care nor the right to refuse it, although exceptions for emancipated minors exist.

- Violent patients may be restrained using physical or chemical means if they are a danger to themselves or others. Always follow local medical and law enforcement protocols when addressing the needs of violent or potentially violent patients.

- Allocation of resources and triage challenges can present serious ethical dilemmas to paramedics. In such circumstances, well-established protocols and professional ethics should take precedence over any personal feelings or ethics of the paramedic.

- Negligence occurs only when the following four processes have occurred:
  - Duty to act. The paramedic must have had a duty to act.
  - Breach of duty. The paramedic did not fulfill that duty.
  - Proximate cause. The paramedic's breach of duty caused the plaintiff's injury.
  - Injury resulted. An injury occurred as a result of the above.

- Negligence can be categorized as acts of commission (malfeasance and misfeasance) or acts of omission (nonfeasance).

- As the highest level of prehospital care providers, paramedics must ensure that they do not abandon their patients. Abandonment can occur anytime paramedics turn over their patients inappropriately or to a level of care lesser than themselves.

- Documentation is the only methodology to prevent the appearance of abandonment.

- Patients have the right to determine their own care. Paramedics must understand their legal limitations based on any advance directives issued by the patient.

- Do not resuscitate (DNR) orders are a specific form of advance directive that generally define the care a patient wants when lifesaving procedures are required. A DNR order is *not* a "do-not-care-for-the-patient" order.

- Patients often decide on medical care and treatment issues prior to an emergency. Paramedics need to be familiar with DNR orders, living wills, health care powers of attorney, surrogate decisions, and organ donations.

- Futile resuscitation efforts, which you may encounter, need to be addressed and considered prior to an emergency event. Weighing various ethical issues prior to their occurrence can help prevent and reduce suffering in your patient population.

- You may provide care when off duty and in most jurisdictions be protected under the Good Samaritan laws. Paramedics must remember that they are only protected if they perform within their training and education and if they do not receive any compensation.

- You can be protected under certain governmental immunity clauses. These protections may not be valid if the paramedics have committed negligence or if the paramedics are deemed to be personally liable.

- Two common legal defenses are the statute of limitations (time in which to file a lawsuit) and contributory negligence, when a plaintiff has contributed to the negative outcome by committing an act or failing to disclose relevant information to medical practitioners.

- Several federal and state laws affect the relationship between the paramedic and his or her employer. These laws promote a healthier, safer workplace by addressing topics such as discrimination, sexual harassment, family leave, and occupational safety regulations.

Vital Vocabulary

abandonment Termination of care for the patient without giving the patient sufficient opportunity to find another suitable health care professional to take over his or her medical treatment.

advance directive A written document or oral statement that expresses the wants, needs, and desires of a patient in reference to future medical care; examples include living wills, do not resuscitate (DNR) orders, and organ donation choices.

assault To create in another person a fear of immediate bodily harm or invasion of bodily security.

battery Any act of touching another person without that person's consent.

civil suit An action instituted by a private person or corporation against another private person or corporation.

consent Agreement by the patient to accept a medical intervention.

contributory negligence Act(s) committed by plaintiff that contributes to adverse outcomes.

criminal prosecution An action instituted by the government against a private person for violation of criminal law.

damages Compensation for injury awarded by a court.

decision-making capacity The patient's ability to understand and process the information you give him or her about your proposed plan of care.

defamation Intentionally making a false statement, through written or verbal communication, which injures a person's good name or reputation.

defendant In a civil suit, the person against whom a legal action is brought.

do not resuscitate (DNR) order A type of advance directive that describes which life-sustaining procedures should be performed in the event of a sudden deterioration in a patient's medical condition.

due process A right to a fair procedure for a legal action against a person or agency; has two components: Notice and Opportunity to be Heard.

duty Legal obligation of public and certain other ambulance services to respond to a call for help in their jurisdiction.

emancipated minor A person who is under the legal age in a given state, but is legally considered an adult because of other circumstances.

EMTALA The Emergency Medical Treatment and Active Labor Act enacted in 1986 to combat the practice of patient dumping (hospitals refusing to admit seriously ill patients or women in labor who could not pay, forcing EMS providers to dump the patients at another hospital). EMTALA regulates hospitals that receive Medicare funding and severely fines hospitals or doctors who violate its provisions.

ethics A set of values in society that differentiates right from wrong.

expressed consent A type of informed consent that occurs when the patient does something, either through words or by taking some sort of action, that demonstrates permission to provide care.

false imprisonment The intentional and unjustified detention of a person against his or her will.

Good Samaritan law A statute providing limited immunity from liability to persons responding voluntarily and in good faith to the aid of an injured person outside the hospital.

gross negligence Negligence that is willful, wanton, intentional, or reckless; a serious departure from the accepted standards.

health care power of attorney A legal document that allows another person to make health care decisions for the patient, including withdrawal or withholding of care, when the patient is incapacitated.

HIPAA The Health Insurance Portability and Accountability Act that was enacted in 1996, providing for criminal sanctions as well as for civil penalties for releasing a patient's protected health information (PHI) in a way not authorized by the patient.

hostile environment Situation in which an employer or an employer's agent either creates or allows to continue an offensive practice related to sex that makes it uncomfortable or impossible for an employee to continue working.

immunity Legal protection from penalties that could normally be incurred under the law.

implied consent Assumption on behalf of a person unable to give consent that he or she would have done so.

in loco parentis Phrase used to describe situations in which a designated authority figure makes medical treatment and transport decisions for a minor child when a parent is not available.

informed consent A patient's voluntary agreement to be treated after being told about the nature of the disease, the risks and benefits of the proposed treatment, alternative treatments, or the choice of no treatment at all.

involuntary consent An oxymoron, as consent is never involuntary; often used to describe a figure of authority dictating medical care be given to someone in custody, incapacitated, or a minor.

liability A finding in civil cases that the preponderance of the evidence shows the defendant was responsible for the plaintiff's injuries.

libel Making a false statement in written form that injures a person's good name.

living will A type of advance directive, generally requiring a precondition for withholding resuscitation when the patient is incapacitated.

malfeasance Unauthorized act committed outside the scope of medical practice defined by law.

Medical Practice Act An act that usually defines the minimum qualifications of those who may perform various health services, defines the skills that each type of practitioner is legally permitted to use, and establishes a means of licensure or certification for different categories of health care professionals.

misfeasance Appropriate act performed in an improper manner, such as a medication administered at the wrong dose.

morality Pertaining to conscience, conduct, and character.

negligence Professional action or inaction on the part of the health care worker that does not meet the standard of ordinary care expected of similarly trained and prudent health care practitioners and that results in injury to the patient.

negligence per se Inexcusable violation of a statute, such as practicing without a valid license or certification.

nonfeasance Failing to perform a required or expected act.

ordinary negligence Negligence that is a failure to act, or a simple mistake that causes harm to a patient.

palliative care A type of care intended to provide comfort and relief from pain.

patient autonomy The right to direct one's own care, and to decide how you want your end-of-life medical care provided.

plaintiff In a civil suit, the person who brings a legal action against another person.

proximate cause The specific reason that an injury occurred; one of the items that must be proven in order for a paramedic to be held liable for negligence.

punitive damages Compensation, usually monetary, awarded to a plaintiff for intentional or reckless acts committed by the defendant.

qualified immunity Protection in which the paramedic is only held liable when the plaintiff can show that the paramedic violated clearly established law of which he or she should have known.

quid pro quo Circumstance in which a person in authority attempts to exchange some work-related benefit, such as a raise or promotion, for sexual favors.

res ipsa loquitur Theory of negligence that assumes an injury can only occur when a negligent act occurs.

scope of practice What a state permits a paramedic practicing under a license or certification to do.

slander Verbally making a false statement that injures a person's good name.

standard of care What a reasonable paramedic with training would do in the same or a similar situation.

statutes of limitations Laws that limit the time within which a lawsuit may be filed.

surrogate decision maker A person designated by a patient to make health care decisions as the patient would want when the patient becomes incapable of making decisions.

tort A wrongful act that gives rise to a civil suit.

triage Process of establishing treatment and transportation priorities according to severity of injury and medical need.

Assessment in Action

You are dispatched to 745 Reader Street for a possible suicide attempt. This is a residential neighborhood and the dispatcher tells you that the patient is a man with a gun in the back bedroom. A police officer is on the phone with the patient, who says he will kill anyone who tries to stop him. The police have set up a perimeter around the house and ask that you stand by at a nearby intersection.

You are posting at the intersection when the dispatcher notifies you that shots have been fired. Police are requesting that you come in—the subject has shot himself and the scene is secure. As you reach the house, a police officer asks that only one paramedic enter the scene to determine whether anything can be done to save the patient.

You follow the police officer to the bedroom and are presented with a middle-aged man lying supine across the bed with his legs hanging off the end. The shotgun has fallen to the side and it is obvious that he had the barrel in his mouth when he pulled the trigger. The top of his head is missing and there is brain matter on the wall and ceiling. He has no pulse and you determine that he is not viable.

1. How should you respond in situations where you are unsure of whether or not to attempt resuscitation?
   A. Contact medical control.
   B. Wait for your partner to make a decision.
   C. Start resuscitation if you are unsure.
   D. Consult law enforcement personnel.

2. As you are leaving the scene you are approached by a reporter who asks that you give him only the patient's age and sex and to tell him if he is still alive. He has been listening to a scanner and knows most of the story. To give him this information would be a(n) _____ violation.
   A. ethical
   B. HIPAA
   C. civil
   D. EMTALA

3. If you make the decision to treat this patient, what type of consent would be used?
   A. Implied consent
   B. Informed consent
   C. Consent as an emancipated minor
   D. Expressed consent

4. You have determined that the patient is not viable. How should you proceed?
   A. Cover him with a sheet.
   B. Immediately leave the scene.
   C. Preserve the crime scene.
   D. Roll the patient to look for any other injuries.

5. Your best protection in court is thorough and accurate documentation. Which characteristic of an effective PCR describes your assessment for justifying your actions for this patient?
   A. Date and times
   B. History
   C. Physical examination
   D. Treatment

6. There are four components to prove negligence. If you have not met the standard of care in treating this patient, which requirement for proving negligence does this fulfill?
   - **A.** Duty
   - **B.** Breach of duty
   - **C.** Proximate cause
   - **D.** Harm

7. The family has decided to sue for lack of care because they feel he may have had a chance had he received prompt care. This sort of legal action is known as:
   - **A.** a civil suit.
   - **B.** slander.
   - **C.** defamation.
   - **D.** a tort.

Additional Questions

8. Prior to accepting a patient's consent or refusal of treatment, you must evaluate the patient's decision-making capacity. How is this accomplished?

9. You are called to the scene of a violent diabetic patient who is hypoglycemic. His wife tells you that she was able to check his blood glucose just prior to calling and it was 34 mg/dL. He is refusing to allow anyone near him and will not eat anything. How will you proceed?

EMS Communications

National EMS Education Standard Competencies

Preparatory

Integrates comprehensive knowledge of the EMS system, safety/well-being of the paramedic, and medical/legal and ethical issues which is intended to improve the health of EMS personnel, patients, and the community.

EMS System Communication

Communication needed to

- Call for resources (p 129)
- Transfer care of the patient (p 130)
- Interact within the team structure (p 130)
- EMS communication system (p 121)
- Communication with other health care professionals (p 130)
- Team communication and dynamics (pp 130, 131)

Therapeutic Communication

Principles of communicating with patients in a manner that achieves a positive relationship

- Interviewing techniques (pp 134-135)
- Adjusting communication strategies for age, stage of development, patients with special needs, and differing cultures (pp 137-141)
- Verbal defusing strategies (p 138)
- Family presence issues (pp 133, 134, 139, 140)
- Dealing with difficult patients (pp 137-138)
- Factors that affect communication (p 126)

Medical Terminology

Integrates comprehensive anatomic and medical terminology and abbreviations into written and oral communication with colleagues and other health care professionals.

Knowledge Objectives

1. Identify the importance of communications when providing EMS. (p 121)
2. Identify the role of verbal and electronic communications in the provision of EMS. (p 121)
3. Describe the phases of communications necessary to complete a typical EMS event. (p 130)
4. Identify the importance of proper terminology when communicating during an EMS event. (p 130)
5. List factors that impede effective verbal communications. (p 126)
6. List factors that enhance verbal communications. (pp 132-134)
7. Identify technology used to collect and exchange patient and/or scene information electronically. (pp 122-126)

8. Recognize the legal status of patient medical information exchanged electronically. (p 127)
9. Identify the components of the local EMS communications system and describe their function and use. (pp 121-122)
10. Identify and differentiate among the following communications systems
    a. Simplex (p 123)
    b. Multiplex (p 123)
    c. Duplex (p 123)
    d. Trunked (p 123)
    e. Digital communications (p 123)
    f. Cellular telephone (p 124)
    g. Computer (pp 123, 124)
11. Identify components of the local dispatch communications system and describe their function and use. (pp 121-122)
12. Describe the functions and responsibilities of the Federal Communications Commission. (pp 123, 126)
13. Describe how an EMS dispatcher functions as an integral part of the EMS team. (pp 131-132)
14. Identify the role of the emergency medical dispatcher in a typical EMS event. (pp 131-132)
15. Identify the importance of prearrival instructions in a typical EMS event. (p 132)
16. Describe the purpose of verbal communication of patient information to the hospital. (p 129)
17. List information that should be included in patient assessment information verbally reported to medical direction. (pp 129-130)
18. Identify internal and external factors that affect a patient/bystander interview conducted by a paramedic. (pp 132-133)
19. Discuss the strategies for developing patient rapport. (pp 133-134)
20. Provide examples of open-ended and closed-ended questions. (p 134)
21. Discuss common errors made by paramedics when interviewing patients. (p 137)
22. Identify the nonverbal skills that are used in patient interviewing. (p 137)
23. Discuss strategies to obtain information from a patient. (pp 136-137)
24. Summarize the methods to assess mental status based on interview techniques. (p 135)
25. Differentiate the strategies a paramedic uses when interviewing a patient who is hostile compared with one who is cooperative. (p 138)
26. Summarize developmental considerations of various age groups that influence patient interviewing. (pp 138-139)
27. Discuss unique interviewing techniques necessary to employ with patients who have special needs. (p 139)
28. Discuss interviewing considerations used by paramedics in cross-cultural communications. (pp 139-141)

Skills Objectives

There are no skills objectives for this chapter.

Introduction

In EMS communication, relaying information from one person to another becomes extremely urgent in the short time that you will have to care for a patient. That information needs to move rapidly, efficiently, and effectively. As a paramedic, you must be able to communicate with many other people effectively.

You need to know what constitutes an EMS communications system, who needs to be able to talk with whom, what technical resources are available to you to make those conversations possible, and what you can do to make communications as efficient as possible. You also need to understand the crucial role of the **emergency medical dispatcher (EMD)** in facilitating all phases of EMS communications. You need to know how to organize patient information into a brief, orderly verbal report that can be transmitted by radio or by telephone.

Just as important as communicating with the dispatcher and fellow health care professionals is communicating with the patient. This is called **therapeutic communication** and it involves the art and skill of communicating with people on what may be one of the worst days of their life. Being a good paramedic entails putting forth your best efforts at service—what the "S" in EMS stands for. A professional demeanor and skilled communication techniques are key components of a successful patient-paramedic interaction.

EMS Communications System

Communication during an emergency call will require the use of specialized equipment. Although the digital revolution is improving communications, most EMS communications systems today are based on the use of radios, so it is important for you to learn about radio signals and what equipment is available for sending and receiving them.

You must have a reliable method of sending and receiving information back and forth to medical direction. Although this communication has mainly been accomplished by radio in the past, cellular devices and mobile data terminals are now helping in this endeavor. The EMS system must be configured to allow 24-hour methods of contact with medical direction at local and regional facilities.

Although these communication systems are relatively dependable, a backup communication system is also needed. For example, if the primary method is digital radio, a secondary means might include the use of cellular phones or a satellite phone, or a mobile data terminal. Having backup communication systems in place ensures that there will always be a method to access medical direction, in any circumstance, 24 hours per day.

Backup communications are even more critical in times of disaster or multiple-casualty incidents. In these situations, primary methods of communications may be disabled. Towers may be damaged, cell sites may be disabled, and computer data servers may be crippled. In these circumstances, disaster communications are often established by amateur radio groups. Most of the equipment for this type of communication is available after a major incident through your local emergency management office.

Communications System Components

Although EMS communications systems vary considerably among one another, most systems serving moderate to large populations are constructed of the following components.

Base Stations

The **base station** is a collection of radio equipment consisting, at minimum, of a transmitter, receiver, and antenna. The base station serves as a **dispatch** and coordination area and ideally should be in contact with all other elements of the system. Base stations generally use relatively high power output (45 to 275 W); the maximum allowable power is determined by the Federal Communications Commission (FCC) and printed on the station's license.

The base station must be equipped with an antenna sited in suitable terrain, preferably on a hill or high building, close to the base. The antenna system has a vital part in transmission and reception efficiency. A good antenna system can compensate for FCC limits on power output and human-made signal distortion in the area.

YOU *are the Medic* **PART 1**

Your unit is dispatched to a local residence for a man who is not feeling well. Your crew is met at the door by an elderly woman who tells you that her husband is ill with cancer and that he is not feeling well. After ensuring that the scene is safe, you enter the residence. You see a frail-looking elderly man sitting in a recliner. The room is immaculately clean. There is a television set playing loudly in the corner of the room. The wife tells you her husband does not hear well.

1. How will you open communication with this patient?
2. Is the television set a consideration in your assessment?

Mobile Transmitter/Receivers (Transceivers)

A mobile transmitter/receiver, or mobile transceiver, is a two-way radio mounted in a vehicle. Mobile transmitter/receivers come in a variety of power ranges, and the power output largely determines the distance over which the signal can be effectively transmitted. A transmitter around 7.5 W, for example, will transmit for distances of 10 to 12 miles over slightly hilly terrain. Transmission distances are greater over water or flat terrain and reduced in mountainous areas or where there are many tall buildings. Mobile transmitters with higher outputs have proportionally greater transmission ranges. Today, the typical mobile transmitter operates at between 20 and 50 W.

Portable Transmitter/Receivers

Portable, hand-held radios are useful when paramedics must work at a distance from their vehicle but need to stay in communication with the base or with one another Figure 1 . Portable units may also be used by physician consultants when not stationed at the hospital. Portable units usually have power outputs of up to 5 W and, thus, have limited range by themselves, although the signal of a hand-held transmitter can be boosted by retransmission through the vehicle.

Repeaters

A repeater is a miniature base station used to extend the transmitting and receiving range of a telemetry or voice communications system. Repeaters may be stationary in one location (fixed repeaters) or carried in emergency vehicles (mobile repeaters). A repeater picks up a weak signal and retransmits it at a higher power on another frequency, so it extends the range of low-power portable radios and allows more members of the system to hear one another. This is how a trooper on the side of the state highway can talk to a supervisor on the other end of the state.

Remote Consoles

A remote console, usually located in the emergency department of a hospital, is a terminal that receives transmissions of

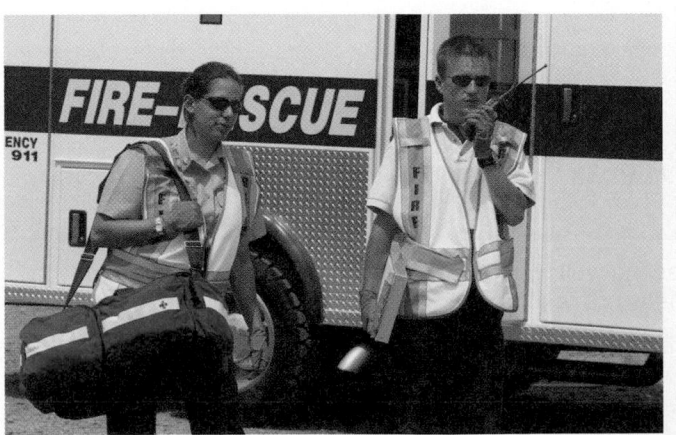

Figure 1 A portable radio is essential if you need to communicate with the dispatcher or medical control when you are away from the ambulance.

telemetry and voice from the field and transmits messages back, usually through the base station. Remote consoles are connected to the base station by dedicated telephone lines, microwave, or radio. They contain an amplifier and speaker for incoming voice reception, a decoder for translating the telemetry signal into an oscilloscope tracing or printout, and a microphone for voice transmission.

■ Radio Communications

A radio transmits signals by electromagnetic waves. When energy is emitted in the form of waves, the energy can be characterized by the length of the waves it produces. Energy of a relatively long wavelength produces audible sound; energy of a shorter wavelength is in the infrared light spectrum. Between sound and infrared light are the wavelengths for radio transmission. Radio wavelengths are used for tuning by adjusting your radio to the proper frequency—how frequently the wave recurs in a given time (usually 1 second). Short wavelengths are repeated more often (ie, with higher frequency) than longer wavelengths. Radio frequencies are designated by their cycles per second, or hertz (Hz) (named for the man who first described the propagation of electromagnetic waves). The following abbreviations are commonly used:

- hertz (Hz)—cycles per second
- kilohertz (kHz)—1,000 cycles per second
- megahertz (MHz)—1 million cycles per second
- gigahertz (GHz)—1 billion cycles per second

Radio waves are confined to the part of the electromagnetic frequency spectrum extending from 3 kHz to about 3,000 GHz. A normal voice channel requires a minimum of 3 kHz. Frequency bands are portions of the radio frequency spectrum assigned for specific uses. The most commonly used bands for medical communications are the very high frequency (VHF) band and the ultrahigh frequency (UHF) band. The VHF band extends from roughly 30 to 175 MHz and has been arbitrarily divided into a low band (30 to 50 MHz) and a high band (150 to 175 MHz). The low-band frequencies may have ranges up to 2,000 miles but are unpredictable because changes in ionospheric (about 30 miles [50 km] into the atmosphere) conditions may cause "skip interference," with patchy losses in communication. The high-band frequencies are almost wholly free of skip interference, but have a much shorter transmission range. The most commonly used of the VHF high-band frequencies for emergency medical purposes are in the 150-to 160-MHz range. This has historically been the main radio band assigned by the FCC. In the late 1970s, however, the ultra-high frequency (UHF) band was assigned to EMS in the form of the MED channels. The UHF band extends from 300 to 3,000 MHz, with most medical communications occurring around 450 to 470 MHz. At these frequencies, communications are entirely free of skip interference and have minimal noise (signal distortion). The UHF band has better penetration in dense metropolitan areas, and UHF reception is usually quite adequate inside buildings. The UHF band, however, has a shorter range than the VHF band, and energy at UHF is more readily absorbed by rain and environmental objects, such as trees and brush.

Radios that operate at 800 MHz are common in EMS systems. This frequency offers excellent penetration of buildings and has minimal interference and reduced channel noise. Because of this, it works quite well in metropolitan areas; 800 MHz also allows for trunking, in which multiple agencies or systems can share frequencies. An 800-MHz radio can also be linked to a computer system to transmit voiceless communications. The use of trunked systems allows the dispatcher to reprogram the radios so that agencies that do not routinely talk to each other can easily do so at the scene of a multiple-casualty incident, a rescue, a hazardous materials incident, or other special operations.

The Federal Communications Commission (FCC), which controls frequency allocation in the United States, has set aside medical VHF band assignments for general emergency radio communications and UHF band assignments for ambulance-to-hospital telemetry systems, especially where communications from physicians to rescue personnel are needed to consult or direct patient care activities. Those band assignments will be given to you by your EMS system.

Routine radio system checks are necessary to ensure communication lines are in place. This is especially true at hospitals, where radio use and maintenance may not be familiar to some staff. The EMS system must perform a communications check (COMM CHEK) at routine times. Some systems do these checks daily or weekly, but these checks should be done at least once a month. The communications check consists of a simple voice transmission check ("Rampart ER this is John's County Communications, radio check. Do you copy?"). If the transmission was successful, a voice and data check by an EMS unit should follow to confirm ability to send and receive voice and ECG. This confirmation can be done by a simple return transmission ("Rampart, this is EMS 1 calling on 155.340. Do you copy?"). If the communication is confirmed, then a sample ECG can be sent, with the emergency department radioing back receipt.

Once each test is performed, it is important to log the success or failure. This gives the system a method of communications quality control. These checks are most effective when they are made a standard part of operations policy.

Modes of Radio Operation

Assigned radio frequencies may be used in a variety of systems. In a simplex system, portable units can transmit only in one mode (voice or telemetry) or receive (voice) at any given time. A simplex system requires only a single radio frequency. A network that uses two different frequencies at the same time, to permit simultaneous transmission and reception (like a telephone), is referred to as duplex. Another alternative is to combine, or multiplex, two or more signals—such as the paramedic's voice and the patient's ECG—for simultaneous transmission on one frequency.

Suppose that an ambulance service wanted the possibility of voice communications and continuous telemetry (discussed later in this chapter). There are at least four ways to design the communications system to meet those requirements:

- The ambulance could transmit on two frequencies of a UHF-frequency pair (channel) allocated for telemetry (duplex). One frequency would transmit the voice signal and the other, the telemetry signal. Such a system requires that the ambulance have two UHF transmitters (one for voice, one for telemetry) and one receiver (voice).
- The ambulance service could multiplex (combine) telemetry and voice on one frequency of the allocated UHF pair and receive voice communications on the other frequency of the pair. That requires only one UHF transmitter on the vehicle, but the base station must be fitted with demultiplexing equipment to separate the two signals coming in on one frequency.
- The ambulance could transmit telemetry data on one frequency of the allocated telemetry pair and transmit voice data on a VHF frequency. That requires a UHF and a VHF transmitter on the vehicle (two simplex systems).
- There is an increasing trend toward using cellular telephones for ECG telemetry. Cellular phones have full duplex capability, a multitude of available channels, a high-quality signal that is unlikely to degrade over distance, and a much lower capital and maintenance cost.

Digital Radio and Trunked Systems

Digital radio has helped clear up distorted or lost transmissions. Conventional radios operate on fixed radio frequency (RF) channels. In the case of radios with multiple channels, they operate on one channel at a time and the proper channel is selected by a user. The user operates a channel selector or buttons on the radio control panel to pick the channel. In the case of digital radio, instead of using multiple channels, digital trunked radios are related by groups. These can be thought of as virtual channels that appear and disappear as conversations occur. Digital trunked systems may carry simultaneous conversations on one physical channel.

Digital systems may also communicate text from computer-aided dispatch (CAD). CAD is a computerized method of call handling in which a computer collects and manages the call information and makes recommendations for which EMS unit is closest based on existing dispatch policy. As it does this, the data for dispatch can be sent directly to the individual EMS unit by data transfer. The result is that the EMS unit will see what is seen on the CAD terminal. For example, a display in an ambulance may give a textual location for a call and any related details including mapping and directions to a call. The driver may press an acknowledge button, sending data in the opposite direction and flagging the call as received by the driver, thus allowing dispatch and call response information exchange on the mobile display.

In addition to managing call dispatch and location information, the CAD can recommend emergency actions to the dispatcher for relay to the patient or bystanders at the emergency scene. This is referred to as prearrival instructions (PAI), and allows care to begin before the ambulance arrives on the scene. The CAD operator has access to emergency aid information relating to almost every possible EMS-related emergency. These protocols are typically developed by a major supplier, and then reviewed by a physician. Upon installation, the protocols must then be reviewed and approved by local medical direction and the EMS system.

■ Cellular Telephones

<u>Cellular telephones</u> operate on 3 W of power or less. Mobile antennas are much closer to the ground than base station antennas, so communications from the unit are typically limited to 10 to 15 miles over average terrain. Base station antennas are usually located on high sites to increase the coverage area.

Cellular telephones are commonly used in EMS communications systems Figure 2 . These telephones are simply low-power portable radios that communicate through a series of interconnected repeater stations called "cells" (hence the name "cellular"). Cells are linked by a sophisticated computer system and connected to the telephone network. Cellular telephones are also popular with other public safety agencies, particularly as more cell sites are constructed in rural areas.

The use of cellular telephones requires that the paramedic be familiar with important and commonly used telephone numbers, such as medical control, local hospital EDs, and dispatch centers. Also, because cellular deadspots can cripple effective communications, the paramedic should know the locations of cellular deadspots in the area.

Many cellular systems make equipment and air time available to EMS systems at little or no cost as a public service. The public is often able to call 9-1-1 or other emergency numbers on a cellular telephone free of charge. However, this easy access may result in overloading and jamming of cellular systems in a multiple-casualty incident (MCI) and disaster situations, and you should have a backup communications plan in your service to circumvent these overloads.

Most newer cell phones have a global positioning system (GPS) built in specifically for emergencies. This helps the CAD

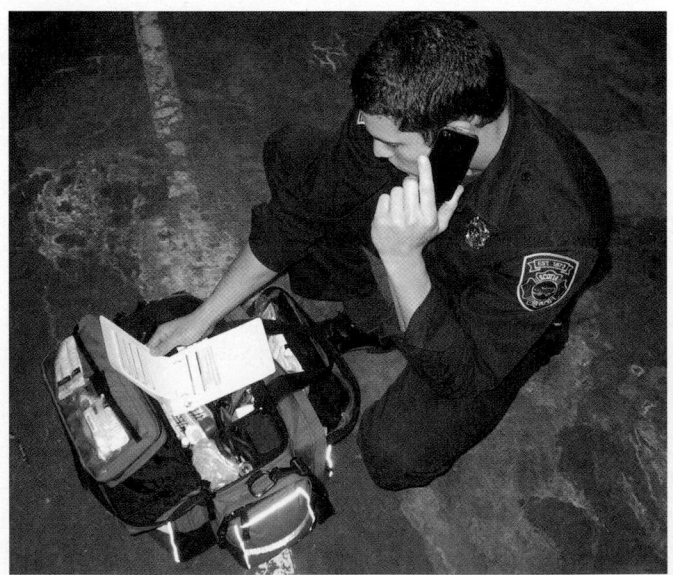

Figure 2 Cellular telephones allow EMS communications over a wide geographic area.

operator know exactly where the cell call is originating. In the past, when a cell phone call was made by a person who was experiencing some type of emergency, rescuers would often search blindly because many patients became unconscious or did not know their location. Many vehicles also have vehicle locator and navigation systems that notify emergency services when a crash has occurred. These, too, are based on GPS technology. Typically, cell phone calls for emergency services go through a routing center rather than directly to the local dispatch center. The 9-1-1 cellular calls often go through a regional or statewide agency such as the state police. The National Emergency Number Association estimates that more than 75% of the nation's population resides in areas where wireless 9-1-1 services deliver the caller's call-back number and location to the appropriate public safety answering point (PSAP).

■ Backup Communications Systems

In addition to radio communications, most systems use <u>landline</u> (telephone) backup to link various fixed components of the system, such as hospitals, public safety services, and poison control. Telephones may also be patched into radio transmissions through the base station, enabling, for example, communication between paramedics using radios in the field and a physician using his or her telephone at home. Finally, as mentioned earlier, cellular telephones are becoming an increasingly important part of EMS communications, overcoming many of the problems of overcrowded EMS radio frequencies. Cellular phones are less expensive than radios and generally give a much clearer signal. Furthermore, they enable a paramedic in the field to communicate with anyone who has a telephone—the patient's family physician, an injured child's parent, an expert in another state who can advise on a hazardous materials situation. The limitation of using cellular communications as backup is that of disasters. If a disaster affects your primary communications system (such as widespread power outages or tower damages), your cell towers may also be affected. In addition, in times of widespread unrest such as in MCIs or disasters, the cell sites are commonly busy with civilian traffic. The cellular computer that assigns channels does not recognize your phone over another user and you may be delayed in getting a channel.

In these situations, it is commonly found that older low-band and high-band simplex systems are still licensed and are operable just for redundancy. In the case of disasters or power failures, older systems can still transmit and receive because most base stations have generators and EMS units operate off batteries. Because no power supply is necessary at a cell site or repeater site miles away, the older radios continue to allow communication.

■ Biotelemetry

<u>Biotelemetry</u> is the capability of measuring vital life signs and transmitting them to a distant terminal. Biotelemetry started with ECGs but often is used for other measurements. Even the US

space program uses telemetry to send the pulse and respiratory rate of astronauts from space to a receiving station on earth.

The term *biotelemetry* in emergency medical care is usually shortened to *telemetry*. Most often, telemetry is a short way of saying that you are transmitting an ECG signal from your patient to a distant receiving station. The standard ECG is composed of low-frequency signals (100 Hz or less), which would be filtered out by a voice communications system. To make sure voice communication does not filter out the ECG, the ECG signal must be <u>encoded</u> if it is to be sent over the same radio channels used to transmit voice. ECG telemetry over UHF frequencies is confined to one lead of a 12-lead ECG, so it can be used to interpret cardiac rhythms. For a more complete diagnosis of an ECG, such as in the case of examining the ECG of a patient with suspected acute coronary syndrome, the information from all 12 leads of the ECG must be examined. Most newer systems use facsimile technology to allow transmission of ECGs, including 12-lead ECGs, to receiving hospitals before the arrival of the ambulance at the facility.

Distortion of the ECG signal by extraneous spikes and waves is known as noise and may arise from a variety of sources:

- Muscle tremor
- Loose ECG electrodes
- Sources of 60-cycle alternating current (AC), such as transformers, power lines, and electric equipment
- Attenuation (reduction) of transmitter power, caused by weak batteries or transmission beyond the range of the transmitter

ECG telemetry, begun in Miami, Florida, by Eugene Nagel, MD, during the early 1970s, had an important role in establishing the paramedic profession—it made it possible for doctors in the hospital to supervise paramedics caring for patients in the field. It was the technical feasibility of such supervision that convinced the medical community and the public to accept the idea of paramedics carrying out procedures such as defibrillation and administration of cardiac drugs, and many states made it mandatory for all ALS units to have telemetry capabilities.

In the last decade, as paramedics have become more and more skilled in dysrhythmia recognition, the trend has been to make less and less use of ECG telemetry; rather, most systems rely solely on the paramedic's assessment of the patient's cardiac rhythm and rarely require confirmation of the assessment by a physician. However, just as use of ECG telemetry seemed to be declining, two developments occurred to bring about a reassessment of prehospital ECG telemetry. First, conclusive research on the use of fibrinolytic agents indicated that the earlier the agents were given during an acute myocardial infarction, the better the chances of myocardial reperfusion. Second, cellular telephone and facsimile technology made it possible to transmit a 12-lead ECG from a moving ambulance to a hospital and, therefore, to diagnose myocardial infarction before the patient reaches the hospital. Such early diagnosis enables the hospital to prepare for the administration of fibrinolytic therapy or coronary cauterization immediately as the patient arrives; and in some EMS systems, the fibrinolytics are actually administered in the prehospital setting. Because technology can facilitate assessment and treatment in the prehospital setting, it is probable that telemetry in one form or another will remain a part of emergency care for some time. Information other than ECGs may also be transmitted to the receiving hospital before the patient arrives. Because advancements in technology are occurring rapidly, EMS systems must keep up with the technology that will allow better methods for communication of patient information.

The old telemetry system can still be used; however, it requires a functional biotelemetry system. In some cases, older radio biotelemetry systems were discarded to make way for

YOU *are the Medic* | **PART 2**

You bend down to the patient's eye level and introduce yourself and your partner. The patient looks at you and smiles. You ask the patient for his name. The patient continues to smile and looks to his wife. The wife states her husband's name is John Smith. She leans over to her husband's left ear and yells, "They wanted to know your name, John." Mr. Smith nods in acknowledgment. You continue with your assessment and ask, "May we call you John?" Mrs. Smith answers the question for her husband, "Yes, he goes by John."

Recording Time: 2 Minutes	
Appearance	Frail
Level of consciousness	Alert and oriented
Airway	Open
Breathing	Adequate
Circulation	Adequate

3. What does it mean to "get on the same level as the patient"? What is the importance of this?

4. How can you address the problem of a family member answering questions for the patient?

newer technology, such as fax or digital transmission. In some services, a facsimile (fax) of the ECG is transmitted directly by cellular phone to the coronary catheterization laboratory to help the staff determine the best treatment, such as preparing for fibrinolytic therapy or a catheterization procedure. In these situations, the ECG is captured on the heart monitor and then stored in the machine in a data file. This data file can then be transmitted to the hospital via a cell phone link from a connective Bluetooth device from the heart monitor to a cell phone. In other services, direct transmission of the data by email can do the same thing. The heart monitor transmits data to the computer by Bluetooth, and then it retransmits the data over mobile data links to the hospital, using the Internet. There are even systems that will "dump" patient data directly into hospital patient charts, enabling the immediate transmission of the information, along with electronic filing of the data to the patient's record.

Factors That May Affect Communications

In communication, many things may go wrong, and not all of them are equipment failures. You need to be prepared for such situations. Radio communication is technical and technology-driven. At times, systems may have problems, such as radio tower issues, computer crashes, telemetry failure, and audio problems. In these situations, you must be able to troubleshoot the device quickly and, if you cannot fix it, use your planned redundancy. Follow your local protocols regarding radio failure.

Communicating by Radio

The effectiveness of an EMS communications network depends on the technical hardware and on the people who use it. Communicating effectively by radio under emergency conditions requires skill and experience. Some paramedics "freeze" at the microphone, whereas others find themselves talking excessively, providing unlimited streams of patter. Neither behavior is appropriate or useful. Effective radio communication in EMS requires knowledge of the rules that govern the communications and an understanding of conventions for transmitting medical information by radio. It is not complicated if you bear in mind that the purpose of talking on the radio is to transmit pertinent information. Keep communications simple, brief, and direct.

You should practice effective communications skills and be familiar with all of the various methods of communication that will be required through your radio. As part of your job, you will need to demonstrate how to communicate effectively with your dispatcher for the call, from call receipt to call end. In addition, you must be able to communicate effectively with the receiving medical facility and deliver a precise and direct radio report in an organized and systematic manner.

FCC Regulations

As mentioned earlier, the FCC is the agency of the US government that regulates all radio and television communications in the United States. For radio, the FCC issues licenses, allocates frequencies, establishes technical standards, and establishes and enforces rules and regulations for the operation of radio equipment. FCC officials monitor transmissions on various frequencies and conduct spot checks of base stations to ensure that they are properly licensed. Fines can be imposed for failing to follow the FCC rules and regulations.

The FCC requires that communications over frequencies allocated for emergency medical use be confined to that use. The use of obscenities and the transmission of messages unrelated to the provision of medical services are forbidden by the FCC. When it is necessary to communicate a personal message to a paramedic in the field, it is best simply to notify him or her by radio to contact the base by phone. Similarly, a paramedic with a personal request of the dispatcher should use a telephone, not a two-way radio, to communicate that message **Figure 3**.

All EMS radio communications are regulated by the Special Emergency Radio Service provisions of the FCC Rules and Regulations, Part 90, and a copy of the Part 90 regulations should be available for reference at every base station.

Clarity of Transmission

The basic model of communication, whether by radio, intercom, telephone, or face-to-face involves a *sender*, a clear message, a *receiver*, and a *feedback loop* (repeating the information for confirmation) to ensure that the exact message that was sent is received and interpreted properly by the receiver. For example, if the emergency department orders 100 mg of lidocaine given IV push, you should repeat the order for confirmation (eg, EMS unit 1, I understand, give the patient 100 mg of lidocaine, IV push, correct?). The purpose of communications equipment is to permit communication. That sounds obvious, yet it is often forgotten. Simply blurting something into a microphone is not communicating. For communication to occur, someone at the

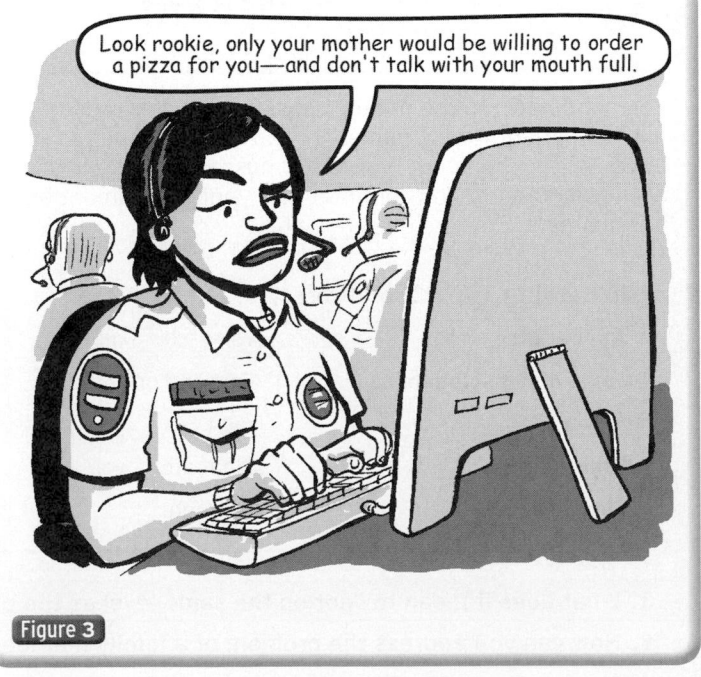

Figure 3

other end of the radio has to be able to hear and understand what you say. The first principle of communicating by radio is clarity.

A number of guidelines can help you improve the clarity of your transmissions:

- Before you begin to transmit, check the volume, and then listen to make sure the channel is clear. If another radio transmission is in progress, wait until the parties have finished transmitting before you try to get on the air. Cutting in on someone else's transmission will only ensure that neither of you will be adequately heard.

- Once the channel is quiet, press the transmit key for at least 1 second before you start speaking to ensure that the beginning of your message is not lost.

- Start your transmission with the identifying information: give the number or the name of the unit being called first, then your own identification (for example, "Williamsburg Hospital, this is Medic 3"). That way, the unit being called is alerted immediately and will be listening when you give your own identification, so they can reply at once, "Go ahead, Medic 3." If you do say, for example, "Medic 3 calling Williamsburg Hospital," the recipients might listen only when you have mentioned their identification and, therefore, will miss your identification. What inevitably happens then is, "This is Williamsburg Hospital. What unit is calling?" That extra transmission wastes time.

- Keep your mouth close to the microphone, but not too close. About 2″ to 3″ is usually ideal.

- Speak clearly and distinctly, pronouncing each word carefully.

- Do not shout! Shouting distorts the signal. Speak in a normal pitch; high- and low-pitched sounds do not transmit well. Whispering is not effective for transmitting.

- Do not talk with your mouth full. It muffles transmission.

- Keep calm and keep your voice free from emotion. You do not have to imitate a talking computer; a normal conversational tone is fine. Just keep your voice and mind free of panic, anger, excitement, and other feelings that can distort your transmission and your judgment.

- Keep your transmissions brief. Air time is precious, and emergency medical frequencies are not the place for long dialogues. Try having your radio reports taped at some point to critique your own transmissions and perfect your style.

- If you have a long message to transmit, break the message into 30-second segments, checking at the end of each segment to determine whether it was received and understood.

- Do not waste air time with unnecessary phrases, such as "be advised." Also bear in mind that courtesy is taken for granted; there is no need to use air time for social graces such as "please," "thank you," and "how nice to hear your voice."

- When speaking a word or name that might be misunderstood, spell it out, using the international radiotelephony spelling alphabet (or NATO phonetic alphabet) Table 1 or a similar system. Suppose, for example, you are asking the hospital to notify the patient's family doctor whose name might be mistaken for that of another doctor on the staff; you might say, "Notify Dr. Wilby. That's Dr. WHISKEY-INDIA-LIMA-BRAVO-YANKEE, Wilby."

Table 1	International Radiotelephony Spelling Alphabet		
A	Alpha	J Juliet	S Sierra
B	Bravo	K Kilo	T Tango
C	Charlie	L Lima	U Uniform
D	Delta	M Mike	V Victor
E	Echo	N November	W Whiskey
F	Foxtrot	O Oscar	X X-ray
G	Golf	P Papa	Y Yankee
H	Hotel	Q Quebec	Z Zulu
I	India	R Romeo	

- When presenting numbers that might be misunderstood, transmit the number as a whole, then digit by digit. For example, if the respirations are 16, you would say, "The respirations are sixteen, that is, one-six."

Content of Transmissions

Radio transmissions for EMS should be brief, to the point, and professional in tone Figure 4 . Here are some guidelines about what you should and should not include in EMS radio communications:

- The first thing to remember when you get "on the air" is that your words are, quite literally, in the air, floating around for anyone to hear. Remember, anyone may be listening.

  The medical staff at the local ED, a patient signing in at the front desk of another ED, a 12-year-old radio buff playing with his scanner at home . . . any of them may be listening with great attention to your transmission. Therefore, it is essential to protect the privacy of the patient at all times. Do not use the patient's name on the air, and do not transmit personal information about the patient. It is an issue that relates to the Health Information Portability and Accountability Act (HIPAA) guidelines on confidentiality. Also, check local laws applicable to your EMS system. Certain types of cases, such as rape or psychiatric problems and confidential communicable disease history (such as HIV status), are best identified on the air by an established code or given in face-to-face communications when you arrive in the ED.

  Do not assume that your cellular telephone offers you protected conversations. There are scanners on the market that can tune into the

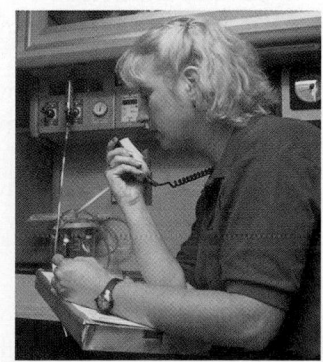

Figure 4 The patient report should be given in an objective, accurate, professional manner.

local cellular frequencies. Do not say anything on the radio or the cellular phone that you do not want others to hear.

- The agency being called must signal that it is ready to receive the information. A simple "Rampart Hospital standing by to copy" will let the sender know the agency is ready to receive the information.
- Be impersonal. Use "we," not "I," to refer to yourself, and use proper names and titles ("Paramedic Smith," not "Billy") to refer to others when necessary.
- Always use clear text; do not use codes or signals.
- Reduce background noise; roll up windows to limit interference.
- Do not try to be a comedian or a critic. There is no place for unprofessional behavior, sarcasm, or other poor conduct on emergency medical radio frequencies.
- Do not use profane language on the air. Aside from the reflection on your professional character, the FCC might issue civil monetary penalties, revoke a license, or deny a renewal application. In addition, violators of the law, if convicted in a federal district court, are subject to criminal fines and/or imprisonment for not more than 2 years.
- Use professional language, but do not show off. Once again, remember that the object of the exercise is to communicate information, so although it is advisable for you to use proper medical terminology, it must be used correctly.
- Avoid using words that are difficult to hear. The word "yes," for example, is easily lost in transmission; use "affirmative" instead. Similarly, use "negative" instead of "no."
- Use standard formats agreed on by your EMS service for transmission of information. The patient's history, for example, should always be presented in the same order. When the listeners know what they are listening for, they are less likely to miss parts of the transmission.
- When you finish transmitting, notify the receiver that the transmission is finished. This can be a simple, "Over," or "end of transmission."
- Obtain confirmation that the transmission was received. When you receive instructions by radio from the dispatcher or from medical control, echo the order back to make certain you have understood it correctly. For example, if the physician instructs you to administer 75 mg of lidocaine slowly IV, you would respond, "That is lidocaine, 75 milligrams, repeat, 75 milligrams, slowly IV. Is that confirmed?"
- Question any orders you did not hear clearly or did not understand.
- Use EMS frequencies only for emergency medical communications.

Codes

Some ambulance services still use radio codes; most do not. Codes were used for several reasons:

- To maintain security of communication
- To keep air time as brief as possible
- To diminish the likelihood of misunderstanding or noise
- To prevent the patient, family, and bystanders from understanding what is being said

The last-mentioned reason is particularly important when the information you need to convey to the dispatcher or physician could alarm the patient. Suppose that you want to tell the physician that your patient is probably having an acute myocardial infarction and is in serious condition. It is preferable that the patient not hear that assessment because it could increase anxiety and possibly worsen the patient's condition. In fact, it is best not to be sitting right next to the patient when transmitting your report to the emergency department.

For a code to be of any use, everyone using the radio must know the meaning of the code words. When codes are used, therefore, they should be simple and standardized within a given region, and a copy of the code should be posted at every radio terminal.

The **ten-code** system, once commonly used, has been phased out in many EMS systems, and use is not recommended in the National Incident Management System (NIMS), which is discussed further in the chapter, *Incident Management and Multiple-Casualty Incidents*. If codes are still used in your agency, be sure to learn the code system used.

When and if you use codes, remember that one of their main purposes is to shorten air time. Codes should be kept simple and reserved for situations in which they are really needed. During MCIs, when personnel unfamiliar with the codes may be staffing radios and when everyone is apt to be anxious, it is usually best to abandon codes and to use words that all personnel understand. Most services use standard terms rather than codes for regular day-to-day operations as well.

Response to the Scene

When a call is received requesting EMS response, you should follow a standard method of communications. This methodology is usually standardized for the individual agency; although different agencies may have differing methods, most are similar in content. When you are alerted by dispatch, record the location and call information as it is given. This is important to ensure you fully understand the transmission. After the call is dispatched and you have recorded the details, respond back to the dispatcher that you have received the information.

A standard sequence is illustrated as follows:

Dispatch: *Attention Medic 2, respond emergency traffic to Second Street at Main Street, reference motor vehicle crash. Possibly two patients. Time 21:04.*

Medic 2: *Medic 2 received, responding to Second Street at Main Street, reference motor vehicle crash, two victims.*

This exchange shows dispatch that you have received the message and are responding to the alert. Further, it confirms the location and call reference, ensuring that there has been an effective and accurate transfer of information between the dispatcher and the EMS unit. This establishes your dispatch time.

Next, the EMS unit leaves its location and begins the trip to the scene. This should be documented by contacting dispatch and announcing your action. This establishes your en route time. This exchange could be as follows:

Medic 2: *Medic 2 en route to Second Street at Main Street. Emergency traffic.*

Dispatch: *Medic 2, received. En route time 21:05.*

The next transmission should be your arrival on scene. Dispatch must be notified. This allows a time stamp to document the EMS unit arrival and can also be used to record your observations and findings regarding the scene. Your notification can be as follows:

Medic 2: *Medic 2, on scene. Confirm two vehicles, moderate damage; both occupants are still in vehicles. Dispatch, can you notify any other responders that access to Second Street is blocked and they need to approach from the north side of the street?*

Dispatch: *Medic 2, received. Two vehicles, occupants inside, approach to Second Street is blocked. On scene time is 21:10.*

In this simple exchange, you have confirmed arrival, the number of vehicles, and that occupants are inside the vehicles. Further, you have given important prearrival instructions to the other responding agencies, without using valuable radio time. Also, this is a perfect opportunity to call for additional resources if needed.

Then, after you have treated your patients and are ready to provide transport, you need to contact dispatch again to confirm your actions. This establishes a time stamp for departing the scene. The radio exchange may be as follows:

Medic 2: *Medic 2, leaving Second and Main, en route to Municipal Hospital, two patients on board, nonemergency traffic.*

Dispatch: *Medic 2, received. I show you en route to Municipal Hospital, nonemergency traffic with two patients. Time 21:34.*

This series of transmissions documents the fact that you have completed operations at the scene and are on the way to the hospital, and the response is nonemergency. Again, a time stamp is generated for the record. If you are not able to communicate with dispatch while on scene, it is imperative that you maintain a list of procedure times and event times while on scene. These can be logged by responders or jotted down on a notepad for later communication to dispatch. When given to dispatch after the call, make sure to inform them to note in the record your times for documentation purposes.

The next radio transmission to dispatch is to notify them of your arrival at the medical facility. This can be as follows:

Medic 2: *Medic 2, arrived at Municipal, out of service.*

Dispatch: *Medic 2 received. I have you out at Municipal and unavailable for service. Time 21:45.*

In this exchange, the EMS unit confirms arrival at the hospital and establishes its status. This is important because it documents the unit's unavailability for further service at this time.

The last transmission confirms call completion and establishes status. If the unit is available, it means that they can respond to another call. If not, it establishes their status and intent. For example:

Medic 2: *Medic 2, we are clear of Municipal Hospital, but unavailable for service due to need to resupply. We will be en route to headquarters to pick up equipment.*

Dispatch: *Medic 2 received. I show you unavailable for calls and en route to headquarters for resupply. Time 21:59.*

This exchange indicates the unit's inability to respond because of equipment needs. As soon as the unit is resupplied and available, the unit should notify dispatch. For example:

Medic 2: *Medic 2, we are available at headquarters, ready to respond.*

Dispatch: *Medic 2, I show you now as available and ready to respond. Time 22:12.*

Radio transmissions for EMS should be brief, to the point, and professional in tone, as illustrated here. Never assume that dispatch knows your status. Always notify them of your status and confirm their receipt of transmission.

Relaying Information to Medical Control

Radio communications between paramedics in the field and their medical control physician need to be concise and accurate. A standard format for communicating patient information over the radio will ensure that significant information is relayed in a consistent manner and that nothing is omitted Figure 5. The standard format following works when medical control is at the facility receiving the patient. If the patient is being received at a different facility (such as per patient request), however, provide the same information but specify that the patient has requested to go to a different facility and name the facility.

It is not uncommon in larger EMS systems for the paramedic to need to go to a different facility than medical control. In these cases, always follow local protocol and notify both facilities of your destination. Medical control orders that come from another facility will usually be accepted by the receiving facility. See your local protocols and system requirements for details.

Format for Reporting Medical Information

The following list shows the items that should be included when reporting medical information:

- The patient's age and sex
- The patient's chief complaint
- A brief, pertinent history of the present illness or injury

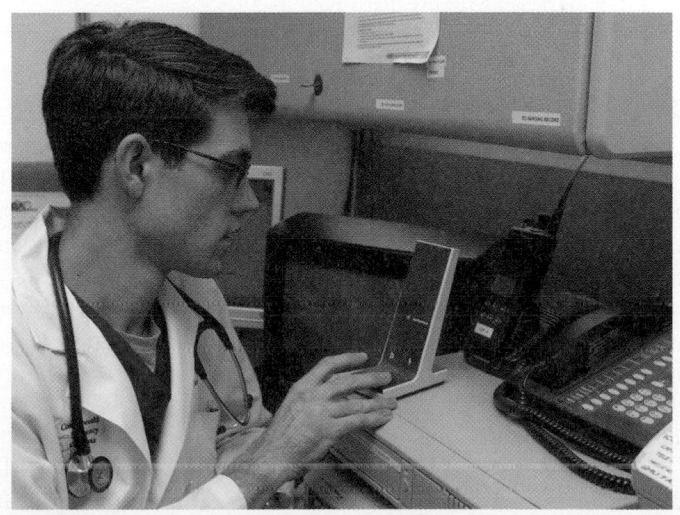

Figure 5 Use a standard format for communicating patient information to medical control.

- Anything the physician needs to know about the patient's other medical history relative to the current situation, including major underlying medical conditions, medications, and important allergies
- The patient's level of consciousness and degree of distress
- The patient's mental status
- The patient's vital signs
- The pertinent physical findings in head-to-toe order
- ECG findings
- Treatment given so far and response to treatment
- Estimated time of arrival at receiving facility

For example, here is a transmission regarding a patient in congestive heart failure: "We have a 53-year-old man reporting severe shortness of breath, which wakened him from sleep and is worse when he is lying down. He has a history of hypertension and takes chlorothiazide (Diuril). He is alert but in significant respiratory distress, with a pulse of 130 and regular, respirations 36 and labored, and a BP of 190/120. Physical exam reveals no JVD but crackles and wheezes in both lung fields. He has 2+ pitting ankle edema. We are sending you a 12-lead ECG."

The preceding transmission can be relayed in less than 30 seconds, and any physician hearing that information will immediately recognize that this is a hypertensive patient in moderately severe left-sided heart failure.

When paramedics call in without a standard reporting format, the physician might have to spend time gleaning the information needed to know what is going on. Consider the following dialogue:

Paramedic: *We have a patient with a pulse of 130, a blood pressure of 190/120, and respirations of 30. We're sending you a strip.*
Physician: *Fine, but what's his problem?*
Paramedic: *He's short of breath.*
Physician: *How long has this been going on?*
Paramedic: *Just a minute (pause). He says it woke him up from sleep about an hour ago.*
Physician: *Does he have any underlying medical problems?*
Paramedic: *He takes medicine for hypertension.*
Physician: *Is he in any distress?*
Paramedic: *Yes, he's having a hard time breathing.*
Physician: *What do his lungs sound like?*
Paramedic: *He has crackles and wheezes all over.*

Disorganized and incomplete communication is not efficient. It is a waste of time and causes frustration. The physician might respond to transport the patient immediately rather than try to get more complete information. To avoid ineffective dialogues, gather your information thoroughly at the scene, organize it clearly in your mind, and only then get on the air to the physician. Because even the best paramedics can be rattled under pressure, it is a good idea for you to write your reporting format on a card and affix the card to your hand-held transmitter or the dashboard of the ambulance so you may refer to it while reporting in.

As always, it is important to continue assessment of the patient. Once the report is given, reassess your patient according to protocol. Any changes should be reported in an update to the receiving facility.

Communication With Health Care Professionals

Phases of Communication

Communication during an emergency call has several phases that are essential to appropriate patient care and transportation. You will be exchanging information with many people, including the patient, bystanders with valuable information, the patient's family, medical control, the receiving medical facility staff, your dispatch center, law enforcement officials, and other members of the EMS team. One paramount responsibility in an emergency is communication with your partner. Staying in constant touch will keep each of you on top of your responsibilities and working effectively as a team while caring for your patient.

Each phase of the communication process requires using terminology understood by the people with whom you are communicating. Patients might need you to explain their medical condition in terms they understand. When you relay information to the receiving medical facility, you can use the medical terminology you have learned to make your radio report clear. Using medical terminology and avoiding slang terms shows your professionalism and respect for everyone you work with.

Medical Terminology

Using medical terminology correctly is essential to EMS communications. You should learn the established and accepted medical terms and abbreviations for your EMS operations. Some EMS systems have specific approved lists of medical abbreviations and terms that must be used.

Medical terminology may seem to be a foreign language, and in a sense it is. Most terminology comes from the ancient Roman language, Latin. In addition, some common expressions used in EMS such as "packaging a patient for transport" or "bagging the patient during airway management" might be used. Be sure to know acceptable terms and words used in your EMS agency. An ongoing review of the anatomy and physiology and documentation chapters can help you become familiar with medical terminology.

In-Person Report

When you are relaying medical information in person, such as when a bedside transfer of patient care occurs, be mindful of the information you are supplying, many times in the presence of the patient `Figure 6`. At times, it may be more practical to step outside the patient care room or to speak in a softer tone to provide the history and transferring information to the receiving medical practitioner. In addition, be brief. At this time, additional information should be shared that may not have been given in the radio report to the receiving facility. Ensure you are providing this information in person to a medical practitioner of an equal or a higher level of care to avoid abandonment and confidentiality issues and to ensure continuity of care.

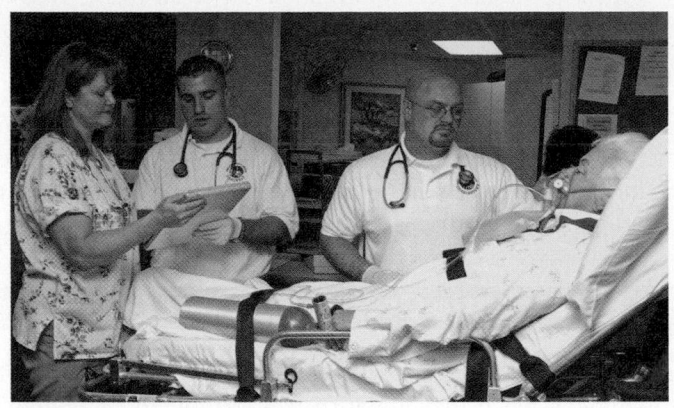

Figure 6 Be mindful of how you provide your report when the patient or family members are present.

Dispatching

The verb "to dispatch" means "to send out on a mission," but the EMD does a lot more than just send ambulances to emergencies. The EMD functions as a vital part of the paramedic team who obtains as much information as possible about the emergency, then directs the appropriate vehicle to the scene, and provides the caller with whatever advice may be needed to manage the situation until help arrives. The EMD also monitors and coordinates communication with the field and maintains written records pertaining to the response to the call.

The next section discusses the EMD's tasks in each phase of the call.

Receipt of the Call for Help

Whenever someone telephones for an ambulance, the EMD has to assume that the caller needs help, even if the caller is too upset to be clear about the nature of the problem. The EMD, therefore, has to be able to put himself or herself in the caller's place and understand the caller's distress. That means the EMD must do the following:

- *Answer the telephone promptly*, within two or three rings; each ring may seem like an eternity to a panicky person.
- *Identify himself or herself and the agency*. The caller needs immediate confirmation of having reached the right number.
- *Speak directly into the mouthpiece*, clearly and without mumbling.
- *Observe telephone courtesy*. The EMD must be calm and professional, informing the caller exactly what is being done and how soon assistance can be expected. As mentioned earlier, in some cases, EMDs provide prearrival instructions such as in the form of **emergency medical dispatch**—the EMD relays vital first aid information to the caller, who can then apply the aid techniques while waiting for the ambulance to arrive.
- *Take charge of the conversation*. Once the EMD has identified the ambulance service, he or she must start asking the

caller questions to which immediate answers are needed. Questions pertaining to safety issues are a priority. Additional useful information may also be obtained, such as specific situations the EMS crew might encounter: Is the residence door locked? What pets does the patient have? These pieces of information are invaluable in the field.

Information Gathering

The method used to gather information from a caller is most often a series of short questions asked by the EMD. When a call for EMS comes in, the EMD should elicit the following minimum information:

- The exact location of the patient(s), including the street name and number; the proper geographic designation (such as whether the street is East Maple or West Maple), and the name of the community (adjacent towns may have streets by the same name). If the call comes from a rural area, the dispatcher should try to establish landmarks (such as the nearest cross street or business establishment, water tower, or antenna).
- The telephone number (call-back number) of the caller, in case the call is disconnected or there is a need to phone the caller for more information. It is not uncommon for paramedics not to be able to find the address and to ask for help from the original caller. Asking for the caller's telephone number also helps discourage nuisance calls to EMS because prank callers are reluctant to supply their phone numbers. In services equipped with an **enhanced 9-1-1 system**, a lot of the information mentioned—such as the phone number and location of the caller—is recorded automatically through sophisticated telephone technology, and the EMD need only confirm the information on the screen.
- The caller's perception of the nature of his or her or the patient's problem.
- Specific information concerning the patient's condition that will help the EMD evaluate the urgency of the situation and decide if he or she needs to provide the caller with prearrival instructions by phone. The EMD should ask specifically:
  - Is the patient conscious?
  - If not, is the patient breathing?
  - Is the patient bleeding badly?
- If the emergency is a motor vehicle crash, further important information should be obtained:
  - The kinds of vehicles involved (that is, cars, trucks, motorcycles, buses). If a truck is involved, is there any indication of the cargo it is carrying? A truck carrying dynamite requires a different approach from one carrying bananas.
  - The number of persons injured and an estimate of the extent of injuries. This information will enable the EMD to estimate the magnitude of the problem.
  - Apparent hazards at the scene, such as heavy traffic, downed power lines, fire, spilled chemicals, and peculiar odors.

Information about such hazards enables the EMD to contact other agencies that may have to be involved, such as utility workers to take care of downed wires or an engine company to deal with spilled fuel. In most modern dispatch centers, the EMD has a computer screen with visual prompts that list the key questions to ask the caller.

Dispatch

At the point when your EMD has obtained the address of the emergency, the telephone number of the caller, and the apparent problem, the EMD should ask the caller to wait on the line. The EMD must then decide, assuming the call is a medical emergency within the service's jurisdiction, which crew(s) and vehicle(s) will be dispatched. That decision will be governed by the nature and location of the call and the availability of various units at the time. The appropriate crew is contacted and informed of the nature of the call and its exact location ("Medic 5, possible heart attack at 573 East Main Street, that's five-seven-three East Main Street with Jones Drive on the cross"). Once the ambulance is dispatched, the EMD may return to the telephone to obtain the rest of the information previously outlined. Further questioning may reveal special conditions that might affect your travel to the scene or your actions at the scene. If so, that information should be relayed to you while you are en route, for two reasons:

- So that you may know if the response requires travel under emergency conditions, using emergency warning devices
- So that while en route you may anticipate and prepare for tasks to be performed at the scene: assembling the equipment to deliver a baby or transmitting cardiac information to the receiving hospital

The EMD might also remind you to fasten your seat belts en route to the scene because this is usually the most dangerous part of the call.

Advice to the Caller

After directing you and any rescue crew(s) to the scene and alerting all of you to any special conditions, your EMD should return to the telephone and tell the caller what is being done ("An ambulance is on the way and should be there in about 5 minutes."). If your EMD suspects your patient has a life-threatening emergency, your EMD should also provide instructions to the caller in simple terms about emergency care techniques (such as airway maintenance, Heimlich maneuver, hands-only CPR, hemorrhage control). The caller is likely to be in an agitated state, so instructions must be clear and simple.

Excellent protocols have been developed for giving such instructions by telephone, and all EMDs should undergo training in those procedures. Most often, this training will be based on the original medical priority dispatch system designed by Jeff Clawson, MD, in Salt Lake City, Utah, in the early 1980s. The system is used throughout the world.

Ongoing Communications With the Field

It is important for your EMD to monitor the communications of the ambulance and to be aware of what is occurring in the field. Your EMD must coordinate communications between the ambulance and medical control and contact any other agencies (such as fire and police) whose presence may be required at the scene.

The phases of the EMD's work are summarized in Table 2.

In general, it is routine practice to use standard military time when documenting times for calls. Most dispatchers use this format when providing times over the radio as well. Standard military time is discussed in the chapter, *Documentation*.

Therapeutic Communication

As a paramedic, your job will involve daily interactions with people, often when they are at their worst or most vulnerable. At least half of the calls you will run as a paramedic will take you into people's homes, day and night, and in the most private moments of their lives. Try to see every invitation into the home of someone else as a personal honor in a time and place where no one else would be welcome Figure 7.

If you want people to tell you about their problems, convince them you want to hear what they have to say. Give patients your undivided attention; do not treat them like nuisances. There is nothing worse than talking about someone in his or her presence, as though he or she is an inanimate object—or worse, as though the person does not even exist. And it is unforgivable to ask someone a question you are just going to repeat later because you did not pay attention to the answer the first time. Jot it down. When it is time to communicate, *communicate*. That means listen, do not just talk. Listening is part of communicating too, in that it transmits information.

Table 2 Phases of Dispatch	
Information Gathered	**Dispatcher Action**
Answers telephone promptly Identifies agency Address of incident Call-back number Perceived problem Patient's name	Dispatches (first) ambulance

Patient's condition
For road accident:
    Number of vehicles
    Kinds of vehicles
    Number of victims
	Gives patient care instructions by phone if required

Hazards at the scene	Notifies responding ambulance(s) of special situations Dispatches additional ambulances as needed Contacts other agencies as needed Monitors communications from the field

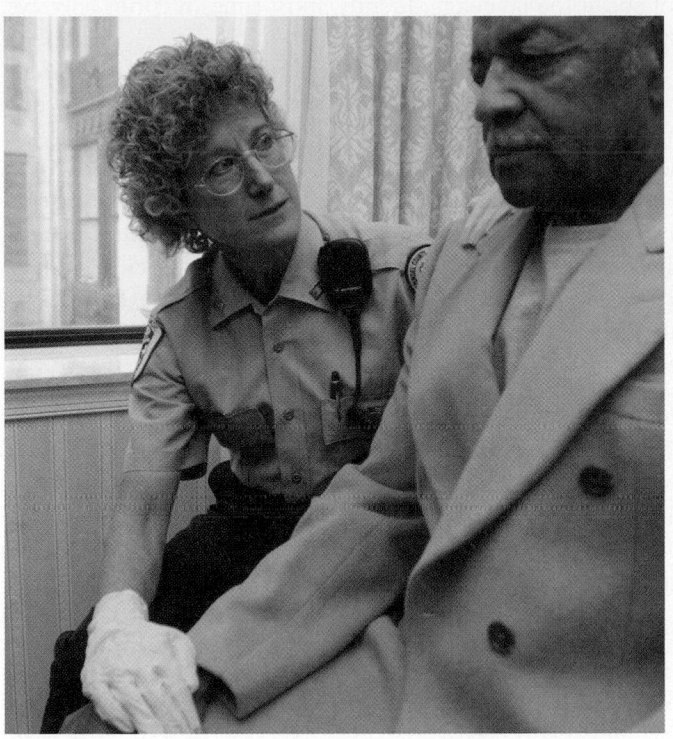

Figure 7 Think of it as an honor to be asked into a patient's home. Be respectful, and always be kind.

An excellent way to convince someone that you are really listening to him or her is a technique called "active listening." Almost all professional interviewers use it routinely. Active listening is repeating the key parts of a patient's responses to questions. Especially when you are taking notes at the same time, repeating key parts of the patient's responses helps you to assure the patient that you really want to hear what he or she is saying. Active listening also helps confirm the information patients are providing. This ensures there is no misunderstanding between you and your patients.

Some specific expressions that are helpful are as follows:

- When patients thank you, say, "You're welcome!" (not "No problem." "No problem" implies, "That's OK; you aren't too much of a nuisance." It's definitely not as nice as saying, "You're welcome.")
- When patients apologize to you because they are incontinent or vomiting or because you have to carry them down a flight of stairs, tell them something like, "It's OK; you don't need to be sorry. This is what we do, *and we're here because we want to be.*"

If you like serving people, these kinds of expressions will feel natural to you, and no doubt you will find your colleagues imitating you and saying the same types of responses.

Some scenes are noisy, but try hard not to shout. When you shout, so does everyone else. And when people are shouting, they tend to get excited. If you are answering a call in a noisy place such as a bar, ask the bartender to help by turning off the music, turning up the lights, and keeping an eye on the other patrons. (In this type of situation, get your patient out of

there as soon as you can.) Move the patient to the back of the ambulance. If you must use a compressor or run a noisy diesel engine on the scene, shut it off as soon as you can to cut down on the noise level. Meanwhile, try to talk close to your patient's ears in a calm voice. It lets him or her know that you have your emotions under control, which helps him or her stay calm as well. Try managing your history taking all at one time. Taking the patient's medical and health history helps you stay organized and encourages people to take your questions seriously.

If you want reliable answers to personal questions, try to manage your scene so you can ask these kinds of questions quietly and in private. Even if you do earn a patient's trust, there are things people just do not want to talk about in front of others. Do not forget to ask a few payoff questions—questions that do not fall under the category of routine medical history but that, time after time, will net you information that is critical to a presumptive diagnosis. Some payoff questions are listed and explained later in this chapter.

Some scenes are easy to manage; however, paramedics often work in bizarre, noisy, chaotic, and sometimes dangerous environments that are challenging at best. Under these circumstances, communicating with patients (and their family members) is especially critical to the skills of assessment and the art of bringing about calm (and therefore healing).

Developing Rapport

It is crucial that as soon as you meet the patient, you try to develop a good rapport because it is important for the flow of information. To be able to treat a patient effectively, you must obtain information relating to the condition and disorders of the patient. Start by trying to set an atmosphere of trust and comfort. Try to put the patient at ease. Reassure the patient with remarks like "we are here to take care of you, but we need some information to do that."

People in crisis are highly perceptive, and there is no greater crisis than being terribly frightened that you are about to lose someone you love. Your most essential challenge as a therapeutic communicator is to convey calm, unmistakable, genuine concern for someone you have never met. People in crisis do much better if someone can relieve their fear.

Obtaining information is a learned skill. Even under the best circumstances, getting necessary information can be a difficult task. Some patients are resistant to giving details about themselves. Others have trouble focusing on you, possibly due to the chaos of the scene, but they may also be numbed by the physical condition they are experiencing. The patient may also feel threatened by you or by others at the scene.

For patients who are reluctant to share personal information, start by explaining why you need their name and date of birth. Reassure them that all the information is confidential and must be protected as mandated by federal law. Due to the chaos at the scene, getting patients to focus is another issue. If you can safely move the patient to the ambulance, do so. Sometimes this will help create a less chaotic atmosphere for the patient and make talking and listening easier. If the patient is reluctant to communicate because he or she feels threatened, cautiously approach the patient and use open posturing. Smile and be calm. Reassure the patient and if possible, take things a little slower than usual. All of these actions can promote a less threatening environment.

Here are some tips for more positive communications:

1. Introduce yourself and obtain the patient's first name, then use it.
2. Make and keep eye contact.
3. Position yourself at their level, or slightly lower, but maintain safety.
4. Be honest.
5. Use language the patient can understand.
6. Be aware of your body language.
7. Speak calmly and clearly.
8. If the patient has hearing deficits, make sure your lips are visible.
9. Allow the patient time to answer.
10. Always act confident and professional.

Words of Wisdom

Patients will pick up on how you treat or are treated by other EMS officials at the scene. If you are treated with respect, and if you treat the other EMS officials with respect, the patient will see this and will have more confidence in you as well.

Introductions

To communicate better with patients, you may apply a few principles to help bridge communication gaps. **Interpersonal communications** is the exchange of information between two or more persons. The first step in promoting good communications is the introduction.

As soon as is reasonably possible, you should begin patient interaction by introducing yourself. This does not entail any special social skills or societal standard. Rather, a simple "Good afternoon, my name is Mark. I am a paramedic with the fire department. What is your name?" will usually suffice. This simple exchange offers comfort and promotes an atmosphere of "we are in this together."

Be sure you make eye contact and maintain it, for a few reasons. First, it reinforces trust and honesty. Second, it allows you to evaluate the patient's neurologic status, because certain conditions can relay neurologic information via the person's gaze. A vague, far-off stare may suggest mental dullness, which could be the result of physical issues or substance abuse. Third, the eyes may signal a person's behavioral unrest, as in certain psychiatric conditions.

Next, if there is no threat evident, try to get on the same level as the patient. This promotes trust and alleviates anxiety. This is especially true when dealing with children. Position yourself where the patient can easily see you, and so that those with hearing impairment may better observe your lips and facial expressions. Be aware of your own body language, because this can put patients at ease or make them uncomfortable. Use open-handed gestures, do not cross your arms, and do not react to answers with skepticism.

Use the patient's name in all interactions. Speak slowly and calmly. Always be honest; a falsehood can permanently damage a relationship. Finally, if the patient is from another country or culture, try and get a family member to help interpret. If you do

not speak the language fluently, most times it is not effective to try to speak their language.

Sometimes even with the best techniques, it is difficult to communicate with the patient. There are two basic factors necessary to improve communications. First, remember that external factors such as noise, disruptive scenes, language barriers, and sensory impairment will make communications difficult. Second, be aware of the internal factors that affect communications. The biggest factors are acceptance of others, lack of empathy, poor listening skills, and interrupting the patient. Remember to take good notes. Even persons with an excellent memory will miss things if they are not written down.

Respect and Protect People's Modesty

Modesty matters—no matter how acute the medical condition. It is especially important to the elderly, adolescents, and sometimes, the very young. If the patient is not personally sensitive to modesty (because of an impaired mental state, for example), family members most certainly are Figure 8 .

Conducting the Interview

Interviewing techniques are an important skill to develop and maintain. Remember, there are two types of questions used in effective interviewing. The first is the **open-ended question**. Always use open questions when interviewing patients. This allows the patient to give you feedback and not only gives you information, but allows you to gauge mentation. An example of an open-ended question is "How are you feeling at this moment?" or "Can you tell me how this all started?"

The second type of question is the **closed-ended question** or direct question. In this type of question you are eliciting a specific answer. Examples are: "What year were you born?" or "Does your arm hurt here?" (as you palpate the injured area). In fact, it is a good idea to develop a standard set of questions concerning medical history that you ask almost all patients. Avoid talking

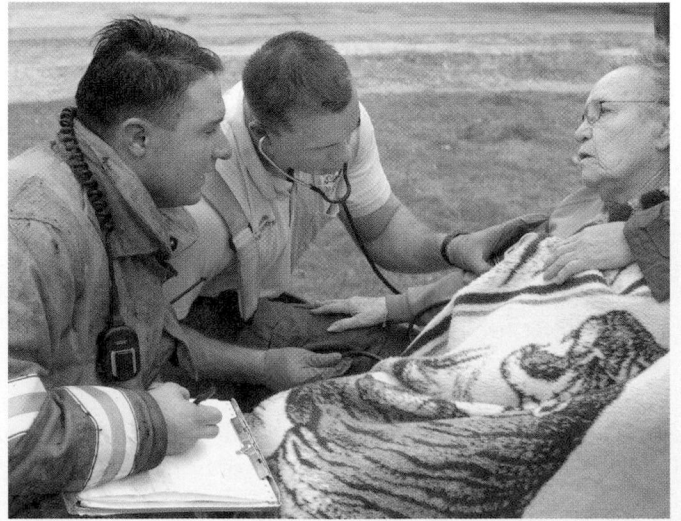

Figure 8 Show your patient the same respect you would want others to show your father or brother or your mother or sister. Protect a patient's modesty with a blanket or towel.

down to them (which is insulting), but avoid using medical terms. Instead, try using words that people without medical training can understand. Your standard questions may include the following:

- Have you ever had any heart problems?
- Any lung problems?
- Any high or low blood pressure?
- Diabetes?
- Seizures?
- Fainting spells?
- Any prior head injury?
- Do you have both lungs and both kidneys?

If the patient is female and of childbearing age (generally, ages 12 to 50 years), be sure to ask about her history of pregnancies, deliveries, and abortions, when her last menstrual period was and if it was normal, and if she has had any gynecologic surgeries.

Most seasoned paramedics have developed their own repertoire of additional questions for patients in specific circumstances. We call them payoff questions because they are like icebergs—tiny questions that can reveal huge subsurface issues. Sometimes these issues are the hidden reason that EMS has been called to help someone. Some examples of payoff questions are as follows:

- Have you ever felt like this before?
- Have you been upset about anything lately?
- Are you afraid of someone? (Save this one for the privacy of the ambulance.)
- Have you been thinking about hurting yourself?
- What happened the last time you felt this way?

It is important not to use leading questions when interviewing a patient because this may produce an aberrant answer. For example, "You said your neck hurt and your back hurt; is your head hurting also?" Always pose your questions clearly and in an even tone. Ask one question at a time and do not rush the patient. Let patients answer at their own pace and do not lead them.

■ Assessing Mental Status

A patient's mental status is often a prime indicator of the extent of the illness or injury. Changes in mentation are often the first clue to a patient's impending crash. Because the brain is the central coordination control of the body systems, changes in mental status can provide an early warning signal.

One of the quickest methods of establishing mental status is the AVPU method. This procedure checks the patient's level of response: **A**lert to person, place, and day; **V**erbal response; **P**ain response; and **U**nresponsiveness.

The AVPU procedure begins by assessing whether the patient can answer questions that everyone should be able to answer, such as "what day is today?" or "Do you know where you are?" and "What is your name?" An appropriate answer to these questions establishes the "alert" category.

If the answer is not appropriate, assess the patient's response to verbal commands. Tell him or her to "Raise your left arm," or "move your feet," or "blink your eyes twice." Appropriate response to these commands, although the patient is not alert, establishes the "verbal" response level and shows a lesser degree of mental acuity.

If neither of these assessments produces appropriate results, then you can determine the response to pain. Pinch the finger-web, or squeeze the finger hard enough to elicit a movement of withdrawal in normal people. If the patient withdraws, he or she is termed "responsive to pain stimulus." If the patient does not respond, however, then he or she is deemed "unresponsive."

There are many useful techniques for assessing mental status during the interview. It is vital that you use your observation and conversation skills to assess how alert your patients are. Patients should be able to tell you quickly and accurately who they are and who you are, where they are, what day of the week it is, and what happened that necessitated your being called (orientation). You can further assess the mental status if

YOU are the Medic   PART 3

Your partner asks Mrs. Smith to please take her to John's medications so she can make note of them. Mrs. Smith happily complies. You are still on the same level as John and you slowly ask in a slightly louder voice, "Can you understand me John?" After a pause, John answers "Yes."

Recording Time: 5 Minutes	
Respirations	14 breaths/min
Pulse	76 beats/min, strong and regular
Skin	Pale, cool, dry
Blood pressure	110/66 mm Hg
Oxygen saturation (Spo$_2$)	98% room air
Pupils	Equal and reactive

5. Give some examples of effective communication techniques for persons with hearing impairment.

6. How can your body language affect your assessment of this patient?

you get a response by judging the speech: Is it impaired? Is it clear? Does the person seem to make logical sentences? Can he or she understand further questions? Inappropriate responses may indicate mental slowing due to injury/illness.

Strategies to Elicit Useful Reponses to Questions

For you to get the right answers, it is not always enough just to ask the right questions. This is because when people are in crisis, some of them experience a breakdown in their ability to communicate. It can be almost impossible to think and organize your thoughts when you are terrified. Fortunately, good interviewers also have the following tools to use to get informative answers.

Reflection

Reflection is the repetition of a word or phrase that a patient has used in previous statements to encourage more detail. For example, your patient may have said, "I can't catch my breath."

You could probe, "You say you can't catch your breath, sir?"

Then the patient may respond, "Well, my chest felt tight, and I could not breathe fully."

Then you could ask, "What were you doing when this occurred? Were you exerting yourself?"

Then the patient says, "No, I was in my chair, and it started all of a sudden."

This technique has given you vital information. Now you are aware that the onset was sudden and did not result from exertion or strain, much more information than was originally communicated by the patient.

Empathy

Empathy is described as "feeling what the patient is feeling;" in other words, putting yourself in the patient's position. For example, you ask, "Why did you call us tonight, Mr. Smith?"

He answers, "I just feel so sad and depressed. I cannot seem to function."

You ask, "What do you think is making you feel this way, sir?"

He says, "I just have not been normal since my wife died of cancer last week. I just don't have the spirit to continue."

You respond, "I am terribly sorry Mr. Smith. That is so unfair. I don't know how I would feel in your situation, but I am sure I would feel similar."

This patient may or may not have other issues affecting his health, but he is in need of help. Concern and caring followed up by a suggestion to let you take him to the hospital might be what keeps this patient alive and well.

Confrontation

Confrontation is described as making your patients aware that you understand that something is not "right" or "consistent" with their story. You must balance this tool with statements that could provoke the patient. The key is to remain professional and nonjudgmental. For example, Mr. Jones tells you, "My whole life sucks. I am tired of living."

You respond, "You sound so negative; are you considering suicide?"

Mr. Jones, "I might be; I just might."

You ask, "What makes you think that would be the answer? Have you made plans to do something harmful to yourself? If so, how do you plan to do it?"

Mr. Jones, "I don't know. I just don't know."

Whereas this conversation may indicate that the patient is not happy, he may not yet be distressed enough to take his life. With that in mind, it gives you more opportunities to suggest help and to gauge his aggressiveness.

Interpretation

If you are not sure what a patient is trying to tell you, sometimes it helps to vocalize what you think he or she said and invite him or her to correct you.

Interpretation can also be used when a patient refuses to give information that you need to determine a course of treatment.

In this method, you begin by diplomatically telling the patient what you think is going on, and then asking him or her if you are right. For example, you are with a patient who is 16 years old. Her parents have called you because she was "acting depressed and we think she is on drugs." You remove her to the ambulance for transport, and she says, "I don't know how I got in this mess."

You ask, "What mess?"

She says, "I can't say. I so don't want to hurt my parents."

You inquire, "Why do you think you are hurting your parents?"

She says, "They never liked my boyfriend, and now, I'm in trouble."

You ask, "Did your boyfriend hurt you?"

She replies, "No, but I cannot tell them what is wrong."

You ask, "This may be totally wrong, but I must ask the question so I can inform the doctor for your well-being: Do you think you are pregnant?"

She says, starting to cry, "I don't know, but I think I may be."

The skill of interpretation requires you to use your best intuition and diplomatic skills. One of the best phrases to begin with is, "So, if I understand what you are saying correctly, . . ."

Facilitation

If patients hesitate to answer questions completely, encourage them to provide you with more information. One useful expression is simply, "Please say more." Another is, "Please feel welcome to tell me about that."

Being Quiet

If you sense that patients are trying to put something into words but are having trouble expressing themselves, try this famous tip: "Never miss a good opportunity to shut up." Be patient. Do not say anything at all for a few seconds. Let the patient talk.

Clarification

If you do not understand what patients have told you, ask them to explain what they mean. This communicates that you are listening and taking their comments seriously. It may also help you understand what they are trying to tell you.

Redirection

Sometimes patients will mention something in passing or will avoid answering a specific question. You can politely redirect their attention to that question (several times, if necessary) until you get them to answer it.

Simplification and Summarization

Some patients have a hard time speaking plainly, no matter how hard they try. It can be difficult to communicate with people who have psychiatric problems, who fabricate their diseases, and who are afraid or upset. If patients give you a confusing or disorganized response, try putting their comments into simpler terms and see if they agree with your synopsis. This method can help them focus their thoughts and help you as an interviewer.

Common Interviewing Errors

In addition to good interviewing techniques, there are some errors that can be considered "traps." First, never provide false assurance or make claims that are not likely to be borne out. Your job is to be neutral and objective, not falsely supportive. You cannot possibly see in advance what is going to happen to someone. Assuring someone that he or she will be fine seems like a simple and caring statement. However, if that patient worsens, your statement can be devastating.

Second, do not give advice. Remember your role. You are not a physician or counselor. A simple statement like, "I don't think you are having a heart attack; it may just be that spicy food you ate" can prove to be wrong. Statements such as this can result in a patient not seeking medical help. Remember, most patients do not want to go to the emergency department. A statement like this can lead them to reject transport, and if they are actually having a myocardial infarction, this decision can be life threatening to the patient.

Third, do not consider yourself an authority. You may have finished at the top of your class, but you are lacking in overall medical education. Physicians attend school for years and practice under close scrutiny before they are licensed to give advice and act as an authority.

Do not use avoidance language. Be direct and honest. In addition, stay away from professional jargon as much as possible; it may be tempting to use complicated medical terms, but the average person will not understand them. Use clear, concise terms. Also, do not interrupt the patient or talk too much; you need to hear what the patient has to say.

Nonverbal Skills

There are some nonverbal communication skills that you need to master. First, remember the old adage, "You only get one chance to make a first impression." People often form opinions of others at the first observation. If you look slovenly and unkempt, the patient may form the impression that your skills likely are that way also. A professional appearance and demeanor is likely to instill confidence in patients.

Be patient. An impatient paramedic will make the patient feel uncomfortable and stressed. It is understood that most emergencies require quick actions; however, you can still be efficient and quick while displaying an air of patience and calm.

Try to avoid gestures, facial expressions, and "closed posture" because this sends negative signals. Do not frown or smirk at answers. Do not roll your eyes at your partner. Maintain constant, nonjudgmental eye contact. Keep your voice calm and neutral, and encourage answers; do not demand them.

Some people do not like to be touched at all; to others, it is a valuable assurance that someone cares about them. Try gently touching patients on a neutral part of the body, such as a shoulder or arm, especially when you are trying to reassure them or to mitigate their fear **Figure 9**. Watch how they react, however. If they pull away from you, it is likely that touch in this instance will not be a valuable strategy. If they react positively (for instance, by leaning toward you or seeming to relax), then touch as a form of reassurance will work with them.

Special Interview Situations

There are situations in paramedic practice that may require special communication techniques. Some of these may include uncommunicative patients, hostile patients, elderly or very young patients, and patients with special needs. Stereotyping any of these groups of patients, however, will only work against effective communication. A good paramedic is never judgmental about his or her patients.

Sometimes you will encounter difficult or potentially violent patients. These patients present quite a challenge to the paramedic. Patients may be difficult for a variety of reasons. They may be scared or panicked. They may be under the influence of drugs or alcohol. They may have behavioral or mental issues. Or they may just be having a bad day. When you are caring for these patients, you need to use patience, persistence, and persuasion.

The following are some broad tips for caring for difficult patients:

1. Approach the patient cautiously, while maintaining eye contact.
2. Begin by introducing yourself and asking for the patient's name.
3. Use open-ended questions.
4. Provide positive feedback.
5. Make sure the patient understands you.
6. Continue to ask questions, rephrasing if necessary.

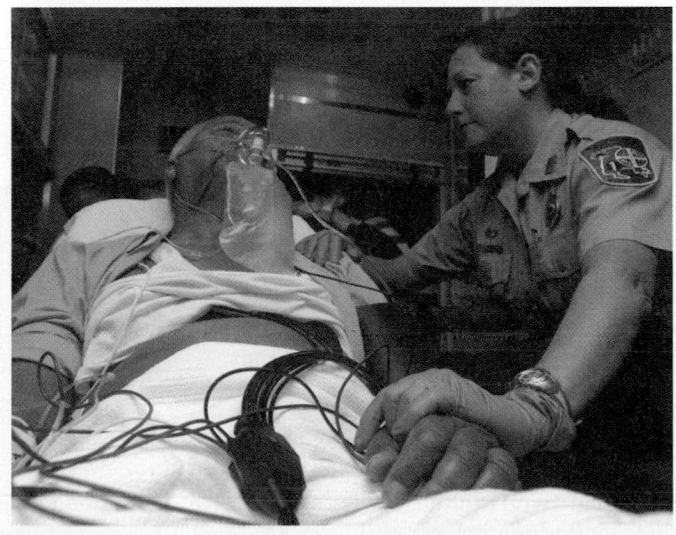

Figure 9 A gentle touch on the hand, arm, or shoulder can comfort someone who is sick or hurt and scared.

People Who Are Hostile

Emergency situations can be emotional for the people involved, particularly patients and their loved ones. This heightened emotion may cause some people to become hostile, even toward the paramedic trying to help. It is important to acknowledge the hostile person's concerns and to empathize with him or her. Remain calm and try to understand the person's arguments. Use questioning, clarification, and summary to help the person feel heard and understood.

Remember, just like you cannot fix everybody medically, you cannot fix everybody emotionally, either. Consider the possibility that you may not be able to defuse an angry person, in which case you may have to defer to law enforcement personnel.

You are guaranteed to receive some unpleasant insults from people who are in crisis, and that will probably happen on a near-daily basis. It is especially predictable when you are dealing with people who are chemically impaired. Discipline yourself never to respond in kind. Nothing escalates a situation faster than trading insults with people, and very often when it involves a patient there are plenty of witnesses. It makes no sense, it is unprofessional, and it can be dangerous.

Hostile or angry patients may present a threat to you and others. Always approach hostile or angry patients with caution and maintain eye contact. Try not to interview an angry patient by yourself. It is a good idea for your partner to be present, but have him or her stay a little farther back to prevent the patient from feeling crowded. The following are some additional tips for dealing with potentially violent patients:

1. As you enter the scene, identify escape routes.
2. Approach the patient from the front, with your hands visible and open.
3. If safe to do so, assume the patient's level.
4. Ask permission to ask questions and touch the patient.
5. Always be honest.
6. Be wary for signs of impending attack such as clenched fists, violent language, tensed neck and face muscles, and threatening gestures.
7. Always be prepared to escape if necessary.

Words of Wisdom

Make it part of your routine to look for aggressive body language that signals increased anger and a possible attack. These signs include clenched fists, intense staring directed at you, and breathing heavily through clenched teeth.

Sexually Aggressive Patients

Occasionally, you will encounter a patient who is more aggressive sexually than others. If this occurs, make sure you follow your agency's policies. You can begin by making sure you have someone present at all times when you are with the patient. Communicate professionally and politely. Make sure your words are not sexually ambiguous. Most of all, maintain professionalism at all times. Document your encounter meticulously and get witness names and signatures on the patient notes.

Special Considerations of Age

Try not to presume that older people are any harder to communicate with than anyone else just because they are older. When they get sick, their illnesses do tend to be more complex than the illnesses of younger people because they may have more than one disease process and they may be taking more kinds of medications concurrently. You may note individual differences among the geriatric population related to hearing, eyesight, mentation, and mobility; and you will need to adapt to them. The fact remains, however, that geriatric patients are people and those differences are individual.

Children can be difficult patients because they pose communication challenges even to the best paramedics. They tend to protest pain vigorously, they may be afraid of strangers, they can panic when separated from their parents, and their bodies may seem unfamiliar to you. (Many paramedics are not as experienced at taking children's vital signs, starting IV lines, or intubating tracheas as they might be in the case of adults.) However, with a little practice you can become comfortable with these skills.

Equipment (like stethoscopes and needles) is not as important early in your contact with children as friendly eye contact; smiles; and calm, subdued explanations geared to match the child's age. Discipline yourself to minimize your movements, lower your voice, and touch as gently as you can. Try keeping your eye level at or below the child's level, for instance by sitting on the floor and placing the child on the cot or on a parent's lap **Figure 10**. If possible, involve a parent in the hands-on care of a conscious small child (for instance, by holding an extremity while you insert an IV line). This is more important with infants and toddlers, and less helpful with older children.

When parents are not available, toys are useful for bridging the space between paramedics and some children. Many crews stock their ambulances with teddy bears for toddlers. Short of

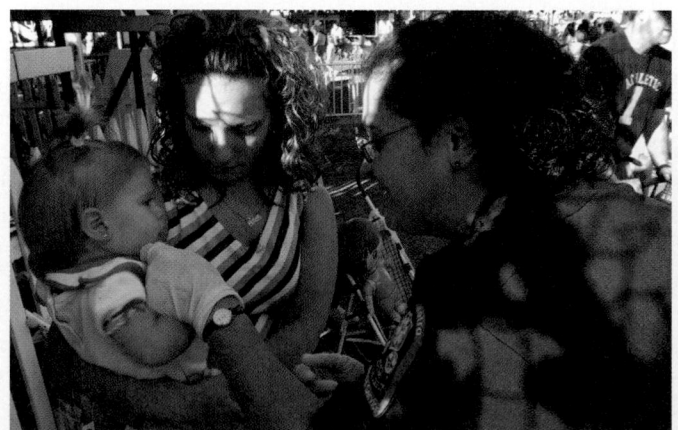

Figure 10 When you are examining a young child, involve the parents. Have a parent hold the child on his or her lap, or ask the parent to keep the child occupied while you work.

those, you can make a serviceable chicken out of an exam glove by inflating the glove and marking its eyes with a felt marker Figure 11 . You are more likely to connect with the child if you do this right in front of them than if you ask someone else to do it.

Adolescents (beginning at around age 12) may not want their parents present at all during questioning or examination. In fact, an adult who insists on monitoring your conversation with an adolescent should raise concern in your mind. Do not refuse that prerogative of a parent, but be sure you communicate the situation to the emergency department physician. Generally, it is a good idea to deal with adolescents as adults, gaining better cooperation by offering them options and honoring their choices. (Hint: Never offer an option you know you cannot honor.) Make special efforts to protect the modesty of patients older than age 2 years, and of adolescents in particular. Patients in this age grouping are becoming more aware of their bodies and may be especially embarrassed during physical examination. Try to avoid disrobing the patient unless necessary.

People Who Live With Special Challenges

It would be a mistake to overlook the needs of people with speech, hearing, sight, and other kinds of communication disorders. Many caregivers enroll in classes on sign language and lip reading to facilitate communication with these patients.

When you encounter a patient who has trouble communicating, remember that family members or primary caretakers who know these patients well can facilitate your efforts. Just as importantly, they can also help you alleviate the patient's fear. If a patient wears glasses or a hearing aid, ensure that those items are available; they could facilitate communication and reduce the patient's fear.

Many caregivers find that touch and eye contact are helpful bridging mechanisms when caring for these kinds of patients. For example, a light touch on a patient's shoulder can convey kindness, while a firm grasp can express reassurance. Some patients respond well to brief, one-armed hugging. In other situations, you can grasp a patient's face between your hands and use your eyes to convey concern or to calm them down.

Another group of patients paramedics are beginning to encounter more often are those with autism. Autism can vary in severity and falls under a broader category known as **pervasive developmental disorders (PDDs)**. PDDs cause delays in many areas of childhood development, such as the development of skills to communicate and interact socially, and the effects can be lifelong.

Children with autism may have difficulty developing language skills and understanding what others say to them. They also may have difficulty communicating nonverbally, such as through hand gestures, eye contact, and facial expressions. Not every person with an autism spectrum disorder will have a language problem, however. A person's ability to communicate will vary depending on his or her intellectual and social development. Some people with autism may be unable to speak. Others may have rich vocabularies and be able to talk about specific subjects in great detail. Most children with autism have little or no problem pronouncing words. The majority, however, have difficulty using language effectively, especially when they talk to other people. Many have problems with the meaning and rhythm of words and sentences. They also may be unable to understand body language and the nuances of vocal tones.

Often, children with autism who can speak will say things that have no meaning or that seem out of context in conversations with others; for example, they may use continuous repetition. When communicating with an autistic patient, it may be best to address questions to the caregiver. Most caregivers have developed knowledge of the patient's needs through years of working with the patient. They are your best resource for communicating with the autistic patient.

Documentation and Communication

Many hospitals and 9-1-1 dispatch centers have interpreter capabilities and are a good resource for communicating with patients who speak a language that is different from yours. Know what resources are available for patients who use sign language as a means of communication as well.

Cross-Cultural Communication

Communicating with people of cultures not your own can be challenging. Diversity exists in our everyday lives. You have the opportunity to interact with many different people, and in these interactions you are exposed to people of differing races and religions. You are called to help people of different genders, classes, and lifestyles. In all interactions, remain considerate and professional with all patients, even those whose culture you do not understand.

It is always considered a mark of your respect for them if you make an effort to learn their language (remember who is serving whom). If your service area features one or more populations whose culture differs from your own, learn as much as you

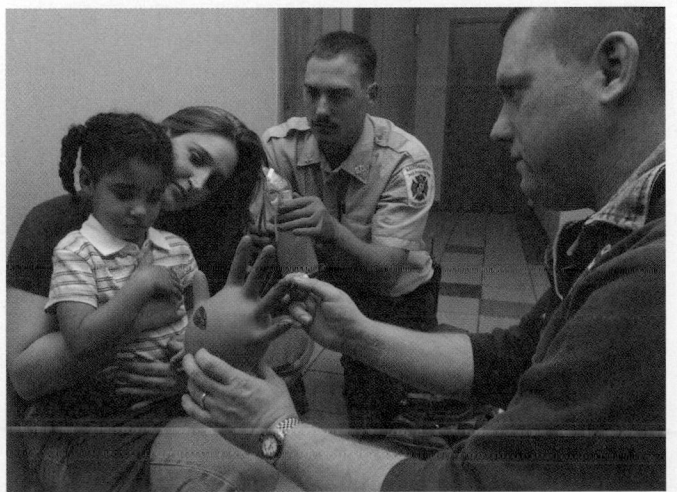

Figure 11 An exam-glove chicken can put a youngster at ease.

can about them. In other words, "know your audience." Good eye contact demonstrates that you are actively listening to the patient. However, some cultures may consider this disrespectful.

Cultural sensitivity and cultural diversity have become important terms. There are many classes and seminars designed to teach how to deal with cultural differences between employees and contacts. These classes and seminars ultimately teach students and attendees to show respect, interest, and concern for other cultures. This sounds simple, but in practice it is difficult. Many people have difficulty conveying basic respect in normal interactions. Often people offend each other with the abruptness in their behavior.

Whereas the social purposes, mannerisms, etiquette, and idiosyncrasies of all cultures are too numerous to list in this book, it is highly important that you be open to educating yourself. It is your responsibility to research various groups in your community and to learn how to communicate respectfully with each of them. Remember, too, that a patient may not share the beliefs of his or her family or ethnic background and therefore disagree with family or bystanders regarding his or her condition and treatment. Some cultures have beliefs about treatment and medical care that may affect your care plan. Certain religions prohibit certain medical procedures. Some do not allow blood transfusions or other standard treatments. Always remain sensitive to the patient's religious, cultural, and sociological beliefs. Also remember that even if you and the patient disagree about what may be causing an illness, the patient may still accept treatment.

Manners Manners are also important, but are not uniform across cultures. Take, for instance, the baseball cap. In the past, it was considered rude for a man to wear a cap indoors, when a woman walked by, or even in a bar. Today, many people wear them inside, outdoors, backwards, and sideways. Some people wear them with remarks or pictures on them that are designed to shock. Although wearing a baseball cap has become an

Documentation and Communication

Cultural diversity is found in EMS every day. If you are not familiar with the various cultures present in your community, consider a training session in which leaders from various cultural organizations in your community are invited to meet members of your organization. This could open up dialogue for both groups and could create an avenue for growth and development to reduce communication barriers in EMS calls. In addition, training members of your EMS organization to speak other languages that are spoken in your area may also be of significant benefit to your community.

accepted practice in some places in the United States, some people are offended by this practice. In other cultures, however, wearing a hat has religious connotations. It is important for you to know the difference in cultures' perceptions of manners.

Forms of address are another important element. Do not refer to patients as "dude," or "man." Do not respond to patients' questions using "nope," "yep," "yeah," or "uh huh." This is slang and it is not professional. Instead, address patients with words such as "yes sir," "no sir," "no, ma'am," "thank you," and "please." These niceties will go far in instilling confidence and respect and establishing a professional relationship for you.

Using phrases like "may I" or "could I" are equally important. Most people like to give permission before being touched. Lack of address and assumption of permission is particularly demeaning to an elderly patient. You are nonverbally communicating to them "You are not important enough or mentally competent enough to be asked for permission."

Hand Gestures Another American usage that may cause miscommunication is hand gestures. The "thumbs up" sign that Americans use to illustrate "everything is OK" or "ready to go"

YOU *are the Medic*   PART 4

You find John is able to hear you with some minor adjustments on your part. He tells you that he feels weak. He states his doctor put him on a new "heart pill" within the last week. He thinks it is making him sick and he cannot remember the name of it. You assemble oxygen via nasal cannula for the patient. When you go to put the cannula on the patient, he pushes your hand away and turns his head. You state, "John, it is just a cannula." He reluctantly lets you apply it.

Recording Time: 10 Minutes	
Respirations	14 breaths/min
Pulse	78 beats/min
Skin	Pale, cool, dry
Blood pressure	110/64 mm Hg
Oxygen saturation (Spo$_2$)	98% on 4 L/min via nasal cannula
Pupils	Equal and reactive

7. How can you overcome the reaction presented to the nasal cannula? Could you have prevented this reaction?

is actually the equivalent of the middle finger in some Arabic and Latin countries. The OK sign, made by circling the thumb and forefinger, with the other fingers extended, is the standard American for "good to go." In Latin countries, however, it is a reference to a circular orifice located posteriorly. It also has this same meaning in Germany, Russia, and Italy. In France it can mean zero or worthless. In other cultures it can reference the "evil eye." In Japan it indicates that money is needed or that coins are preferred. Conversely in Japan, the middle finger gesture is a form of pointing. To an American, it refers to being "flipped off." This illustrates how the same gesture can have widely disparate meanings in different cultures.

Body Language Body language and gestures are common the world over. But an innocent gesture in one country may be a serious insult in another. Perhaps the most cross-cultural gesture, and the most easily remembered one, is the smile. A smile is readily received by most every culture and has the tendency to convey goodwill. Use it often when dealing with patients.

Every culture has its own peculiarities and social and religious practices that are unique. The following list is by no means all inclusive; it just illustrates some of the differences you may encounter when providing care for persons from cultures other than your own.

- **Bowing:** Bowing shows rank and status in Japan. The deeper the bow, the more respect is communicated.
- **Touching the head:** Many Asians do not touch the head. The head is considered to be the most sacred part of the body and is the residence of the soul. Touching the head may put the soul in jeopardy.
- **Touching with the left hand:** Islamic and Hindu cultures avoid touching with the left hand because traditionally this hand was used for unclean functions. It is considered rude and offensive to use the left hand in greeting.
- **Feet:** Showing the bottom of the feet is considered offensive in the Muslim nations as well as most of Thailand. To point the soles of your shoes or the soles of your feet at someone is to say "you are beneath my feet" or "you are worth less than dirt."
- **Slouching:** Considered rude in Japan and Northern European areas.
- **Hands in pockets:** Disrespectful in Turkey.
- **Sitting with legs crossed:** This position is considered disrespectful in Turkey and Ghana.
- **Hands on hips:** This can be a sign of hostility in Mexico and Argentina.
- **Eye contact:** Avoiding direct eye contact shows respect in some Asian, African, Latin American, and Caribbean countries (Somalia and Brazil are exceptions). Prolonged eye contact is acceptable in Arab, Somali, and Brazilian cultures because it communicates honesty and interest.
- **Nodding:** Indian and Arabic cultures may signal agreement by moving the head from side to side (the Western "no"). They may indicate "no" by tipping the head backward and clicking the tongue against the roof of the mouth.

YOU are the Medic | SUMMARY

1. How will you open communication with this patient?

As soon as is reasonably possible, you should begin a patient interaction by introducing yourself. This does not entail any special "social skills" or societal standard. Rather, a simple "Good afternoon, my name is Mark. I am a paramedic with the fire department. What is your name?" will usually suffice. This simple exchange offers comfort and promotes a feeling that "we are in this together."

Be sure you make eye contact and maintain it, for a few reasons. First, it reinforces trust and honesty. Second, it allows you to evaluate the neurologic status, because certain conditions can relay abnormal information through the person's gaze. A vague, far-off stare may suggest mental dullness, which could be the result of physical issues or substance abuse. Third, the eyes may signal a person's behavioral unrest, as in psychiatric conditions.

2. Is the television set a consideration in your assessment?

Sometimes, even with the best techniques, it is difficult to communicate with the patient. There are two basic factors necessary to improve communication. First, remember that external factors such as noise, disruptive scenes, language barriers, and sensory impairment can make communication difficult. In this situation, the television may interfere with effective communication with the patient. Resist the urge to walk over and simply turn it off.

You are a guest in the patient's home. Whenever possible, ask permission before moving furniture or turning off appliances. The respect you demonstrate will go a long way to improving overall communications with your patient.

3. What does it mean to "get on the same level as the patient"? What is the importance of this?

If there is no threat evident, you should try to get on the same level as the patient. This means placing yourself in a position in which the patient will not have to look up at you. This promotes trust and alleviates anxiety. This is especially true when dealing with children. In essence, you are demonstrating a stance of equality through physical orientation.

4. How can you address the problem of a family member answering questions for the patient?

When this type of problem occurs, do not become irritated with the family member. This method of communication may work well for this couple because the patient has a hearing impairment. You have a number of options available to you. You can politely ask the family member to allow the patient to speak so you can hear his or her voice. You can also ask the family member to perform another function, like gathering medications. Whatever you

YOU are the Medic   SUMMARY, continued

choose to do, do it tactfully and understand that you are treading on a relationship.

5. Give some examples of effective communication techniques for persons with hearing impairment.

There are differing levels of hearing impairment. These range from minimal deficit to total deafness. Do not raise your voice into a yell because the patient may have a hearing problem. Take your cues from family members. In this case, Mrs. Smith leaned close to the patient's left ear and spoke to him. Alternately, you should position yourself so the patient can clearly see you; speak slowly and clearly to the patient. Many people who are hearing impaired are able to read lips and facial expressions. You may also try writing your questions and allowing the patient to write his or her answer. Lastly, American Sign Language (ASL) may be necessary when working with people who are deaf.

6. How can your body language affect your assessment of this patient?

You should try to avoid gestures, facial expressions, and "closed posture" because these mannerisms send negative signals. Do not frown or smirk at answers. Rolling your eyes at your partner is also not appropriate because it could provoke a fight from

a patient with a behavioral issue. Maintain constant, nonjudgmental eye contact. Keep your voice calm and neutral, and encourage answers; do not demand them. Demonstrate patience to the patient. Use open-handed gestures to demonstrate openness. Do not show a closed posture, such as crossing your arms. It is crucial that as soon as you meet the patient, you try to develop a good rapport.

7. How can you overcome the reaction presented to the nasal cannula? Could you have prevented the reaction?

Are you sure the patient knows what item you are trying to place on his or her face? It can be frightening when someone reaches over your face with a piece of equipment that has not been explained to you. In the scenario, the crew member tells the patient, "It is just a cannula." Does the patient know what a cannula is and what it is designed to do?

Before touching a patient, you need to educate and communicate what you are trying to do for a patient. Depending on the severity of the patient's condition, this may not always be possible. Do not assume a patient has worn an oxygen cannula before. Explain what it does, how it is worn, and how it will help before placing it on the patient's face. The same is true for any item you place on the patient.

EMS Patient Care Report (PCR)

Date: 07-01-11	Incident No.: 876	Nature of Call: General medical		Location: 450 Maple Street	
Dispatched: 0810	En Route: 0812	At Scene: 0816	Transport: 0836	At Hospital: 0845	In Service: 0855

Patient Information

Age: 86 Sex: M Weight (in kg [lb]): 59 kg (130 lb)	Allergies: No known drug allergies Medications: Numerous—see attached list Past Medical History: Pancreatic cancer, A-fib Chief Complaint: General weakness

Vital Signs

Time: 0821	BP: 110/66	Pulse: 76	Respirations: 14	Spo$_2$: 98% on room air
Time: 0826	BP: 110/64	Pulse: 78	Respirations: 14	Spo$_2$: 98% on 2 L/min NC
Time:	BP:	Pulse:	Respirations:	Spo$_2$:

EMS Treatment
(circle all that apply)

Oxygen @ __4__ L/min via (circle one): (NC) NRM Bag-mask device	Assisted Ventilation	Airway Adjunct	CPR
Defibrillation	Bleeding Control	Bandaging	Splinting	Other

Narrative

Arrived at this residence for a general medical event. Pt is an 86-year-old male reporting weakness. Pt states his physician changed a medication within the last week and pt believes this may be causing the weakness. Pt is alert and oriented x4, sitting in a recliner. Pt denies chest pain, dizziness, and nausea/vomiting. Extensive medication list attached to this report. Pt placed on 2 L/min O$_2$ NC prior to transport. Pt lifted from recliner to stretcher and secured. Pt transported without change to regional hospital. Report to Shari RN upon arrival. **End of report**

Prep Kit

Ready for Review

- You must be able to communicate rapidly, efficiently, and effectively when responding to a call to fulfill your role as a paramedic.
- The phases of communication include notification, potential prearrival instructions for the caller, dispatch, communication during on-scene care, and communication with the receiving facility while en route.
- The dispatcher communicates with people who call in an emergency, and with the EMS unit in sending it to the scene. Most of his or her telecommunication is done through digital technology.
- The dispatcher identifies the exact location of the patient, the telephone number, the nature of the problem, and specific information about the patient's condition and emergency, such as the types of vehicles involved in a motor vehicle crash or hazards at the scene.
- The dispatcher is also responsible for monitoring communications with the ambulance, coordinating communication with medical control and other agencies, and recording the times when the various phases of the call occurred.
- Emergency medical dispatch requires special training that teaches dispatchers to provide basic medical instructions to emergency callers over the phone. Updates resulting from this prearrival care can be communicated to the EMS crew as they are en route.
- Radio is one of the main methods of communication in EMS. The most commonly used bands for medical communications are the very high frequency (VHF) and ultrahigh frequency (UHF) band. The higher the band, the less interference there is, but the shorter the transmission range.
- Trunking is the ability for multiple agencies or systems to share frequencies. This allows the dispatcher to reprogram radios so that agencies that do not normally talk to each other are able to, if necessary, such as in a multiple-casualty incident.
- The Federal Communications Commission controls frequency allocation and licensing in the United States. It also establishes technical standards for radio equipment, establishes and enforces rules and regulations for the operation of radio equipment, and monitors transmissions. Communications over frequencies allotted for medical purposes are supposed to be used strictly for that purpose.
- Telemetry is used to transmit vital life signs to a distant terminal. In EMS, it is usually used for transmitting an ECG. This can be useful in diagnosing myocardial infarction and can allow the hospital to prepare to administer fibrinolytic therapy.
- Cellular telephones are becoming more common in EMS communications systems. Many newer cell phones have global positioning systems built in, which aid the enhanced 9-1-1 operator to determine exactly where the call is being made.

- Systems used for radio transmission include simplex, duplex, and multiplex. Simplex operates on one frequency and allows the transmission to go one way. Duplex operates on two frequencies and allows simultaneous transmission and reception. Multiplex operates on two or more frequencies and allows for more than one transmission simultaneously.

- An EMS communications system consists of a base station, mobile and portable transmitters or receivers, a repeater, a remote console, and a landline or backup communications system.

- Keep radio communication simple, brief, and direct. One of the main goals is clarity. Use the international radiotelephony spelling alphabet to aid transmission of spellings.

- Remember that your words can be heard by anyone who is listening. Keep your communications professional at all times. Do not transmit a patient's name or personal information over the radio; this would be in violation of HIPAA.

- Most ambulance systems use plain English in radio communications, but some use radio codes. If your agency uses codes, be sure to learn them.

- When reporting medical information, include the patient's age and sex, chief complaint, brief history, level of consciousness, degree of distress, vital signs, mental status, physical findings, ECG findings, treatment, and response to treatment.

- Most of the people you will meet during responses will be in crisis and having the worst day of their lives.

- At least half of the calls you will run as a paramedic will take you into people's homes, day and night, and in the most private moments of their lives. Try to see every invitation into the home of someone else as a personal honor in a time and place where no one else would be welcome.

- If you want people to tell you about their problems, convince them you want to hear what they have to say. Give them your undivided attention.

- Active listening is repeating the key parts of a patient's responses to questions. It helps confirm the information the patient is providing and ensures there is no misunderstanding.

- A therapeutic communicator's most essential challenge is to convey calm, unmistakable, genuine concern for someone he or she has never met.

- When you first meet your patients, introduce yourself and ask them for their name. This communicates your respect for them.

- Even if you are not convinced that patients are in real trouble, consider the possibility that they are terribly frightened.

- External factors, such as noise, lighting, distracting equipment, and interruptions, can make communication with a patient difficult.

- Patient modesty matters, no matter how acute the medical condition. If the patient is not personally sensitive to it, family members most certainly are.

- When you need to know how patients feel, try asking open-ended questions—questions that do not have a yes or no answer, and which do not give them specific options from which to choose.

- When you are trying to find facts (for example, a medical history), use closed-ended or direct questions.

- If you sense that patients are trying to put something into words, but are having trouble, be patient. Do not say anything at all for a few seconds. Let them talk.

- If you have tried clarification and you are still not sure what patients are trying to tell you, sometimes it helps to vocalize what you think they have said and invite them to correct you.

- Nonverbal communication can be as powerful as words.

- Direct eye contact generally communicates honesty and concern.

- Posture is important. Try to position your eyes at the same level or below the level of the patient's eyes.

- Some people do not like to be touched at all; to others, it is a valuable assurance that someone cares about them. You should try gently touching patients on a neutral part of the body, such as a shoulder or arm, especially when you are trying to reassure them or to mitigate their fear.

- Hostile or angry patients may present a threat to you and others. Always approach with caution and maintain eye contact. Try not to interview them by yourself.

- Try not to presume that older people are any harder to communicate with than anyone else, just because they are older.

- Children can pose treatment and communication challenges even to the best EMS personnel. Minimize your movements, lower your voice, and touch them as gently as you can. Try keeping your eye level at or below the child's by sitting on the floor and placing the child on the cot or on a parent's lap.

- When you encounter a patient who has trouble communicating, remember that family members or primary caregivers who know these patients well can facilitate your efforts. Just as importantly, they can also help you alleviate fear.

- Dealing with people of cultures different from your own can be challenging. It is always considered a mark of your respect if you make an effort to learn about their language and culture.

- Manners, hand gestures, and body language may differ among cultures. Remember that another person's culture may have different rules for polite behavior from your own.

Vital Vocabulary

<u>base station</u> Assembly of radio equipment consisting of at least a transmitter, receiver, and antenna connection at a fixed location.

<u>biotelemetry</u> Transmission of physiologic data, such as an ECG, from the patient to a distant point of reception (commonly referred to in EMS as "telemetry").

cellular telephones Low-power portable radios that communicate through an interconnected series of repeater stations called "cells."

closed-ended question A question that is specific and focused, demanding either a yes or no answer or an answer chosen from specific options.

digital radio The microwave transmission of digital signals through space or the atmosphere instead of transmission by radio waves.

dispatch To send to a specific destination or to send on a task.

duplex Radio system using more than one frequency to permit simultaneous transmission and reception.

emergency medical dispatch First aid instructions given by specially trained dispatchers to callers over the telephone while an ambulance is en route to the call.

emergency medical dispatcher (EMD) A person who receives information and relays that information in an organized manner during the emergency.

encoded A message is put into a code before it is transmitted.

enhanced 9-1-1 system An emergency call-in system in which additional information such as the phone number and location of the caller is recorded automatically through sophisticated telephone technology and the dispatcher need only confirm the information on the screen.

Federal Communications Commission (FCC) The federal agency that has jurisdiction over interstate and international telephone and telegraph services and satellite communications, all of which may involve EMS activity.

frequency In radio communications, the number of cycles per second of a signal; inversely related to the wavelength.

hertz (Hz) Unit of frequency equal to 1 cycle per second.

interpersonal communications The exchange of information between two or more persons.

landline Communications system linked by wires, usually in reference to a conventional telephone system.

multiplex Method by which simultaneous transmission of voice and ECG signals can be achieved over a single radio frequency.

noise In radio communications, interference in a radio signal.

open-ended question A question that does not have a yes or no answer, and that does not give the patient specific options from which to choose.

pervasive developmental disorders (PDDs) A group of disorders that cause delays in many areas of childhood development, such as the development of skills to communicate and interact socially, and may include repetitive body movements and difficulty with changes in routine; includes autism and Asperger syndrome, among others.

remote console A terminal that receives transmissions of telemetry and voice from the field and transmits messages back, usually through the base station.

repeater Miniature transmitter that picks up a radio signal and rebroadcasts it, extending the range of a radio communications system.

simplex Method of radio communication using a single frequency that enables transmission reception of voice or an ECG signal but is incapable of simultaneous transmission and reception.

ten-code A radio code system using the number 10 plus another number.

therapeutic communication Communicating with the patient.

transceiver A radio transmitter and receiver housed in a single unit; a two-way radio.

trunking Sharing of radio frequencies by multiple agencies or systems.

ultrahigh frequency (UHF) band The portion of the radio frequency spectrum between 300 and 3,000 mHz.

very high frequency (VHF) band The portion of the radio frequency spectrum between 30 and 150 mHz.

wavelength The distance in a propagating wave from one point to the corresponding point on the next wave.

Assessment in Action

Y ou are dispatched to a local hotel for a "CPR in progress." Your dispatcher informs you that CPR instructions are being given for a 55-year-old man. The patient is located in Room 450 at the Downtown Inn on Bay Street. You read the notes field on your Mobile Data Terminal and find the patient's son is performing CPR and is certified. The patient's wife is hysterical in the background. The hotel manager will meet your crew at the main entrance and direct you to the room in question.

1. What is the first stage of EMS response?
   A. When units are notified via radio to respond
   B. When someone calls and reports an emergency to EMS
   C. When the call information is entered into the computer-aided dispatch system
   D. When the emergency unit leaves the station

2. At what point should the dispatcher send units to the call?
   A. After all medical questioning is completed
   B. After the location of the patient, telephone number, and chief complaint are obtained
   C. After all medical questioning and prearrival instructions are given
   D. When a unit becomes available to respond to the call

3. What is the minimum amount of data an EMD will need to obtain prior to beginning medical questioning?
   A. Exact location from which the call is made, the telephone number, and the chief complaint
   B. Exact location where the patient is located, the telephone number, and the chief complaint
   C. The patient's name and the exact location from which the call is made
   D. The telephone number only

4. What information is automatically available with enhanced 9-1-1?
   A. Patient name and phone number
   B. Caller address, phone number, and chief complaint
   C. Caller address and phone number
   D. Current location of the patient

5. After determining the location of a patient with a medical complaint, what specific information concerning the patient is obtained by the EMD?
   A. Level of responsiveness and breathing
   B. Breathing and bleeding
   C. Level of responsiveness and pulse
   D. Level of responsiveness, breathing, and bleeding

Additional Questions

6. Should you be concerned with how other cultures may react to you?

7. How can you handle a hostile patient more effectively?

Documentation

National EMS Education Standard Competencies

Preparatory

Integrates comprehensive knowledge of the EMS system, safety/well-being of the paramedic, and medical/legal and ethical issues, which is intended to improve the health of EMS personnel, patients, and the community.

Documentation

- Recording patient findings (p 149)
- Principles of medical documentation and report writing (p 149)

Medical Terminology

Integrates comprehensive anatomic and medical terminology and abbreviations into written and oral communication with colleagues and other health care professionals.

Knowledge Objectives

1. Describe the purpose of documentation. (pp 151-152)
2. Identify the information required in a patient care report. (PCR) (pp 153-154, 158-159, 163)
3. Explain the legal implications of the patient care report. (pp 149-150)
4. Discuss the implications of the Health Insurance Portability and Accountability Act of 1996 as they relate to documentation. (pp 150-151)
5. List standard items that must be documented for every emergency call. (pp 153, 163)
6. Discuss the process for documenting transfer of care, and special considerations surrounding documentation. (pp 154-158)
7. Discuss state and/or local special reporting requirements, including multiple-casualty incidents, exposure situations, involvement of other agencies, workplace injuries, interfacility transfers, and potential abuse or neglect. (pp 156-158)
8. Understand how to document refusal of care, including the legal implications. (pp 154-156)
9. Compare handwritten reporting with electronic reporting, and discuss the pros and cons of each. (pp 152-154)
10. Discuss various types of formats for the narrative portion of the patient care report. (pp 158-160)
11. Discuss why it is important that documentation be accurate, legible, and professional. (pp 159-161)
12. Explain the procedure to follow should an error occur during or after creating a patient care report. (pp 161-162)
13. Discuss the consequences of intentional falsification of documentation. (pp 161-162)
14. Discuss the importance of being familiar with medical terminology. (pp 163-164)

Skills Objectives

1. Demonstrate completion of a patient care report. (pp 158-161)

Introduction

Although the EMS documentation report may not be the first item that comes to mind when you are thinking of pursuing a career in EMS, it is an important part of the patient care process. Thorough documentation pulls the run together for all parties involved. The adage, "No job is finished until the paperwork is done" is especially true in EMS. Your report, most commonly referred to as the **patient care report (PCR)**, is also sometimes called the prehospital care report, and is the only written record of the events that transpired during the call for service. Writing an accurate and proper PCR is one of the most important skills you will learn as a paramedic. The PCR is the legal record for the call and will be a part of the patient's medical record and the hospital's emergency department chart. A complete patient care documentation report will not only allow other health care providers to obtain information about what has occurred from the start of the call to its conclusion, but will also help guide future patient care via research and quality assurance Figure 1. As a paramedic, you must be able to create a patient care report thoroughly and efficiently.

You need to know what constitutes an EMS documentation report, what information must be included, who might read the report, when the report must be completed, and what terminology may be used. Learning to write effectively and accurately is an important paramedic skill. Information may be categorized as objective or subjective. **Objective information** includes the measurable signs that you observe and record, such as blood pressure. **Subjective information** includes information that is told to you, but which cannot be seen, such as the symptoms patients describe—the degree of pain, for example. You must record objective *and* subjective information and the details of patient care for

every call in a written or computer-based report, and in some cases, both. This report needs to be complete, accurate, and legible because it can provide the basis of defense in legal proceedings and is of vital importance to your service or agency for many other reasons as well, including facilitation of quality care, continuity, and billing insurance. Your report should "paint a picture" of the entire call that is accurate and clear to the reader.

Legal Issues of a Patient Care Report

Although you may include subjective information from the patient, such as statements from him or her about symptoms, no bias or personal opinions (subjectivity) of yours should be contained within your report. An example of such would be if you

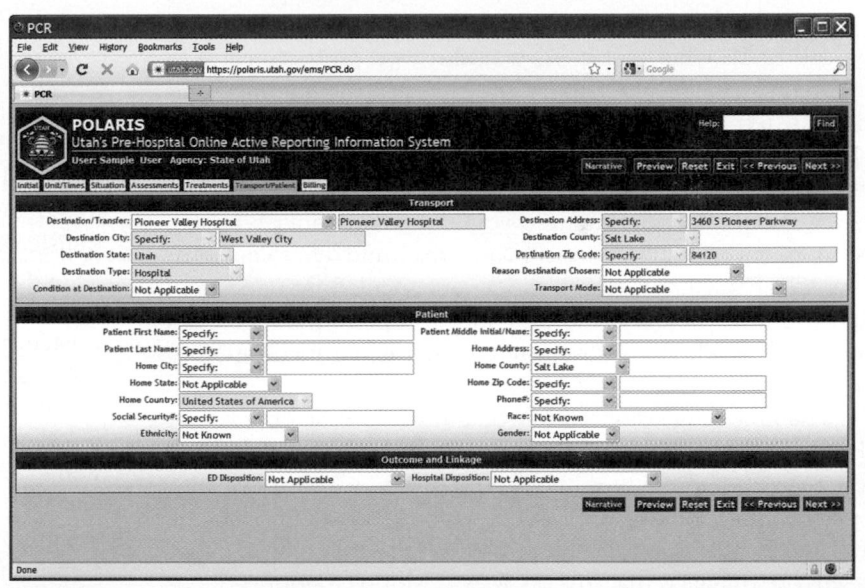

Figure 1 Electronic patient care reports are the standard in EMS documentation. An online patient care report is shown here.

YOU *are the Medic*   **PART 1**

Your unit has been dispatched to a single-vehicle collision involving a pole near the county courthouse at approximately 1300 hours on a weekday. On arrival, you ensure that the scene is safe before you exit the ambulance. The vehicle appears to have light damage to the front bumper and hood. You don your personal protective equipment and approach the vehicle. As you are walking up, a man opens the door of the vehicle and attempts unsuccessfully to stand up. The man falls back down on the seat exclaiming in a loud, slurred voice, "I need my lawyer." You look past the patient into the passenger compartment and see that the air bags have deployed.

1. What is your first consideration in regard to this patient?

2. What is your first consideration in regard to the scene?

documented "the patient was drunk and out of control" versus "the patient had an altered mental status and stated he had eight beers today." Poorly written, inappropriately documented PCRs could have adverse implications for patient care and for your career. Omissions or errors in your report could lead to further errors in care. Improper and inadequate reports also could result in litigation, loss of job or position, a negative reflection on one's reputation as an EMS professional, and more.

No matter your particular writing style, your report should be complete, well written, legible, professional, and your sole source of information about the call. Your report may also be used in legal proceedings against you or someone else. In some cases, it may be your only defense against a complaint about a call—if you document what happened, you will have solid evidence of your conduct and what transpired on the call. Your memory may not serve you well 5 to 7 years from now, but your written report will remain as a record. If it is well written, it will jog your memory and should provide a picture of the events of the call to all who read it. As a health care professional, it is important that you use proper spelling, proper grammar, and accurate terminology in your report. Do not attempt to use medical terms and abbreviations if you do not fully understand their meaning. Never make up your own abbreviations because they will only be meaningful to you and could confuse others. Doing so could result in patient care errors and leave your professional character at stake if the report is called into question. Your report is the only record of why you performed a certain procedure or why you administered a particular medication to a patient.

The following is an example that illustrates the importance of neat and accurate documentation. A town's EMS agency was being sued for providing inappropriate care to a patient with a spine injury. During the discovery phase of the lawsuit, the attorney for the town decided to settle the case out of court based on the fact that the PCR was sloppy (sloppy documentation implies sloppy care) and incomplete (not clearly documenting whether distal pulses, and motor and sensory functions [PMS] were assessed before and after immobilization of the patient).

Another example of poor documentation was a case where a 15-year-old boy had been involved in a motor vehicle crash and the paramedic crew had to secure his airway because of head trauma. The patient was transferred to a trauma center, where the emergency department (ED) physician found the patient to be extubated. The patient survived but sustained a significant brain injury. The family sued the paramedic crew, claiming that their son was brain damaged from the hypoxia caused by the failed intubation and not the significant head trauma. The crew testified that they had continuous capnography indicating a secured airway throughout transport, yet they had failed to document such readings in their narrative. Although it was likely that the patient was extubated while being moved to the ED exam bed, the crew's failure to document their readings resulted in a finding for the family. The agency lost a significant monetary amount as a result.

Confidentiality and HIPAA

The Health Insurance Portability and Accountability Act (HIPAA) was passed in 1996. Many people are confused about the legal issues surrounding HIPAA and feel that any release of a patient's private medical information may result in penalties. HIPAA was an attempt to protect a patient's privacy, but it also attempts to permit disclosure of patient care information and other processes for the purposes of treatment, payment, or operations. The HIPAA Privacy Rule, which is the most relevant part of HIPAA for health care providers, is enforced by the Office for Civil Rights. The HIPAA Privacy Rule protects a person's identifiable health information. Additionally, the HIPAA Security Rule is the portion of HIPAA that pertains to protecting electronic health information.

HIPAA was not created to stop the flow and continuity of a patient's health care information, but to control the distribution of information to ensure that a person's privacy is kept. In essence, HIPAA mandates that patient information shall not be shared with entities or persons not involved in the care of the patient. For example, EMS providers may be confused about how HIPAA affects the area of patient follow-up. When you treat and transport a patient to the receiving facility, you may inquire as to what further care your patient required once you transferred care.

One final note on the importance of HIPAA regulations has come about in recent years as social media networks came into existence and gained popularity. Many agencies have created policies to address issues associated with patient care information being shared over Internet media. Some have gone as far as not allowing cellular phones with a camera to be in the possession of EMS providers while on duty. As a paramedic, you must take the first step to ensure that everyone on your call recognizes the importance of not posting any patient information (photos, comments, data, etc) on any social media network.

HIPAA rules and regulations should be taught to all entities involved. Each agency in the United States that is a covered entity defined by the U.S. Department of Health and Human Services should follow HIPAA guidelines to help protect the patient and the provider. Each agency, in compliance with HIPAA, shall have a designated officer who can help you better understand all of the rules and regulations associated with HIPAA and your role in EMS.

Special HIPAA Circumstances

There are times that the HIPAA Privacy Rule acknowledges that patient information must be shared for the betterment of society

Documentation and Communication

To help protect patient information, do not leave PCRs or assessment cards on counters or any other area that is not secured. Many agencies use lockboxes as the location where completed PCRs should be placed.

as a whole. The Privacy Rule permits covered entities to disclose protected health information, without authorization, to public health authorities who are legally authorized to receive such reports for the purpose of preventing or controlling disease, injury, or disability. Some of the areas that are included for such information release are births, deaths, disease, or injury that are being investigated or are at risk of causing a public epidemic, and abuse cases. Exchange of health information for a medical need is allowed under HIPAA, and is in fact ethical and necessary. For example, electronic transfer of health information from your electronic documentation report to the receiving hospital is perfectly appropriate. A physician dictating patient information into a dictaphone which is then transcribed into the patient's record is also appropriate. Furthermore, it is perfectly acceptable and permissible under HIPAA for hospitals to share information with the EMS providers about patient outcome for the purposes of quality assurance, quality improvement, and education. It is clearly important and necessary for you to understand the outcome of your interventions so that you can learn. Finally, exchange of health information for insurance and billing purposes is appropriate, although in most cases the billing agency must sign an agreement indicating that the health information will be used for billing purposes only, and will not be shared with outside parties.

Purposes of Documentation

Continuity of Care

The PCR serves as a record of the patient's condition on your arrival at the scene, the care that was provided, any changes in the patient's condition en route, and condition on arrival at the hospital. It is critical that you document everything as clearly as possible because the report will help other health care providers at the hospital understand the particular emergency and assessments and treatments performed thus far. Accurate reporting helps paint a picture of the environment the patient was taken out of, the mechanism of injury, and ultimately leads to better patient care.

Minimum Requirements and Billing

Billing and administration are significant reasons why PCR writing needs to be accurate and complete. Most EMS agencies now need to bill for services to recover the costs of providing patient care. For complete and accurate revenue recovery, you must ensure that all procedures performed are documented, insurance codes obtained, and the appropriate **medical necessity** signature obtained (where required). You need to document why a patient may have needed emergency care, especially in the case of private or scheduled transports, to ensure your service's billing information will result in payment from the responsible insurer, agency, or private payer. It is imperative for you to be accurate and complete in your documentation so that time is not spent correcting the documentation, thus delaying billing processing. You will often be trained by your agency and

its billing company about what additional forms you need to complete as a part of each EMS response. EMS providers must understand that completing billing paperwork and supplying the most accurate and defensible information to the EMS agency are necessary portions of the call.

Medicare sets the standard for medical necessity. The chart shown in **Table 1** gives some of the significant findings that are required to show that the patient needed to be transported by an ambulance rather than by other means of transportation.

EMS Research

Just as billing has become necessary in EMS, so has research. As mentioned in the chapter, *EMS Systems*, proper documentation done by all EMS providers results in compiled data that are reviewed by researchers who then use that data to justify innovative, lifesaving techniques. Many states now require EMS agencies to submit data to their state EMS office to verify call volumes and skills used. This data may include the number of calls an agency responds to, the types of calls, care provided, and patient outcomes. Such patient care data collection can lead to improvement of the EMS system as a whole.

The National Emergency Medical Services Information System (NEMSIS) stores standardized EMS data from each individual state. This central repository will help assist states in collecting comparable data elements so the entire nation can benefit from research and use the trends for future curriculum development. The goal of NEMSIS is to define EMS care by collecting data to improve patient care, indicating equipment needs, and defining a standard of care across the nation.

Incident Review and Quality Assurance

On occasion, EMS reports may be requested for medical audits and other educational activities. Run reviews, or sessions in which peers and other medical professionals review care reports for adherence to local protocols, quality assurance, and quality monitoring, may occur. Your reports may be used to calculate

Table 1 Significant Findings that Indicate Medical Necessity for Ambulance Transport

- Patient is transported in an emergency fashion (Code 3).
- Patient is in shock.
- Patient needs to be restrained.
- Patient requires emergency treatment while being transported (eg, oxygen therapy, IV therapy).
- Patient must be immobilized for transport or fracture management.
- Patient is experiencing an acute myocardial infarction (AMI) or stroke.
- Patient has uncontrollable hemorrhage.
- Patient is only able to be moved by a stretcher because of a condition.

the number of times you have performed a specific skill, such as medication administration or oral intubation. Always accurately document all skills attempted and performed with patient care.

Documentation and Communication

EMS agencies and departments should have a process to ensure that all reports are well written and a quality assurance program to ensure that what was written in the PCR actually occurred as stated on the call.

■ Types of Patient Care Reports

EMS has entered an age in which electronic documentation has become the standard. Although some services still use paper documentation, you will most likely document your emergency calls and other reports electronically. Electronic documentation has many benefits as discussed later in this section. Perhaps the most significant benefit is the ability for electronic data to be shared—between the facilities and personnel involved in a patient's care, thereby improving continuity and efficiency, but also among state and national databases to improve national data collection and further the advancement of evidence-based practice.

A multitude of patient care report designs exist throughout the United States and range from half-page notes to complete and thorough reports. EMS patient care reporting has evolved over the years because the field of medicine has recognized the necessity for information about the patient's condition and interventions performed in the field. The old adage of "it didn't happen unless it was written down" has pressured some services to create run reports that nearly eliminate the narrative section (the

section that allows for free-form writing) and replace the space with check boxes, or with electronic dropdown menus with predetermined terms. You may encounter some reports that have hundreds of check boxes allowing for you to mark every action you took. The problem with these types of reports is that the format increases the risk of errors when your eyes become overwhelmed by so many boxes and the wrong boxes are filled in. It is important that, regardless of what form of patient reporting your service may use, that the proper information is obtained and documented.

Paper reporting is becoming a thing of the past because it is a duplication of work in the health care system. To fulfill EMS data collection requirements, handwritten reports must be entered into an electronic system, either by health care agencies or outsourced to separate companies. Along with the additional data entry needs, a paper system also requires space to store the records, possibly for a lengthy period of time depending on state laws. The final reason there is a major shift away from paper reporting systems is error reduction. Oftentimes penmanship and spelling errors lead to medical mistakes when it comes to medication doses and orders; an electronic system minimizes these issues.

With today's technology, a multitude of companies have created a variety of electronic patient care reports. These services range from scanning of paper forms to computer-based programs for desktops, tablets, and laptops, allowing for a more accurate and legible report **Figure 2**.

Modern data systems can incorporate data from various sources, such as multiple facilities—a feature that is in line with the major effort to improve the quality of cardiac, stroke, and diabetic care, and improve the success of resuscitation efforts. Such cutting-edge systems are being used by hospitals and physicians, and will ultimately involve EMS documentation so

YOU *are the Medic*   PART 2

The engine company that was dispatched with you arrives on scene, parking to ensure scene safety. Your crew directs the engine company to make sure the vehicle is secure while you and your partner attempt to speak to the patient. The patient yells at you to leave him alone. Your partner taps your shoulder and asks you if you smell alcohol and you reply that you do. She also points to an empty vodka bottle on the floor of the vehicle. The patient yells, "You don't know who I am, do you? You're going to pay!" You hear a bystander standing behind you say, "Isn't that Assemblyman Taylor?"

Recording Time: 0 Minutes	
Appearance	Awake
Level of consciousness	Alert
Airway	Open
Breathing	Adequate
Circulation	Appears normal

3. Why is it not acceptable to document the patient's appearance as "drunk" on a PCR?

4. Would it be acceptable to document that the patient is "yelling" for the breathing description on a PCR?

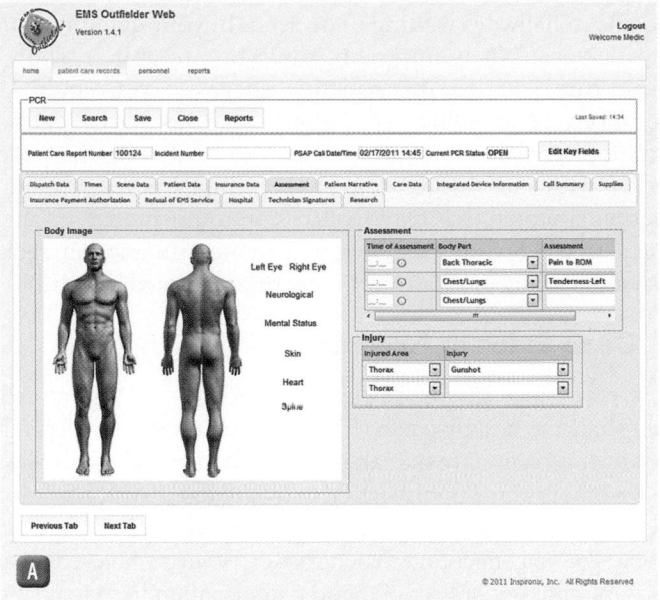

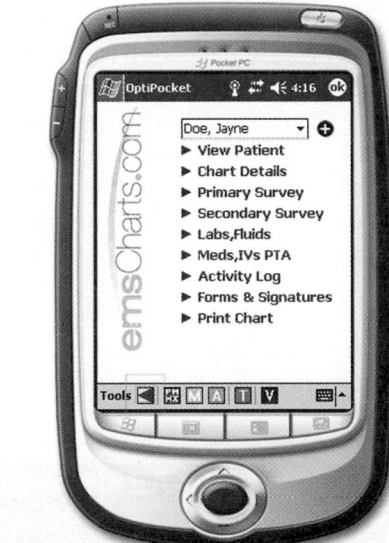

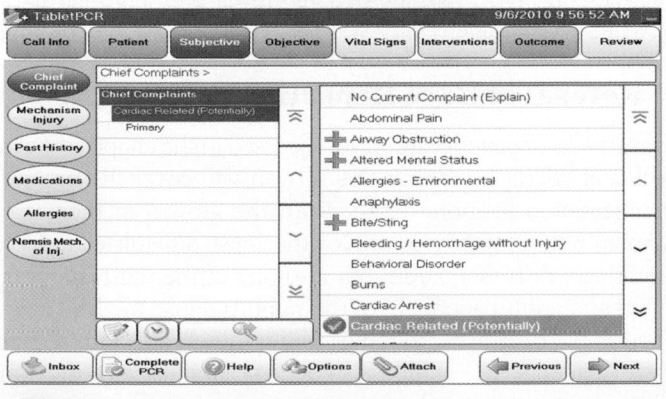

Figure 2 A variety of software programs exist for creating electronic patient care reports, allowing EMS personnel to clearly document details of the call.

that the patient care report contains prehospital information documented in the field, and further data from the hospitals or facilities where the patient was treated, resulting in one comprehensive record of the care the patient received.

Programs for computer-based PCRs should be NEMSIS-compliant to ensure that data can be shared on a national level. As mentioned, data submission to NEMSIS is important for EMS research, and to assess and improve EMS care throughout the country. NEMSIS' goal is to facilitate submission of EMS data from all states, and part of that is to implement electronic documentation systems in all states. The majority of US states and territories are submitting electronic data to NEMSIS, or are actively working toward achieving this in the near future.

Some of the benefits of the electronic reporting system are the ease of data collecting, merging data into hospital systems, and a decrease in patient medication errors. With the growing environment of lawsuits, the electronic report eliminates many of the spelling and legibility issues that have arisen in the past. Regardless of agency size, the major obstacle that often stands in the way of agencies switching from paper format to an electronic format is the cost of purchasing computers and software and yearly maintenance for the electronic PCR; however, most services that bill insurance, Medicare, or the patient noted that though the upfront costs of going to an electronic system were expensive, collection improved significantly once the system became computerized. Another possible obstacle in electronic reporting is that it relies on technology, which is not always reliable. Also, systems need to be interchangeable so data can easily transfer into the hospital ED systems.

Documentation for Every EMS Call

Every EMS call requires documentation. There are standard items that you will document on every call, which are called the **minimum data set**. The minimum data set is the mandatory clinical assessment standard information that must be documented on every emergency call as set by Medicare and Medicaid, and per the National Highway Traffic Safety Administration (NHTSA) for the purpose of the national data system. The minimum data set is divided into two sections: run data and patient data. Run data consist of such information as incident times, locations, responding units, and crew members working at the incident. Patient data includes basic patient information collected on a PCR, documenting the following:

- Chief complaint
- Level of consciousness (according to the AVPU scale) or mental status
- Vital signs
- Assessment
- Patient demographics (age, gender, ethnic background)

The PCR should contain your objective observations of the scene, as well as the treatments provided, their effects, and any changes that occurred in the patient's condition during the

Documentation and Communication

To understand how electronic data collection can improve operations, consider the following two methods (paper versus electronic).

Paper

- Citizen calls for assistance.
- Dispatcher handwrites the information.
- Ambulance is dispatched with the information given over the radio. Information may need to be reconfirmed two or three times.
- The crew treats the patient and transports to the hospital.
- At the hospital, a handwritten PCR is generated.
- A copy is left at the hospital and the original logged and stored at the station.
- The paperwork is picked up and taken to the head-quarters station (sometimes located far away) where it is reviewed, sorted, and coded by the supervisor.
- The paperwork is forwarded to the business office where it is entered into a computer system for billing.
- The supervisor in charge of quality assurance/quality improvement manually sorts through PCRs for review.

Electronic

- Citizen calls for assistance.
- Dispatcher electronically enters information while on the phone with the caller.
- Dispatcher assigns the call to an ambulance in the computer-aided dispatch, immediately pulling up a map on the computer screen showing the exact location of the call.
- Dispatcher pages the crew; crew steps into ambulance.
- If a mobile data terminal is installed in the ambulance, the problem, any hazards associated with the address, and the street address with a location on a computer map are right there.
- EMS arrives on scene and treats the patient. Transport to the hospital is completed.
- The crew fills out a short paper form with the basics of demographics and treatments given. This form is left with the emergency department staff.
- The crew synchronizes its laptop with the server through a Wi-Fi (wireless-fidelity) connection. Information gathered by the dispatcher is downloaded into the patient record.
- En route to the station, the crew uses a touch screen to select information for the PCR, which reduces the narrative required and allows for drawing injuries and complaints on an anatomic model.

emergency call Figure 3 . Depending on your transport service type, you may need to differentiate the treatments between those that were scheduled, such as in a transfer transport, and those that were unexpected because of changes in a patient's condition.

Transfer of Care

As the growing need for medical care begins to exceed that which is available, EMS personnel are seeing overwhelmed emergency departments and often find themselves leaving patients in hallways waiting to be seen. In your documentation of patient care, it is important that you are able to show in whose care you left the patient; otherwise, you could face allegations of abandonment. Some agencies have begun to require physician or nurse signatures to verify that the patient was left with a medical professional of a higher level of training. Another situation that may require you to document a transfer of care is when you hand over your patient to another agency such as a paramedic transport crew or an air medical team.

Care Prior to Arrival

More emergency dispatch centers are going to a system called emergency medical dispatch (EMD), which allows the dispatcher to provide directions to the caller for medical care. These programs are becoming very sophisticated, allowing the dispatcher to provide detailed medical care and medication administration via the phone. You may encounter such cases in your response area and it is important not only to obtain the information from the patient or caller as to what care they have provided prior to your arrival, but to also document such findings. A good example of this delivery of care is when a person calls 9-1-1 to an EMD center and tells the dispatcher that he or she is experiencing chest pain. After detailed questioning, the dispatcher may have the patient take 324 mg of aspirin, for example. If you fail to obtain such information from the patient and then relay that information to the hospital via your report, the patient could accidentally be given the same medication again, increasing the risk of complications.

You may also encounter off-duty health care providers and lay personnel providing emergency care prior to EMS arrival. Be sure to include their procedures in your report with specific notations that this care was provided prior to your arrival and by whom it was provided.

Situations Requiring Additional Documentation

There are special situations that require additional or different reporting procedures. These are discussed in the next sections.

Refusal of Care Reporting

Legal aspects of patient care were discussed in the chapter, *Medical, Legal, and Ethical Issues*, but this section will cover the necessary documentation in more depth. With the growth in malpractice lawsuits, refusal of care is one of the most difficult elements of patient care documentation, but also one of the most important. Competent adult patients have the right to refuse medical care or to consent to treatment. You must know and understand the rights of your patients. You should also be very familiar with the applicable laws in your state about patient care and who has the right to refuse such care. For a person to refuse care, the decision must be based on the patient's knowledge of his or her situation.

Your most important job is to ensure that your patient is fully informed about his or her current situation, the right to receive and refuse medical care, and the consequences of such a refusal of care. You should have explained and the patient must understand,

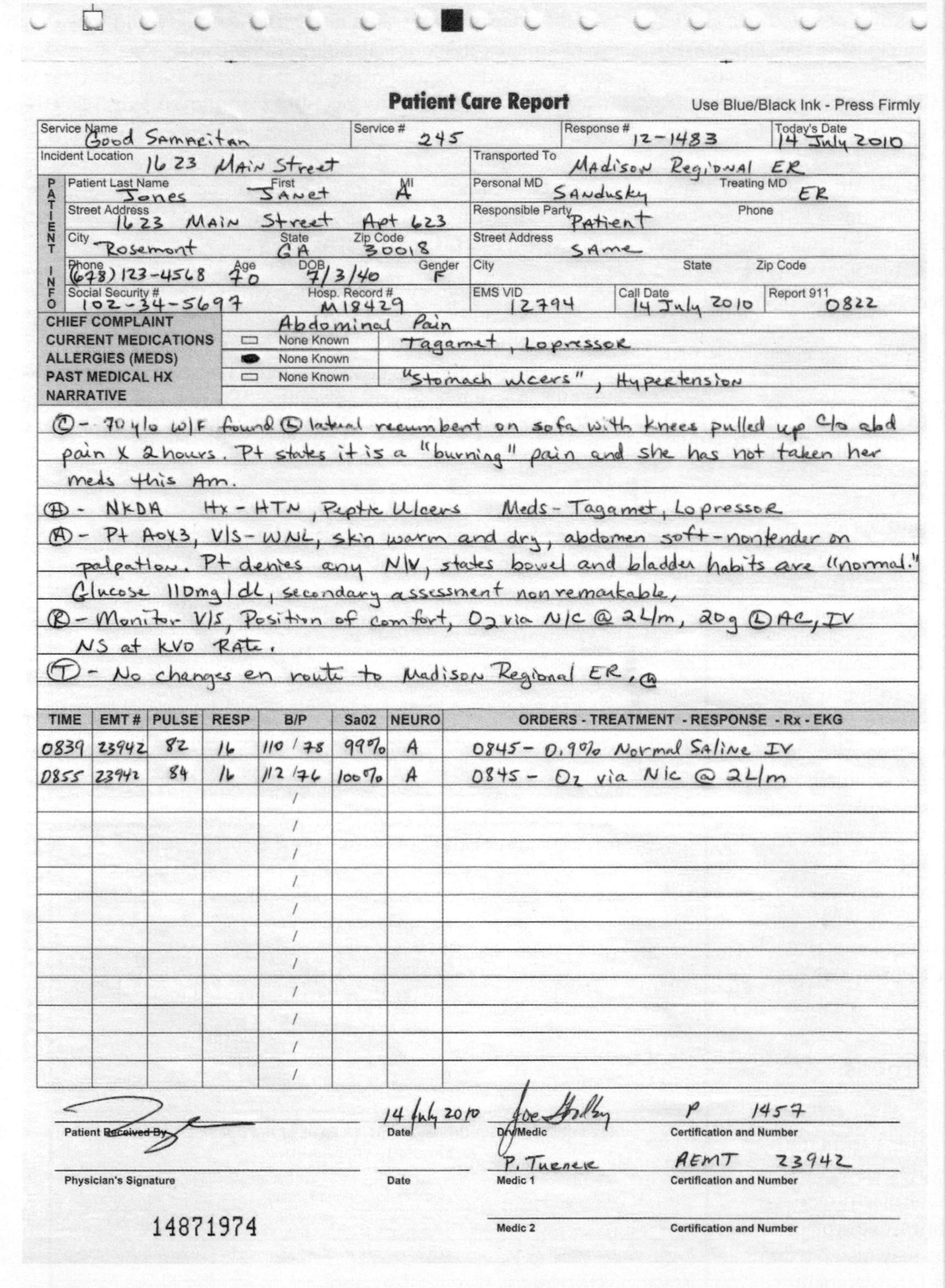

Patient Care Report   Use Blue/Black Ink - Press Firmly

Service Name: Good Samaritan	Service #: 245	Response #: 12-1483	Today's Date: 14 July 2010
Incident Location: 1623 Main Street	Transported To: Madison Regional ER		

Patient Last Name: Jones First: Janet MI: A	Personal MD: Sandusky	Treating MD: ER
Street Address: 1623 Main Street Apt 623	Responsible Party: Patient	Phone:
City: Rosemont State: GA Zip Code: 30018	Street Address: Same	
Phone: (678) 123-4568 Age: 70 DOB: 7/3/40 Gender: F	City: State: Zip Code:
Social Security #: 102-34-5697 Hosp. Record #: M18429	EMS VID: 12794 Call Date: 14 July 2010 Report 911: 0822

CHIEF COMPLAINT		Abdominal Pain
CURRENT MEDICATIONS	☐ None Known	Tagamet, Lopressor
ALLERGIES (MEDS)	☒ None Known	
PAST MEDICAL HX	☐ None Known	"Stomach ulcers", Hypertension
NARRATIVE		

Ⓒ - 70 y/o W/F found Ⓛ lateral recumbent on sofa with knees pulled up C/o abd pain X 2 hours. Pt states it is a "burning" pain and she has not taken her meds this Am.

Ⓗ - NKDA   Hx - HTN, Peptic Ulcers   Meds - Tagamet, Lopressor

Ⓐ - Pt AOx3, V/S - WNL, skin warm and dry, abdomen soft - nontender on palpation. Pt denies any N/V, states bowel and bladder habits are "normal." Glucose 110mg/dl, secondary assessment nonremarkable.

Ⓡ - Monitor V/S, Position of comfort, O₂ via N/c @ 2L/m, 20g Ⓛ AC, IV NS at KVO Rate.

Ⓣ - No changes en route to Madison Regional ER. Ⓐ

TIME	EMT #	PULSE	RESP	B/P	Sa02	NEURO	ORDERS - TREATMENT - RESPONSE - Rx - EKG
0839	23942	82	16	110/78	99%	A	0845 - 0.9% Normal Saline IV
0855	23942	84	16	112/76	100%	A	0845 - O₂ via N/c @ 2L/m
				/			
				/			
				/			
				/			
				/			
				/			
				/			
				/			
				/			
				/			
				/			
				/			

Patient Received By: _____   Date: 14 July 2010   Dr/Medic: Joe Godby   P   Certification and Number: 1457

Physician's Signature: _____   Date: _____   Medic 1: P. Turner   AEMT   Certification and Number: 23942

Medic 2: _____   Certification and Number: _____

14871974

Figure 3 The minimum data set includes both patient information and administrative information.

refusal section of the PCR. The refusal documentation should clearly show the process you went through, how was it was documented, and who witnessed it. It is not merely about getting the patient to sign the refusal section.

Unresponsive patients may be treated under implied consent. All paramedics should be familiar with the laws of their state regarding the age of consent, care of minors, emancipated minors, and people with mental or cognitive impairments, such as mental illness or the effects of drug or alcohol use. Above all else, you need to confirm that every reasonable effort has been made to ensure the patient's welfare and best interests.

If the person refusing care has an obvious injury or medical condition that requires immediate medical attention, you should involve online medical control for further guidance and assistance. In such cases where you, the provider, do not agree with the refusal, you should have a protocol or policy in place of what your next steps should be—for example, contact your supervisor, involve law enforcement, or involve medical control. If contact is made with any of those parties, it should be documented on the PCR, including the events that transpired.

It is essential that you have a witness to the process to ensure that your patient has sufficient knowledge of the situation to make an informed choice. If the patient refuses to sign the form for refusing treatment, your witness

in great detail, the potential consequences of refusing medical care when it may be warranted, including the possibility of death. This information needs to be conveyed in a language that the person understands, and this information must be subsequently documented on the PCR. Some agencies will write this on the PCR and have a witness observe them reading it to the patient, and will ask the patient to initial the statement followed by a signature on the

should also be present. The observations of the witness should be documented, and the name and contact information of the witness should be included.

A complete history and assessment should be performed or attempted when possible and practical. This includes obtaining a full set of baseline vital signs. A patient's refusal to allow such an assessment should be well documented on the PCR. Be sure to evaluate the patient's mental status. A person's mental status may be considered impaired if the person is not oriented to person, time, or place or makes nonsensical statements. The impairment can be a result of an injury, a medical condition, such as electrolyte imbalance or hypoglycemia, mental illness, or drugs or alcohol.

You should always politely and tactfully explain to patients that they have the right to change their mind and may recall EMS later. Such an exchange of information should be witnessed and documented with signatures and identifying information such as phone numbers of the witnesses involved, who frequently may be law enforcement personnel or others at the scene. Clearly document the care that you intended to provide if the patient had not refused care. Also, be sure that you have proposed all potential methods of care, including alternatives that may be options, even if they are not your first choice of treatment. An example of an alternative could be that the patient is going to be taken to the hospital for further care by a family member. Although that may not be the ideal situation, ultimately the patient will at least be seen at the hospital. Always encourage transport via ambulance because a patient's condition can change at any time, and without medical personnel there to assist, the change could have serious consequences.

The PCR should be thoroughly completed and well documented for all patient refusals of care **Figure 4** . At times, patients may agree to transport but refuse a particular procedure such as IV therapy or backboarding procedures. In such cases, refusal of the specific procedure(s) should be handled as if it is a refusal of care, including an explanation of associated risks and complications of refusal, a signature by the patient acknowledging refusal of a portion of care, a witness, and complete and accurate documentation.

Table 2 provides a reasonable list of items that should be included within the PCR of a patient refusal.

Workplace Injury and Illness Documentation

With the growing budgetary restrictions in many workplaces, a paramedic often provides workplace medical care rather than a traditional nurse providing it. According to OSHA guidelines, workplace injuries must be logged. Institutions may also have their own forms and requirements for documenting workplace injuries. Many injuries are minor, requiring only basic first aid and thus do not require an OSHA record; however, local documentation may still be required by the company. When documenting workplace injury or illness, be sure to document what precautions were taken and what protective equipment was being worn by the person involved. Companies can be fined heavily for safety violations, so it is important from the employer's and OSHA's point of view that proper

documentation occurs. It is important to note that reporting regulations vary from state to state, and you should make yourself familiar with your state's requirements. Paramedics may also perform medical monitoring for hazardous materials (HazMat) teams, may respond to other public employee workplace injuries, or may experience on-the-job injuries or illnesses themselves, which will need to be appropriately documented and reported to supervisors for workers' compensation follow-up.

Special Circumstances

There are many circumstances that you may encounter during your career that can puzzle you with the documentation requirements. Some of those situations could be a multiple-casualty incident (MCI), occupational exposure reports, abuse and neglect cases, and when a physician arrives on the scene of a call. Each of these situations may require specialized forms per your state or local

Figure 4 A competent adult patient has the right to refuse medical treatment, but it is essential that the paramedic fully inform the patient of potential consequences.

Table 2 Components of a Thorough Patient Refusal Document

Evidence the patient is able to make a rational, informed decision.

Documentation of complete assessment. If the patient refused care or did not allow a complete assessment, document that the patient did not allow for proper assessment and document whatever assessments were completed.

Discussion with the patient as to what care/transportation the provider would like to do.

Discussion with the patient as to what may happen if he or she does not allow care or transportation. Typically these consequences should be listed clearly and should include the possibility of severe illness/injury or death if care or transportation is refused.

Discussion with family/friend/bystanders to try to encourage the patient to allow care.

Discussion with medical direction according to local protocol.

Providing the patient with other alternatives: Going to see his or her family doctor, having a family member drive him or her to the hospital.

Willingness of EMS to return.

Signatures: Have a family member, police officer, or bystander sign the form as a witness. If the patient refuses to sign the refusal form, have a family member, police officer, or bystander sign the form verifying that the patient refused to sign.

agency, so it is in your best interest to become familiar with these local forms of documentation and their requirements for use.

In an MCI, the patient load can very easily overwhelm providers and, in the best interest of patient care, documentation often occurs initially on triage tags. Rather than waiting until an MCI occurs, become familiar with the triage tags, learn where they are stored, the information needed on the tags, and situations that may warrant their use in your agency or department. Although the MCI tag is designed to relay information, it is important for each emergency responder completing the tags to supply as much information as possible on them. When the time comes to transport the patient, the crew in the ambulance should complete a PCR on each patient. Although the information will be limited on the PCR, it is still imperative to complete the report to the best of your ability.

During the course of your work as a paramedic, you will be exposed to many body fluids. If your barrier devices fail or do not offer enough protection, an occupational exposure report should be completed. Because each agency or state creates their own forms for these exposures, it is important that you make yourself familiar with the requirements. Keep in mind that if you treat and/or transport a coworker for an occupational exposure, you should complete a full PCR along with the occupational exposure form.

Additional specialized documentation can be encountered when you are called to scenes of alleged neglect or abuse. It is imperative that you supply as much detail as possible about these circumstances because your initial findings may be the focus of an investigation. Some providers do not document their suspicions of abuse and neglect for fear of allegations from

YOU are the Medic PART 3

You and your partner attempt to reason with the patient to allow you to do an assessment for injuries. The patient tries to push you away and says slurring, "Keep your hands off me! I have rights!" You contact your dispatcher to confirm that law enforcement officers are en route to your location.

Recording Time: 5 Minutes	
Respirations	Unable to measure; appear adequate, approximately 20 to 24 breaths/min
Pulse	Unable to measure
Skin	Unable to measure; appears pink
Blood pressure	Unable to measure
Oxygen saturation (Spo$_2$)	Unable to measure
Pupils	Unable to measure

5. How should you document that the patient has directed you to "keep your hands off," as well as account for not being able to obtain the patient's vital signs?

6. Does this patient have the right to refuse treatment?

the patient or the abuser of <u>slander</u>. You must document your objective findings and allow the legal system to investigate and make the ultimate determination of abuse or neglect.

When a physician of any specialty arrives or is on the scene of your call, he or she may have the authority under local protocol to interject with patient care and give directives. Most protocols require that once a physician begins care that is beyond the paramedic's scope, he or she must accompany the patient to the hospital to avoid being accused of abandonment. When completing your documentation of such a run, document all orders and actions given by the physician.

You should also document the use of mutual aid services such as helicopters, specialized rescue teams, and other agencies called in to assist. Unusual occurrences should be documented as well, including having to secure the patient with restraining devices for safe transport or other unusual circumstances that arise. If you need to summon an additional crew or specialty vehicle for lifting a heavy patient or if you will have an extended scene time owing to a prolonged extrication, this information should be clearly documented to explain why "something out of the ordinary" occurred. In the event that severe weather conditions delay your response, this should also be documented.

Another special circumstance would be the appropriate documentation, as defined by medical control and your state's laws, concerning drawing a blood sample as evidence for law enforcement personnel who have a driver suspected of being under the influence in their custody. Always follow the policy of your medical director in these special circumstances.

Finally, with the increasing presence of controlled substances in the field of EMS, the paramedic is held responsible for the security and accountability of these medications. Most services require a double signature system any time a controlled substance is checked, used, discarded, or replaced. Documentation of the amount used versus wasted, the patient to whom it was given, date and time, and by whom it was given should all be documented in the PCR along with any specialized accountability forms your agency uses.

Completing a Patient Care Report

Paramedics must know and understand that EMS documentation is a required and necessary element of patient care. Just as you take pride in your patient care skills, you should take pride in your documentation skills. Now that you have been given an overview of the various aspects of the PCR along with special situations to document, you will learn how to complete the patient care report.

The PCR Narrative

As mentioned earlier, the PCR contains check boxes as well as a narrative portion. The narrative portion of the PCR should be a detailed segment indicating the elements of the call. It should be written in a format accepted by your agency and should be accurate and complete. Simply writing "followed ACLS protocols" may not be sufficient documentation for

your agency or medical director. Specifics of the call should be recorded such as "the patient was intubated with a 7.5 ET tube and ventilatory assistance provided with supplementary oxygen at 15 L/min. ET tube placement was confirmed by breath sounds, chest rise, and a tube check, before securing the ET tube at the mark of 22 at the teeth. The end-tidal CO_2 detector and pulse oximeter were placed immediately and their readings were: SpO_2 94% and $SQECO_2$ 35 mm Hg." (Always be sure to clarify which is which.) Also, some services will attach a copy of the reading to their documentation; you may wish to do this. **Table 3** provides guidelines on how to write the narrative portion of your report.

Any medical control orders received and medical advice given should be documented in the narrative section. In some EMS systems, items such as consultations, orders requested or received from medical control, and any refusal situations in which medical control has been consulted should be documented in detail in the narrative section. Simply writing "see refusal on back" is not an effective method of patient care documentation.

Many methods for narrative documentation exist. Your EMS agency or medical director may prefer a specific method to be used when documenting PCRs. Be familiar with the approved methods and all required elements for report writing for your agency. Some examples of narrative writing styles for reports are as follows:

- **Chronological order.** This is telling the narrative in a story format from the time of the initial dispatch until the call was completed. This format allows you to explain the call from start to finish **Figure 5** .
- <u>SOAP method:</u> **Subjective, Objective, Assessment, and Plan (for treatment).** Simple and logical method used to document various aspects of the patient care encounter **Figure 6** .
- <u>CHARTE method:</u> **Chief complaint, History, Assessment, Treatment (Rx), Transport, and Exceptions.** This is similar to the SOAP method, but allows you to break the narrative down into logical sections similar to that of your EMS assessment **Figure 7** .
- **Body systems/parts approach.** In this format, assessment of each body system is documented from head to toe. This method of report writing may be difficult to apply in EMS and may be too time-consuming for paramedics.

Regardless of the style of narrative report writing you and your service agree on, be sure to follow it routinely. Switching from one format to another or attempting to change formats during report writing may cause you to forget certain elements or essential details that should have been included. Proper grammar and spelling are essential when writing reports. You might consider carrying a pocket guide, reference, or medical terminology book in your ambulance to avoid spelling errors.

<u>Pertinent negatives</u> should be documented when writing your EMS report. This is a record of negative findings that warrant no care or intervention but indicate that a thorough and complete examination and history were performed. For example, "The patient denies any shortness of breath with his chest pain, patient denies any radiation of the chest pain to

Table 3 How to Write a Narrative

Topic	Items to Include
Standard precautions	Were standard precautions initiated? If so, state which precautions you used and why.
Scene safety	Did you have to make your scene safe? If so, what did you do and why did you do it? Did this create a delay of patient care?
Mechanism of Injury/Nature of Illness	Simply state. For example, "motor vehicle crash" or "difficulty breathing."
Number of patients	Record only when more than one patient is present. "This is patient 2 of 3."
Additional help	Did you call for help? If so, state why, at what time, and what time the help arrived. Was transport delayed?
Cervical spine	State what cervical spine precautions were initiated. You may want to include why; "Due to the significant MOI . . ."
Initial general impression	Simply record, if not already documented on the PCR.
Level of consciousness	Be sure to report LOC, any changes in LOC, and at what time changes occurred.
Chief complaint	Note and quote pertinent statements made by the patient and/or bystanders. This includes any pertinent denials; "Patient denies chest pain . . ."
Life threats	List all interventions and how the patient responded; "Assisted ventilations with oxygen (15 L/min) at 20 breaths/min with no change in LOC."
ABCs	Document what you found, and again, any interventions performed.
Oxygen	Record if oxygen was used, how it was applied, and how much was administered.
Primary and secondary assessment, patient history, or reassessment	State the type of assessment used and any pertinent findings; "Secondary assessment revealed unequal pupils, crepitus to right ribs, and an apparent closed fracture of the left tibia." Note the time each assessment was made and the findings.
SAMPLE/OPQRST	Note and quote any pertinent answers.
Vital signs	Your service may want you to record vital signs in the narrative portion, as well as other places in the PCR. Record the times when vital signs were taken, and the findings.
Medical direction	Quote any orders given to you by medical control and who gave them.
Management of secondary injuries/treat for shock	Report all interventions, at what time they were completed, and how the patient responded.

Abbreviations: ABCs, airway, breathing, and circulation; LOC, level of consciousness; MOI, mechanism of injury; OPQRST, mnemonic used to evaluate a patient's pain; PCR, patient care report; SAMPLE, mnemonic used to facilitate obtaining a brief patient history.

Reprinted with permission. Courtesy of Jay C. Keefauver.

other parts of the body." This would indicate that you not only obtained the information about the chest pain, but also inquired about shortness of breath and radiation of the pain.

The use of pertinent spoken accounts made by your patient and others on scene may be essential to the continuum of patient care. If you use any spoken accounts made by the patient or others, be sure to indicate who made the statement and place the exact words in quotation marks.

This may include statements about the patient's behavior, the mechanism of injury (MOI), and safety-related information such as the use of weapons. Information that may be useful to criminal investigators as a part of their investigation, disposition of valuables, admissions of suicidal intentions made by a patient, or any first aid interventions provided by bystanders before the arrival of EMS can also be useful to list in the narrative section.

Elements of a Properly Written Report

Documentation accuracy depends on all information being provided, such as times, narrative information, and check boxes, and it must be comprehensive and precise. All sections should show that you have completed them, even if a section was not applicable to the call. For example, if your PCR has a section of check boxes for specific information on cardiac arrest calls but the call you are documenting was not a cardiac arrest call, note that on the report in a manner that is approved by your agency. Simply leaving the boxes blank may raise questions about the completeness of the report.

When using a handwritten report, all reports should be legible and written in ink. The color of ink used may be determined by your EMS agency. Standard ink colors of black and blue are most commonly selected. Handwriting, especially in

Squad called to residence for ill man. On arrival found an alert and oriented 78 yo man sitting on the couch reporting CP. Pt sts this began approximately 30 min prior when he was mowing the lawn. Pt denies any radiation of the pain and rates it at a "7" out of 10 on pain scale. Pt has a known cardiac history with an MI 2 years prior. Pt is compliant with all meds as listed above. Pt denies any SOB or N/V with this episode. V/S stable, lungs CTA, SpO_2 96% RA, Skin pale/warm/dry to touch, PEARRL 4 mm, GCS 15. Pt placed on O_2 @ 15 L/min via NRB. Monitor showed RSR @ 88 bpm without ectopy. IV of NS was established in L AC with 18 g @ TKO (medic 785). 2 × 81 mg ASA were given PO @ 1501 (medic 785). Pt was given 1 SL 0.4 mg nitro @ 1503 with relief down to a "4" on scale (medic 785). V/S still stable. Secondary exam showed negative new findings. Med control contacted with negative orders. Left pt in care of ED staff with report in room 7.

Figure 5 Example of a narrative written in chronological order.

Note: In this example, "(medic 785)" identifies which provider performed the intervention. His or her initials may also be used. It is important to document who performed the procedure, because the person who is writing the narrative may not have been the crew member to perform the procedure or administer the medication.

(S) Called to scene for 78 yo man complaining of chest pain. Pt states pain began approximately 30 min prior to arrival when he was mowing the lawn. Pt denies any radiation of pain. States pain is "7" out of 10 on pain scale. Pt has known cardiac hx with an MI 2 yrs prior. Pt denies SOB or N/V. Pt has no allergies and is compliant with all meds listed above.

(O) U/A found Pt sitting on the couch. Pt alert and oriented with NARD and strong radial pulse. Pt calm and cooperative. Skin: Pale/warm/dry. Pupils PEARRL 4 mm, GSC 15. Lungs CTA. No noted JVD. Abd soft and nontender. PMS × 4. Secondary exam unremarkable.

(A) Possible MI.

(P) Primary, secondary Hx, V/S as listed above. Assisted pt to cot. Cardiac monitor: showed RSR @ 88 bpm without ectopy. IV: NS 18 g in L AC @ TKO (BW); SpO_2 – 96% RA, O_2 @ 15 L/min via NRB – 100%; 2 × 81 mg ASA given PO, 1 SL 0.4 mg nitro (BW) – pain down to "4". Transported to _____. Pt care transferred to ED with report.

Figure 6 Example of a narrative written with the SOAP method.

(C) 78 yo man complaining of chest pain without radiation. Pt sts pain is a "7" out of 10 on pain scale.

(H) Pt has a known cardiac history with an MI 2 years prior.

(A) Pt denies any SOB or nausea/vomiting with this episode. Vital signs stable, lungs clear to auscultation, SpO_2 96% RA, skin pale/warm/dry to touch, PEARRL 4 mm, GCS 15. Monitor showed RSR @ 88 bpm without ectopy.

(R) Pt placed on O_2 @ 15 L/min via NRB. IV of NS was established in L AC with 18 g @ TKO (medic 785). 2 × 81 mg ASA were given PO @ 1501 (medic 785). Pt was given 1 SL 0.4 mg nitro @ 1503 (medic 785).

(T) Pt improved during transport, pain went down to a "4" on the scale, V/S remained stable, and patient care was transferred to ED staff.

(E) None.

Figure 7 Example of a narrative written in the CHARTE method.

the narrative portion of the report, needs to be neat and easily read by others. In addition, take great care to not contaminate your written reports with any liquids found in the field. Place all your completed reports in a secure location agreed on by you and your partner that protects the patient's privacy, until they can be secured in the proper place at your EMS agency office or headquarters.

The PCR needs to be timely, even in EMS systems where call volume is high. If you respond to multiple calls without accurately completing PCRs before proceeding to the next call, details may be forgotten and important information left out, or worse, inaccurate information may be written. Your EMS agency should allow you a reasonable amount of time to complete your reports, replenish supplies, and clean and disinfect vehicles *before* returning them to service. Many paramedics use assessment cards during their calls to take notes, and use the ECG monitor to note times and vital signs; then after the call, they complete the PCR (rather than on the bumpy ride to the hospital). Time should be set aside at the hospital to neatly complete all documentation. If you do not have time to complete the full PCR while at the hospital, a written record still must be left with the patient. In these cases, most systems will have a "drop report" or "transfer report" **Figure 8**. These single-page, abbreviated forms are used as a memory aid during an EMS call. If you are unable to remain at the hospital to complete the PCR, copy these documents and leave them with the nurse or physician. Some states require that copies of written reports be supplied to the receiving facility or hospital within a specific time frame, such as 24 hours. Know the applicable laws and requirements of your state and EMS system. In some systems, EMS providers fax the completed form to the emergency department because the hospital has a secure fax location that meets HIPAA requirements. You should consider your call incomplete until you have completed the documentation process.

As mentioned previously, all PCRs should be free of jargon, slang, and opinions of the EMS provider. Be certain that your documentation is not libelous. **Libel** is writing a false statement that could be harmful to a person's current or future reputation. Only true and accurate statements should be documented. If quotes of bystanders or statements made by the patient are used, be sure to indicate who made them and place the exact words in quotation marks on the report.

All reports should be reviewed by the paramedic who authored them before submitting them to the receiving medical facility and to the paramedic's EMS agency. Always reviewing your PCR for completeness, accuracy, grammar, spelling, and

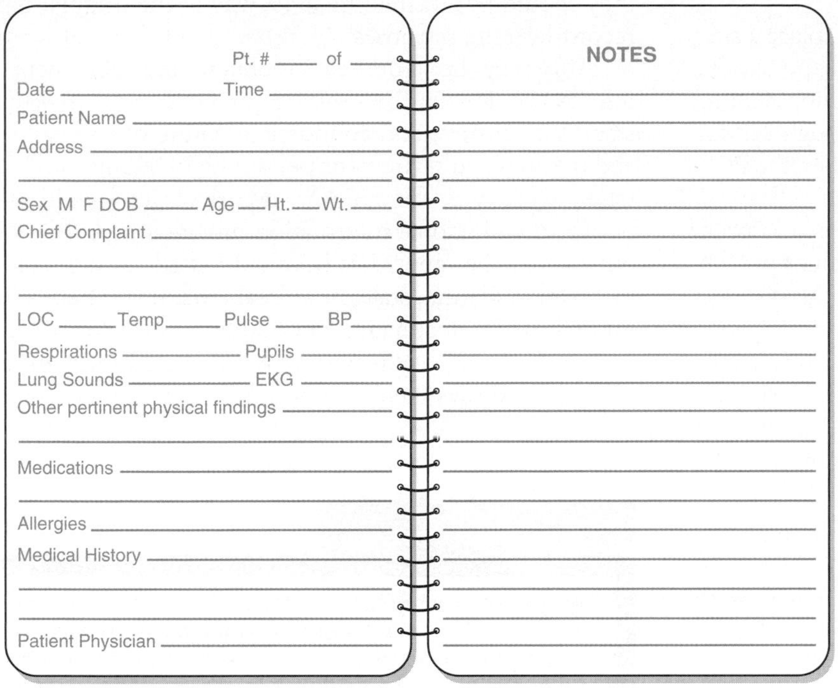
Pt. # ___ of ___
Date ___ Time ___
Patient Name ___
Address ___
Sex M F DOB ___ Age ___ Ht. ___ Wt. ___
Chief Complaint ___
LOC ___ Temp ___ Pulse ___ BP ___
Respirations ___ Pupils ___
Lung Sounds ___ EKG ___
Other pertinent physical findings ___
Medications ___
Allergies ___
Medical History ___
Patient Physician ___
NOTES

Figure 8 A sample prehospital notepad, also called a drop report or transfer report.

Documentation and Communication

Remember to document problems encountered when responding to or during the call (eg, an infectious disease exposure, a delayed response, a conflict at the scene with family or other response agencies, an MCI, an injury to an EMS provider that happened while providing care to the patient, etc).

proper use of medical terminology and abbreviations will help ensure you have a well-written and well-documented report.

Too often, the importance of report writing and documentation in EMS is ignored. Always remember that the report that you write reflects directly on you. When you file a complete, well-documented, legible report, you have done the most important part of the completion of your call.

The Effects of Poor Documentation

Documentation may affect the quality of care provided after you have delivered the patient to the hospital. Inappropriate, inaccurate, and poor documentation can adversely affect the quality of care received by patients after arrival at the hospital. For example, you administered a breathing treatment en route to the hospital but forgot to document the medication and procedure and the administration times. The hospital would not be aware of this and the patient could be treated inappropriately because of your failure to document the care you provided. Another example is to remember to document the specific time a suspected stroke patient was last seen "normal" by family members; this is important to the window of time for treatment using fibrinolytics in a stroke center. Documenting what the patient or family members tell you and your findings from examining the patient enhances the quality of care. For example, if hospital personnel know that a patient has a seizure disorder or that a patient who has had transient ischemic attacks in the past had symptoms of stroke en route to the hospital, proper care can be planned.

As mentioned previously, there are legal implications of documentation. Poorly written, inaccurate, or illegible reports might lead a judge or jury to decide in favor of the plaintiff. Conversely, a lawyer may decide not to pursue a case when the documentation reveals a correctly written and well-documented report.

Poor documentation skills can also affect a paramedic's reputation. Poorly written, inappropriate, or inaccurate reports might make others question the care provided, whereas a well-written report shows organizational skills, knowledge of patient conditions and needs, and respect for organizational policies and procedures. Part of being a good paramedic is completing the paperwork and reports as required. If you find it difficult to write reports, seek additional classes or study report writing skills to enhance your abilities. Your agency or service might have an educational program to assist you with such education and training.

Errors and Falsification

At times, it may be necessary to revise or correct your PCR. Although every attempt should be made to create an accurate and legible initial report, if a report has to be revised or corrected, you must note the date and time of the revised report and the purpose for writing the revision or making the correction. Never discard or destroy the original PCR.

Only the person who wrote the original report can revise it. Additions or notations added by others after the completion of the report may raise questions about the authenticity of the report and the confidentiality practices of your agency. Routine administrative report handling and reviews are necessary for entering information into computer databases, billing for services, and quality assurance monitoring. At no time should administrative activities involve altering or rewriting the report or portions of it.

When writing your report, if you make an error, place a single line through the error and initial and date the line, preferably in a different color ink. Write the corrected information next to it **Figure 9**. Do not erase information, scribble through errors, use correction fluid, or use correction tape. Remember, the PCR is a legal document.

If an error is discovered after an electronic report has been submitted, most systems will allow for amendments but will prevent erasure in a completed document. Refer to the system's directions as to how to make an amendment to the original document. In the event that there is no way to electronically change the report, the same procedure should be followed as for a written document. Simply follow the correction method used for a handwritten report on a printout of the electronic report. Most electronic PCR systems keep good records of who made an alteration to the report and when it was made.

If you forgot to include important information, you may need to write an addendum to your report. You may also need to write an addendum if you are asked to write statements of events for matters related to quality assurance or risk management and to answer complaints. An addendum added to your original report should be noted as added to the original and the reason for the late entry and should include the date of entry, the time of entry, and signature of the author.

Supplemental narratives also may be needed if additional information becomes available after the original report has been written. Such reports should be documented with the date, the time, and the reason for the added information and should be signed by the author. Some EMS services use a supplemental report to write lengthy information when space on the original report is limited. Follow your service's policies for using supplemental reports and the procedures for writing them. Regardless of when the supplemental reports are added, they should be attached in some way to the original report for record-keeping purposes.

You may be required to obtain and document billing information for the EMS service provided. You need to understand the sensitive and confidential nature of such information and the laws and regulations pertaining to billing and documentation security under HIPAA. EMS agencies should take care not to add additional information provided by billing clerks or others after the report has been submitted. Doing so might be in violation of local, state, or federal laws. If you have additional information to document after handing in the form, follow the policy of your agency regarding whether a supplementary form is needed. Always be honest and thorough in your documentation process.

Controversies

Because of strict guidelines for what is considered a medical necessity for emergency ambulance transportation, some agency leaders urge providers not to document certain findings with the patient, such as the patient's ability to ambulate. Other leaders have urged field personnel to document findings that meet the medical necessity standards to help bring in revenue. Intentionally documenting inaccurate or fraudulent information is unethical, as well as illegal, and could lead to the loss of your certification.

Lost reports pose huge legal implications for paramedics, EMS agencies and departments, and medical directors. All paramedics are responsible for ensuring that their reports are completed and turned in as required by policy or procedure. (Do not keep copies of your reports—if you need to document numbers of procedures or ages of patients for your paramedic internship, follow the specific policy of your training center.) If lost reports are an ongoing problem for an agency or provider, steps should be taken to correct the problem. Know that attempting to recreate PCRs is irresponsible and possibly illegal. Also, record keeping may be a legal requirement in your state, and there may also be a specified time requirement for submission of reports.

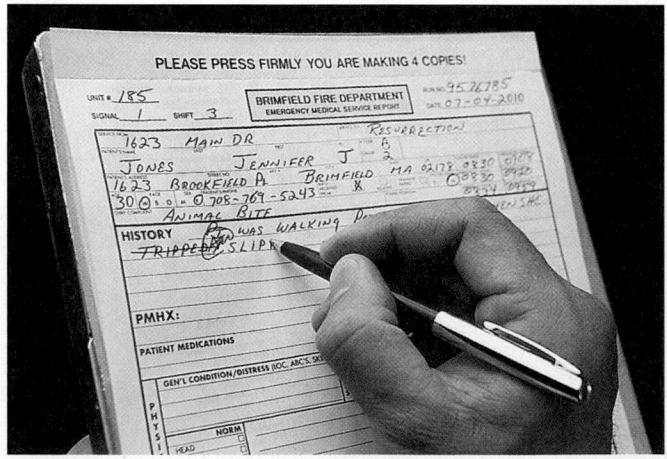

Figure 9 If you make a mistake in writing your report, the proper way to correct it is to draw a single horizontal line through the error, initial it, and write the correct information next to it.

Documentation and Communication

Reports should be complete to the point that people reviewing them, whether your medical director or the administrative office clerk billing for the service provided, can read them and understand exactly what transpired on the EMS call. If your report does not paint a clear picture of what happened, it is not written well. Remember, your report is a reflection of your actions and your professionalism.

Documenting Incident Times

Keeping good records of time is essential to all EMS operations. The role of timekeeper falls to dispatchers. You must also keep track of time during your documentation of the incident. You should compare your times with those of the dispatcher to ensure accuracy and proper timekeeping, and ensure that your and your dispatcher's clocks are synchronized. If your ECG monitor reports or documentation times are not in sync with the dispatcher's time, this could create a controversy in the courtroom. It is important that the reported times of all the events are accurate.

Several times are absolutely vital to be kept and documented for accurate report writing. The vital incident times to track are as follows:

- **Time of call.** Time when the call for help is placed or requested
- **Time of dispatch.** Time when call is toned or alerted for a response
- **Time of arrival at the scene.** Time when EMS unit arrives on scene
- **Time with patient.** Time recorded when patient contact is made (this may not be the same as time of arrival, for example, when responding to a patient on the 17th floor of a high-rise building; should include the time it takes to physically get to the patient)
- **Time of medication administration.** Time when medications are administered for adherence to protocols (1 × 0.4 mg of nitroglycerin was given SL at 1804 without relief [medic 785])
- **Time of medical procedure.** Time when a procedure is conducted on the patient such as when vital signs are taken, when a patient is intubated, or when a child is delivered. (Example: Pt was intubated with a 7.5 fr endotracheal tube with confirmation of negative epigastric sounds, clear bilateral lung sounds in all fields, and a wave-form capnography reading of 35 mm Hg at 1807 [medic 785])
- **Time of departure from scene.** Time recorded when EMS unit leaves the scene
- **Time of arrival at medical facility.** Time when arriving at medical facility (if a patient is transported)
- **Time of transfer of care.** Time when care was transferred to another health care professional at the receiving facility (if a patient is transported)
- **Time back in service.** Time when EMS unit and crew are ready for return to service

It is standard procedure to use military time in EMS documentation. This ensures that each time is unique; for example, 1 AM cannot be confused with 1 PM. Military times are shown in Table 4 .

Medical Terminology

Using medical terminology correctly is essential to EMS communications. You should learn the established and accepted medical terms and abbreviations for your EMS operations. Some EMS systems have specific approved lists of medical abbreviations and terms that must be used.

Medical terminology may seem to be a foreign language; however, most terminology comes from the ancient Roman language, Latin. In addition, you may encounter some common slang terms used in EMS such as "packaging a patient for transport" or "bagging the patient during airway management." Be sure to know acceptable terms and words used in your EMS agency. The wider your vocabulary base, the more competent you will seem to the rest of the medical community and the better the patient care you will be able to provide. An ongoing review of the anatomy and physiology chapter can help you become familiar with medical terminology. Understanding terminology involves breaking words down into their separate components of prefix, suffix, and root word and having a good working knowledge of those parts. The next section provides a more in-depth look at commonly used medical terms and their meanings.

Prefixes

A prefix appears at the beginning of a word and generally describes location or intensity. Prefixes are frequently found in general language (ie, autopilot, submarine, tricycle), as well as in medical and scientific terminology. When a medical word (ventilation) contains a prefix (hyper), the meaning of the word is altered (hyperventilation). Not all medical terms have prefixes.

By learning to recognize a few of the more commonly used medical prefixes, you can figure out the meanings of terms that may not be immediately familiar to you. Table 5 lists common prefixes.

Table 4 Military Times

Regular Time	Military Time	Regular Time	Military Time
Midnight	0000	Noon	1200
1:00 AM	0100	1:00 PM	1300
2:00 AM	0200	2:00 PM	1400
3:00 AM	0300	3:00 PM	1500
4:00 AM	0400	4:00 PM	1600
5:00 AM	0500	5:00 PM	1700
6:00 AM	0600	6:00 PM	1800
7:00 AM	0700	7:00 PM	1900
8:00 AM	0800	8:00 PM	2000
9:00 AM	0900	9:00 PM	2100
10:00 AM	1000	10:00 PM	2200
11:00 AM	1100	11:00 PM	2300

Suffixes

Suffixes are placed at the end of words to change the original meaning. In medical terminology, a suffix usually indicates a procedure, condition, disease, or part of speech. A commonly used suffix is -itis, which means "inflammation." When this suffix is paired with the root word arthro-, meaning "joint", the resulting word is arthritis, an inflammation of the joints. Sometimes it is necessary to change the last letter or letters of the root word or prefix when a suffix is added to make pronunciation easier. Table 6 lists common suffixes.

Root Words

The main part or stem of a word is called a root word. A root word conveys the essential meaning of the word and frequently indicates a body part. With a combining form, the root word and a combining vowel such as i, e, o, or a may be combined with another root word, a prefix, or a suffix to describe a particular structure or condition.

A frequently used term in EMS is CPR, which stands for cardiopulmonary resuscitation. When the word is broken down, cardio is a root word meaning "heart," and pulmonary is a root word meaning "lungs." When you perform CPR, you are introducing air into the lungs and circulating blood by compressing the heart to resuscitate the patient. Some root words may also be used as prefixes or suffixes; those already appear in the earlier tables. Table 7 lists common root words.

Medical Abbreviations

Medical abbreviations can be very useful for documentation purposes, but you must be certain the abbreviations you are using are consistent with approved medical abbreviations in your EMS system. Incorrect or inappropriate medical abbreviations can cause confusion and, in the worst cases, could lead to medication and treatment errors. You should learn the approved medical abbreviations for your service area before you use them in a report. For example, some agencies do not use "SOB" to abbreviate "shortness of breath." Each EMS system should have a list of approved medical abbreviations available for use and documentation purposes. Once again, accuracy, neatness, and completeness reflect a professional writing style. Note that many abbreviations have more than one meaning, so extreme care is needed when using them. (For patient safety reasons, hospitals are required by The Joint Commission to have a list of approved abbreviations; certain abbreviations are prohibited by the commission.) Table 8 lists commonly used medical abbreviations. It is important that you learn your agency's approved terminology.

It is important for you to be familiar with abbreviations that have a significant potential to be misunderstood. In 2004, the Joint Commission identified abbreviations that lead to errors, and should therefore not be used. Table 9 lists those abbreviations, as well as others that can be confusing and therefore should not be used. In most instances, the term should be written out in full; for example, rather than using the "at" symbol (@), write out "at."

YOU are the Medic   PART 4

Law enforcement officers arrive on scene. At about that time the patient yells, "Great! Officers, arrest these people. They're harassing me!" One officer tells the patient to relax and do what the EMS crew asks, saying, "All they are trying to do is make sure you're OK." The officer asks the patient, "Have you been drinking today?" The patient replies, "I had a few at lunch is all. I'm just fine." The officer asks for, and receives, the patient's driver's license. He says to the patient, "I'm sure you are aware Assemblyman Taylor, there are laws that you have to obey and it would look much better to your constituents if you cooperated. Going to the hospital in an ambulance is much better than in a police cruiser." The patient agrees and you can finally assess the patient and prepare for transport.

Recording Time: 15 Minutes	
Respirations	16 breaths/min with adequate tidal volume
Pulse	100 beats/min, strong and regular
Skin	Warm, dry, pink
Blood pressure	130/80 mm Hg
Oxygen saturation (Spo_2)	97% on room air
Pupils	Equal and react to light

7. Is it important to document the interaction between the patient and law enforcement officers when there is no patient care involved?

8. What is the legal basis to determine whether a patient is competent to refuse care?

Table 5   Common Prefixes

Prefix	Meaning	Prefix	Meaning	Prefix	Meaning
a-	without, lack of	dermat(o)-	pertaining to the skin	lith(o)-	pertaining to a stone
ab-	away from	di-	twice, double	macro-	large
abdomi(n)-	abdomen	dia-	through, completely	mal-	bad or abnormal
acr(o)-	to, toward	dys-	difficult, painful, abnormal	medi-	middle
aden(o)-	pertaining to a gland	ect(o)-	out from	mega-	large
an-	without, lack of	electro-	pertaining to electricity	melan-	black
ana-	up, back, again	end(o)-	within	mening(o)-	pertaining to a membrane, particularly the meninges
angio-	vessel	enter(o)-	pertaining to the intestines	micro-	small
ante-	before, forward	epi-	upon, on	mono-	one
anti-	against, opposed to	erythr(o)-	pertaining to anything red or to erythrocytes (red blood cells)	myel(o)-	pertaining to the spinal cord, the bone marrow, or myelin
arteri(o)-	artery	eu-	easy, good, normal	my(o)-	pertaining to muscle
arthro-	pertaining to a joint	ex(o)-	outside	nas(o)-	pertaining to the nose
auto-	self	extra-	outside, in addition	ne(o)-	new
bi-	two	gastr(o)-	pertaining to the stomach	nephr(o)-	pertaining to the kidney
bi(o)-	pertaining to life	glyc(o)-	sugar	neur(o)-	pertaining to a nerve or the nervous system
blast(o)-	germ or cell	gynec(o)-	pertaining to females or the female reproductive organs	noct-	night
blephar(o)-	pertaining to an eyelid	hemat(o)-	pertaining to blood	olig(o)-	little, deficient
brady-	slow	hemi-	half	oophor(o)-	pertaining to the ovary
calc-	stone; also heel	hem(o)-	pertaining to blood	ophthalm(o)-	pertaining to the eye
cardi(o)-	pertaining to the heart	hepat(o)-	pertaining to the liver	orchid(o)-	pertaining to the testicles
cephal(o)-	pertaining to the head	heter-	other, different	orchi(o)-	pertaining to the testicles
cerebr(o)-	pertaining to the cerebrum, a part of the brain	hom-	same or like	oro-	pertaining to the mouth
cervic(o)-	pertaining to the neck or the uterine cervix	hydr(o)-	water	ortho-	straight or normal
chole-	pertaining to bile	hyper-	over, excessive	oste(o)-	pertaining to bone
chondr(o)-	pertaining to cartilage	hypo-	under, deficient	ot(o)-	pertaining to the ear
circum-	around, about	hyster(o)-	pertaining to the uterus	para-	by the side of
contra-	against, opposite	infra-	below	path(o)-	pertaining to disease
cost(o)-	pertaining to a rib	inter-	between	per-	through
cyan(o)-	blue	intra-	within	peri-	around
cyst(o)-	pertaining to the bladder or any fluid-containing sac	iso-	equal	phag(o)-	pertaining to eating, ingesting, or engulfing
cyt(o)-	pertaining to a cell	latero-	side	pharyng(o)-	pertaining to the throat, or pharynx
de-	down from	leuk(o)-	pertaining to anything white or to leukocytes (white blood cells)	phleb(o)-	pertaining to a vein

Continues

Table 5   Common Prefixes, continued

Prefix	Meaning	Prefix	Meaning	Prefix	Meaning
pneum(o)-	pertaining to respiration, the lungs, or air	pyel(o)-	pertaining to the kidney or pelvis	sub-	under, moderately
poly-	many	py(o)-	pertaining to pus	super-	above, excessive, or more than normal
post-	after, behind	quadr(i)-	four	supra-	above
pre-	before	quar-	four	tachy-	fast
pro-	before, in front of	quat-	four	therm-	pertaining to temperature
proct(o)-	pertaining to the rectum	retr(o)-	backward or behind	thorac(o)-	pertaining to the chest
pseud(o)-	false	rhin(o)-	pertaining to the nose	trans-	across
psych(o)-	pertaining to the mind	salping(o)-	pertaining to a tube	tri-	three
pulm(o)-	pertaining to the lung	scler(o)-	hard; also means pertaining to the sclera	uni-	one
pur-	pertaining to pus	semi-	half or partial	vas(o)-	vessel

Table 6   Common Suffixes

Suffix	Meaning	Suffix	Meaning	Suffix	Meaning
-algia	pertaining to pain	-megaly	enlargement of	-ptosis	drooping
-asthen(o)	weakness	-ology	science of	-rrhage	abnormal or excessive flow or discharge
-blast	immature cell	-oma	tumor	-rrhagia	abnormal or excessive flow or discharge
-cele	pertaining to a tumor or swelling	-osis	pertaining to a disease process (see also -sis)	-rrhaphy	suture of; repair of
-centesis	pertaining to a procedure in which an organ or body cavity is punctured, often to drain excess fluid or obtain a sample for analysis	-ostomy	surgical creation of an opening, or hole	-rrhea	flow or discharge
-cyte	cell	-otomy	surgical incision	-scope	instrument for examination
-ectomy	surgical removal of	-pathy	disease or a system for treating disease	-scopy	examination with an instrument
-emia	pertaining to the presence of a substance in the blood	-phagia	pertaining to eating or swallowing	-sis	a process, action, or condition
-genic	causing	-phasia	pertaining to speech	-taxis	order, arrangement of
-gram	record	-phobia	pertaining to an irrational fear	-trophic	pertaining to nutrition
-graph	a record or the instrument used to create the record	-plasty	plastic surgery	-uria	pertaining to a substance in the urine or the condition so indicated
-itis	inflammation	-plegia	paralysis		
-lysis	decline, disintegration, or destruction	-pnea	pertaining to breathing		

Table 7   Common Root Words

Root Word	Meaning	Root Word	Meaning	Root Word	Meaning
acou-	hear	digit	finger or toe	pleur-	rib, side
adip-	fat	ede-	swelling	pod-	foot
alb-	white	-esthesi(o)-	pertaining to sensation or perception	pto-	fall
alges-	pain	febr-	fever	ptyal-	saliva
andr-	male	flex	bend	pyr-	fire
aorta	large artery exiting from the left ventricle of the heart	foramen	opening	radius	the forearm bone on the thumb side; also a line from the center of a circle or sphere to the edge
aqua	water	fract	break	ren	kidney
asphyxia	lack of oxygen or excess of carbon dioxide in the body that results in unconsciousness	gest-	carry, produce, congestion	retina	inner nerve-containing layer of the eye
asthen-	weak	gno-	know	sangui(n)-	blood
audi-	to hear	-gram	something written or recorded	sebum	a fatty secretion of the sebaceous glands
bronch-	windpipe	graph-	write, record	sect-	cut
bucc-	cheek	humerus	the bone in the upper arm	sepsis	the presence of microorganisms or their toxins in the blood; also the toxic condition caused by such presence
bursa	pouch or sac	idi-	separate, distinct	sept-	wall, divider; also seven
callus	hard, thick skin; also a meshwork of connective tissue that forms during the healing process after a fracture	iod(o)-	iodine	serum	the clear portion of body fluids, including blood
carcin-	cancer	lact-	milk	sinus	cavity, channel, or hollow space
carotid	great arteries of the neck	lingu-	tongue	som(a)-	body
carpus	wrist	men-	month	spir-	coil
cent-	a fraction in the metric system; one hundredth or 100	ocul-	eye	stasis	slowing or stopping of the normal flow of a fluid, such as blood
cente-	to puncture (a body cavity)	ov-	egg	stature	height
cili-	eyelid	palpate	to examine by touch	stern(o)-	sternum (breastbone)
cleid(o)-	clavicle	ped-	child or foot	stoma	any small opening on the surface of the body, such as a pore; also, the opening created in the abdominal wall for the passage of urine or feces
cubitus	elbow	percuss	to examine by striking	tact-	touch
cycl-	circle or cycle	phot-	light	tetra-	four

Continues

Table 7 Common Root Words, continued

Root Word	Meaning	Root Word	Meaning	Root Word	Meaning
tom-	cut	varic-	varicose vein	xen-	foreign (material)
toxic	poisonous	vertigo	a disordered sensation in which one's own body or the surroundings are perceived as moving	xer-	dry
trich-	hair	viscer-	internal organs		
ur-	urine	viscous	sticky		

Table 8 Common Abbreviations*

Abbreviation	Meaning	Abbreviation	Meaning	Abbreviation	Meaning
A&P	anatomy and physiology	A-line	arterial line	AV, A-V	atrioventricular, arteriovenous
ā	before	ALS	advanced life support	AVPU	alert, verbal, pain, unresponsive
āā	of each (used in writing prescriptions)	AMA	against medical advice	BBB	bundle branch block
ABC	airway, breathing, circulation	amb	ambulatory	BG	blood glucose
abd	abdomen	AMI	acute myocardial infarction	BGL	blood glucose level
ABG	arterial blood gas	AMS	altered mental status	bid	twice daily
ac	before meals	ant	anterior	bilat	bilaterally
AC	antecubital fossa	AO×3	alert and oriented to person, time, and place	BKA	below the knee amputation
ACLS	advanced cardiac life support	AOB	alcohol on breath	BLS	basic life support
ad lib	as much as desired	AP	anteroposterior, front-to-back, action potential, angina pectoris, anterior pituitary, arterial pressure	BM	bowel movement
ADL	activity of daily living	APAP	acetaminophen	BP	blood pressure
AED	automated external defibrillator	APC	atrial premature complex, activated protein C, aspirin-phenacetin-caffeine	bpm	beats per minute
AF	atrial fibrillation	Aq	water	BS	blood sugar, breath sounds, bowel sounds, bachelor of science (degree)
AICD	automated internal cardiac defibrillator	ARDS	acute respiratory distress syndrome	BSA	body surface area
AIDS	acquired immunodeficiency syndrome	ASA	aspirin (acetylsalicylic acid)	bx	biopsy
AK	above the knee	ASAP	as soon as possible	c̄	with
AKA	above the knee amputation	ASHD	arteriosclerotic or atherosclerotic heart disease	°C	degrees Celsius (centigrade)

Continues

Table 8 Common Abbreviations*, continued

Abbreviation	Meaning	Abbreviation	Meaning	Abbreviation	Meaning
C2	code 2 (nonemergent)	CP	chest pain, chemically pure, cerebral palsy	DOS	dead on scene
C3	code 3 (emergent)	CPR	cardiopulmonary resuscitation	DPT	diphtheria and tetanus toxoids and pertussis vaccine
Ca	calcium	CRNA	certified registered nurse anesthetist	DSD	dry sterile dressing
CA	cancer, cardiac arrest, chronological age, coronary artery, cold agglutinin	CRT	capillary refill time, cathode ray tube	DtaP	diphtheria and tetanus toxoids and acellular pertussis vaccine
CABG	coronary artery bypass graft	CSF	cerebrospinal fluid	DTP	diphtheria and tetanus toxoids and pertussis vaccine
CAD	coronary artery disease	CSM	carotid sinus massage, cerebrospinal meningitis	DTs	delirium tremens
CAO	conscious, alert, and oriented	c-spine	cervical spine	DVT	deep venous thrombosis
CBC	complete blood count	CT	computerized tomography (CAT scan)	Dx	diagnosis
CC or C/C	chief complaint	CTA	clear to auscultation	ECG	electrocardiogram
CCT	critical care transport	CTL	cervical, thoracic, lumbar spine	ED	emergency department
CCU	coronary care unit	CVA	cerebrovascular accident	EDC	estimated date of confinement
CHB	complete heart block	CVP	central venous pressure	EEG	electroencephalogram
CHF	congestive heart failure	Cx	chest	eg	for example
CHI	closed head injury	CXR	chest x-ray	EKG	electrocardiogram
Cl$^-$	chloride	D$_{50}$	dextrose 50%	EMS	emergency medical services
clr	clear	D$_5$W	dextrose 5% in water	ENT	ears, nose, and throat
cm	centimeter	D&C	dilation and curettage	ER	emergency room
cm^3	cubic centimeter	defib	defibrillation	ET	endotracheal tube, endotracheal
CMS	circulation, movement, sensation	diff	differential	ETA	estimated time of arrival
CNS	central nervous system	dig	digoxin	ETOH	ethyl alcohol
c/o	complaining of	DKA	diabetic ketoacidosis	ETT	endotracheal tube
CO	cardiac output, carbon monoxide	DM	diabetes mellitus	Exp	expansion
CO$_2$	carbon dioxide	DOA	dead on arrival	°F	degrees Fahrenheit
COLD	chronic obstructive lung disease	DOE	dyspnea on exertion	FA	forearm
COPD	chronic obstructive pulmonary disease	DON	director of nursing	FBS	fasting blood sugar

Continues

Table 8 Common Abbreviations*, continued

Abbreviation	Meaning	Abbreviation	Meaning	Abbreviation	Meaning
Fe	iron	Hb	hemoglobin	IVP	intravenous push
FHR	fetal heart rate	HB	heart block	J	joule
FHT	fetal heart tones	Hct	hematocrit	JVD	jugular venous distention
FHx	family history	HEENT	head, ears, eyes, nose, throat	K+	potassium
F_{IO_2}	fraction of inspired oxygen	Hg	mercury	KCl	potassium chloride
fL	femtoliter	Hgb	hemoglobin	KED	Kendrick extrication device
fl	fluid	HH	hiatal hernia	kg	kilogram
fld	fluid	HI	head injury	KUB	kidneys, ureters, and bladder
FSH	follicle-stimulating hormone	HIV	human immunodeficiency virus	KVO	keep vein open
fx	fracture	H_2O	water	L	liter
g	gram	H_2O_2	hydrogen peroxide	LAC	laceration, laparoscopic-assisted colectomy
GB	gallbladder	hosp	hospital	LAD	left anterior descending, left axis deviation
GCS	Glasgow Coma Scale	HPI	history of present illness	LAH	left anterior hemiblock
GERD	gastroesophageal reflux disease	hr	hour	lb	pound
GI	gastrointestinal	HR	heart rate	LBB	left bundle branch block
gm	gram	HTN	hypertension	LE	lower extremity, left eye, lupus erythematosus
gr	grain	Hx	history	LGL	Lown-Ganong-Levine syndrome
GSW	gunshot wound	Hz	hertz	LLL	left lower lobe of the lung
gtt	drop(s)	I&O	intake and output	LLQ	left lower quadrant of the abdomen
GTT	glucose tolerance test	IC	intracardiac, inspiratory capacity, irritable colon	L/M	liters per minute
GU	genitourinary	ICP	intracranial pressure	LMP	last menstrual period
gyn	gynecology	ICS	intercostal space	LOC	level of consciousness, loss of consciousness
h	hour	ICU	intensive care unit	LPH	left posterior hemiblock
(H)	hypodermic	IDDM	insulin-dependent diabetes mellitus	LPM	liters per minute
H	hypodermic	IM	intramuscular	LPN	licensed practical nurse
H&H	hemoglobin and hematocrit	IO	intraosseous	LR	lactated Ringer's
H&P	history and physical	IPPB	intermittent positive pressure breathing	LS	lung sounds
H/A	headache	IUD	intrauterine(contraceptive) device	LSB	long spineboard
H/P	history and physical	IV	intravenous	LSD	lysergic acid diethylamide

Continues

Table 8 Common Abbreviations*, continued

Abbreviation	Meaning	Abbreviation	Meaning	Abbreviation	Meaning
LUL	left upper lobe of the lung	MVP	mitral valve prolapse	N/V/D	nausea, vomiting, and diarrhea
LUQ	left upper quadrant of the abdomen	N	normal	NVD	neck vein distention
LVN	licensed vocational nurse	Na	sodium	O_2	oxygen
m	meter	NA, N/A	not applicable	OB	obstetrics
mA	milliamps	NaCl	sodium chloride	OBS	organic brain syndrome
MAE	moves all extremities	NAD	no apparent distress, no appreciable disease	Occ	occipital
MAEW	moves all extremities well	$NaHCO_3$	sodium bicarbonate	OETT	oral endotracheal tube
MAP	mean arterial pressure	NARD	no apparent respiratory distress	OM	otitis media
MAST	medical antishock trouser	NATO	not able to obtain	OP	outpatient
MCA	motorcycle accident	NEB	nebulizer	OPA	oropharyngeal airway
mcg	microgram	NETT	nasal endotracheal tube	OR	operating room
MCL	midclavicular line, modified chest lead	NC	nasal cannula	OS	left eye
meds	medications	NG	nasogastric	OU	both eyes
mEq	milliequivalents	NICU	neonatal intensive care unit	oz	ounce
mg	milligram (mgm is a former symbol)	NIDDM	non-insulin-dependent diabetes mellitus	$\bar{p}$	after
MI	myocardial infarction	NKA	no known allergies	PA	physician assistant
MICU	mobile intensive care unit; medical intensive care unit	NKDA	no known drug allergies	PAC	premature atrial contraction
min	minute	NL	nonlabored	palp	palpation
mL	milliliter	NP	nasopharyngeal	PASG	pneumatic antishock garment
mm	millimeter	NPA	nasopharyngeal airway	pc	after meals
mm Hg	millimeters of mercury	NPO	nil per os (nothing by mouth)	P_{CO_2}	partial pressure of carbon dioxide
MOE	movement of extremity	NRB	nonrebreathing mask	PDR	*Physician's Desk Reference*
MOI	mechanism of injury	NS	normal saline	PE	pulmonary embolism, physical examination
MRI	magnetic resonance imaging	NSR	normal sinus rhythm	PEA	pulseless electrical activity
MVA	motor vehicle accident	NTG	nitroglycerin	PEARL	pupils equal and reactive to light
MVC	motor vehicle crash	N/V	nausea and vomiting	ped(s)	pediatric

Continues

Table 8 Common Abbreviations*, continued

Abbreviation	Meaning	Abbreviation	Meaning	Abbreviation	Meaning
PEEP	positive end-expiratory pressure	PTA	prior to admission, plasma thromboplastin antecedent	RSI	rapid sequence intubation
PERL	pupils equal and reactive to light	PTSD	posttraumatic stress disorder	RUL	right upper lobe of the lung
PERRL	pupils equal, round, and reactive to light	PTT	partial thromboplastin time	RUQ	right upper quadrant of the abdomen
PG	pregnant	PVC	premature ventricular complex, polyvinyl chloride	Rx	prescription
P#/G#	para #/gravida # (Example: P1G1)	PVD	peripheral vascular disease	s̄	without
pH	hydrogen ion concentration	Px	pain	Sao$_2$	oxygen saturation
PID	pelvic inflammatory disease	q	every	sec	second
PJC	premature junctional contraction	RA	rheumatoid arthritis, right atrium, room air	SICU	surgical intensive care unit
PMS	pulse, movement, sensation	RAD	reactive airway disease, right axis deviation, radial pulse	SIDS	sudden infant death syndrome
PN	pneumonia	RBB	right bundle branch block	SL	sublingual
PND	paroxysmal nocturnal dyspnea	RBC	red blood cell	SMOE	sensory, movement of extremity
po	per os (by mouth)	RCA	right circumflex artery	SOB	shortness of breath
PO	postoperative, "post op"	resp	respiration	s/p	status post
Po$_2$	partial pressure of oxygen	Rh	Rhesus blood factor, rhodium	Spo$_2$	oxygen saturation
POP	pain on palpation	RHD	rheumatic heart disease	SQETCO$_2$	semi-quantitative end-tidal CO$_2$
post	posterior	RL	Ringer's lactate	S/S	signs and symptoms
PR	per rectum; rectally	RLL	right lower lobe of the lung	ST	S-T segment elevation (relative to ECG)
PRI	P-R interval (relating to ECG)	RLQ	right lower quadrant of the abdomen	stat	immediately
PRN	pro re nata (as needed)	RN	registered nurse	STD	sexually transmitted disease
psi	pounds per square inch	R/O	rule out	Sub Q	subcutaneous
PSVT	paroxysmal supraventricular tachycardia	ROM	range of motion, rupture of membranes	sux	succinylcholine
pt	patient	ROSC	return of spontaneous circulation	SVT	supraventricular tachycardia
PT	physical therapy	RR	respiratory rate	Sx	symptoms

Continues

Table 8 Common Abbreviations*, continued

Abbreviation	Meaning	Abbreviation	Meaning	Abbreviation	Meaning
sym	symptoms	UA	urinalysis	wt	weight
synch	synchronous (switch on defibrillator)	UE	upper extremity	yo	year old
sz	seizure	UGI	upper gastrointestinal	x̄	except
TA	traffic accident	URI	upper respiratory infection	1°	first, first degree, primary
tab	tablet	USP	United States Pharmacopeia	2°	secondary, second degree
TB	tuberculosis	UTI	urinary tract infection	↑	increase(d)
TBA	to be admitted, to be announced	V	volt	↓	decrease(d)
tbsp	tablespoon	VD	venereal disease	®	right
TCA	tricyclic antidepressant	VF	ventricular fibrillation	Ⓛ	left
TCP	transcutaneous pacemaker	V fib	ventricular fibrillation	α	alpha
tech	technician, technologist	vol	volume	β	beta
temp	temperature	VS	vital signs	~	approximately
TIA	transient ischemic attack	VT	ventricular tachycardia	×2	times two
tid	three times a day	V tach	ventricular tachycardia	/	per
TKO	to keep open	w/	with	≠	not equal
TPR	temperature, pulse, respiration	WBC	white blood cell	?	questionable, possible
trans	transport	W/D/G	warm, dry, good skin	Δ	change
tsp	teaspoon	WNL	within normal limits	−	negative
Tx	treatment	w/o	without	♀	female
U/A	upon arrival	WPW	Wolff-Parkinson-White syndrome	♂	male

Sometimes abbreviations are written with periods (for example, abd. and a.c.), and sometimes different capitalization might be used and might convey a different meaning. Not all possible meanings for the abbreviations in this table are given here. Unless you are certain about the meaning, ask the person who used the abbreviation.

Table 9 Abbreviations That Lead to Errors (DO NOT USE)

Abbreviation	Intended Meaning	Possible Error; Solution	Abbreviation	Intended Meaning	Possible Error; Solution
BT	bedtime	Confused with BID (twice daily); write out	D/C	discontinue, discharge	Multiple meanings can lead to premature discontinuation or premature discharge; write out
cc	cubic centimeter	Confused with U; write mL	hs	at bedtime, half-strength	Meanings confused for each other; write out

Continues

Table 9 Abbreviations That Lead to Errors (DO NOT USE), continued

Abbreviation	Intended Meaning	Possible Error; Solution	Abbreviation	Intended Meaning	Possible Error; Solution
IJ	injection	Confused with IV; write out	U	unit	Mistaken for number "0"; write out
IU	international unit	Can be mistaken for IV; write out, or use "units"	Ø	no, not, none	Mistaken for other numbers; write out
MgSO$_4$	magnesium sulfate	Can be confused with morphine sulfate; write out	@	at	Confused with the number 2; write out
MS	morphine sulfate, magnesium sulfate, multiple sclerosis	Multiple meanings can be confusing; write out	μ	micro	Confused with "m" (milli-), causing possible overdose; use "mc"
MSO$_4$	morphine sulfate	Can be confused with magnesium sulfate; write out	/	(slash mark)	Mistaken for number "1"; write "per"
nitro drip	nitroglycerin infusion, sodium nitroprusside infusion	Confused for each other; write out	&	(and)	Mistaken for number "2"; write out
OD	overdose, once daily, right eye, optical density, outside diameter, doctor of optometry	Mistaken for each other; write out	+	(plus, and)	Mistaken for the number "4"; write out
qd	every day	Mistaken for other similar abbreviations (qh, qid, qod); write out	>	greater than	Confused with various numbers or letters (such as the number 7); write out
qh	every hour	Mistaken for other similar abbreviations (qd, qid, qod); write out	≥	greater than or equal to	Confused with various numbers or letters; write out
qid	four times a day	Mistaken for other similar abbreviations (qd, qh, qod); write out	<	less than	Confused with various numbers or letters (such as the letter L); write out
qod	every other day	Mistaken for other similar abbreviations (qd, qh, qid); write out	≤	less than or equal to	Confused with various numbers or letters; write out
SC	subcutaneous, secretory component	Mistaken for "SL"; write out	Abbreviations for drug names		Misinterpreted due to various abbreviations; write out full drug names
SQ	subcutaneous	Mistaken for "5 every"; write out	Apothecary units		Uncommon, not understood; use metric units
ss	half	Mistaken for "55"; write out	Inclusion of period after units	Example: mg.	Period mistaken for the number "1"; do not include period after units

Continues

Table 9 Abbreviations That Lead to Errors (DO NOT USE), continued

Abbreviation	Intended Meaning	Possible Error; Solution	Abbreviation	Intended Meaning	Possible Error; Solution
Lack of commas in drug dosages	Example: 100000	Number of zeros mistaken; include comma in proper location or spell out (in this example, 100,000, or 100 thousand)	Trailing zero	Example: 2.0 mg	Decimal point is missed (this example would be misinterpreted as 20 mg); write whole number only (change this example to 2 mg)
Lack of preceding zero	Example: .4 mg	Decimal point is missed (this example would be misinterpreted as 4 mg); include a zero before the decimal point (change this example to 0.4 mg)			

Data sources: Facts About the Official "Do Not Use" List. The Joint Commission. Available at http://www.jointcommission.org/assets/1/18/Official_Do%20Not%20Use_List_%206_10.pdf. Accessed April 21, 2011.
ISMP's List of Error-Prone Abbreviations, Symbols, and Dose Designations. Institute for Safe Medication Practices. Available at http://www.ismp.org/tools/errorproneabbreviations.pdf. Accessed April 21, 2011.

YOU are the Medic   SUMMARY

1. What is your first consideration in regard to this patient?

The patient is not well enough to stand up when he attempts to exit the vehicle under his own power and appears to have inadequate balance. At this point you do not know whether the patient has been drinking. The patient's behavior could be the result of medical conditions such as diabetes, an allergic reaction, or cardiac insufficiency. Trauma may also be present. The patient may have struck his head, which could be affecting his balance. He also may have something as simple as a foot injury that is painful to stand on. Slurred speech may be caused by loose teeth or dentures from the crash. Do not assume a patient has been drinking. You must obtain more information in order to make the determination.

2. What is your first consideration in regard to the scene?

The visible damage to the vehicle appears to be minor, but there may still be hazards ranging from leaking fluids to sharp, torn metal. Because of potential hazards, it is essential that all responders wear personal protective equipment to ensure their safety, even if the scene initially appears to be safe. The county courthouse would be a busy place at 1300 hours on a weekday, and you should be concerned with traffic control as well as crowd control. Ensure that a law enforcement response has been dispatched to the incident.

3. Why is it not acceptable to document the patient's appearance as "drunk" on a PCR?

Document only the facts. Do not describe the situation according to your first suspicions, such as describing the patient as "Awake

and appears drunk." Statements such as this will come back to haunt you. Perform a thorough assessment before determining whether a patient is intoxicated.

4. Would it be acceptable to document that the patient is "yelling" for the breathing description on a PCR?

The patient is obviously breathing since he is attempting to extricate himself from the vehicle. You do not have the other points of direct assessment to determine rate, rhythm, and quality. You are directly witnessing the patient yelling, which is an accurate description of your initial observation, so you could document this.

5. How should you document that the patient has directed you to "keep your hands off," as well as account for not being able to obtain the patient's vital signs?

You should use the patient's words as much as possible. It would be acceptable to write, "When attempting to approach the patient to begin an assessment, the patient stated, 'Keep your hands off of me.' We were unable to assess pulse, respiration, blood pressure, pupils, SpO_2 or skin signs other than visually until after the intervention of law enforcement." Review the chapter, *Medical, Legal, and Ethical Issues*, for information on the concepts of patient consent and refusal.

6. Does this patient have the right to refuse treatment?

The patient is exhibiting signs associated with being intoxicated. The patient told the officer that he had had a few drinks at lunch. You also saw an empty bottle of alcohol on the floor of the car.

YOU are the Medic   SUMMARY, continued

Because the patient's decision-making ability has been impaired, you should not accept a refusal request. You also need to further assess the patient's level of orientation to person, time, and place.

7. Is it important to document the interaction between the patient and law enforcement officers when there is no patient care involved?

It is essential that you document the interaction between the law enforcement officer and the patient. Usually state laws allow officers to detain people if they are a "danger to themselves or others." Please review the rights of law enforcement officers in relation to patients for your area. In this case, the officer appealed to the patient's sense of self to convince him of the better of two courses of action so detaining the patient was not necessary. When you are documenting interaction

between law enforcement personnel and a patient, make sure to document the officer's name, badge number, and agency on your form. This will help you and your agency if you should need more information on the call.

8. What is the legal basis to determine whether a patient is competent to refuse care?

All paramedics should be familiar with the laws of their state regarding the age of consent, care of minors, emancipated minors, and people with mental or cognitive impairments, such as mental illness or the effects of drug or alcohol use. Above all else, you need to ensure that every reasonable effort has been made for the patient's welfare and best interests. Do not assume the patient is "just drunk," and always provide the highest level of care.

EMS Patient Care Report (PCR)

Date: 06-01-11	**Incident No.:** 890	**Nature of Call:** MVC		**Location:** 200 First Street	
Dispatched: 1300	**En Route:** 1301	**At Scene:** 1305	**Transport:** 1335	**At Hospital:** 1345	**In Service:** 1350

Patient Information

Age: 60 **Sex:** M **Weight (in kg [lb]):** 113 kg (250 lb)	**Allergies:** No known drug allergies **Medications:** None **Past Medical History:** None **Chief Complaint:** MVC

Vital Signs

Time: 1320	**BP:** 130/80	**Pulse:** 100	**Respirations:** 16	**Spo$_2$:** 97%
Time:	**BP:**	**Pulse:**	**Respirations:**	**Spo$_2$:**
Time:	**BP:**	**Pulse:**	**Respirations:**	**Spo$_2$:**

EMS Treatment
(circle all that apply)

Oxygen @ _____ L/min via (circle one): NC NRM Bag-mask device	**Assisted Ventilation**	**Airway Adjunct**	**CPR**
Defibrillation	**Bleeding Control**	**Bandaging**	**Splinting**	**Other**

Narrative

Arrived on scene to find a single-vehicle crash involving a pole in front of the county courthouse. On exiting our unit, we witnessed a man open the driver's door of the vehicle involved in the crash and attempt to exit the vehicle without assistance. He could not keep his balance and sat back down on the driver's seat. Once we approached the vehicle, we determined that the air bag system had deployed on impact. There is minimal visible damage to the front of the vehicle. When attempting assessment of the pt's blood pressure, pulse, respiration, and Spo$_2$ level, the pt, in slurred speech, stated "I need my lawyer" and "Keep your hands off me." The pt exhibited signs associated with being intoxicated. Open empty vodka bottle was clearly visible on the floor of the vehicle. Confirmed that law enforcement was en route. Officer B.D. Smith, Badge 1345, Downtown Police Dept, and officer Jenkins, Badge 1429, also from Downtown, arrived to assist. Officer Smith was able to convince the pt to allow our assessment, treatment, immobilization, and transport without further incident. This accounts for the initial delay in obtaining vital signs on this pt. Pt was cooperative and his condition remained unchanged during transport. Primary and secondary assessment findings were normal. Radio report called in to Downtown Hospital during transport and verbal report given to Shelley RN on pt transfer. **End of report**

Prep Kit

■ Ready for Review

- For each emergency call, you must complete a formal written report before you leave the hospital. This action is a vital part of providing emergency medical care and ensuring the continuity of patient care. This information guarantees the proper transfer of responsibility, complies with the requirements of health departments and law enforcement agencies, and fulfills administrative needs.

- Your written report, or patient care report, is the only record of events that transpired during the call and serves as a legal record. It should be complete, well-written, legible, and professional.

- Your report may be used in legal proceedings against you or someone else, and is the only record of the care you provided and why.

- The Health Insurance Portability and Accountability Act of 1996 (HIPAA) was designed to protect a person's health information, but permits disclosure of patient care information when necessary for the betterment of society as a whole, such as when data are used to protect or improve public health.

- The patient care report (PCR) may be handwritten or electronically written. Either way, it will include a checklist and a narrative portion. The report should be objective, accurate, and neat; this reflects good patient care.

- If a patient refuses care, ensure that you have obtained vital signs and a complete history, fully inform the patient of the situation, involve medical control if needed, and thoroughly document the situation.

- Special situations that may require filling out different or additional forms include injuries that occur in the workplace, multiple-casualty incidents, exposure to potentially infectious diseases, cases that involve potential abuse or neglect, transfer of care to an on-scene physician, interfacility transports, calls involving controlled substances, cancelled emergency calls, and calls involving other agencies. Reporting regulations vary from state to state, and you should make yourself familiar with your state's requirements.

- There are many methods for writing the narrative in your patient care report, including chronological order, the SOAP method, the CHARTE method, and the body systems approach. Learn the method used by your system.

- The patient care report needs to be filled out in a timely manner. Be sure to fill it out directly after the call.

- If you must revise or correct your patient care report, note the date, time, and purpose for the correction. Place a single line through the error and write the correct information next to it. Write down what did or did not happen and the steps that were taken to correct the situation.

- Falsifying information on the patient care report may result in suspension and/or revocation of your certification/license.

- Inaccurate or poor documentation could lead to subsequent caregivers providing inappropriate care to the patient. It could also be detrimental for you if a lawsuit is initiated, and could negatively affect your reputation.

- Proper use of terminology is essential. Learn common medical abbreviations.

Vital Vocabulary

CHARTE method A narrative writing method that allows the narrative to be broken down into logical sections similar to the steps of the EMS assessment; components include chief complaint, history, assessment, treatment, transport, and exceptions.

Health Insurance Portability and Accountability Act (HIPAA) The law enacted in 1996 that provides for criminal sanctions as well as civil penalties for releasing a patient's protected health information (PHI) in a way not authorized by the patient.

libel Making a false statement in written form that injures a person's good name.

medical necessity A standard used by Medicare to determine whether a patient's condition requires ambulance transport in a particular situation.

minimum data set The mandatory clinical assessment standard information that must be documented on every emergency call as set by Medicare and Medicaid, and per the National Highway Traffic Safety Administration (NHTSA) for the purpose of the national data system.

objective information Information that you observe and that is measurable, such as a patient's blood pressure.

patient care report (PCR) A written record of the incident that describes the nature of the patient's injuries or illness at the scene and the treatment provided; also known as the prehospital care report.

pertinent negatives Findings that warrant no medical care or intervention, but which, by seeking them, show evidence of the thoroughness of the patient examination and history.

slander Verbally making a false statement that injures a person's good name.

SOAP method A narrative writing method in which information is organized into four categories, including subjective information, objective information, assessment, and treatment plan.

subjective information Information that is told to you, but which cannot be seen, such as the symptoms a patient describes.

Assessment in Action

You and your partner are dispatched to a local stadium where a football game is in progress. A player is unresponsive after being tackled. On arrival, your unit is directed onto the field by security. As your vehicle approaches the area where the player went down, you see numerous flashes apparently coming from cameras. A law enforcement officer walks up to your vehicle and tells you that the scene is safe and the crowds and press are under the control of law enforcement personnel. You exit the vehicle and wade into the press to get to the patient. The athletic team trainers as well as the team physician are taking care of the patient by placing him in full spinal precautions. As you bend down to the patient, a reporter sticks a microphone in front of you and asks, "Is this kid's career over?" You look over your shoulder for your partner, who is making his way toward you through the reporters.

1. During patient care activities in a chaotic environment, it is most important to maintain effective communication with:
   A. the dispatcher.
   B. law enforcement personnel.
   C. your partner.
   D. medical control.

2. What is the term used to describe documentation of a false statement that injures a person's reputation?
   A. Slander
   B. Ethics violation
   C. Verbal assault
   D. Libel

3. Which aspect of the Health Insurance Portability and Accountability Act (HIPAA) is the most important to pre-hospital care?
   A. Ensuring that patient privacy is protected
   B. Recovering patient care information from the archive
   C. Ensuring that crew privacy is protected
   D. Ensuring that all documentation is complete and accurate

4. What does the HIPAA Privacy Rule of Operations allow EMS providers access to?
   A. Insurance and billing information
   B. Patient name, birth date, address, and next of kin
   C. Patient files and records at the receiving facility
   D. Patient care required after the patient was in the care of the facility

5. Documentation of the chief complaint, vital signs, level of consciousness, patient demographics, and assessment information is referred to as the:
   A. minimum data set.
   B. maximum data set.
   C. HIPAA data set.
   D. patient care report.

6. What information is generally allowed to be disclosed without authorization to public health officials under the HIPAA Privacy Rule?
   A. Information concerning preventing or controlling disease
   B. Information concerning prevention of injuries
   C. Information concerning prevention of disability
   D. All of the above

Additional Questions

7. Referring back to the scenario, if you answered the reporter about the future of the patient's sports career, are you in violation of HIPAA?

8. How is the right of the press to cover stories balanced with HIPAA requirements for privacy?

The Human Body and Human Systems

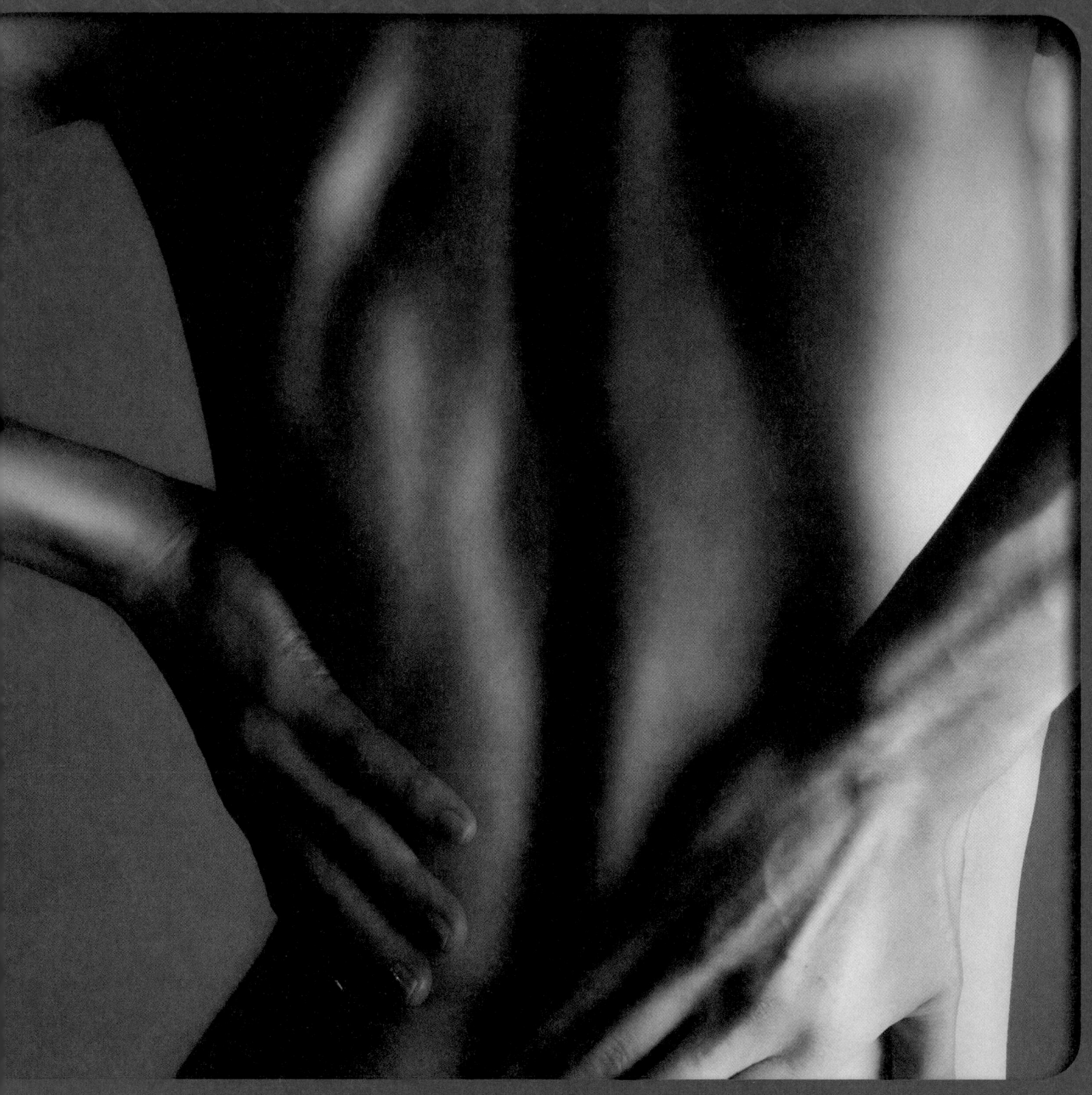

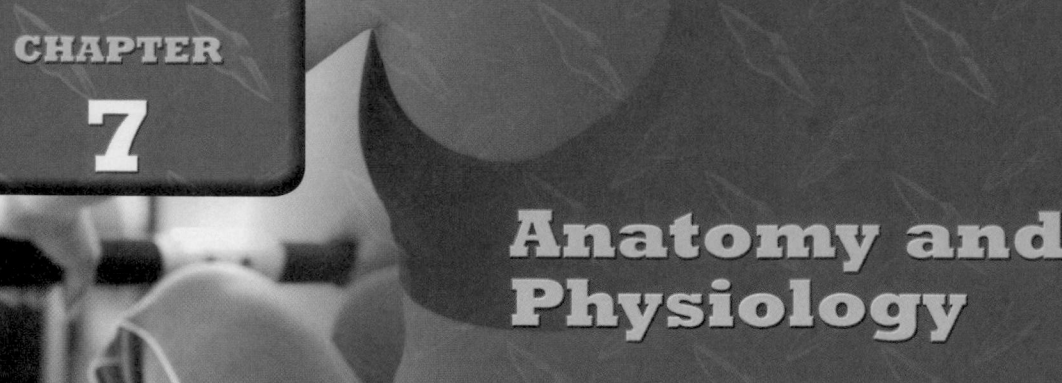

National EMS Education Standard Competencies

Anatomy and Physiology

Integrates a complex depth and comprehensive breadth of knowledge of the anatomy and physiology of all human systems.

Knowledge Objectives

1. Understand the body's topographic anatomy, including the anatomic position and the planes of the body. (p 183)

2. List the planes and sections of the body, including frontal, sagittal, midsagittal, transverse, cross section, and longitudinal. (p 183)

3. List and define terms related to specific areas of the body. (pp 183-184)

4. Explain the following directional terms: right, left, superior, inferior, lateral, medial, proximal, distal, superficial, deep, anterior (ventral), posterior (dorsal), palmar, plantar, and apex. (pp 185-186)

5. Describe movement and positional terms including abduction, adduction, hyperflexion, and hyperextension. (pp 186-187)

6. Describe the prone, supine, Trendelenburg shock, Fowler, and recovery positions of the body. (pp 187-188)

7. Describe the topography of the abdominal region, including the four abdominal quadrants and the nine abdominal regions. (pp 187-188)

8. Discuss the atomic composition of the body, including bonding and chemical reactions. (pp 188-190)

9. Discuss the chemical composition of the body, including key substances: enzymes, carbohydrates, lipids, proteins, nucleic acids, and trace elements. (pp 190-194)

10. Discuss cell structure and function as it relates to the practice of paramedicine. (pp 194-198)

11. Describe the anatomy and physiology of the cell, as well as the cellular environment. (pp 194-198)

12. Discuss cell transport mechanisms, including diffusion, osmosis, facilitated diffusion, active transport, endocytosis, and exocytosis. (pp 198-200)

13. Discuss the life cycle of a cell, including interphase, mitosis, cytokinesis, and differentiation. (pp 200-201)

14. List and describe the types of tissues found in the body: epithelial tissue, connective tissue, muscle tissue, neural tissue, and membranes. (pp 201-208)

15. Discuss the anatomy and the physiology of the skeletal system, including types of bones, embryonic skeleton maturation, bone growth and maintenance and related hormones, major subdivisions of the skeleton, components of the skeleton, and classification and types of joints. (pp 208-226)

16. Discuss the anatomy and physiology of the muscular system, including gross and microscopic anatomy, actions of muscles, contraction of skeletal muscle fiber, and major muscles of the body. (pp 226-232)

17. Discuss the anatomy and physiology of the respiratory system, including the structure and function of the nasal cavities, pharynx, larynx, speaking mechanism, trachea, bronchial tree, lungs, alveoli, and pulmonary capillaries. (pp 232-240)

18. Describe the process of gas exchange in the alveoli. (p 236)

19. Discuss the concept of respiration. (pp 236-238)

20. Discuss acid/base balance and how it relates to respiration. (pp 236-238)

21. Describe the concept of hypoxic drive. (p 237)

22. Discuss the concept of ventilation, including pulmonary volumes and diffusion of gases. (pp 238-239)

23. Explain the brainstem's role in regulating respiration. (p 238)

24. Explain how the level of carbon dioxide in the blood and the blood's pH relate to ventilation. (pp 236-240)

25. Discuss the anatomy and physiology of the circulatory system, including the composition and function of blood, the heart, and the blood vessels, as well as the blood groups. (pp 240-255)

26. Discuss the concepts of afterload, stroke volume, and cardiac output. (p 244)

27. Discuss the Frank-Starling mechanism. (p 244)

28. Discuss the anatomy and physiology of the lymphatic and immune system, including the formation of lymph, the locations and function of lymph nodes and the spleen, innate versus adaptive immunity, humoral versus cell-mediated immunity, acquired versus genetic immunity, and other mechanisms of protection including B cells, T cells, vaccinations, and flora. (pp 255-261)

29. Discuss the anatomy and physiology of the nervous system, including the central and peripheral nervous systems, as well as sensory function. (pp 261-275)

30. Describe the anatomy and physiology of the integumentary system, including function, layers of the skin, and other structures present in the skin. (pp 275-277)

31. Explain the anatomy and physiology of the digestive system, including general function, organs and structures involved in digestion, and the process of digestion. (pp 277-281)

32. Discuss the anatomy and physiology of the endocrine system, including endocrine and exocrine glands, chemistry of hormones, regulation of hormone secretion, and the roles of hormones in various processes in the body. (pp 281-286)

33. Describe the anatomy and physiology of the urinary system, including its components, general function, the process of urine formation, and the role of the kidneys in maintaining blood volume, blood pressure, pH, and electrolyte balance. (pp 286-292)

34. Explain the concept of fluid balance, as well as the purpose and mechanisms for maintaining homeostasis. (p 292)

35. Discuss the anatomy and physiology of the genital system, including the hormones and structures involved in reproduction, the menstrual cycle, spermatogenesis and oogenesis, gestational changes, and fetal circulation and respiration. (pp 292-302)

36. Discuss the relationship between nutrition, metabolism, and body temperature, including methods of heat generation and loss, fever, the role of the hypothalamus, and cellular metabolism. (pp 302-310)

Skills Objectives

There are no skills objectives for this chapter.

Introduction

Knowledge of anatomy and physiology is a fundamental portion of the education of any health care provider and is paramount for successful practice as a paramedic. In every patient encounter, you will call on your knowledge of anatomy and physiology to help you understand the patient's presentation, anticipate or understand the suspected disease process, and make a decision regarding the care you will provide. A strong foundation of anatomy and physiology is also required to help you fully understand the concepts you will learn in many other chapters of this text, including patient assessment, pharmacology, and the sections describing specific disease processes. <u>Anatomy</u> is the study of the structure and makeup of the organism. This knowledge can be divided into gross anatomy, which studies organs and their location in the body, and microscopic anatomy, which studies the tissue and cellular components that cannot be seen with the naked eye. <u>Physiology</u> is the study of the processes and functions of the body. These systems, operating simultaneously and relying on a myriad of interactions, all work to maintain a state of balance in which organs and systems can function effectively, known as <u>homeostasis</u>. Maintaining homeostasis preserves a range of temperature, acid/base balance, gas and mineral concentrations, and other conditions necessary for normal life processes to function correctly.

Adding the prefix *patho–*, meaning "disease," forms the term "pathophysiology," which is the study of how body functions change and react when the body encounters disease or when homeostasis is otherwise disturbed. See the *Pathophysiology* chapter of this text for more information.

Topographic Anatomy

The surface of the body has many definite visible features that serve as guides or landmarks to the structures that lie beneath them. You must be able to identify the superficial landmarks of the body—its <u>topographic anatomy</u>—to perform an accurate assessment.

To accomplish this, the terms that are used to describe the topographic anatomy are applied to the body when it is in the <u>anatomic position</u>. This is a position of reference in which the patient stands facing you, arms at the side, with the palms of the hands forward. The anatomic position is used as a common starting point so that everyone is referring to the body in the same way. For example, you are looking at a person who reports pain in his arm. Which left or right do you use? To be consistent, health care providers use the patient's left and right as the reference point.

The Planes of the Body

The anatomic planes of the body are imaginary straight lines that divide the body Figure 1 . There are three main axes of the body depending on how it is sliced. Slicing the body so that you have a front and back portion creates the frontal or <u>coronal plane</u>. If the body is sliced so the result is a top and bottom portion, this is referred to as the <u>transverse (axial) plane</u>. If the body is sliced so that you have a left and right portion, a <u>sagittal (lateral) plane</u> is formed.

The <u>midsagittal plane (midline)</u> is a special type of sagittal plane where the body is cut in half, leaving equal left and right halves. Your nose and navel are found along this imaginary line. A <u>cross section</u> is the product of slicing an object across or perpendicular to its long axis, as you would do if you wanted to count the rings in a tree trunk. A <u>longitudinal section</u>, in contrast, is a view of an object cut along its long axis.

These planes help you to identify the location of internal structures and understand the relationships between and among the organs Table 1 .

Specific Areas of the Body

In addition to using planes and topographic landmarks, many body areas are given specific names that are important to learn. Becoming familiar with these names will not only help you communicate with other professionals, but will also help in breaking down other names, because many of these terms are used as root words. For example, "sternocleidomastoid" is a combination of *sterno–*, *cleido–*, and *–mastoid*, which refer to the sternum,

YOU *are the Medic* PART 1

You and your partner are dispatched to a motor vehicle crash on a major roadway. Prior to entering the scene, you and your partner don protective gear and reflective safety vests. You assess the scene as safe and approach a single passenger car that had frontal impact with a concrete bridge support. The patient has been removed from the vehicle prior to your arrival by six bystanders who feared the vehicle would start on fire. Your patient is positioned face up on the pavement and appears to be unresponsive. Five of the bystanders are walking around the damaged vehicle and one is trying to place an item under the patient's head to make him more comfortable.

1. Since the patient has been removed from the vehicle, how can you assess the mechanism of injury?

2. After scene safety and protection of yourself and your partner, what is your first concern?

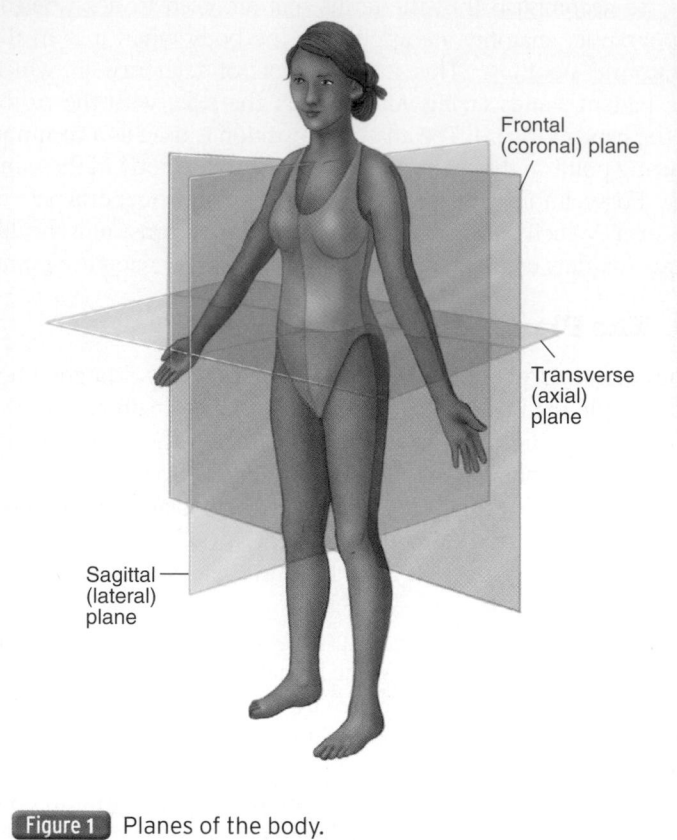

Frontal
(coronal) plane

Transverse
(axial)
plane

Sagittal
(lateral)
plane

Figure 1   Planes of the body.

Table 1   Planes of the Body

Plane of the Body	Description
Coronal	Front and back
Transverse	Top and bottom
Sagittal	Left and right
Midsagittal (midline)	Left and right–equal halves

Words of Wisdom

When a patient experiences an injury, the anatomic planes, body surfaces, and imaginary lines are often used by the paramedic to describe the location of the injury.

clavicle, and mastoid process, respectively. By understanding those roots, you will be able to locate the origin and insertion of this large neck muscle.

The remainder of the body is classified into regions that clinically describe them. The most common body regions are described in **Table 2**.

Table 2   Terminology Related to Specific Areas of the Body

Term	Definition
Axillary	pertaining to the armpit
Brachial	pertaining to the upper arm
Buccal	pertaining to the cheek
Cardiac	pertaining to the heart
Cervical	pertaining to the neck
Cranial	pertaining to the skull or cranium
Cutaneous	pertaining to the skin
Deltoid	pertaining to the shoulder muscle
Femoral	pertaining to the thigh
Gastric	pertaining to the stomach
Gluteal	pertaining to the buttocks
Hepatic	pertaining to the liver
Inguinal	pertaining to the groin (depressions of abdominal wall near thighs)
Lumbar	pertaining to the loin (lower back, between ribs and pelvis)
Mammary	pertaining to the breast
Nasal	pertaining to the nose
Occipital	pertaining to the inferior posterior region of the head
Orbital	pertaining to the bones surrounding the eye
Parietal	pertaining to the superior posterior region of the head
Patellar	pertaining to the front of the knee (kneecap)
Pectoral	pertaining to the chest
Perineal	pertaining to the perineum; between the sacrum and pubis
Plantar	pertaining to the sole of the foot
Popliteal	pertaining to the posterior knee
Pulmonary	pertaining to the lungs
Renal	pertaining to the kidneys
Sacral	pertaining to the inferior most portion of the spine
Temporal	pertaining to temples of the skull
Umbilical	pertaining to the navel
Volar	pertaining to the sole of the foot or palm of the hand

■ Directional Terms

Directional terms used in the study of anatomy include words that describe relative positions of body parts as well as imaginary anatomical divisions. When you are discussing where an injury is located or how a pain radiates in the body, you need to know the correct directional terms Figure 2 . Table 3 provides the basic terms used in medicine. Notice how directional terms are paired as "opposites."

Right and Left

The terms "right" and "left" refer to the patient's right and left sides, not to your right and left sides.

Superior and Inferior

The superior part of the body, or any body part, is the portion nearer to the head from a specific reference point. The part

Table 3   Common Directional Terms

Common Term	Directional Term	Definition
Right and left	Right	The patient's right
	Left	The patient's left
Top and bottom	Superior	Closest to the head
	Inferior	Closest to the feet
Middle and side	Medial	Closest to the midline
	Lateral	Farthest from the midline
Closest and farthest	Proximal	Closest to the point of attachment
	Distal	Farthest from the point of attachment
In and out	Superficial	Closest to the surface of the skin
	Deep	Farthest from the surface of the skin
Front and back	Anterior (ventral)	The front surface of the body
	Posterior (dorsal)	The back surface of the patient

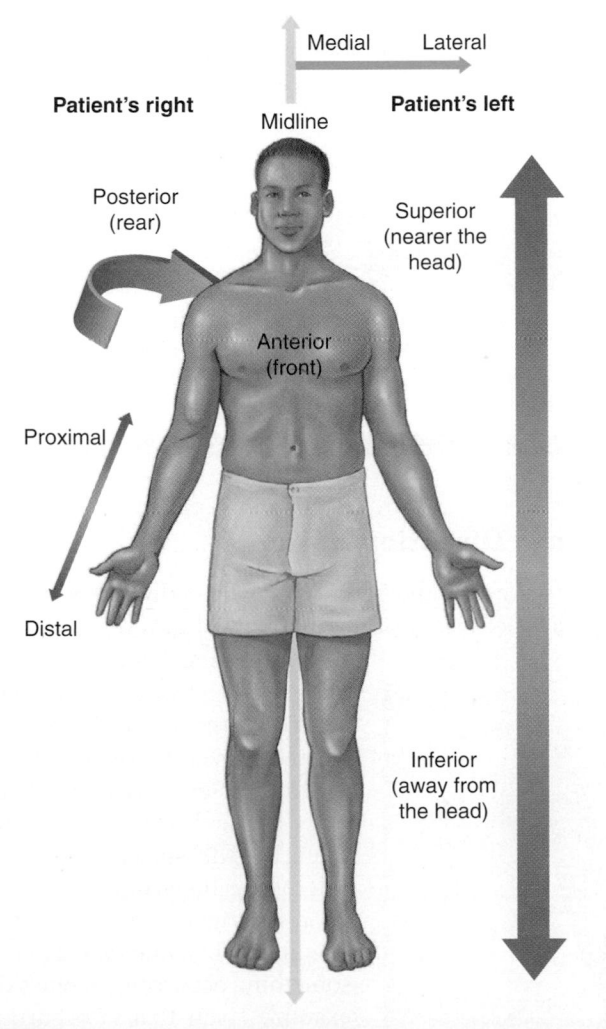

Figure 2   Directional terms indicate distance and direction from the midline.

nearer to the feet is the inferior portion. These terms are also used to describe the relationship of one structure to another. For example, the knee is superior to the foot and inferior to the pelvis.

Lateral and Medial

Parts of the body that lie farther from the midline are called lateral (outer) structures. The parts that lie closer to the midline are called medial (inner) structures. For example, the knee has medial (inner) and lateral (outer) aspects (surfaces).

Proximal and Distal

The terms "proximal" and "distal" are used to describe the relationship of any two structures on an extremity. Proximal describes structures that are closer to the trunk. Distal describes structures that are farther from the trunk or nearer to the free end of the extremity. For example, the elbow is distal to the shoulder and proximal to the wrist and hand.

Superficial and Deep

Superficial means closer to or on the skin. Deep means farther inside the body and away from the skin.

Anterior and Posterior

Anterior refers to the belly side of the body. Another term for anterior is ventral. Posterior refers to the spinal side of the body, including the back of the hand. Another term for posterior is dorsal. The terms anterior and posterior are more commonly used than the terms ventral and dorsal.

Palmar and Plantar

The front region of the hand is referred to as the palm or **palmar** surface. The bottom of the foot is referred to as the **plantar** surface.

Apex

The **apex** (the plural is apices) is the tip of a structure. For example, the apex of the heart is the bottom (inferior portion) of the ventricles in the left side of the chest.

■ Movement and Positional Terms

All movements of the body, from the simplest grasp to the most complicated ballet maneuver, can be broken down into a series of simple components and described with specific terms. As with the terms for anatomic positions, an accepted set of terms describes body movements. These are particularly useful in describing how an injury occurred.

Range of motion is the full distance that a joint can be moved. In the anatomic position, moving a distal point of an extremity toward the trunk is usually called flexion. **Flexion** of the elbow brings the hand closer to the shoulder, flexion of the knee brings the foot up to the buttocks, and flexion of the fingers forms the hand into a fist. In certain cases, specific terms are used to clarify the movement, such as in the foot. Dorsiflexion is movement of the foot toward the dorsal aspect, while plantar flexion describes movement toward the sole. **Extension** is the motion associated with the return of a body part from a flexed position to the anatomic position. In the anatomic position, all extremities are in extension. **Abduction** of an extremity moves it away from the midline. **Adduction** moves the extremity toward the midline **Figure 3**. A patient's neck can be in one of several positions when the patient is found in the supine position **Figure 4**.

The prefix *hyper* often is added to the terms flexion or extension to indicate a mechanism of injury. "Hyper" implies that the normal range of motion for the particular movement was maximized or even exceeded, potentially resulting in injury. This prefix is used commonly in clinical literature, as well as in written and verbal communication among health care providers. The term **hyperflexion** refers to a body part that was flexed to the maximum level or even beyond the normal range of motion. **Hyperextension** refers to a body part that was extended to the maximum level or even beyond the normal range of motion. A hyperextension injury occurs when a person falls on an outstretched hand, resulting in a distal radius fracture **Figure 5**. A hyperflexion injury to the back can occur while bending. Wrist injuries can also be described using the terms **supination** and **pronation**. Turning the palms upward (toward the sky) constitutes supination of the forearm. Turning the palms downward (toward the ground) is described as pronation of the forearm.

Internal rotation describes turning the anterior portion of an extremity toward the midline. The lower extremity is internally rotated when the toes are turned inward. **External rotation** describes turning an extremity away from the midline. Often, when you are comparing an injured extremity with the uninjured extremity, you will note rotational deformities. A hip can be dislocated anteriorly or posteriorly. In an anterior hip dislocation, the foot is externally rotated and the head of the femur is palpable in the inguinal area (the lower lateral regions of the abdomen and the groin). In the more common posterior hip dislocation, the knee and foot usually are flexed and internally rotated. The term rotation also can be applied to the spine. The spine is rotated when it twists on its axis. Placing the chin on the shoulder rotates the cervical spine.

Words of Wisdom

Using the correct anatomic terminology in your patient care report (PCR) improves patient care by making the report more useful to hospital personnel and enhances your professional image as a paramedic.

■ Other Directional Terms

Many structures of the body occur bilaterally. A body part that appears on both sides of the midline is **bilateral**. For example, the eyes, ears, hands, and feet are bilateral structures. This is also true for structures inside the body, such as the lungs and kidneys. Structures that appear on only one side of the body are said to be **unilateral**. For example, the spleen is on the left side of the body only, and the liver is on the right side. The terms unilateral and bilateral can also refer to something occurring on one side; for example, pain that is occurring on only one side of the body could be called unilateral pain.

As part of the assessment process, you will palpate the abdomen and report your findings. Therefore,

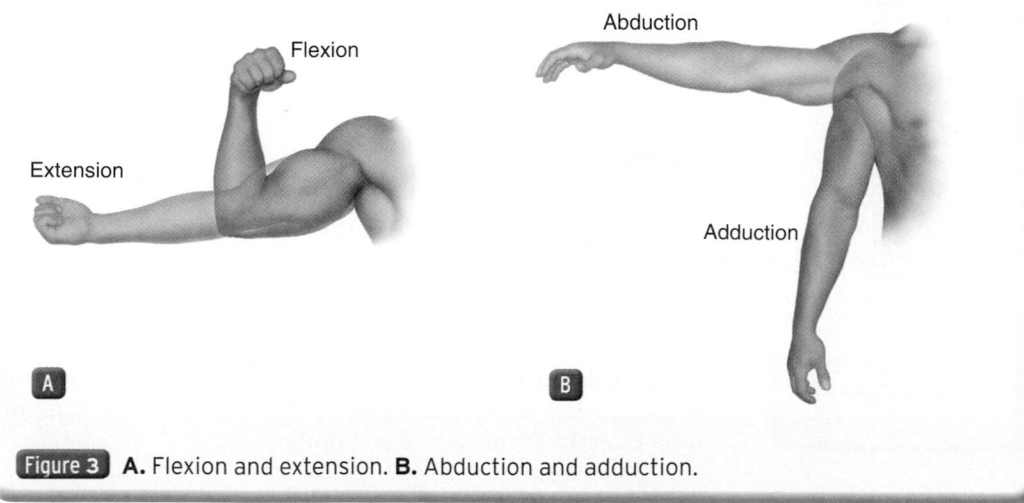

Figure 3 **A.** Flexion and extension. **B.** Abduction and adduction.

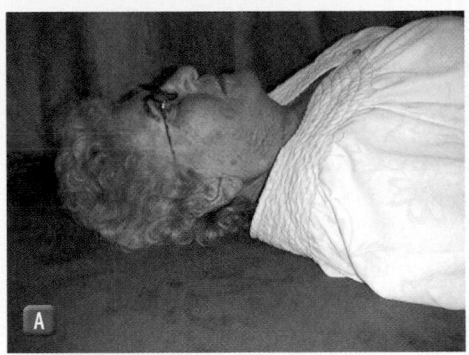 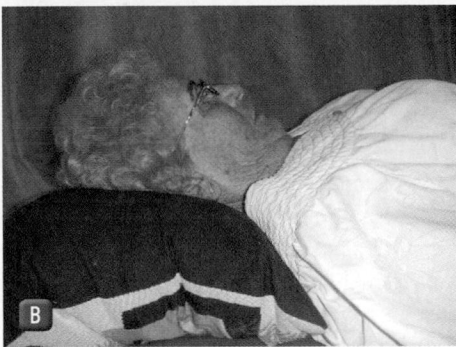 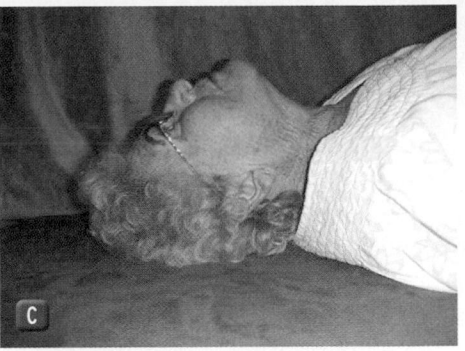

Figure 4 Positions of the neck in a patient found in a supine position. **A.** Neutral. **B.** Flexed. **C.** Extended.

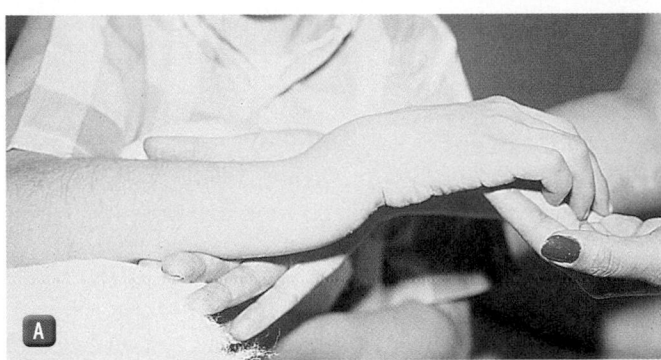

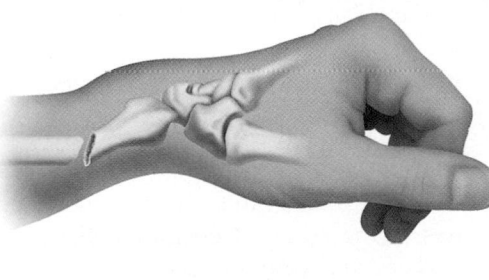

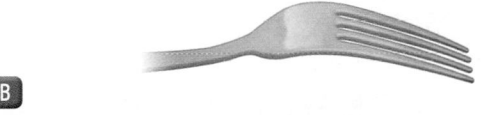

Figure 5 **A.** Exceeding the range of motion of an extremity can result in a fracture. **B.** Fractures of the distal radius produce a characteristic silver fork deformity and can result from hyperextension at the wrist secondary to falling on an outstretched hand.

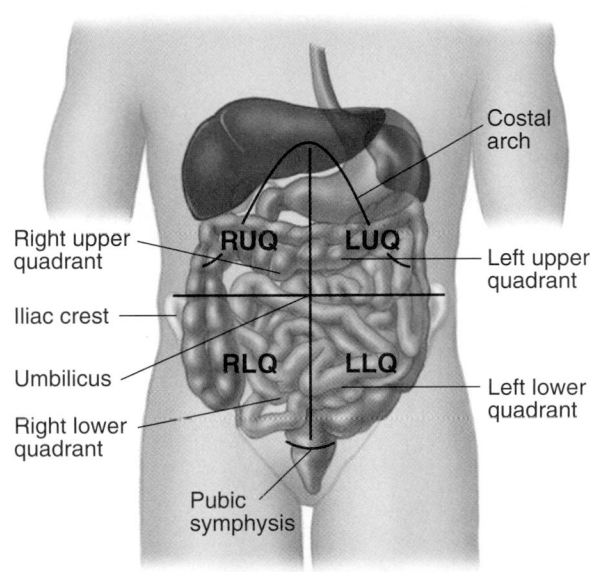

Figure 6 The abdomen is divided into four quadrants. RUQ indicates right upper quadrant; LUQ, left upper quadrant; RLQ, right lower quadrant; and LLQ, left lower quadrant.

it is important that you are able to describe the exact location of areas of the abdomen. The way to describe the sections of the abdominal cavity is by **quadrants**. Imagine two lines intersecting at the umbilicus, dividing the abdomen into four equal areas Figure 6. These are referred to as the right upper quadrant, left upper quadrant, right lower quadrant, and left lower quadrant. Remember that here, too, right and left refer to the patient's right and left, not yours. Pain or injury in a given

quadrant usually arises from or involves the organs that lie in that quadrant.

The abdomen can also be divided into nine regions for assessment Figure 7.

It is important for you to learn all of these terms and concepts so that you can describe the location of any injury or assessment findings. When you use these terms properly, any other medical personnel who care for the patient will know immediately where to look and what to expect.

Anatomic Positions

You will use these terms to describe the position of the patient as you find him or her or when you are ready to transport the patient to the emergency department Figure 8.

Prone and Supine

The terms prone and supine describe the position of the body. The body is in the **prone** position when lying face down; the body is in the **supine** position when lying face up.

Trendelenburg Position

The **Trendelenburg position** was named after a German surgeon, Friedrich Trendelenburg, at the turn of the 20th century. Dr Trendelenburg frequently placed his patients in a supine position on an incline with their feet higher than their head to keep blood in the core of the body. The Trendelenburg position is a position in which the patient is on a backboard or stretcher with the feet 6″ to 12″ higher than the head.

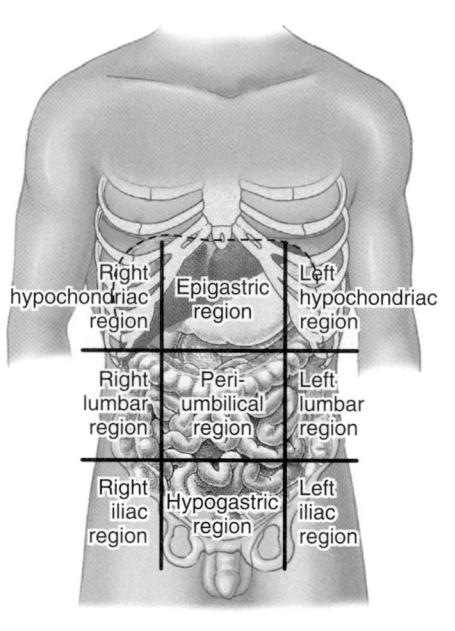

 Figure 7 Abdominal regions.

Shock Position

In the **shock position**, or modified Trendelenburg position, the head and **torso** (the trunk without the head and limbs) are supine, and the lower extremities are elevated 6″ to 12″ to help increase blood flow to the brain. The chapter, *Bleeding*, discusses body positioning and treatment of shock in more depth.

Relative contraindications to the shock position include the following:

- Pelvic fracture or significant lower extremity injury
- Severe chest injury
- Severe head injury

Fowler Position

The **Fowler position** was named after a US surgeon, George R. Fowler, MD, at the end of the 19th century. Dr Fowler placed his patients in a semireclining position with the head elevated to help them breathe easier and to control the airway. A patient who is sitting up with the knees bent or straight is therefore said to be in the Fowler position.

Recovery Position

The recovery position is used to help maintain a clear airway in an unresponsive patient. In this position, the patient is lying on his or her left side and the bottom arm is extended straight with the head lying on it. The top knee is bent, angling the patient's body slightly toward the floor. This position is also referred to as the left lateral recumbent position. This position helps prevent the aspiration of vomitus and is discussed in more detail in the chapter, *Airway Management and Ventilation*.

▪ Atoms, Molecules, and Chemical Bonds

The composition of matter and changes in its composition are the focuses of the study of chemistry. If you understand the basics of chemistry, your understanding of anatomy and

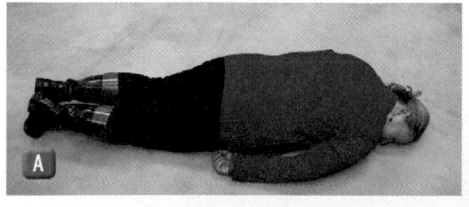
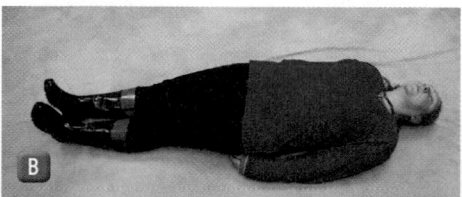
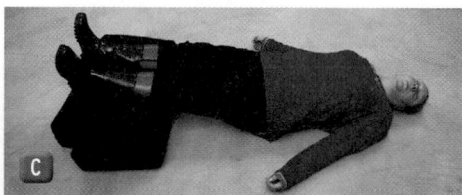
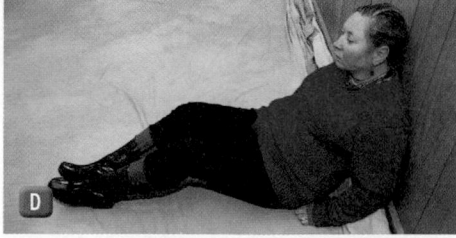
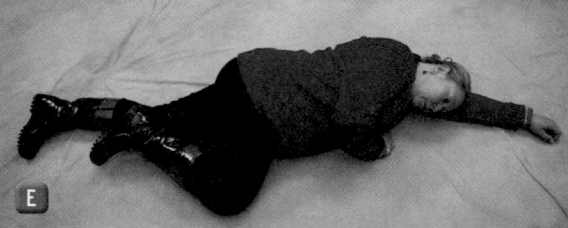

Figure 8 Anatomic positions. **A.** Prone. **B.** Supine. **C.** Modified Trendelenburg position. **D.** Fowler position. **E.** Recovery position.

physiology will be improved. Chemical changes within cells influence body functions and the status of the body's structures. Chemicals of the body include water, proteins, carbohydrates, lipids, nucleic acids, and salts, as well as foods, drinks, and medications.

Matter is defined as anything that takes up space and has mass. Mass is a physical property that determines an object's weight, based on the earth's gravitational pull. Matter includes liquids, gases, and solids both inside and outside of the human body. Elements are fundamental substances that compose matter. Copper, iron, gold, silver, aluminum, carbon, hydrogen, and oxygen are all examples of elements. Most living organisms need about 20 elements to survive. Table 4 lists the major and trace elements required by the human body.

Atoms are tiny particles that compose elements. Atoms are the smallest complete units of an element, and vary in size, weight, and interaction with other atoms. The characteristics of living and nonliving objects result from the atoms that they contain, as well as how those atoms combine and interact. Thus, by forming chemical bonds, atoms can combine with other atoms that are not similar to them.

Table 4 Elements of the Human Body

Major Elements (totaling 99.9%)	Percentage in the Body
Oxygen (O)	65%
Carbon (C)	18.5%
Hydrogen (H)	9.5%
Nitrogen (N)	3.2%
Calcium (Ca)	1.5%
Phosphorus (P)	1%
Potassium (K)	0.4%
Sulfur (S)	0.3%
Chlorine (Cl)	0.2%
Sodium (Na)	0.2%
Magnesium (Mg)	0.1%
Trace Elements (totaling 0.1%)	
Chromium (Cr)	–
Cobalt (Co)	–
Copper (Cu)	–
Fluorine (F)	–
Iodine (I)	–
Iron (Fe)	–
Manganese (Mn)	–
Zinc (Zn)	–

Atomic Structure

Atoms are composed of subatomic particles. Each atom consists of protons, neutrons, and electrons. Protons and neutrons are similar in size and mass; however, protons bear a positive electrical charge whereas neutrons are electrically neutral (uncharged). Electrons bear a negative electrical charge. An atom's mass is determined mostly by the number of protons and neutrons in its nucleus. The mass of a larger object, such as the human body, is the sum of the masses of all of its atoms.

Electrons orbit an atom's nucleus at high speed, forming a spherical electron cloud. Atoms normally contain equal numbers of protons and electrons. The number of protons in an atom is known as its atomic number. Thus, hydrogen (H), the simplest atom, has one proton, giving it the atomic number 1, while magnesium, with 12 protons, has the atomic number 12.

The atomic weight of an element's atom equals the number of protons and neutrons in its nucleus. For example, oxygen has eight protons and eight neutrons, so its atomic weight is 16. An isotope is defined as when an element's atoms have nuclei containing the same number of protons, but different numbers of neutrons. Isotopes may or may not be radioactive. Radioactivity is the emission of energetic particles known as radiation, which occurs because of instability of the atomic nuclei.

The nuclei of certain isotopes (radioisotopes) spontaneously emit subatomic particles or radiation in measurable amounts. The process of emitting radiation is called radioactive decay. Strong radioactive isotopes are dangerous because their emissions can destroy molecules, cells, and living tissue. For diagnostic procedures, weaker radioactive isotopes are used to diagnose structural and functional characteristics of internal organs. Radiation is basically identified as one of three common forms: alpha (α), beta (β), or gamma (γ). Gamma radiation is the most penetrating type, and is similar to X-ray radiation.

Molecules

The term molecule is defined as any chemical structure that consists of atoms held together by covalent bonds (involving the sharing of electrons between atoms). When two atoms that are of the same element bond, they produce molecules of that element, such as hydrogen, oxygen, or nitrogen molecules.

Chemical Bonds

Atoms can bond with other atoms by using chemical bonds that result from interactions between their electrons. During this process, the atoms may gain, lose, or share electrons. Chemically inactive atoms are known as *inert* atoms. An example of a chemical that is made up of inert atoms is helium. Atoms that either gain or lose electrons are called ions. These atoms are electrically charged. An example of an electrically charged atom, or ion, is sodium (Na).

Ionic Bonds

Ionic bonds form between ions. Ions with a positive charge (+) are called cations, and those with a negative charge (−) are called anions. Oppositely charged ions attract each other to form an ionic bond. This is a chemical bond that forms arrays (indiscreet molecules) such as crystals. An example is when sodium forms an ionic bond with chloride to create sodium chloride (table salt).

Covalent Bonds

Some atoms can complete their outer electron shells by sharing electrons to create a <u>covalent bond</u>. They do not gain or lose electrons. In a covalent bond, each atom achieves a stable form. An example of a covalent bond is when two hydrogen atoms bond to form a hydrogen molecule Figure 9 .

If a single pair of electrons is shared, the result is a single covalent bond. If two pairs are shared, the result is a double covalent bond. Some atoms can even form triple covalent bonds. Some covalent bonds do not share electrons equally, resulting in a polar molecule—one that has an uneven distribution of charges. Polar molecules have equal numbers of protons and electrons, but one end of the molecule is slightly negative while the other end is slightly positive. An example of a polar molecule is water, created by hydrogen and oxygen atoms.

When the positive hydrogen end of a polar molecule is attracted to the negative nitrogen or oxygen end of another polar molecule, the attraction is called a <u>hydrogen bond</u>. These bonds are weak at body temperature, and may change form, from water to ice and back again. Hydrogen bonds are important in protein and nucleic acid structure, forming between polar regions of different parts of a single, large molecule.

Molecules made up of different bonded atoms are called <u>compounds</u>. Examples of compounds include water (a compound of hydrogen and oxygen), table sugar, baking soda, alcohol as used in beverages, natural gas, and most medicinal drugs. A molecule of a compound has specific types and amounts of atoms. For example, water consists of two hydrogen atoms and one oxygen atom. When two hydrogen atoms bind with two oxygen atoms, they form hydrogen peroxide instead of water.

The numbers and types of atoms in a molecule are represented by a molecular formula. The molecular formula for water is H_2O, signifying the two atoms of hydrogen and the one atom of oxygen. Structural formulas are used to signify how atoms are joined and arranged inside molecules. Single bonds are represented by single lines, and double bonds are represented by double lines. When structural formulas are represented in three-dimensional models, different colors are used to show different types of atoms.

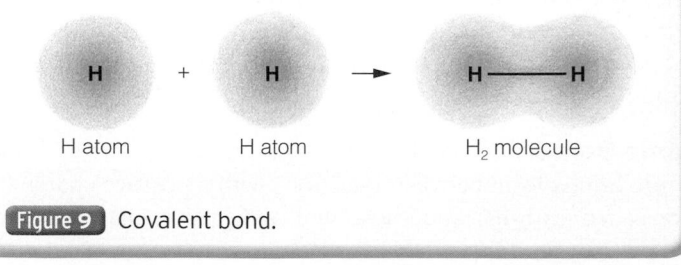

H atom   H atom H_2 molecule

Figure 9 Covalent bond.

Types of Chemical Reactions

Four types of chemical reactions are important to the study of physiology: synthesis reactions, decomposition reactions, exchange reactions, and reversible reactions.

Synthesis Reactions

Chemical reactions change the bonds between atoms, molecules, and ions to generate new chemical combinations. <u>Synthesis reaction</u> occurs when two or more reactants (atoms) bond to form a more complex product or structure. The formation of water from hydrogen and oxygen molecules is a synthesis reaction. Synthesis always involves the formation of new chemical bonds, whether the reactants are atoms or molecules. Synthesis requires energy, and it is important for growth and the repair of tissues.

Synthesis is symbolized as follows:

$$A + B \rightarrow AB$$

Decomposition Reactions

<u>Decomposition reaction</u> is a reaction that occurs when bonds within a reactant molecule break, forming simpler atoms, molecules, or ions. For example, a typical meal contains molecules of sugars, proteins, and fats that are too large and too complex to be absorbed and used by the body. Decomposition reactions in the digestive tract break these molecules down into smaller fragments before absorption begins.

Decomposition is symbolized as follows:

$$AB \rightarrow A + B$$

Exchange Reactions

In an <u>exchange reaction</u>, parts of the reacting molecules are shuffled around to produce new products. An example of an exchange reaction is the reaction of an acid with a base, which forms water and a salt.

Exchange reactions are symbolized as follows:

$$AB + CD \rightarrow AD + CB$$

Reversible Reactions

A <u>reversible reaction</u> is one wherein the products of the reaction can change back into the reactants they originally were. These reactions can proceed in opposite directions, depending on the relative proportions of reactants and products, as well as how much energy is available.

So, if $A + B \rightleftarrows AB$, then $AB \rightleftarrows A + B$. Many important biologic reactions are freely reversible.

Enzymes

<u>Enzymes</u> promote chemical reactions by lowering the activation energy requirements. Activation energy is the energy that must be overcome in order for a chemical reaction to occur.

Therefore, enzymes make chemical reactions possible. Enzymes belong to a class of substances called catalysts (compounds that accelerate chemical reactions without themselves being permanently changed or consumed). A cell makes an enzyme molecule to promote a specific reaction. Enzymatic reactions, which are reversible, can be written as:

$$\text{A} + \text{B} \overset{\text{enzyme}}{\rightleftarrows} \text{AB}$$

Acids, Bases, and the pH Scale

Electrolytes are substances that release ions in water. When they dissolve in water, the negative and positive ends of water molecules cause ions to separate and interact with water molecules instead of each other. The resulting solution contains electrically charged particles (ions) that will conduct electricity. Acids are electrolytes that release hydrogen ions in water. An example of an acid is hydrochloric acid, made up of hydrogen and chloride ions. Bases are electrolytes that release ions that bond with hydrogen ions. An example of a base is sodium hydroxide, made up of sodium, oxygen, and hydrogen ions. In body fluids, the concentrations of hydrogen and hydroxide ions greatly affect chemical reactions. These reactions control certain physiologic functions such as blood pressure and breathing rates.

Hydrogen ion concentrations can be measured by a value called pH. The hydrogen ion concentration in body fluids is vital. It is expressed in a type of mathematical shorthand based on concentrations calculated in moles per liter (with a mole representing an amount of solute in a solution). The pH of a solution is defined as the level of acidity or alkalinity. The pH scale ranges from 0 to 14, with 7 being the midpoint (meaning it has equal numbers of hydrogen and hydroxide ions). Pure water has a pH of 7, and this midpoint is considered to be neutral (neither acidic nor alkalinic). Measurements of less than 7 pH are considered acidic, meaning that there are more hydrogen ions than hydroxide ions. Measurements of more than 7 pH are considered basic, also known as alkaline, meaning that there are more hydroxide ions than hydrogen ions.

The pH of blood usually ranges from 7.35 to 7.45. Abnormal fluctuations in pH can damage cells and tissues, change the shapes of proteins, and alter cellular functions. Acidosis is an abnormal physiologic state caused by blood pH that is lower than 7.35. If pH falls below 7, coma may occur. Alkalosis results from blood pH that is higher than 7.45. If pH rises above 7.8, it generally causes uncontrollable and sustained skeletal muscle contractions.

Chemicals that resist pH changes are called buffers. They combine with hydrogen ions when these ions are excessive and contribute hydrogen ions when these ions are reduced. Figure 10 shows the pH values of acids and bases.

Chemical Constituents of Cells

Chemicals can basically be divided into two main groups: organic and inorganic. Organic chemicals are those that always contain the elements carbon and hydrogen, and generally oxygen as well. Inorganic chemicals are any chemicals that do not. Inorganic substances release ions in water and are also called electrolytes. Though many organic substances also dissolve in water, they dissolve to greater effect in alcohol or ether. Organic substances that dissolve in water usually do not release ions and are known as nonelectrolytes.

Inorganic Substances

Inorganic substances in body cells include oxygen, carbon dioxide, compounds that are known as salts, and water. The most abundant compound in the human body is water, accounting for nearly two thirds of body weight. Any substance that dissolves in water is called a solute. Because solutes dissolved in water are more likely to react with each other as they break down into smaller particles, most metabolic reactions occur in water. In the blood, the watery (aqueous) portion carries vital substances such as oxygen, salts, sugars, and vitamins among the digestive tract, respiratory tract, and the cells.

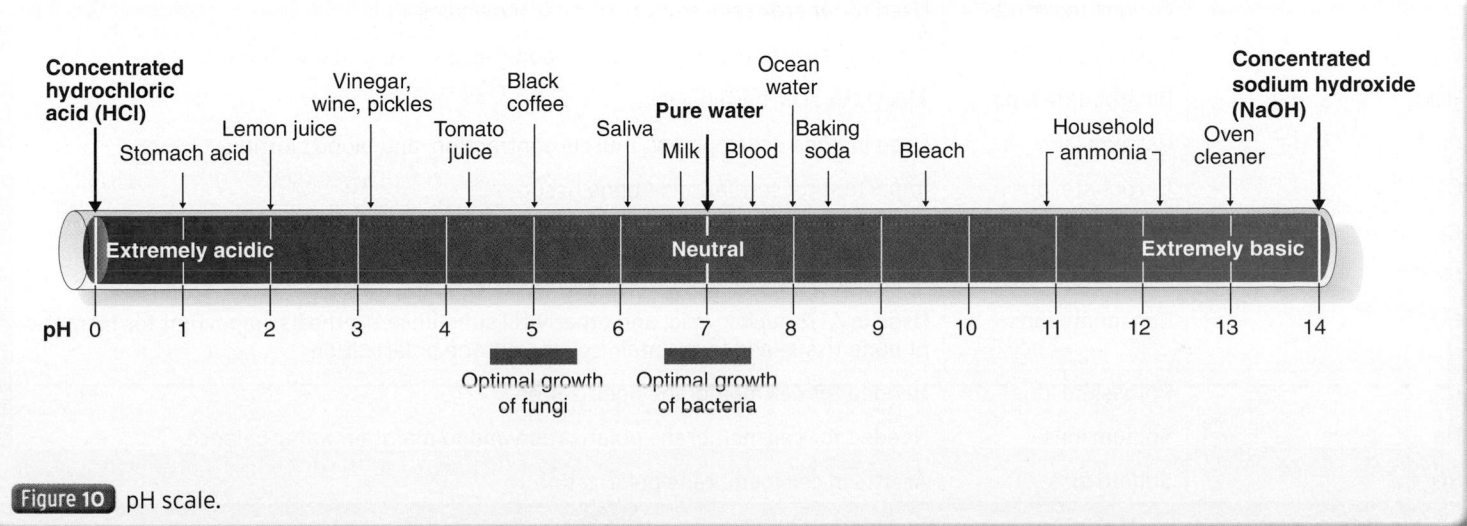

Figure 10 pH scale.

Oxygen enters the body through the respiratory organs and is transported in the blood. The red blood cells bind and carry the largest amount of oxygen. Organelles inside the cells use oxygen for energy release from nutrients such as glucose (sugar) to drive cellular metabolic activities. Carbon dioxide is an inorganic compound produced as a waste product when some metabolic processes release energy. It is exhaled via the lungs.

Salts are compounds of oppositely charged ions that are abundant in tissues in fluids. Many ions required by the body are supplied in salts, including sodium, chloride, calcium, magnesium, phosphate, carbonate, bicarbonate, potassium, and sulfate. Salt ions are important for transporting substances to and from the cells, as well as for muscle contractions and nerve impulse conduction. Common inorganic molecules are summarized in Table 5.

Organic Substances

Organic substances include carbohydrates, lipids, proteins, and nucleic acids. Many organic molecules are made up of long chains of carbon atoms linked by covalent bonds. The carbon atoms usually form additional covalent bonds with hydrogen or oxygen atoms and, less commonly, covalent bonds with nitrogen, phosphorus, sulfur, or other elements.

Carbohydrates

Carbohydrates provide much of the energy required by the body's cells, as well as help to build cell structures. Carbohydrate molecules consist of carbon, hydrogen, and oxygen molecules. The carbon atoms they contain join in chains that vary with the type of carbohydrate. Carbohydrates with shorter chains are called sugars.

Simple sugars have 6 carbon atoms, 12 hydrogen atoms, and 6 oxygen atoms ($C_6H_{12}O_6$). They are also known as mono-saccharides. Simple sugars include glucose, fructose, galactose, ribose, and deoxyribose. Ribose and deoxyribose differ from the others in that they each contain five atoms of carbon. Complex carbohydrates include sucrose (table sugar) and lactose (milk sugar). Some of these carbohydrates are double sugars or disaccharides. Adding more sugar chains creates an oligosaccharide. Other types of complex carbohydrates contain many simple joined sugar units, such as plant starch, and are known as polysaccharides. Some polysaccharides cannot be broken down for nutrition in humans but play important roles in digestion as they pass through the gastrointestinal tract. For example, cellulose is a polysaccharide that makes up plant cell walls but is indigestible to humans. Humans and other animals synthesize a polysaccharide called glycogen Figure 11, sometimes known as animal starch, to store energy for later use. Understanding the function of this compound will enable you to better comprehend what processes are occurring in diabetic emergencies.

Lipids

Lipids are not soluble in water. They may dissolve in other lipids, oils, ether, chloroform, or alcohol. Lipids include a variety of compounds with vital cell functions. These compounds include fats, phospholipids, and steroids. Fats are the most common type of lipids. Like carbohydrates, fat molecules also contain carbon, hydrogen, and oxygen, but they have far fewer oxygen atoms than do carbohydrates.

Fatty acids and glycerol are the building blocks of fat molecules. A single fat molecule consists of one glycerol molecule bonded to three fatty acid molecules. These fat molecules are known as triglycerides, a subcategory of lipids that includes

Table 5 Inorganic Substances in Cells

Formula or Symbol	Molecule or Ion	Function
H_2O	Water molecule	Major component of body fluids, biochemical reactions, chemical transport, and temperature regulation
O_2	Oxygen molecule	Used for energy release from glucose molecules
CO_2	Carbon dioxide	Metabolic waste product; forms carbonic acid via reaction with water
HCO_3^-	Bicarbonate ions	Assists in acid-base balance
Ca^{+2}	Calcium ions	Used in bone development, muscle contraction, and blood clotting
CO_3^{-2}	Carbonate ions	Important for formation of bone tissue
Cl^-	Chloride ions	Assists in maintaining water balance
Mg^{+2}	Magnesium ions	Important for formation of bone tissue and certain metabolic processes
PO_4^{-3}	Phosphate ions	Used in ATP, nucleic acid, and other vital substance synthesis; important for formation of bone tissue and to maintain cell membrane polarization
K^+	Potassium ions	Needed for cell membrane polarization
Na^+	Sodium ions	Needed for cell membrane polarization and to maintain water balance
SO_4^{-2}	Sulfate ions	Assists in cell membrane polarization

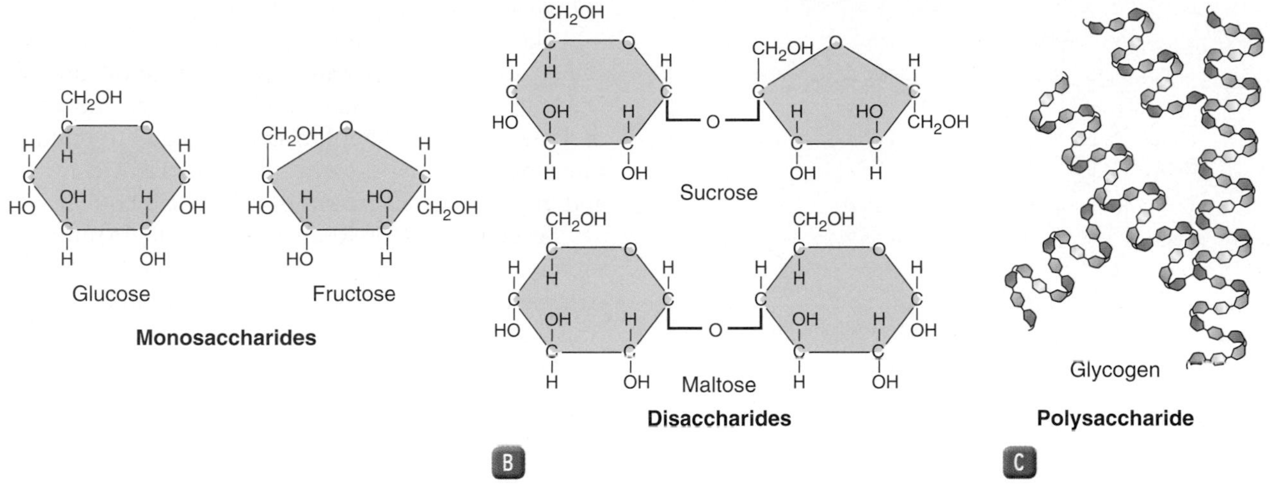

Glucose   Fructose

Monosaccharides

Sucrose

Maltose

Disaccharides

Glycogen

Polysaccharide

A   B   C

Figure 11 Composition of simple sugars. **A.** Monosaccharides, based on a single ring of carbons each. **B.** Disaccharides, composed of two linked monosaccharides. **C.** Polysaccharides, composed of many linked saccharides.

fat and oil. These molecules are formed by the condensation of one molecule of glycerol, which is a three-carbon alcohol. Glycerol contains three fatty acid molecules. Triglycerides contain different saturated and unsaturated fatty acid combinations. Those with mostly saturated fatty acids are called saturated fats **Figure 12**. Those with mostly unsaturated fatty acids are called unsaturated fats.

Saturated fat is defined as containing carbon atoms that are bound to as many hydrogen atoms as possible, becoming saturated with them. Fatty acid molecules with double bonds only are called unsaturated. Fatty acid molecules with many double-bonded carbon atoms are called polyunsaturated.

Similar to a fat molecule, a **phospholipid** consists of a glycerol portion with fatty acid chains. Phospholipids are structurally related to glycolipids. Human cells can synthesize both types of lipids, primarily from fatty acids. A phospholipid includes a phosphate group that is soluble in water and a fatty acid portion that is not. Phospholipids are an important part of cell structures.

Steroid molecules are large lipid molecules that share a distinctive carbon framework. Steroids have four connected rings of carbon atoms. All steroid molecules have the same basic structure: three 6-carbon rings joined to one 5-carbon ring. They include cholesterol, estrogen, progesterone, testosterone, cortisol, and estradiol **Figure 13**.

Proteins

Proteins are the most abundant organic components of the human body, and in many ways the most important. Proteins are vital for many body functions, including structures and their functions, energy, enzymatic function, defense (antibodies), and hormonal requirements. On cell surfaces, some proteins combine with carbohydrates to become glycoproteins.

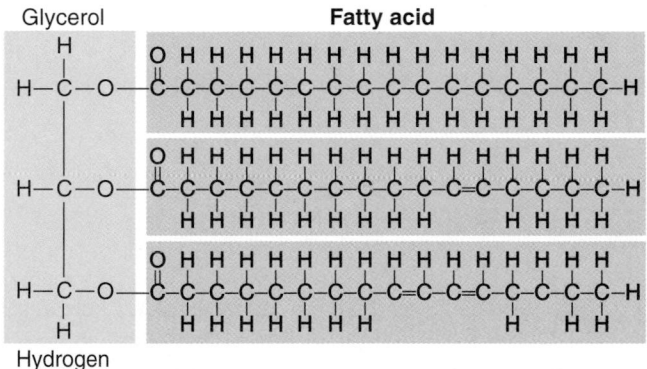

Glycerol   **Fatty acid**

Hydrogen

Figure 12 Saturated fats (top). Note that almost all of the carbon atoms are bonded together with single bonds due to being saturated with hydrogen atoms. Unsaturated fats (bottom). Note that several less hydrogen atoms are present and some pairs of carbon atoms are joined with double bonds.

They allow cells to respond to certain molecules that bind to them.

There are more than 200,000 types of proteins in the human body. Antibodies are proteins that detect and destroy foreign substances. All proteins contain carbon, hydrogen, oxygen, and nitrogen atoms, with small quantities of sulfur also present. Proteins always contain nitrogen atoms. Twenty-two different amino acids make up the proteins that exist in humans and most other living organisms. Protein molecules consisting of amino acids held together by peptide bonds are called **peptides**. A **polypeptide** is formed from many amino acids bound into a chain. Polypeptides usually have specialized functions.

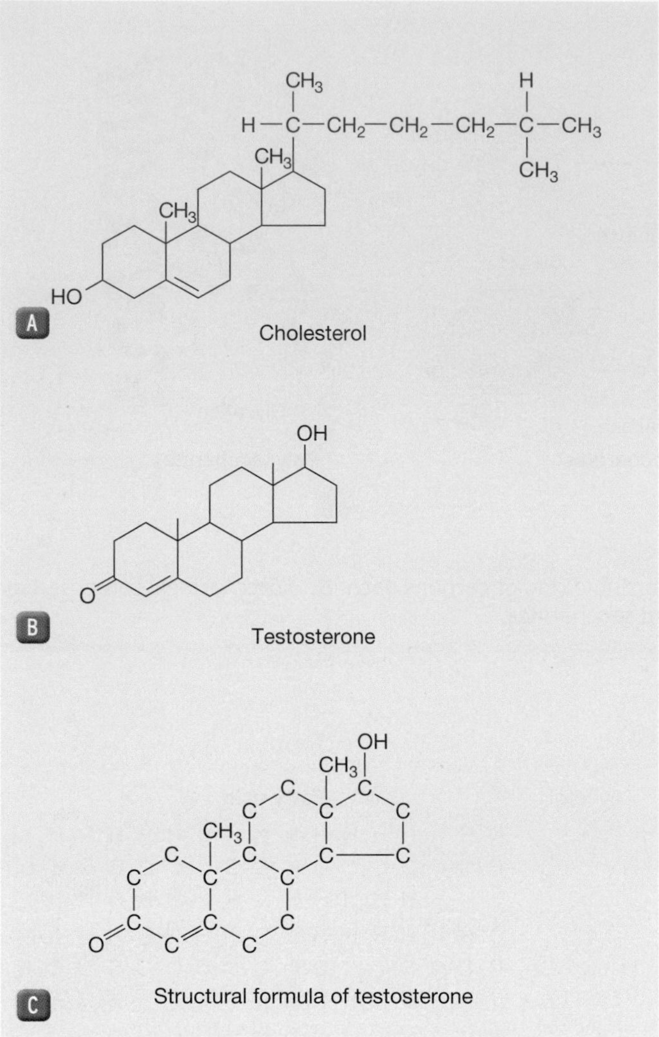

Figure 13 Various types of steroid molecules. **A.** Cholesterol. **B.** Testosterone. **C.** Structural formula of testosterone.

When a polypeptide has more than 100 molecules, it is considered to be a protein. Certain protein molecules have more than one polypeptide.

Other types of proteins include structural proteins such as collagen, which gives strength to ligaments and connective tissues, and keratin, which functions to prevent water loss through the skin. More active proteins include antibodies and enzymes. Cell membrane proteins may serve as receptors and carriers for specific molecules.

Nucleic Acids

Nucleic acids are large organic molecules (macromolecules) that carry genetic information or form structures within cells. They are composed of carbon, hydrogen, oxygen, nitrogen, and phosphorus. Nucleic acids store and process information at the molecular level, inside the cells. The two classes of nucleic acids are deoxyribonucleic acid (DNA) and ribonucleic acid (RNA). Nucleic acids are found in all living things, cells, and viruses.

The DNA in your cells determines your inherited characteristics, including hair color, eye color, and blood type. DNA affects all aspects of body structure and function. DNA molecules encode the information needed to build proteins. By directing structural protein synthesis, DNA controls the shape and physical characteristics of the human body.

Several forms of RNA cooperate to manufacture specific proteins by using the information provided by DNA. Important structural differences distinguish RNA from DNA. An RNA molecule consists of a single chain of nucleotides.

Human cells have three types of RNA:

1. Messenger RNA (mRNA)
2. Transfer RNA (tRNA)
3. Ribosomal RNA (rRNA)

A DNA molecule consists of a pair of nucleotide chains Figure 14 . The two DNA strands twist around each other in a double helix that resembles a spiral staircase.

Cell Physiology

Cells are the foundation of the human body. Billions of cells compose the human body. Some cells make hair, other cells are involved in storing memory, and others help to move your eyes as you read this page. Cells with a common job grow close to each other and are called tissues. Groups of tissues that all perform interrelated jobs form organs. A series of organs working together make up the body systems that are discussed in this chapter.

Structure of the Cell

The human body contains two general classes of cells: sex cells and somatic cells. Sex cells (also called germ cells or reproductive cells) are either the sperm of males or the oocytes of females. Somatic cells (derived from the term soma, meaning "body") include all the other cells in the human body. This section focuses on somatic cells.

There are three basic parts to a cell: the cell membrane, the nucleus, and the cytoplasm. The cell membrane encloses the cell, its nucleus, various organelles, and its cytoplasm. The nucleus contains the cell's genetic material and controls its activities. The cytoplasm fills out the cell and its shape. Organelles are microscopic, specialized cell structures that perform specific functions required by the cell Figure 15 .

Cell Membrane

The cell membrane (also called the plasma membrane) controls movement of substances both into and out of the cell. The cell membrane allows selective communication between the

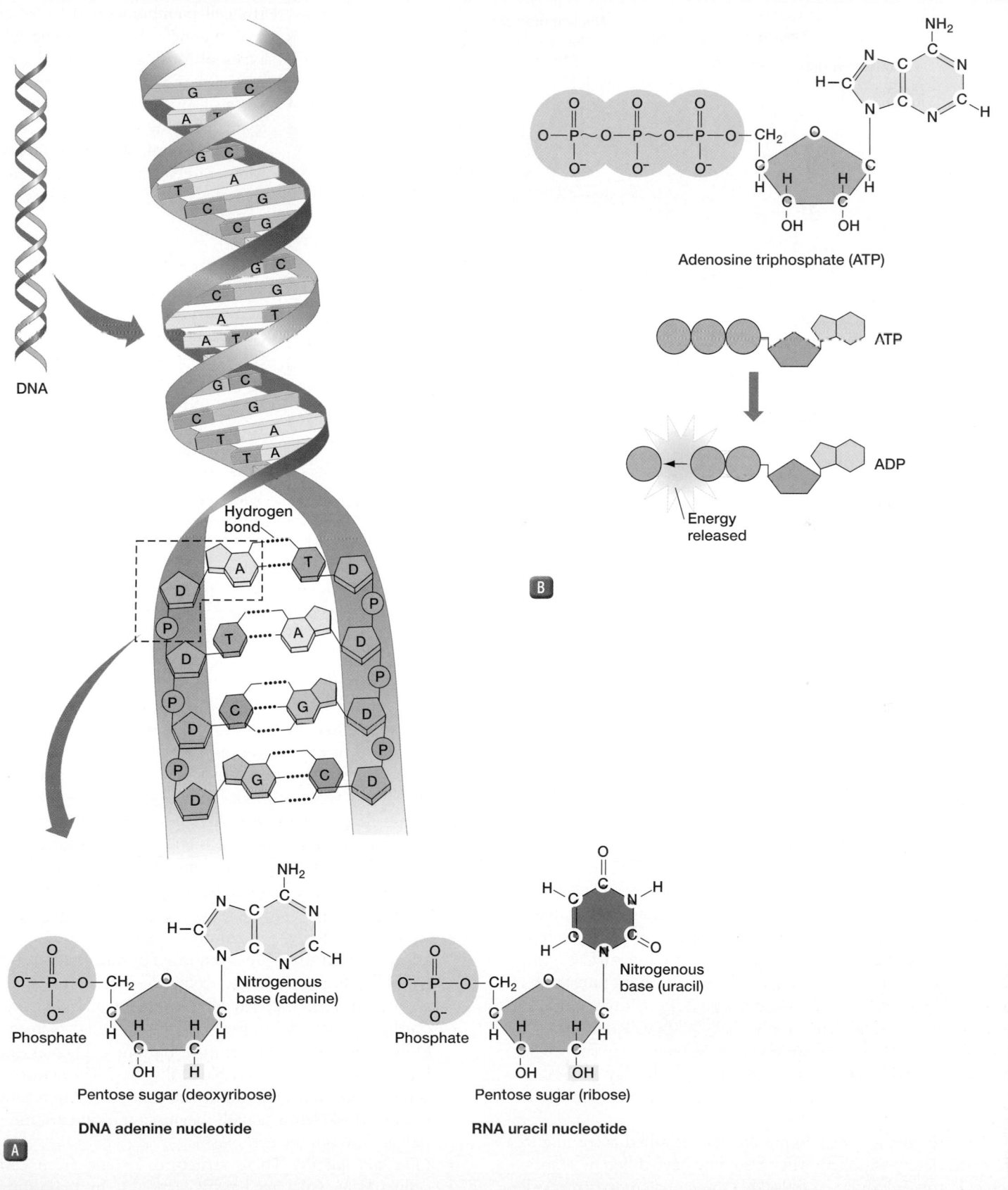

Adenosine triphosphate (ATP)

ATP

ADP

Energy released

B

DNA

Hydrogen bond

A

NH₂

Nitrogenous base (adenine)

Phosphate

Pentose sugar (deoxyribose)

DNA adenine nucleotide

Nitrogenous base (uracil)

Phosphate

Pentose sugar (ribose)

RNA uracil nucleotide

Figure 14 **A.** Nucleic acids, DNA, a DNA nucleotide, and an RNA nucleotide. **B.** Adenosine triphosphate (ATP).

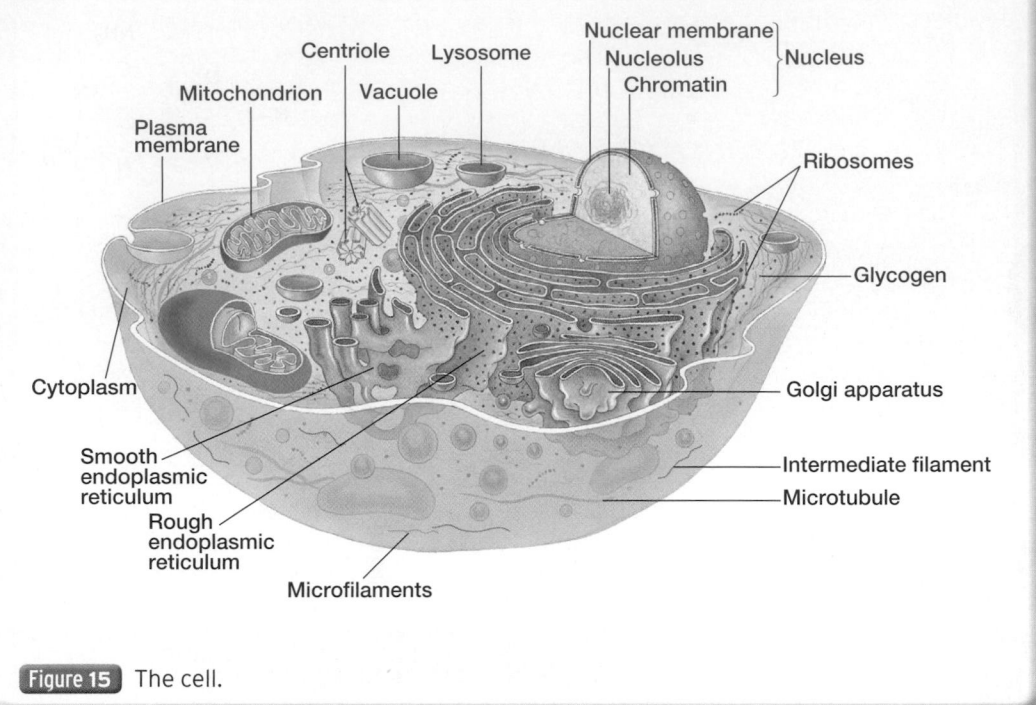

Centriole   Lysosome   Nuclear membrane
Mitochondrion   Vacuole   Nucleolus
Plasma   Chromatin   Nucleus
membrane
Ribosomes
Glycogen
Cytoplasm
Golgi apparatus
Smooth   Intermediate filament
endoplasmic   Microtubule
reticulum
Rough
endoplasmic
reticulum
Microfilaments

Figure 15 The cell.

factors, transport substances across the cell membrane, and form selective channels that determine which types of ions can enter or leave the cell. On the cell membrane's outer surface, proteins may extend outward, marking the cell as a component of a particular tissue or organ. Many proteins are attached to carbohydrates to form glycoproteins.

Cytoplasm

Cytoplasm is the substance that contains all the cellular contents between the cell membrane and the nucleus. It serves as a matrix substance in which chemical reactions occur. Cytoplasm makes up most of each cell's volume, and is a gel-like material suspending the cell's organelles. It usually appears clear with scattered "specks," though more powerful magnification reveals that it contains membranous networks, protein frameworks, and a cytoskeleton (cell skeleton).

intracellular and extracellular compartments while aiding in cellular movement. It gives form to the cell and is also where much of the cell's biologic activities are conducted. Molecules in the cell membrane form pathways that allow the signals from outside the cell to be detected and transmitted inside. When cells form tissues, the cell membrane assists by adhering the cell to other cells.

Each cell's membrane is extremely thin and delicate, able to stretch to differing degrees. There are usually tiny folds on the surface, which help to increase its surface area. Cell membranes can be differentially permeable or semipermeable. A semipermeable membrane allows certain elements to pass through while not allowing others to do so. In some instances, and often depending on various factors, only certain substances can enter or leave each cell (a condition known as selective permeability).

Lipids and proteins are the primary substances that make up cell membranes, usually in a double layer of phospholipid molecules. The phosphate portion forms the outer surface, with the fatty acid portion forming the inner surface. Substances such as oxygen and carbon dioxide, which are soluble in lipids, can easily pass through this double layer (also called a bilayer). Other substances, such as amino acids, proteins, nucleic acids, certain ions, and sugars cannot pass through this layer. Cholesterol in the inner cell membrane helps to keep the membrane stable.

The proteins in a cell membrane are classified according to where they are positioned. They also may have different shapes, such as fibrous, globular, or rod-like. Proteins can move in the cell membrane because they are enclosed in an oily background. Cell membrane proteins may form receptors for hormones or growth

Cytoplasm consists of cytosol and organelles (excluding the nucleus), which are subcellular structures that perform specific functions. Cytosol is the fluid portion of cytoplasm, containing mostly water, as well as glucose, amino acids, fatty acids, ions, lipids, proteins, adenosine triphosphate (ATP), and waste products. Cytosol is the site of many chemical reactions that are required for cells to exist. It is the part of the cytoplasm that cannot be removed by centrifugation.

The cytoplasm receives, processes, and uses nutrients. It contains various types of organelles. Organelles perform most of the tasks that keep the cell alive and functioning normally. Each organelle accomplishes specific tasks related to cell structure, growth, maintenance, and metabolism. The following organelles have specific actions that help the cell to carry out its activities:

- *Centrioles:* Cell division requires a pair of centrioles, which are cylindrical structures composed of short microtubules. During cell division, the centrioles form the spindle-shaped structure needed for movement of DNA strands. Cardiac muscle cells, skeletal muscle cells, mature red blood cells, and typical neurons have no centrioles; therefore, these cells are incapable of dividing. The centrosome is the cytoplasm surrounding the centrioles. Microtubules of the cytoskeleton usually begin at the centrosome and radiate through the cytoplasm.

- *Cilia and flagella:* These structures extend from certain cell surfaces. Cilia are hair-like, moving in a coordinated sweeping motion to move fluids over the surface of tissues. They are found on cells lining the respiratory tract and on cells lining the reproductive tract. Flagella are longer than cilia, and often exist as only a single flagellum (an example of which is the flagellum that appears as the "tail" of a sperm cell).

- *Ribosomes:* Sites on the outer membrane of the endoplasmic reticulum where protein synthesis occurs; they may also be scattered through the cytoplasm. Ribosomes are composed of protein and RNA. Their functions involve the formation of proteins, and they are therefore called the "protein factories" of the cell.

- *Endoplasmic reticulum (ER):* The ER is a network of intracellular membranes connected to the nuclear envelope, which surrounds a cell's nucleus. There are two types of ER: the smooth endoplasmic reticulum (SER) and the rough endoplasmic reticulum (RER). The SER does not have ribosomes on its outer surface, whereas fixed ribosomes appear on the RER's outer surface **Figure 16**. The SER can synthesize phospholipids and cholesterol, which are needed for the cell membrane's growth and maintenance. The RER can synthesize proteins. Both free and fixed ribosomes synthesize proteins via instructions from messenger RNA.

- *Golgi apparatus:* This apparatus, also called the Golgi complex, consists of a stack of several flattened sacs. These

"pancake-like" structures are hollow, with cavities called cisternae inside them. The Golgi apparatus deals primarily with proteins synthesized on the ribosomes. The end of the Golgi apparatus is specialized to receive glycoproteins, modifying them by removing or adding sugar molecules. The Golgi apparatus has three main functions: (1) modifying and packaging secretions (such as hormones or enzymes) that are released via exocytosis, (2) packaging special enzymes inside vesicles for use in the cytosol, and (3) renewing or modifying the cell membrane.

- *Lysosomes:* These tiny sacs dispose of cell wastes, using enzymes to break down nutrients or foreign particles (such as bacteria). They also destroy older, worn-out parts of the cell. This breakdown process requires the use of powerful enzymes. It often generates toxic chemicals capable of damaging or killing the cell. Lysosomes are specialized vesicles that provide an isolated environment for potentially dangerous chemical reactions. They are produced close to the Golgi apparatus and contain digestive enzymes.

- *Microfilaments:* The smallest of the cytoskeletal elements, microfilaments are composed of the proteins actin and myosin. They are typically found in muscle cells. Microfilaments provide cell movement and contraction via interaction with actin and myosin. This process can also change the shape of the entire cell.

- *Mitochondria:* All cells in the body, with the exception of mature red blood cells, have between a hundred and a few thousand organelles called mitochondria (singularly called a mitochondrion). Mitochondria have double membranes that play the central role in the production of energy (via ATP). Mitochondria are the "powerhouses" of cells. The liver, kidneys, and muscles have a large number of mitochondria in their cells because they use ATP at a high rate. A mitochondrion is surrounded by two membranes that are similar in structure to the plasma membrane. The outer mitochondrial membrane is smooth. The inner mitochondrial membrane has a series of folds called cristae. The central fluid-filled cavity is called the matrix, and is enclosed by the inner membrane and cristae.

The number of mitochondria in a particular cell varies, based on the cell's energy demands. They can migrate through the cytoplasm of a cell, and are able to reproduce themselves. Mitochondria contain their own DNA, but in a more primitive form than that found within the cell nucleus.

- *Peroxisomes:* These sacs have enzymes that speed up many biochemical reactions. They are abundant in the liver and kidney cells, and their diverse actions include synthesis of bile acids, detoxification of hydrogen peroxide or alcohol, and breaking down lipids and biochemicals.

- *Thick filaments:* Relatively massive bundles of subunits composed of the protein myosin. Thick filaments appear in muscle cells only, where they interact with actin filaments to produce powerful contractions.

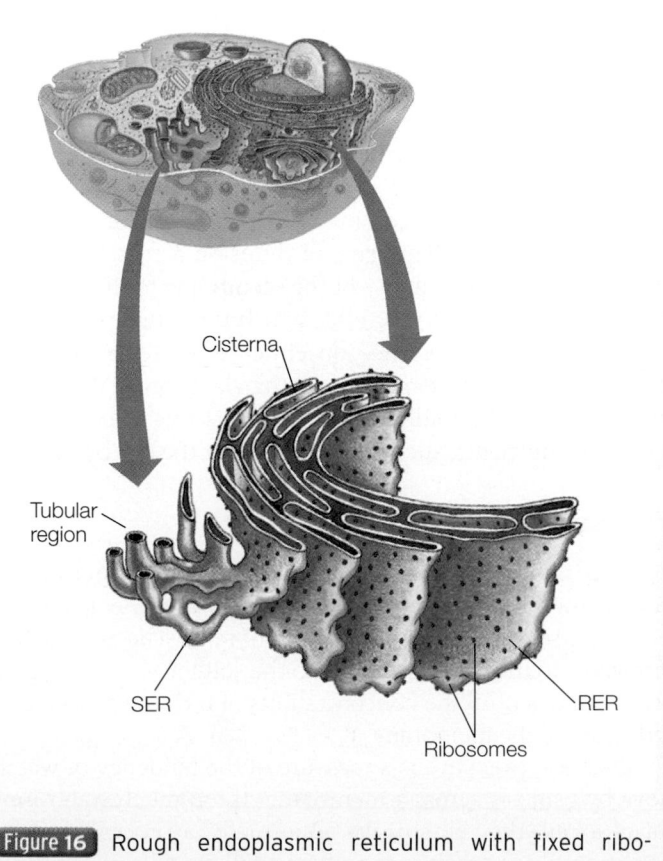

Cisterna

Tubular region

SER

RER

Ribosomes

Figure 16 Rough endoplasmic reticulum with fixed ribosomes on its outer surface.

- *Vesicles:* Also known as vacuoles, these sacs are formed when a part of a cell membrane folds inward, establishing a bubble-like structure within the cytoplasm. Vesicles contain various liquid or solid materials that formerly existed outside of the cell membrane.

Nucleus

The <u>nucleus</u> is usually the largest, most visible structure inside a cell. The nucleus serves as the control center for cellular operations. It contains DNA, or genetic material, that controls cell activities. A single nucleus stores all required information that directs the synthesis of the 100,000 proteins in the human body. A cell without a nucleus cannot repair itself. It will disintegrate within 3 to 4 months. The nucleus contains the genetic instructions needed to synthesize the proteins that determine cell structures and functions. These instructions are stored in the chromosomes. These structures consist of DNA and various proteins that control and access genetic information. Most cells contain a single nucleus, with the exception of skeletal muscle cells (with numerous nuclei) and mature red blood cells (with no nuclei).

The nucleus of a cell is usually round, and is enclosed in a double nuclear envelope, with inner and outer lipid membranes. This envelope also has a protein lining, allowing certain molecules to exit the nucleus. Inside the nucleus is a fluid called nucleoplasm that suspends the following structures:

- *Nucleolus:* A "mini nucleus" made up mostly of RNA and protein molecules, with no surrounding membrane. Ribosomes form in the nucleolus and migrate out to the cell's cytoplasm.
- *Chromatin:* Loosely coiled DNA and protein fibers that condense, forming <u>chromosomes</u>. The DNA controls protein synthesis, and when the cell starts to divide, the chromatin fibers coil tightly to form the chromosomes.

■ Cellular Transport Mechanisms

It is important for you to understand cell transport mechanisms, or how materials enter and exit the cell, because this relates to fluid administration, a paramedic skill. This section discusses some basic cell transport concepts. These concepts are discussed in more detail in the chapter, *Medication Administration.*

■ Cell Membrane Permeability

The cell membrane (the cell wall) is described as being selectively permeable, which means that it allows some substances to pass through it, but not others Figure 17 .

Selective permeability allows normal differences in concentrations between intracellular and extracellular environments to be maintained. The separation of the extracellular and intracellular areas by a selectively permeable membrane helps to maintain homeostasis, the maintenance of a stable internal physiologic environment including a stable temperature, fluid balance, and pH balance. Various enzymes, sugar molecules,

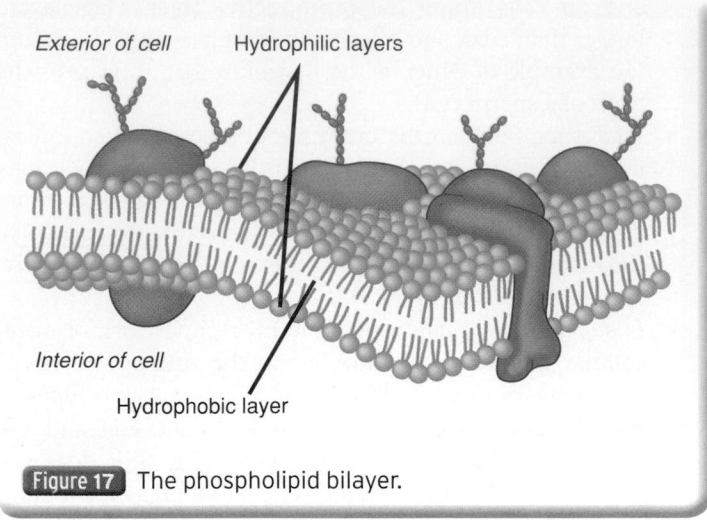

Exterior of cell Hydrophilic layers

Interior of cell

Hydrophobic layer

Figure 17 The phospholipid bilayer.

and electrolytes freely pass in and out of the cell. Electrolytes are chemicals that are dissolved in the blood and are made up of salt or acid substances that become ionic conductors when dissolved in a solvent such as water.

Several mechanisms, such as diffusion, osmosis, facilitated diffusion, active transport, endocytosis, and exocytosis allow material to pass through the cell wall Figure 18 .

■ Diffusion

Particles such as molecules and ions live in water, which creates a solution. Water is the most common solvent or substance in which other substances or solutes will dissolve. <u>Diffusion</u> is the movement of <u>solutes</u>, particles such as salts that are dissolved in a solvent, from an area of high concentration to one of low concentration, to produce an even distribution of particles in the space available. The degree of diffusion across a membrane depends on the permeability of the membrane to that substance and the <u>concentration gradient</u>, which is the difference in concentrations of the substance on either side of the membrane. Small molecules diffuse more easily than large ones. Watery solutions diffuse more rapidly than thicker, viscous solutions. Many of the cell's nutrients, such as oxygen, enter the cell by diffusion.

■ Osmosis

<u>Osmosis</u> is the movement of a solvent, such as water, from an area of low solute concentration to one of high concentration through a selectively permeable membrane. The membrane is permeable to the solvent but not to the solute. Movement generally continues until the concentrations of the solute equalize on both sides of the membrane.

<u>Osmotic pressure</u> is a measure of the tendency of water to move by osmosis across a membrane. If too much water moves out of a cell, the cell shrinks abnormally, a process known as <u>crenation</u>. If too much water enters a cell, it will swell and burst, a process known as <u>lysis</u>.

If the concentration of solute is higher within the cell than outside, the cell is said to by <u>hypertonic</u>. If the opposite is true,

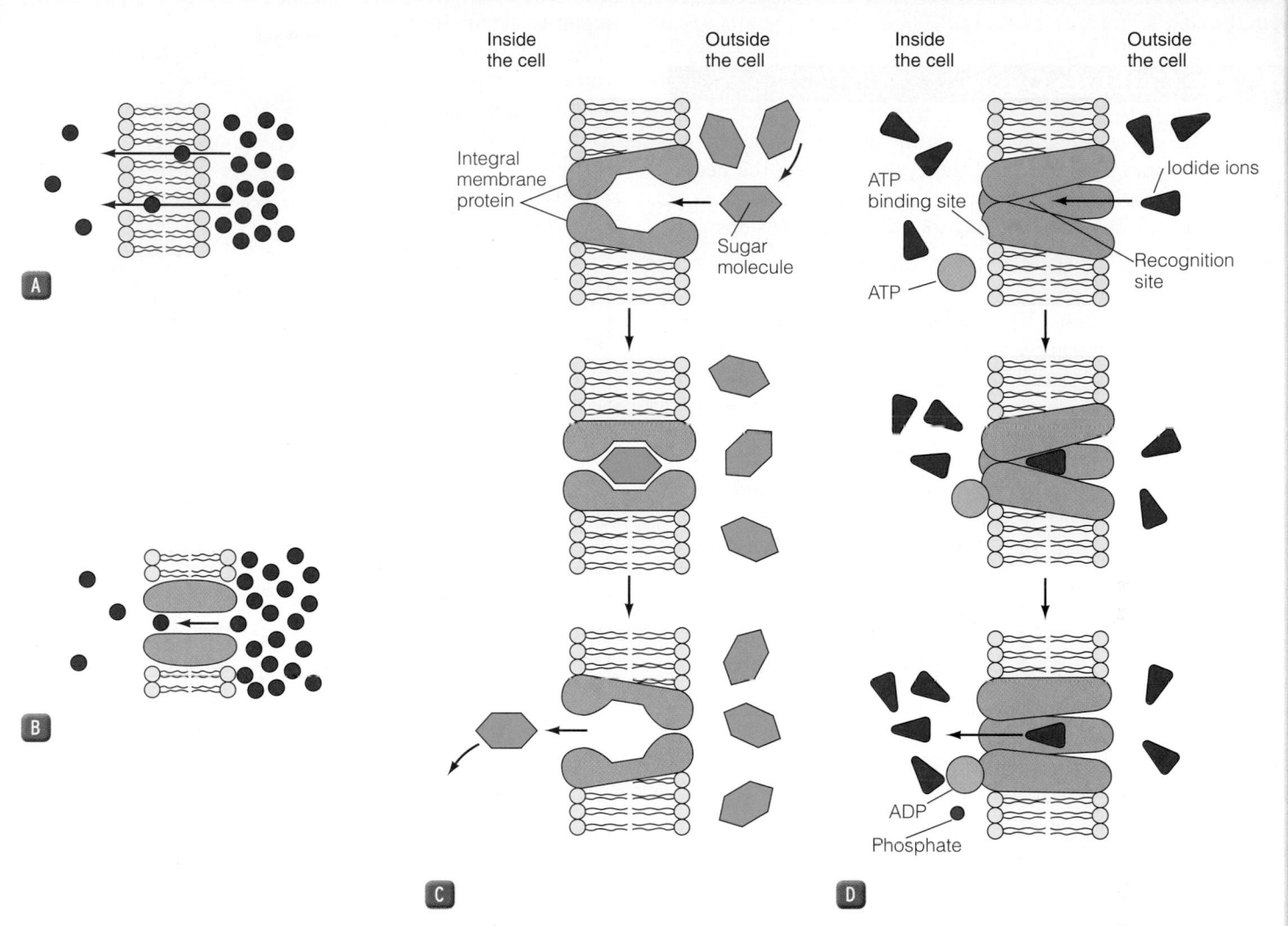

Figure 18 Methods of material transport through the cell wall. **A.** Simple diffusion. **B.** Diffusion through protein pores. **C.** Facilitated diffusion. **D.** Active transport.

where less solute is present within the cell than outside, the cell is said to by <u>hypotonic</u>. The degree of difference between the two concentrations determine how much osmotic pressure is present and how quickly the two concentrations will tend to equalize. When the concentrations on either side of the membrane are equal, they are said to be <u>isotonic</u>.

Facilitated Diffusion

<u>Facilitated diffusion</u> is the process in which a carrier molecule moves substances in or out of cells from areas of high concentration to areas of lower concentration (see Figure 18). Energy is not required; the number of molecules transported is directly proportional to the amount of concentration.

Active Transport

<u>Active transport</u> is the movement of a substance against a concentration or gradient such as the cell membrane. Active transport requires energy as well as some type of carrier mechanism and is a movement opposite that of the normal movement of diffusion. Both glucose and amino acids are absorbed via active transport. At times, the active transport mechanism may exchange one substance for another. Endocytosis and exocytosis both use energy from the cell to move substances into or out of the cell without crossing the cell membrane. In endocytosis, a secretion from the cell membrane moves particles too large to enter the cell by other processes within a vesicle of the cell. There are three forms of endocytosis: pinocytosis, phagocytosis, and receptor-mediated endocytosis. Pinocytosis ("cell drinking") involves cells taking in small liquid droplets from the surrounding cell environment with a small indentation of the cell membrane. Phagocytosis ("cell eating") involves cells taking in solids instead of liquids. Receptor-mediated endocytosis involves the movement of specific kinds of particles into the cell, with protein molecules extending through part of the cell membrane to the outer surface. The opposite process to endocytosis

is exocytosis, in which a substance stored in a vesicle is secreted from the cell.

The Cell Life Cycle

The cell's life cycle is regulated via stimulation from hormones or growth factors. Disruption of the cycle can affect the health of the body. Most human cells divide from 40 to 60 times before they die. The life cycle of a cell includes the following steps:

- *Interphase:* The cell obtains nutrients to grow and duplicate.
- *Cell division (mitosis):* The nucleus divides.
- *Cytoplasmic division (cytokinesis):* The cytoplasm divides.
- *Differentiation:* The cell becomes specialized.

Interphase

A cell must grow and duplicate most of its contents before it can actively divide. Interphase describes this period of preparation to divide. During interphase, the cell manufactures new living material, duplicating membranes, lysosomes, mitochondria, and ribosomes. It also replicates its own genetic material.

Cell Division and Cytoplasmic Division

There are two types of cell division: meiosis and mitosis/cytokinesis. **Meiosis** is part of gametogenesis (the formation of egg or sperm cells depending on gender). Meiosis reduces by half the number of chromosomes, from 46 to 23, in eggs and sperm so that when they unite, the fertilized egg will have the proper total of 46 chromosomes.

In the rest of the body, cell numbers are increased by **mitosis**, the division of the nucleus of a cell, and **cytokinesis**, the division of the cytoplasm of a cell. All cells except egg and sperm cells can be divided by mitosis. When the nucleus divides, it must be precise so that an accurate copy of the DNA information can be made by the new cell. There are several stages of mitosis **Figure 19** :

- *Prophase:* The two new centriole pairs move to opposite ends of the cell.
- *Metaphase:* The chromosomes line up near the middle portion (equatorial plane) between the centrioles, and spindle fibers attach to them.
- *Anaphase:* The centromere sections of each chromosome are pulled apart to become individual chromosomes, and move toward opposite ends of the cell.
- *Telophase:* The chromosomes lengthen and unwind, with a nuclear envelope forming around them and nucleoli appearing in each newly formed nucleus.

Cytoplasmic division (cytokinesis) begins during anaphase, when the cell membrane constricts down the middle portion of the cell. This continues through telophase to divide the cytoplasm. The two newly formed nuclei are then separated and nearly half of the organelles are distributed into each new cell.

Differentiation

Differentiation, the process of specialization of a cell, makes each cell unique. New cells must be generated in order for growth and tissue repair to occur. **Stem cells** are those that can divide repeatedly without specializing. They either can divide into two identical daughter cells or can divide so that one daughter cell becomes partially specialized (progenitor cells). In the human body, all differentiated cell types are created because of the variance of stem and progenitor cells.

Stem cells in certain organs may have the ability to heal the body in the future, even though they were differentiated when the organism was still an embryo or fetus. As the body continually develops, cells use different parts of complete genetic instructions so that they can become specialized. Genes may be activated in various types of cells. For example, stem cells differentiate into islet cells in the pancreas. Islet cells produce insulin, but in diabetes, the islet cells do not function. Research is being done into whether stem cells can be used to replace islet cells. The possibility of repairing damaged spinal cords via the use of stem cells is also being researched.

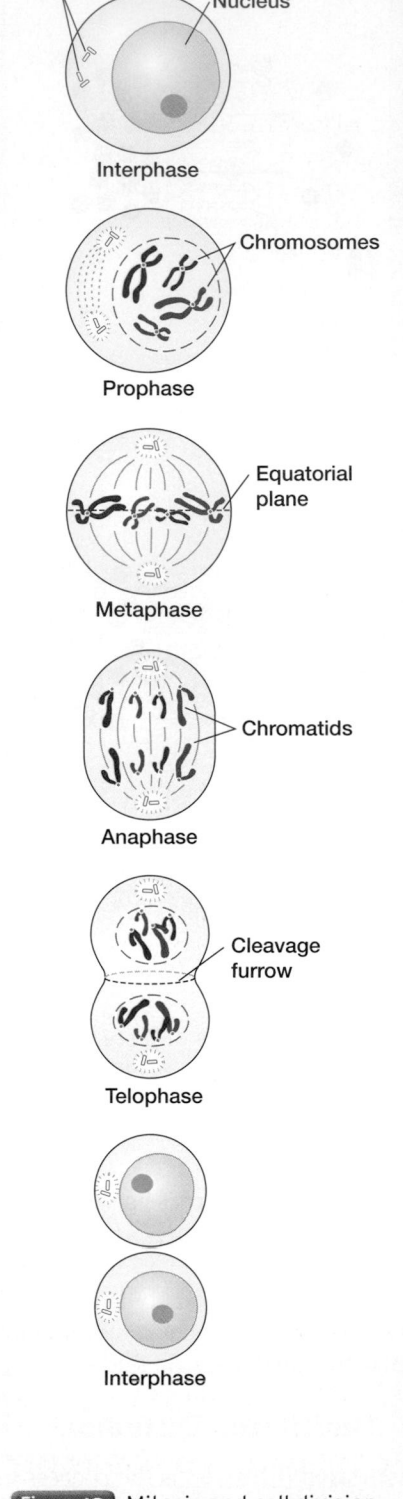

Figure 19 Mitosis and cell division.

Cell Division and Cancer

Cell division and growth normally occurs at approximately the same rate as cell death. However, when cell division and growth are higher than the cell death rate, tissues enlarge. A neoplasm or tumor is a mass of tissue produced by abnormal cell growth and division. A tumor is called benign when it remains within the epithelium or a capsule made of connective tissue. This type of tumor seldom becomes life threatening and can usually be surgically removed if it affects tissue function.

Malignant tumors spread into surrounding tissues in a process called invasion. The tumor of origin (the primary tumor or primary neoplasm) may result in malignant cells traveling to other organs or tissue to establish secondary tumors. This process, called metastasis, is not easily controlled. Cancer develops, and exhibits mutations disrupting normal cell growth. Usually, all tumor cells are daughter cells of just one malignant cell. Malignancy often occurs when a normal gene mutates. These modified genes are called oncogenes. Cancer often begins where stem cells divide. This is because there is a greater chance of error the more frequently that chromosomes are copied for cell division.

Cancer cells change shape as they grow and gradually resemble normal cells less and less. Tumor cells escape the primary tumor to invade surrounding tissue—this is the manner in which metastasis begins. If tumor cells penetrate blood vessels, they circulate throughout the body. If they enter the lymphatic system, they accumulate in lymph nodes. The presence of tumor cells stimulates the growth of new blood vessels where the cells situate themselves. This supplies them with more nutrients and accelerates their growth and further metastasis.

As metastasis increases, organ function changes. Cancer cells grow and multiply by taking nutrients and space from normal cells, causing weight loss in most cancer patients as the normal cells deteriorate. When cancer cells compress vital organs or have replaced healthy cells in vital organs, death may occur.

Facilitating Cellular Metabolism

The body's cells, tissues, and organs, regardless of their function, all require oxygen, nutrients, and the removal of wastes to perform their job. Oxygen is brought to the cells through the respiratory and circulatory systems. Nutrients are made available to the body after we eat. The digestive system takes the food we eat and breaks it down into, among other things, glucose. Glucose is the primary fuel of the body. The circulatory system is the carrier of these supplies and wastes through the process of perfusion. If interference occurs in this delivery system, cells will become damaged or die.

The human body is designed to be able to handle a wide array of metabolic disturbances. Oxygen is a critical component for cells. Cells use oxygen to take the available nutrients and turn them into chemical energy. **Adenosine triphosphate (ATP)** is involved in energy metabolism and is used to store energy. Cells prefer to operate using oxygen because it provides the cells with 15 times as much ATP as when they operate without oxygen. The process that uses oxygen is called aerobic (meaning with air) metabolism. The waste products of **aerobic metabolism** are carbon dioxide and water. Some cells, such as those of the brain and heart, have become so specialized that they are unable to survive without constant supplies of oxygen. Without oxygen, brain cells will begin to die within 4 to 6 minutes.

Most cells in the body are able to continue to function, even without oxygen. This anaerobic (without air) state allows cells to operate despite no available oxygen. When illness or injury occurs, the body needs to shift available resources to areas in need while ensuring that critical areas, such as the brain and heart, have an uninterrupted supply of resources. Any time that available oxygen is limited to portions of the body, cells will switch to **anaerobic metabolism**. This occurs anytime you exercise vigorously and begin to feel a burning sensation. In this state, very limited amounts of energy are able to be released so the body must quickly correct the oxygen deficiency or risk cellular death. The most well-known by-product of anaerobic metabolism is lactic acid, which is the material that causes muscle burning during anaerobic exercise. **Lactic acid** is converted back to a useful energy source once oxygen is available. Anaerobic metabolism can be supported in most cells for only 1 to 3 minutes.

Words of Wisdom

When cells function with oxygen, they use aerobic metabolism. They generate large amounts of ATP (cellular energy) and produce wastes of carbon dioxide and water.

When cells function without oxygen, they use anaerobic metabolism. They generate small amounts of ATP (cellular energy) and produce waste of lactic acid.

■ Types of Tissue

The human body is primarily made up of four major types of tissue: epithelial, connective, muscle, and nervous tissues. **Epithelial tissues** cover body surfaces, cover and line internal organs, and make up the glands. **Connective tissues** are widely distributed throughout the body, filling the internal spaces, and function to bind, support, and protect body structures. **Muscle tissues** are specialized for contraction, and include the skeletal muscles of the body, the heart, and the muscular walls of hollow organs. Skeletal muscles are attached to bones, and are used for movement of the body. **Nervous tissues** carry information from one part of the body to another via electrical impulses. They are found in the brain, spinal cord, and nerves.

Epithelial Tissues

Epithelial tissues include epithelia and glands. Epithelium covers the surface of the skin and organs, forms the inner lining of the body's cavities, and also lines hollow organs. Epithelial tissues throughout the body are anchored to connective tissue by a **basement membrane**. An epithelium is an **avascular** layer of cells that forms a barrier providing protection and regulating permeability. Glands are secretory structures derived from epithelia.

Epithelial cells divide quickly, aiding in wound healing and replacement of cells when damage occurs. Tightly packed epithelial cells protect body structures such as the outer skin and the lining of body cavities such as the mouth. Epithelial tissues are involved in secretion, absorption, and excretion. They also provide sensation. They are classified according to the shape of their cells and the number of cell layers that exist. Table 6 summarizes the different types of epithelial tissues.

Epithelia perform four essential functions:

1. *Physical protection:* Epithelia protect exposed and internal surfaces from abrasion, dehydration, and destruction from biologic or chemical agents.

2. *Permeability:* Any substance entering or leaving the body must cross an epithelium, so the epithelia control permeability. Some epithelia are relatively impermeable whereas others are crossed easily by compounds of various sizes. In response to stimuli, the epithelial barrier may be modified and regulated. Hormones can affect ion and nutrient transport through epithelial cells. Physical stress can also alter the structure and properties of epithelia. An example is the formation of calluses on the hands after repeated manual labor.

3. *Sensation:* Most epithelia are very sensitive to stimulation because they have a large sensory nerve supply.

4. *Specialized secretions:* Epithelial cells that produce secretions are called gland cells, and individual cells of this type are scattered among other types of cells in an epithelium. Most or all of the epithelial cells in a glandular epithelium produce secretions, which are either discharged onto the surface of the epithelium or released into the surrounding interstitial fluid and blood.

The following are the various forms of epithelial tissues:

- **Simple squamous epithelium**: Consists of a single layer of thin and flattened cells with broad, thin nuclei. It lines the alveoli of the lungs, forms capillary walls, lines blood and lymph vessels, and covers membranes that line body cavities Figure 20 .

- **Simple cuboidal epithelium**: Consists of a single layer of cube-shaped cells with round nuclei. It covers the ovaries, lines many kidney tubules and glandular ducts, and functions in secretion and absorption.

- **Simple columnar epithelium**: Consists of cells that are longer than wide, composed of a single cellular layer with elongated nuclei, located near the basement membrane, and may have cilia on their surfaces. It is found in the female reproductive tubes, uterus, and most digestive tract organs, being involved in secretion and absorption. Simple columnar cells, specialized for absorption, usually have tiny, cylinder-shaped processes (microvilli) that extend from their surfaces and increase the surface area of the cell membrane. Often, special flask-shaped glandular cells (goblet cells) are scattered among the columnar cells, secreting mucus on the tissue surface.

- **Pseudostratified columnar epithelium**: Appear as if they are layered due to the nuclei being located at different levels. The cells vary in shape and usually reach the basement membrane. Pseudostratified columnar epithelium usually has cilia and lines respiratory system passages, as well as being involved in secretion. Goblet cells, which secrete mucus, are found throughout this tissue Figure 21 .

- **Stratified squamous epithelium**: A thick layer with cells that flatten as they are pushed outward. It forms the epidermis, with cells hardening as they age (keratinization). It also lines the mouth, esophagus, vagina, and anus, where the cells do not harden but remain soft and moist.

- **Stratified cuboidal epithelium**: Consists of up to three layers of cubed cells. It lines the mammary gland ducts, sweat glands, salivary glands, pancreas, and the developing ovaries and seminiferous tubules.

Table 6 Types of Epithelial Tissues

Type	Location	Function
Simple squamous epithelium	Air sacs of lungs, capillary walls, linings of lymph, and blood vessels	Diffusion, filtration, osmosis, covering of surfaces
Simple cuboidal epithelium	Ovary surfaces, kidney tubule linings, linings of ducts of certain glands	Absorption, secretion
Simple columnar epithelium	Intestine, stomach, and uterus linings	Absorption, protection, secretion
Pseudostratified columnar epithelium	Respiratory passage linings	Movement of mucus, protection, secretion
Stratified squamous epithelium	Outer layer of skin, linings of anal canal, oral cavity, throat, and vagina	Protection
Stratified cuboidal epithelium	Linings of larger mammary gland ducts, pancreas, salivary glands, sweat glands	Protection
Stratified columnar epithelium	Part of male urethra and parts of the pharynx	Protection, secretion
Transitional epithelium	Inner urinary bladder lining, linings of ureters, and part of urethra	Distensibility, protection
Glandular epithelium	Endocrine, salivary, and sweat glands	Secretion

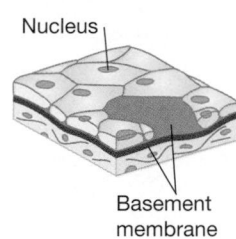

Nucleus

Basement
membrane

Simple squamous epithelium

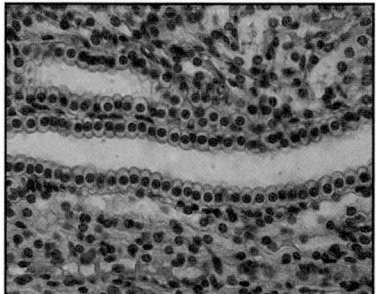

Simple cuboidal epithelium

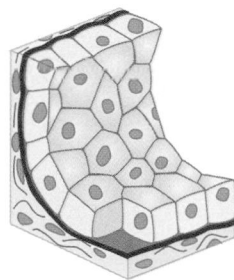

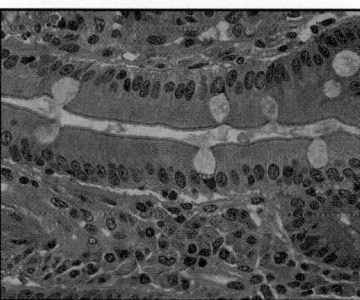

Simple columnar epithelium

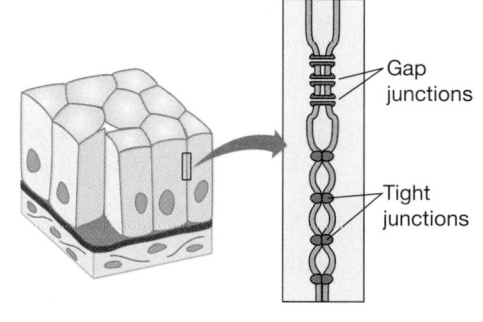

Gap
junctions

Tight
junctions

Figure 20 Shapes of epithelial cells.

- **Stratified columnar epithelium**: Consists of several layers of either columnar or cubed shapes. It is found in the male urethra, ductus deferens, and areas of the pharynx.
- **Transitional epithelium**: Changes in appearance in response to tension. It lines the urinary bladder, ureters, and superior urethra, and prevents urinary tract contents from diffusing back into the internal body environment.
- **Glandular epithelium**: Consists of specialized cells that produce and secrete substances into ducts or body fluids. It is usually found in **exocrine glands** (which open onto surfaces or into the digestive tract) or in endocrine glands (which secrete into tissue fluid or blood). There are three types of exocrine glands: merocrine, apocrine, and holocrine **Figure 22**. Merocrine glands release fluid by exocytosis. Apocrine glands lose parts of their cell bodies during secretion. Holocrine glands release entire cells that disintegrate to release secretions.

Connective Tissues

The cells that make up connective tissues are farther apart than those of epithelial tissues. These tissues bind body structures, provide support and protection, create frameworks, fill body spaces, store fat, produce blood cells, transport fluids and dissolved materials, repair damaged tissues, and protect the body from infection. Connective tissues vary greatly in appearance and function, but have three basic components:

1. Specialized cells
2. Extracellular protein fibers
3. A fluid known as a ground substance

Together, the extracellular protein fibers and ground substance constitute the **matrix**, which surrounds the cells. Although cells make up the majority of epithelial tissue, the matrix usually accounts for the majority of connective tissue.

Most connective tissue cells divide, have good blood supply, and require large amounts of nourishment. Connective tissues include those of bone, cartilage, and fat. Connective tissues contain different types of cells, including those that are fixed or wandering. The most common type of fixed cell is the star-shaped **fibroblast**, which produces fibers via protein secretion into the extracellular matrix. **Table 7** summarizes the major cells and tissue fibers of connective tissue.

Fibroblasts produce three connective tissue fibers:

1. *Collagenous fibers:* Important for body parts that hold structures together (ligaments and tendons); collagenous fibers are also called dense connective tissue or white fibers.
2. *Elastic fibers:* Common in body parts that are often stretched, such as the vocal cords; they are composed of a protein called elastin, and are also called yellow fibers.
3. *Reticular fibers:* Form delicate supporting networks in the spleen and other tissues.

The other types of cells found in connective tissue include mast cells, macrophages, adipocytes, and melanocytes. **Mast cells** are distributed throughout connective tissues, usually near blood vessels, and release both heparin (to prevent blood clotting) and histamine (for the inflammatory and allergic response). **Macrophages** are responsible for phagocytosis.

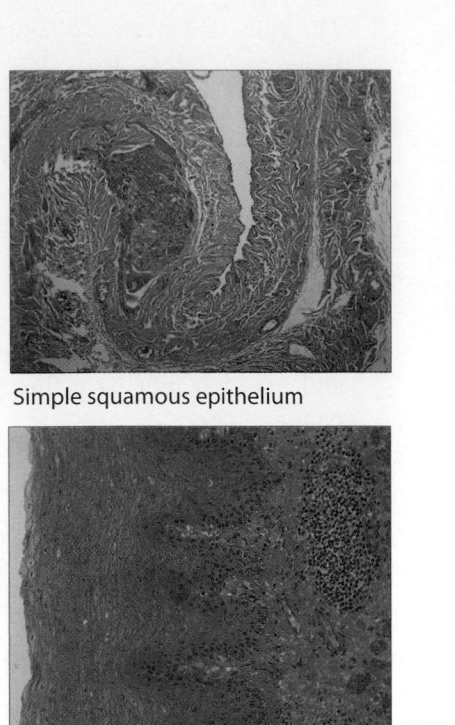

Simple squamous epithelium

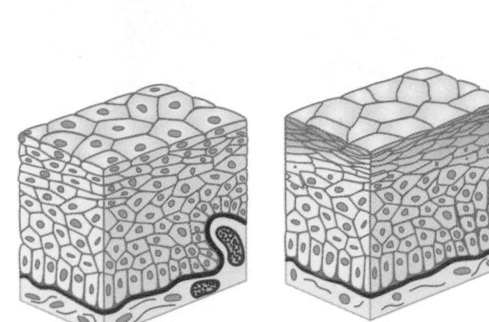

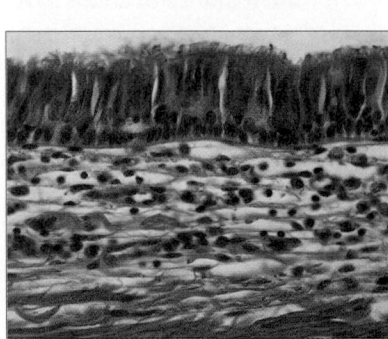

Stratified squamous epithelium

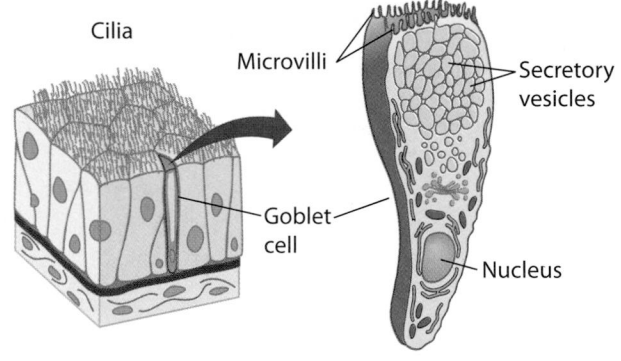

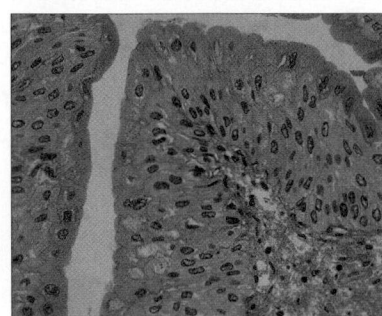

Pseudostratified columnar
epithelium

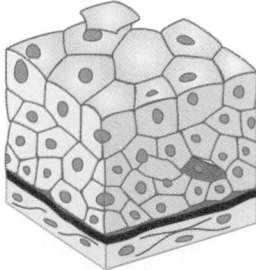

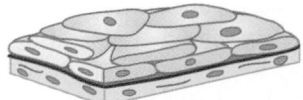

Transitional epithelium

Figure 21 Organizational arrangement and surface modification of epithelial cells.

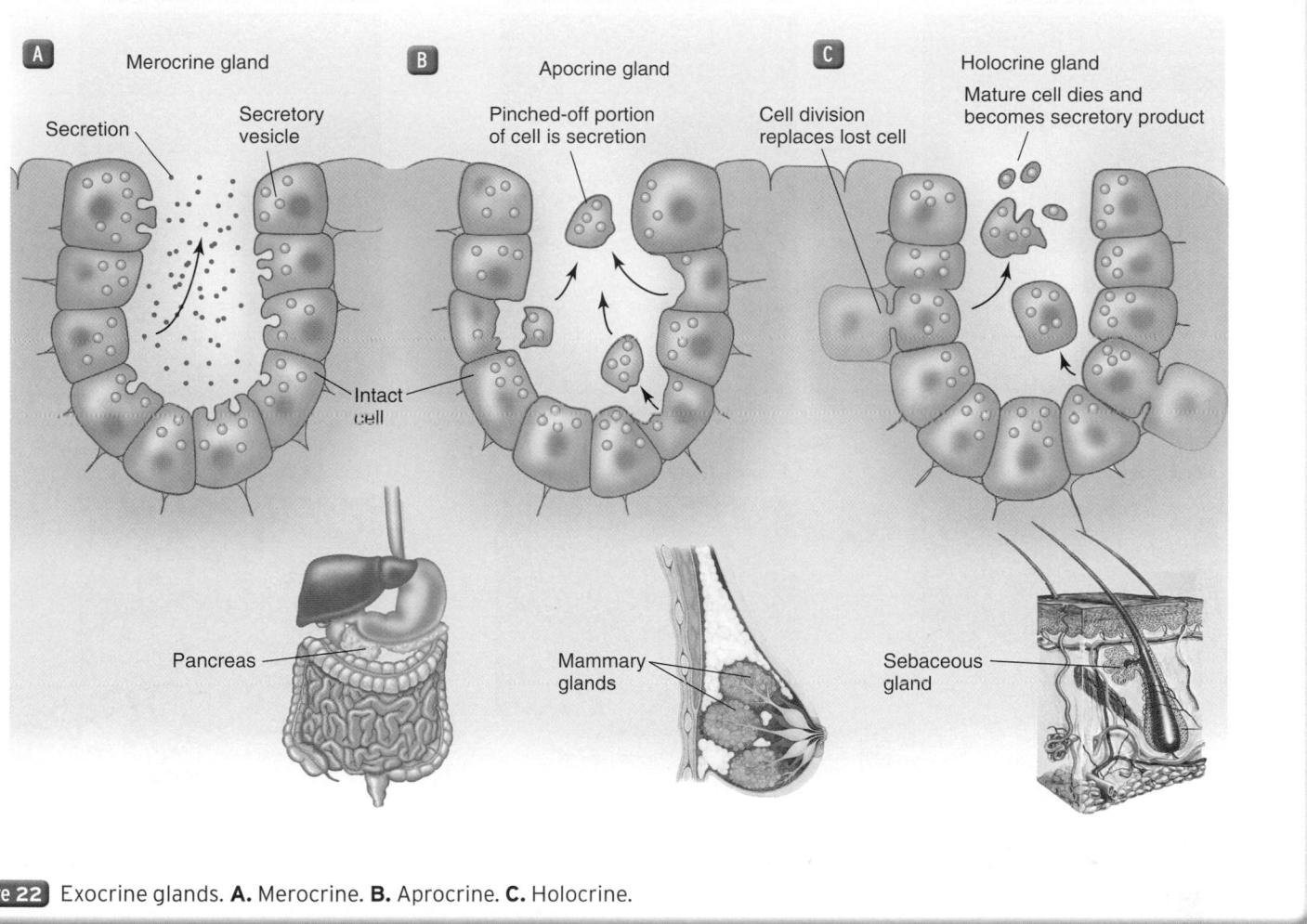

Figure 22 Exocrine glands. **A.** Merocrine. **B.** Aprocrine. **C.** Holocrine.

Table 7 Connective Tissue Cells and Tissue Fibers

Tissue Cell Type	Action
Fibroblasts	Produce fibers
Macrophages	Engulf and devour unwanted microorganisms
Mast cells	Secrete histamine and heparin

Tissue Fiber Type	Action
Collagenous	Bind structures together with high tensile strength
Elastic	Ease of stretching
Reticular	Form delicate support networks

Adipocytes (fat cells) store body fat. Melanocytes are specialized cells in the deeper epithelium of the skin that are responsible for the production of melanin.

Classifications of Connective Tissues

Connective tissues are classified based on their physical properties. The three general categories of connective tissue are connective tissue proper, supporting connective tissues, and fluid connective tissues:

1. Connective tissue proper includes those connective tissues with many types of cells and extracellular fibers in a syruplike ground substance. They are divided into dense connective tissue and loose connective tissue.

   - <u>Dense connective tissue</u> contains many collagenous fibers, and appears white. Its fine network of elastic fibers contains few cells and is very strong Figure 23 . In the tendons and ligaments, dense connective tissue binds muscles to bones and bones to other bones. It also exists in the eyeballs and deep skin layers. Dense connective tissue has poor blood supply and is repaired very slowly as a result.

   - <u>Loose connective tissue</u> includes adipose (fat) tissue, areolar tissue, and reticular connective tissue. <u>Adipose tissue</u> lies beneath the skin, between muscles, around the kidneys, behind the eyes, in certain

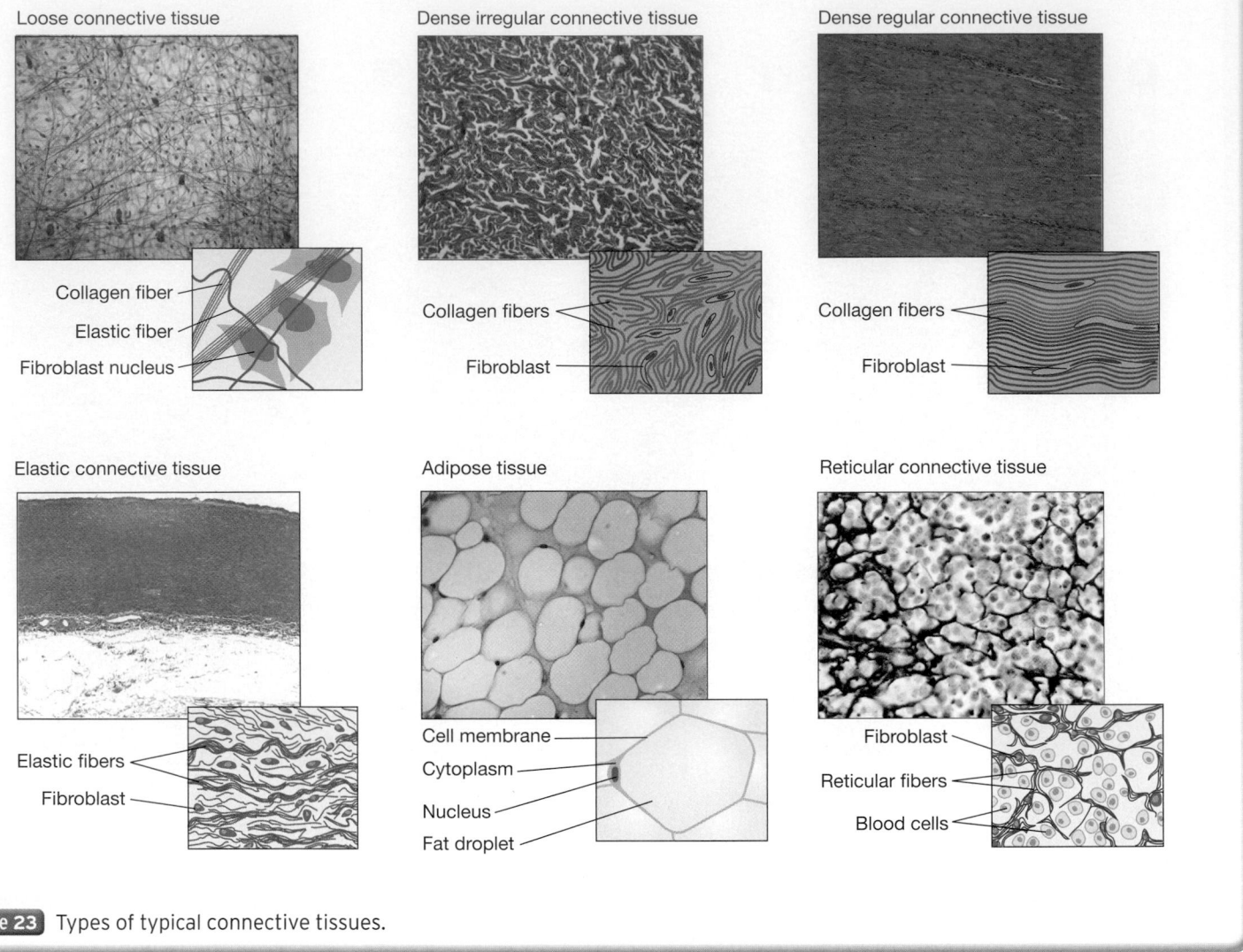

Figure 23 Types of typical connective tissues.

membranes of the abdomen, on the heart's surface, and around some of the body's joints. It functions as a cushion for these body parts. Adipose tissue is also important for storing energy in fat molecules (triglycerides). **Areolar tissue** binds skin to underlying organs and fills in spaces between muscles. It is found beneath most layers of the epithelium. **Reticular connective tissue** helps to create a framework inside internal organs such as the spleen and liver.

2. Supporting connective tissue differs from connective tissue proper because it has a less diverse cell population and a matrix that contains many more densely packed fibers. Supporting connective tissue protects soft tissues and some or all of the body's weight. The two types of supporting connective tissue are cartilage and bone.

  ▪ **Cartilage** is a rigid connective tissue with a gelatinous matrix that contains an abundance of fibers. It supports, frames, and attaches to many underlying tissues and bones. Cartilage cells are known as chondrocytes, and they lie totally inside the extracellular matrix. Cartilage is enclosed in a covering called the perichondrium,

which provides nutrients via diffusion. It has no direct blood supply, so cartilage heals very slowly.

The three major types of cartilage are as follows **Figure 24** :

  - **Hyaline cartilage**: On the ends of bones in many joints, the soft portion of the nose, and in the respiratory passages' supporting rings. It is important for bone growth. Hyaline cartilage is the most common type of cartilage.

  - **Elastic cartilage**: This flexible cartilage provides framework for the ears and larynx.

  - **Fibrocartilage**: This tough form of cartilage absorbs shock in the spinal column, knees, and pelvic girdle.

  ▪ **Bone** is the most rigid type of connective tissue, with a high mineral content that makes it harder than other types. Bone tissue establishes the framework of the body. Bone consists of a matrix of connective tissue, blood vessels, and minerals (particularly calcium and phosphorus).

  - Bone marrow is the soft tissue that fills the inside of bones, and is the site of production of red blood cells, platelets, and most white blood cells.

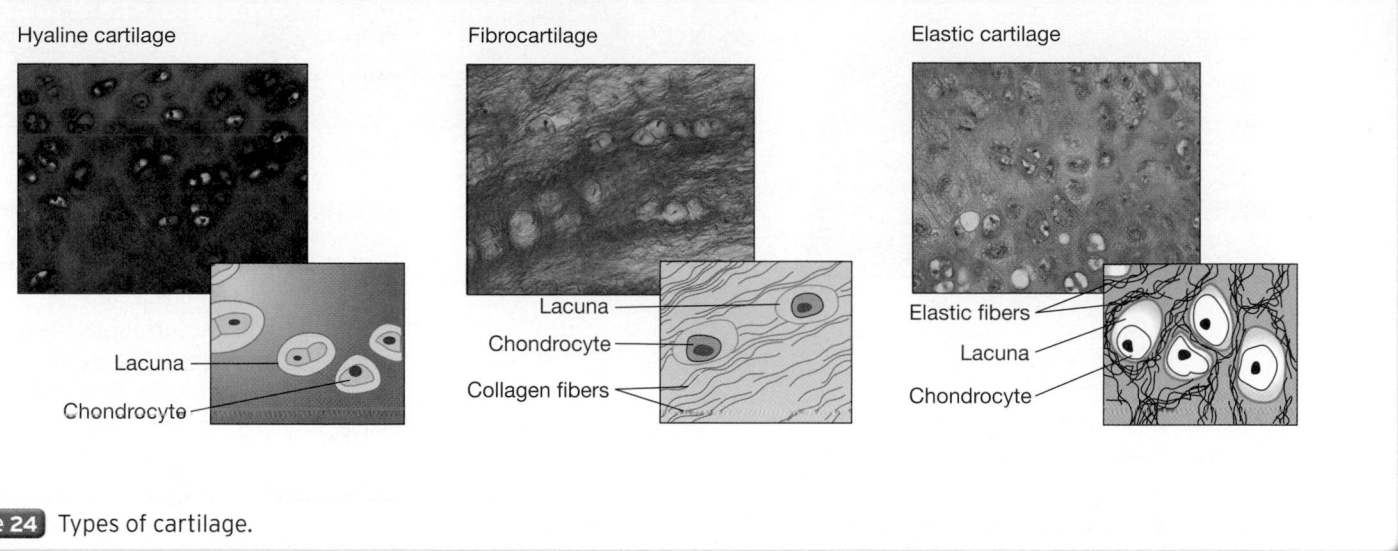

Hyaline cartilage

Fibrocartilage

Elastic cartilage

Lacuna

Chondrocyte

Lacuna

Chondrocyte

Collagen fibers

Elastic fibers

Lacuna

Chondrocyte

Figure 24 Types of cartilage.

- Bone cells, or <u>osteocytes</u>, contain a small amount of ground substance, but actually consist of a dense and mineralized matrix. The osteocytes, and layers of the extracellular matrix, form a cylinder-shaped osteon (also called a Haversian system). Many osteons that are cemented together form the substance of bone. The matrix consists of calcium salts and collagen fibers. Bones attach to muscles, and protect as well as support vital body structures.

3. Fluid connective tissues have distinctive populations of cells suspended in a water matrix. This contains dissolved proteins, and may be of two types: either blood or lymph. Blood and lymph are fluid connective tissues that contain distinctive collections of cells in a fluid matrix. They transport many materials between interior body cells and other cells that exchange substances with the external environment, maintaining a stable internal environment. Blood contains formed elements (red blood cells, white blood cells, and platelets), which are suspended in a liquid extracellular matrix known as blood plasma. Together, the formed elements and blood plasma make up the blood. Most blood cells are formed in the red bone marrow. Lymph forms as interstitial fluid enters the lymphatic vessels, which return the lymph to the cardiovascular system.

Muscle Tissues

Muscle tissues can contract by shortening their elongated muscle fibers. This action moves body parts. The three types of muscle tissue are skeletal muscle tissue, smooth muscle tissue, and cardiac muscle tissue.

1. <u>Skeletal muscle tissue</u>: Known as voluntary muscle tissue because it is found in muscles controlled by conscious effort; it attaches to bones and is composed of long thread-like cells that have light and dark markings called striations **Figure 25** . These multinucleated muscle cells

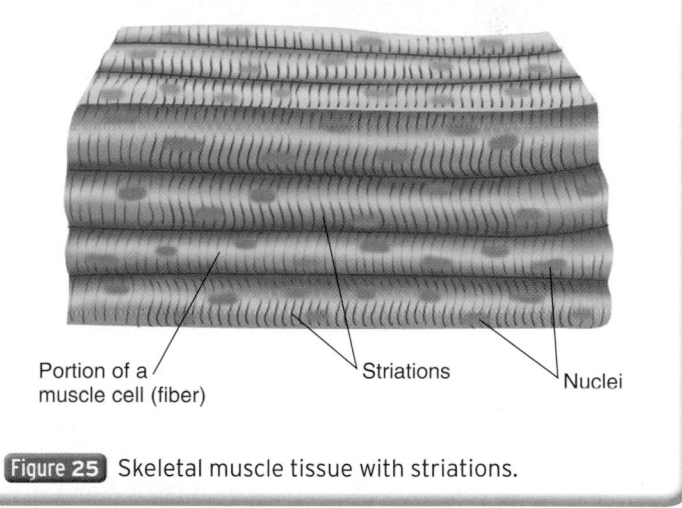

Portion of a muscle cell (fiber)

Striations

Nuclei

Figure 25 Skeletal muscle tissue with striations.

contract when stimulated by nerve cells. Skeletal muscle tissue moves the head, trunk, and limbs, allowing all voluntary movements in these body areas.

2. <u>Smooth muscle tissue</u>: Composed of elongated, spindle-shaped cells in muscles not under voluntary control. Smooth muscle fibers are shorter than striated fibers, having only one nucleus per spindle-shaped fiber. They are also called nonstriated involuntary muscles or unstriated muscles **Figure 26** . Smooth muscle cells can divide; therefore, they regenerate after being injured. Smooth muscle tissue composes hollow internal organ walls (such as the intestines, stomach, urinary bladder, blood vessels, and uterus). Smooth muscle cannot, in most cases, be controlled by conscious effort. This type of tissue moves food through the digestive tract, empties the urinary bladder, and constricts blood vessels.

3. <u>Cardiac muscle tissue</u>: Also called myocardium; it is a thick contractile middle layer of the heart wall. The contractile tissue of the myocardium is composed of fibers with

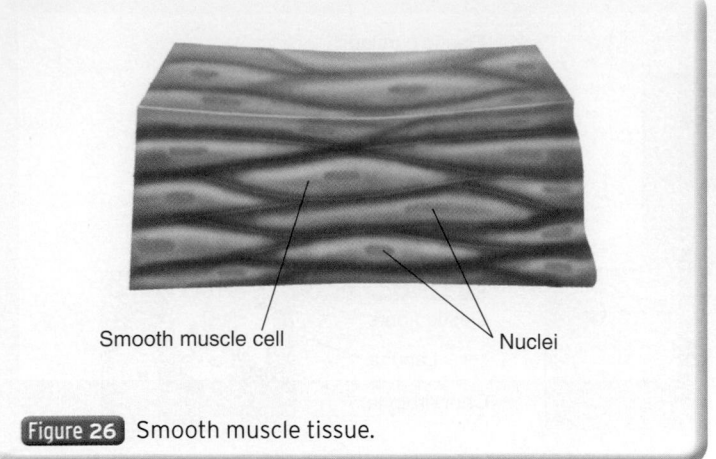

Figure 26 Smooth muscle tissue.

the characteristic cross-striations of muscular tissue. These striations branch frequently and are interconnected, forming a network. Myocardial muscle contains less connective tissue than skeletal muscle. Cardiac muscle is involuntary, and makes up most of the heart. Cardiac muscle relies on pacemaker cells or nodes of tissue in the conduction system for regular contraction. Under the right circumstances each cardiac tissue has the ability to generate an impulse. This property is known as automaticity and may be caused by hypoxia or electrolyte imbalance in the cardiac cells.

Nervous Tissues

Nervous tissues are specialized for the conduction of electrical impulses from one region of the body to another. Nervous tissues contain two basic types of cells: (1) neurons, and (2) several kinds of supporting cells, collectively called neuroglia, or glial cells. Nervous tissues are found in the brain, peripheral nerves, and spinal cord; the basic cells of these tissues are the neurons (nerve cells). **Neurons** are the basic structure of neural tissue that respond to environmental changes by transmitting impulses along axons (cellular processes) to other neurons, to muscles, or to glands. Neurons coordinate, integrate, and regulate a wide variety of functions in the body.

Neuroglial cells are crucial to neuronal functioning. These cells divide and support nervous tissue components. Neuroglial cells also phagocytize other cells and supply nutrients to neurons and help in communications between cells. The four types of neuroglia are astrocytes, oligodendroglia, microglia, and ependymal cells.

Types of Membranes

Membranes form a barrier or an interface. **Epithelial membranes** are thin structures made up of epithelium and underlying connective tissue. They cover body surfaces and line body cavities. The four types of membranes are as follows (Table 8):

1. **Serous membrane**: Lines body cavities that lack openings to the outside of the body. They form a fluid called a transudate. Serous membranes line the thorax and

Table 8 Membranes or Covering of the Body's Organs

Type	Name	Location
Serous membrane	Visceral pleura	Inner lining covering the lungs
	Parietal pleura	Outer lining separating the visceral pleura and the interior of the chest wall
	Pericardium	Surrounds the heart
	Peritoneum	Surrounds the abdominal organs
	Meninges	Coverings between the brain and skull
Synovial membrane	Knee capsule	Surrounds the synovial fluid contained in the knee joint
Mucous membrane	Oral mucosa	Soft, mucus-producing membranes lining the nose and mouth
Cutaneous membrane	Skin	All exterior surfaces of the body
	Periosteum	Surrounds mature bone
	Perichondrium	Surrounds developing bone

abdomen, as well as forming the visceral pleura and visceral peritoneum. Serous membranes consist of simple squamous epithelium and loose connective tissue, and secrete serous fluid, which lubricates membrane surfaces.

2. **Mucous membrane**: Lines body cavities that open to the outside of the body including the nose and mouth as well as digestive, respiratory, urinary, and reproductive tubes. Mucous membranes consist of epithelium above loose connective tissue, with goblet cells that secrete mucus.

3. **Cutaneous membrane**: The skin, which covers the body surface.

4. **Synovial membrane**: Forms an incomplete lining within the cavities of the synovial joints. It is entirely made up of connective tissues.

Organ Systems

In each organ system of the human body, organs work together to maintain homeostasis. These organ systems include the skeletal, muscular, respiratory, circulatory, lymphatic, nervous, integumentary, digestive, endocrine, urinary, and genital systems (Figure 27).

The Skeletal System: Anatomy

The **skeleton** gives us our recognizable human form and protects our vital internal organs. Bones constitute the major structure

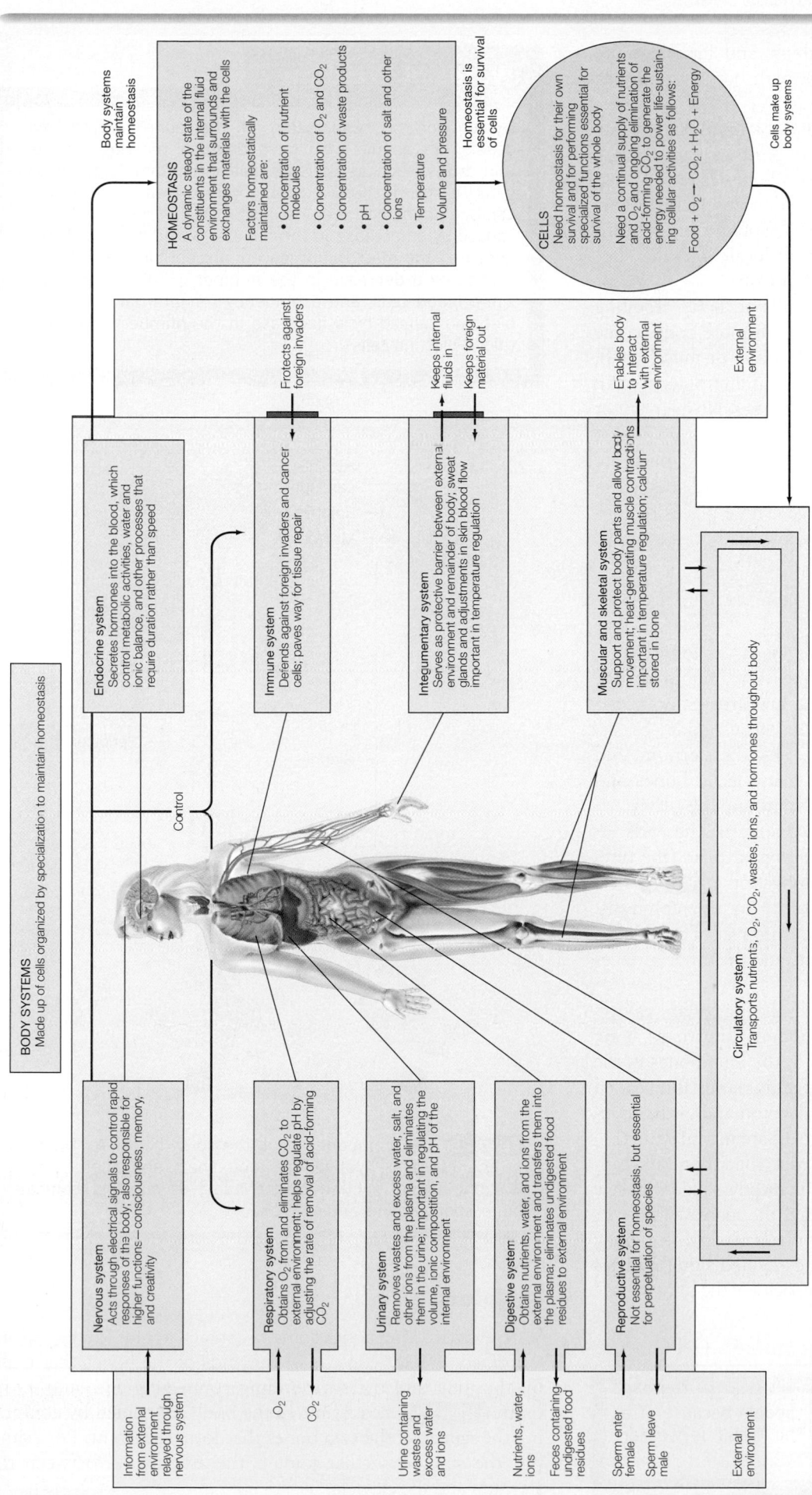

Figure 27 Systems of the body.

of the skeletal system. Cartilage, tendons, and ligaments are important connective tissues that work with bones to provide the support framework of the skeleton.

Tendons are specialized tough cords or bands of dense white connective tissue that connect muscles to bones. Ligaments are tough white bands of tissue that connect bones to each other. Tendons and ligaments are composed of densely packed fibers of collagen, a twisted rope-like protein. A sprain occurs when the bone ends partially or temporarily dislocate and the supporting ligaments are partially stretched or torn.

When a muscle contracts, tendon pulls on bone, resulting in motion at the joint, the point where two or more bones come together, allowing movement to occur. A strain, or muscle pull, occurs when a muscle is stretched or torn. A strain results in pain, swelling, and bruising of surrounding soft tissues. No ligament or joint damage occurs with a strain. Sprains and strains are graded based on their severity and physical findings during examination.

Cartilage covers the ends of the bones where they form joints and is known as articular cartilage. These pieces of connective tissue provide cushioning and allow the bones to move smoothly against each other.

■ Overview of Bones

Bones are classified according to their shape, as long bones, short bones, flat bones, and irregular bones. Long bones include the femur, tibia, fibula, ulna, radius, and humerus. Short bones include the carpal (wrist) bones and the tarsal (ankle) bones. Flat bones include certain skull bones, ribs, the sternum, and the scapulae. Irregular bones include many facial bones and those that make up the vertebrae in the spine and the pelvis.

Long bones consist of a shaft, the diaphysis; the ends, or epiphyses; and the growth plate or epiphyseal plate (the physis), which is the major site of bone elongation **Figure 28**. The epiphyseal plate is located just proximal to the epiphysis. The periosteum, which consists of a double layer of connective tissue, lines the outer surface of the bone, and the inner surfaces are lined with endosteum.

The diaphysis of many bones includes the medullary cavity, an internal cavity that contains a substance known as bone marrow. In adults, most bone marrow in the long bones in the extremities contains adipose (fat) tissue and is, therefore, called yellow marrow. The bones of the axial skeleton and girdles contain red marrow, where most red blood cells are manufactured.

The two main types of bone are compact (solid) bone and cancellous (spongy) bone. Compact bone is mostly solid, with few spaces and contains a central space called the marrow cavity or marrow canal. Cancellous bone consists of a lacy network of bony rods called trabeculae. The trabeculae are oriented along the lines of stress to increase the weight-bearing capacity of the long bones.

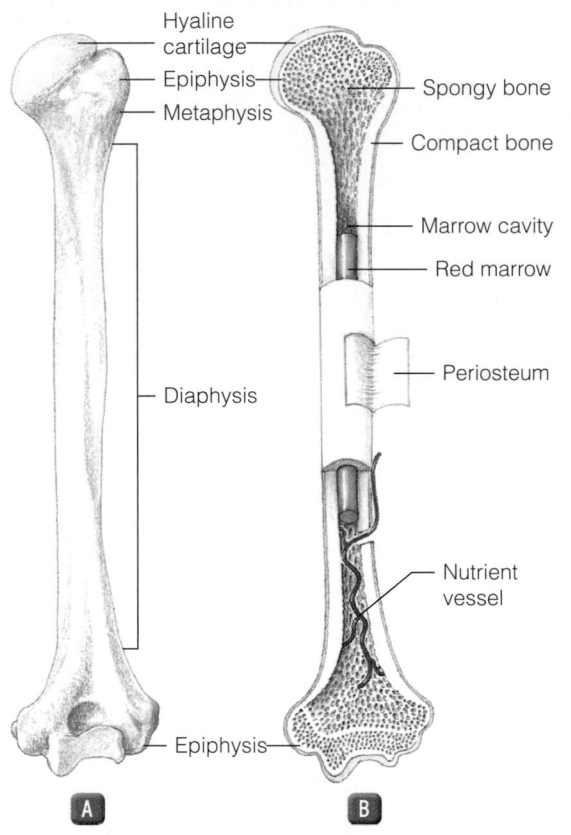

Figure 28 The components of the long bone. **A.** Drawing of the humerus. Notice the long shaft and dilated ends. **B.** Longitudinal section of the humerus showing compact bone, spongy bone, and marrow.

■ Joints

Wherever two long bones come in contact, a joint (articulation) is formed. A joint consists of the ends of the bones that make up the joint and the surrounding connecting and supporting tissue **Figure 29**. Most joints in the body are named by combining the names of the two bones that form that joint. For example, the sternoclavicular joint is the articulation between the sternum and the clavicle.

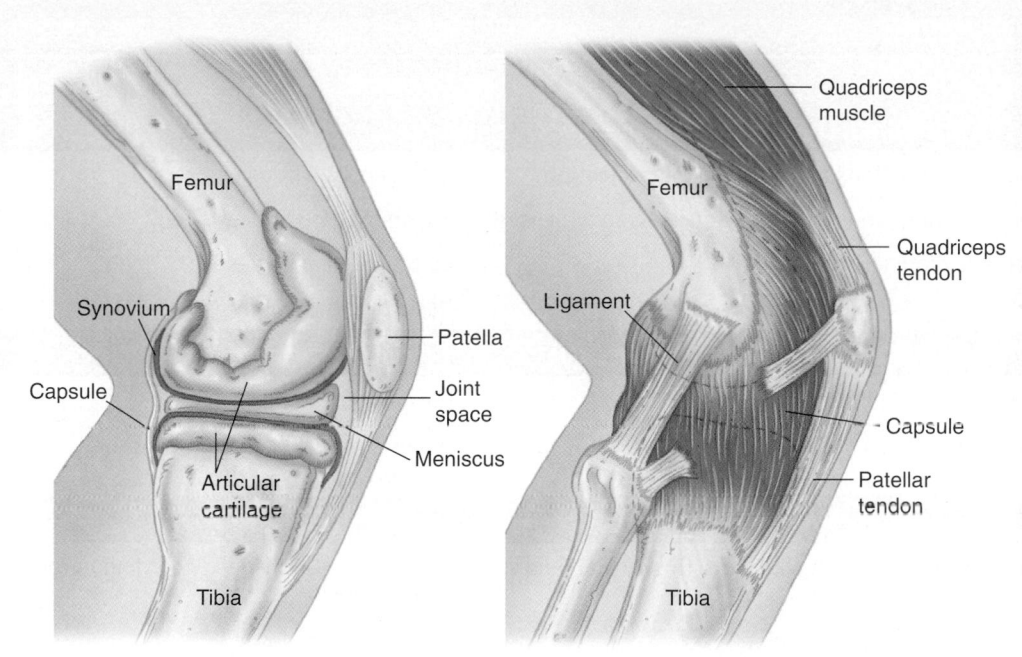

Figure 29 A joint consists of bone ends, the fibrous joint capsule, the synovial membrane, and ligaments. The degree to which a joint can move is determined by how the ligaments hold the bone ends and by the configuration of the bones themselves.

Joints are classified as slightly moveable (amphiarthrotic), freely movable (diarthrotic), or immovable (synarthrotic). Most joints allow motion—for example, the knee, hip, and elbow—whereas some bones fuse with one another at joints to form a solid, immobile, bony structure. For example, the skull is composed of several bones that fuse as a child grows. Some joints have slight, limited motion in which the bone ends are held together by fibrous tissue. Such a joint is called a **symphysis**.

Joints can also be grouped according to the type of tissue binding them at their junctions. These groups include fibrous, cartilaginous, and synovial joints. **Table 9** shows functional classification of joints.

The 230 joints in the human body are summarized as follows:

- **Fibrous joints**: Lying between bones that closely contact each other, they are joined by thin, dense connective tissue **Figure 30**. An example of a fibrous joint is a suture between flat bones of the skull. No real movement takes place in most fibrous joints, making them synarthrotic in classification. Those with limited movement (amphiarthrotic) include the joint between the distal tibia and fibula.
- **Cartilaginous joints**: Connected by hyaline cartilage, or fibrocartilage, these joints include those that separate the vertebrae. Each intervertebral disk is an example of a cartilaginous joint, and has slight flexibility.
- **Synovial joints**: These joints allow free movement (diarthrotic) and are more complex than other types of joints. They have an outer layer of ligaments (the joint capsule) and an inner lining of synovial membrane that secretes synovial fluid, which lubricates the joint **Figure 31**. Some

synovial joints have shock-absorbing fibrocartilage pads called menisci. They may also have fluid-filled sacs (bursae), commonly located between tendons and underlying bony prominences such as in the knee or elbow.

Synovial joints are classified as follows **Figure 32**:

- *Ball-and-socket joints: Such as in* the shoulders and hips
- *Condyloid (ellipsoidal) joints:* Such as between the metacarpals and phalanges
- *Gliding (plane) joints:* Such as in the wrists and ankles
- *Hinge joints:* Such as in the elbow and phalanges
- *Pivot joints:* Such as between the proximal ends of the radius and ulna
- *Saddle joints:* Such as between the carpal and metacarpal bones of the thumb

The bone ends of a joint are held together by a fibrous sac called the **joint capsule**. This sac is composed of ligaments (bone to bone). At certain points around the circumference of the joint, the capsule is lax and thin so motion can occur. In other areas, it is quite thick and resists stretching or bending. A joint that is virtually surrounded by tough, thick ligaments will have little motion, whereas a joint such as the shoulder, with few ligaments, will be free to move in almost any direction (and will, as a result, be more prone to dislocation). On the inner lining of the joint capsule is the synovial membrane. This special tissue makes a thick lubricant called **synovial fluid**. This "oil" allows the ends of the bones to glide over each other as opposed to rubbing and grating over each other. Synovial fluid contains white blood cells to fight infections and provides nourishment to the cartilage covering the bone.

Growth and Development of Bones

Bones begin to form in utero during the first 6 weeks after fertilization. Intramembranous bones originate between layers of connective tissues that are sheet-like in appearance. Examples of intramembranous bones are the flat, broad bones of the skull. These bones begin development when unspecialized connective tissues form at the sites where future bones will be developed. Bone-forming cells (**osteoblasts**) develop, depositing bony matrix around them. When extracellular matrix has surrounded the osteoblasts, they are termed osteocytes. The surrounding membranous tissues begin to form the periosteum, or membrane that lines the surface of all bones. Inside the periosteum, the osteoblasts form a compact bone layer over the new spongy bone.

Endochondrial bones begin as cartilaginous masses that are eventually replaced by bone tissue. These bones develop

Table 9 Functional Classification of Joints

Category and Type	Description	Example
Amphiarthrosis (little movement)		
Fibrous: Suture	Fibrous connections and interlocking projections	Between skull bones
Fibrous: Gomphosis	Fibrous connections and insertion in alveolar process	Between teeth and jaws
Cartilaginous: Synchondrosis	Cartilage plate interposed	Epiphyseal cartilages
Bony fusion: Synostosis	Conversion of other joint forms to a solid bone mass	Parts of skull, epiphyseal lines
Diarthrosis (free movement)		
Fibrous: Syndesmosis	Connections of ligaments	Between tibia and fibula
Cartilaginous: Symphysis	Connections via a fibrocartilage pad	Between pubic bones of pelvis; between vertebrae
Synarthrosis (no movement)		
Synovial	Complex joint in a joint capsule with synovial fluid	Numerous; subdivided according to range of movement
Monaxial	Allows movement in one plane	Elbows and ankles
Biaxial	Allows movement in two planes	Ribs and waist
Triaxial	Allows movement in all three planes	Shoulders and hips

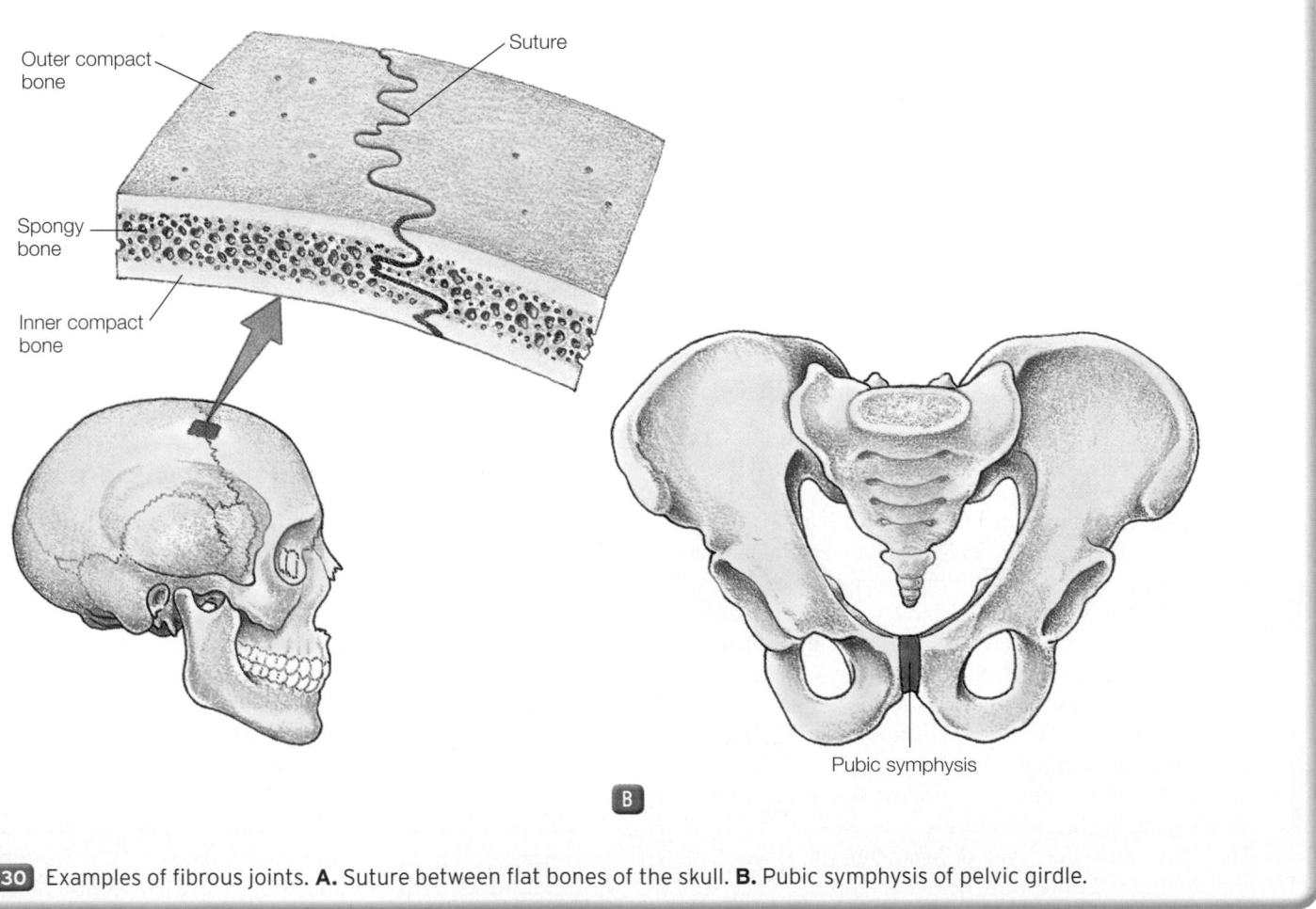

Figure 30 Examples of fibrous joints. **A.** Suture between flat bones of the skull. **B.** Pubic symphysis of pelvic girdle.

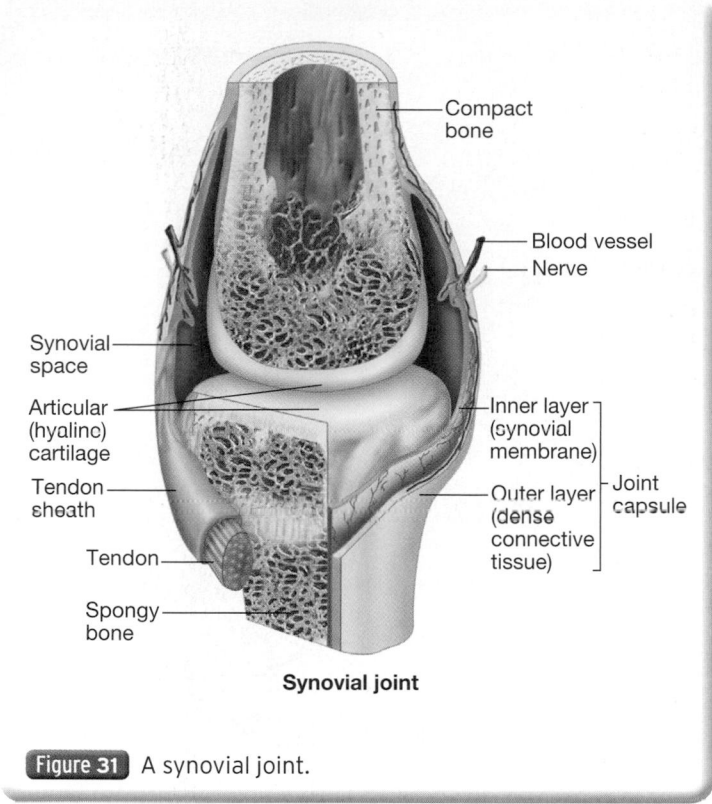

Figure 31 A synovial joint.

Labels on Figure 31:
- Compact bone
- Blood vessel
- Nerve
- Synovial space
- Articular (hyaline) cartilage
- Inner layer (synovial membrane)
- Tendon sheath
- Outer layer (dense connective tissue)
- Joint capsule
- Tendon
- Spongy bone

Synovial joint

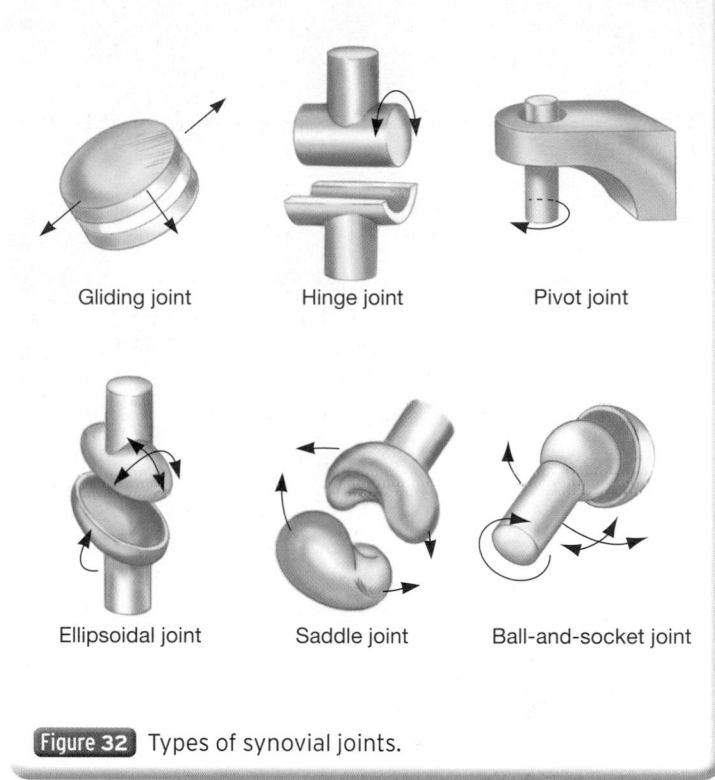

Figure 32 Types of synovial joints.

Labels on Figure 32:
- Gliding joint
- Hinge joint
- Pivot joint
- Ellipsoidal joint
- Saddle joint
- Ball-and-socket joint

from hyaline cartilage that is shaped similarly to the bones they will become. They grow rapidly at first, and then begin to change in appearance. When spongy bone begins to replace the original cartilage, a primary ossification center is created, with bone tissue developing outward toward the ends of the structure. Eventually, secondary ossification centers will appear in the epiphyses, forming more spongy bone.

During the first 6 weeks of fetal development, the skeleton is cartilaginous. The bones increase greatly in size as the fetus develops, and throughout childhood **Figure 33**. Bone growth continues through adolescence. The process of replacing other tissues with bone is called **ossification**, which involves the deposition of calcium salts.

Osteogenesis is defined as the formation of bone. Long bones are first formed of hyaline cartilage, and later replaced by bony tissue that becomes compact bone. This process begins with the diaphysis and ends with the epiphyses of each long bone. This process of bone formation is called **endochondrial ossification**.

Flat bones are not formed in this manner. These bones develop from connective tissue membranes that are replaced by spongy bone, and then compact bone. This process is called **intramembranous ossification**. In infants, fontanelles or "soft spots" are sheets of tough connective tissue between the flat bones of the skull; they are gradually replaced as the bones of the skull fuse together **Figure 34**.

When the bones are growing, the diaphyses meet the epiphyses at the epiphyseal plate. It is made of four cartilage layers: reserve cartilage, proliferating (hyperplastic) cartilage, hypertrophic cartilage, and the calcified matrix. Growth of long

bones depends on good nutrition and several hormones, including human growth hormone. Other hormones involved in long bone growth include thyroid hormone, estrogen, and testosterone **Table 10**. Once the epiphyseal plate experiences closure, the long bones can no longer grow **Figure 35**. Length of bone is balanced by increased bone width. Osteoblast and **osteoclast** activity is balanced in the body so that the bones grow with uniformity.

Bone development, growth, and repair are influenced by heredity, nutrition, hormones, and exercise. Vitamin D is required for the absorption of calcium in the small intestine. Without it, calcium is not absorbed well, softening bones and potentially causing deformity. Growth hormone from the pituitary gland stimulates cell division in the epiphyseal plates, and sex hormones stimulate ossification of these plates. Exercise stresses the bones, stimulating them to become thickened and strong.

■ The Axial Skeleton

The skeletal system is divided into two main portions: the **axial skeleton** and the **appendicular skeleton**. The axial skeleton forms the foundation on which the arms and legs are hung. The axial skeleton is composed of the skull, face, **thoracic cage**, and vertebral column. The arms and legs, their connection points, and the pelvis make up the appendicular skeleton. The brain lies within the skull. The heart, lungs, and great vessels are enclosed in the **thorax**, also called the thoracic cavity, which is part of the torso. Much of the liver and spleen are protected by the lower ribs. The spinal cord is contained within and protected by a bony spinal canal formed by the vertebrae.

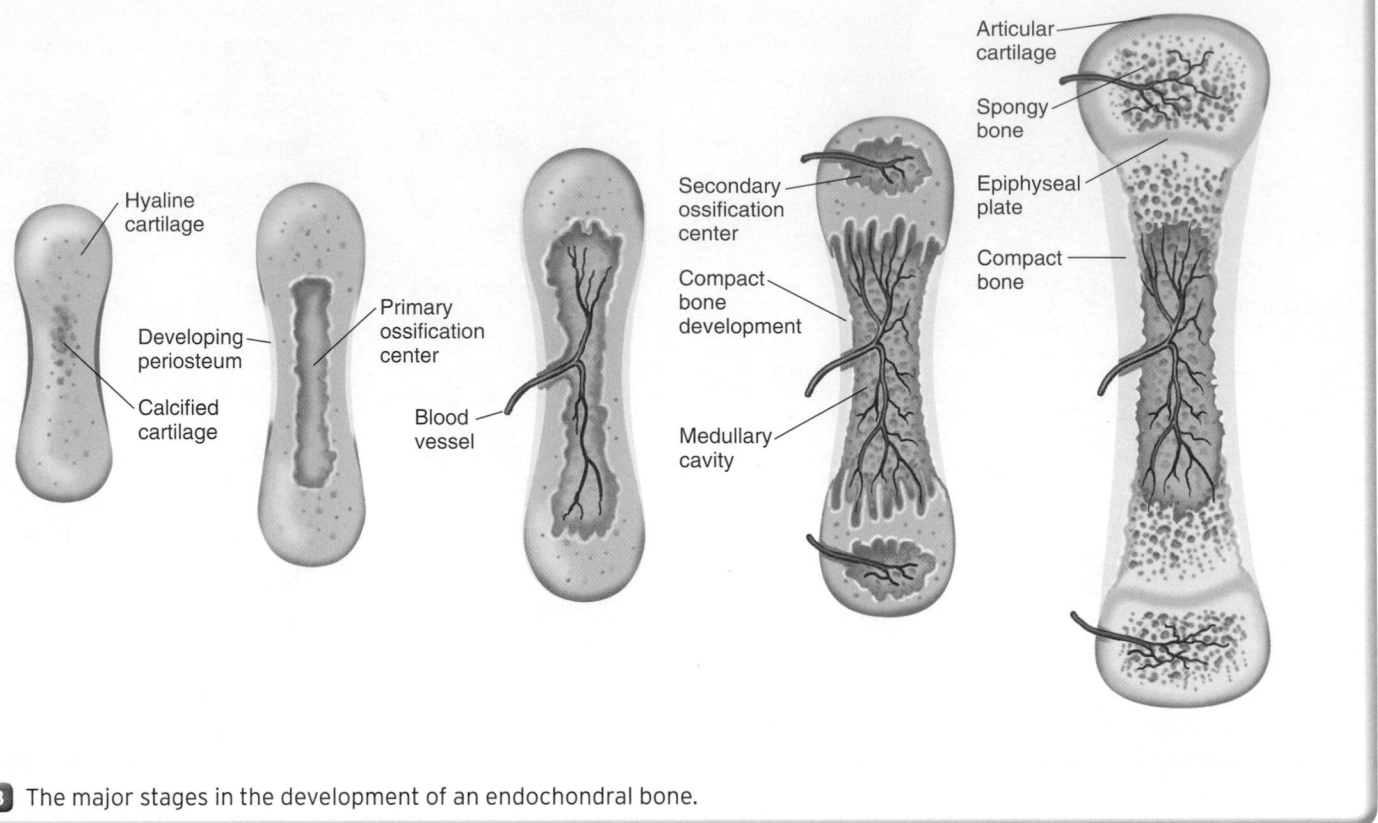

Figure 33 The major stages in the development of an endochondral bone.

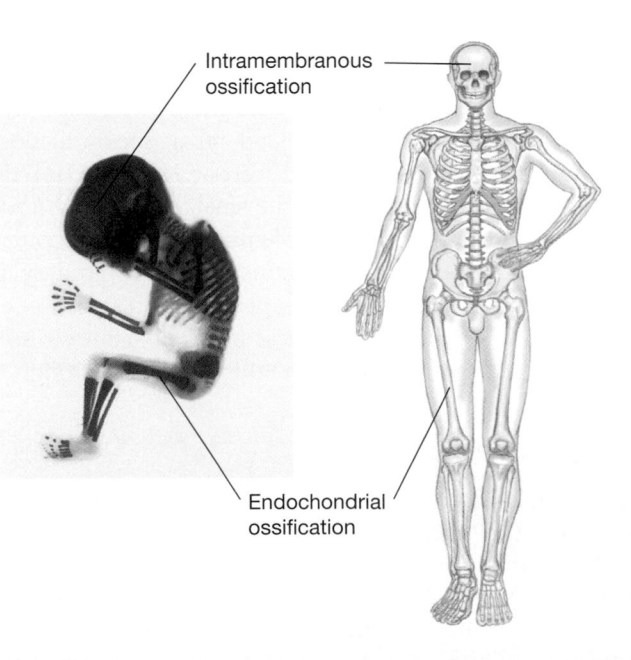

Figure 34 Intramembranous ossification results in the development of flat bones. Endochondral ossification results in the production of long bones.

Table 10 Hormones Involved in Bone Growth and Maintenance
• Human growth hormone
• Thyroxine
• Insulin
• Parathyroid hormone
• Calcitonin
• Estrogen
• Testosterone

The 206 bones of the skeleton provide a framework for the attachment of muscles **Figure 37**. The skeleton is also designed to allow motion of the body. Bones come into contact with one another at joints where, with the help of muscles, the body is able to bend and move.

The Skull

At the top of the axial skeleton is the <u>skull</u>, which consists of 28 bones in three anatomic groups: the auditory ossicles, the cranium, and the face. The six <u>auditory ossicles</u> function in hearing and are located, three on each side of the head, deep

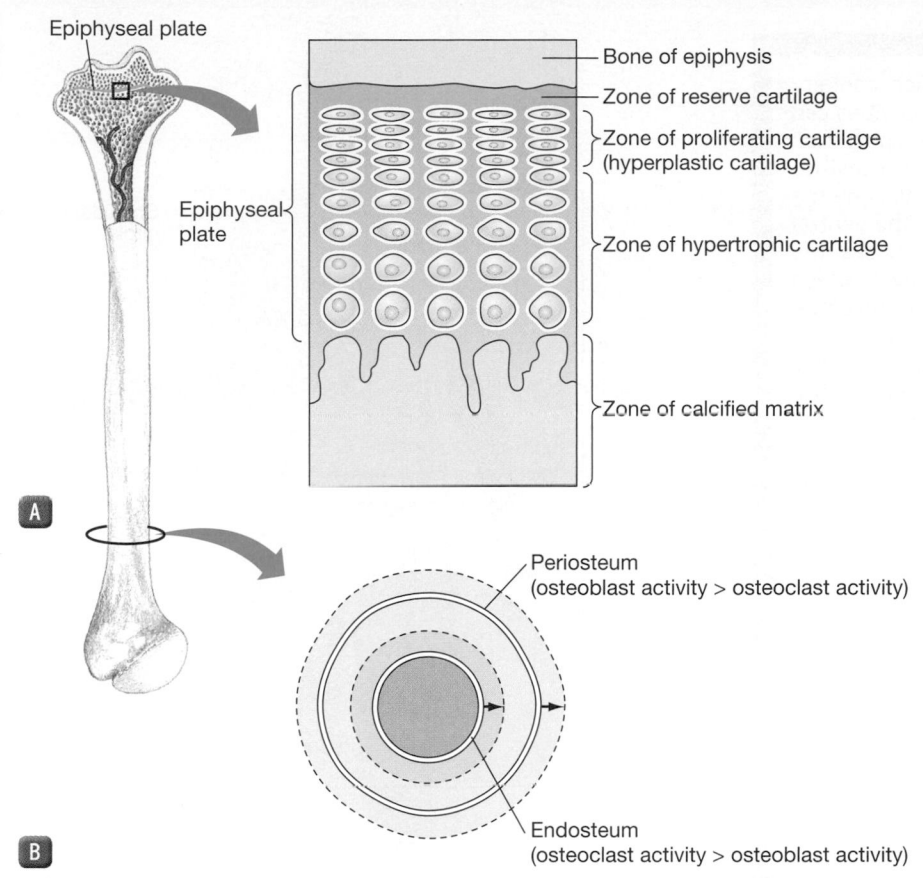

Epiphyseal plate

Epiphyseal plate

Bone of epiphysis

Zone of reserve cartilage

Zone of proliferating cartilage (hyperplastic cartilage)

Zone of hypertrophic cartilage

Zone of calcified matrix

A

Periosteum (osteoblast activity > osteoclast activity)

Endosteum (osteoclast activity > osteoblast activity)

B

Figure 35 **A.** Lengthwise growth occurs in the epiphyseal plate until puberty when the epiphyseal plate closes, becoming the epiphyseal line. **B.** Growth in diameter involves altered rates of osteoclast and osteoblast activity at the periosteum and endosteum.

The Floor of the Cranial Vault Viewed from above, the floor of the interior of the skull, or cranial vault, is divided into three compartments: the anterior fossa, middle fossa, and posterior fossa **Figure 40**.

The **crista galli** forms a prominent bony ridge in the center of the anterior fossa and is the point of attachment of the meninges, the three layers of membranes—the dura mater, arachnoid, and pia mater—that surround the brain. On either side of the crista galli is the **cribriform plate** of the ethmoid bone, the horizontal bone that is perforated with numerous openings (**foramina**) for the passage of the olfactory nerve filaments from the nasal cavity. The **olfactory bulb**, the cranial nerve for smell, sends projections through the foramina in the cribriform plate and into the **nasal cavity**, the chamber inside the nose that lies between the floor of the cranium and the roof of the mouth.

The Facial Bones The frontal and ethmoid bones are part of both the cranial vault and the face. The 14 facial bones form the structure of the face, without contributing to the cranial vault. These bones include the **maxillae**, mandible, **zygoma**, palatine, nasal, lacrimal, vomer, and inferior nasal concha bones.

within cavities of the temporal bone. The remaining 22 bones comprise the **cranium** and the face **Figure 38**.

The **cranial vault** consists of the eight bones that encase and protect the brain: the parietal, temporal, frontal, occipital, sphenoid, and ethmoid bones. The brain and the spinal cord are connected through a large opening at the base of the skull called the **foramen magnum**.

The bones of the skull are connected together at special joints known as **sutures** **Figure 39**. The paired parietal bones join together at the sagittal suture. The parietal bones abut the frontal bone at the coronal suture. The occipital bone attaches to the parietal bones at the lambdoid suture. Fibrous tissues called **fontanelles**, which soften and expand during childbirth, link the sutures. The tissue felt through the fontanelles are layers of the scalp and thick membranes overlying the brain. Under normal conditions, the brain may not be felt through the fontanelles. By the time a child reaches age 2 years, the sutures should have solidified and the fontanelles closed.

At the base of the temporal bone is a cone-shaped section of bone known as the **mastoid process**. This area is an important site for attachment of various muscles.

Words of Wisdom

Fractures of the cribriform plate result in leakage of cerebrospinal fluid (CSF) from the nose. CSF is the fluid that bathes and provides hydraulic cushioning to the brain and spinal cord. Leakage of clear, watery fluid from the nose following head trauma suggests leakage of CSF. The patient found in the seated position may complain of a salty taste in his or her throat. This is due to the high salt content of the CSF.

The facial bones protect the eyes, nose, and tongue and provide attachment points for the muscles that allow chewing. The zygomatic process of the temporal bone and the temporal process of the zygomatic bone form the zygomatic arch **Figure 41**. The zygomatic arch lends shape to the cheeks.

Bones of the Orbit The **orbits** are cone-shaped fossae that enclose and protect the eyes. In addition to the eyeball and muscles that move it, the orbit contains blood vessels, nerves,

Words of Wisdom

The human body contains several cavities, each containing various organs and other structures. These cavities can be grouped into dorsal cavities, which are more posterior, and ventral cavities, which are anterior. The dorsal cavities include the cranial cavity, which contains the brain, and the spinal cavity, which surrounds the spinal cord. The ventral cavities include the thoracic cavity, which encloses the heart, lungs, and great vessels; the abdominal cavity, which holds several digestive and endocrine organs; and the pelvic cavity, which also contains many digestive organs as well as the female reproductive organs. The abdominal and pelvic cavities can be referred to together as the abdominopelvic cavity **Figure 36** . Another cavity is the retroperitoneal cavity, which is separate from and lies posterior to the abdominal cavity and contains fewer organs, most notably the kidneys.

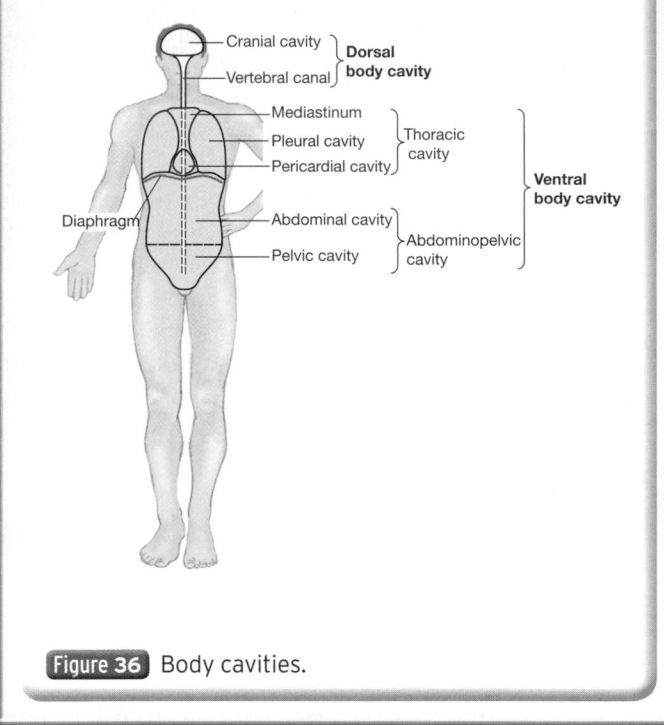

Figure 36 Body cavities.

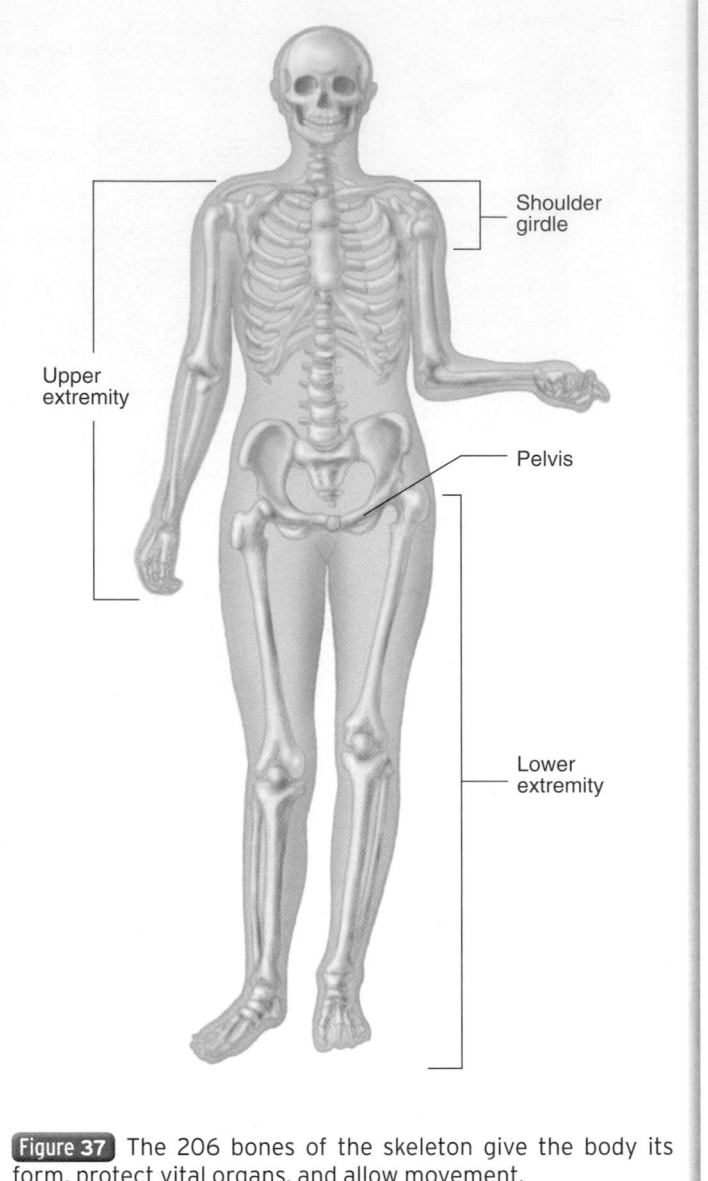

Figure 37 The 206 bones of the skeleton give the body its form, protect vital organs, and allow movement.

and fat. The frontal, sphenoid, zygomatic, maxilla, lacrimal, ethmoid, and palatine bones each form portions of the orbits.

A blow to the eye may result in fracture of the floor of the orbit. This bone is extremely thin and breaks easily. The result is transmission of forces away from the eyeball itself to the bone. Blood and fat then leak into the maxillary sinus below. This type of fracture is called a blowout fracture.

Bones of the Nose The nasal cavity comprises portions of several of the facial bones, including the frontal, nasal, sphenoid, ethmoid, inferior nasal concha, maxilla, palatine, and vomer bones. The <u>nasal septum</u> is the separation between the nostrils and is

located in the midline. Often, it bulges slightly to one side or the other. The external portion of the nose is formed mostly of cartilage.

Several of the bones associated with the nose contain cavities known as the <u>paranasal sinuses</u>, or sinuses. These hollowed sections of bone decrease the weight of the skull as well as provide resonance for the voice. The contents of the sinuses drain into the nasal cavity. Lining the inside of the sinuses and nasal cavity is ciliated epithelium, which helps to trap foreign material and move it down to the throat where it can be entered into the digestive system. Sinusitis is an inflammation of the paranasal sinuses that is relatively common. Sinusitis may range in severity from a simple upper respiratory tract infection consisting of headache and nasal drainage to a potentially life-threatening brain infection, depending on the extent of the infection and which sinuses are affected.

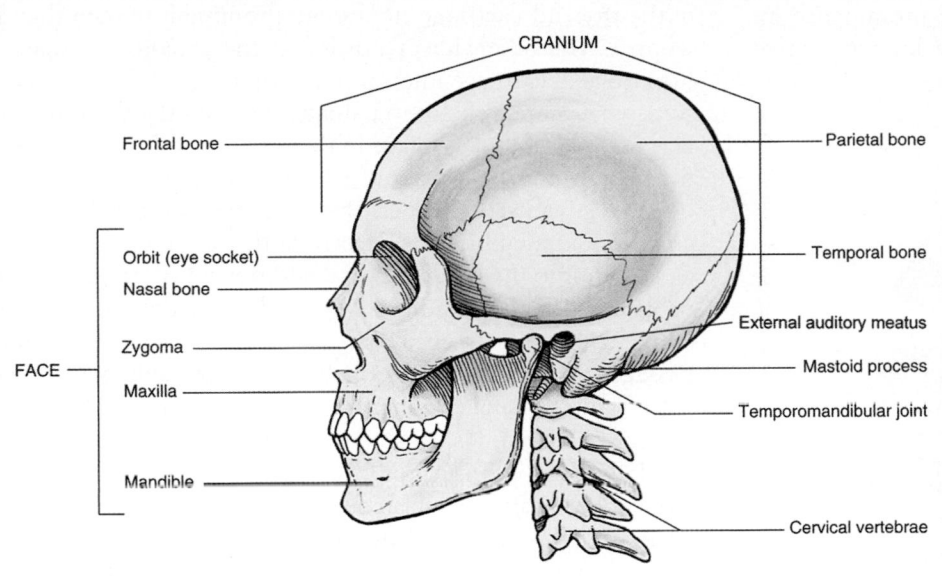

Figure 38 The skull consists of 28 bones in three anatomic groups: the auditory ossicles, the cranium, and the face.

The Mandible and Temporomandibular Joint The <u>mandible</u> is the large movable bone comprising the lower jaw and containing the lower teeth. Numerous muscles of chewing attach to the mandible. The posterior condyle of the mandible articulates with the temporal bone at a condyloid joint known as the <u>temporomandibular joint (TMJ)</u>. This joint, which is formed when a rounded bone fits into a similarly curved fossa, allows many different movements of the mandible.

The Hyoid Bone The <u>hyoid bone</u> "floats" in the superior aspect of the neck just below the mandible. It is not actually part of the skull, but it supports the tongue and serves as a point of attachment for many important neck and tongue muscles. When damaged by a blow to the anterior neck, the patient may have a hoarse and low volume voice due to airway swelling.

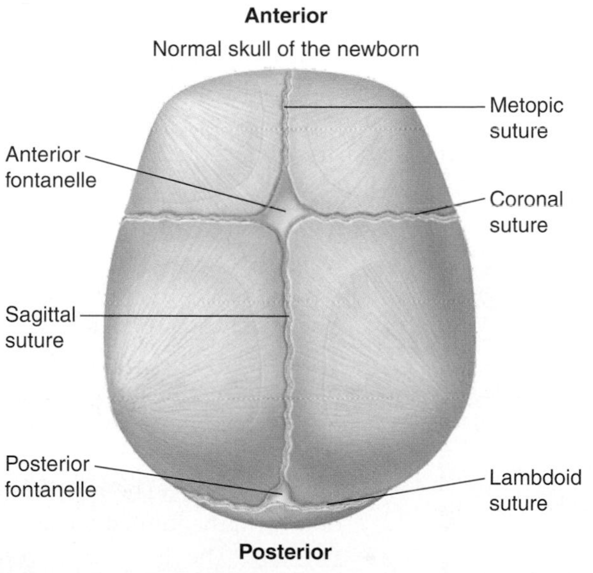

The Neck

The neck contains many important structures. It is supported by the cervical spine, or the first seven vertebrae in the spinal column (C1 through C7). The spinal cord exits from the foramen magnum and lies within the spinal canal formed by the vertebrae. The upper part of the esophagus and the trachea (windpipe) lie in the midline of the neck. The carotid arteries are found on either side of the trachea, along with the jugular veins and several nerves.

Figure 39 The sutures of the skull.

Bones of the Ear Contained within the middle ear are the ossicles, three tiny auditory bones responsible for converting sound waves collected by the eardrum into pressure waves transmitted to the cochlea. These bones are known as the hammer, anvil, and stirrup for their shapes, or by the Latin names for their shape, the malleus, incus, and stapes, respectively.

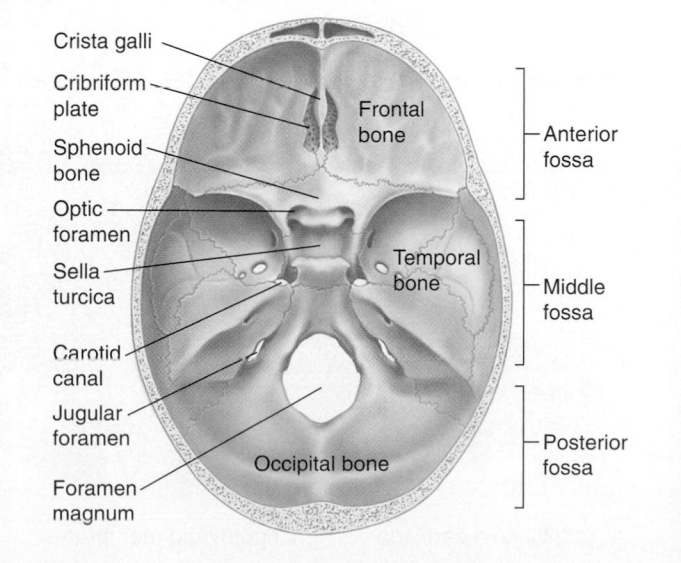

Figure 40 The floor of the cranial vault and its anatomy.

Several useful landmarks can be palpated and seen in the neck Figure 42 . The most obvious is the firm prominence in the center of the anterior surface commonly known as the Adam's apple. Specifically, this prominence is the upper part of the **thyroid cartilage**. It is more prominent in men than in women. The other, lower portion is the **cricoid cartilage**, a firm ridge of cartilage inferior to the thyroid cartilage, which is somewhat more difficult to palpate. Between the thyroid cartilage and the cricoid cartilage in the midline of the neck is a soft depression, the **cricothyroid membrane**. This is a thin sheet of connective tissue (**fascia**) that joins the two cartilages. The cricothyroid membrane is covered at this point only by skin.

Inferior to the larynx, several additional firm ridges are palpable in the anterior midline. These ridges are the cartilage rings of the trachea. The trachea connects the larynx with the main air passages of the lungs (the bronchi). On either side of the lower larynx and the upper trachea lies the thyroid gland. Unless it is enlarged, this gland is usually not palpable.

Pulsations of the carotid arteries are easily palpable in a groove about half an inch lateral to the larynx. Lying immediately adjacent to these arteries, but not palpable, are the internal jugular veins and several important nerves. Lateral to these vessels and nerves lie the **sternocleidomastoid muscles**, which allow movement of the head. These muscles originate from the mastoid process of the cranium and insert into the medial border of each collarbone and the **sternum** (breastbone) at the base of the neck.

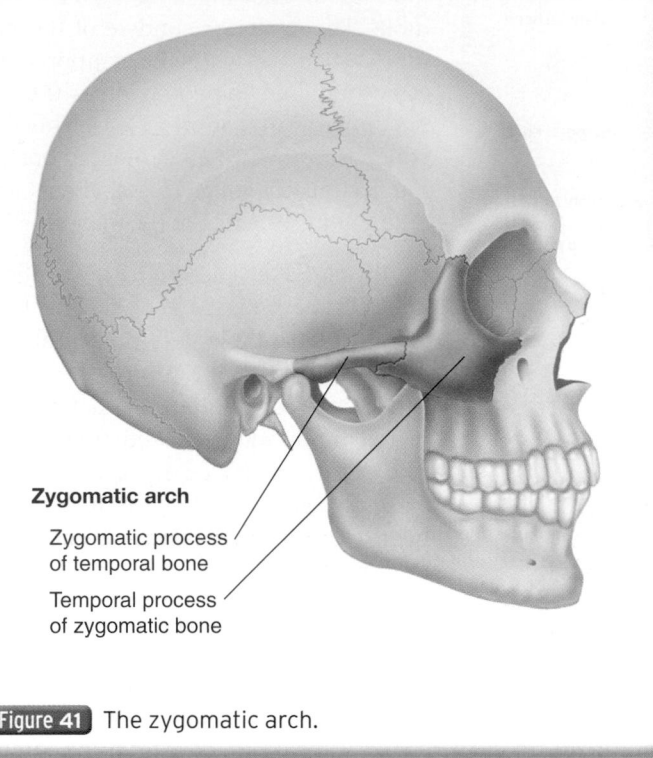

Zygomatic arch

Zygomatic process of temporal bone

Temporal process of zygomatic bone

Figure 41 The zygomatic arch.

Thyroid cartilage

Carotid arteries

Sternocleido-mastoid muscle

Cricoid cartilage

Cricothyroid membrane

Trachea

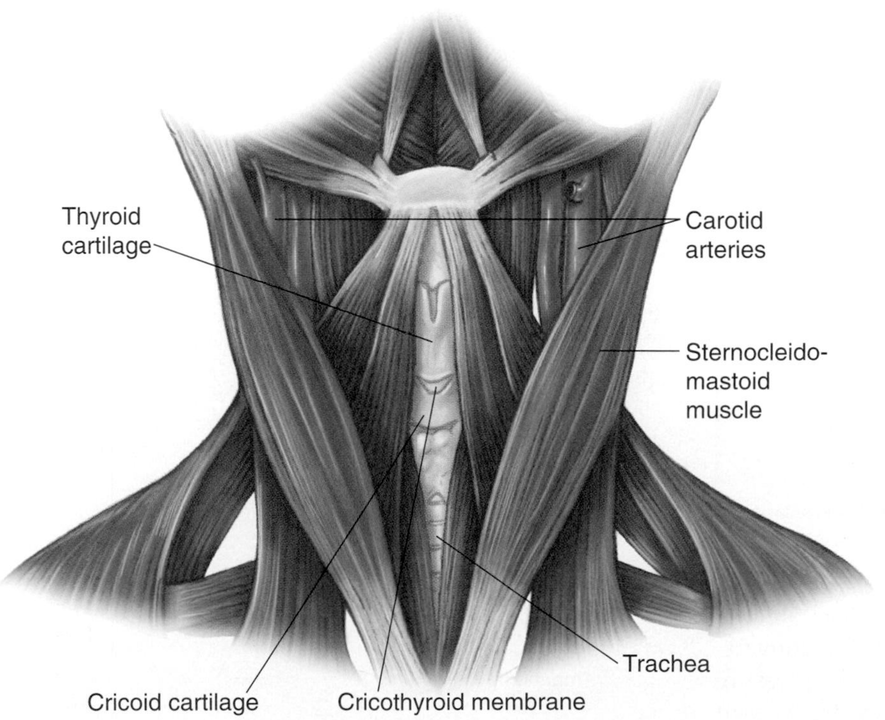

Figure 42 The principal structures of the neck include the trachea, along with many blood vessels, muscles, and nerves.

The Spinal Column

The spinal column, or **vertebral column**, is the central supporting structure of the body and is composed of 33 bones, each called a vertebra. The **vertebrae** are named according to the section of the spine in which they lie and are numbered from top to bottom Figure 43 . From the top down, the spine is divided into five sections:

- **Cervical spine**. The first seven vertebrae (C1 through C7) in the neck form the cervical spine. The skull rests on the first cervical vertebra (the atlas) and articulates with it.
- **Thoracic spine**. The next 12 vertebrae make up the thoracic spine. One pair of ribs is attached to each of the thoracic vertebrae.
- **Lumbar spine**. The next five vertebrae form the lumbar spine.
- **Sacrum**. The five sacral vertebrae are fused together to form one bone called the sacrum. The sacrum is joined to the iliac bones of the pelvis with strong ligaments at the sacro-iliac joints to form the pelvis.
- **Coccyx**. The last four vertebrae, also fused together, form the coccyx, or tailbone.

The first cervical vertebra (C1) is called the **atlas**. The atlas is located directly beneath the skull and provides support for the head. The atlas articulates with the occipital condyles at the base of

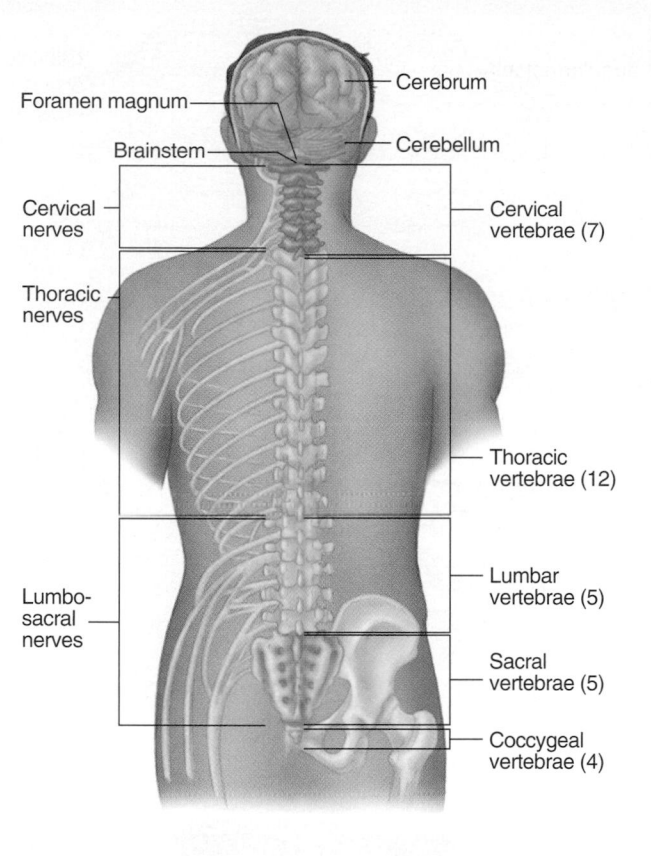

Figure 43 The spinal column is composed of 33 bones divided into five sections.

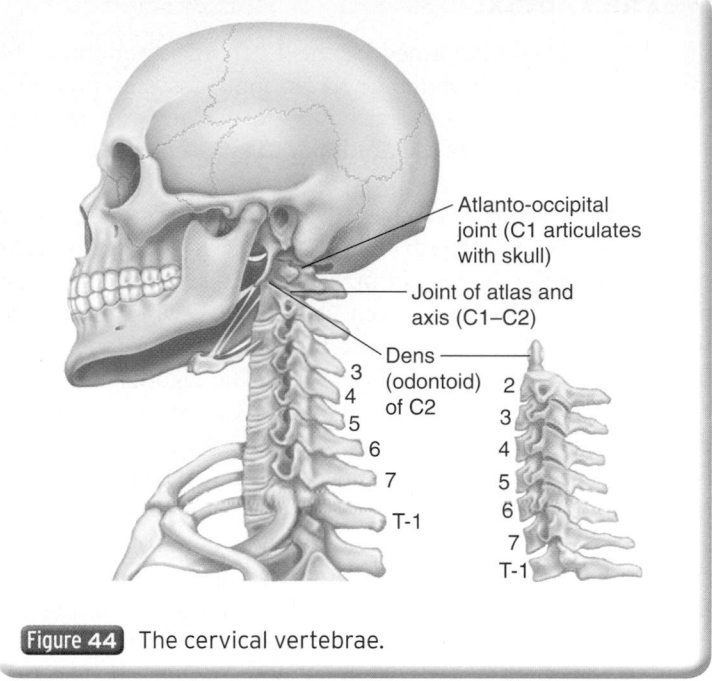

Figure 44 The cervical vertebrae.

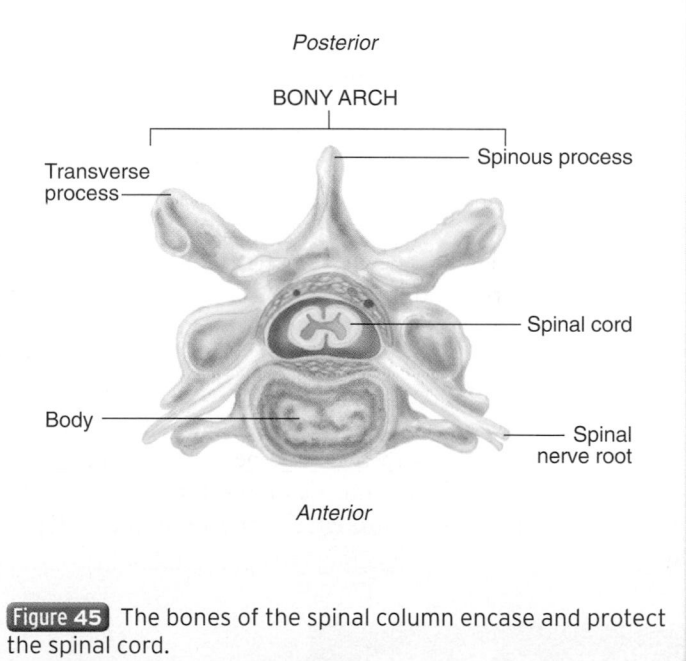

Figure 45 The bones of the spinal column encase and protect the spinal cord.

the skull at the **atlanto-occipital joint**. The only motions of this joint are flexion and extension and lateral bending.

The second cervical vertebra (C2) is known as the **axis** and is the point at which the head rotates, such as when moving the head from left to right. A large offshoot of C2 is the dens, or odontoid process, which fits into the enlarged vertebral foramen of the atlas. The atlas rotates around the axis at the dens. The cervical vertebrae numbered C3 through C6 form the cervical curve. C7, called the vertebra prominens, is different. It has a large spinous process that may be seen and felt at the base of the neck **Figure 44**.

The spinal cord is an extension of the brain, composed of virtually all the nerves that carry messages between the brain and the rest of the body. It exits through a large hole in the base of the skull called the foramen magnum and is contained within and protected by the vertebrae of the spinal column. The spinal column is virtually surrounded by muscles. However, the posterior spinous process of each vertebra can be felt as it lies just under the skin in the midline of the back.

The anterior part of each vertebra consists of a round, solid block of bone called the body. The posterior part of each vertebra forms a bony arch. This series of arches from one vertebra to the next forms a tunnel that runs the length of the spine called the spinal canal. The bones of the spinal canal encase and protect the spinal cord **Figure 45**. Nerves branch from the spinal cord and exit from the spinal canal between each vertebra to form the motor and sensory nerves of the body.

The vertebrae are connected by ligaments, and between each vertebra is a cushion called the intervertebral disk. These ligaments and disks allow some motion so the trunk can bend forward (flex) and back (extend), and they allow for rotation and lateral movement. However, they also limit motion of the vertebrae so that the spinal cord will not be injured. An injury to the spine may damage part of the spinal cord and its nerves that may not be protected by the vertebrae. Therefore, until the injury is stabilized, you must use extreme caution in caring for the patient to prevent injury to the spinal cord.

■ The Thorax

The thorax (chest) is formed by the 12 thoracic vertebrae (T1 through T12). These vertebrae have long transverse processes that, along with the vertebral bodies, articulate with the first 10 ribs. The presence of the ribs limits the movement of the thoracic spine.

One pair of ribs is attached to each thoracic vertebra. These 12 pairs of ribs form the rib cage Figure 46 . The rib cage protects organs within the thorax and prevents collapse of the chest during breathing. The upper seven pairs of ribs, which are called the true ribs, articulate with the thoracic vertebrae and attach directly to the sternum, or breastbone. The eighth, ninth, and tenth ribs attach to the inferior portion of the preceding rib's cartilage instead of the sternum itself. These are referred to as false ribs. The remaining two pairs of ribs, called floating ribs, are held in place by cartilage and have no attachment to the sternum.

Anteriorly, in the midline of the chest is the sternum. The superior border of the sternum forms the easily palpable jugular notch. This is the location where the trachea is entering the chest. The sternum has three components: the manubrium, the elongated body, and the xiphoid process. The upper section of the sternum is called the **manubrium**. The body comprises the rest of the sternum except for a narrow, cartilaginous tip inferiorly, which is called the **xiphoid process** Figure 47 .

Within the thoracic cage, the largest structures are the heart, lungs, and great vessels Figure 48 . The heart lies immediately behind the sternum (retrosternal). It extends from the second to the sixth ribs anteriorly and from the fifth to the eighth thoracic vertebrae posteriorly. The inferior border of the heart extends into the left side of the chest. Diseased hearts may be larger or smaller. The major blood vessels that travel to and from the heart also lie in the chest cavity. On the right side of the spinal column, the superior and inferior venae cavae carry blood to the heart.

Just beneath the manubrium of the sternum, the arch of the aorta and the **pulmonary artery** exit the heart. The arch of the aorta passes to the left and lies along the left side of the spinal column as it descends into the abdomen. The esophagus lies behind the great vessels and directly on the anterior aspect of the spinal column as it passes through the chest into the abdominal cavity.

Words of Wisdom

Pay attention to spelling to prevent misunderstandings. Even though *ilium* and *ileum* are pronounced the same, they refer to two different parts of the body.
- Ilium = the bony prominences of the pelvis
- Ileum = the lower 3/5 of the small intestine

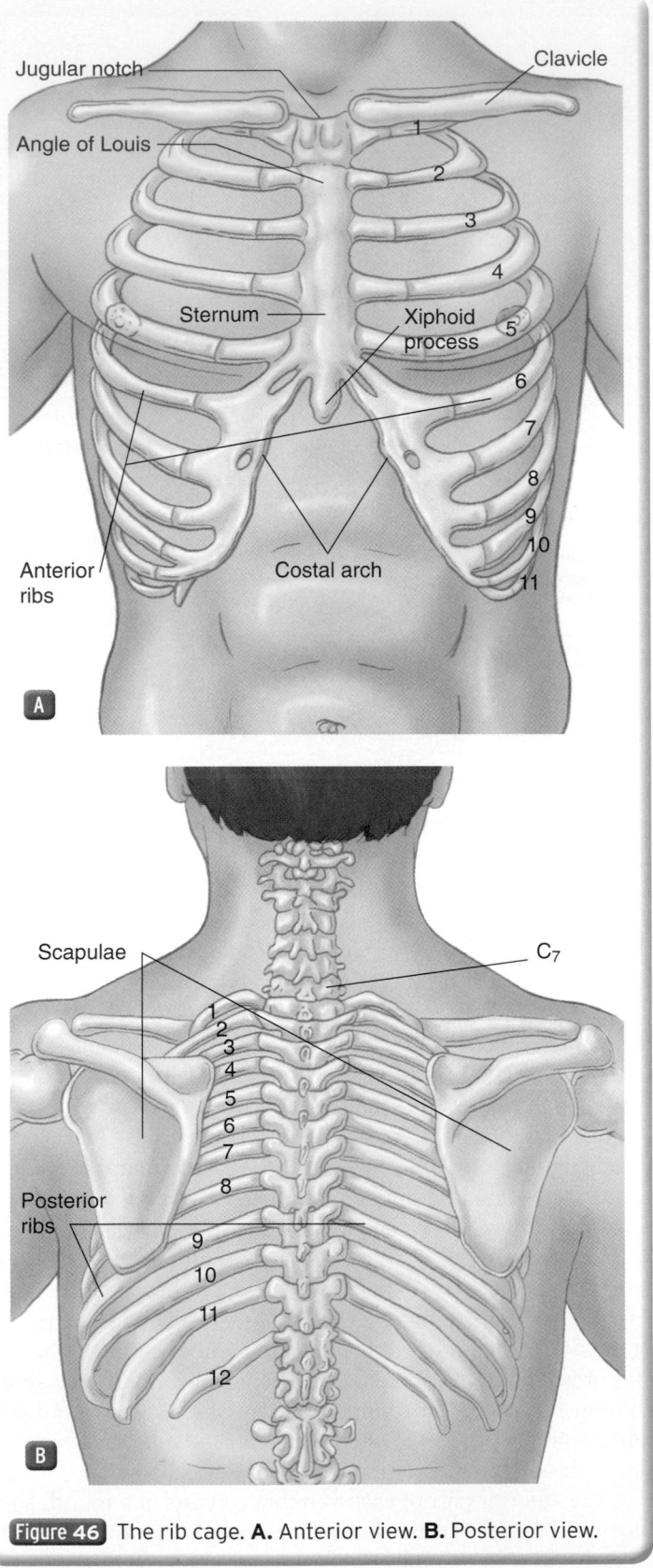

Figure 46 The rib cage. **A.** Anterior view. **B.** Posterior view.

All space within the chest that is not occupied by the heart, great vessels, and esophagus is occupied by the lungs. Anteriorly, the lungs extend down to the surface of the diaphragm at the level of the xiphoid process. Posteriorly, the lungs extend farther inferiorly to the surface of the diaphragm at the level of the 12th thoracic vertebra.

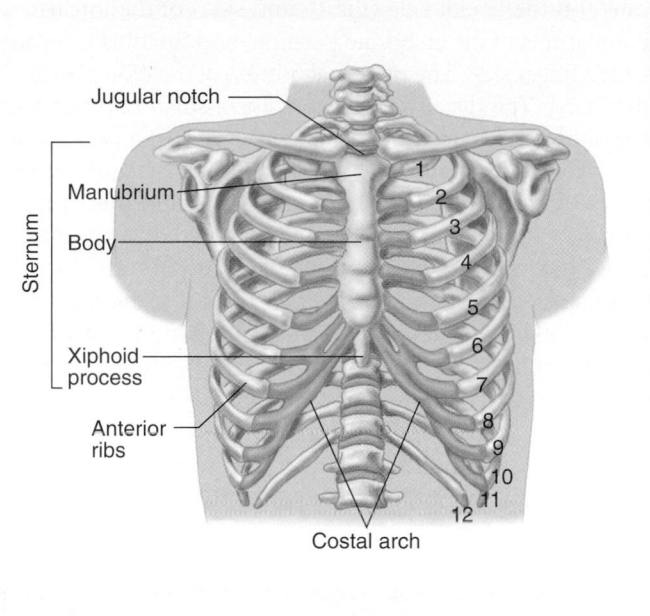

Figure 47 Thoracic cavity.

The Appendicular Skeleton

The Shoulder Girdle

The **shoulder girdle** attaches the upper extremity to the body. The two components of the shoulder girdle are the triangular shaped **scapula** (shoulder blade) and the **clavicle** (collarbone).

The **acromion process** protects the shoulder joint and provides a site of attachment for both the clavicle and various shoulder muscles **Figure 49**. Important muscles of the shoulder, including those of the rotator cuff, originate here.

The clavicle is an S-shaped bone that is easily felt on either side of the jugular notch. The lateral end of the clavicle articulates with the acromion and the medial end with the manubrium.

The Shoulder Joint

The shoulder joint is a ball-and-socket joint in which the head of the humerus articulates with the **glenoid fossa**, which is part of the scapula. The hip and shoulder are typical ball-and-socket joints.

Four ligaments attach the humeral head to the glenoid fossa. A fibrocartilage ring surrounds the glenoid rim and provides a

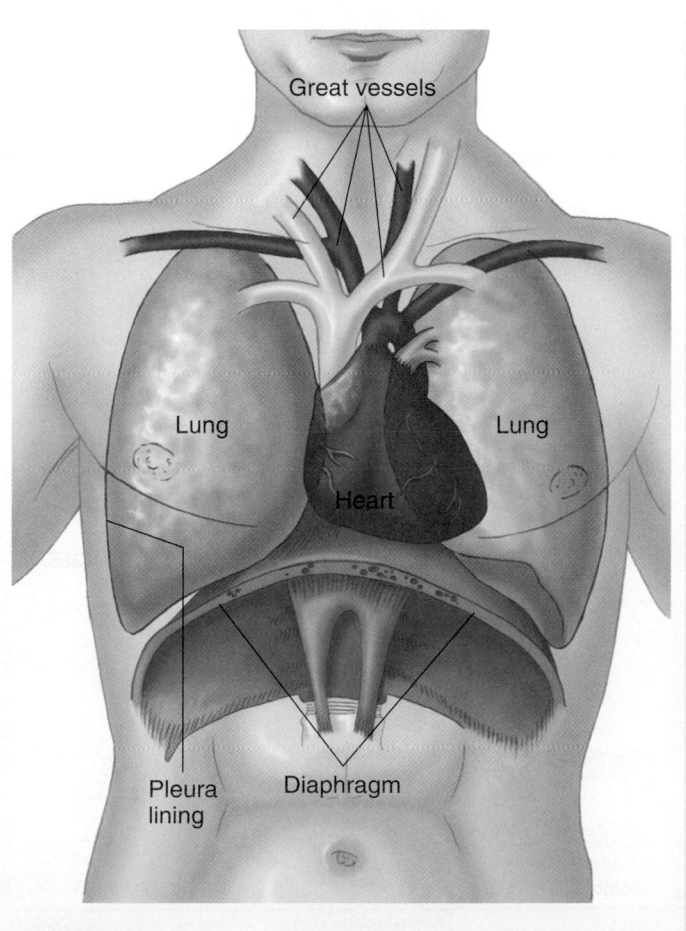

Figure 48 The anterior aspect of the thorax shows the relative positions of the principal organs beneath the surface.

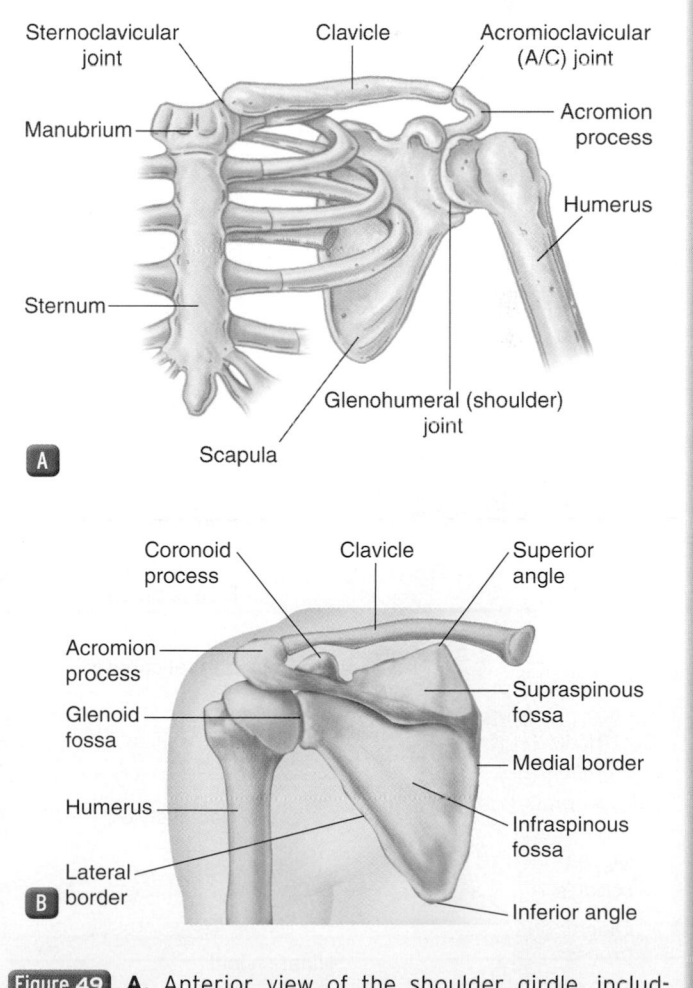

Figure 49 **A.** Anterior view of the shoulder girdle, including the clavicle. **B.** Posterior view of the shoulder girdle, including the scapula.

point of attachment for the capsule, which is made up of fibrous connective tissue. A <u>bursa</u> is a fluid-filled sac situated between a tendon and a bone that cushions and protects joints such as the shoulder, hip, or knee.

Words of Wisdom

<u>Acromioclavicular separation (AC separation)</u>, also called a separated shoulder, occurs when any of the four ligaments of the AC joint are partially or completely torn. In partial tears, no deformity is noted unless the patient attempts to hold a weight with the arm directed downward. In this case, the weakened joint is transiently widened, a finding visible on radiographs. In patients with complete separation, in which all four ligaments are severely damaged, the clavicle essentially lies above the acromion, causing a visible deformity in the patient's shoulder area.

The Upper Extremity

The upper extremity consists of the arm (more commonly thought of as the upper arm), forearm, wrist, hand, and fingers.

The <u>humerus</u> is the bone of the upper arm Figure 50. It articulates proximally with the glenoid fossa and distally with the radius and ulna at the elbow joint. The elbow joint is a hinge joint, permitting motion in one plane only. Several ligaments connect the humerus, radius, and ulna at the elbow joint, and a fluid-filled bursa cushions and protects the joint posteriorly.

The Forearm and Wrist

The forearm extends from the elbow to the wrist. The forearm contains two bones, the <u>radius</u> and <u>ulna</u>. The radius is the bone located on the lateral side (the thumb side) of the forearm when the forearm is in the anatomic position, and the ulna is located on the little finger side. The proximal portion of the radius is called the radial head. The distal portion contains a small bony protrusion, the styloid process, to which ligaments of the wrist are attached.

The wrist is made of a group of eight irregularly shaped bones, called the carpals. The carpals include the triquetrum, pisiform, capitate, lunate, hamate, trapezoid, trapezium, and scaphoid (carpal navicular) bones. The carpal tunnel is formed by the space bounded by the trapezium and hamate dorsally and the flexor retinaculum, a sheath of tough connective tissue that forms the roof of the carpal tunnel, on the palmar side. Tendons, nerves, and blood vessels lie within the carpal tunnel. Structures within the carpal tunnel include the long flexor tendon to the fingers and the median nerve, which supplies sensory and motor function to the radial half of the palm of the hand.

The Hand

The <u>metacarpals</u> are the bones that form the hand. The <u>phalanges</u> are a series of small bones that exist in each finger. The phalanges in the fingers form hinge joints. Each finger has three phalanges, except the thumb, which has only two Figure 51. The <u>carpometacarpal joint</u> of the thumb is a <u>saddle joint</u>, consisting of two saddle-shaped articulating surfaces that are oriented at right angles to one another so that the complementary surfaces articulate with each other. Movement in these joints can occur in two planes. Arthritis commonly affects the carpometacarpal joint, resulting in stiffness and deformity.

The Pelvic Girdle

The <u>pelvis</u>, or pelvic girdle, attaches the lower limbs to the axial skeleton Figure 52. The pelvis contains a ring of bones formed by the sacrum and the coxal, or pelvic bones; the sacrum is

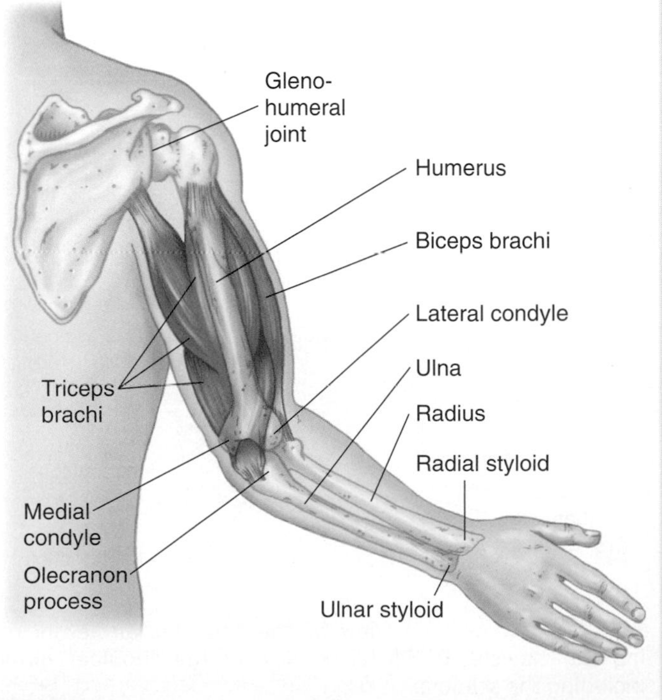

Figure 50 The upper arm contains the humerus; the forearm contains the radius and ulna.

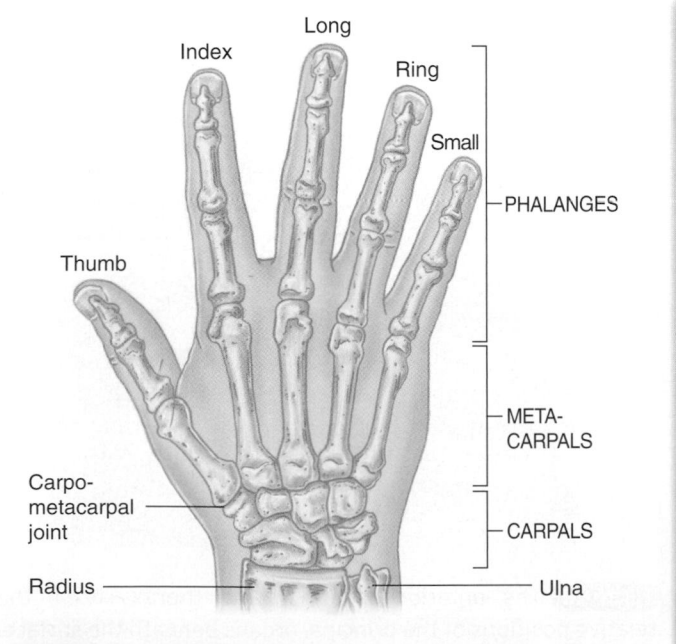

Figure 51 The principal bones in the wrist and hand include the carpals, the metacarpals, and the phalanges.

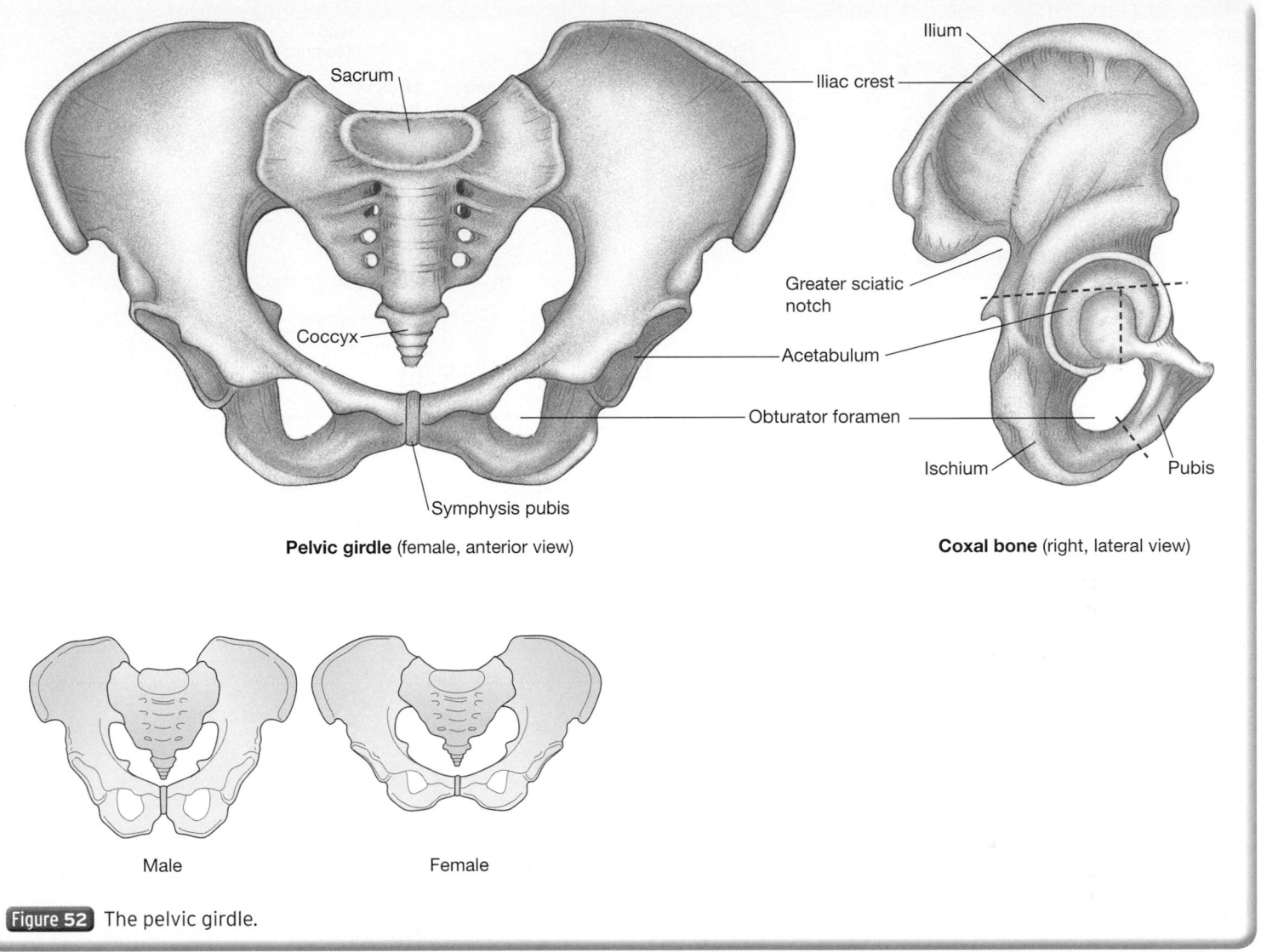

Pelvic girdle (female, anterior view)

- Sacrum
- Coccyx
- Symphysis pubis

Coxal bone (right, lateral view)

- Ilium
- Iliac crest
- Greater sciatic notch
- Acetabulum
- Obturator foramen
- Ischium
- Pubis

Male

Female

Figure 52 The pelvic girdle.

posterior and the coxal bones are on each side. Each coxa consists of three fused bones: the ilium, ischium, and pubis:

- <u>Ilium</u>: The largest portion of the hip bone, it forms the prominence of the hip. The margin of the prominence is called the iliac crest. The ilium joins the sacrum at the sacroiliac joint. A projection from the ilium provides attachments for ligaments and muscles.
- <u>Ischium</u>: The lowest portion of the hip bone, it is L-shaped. It supports the weight of the body when sitting. Its angle, the ischial tuberosity, points downward and posteriorly.
- <u>Pubis</u>: The anterior portion of the hip bone, it forms an angle known as the pubic arch. The two pubic bones join at the symphysis pubis, the upper margin of which (the pelvic brim) separates the lower pelvis from the upper portion. A large opening, known as the obturator foramen, lies between the pubis and ischium.

The pelvis contains three joints: the two posterior <u>sacroiliac joints</u> and the interior midline <u>pubic symphysis</u>. The location where the ilium connects with the sacrum is the sacroiliac joint. The pubic symphysis is the lower midportion of the pelvic ring where the left and right sides fuse together. The superior portion

of the ilium is the iliac crest. The obturator foramen is an opening between the ischium and pubis that contains several important nerves and muscles. The pelvic girdle supports the body weight and protects the internal organs. In a pregnant woman, the bones protect the developing fetus and provide a passageway through which the infant passes during delivery.

■ The Lower Extremity

The lower extremity is made of the thigh, knee, leg, ankle, foot, and toes **Figure 53**. The <u>acetabulum</u> is the socket of the ball-and-socket joint that connects the pelvic girdle with the lower extremity. The thigh is the part of the lower extremity that extends from the hip to the knee and contains the <u>femur</u>, which is the longest and strongest bone in the body. The uppermost portion of the femur, the <u>femoral head</u>, articulates with the pelvic girdle at the acetabulum. In addition to the femoral head, the proximal femur consists of the neck, <u>greater trochanter</u>, and <u>lesser trochanter</u>. The greater trochanter arises lateral to the juncture of the neck and shaft and is clinically considered as part of the hip. Several ligaments and muscle tendons provide integrity to the hip joint. The articular capsule is supported by

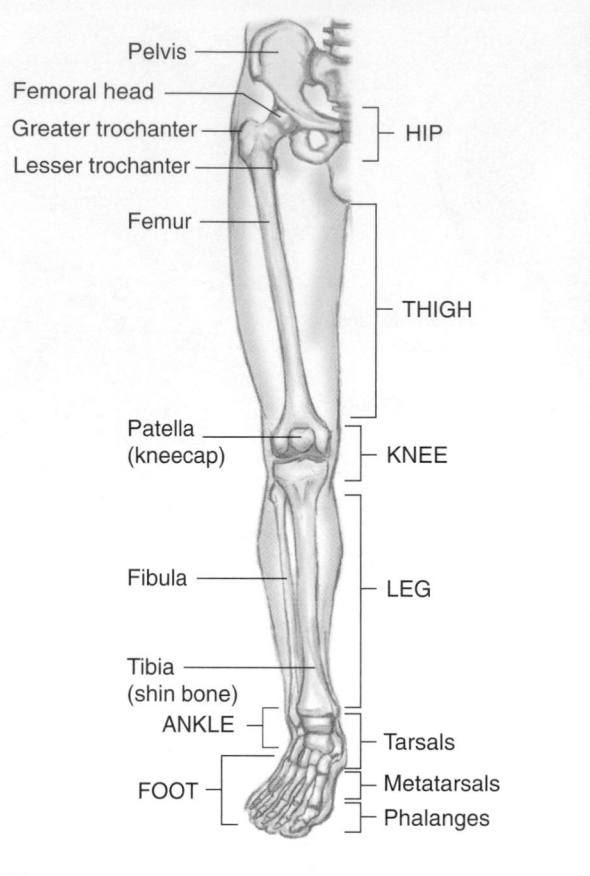

Figure 53 The principal parts of the lower extremity, including the femur, femoral head, greater and lesser trochanters, patella, tibia, and fibula.

three ligaments that are quite strong; they support much of the body's weight.

The Leg

At the distal end of the femur, the lateral and medial condyles articulate with the proximal tibia at the knee **Figure 54**. These are important sites of muscle and ligament attachment. The **patella**, or kneecap, lies within the major anterior tendon of the thigh muscles and articulates with the femur.

The leg is made of the tibia and fibula, and extends from the knee to the ankle. The **tibia** is the longer and thicker of the two bones and is situated on the anterior surface of the leg. The anterior portion of the tibia, covered only by skin, is commonly called the shin. The flat medial and lateral condyles of the proximal tibia articulate with the condyles of the femur at the knee. The **medial malleolus**, which forms the medial side of the ankle joint, lies at the distal end of the tibia.

The second of the two leg bones, the **fibula**, is posterior to the tibia and does not articulate directly with the femur, but rather with the tibia at the head. An enlargement of the distal end of the fibula forms the lateral wall of the ankle joint, the **lateral malleolus**.

The Knee

The knee joint is traditionally classified as a hinge joint and is unusual because it contains ligaments within the joint. Thick

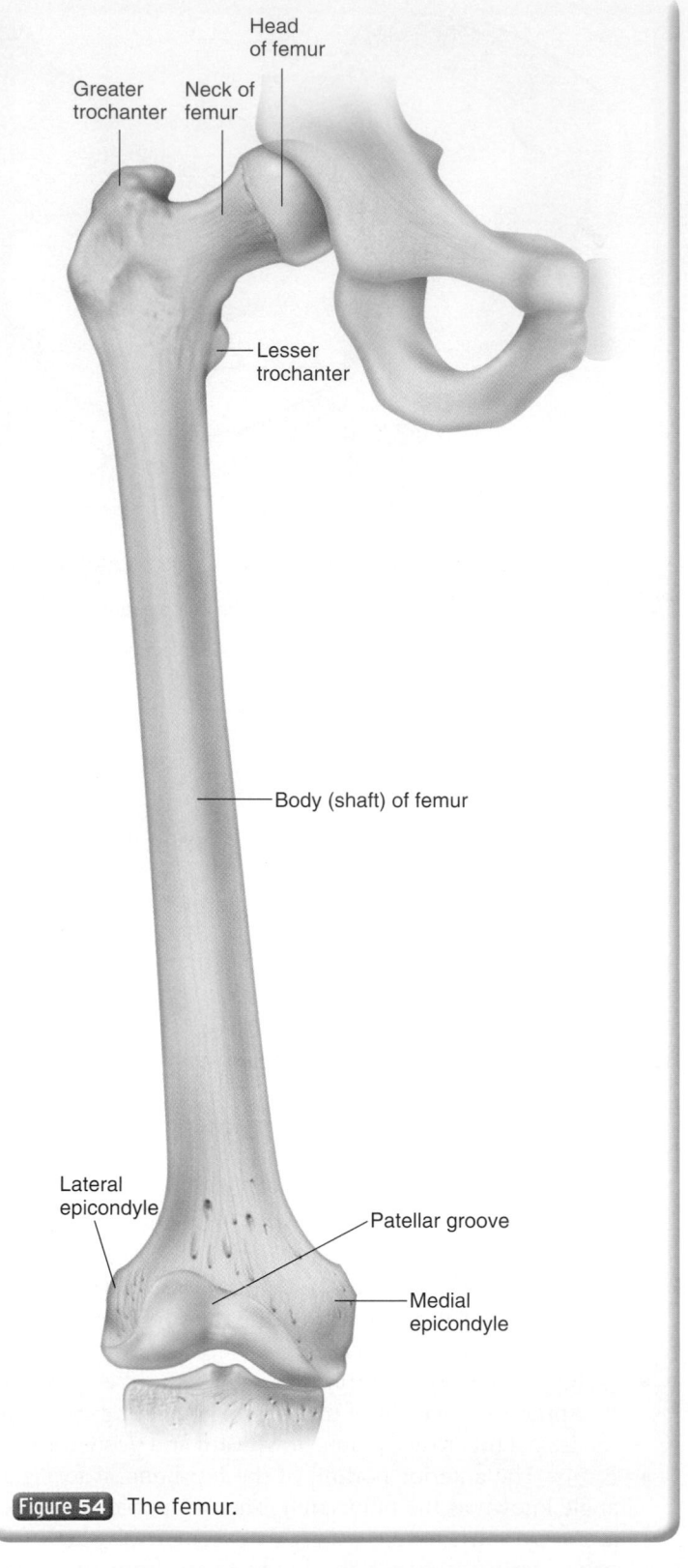

Figure 54 The femur.

crescent-shaped articular disks, menisci, cover the margins of the tibia to cushion the articular surface. The anterior cruciate ligament (ACL), which extends between the tibia and femur, prevents abnormal anterior movement (hyperextension) of the tibia. The posterior cruciate ligament (PCL) prevents abnormal posterior displacement of the tibia. Several tendons, as well as collateral ligaments, lend further strength to the knee joint. The knee is surrounded by several fluid-filled bursae Figure 55.

The Ankle

The <u>talus</u> articulates with the tibia and fibula to form the ankle Figure 56. The ankle (tarsus) is made up of seven bones called <u>tarsals</u> that are arranged so that the talus bone moves freely where it joins the leg bones.

The <u>calcaneus</u>, or heel bone, lies inferior and lateral to the talus, providing additional support. A fibrous capsule surrounds the ankle joint; the medial and lateral portions are thickened to form ligaments. Movements include dorsiflexion and plantar flexion, as well as limited inversion and eversion.

The <u>metatarsals</u> and phalanges of the foot are arranged much like the bones of the hand. The toes have three phalanges each, except the big toe, which has two phalanges. The ball of the foot is the junction between the metatarsals and the phalanges.

◼ The Skeletal System: Physiology

The skeletal system is responsible for several functions. Bones protect internal organs and, with muscles, enable movement. Bone also serves as a storage site for minerals, particularly calcium, and has a role in the formation of blood cells and platelets. Calcium is the main element the various bones cells use to create a structure that is hard and resilient. Bones store and release calcium, which is important for other body systems.

Bones consist of collagen and the mineral hydroxyapatite, a compound that contains calcium and phosphate. The collagen fibers in bone act much like reinforcing rods in a concrete structure, lending flexible strength to the bone. The mineral components of the bone supply strength for bearing weight, much like concrete does in a structure. Bone without the necessary amount of mineral is flexible; bone without enough collagen is extremely brittle.

The skeletal system also helps with the creation of various types of blood cells. In the marrow of certain types of bones, special cells are present that can transform themselves into red blood cells, white blood cells, and platelets. The cells, when stimulated, help to replace worn-out cells in the blood.

Bones are a living substance with cells requiring a blood supply. During a person's life, bones are constantly remodeled to

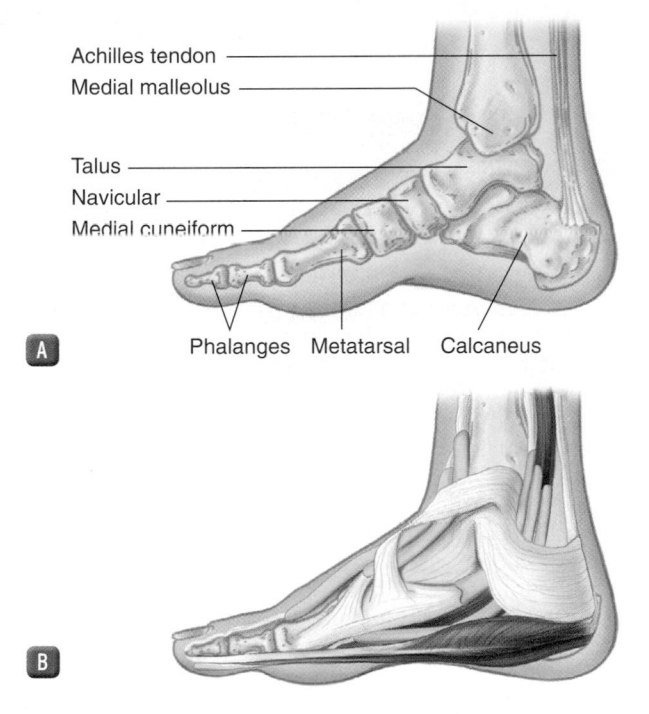

Figure 56 **A.** The surface landmarks of the foot, including the talus, the calcaneus, and the phalanges. **B.** Soft tissue of the ankle.

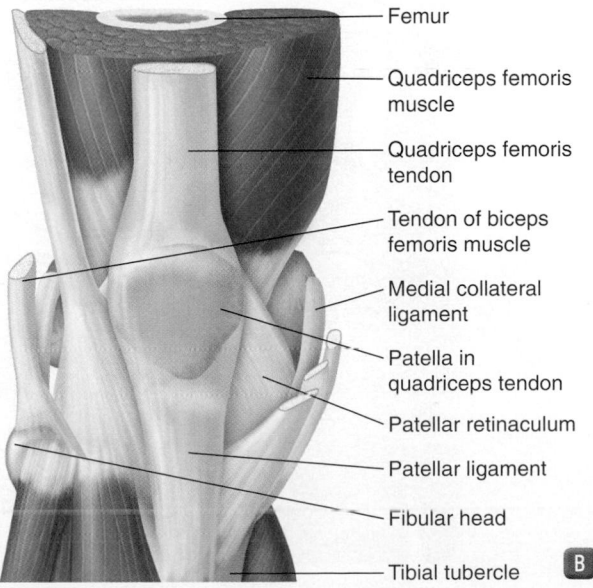

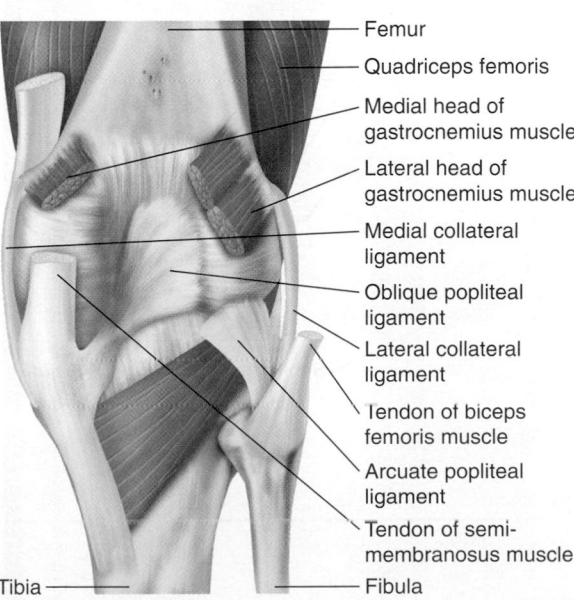

Figure 55 **A.** Anterior view of the knee. **B.** Posterior view of the knee.

meet the stresses that are placed on them. The level of a person's activity directly affects how the bones are remodeled.

The Musculoskeletal System: Anatomy

The human body is a well-designed system whose form, upright posture, and movement are provided by the **musculoskeletal system**. The term musculoskeletal refers to the bones and voluntary muscles of the body. The musculoskeletal system also protects the vital internal organs of the body. Muscles are a form

of tissue that allows body movement. There are more than 600 muscles in the musculoskeletal system. The type of muscle found here is called skeletal muscle. As you know, other types of muscle outside of the musculoskeletal system include smooth muscle (**involuntary muscle**) and cardiac muscle Figure 58 .

Skeletal Muscle

Skeletal muscle, so named because it attaches to the bones of the skeleton, forms the major muscle mass of the body. It is also called **voluntary muscle**, because all skeletal muscle is under direct voluntary control of the brain and can be stimulated to contract or relax at will. Movement of the body, like waving or

Special Populations

Hip fractures actually are fractures of the proximal portion of the femur near or at the site of articulation with the acetabulum. These fractures are classified based on the structures of the femur involved Figure 57 .

Hip fractures account for nearly 30% of orthopaedic hospital admissions. Up to 80% of hip fractures occur in women. Results often are disabling because many patients are elderly and have underlying cardiac disease, osteoporosis, and senility. Mortality from all causes is 20% in the first 6 months following a hip fracture. Treatment depends on the portion of the proximal femur that is injured.

Dislocations of the hip joint commonly occur from a fall or during a motor vehicle crash in which the knee impacts the dashboard. The force of the impact is transmitted posteriorly to the hip, resulting in posterior dislocation. Anterior hip dislocations are less common.

Words of Wisdom

As you gain a better understanding of the anatomy and physiology of the body, it is important to remember that body systems work together and not in isolation. A person who falls and breaks a leg has an isolated injury. It may appear to you that the skeletal system is the only system that is involved. But then ask yourself the following questions: Is there bleeding inside the leg? Is there damage to the nerves, tendons, or ligaments? Has the injury broken the skin and is there now a risk of infection? A seemingly simple illness or injury can involve several body systems. Give each patient a thorough assessment.

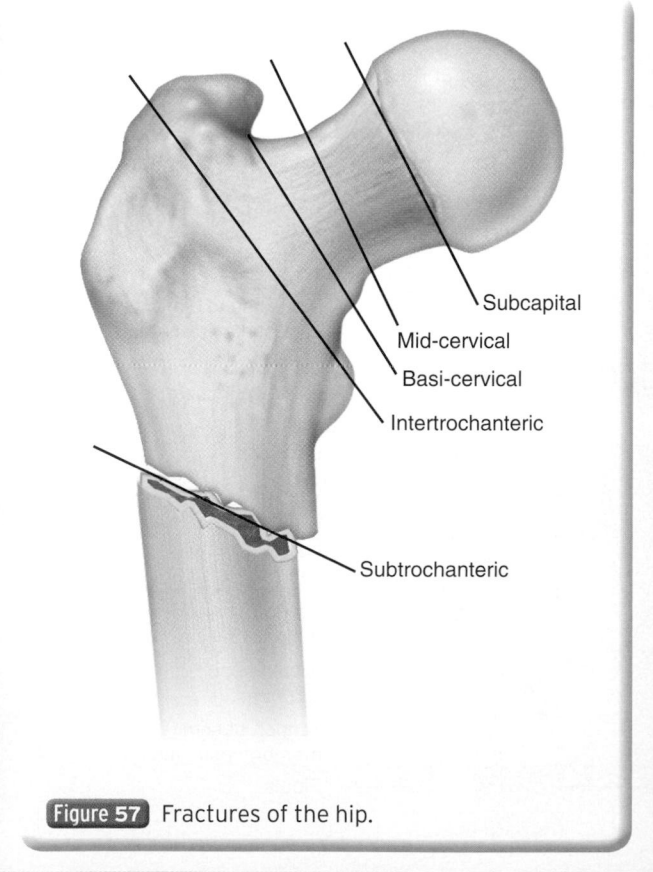

Subcapital
Mid-cervical
Basi-cervical
Intertrochanteric

Subtrochanteric

Figure 57 Fractures of the hip.

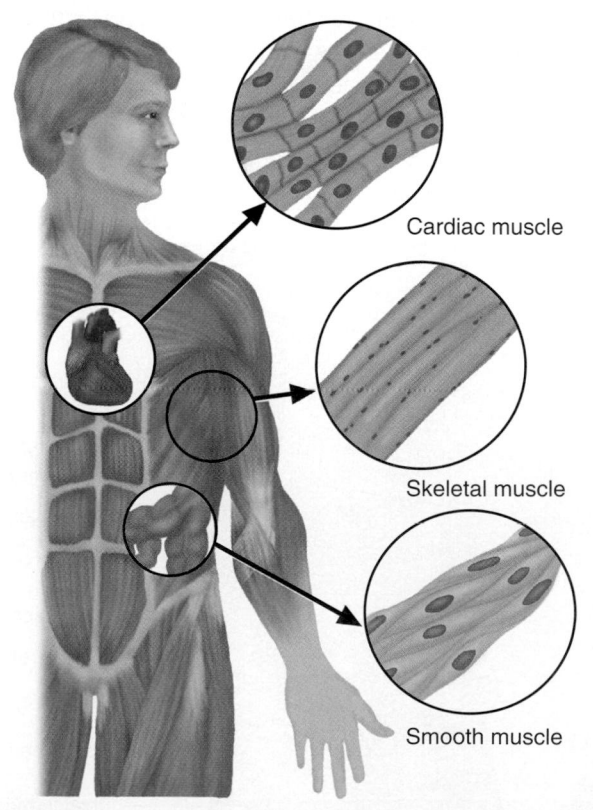

Cardiac muscle

Skeletal muscle

Smooth muscle

Figure 58 The three types of muscle are skeletal, smooth, and cardiac.

walking, results from skeletal muscle contraction or relaxation. Usually, a specific motion is the result of several muscles contracting and relaxing simultaneously. Individual skeletal muscles are separated from other muscles and held in position by layers of fibrous connective tissue known as fascia.

Coverings of Connective Tissue

Fascia surrounds every muscle and may form cord-like tendons beyond each muscle's end. Tendon fibers may intertwine with bone fibers in order to attach muscle to bones. Broad sheets of fibers that may attach to bones or to the coverings of other muscles are known as aponeuroses.

Skeletal muscles are closely surrounded by a layer of connective tissue known as an epimysium. The muscle is separated into small compartments by another layer known as the perimysium. Inside these compartments are fascicles, which are bundles of skeletal muscle fibers. Inside the fascicles, muscle fibers are contained within connective tissue layers. These layers form a thin covering (endomysium). The many layers of connective tissue that enclose and separate skeletal muscles allow a great deal of independent movement.

Structure of Skeletal Muscle Fibers

A single cell that contracts in response to stimulation and relaxes when the stimulation ceases is known as a skeletal muscle fiber. These fibers are thin, elongated cylinders with rounded ends. The cell membrane (sarcolemma) lies above the cytoplasm (also known as sarcoplasm), with many small, oval-shaped mitochondria and nuclei. The sarcoplasm is made up of many threadlike myofibrils arranged parallel to each other.

Myofibrils have thick protein filaments composed of myosin, and thin protein filaments mostly composed of actin. These filaments are organized so that they appear as striations—areas of alternating colored bands of skeletal muscle fiber. The repeating patterns of striation units that appear along each muscle fiber are referred to as sarcomeres. Muscles are basically considered to be collections of sarcomeres.

There are two main parts of the striation pattern of skeletal muscle fibers. The light bands (I bands) are made up of thin filaments of actin attached to Z lines. The dark bands (A bands) are made up of thick filaments of myosin that overlap thin filaments of actin. There is a central region (H zone) of thick filaments, with a thickened area (the M line) that consists of proteins holding them in place. Sarcomeres extend from one Z line to another Z line, as shown in **Figure 59**.

Inside the sarcoplasm of a muscle fiber, a network of channels surrounds each myofibril. These membranous channels form the sarcoplasmic reticulum. Transverse tubules (T-tubules) are other membranous channels extending inward and passing through the fiber. These tubules open to the outside of the muscle fiber, and contain extracellular fluid. Each tubule lies between enlarged structures called cisternae, near the point where actin and myosin filaments overlap. Together, the sarcoplasmic reticulum and T-tubules activate muscle contraction when stimulated.

Neurologic Structures

Neurons (nerve cells) conduct nerve impulses. **Motor neurons** control effectors, which include skeletal muscle. Each skeletal muscle fiber is connected in a functional manner to the axon of a motor neuron. These pass outward from the brain or spinal cord. Each functional connection is called a synapse. At the synapses, neurons communicate with other cells by releasing **neurotransmitters** (chemicals that enable communication). Skeletal muscle fibers usually contract when stimulated by motor neurons.

A **neuromuscular junction** is the connection between a motor neuron and a muscle fiber **Figure 60**. A **motor end plate** is formed by specialized muscle fiber membranes. Motor end plates have abundant mitochondria and nuclei, with greatly folded sarcolemmas.

Motor neurons branch out and project into muscle fiber membrane recesses. Cytoplasm at these distal ends have many mitochondria and tiny synaptic vesicles that contain neurotransmitters. On receiving impulses, the vesicles release neurotransmitters into the synaptic cleft between the neuron and motor end plate, stimulating muscle contraction.

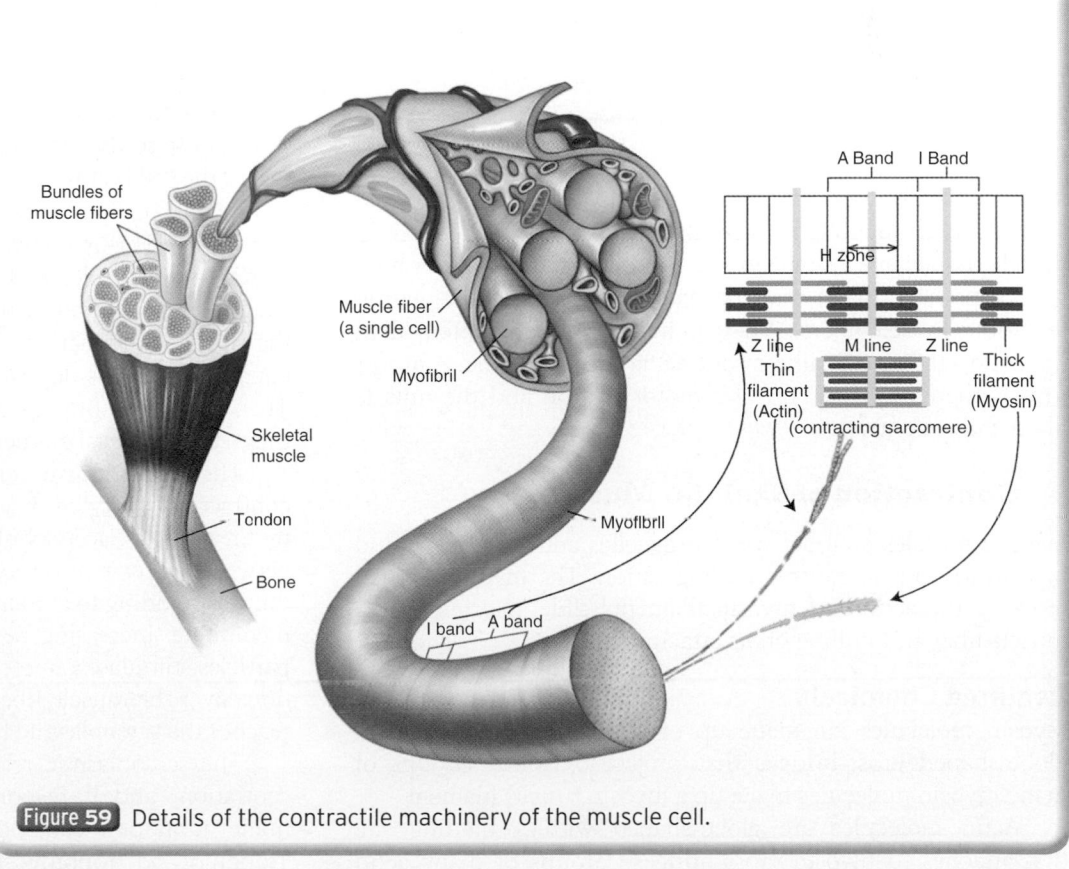

Figure 59 Details of the contractile machinery of the muscle cell.

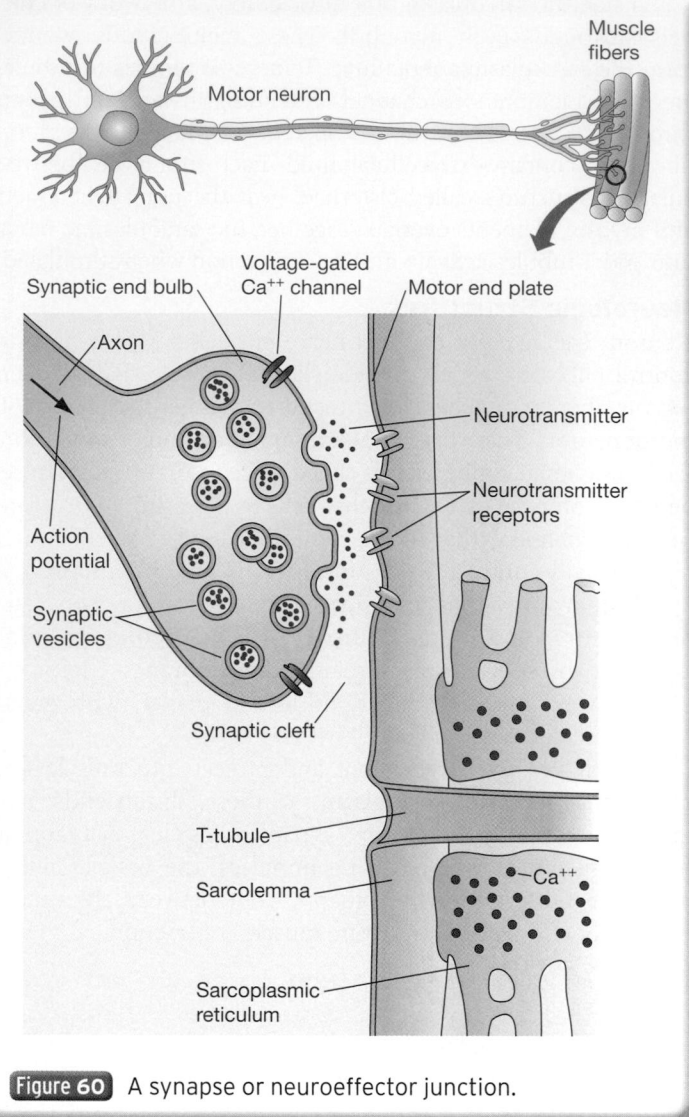

Figure 60 A synapse or neuroeffector junction.

Motor Units

Each of the numerous muscle fibers that make up a piece of muscle tissue have a single motor end plate, though motor neuron axons have many branches connecting the motor neuron to various muscle fibers. When an impulse is transmitted, all of the connected muscle fibers contract at the same time. A **motor unit** is therefore made up of a motor neuron and the muscle fibers that it controls.

■ Contraction of Skeletal Muscles

Skeletal muscles contract when organelles and molecules bind myosin to actin to cause a pulling action. The myofibrils then move as the actin and myosin filaments slide, shortening the muscle fiber and pulling on its attachments.

Required Chemicals

Myosin molecules are made up of two protein strands with globe-shaped cross-bridges that project outward. Groups of many myosin molecules make up a myosin (thick) filament.

Actin molecules are globe-shaped with a binding site that attaches to myosin cross-bridges. Groups of many actin molecules twist in double strands (helixes) to form an actin (thin) filament, which includes the proteins known as **troponin** and **tropomyosin** **Figure 61**.

Strands of tropomyosin prevent actin–myosin interaction. One subunit of the troponin molecule binds to tropomyosin, forming the troponin–tropomyosin complex. Another subunit binds to G actin to hold the complex in position. A third subunit has a receptor binding a calcium ion. When the muscle is at rest, intracellular calcium is low, and the binding site is empty. Contractions cannot occur unless the position of the troponin–tropomyosin complex changes to expose the active sites on F actin. The position change occurs when calcium ions bind to receptors on the troponin molecules.

The functional unit of skeletal muscle is the sarcomere. When sarcomeres shorten within a skeletal muscle fiber, a skeletal muscle contracts. This occurs because of the cross-bridges pulling on the thin filaments of actin. The **sliding filament model** is so named because of the way sarcomeres shorten, with thick and thin filaments sliding past each other toward the center of the sarcomere, from both ends.

Myosin filaments contain the enzyme ATPase in their globe-shaped portions. This enzyme catalyzes the breakdown of ATP to both adenosine diphosphate (ADP) and phosphate, releasing energy. The myosin cross-bridges assume a "cocked" position, binding to actin to pull on the thin filament. After the pulling occurs, the cross-bridge is released from actin before the ATP splits. The cycle repeats as long as there is enough ATP for energy, and muscular stimulation occurs.

Contraction Stimulus

The impulse that causes contraction of skeletal muscle is transmitted through motor neurons as a **nerve impulse**. These impulses are also known as **action potentials**, and are transmitted from one cell to another in the nervous system, causing each successive cell in the chain to "fire." The process by which cells activate in response to the action potential is known as **depolarization**. When the cell is at rest, ions are actively transported into and out of the cell to create an electrochemical gradient across the cell membrane. This is known as being **polarized**. When the cell is activated by the release of a neurotransmitter, proteins in the cell wall open rapidly, allowing a rapid influx of ions that equalizes the charges on either side of the cell wall. When the charges are equal, the cell has depolarized, and the protein channels close. Then begins the process of **repolarization**, which again creates the electrochemical gradient so the cell can "fire" again.

The neurotransmitter that stimulates skeletal muscle to contract is **acetylcholine**. Synthesized in the cytoplasm of motor neurons, acetylcholine is released into the synaptic clefts between motor neuron axons and motor end plates. It rapidly diffuses, binding to certain protein receptors in the muscle fiber membrane, increasing permeability to sodium. These charged particles stimulate a **muscle impulse** that passes in many directions over the muscle fiber membrane. This impulse eventually reaches the sarcoplasmic reticulum.

The sarcoplasmic reticulum has a high calcium ion concentration, and it responds by making the cisternae membranes more permeable, diffusing calcium into the sarcoplasm. Troponin and tropomyosin interact to form linkages between

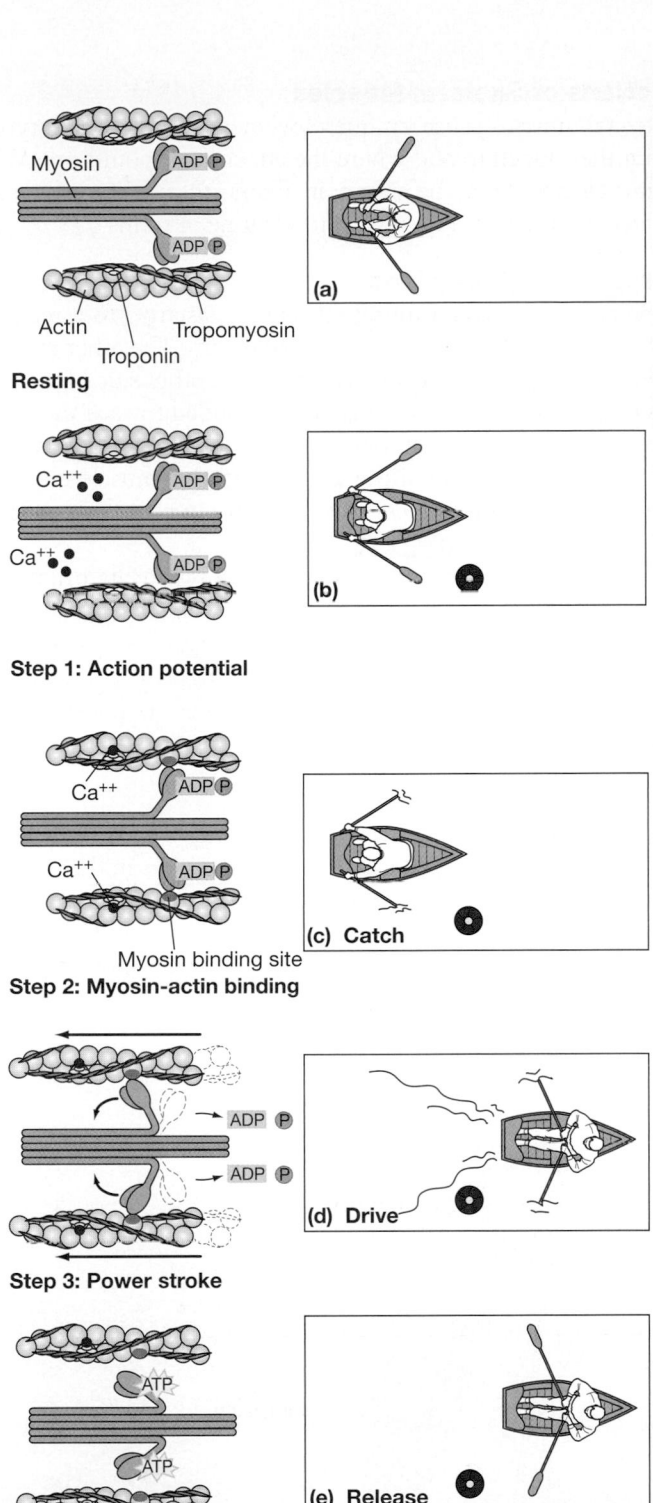

Resting

Step 1: Action potential

Step 2: Myosin-actin binding

Myosin binding site

Step 3: Power stroke

Step 4: ATP binding and actin-myosin release

Step 5: ATP cleavage

(a)

(b)

(c) Catch

(d) Drive

(e) Release

(f) Recover

Figure 61 The sliding filament theory: how muscle fibers contract.

actin and myosin filaments. The muscular contraction also requires ATP and continues as long as acetylcholine is released.

Muscle relaxation is caused by the decomposition of acetylcholine via the enzyme **acetylcholinesterase**. It prevents a single nerve impulse from stimulating the muscle fiber continuously. When the stimulus ceases, calcium ions are transported back to the sarcoplasmic reticulum. The actin and myosin linkages break, and the muscle relaxes.

Energy Sources

Muscle fibers have just enough ATP for short-term contraction. ATP must be regenerated when fibers are active, using existing ATP molecules in the cells. ATP is regenerated from ADP and phosphate. **Creatine phosphate** accomplishes this with high-energy phosphate bonds. It is between four and six times more abundant in muscle fibers than ATP; however, it does not directly supply energy. It stores excess energy from the mitochondria in the phosphate bonds.

When ATP breaks down, energy from creatine phosphate is transferred to ADP molecules to convert them back into ATP. Creatine phosphate stores are exhausted rapidly when muscles are active; therefore, the muscles use cellular respiration of glucose as energy to synthesize ATP.

Oxygen Use and Debt

Oxygen is required for the breakdown of glucose in the mitochondria. Red blood cells carry oxygen, bound to hemoglobin molecules. **Hemoglobin** is the pigment that makes blood appear red. The pigment **myoglobin** is synthesized in the muscles to give skeletal muscles their reddish-brown color. Myoglobin can also combine with oxygen and temporarily store it in order to reduce muscular requirements for continuous blood supply during contraction.

When skeletal muscles are used for a minute or more, anaerobic respiration is required for energy. In one type of anaerobic respiration, glucose is broken down via glycolysis to yield pyruvic acid, which reacts by producing lactic acid. Lactic acid can accumulate in muscles, but diffuses in the bloodstream, reaching the liver, where it is synthesized into glucose.

When a person is exercising strenuously, oxygen is used mostly to synthesize ATP. As lactic acid increases, an **oxygen debt** develops. Oxygen debt is equivalent to the amount of oxygen that liver cells require to convert the lactic acid into glucose, as well as the amount needed by muscle cells to restore ATP and creatine phosphate levels.

It may take several hours for the body to convert lactic acid back into glucose. Muscles may experience a change in their metabolic activity as exercise levels change. Increased exercise raises the muscles' capacity for glycolysis. Aerobic exercise increases the muscles' capacity for aerobic respiration. This process is summarized in Table 11.

Muscle Fatigue

Prolonged exercise may cause a muscle to become unable to contract. This condition is called fatigue, and it may also occur because of interruption of muscular blood supply, or occasionally a lack of acetylcholine in the motor neuron axons. Lactic acid accumulation is the usual cause of muscular fatigue.

Table 11	Changes in Muscular Metabolism		
Variety of Exercise	**Pathway Needed**	**Production of ATP**	**Result**
Low to moderate intensity: blood flow provides enough oxygen for the cells' needs	Glycolysis, which leads to formation of pyruvic acid and aerobic respiration	For skeletal muscle, 36 ATP per glucose	Exhalation of carbon dioxide
High intensity: oxygen supply is not enough for the cells' needs	Glycolysis, which leads to formation of lactic acid	2 ATP per glucose	Accumulation of lactic acid

As lactic acid lowers pH levels, muscle fibers cannot respond to stimulation. When a muscle becomes fatigued and cramps, it experiences a sustained, involuntary contraction. Though not fully understood, muscle cramps appear to be caused by changes in the extracellular fluid surrounding muscle fibers and motor neurons.

Production of Heat

Most of the energy released in cellular respiration becomes heat. Muscle tissue generates a significant amount of heat because muscles form so much of the total body mass. Body temperature is partially maintained by the blood transporting heat generated by the muscle to other body tissues.

Muscle Responses

Muscle contractions can be observed by using a myogram to "see" muscle twitches. This requires electrical signals that can cause various strengths and frequencies of responses. A muscle fiber will remain unresponsive until a certain strength of stimulation (the threshold stimulus) is applied. An action potential is then generated that results in an impulse that spreads throughout the fiber, releasing calcium and activating cross-bridge binding. This causes contraction.

The contractile response of a fiber to an impulse is called a twitch, and it consists of a period of contraction followed by a period of relaxation. A myogram records this pattern of events. There is a brief delay between the stimulation time and the beginning of contraction. This is known as the latent period, and may last less than 2 milliseconds. A myogram results from the combined twitches of muscle fibers taking part in contraction. There are two types of twitches: the fatigue-resistant slow twitch and the fatigable fast twitch.

The force of individual twitches combines via the process of summation. When sustained contractions have no relaxation at all, they are referred to as either tetanic contractions or the condition known as tetany. High intensities of stimulation can activate many motor units (recruitment).

Actions of Skeletal Muscles

Skeletal muscles cause unique movements based on the type of joint they attach to and where the attachment points are. When a muscle appears to be at rest, its fibers still undergo some sustained contraction, known as muscle tone or tonus.

Origins and Insertions

One end of a skeletal muscle usually is fastened to a relatively immovable part (**origin**) at a moveable joint. The other end connects to a movable part (**insertion**) on the other side of the joint. As contraction occurs, the insertion is pulled toward the origin. There may be more than one origin or insertion, such as in the biceps brachii muscle of the arm. When this muscle contracts, the insertion being pulled toward its origin causes the forearm to flex at the elbow `Figure 62`.

The head of a muscle is the part closest to its origin. The term flexion describes a decrease in the angle of a joint; for example, a movement of the forearm that causes it to bend at the elbow. The term extension describes an increase in the angle of a joint; for example, a movement of the forearm that straightens the elbow.

Skeletal Muscle Interactions

Skeletal muscles usually function in groups, with the nervous system stimulating the desired muscles to perform the intended function. A muscle that contracts to provide most of the desired movement is called a prime mover or agonist. Other muscles, known as synergists, work with a prime mover to make

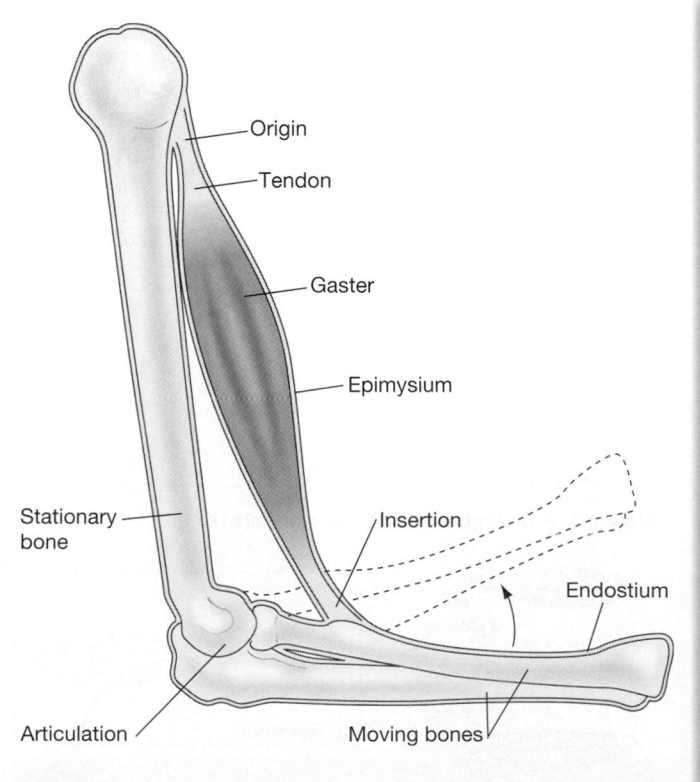

Figure 62 The parts of a muscle. The actual origin of the muscle shown is in the scapula. Origin on humerus is shown for clarity.

its action more effective. For example, when you bend your forearm, the agonist muscles are the biceps, while the synergists are the triceps.

Other muscles act as antagonists to prime movers. They cause movement in the opposite direction. In the above example, the triceps would be the antagonists to the biceps. Smooth body movement depends on antagonists relaxing while prime movers contract. Muscles may work opposite to each other or together in order to control various movements.

There are some important muscle groups to know. **Figure 63** and **Table 12** show the major muscles, their locations, and their functions.

■ The Musculoskeletal System: Physiology

The musculoskeletal system has several functions. A person's ability to move and be able to manipulate his or her environment is made possible by the contraction and relaxation of this system. A by-product of this movement is heat. When you get cold, you involuntarily shake your muscles, or shiver, to produce heat. Shivering is an essential function. Another function of muscles is to protect the structures under them, such as the intestines, which are protected by the rectus abdominus muscles.

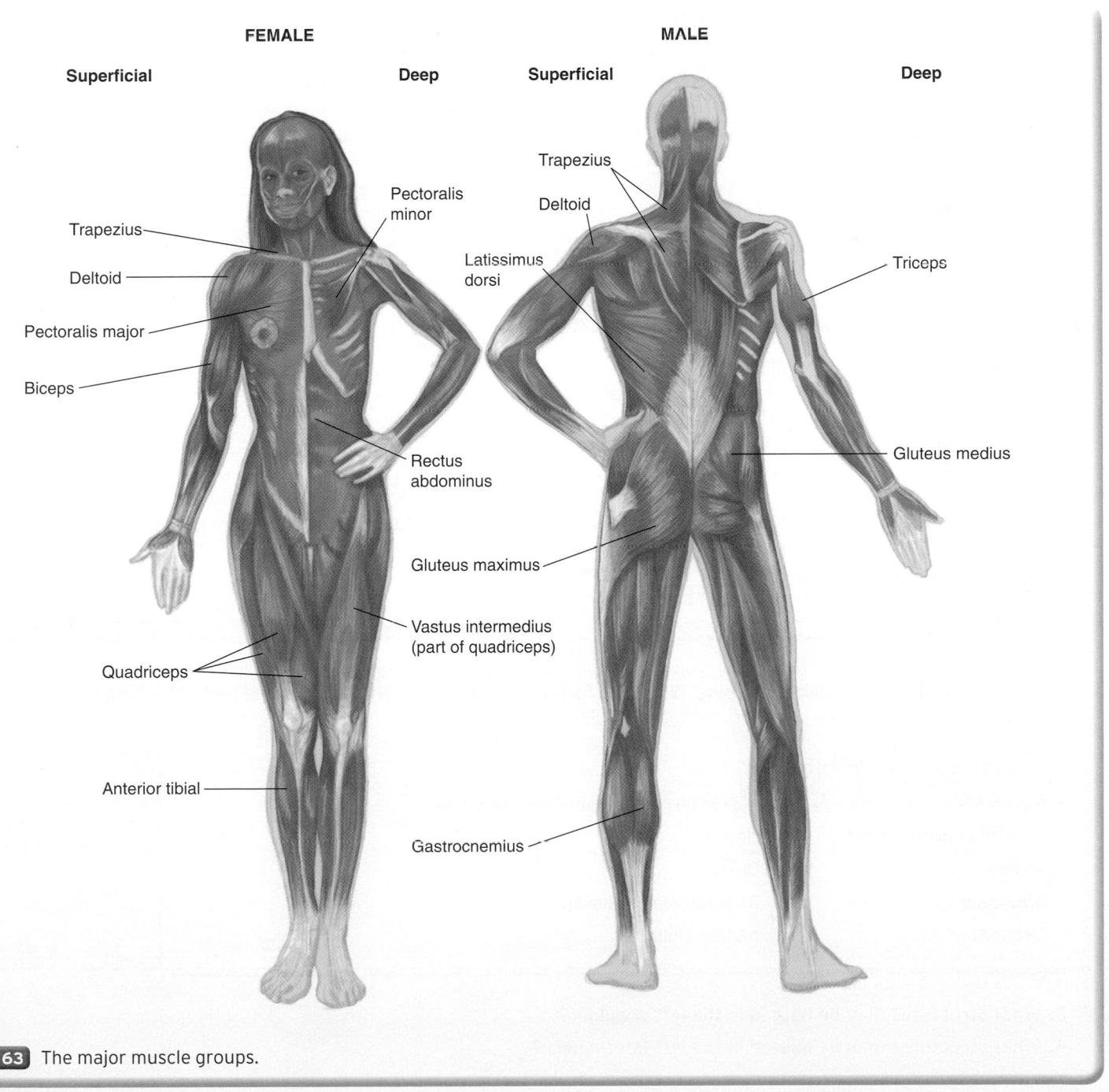

FEMALE

Superficial   **Deep**

Pectoralis minor

Trapezius

Deltoid

Pectoralis major

Biceps

Rectus abdominus

Gluteus maximus

Vastus intermedius (part of quadriceps)

Quadriceps

Anterior tibial

MALE

Superficial   **Deep**

Trapezius

Deltoid

Latissimus dorsi

Triceps

Gluteus medius

Gastrocnemius

Figure 63 The major muscle groups.

Table 12   Muscles: Locations and Functions

Muscle Name	Location	Function
Biceps	Anterior, humerus	Flexes lower arm
Triceps	Posterior, humerus	Extends lower arm
Pectoralis	Anterior, thorax	Flexes and rotates arm
Latissimus dorsi	Posterior, thorax	Extends and rotates arm
Rectus abdominis	Anterior, abdomen	Flexes and rotates spine
Tibialis anterior	Anterior, tibia	Points toes toward head
Gastrocnemius	Posterior, tibia	Points toes away from head
Quadriceps (four separate muscles)	Anterior, femur	Extends lower leg
Biceps femoris	Posterior, femur	Flexes lower leg
Gluteus (three separate muscles)	Posterior, pelvis	Extends and rotates leg

The Respiratory System: Anatomy

The respiratory system consists of all the structures of the body that contribute to respiration, or the process of breathing Figure 64 . It includes the nose, mouth, throat, larynx, trachea, bronchi, and bronchioles, which are all air passages or airways. The system also includes the lungs, where oxygen is passed into the blood and carbon dioxide removed. Finally, the respiratory system includes the diaphragm, the muscles of the chest wall, and

Words of Wisdom

A cough is the perfect mechanism for aerosolizing infectious materials. Whenever possible, minimize the risk of exposure by placing an oxygen mask on a patient with a cough.

accessory muscles of breathing, which permit normal respiratory movement. In this text, the term "airway" usually refers to the upper airway or the passage above the larynx (voice box).

The Upper Airway

The structures of the upper airway are located anteriorly and at the midline. The upper airway includes the nose, mouth, tongue, jaw, oral cavity, larynx, and pharynx. Inspired air flows into the body through the mouth or nose. The nasal cavity is referred to as the nasopharynx and the oral cavity is referred to as the oropharynx. These two cavities connect posteriorly to form a common cavity called the pharynx (throat). The pharynx is a funnel-shaped structure that opens into the nose and mouth anteriorly and joins below with the larynx. The larynx, or voice box, is a rigid, hollow structure made of cartilage. The larynx plays an important role in swallowing.

The pharynx is composed of the nasopharynx, oropharynx, and the laryngopharynx. The nasopharynx and the nasal passages, which include the turbinates (three curved bone shelves inside each nasal passage that force inhaled air to flow in a steady pattern across the largest possible surface of the cilia and tissue that controls climate), warm, filter, and humidify air as a person breathes. The nasal mucosa is the mucous membrane that lines the nasal cavity. Olfactory receptors located in the epithelium in the nasal cavity are responsible for recognizing odors. Air enters through the mouth more rapidly and directly. As a result,

YOU are the Medic   PART 2

You approach the patient and determine that the patient has a rapid pulse and his breathing is shallow. You direct the next crew that has arrived to stabilize the spine. When you further assess the patient you find substantial bruising to the left shoulder and left lateral neck, anterior chest, and left lateral abdomen.

Recording Time: 3 Minutes	
Appearance	Supine on roadway, no visible bleeding
Level of consciousness	Unresponsive
Airway	Open
Breathing	22 breaths/min, shallow
Circulation	118 beats/min

3. What structures may be injured in the left shoulder?

4. What structures may be injured in the left lateral neck?

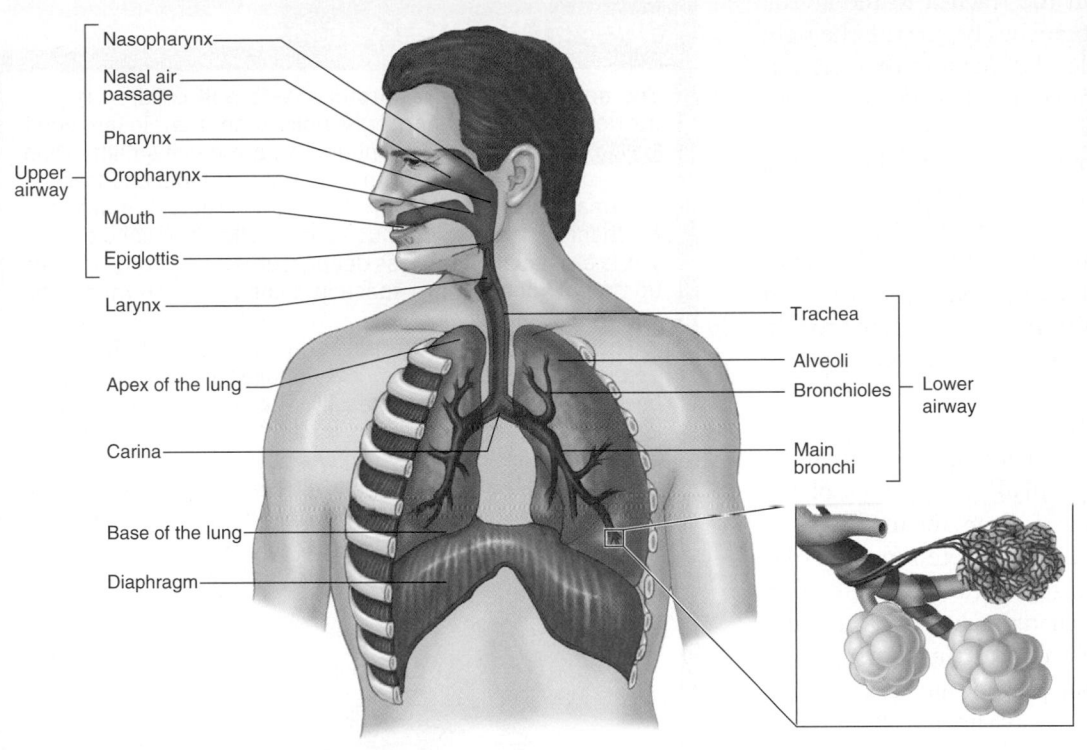

Figure 64 The respiratory system consists of all structures of the body that contribute to the process of breathing.

it is less moist than air that enters through the nose. Air inhaled through the mouth passes through the oropharynx, which is separated from the nasopharynx by the hard palate anteriorly and the soft palate posteriorly. Once through the nasopharynx and oropharynx, air then enters the laryngopharynx, also known as the hypopharynx because it is the inferiormost passage of the upper airway.

Two passageways are located at the bottom of the pharynx: the **esophagus** behind and the **trachea** (windpipe) in front. Food and liquids enter the pharynx and pass into the esophagus, which carries them to the stomach. Air and other gases enter the trachea and go to the lungs.

Protecting the opening of the trachea is a thin, leaf-shaped valve called the **epiglottis**. This valve allows air to pass into the trachea but prevents food and liquid from entering the airway under normal circumstances. Air moves past the epiglottis into the larynx and the trachea. The glottis or glottic opening is the space between the vocal cords where air enters the trachea.

▇ The Lower Airway

The Adam's apple, or thyroid cartilage, is easily seen in the middle of the front of the neck. The thyroid cartilage is actually the anterior part of the larynx. Tiny muscles open and close the vocal cords and control tension on them. Sounds are created as air is forced past the vocal cords, making them vibrate. These vibrations make the sound. The pitch of the sound changes as the cords open and close. You can feel the vibrations if you place your fingers lightly on the larynx as you speak

or sing. The vibrations of air are shaped by the tongue and muscles of the mouth to form understandable sounds.

As mentioned earlier, immediately below the thyroid cartilage is the palpable cricoid cartilage. Between the thyroid and cricoid cartilage lies the cricothyroid membrane, which can be felt as a depression in the midline of the neck just inferior to the thyroid cartilage.

Below the cricoid cartilage is the trachea. The trachea extends downward into the thoracic cavity where it splits into the right and left **mainstem bronchi**. The trachea is approximately 5″ long and is a semirigid, enclosed air tube made up of rings of cartilage that are open in the back. This enables food to pass through the esophagus, which lies right behind the trachea. The rings of cartilage keep the trachea from collapsing when air moves into and out of the lungs.

Words of Wisdom

Acute asthma is a recurring condition of reversible acute airflow obstruction in the lower airway. It is the most common chronic disease of childhood. Four distinct events occur in an asthma attack. Smooth muscle spasm occurs when the muscle layers around the airways constrict (**bronchospasm**), resulting in narrowing of the airway diameter. Increased secretion of mucus causes mucus plugging, further decreasing the airway diameter, and finally, inflammatory cell proliferation occurs. White blood cells accumulate in the airway and secrete substances that worsen the muscle spasm and increase mucus production.

The most common cause of an asthma attack is an upper respiratory infection, such as bronchitis or a cold. Other causes include changes in environmental conditions; emotions, especially stress; allergic reactions to pollens, foods (chocolate, shellfish, milk, nuts) or drugs (sulfa, penicillin, lidocaine, and other local anesthetics); and occupational exposures.

The severity of asthma attacks varies among patients. In severe cases (status asthmaticus), the patient may die as a result of respiratory failure. In other cases, treatment may produce rapid improvement and resolution of the asthmatic crisis.

Branched airways leading from the trachea to the alveoli make up the bronchial tree. These branches begin with the right and left primary bronchi, near the level of the fifth thoracic vertebra. Each primary bronchus divides into a secondary bronchus, tertiary bronchi, and even finer tubes.

At the level of the fifth thoracic vertebra, the trachea branches into the right and left mainstem bronchi at the carina, a projection of the lowest portion of the tracheal cartilage.

Beyond the carina, air enters the lungs through the mainstem bronchi. The point of entry for the bronchi, vessels, and nerves into each lung is called the <u>hilum</u>. The mainstem bronchi divide into the <u>secondary bronchi</u>, each one going to a separate lobe of the lung (Figure 65).

Secondary bronchi branch into <u>tertiary bronchi</u>, which continue to branch several times. After several generations of successive branching, <u>bronchioles</u>, small subdivisions of the bronchi, are formed. Bronchioles develop from the final branching of the bronchiole. Each bronchiole divides to form <u>alveolar ducts</u>. Each alveolar duct ends in clusters known as <u>alveoli</u>, tiny sacs of lung tissue in which gas exchange takes place. Pulmonary <u>surfactant</u> found in the alveoli reduces surface tension to increase pulmonary compliance and prevent atelectasis at the end of expiration. The lung contains approximately 300 million alveoli; each alveolus is about 0.33 mm in diameter. Capillaries cover the alveoli. The <u>alveolocapillary membrane</u> lies between the alveolus and the capillary and is thin, consisting of only one cell layer. Respiratory exchange between the lung and blood vessels occurs in the alveoli at the alveolocapillary membrane.

Lungs

The <u>lungs</u> are the primary organs of breathing. The right lung contains three lobes (the upper, middle, and lower lobes); the

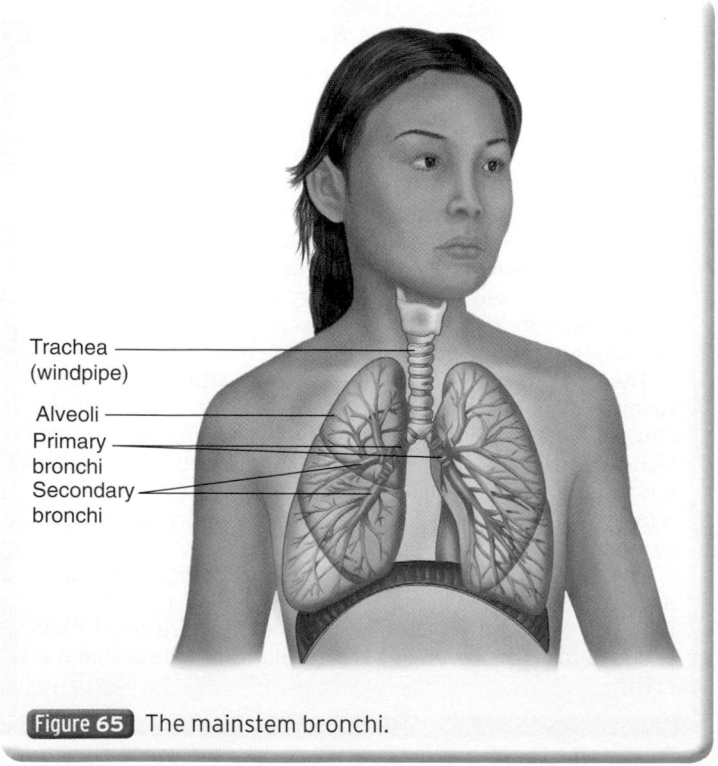

Trachea
(windpipe)

Alveoli

Primary
bronchi

Secondary
bronchi

Figure 65   The mainstem bronchi.

The anatomy of the respiratory system in children is proportionally smaller and less rigid than that in an adult Figure 66 . A child's nose and mouth are much smaller than those of an adult. The larynx, cricoid cartilage, and trachea are smaller, softer, and more flexible as well. This makes the mechanics of breathing much more delicate. A child's pharynx is also smaller and less deeply curved. The tongue takes up proportionally more space in a child's mouth than in an adult's mouth.

These anatomic differences are important for your assessment. For example, the smaller larynx of a child becomes obstructed more easily. The chest wall in children is softer. Therefore, children depend more heavily on the diaphragm for breathing. You will notice that the abdomen moves in and out considerably with each breath, especially in an infant. Young infants do not know how to breathe through the mouth. Therefore, as you assess an infant or a child, you must carefully consider these differences.

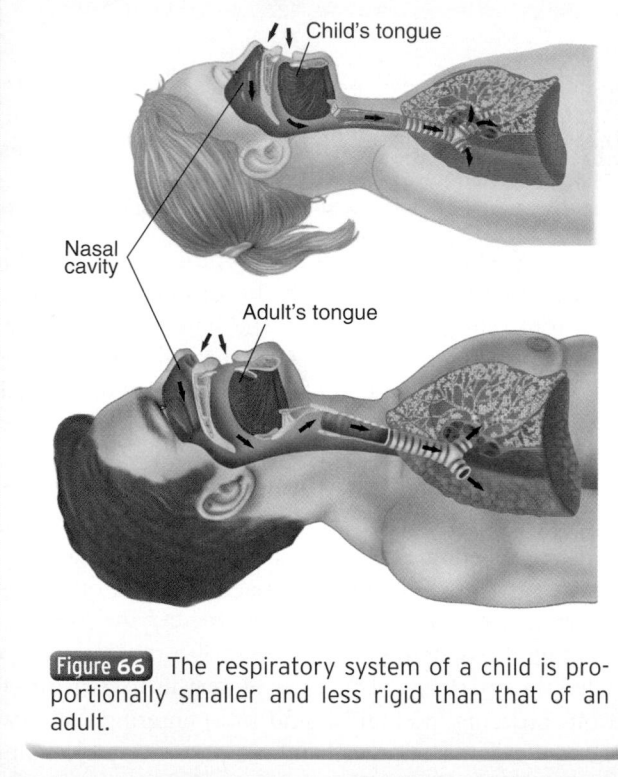

Child's tongue

Nasal
cavity

Adult's tongue

Figure 66   The respiratory system of a child is proportionally smaller and less rigid than that of an adult.

left lung contains only two (the upper and lower lobes). The lungs are surrounded by a membrane of connective tissue known as <u>pleura</u>.

The <u>visceral pleura</u> is the pleural membrane that covers the lung and folds back to become the <u>parietal pleura</u>. A potential space known as the <u>pleural space</u> exists between the visceral and parietal pleura. Normally, the two membranes are close together and a space does not exist. Both layers of pleura work together to help maintain normal expansion and contraction of the lung. Under certain disease conditions or following trauma, fluid and/or air may accumulate in the pleural space, potentially causing respiratory problems **Figure 67** .

The lungs receive blood in two ways. Deoxygenated blood flows from the right ventricle via the pulmonary arteries. This blood flows through pulmonary capillaries, is reoxygenated at the alveoli, and then returns to the heart via the pulmonary veins.

In addition, bronchial arteries branch off of the thoracic aorta and supply the lung tissues themselves with blood. Deoxygenated blood returns to the heart via the bronchial veins. Peripherally in the lungs, venous blood from the bronchi enters the pulmonary veins, returning with oxygenated blood from the alveoli.

Muscles of Breathing

Respiration consists of ventilation, which is the movement of air from outside the body into and out of the bronchial tree and alveoli. There are several muscles involved in making the lungs expand and contract. The primary muscle is called the **diaphragm**. Contraction of the diaphragm, along with that of the chest wall muscles, assists with allowing air to be drawn into the lungs. Anteriorly, it attaches to the costal arch; posteriorly, it attaches to the lumbar vertebrae. The diaphragm cannot be seen or palpated.

The diaphragm is unique because it has characteristics of voluntary (skeletal) and involuntary (smooth) muscle. It is a dome-shaped muscle that divides the thorax from the abdomen and is pierced by the great vessels and the esophagus **Figure 68** . It acts like a voluntary muscle when you take a deep breath, cough, or hold your breath. You control these variations in the way you breathe.

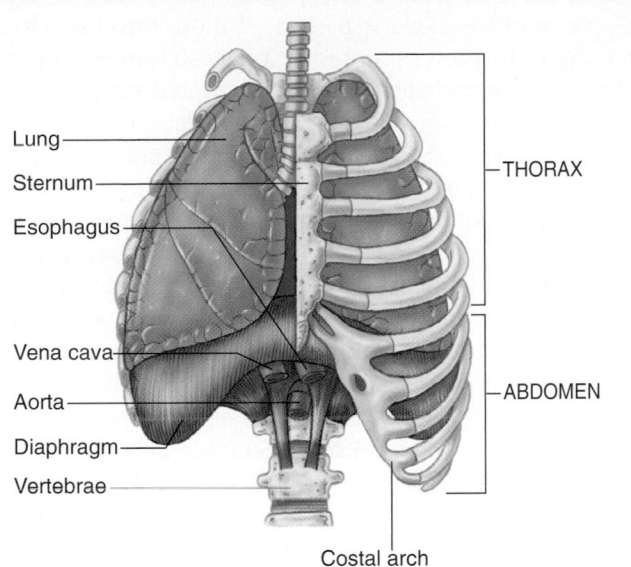

Figure 68 The dome-shaped diaphragm divides the thorax from the abdomen. It is pierced by the great vessels and the esophagus.

However, unlike other skeletal or voluntary muscles, the diaphragm performs an automatic function. Breathing continues during sleep and at all other times. Even though you can hold your breath or temporarily breathe faster or slower, you cannot continue these variations in breathing pattern indefinitely. When the concentration of carbon dioxide becomes too high, automatic regulation of breathing resumes. Therefore, although the diaphragm looks like voluntary skeletal muscle and is attached to the skeleton, it behaves, for the most part, like an involuntary muscle.

The other muscles involved in breathing are the internal and external intercostal muscles, the abdominal muscles, and the pectoral muscles. Muscles of the chest wall are innervated by the intercostal nerves, while the diaphragm is innervated by the phrenic nerve. During inhalation or inspiration, the diaphragm and external intercostal muscles between the ribs contract. When the diaphragm contracts, it moves down slightly, enlarging the thoracic cage from top to bottom. When the external intercostal muscles contract, they move the ribs up and out. These actions combine to enlarge the chest cavity in all dimensions. Pressure in the cavity then falls, making it lower than atmospheric pressure, and air rushes into the lungs. This is referred to as negative pressure breathing because air is essentially sucked into the lungs. This part of the cycle is active, requiring the muscles to contract.

During exhalation or expiration, the diaphragm and the intercostal muscles relax. Unlike inhalation, exhalation does not normally require muscular effort. As these muscles relax, all dimensions of the thorax decrease, and the ribs and muscles assume a normal resting position. When the volume of the chest cavity decreases, air in the lungs is compressed into a smaller space and pressure is greater than atmospheric pressure. Intrapulmonic pressure, which is the pressure within the lungs and

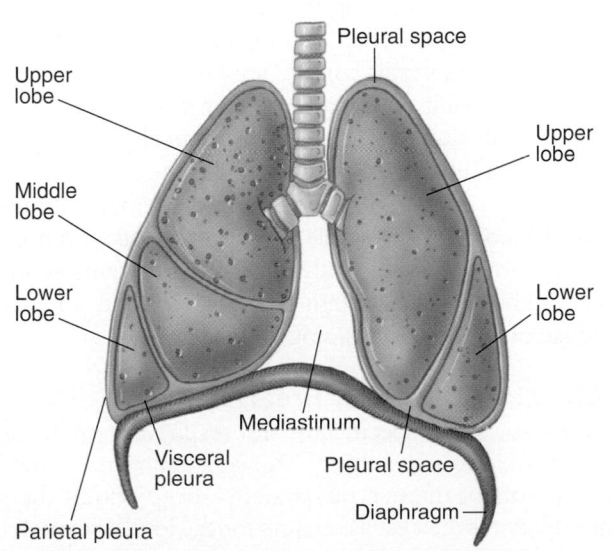

Figure 67 The pleura lining the chest wall and covering the lungs is an essential part of the breathing mechanism. The pleural space is not an actual space until blood or air leaks into it, causing the pleural surfaces to separate.

airways, is increased, and air is pushed out through the trachea. This phase of the cycle is passive. If more forceful exhalation is required, the posterior internal intercostals muscles contract, pulling the ribs and sternum downward and inward to further increase the pressure in the lungs. Exhalation ends when the intrapleural pressure is equal to the atmospheric pressure, at which point air stops flowing from the lungs to the outside. At the point of equilibration, all pressures in the respiratory system are exactly equal to atmospheric pressure except the intrapleural pressure, which is the pressure between the pleura of the lungs, and which stays just slightly negative as the visceral pleura is pulled inward by the tendency of the lungs to collapse and the parietal pleura is pulled outward by its adhesion to the chest wall. This negative pressure will be studied later because it is the primary cause of accumulations of air known as a pneumothorax.

The process of breathing is typically easy and requires little muscular effort. But, now imagine breathing through a straw and suddenly the diameter of the straw decreases. The smaller the diameter of the straw, the more effort you will now have to exert to move air. As the resistance in the airway increases, you will begin to use more muscle groups, namely your abdominal and pectoral muscles, to assist the diaphragm in moving that air.

Words of Wisdom

Chronic obstructive pulmonary disease (COPD) is a progressive, irreversible disease of the airway marked by decreased inspiratory and expiratory capacity of the lungs. COPD may result from chronic bronchitis (excess mucus production) or emphysema (lung tissue damage with loss of elastic recoil of the lungs). Patients with COPD usually have a combination of both problems and generally function at a certain baseline level until an event occurs that causes an acute episode.

Chronic bronchitis results from overgrowth of the airway mucous glands and excess secretion of mucus, which blocks the airway. Patients have a chronic productive cough. Emphysema results from destruction of the alveolar walls, which creates resistance to expiratory airflow. The major cause of COPD is cigarette smoking. Industrial inhalants (such as asbestos and coal dust), air pollution, and tuberculosis can also lead to COPD. The patient who is experiencing an acute COPD episode will report shortness of breath with gradually increasing symptoms over a period of days. This concept is discussed in greater detail in the chapter, *Respiratory Emergencies*.

The Respiratory System: Physiology

The primary function of the respiratory system is to exchange gases at the alveolocapillary membrane, or conduct **respiration**. Oxygen is essential for the body to function. The amount of oxygen in inspired air is approximately 21%. The blood does not use all the inhaled oxygen as it passes through the body. Exhaled air contains 16% oxygen and 3% to 5% carbon dioxide; the rest is nitrogen. This 16% concentration of oxygen is adequate to support artificial ventilation. **Ventilation** is the process of moving air in and out of the lungs. So as you provide artificial ventilations to a patient who is not breathing, the patient is receiving a 16% concentration of oxygen with each ventilation.

Respiration

At the alveolocapillary exchange surface, the alveolus and the red blood cells are located close together. Diffusion is the process by which a gas dissolves in a liquid. Through the process of diffusion, the gases move from a higher concentration to a lower concentration. Therefore, oxygen moves across the membrane into the capillaries where it attaches to the hemoglobin. Likewise, carbon dioxide moves into the alveoli where the concentration is lower. Oxygenated blood enters the left side of the heart and is pumped to the tissues. Oxygen is "offloaded" from the red blood cells to the tissues as carbon dioxide and waste products from the tissues are "loaded" into the bloodstream. Venous blood returns to the right side of the heart and the pulmonary capillary bed (via the pulmonary arteries). The carbon dioxide diffuses into the alveoli and is released into the atmosphere as the person exhales **Figure 69**. The primary waste product of metabolism is carbon dioxide, which is carried in the blood to the lungs.

Because there are so many alveoli, a fairly large surface area exists for respiratory exchange to occur in the context of the relatively limited size of the thoracic cavity. The total surface area created around the alveoli is more than 85 m². This is significantly more than would exist if each lung consisted of only a single sphere, like a large balloon. In that case, the surface area would be only 0.01 m² (1 m equals 39.37″).

In normal physiology, the amount of surface area available for ventilation, symbolized by the letter V, is well matched with the amount of blood flowing through the alveoli and available for gas exchange, also termed perfusion, symbolized by the letter Q. Disturbances in this balance are known as V̇/Q̇ mismatch, and can be the result of severe illness or injury. For example, a pulmonary contusion reduces the amount of alveoli available for gas exchange, inhibiting gas exchange despite a normal amount of blood flow. Conversely, a pulmonary embolus limits the amount of blood flow available for gas exchange, even though there are a normal amount of alveoli capable of being ventilated. V̇/Q̇ mismatches are difficult to diagnose without an excellent knowledge of the pathophysiology involved.

The Chemical Control of Breathing

The brain—or more specifically, the respiratory center in the brainstem—controls breathing. This area is in one of the best-protected parts of the nervous system—deep within the skull. The nerves in this area act as sensors for the level of carbon dioxide in the blood and subsequently the spinal fluid. The brain automatically controls breathing if the level of carbon dioxide or oxygen in the arterial blood is too high or too low. In fact, adjustments can be made in just one breath. For these reasons, you cannot hold your breath indefinitely or breathe rapidly and deeply indefinitely.

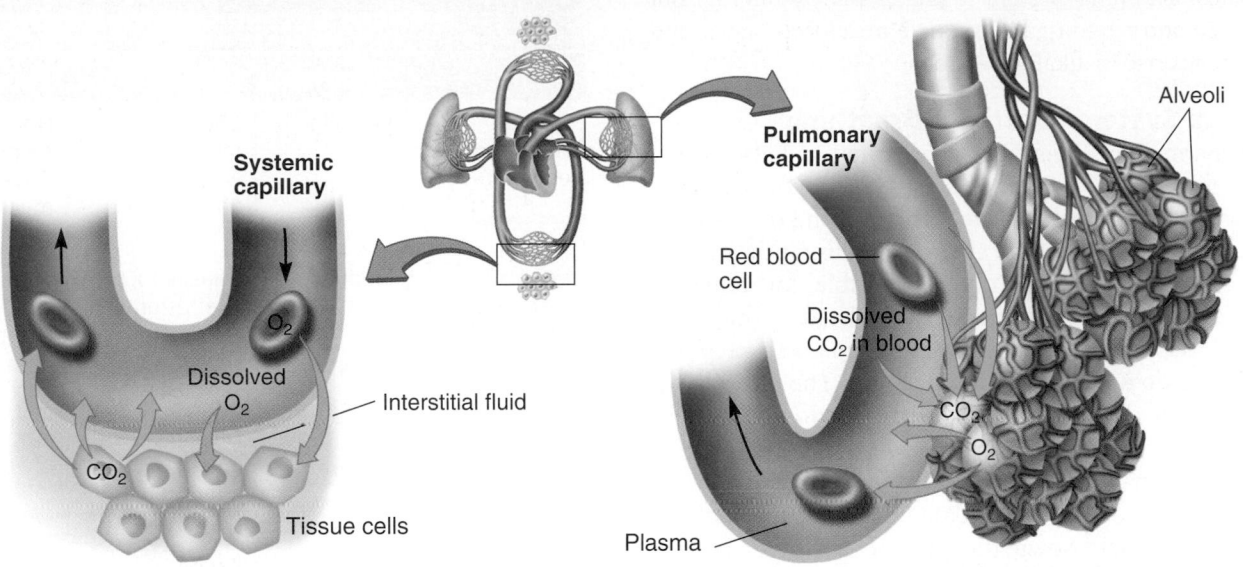

Systemic capillary

Dissolved O$_2$

O$_2$

Interstitial fluid

CO$_2$

Tissue cells

Pulmonary capillary

Alveoli

Red blood cell

Dissolved CO$_2$ in blood

CO$_2$

O$_2$

Plasma

Figure 69 In the capillaries of the lungs, oxygen (O$_2$) passes from the blood to the tissue cells, and carbon dioxide (CO$_2$) and waste pass from the tissue cells to the blood. Diffusion occurs when molecules move from an area of higher concentration to an area of lower concentration.

A complicated interaction of signals provides feedback to the respiratory center, allowing it to continuously control respiration. The main respiratory stimulus is accumulation of carbon dioxide in the blood. Typically, this is measured as the Paco$_2$ on the arterial blood gases. Increases in the Paco$_2$ result in decreased pH levels in the respiratory center, which triggers an increase in ventilation. Decreases in the Paco$_2$ result in increased pH levels in the respiratory center and a decrease in ventilation. Low blood oxygen levels also stimulate breathing, but normally have much less of an effect than does the Paco$_2$.

Words of Wisdom

Measurements of oxygen and carbon dioxide levels in the blood are called the __partial pressure of oxygen (Pao$_2$)__ and the __partial pressure of carbon dioxide (Paco$_2$)__. These values are not always available to paramedics, but are useful for paramedics to understand. pH is the degree of acidity or alkalinity. Deviations from normal Pao$_2$, Paco$_2$, and pH values occur in many different disease states.

Essentially, Paco$_2$ acts as "respiratory acid." Changes in the Paco$_2$ value rapidly change the pH levels, either making it more basic (increased) or more acidic (decreased). Changes in the Paco$_2$ can result from diseases such as asthma or COPD exacerbation, drug overdose, or can be a response to a change in the blood pH because of a metabolic problem. A decrease in the pH of the arterial blood that is caused by an elevation in the Paco$_2$ is called a primary __respiratory acidosis__, whereas an increase in the pH of the blood that is caused by excessive exhalation of co$_2$ is called a primary __respiratory alkalosis__. Conversely, changes in the Paco$_2$ that occur in response to primary metabolic problems (__metabolic alkalosis__ or __metabolic acidosis__) are called compensatory changes.

The body also has a "backup system" to control respiration called the __hypoxic drive__. When the oxygen level falls, this system will also stimulate breathing. There are areas in the brain, the walls of the aorta, and the carotid arteries that act as oxygen sensors. These sensors are easily satisfied by minimal levels of oxygen in the arterial blood. Therefore, the backup system, the hypoxic drive, is much less sensitive and less powerful than the carbon dioxide sensors in the brainstem.

Buffer Systems A __buffer__ is a substance that can absorb or donate hydrogen (H$^+$). Buffers absorb hydrogen ions when they are in excess and donate hydrogen ions when they are depleted. Therefore, __buffer systems__ act as rapid defenses for acid-base changes, providing almost immediate protection against changes in the hydrogen ion concentration of the extracellular fluid. The generic reaction between a hydrogen ion and a buffer is expressed as follows:

$$H^+ + \text{Buffer} \leftrightarrow \text{H-Buffer}$$

Free H$^+$ (acid) binds with the buffer to form a weak acid (H–Buffer). This reaction can shift to the right or left depending on the hydrogen ion concentration. When the H$^+$ concentration increases and buffer is available, the reaction is forced to the right and more H–Buffer is formed. When the H$^+$ concentration decreases, the reaction shifts toward the left, and H$^+$ disassociates from the buffer, leaving H$^+$ and buffer.

The respiratory system and the renal system work in conjunction with the bicarbonate buffer to maintain homeostasis. The fastest way the body can get rid of excess acid is through the respiratory system. Excess acid can be expelled as co$_2$ from the lungs. Conversely, slowing respirations will increase co$_2$ in alkalotic states. The renal system regulates pH by filtering out more hydrogen and retaining bicarbonate in acidotic states, and doing just the reverse in alkalotic states.

The Nervous System Control of Breathing

The exact way breathing occurs is complicated and also poorly understood by science. It is known that the medulla oblongata—the lower half of the brainstem that, among others, controls those autonomic functions such as breathing, heart rate, and blood pressure—is primarily responsible for initiating the ventilation cycle and is primarily stimulated by high carbon dioxide levels. The function of the medulla is to keep you breathing so you do not have to think about it. The medulla has two main portions that control breathing: the <u>dorsal respiratory group (DRG)</u> and the <u>ventral respiratory group (VRG)</u>. The DRG is the main pacemaker for breathing and is responsible for initiating inspiration. It sets the base pattern for respirations. The DRG sends signals down the phrenic nerve to the diaphragm. The diaphragm contracts, and inspiration begins. The DRG shuts off, the diaphragm relaxes, and expiration begins. The VRG helps to provide for forced inspiration or expiration as needed.

The pons, another area within the brainstem, helps regulate the DRG activities. The pons has two areas. The <u>pneumotaxic (pontine) center</u>, located in the superior portion of the pons, helps shut off the DRG, resulting in shorter, faster respirations. The <u>apneustic center</u>, located in the inferior portion of the pons, stimulates the DRG, resulting in longer, slower respirations. Both areas of the pons are used to help augment respirations during emotional or physical stress. The two areas of the medulla and the two areas of the pons work together to help you get the right amount of air when you need it.

The VRG, pneumotaxic center, and apneustic center are involved in changing the depth of inspiration, expiration, or both. How does the body know when to stop breathing in or out? When the VRG is causing you to take a forced inspiration, what prevents you from taking in so much air that you pop your lungs like a balloon? The answer is the <u>Hering-Breuer reflex</u>. Special stretch receptors in the chest wall are able to detect if the lungs are too full or too empty. The Hering-Breuer reflex stops the VRG, pneumotaxic center, and apneustic centers from accidentally causing lung trauma. **Table 13** summarizes the nervous system functions regarding respirations.

◼ Ventilation

A substantial amount of air can be moved within the respiratory system. **Figure 70** shows the typical volumes. An adult male has a total lung capacity of 6,000 mL (equivalent to three 2-liter bottles of soda). An adult female has about one third less total capacity because the lung size is smaller.

As you are reading this book, unless you just finished exercising, the amount of your air movement is approximately 500 mL. This is called <u>tidal volume</u>. Tidal volume is the amount of air that is moved into or out of the lungs during a single breath. <u>Inspiratory reserve volume</u> is the deepest breath you can take

Table 13	Nervous System Control of Breathing		
Name	**Location**	**Function**	**Timing**
Dorsal respiratory group (DRG)	Medulla	Causes inspiration when stimulated	Normal, resting respirations. Rhythmic, mechanical pattern
Ventral respiratory group (VRG)	Medulla	Causes forced expiration or inspiration	Speech, increased emotional or physical stress
Pneumotaxic (pontine) center	Pons	Inhibits the DRG; increases speed and depth of respirations	Increased emotional or physical stress
Apneustic center	Pons	Excites the DRG; prolongs inspiration, decreases rate	Increased emotional or physical stress
Hering-Breuer inflation reflex (stretch reflex)	Chest	Detects lung expansion to a point and then tells VRG and pneumotaxic and apneustic centers to stop	Increased emotional or physical stress
Hering-Breuer deflation reflex	Chest	Detects potential lung collapse and then tells VRG and pneumotaxic and apneustic centers to stop	Increased emotional or physical stress

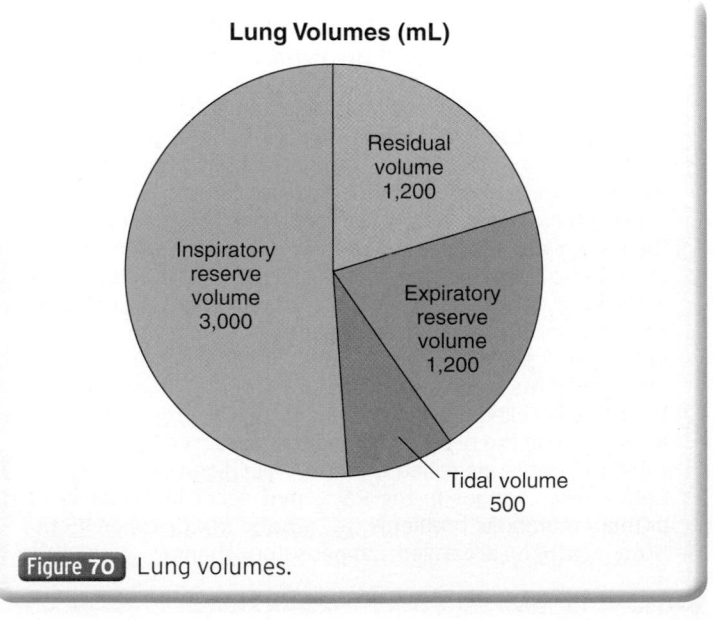

Lung Volumes (mL)

Residual volume 1,200

Inspiratory reserve volume 3,000

Expiratory reserve volume 1,200

Tidal volume 500

Figure 70 Lung volumes.

after a normal breath. Conversely, <u>expiratory reserve volume</u> is the maximum amount of air that you can forcibly breathe out after a normal breath. Gas remains in the lungs simply to keep the lungs open. This is called the <u>residual volume</u>. This gas does not move during ventilation. Some residual volume is lost when a person is hit in the chest and has the "wind knocked out of him." <u>Vital capacity</u> is the amount of air moved in and out of the lungs with maximum inspiration and expiration.

When you assist a patient's breathing, you move air in and out of the lungs. You will use a bag-mask device—a large bag filled with air that, when squeezed, pushes air out one end. The typical bag-mask device holds approximately 1,000 to 1,200 mL of air. Note that although a person's resting tidal volume is 500 mL, you need to use a bag-mask device that provides more than twice that volume. This is because of dead space.

<u>Dead space</u> is the portion of the respiratory system that has no alveoli, and, therefore, little or no exchange of gas between air and blood occurs. The mouth, trachea, bronchi, and bronchioles are all considered dead space. When you ventilate a patient with any device, you create more dead space. Gas must first fill the device before it can be moved into the patient.

When you are assessing your patient, you need to accurately determine whether he or she is having trouble breathing. The patient's respiratory rate provides only part of the information that is needed. The depth of each breath is critical information to know when assessing ventilation. There is another measurement called minute volume that provides you with a more accurate determination of effective ventilation. <u>Minute volume</u>, also referred to as minute ventilation or minute respiratory volume (MRV), is easy to understand; it is the amount of air that moves in and out of the lungs in 1 minute minus the dead space.

Minute Volume = Respiratory Rate × Tidal Volume

This calculation helps you to determine how deeply a patient is breathing. While riding in the ambulance it will be difficult to determine the patient's exact tidal volume, but you will be able to estimate it. Consider the scenario of a patient who is breathing at a normal rate of 20 breaths/min. Yet, when you look at the patient's chest, it is barely moving. When you feel for air movement out of the mouth, you find little movement. The patient is in trouble and needs your assistance now! Even though the patient's respiratory rate is normal, the amount of air being moved is inadequate. The minute volume is too low, and the patient needs ventilatory assistance. You will need to always evaluate the amount of air being moved with each breath when you are assessing a patient's respirations.

Characteristics of Normal Breathing

You can think of a normal breathing pattern as a bellows system. Normal breathing should appear easy, not labored. As with a bellows that is used to move air to start a fire, breathing should be a smooth flow of air moving into and out of the lungs.

Normal breathing has the following characteristics:

- Adequate rate and depth (tidal volume)
- A regular rhythm or pattern of inhalation and exhalation
- Audible breath sounds on both sides of the chest
- Regular rise and fall movement on both sides of the chest
- Movement of the abdomen
- Silent and effortless

Inadequate Breathing Patterns in Adults

An adult who is awake, alert, and talking to you has no immediate airway or breathing problems. However, you should keep supplemental oxygen on hand to assist with breathing should it become necessary. An adult who is not breathing well will appear to be working hard to breathe. This type of breathing pattern is called <u>labored breathing</u>. Labored breathing requires effort and may involve the accessory muscles. The person may also be breathing much slower (fewer than 12 breaths/min) or much faster (more than 20 breaths/min) than normal. An adult who is breathing normally and is at rest will have respirations of 12 to 20 breaths/min Table 14 .

With a normal breathing pattern, the accessory muscles are not being used. With inadequate breathing, a person, especially a child, may use the accessory muscles of the chest, neck, and abdomen. Other signs that a person is not breathing normally include the following:

- Muscle retractions above the clavicles, between the ribs, and below the rib cage, especially in children
- Pale or cyanotic (blue) skin
- Cool, damp (clammy) skin
- Tripod position Figure 71 (a position in which the patient is leaning forward onto two arms stretched forward)

Table 14	Normal Respiratory Rate Ranges
Adults	12 to 20 breaths/min
Children	15 to 30 breaths/min
Infants	25 to 50 breaths/min

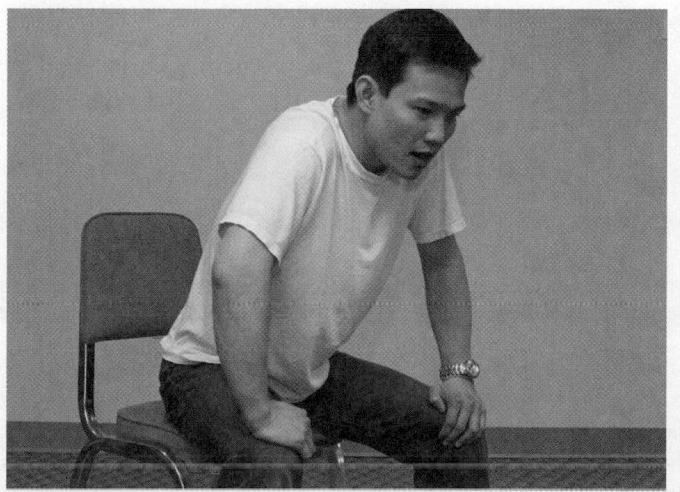

Figure 71 A patient in the tripod position will sit leaning forward on outstretched arms with the head and chin thrust slightly forward.

A patient may also appear to be breathing after the normal respiration has stopped. These occasional, gasping breaths are called **agonal gasps**. Agonal gasps occur when the respiratory center in the brain continues to send signals to the breathing muscles. These respirations are not adequate because they are slow and generally shallow. You should assist ventilations of patients with agonal gasps.

Special Populations

Normal breathing patterns in infants and children are essentially the same as those in adults. However, infants and children breathe faster than adults. An infant who is breathing normally will have respirations of 25 to 50 breaths/min. A child will have respirations of 15 to 30 breaths/min. Like adults, infants and children who are breathing normally will have smooth, regular inhalation and exhalation, equal breath sounds, and regular rise and fall movements on both sides of the chest.

Breathing problems in infants and children often appear the same as breathing problems in adults. Signs such as increased respirations, an irregular breathing pattern, unequal breath sounds, and unequal chest expansion indicate breathing problems in adults and children. Other signs that an infant or child is not breathing normally include the following:

- Accessory muscle use, in which the muscles of the abdomen, shoulders, and neck are also used for breathing
- Retractions, in which the skin between the ribs (intercostals retractions), above the sternum or clavicles (suprasternal or supraclavicular retractions), or below the costal margins (subcostal retractions) is sunken or pulled inward as the child struggles to inhale
- Nasal flaring, in which the nostrils flare out as the child inhales
- Seesaw respirations in infants, in which the chest and abdominal muscles alternately contract to look like a seesaw

Exhalation becomes active when infants and children have trouble breathing. Normally, inhalation alone is the active, muscular part of breathing, as described earlier. However, with labored breathing, both inhalation and exhalation are hard work. With labored breathing, exhalation is not passive. Instead, air is forced out of the lungs during exhalation, and the child will often begin to wheeze. This type of labored breathing may involve the use of the accessory muscles of breathing.

The Circulatory System: Anatomy

The **circulatory system** includes the heart and a complex arrangement of connected tubes, including the arteries, arterioles, capillaries, venules, and veins Figure 72 . Another name for this system is the cardiovascular (heart/blood vessels) system. The circulatory system is entirely closed. There are two circuits in the body: the **systemic circulation**, which travels throughout the body, and the **pulmonary circulation**, which travels only between the heart and lungs. The systemic circulation carries oxygen-rich blood from the left ventricle through the body and back

to the right atrium. In the systemic circulation, as blood passes through the tissues and organs, it gives up oxygen and nutrients and absorbs cellular wastes and carbon dioxide. The cellular wastes are eliminated as blood passes through the liver and kidneys. The pulmonary circulation carries oxygen-poor blood from the right ventricle through the lungs and back to the left atrium. In the pulmonary circulation, as blood passes through the lungs, it is refreshed with oxygen and gives up carbon dioxide.

The Heart

Location and Major Structures of the Heart

The **heart** is a muscular organ that pumps blood throughout the body. Heart muscle is called **myocardium**. The term "myo" means muscle and "cardium" means heart. The heart is located behind the sternum and is about the size of the closed fist of the person it belongs to, roughly 5″ long, 3″ wide, and 2″ thick. It weighs 10 to 12 oz in male adults and 8 to 10 oz in female adults. Approximately two thirds of the heart lies in the left part of the **mediastinum**, the area between the lungs that also contains the great vessels.

The **pericardium**, also called the pericardial sac, is a thick, fibrous membrane that surrounds the heart. The pericardium anchors the heart within the mediastinum and prevents overdistention of the heart. It has an outer, fibrous membrane (parietal), and an inner membrane (visceral). The fibrous pericardium is made of dense connective tissue. This is attached to the central diaphragm, posterior sternum, vertebral column, and large blood vessels connected to the heart. An inner, double-layered visceral pericardium (epicardium) covers the heart as well. At the base of the heart, the visceral pericardium folds back to become the parietal pericardium. Between the parietal and visceral layers is the pericardial cavity, containing a small volume of serous fluid (about 5 mL) that reduces friction between the pericardial membranes as the heart moves within them.

The three layers composing the wall of the heart are the outer epicardium, middle myocardium, and inner endocardium. The **epicardium** protects the heart by reducing friction, and is the visceral portion of the pericardium on the surface of the heart. It consists of connective tissue and some deep adipose tissue. The thick myocardium is made mostly of cardiac muscle tissue that is organized in planes and richly supplied by blood capillaries, lymph capillaries, and nerve fibers. It pumps blood out of the chambers of the heart. The **endocardium** is made up of epithelium and connective tissue with many elastic and collagenous fibers. It also contains blood vessels and specialized cardiac muscle fibers known as **Purkinje fibers**.

The normal human heart consists of four chambers: two atria and two ventricles. The upper chambers are the atria, and the lower chambers are the ventricles. Each side of the heart contains

Words of Wisdom

Complete blockage of an artery that supplies oxygen to the heart results in interruption of blood flow to a portion of the myocardium, called a **myocardial infarction**.

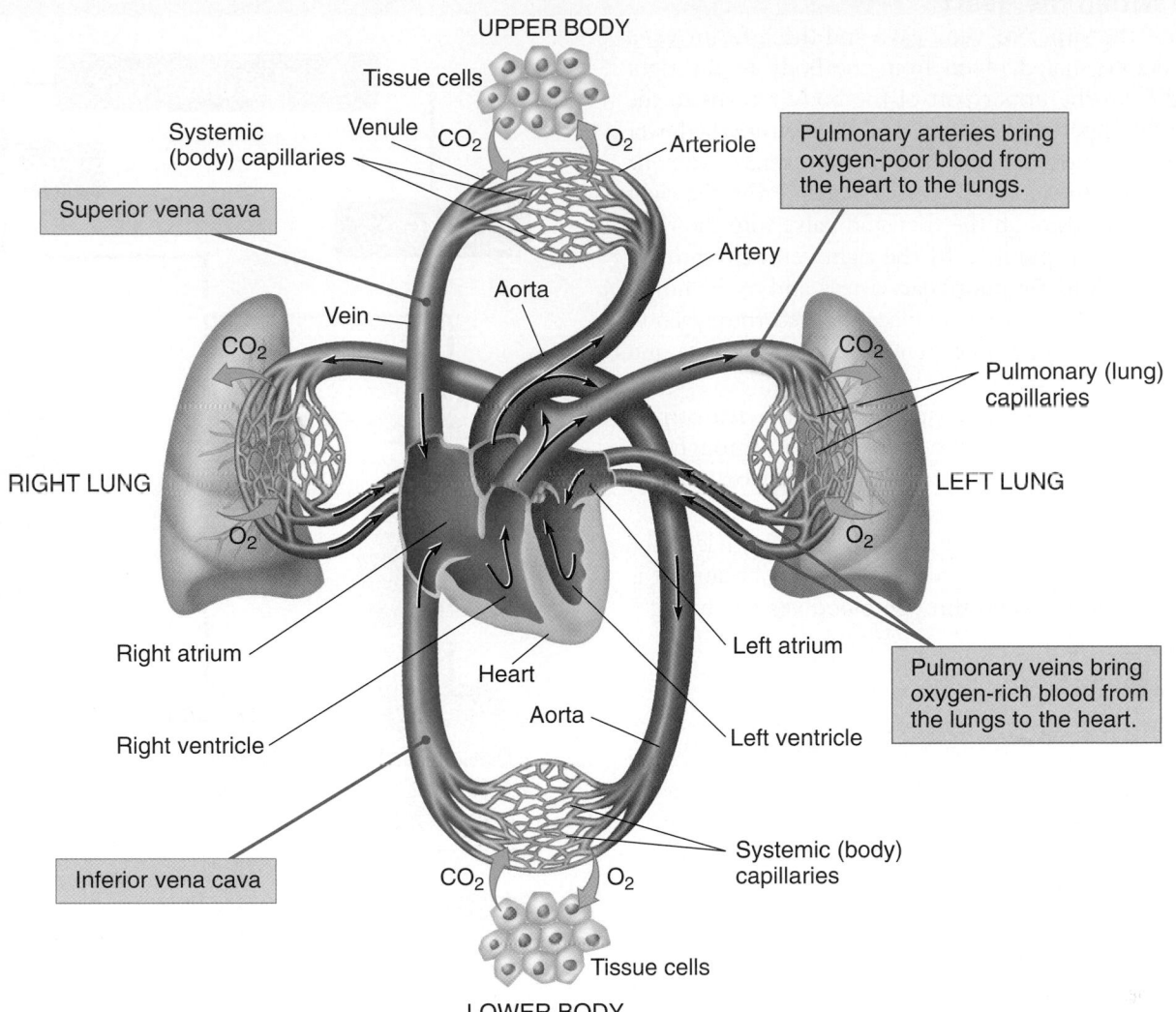

UPPER BODY

Tissue cells

Systemic (body) capillaries — Venule — CO_2 — O_2 — Arteriole

Superior vena cava

Pulmonary arteries bring oxygen-poor blood from the heart to the lungs.

Artery

Aorta

Vein

CO_2

CO_2

Pulmonary (lung) capillaries

RIGHT LUNG

O_2

O_2

LEFT LUNG

Right atrium

Left atrium

Heart

Aorta

Pulmonary veins bring oxygen-rich blood from the lungs to the heart.

Right ventricle

Left ventricle

Systemic (body) capillaries

Inferior vena cava

CO_2

O_2

Tissue cells

LOWER BODY

Figure 72 The circulatory system includes the heart, arteries, veins, and interconnecting capillaries. The capillaries are the smallest vessels and connect venules and arterioles. At the center of the system, and providing its driving force, is the heart. Blood circulates through the body under pressure generated by the two sides of the heart.

one atrium and one ventricle. A membrane, the <u>interatrial septum</u>, separates the two atria; a thicker wall, the <u>interventricular septum</u>, separates the right and left ventricles. Each <u>atrium</u> receives blood that is returned to the heart from other parts of the body and contracts to ensure its corresponding ventricle is filled completely; each <u>ventricle</u> pumps blood out of the heart. The upper and lower portions of the heart are separated by the atrioventricular valves, which prevent blood from flowing backward. There are also valves located between the ventricles and the arteries into which they pump blood. These are called the semilunar valves.

Blood enters the right atrium via the superior and inferior venae cavae and the <u>coronary sinus</u>, which consists of veins that collect blood that is returning from the walls of the heart. Blood from four <u>pulmonary veins</u> enters the left atrium. Between the right and left atria is a depression, the <u>fossa ovalis</u>, which represents the former location of the <u>foramen ovale</u>, an opening between the two atria that is present in the fetus.

Valves of the Heart

Blood passing from the atria to the ventricles flows through one of two <u>atrioventricular valves</u>. The <u>tricuspid valve</u> separates the right atrium from the right ventricle, and the <u>mitral valve</u>, a bicuspid valve, separates the left atrium from the left ventricle. The valves consist of flaps called <u>cusps</u>. <u>Papillary muscles</u> attach to the ventricles and send small muscular strands called <u>chordae tendineae</u> to the cusps. When the papillary muscle contracts, these strands tighten, preventing backflow of blood through the valves from the ventricles to the atria.

Two <u>semilunar valves</u>, the aortic valve and the pulmonic valve, divide the heart from the aorta and the pulmonary artery. The <u>pulmonic valve</u> regulates blood flow from the right ventricle to the pulmonary artery. The <u>aortic valve</u> regulates blood flow from the left ventricle to the aorta. The semilunar valves are not attached to papillary muscles. When these valves close, they prevent backflow from the aorta and pulmonary artery into the left and right ventricles, respectively.

Blood Flow Within the Heart

Two large veins, the <u>superior vena cava</u> and the <u>inferior vena cava</u>, return deoxygenated blood from the body to the right atrium. Blood from the upper part of the body returns to the heart through the superior vena cava, and blood from the lower part of the body returns through the inferior vena cava. The inferior vena cava is the larger of the two veins. From the right atrium, blood passes through the tricuspid valve into the right ventricle. Blood is then pumped by the right ventricle through the pulmonic valve into the pulmonary artery and to the lungs. In the lungs, various processes take place that return oxygen to the blood, and at the same time, remove carbon dioxide and other waste products.

Freshly oxygenated blood is returned to the left atrium through the pulmonary veins. Blood then flows through the mitral valve into the left ventricle, which pumps the oxygenated blood through the aortic valve, into the <u>aorta</u>, the body's largest artery, and then to the entire body. The left ventricle is the strongest and largest of the four cardiac chambers because it is responsible for pumping blood through blood vessels throughout the body.

Heart Sounds

Heart sounds are created by the contraction and relaxation of the heart and flow of blood. These sounds can be heard during auscultation with a stethoscope. Normal heart sounds are often described as sounding like "lub-DUB, lub-DUB, lub-DUB…." The "lub" is called the first heart sound or S_1, and the "DUB" is called the second heart sound or S_2 **Figure 73** . S_2 ("DUB") is often louder than S_1 ("lub"). The sudden closure of the mitral and tricuspid valves at the start of ventricular contraction causes S_1. The closure of both the aortic and pulmonic valves at the end of a ventricular contraction causes S_2.

Two other heart sounds, S_3 and S_4, usually are not heard in people with normal heart sounds **Figure 74** . The S_3 or the third heart sound is a soft, low-pitched heart sound that occurs about one third of the way through diastole (the period during which the ventricles are relaxed). When an S_3 sound is present, the heart beat cycle is described as sounding like "lub-DUB-da." This sound may correlate to a period of rapid ventricular filling. Although the S_3 sound sometimes is present in healthy young people, it most commonly is associated with abnormally increased filling pressures in the atria secondary to moderate to severe heart failure.

The S_4 heart sound is a medium-pitched sound that occurs immediately before the normal S_1 sound. When an S_4 sound is present, the heart contraction cycle sounds like "bla-lub-DUB." The S_4 sound represents either decreased stretching (compliance) of the left ventricle or increased pressure in the atria. An S_4 heart sound almost always is abnormal.

Other sounds, all abnormal, may be heard when you are auscultating the heart and great vessels. Some of these sounds are easy to auscultate; others may require years of experience to identify. These include murmurs, bruits, ejection clicks, and opening snaps. A <u>murmur</u> is an abnormal "whooshing-like" sound heard over the heart that indicates turbulent blood flow through the heart valves.

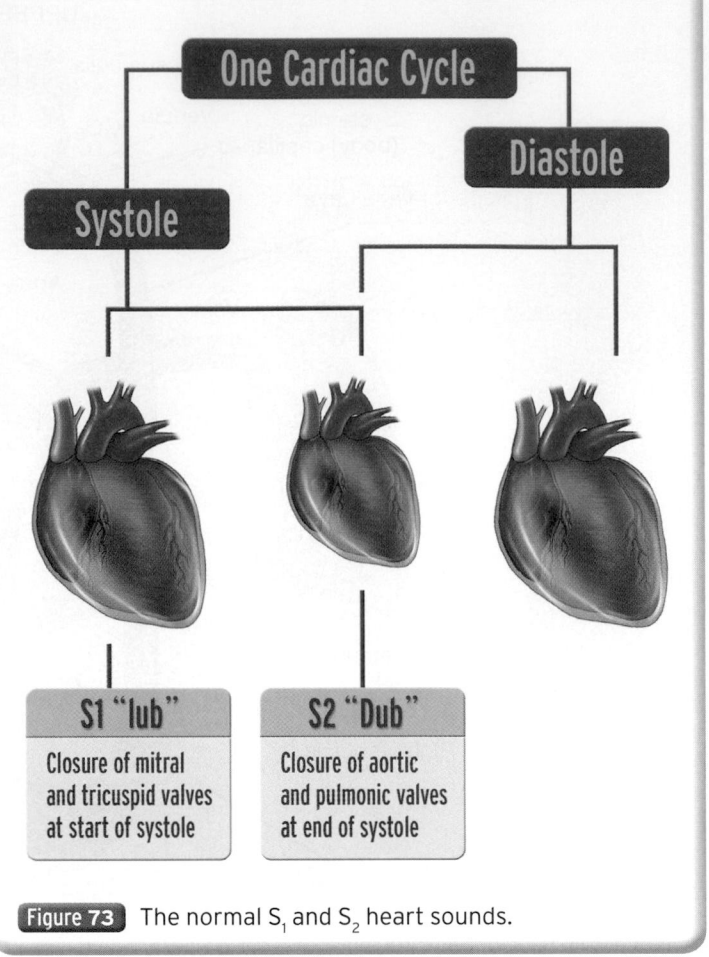

Figure 73 The normal S_1 and S_2 heart sounds.

Although many murmurs are "functional" (benign) and often go away, several are characteristic of heart disease. A <u>bruit</u> is an abnormal "whooshing-like" sound heard over a main blood vessel that indicates turbulent blood flow within the blood vessel. A bruit often indicates localized atherosclerotic disease (plaque formation in the arteries). Both ejection clicks and opening snaps indicate abnormal cardiac valve function. They occur at different times in the cardiac cycle, depending on which valve is diseased. Although these sounds are significant, most of these sounds are fleeting and difficult to hear. See the chapter, *Cardiovascular Emergencies* for more information on abnormal heart sounds.

The Electrical Conduction System

The mechanical pumping action of the heart can only occur in response to an electrical stimulus. This impulse causes the heart to beat via a set of complex chemical changes within the myocardial cells. The central nervous system and the endocrine system can influence the rate, strength, and speed of contraction. The myocardium is the only muscle that has the property of automaticity, or the ability to generate its own electrical impulses. Therefore, the contractions are initiated within the heart itself, in a group of complex electrical tissues that are part of an <u>electrical conduction system</u>. The cardiac conduction system consists of six parts: the sinoatrial (SA) node, the atrioventricular (AV)

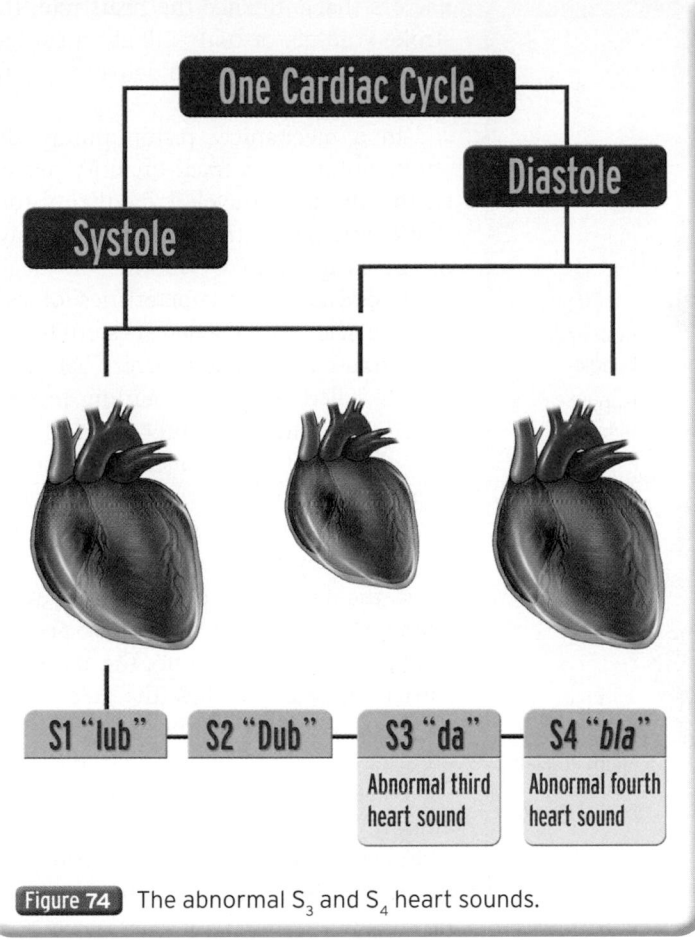

Figure 74 The abnormal S₃ and S₄ heart sounds.

heart tissue. Receptors in the blood vessels, kidneys, brain, and heart constantly monitor body functions to help maintain homeostasis. Baroreceptors and chemoreceptors, found in the carotid sinus and aortic arch, are also involved in regulation of heart function. **Baroreceptors** respond to changes in pressure, usually within the heart or the main arteries. **Chemoreceptors** sense changes in the chemical composition of the blood. If either of these types of receptors sense abnormalities, they transmit nerve signals to the appropriate organs. As a result, hormones or neurotransmitters are released to correct the situation. The transmission of nerve signals stops when conditions return to normal.

Stimulation of receptors often causes activation of either the parasympathetic or sympathetic branches of the autonomic nervous system, affecting both the **heart rate** and the strength of heart muscle contraction (**contractility**). Parasympathetic stimulation slows the heart rate, primarily by affecting the AV node. Sympathetic stimulation has two potential effects, alpha effects or beta effects, depending on which nerve receptor is stimulated. Both alpha and beta stimulation result in a range of effects on the body as a whole. **Alpha effects** occur when alpha receptors are stimulated, and in the cardiovascular system, this results mainly in vasoconstriction. **Beta effects** occur when beta receptors are stimulated, which causes increased inotropic, dromotropic, and chronotropic states in the cardiovascular system in addition to other effects elsewhere in the body.

Epinephrine and norepinephrine, also referred to as **catecholamines**, are naturally occurring hormones that also may be given as cardiac drugs. Epinephrine has a greater stimulatory effect on beta receptors, and norepinephrine has predominant stimulatory actions on alpha receptors. Many other emergency medications have primary or side effects on the adrenergic nervous system. You should know these drugs well because they can have significant effects on a wide range of patients.

node, the bundle of His, the right and left bundle branches, and the Purkinje fibers **Figure 75**.

The **sinoatrial (SA) node** is a nonspecific cell or group of cells located high in the right atrium and is the normal site of origin of the electrical impulse. Like all cardiac cells, the SA node's cells can reach threshold on their own, initiating impulses through the myocardium, stimulating contraction of cardiac muscle fibers. Because it creates these impulses more frequently than other sites in the heart, the SA node is the most common natural pacemaker. The impulse then travels to the **atrioventricular (AV) node**, located in the AV junction adjacent to the septum, where it transiently slows. Electrical stimulation of the heart muscle then continues toward the **bundle of His**, which is a continuation of the AV node. From here, it proceeds rapidly to the right and left bundle branches, stimulating the intraventricular septum. The impulse then spreads out, via the Purkinje fibers, to the left, then the right ventricular myocardium, resulting in ventricular contraction or systole.

Regulation of Heart Function

The heart's **chronotropic effect** (effect of the rate of contraction), **dromotropic effect** (effect of the rate of electrical conduction), and **inotropic effect** (effect of the strength of contraction) are provided by the brain via the autonomic nervous system, the hormones of the endocrine system, and the

The Cardiac Cycle

The process that creates the pumping of the heart is known as the **cardiac cycle**. One cycle begins with myocardial contraction and concludes at the beginning of the next contraction. The heart's contraction results in pressure changes within the cardiac chambers, resulting in the movement of blood from areas of high pressure to areas of low pressure.

Systole is a term that refers to the contraction of the ventricular mass and the pumping of blood into the systemic and pulmonary circuits. During systole, a pressure is created within the arteries that can be recorded and is known as the systolic blood pressure. A normal systolic blood pressure in an adult at rest is between 110 and 140 mm Hg. A pressure also exists in the vessels during **diastole**, the relaxation phase of the heart cycle, and is called the diastolic blood pressure. A normal diastolic blood pressure in an adult is between 70 and 90 mm Hg. The **pulse pressure** is the difference between the systolic and diastolic pressures:

Pulse pressure = Systolic pressure − Diastolic pressure

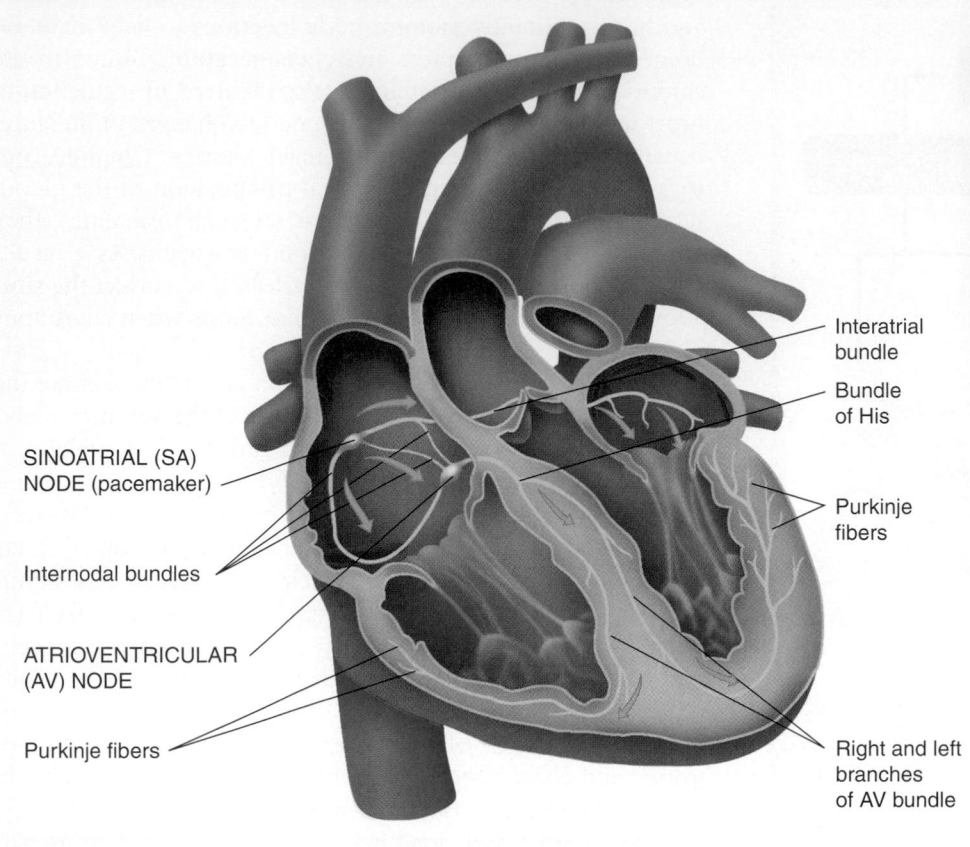

SINOATRIAL (SA)
NODE (pacemaker)

Internodal bundles

ATRIOVENTRICULAR
(AV) NODE

Purkinje fibers

Interatrial
bundle

Bundle
of His

Purkinje
fibers

Right and left
branches
of AV bundle

Figure 75 The cardiac conduction system. Specialized groups of cardiac muscle cells initiate an electrical impulse throughout the heart. The conduction pathway travels through the six parts of the cardiac conduction system, starting at the sinoatrial node.

Blood pressure is noted as a fraction, and the systolic reading is placed above the diastolic reading (for example, a systolic reading of 140 and a diastolic reading of 70 would be noted as 140/70 mm Hg). The unit of measure mm Hg refers to millimeters of mercury and describes the height, in millimeters, to which the blood pressure elevates a column of liquid mercury in a glass tube. Although many blood pressure measurement devices now use dials, blood pressure is still described in millimeters of mercury.

The pressure in the aorta against which the left ventricle must pump blood is called the **afterload**. The greater the afterload, the harder it is for the ventricle to eject blood into the aorta, reducing the **stroke volume (SV)**, or the amount of blood ejected per contraction. To a large degree, afterload is governed by arterial blood pressure. Afterload is greater with vasoconstriction and less with vasodilation.

Cardiac output is the amount of blood pumped through the circulatory system in 1 minute. Cardiac output is expressed in liters per minute (L/min). The cardiac output equals the heart rate multiplied by the stroke volume:

Cardiac Output = Stroke Volume × Heart Rate

Factors that influence the heart rate, the stroke volume, or both will affect cardiac output and, thus, oxygen delivery (perfusion) to tissue.

In a mechanical piston pump, the stroke volume is a fixed quantity related to the distance traveled by the piston. The heart, by contrast, has several ways of increasing stroke volume. To begin with, one of the characteristics of cardiac muscle is that when it is stretched, it contracts with greater force. That property is called the Frank-Starling mechanism, or Starling's law, after the man who first described it. If for any reason an increased volume of blood is returned from the systemic veins to the right heart, or from the pulmonary veins to the left heart, the muscle surrounding the cardiac chambers will have to stretch to accommodate the larger volume; the more the cardiac muscle stretches, the greater will be the force of its contraction, the more completely it will empty, and therefore the greater will be the stroke volume. The amount of blood returning to the right atrium may vary somewhat from minute to minute, but the normal heart continues to pump out the same percentage of blood returned. This is called the **ejection fraction**.

If you recall the previous equation:

Cardiac Output = Stroke Volume × Heart Rate

it is clear that any increase in stroke volume, with the heart rate held constant, will cause an increase in the overall cardiac output. The pressure under which a ventricle fills is called the **preload** and is influenced by the volume of blood returned by the veins to the heart. In situations of increased oxygen demand, the body returns more blood to the heart (preload increases), and cardiac output therefore increases through the Frank-Starling mechanism. In the diseased heart, the same mechanism is used to achieve a normal resting cardiac output (that is why some diseased hearts become enlarged).

Words of Wisdom

Starling's law states that primarily the length of fibers constituting the heart's muscular wall determines the force of the heartbeat. In other words, an increase in diastolic filling increases the force of the contraction.

Think of stretching a rubber band: the further it is stretched, the greater the strength of the recoil.

The Vascular System

Blood is transported through the body in the arteries, which carry blood away from the heart, and veins, which carry blood back to the heart. Arteries become smaller as they get farther from the heart. Eventually, they branch into many small arterioles that divide even further into capillaries, which are microscopic, thin-walled blood vessels. Oxygen and nutrients pass out of the capillaries into the cells, and carbon dioxide and waste products pass from the cells into the capillaries by diffusion Figure 76 .

Once oxygenated blood has been delivered in the capillaries, deoxygenated blood is returned to the heart, starting from the capillaries. The capillaries eventually enlarge to form venules, which merge together and form veins. Eventually the veins empty into the heart, where blood is reoxygenated and the process begins again.

The walls of the blood vessels are composed of three layers of tissue Figure 77 . The smooth, thin, inner lining is called the tunica intima, or endothelium. The middle layer, the tunica media, is composed of elastic tissue and smooth muscle cells that allow the vessels to expand or contract in response to changes in blood pressure and tissue demand. It is the thickest of the three tissue layers. The outer layer of tissue is called the tunica adventitia and consists of elastic and fibrous connective tissue.

Although each blood vessel may hold only a small amount of blood, the total volume of all vessels in the body forms a large container when considered together. It is important to understand that the size of this container is dynamic—that is, it changes in response to conditions present within and outside of the body. For example, if the body is moderately or severely dehydrated, the amount of circulating blood volume falls. If the total volume of the circulatory system (the container) were to remain constant, then the patient's stroke volume, blood pressure, and cardiac output may drop significantly. To prevent this, the blood vessels receive constant feedback from the autonomic nervous system. If baroreceptors in the central circulation detect a drop in pressure, the blood vessels constrict to shrink the size of the container proportionally. These adjustments are coordinated by a wide array of feedback mechanisms to maintain homeostasis. In some cases, the autonomic nervous system also changes the distribution of blood by constricting peripheral blood vessels to a greater degree than those supplying the vital organs. This process is known as shunting and is a hallmark sign of shock.

Circulation to the Heart

The heart, like any other muscle, requires oxygen and nutrients. These are supplied via the coronary arteries, which arise from the aorta shortly after it leaves the left ventricle. Coronary arteries receive their blood supply during the diastolic phase. The coronary circulation emanates from the left and right coronary arteries Figure 78 .

The right coronary artery divides into nine important branches. Not all branches are always present in all people. These branches supply blood to the walls of the right atrium and ventricle, a portion of the inferior part of the left ventricle, and portions of the conduction system (the sinus and AV nodes). When vessels to the conduction system fail to arise from the right coronary artery, they originate from the left side instead.

The left main coronary artery is the largest and shortest of the myocardial blood vessels. It rapidly divides into two branches, the left anterior descending (LAD) artery and the circumflex coronary arteries. These arteries subdivide further,

YOU are the Medic   PART 3

As your partner is placing high-flow oxygen on the patient, you begin your rapid scan. When you assess the chest, you feel instability and a grating sensation as you palpate. The chest does not rise and fall equally on both sides. Your patient moves slightly and groans audibly. It is extremely difficult to obtain lung sounds due to traffic and running diesel engines.

Recording Time: 5 Minutes	
Respirations	24 breaths/min, shallow
Pulse	120 beats/min
Skin	Pale, moist, and hot (comparable to ambient temperature)
Blood pressure	106/70 mm Hg
Oxygen saturation (SpO$_2$)	93% on high-flow oxygen
Pupils	Equal and reactive to light

5. What is the obvious injury you find to the patient's chest?

6. What are the potential hidden injuries you should consider?

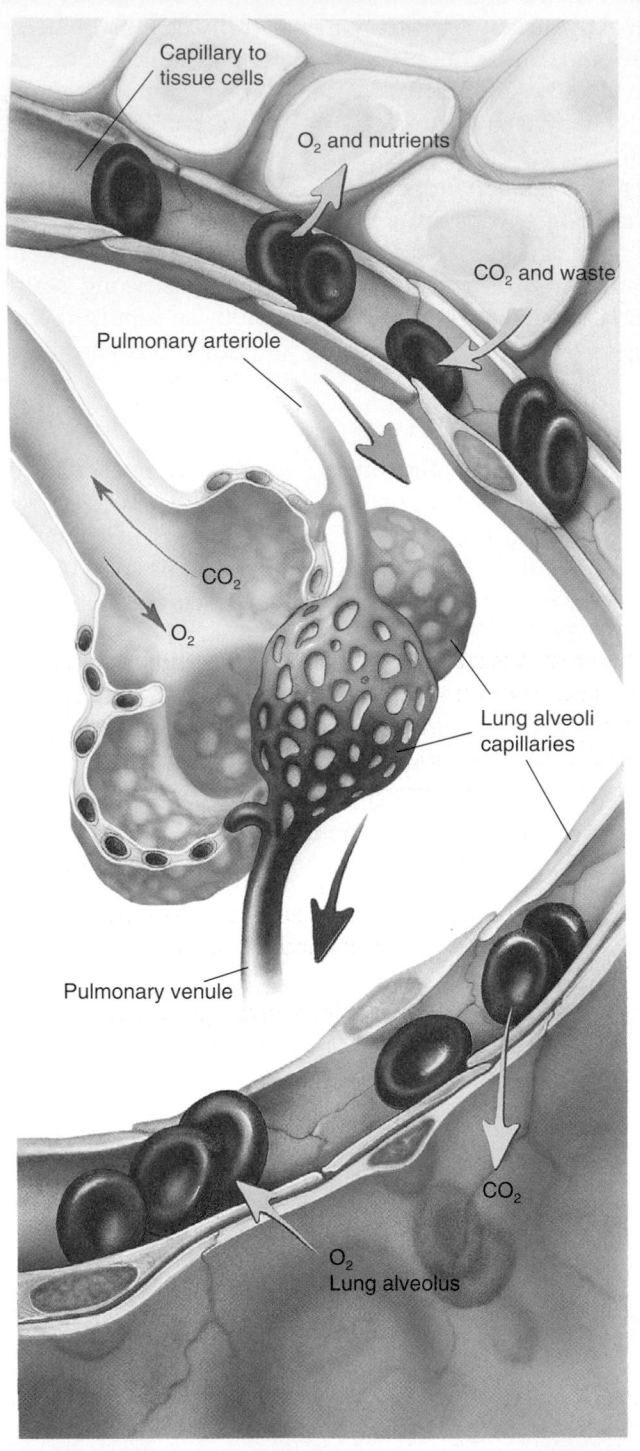

Figure 76 Diffusion. Oxygen and nutrients pass easily from the capillaries into the cells, and waste and carbon dioxide pass from the cells into the capillaries.

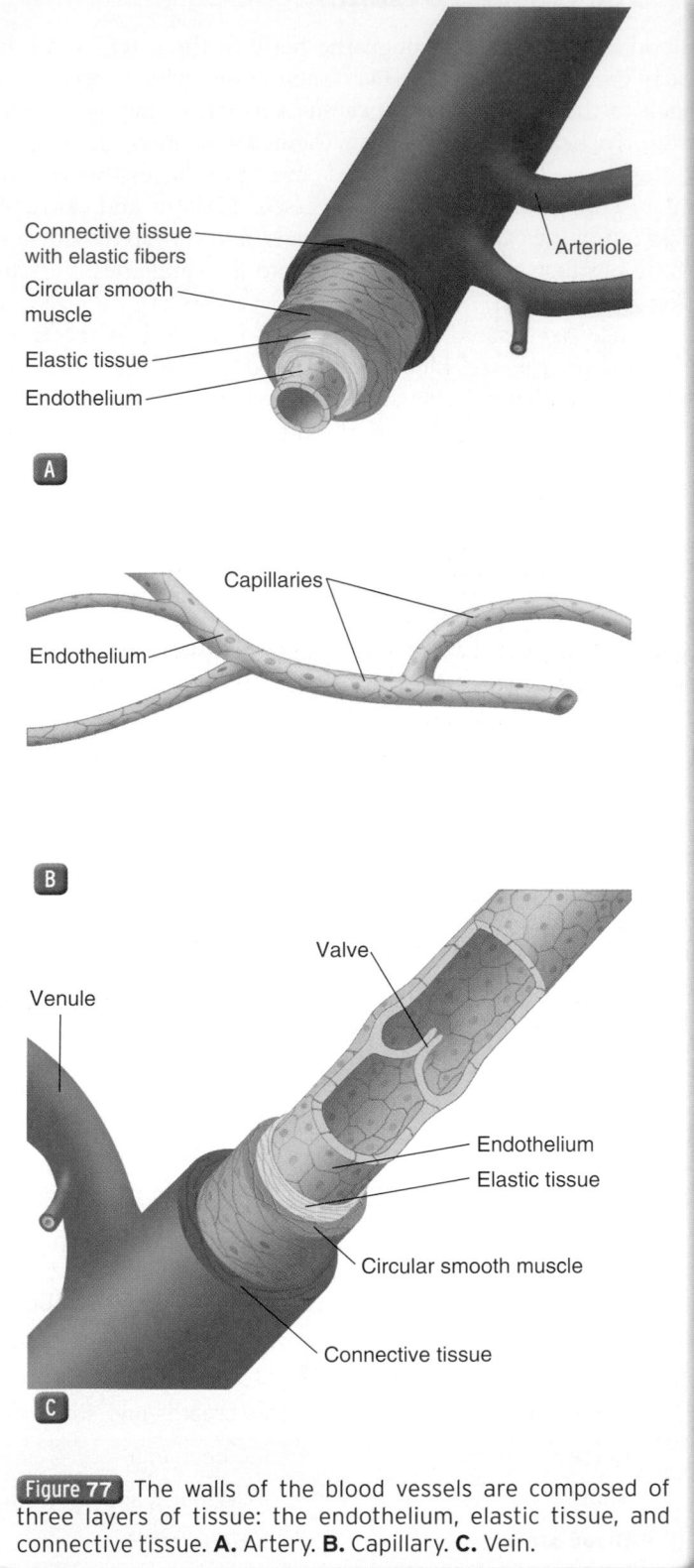

Figure 77 The walls of the blood vessels are composed of three layers of tissue: the endothelium, elastic tissue, and connective tissue. **A.** Artery. **B.** Capillary. **C.** Vein.

supplying blood to most of the left ventricle, the intraventricular septum, and, at times, the AV node.

Pulmonary Circulation
Within the body, the pulmonary circulation carries blood from the right side of the heart to the lungs and back to the left side of the heart, and the systemic circulation is responsible for

blood flow throughout the body. Deoxygenated blood from the right ventricle is pumped through the pulmonic valve into the pulmonary artery. This artery rapidly divides into the right and left pulmonary arteries. These arteries transport the blood to the right and left lungs. Inside the lungs, the arteries branch, becoming smaller and smaller. At the level of the capillary, waste products are exchanged and the blood is reoxygenated.

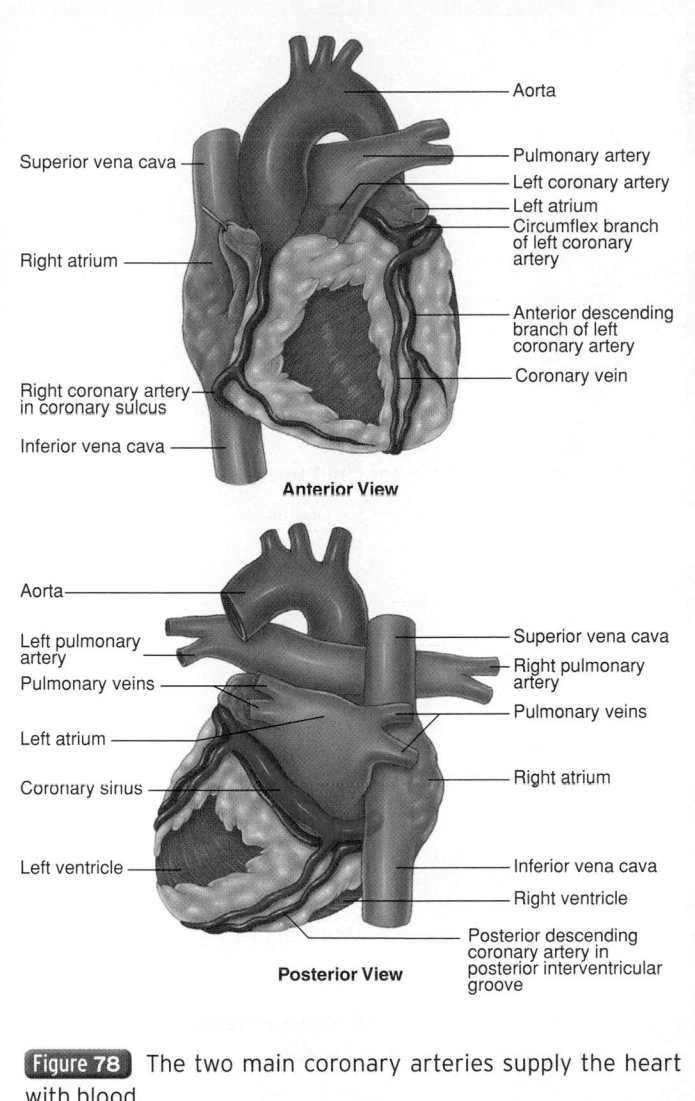

Anterior View

Posterior View

Figure 78 The two main coronary arteries supply the heart with blood.

The reoxygenated blood travels through venules into the pulmonary veins. The four pulmonary veins empty into the left atrium, two from each lung (see Figure 72).

Systemic Arterial Circulation

Oxygenated blood leaves the heart through the aortic valve and passes into the aorta. From the aorta, blood is distributed to all parts of the body **Figure 79**. All arteries of the body are derived from the aorta. The aorta is divided into three portions: the ascending aorta, the aortic arch, and the descending aorta.

The **ascending aorta** arises from the left ventricle and withstands the highest pressures of any vessel in the body. The aorta then arches posteriorly and to the left, forming the aortic arch. Three major arteries arise from the **aortic arch**: the brachiocephalic (innominate) artery, the left common **carotid artery**, and the left subclavian artery.

The **descending aorta** is the longest portion of the aorta and is subdivided into the thoracic aorta and the abdominal aorta. The descending aorta extends through the thorax and abdomen into the pelvis. In the pelvis, the descending aorta divides into

the two common iliac arteries, which further divide into the internal and external iliac arteries.

The Head and Neck The brachiocephalic artery is the first vessel to branch from the aortic arch. It is relatively short and rapidly divides into the right common carotid artery and the right subclavian artery. The carotid arteries transport blood to the head and neck, whereas the subclavian arteries transport blood to the upper extremities.

Each common carotid artery branches at the angle of the mandible into the internal and external carotid arteries. This point of division is called the **carotid bifurcation**. Here, a slight dilation, the carotid sinus, contains structures that are important in regulating blood pressure. Branches of the external carotid artery supply blood to the face, nose, and mouth. The internal carotid arteries, together with the vertebral arteries (branches of the subclavian arteries), supply blood to the brain **Figure 80**.

The Upper Extremity The **subclavian artery** supplies blood to the brain, neck, anterior chest wall, and shoulder. Shortly after its point of origin, the subclavian artery gives rise to the vertebral arteries. The subclavian system then continues from the thorax into the upper extremity. At the shoulder joint, it becomes the axillary artery, then the **brachial artery** below the head of the humerus. The brachial artery divides into the ulnar and radial arteries **Figure 81**.

The Thoracic Aorta Two types of branches of arteries make up the thoracic aorta: the visceral arteries and the parietal arteries. Visceral arteries supply blood to the thoracic organs, and parietal arteries supply blood to the thoracic wall.

Intercostal arteries run along the ribs and provide circulation to the chest wall. Intercostal arteries branch into anterior and posterior intercostal arteries. The anterior intercostal arteries originate as branches of the subclavian system. The posterior intercostal arteries arise directly from the aorta. Visceral branches of the thoracic aorta supply the bronchial arteries in the lungs and the esophageal arteries.

The Abdominal Aorta Like their thoracic counterpart, branches of the abdominal aorta are divided into visceral and parietal portions. The visceral arteries are subdivided into paired and nonpaired arteries. The three major unpaired branches of the abdominal aorta's visceral arteries include the celiac trunk, the superior mesenteric, and the inferior mesenteric arteries **Figure 82**. The celiac trunk supplies blood to the esophagus, stomach, duodenum, spleen, liver, and pancreas **Figure 83**. The superior mesenteric artery and its branches supply blood to the pancreas, small intestine, and colon. The inferior mesenteric artery and its branches supply blood to the descending colon and rectum. Paired branches of the visceral abdominal aorta supply blood to the kidneys, adrenal gland, and gonads. The parietal branches supply blood to the diaphragm and abdominal wall.

The Pelvis and Lower Extremity At the level of the fifth lumbar vertebra, the aorta divides into the two common iliac arteries. These arteries further divide into the internal iliac arteries,

Major Arteries

Major Veins

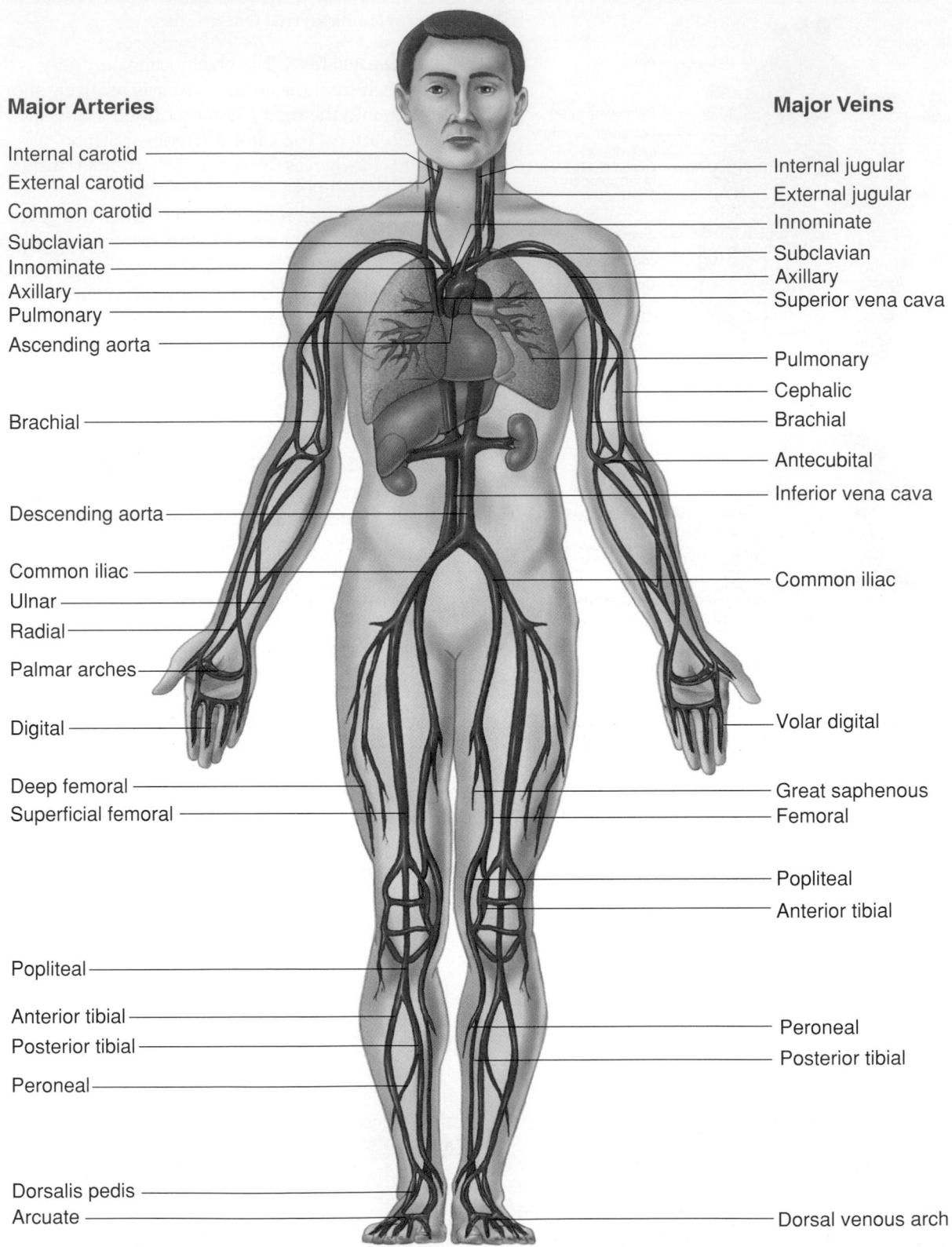

Internal carotid

External carotid

Common carotid

Subclavian

Innominate

Axillary

Pulmonary

Ascending aorta

Brachial

Descending aorta

Common iliac

Ulnar

Radial

Palmar arches

Digital

Deep femoral

Superficial femoral

Popliteal

Anterior tibial

Posterior tibial

Peroneal

Dorsalis pedis

Arcuate

Internal jugular

External jugular

Innominate

Subclavian

Axillary

Superior vena cava

Pulmonary

Cephalic

Brachial

Antecubital

Inferior vena cava

Common iliac

Volar digital

Great saphenous

Femoral

Popliteal

Anterior tibial

Peroneal

Posterior tibial

Dorsal venous arch

Figure 79   The principal arteries supply blood to a vast network of smaller arteries and arterioles. Venules deliver oxygen-poor blood to the veins that return blood to the heart.

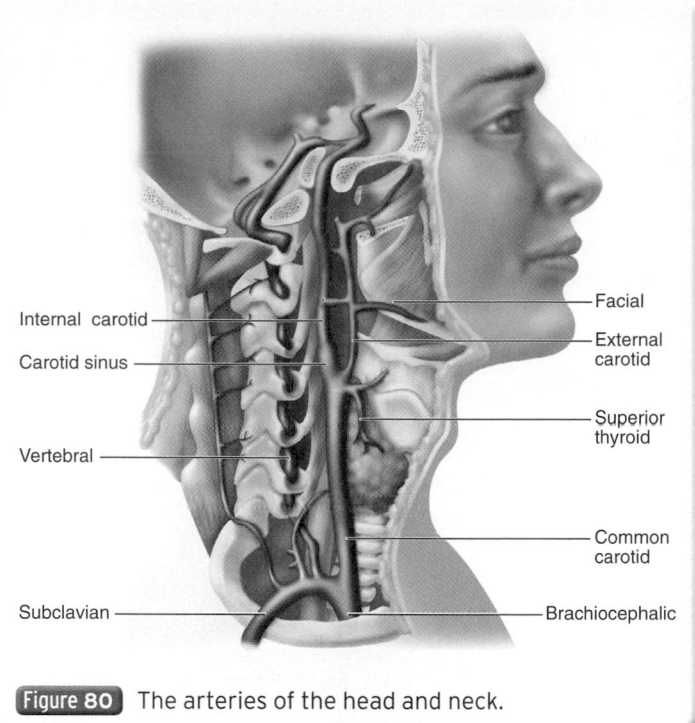

Figure 80 The arteries of the head and neck.

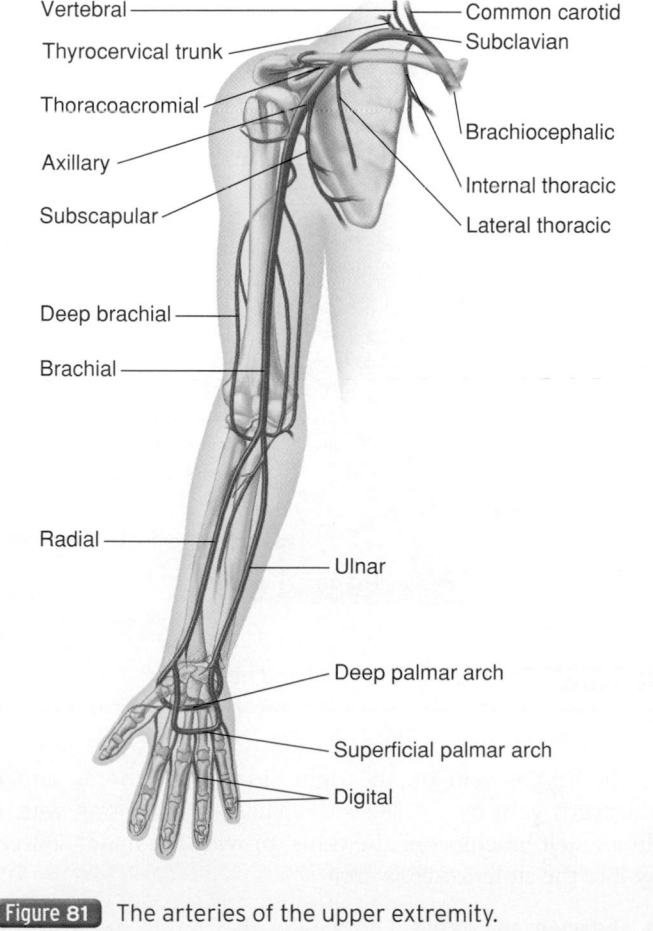

Figure 81 The arteries of the upper extremity.

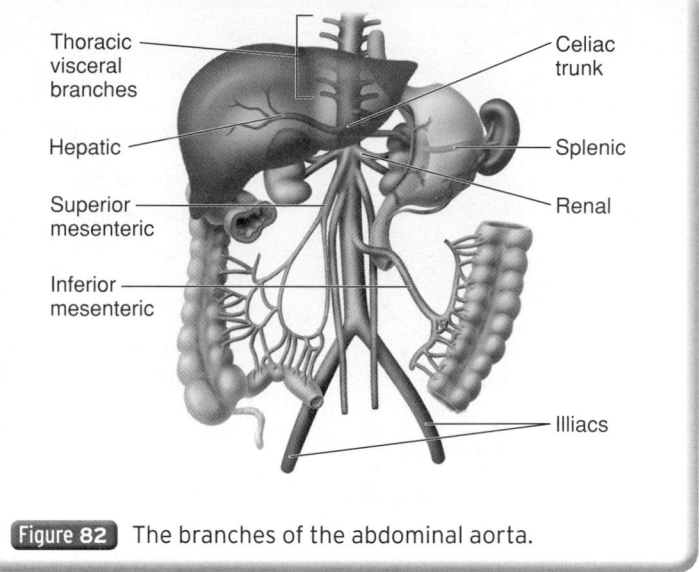

Figure 82 The branches of the abdominal aorta.

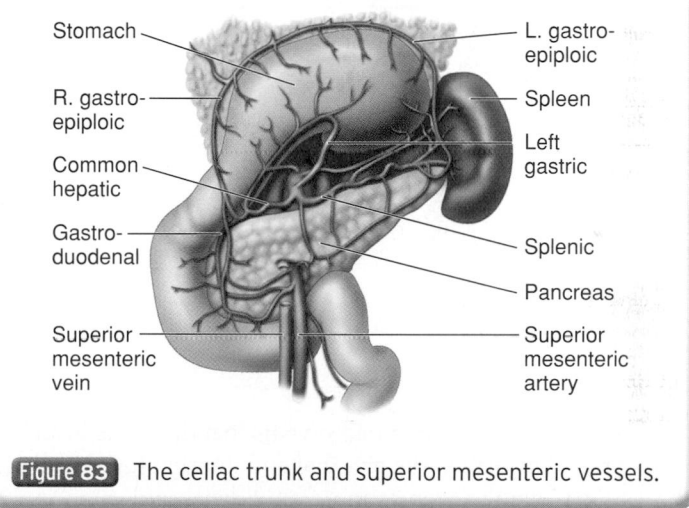

Figure 83 The celiac trunk and superior mesenteric vessels.

which supply blood to the pelvis, and the external iliac arteries, which enter the lower extremity **Figure 84**. The internal iliac artery sends out visceral branches to the rectum, vagina, uterus, and ovary. Parietal branches supply blood to the sacrum, gluteal muscles of the buttocks region, the pubic region, rectum, external genitalia, and proximal thigh.

Like the upper extremity, the vessels of the lower extremity form a continuum. The external iliac arteries become the <u>femoral arteries</u>. Each femoral artery supplies blood to the thigh, external genitalia, anterior abdominal wall, and knee. The femoral artery becomes the <u>popliteal artery</u> in the lower thigh. Each popliteal artery then branches into the anterior tibial, posterior tibial, and peroneal arteries. At the foot, the anterior tibial artery becomes the <u>dorsalis pedis artery</u>. Plantar arteries arise from the <u>posterior tibial artery</u> and subdivide into digital branches that supply blood to the toes **Figure 85**.

The Systemic Venous Circulation

As a rule, veins accompany the major arteries. Many veins have the same names as the arteries they accompany.

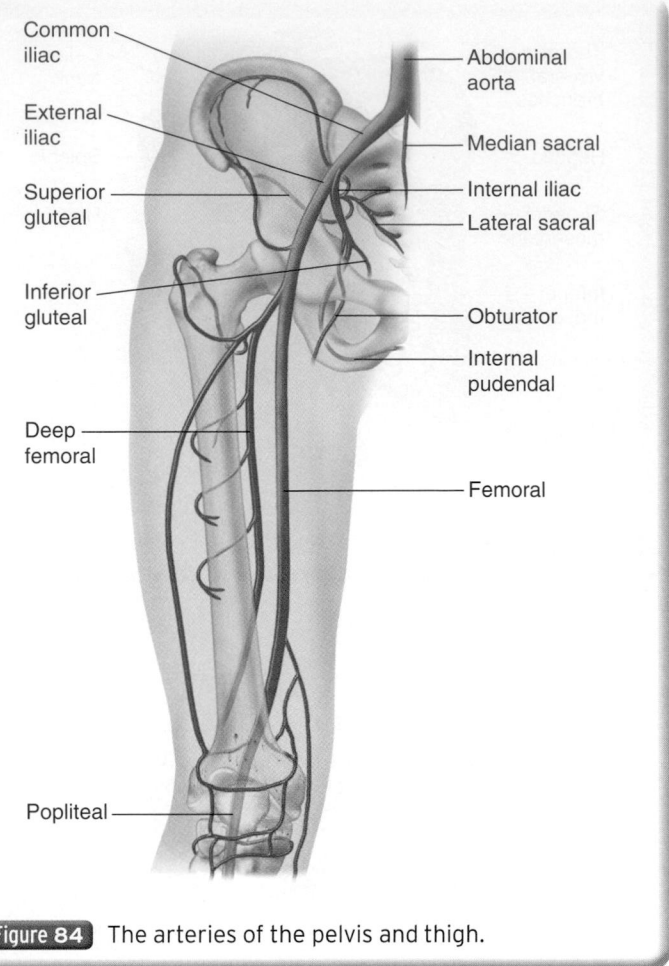

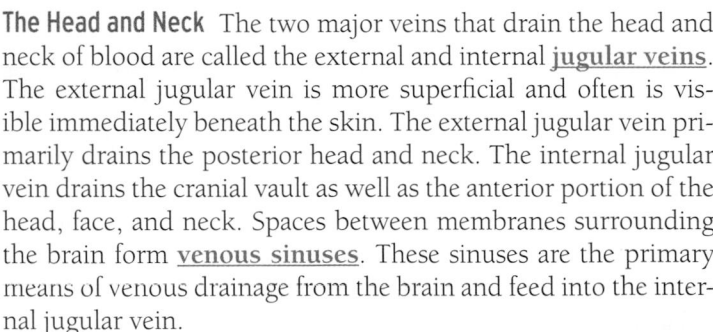

The arteries of the pelvis and thigh.

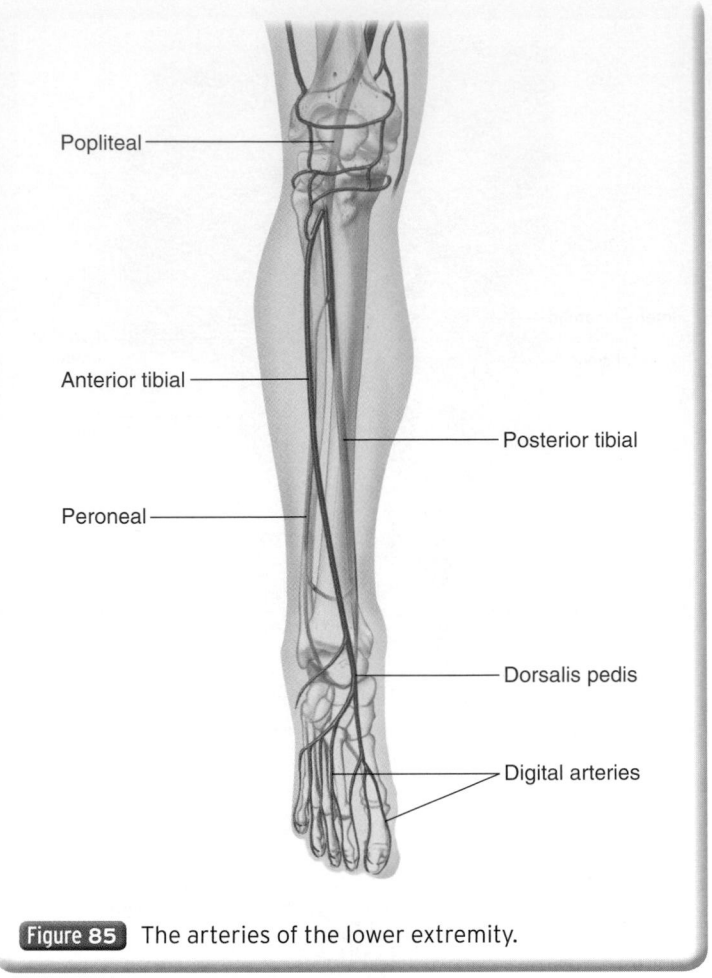

The arteries of the lower extremity.

The Head and Neck The two major veins that drain the head and neck of blood are called the external and internal **jugular veins**. The external jugular vein is more superficial and often is visible immediately beneath the skin. The external jugular vein primarily drains the posterior head and neck. The internal jugular vein drains the cranial vault as well as the anterior portion of the head, face, and neck. Spaces between membranes surrounding the brain form **venous sinuses**. These sinuses are the primary means of venous drainage from the brain and feed into the internal jugular vein.

The external and internal jugular veins join the **subclavian veins** (the proximal part of the main vein of the arm) **Figure 86** to form the brachiocephalic veins, which drain into the superior vena cava.

The Upper Extremity The veins of the upper extremity vary somewhat from person to person **Figure 87** . The names of the veins of the hands, wrists, and forearm follow the arteries of the same name. In the upper forearm, these veins combine to form the **basilic vein** and the **cephalic vein**, the major veins of the arm. The basilic and cephalic veins combine to form the **axillary vein**, which drains into the subclavian vein.

The Thorax In the thorax, venous drainage begins at the anterior and posterior intercostal veins. The intercostal veins empty

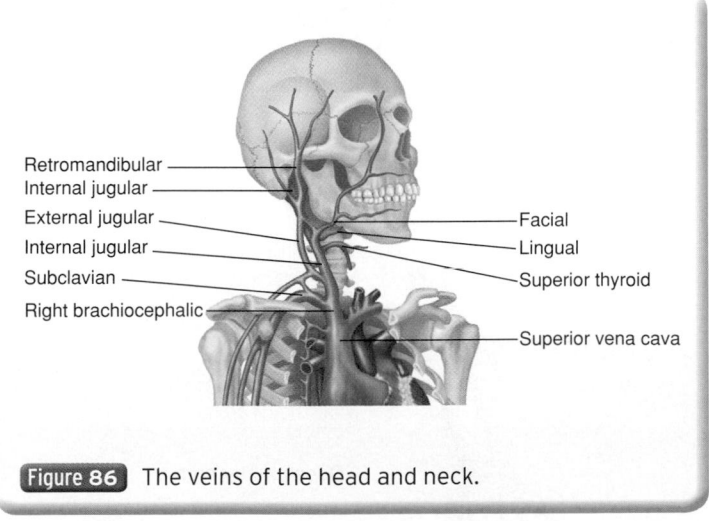

The veins of the head and neck.

into the azygos vein on the right side of the thorax and the hemiazygos vein on the left side. These veins, along with the right and left brachiocephalic veins, provide the major source of flow into the superior vena cava.

The Abdomen and Pelvis Ultimately, all venous drainage from the lower part of the body passes through the inferior vena cava.

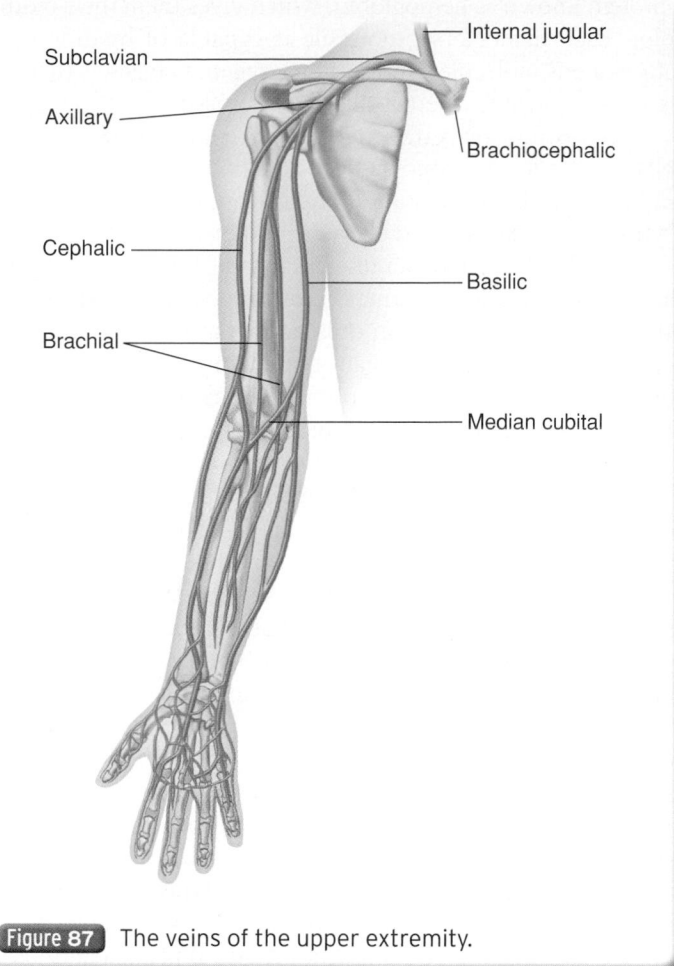

Figure 87 The veins of the upper extremity.

respective arteries, uniting at the knee to form the **popliteal vein**. The popliteal vein ascends through the thigh, becoming the femoral vein **Figure 89** .

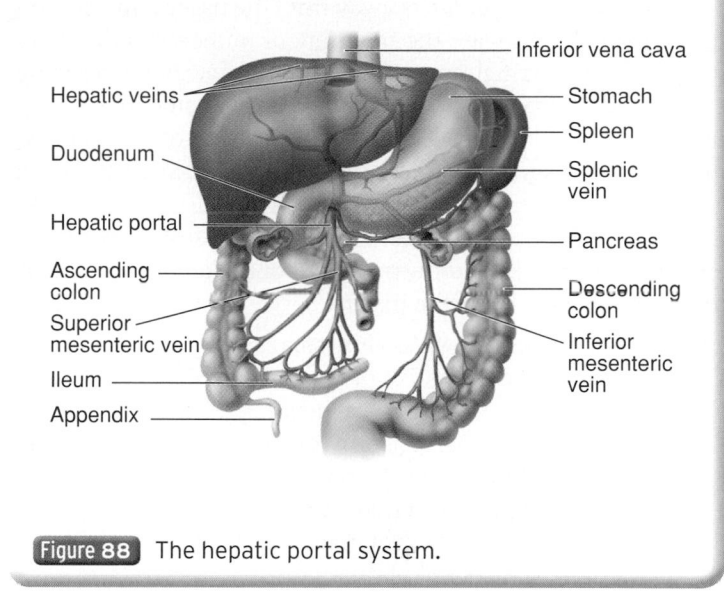

Figure 88 The hepatic portal system.

The inferior vena cava returns deoxygenated blood from the lower parts of the body to the right atrium for oxygenation. Within the abdominal and pelvic cavities, veins of the same name accompany the major arteries, providing venous drainage from structures including the kidney, adrenal glands, gonads, and diaphragm. The internal iliac veins drain the pelvis, and the external iliac veins drain the lower limbs. The internal and external iliac veins combine together in the pelvis, forming the common iliac veins, which combine to form the inferior vena cava.

The **hepatic portal system** is a specialized part of the venous system that drains blood from the liver, stomach, intestines, and spleen **Figure 88** . Blood from the system flows first through the liver, where blood collects in sinusoids. In the sinusoids, the liver extracts nutrients, filters the blood, and metabolizes various drugs. The blood then empties into the **hepatic veins**, which join the inferior vena cava.

The Lower Extremity The longest vein in the body is the great **saphenous vein**. It drains the foot, leg, and thigh. The saphenous vein originates over the dorsal and medial side of the foot, ascends along the medial side of the leg and thigh, and empties into the **femoral vein**, which then drains into the external iliac vein. Laterally, the small saphenous vein helps drain the leg and lateral side of the foot. The veins of the feet also drain into the anterior and posterior tibial veins, which accompany their

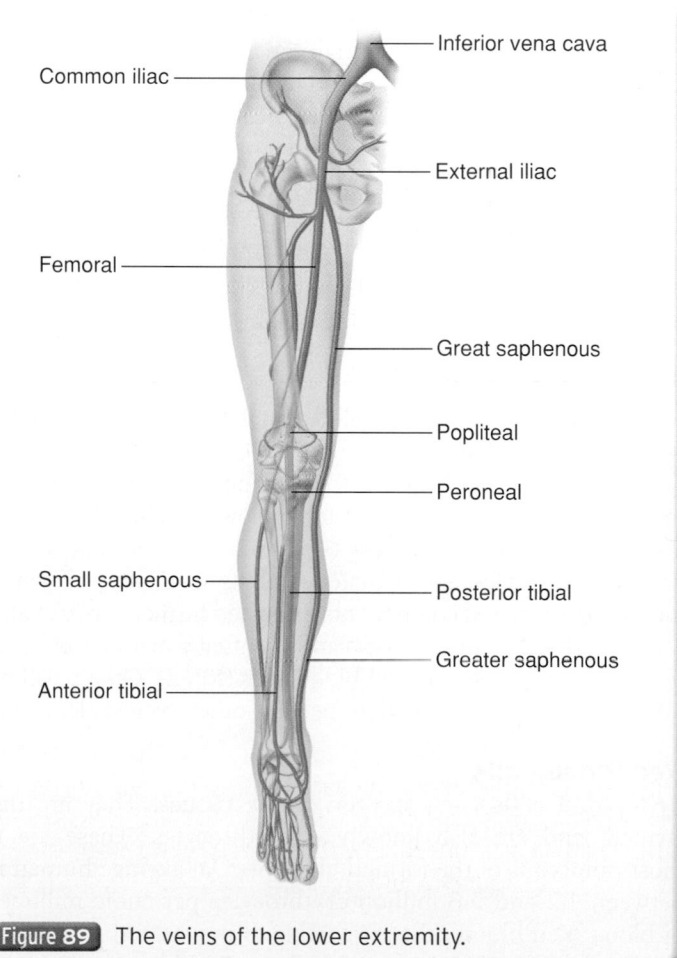

Figure 89 The veins of the lower extremity.

Blood Composition

Blood is the substance that is pumped by the heart through the arteries, veins, and capillaries. Blood consists of plasma and formed elements or cells that are suspended in the plasma. These cells include red blood cells, white blood cells, and platelets. The purpose of blood is to carry oxygen and nutrients to the tissues and carry cell waste products away from the tissues. In addition, the formed elements are the mainstay of numerous other body functions such as fighting infection and controlling bleeding. Human adult male bodies contain approximately 70 mL/kg, or about 5 L, of blood, whereas female bodies contain approximately 65 mL/kg. Plasma is a watery, straw-colored fluid that accounts for more than half of the total blood volume. Plasma is made up of 92% water and 8% dissolved substances such as chemicals, minerals, and nutrients. All of the other components together make up 1% of the plasma:

- **Water:** Constitutes 92% of plasma
- **Proteins:** Constitutes 7% of the plasma.
  - Albumins: Make up the majority of the plasma proteins. Albumins function mainly to regulate oncotic pressure, and thereby control the movement of water into and out of the circulation.
  - Globulins: Antibodies made by the liver that make up around 36% of the plasma proteins.
  - Fibrinogen: Important for blood coagulation, makes up about 4% of the plasma proteins.
- **Oxygen:** Little oxygen is dissolved in the plasma, almost all oxygen is bound to hemoglobin
- **Carbon dioxide:** Transported as bicarbonate in the plasma
- **Nitrogen:** The air that you breathe is mostly nitrogen; therefore, this gas is dissolved within the plasma
- **Nutrients:** Fuel for the cells
- **Cellular wastes:** Lactic acid, carbon dioxide, etc
- **Others:** Hormones, other cellular products

Water enters the plasma from the digestive tract, from fluids between cells, and as a by-product of metabolism.

Formed Elements

All formed elements are created through a process known as hematopoeisis. Through a series of transformations, most of which begin in the bone marrow in mature humans, a type of stem cell specific to the circulatory system, known as a hematocytoblast, forms and begins the process of maturation. Through multiple changes and stages, the hematocytoblasts gradually differentiate into one of the blood components discussed further in this chapter. Some will become normoblasts and eventually mature into reticulocytes, the precursors to red blood cells (RBCs). Others will randomly follow a different path to become other formed elements.

Red Blood Cells

Red blood cells carry oxygen to the tissues. They are disk-shaped, and are also known as erythrocytes. These are the most numerous of the formed elements. An average human has between 4.2 and 5.8 million erythrocytes per cubic millimeter of blood. Red blood cells are unable to move on their own; the flowing plasma passively propels them. Red blood cells contain a protein known as hemoglobin, which gives them their reddish color. Each hemoglobin molecule is capable of binding up to four gaseous molecules, most often oxygen. Oxygen is then carried to end organs, where it diffuses into tissues.

Erythropoiesis is the ongoing process by which red blood cells are made. Approximately 25 trillion red blood cells are contained in the normal adult circulation; of these, 2.5 million erythrocytes are destroyed every second.

Red blood cells have a finite life span of 120 days. Those cells that are destined for destruction decompose in the spleen and other tissues that are rich in cells known as macrophages. Macrophages protect the body against infection. The body "recycles" some components of hemoglobin, such as the protein, globin, and iron. The part of hemoglobin that is not recycled is converted to bilirubin, which is a waste product that undergoes further metabolism in the liver. Normally, a chemical derivative of bilirubin, urobilinogen, is excreted in the stool and in the urine.

Red blood cells contain antigens on their surface, which are proteins recognized by the immune system. Within the plasma are antibodies, which are proteins that react with antigens. People are classified as having one of four blood types based on the presence or absence of these specific antigens. This process of classification is referred to as blood typing, or determining the ABO blood group.

Type A blood contains red blood cells with type A surface antigens and plasma containing type B antibodies; type B blood contains type B surface antigens and plasma containing type A antibodies. Type AB blood contains both types of antigens but the plasma contains no ABO antibodies. Type O contains neither A nor B antigens but contains both A and B plasma antibodies. A person's blood type determines which type of blood he or she may receive in a blood transfusion.

Rh blood groups involve a complex of antigens first discovered in rhesus monkeys. The presence of any of the 18 separate Rh antigens makes a person's blood Rh positive. If a person with Rh-negative blood were to be exposed to Rh-positive blood, antibodies to the antigens could be produced.

When blood flow to the kidneys decreases or the oxygen content of the air in the lungs declines, oxygen concentrations in the blood are low. This situation may occur because of disease, high altitude, and because of anemia. This condition is known as hypoxia. During hypoxia especially, kidneys produce erythropoietin, which is also called erythropoiesis-stimulating hormone. Erythropoietin stimulates production of erythroblasts from bone marrow. Therefore, bone marrow can increase the rate of red blood cell formation by approximately ten times— about 30 million cells per second.

Words of Wisdom

Any decrease in the number of red blood cells in the body is called anemia. Anemia may be caused by inadequate nutrition (such as iron deficiency), inadequate production of red blood cells by bone marrow, increased destruction of red blood cells by the body (hemolysis), or bleeding.

White Blood Cells

White blood cells are also known as leukocytes. Normally there are 4,500 to 10,000 white blood cells in a microliter of human blood. There are several different types of white blood cells and each has a different function. The primary function of all white blood cells is to fight infection. Antibodies to fight infection may be produced, or white blood cells may directly attack and kill bacterial invaders. White blood cells are larger than red blood cells. Most white blood cells are motile and leave the blood vessels by a process known as **diapedesis** to move toward the tissue where they are needed most.

White blood cells are named according to their appearance in a stained preparation of blood. In general, **granulocytes** have large cytoplasmic granules that are easily seen with a simple light microscope; **agranulocytes** are white blood cells that lack these granules. There are three types of granulocytes (neutrophils, eosinophils, and basophils) and two types of agranulocytes (monocytes and lymphocytes).

Neutrophils are normally the most common type of granulocyte in the blood. Neutrophils destroy bacteria, antigen-antibody complexes, and foreign matter. **Eosinophils** are granulocytes that contain granules that stain bright red with the acidic stain, eosin. Eosinophils function in the body's allergic response and are, thus, increased in people with allergies. Certain parasitic infections, such as trichinosis, also result in an increase in the number of eosinophils present. **Basophils** are the least common of all granulocytes and play a role in both allergic and inflammatory reactions. Basophils contain large amounts of **histamine**, a substance that increases tissue inflammation, and **heparin**, a substance that inhibits blood clotting.

Lymphocytes are the smallest of the granulocytes. Lymphocytes originate in the bone marrow but migrate through the blood to the lymphatic tissues. Most lymphocytes are located in the lymph nodes, spleen, tonsils, lymph nodules, and thymus.

Monocytes and macrophages are one of the first lines of defense in the inflammatory process. Monocytes migrate out of the blood and into the tissues in response to an infection. They engulf microbes and digest them in a process called phagocytosis. Unlike their counterparts, the neutrophils, which are short-lived, once in the tissues monocytes mature into long-lived macrophages.

Platelets and Blood Clotting

Platelets are small cells in the blood that are necessary for the series of chemical reactions that occur to form a clot. Usually, platelet counts range from 150,000 to 500,000 per microliter of blood. The blood clotting or coagulation process is a complex set of events involving platelets, clotting proteins in the plasma (clotting factors), other proteins, and calcium. The process begins with platelets clumping together. Then clotting proteins produced by the liver solidify the remainder of the clot, which eventually includes red and white blood cells.

Following injury to a blood vessel wall, a predictable series of events takes place, resulting in **hemostasis** (cessation of bleeding) and formation of the final blood clot. Chemicals released from the vessel wall cause local vasoconstriction, as well as activation of the platelets. The combination of vessel contraction and loose platelet aggregation forms a temporary "plug." Clotting is a chain reaction stimulated by the release of a chemical called **thromboplastin** from injured cells lining damaged blood vessels. Thromboplastin acts on an inactive plasma enzyme in the blood known as **prothrombin** (produced by the liver). Thromboplastin causes prothrombin to be converted into its active form, **thrombin**. Thrombin, in turn, acts on another blood protein fibrinogen, also produced by the liver. When activated, fibrinogen is converted into fibrin. **Fibrin** are long, branching fibers that produce a weblike network in the wall of the damaged blood vessel. Fibrin binds to the platelet plug, forming a plug that stops the flow of blood to the tissue.

The body also has two systems to counterbalance the clotting system. One, the fibrinolytic system, lyses or disrupts clots that already have formed. The main steps in the fibrinolytic system are the activation of **tissue plasminogen activator (t-PA)**, which then converts plasminogen to **plasmin**.

Together, the fibrinolytic system and the body's own anticoagulants attempt to provide a balance between clotting and bleeding; however, neither system is absolutely effective (for example, in patients in which formation of clots is creating problems, such as myocardial infarction or stroke, as well as in patients with spontaneous bleeding, such as subarachnoid hemorrhage).

■ The Circulatory System: Physiology

The **pulse**, which is palpated most easily at the neck, wrist, or groin, is a pressure wave created by the forceful pumping of blood out the left ventricle and into the major arteries. It is present throughout the entire arterial system. It can be felt most easily where the larger arteries are near the skin. The central pulses are the carotid artery pulse, which can be felt at the upper portion of the neck, and the femoral artery pulse, which is felt in the groin. The peripheral pulses are the radial pulse, which is felt at the wrist at the base of the thumb; the brachial artery pulse, which is felt on the medial aspect of the arm, midway between the elbow and shoulder; the posterior tibial artery pulse, which is felt posterior to the medial malleolus; and the dorsalis pedis artery pulse, which is felt on the top of the foot Figure 90 .

Blood pressure is the pressure that the blood exerts against the walls of the arteries as it passes through them. As mentioned earlier, systole and diastole are the phases that occur when the left ventricle contracts and when the ventricle relaxes, respectively. The pulsed forceful ejection of blood from the left ventricle of the heart into the aorta is transmitted through the arteries as a pulsatile pressure wave. This pressure wave keeps the blood moving through the body. The high and low points of the wave can be measured with a **sphygmomanometer** (blood pressure cuff) and are expressed numerically in millimeters of mercury (mm Hg).

The state of the blood vessels, how dilated or constricted they are, is referred to as the **systemic vascular resistance (SVR)**. SVR is the resistance to blood flow within all of the blood vessels except the pulmonary vessels. The relationship between the size of the vessels and shock is important to understand.

In some types of shock, blood vessels dilate and the patient's blood pressure falls dramatically Table 15 .

The average adult has approximately 5 L of blood in the vascular system. Children have less, 2 to 3 L, depending on their age and size. Infants have only about 300 mL. The loss of an amount of blood that may be negligible for an adult could be fatal for an infant.

Normal Circulation in Adults

In all healthy people, the circulatory system is automatically adjusted and readjusted constantly so 100% of the capacity

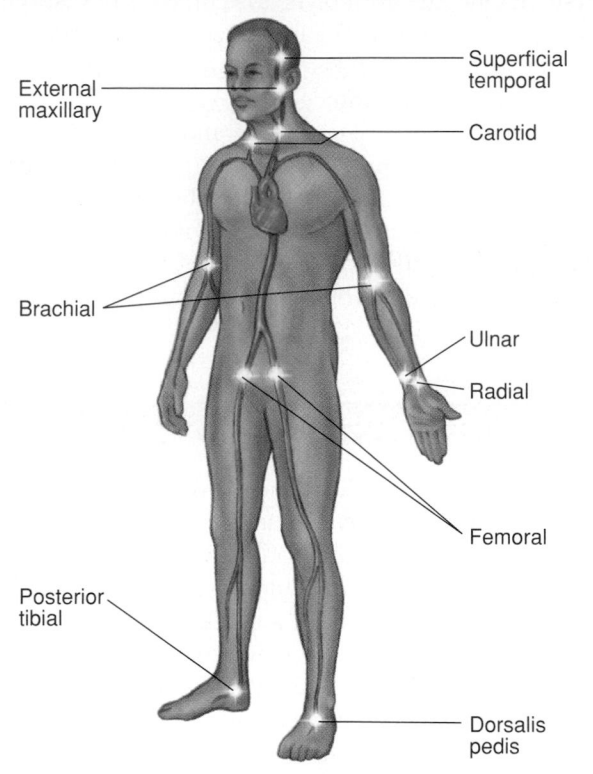

Figure 90 The central and peripheral pulses can be felt where the large arteries are near the skin.

Table 15	Effects of Blood Vessel Diameter on Blood
State	**Effects**
Constricted blood vessel	Decreased size of container Increased pressure within container
Normal diameter	Balance of size and pressure
Dilated blood vessel	Increased size of container Decreased pressure within container

of the arteries, veins, and capillaries holds 100% of the blood at that moment. All of the vessels are never fully dilated or constricted. The size of arteries and veins is controlled by the nervous system, according to the amount of blood that is available and many other factors, to keep blood pressure normal at all times. The feedback mechanisms in place maintain the system in such a way that delivers adequate circulation to all body areas without overtaxing any part of the system.

Perfusion is the circulation of blood in an organ or tissue in adequate amounts to meet the cells' current needs. Blood enters an organ or tissue through the arteries and leaves it through the veins Figure 91 . Loss of normal blood pressure is an indication that blood is no longer circulating efficiently to every organ in the body. (However, a "good blood pressure" does not indicate that it is reaching all parts of the body.) There are many reasons for loss of blood pressure. The result in each case is the same: Organs, tissues, and cells are no longer adequately perfused or supplied with oxygen and food, and wastes can accumulate. Under these conditions, cells, tissues, and whole organs may die. The state of inadequate circulation, when it involves the entire body, is called <u>shock</u>, or hypoperfusion.

Inadequate Circulation in Adults

When a patient loses a small amount of blood, the arteries, veins, and heart automatically adjust to the smaller new volume. The

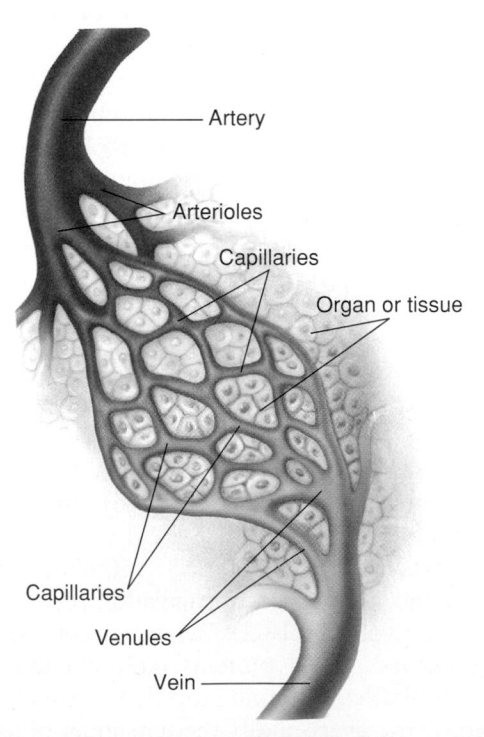

Figure 91 Blood enters an organ or tissue through the arteries and leaves through the veins. This process, called perfusion, provides adequate blood flow to the tissue to meet the cells' needs.

adjustment occurs in an effort to maintain adequate pressure throughout the circulatory system and maintain circulation for every organ. The adjustment occurs rapidly after the loss, usually within minutes. Specifically, the vessels constrict to provide a smaller bed for the reduced volume of blood to fill. The heart then pumps more rapidly to circulate the remaining blood more efficiently. As the blood pressure falls, the pulse increases in an attempt to keep the cardiac output constant at 5 to 6 L per minute. If the loss of blood is too great, the adjustment fails, and the patient goes into shock.

Words of Wisdom

If a patient is bleeding or severely dehydrated, baroreceptors sense the abnormally low volume. Although several different body responses occur at once, a major response is the release of epinephrine and norepinephrine from the adrenal glands, causing sympathetic (adrenergic) stimulation, resulting in an increased heart rate, as well as increased myocardial contractility.

The Distribution of Blood

Most blood is unevenly distributed throughout the body. Approximately 30% of blood is found within the heart, arteries, and capillaries. Seventy percent of blood is found within the veins and venules. This may seem confusing, but if you remember that the heart and arteries are high-pressure systems and veins are low-pressure systems, it becomes clearer. As blood pressure falls, blood flow slows down and there is more blood in the veins. The blood flows away from the left ventricle and moves back to the right atria.

Consider the movement of blood and its ultimate function of perfusion. You know that capillaries are the smallest portions of the circulatory system where materials are able to exit and enter the bloodstream. Nutrients move from the capillaries into the interstitial space and into the cells. The **interstitial space** is the space between the cells. Wastes move from the cells through the interstitial space and into the capillaries.

Here is a simplified version of what is happening inside the capillary. The two main forces at work inside the capillary are **hydrostatic pressure** and **oncotic pressure**. Hydrostatic pressure is pressure exerted by a liquid and occurs when blood is moved through the artery at relatively high pressures. When that blood meets the capillary walls, the pressure of the fluid pushes against the walls to force fluid out of the capillary. The opposing force is oncotic pressure. Oncotic pressure is a form of osmotic pressure exerted by proteins in the blood plasma that usually tends to pull water into the circulatory system. These proteins tend to make the blood thicker. This thickness means that relative to the interstitial space, there is more water outside the capillary than inside. Diffusion occurs, and water seeks to move into the capillary.

Here is the entire process **Figure 92**. Blood flows into the arterial side of the capillary. Plasma is trying to enter the capillary from the interstitial space, but hydrostatic pressure on the arterial side of the capillary is higher, so plasma, carrying nutrients, leaves the capillary and enters the interstitial space. The hydrostatic pressure is greatly diminished by the time the fluid reaches the venous side of the capillary because the effort of pushing the fluid out of the capillary decreased its force. This decrease in pressure is beneficial because now oncotic pressure can push fluid into the capillary; plasma, with all of the wastes from the cells, enters the venous side of the capillary. These wastes are then carried away.

As mentioned, another function of blood is the ability to clot. Coagulation, or clotting, occurs as the result of a complex chemical process that creates small fibers near the injured blood vessel, trapping red blood cells. This chemical process involves platelets and clotting factors that are in the bloodstream. **Table 16** outlines the major functions of the blood.

The Lymphatic System

The primary function of the lymphatic system is the production, maintenance, and distribution of lymphocytes. Another major function is to transport excess fluid out of interstitial spaces in tissues and return it to the bloodstream. The **lymphatic system** transports lymph by passive circulation. **Lymph** is a thin plasma-like fluid formed from interstitial or extracellular fluid that bathes the tissues of the body. Lymphatic capillaries pick up the lymph and drain it into larger vessels. Lymph circulates through the body in thin-walled **lymph vessels** that travel close to the major arteries and veins **Figure 93**. Like veins, lymphatic vessels contain valves that limit backflow. Foreign material such as debris or bacteria is filtered from the lymph in the **lymph nodes**, round or bean-shaped structures that are interspersed along the course of the lymph vessels, and returns to the main circulatory system via the **thoracic duct**, one of two great lymph vessels, which empties into the junction of the left subclavian vein and the left internal jugular vein. The lymphatic system helps absorb fat from the digestive tract, maintain fluid balance in the body, and fight infection. The movement of lymph is influenced by muscular activity.

Lymphatic Vessels

Lymphatic vessels only carry fluid away from the tissues. In the lymphatic capillaries, the epithelial cells contain one-way valves that allow fluid to enter the vessel but prevent it from flowing back into the tissues. Lymphatic capillaries are present in all tissues except the central nervous system, bone marrow, cartilage, epidermis, and cornea. Generally, fluid flows from the blood capillaries to the tissues, then out of the tissue spaces into lymph capillaries. In the major blood capillary beds of the body, the internal hydrostatic pressure allows a normal and continuous leak of a total of 3 to 4 mL/min of fluid into

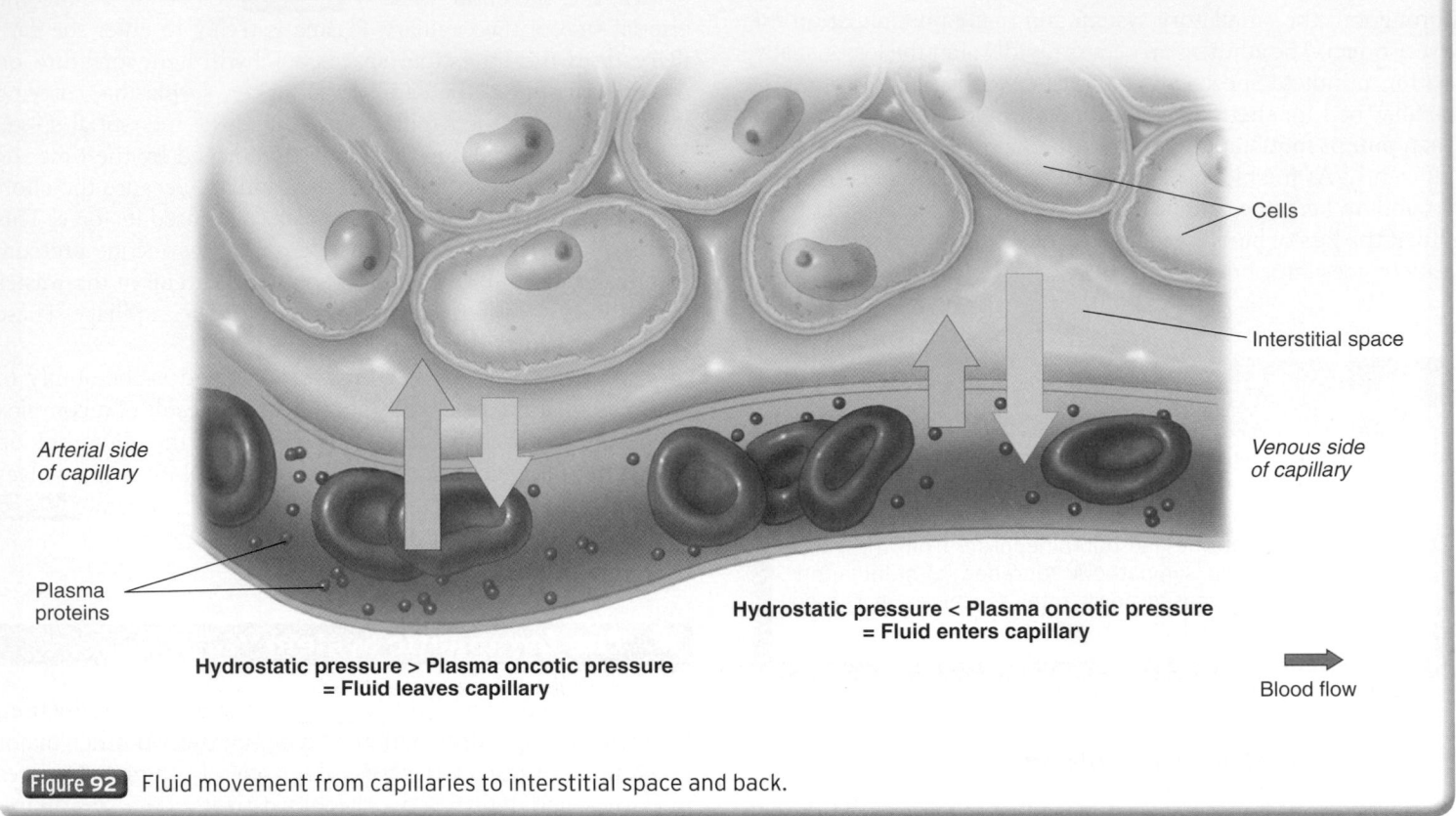

Cells

Interstitial space

Arterial side
of capillary

Venous side
of capillary

Plasma
proteins

**Hydrostatic pressure < Plasma oncotic pressure
= Fluid enters capillary**

Blood flow

**Hydrostatic pressure > Plasma oncotic pressure
= Fluid leaves capillary**

Figure 92 Fluid movement from capillaries to interstitial space and back.

Table 16 Functions of the Blood and the Components of Blood in Use	
Function	**Component of the Blood in Use**
Fighting infection	White blood cells
Transporting oxygen	Red blood cells (hemoglobin)
Transporting carbon dioxide	Plasma
Controlling (buffering) pH	Chemicals within the plasma
Transporting wastes and nutrients	Plasma (water)
Clotting (coagulation)	Platelets and clotting factors in the plasma

the interstitial spaces. To prevent the tissues from becoming edematous, the lymphatic vessel must absorb this excess fluid and return it to the central venous circulation.

The Thymus

The **thymus** is located in the thorax, anterior to the aorta and posterior to the upper sternum. It is soft, and consists of two lobes that are enclosed in a connective tissue capsule **Figure 94**. Although relatively large in infancy and early childhood, it shrinks

after puberty, becoming much smaller in adults. Its lymphatic tissue is replaced during the later years of life by adipose and connective tissues.

The thymus is divided into lobules by inward-extending connective tissues. The lobules contain large amounts of lymphocytes, including primarily inactive thymocytes, which formed from stem cells in the bone marrow and settled in the thymus. Some thymocytes mature into T lymphocytes, which leave the thymus after 3 weeks and provide immunity in the body. T lymphocytes are discussed later in this chapter. Thymosins are secreted by the thymus's epithelial cells. This hormone causes T lymphocytes to mature.

The Spleen

The **spleen** is located in the upper left abdominal cavity, inferior to the diaphragm and posterior and lateral to the stomach. It is the body's largest lymphatic organ, resembling a large, subdivided lymph node. The spleen contains the largest amount of lymphatic tissue in an adult's body. It differs from lymph nodes in that its venous sinuses are filled with blood, not lymph. There are two types of tissues inside the splenic lobules. White pulp is located throughout the spleen in small "islands," made up of splenic nodules containing many lymphocytes. The remainder of the lobules are filled by red pulp, which contains many red blood cells, lymphocytes, and macrophages.

The blood capillaries of the red pulp are extremely permeable, and red blood cells easily squeeze through the capillary

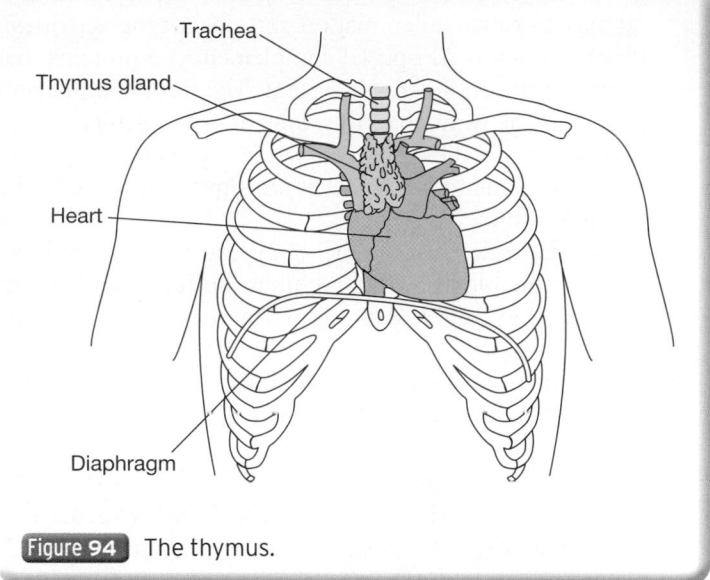

Figure 94 The thymus.

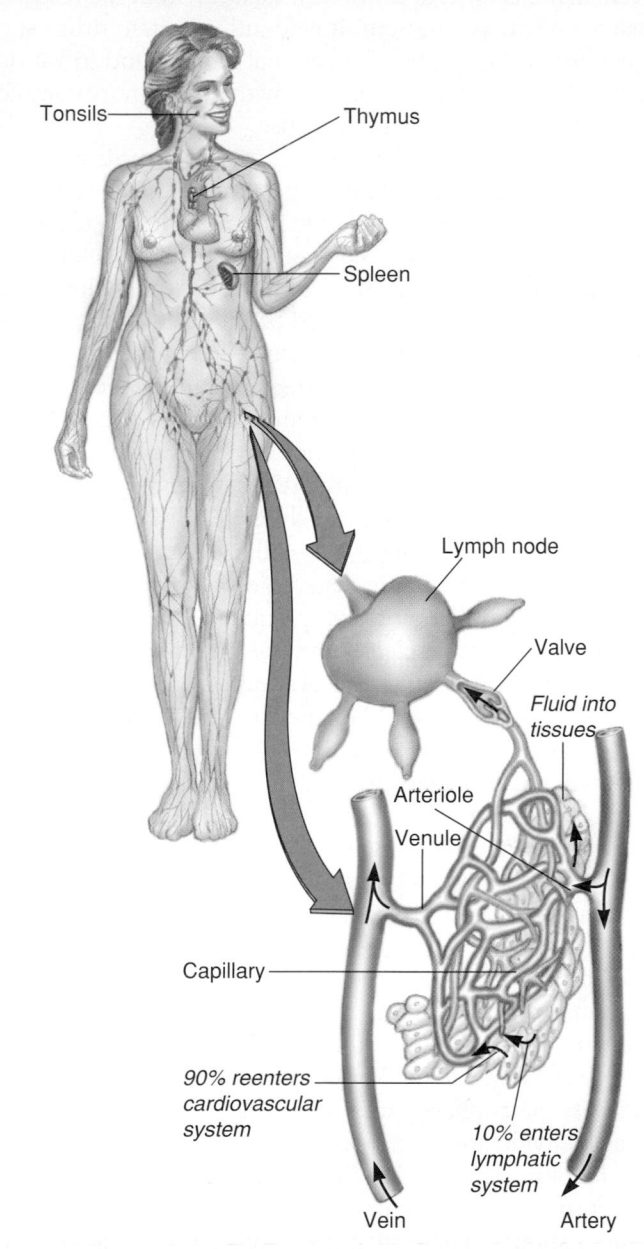

Figure 93 The lymphatic vessel. The enlarged diagram of a lymph node and vessels shows the path of the excess fluid that leaves the capillary, enters the adjacent tissue spaces, and is absorbed by lymphatic capillaries.

walls to enter the venous sinuses. Older red blood cells may be damaged during this process, so they are engulfed by macrophages inside the splenic sinuses. Via the action of macrophages and lymphocytes, the spleen filters blood similarly to the way that lymph nodes filter lymph.

Body Defenses and Fighting Infection

The human body has multiple defense mechanisms that work together to provide resistance, which is the ability to fight disease, illness, and infection. An infection may be caused by the presence and multiplication of a disease-causing agent

(pathogen), which can be a virus, bacterium, fungus, or protozoan. Body defenses can be divided into two general categories: innate (nonspecific) and adaptive (specific) defenses. <u>Innate (nonspecific) defense</u> defends against many different types of pathogens. This type of defense, which is present at birth, includes mechanical barriers, chemical barriers, natural killer cells (NK cells), inflammation, phagocytosis, fever, and species resistance.

Specific defenses are more precise, and target specific pathogens to provide <u>adaptive (specific) defense</u> or <u>immunity</u>. In this type of defense, specialized lymphocytes recognize foreign molecules and act against them. Both innate and adaptive defense mechanisms work together to fight infection. Innate defenses act more rapidly than adaptive defenses. Specific defenses depend on the activity of lymphocytes.

Innate (Nonspecific) Defenses

Nonspecific defenses prevent or limit microorganisms and other environmental hazards from approaching, entering, or spreading. Nonspecific defenses are classified as follows, with mechanical barriers being the first line of defense and the others being second lines of defense:

- *Mechanical barriers:* Also known as physical barriers, they include the skin and the mucous membranes that line the respiratory, digestive, urinary (basement membranes), and reproductive passageways. They protect against certain infectious agents. The body's hair, sweat, and mucus also act as mechanical barriers.
- *Chemical barriers:* Provided by enzymes and other chemical substances in body fluids; these include pepsin and hydrochloric acid in the stomach, tears, lysozyme (which is present in tears, saliva, breast milk, and mucus), salt (which exists in perspiration), <u>interferons</u> (hormone-like peptides) that bind to uninfected cells and stimulate them to make protective proteins, and <u>complement</u> (a

group of proteins in plasma and other body fluids that interact to cause inflammation and phagocytic activities). Plasma contains 11 special complement (C) proteins that comprise the complement system. The term complement refers to the way that this system "complements" the action of antibodies. The complement proteins interact in chain reactions (cascades) that are similar to those of the clotting system.

- *Fever:* Elevation of body temperature that reduces iron in the blood, which inhibits bacterial and fungal reproduction; fever also causes increased phagocytosis (macrophages).
- *Inflammation:* A tissue response to injury or infection that may include redness, swelling, heat, and pain; infected cells attract white blood cells, which engulf them. Masses of leukocytes, bacterial cells, and damaged tissue may form a thick fluid called pus. The body may react to inflammation by forming a network of fibrin threads where the infection is centered. This closes off the infected area to inhibit the spread of pathogens. An inflammatory response is triggered when mast cells and basophils release histamine, serotonin, and heparin. The inflammatory response is a tissue-level reaction, and is therefore related to the tissues and integumentary system.
- *Immunologic surveillance:* The constant monitoring, recognizing, and destruction of abnormal cells by natural killer (NK) cells in peripheral tissues. NK cells defend the body against cancer cells and various viruses.
- *Langerhans cells (antigen-presenting cells):* Detect, process, and present foreign materials or germs to other parts of the immune system, stimulating an immune response.
- *Phagocytosis:* Injured tissues attract neutrophils and monocytes, which engulf and digest particles (pathogens and cell debris); monocytes influence the development of macrophages that attach to blood and lymphatic vessels. Together, these various phagocytic cells make up the **mononuclear phagocytic system** to remove foreign particles from the lymph and also the blood.

A final form of innate (nonspecific) defense is species resistance. In this example, a human being may be resistant to certain diseases that affect other species of animals. A pathogen effective against a dog, for example, may be unable to survive in a human. In reverse, humans can be infected with measles, gonorrhea, mumps, and syphilis, none of which affect other animal species.

Immunity (Specific Defenses)

Immunity is also known as the third line of defense. It is defined as resistance to specific pathogens or their toxins and metabolic by products. Adaptive immune responses are carried out by lymphocytes and macrophages that recognize and remember certain foreign molecules. Antigens include proteins, polysaccharides, glycoproteins, and glycolipids that are commonly found on cell surfaces. As a fetus develops, cells learn to recognize proteins and large molecules as being "self." The lymphatic system, as it develops, responds to "nonself" (foreign) antigens, and does not respond to "self" antigens, if the system is normal.

A small molecule that cannot stimulate an immune response by itself is known as a **hapten**. It is found in certain drugs such as penicillin, in dust particles, in animal dander, and in various chemicals. Haptens usually combine with larger, more complex molecules to elicit an immune response.

There also exist a large number of minute organisms whose presence in the body in normal proportions and expected locations is not only harmless, but in many cases, helps or enables the body's normal functions. For example, certain bacteria normally inhabit the lower digestive tract and without their presence, digestion of some foods would be impaired or impossible. Other normal flora help maintain the mucosal linings of various body orifices. However, when these organisms are spread to unfamiliar locations in the body or are present in unusually low or high proportions, disease can and often does result.

Before birth, red bone marrow releases lymphocyte precursors, about half of which reach the thymus. They specialize into transitioning to **T lymphocytes (T cells)**, which later make up between 70% and 80% of circulated blood lymphocytes. Other T cells exist in lymphatic organs, particularly in lymph nodes, the white pulp of the spleen, and the thoracic duct. Others remain in the red bone marrow, eventually differentiating into **B lymphocytes (B cells)**. They are distributed by the blood, and make up between 20% and 30% of the circulating lymphocytes. B cells are abundant in the lymph nodes, bone marrow, intestinal lining, and spleen.

T cells attach to foreign, antigen-bearing cells such as bacterial cells, and interact with direct cell-to-cell contact. This is known as **cellular immune response** or cell-mediated immunity. T cells, along with some macrophages, also synthesize polypeptides called cytokines that enhance responses to antigens. Interleukin-1 and interleukin-2 stimulate synthesis of cytokines from other T cells. Other cytokines called colony-stimulating factors (CSFs) stimulate leukocyte production in red bone marrow, activate macrophages, and cause B cells to grow.

B cells divide and differentiate into **plasma cells**, producing antibodies (immunoglobulins) that react to destroy antigens or antigen-containing particles. This is called the **humoral immune response**. There are millions of different types of T and B cells. Each variety originates from a single early cell to form a clone of cells (identical to the original cell). Each variety has a certain antigen receptor responding to only a specific antigen. Table 17 compares characteristics of T and B cells.

Before a lymphocyte can respond to an antigen, it must be activated. T cells are activated by the presence of processed antigen fragments attached to the surface of an antigen-presenting cell (accessory cell), which may be macrophages, B cells, or other types of cells. When a macrophage phagocytizes a bacterium and digests it in its lysosomes, T cell activation begins. Some bacterial antigens then move to the surface of the macrophage. They are displayed near certain protein molecules that make up the major histocompatibility complex (MHC). MHC antigens help T cells recognize foreign antigens. Helper T cells contact displayed foreign antigens. If the antigen combines with the helper T cell's antigen receptors, it becomes activated and stimulates a B cell to produce antibodies specific for the displayed antigen.

Table 17 T and B Cells

T Cells	B Cells
Originate in red bone marrow	Originate in red bone marrow
Differentiate in the thymus	Differentiate in red bone marrow
Primarily located in lymphatic tissues	Primarily located in lymphatic tissues
Make up 70% to 80% of circulating lymphocytes	Make up 20% to 30% of circulating lymphocytes
Provide cellular immune response	Provide humoral immune response
Interact directly with antigens or antigen-bearing agents to destroy them	Interact indirectly to produce antibodies that destroy antigens or antigen-bearing agents

Table 18 Antibody Production by B and T Cells

B Cell	T Cell
Antigen-bearing agents enter tissues.	Antigen-bearing agents enter tissues.
An antigen that fits antigen receptors is encountered.	An accessory cell phagocytizes the antigen-bearing agent and lysosomes digest the agent.
Activation occurs, and the B cell proliferates, enlarging its clone.	Antigens are displayed on the membrane of the accessory cell.
Further differentiation occurs as B cells become plasma cells.	A helper T cell activates when it encounters a displayed antigen fitting its antigen receptors.
Plasma cells synthesize and secrete antibodies with molecular structure similar to that of activated B cell antigen receptors.	The activated helper T cell releases cytokines when encountering a B cell that has combined with an identical antigen-bearing agent.
Antibodies combine with antigen-bearing agents to help destroy them.	Cytokines stimulate B cell proliferation. Some newly formed B cells give rise to cells differentiating into antibody-secreting plasma cells. Antibodies combine with antigen-bearing agents to help destroy them.

A cytotoxic T cell recognizes and combines with foreign antigens displayed on cell surfaces near certain MHC proteins. This is common with cancer cells or virally infected cells. Cytotoxic T cells are activated via cytokines from helper T cells. They bind to antigen-bearing cells and release a protein that cuts openings into these cells to destroy them. Cytotoxic T cells continually recognize and eliminate tumor cells and virally infected cells. They are effective in fighting human immunodeficiency virus (HIV) infection, but are often killed by the viruses they combat. Some T cells act as memory cells, immediately dividing to yield more cytotoxic T cells and helper T cells when reexposed to the same antigen.

B cells may activate when encountering an antigen whose shape fits the B cell's antigen receptor shape, dividing repeatedly and expanding its clone. However, B cells usually require T cells in order to activate. T cells that encounter B cells bound to identical foreign antigens release cytokines that stimulate the B cells. The cytokines attract macrophages and leukocytes. Some of the B cell's clones differentiate into more memory cells. These memory B cells respond quickly to reexposure to specific antigens. Other B cell clones differentiate into antibody-secreting plasma cells, which can combine with their corresponding foreign antigens and react against them.

Table 18 summarizes B cell and T cell antibody production activities.

B cells can produce between 10 million and 1 billion varieties of antibodies, each specific to an antigen. Antibody response therefore defends against many pathogens. Antibodies are round, soluble proteins making up the gamma globulin part of the plasma proteins. There are five major types of antibodies:

Immunoglobulin G (IgG): A single molecule in plasma and tissue fluids; effective against bacteria, viruses, and toxins. It activates complement.

Immunoglobulin A (IgA): In exocrine gland secretions, breast milk, tears, nasal fluid, gastric juice, intestinal juice, bile, and urine.

Immunoglobulin M (IgM): Composed of five single molecules found together, it is the first antibody to be produced in response to infection. IgM in plasma responds to certain antigens in foods or bacteria. The antibodies known as anti-A and anti-B are examples of IgM. This antibody also activates complement.

Immunoglobulin D (IgD): On the surfaces of most B cells, especially in infants; important in the activation of B cells. It may play a role in regulation of the humoral immune response.

Immunoglobulin E (IgE): Attaches to mast cells and basophils, and is involved in allergic reactions.

Antibodies commonly attack antigens directly, activate complement, or stimulate inflammation. They combine with antigens, causing clumping (agglutination) or forming insoluble substances (precipitation). Phagocytosis then can occur more easily. Sometimes antibodies neutralize the toxic effects of antigens. Complement activation is generally more important in protecting against infection than direct antibody attack, however.

When some IgM or IgG antibodies combine with antigens, they trigger many reactions that lead to the activation of the complement proteins. Effects include coating the antigen–antibody complexes (opsonization), attracting macrophages and neutrophils (chemotaxis), making the complexes more susceptible to phagocytosis, clumping antigen-bearing cells, rupturing foreign cell membranes (lysis), and altering viral molecular structures to make them harmless.

A primary immune response is constituted by activation of B cells or T cells after they first encounter the antigens for which they are specialized to react. Plasma cells release IgM into the lymph, followed by IgG. The antibodies are transported to the blood and throughout the body to help destroy antigen-bearing agents. This continues for several weeks.

Some of the B cells then remain as memory cells so that if the identical antigen is reencountered, clones of these memory cells enlarge and send IgG to the antigen. These memory B cells, along with memory T cells, produce a secondary immune response. After a primary immune response, detectable concentrations of antibodies appear in the blood plasma, usually 5 to 10 days after exposure to antigens, and a secondary immune response can then occur within 1 to 2 days. Memory cells live much longer than newly formed antibodies (which live between a few months and a few years). Secondary immune responses may last a long time.

Adaptive (acquired) immunity can be caused by natural events or by administration (oral or injected) of suspensions of killed or weakened pathogens or their molecules. This type of immunity may be active or passive. Active immunity is long-lasting, and occurs when a patient produces an immune response to an antigen. Passive immunity occurs when antibodies produced by another person are received by a patient; it has only short-term effects. Naturally acquired active immunity occurs when a person develops a disease from exposure to a pathogen. Resistance then occurs as a result of the primary immune response.

A preparation known as a vaccine produces another type of active immunity. A vaccine may consist of killed or weakened bacteria or viruses, or pathogenic molecules. It cannot cause serious infections or diseases. Vaccines can also be made of a toxoid, with a toxin from an infectious organism chemically altered so that it is not dangerous. Vaccines cause patients to develop artificially acquired active immunity.

If a patient has been exposed to a disease-causing microorganism, but there is not enough time to develop active immunity, an injection of antiserum may be given. Antiserum consists of ready-made antibodies that can be obtained from gamma globulin acquired from people who are already immune to the same disease. Injection of such gamma globulin provides artificially acquired passive immunity.

IgG antibodies pass from maternal blood to the fetus during pregnancy, giving the fetus limited immunity against pathogens that the mother is immune to. The fetus therefore has naturally acquired passive immunity, which lasts from 6 months to 1 year after birth. **Table 19** explains the various types of acquired immunity.

When an immune response occurs because of a nonharmful substance, it is called an allergic response. These reactions create many of the same responses as a beneficial immune response, but are created by a hypersensitivity to a given substance that causes an inappropriate effect. An **allergen** is an antigen that triggers an allergic response. Allergic responses are classified as:

- *Delayed-reaction allergy:* Results from repeated exposure of the skin to certain chemicals; it usually takes about 48 hours to occur
- *Immediate-reaction allergy:* Affects people with inherited tendencies to overproduce IgE antibodies because of certain

Table 19 Types of Acquired Immunity

Type	Exposure	Outcome
Artificially acquired active immunity	Exposure to vaccine containing weakened or killed pathogens or their components	Immune response is stimulated without severe disease symptoms
Artificially acquired passive immunity	Injection of gamma globulin containing antibodies	Short-term immunity without an immune response
Naturally acquired active immunity	Exposure to live pathogens	Immune response is stimulated with disease symptoms
Naturally acquired passive immunity	Antibodies passed from mother who has active immunity to her fetus, or to newborn via breast milk from mother who has active immunity	Short-term immunity for newborn without an immune response

antigens; it takes only a few minutes to occur, and subsequent reexposure continues to trigger allergic reactions

Another type of reaction concerns transplantation and tissue rejection. When a body part is transplanted from one person to another, the receiving patient's immune system may recognize the transplanted part as foreign and attempt to destroy its tissues, causing a tissue rejection reaction. The greater the difference between the antigens on cell surface molecules of the donor and recipient, the greater and more rapid the rejection reaction. Therefore, donor and recipient tissues must be matched to minimize these reactions. Immunosuppressive drugs are used to reduce tissue rejection. Although they reduce the immune response by suppressing antibody and T cell formation, they weaken the recipient's immune system. Frequently, transplant patients survive the transplant but die from an infection caused by a weakened immune system.

When the immune system fails to distinguish self from nonself, it may produce autoantibodies as well as cytotoxic T cells that attack and damage the body's tissues and organs. This "attack against self" is called autoimmunity. About 5% of all people have an autoimmune disorder. It is believed that this type of condition occurs in one of three ways:

- When a replicating virus "borrows" proteins from a host cell, incorporating them onto its own surface, the immune system "learns" the surface of the virus to destroy it, and also begins to attack the original cells bearing the same proteins.

- T cells may not learn to distinguish self from nonself.
- A nonself antigen happens to resemble a self antigen, such as when a *Streptococcus* bacterial infection triggers inflammation of the heart valves.

The Effects of Aging on the Lymphatic System and Immunity

The lymphatic system becomes less effective at fighting disease as a person ages, resulting in lowered immunity. T cells weaken, and fewer of them can respond to infections. As the thymus shrinks with age, there are lower circulating levels of thymic hormones. The number of helper T cells is reduced, B cells are less responsive, and antibody levels do not rise after exposure to antigens with the same speed they used to. Viral and bacterial infections are able to proliferate more. This is why vaccinations for diseases such as influenza and pneumococcal pneumonia are recommended for elderly patients. With decreased immunity, tumor cells are not eliminated as effectively, and cancer rates increase with age.

The Nervous System: Anatomy and Physiology

The nervous system is perhaps the most complex organ system within the human body. It is composed of two major structures, the brain and the spinal cord, and thousands of nerves that allow every part of the body to communicate. This system is responsible for fundamental functions such as controlling breathing, pulse rate, and blood pressure. However, what makes the nervous system so special is that it allows the performance of higher level activity, such as memory, understanding, and thought.

The nervous system is divided into two main portions: the central nervous system (CNS) and the peripheral nervous system (PNS). The somatic nervous system is the part of the peripheral nervous system that regulates activities over which there is voluntary control, such as walking, talking, and writing. The autonomic nervous system (ANS) controls the many body functions that occur without voluntary control. These activities include body functions such as

digestion, dilation and constriction of blood vessels, sweating, and all other involuntary actions that are necessary for basic body functions. Thus, the nervous system as a whole can be divided anatomically into the central and peripheral nervous systems and functionally into somatic (voluntary) and autonomic (involuntary) components Figure 95 .

The nervous system is composed of specialized tissue that conducts electrical impulses between the brain and the rest of the body. Neural tissue contains two basic types of cells: nerve cells, which are known as neurons and contain projections called axons and dendrites that make connections between adjacent cells Figure 96 , and neuroglia, which are supporting cells

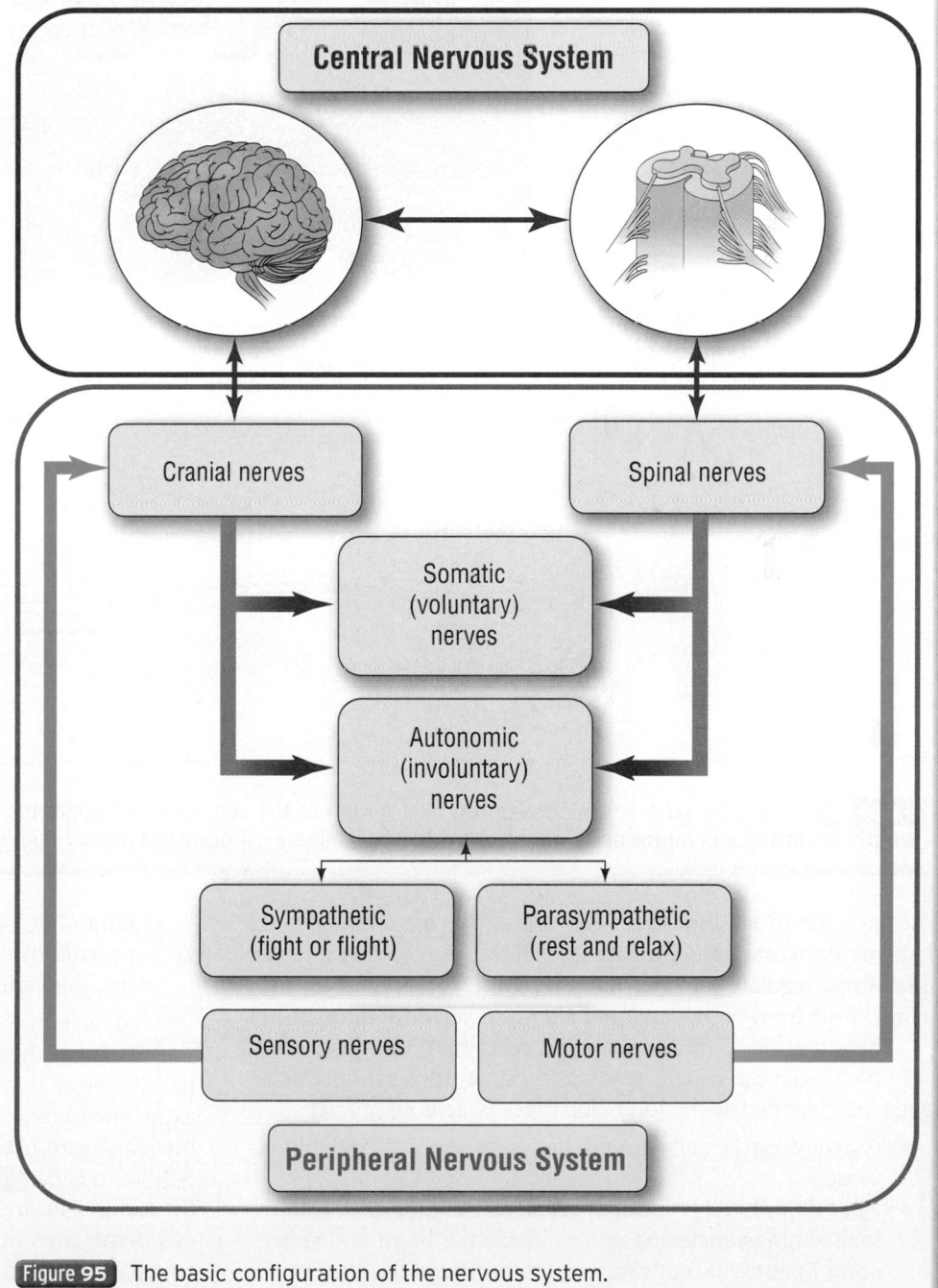

Figure 95 The basic configuration of the nervous system.

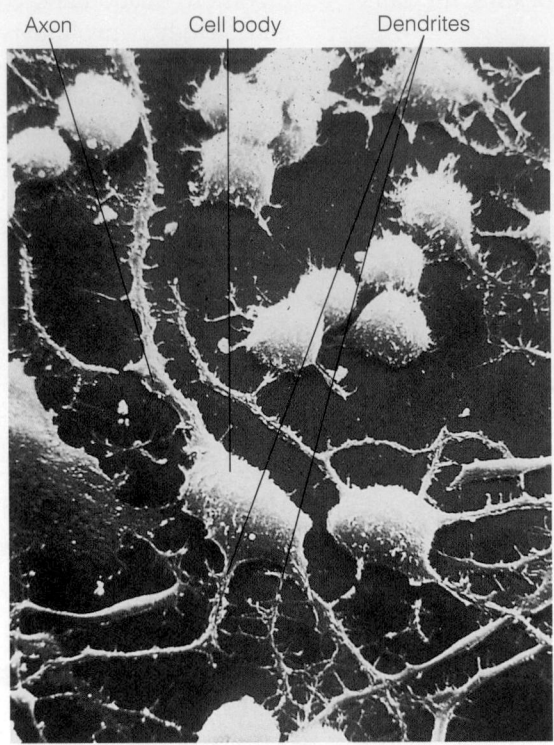

Axon · Cell body · Dendrites

A

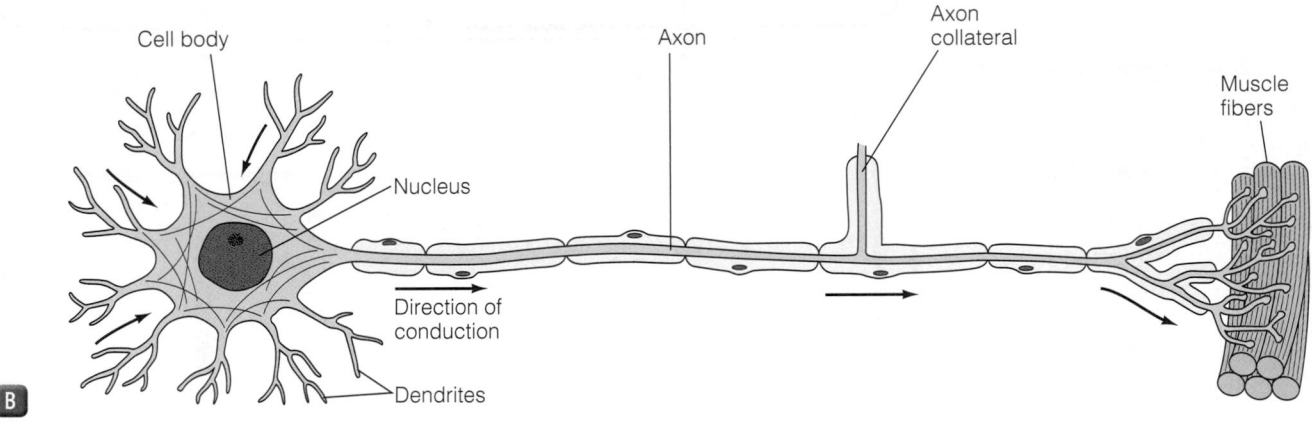

Cell body · Axon · Axon collateral

Muscle fibers

Nucleus

Direction of conduction

Dendrites

B

Figure 96 A neuron. **A.** A scanning electron micrograph of the cell body and dendrites. **B.** Collateral branches may occur along the length of the axon. In motor neurons, when the axon terminates, it branches many times, ending on individual muscle fibers.

that have four basic functions. <u>Neuroglia</u> provide a supporting skeleton for neural tissue, isolate and protect the cell membranes of neurons, regulate the composition of interstitial fluid, defend neural tissue from pathogens, and aid in the repair of injury.

There are many more neuroglial cells than neurons in the body. Neuroglia can divide, whereas most neurons cannot. Neuroglia are classified as the following types of cells **Figure 97** :

- <u>Astrocytes</u>: Usually found between neurons and blood vessels.
- <u>Ependymal cells</u>: Cover specialized brain parts and form inner linings enclosing spaces inside the brain and spinal cord. Ependymal cells secrete cerebrospinal fluid.
- <u>Microglial cells</u>: Found throughout the central nervous system, they phagocytize bacterial cells and cellular debris.

- <u>Oligodendrocytes</u>: Found aligned along nerve fibers, they provide insulating layers of myelin around axons within the brain and spinal cord.

Axons may or may not be surrounded by a membrane sheath. In unsheathed or unmyelinated axons, action potential electrical signals in the nerves propagate along the entire axon membrane. Myelinated nerves are surrounded by a myelin sheath manufactured by a form of nervous tissue called <u>Schwann cells</u> **Figure 98** . These cells are wound tightly around the axons. The areas of the Schwann cells containing most of the cytoplasm and nuclei are located outside the myelin sheath, comprising a neurilemma (or neurilemmal sheath). There are narrow gaps between the Schwann cells known as <u>nodes of Ranvier</u>.

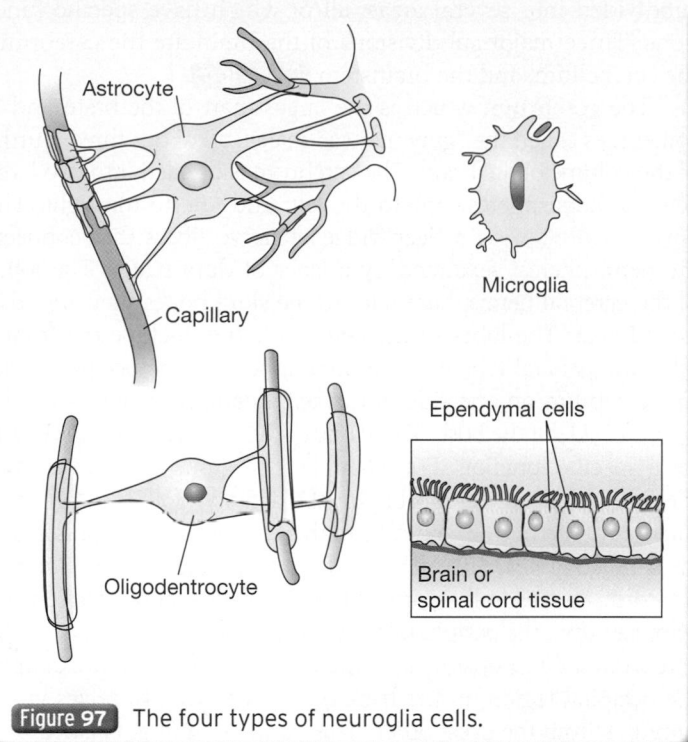

Figure 97 The four types of neuroglia cells.

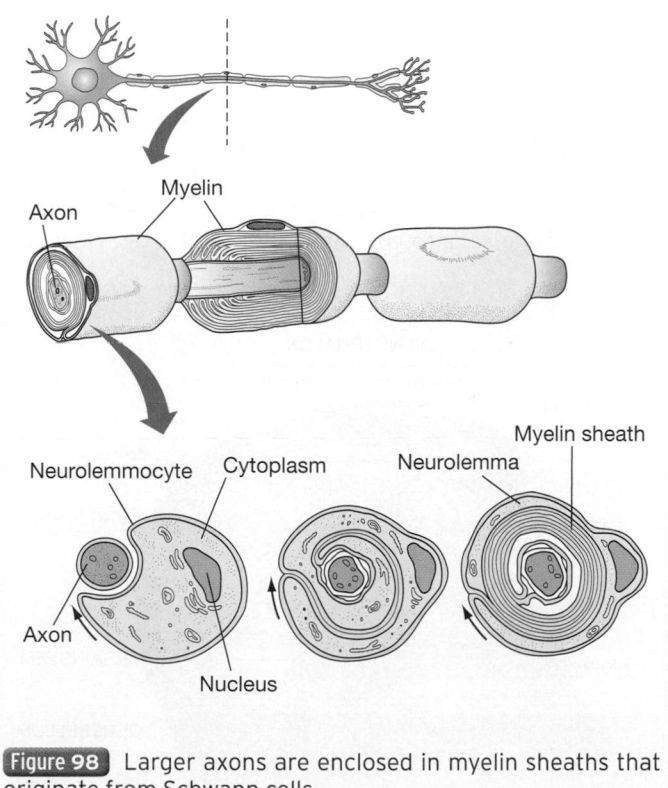

Figure 98 Larger axons are enclosed in myelin sheaths that originate from Schwann cells.

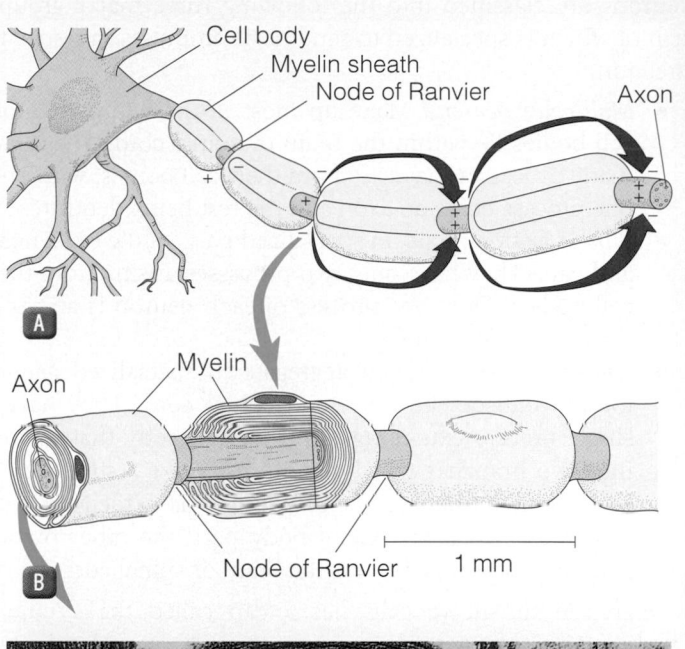

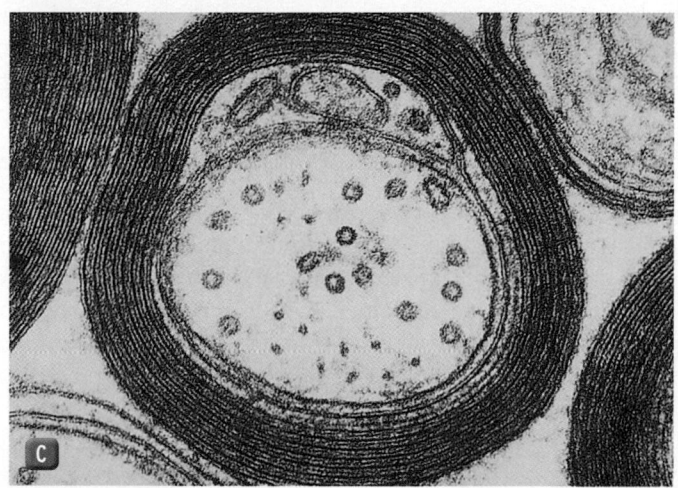

Figure 99 A myelinated nerve. **A.** The myelin sheath allows impulses to "jump" from node to node, greatly accelerating the rate of transmission. **B.** The node of Ranvier. **C.** A transmission electron micrograph of an axon in a cross section, showing a myelin sheath.

Nodes of Ranvier are located between the individual Schwann cells at intervals of approximately 1 to 1.5 mm **Figure 99**. In myelinated nerves, the action potential jumps between these regions in a process called saltatory conduction, resulting in increased speed of transmission of the impulse. Bundles of myelinated nerves are referred to as **white matter**.

There are a variety of neurons; the following list groups them by their functions:

- *Sensory neurons (afferent neurons):* Carry nerve impulses from the peripheral body parts into the brain or spinal cord; most sensory neurons are unipolar, although some are bipolar. They may have receptor ends at the tips of the dendrites or receptor cells that are associated with the dendrites in the sensory organs or the skin.
- *Interneurons (association or internuncial neurons):* Within the brain and spinal cord; they are multipolar. The cell bodies of some interneurons form masses called *nuclei*, which are similar to ganglia.
- *Motor neurons (efferent neurons):* Carry impulses out of the brain or spinal cord to effectors; they are multipolar.

Neurons are classified into the following three major groups, each of which is specialized to send nerve impulses in a specific direction:

- *Multipolar neurons:* Make up most of the neurons whose cell bodies lie within the brain or spinal cord. They have many processes that arise from their cell bodies, with only one process being an axon and the rest being dendrites.
- *Bipolar neurons:* Exist in specialized parts of the eyes, nose, and ears. They have only two processes arising from their cell bodies. Only one process of each neuron is an axon; the rest are dendrites.
- *Unipolar neurons:* Often aggregate in specialized ganglia located outside the brain and spinal cord. They have a single process extending from the cell body that divides into two branches that function more like a single axon. One branch (the peripheral process) is associated with dendrites near a peripheral body part; the other branch (the central process) enters the brain or spinal cord.

Between the nerve cells lies a gap called the synapse, which consists of a terminal bouton or other type of axon terminal, the synaptic cleft, and the membrane of the postsynaptic cell. The presynaptic terminal is at one end of a nerve. The synaptic cleft is the space between neurons. Opposite of the presynaptic terminal, across the synaptic cleft, is the postsynaptic terminal. Electrical impulses travel down the nerve and trigger the release of chemicals known as neurotransmitters from the presynaptic terminal. These neurotransmitters cross the synaptic cleft to stimulate an electrical reaction in adjacent neurons. Neurotransmitters are contained within synaptic vesicles and are released into the synaptic cleft at the presynaptic terminal. This electrical reaction passes through the neuron to the next synapse, and the process is repeated.

Groups of nerve cells are bundled together to form nerve fibers. Groups of nerve fibers are bundled together to form a nerve, which is tissue that connects the nervous system with body parts or organs. The nervous system is divided into the central nervous system (CNS), the peripheral nervous system (PNS), and the autonomic nervous system (ANS). The CNS is composed of the brain and spinal cord. The CNS includes the 12 pairs of cranial nerves that branch directly from the brain. The 31 pairs of spinal nerves that exit the spinal cord via the vertebral column are part of the PNS. The ANS controls smooth muscle and is responsible for the "fight-or-flight" response. Autonomic functions are not under conscious control and include such activities as maintaining heart rate and blood pressure, intestinal motility, and pupillary response.

The Central Nervous System

Brain

The brain is the controlling organ of the body. It is the center of consciousness. It is responsible for all of your voluntary body activities, your perception of your surroundings, and the control of your reactions to the environment. In addition, the brain enables you to experience all the fine shadings of thought and feeling that make each of us an individual. The brain is

subdivided into several areas, all of which have specific functions. Three major subdivisions of the brain are the cerebrum, the cerebellum, and the brainstem **Figure 100** .

The cerebrum, which is the largest part of the brain and is sometimes called the "gray matter," makes up about three fourths of the volume of the brain. The cerebrum is divided into two large cerebral hemispheres, one to the left, and one to the right. The corpus callosum is a deep ridge of nerve fibers that connects the hemispheres, separated by a layer of dura mater. The lobes of the cerebral hemisphere refer to the skull bones they are positioned near. The lobes of the cerebral cortex include the frontal lobe, the parietal lobe, the temporal lobe, and the occipital lobe. The cerebrum on one side of the brain controls activities on the opposite side of the body. Each lobe of the cerebrum is responsible for a specific function. For example, one group of brain cells in the frontal lobe is responsible for the activity of all the voluntary muscles of the body. Brain cells in this area generate impulses that are sent along nerve fibers that extend from each cell into the spinal cord. An area in the parietal lobe has cells that receive sensory impulses from the peripheral nerves of the body. Other parts of the cerebrum are responsible for other body functions. For example, the occipital region, in the back of the cerebrum, receives visual impulses from the eyes; other areas control hearing, balance, and speech. Still other parts of the cerebrum are responsible for emotions and other characteristics of a person's personality **Figure 101** .

Several masses of gray basal nuclei (basal ganglia) lie deep inside each cerebral hemisphere. These include the caudate nucleus, globus pallidus, and putamen. The basal nuclei help to control skeletal muscle activities. **Figure 102** show the basal nuclei (basal ganglia) and nearby structures.

The cerebellum, which is located underneath the great mass of cerebral tissue, is sometimes called the "little brain." The major function of this area is to coordinate the various activities of the

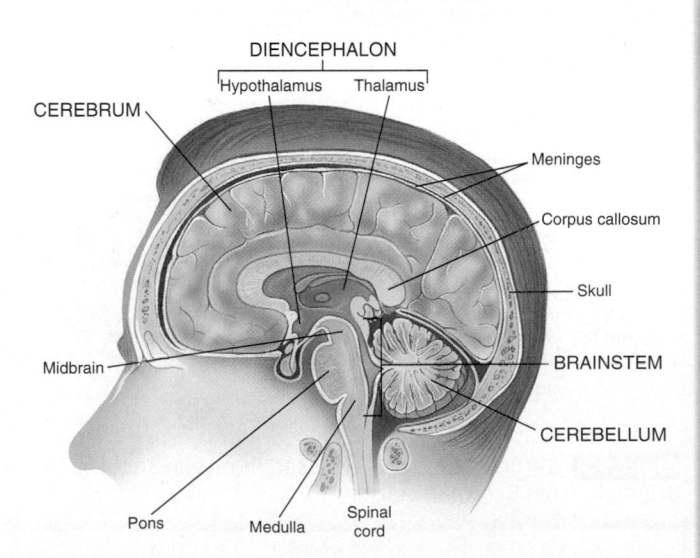

Figure 100 The brain lies well protected within the skull. Its principal subdivisions are the cerebrum, the cerebellum, and the brainstem.

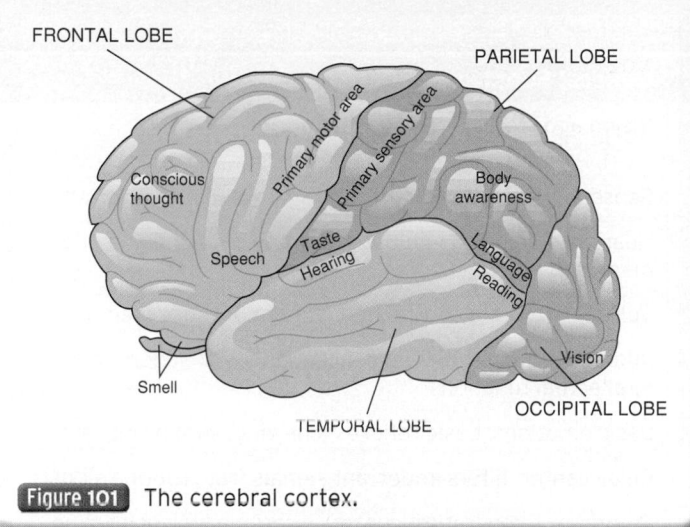

Figure 101 The cerebral cortex.

FRONTAL LOBE

PARIETAL LOBE

Primary motor area

Primary sensory area

Conscious thought

Body awareness

Speech

Taste

Hearing

Language

Reading

Smell

Vision

TEMPORAL LOBE

OCCIPITAL LOBE

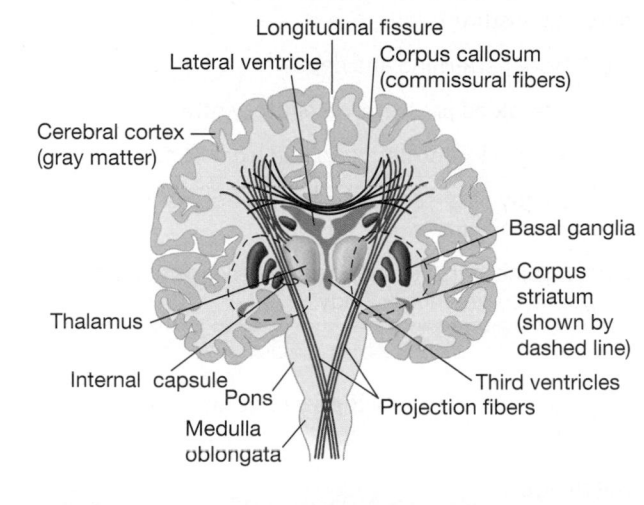

Figure 102 A coronal section of the cerebrum indicating deep cerebral structures.

Longitudinal fissure

Lateral ventricle

Corpus callosum (commissural fibers)

Cerebral cortex (gray matter)

Basal ganglia

Corpus striatum (shown by dashed line)

Thalamus

Internal capsule

Pons

Third ventricles

Medulla oblongata

Projection fibers

body, particularly body movements. Without the cerebellum, specialized muscular activities such as writing would be impossible.

The **brainstem** is so called because the brain appears to be sitting on this portion of the CNS as a plant sits on its stem. The brainstem is the most primitive part of the CNS. It lies deep within the cranium and is the best-protected part of the CNS. The brainstem is the controlling center for virtually all body functions that are absolutely necessary for life. Cells in this part of the brain control cardiac, respiratory, and other basic body functions. The brainstem comprises three areas: the **midbrain**, the **pons**, and the **medulla oblongata**. One of the interesting operations of the brainstem is the regulation of consciousness. The **reticular activating system** in the midbrain keeps you conscious.

The brain has many other anatomic areas, all of which have specific and important functions. The brain receives a vast amount of information from the environment, sorts it all out, and directs the body to respond appropriately. Many of the responses involve voluntary muscle action; others are automatic

and involuntary. **Table 20** summarizes the major portions of the nervous system and their functions.

Interconnected cavities known as ventricles exist within the cerebral hemispheres and brainstem. They are continuous with the spinal cord's central canal, and also contain cerebrospinal fluid (CSF). The two large lateral ventricles are located inside the frontal, occipital, and temporal lobes. The third ventricle is under the corpus callosum in the brain's midline. The fourth ventricle is in the brainstem, and a narrow cerebral aqueduct joins it to the third ventricle. Figure 102 shows the ventricles in the brain.

Words of Wisdom

In the brainstem, most nerves cross from one side to the other. Motor and sensory nerves on the left side of the brain, for example, serve the right side of the body. This is why a person who has had a stroke or trauma in one hemisphere has nerve deficits on the opposite side of the body. Because the cranial nerves do not cross over, their function will be affected on the same side of the face as the injury or stroke.

Small red choroid plexuses (specialized capillaries) secrete CSF and project into the ventricles. The majority of CSF is formed in the lateral ventricles. CSF also enters the meninges' subarachnoid space and is reabsorbed into the blood. CSF surrounds the brain and spinal cord, maintaining a stable ionic concentration and protecting CNS structures.

Spinal Cord

The **spinal cord** is an extension of the brainstem **Figure 103** . Like the brain, the spinal cord contains nerve cell bodies, but the major portion of the spinal cord is made up of nerve fibers that extend from the cells of the brain. These nerve fibers transmit information to and from the brain. All fibers join together just below the brainstem to form the spinal cord. The spinal cord exits through a large opening at the base of the skull called the foramen magnum. It is encased within the spinal canal down to the level of the second lumbar vertebra. The spinal canal is created by an opening through the vertebrae, stacked one on another. Each vertebra surrounds the cord, and together the vertebrae form the bony spinal canal.

The principal function of the spinal cord is to transmit messages between the brain and the body. These messages are passed along the nerve fibers as electrical impulses, just as messages are passed along a telephone cable. The nerve fibers are arranged in specific bundles within the spinal cord to carry the messages from one specific area of the body to the brain and back.

In some cases, humans have developed "pre-wired" reflexes that protect the body from harm. The advantage is that the body has the ability to respond to a stimulus without waiting for the brain to process the stimulus, select a corrective action, and transmit messages to the necessary motor nerves to effect the protective action. An irritating stimulus to the sensory nerve, such as heat, will be transmitted from the sensory nerve along the connecting nerve, which directly activates the associated

Table 20   Structures of the Nervous System and General Functions

System	Major Structure	Subdivision	General Function
Central nervous system	Brain	Occipital lobe	Vision and storage of visual memories
		Parietal lobe	Sense of touch and texture; storage of those memories
		Temporal lobe	Hearing, smell, and language; storage of sound and odor memories
		Frontal lobe	Voluntary muscle control and storage of those memories
		Prefrontal area	Judgment and predicting consequences of actions, abstract intellectual functions
		Limbic system	Basic emotions, basic reflexes (chewing, swallowing, etc)
		Diencephalon (thalamus)	Relay center; filters important signals from routine signals
		Diencephalon (hypothalamus)	Emotions, temperature control, interface with endocrine system (hormone control)
	Brainstem	Midbrain	Level of consciousness, reticular activating system, muscle tone, and posture
		Pons	Respiratory patterning and depth
		Medulla oblongata	Heart rate, blood pressure, respiratory rate
	Spinal cord		Reflexes, relays information to and from body
Peripheral nervous system	Cranial nerves		Brain to body part; special peripheral nerves that connect directly to body parts
	Peripheral nerves		Brain to spinal cord to body part; receive stimulus from body, send commands to body

motor nerve in what is known as a **reflex arc**. The muscle responds promptly, withdrawing the limb from the irritating stimulus even before this information can be transmitted to the brain. Technically, you do not "feel" the heat of the fire before you move your hand away. This process, an example of a flexor reflex, is in place to limit damage to the body. When a physician taps your knee with a reflex hammer, he or she is testing to see whether your reflex arc is intact.

Other reflexes are also present. For example, when a muscle is stretched, such as when a basketball player's arm is pulled into extension, a stretch receptor in the muscle being stretched will activate a sensory pathway that synapses with a motor neuron in the spinal cord. The effect is to make the muscle involuntarily contract, which helps prevent the arm from being hyperex-tended or the muscle from being strained or torn. This is known as a stretch reflex.

The Meninges

The entire CNS is enclosed by a set of three tough membranes known as the **meninges** **Figure 104**. The outer membrane is the **dura mater** and is the toughest membrane. The second layer is called the **arachnoid** because the blood vessels it contains appear like a spider web. The innermost layer, resting directly on the brain or spinal cord, is the **pia mater**. When a hematoma develops, it can be classified according to its location in respect to the meninges (an epidural or a subdural hematoma). The meninges float in **cerebrospinal fluid (CSF)**, which is manufactured in the ventricles of the brain and flows in the **subarachnoid space**. The subarachnoid space is located between the pia mater and the arachnoid membrane.

CSF is manufactured by specialized cells within the **choroid plexus** in the ventricles, specialized hollow areas in the brain. These areas normally are interconnected, and CSF flows freely between them. CSF is similar in composition to plasma. The meninges and CSF form a fluid-filled sac that cushions and protects the brain and spinal cord.

■ The Peripheral Nervous System

Many of the cells in the CNS have long fibers that extend from the cell body out through openings in the bony covering of the

Words of Wisdom

Cerebrospinal fluid is a clear body fluid that can carry the same infectious diseases as blood. The risk of exposure to infectious agents from cerebrospinal fluid can be even greater than from blood because its presence is not as obvious as blood at first sight. To avoid exposure to infectious agents, ALWAYS wear gloves when you are making patient contact.

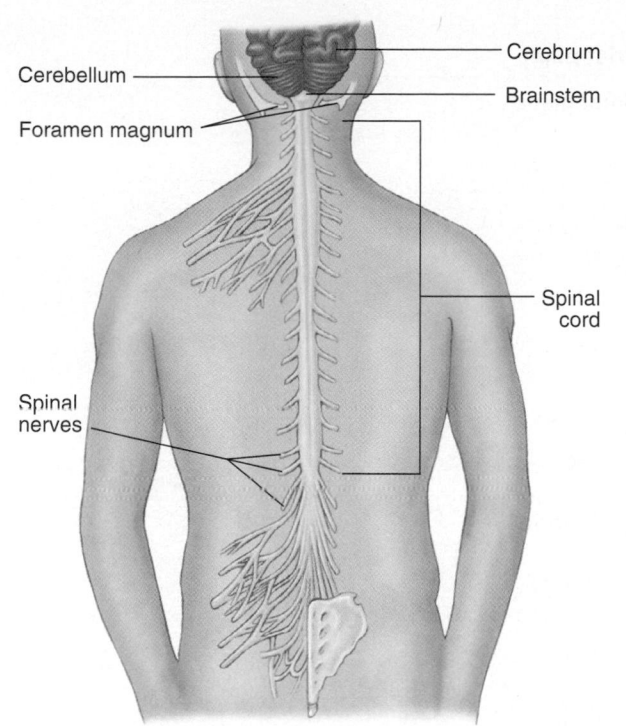

Figure 103 The spinal cord is a continuation of the brainstem. It exits the skull at the foramen magnum and extends down to the level of the second lumbar vertebra.

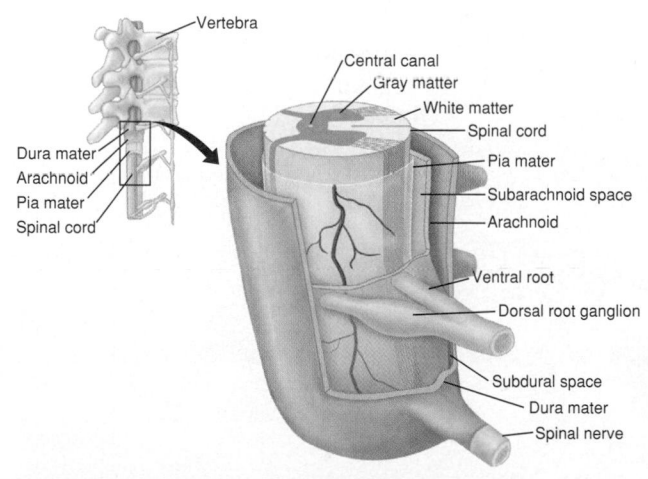

Figure 104 Components of the spinal cord. The meninges enclose the brain and the spinal cord.

spinal canal to form a cable of nerve fibers that link the CNS to the various organs of the body. These cables of nerve fibers make up the peripheral nervous system (PNS). The PNS is divided into two portions. The first is the somatic nervous system that transmits signals from the brain to the voluntary muscles. As you turn the page of a text, you are accessing your somatic nervous system.

The other portion of the PNS is the autonomic nervous system, which, in turn, is split into two areas. The <u>sympathetic nervous system</u> is responsible for the "fight-or-flight" response, enabling you to fight if you find yourself in a dangerous situation or to run away. This fight-or-flight response generally increases the activities within your body so that your muscles are able to perform more effectively when presented with an extreme situation. However, stimulation of these receptors can also occur during periods of acute stress or any other time you feel threatened. Stimulation of the sympathetic nervous system activates the adrenal glands to produce adrenaline to influence cardiovascular functions, norepinephrine to constrict peripheral blood vessel, and endorphins to increase pain tolerance. End organ effects include shunting of blood from the skin and periphery to the vital organs, improved skeletal muscle strength and endurance, increasing the force and rate of the heartbeat, increasing respirations, increasing blood pressure, dilation of the pupils, and reduction of digestive system activity.

The <u>parasympathetic nervous system</u>, the other half of the autonomic nervous system, generally slows down the cardiovascular and respiratory functions. Parasympathetic effects are commonly remembered as the "feed and breed" functions. When you are eating, your blood supply needs to move to your stomach and intestines so the food you eat can be processed. The parasympathetic responses include slowing the heart and respiratory rates, lowering the blood pressure, constricting the pupils, and increasing digestive system activity **Figure 105**. Parasympathetic stimulation is also responsible for many reproductive functions, including mediating arousal in males and females.

There are two types of nerves within the peripheral nervous system. <u>Sensory nerves</u> carry information from the body to the CNS. <u>Motor nerves</u> carry information from the CNS to the muscles of the body.

Sensory Nerves

Sensory nerves of the body are quite complex. There are many types of sensory cells in the nervous system. One type forms the retina of the eye; others are responsible for the hearing and balancing mechanisms in the ear. Other sensory cells are located in the skin, muscles, joints, lungs, and other organs of the body.

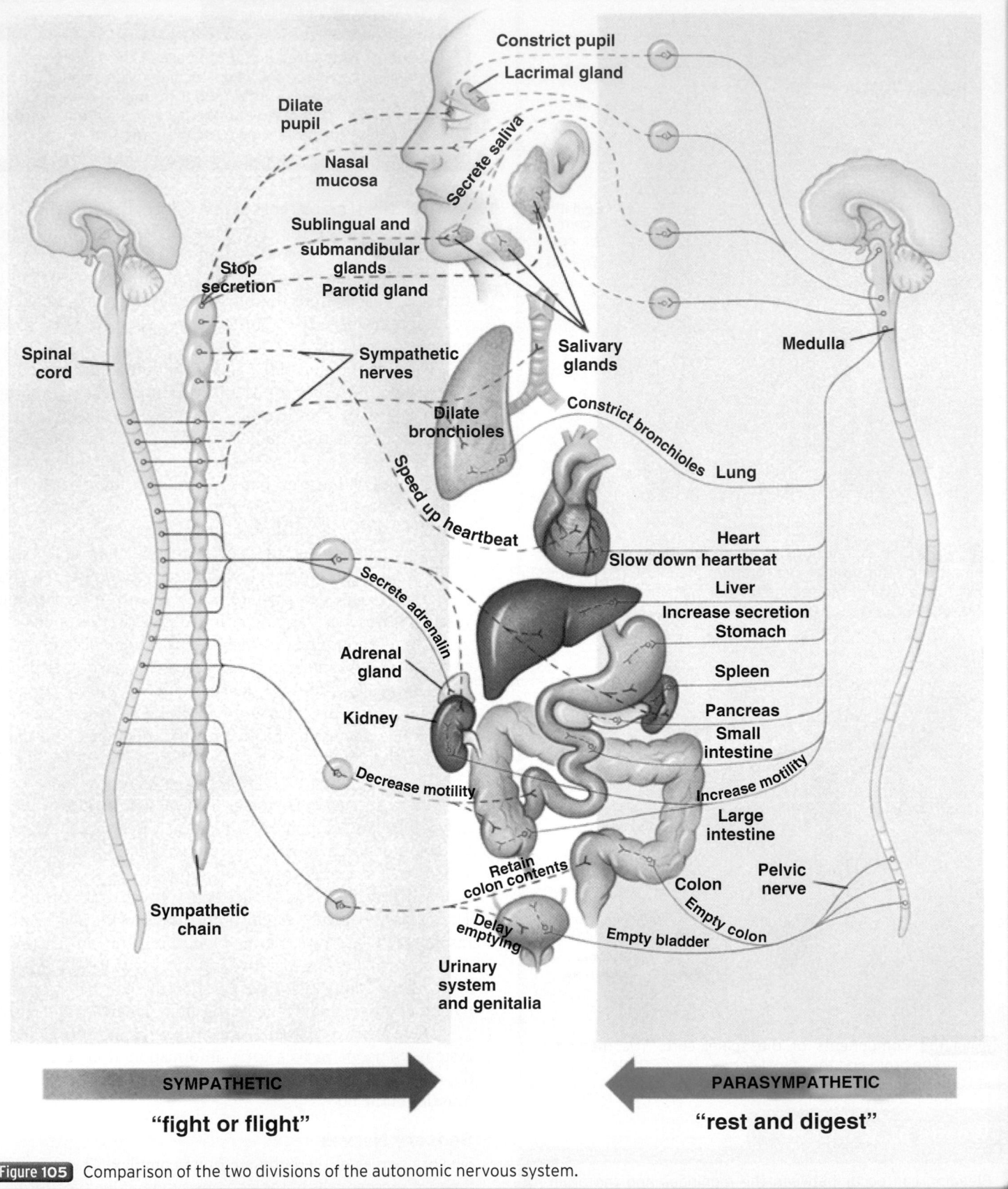

Figure 105 Comparison of the two divisions of the autonomic nervous system.

When a sensory cell is stimulated, it transmits its own special message to the brain. There are special sensory nerves to detect heat, cold, touch, position, motion, pressure, pain, balance, light, taste, smell, hearing, vision, balance, as well as other sensations. Specialized nerve endings are adapted for each cell so it perceives only one type of sensation and transmits only that message.

The sensory impulses constantly provide information to the brain about what the different parts of the body are doing in relation to their surroundings. Thus, the brain is continuously made aware of its surroundings. The cranial nerves supply sensations directly to the brain. Visual sensations (what you see) reach the brain directly by way of the optic nerve (the second cranial nerve) in each eye. The nerve endings for the optic nerve lie in the retina of the eye. The nerve endings are stimulated by light, and the impulses are carried along the nerve that passes through a hole in the back of the eye socket and carries impulses to the occipital portion of the brain.

When sensory nerve endings in the extremities are stimulated, the impulses are transmitted along a peripheral nerve to the spinal cord. The cell body of the peripheral nerve lies in the spinal cord. The impulse is then transmitted from that cell body to another nerve ending in the spinal cord and from there up the spinal cord to the sensory area in the parietal lobe of the brain, where the sensory information can be interpreted and acted on by the brain.

Motor Nerves

Each muscle in the body has its own motor nerve. The cell body for each motor nerve lies in the spinal cord, and a fiber from the cell body extends as part of the peripheral nerve to its specific muscle. Electrical impulses that are produced by the cell body in the spinal cord are transmitted along the motor nerve to the muscle and cause it to contract. The cell body in the spinal cord is stimulated by an impulse produced in the motor strip of the cerebral cortex. This impulse is transmitted along the spinal cord to the cell body of the motor nerve.

Cranial Nerves

Twelve pairs of cranial nerves arise from the base of the brain. All but two pairs, the olfactory nerves and the optic nerves, exit from the brainstem Figure 106 .

Some of the cranial nerves carry only sensory fibers (I, II, and VIII), and others carry only motor fibers (III, IV, VI, XI, and XII). Many carry a combination of sensory fibers and motor fibers (V, VII, IX, and X). Some cranial nerves also carry nerves of the parasympathetic nervous system in combination with motor, sensory, or both types of nerves (III, VII, IX, and X). Each nerve passes from the brain through a foramen in the skull to reach its end point.

The olfactory nerve (I) provides the sense of smell. The optic nerve (II) provides the sense of vision.

The oculomotor nerve (III) innervates the muscles that cause motion of the eyeballs and upper lid. The oculomotor nerve also carries parasympathetic nerve fibers that cause constriction of the pupil (sphincter muscle), and accommodation of the lens (ciliary muscle).

The trochlear nerve (IV) innervates the superior oblique muscle of the eyeball, which allows a downward gaze. The trigeminal nerve (V) supplies sensation to the scalp, forehead, face, and lower jaw via three branches: the ophthalmic, maxillary, and mandibular divisions. The trigeminal nerve also provides motor innervation to the muscles of mastication (chewing), the throat, and the inner ear.

The abducens nerve (VI) supplies the lateral rectus muscle of the eyeball (lateral movement). The facial nerve (VII) supplies motor activity to all muscles of facial expression, the sense of taste to the anterior two thirds of the tongue, and cutaneous sensation to the external ear, tongue, and palate. The facial nerve also carries parasympathetic stimulation to the salivary glands, lacrimal gland, and the glands of the nasal cavity and palate.

The vestibulocochlear nerve (VIII) passes through the internal auditory meatus and provides the senses of hearing and balance. The glossopharyngeal nerve (IX) supplies motor fibers to the pharyngeal muscles. It provides taste sensation to the posterior portion of the tongue and carries parasympathetic fibers to the salivary glands (parotid glands) located on each side of the face.

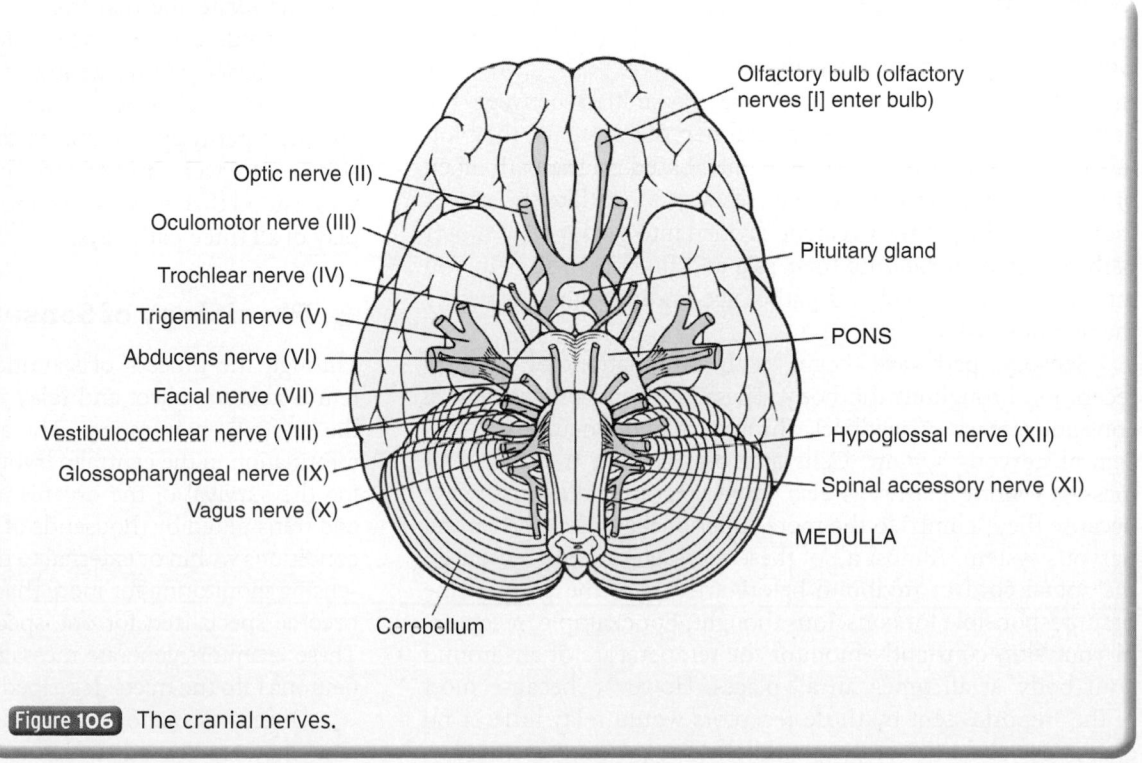

Figure 106 The cranial nerves.

The vagus nerve (X) provides motor functions to the soft palate, pharynx, and larynx (voice). The vagus nerve carries sensory fibers from the inferior pharynx, larynx, thoracic, and abdominal organs, taste bud fibers from the posterior tongue, and parasympathetic fibers to thoracic and abdominal organs.

The spinal accessory nerve (XI) provides motor innervation to the muscles of the soft palate and the pharynx and to the sternocleidomastoid and trapezius muscles. The spinal accessory nerve controls swallowing, speech, and head and shoulder movements. The hypoglossal nerve (XII) provides motor function to the muscles of the tongue and throat.

Spinal Nerves

The spinal nerves consist of 31 pairs of nerves arising bilaterally from between the vertebrae of the spine. Each pair is responsible for sending and receiving sensory and motor messages to and from the CNS from a portion of the body. These areas of innervations can be mapped out and are identified as that nerve's dermatome. This information can be useful to you because a loss of sensation at a given point on the body can indicate the level of the spinal cord that may be injured. These nerve pairs share similar distribution and names as the vertebrae, although they differ slightly. There are 8 cervical pairs, 12 thoracic pairs, 5 lumbar pairs, 5 sacral pairs, and 1 coccygeal pair.

Nerve Plexuses

In some locations, as nerves exit the spinal cord and follow similar tracts through the body, they may combine to form a nerve plexus. This commonly occurs when nerves that innervate similar or contiguous areas and whose functions are similar approach the spine. For example, the brachial plexus, made up of the ventral roots of spinal nerves C5–C8 and T1, gives rise to the major nerves of the shoulder and arm. Plexuses also play a role in coordination of reflexes.

Sensory and Motor Pathways

As millions of action potentials are transmitted between the nerves of the central and peripheral nervous systems, they follow common pathways that are named based on the path taken or the beginning and end of the pathway. Much like the nerves themselves, the pathways can be divided into sensory and motor pathways. Understanding their role and function will help you interpret many normal and pathologic findings when assessing the nervous system.

Sensory pathways begin with stimulation of sensory receptors throughout the body. These cells and organs send a constant stream of feedback through afferent neurons to the central nervous system. Cells and organs then transmit their messages along pathways also known as ascending pathways because they "climb" to the more superior regions of the central nervous system. Almost all of these messages are filtered out in the spinal cord or midbrain before arriving at the parts of the brain responsible for conscious thought. For example, receptors in your skin constantly monitor the temperature of air around your body, at all times, in all places. However, because most of the "reports" sent by those receptors would relay little or no change in conditions and are unlikely to require any action, few

if any messages make it into your thoughts until there is a rapid change or significant condition of which to be aware.

The specific functions of these pathways can be studied. The posterior column pathway is responsible for sending information about localized fine touch, pressure, vibration, and proprioception to the brain. This pathway stretches from the sensory receptors throughout the body, through the dorsal roots of spinal nerves, up the spinal cord, and eventually into the primary sensory cortex. Interestingly, like most pathways, it crosses over from one side of the body to the other at the level of the thalamus. The fact that almost all nerves cross over in this manner is the reason that a stroke on one side of the brain will commonly affect the sensation or motor function of the opposite side of the body.

The spinothalamic pathway is so named because it originates in the spine and relays messages to the thalamus. This tract conducts messages regarding pain, temperature, itching, and nonspecific touch—some of the senses that the thalamus is primarily responsible for. Similarly, the spinocerebellar pathway transmits information that the cerebellum needs to perform its functions: namely, limb and joint position and proprioception, which is necessary for the cerebellum to maintain balance and overall coordination.

Motor pathways are those by which commands issued by the central nervous system are carried out. These may result in a range of effects from voluntary or involuntary movement to activation of the effects of the "fight-or-flight" sympathetic response. These can be divided into separate pathways similarly to the sensory nerves, but are also commonly divided into the pyramidal and extrapyramidal systems. The pyramidal system uses the corticospinal pathway to communicate messages from a triangular group of cells in the cerebral cortex, for which the pathway is named, down the spinal cord to motor neurons to create voluntary movement, again crossing to the opposite side just inferior to the thalamus. The medial and lateral pathways were considered a separate system because they primarily control involuntary movement and things like posture and resting muscle tone. They were named extrapyramidal because they included pathways excepting those involved in the pyramidal system and were thought to function independently. It is now understood that all muscle control is exerted as a complex interplay of all three pathways.

▋ Physiology of Sensation

Through the process of sensation, the peripheral nervous system is able to collect and relay information about the body and the external environment. The ability to gather and process this information in the central nervous system is paramount in ensuring the survival of the organism. These messages are generated and transmitted by thousands of sensory receptors that monitor conditions within or external to the body. Receptors are capable of sensing monitoring for more than one type of sensation but often become specialized for one specific or a few related sensations. These receptors generate messages and pass them along sensory neurons into the tracts described in the preceding section.

Once these action potentials reach the central nervous system, they are routed to the specific center with responsibility for interpreting that stimulus, where the message is processed and either is brought to conscious thought through <u>perception</u>, generates an automatic response through reflexes or other mechanisms, or is discarded as unimportant. The intensity of the stimulus is determined by how many nerve endings are activated, how frequently the action potentials are created and propagated, and how many messages are received by the CNS. However, through <u>adaptation</u>, the CNS may temporarily or permanently reduce sensitivity to a particular stimulus. For example, when you are walking into a crowded restaurant, the noise of a bustling waitstaff and dozens of conversations being held over background music may initially strike you as loud and may rise to your consciousness so that you might even mention it to the rest of your party. However, over the next several minutes, the cerebral cortex adjusts to that level of noise and after that, the noise level may not enter your thoughts again until you walk out of the restaurant into the much quieter environment. In some cases, the perception of the stimuli may still be present after the stimuli is removed; this is known as an <u>after-image</u>.

The General Senses

Some sensations are monitored throughout the body by receptors scattered throughout many different tissues. These are known as the <u>general senses</u> and their receptors are named for the sensation they produce. Nociceptors monitor for pain, thermoreceptors monitor temperature, chemoreceptors monitor levels of chemicals found in the body, and mechanoreceptors monitor for physical changes such as touch, pressure, and position.

Nociceptors are of particular interest because the perception of pain is a common and useful finding when you are gathering a patient's history and performing examinations. Although nociceptors may be stimulated by any of several mechanisms such as physical forces or cell death, they transmit their activation potential along the same pathways and to the same areas of the central nervous system. Therefore, sensations that activate nociceptors for different reasons may create perceptions of pain that are similar. In other cases, stimulation of nociceptors in the internal organs may produce sensation of pain at the body surface area that shares the same spinal nerve pathway. In a classic example, an injury to the spleen may cause pain to be felt at the left shoulder. This is known as <u>referred pain</u>. Although the exact mechanism is not well understood, referred pain occurs in known and predictable patterns across the human body, and therefore can be of great value when you are assessing your patient. In patients who have undergone amputations, a common finding is <u>phantom pain</u>, in which the patient feels the sensation of pain in a part of the body that is no longer present.

Mechanoreceptors monitor for changes in physical properties. Among them are tactile receptors that sense touch, proprioceptors responsible for tracking position in space, and baroreceptors that measure changes in pressure. Tactile receptors form the cutaneous senses of touch, pressure, and vibration, through a mix of <u>encapsulated nerve endings</u>, which are fewer and sense only substantial changes, and the more numerous and fine <u>free nerve endings</u>, which are responsible for sensing light touch and smaller vibrations. Damage to any of these nerve endings may result in <u>neuropathy</u>, or more properly peripheral neuropathy, which can cause a wide range of symptoms from weakness to tremors and from mild pain or "pins and needles" to such hypersensitivity that some parts of the body cannot be touched.

Baroreceptors play an especially important role in many autonomic functions. The most important of these may be measuring the "stretch" produced in the great vessels. The autonomic nervous system uses this information to regulate various cardiovascular functions to maintain sufficient cardiac output. Similarly, chemoreceptors measure the content of various chemicals in the body and/or bloodstream. By sending messages regarding the amount of carbon dioxide, for example, the autonomic nervous system can regulate the respiratory rate and depth to ensure proper levels.

The Special Senses

Whereas the general senses collect and transmit general information about the body at all times and all areas, the special senses each relay information from specialized organs related to specific interactions with the environment. Despite these differences, the senses of taste, smell, sight, hearing, and balance are composed of the same basic structures and follow the same basic physiologic processes.

Sense of Taste Located in various areas of the mouth, <u>taste receptors</u> respond to four <u>primary taste sensations</u>: sweet, salty, sour, and bitter. These cells, located on the taste buds, help a person to identify foods that are satiating and, sometimes, substances that are potential poisons (for example, poisons that taste unpalatable). The distribution of over 10,000 taste buds and variations in their sensitivity vary between areas of the mouth, but all respond to each of the primary taste sensations. Most taste buds are found on the surface of the tongue with tiny elevations called papillae **Figure 107**. Dissolved chemicals from the substance introduced into the mouth combine with specific receptors and cause an action potential that is transmitted to the thalamus for further processing.

Sense of Smell The upper nasal cavity contains smell (olfactory) receptors. Similar to taste receptors, the <u>olfactory cells</u> contained in the superior nasopharynx respond to chemicals dissolved in the mucus covering these cells **Figure 108**. Once those chemicals reach a threshold level, which may be attained by sniffing to introduce more airflow and therefore more of the substance to be smelled, the chemicals bind with proteins in the olfactory receptors and cause a change in membrane permeability that creates an action potential. Unlike other senses, however, olfactory signals are transmitted directly to the cerebral cortex without first being filtered by the thalamus. This creates a close connection to the emotional centers in the brain, and is why you can often recall a feeling or mood associated with a smell even before you remember from where you recognize it. The sense of smell is also important in helping you decipher the taste signals sent by the taste buds. You have probably noticed that when your sense of smell is hampered, such as when you have a cold, foods that normally have mild flavors may have none at all, and others require a much stronger taste stimulus to trigger a response.

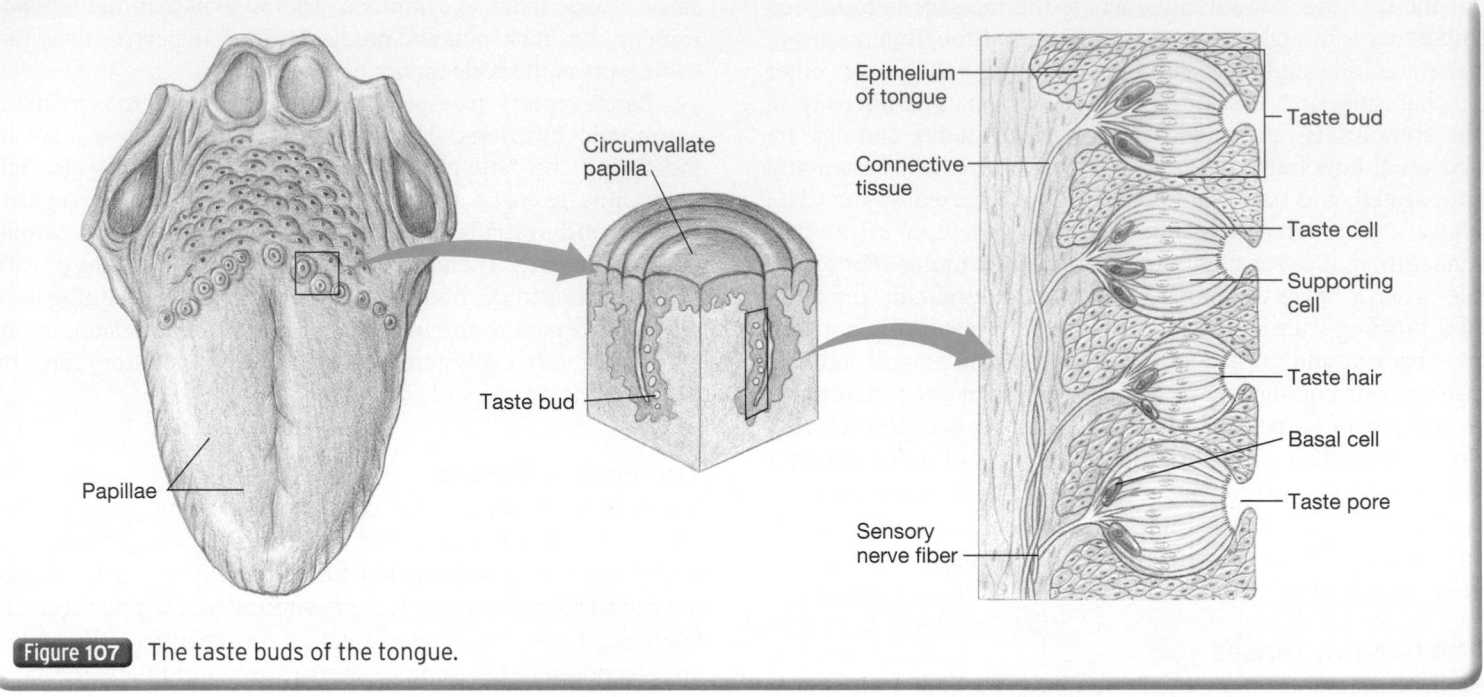

Figure 107 The taste buds of the tongue.

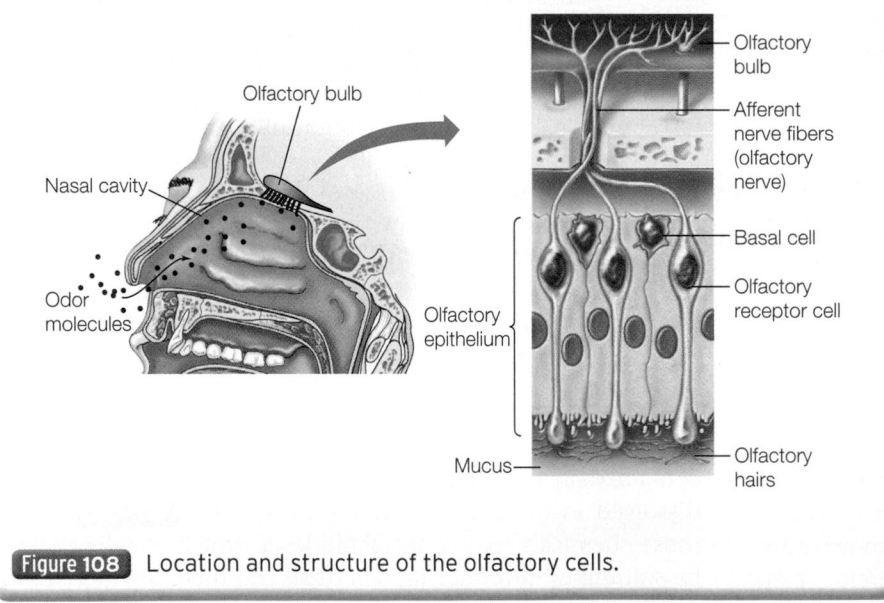

Figure 108 Location and structure of the olfactory cells.

Sense of Sight Because of the nature of the sensory information and the complexity involved in obtaining that information, the sense of sight is much more complex to understand. In order to produce vision, many small and intricate structures must work together to create one of your most vital sources of information about your environment.

The eyeball, or <u>globe</u>, is the source of the information the brain processes into pictures. It is imperfectly round and fills the space of the orbit along with the external muscles and a layer of orbital fat that provides cushioning and support. The globe is hollow and can be divided into the <u>anterior cavity</u> and the <u>posterior cavity</u>. The posterior cavity is also known as the vitreous chamber and is filled with <u>vitreous humor</u>, a jellylike fluid that helps the globe maintain its shape without distorting light. The anterior cavity is filled with the more fluid-like <u>aqueous humor</u>. The amount of aqueous humor determines the intraocular pressure, which is critical to sight, and regulated by the <u>Schlemm's canal</u>, which drains extra aqueous humor into the bloodstream. If this pressure is not controlled, high pressures may cause pressure on the optic nerve, known as <u>glaucoma</u>, which can cause permanent nerve damage and vision loss. The anterior cavity is further divided into the anterior chamber and the posterior chamber. The globe is controlled and directed within the orbit by six <u>extrinsic muscles</u>, which attach to the exterior of the globe and are controlled by the cranial nerves.

As light passes into the globe, it enters a series of transparent structures that create a <u>refracting system</u> responsible for miniaturizing and focusing the image onto the specialized nerve endings of the eye. This is accomplished through redirecting, or refracting light as it passes through mediums of different densities. A classic demonstration of this concept occurs when you attempt to retrieve an object from shallow water—for example, retrieving an item at the beach. Because the light is refracted, putting your hand exactly where you see the object will result in a failed attempt to grab the object because the light's direction is changed as it goes from water to air, leading to a misperception of the object's actual position in space. By altering the shape and thickness of the <u>lens</u>, it is possible for the eye to bring an image into focus.

The lens is normally transparent, but can develop <u>cataracts</u>, which can cause varying levels of obstruction ranging from a light film to complete obstruction. The lens is anchored to the <u>cornea</u>, a protective structure, by <u>suspensory ligaments</u>, which allow the various muscles of the eye to pull the lens into varying degrees of refraction. The image focused on the retina is actually an upside-down, miniature version of the environment in front of the eye. In some cases, the shape of the lens is distorted enough that it cannot adequately bring an object at a given distance into focus onto the retina, resulting in poor vision. When a person can see objects that are close by but has difficulty seeing objects far away, he or she is said to be nearsighted, a condition known as <u>myopia</u>. In the opposite scenario, <u>hyperopia</u>, the person can see distant objects but may have difficulty focusing on objects that are close by. The increased difficulty in focusing that occurs with aging is termed <u>presbyopia</u>, although there is debate as to the actual mechanism. In <u>astigmatism</u>, irregularities in the shape of the lens create similar problems because parts of the image are out of focus when other parts are in focus.

The walls of the globe are composed of three layers of elastic and fibrous connective tissue that allow the shape of the globe to vary slightly to help with focusing **Figure 109**. The outermost layer, known as the fibrous tunic, is composed of the white <u>sclera</u> and transparent cornea, which surround and protect the internal structures. The <u>conjunctiva</u> are a layer of soft mucous membranes lining the inside of the eyelid that cushion and allow smooth movement. Infection of the conjunctiva, known as <u>conjunctivitis</u>, is commonly known as "pink eye" and results in inflammation and pain. The <u>lacrimal glands</u> provide nourishment and lubrication through the provision of tears **Figure 110**. The act of blinking, whether voluntary or involuntary, uses tears

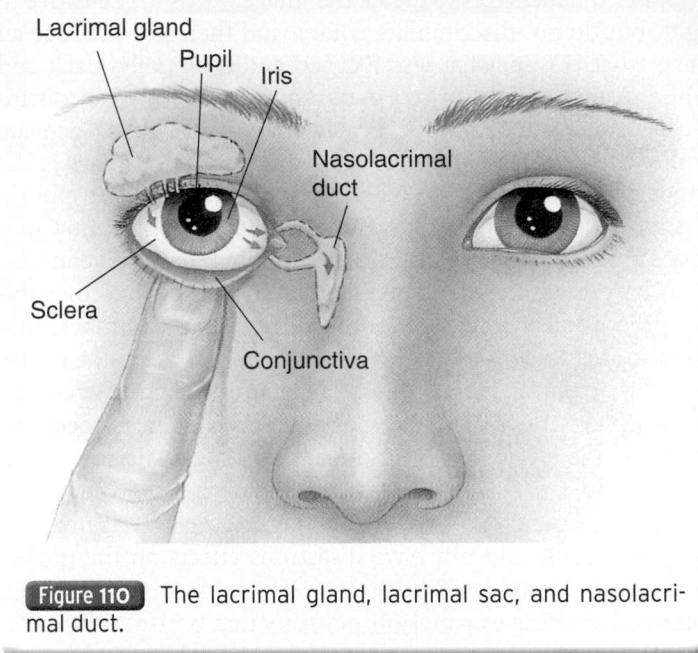

Figure 110   The lacrimal gland, lacrimal sac, and nasolacrimal duct.

to sweep debris, bacteria, or other material from the surface of the eye to the <u>lacrimal sac</u> for disposal. Tears also contain lysozyme, an enzyme that breaks down cell walls of potential bacterial invaders. Excess tears are carried away via the nasolacrimal duct.

The middle layer of the three, the vascular tunic, is aptly named because it contains the blood vessels that supply the eye tissues, as well as the lymph vessels and intrinsic eye muscles. These vessels are contained in a layer known as the <u>choroid</u>. Folds of tissue in the choroid layer form the <u>ciliary body</u>. This layer is also responsible for altering and maintaining the shape of the lens as well as maintaining the size of the <u>pupil</u>, which regulates the amount of light entering the eye. The <u>iris</u>, which gives the eye its color, contains two sets of muscles to change the size of the pupil. The pupil is not actually a structure itself; its boundaries are simply the empty space left by changing the size of the iris.

The innermost layer is known as the neural tunic or <u>retina</u>, and contains the nerve cells responsible for generating nerve impulses to be conducted through the optic nerves. The retina contains two types of photoreceptors, which contribute different information to the vision center which must

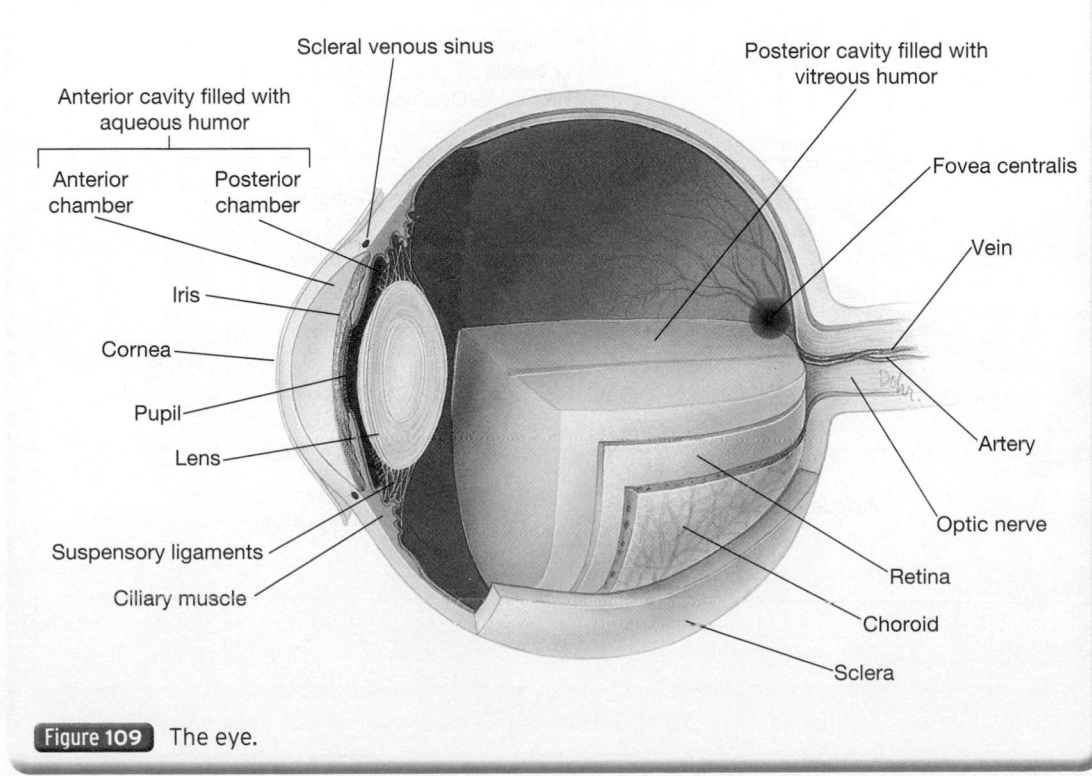

Figure 109   The eye.

decipher the messages to create the image. <u>Rods</u> are sensitive to light, but do not discriminate colors, and therefore produce an image that is somewhat less focused and essentially black and white. A separate set of receptors known as <u>cones</u> can distinguish colors, but require a greater amount of light to activate and create an image. Absence of or dysfunction of cones is the cause of color blindness. When light is refracted onto photoreceptors, the protein rhodopsin changes shape, the first in a series of reactions that causes a nerve impulse to be generated.

Photoreceptors are found across the retina but in varying proportions. Cones are found in the greatest numbers in a specific area known as the <u>fovea centralis</u>, found in the center of the <u>macula</u>, or macula lutea. When you strain to focus on an object, your eyes reshape the refractory system to focus the image on the fovea, which produces the clearest and most vivid image possible. This area gives the disease macular degeneration its name, and explains why damage to this area is immediately noticeable and can have disastrous effects on the quality of vision. Each rod and cone transmits its information through intermediary cells to <u>ganglion neurons</u> that transmit the information through the optic nerve. The point where these many nerves penetrate the posterior globe to form the base of the optic nerve is a structure known as the <u>optic disk</u>. The optic disk contains no rods or cones and therefore creates a blind spot in the visual field of each eye.

As these signals follow the optic nerve toward the CNS, they pass through the <u>optic chiasm</u>, where approximately half of the nerve fibers from each eye cross over to the opposite side of the brain. The vision centers on each side of the brain interpret information separately but then combine those signals to create one image that the brain "sees." This merging of two images into one is known as <u>binocular vision</u>. Binocular vision creates the perception of depth when both eyes are able to focus on the same target. In <u>strabismus</u>, however, there is a loss of perception of depth and overlapping or doubled images because the eyes fail to coordinate their movement and may become "crossed" or separated. The opposite problem is also possible. In <u>amblyopia</u>, known by the layman's term lazy eye, the eyes may be oriented correctly but one fails to send adequate signals to the vision centers, also causing a loss of depth perception and poor-quality images.

Sense of Hearing The sense of hearing is made possible by special-purpose structures paired with specialized sensory receptors. The external ear, also known as the auricle or <u>pinna</u>, is a formation of cartilage that protects the ear and collects sounds into the ear canal, while allowing some perception of the direction from which the sound comes Figure 111. From there, sound waves travel through the <u>ear canal</u> to the <u>tympanic membrane</u>, or eardrum. This thin membrane separates the ear canal from the middle ear, which contains the auditory ossicles, three small and delicate bones that link together to convert sound waves into exaggerated physical motion. As described earlier in the chapter, they are known by their Latin names, which refer to their shapes—the malleus (mallet or hammer), the incus (anvil), and the stapes (stirrup). The middle ear also contains a passage known as the

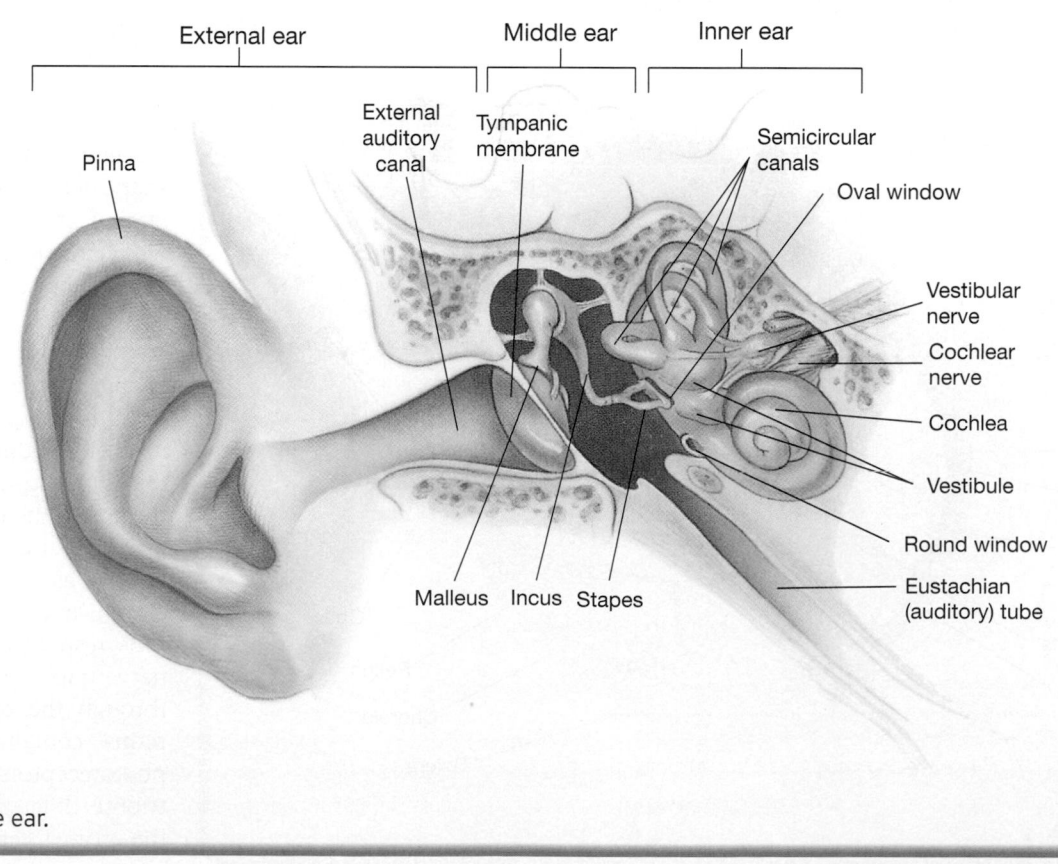

Figure 111   The ear.

eustachian tube, which opens into the posterior pharynx and allows equalization of pressure on each side of the tympanum.

The medial end of the stapes is attached to another membrane, the oval window, that separates the middle ear from the entrance to the cochlea, which encases the primary receptor for sound. Sound is amplified by the middle ear and transmitted through this membrane to the delicate structures of the inner ear, which are filled with fluid. This movement of fluid within an enclosed space is made possible by the round window, which allows fluid to move in minute amounts as it flexes out of the canal.

The structures of the inner ear are quite sensitive and therefore are surrounded by the bony labyrinth to provide protection from damage and from extraneous stimulation. The bony labyrinth is filled with a fluid called perilymph, which surrounds the membranous labyrinth, a collection of passageways and reservoirs filled with a fluid known as endolymph and containing the actual nerve receptors. The cochlea is a bony, spiral shell shape containing the cochlear duct. It is within this duct that the organ of Corti is contained. This organ is the primary receptor for sound, and is made up of thousands of individual cilia, each with their own associated nerve. As fluid in the ear reacts to the vibration transmitted through the ear by sound waves, the cilia are disturbed, activating the nerve cells. Interpretation of those signals becomes the sense of hearing.

Any condition that results in the partial or complete loss of hearing is known as deafness. This can result from many causes. If any of the structures that normally transmit, or conduct, the vibration of sound from the outer ear to the inner ear fail to do so, this is termed a conductive deafness. If, instead, the sound is transmitted correctly by the physical structures but some dysfunction or malformation of the organ of Corti or the receptor cells is present, this is known as a nerve deafness. In the least common case, the nerve impulses may reach the auditory cen-ters of the brain appropriately, but the brain may have a damaged ability to interpret those signals. This is termed central deafness.

Sense of Balance Also contained within the inner ear is the vestibular system, composed of a pair of fluid-filled sacs known as otoliths and three more fluid-filled, looping passageways known as semicircular canals. These formations have no effect on hearing, but instead are used by the CNS to collect information about movement and orientation in space. The semicircular canals use the movement of fluid to sense rotational movement in each of three planes. The saccule gathers information from its mass of fluid to capture linear movements, while the utricle monitors the degree of head tilt. By processing all of these sensations simultaneously, the vestibular system keeps you upright and aware of your position in space, known as proprioception.

■ The Integumentary System (Skin): Anatomy

The skin is the largest organ of the human body and serves as the interface between the body and the outside world. The skin is divided into two parts, the epidermis and dermis. Below the skin lies the subcutaneous tissue layer Figure 112 . The cells of the epidermis are sealed to form a watertight protective covering for the body. The subcutaneous tissue is composed largely of fat. The fat serves as an insulator for the body and as a reservoir to store energy. The amount of subcutaneous tissue varies greatly from person to person. Beneath the subcutaneous tissue lie the muscles and the skeleton. The subcutaneous layer helps to anchor the skin to the structures below. As a person ages, the loss of the subcutaneous layer causes the skin to have limited support. This is why wrinkles form in the skin.

YOU *are the Medic* PART 4

You continue your assessment of the patient's abdomen by checking the four quadrants. The extensive bruising is located on and lateral to the left upper quadrant. The patient again groans audibly during your assessment.

Recording Time: 10 Minutes	
Respirations	24 breaths/min, shallow
Pulse	118 beats/min
Skin	Pale, moist, and hot (comparable to ambient temperature)
Blood pressure	102/66 mm Hg
Oxygen saturation (Spo$_2$)	93% with high-flow oxygen
Pupils	Equal and reactive to light

7. What structures are located in the abdominal area under the noted bruising?

8. How can you determine what structures are actually injured in the abdominal cavity?

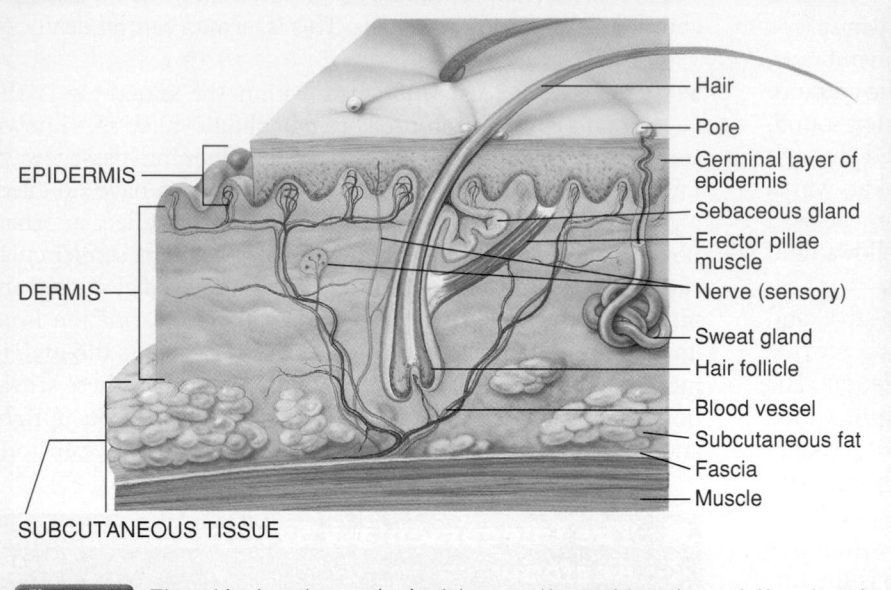

EPIDERMIS

DERMIS

SUBCUTANEOUS TISSUE

Hair

Pore

Germinal layer of epidermis

Sebaceous gland

Erector pillae muscle

Nerve (sensory)

Sweat gland

Hair follicle

Blood vessel

Subcutaneous fat

Fascia

Muscle

Figure 112   The skin has two principal layers: the epidermis and the dermis. Below the skin is a layer of subcutaneous tissue.

The skin covers the entire external surface of the body. The various orifices—including the mouth, nose, anus, and vagina—are not covered by skin. Orifices are lined with mucous membranes. Mucous membranes are quite similar to skin in that they provide a protective barrier against bacterial invasion. Mucous membranes differ from skin in that they secrete <u>mucus</u>, a watery substance that lubricates the openings. Thus, mucous membranes are moist, whereas the skin is dry. A mucous membrane lines the entire gastrointestinal tract from the mouth to the anus.

Epidermis

The <u>epidermis</u> is the most superficial layer of the skin and varies in thickness in different areas of the body. On the soles of the feet, the back, and the <u>scalp</u>, it is quite thick, but in some areas of the body, the epidermis is only two or three cell layers thick. The epidermis is actually composed of several layers of cells. These layers can be separated into two regions. At the base of the epidermis is the <u>germinal layer</u>, also known as the stratum basale or stratum germinativum, which continuously produces new cells that germinate and gradually rise to the surface. On the way to the surface, these cells die and enter the <u>stratum corneal layer</u>. This is the dead layer of skin. Whereas the germinal layer has a blood supply, the stratum corneal layer does not. The journey from the germinal layer to the surface takes about 4 weeks. The outermost cells of the epidermis are constantly rubbed away and replaced by new cells produced by the germinal layer. The germinal layer also contains cells bearing melanin granules, known as melanocytes. The darkness of a person's skin is directly proportional to the amount of melanin present.

Dermis

Below the germinal layer is the <u>dermis</u>. Within the dermis lie many of the special structures of the skin: sweat glands, sebaceous (oil) glands, nails, hair follicles, blood vessels, and specialized nerve endings.

■ Accessory Structures

The accessory structures of the integumentary system include nails, hair follicles, and sebaceous and sweat glands.

Nails

Nails protect the ends of the fingers and toes, consisting of a nail plate above a skin surface called the nail bed. The part of the nail plate that grows most actively is covered by a whitish, half moon-shaped lunula, where epithelial cells divide and become keratinized. The nail cells push forward over the nail bed, causing the nail to continually grow outward. The nail of the middle finger grows fastest whereas the nail of the thumb grows slowest.

Hairs

<u>Hair follicles</u> are the small organs that produce hair. The hair grows from the follicle along a shaft until it reaches the epidermal surface. A sebaceous gland is located along the hair shaft. Connected to the hair is a small muscle. The muscle pulls the hair into an erect position when a person is cold or frightened. Hair goes through stages of growth and rest. Blood vessels provide nutrients and oxygen to the skin. The blood vessels lie in the dermis. Small branches extend up to the germinal layer. A complex array of nerve endings also lies in the dermis. These specialized nerve endings are sensitive to environmental stimuli; they respond to these stimuli and send impulses along the nerves to the brain.

Glands in the Skin

<u>Sweat glands</u> produce sweat for cooling the body. The sweat is discharged onto the surface of the skin through small pores, or ducts, that pass through the epidermis. The skin contains two kinds of sweat glands: merocrine and apocrine sweat glands. Merocrine (eccrine) glands are the predominant type of sweat glands, responding to body temperature, and are present at birth. Adult skin contains 2 to 5 million merocrine sweat glands. They are found on the forehead, neck, and back, though the palms and soles have the highest numbers. Apocrine glands are sweat glands that become active at puberty. They are found mostly in the armpits and groin, with the sweat excreted at these places developing a scent as it comes into contact with skin bacteria. Modified sweat glands include the ceruminous glands of the external ear (which produce earwax) and the mammary glands (which produce milk).

The sebaceous glands produce sebum, the oily material that seals the surface epidermal cells. The <u>sebaceous glands</u> lie next to hair follicles and secrete sebum along the hair follicle to the skin surface. In addition to providing waterproofing for the skin, sebum keeps the skin soft so it does not crack.

The Integumentary System (Skin): Physiology

The skin serves three major functions: to protect the body in the environment, to regulate the temperature of the body, and to transmit information from the environment to the brain.

The protective functions of the skin are numerous. Water makes up a large portion of the body. This water contains a delicate balance of chemical substances in solution. The skin is watertight and serves to keep this balanced internal solution intact. The skin also protects the body from the invasion of infectious organisms: bacteria, viruses, and fungi. These organisms are everywhere and are routinely found lying on the skin surface. However, they never penetrate the skin unless it is broken by injury; thus, the skin provides a constant protection against outside invaders.

The major organ for regulation of body temperature is the skin. Blood vessels in the skin constrict when the body is in a cold environment and dilate when the body is in a warm environment. In a cold environment, constriction of the blood vessels shunts the blood away from the skin to decrease the amount of heat radiated from the body surface. When the outside environment is hot, the vessels in the skin dilate, the skin becomes flushed or red, and heat radiates from the body surface.

Also, in a hot environment, sweat is secreted to the skin surface from the sweat glands. Evaporation of the sweat requires energy. This energy, as body heat, is taken from the body during the evaporation process, which causes the body temperature to fall. Sweating alone will not reduce body temperature; evaporation of the sweat must also occur.

Information from the environment is carried to the brain through a rich supply of sensory nerves that originate in the skin. Nerve endings that lie in the skin are adapted to perceive and transmit information about heat, cold, external pressure, pain, and the position of the body in space. The skin thus recognizes any changes in the environment. The skin also reacts to pressure, pain, and pleasurable stimuli.

The integument responds to injuries and wounds with inflammation, which causes redness, increased warmth, and painful swelling. The blood vessels of the wounded area dilate and allow fluids to leak into the damaged tissues. This provides more nutrients and oxygen to the tissues, aiding in healing.

The Digestive System: Anatomy

The mechanical and chemical breakdown of foods and the absorption of resulting nutrients by the body's cells are known as digestion. The alimentary canal extends from the mouth to the anus. It includes the mouth, pharynx, esophagus, stomach, small intestine, large intestine, rectum, and anus. The walls of the alimentary canal consist of four layers, specialized in certain regions for particular functions, as follows Figure 113 :

- *Mucosa (mucous membrane):* Surface epithelium, underlying connective tissue, and a small amount of smooth muscle; it is folded in some regions, with projections extending into the lumen that increase its absorptive surface. The mucosa carries out secretion and absorption.
- *Submucosa:* Loose connective tissue with glands, blood vessels, lymphatic vessels, and nerves; it nourishes surrounding tissues and carries away absorbed materials.
- *Muscular layer:* Produces movements of the tube, and is made of two smooth muscle tissue coats: circular fibers of the inner coat encircle the tube, causing contraction, and longitudinal fibers run lengthwise, causing shortening of the tube.
- *Serosa (serous layer):* Composed of a visceral peritoneum on the outside and connective tissue beneath; it protects underlying tissues and secretes serous fluid so that abdominal organs slide freely against each other.

The accessory organs of the alimentary canal include the teeth, tongue, salivary glands, liver, gallbladder, and pancreas. The secretions from these accessory organs empty via ducts into the digestive tract. The organs of the digestive system are found within the abdomen.

The Abdomen

The abdomen is the second major body cavity; it contains the major organs of digestion and excretion. The diaphragm separates the thoracic cavity from the abdominal cavity. Anteriorly and posteriorly, thick muscular abdominal walls create the boundaries of this space. Inferiorly, the abdomen is separated from the pelvis by an imaginary plane that extends from the pubic symphysis through the sacrum Figure 114 . Some organs lie in the abdomen and the pelvis, depending on the posture of the patient.

The simplest and most common method of describing the portions of the abdomen is by quadrants, the four equal areas formed by two imaginary lines that intersect at right angles at the umbilicus. On the anterior abdominal wall, the quadrants thus formed are the right upper, right lower, left upper, and left lower. The terms "right quadrant" and "left quadrant" refer to the patient's right and left. Pain or injury in a given quadrant usually arises from or involves the organs that lie in that quadrant. This simple means of designation allows you to identify injured or diseased organs that require emergency attention.

In the right upper quadrant (RUQ), the major organs are the liver, the gallbladder, and a portion of the colon and small intestine. Most of the liver lies in this quadrant, almost entirely under the protection of the 8th to 12th ribs. The liver fills the entire anteroposterior depth of the abdomen in this quadrant. Therefore, injuries in this area are frequently associated with injuries of the liver.

In the left upper quadrant (LUQ), the principal organs are the stomach, the spleen, and a portion of the colon and small intestine. The spleen is almost entirely under the protection of the left rib cage, whereas the stomach may sag well down into the left lower quadrant when full. The spleen lies in the lateral and posterior portion of this quadrant, under the diaphragm and immediately in front of the 9th to 11th ribs. The spleen is frequently injured, especially when these ribs are fractured.

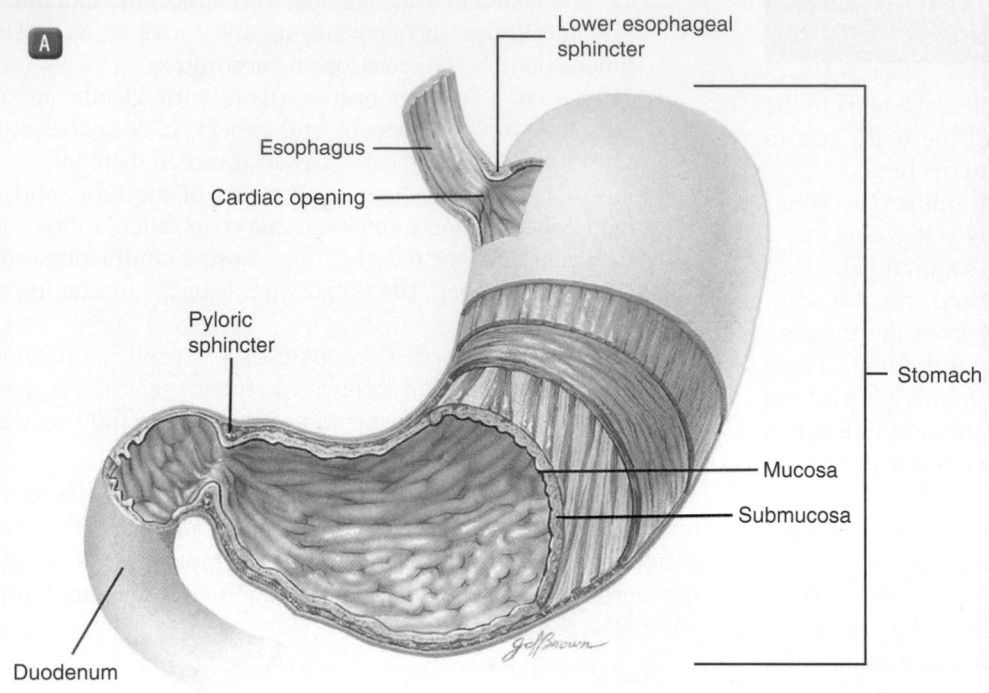

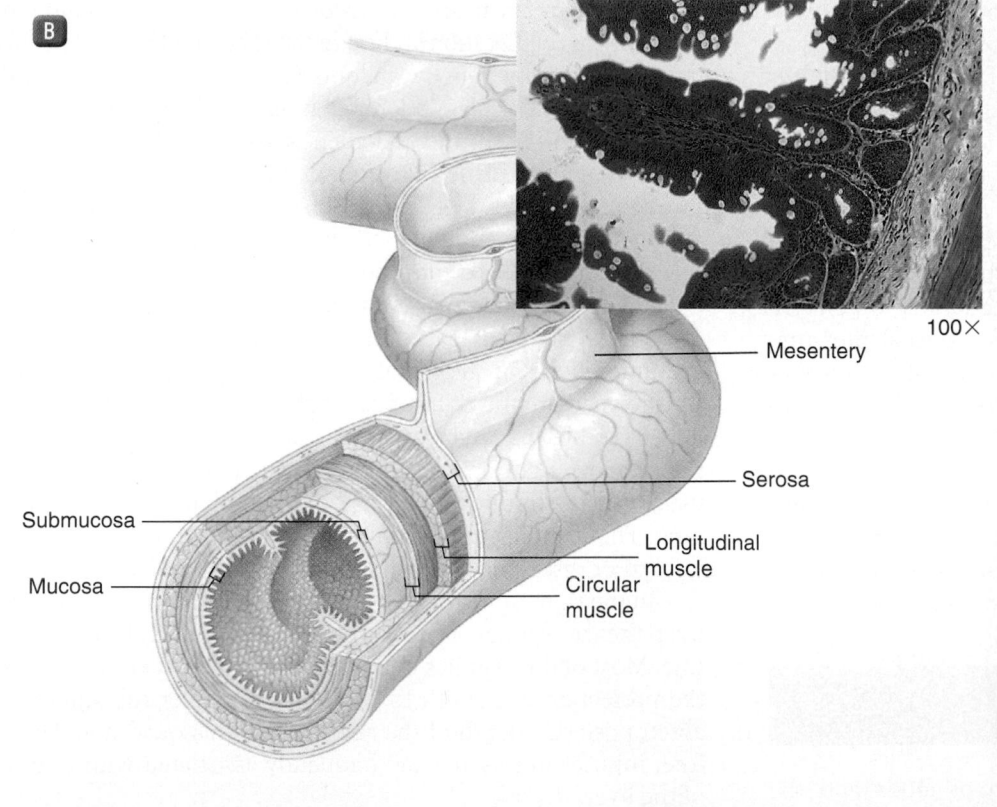

Figure 113 The layers of the alimentary canal. **A.** Layers of the stomach. **B.** Layers of the intestines.

tenderness and pain in this region. In the left lower quadrant (LLQ) lie the descending and the sigmoid portions of the colon.

As mentioned early in this chapter, several organs lie in more than one quadrant. The small intestine, for example, occupies the central part of the abdomen around the umbilicus, and parts of it lie in all four quadrants. The pancreas lies just behind the abdominal cavity on the posterior abdominal wall in both upper quadrants. The large intestine also traverses the abdomen, beginning in the RLQ and ending in the LLQ as it passes through all four quadrants. The urinary bladder lies just behind the pubic symphysis in the middle of the abdomen and therefore lies in both lower quadrants and also in the pelvis.

The kidneys are called **retroperitoneal** organs because they lie behind the abdominal cavity **Figure 115**. They are above the level of the umbilicus, extending from the 11th rib to the 3rd lumbar vertebra on each side. They are approximately 5 ″long and lie just anterior to the costovertebral angle.

■ Mouth

The mouth consists of the lips, cheeks, gums, teeth, and tongue. A mucous membrane lines the mouth. The roof of the mouth is formed by the hard and soft palates. The hard palate is a bony plate lying anteriorly; the soft palate is a fold of mucous membrane and muscle that extends posteriorly from the hard palate into the throat. The soft palate is designed to hold food that is being chewed within the mouth and to help initiate swallowing.

Salivary Glands

There are two **salivary glands** located under the tongue, one on each side of the lower jaw, and one inside each cheek. They produce nearly 1.5 L of saliva daily. Saliva is approximately 98% water. The remaining 2% is composed of mucus, salts, and organic compounds. Saliva serves as a binder for the chewed food that is being swallowed and as a lubricant within the mouth. Saliva also contains certain digestive enzymes.

The right lower quadrant (RLQ) contains two portions of the large intestine: the **cecum**, the first portion into which the small intestine (ileum) opens, and the ascending colon. The **appendix** is a small tubular structure that is attached to the lower border of the cecum. Appendicitis is the most frequent cause of

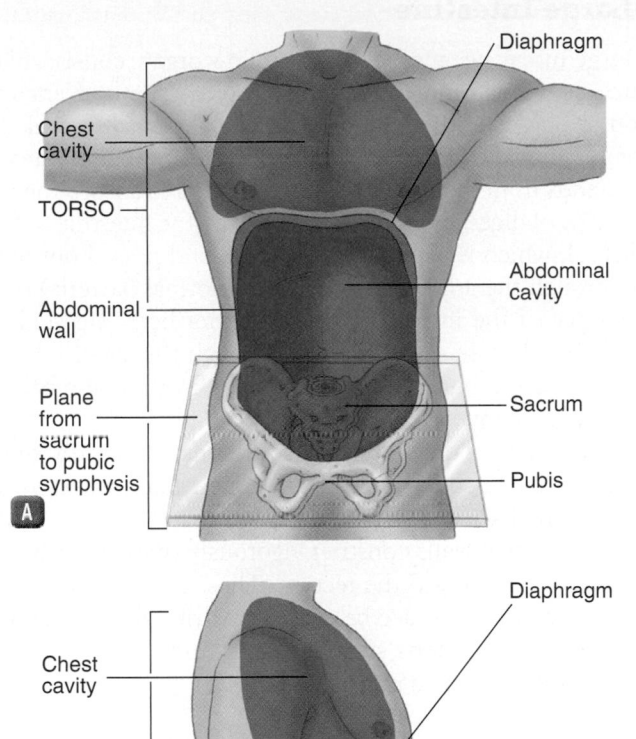

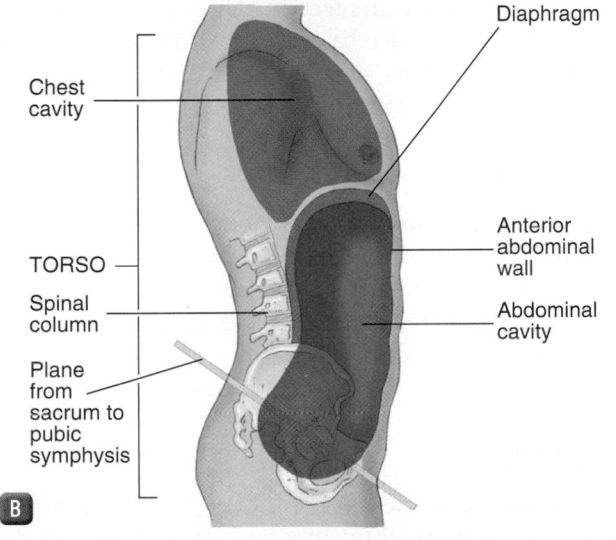

Figure 114 The boundaries of the abdomen are the anterior and posterior abdominal cavity walls, the diaphragm, and an imaginary plane from the pubic symphysis to the sacrum. **A.** Anterior view. **B.** Lateral view.

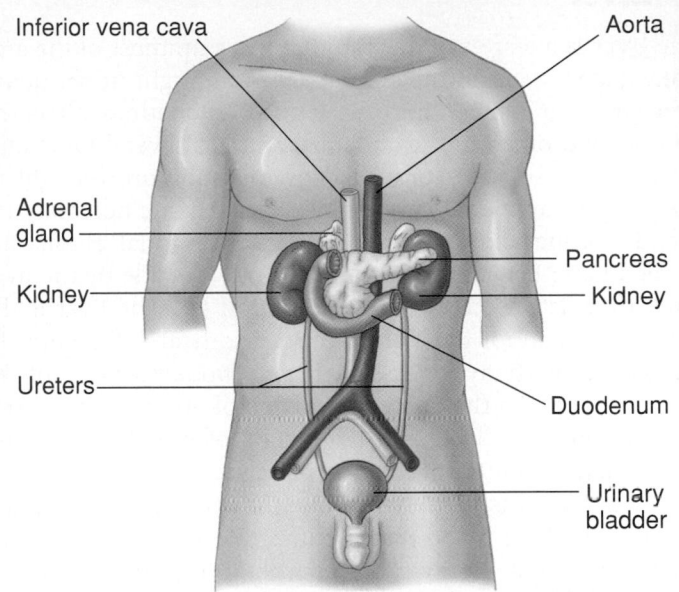

Figure 115 The major organs of the retroperitoneal space lie behind the abdominal cavity, above the level of the umbilicus, and extend from the 11th rib to the 3rd lumbar vertebra. Note that the bladder, inferior vena cava, and aorta also lie in this plane.

Oropharynx

The oropharynx is a tubular structure that extends vertically from the back of the mouth to the esophagus and trachea. An automatic movement of the pharynx during swallowing lifts the larynx to permit the epiglottis to close over it so that liquids and solids are moved into the esophagus and away from the trachea.

Esophagus

The esophagus is a collapsible tube about 10″ long that extends from the end of the pharynx to the stomach and lies just anterior to the spinal column in the chest. Contractions of the muscle in the wall of the esophagus propel food through it to the stomach. Liquids pass with little assistance.

Stomach

The stomach is a hollow organ located in the left upper quadrant of the abdominal cavity, largely protected by the lower left ribs. Muscular contractions in the wall of the stomach and gastric juice, which contains a lot of mucus, convert ingested food to a thoroughly mixed semisolid mass, called <u>chyme</u>. The stomach produces approximately 1.5 L of gastric juice daily for this process. The principal function of the stomach is to receive food in large quantities intermittently, store it, and provide for its movement into the small bowel in regular, small amounts. In 1 to 3 hours, the semisolid food mass derived from one meal is propelled by muscular contraction into the duodenum, the first part of the small intestine.

Pancreas

The <u>pancreas</u>, a flat, solid organ, lies below and behind the liver and stomach and behind the peritoneum. It is firmly fixed in position, deep within the abdomen, and is not easily damaged. It contains two kinds of glands, and the two portions of the pancreas are intertwined. One portion is exocrine, and it secretes nearly 2 L of pancreatic juice daily. This juice contains many enzymes that aid in the digestion of fat, starch, and protein. Pancreatic juice flows directly into the duodenum through the pancreatic ducts. The other portion of the gland is endocrine. It is called the islets of Langerhans, and this is where insulin is produced. Insulin regulates the amount of glucose in the blood.

■ Liver

The <u>liver</u> is a large, solid organ that takes up most of the area immediately beneath the diaphragm in the right upper quadrant and also extends into the left upper quadrant. It is the largest solid organ in the abdomen and has several functions. Poisonous substances produced by digestion are brought to the liver and rendered harmless. Factors that are necessary for blood clotting and for the production of normal plasma are formed here. Between 0.5 and 1 L of bile is made by the liver daily to assist in the normal digestion of fat. The liver is the principal organ for the storage of sugar or starch for immediate use by the body for energy. It also produces many of the factors that aid in the proper regulation of immune responses. Anatomically, the liver is a large mass of blood vessels and cells, packed tightly together. It is fragile and, because of its size, relatively easily injured. Blood flow in the liver is high, because all of the blood that is pumped to the gastrointestinal tract passes into the liver, through the portal vein, before it returns to the heart. In addition, the liver has a generous arterial blood supply of its own. Ordinarily, approximately 25% of the cardiac output of blood (1.5 L) passes through the liver each minute.

Bile Ducts

The liver is connected to the intestine by the <u>bile ducts</u>. The <u>gallbladder</u> is an outpouching from the bile ducts that serves as a reservoir and concentrating organ for bile produced in the liver. Together, the bile ducts and the gallbladder form the biliary system. The gallbladder discharges stored and concentrated bile into the duodenum through the common bile duct. The presence of food in the duodenum triggers a contraction of the gallbladder to empty it. The gallbladder usually contains about 60 to 90 mL of bile.

■ Small Intestine

The <u>small intestine</u> is the major hollow organ of the abdomen. The cells lining the small intestine produce enzymes and mucus to aid in digestion. Enzymes from the pancreas and the small intestine carry out the final processes of digestion. More than 90% of the products of digestion (amino acids, fatty acids, and simple sugars), together with water, ingested vitamins, and minerals are absorbed across the wall of the lower end of the small intestine into veins to be transported to the liver. The small intestine is composed of the duodenum, the jejunum, and the ileum. The duodenum, which is about 12″ long, is the part of the small intestine that receives food from the stomach. Here, food is mixed with secretions from the pancreas and liver for further digestion. Bile, produced by the liver and stored in the gallbladder, is emptied as needed into the duodenum. It is greenish black, but through changes during digestion, it gives feces its typical brown color. Its major function is in the digestion of fat. The jejunum and ileum together measure more than 20′ on average to make up the rest of the small intestine.

■ Large Intestine

The <u>large intestine</u>, another major hollow organ, consists of the cecum, the colon, and the rectum. About 5′ long, it encircles the outer border of the abdomen around the small bowel. The major function of the colon, the portion of the large intestine that extends from the cecum to the rectum, is to absorb the final 5% to 10% of digested food and water from the intestine to form solid stool, which is stored in the rectum and passed out of the body through the anus. Intestinal flora (normal bacteria) break down some of the molecules that have not been digested. An example is cellulose, which moves through the small intestine with little change, but can be broken down by the colon bacteria to be used as energy.

The mixing actions of the large intestine are usually slower than those of the small intestine. The peristaltic waves of the large intestine happen only between twice and three times per day. The intestinal walls constrict vigorously (mass movements) to force contents toward the rectum. These movements usually follow a meal, but may also be caused by irritations of the intestinal mucosa. Conditions such as colitis (inflamed colon) may also cause frequent mass movements.

■ Appendix

The appendix is a tube 3″ to 4″ long that opens into the cecum (the first part of the large intestine) in the right lower quadrant of the abdomen that contains many bacteria. It may easily become obstructed and, as a result, inflamed and infected. Appendicitis, which is the term for this inflammation, is one of the major causes of severe abdominal distress.

■ Rectum

The lowermost end of the colon is the <u>rectum</u>. It is a large, hollow organ that is adapted to store quantities of feces until it is expelled. At its terminal end is the anus, a 2″ canal lined with skin. The rectum and anus are supplied with a complex series of circular muscles called <u>sphincters</u> that control, voluntarily and automatically, the escape of liquids, gases, and solids from the digestive tract. **Table 21** provides a summary of the organs and functions of the digestive system.

■ The Digestive System: Physiology

Digestion of food, from the time it is taken into the mouth until essential compounds are extracted and delivered by the circulatory system to nourish all of the cells in the body, is a complicated process. The functions of the digestive system consist of a series of steps, which include:

- *Ingestion:* Materials enter the digestive tract via the mouth.
- *Mechanical processing:* Materials are crushed and broken into smaller fragments, making them easier to move through the digestive tract; enzymes begin to attack the particles during chewing, as the teeth and tongue are used to tear and mash food; additional mechanical processing

Table 21 Digestive Organs and Functions

Organ/Structure	Function
Mouth	Mechanically breaks down food; begins chemical breakdown with saliva
Esophagus	Moves food from the mouth to the stomach; muscular and vascular structure
Stomach	Performs mechanical and chemical breakdown of food: food in, chyme out
Small intestine: duodenum, jejunum, and ileum	Major site for chemical breakdown of food; major absorption of water, fats, proteins, carbohydrates, and vitamins
Large intestine	Water absorption; formation of feces; bacterial digestion of food
Anus/rectum	Last portion of large intestine; sphincter to control release of feces
Liver	Production of bile; assists with carbohydrate, protein, and fat metabolism of nutrients within the bloodstream; vitamin storage and manufacture; detoxification of blood; elimination of waste
Pancreas	Exocrine: enzymes for protein, carbohydrate, and fat breakdown within the duodenum Endocrine: insulin and glucagon
Gallbladder	Storage of bile

is provided by the mixing motions of the stomach and intestines.

- *Digestion:* The chemical breakdown of food into particles that are small enough to be absorbed by the digested epithelium; simple molecules such as glucose are absorbed intact while others (polysaccharides, proteins, triglycerides) must first be broken down before they can be absorbed.
- *Secretion:* Release of water, acids, buffers, enzymes, and salts by the epithelium and glandular organs of the digestive tract.
- *Absorption:* The movement of organic substrates (molecules acted on by enzymes), electrolytes, vitamins, and water across the epithelium of the digestive tract, into the interstitial fluid.
- *Excretion:* The removal of waste products from body fluids via secretions from the digestive tract and glandular organs; after mixing with residue that cannot be digested, these waste products become feces, which is eliminated during the process of defecation.

In succession, different secretions, primarily enzymes, are added to the food by the salivary glands, the stomach, the liver, the pancreas, and the small intestine to convert the food into basic sugars, fatty acids, and amino acids. These basic products of digestion are carried across the wall of the intestine and transported through the portal vein to the liver. In the liver, the products are processed further and stored or transported to the heart through veins draining the liver. The heart then pumps the blood with these nutrients throughout the arteries to the capillaries, where the nutrients pass through the capillary walls to nourish the body's individual cells.

In normal routine activity, without any food or fluid ingestion at all, between 8 and 10 L of fluid is secreted daily into the gastrointestinal tract. This fluid comes from the salivary glands, stomach, liver, pancreas, and small intestine. In a healthy adult, about 7% of the body weight is delivered as fluid daily to the gastrointestinal tract. If significant vomiting or diarrhea occurs for more than 2 or 3 days, the person will lose a substantial portion of body composition and become severely ill.

■ The Endocrine System: Anatomy and Physiology

The endocrine system is made up of various glands located throughout the body. Through endocrine glands, the endocrine system releases hormones such as insulin into the bloodstream. Hormones help regulate metabolism, controlling chemical reactions, transporting substances, regulating water and electrolyte balances, and aiding in reproduction, growth, and development. Each endocrine gland secretes one or more hormones. Each hormone has a specific effect on some organ, tissue, or process. The major endocrine glands include the pituitary gland, thyroid gland, parathyroid glands, adrenal glands, pancreas, pineal gland, thymus gland, and reproductive glands Figure 116 . Exocrine glands are those that secrete outside the body through ducts (such as tears) and include the sweat glands.

The majority of hormones are either steroids (or steroid-like substances), which are made from cholesterol, or nonsteroidal, including amines, glycoproteins, peptides, or proteins made from amino acids. Even low concentrations of hormones can stimulate target cell changes. Table 22 lists various types of hormones.

Steroid hormones are insoluble in water but soluble in lipids (fats). Therefore, they can easily diffuse into nearly any cell in the body because lipids make up the majority of cell membranes. The following steps are involved in a steroid hormone entering a target cell:

1. The steroid hormone diffuses through the cell membrane.
2. It binds to a specific protein molecule, which is its receptor.
3. The resulting complex binds inside the nucleus to certain parts of the target cell's DNA, activating transcription of specific genes into messenger RNA molecules.
4. These molecules, referred to as *mRNA*, leave the nucleus and enter the cytoplasm.
5. The mRNA molecules are associated with ribosomes, directing the synthesis of certain proteins.

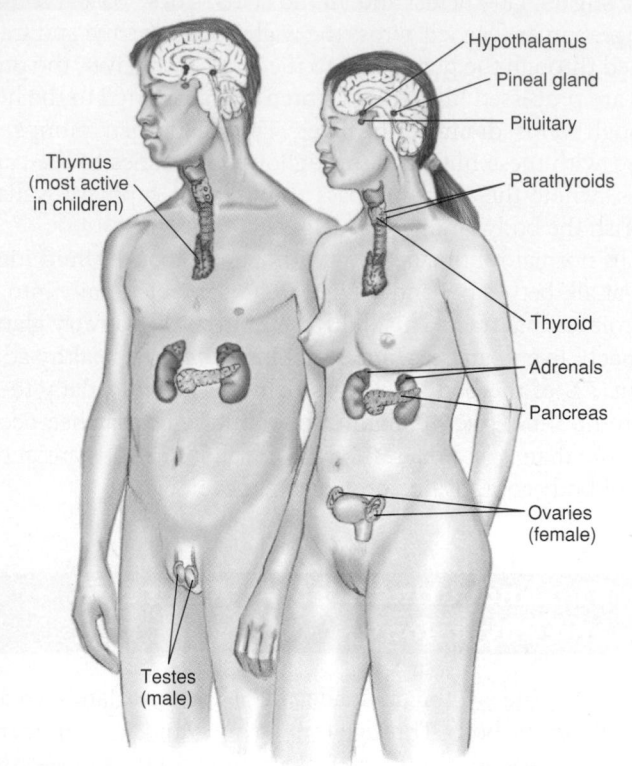

Hypothalamus

Pineal gland

Pituitary

Thymus
(most active
in children)

Parathyroids

Thyroid

Adrenals

Pancreas

Ovaries
(female)

Testes
(male)

Figure 116 The endocrine system controls the release of hormones in the body.

Table 22   Types of Hormones

Type	Examples	Derived From
Steroids	Aldosterone, cortisol, estrogen, testosterone	Cholesterol
Amines	Epinephrine, norepinephrine	Amino acids
Glycoproteins	Follicle-stimulating hormone (FSH), luteinizing hormone (LH), thyroid-stimulating hormone (TSH)	Carbohydrates and proteins
Peptides	Antidiuretic hormone (ADH), oxytocin (OT), thyrotropin-releasing hormone (TRH)	Amino acids
Proteins	Growth hormone (GH), parathyroid hormone (PTH), prolactin (PRL)	Amino acids

The nonsteroidal hormones, listed in Table 22, usually bind to specific receptors in target cell membranes. The activity site of a hormone is where it exerts its effects. Receptor binding can alter enzyme function and membrane transport mechanisms. The first messenger is the hormone that triggers this chain of

biochemical activity. Second messengers are biochemicals in the cell that cause changes in response once the hormone binds to the receptor. Signal transduction describes the entire process of chemical communication from outside cells to inside them. Cyclic adenosine monophosphate (also known as cyclic AMP or cAMP) is the second messenger associated with one group of hormones. **Figure 117** shows how it works, following the steps listed below:

1. A hormone binds to its receptor.
2. The resulting complex activates a G protein.
3. This activates the enzyme adenylate cyclase, which is a membrane protein.
4. This catalyzes the circularization of adenosine triphosphate (ATP) into cAMP.
5. This activates enzymes called protein kinases to cause phosphorylation, altering the shapes of and activating substrate molecules.

Cellular processes are then altered by these steps to cause the hormone's effects, based on the kinds of protein substrate molecules present. The enzyme phosphodiesterase then inactivates the cAMP quickly. Because of this, a target cell's continuing response requires a continuing signal from hormone molecules that bind the target cell's membrane receptors. Other second messengers include diacylglycerol (DAG) and inositol triphosphate (IP_3).

Prostaglandins are lipids made from arachidonic acid in cell membranes of the kidneys, heart, liver, lungs, pancreas, brain, reproductive organs, and thymus. They usually act more locally than hormones, and are potent in small quantities. They are made just before release and are rapidly inactivated. They often have diverse or opposite effects. Prostaglandins stimulate hormone secretions and influence sodium and water movements in the kidneys, helping to regulate blood pressure.

Hormones act on the body's cells by increasing or decreasing the rate of cellular metabolism. They transfer information from one set of cells to another to coordinate bodily functions, such as the regulation of mood, growth and development, metabolism, tissue function, and sexual development and function.

Many cells contain multiple receptors and act as targets for several hormones—or for molecules introduced into the body as therapy. **Agonists** are molecules that bind to a cell's receptor and trigger a response by that cell; they produce some kind of action or biologic effect. **Antagonists** are molecules that bind to a cell's receptor and block the action of agonists. Hormone antagonists are widely used as drugs.

Hormones, regardless of their source, act by binding to receptors. Steroids and thyroid hormones bind to receptors located within cells. All other hormones, as a rule, bind to receptors located on the surface of cells. Hormones stimulate the production of intracellular proteins and other substances that carry out the next task in whatever body process the particular hormone is involved.

The Pituitary Gland and the Hypothalamus

The **pituitary gland** is often referred to as the "master gland" because its secretions control the secretions of other endocrine glands. It is located at the base of the brain and is about the size

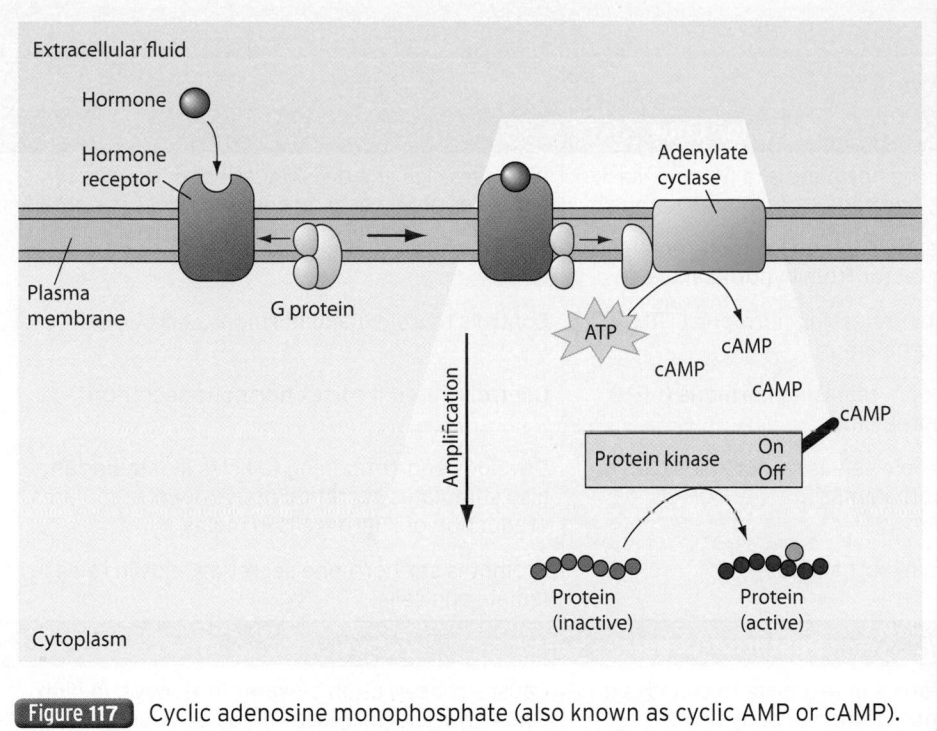

Figure 117 Cyclic adenosine monophosphate (also known as cyclic AMP or cAMP).

by the kidneys. Decreased levels of ADH causes polyuria and diabetes insipidus.

Osmoreceptors sense increases in osmotic pressure due to dehydration and use ADH to signal the kidneys to produce less urine. If too much water is in the body, ADH release is inhibited, and urine production increases. Oxytocin is important to stimulate uterine contractions during childbirth. It stimulates milk let-down, which is the ejection of milk from the breast glands soon after suckling begins. **Table 23** discusses the pituitary gland hormones in greater detail.

The Thyroid Gland

The large gland at the base of the neck is called the **thyroid gland**. It consists of two lobes that are connected by a narrow band of tissue, and is covered by a capsule of connective tissue with secretory parts called follicles. The thyroid is filled with a clear substance called colloid, which stores hormones produced by the follicles. The thyroid gland manufactures and secretes hormones that have a role in growth, development, and metabolism.

Two hormones are synthesized here: thyroxine (also known as tetraiodothyronine or T_4) and triiodothyronine (T_3). The num-

of a grape. The **hypothalamus** is a small region of the brain (not a gland) that regulates the function of the pituitary gland. The hypothalamus is the primary link between the endocrine system and the nervous system. The pituitary is attached to the hypothalamus by a thin piece of tissue.

The pituitary gland is divided into two portions. The anterior pituitary has five types of secretory cells, four of which (growth hormone [GH], prolactin [PRL], thyroid-stimulating hormone [TSH], and **adrenocorticotropin hormone [ACTH]**), secrete a single hormone. The fifth type secretes both follicle-stimulating hormone (FSH) and luteinizing hormone.

The posterior pituitary secretes two hormones (antidiuretic hormone [ADH] and oxytocin) but does not produce them **Figure 118**. ADH and oxytocin are synthesized in hypothalamic neurons but are stored in the posterior pituitary gland until the hypothalamus sends nerve signals to the pituitary to release them. ADH is also called vasopressin, and is discussed in more detail in the chapter, *Emergency Medications*. Nerve impulses from the hypothalamus release these hormones into the blood. A diuretic is a chemical that increases urine production, whereas an antidiuretic decreases urine formation. ADH regulates the water concentration of body fluids by reducing water excretion

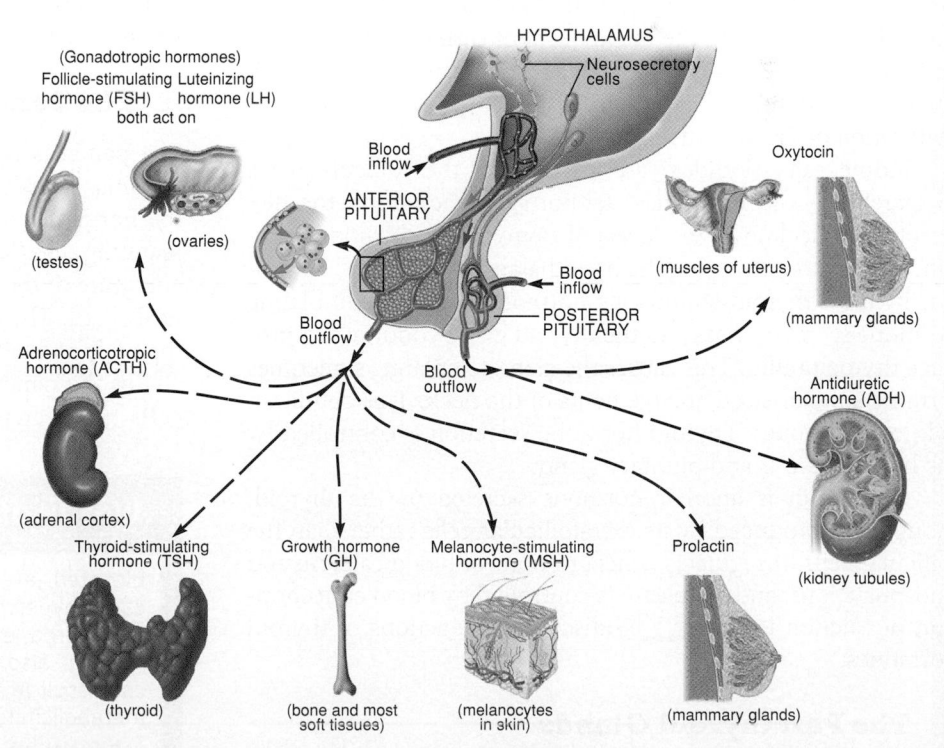

Figure 118 The pituitary gland secretes hormones from its two regions, the anterior pituitary lobe and the posterior pituitary lobe.

Table 23 Pituitary Gland Hormones

Hormone	Source	Action
Anterior Lobe		
Growth hormone (GH)	GH-releasing hormone and GH-release-inhibiting hormone from hypothalamus	Increases size and division rate of body cells, enhances amino acid movement across membranes
Prolactin (PRL)	PRL release-inhibiting hormone and PRL-releasing factor from hypothalamus	Sustains milk production after birth
Thyroid-stimulating hormone (TSH)	Thyrotropin-releasing hormone (TRH) from hypothalamus	Controls thyroid gland hormone secretion
Adrenocorticotropic hormone (ACTH)	Corticotropin-releasing hormone (CRH) from hypothalamus	Controls adrenal cortex hormone secretion
Follicle-stimulating hormone (FSH)	Gonadotropin-releasing hormone (GRH) from hypothalamus	Develops egg-containing follicles in females and also stimulates secretion of estrogen; stimulates production of sperm cells in males
Luteinizing hormone (LH)	GRH from hypothalamus	Promotes sex hormone secretion; aids in release of female egg cells
Posterior Lobe		
Antidiuretic hormone (ADH)	Hypothalamus in response to changes in water concentration in body fluids	Causes conservation of water in kidneys; in high concentrations increases blood pressure
Oxytocin (OT)	Hypothalamus in response to stretching of uterine and vaginal walls, and stimulation of breasts	Contracts uterine wall muscles; contracts milk-secreting gland muscles

ber of each of these indicates the number of atoms of iodine. The thyroid hormones regulate metabolism of carbohydrates, lipids, and proteins, determining the body's basal metabolic rate (BMR). Thyroid hormones are required for growth, development, and maturation of the nervous system.

Iodine salts (iodides) are needed by the follicular cells to secrete thyroid hormones. A shortage of iodide in the diet results in a decline in the levels of thyroxine and triiodothyronine in the blood, causing the hypothalamus to respond by producing more thyroid-stimulating hormone. Thyroid-stimulating hormone secretion rises and the thyroid gland continues to produce thyroglobulin. This causes the gland to enlarge, sometimes forming softball-sized enlargements of the neck. This condition is known as goiter. Thyroid hormone secretion is controlled by the hypothalamus and pituitary gland.

Calcitonin is another hormone secreted by the thyroid, though it is produced by its extrafollicular cells rather than the follicular cells. It regulates concentrations of blood calcium and phosphate ions, and its release is controlled by blood concentration of calcium ions. Table 24 discusses the actions of thyroid hormones.

The Parathyroid Glands

The parathyroid glands are embedded in the posterior portion of each lobe of the thyroid. They produce and secrete parathyroid hormone (PTH), which maintains normal levels of calcium in the blood and normal neuromuscular function. Parathyroid hormone effects are opposite to those of calcitonin.

The Pancreas

The pancreas is an organ of both the endocrine and digestive systems. It functions as two glands: an endocrine gland releasing the hormones insulin and glucagon, and as an exocrine gland secreting digestive juices. The pancreas lies between the greater curvature of the stomach and the duodenum in the retroperitoneal space. The head of the pancreas rests near the duodenum; the body and tail of the pancreas project toward the spleen.

In the pancreas, within each islet of Langerhans are alpha cells that secrete glucagon and beta cells that secrete insulin.

Words of Wisdom

Elevated levels of thyroxine are indicative of a condition called hyperthyroidism or Graves' disease.

Lowered levels of thyroid hormones can result in myxedema, also known as hypothyroidism. This condition can result in a wide variety of symptoms ranging from low metabolism to depression.

Cretinism is a disease caused by lack of thyroid hormone during pregnancy; it results in severely stunted physical and mental development.

Table 24   Thyroid Gland Hormones

Hormone	Source	Action
Thyroxine (T$_4$)	TSH from anterior pituitary	Increases energy release from carbohydrates; increases protein synthesis; accelerates growth; stimulates nervous system activity
Triiodothyronine (T$_3$)	TSH from anterior pituitary	Same as T$_4$, but five times more potent
Calcitonin	Blood calcium concentration	Lowers blood calcium and phosphate ion concentrations by inhibiting calcium and phosphate ion release from bones, and by increasing kidney excretion of these ions

Insulin and glucagon perform opposite functions. Insulin causes substances such as sugar, fatty acids, and amino acids to be taken up and metabolized by cells. Insulin also stimulates the storage of unmetabolized food and the conversion of glucose into glycogen.

Glucagon stimulates the breakdown of glycogen to glucose by a process known as glycogenolysis. In addition, glucagon stimulates both the liver and the kidneys to produce glucose from noncarbohydrate molecules by a process known as gluconeogenesis. In addition, glucagon activates the breakdown of triglycerides into free fatty acids and glycerol. Depending on the metabolic needs of the body, the free fatty acids and glycerol may be metabolized directly or converted to ketones. In small amounts, ketone production is normal. In disease states, such as diabetic ketoacidosis, increased plasma glucagon concentrations and unopposed glucagon activity lead to excessive production, resulting in possible harm to the patient.

Through the actions of insulin and glucagon, among others, the endocrine system regulates the amount and distribution of glucose throughout the body. This system, however, is not without its failures. Patients who fail to take in enough nutrients suffer from malnutrition, and patients who exert themselves too strenuously may suffer from hypoglycemia, commonly resulting in an altered mental status that may quickly lead to coma if untreated. Other patients, especially those who cannot produce enough insulin, may instead be found in hyperglycemia, which can result in vomiting, and dehydration, and can also lead to coma, but has a much more gradual onset. The most prevalent disturbance in this system is diabetes mellitus, in which the patient either does not produce enough insulin or lacks the ability to use it effectively. The effects of diabetes mellitus are among the most frequent calls for service in EMS.

Also contained in the pancreas are several other types of cells that produce other hormones not directly related to glucose levels. The most important of these are the delta cells, which produce somatostatin. Somatostatin helps to regulate the endocrine system with a wide range of effects throughout the body.

The Adrenal Glands

The adrenal glands are located on top of each kidney. The adrenal glands manufacture and secrete certain sex hormones, as well as other hormones that are vital in maintaining the body's water and salt balance. These glands produce adrenaline (also called epinephrine), which mediates the "fight-or-flight" response of the sympathetic nervous system when the body is under stress.

The inner portion, or medulla, of the adrenal glands produces epinephrine and norepinephrine. These hormones are vital in the function of the sympathetic nervous system. The remainder of adrenal tissue is known as the adrenal cortex Figure 119.

The adrenal cortex produces several hormones, called corticosteroids, as well as more than 30 steroids. Some of these hormones are vital for survival, especially aldosterone, cortisol, and some sex hormones.

The outer adrenal cortex synthesizes aldosterone, a mineralocorticoid that helps regulate mineral electrolyte concentrations. Aldosterone helps the kidneys to balance sodium and potassium, and stimulates water retention via the process of osmosis. This mechanism is an excellent example of the complex interplay of multiple hormones found in many areas of the body. In this instance, if blood sodium decreases or blood potassium increases, the adrenal cortex secretes renin. Renin stimulates an increase in angiotensin I, which is then converted into angiotensin II. The presence of increased levels of angiotensin II stimulates the production of aldosterone, as well as several other endocrine functions that help preserve water balance and improve perfusion. Conversely, many stimuli from many systems can also produce this reaction. Because of the multitude of interactions, the endocrine system is constantly adjusting to maintain homeostasis and is considerably complex.

Cortisol is a glucocorticoid produced in the middle adrenal cortex that

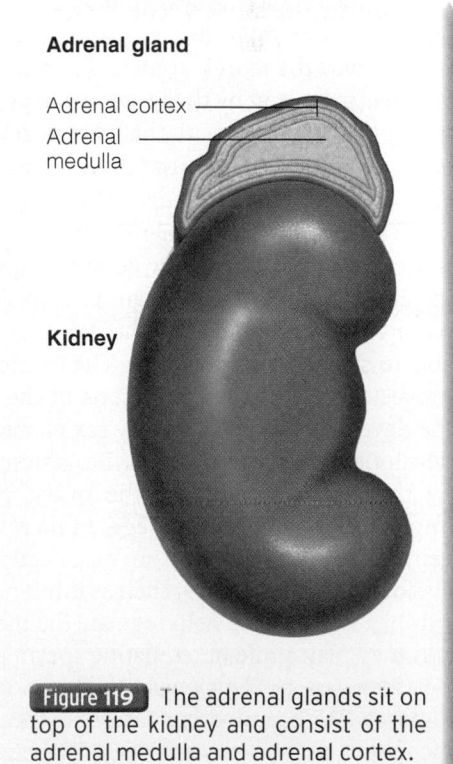

Figure 119 The adrenal glands sit on top of the kidney and consist of the adrenal medulla and adrenal cortex.

also influences protein and fat metabolism. It inhibits protein synthesis, promotes fatty acid release, and stimulates the liver to synthesize glucose from noncarbohydrates. Cortisol helps balance blood glucose and is controlled by negative feedback; stress plays an important part in triggering cortisol release. Cortisol also helps regulate the immune response by decreasing histamine response, which results in lessened swelling, as well as protecting healthy tissues from unnecessary lysosome activation.

The adrenal medulla produces hormones called catecholamines (epinephrine and norepinephrine), which assist the body in coping with physical and emotional stress by increasing the heart and respiratory rates and the blood pressure.

Diseases of the adrenal cortex include Addison's disease and Cushing's syndrome. Most cases of Addison's disease are thought to be autoimmune reactions in which the cells of the adrenal cortex are recognized as foreign and are then destroyed by the body's own immune system. Addison's disease is characterized by a variety of symptoms caused by the loss of hormones from the adrenal cortex. These include loss of appetite, weight loss, fatigue, and weakness.

Cushing's syndrome generally results from pharmacologic doses of cortisone—that is, from injections of large amounts of cortisone. It is used to treat rheumatoid arthritis and asthma. These patients suffer from persistent hyperglycemia because of the presence of high levels of glucocorticoid. Bone and muscle protein may also decline sharply because glucocorticoids stimulate the breakdown of protein. Patients report weakness and fatigue.

The Reproductive Glands and Hormones

Finally, the endocrine system includes reproductive glands. The gonads are the reproductive glands and consist of the ovaries in women and the testes in men. Testosterone is the major androgen manufactured by the testes. Testosterone also is produced in small amounts in the adrenal glands and in the ovaries. Testosterone is responsible for the development of male secondary sex characteristics, such as a deep voice and facial hair.

The three major female hormones are estrogen, progesterone, and human chorionic gonadotropin (hCG). The developing embryo in the uterus manufactures hCG if conception takes place to keep the lining of the uterus (endometrium) thick and able to sustain the pregnancy. The ovaries produce estrogen and progesterone. Estrogen functions in the menstrual cycle and in the development of secondary sex characteristics, such as breast development in adolescence. Progesterone, which is produced by the corpus luteum of the ovary, prepares the uterus for implantation of a fertilized egg. In men, small amounts of estrogen and progesterone also are produced in the testes and adrenal glands. Other hormones, such as inhibin, are poorly understood. Inhibin is known to help regulate the menstrual cycle in females and may play a role in regulating sperm production in the male.

Excesses or deficiencies in hormone levels cause various diseases. With endocrine diseases, specific body functions are increased, decreased, or absent. Diabetes mellitus is a common problem. Because production of the hormone insulin is deficient,

the body is unable to use glucose normally. Insulin is responsible for rapidly moving glucose into cells. Without insulin, glucose moves slowly. This creates a series of complications as the body struggles to find a more readily available fuel for its cells. People with diabetes begin to burn fats and proteins to create the glucose that cells need. Interestingly, the end result is higher and higher blood glucose levels as glucose accumulates, unable to be moved efficiently into the cells. The chapter, *Endocrine Emergencies*, discusses how high blood glucose levels affect the body.

The Urinary System: Anatomy and Physiology

The urinary system controls the discharge of certain waste materials filtered from the blood by the kidneys. In the urinary system, the kidneys are solid organs; the ureters, bladder, and urethra are hollow organs **Figure 120**. The main functions of the urinary system are (1) to control fluid balance in the body, (2) to filter and eliminate wastes, and (3) to control pH balance.

The body has two kidneys that lie on the posterior muscular wall of the abdomen behind the peritoneum in the retroperitoneal space. These organs rid the blood of toxic waste products and control its balance of water and salt. Blood flow in the kidneys is high. Nearly 20% of the output of blood from the heart passes through the kidneys each minute. Large vessels attach the kidneys directly to the aorta and the inferior vena cava. Waste products and water are constantly filtered from the blood to form urine. The kidneys continuously concentrate this filtered urine by reabsorbing the water as it passes through a system of specialized tubes within them. The tubes finally unite to form the renal pelvis, a cone-shaped collecting area that connects the ureter and the kidney.

Each kidney has an inner renal medulla and an outer renal cortex. The renal medulla is made of conical tissue called renal pyramids, and has striations. The renal cortex encloses the medulla, dipping into it between the renal pyramids to form renal columns. The cortex appears to have granules due to tiny tubules associated with the functional units of the kidneys, the nephrons.

The kidneys help to maintain homeostasis by regulating the composition, pH, and volume of the extracellular fluid. This is accomplished by their removal of metabolic wastes from the blood and diluting them with water and electrolytes. This process forms urine, which the kidneys excrete. The other important functions of the kidneys include the following:

- Secretion of the hormone erythropoietin, which helps to control red blood cell production
- Help with the activation of vitamin D
- Help to maintain blood volume and pressure via secretion of the enzyme renin

The kidneys are supplied with blood from the renal arteries, which arise from the abdominal aorta. These arteries transport large volumes of blood. While a person rests, the renal arteries carry between 15% and 30% of the total cardiac output into the kidneys.

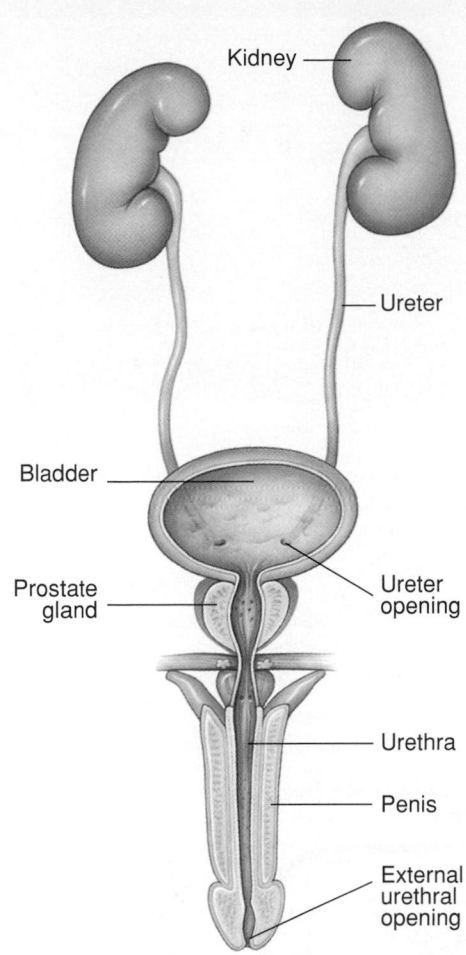

Kidney

Ureter

Bladder

Prostate gland

Ureter opening

Urethra

Penis

External urethral opening

Figure 120 The urinary system lies in the retroperitoneal (behind the peritoneum) space behind the organs of the digestive system. The urinary system in males and females includes the kidneys, ureters, bladder, and urethra. This diagram shows the male urinary system.

The renal arteries branch off inside the kidneys into interlobar arteries, arcuate arteries, and interlobular arteries. The final branches of the interlobular arteries lead to the nephrons, and are called **afferent arterioles** **Figure 121**. Corresponding, in general, with the arterial pathways, the venous blood returns through a similar series of vessels. The **renal vein** then joins the inferior vena cava. Venous blood returns through a series of vessels that correspond generally to arterial pathways.

The Nephrons

There are about 1 million nephrons in a kidney, each consisting of a **renal corpuscle** and a **renal tubule**. Fluid moves through the renal tubules as it moves toward exiting the body. A **glomerulus** is a tangled cluster of blood capillaries that comprises a renal corpuscle. The first step in urine formation is the filtering of fluid via the glomerular capillaries. The glomerulus is surrounded by a sac-like structure called a **glomerular capsule** **Figure 122**. It is located at the proximal end of a renal tubule and

receives filtered fluid from the glomerulus. The renal tubule then leads away from the glomerular capsule, coiling into the proximal convoluted tubule.

The proximal convoluted tubule dips toward the renal pelvis to form the descending limb of the nephron loop, also called the loop of Henle. It then curves toward the renal corpuscle to form the ascending limb of the nephron loop. This returns to the renal corpuscle region, coiling tightly to become the distal convoluted tubule. Therefore, the loop of Henle has a horseshoe shape. These tubules, from several nephrons, merge to form collecting ducts in the renal cortexes. They pass into the renal medulla, resulting in tubes that empty into the minor calyces through openings in the renal papillae.

Glomerular capillaries arise from afferent arterioles, with blood (minus filtered fluids) entering an **efferent arteriole**. Efferent arterioles are smaller in diameter than afferent arterioles. The efferent arterioles resist blood flow slightly and back up into the glomeruli, increasing glomerular capillary pressure. Efferent arterioles branch into complex, interconnected capillary networks, each called a **peritubular capillary**. This structure surrounds the renal tubule. Blood in this capillary system is under low pressure, and eventually enters the venous system of the kidney.

The distal convoluted tubule contacts the afferent and efferent arterioles while passing between them. The densely packaged, narrow distal tubule epithelial cells form the macula densa. Enlarged smooth muscle cells (juxtaglomerular cells), along with the macula densa, constitute the **juxtaglomerular apparatus** (juxtaglomerular complex).

■ Formation of Urine

Glomerular filtration initiates urine formation. The plasma is filtered by the glomerular capillaries, with most of this fluid reabsorbed into the bloodstream via the colloid osmotic pressure of the plasma. Using two capillaries in series, the nephrons use this process to help produce urine. The first capillary bed filters instead of forming interstitial fluid, with the filtrate moving into the renal tubule to form urine.

Every 24 hours, glomerular filtration produces 180 liters of fluid—this is more than four times the amount of total body water. Two other processes contribute to urine formation. **Tubular reabsorption** moves substances from the tubular fluid into the blood, within the peritubular capillary **Figure 123**. The kidney reclaims the correct amounts of water, electrolytes, and glucose as required by the body. **Tubular secretion** moves substances from the blood in the peritubular capillary into the renal tubule. Some substances that the body must excrete, such as hydrogen ions and some toxins, are removed more quickly than through filtration.

Urine is the final product of the above processes. The amount of a given substance excreted in the urine is calculated as follows:

Amount filtered at the glomerulus – Amount reabsorbed by the tubule + Amount secreted by the tubule = Amount excreted in the urine

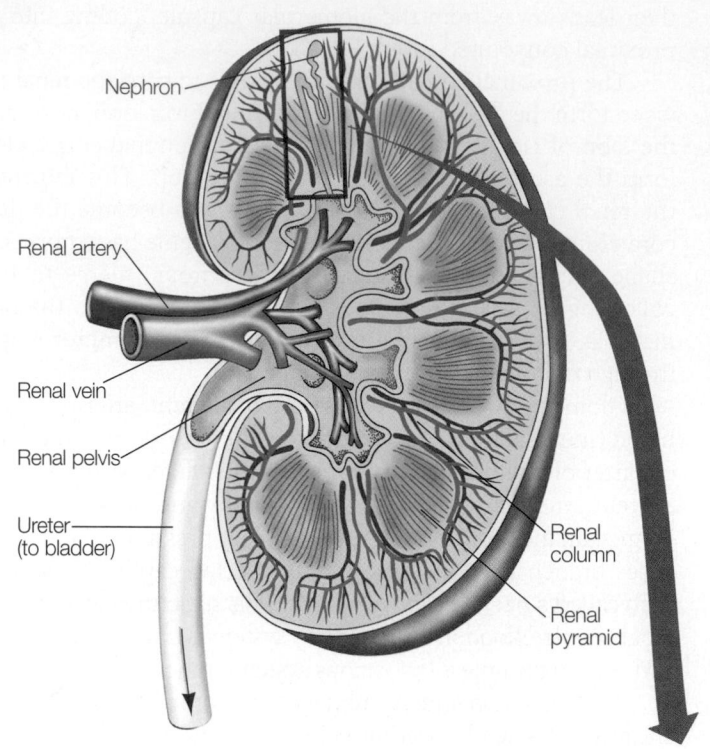

Nephron

Renal artery

Renal vein

Renal pelvis

Ureter
(to bladder)

Renal
column

Renal
pyramid

A

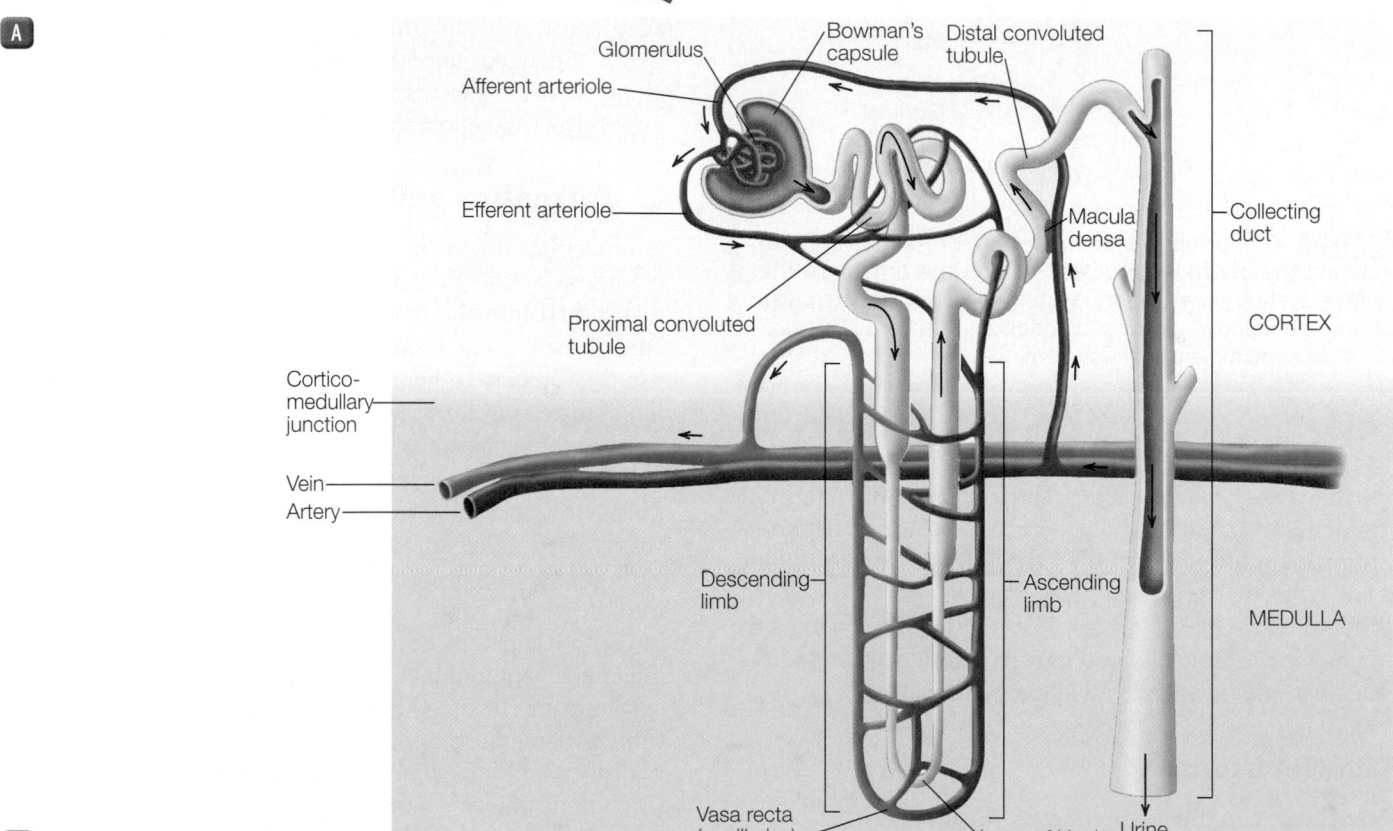

Glomerulus

Afferent arteriole

Efferent arteriole

Proximal convoluted
tubule

Bowman's
capsule

Distal convoluted
tubule

Macula
densa

Collecting
duct

CORTEX

Cortico-
medullary
junction

Vein

Artery

Descending
limb

Ascending
limb

MEDULLA

Vasa recta
(capillaries)

Loop of Henle

Urine

B

Figure 121 The main branches of the renal artery and renal vein. **A.** Blood flow within the kidney. **B.** Blood flow through a nephron.

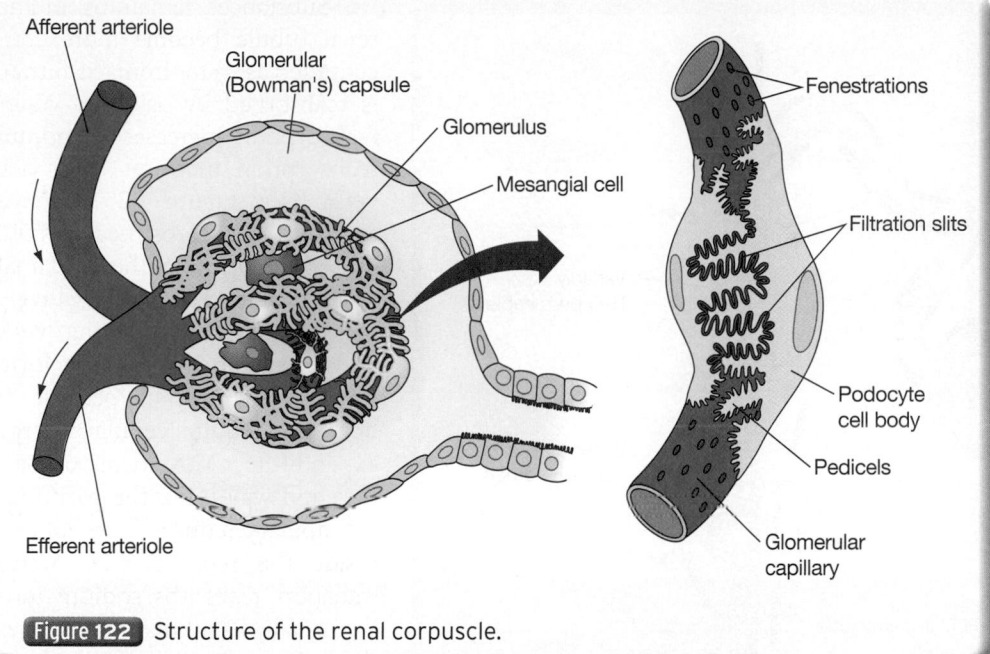

Afferent arteriole

Glomerular (Bowman's) capsule

Glomerulus

Mesangial cell

Efferent arteriole

Fenestrations

Filtration slits

Podocyte cell body

Pedicels

Glomerular capillary

Figure 122 Structure of the renal corpuscle.

When water and dissolved substances are filtered out of the glomerular capillaries into the glomerular capsules, urine formation begins. This type of filtration is similar to filtration at the arteriolar ends of other capillaries. Tiny openings (fenestrae) in glomerular capillary walls make them more permeable than the capillaries of other tissues. Cells called podocytes cover these capillaries, helping to make them impermeable to plasma proteins.

The resulting **glomerular filtrate** is received by the glomerular capsule. It is similar to filtrate that becomes tissue fluid throughout the body. Glomerular filtrate is mostly water with the same components as blood plasma, except for large protein molecules. **Table 25** compares concentrations of substances in glomerular filtrate, plasma, and urine.

The hydrostatic pressure of blood forces substances through the glomerular capillary wall; this action is also influenced by plasma osmotic pressure and hydrostatic pressure in the glomerular capsule. When one of these pressures increases, movement out of the capillary is opposed and filtration is reduced. The **net filtration pressure** forces substances out of the glomerulus, and is usually positive pressure **Figure 124**. Net filtration pressure is directly proportional to the glomerular filtration rate. All the factors related to the glomerular filtration rate affect the net filtration pressure. Any changes in afferent or efferent arteriole diameters alter the glomerular filtration rate. During filtration through capillary walls, proteins in the plasma raise colloid osmotic pressure with the glomerular capillaries. Anything that decreases plasma colloid osmotic pressure increases the filtration rate.

When a ureter is obscured by a stone or an enlarged prostate gland presses on the urethra, fluids back up into the renal tubules, raising the hydrostatic pressure in the glomerular capsule. This may significantly decrease the filtration rate. Normally, while at rest, the kidneys receive 25% of the cardiac output, with about 20% of blood plasma being filtered while moving through the glomerular capillary. Therefore, an average adult's glomerular filtration rate is about 180 liters (45 gallons) in just 24 hours. Only a small amount of this is excreted as urine; most fluid passing through the renal tubules is reabsorbed into the plasma.

The glomerular filtration rate may increase when body fluids are excessive, and decrease when fluid conservation is required. It can respond to sympathetic nervous system reflexes. The enzyme renin also controls filtration rate. Secretion of renin responds to three types of stimuli:

- When special afferent arteriole cells sense a drop in blood pressure
- In response to sympathetic stimulation
- When the macula densa senses decreased chloride, potassium, and sodium ions that reach the distal tubule

Renin in the bloodstream reacts with the plasma protein angiotensinogen, forming angiotensin I. In the lungs and blood plasma, angiotensin-converting enzyme (ACE) converts angiotensin I to angiotensin II.

Angiotensin II helps maintain sodium and water balance as well as blood pressure. It vasoconstricts the efferent arteriole, raising glomerular capillary hydrostatic pressure. This helps the decrease in glomerular filtration rate. Angiotensin II stimulates the kidneys to secrete aldosterone, encouraging tubular reabsorption of sodium.

Atrial natriuretic peptide (ANP) is a hormone secreted by the heart when blood volume increases. It increases sodium excretion by increasing the glomerular filtration rate, among other methods. Composition of glomerular filtrate and urine differs.

The glomerular filtrate, for example, contains glucose, but urine does not. Tubular reabsorption greatly influences these differences. It transports substances out of the tubular fluid, through the renal tubule, into the interstitial fluid, diffusing into the peritubular capillaries. Substances must first cross cell membranes facing the inside of the tubules, and then cross those facing the interstitial fluid. Substances moving down a concentration gradient must be soluble in lipids, or a carrier or channel for that substance must exist in the renal tubular cells. Peritubular blood is under relatively low pressure, enhancing the rate of fluid reabsorption from the renal tubule. It occurs mostly in the proximal convoluted portion of the tubule, where microvilli form a brush border that increases the surface area exposed to glomerular filtrate (enhancing reabsorption). **Figure 125** shows how tubular reabsorption transports substances into the blood within the peritubular capillary, as well as from the blood within the peritubular capillary into the renal tubule.

Substances remaining in the renal tubule become more concentrated as water from the filtrate is reabsorbed by osmosis. Water reabsorption increases if sodium reabsorption increases, and vice versa (see Figure 125). Active transport reabsorbs nearly 70% of sodium ions in the proximal renal tubule. Passive, negatively charged ions move along with the sodium ions. This is a form of passive transport because it does not require cellular energy expenditure. Movement of solutes and water into the peritubular capillary reduces fluid volume inside the renal tubule. Active transport reabsorbs sodium ions continually as tubular fluid moves through the nephron loop, distal convoluted tubule, and collecting duct. Nearly all sodium ions and water from the renal tubule via the glomerular filtrate are reabsorbed before urine excretion.

In tubular secretion, some substances move from the blood plasma into the fluid of the renal tubule. The renal tubule secretes hydrogen ions, regulating the pH of body fluids. Most potassium ions are reabsorbed. Because positively charged potassium and hydrogen ions are attracted to negatively charged ions (such as chloride or sulfate), they move passively through the tubular epithelium to enter the tubular fluid.

Urine formation is summarized as follows:

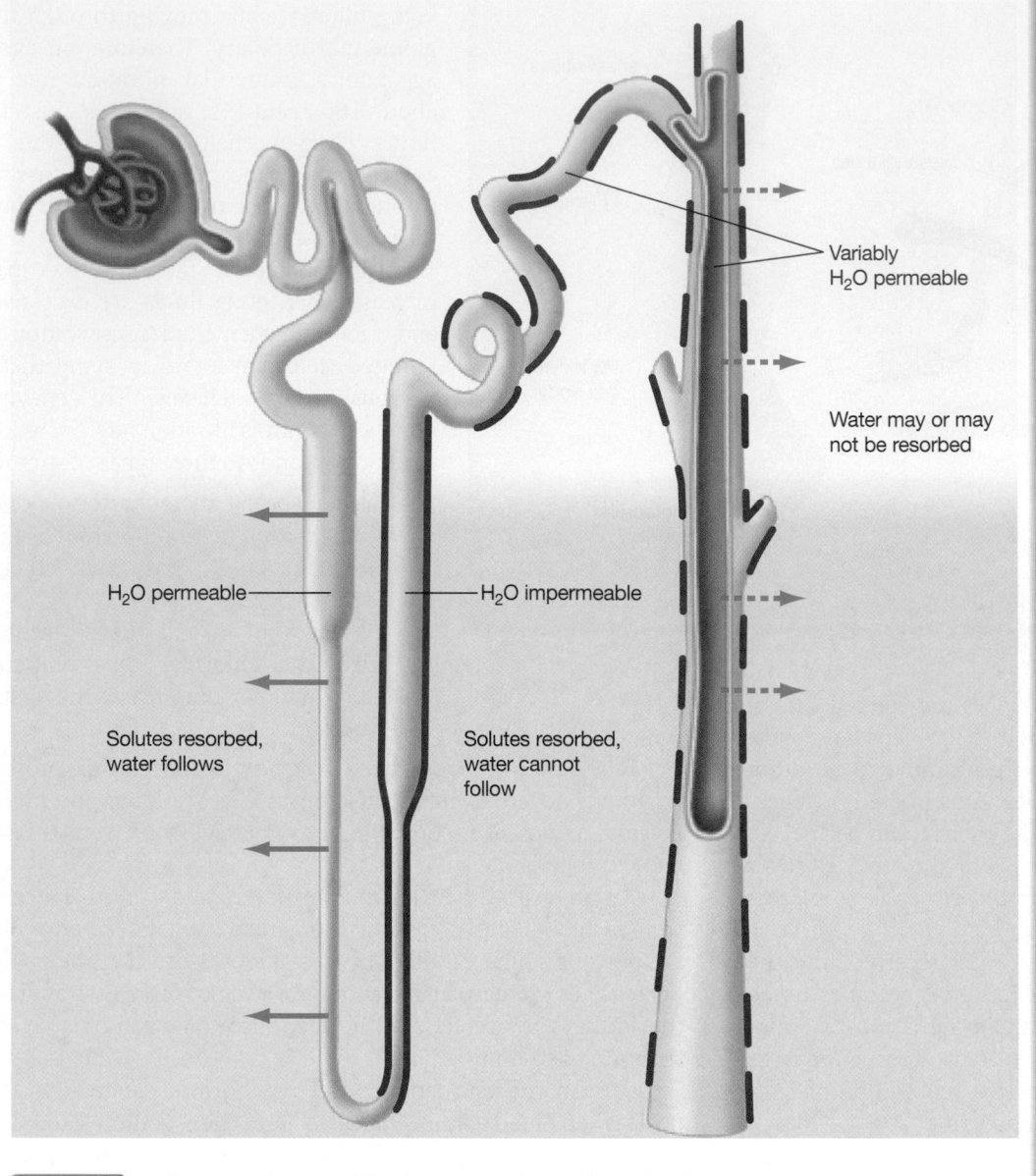

Figure 123 A single nephron and the tubular reabsorption of water.

Labels within figure:
- Variably H₂O permeable
- Water may or may not be resorbed
- H₂O permeable
- H₂O impermeable
- Solutes resorbed, water follows
- Solutes resorbed, water cannot follow

Active transport requires carrier molecules from cell membranes to transport certain molecules across the membrane, release them, and then begin the process again. This process has only a limited transport capacity, meaning that because the number of carriers is limited, only a certain amount of molecules can be transported over a given period of time.

When plasma glucose reaches the renal plasma threshold, more glucose molecules exist in the filtrate than can be actively transported. Therefore, some glucose remains in the tubular fluid, which is excreted in the urine. Amino acids enter the glomerular filtrate for reabsorption in the proximal convoluted tubule. Glomerular filtrate has no protein except for traces of albumin. Other substances reabsorbed by the proximal convoluted tubule include creatine, acids (citric, lactic, ascorbic, and uric), and ions (phosphate, calcium, potassium, sodium, and sulfate).

- *Glomerular filtration:* Materials from blood plasma
- *Reabsorption of substances:* Glucose, water, creatine, amino acids, lactic/citric/uric acids, phosphate/sulfate/calcium/potassium/sodium ions
- *Secretion of substances:* Hydrogen ions (H⁺), potassium ions (K⁺), ammonia (NH₃), and some drugs

Aldosterone may stimulate additional reabsorption of sodium, and ADH does the same for water. Aldosterone stimulates reabsorption of sodium and secretion of potassium from the distal convoluted tubule. When ADH reaches the kidney, it increases water permeability, moving water via osmosis out of the distal convoluted tubule and collecting duct. **Table 26** summarizes how ADH helps regulate urine concentration and volume. Other hormones also influence the retention or secretion of various substances. For example, parathyroid hormone

Table 25   Concentrations of Different Substances

Substance	Glomerular Filtrate	Plasma	Urine
Concentrations in mEq/L			
Sodium (Na^+)	142	142	128
Chloride (Cl^-)	103	103	134
Bicarbonate (HCO_3^-)	27	27	14
Potassium (K^+)	5	5	60
Calcium (Ca^{+2})	4	4	5
Magnesium (Mg^{+2})	3	3	15
Phosphate (PO_4^{-3})	2	2	40
Sulfate (SO_4^{-2})	1	1	33
Concentrations in mg/100 mL			
Glucose	100	100	0
Urea	26	26	1820
Uric acid	4	4	53

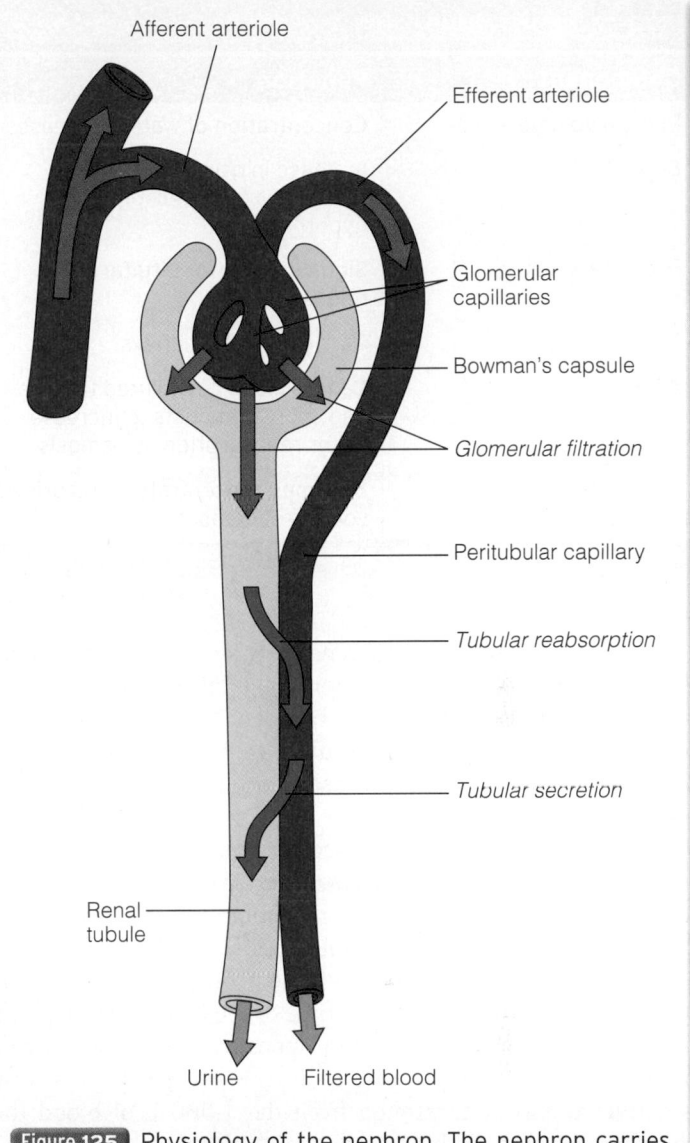

Figure 125 Physiology of the nephron. The nephron carries out three processes: (1) glomerular filtration, (2) tubular reabsorption, and (3) tubular secretion. All contribute to the filtering of the blood.

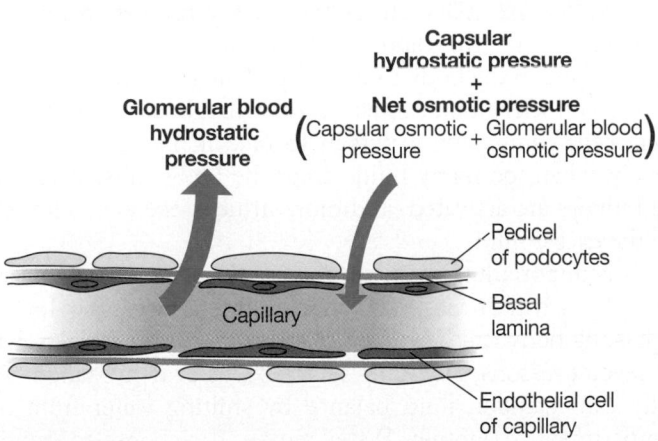

Figure 124 The presence of an efferent arteriole results in a high glomerular blood hydrostatic pressure. This pressure exceeds the sum of the pressures that oppose the movement of fluid through the glomerular filtration membrane. Filtration is the outcome of this balance of pressures.

(PTH) causes an decrease in the amount of calcium excreted in the urine.

<u>Urea</u> is a result of amino acid catabolism, and its plasma concentration reflects the amount of protein in the diet. Urea filters into the renal tubule, with about 80% reabsorbed while the remainder is excreted in the urine. <u>Uric acid</u> is a result of metabolism of certain organic bases in nucleic acids. Active transport reabsorbs most of the uric acid present in the glomerular filtrate.

The composition of urine is related to water volume and the amount of solutes that the kidneys must eliminate or retain to maintain homeostasis. Urine is about 95% water, and usually contains urea and uric acid. It is slightly heavier than water, with a specific gravity of 1.003 to 1.035. Its pH is usually close to neutral, but can vary widely depending on many factors, not the least of which being what the patient has eaten. It can be clear to "straw-colored," but darker color usually indicates a concentration of solutes that may indicate dehydration or some other malady. It may have traces of amino acids and electrolytes. Urine production varies between 0.6 and 2.5 liters per day. Urine production of 50 to 60 mL per hour is normal, with output of less than 30 mL per hour possibly indicating kidney failure.

Table 26 ADH and Urine

Component	Function
Plasma volume	Concentration of water decreases
Body fluids	Increase in osmotic pressure stimulates osmoreceptors in hypothalamus
Hypothalamus	Signals posterior pituitary to release ADH
Blood	Carries ADH to kidneys
ADH	Causes distal convoluted tubules and collecting ducts to increase water reabsorption by osmosis
Urine	Becomes concentrated, and urine volume decreases

A ureter passes from the renal pelvis of each kidney along the surface of the posterior abdominal wall behind the peritoneum to drain into the urinary bladder. The ureters are small (0.2″ in diameter), hollow, muscular tubes. Peristalsis, a wave-like contraction of smooth muscle, occurs in these tubes to move the urine to the bladder.

The urinary bladder is located immediately behind the pubic symphysis in the pelvic cavity and is composed of smooth muscle with a specialized lining membrane. The two ureters enter posteriorly at its base on either side. The bladder empties to the outside of the body through the urethra. In the male, the urethra passes from the anterior base of the bladder through the penis. In the female, the urethra opens in front of the vagina. A healthy adult forms 1.5 to 2 L of urine every day. This waste is extracted and concentrated from the 1,500 L of blood that circulates through the kidneys daily.

Words of Wisdom

The kidneys also are important in the regulation of the body's fluid balance and blood pressure. They perform these vital functions in conjunction with complex hormone-driven mechanisms. Fluid balance is controlled by the effects of ADH on the kidney. The blood pressure effects are influenced by the renin-angiotensin system, of which the kidneys are an important part.

■ Body Fluid Balance

The total body water content of the average adult ranges from 50% to 70% of total body weight, depending on age and sex. A newborn's total body water content may be as high as 75% to 80% of total body weight.

Body fluid is divided into two main compartments: intracellular fluid and extracellular fluid. Intracellular fluid (ICF)

exists within individual cells and equals approximately 40% to 45% of total body weight. The intracellular fluid makes up approximately 75% of all body fluid. Extracellular fluid (ECF) exists outside of the cell membranes. It equals approximately 15% to 20% of the total body weight, or 25% of all body fluid. Examples of extracellular fluids include plasma, lymph, synovial fluid, cerebrospinal fluid, and the aqueous humor of the eye. Extracellular fluid is further divided into intravascular fluid and interstitial fluid. Intravascular fluid (plasma), the fluid portion of blood, is found within the blood vessels and accounts for approximately 4.5% of total body weight. Interstitial fluid is located outside of the blood vessels, in the spaces between the body's cells. It accounts for approximately 10.5% of total body weight. There is a delicate balance among the various fluid compartments of the body that is essential to maintain homeostasis. If fluid is lost from anywhere in the body, there can be serious ramifications because this disturbs the balance among various fluid compartments (homeostasis). Under normal conditions, the total volume of water in the body and its distribution in the body compartments remain relatively constant, even though there are fluctuations in the amount of water that enters and is excreted from the body each day. Fluid balance is the process of maintaining homeostasis through equal intake (water taken into the body) and output (water excreted from the body) of fluids.

There are mechanisms in the body that maintain the balance between what is taken in and what is excreted. For example, when the fluid volume drops, the pituitary gland secretes ADH Figure 126 . ADH causes the kidney tubules to reabsorb more water into the blood and excrete less urine, allowing fluid volume in the body to build up. Thirst also regulates fluid intake. The sensation of thirst occurs when body fluids become decreased, stimulating a person to take in more fluids. Conversely, when too many fluids enter the body, thirst decreases, the kidneys are activated, and more urine is excreted, eliminating the excess fluid.

It is important to maintain the proper balance of fluids and electrolytes within the body, because this is necessary for life. A person's body can become depleted of fluids and electrolytes for several reasons, including severe burns or dehydration. The body can maintain fluid balance by shifting water from one compartment to another. Water moves in response to osmotic forces as well as hormonal stimuli such as ADH. By moving unequal amounts of electrolytes into and out of the cells, it is also possible for the body to balance other properties of intracellular fluid. For a patient whose fluids or electrolytes are depleted, rapid restoration of fluid balance may mean the difference between life and death Table 27 .

■ The Genital System: Anatomy and Physiology

The genital system controls the reproductive processes by which life is created. The reproductive systems of both males and females contain organs and glands that create sex cells and transport them to areas where fertilization can occur. The male

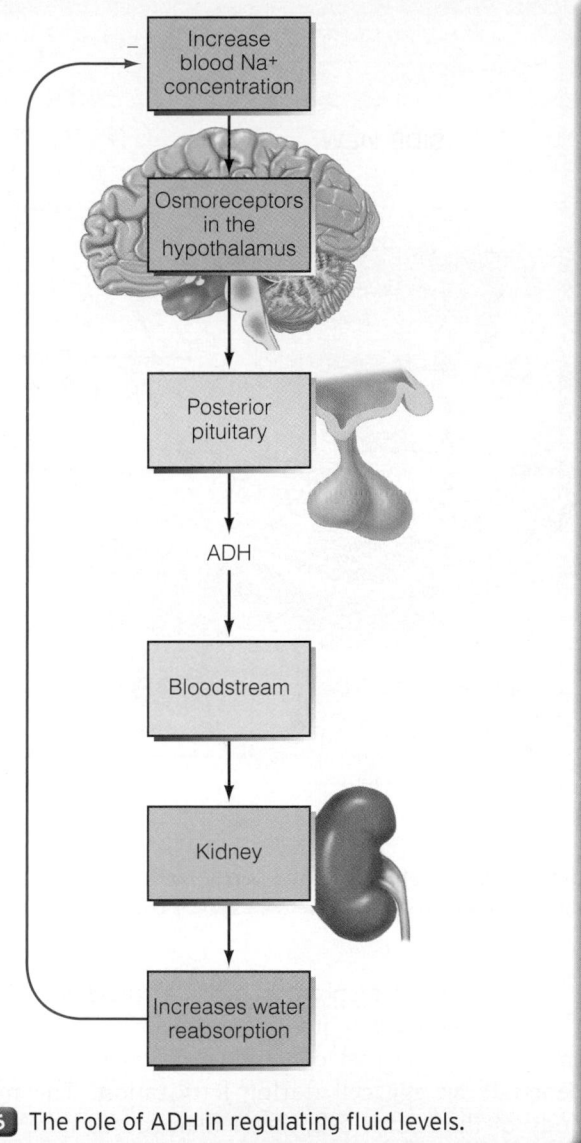

Figure 126 The role of ADH in regulating fluid levels.

Table 27   Major Mechanisms for Fluid Homeostasis
■ Antidiuretic hormone (ADH)
■ Thirst
■ Kidneys
■ Water shifts

and female reproductive systems are functionally very different, but the first step in reproduction for each is to produce cells specially created to combine with a partner's to create a new organism. These cells are known as sex cells or <u>gametes</u>. Male gametes are called <u>sperm</u>. Female gametes are called <u>oocytes</u> or eggs. Gametes are described as <u>haploid cells</u> because they carry genetic instructions via 23 individual chromosomes. When sex cells from a male and female unite during fertilization, the

chromosomes from each partner unite with their accompanying chromosome from the opposite gamete, called a <u>homologous chromosome</u>, to form 23 pairs of chromosomes, for a total of 46 chromosomes. This first fertilized cell, from which all other body cells are created, is known as the <u>zygote</u>. It, and all other cells besides the gametes, are described as <u>diploid</u> because they carry two of each of the 23 chromosomes—one from the father and one from the mother. Among these, 22 are <u>autosomes</u>, which have a corresponding homologous chromosome in both males and females. The 23rd chromosome pair is made up of <u>sex chromosomes</u>—one labeled "X," which both males and females have, and the other being either a second copy of the X chromosome or a Y chromosome. If the 23rd pair in the zygote is XX, the organism will be biologically female; if it is XY, a male will develop.

It is crucial to understand how critical these chromosomes are and how far-reaching their effects can be on the developing organism. These chromosomes contain the entire sequence of genetic information the organism will have throughout its entire life (unless some artificial change is effected). As you learned already, this genetic information contains the instructions for every structure and process in the body. They also contain sequences that will determine or influence various characteristics such as hair color, skin color, body composition, height, and predisposition to certain diseases. These traits are determined through the action of dominant and recessive <u>alleles</u> of the same gene. For example, the allele that contains instructions for red hair color is recessive. If it is paired with an allele from the other parent that is dominant, the cell is said to be heterozygous, and hair color will be dictated by the dominant allele (the allele for red hair will be overridden by the dominant allele). If, however, it is paired with another "redhead" allele, the cell is said to be homozygous, and the new organism's hair color will be red. The arrangement of genes and their characteristics is known as the person's <u>genotype</u>, whereas the set of characteristics that results from expression of those genes is known as a <u>phenotype</u>.

The Male Reproductive System and Organs

Sperm cells are produced and maintained by the male reproductive organs, which also transport these cells to the outside of the body, as well as secreting male sex hormones. The primary sex organs (gonads) of the male consist of the two testes, in which sperm cells and male sex hormones are formed. The accessory sex organs are the internal and external reproductive organs. The male genitalia, except for the <u>prostate gland</u> and the <u>seminal vesicles</u>, lie outside the pelvic cavity **Figure 127** .

Testes

The testes are oval-shaped structures about 5 cm long and 3 cm in diameter. They are located within the cavity of the <u>scrotum</u>.

Each testis is enclosed in a tough, fibrous, white capsule. The posterior border of the capsule has thickened connective tissue that extends into the testis. This forms thin septa, dividing the testis into approximately 250 lobules. Each lobule

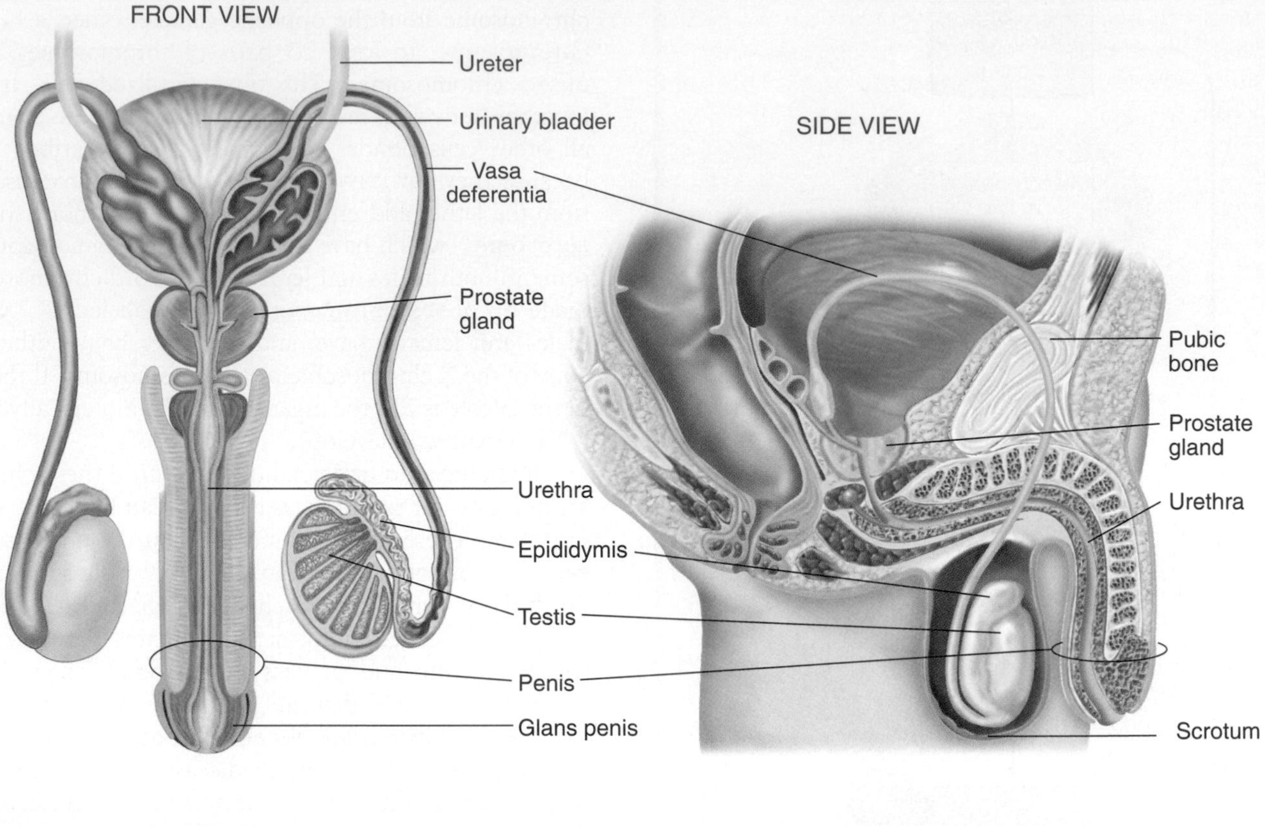

FRONT VIEW

Ureter

Urinary bladder

SIDE VIEW

Vasa deferentia

Pubic bone

Prostate gland

Prostate gland

Urethra

Urethra

Epididymis

Testis

Penis

Glans penis

Scrotum

Figure 127   The male reproductive system consists of the testicles, epididymis, vasa deferentia, and penis.

contains up to four highly coiled <u>seminiferous tubules</u> that, when uncoiled, may reach 80 cm in length. A normal testis contains nearly a half mile of seminiferous tubules. Each of these tubules forms a loop that is connected to a network of passageways known as the rete testis. Fifteen to 20 large efferent ductules connect the rete testis to the epididymis. This tube coils on the outer surface of the testis and becomes the ductus deferens.

Spermatogenic cells form sperm cells and line the seminiferous tubules. Interstitial cells, also known as the cells of Leydig, lie in spaces between the seminiferous tubules. Male sex hormones are produced and secreted by these interstitial cells.

The epithelium that makes up the seminiferous tubules contains supporting sustentacular (Sertoli) cells and spermatogenic cells. These cells provide a framework that nourishes and regulates sperm cells, which are continually produced beginning at puberty. Sperm cells collect in the lumen of each tubule, pass to the epididymis, and then mature. Each mature sperm cell is about 0.06 mm (60 micrometers) in length, and appears like a tiny tadpole. It has a flattened "head," a cylinder-shaped "body," and a long "tail" **Figure 128**.

The head of a sperm cell has a nucleus and compacted chromatin containing its 23 chromosomes. The acrosome is a small protrusion that contains enzymes needed to help it to penetrate an egg cell during fertilization. The midpiece, or body of the sperm cell, has a filamentous core and spiraled mitochondria. The tail, or flagellum, consists of microtubules in an extension of the cell membrane. The tail moves via adenosine triphosphate (ATP) from the mitochondria, propelling the sperm cell through its containing fluid. Normal development of spermatozoa in the testes requires temperatures that are about 1.1°C, or 2°F lower than temperatures found elsewhere in the body.

A mature spermatozoan lacks an endoplasmic reticulum, a Golgi apparatus, lysosomes, peroxisomes, and many other intracellular structures. The loss of these organelles reduces the

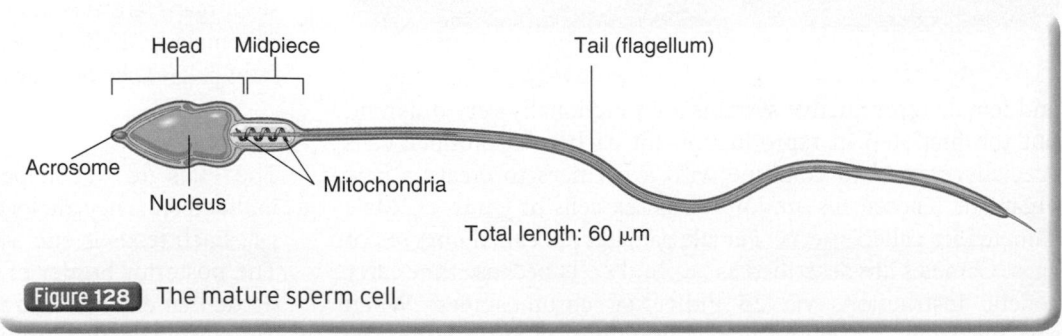

Head   Midpiece   Tail (flagellum)

Acrosome

Nucleus   Mitochondria

Total length: 60 μm

Figure 128   The mature sperm cell.

cell's size and mass. Spermatozoa are basically mobile carriers for the enclosed chromosomes and can be slowed down by extra weight. Because the sperm cell lacks glycogen and other energy reserves, it must absorb nutrients (mostly fructose) from the surrounding fluid.

Spermatogenesis

Spermatogenesis is the process by which sperm cells are formed. In a male embryo, spermatogenic cells are undifferentiated. They are also called spermatogonia, and contain 46 chromosomes. During embryonic development, spermatogonia undergo mitosis, creating two daughter cells. One of these is a new "type A" spermatogonium that maintains supplies of undifferentiated cells; the other is a "type B" spermatogonium that enlarges to become a primary spermatocyte.

During puberty, primary spermatocytes reproduce via meiosis, a type of cell division that includes first and second meiotic divisions. Meiosis I (the first division) separates chromosome pairs that are homologous, meaning "gene for gene." This does not mean they are identical because genes may vary due to hereditary factors. Each homologous chromosome is replicated before meiosis I occurs, so that it consists of two complete DNA strands (chromatids). These attach at areas called centromeres, and carry all of the genetic information associated with that specific chromosome.

Meiosis II causes one member of each homologous pair to separate its chromatids. This produces other haploid cells

(with one set of chromosomes), but with the chromosomes no longer in the replicated form. Meiosis II causes each of the chromatids to become an independent chromosome. Each primary spermatocyte divides into two secondary spermatocytes; these divide again to form two spermatids, which mature. For each primary spermatocyte that undergoes meiosis, four sperm cells, with 23 chromosomes in each of their nuclei, are formed **Figure 129**.

Male Internal Accessory Organs

The structures of the male reproductive system include two epididymides, two vasa deferentia (ductus deferentia), two ejaculatory ducts, the urethra, two seminal vesicles, the prostate gland, and two bulbourethral glands. The epididymides are tightly coiled tubes about 6 meters in length, connected to the posterior border of the testes. Each of them emerges from the top of the testis to descend along its posterior surface, and then course upward to become the vas deferens. Immature sperm cells are nonmotile when they reach the epididymis; therefore, rhythmic peristaltic contractions move them through the duct as they mature. Once mature, sperm cells can move independently to fertilize egg cells, but usually do not actually "swim" until after ejaculation.

The epididymis can be felt through the skin of the scrotum. It is nearly 7 meters in length, and is coiled and twisted so that it takes up only a small amount of space. The epididymis controls the composition of the fluid that is produced by

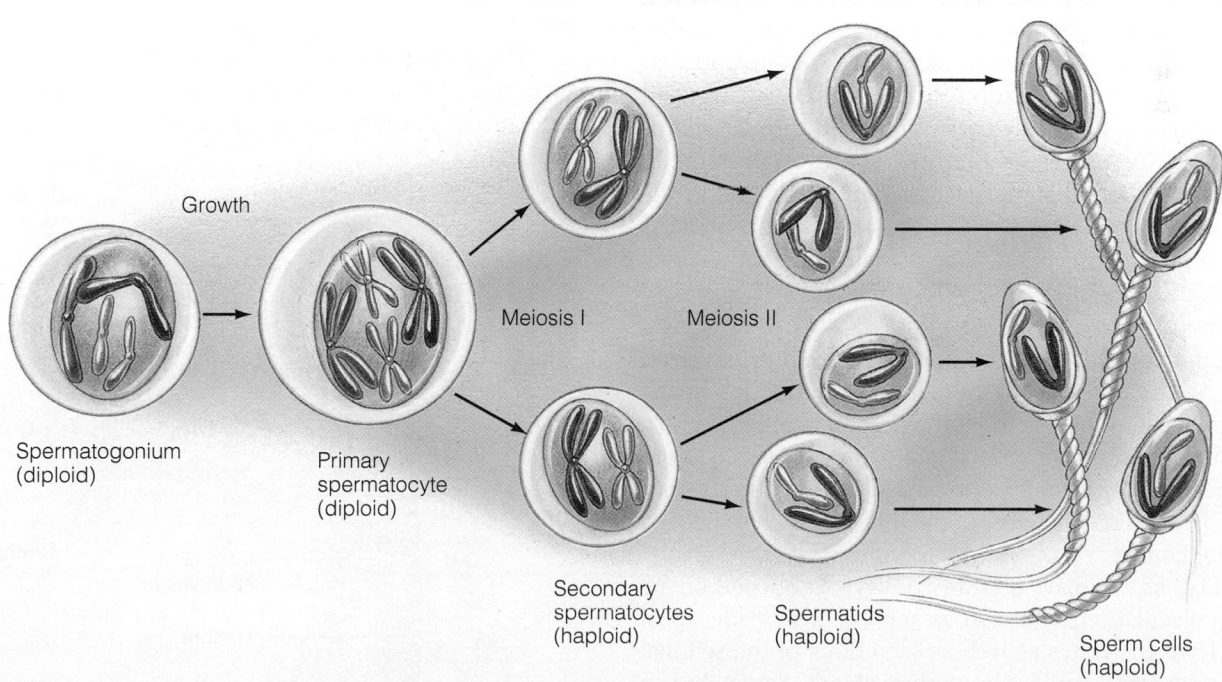

Growth

Meiosis I   Meiosis II

Spermatogonium (diploid)

Primary spermatocyte (diploid)

Secondary spermatocytes (haploid)

Spermatids (haploid)

Sperm cells (haploid)

Figure 129 Meiosis II causes one member of each homologous pair, via a condition called haploid, to separate its chromatids. This produces other haploid cells (with one set of chromosomes), but with the chromosomes no longer in the replicated form. Meiosis II causes each of the chromatids to become an independent chromosome. Each primary spermatocyte divides into two secondary spermatocytes, then dividing again to form two spermatids, which mature. For each primary spermatocyte that undergoes meiosis, four sperm cells, with 23 chromosomes in each of their nuclei, are formed.

the seminiferous tubules. It also absorbs and recycles damaged spermatozoa, while also absorbing cellular debris. The products of the breakdown of enzymes are released into the surrounding interstitial fluids for pickup by the epididymal blood vessels. The epididymis also stores and protects spermatozoa and facilitates their functional maturation.

The <u>vasa deferentia</u> are muscular tubes approximately 45 cm in length. They each pass upward along the medial side of a testis, through the inguinal canal in the lower abdominal wall to enter the pelvic cavity. They end behind the urinary bladder, uniting just outside the prostate gland with the duct of a seminal vesicle. This forms an <u>ejaculatory duct</u>, passing through the prostate gland to empty into the urethra.

The seminal vesicles are sac-like structures approximately 5 cm in length that attach to the vas deferens near the base of the urinary bladder. Each seminal vesicle is a tubular gland having a total length of about 15 cm. They have glandular tissue linings that contribute nearly 60% of semen volume. The seminal vesicles secrete a slightly alkaline fluid. This helps to regulate the pH of the tubular contents as sperm cells travel to outside the body. These secretions contain fructose, a monosaccharide that provides energy for sperm cells, as well as prostaglandins that stimulate muscular contractions within the female reproductive organs. These contractions aid the movement of sperm cells toward the egg cell.

The secretions of the seminal vesicles are discharged into the ejaculatory duct at emission (when peristaltic contractions are occurring in the vas deferens, seminal vesicles, and prostate gland). These contractions are controlled by the sympathetic nervous system. The prostate gland surrounds the proximal portion of the urethra, slightly inferior to the urinary bladder. It is a chestnut-shaped, muscular structure that is approximately 4 cm in width and 3 cm in thickness. It is surrounded by connective tissue and made up of branched tubular glands with ducts that open into the urethra. The prostate secretes a milky fluid with an alkaline pH that neutralizes the acidic fluid that contains the sperm cells. Prostatic fluid enhances the motility of the sperm cells and helps neutralize the vagina's acidic secretions.

The <u>bulbourethral glands</u>, also known as Cowper glands, are about 1 cm in diameter, and lie inferior to the prostate gland surrounded by the external urethral sphincter muscle's fibers. These glands have tubes with epithelial linings secreting a mucus-like fluid as a response to sexual stimulation. The fluid lubricates the end of the penis to prepare for sexual intercourse, even though females secrete most of the lubricating fluid needed for sexual intercourse.

The fluid that the male urethra conveys to outside of the body during ejaculation is known as <u>semen</u>. It is made up of sperm cells from the testes as well as secretions of the seminal vesicles, prostate gland, and bulbourethral glands. Semen has an alkaline pH of 7.5, and includes prostaglandins and nutrients. Between 2 and 5 mL of semen is released at one time, with about 120 million sperm per milliliter.

Sperm cells begin to swim as they mix with accessory gland secretions. They acquire the ability to fertilize a female egg cell once they are inside the female reproductive tract. This ability is called capacitation. It is due to the weakening of the sperm cells' acrosomal membranes.

Male External Reproductive Organs

The male external reproductive organs consist of the scrotum (enclosing the testes) and the penis (through which the urethra passes). The scrotum consists of a pouch of skin and subcutaneous tissue hanging from the lower abdominal region, posterior to the penis. A medial septum subdivides it into two chambers, each enclosing a testis. Each testis is also enclosed in a serous membrane so that it moves smoothly inside the scrotum. The scrotum protects and controls the temperature of the testes, which is important for sex cell production.

When environmental temperatures are cold, the scrotum contracts and wrinkles, moving the testes closer to the pelvic cavity to absorb heat. When it is warmer outside, the scrotum relaxes and hangs loosely to ensure that the testes are about 5°F lower than body temperature. This cooler temperature is better for the sperm cells to be produced and to survive.

The <u>penis</u> is cylindrical in shape, and conveys urine and semen through the urethra. When erect, it stiffens and enlarges, enabling insertion into the vagina during sexual intercourse. The penis is divided into three regions: the root, body, and glans. The root of the penis is the fixed portion that attaches the penis to the body wall. The shaft (or body) of the penis is the tubular, movable portion of the organ. It contains three columns of erectile tissue. It has two dorsal corpora cavernosa and one ventral corpus spongiosum **Figure 130**. Dense connective tissue surrounds each column in a capsule. The penis is enclosed by a layer of connective tissue, a thin layer of subcutaneous tissue, and skin.

The <u>glans penis</u> is the expanded distal end of the penis that surrounds the external urethral orifice. This structure covers the ends of the corpora cavernosa and opens as the external ure-

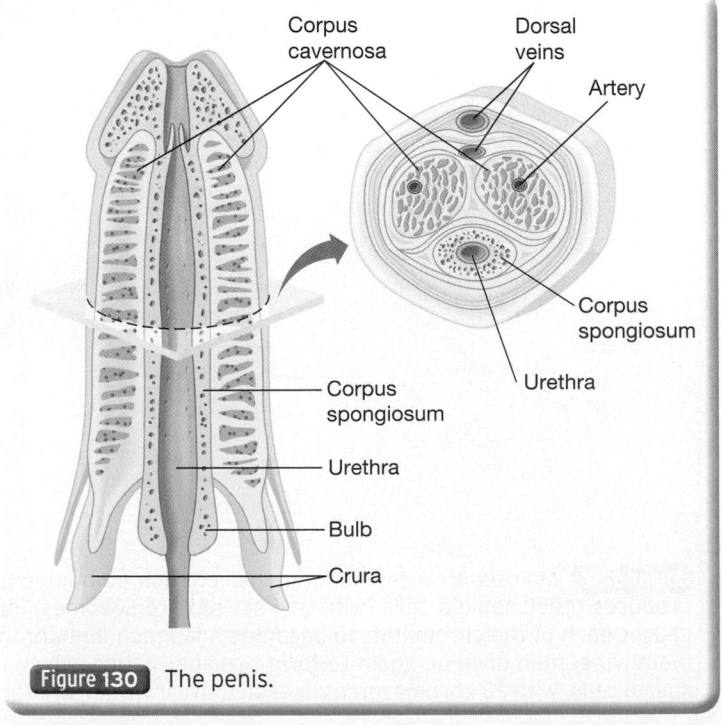

Figure 130   The penis.

thral orifice. Skin in this area is thin and hairless, with sensory receptors for sexual stimulation. Males are born with a loose fold of skin called the foreskin (prepuce) that extends to cover the glans, as a sheath. It is often removed by a surgical procedure called circumcision.

When sexual stimulation occurs, parasympathetic nerve impulses from the sacral area of the spinal cord release nitric oxide (NO), which dilates the arteries leading into the penis. Arterial pressure in the erectile tissue compresses the veins to reduce blood flow away from the penis. The erectile tissues expand with blood and the penis swells and elongates to produce an erection. Physiologic and psychological release, known as an orgasm, is the culmination of sexual stimulation. Male orgasm is accompanied by emission and ejaculation.

The movement of sperm cells from the testes and secretions of the prostate gland and seminal vesicles into the urethra is known as emission. In the urethra, all of these components mix to form semen. Emission occurs as a result of spinal sympathetic nerve impulses that stimulate peristaltic contractions in the testicular ducts, epididymides, vasa deferentia, and ejaculatory ducts. Other sympathetic impulses simultaneously cause rhythmic contractions of the seminal vesicles and prostate gland.

The urethra fills with semen as sensory impulses pass into the sacral portion of the spinal cord. Motor impulses are then transmitted to certain skeletal muscles, causing the penile erectile columns to contract rhythmically. This increases pressure inside the erectile tissues, helping to force semen through the urethra to outside of the body (ejaculation).

Fluid from the bulbourethral glands is expelled first during emission and ejaculation, followed by fluid from the prostate gland, passage of sperm cells, and lastly, fluid from the seminal vesicles. After ejaculation, the arteries of the erectile tissue immediately constrict. Smooth muscles in the vascular spaces contract partially, and veins of the penis carry away excess blood, gradually returning the penis to its flaccid state. Table 28 summarizes the functions of the male reproductive organs.

Male Sex Hormones

Male reproductive functions are controlled by hormones from the hypothalamus, anterior pituitary gland, and testes. The hormones begin and maintain sperm cell production, overseeing development and maintenance of secondary sex characteristics. Before puberty, the male body cannot reproduce, and its spermatogenic cells are undifferentiated. The hypothalamus controls the changes during puberty that make a male's body able to reproduce.

The hypothalamus secretes gonadotropin-releasing hormone, and the anterior pituitary secretes the gonadotropins known as luteinizing hormone (LH) and follicle-stimulating hormone (FSH). LH is also known as interstitial cell–stimulating hormone (ICSH), and promotes development of testicular interstitial cells that secrete male sex hormones. FSH stimulates seminiferous tubule cells to respond to the male sex hormone testosterone. These supporting cells cause spermatogenic cells to undergo spermatogenesis, creating sperm cells. Another hormone, inhibin, is secreted, inhibiting the anterior pituitary gland from oversecreting FSH via negative feedback.

Table 28 The Male Reproductive Organs

Organ	Function
Testis (testes)	
Interstitial cells	Produce and secrete sex hormones
Seminiferous tubules	Produce sperm cells
Epididymis	A coiled duct that connects the rete testis to the vas deferens; it is the site of functional maturation of spermatozoa
Vas deferens	Transfers sperm cells to the ejaculatory duct
Seminal vesicle	Generates an alkaline fluid that contains prostaglandins and nutrients; this fluid helps to neutralize the acidic components of the semen
Prostate gland	The alkaline fluid secreted helps to neutralize the acidity of the semen to enhance motility of sperm cells
Bulbourethral gland	Located at the base of the penis, it secretes fluids into the penile urethra
Scrotum	Regulates the temperature of the testes by enclosing and protecting them
Penis	The copulatory organ that surrounds the urethra and serves to introduce semen into the female vagina

Androgens (male sex hormones) are mostly produced by the testicular interstitial cells, though the adrenal cortex synthesizes small amounts of them. Testosterone is the most important androgen, loosely attaching to plasma proteins for secretion and transport via the blood. Secretion begins during fetal development, continues for several weeks after birth, and almost stops completely during childhood. Between ages 13 and 15 years, its secretion restarts, producing testosterone at a rapid rate, making the body reproductively functional (puberty). Secretion continues after puberty throughout the life of males.

Testosterone enlarges the testes and accessory reproductive organs, and develops the male secondary sex characteristics. These characteristics include the following:

- Increased body hair on the face, chest, armpits, and pubic region
- Sometimes, decreased hair growth on the scalp
- Enlargement of the larynx and thickening of the vocal folds, which lower the pitch of the voice
- Thickening of the skin
- Increased muscular growth, broadening of the shoulders, and narrowing of the waist
- Thickening and strengthening of the bones

Testosterone also increases cellular metabolism and red blood cell production. Males usually have more red blood cells in a microliter of blood than females do because of the actions of testosterone. It also affects the brain, stimulating sexual activity.

The more testosterone received by the interstitial cells, the greater the speed at which the male secondary sex characteristics develop. Testosterone output is regulated by a negative feedback system in the hypothalamus. More testosterone in the blood inhibits the hypothalamus, decreasing gonadotropin-releasing hormone (GnRH) secretion from the anterior pituitary. As LH secretion also falls, testosterone release from the interstitial cells decreases. Decreasing blood testosterone causes the hypothalamus to stimulate the anterior pituitary to release LH. Then the interstitial cells release more testosterone, and the blood testosterone levels increase again. A period in a male's life known as the male climacteric marks a decrease in testosterone level and a decline in sexual function.

The Female Reproductive System and Organs

The female reproductive organs produce and maintain the egg cells (oocytes), which are the female sex cells. The organs also transport them to the site of fertilization, provide a strong environment for the developing fetus, give birth to a fetus, and produce female sex hormones. The principal organs of the female reproductive system (besides the ovaries) are the fallopian (uterine) tubes, uterus, vagina, and the components of the external genitalia. The primary sex organs (gonads) are the two ovaries, which reproduce female sex cells and sex hormones. The accessory sex organs are the internal and external reproductive organs **Figure 131** . As in males, a variety of accessory glands release secretions into the female reproductive tract.

Ovaries

The ovaries are oval-shaped, solid structures about 3.5 cm in length, 2 cm in width, and 1 cm in thickness. They lie in shallow depressions in the lateral pelvic cavity wall. Ovarian tissues consist of an inner medulla and an outer cortex. The medulla is made up of loose connective tissue with many blood and lymphatic vessels as well as nerve fibers. The cortex has more compact tissue with a granular appearance because of masses of ovarian follicles. The ovary's free surface is covered with cuboidal epithelium above a layer of dense connective tissue. The ovaries perform three main functions: (1) production of immature female gametes (oocytes), (2) secretion of female sex hormones (including estrogens and progestins), and (3) secretion of inhibin (involved in the feedback control of pituitary FSH production).

Before birth, a female fetus develops small cell groups in the outer ovarian cortex that form several million **primordial follicles**. Each follicle consists of a primary oocyte surrounded by follicular cells. The primary oocytes begin to undergo meiosis early in development, but then the process stops and does not restart until puberty. No new primordial follicles form after the initial ones form, and oocytes degenerate. Although several million oocytes form in the female embryo, only about 1 million remain at birth, with only 400,000 left at puberty. The ovary releases less than 400 to 500 oocytes during a female's reproductive life.

Oogenesis is the process of egg cell formation, which begins at puberty. During this time, some primary oocytes continue meiosis, with 23 chromosomes in their nuclei like their parent cells. When they divide, the distribution of the oocyte cytoplasm is unequal. The cells that result are different in size. The secondary oocyte is large whereas the first polar body is small **Figure 132** . The large secondary oocyte can be fertilized by a sperm cell. When this occurs, it divides unequally, producing a tiny second polar body and a large fertilized egg cell (zygote).

The polar bodies soon degenerate. They allow for production of egg cells with massive amounts of cytoplasm and

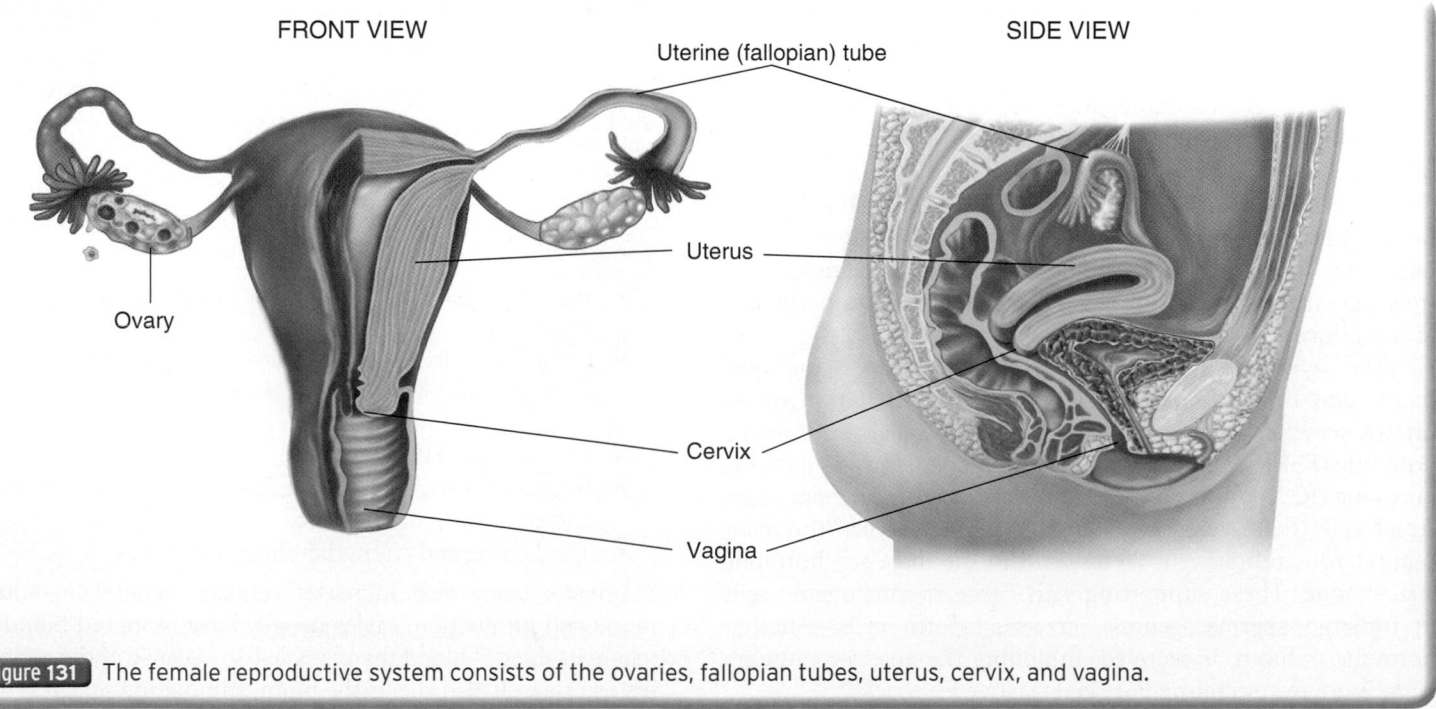

FRONT VIEW   SIDE VIEW

Uterine (fallopian) tube

Ovary

Uterus

Cervix

Vagina

Figure 131 The female reproductive system consists of the ovaries, fallopian tubes, uterus, cervix, and vagina.

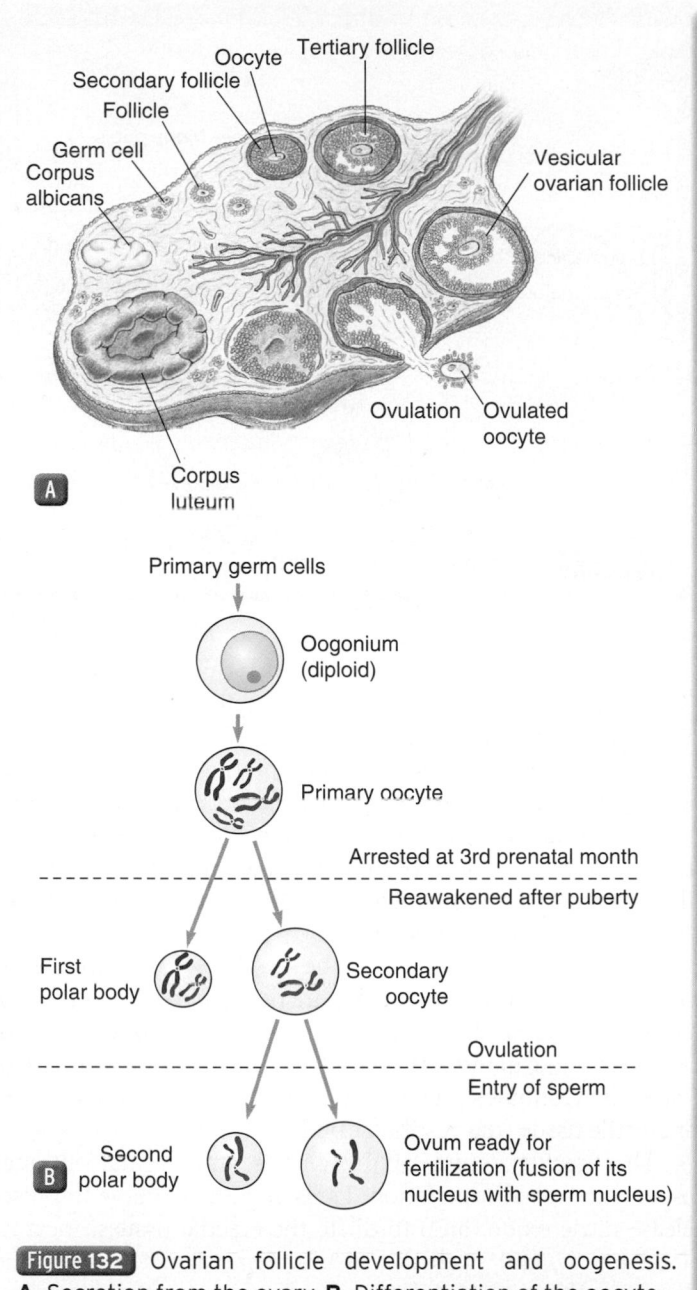

Figure 132 Ovarian follicle development and oogenesis. **A.** Secretion from the ovary. **B.** Differentiation of the oocyte.

radiata). The follicular cells have processes extending through the zona pellucida that supply the secondary oocyte with nutrients. Up to 20 primary follicles mature at once, but one follicle usually grows larger than the others. Usually just the dominant follicle develops fully while the others degenerate.

The primary oocyte undergoes oogenesis, developing a secondary oocyte and first polar body (<u>ovulation</u>). This process releases these developed structures along with one or two layers of follicular cells from the mature follicle. Anterior pituitary gland hormones trigger ovulation, swelling the mature follicle while weakening its wall. The wall ruptures, allowing the fluid and secondary oocyte to ooze from the ovary's surface. After the process is completed, the secondary oocyte and follicular cells are usually moved to the opening of a nearby fallopian tube. If not fertilized within a short time, the oocyte degenerates.

Female Internal Accessory Organs

The female reproductive system includes accessory structures, including two fallopian tubes, a uterus, and a vagina. The <u>uterine tubes</u> (fallopian tubes or oviducts) open near the ovaries, and are each about 10 cm long. They pass medially to the uterus, penetrating its wall, and opening into the uterine cavity. Near the ovaries, each tube expands into a funnel-shaped infundibulum that partially encircles the ovary. Finger-like fimriae surround its margin with one of the larger extensions connecting with the ovary.

The epithelium lining the uterine tube is composed of ciliated columnar epithelial cells, with scattered mucin-secreting cells. The mucosa is surrounded by concentric smooth muscle layers. The transport of occytes involves a combination of ciliar movement and peristaltic contractions in the fallopian tube walls.

If the secondary oocyte is fertilized to become a zygote, the <u>uterus</u> receives the developing embryo, sustaining its development. The uterus is hollow and muscular, shaped slightly like an inverted pear. Its size changes during pregnancy, from about 7.5 cm by 5 cm by 2.5 cm to much larger, able to hold the developing fetus up until birth. In a nonpregnant state, the uterus weighs 30 to 40 grams. The uterus is located in the anterior pelvic cavity, superior to the vagina, usually bending over the urinary bladder. The uterine body (corpus) is the largest portion of the uterus. The fundus is the rounded portion of the corpus, and is superior to the attachment of the uterine tubes. It ends at a constriction known as the isthmus of the uterus. The <u>cervix</u> is the inferior portion of the uterus, extending from the isthmus to the vagina. The cervix surrounds the cervical orifice, where the uterus opens to the vagina.

The uterine wall is thick, with three layers. The <u>endometrium</u> is the inner mucosal layer, covered with columnar epithelium and many tubular glands. Controlled by estrogen, the uterine glands, blood vessels, and epithelium change with the phases of the monthly uterine cycle. The <u>myometrium</u> is the thickest portion of the uterine wall, making up the muscular middle layer, with bundles of smooth muscle fibers. During the female reproductive cycle and during pregnancy, the endometrium and myometrium change greatly. The <u>perimetrium</u> is the outer serosal layer covering the body of the uterus and part of the cervix.

abundant organelles that carry the zygote through its first cell divisions, still with the right number of chromosomes.

During puberty, the anterior pituitary gland secretes higher amounts of FSH, enlarging the ovaries. The primordial follicles mature into <u>primary follicles</u>. During maturation, a primary oocyte enlarges and the surrounding follicular cells proliferate via mitosis. They organize into layers, with a cavity (antrum) appearing in the cellular mass. Clear follicular fluid fills the cavity to bathe the primary oocyte. The cavity moves the primary oocyte to one side.

Eventually, the mature follicle becomes 10 mm or greater in diameter, bulging outward on the ovary surface. The secondary oocyte is large and round, surrounded by a glycoprotein (the zona pellucida) and attached to follicular cells (the corona

The uterus is supported and held in place by suspensory ligaments, which stabilize its position. These include the following:

- *The broad ligaments:* These attach to the entire body of the uterus laterally, and superiorly to the uterine tubes.
- *The uterosacral ligaments:* These extend from the lateral uterus surfaces to the anterior face of the sacrum; they keep the body of the uterus from moving inferiorly and anteriorly.
- *The round ligaments:* These arise on the lateral margins of the uterus just posterior and inferior to the attachments of the uterine tubes; they extend through the inguinal canal to end in the connective tissues of the external genitalia, primarily restricting posterior movement of the uterus.
- *The lateral ligaments:* These extend from the base of the uterus and vagina to the lateral walls of the pelvis; they tend to prevent inferior movement of the uterus, with additional support provided by the pelvic floor muscles and fascia.

The **vagina** is a fibromuscular tube, about 7.5 to 9 cm in length, extending from the cervix to the outside of the body. It conveys uterine secretions, receives the erect penis during intercourse, and provides the open channel for birth. The vagina extends up and back into the pelvic cavity, and lies posterior to the urinary bladder and urethra, but anterior to the rectum. It is attached to these other structures by connective tissues. The **hymen** is a thin membrane of connective tissue and epithelium that partially covers the vaginal orifice. It has a central opening that allows uterine and vaginal secretions to pass to the outside of the body. The three major functions of the vagina include: (1) serving as a passageway for the elimination of menstrual fluids, (2) receiving the penis during sexual intercourse, and (3) holding the spermatozoa prior to their passage into the uterus. The vagina forms the interior portion of the birth canal, through which the fetus passes during delivery.

The vaginal wall has three layers:

- *Inner mucosal layer:* Stratified squamous epithelium with no mucous glands
- *Middle muscular layer:* Mostly smooth muscle fibers; helps to close the vaginal opening
- *Outer fibrous layer:* Dense connective tissue and elastic fibers

Female External Reproductive Organs

The external accessory organs of the female reproductive system include the labia majora, labia minora, clitoris, and vestibular glands **Figure 133**. They surround the openings of the urethra and vagina, composing the **vulva**.

The **labia majora** enclose and protect the other external reproductive organs. They are made up of rounded folds of adipose tissue and thin smooth muscle covered by skin. They lie close together, with a cleft that includes the urethral and vaginal openings separating the labia longitudinally. They merge at their anterior ends to form a medial, rounded elevation called the mons pubis, overlying the symphysis pubis.

The **labia minora** lie between the labia majora, and are flattened, longitudinal folds composed of connective tissue. They have a rich blood supply, and therefore, a pinkish appearance.

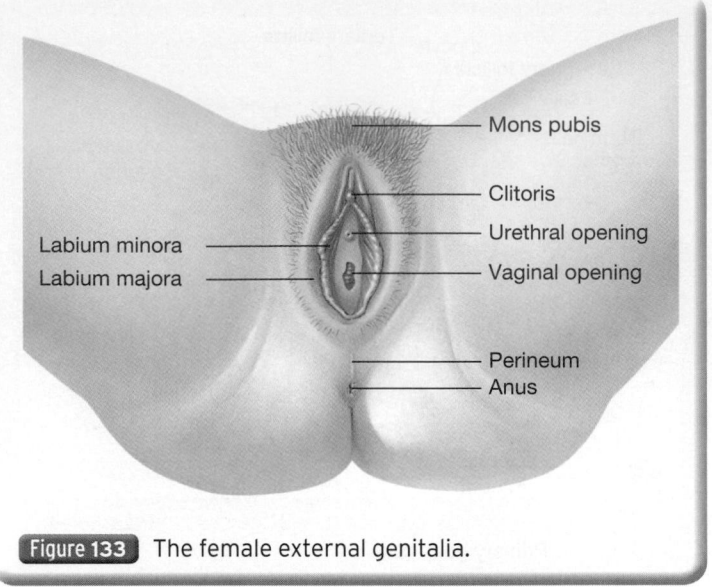

Figure 133   The female external genitalia.

They merge posteriorly with the labia majora. Anteriorly, they converge to form the hood-like covering of the clitoris.

The **clitoris** projects from the anterior end of the vulva between the labia minora. It is usually about 2 cm in length and 0.5 cm in diameter. It corresponds to the penis in males, with a similar structure. It is made up of two columns of erectile tissue (the corpora cavernosa) and forms a glans at its anterior end that has many sensory nerve fibers.

The labia minora encloses the **vestibule**, into which the vagina opens posteriorly. The urethra opens into the vestibule in the midline, about 2.5 cm posterior to the glans of the clitoris. One **vestibular gland** lies on each side of the vaginal opening. Under the vestibule's mucosa, on either side, is a mass of vascular erectile tissue (the vestibular bulb).

The erectile tissues of the clitoris and vaginal entrance respond to sexual stimulation. Parasympathetic nerve impulses release nitric oxide (NO) to dilate the erectile tissues, increase blood inflow, and swell the tissues. The vagina expands and elongates. If sexual stimulation is sufficiently intense, parasympathetic impulses cause the vestibular glands to secrete mucus into the vestibule, moistening and lubricating the surrounding tissues and lower vagina. This facilitates insertion of the penis.

The clitoris responds to local stimulation, culminating in an orgasm if stimulation is sufficient. Just before orgasm, the outer one third of the vagina is engorged with blood. This increases friction on the penis, with orgasm initiating reflexes directed by the sacral and lumbar spinal cord. The muscles of the perineum and walls of both the uterus and uterine tubes contract rhythmically. This helps transport sperm through the female reproductive tract toward the upper uterine tubes. **Table 29** summarizes the functions of the female reproductive organs.

Female Sex Hormones

The female reproductive system is controlled by hormones, involving an interplay between pituitary gland and gonadal secretions. Female hormonal regulation is much more complicated

Table 29   Functions of the Female Reproductive Organs

Organ	Function
Ovary (ovaries)	The female reproductive organ that produces oocytes and sex hormones
Uterine (Fallopian) tube(s)	Transports secondary oocytes in the direction of the uterus; fertilization occurs here, with the developing embryo conveyed to the uterus
Uterus	The muscular organ of the female reproductive tract, in which implantation, placenta formation, and fetal development occur
Vagina	Transports uterine secretions to outside of the body, receives the erect penis during intercourse; the fully developed fetus passes through the vagina during normal delivery
Labia majora	Protects and encloses the external reproductive organs
Labia minora	Protects the openings of the vagina and urethra
Clitoris	Gives pleasurable sensations during sexual stimulation
Vestibule	Contains the vaginal and urethral openings
Vestibular glands	Moisten and lubricate the vestibule with a secretion

than male hormonal regulation because it coordinates both the ovarian and uterine cycles.

The maturation of female sex cells, development and maintenance of secondary sex characteristics, and changes during the monthly reproductive cycle are controlled by the hypothalamus, anterior pituitary gland, and ovaries. Until about age 10 years, the female body is reproductively immature. When the hypothalamus begins to secrete more GnRH, the anterior pituitary releases FSH and LH, controlling female sex cell maturation and producing female sex hormones. The ovaries, adrenal cortices, and placenta (during pregnancy) secrete sex hormones that include estrogens and progesterone. The most abundant of the estrogens is estradiol, followed by estrone and estriol.

In nonpregnant females, the ovaries are the main source of estrogens, and they secrete increasing amounts of estrogens beginning at puberty. These hormones stimulate enlargement of accessory sex organs, and develop and maintain the female secondary sex characteristics:

- Development of breasts and the mammary gland ductile systems
- Increasing adipose tissue deposition in the subcutaneous layer, breasts, thighs, and buttocks
- Increasing skin vascularization

The ovaries are also the main source of progesterone (in nonpregnant females), which promotes uterine changes during the monthly cycle, affects the mammary glands, and helps regulate gonadotropin secretion. Concentrations of androgen in females at puberty produce different changes. These include increased hair growth in the pubic region and armpits. The female skeleton responds to low androgen concentration by narrowing the shoulders and widening the hips.

The female reproductive cycle involves regular, recurring changes in the uterine lining as well as menstrual bleeding (menses). This monthly cycle usually begins around age 13 years, continues into middle age, and then ceases (menopause). A female's first reproductive cycle is called __menarche__. It occurs once the ovaries and other reproductive organs have matured and started responding to specific hormones. Secretion of GnRH stimulates threshold levels of FSH and LH to be released. FSH stimulates maturation of ovarian follicles. Follicular cells produce increased estrogens and some progesterone. LH stimulates some ovarian cells to secrete precursors, such as testosterone, which are used to produce estrogens.

In younger females, estrogens stimulate development of the secondary sex characteristics. They maintain and develop these characteristics as time passes. Increased estrogens during the first week of a reproductive cycle thicken the glandular endometrium of the uterine lining. This is known as the proliferative phase. **Figure 134** shows the various phases of the female reproductive cycle.

The developing follicle matures, and by approximately day 14 of the cycle, it appears on the surface of the ovary as a blister-like bulge. Follicular cells inside the follicle loosen and follicular fluid accumulates. The maturing follicle secretes estrogens that inhibit the anterior pituitary from releasing LH, but allow it to be stored. Anterior pituitary cells become more sensitive to GnRH secreted from the hypothalamus in rhythmic pulses. The stored LH is released, weakening and rupturing the bulging follicular wall. This sends the secondary oocyte and fluid from the ovary (ovulation). The space containing the follicular fluid fills with blood, which clots. The follicular cells enlarge to form a temporary __corpus luteum__.

Corpus luteum cells secrete large amounts of progesterone and estrogens during the last half of the cycle, and blood progesterone concentration increases sharply. Progesterone causes the endometrium to become more vascular and glandular while stimulating uterine gland secretion of more lipids and glycogen. This is known as the secretory phase. Endometrial tissues fill with fluids (made up of nutrients and electrolytes), which support embryo development.

LH and FSH release is then inhibited, and no other follicles develop when the corpus luteum is active. If no egg cell is fertilized, on the 24th day of the cycle the corpus luteum begins to degenerate, to be replaced by connective tissue. The leftover remnant is called a corpus albicans. Then, estrogens and progesterone levels decline, and the endometrium constricts its blood vessels. The uterine lining starts to disintegrate and slough off. Damaged capillaries create a flow of blood and cellular debris, which passes through the vagina (the menstrual flow). It usually

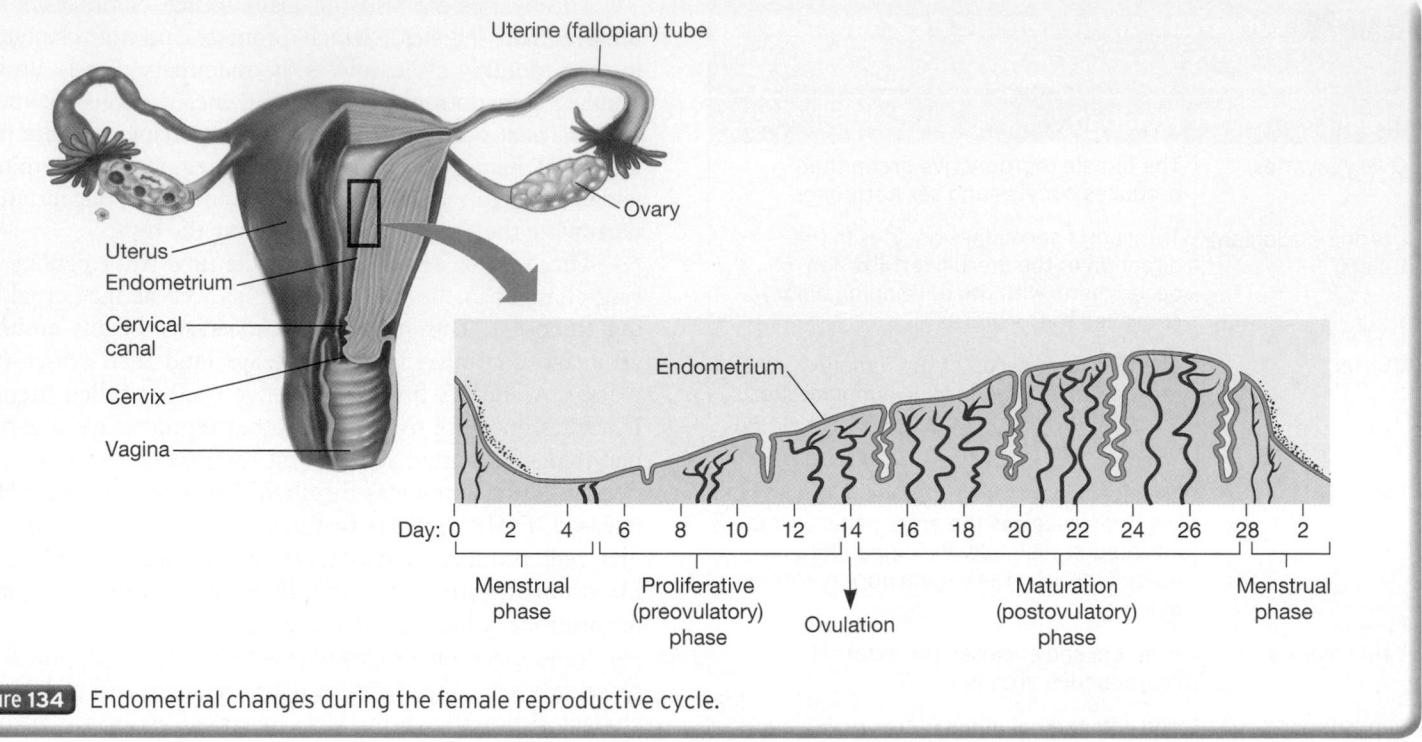

Figure 134 Endometrial changes during the female reproductive cycle.

begins approximately on the 28th day of the cycle, continuing for 3 to 5 days while estrogen concentrations are low. Table 30 summarizes the female reproductive cycle.

The female body undergoes many major changes during pregnancy, including development of the placenta, umbilical cord, and of course, the fetus. These changes, as well as fetal circulation, fetal respiration, stages of labor, and physiologic changes in the infant after birth are covered in the chapter, *Obstetrics*, and in the chapter, *Neonatal Care*.

Nutrition, Metabolism, and Body Temperature

Throughout this discussion of human anatomy and physiology, you have learned about numerous chemical and biologic processes that run continuously as long as the organism is living, and some that continue after the organism has died. The sum total of all of these reactions is called **metabolism**. Laypersons use the term to describe the rate at which your body processes food. For example, someone with a "high metabolism" burns more calories at rest than those with a "low metabolism." This is overly simplistic but essentially true, because a large part of the body's resting metabolism is devoted to the intake, processing, and use of nutrients, the substances on which the "engine" of each individual cell runs. The correct term for the rate at which nutrients are consumed in the body is the **basal metabolic rate**.

The body obtains nutrients through a variety of processes, but the most common are through inhalation, as is the case with oxygen, and ingestion, as in the food you eat. The various systems of the body break down these substances into usable forms. The amount of energy that can be obtained from the nutrients you eat is measured in **kilocalories**, which are commonly known as calories. If the amounts of nutrients are more abundant than the body's needs, some nutrients can be stored, as in the case of lipids, which are stored as fatty tissue. In this way, the body can be prepared for times when nutrients are not plentiful and draw on those reserves. In other cases, excesses cannot be stored and are simply excreted through waste elimination. When the amount of nutrients consumed by the body exceeds the amount of nutrients available, body structures may be metabolized to sustain life.

Digestion and Absorption of Nutrients

Typical meals contain carbohydrates, lipids, proteins, water, electrolytes, and vitamins. The digestive system handles each of these components differently. Digestion involves breaking down large organic molecules before absorption can occur. Water, electrolytes, and vitamins can be absorbed without preliminary breakdown, but may require special transport mechanisms. Discussion of the various types of nutrients is essential to help you understand their actions within the digestive system.

The study of nutrients and how the body uses them is known as nutrition. **Nutrients** include carbohydrates, lipids, proteins, vitamins, minerals, and water. They are grouped as follows:

- *Macronutrients:* Those required in large amounts (carbohydrates, lipids, and proteins); they provide energy and have other specific functions. Potential energy is expressed in calories (units of heat).

Table 30   Steps of the Female Reproductive Cycle

Structure	Function
Anterior pituitary gland	Secretes FSH and LH
Follicle	Maturation is stimulated by FSH
Follicular cells	Produce and secrete estrogens
	Estrogens maintain secondary sex characteristics
Endometrium	Estrogens cause it to thicken
Anterior pituitary gland	Releases a surge of LH, stimulating ovulation
Follicular cells	Become corpus luteum cells, secreting estrogens and progesterone
Uterine wall	Estrogens continue to stimulate its development
Endometrium	Progesterone stimulates it to become more glandular and vascular
Anterior pituitary gland	Estrogens and progesterone inhibit it from secreting LH and FSH
Corpus luteum	If the egg cell is not fertilized, the corpus luteum degenerates and no longer secretes estrogens and progesterone
Blood vessels in the endometrium	As concentrations of estrogens and progesterone decline, these vessels constrict
Uterine lining	Disintegrates and sloughs off, producing menstrual flow
Anterior pituitary gland	No longer inhibited, it again secretes FSH and LH—and the reproductive cycle repeats

- *Micronutrients:* Those required in much smaller amounts (vitamins and minerals); they do not directly provide energy, but allow biochemical reactions that extract energy from macronutrients.

A **calorie** is the amount of heat needed to raise the temperature of a gram of water by 1°C. The calorie used to measure food energy is greater, by 1,000 times. Though referred to commonly as a calorie, it is technically referred to as a kilocalorie.

Cellular oxidation causes the following calorie releases:

- 1 gram of carbohydrate yields about 4 calories.
- 1 gram of protein yields about 4 calories.
- 1 gram of fat yields about 9 calories.

Digestion breaks down nutrients so they can be absorbed and transported via the bloodstream. Essential nutrients are those that human cells cannot synthesize (such as certain amino acids).

Carbohydrates include sugars and starches, and are organic compounds. Energy from carbohydrates mostly is used to power cellular processes. They are ingested in forms that include grains, vegetables, glycogen (from meats), disaccharides (from cane sugar, beet sugar, and molasses), and monosaccharides (from fruits and honey). Digestion breaks carbohydrates down into monosaccharides (which include fructose, galactose, and glucose) for easy absorption. Liver enzymes convert fructose and galactose into glucose, which is the form of carbohydrate most commonly oxidized for use as cellular fuel.

Cellulose is a complex carbohydrate not digestible by humans. It provides bulk (fiber, or roughage) that helps the muscular digestive system walls to push food through its tubes. Many cells get their energy by oxidizing fatty acids, though neurons require continuous glucose in order to survive. The nervous system can be seriously impaired by a lack of glucose. When carbohydrates are not consumed sufficiently, the liver may convert amino acids (from proteins) into glucose.

Some excess glucose is changed to glycogen, which is stored in the liver and muscles. Glucose can be rapidly mobilized from glycogen, but only a certain amount of glycogen can be stored. Excess glucose is usually converted into fat and stored in adipose tissue. For energy, the body first metabolizes glucose, then glycogen into glucose, and lastly, fats and proteins.

Carbohydrates are used by cells to synthesize vital biochemicals such as ribose and deoxyribose (which are needed to produce the nucleic acids RNA and DNA). They are also needed to synthesize the disaccharide lactose (milk sugar) during breast milk secretion. Physically active people need more fuel than others who are more sedentary, but eating excess carbohydrates may cause obesity and increased cardiovascular disease risks. Carbohydrate intake differs for each person, but current estimates state that between 125 and 175 grams of carbohydrates should be consumed daily in order to avoid protein breakdown as well as metabolic disorders that result from the use of excess fat.

Lipids include fats, fat-like substances, and oils. They supply energy for body processes and building of certain structures. As described earlier in the chapter, lipids include fats, steroids (which includes cholesterol), and phospholipids. The most common lipids found in the diet are fats known as triglycerides. They are found in both plant and animal-based foods. Saturated fats are found mostly in meats, eggs, milk, animal fat (lard), palm oil, and coconut oil. These fats, when consumed excessively, are a risk factor for cardiovascular disease. Unsaturated fats exist in nuts, seeds, and plant oils. Monounsaturated fats are found in olive, peanut, and canola oils, and they are the healthiest type of fats. Cholesterol is found in animal products, including liver, egg yolk, whole milk, butter, cheese, and meats. It is not present in foods of plant origin.

Lipids have many functions, but mostly they supply energy. Triglyceride molecules must first undergo hydrolysis (breakdown in the presence of water) before they can release energy. When this occurs, fatty acids and glycerol are released, absorbed, and transported in lymph and blood to the tissues. Some fatty acid portions react to form molecules of acetyl coenzyme A via reactions known as beta oxidation. Excess amounts of this coenzyme convert into ketone bodies such as acetone, and can be reconverted in reverse.

Certain fatty acids cannot be synthesized by the liver. These are known as essential fatty acids. For example, linoleic acid (needed for phospholipid synthesis, cell membrane formation, and transport of lipids) is an essential fatty acid found in corn, cottonseed, and soy oils. Another essential fatty acid is linolenic acid.

Free fatty acids are used by the liver to synthesize triglycerides, phospholipids, and lipoproteins. Lipids are less dense than proteins; therefore, the proportion of lipids in a lipoprotein increases as the density of the particle decreases. The reverse is also true. Very low-density lipoproteins have a relatively high concentration of triglycerides. Low-density lipoproteins have a relatively high concentration of cholesterol. High-density lipoproteins have a relatively high concentration of proteins.

The liver controls cholesterol in the body. It synthesizes cholesterol and releases it into the bloodstream, or removes it from the bloodstream to be excreted via bile, or to produce bile salts. Cholesterol does not create energy but provides structural materials for cell membranes, as well as being important to synthesize certain sex hormones and adrenal hormones. Triglycerides are stored in adipose tissue, and may be hydrolyzed into free fatty acids and glycerol when blood lipid concentration drops, such as during fasting.

Lipids vary in how they may be required for health. Fat intake must be enough to carry the fat-soluble vitamins. Lipids also make foods taste more appetizing. It is recommended that lipid intake not exceed 30% of daily calories.

Proteins are created from amino acids, and include enzymes, plasma proteins, muscle components (actin and myosin), hormones, and antibodies. After digestion breaks proteins down into amino acids, they may also supply energy. They are transported to the liver, where deamination occurs, which is the loss of their nitrogen-containing portions. They react to form the waste urea, excreted in urine.

Foods rich in protein include meats, fish, poultry, cheese, nuts, milk, eggs, and cereals, and in lesser amounts, legumes (including beans and peas). All except nine of the required amino acids can be synthesized by an adult's body. Essential amino acids are those that the body cannot synthesize on its own. The body requires all of these amino acids for proper growth and tissue repair.

The three classes of proteins are complete, incomplete, and partially complete proteins. Complete proteins (found in milk, meats, and eggs) have adequate amounts of the essential amino acids. Incomplete proteins (such as those in corn) have too little tryptophan and lysine to maintain human tissues or support growth and development. A partially complete protein (such as gliadin, found in wheat) does not have enough lysine to promote growth, but does have enough to maintain life.

Proteins supply the essential amino acids and provide nitrogen and other elements. Protein requirements differ based on body size, metabolism, activity levels, and other factors. Nutritionists recommend a daily protein intake of 0.8 grams per kilogram of body weight; therefore, most average adults should consume 60 to 150 grams of protein per day.

Vitamins are other organic compounds that are required for normal metabolism. Body cells cannot synthesize adequate amounts of vitamins, so they must come from foods. They are classified by their solubility. Fat-soluble vitamins include A, D, E, and K. Water-soluble vitamins include the B vitamin group and vitamin C.

Bile salts in the small intestine promote absorption of fat-soluble vitamins. They accumulate in various tissues and intake must be controlled. For example, when too much vitamin A is consumed, the body receives too much beta carotene, and the skin may appear orange in color. **Table 31** explains the fat-soluble vitamins, including their adult recommended daily allowance (RDA).

The water-soluble vitamins include the B vitamins and vitamin C. The B vitamins consist of compounds essential for normal metabolism, and help to oxidize carbohydrates, lipids, and proteins. They are often present together in foods, hence they are referred to as the vitamin B complex. Cooking and food processing destroy some of these vitamins. Vitamin C (ascorbic acid) is one of the least stable vitamins. It is found in many plant foods, and is necessary for the body to produce collagen, convert folacin to folinic acid, and metabolize certain amino acids. Vitamin C also promotes synthesis of hormones from cholesterol and is vital for iron absorption.

Minerals are inorganic elements essential for human metabolism. Humans obtain minerals from plant foods, or from animals that have eaten plants. Minerals are most concentrated in the bones and teeth, and make up about 4% of body weight. Certain minerals are often incorporated into organic molecules, such as phosphorus (found in phospholipids), iron (in hemoglobin), and iodine (in thyroxine). Others are part of inorganic compounds, such as calcium phosphate (in bone). Still others are free ions (sodium, chloride, and calcium) in blood.

Minerals make up part of every cell's structure, and are present in enzymes, affect osmotic pressure, and are required for nerve impulse conduction. Other functions that rely on minerals include blood coagulation, muscle fiber contraction, and pH of body fluids. The minerals calcium and phosphorus make up almost 75% (by weight) of the body's mineral elements. These are called major minerals.

Trace elements are essential minerals that are found in small amounts. Each makes up less than 0.005% of adult body weight.

When a person's diet lacks essential nutrients, malnutrition results. This may be due to either undernutrition or overnutrition. Causes can include lack of food, poor-quality food, overeating, or taking too many vitamin supplements. Overeating, as well as insufficient exercise, results in the body becoming overweight, and potentially obese (defined as having a body mass index of 30 or more). A person's body mass index (BMI) is used to determine adequate weight, being overweight, or being obese. BMI is calculated by dividing a person's weight in kilograms (1 kg = 2.2 lb) by height in meters squared (1 ft = 0.3 m). For example, a person who is 5′ 6″ tall is equivalent to 1.65 m tall. If this person weighs 180 lb, that is equivalent to 82 kg. By dividing 82 kg by 1.65 m², a BMI of 29 is found, which is considered overweight but not obese.

Table 31 Fat-Soluble Vitamins

Vitamin	Source	Adult RDA	Characteristics	Functions
A	Liver, fish, whole milk, butter, eggs, leafy green vegetables, yellow and orange vegetables, and fruits	4,000 to 5,000 international units (IU)	Several forms; synthesized from carotenes; stored in liver; stable in heat, acids, and bases; unstable in light	Necessary for synthesis of visual pigments, mucoproteins, and mucopolysaccharides; for normal development of bones and teeth; and for maintenance of epithelial cells
D	Produced when skin is exposed to ultraviolet light; also exists in milk, egg yolk, fish liver oils, and fortified foods	400 IU	A group of steroids; resistant to heat, oxidation, acids, and bases; stored in liver, skin, brain, spleen, and bones	Promotes absorption of calcium and phosphorus, as well as development of teeth and bones
E	Oils from cereal seeds, salad oils, margarine, shortenings, fruits, nuts, and vegetables	30 IU	A group of compounds; resistant to heat and visible light; unstable in presence of oxygen and ultraviolet light; stored in muscles and adipose tissues	An antioxidant; prevents oxidation of vitamin A and polyunsaturated fatty acids; may help maintain stability of cell membranes
K	Leafy green vegetables, egg yolk, pork liver, soy oil, tomatoes, cauliflower	55 to 70 micrograms	Occurs in several forms; resistant to heat, but destroyed by acids, bases, and light; stored in the liver	Required for synthesis of prothrombin, which functions in blood clotting

After digestion, individual cells are supplied these nutrients and use them in various processes. The term that encompasses all of the processes occurring within the cell is <u>cellular metabolism</u>. Within these processes, nutrients can be broken down from complex to simpler forms or complex forms can be built from those building blocks. When complex molecules are broken down, energy is released that may be used for other cellular processes.

■ Cellular Metabolism

Metabolism consists of the chemical changes that take place inside living cells. As a result of metabolism, organisms grow, maintain body functions, release or store energy, produce and eliminate waste, digest nutrients, or destroy toxins. These reactions alter the chemical nature of a chemical substance, maintaining homeostasis.

Two major types of metabolic reactions control how cells use energy. The buildup of larger molecules from smaller molecules is called anabolism. The breakdown of larger molecules into smaller ones is called catabolism. Each of these actions requires the use of energy.

Anabolism

<u>Anabolism</u> is the process of building complex molecules in the body from simpler materials. When a person is healthy and has adequate nutrition, simple nutrients (such as amino acids, fats, and glucose) are used by the body to build the basic chemicals that support cellular functioning and sustain life.

Anabolism supplies biochemicals needed for cells to grow and repair themselves. An example of anabolism is when simple sugar molecules (monosaccharides) are linked to form a chain, making up molecules of glycogen (a carbohydrate). This anabolic process is called dehydration synthesis. As the links in this chain are formed, an OH (hydroxyl group) is removed from one molecule while an H (hydrogen atom) from another is removed. Together the OH and H produce a water molecule (H_2O). The monosaccharides are then joined by a shared oxygen atom, making the chain grow.

Dehydration synthesis, which links glycerol and fatty acid molecules in adipose (fat) cells, forms fat molecules (triglycerides). This occurs when three hydrogen atoms are removed from a glycerol molecule. An OH group is removed from each of three fatty acid molecules. This creates three water molecules and one fat molecule. Oxygen atoms are then shared between the glycerol and fatty acid portions.

Cells also use dehydration synthesis to join amino acid molecules, eventually forming protein molecules. As two amino acids unite, one OH molecule is removed from one of them, while one H molecule is removed from the NH_2 group of another. This forms a water molecule. The amino acid molecules are then joined by a bond created between a nitrogen atom and a carbon atom (a peptide bond).

A dipeptide is formed from two amino acids bound together, and a polypeptide is formed from many amino acids bound into a chain. Polypeptides usually have specialized functions. When a polypeptide has more than 100 molecules, it is considered to be a protein. Certain protein molecules have more than one polypeptide.

Catabolism

<u>Catabolism</u> can be defined as the metabolic breakdown of stored carbohydrates, fats, or proteins in order to provide energy. It occurs continuously to differing degrees. Excessive catabolism

leads to wasting of tissues. An example of catabolism is the process of hydrolysis, which is actually the opposite of dehydration synthesis. This involves the decomposition of carbohydrates, lipids, and proteins.

Hydrolysis splits a water molecule; for example, hydrolysis of sucrose (a disaccharide) gives off glucose and fructose (two monosaccharides) as the water molecule splits. The equation is as follows:

$$C_{12}H_{22}O_{11} + H_2O \rightarrow C_6H_{12}O_6 + C_6H_{12}O_6$$
(Sucrose) (Water) (Glucose) (Fructose)

As shown in the equation, inside the sucrose molecule, the bond between the simple sugars breaks. The water molecule supplies a hydrogen atom to one of the sugar molecules while supplying a hydroxyl group to the other.

Both dehydration synthesis and hydrolysis are reversible, and are summarized in the following equation:

Hydrolysis → Disaccharide + Water ↔ Monosaccharide + Monosaccharide ← Dehydration synthesis

During digestion, hydrolysis breaks down carbohydrates into monosaccharides. It also breaks down fats into glycerol and fatty acids, nucleic acids into nucleotides, and proteins into amino acids.

Control of Metabolic Reactions

Nerve, muscle, and blood cells are specialized to carry out distinctive chemical reactions; however, every type of cell performs basic chemical reactions. These include the buildup and breakdown of carbohydrates, lipids, nucleic acids, and proteins. Enzymes coordinate hundreds of rapid chemical changes to control metabolic reactions.

Enzymes and Their Actions

As mentioned earlier, an enzyme is a protein that catalyzes biochemical reactions. Enzymes are among the most important of all the body's proteins. They catalyze the reactions that sustain life. Nearly everything that occurs in the human body relies on a specific enzyme. In the body, enzymes assist in the digestion of food, drug metabolism, protein formation, and many other types of reactions. Enzymes make metabolic reactions possible inside cells by controlling temperature conditions that otherwise would be too mild for them to occur.

Enzymes are complex molecules. They lower the amount of activation energy needed for metabolic reactions. This speeds up the rates of the reactions in a process called catalysis. Enzyme molecules that are not used in the reactions they catalyze are recycled. Activation energy is defined as the excess energy that must be added to an atomic or molecular system to allow a particular process to take place.

Enzymes catalyze specific reactions. Each enzyme acts on a <u>substrate</u>, which is a particular chemical affected by the enzyme. Enzymes are often named after their substrates using

the suffix -ase. For example, a lipid is catalyzed by an enzyme called a lipase. Another enzyme, called a catalase, breaks down hydrogen peroxide into water and oxygen. Hydrogen peroxide is a toxic substance that results from certain metabolic reactions.

Every cell holds hundreds of various enzymes, each of which recognizes its specific substrates. Enzyme molecules have three-dimensional shapes (conformations) that allow them to identify their substrates. The coiled and twisted polypeptide chain of each enzyme fits the shape of its substrate. The active site of an enzyme molecule combines with portions of its substrate molecules temporarily. This forms an enzyme–substrate complex.

When enzyme–substrate complexes are formed, some chemical bonds within the substrates are distorted or strained. Requiring less energy as a result, the enzyme is released as it was originally configured. Enzyme-catalyzed reactions can be summarized as follows:

Substrate molecules +	Enzyme molecule →	Enzyme-substrate complex →	Produce (changed substrates)	Enzyme + molecule

These reactions are often reversible. Sometimes, the same enzyme catalyzes the reaction in both directions. The reactions occur at differing rates, based on the number of molecules of the enzyme and its substrate. Some enzymes process a few substrate molecules every second, whereas others can process thousands in the same length of time.

Altering of Enzymes

Enzymes are most often proteins that can change due to exposure to heat, electricity, chemicals, radiation, or fluids that have extreme pH levels. Many enzymes are inactive at 45°C (111°F), and most of them are denatured at 55°C (131°F). Denaturing is defined as changing or altering some of the structures of the enzyme. Poisons such as potassium cyanide denature enzymes to achieve their effects. The poison stops the cells from being able to release energy from nutrient molecules.

Some enzymes must combine with a non-protein component in order to be active. These non-protein components are referred to as cofactors, and may be an element's ion (such as calcium, magnesium, copper, iron, or zinc). They may also be small (non-protein) organic molecules called coenzymes. The human body converts many vitamins into essential coenzymes. An example of a coenzyme is coenzyme A, which is involved in cellular respiration.

Chemical Energy

The ability to do work, and to change or move matter, is called energy. Most metabolic processes use chemical energy. Other forms of energy include heat, light, electrical energy, mechanical energy, and sound.

Chemical Energy Release

When the bonds between the atoms of molecules are broken, chemical energy is released. When a substance is burned, for example, bonds break and energy escapes as both light and heat. During the process of <u>oxidation</u>, cells "burn" molecules of glucose to release chemical energy that fuels the process of anabolism; however, oxidation is different from the burning of substances that exist outside cells.

Inside the cells, enzymes reduce the amount of activation energy needed for oxidation as part of cellular respiration. Energy is released in the bonds of nutrient molecules. The cells then transfer about 40% of the released energy to special energy-carrying molecules. The remaining energy escapes as heat, helping the body to remain at a normal temperature.

■ Cellular Respiration

<u>Cellular respiration</u> is a process that releases energy from organic compounds. This process requires three types of reactions: glycolysis, the citric acid cycle, and the electron transport chain. In cellular respiration, glucose and oxygen are needed. The products of these reactions include carbon dioxide, water, and energy. Therefore, in cellular respiration, the presence of oxygen is vital to produce a significant amount of energy.

Glycolysis

<u>Glycolysis</u> is a process that involves a series of enzymatically catalyzed reactions in which glucose is broken down to yield lactic acid or pyruvic acid. The breakdown releases energy as adenosine triphosphate (ATP) **Figure 135** . The six-carbon sugar glucose is broken down in the cytosol; it becomes 2 three-carbon pyruvic acid molecules, gaining two ATP molecules and releasing high-energy electrons.

Glycolysis begins the process of cellular respiration. It occurs in the cytosol (the liquid portion of the cytoplasm). Glycolysis does not require oxygen and is occasionally referred to as the anaerobic phase. If oxygen is present in the right amounts, pyruvic acid, which is generated by glycolysis, can enter the more energy-efficient pathways of aerobic respiration. These pathways are located in the mitochondria.

Aerobic reactions yield as many as 36 ATP molecules per glucose molecule. Completely decomposed glucose molecules can produce up to 38 molecules of ATP. Most result from the aerobic phase, with only two resulting from glycolysis. Approximately half of the released energy is used for ATP synthesis, while the rest becomes heat. The oxidation of glucose also produces carbon dioxide (which is exhaled) and water (which is absorbed into the internal body environment). The volume of water produced by metabolism is lower than the requirements of the body, so the drinking of water is necessary for survival.

Citric Acid Cycle

The citric acid cycle is also called the tricarboxylic acid cycle or the TCA cycle. It is a sequence of enzymatic reactions involving the metabolism of carbon chains of glucose, fatty acids, and amino acids to yield carbon dioxide, water, and high-energy phosphate bonds (ATP). The three-carbon pyruvic acids enter the mitochondria, each losing a carbon. They then combine with a coenzyme to form a two-carbon acetyl coenzyme A, and

release more high-energy electrons; then, each acetyl coenzyme A combines with a four-carbon oxaloacetic acid to form a six-carbon citric acid.

A series of reactions removes two carbons, synthesizes one ATP molecule, and releases more high-energy electrons **Figure 136** . When food is ingested, large macromolecules are broken down to simple molecules. Proteins are broken down into amino acids, carbohydrates are broken down into simple sugars (glucose), and fats are broken down into both glycerol and fatty acids. The breakdown of simple molecules to acetyl coenzyme A is accompanied by the production of limited amounts of ATP (via glycolysis) and high-energy electrons.

Glucose, through glycolysis, is converted into pyruvic acid. Glycerol and amino acids are also broken down into pyruvic acid. Actually, all of these processes result, in differing ways, in acetyl coenzyme A. Complete oxidation of acetyl coenzyme A to H_2O and CO_2 produces high-energy electrons, which yield greater amounts of ATP via the electron transport chain. In the TCA cycle, the process of oxidation provides more molecules of ATP.

Electron Transport Chain

In the electron transport chain, the high-energy electrons still contain most of the chemical energy of the original glucose molecule. Special carrier molecules bring them to enzymes that store most of the remaining energy in more ATP molecules; heat and water are also produced. Oxygen is the final electron acceptor in this step; therefore, the overall process is termed aerobic respiration.

For cellular respiration, glucose and oxygen are required. This process produces carbon dioxide, water, and energy. Nearly half of the energy is recaptured as high-energy electrons stored in the cells through the synthesis of ATP.

Each ATP molecule has a chain of three chemical groups. These groups are called phosphates. Some of the energy is recaptured in the bond of the end phosphate. When energy is later needed, the terminal phosphate bond breaks to release the stored energy. Cells use ATP for many functions, including active transport and the synthesis of needed compounds.

When an ATP molecule has lost its terminal phosphate, it becomes an ADP (adenosine diphosphate) molecule. ADP can be converted back into ATP by adding energy and a third phosphate. ATP and ADP molecules shuttle between the energy-releasing reactions of cellular respiration and the energy-using reactions of the cells **Figure 137** .

Metabolic Pathways

There are a number of steps in each of the processes of cellular respiration, anabolic reactions, and catabolic reactions. A specific sequence of enzymatic actions controls these reactions; therefore, the enzymes are organized in the exact same sequence as the reactions they control. Each sequence of enzyme-controlled reactions is called a metabolic pathway.

An enzyme-controlled reaction usually increases its rate if the number of substrate molecules or enzyme molecules increases; however, the rate is often determined by

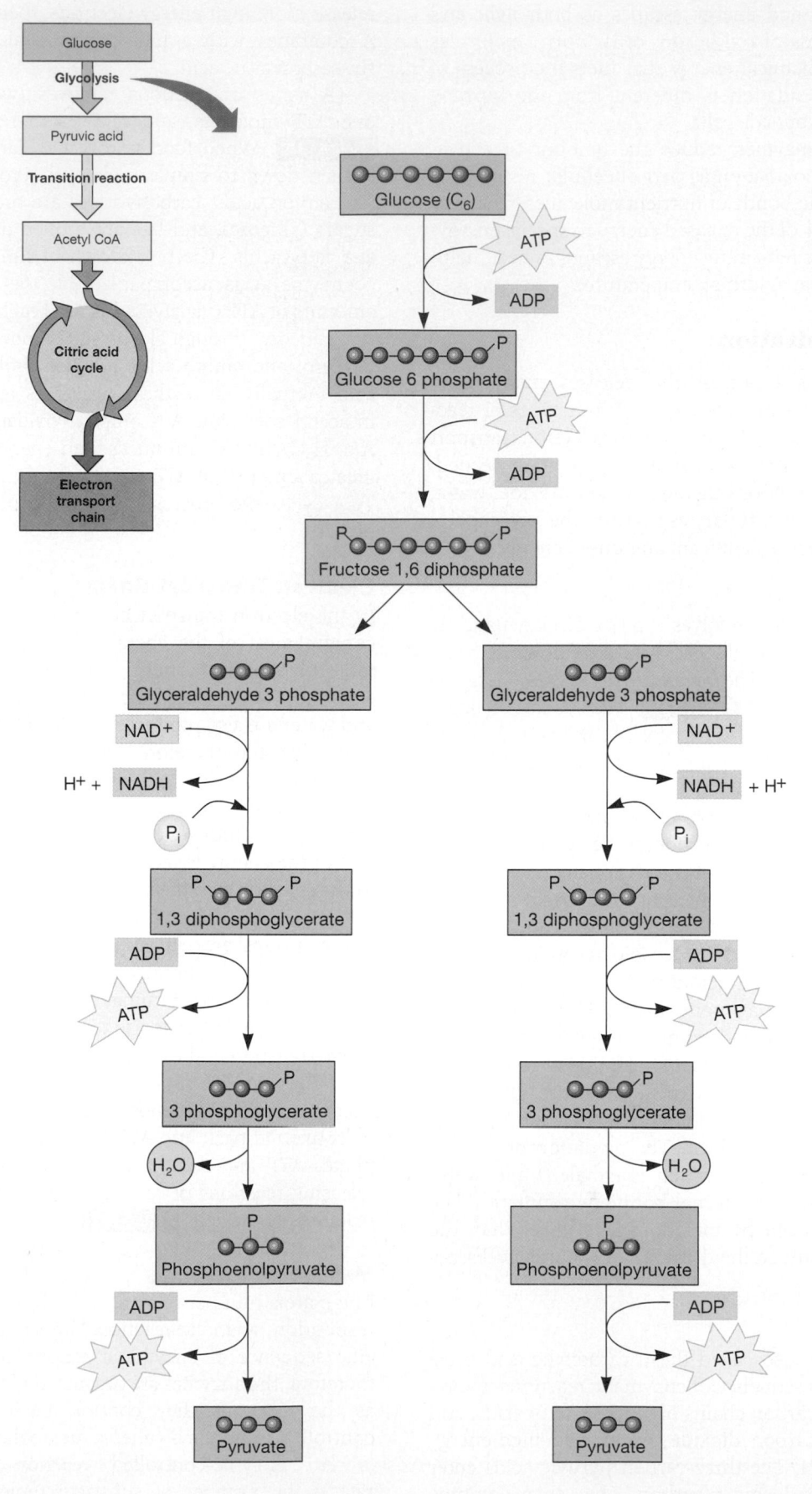

Figure 135 Glycolysis.

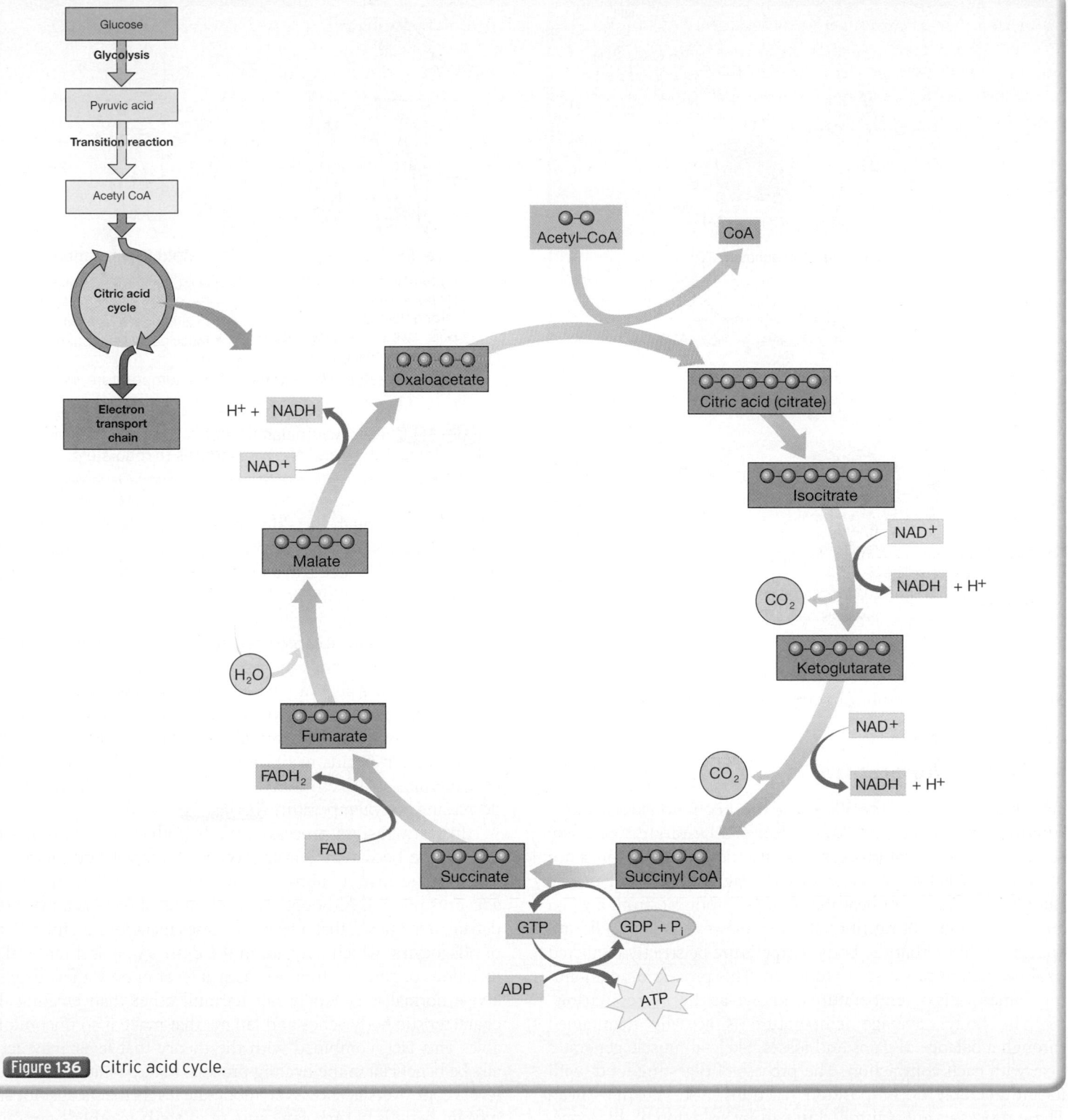

Figure 136 Citric acid cycle.

an enzyme that regulates one of the reaction's steps. Regulatory enzyme molecules are limited, and when the substrate concentration exceeds a certain level, the enzyme supply can become saturated. When this occurs, increasing substrate molecules will no longer have any effect on the reaction rate. Because of this, just one enzyme can control the entire pathway.

A rate-limiting enzyme is usually the first enzyme in a series. Being first is critical because if a rate-limiting enzyme were located somewhere else in the chemical pathway, an intermediate chemical could accumulate at that point. Fats and proteins, as well as glucose, can be broken down to release energy needed to synthesize ATP. In all three cases, aerobic

Adenosine triphosphate (ATP)

ATP

ADP

Energy
released

Figure 137 ATP and ADP molecules.

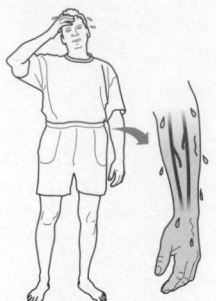
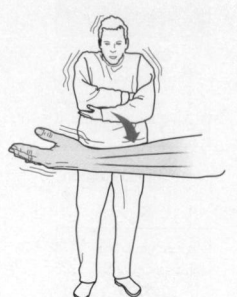

Hot Environment
- Hypothalamus stimulated
- Blood vessels dilate, maximizing heat loss from skin
- Body sweats, causing evaporation and cooling

Body temperature *decreases*

Cold Environment
- Hypothalamus stimulated
- Blood vessels constrict, minimizing heat loss from skin
- Muscles shiver, generating heat

Body temperature *increases*

Figure 138 The hypothalamus notes a rise or fall in core body temperature and elicits responses to regulate it.

respiration is still the final result of these breakdown processes. The most common point of entry is into the citric acid cycle as acetyl coenzyme A.

Body Temperature

Temperature is one of the oldest and most common factors measured when assessing the body. Heat is a by-product of many cellular and chemical processes, so it follows that the presence of body heat is one of the most basic signs of life. In fact, the calorie is a measure of heat that may be produced from a given amount of food, not nutritional value. However, many cells and enzymes require that the body temperature be strictly regulated to allow certain processes to function. This process of maintaining homeostasis of temperature is known as <u>thermoregulation</u>.

The body's average temperature is actually maintained through a balance of gains and losses. Skeletal muscle generates heat with each contraction. The process of digesting food, with its innumerable decomposition reactions, also generates heat. These processes are controlled in part by secretion of thyroxine, which has many functions, one of which being regulation of body temperature. They can also be influenced by activation of the sympathetic nervous system. The body also has means for releasing heat. The simplest of these mechanisms can be seen when a person exercises in warm atmospheres: The pulse quickens, circulating more blood to the periphery, where it can

give off heat through the skin; the skin itself begins to perspire, which amplifies heat loss through evaporation; and the respirations accelerate, which exchanges warmed air for cooler air with each breath. Inhibition of digestion and other mechanisms of heat generation also contribute to net heat loss.

The commonly accepted average body temperature is 37°C, or 98.6°F. However, body temperature can vary slightly from person to person and also vary based on conditions without causing any adverse effect on the body; therefore, these variances are not necessarily considered abnormal or pathologic. Body temperature regulation begins in the hypothalamus, which acts similar to a thermostat in activating the mechanisms for increasing or decreasing body temperature **Figure 138**.

In many disease processes, the hypothalamus is influenced to raise the body temperature. When the target body temperature is more than 1° above the patient's "normal" temperature, a fever is present. Although the usefulness of fever is a matter of debate, it is known that a fever increases metabolism and activity of phagocytes, which may aid in the destruction and removal of infectious organisms. In most cases, a fever of only a few degrees above normal is generally not harmful other than creating the characteristic body aches and fatigue that make it so uncomfortable. This fact, combined with the theory that fever may actually be beneficial in the healing process, makes treatment of mild fevers controversial. However, moderate fevers that persist for significant periods of time can cause or exacerbate other symptoms and effects of illness, such as dehydration. High fevers can cause febrile seizures in children and, if they persist, have the potential to cause long-term CNS damage in children and adults. For this reason, moderate to high fevers are usually treated with antipyretics such as acetaminophen or ibuprofen, and dangerously high fevers are sometimes treated with active cooling measures.

YOU *are the Medic* | SUMMARY |

1. Since the patient has been removed from the vehicle, how can you assess mechanism of injury?

Because the vehicle in which the patient was injured is still on scene, have a crew member assess its interior. Look for intrusion into the patient compartment, evidence of air bag deployment, and seat belt use (if possible). If the glass is shattered, note the location of the glass and how it may relate to the patient's location in the vehicle. If the glass is only partially shattered, in which direction did the glass dent? If it dented outward, look for something inside the vehicle that may have struck the glass on impact. If the glass is dented inward, look for the source of the impact from the outside. Look for and document findings such as blood and/or tissue, hair, and the position of the seats.

2. After scene safety and protection of yourself and partner, what is your first concern?

Scene safety for yourself and your partner/crew is the primary concern. After you ensure your safety, your next concern is to move the bystanders away from the patient and away from danger. In this instance the roadway is described as "major," which may indicate heavy traffic or higher speeds. Keeping everyone safe is vitally important.

Preventing further manipulation of the patient by bystanders is also a priority, especially because one bystander is placing a cushion under the patient's head. Determine if more than one person was inside the vehicle at the time of the collision. If the bystanders are unsure, look for evidence of a second person inside the vehicle, such as drinks, clothing, or toys.

3. What structures may be injured in the left shoulder?

The bony structures that may be injured include the scapula, clavicle, upper ribs, and the proximal end of the humerus. Underneath these structures, the following may be injured: the upper lobe of the left lung and the subclavian arteries and veins. Remember, when an object comes into contact with the body, the bones are not the only area of injury. Structures protected by bones continue to travel with momentum and will make impact within the affected cavity.

4. What structures may be injured in the left lateral neck?

The bony structures that may be injured include the cervical spine, the base of the skull, and possibly the mandible. Spinal injury should also be suspected. Possible injuries to the left carotid artery and jugular vein should also be suspected. A significant hematoma in the area of the carotid artery may occlude the artery. The patient's upper airway may have been injured in the impact. Observe the entire neck anteriorly and posteriorly prior to placing a cervical spine stabilization collar.

5. What is the obvious injury you find to the patient's chest?

There is an injury to the true and false ribs anteriorly, and possibly to the sternum/xiphoid process/manubrium.

6. What are the potential hidden injuries you should consider?

With the findings of unequal chest rise and fall as well as a grating sensation, there may be substantial injury to the lungs and upper and lower airways. The heart and great vessels located in the chest cavity may have also been injured. Injury to the upper abdominal structures should also be considered.

7. What structures are located in the abdominal area under the noted bruising?

The upper left lateral quadrant of the abdomen contains the left lobe of the liver, spleen, pancreas, adrenal gland, portions of the left kidney, and parts of the colon. Abdominal injuries can be difficult to assess. During your assessment, gently palpate the entire abdomen starting at the location furthest from the apparent injury site. You are looking for guarding, which is the voluntary tensing of muscles. Assessment of reaction to pain will also be essential. You may also find rigidity, which could indicate internal bleeding. As blood and other fluids collect in the abdominal cavity, it will eventually feel rigid.

8. How can you determine what structures are actually injured in the abdominal cavity?

The short answer is that unless the injury is an open injury where structures are visible, you cannot determine internal injuries. Knowledge of anatomy, physiology, and signs/symptoms of internal injury will be the key to treating your patient.

YOU *are the Medic*   **SUMMARY,** *continued*

EMS Patient Care Report (PCR)

Date: 04-02-11	Incident No.: 245	Nature of Call: MVC		Location: N/B I-95 @ county line	
Dispatched: 1430	En Route: 1430	At Scene: 1440	Transport: 1450	At Hospital: 1507	In Service: 1515

Patient Information

Age: 22 **Sex:** M **Weight (in kg [lb]):** 91 kg (200 lb)	**Allergies:** Unknown **Medications:** Unknown **Past Medical History:** Unknown **Chief Complaint:** Unresponsive from MVC

Vital Signs

Time: 1445	BP: 106/70	Pulse: 120	Respirations: 24	Spo$_2$: 93%
Time: 1450	BP: 102/66	Pulse: 118	Respirations: 24	Spo$_2$: 93%
Time: 1455	BP: 100/58	Pulse: 122	Respirations: 24	Spo$_2$: 92%
Time: 1500	BP: 95/50	Pulse: 128	Respirations: 24	Spo$_2$: 91%

EMS Treatment
(circle all that apply)

Oxygen @ __15__ L/min via (circle one): NC (NRM) Bag-mask device	Assisted Ventilation	Airway Adjunct:	CPR
Defibrillation	Bleeding Control	(Bandaging)	(Splinting)	Other

Narrative

Crew dispatched to a passenger vehicle that struck a concrete bridge support at high speed. On arrival, found pt unresponsive, lying supine on the pavement after reportedly being removed from the vehicle by bystanders. Heavy damage noted to the front of the vehicle and driver's door with intrusion into the patient compartment. Pt's spine immobilized manually immediately and placed in full spinal precautions per protocol. Pt responsive to painful stimuli only. Physical exam revealed extensive bruising to the left lateral neck, left shoulder, anterior chest, and left lateral abdomen. Chest is unstable and appears to have a flail segment. Pt vital signs as noted above. Chest stabilized with padding and longboard straps. Lung sounds remain unchanged before and after stabilization. Pt condition remained unchanged during transport to Regional Trauma Center. Reported on arrival to Dr. Warren. **End of report**

Prep Kit

■ Ready for Review

- To care for your patients properly, you must have a thorough understanding of human anatomy and physiology so you can assess the patient's condition and communicate with hospital personnel and other health care providers.

- You must be able to identify superficial landmarks of the body and know what lies underneath the skin so that you can perform an accurate patient assessment.

- If you understand the basics of chemistry, your understanding of anatomy and physiology will be improved. Chemical changes within cells influence body functions and the status of the body's structures.

- Chemicals can basically be divided into two main groups: organic and inorganic. Organic substances include carbohydrates, lipids, proteins, and nucleic acids. Inorganic substances in body cells include oxygen, carbon dioxide, compounds that are known as salts, and water.

- Cells are the foundation of the human body. Cells with a common job grow close to each other and are called tissues. Groups of tissues that all perform interrelated jobs form organs.

- Cell transport mechanisms, or how materials enter and exit cells, relates to fluid administration. Several mechanisms, such as diffusion, osmosis, facilitated diffusion, active transport, endocytosis, and exocytosis allow material to pass through the cell wall.

- The cell's life cycle is regulated via stimulation from hormones or growth factors. The life of a cell includes interphase, cell division or mitosis, cytoplasmic division, and differentiation.

- The human body is primarily made up of four major types of tissue: epithelial, connective, muscle, and nervous tissues.

- Membranes form a barrier or an interface. The four types of membranes are serous membranes, mucous membranes, cutaneous membranes, and synovial membranes.

- Organs systems include the integumentary, skeletal, muscular, nervous, endocrine, cardiovascular, lymphatic, digestive, respiratory, urinary, and reproductive systems.

- The skeleton gives the body its recognizable human form through a collection of bones, ligaments, tendons, and cartilage.

- Bones are classified according to their shape, as long bones, short bones, flat bones, and irregular bones. The bones increase greatly in size as the fetus develops and throughout adolescence.

- Joints are classified as immovable (synarthrotic), slightly moveable (amphiarthrotic), or freely movable (diarthrotic). Most joints allow motion (knee, hip, elbow), and some bones fuse with one another at joints to form a solid, immobile, bony structure (skull).

- The 230 joints in the human body are fibrous, cartilaginous, or synovial.

- The human body contains several cavities that can be grouped into dorsal cavities (posterior) and ventral cavities (anterior).

- The axial skeleton forms the foundation on which the arms and legs are hung. The arms and legs, their connection points, and the pelvis make up the appendicular skeleton.

- The skeletal system is responsible for several functions. Bones protect internal organs and muscles enable movement. Bone also serves as a storage site for minerals, particularly calcium, and has a role in the formation of blood cells and platelets.

- Smooth muscle is found within blood vessels and intestines, and controls involuntary functions. Skeletal muscle, so named because it attaches to the bones of the skeleton, forms the major muscle mass of the body. It is also called voluntary muscle, because all skeletal muscle is under direct voluntary control.

- The contraction and relaxation of the musculoskeletal system gives the body its ability to move. Skeletal muscles contract when organelles and molecules bind myosin to actin to cause a pulling action.

- Cardiac muscle is different from skeletal and smooth muscle because it has the property of "automaticity"; it can generate and conduct electricity without influence from the brain.

- The respiratory system consists of all the structures of the body that contribute to the process of breathing. It includes the nose, mouth, throat, larynx, trachea, bronchi, and bronchioles. The system also includes the lungs, diaphragm, the muscles of the chest wall, and the accessory muscles of breathing.

- The primary function of the respiratory system is to conduct respiration. Oxygen is essential for the body to function. Gas exchange of oxygen into the blood and carbon dioxide out of the blood occurs at the alveoli of the lungs via diffusion.

- The respiratory center in the brainstem controls breathing. Nerves in this area sense the level of carbon dioxide in the blood and spinal fluid. The brain adjusts breathing as needed if the level of carbon dioxide or oxygen in the arterial blood is too high or too low.

- Increases in the level of carbon dioxide in the blood (Pa_{CO_2}) cause decreased pH levels in the respiratory center, which triggers an increase in ventilation. Decreases in the Pa_{CO_2} result in increased pH levels in the respiratory center and a decrease in ventilation.

- Hypoxic drive is a backup system the body uses to control respiration. Areas in the brain, walls of the aorta, and carotid arteries act as oxygen sensors and stimulate breathing if the oxygen level falls.

- The medulla oblongata is primarily responsible for initiating the ventilation cycle and is primarily stimulated by high carbon dioxide levels.

- The medulla has two main portions that control breathing: the dorsal respiratory group (DRG) and the ventral respiratory group (VRG). The DRG is the main pacemaker for breathing and is responsible for initiating inspiration. The VRG helps to provide for forced inspiration or expiration as needed.

- The circulatory system is a complex arrangement of connected tubes, including the arteries, arterioles, capillaries, venules, and veins.

- The cardiac cycle begins with myocardial contraction and concludes at the beginning of the next contraction. The heart's contraction results in pressure changes within the cardiac chambers, resulting in the movement of blood from areas of high pressure to areas of low pressure.

- The pressure in the aorta against which the left ventricle must pump blood is called the afterload. The greater the afterload, the harder it is for the ventricle to eject blood into the aorta. This reduces the stroke volume—the amount of blood ejected per contraction.

- Cardiac output is the amount of blood pumped through the circulatory system in 1 minute. Cardiac output is expressed in liters per minute (L/min). The cardiac output equals the heart rate multiplied by the stroke volume.

- Increased venous return to the heart stretches the ventricles, resulting in increased cardiac contractility. This relationship is known as the Frank-Starling mechanism.

- Blood consists of plasma and formed elements or cells that are suspended in the plasma. These cells include red blood cells, white blood cells, and platelets.

- Blood has many functions including fighting infection, transporting oxygen and carbon dioxide, controlling pH, transporting wastes and nutrients, and clotting.

- The lymphatic system helps absorb fat from the digestive tract, maintain fluid balance in the body, and fight infection. The spleen is the body's largest lymphatic organ.

- Body defenses can be divided into two general categories: innate (nonspecific) and adaptive (specific) defenses. Immunity is known as the third line of defense.

- The nervous system is perhaps the most complex organ system within the human body. It consists of the brain, spinal cord, and nerves.

- The nervous system is responsible for fundamental functions such as controlling breathing, heart rate, and blood pressure. This system also allows the performance of higher level activity, such as memory, understanding, and thought.

- The nervous system is divided into the central nervous system (CNS) and the peripheral nervous system. The CNS includes the brain and the spinal cord. The somatic nervous system is the part of the peripheral nervous system that regulates activities over which there is voluntary control, such as walking, talking, and writing. The autonomic nervous system is the part of the peripheral nervous system that controls the many body functions that occur without voluntary control such as digestion, dilation and constriction of blood vessels, and sweating.

- The autonomic nervous system is split into two areas. The sympathetic nervous system is responsible for fight-or-flight response, and the parasympathetic nervous system is responsible for moving blood to the stomach and intestines after eating and for many reproductive functions.

- There are two types of nerves within the peripheral nervous system, sensory nerves and motor nerves.

- The integumentary system is the skin. The skin is divided into two parts: the superficial epidermis, which is composed of several layers of cells including the germinal layer and the stratum corneal layer, and the deeper dermis, which contains the specialized skin structures such as sweat glands, sebaceous (oil) glands, nails, hair follicles, blood vessels, and specialized nerve endings.

- Subcutaneous tissue is below the skin and is composed largely of fat, serving as an insulator for the body and as a reservoir to store energy. The subcutaneous layer also helps to anchor the skin to the structures beneath it.

- The skin, the largest single organ in the body, serves three major functions: to protect the body in the environment, to regulate the temperature of the body, and to transmit information from the environment to the brain.

- The functions of the digestive system consist of a series of steps, which include ingestion, mechanical processing, digestion, secretion, absorption, and excretion.

- The alimentary canal extends from the mouth to the anus. It includes the mouth, pharynx, esophagus, stomach, small intestine, large intestine, rectum, and anus. The accessory organs of the alimentary canal include the teeth, tongue, salivary glands, liver, gallbladder, and pancreas.

- The endocrine system is made up of various glands located throughout the body.

- Endocrine glands help regulate metabolism, control chemical reactions, transport substances, regulate water and electrolyte balances, and aid in reproduction, growth, and development.

- The major endocrine glands include the pituitary gland, thyroid gland, parathyroid glands, adrenal glands, pancreas, pineal gland, thymus gland, and reproductive glands.

- The main functions of the urinary system are to control fluid balance in the body, to filter and eliminate wastes, and to control pH balance.

- In the urinary system, the kidneys are solid organs; the ureters, bladder, and urethra are hollow organs.

- The kidneys rid the blood of toxic waste products and control its balance of water and salt.

- The total body water content of the average adult ranges from 50% to 70% of total body weight, depending on age and sex.

- Body fluid is divided into intracellular and extracellular fluid compartments. Intracellular fluid exists within individual cells and makes up approximately 75% of all body fluid. Extracellular fluid exists outside of the cell membranes. The body can maintain fluid balance by shifting water from one compartment to another.

- The reproductive systems of both males and females contain organs and glands that create sex cells and transport them to areas where fertilization can occur.

- Chromosomes contain the entire sequence of genetic information the organism will have throughout its entire life. This genetic information contains the instructions for every structure and process in the body. They also contain sequences that will determine or influence various characteristics such as hair color, skin color, body composition, height, and predisposition to certain diseases.

- The primary sex organs (gonads) of the male consist of the two testes, in which sperm cells and male sex hormones are formed.

- Male reproductive functions are controlled by hormones from the hypothalamus, anterior pituitary gland, and testes.

- Testosterone enlarges the testes and accessory reproductive organs, and develops the male secondary sex characteristics. These characteristics include increased amount of body hair; enlargement of the larynx and thickening of vocal folds, which lowers the pitch of the voice; thickening of the skin; increased muscular growth; and thickening and strengthening of bones.

- The female reproductive organs produce and maintain the oocytes, which are the female sex cells.

- The primary sex organs (gonads) of the female are the two ovaries, which reproduce female sex cells and sex hormones.

- The hypothalamus, anterior pituitary gland, and ovaries control the maturation of female sex cells, development and maintenance of secondary sex characteristics, and changes during the monthly reproductive cycle.

- In nonpregnant females, the ovaries are the main source of estrogens, and they secrete increasing amounts of estrogens beginning at puberty. These hormones stimulate enlargement of accessory sex organs and develop and maintain the female secondary sex characteristics including development of breasts and mammary gland systems.

- The female reproductive cycle involves regular, recurring changes in the uterine lining as well as menstrual bleeding (menses).

- The body obtains most nutrients through ingestion (food) and inhalation (oxygen).

- Nutrients include carbohydrates, lipids, proteins, vitamins, minerals, and water.

- Digestion breaks down nutrients so they can be absorbed and transported via the bloodstream.

- Individual cells are supplied the nutrients and use them in various processes. As a result of cellular metabolism, organisms grow, maintain body functions, release or store energy, produce and eliminate waste, digest nutrients, or destroy toxins. These reactions alter the chemical nature of a chemical substance, maintaining homeostasis.

- In the body, enzymes assist in the digestion of food, drug metabolism, protein formation, and many other types of reactions.

- Cellular respiration is a process that releases energy from organic compounds. This process requires three types of reactions: glycolysis, the citric acid cycle, and the electron transport chain.

- Heat is a by-product of many cellular and chemical processes; the presence of body heat is one of the most basic signs of life.

- Body temperature regulation begins in the hypothalamus, which acts similar to a thermostat in activating the mechanisms for increasing or decreasing body temperature.

■ Vital Vocabulary

abdomen The body cavity that contains the major organs of digestion and excretion. It is located below the diaphragm and above the pelvis.

abduction Motion of a limb away from the midline.

acetabulum The depression on the lateral pelvis where its three component bones join, in which the femoral head fits snugly.

acetylcholine An excitatory neurotransmitter used in the peripheral and central nervous systems.

acetylcholinesterase The enzyme that causes muscle relaxation by the decomposition of acetylcholine.

acid A substance that increases the concentration of hydrogen ions in a water solution.

acidosis A pathologic condition resulting from the accumulation of acids in the body.

acromioclavicular separation (AC separation) An injury caused by distraction of the clavicle away from the acromion process of the scapula.

acromion process The tip of the shoulder and the site of attachment for both the clavicle and various shoulder muscles.

action potentials An electrochemical event where stimulation of a nearby cell could cause excitation of another cell.

active transport Any of a number of transport methods used to move compounds across a cell membrane to create or maintain an imbalance of charges, usually against a concentration gradient and requiring the expenditure of energy.

Adam's apple The firm prominence in the upper part of the larynx formed by the thyroid cartilage. It is more prominent in men than in women.

adaptation The temporary or permanent reduction of sensitivity to a particular stimulus.

adaptive (specific) defense Immunity; it targets specific pathogens and acts more slowly than innate defenses.

adduction Motion of a limb toward the midline.

adenosine triphosphate (ATP) The nucleotide involved in energy metabolism; used to store energy.

adipose tissue Fat tissue that lies beneath the skin, between muscles, around the kidneys, behind the eyes, in certain abdominal membranes, on the heart's surface, and around certain joints.

adrenal cortex The outer layer of the adrenal gland; it produces hormones that are important in regulating the water and salt balance of the body.

adrenal glands Endocrine glands located on top of the kidneys that release adrenaline when stimulated by the sympathetic nervous system.

adrenaline Hormone produced by the adrenal glands that mediates the "fight-or-flight" response of the sympathetic nervous system; also called epinephrine.

adrenocorticotropin hormone (ACTH) Hormone that targets the adrenal cortex to secrete cortisol (a glucocorticoid).

aerobic metabolism Metabolism that can proceed only in the presence of oxygen.

afferent arterioles The final branches of the interlobular arteries of the kidneys; they lead to the nephrons.

after-image The perception of a stimuli is still present after the stimuli is removed.

afterload The pressure in the aorta against which the left ventricle must pump blood.

agonal gasps Slow, gasping respirations, indicating life-threatening cerebral injury or ischemia.

agonist A substance that mimics the actions of a specific neurotransmitter or hormone by binding to the specific receptor of the naturally occurring substance.

agranulocytes Leukocytes that lack granules.

albumins The smallest of plasma proteins; they make up around 60% of these proteins by weight.

alkalosis A pathologic condition resulting from the accumulation of bases in the body.

alleles Variant forms of a gene, which can be identical or slightly different in DNA sequence.

allergen A substance that causes an allergic reaction; also referred to as an antigen.

alpha cells Cells located in the islets of Langerhans that secrete glucagon.

alpha effects Stimulation of alpha receptors that results in vasoconstriction.

alveolar ducts Ducts formed from division of the respiratory bronchioles in the lower airway; each duct ends in clusters known as alveoli.

alveoli The air sacs of the lungs in which the exchange of oxygen and carbon dioxide takes place.

alveolocapillary membrane The very thin membrane, consisting of only one cell layer, that lies between the alveolus and capillary, through which respiratory exchange between the alveolus and the blood vessels occurs.

amblyopia Lazy eye; the eyes may be oriented correctly but one fails to send adequate signals to the vision centers, also causing a loss of depth perception and poor-quality images.

anabolism The synthesis of larger molecules from smaller ones.

anaerobic metabolism The metabolism that takes place in the absence of oxygen; the principal product is lactic acid.

anatomic position The position of reference in which the patient stands facing you, arms at the side, with the palms of the hands forward.

anatomy The study of the structure of an organism and its parts.

androgens Male sex hormones mostly produced by the testicular interstitial cells.

anions Ions with a negative charge.

antagonist A molecule that blocks the ability of a given chemical to bind to its receptor, preventing a biologic response.

anterior The front surface of the body; the side facing forward in the anatomic position.

anterior cavity Aqueous chamber; portion of the eyeball filled with aqueous humor, a fluid whose quantity determines the intraocular pressure, which is critical to sight.

antibodies (immunoglobulins) Proteins within plasma that react with antigens.

antigens Substances or molecules that causes a response of the immune system.

aorta The principal artery leaving the left side of the heart and carrying freshly oxygenated blood to the body.

aortic arch One of the three described portions of the aorta; the section of the aorta between the ascending and descending portions that gives rise to the right brachiocephalic (innominate), left common carotid, and left subclavian arteries.

aortic valve The semilunar valve that regulates blood flow from the left ventricle to the aorta.

apex (plural apices) The pointed extremity of a conical structure.

apneustic center A portion of the pons that assists in creating longer, slower respirations.

appendicular skeleton The portion of the skeletal system that comprises the arms, legs, pelvis, and shoulder girdle.

appendix A small tubular structure that is attached to the lower border of the cecum in the lower right quadrant of the abdomen.

aqueous humor Watery fluid filling the anterior eye cavity; the quantity determines the intraocular pressure, which is critical to sight.

arachnoid The middle membrane of the three meninges that enclose the brain and spinal cord.

areolar tissue The type of tissue that binds skin to underlying organs and fills in spaces between muscles.

arteries The blood vessels that carry blood away from the heart.

arterioles The smallest branches of arteries leading to the vast network of capillaries.

ascending aorta The first of three portions of the aorta; originates from the left ventricle and gives rise to two arteries, the right and left main coronary arteries.

astigmatism Condition where parts of the image are out of focus and others are in focus; caused by irregularities in the shape of the eye lens.

astrocytes Neuroglia found usually between neurons and blood vessels.

atlanto-occipital joint The location where the atlas articulates with the occipital condyles.

atlas The first cervical vertebra (C1), which provides support for the head.

atomic number A whole number representing the number of positively charged protons in the nucleus of an atom.

atomic weight The total number of protons and neutrons in the nucleus of an atom.

atoms The smallest complete units of an element that have the element's properties; they vary in size, weight, and interaction with other atoms.

atrioventricular (AV) node The site located in the AV junction that is responsible for transiently slowing electrical conduction.

atrioventricular valves The mitral and tricuspid valves through which blood flows from the atria to the ventricles.

atrium One of the two upper chambers of the heart.

auditory ossicles The bones that function in hearing and are located deep within cavities of the temporal bone.

autonomic nervous system (ANS) The part of the nervous system that regulates functions, such as digestion and sweating, that are not controlled voluntarily.

autosomes The chromosomes that do not carry genes that determine sex.

avascular Lacking blood vessels.

axial skeleton The part of the skeleton comprising the skull, spinal column, and rib cage.

axillary vein The vein that is formed from the combination of the basilic and cephalic veins; it drains into the subclavian vein.

axis The second cervical vertebra; the point that allows the head to turn.

axons Extensions from neurons that send out electrochemical messages.

B lymphocytes (B cells) Lymphocytes that exist in the blood, and are abundant in the lymph nodes, bone marrow, intestinal lining, and spleen.

baroreceptors Receptors in the blood vessels, kidneys, brain, and heart that respond to changes in pressure in the heart or main arteries to help maintain homeostasis.

basal metabolic rate The rate at which nutrients are consumed in the body.

base A substance that decreases the concentration of hydrogen ions.

basement membrane Anchors epithelial tissue to connective tissue.

basilic vein One of the two major veins of the arm; it combines with the cephalic vein to form the axillary vein.

basophils White blood cells that work to produce chemical mediators during an immune response.

beta cells Cells located in the islets of Langerhans that secrete insulin.

beta effects Stimulation of beta receptors that results in inotropic, dromotropic, and chronotropic states.

bilateral In anatomy, a body part that appears on both sides of the midline.

bile ducts The ducts that convey bile between the liver and the intestine.

bilirubin A waste product of red blood cell destruction that undergoes further metabolism in the liver.

binocular vision The merging of two images into one.

blood The fluid tissue that is pumped by the heart through the arteries, veins, and capillaries and consists of plasma and formed elements or cells, such as red blood cells, white blood cells, and platelets.

blood pressure The pressure that the blood exerts against the walls of the arteries as it passes through them.

bone The most rigid type of connective tissue, with high mineral content that makes it harder than the other types.

bone marrow A substance that manufactures most red blood cells.

bony labyrinth The collection of hollows in the bone of the inner ear that provide protection to the structures of the inner ear from damage and from extraneous stimulation.

brachial artery The major vessel in the upper extremity that supplies blood to the arm.

brain The controlling organ of the body and center of consciousness; functions include perception, control of reactions to the environment, emotional responses, and judgment.

brainstem The area of the brain between the spinal cord and cerebrum, surrounded by the cerebellum; controls functions that are necessary for life, such as respiration.

bronchioles Fine subdivisions of the bronchi that give rise to the alveolar ducts.

bronchospasm Constriction of the airway passages of the lungs that accompanies muscle spasms.

bruit An abnormal "whooshing-like" sound indicating turbulent blood flow within a blood vessel.

buffer Any substance that can reversibly bind H^+.

buffer system Fast-acting defenses for acid-base changes, providing almost immediate protection against changes in the hydrogen ion concentration of extracellular fluid.

bulbourethral glands Cowper's glands; glands that lie inferior to the prostate gland and secrete a lubricating fluid that prepares the penis for sexual intercourse.

bundle of His Part of the conduction system of the heart; a continuation of the atrioventricular node.

bursa A small fluid-filled sac located between a tendon and a bone that cushions and protects the joint.

calcaneus The heel bone.

calcitonin A hormone produced by the parafollicular cells of the thyroid gland that is important in the regulation of calcium levels in the body.

calorie The amount of heat needed to raise the temperature of a gram of water by 1°C.

cancellous bone A type of bone that consists of a lacy network of bony rods called trabeculae.

capillaries The tiny blood vessels between the arterioles and venules that permit transfer of oxygen, carbon dioxide, nutrients, and waste between body tissues and the blood.

carbohydrates Substances (including sugars and starches) that provide much of the energy required by the body's cells, as well as helping to build cell structures.

cardiac cycle The repetitive pumping process that begins with the onset of cardiac muscle contraction and ends just prior to the beginning of the next contraction.

cardiac muscle tissue A special striated muscle of the myocardium, containing dark intercalated disks at the junctions of abutting fibers.

cardiac output The volume of blood pumped through the circulatory system in 1 minute.

carotid artery The major artery that supplies blood to the head and brain.

carotid bifurcation The point of division at which the common carotid artery branches at the angle of the mandible into the internal and external carotid arteries.

carpometacarpal joint The joint between the wrist and the metacarpal bones; the thumb joint.

cartilage The support structure of the skeletal system that provides cushioning between bones; also forms the nasal septum and portions of the outer ear.

cartilaginous joints Those connected by hyaline cartilage, or fibrocartilage, such as the joints that separate the vertebrae.

catabolism The breakdown of larger molecules into smaller ones.

cataract Clouding of the lens of the eye or its surrounding transparent membrane.

catecholamines Hormones produced by the adrenal medulla (epinephrine and norepinephrine) that assist the body in coping with physical and emotional stress by increasing the heart and respiratory rates and the blood pressure.

cations Ions with a positive charge.

cecum The first part of the large intestine, into which the ileum opens.

cell membrane The cell wall; a selectively permeable layer of cells that surround intracellular contents and control movement of substances into and out of the cell.

cellular immune response Cell-mediated immunity; it occurs when T cells attach to foreign, antigen-bearing cells such as bacterial cells, and interact with direct cell-to-cell contact.

cellular metabolism Process within a cell where nutrients can be broken down from complex to simpler forms or complex forms can be built from those building blocks.

cellular respiration A biochemical process resulting in the production of energy in the form of ATP.

central nervous system (CNS) The brain and spinal cord.

cephalic vein One of the two major veins of the arm that combine to form the axillary vein.

cerebellum One of the three major subdivisions of the brain, sometimes called the "little brain"; coordinates the various activities of the brain, particularly fine body movements.

cerebrospinal fluid (CSF) Fluid produced in the ventricles of the brain that flows in the subarachnoid space and bathes the meninges.

cerebrum The largest part of the three subdivisions of the brain, sometimes called the "gray matter"; made up of several lobes that control movement, hearing, balance, speech, visual perception, emotions, and personality.

cervical spine The portion of the spinal column consisting of the first seven vertebrae that lie in the neck.

cervix The lower one third or neck of the uterus.

chemoreceptors Receptors in the blood vessels, kidneys, brain, and heart that respond to changes in chemical composition of the blood to help maintain homeostasis.

chordae tendineae Thin bands of fibrous tissue that attach to the valves in the heart and prevent them from inverting.

choroid The vascular, pigmented middle layer of the eye wall.

choroid plexus Specialized capillaries within hollow areas in the ventricles of the brain that produce cerebrospinal fluid.

chromosomes Structures formed from condensed DNA fibers and protein; they are thread-like, and are contained within the nucleus of the cells.

chronic obstructive pulmonary disease (COPD) A progressive and irreversible disease of the airway marked by decreased inspiratory and expiratory capacity of the lungs.

chronotropic effect Related to the effect of the heart's rate of contraction.

chyme The name of the substance that leaves the stomach. It is a combination of all of the eaten foods with added stomach acids.

ciliary body The structure associated with the choroid layer of the eye that secretes aqueous humor and contains the ciliary muscle.

circulatory system The complex arrangement of connected tubes, including the arteries, arterioles, capillaries, venules, and veins, that moves blood, oxygen, nutrients, carbon dioxide, and cellular waste throughout the body.

circumflex coronary arteries One of two branches of the left main coronary artery.

clavicle The collarbone; it is lateral to the sternum and anterior to the scapula.

clitoris In females, the small erectile body partially hidden by the labia minora.

coccyx The last three or four vertebrae of the spine; the tailbone.

cochlea The portion of the inner ear that has hearing receptors.

compact bone A type of bone that is mostly solid.

complement A group of proteins in plasma and other body fluids that interact to cause inflammation and phagocytic activities.

compounds Molecules made up of different bonded atoms.

concentration gradient The difference in concentrations of a substance on either side of a selectively permeable membrane.

cones One of two photoreceptors of the retina that can distinguish colors, but requires a greater amount of light to activate and create an image.

conjunctiva The membranous covering on the anterior surface of the eye that also lines the eyelids.

conjunctivitis Inflammation of the conjunctiva.

connective tissues Tissues that bind, support, protect, frame, and fill body structures; they also store fat, produce blood cells, repair tissues, and protect against infection.

contractility The strength of heart muscle contraction.

cornea The transparent tissue layer in front of the pupil and iris of the eye.

coronal plane An imaginary plane where the body is cut into front and back parts.

coronary arteries Arteries that arise from the aorta shortly after it leaves the left ventricle and supply the heart with oxygen and nutrients.

coronary sinus Veins that collect blood that is returning from the walls of the heart.

corpus callosum A deep bridge of nerve fibers connecting the brain hemispheres.

corpus luteum Yellow body; a temporary glandular structure created from enlarged follicular cells because of the release of luteinizing hormone.

corticosteroids Any of several steroids secreted by the adrenal gland.

cortisol A glucocorticoid of the middle adrenal cortex that influences protein and fat metabolism and stimulates glucose to be synthesized from noncarbohydrates.

covalent bond A chemical bond where atoms complete their outer electron shells by sharing electrons.

cranial nerves The 12 pairs of nerves that arise from the base of the brain.

cranial vault The bones that encase and protect the brain, including the parietal, temporal, frontal, occipital, sphenoid, and ethmoid bones.

cranium The area of the head above the ears and eyes; the skull. The cranium contains the brain.

creatine phosphate An organic compound in muscle tissue that can store and provide energy for muscle contraction.

crenation Shrinkage of a cell that results when too much water leaves the cell through osmosis.

cretinism A disease caused by lack of thyroid hormone during pregnancy; it results in severely stunted physical and mental development.

cribriform plate A horizontal bone perforated with numerous foramina for the passage of the olfactory nerve filaments from the nasal cavity.

cricoid cartilage A firm ridge of cartilage that forms the lower part of the larynx.

cricothyroid membrane A thin sheet of fascia that connects the thyroid and cricoid cartilages that make up the larynx.

crista galli A prominent bony ridge in the center of the anterior fossa to which the meninges are attached.

cross section The product of slicing an object across or perpendicular to its long axis.

cusps The flaps that comprise the heart valves.

cutaneous membrane The skin; it covers the entire surface of the body.

cytokinesis The division of the cytoplasm of a cell.

cytoplasm The gel-like material that fills out a cell; it makes up most of the cell's volume, and suspends the cell's organelles.

cytosol The clear liquid portion of the cytoplasm.

dead space Any portion of the airway that contains air and cannot participate in gas exchange, such as the trachea and bronchi.

decomposition reaction A reaction that occurs when bonds within a reactant molecule break, forming simpler atoms, molecules, or ions.

deep Further inside the body and away from the skin.

delta cells Cells within the pancreas that produce somatostatin, which helps to regulate the endocrine system.

dendrites Extensions from neurons that receive electrochemical messages.

dense connective tissue White fibrous tissue that makes up tendons and ligaments, and exists in the eyeballs and deep skin layers.

depolarization The process by which cells activate in response to the action potential.

dermatome The area of the body served by a given nerve.

dermis The inner layer of the skin, containing hair follicles, sweat glands, nerve endings, and blood vessels.

descending aorta One of the three portions of the aorta, it is the longest portion and extends through the thorax and abdomen into the pelvis.

diabetes mellitus A metabolic disorder in which the ability to metabolize carbohydrates (sugar) is impaired due to lack of insulin or failure of the cells to use insulin properly.

diapedesis A process whereby leukocytes leave blood vessels to move toward tissue where they are needed most.

diaphragm A muscular dome that forms the undersurface of the thorax, separating the chest from the abdominal cavity. Contraction of the diaphragm (and the chest wall muscles) brings air into the lungs. Relaxation allows air to be expelled from the lungs.

diastole The relaxation, or period of relaxation, of the heart, especially of the ventricles.

differentiation The process of specialization of a cell.

diffusion Movement of a gas from an area of higher concentration to an area of lower concentration.

digestion The mechanical and chemical breakdown of foods and the absorption of resulting nutrients by the body's cells.

diploid Cells that carry two of each of the 23 chromosomes—one from the father and one from the mother.

disaccharides A simple sugar comprised of two monosaccharides.

distal Farther from the trunk or nearer to the free end of the extremity.

dorsal The posterior surface of the body, including the back of the hand.

dorsal respiratory group (DRG) A portion of the medulla oblongata where the primary respiratory pacemaker is found.

dorsalis pedis artery The artery on the anterior surface of the foot between the first and second metatarsals.

dromotropic effect Related to the effect of the heart's conduction rate.

dura mater The outermost of the three meninges that enclose the brain and spinal cord; it is the toughest membrane.

ear canal The cavity leading from the exterior atmosphere to the tympanum.

efferent arteriole Receives blood that has had fluids filtered from it via the glomerular capillaries, which arise from the afferent arterioles.

ejaculation The forcing of semen through the urethra to outside of the body.

ejaculatory duct A structure formed by the vasa deferentia uniting with the duct of a seminal vesicle; this type of duct passes through the prostate gland to empty into the urethra.

ejection fraction The portion of the blood in the left ventricle ejected during systole, expressed as a percentage.

elastic cartilage A flexible type of cartilage that provides framework for the ears and larynx.

electrical conduction system A group of complex electrical tissues within the heart that initiate and transmit stimuli that result in contractions of myocardial tissue.

electrolytes Salt or acid substances that become ionic conductors when dissolved in a solvent (ie, water); chemicals dissolved in the blood.

electrons Single, negatively charged particles that revolve around the nucleus of an atom.

elements Fundamental substances, such as carbon, hydrogen, and oxygen, that compose matter.

emission The movement of sperm cells from the testes, and secretions of the prostate gland and seminal vesicles, into the urethra.

encapsulated nerve endings Nerve endings in the skin surrounded by connective tissue that measure mechanical inputs.

endocardium The thin membrane lining the inside of the heart.

endochondrial ossification The process of bone formation.

endocrine glands Glands that secrete or release hormones that are used inside the body.

endocrine system The complex message and control system that integrates many body functions, including the release of hormones.

endolymph The fluid containing nerve receptors that resides inside the membranous labyrinth. Sound waves converted into pressure waves are transmitted through this fluid to the auditory nerves.

endometrium The inner layer of the uterine wall.

endosteum A layer that lines the inner surfaces of bone.

enzymes Substances designed to speed up the rate of specific biochemical reactions.

eosinophils A leukocyte that may play a role following infection in various areas in the body.

ependymal cells Neuroglia that cover specialized brain parts and form inner linings enclosing spaces inside the brain and spinal cord; they secrete cerebrospinal fluid.

epicardium The layer of the serous pericardium that lies closely against the heart; also referred to as the visceral pericardium.

epidermis The outer layer of skin, which is made up of cells that are sealed together to form a watertight protective covering for the body.

epididymides Tightly coiled tubes connected to ducts within a testis; they become the vas deferens.

epiglottis A thin, leaf-shaped valve that allows air to pass into the trachea but prevents food and liquid from entering.

epinephrine A hormone produced by the adrenal medulla that has a vital role in the function of the sympathetic nervous system.

epiphyses The growth plate of a long bone; also called the epiphyseal plate.

epithelial membranes Membranes that cover body surfaces and line body cavities.

epithelial tissues Body tissues that cover organs, form the inner lining of cavities, and line hollow organs.

erection The swelling and elongation of the penis in preparation for sexual intercourse.

erythropoiesis The process by which red blood cells are made.

esophagus A collapsible tube that extends from the pharynx to the stomach; contractions of the muscle in the wall of the esophagus propel food and liquids through it to the stomach.

estrogen A hormone released from the ovaries that stimulates the uterine lining during the menstrual cycle.

eustachian tube A branch of the internal auditory canal that connects the middle ear to the oropharynx.

exchange reaction A chemical reaction where parts of the reacting molecules are shuffled around to produce new products.

exocrine glands Glands that secrete chemicals for elimination.

expiratory reserve volume The amount of air that can be exhaled following a normal exhalation; average volume is about 1,200 mL.

extension The straightening of a joint.

external rotation Rotating an extremity at its joint away from the midline.

extracellular fluid (ECF) Fluid outside of the cell, in which most of the body's supply of sodium is contained.

extrinsic muscles Referring to the eye; six muscles that attach to the exterior of the globe and are controlled by the cranial nerves.

facilitated diffusion Process whereby a carrier molecule moves substances in or out of cells from areas of higher to lower concentration.

fascia A sheet or band of tough fibrous connective tissue that covers, supports, and separates muscles.

femoral artery The principal artery of the thigh, a continuation of the external iliac artery. It supplies blood to the lower abdominal wall, external genitalia, and legs. It can be palpated in the groin area.

femoral head The proximal end of the femur, articulating with the acetabulum to form the hip joint.

femoral vein A continuation of the saphenous vein that drains into the external iliac vein.

femur The thighbone; the longest and one of the strongest bones in the body.

fibrin A white insoluble protein formed in the clotting process.

fibrinogen A plasma protein that is important for blood coagulation.

fibroblast A star-shaped fixed cell that produces fibers via protein secretion into the extracellular matrix.

fibrocartilage A tough type of cartilage that absorbs shock in the spinal column, knees, and pelvic girdle.

fibrous joints Those that lie between bones that closely contact each other, joined by thin, dense connective tissue.

fibula The long bone on the lateral aspect of the lower leg.

flexion The bending of a joint.

fluid balance The process of maintaining homeostasis through equal intake and output of fluids.

fontanelles The soft spots in the skull of a newborn and infant where the sutures of the skull have not yet grown together.

foramen magnum A large opening at the base of the skull through which the brain connects to the spinal cord.

foramen ovale An opening between the two atria that is present in the fetus but normally closes shortly after birth.

foramina Small openings, perforations, or orifices in the bones of the cranial vault.

fossa ovalis A depression between the right and left atria that indicates where the foramen ovale had been located in the fetus.

fovea centralis The region of the retina of the eye that has densely packed cones and provides the greatest visual activity.

Fowler position The position in which the patient is sitting up with the knees bent or straight.

free nerve endings Fine receptors responsible for sensing light touch and smaller vibrations.

gallbladder A sac on the undersurface of the liver that collects bile from the liver and discharges it into the duodenum through the common bile duct.

gametes Sex cells; in humans, sperm and ovaries.

ganglion neurons Responsible for transmitting information from the rods and cones of the eye through the optic nerve.

general senses Sensations monitored throughout the body by receptors scattered throughout many different tissues.

genital system The reproductive system in males and females.

genotype The arrangement of a person's genes and their characteristics is based on the combination of alleles, for one gene or many.

germinal layer The deepest layer of the epidermis where new skin cells are formed.

glandular epithelium Specialized tissue that produces and secretes substances into ducts or body fluids.

glans penis The cone-shaped end of the penis that covers the ends of the corpora cavernosa and opens as the external urethral orifice.

glaucoma A disease of the eye caused by an increase in intraocular pressure; when severe enough, this may damage the optic nerve and potentially cause permanent loss of vision.

glenoid fossa The part of the scapula that forms the socket in the ball-and-socket joint of the shoulder.

globe The eyeball.

globulins Antibodies made by the liver or lymphatic tissues that make up around 36% of the plasma proteins.

glomerular capsule A sac-like structure that surrounds the glomerulus, from which it receives filtered fluid.

glomerular filtrate Mostly water, it has the same components as blood plasma except for large protein molecules; it is received by the glomerular capsule.

glomerular filtration The process that initiates urine formation.

glomerulus A tangled cluster of blood capillaries that comprises a renal corpuscle.

gluconeogenesis A process that stimulates both the liver and the kidneys to produce glucose from noncarbohydrate molecules.

glycogen A long polymer from which glucose is converted in the liver (animal starch).

glycogenolysis The breakdown of glycogen to glucose.

glycolysis A process that involves a series of enzymatically catalyzed reactions in which glucose is broken down to yield lactic acid or pyruvic acid.

gonadotropins Hormones secreted by the anterior pituitary gland, which include luteinizing hormone and follicle-stimulating hormone.

gonads The reproductive glands.

granulocytes A type of leukocyte that has large cytoplasmic granules that are easily seen with a simple light microscope.

greater trochanter A bony prominence on the proximal lateral side of the thigh, just below the hip joint.

hair follicles The small organs that produce hair.

haploid cells Cells that carry genetic instructions via 23 individual chromosomes.

hapten A small molecule that cannot stimulate an immune response by itself; found in certain drugs, dust particles, animal dander, and various chemicals.

heart A hollow muscular organ that pumps blood throughout the body.

heart rate The number of heartbeats per minute.

hematopoeisis The creation of all formed elements.

hemoglobin An iron-containing pigment found in red blood cells, carries 97% of oxygen.

hemostasis Control of bleeding by formation of a blood clot.

heparin A substance found in large amounts in basophils that inhibits blood clotting.

hepatic portal system A specialized part of the venous system that drains blood from the stomach, intestines, and spleen.

hepatic veins The veins to which blood empties after liver cells in the sinusoids of the liver extract nutrients, filter the blood, and metabolize various drugs.

Hering-Breuer reflex A protective mechanism that terminates inhalation, thus preventing overexpansion of the lungs.

hilum The point of entry for the bronchi, vessels, and nerves into each lung.

histamine A substance found in large amounts in basophils that increases tissue inflammation.

homeostasis A tendency to constancy or stability in the body's internal environment.

homologous chromosome A chromosome of the same numbered pair from the opposite parent.

hormones Substances formed in specialized organs or glands and carried to another organ or group of cells in the same organism.

Hormones regulate many body functions, including metabolism, growth, and body temperature.

human chorionic gonadotropin (hCG) One of three major female hormones; it is produced by a developing embryo after conception.

humerus The supporting bone of the upper arm.

humoral immune response When antibodies react to destroy antigens or antigen-containing particles.

hyaline cartilage The type of cartilage on the ends of bones in many joints, the soft portion of the nose, and in the respiratory passages' supporting rings; it is the most common type of cartilage.

hydrogen bond The attraction of the positive hydrogen end of a polar molecule to the negative nitrogen or oxygen end of another polar molecule.

hydrostatic pressure The pressure of water against the walls of its container.

hymen A fold of mucous membrane that partially covers the entrance to the vagina.

hyoid bone A bone at the base of the tongue that supports the tongue and its muscles.

hyperextension When a body part is extended to the maximum level or beyond the normal range of motion.

hyperflexion When a body part is flexed to the maximum level or beyond the normal range of motion.

hyperglycemia Abnormally high glucose level in the blood.

hyperopia Farsighted; the ability to see distant objects with difficulty focusing on objects close.

hypertonic Concentration of solute is higher within the cell as compared to outside the cell.

hypoglycemia Abnormally low blood glucose level in the blood.

hypothalamus The basal part of the diencephalons; it regulates the function of the pituitary gland.

hypothyroidism Myxedema; lowered levels of thyroid hormones.

hypotonic Concentration of solute is lower within the cell as compared to outside the cell.

hypoxic drive A "backup system" to control respiration; senses drops in the oxygen level in the blood.

ilium One of three bones that fuse to form the pelvic ring.

immunity The body's ability to protect itself from acquiring a disease.

inferior Below a body part or nearer to the feet.

inferior vena cava One of the two largest veins in the body; carries blood from the lower extremities and the pelvic and the abdominal organs to the heart.

inhibin Hormone that helps to regulate the menstrual cycle in females and may play a role in regulating sperm production in the male.

innate (nonspecific) defense One that protects the body from pathogens involving mechanical barriers, chemical barriers, natural killer cells, inflammation, phagocytosis, fever, or species resistance.

inorganic Not having both carbon and hydrogen atoms.

inotropic effect Related to the strength of the heart's contraction.

insertion A moveable part of the body to which a skeletal muscle is fastened at a moveable joint; its action opposes that of an origin.

inspiratory reserve volume The amount of air that can be inhaled after a normal inhalation; the amount of air that can be inhaled in addition to the normal tidal volume.

interatrial septum A membrane that separates the right and left atria.

interferons Hormone-like peptides that bind to uninfected cells and stimulate them to make protective proteins.

internal rotation Rotating the anterior surface of an extremity toward the midline.

interstitial cells The cells of Leydig; they lie in spaces between the seminiferous tubules, producing and secreting male sex hormones.

interstitial fluid The fluid located outside of the blood vessels in the spaces between the body's cells.

interstitial space The space in between the cells.

interventricular septum A thick wall that separates the right and left ventricles.

intracellular fluid (ICF) Fluid within cells in which most of the body's supply of potassium is contained.

intramembranous ossification Process where bones develop from connective tissue membranes, are replaced by spongy bone, and then compact bone, to form flat bones.

intravascular fluid (plasma) The noncellular portion of blood found within the blood vessels; also called plasma.

involuntary muscle The muscle over which a person has no conscious control. It is found in many automatic regulating systems of the body.

ionic bond A chemical bond where oppositely charged ions attract each other.

ions Atoms that either gain or lose electrons.

iris The muscle and surrounding tissue behind the cornea that dilate and constrict the pupil, regulating the amount of light that enters the eye; pigment in this tissue gives the eye its color.

ischium One of three bones that fuse to form the pelvic ring.

isotonic Concentrations on either side of the membrane are equal.

isotope One of two (or more) forms of an element having the same number of protons and electrons, but different numbers of neutrons; they may or may not be radioactive.

joint (articulation) The place where two bones come into contact.

joint capsule The fibrous sac that encloses a joint.

jugular vein The two main veins that drain the head and neck.

juxtaglomerular apparatus Also called a juxtaglomerular complex; it is made up of enlarged smooth muscle cells along with the macula densa.

kidneys Two retroperitoneal organs that excrete the end products of metabolism as urine and regulate the body's salt and water content.

kilocalories Commonly known as calories, the amount of energy that can be obtained from the nutrients you eat.

labia majora Two prominent, rounded folds of skin lateral to the labia minora of the female external genitalia.

labia minora A pair of skin folds in the female external genitalia that border the vestibule.

labored breathing The use of muscles of the chest, back, and abdomen to assist in expanding the chest; occurs when air movement is impaired.

lacrimal glands The glands that produce fluids to keep the eye moist; also called tear glands.

lacrimal sac Depository for debris, bacteria, or other material that is swept from the surface of the eye.

lactic acid A metabolic end product of the breakdown of glucose that accumulates when metabolism proceeds in the absence of oxygen.

large intestine The portion of the digestive tube that encircles the abdomen around the small bowel, consisting of the cecum, the colon, and the rectum; it helps regulate water balance and eliminate solid waste.

larynx A complete structure formed by the epiglottis, thyroid cartilage, cricoid cartilage, arytenoid cartilage, corniculate cartilage, and cuneiform cartilage; the voice box.

lateral In anatomy, parts of the body that lie farther from the midline; also called outer structures.

lateral malleolus An enlargement of the distal end of the fibula, which forms the lateral wall of the ankle joint.

left anterior descending (LAD) artery One of the two branches of the left main coronary artery that is the largest and shortest of the myocardial blood vessels; this vessel and the circumflex coronary arteries supply blood to the left ventricle and other areas.

lens The transparent part of the eye through which images are focused on the retina.

lesser trochanter The projection on the medial/superior portion of the femur.

ligament A band of fibrous tissue that connects bones to bones. It supports and strengthens a joint.

lipids Fats, fat-like substances (cholesterol and phospholipids), and oils that supply energy for body processes and building of certain structures.

liver A large solid organ that lies in the right upper quadrant immediately below the diaphragm; it produces bile, stores glucose for immediate use by the body, and produces many substances that help regulate immune responses.

longitudinal section The view of an object cut along its long axis.

loose connective tissue Adipose, areolar, and reticular connective tissue.

lumbar spine The lower part of the back, formed by the lowest five nonfused vertebrae; also called the dorsal spine.

lungs The two primary organs of breathing.

lymph A thin, plasma-like liquid formed from interstitial or extracellular fluid that bathes the tissues of the body.

lymph nodes Round or bean-shaped structures interspersed along the course of the lymph vessels, which filter the lymph and serve as a source of lymphocytes.

lymph vessels Thin-walled vessels through which lymph circulates through the body; they travel close to the major veins.

lymphatic system A passive circulatory system that transports a plasma-like liquid called lymph, a thin fluid that bathes the tissues of the body.

lymphocytes The smallest of the agranulocytes, they originate in the bone marrow but migrate through the blood to the lymphatic tissues.

lysis The process of disintegration or breakdown of cells that occurs when excess water enters the cell through osmosis.

macrophages Cells that are responsible for protecting the body against infection.

macula Also known as the macula lutea; a yellowish depression in the retina where acute vision arises.

mainstem bronchi The part of the lower airway below the larynx through which air enters the lungs.

mandible The bone of the lower jaw.

manubrium The upper quarter of the sternum.

mast cells Cells located in the tissues that release chemical mediators in response to an antigen-antibody reaction.

mastoid process A prominent bony mass at the base of the skull behind the ear.

matrix A combination of connective tissue, blood vessels, and minerals that compose bone.

matter Liquids, gases, and solids both inside and outside of the human body; it takes up space and has weight.

maxillae The upper jawbones that assist in the formation of the orbit, the nasal cavity, and the palate and hold the upper teeth.

medial Parts of the body that lie closer to the midline; also called inner structures.

medial malleolus The distal end of the tibia, which forms the medial side of the ankle joint.

mediastinum The space between the lungs, in the center of the chest, that contains the heart, trachea, mainstem bronchi, part of the esophagus, and large blood vessels.

medulla oblongata Nerve tissue that is continuous inferiorly with the spinal cord; serves as a conduction pathway for ascending and descending nerve tracts; coordinates heart rate, blood vessel diameter, breathing, swallowing, vomiting, coughing, and sneezing.

medullary cavity An internal cavity that contains bone marrow.

meiosis A type of cell division that includes first and second divisions.

membranous labyrinth A collection of passageways and reservoirs within the bony labyrinth of the inner ear.

menarche The first menstrual cycle; the onset of menses.

meninges A set of three tough membranes, the dura mater, arachnoid, and pia mater, that enclose the entire brain and spinal cord.

metabolic acidosis A pathologic condition characterized by a blood pH of less than 7.35, and caused by accumulation of acids in the body from a metabolic cause.

metabolic alkalosis A pathologic condition characterized by a blood pH of greater than 7.45, and resulting from the accumulation of bases in the body from a metabolic cause.

metabolism The chemical processes that provide the cells with energy from nutrients.

metacarpals The bones of the palms of the hand.

metatarsals The bones of the soles of the feet; they form the foot arches.

microglial cells Neuroglia found throughout the central nervous system.

midbrain The part of the brain that is responsible for helping to regulate the level of consciousness.

midsagittal plane (midline) An imaginary vertical line drawn from the middle of the forehead through the nose and the umbilicus (navel) to the floor.

minerals Inorganic elements essential for human metabolism.

minute volume The amount of air that moves in and out of the lungs per minute minus the dead space. Also called minute ventilation.

mitosis The division of chromosomes in a cell nucleus.

mitral valve The valve in the heart that separates the left atrium from the left ventricle.

molecule Particles made up of two or more joined atoms.

monocytes White blood cells that migrate out of the blood and into the tissues in response to an infection.

mononuclear phagocytic system Phagocytic cells that remove foreign particles from the lymph and blood.

monosaccharides The most simple carbohydrate molecule.

motor end plate The flattened end of a motor neuron that transmits neural impulses to a muscle.

motor nerves Nerves that carry information from the CNS to the muscles of the body.

motor neurons Nerve cells that transmit instructions from the CNS to the end organs; also known as efferent neurons.

motor pathways In the peripheral nervous system, common routes by which motor nerve impulses are transmitted.

motor unit A motor neuron and the muscle fibers that it controls.

mucous membranes The lining of body cavities and passages that communicate directly or indirectly with the environment outside the body.

mucus The opaque, sticky secretion of the mucous membranes that lubricates the body openings.

murmur An abnormal heart sound, heard as a "whooshing-like" sound indicating turbulent blood flow within the heart.

muscle impulse One that passes in many directions over a muscle fiber membrane after stimulation by acetylcholine.

muscle tissues Contractile tissue consisting of filaments of actin and myosin, which slide past each other, shortening cells.

musculoskeletal system The bones and voluntary muscles of the body.

myocardial infarction Blockage of the arteries that supply oxygen to the heart, resulting in death to a portion of the myocardium.

myocardium The heart muscle.

myoglobin A pigment synthesized in the muscles to give skeletal muscles their reddish-brown color.

myometrium The thick muscular middle layer of the uterine wall.

myopia Nearsighted; the ability to see objects close with difficulty seeing objects far away.

myxedema Hypothyroidism; lowered levels of thyroid hormones.

nasal cavity The chamber inside the nose that lies between the floor of the cranium and the roof of the mouth.

nasal septum The separation between the right and left nostrils.

nasopharynx The part of the pharynx that lies above the level of the roof of the mouth, or palate.

nephrons The functional units of the kidneys.

nerve impulse Electrochemical changes transmitted by neurons to other neurons and to cells outside the nervous system.

nerve plexus Nerves that exit the spinal cord and follow similar tracts through the body.

nervous system The system that controls virtually all activities of the body, both voluntary and involuntary.

nervous tissues Neurons and neuroglia.

net filtration pressure Usually a positive pressure, it forces substances out of the glomerulus.

neuroglia Supporting cells that provide a supporting skeleton for neural tissue, isolate and protect the cell membranes of neurons, regulate the composition of interstitial fluid, defend neural tissue from pathogens, and aid in the repair of injury.

neuroglial cells The supporting tissue cells of the nervous system that provide insulation, physical support, and nutrients to neurons.

neuromuscular junction The connection between a motor neuron and a muscle fiber.

neurons The basic nerve cells of the nervous system, containing a nucleus within a cell body and extending one or more processes; they exist in masses to form nervous tissue.

neuropathy Damage to nerve endings causing a wide range of symptoms including weakness, tremors, mild pain or "pins and needles," to such hypersensitivity that some parts of the body cannot be touched; also referred to as peripheral neuropathy.

neurotransmitters Chemicals that enable neurons to communicate.

neutrons Uncharged or "neutral" particles in the nucleus of an atom.

neutrophils One of the three types of granulocytes; they have multi-lobed nuclei that resemble a string of baseballs held together by a thin strand of thread; they destroy bacteria, antigen-antibody complexes, and foreign matter.

nodes of Ranvier Narrow gaps between Schwann cells.

norepinephrine A neurotransmitter and drug sometimes used in the treatment of shock; produces vasoconstriction through its alpha-stimulator properties.

nucleic acids Large organic molecules, or macromolecules, that carry genetic information or form structures within cells, and include DNA and RNA.

nucleus The central portion of an atom that contains protons and neutrons.

nutrients Carbohydrates, lipids, proteins, vitamins, minerals, and water.

oculomotor nerve The cranial nerve (III) that innervates the muscles that cause motion of the eyeballs and upper lid.

olfactory bulb The cranial nerve for smell.

olfactory cells Cells in the superior nasopharynx that respond to smell.

oligodendrocytes Neuroglia found aligned along nerve fibers.

oligosaccharide A simple sugar composed of 2 to 10 monosaccharides.

oncotic pressure The pressure of water to move, typically into the capillary, as the result of the presence of plasma proteins.

oocytes Eggs; female sex cells; they are formed in the ovaries.

oogenesis The process of egg cell formation, which begins at puberty.

optic chiasm Location where approximately half of the nerve fibers from each eye cross over to the opposite side of the brain.

optic disk Area of the retina where nerve fibers (axons) exit to become part of the optic nerve.

orbit The eye socket, made up of the maxilla and zygoma.

organ of Corti The organ that is the primary receptor for sound, and is made up of thousands of individual cilia, each with their own associated nerve.

organelles Structures within cells that have specialized functions.

organic Having both carbon and hydrogen atoms.

orgasm Physiologic and psychological release that is the culmination of sexual stimulation; accompanied by emission and ejaculation—in females there is a lesser expulsion of fluid.

origin A relatively immovable part of the body where a skeletal muscle is fastened at a moveable joint; its action opposes that of an insertion.

oropharynx A tubular structure that extends vertically from the back of the mouth to the esophagus and trachea.

osmosis The movement of a solvent, such as water, from an area of low solute concentration to one of high concentration through a selectively permeable membrane to equalize concentrations of a solute on both sides of the membrane.

osmotic pressure The tendency of water to move by osmosis across a membrane.

ossification The formation of bone by osteoblasts.

osteoblasts Cells involved in the formation of bony tissue.

osteoclasts Macrophages of the bone surface that dissolve the matrix and return minerals to the extracellular fluid.

osteocytes Mature bone cells.

otoliths A pair of fluid-filled sacs within the inner ear that are used by the CNS to collect information about movement and orientation in space.

oval window The opening between the stapes and inner ear.

ovaries Female glands that produces sex hormones and ova (eggs).

ovulation The development of a secondary oocyte and first polar body via oogenesis of the primary oocyte.

oxidation The process by which oxygen combines with another chemical, is involved in the removal of hydrogen, or loses electrons.

oxygen debt The amount of oxygen that liver cells need to convert lactic acid into glucose, as well as the amount needed by muscle cells to restore ATP and creatine phosphate levels.

palmar The forward facing part of the hand in the anatomic position.

pancreas A flat, solid organ that lies below the liver and the stomach; it is a major source of digestive enzymes and produces the hormone insulin.

papillary muscles Specialized muscles that attach the ventricles to the cusps of the valves by muscular strands called chordae tendineae.

paranasal sinuses The sinuses, or hollowed sections of bone in the front of the head, which are lined with mucous membrane and drain into the nasal cavity.

parasympathetic nervous system A subdivision of the autonomic nervous system, involved in control of involuntary, vegetative functions, mediated largely by the vagus nerve through the chemical acetylcholine.

parathyroid glands Four glands that are embedded in the posterior portion of each lobe of the thyroid; they produce and secrete parathyroid hormone.

parathyroid hormone (PTH) Hormone produced and secreted by the parathyroid glands; it maintains normal levels of calcium in the blood and normal neuromuscular function.

parietal pleura The pleural membrane that lines the pleural cavity.

partial pressure of carbon dioxide (Paco$_2$) A measurement of the amount of carbon dioxide in the blood.

partial pressure of oxygen (Pao$_2$) A measurement of the amount of oxygen in the blood.

patella The kneecap; a specialized bone that lies within the tendon of the quadriceps muscle.

pelvis The attachment of the lower extremities to the body, consisting of the sacrum and two pelvic bones.

penis The cylindrical male sex organ, it conveys urine and semen through the urethra.

peptides Protein molecules consisting of amino acids held together by peptide bonds.

perception Brought to conscious thought.

perfusion The circulation of oxygenated blood within an organ or tissue in adequate amounts to meet the cells' current needs.

pericardium The serous membranes that surround the heart.

perilymph Fluid within the bony labyrinth that surrounds and protects the membranous labyrinth while allowing transmission of pressure waves caused by sound.

perimetrium The outer serosal layer of the uterine wall.

periosteum A double layer of connective tissue that lines the outer surface of the bone.

peripheral nervous system (PNS) The part of the nervous system that consists of 31 pairs of spinal nerves and 12 pairs of cranial nerves. These peripheral nerves may be sensory nerves, motor nerves, or connecting nerves.

peristalsis The wavelike contraction of smooth muscle by which the ureters or other tubular organs propel their contents.

peritubular capillary One of many complex, interconnected capillary networks that branch off of efferent arterioles.

pH The measure of acidity or alkalinity of a solution.

phalanges The small bones of the digits of the fingers and toes.

phantom pain A sensation of pain in a part of the body that is no longer present.

pharynx The cavity lying posterior to the mouth connecting to the esophagus; it has both oral and nasal usages.

phenotype The appearance, health condition, or other characteristics associated with a particular genotype.

phospholipid A type of lipid molecule that comprises the cell membrane.

physiology The study of the body functions of the living organism.

pia mater The innermost of the three meninges that enclose the brain and spinal cord; it rests directly on the brain and spinal cord.

pinna Auricle; a formation of cartilage within the inner ear that protects the ear and collects sounds into the ear canal, while allowing some perception of the direction from which the sound comes.

pituitary gland An endocrine gland, located in the sella turcica of the brain, responsible for directly or indirectly affecting all body functions.

plantar The bottom surface of the foot.

plasma A sticky, yellow fluid that carries the blood cells and nutrients and transports cellular waste material to the organs of excretion.

plasma cells Cells that produce antibodies (immunoglobulins) to destroy antigens or antigen-containing particles; formed from divided and differentiated B cells.

plasmin An enzyme that dissolves the fibrin in blood clots.

platelets Tiny, disk-shaped elements that are much smaller than the cells; they are essential in the initial formation of a blood clot, the mechanism that stops bleeding.

pleura The serous membranes covering the lungs and lining the thoracic cavity, completely enclosing a potential space known as the pleural space.

pleural space The potential space between the parietal pleura and the visceral pleura. It is described as "potential" because under normal conditions, the space does not exist.

pneumotaxic (pontine) center A portion of the pons that assists in creating shorter, faster respirations.

polarized When a cell is at rest, ions are actively transported into and out of the cell to create an electrochemical gradient across the cell membrane.

polypeptide Formed from many amino acids bound into a chain. When a polypeptide has more than 100 molecules, it is considered to be a protein. Certain protein molecules have more than one polypeptide.

polysaccharides Complex carbohydrates that contain many simple joined sugar units, such as plant starch. Some polysaccharides such as cellulose cannot be broken down for nutrition in humans but play important roles in digestion.

pons An organ that lies below the midbrain and above the medulla and contains numerous important nerve fibers, including those for sleep, respiration, and the medullary respiratory center.

popliteal artery A continuation of the femoral artery at the knee.

popliteal vein The vein that forms when the anterior and posterior tibial veins unite at the knee.

posterior In anatomy, the back surface of the body; the side away from you in the standard anatomic position.

posterior cavity Vitreous chamber; portion of the eyeball filled with vitreous humor, a jellylike fluid that helps the globe maintain its shape without distorting light.

posterior column pathway Sensory pathway responsible for sending information about localized fine touch, pressure, vibration, and proprioception to the brain.

posterior tibial artery The artery just behind the medial malleolus; supplies blood to the foot.

postsynaptic terminal Portion of the postsynaptic cell that contains receptor sites and receives the neurotransmitter.

preload The volume of blood returned to the heart.

presbyopia The increased difficulty in focusing on objects that occurs with aging.

presynaptic terminal Portion of the presynaptic cell that contains and releases the neurotransmitter.

primary follicles Matured primordial follicles; the site of gene transcription in the growth of the oocyte.

primary taste sensations Sweet, salty, sour, and bitter.

primordial follicles Structures in developing female fetuses that contain a primary oocyte surrounded by follicular cells.

progesterone A hormone released from the ovaries that stimulates the uterine lining during the menstrual cycle.

pronation Turning the palms downward (toward the ground).

prone Lying flat, and face down.

proprioception Ability to be upright and aware of position in space.

prostaglandins Lipids made from arachidonic acid that usually act more locally than hormones, are very potent, stimulate hormone secretions, and help to regulate blood pressure.

prostate gland A small gland that surrounds the male urethra where it emerges from the urinary bladder; it secretes a fluid that is part of the ejaculatory fluid.

proteins Created from amino acids, they include enzymes, plasma proteins, muscle components (actin and myosin), hormones, and antibodies.

prothrombin An alpha globulin made in the liver that is converted into thrombin.

protons Single, positively charged particles inside the nucleus of an atom.

proximal Closer to the trunk

pseudostratified columnar epithelium Tissue that lines respiratory system passages and is layered in appearance and involved in secretion.

puberty The time during development when the body becomes reproductively functional.

pubic symphysis A hard bony and cartilaginous prominence found at the midline in the lowermost portion of the abdomen where the two halves of the pelvic ring are joined by cartilage at a joint with minimal motion.

pubis One of three bones that fuse to form the pelvic ring.

pulmonary artery The major artery leading from the right ventricle of the heart to the lungs; it carries oxygen-poor blood.

pulmonary circulation The flow of blood from the right ventricle through the pulmonary arteries and all of their branches and capillaries in the lungs and back to the left atrium through the venules and pulmonary veins; also called the lesser circulation.

pulmonary veins The four veins that return oxygenated blood from the lungs to the left atrium of the heart.

pulmonic valve The semilunar valve that regulates blood flow between the right ventricle and the pulmonary artery.

pulse The wave of pressure created as the heart contracts and forces blood out the left ventricle and into the major arteries.

pulse pressure The difference between the systolic and diastolic pressures.

pupil The opening in the iris through which light enters the eye.

Purkinje fibers A system of fibers in the ventricles that conducts the excitatation impulse from the bundle branches to the myocardium.

quadrants The way to describe the sections of the abdominal cavity. Imagine two lines intersecting at the umbilicus dividing the abdomen into four equal areas.

radioisotopes Also known as radioactive isotopes or radionuclides, they are atoms with unstable nuclei.

radius The bone on the thumb side of the forearm.

range of motion The arc of movement of an extremity at a joint in a particular direction.

rectum The lowermost end of the colon.

red blood cells Cells that carry oxygen to the body's tissues; also called erythrocytes.

referred pain Pain that feels as if it is originating from a body part other than the site being stimulated.

reflex arc The simplest type of nerve pathway, consisting of only a few neurons.

refracting system A series of transparent structures within the eye that redirect light as it passes through mediums of different densities.

renal arteries The vessels that supply the kidneys with blood for filtration; they arise from the abdominal aorta.

renal corpuscle The initial blood-filtering component of the nephron.

renal cortex The outer portion of each kidney; it forms renal columns and has tiny tubules associated with the nephrons.

renal medulla The inner portion of each kidney; it is made of conical renal pyramids, and has striations.

renal pelvis A cone-shaped collecting area that connects the ureter and the kidney.

renal tubule The portion of the nephron containing the tubular fluid filtered through the glomerulus.

renal vein The vessel from the kidneys that joins the inferior vena cava.

renin-angiotensin system System that helps to regulate fluid balance and blood pressure through actions in the kidney.

repolarization The process by which ions are moved across the cell wall to return to a polarized state.

residual volume The air that remains in the lungs after maximal expiration.

respiration The inhaling and exhaling of air; the physiologic process that exchanges carbon dioxide from fresh air.

respiratory acidosis A pathologic condition characterized by a blood pH of less than 7.35, and caused by accumulation of acids in the body from a respiratory cause.

respiratory alkalosis A pathologic condition characterized by a blood pH of greater than 7.45, and resulting from the accumulation of bases in the body from a respiratory cause.

respiratory system All the structures of the body that contribute to the process of breathing, consisting of the upper and lower airways and their component parts.

reticular activating system Located in the upper brainstem; responsible for maintenance of consciousness, specifically one's level of arousal.

reticular connective tissue The type of tissue that helps to create a framework inside internal organs such as the spleen and liver.

retina The inner layer of the eye wall, including the visual receptors.

retroperitoneal Behind the abdominal cavity.

reversible reaction A chemical reaction where the products of the reaction can change back into the reactants they originally were.

rods One of two photoreceptors of the retina sensitive to light, but does not discriminate colors, producing a picture that is somewhat less focused and essentially black and white.

saccule An enlarged region of the membranous labyrinth of the inner ear.

sacroiliac joint The connection point between the pelvis and the vertebral column.

sacrum One of three bones (sacrum and two pelvic bones) that make up the pelvic ring; consists of five fused sacral vertebrae.

saddle joint Two saddle-shaped articulating surfaces oriented at right angles to each other so that complementary surfaces articulate with each other, such as is the case with the thumb.

sagittal (lateral) plane An imaginary line where the body is cut into left and right parts.

salivary glands The glands that produce saliva to keep the mouth and pharynx moist.

saphenous vein The longest vein in the body, it drains the leg, thigh, and dorsum of the foot.

scalp The thick skin covering the cranium, which usually bears hair.

scapula The shoulder blade.

Schlemm's canal Responsible for maintaining the proper pressure of aqueous humor, draining excess into the bloodstream.

Schwann cells Neuroglial cells in the peripheral nervous system that form a myelin sheath around axons.

sclera The white, fibrous outer layer of the eyeball.

scrotum A pouch of skin and subcutaneous tissue hanging from the lower abdominal region, posterior to the penis.

sebaceous glands Glands that produce an oily substance called sebum, which discharges along the shafts of the hairs.

secondary bronchi Airway passages in the lungs that are formed from the division of the right and left mainstem bronchi.

semen Seminal fluid ejaculated from the penis and containing sperm.

semilunar valves The two valves, the aortic and pulmonic valves, that divide the heart from the aorta and pulmonary arteries.

seminal vesicles Storage sacs for sperm and seminal fluid, which empty into the urethra at the prostate.

seminiferous tubules Highly coiled structures inside each lobule of a testis; they form a network of channels, then ducts, which join the epididymis.

semipermeable Property of the cell membrane that describes the ability to allow certain elements to pass through while not allowing others to do so.

sensory nerves The nerves that carry sensations of touch, taste, heat, cold, pain, and other modalities from the body to the central nervous system.

sensory receptors Structures located in the dermis that initiate nerve impulses that can reach our conscious awareness.

serous membrane Membranes that line body cavities that lack openings to the outside.

sex cells Germ (reproductive) cells; in males they are known as sperm and in females are known as oocytes (eggs).

sex chromosomes The X and Y chromosomes, which determine sex.

shock An abnormal state associated with inadequate oxygen and nutrient delivery to the metabolic apparatus of the cell.

shock position The position that has the head and torso (trunk) supine and the lower extremities elevated 6″ to 12″. This helps to increase blood flow to the brain; also referred to as the modified Trendelenburg position.

shoulder girdle The proximal portion of the upper extremity, made up of the clavicle, the scapula, and the humerus.

simple columnar epithelium Single-layer tissue found in female reproductive tubes, the uterus, and most digestive tract organs; involved in secretion and absorption.

simple cuboidal epithelium Single-layer tissue covering the ovaries and lining kidney tubules and glandular ducts; involved in secretion and absorption.

simple squamous epithelium Single-layer tissue lining the alveoli, capillary walls, blood and lymph vessels, and body cavities.

sinoatrial (SA) node The normal site of the origin of electrical impulses; located high in the right atrium, it is the heart's natural pacemaker.

skeletal muscle tissue Voluntary muscle tissue attached to bones and composed of long thread-like cells that have light and dark striations.

skeleton The framework that gives the body its recognizable form; also designed to allow motion of the body and protection of vital organs.

skull The structure at the top of the axial skeleton that houses the brain and consists of the 28 bones that comprise the auditory ossicles, the cranium, and the face.

sliding filament model A method of action of muscle contraction involving how sarcomeres shorten, with thick and thin filaments sliding past each other toward the center of the sarcomere from both ends.

small intestine The portion of the digestive tube between the stomach and the cecum, consisting of the duodenum, jejunum, and ileum.

smooth muscle tissue Unstriated, involuntary muscle tissue with a "spindle"-shaped appearance; it composes hollow internal organ walls.

solute A particle, such as salt, that is dissolved in a solvent.

somatic cells All of the other cells in the human body besides the sex cells.

somatic nervous system The part of the nervous system that regulates activities over which there is voluntary control.

somatostatin Hormone produced by delta cells that helps to regulate the endocrine system with a wide range of effects throughout the body.

sperm Male sex cells; they are formed in the testes.

spermatogenesis The process by which sperm cells are formed.

spermatogenic cells Those that form sperm cells and line the seminiferous tubules.

spermatogonia Undifferentiated spermatogenic cells in a male embryo.

sphincters Muscles arranged in circles that are able to decrease the diameter of tubes. Examples are found within the rectum, bladder, and blood vessels.

sphygmomanometer A device used to measure blood pressure.

spinal cord An extension of the brain, composed of virtually all the nerves carrying messages between the brain and the rest of the body. It lies inside of and is protected by the spinal canal.

spinal nerves 31 pairs of nerves each responsible for sending and receiving sensory and motor messages to and from the CNS from a portion of the body.

spleen The largest lymphatic organ; filters the blood via the actions of lymphocytes and macrophages.

stem cells Cells that retain the ability to divide repeatedly without specializing, and that allow for continual growth and renewal.

sternocleidomastoid muscles The muscles on either side of the neck that allow movement of the head.

sternum The breastbone.

steroid Molecules with four connected rings of carbon atoms, including cholesterol, estrogen, progesterone, testosterone, cortisol, and estradiol.

strabismus Loss of perception of depth and overlapping or doubled images.

stratified columnar epithelium Thick tissue found in the male urethra, vas deferens, and areas of the pharynx.

stratified cuboidal epithelium Thick tissue that lines the mammary gland ducts, sweat glands, salivary glands, pancreas, ovaries, and seminiferous tubules.

stratified squamous epithelium Thick tissue that forms the epidermis and lines the mouth, esophagus, vagina, and anus.

stratum corneal layer The outermost or dead layer of the skin.

stroke volume (SV) The volume of blood pumped forward with each ventricular contraction.

subarachnoid hemorrhage A hemorrhage between the arachnoid membrane and the pia mater.

subarachnoid space The space located between the pia mater and the arachnoid membrane.

subclavian artery The proximal part of the main artery of the arm, which supplies the brain, neck, anterior chest wall, and shoulder.

subclavian vein The proximal part of the main vein of the arm, which unites with the internal jugular vein.

subcutaneous tissue Tissue, largely fat, that lies directly under the dermis and serves as an insulator of the body.

substrate The target of enzyme action.

superficial Closer to or on the skin.

superior Above a body part or nearer to the head.

superior vena cava One of the two largest veins in the body; carries blood from the upper extremities, head, neck, and chest into the heart.

supination Turning the palms upward (toward the sky).

supine The position in which the body is lying face up.

surfactant A liquid protein substance that coats the alveoli in the lungs, decreases alveolar surface tension, and keeps the alveoli expanded; a low level in a premature baby contributes to respiratory distress syndrome.

suspensory ligaments Ligaments that anchor the lens to the cornea allowing the various muscles of the eye to pull the lens into varying degrees of refraction.

sutures Attachment points in the skull where the cranial bones join together.

sweat glands The glands that secrete sweat, located in the dermal layer of the skin.

sympathetic nervous system Subdivision of the autonomic nervous system that governs the body's fight-or-flight reactions by inducing smooth muscle contraction or relaxation of the blood vessels and bronchioles.

symphysis A type of joint that has grown together forming a very stable connection.

synapse A functional connection where neurons communicate with other cells.

synaptic cleft The space between neurons.

synaptic vesicles Vesicles that contain neurotransmitters.

synovial fluid The small amount of liquid within a joint used as lubrication.

synovial joints Complex joints that allow free movement and are lubricated with synovial fluid.

synovial membrane The lining of a joint that secretes synovial fluid into the joint space.

synthesis reaction A reaction that occurs when two or more reactants (atoms) bond to form a more complex product or structure.

systemic circulation The portion of the circulatory system outside of the heart and lungs.

systemic vascular resistance (SVR) The resistance that blood must overcome to be able to move within the blood vessels. SVR is related to the amount of dilation or constriction in the blood vessel.

systole The contraction, or period of contraction, of the heart, especially that of the ventricles.

T lymphocytes (T cells) Specialized lymphocyte precursors that make up the majority of circulated blood lymphocytes.

talus The bone that articulates with the tibia and fibula to form the ankle.

tarsals The bones of the ankles.

taste receptors Receptors on the taste buds that respond to sweet, salty, sour, and bitter; help us to identify foods that are satiating and substances that are potential poisons.

temporomandibular joint (TMJ) The joint where the mandible meets with the temporal bone of the cranium just in front of each ear.

tendons The fibrous connective tissue that attaches muscle to bone.

tertiary bronchi Airway passages in the lungs that are formed from branching of the secondary bronchi.

testes The male reproductive organs that produce sperm and secrete male hormones; also called testicles.

testosterone The most important male sex hormone (androgen).

thermoregulation The process of maintaining homeostasis of temperature.

thoracic cage The chest or rib cage.

thoracic duct One of two great lymph vessels; it empties into the superior vena cava.

thoracic spine The 12 vertebrae that lie between the cervical vertebrae and the lumbar vertebrae. One pair of ribs is attached to each of the thoracic vertebrae.

thorax The chest cavity that contains the heart, lungs, esophagus, and great vessels.

thrombin An enzyme that causes the conversion of fibrinogen to fibrin, which binds to the platelet plug, forming the final mature clot.

thromboplastin A chemical that stimulates clotting of blood.

thymus A gland that is larger in children but shrinks with age; it secretes thymosins, which are important in early immunity by affecting production and differentiation of lymphocytes.

thyroid cartilage A firm prominence of cartilage that forms the upper part of the larynx; the Adam's apple.

thyroid gland A large endocrine gland that is located at the base of the neck and produces and excretes hormones that influence growth, development, and metabolism.

tibia The shin bone, the larger of the two bones of the lower leg.

tidal volume The amount of air moved in and out of the lungs in one relaxed breath; about 500 mL for an adult.

tissue plasminogen activator (t-PA) A major component in the fibrinolytic system, in which clots that have already formed are lysed or disrupted, converting plasminogen to plasmin.

topographic anatomy The superficial landmarks of the body that serve as guides to the structures that lie beneath them.

torso The trunk without the head and limbs.

trabeculae Bony rods that form the lacy network in cancellous bones and are oriented to increase weight-bearing capacity of long bones.

trace elements Essential minerals found in very small amounts; include chromium, cobalt, copper, fluorine, iodine, iron, manganese, selenium, and zinc.

trachea The windpipe; the main trunk for air passing to and from the lungs.

transitional epithelium Tissue that changes in appearance due to tension; it lines the urinary bladder, ureters, and superior urethra.

transverse (axial) plane An imaginary line where the body is cut into top and bottom parts.

Trendelenburg position The position in which the body is supine with the head lower than the feet.

tricuspid valve The heart valve that separates the right atrium from the right ventricle.

triglycerides A subcategory of lipids that includes fat and oil.

tropomyosin An actin-binding protein that regulates muscle contraction and other actin-related mechanical functions of the body.

troponin A regulatory protein in the actin filaments of skeletal and cardiac muscle that attaches to tropomysin.

tubular reabsorption The process that moves substances from the tubular fluid into the blood, within the peritubular capillary.

tubular secretion The process that moves substances from the blood in the peritubular capillary into the renal tubule.

tunica adventitia The outer layer of tissue of a blood vessel wall, composed of elastic and fibrous connective tissue.

tunica intima The smooth, thin, inner lining of a blood vessel.

tunica media The middle and thickest layer of tissue of a blood vessel wall, composed of elastic tissue and smooth muscle cells that allow the vessel to expand or contract in response to changes in blood pressure and tissue demand.

tympanic membrane The eardrum; a thin membrane that separates the ear canal from the middle ear.

ulna The inner bone of the forearm, on the side opposite the thumb.

unilateral Occurring on only one side of the body.

urea The result of amino acid catabolism; it filters into the renal tubule, with most of it reabsorbed and the balance excreted in the urine.

ureter A small, hollow tube that carries urine from the kidneys to the bladder.

urethra The canal that conveys urine from the bladder to outside the body.

uric acid The result of metabolism of certain organic bases in nucleic acids, mostly reabsorbed via active transport from the glomerular filtrate.

urinary bladder A sac behind the pubic symphysis made of smooth muscle that collects and stores urine.

urinary system The organs that control the discharge of certain waste materials filtered from the blood and excreted as urine.

urine The final product of tubular reabsorption and secretion; it is a clear, yellow-colored fluid that carries wastes out of the body.

uterine tubes Fallopian tubes, or oviducts; they open near the ovaries, penetrate the uterus, and open into the uterine cavity.

uterus A muscular inverted pear-shaped organ that lies situated between the urinary bladder and the rectum.

utricle An enlarged portion of the labyrinth of the inner ear.

vagina A muscular distensible tube that connects the uterus with the vulva (the external female genitalia); also called the birth canal.

vagus nerve The cranial nerve (X) that provides motor functions to the soft palate, pharynx, and larynx and carries taste bud fibers from the posterior tongue, sensory fibers from the inferior pharynx, larynx, thoracic, and abdominal organs, and parasympathetic fibers to thoracic and abdominal organs.

vasa deferentia The spermatic duct of the testicles; also called vas deferens.

veins The blood vessels that transport blood back to the heart.

venous sinuses Spaces between the membranes surrounding the brain that are the primary means of venous drainage from the brain.

ventilation The movement of air between the lungs and the environment.

ventral The anterior surface of the body.

ventral respiratory group (VRG) A portion of the medulla oblongata that is responsible for modulating breathing during speech.

ventricle One of two lower chambers of the heart.

vertebrae The 33 bones that make up the spinal column.

vertebral column The spine or primary support structure of the body that houses the spinal cord and the peripheral nerves.

vestibular gland One of two glands that lies on each side of the vaginal opening; it secretes mucus into the vestibule to moisten and lubricate the vagina for insertion of the penis.

vestibular system A system within the inner ear composed of a pair of fluid-filled sacs (otoliths) and three fluid-filled, looping passageways (semicircular canals) used by the central nervous system to collect information about movement and orientation in space.

vestibule The structure into which the vagina opens posteriorly, and the female urethra opens into in the midline. The central part of the labyrinth, behind the cochlea and in front of the semicircular canals, is also called the vestibule.

visceral pleura The pleural membrane that covers the lungs.

vital capacity The amount of air moved in and out of the lungs with maximum inspiration and exhalation.

vitamins Organic compounds required for normal metabolism.

vitreous humor A jellylike fluid filling the posterior eye cavity that helps the globe maintain its shape without distorting light.

voluntary muscle Muscle that is under direct voluntary control of the brain and can be contracted or relaxed at will; skeletal, or striated, muscle.

vulva The external accessory female organs, including the labia majora, labia minora, clitoris, and vestibular glands; they surround the openings of the urethra and vagina.

white blood cells Blood cells that have a role in the body's immune defense mechanisms against infection; also called leukocytes.

white matter Bundles of myelinated nerves.

xiphoid process The narrow, cartilaginous lower tip of the sternum.

zygomas The quadrangular bones of the cheek, articulating with the frontal bone, the maxillae, the zygomatic processes of the temporal bone, and the great wings of the sphenoid bone.

zygote A large fertilized egg cell produced after contacting a male sperm cell; the first cell of a future offspring, it contains 23 chromosomes from the father and 23 chromosomes from the mother.

Assessment in Action

You are dispatched to a patient who fell from a third floor balcony of a local hotel. When you arrive at the patient's side, you find her to be responsive and breathing. She has no sensation below the level of her umbilicus. She cannot move her legs or flex her hips. You and your partner take full spinal precautions with this patient because the fall was from a substantial height.

1. What are the two main divisions of the nervous system?
   - A. Internal and external
   - B. External and central
   - C. Central and peripheral
   - D. Peripheral and cerebral

2. How would you describe the patient's positioning if she was found face down?
   - A. Supine
   - B. Prone
   - C. Lateral
   - D. Dorsal

3. How many pairs of spinal nerves exist in the normal human body?
   - A. 28
   - B. 29
   - C. 30
   - D. 31

4. What do afferent nerves do?
   - A. Carry information to the CNS
   - B. Carry information away from the CNS
   - C. Control respiration
   - D. Control thermoregulation

5. You decide to use a dermatome due to the lack of sensation in the patient's lower body. What is a dermatome designed to do?
   - A. It determines how the internal organs function.
   - B. It measures the degree of burn injury on the body.
   - C. It helps determine a level of spinal injury on the body.
   - D. It assesses level of consciousness.

6. The vagus nerve has action on which body functions?
   - A. Movement of the eyes and pupils
   - B. Visceral muscle movement and sensation
   - C. Sense of smell and taste
   - D. Sense of hearing

7. If this patient was found not breathing, what would you expect the patient's blood pH to be?
   - A. Higher than 7.35
   - B. Lower than 7.35
   - C. At 7.35
   - D. None of the above

Additional Questions

8. What are the two main fluid compartments in the human body? Why is this information essential to a paramedic?

9. Discuss the difference between aerobic and anaerobic respiration. How will this concept affect this patient?

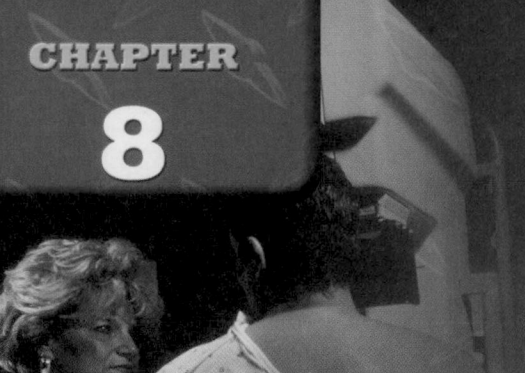

Pathophysiology

National EMS Education Standard Competencies

Pathophysiology

Integrates comprehensive knowledge of pathophysiology of major human systems.

Knowledge Objectives

1. Define pathophysiology, and discuss its scope. (p 335)

2. Explain the function of each of the three main components of a human cell: the cell membrane, the cytoplasm, and the nucleus. (pp 335–336)

3. Discuss how the body maintains homeostasis. (p 337)

4. Describe the characteristics of the four basic tissue types–epithelial, connective, muscle, and nerve tissue–and specify where each is found in the body. (pp 336–337)

5. Explain the function of common ligands, including medications, hormones, neurotransmitters, and electrolytes. (p 339)

6. Compare atrophy, hypertrophy, hyperplasia, dysplasia, and metaplasia as means of cellular adaptation. (pp 339–340)

7. Analyze the functions of water in the body. (pp 340–341)

8. Explain the concepts of osmotic pressure and membrane permeability. (p 341)

9. Explore the causes, clinical manifestations, assessment, and management of edema. (p 342)

10. Survey the mechanisms by which fluid and electrolyte balance are maintained in the body. (p 342)

11. Explain the physiologic consequences of imbalances in sodium, potassium, calcium, phosphate, and magnesium. (pp 342–346)

12. Become familiar with the concepts of acid, base, and pH. (p 347)

13. Explain how proteins, phosphate ions, and bicarbonate (Hco_3^-) buffer pH imbalances in the body. (pp 347–349)

14. Compare the four main clinical presentations of acid-base disorders: respiratory acidosis, respiratory alkalosis, metabolic acidosis, and metabolic alkalosis, and describe the clinical presentation that might be associated with a mixed acid-base disorder. (pp 349–352)

15. Outline how cellular injury occurs in patients with hypoxia, chemical exposures, infection (sepsis), immunologic exposures (hypersensitivity reactions), inflammatory conditions, genetic disorders, nutritional imbalances, physical damage (mechanical injury), and other harmful exposures, such as extremes of hot and cold. (pp 352–356)

16. Examine the concept of apoptosis. (p 356)

17. Analyze the controllable and uncontrollable risk factors that intersect in order to cause disease. (p 357)

18. Outline how incidence, prevalence, morbidity, and mortality data are used in analyzing disease risk. (p 357)

19. Become familiar with autosomal dominant and autosomal recessive patterns of inheritance. (pp 358, 359)

20. Analyze risk factors for cancer and cardiovascular disease. (pp 359–360, 362–363)

21. Describe how the body synthesizes hemoglobin. (p 361)

22. Identify several common renal, gastrointestinal, and neuromuscular disorders. (pp 363–365)

23. Define perfusion, and explain the physiologic consequences of hypoperfusion. (p 366)

24. Analyze the mechanisms by which the body compensates for hypoperfusion. (p 366)

25. Discuss the causes of central and peripheral shock, including cardiogenic, obstructive, hypovolemic, and distributive shock. (pp 366–369)

26. Outline the management of a patient in shock. (p 369)

27. Describe multiple organ dysfunction syndrome. (pp 369–370)

28. Examine the body's three lines of defense against pathogens: anatomic barriers, the immune response, and the inflammatory response. (pp 370–383)

29. List the functions of the five general types of white blood cells: basophils, eosinophils, monocytes, neutrophils, and lymphocytes. (pp 372, 373)

30. Describe the function of macrophages. (p 372)

31. Describe the function of mast cells. (p 373)

32. Compare humoral immunity with cell-mediated immunity. (pp 374–378)

33. Explain how plasma protein systems–the complement system, the coagulation (clotting) system, and the kinin system–modulate the inflammatory response. (p 380)

34. Compare wound healing by primary intention with wound healing by secondary intention. (pp 381, 383)

35. Explain why hypersensitivity reactions sometimes occur, and outline the four types of hypersensitivity reactions. (pp 383, 384)

36. List several autoimmune reactions, and explain blood group incompatibility. (pp 385, 386)

37. Compare inherited and acquired immunodeficiencies. (pp 386, 387)

38. List the stages of the general adaptation syndrome, and explore the relationship between stress and disease. (pp 387–389)

Skills Objectives

There are no skills objectives in this chapter.

Introduction

The human body is made up of cells, tissues, and organs, which function in a constantly changing microenvironment. The study of living organisms with regard to their origin, growth, structure, behavior, and reproduction is known as biology. The word **pathophysiology** refers to the study of the functioning of an organism in the presence of disease. It is derived from the Greek words *pathos*, meaning "suffering", and *phýsis*, meaning "form." When the normal condition or functioning of a cellular system breaks down in response to stressors and the system can no longer maintain homeostasis, disease may result. Determining the cause of the disease process often helps paramedics identify a reasonable approach to evaluation and initial treatment of patients.

To understand how disease may alter cellular function, it is necessary to understand normal cellular structure and function. This chapter begins by reviewing the structure and function of the cellular systems and environment. Following that review is a discussion of how alterations of the environment and its normal state of homeostasis may lead to disease. Next, the chapter describes the effect of genetics in the development of disease and the role of immunity and defense mechanisms in protecting the organism from disease. Finally, the influence of inflammation, shock, and stress in disease development is considered in detail.

Review of the Basic Cellular Systems

Cells

The cell is the basic self-sustaining unit of the human body. As cells—neurons, epithelial cells, ciliated lung cells, contractile muscle cells, erythrocytes, and so on—grow and mature, they become specialized through the process of differentiation. Cells may perform one function, or may work with other cells to perform a function that is best not performed by one cell alone (in this way they act similar to a multicellular organism). Groups of cells form tissues, various types of tissues make up organs, and groups of organs constitute organ systems. There are as many classes of cells as there are organ systems in the human body, and each organ system has multiple types of cells within its class.

Nearly all cells of higher organisms, except mature red blood cells and platelets, have three main components:

1. Cell membrane
2. Cytoplasm, which contains the cell's internal components, or organelles
3. Nucleus

The cell membrane consists of fat and protein. It surrounds the cell and protects the nucleus and the **organelles**, functional structures within the cell's cytoplasm (fluid). The organelles operate in a cooperative and organized manner to maintain the life of the cell. They include the following components Figure 1 :

- *Ribosomes* contain **ribonucleic acid (RNA)** and protein. RNA is responsible for controlling cellular activities. Ribosomes interact with RNA from other parts of the cell, joining amino acid chains together to form proteins. When ribosomes attach to endoplasmic reticulum, they create rough endoplasmic reticulum.
- The *endoplasmic reticulum* is a network of tubules, vesicles, and sacs. Rough endoplasmic reticulum is involved in building proteins. Smooth endoplasmic reticulum is involved in building lipids (fats), such as those found in the cell membranes.
- The *Golgi complex* is located near the nucleus of the cell. It is involved in the synthesis and packaging of various carbohydrates (sugars) and complex protein molecules, such as enzymes.
- *Lysosomes* are membrane-bound vesicles that contain digestive enzymes. These enzymes function as an intracellular digestive system, breaking down organic debris, such as bacteria, that has been taken into the cell.
- Similar to lysosomes, *peroxisomes* are found in high concentrations in the liver and neutralize toxins such as alcohol.

YOU *are the Medic* **PART 1**

You and your partner are dispatched to a single-family residence for a report of a 72-year-old man with difficulty breathing. On arrival, you are met at the door by a neighbor. The neighbor tells you that the resident of the home lives alone, has had numerous heart attacks, and is not doing well. As you approach the patient, you assess his surroundings. You find a large number of used facial tissues on the side table and numerous prescription medication bottles. The patient is sitting upright in a chair, wearing a nasal cannula that is attached to a home oxygen unit. He is able to speak only a few words at a time. The patient tells you he cannot breathe, and his skin color is pale.

1. What is your general impression of the patient?
2. What could his surroundings indicate to you?

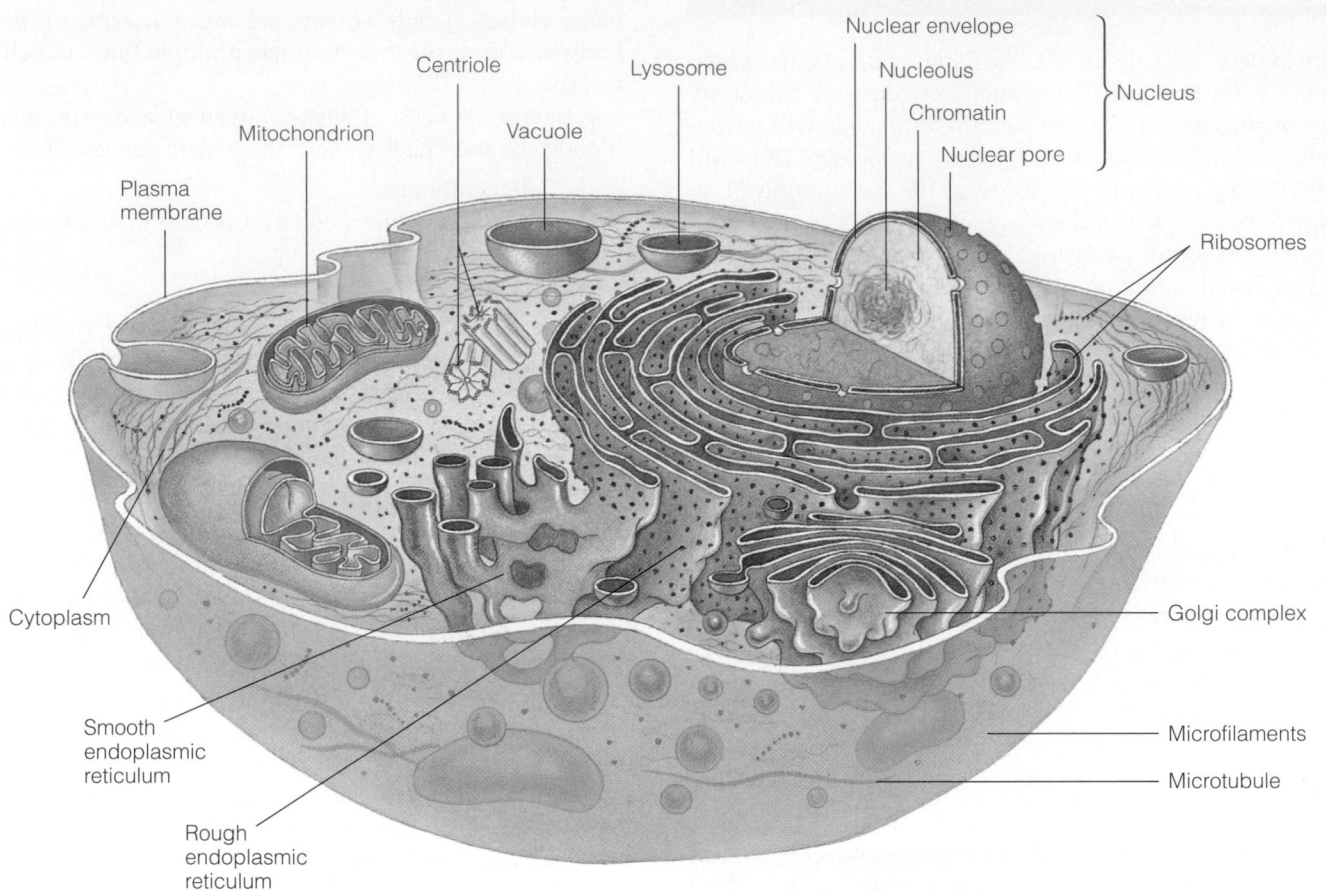

Figure 1 The structure of a cell. The cell is divided into nuclear and cytoplasmic compartments. The cytoplasm is packed with organelles, the structures with which the cell carries out many functions.

- **Mitochondria** are small organelles that may be rodlike or spherical in shape. They function as the metabolic center of the cell, and produce adenosine triphosphate (ATP), the major energy source for the cell.
- The **nucleus** contains two different types of genetic material. Deoxyribonucleic acid (DNA) is contained in the chromosomes, which are long and thin in the nondividing cell and cannot be identified as distinct structures. Instead, they appear as a network of granules called nuclear chromatin. RNA is contained in spherical intranuclear structures called nucleoli. The nucleus is surrounded by a membrane called the nuclear envelope; the nucleus itself is embedded in the cytoplasm.

Words of Wisdom

Chemically, fatty compounds, such as those in the cell membrane, are neutral (uncharged), whereas electrolytes (sodium and potassium) are water based (charged). Thus, for a charged molecule to permeate a cell membrane, it has to travel through a special pathway. These transport channels—the so-called ion channels—consist of protein-lined pores specifically sized for each substance (for example, calcium and potassium). Local anesthetics (such as lidocaine) and antidysrhythmic drugs (such as amiodarone) exert their effects by blocking ion channels.

Tissues

Tissues are composed of groups of similar cells that work together to perform a common function. There are four basic types of tissues: epithelial, connective, muscle, and nerve tissue.

Epithelial Tissue

Epithelial tissue, or **epithelium**, covers the external surfaces of the body and lines hollow organs within the body, such as the intestines, blood vessels, and bronchial tubes. In addition to providing a protective barrier, epithelial tissue is necessary for the absorption of nutrients in the intestines and the secretion of various body substances. For example, sweat glands in the dermis layer of the skin—specifically, stratified squamous epithelial cells within the dermis—produce a solution containing urea and salt, ultimately secreted as sweat. In contrast, the simple columnar epithelium that lines the small intestine absorbs nutrients from food. The epithelial cells that line the blood vessels are called <u>endothelial cells</u>; they help regulate the flow of blood through the vessel and have a role in blood clotting (coagulation).

Connective Tissue

<u>Connective tissue</u> binds the other types of tissue to one another. Connective tissue cells are separated by a nonliving extracellular matrix consisting of protein fibers, nonfibrous protein, and fluid. Collagen is the main protein within the extracellular matrix. At least 12 types of collagen exist, with types I, II, and III being the most abundant. Alteration of collagen structure caused by abnormal genes or abnormal processing of collagen proteins occurs in diseases such as scurvy. Bone and cartilage are subtypes of connective tissue. <u>Adipose tissue</u> is a special type of connective tissue that contains large amounts of lipids (fat). Blood is also considered a connective tissue.

Muscle Tissue

Muscle tissue is characterized by its ability to contract. It is enclosed by fascia, an envelope of fibrous connective tissue that encapsulates individual muscles. Muscles overlie the framework of the skeleton and are classified in terms of their structure and their function. Structurally, muscle tissue in which microscopic bands, or striations, can be seen is called striated muscle; muscle tissue without such bands is called smooth muscle. Functionally, muscle is voluntary (consciously controlled) or involuntary (not normally under conscious control).

These structural and functional classifications are combined in the categorization of muscle into three types:

1. **Skeletal muscle (striated voluntary).** Most of the muscles used voluntarily in day-to-day activities are skeletal muscles.
2. **Cardiac muscle (striated involuntary).** The heart consists of cardiac muscle and has contractile ability and the ability to generate electrical impulses.
3. **Smooth muscle (nonstriated involuntary).** Smooth muscle lines most glands, digestive organs, lower airways, and vessels. When a patient's brain senses the need to respond to an environmental stimulus by vasoconstriction, the vessels in the periphery react. For example, the smooth muscle of the bronchioles may constrict during an asthma attack, causing the person to wheeze and making it difficult for him or her to expel air from the lungs. Smooth muscle in the iris is responsible for constriction and dilation of the pupil in response to changing light conditions.

Nerve Tissue

Nerve tissue is characterized by its ability to transmit nerve impulses. The central nervous system (CNS) consists of the brain and the spinal cord. <u>Peripheral nerves</u> extend from the brain and spinal cord, exiting from between the vertebrae to various parts of the body.

Neurons are the main conducting cells of nerve tissue, and the cell body of the neuron is the site of most cellular functions. <u>Dendrites</u> receive electrical impulses from the axons of other nerve cells and conduct them toward the cell body, whereas <u>axons</u> typically conduct electrical impulses away from the cell body. Each neuron has only one axon, but it may have several dendrites. Nerve cells are separated by a gap called the synapse. Electrical impulses travel down the nerve and trigger the release of neurotransmitters, which carry the impulse from axon to dendrite.

■ Homeostasis

Adaptive responses to various stimuli allow the cells and tissues to respond and function in stressful environments, in a constant effort to preserve a degree of stability or equilibrium. This adaptation process is known as <u>homeostasis</u> (from the Greek words for "same" and "steady"); it is also called the *dynamic steady state*. Physiologic cell turnover refers to the process in which older cells are eliminated and replaced by newer cells. This occurs via <u>apoptosis</u>, which is normal cell death. This is genetically programmed into the cell as a part of normal development, organogenesis, immune function, and tissue growth. It has a normal role in aging, early development, menses, lactating breast tissue, thymus involution, and red blood cell turnover. This process is discussed later in the chapter. Appropriate cell turnover is one component of homeostasis; for example, it allows damaged cells to be replaced so that proper tissue function can continue.

Homeostasis is maintained in the body because normal regulatory systems are counterbalanced by counterregulatory systems. Thus, for every cell, tissue, or organ that performs one function, there is always at least one component that performs the opposing function. For example, the autonomic nervous system consists of the sympathetic and parasympathetic components, which act to speed up or slow down the activity of target organs. Other homeostatic mechanisms include the body's control of its internal temperature despite fluctuations in the external temperature, the regulation of pH and acid-base balance in the body, and the balance of water or hydration in the cells and body of the organism.

Regulatory systems communicate within the body mainly at the cellular level. Cells communicate electrochemically through a process called <u>cell signaling</u>, in which they release molecules (such as hormones) that bind to protein receptors on the cell surface. This signaling triggers chemical reactions in the receptor cells that initiate a biologic action. When the action has been completed, the opposing system is alerted to discontinue the action through a process called <u>feedback inhibition</u> or <u>negative feedback</u> **Figure 2**.

Receptors in the body are specialized, depending on the role they perform. <u>Adrenergic receptors</u> are associated with the sympathetic nerves and are stimulated by epinephrine and norepinephrine. Activation of an adrenergic receptor causes a sympathetic response, such as vasoconstriction or vasodilation. Alpha receptors and beta receptors are in the adrenergic class.

Baroreceptors and chemoreceptors are involved in regulation of heart function. <u>Baroreceptors</u> respond to changes in pressure, usually within the heart or the main arteries. <u>Chemoreceptors</u> sense changes in the chemical composition of the blood, especially reduced oxygen levels and elevated carbon dioxide levels. If either of these types of receptors sense

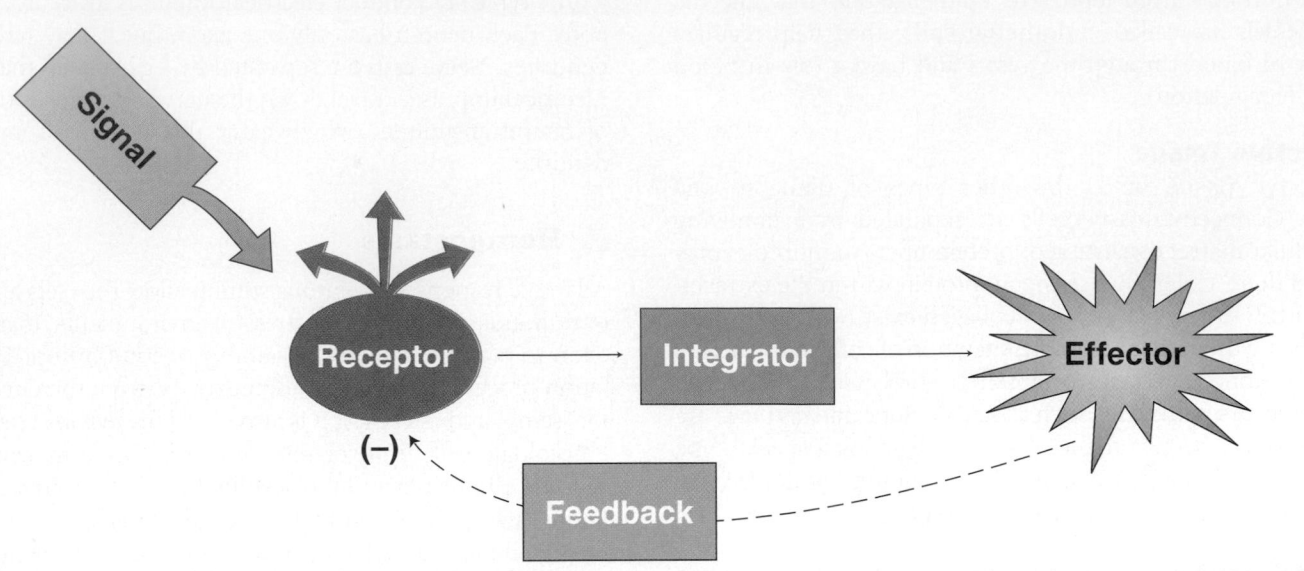

Figure 2   Most cellular communication includes a component of negative feedback in which the product of a reaction returns information about its own manufacture, thereby stopping its own production.

abnormalities, they transmit nerve signals to the appropriate organs. As a result, hormones or neurotransmitters are released to correct the situation, for example through changes to respiration and blood pressure.

The thermostat mechanism in a home is a good example of a feedback mechanism. In the middle of the winter, heat is continually lost through drafty windows, doors, and poorly insulated areas such as the roof or walls. The thermostat detects decreases in temperature and signals the furnace to produce heat to rewarm the house. Once the temperature has risen to a certain point, the thermostat gives negative feedback to the furnace, causing it to shut down to prevent overheating. This feedback process keeps the temperature of the house within a selected range **Figure 3**. Similarly, the body constantly generates heat through cellular processes. Five primary mechanisms help the body reduce excess temperature or eliminate heat: convection, conduction, radiation, evaporation, and respiration. In short, the body's thermostat balances the generation of heat with the elimination of heat.

The human body maintains homeostasis by balancing what it takes in with what it puts out. For example, the body takes in chemicals and electrolytes, food, and water. It utilizes the nutrients, proteins, sugars, and oxygen and then eliminates the unnecessary chemicals and by-products through respiration (carbon dioxide), sweating (excess liquids), urination, and defecation (feces). **Figure 4** illustrates this normal balance.

When normal cell signaling is interrupted, disease occurs. The body's counterregulatory mechanisms are rendered ineffective, and its regulatory systems begin to operate autonomously. The system stops providing critical negative feedback; instead, it gives unopposed positive feedback.

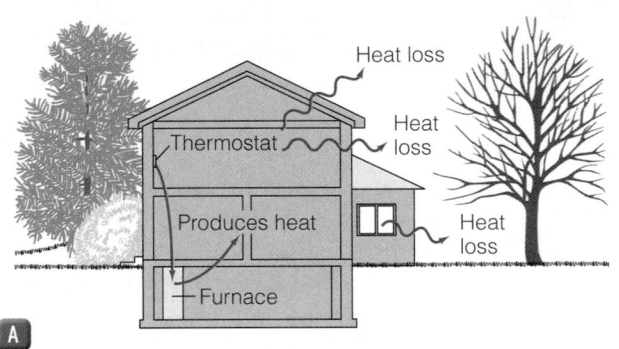

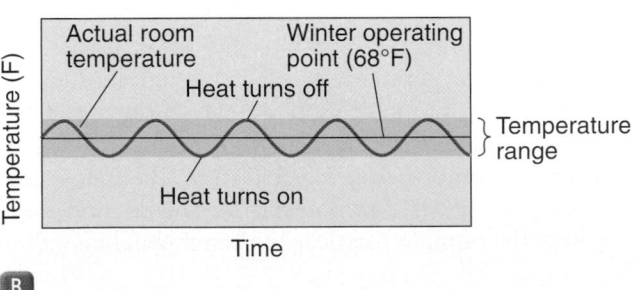

Figure 3   Homeostasis and the house. **A.** Heat is maintained in a house by a furnace, which compensates for heat loss. The thermostat monitors the internal temperature and switches the furnace on and off in response to temperature changes. **B.** A hypothetical temperature graph showing temperature fluctuation around the set point.

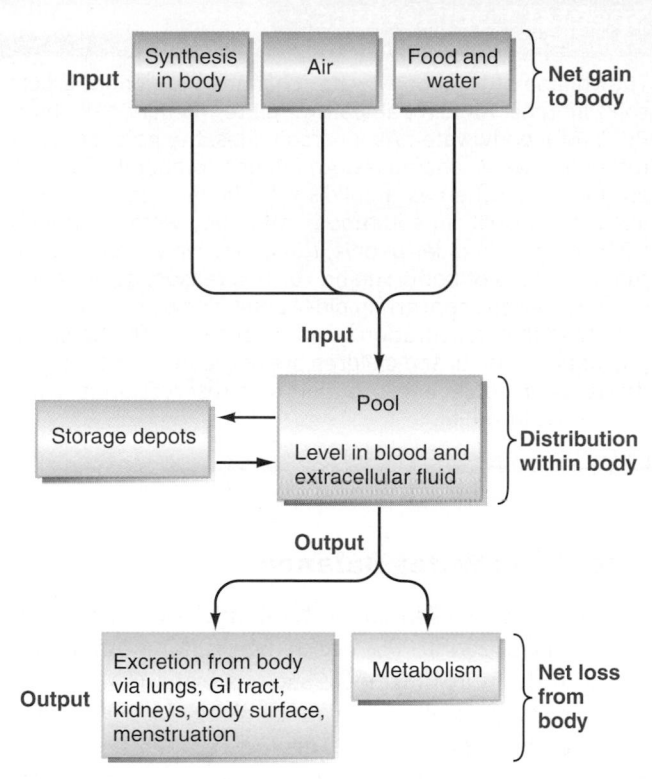

Figure 4 Generalized view of the homeostatic system. Inputs and outputs are balanced to maintain more or less constant chemical and physical parameters.

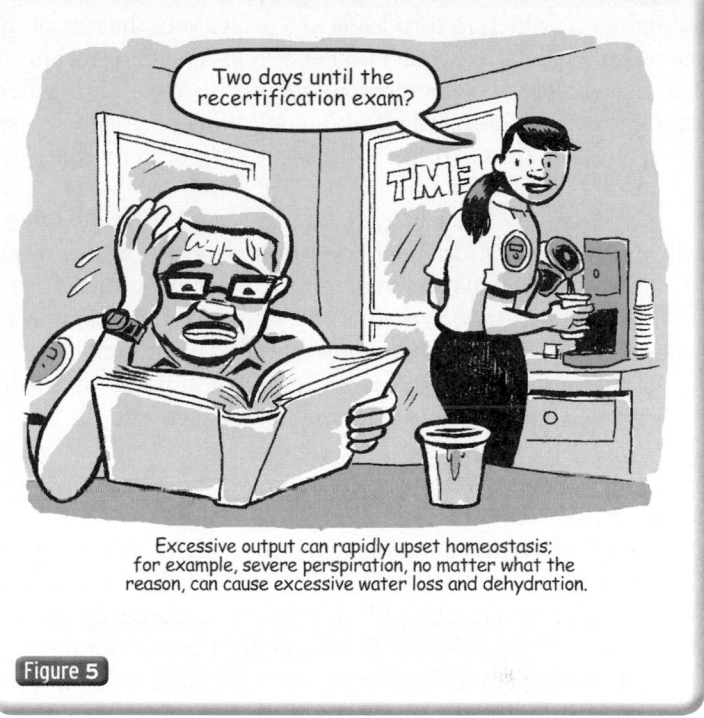

Excessive output can rapidly upset homeostasis; for example, severe perspiration, no matter what the reason, can cause excessive water loss and dehydration.

Figure 5

Excessive output can rapidly upset homeostasis. Severe diarrhea, for example, kills millions of children each year in some nations. Even profuse perspiration can cause excessive water loss and dehydration. Likewise, changes in water intake can alter homeostasis. Going without water for 3 or more days is life threatening **Figure 5**. In addition, excessive salt intake can cause hypertension.

The degree of fluid imbalance required to upset homeostasis and cause illness depends on the patient's size, age, and underlying medical conditions. In healthy adults, loss of more than 30% of total body fluid is required, but a loss of only 10% to 15% of total body fluid in a small child could easily produce symptoms. For this reason, fluid therapy is one of the basics of resuscitation.

Ligands

The word *ligand* comes from the Latin verb *ligare*, meaning "to tie or bind." The word *ligament* is derived from the same root. Just as ligaments connect bones, <u>ligands</u> are molecules that bind to receptors in the body to form more complex structures. Ligands can be produced by the body (endogenous ligands) or administered as drugs (exogenous ligands). In addition to medications, common ligands include hormones, neurotransmitters, and electrolytes.

<u>Hormones</u> are substances formed in tiny amounts by one specialized organ or group of cells and then carried to another organ or group of cells in the same organism to perform regulatory functions. For example, adrenocorticotropic hormone, produced by the anterior pituitary gland, stimulates the adrenal glands to secrete cortisol. <u>Endocrine hormones</u> (such as thyroid hormones and adrenal steroids) are carried to their target organ or cell group in the blood. <u>Exocrine hormones</u> reach their target via a specific duct that opens into an organ; examples of exocrine secretions include stomach acids and perspiration. <u>Paracrine hormones</u> (such as histamine, the hormone released during allergic and inflammatory reactions) diffuse through intracellular spaces to reach their target. A hormone that acts on the cell from which it has been secreted is called an <u>autocrine hormone</u>.

<u>Neurotransmitters</u> are proteins that affect signals between cells of the nervous system. For example, acetylcholine, which aids in the movement of nerve impulses from neuron to neuron, is a neurotransmitter.

Electrolytes are dissolved mineral salts that dissociate in solution, yielding <u>ions</u>. Examples of electrolytes commonly found in the body include sodium, potassium, calcium, and chloride. Electrolytes have an important role in cell signaling and in generating the nervous system's action potential. Ions can be positively charged (<u>cations</u>) or negatively charged (<u>anions</u>). Body fluids are electrically neutral; the sum of positively charged ions in a solution is always balanced by the sum of negatively charged ions. In disease, the concentrations of the individual ions may vary, but electrical neutrality is always maintained.

Adaptations in Cells and Tissues

When cells are exposed to adverse conditions, they undergo a process of adaptation in an attempt to protect themselves from injury. In some situations, the cells change permanently; in others, they change their structure or function only temporarily.

<u>Atrophy</u> is a decrease in cell size due to a loss of subcellular components, which in turn leads to a decrease in the size of the tissue and organ. The actual number of cells remains unchanged. The decreased size represents an attempt to cope with a new steady state in less-than-favorable conditions or a lack of use. For example, a casted, immobilized limb shrinks in muscle mass as a result of disuse atrophy.

<u>Hypertrophy</u> is an increase in the size of the cells due to synthesis of more subcellular components, which in turn leads to an increase in tissue and organ size. For example, the left ventricle in the heart may hypertrophy owing to chronic high resistance pressures from hypertension (elevated blood pressure).

<u>Hyperplasia</u> is an increase in the actual number of cells in an organ or tissue, usually resulting in an increase in the size of the organ or tissue. For example, a callus represents hyperplasia of the keratinized layer of the epidermis of the foot in response to increased friction or trauma.

<u>Dysplasia</u> is an alteration of the size, shape, and organization of cells. It is most often found in epithelial cells that have undergone irregular, atypical changes in response to chronic irritation or inflammation. For example, the development of cervical dysplasia in women is strongly associated with exposure to certain human papillomaviruses.

<u>Metaplasia</u> refers to the reversible cellular adaptation in which one adult cell type is replaced by another adult cell type. For example, in squamous metaplasia, the ciliated epithelium in the airways of smokers may be replaced by metaplastic epithelium.

The Cellular Environment

Distribution of Body Fluids

The cellular environment refers to the distribution of cells, molecules, and fluids throughout the body. This environment changes with aging, exercise, pregnancy, medications, disease, and injury. Body fluids contain water, sodium, chloride, potassium, calcium, phosphorus, magnesium, and other substances.

Approximately 50% to 70% of the total body weight is fluid (a component also known as the total body water). An average man is 60% fluid; an average woman is 50% fluid. Body fluid is classified into two main types: intracellular fluid (45% of body weight) and extracellular fluid (15% of body weight). (In terms of the total body water volume—compared with body weight— approximately 75% of the body's fluid is intracellular, and the remaining 25% is extracellular.) The extracellular fluid can be further classified into interstitial fluid (10.5% of body weight; see **Figure 6**), which surrounds tissue cells and includes cerebrospinal fluid and synovial fluid, and intravascular fluid (4.5% of body weight), which is found within the blood vessels but outside the cells.

Special Populations

The volume of total body water changes throughout a person's lifetime. At birth, a healthy, full-term infant has about 80% total body water. As a person ages, the percentage of total body water decreases. An infant's total body water is around 70%, whereas a child's total body water is generally around 60%. In adulthood, total body water is around 50% to 60%. In older people, total body water may constitute only 45% of body weight. For this reason, dehydration can be a serious concern in older adults; however, this does not mean that dehydration is not a concern in the pediatric population. Infants and children are at greater risk for dehydration than adults because their fluid reserves are smaller than those in adults.

Fluid and Water Balance

An average adult takes in about 2,500 mL of water per day. Of this fluid intake, about 60% occurs by drinking. Another 30% comes from the water in foods, such as fruits. The remaining 10% is a by-product of cellular metabolism. Most water (60%) is lost in the form of urine; 28% is lost through the lungs (via respiration) and the skin; 6% is lost in the feces; and 6% is lost through sweat. The amount of water lost through sweating is

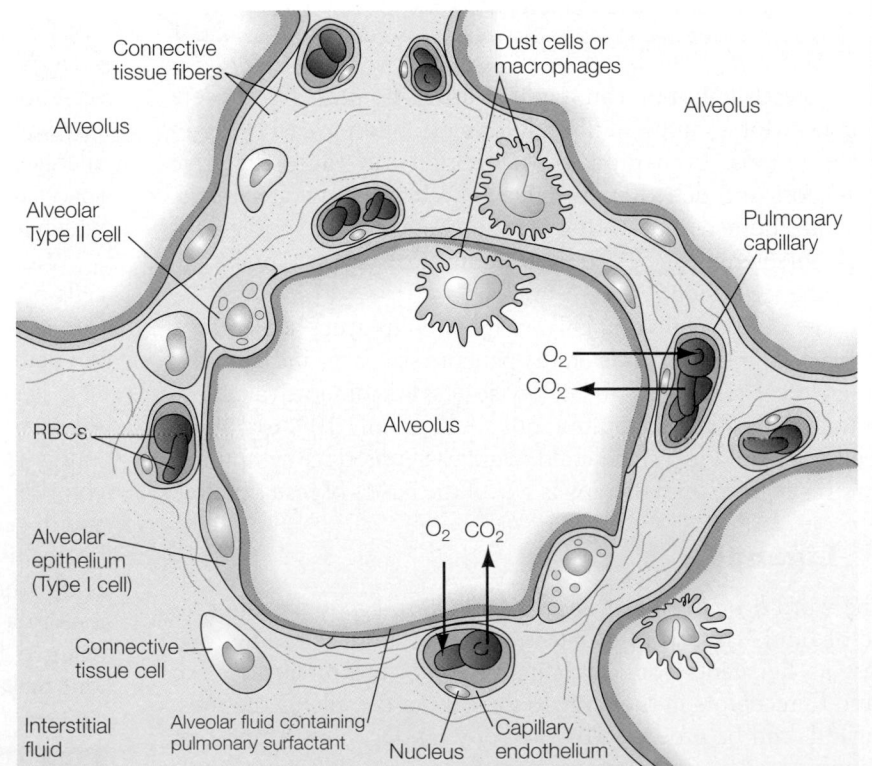

Figure 6 Close-up of the alveolus. Oxygen diffuses out of the alveolus and into the capillary. Carbon dioxide diffuses in the opposite direction, entering the alveolar air that is expelled during exhalation. Note the location of the interstitial fluid.

Table 1 Movement of Molecules

Method	Movement
Passive transport	Movement of a substance by diffusion from an area of higher concentration to an area of lower concentration
Facilitated diffusion	The easing of the passage of a substance from an area of higher concentration to an area of lower concentration by a transport (helper) molecule within the membrane
Osmosis	The movement of a solvent, such as water, from an area of low solute concentration to one of high concentration through a selectively permeable membrane to equalize the solute concentration on both sides of the membrane
Filtration	The movement of water and a dissolved substance from an area of high pressure to an area of low pressure
Active transport	Movement via transport molecules, or pumps, that require energy to move substances from an area of low concentration to an area of high concentration

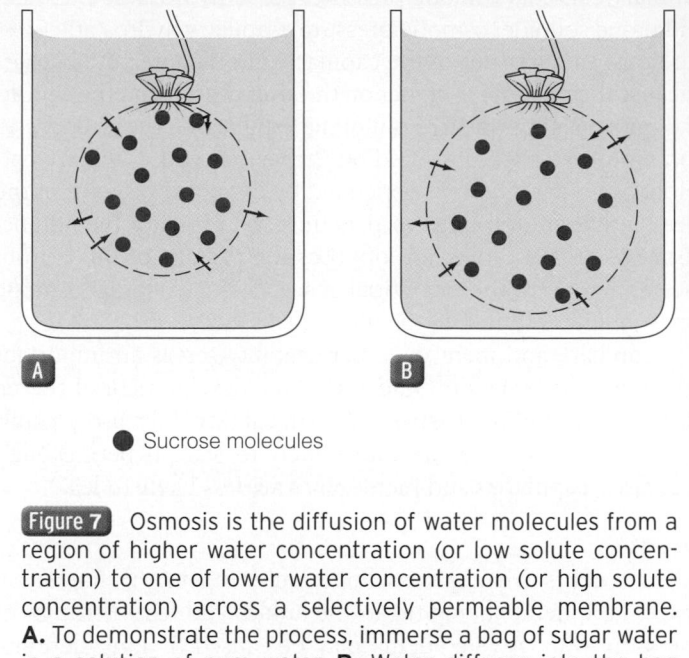

● Sucrose molecules

Figure 7 Osmosis is the diffusion of water molecules from a region of higher water concentration (or low solute concentration) to one of lower water concentration (or high solute concentration) across a selectively permeable membrane. **A.** To demonstrate the process, immerse a bag of sugar water in a solution of pure water. **B.** Water diffuses into the bag (toward the lower water concentration).

highly variable—for example, in hot environmental conditions or during periods of rigorous exercise, it is possible to lose large amounts of fluid.

Water (solvent) and dissolved particles (solutes) move between cells and between blood vessels and connective tissues. The two general methods of movement are passive transport and active transport Table 1 .

Water moves between intracellular and extracellular fluid by osmosis. **Osmosis** is the movement of water or another solvent across a membrane from a region of higher water concentration (or low solute concentration) to one of lower water concentration (or high solute concentration). Osmotic pressure develops when two solutions of different concentrations are separated by a semipermeable membrane. Water moves from the region of low osmotic pressure to the region of higher osmotic pressure Figure 7 . The solution with a higher solute concentration has a higher osmotic pressure and is referred to as a **hypertonic solution**. The solution with a lower solute concentration has a lower osmotic pressure and is referred to as a **hypotonic solution**. Solutions with equal solute concentrations are called **isotonic solutions** (such as normal saline [0.9% NaCl] and lactated Ringer's solution).

Intracellular fluid volume is controlled in two ways: by the proteins and organic compounds that cannot escape through the cell membrane and by the sodium–potassium (Na^+/K^+)

membrane pump. Most intracellular substances are negatively charged and so attract positively charged ions, including potassium. Because all of these substances are osmotically active, they can pull water into the cell—even until the cell ruptures. The Na^+/K^+ pump is responsible for keeping this situation in check and maintaining the cell's electrical potential by continuously removing three Na^+ ions from the cell for every two K^+ ions that are moved back into the cell. If this pump is impaired due to insufficient potassium in the body, sodium accumulates and causes the cells to swell.

Words of Wisdom

A hypertonic solution, such as mannitol, contains more solute than in the interstitial or tissue fluid in the brain. Its administration causes excess fluid to be drawn into the blood, potentially decreasing swelling in the brain.

Plasma

Plasma, which makes up about 55% of the blood, is composed of 91% water and 9% plasma proteins. Plasma proteins include albumin, which maintains osmotic pressure; globulin; and fibrinogen and prothrombin, which assist with clotting. Water moves between plasma and interstitial fluid according to principles explained by the Starling hypothesis. Under normal conditions, the amount of fluid filtering outward through the arterial ends of the capillaries equals the amount of fluid that is returned to the circulation by reabsorption at the venous ends of the capillaries.

The equilibrium between the capillary and the interstitial space is controlled by four forces: capillary hydrostatic pressure, capillary colloidal osmotic pressure, tissue hydrostatic pressure, and tissue colloidal osmotic pressure. Capillary hydrostatic pressure pushes water out of the capillary into the interstitial space. Because the pressure is higher on the arterial end than the venous end, more water is pushed out of the capillary on the arterial end and more water is reabsorbed on the venous end. Capillary colloidal osmotic pressure is generated by dissolved proteins in the plasma that are too large to penetrate the capillary membrane. Tissue hydrostatic pressure opposes the passage of fluids from the capillary into the interstitial space. Tissue colloidal osmotic pressure draws fluid into the interstitial space.

Capillary and membrane permeability serves an important role in the movement of fluid and in the development of edema in the surrounding tissues. If permeability increases, capillaries and membranes are more likely to leak. If permeability decreases, capillaries and membranes are less likely to leak.

Edema

Edema occurs when excess fluid builds up in the interstitial space. Peripheral edema (as in the ankles and feet) is the most common form. Severe edema may be caused by long-standing lymphatic obstruction. If a person is unable to get out of bed for an extended period, edema may occur in the sacral area (sacral edema). Ascites is the abnormal accumulation of fluid in the peritoneal cavity.

Causes Edema may have any of several causes:

- Increased capillary hydrostatic pressure from any of the following:
  - Arteriolar dilation (for example, from allergic reactions or inflammation)
  - Venous obstruction (for example, hepatic obstruction, heart failure, or thrombophlebitis)
  - Increased vascular volume, as occurs in patients with heart failure
  - An increased level of adrenocortical hormones
  - Premenstrual sodium retention
  - Pregnancy
  - Environmental heat stress
  - The effects of gravity from prolonged standing
- Decreased colloidal osmotic pressure in the capillaries from any of the following:
  - Decreased production of plasma proteins, such as occurs in starvation and in patients with liver disease or severe protein deficiency
  - Increased loss of plasma proteins attributable to protein-losing kidney diseases, extensive burns, or other causes
- Lymphatic vessel obstruction attributable to infection or to disease of the lymphatic structures or their removal (for example, mastectomy and removal of lymph nodes may lead to edema in an upper extremity). In this case, the amount of fluid leaving the arterial end of capillaries does not equal the amount of fluid returned from the venous side. Hence, more fluid leaves the arterial side, where the mean forces favoring outward movement are slightly higher; therefore, the additional fluid is picked up by the lymphatic system.

Clinical Manifestations The clinical manifestations of edema may be local or generalized. Patients may have pulmonary edema for cardiac reasons, or edema may present following near-drowning (submersion) or a narcotic overdose. Excess fluid in the lungs (such as acute pulmonary edema) impairs the diffusion of oxygen into pulmonary capillaries, making the patient hypoxic. Patients can drown in their own fluids if they do not receive proper care.

Assessment and Management Paramedics must perform an in-depth physical assessment that includes auscultation of breath sounds, evaluation for pedal and sacral edema and jugular venous distention, an electrocardiogram (ECG), and vital signs. Along with a thorough exam, it is important to determine a patient's medical history and his or her current and past medications. Often treatment is dictated by the patient's chief complaint and presenting problem and is limited to treating immediately life-threatening conditions in the prehospital setting. Treatment may include diuretics, nitrates, continuous positive airway pressure, high-flow oxygen, and advanced airway placement.

■ Fluid and Electrolyte Balance

Water balance in the body is maintained through a variety of factors, of which the thirst mechanism and release of **antidiuretic hormone (ADH)**, also known as vasopressin, are the most important. The **renin-angiotensin-aldosterone system (RAAS)** also has a role in water homeostasis. The body's state of hydration is monitored continuously by the following three types of receptors:

- *Osmoreceptors* monitor extracellular fluid osmolarity. Sensors for these receptors are located primarily in the hypothalamus. When the extracellular fluid osmolarity is too high, they stimulate the production of ADH.
- *Volume-sensitive receptors* are located in the atria. When the intravascular fluid volume increases, the atria are stretched, leading to the release of atrial natriuretic proteins.
- *Baroreceptors* are found primarily in the carotid artery, aorta, and kidneys. They are sensitive to changes in blood pressure.

The most potent stimulation for the release of ADH is an increase in blood **osmolarity**. When osmolarity increases, the pituitary gland releases ADH; ADH stimulates the kidneys to resorb water, decreasing the osmolarity of the blood.

Regulation of Sodium, Chloride, and Water Balance

Sodium is the most common cation, or positively charged ion, in the body. An average adult has 60 mEq of sodium for each kilogram of body weight (2.2 lb = 1 kg). Most of the body's sodium is found in the extracellular fluid, but a small amount is found in the intracellular fluid. Intracellular sodium is transported out of the cell by the sodium-potassium pump because a resting cell membrane is relatively impermeable to sodium. Sodium also has an important role in the regulation of the body's acid-base balance (sodium bicarbonate buffer system).

Sodium is taken in with foods. As little as 500 mg/d meets the body's needs. In the United States, an average adult ingests around 3,400 mg of sodium per day (the American Heart Association recommends that this be trimmed back to a maximum of 1,500 mg/d for an adult).

The sodium level is regulated primarily by the RAAS and by natriuretic peptides. Natriuretic peptides are a type of protein that causes excretion of sodium, among other effects, which ultimately helps regulate blood pressure and volume. The RAAS is a complex feedback mechanism responsible for the kidney's regulation of the sodium level in the body. When sodium is present in excess, it is excreted into the urine; when the body's sodium level is low, the kidneys resorb sodium.

Renin is a protein that is released by the kidneys into the bloodstream in response to changes in blood pressure, blood flow, the amount of sodium in the tubular fluid, and the glomerular filtration rate. When renin is released, it converts the plasma protein angiotensinogen to angiotensin I. In the lungs, angiotensin I is converted rapidly to angiotensin II

by angiotensin-converting enzyme. Angiotensin II, in turn, stimulates sodium resorption by the renal tubules. It also constricts the renal blood vessels, slowing kidney blood flow and decreasing the glomerular filtration rate. As a result, less sodium is filtered into the urine and more sodium is resorbed in the blood. **Figure 8** illustrates the role of the kidneys in the regulation of blood pressure and blood volume.

Angiotensin II is also responsible for stimulating the secretion of the adrenal hormone aldosterone. Aldosterone acts on the kidneys to increase the reabsorption of sodium into the blood and enhance the elimination of potassium in the urine. In addition to the stimulation by angiotensin II, aldosterone release is stimulated by an increased extracellular potassium level, a decreased extracellular sodium level, and release of adrenocorticotropic hormone from the pituitary gland.

Whereas activation of the RAAS leads to retention of sodium and water, production of natriuretic proteins increases when the

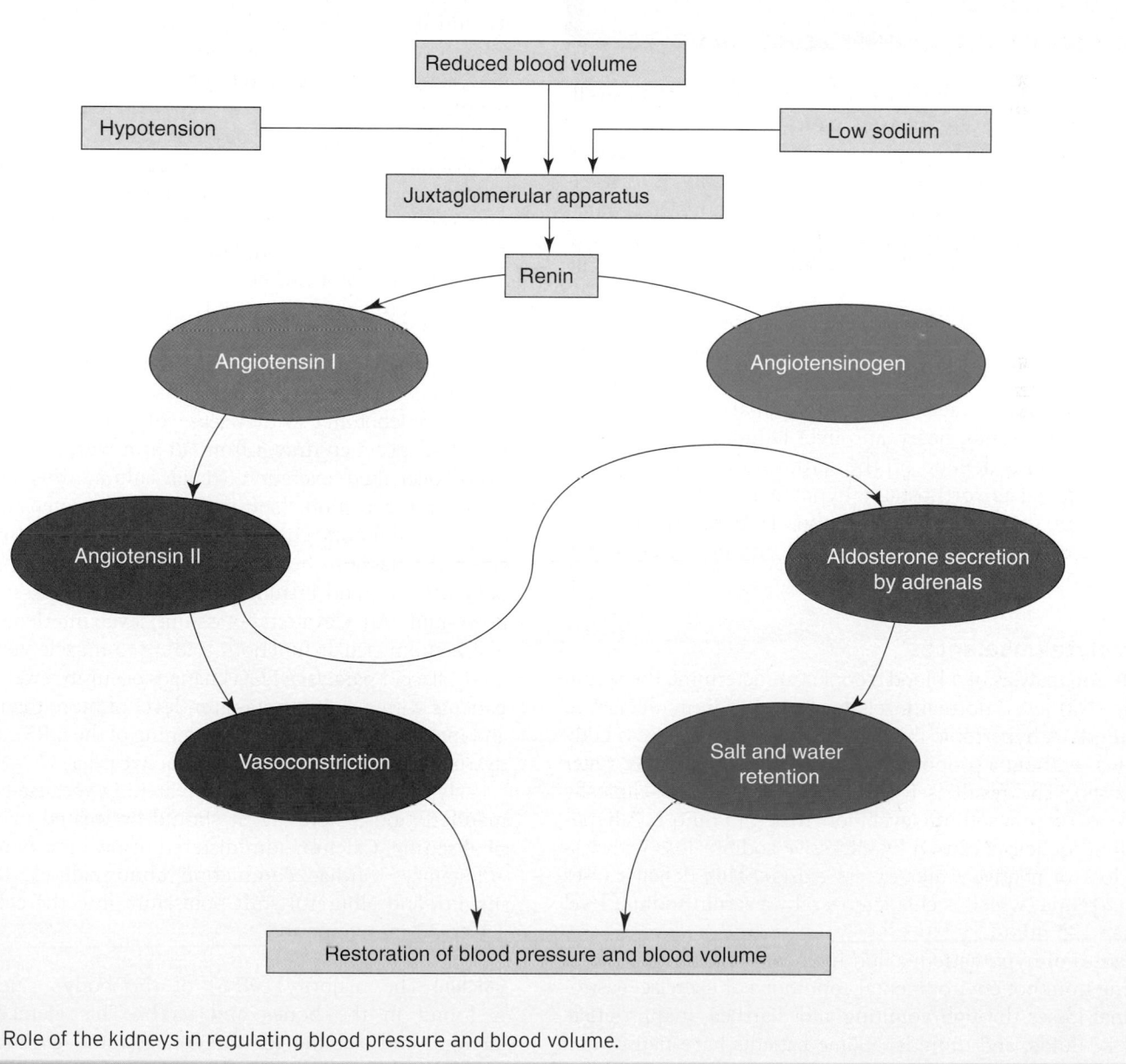

Figure 8 Role of the kidneys in regulating blood pressure and blood volume.

body contains too much sodium and water. Natriuretic proteins inhibit ADH and promote excretion of sodium and water by the kidneys.

Chloride is an important anion, or negatively charged ion, that makes ordinary table salt when combined with sodium. When placed in water, the compound separates into its original ionic form. It assists in regulating the acid-base balance, especially the pH of the stomach, and is involved in the osmotic pressure of the extracellular fluid. Table salt, milk, eggs, and meats all contain chloride. It is often the case that where sodium goes, chloride follows.

Words of Wisdom

When you eat a bag of potato chips, you ingest a large quantity of salt. Acutely, the body responds by holding on to water (hence, urine output temporarily declines). In healthy people, the kidneys and other regulatory mechanisms soon straighten things out.

Changes in water content can cause a cell to shrink or swell. Tonicity refers to the tension exerted on a cell as a result of water movement across the cell membrane. When cells are placed in an isotonic solution (one with the same osmolarity as intracellular fluid—280 mOsm/L), they neither shrink nor swell. When cells are placed in a hypertonic solution, water is pulled out of the cells and they shrink. When cells are placed in a hypotonic solution, they swell.

An isotonic fluid deficit is a decrease in extracellular fluid with proportionate losses of sodium and water. An isotonic fluid excess is a proportionate increase in sodium and water in the extracellular fluid compartment; common causes include kidney, heart, and liver failure. Manifestations of these problems depend on the serum sodium level. When dehydration exists, orthostatic hypotension and decreased urine output (oliguria) are common. Hyperthermia, delirium, and coma may be seen when the sodium level is very high (> 160 mEq/L).

Electrolyte Imbalances

Sodium An analysis of a blood sample can determine the serum sodium (Na) level; normal levels for serum sodium are 136 to 144 mEq/L. A hypertonic fluid deficit is caused by excess body water loss without a proportionate sodium loss (a relative water loss exists). The result is hypernatremia, which is clinically defined as a serum sodium level more than 145 mEq/L. A hypotonic fluid deficit is caused by excessive sodium loss with less water loss (a relative water excess exists). This deficit causes hyponatremia, which is characterized by a serum sodium level less than 135 mEq/L.

Causes of hypernatremia and hyponatremia include excess sweating from hot environmental conditions or exercise, gastrointestinal losses through vomiting and diarrhea, inappropriate use of IV fluids, and diuretics. Some patients have nausea and headaches, and in others, seizures and coma develop. Clinical findings typically depend not only on the absolute sodium level, but also on the period during which the abnormality developed. People who become hyponatremic during a period of days tend to have fewer symptoms than people in whom the abnormality develops acutely.

Potassium Potassium (K⁺), as the major intracellular cation, is critical to many functions of the cell. Potassium is necessary for neuromuscular control, regulation of the three types of muscles (skeletal, smooth, and cardiac), acid-base balance, intracellular enzyme reactions, and maintenance of intracellular osmolarity. The normal serum level of potassium is in the range of 3.5 to 5 mEq/L.

Hypokalemia is defined as a decreased serum potassium level. Common causes include decreased potassium intake, potassium shifts into the cells (related to insulin, alkalosis, or beta-adrenergic stimulation such as with epinephrine), renal potassium losses (such as with increased aldosterone activity and diuretic use), and extrarenal potassium losses (such as with vomiting, diarrhea, and laxative use). Muscular weakness, fatigue, and muscle cramps are the most frequent complaints in mild to moderate hypokalemia. Flaccid paralysis, hyporeflexia, and tetany may occur with a very low level of potassium (< 2.5 mEq/L). The ECG shows decreased amplitude and broadening of T waves, prominent U waves, premature ventricular contractions and other dysrhythmias (such as torsades de pointes), and depressed ST segments. Although acute hypokalemia can be treated with IV potassium supplementation, this therapy is rarely undertaken in the prehospital setting.

Hyperkalemia is an elevated serum potassium level. Common causes include spurious causes (repeated fist-clenching during phlebotomy, with release of potassium from forearm muscles; specimen drawn from an arm with a potassium infusion), decreased excretion (renal failure, drugs that inhibit potassium excretion [spironolactone, angiotensin-converting enzyme inhibitors, nonsteroidal anti-inflammatory drugs]), shifts of potassium from within the cell (as with burns, metabolic acidosis, and insulin deficiency), and excessive intake of potassium. An elevated potassium level interferes with normal neuromuscular function, leading to muscle weakness and, rarely, flaccid paralysis. ECG changes occur in fewer than half of patients with a serum potassium level of more than 6.5 mEq/L and include peaked T waves, widening of the QRS complex, and dysrhythmias such as ventricular tachycardia.

Hyperkalemia can be life threatening because of its cardiac manifestations; therefore, it should be treated in the prehospital setting. Calcium administered intravenously immediately antagonizes cardiac conduction abnormalities. Bicarbonate, insulin, and albuterol shift potassium into the cells during a 15- to 30-minute period.

Calcium The majority (98%) of the body's calcium (Ca⁺⁺) is found in the bones and teeth. This element provides strength and stability for the collagen and ground substance that forms the matrix of the skeletal system. Calcium enters the body through the gastrointestinal tract and is absorbed from the intestine in a process that depends on the presence of vitamin D **Figure 9**. Vitamin D is largely obtained through exposure to sunlight, stored in the bone, and ultimately excreted by the kidney. The normal serum calcium level is 8.5 to 10.5 mg/dL.

<u>Hypocalcemia</u> is a decreased serum calcium level. Causes of hypocalcemia include decreased intake or absorption (as in malabsorption and vitamin D deficit), increased loss (as in alcoholism and diuretic therapy), endocrine disease (such as hypoparathyroidism), and sepsis. Symptoms reflect the increased excitation of the neuromuscular and cardiovascular systems. Spasm of skeletal muscle causes cramps and tetany. Laryngospasm with stridor can obstruct the airway. Seizures can occur, as can abnormal sensations (paresthesias) of the lips and extremities. Prolongation of the QT interval predisposes to the development of ventricular dysrhythmias.

<u>Hypercalcemia</u> is an increased serum calcium level. Causes include increased intake or absorption (such as excess antacid ingestion), endocrine disorders (such as primary hyperparathyroidism and adrenal insufficiency), neoplasms (cancers), and miscellaneous causes (such as diuretics and sarcoidosis). Symptoms include constipation and frequent urination (<u>polyuria</u>). Stupor, coma, and renal failure may develop in severe cases. Treatment of the underlying cause is the mainstay of dealing with hypercalcemia. On an acute basis, volume replacement with boluses of 0.45% or 0.9% sodium chloride solution may be helpful.

Phosphate Phosphate (PO_4^{3-}) is primarily an intracellular anion and is essential to many body functions.

<u>Hypophosphatemia</u> is characterized by a decrease in the level of serum phosphate. Causes include the following:

- Decreased supply or absorption, as can occur in starvation, malabsorption, or blocked absorption (such as with aluminum-containing antacids)
- Excessive loss of phosphate ion through use of diuretics or in cases of hyperparathyroidism, hyperthyroidism, or alcoholism

LOW BLOOD CALCIUM		HIGH BLOOD CALCIUM	
Increase PTH secretion and calcitriol formation	Thyroid/Parathyroid	**Secrete calcitonin**	**Decrease PTH secretion and calcitriol formation**
Parathyroid gland secretes PTH. Increased PTH levels stimulate calcitriol (vitamin D₃) production in the kidney	Thyroid · Parathyroid (embedded in the thyroid)	Thyroid gland secretes calcitonin	PTH formation slows and PTH levels drop. Decreased PTH levels slow calcitriol formation
Absorb more dietary calcium	Small intestine 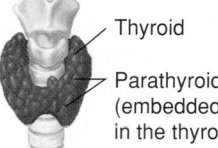	**Absorb less dietary calcium**	
Calcitriol increases intestinal absorption of calcium and phosphorus		No major effect—calcitonin slightly inhibits calcium absorption	Decreased calcitriol slows intestinal absorption of calcium and phosphorus
Retain calcium	Kidney 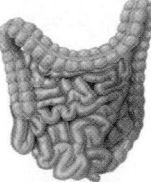	**Excrete calcium**	
PTH and calcitriol increase calcium reabsorption in the kidney, thus decreasing calcium excretion		No major effect—calcitonin slightly increases calcium excretion	Decreased PTH and calcitriol levels increase calcium excretion
Move calcium from bone to bloodstream	Bone 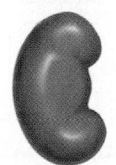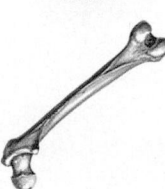	**Move calcium from bloodstream to bone**	
PTH and calcitriol work together to stimulate osteoclast activity. The osteoclasts resorb bone, releasing calcium into the bloodstream		Calcitonin inhibits the activity of osteoclasts, shifting the balance toward the deposition of calcium in bone	Decreased PTH and calcitriol levels slow osteoclast activity and breakdown of bone
RAISE BLOOD CALCIUM		**LOWER BLOOD CALCIUM**	

Figure 9 Regulation of the blood calcium level. Calcitonin has only a weak effect on calcium ion concentration. It is fast-acting, but any decrease in calcium ion concentration triggers the release of parathyroid hormone (PTH), which almost completely overrides the calcitonin effect. In a patient with a prolonged calcium excess or deficiency, the parathyroid mechanism is the most powerful hormonal mechanism for maintaining a normal blood calcium level.

- Intracellular shift of phosphorus (for example, after administration of glucose, anabolic steroids, or oral contraceptives or in patients with respiratory alkalosis or salicylate poisoning)
- Electrolyte abnormalities such as hypercalcemia and hypomagnesemia
- Abnormal losses followed by inadequate repletion, as can occur in patients with diabetic ketoacidosis or chronic alcoholism

Symptoms include muscle weakness, decreased deep tendon reflexes, mental obtundation, and confusion. Weakness is common. Acute, severe hypophosphatemia can lead to acute hemolytic anemia and increased susceptibility to infection. The breakdown of muscle fibers (rhabdomyolysis) may also occur. Treatment involves oral replenishment in mild to moderate cases. Severe cases and symptomatic patients require IV phosphate replacement.

Hyperphosphatemia is an increased serum phosphate level. Causes include massive loading of phosphate into the extracellular fluid (such as with the use of excess vitamin D, laxatives or enemas containing phosphate, and IV phosphate supplements; chemotherapy; and metabolic acidosis) and decreased excretion into the urine (such as in renal failure and hypoparathyroidism and with excessive growth hormone [which results in acromegaly]).

Symptoms vary widely but may include tremor, paresthesia, hyporeflexia, confusion, seizures, muscle weakness, stupor, coma, hypotension, heart failure, and prolonged QT interval. Treatment of the underlying cause and of any accompanying hypocalcemia is the most common therapeutic approach. Saline boluses (forced diuresis) are often helpful.

Magnesium Magnesium (Mg^{++}) is the second most abundant intracellular cation, after potassium. About 50% of the body's magnesium is stored in the bones, 49% in the body cells, and the remaining 1% in the extracellular fluid. The normal range of serum magnesium is 1.5 to 2 mEq/L.

Hypomagnesemia is a decreased serum magnesium level. Causes include diminished absorption or intake (as in malabsorption, chronic diarrhea, laxative abuse, and malnutrition), increased renal loss (related to diuretics, hyperaldosteronism, hypercalcemia, volume expansion), and miscellaneous causes (such as diabetes, respiratory alkalosis, and pregnancy). Common symptoms are weakness, muscle cramps, and tremor. Marked neuromuscular and CNS hyperirritability, with tremors and jerking, develop. Hypertension, tachycardia, or ventricular dysrhythmia may occur, and confusion and disorientation can be pronounced. Treatment consists of IV fluids containing magnesium.

Hypermagnesemia is an increased serum magnesium level. It is almost always the result of kidney insufficiency and the inability to excrete the amount of magnesium taken in from food or drugs, especially antacids and laxatives. Symptoms include muscle weakness, decreased deep tendon reflexes, mental obtundation, and confusion. Weakness is common, and respiratory muscle paralysis and cardiac arrest are possible.

Table 2 summarizes the major electrolytes of the body.

YOU are the Medic   PART 2

You ask your partner to remove the nasal cannula, give the patient high-flow oxygen, and obtain baseline vital signs. While your partner is setting up her equipment, you ask the patient about his past medical history. The patient with great difficulty tells you, "heart failure."

Recording Time: 1 Minute	
Appearance	Awake, in distress, anxious
Level of consciousness	Alert (oriented to person, place, and day)
Airway	Open
Breathing	Elevated rate; accessory muscle use; productive cough
Circulation	Weak radial pulses; moist, pale, cool skin

3. What is the body trying to do through the use of accessory muscles of breathing?

4. What could the productive cough indicate in relation to the level of difficulty breathing?

Table 2 Major Electrolytes

Electrolyte	Symbol	Normal Serum Level (mEq/L)
Sodium	Na	136-144
Chloride	Cl^-	98-108
Potassium	K^+	3.5-5
Calcium	Ca^{++}	8.5-10.5
Phosphate	PO_4^{3-}	2.3-4.7
Magnesium	Mg^{++}	1.5-2

Acid-Base Balance

An <u>acid</u> is any molecule that can give up a hydrogen ion (H^+). A <u>base</u>, or alkali, is any molecule that can accept a hydrogen ion (OH^-). The acidity or basicity (alkalinity) of a solution is determined by the amount of free hydrogen in the solution.

The <u>pH</u> of a solution is a measurement of the level of its acidity or alkalinity **Figure 10**. An acidic solution is one with a pH less than 7. An alkaline (base) solution is one with a pH greater than 7. Normal physiologic functions can be optimally performed within a very narrow range of pH: between 7.35 and 7.45. Hypoventilation, hyperventilation, and hypoxia can disrupt the acid-base balance. Cellular function deteriorates and death occurs when the pH drops below 6.9 or rises above 7.8.

One important point is that changes in the pH are exponential, not linear. For example, a change in the pH from 7.40 to 7.20 yields a 10^2 change—that is, a 100-fold increase—in acid concentration.

Disturbance of Acid-Base Balance

Acids and bases neutralize each other and must remain in balance to maintain homeostasis in the body. In other words, the

ionic charge inside and outside the cell must in balance. An increase in extracellular H^+ ions results in <u>acidosis</u>; a decrease in extracellular H^+ ions results in <u>alkalosis</u>.

↓ pH Means ↑ H^+ Concentration = Acidosis
↑ pH Means ↓ H^+ Concentration = Alkalosis

If intracellular pH is low, an excessive concentration of H^+ ions exists in the extracellular fluid (the fluid outside the cell), signaling H^+ ions to move into the cell, giving it an overall positive charge. To return its charge to neutral, the cell begins to shift cations (positively charged ions) such as potassium into the interstitial fluid.

Disturbances of acid-base balance are associated with disturbances in potassium balance, in part because of the kidney transport system that moves H^+ and K^+ in opposite directions. In acidosis, the kidneys excrete H^+ and resorb K^+. Conversely, when the body goes into a state of alkalosis, the kidneys resorb H^+ and excrete K^+. A potassium imbalance usually shows up as a disturbance in excitable tissues, especially the heart.

In addition, calcium ions shift out of the cell in response to the influx of hydrogen. A high serum calcium level (hypercalcemia) decreases the rate of neural transmission, the speed at which an impulse is conveyed by the neuron. This reaction will cause some minimal ECG changes, but seldom causes dysrhythmias. A low serum calcium level (hypocalcemia), on the other hand, leads to hypersensitive neurons and an accelerated rate of neural transmission. Effects of hypocalcemia include wheezing, stridor, bradycardia, crackles, and an S_3 heart sound. It also causes ECG changes and can lead to dysrhythmias.

Buffer Systems

To maintain the delicate acid-base balance, the body relies on its buffer systems. <u>Buffers</u> are molecules or compounds that modulate changes in pH by neutralizing excessive acids or bases. In the absence of buffers, the rapid buildup of acid can cause an

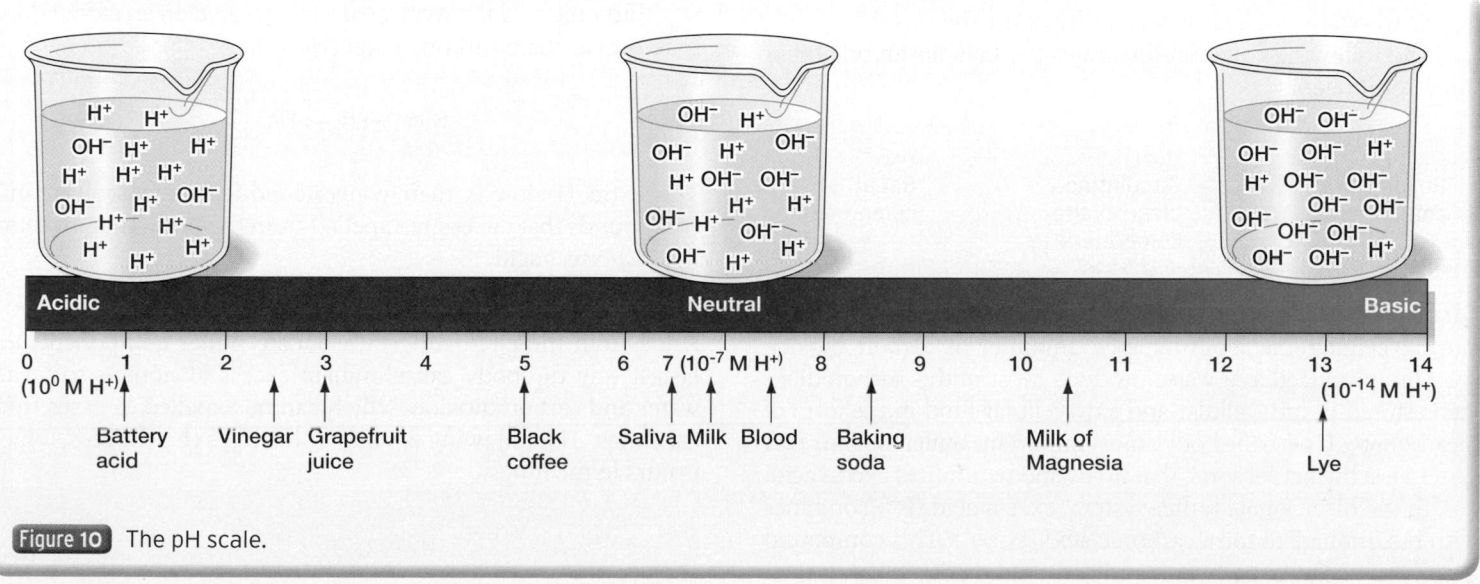

Figure 10 The pH scale.

abrupt change in pH. Buffers regulate changes in pH to avert such precipitous fluctuations. For example, bone acts as a buffer by absorbing excess acids and bases and by releasing calcium into the circulation.

The pH scale ranges from 0 to 14. An acid or base can be classified as strong or weak, depending on how completely it **dissociates** in water. Any solution approaching a pH of 14, such as the fluid used to flush clogged drains, is said to be a strong base, whereas any solution close to the other end of the scale, such as stomach acid, is said to be a strong acid. Solutions near the midpoint of the pH scale, such as milk, are said to be neutral. Not surprisingly, water has a pH of 7.

The ability of weak acids to bond weakly to H^+ ions makes them ideal buffers because they can accept or donate H^+ ions, depending on the needs of the body. Buffer systems include proteins, phosphate ions, and bicarbonate (HCO_3^-). Because acid production is the major challenge to pH homeostasis, most physiologic buffers combine with H^+. Protein buffering refers to the fact that charged proteins in the cells can accept or donate hydrogen ions, thereby helping to regulate acid-base balance by moving hydrogen into or out of the blood.

The body responds to normal shifts in the pH level by absorbing a small quantity of acid from the blood or by releasing the necessary amount of acid into the blood. Problems occur when the amount of acid in circulation is too great for the buffer system to accommodate. To grasp this concept, it is helpful to imagine the buffer system as a bucket that contains the acid in the body **Figure 11**. Like a bucket, the buffer system can hold only a certain amount before it overflows.

Three primary buffer systems help the body maintain pH within the optimal range: the circulating bicarbonate (HCO_3^-) buffer component, the respiratory system, and the renal system. The body's fastest means of restoring acid-base balance is the so-called blood buffer—the bicarbonate content of intracellular and extracellular fluid. When an excessive level of acid builds up, it is eliminated through the respiratory system, when carbon dioxide is expelled from the lungs. Conversely, slowing the rate of respiration encourages the retention of carbon dioxide. The renal system regulates pH by filtering out hydrogen and retaining bicarbonate when necessary, or by doing the reverse.

The following equation illustrates the balance among these three components:

| $CO_2 + H_2O$ | $\leftrightarrow$ | H_2CO_3 | $\leftrightarrow$ | HCO_3^- |
| Respiratory component | | Circulating bicarbonate component | | Renal component |

Circulating Bicarbonate Buffer Component

During cellular metabolism, large amounts of carbon dioxide (CO_2) are produced as a waste product. Most of this carbon dioxide is stored in intracellular and extracellular fluid in the form of bicarbonate (HCO_3), the body's most important buffer system. This system is a bucket, of sorts, that holds and neutralizes excess acid.

In the bicarbonate buffer system, excess acid (H^+) combines with bicarbonate to form carbonic acid (H_2CO_3). This compound rapidly dissociates into water and carbon dioxide, which is then

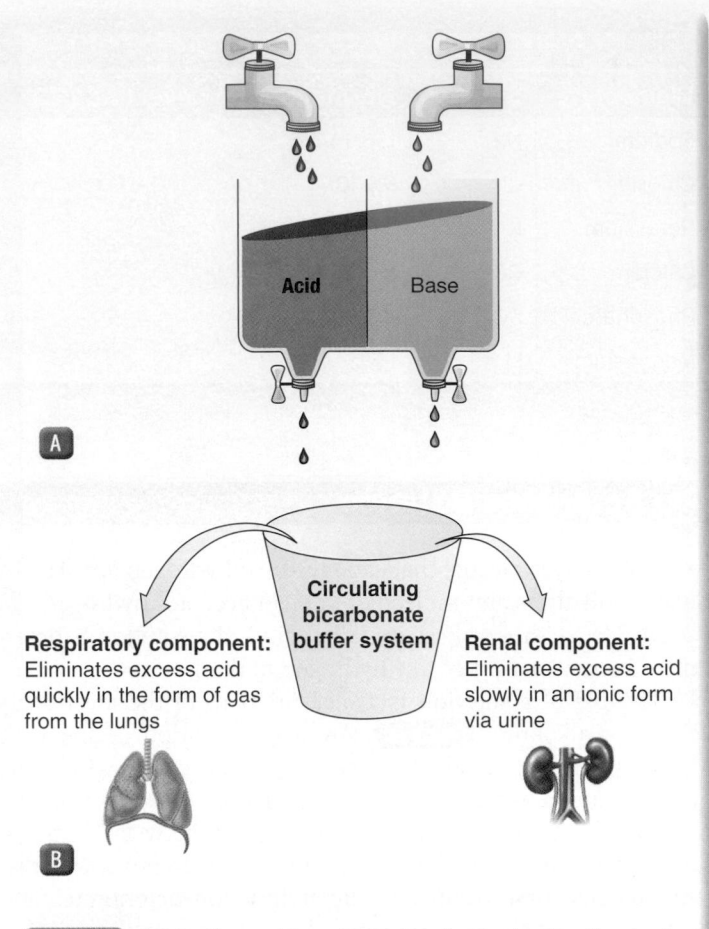

Figure 11 **A.** As the acid or base levels fluctuate, the body must work to ensure that the acid-base balance is maintained. **B.** The respiratory component and the renal component are two systems for eliminating excess acid.

exhaled. Because the acid is eliminated as water and carbon dioxide, the total pH does not change significantly. A similar process occurs with the production of metabolic base (bicarbonate).

Carbonic acid is a weak acid that can give up an extra H^+ ion to reform as the bicarbonate ion (HCO_3^-):

$$H_2CO_3 \leftrightarrow H^+ \leftrightarrow HCO_3^-$$

The extra H^+ ion is then converted during metabolism into compounds that are easily expelled from the body, thereby eliminating excess acid.

Respiratory Buffer Component

Aside from the circulating bicarbonate buffer component, the fastest way the body can eliminate excess H^+ ions is to create water and carbon dioxide, which can be expelled as gases from the lungs. The following equation illustrates this process, which occurs in the lungs:

$$H_2CO_3 \leftrightarrow CO_2 + H_2O$$

The function of the respiratory system is simple: to distribute oxygen to the body for aerobic metabolism and to remove excess carbon dioxide from the blood. Carbonic acid is created when carbon dioxide combines with circulating water in the blood. Chemoreceptors in the brain sense the rising level of carbonic acid and signal the respiratory center to increase the respiratory rate in order to reduce the amount of circulating carbon dioxide. Although the respiratory buffer reacts within minutes, it is much slower to respond than the circulating bicarbonate buffer component.

Any inhibition of respiratory function can lead to acid retention and acidosis. Any time a patient is in respiratory distress or is unable to breathe, acidosis quickly develops:

$$\uparrow H^+ \rightarrow H_2co_3 \rightarrow \uparrow co_2 \rightarrow \text{Tachypnea}$$

Acidosis can develop as a result of abnormal respiratory function, including bradypnea, tachypnea, labored breathing, or shallow breathing (reduced tidal volume). The following equation demonstrates this:

$$\downarrow \text{Respirations} \rightarrow \uparrow co_2 \rightarrow \uparrow H_2co_3 \rightarrow \text{Acidosis}$$

At the other end of the acid-base spectrum, alkalosis can develop if the respiratory rate is too high or the volume too large, as shown in the following equation:

$$\uparrow \text{Respirations} \rightarrow \downarrow co_2 \rightarrow \downarrow H_2co_3 \rightarrow \text{Alkalosis}$$

Renal Buffer Component

The kidneys filter each molecule, ion, and electrolyte in the circulatory system; they maintain homeostasis by retaining certain products and filtering out others. This system, however, responds more slowly than the bicarbonate and respiratory buffer components to an increasing acid level. It could take hours or even days for the renal buffer system to restore the body's pH to normal.

As with the respiratory system, the renal system can control the increasing acid level in the blood by excreting the acid. The respiratory system expels acid as a gas, whereas the kidneys excrete acid in an ionic form (Hco_3^-) in the urine:

$$H_2co_3 \leftrightarrow H^+ + Hco_3^-$$

If a patient's urine output drops, excess acid cannot be removed from the blood, and acidosis can develop:

$$\downarrow \text{Renal output} \rightarrow \uparrow H^+ \rightarrow \text{Acidosis}$$

If urine output becomes excessive, alkalosis can develop:

$$\uparrow \text{Renal output} \rightarrow \downarrow H^+ \rightarrow \text{Alkalosis}$$

Types of Acid-Base Disorders

Fluctuations in pH due to the level of bicarbonate in the body result in metabolic acidosis or alkalosis, whereas fluctuations in pH due to respiratory disorders result in respiratory acidosis or alkalosis. When an acid-base disorder is not immediately correctable by the body's buffering systems, the body initiates compensatory mechanisms to help restore the normal balance. For example, metabolic acidosis may create respiratory alkalosis as a compensatory response. Thus, patient management often involves treating more than one form of acid-base imbalance.

There are four main clinical presentations of acid-base disorders: respiratory acidosis, respiratory alkalosis, metabolic acidosis, and metabolic alkalosis.

Words of Wisdom

Respiratory compensation for metabolic problems (acidosis or alkalosis) occurs rapidly and is relatively predictable. Metabolic compensation for respiratory problems (acidosis or alkalosis), if it occurs at all, takes hours or even days. Compensation brings the pH closer to normal. Acute compensation is never complete. Chronic compensation, such as that which occurs in patients with chronic obstructive pulmonary disease, often returns the pH to normal.

Respiratory Acidosis

Recall the following equation from earlier in this section, which demonstrates how a diminished rate of respiration can result in acidosis:

$$\downarrow \text{Respirations} \rightarrow \uparrow co_2 \rightarrow \uparrow H_2co_3 \rightarrow \text{Acidosis}$$

Respiratory acidosis is always related to hypoventilation. Because the acidosis is attributable to inadequate breathing, the compensatory mechanism initiated is the slower-reacting renal buffer system. Some causes of respiratory acidosis include the following:

- Airway obstruction
- Cardiac arrest
- Overdose of a CNS depressant drug such as heroin
- Near-drowning (submersion)
- Respiratory arrest
- Pulmonary edema
- Closed head injury
- Chest trauma
- Carbon monoxide poisoning

Hypoventilation associated with any of these conditions is a life-threatening condition. It devolves quickly into an overwhelming, potentially fatal acidosis, making it impossible for the slower-reacting renal system to compensate in time to accomplish a pH shift. The release of potassium ions into the extracellular fluid can cause a potentially fatal cardiac dysrhythmia.

The discharge of calcium into extracellular spaces causes hypercalcemia, characterized by lethargy, a decreasing level of consciousness, and a generalized slowing of the nervous system. This nervous system inhibition may be evidenced by a delayed pupillary response or a weakened or delayed response to painful stimuli.

Signs and symptoms of respiratory acidosis include the following:

- Systemic or cerebral vasodilation (or both)
- Headaches
- Red, flushed skin
- CNS depression
- <u>Bradypnea</u> (slow respiratory rate)
- Nausea and vomiting
- Hypercalcemia

Chronic obstructive pulmonary disease (COPD) creates respiratory acidosis over time, as gradual destruction of lung tissue inhibits the exchange of oxygen and carbon dioxide **Figure 12**. In patients with COPD, the normal stimulus for this exchange is absent. Carbon dioxide retention leads to an increased level of carbonic acid. Chemoreceptors eventually become unable to detect the presence of metabolic acids. The hypoxic drive is then the only remaining stimulus for breathing. The hypoxic drive stimulates breathing by sensing a decreased oxygen level in the blood.

The slow onset of this form of respiratory acidosis in patients with COPD makes it survivable. The renal system slowly moderates the acidosis, preventing the life-threatening cardiac dysrhythmias often associated with acute acidosis.

Respiratory Alkalosis

Recall the following equation from earlier in this section, which demonstrates how an increased respiratory rate can lead to alkalosis:

$$\uparrow \text{Respirations} \rightarrow \downarrow CO_2 \rightarrow \downarrow H_2CO_3 \rightarrow \text{Alkalosis}$$

<u>Respiratory alkalosis</u> is always caused by hyperventilation. Although that may not sound worrisome, life-threatening events such as pulmonary embolism and acute myocardial infarction and dangerous states such as sepsis and diabetic ketoacidosis may be responsible for hyperventilation.

In respiratory alkalosis, the carbon dioxide level drops in the blood, forcing a reduction of circulating carbonic acid. The renal system then begins to retain H^+ ions to rebalance the depleted acid level. As this is happening, H^+ ions begin to shift from the extracellular fluid compartment to the intracellular fluid. Calcium shifts into the intracellular fluid to rebalance the depleted hydrogen level. The resulting hypocalcemia causes muscle contractions; hyperventilation accompanied by carpopedal spasm is the classic sign of respiratory alkalosis.

Some causes of hyperventilation and respiratory alkalosis include the following:

- Drug overdose, especially aspirin
- Fever
- Overzealous bag-mask ventilation

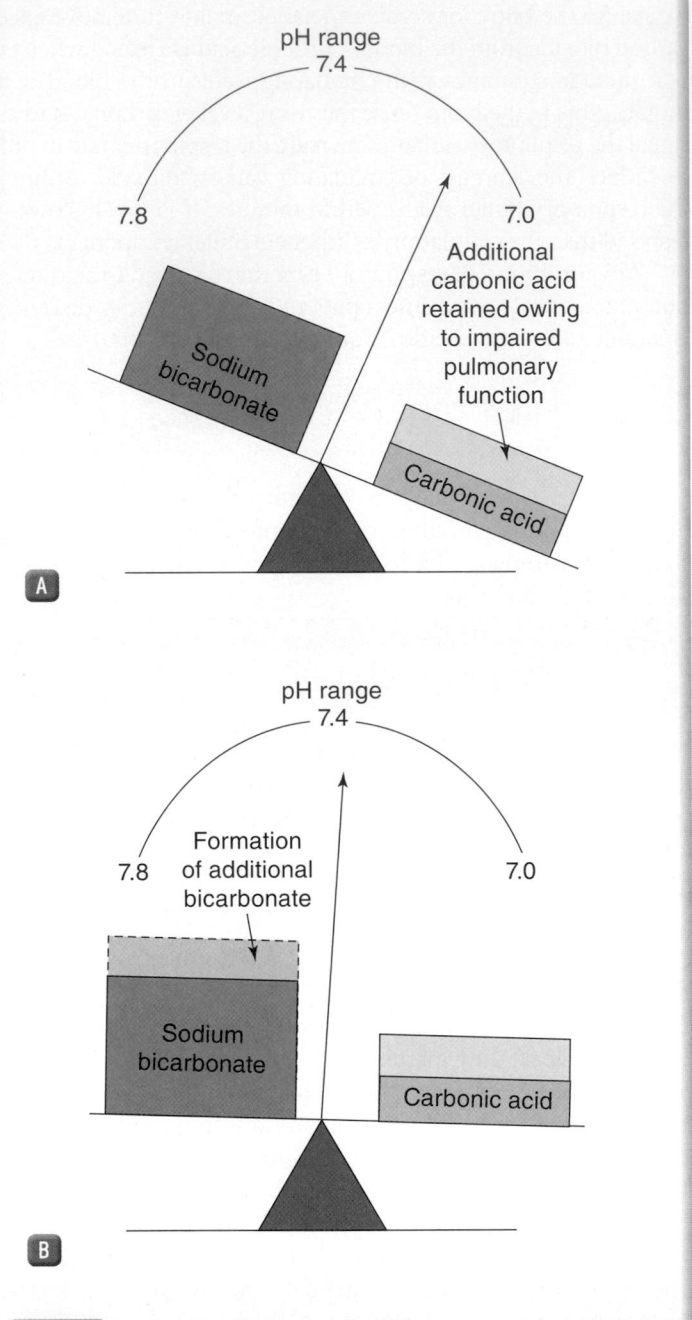

Figure 12 **A.** Derangement of acid-base balance in respiratory acidosis. **B.** Compensation by formation of additional bicarbonate.

Some signs and symptoms of respiratory alkalosis include the following:

- Diminished level of consciousness
- Light-headedness
- Carpopedal spasm
- Tingling lips and face
- Chest tightness
- Confusion
- Vertigo
- Blurred vision

- Hypocalcemia
- Nausea and vomiting

Metabolic Acidosis

The following equation demonstrates how an increased carbonic acid level can result in **metabolic acidosis**:

$$\uparrow H_2CO_3 \rightarrow \uparrow H^+ + HCO_3^- \rightarrow Acidosis$$

Any acidosis that is not related to the respiratory system is considered metabolic. Increased respiration (tachypnea) is the compensatory mechanism for this condition. It is the body's attempt to restore acid-base balance by eliminating carbon dioxide through the respiratory system. For example, patients with diabetic ketoacidosis often experience *Kussmaul respirations* (deep, closely spaced, sighing breaths), in which the body hyperventilates in an attempt to "blow off" carbon dioxide and decrease the acidosis.

As with any acidosis, the extracellular hydrogen level increases and the extracellular buffers attempt to neutralize the excess acid. Ion shifts occur, hydrogen leaks into the cell, and potassium shifts into the extracellular spaces, raising the serum potassium level, which can cause a life-threatening dysrhythmia. Calcium also shifts into the extracellular spaces. The resulting hypercalcemia obstructs impulses to neurons in muscle and other tissues, and the patient becomes lethargic, with a decreased level of consciousness.

Causes of metabolic acidosis include the following:

- **Lactic acidosis.** <u>Lactic acidosis</u> is caused by anaerobic cellular respiration due to hypoperfusion of tissues and organs, as seen in shock and cardiac arrest.
- **Ketoacidosis.** <u>Ketoacidosis</u> develops when cells are forced to switch to begin metabolizing fatty acids for energy because they are unable to use glucose due to insulin deficiency or desensitization of the cells to insulin. The by-products of fat metabolism are **ketones**, compounds that are extremely acidic.
- **Aspirin (acetylsalicylic acid) overdose.** A dose of 10 to 30 g in an adult constitutes an aspirin overdose. Aspirin directly stimulates the respiratory centers in the brain, creating tachypnea, which leads to respiratory alkalosis. Initiation of renal compensatory mechanisms leads to metabolic acidosis.
- **Alcohol ingestion.** Ingestion of ethyl alcohol can lead to <u>alcoholic ketoacidosis</u>. Methanol (wood alcohol) and ethylene glycol (antifreeze) can produce fatal forms of acidosis, often with amounts as small as 30 mL.
- **Gastrointestinal losses.** Diarrhea, for example, removes bases from the lower intestinal tract.

The clinical presentation of metabolic acidosis is similar to that of respiratory acidosis. Signs and symptoms of metabolic acidosis include the following:

- Vasodilation
- CNS depression
- Headaches

- Hot, flushed skin
- Hypercalcemia
- Tachypnea
- Nausea and vomiting
- Cardiac dysrhythmia

Metabolic Alkalosis

The following equation demonstrates how a decreased concentration of hydrogen ions can result in alkalosis:

$$\downarrow H^+ \rightarrow \downarrow H_2CO_3 \rightarrow Alkalosis$$

<u>Metabolic alkalosis</u> occurs when there is an excessive loss of acid from increased urine output or from a decreased acid level in the stomach. It is rarely seen as an acute condition, but is common among chronically ill patients, especially patients undergoing nasogastric suctioning.

Several factors related to upper gastrointestinal losses can lead to metabolic alkalosis:

- Excessive vomiting
- Excessive water intake
- Nasogastric suctioning
- Excessive intake of alkaline substances
- Eating disorders

Causes of metabolic alkalosis include the following:

- **Upper gastrointestinal losses of acid resulting from illness or an eating disorder such as anorexia nervosa or bulimia.** When a patient expels a great deal of acid from the stomach, a complex metabolic pathway can lead to metabolic alkalosis.
- **Drinking large amounts of water during vigorous exercise.** Water not only dilutes the stomach acid, it also stimulates the digestive system to prepare for incoming food from the stomach. This stimulation causes an outpouring of very alkaline digestive enzymes into the lower gastrointestinal tract, exacerbating the acid-base imbalance.

  As with respiratory alkalosis, calcium shifts out of the cell, resulting in hypercalcemia and overstimulating the nervous system, which leads to muscle cramping. This cramping is analogous to carpopedal spasm, except it occurs in the abdominal area and is referred to as heat cramps. If alkalosis is severe, muscle twitches turn into sustained contractions (tetany) that paralyze respiratory muscles.
- **Excessive intake of alkaline substances, such as antacids.** This cause is important to remember when assessing patients with cardiac disease who might report having self-medicated for hours or days with over-the-counter antacids. Another cause of excessive intake of bases is the excessive administration of sodium bicarbonate during resuscitation. Introducing excessive amounts of sodium bicarbonate into the circulatory system can severely alter the pH level.

The compensatory mechanism for metabolic alkalosis is the respiratory system. To correct the reduced hydrogen ion level, bradypnea develops as a means of retaining carbon dioxide and driving up levels of circulating acids.

Signs and symptoms of metabolic alkalosis include the following:

- Confusion
- Muscle tremors and cramps
- Bradypnea
- Hypotension

Mixed Acid-Base Imbalance

Finally, recall that metabolic acidosis may create respiratory alkalosis as a compensatory response. <u>Mixed acidosis</u> involves a low pH, an elevated pco_2 level, and a low Hco_3^- level. This occurs when both respiratory and metabolic acidosis are present at the same time in the patient. Severe trauma, cardiogenic shock, or a drug overdose are common situations where this may occur.

<u>Mixed alkalosis</u> involves an elevated pH, a low pco_2 level, and an elevated Hco_3^- level. This may occur when two seemingly unrelated medical issues manifest at the same time in the patient. For example, a patient with chronic respiratory alkalosis who experiences a gastrointestinal emergency may have respiratory alkalosis combined with metabolic alkalosis and therefore demonstrate mixed alkalosis. **Figure 13** shows conditions that are related to mixed acid-base disorders.

A patient with one of these conditions may present as uncompensated, partially compensated, or well compensated, but not overcompensated unless two pathologic conditions are simultaneously present. Practice is essential to developing comfort in the identification of complex acid-base disorders.

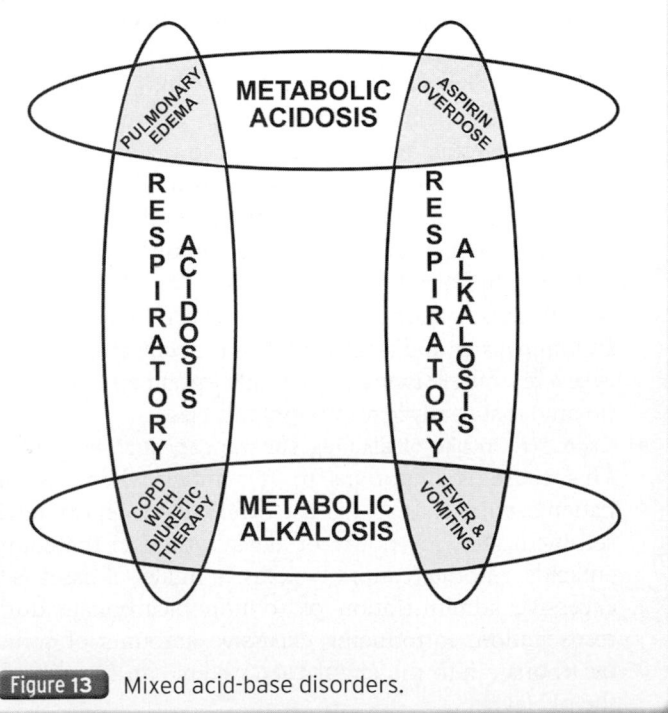

Figure 13 Mixed acid-base disorders.

Cellular Injury

Cellular injury may result from various causes, such as hypoxia (lack of oxygen), ischemia (lack of blood supply), chemical injury, infectious injury, immunologic (hypersensitivity) injury, physical damage (mechanical injury), and inflammatory injury. The manifestations of cellular injury and death depend on how many cells and which types of cells are damaged.

Manifestations of cellular injury occur at the microscopic (structural) and the functional levels. Common microscopic abnormalities (such as injuries in cardiac cells undergoing necrosis from hypoxemia for an extended period) include cell swelling, rupture of cell membranes or nuclear membranes, and breakdown of nuclear material (such as chromosomes) **Figure 14**. This damage often initiates a change in cell shape and function. Functional changes may include an inability to use oxygen appropriately, development of intracellular acidosis, accumulation of toxic waste products, and an inability to metabolize nutrients.

Damage and functional changes in individual cells often have an effect on the entire organism. In some cases, only minor systemic abnormalities are noted, such as fever. At other times, entire organ systems fail and the patient's situation becomes critical, such as when renal system failure occurs. Because all body systems are connected in some manner, dysfunction in one system inevitably affects other systems. When the homeostatic balance in the body is upset, the scales can tip in an unfavorable direction.

Cellular injury may, up to a point, be repaired with proper treatment. When irreversible injury occurs, no treatment will help. Cell death is followed by necrosis, a process in which the cell breaks down. The cell membrane becomes abnormally permeable, leading to an influx of electrolytes and fluids. The cell and its organelles swell. Lysosomes also release enzymes that destroy intracellular components. These processes occur during and after cell death.

Hypoxic Injury

Hypoxic injury is a common—and often deadly—cause of cellular injury. It may result from decreased amounts of oxygen in the air or loss of hemoglobin function (such as in carbon monoxide poisoning), a decreased number of red blood cells (as from bleeding), disease of the respiratory or cardiovascular system (such as COPD), or loss of cytochromes (mitochondrial proteins that convert oxygen to ATP, like that seen in cyanide poisoning).

Although hypoxia has deleterious effects on cells, the damage does not stop there. Cells that are hypoxic for more than a few seconds produce mediators (substances) that may damage other local or distant body locations. The result is a positive feedback cycle in which mediators lead to more cell damage, which leads to more hypoxia, which leads to further mediator production, and so forth.

The earliest and most dangerous mediators produced by cells in response to hypoxia are <u>free radicals</u>. These molecules

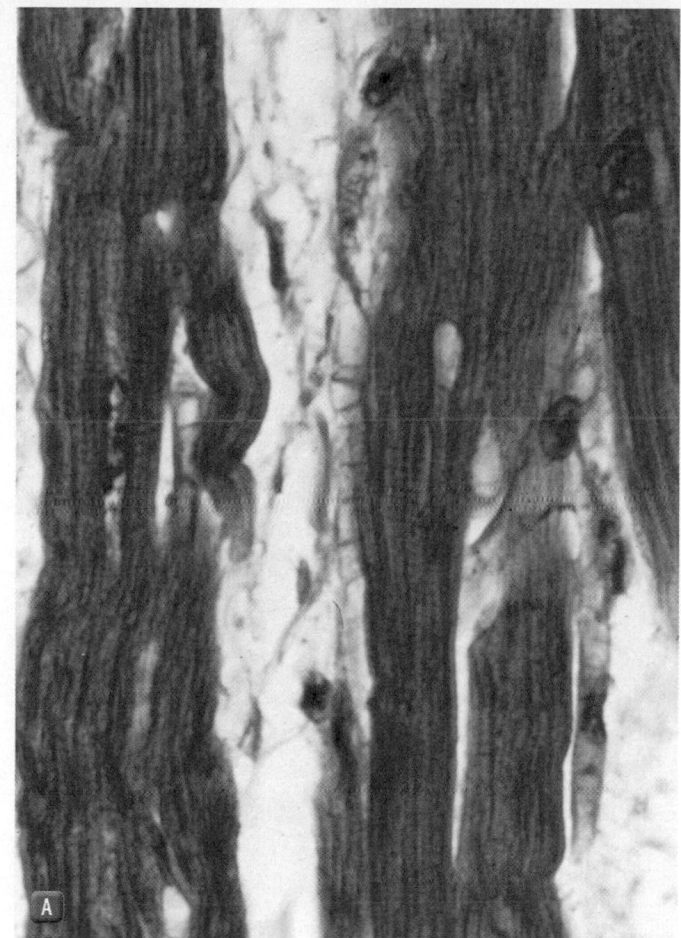
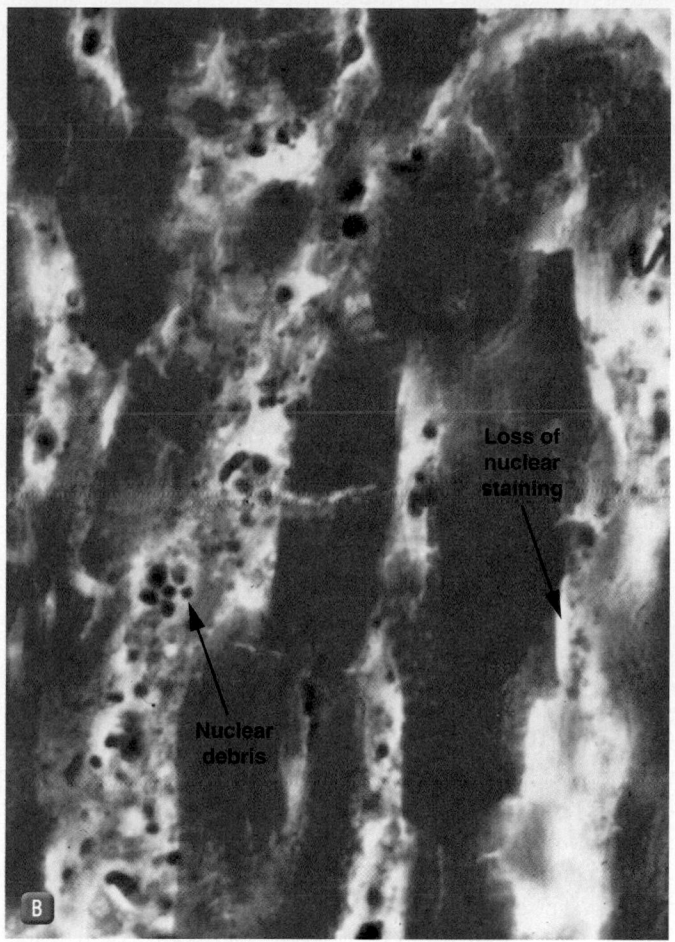

Figure 14 Comparison of cardiac muscle fibers. **A.** With necrotic fibers. **B.** Note fragmentation of fibers, loss of nuclear staining, and fragmented bits of nuclear debris. When the cell is injured it swells, resulting in nuclear membrane rupture and breakdown of the nuclear material (original magnification × 400).

are missing one electron in their outer shell. The presence of an odd, unpaired electron causes chemical instability Figure 15 as free radicals randomly attack cells and membranes in an attempt to steal back the missing electron. The result is widespread and potentially deadly tissue damage.

Chemical Injury

A variety of chemicals, including poisons, lead, carbon monoxide, ethanol, and pharmacologic agents, may injure and ultimately destroy cells. Common poisons include cyanide and pesticides. Cyanide induces cell hypoxia by blocking oxidative phosphorylation in the mitochondria and preventing the metabolism of oxygen. Pesticides block an enzyme, acetylcholinesterase, thereby preventing proper transmission of nerve impulses.

Long-term ingestion of lead, such as that caused by chewing on windowsills painted with lead-based paint, leads to brain injury and neurologic dysfunction. The ability of lead

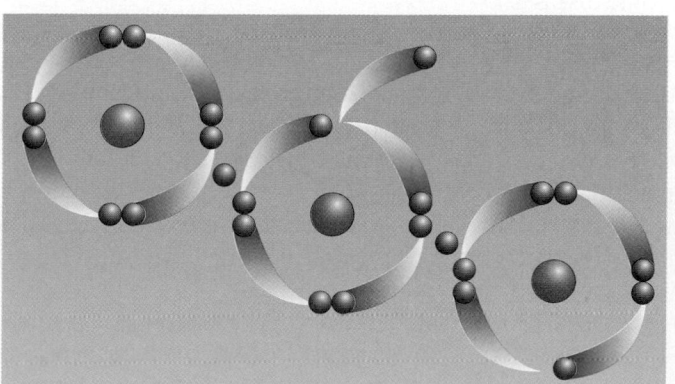

Figure 15 Free radicals are missing one electron in their outside orbit. This molecular structure causes chemical instability. Each black dot represents an electron in the outer shell.

to substitute for calcium (molecules of lead and calcium are a similar size) is a common factor in many of its toxic actions. Mostly likely, lead is mistaken for calcium in vital biochemical reactions, leading to abnormal results and dysfunction.

Carbon monoxide binds to hemoglobin, preventing adequate oxygenation of the tissues. A low level causes nausea, vomiting, and headache. A higher level can be fatal in less than 2 hours.

At lower doses, ethanol causes the well-known effects of inebriation. Higher doses produce severe CNS depression and hypoventilation, sometimes precipitating cardiovascular collapse.

Some pharmacologic agents produce toxic products when they are metabolized in the body, especially in overdose conditions. For example, acute overdose occurs when an excessive dose of acetaminophen (Tylenol) is ingested. If an adult takes a dose of more than 140 mg/kg, or 4 g, the toxins that accumulate can poison the liver and can sometimes be fatal.

Infectious Injury

Infectious injury to cells occurs as a result of an invasion of bacteria, fungi, or viruses. Bacteria may cause injury by direct action on cells or by the production of toxins. Viruses often initiate an inflammatory response that leads to cell damage and patient symptoms.

Virulence measures the disease-causing ability of a microorganism. The pathogenicity of any particular microorganism is a function of its ability to reproduce and cause disease within the human body. In particular, the growth and survival of bacteria in the body depend on the effectiveness of the body's own defense mechanisms and on the bacteria's ability to resist the mechanisms. A depressed immune system is less capable of fighting off microorganisms that the body perceives as harmful; populations with weaker immune systems include newborn infants, older adults, people with diabetes, and people with cancer or other chronic diseases.

Bacteria

Many bacteria have a capsule that protects them from ingestion and destruction by **phagocytes**—cells (that is, white blood cells) that engulf and consume foreign material such as microorganisms and cellular debris **Figure 16** . Not all bacteria are encapsulated, however. *Mycobacterium tuberculosis*, for example, lacks a capsule, yet stubbornly resists destruction; it can be transported by phagocytes throughout the body.

Bacteria can be categorized depending on the results of Gram staining. In Gram staining, a dried, fixed suspension of bacteria, prepared on a microscopic slide, is stained first with a purple dye and then with an iodine solution. Next, the slide is decolorized with alcohol or another solvent; it is then stained with a red dye. Bacteria that resist decolorization and retain the purple stain are called **gram-positive** bacteria, whereas those that have been decolorized and accept the red counterstain are termed **gram-negative** bacteria. Gram-positive bacteria are distinguished by thick cell walls composed of many layers of

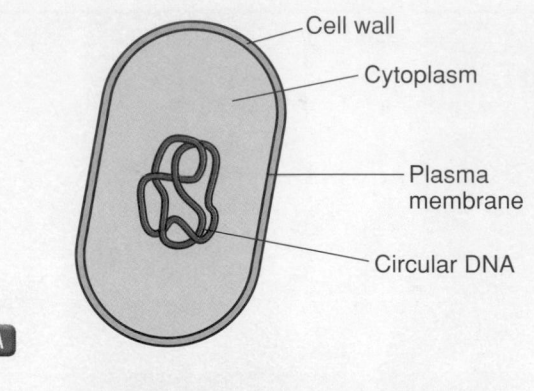

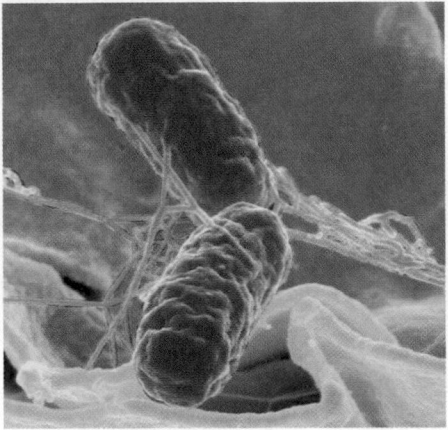

Figure 16 General structure of a bacterium. **A.** Bacteria come in many shapes and sizes, but all have a circular strand of deoxyribonucleic acid (DNA), cytoplasm, and a plasma membrane. A cell wall surrounds the membrane in many bacteria. **B.** An electron micrograph of *Salmonella* bacteria. Many bacteria have a capsule that protects them from ingestion and destruction by phagocytes.

peptidoglycan (amino acids and sugar); conversely, the cell walls of gram-negative bacteria consist largely of lipids. The pathogenic qualities of gram-negative bacteria, which include the microorganism that causes bubonic plague, make them especially problematic for humans.

Bacteria also produce exotoxins or endotoxins—substances such as enzymes or toxins—that can injure or destroy cells. Staphylococci, streptococci, and *Clostridium tetani*, for example, secrete exotoxins into the medium surrounding the cell. Exotoxins are produced within the cell and are released into surrounding tissues or fluids (blood or lymph). They are poisonous and their actions vary depending on the organism; for example, neurotoxins damage nervous tissue, enterotoxins affect the tissues of the gastrointestinal tract, and cytotoxins damage a variety of host tissues. Inactive exotoxins are sometimes used as the basis for vaccines.

Endotoxins are lipopolysaccharides that are part of the cell walls of gram-negative bacteria. Endotoxins cause inflammation, fever, chills, and malaise, as well as effecting vascular tone. When large amounts of endotoxins are present in the body, septic shock may develop. Endotoxins remain active even after the bacteria are destroyed, which may be one reason why there is a delay in seeing the effects of antibiotics.

When cells are injured, circulating white blood cells are attracted to the site of injury. White blood cells release endogenous **pyrogens**, which then cause a fever to develop. Indeed, the body's most common reaction to the presence of bacteria is inflammation. Some bacteria have the ability to produce hypersensitivity reactions. The presence of bacteria in the blood is called bacteremia; septicemia (sepsis) is systemic disease, which may be life threatening, caused by the proliferation of microorganisms (or their toxins) in the blood.

Viruses

Viruses are among the most common causes of afflictions. They are intracellular parasites that take over the metabolic processes of the host cell and use the cell to help them replicate. A virus consists of a nucleic acid core of RNA or DNA. Surrounding the viral core is a protein coat known as the capsid, which protects the virus from phagocytosis. Some viruses have an additional protective coat known as the envelope.

The replication of a virus occurs inside the host cell because viruses do not have their own organelles. Viral infection of a host cell leads to a decreased synthesis of macromolecules that are vital to the host cell. Unlike bacteria, however, viruses do not produce exotoxins or endotoxins.

A symbiotic relationship may exist between a virus and normal cells that allows the virus to persist without causing an active infection. Viruses such as the human immunodeficiency virus (HIV) can elicit a strong immune response, rapidly producing an irreversible, lethal injury in susceptible cells.

■ Immunologic and Inflammatory Injury

Inflammation is a protective response that can occur even without bacterial invasion. Infection is characterized by an invasion of microorganisms that causes cell or tissue injury, which leads to the **inflammatory response**. The inflammatory response can be triggered by an agent that is physical (heat or cold), chemical (such as concentrated acid or alkali or another caustic chemical), or microbiologic (such as a bacterium or virus). The inflammatory response is characterized by both local and systemic effects, as shown in **Figure 17**.

Local effects consist of dilatation (expansion) of blood vessels and increased vascular permeability. Leukocytes (white blood cells) are attracted to the site of injury. They adhere to the endothelium of the small blood vessels, force their way through the walls, and migrate to the area of tissue damage. The characteristic signs of inflammation are heat, redness, tenderness, swelling, and pain. The increased warmth and redness of the inflamed tissues are caused by dilatation of capillaries and slowing of blood flow

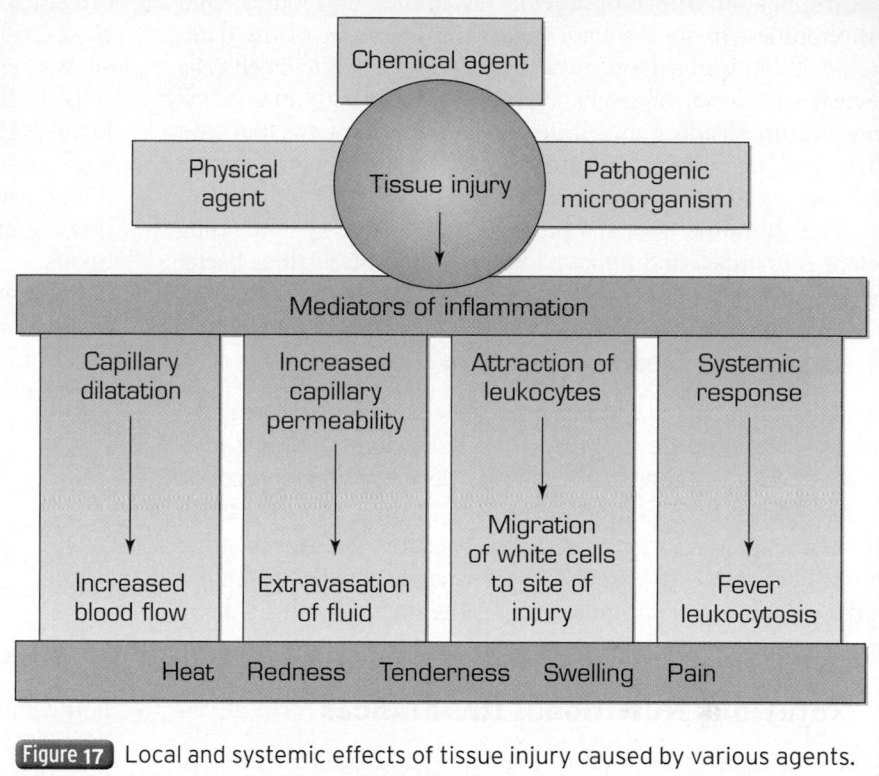

Figure 17 Local and systemic effects of tissue injury caused by various agents.

through the vessels. Swelling occurs because the extravasation (leakage) of plasma from the dilated and more permeable vessels causes the volume of fluid in the inflamed tissue to increase. The tenderness and pain are secondary to irritation of sensory nerve endings at the site of the inflammatory process.

If the inflammatory process is severe, systemic effects become evident. The person feels ill, and the temperature is elevated. The bone marrow accelerates its production of leukocytes so that the number of leukocytes circulating in the bloodstream increases; this increase in the number of leukocytes in the blood is called **leukocytosis**. The liver produces several proteins called acute phase proteins that are released into the bloodstream in response to tissue injury or inflammation, which help protect the body from the tissue injury caused by the inflammation. The best known of these proteins is called C-reactive protein, which is often measured to monitor the activity of diseases characterized by tissue inflammation.

The outcome of an inflammation depends on the amount of tissue damage. If the inflammation is mild, it soon subsides, and the tissues return to normal. If the inflammatory process is more severe, tissue is destroyed to some extent and must be repaired. During healing, damaged cells are replaced, and the framework of the injured tissue is repaired as an ingrowth of cells produces connective-tissue fibers and new blood vessels. Scar tissue replaces large areas of tissue destruction. Sometimes, the scarring subsequent to a severe inflammation is so severe that function is seriously disturbed.

Cellular membranes may be injured when they come in direct contact with the cellular and chemical components of the immune or inflammatory process, such as phagocytes (neutrophils and macrophages), histamine, antibodies, and lymphokines. In such a case, potassium leaks out of the damaged cell and water flows inward, causing the cell to swell. The nuclear envelope, organelle membranes, and cell membrane may rupture, leading to cell death. The degree of swelling and chance of membrane rupture depend on the severity of the immune and inflammatory responses.

The immune system protects the body by providing defenses to attack and remove foreign organisms such as bacteria and viruses.

Injurious Genetic Factors

Genetic factors that may damage cells include chromosomal disorders, premature development of atherosclerosis, and, sometimes, obesity. An abnormal gene may develop in person in one of three ways: by mutation of the gene during meiosis, which affects the newly formed fetus; by heredity; or due to other causes later in life. In trisomy 21 (Down syndrome), the child is born with an extra chromosome 21. Rheumatoid arthritis has a genetic link as well.

Injurious Nutritional Imbalances

Good nutrition is required to maintain good health and assist the cells in fighting disease. Injurious nutritional imbalances that can injure cells and the organism as a whole include obesity, malnutrition, vitamin excess or deficiency, and mineral excess or deficiency. These conditions can lead to alterations in physical growth, mental and intellectual retardation, and even death.

Injurious Physical Agents or Conditions

Physical agents, such as heat, cold, and radiation, may also cause cell injury—for example, burns, frostbite, radiation sickness, and tumors. The degree of cell injury that results is determined by the strength of the agent and the length of exposure.

Apoptosis

As mentioned earlier, apoptosis is normal cell death. It is unique in that it is genetically programmed into the cell as a part of normal development, organogenesis, immune function, and tissue growth. It has a normal role in aging, early development, menses, lactating breast tissue, thymus involution, and red blood cell turnover.

During apoptosis, cells exhibit characteristic nuclear changes, and they typically die in well-defined clusters rather than in a random manner. The molecular mechanism underlying apoptosis involves the activation of genes that encode for proteins known as caspases (cysteine-aspartic proteases). These proteins are essentially cellular cyanide—in essence, their production leads to

cell suicide. Unlike in the case of cell death from disease processes, proteins and DNA undergo controlled degradation that allows their remnants to be taken up and reused by neighboring cells. In this way, apoptosis allows the body to eliminate a cell but recycle many of its components. Pathologically, areas that have undergone apoptotic death do not show any evidence of inflammation. In contrast, an inflammatory response is typically observed when cells undergo necrosis from hypoxia or cellular toxins.

Apoptosis can be activated prematurely by pathologic factors such as cell injury. This sort of premature stimulation, which occurs in some forms of heart failure, causes early cell death. Another example of pathologic apoptosis is the death of hepatocytes (liver cells) in patients with viral hepatitis. The dying cells form lumps of chromatin known as Councilman bodies. Inhibition of the normal course of apoptosis allows destructive cellular proliferation, such as in cancer and rheumatoid arthritis (uncontrolled synovial tissue proliferation). **Figure 18** illustrates the process by which cancerous cells develop from normal cells.

Abnormal Cell Death

If the injury leading to cellular degeneration is of sufficient intensity and duration, irreversible cell injury leads to cell death. **Necrosis** is the result of the morphologic changes that occur following cell death in living tissues. It may be simple necrosis (coagulation) or derived necrosis.

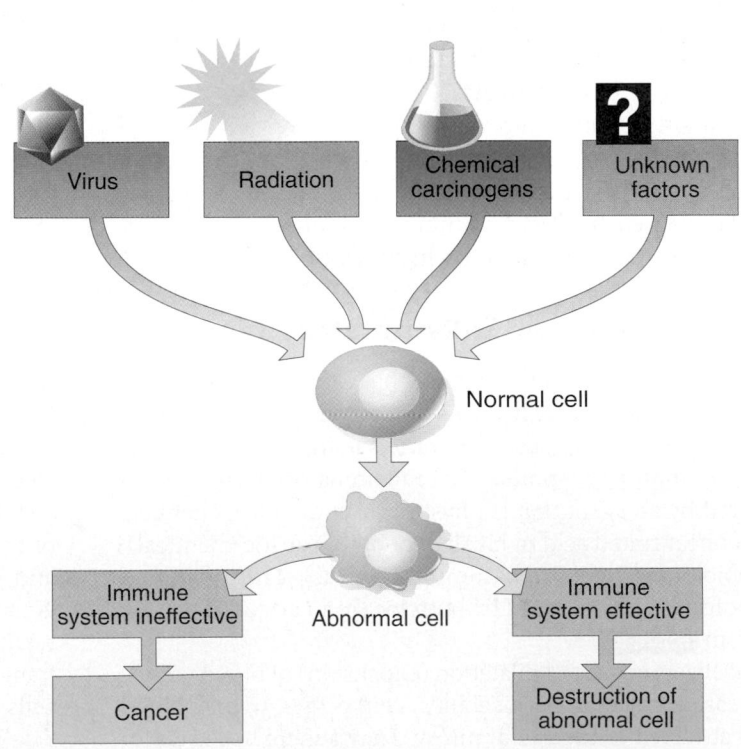

Figure 18 The onset of cancer. Viruses and other factors induce a normal cell to become abnormal. When the immune system is working effectively, it destroys the abnormal cells, so no cancer develops. When abnormal cells evade the immune system, they form a tumor and may become a spreading cancer.

Simple necrosis refers to areas of necrosis where the gross and microscopic tissue and some of the cells are recognizable. It may be caused by acute ischemia, acute toxicity (such as from heavy metals), or direct physical injury (such as from caustic chemicals and burns).

Derived necrosis includes caseation necrosis, dry gangrene, fat necrosis, and liquefaction necrosis. Caseation necrosis is manifested by the loss of all features of the tissue and cells, so that they come to resemble cheese when viewed through a microscope. Dry gangrene results from invasion and putrefaction of necrotic tissue, after the blood supply is compromised and the tissue undergoes coagulation necrosis. Fat necrosis results from the destruction of fat cells, usually by enzymes (such as pancreatic proteases and lipases). Liquefaction necrosis results from coagulation necrosis followed by conversion of tissues into a liquid form and invasion by putrefying bacteria that grow rapidly in a warm moist environment; the bacteria produce lytic enzymes and gas.

Factors That Cause Disease

Genetic, environmental, age-related, and sex-associated factors can cause or contribute to disease. Genetic factors are present at birth and are passed on through a person's genes to future generations. Environmental factors include microorganisms, immunologic vulnerabilities, personal habits and lifestyle, exposures to chemicals and other toxins, the physical environment, and the psychosocial environment. Family violence, for example, might be a key factor in causing depression or substance abuse, perhaps even years later. A sedentary lifestyle and a high-fat diet can cause or contribute to obesity, diabetes, heart disease, stroke, and other diseases.

Disease can also have anatomic causes. For example, malrotation of the colon is a disease in which the colon does not form properly, resulting in partial blockage. Another example is degenerative diseases of the spine; as intervertebral disks age, they may degenerate to the extent that the patient experiences pain due to nerve compression. Aortic stenosis is a condition in which the aortic valve becomes very tight and narrowed, resulting in chest pain from decreased perfusion of the coronary arteries or congestive heart failure.

Finally, an immunologic reaction may result in disease. An example is exposure to an agent that triggers an abnormal immune response against myelin, leading to the development of multiple sclerosis.

Controllable Versus Uncontrollable Risk Factors

Some uncontrollable factors, such as genetics and race, influence the development of disease, but many other factors can be controlled. For example, behaviors such as smoking, drinking alcohol, inadequate nutrition (excessive fat, salt, and sugar intake or insufficient intake of protein, fruits, vegetables, and fiber), lack of physical activity, and stress can be modified.

Age-Related Risk
The risk of a particular disease often depends on a person's age. For example, newborns are at greater risk of certain diseases because

their immune systems are not fully developed (see the chapter, *Neonatal Care*). Teenagers are at high risk of other diseases due to trauma and use of drugs and alcohol. The older a person becomes, the greater the risk of cancer, heart disease, stroke, and Alzheimer disease (see the chapter, *Geriatric Emergencies*).

Sex-Associated Factors
In some cases, sex is related to the risk of having a certain disease. Some diseases occur more often in men, and others occur more often in women. Diseases such as lung cancer, gout, and Parkinson disease, are more prevalent in men. Women are more likely to have diseases such as osteoporosis, rheumatoid arthritis, and breast cancer.

Some diseases present differently in women compared with men (ie, presentation of AMI). For example, the hormones found in a premenopausal woman have been shown to have a protective effect in major head trauma and certain cardiac conditions. Studies are under way to investigate this finding, which could lead to the possibility of administering female sex hormone to male cardiac arrest patients to improve survival.

Finally, genetic disorders are related to a person's sex when a defective gene is located on a sex chromosome. Most sex-linked disorders are X linked. X-linked disorders may be either recessive or dominant. Because females have two X chromosomes, those with a defective X gene may or may not have the disorder; if the disorder is recessive, the X chromosome without the defect will "mask" the defective X chromosome. Men with a defective X gene will always be affected because they only have one X chromosome; the defect cannot be masked.

Analysis of Disease Risk

Analyzing disease risk involves consideration of disease rates and disease risk factors (causal and noncausal). Risk factors that can directly cause a disease to develop are called causal risk factors. For example, *Mycobacterium tuberculosis* is a causal risk factor for a person becoming infected with tuberculosis. Risk factors that are associated with risk for a disease but not a direct cause are called noncausal risk factors. For example, poverty is a noncausal risk factor for tuberculosis.

All studies of a disease should consider the incidence, prevalence, and mortality of the disease. The **incidence** is the number of new cases of a disease in a population (for example, six cases of West Nile virus infection were identified in the county). **Prevalence** refers to the number of cases of a disease or condition in a particular population within a particular period (for example, last year, more than 100,000 patients had this disease). **Morbidity** refers to the presence of disease or to the incidence or prevalence of a disease. **Mortality** is most often discussed as the mortality rate, which is the number of deaths from a disease in a given population, expressed as a proportion (for example, 1 in 50 affected people in the United States). **Table 3** illustrates how the concepts of incidence, prevalence, morbidity, and mortality might be expressed, using statistics on diabetes as an example.

Interaction of Risk Factors
Risk factors, age, and sex differences often interact. For example, suppose a person has a genetic tendency toward coronary

Table 3 Incidence, Prevalence, Morbidity, and Mortality Rate of Diabetes in the United States

Incidence	In 2010, 1.9 million people 20 years or older were newly diagnosed with type 1 or type 2 diabetes.
Prevalence	A total of 8.3% of the total US population (adults and children) had diabetes in 2010.*
Morbidity	In 2010, 25.8 million adults and children in the United States had diabetes (18.8 million diagnosed and an estimated 7 million undiagnosed).*
Mortality rate	In 2007, diabetes was responsible for or a key contributor to the deaths of 231,404 people,* or 22.5 deaths per 100,000 population.†

*National Diabetes Information Clearinghouse, National Institute of Diabetes and Digestive and Kidney Diseases, National Institutes of Health: National Diabetes Statistics, 2011. http://diabetes.niddk.nih.gov/dm/pubs/statistics/index.aspx. Accessed September 9, 2011.

† Xu J, Kochanek KD, Murphy SL, et al. Deaths: final data for 2007. *Natl Vital Stat Rep.* 2010; 58(19):1-138. Table 29: www.cdc.gov/nchs/data/nvsr/nvsr58/nvsr58_19.pdf. Accessed September 9, 2011.

artery disease; the risk of myocardial infarction or sudden death is higher in this person even if he or she exercises regularly and has no other risk factors. A person who smokes heavily but has no other risk factors may have a similarly elevated risk. Table 4 shows the interplay of various risk factors in causing respiratory disease.

Common Familial Diseases and Associated Risk Factors

The terms *genetic risk* and *familial tendency* are often used interchangeably. A true genetic risk is one that is passed through generations by inheritance of a gene. In contrast, with a familial tendency, diseases seem to cluster in family groups despite lack of evidence for heritable gene-associated abnormalities.

Table 5 lists some of the traits and diseases carried on human chromosomes. **Autosomal recessive** is a pattern of inheritance that involves genes located on autosomes (any chromosome other than sex chromosomes). A person needs to inherit two copies of a particular form of such a gene to show that trait. A parent who carries the gene for an autosomal recessive trait but does not display the trait has a 25% chance of passing the inherited condition to his or her child if the other parent is also a carrier for the trait. If both parents *have* the inherited condition, all of their children will have the condition. Hemochromatosis,

Table 4 Common Respiratory Diseases

Disease	Pathology and/or Symptoms	Causes and Possible Contributing Causes
Emphysema	Breakdown of alveoli, shortness of breath	Smoking Air pollution Possible genetic susceptibility Exacerbated by obesity
Chronic bronchitis	Coughing, shortness of breath	Smoking Air pollution Possible genetic susceptibility Exacerbated by obesity
Acute bronchitis	Inflammation of the bronchi; yellowish mucus coughed up, shortness of breath	Many viruses and bacteria Possible genetic susceptibility Smoking Exacerbated by obesity
Sinusitis	Inflammation of the sinuses; characterized by mucus discharge, blockage of nasal passageways, and headache	Many viruses and bacteria Poor general health
Laryngitis	Inflammation of larynx and vocal cords, sore throat, hoarseness, mucus buildup, and cough	Many viruses and bacteria Poor general health
Pneumonia	Inflammation of the lungs, ranging from mild to severe; cough and fever, shortness of breath at rest, chills, sweating, chest pain, blood-tinged mucus	Bacteria, viruses, fungi, or inhalation of irritating gases Lack of physical activity
Asthma	Constriction of bronchioles, mucus buildup in bronchioles, periodic wheezing, difficulty breathing	Allergy to pollen, some foods, food additives; dander (dead skin cells and other debris shed by dogs, cats, or birds) Physical activity (exercise-induced asthma) Probable genetic link

Table 5 Traits and Diseases Carried on Human Chromosomes

Autosomal Recessive	
Albinism	Lack of pigment in eyes, skin, and hair
Cystic fibrosis	Pancreatic failure, mucus buildup in lungs
Sickle cell anemia	Abnormal hemoglobin characterized by sickle-shaped red blood cells that obstruct vital capillaries
Tay-Sachs disease	Improper metabolism of gangliosides in nerve cells
Phenylketonuria	Accumulation of phenylalanine in blood; causes mental retardation
Attached earlobe	Earlobe attached to skin of the neck
Hyperextensible thumb	Thumb bends past 45° angle

Autosomal Dominant	
Achondroplasia	Dwarfism resulting from a defect in the epiphyseal plates that interferes with the formation of long bones
Marfan syndrome	Defect of connective tissue resulting in excessive growth and a high risk of aortic rupture
Widow's peak	Hairline coming to a point on forehead
Huntington disease	Progressive deterioration of the nervous system beginning in late 20s or early 30s; causes mental deterioration and early death
Brachydactyly	Disfiguration of hands, shortened fingers
Freckles	Permanent aggregations of melanin in the skin

which causes the accumulation of too much iron in the body, has an autosomal recessive pattern of inheritance—a person must inherit a copy of the hemochromatosis gene from each parent for the disease to develop.

In **autosomal dominant** inheritance, a person needs to inherit only one copy of a particular form of a gene to show that trait; it does not matter which form of the gene is inherited from the other parent. A parent has at least a 50% chance of passing on an autosomal dominant inherited condition to his or her child. Familial adenomatous polyposis, which places people at extremely high risk for the development of colon cancer, has an autosomal dominant pattern of inheritance.

Immunologic Disorders

Immunologic diseases are caused by hyperactivity or hypoactivity of the immune system. Most immunologic diseases that exhibit familial tendencies involve an overactive immune system—for example, allergies, asthma, and rheumatic fever.

Often significant overlap exists among causative factors, including the person's environment.

Allergies are acquired following initial exposure to a stimulant, known as an **allergen**. Repeated exposures cause the immune system to react to the allergen **Figure 19**. Although the clinical presentation varies, it usually includes swelling and itching, runny nose, coughing, sneezing, wheezing, and nasal congestion. A person who has an allergic tendency is said to be **atopic**. Environmental conditions may also increase a person's susceptibility to an allergic reaction.

Asthma is a chronic inflammatory condition resulting in intermittent wheezing and excess mucus production. Nearly 60% of attacks are precipitated by viral infections. Allergies account for another 20% of asthma attacks, with stress and emotions causing the remainder. In addition to the familial component, chromosomal differences in certain persons may enhance their susceptibility to asthma.

Special Populations

Rheumatic fever is an inflammatory disease that occurs primarily in children. This disease results from a delayed reaction to an untreated streptococcal infection of the upper respiratory tract (such as strep throat). Symptoms, which appear several weeks after the acute infection, may include fever, abdominal pain, vomiting, arthritis, palpitations, and chest pain. Recurrent episodes of rheumatic fever may cause permanent myocardial damage, especially to the cardiac valves. A family history of acute rheumatic fever may predispose a person to the disease.

Cancer

Cancer includes a large number of malignant growths (neoplasms). The prognosis often depends on the extent of its spread (metastasis) and the effectiveness of treatment.

Lung cancer is the leading cause of death due to cancer in the United States. The major risk factor is cigarette smoking. Research has identified eight alterations in the genetic material of lung cancers that suggest a genetic tendency to develop the disease. Other predisposing factors include exposure to asbestos, coal products, and other industrial and chemical products. Symptoms include cough, difficulty breathing, blood-tinged sputum, and repeated infections. Treatment depends on the type, site, and extent of the cancer and may include surgery, chemotherapy, and/or radiotherapy.

Breast cancer is the most common type of cancer occurring among women and accounts for as many as 178,700 newly diagnosed cases and 48,000 deaths each year in the United States. Women whose first-degree relatives (that is, parent, sister, or daughter) have breast cancer are 2.1 times more likely to have the disease. Risk varies with the age at which the affected relative was diagnosed; the younger the age at occurrence, the greater the risk posed to relatives. Approximately 5% to 10% of patients with breast cancer have a pattern of autosomal dominant inheritance, in which cancer predisposition is transmitted from generation to generation. The susceptibility may be inherited through the mother's or the father's side of the family.

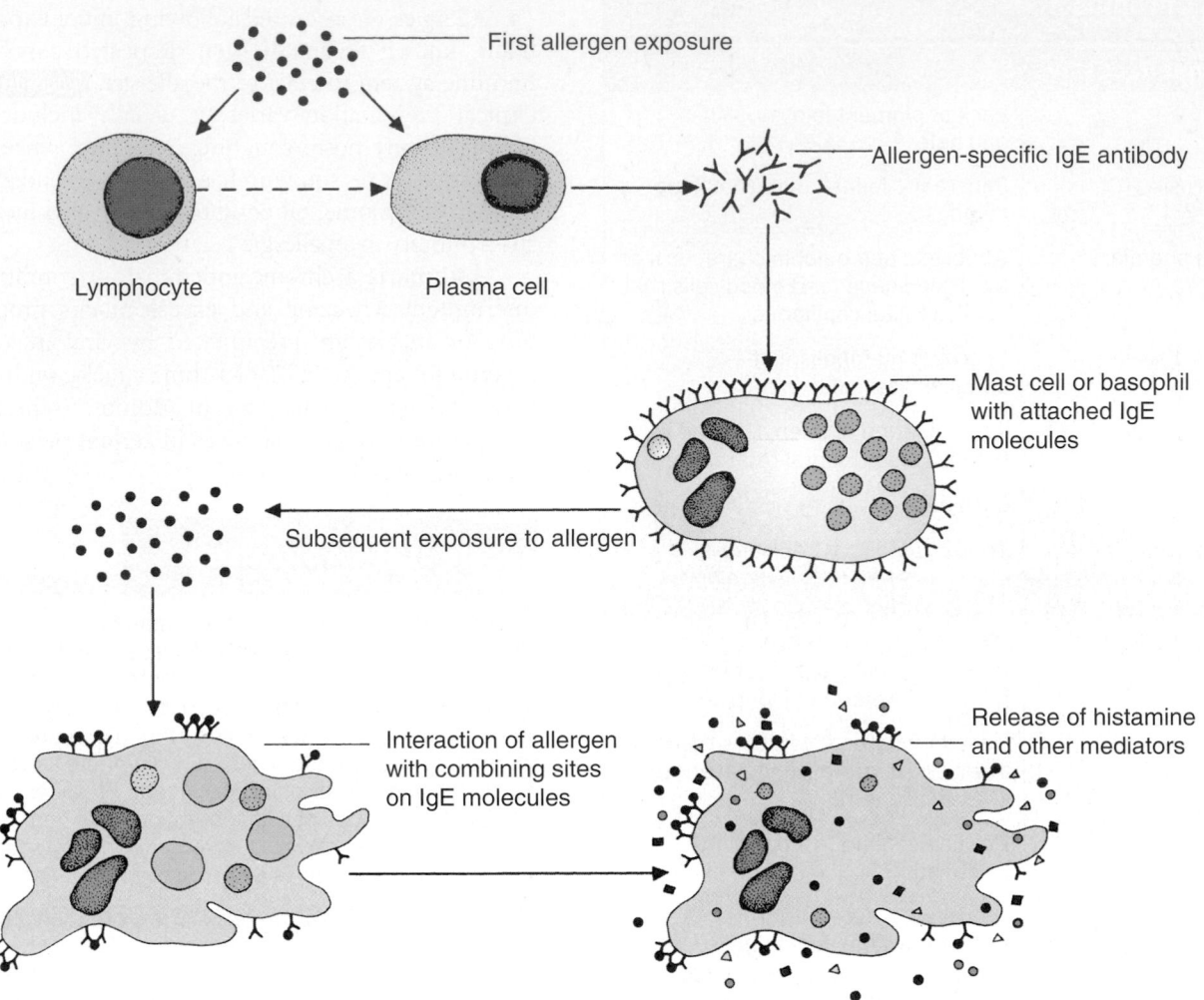

First allergen exposure

Allergen-specific IgE antibody

Lymphocyte

Plasma cell

Mast cell or basophil with attached IgE molecules

Subsequent exposure to allergen

Interaction of allergen with combining sites on IgE molecules

Release of histamine and other mediators

Figure 19 Pathogenesis of allergy. First, exposure to an allergen induces formation of specific IgE antibodies in susceptible persons, which then bind to mast cells and basophils by the nonantigen receptor end of the molecule. Subsequent exposure to the same allergen leads to antigen-antibody interaction, liberating histamine and other mediators from mast cells and basophils. These mediators induce allergic manifestations.

Early symptoms of breast cancer are usually detected by the woman during breast self-examination and include a small, painless lump, thick or dimpled skin, or a change in the nipple **Figure 20**. Later symptoms include nipple discharge, pain, and swollen lymph glands in the axilla. Treatment depends on the location, size, and metastasis of the tumor.

Colorectal cancer is the third most common type of cancer in men and women, accounting for a combined 131,600 newly diagnosed cases and 55,000 deaths in the United States each year. Relatives of people who have had colorectal cancer are more likely to have the disease themselves, and parents can pass on to their children changes in certain genes that can lead to colorectal cancer. Symptoms may be minimal, consisting only of small amounts of blood in the stool. Treatment involves surgery and sometimes chemotherapy. Periodic rectal examinations

and colonoscopy are recommended for adults age 50 years and older to detect the disease at an early stage.

Endocrine Disorders

Diabetes mellitus is one of the most significant endocrine diseases. This chronic disorder of metabolism is associated with partial insulin secretion or total lack of insulin secretion by the pancreas, which in turn affects the body's ability to use glucose. Symptoms include excessive thirst and urination, weight abnormalities, and the presence of excessive glucose in the urine and the blood.

Ketoacidosis-prone (type 1) diabetes is also known as insulin-dependent diabetes mellitus because patients need exogenous insulin to survive. Non–ketoacidosis-prone (type 2) diabetes is called non–insulin-dependent diabetes, even though many people with type 2 diabetes require exogenous insulin injections. Both forms have a hereditary predisposition. Type 1 diabetes has no known cure (other than pancreas transplantation) at the present time; type 2 diabetes can occasionally be brought under control with weight loss and medications.

Hematologic Disorders

<u>Hemolytic anemia</u> is characterized by increased destruction of red blood cells. This disorder has a number of causes, such as an Rh factor blood transfusion reaction (which would most likely occur in the neonate population), a disorder of the immune system, and exposure to bacterial toxins or chemicals such as benzene. **Figure 21** depicts how the body handles iron. Hemolytic anemia following aspirin overdose or penicillin treatment is rare; it is much more common, albeit still rare, with sulfa drugs used to treat urinary tract infection, such as the trimethoprim sulfamethoxazole combination (known as Septra and Bactrim). An inherited enzyme deficiency (glucose-6-phosphatase dehydrogenase deficiency) markedly increases a person's susceptibility to sulfa drug–induced hemolytic anemia.

<u>Hemophilia</u> is an inherited disorder characterized by excessive bleeding. It is a sex-linked condition, occurring only in males, and is passed from asymptomatic mothers to sons. In this disorder, one of the blood-clotting proteins (usually factor VIII) necessary for normal blood coagulation is missing or is present in abnormally low amounts. Patients experience greater than usual blood loss in dental extractions and following simple injuries. They may also have bleeding into joints and, rarely, into the brain. Treatment consists of administration of the missing blood-clotting factors.

<u>Hemochromatosis</u> is an inherited (autosomal recessive) disease in which the body absorbs more iron than it needs. The excess iron is stored in various organs, including the liver, kidneys, and pancreas. Hemochromatosis can lead to diabetes,

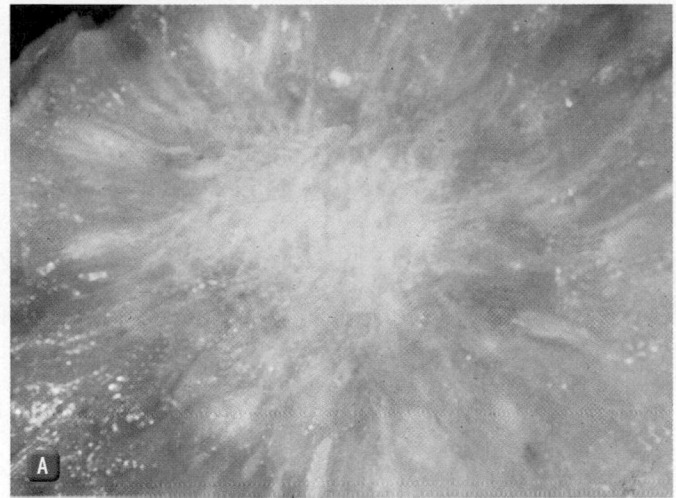

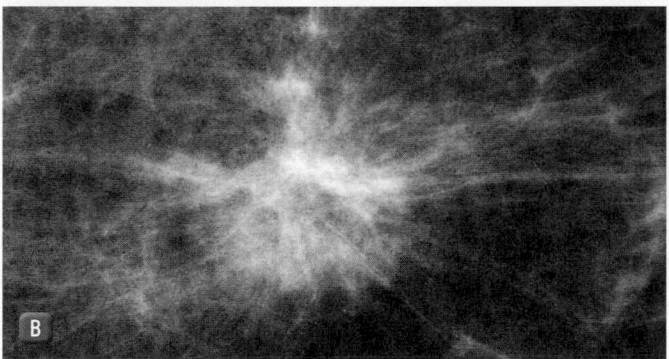

Figure 20 Breast carcinoma. **A.** Cross-section of breast biopsy specimen. The tumor appears as a firm, poorly circumscribed mass that infiltrates the surrounding fatty breast tissue. **B.** Appearance of breast carcinoma in a mammogram. The tumor appears as a white area with infiltrating margins.

YOU are the Medic   PART 3

Your partner is administering high-flow oxygen, assessing vital signs, placing the cardiac monitor, and setting up an IV line. You auscultate lung sounds and hear little air movement. You hear coarse crackles (rales) bilaterally in all fields. The patient coughs, and you notice pink, foamy sputum. You ask your partner to assess the medications on the side table while you establish the IV.

Recording Time: 2 Minutes	
Respirations	22 breaths/min; shallow
Pulse	110 beats/min
Skin	Cool, moist, and pale
Blood pressure	140/90 mm Hg
Oxygen saturation (Spo$_2$)	89% before high-flow oxygen administration
Pupils	Equal and reactive to light

5. On the basis of what you know about physiology, what is causing the pink, foamy sputum?

6. How do you account for the decreased Spo$_2$ level based on physiology?

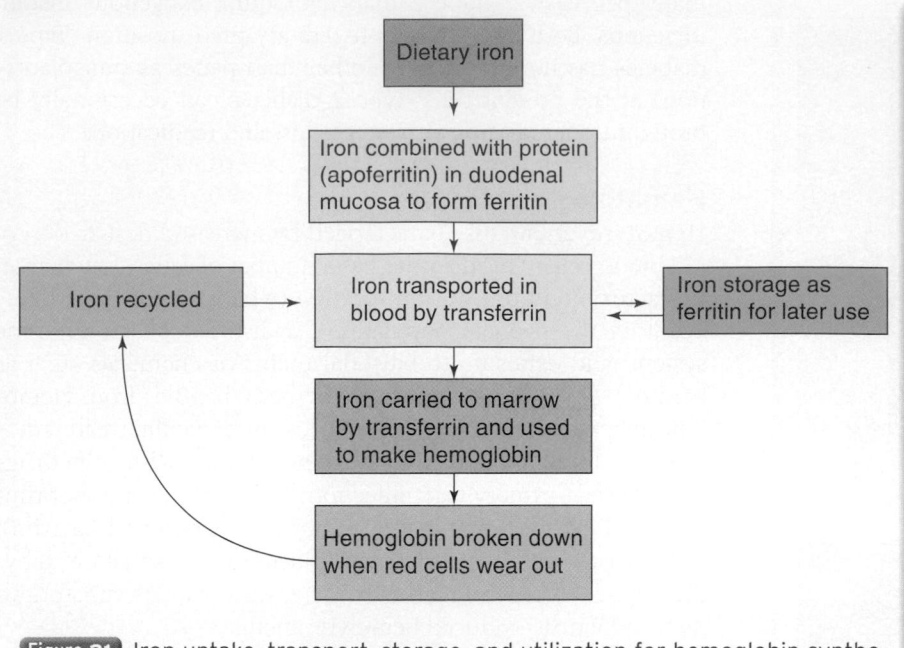

Figure 21 Iron uptake, transport, storage, and utilization for hemoglobin synthesis. Most of the iron used for hemoglobin synthesis is recycled from worn-out red blood cells. Chronic blood loss removes iron-containing cells from the circulation, and the iron contained in the red blood cells can no longer be recycled to make hemoglobin, leading to iron deficiency anemia.

heart disease, liver disease, arthritis, impotence, and a bronzed skin color. These symptoms can be avoided by regularly drawing blood (phlebotomy).

Cardiovascular Disorders

Several cardiovascular disorders are known to follow specific patterns of inheritance. Still others have strong familial tendencies (such as coronary heart disease).

Long QT Syndrome Long QT syndrome is a cardiac conduction system abnormality characterized by prolongation of the QT interval on the ECG. Because most cases of long QT syndrome are inherited in an autosomal dominant manner, all first-degree relatives of affected people must be screened. Sometimes these syndromes are associated with congenital hearing loss, hypertrophic cardiomyopathy, or mitral valve prolapse (MVP). Patients are at risk for palpitations and ventricular dysrhythmias, especially torsades de pointes. Many patients are asymptomatic until they have a dysrhythmia, causing syncope or sudden death. Always consider syncope under the following conditions to be due to a life-threatening dysrhythmia until proven otherwise:

- Exercise-induced syncope
- Syncope associated with chest pain
- A history of syncope in a close family member (that is, parent, sibling, or child)
- Syncope associated with startle (for example, loud noises such as phones or alarm clocks)

Cardiomyopathy Cardiomyopathy is a general term for diseases of the myocardium (heart muscle) that ultimately progress to heart failure, acute myocardial infarction, or death. These diseases cause the heart muscle to become thin, flabby, dilated, or enlarged. One variant, hypertrophic cardiomyopathy, is genetically autosomal dominant. The main feature of hypertrophic cardiomyopathy is an excessive thickening of the heart muscle (hypertrophy means to thicken or grow excessively) **Figure 22**. In addition, microscopic examination of the heart muscle shows that it is abnormal. Patients may have shortness of breath, chest pains, palpitations, or syncope; sudden cardiac death is also possible. Beta blockers are effective treatment in some patients. Others require surgery or an automatic implantable cardiac defibrillator designed to deliver a shock to the heart.

Mitral Valve Prolapse Also referred to as a floppy mitral valve, MVP is relatively common, affecting 2.5% of males and 7.6% of females. A familial tendency toward MVP exists, but the condition is usually associated with other cardiovascular conditions. The mitral valve leaflets balloon into the left atrium during systole. Although MVP is often benign and asymptomatic, some patients have chest pain, fatigue, dizziness, dyspnea, or palpitations. Generally, the only physical finding is a clicking sound heard during cardiac auscultation. Cardiac dysrhythmias develop in a small number of patients.

Sometimes MVP leads to mitral regurgitation (also called mitral insufficiency), in which a large amount of blood leaks backward through the defective valve. Mitral regurgitation can lead to thickening or enlargement of the heart wall, caused by the extra pumping of the heart to make up for the backflow of blood. It sometimes causes people to feel tired or short of breath. Mitral regurgitation usually can be treated with medication, but some people need surgery to repair or replace the defective valve.

Coronary Heart Disease Coronary heart disease, often called coronary artery disease, is caused by impaired circulation to the heart. Typically, patients have occluded coronary arteries from atherosclerotic plaque buildup. The effects can range from ischemia to infarction and necrosis (death) of the myocardium. Almost half of all cardiovascular deaths are caused by coronary heart disease. This condition has a familial tendency; significant risk factors for coronary artery disease development include having a father who had an acute myocardial infarction or died suddenly before 55 years of age or having a mother who had an acute myocardial infarction or died suddenly before 65 years of age. Other risk factors include hypercholesterolemia, cigarette smoking, hypertension (high blood pressure), age (as age increases, the risk for coronary heart disease increases), and diabetes.

Hypercholesterolemia is an elevation of the blood cholesterol level. The blood cholesterol level is divided into high-density lipoprotein ("good cholesterol") and low-density lipoprotein ("bad cholesterol"). Despite having a normal total cholesterol level, having an abnormally low level of high-density lipoprotein

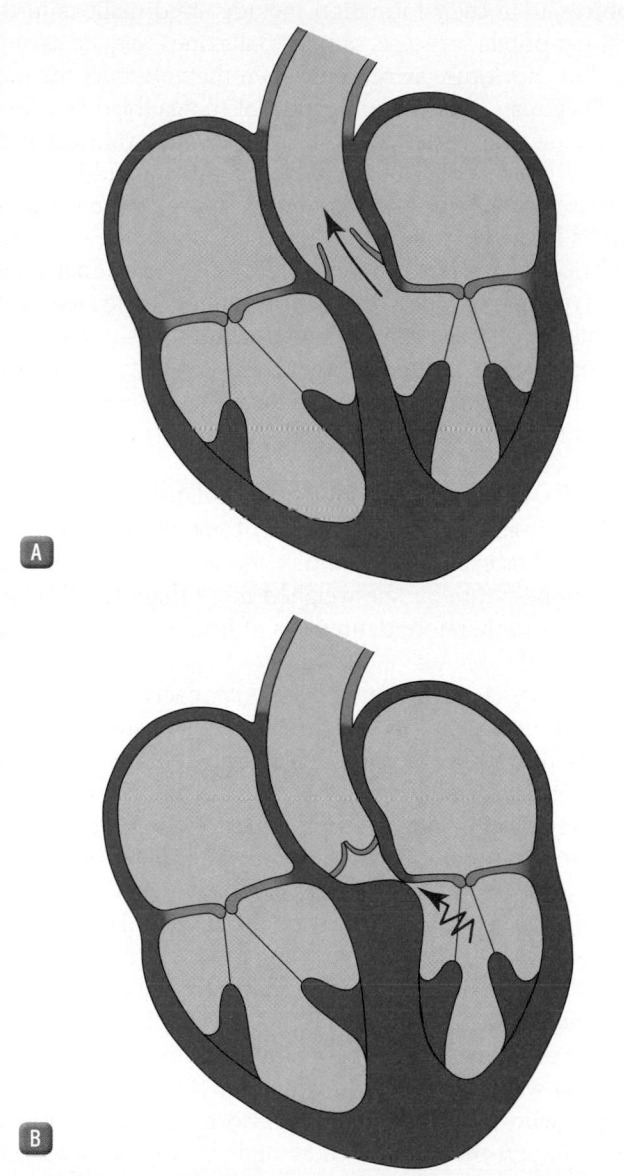

Figure 22 Comparison of normal cardiac function with malfunction characteristic of hypertrophic cardiomyopathy. **A.** Normal heart, illustrating unobstructed flow of blood from left ventricle into aorta during ventricular systole. **B.** Hypertrophic cardiomyopathy, illustrating obstruction to outflow of blood from left ventricle by hypertrophied septum, which impinges on the anterior leaflet of mitral valve.

and/or an elevation of low-density lipoprotein increases the risk of coronary heart disease.

Hypertension and Stroke Hypertension (high blood pressure) is associated with an increased risk of coronary artery disease and is also strongly associated with an increased risk of stroke. Risk factors for developing hypertension can be categorized as genetic or lifestyle-related and include age (as age increases, the risk increases), race (more common in African Americans), sex (men are more likely to experience hypertension), family history, obesity or being overweight, sedentary lifestyle, tobacco use, diet (too much salt, too little potassium, too little vitamin D, too much alcohol), and stress.

Stroke risk factors are also either genetic or lifestyle-related, and include age (persons 55 years or older are at increased risk), race (more common in African Americans, Hispanics, and American Indian/Alaska Natives), sex (men are more likely to have a stroke), family history, obesity or being overweight, sedentary lifestyle, hypertension, hypercholesterolemia, cigarette smoking, diabetes, cardiovascular disease, using birth control pills or hormone therapies, and excessive alcohol consumption.

Renal Disorders

Gout Gout is an abnormal accumulation of uric acid due to a defect in metabolism. As a result of this defect, uric acid accumulates in the blood and joints, causing pain and swelling of the joints, especially the big toe. Often, the patient has fever and chills. Gout is more common among men than women and usually has a genetic basis. If left untreated, it causes destructive tissue changes in the joints and kidneys. Treatment includes diet and drugs to reduce inflammation and to increase the excretion of uric acid or decrease its formation.

Kidney Stones Kidney stones are small masses of uric acid or calcium salts that form in any part of the urinary system (kidney, ureter, or bladder). Often—although not always—stones cause severe pain, nausea, and vomiting when the body attempts to pass them. Although most stones are small, occasionally they become large enough to adopt the internal contours of the kidney **Figure 23**. Researchers have found a gene that causes the

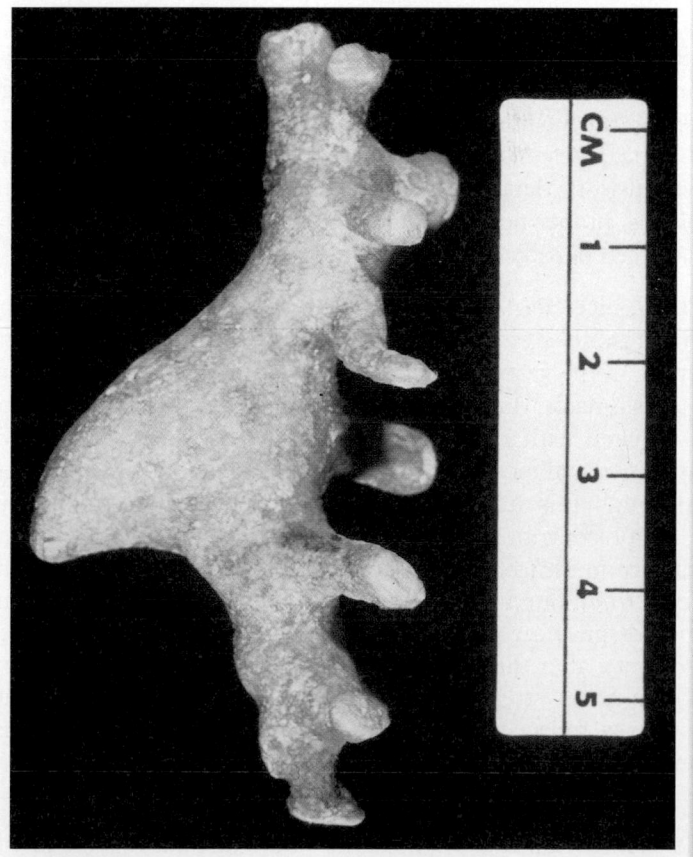

Figure 23 Large staghorn-shaped kidney stone.

intestines to absorb too much calcium, which can lead to the formation of kidney stones. Uric acid stones also often have a genetic basis. Some are small enough to pass in the urine, with or without pain; others must be removed surgically.

Gastrointestinal Disorders

Malabsorption Disorders Malabsorption disorders are caused by defects in the function of the bowel wall that prevent adequate nutrient absorption. The result is a complex of symptoms, including loss of appetite, bloating, weight loss, muscle pain, and stools with high fat content. Diarrhea, which may be bloody, may also be a prominent symptom.

Lactose intolerance is caused by a defect or deficiency of the enzyme lactase, resulting in an inability to digest lactose (milk sugar). Lactase deficiency, which seems to be due to an abnormal gene, affects between 30 and 50 million people in the United States, and nearly three fourths of the world's population is believed to be lactose intolerant. Symptoms include bloating, flatulence, abdominal discomfort, nausea, and diarrhea after ingestion of milk or milk products.

Ulcerative colitis is a serious chronic inflammatory disease of the large intestine and rectum. This disease, which shows a familial tendency, is characterized by recurrent episodes of abdominal pain, fever, chills, and profuse diarrhea, with stools containing pus, blood, and mucus. Treatment consists of anti-inflammatory agents, including corticosteroids. Patients with severe cases may require surgery to remove parts of the intestinal tract. Patients are at increased risk for the development of colon cancer.

Crohn disease is a serious chronic inflammatory condition affecting the colon and/or the terminal portion of the small intestine. It is believed to be associated with as-yet-undetermined gene abnormalities. Symptoms include frequent episodes of diarrhea, melena, abdominal pain, nausea, fever, weakness, and weight loss. Management is by anti-inflammatory agents, antibiotics, proper nutrition, and sometimes surgery to remove the damaged portion of the bowel, fistulas, or scar tissue.

Peptic Ulcer Disease Peptic ulcer disease is characterized by circumscribed erosions (ulcerations) of the mucous membrane lining of the gastrointestinal tract—specifically, in the esophagus, stomach, duodenum, or jejunum. Peptic ulcers may be associated with excess acid production or from a breakdown in the normal mechanisms protecting the mucous membranes. Although this disease seems to have a genetic component, a major contributor to its development is infection with the bacterium *Helicobacter pylori*—the observed familial patterns seem to be due to shared infections with *H pylori*. Symptoms include gnawing pain, which is often worse when the stomach is empty, after the person eats certain foods, or when the person is under stress. Treatment includes avoidance of irritants (such as tobacco, alcohol, and irritating foods), antibiotics, and drugs to decrease acidity. In refractory cases, surgery may be necessary.

Gallstones Gallstones (choleliths) are stonelike masses in the gallbladder or its ducts caused by precipitation of substances contained in bile (such as cholesterol and bilirubin). Factors that contribute to their formation include abnormalities in the composition of bile, or stasis of bile. Gallstones may be asymptomatic, but they cause symptoms when they obstruct the flow of bile. They may cause inflammation of the gallbladder. Small stones that are able to pass into the common duct produce indigestion and biliary colic. Biliary colic pain has a sudden onset and increases steadily to its maximum in approximately 1 hour. The pain is located in the upper right quadrant or the epigastric area and may be referred to the back. Larger stones may cause jaundice (yellow skin and sclerae). Although genetic factors are responsible for at least 30% of symptomatic gallstone disease, heredity probably has an even larger role in gallstone pathogenesis. Data based on symptomatic gallbladder disease underestimate the true prevalence in the population.

Obesity <u>Obesity</u> is an unhealthy accumulation of body fat, and is defined as a body mass index of greater than or equal to 30 kg/m^2. For example, an adult who is 5′ 9″ tall would be considered obese if he or she weighed more than 203 lb. Body mass index, and therefore definitions of obesity, is different for children and adolescents.

Obesity has a significant negative impact on a person's health and life span; simply put, it has been statistically proven that obesity decreases a person's life span by an average of 8 to 13 years. Obesity has become an epidemic among adults and children in the United States. Approximately one third of adults in the United States are obese. Approximately 17% of children and adolescents in the United States are obese.

<u>Morbid obesity</u> is defined as a body mass index of greater than or equal to 40 kg/m^2. Again using the example of an adult who is 5′ 9″ tall, he or she would be morbidly obese if he or she weighed more than 270 lb. Morbid obesity includes all of the health risks associated with obesity, but also makes basic functions such as walking or breathing difficult.

People who are overweight are also at increased risk for disease, although the risk is not as high as for those who are obese. Being <u>overweight</u> is defined as a body mass index of 25 to 29.9 kg/m^2. Using the previous example of an adult who is 5′ 9″ tall, he or she would be overweight if he or she weighed between 169 and 202 lb.

Obesity has many deleterious effects, both medical and social. Health risks associated with obesity include hypertension, hyperlipidemia, cardiovascular disease, glucose intolerance, insulin resistance, diabetes, gallbladder disease, infertility, and cancer of the endometrium, breast, prostate, and colon. Social and psychological effects of obesity include depression, anxiety, shame, rejection, and discrimination in various environments including school and the workplace.

Although some people likely have a genetic predisposition to obesity, the roles of specific genes in its development have yet to be determined. Behavioral and environmental factors are better known. Behavioral factors that contribute to obesity include choosing a sedentary lifestyle, overeating, or choosing foods high in calories and low in nutritional value, such as fast food and soda. A person's community or work environment may make it difficult to choose to be physically active or to eat properly. For example, a lack of sidewalks in a community would contribute to the risk of members of that community becoming obese. Large portion sizes offered by restaurants contribute to a lack of understanding of what is a proper portion size. Finally, television and technological media take time away from physical activity and promote unhealthy products. Because people tend to snack while watching TV or using a computer, they consume unnecessary additional calories.

Neuromuscular Disorders

Although environmental contributions are highly likely, certain neuromuscular disorders have a familial and genetic basis. The next few sections present several of the better known and more worrisome disorders in this category.

Huntington Disease Huntington disease (also called Huntington chorea), for example, is a hereditary condition (autosomal dominant) characterized by progressive chorea (involuntary rapid, jerky motions) and mental deterioration, leading to dementia. Symptoms usually first appear in the third or fourth decade of life and progress to death, often within 15 years.

Muscular Dystrophy Muscular dystrophy is a generic term for a group of hereditary diseases of the muscular system characterized by weakness and wasting of groups of skeletal muscles, leading to increasing disability. The various forms differ in age of onset, rate of progression, and mode of genetic transmission. Duchenne muscular dystrophy is a sex-linked recessive disease (affecting only males); symptoms first appear around the age of 4 years. Progressive wasting of leg and pelvic muscles produces a waddling gait and abnormal curvature of the spine. Usually by age 12, the person becomes unable to walk and begins to use a wheelchair. No known treatment exists, and the person often dies, most often of a heart disorder, by 20 years.

Multiple Sclerosis Multiple sclerosis is a progressive disease in which nerve fibers of the brain and spinal cord lose their protective sheaths of myelin. Although the disease is not directly inherited, some patients have a familial predisposition, suggesting a genetic influence on susceptibility. The disease usually begins in early adulthood and progresses slowly, with periods of remission and exacerbation. Early symptoms include abnormal sensations in the face or extremities, weakness, and visual disturbances (such as double vision), which progress to ataxia (lack of coordination), abnormal reflexes, tremors, difficulty in urination, and difficulty in walking. Depression is also common. No specific treatment or cure has been developed, but corticosteroids and other drugs are used to treat symptoms.

Alzheimer Disease Alzheimer disease affects nearly 4 million Americans. Although its cause is unknown, the disease is characterized by cortical atrophy and loss of neurons in the frontal and temporal lobes of the brain; in addition, the ventricles become enlarged as brain tissue is lost. Histologic changes in the brain of a person with Alzheimer disease include neurofibrillary tangles and senile plaques **Figure 24**. Studies of the genetics of inherited early-onset Alzheimer disease have been linked to mutations on three genes.

Alzheimer disease is progressive. Early in its progression, it is characterized by memory loss, lack of spontaneity, subtle

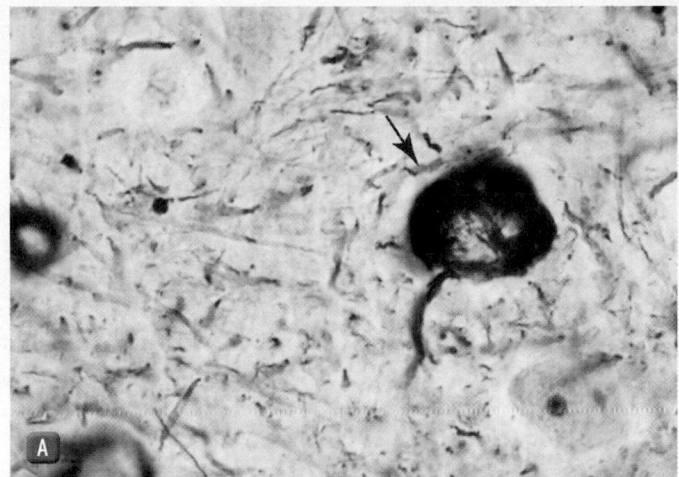
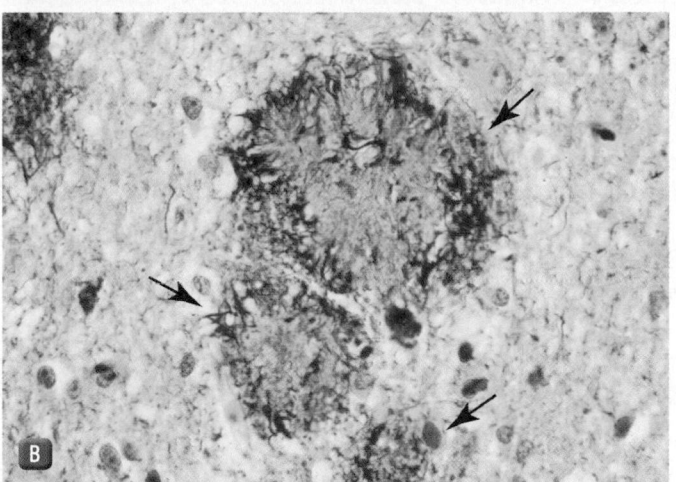

Figure 24 Alzheimer disease. **A.** Thickened neurofilaments encircle and obscure the nuclei of nerve cells (arrow), forming a neurofibrillary tangle (original magnification, ×400). **B.** Three senile plaques (arrows) composed of broken masses of thickened neurofilaments (original magnification, ×100).

personality changes, and disorientation to time and date. It may then progress to including impaired cognition and abstract thinking, restlessness and agitation, wandering, inability to carry out activities of daily living, impaired judgment, and inappropriate social behavior. Advanced Alzheimer disease involves indifference to food, inability to communicate, urinary and fecal incontinence, and seizures.

Special Populations

Never assume that new or worsening confusion in an older adult is due purely to Alzheimer disease, without first considering potentially correctable causes such as new medications, infections, or myocardial infarction. An apparent emotional, psychological, or behavioral problem may have an organic cause, especially in the older adult population.

Psychiatric Disorders

Some common psychiatric disorders seem to have a familial and perhaps even genetic component. Two of the most important are schizophrenia and bipolar disorder.

Schizophrenia Schizophrenia comprises a group of mental disorders characterized by gross distortions of reality (psychoses), withdrawal from social contacts, and disturbances of thought, language, perception, and emotional response. Its symptoms are highly varied but may include apathy, catatonia or excessive activity, bizarre actions, hallucinations, delusions, and rambling speech. Although the cause of schizophrenia has not been identified, a combination of hereditary or genetic predisposing factors is likely in most cases.

Bipolar Disorder Bipolar disorder (formerly known as manic-depressive disorder or manic-depressive psychosis) is a mental disorder characterized by episodes of mania and depression. One or the other phase may be dominant at any given time, the phases may alternate, or aspects of both phases may be present at once. The higher rates of bipolar disorder among relatives, identical twins, and biologic parents versus adoptive parents have been cited as evidence of the role of genetics in this disorder; the risk within the general population as a whole is approximately 1%. Treatment consists of psychotherapy plus antidepressants and tranquilizers.

■ Hypoperfusion

Perfusion is defined as the delivery of oxygen and nutrients and removal of wastes from the cells, organs, and tissues by the circulatory system. Evaluation of a patient's level of organ perfusion is important in emergency care, especially in diagnosing shock. Hypoperfusion occurs when the level of tissue perfusion decreases below normal.

When the body senses tissue hypoperfusion, it sets compensatory mechanisms into motion. In some cases, this action is sufficient to stabilize the patient's condition. In other cases, the hypoperfusion overwhelms the normal compensatory mechanisms and the patient's condition progressively deteriorates Table 6 .

In response to hypoperfusion, the body releases catecholamines (epinephrine and norepinephrine), which produce vasoconstriction and, consequently, increase systemic vascular resistance. In addition, the RAAS is activated and antidiuretic hormone is released from the pituitary gland. Together, these actions trigger salt and water retention and peripheral vasoconstriction, thereby increasing blood pressure and cardiac output. Depending on the severity of the insult, variable amounts of fluid will shift from the interstitial tissues into the vascular compartment. The spleen also releases some red blood cells that are normally sequestered there, to augment the oxygen-carrying capacity of the blood. The overall response of the initial compensatory mechanisms is to increase the preload (venous return), stroke volume, and heart rate so that blood volume is adequate. The result is usually an increase in cardiac output and myocardial oxygen demand.

Table 6 Signs and Symptoms of Compensated and Decompensated Hypoperfusion	
Compensated	**Decompensated**
Agitation, anxiety, restlessness	Altered mental status (verbal to unresponsive)
Sense of impending doom	Hypotension
Weak, rapid (thready) pulse	Labored or irregular breathing
Clammy (cool, moist) skin	Thready or absent peripheral pulses
Pallor with cyanotic lips	Ashen, mottled, or cyanotic skin
Shortness of breath	Dilated pupils
Nausea, vomiting	Diminished urine output (oliguria)
Delayed capillary refill time in infants and children	Impending cardiac arrest
Thirst	
Normal blood pressure	

As hypoperfusion persists, the myocardial oxygen demand continues to increase. Eventually, the above-normal compensatory mechanisms can no longer keep up with the demand. Myocardial function worsens, with decreased cardiac output and ejection fraction. Tissue perfusion decreases, leading to impaired cell metabolism. Often, the blood pressure decreases, especially in progressive hypoperfusion. Fluid may leak from the blood vessels, causing systemic and pulmonary edema. At this point, other signs of hypoperfusion may be present, such as dyspnea, dusky skin, low blood pressure, oliguria, and impaired mentation.

Documentation and Communication

The terms shock and hypoperfusion are usually synonymous, at least when they are applied to multiple body systems. Localized hypoperfusion, such as from arterial occlusion, is not shock.

■ Types of Shock

Shock is an abnormal state associated with inadequate oxygen and nutrient delivery to the metabolic apparatus of the cell, resulting in impairment of cellular metabolism and inadequate perfusion of vital organs. Once a certain level of tissue hypoperfusion has been reached, cell damage proceeds in a similar manner regardless of the type of initial insult. Impairment of cellular metabolism prevents the body from properly using oxygen and glucose at the cellular level. Cells revert to anaerobic metabolism, which causes increased lactic acid production and metabolic acidosis, decreased oxygen affinity for hemoglobin, decreased ATP production, changes in cellular electrolyte levels, cellular edema, and release of lysosomal enzymes. Glucose impairment raises the level of blood glucose as catecholamines and cortisol are released. In addition, fat breakdown (lipolysis) with ketone formation may occur.

Shock can occur due to inadequacy of the central circulation (the heart and the great vessels) or of the peripheral circulation (the remaining vessels, including the microscopic circulation—that is, arterioles, venules, and capillaries, as illustrated in **Figure 25**). From a mechanistic approach, two types of shock are distinguished: central and peripheral. <u>Central shock</u> consists of cardiogenic shock and obstructive shock. <u>Peripheral shock</u> includes hypovolemic shock and distributive shock.

The following sections contain an overview of types of shock. These topics are also discussed in later chapters.

■ Central Shock

Cardiogenic Shock
<u>Cardiogenic shock</u> occurs when the heart cannot circulate enough blood to maintain adequate peripheral oxygen delivery. In the case of ischemic heart disease, this requires loss of 40% or more of functioning myocardium. The most common cause of cardiogenic shock is myocardial infarction, as a single event or by cumulative damage. Other forms of cardiac dysfunction may also precipitate cardiogenic shock (such as a large ventricular septal defect or hemodynamic significant dysrhythmias) (see the chapter, *Cardiovascular Emergencies*).

Obstructive Shock
<u>Obstructive shock</u> occurs when blood flow becomes blocked in the heart or great vessels. In <u>pericardial tamponade</u> **Figure 26**,

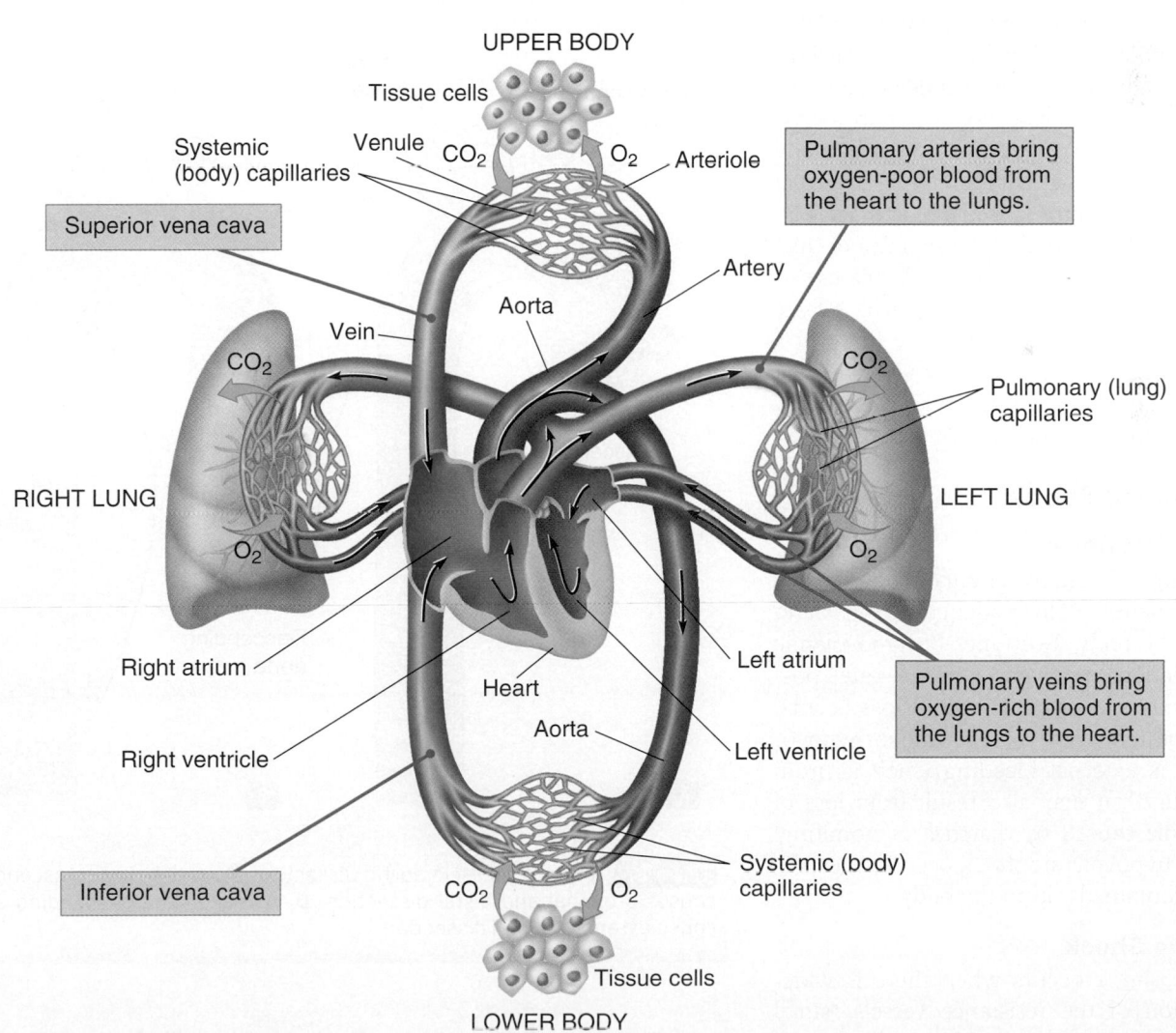

Figure 25 The circulatory system includes the heart, arteries, veins, and interconnecting capillaries. The capillaries—the smallest vessels—connect with venules and arterioles. The heart is the center of the system and is its driving force.

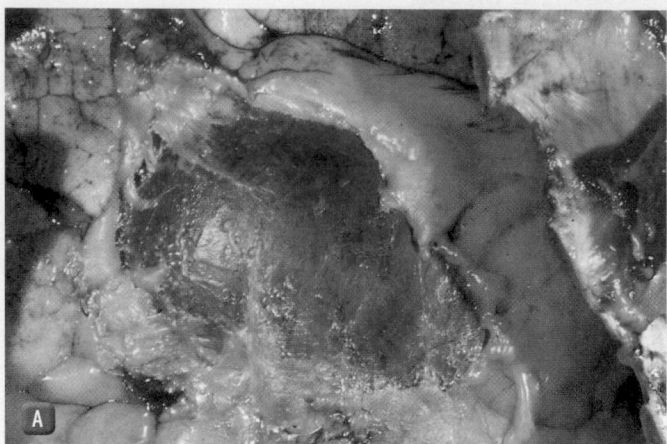
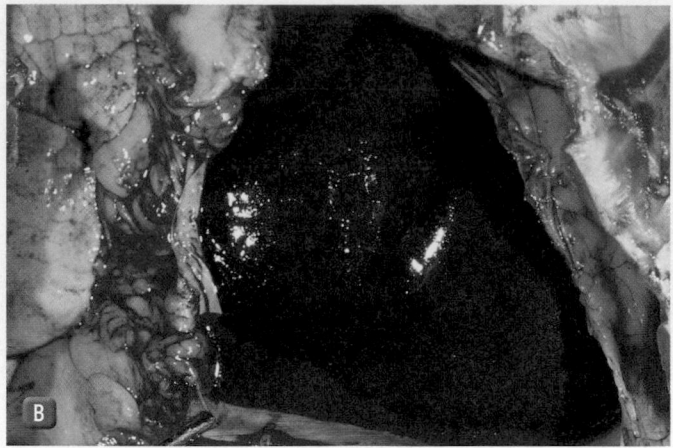

Figure 26 Cardiac tamponade following myocardial rupture. **A.** Distended pericardial sac. **B.** Pericardial sac opened, showing clotted blood surrounding the heart, which compressed the heart and prevented filling of the right ventricle in diastole.

diastolic filling of the right ventricle is impaired due to significant amounts of fluid in the pericardial sac surrounding the heart, leading to a decrease in the cardiac output. Aortic dissection leads to a false lumen (aortic opening), with loss of normal blood flow **Figure 27**. A left atrial tumor may obstruct flow between the atrium and ventricle and decrease cardiac output. Obstruction of the superior or inferior vena cava (vena cava syndrome) decreases cardiac output by decreasing venous return. A large pulmonary embolus (blood clot in the lung) or a tension pneumothorax (lung collapse) may prevent adequate blood flow to the lungs, resulting in inadequate venous return to the left side of the heart.

▇ Peripheral Shock

Hypovolemic Shock

In **hypovolemic shock**, the circulating blood volume is insufficient to deliver adequate oxygen and nutrients to the body. Two types of hypovolemic shock—exogenous and endogenous—are possible, depending on where the fluid loss occurs. The most common type of exogenous hypovolemic shock is external bleeding (such as from an open wound); it may also result from loss of plasma volume caused by diarrhea or vomiting. Endogenous hypovolemic shock occurs when the fluid loss is contained within the body.

Distributive Shock

Distributive shock occurs when there is widespread dilation of the resistance vessels (small arterioles), the capacitance vessels (small venules), or both. The circulating blood volume then pools in the expanded vascular beds, and tissue perfusion decreases. The three most common types of distributive shock are anaphylactic shock, septic shock, and neurogenic shock **Figure 28**.

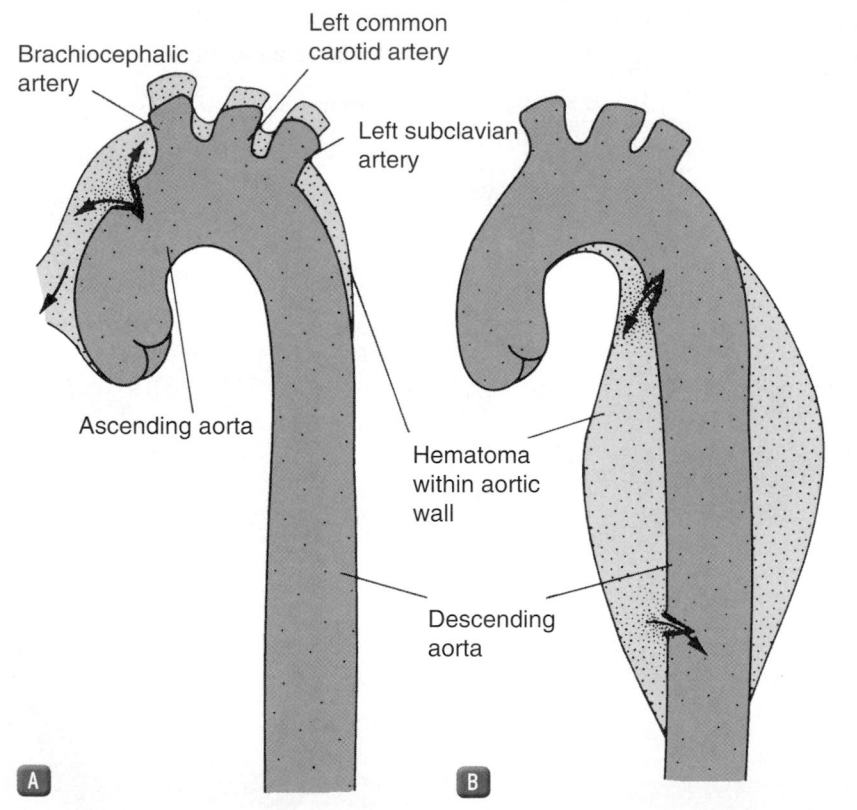

Figure 27 Sites of thoracic aortic dissection. **A.** A tear in the ascending aorta causes proximal and distal dissection. **B.** A tear in the descending aorta may cause extensive distal dissection.

In **anaphylactic shock** (also called anaphylaxis), histamine and other vasodilator proteins are released on exposure to an allergen. Anaphylactic shock is also accompanied by wheezing and **urticaria** (hives). The result is widespread vasodilation that causes distributive shock and blood vessels that continue

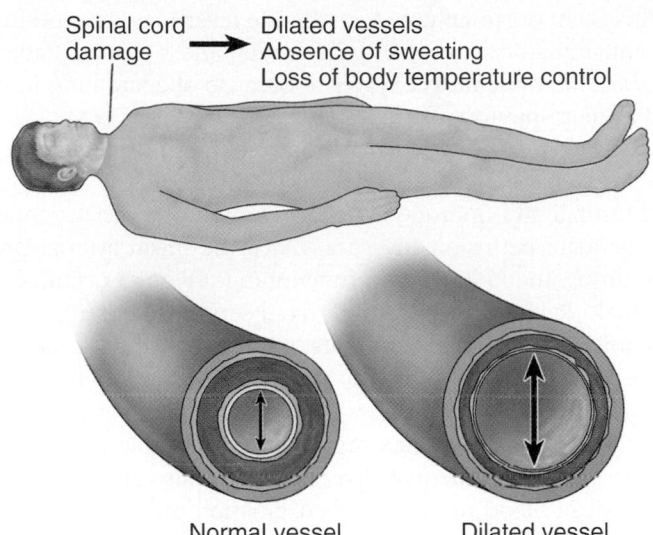

Spinal cord damage → Dilated vessels
Absence of sweating
Loss of body temperature control

Normal vessel   Dilated vessel

Figure 28 Damage to the spinal cord can cause significant injury to the part of the nervous system that controls the size and muscle tone of blood vessels. If the muscles in the blood vessels are cut off from their impulses to contract, the vessels dilate widely, increasing the size and capacity of the vascular system. The blood in the body can no longer fill the enlarged vessels, resulting in inadequate perfusion and neurogenic shock.

to leak. Fluid leaks out of the blood vessels into the interstitial spaces, resulting in intravascular hypovolemia.

Septic shock occurs as a result of widespread infection, usually bacterial. Complex interactions occur between the bacterial invader and the body's defense systems. Initially, the body's own defense mechanisms may keep the infection at bay. If the normal immune mechanisms become overwhelmed, the body produces a multitude of substances that cause vasodilation and decreased cardiac output. If left untreated, the result is multiple organ dysfunction syndrome (discussed later) and often death.

Words of Wisdom

Typically the earliest signs of shock are restlessness and anxiety. The patient looks scared!

Neurogenic shock usually results from spinal cord injury. The effect is loss of normal sympathetic nervous system tone and vasodilation. Often patients have fluid-refractory hypotension due to the degree of vasodilation.

■ Management of Shock

Most types of shock are characterized by reduced cardiac output, circulatory insufficiency, and rapid heartbeat. Although low blood pressure is classically associated with shock, it is a late sign, especially in children. In compensated shock, the systolic

Words of Wisdom

In anaphylaxis, interstitial fluid may cause significant swelling. In some cases, this swelling may occlude the upper airway, resulting in a life-threatening condition. Recurrent large areas of subcutaneous edema of sudden onset, usually disappearing within 24 hours, are called angioedema. This condition is seen mainly in young women, frequently as a result of allergy to food or drugs.

blood pressure is within the normal range; in decompensated shock, the systolic blood pressure is less than the fifth percentile for the age.

Clinically, determining the presence or absence of shock requires the evaluation of the presence and volume of the peripheral pulses and assessment of end-organ perfusion and function. Strength of the peripheral pulses is related to stroke volume of the heart and pulse pressures. Peripheral pulses should be readily palpable if the person is not in shock, although cold environments or obesity may compromise the presence or strength of these pulses. Normal skin perfusion is indicated by warm, dry, pink extremities, fingers, and toes, whereas a slow, delayed, or prolonged **capillary refill time** indicates shock (although this technique is more reliable in children). To test the capillary refill time, briefly squeeze the toenail or fingernail, and then look for return of color. A normal capillary refill time is less than 2 seconds after blanching of the toe or finger, whereas a person in shock may have a capillary refill time of more than 2 seconds. Mottling, pallor, peripheral or central cyanosis, and delayed capillary refill may signal the presence of shock, whereas altered mental status is an indication of inadequate brain tissue perfusion. Note that the accuracy of capillary refill measurement decreases after age 6 years; it is most useful in young children but not as useful in the adult population.

Treatment primarily addresses the underlying condition (see the chapter, *Bleeding*).

Words of Wisdom

Neurogenic shock can involve bradycardia if the injury is in the high thoracic region because of disruption in the sympathetic autonomic pathway. Cardiogenic shock can involve bradycardia when myocardial infarction is the cause and there is a disruption in the electrophysiologic pathway.

■ Multiple Organ Dysfunction Syndrome

Multiple organ dysfunction syndrome (MODS), first described in 1975, is a progressive condition that occurs in some critically ill patients. It is characterized by the concurrent failure of two or more organs or organ systems that were initially unharmed by the acute disorder or injury that caused the patient's current illness. Six organ systems are surveyed in diagnosing MODS: respiratory,

Words of Wisdom

A possible exception to the standard use of IV fluid therapy to treat shock is hypovolemic shock caused by ongoing bleeding. Some studies suggest that fluid therapy to maintain the systolic blood pressure at around 80 to 90 mm Hg may be safer than attempting restoration of normotension, which may aggravate ongoing bleeding. As always, follow your local protocols.

hepatic, renal, hematologic, neurologic, and cardiovascular. Each system is assigned a score to determine the patient's overall risk. For example, the Glasgow Coma Scale score is used to score the patient's neurologic system function.

In MODS, the overall mortality rate is 60% to 90%. Nevertheless, despite the inevitability its name suggests, the condition is often reversible, particularly in patients who were healthy before the physiologic insult occurred. A patient with two failing organ systems has a 20% to 50% chance of survival. When four or more organ systems become dysfunctional, however, the mortality rate is nearly 100%. Multiple organ dysfunction syndrome is the major cause of death following sepsis, trauma, and burn injuries.

Primary MODS is a direct result of an insult, such as a pulmonary contusion from striking the chest on the steering wheel during a collision. Secondary MODS is a slower, more progressive organ dysfunction.

When injury or infection (septic shock) triggers a massive systemic immune, inflammatory, and coagulation response accompanied by endotoxin release, MODS results. Overactivation of the complement system further increases inflammation and cellular damage. Vascular endothelial damage triggers overactivation of the coagulation system, which leads to uncontrolled coagulation in the venules and arterioles. This coagulation, in turn, causes microvascular thrombus formation and tissue ischemia. In addition, MODS activates the kallikrein-kinin system, stimulating the release of bradykinin, a potent vasodilator. Kallikrein is an inactive enzyme of the pancreas. When it becomes activated, it can dilate blood vessels, influence blood pressure, modulate salt and water excretion by the kidneys, and influence cardiac remodeling after acute myocardial infarction. Bradykinin increases vascular permeability, dilates blood vessels, contracts smooth muscle, and causes pain when injected into the skin. Vasodilation leads to tissue hypoperfusion and may also contribute to hypotension.

The net outcome of the activation of these systems is maldistribution of systemic and organ blood flow. Often the body attempts to compensate for this problem by accelerating tissue metabolism. The result is an imbalance in oxygen supply and demand that causes tissue hypoxia, initiating a cascade of ill effects including tissue hypoperfusion, exhaustion of the cells' fuel supply (ATP), metabolic failure, lysosome breakdown, anaerobic metabolism, and acidosis and impaired cellular function.

Typically, MODS develops hours or days following resuscitation. The signs and symptoms include hypotension, insufficient tissue perfusion, uncontrollable bleeding (coagulopathy), and multisystem organ failure. A low-grade fever may develop from the inflammatory response, tachycardia, and dyspnea. Patients may also be difficult to oxygenate because of acute lung injury and acute respiratory distress syndrome.

During a 14- to 21-day period, renal and liver failure can develop in patients with MODS, along with collapse of the gastrointestinal and immune systems. The kidneys are dependent on adequate perfusion pressure. Once the mean arterial pressure drops, the kidneys stop functioning. Oliguria occurs early in shock. Renal studies show elevated serum urea nitrogen and creatinine levels. Many patients require continuous bedside dialysis. Renal failure accompanying MODS increases the risk of death by 30%.

The liver is a complex organ with a key role in excreting wastes and toxins. Adequate liver function is also essential for the synthesis of blood proteins and coagulation proteins, as well as the storage of glycogen, iron, and vitamins. Patients with MODS have elevated levels of total bilirubin and of the liver enzymes aspartate aminotransferase and alanine aminotransferase. Unfortunately, there are no definitive treatments for liver failure. Treatment focuses on minimizing the effects of liver damage.

The brain, adrenal glands, and heart are also affected early in MODS. The level of consciousness deteriorates quickly in hypoxic states, but it declines precipitously in patients with MODS. As a peripheral organ, the brain is not above sacrificing itself for the sake of maintaining adequate blood pressure. Cerebral hypoxia and subsequent ischemia can cause permanent deficits as a result of anoxic brain injury.

Perhaps the heart suffers more than any other organ in a patient with MODS. As it struggles to maintain arterial perfusion pressure, it too becomes hypoxic. Hypotension cannot be controlled despite the administration of fluids and vasopressors. Compensatory tachycardia consumes even more oxygen, and dysrhythmias such as bradycardia, ventricular tachycardia, and ventricular fibrillation develop. As the pancreas becomes ischemic, it releases myocardial depressant factor, further impairing the ability of the myocardium to contract. Cardiovascular collapse and death typically occur within days to weeks of the initial insult.

The Body's Self-Defense Mechanisms

The **immune system** includes all structures and processes associated with the body's defense against foreign substances and disease-causing agents. The body has three lines of defense: anatomic barriers, the immune response, and the inflammatory response.

Anatomic Barriers

Several anatomic barriers decrease the chances of invasion of the body by foreign substances. The skin serves as a major deterrent. Hairs in the upper respiratory tract (the nose) and the lining of the lower respiratory tract (cilia-covered epithelial cells) help repel foreign matter, especially small particles and some bacteria. Acid in the stomach prevents many infectious agents from entering the body via the gastrointestinal tract.

Immune Response

The <u>immune response</u> is the body's defense reaction to any substance that is recognized as foreign. Often, this response is directed toward invading microbes, such as bacteria or viruses. It is also triggered by foreign bodies, such as a splinter, and even abnormal cell growths, such as tumors. The immune response involves only one type of white blood cells, namely lymphocytes.

Not all invaders can be destroyed by the body's immune system. In some cases, the best compromise the body can reach is to control the damage and keep the invader from spreading. Often, the immune system succeeds in preventing severe disease following infection. When the normal systems become overwhelmed or fail, serious disease occurs.

Anatomy of the Immune System

The <u>lymphatic system</u> is a network of capillaries, vessels, ducts, nodes, and organs that help maintain the fluid environment of the body by producing lymph and conveying it through the body `Figure 29`. The immune system has two anatomic components: the lymphoid tissues and the cells that are responsible for the immune response.

Lymphoid tissues are distributed throughout the body. The two primary lymphoid tissues are bone marrow and the thymus gland. <u>Bone marrow</u> is specialized soft tissue found within bone. Red bone marrow, which is widespread in the bones of children and is found in some adult bones (in the sternum and ribs), is essential for formation of mature blood cells; it produces B lymphocytes. T lymphocytes originate from

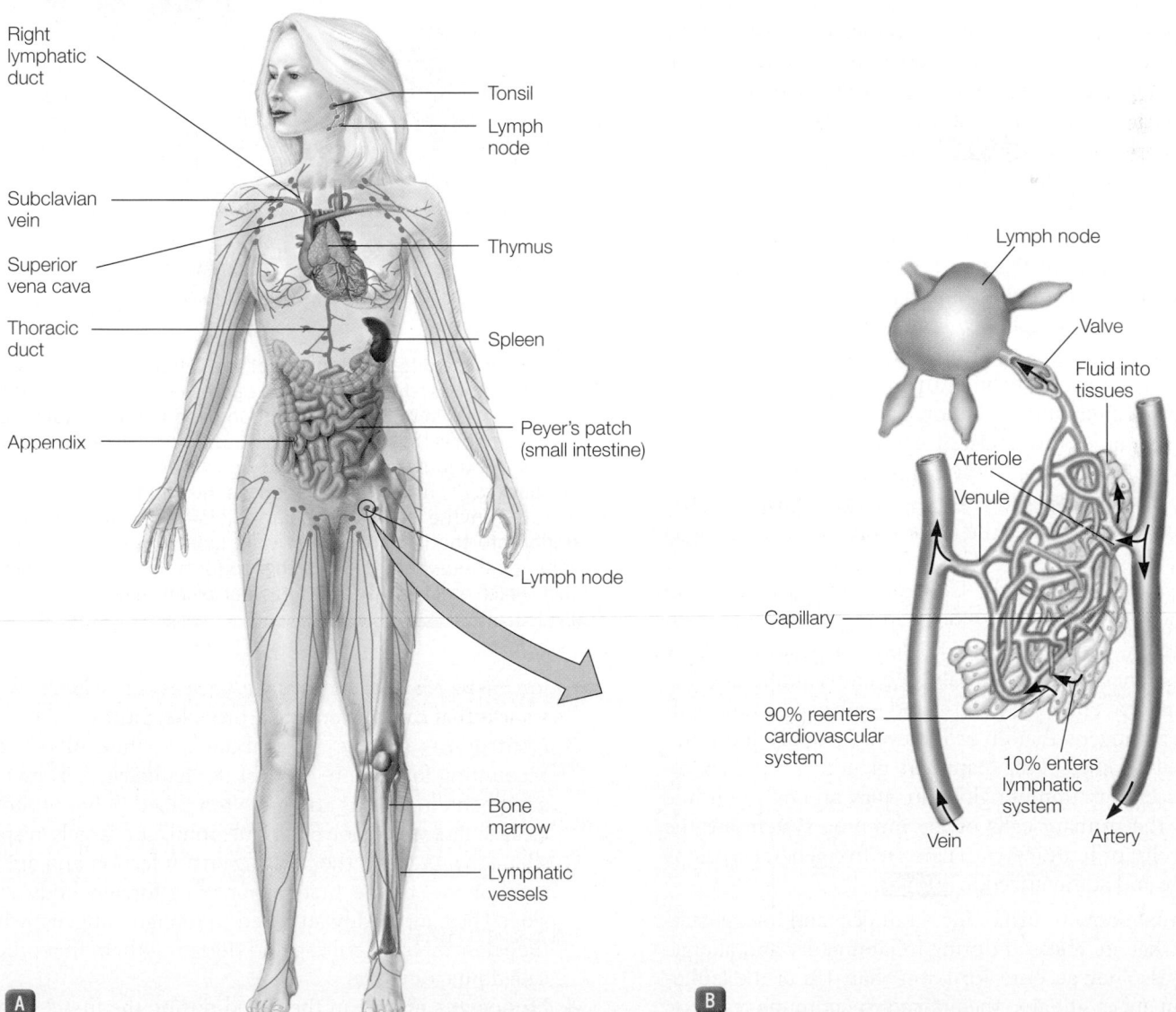

Figure 29 The lymphatic system. **A.** The lymphatic system consists of vessels that transport lymph and excess tissue fluid back to the circulatory system. **B.** Lymph is picked up by lymphatic capillaries that drain into larger vessels. Like the veins, the lymphatic vessels contain valves that prohibit backflow. Lymph nodes are interspersed along the vessels and filter the lymph.

precursor cells in the bone marrow, leave the bone marrow, and mature in the thymus gland. This bilobed gland—located below the thyroid gland and behind the sternum—is prominent at birth, increases in size until the body reaches puberty, and then shrinks and decreases in functional activity during adulthood.

In secondary lymphoid tissues (that is, encapsulated and unencapsulated diffuse lymphoid tissues), mature immune cells interact with invaders and initiate a response. Encapsulated lymphoid tissues consist of the lymph nodes and the spleen. Lymph nodes (lymph glands) are small structures that filter lymph and store lymphocytes; they are concentrated in areas of the body such as the axillae, groin, and neck. The spleen is located on the left side of the body, posterior and lateral to the stomach (left upper quadrant); it monitors the blood, destroys worn-out red blood cells, and traps foreign invaders. The diffuse lymphoid tissues are scattered throughout the body.

Lymph is a thin, watery fluid that bathes the tissues of the body; it circulates through lymph vessels and is filtered in lymph nodes. Lymphatic capillaries unite to form the lymph vessels, which eventually coalesce and empty their contents into the central venous circulation **Figure 30**. Most lymph empties into the superior vena cava via the thoracic duct, located on the left side of the thorax. The remaining lymph enters the right subclavian vein via three or four lymphatic ducts.

Clusters of lymphoid tissue are associated with the skin and the respiratory, urinary, gastrointestinal, and reproductive tracts. clusters of lymphoid tissue, which are collectively termed **mucosa-associated lymphoid tissue**, contain immune cells that are in a position to intercept pathogens before they reach the general circulation. The tonsils are perhaps the best-known type of mucosa-associated lymphoid tissue. Unencapsulated lymphoid tissue is particularly prominent in the gastrointestinal tract. Called the **gut-associated lymphoid tissue**, this tissue lies just under the inner lining of the esophagus and intestines.

The salivary glands and the lacrimal glands play a role in the immune system as well; the salivary and lacrimal glands produce an antibody, secretory immunoglobulin A, which bathe mucous membranes. As a result, saliva contains antibodies that fight pathogens that enter the mouth, and tears contain antibodies that fight pathogens that enter the eye. Secretory immunoglobulin A is also found in the mammary glands.

Though secretory immunoglobulins play an important role in immunity, the primary cells of the immune system are the white blood cells, or **leukocytes**. There are five general types, as described here and summarized in **Table 7**:

1. **Basophils** contain histamine granules and other substances that are released during inflammatory and allergic responses. They account for fewer than 1% of the leukocytes but are essential to the nonspecific immune response to inflammation because they release histamine and other chemicals that dilate blood vessels.

2. **Eosinophils** release substances that damage or kill parasitic invaders. They also have a major role in mediating the allergic response. These white blood cells, which account

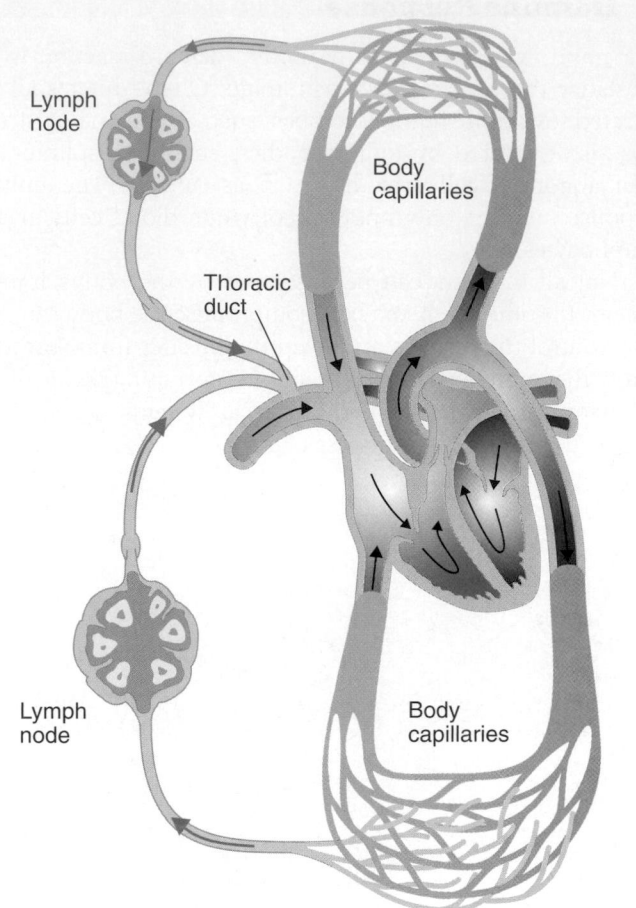

Figure 30   The interrelationship of the lymphatic system and the circulatory system. Blood fluid passes out of the arteries in the upper and lower parts of the body and enters a system of lymphatic ducts that arise in the tissues. The fluid, called lymph, passes through lymph nodes and on the right side makes its way back to the general circulation via the thoracic duct. Lymph vessels from the left upper quadrant join the thoracic duct and empty into the left subclavian vein. Lymph vessels from the right upper quadrant join together to form the right lymphatic duct, which empties into the right subclavian vein.

for 1% to 3% of the leukocytes, release chemoactive substances that can trigger severe bronchospasm.

3. **Neutrophils** are the most abundant white blood cells, accounting for 55% to 70% of the leukocytes. They have a segmented nucleus and are often called polymorphonuclear leukocytes ("polys"). Neutrophils are largely responsible for protecting the body against infection and are key components of the first response to foreign body invasion. They are readily attracted to foreign antigens, which they destroy by engulfing and digesting them in a process called **phagocytosis**.

4. **Monocytes** mature in the blood during the first 24 hours after they are generated. They then travel to the tissues, where they differentiate into **macrophages**. Macrophages function primarily as scavengers for the tissues. Monocytes and macrophages represent one of the first lines of defense in the inflammatory process.

Table 7 Primary Types of White Blood Cells

Type	Description	Concentration (number of cells/mm³)	Life Span	Function
Neutrophil	Approximately twice the size of a red blood cell; multilobed nucleus; clear-staining cytoplasm	3,000–7,000	6 hours to a few days	Phagocytizes bacteria
Eosinophil	Approximately the same size as a neutrophil; large pink-stained granules; bilobed nucleus	100–400	8–12 days	Phagocytizes antigen-antibody complex; attacks parasites
Basophil	Slightly smaller than a neutrophil; contains large purple cytoplasmic granules	20–50	A few hours to a few days	Releases histamine during inflammation
Monocyte	Larger than a neutrophil; cytoplasm grayish blue; no cytoplasmic granules; U- or kidney-shaped nucleus	100–700	Lasts many months	Phagocytizes bacteria, dead cells, and cellular debris
Lymphocyte	Slightly smaller than a neutrophil; large, relatively round nucleus that fills the cell	1,500–3,000	Can persist many years	Involved in immune protection, attacking cells directly or producing antibodies

Table 8 Other Immune System Cells

Type of Cell	Description
Macrophage	White blood cells within tissues, produced by differentiation of monocytes. Functions include phagocytosis and stimulating lymphocytes and other immune cells to respond to pathogens; one of the first lines of defense in the inflammatory process.
Mast cells	Cells found in the connective tissues, beneath the skin, in the gastrointestinal mucosa and in the mucosal membranes of the respiratory system. Functions relate to allergic reactions, immunity, and wound healing.
Plasma cells	White blood cells that develop from B cells and produce large volumes of specific antibodies.
B cells (B lymphocytes)	Cells that mature in the bone marrow where they differentiate into memory cells or immunoglobulin-secreting (antibody) cells. Functions including eliminating bacteria, neutralizing bacterial toxins, preventing viral reinfection, and producing immediate inflammatory response.
Helper B cells	A type of regulator cell that activates B cells to produce antibodies.
Memory B cells	A type of B cell that aids quick response to subsequent exposures to an antigen because memory cells recall the antigen as foreign. These cells rapidly produce antibodies.
T cells (T lymphocytes)	Cells produced in the bone marrow and which mature in the thymus. Two major types work to destroy antigens—regulator cells and effector cells.
Killer T cells	A type of T cell that destroys cells infected with viruses by releasing lymphokines that destroy cell walls; also called cytotoxic or effector cells.

5. **Lymphocytes** and their derivatives mediate the acquired immune response. Although most lymphocytes are found in the lymphoid tissues, many are found in circulating lymph and blood as well. There are two basic types: B lymphocytes and T lymphocytes.

Mast cells resemble basophils but do not circulate in the blood. They are found in the connective tissues, beneath the skin, in the gastrointestinal mucosa, and in the mucosal membranes of the respiratory system. Mast cells have a role in allergic reactions, immunity, and wound healing.

Table 8 summarizes other types of immune system cells that will be discussed in later sections.

Characteristics of the Immune Response
The native and acquired immune responses protect the body from infectious agents such as viruses and bacteria and from foreign substances that have gained access to the body through the skin or the lining of internal organs.

Natural immunity, also called native immunity, is a nonspecific cellular and humoral (antibody) response that operates as the first line of defense against pathogens. Most natural immunity is associated with the initial inflammatory response.

Acquired immunity (also called adaptive immunity) is a highly specific, inducible, discriminatory method by which armies of cells respond to an immune stimulant, such that the immune system will never fail to recognize the same stimulant when it is subsequently encountered, even years later. It arises when the body is exposed to a foreign substance or disease and produces antibodies to the invader. Passively acquired immunity is the receipt of preformed antibodies to fight or prevent infection. Passively acquired immunity lasts for a much shorter period than actively acquired immunity. Examples of passively acquired immunity include the transplacental passage of antibodies and the passage of antibodies in colostrum (the mother's initial milk to her infant), which protects the newborn infant until his or her own immune system matures sufficiently to take over. The injection of immunoglobulin (a concentrated form of antibodies obtained from donors) is also a form of passively acquired immunity.

The primary (initial) immune response takes place during the first exposure to an antigen (a foreign substance; a neoantigen is an antigen associated with cancerous cells). Clinical symptoms might or might not be apparent. Sometimes, the body's initial response is to produce an antibody that triggers symptoms on subsequent exposures. The secondary (amnestic) immune response occurs with reexposure to a foreign substance. The body has already developed a memory, of sorts, for that substance, so a reaction occurs on reexposure to it.

The beginning (induction) phase of the immune response occurs when a part of the immune system recognizes an antigen. Antigens may be immunogenic (elicit an immune response) or nonimmunogenic (do not elicit an immune response).

An antibody binds a specific antigen so that the complex can attach itself to specialized immune cells that ingest the complex to destroy it or release biologic mediators such as histamine to induce an allergic or inflammatory response. The specific features of the antigen-antibody interaction depend on the foreign substance involved Figure 31 .

An immunogen is an antigen capable of generating an immune response. Thus, an immunogen is an antigen, but an antigen is not necessarily an immunogen. Antigens and immunogens can be categorized by size. Proteins, polysaccharides, and nucleic acids are larger, whereas amino acids, monosaccharides, and fatty acids are smaller. A hapten is a substance that normally does not stimulate an immune response but that can be combined with an antigen and, at a later time, initiate a specific antibody response on its own.

Humoral Immune Response

In humoral immunity, B-cell lymphocytes produce antibodies called immunoglobulins, which recognize a specific antigen and then react

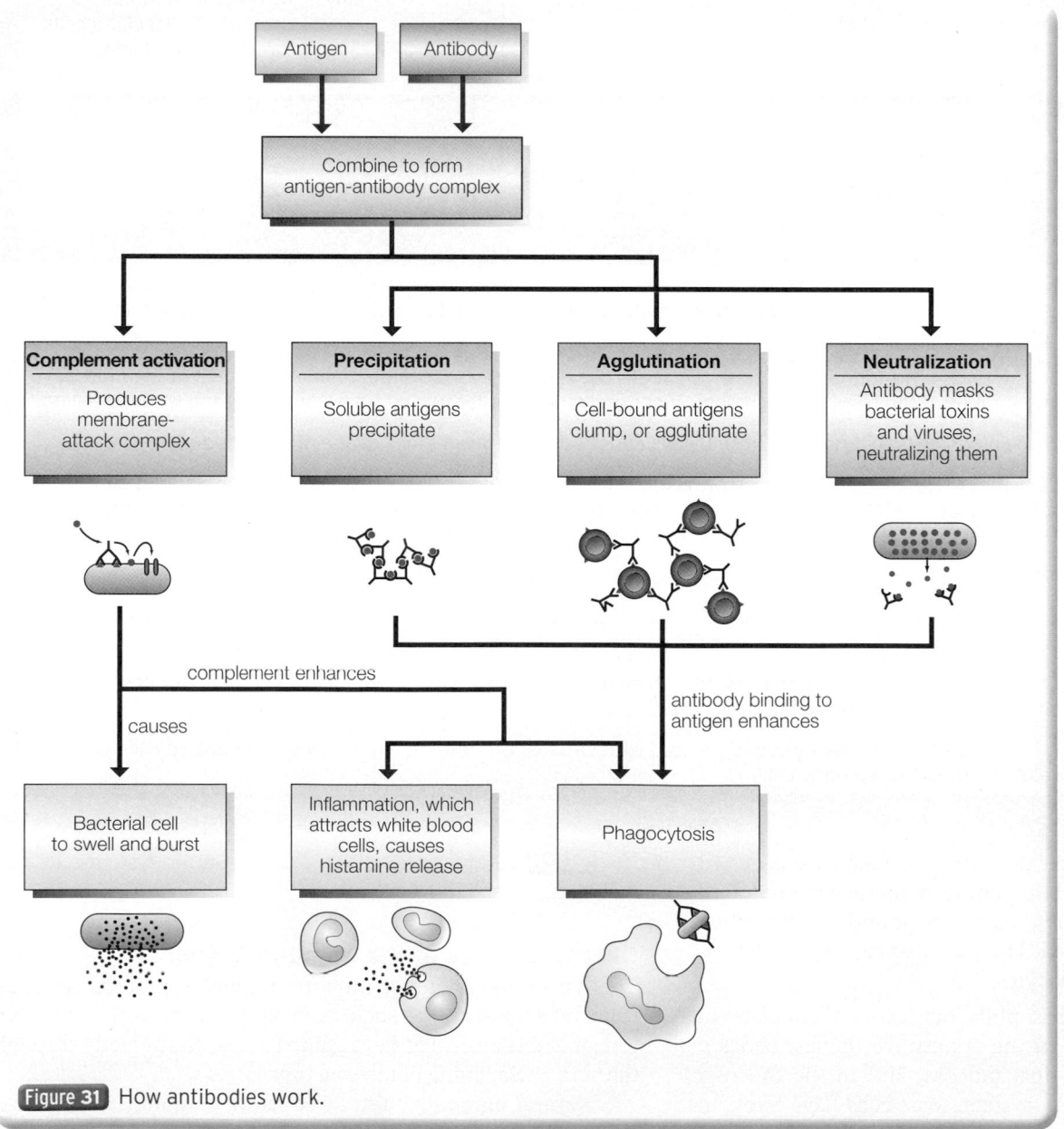

Figure 31 How antibodies work.

with it, as shown in **Figure 32**. This differs from cell-mediated immunity, discussed later, in which macrophages and T cells attack and destroy pathogens or foreign substances.

B Lymphocytes Like all blood cells, B cells are born in the bone marrow, where they are descended from stem cells. The clonal selection theory holds that each B cell makes antibodies that

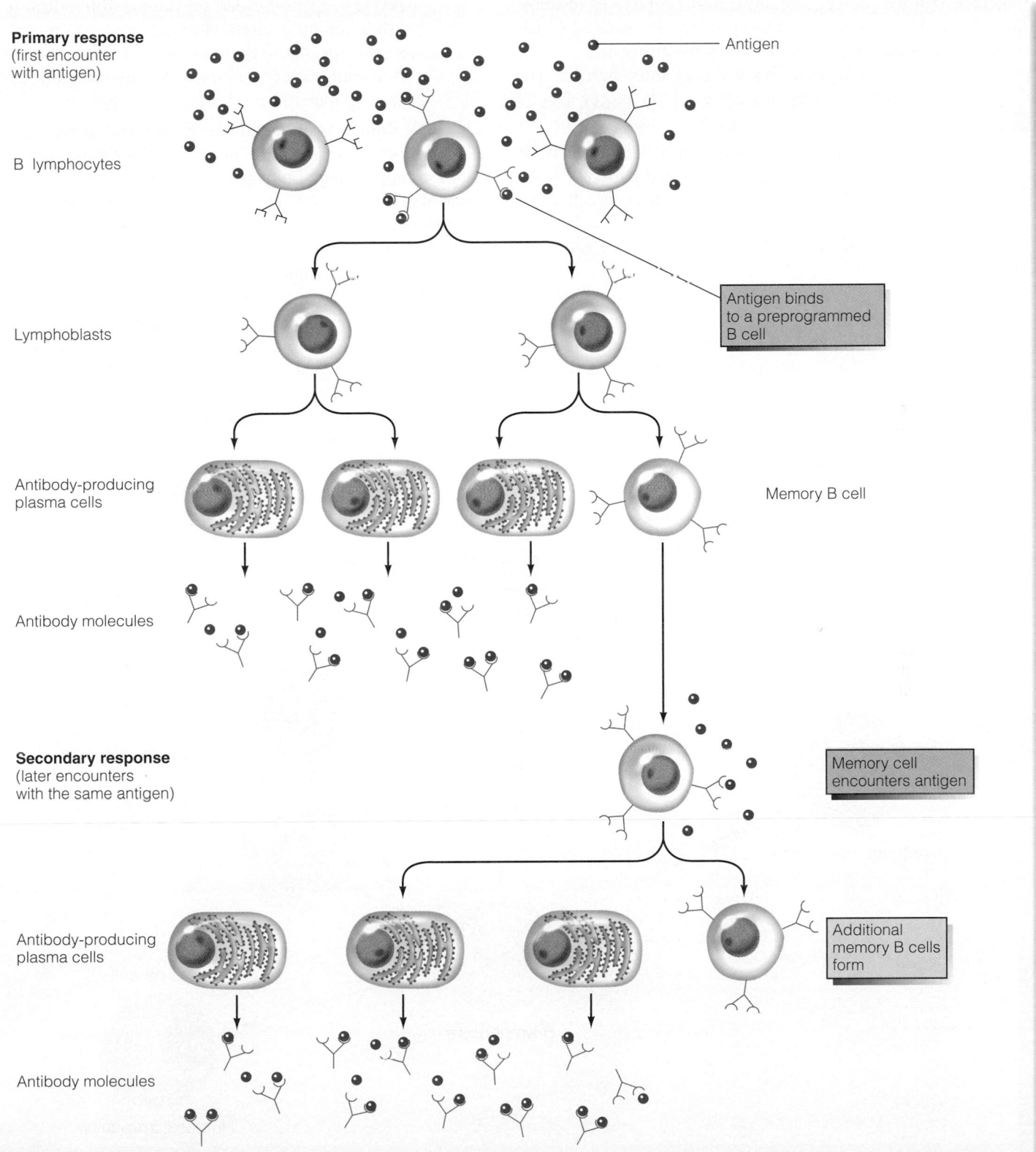

Figure 32 B-cell activation. Immunocompetent B cells are stimulated by the presence of an antigen, producing an intermediate cell, the lymphoblast. The lymphoblasts divide, producing plasma cells and some memory B cells. Memory B cells respond to subsequent antigen encroachment, yielding a rapid secondary response.

have only one type of antigen-binding region and, therefore, are specific for a particular antigen, known as the cognate antigen. Antibodies are found on the surface of B cells, where they are able to recognize the presence of their cognate antigens. When a B cell recognizes the cognate antigen, it proliferates to make more identical B cells in an exponential manner, each of which can make antibodies that recognize the same antigen.

For B cells to produce antibodies, they must first be activated. The most common way this occurs is via **helper T cells** (**Figure 33**):

1. A macrophage engulfs the antigen via phagocytosis. It digests the antigen, pushing the discarded particles to the cell surface. These remnants interact with the B cell and a helper T cell.
2. The antigen binds to the B cell and the helper T cell, activating both.
3. The activated helper T cell secretes a lymphokine, a substance that stimulates the B cells to produce a clone. A clone is a group of identical cells formed from the same

parent cell. The clone comprises two types of identical cells that have different functions: plasma cells, which make the antibodies, and memory cells, which "remember" the initial encounter with the antigen. B cells produce many such clones, called polyclonal antibodies. It is also possible for monoclonal antibodies to be created. These are very specific antibodies used in laboratory research and in some cancer therapies, but are not particularly relevant to paramedic field practice.

The human body distinguishes between foreign substances and its own cells and tissues by means of the major histocompatibility complex, a group of genes located on a single chromosome that permits a person who is capable of generating an immune response to distinguish *self* from *nonself* (namely, what is foreign). The human leukocyte antigen gene complex is the human major histocompatibility complex and is present in all nucleated human cells. It encodes for numerous antigens that are unique to a person. When the immune system encounters these particular antigens, it recognizes them as self, and no immune response occurs.

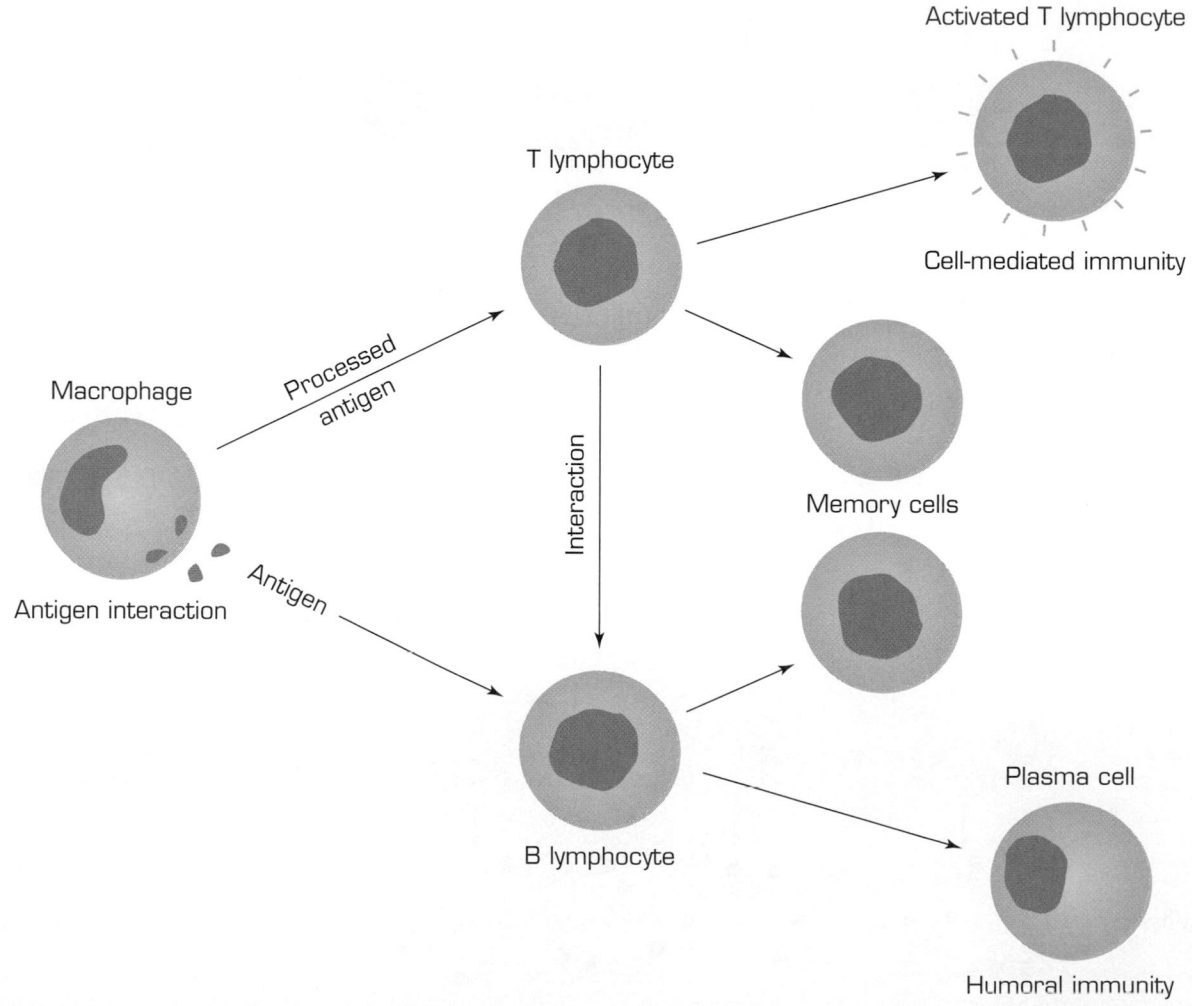

Figure 33 Interaction of cell-mediated and humoral immunity. A macrophage presents processed antigen fragments to the T lymphocyte. The B lymphocyte processes the intact antigen and displays fragments of the same antigen on its cell membrane. The T lymphocyte, which has responded to the same antigen, stimulates the B lymphocyte to proliferate, mature into plasma cells, and make antibodies.

Immunoglobulins The antibodies secreted by B cells are called <u>immunoglobulins</u> (this text uses the terms *immunoglobulins* and *antibodies* interchangeably, unless otherwise stated). These Y-shaped proteins consist of a crystallizable fragment (Fc) portion and two antigen-binding fragment (Fab) regions that bind only a specific antigen. The basic antibody molecule has four chains linked into a Y shape. Each side of the Y is identical, with one light chain attached to one heavy chain [Figure 34]. The two arms, or Fab regions, contain antigen-binding sites. The stem, or Fc region, determines to which of the five immunoglobulin classes an antibody belongs [Figure 35].

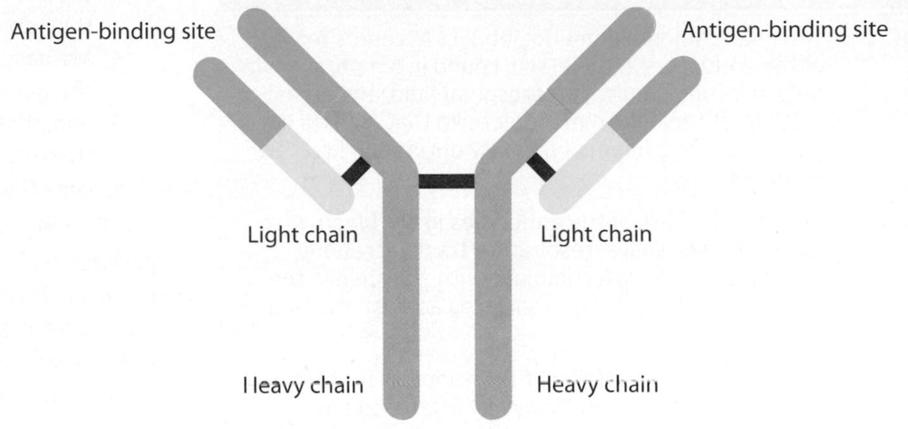

There are three main categories of antigens on antibodies: isotypic, allotypic, and idiotypic. An isotypic antigenic marker occurs in all members of a subclass of an immunoglobulin class. An allotypic antigenic marker is found on some members of a subclass of an immunoglobin class, but not on all of them. An idiotypic antigenic determinant is a unique structure that is created on the light and heavy chains of an immunoglobulin molecule. Some of these structures are involved in immune regulation.

Most antibodies are found in the plasma, where they make up about 20% of the plasma proteins in a healthy person. Antibodies make antigens more visible to the immune system in three ways:

- Antibodies act as opsonins. In <u>opsonization</u>, an antibody coats an antigen to facilitate its recognition by immune cells. Antibodies themselves are not toxic, but they label antigens so that other immune cells will attack them.
- Antibodies cause antigens to clump (precipitate, also known as agglutinate) for easier phagocytosis.
- Antibodies bind to and inactivate some toxins produced by bacteria. Macrophages can then ingest and destroy the inactivated toxins.

Antibodies are divided into five general classes of immunoglobulins [Table 9]. Fetal immunity is a passively acquired immunity that is derived primarily from maternal IgG and IgM antibodies. As a fertilized ovum grows, its peripheral cells differentiate into a group of cells called the trophoblast. The trophoblast forms the placenta and other structures that will support and nourish the embryo. The pregnant woman's immunity passes through the trophoblast. In fact, the

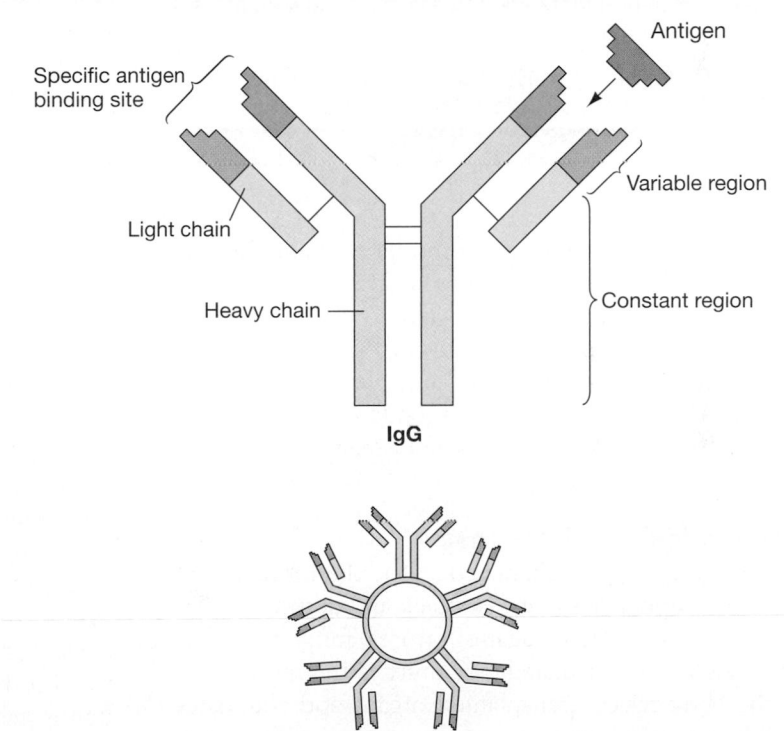

[Figure 34] Structure of an immunoglobulin molecule.

[Figure 35] General structure of an antibody. Note that IgG is a monomer; it is one molecule. IgM is a pentamer; it is a cluster of five antibodies and is effective in combining with foreign antigens. Also note that the antigen fits exactly into the antigen–binding site (if it did not, it would not be able to bind). Antigen binding sites therefore have different structures depending on the antigen to which they are designed to bind.

umbilical cord's blood cells contain immunologic properties and have been used in medical treatment, which is a reason why some people decide to store their child's umbilical cord blood. The fact that the umbilical cord contains immunologic properties relates to paramedicine in that, when cutting the umbilical

Table 9   General Classes of Immunoglobulins

IgG	The most common immunoglobulin. Accounts for 75% of the antibodies in the blood. Found in lymph, synovial fluid, peritoneal fluid, cerebrospinal fluid, and breast milk. IgG is the only immunoglobulin that crosses the placenta, giving infants immunity during the first few months of life.
IgA	Accounts for 15% of the antibodies in the blood. Also found in tears, saliva, respiratory tract secretions, and the stomach. IgA combines with a protein in the mucosa and defends body surfaces against invading microorganisms.
IgM	Accounts for 5% to 10% of the antibodies in the blood and is the dominant antibody in ABO (blood type) incompatibilities. IgM is the initial antibody formed in most infections.
IgE	Accounts for less than 1% of the antibodies in the blood and is associated with allergic reactions. When mast cell receptors combine with IgE and antigen, the mast cells degranulate and release chemical mediators such as histamine.
IgD	Accounts for less than 1% of the antibodies in the blood. The physiologic role of IgD is unclear.

cord, the position of the newborn is important; ensure that the newborn is not held too high or too low relative to the mother; otherwise the newborn could lose or gain an excess of blood and, therefore, immunity. Following delivery, the antibodies that were passed to the fetus persist until the neonate's own B cells take over. A substantial number of antibodies are also transferred through breast milk, which is one of many reasons that many experts favor breastfeeding.

Cell-Mediated Immune Response

Cell-mediated immunity is characterized by the formation of a population of lymphocytes that can attack and destroy foreign material. It is the main defense against viruses, fungi, parasites, and some bacteria. Cell-mediated immunity is the mechanism by which the body rejects transplanted organs and eliminates the abnormal cells that sometimes arise spontaneously in cell division.

In cell-mediated immunity, T-cell lymphocytes recognize antigens and contribute to the immune response in two major ways: (1) by secreting cytokines that attract other cells or (2) by becoming cytotoxic and killing infected or abnormal cells. There are five subgroups of T cells:

1. **Killer T cells.** Killer T cells (also called cytotoxic T cells) destroy the antigen. Killer T cells help rid the body of cells that have been infected by viruses and cells that have been transformed into cancer cells. They are also responsible for the rejection of tissue and organ grafts.
2. **Helper T cells.** Helper T cells activate many immune cells, including B cells and other T cells (also called T4 or CD4+ cells).

3. **Suppressor T cells.** Suppressor T cells (also called T8 or CD8+ cells) suppress the activity of other lymphocytes so they do not destroy normal tissue.
4. **Memory T cells.** Memory T cells remember the reaction for the next time it is needed.
5. **Lymphokine-producing cells.** Secreted by lymphocytes, these cells work to damage cells; for example, they destroy cells that have been infected with a virus.

During the cell-mediated response, macrophages ingest pathogens. When a macrophage digests a pathogen, it releases small particles of antigen. This antigen pushes its way to the macrophage surface, where it is recognized by specific T cells. Other T cells, such as helper T cells and killer T cells, bind to the antigen and macrophage, destroying the invader.

Cellular Interactions in the Immune Response

The body responds to different kinds of immune challenges in remarkably similar ways. Although the details depend on the particular challenge, the basic pattern is the same—the innate response starts first and is then reinforced by the more specific acquired response. These two pathways are interconnected.

Consider what happens when bacteria enter the body. If the bacteria are not encapsulated, macrophages begin to ingest them immediately. If the bacteria are encapsulated, antibodies (opsonins) must coat the capsule before they can be ingested by phagocytes.

Components of the cell wall then activate the complement system. Some components of the activated complement system, termed **chemotaxins**, attract leukocytes from the circulation to help fight the infection. The complement cascade ends with the formation of a set of proteins called the **membrane attack complex**. These molecules insert themselves into the bacterial membrane, weakening those areas in the membrane. Ions and water enter the cell through the weakened areas, leading to lysis of the bacterium (a chemical process that does not involve immune cells).

If antibodies to the bacteria are already present in the body, they will assist the innate response by acting as opsonins and neutralizing bacterial toxins. Although it often takes several days, memory B cells attracted to the infection site will be activated if they encounter an antigen they recognize. If the infection is new to the body—that is, preexisting antibodies are not present—B cells will be activated. Combined with helper T cells and cytokine release, antibodies are produced and memory B and T cells are formed.

Special Populations

> T-cell and B-cell function is deficient in older people. Depressed lymphocyte function is accompanied by a decrease in macrophage activity. Therefore, older people are more prone to experience infections and recover slowly. In addition, older adults have an increased level of **autoantibodies** (antibodies directed against the self), which partly explains why older people are prone to autoimmune disease.

Inflammatory Response

The inflammatory response is a response of the tissues of the body to irritation or injury. It is characterized by pain, swelling, redness, and heat. White blood cells of various types are a major component of this response.

The inflammatory reaction and the immune response are independent processes, although they often occur simultaneously. Inflammation can be present without activation of the immune response, and vice versa. Inflammation is a dynamic process that, once initiated, triggers a complex cascade involving local and systemic events. The two most common causes of inflammation are infection (such as bacterial or viral) and injury.

Acute Inflammation

The acute inflammatory response involves vascular and cellular components. After transient arteriolar constriction, the arterioles dilate, allowing an influx of blood under increased pressure. This <u>active hyperemia</u> (leading to increased intravascular pressure) causes the blood vessel to expand; as in a balloon that is being inflated, the vessel walls become thinner. The higher pressure combined with increased vessel wall permeability causes fluid to leak into the interstitial spaces (edema). When enough fluid has escaped into the surrounding area and the intravascular pressure has been released, the vessel wall contracts and the outflow slows, leading to stasis of blood in the capillaries.

A variety of blood cells participate in tissue inflammatory reactions: white blood cells (leukocytes), platelets, mast cells, and plasma cells (B lymphocytes that create antibodies). Specific cell types include neutrophils, monocytes, lymphocytes, eosinophils, basophils, and activated platelets. Chemical mediators, primarily produced by the mast cells, account for the vascular and cellular events that occur during the acute inflammatory response. Cell-derived mediators include histamine, arachidonic acid derivatives, and cytokines such as interleukins and tumor necrosis factor.

Words of Wisdom

Corticosteroids can decrease the initial inflammatory response, which is a necessary part of wound healing. As immunosuppressants, however, they also increase the risk of wound infection. This consideration is important in patients with diabetes because of their propensity to develop such infections.

Mast Cells Mast cells have a major role in inflammation. During inflammation, they degranulate and release a variety of substances. The primary stimuli for the degranulation of mast cells during the inflammatory response are physical injury (trauma), chemical agents (for example, bacterial toxins), and immunologic substances (for example, interaction of an antigen and an IgE antibody).

Following their degranulation, mast cells release <u>vasoactive amines</u>. The most important of these substances, <u>histamine</u> and <u>serotonin</u>, increase vascular permeability, cause vasodilation, and can cause bronchoconstriction, nausea, and vomiting. Because histamine is a preformed vasodepressor amine stored in mast cells, it can be released quickly, so its actions are seen early in the inflammatory response. Mast cells also synthesize chemotactic factors that attract neutrophils (neutrophil chemotactic factor) and eosinophils (eosinophilic chemotactic factor).

Mast cells also synthesize leukotrienes. <u>Leukotrienes</u>—also known as <u>slow-reacting substances of anaphylaxis</u>—are a family of biologically active compounds derived from arachidonic acid. The clinically important leukotrienes participate

---

YOU *are the Medic* | PART 4 |

Your partner reports that all of the medication bottles are out of date and empty. You ask the patient about this and he states that he does not have the means necessary to buy the medications. When you look at the list of medications, you find one for a diuretic. Your cardiac monitor indicates a sinus tachycardia matching the pulse rate. No ectopy is noted.

Recording Time: 7 Minutes	
Respirations	24 breaths/min; shallow
Pulse	114 beats/min
Skin	Cool, pale, and moist
Blood pressure	138/88 mm Hg
Oxygen saturation (Spo₂)	92% with high-flow oxygen administration
Pupils	Equal and reactive to light

7. Why would a diuretic be prescribed for a patient with congestive heart failure?

8. Why would this patient have a normal or slightly high blood pressure?

in host defense reactions and pathophysiologic conditions that paramedics commonly see in the field, such as immediate hypersensitivity and inflammation. Leukotrienes have potent actions on many parts of the body, including the cardiovascular, pulmonary, immune, and central nervous systems and the gastrointestinal tract.

Leukotrienes are primarily endogenous mediators of inflammation. They contribute to the signs and symptoms seen in acute inflammatory responses, including responses resulting from the interaction of allergens with IgE antibodies on mast cells. Certain leukotrienes are bronchoconstrictors, stimulate airway mucus secretion, and are very effective at increasing the permeability of postcapillary venules (including those in the bronchial circulation), thereby causing plasma protein exudation (oozing out of the tissue) and edema. Certain leukotrienes may also promote eosinophil migration into the airways of animals and persons with asthma, and they may also increase bronchial hyperresponsiveness through an action on sensory nerves.

Finally, mast cells synthesize <u>prostaglandins</u>. These substances, which are derived from arachidonic acid, comprise a group of about 20 lipids that are composed of modified fatty acids attached to a five-member ring. Prostaglandins are found in many vertebrate tissues, where they act as messengers in reproduction, the inflammatory response to infection, and pain perception. Aspirin and nonsteroidal anti-inflammatory drugs inhibit prostaglandin synthesis, leading to reduced inflammation and pain.

Plasma Protein Systems The plasma-derived mediators that modulate the inflammatory process are called plasma protein systems. They include the complement system, the coagulation (clotting) system, and the kinin system. The interaction of these systems is vital to a normal inflammatory response. Each system consists of a cascade of biochemical reactions such that as one compound is produced, it catalyzes the formation of the next compound—much like knocking over a line of dominoes.

- **Complement system.** The <u>complement system</u> is a group of plasma proteins that attract white blood cells to sites of inflammation, activate white blood cells, and directly destroy cells. The central compound in this complement cascade is called C3. C3 is produced by one of the two complement pathways: the classic pathway or the alternative pathway. The classic pathway starts when an antigen-antibody complex binds to a complement component (C1); activation of this pathway is dependent on the presence of antibodies. The alternative pathway can be triggered by bacterial toxins and does not need antibodies to be activated.

  Regardless of which pathway is taken, the main products are the same: C3b, anaphylatoxins, and the membrane attack complex. C3b coats bacteria, making it easier for macrophages to engulf them. Anaphylatoxins (C3a, C4a, and C5a) stimulate smooth-muscle contraction and increase vascular permeability by stimulating the release of histamine from mast cells and platelets. The membrane attack complex is a set of complement proteins (C5b, C6, C7, C8, and C9) that bind to form a hollow tube, much like a short straw, that can puncture into the plasma membrane of a cell. In this way, transmembrane channels are formed that allow ions, water, and other small molecules to pass through, resulting in loss of cellular osmolarity and death of the cell.

- **Coagulation system.** The <u>coagulation system</u> serves a vital role in the formation of blood clots in the body and facilitates repair of the vascular tree. Inflammation triggers the coagulation cascade, initiating a complex series of reactions that encourage fibrin formation. <u>Fibrin</u> is the protein that polymerizes (bonds) to form the fibrous component of a blood clot. The various coagulation factors are counterbalanced by a variety of inhibitors, so that the coagulation is restricted to one area. Simultaneously, the <u>fibrinolysis cascade</u> is activated to dissolve the fibrin and create fibrin split products (namely, fragments of the dissolving clot).

- **Kinin system.** The <u>kinin system</u> leads to the formation of the vasoactive protein bradykinin from kallikrein. Kallikrein is an enzyme that is normally found in blood plasma, urine, and body tissue in an inactive state. When it becomes activated, it can dilate blood vessels, influence blood pressure, modulate salt and water excretion by the kidneys, and influence cardiac remodeling after acute myocardial infarction. Bradykinin increases vascular permeability, dilates blood vessels, contracts smooth muscle, and causes pain when injected into the skin.

  The kinin system is spurred into action by the activation of Hageman factor (coagulation factor XII). (**Table 10** lists the various coagulation factors.) In addition to its role in the kinin system, Hageman factor participates in the clotting, fibrinolytic, and complement cascades. Its activators include bacterial lipopolysaccharides and endotoxin. Activated factor XII triggers the intrinsic clotting cascade, which occurs when blood is exposed to collagen or other substances. For example, when a blood vessel is cut, the skin cells are damaged and the blood comes in contact with collagen. The extrinsic clotting cascade is activated by substances released from injured cells when tissue damage occurs.

Cellular Components of Inflammation The goal of the cellular components of the acute inflammatory response is for inflammatory cells—namely, <u>polymorphonuclear neutrophils</u> <u>(PMNs)</u>—to arrive at the sites in the tissue where they are needed. This process involves two major stages: an intravascular phase and an extravascular phase. During the intravascular phase, leukocytes move to the sides of blood vessels and attach to the endothelial cells. During the extravascular phase, leukocytes travel to the site of inflammation and kill organisms. The cellular event sequence is as follows:

1. <u>Margination</u>. Loss of fluid from the blood vessels into the inflamed or infected tissue gives the blood that remains in the vessels increased viscosity, which slows the flow of blood and produces stasis. PMNs, which usually travel toward the center of the vessel, settle toward the sides as the blood flow slows. As stasis develops, leukocytes also move (marginate) toward the sides of the vessels, where they bump into the endothelial cells and bind to them.

Table 10 Coagulation Factors

Factor Number	Name	Description
I	Fibrinogen	Protein synthesized in liver; converted into fibrin in stage 3
II	Prothrombin	Protein synthesized in liver (requires vitamin K); converted into thrombin in stage 2
III	Tissue thromboplastin	Released from damaged tissue; required in extrinsic stage 1
IV	Calcium ions	Required throughout entire clotting sequence
V	Proaccelerin (labile factor)	Protein synthesized in liver; required to form prothrombin activator in intrinsic and extrinsic stage 1
VII	Serum prothrombin conversion accelerator (stable factor, proconvertin)	Protein synthesized in liver (requires vitamin K); functions in extrinsic stage 1
VIII	Antihemophilic factor (antihemophilic globulin)	Protein synthesized in liver; required for intrinsic stage 1
IX	Plasma thromboplastin component	Protein synthesized in liver (requires vitamin K); required for intrinsic stage 1
X	Stuart factor (Stuart-Prower factor)	Protein synthesized in liver (requires vitamin K); required to form prothrombin activator in intrinsic and extrinsic stage 1
XI	Plasma thromboplastin antecedent	Protein synthesized in liver; required for intrinsic stage 1
XII	Hageman factor	Protein required for intrinsic stage 1
XIII	Fibrin-stabilizing factor	Protein required to stabilize the fibrin strands in stage 3

Stress can lead to demargination of some white blood cells, which stimulates the bone marrow to produce more, in turn increasing the white blood cell count.

2. <u>Activation</u>. Mediators of inflammation trigger the appearance of selectins and integrins on the surfaces of endothelial cells and PMNs, respectively.
3. <u>Adhesion</u>. PMNs attach to endothelial cells, as mediated by selectins and integrins.
4. <u>Transmigration (diapedesis)</u>. The PMNs permeate the vessel wall, passing into the interstitial space.
5. <u>Chemotaxis</u>. The PMNs move toward the site of inflammation in response to chemotactic factors released by bacteria or formed from activated complement, chemokines, or arachidonic acid derivatives (such as leukotrienes) in response to cell injury. **Figure 36** illustrates the inflammatory response.

Cellular Products of Inflammation <u>Cytokines</u> are products of cells that affect the function of other cells. Monocytes release monokines, and lymphocytes release lymphokines.

<u>Interleukins</u> include IL-1 (interleukin-1) and IL-2 (interleukin-2), which attract white blood cells to the sites of injury and bacterial invasion. <u>Interferon</u> is a protein produced by cells when they are invaded by viruses. This cytokine is released into the bloodstream or intercellular fluid to induce healthy cells to manufacture an enzyme that counters the infection.

<u>Lymphokines</u> stimulate leukocytes. Macrophage-activating factor stimulates macrophages to help engulf and destroy foreign substances. Migration inhibitory factor keeps white blood cells at the site of infection or injury until they can perform their designated task.

Injury Resolution and Repair

Normal wound healing involves four steps—repair of damaged tissue, removal of inflammatory debris, restoration of tissues to a normal state, and regeneration of cells. Healing after tissue injury or loss caused by inflammation depends on the type of cells that make up the affected organ. Labile cells divide continuously, so organs derived from these cells (such as skin and intestinal mucosa) heal completely. Stable cells are replaced by regeneration of remaining cells, which are stimulated to enter mitosis. These cells are found in the liver and kidney. Permanent cells, such as nerve cells and cardiac myocytes, cannot be replaced; scar tissue is laid down instead. However, research is being done on the use of stem cells to replace damaged nerve cells.

Wounds may heal by primary or secondary intention. Healing by primary intention occurs in clean wounds with opposed margins (such as clean surgical wounds or surgically débrided wounds). First, blood fills the defect and coagulates, forming a scab, which is a meshlike structure composed of fibrin and fibronectin. If the inflammatory process was severe, tissue may be destroyed and require repair. Next, macrophages remove cellular debris and secrete growth factors. These growth factors stimulate angiogenesis and growth of fibroblasts, encouraging the formation of granulation tissue. The epithelium then regenerates, covering the surface defect. Deposition of collagen produces fibrous union. By the end of the first week, 10% of the preinjury strength is regained. Scar maturation occurs as collagen cross-linking takes place. By the end of 3 months, 80% of the normal tensile strength of the tissue has been restored.

Healing by secondary intention occurs in large, gaping or infected wounds. Wounds that heal by secondary intention

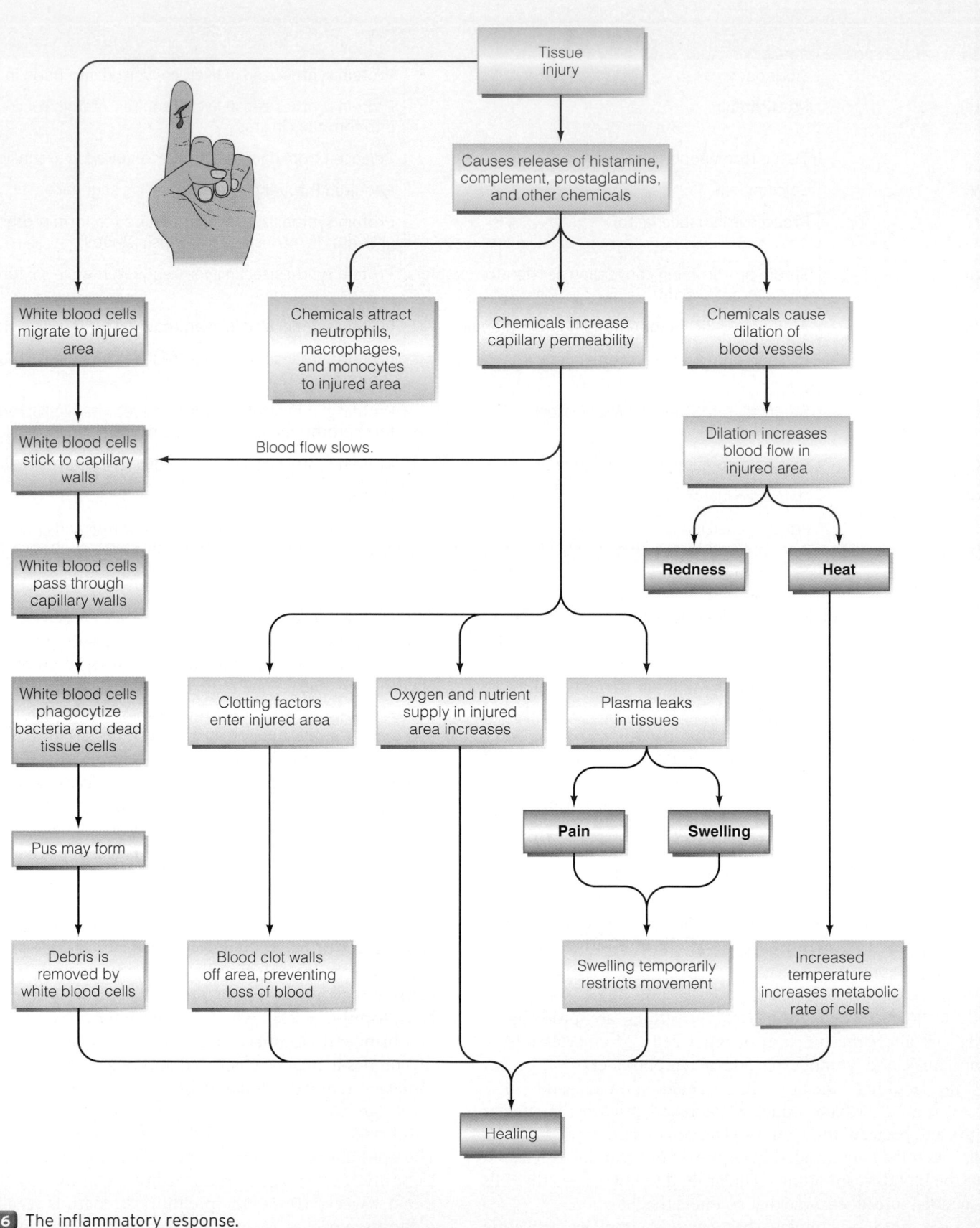

Figure 36 The inflammatory response.

have a more pronounced and prolonged inflammatory phase, causing the neutrophils to persist for days. They also have more abundant granulation tissue. Wound contraction is mediated by myofibroblasts, which help to draw the margins of the wound closer to each other as time passes.

Dysfunctional Wound Healing Factors that can lead to dysfunctional wound healing may be local or systemic. Local factors include infection (when the body's healing efforts are diverted to fight off the cause of the infection); an inadequate blood supply (as in diabetes) that produces tissue hypoxia, which slows wound healing and may promote infection; and foreign bodies (when present in a wound, they stimulate acute and chronic inflammation, both of which interfere with wound healing).

There are several systemic factors that influence the healing of wounds. Collagen is necessary for wound healing, but inadequate nutritional intake can lead to insufficient levels of collagen, which in turn can lead to inadequate scar formation and suppression of the immune system. Anything that interferes with epithelialization (the process during which epithelial cells begin to form a scab that protects the wound from the outside world) will prevent proper wound healing. Wound contraction is the process during which the size of the wound becomes smaller, as part of healing. Anything that interferes with wound contraction can also prevent healing.

Additional systemic factors that disrupt wound healing include hematologic abnormalities (proper wound healing requires the presence of adequate numbers of white blood cells). Patients who have impaired bone marrow stores of white blood cells are susceptible to infection and their wounds often heal more slowly. Diabetes and AIDS affect the cells of the immune system, which has a direct role in wound healing, and increase the likelihood of wound infection. Corticosteroids suppress the initial inflammatory response required for the proper formation of scar tissue and increase the risk of wound infection by slowing the immune system response.

Finally, if a wound separates, for example from stress, this will slow down the healing process as healing needs to start over, at least to some extent.

Special Populations

Neonates and older adults often have relative impairment of their immune systems, potentially slowing their inflammatory response. As a consequence, signs of inflammation may be more subtle in these populations. In addition, wound healing often takes longer, especially in older patients. The immune system is not fully developed until a child is between 2 and 3 years old. Therefore, investigation of a fever in younger children must be aggressive and thorough. Many experts recommend hospital admission for a temperature greater than 100.4°F in a child younger than 3 months.

Chronic Inflammatory Responses

Chronic inflammatory responses are usually caused by an unsuccessful acute inflammatory response to a foreign body, a persistent infection, or the presence of an antigen. They are associated with an infiltrate (pus) containing monocytes and lymphocytes and usually involve tissue destruction and repair (or scar formation). The vascular events are similar to those that take place in acute inflammation but also include the growth of new blood vessels (a process known as **angiogenesis**).

Variances in Immunity and Inflammation

Hypersensitivity

Hypersensitivity is any response of the body to any substance to which a patient has increased sensitivity. It is a generic term for a variety of reactions. **Allergy** is a hypersensitivity reaction to the presence of an agent (allergen). **Autoimmunity** is the production of antibodies or T cells that work against the tissues of one's own body, producing hypersensitivity reactions or autoimmune disease (as in systemic lupus erythematosus [SLE]). **Isoimmunity** is the formation of T cells or antibodies directed against the antigens on another person's cells (typically after the transplantation of an organ or tissues). A blood transfusion reaction is an example of an isoimmune reaction to another person's red blood cells. The destruction of cells by antibodies or T cells may be an autoimmune or an isoimmune reaction.

Transient neonatal diseases are those that are present at birth, but which eventually resolve. There are many examples; some include transient neonatal hyperglycemia, transient neonatal myasthenia gravis, and transient neonatal neutropenia. Transient neonatal diseases occur due to pathogenic immunoglobulins passing from the pregnant woman to the fetus during pregnancy. In some cases the disease can become permanent, for example if pathogenic immunoglobulins develop in the infant.

Types of Hypersensitivity Reactions

A hypersensitivity reaction may be immediate, occurring within seconds to minutes, or delayed, occurring hours to days after exposure to an antigen. The speed of symptom evolution depends on the antigen and the type of response the body mounts against it. Hypersensitivity reactions are typically classified based on how the immune system caused the injury. **Table 11** describes the four types of injuries.

Type I: Immediate Hypersensitivity Reactions A type I hypersensitivity reaction is an acute reaction that occurs in response to a stimulus (such as a bee sting, penicillin, or shellfish). The mechanism involves interaction between the stimulus (antigen) and a preformed antibody of the IgE type. At first exposure to a specific antigen, specific IgE antibodies bind to mast cells via the nonspecific region (Fc) portion. On secondary exposure to the same antigen, these bound antibodies are cross-linked by the

Table 11   Mechanisms of Immunologic Injury

Type	Mechanism	Examples
I: Immediate hypersensitivity	IgE antibodies fix to mast cells and basophils. Later contact with a sensitizing antigen triggers mediator release and clinical manifestations.	Localized response: hay fever, food allergy Systemic response: bee sting, penicillin anaphylaxis
II: Cytotoxic hypersensitivity reactions	Antibody binds to cell or tissue antigen, and complement is activated, which damages cell, causes inflammation, and promotes destruction of antibody-coated cell by phagocytosis.	Autoimmune hemolytic anemia Blood transfusion reactions Rh hemolytic disease Some types of glomerulonephritis
III: Immune complex disease	Circulating antigen-antibody complexes form, which activate complement and cause inflammatory reaction	Some types of glomerulonephritis Lupus erythematosus Rheumatoid arthritis
IV: Delayed (cell-mediated) hypersensitivity	Sensitized (delayed hypersensitivity) T cells release lymphokines that attract macrophages and other inflammatory cells.	Tuberculosis Fungus and parasitic infections Contact dermatitis

antigen, resulting in degranulation of the mast cell and release of histamine and other mediators **Figure 37**. The released histamine feeds back on mast cells and eosinophils, leading to the release of additional histamine and other mediators. The severity of the symptoms that develop in a particular patient depends on the extent of mediator release.

The degree of severity of hypersensitivity reactions varies from severe, life-threatening reactions, such as anaphylaxis, to milder reactions, such as allergic rhinitis (edema and irritation of the nasal mucosa), bronchial asthma (bronchial constriction, mucus production, and airway inflammation), wheal and flare (such as an insect bite leading to vasodilation and swelling), and mild food allergy (leading to diarrhea, gastrointestinal distress, and vomiting). A propensity to type I reactions may be diagnosed through skin tests (such as the patch test and scratch test) and other laboratory procedures (measurement of specific IgE antibody levels). Treatment is avoidance of the antigen, but desensitizing injections may be helpful in severe cases.

It is impossible to predict the severity of any given reaction. If a person has had a severe reaction in the past, he or she is at an increased risk for another one with subsequent antigen exposures. You should always assume that an IgE-mediated reaction could rapidly become a life-threatening event. These reactions need to be treated quickly in the field, and most prehospital providers are trained to administer epinephrine by using an EpiPen auto-injector or by giving a subcutaneous injection.

Type II: Cytotoxic Hypersensitivity

Type II hypersensitivity reactions are cytotoxic (cell destructive) and classically involve the combination of IgG or IgM antibodies with antigens on the cell membrane. Cells are lysed (destroyed) by complement fixation or by other antibodies. This process also destroys many of the body's healthy cells. Histamine release from mast cells is not involved, and IgG-mediated allergic responses occur within a few hours of antigen exposure. Examples of IgG-mediated responses include transfusion reactions and newborn hemolytic disease.

Type III: Tissue Injury Caused by Immune Complexes

Type III hypersensitivity responses involve primarily IgG antibodies that form immune complexes with antigen to recruit phagocytic cells, such as neutrophils, to a site where they can release inflammatory cytokines. Because histamine release from mast cells is not involved, IgG-mediated allergic responses occur within a few hours of antigen exposure. Reactions may be systemic or localized.

The systemic form is called **serum sickness** and results from a large, single exposure to an antigen, such as horse antibody serum. Antigen–antibody complexes formed in the bloodstream are then deposited in sites around the body, most notably in the kidney, with resultant inflammatory reactions (such as serum sickness from penicillin). Signs and symptoms of serum sickness may include fever, malaise, rashes, joint aches, lymphadenopathy, and splenomegaly.

The localized form of a type III response is called an **Arthus reaction**. Arthus reactions consist of a circumscribed area of vascular inflammation (**vasculitis**). An example of an Arthus reaction is farmer's lung (a hypersensitivity pneumonitis), which is a local hypersensitivity reaction in the lung to molds that grow on hay.

Type IV: Delayed (Cell-Mediated) Hypersensitivity

Type IV allergic responses, also known as cell-mediated hypersensitivity, are primarily mediated by soluble molecules that are released by specifically activated T cells. These reactions are classified into two subtypes: delayed hypersensitivity and cell-mediated cytotoxicity.

Delayed hypersensitivity involves lymphocytes and macrophages. T cells respond to an antigen and activate CD4 (a helper T cell) lymphocytes. These lymphocytes release mediators that are designed to destroy the foreign substance. Examples include contact hypersensitivity to poison ivy and the local induration due to mononuclear cell infiltrates from a tuberculin skin test.

Cell-mediated cytotoxicity involves only sensitized T cells (CD8 lymphocytes or **T killer cells**). These cells kill the

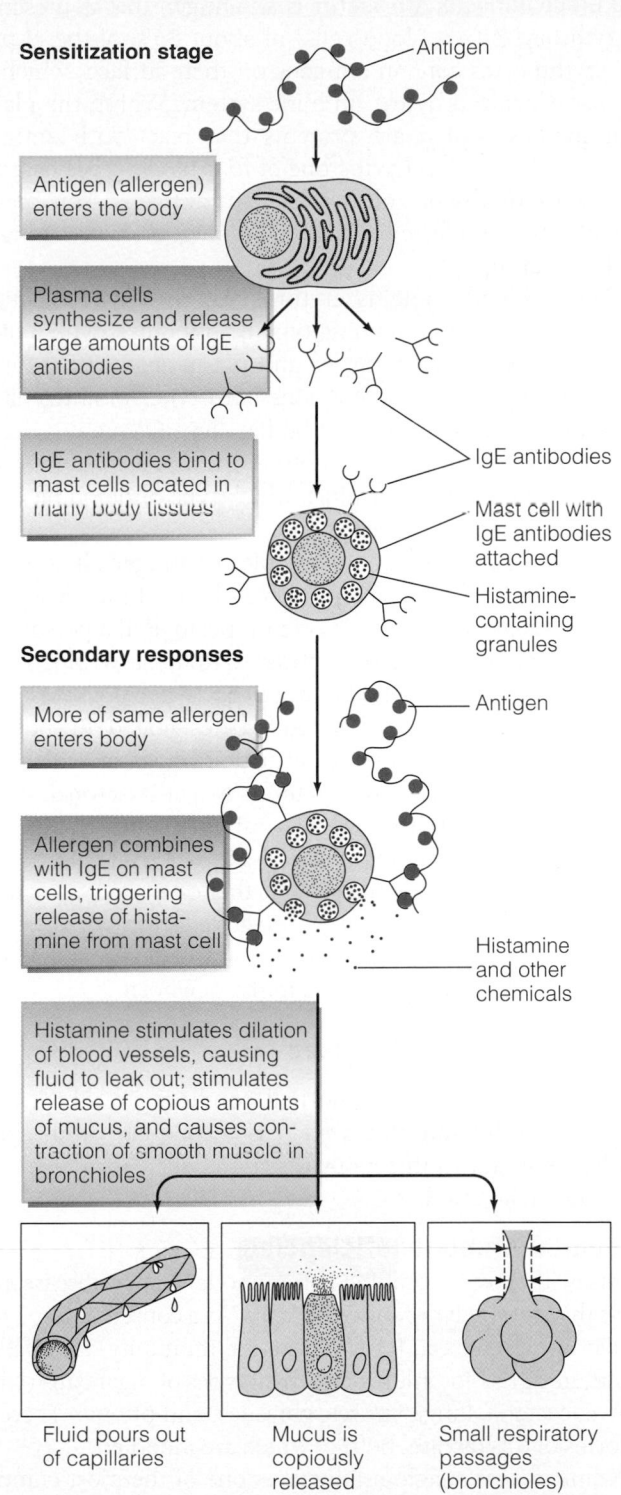

Sensitization stage

Antigen

Antigen (allergen) enters the body

Plasma cells synthesize and release large amounts of IgE antibodies

IgE antibodies bind to mast cells located in many body tissues

IgE antibodies

Mast cell with IgE antibodies attached

Histamine-containing granules

Secondary responses

More of same allergen enters body

Antigen

Allergen combines with IgE on mast cells, triggering release of histamine from mast cell

Histamine and other chemicals

Histamine stimulates dilation of blood vessels, causing fluid to leak out; stimulates release of copious amounts of mucus, and causes contraction of smooth muscle in bronchioles

Fluid pours out of capillaries

Mucus is copiously released

Small respiratory passages (bronchioles) constrict

Figure 37 Type I allergic reaction. The antigen stimulates the production of massive amounts of IgE, a type of antibody produced by plasma cells; the IgE, in turn, attaches to mast cells. This is a sensitization stage. When the antigen enters again, it binds to the IgE antibodies on the mast cells, triggering a massive release of histamine and other chemicals. Histamine causes blood vessels to dilate and become leaky, and it promotes increased production of mucus in the respiratory tract. Mast cell degranulation may also cause bronchospasm in some people.

antigen-bearing target cells rather than activating the CD4 lymphocyte to do so. Examples include the body's response to viral infections, tumor immune surveillance, and the mechanism by which transplant rejection occurs.

Targets of Hypersensitivity Reactions

The immune system targets different molecules, depending on the type of hypersensitivity reaction. In allergic reactions, the target is an antigen or allergen. Allergens are substances that cause a hypersensitivity reaction, such as those listed in **Table 12**.

Autoimmune Reactions In autoimmune reactions, the target is a person's own tissues. For reasons that are unclear, normal tolerance of "self" tissues breaks down and the immune system treats the body's own tissues as foreign.

Graves disease is an autoimmune disease caused by thyroid-stimulating or thyroid-growth immunoglobulins. These antibodies activate receptors for thyroid-stimulating hormone, causing increased activity by the thyroid gland. In addition to hyperthyroidism, Graves disease is associated with characteristic eye changes—lid retraction, stare, and exophthalmos (protrusion of the eyes)—and skin changes (pretibial myxedema—localized edematous skin in the pretibial area).

Type 1 diabetes mellitus is also considered an autoimmune disease. Although the exact insult is unknown (but is suspected to be a viral infection), some agent stimulates the body to produce autoantibodies against beta cells in the pancreas that produce insulin. The results are a deficiency of insulin and, therefore, diabetes.

Rheumatoid arthritis is a chronic systemic disease that affects the entire body. One of the most common forms of arthritis, it is characterized by inflammation of the synovium (the connective tissue membrane lining the joint) with resulting pain, stiffness, warmth, redness, and swelling. Inflammatory cells release enzymes that cause damage to bone and cartilage. The involved joint can lose its shape and alignment, resulting in pain and loss of movement. Rheumatoid arthritis is associated with the formation of rheumatoid factor—that is, IgM antibodies to tissue IgG. In the joints, the synovial membrane is thickened due to infiltration of inflammatory cells (lymphocytes).

Myasthenia gravis is an acquired autoimmune disease that is characterized by autoimmune attack on the nerve-muscle

Table 12 Allergens That Can Cause Hypersensitivity Reactions

Type	Examples
Inhalants	Pollen, dust, smoke, fungi, plastic, odors
Food	Eggs, milk, wheat, chocolate, strawberries
Drugs	Aspirin, antibiotics, serums, codeine
Infectious agents	Bacteria, viruses, fungi, animal parasites
Contactants	Animals, plants, metals, chemicals
Physical agents	Light, pressure, radiation, heat and cold

junction. The circulating autoantibodies cause abnormal muscle fatigability and typically involve the smallest motor units first, such as the extraocular muscles. This produces ptosis (droopy eyelid) and diplopia (double vision). Other muscles may be involved, causing problems with swallowing (dysphagia). Characteristically, repeated contraction of the affected muscles makes the symptoms worse. Two thirds of people with myasthenia gravis have thymic abnormalities, with the most common being thymic hyperplasia. A minority of people have a tumor of the thymus, called a thymoma.

Neutropenia refers to a decrease in circulating neutrophils. Neutrophils are usually the first to arrive at the scene of an infection and serve to scavenge pathogenic microorganisms so that infection cannot spread. Once the neutrophils are fully used, they die and become part of the yellowish wound drainage (pus). When a patient has neutropenia, an insufficient level of neutrophils decreases the body's ability to fight infection. Isoimmune neutropenia is the term that refers to this condition in a neonate; the condition develops when a pregnant woman produces antibodies against neutrophils, which then cross the placenta and cause neutropenia in the fetus.

Immune thrombocytopenic purpura (ITP) is a blood disorder in which antibodies form to blood platelets that cause their destruction. Thrombocytopenia describes a decrease in blood platelets; purpura is purplish areas of the skin and mucous membranes (such as the lining of the mouth) where bleeding has occurred as a result of decreased numbers of or ineffective platelets. Some cases of ITP are caused by drugs, whereas others are associated with infection, pregnancy, or immune disorders such as SLE. About half of all cases are classified as idiopathic (the cause is unknown).

Bleeding is the main symptom of ITP and can include bruising and tiny red dots on the skin or mucous membranes. In some cases, bleeding from the nose, gums, and digestive or urinary tracts may occur. Rarely, the patient has bleeding within the brain.

Treatment of idiopathic ITP is based on the severity of the symptoms and the patient's platelet count. In some cases, no therapy is needed. In most cases, drugs that alter the immune system's attack on the platelets are prescribed, such as corticosteroids (for example, prednisone) and IV infusions of immunoglobulin. Another treatment that usually increases the number of platelets is removal of the spleen, the organ that destroys antibody-coated platelets.

Systemic lupus erythematosus is a chronic autoimmune disease with many manifestations. In SLE, the body's own immune system is directed against the body's own tissues. The cause of SLE is not known. Although SLE is more common in young women, it can occur in either sex at any age. The production of autoantibodies leads to immune complex formation. These immune complexes can then be deposited in glomeruli, skin, lungs, synovium, and mesothelium, among other places. Symptoms include arthritis, a red rash over the nose and cheeks, fatigue, weakness, fever, and photosensitivity. Glomerulonephritis (kidney disease), pericarditis, anemia, and neuritis may develop. In addition, many people with SLE have renal complications.

Blood Group Antigens Rh factor is an antigen that is present in the erythrocytes (red blood cells) of about 85% of the population. Erythrocytes contain antigens on their surface, which are proteins recognized by the immune system. Within the plasma are antibodies, which are proteins that react with antigens. People are classified as having one of four blood types based on the presence or absence of these specific antigens. This process of classification is referred to as blood typing, or determining the ABO blood group.

Type A blood contains erythrocytes with type A surface antigens and plasma containing type B antibodies; type B blood contains type B surface antigens and plasma containing type A antibodies. Type AB blood contains both types of antigens but the plasma contains no ABO antibodies. Type O contains neither A nor B antigens but contains both A and B plasma antibodies. A person's blood type determines which type of blood he or she may receive in a blood transfusion.

Rh blood groups involve a complex of antigens first discovered in rhesus monkeys. The presence of any of the 18 separate Rh antigens makes a person's blood Rh positive. If a person with Rh negative blood were to be exposed to Rh positive blood, antibodies to the antigens could be produced.

Persons who have the factor are designated Rh-positive; those who lack the factor are termed Rh-negative. Blood for transfusions must be classified in terms of its Rh factor, as well as the ABO blood group, to prevent possible incompatibility reactions. An issue relating to Rh factor arises when and Rh-positive fetus has an Rh-negative mother. In this case, the woman can develop antibodies against the Rh-positive factor, which in subsequent pregnancies can cause hemolysis of fetal or neonatal red blood cells and hemolytic disease in the newborn.

■ Immune Deficiencies

Immunodeficiency is an abnormal condition in which some part of the body's immune system is inadequate, and, consequently, resistance to infectious disease is decreased. It may be congenital or acquired.

Congenital Immunodeficiencies

Patients with severe combined immunodeficiency disease have defects that involve lymphoid stem cells. As a consequence, T cells (cellular immunity) and B cells (humoral immunity) are affected. Patients are at risk for infection with all types of organisms (bacteria, mycobacteria, fungi, viruses, parasites, and prions). There are two forms of this disease, both of which are inherited.

X-linked agammaglobulinemia is one of the most common forms of primary immunodeficiency. This disease, which affects male infants, is caused by a defect in the differentiation of pre-B cells into B cells. The result is a markedly decreased level of all immunoglobulins and of mature B lymphocytes. T lymphocytes, however, function normally. Recurrent pyrogenic infections develop, but patients have no problems with fungal and viral infections because their cell-mediated immunity is unaffected. These infections first emerge in affected infants at about 6 months of age, when the level of maternal immunoglobulin has decreased.

Isolated deficiency of IgA is probably the most common form of immunodeficiency. This disease results from a block in the terminal differentiation of B lymphocytes. Most patients are asymptomatic, but in some, chronic sinus infections may develop. Patients also have an increased incidence of autoimmune disease.

Acquired Immunodeficiencies

Any nutritional deficiency can hamper normal immune function and the inflammatory response. Nutritional deficiencies may depress bone marrow function and diminish white blood cell development **Figure 38**. A lack of protein in the diet, for example, decreases the liver's ability to manufacture inflammatory mediators and plasma proteins.

The stress of trauma can also cause immunodeficiency. Other contributors to this condition may include hypoperfusion or shock, mediator production, damage to vital organs, and the decreased nutrition occurring during trauma states.

Iatrogenic (treatment-induced) immunodeficiency is most often caused by drugs. Corticosteroids, whether taken orally or inhaled, suppress the immune system. Often, this immune system suppression is of therapeutic benefit. In a small number of patients, however, the resulting immunosuppression leads to other diseases, such as tuberculosis. Because of its potential for adverse effects, physicians are usually cautious about prescribing this therapy for a prolonged period. In addition, idiosyncratic reactions to antibiotics may cause bone marrow suppression. Bone marrow suppression in cancer is often a direct side effect of chemotherapy and not a true idiosyncratic reaction.

Physical or mental stress has been shown to decrease white blood cell and lymphocyte function. It may also lead to decreased production of various antibodies.

AIDS is an immunodeficiency disease that is caused by the RNA retrovirus HIV. HIV binds to the CD4 surface protein of helper T cells, infects these cells, and kills them. Their destruction causes decreased humoral and cell-mediated reactions.

Treatment of Immunodeficiencies

Replacement therapy is available for immunodeficiencies such as common variable immunodeficiency. Intravenous gamma globulin has been used in the therapy for a number of immunologic disorders of the nervous system, especially myasthenia gravis and inflammatory neuropathies, with considerable success. Bone marrow transplantation may restore immune competence in persons with acquired causes of immunodeficiency, such as following chemotherapy for cancer. Transfusion is another form of replacement therapy for immunodeficiencies. In the future, gene therapy may be useful for treatment of congenital and acquired causes of immunodeficiency.

■ Stress and Disease

Stress is the medical term for a wide range of strong external stimuli, physiologic and psychological, that can cause a physiologic response. Physiologic stress is defined as a change that makes it necessary for the cells of the body to adapt. **Figure 39** shows the series of events that occur when the body responds to a stimulus or stressor. Three concepts related to physiologic stress include the stressor itself, its effect in the body, and the body's response to the stress.

The brain and CNS constantly interact with a person's consciousness. Scientific studies have shown a strong connection between the human psyche and brain physiology. When a person experiences stress, the body's defense mechanisms are activated. Usually, the response to stress is appropriate and beneficial. However, an unchecked stress response can have deleterious outcomes, including chemical dependency, heart attack, stroke, depression, headache, and abdominal pain.

■ General Adaptation Syndrome

The general adaptation syndrome, a term introduced by Hans Selye in the 1920s, characterizes a three-stage reaction to stressors, physical (such as injury) and emotional (such as loss of a loved one).

Stage 1: Alarm

The body reacts to stress first by releasing catecholamines, chemical compounds derived from the amino acid tyrosine that act as hormones or neurotransmitters. They are produced mainly from the adrenal medulla and the postganglionic fibers of the sympathetic nervous system. Catecholamines are soluble, so they circulate dissolved in blood. The most abundant catecholamines are epinephrine (adrenaline), norepinephrine (noradrenaline), and dopamine. Adrenaline acts as a neurotransmitter in the CNS and as a hormone in the blood. Noradrenaline is primarily a neurotransmitter of the peripheral sympathetic nervous system but is also present in the blood (mostly through spillover from the synapses of the sympathetic system).

As shown in Figure 39, stress causes the sympathetic nervous system to be stimulated. When the body senses stress,

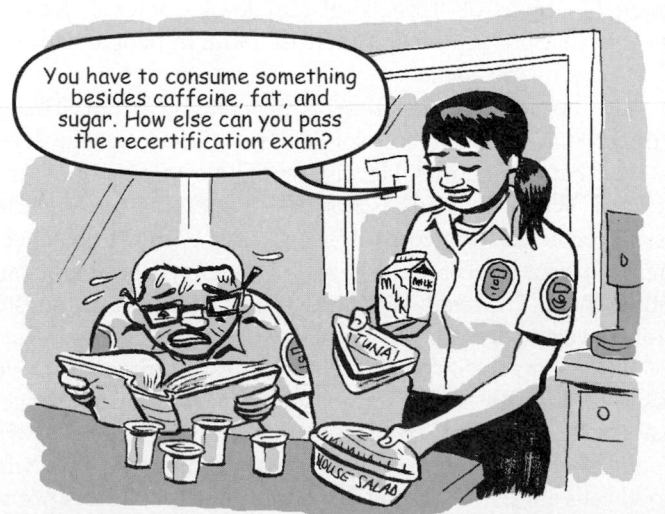

Nutritional deficiencies have been shown to result in depression of bone marrow function and reduction in white blood cell development.

Figure 38

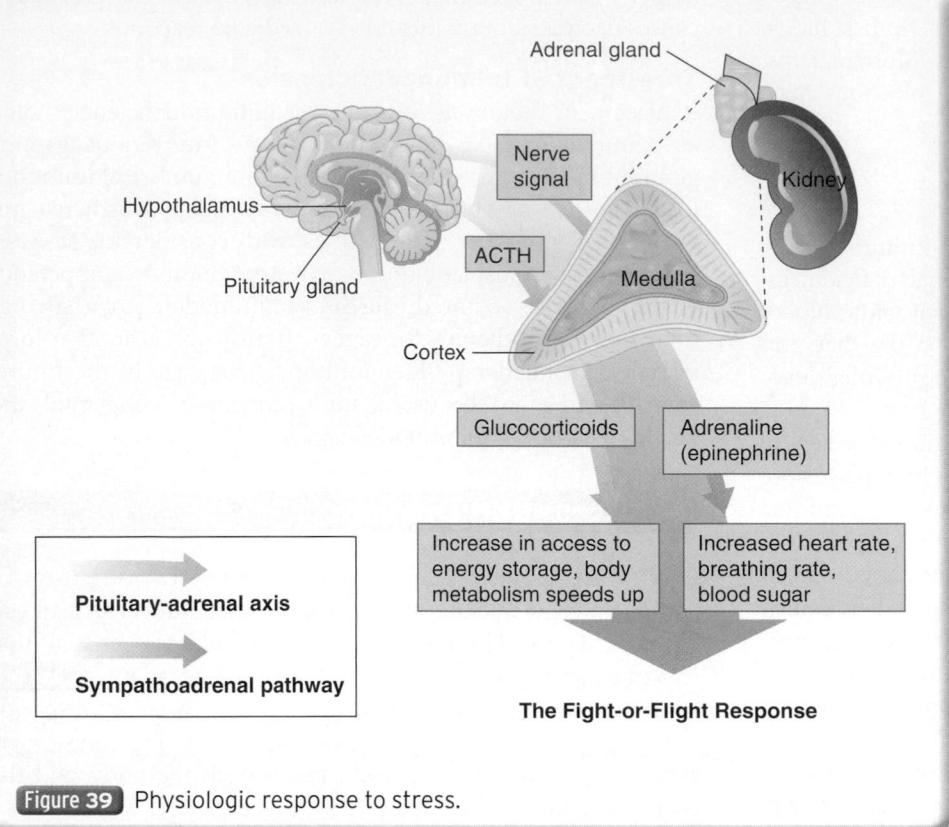

Figure 39 Physiologic response to stress.

During times of stress, the hypothalamus secretes a hormone that stimulates the anterior pituitary to release adrenocorticotropic hormone (ACTH) **Figure 40**. ACTH targets the adrenal cortex, resulting in cortisol secretion. Cortisol stimulates body cells to increase their energy production in response to increased stressors; cortisol increases serum glucose levels and impairs the use of glucose by peripheral tissues. It also decreases protein reserves and permits mobilization of fatty acids by epinephrine and growth hormone. It reduces inflammation when inflammation has served its purpose; therefore, it has a role in wound healing. Cortisol also increases red blood cell production and affects electrolyte levels. However, it also decreases the size of lymphoid tissue. Since the lymphatic system has an important role in immunity, this may explain why stress and disease are linked.

Other hormones related to stress include endorphins, which are neurotransmitters released during times of stress. Endorphins help reduce pain and stress by activating opiate receptor sites. They essentially produce a type of analgesia.

Additional hormones include growth hormone, prolactin, and testosterone. Growth factor is a hormone that promotes cell and tissue growth and repair. In the context of stress, growth factor is reduced. Since growth factor correlates to the body's ability to heal, this means that there is a reduced ability to heal when the body is under chronic stress.

Prolactin is a hormone that stimulates production of breast milk, and which is also believed to play a role in the immune system. In times of stress, prolactin levels increase. Research suggests that prolactin levels increase more in people with ineffective coping mechanisms.

The hormone testosterone is affected by stress. There is a direct link between cortisol levels and testosterone levels; namely, that when cortisol levels are high, testosterone levels are reduced. When the body is not under stress, testosterone levels are protected from cortisol by an enzyme. In the presence of stress, cortisol levels are too high for the enzyme to sufficiently handle them. The result is that the excess cortisol causes testosterone levels to decrease.

It was once believed that elevated testosterone levels were linked to a suppressed immune system. Now, research suggests that testosterone may be related to the distribution of white blood cells in the body. It is thought that in times of stress, white blood cells are sent to the skin in order to protect against wound infection. But in the context of chronic stress, this would mean fewer white blood cells in other parts of the body on a regular basis, making those parts more susceptible to infection.

Cortisol levels and the sympathetic nervous system return to normal during this resistance stage, causing fight-or-flight symptoms to disappear. Continuation of stress and

the brain causes the adrenal medulla of the endocrine system to send catecholamines (the hormones epinephrine and norepinephrine) that activate the sympathetic nervous system by binding to <u>receptor</u> sites. In the sympathetic nervous system, the receptors that allow certain responses to be activated are called alpha and beta receptors. Whenever one of these is activated, a predictable sequence of responses will occur. Activation of alpha receptors results in vasoconstriction, while activation of beta receptors results in increased heart rate, increased force of contraction, and increased conduction velocity. Beyond those cardiac effects of catecholamines, other physiologic effects include an increase in respiratory rate, decreased blood flow to the skin, smooth-muscle constriction, and various effects on the liver that increase the body's use of glucose.

Normally, the fight-or-flight response that occurs in the alarm reaction prepares the body to deal with stress, but it can also weaken the immune system, leading to infection.

Stage 2: Resistance

Stage 2, the resistance stage, is the body's way of adapting to stressors. It does so primarily by stimulating the adrenal gland to secrete two types of corticosteroid hormones that increase the blood glucose level and maintain blood pressure: glucocorticoids and mineralocorticoids. The most significant glucocorticoid in the body is cortisol, which controls carbohydrate, fat, and protein metabolism. Cortisol also has potent anti-inflammatory actions. Mineralocorticoids (predominantly aldosterone) control electrolyte and water levels in the body, mainly by promoting sodium retention by the kidneys.

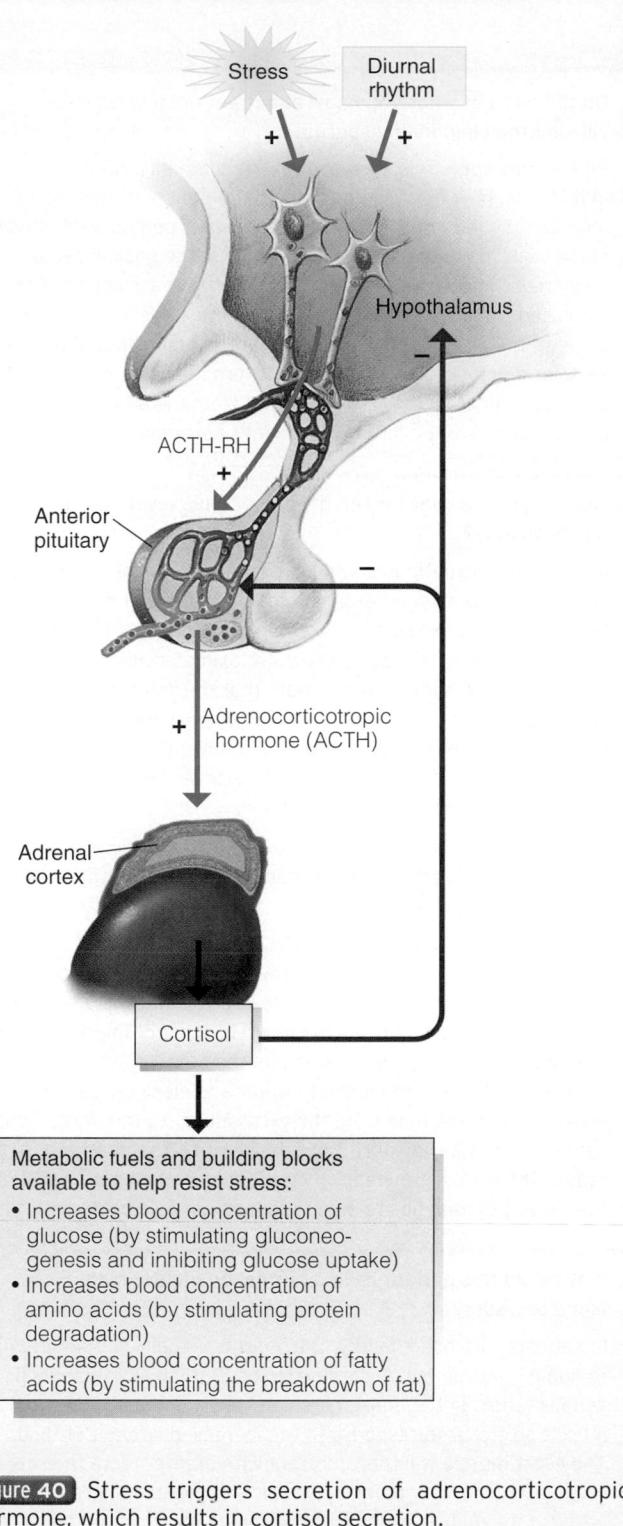

Stress

Diurnal rhythm

+   +

Hypothalamus

−

ACTH-RH

+

Anterior pituitary

−

+ Adrenocorticotropic hormone (ACTH)

Adrenal cortex

Cortisol

Metabolic fuels and building blocks available to help resist stress:
- Increases blood concentration of glucose (by stimulating gluconeo-genesis and inhibiting glucose uptake)
- Increases blood concentration of amino acids (by stimulating protein degradation)
- Increases blood concentration of fatty acids (by stimulating the breakdown of fat)

Figure 40 Stress triggers secretion of adrenocorticotropic hormone, which results in cortisol secretion.

accompanying corticosteroid release eventually lead to fatigue, lapses in concentration, irritability, lethargy, depression, and a depressed immune system.

Stage 3: Exhaustion

After a long period of stress, the person enters the exhaustion stage. The adrenal glands become depleted, diminishing the level of blood glucose. The result is decreased stress tolerance,

progressive mental and physical exhaustion, illness, and collapse. At this point, the body's immune system is compromised, significantly reducing a person's ability to resist disease. Heart attack, high blood pressure, or severe infection may result.

Effects of Chronic Stress

The <u>hypothalamic-pituitary-adrenal axis</u> is a major part of the neuroendocrine system that controls reactions to stress. The hypothalamic-pituitary-adrenal axis triggers a set of interactions among the glands, hormones, and parts of the midbrain that mediate the general adaptation syndrome. Continued stress, however, leads to loss of these normal control mechanisms. As a result, the adrenals continue to produce cortisol, which exhausts the stress mechanism and leads to fatigue and depression. Cortisol also interferes with serotonin activity, furthering the depressive effect.

A consistently high cortisol level suppresses the immune system by increasing production of interleukin-6, an immune system messenger. Not surprisingly, then, research indicates that stress and depression have a negative effect on the immune system. Reduced immunity makes the body more susceptible to everything from colds and flu to cancer. For example, the incidence of serious illness, including cancer, is significantly higher among people whose spouse has died during the past year.

Although severe, prolonged stress does not cause death directly, it does cause the body to lose its ability to fight disease in its effort to manage the stress. Stress also encourages the body to release fat and cholesterol into the bloodstream, which in turn block the arteries and can eventually cause a heart attack or stroke. Many people start drinking alcohol to excess to combat their stress. Other diseases and conditions related to chronic stress include depression, headaches, insomnia, ulcers, diuresis, acne, diabetes mellitus, rheumatoid arthritis, and asthma. The variety in this list shows that stress affects most every organ system in the body.

However, it is important to note that a person's reaction to stressful events correlates to elevation or reduction in hormone levels. Therefore, coping mechanisms play a role in the physiologic response to stress. When a healthy person experiences stress, he or she may be able to manage the stress with minimal negative effects to the immune system if he or she has effective coping mechanisms. But in any patient, ineffective coping mechanisms will have deleterious effects on immune status. Effects will be worst in those whose immune systems are already compromised and who do not have effective coping mechanisms to combat the stress. Conversely, effective coping mechanisms can go a long way in helping a patient improve his or her immune system's response. Finally, a person's outlook has been shown to relate to the effectiveness of his or her medical treatment; much like a placebo effect, if a patient believes that the treatment will be effective, it is more likely to be effective.

Fortunately, this immune suppression process can be corrected with psychotherapy, medication, or any number of other positive influences that restore hope and a feeling of self-esteem. The ability of human beings to recover from adversity is remarkable.

YOU *are the Medic*   SUMMARY

1. What is your general impression of the patient?

The patient is in obvious respiratory distress because he is not able to speak complete sentences without taking a breath. This finding is very important in the assessment of your patient because it indicates there is not enough oxygen available to the patient to speak effectively. Assessing the respiratory system includes opening the airway, if it is not self-maintained. In this presentation, the patient is maintaining his own open airway. The next step is to count the number of respirations in 1 minute. While counting the rate, assess whether the rhythm of the respirations is regular, irregular, or intermittent. Before auscultating lung sounds, listen to your patient. Is breathing quiet or noisy? Look for accessory muscle use such as nasal flaring or retractions of chest muscles. Sitting upright or leaning slightly forward places the patient's airway in alignment, which increases airflow.

2. What could his surroundings indicate to you?

The scene assessment gives numerous indications that the patient has a significant medical history. The first significant finding is that you were met at the door by a neighbor. The neighbor tells you the patient has had medical issues and lives alone. Once you enter the residence, take in the overall picture. Is the room clean or cluttered? Is the heat or air conditioning appropriate to ambient temperature outside? Are there medical items visible? Do you smell anything abnormal? In this scenario, there are multiple medication containers noted and an abundance of used facial tissues adjacent to the patient. These need to be investigated further. The patient is also wearing a nasal cannula attached to a home oxygen unit, which indicates a preexisting respiratory condition.

3. What is the body trying to do through the use of accessory muscles of breathing?

As you have learned, the act of breathing relies on positive and negative pressures. The chest and other related muscles expand and contract to create the pressure. When the act of breathing becomes difficult, accessory muscles assist with the mechanical aspect breathing. The nasal passages will flare in an attempt to gain as much space as possible to increase airflow into the airways. Musculature in the chest will work visibly harder to move the chest wall and diaphragm to assist in creating the pressure gradient necessary for breathing. Sitting upright aligns the airway to decrease the amount of pressure needed within the chest.

4. What could the productive cough indicate in relation to the level of difficulty breathing?

The productive cough could indicate many disease processes. The color of the sputum is of particular interest in your assessment. Thick green, brown, or yellow sputum may indicate infection. Pink frothy sputum indicates pulmonary edema. Hemoptysis may indicate trauma or carcinoma. After assessing the color, how much of it is present? In this case there are numerous used facial tissues that could indicate an amount.

5. On the basis of what you know about physiology, what is causing the pink, foamy sputum?

Pink, foamy sputum is an indication of pulmonary edema that, in this case, may be a sign of exacerbation of congestive heart failure. If the left ventricle of the heart is not pumping effectively, blood backs up in the system. The result of the backup causes an increase in pressure within the pulmonary vasculature. The increased pressure forces fluid through the alveolar membrane and into the alveoli. Blood will enter the alveoli through the alveolar membrane in small amounts, producing a pink rather than red appearance. The froth comes from the additional fluid being exposed to the air in the patient's lungs and airways.

6. How do you account for the decreased Spo_2 level based on physiology?

In this case, the patient would have a decreased amount of surface area for oxygen exchange due to pulmonary edema. Less surface area means less oxygen will "saturate" the cells, which will in turn be read by the pulse oximeter as a decrease in saturation. It is important to note that the saturation amount shown on the electronic device represents any gas that is saturating the cells. Oxygen is one of many gases that can affect the reading. In addition, saturation levels may be compromised by the patient's own lack of circulation.

7. Why would a diuretic be prescribed for a patient with congestive heart failure?

If a patient has congestive heart failure, the heart is not pumping blood effectively. This causes a backup within the circulatory system, which in turn causes fluid to back up into the pulmonary vasculature. A diuretic helps to eliminate some of the fluid from the system to lessen the workload on the heart. Most diuretics work on the kidneys to eliminate water and electrolytes. The elimination moves fluid from the extracellular to the intravascular space, which will transport it out of the body. The goal is to reduce the cardiac preload, which will reduce the amount of work the cardiac system has to do and reduce the fluid backup.

8. Why would this patient have a normal or slightly high blood pressure?

In patients with heart failure, the heart is actually working harder to pump fluid volume. According to the Starling law, increased venous return to the heart increases cardiac preload. The heart muscle stretches in response to the increased amount of fluid. The heart muscle will then contract with greater force to expel the fluid. This accounts for a normal or higher blood pressure because the body is trying to compensate for a lack of the heart's muscular ability.

YOU are the Medic   SUMMARY, continued

EMS Patient Care Report (PCR)

Date: 03-01-11	Incident No.: 1234	Nature of Call: Difficulty breathing	Location: 420 Beach Street		
Dispatched: 2041	En Route: 2041	At Scene: 2045	Transport: 2052	At Hospital: 2107	In Service: 2122

Patient Information

Age: 72	Allergies: No known drug allergies
Sex: M	Medications: Numerous
Weight (in kg [lb]): 79.5 kg (177 lb)	Past Medical History: Congestive heart failure
	Chief Complaint: Difficulty breathing

Vital Signs

Time: 2047	BP: 140/90	Pulse: 110	Respirations: 22	Spo$_2$: 89%
Time: 2052	BP: 138/88	Pulse: 114	Respirations: 24	Spo$_2$: 92%
Time:	BP:	Pulse:	Respirations:	Spo$_2$:

EMS Treatment
(circle all that apply)

Oxygen @ __15__ L/min via (circle one): NC (NRM) Bag-mask device	Assisted Ventilation	Airway Adjunct	CPR
Defibrillation	Bleeding Control	Bandaging	Splinting	Other

Narrative

Arrived to find this 72-year-old man being attended by his neighbor. Pt lives alone in this residence. Pt alert (oriented to person, place, and day) pt unable to speak in completed sentences due to respiratory effort. Pt states he has not been compliant with his medications for a time. Pt states he has a history of "heart failure" and is using 2 L/min O_2 via cannula. Assessment shows vital signs as above; lung sound assessment shows coarse crackles in all fields. Pt has productive cough with pink foamy sputum. O_2 via NRM applied at 15 L/min on scene and throughout transport. IV of NS established TKO, ECG shows sinus tach @114, no ectopy noted. Treatment per local protocol, radio report during transport, and verbal report to Halifax Health on arrival. Pt transferred to room A-20. **End of report**

Prep Kit

- Pathophysiology is the study of the functioning of an organism in the presence of disease.

- All cells except red blood cells and platelets have three main components: a nucleus, cytoplasm, and a cell membrane.

- There are four major tissue types: epithelial tissue, connective tissue, muscle tissue, and nervous tissue.

- When cells are exposed to adverse conditions, they undergo a process of temporary or permanent adaptation to protect themselves from injury. Examples of adaptation include atrophy, hypertrophy, hyperplasia, dysplasia, and metaplasia.

- The cellular environment refers to the distribution of cells, molecules, and fluids throughout the body. It is controlled by variables such as age, exercise, pregnancy, medications, nutrition and hydration, disease, and injury.

- Electrolytes in body fluids include sodium, chloride, potassium, calcium, phosphorus, and magnesium.

- pH is a measurement of the hydrogen ion concentration—that is, the acidity or alkalinity—of a solution, such as the blood. Normal body functioning depends on maintaining an acid-base balance within the normal physiologic pH range of 7.35 to 7.45.

- Cellular injury is caused by factors such as hypoxia, chemical exposure, infectious agents, inappropriate immunologic responses, inflammatory responses, genetic factors, nutritional imbalances, physical agents such as radiation, and adverse conditions such as extreme cold.

- Inflammatory response is characterized by both local and systemic effects. Local effects consist of dilatation (expansion) of blood vessels and increased vascular permeability. If the inflammatory process is severe, systemic effects such as fever become evident. The outcome of an inflammation depends on how much tissue damage has resulted from the inflammation.

- Age- and sex-associated factors interact with a combination of genetic and environmental factors, lifestyle, and anatomic or hormonal differences to cause disease.

- Analyzing disease risk involves consideration of disease rates (incidence, prevalence, morbidity, and mortality) and controllable and uncontrollable disease risk factors (causal and noncausal). These risk factors, age, and sex differences interact to influence a person's level of risk.

- A true genetic risk is passed through generations on a gene. In contrast, a familial tendency may cluster in family groups despite lack of evidence for heritable gene-associated abnormalities. In autosomal dominant inheritance, a person needs to inherit only one copy of a particular form of a gene to show the trait. In autosomal recessive inheritance, the person must inherit two copies of a particular form of a gene to show the trait.

- Immunologic diseases occur because of hyperactivity or hypoactivity of the immune system. Allergies are acquired following initial exposure to a stimulant known as an allergen. Repeated exposures generate an immune system reaction to the allergen.

- Perfusion is the delivery of oxygen and nutrients to cells, organs, and tissues through the circulatory system. Hypoperfusion occurs when the level of tissue perfusion falls below normal.

- Shock is an abnormal state associated with inadequate oxygen and nutrient delivery to the metabolic apparatus of the cell, resulting in an impairment of cellular metabolism.

- Central shock consists of cardiogenic shock and obstructive shock. Cardiogenic shock occurs when the heart cannot circulate enough blood to maintain adequate peripheral oxygen delivery. Obstructive shock occurs when blood flow within the heart or great vessels (aorta and pulmonary vein) becomes blocked.

- Peripheral shock includes hypovolemic shock and distributive shock. In hypovolemic shock, the circulating blood volume is insufficient to deliver adequate oxygen and nutrients to the body. Distributive shock occurs when there is widespread dilation of the resistance vessels (small arterioles), the capacitance vessels (small venules), or both.

- Multiple organ dysfunction syndrome (MODS) occurs in acutely ill patients and is characterized by the dysfunction of two or more organs that were not affected by the physiologic insult for which the patient was initially being treated. Six organ systems are surveyed to determine whether a patient has MODS and, if so, how high a risk of mortality he or she faces: respiratory, hepatic, renal, hematologic, neurologic, and cardiovascular.

- The immune system includes all of the structures and processes that mount a defense against foreign substances and disease-causing agents.

- The body has three lines of defense: anatomic barriers, the inflammatory response, and the immune response.

- The two anatomic components of the immune system are the lymphoid tissues and the cells responsible for mounting an immune response.

- The primary cells of the immune system are the white blood cells, or leukocytes.

- There are two general types of immune response: native and acquired.

- Immunity may be humoral or cell-mediated.

- Important white blood cells in the immune system include neutrophils, eosinophils, basophils, monocytes, and lymphocytes. Other important cells of the immune system include macrophages, mast cells, plasma cells, B cells, and T cells.

- The antibodies secreted by B cells are called immunoglobulins. Antibodies make antigens more visible to the immune system in three ways: by acting as opsonins, by making antigens clump, and by inactivating bacterial toxins.

- The inflammatory response is the reaction of the body's tissues to cellular injury. It is characterized by pain, swelling, redness, and heat.
- The two most common causes of inflammation are infection and injury.
- The plasma protein systems that modulate the inflammatory process include the complement system, the coagulation (clotting) system, and the kinin system.
- Cytokines are products of cells that affect the functioning of other cells; they include interleukins, lymphokines, and interferon.
- Chronic inflammatory responses are usually caused by an unsuccessful acute inflammatory response after the invasion of a foreign body, a persistent infection, or an antigen.
- Normal wound healing involves four steps: repair of damaged tissue, removal of inflammatory debris, restoration of tissues to a normal state, and regeneration of cells.
- Wounds may heal by primary or secondary intention. Healing by primary intention occurs in clean wounds with opposed margins. Wounds that heal by secondary intention have a prolonged inflammatory phase and more abundant granulation tissue.
- Hypersensitivity is an increased response of the body to any substance to which the person is abnormally sensitive. A hypersensitivity reaction may be immediate, occurring within seconds to minutes, or delayed, occurring hours to days after exposure to the antigen.
- Hypersensitivity reactions may be classified as autoimmune, idiopathic, or blood incompatibility reactions.
- Immunodeficiency may be congenital or acquired.
- Stress does not cause death directly, but it can permit diseases to flourish, ultimately leading to death.
- The general adaptation syndrome describes the body's short-term and long-term reactions to stress.
- Stress causes the sympathetic nervous system to be stimulated. This occurs through release of catecholamines that activate the sympathetic nervous system by binding to alpha and beta receptor sites, resulting in effects categorized as fight-or-flight response.
- Stress also causes secretion of cortisol, which has many useful effects such as increasing serum glucose levels, decreasing protein reserves, and permitting mobilization of fatty acids. However, continuous secretion of cortisol has deleterious effects.

■ Vital Vocabulary

acid Any molecule that can give up a hydrogen ion (H^+).

acidosis A blood pH of less than 7.35.

acquired immunity The immunity that occurs when the body is exposed to a foreign substance or disease and produces antibodies to the invader.

activation Mediators of inflammation trigger the appearance of molecules known as selectins and integrins on the surfaces of endothelial cells and polymorphonuclear neutrophils, respectively.

active hyperemia The dilation of arterioles after transient arteriolar constriction, which allows influx of blood under increased pressure.

adhesion The attachment of polymorphonuclear neutrophils to endothelial cells, mediated by selectins and integrins.

adipose tissue A connective tissue containing large amounts of lipids.

adrenergic receptor A type of receptor that is associated with the sympathetic nerves and which is stimulated by epinephrine and norepinephrine; activation causes a sympathetic response.

alcoholic ketoacidosis The metabolic acidotic state that manifests because of the inadequate nutritional habits associated with chronic alcohol abuse. The liver and body experience inadequate fuel reserves of glycogen and, thus, have to switch to fatty acid metabolism.

alkalosis A blood pH greater than 7.45.

allergen Any substance that causes a hypersensitivity reaction.

allergy A hypersensitivity reaction to the presence of an agent (allergen) that is intrinsically harmless.

anaphylactic shock A severe hypersensitivity reaction that involves bronchoconstriction and cardiovascular collapse.

angiogenesis The growth of new blood vessels.

anions Negatively charged ions.

antibody A protein secreted by certain immune cells that bind antigens to make them more visible to the immune system.

antidiuretic hormone (ADH) One of the two main hormones responsible for adjustments to the final composition of urine; causes ducts in the kidney to become more permeable to water.

antigen A foreign substance recognized by the immune system.

apoptosis Normal, genetically programmed cell death.

Arthus reaction A localized reaction involving vascular inflammation in response to an IgG-mediated allergic response.

asthma A chronic inflammatory lower airway condition resulting in intermittent wheezing and excess mucus production.

atopic The medical term for having an allergic tendency.

atrophy A decrease in cell size due to a loss of subcellular components.

autoantibodies Antibodies directed against the person's own proteins.

autocrine hormone A hormone that acts on the cell from which it has been secreted.

autoimmunity The production of antibodies or T cells that work against the tissues of a person's own body, producing autoimmune disease or a hypersensitivity reaction.

autosomal dominant A pattern of inheritance that involves genes that are located on autosomes or the nonsex chromosomes.

Inheritance of only one copy of a particular form of a gene is needed to show the trait.

autosomal recessive A pattern of inheritance that involves genes located on autosomes or the nonsex chromosomes. Inheritance of two copies of a particular form of a gene is needed to show the trait.

axons The part of neurons that conduct the impulses away from the cell body.

baroreceptor A type of receptor that responds to changes in pressure, usually within the heart or the main arteries.

base Any molecule that can accept a hydrogen ion (OH^-).

basophils Approximately 1% of the leukocytes, they are essential to nonspecific immune response to inflammation due to their role in releasing histamine and other chemicals that dilate blood vessels.

bone marrow Specialized tissue found within bone.

bradypnea A slow respiratory rate.

buffers Molecules that modulate changes in pH to keep it in the physiologic range.

capillary refill time A test done on the fingernails or toenails by briefly squeezing the toenail or fingernail and evaluating the time it takes for the color to return.

cardiogenic shock A condition caused by loss of 40% or more of the functioning myocardium; the heart is no longer able to circulate sufficient blood to maintain adequate oxygen delivery.

cations Positively charged ions.

cell-mediated immunity The immune process by which T-cell lymphocytes recognize antigens and then secrete cytokines (specifically lymphokines) that attract other cells or stimulate the production of cytotoxic cells that kill the infected cells.

cell signaling The process by which cells communicate with one another.

central shock A type of shock caused by central pump failure, including cardiogenic shock and obstructive shock.

chemoreceptor A type of receptor that senses changes in the chemical composition of the blood, especially reduced oxygen levels.

chemotaxins Components of the activated complement system that attract leukocytes from the circulation to help fight infections.

chemotaxis The movement of additional white blood cells to an area of inflammation in response to the release of chemical mediators, such as neutrophils, injured tissue, and monocytes.

coagulation system The system that forms blood clots in the body and facilitates repairs to the vascular tree.

complement system A group of plasma proteins whose function is to do one of three things: attract leukocytes to sites of inflammation, activate leukocytes, and directly destroy cells.

connective tissue The type of tissue that binds various tissue types together.

cytokines The products of cells that affect the function of other cells.

dendrites The parts of neurons that receive impulses from the axon and contain vesicles for release of neurotransmitters.

dissociates Process of losing a hydrogen atom in the presence of water. Acids are classified as strong or weak, depending on how completely they dissociate.

distributive shock The type of shock that occurs when there is widespread dilation of the resistance vessels (small arterioles), the capacitance vessels (small venules), or both.

dysplasia An alteration in the size, shape, and organization of cells.

endocrine hormones The hormones that are carried to their target or cell group in the bloodstream.

endothelial cells Specific types of epithelial cells that line the blood vessels.

eosinophils White blood cells with a major role in allergic reactions and bronchoconstriction during an asthma attack; make up approximately 1% to 3% of leukocytes.

epithelium A type of tissue that covers all external surfaces of the body.

exocrine hormones The hormones that are secreted through ducts into an organ or onto epithelial surfaces.

feedback inhibition Negative feedback resulting in the decrease of an action in the body.

fibrin A whitish, filamentous protein formed by the action of thrombin on fibrinogen; the protein that polymerizes (bonds) to form the fibrous component of a blood clot.

fibrinolysis cascade The breakdown of fibrin in blood clots and the prevention of the polymerization of fibrin into new clots.

free radicals Molecules that are missing one electron in their outer shell.

general adaptation syndrome A three-stage description of the body's short-term and long-term reactions to stress.

gram-negative A reaction of bacteria to a Gram stain in which the bacteria do not retain the dark purple stain; this type of bacteria has cell walls that consist largely of lipids, and have pathogenic qualities that make them especially problematic for humans.

gram-positive A reaction of bacteria to a Gram stain in which the bacteria retain the dark purple stain; this type of bacteria has thick cell walls composed of many layers.

gut-associated lymphoid tissue The lymphoid tissue that lies under the inner lining of the esophagus and intestines.

hapten A substance that normally does not stimulate an immune response but can be combined with an antigen and at a later point initiate an antibody response.

helper T cells A type of T lymphocyte that is involved in cell-mediated and antibody-mediated immune responses. It secretes cytokines that stimulate the B cells and other T cells.

hemochromatosis An inherited disease in which the body absorbs more iron than it needs and stores it in the liver, kidneys, and pancreas.

hemolytic anemia A disease characterized by increased destruction of the red blood cells. It can occur from an Rh factor reaction (primarily in Rh-positive neonates born to sensitized Rh-negative mothers), exposure to chemicals, or a disorder of the immune system.

hemophilia An inherited sex-linked disorder characterized by excessive bleeding.

histamine A vasoactive amine that increases vascular permeability and causes vasodilation.

homeostasis The adaptive process by which the body maintains internal balance.

hormones Proteins formed in specialized organs or glands and carried to another organ or group of cells in the same organism. Hormones regulate many body functions, including metabolism, growth, and temperature.

humoral immunity The immunity that uses antibodies made by B-cell lymphocytes.

hypercalcemia An elevated blood calcium level.

hypercholesterolemia An elevated blood cholesterol level.

hyperkalemia An elevated serum potassium level.

hypermagnesemia An increased serum magnesium level.

hypernatremia A serum sodium level greater than 145 mEq/L.

hyperphosphatemia An elevated serum phosphate level.

hyperplasia An increase in the actual number of cells in an organ or tissue, usually resulting in an increase in the size of the organ or tissue.

hypersensitivity A generic term for responses of the body to a substance to which a patient has increased sensitivity.

hypertonic solution A solution with a higher solute concentration than another solution to which it is compared.

hypertrophy An increase in the size of the cells due to synthesis of more subcellular components, leading to an increase in tissue and organ size.

hypocalcemia A decreased serum calcium level.

hypokalemia A decreased serum potassium level.

hypomagnesemia A decreased serum magnesium level.

hyponatremia A serum sodium level that is less than 135 mEq/L.

hypoperfusion A condition that occurs when the level of tissue perfusion decreases below that needed to maintain normal cellular functions.

hypophosphatemia A decreased serum phosphate level.

hypothalamic-pituitary-adrenal axis A major part of the neuroendocrine system that controls reactions to stress. It is the mechanism for a set of interactions among glands, hormones, and parts of the midbrain that mediate the general adaptation syndrome.

hypotonic solution A solution with a lower solute concentration than another solution to which it is compared.

hypovolemic shock A condition that occurs when the circulating blood volume is inadequate to deliver adequate oxygen and nutrients to the body.

immune response The body's defense reaction to any substance that is recognized as foreign.

immune system The body system that includes all of the structures and processes designed to mount a defense against foreign substances and disease-causing agents.

immunodeficiency An abnormal condition in which some part of the body's immune system is inadequate, and, consequently, resistance to infectious disease is decreased.

immunogen An antigen that is capable of generating an immune response.

immunoglobulins Antibodies secreted by the B cells.

incidence The number of new cases of a disease in a population.

inflammatory response A reaction by tissues of the body to irritation or injury, characterized by pain, swelling, redness, and heat.

interferon A protein produced by cells in response to viral invasion that is released into the bloodstream or intercellular fluid to induce healthy cells to manufacture an enzyme that counters the infection.

interleukins Chemical substances that attract white blood cells to the sites of injury and bacterial invasion.

ions Atoms that have become positively or negatively charged by giving up or acquiring an electron.

isoimmunity The formation of antibodies or T cells that are directed against antigens or another person's cells.

isotonic solutions Solutions with the same osmolarity as intracellular fluid (280 mOsm/L).

ketoacidosis An acidotic state created by the production of ketones via fat metabolism.

ketones Acidic by-products of fat metabolism.

kinin system A general term for a group of polypeptides that mediate inflammatory responses by stimulating visceral smooth muscle and relaxing vascular smooth muscle to produce vasodilation.

lactic acidosis Anaerobic cellular respiration due to hypoperfusion of tissues and organs.

leukocytes The white blood cells responsible for fighting infection.

leukocytosis Elevation of the white blood cell count, often due to inflammation.

leukotrienes Arachidonic acid metabolites that function as chemical mediators of inflammation; also known as slow-reacting substances of anaphylaxis.

ligands Any molecules that bind to a receptor to form a more complex structure.

lymph A thin, watery fluid that bathes the tissues of the body.

lymphatic system A network of capillaries, vessels, ducts, nodes, and organs that helps to maintain the fluid environment of the body by producing lymph and transporting it through the body.

lymphocytes The white blood cells responsible for a large part of the body's immune protection.

lymphokines Cytokines released by lymphocytes, including many of the interleukins, gamma interferon, tumor necrosis factor beta, and chemokines.

macrophages Cells that develop from the monocytes that provide the body's first line of defense in the inflammatory process.

margination The loss of fluid from the blood vessels into the tissue, causing the blood left in the vessels to have increased viscosity, which in turn slows the flow of blood and produces stasis.

mast cells The cells that resemble basophils but do not circulate in the blood; have a role in allergic reactions, immunity, and wound healing.

membrane attack complex Molecules that insert themselves into the bacterial membrane, leading to weakened areas in the membrane.

metabolic acidosis A pathologic condition characterized by a blood pH of less than 7.35 and caused by an accumulation of acids in the body from a metabolic cause.

metabolic alkalosis A pathologic condition characterized by a blood pH of greater than 7.45 and caused by an accumulation of bases in the body from a metabolic cause.

metaplasia A reversible, cellular adaptation in which one adult cell type is replaced by another adult cell type.

mitochondria The metabolic center or powerhouse of the cell; small and rod-shaped organelles.

mixed acidosis A pathologic condition in which there is a low pH, an elevated P_{CO_2} level, and low bicarbonate level, and which occurs when there is both a respiratory and metabolic cause present at the same time.

mixed alkalosis A pathologic condition in which there is an elevated pH, a low P_{CO_2} level, and an elevated bicarbonate level, which occurs when there is both a respiratory and metabolic cause present at the same time.

<u>monocytes</u> Mononuclear phagocytic white blood cells derived from myeloid stem cells that circulate in the bloodstream for about 24 hours and then move into tissues to mature into macrophages.

<u>morbidity</u> Number of nonfatally injured or disabled people; usually expressed as a rate, meaning the number of nonfatal injuries in a certain population in a given time period divided by the size of the population.

<u>morbid obesity</u> An excessively unhealthy accumulation of body fat, defined as a body mass index of greater than or equal to 40 kg/m^2.

<u>mortality</u> The quality of being mortal; number of deaths from a disease in a given population.

<u>mucosa-associated lymphoid tissue</u> The lymphoid tissue associated with the skin and the respiratory, urinary, and reproductive traits as well as the tonsils.

<u>multiple organ dysfunction syndrome (MODS)</u> A grave but sometimes reversible condition in an acutely ill patient characterized by the progressive dysfunction of two or more organs or organ systems not affected by the patient's initial illness or injury.

<u>natural immunity</u> A nonspecific cellular and humoral response that operates as the body's first line of defense against pathogens; also called native immunity.

<u>necrosis</u> The death of tissue, usually caused by a cessation of the blood supply.

<u>negative feedback</u> The concept that once the desired effect of a process has been achieved, further action is inhibited until it is needed again; also called feedback inhibition.

<u>neurogenic shock</u> A type of shock that usually results from spinal cord injury; loss of normal sympathetic nervous system tone and vasodilation occur.

<u>neurotransmitters</u> Proteins that affect signals between cells of the nervous system.

<u>neutrophils</u> Cells that make up approximately 55% to 70% of the leukocytes responsible in large part for the body's protection against infection; they are readily attracted by foreign antigens and destroy them by phagocytosis.

<u>nucleus</u> A cellular organelle that contains the genetic information; controls the function and structure of a cell.

<u>obesity</u> An unhealthy accumulation of body fat, defined as a body mass index of greater than or equal to 30 kg/m^2.

<u>obstructive shock</u> The type of shock that occurs when blood flow to the heart or great vessels is obstructed.

<u>oliguria</u> Decreased urine output.

<u>opsonization</u> The process by which an antibody coats an antigen to facilitate its recognition by immune cells.

<u>organelles</u> The internal cellular structures that carry out specific functions for the cell.

<u>osmolarity</u> The concentration of osmotically active particles in solution expressed as osmoles of solute per liter of solution.

<u>osmosis</u> Movement of water or another solvent across a membrane from a region of higher water concentration (or low solute concentration) to one of lower water concentration (or high solute concentration).

<u>overweight</u> An unhealthy accumulation of body fat, defined as a body mass index of 25 to 29.9 kg/m^2.

<u>paracrine hormones</u> The hormones that diffuse through intracellular spaces to their target.

<u>pathophysiology</u> The study of how normal physiologic processes are affected by disease.

perfusion The delivery of oxygen and nutrients to the cells, organs, and tissues of the body; also involves the removal of wastes.

pericardial tamponade The impairment of diastolic filling of the right ventricle due to significant amounts of fluid in the pericardial sac surrounding the heart, leading to a decrease in the cardiac output.

peripheral nerves All of the nerves of the body extending from the brain and spinal cord.

peripheral shock A term that describes shock caused by peripheral circulatory abnormalities; includes hypovolemic shock and distributive shock.

pH The measure of acidity or alkalinity of a solution.

phagocytes The cells that engulf and consume foreign material such as microorganisms and debris.

phagocytosis The process in which one cell "eats" or engulfs a foreign substance to destroy it.

polymorphonuclear neutrophils (PMNs) The type of white blood cells formed by bone marrow tissue that have a nucleus consisting of several parts or lobes connected by fine strands.

polyuria Frequent and plentiful urination.

prevalence The number of cases of a disease in a specific population within a given period.

prostaglandins A group of lipids that act as chemical messengers.

pyrogens Chemicals or proteins that travel to the brain and affect the hypothalamus and stimulate a rise in the body's core temperature.

receptor A specialized area in tissue that initiates certain actions after specific stimulation.

renin-angiotensin-aldosterone system (RAAS) A complex feedback mechanism responsible for the regulation of sodium in the body by the kidneys.

respiratory acidosis A pathologic condition characterized by a blood pH of less than 7.35 and caused by an accumulation of acids in the body from a respiratory cause.

respiratory alkalosis A pathologic condition characterized by a blood pH of less than 7.35 and caused by an accumulation of bases in the body from a respiratory cause.

Rh factor An antigen present in the erythrocytes (red blood cells) of about 85% of people.

ribonucleic acid (RNA) A nucleic acid associated with controlling cellular activities.

septic shock The type of shock that occurs as a result of widespread infection, usually bacterial; untreated, the result is multiple organ dysfunction syndrome and often death.

serotonin A vasoactive amine that increases vascular permeability to cause vasodilation.

serum sickness A condition in which antigen-antibody complexes formed in the bloodstream deposit in sites around the body, most notably the kidneys, with resultant inflammatory reactions.

slow-reacting substances of anaphylaxis Biologically active compounds derived from arachidonic acid called leukotrienes.

T killer cells The cells released during a type IV allergic reaction that kill antigen-bearing target cells.

tonicity The tension exerted on a cell due to water movement across the cell membrane.

transmigration (diapedesis) The polymorphonuclear neutrophils permeate through the vessel wall, moving into the interstitial space.

urticaria Multiple small, raised areas on the skin that may be one of the warning signs of impending anaphylaxis; also known as hives.

vasculitis An inflammation of the blood vessels.

vasoactive amines Substances such as histamine and serotonin that increase vascular permeability.

virulence A measure of the disease-causing ability of a microorganism.

Assessment in Action

Y ou are dispatched to a local park for a 20-year-old woman who was stung by a bee. On arrival, you are met by a law enforcement officer who directs you to the patient. The patient is sitting upright on a park bench in obvious distress. You can see urticaria covering her arms, legs, and face. Her tongue is swollen, and she points to a medical alert bracelet that says, "Allergic to bee stings." You can hear wheezing in all fields when assessing lung sounds. When you assess her pulse, you find it weak at the radial site.

1. The strength of a person's peripheral pulses is related to:
   A. heart rate and preload.
   B. stroke volume.
   C. physical size.
   D. mast cells.

2. Anaphylactic shock is characterized by:
   A. hypertension and vasoconstriction.
   B. wheezing and widespread vasodilation.
   C. hypotension and hives.
   D. crackles (rales) and stridor.

3. When oxygen does not reach the cell, the cell reverts to:
   A. anaerobic metabolism.
   B. aerobic metabolism.
   C. production of ketones.
   D. production of bicarbonate.

4. Distributive shock occurs when:
   A. blood moves from the core of the body.
   B. blood pools in expanded vascular structures.
   C. microorganisms attack the body.
   D. a significant decrease in stroke volume occurs.

5. How does the body respond to hypoperfusion?
   A. Decreased preload and heart rate
   B. Increased systemic vascular resistance
   C. Systemic hypoxia increases vascular resistance
   D. A decreased cardiac oxygen demand

6. The worst respiratory sign in a patient with anaphylactic shock is:
   A. diminished lung sounds.
   B. loud expiratory wheezing.
   C. diffuse coarse crackles.
   D. labored breathing.

Additional Questions

7. In arterial blood gas analysis, a patient has a low pH and a high Pa_{CO_2}. What type of acidosis or alkalosis does the patient have?

8. Will a patient who has been hyperventilating have signs and symptoms of respiratory acidosis or respiratory alkalosis?

Life Span Development

National EMS Education Standard Competencies

Life Span Development

Integrates comprehensive knowledge of life span development.

Knowledge Objectives

1. Understand the terms used to designate the following age groups: infants, toddlers, preschoolers, school-age children, adolescents (teenagers), early adults, middle adults, and late adults. (pp 401, 405, 407, 408, 409, 410)
2. Describe the major physiologic and psychosocial characteristics of an infant's life. (pp 401-405)
3. Describe the major physiologic and psychosocial characteristics of a toddler and preschooler's life. (pp 405-407)
4. Describe the major physiologic and psychosocial characteristics of a school-age child's life. (pp 407-408)
5. Describe the major physiologic and psychosocial characteristics of an adolescent's life. (pp 408-409)
6. Describe the major physiologic and psychosocial characteristics of an early adult's life. (p 409)
7. Describe the major physiologic and psychosocial characteristics of a middle adult's life. (pp 409-410)
8. Describe the major physiologic and psychosocial characteristics of a late adult's life. (pp 410-414)

Skills Objectives

There are no skills objectives for this chapter.

Introduction

One of the most interesting things about humans is that we evolve as people over our life span. Paramedics must be aware of the obvious and subtle changes that a person undergoes physically and mentally at various stages of life and understand how these changes might alter the approach to patient care.

Infants

As any parent can attest, <u>infants</u> develop at a startling rate Figure 1 . In medicine, an infant is defined as a baby who is age 1 month to 1 year. Babies younger than age 1 month are categorized as either newborn or neonate depending on their age, and are covered in detail in the chapter, *Neonatal Care*.

Physical Changes

Vital Signs
Table 1 lists the normal ranges of vital signs for various age groups. The younger the person, the faster the pulse rate and

respirations. At birth, a pulse rate of 100 to 180 beats/min and a respiratory rate of 30 to 60 breaths/min are considered normal. After about half an hour, an infant's pulse rate often drops to around 120 beats/min and the respiratory rate adjusts to between 30 to 40 breaths/min. Tidal volume in infants starts at 6 to 8 mL/kg. By age 1 year, the volume increases to 10 to 15 mL/kg.

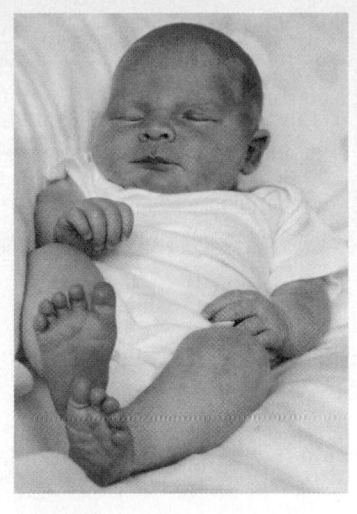
Figure 1 An infant.

Blood pressure directly corresponds to the patient's weight, so it typically increases with age. At birth, the average systolic blood pressure of an infant is 50 to 70 mm Hg. By 1 year of age, it is in the range of 70 to 95 mm Hg.

Table 1 Vital Signs at Various Ages

Age	Pulse Rate (beats/min)	Respirations (breaths/min)	Blood Pressure (mm Hg, systolic)	Temperature (°F)
Newborn (0 to 1 mo)	100 to 180	30 to 60	50 to 70	98 to 100
Infant (1 month to 1 y)	100 to 160	25 to 50	70 to 95	96.8 to 99.6
Toddler (1 to 3 y)	90 to 150	20 to 30	80 to 100	96.8 to 99.6
Preschool age (3 to 5 y)	80 to 140	20 to 25	80 to 100	98.6
School age (6 to 12 y)	70 to 120	15 to 20	80 to 110	98.6
Adolescent (13 to 17 y)	60 to 100	12 to 20	90 to 110	98.6
Early adult (18 to 40 y)	60 to 100	12 to 20	90 to 140	98.6
Middle adult (41 to 60 y)	60 to 100	12 to 20	90 to 140	98.6
Late adult (61 y and older)	Depends on health	Depends on health	Depends on health	98.6

YOU *are the Medic*   PART 1

Your unit is dispatched to a private residence for a 3-year-old boy who has fallen in the back yard. The dispatcher tells you the child was running and fell, striking his head on the deck. The dispatcher states that the child is crying audibly over the phone. As you arrive in front of the residence, the father runs toward your vehicle to meet you, carrying the child in his arms. The child appears to be vigorously struggling to be set down and is crying loudly.

1. What is your first concern at this scene?
2. What stage of development describes a 3-year-old child and how will this affect your assessment?

Weight

An infant usually weighs 6 to 8 lb (3 to 3.5 kg) at birth. After birth, infants usually lose 5% to 10% of their birth weight due to the loss of fluid in the first week. Then they normally gain weight in their second week of life. From here on, infants grow at a rate of about 30 g per day, doubling their weight by 4 to 6 months and tripling it by age 1 year.

Cardiovascular System

Prior to birth, fetal circulation occurs through the placenta. Just after birth, cardiovascular physiologic changes take place that allow independent circulation via the newborn's own vasculature. This process will be covered in detail in the chapter, *Neonatal Care*.

Pulmonary System

Prior to an infant's first breath, the lungs have never been inflated. An infant's first breath is therefore forceful—it has to be!

Infants are primarily "nose breathers" for the first month of their lives. Infants younger than 6 months are particularly prone to nasal congestion, which can cause viral upper respiratory infections. If you receive a call for a baby choking, always make sure the infant's nasal passages are clear and unobstructed by mucus.

The rib cages of infants are less rigid than those of older humans, and the ribs sit horizontally. This explains the diaphragmatic breathing ("belly breathing") in infants. Owing to the immaturity of the accessory muscles, fatigue sets in quickly.

Two other important anatomic points related to an infant's airway, when compared with an adult's, are the proportionally large size of the tongue and the proportionally shorter and narrower airway. As a result of these factors, the airway in infants can be occluded much more easily than the airway in older children or adults. There are also fewer alveoli in the lungs, which decreases the surface area for gas exchange.

When providing bag-mask ventilations to an infant, you need to be aware that an infant's lungs are fragile. Ventilations that are delivered with excessive force or excessive volume can result in trauma from pressure, or **barotrauma** Figure 2.

Renal System

Infants can become easily dehydrated because their kidneys usually cannot produce concentrated urine. An infant's urine consists mainly of water, which can cause the child to develop electrolyte imbalances.

Immune System

While in the womb, infants collect antibodies from the maternal blood. For the first year of life, the infant maintains some of the mother's immunities, so he or she has naturally acquired passive immunities. Infants can also receive antibodies via breastfeeding, further bolstering their immune system.

Nervous System

Although an infant's nervous system is developed at birth, its evolution continues after birth. For example, a newborn lacks the ability to localize and isolate a particular response to sensation. Motor and sensory development are most developed in the cranial nerves, which control blinking, sucking, and gag reflexes.

An infant is born with certain reflexes. The **moro reflex** (startle reflex) occurs when an infant is caught off guard by something or someone; the infant opens his or her arms wide, spreads the

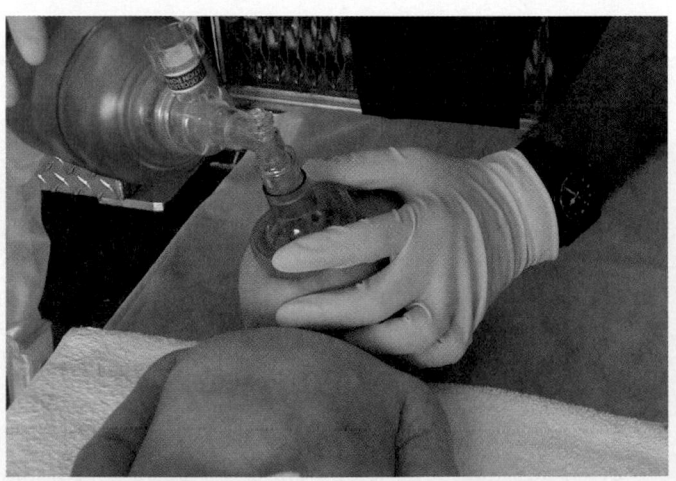

Figure 2 An infant's lungs are fragile. Use caution when providing bag-mask ventilations to avoid barotrauma.

fingers, and seems to grab at things. A <u>palmar grasp</u> occurs when an object is placed into the infant's palm. The <u>rooting reflex</u> occurs when something touches an infant's cheek; the infant will instinctively turn his or her head toward the touch. In conjunction with the <u>sucking reflex</u>, which occurs when an infant's lips are stroked, these reflexes are often tested when feeding.

An infant's <u>fontanelles</u> allow the head to be molded **Figure 3**—for example, when the newborn passes through the birth canal. These three or four bones of the skull eventually bind together and form suture joints within 18 months of birth. If the anterior fontanelle is sunken, the infant is most likely dehydrated.

Perhaps the neurologic development that is of most interest to parents is the development of a sleep pattern.

Some physicians suggest that parents wake infants every few hours for both feeding and safety (eg, to guard against sudden infant death syndrome [SIDS]). Others suggest that infants should be left to sleep so that they can adjust to family life and develop a circadian rhythm, ideally within 4 months after birth. (For more information on SIDS, see the chapter, *Pediatric Emergencies*.)

Musculoskeletal System

<u>Growth plates</u>, located on either end of an infant's bone, aid in lengthening a child's bones. Epiphyseal plates, or secondary bone-growing plates, are also present. Bones grow in thickness by building on themselves. In contrast, an infant's muscles account for approximately 25% of his or her

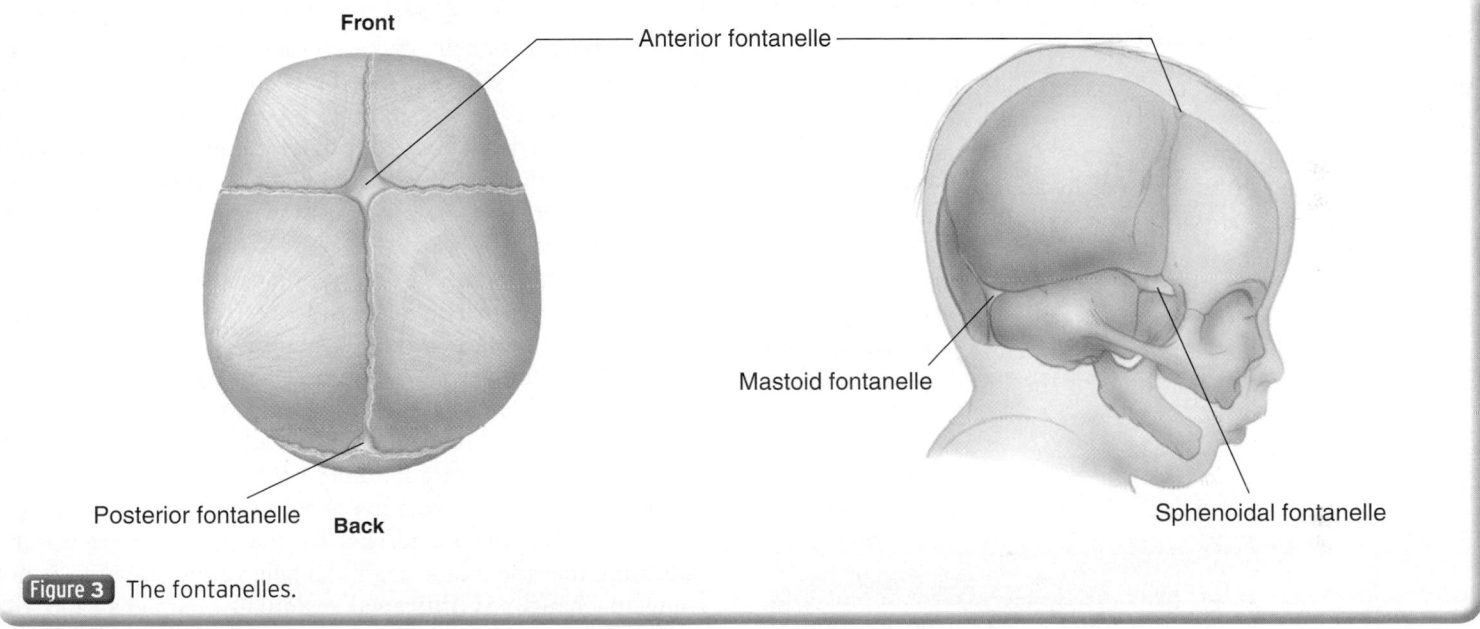

Figure 3 The fontanelles.

YOU are the Medic — PART 2

You and your partner convince the mother and father to sit down on the front steps of the residence rather than immediately climb up into your vehicle. You ask the child his name and he buries his face in his father's chest. The mother tells you his name is Shane. The father tries to forcefully turn Shane so he will face you and the child clings to him even harder and cries louder.

Recording Time: 2 Minutes	
Appearance	Actively moving and crying
Level of consciousness	Conscious and agitated
Airway	Open
Breathing	Loud crying
Circulation	Adequate

3. Why is Shane clinging to his father and turning away from your voice?

4. What are some of the measures you can take to alleviate the child's reaction?

total weight. Growth charts are used to track the growth of an infant or child and provide percentiles comparing the child's growth to the growth that is expected for an average child of that age.

Dental System

Teething often starts between 4 and 7 months of age and can be a challenge to both parents and infants. As with many of the changes in life, this time frame is an estimate, and some children will have teeth erupt (break through the gums) as early as 1 month, and some may have to wait as long as 1 year. Teeth usually erupt in a predetermined order, and a child should have a full set by the age of 3 years. The child will usually keep this set of "baby teeth" until around the age of 6 years, when permanent teeth start to come in.

Psychosocial Changes

An infant's psychosocial development begins at birth and continues to evolve as the infant interacts with and reacts to the environment. Parents are often concerned about whether their child is developing within the socially accepted norms. **Table 2** outlines typical ages at which major psychosocial changes are noticed.

One key to having a happy, healthy infant is spending time with the child. Nevertheless, infants often have their own timetable as to when they will become attached to their parents and other family members. Bonding, or the formation of a close,

Table 2	Noticeable Characteristics at Various Ages
Age	**Characteristics**
2 months	Can recognize familiar faces; able to track objects with the eyes
3 months	Can bring objects to the mouth; can smile and frown
4 months	Reaches out to people; drools
5 months	Sleeps through the night; can tell family from strangers
6 months	Teething begins, sits upright in a chair, one-syllable words spoken
7 months	Afraid of strangers, mood swings
8 months	Responds to "no"; can sit alone; plays peek-a-boo
9 months	Pulls himself or herself up; places objects in mouth to explore them
10 months	Responds to his or her name; crawls efficiently
11 months	Starts to walk without help; frustrated with restrictions
12 months	Knows his or her name; can walk

personal relationship, is usually based on a **secure attachment**. A secure attachment occurs when an infant understands that parents or caregivers will be responsive to his or her needs. This realization encourages a child to reach out and explore, knowing that his or her parents will provide a "safety net."

Another type of attachment, referred to as **anxious avoidant attachment**, is observed in infants who are repeatedly rejected. These children develop an isolated lifestyle in which they do not have to depend on the support and care of others. Child neglect will be covered in more detail in the chapter, *Pediatric Emergencies*.

In most infants, the primary method of communicating distress is through crying. Infants will cry to express anything. Parents can often tell what is upsetting their child simply by listening to the tone of the child's crying—that is, they know the difference between a basic cry (which conveys hunger, discomfort, frustration, or sleepiness) and one that conveys anger or pain. Infants occasionally make another distinct cry—an alarming distressed cry. This cry may be heard when an unexpected event occurs, causing a **situational crisis** for the infant.

Infants who have bonded well with their parents and have good relationships will usually respond predictably when a situational crisis (crisis caused by a specific set of circumstances) occurs. The most prevalent example of a situational crisis is being separated from a parent. Separation anxiety is common and normal in older infants. The normal reaction peaks between 10 and 18 months and involves clingy behavior and fear of unfamiliar places and people. An infant's reaction to a situational crisis is classified into three phases. The **protest phase** can start immediately and usually lasts about a week. It is easily recognized by loud crying, irritability, restlessness, and rejection of other caregivers' efforts. The **despair phase** follows, which is characterized by the monotonous wailing indicating that the infant begins to believe the situation is not going to change. **Withdrawal** eventually happens, and the infant becomes almost apathetic and appears bored by his or her surroundings.

As infants become accustomed to their homes and families, they begin to need the security of a predictable environment. If an infant's environment is too unpredictable, the infant may despair and become withdrawn, which may lead to problems in the development of trust. **Trust and mistrust** refers to a stage of development from birth to about 18 months of age. Most infants desire that their world be planned, organized, and routine. When their caregivers and parents provide this environment for them, the infant gains trust in them. The opposite also holds true; if an infant perceives that his or her parents or caregivers will not provide an organized, routine environment, the infant can develop behavioral problems.

Infants respond well to an instructional technique called **scaffolding**. Scaffolding is a technique in which a person builds on what has already been learned. Paramedic students can also benefit from this technique! For example, the basic assessment skills that students learned in their EMT course will now be used as building blocks for the advanced assessments taught in this paramedic course.

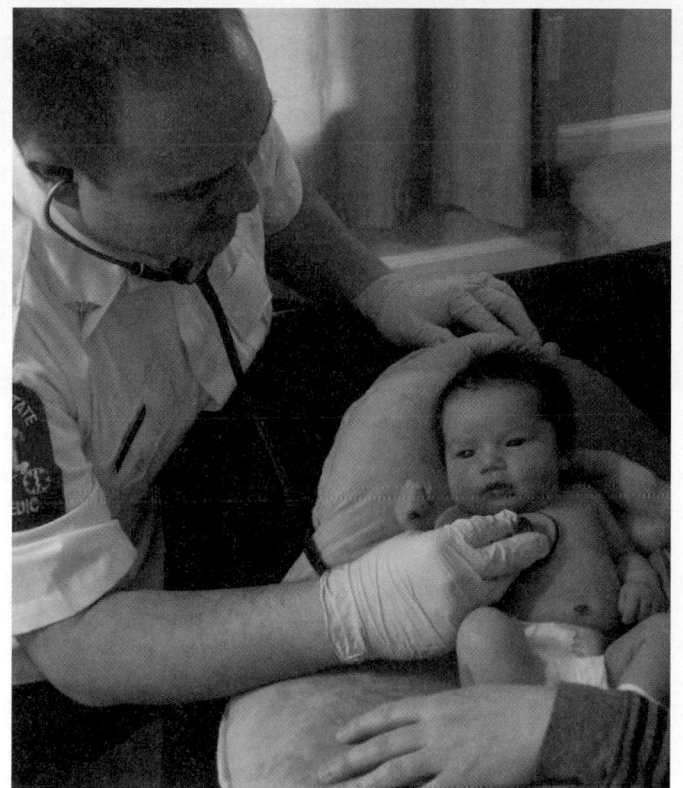

Figure 4 Have the parent or caregiver hold the infant while you perform your assessment and treatment, if possible.

Temperament

With regard to temperament, children are classified as being easy, difficult, or slow to warm up. Easy children are characterized by the relative ease by which they adapt to their surroundings and lifestyle. Their body functions are working properly, they have low-intensity reactions, and they accept new surroundings well. A difficult child will have intense reactions, and does not acclimate to new surroundings well. A child who is slow to warm up usually has a low-intensity reaction but generally is in a negative mood.

As a paramedic, you can adjust your approach according to the developmental stage of your patient. Effective techniques include having the caregiver hold the infant and allowing the infant to hold a toy **Figure 4**. In fact, physical assessment of an infant should be completed with the infant in the caregiver's arms unless the child is in respiratory failure, in need of spinal immobilization, or has a reduced level of consciousness. You may also distract the child and save the most difficult part of the assessment and treatment for last.

■ Toddlers and Preschoolers

▌ Physical Changes

In <u>toddlers</u> (ages 1 to 3 years **Figure 5**) and <u>preschoolers</u> (ages 3 to 5 years **Figure 6**), the pulse rate and respiratory rate are slower than the corresponding vital signs in infants, whereas the systolic blood pressure is higher (approximately 100 mm Hg). At the same time, weight gain should level off.

A toddler's cardiovascular system is not dramatically different from that of an adult. A toddler's lungs continue to develop more bronchioles and alveoli. Although toddlers and preschoolers have more lung tissue, they do not have well-developed lung musculature, which prevents them from sustaining deep or rapid respirations for an extended period of time.

The loss of passive immunity in the immune system is possibly the most obvious development at this stage of human life. "Colds" often develop that may manifest as gastrointestinal distress or upper respiratory tract infections. As toddlers spend more time around playmates and classmates, they acquire their own immunity as the body is exposed to various pathogens.

Neuromuscular growth also makes considerable progress at this age. Toddlers and preschoolers spend a great deal of time finding out exactly how to use their expansive nervous system and the muscles it controls by walking, running, jumping, and playing catch **Figure 7**. Watching children play as they age from 1 to 5 years demonstrates how they move from gross motor activities (grabbing an object with the full palm) to fine motor activities (picking up a crayon). By the end of this stage, preschoolers will have a brain that weighs 90% of its final adult weight. In addition, all of this playing places stress on the muscles and bones. Consequently, muscle mass increases, as does bone density.

This stage also includes the continued development of the renal system and perhaps the most anticipated event of

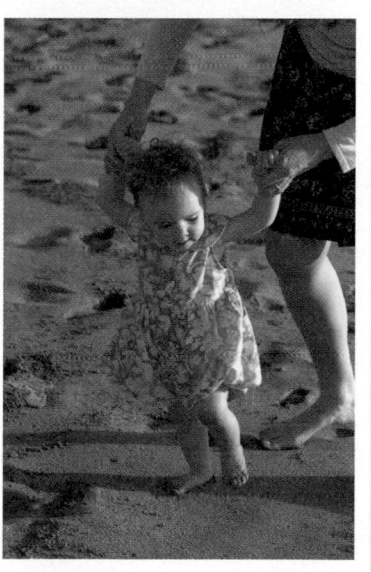

Figure 5 A toddler.

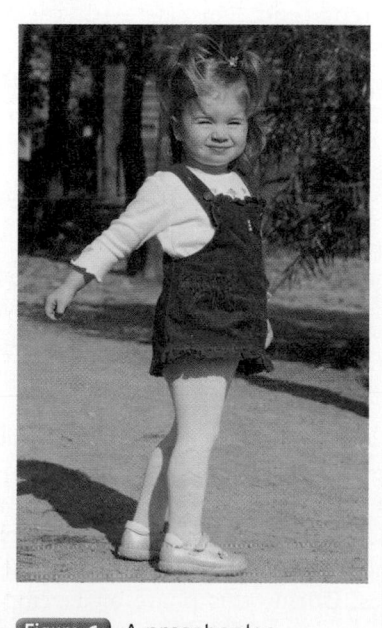

Figure 6 A preschooler.

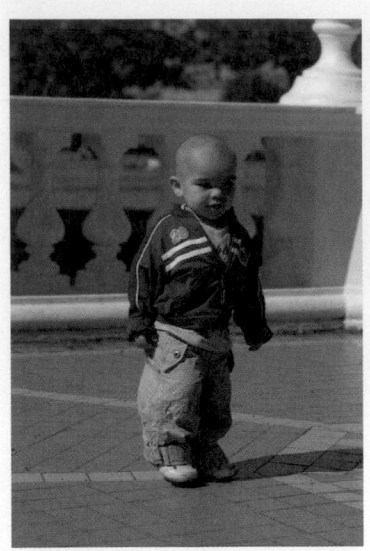

Figure 7 Toddlers learn to walk, one of the major milestones in life.

this stage of life—toilet training! Physiologically, toddlers have the neuromuscular control needed for bladder control and can feel when the bladder is full by 12 to 15 months of age. On average, the 18-month-old child has the ability to control his or her muscles to delay excretion for a short period of time. However, the child may not be psychologically ready until 18 to 30 months of age. There might not be any greater satisfaction for a child of this age than to run up to his parents and tell them, "I'm a big boy now, I used the potty!"

Other developments that continue during this time frame include the emergence of "baby" teeth. Teething (ie, "breaking teeth" through the gums) can be painful and accompanied by fever. In addition, parents and toddlers are enthralled with sensory development—for example, tickling.

Psychosocial Changes

This period of development is often exciting for parents. Toddlers or preschoolers are learning to speak and express themselves, thereby taking a major step toward independence. At the same time, toddlers are very attached to their parents and feel safe with them. Separation anxiety peaks between 10 and 18 months of age. It is fascinating to watch a child struggle through the conflict of wanting to play, yet also wanting to be protected.

In most toddlers, basic language is mastered at 36 months of age. Refinement of this skill is continued throughout childhood. By the age of 3 or 4 years, most children can use and understand full sentences. As they progress through this stage of their life, they will go from using language to communicate what they want to using language creatively and playfully.

This is also the time when toddlers begin to interact with other playmates and start to play games. Playing games teaches control, following rules, and even competitiveness. A lot of learning and development take place when children watch their peers during group outings, such as "play dates." Of course, behavior observed on television and computers can also be learned, which is why some parents limit their children's viewing choices or the amount of time they devote to these activities. During this phase of development, children also learn to recognize sexual differences by observing their role models and siblings.

Words of Wisdom

When you are dealing with patients who are very young, try to keep their routine the same by keeping family and familiar items nearby.

With toddlers and preschoolers, you might try to "break the ice" by giving them a teddy bear and explaining what you are going to do by showing them on the teddy bear. Such children may be able to understand by show-and-tell more clearly than using only a verbal description. Be sure that the toy has no removable parts, and store it in a clean plastic bag between calls.

As with infants, it is important to include the parent or caregiver when working with a toddler or preschool-age child. Also, be sure to position yourself at the child's level so that you are making eye contact. Explain to the child what you are going to do before you do it, and allow the child to make choices when possible. As with infants, save the most difficult part of the assessment and treatment for last.

Another tip—do not try to reason with a child as to why a procedure (such as establishing an IV line) has to be done. Explain it briefly at a level they can understand, make sure they are secure, and then do it! Often the psychological experience can be worse than the physical one if you give them too much time to worry about a minor procedure.

Documentation and Communication

When documenting your assessment of a young child or infant, it is often best to avoid struggling with a stable patient to obtain a blood pressure. Simply documenting lung sounds, an apical pulse, and the child's interactions with his or her surroundings can more than adequately describe your patient's condition.

Parenting Styles

A child's development is affected by the parenting style employed by his or her parents. Although the process of parenting is a complex behavior, rarely well defined in any one individual, three idealized approaches may be examined. An <u>authoritarian</u> parenting style demands absolute obedience from a child no matter what the situation. This style of parenting shows no regard for the child's personal freedoms, for example, when a child is punished for simply questioning a parent. Children who are raised in this manner often develop self-esteem problems; females are more likely to become shy and males are more likely to become argumentative or hostile.

<u>Authoritative</u> parenting is based on respect for parental authority and balance with individual freedom of the child. These parents regularly respond to the personal needs of the child. They set rules and enforce them fairly; however, they believe that children need certain freedoms and attempt

to maintain a balance between the two. This style can allow children to develop into adults who are independent, well-socialized, and easy going.

Permissive parenting does not impose many rules, if any, on the child. The child is in control and the parent takes a very tolerant approach to the child's behavior, including socially unacceptable behaviors. Permissive parenting is broken into two subcategories—indifferent and indulgent. The former style describes parents who just do not care; the latter style describes parents who are excessively lenient. Permissive parents rarely, if ever, punish their children, and therefore their children may grow up to be considered spoiled. These children often become adults who are immature, irresponsible, and lack self-control.

Divorce

More than half of the marriages in the United States result in divorce. No matter what stage of life a child is in, a divorce will have a profound effect. Children naturally question if the divorce was their fault, may second-guess themselves as to what they could have done to prevent it, and experience pain from having their environment changed. Many parents respond to their child's feelings and needs together, and by doing so, they assure their children that although their life will experience some changes, they will always have a mommy and daddy who love them very much. Unfortunately, divorce has almost become commonplace. Nonetheless, as long as both parents maintain their children as their priority, most children adapt relatively easily to the social changes a divorce brings upon a family.

School-Age Children

Physical Changes

From ages 6 to 12 years, a school-age child's vital signs and body gradually approach those observed in adulthood Figure 8 . Obvious physical traits and body function changes become apparent as most children grow about 4 lb (2 kg) and 2½″ (6 cm) each year. Brain function develops further in both hemispheres, and permanent teeth also come in during this period. Also, the onset of puberty may begin in elementary school-age children and has been documented at age 10 years or younger.

Psychosocial Changes

Children are engaged in a great deal of psychosocial growing up during the school years, though the pace of development varies from child to child. Parents as a whole do not devote as much

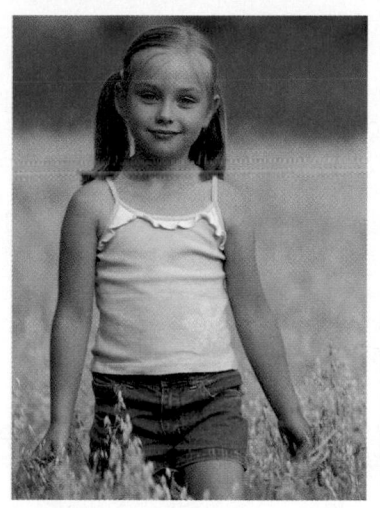
Figure 8 A school-age child.

YOU *are the Medic* | **PART 3**

Your partner asks the mother what Shane's favorite item is and she answers, "his blanket." Your partner asks the mother to retrieve the blanket and to show her where the fall occurred. The mother agrees and both enter the residence. The father is still struggling with the child and you ask him to loosen his embrace and allow the child to pick his position of comfort. Your partner and the mother return with the child's blanket. Your partner sits down on the ground slightly lower than the child and offers him the blanket. Shane takes the blanket from her and appears to calm down considerably. You begin your assessment carefully.

Recording Time: 7 Minutes	
Respirations	Crying
Pulse	130 beats/min
Skin	Hot, dry, red
Blood pressure	Unable to obtain
Oxygen saturation (Spo$_2$)	Unable to obtain
Pupils	Reactive

5. Measurement of Spo$_2$ and blood pressure requires equipment. How can you gain the child's trust in order to use your equipment?

6. What is the expected normal range for a 3-year-old child's pulse and respiratory rate?

time to their children during this phase. Nevertheless, it is at this critical time in human development that children learn various types of reasoning. In **preconventional reasoning**, children act almost purely to avoid punishment and to get what they want. In **conventional reasoning**, they look for approval from their peers and society. In **postconventional reasoning**, children make decisions guided by their conscience.

During this stage, children begin to develop their **self-concept** and **self-esteem**. Self-concept is a person's perception of himself or herself; self-esteem is how a person feels about himself or herself, and how a person feels about how he or she fits in with peers.

When you are working with a school-age child, use the same techniques employed for a preschool-age child (position yourself at the child's level, explain what you are going to do, and give choices). Always be honest about what you are doing. For example, if a procedure might hurt, say that to your patient. The biggest issue with school-aged children is trust. You have to earn it quickly through open and honest communication and you must never lose it through lies or "sneaky" maneuvers. Be direct with them, remain assertive, and they will respond well most of the time.

Adolescents (Teenagers)

Physical Changes

The vital signs of **adolescents** (ages 13 through 17 years Figure 9) begin to level off within the adult ranges, with a systolic blood pressure of generally between 90 and 110 mm Hg, a pulse rate between 60 and 100 beats/min, and respirations in the range of 12 to 20 breaths/min.

Adolescence is also the time of life when humans experience a rapid, 2- to 3-year growth spurt (that is, an increase in muscle and bone growth) as well as changes in blood chemistry. Growth begins with the hands and feet, then moves to the long bones of the extremities, and finishes with growth of the torso. As a whole, boys experience this stage of development later in life than girls do. When this period of growth has finished, however, boys are generally taller and stronger than girls. Muscle mass and bone density are nearly at adult levels.

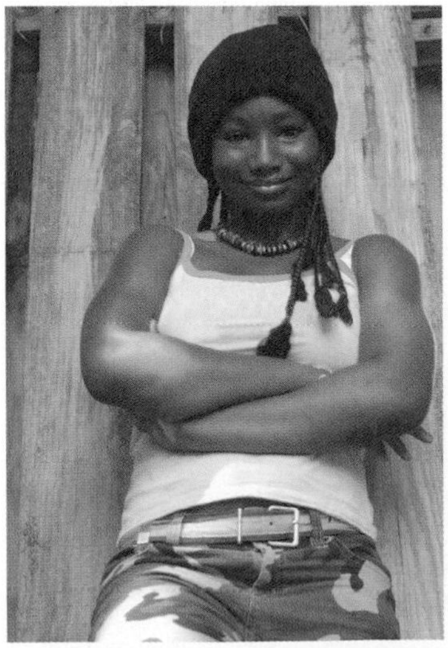

One of the more subtle changes during this phase of life is the maturation of the human reproductive system. Secondary sexual development begins, along with enlargement of the external sex organs. Pubic hair and axillary hair begin to appear. Voices start to change in range and depth. In females, the breasts and thighs increase in size as adipose tissue is deposited there. Menstruation begins during this time; however, **menarche** (the first menstrual bleeding) is starting to occur at increasingly younger ages, so it is not uncommon to begin menstruation prior to becoming a teenager.

Another key development in female teenagers is the release of follicle-stimulating hormone and luteinizing hormone, both of which increase estrogen and progesterone production. In contrast, the hormone gonadotropin is secreted in males and results in the production of testosterone. Acne can occur due to hormonal changes.

These changes in the endocrine and reproductive systems provide the platform for reproduction. By the middle of adolescence, boys are able to produce sufficient sperm and girls are able to develop eggs for reproduction to take place.

Psychosocial Changes

Adolescents and their families often deal with conflict as teenagers try to gain control of their lives from their parents. Privacy becomes an issue among adolescents, their siblings, and their parents. Self-consciousness also increases. Adolescents may struggle to create their own identity—to define who they are Figure 10 , for example, by dressing in a certain style of clothing to fit their personality. Adolescents use the feedback from their family and peers to help create their adult image. Adolescents are often caught between two worlds. They want to be treated like adults yet want to be cared for like younger children.

Figure 9 An adolescent.

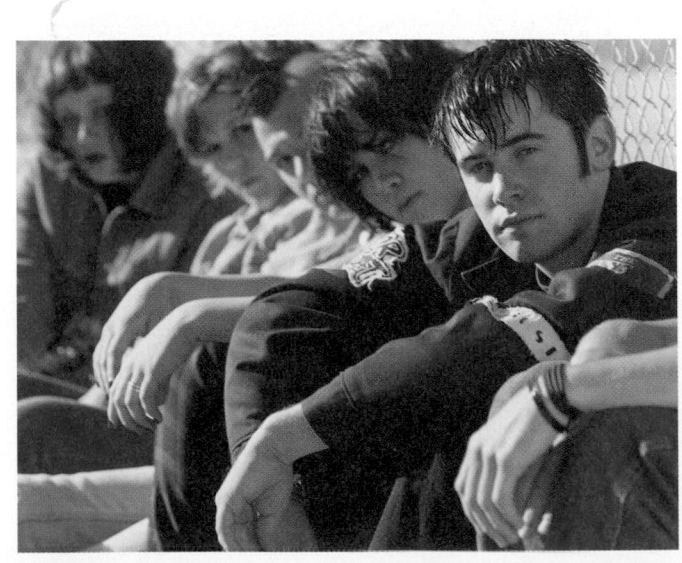

Figure 10 Adolescents want to fit in and may struggle to create an identity.

Rebellious behavior can be part of an adolescent trying to find his or her own identity. Adolescents continually compare themselves with their peers, which makes peer pressure a major factor in the psychological growth of an adolescent. Antisocial behavior peaks during the eighth or ninth grade. Adolescence is also a time when eating disorders may develop as teenagers become obsessed with body image. Self-destructive behaviors such as smoking, drinking, and experimenting with drugs may begin. Although these behaviors can be very troubling to parents, the adolescent is trying to determine if he or she is ready to take control of his or her own life. An adolescent's struggle toward independence may include setbacks that can be devastating. Patience and support from family and friends are essential in assisting an adolescent's transition into adulthood.

Adolescents may also show greater interest in sexual relations. Many adolescents are fixated on their public image and are terrified of being embarrassed. At this age, a code of personal ethics is developed, based partly on the ethics and values of the parents and partly on the influence of the teenager's environment. At this tumultuous time, teenagers are at a higher risk than other populations for suicide and depression.

When you are working with adolescents, be respectful and discreet. Privacy is important to adolescents. If possible, have your partner speak with the parent in a separate area while you talk with the patient **Figure 11**. This may make the adolescent more comfortable and provide you more accurate answers than you would receive in the presence of a parent.

Words of Wisdom

It is best to ask adolescent patients certain questions in total privacy, where they feel they can answer without constraint.

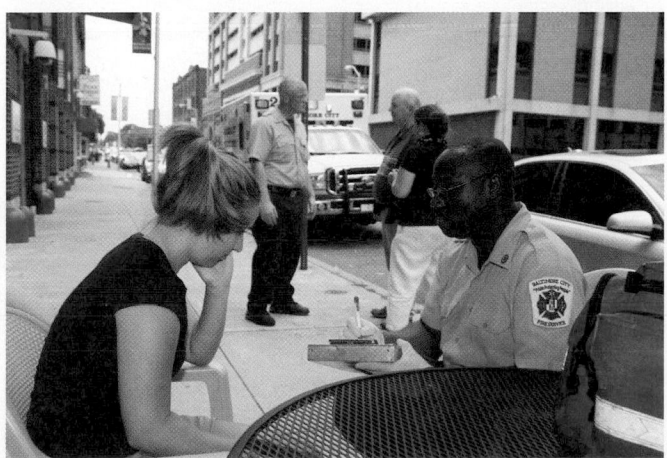

Figure 11 Try to interview adolescent patients in privacy, if possible.

Early Adults

Physical Changes

<u>Early adults</u> range in age from 18 to 40 years **Figure 12**. Their vital signs do not vary greatly from those seen throughout adulthood. Ideally, the human pulse rate will stay around 70 beats/min, the respiratory rate will stay in the range of 12 to 20 breaths/min, and the systolic blood pressure will be approximately 120/80 mm Hg.

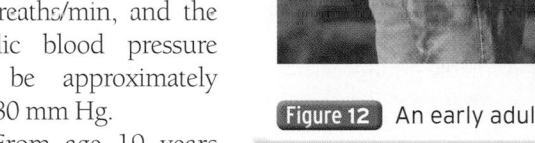

Figure 12 An early adult.

From age 19 years to just a little after 25 years, the human body should be functioning at its optimal level. After this point, the disks in the spine begin to settle, and height can sometimes be affected, causing a "shrinking." Fatty tissue increases, which leads to weight gain. Muscle strength decreases, and the reflexes slow. For all these reasons, accidents are common causes of death in this age group.

Psychosocial Changes

Three words best describe a human's world during this stage of life: work, family, stress. During this period, humans strive to create a place for themselves in the world, and many do everything they can to "settle down." As early adults struggle to find stability in their careers, stress on the job becomes high. Along with this natural tendency to settle come the experiences of romantic and affectionate love. Childbirth is most common in this age group. Despite all of this stress and change, this age group enjoys one of the more stable periods of life. People in early adulthood generally experience fewer psychological problems related to well-being.

Middle Adults

Physical Changes

<u>Middle adults</u> are ages 41 to 60 years **Figure 13**. Even though the body is still functioning at a high level, this age group is vulnerable to vision and hearing loss along with other varying degrees of degradation. Cardiovascular health also becomes an issue in many people in this age group. Cardiac output decreases, while cholesterol levels increase, leading to higher incidences of cardiovascular disease. Owing to the decrease in metabolism, it becomes more difficult for middle adults to control weight. Middle adults also experience a greater incidence of cancer. In women, menopause—the cessation of menstruation—begins in the late 40s or early 50s.

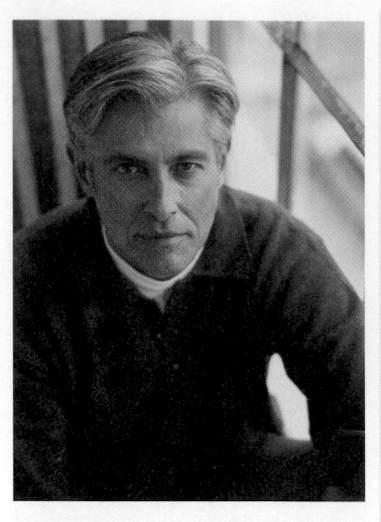

Figure 13 A middle adult.

This change can result in both the loss of bone density and the development of cardiovascular disease. Subsequently, these women are at a higher risk for fractures and cardiac problems.

Psychosocial Changes

Middle adults tend to focus on achieving their life's goals, as they realize that they are past the halfway point in human life expectancy. After years of nurturing and living with children, parents must readjust their lifestyle as their children leave the home, commonly called the "empty nest" syndrome. Finances may become a worrisome issue, as people plan for retirement while still managing everyday financial demands. During this time, people often view crisis as a challenge to be overcome rather than a threat to be avoided.

Late Adults

Physical Changes

Late adults include those ages 61 and older **Figure 14**. Life expectancy is constantly changing. When the first edition of this text was printed in 1979, life expectancy was about 73 years. It

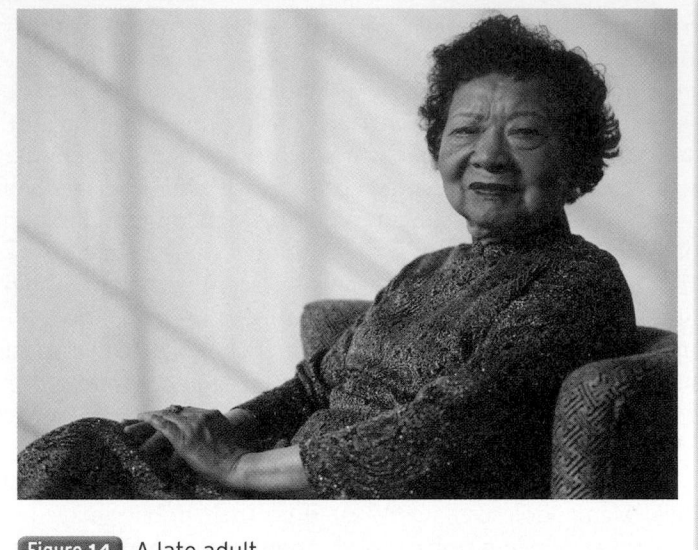

Figure 14 A late adult.

is now approximately 78 years, with maximum life expectancy estimated at 120 years.

Later in life, the vital signs depend on the patient's overall health, medical conditions, and medications taken. Today's late adults are staying active longer than their ancestors did. Thanks to medical advances, they are often able to overcome numerous medical problems, but may need multiple medications to do so **Figure 15**.

Cardiovascular System

Cardiac function declines with age consequent to anatomic and physiologic changes that are largely related to atherosclerosis. In this disorder, which most commonly affects coronary vessels, cholesterol and calcium build up inside the walls of blood

---

YOU *are the Medic* | **PART 4**

You and your partner are slowly gaining the trust of your patient. You are finally able to see a ½″ laceration on the child's forehead with a corresponding abrasion and hematoma. The wound is not actively bleeding.

Recording Time: 17 Minutes	
Respirations	20 breaths/min
Pulse	118 beats/min
Skin	Hot, dry, pink
Blood pressure	Unable to obtain
Oxygen saturation (Spo$_2$)	99% room air
Pupils	Reactive

7. You need to bandage your patient's laceration. Offer some ideas to make this more acceptable to the patient.

8. How should this patient be transported?

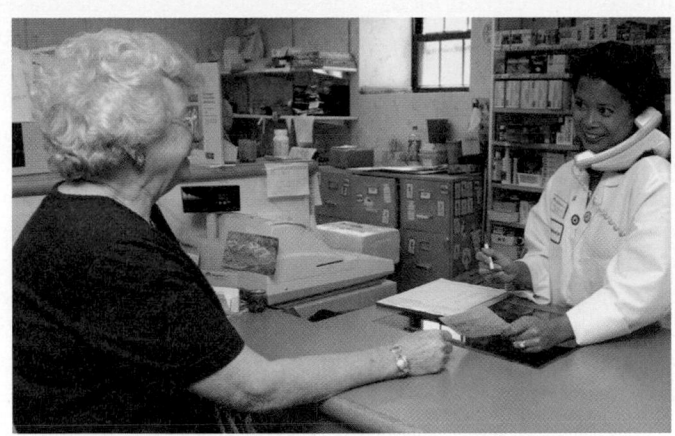

Figure 15 Older people are often on multiple medications to help them stay active.

vessels, forming plaque. The accumulation of plaque eventually leads to partial or complete blockage of blood flow. Atherosclerosis can also contribute to development of an **aneurysm**, or weakening and bulging of the blood vessel wall; an aneurysm may potentially rupture if it is subjected to high stretching forces. More than 60% of people older than age 65 have atherosclerotic disease.

Other age-related changes typically include a decrease in pulse rate, a decline in cardiac output (the amount of blood circulated each minute), and the inability to elevate cardiac output to match the demands of the body. This translates into a heart that is less able to respond to exercise or disease (for example, by an increased pulse rate). In the event of a life-threatening illness, the body typically needs to increase the pulse rate to ensure adequate blood pressure. Because heart muscle may be weakened with age, the increase in pulse rate can actually cause damage to the heart itself.

The vascular system also becomes "stiff." Because of this change, the diastolic blood pressure increases with age. The left ventricle must then work harder to move blood effectively, so it becomes thicker, losing its elasticity in this process. The thickening and stiffening of this muscle hinders filling in the ventricle, thereby decreasing cardiac output. Similar stiffening occurs in the heart valves, which may impede normal blood flow into and out of the heart. As the blood passes through these stiffened valves, a heart murmur may be heard, even in the absence of disease. Decreases in elastin and collagen in blood vessel walls reduce the elasticity of the peripheral vessels by as much as 70%. Compensation for blood pressure changes will be hampered because these vessels are less able to distend and contract.

Blood cells are also affected by aging. The body's cells originate from within the bone marrow. As a person ages, more of the bone marrow is replaced with fatty tissue. This replacement decreases the ability of the bones to manufacture more blood cells when needed. Although typically by itself the fatty tissue does not pose a problem, if an elderly person sustains trauma, the ability of the body to produce blood cells to replace those

lost is diminished. Finally, functional blood volume gradually declines over time.

Respiratory System

In late adults, the size of the airway increases and the surface area of the alveoli decreases. Metabolic changes cause the natural elasticity of the lungs to decrease, forcing people to increasingly rely on their intercostal muscles to breathe. In addition, the chest becomes more rigid because of calcification of the ribs to the sternum, which adds to the difficulty of breathing. As the elasticity of the lungs decreases, the overall strength of the intercostal muscles and diaphragm also decreases. These factors together make breathing more labor-intensive for elderly people. You might think that a rigid chest would be more protecting, but this rigidity actually makes the chest more fragile. Overall, the bone structure of late adults is weakened. Instead of the chest being able to bend and give if struck, the calcified bony structure of the chest can fracture. As with all of the physical changes related to aging, however, the changes in the respiratory system are often gradual and go unnoticed until a severe, life-threatening condition occurs. An older person will then have less respiratory reserve to maintain adequate breathing.

Within the mouth and nose, there is a gradual loss of the mechanisms that protect the upper airway. This loss leads to decreased ability to clear secretions and decreased cough and gag reflexes. The number of cilia that line the airways diminishes with age; this results in decreased sensation to foreign objects such as dust or smoke, and less responsiveness when structures of the airway are innervated. With a lesser ability to maintain upper airway function, aspiration and obstruction become more likely.

When a younger patient inhales, the airway maintains its shape, allowing air to enter. As the smooth muscles of the lower airway weaken with age, strong inhalation can make the walls of the airway collapse inward and cause inspiratory wheezing **Figure 16**. The collapsing airways result in low flow rates, because less air can move through the smaller airways, and air trapping, because air does not completely exit the alveoli (incomplete expiration).

By age 75 years, the vital capacity (the volume of air moved during the deepest inspiration and expiration) may amount to only 50% of the vital capacity noted in young adulthood. Factors contributing to this decline include loss of respiratory muscle mass, increased stiffness of the thoracic cage, and decreased surface area available for the exchange of air.

Physiologically, vital capacity decreases and residual volume (the amount of air left in the lungs after expiration of the maximum possible amount of air) increases with age. As a consequence, stagnant air remains in the alveoli and hampers gas exchange. This effect can produce **hypercarbia** (increased carbon dioxide in the bloodstream) and acidosis, even when the person is at rest.

Endocrine System

As with other systems of the body, the function of the endocrine system gradually declines. As people get older, they tend to slow their physical activity. Unfortunately, many do not decrease their

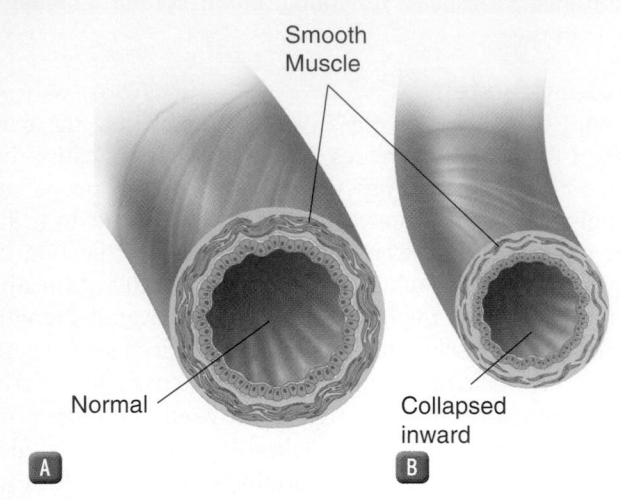

Smooth
Muscle

Normal

A

Collapsed
inward

B

Figure 16 **A.** Healthy muscle in a younger patient's airway helps maintain the open airway during the pressures of inhalation. **B.** Muscle weakening with age can lead to airway collapse that may produce wheezing.

food intake. When a person gains weight, more insulin is needed to control the body's metabolism and blood glucose (sugar) level. However, insulin production and glucose metabolism decrease, so late adults are more prone to the development of diabetes mellitus. Changes in a late adult's mental status may also be the result of changes in his or her blood glucose level. The reproductive systems of both men and women change with age. Men are able to produce sperm long into their 80s but the rigidity of the penis tends to decrease over time. It is unclear whether this decrease is due to aging itself or other conditions such as cardiovascular disease. During menopause, decreased production of regulating hormones results in atrophy of the woman's reproductive organs. The uterus and vagina both decrease in size. Hormone production for both sexes gradually decreases as people age. Sexual desire may diminish with age but does not cease.

Renal and Gastrointestinal Systems

In the kidneys, both structural and functional changes occur in the late adult. The filtration function of these organs, for example, declines by 50% between the ages of 20 and 90 years. Kidney mass decreases by 20% over the same span of time. The number of **nephrons**—the sophisticated capillaries that are basic filtering units in the kidneys—also declines between the ages of 30 and 80 years. One portion of the nephron is the glomeruli. The decreased blood supply causes more abnormal glomeruli to be present as a person ages. Aging kidneys respond less efficiently to hemodynamic stress (ie, stress relating to the circulation of blood) and to fluid and electrolyte imbalances. Therefore, there is a decrease in the body's ability to eliminate wastes and a decreased ability to conserve fluids when needed.

Changes in gastrointestinal function may inhibit nutritional intake and utilization in older adults, resulting in vitamin and mineral deficiencies. In the mouth, for example, taste bud sensitivity to salty and sweet sensations decreases. Teeth become weaker during this phase of life, making it more difficult for late

adults to chew certain foods. The secretion of saliva decreases, which reduces the body's ability to process complex carbohydrates. Gastric motility slows with age because of the loss of intestinal tract neurons, which can lead older adults to feel constipated or not hungry. Likewise, gastric acid secretion diminishes. Blood flow in the vessels supplying the mesentery (membranes that connect organs to the abdominal wall) may drop by as much as 50%, decreasing the ability of the intestines to extract nutrients from digested food. Gallstones become increasingly common with age, and anal sphincter changes reduce elasticity and can produce fecal incontinence. Believe it or not, this is often a great concern to many patients in this age group. Many patients keep meticulous track of their bowel movements and can become quite concerned should they not have a bowel movement for a day or two. Whereas this situation does not necessarily constitute an emergency, it can still be a valid fear that the patient has. A good paramedic always asks about bowel habits during their interview and remembers that the patient has the right to define their own emergency.

Nervous System

Nervous system changes can result in the most debilitating of age-related ailments. In the central nervous system, the brain weight may shrink 10% to 20% by age 80 years. A selective loss of 5% to 50% of neurons occurs, and the surviving neurons shrink in size. The frontal lobe may lose as much as 20% of its synapses (the junctions between neurons) during the course of a person's life. Motor and sensory neural networks become slower and less responsive. The metabolic rate in the older brain does not change, however, and oxygen consumption remains constant throughout life.

One natural consequence of aging is a change in sleep patterns. For example, instead of sleeping through the night, elderly people may take a nap during the day and be up late at night. Their sleep cycle may move into a biphasic (two-phased) sleep cycle—for example, sleep from 1 AM to 6 AM and nap from 12 PM to 3 PM.

The brain, which is surrounded by the meninges, takes up almost all of the space in the skull. Cerebrospinal fluid protects the brain inside these membranes. Unfortunately, age-related shrinkage creates a void between the brain and the outermost layer of the meninges, which provides room for the brain to move when stressed. This shrinkage also stretches the bridging veins that return blood from inside the brain to the dura mater. If trauma moves the brain forcibly, the bridging veins can tear and bleed **Figure 17**. Bleeding can empty into this void, resulting in a subdural hematoma, which may go unnoticed for some time in this age group. Increased intracranial pressure is required for signs of head trauma to be present; the intracranial pressure will not rise—and, therefore, its signs will not be present—until the void has been filled and pressurized. (For more information, see the chapter, *Head and Spine Trauma*.)

Functioning of the peripheral nervous system also slows with age. Sensation becomes diminished and misinterpreted. The ability to know where the body is in space (proprioception) can be diminished. Increased reaction times cause longer delays between stimulation and motion. The resulting slowdown in

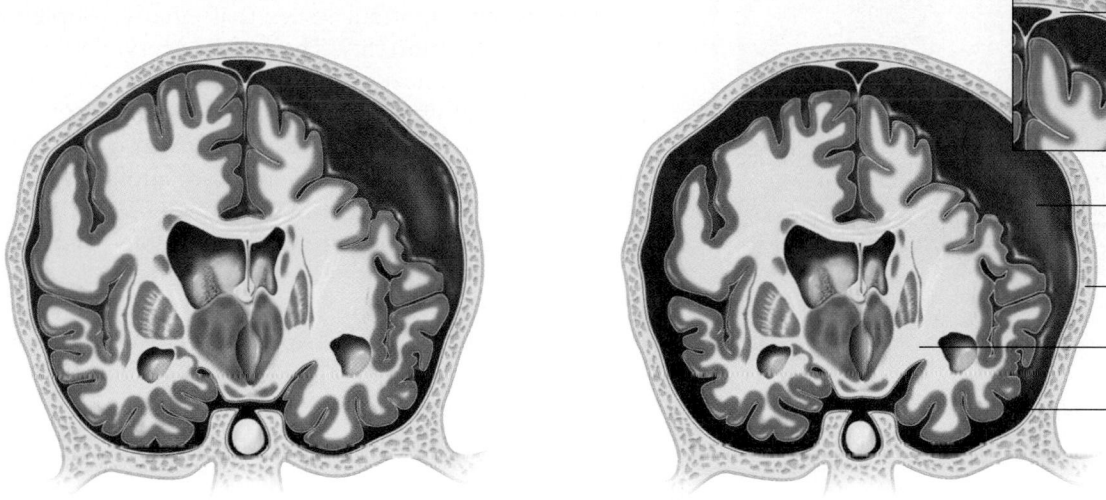

Meninges (dura mater)

Subdural hematoma

Skull

Brain

CSF

Younger adult

Older adult

Figure 17 Age-related atrophy or shrinkage of the brain results in a space between the brain and its cover, the dura mater. Bleeding into this area can occur more easily from trauma because veins are stretched. Because of the additional space, bleeding in an older brain does not always produce immediate signs of increased intracranial pressure.

reflexes and decreased kinesthetic sense may contribute to the incidence of falls and trauma. Nerve endings deteriorate, and the ability of the skin to sense the surroundings becomes hindered. Hot, cold, sharp, and wet items can all create dangerous situations because reaction time and pain perception are both diminished in late adults.

Sensory Changes

In addition to a diminished sensation of touch, the other senses are also affected by aging. Often it is assumed that elderly people are hard of hearing and have difficulty seeing. It is true that in all late adults, there are changes that diminish the effectiveness of the eyes and ears; however, most elderly people can still hear well and are able to see clearly. They may need glasses or hearing aids, but it is wrong to assume that your older patient is deaf and nearly blind. Pupillary reaction and ocular movements become more restricted with age. The pupils are generally smaller in older patients, and the opacity of the eye's lens diminishes visual acuity and makes the pupils sluggish when responding to light. Visual distortions are also common in older people. Thickening of the lens makes it harder for the eye to focus, especially at close range. Peripheral fields of vision become narrower, and a greater sensitivity to glare constricts the visual field.

Hearing loss is about four times more common than loss of vision in late adults. Changes in several hearing-related structures may lead to a loss of high-frequency hearing, or even deafness.

Finally, loss of taste bud sensation and a decline in olfactory (sense of smell) perception are normal occurrences. Unfortunately, these changes make eating less pleasurable, which can contribute to an older person's lack of adequate nutrition.

Psychosocial Changes

Paramedics should treasure their opportunities to spend time with and communicate with late adults. Many of them have amazing stories and experiences to share with us, yet we often take them for granted. Older people have a great amount of wisdom to share, and we need to remind them of their worth. Indeed, until about 5 years before death, most late-stage adults retain high brain function. In the 5 years preceding death, however, mental function is presumed to decline, a theory referred to as the **terminal drop hypothesis**.

As the elderly population continues to grow, we have the responsibility to seek out unique ways to accommodate their needs during their last 20 to 40 years of life. Statistics indicate that 95% of elderly people live at home. They certainly may have the assistance of family, friends, or home health care, but they are relatively healthy, active, and independent. Although most older adults live at home, the number of assisted-living communities is growing across the nation. These facilities allow older adults to live in campus-based communities with people in their own age group, while enjoying the privacy of their own apartment and the security of nursing care, maintenance, and food preparation, if desired **Figure 18** . Unfortunately, these facilities can be expensive.

Most people need to deal with financial issues throughout their lives. Few things in life produce more worry and stress than money problems. Late adults, in particular, may constantly worry about rising costs of health care and are often forced to make decisions such as whether to pay for groceries or their medication. Modern families often take less responsibility for their elderly family members than earlier generations did. Today, more than 50% of all single women in the United States who are

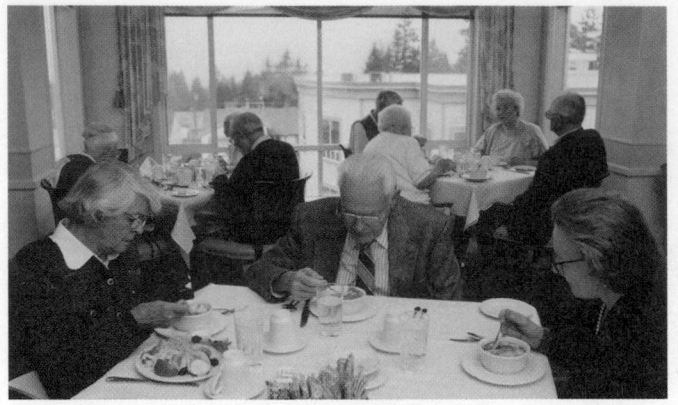

Figure 18 Many older adults live in assisted-living facilities.

60 years of age or older are living at or below the poverty level. This problem remains to be resolved.

One of the important issues that elderly people need to face is their own mortality. The fact is, everyone dies. Yet for most of us, this concept is an intellectual exercise with a distant connection to reality. It is difficult for late adults to watch as their friends, relatives, and companions grow older and die, leaving them seemingly alone. Late adults may feel useless or worry about being a burden to their families as their health declines and they are no longer able to take care of themselves. Isolation and depression are challenges for elderly people.

Many elderly people are happy and actively participating in life. With good financial resources and a good support system of family and friends, elderly people in their 80s and beyond can enjoy life and continue to feel productive.

YOU are the Medic   SUMMARY

1. What is your first concern at this scene?

With the family actively moving toward your vehicle, scene safety is the primary concern. The mother and father may try to open doors to get their son inside for your care. There may be a fall or other unintended injury as a result. Remember, in this case you actually have three patients to care for until you can gain control of the situation.

2. What stage of development describes a 3-year-old child and how will this affect your assessment?

This child is on the older end of the toddler phase of development, which ranges in age from 1 to 3 years old. By 3 years of age, bone density and muscle mass increase to become more adult-like. On impact, older toddlers are less flexible because they have less cartilage and fat storage.

3. Why is Shane clinging to his father and turning away from your voice?

Fear of strangers is pronounced in toddlers and preschoolers. Shane has also had an interruption in his normal routine and a loss of control over his environment. The toddler may also be sensing his parents' sense of urgency, reinforcing the thought, "There is something really wrong here." These are all issues that will need to be overcome in the successful treatment of this child.

4. What are some of the measures you can take to alleviate the child's reaction?

Gaining the trust of the father and mother is paramount in order to gain the trust of the toddler. Once you gain the support of the caregiver, approach the toddler in a calm, friendly manner. If you can find a favorite toy or object that will normally comfort the child, use it. In this case the father is actively fighting his son to turn him around to face you. The toddler age group looks for the caregiver to protect them from harm, not hurt them. Allowing the toddler to move as he wishes (condition permitting), rather than being physically forced is always preferred.

5. Measurement of Spo$_2$ and blood pressure requires equipment. How can you gain the child's trust in order to use your equipment?

Unfamiliar equipment can be especially frightening for a child. Any item that attaches to the child may present a problem. One of the best methods to overcome the fear is to show the equipment to the child. Show the child what it is, how it is used, and let the child touch it prior to using it (condition permitting). If any part of your examination or treatment is going to hurt, never lie and say it will not. It will completely eliminate any trust that you have built.

6. What is the expected normal range for a 3-year-old child's pulse and respiratory rate?

A normal pulse rate for toddlers ranges from 90 to 150 beats/min, depending on the child's level of physical development. Respiratory rates range from 20 to 30 breaths/min.

7. You need to bandage your patient's laceration. Offer some ideas to make this more acceptable to the patient.

As mentioned earlier, it is important to explain what you are going to do before you do it. In this case you need to bandage a laceration on the toddler's forehead. If conditions allow, ask the parents to assist with the bandaging. Allow the child to hold a toy or other special item during bandaging so the situation will be less scary.

8. How should this patient be transported?

Most EMS providers have a policy on family members accompanying patients to the hospital. Please make sure you are familiar with this policy. Younger children have a strong fear of being left alone or of being taken away from their family. It is preferable to have one of the parents ride in the patient compartment with the child for comfort. This is only advisable if the family member can be properly seated with an acceptable automotive restraint firmly fastened.

SUMMARY, *continued*

EMS Patient Care Report (PCR)

Date: 05-01-11	**Incident No.:** 0909	**Nature of Call:** Fall		**Location:** 215 Shady Glen Way	
Dispatched: 1400	**En Route:** 1400	**At Scene:** 1407	**Transport:** 1429	**At Hospital:** 1449	**In Service:** 1459

Patient Information

Age: 3 years **Sex:** M **Weight (in kg [lb]):** 13.6 kg (30 lb)	**Allergies:** Family denies **Medications:** Family denies **Past Medical History:** Family denies **Chief Complaint:** Laceration & abrasion to forehead

Vital Signs

Time: 1407	**BP:** Unable to obtain	**Pulse:** 130	**Respirations:** Crying	**Spo₂:** Unable to obtain
Time: 1417	**BP:** Unable to obtain	**Pulse:** 118	**Respirations:** 20	**Spo₂:** 99% room air
Time:	**BP:**	**Pulse:**	**Respirations:**	**Spo₂:**

EMS Treatment
(circle all that apply)

Oxygen @ _____ L/min via (circle one): NC NRM Bag-mask device	Assisted Ventilation	Airway Adjunct	CPR
Defibrillation	Bleeding Control	(Bandaging)	Splinting	Other

Narrative

Arrived in front of this residence to find the father carrying the 3-year-old male to this unit. Mother is also present. The child appears to be actively resisting the father who is trying to hold him. Family asked to move from the roadway to the front steps of the residence. Father allowed to hold the child who is actively crying. The mother states the child was running in the back yard of this residence when he fell forward, striking his head on the deck. Assessment of the injured area shows a ½" laceration approx 1" superior to the right eye. There is a corresponding hematoma and area of abrasion around the laceration. Pt initially resisted attempts at assessment but was able to be calmed sufficiently. Area of injury successfully bandaged with assistance from family. Pt transported to Children's Hospital with further calming noted during transport. Father allowed per policy in the patient compartment with seat belts in place. Report to Jim RN on arrival at Children's Hospital. **End of report**

Prep Kit

- Developmental stages of life include the following: infant, toddler, preschool-age, school-age, adolescence, early adulthood, middle adulthood, and late adulthood.
- Each developmental stage is marked by different physical and psychological changes and characteristics.
- The vital signs of toddlers (ages 1 to 3 years) and preschoolers (ages 3 to 5 years) differ somewhat from those of an infant.
- From ages 6 to 12 years, the school-age child's vital signs and body gradually approach those observed in adulthood.
- The vital signs of adolescents (ages 13 to 17 years) begin to level off within the adult ranges.
- Vital signs do not vary greatly through adulthood; however, the vital signs of late adults do vary depending on each person's health.
- Infants (1 month to 1 year of age) develop at a startling rate, experiencing specific developmental milestones during every month of the first year of life.
- Two important points regarding an infant's airway are that an infant's tongue can more easily occlude the airway, and the lungs are fragile.
- Infants are classified as an easy child, difficult child, or slow to warm up. Their primary means of communication is crying.
- Toddlers and preschoolers learn to speak and express themselves. Toilet training is usually accomplished around age 28 months.
- A child's development is affected by the parenting style employed by his or her parents. Types of parenting styles include authoritarian, authoritative, and permissive. Divorce may begin to affect children when they are toddlers.
- School-age children (6 to 12 years) develop self-esteem and reasoning abilities and receive their permanent teeth.
- Adolescents (13 to 17 years) undergo significant reproductive development. They also focus on creating their self-image and are self-conscious. They also may engage in self-destructive behavior.
- Early adults (18 to 40 years) focus on work and family. The body should function at an optimal level, and lifelong habits are developed.
- Middle adults (41 to 60 years) focus on achieving life goals. During this stage, medical problems such as diabetes, hypertension, and cancer become more common.
- Late adults (61 years and older) undergo significant physical changes. They also focus on their mortality. Suicide and depression are concerns in this age group.

■ Vital Vocabulary

<u>adolescents</u> Persons who are 13 to 17 years of age.

<u>aneurysm</u> A swelling or enlargement of part of a blood vessel, resulting from weakening of the vessel wall.

<u>anxious avoidant attachment</u> A bond between an infant and his or her parent or caregiver in which the infant is repeatedly rejected and develops an isolated lifestyle that does not depend on the support and care of others.

<u>atherosclerosis</u> A disorder in which cholesterol and calcium build up inside the walls of the blood vessels, forming plaque, which eventually leads to partial or complete blockage of blood flow.

<u>authoritarian</u> A parenting style that demands absolute obedience.

<u>authoritative</u> A parenting style that balances parental authority with the child's freedom by setting and enforcing rules, but also allowing the child to have some freedom.

<u>barotrauma</u> Trauma resulting from increased pressure, for example from too much pressure in the lungs.

<u>bonding</u> The formation of a close, personal relationship.

<u>conventional reasoning</u> A type of reasoning in which a child looks for approval from peers and society.

<u>despair phase</u> The second phase of an infant's response to a situational crisis; characterized by monotonous wailing.

<u>early adults</u> Persons who are 18 to 40 years of age.

<u>fontanelles</u> Areas where the infant's skull has not fused together; usually disappear at approximately 18 months of age.

<u>growth plates</u> Structures located on either end of an infant's bone that aid in lengthening bones as the child grows.

<u>hypercarbia</u> Increased carbon dioxide levels in the bloodstream.

<u>infants</u> Persons who are from 1 month to 1 year of age.

<u>late adults</u> Persons who are 61 years old or older.

<u>life expectancy</u> The average amount of years a person can be expected to live.

<u>menarche</u> The beginning phase of a woman's life cycle of menstruation.

<u>middle adults</u> Persons who are 41 to 60 years of age.

<u>moro reflex</u> An infant reflex in which, when an infant is caught off guard, the infant opens his or her arms wide, spreads the fingers, and seems to grab at things.

<u>nephrons</u> The basic filtering units in the kidneys.

<u>palmar grasp</u> An infant reflex that occurs when something is placed in the infant's palm; the infant grasps the object.

<u>permissive</u> A parenting style in which the parent does not impose many rules, if any, on the child; two subcategories include indifferent and indulgent.

<u>postconventional reasoning</u> A type of reasoning in which a child bases decisions on his or her conscience.

<u>preconventional reasoning</u> A type of reasoning in which a child acts almost purely to avoid punishment to get what he or she wants.

<u>preschoolers</u> Persons who are 3 to 5 years of age.

protest phase An infant's initial response to a situational crisis; characterized by loud crying.

rooting reflex An infant reflex that occurs when something touches an infant's cheek, and the infant instinctively turns his or her head toward the touch.

scaffolding An instructional technique that builds on what has already been learned.

school age A person who is 6 to 12 years of age.

secure attachment A bond between an infant and his or her parent or caregiver, in which the infant understands that parents or caregivers will be responsive to his or her needs and provide care when help is needed.

self-concept A person's perception of himself or herself.

self-esteem How a person feels about himself or herself, and how a person feels about how he or she fits in with peers.

situational crisis A crisis caused by a specific set of circumstances.

sucking reflex An infant reflex in which the infant starts sucking when his or her lips are stroked.

terminal drop hypothesis The theory that a person's mental function declines in the last 5 years of life.

toddlers Persons who are 1 to 3 years of age.

trust and mistrust A phrase that refers to a stage of development from birth to approximately 18 months of age, during which infants gain trust of their parents or caregivers if their world is planned, organized, and routine.

withdrawal In the context of infant behavior, the final phase of an infant's response to a situational crisis; characterized by apathy and boredom.

Assessment in Action

Your unit has arrived at an apartment complex for a call involving childbirth. Once inside the apartment, you find the mother lying supine on the bed. She is alone in the residence. The baby has already been delivered and is lying between her legs. The baby is crying loudly and is wet. You and your partner quickly assemble your equipment and begin your assessment of both patients.

1. A age of a neonate is classified as:
   A. birth through the first hour of life.
   B. birth through 1 month of life.
   C. birth through 1 year of life.
   D. birth through 6 months of life.

2. Where are the fontanelles located in a neonate?
   A. The heart
   B. The head
   C. The spine
   D. The chest

3. The expected normal pulse rate for a newborn at birth is:
   A. 60 to 80 beats/min.
   B. 90 to 100 beats/min.
   C. 100 to 120 beats/min.
   D. 100 to 180 beats/min.

4. The expected normal respiratory rate for a newborn at birth is:
   A. 10 to 20 breaths/min.
   B. 20 to 30 breaths/min.
   C. 30 to 60 breaths/min.
   D. 60 to 70 breaths/min.

5. Infants younger than 6 months old are primarily:
   A. nose breathers.
   B. mouth breathers.
   C. chest breathers.
   D. All of the above

Additional Questions

6. What information can you gather from an infant who is crying?

7. Why are infants called "belly breathers"?

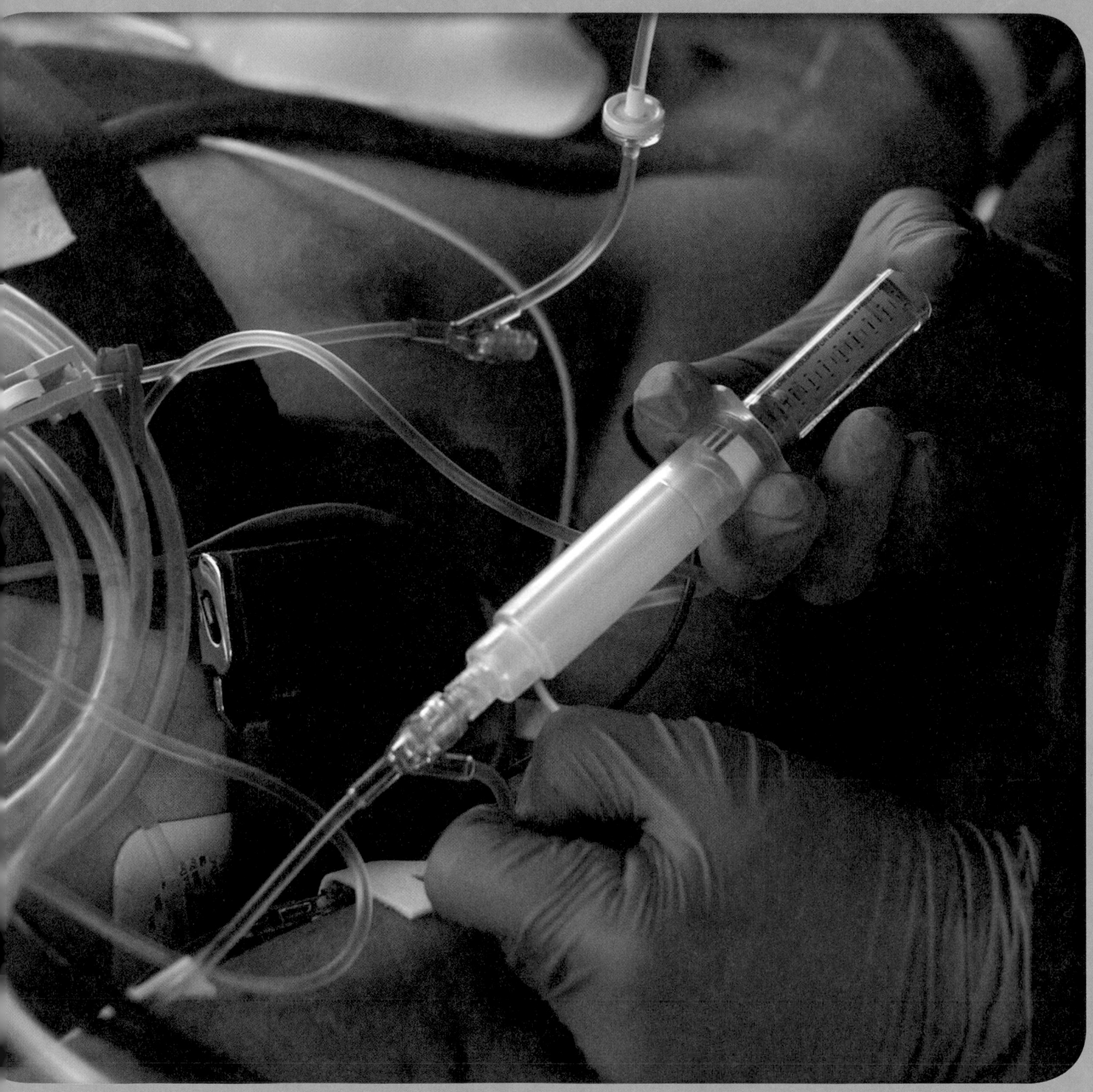

Principles of Pharmacology

National EMS Education Standard Competencies

Pharmacology

Integrates comprehensive knowledge of pharmacology to formulate a treatment plan intended to mitigate emergencies and improve the overall health of the patient.

Principles of Pharmacology

- Medication safety (pp 423-424)
- Medication legislation (pp 423-424)
- Naming (pp 425-426)
- Classifications (p 424)
- Schedules (p 424)
- Pharmacokinetics (pp 427, 436)
- Storage and security (pp 426-427)
- Autonomic pharmacology (pp 452-454)
- Metabolism and excretion (pp 430-431)
- Mechanism of action (pp 427, 436)
- Phases of medication activity (p 427)
- Medication response relationships (pp 433-436)
- Medication interactions (p 436)
- Toxicity (p 427)

Knowledge Objectives

1. Explain how pharmacology relates to paramedic clinical practice. (p 423)
2. Describe the regulatory measures affecting medications administered in the prehospital setting. (pp 423-424)

3. Outline reliable sources of medication information available to paramedics. (p 426)
4. Discuss requirements for medication storage, security, and accountability. (pp 426-427)
5. Describe the pharmacokinetic and pharmacodynamic properties of medications in general as well as those routinely administered by paramedics. (pp 427-430, 436)
6. Identify situations where medication effects will be altered by the age, sex, weight, and other characteristics of a particular patient. (pp 430-433)
7. Present steps to reduce the incidence of medication errors and limit the severity of harmful effects associated with medication administration. (pp 443-444)
8. Select the optimal medication and method of medication administration for patients with a particular clinical condition or situation. (pp 437-441)
9. Discuss the prevention, recognition, and management of adverse medication reactions. (pp 433-436)
10. Describe specific medications used by paramedics in the prehospital setting. (pp 445-455)
11. List notable classes of medications that may be taken by patients in the prehospital setting. (pp 445-447)

Skills Objectives

There are no skills objectives for this chapter.

Introduction

Medication administration is a defining element of paramedic clinical practice. When given appropriately, medications have the unique ability to correct or decrease the severity of an illness or injury, manage many life-threatening conditions, and substantially reduce patient discomfort. If paramedics administer the incorrect medication, use the incorrect route, select an inappropriate dose, or fail to follow the correct technique for administration, severe and often life-threatening consequences are likely. This chapter will assist paramedics and paramedic students in minimizing the risks associated with medication administration while providing patients with a large variety of benefits available from pharmacologic interventions.

Pharmacology is the scientific study of how various substances interact with or alter the function of living organisms. Paramedics use the science of pharmacology in a variety of ways, for example when treating patients who already receive medications on an intermittent or long-term basis. Prehospital providers will encounter patients who are experiencing adverse effects of medications taken at home, so it is crucial to obtain a medication history during patient assessment. Paramedics must also understand pharmacology when administering medications to treat patient symptoms during an EMS response or while treating a patient who has been exposed to a potentially toxic chemical, drug, or medication.

Historical Perspective on Medication Administration

Chemicals, primarily derived from plants or animals, have been used for many centuries to cure disease or relieve symptoms. Early Chinese, Mesopotamian, and Egyptian societies used chemical remedies to treat everything from pain to baldness. Diseases were poorly understood, and natural remedies were directed toward various symptoms rather than the disease process itself. Formal scientific study of the effects of medication on the body began to emerge during the late 17th and 18th centuries. Today, the science of pharmacology has evolved into a highly profitable and highly regulated industry. Many unique subspecialties such as genetic manipulation and toxicology continue to blur the line between pharmacology, medicine, and a variety of other scientific fields. Although the science of pharmacology has evolved into a sophisticated area of health care, certain medications discovered in ancient times are still in use.

Medication selection and administration is no longer random or anecdotal as it was in previous centuries. Evidence-based guidelines assist clinicians using pharmacologic interventions across the spectrum of medical specialties. Medications now undergo extensive testing and numerous clinical trials before widespread use is permitted. Despite the advanced science of pharmacology, adverse reactions are commonplace.

Medication and Drug Regulation

The United States has implemented a comprehensive system of medication and drug regulation. The first significant regulation was enacted in 1906 with the passage of the Pure Food and Drug Act. As its name implies, this act prohibited altering or mislabeling medications. In 1909, opium was prohibited from being imported under the Opium Exclusion Act. The Harrison Narcotic Act became law in 1914, restricting the use of various opiates and cocaine.

Under the Food, Drug, and Cosmetic Act (1938), the United States Food and Drug Administration (FDA) was given enforcement authority for rules requiring that new drugs were safe and pure. The FDA remains the federal agency responsible for approving new medications and removing unsafe medications from use. Approval of a new medication typically takes several years. Occasionally, breakthrough medications for life-threatening conditions may receive preferential expedited consideration. Only a small fraction of medications submitted to the FDA are approved, and many medications, once approved, are used "off-label," that is, for

---

YOU *are the Medic*   **PART 1**

It is 11:00 AM and you and your partner are dispatched to a 22-year-old woman who complains of lightheadedness. You have a response time of 5 minutes. You pull up to a large office building and are met outside by a staff member.

1. What are some possible causes of lightheadedness in a young adult?

2. What are your priorities for the initial patient contact?

a purpose not approved by the FDA, at doses different from the recommended doses, or by a route of administration not approved by the FDA. This practice is extremely common in health care, but a physician medical director or paramedic may have an increased risk of liability for ill-advised, off-label use of a medication that results in a bad outcome for a patient. Medications should be administered off-label only when they are specifically approved for this use by the service medical director or agency/regional protocol.

Paramedics need to be familiar with the rules and regulations implemented under the Controlled Substances Act (also known as the Comprehensive Drug Abuse Prevention and Control Act) of 1970. This act classifies certain medications with the potential of abuse into five categories (schedules) with corresponding security, dispensing, and record-keeping requirements Table 1. The US Drug Enforcement Agency is responsible for enforcing this act.

Schedule I medications may not be prescribed, dispensed, used, or administered for medical use. Marijuana, prescribed for medical purposes, remains a controversial Schedule I controlled substance. Various states permit prescription marijuana for certain medical conditions, which is in conflict with federal controlled substances regulation.

Paramedics are likely to carry and administer Schedule II medications such as fentanyl (Sublimaze) and morphine sulfate, and Schedule IV medications such as midazolam (Versed), diazepam (Valium), and lorazepam (Ativan). All Schedule II through V medications require locked storage, significant record keeping, and controlled wasting procedures. State EMS, pharmacy, or law enforcement agencies may impose additional requirements for the security and accountability of these controlled substances.

Words of Wisdom

Careful accountability of controlled substances protects the paramedic and the EMS organization. Tampering and diversion will be less likely to adversely impact patient care.

◼ Sources of Medication

Medications can be derived or manufactured from a wide variety of possible sources. Ancient societies used medications isolated from the roots, leaves, or bark of certain plants. Animals, particularly animal endocrine systems, are used as the source of other medications. Minerals provide yet another source of many medications used for a wide variety of clinical conditions. Microorganisms such as bacteria, fungi, and mold, too, are used for the manufacture of medication. Table 2 lists sources of many common medications.

Many other medications are either synthetic (made completely in a laboratory setting) or semisynthetic (made from chemicals derived from plant, animal, or mineral sources that have been chemically modified in a laboratory setting). Genetic engineering is also used to manufacture certain medications that cannot otherwise be obtained from natural sources.

During the manufacturing process, pharmaceutical companies tightly control the concentration, purity, preservatives, and other ingredients present in medications. The USP-NF (discussed later) is a great source of information regarding the manufacturing details of a particular medication. Paramedics will notice a manufacturing lot number and expiration date on every medication carried and administered in the prehospital setting.

◼ Forms of Medication

Paramedics use and administer medication in various forms. The vast majority of medications are administered as sterile injectable solutions. These solutions require careful handling and aseptic technique during administration to avoid contamination with microorganisms or other harmful substances. These solutions are supplied in larger IV bags, vials, ampules, and occasionally in glass bottles for medications such as nitroglycerin or ethanol. Other forms of medication are outlined in Table 3.

Table 1 Classification of Medications Considered Controlled Substances

Schedule	Description	Examples
I	High abuse potential; no recognized medical purpose	Heroin, marijuana, LSD
II	High abuse potential; legitimate medical purpose	Fentanyl (Sublimaze), methylphenidate (Ritalin), cocaine
III	Lower potential for abuse than Schedule II medications	Hydrocodone (Vicodin), acetaminophen with codeine, ketamine
IV	Lower potential for abuse than Schedule III drugs	Diazepam (Valium), lorazepam (Ativan)
V	Lower potential for abuse than Schedule IV drugs	Narcotic cough medicines

Abbreviation: LSD, lysergic acid diethylamide.

Table 2 Sources of Medication

Source	Example
Plant	Atropine, aspirin, digoxin, morphine
Animal	Heparin, antivenom, thyroid preparations, insulin
Microorganism	Streptokinase, numerous antibiotics
Minerals	Iron, magnesium sulfate, lithium, phosphorus, calcium

Table 3   Forms of Medication

Form	Description	Example
Capsule	Powdered or solid medication enclosed in a dissolvable cylindrical gelatin shell	Acetaminophen (Tylenol), ibuprofen (Motrin), diphenhydramine (Benadryl)
Tablet	Solid medication particles bound into a shape designed to dissolve or be swallowed	Aspirin (ASA), nitroglycerin SL
Powder	Small particles of medication designed to be dissolved or mixed into a solution or liquid	Glucagon, vecuronium (Norcuron)
Drops	Sterile solution or nonsterile liquid intended for direct administration into nose or ear	Neosynephrine (Afrin), tetracaine
Skin preparation	Gel, ointment, or paste substance designed to permit transdermal (through the skin) absorption	Nitroglycerin paste, fentanyl patch
Suppository	Medication in a waxlike material that dissolves in the rectum or other body cavity	Promethazine (Phenergan), acetaminophen (Tylenol)
Liquid	Medication dissolved or suspended in liquid intended for oral consumption	Infant acetaminophen (Tylenol), cough syrup
Inhaler/spray	Medication in gas or fine mist form intended for inhalation and absorption through lung, airway, or oral tissues	Albuterol (Ventolin), nitroglycerin spray

Words of Wisdom

If glass bottles are being used during interfacility transport, carefully secure them to prevent injury to the patient or yourself in the event of a crash.

Medication Management for Paramedics

Medication Names

Every medication in the United States is given three distinct names. During initial development, medications are given a chemical name, which is often long and difficult to pronounce and may contain specific letters or numbers according to their chemical composition. The chemical name is rarely used in clinical practice by paramedics, pharmacists, nurses, or physicians. Sodium bicarbonate, potassium chloride, and certain others are the few exceptions in which the chemical name is used in clinical practice. The majority of medication reference sources used by paramedics do not publish the chemical name or structure of a medication.

Every medication also receives a nonproprietary, or generic, name. The generic name is proposed by the manufacturer and needs to be approved by the US Adopted Names Council and the World Health Organization. The generic name is regulated internationally to promote consistency and avoid duplication in drug names. Generic names typically include a "stem" that links them to other medications in the same class. Often the stem is at the end of the name, but it may also appear at the beginning or within the drug name. Many benzodiazepine medications, such

as midazolam, diazepam, and lorazepam have the stem "am." Angiotensin-converting enzyme (ACE) inhibitor medications, such as enalapril (Vasotec), captopril (Capoten), and lisinopril (Prinivil, Zestril), have the stem "pril" that signifies that each medication is a member of the ACE inhibitor class. Numerous other examples exist.

Paramedics should not rely entirely on a stem when attempting to determine the class of a medication because different classes might have the same stem. Tricyclic antidepressants, such as amitriptyline (Elavil) and desipramine (Norpramin), have the same stem as certain selective serotonin reuptake inhibitors (SSRIs) such as fluoxetine (Prozac) and paroxetine (Paxil). An overdose of a tricyclic antidepressant is often life threatening, whereas an overdose of an SSRI medication does not typically have the same risk. Besides knowing that stems provide information about the class of drugs, paramedics need to know the specific names of and indications for the drugs they administer.

The final type of medication name is the brand name, which is chosen by the manufacturer and approved by the FDA. The brand name does not have the same functional requirements as the generic name, but it must meet certain minimum criteria set by the FDA. Brand names are often selected for marketing purposes. Creative examples are sometimes linked to a particular condition. Metoprolol, a beta-adrenergic blocking agent, has the brand name Lopressor, which may be a subtle reference to lowering the (blood) pressure. Oseltamivir has the brand name "Tamiflu" and is used to treat influenza. The three distinct medication names are illustrated with the following example of a medication commonly administered by paramedics:

Chemical name: 4-chloro-N-furfuryl-5-sulfamoylanthranilic acid
Generic name: furosemide
Brand name: Lasix

Paramedics may also notice that many reference sources now use "tall man" lettering when the names of certain medications are printed. The capitalized letters highlight a portion of the name in medications with similar names. One example is DOBUTamine and DOPamine, and another is diphenhydrAMINE and dimenhyDRINATE. This approach is intended to avoid confusion among medications with similarly spelled names.

Medication Reference Sources

Paramedics have a vast array of medication reference sources available. When selecting a reference source to use or purchase, paramedics must consider a variety of factors: reliability of the reference source; whether the source is printed, electronic, or both; the depth of information needed or provided; accessibility; cost; availability of updates; and size or materials used.

Medication information is typically compiled in a format called a **medication monograph** or medication profile. The detail may vary dramatically between reference sources, but the basic structure remains consistent. **Table 4** highlights common components of medication profiles.

The *United States Pharmacopeia–National Formulary* (USP-NF) and *Physicians' Desk Reference* (PDR) provide a wealth of reliable, detailed information about thousands of medications. The information includes graphic diagrams of the chemical structure and other specific chemical properties. The printed forms of

Table 4 Components of Medication Profiles
Medication names
Category or class of medication
Uses/indications
Mechanism of action (pharmacodynamics)
Pregnancy risk factors
Contraindications
Available forms
Dosages (often differentiated based on age or indication)
Administration and monitoring considerations
Potential incompatibility
Adverse effects
Pharmacokinetics

these sources are impractical in prehospital settings because of their size and amount of information. Much of the information in these sources is not needed in prehospital settings, and it may be difficult for paramedics to locate needed information rapidly. The electronic versions of the USP-NF and the PDR may be helpful to EMS educators and administrators developing agency-specific medication protocols or creating training materials.

Manufacturers provide written materials with every package of medication distributed. These "package inserts" are written by manufacturers and approved by the FDA. The package inserts include information on dosing, route of administration, contraindications, adverse effects, and a variety of other factors.

Hospital pharmacies often compile medication information into formularies that are specific to the information needs of specific hospitals. The hospital formulary typically includes much of the same information as in the medication package insert, USP-NF, or PDR, but it is tailored to the needs of prescribers in the hospital. Paramedics in hospital-based or hospital-affiliated EMS systems may have access to the hospital formulary.

The American Medical Association (AMA) publishes another reliable source of medication information. *AMA Drug Evaluations* provides great detail about medication selection and administration. It contains much of the same information as the USP-NF and PDR, with additional discussion of investigational medications. Paramedics must use caution when referencing the AMA publication because not every medication in the compendium has received FDA approval.

Paramedics have many other choices for commercially published medication information references. Some resources are specifically for prehospital or critical care transport providers with an emphasis on medication selection, dosing, and administration for patient conditions encountered by paramedics. Other references focus exclusively on IV medications or emphasize only information needed during hands-on patient care. With the advancements in portable electronic devices and "smart" cellular telephones, many medication references can be accessed electronically, making vast amounts of information available without requiring additional space or weight in an ambulance. State EMS agencies and individual fire and EMS organizations frequently compile information on approved medications given by paramedics in a particular setting through specific protocols or a medication formulary.

Medication Storage

Medication storage is an important consideration for paramedics. The uncontrolled prehospital environment is a difficult place to maintain the safety and integrity of medication packages. Paramedics must keep medication in a location that provides adequate protection for medication supplies yet is convenient enough to allow quick access in emergency situations. Devices such as medication refrigerators and secure cabinets are impractical in many prehospital settings or response vehicles.

The most basic concern regarding medication storage is the integrity of the medication container. Medication should be stored in a manner that prevents physical damage to the medication vial, ampule, solution, or tablets. In many instances it is necessary to remove most of the packaging provided by the manufacturer, leaving only the bare medication container in the vehicle or response bag. Because drug boxes or bags may be dropped accidentally during a call, medication containers should be placed in protective bins or surrounded by enough padding to avoid damage during response or patient care at the scene. Paramedics should organize medication containers in a manner that facilitates quick, accurate identification of the medication during emergency situations. Needs of individual EMS organizations dictate the type and quantity of medications that are available on a particular response vehicle or in a provider's bag. Excessive quantities of medication may make storage difficult or cause unnecessary waste due to expiration. Insufficient quantities may undermine patient care or necessitate frequent restocking.

Direct sunlight, extremes of heat and cold, and physical damage to medication containers can make medications ineffective or unsafe for use. Temperature extremes hasten the expiration of many medications. Medications in general require secure storage in a climate-controlled environment. Special medication warmers or refrigerators may be necessary if safe temperatures cannot be maintained in an ambulance or EMS response vehicle. A recent multicenter study demonstrated that ambulance interiors in a variety of geographic regions had temperature extremes outside the USP recommended 15°C to 30°C (55°F–86°F) range for the storage of most medications used in the prehospital setting. Paramedics may need to remove from service medication that has been exposed to extremes of temperature. EMS agencies in environments where temperature extremes are common may need to invest in equipment such as heaters, coolers, and refrigerators for transport vehicles to ensure the safety and integrity of the medications they carry.

■ Medication Security

Controlled substances (as in Table 1) require additional security, record keeping, and disposal precautions. These medications must be in locked storage or continuously held by an (on-duty) EMS provider responsible for administration. Disposal of partially used or damaged medication containers requires verification by a witness or return of the damaged or unused portion to the department responsible for dispensing the medication. EMS agencies and individual paramedics are jointly responsible for adhering to all federal, state, and local regulations regarding the security and accountability of controlled substances. These regulations vary slightly from region to region. In general, every last milliliter or milligram of a controlled substance needs to be documented from ordering, to receipt by the EMS agency, to administration by the EMS provider (and quantity discarded as waste). The particular forms and procedures may vary from place to place, but the standard for accountability remains constant.

Controlled substances are often the target of tampering or diversion. Inspect medication vials, ampules, and the like for subtle signs of tampering that may be as small as a pinhole. Suspect tampering in situations in which appropriate doses of analgesic or sedative medications seem ineffective, especially when patient tolerance is unlikely.

■ The Physiology of Pharmacology

Paramedics administer medications to produce a desired effect in the body, usually in response to a particular illness, injury, or medical condition, but occasionally to prevent a specific harmful situation. As a medication is administered, it begins to alter a function or process within the body. This action is known as **pharmacodynamics**.

Any medication capable of beneficial clinical effects can cause toxic effects when given at an excessive dose. Toxic effects may also occur if a medication is given by an incorrect route or when a delivery device, such as an IV catheter or intraosseous (IO) needle, malfunctions. In other cases, medications may become ineffective when given at an inadequate dose or through the incorrect route. Even in the absence of error, many factors related to the patient, patient condition, and particular medication may cause toxicity or adverse effects.

The human body simultaneously begins the process of **absorption**, **distribution**, possibly **biotransformation**, and, ultimately, **elimination** of a medication or chemical following administration. The action of the body on a medication is known as **pharmacokinetics**. Paramedics must consider the principles of pharmacodynamics and pharmacokinetics when deciding whether to administer a particular medication.

■ Principles of Pharmacodynamics

Scientific research has demonstrated the presence of **receptor** sites in proteins connected to cells throughout the body. Various receptors are activated by **endogenous** chemicals, those occurring naturally within the body, and by the presence of medications and chemicals absorbed into the body. Activation of these receptors produces a specific response by individual cells, tissues, organs, and, ultimately, body systems. When a medication binds with a receptor site, one of four possible actions will occur:

1. Channels permitting the passage of **ions** (charged particles) in cell walls may be opened or closed.
2. A biochemical messenger becomes activated, initiating other chemical reactions within the cell.
3. A normal cell function is prevented.
4. A normal or abnormal function of the cell begins.

For purposes of this chapter, **exogenous** (from outside the body) chemicals will be referred to as medications, even though exposure to chemicals in the environment can cause effects similar to those of medications, including adverse effects. Clandestine methamphetamine laboratories are a great example of environmental exposure to a chemical. Law enforcement officers and other emergency responders may experience accidental inhalation or dermal exposure to methamphetamines during an emergency response and demonstrate identical clinical effects to those who intentionally abuse these substances. In another example, toddlers who accidentally ingest certain mouse poisons have clinical effects identical to the therapeutic administration of warfarin (Coumadin). In each instance, the exposure is different from normal therapeutic administration, yet the clinical effects are identical.

Later sections of this chapter will discuss specific medications and chemicals used by paramedics and introduce the properties of various classes of medications pertinent to prehospital care. The *Toxicology* chapter discusses the adverse properties of commonly abused drugs. Functionally, the distinction among therapeutic medications, exogenous chemicals, and illicit drugs is largely irrelevant. These terms reflect substances that follow similar (and often predictable) patterns when interacting with the body.

Medications are developed to reach and bind with particular receptor sites of target cells. Newer medications are designed to target only specific receptor sites on certain cells in an attempt to minimize the adverse effects. Many older medications, including those used by paramedics, affect cells and tissues totally unrelated to the condition being treated, causing adverse effects throughout the body.

Two types of medications or chemicals directly affect cellular activity by binding with receptor sites on individual cells. **Agonist medications** initiate or alter a cellular activity by attaching to receptor sites, prompting a cell response.

Antagonist medications prevent endogenous or exogenous agonist chemicals from reaching cell receptor sites and initiating or altering a particular cellular activity **Figure 1**. Certain notable agonist/antagonist pairs are discussed at various points later in the chapter. Opiate medications such as morphine sulfate and fentanyl (Sublimaze) are agonist chemicals causing analgesia and respiratory depression. The effects of these chemicals can be reversed by the opiate antagonist naloxone (Narcan). In certain circumstances, the clinical effects from benzodiazepine agonist medications can be reversed by the benzodiazepine antagonist medication flumazenil (Romazicon).

Agonist Medications

The dose of a particular medication, the route of administration, and a large number of other factors determine the concentration of a medication present at target cell receptor sites. **Affinity** is the ability of a medication to bind with a particular receptor site. Medication concentration and affinity determine the number of receptor sites bound by that medication. Agonist medications bind with receptor sites, initiating or altering an action by the cell **Table 5**.

A certain minimum concentration of agonist medication must be present for cellular activity to be initiated or altered. As the concentration of the medication increases and crosses the **threshold level**, initiation or alteration of cellular activity begins. Increasing concentrations of medication cause increased effects until all receptor sites become occupied or the maximum capability of the cell is reached. The concentration of the medication required to initiate a cellular response is known as the medication's **potency**. As the potency of a medication increases, the concentration or dose required for a particular cellular response decreases. Conversely, a higher concentration is required when the potency of a medication is low. The ability to initiate or alter cell activity in a therapeutic or desired manner is referred to as **efficacy**. Once all the cellular receptor sites become bound with agonist medications, cellular activity plateaus and no increase or further change in activity is possible. At this point, the effect of the medication has peaked and additional doses or higher concentrations of the medication will not cause additional cellular action. The **dose-response**

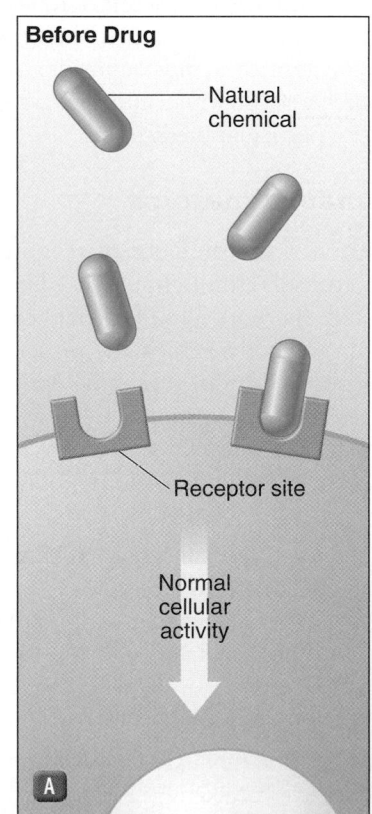
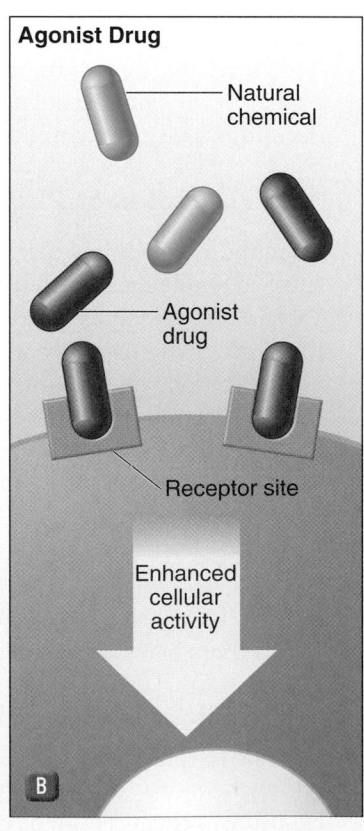
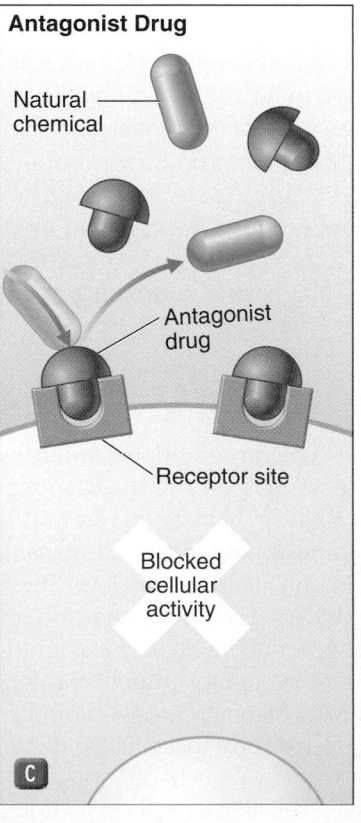

Figure 1 **A.** Normally, natural chemicals bind to receptor sites to cause actions. **B.** When an agonist drug is present, it binds to the receptor site and enhances cellular activity. **C.** When an antagonist drug is present, it binds to the receptor site and blocks cellular activity.

Table 5	Important Receptor Sites Within the Body
Receptor	**Agonist Effect**
Alpha (α)-1	Vasoconstriction of arteries and veins
Alpha (α)-2	Insulin restriction Glucagon secretion Inhibition of norepinephrine release
Beta (β)-1	Increased heart rate (chronotropic effect) Increased myocardial contractility (inotropic effect) Increased myocardial conduction (dromotropic effect) Renin secretion for urinary retention
Beta (β)-2	Bronchus and bronchiole relaxation Insulin secretion Uterine relaxation Arterial dilation in certain key organs
Dopaminergic	Vasodilation of renal and mesenteric arteries (Numerous receptor subtypes exist.)
Nicotinic	Present at neuromuscular junction, allowing acetylcholine (ACh) to stimulate muscle contraction
Muscarinic-2	Present in the heart; activated by ACh to offset sympathetic stimulation, decreasing heart rate, contractility, and electrical conduction velocity

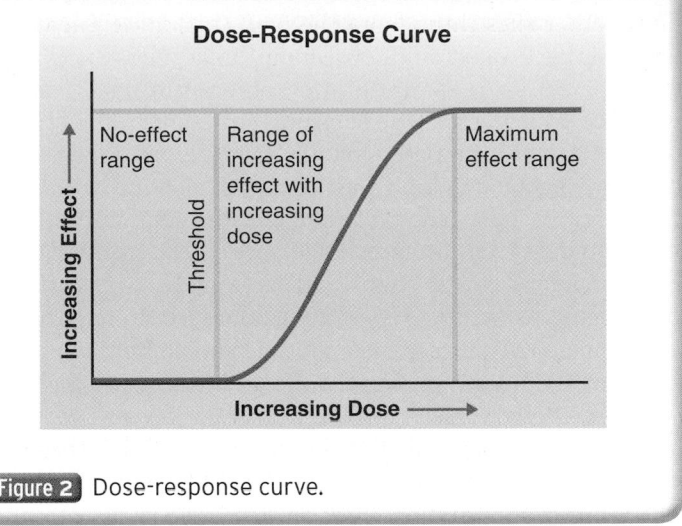

Figure 2 Dose-response curve.

curve illustrates the relationship of medication dose (or concentration) and efficacy. Relative potency is demonstrated when the dose-response curves of two different medications causing the same effect are compared. The threshold dose is lower for medications with a higher potency **Figure 2** .

Antagonist Medications

Antagonist medications bind with receptor sites to prevent a cellular response to agonist chemicals. Antagonists may be used to inhibit normal cellular activation by naturally occurring agonist chemicals within the body. Antagonist medications may also be used to treat the harmful agonist effects of exogenous medications or chemicals, possibly following an overdose or a toxic exposure.

Antagonists may be competitive or noncompetitive. <u>Competitive antagonists</u> temporarily bind with cellular receptor sites, displacing agonist chemicals. The efficacy of a competitive antagonist medication is directly related to its concentration near the receptor sites. As the concentration of a competitive antagonist increases near the receptor sites, it is able to prevent a greater number of agonist chemicals from reaching the receptor, thus decreasing cellular action. This can apply to a large quantity of one particular agonist chemical or the presence of multiple chemicals with similar agonist effects. As the competitive antagonist concentration falls (due to elimination of the drug or substance such as through the kidneys) or when the concentration of agonist chemicals increases, a greater number of agonist chemicals bind with receptor sites and continue or resume cellular activation.

The efficacy of a competitive antagonist medication is also related to its affinity (ability to bind at a receptor site) compared with the affinity of the agonist chemicals present. Competitive antagonist medications with a lower affinity require a higher concentration to be effective.

<u>Noncompetitive antagonists</u> permanently bind with receptor sites and prevent activation by agonist chemicals. Effects of noncompetitive antagonist medications continue until new receptor sites or new cells are created, which may be a long time after the last dose of antagonist medication was given. Ketamine (discussed later) is a noncompetitive antagonist of the agonist glutamate on N-methyl-D-aspartate receptors in the CNS. Effects of ketamine last for only approximately 25 minutes. Aspirin (also discussed later) is a noncompetitive antagonist that binds to the enzyme cyclooxygenase, causing antiplatelet effects that last up to 10 days when platelets are regenerated. Even increased doses of agonist chemicals will not overcome the presence of noncompetitive antagonist chemicals on cellular receptor sites.

Partial Agonist Chemicals

It is also possible to have a <u>partial agonist</u> chemical attach to cellular receptor sites. Partial agonists bind to the receptor site but do not initiate as much cellular activity or change as do other agonists. Partial agonists effectively lower the efficacy of other agonist chemicals that may be present at the cells. Buprenorphine (Buprenex, Subutex) is a partial agonist medication used for both analgesia and the management of opioid addiction. Buprenorphine has a high affinity for binding to the mu opioid receptors, preventing agonism by other opioid chemicals. Buprenorphine provides some degree of agonism, causing analgesia and euphoria, but has a "ceiling effect" that allows only partial activation of the opioid receptors, minimizing the risk of toxicity and physical dependence. The maximum effects possible from buprenorphine are much less than other opioid chemicals.

Alternative Mechanisms of Drug Action

It is possible for medications to alter cell, tissue, organ, and system function in the body without directly interacting with receptors on individual cells. Medications are engineered to target other sites throughout the body, including microorganisms, lipids, water, and exogenous toxic substances. Antimicrobials, such as antibiotics and antifungals, may be designed to target specific substances present in the cell walls of a particular bacteria or fungus. Other medications, known as chelating agents, bind with heavy metals such as lead, mercury, and arsenic in the body and create a compound that can be eliminated. Sodium bicarbonate (discussed in detail later in this chapter), a medication used for a wide variety of medical conditions, breaks down after administration, producing bicarbonate ions. Bicarbonate ions are able to bind with excess hydrogen (H^+) ions, raising the pH and decreasing the acidity of various body fluids.

Mannitol (Osmitrol) is a diuretic medication, designed to distribute into water in the body, creating osmotic changes that alter the distribution of fluids and electrolytes. The resulting diuretic effect draws excess water from certain body tissues, including the brain and eyes, while enhancing excretion of urine by the kidneys. Plasma expanders and bulk laxatives target water in the body and alter the distribution of various body fluids.

Electrolyte-based medications such as magnesium, potassium, and calcium change the concentration and distribution of ions in cells and fluids throughout the body, affecting a wide variety of cell activities. An alteration in the concentration of certain electrolytes at the cellular level affects the ability of various cells to function. Alterations of cell function occur without chemicals directly binding to cell receptor sites.

Factors Affecting Response to Medications

A wide variety of factors determine how a particular medication will affect a patient. These factors may influence the choice of medication, dose, route, timing, manner of administration, and monitoring necessary after a patient receives a medication. Even weight-based medication dosing, which is common in the prehospital setting, produces profound differences in how a medication affects an individual patient because of the factors described in the following sections.

Age The distribution, metabolism, and elimination of medication continue to change throughout the human life span. Elderly and pediatric patients have a response to a variety of medications that is much different from responses in adolescents and adults. Paramedics may need to adjust the dose of medication for infants, children, and elderly patients to obtain the desired response.

Medications distribute into three primary types of body substances (water, lipids or fat, and protein) following administration. The percentage of body fat is lowest in preterm infants, increases significantly in toddlers, decreases through adolescence, and increases in adults, including elderly people. The percentage of body water is highest in newborns and steadily decreases throughout the life span. The percentage of body protein varies throughout the life span, generally peaking in preteens, adolescents, and adults. Infants and elderly people have the lowest percentage of body protein. If a medication is water-soluble, higher weight-based doses must be administered to infants (with a higher percentage of body water) than to adults and elderly people. Fat- and lipid-soluble medications require higher weight-based doses in elderly people because of their higher body fat percentage and increased fat distribution.

When you are treating pediatric or elderly patients with altered percentages of body water, fat or lipid, and protein, consider careful titration of medication rather than simply administering a weight-based bolus. Water-soluble and lipid-soluble medications may require increased initial doses to overcome widespread distribution. Elderly patients, for example, generally have a lower percentage of body water. Therefore, water-soluble medications, such as digoxin, cause higher serum levels in elderly patients compared with other patients who weigh the same and are given the same dose. There is less body water for the digoxin to spread into, causing a greater concentration in the body water present, particularly in the blood (serum). Elderly patients also generally have a higher percentage of body fat. Lipid-soluble medications such as diazepam (Valium) initially produce much lower serum levels for a given dose, but take much longer for the body to eliminate, dramatically prolonging the effects of the medications. Without careful monitoring, it is easy to exceed therapeutic serum levels when administering repeated doses, causing adverse or toxic effects that may persist for hours to days. Solubility is typically included with other information in medication reference materials.

Alteration of metabolism and elimination in pediatric and elderly patients may prolong the effects of medications or result in higher medication concentrations in various tissues. Medication metabolism in the liver is affected by the cytochrome P-450 system (discussed later in this chapter). This system works differently on different types of medications, is extremely variable in infants and children, and has a functional decline in elderly people. Hepatic metabolism is also generally impaired in elderly people due to decreased blood flow to the liver. A decline in liver or kidney function, due to aging or other cause, requires a decrease in the dosage of many medications because elimination from the body is impaired.

Patients at extremes of age are disproportionately prone to paradoxical medication reactions. In paradoxical medication reactions, patients experience clinical effects opposite from the intended effects of the medication. Normally, sedative medications produce profound excitement or agitation. Barbiturates can cause unexpected excitement or agitation in elderly patients. Promethazine (Phenergan), diphenhydramine (Benadryl), chloral hydrate, and various benzodiazepines, such as midazolam, can cause paradoxical excitement or agitation in children. Paradoxical reactions frequently complicate an already delicate clinical situation in which patients who need sedation become even more excited, agitated, or combative.

Weight Many medications used in prehospital care and critical care transport are administered using weight-based dosing. A quantity of medication (usually grams, milligrams, micrograms, or milliliters) is multiplied by the patient's weight in kilograms to obtain the recommended dose for the individual

Special Populations

When you are caring for a pediatric patient, ask the parents whether the child has had a previous reaction, such as a paradoxical reaction, prior to administering any medication.

patient. This method of medication dosing has advantages and limitations. The major advantage of this method is that the amount of medication administered is proportional to the size of the patient. Medication manufacturers and clinicians have already calculated factors affecting absorption, distribution, metabolism, rates of elimination, and desired quantity present at target cells or tissues when giving a particular medication at a weight-based dose. Paramedics can use the weight-based formula to calculate the appropriate medication dose for patients ranging from preterm neonates through large adults.

There are several limitations associated with this method as well. To calculate a weight-based medication dose, the patient's weight in kilograms is needed. In emergency situations, a patient's weight must be estimated and, often, converted from pounds to kilograms. Even in controlled settings, health care providers might have difficulty accurately estimating patient weights. A recent study revealed that a significant portion of health care providers' estimates of patient weight were off by more than 10% to 15%. Patients are generally more accurate at estimating their own weight than are health care providers. An inaccurate estimate of a patient's weight, depending on the degree of inaccuracy, could result in administration of an incorrect dose of medication. Multiplication of numbers in the formula during a stressful situation or at an uncontrolled scene may also lead to dosing errors. Using a calculator or a preprinted medication dose chart when administering weight-based medications can help reduce errors.

The weight-based method of dose calculation does not consider the various alterations in distribution, metabolism, and elimination discussed earlier. Data regarding the percentages of body water, fat, and protein at various ages become less reliable as obesity and malnutrition affect society. Weight-based medication doses can be calculated by using the patient's actual body weight or ideal body weight. For example, lidocaine, an antidysrhythmic medication, is administered based on a patient's actual body weight. The cardiac medication digoxin is given based on a patient's ideal body weight. Unfortunately, many reference sources do not provide guidance about whether the patient's actual or ideal body weight should be used for medication dose calculations. The formulas for ideal body weight in adults are as follows:

For men: Ideal Weight (kg) = 50 + (2.3 times patient's height in inches over 5 feet)

For women: Ideal Weight (kg) = 45.5 + (2.3 times patient's height in inches over 5 feet)

For example, the ideal weight for a 6′ tall man would be 77.6 kg [50 + (2.3 × 12)], and the ideal weight for a 5′5″ woman would be 57 kg [45.5 + (2.3 × 5)].

Environment Hyperthermia and hypothermia can affect medication absorption, metabolism, and efficacy. Fever causes tachycardia that may increase hepatic blood flow, theoretically increasing the initial metabolism of drugs in the liver and reducing the amount of drug returned to circulation by the liver. Fever also suppresses the function of the cytochrome P-450 system in the liver, which ultimately decreases the rate of metabolism of certain classes of medications. Individual patient responses may vary from the expected response.

Hypothermia is known to impair the effectiveness of medications used in traditional advanced cardiac life support (ACLS). Atropine sulfate and lidocaine are generally viewed as ineffective and are not indicated for hypothermic cardiac arrest. Epinephrine and vasopressin have demonstrated the ability to maintain coronary perfusion pressure during hypothermic cardiac arrest, but are not specifically recommended during cardiac arrest resulting from hypothermia.

Genetic Factors Paramedics should be extremely careful when deciding whether to administer medications to patients with specific genetic disorders. Primary pulmonary hypertension, sickle cell disease, and glucose-6-phosphate dehydrogenase deficiency require special consideration and may exclude certain medications frequently used by paramedics. Patients with primary pulmonary hypertension may have acute decompensation when vasopressor medications are used. Salicylate medications such as aspirin (acetylsalicylic acid) may precipitate hemolysis in patients with glucose-6-phosphate dehydrogenase deficiency. Patients with sickle cell disease require adequate hydration and intravascular fluid volume. Medications that cause diuresis, such as furosemide (Lasix), or vasoconstriction, such as epinephrine or dopamine, may cause or worsen potentially fatal complications of sickle cell disease. Many other genetically linked conditions require careful consideration when administering medications in the prehospital setting.

Patients with genetic disorders and their family members are often excellent sources of information specific to the disorder. Paramedics should use the knowledge of patients and family members about genetic conditions; admitting a lack of knowledge about an unusual genetic condition and treating patients and families as experts on the genetic condition can help build their confidence in paramedics.

Pregnancy Pregnancy causes an array of physiologic changes in the body, which can affect medication decisions significantly. Cardiac output and intravascular volume increase dramatically, each by about 40% above baseline. The **hematocrit**, or the percentage of red blood cells (RBCs) in the intravascular space, decreases in response to an increase in overall blood plasma volume. Respiratory tidal volume and minute volumes increase, while the inspiratory and expiratory reserve volumes decrease. Gastrointestinal (GI) motility decreases as pregnancy progresses. Renal blood flow and urinary elimination increase, roughly in proportion to cardiac output and intravascular volume. Pregnant patients have better renal function in a supine position than when upright. The majority of endocrine glands undergo some degree of change during pregnancy, causing emotional instability, altered glucose metabolism, thyroid-generated tachycardia, and other problems.

Each of these changes can affect the absorption, distribution, or elimination of medications during pregnancy. The stress imposed on the body during pregnancy from these changes can also exacerbate an underlying disease process, potentially threatening the life or health of the patient and fetus. In addition to considering maternal alterations during pregnancy, paramedics must also consider potential harmful effects on the developing fetus when administering medication to a pregnant patient. During the research, approval, and marketing process, medications are assigned into one of five possible FDA pregnancy risk categories based on potential harm to the fetus. Table 6 outlines the level of risk associated with each category. In general, medications and interventions that protect the life and health of the mother are usually in the best interest of the dependent fetus. The majority of medications given by paramedics do not pose an unacceptable risk to a fetus. Paramedics should avoid medications known to cause harm to the fetus in all but the most extreme, life-threatening situations for the mother. Most commercial reference sources provide the FDA pregnancy risk category for each medication. Aspirin and certain benzodiazepines such as diazepam (Valium) and midazolam (Versed) are common prehospital medications known to cause fetal harm.

Special Populations

Treat every female of childbearing age as though she could be pregnant.

Psychosocial Factors Paramedics should be aware of the role of psychosocial factors in the effectiveness of medications when they select and administer medications. Pain, anxiety, and overall discomfort can vary dramatically among individual patients with the same illness or injury. Unlike measurable vital signs and readily observable clinical findings, patient perceptions and responses to discomfort remain largely subjective. Psychological, cultural, emotional, and situational factors may influence the amount of discomfort reported by patients in relation to the underlying medical condition, positioning, environmental stressors, and the interventions performed by paramedics during treatment. Paramedics should be alert to verbal and nonverbal cues when assessing for discomfort and administering medications for anxiety, pain, and sedation. Nonverbal cues may be indicated by vital sign changes, facial expression, posture and movement changes, altered respiratory patterns, tears or crying, and other behaviors. The cues provide potentially useful information about patient pain, anxiety, or discomfort but can have different meanings to different people, so interpretations of the cues should be confirmed with patients.

Medication administration is further complicated by the **placebo effect**. Numerous studies have demonstrated that patients experience measurable clinical improvement or have unexplained adverse effects after receiving a medication with no pharmacologic properties. Placebos were used heavily in 17th and 18th century medical practice, and use continued until the early 1900s. Pharmacologically inactive medications continue to be used by health care researchers to validate the efficacy or adverse effects of investigational medications by quantifying the placebo effect present in the particular study. The physiologic mechanism of the placebo effect remains under speculation. Pain relief from a placebo may be from endorphins released by the brain in anticipation of pain relief from the placebo. Adverse effects following placebo administration may somehow be linked to negative expectations or anxiety, but this mechanism remains uncertain. The efficacy of a placebo may be related to the timing of administration in relation to medications that are pharmacologically active.

Table 6   FDA Pregnancy Category Classification

Pregnancy Category	Implications
A	Controlled studies in women fail to demonstrate a risk to the fetus in the first trimester (and there is no evidence of a risk in later trimesters), and the possibility of fetal harm appears remote.
B	Either animal-reproduction studies have not demonstrated a fetal risk but there are no controlled studies in pregnant women, or animal-reproduction studies have shown an adverse effect (other than a decrease in fertility) that was not confirmed in controlled studies in women in the first trimester (and there is no evidence of a risk in later trimesters).
C	Either studies in animals have revealed adverse effects on the fetus (teratogenic or embryocidal or other) and there are no controlled studies in women, or studies in women and animals are not available. Drugs should be given only if the potential benefit justifies the potential risk to the fetus.
D	There is positive evidence of human fetal risk, but the benefits from use in pregnant women may be acceptable despite the risk (eg, if the drug is needed in a life-threatening situation or for a serious disease for which safer drugs cannot be used or are ineffective).
X	Studies in animals or human beings have demonstrated fetal abnormalities, there is evidence of fetal risk based on human experience, or both, and the risk of the use of the drug in pregnant women clearly outweighs any possible benefit. The drug is contraindicated in women who are or may become pregnant.

Data source: FDA, Title 21: Food and Drugs, Code of Federal Regulations, Title 21, Volume 4, Part 200 to 299. Revised as of April 1, 1997.

It may be tempting to exploit the placebo effect by administering inactive substances to a patient as an alternative to pharmacologic treatment. This practice is demeaning to patients and may lead to discipline or criminal prosecution if the act involves the diversion of controlled substances. Placebo use by paramedics violates ethical principles, deceives patients, and undermines the credibility of the EMS profession.

Types of Medication Responses

Every medication capable of a therapeutic benefit also has the potential for adverse or toxic effects at excessive doses. Even at appropriate doses, many medications produce harmful or undesired effects in susceptible persons. Paramedics may prevent or minimize adverse effects by properly selecting the correct medication, route, dose, method of administration, and supportive treatment necessary for each individual patient.

Therapeutic (Desired) Response

Paramedics select pharmacologic interventions based on a patient's actual or anticipated illness, injury, presenting complaint, sign, or symptom. This condition should match the "Use/Indication" listed on the profile for the specific medication. EMS agencies and organizations often formulate protocols that specify which medications should or can be administered in certain situations. Medical directors may authorize off-label uses (discussed earlier) for approved medications when this use reflects accepted medical practice. When protocols or guidelines do not seem appropriate for the needs of a patient, paramedics in many EMS systems may be able to contact online medical control for advice or authorization for medication administration.

Medication is administered in a dose intended to produce a desired clinical response for the patient. The response may be complete resolution of the problem following one dose of medication. Paramedics may also need to administer multiple doses of the same medication to obtain a desired response. Certain medications require frequent repeated dosing, careful titration, or continuous administration to obtain or maintain the desired response. These medications are capable of demonstrating **cumulative action**. Several smaller doses of a medication produce the same desired clinical effect as a larger, single dose of that same medication. This approach allows the same therapeutic benefit while decreasing any risks associated with administering too much of a medication by a single, larger dose. Not every medication or situation allows cumulative action. Many medications require a minimum threshold concentration to cause a clinical effect. Metabolism and elimination (discussed later) may remove medication molecules before the threshold concentration is reached if the doses are too small or infrequent. The clinical situation and medication choice determine which manner of medication administration is necessary or optimal.

Adverse Medication Effects

Adverse and toxic effects are important considerations during medication selection and administration. Pharmaceutical researchers and manufacturers attempt to develop medications that target only specific receptor sites on particular types of cells. Unfortunately, the vast number of possible receptor sites within the body makes medications selective (rather than specific) at best. Even medications that bind with a limited group of receptor sites cause undesired responses in a variety of cells.

YOU are the Medic | PART 2

You make contact with the patient, who is surrounded by her coworkers. The patient is responsive to your questions and states that she suddenly became nauseous and lightheaded. Her coworkers tell you that she was walking to her desk when they suddenly realized she was on the ground. You ask the patient about her morning, and she replies that she had toast and a large cup of coffee and came to work. The patient states that she takes a daily vitamin.

Recording Time: 0 Minutes	
Appearance	Slightly pale and anxious
Level of consciousness	Alert
Airway	Open and maintained
Breathing	Clear breath sounds
Circulation	Pulse weak and very rapid

3. Given the information, what are some of your concerns?

4. The patient reports taking a vitamin each day; can a vitamin be the cause of her problem?

The term *side effect* is often used to mean *adverse effect*. Although both terms are usually used to mean harmful or potentially harmful effects, the term *adverse effect* more clearly indicates the possibility of serious consequences. Some side effects can be beneficial (such as a physician prescribing a specific antidepressant to treat postmenopausal symptoms, such as "hot flashes," because a positive side effect of the drug had been identified). Various sources may also refer to adverse effects as **untoward effects**. Both adverse and untoward effects are clinical changes, caused by medication, that are not desired and that cause some degree of harm or discomfort to the patient.

Undesired or harmful responses to a medication may be directly related to the intended cellular response or to random activation of unrelated cells throughout the body. Examples of undesired or harmful responses include hypoglycemia after the administration of insulin (exaggerated "therapeutic" effect); profound bradycardia after taking metoprolol, a beta-adrenergic antagonist medication (exaggerated therapeutic effect); and an allergic reaction to a medication (not a therapeutic effect). Common adverse effects include nausea, vomiting, sedation, palpitations, hypotension, hypertension, bradycardia, tachycardia, respiratory depression, endocrine abnormalities, dizziness, and a variety of others. Medication reference sources often categorize adverse effects by body system, frequency of occurrence, or severity.

When you are selecting medications, possible adverse effects should be considered in relation to the patient's condition. For example, the respiratory depressant properties of opioid analgesics, such as morphine sulfate, are unlikely to adversely affect a patient with burns who is intubated and being mechanically ventilated; however, an immediate threat to life might result if morphine is given to a patient becoming fatigued during an asthma attack. Another example involves the choice between two or more medications that can be given for the same condition, such as ondansetron (Zofran) and promethazine (Phenergan), antiemetic medications. Promethazine (Phenergan) causes significant hemodynamic and electrocardiographic changes that are not known to occur with ondansetron. Ondansetron may prove to be a safer antiemetic medication for patients who are particularly susceptible to adverse effects known to be associated with promethazine. In general, a medication should be avoided or used with caution in patients who are particularly susceptible to adverse effects associated with that medication.

Patients with certain chronic medical conditions are generally more susceptible to the adverse effects of medications than patients without such conditions. Significant cardiovascular disease, diabetes, impaired immunity, and renal failure are more often associated with greater severity or frequency of adverse effects. Many adverse effects of medications directly relate to these conditions; for example, renal failure hinders the ability of the kidneys to eliminate medications properly. In addition, patients with respiratory distress, shock, multiple trauma, or other life-threatening conditions may be unable to tolerate even mild adverse effects. Paramedics should use caution when selecting medications for patients with these conditions. Paramedics also need to be alert for adverse effects once medications have been given.

Adverse effects may range in severity from barely perceptible by patients and paramedics to an immediately life-threatening condition, requiring aggressive intervention. Cardiomyopathy, a disease of the heart muscle, can be caused by certain antidepressant medications. Certain antibiotics and antiseizure medications are known to cause **Stevens-Johnson syndrome**, a severe, possibly fatal medication reaction that mimics a burn. A wide variety of medications are known to cause anemia (low RBC count) through bone marrow suppression or direct **hemolysis**.

An adverse effect of a medication can be desirable in certain situations and harmful in others. For example, benzodiazepines are used to treat seizure activity and are known to cause sedation. Sedation may be desirable for a combative patient with a head injury but could also jeopardize the life of the same patient if he or she is vomiting.

Adverse effects occasionally occur that are completely unexpected and not previously known to occur with a particular medication. These effects are **idiosyncratic** medication reactions. Idiosyncratic medication reactions involve abnormal susceptibility to a medication, possibly due to genetic traits or dysfunction of a metabolic enzyme, that is peculiar to an individual patient.

Therapeutic Index

Pharmaceutical companies and scientists evaluate the safety and effectiveness of a potential medication before it is made available to the public. Animal testing establishes the **median lethal dose (LD_{50})**, which is the weight-based dose of a medication that causes death in 50% of the animals tested. Manufacturers determine the **median toxic dose (TD_{50})** for a particular adverse effect of the medication, which means that 50% of the animals tested had toxic effects at or above this weight-based dose. Human or animal testing also reveals the **median effective dose (ED_{50})** for a particular use or indication of the medication. The relationship between the median effective dose and the median lethal dose or median toxic dose is known as the **therapeutic index**, or therapeutic ratio. If there is a large difference between the median effective dose and the median toxic dose or median lethal dose, the medication is considered safe or possibly nontoxic. If the ratio is relatively small, careful patient selection, medication use, and monitoring of the medication are essential. A relatively unsafe medication may still be used in clinical practice if it is the only choice available for an otherwise fatal medical condition.

Immune-Mediated Medication Response

Medications and substances present in the environment have the potential to trigger an exaggerated response from the body's immune system. This response is described generally as an allergic reaction. It can range from mild skin changes to a multisystem, life-threatening reaction. Paramedics may encounter patients with this condition who request EMS assistance or encounter it immediately after medication administration to a patient being treated for an unrelated condition.

Patients who are genetically predisposed have an initial exposure and sensitization to a particular allergen. Various components of the body's immune system evolve into antibodies that specifically target this type of allergen. When the patient is reexposed to this type of allergen, a potentially massive cascade of immune system activity, known as <u>anaphylaxis</u>, begins. In severe cases, this reaction dramatically alters the function of the skin, GI, respiratory, and cardiovascular systems, ultimately manifesting as shock and respiratory failure. The chapter, *Immunologic Emergencies*, includes additional discussion of the pathophysiology and management of an immune-mediated medication response.

Patients predisposed to an allergic reaction, anaphylaxis, or other immune-mediated medication response may report previous reactions to medications, latex, foods, or other substances in the environment. Aspirin and antibiotics, most commonly penicillin and sulfa-based antibiotics, are the major culprits in immune-mediated medication responses. It is possible for a very small amount of any medication to cause this reaction. An immune-mediated reaction can occur days or weeks after initiating a medication.

Patients may also have <u>medication sensitivity</u> that is not related to an exaggerated immune system response. A mild to severe reaction may occur after the first exposure to a medication or other substance, often with many of the same signs and symptoms as an immune-mediated reaction. The treatment for medication sensitivity is similar to the treatment for an immune-mediated response. Paramedics should avoid administering medications to patients who have had a serious reaction to the specific medication (or a medication in the same class), unless the adverse effect was clearly dose-related and can be mitigated by judicious administration and careful monitoring.

Words of Wisdom

Do not be afraid to ask the same patient about allergies more than once if multiple medications are being administered.

Medication Tolerance

Certain medications are known to have decreased efficacy or potency when taken repeatedly by a patient, a state known as <u>tolerance</u>. Theories suggest that tolerance results from a mechanism reducing available cell receptors for a particular medication, a process known as <u>down-regulation</u>. The body also compensates for the effects associated with a medication by increasing the metabolism and/or elimination of the medication, resulting in a decreased concentration of the medication present near receptor sites. In certain cases, the desirable effects continue while other unintended or adverse effects decrease. In other situations, adverse effects persist or increase while additional medication is required to achieve the same therapeutic goal.

Repeated exposure to a medication within a particular class, such as opioids or benzodiazepines, has the potential to cause a tolerance to other medications in the same class. This phenomenon is known as <u>cross-tolerance</u>. Cross-tolerance becomes problematic when patients use or abuse medications, drugs, or chemicals on a regular basis and then require medications in

the class for a legitimate medical purpose. It becomes extremely difficult to determine the appropriate dose for the patient, often resulting in inadequate or excessive doses of therapeutic medications.

A similar condition, known as <u>tachyphylaxis</u>, occurs with certain medications. Repeated doses of medication within a short time rapidly cause tolerance, making the medication virtually ineffective. Tachyphylaxis is prone to occur with certain sympathomimetic medications (discussed later) and may occur with other medications paramedics may administer: nitroglycerin, dobutamine, and metoclopramide.

Words of Wisdom

Consider patient tolerance, IV infiltration or disconnect, or possible medication tampering every time a controlled substance does not demonstrate the expected clinical effect.

Medication Abuse and Dependence

Certain classes of medications, along with similar groups of illicit chemicals, have serious potential for misuse and abuse. People may choose to experience many of the desirable clinical effects from medications or chemicals without the presence of an underlying medical condition or symptom. Patients who receive certain medications for legitimate medical conditions may continue to use these medications long after the legitimate medical condition has resolved. In many instances it is difficult to determine whether an appropriate medical indication for certain medications continues to exist. Paramedics will undoubtedly encounter patients who misuse or abuse medications, illicit drugs, and other chemicals.

Two distinct groups of medications and chemicals are prone to misuse and abuse: stimulants and depressants. <u>Stimulant</u> chemicals cause a transient increase in physical, mental, or emotional performance. Caffeine, cocaine, and amphetamines are stimulants that have serious potential for misuse or abuse. In general, these medications increase a person's level of alertness, increase the heart rate, increase blood pressure, and otherwise activate the sympathetic nervous system. The immediate or long-term effects of stimulant medications have the potential to become life-threatening.

<u>Depressant</u> medications and chemicals, in contrast to stimulants, reduce CNS and sympathetic nervous system functioning, causing sedation, anxiolysis, respiratory depression, bradycardia, hypotension, and a variety of similar clinical symptoms. Benzodiazepines, alcohol, and opioid chemicals are common depressant substances. Toxicity from depressant substances is also potentially life-threatening following acute or long-term exposure.

Repeated exposure to certain medications or chemicals causes a patient to experience <u>habituation</u>, the abnormal tolerance to adverse or therapeutic effects associated with a substance. In essence, the body adapts to accommodate the exposure and protect itself from the severity of clinical changes associated with a substance. Prolonged or significant exposure to depressants, stimulants, and other medications and chemicals can cause some degree of <u>dependence</u>. Dependence is the physical, emotional, or behavioral need for these substances to maintain a certain level of "normal" function. The person has adapted to the frequent presence of the substance. In absence of the substance, adverse clinical effects occur. In severe cases, abrupt withdrawal from a substance can precipitate life-threatening clinical changes.

Medication Interactions

Patients receiving multiple medications, drugs, or other chemicals are at risk of an unintended interaction between or among the various substances, possibly with unexpected results. Undesirable medication interactions are referred to as medication <u>interference</u>. Paramedics must consider the possibility of illicit drugs, over-the-counter and prescribed medications, and herbal remedies interacting with any medication that might be given to a patient. As patients are prescribed a greater number of medications to treat chronic medical conditions, the risk of a medication interaction increases dramatically.

The most obvious concern with medication interactions is incompatibility during administration. When given simultaneously through the same IV tubing, certain medications will change chemical composition, possibly creating solid particles in the tubing, which then travel into the patient. Other medication combinations will deactivate one or more of the medications, making them ineffective. Medications require the proper IV solution. Various medications can be mixed only in normal saline or dextrose-containing solutions. Paramedics should consult a reliable medication reference source before administering multiple medications, especially continuous medication infusions, through the same IV tubing. Sodium bicarbonate and furosemide are two medications used frequently in the prehospital setting that are incompatible with several other common prehospital medications.

It is possible for a medication to increase the effect, decrease the effect, or alter the effect of another medication within the body. **Table 7** describes various types of medication interactions.

Principles of Pharmacokinetics

Paramedics must carefully consider the pharmacokinetic properties of any medication they are considering administering to a patient. As a medication is administered, the body begins a complex process of moving the medication, possibly altering the structure of the medication, and ultimately removing the medication from the body. The medication dose, route of administration, and clinical status of a patient will largely determine the duration and effectiveness of the medication (pharmacodynamics, discussed earlier in this chapter). Actions of absorption, distribution, metabolism, and elimination are discussed in detail in the following text.

The pharmacokinetics section of medication profiles typically states the <u>onset</u>, <u>peak</u>, and <u>duration of effect</u> for most medications. These values vary by route of administration and may have a broad range, depending on characteristics of individual patients. The onset and peak of a medication are generally related to absorption and distribution. A minimum dose or concentration of medication must be present at certain sites in the body for clinical effects to occur (see earlier discussion of pharmacodynamics).

The duration of effect is generally related to medication metabolism and elimination. As the amount of a medication near cell receptors (or other site of action) decreases, the clinical effects caused by the medication begin to decrease and normal function resumes.

If a medication permanently binds with a receptor site or irreversibly alters the function of a cell, the duration of the medication is determined by the body's ability to regenerate cells. In these cases, the duration of effect of a medication may be almost entirely unrelated to the dose or concentration present in the body. A single dose of aspirin, for example, is rapidly eliminated by the body, usually within several hours, but can cause an inhibition of platelet activity lasting for 3 to 10 days.

Documentation and Communication

Communicating the time of onset and peak of a medication to the patient will build trust and credibility.

Routes of Medication Administration

Absorption

Medication must enter the body to provide a clinical benefit. Consequently, paramedics must select a route of administration capable of delivering an appropriate amount of medication to the correct location within a patient's body. The route of administration is determined by the physical and chemical properties of the medication, the routes of administration available for a specific patient, and how quickly the effects of the medication are needed.

The chosen route of administration determines the percentage of the unchanged medication that reaches systemic circulation. This percentage, known as <u>bioavailability</u>, varies significantly from one medication to another, except when administered by the IV route. Medications administered by the IV route, by definition, have 100% bioavailability. Bioavailability is irrelevant for medications that are sequestered in the GI tract, such as activated charcoal and certain cathartic medications. Bioavailability is a critical consideration for other medications that are poorly absorbed by certain routes or subject to immediate metabolism by the liver before reaching systemic circulation. A number of important medication groups, such as beta blockers and calcium channel blockers, have a relatively low bioavailability when taken orally. The IV doses of these medications are many times lower than the oral doses when given for the same indication. Lidocaine and fentanyl are generally not given orally because of their low bioavailability with this route. Various routes of administration available to paramedics are discussed in the following sections.

Oral, Orogastric Tube, and Nasogastric Tube

A large number of medications prescribed for chronic medical conditions and several important prehospital medications

Table 7 Medication Interactions

Type of Interaction	Description	Example
Addition or summation	Two medications with a similar effect combine to produce an effect greater than that of either medication individually.	The antipyretic properties of acetaminophen (Tylenol) and the antipyretic properties of ibuprofen (Motrin, Advil) combine to reduce a fever in patients with fevers that could not be controlled by either medication alone.
Synergism	Two medications with a similar effect combine, and the resulting effect is greater than the sum of the effects of the medications (ie, 1 + 1 = 6).	Patients experience profound sedation when IV opioid medications such as fentanyl (Sublimaze) are given with IV benzodiazepines such as midazolam (Versed), greater than the expected sum of these two medications.
Potentiation	The effect of one medication is greatly enhanced by the presence of another medication, which does not have the ability to produce the same effect.	Promethazine (Phenergan) is given to increase the effects of codeine or other antitussives (cough suppressants) for more improved relief of cough than antitussive alone.
Altered absorption	The action of one medication increases or decreases the ability of another medication to be absorbed by the body. For example, medications that increase or decrease the gastrointestinal pH or motility may increase or decrease the absorption of other medications that are taken orally.	Ranitidine (Zantac), an H_2-blocker, can reduce absorption of ketoconazole (an antifungal) or certain cephalosporin antibiotics.
Altered metabolism	The action of one medication increases or decreases the metabolism of one medication within the body. For example, many medications (and certain foods) alter the performance of the cytochrome P-450 system in the liver, which is responsible for the metabolism of a variety of other medications.	Ethanol is administered to patients who have been poisoned with ethylene glycol (antifreeze). The presence of ethanol alters the metabolism of ethylene glycol in the liver, decreasing the severity of metabolic acidosis.
Altered distribution	The presence of one medication alters the area available for the distribution of another medication in the body, which becomes important when both medications are bound to the same site, such as plasma proteins. If proteins are already occupied by one medication, toxic levels of the other medication may develop.	The anticonvulsant medication valproic acid (Depakote, Depakene) competes with another anticonvulsant medication, phenytoin (Dilantin), causing potentially increased or decreased serum levels and possibly unpredictable clinical effects.
Altered elimination	Medications may increase or decrease the functioning of the kidneys or other route of elimination, influencing the amount of or duration of effect of another medication in the body.	Ethanol decreases the metabolism of warfarin (Coumadin), which may predispose the patient to bleeding risk.
Physiologic (drug) antagonism	Two medications, each producing opposite effects, are present simultaneously, resulting in minimal or no clinical changes.	Sodium nitroprusside (Nipride) and dobutamine (Dobutrex) are often given simultaneously for cardiogenic shock. By itself, dobutamine increases cardiac output, possibly causing an elevated blood pressure. Sodium nitroprusside causes vasodilation and possibly hypotension. When given together, these medications can be titrated to maintain a normal patient blood pressure.
Neutralization	Two medications bind together in the body, creating an inactive substance.	Digoxin-specific antibodies (Digibind, Digifab) are administered to patients with toxicity to the medication digoxin. These medications combine, rendering digoxin molecules inactive.

are administered into the GI system. This route requires that a patient is conscious, is able to swallow, or has a nasogastric tube or an orogastric tube in place. Aspirin, antipyretic medications, activated charcoal, diphenhydramine, and oral glucose are prehospital medications that may be administered into the GI system. Once administered, medication absorption varies depending on several factors Table 8.

In addition to these factors, GI medications may be subject to first-pass metabolism. Medication passes from the GI tract into the portal vein and travels directly into the liver. Once in

Table 8 GI Medication Absorption

Factor	Medication Absorption
GI motility	Ability of medication to pass through the GI tract into the bloodstream
GI pH	Perfusion of the GI system (may be decreased during systemic trauma or shock)
Presence of food, liquids, or chemicals in the stomach	Injury or bleeding in the GI system (both can alter GI motility, decreasing the time that oral medications can be absorbed)

Abbreviation: GI indicates gastrointestinal.

the liver, metabolism occurs, altering and potentially inactivating the medication before it ever reaches systemic circulation. First-pass metabolism can be exploited if metabolism changes a previously inactive medication into an active medication. Codeine, for example, undergoes a significant first-pass effect and a portion of the medication can be converted to morphine, a more potent analgesic, by the liver. Metabolism of a medication may also occur within the GI tract and as the medication enters the bloodstream. Bioavailability of medications given orally or through a nasogastric or an orogastric tube can range from 5% to 100%, depending on the particular medication and the effect of first-pass metabolism. Several important cardiac medications such as metoprolol (Lopressor) and verapamil (Calan) are subject to significant first-pass metabolism when taken orally. The reduction in bioavailability due to first-pass hepatic metabolism is already calculated into oral dosing, explaining why the oral dose of these medications is significantly higher than the IV doses of these medications for the same purpose. Patients with hepatic (liver) dysfunction are at risk of toxicity of these medications when given orally, even at conventional doses, because first-pass effect is impaired and a greater quantity of this medication reaches systemic circulation.

Endotracheal

The endotracheal route is no longer considered a reliable method of medication administration. The ACLS protocols deemphasize the usefulness of medication administration via the endotracheal tube. If endotracheal medications must be given, sources recommend administering at least 2 to 2.5 times the IV dose for medications approved for this route, followed by a 5- to 10-mL flush with sterile water or normal saline. With improved IO techniques and devices that have superior medication uptake, it is likely that use of the endotracheal route of medication administration will become increasingly limited. Paramedics may still administer bronchodilators or mucolytic medications in certain critical care settings via the endotracheal route.

Intranasal

The intranasal route of medication administration seems to be gaining popularity in the prehospital setting. Liquid medications are converted into a fine mist that is sprayed into one or both nostrils. Fentanyl (Sublimaze), midazolam (Versed), and naloxone (Narcan) can be administered using this route, often with effectiveness equal to or better than conventional methods. Medication absorption is rapid, and the bioavailability of intranasal medications appears close to 100% in certain studies. Other studies suggest that this method is superior to the IV and rectal routes of administration for a variety of reasons. Nasal medication administration can occur almost immediately, without delay for initiating an IV line, especially in situations where IV access is difficult or impossible to obtain. Additionally, nasal administration does not place the paramedic at risk for a needlestick injury when treating uncooperative patients.

Intravenous

The IV route remains the preferred method for the administration of the majority of medications used in the prehospital setting. A small-diameter catheter is inserted into a peripheral or external jugular vein, allowing medications to be administered directly into systemic circulation. Paramedics in special situations may also be permitted to use permanent indwelling venous catheters or large-bore catheters that have already been inserted into central veins by other health care professionals. The bioavailability of medication is 100% by definition. Medications administered by the IV route have an onset of action that is significantly quicker than medications given orally or through an orogastric or nasogastric tube, allowing an often immediate response or creating the ability to titrate a medication carefully in a rapidly evolving clinical situation.

There are several important limitations regarding the IV route of medication administration. Access is difficult in several noteworthy groups of patients: patients who have abused IV drugs, patients in profound shock or having cardiovascular collapse, and patients with certain chronic medical conditions such as diabetes and renal failure. The IV access procedure (discussed in the *Medication Administration* chapter) has the potential to cause pain or infection and is somewhat time-consuming. Uncontrolled scenes, environmental extremes, and movement of the transport vehicle make IV access challenging in the prehospital setting.

The infiltration of IV medication into tissues around the blood vessel is a significant concern for paramedics. Certain classes of medications such as **sympathomimetics** and electrolyte solutions can cause significant pain and tissue damage when they accumulate in surrounding tissues. In extreme cases, tissue death will occur in affected areas, leaving a large area of necrotic tissue or skin.

Words of Wisdom

Frequently reassess the IV site for infiltration or tubing disconnect during transport. Confirm that the IV is still working properly during patient turnover, especially if the medication being administered has a high potential to cause an adverse effect.

Intraosseous

The IO route of medication administration provides a viable alternative when IV access cannot be obtained in the prehospital setting. A needle is inserted through the patient's skin and into the bone. The tip of the needle pierces the hard, outer layer of bone and enters the softer bone marrow. Vascular uptake from the bone marrow provides a reliable route for medications and IV fluids (Table 9). The *Medication Administration* chapter describes the technique for IO access in greater detail.

Any medication that can be administered by the IV route can also be administered by the IO route. Infusion rates for IO fluids are comparable to IV rates when a pressure bag or mechanical infusion device is used. The IO devices can generally be left in place for up to 24 hours, allowing a route of medication or fluid administration until IV access can be obtained.

Administration by the IO route is contraindicated in bones that are fractured. It is also discouraged when patients have various bone diseases or a skin infection over a possible insertion site. Newer devices allow IO insertion in a variety of anatomic locations and across the spectrum of patient age and weight.

Intramuscular

Various medications used in the prehospital setting can be administered by the intramuscular (IM) route. Sterile medication is drawn into a syringe attached to a needle and injected into one of a patient's larger muscles. This route is used when IV access cannot be established or when the clinical situation requires immediate medication administration that cannot wait for IV access. Medications have a bioavailability from 75% to 100% following IM administration. The absorption rate is determined by the accuracy of the injection landmark and the perfusion to the chosen muscle.

Paramedics should use caution when performing an IM injection. Uncooperative patients may move suddenly, placing paramedics or other responders at risk for a contaminated needle stick. Auto-injection devices, such as the EpiPen and Mark-1 Kit, are commercially available, are spring-loaded, and deliver a predetermined quantity of medication. These devices usually do not retract the needle following administration, so risks to paramedics are still present.

Paramedics should confirm that a medication is appropriate for IM use before administering it. Even if a medication is safe for IM use, medication reference sources may indicate that a particular muscle should be used or recommend a particular technique for the injection. Many medications are safe for IV use but cause significant injury if given by the IM route. Certain medications are indicated only for IM use and cause a variety of complications if given by the IV route.

Subcutaneous

Subcutaneous (SC) medication administration is similar to IM administration. A sterile medication solution is drawn into a syringe attached to a needle. The medication is then injected into various SC tissue sites throughout the body. The anterior part of the abdomen, just outside the umbilicus, and the skin overlying the triceps muscle are common sites for SC injection. The needles for SC administration are shorter and have a smaller diameter than IM needles. The techniques for SC and IM medication administration are discussed in greater detail in the chapter, *Medication Administration*. Certain medications may be indicated for SC use only and should not be given by the IV route, even if a patent IV is already in place. Slower absorption through the SC tissue may prevent adverse cardiovascular effects compared with IV administration of the medication. Consult ALS protocols or a reliable medication reference for specific information about the SC administration of a medication.

Dermal and Transdermal

Paramedics may encounter patients in the prehospital setting who are receiving medication via the transdermal route. Patches commonly containing nicotine, antiemetics, analgesics, nitroglycerin, or other medications are placed in various locations on the body. Transdermal medications may alter a patient's clinical presentation or interfere with medications administered by a paramedic. It is often helpful to ask a patient or family member if a transdermal medication patch is in place while obtaining a medication history for the patient. Transdermal patches deliver a relatively constant dose of medication during a long period. Changes in patient temperature or perfusion may alter the delivery of medication to the patient, potentially causing significant clinical changes. Paramedics should also be aware that transdermal patches often contain a large quantity of medication. If these patches are chewed or ingested, particularly by children, life-threatening toxic effects are possible.

Sublingual

Nitroglycerin is frequently given to patients by paramedics using the sublingual (SL) route of administration. Nitroglycerin tablets are placed under a patient's tongue or nitroglycerin is sprayed under the patient's tongue, where it is absorbed rapidly by the mucous membranes, resulting in a relatively quick onset. Bioavailability of nitroglycerin administered sublingually is quite low. Relatively large doses of SL nitroglycerin are required compared with an IV infusion, close to 100 times larger for initial dosing. Patients must be conscious and alert to receive SL medications. In addition, a lack of moisture or saliva in a patient's mouth may significantly delay the absorption of SL medications. In this case, the spray formulation is preferable over SL tablets. Paramedics may also encounter patients receiving certain analgesic medications by lozenges and other

Table 9 Veins Used During IO Infusion	
Intraosseous Site	**Vein**
Proximal tibia	Popliteal vein
Femur	Femoral vein
Distal tibia (medial malleolus)	Great saphenous vein
Proximal humerus	Axillary vein
Manubrium (sternum)	Internal mammary and azygos veins

medications administered sublingually using lollipops, gums, and orally dissolving tablets.

Inhaled or Nebulized

The respiratory system is an extremely important route of medication administration for paramedics. In the prehospital setting, medications may be inhaled or nebulized into the respiratory tract. Inhaled prehospital medications are limited to oxygen and, possibly, the antidote, amyl nitrate, which is given in laboratory and industrial settings for cyanide exposure. Paramedics may also administer or assist patients administering respiratory medication using a metered-dose inhaler (MDI), typically for asthma or chronic obstructive pulmonary disease (COPD). Activation of the MDI converts liquid medicine into a gas, allowing the medication to pass into the patient's lungs. When used with an aerochamber, MDIs are at least as effective as nebulizers for the administration of bronchodilator medications.

Medication in liquid form may also be nebulized (converted into a fine spray) for administration directly into the respiratory system. Tubing with oxygen or compressed air is attached to a small chamber, creating a mist as the gas passes through the liquid medication. The chamber is attached to a mouthpiece or a mask, allowing patients to receive droplets of medication with each inspired breath. Unfortunately, a portion of the medication is lost during exhalation and during any pauses in patient respiration. Nebulized medications are typically administered by paramedics for the treatment of bronchospasm or airway edema. Racemic epinephrine, albuterol, levalbuterol (Xopenex), and ipratropium bromide (Atrovent) are nebulized medications available in the prehospital setting. Paramedics may occasionally be asked to administer unusual medications by nebulizer. Calcium gluconate may be nebulized following inhalation exposure to hydrofluoric acid. Paramedics must be aware that nebulized medications have the potential to cause bronchospasm and should not routinely administer calcium, lidocaine, or other nontraditional medications by nebulizer without approval from medical control.

Rectal

Certain medications used in the prehospital setting may be administered by the rectal route. The rectal route is preferred over the oral route for several reasons. The rectal route can be used when the patient is unconscious, having seizures, vomiting, or unable to swallow oral medications. In addition, rectal medications are usually not subject to first-pass metabolism, which decreases the bioavailability of many oral medications. Certain medications administered rectally may have greater than 90% bioavailability. If a medication is administered into the proximal rectum, some first-pass effect is still possible. Medications administered into the lower rectum are less likely to have any dose reduction due to first-pass effect. Whenever possible, medications should be administered into the lower, rather than proximal, rectum.

Rectal medications are manufactured in suppository form, which is a waxlike substance molded into a shape similar to a bullet. The suppository is lubricated and inserted into the patient's rectal cavity. Antiemetics and antipyretic medications are often available in suppository form. Absorption of rectal medications can be unpredictable, often related to the specific site of absorption within the rectum. The rectal dose of a medication is often higher than the oral or IV dose.

Paramedics may administer or assist with the administration of rectal diazepam for the emergency control of seizures, particularly in children. This method has been proven effective, with minimal risk of subsequent respiratory depression. Paramedics may administer the IV solution rectally, using a commercial device for this purpose, a lubricated feeding tube attached to a syringe, or a lubricated small-diameter syringe, such as a tuberculin syringe with the needle removed. (Never insert a needle into a patient's rectum; doing so may cause trauma, bleeding, or perforation into the abdominal cavity.)

Ophthalmic

EMS systems may approve the administration of medications by the ophthalmic route. In the prehospital setting, the ophthalmic route is generally limited to ocular anesthetic agents given to facilitate the irrigation of eyes following a chemical exposure. Although the role of ophthalmic medications in the prehospital setting is generally limited, paramedics should be aware that it is possible for medications to cause systemic toxic effects following ophthalmic administration.

Other Methods of Medication Administration

Hemodialysis is one of the rare exceptions in which medications produce their beneficial effects outside the patient's body. Blood from a patient is pumped through a dialysis machine, exposing the blood to dialysate solution that removes toxins, excess electrolytes, and other chemicals from the blood before returning it to the patient. It is doubtful that paramedics working in the prehospital setting will use this method.

Paramedics may encounter patients receiving medication through a variety of other routes. These methods are not generally used in the prehospital setting and may cause serious or life-threatening complications if used by untrained personnel. Paramedics should not use any unfamiliar catheters, lines, tubes, or other devices for medication or fluid administration unless they have received appropriate training and authorization.

■ Distribution of Medication

Chemical and physical properties of a medication determine how the medication moves through the body. Many medication factors such as the size of medication molecules, the ability to bind with other substances within the body, and the ability to dissolve in certain body fluids determine which cells, tissues, and organs a particular medication will reach. Individual patient factors such as fat, water, and protein content will also determine how much of a medication is available to cause physiologic changes at a given dose.

The human body has an elaborate system of barriers designed to prevent the introduction of foreign substances into the body and into specific cells, tissues, and organs. Medication molecules need to pass through various barriers to reach target sites within the body. To cross these barriers, medication molecules must move through spaces between individual cells or pass directly through the center of individual cells.

Paramedics use the process of __osmosis__ to enhance the distribution of certain medications, electrolytes, and IV fluids. During osmosis, free water along with certain particles such as sodium and potassium can pass through a semipermeable membrane to equalize the concentration of the water and other particles on each side of the membrane. This process allows IV fluids to leave the intravascular space and enter various tissues and cells. Osmosis is also one of the mechanisms that the kidneys use to regulate the fluid balance within the body.

__Filtration__ is a process within the body, similar to osmosis, that is used to redistribute water and other particles. Most discussion of filtration within the body focuses on renal sodium and water filtration in the glomerular capillaries. Hydrostatic pressure forces various body fluids against semipermeable membranes, causing the passage of certain substances into an adjacent compartment.

The skin, GI tract, eyes, and urinary tract contain epithelial cells that create a continuous barrier. This barrier prevents the movement of medication molecules between the epithelial cells. For medications to cross the epithelial barrier, the medication molecules must pass directly through cells to enter the body. Small medication molecules that are __nonionic__ (uncharged) and __lipophilic__ (attracted to fats and lipids) pass easily through cell membranes. All but the largest lipid-soluble medications can pass easily through cell membranes.

Larger, __hydrophilic__ (attracted to water molecules) and ionic (charged) medication molecules must find another route of entry into cells. For larger medication molecules, cells use a process called __pinocytosis__ to ingest extracellular fluids and their contents. Medication molecules may also bind with carrier proteins for transport into cells. This process of binding with carrier proteins is called __facilitated diffusion__ when no energy is expended and is called __active transport__ when energy is used to move the molecules against a concentration gradient.

In addition to the epithelial barrier, the human body has capillary barriers near specific tissues. Once inside blood vessels, medication molecules must pass through capillary walls to reach target cells or other sites. The blood-brain barrier, the blood-placenta barrier, and the blood-testes barrier are areas where capillary cells form a continuous barrier, preventing the passage of medication molecules through openings in capillary walls. These three anatomic barriers prevent various medication molecules from reaching underlying tissues. Only certain medications are able to pass through cell membranes in these areas and enter adjacent tissues.

Capillaries in the kidney, thyroid, pancreas, and others areas allow medication molecules to pass freely through the capillary walls into surrounding tissues. Only protein-bound medications have difficulty passing through the capillaries in these areas. The lungs and peritoneum also permit medication molecules to enter and exit easily through capillary walls.

__Plasma protein binding__ significantly alters the distribution of certain medications within the body. Medication molecules temporarily attach to proteins in the blood plasma. Albumin and other plasma proteins effectively store a quantity of medication largely independent of the concentration of the medication present in the blood or other body tissues. Patient age,

YOU *are the Medic* | PART 3 |

You give the patient oxygen by nonrebreathing mask. Your partner obtains the patient's vital signs and a blood glucose reading as you apply the heart monitor. The heart monitor shows a narrow, rapid rhythm with no other ectopy and no discernable P waves. The patient states she has history of cardiac problems and that this situation has not happened before. She states that she does not take any medications, except the vitamin mentioned earlier.

Recording Time: 5 Minutes	
Respirations	24 breaths/min
Pulse	198 beats/min; rapid and weak
Skin	Slightly pale
Blood pressure	100/40 mm Hg
Oxygen saturation (Spo$_2$)	99% on oxygen
Pupils	Equal and reactive
Blood glucose level	100 mg/dL
ECG	Supraventricular tachycardia

5. What medication classifications can slow the heart rate?

6. In what form do the medications come, what is the route of administration, and what effect do they have?

nutritional status, and medical condition influence the amount of plasma protein present in the body. As plasma protein levels change or when another medication that binds with plasma proteins is introduced, the concentration of the original medication in blood and body tissues may change significantly.

Protein binding increases the amount of medication necessary for a desired clinical effect. This reversible process also releases medication as circulating levels of a particular medication begin to fall, leading to a longer duration of action for the medication. It is possible for a patient to have a therapeutic (safe) level of a protein-bound medication until a second protein-bound medication with greater affinity is administered. The second medication displaces the original medication attached to plasma proteins, causing a dramatic increase in the amount of the original medication present in circulation and subsequent toxic effects.

Fat tissue is another site of medication distribution that alters the amount of medication available for action within the body. Large quantities of lipophilic medications can be sequestered in the fat tissues of obese persons. The medication is released slowly, causing prolonged effects compared with the same dose in lean persons. As the percentage of body fat increases, the same weight-based dose of a hydrophilic medication results in a higher concentration in the plasma and water throughout the body.

■ Volume of Distribution

The **volume of distribution** for a medication describes the extent to which a medication will spread within the body. Certain medications do not readily leave the plasma. Other medications spread into water throughout the body. Still other medications readily bind with bone, teeth, or other tissues, resulting in a relatively low concentration in the blood. The volume of distribution relates medication dose to the anticipated plasma level of a given medication in an "average" patient. Medications with a lower volume of distribution have higher levels present in the plasma at a given dose than do medications with a higher volume of distribution. In the alternative, if a medication has a high volume of distribution, a larger total dose is needed to obtain a certain level in the plasma than with a medication with a lower volume of distribution. It is also possible to estimate the amount of a medication or chemical present in the body by knowing the level of the medication present in the plasma and the known volume of distribution for a particular medication. This value may help explain why a large dose of additional medication may cause only a modest increase of available medication.

■ Medication Metabolism

Many medications undergo some degree of chemical change by the body, known as biotransformation. As a medication undergoes biotransformation, it becomes known as a metabolite. Metabolites can either be active or inactive. **Active metabolites** remain capable of some pharmacologic activity, such as altering a cell process

or body function. It is possible for active metabolites to go from helpful or therapeutic to harmful. **Inactive metabolites**, however, no longer possess the ability to alter a cell process or body function. Biotransformation is a process that has four possible effects on a medication absorbed into the body:

1. An inactive substance can become active, capable of producing desired or unwanted clinical effects (active metabolite).
2. An active medication can be changed into another active medication (active metabolite).
3. An active medication can be completely or partially inactivated (inactive metabolite).
4. A medication can be transformed into a substance (active or inactive metabolite) that is easier for the body to eliminate.

Most biotransformation occurs in the liver. The cytochrome P-450 system in the liver uses a complex, enzyme-based process to alter the chemical structure of a medication or other chemical. Separate pathways within the cytochrome P-450 system are responsible for the metabolism of different medication groups. These pathways can be selectively influenced by other medications, chemicals, and diet choices, altering the metabolism of certain groups of medications. Ethanol, oral contraceptives, and grapefruit juice are known to cause potentially life-threatening alterations in the cytochrome P-450 metabolism of certain medications.

The kidneys, skin, lungs, GI tract, and many other body tissues have some ability to cause biotransformation as well. Microorganisms present in the GI tract begin biotransformation of certain medications taken orally. In general, biotransformation makes medications and chemicals more water-soluble and easier for the kidneys and other organs to eliminate from the body. Paramedics should suspect altered metabolism of medications in patients with chronic alcoholism, liver disease, or any condition known to affect the liver.

■ Medication Elimination

Medications and other chemicals are primarily removed from the body by the kidneys. The original medication or its metabolite (the chemical produced following biotransformation) is filtered by the kidneys and excreted into the urine. A variety of factors influences how quickly medication is eliminated from the body. Kidney dysfunction or disease impairs elimination of many substances. Patients with acute or chronic renal failure are at significant risk for toxic effects of medications or metabolic waste products in the body. Renal blood flow, urinary tract obstruction, and alterations in the pH of urine affect the ability of the kidneys to remove medication and toxins from the body.

Medications and chemicals in the body follow two distinct patterns of metabolism and elimination: zero-order elimination and first-order elimination. Under **zero-order elimination**, a fixed amount of a substance is removed during a certain period, regardless of the total amount in the body. Ethanol is a classic example of zero-order elimination. Chronic consumption of ethanol increases the liver's ability to metabolize ethanol because of enhanced activation of the cytochrome P-450 system. Despite the increased rate of elimination, only a fixed amount of ethanol will be eliminated each hour, regardless of initial plasma levels. The duration of intoxication is directly related to the initial plasma level.

The majority of medications and chemicals undergo **first-order elimination**. The rate of elimination is directly influenced by the plasma levels of the substance. In essence, the more substance in the plasma, the more the body works to eliminate the substance. First-order elimination is quantified as a medication **half-life** on the medication profile. The half-life of a medication is the time needed in an average person for metabolism or elimination of 50% of the substance in the plasma. It takes much longer than two half-lives to eliminate a medication completely, despite the literal connotation of the term. A medication half-life is altered by factors such as disease states, changes in perfusion, and medication interactions. Consider the following example of half-life calculations:

> *Patient A has taken an overdose of medication X, which has a half-life of 2 hours. The plasma level of the medication on arrival to the emergency department was 100 µg/mL. After 2 hours, the plasma level will be 50 µg/mL. Four hours after arrival, the plasma level will be 25 µg/mL. Two hours later, the plasma level will be 12.5 µg/mL.*

A medication half-life pertains only to the quantity of medication within the body, not necessarily to the clinical effects of the medication. Aspirin, as discussed earlier, has a half-life of only 15 to 20 minutes, but it causes antiplatelet effects that last for 3 to 10 days. Adenosine, a medication given in the prehospital setting for dysrhythmias, has a half-life of less than 10 seconds, but it may permanently resolve supraventricular tachycardia. The benzodiazepine clonazepam (Klonopin) has a long half-life—19 to 50 hours in adults. Patients often remain sedated for several days following an intentional overdose.

Physicians and other health care providers attempt to create a steady state of certain medications. Medications are administered at a dose and frequency that equals the body's rate of elimination, resulting in a constant level of medication within the body. A medication steady state is desirable for anticoagulants, antibiotics, antiseizure medications, and certain antidysrhythmic medications. Paramedics should suspect alterations in the steady state of a medication when patients manifest symptoms of an underlying disease (such as seizures or a dysrhythmia) that is usually well controlled by long-term medications.

Smaller amounts of medication can be eliminated through other body systems. Medication, medication metabolites, and other chemicals can be eliminated in expired air from the lungs, stool, saliva, breast milk, and perspiration. When given orally, activated charcoal (discussed in the *Toxicology* chapter) is capable of binding with oral toxins (and several chemicals present in the bloodstream) and eliminating them through the GI tract.

Reducing Medication Errors

Paramedics have the difficult tasks of assessing patients, performing invasive procedures, and administering medications in the uncontrolled prehospital setting. In this environment, patient history is often limited, inaccurate, or nonexistent. Paramedics do not always have the time or resources for a careful evaluation of the risks and benefits associated with medications that they are considering administering to a patient. Medication decisions are often based on memory and frequently occur in the context of a stressful, life-threatening patient situation. Paramedics are constantly at risk for a cognitive error, such as choosing the wrong medication or dose, or a technical error, such as administering more volume of medication than was intended. **Table 10** lists the six rights of medication administration.

Paramedics should use a current, reliable medication reference source whenever administering potentially unfamiliar medications or whenever an unusual dose or route of administration is being considered. Technical errors can be avoided by having a partner confirm the volume in a syringe or a weight-based medication calculation. Many health care settings require that two providers check pediatric and high-risk medication calculations. Paramedics should also evaluate for a patient medication allergy or hypersensitivity before each medication administration.

The Institute for Safe Medication Practices (IMSP) has developed a list of error-prone medication abbreviations. When these symbols and abbreviations are used by physicians, paramedics, and other health care providers, there is an increased likelihood of a medication error due to miscommunication. The full list is exhaustive. **Table 11** lists several important error-prone items relevant to the prehospital setting.

Important Medications in the Prehospital Setting

It is essential that paramedics understand the indications and limitations of several important groups of medications. The following sections contain an overview of medications and medication groups used to treat medical conditions primarily affecting certain body systems. Many medication groups have indications for a wide range of medical conditions, including outside the context of a particular body system **Table 12**.

Medications Used in Airway Management

Paramedics in certain EMS systems may be permitted to use a variety of medications for airway management. Rapid-sequence intubation and medication-facilitated airway placement are controversial procedures in the prehospital setting and are not permitted in many locations. When these procedures are performed, paramedics use various sedative medications with or without chemical paralytic medications to secure an artificial airway in patients with an intact gag reflex and some degree of responsiveness. Patients become adequately sedated, the gag reflex disappears, and trismus or other facial muscle

Table 10   The Six Rights of Medication Administration

1. Right patient

Although you will typically treat one patient at a time, sometimes you may have to manage multiple patients. It is essential to confirm the identity of a patient before administering any medication—especially when patients are unconscious or are unable to communicate (because of extremes of age, altered consciousness, or other factors). Always make an attempt to have the patient confirm his or her identity verbally, or confirm the identity of the patient yourself through identification devices (such as bracelets or ID cards), to the extent possible. A critical issue, as identified in the SAMPLE history, is to ensure that the patient does not have allergies to the medication(s) you intend to give Figure 3 .

2. Right medication

Administration of the wrong medication is the most common pharmacology-related error. Several factors may lead to "wrong medication" errors, including similar packaging and labeling, similar names and storage practices, and ineffective communication. Always repeat (echo) the medication order, and confirm that the packaging matches the intended order. Avoid using abbreviations, and always recheck the order before administration.

3. Right dose

Doses of nearly every medication depend on patient-specific factors (such as condition, weight, and age); the actual dose needed is often not equal to the amount supplied in an ampule or a prefilled syringe in the prehospital setting. Therefore, you will have to calculate the patient-specific dose. When calculating the correct dose, always recheck your math, and, if possible, have your partner recheck and verify the final dose.

4. Right route

Many medications can be administered by a variety of routes; the optimal route depends on the patient's condition and the speed with which the medication needs to take effect. Errors can occur when medication doses and routes are confused. For example, IV drip doses can be different from doses for the same medication injected into an IV as a bolus. Another important route-related issue is the patient's condition. If a patient is in profound shock, you must consider how well the medication will be absorbed and distributed to target issues. Choosing the right route helps enable the medication to have the correct effect. Always verify the route of administration.

5. Right time

Because all medications take a certain amount of time to take effect and may have the potential to interfere with other medications, you must always follow the recommended guidelines for the proper frequency of medication administration. Evaluate the patient's condition before and after you administer any medication, and document any noted response or change in the patient's condition. Also remember that some medications require a specific administration frequency to maintain a therapeutic level.

6. Right documentation and reporting

Because paramedics frequently transfer care of a patient to other health care providers, it is critical to document in writing the medications administered, the dose, when they were administered, and the effects the patient experienced. Whenever possible, communicate this information in writing, on the PCR, and in a verbal report to the next level of care.

Table 11   Errors and Misinterpretations in Reporting

Item	Intended Meaning	Possible Misinterpretation	Correction
Trailing zero after the decimal point (eg, 4.0 mg)	4 mg	40 mg	Avoid trailing zeros when decimal place is not needed.
No leading zero before decimal point (eg, .8 mg)	0.8 mg	8 mg	Use a zero before the decimal point when the dose is less than 1 unit.
MSO_4	Morphine sulfate	Magnesium sulfate	Write out "morphine sulfate."
$MgSO_4$	Magnesium sulfate	Morphine sulfate	Write out "magnesium sulfate."
SC	Subcutaneous	May be interpreted as SL (sublingual)	Write out "subcutaneous."
IN	Intranasal	May be interpreted as IV (intravenous) or IM (intramuscular)	Write out intranasal.

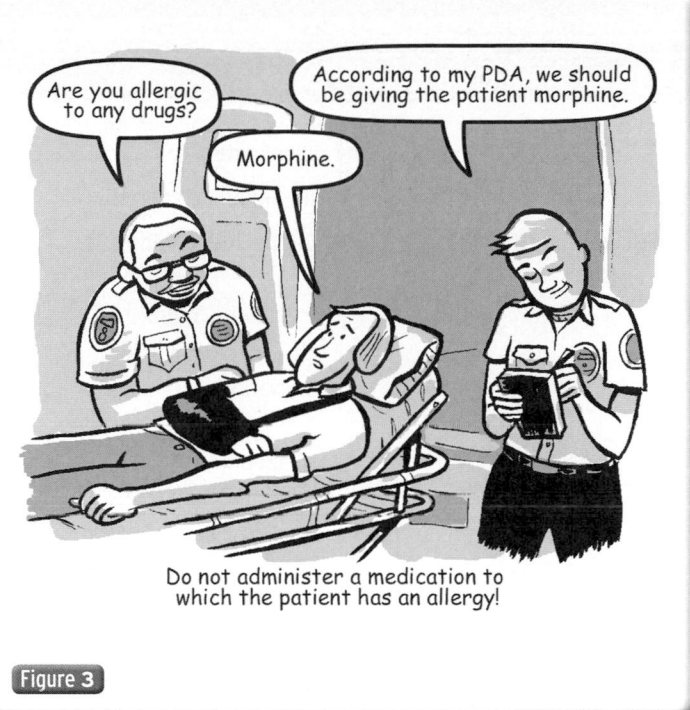

Do not administer a medication to which the patient has an allergy!

Figure 3

tension ceases following the correct use and sequence of airway medication. If performed correctly, patients have no awareness or memory of the procedure.

Sedative-Hypnotic Agents Used in Airway Management

Etomidate (Amidate) and ketamine (Ketalar) are two ultra–short-acting sedative medications used to facilitate airway placement. Etomidate is an imidazole derivative that works as a single-dose profound sedative. It is preferred for its minimal effect on blood pressure and other hemodynamic parameters. Etomidate begins working in 30 to 60 seconds, peaks in approximately 60 seconds, and lasts approximately 5 minutes. The short duration is usually desirable for airway procedures, but paramedics need to resedate patients promptly with an alternative sedative medication during or immediately after inserting an airway device. Etomidate causes adrenal suppression (if multiple doses are given) that has the potential to further compromise the condition of an already critically ill patient. No more than one dose of etomidate should be given.

Ketamine is another possible adjunct to airway placement. It has a chemical composition similar to that of phencyclidine and causes profound dissociation and general anesthesia. Ketamine

Table 12 Notable Medication Groups Affecting Prehospital Patient Care			
Medication Class	**Common Indications or Purposes**	**Primary Body System Affected**	**Examples**
Alkalinizing agents	Increase serum or urine pH	Renal	Sodium bicarbonate
Antacids	Neutralize excess acids present in stomach	Gastrointestinal	Sucralfate (Carafate), aluminum salts, calcium carbonate
Anthelmintics	Treat intestinal parasites	Gastrointestinal	Mebendazole (Vermox)
Antibiotics	Treat bacterial infection	Varied	Penicillin, ciprofloxacin (Cipro)
Anticoagulants	Reduce efficacy of clotting factors present in the blood	Hematologic	Heparin, warfarin (Coumadin)
Antidiarrheals	Decrease gastrointestinal motility, alter gastrointestinal secretion activity	Gastrointestinal	Loperamide (Imodium), diphenoxylate-atropine combination (Lomotil)
Antidysrhythmics	Prevent or control various cardiac dysrhythmias	Cardiovascular	Lidocaine, amiodarone (Cordarone)
Antiemetics	Treat or prevent nausea and vomiting	Gastrointestinal, CNS	Promethazine (Phenergan), ondansetron (Zofran)
Antiflatulents	Prevent or treat excess intestinal gas	Gastrointestinal	Simethicone, lactase
Antifungals	Treat fungal infections	Varied	Fluconazole (Diflucan), ketoconazole (Nizoral)
Antiglaucoma agents (usually eye drops)	Treat glaucoma	Varied	Brinzolamide (Azopt), bimatoprost (Lumigan)
Antihistamines	Block histamine receptors, dry mucous membranes, inhibit immune response in allergic reactions	Varied	Diphenhydramine (Benadryl), loratadine (Claritin)

Continues

Table 12 Notable Medication Groups Affecting Prehospital Patient Care, continued

Medication Class	Common Indications or Purposes	Primary Body System Affected	Examples
Antihyperlipidemics	Decrease blood cholesterol, sequester cholesterol chemicals in bile	Hematologic, cardiovascular	Cholestyramine (Questran), colesevelam (Welchol)
Antiparasitic agents	Treat parasitic infections	Varied	Nitazoxanide (Alinia)
Antipsychotics	Treat psychoses, including schizophrenia	Sympathetic nervous system	Haloperidol (Haldol), olanzapine (Zyprexa)
Antivirals	Treat viral infections	Varied	Acyclovir (Zovirax), famciclovir (Famvir)
Barbiturates	Reduce or prevent seizures, provide sedation	CNS	Phenobarbital
Benzodiazepines	Treat anxiety and seizures, provide sedation	CNS	Lorazepam (Ativan), diazepam (Valium), oxazepam (Serax)
Beta-agonists	Bronchodilation	Respiratory	Albuterol; levalbuterol (Xopenex)
Beta-blocking agents	Reduce heart rate and blood pressure	Cardiovascular	Metoprolol (Lopressor), atenolol (Tenormin)
Calcium channel blockers	Reduce heart rate and blood pressure	Cardiovascular	Diltiazem (Cardizem), verapamil (Calan)
Cardiac glycosides	Decrease heart rate and improve contractility	Cardiovascular	Digoxin (Lanoxin)
Chemotherapeutic agents	Treat cancer or malignancy	Varied	Vincristine (Oncovin, Vincasar), cisplatin (Platinol)
Cholesterol synthesis inhibitors	Prevent cholesterol conversion in the liver	Gastrointestinal	Atorvastatin (Lipitor), simvastatin (Zocor)
Cholinergics	Activate secretory glands in eyes and gastrointestinal tract; improve muscle weakness in myasthenia gravis	Parasympathetic nervous system	Pilocarpine (Isopto); pyridostigmine (Mestinon)
Corticosteroids	Decrease inflammation; immunosuppressant	Endocrine and immune	Prednisone, dexamethasone (Decadron)
Cough suppressants	Decrease bronchial irritation causing cough	CNS	Codeine, dextromethorphan
Digestants	Enhance digestion of food; may include supplemental pancreatic enzymes	Gastrointestinal	Glutamine
Diuretics	Promote excretion of urine; manage fluid overload	Renal	Mannitol (Osmitrol), furosemide (Lasix)
Fibrinolytics	Dissolve clots present in blood vessels or vascular access devices	Hematologic	Tissue plasminogen activator (tPA), tenecteplase (TNKase)
Glucocorticoids	Replacement or maintenance therapy, treat systemic inflammation, numerous other uses	Endocrine and immune	Hydrocortisone, beclomethasone (Beconase)
Glycoprotein IIb/IIIa inhibitors	Deactivate proteins involved in platelet aggregation	Hematologic	Tirofiban (Aggrastat), eptifibatide (Integrilin)
Histamine-2 receptor antagonists	Block histamine receptors, including those responsible for gastric acid secretion	Gastrointestinal and immune	Ranitidine (Zantac), famotidine (Pepcid)
Hormone replacement drugs	Replace hormones, improve bone density that has decreased due to aging and hormone loss	Endocrine	Estrogen, progesterone

Continues

Table 12 Notable Medication Groups Affecting Prehospital Patient Care, continued

Medication Class	Common Indications or Purposes	Primary Body System Affected	Examples
Immunomodulators	Inhibit or enhance functioning of the immune system	Immune	Interferon, levamisole (Ergamisol)
Immunosuppressants	Prevent rejection of transplanted organs and tissues; treat rheumatoid arthritis	Immune	Cyclosporine (Gengraf), tacrolimus (Prograf)
Insulin	Positive inotropic effects, allows cellular glucose uptake, treat hyperkalemia	Endocrine	Insulin
Laxatives	Increase gastrointestinal motility	Gastrointestinal	Bisacodyl (Dulcolax), docusate (Colace)
Mineralocorticoids	Promote sodium and water retention	Endocrine and immune	Fludrocortisone (Florinef)
Mucolytics	Assist with elimination of mucous in the respiratory tract	Pulmonary	Acetylcysteine (Mucomyst)
Mydriatics	Dilate pupils for ocular diagnostic and treatment procedures	Ocular and parasympathetic nervous system	Cyclopentolate (Cyclogyl)
Narcotic analgesics	Relieve pain and relieve or suppress cough	CNS	Morphine, oxycodone
Nasal decongestants	Decrease upper airway mucous secretion	Sympathetic nervous system	Pseudoephedrine (Sudafed), phenylephrine (Neo-Synephrine)
Neuromuscular blocking agents	Provide chemical paralysis in intubated and ventilated patients	Peripheral nervous system and musculoskeletal	Succinylcholine (Anectine), rocuronium (Zemuron)
Nonsteroidal anti-inflammatory drugs	Treat pain and inflammation	Endocrine	Ibuprofen (Motrin, Advil), ketorolac (Toradol), indomethacin (Indocin)
Oral contraceptives	Prevent conception (pregnancy)	Endocrine and genitourinary	Estrogen, progesterone
Oral hypoglycemic agents	Manage type 2 diabetes mellitus	Endocrine	Glyburide (Diabeta), metformin (Glucophage), glipizide (Glucotrol)
Phosphodiesterase inhibitors	Treat erectile dysfunction	Cardiovascular	Sildenafil (Viagra), tadalafil (Cialis)
Platelet inhibitors	Decrease platelet aggregation in patients at risk of thrombus formation	Hematologic	Aspirin, clopidogrel (Plavix)
Protein pump inhibitors	Suppress activity of parietal cell acid secretion	Gastrointestinal	Omeprazole (Prilosec), esomeprazole (Nexium)
Selective serotonin reuptake inhibitors	Treat depression, anxiety, and related conditions	CNS	Paroxetine (Paxil), sertraline (Zoloft)
Sympathomimetics	Increase blood pressure, heart rate, and cardiac output; constrict blood vessels	Cardiovascular	Epinephrine (Adrenalin), phenylephrine (Neo-Synephrine)
Tocolytics	Decrease or eliminate uterine contractions during preterm labor	Endocrine and genitourinary	Magnesium sulfate
Tricyclic antidepressants	Treat depression, neuropathy, and chronic pain syndromes	CNS	Amitriptyline (Elavil), doxepin, desipramine (Norpramin)
Xanthines	Bronchodilation	Respiratory	Theophylline (Uniphyl)

Abbreviation: CNS indicates central nervous system.

can maintain the blood pressure and heart rate, but it also raises intracranial pressure, making it less than optimal for patients with head injury who require airway placement. Ketamine causes some degree of bronchodilation, which is potentially helpful in patients with asthma or another COPD who require airway placement for respiratory failure. An emergence reaction with brief psychosis, disorientation, hallucinations, and other effects is possible following ketamine administration. Many paramedic agencies have moved away from the use of this drug. Check with your medical director on his or her thoughts on this medication. Emergence reactions may be eliminated or reduced by administering benzodiazepine medications with ketamine during airway procedures.

Benzodiazepines

Benzodiazepine medications are widely used in the prehospital setting. This group of medications includes diazepam (Valium), lorazepam (Ativan), and midazolam (Versed). Patients may be prescribed other benzodiazepines such as clonazepam (Klonopin) and temazepam (Restoril) for use on a long-term basis. Benzodiazepines have potent antiseizure, anxiolytic, and sedative properties, making them desirable in many situations. It is possible for benzodiazepine to be used as the primary sedative for airway placement procedures, but high doses of these medications are required to achieve adequate sedation. At high doses, benzodiazepines cause hypotension, further complicating the conditions of patients with shock or multiple trauma. Benzodiazepines are best used for maintenance sedation following airway placement. Benzodiazepines provide some degree of seizure protection in patients with head injuries. Active seizures can be treated initially with IV, IM, intranasal, and rectal administration of benzodiazepines. Lower doses of benzodiazepines may also be helpful to reduce anxiety, although this use is not approved in all EMS systems. Paramedics should be aware that the three prehospital benzodiazepine medications are pregnancy class D, which means they have demonstrated potential harm to the fetus. These medications should be administered to pregnant patients only during life-threatening situations when no safer alternative medications are available.

Flumazenil (Romazicon) is a competitive benzodiazepine antagonist available in certain health care settings. Unlike the reversal of opiates with naloxone, the reversal of benzodiazepines with flumazenil has the serious potential of exposing patients to numerous life-threatening conditions. There are several important contraindications to flumazenil that require careful consideration before it can be administered. Death from isolated benzodiazepine toxicity is rare. The risks associated with flumazenil outweigh its potential benefits in most clinical situations. Flumazenil can precipitate benzodiazepine withdrawal symptoms in patients who receive benzodiazepines on a long-term basis. Reversal of benzodiazepine sedation may cause combative behavior, anxiety, and possibly elevated ICP in susceptible patients. Additionally, if seizures occur following flumazenil administration, benzodiazepine anticonvulsant medications will be minimally effective or ineffective in controlling seizure activity and other effective anticonvulsant medications may not be immediately available.

Chemical Paralytic Agents

Two classes of chemical paralytic agents may be used in the prehospital setting. These medications provide muscle relaxation that facilitates airway device placement and prevents patient-ventilator asynchrony during mechanical ventilation. Paralytic agents allow better visualization of airway structures than when only sedative medications are used. The onset and duration of muscle relaxation is largely influenced by the class of chemical paralytic agent used.

Under normal circumstances, nerve cells release acetylcholine (ACh), which binds to nicotinic receptor sites on muscle cells, causing muscle contraction. Chemical paralytic (neuromuscular blocking) medications bind with nicotinic receptor sites on muscle cells, antagonizing (preventing activation by) ACh Figure 4 .

Succinylcholine (Anectine) is a **competitive depolarizing** paralytic agent. It reaches the neuromuscular junction, binds with nicotinic receptors on muscles, causes a brief activation known as **fasciculation**, and prevents additional activation by ACh. Succinylcholine is preferred by many health care providers because of its rapid onset (30 to 60 seconds) and relatively brief duration (3 to 8 minutes). Succinylcholine has several important adverse effects. It may cause or worsen hyperkalemia (elevated potassium level), cause bradycardia (especially in children), and elevate intraocular pressure in susceptible patients. Malignant hyperthermia is a rare, but immediately life-threatening, adverse reaction to succinylcholine. This disorder is characterized by severe hyperthermia (elevated temperature), muscle rigidity, and metabolic acidosis. Other anesthetic agents can cause this disorder as well. Patients able to communicate should be screened for personal or family reactions to anesthesia before administering succinylcholine.

Several **nondepolarizing** paralytic agents are used in the prehospital or critical care transport setting. Nondepolarizing agents compete with ACh at nicotinic receptor sites. They occupy but do not activate receptor sites, preventing activation by ACh. These medications generally have a longer duration than succinylcholine and fewer adverse effects. Rocuronium (Zemuron) has the most rapid onset (1 to 3 minutes) combined with a shorter duration (15 to 60 minutes), making it an appropriate nondepolarizing agent for placement of airway devices in emergency situations. Vecuronium (Norcuron) may also be administered either as an adjunct or sole chemical paralytic agent for emergency airway procedures. The onset of vecuronium is slightly longer than rocuronium, but it is available as a powder for reconstitution, giving it a longer room-temperature shelf-life than rocuronium.

Depolarizing and nondepolarizing chemical paralytic agents create an immediate threat to life if they are administered by paramedics who are not able to secure an artificial airway. Paramedics who are authorized to administer these medications must be proficient with bag-mask ventilation and skilled with the placement of backup airway devices. If paramedics are not able to oxygenate and ventilate a patient adequately following administration of a chemical paralytic agent, potentially fatal complications are likely.

Other Airway Medications

Paramedics also use medication to treat upper airway edema in patients who are conscious and spontaneously breathing. Corticosteroid, vasoconstrictor, and bronchodilator medications

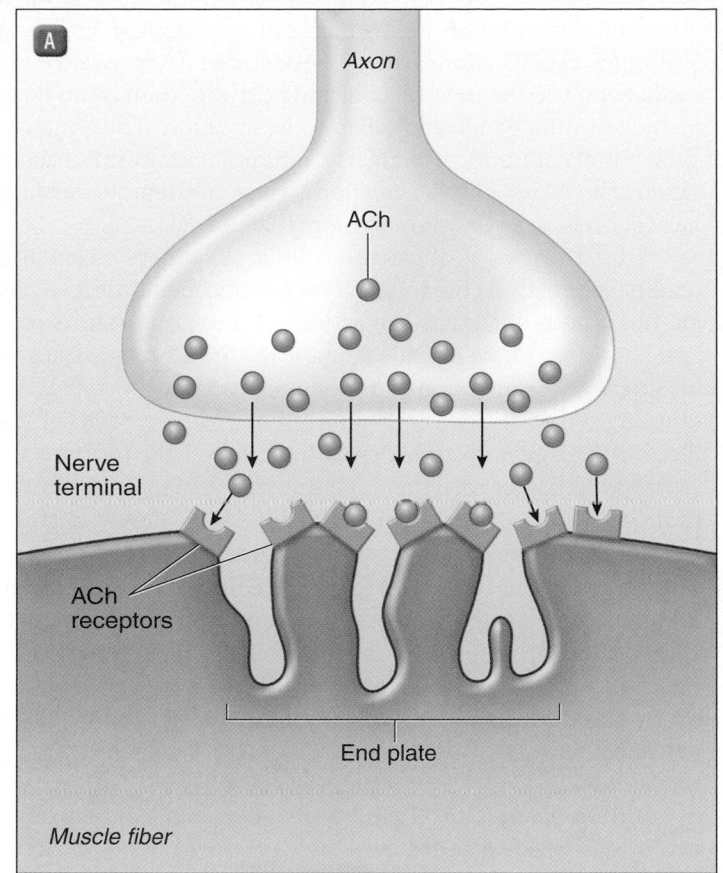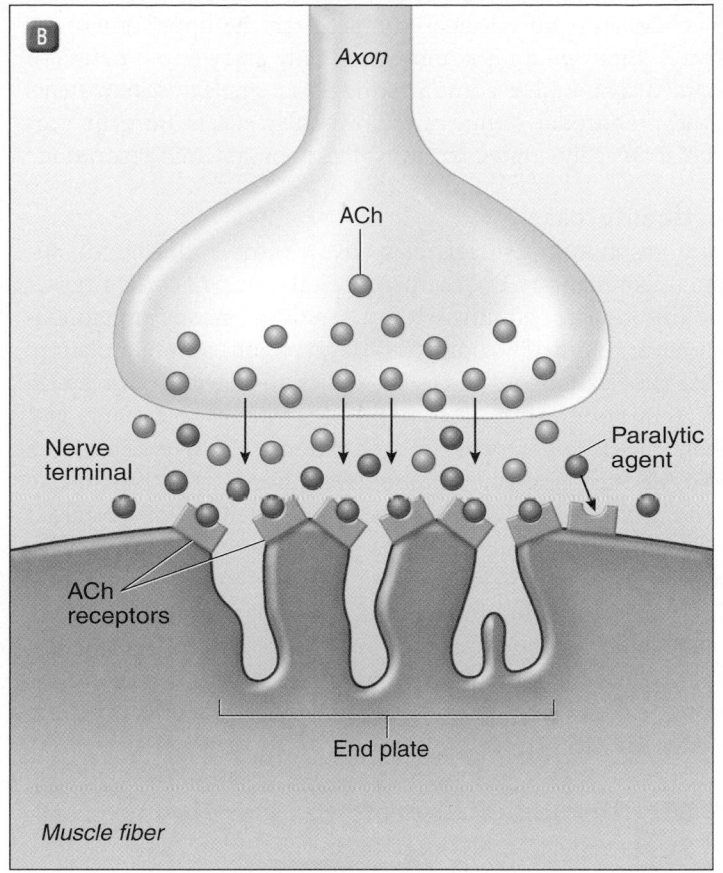

Figure 4 Chemical paralytic medications bind with nicotinic receptor sites on muscle cells, antagonizing acetylcholine (ACh).

may be used when upper airway edema is present. These medications are discussed later in this chapter.

Medications Used in Respiratory Management

Effective respiration requires adequate oxygenation and ventilation. Respiratory emergencies can be a primary complaint or the manifestation of a disease process in another body system. Medication groups discussed in this section relate to primary respiratory conditions such as asthma and COPD.

Beta-Agonist Medications

Beta-adrenergic agonist medications remain the primary treatment for acute bronchospasm associated with asthma, COPD, and a variety of other conditions. The walls of lower airways contain smooth muscles that contract (causing a smaller airway lumen) or relax (increasing the airway lumen) in response to biochemical changes and external irritants. Beta-2 receptor sites on bronchial smooth muscle cause muscle relaxation and bronchodilation when activated by beta-2 agonist chemicals. Norepinephrine and epinephrine are naturally occurring beta-2 agonists in the body. Paramedics are able to administer a variety of beta-2 agonist medications for patients experiencing bronchospasm.

Beta-agonist medications can be selective, targeting only beta-2 receptor sites, or nonselective, affecting beta-1 and beta-2.

Despite advertised selectivity, many beta-2 agonist medications demonstrate some degree of beta-1 activation. Albuterol (Ventolin, Proventil) is a selective beta-2 agonist medication used in the prehospital setting and throughout health care. This medicine is typically nebulized or administered using an MDI for the emergency treatment of bronchospasm. Albuterol may cause varying degrees of tachycardia, especially during prolonged administration. Metabolic acidosis may also develop if patients receive prolonged, continuous administration of nebulized albuterol. Albuterol can promote cellular uptake of potassium, making it a potential temporary treatment for hyperkalemia until definitive potassium removal occurs.

Levalbuterol is structurally similar to albuterol, without many of the reported beta-1 effects. Terbutaline (Brethaire) and epinephrine are additional beta-agonist medications that may be used for the emergency treatment of bronchospasm in the prehospital setting. Racemic epinephrine is the nebulized form of epinephrine engineered to limit cardiovascular effects. Paramedics should exercise caution and carefully monitor for adverse cardiovascular effects when administering racemic epinephrine and other beta-agonist medications.

Mucokinetic and Bronchodilator Medications

Paramedics may supplement beta-agonist medications with ipratropium bromide (Atrovent) or a similar medication when treating patients with bronchospasm or reactive airway disease.

Ipratropium bromide antagonizes muscarinic receptors, causing bronchodilation and decreased mucous in the upper and lower airways. Ipratropium is administered only every 6 to 8 hours, so paramedics should be administering only a single dose to patients in the prehospital setting. Cardiovascular effects from ipratropium are usually limited because of its poor systemic absorption.

Corticosteroids

Many respiratory emergencies involve some degree of airway inflammation. In the prehospital setting, corticosteroid medications are administered to reduce airway inflammation and, ultimately, improve oxygenation and ventilation. These medications significantly reduce the severity of respiratory compromise from asthma, COPD, allergic reactions, and other causes of airway inflammation. Methylprednisolone (Solu-Medrol), dexamethasone (Decadron), and prednisone are administered in certain prehospital systems. Corticosteroid medications have immunosuppressant properties and can alter a vast array of endocrine functions. These medications have a wide variety of contraindications and adverse effects, so EMS agencies and organizations may limit or restrict the use by paramedics. If paramedics are permitted to administer these medications, care should be taken to evaluate the potential risks and benefits for each individual patient.

■ Medications Affecting the Cardiovascular System

The cardiovascular system is divided into three functional components: the pump (heart), the plumbing (arteries, veins, and capillaries), and the blood. Many medications are used to affect one or more of these three components. Blood products and medications affecting the functions of the blood are discussed separately later in the chapter. Antidysrhythmic medications specifically target cells within the heart to resolve a dysrhythmia or suppress ectopic foci (sites of electrical impulse generation other than normal pacemaker cells). Many antidysrhythmic medications affect cells in other parts of the cardiovascular system or throughout the body. Other cardiovascular medications alter the activity of the heart or change the tone of blood vessels.

Several of the medications discussed in this section are not generally used in the prehospital setting. Paramedics may encounter these medications during interfacility transport or while responding to an emergency in a health care setting outside of a hospital.

Antidysrhythmic Medications

A variety of medications have the ability to improve or correct abnormalities in a patient's cardiac rhythm. Many of the medications used to treat cardiac dysrhythmias have a similar ability to cause cardiac dysrhythmias and a large number of adverse effects in patients receiving these medications. Paramedics must carefully consider the risks and benefits of a particular medication in the context of an individual patient. In many cases, paramedics will benefit from the expert guidance of a physician through online medical control when treating patients in hemodynamically stable condition with a cardiac dysrhythmia.

Medications used to treat cardiac dysrhythmias are grouped into four classes according to mechanism using the **Vaughan-Williams** classification scheme. Adenosine (Adenocard) is a medication used to treat certain cardiac dysrhythmias but is not included in the Vaughan-Williams classification. The Vaughan-Williams classification scheme is based on mechanism of action rather than on specific medication groups. Certain medications have a mechanism of action in more than one class.

A brief overview of cardiac cellular activity is essential to understanding the action of antidysrhythmic medications. There are five phases of cardiac cell activity, 0 through 4. The cardiac cycle begins at phase 4. During phase 4, cardiac cells are at rest, waiting for the generation of a spontaneous impulse from within (**automaticity**) or transfer of an impulse from an adjacent cardiac cell. This period coincides with diastole of the heart.

Phase 0 begins with the rapid influx of sodium ions through channels in the cardiac cell. Potassium ions slowly begin to exit the cell, and **depolarization** occurs, altering the electrical charge present in the cell **Figure 5**. During phase 1, sodium influx decreases while potassium continues to exit the cell slowly. Phase 2 begins movement of calcium into the cell while potassium continues to leave the cell. During phase 3, calcium movement ceases with continued outflow of potassium. Repolarization and myocardial contraction are occurring through phases 2 and 3.

During phases 0, 1, 2, and 3, no additional depolarization may occur because of external stimuli. This protection limits the potential maximum heart rate by ensuring that a certain amount of time elapses between myocardial contractions. This period is known as the **absolute refractory period** or effective refractory period. Immediately following the absolute (effective) refractory period, there is a brief window for an unusually powerful stimulus to initiate depolarization, known as the **relative refractory period**.

It is possible for nonpacemaker cells to initiate electrical activity spontaneously. During periods of cellular hypoxia, certain ion channels become altered. These changes permit calcium

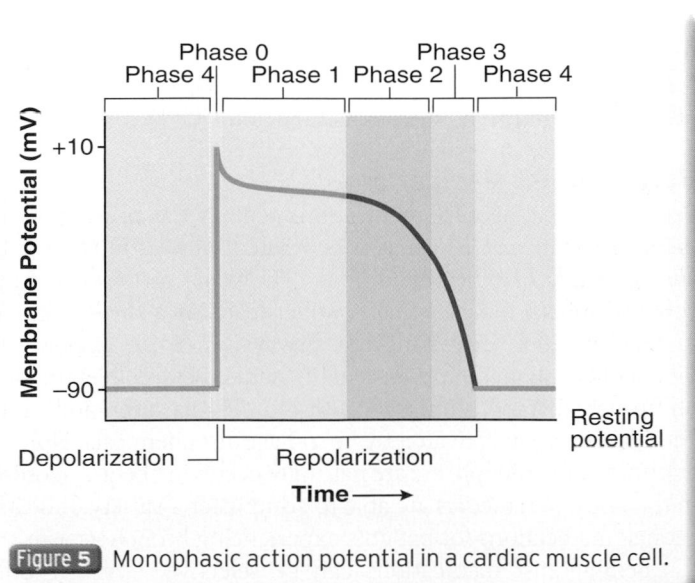

Figure 5   Monophasic action potential in a cardiac muscle cell.

(instead of sodium) to initiate depolarization, resulting in ectopic beats that frequently accompany myocardial ischemia.

Class I Antidysrhythmic Medications

Class I antidysrhythmic medications slow the movement of sodium through channels in certain cardiac cells. Procainamide (Pronestyl) is a class IA medication that can suppress activity of ectopic foci and slow conduction velocity. This action has the potential to prolong the QRS and QT intervals. This medication is effective for a variety of atrial and ventricular dysrhythmias but requires careful administration and monitoring.

Lidocaine was a popular class IB antidysrhythmic medication used in the prehospital setting for many years. Today there are more effective agents. It blocks sodium channels in the Purkinje fibers and ventricle, effectively resolving various ventricular dysrhythmias and suppressing ectopic foci. Lidocaine is poorly absorbed orally and quickly metabolized by the liver. Administration typically involves a larger bolus dose, followed by a continuous infusion. Paramedics may also see lidocaine used as a local anesthetic during soft-tissue repair and as an adjunct to sedation in patients who are at risk of increases in intracranial pressure during intubation attempts. Lidocaine has numerous significant medication interactions and should be used with caution in patients with liver or kidney disease.

Class II Antidysrhythmic Medications/Beta-Adrenergic Blocking Agents

Beta-adrenergic blocking agents (beta blockers) constitute the second major class of antidysrhythmic agents. Beta blockers competitively inhibit catecholamine (epinephrine and norepinephrine) activation of beta receptor sites. At therapeutic doses, certain beta blockers are capable of some beta-1 selectivity, affecting heart rate, contractility, or cardiac conduction velocity, without substantial impact on beta-2 receptors in the lungs. Selectivity is lost when higher doses or nonselective beta blockers are administered. Toxic effects from beta blockers typically include bradycardia, hypotension, conduction delays, and a variety of other cardiovascular effects. Beta blockers should be used with extreme caution in patients with reactive airway disease because of the potential beta-2 antagonism causing bronchospasm. Beta blockers may also cause massive conduction abnormalities when given simultaneously with calcium channel blockers or other medications that slow atrioventricular node conduction.

Metoprolol (Lopressor) is a beta-blocking agent used to reduce the heart rate during myocardial ischemia and in certain atrial tachycardias. This medication decreases the heart rate with a modest reduction in blood pressure. In the setting of myocardial ischemia, metoprolol is used to decrease the heart rate, resulting in lower myocardial oxygen consumption. Paramedics in certain EMS systems may carry and administer metoprolol. It is essential to monitor patient heart rate and blood pressure carefully while slowly administering metoprolol in select situations.

Class III Antidysrhythmic Medications

Class III antidysrhythmic medications increase the duration of phases 1, 2, and 3 of the cardiac cycle. By extending the cellular action potential, these medications prolong the absolute refractory period, treating atrial or ventricular tachycardias. In certain class III medications, the degree of prolongation of action potential is inversely proportional to the baseline heart rate, essentially making the medications less effective for treating extremely rapid heart rates while dramatically decreasing relatively slower baseline heart rates.

Amiodarone (Cordarone) is a class III antidysrhythmic medication that has gained popularity in recent years. Amiodarone is useful for treating atrial and ventricular tachycardia. The role of amiodarone in the treatment of Wolff-Parkinson-White syndrome remains controversial. It is recommended in the ACLS algorithm, but several studies suggest that the risks of amiodarone for the treatment of Wolff-Parkinson-White syndrome outweigh potential benefits. Amiodarone is administered by the IV route in the prehospital or critical care setting and can be continued orally for long-term maintenance. Amiodarone is widely distributed throughout the body, potentially causing a wide range of adverse effects. In addition to severe adverse cardiovascular effects, amiodarone causes various life-threatening pulmonary conditions in up to 17% of patients.

Class IV Antidysrhythmic Medications/Calcium Channel Blockers

Calcium channel blockers have a variety of potential uses in the prehospital setting. These medications can be used for reducing blood pressure and controlling the heart rate and may increase myocardial oxygen delivery during periods of ischemia. In addition, these medications may be used to inhibit uterine contractions during preterm labor, for long-term management of migraines, and for the treatment of cardiomyopathy.

Calcium channel blockers displace calcium at certain receptor sites or enter smooth muscle cells in place of calcium. This action relaxes smooth muscle present in the heart, blood vessels, GI tract, and uterus. Calcium channel blockers slow conduction through the atrioventricular node, decrease the automaticity of ectopic foci within the heart, and decrease the velocity of cardiac contraction. Cardiac workload and oxygen consumption are decreased by lowering peripheral vascular resistance (afterload) while simultaneously reducing cardiac output.

Verapamil (Calan) and diltiazem (Cardizem) are two calcium channel blockers commonly used in prehospital and critical care transport settings. In most cases, these medications are used for the control of the heart rate in patients with atrial fibrillation or atrial flutter. Diltiazem appears to have less effect on blood pressure, making it more desirable for patients at risk for hypotension. Many EMS agencies stock verapamil rather than diltiazem because it has a longer room-temperature shelf-life and lower cost. Intravenous calcium preparations such as calcium chloride and calcium gluconate may mitigate hypotension or bradycardia following an overdose of or toxicity from a calcium channel blocker. Both medications are administered IV over at least 2 minutes with continuous electrocardiographic and frequent blood pressure monitoring.

Adenosine

Adenosine is the only member of the fifth (unnamed) class of antidysrhythmic medications that is used routinely in the prehospital setting. Adenosine can be used to treat paroxysmal supraventricular tachycardia or to assist in diagnosis when the origin or pattern cannot be determined on an ECG because of an unusually fast heart rate. It is difficult to identify the presence and morphology of P-waves on an ECG when the patient's heart rate is elevated. Immediately after administration, adenosine decreases cardiac conduction velocity and prolongs the effective refractory period, producing a several-second pause in cardiac activity. One or two doses of adenosine are often successful in resolving an episode of paroxysmal supraventricular tachycardia. For diagnosis, paramedics and other health care providers use adenosine to evaluate the ECG tracing as cardiac electrical activity terminates and resumes to determine the presence of P waves, flutter waves, or other evidence of supraventricular activity, especially when a wide (> 0.12 seconds) QRS complex is present. This technique may distinguish between ventricular tachycardia and atrial tachycardia with aberrancy. Adenosine is occasionally used in cardiac and neurologic surgical settings to produce a brief, predictable cessation of cardiac activity during blood vessel repair.

Patients and health care providers often experience similar levels of anxiety during the 5- to 15-second pause in electrical and mechanical cardiac activity caused by adenosine. Adenosine has a rapid onset, a brief duration, and a half-life of less than 10 seconds. Paramedics should administer adenosine through a large-bore proximal IV site, immediately followed by a 10-mL normal saline flush. This technique often requires planning and coordination, possibly with two providers, to maximize adenosine's clinical effects. Paramedics should run a continuous paper ECG recording during any time adenosine is being administered. Doing so will assist paramedics and other health care providers with dysrhythmia identification if conversion with adenosine is unsuccessful.

■ Additional Cardiovascular Medications

Alpha-Adrenergic Receptor Antagonists

Alpha-adrenergic receptor antagonists (alpha-blockers) prevent endogenous catecholamines from reaching alpha receptors, primarily in the smooth muscle of blood vessels. In general, these medications lower blood pressure (particularly diastolic) and decrease systemic vascular resistance. Nonselective blockade of alpha-2 receptors causes a "reflex" tachycardia by allowing an increase of norepinephrine secretion from the sympathetic nervous system.

Patients taking alpha-blocking medications at home are frequently prone to postural hypotension (hypotension related to sudden position changes) and tachycardia. Alpha-adrenergic receptor antagonists are prescribed for patients with hypertension, an enlarged prostate gland, and glaucoma. Alpha-receptor antagonism occurs frequently as a seemingly unrelated adverse effect of other medications.

It is conceivable that paramedics may administer one of three alpha-adrenergic medications in the prehospital or critical care transport settings. Clonidine (Catapres) is a primarily alpha-2 receptor agonist, often given orally for emergency treatment of hypertension. By activating alpha-2 receptors, clonidine suppresses the release of norepinephrine, a potent vasoconstrictor, causing vasodilation. Paramedics may also administer phentolamine (Regitine). Catecholamines and sympathomimetics (discussed later) can cause profound tissue necrosis if **extravasation**

(seepage of blood and medication into the tissue surrounding the blood vessel) occurs during administration through a peripheral IV line. As extravasation occurs, blood vessels in the skin and soft tissue constrict, cutting off blood flow to cells in the affected area. Phentolamine can be subcutaneously injected to reverse vasoconstriction in affected soft tissue, preventing tissue death.

Paramedics may also administer labetalol (Trandate), a relatively novel medicine with alpha-1, beta-1, and beta-2 antagonism properties. It is administered in emergency settings for hypertension. The IV form has a far greater effect on beta-1 and beta-2 receptors than alpha-1 receptors. Patients at risk for unopposed alpha stimulation, such as patients with a pheochromocytoma or cocaine overdose, should receive another alpha-adrenergic antagonist before receiving labetalol for a hypertensive emergency. In this case, a declining cardiac output from the beta-1 antagonism prompts the secretion of endogenous catecholamines, causing potentially uncontrolled hypertension.

Angiotensin-Converting Enzyme Inhibitors

The medications known as ACE inhibitors alter the function of the renin-angiotensin system in the body. This system causes vasoconstriction and fluid retention in response to hypotension or hypoperfusion. When the conversion of angiotensin I to angiotensin II is altered by the use of ACE inhibitor medications, a variety of clinically beneficial effects occur. Blood pressure is reduced and cardiac afterload is decreased without significantly altering cardiac output or causing an increased heart rate. These medications are useful for treating hypertension, cardiomyopathy, and congestive heart failure (CHF). In addition, they protect kidney function in certain groups of susceptible persons.

Patients taking ACE inhibitors are known to have a chronic, dry cough that is thought to be linked to an accumulation of chemicals from the now-altered renin-angiotensin system. Patients taking ACE inhibitors may experience sudden, life-threatening angioedema. This swelling of the mouth, face, and airway is a result of a rapid increase in subdermal and submucosal vascular permeability. When angioedema occurs, normal treatments such as epinephrine and antihistamines are not as effective. Paramedics should expect to provide close monitoring and supportive treatment or, in severe situations, prepare for an extremely difficult endotracheal intubation.

Anticholinergic Medications

Anticholinergic medications are used in prehospital and other health care settings for several important clinical purposes. The parasympathetic and sympathetic nervous systems continually respond to internal and external stimuli by releasing various biochemicals. These chemicals enhance or suppress the function of many tissues, organs, and body systems. Throughout the day, activity of the sympathetic or the parasympathetic nervous system will predominate, depending on perceived needs of the body. The sympathetic nervous system predominates in response to stress, releasing catecholamines to improve cardiovascular performance, enhance respiration, and retain body water. As the stressful stimulus disappears, the parasympathetic nervous system predominates, allowing vital functions such as rest, digestion, and urination to resume.

The vagus nerve (cranial nerve X) is a major component of the parasympathetic nervous system. This nerve controls parasympathetic stimulation of receptor sites in the heart, lungs, digestive system, and throughout the chest and abdomen. The vagus nerve releases ACh that acts on muscarinic-2 receptors in the heart to decrease heart rate and contractility and cardiac conduction velocity. Excessive activation of muscarinic-2 receptors in the heart by ACh causes bradycardia and conduction delays. Excessive activation of other muscarinic receptors causes increased salivation, bronchoconstriction, pulmonary secretions, vomiting, emesis, diarrhea, tearing, and a vast array of unwanted clinical effects. Many of these symptoms are present when patients are exposed to acetylcholinesterase inhibitors in pesticides and nerve agents, which permits excessive release of ACh and leads to elevated ACh levels in the body. Atropine sulfate is used in the prehospital and other health care settings to treat many cholinergic symptoms associated with excessive release of ACh.

Atropine is considered a competitive muscarinic receptor antagonist. The effectiveness of atropine is largely related to its concentration at receptor sites compared with ACh. When ACh increases dramatically due to inhibition of acetylcholinesterase (the enzyme that breaks down ACh), massive doses of atropine may be required.

Atropine is used for the treatment of bradycardia when vagal (vagus nerve) stimulation of muscarinic-2 receptors is suspected. This condition may occur when a patient strains to defecate or has mechanical pressure applied to his or her neck or when another event causes the vagus nerve to release excessive ACh. In many cases, atropine is administered empirically to exclude the possibility of vagal stimulation during episodes of bradycardia with an unidentified cause. As atropine is administered for bradycardia, ACh activation of muscarinic-2 receptors is prevented, allowing underlying sympathetic stimulation to predominate. Atropine is unlikely to be effective for the treatment of bradycardia caused by blocked cardiac conduction such as in second- and third-degree atrioventricular blocks.

Atropine is used before airway manipulation, especially in children. Laryngoscopy can stimulate the vagus nerve, causing ACh-induced bradycardia. In addition to preventing bradycardia, atropine can suppress the release of saliva and other secretions in the patient's airway. Low doses (< 0.1–0.2 mg) of atropine can cause central nervous system stimulation and paradoxical bradycardia.

Atropine is the lifesaving antidote for acetylcholinesterase inhibitor toxicity. When patients are exposed to pesticides and nerve agents, atropine is continuously administered until respiratory and hemodynamic status improves, regardless of the total dose required. Ambulance and hospital atropine supplies can be quickly exhausted following severe exposures, especially when multiple patients are involved. Atropine does not bind with nicotinic receptors so consequently it will not improve muscle weakness, fasciculations, or paralysis from cholinergic poisoning.

Catecholamines and Sympathomimetics

Catecholamines are naturally occurring chemicals in the body that stimulate receptor sites in the sympathetic nervous system. These chemicals contain two structures: the catechol group and the monoamine oxidase group. Endogenous catecholamines include epinephrine, norepinephrine, and dopamine. These chemicals stimulate alpha, beta, and dopaminergic receptor sites, causing the "fight-or-flight" response to stressful stimuli. These three chemicals are manufactured commercially for administration to patients with certain medical conditions. Catecholamines are rapidly metabolized by monoamine oxidase and catechol O-methyltransferase (an enzyme), resulting in a brief duration of action after administration. Paramedics may encounter certain catecholamine and sympathomimetic medications in the prehospital setting. Other medications in this category may be encountered during critical care transport.

Sympathomimetic chemicals are not found naturally within the body. These synthetic chemicals mimic naturally occurring catecholamines, activating receptor sites in the sympathetic nervous system. Various amphetamines, albuterol, phenylephrine (Neo-Synephrine), and cocaine have sympathomimetic properties. Sympathomimetic medications do not undergo the same metabolism as catecholamines, thus allowing for a longer duration of action following administration.

Epinephrine (Adrenalin), also known as adrenaline (note the similarity with the brand name), is a catecholamine used in the prehospital setting. Epinephrine stimulates alpha, beta-1, and beta-2 receptor sites, causing potent vasoconstriction; a marked increase in heart rate, contractility, and cardiac output; and powerful bronchodilation. Epinephrine can be administered by the IV, IO, IM, SC, endotracheal, and nebulized routes, depending on the clinical situation and type of medication access available. Nebulized epinephrine is used for airway edema and bronchospasm from various causes. Epinephrine may be given by the IM and SC routes for anaphylaxis and by the IV route in severe cases of anaphylactic shock. Epinephrine is administered by the IV and IO routes and through the endotracheal tube for cardiac arrest. Epinephrine infusions are used for profound hypotension, shock, and refractory bradycardia.

Epinephrine, like many catecholamines and sympathomimetic chemicals, can dramatically increase the cardiac workload and myocardial oxygen demand. These medications should be used with extreme caution in patients with myocardial ischemia, cardiomyopathy, or cardiogenic shock.

Norepinephrine (Levophed) is another naturally occurring catecholamine that has been manufactured commercially for use in health care. This medication stimulates beta-1 and alpha receptor sites, causing an increase in blood pressure, cardiac contractility, and heart rate. Vasoconstrictor (alpha) effects are usually greater than cardiac (beta-1) effects. Conditions that involve loss of vasomotor tone such as sepsis, neurogenic shock, and anaphylactic shock are the primary indications for norepinephrine as intravascular volume is being restored.

Norepinephrine is administered by continuous IV infusion and titrated according to patient response. Paramedics may administer norepinephrine in the critical care transport setting using an infusion pump. Norepinephrine is not typically used as an initial vasopressor in the prehospital setting. Norepinephrine and other vasopressor medications have the potential to cause tissue necrosis if extravasation occurs during IV administration. Alpha receptor activation causes constriction of blood vessels in the affected area, cutting off the blood supply and leading to tissue death if not treated promptly. Frequent assessment of the IV site is imperative if norepinephrine is being administered through a peripheral IV site. Paramedics who have been appropriately trained should ideally administer norepinephrine and other vasoconstrictor medications through a central venous catheter when available.

Dopamine (Inotropin) is frequently used in the prehospital setting as the primary medication for hypotension refractory to volume resuscitation. Dopamine is administered using a weight-based infusion calculation, typically micrograms per kilogram per minute (µg/kg/min). The clinical effects of dopamine vary dramatically depending on the dose range being administered. There is some overlap among the various receptors being activated. Dopamine has an affinity for dopaminergic receptor sites that is greater than the affinity for beta receptor sites and a greater affinity for beta receptor sites than for alpha sites. Dopaminergic receptor sites are activated at a dose of 2.5 to 5 µg/kg/min, causing renal and mesenteric artery vasodilation. At 5 to 10 µg/kg/min, dopamine activates beta-1 receptor sites, causing an increased heart rate and increased contractility. Some activation of dopaminergic receptor sites continues in this dose range as well. From 10 to 20 µg/kg/min, alpha effects predominate, causing profound vasoconstriction.

Dobutamine is a synthetically manufactured catecholamine that is similar to dopamine. It activates beta-1 and, to a lesser degree, beta-2 and alpha receptor sites. Dopaminergic receptors are not activated. Dobutamine may slightly increase heart rate, while providing a significant improvement in inotropic effects (force of cardiac contraction). When used for the treatment of cardiogenic shock, dobutamine is frequently combined with an IV vasodilator medication to increase inotropic effects and decrease afterload, resulting in improved cardiac output. A dobutamine infusion is not routinely initiated in the prehospital setting. During use in a hospital or critical care transport, dobutamine is administered with an infusion pump with careful cardiac and hemodynamic monitoring. Hypotension is possible, especially when initiating a dobutamine infusion. Some clinicians recommend briefly using another beta-1 agonist medication while initiating a dobutamine infusion or temporarily delaying administration of a vasodilator medication if patient condition permits.

Phenylephrine (Neo-Synephrine) is a synthetic, almost pure, alpha agonist medication. Minimal beta effects may be possible at high doses, but for all purposes, it is a pure alpha agonist medication. It is a potent vasoconstrictor with a longer duration of action than catecholamine medications. Clinically, phenylephrine is used for the treatment of hypotension resulting from a loss of vascular tone. Paramedics may also use phenylephrine as a mucosal vasoconstrictor during artificial airway placement. Phenylephrine may cause reflex tachycardia, and tachyphylaxis (discussed earlier in the Pharmacodynamics section) is relatively likely. Extravasation is a major concern with phenylephrine because of powerful alpha receptor activation. If paramedics are administering phenylephrine during a critical care transport, careful monitoring of the IV site is essential, and phentolamine (discussed earlier) should be available.

Vasopressin (Pitressin; antidiuretic hormone) has emerged as a potent vasopressor medication recommended in ACLS protocols. This naturally occurring hormone is secreted in the body in response to plasma hyperosmolality (elevated concentration of glucose and plasma proteins) or intravascular volume depletion. In clinical situations, vasopressin is administered for the treatment of GI bleeding, diabetes insipidus, shock, and cardiac arrest. A low-dose infusion of vasopressin can be initiated when other catecholamine medications become ineffective in treating shock in a particular patient. In ACLS protocols, a single dose of 40 U of vasopressin replaces the first or second epinephrine dose in certain cardiac arrest algorithms.

Direct Vasodilator Medications

Paramedics use various direct vasodilator medications for the management of uncontrolled hypertension, CHF, myocardial infarction, cardiac ischemia, and cardiogenic shock. These medications act on arteries, veins, or both, causing vascular smooth muscle relaxation and vasodilation. These medications have the potential to reduce cardiac preload and afterload and pulmonary vascular resistance.

Nitroglycerin (Nitro-Bid, Nitrostat) is a direct vasodilator that paramedics administer for a variety of cardiovascular conditions. Nitroglycerin primarily dilates veins and coronary arteries, decreasing cardiac preload, reducing myocardial oxygen demand, and improving coronary circulation. When administered sublingually by tablet or spray, effects begin in 1 to 3 minutes and peak in 4 to 10 minutes. Effects begin almost immediately following IV administration but persist only a few minutes after the IV infusion is discontinued. The rapid physiologic responses associated with the administration of IV nitroglycerin (relief of chest pain, decreased blood pressure) makes it a relatively safe medication to titrate to desired clinical effect. The IV doses begin at 5 µg/min in adults and can be increased to 200 µg/min if symptoms persist and an acceptable blood pressure is maintained. As mentioned earlier in this chapter, the SL dose of nitroglycerin is substantially higher than the IV dose. Nitroglycerin is prone to causing tolerance after 24 to 48 hours of continuous IV infusion. Some clinicians recommend obtaining a 15-lead ECG (12-lead ECG with additional evaluation for ischemia of the right side of the heart) prior to initiating treatment with nitroglycerin. Right-sided myocardial infarction requires an adequate preload to maintain adequate cardiac output, which may be compromised by the administration of nitroglycerin.

Sublingual nitroglycerin tablets are prone to degradation. Store tablets in a closed, light-protected container. Nitroglycerin binds with the plastic of containers and IV fluids or tubing. Glass bottles should be used for IV administration as safety and availability permit. The use of nitroglycerin should be avoided in patients taking phosphodiesterase-5 inhibitors used for erectile dysfunction, such as sildenafil (Viagra) and tadalafil (Cialis). When combined, nitroglycerin and phosphodiesterase-5 inhibitors may cause severe, refractory hypotension Figure 6 . (Note: *Nitroglycerin is a component of dynamite, but medical preparations of nitroglycerin have no explosive hazards.*)

Sodium nitroprusside (Nipride) is a potent IV vasodilator, affecting the smooth muscle of veins and arteries. Frequently, it is used in conjunction with inotropic medications for the management of cardiogenic shock. Sodium nitroprusside is

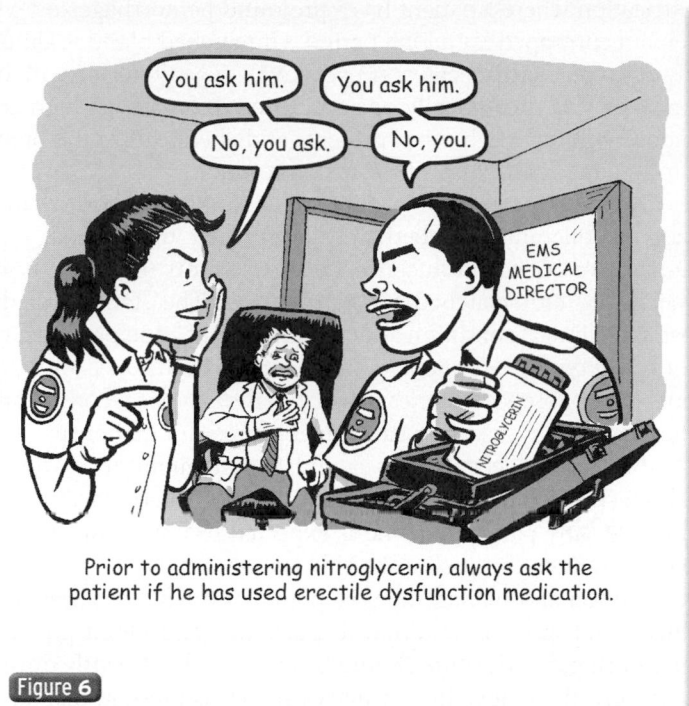

Prior to administering nitroglycerin, always ask the patient if he has used erectile dysfunction medication.

Figure 6

used for malignant hypertension and in situations where intentional hypotension is desired, such as with an unstable vascular aneurysm. The IV infusion rates can be adjusted to maintain optimal blood pressure and cardiac output.

Sodium nitroprusside is administered by continuous IV infusion with frequent or constant blood pressure monitoring. Effects from sodium nitroprusside decrease rapidly once the infusion is discontinued. Sodium nitroprusside is metabolized into cyanide and thiocyanate, which can cause toxicity during a prolonged infusion. When it is administered in the critical care transport setting, paramedics should ask about obtaining plasma cyanide and thiocyanate levels before departure with the patient.

Hydralazine (Apresoline) is a direct vasodilator that paramedics may administer for hypertensive emergencies, for pulmonary hypertension, or, in pregnant patients, for eclampsia or preeclampsia. This medication dilates arterioles, lowering pulmonary and systemic vascular resistance. In emergency situations, an IV bolus dose is administered over at least 1 minute and repeated (or increased) up to every 20 to 30 minutes as clinically indicated.

Diuretic Medications

Paramedics administer diuretic medications to correct volume overload, manage CHF, and improve respiration in patients experiencing pulmonary edema. Diuretic medications also have the potential to preserve kidney function when large quantities of by-products from cellular destruction, such as from muscle breakdown or blood cell hemolysis, are released. Diuretic medications are used to eliminate certain toxins from the body and to promote the excretion of excess electrolytes.

Furosemide is a diuretic medication frequently used in the prehospital setting. People may also take furosemide on a long-term basis for the management of hypertension, CHF, liver disease, or kidney dysfunction. Paramedics generally administer furosemide for the treatment of pulmonary edema, often related to cardiac dysfunction. Careful consideration is necessary before administering furosemide to patients with hemodynamic instability and known electrolyte disturbances. Furosemide is administered by the IV route over 1 to 2 minutes per 40-mg dose. In emergency situations, furosemide can be administered by the IM route, although effects are significantly delayed compared with the IV route. Some research studies suggest that furosemide

YOU are the Medic   PART 4

You insert an 18-gauge catheter in the patient's left antecubital space, with normal saline hooked up with a 10-gtt set and a 1-L bag. You administer a 250-mL fluid bolus and have the patient bear down (vagal maneuver). The patient states no difference in how she feels. You tell your partner to prepare adenosine, 6 mg, and a 10-mL flush. You recall that adenosine is naturally occurring in the body and, therefore, the cells absorb it very quickly, causing it to have a very short half-life.

Recording Time: 10 Minutes	
Respirations	24 breaths/min
Pulse	196 beats/min
Skin	Slightly pale
Blood pressure	98/44 mm Hg
Oxygen saturation (Spo$_2$)	100% on oxygen at 10 L/min
Pupils	Equal and reactive

7. Why is adenosine indicated for this patient?

8. How is adenosine administered?

causes renal artery vasodilation in addition to promoting urinary excretion from the kidneys.

Mannitol is an osmotic diuretic that may or may not be available to paramedics. In critical care settings, mannitol is used to decrease intracranial pressure associated with cerebral edema. Osmotic diuretics can target specific body tissues, removing excess water from the brain and eyes. Osmotic pressure gradients also draw water out of selected body tissues and through the kidneys to maintain urine flow when the kidneys risk becoming clogged with cellular by-products. Many electrolyte disturbances are possible following mannitol administration. Prolonged mannitol infusions have been known to cause a paradoxical increase in intracranial pressure.

Blood Products and Medications Affecting the Blood

In the body, blood acts as the primary transport mechanism for oxygen, carbon dioxide, nutrients, waste products, biochemicals, and medications. Paramedics have the ability to manipulate or enhance many characteristics of the blood for a therapeutic clinical purpose. In certain situations, it is desirable to suppress the clotting ability of the blood to enhance circulation or mitigate the effects of hypoperfusion. In other cases, paramedics need to augment the oxygen-carrying or clotting capability of the blood when these functions become impaired. A variety of medications affecting the blood are used in the prehospital and critical care transport settings. In addition, many EMS systems allow paramedics to initiate or monitor the administration of various blood products in appropriate clinical situations.

Blood Product Administration

The average adult has about 5 L of blood, constituting approximately 7% to 8% of body weight. Blood is roughly 55% plasma. Water makes up approximately 50% of the total intravascular volume. Red blood cells account for approximately 45% of the blood volume. Many chemicals, cells, proteins, and hormones make up the remainder of blood composition. Trauma and a vast array of medical conditions alter the total amount, composition, or performance of the blood. Paramedics may administer several different blood products to correct these abnormalities. Patients receive transfusions of specific components of the blood that are diminished or have impaired function. Whole blood transfusions are no longer used clinically in the United States.

Blood components are unmatched, type-specific to a particular patient, or crossmatched to a particular recipient. Type-specific blood products can be used as soon as the decision has been made and the recipient patient's blood type is known, but there is a somewhat greater risk of an adverse, potentially life-threatening transfusion reaction. Crossmatched blood has a decreased risk of transfusion reaction but requires a blood sample from the patient, followed by careful analysis in the blood bank before the blood product can be released for administration to the patient.

In the prehospital setting, paramedics will most likely use unmatched blood, possibly carried by air-medical crews or when blood products are sent to the scene of a prolonged extrication where a patient has a profound hemorrhage and will remain entrapped for a long period. Unmatched blood is almost always type O, Rh-negative (O negative). Type O-negative blood products can theoretically be administered to patients with any blood type, although other proteins and chemicals in the blood product may still cause a transfusion reaction.

During interfacility patient transports, paramedics may face the dilemma of whether to administer unmatched, type O-negative blood products or delay transport to obtain type-specific or crossmatched blood products. The stability of the patient's clinical condition and the duration of anticipated delays for blood typing or crossmatching often make the decision obvious. In the absence of a clear choice, online medical control and the sending physician are valuable resources for guidance.

Blood products require careful patient monitoring during administration. Many types of transfusion-related reactions are possible. Any paramedic who is expected to initiate or monitor blood product transfusion should become very familiar with the recognition and management of potential transfusion reactions during transport. In addition to pulse rate and blood pressure monitoring, temperature should be reassessed frequently during transport. If an indwelling urinary catheter is present, paramedics should monitor for changes in urine color that may indicate a life-threatening hemolytic transfusion reaction.

Most blood products require special filtered IV tubing. This tubing may become clogged during massive blood product transfusions. Certain IV fluids are incompatible with blood products in the same IV tubing. Normal saline is the preferred IV fluid for Y-site tubing administration during blood product transfusions.

Packed Red Blood Cells

Packed RBCs (PRBCs) can be administered by paramedics to correct anemia resulting from blood loss, inadequate RBC production, or the massive destruction of circulating RBCs, known as hemolysis. Patients without a concurrent serious medical condition may compensate well for profound anemia that has developed during weeks to months. When blood cell loss occurs suddenly from trauma, hemorrhage, or hemolysis, patients are far less able to compensate. In general, the rate of administration of PRBCs should be proportional to the rate of blood cell loss.

A unit of PRBCs contains approximately 225 to 250 mL of concentrated RBCs, along with a preservative. Administration of 1 U of PRBCs will increase the hematocrit value, the percentage of RBCs in the blood, by roughly 3% (less with continued RBC loss). In children and infants, a patient-specific volume of PRBCs is administered. Patients at risk for volume overload, such as patients with renal failure or CHF, require slow PRBC administration and careful monitoring of fluid volume and respiratory status.

Typically, PRBCs are administered over no longer than 4 hours per unit. In patients in critical condition, PRBCs can be administered rapidly through a commercial pressure infuser-warmer or by using pressure bags. Paramedics should use the largest IV catheter possible. In adults, at least a 20-gauge IV catheter should be used, preferably an 18-gauge or larger. Patients with trauma and hemorrhage should have adequate IV fluid resuscitation before or concurrently with PRBC administration. For blood cells, AB is the universal recipient and O the universal donor.

Units of PRBCs usually contain a citrate-based preservative. Hypocalcemia may develop as the citrate binds with calcium in the body. During massive PRBC transfusions, paramedics should monitor for signs of hypocalcemia, such as tetany and a prolonged QT interval on the ECG tracing.

Patients receiving PRBCs are also at risk for hyperkalemia. If PRBCs are stored for a long period or if hemolysis occurs during PRBC administration, large amounts of intracellular potassium are released. In severe situations, hyperkalemia can be life threatening. Peaked T waves on the ECG tracing are highly suggestive of hyperkalemia.

Fresh Frozen Plasma

Impaired blood clotting can be treated by the administration of fresh frozen plasma (FFP). Because FFP contains many clotting factors, it is often given following trauma, hemorrhage, warfarin (Coumadin) toxicity, disseminated intravascular coagulation, and other conditions. Whenever large volumes of other blood components (such as PRBCs) are administered, FFP should also be used. The FFP must be compatible with a patient's blood type but does not need to be Rh compatible. (Rh is the antigen responsible for hemolytic disease of the newborn.)

In general, units of FFP hold the same volume as units of PRBCs (225–250 mL). These units require adequate defrosting before administration. Fresh frozen plasma is used for replacement of clotting factors, not volume expansion. Volume expansion is usually best accomplished with IV fluids and PRBC transfusion.

Cryoprecipitate is a blood product that contains a concentrated assortment of blood clotting factors, without the additional volume present in FFP. It is unlikely that paramedics will administer cryoprecipitate in the prehospital setting. Type AB plasma and cryoprecipitate can be given to patients with any blood type.

Platelets

Paramedics and other health care providers administer platelets to correct thrombocytopenia, a low platelet level in the blood. Thrombocytopenia can be caused by trauma, hemorrhage, various chronic medical conditions, and by certain anticoagulant medications. Patients may also have a normal level of platelets that are dysfunctional because of a clotting disorder or antiplatelet medication. Platelets must be blood type and Rh compatible.

Medications That Alter Blood Performance

Blood platelets combine with clotting or coagulation chemicals in the bloodstream to terminate bleeding when a blood vessel ruptures. This complicated process is essential for human survival. Without this process, spontaneous bleeding would readily occur and otherwise minor trauma would cause death from exsanguination. When blood clotting occurs in a blood vessel, a thrombus (blood clot) is created. This thrombus can occlude the blood vessel, jeopardizing dependent cells, tissues, and organs. During prehospital care and interfacility transport, paramedics administer or monitor several important medications that alter the ability of the blood to form a thrombus, preventing or limiting the injury to vital organs such as the heart and lungs.

Anticoagulant Medications

Anticoagulant medications impair the function of clotting or coagulation chemicals in the bloodstream. Human blood contains a balance of substances that promote the formation of blood clots or are capable of dissolving blood clots. This balance permits the termination of bleeding while simultaneously allowing blood clots to dissolve once blood vessel integrity is restored. Anticoagulant medications enhance the function of substances in the blood that inhibit clot formation. These medications prevent the formation of new blood clots and the growth of existing clots, but they do not dissolve existing blood clots.

Heparin and enoxaparin (Lovenox) are frequently used anticoagulant medications that enhance antithrombin III to inhibit blood coagulation. Both medications are used to treat or prevent acute coronary syndrome, deep vein thrombosis, and pulmonary embolus. These medications are not generally initiated in the prehospital setting, although it is conceivable that paramedics in remote locations or ambitious EMS systems may administer these medications in specific clinical situations. Enoxaparin is administered as a single IV or SC dose, usually every 12 hours. In addition to the possibility of prehospital administration, paramedics may continue an IV heparin infusion during interfacility transport. If only one IV site is available, heparin infusions are compatible with nitroglycerin and several other prehospital medication infusions through Y-site IV tubing. Both heparin and enoxaparin have the potential to cause bleeding, thrombocytopenia, and a variety of other adverse effects.

Antiplatelet Medications

Platelets perform an essential role in blood clotting and thrombus formation. Medications can be used to reduce platelet aggregation (clumping), preventing new thrombus formation or the extension of an existing thrombus. Paramedics may encounter several oral and IV antiplatelet medications.

Aspirin is an oral antiplatelet medication used extensively for the treatment and prevention of thrombus formation. Aspirin is administered in the prehospital setting for treatment of acute coronary syndrome, often suspected in patients reporting chest pain. Aspirin is also indicated for the treatment of a stroke once the presence of hemorrhage has been reliably excluded. Paramedics should carefully assess for the possibility of an occult aneurysm when considering aspirin for a patient with chest pain. Platelet inactivation from aspirin has the potential to seriously complicate any condition associated with bleeding.

When indicated, aspirin is crushed or chewed before swallowing, promoting rapid GI absorption. Aspirin is rapidly eliminated by the body, but the antiplatelet effects persist until all affected platelets are replaced, which may take up to 10 days. Patients may claim an aspirin allergy based on GI upset. Paramedics should ask about the specific circumstances when a patient reports an aspirin allergy or sensitivity and aspirin is otherwise clinically indicated.

Clopidogrel (Plavix) and ticlopidine (Ticlid) are two additional oral antiplatelet medications that paramedics may administer as an aspirin alternative. These medications inhibit platelet aggregation by a mechanism different from that of aspirin. Clopidogrel has been shown to be superior to aspirin in certain clinical situations. Ticlopidine has several serious adverse effects that limit its role in prehospital and long-term treatment. Aspirin, clopidogrel, and ticlopidine cause bleeding in 2% to 3% of patients receiving these medications.

Paramedics may encounter various glycoprotein IIb/IIIa inhibitor medications during interfacility transport. Abciximab (ReoPro), tirofiban (Aggrastat), and eptifibatide (Integrilin) provide potent platelet inhibition in a manner more effective than the aforementioned oral antiplatelet medications. These medications are administered by an IV infusion, which is often continued during interfacility transport to a tertiary cardiac care center. Bleeding and thrombocytopenia are adverse effects observed in up to 5% of patients receiving these medications.

Fibrinolytics

Fibrinolytics (eg, Activase) dissolve blood clots in arteries and veins. These medications are administered for the emergency treatment of acute myocardial infarction and stroke. In addition, fibrinolytics are administered in lower doses to open certain vascular catheters that have become occluded by a presumed blood clot.

Fibrinolytics have the serious potential to cause life-threatening hemorrhage. Careful patient selection and exclusion are essential before these medications are administered. Any condition suggestive of blood clot formation elsewhere in the body, such as recent trauma or surgery, is likely to prevent a patient from receiving fibrinolytics. There are numerous other absolute and relative contraindications to fibrinolytic therapy.

Fibrinolytics remain valuable in remote locations and smaller community hospitals but have a limited role in the treatment of acute myocardial infarction when interventional cardiology services are readily available. Many hospitals have developed rapid diagnostic and treatment procedures to optimize the effectiveness of fibrinolytics for acute ischemic strokes.

Paramedics should avoid multiple IV attempts and unnecessary trauma in any patient who is a likely candidate for fibrinolytics. A careful determination of the time of onset of symptoms will influence the decision about whether fibrinolytics will be administered. Paramedics should not unnecessarily delay patient transport because these medications are indicated only within a short period after the onset of symptoms. Prolonged prehospital time may preclude the administration of fibrinolytics.

Medications Used for Neurologic Conditions

Paramedics encounter and treat a large number of patients with neurologic complaints and conditions. Pain accompanies the vast majority of traumatic injuries and is a common symptom associated with many medical conditions. Seizure activity is another event that frequently triggers EMS activation. Many patients encountered by EMS would benefit clinically from the treatment of anxiety or the administration of sedative medications.

Paramedics rely heavily on opioid (narcotic) medications for analgesia (treatment of pain) in the prehospital setting. These medications are effective at eliminating or reducing pain caused by a variety of conditions. Paramedics also administer naloxone, a powerful reversal agent for patients who have received dangerous amounts of opioid chemicals.

Benzodiazepine medications (discussed earlier in the section about medications used in airway management) are the primary treatment modality for persistent seizure activity. These medications also work well for sedation and the treatment of anxiety. Benzodiazepines are arguably underused in the prehospital setting.

Analgesic Medications

Paramedics administer medications that stimulate opioid receptors in the body to relieve or prevent pain associated with an injury, medical condition, or medically related procedure or movement. The human body contains at least seven types of opioid receptors in the central nervous system, peripheral nervous system, and GI tract. Paramedics use medications that act on mu (μ) opioid receptor sites. Natural endorphins also stimulate (activate) mu receptor sites, causing analgesia, euphoria, constricted pupils, respiratory depression, and decreased GI motility. Opioid medications are also known to suppress the cough reflex, which can be a desirable or an adverse clinical effect.

Opioid chemicals, medications, and illicit drugs are known for causing tolerance, cross-tolerance, and addiction. Patients who receive opioid substances on a long-term basis often require unusually high doses of opioid medications for relief of pain from an acute illness or injury. They may also experience severe withdrawal symptoms if opioid reversal is required following an error during treatment.

Opioid medications can cause profound sedation, respiratory depression, and apnea when excessive doses are administered. Other adverse effects include hypotension, bradycardia, palpitations, dysrhythmias, and noncardiogenic pulmonary edema. The severity or likelihood of adverse effects may vary significantly among different opioid medications.

Paramedics often administer morphine sulfate or fentanyl in the prehospital setting. Meperidine (Demerol), hydromorphone (Dilaudid), and newer synthetic opioid medications may be used in select EMS or critical care transport settings. Depending on the medication chosen, paramedics may use the IV, IM, or intranasal route of administration.

Morphine sulfate is used frequently in EMS. In addition to the aforementioned adverse effects, morphine sulfate is known to cause nausea or vomiting in up to 28% of patients. Paramedics should use extreme caution when administering morphine to patients who are unable to protect their airway. Patients with an altered level of consciousness and patients secured to a backboard may experience a life-threatening airway obstruction if vomiting occurs after morphine administration. Morphine may also prompt a histamine release that causes pruritus (itching), flushing, and diaphoresis. These symptoms are often inaccurately described as an allergic reaction.

Fentanyl (Sublimaze) is gaining popularity as an opioid analgesic in the prehospital setting. Fentanyl is generally not as prone to causing hypotension, making it the preferred analgesic for patients in critical or unstable condition. Fentanyl also does not have the same risk of nausea and histamine release as morphine and it can be administered intranasally.

Opiate Antagonist Medication

Naloxone is a powerful opioid receptor antagonist that is used by paramedics and other health care providers to reverse the effects of excessive opioid chemicals in the body. Naloxone competes with opioid chemicals at opioid receptor sites, causing a complete or partial reversal of the clinical effects of opioids. Efficacy is dose-dependent. Large doses of naloxone are often required to reverse the effects of potent opioid chemicals. In addition, the duration of naloxone in the body is less than that of many opioid chemicals. Recurrent toxic effects are a risk when naloxone is eliminated more rapidly than the opioid chemicals in the body. Severe opioid overdose situations require repeated naloxone administration or continuous IV infusion.

When you are administering naloxone to patients who receive opioids on a long-term basis, only administer enough naloxone to correct life-threatening conditions such as respiratory depression and airway compromise. Complete opioid reversal is likely to cause severe withdrawal symptoms, endangering the patient and health care providers.

Phenytoin and Fosphenytoin

Phenytoin (Dilantin) and fosphenytoin (Cerebyx) are administered to prevent seizure activity. Patients may receive either of these medications on a long-term basis for control of a seizure disorder. Paramedics may also encounter these medications while performing an interfacility transport of patients with a head injury, intracranial hemorrhage, or status epilepticus. Both medications are administered by IV infusion, usually during 10 to 30 minutes, depending on medication and dose. Phenytoin and fosphenytoin decrease the potential for seizure activity by altering sodium channels, limiting cellular sodium in portions of the central nervous system. In general, fosphenytoin has fewer adverse effects than phenytoin, but both medications can cause a wide variety of adverse effects throughout the body.

◾ Medications Affecting the Gastrointestinal System

Paramedics administer two major groups of medications that affect the GI system. Histamine-2 receptor antagonists are administered to reduce the acid in the stomach and GI tract and also augment other medications used in the treatment of allergic reactions. Antiemetic agents are administered to prevent and treat nausea and vomiting.

Histamine-2 Receptor Antagonists

Histamine-2 receptor antagonist medications (H_2 blockers) decrease acid secretion in the stomach. Paramedics may encounter patients who receive H_2 blockers for short-term and episodic treatment of acid-related GI conditions. These medications are also administered in emergency settings to offset histamine release during an immune-mediated medication reaction or other type of allergic reaction. H_2 blockers prevent histamine from stimulating receptor sites on parietal cells in the stomach. Acid secretion is reduced, protecting against ulcers, GI bleeding, acid-aspiration pneumonitis, and a variety of other related

conditions. Ranitidine (Zantac), cimetidine (Tagamet), and famotidine (Pepcid) are available for oral and IV administration.

Antiemetic Medications

Several types of antiemetic medications are available for use in the prehospital setting. Patients may activate EMS with a primary complaint of nausea or vomiting. Nausea and vomiting occur as symptoms associated with events such as head injury, pregnancy, overdose, and myocardial ischemia. In addition to obvious discomfort associated with nausea and vomiting, vomiting may dramatically worsen many serious medical conditions. Protracted vomiting may cause a Mallory-Weiss tear (a tear in the mucous membrane of the lower part of the esophagus or the upper part of the stomach), leading to GI bleeding. Vomiting can raise intracranial and intraocular pressure, adversely affecting patients with head or eye injuries. Vomiting can also cause pulmonary aspiration in patients with an inadequately protected airway because of a decreased level of consciousness or positioning (such as on a backboard or supine). Vomiting with aspiration of activated charcoal, administered following a toxic exposure, is often lethal. Patients with epiglottitis, peritonsilar abscess, or other airway disease may have increased edema due to vomiting. Paramedics are strongly encouraged to use antiemetic medications to prevent nausea and vomiting in at-risk patients.

Promethazine (Phenergan) and prochlorperazine (Compazine) are phenothiazine antiemetic medications used in various health care settings. Phenothiazine medications have antiemetic and antipsychotic properties. These medications activate dopaminergic receptors in the brain, releasing hormones that depress the reticular activating system of the brain and, ultimately, inhibit emesis.

Both medications are available in oral and IV preparations. Promethazine and prochlorperazine have a number of serious adverse effects related to IV administration. Paramedics may administer these medicines, diluted in a large syringe, by the IV route during 1 to 2 minutes. In ideal situations, paramedics should dilute either medication in 50 mL of normal saline and administer during approximately 10 minutes. Promethazine is notorious for tissue injury during IV administration. Prochlorperazine is known for causing hypotension if administered rapidly through an IV line. <u>Dystonic</u> reactions are possible with promethazine and prochlorperazine, causing unusual muscle activity and significant patient discomfort. Dystonic reactions can be treated with IV diphenhydramine. Many other potential adverse effects are possible.

Metoclopramide (Reglan) is a novel antiemetic medication that may be available in the prehospital setting. Metoclopramide increases GI motility by enhancing the effects of ACh at receptor sites in the upper GI tract. Increased GI motility promotes gastric emptying that is useful in a variety of clinical situations. Metoclopramide can be administered orally, by slow IV injection, and by IV infusion. Dystonic reactions are also a possible adverse effect of metoclopramide and are also treated with IV diphenhydramine.

Antiemetic medications that antagonize the 5-HT_3 receptor sites have experienced a recent surge in popularity. The 5-HT_3 receptors are present in the brain and GI tract. These receptors have a prominent role in activation of the vomiting center of the brain. Medications with the ability to occupy these receptor sites prevent certain (but not all) mechanisms that induce vomiting. For example, 5-HT$_3$ antagonists do not prevent vomiting related to motion sickness.

Ondansetron, granisetron (Kytril), and dolasetron (Anzemet) are 5-HT$_3$ receptor antagonists available for clinical use. These medications are available in oral and IV preparations. Adverse effects are minimal but include the potential for QT prolongation shown on an ECG tracing. Paramedics should expect to encounter these medications more frequently as costs decrease and use becomes more widespread.

Octreotide

Paramedics may encounter octreotide (Sandostatin) during interfacility transport of certain patients. Octreotide is not routinely administered in the prehospital setting. This medication is a synthetic version of somatostatin, a hormone that inhibits serotonin release, causing decreased secretion of insulin, glucagons, growth hormones, and various other chemicals. Octreotide has many potential uses. Paramedics may be requested to monitor an IV octreotide infusion during interfacility transport of patients with bleeding esophageal varices. Octreotide decreases blood flow through esophageal blood vessels, reducing bleeding until definitive treatment can be provided. Paramedics should carefully monitor patients for a wide assortment of adverse effects, including bradycardia and chest pain related to octreotide.

◼ Miscellaneous Medications Used in the Prehospital Setting

Certain medications are used widely in the prehospital setting but do not belong to one of the medication classes discussed. Paramedics should expect to use these medications for a variety of clinical situations. Additional dosing and administration information is available in the *Emergency Medications* chapter.

Acetaminophen

Acetaminophen (Tylenol, APAP) is a medication with antipyretic (fever reduction) and mild analgesic properties. Paramedics and other EMS providers may administer acetaminophen as an adjunct to other analgesic medications, to reduce discomfort by treating fever symptoms, or to prevent febrile seizures in pediatric patients. Acetaminophen is not indicated for hyperthermia related to the toxic effects of medications or environmental exposure.

Acetaminophen is available as a tablet and capsule, liquid, and rectal suppository. At least two liquid concentrations are available, which may lead to dose calculation errors if the concentration is not confirmed before administration. Oral administration should be avoided in patients who are at high risk for seizures or airway compromise.

Adverse effects are rare when acetaminophen is given at therapeutic doses. Toxicity from acetaminophen overdose is insidious and often mismanaged by health care providers. Elevated acetaminophen levels can cause severe, potentially fatal liver damage. Toxicity is determined by patient history and evaluation of a serum acetaminophen level, calculated according to the likely time of overdose. Once toxicity has been determined, many providers continue to mistakenly associate toxicity with serum acetaminophen levels. Liver damage will continue to occur from the presence of a harmful metabolite, rather than from the acetaminophen itself.

Calcium Preparations

In the prehospital setting, IV calcium has many potentially life-saving uses. Calcium can be used for all of the following purposes:

- As an antidote to calcium channel blocker overdose
- To treat magnesium (sulfate) toxicity
- To prevent dysrhythmia during severe hyperkalemia
- For calcium repletion in patients with hypocalcemia
- For calcium restoration after hydrofluoric acid exposure
- As a pretreatment to prevent hypotension associated with IV verapamil administration

Calcium is not indicated for routine use during cardiac arrest resuscitation.

Typically, IV calcium is available as calcium chloride or calcium gluconate. Calcium chloride contains approximately three times the amount of elemental calcium per gram as calcium gluconate does. Both medications are known to be extremely irritating to blood vessels and should be diluted for slow IV infusion whenever possible. Carefully monitor IV catheter sites to avoid extravasation. Avoid SC or IM administration. Assess for incompatibility when administering simultaneously with other medications. Precipitation in IV tubing has been known to occur.

Dextrose

Paramedics administer IV dextrose solution to patients with known or presumptive hypoglycemia. In most cases, hypoglycemia is diagnosed with a handheld glucometer, now available on most ALS ambulances. When a glucometer is not immediately available, various clinical clues such as a known history of diabetes, concurrent ethanol intoxication, and altered mental status will prompt an astute paramedic to suspect hypoglycemia.

Once hypoglycemia is diagnosed, dextrose solution is administered through a large IV catheter while the IV site is continually observed for signs of infiltration. Extravasation of IV dextrose can cause tissue destruction and edema. Paramedics are advised to confirm IV placement with an adequate flush or free-flowing IV fluid before administering dextrose.

The initial adult dose for moderate to severe hypoglycemia is 25 g of a 50% dextrose solution for a total volume of 50 mL. Patients with mild hypoglycemia receive a reduced dose. Children receive weight-based doses of a 25% dextrose solution. Infants and smaller children receive weight-based doses of a 10% dextrose solution. Rebound hypoglycemia is possible following dextrose administration. Paramedics should continue to monitor a patient's clinical status and blood glucose level following dextrose administration.

Diphenhydramine

Diphenhydramine (Benadryl) is frequently used by EMS providers for a variety of clinical situations. Diphenhydramine is a competitive histamine-1 receptor antagonist, preventing receptor activation by histamine released during various medical conditions. Diphenhydramine has a wide range of potential uses in the prehospital setting:

- Treatment of anaphylaxis in conjunction with other medications and interventions
- Sole treatment of mild allergic or immune-mediated medication reactions
- Mild sedative
- Mild antitussive (cough suppressant)
- Treatment of dystonic reaction or extrapyramidal symptoms
- Treatment of pruritus from an unknown cause
- Drying of the mucous membranes in patients with symptomatic rhinorrhea

Paramedics typically administer diphenhydramine by the IV or IM route. Oral capsule, tablet, and liquid preparations are also available. Adverse effects from therapeutic doses of diphenhydramine are usually limited to mild sedation, palpitations, and anxiety. Profound toxicity and death are possible following large overdoses.

Glucagon

Glucagon (GlucaGen) is another medication with a variety of potential uses in the prehospital setting. Glucagon is a naturally occurring peptide, secreted by the pancreas, that is also manufactured commercially for the treatment of certain medical conditions.

Paramedics may use glucagon for the treatment of hypoglycemia. Glucagon converts glycogen stores in the liver to circulating blood glucose, which can be used by various cells. This medication is useful when paramedics are unable to initiate IV access in diabetic patients who would otherwise be given glucose. Patients who are combative because of moderate hypoglycemia and unresponsive patients without IV access are likely recipients of glucagon by the IM route. Glucose production takes 5 to 20 minutes following IV administration of glucagon and 30 minutes following IM administration. Blood glucose levels remain increased for only a limited time after glucagon is administered. Paramedics must continually monitor for a return of hypoglycemia. An IV dextrose solution remains the preferred treatment for patients with hypoglycemia.

Glucagon is also used to provide increased heart rate and contractility following a beta-adrenergic antagonist (beta blocker) overdose. It produces positive chronotropic and inotropic effects without directly activating beta-1 receptors. Glucagon is used in the treatment of severe calcium channel blocker overdoses to reverse myocardial depression. These two clinical situations require large amounts of glucagon, often more than 10 mg, which is rarely carried by EMS. In addition, glucagon is supplied as a dry powder in a vial with a separate phenol vial for reconstitution. Large doses of phenol during treatment of beta blocker or calcium channel blocker overdoses will cause phenol toxicity. In these cases, paramedics should reconstitute glucagon with sterile water if more than one vial (1 mg) of glucagon will be administered.

Paramedics may also administer glucagon to patients who present with a foreign body or large food particle lodged in the esophagus. Glucagon relaxes the smooth muscle in the GI tract, possibly allowing the object to pass into the stomach for digestion. Glucagon for this purpose should typically be administered only after consultation with online medical control.

Ketorolac

Certain EMS systems use ketorolac (Toradol) as an alternative or adjunct to opioid analgesic medications. Ketorolac is a nonsteroidal anti-inflammatory drug (NSAID) that inhibits prostaglandin synthesis, treating both pain and inflammation. It is typically administered via IV or IM route, although oral forms are available. Gastrointestinal irritation and headache are the most common adverse effects. Ketorolac is also known to cause pain at the injection site. Avoid or use with caution in any patient known to be susceptible to GI bleeding or a similar disorder.

Magnesium Sulfate

Magnesium sulfate is an IV electrolyte medication with several important clinical indications. Magnesium sulfate is used for the following:

- Emergency treatment of torsades de pointes or similar ventricular dysrhythmia
- Correction of known or presumptive hypomagnesemia, common in patients who are malnourished or consume ethanol on a long-term basis
- Prevention or treatment of seizures in pregnant patients with preeclampsia or eclampsia
- Adjunctive treatment with bronchodilators and other treatments for severe, refractory asthma

In cardiac arrest situations, 1 to 2 g of magnesium sulfate can be given by slow IV push during 1 to 2 minutes. In other emergency situations, magnesium sulfate is administered as an IV infusion during at least 5 minutes, although slower infusion rates are preferred for patients in less critical condition.

Magnesium sulfate replaces magnesium deficiencies in the body. Magnesium is essential for the movement of other electrolytes such as sodium, calcium, and potassium through channels of cell membranes. Hypomagnesemia causes seizure activity and cardiac dysrhythmias. As magnesium sulfate is administered, it decreases the excitability of cell membranes and slows conduction through the atrioventricular node, prolonging conduction time.

Magnesium sulfate acts to relax various smooth muscle tissues. Clinical effects on smooth muscle are most notable in the lower airways, causing bronchodilation, and in the uterus, causing tocolysis. Respiratory depression, decreased muscle tone, and loss of deep tendon reflexes are possible from excessive doses of magnesium sulfate. Toxic effects from magnesium sulfate are treated by discontinuing the infusion and administering an IV calcium preparation.

Sodium Bicarbonate

Sodium bicarbonate is an alkalinizing agent used in the prehospital and other health care settings. Sodium bicarbonate is administered to do the following:

- Raise the blood pH in patients with a severe metabolic acidosis
- Stabilize profound hyperkalemia in an emergency situation
- Provide cardiac cell membrane stabilization following tricyclic antidepressant overdose
- Promote urinary excretion of salicylate chemicals and certain tissue waste products
- Replace bicarbonate lost due to various medical conditions

Sodium bicarbonate can be administered by rapid IV push or added to IV fluids for intermittent or continuous infusion. Paramedics should evaluate potential incompatibility when sodium bicarbonate is administered in the same IV tubing as other prehospital medications. Patients receiving sodium bicarbonate should be monitored for changes in electrolyte and blood pH levels. Excessive bicarbonate administration can cause fluid volume overload, alkalosis, numerous electrolyte abnormalities, and cerebral and pulmonary edema. In many cases, sodium bicarbonate is titrated to maintain a desired arterial or urinary pH value.

Thiamine

Thiamine is a commercial medication preparation of vitamin B_1. Paramedics administer thiamine to correct a presumptive thiamine deficiency before dextrose administration in patients who are malnourished or who consume alcohol on a long-term basis. Thiamine deficiency can cause Wernicke encephalopathy, a neurologic disorder, which may be exacerbated by the sudden administration of IV dextrose. Thiamine is usually administered by the IV route in the prehospital setting, by IV push or added to IV fluids. Toxic and adverse effects are unlikely when therapeutic doses are administered.

YOU are the Medic   SUMMARY

1. What are some possible causes of lightheadedness in a young adult?

A young adult who complains of lightheadedness can be experiencing many different conditions. Some of the more apparent ones, however, are hypoglycemia, supraventricular tachycardia, and dehydration. These are all medical problems that you as a paramedic can treat.

2. What are your priorities for the initial patient contact?

Your priorities are the same as for any other medical patient. Establish the patient's level of consciousness, ensure an open and patent airway, ensure proper breathing rate and quality, make sure the pulse is at the proper rate and quality, and get a good history of the current problem.

3. Given the information, what are some of your concerns?

The patient has some significant medical problems that caused her coworkers to call 9-1-1. Lightheadedness and syncope are concerns regardless of the patient's age. The patient could be pregnant. The patient's heart rate is abnormally fast and could be the cause of her problem. Use caution in administering medications to patients who are, or may be, pregnant.

4. The patient reports taking a vitamin each day; can a vitamin be the cause of her problem?

Vitamins and minerals are necessary substances that allow for normal metabolism, growth and development, and cellular function. Patients may be taking vitamin and mineral supplements to replace deficient items or as a preventive measure. You should ask what type of vitamin the patient is taking and whether she was told to take it by her doctor. Some vitamins can be prescription medications given to resolve a deficiency. Although you should never rule out any cause, vitamin use is not usually known for causing tachycardia.

5. What medication classifications can slow the heart rate?

The common classification of medications that work on heart dysrhythmias is called antidysrhythmics, which are divided into a few subcategories: sodium channel blockers (slow the conduction through the heart), beta blockers (reduce adrenergic stimulation of the beta receptors), potassium channel blockers (increase the heart's contractility [positive inotropic effect] and work against the reentry of blocked impulses), and calcium channel blockers (block the inflow of calcium into the cardiac cells, thereby decreasing the force of contraction and automaticity; may also decrease the conduction velocity). Adenosine is in a separate, unnamed class of antidysrhythmic medications. It occurs naturally in the body and, when given by the IV route, causes a transient heart block in the atrioventricular node, stopping the transmission of impulses and attempting to get the sinoatrial node back on track. This action is sometimes known as chemical cardioversion. Adenosine administration may not be effective for patients who smoke or have high caffeine intake.

6. In what form do the medications come, what is the route of administration, and what effect do they have?

The medications administered to treat a rapid heart rate in the field often come in an IV solution. The effect most commonly related to IV administrations is systemic, occurring after the drug is absorbed by any route and distributed by the bloodstream. The liquid form of many of the medications is preferred in EMS because many patients need immediate relief from their ailment. Administration of many EMS prehospital medications is parenteral, including medications administered via any route other than the alimentary canal (digestive tract), skin, and mucous membrane.

YOU are the Medic — SUMMARY, *continued*

7. Why is adenosine indicated for this patient?

Once you have completed your assessment, you would most likely consider the patient to have stable supraventricular tachycardia. You would choose vagal maneuvers first, and if those do not work, adenosine is the next most likely treatment. Adenosine is naturally occurring in the body and has a very short half-life with minimal side effects. Adenosine can be used as a diagnostic test, slowing the heart rate enough to recognize the underlying rhythm or completely resolving the rhythm. Adenosine has a high success rate in treating supraventricular tachycardia—more than a 75% conversion rate and less than a 5% recurrence rate were shown in recent studies.

8. How is the adenosine administered?

Adenosine has a very short half-life, so it is important to have everything ready before giving the medication. Have the adenosine drawn into a syringe and a flush that is ready to give as soon as the medication is injected into the IV line. Some paramedics prefer to use a two-way stop cock and have both solutions plugged into the ports. The key is to inject the medication as quickly as possible and follow it immediately with a flush so it can reach the heart as quickly as possible. Make sure the cardiac monitor is recording before administering the medication. Some areas require you to contact a medical control physician first. Be sure to adhere to your agency or regional protocol for administration of adenosine.

EMS Patient Care Report (PCR)

Date: 04-01-16	**Incident No.:** 599	**Nature of Call:** Lightheaded/syncope		**Location:** 1 Maxwell Road	
Dispatched: 1510	**En Route:** 1511	**At Scene:** 1516	**Transport:** 1545	**At Hospital:** 1600	**In Service:** 1620

Patient Information

Age: 22 **Sex:** F **Weight (in kg [lb]):** 60 kg (133 lb)	**Allergies:** Penicillin **Medications:** Allegra **Past Medical History:** Environmental allergies **Chief Complaint:** Lightheadedness

Vital Signs

Time: 1521	**BP:** 100/40	**Pulse:** 198	**Respirations:** 24	**Spo$_2$:** 99% on O$_2$
Time: 1526	**BP:** 98/44	**Pulse:** 196	**Respirations:** 24	**Spo$_2$:** 100% on O$_2$
Time: 1548	**BP:** 110/64	**Pulse:** 110	**Respirations:** 20	**Spo$_2$:** 100% on O$_2$

EMS Treatment
(circle all that apply)

Oxygen @ __10__ **L/min via (circle one):** NC **(NRM)** Bag-mask device	**Assisted Ventilation**	**Airway Adjunct**	**CPR**
Defibrillation / **Bleeding Control**	**Bandaging**	**Splinting**	**Other:** Cardiac monitoring

Narrative

On arrival, found 22-year-old woman on floor near her office cubicle. Pt states she suddenly became lightheaded and weak. Pt denies history of this happening in the past. Pt given 100% O$_2$ via nonrebreathing mask. Pt states no deviation from normal morning schedule. Blood glucose checked with a result of 100 mg/dL. Pt vitals taken and noted above. Very rapid pulse noted, and cardiac monitor applied. Monitor shows supraventricular tachycardia at a rate of 198 beats/min. Pt encouraged to bear down, with no change resulting. Fire Department started an IV in the left antecubital space with an 18-gauge catheter. Contacted medical control and gave full report, requested permission to give 6 mg adenosine by IV push, and MD 423 granted request. Normal saline bag hung with 10-drop set at KVO rate. Flush drawn up, and 6 mg of adenosine prepared. The monitor was in recording status, and pt was advised she might feel strange for a brief period. 6 mg of adenosine given at 1530 followed by a 20-mL flush. Pt's rhythm slowed to sinus tachycardia with no ectopy. Pt stated she felt better and the lightheadedness was going away. Pt placed on stretcher and vitals taken. Pt transported to Memorial Hospital without further changes. Pt stated she felt almost completely better. Report given to RN in room 4; IV patent and sinus rhythm shown on the monitor. **End of report**

Prep Kit

■ Ready for Review

- Although the science of pharmacology has evolved into a sophisticated area of health care, certain medications discovered in ancient times are still in use.

- Paramedics need to be familiar with the rules and regulations implemented under the Controlled Substances Act (also known as the Comprehensive Drug Abuse Prevention and Control Act) of 1970.

- Schedule I medications may not be prescribed, dispensed, used, or administered for medical use.

- All Schedule II through V medications require locked storage, significant record keeping, and controlled wasting procedures.

- Every medication in the United States is given three distinct names:
  - Chemical name
  - Generic name
  - Brand name

- The *United States Pharmacopeia–National Formulary* and *Physicians' Desk Reference* provide detail about thousands of medications.

- Direct sunlight, extremes of heat and cold, and physical damage to medication containers can make medications ineffective or unsafe for use.

- Controlled medications require additional security, record keeping, and disposal precautions. They must be in locked storage or continuously held by an (on-duty) EMS provider responsible for administration.

- As a medication is administered, it begins to alter a function or process in the body. This action is known as pharmacodynamics.

- Medications are developed to reach and to bind with particular receptor sites of target cells.

- Newer medications are designed to target only very specific receptor sites on certain cells in an attempt to minimize side effects.

- A wide variety of factors determine how a particular medication will affect a patient and may influence the choice of medication, dose, route, timing, manner of administration, and monitoring necessary after a patient receives a medication.

- The terms *side effect* and *adverse effect* are often used interchangeably, but adverse effect is usually meant in prehospital settings. Adverse effects are the undesired or harmful responses to a medication.

- The relationship between the median effective dose and the median lethal dose or median toxic dose is known as the therapeutic index or therapeutic ratio.

- Repeated exposure to a medication within a particular class has the potential to cause a tolerance affecting other medications in the same class.

- Patients receiving multiple medications, drugs, or other chemicals are at risk of an unintended interaction between or among the various substances, possibly with unexpected results.

- As a medication is administered, the body begins a complex process of moving the medication, possibly altering the structure of the medication, and, ultimately, removing the medication from the body. The medication dose, route of administration, and clinical status of a particular patient will largely determine the duration of action and effectiveness of the medication.

- Many medication factors such as the size of medication molecules, the ability to bind with other substances in the body, and the ability to dissolve in certain body fluids determine which cells, tissues, and organs a particular medication will reach.

- Biotransformation is a process that has four possible effects on a medication absorbed into the body:
  - Can become active, producing wanted or unwanted clinical effects
  - Can be changed into another active medication
  - Can become completely or partially inactivated
  - Can be transformed into a substance that is easier for the body to eliminate

- Paramedics are constantly at risk for a cognitive error (such as choosing the wrong medication or dose) or a technical error (such as administering more volume of medication than intended).

- There are six rights of medication administration:
  - Right patient
  - Right medication
  - Right dose
  - Right route
  - Right time
  - Right documentation and reporting

- Medications and medication groups often used in the prehospital setting are for airway management and respiratory management; for the cardiovascular, gastrointestinal, and neurologic systems; and blood products and medications affecting the blood.

■ Vital Vocabulary

absolute refractory period The early phase of cardiac repolarization, wherein the heart muscle cannot be stimulated to depolarize; also known as the effective refractory period.

absorption The process by which the molecules of a substance are moved from the site of entry or administration into systemic circulation.

acetylcholinesterase An enzyme that breaks down acetylcholine.

active metabolite A medication that has undergone biotransformation and is able to alter a cellular process or body function.

active transport The process of molecules binding with carrier proteins when energy is used to move the molecules against a concentration gradient.

affinity The ability of a medication to bind with a particular receptor site.

agonist medications The group of medications that initiates or alters a cellular activity by attaching to receptor sites, prompting a cellular response.

anaphylaxis An extreme systemic form of an allergic reaction involving two or more body systems.

antagonist medications The group of medications that prevent endogenous or exogenous agonist chemicals from reaching cell receptor sites and initiating or altering a particular cellular activity.

antibiotics The medications used to fight infection by killing the microorganisms or preventing their multiplication to allow the body's immune system to overcome them.

antifungals The medications used to treat fungal infections.

antimicrobials The medications used to kill or suppress the growth of microorganisms.

automaticity A state in which cardiac cells are at rest, waiting for the generation of a spontaneous impulse from within.

bioavailability The percentage of the unchanged medication that reaches systemic circulation.

biotransformation A process with four possible effects on a medication absorbed into the body: (1) An inactive substance can become active, capable of producing desired or unwanted clinical effects. (2) An active medication can be changed into another active medication. (3) An active medication may be completely or partially inactivated. (4) A medication is transformed into a substance (active or inactive) that is easier for the body to eliminate.

chelating agents Medications that bind with heavy metals in the body and create a compound that can be eliminated; used in cases of ingestion or poisoning.

cholinergic A term used to describe the fibers in the parasympathetic nervous system that release a chemical called acetylcholine.

competitive antagonists The medications that temporarily bind with cellular receptor sites, displacing agonist chemicals.

competitive depolarizing A term used to describe paralytic agents that act at the neuromuscular junction by binding with nicotinic receptors on muscles, causing fasciculations and preventing additional activation by acetylcholine.

cross-tolerance A process in which repeated exposure to a medication within a particular class causes a tolerance that may be "transferred" to other medications in the same class.

cumulative action Several smaller doses of a particular medication capable of producing the same clinical effects as a single larger dose of that same medication.

cytochrome P-450 system A hemoprotein involved in the detoxification of many drugs.

dependence The physical, behavioral, or emotional need for a medication or chemical in order to maintain "normal" physiologic function.

depolarization The process of discharging resting cardiac muscle fibers by an electric impulse that causes them to contract.

depressant A chemical or medication that decreases the performance of the central nervous system or sympathetic nervous system.

distribution The movement and transportation of a medication throughout the bloodstream to tissues and cells and, ultimately, to its target receptor.

diuretic A chemical that increases urinary output.

dose-response curve A graphic illustration of the response of a drug according to the dose administered.

dosing The specified amount of a medication to be given at specific intervals.

down-regulation The process in which a mechanism reducing available cell receptors for a particular medication results in tolerance.

duration of effect The time a medication concentration can be expected to remain above the minimum level needed to provide the intended action.

dystonic Pertaining to voluntary muscle movements that are distorted or impaired because of abnormal muscle tone.

ectopic foci Sites of generation of electrical impulses other than normal pacemaker cells.

efficacy In a pharmacologic context, the ability of a medication to produce the desired effect.

elimination In a pharmacologic context, the removal of a medication or its by-products from the body.

endogenous Originating from within the organism (body).

exogenous Originating outside the organism (body).

extravasation Seepage of blood and medication into the tissue surrounding the blood vessel.

facilitated diffusion The process of medication molecules binding with carrier proteins when no energy is expended.

fasciculation Brief, uncoordinated, visible twitching of small muscle groups; may be caused by the administration of a depolarizing neuromuscular blocking agent (namely, succinylcholine).

filtration Use of hydrostatic pressure to force water or dissolved particles through a semipermeable membrane.

first-order elimination The process in which the rate of elimination is directly influenced by plasma levels of a substance.

habituation The unusual tolerance to the therapeutic and adverse clinical effects of a medication or chemical.

half-life The time needed in an average person for metabolism or elimination of 50% of a substance in the plasma.

hematocrit The percentage of red blood cells in a blood sample.

hemolysis The destruction of red blood cells by disruption of the cell membrane.

hydrophilic Attracted to water molecules.

idiosyncratic In a pharmacologic context, abnormal susceptibility to a medication, possibly due to genetic traits or dysfunction of a metabolic enzyme, that is peculiar to an individual patient (and usually unexplained).

inactive metabolite A medication that has undergone biotransformation and now is no longer able to alter a cell process or body function; not pharmacologically active.

ions Charged particles.

interference One medication or chemical taken by a patient that undermines the effectiveness of another medication taken by or administered to a patient.

lipophilic Attracted to fats and lipids.

median effective dose (ED$_{50}$) The weight-based dose of a medication that was effective in 50% of the humans and animals tested.

median lethal dose (LD$_{50}$) The weight-based dose of a medication that caused death in 50% of the animals tested.

median toxic dose (TD$_{50}$) The weight-based dose of a medication that demonstrated toxicity in 50% of the animals tested.

medication monograph A document that gives detailed information about drugs, such as the indications and uses, dosing information, precautions, contraindications, and adverse effects.

medication sensitivity A mild to severe reaction after the first exposure to a medication or other substance, often with many of the same signs and symptoms as an immune-mediated reaction.

noncompetitive antagonists Medications that permanently bind with receptor sites and prevent activation by agonist chemicals.

nondepolarizing A term used to describe drugs that produce muscle relaxation by interfering with impulses between the nerve ending and muscle receptor.

nonionic Uncharged.

onset The time needed for the concentration of the medication at the target tissue to reach the minimum effective level.

osmosis The movement of a solvent, such as water, from an area of low solute concentration to one of high concentration through a selectively permeable membrane to equalize concentrations of a solute on both sides of the membrane.

osmotic Characterized by the movement of a solvent, such as water, across a semipermeable membrane (for example, the cell wall) from an area of lower to higher concentration of solute molecules.

paradoxical Opposite from expected.

partial agonist A chemical that binds to the receptor site but does not initiate as much cellular activity or change as other agonists do; lowers the efficacy of other agonist chemicals present at the cells.

peak In a pharmacologic context, the point of maximum effect of a drug.

pharmacodynamics The biochemical and physiologic effects and mechanism of action of a medication in the body.

pharmacokinetics The fate of medications in the body, such as distribution and elimination.

pharmacology The scientific study of how various substances interact with or alter the function of living organisms.

pinocytosis A process by which cells ingest the extracellular fluid and its contents.

placebo effect In a pharmacologic context, the positive and negative effects of an inactive medication on a person that are related to the person's expectations and other factors.

plasma protein binding A process in which medication molecules temporarily attach to proteins in the blood plasma, significantly altering medication distribution in the body.

potency The relationship between the desired response of a medication and the dose required to achieve the response.

receptor A specialized area in tissues that initiates certain actions after specific stimulation.

relative refractory period The period in the cell-firing cycle at which it is possible but difficult to restimulate the cell to fire another impulse.

Stevens-Johnson syndrome A severe, possibly fatal reaction that mimics a burn; may be due to a medication.

stimulant A medication or chemical that temporarily enhances central nervous system and sympathetic nervous system functioning.

sympathomimetics Medications administered to stimulate the sympathetic nervous system.

tachyphylaxis A condition in which repeated doses of medication within a short period rapidly cause tolerance, making the medication virtually ineffective.

therapeutic index The relationship between the median effective dose and the median lethal dose or median toxic dose; also known as the therapeutic ratio.

threshold level In a pharmacologic context, the concentration of medication at which initiation or alteration of cellular activity begins.

tolerance A condition that develops following repeated use by a patient of a medication that results in decreased efficacy or potency.

untoward effect A clinical change caused by a medication that causes harm or discomfort to a patient; also known as adverse effect.

Vaughan-Williams A classification scheme based on the mechanism of action rather than on specific medication groups.

volume of distribution The extent to which a medication will spread within the body.

water-soluble A property that indicates a material can be dissolved in water.

zero-order elimination A process in which a fixed amount of a substance is removed during a certain period, regardless of the total amount in the body.

Assessment in Action

You arrive at a moderately well-kept apartment of a 76-year-old man who called EMS because of heart palpitations. The patient states that his physician recently prescribed some new medications for an irregular heartbeat and high blood pressure. The new medications are an "ACE inhibitor" and a "calcium channel blocker." He started taking the medication 2 days ago, and the symptoms began this morning. He also takes a low-dose aspirin each day.

The patient says he does not want to go to the hospital; he just wants you to check him out because he is worried. His family members do not visit him often, and he lives alone.

1. The primary action of an ACE inhibitor is to:
   A. suppress the conversion of angiotensin I to angiotensin II.
   B. promote the conversion of angiotensin I to angiotensin II.
   C. block the alpha receptor.
   D. block the beta-1 receptor.

2. On which system does an ACE inhibitor focus?
   A. Sympathetic nervous system
   B. Renin-angiotensin system
   C. Parasympathetic nervous system
   D. Sodium potassium pump

3. Calcium channel blockers have which type(s) of properties?
   A. Antihypertensive
   B. Antidysrhythmic
   C. Antiplatelet
   D. Both A and B

4. Taking a low-dose aspirin helps the patient by:
   A. keeping pain under control.
   B. keeping the blood pressure low.
   C. keeping platelets from coagulating.
   D. helping the patient's mood.

5. The most appropriate route for the patient to take the medication is:
   A. IV.
   B. intramuscular.
   C. transdermal.
   D. oral.

6. Common forms of medications outside the hospital setting include all of the following *except*:
   A. tablets.
   B. ampules.
   C. solutions.
   D. powders.

7. A direct biochemical interaction between two drugs is referred to as which of the following?
   A. Synergism
   B. Interference
   C. Potentiation
   D. Summation effect

Additional Questions

8. You believe your patient overdosed on amitriptyline (Elavil), a tricyclic antidepressant (TCA). Why is the fact that the antidepressant is a tricyclic a cause for concern?

9. You have a patient who intentionally overdosed on night-time acetaminophen (Tylenol PM) and states the pills were ingested 20 minutes ago. Is an acetaminophen overdose fatal?

Medication Administration

National EMS Education Standard Competencies

Pharmacology

Integrates comprehensive knowledge of pharmacology to formulate a treatment plan intended to mitigate emergencies and improve the overall health of the patient.

Medication Administration

- Routes of administration (pp 479-492, 497-501, 508-535)
- Self-administer medication (p 528)
- Peer-administer medication (p 535)
- Assist/administer medications to a patient (pp 479-531)
- Within the scope of practice of the paramedic, administer medications to a patient (pp 469-471)

Knowledge Objectives

1. Explain the "six rights" of medication administration and describe how each one relates to EMS. (pp 469-471)
2. Describe the role of medical direction in medication administration and explain the difference between direct orders (online) and standing orders (off-line). (p 469)
3. Explain why determining what prescription and over-the-counter (OTC) medications a patient is taking is a critical aspect of patient assessment during an emergency. (p 470)
4. Discuss the circumstances surrounding the administration of medication, including patient-assisted medication and paramedic-administered medication. (pp 469-471)
5. Discuss the advantages, disadvantages, and techniques for performing intravenous (IV) therapy. (pp 476-487)
6. Describe complications that can occur as a result of IV therapy. (pp 492-495)
7. Describe special considerations when performing IV therapy on a pediatric or geriatric patient. (pp 491-492)
8. Discuss the advantages, disadvantages, and techniques for establishing an intraosseous (IO) IV line. (pp 497-501)
9. Discuss the systems of weights and measures used when administering medication. (pp 501-503)
10. Explain principles of drug dose calculations, including desired dose, concentration on hand, volume on hand, volume to administer, and IV drip rate. (pp 505-508)
11. Discuss the advantages, disadvantages, and techniques for administering a medication orally. (pp 508-509)
12. Discuss the advantages, disadvantages, and techniques for administering a medication subcutaneously. (pp 517-518)
13. Discuss the advantages, disadvantages, and techniques for administering a medication intramuscularly. (pp 518-520)
14. Discuss the advantages, disadvantages, and techniques for administering a medication sublingually. (pp 526-527)
15. Discuss the advantages, disadvantages, and techniques for administering a medication intranasally. (p 528)
16. Discuss the advantages, disadvantages, and techniques for administering an inhaled medication. (pp 528-531)
17. Discuss the advantages, disadvantages, and techniques for administering a medication via the IV route. (pp 479-490)
18. Discuss the advantages, disadvantages, and techniques for administering a medication via the IO route. (pp 497-501)

Skills Objectives

1. Demonstrate the process a paramedic should follow when following the six rights of medication administration. (pp 469-471)
2. Demonstrate how to spike an IV bag. (p 480, Skill Drill 1)
3. Demonstrate how to obtain vascular access. (pp 486-487, Skill Drill 2)
4. Demonstrate how to gain IO access. (pp 498-500, Skill Drill 3)
5. Demonstrate how to administer oral medication to a patient. (pp 508-509)
6. Demonstrate how to administer medication via a gastric tube. (pp 509-510, Skill Drill 4)
7. Demonstrate how to draw medication from an ampule. (p 513, Skill Drill 5)
8. Demonstrate how to draw medication from a vial. (p 514, Skill Drill 6)
9. Demonstrate how to administer a subcutaneous medication to a patient. (pp 517-518, Skill Drill 7)
10. Demonstrate how to administer an intramuscular medication to a patient. (p 519, Skill Drill 8)
11. Demonstrate how to administer a medication via the IV bolus route. (pp 521-522, Skill Drill 9)
12. Demonstrate how to perform an IO infusion. (pp 524-525, Skill Drill 10)
13. Demonstrate how to administer a sublingual medication to a patient. (p 526, Skill Drill 11)
14. Demonstrate how to administer an intranasal medication to a patient. (p 528)
15. Demonstrate how to administer a medication via inhalation to a patient. (pp 528-531)
16. Demonstrate how to assist a patient with a metered-dose inhaler (MDI). (p 529, Skill Drill 12)
17. Demonstrate how to assist a patient with a small-volume nebulizer. (pp 530-531, Skill Drill 13)

Introduction

Vascular access is often needed in emergency medicine for patients in hemodynamically unstable condition and in need of intravenous (IV) fluids, various medications, or both. A number of techniques are used to gain vascular access in the prehospital setting, including cannulation of a peripheral extremity vein, external jugular vein cannulation, intraosseous access, and long-term vascular access devices. In critically ill or injured patients, survival often depends on your ability to obtain vascular access quickly and effectively. Because these procedures are invasive, you must be proficient, yet cautious. Significant harm to the patient can result from improper technique and/or insufficient knowledge of the medication(s) being administered.

This chapter begins with an overview of fluids and electrolytes—balanced and imbalanced—and the processes of osmosis and diffusion. Next, it discusses the various types of IV solutions used in the prehospital setting and the techniques of IV therapy and intraosseous infusion. It describes the mathematical principles used in pharmacology, and for calculating medication doses (bolus and maintenance infusion).

Paramedics administer medication in different forms. The chapter concludes with a discussion of routes for administering medications.

Medical Direction

Your paramedic education will furnish you with knowledge of anatomy and physiology, pathophysiology, and how pharmacologic treatments will affect your patients. It is your responsibility to administer the appropriate medications and the appropriate dosage when needed, and to determine the most effective route by which to administer them. It is also important to remember that any procedure that is performed by a paramedic must be approved by the medical director. Medication administration is governed by your local protocols and/or online medical direction.

For example, for an unresponsive diabetic patient with a confirmed blood glucose reading of 40 mg/dL, you may be allowed by written protocols (standing orders) to administer 50% dextrose (D_{50}). <u>Standing orders</u> are a form of off-line or indirect medical control where you perform certain predefined procedures before contacting the physician.

Some EMS system medical directors may not allow paramedics to perform certain procedures (for example, administering certain narcotics) before making contact with him or her. This is referred to as <u>online (direct) medical control</u>. When requesting online medical control orders the paramedic should be confident and detailed. All of the patient information should be gathered prior to contacting medical control. The paramedic should be able to paint a picture of the patient to the physician and demonstrate the need for the medication that they are requesting.

Local policies and procedures are designed to guide you in specific situations. When questions or unusual situations arise—even if you function primarily by standing orders—contact medical control for consultation and/or direction. *If you have any doubt as to the correct action, consult with medical control!*

Paramedic's Responsibility Associated With Drug Orders

The danger of something going wrong when you are administering a drug—for example, administering the wrong drug or the wrong dose of a drug—can be minimized by following the "six rights" of medication administration:

1. Right patient
2. Right drug
3. Right dose
4. Right route
5. Right time
6. Right documentation

These principles are included in the following set procedure for administering any medication. These steps also incorporate a number of safety precautions:

1. Obtain an order from medical control. This order may be given to you directly, through online medical control via telephone or radio. Or it may be indirect, through protocols that contain standing orders for the administration of certain medications. For example, your system may use a protocol that describes how the medical director wants you to deal with a patient who is having respiratory difficulties.

YOU *are the Medic*   **PART 1**

You are part of a standby team for a marathon, working at a first aid station. You are asked to respond to the middle of the 26.2-mile course for a runner who is down and in pain. It is a warm, humid day with a temperature of 90°F. You arrive to find a responsive 34-year-old woman who bystanders state fell and may have broken her leg.

1. What are some differential diagnoses for this patient?
2. Is the weather a potential cause for her problem?

Part of this protocol may direct you to use a nonrebreathing mask to deliver oxygen to such a patient at 15 L/min. You may do this without calling online medical control if the patient meets the criteria of the protocol.

When you are communicating with medical control about administering a particular medication, make sure that the medication is indicated for the patient's condition. Knowledge of the indications, contraindications, therapeutic effects, side effects, and appropriate doses for each of the drugs that you carry on your ambulance is critical to safe patient care. On the basis of the patient's clinical presentation, you must know the *right time* to administer a medication (that is, when the medication is indicated). Of equal if not greater importance is knowing when *not* to administer a medication (that is, when the medication is contraindicated). Furthermore, some of the medications you carry on the ambulance have specific intervals for repeated doses; you must be aware of these drugs and the appropriate intervals at which they are administered.

Make sure medical control clearly understands the situation and the reason why you are advocating for specific medical care for your patient. The decision to order the administration of any given drug is complex, involving such considerations as the patient's age, weight, clinical status, allergy history, concomitant medical problems, and other drugs he or she may be taking, including prescription medications, over-the-counter medications, and recreational drugs. Thus, it is critical that you obtain and communicate complete, accurate information about the patient to enable the physician to make prudent, correct decisions about drug administration.

Verify that your patient is indeed the *right patient*. In situations in which there are multiple patients, reconfirm the patient's name and compare it with the wristband or triage tag. If you are assisting a patient with his or her medication, be sure it is prescribed to that patient.

2. Make sure you understand the physician's orders. If the orders are unclear or seem inappropriate for the patient's condition (for example, the dosage is more than the usual range or an unusual route of administration is requested), *ask the physician to repeat the order*.

3. Repeat any orders, word for word, for verification. This will help ensure that you understand the order and that the physician did not inadvertently give you an incorrect dosage order. In the repetition, state the *name of the drug*, the *dose*, and the *route* by which it is to be given. As a paramedic, you are just as responsible for the administration of the drug and its possible consequences as the physician giving the order, so be absolutely certain which drug is to be administered, in what dose, and by which route. If your partner does not hear the exchange of information, you should repeat the order to him or her as an additional safety measure.

4. Inquire about any medication allergies the patient may have. If the patient is unresponsive, try to obtain this information from another reliable source of information. Check for Medic-Alert jewelry or tags as well.

5. Verify the proper medication and prescription. You have received and confirmed the medication order and determined that the patient is still a candidate for the medication. You must now make sure that the medication you are about to give is the correct medication. Carefully read the label. If it is the patient's own prescription, the bottle may show the trade name or the generic name. If you have any questions at all, contact online medical control. Examine the label to confirm that the medication is prescribed to the patient and not to a family member or friend. You should never give a medication to a patient that has been prescribed for someone else. Note the *drug concentration* printed on the label.

Note that you should read the drug label at least three times before administration to ensure that you have the *right drug*:

  - When it is still in the drug box it came in
  - When you prepare the drug for administration
  - Before actually administering the drug to the patient

6. Verify the form, dose, and route of the medication. At this point, you have confirmed your order and verified that the medication is correct. Now you must make sure that the form of the medication, the dose, and the route are all consistent with the order you received. For example, suppose that you are told to administer a sublingual nitroglycerin tablet. The patient's nitroglycerin bottle is empty, but he has another bottle of nitroglycerin capsules. These are to be swallowed four times a day. The medication is the same, but the form, dose, and route of delivery are different from the order given. You may not substitute the capsules for the tablets without specific orders from medical control.

You are responsible for knowing the appropriate doses for the medications you carry on your ambulance. You are also responsible for accurately calculating the appropriate dose of the drug. Always recheck your drug calculations before administration to ensure that you are administering the *right dose*.

It is imperative that you know the *right route* for the drug or drugs that you are about to administer. A drug given by an inappropriate route—even if it is the right drug—could have disastrous and possibly fatal consequences.

7. Check the expiration date and condition of the medication. The last step before administering a medication is to make sure the expiration date has not passed. Prescription and over-the-counter (OTC) medications should have an expiration date on their labels. Check the date. If no date can be found, you should examine the medication with suspicion. Check for defects in the vial, preloaded syringe, or ampule, noting whether the container appears to be cracked or damaged. If the medication looks suspicious in any way, do *not* use it. In addition, if you find discoloration, cloudiness, or particles in a liquid medication, you should not administer it. If a patient with asthma gives you a metered-dose inhaler (MDI) and the expiration date on it is smudged, you should not administer it. Rather, consider using the medication in your drug box.

8. Confirm medication compatibility. If you have orders to administer more than one drug, make sure that the drugs are compatible. Some drugs will not mix with others, which could cause a precipitate to form in the solution. Should any cloudiness occur after a drug has been injected into IV tubing, *clamp the tubing immediately* and replace it with a new administration set.

9. Dispose of any syringes and needles safely. Most over-the-needle catheters have automatic retraction after insertion, and are therefore safer. Regardless of the type of needle you are using, do *not* try to recap a needle because the likelihood of sticking yourself in the process is quite high; rather, immediately dispose of the needle and syringe in a sharps container.

10. Notify the physician when the medication has been administered and advise the physician of any changes in patient condition, whether positive or negative.

11. Monitor the patient for possible adverse side effects. Reassess the vital signs, especially pulse rate and blood pressure, at least every 5 minutes or as the patient's condition warrants.

12. Document. Recall the adage, "If you did not document it, you did not do it." Always document your actions and the patient's response on the patient care report after administering a medication. This includes the:
    - Name of the drug
    - Dose of the drug
    - Time you administered the drug
    - Route of administration
    - Your name or the name of the person who administered the drug
    - Patient's response to the medication, whether positive or negative

    Did the patient's condition improve, get worse, or not change at all? Were there any side effects? If your performance should ever be questioned, documentation is your best defense.

Words of Wisdom

Never guess what the physician has ordered. When in doubt, ask.

Local Drug Distribution System

Before responding to an EMS call, you must ensure that all equipment on the ambulance is fully functional; this verification is made during your check of the ambulance at the beginning of your shift. All medications must be checked to ensure that they are not expired or damaged and that they are readily available in the right quantity. You must be thoroughly familiar with the system used to exchange and replace outdated or damaged drugs in your EMS system.

You are also responsible for the documentation and security of all controlled substances carried on your ambulance, including accounting for all controlled substances that were

Documentation and Communication

If you administer a controlled substance to your patient (eg, morphine, midazolam [Versed], fentanyl [Sublimaze, Duragesic]), document the amount of medication that you gave to the patient and the amount of medication that you wasted (did not give to the patient). Have your partner, nurse or physician from the receiving facility, or supervisor witness (actually see) you wasting the medication. Both of you should sign the form—you as the paramedic who administered and wasted the medication—and the witness who observed you waste the medication.

wasted (ie, residual medication that was not administered to the patient). Follow the specific policies and procedures of your local drug distribution, security, and accountability system.

Medical Asepsis

Medical asepsis is the practice of preventing contamination of the patient by using aseptic technique. This method of cleansing is intended to prevent contamination of a site when you are performing an invasive procedure such as starting an IV line or administering a medication. Medical asepsis may be accomplished through the use of sterilization of equipment, antiseptics, or disinfectants.

Clean Technique Versus Sterile Technique

Some of the equipment you will use in the field has been sterilized for patient safety. For example, some medications have been packaged using sterile technique. Sterile technique refers to the destruction of all living organisms and is achieved by using heat, gas, or chemicals.

In order for a sterile field to exist, multiple pieces of sterile equipment must be used and rules must be followed. You will need to wear sterile sleeves or a gown that covers you from the wrist to 5 cm proximal of the elbow. Then, appropriately sized sterile gloves, using numerical sizes rather than small to extra large sizing, will need to be used. Sterile drapes need to be placed around the procedural area. Anything below the drapes should be considered nonsterile. In order for the area to remain sterile, only sterile items and personnel may enter the sterile field.

Because it may not be feasible to maintain a sterile environment in the field, you must practice medical asepsis to reduce the risk of contamination and infection. Examples of medical asepsis include handwashing, wearing gloves, and keeping equipment as clean as possible. For example, the site on a patient's hand that has been cleaned with iodine and alcohol before starting an IV line is said to be "medically clean."

If you open an IV catheter package and the IV catheter inadvertently falls to the ground or otherwise comes in contact with a contaminated surface, discard it and use a new IV catheter. If you have already cleaned the injection port on the IV tubing where you intend to inject a medication and you inadvertently touch the cleaned injection port, recleanse the port before injecting the medication. You must always make a *conscious* effort to prevent contamination—whether handling equipment, supplies, or the patient. This is the cornerstone of maintaining a medically clean environment.

Words of Wisdom

In addition to ensuring that medications have not expired or become contaminated, you must ensure that the medications are kept at the recommended temperatures while stored in your ambulance. Some medications become inactive in extreme heat or cold conditions. Refer to the package insert for the medication for this information.

Antiseptics and Disinfectants

Antiseptics are used to cleanse an area before performing an invasive procedure such as IV therapy or medication administration. Even though antiseptics are capable of destroying pathogens, they are not toxic to living tissues. Isopropyl alcohol (rubbing alcohol), iodine, and 2% chlorhexidine gluconate (ChloraPrep) are the three most common antiseptics you will use in the field.

Disinfectants, by contrast, are toxic to living tissues; therefore, you should never use them on a patient. Use disinfectants only on nonliving objects such as the inside of the ambulance, laryngoscope blades, and other nondisposable equipment.

Standard Precautions and Contaminated Equipment Disposal

Standard Precautions

The first rule of standard precautions is to treat any body fluid as being potentially infectious. Many patients who harbor infectious diseases may be asymptomatic and/or unaware that they are infected. As a paramedic, you need to protect yourself by taking the proper standard precautions when you are starting an IV line or administering a medication. Minimum standard precautions for these procedures include wearing gloves and protective eyewear (ie, goggles, face shield). If blood splattering is possible, full facial protection is indicated.

According to the Centers for Disease Control and Prevention, handwashing is the *most* effective way to prevent the spread of disease. It should be a routine practice for you, between all patients. Hand sanitizer is becoming common in the prehospital setting because of the lack of handwashing equipment. It is imperative that you remember that if your hands are visibly soiled, hand sanitizer *IS NOT* a substitute for thorough handwashing and that you should wash your hands as soon as you are available to do so. Note, however, that handwashing alone will not prevent you from being infected; use the appropriate standard precautions as dictated by the situation.

Disposal of Contaminated Equipment

After an IV catheter or needle has penetrated a patient's skin, it is contaminated. Considering the fact that accidental needlesticks are the most common route for disease transmission in the health care setting, you must always handle contaminated equipment carefully and dispose of it immediately and properly. Sharps are any contaminated item that can cause injury. Sharps include IV/IM/SQ needles and catheters, broken ampules or vials, and anything else that can penetrate or lacerate the skin.

Immediately dispose of all sharps in a puncture-proof sharps container that bears a biohazard logo **Figure 1**. Sharps containers should be readily accessible; place at least two in the back of the ambulance so that your handling of needles, catheters, and other sharps is kept to a minimum amount of time. In addition, you should have a smaller sharps container in your jump kit for immediate disposal of sharps while not in the ambulance. **Table 1** lists some safe practices that will minimize your risk of an inadvertent needlestick. As always, follow your agency's exposure control plan.

Basic Cell Physiology

Basic cell physiology provides an understanding of how administering fluids to a patient can be beneficial depending on the patient's condition. A human cell can exist only in a special balanced environment. Understanding how this environment is created and maintained will give you the foundation you need to determine how IV therapy will affect the patient and what is needed to protect that delicate homeostasis.

Because the cell is completely enclosed by a cell membrane, compounds must move through the membrane to enter the cell. Small compounds such as water (H_2O), carbon dioxide (CO_2), hydrogen ions (H^+), and oxygen (O_2) can easily pass through the membrane. Larger charged compounds need assistance to cross the cell membrane and enter the cell.

The cell membrane is a **phospholipid bilayer**, which is an important barrier to fluid movement and the acid-base balance. This layer allows the

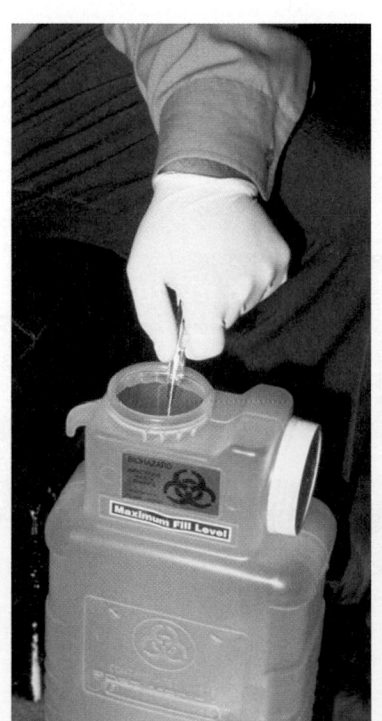

Figure 1 Always dispose of sharp objects or blood-filled items in a puncture-proof sharps container.

Table 1 Minimizing Your Risk of a Needlestick

Use a needleless delivery system. Needleless delivery systems "recap" themselves, which greatly reduces the risk of a needlestick.

Immediately dispose of all sharps in a puncture-proof sharps container. *Do not* drop the sharps on the floor for later disposal, and *do not* attempt to recap a needle and syringe before placing it in the sharps container.

When possible, perform all invasive procedures at the scene. If your patient's condition warrants starting an IV line or administering a medication en route to the hospital, *use extreme caution*. Although most paramedics become proficient at starting IV lines in the back of a moving ambulance, it may be necessary to have your partner briefly stop the ambulance, especially if you are traveling over rough terrain.

Recap needles *only* as an absolute last resort. If you must recap a needle, use the one-handed technique: Place the needle cover on a stationary surface, then slide the needle—with one hand—into the needle cap.

cell membrane to have a characteristic called **selective permeability**—the ability to selectively allow certain compounds into the cell based on the cell's current needs. Everything discussed in this section will in some way be related to the cell membrane barrier and movement across that barrier.

Body Fluid Composition

The human body is composed mostly of water, which provides the environment where the chemical reactions necessary for life take place. Water also serves as a transport medium for nutrients, hormones, and waste materials. The **total body water (TBW)** constitutes 60% of the weight of an adult and is distributed among the following compartments Figure 2:

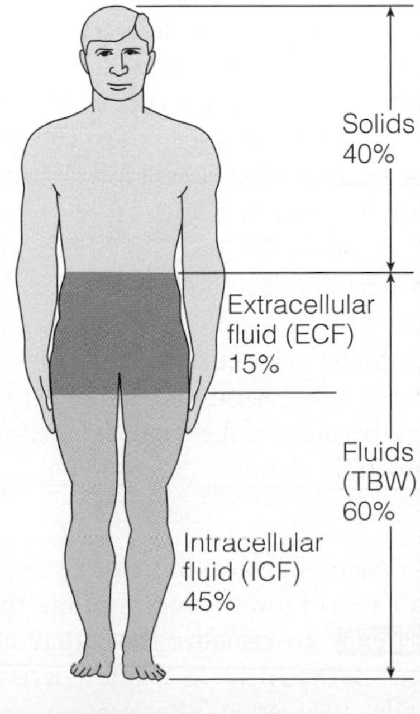

- **Intracellular fluid (ICF)** is the water contained inside the cells; it normally accounts for 45% of body weight.
- **Extracellular fluid (ECF)**, the water outside the cells, accounts for 15% of body weight and is further divided into two types of fluids:

Figure 2 Distribution of water throughout the body.

- **Interstitial fluid**, the water bathing the cells, accounts for about 10.5% of body weight. The interstitial fluid also includes special fluid collections, such as cerebrospinal fluid and intraocular fluid.
- **Intravascular fluid** (plasma), the water within the blood vessels, carries red blood cells, white blood cells, and vital nutrients. Intravascular fluid normally accounts for about 4.5% of body weight.

The fluids in the body are composed of dissolved elements and water, a combination known as a **solution**. A solution is a mixture of two things:

- **Solvent**. The fluid that does the dissolving, or the solution that contains the dissolved components
- **Solute**. The dissolved particles contained in the solvent

Water in the body serves as the universal solvent, dissolving a variety of solutes. These solutes can be classified as electrolytes or nonelectrolytes.

Electrolytes

Atoms carry positive and negative charges. Two or more atoms that bond together form a molecule. When atoms bond together, they share and disperse their charges throughout the molecule. Organic molecules contain carbon atoms—for example, table sugar ($C_6H_{12}O_6$). By contrast, inorganic molecules do not contain carbon—for example, table salt (NaCl). Inorganic molecules give rise to **electrolytes** (so called because of their ability to conduct electricity) when they dissociate in water into their charged components.

Electrolytes, also called **ions**, are reactive and dangerous if left to circulate in the body. The body, however, uses the energy stored in these charged particles. Each electrolyte has a unique property or value to the body. Electrolytes help to regulate everything from water levels to cardiac function and muscle contractions. Water in the body stabilizes the electrolyte charges so that the electrolytes can aid in the **metabolic** functions that are necessary for life.

If the electrolyte has an overall *positive* charge, it is called a **cation**; if it has an overall *negative* charge, it is called an **anion**. The major cations of the body include sodium, potassium, calcium, and magnesium; bicarbonate, chloride, and phosphorus are the major anions.

The unit of measurement for electrolytes is the **milliequivalent (mEq)**; it represents the chemical combining power of the ion and is based on the number of available ionic charges in an electrolyte solution. One milliequivalent of any cation is able to react completely with 1 mEq of any anion. For example, sodium (Na^+) is a singly charged (**monovalent**) cation, and chloride (Cl^-) is a singly charged anion. Thus 1 mEq of Na^+ will react with 1 mEq of Cl^- to form NaCl—ordinary table salt Figure 3. Calcium (Ca^{++}) has two positive charges (**bivalent**); thus the Ca^{++} ion represents 2 mEq and reacts completely with 2 mEq of a singly charged anion Figure 4.

Sodium Sodium (Na^+) is the principal extracellular cation needed to regulate the distribution of water throughout the body in the intravascular and interstitial fluid compartments. Its role in

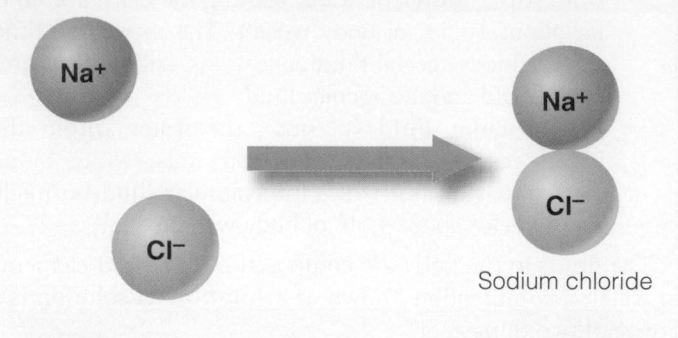

Figure 3 When sodium (Na⁺) and chloride (Cl⁻) unite, they form salt (sodium chloride [NaCl]).

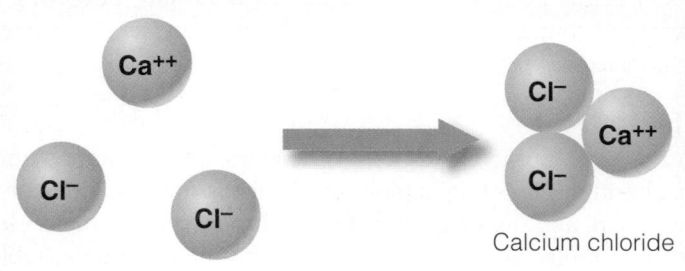

Figure 4 A doubly charged (bivalent) cation such as calcium (Ca⁺⁺) needs two anions in order to be balanced.

maintaining adequate cellular perfusion gives rise to the saying, "Where sodium goes, water follows." Sodium is also a major component of the circulating buffer, sodium bicarbonate ($NaHCO_3$).

Potassium About 98% of all the body's potassium (K^+) is found inside the cells of the body, making it the principal intracellular cation. Potassium plays a major role in neuromuscular function and in the conversion of glucose into glycogen. Cellular potassium levels are regulated by insulin. The <u>sodium-potassium (Na^+-K^+) pump</u> is helped by the presence of insulin and epinephrine. Low potassium levels—<u>hypokalemia</u>—in the serum (blood plasma) can lead to decreased skeletal muscle function, gastrointestinal disturbances, and alterations in cardiac function. High potassium levels in the serum—<u>hyperkalemia</u>—can lead to hyperstimulation of neural cell transmission, resulting in cardiac arrest.

Calcium Calcium (Ca^{++}) is the principal cation needed for bone growth. It also plays an important part in the functioning of heart muscle, nerves, and cell membranes and is necessary for proper blood clotting.

Low serum calcium levels—<u>hypocalcemia</u>—can lead to overstimulation of nerve cells. Signs and symptoms of hypocalcemia include skeletal muscle cramps, abdominal cramps, <u>carpopedal spasms</u>, hypotension, and vasoconstriction.

High serum calcium levels—<u>hypercalcemia</u>—can lead to decreased stimulation of nerve cells. Signs and symptoms of hypercalcemia include skeletal muscle weakness, lethargy, <u>ataxia</u>, vasodilation, and hot, flushed skin.

Magnesium Magnesium (Mg^{++}) has an important role as a coenzyme in the metabolism of proteins and carbohydrates. In addition, it acts in a manner similar to calcium in controlling neuromuscular irritability.

Bicarbonate Bicarbonate (HCO_3^-) levels are a determining factor between metabolic <u>acidosis</u> and <u>alkalosis</u> in the body. Bicarbonate is the primary buffer used in all circulating body fluids.

Chloride Chloride (Cl^-) primarily regulates the pH of the stomach. It also regulates extracellular fluid levels.

Phosphorus Phosphorus (P) is an important component in adenosine triphosphate (ATP), the body's powerful energy source.

Nonelectrolytes

The body also contains solutes that have no electrical charge. These <u>nonelectrolytes</u> include glucose and urea. The normal concentration of glucose in the blood, for example, is 70 to 110 milligrams (mg) per 100 milliliters (mL).

◼ Fluid and Electrolyte Movement

Water and electrolytes move among the body's fluid compartments according to some basic chemical and biologic tenets. One governing principle is that unequal concentrations on different sides of a cell membrane will move to balance themselves equally on both sides of the membrane. Balance across a cell membrane has two components:

- Balance of compounds (for example, water and electrolytes) on either side of the cell membrane
- Balance of charges [the positive (⁺) or negative (⁻) charges carried on the atoms] on either side of the cell membrane

When concentrations of charges or compounds are greater on one side of the cell membrane than on the other side, a gradient is created. The natural tendency for materials is to flow from an area of higher concentration to one of lower concentration, establishing a <u>concentration gradient</u>. Gradients are categorized according to the type of material that flows down them: Chemical compounds flow down chemical gradients; electrical currents flow down electrical gradients. The process of flowing down a gradient depends on whether the cell membrane will allow the material to pass through it. Certain compounds can travel freely across the cell membrane (a kinetically favorable situation that requires little energy), whereas others require active transport across the membrane because of the size of the compound or because of an incompatible charge.

Diffusion

When compounds or charges concentrated on one side of a cell membrane move across it to an area of lower concentration, the process is called <u>diffusion</u> **Figure 5**. To visualize this situation, imagine that too many people show up for a theater performance. The management decides to open another seating area to accommodate the crowd. Patrons (charges or compounds) are concentrated in a small area (the cell) outside the door (the cell membrane) leading to the new seating area. When the theater

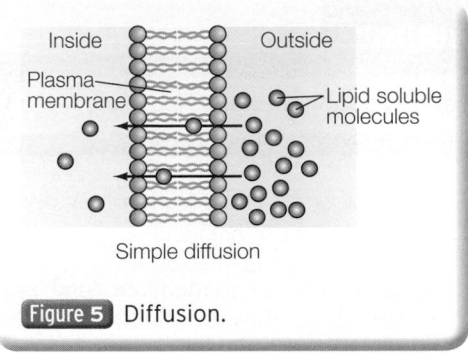

Figure 5 Diffusion.

manager opens the door, patrons can move through it (selective cell membrane permeability) from the congested area (down a concentration gradient). The patrons spread themselves out evenly (diffuse) throughout the total area, with some choosing to stay behind in the original seating area as others move into the new area, until all have an equal amount of room.

Filtration

Filtration, another type of diffusion, is commonly used by the kidneys to clean blood. Water carries dissolved compounds across the cell membranes of the tubules of the kidney. The tubule membrane traps these dissolved compounds but allows the water to pass through. This cleans the blood of wastes and removes the trapped compounds from circulation so they can be flushed out of the body. The **antidiuretic hormone (ADH)** prevents the loss of water from the kidneys by causing its reabsorption into the tubules.

Active Transport

Often, the cell must maintain an imbalance of compounds across its membrane to achieve some metabolic purpose. **Active transport** is a method used to move compounds to create or maintain an imbalance of charges. **Figure 6**. An example of this is the sodium-potassium pump; the cell uses sodium outside the cell and potassium inside the cell for **depolarization**. To maintain this imbalance, the cell must use energy in the form of ATP and actively transport compounds across its membrane. Even though active transport demands a high-energy expenditure, its benefits outweigh the initial use of ATP. Pumping sodium out of the cell and potassium into the cell has the added benefit of moving glucose into the cell at the same time.

Osmosis

Osmosis is movement of water across a cell membrane **Figure 7**. Osmosis occurs when there are different concentrations on each side of a membrane, and equal numbers of molecules on either side are displaced to the other side. As noted earlier, fluid compartments in the body are separated from one another by membranes, such as the cell membranes and the membranes lining blood vessels. The concentration of fluid in those compartments—that is, the number of solute particles—is chiefly influenced by osmosis. If two solutions are separated by a semipermeable membrane (eg, a cell membrane), water will flow across the membrane *from* the solution of *lower* solute concentration *to* the solution of *higher* solute concentration. The net effect is to equalize the solute concentrations on both sides of the membrane.

The effects of osmotic pressure on a cell constitute the **tonicity** of the solution **Figure 8**. Tonicity reflects the

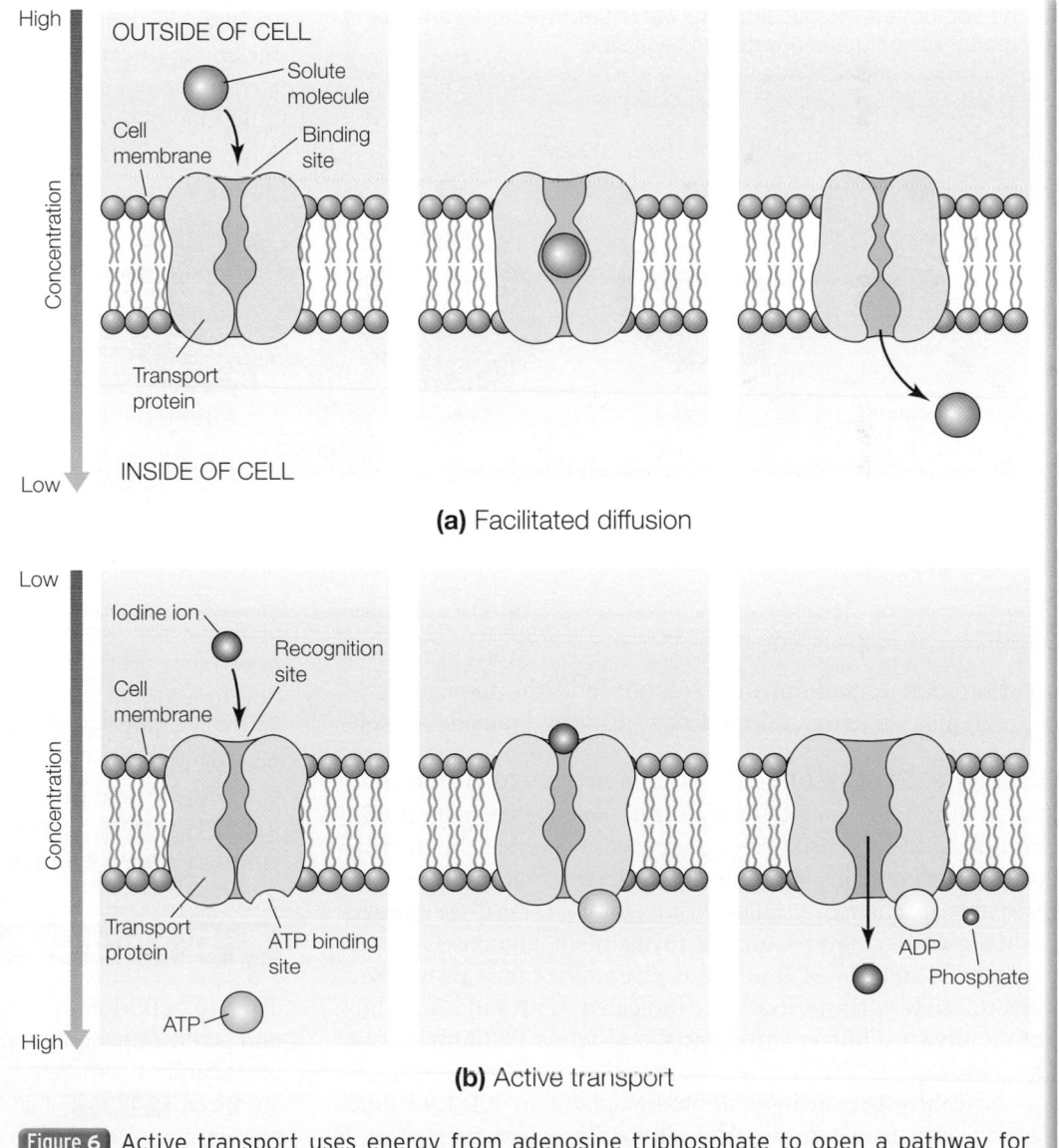

(a) Facilitated diffusion

(b) Active transport

Figure 6 Active transport uses energy from adenosine triphosphate to open a pathway for compounds to move against a concentration gradient.

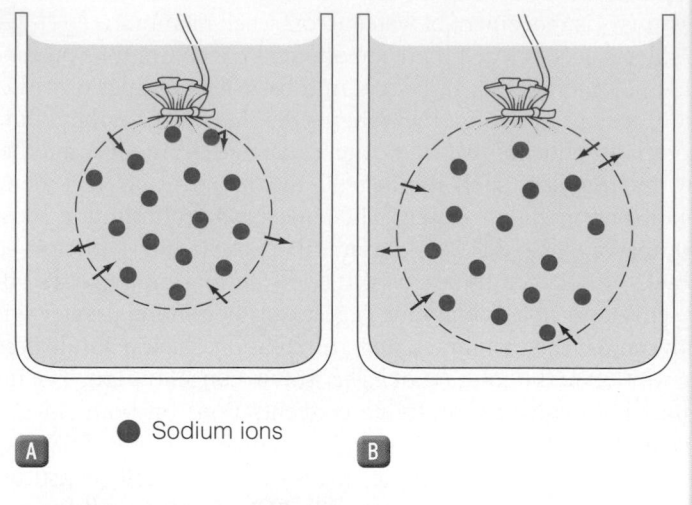

● Sodium ions

Figure 7 **A.** An example of osmosis occurs when a bag of salt water is immersed in a solution of pure water. **B.** Water moves into the bag (toward the area with lower water concentration) and sodium moves out into the water until there is an equal amount of sodium and water on each side.

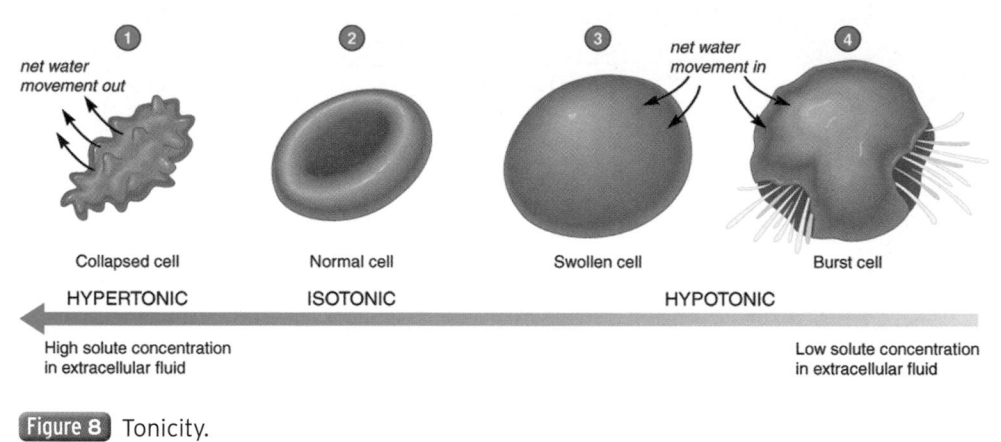

Figure 8 Tonicity.

concentration of sodium in a solution and the movement of water in relation to the sodium levels inside and outside the cell.

Abnormal States of Fluid and Electrolyte Balance

The healthy body maintains a delicate balance between intake and output of fluids and electrolytes, ensuring that the internal environment remains fairly constant. The internal environment's resistance to change is called <u>homeostasis</u>. The ill or injured body, however, may be unable to maintain homeostasis, and excesses or deficits of fluids and electrolytes may occur. You need to know when IV fluids are indicated, what kinds of fluids are required in different situations, and when IV fluids can be dangerous.

A healthy person loses approximately 2 to 2.5 L of fluid daily through urine output, through the lungs (exhalation), and through the skin. These losses are replaced by intake of fluids and by nutrients that are partially converted to water in their

metabolism. In illness, abnormal states of hydration may occur where intake and output are no longer in balance.

Dehydration <u>Dehydration</u> is defined as inadequate total systemic fluid volume. It is usually a chronic condition of the elderly or young persons and may take days to manifest. As fluid is lost from the vascular compartment, the body reacts by shifting interstitial fluid into the vascular area; fluid also shifts from the intracellular to the extracellular compartments. As a consequence, a total systemic fluid deficit occurs.

Signs and symptoms of dehydration include decreased level of consciousness, <u>postural hypotension</u>, tachypnea, dry mucous membranes, decreased urine output, tachycardia, poor skin turgor, and flushed, dry skin. Causes of dehydration include diarrhea, vomiting, gastrointestinal drainage, infections, metabolic disorders such as diabetic ketoacidosis, hemorrhage, environmental emergencies, high caffeine diet, and insufficient fluid intake.

Overhydration When the body's total systemic fluid volume increases, <u>overhydration</u> occurs. Fluid fills the vascular compartment, filters into the interstitial compartment, and is forced from the engorged interstitial compartment into the intracellular compartment. This fluid backup can lead to death **Figure 9** . Overhydration may occur in patients with impaired kidney function, and also when health care professionals administer an amount of fluid that is beyond what the body can excrete. Neonates (children younger than 1 month) are also more likely to experience overhydration because their kidneys are not yet fully developed.

Signs and symptoms of overhydration include shortness of breath, puffy eyelids, edema, polyuria, moist crackles (rales), and acute weight gain. Causes of overhydration include unmonitored IVs (in pediatrics), kidney failure, water intoxication in endurance sports, and prolonged hypoventilation.

■ IV Fluid Composition

The use of IV fluids can significantly alter the patient's condition and facilitate patient treatment. Each bag of IV solution must be sterile and safe; therefore, each bag of IV solution is individually sterilized **Figure 10** . The compounds and ions dissolved in the solutions are identical to the ones found in the body.

Sodium is used as the benchmark to calculate a solution's tonicity. The concentration of sodium in the cells of the body

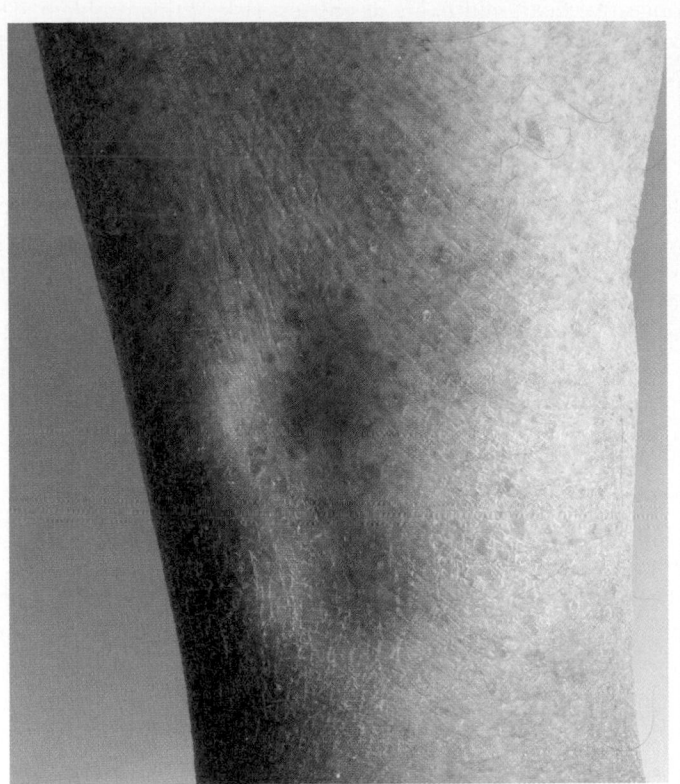

Figure 9 One sign of fluid back up is pitting edema, shown in this patient. Pitting edema occurs when the skin is pressed with a finger and an indentation remains after removal of the finger as seen here.

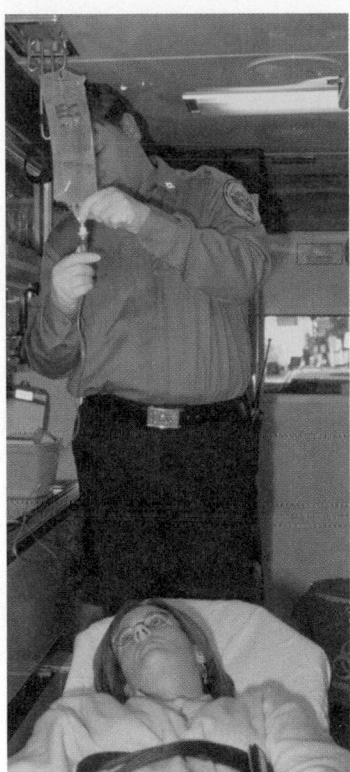

Figure 10 Each bag of IV solution must be sterile, leak-free, clear, and not expired.

When you replace lost volume in a patient, it is imperative to remember that crystalloid solutions cannot carry oxygen. Boluses of 20 mL/kg should be given to maintain perfusion (ie, radial pulses, adequate mental status) but not to raise blood pressure to the patient's normal level. Increasing blood pressure too much with IV solutions not only dilutes remaining blood volume, thereby decreasing the proportion of hemoglobin, but also may increase internal bleeding by interfering with <u>hemostasis</u>—the body's internal blood-clotting mechanism. Blood pressure should be titrated to 90 mm Hg systolic unless otherwise noted by local protocol.

is approximately 0.9%. Altering the concentration of sodium in the IV solution, therefore, can move the water into or out of any fluid compartment in the body.

Types of IV Solutions

IV solutions are categorized in two different ways. They are categorized as crystalloid or colloid based on their dissolved components, or makeup. They are also categorized as isotonic, hypotonic, or hypertonic based on their tonicity. IV fluids use combinations of these solutions to create the desired effects inside the body.

Crystalloid Solutions

<u>Crystalloid solutions</u> are dissolved crystals (eg, salts or sugars) in water. The ability of these fluids to cross membranes and alter fluid levels makes them the best choice for prehospital care of injured patients who need body fluid replacement. When you use an isotonic crystalloid for fluid replacement to support blood pressure after blood loss, remember the 3-to-1 replacement rule: 3 mL of isotonic crystalloid solution is needed to replace 1 mL of patient blood. This amount is needed because approximately two thirds of the infused isotonic crystalloid solution will leave the vascular spaces in about 1 hour. The two thirds of infused crystalloids is either absorbed into the interstitial space or excreted. You should monitor urine output closely when heavy fluid resuscitation occurs. This may alert you to potential kidney abnormalities.

Words of Wisdom

Isotonic crystalloid solutions—normal saline and lactated Ringer's solution (LR)—replace lost volume but do not carry oxygen. Replace lost volume to maintain perfusion, but recognize the need for rapid transport.

Colloid Solutions

<u>Colloid solutions</u> contain molecules (usually proteins) that are too large to pass out of the capillary membranes and, therefore, remain in the vascular compartment. These large protein molecules give colloid solutions a high osmolarity. As a result, they draw fluid from the interstitial and intracellular compartments into the vascular compartments. Colloid solutions work well in reducing edema (eg, in pulmonary or cerebral edema) while expanding the vascular compartment. They could cause dramatic fluid shifts and place the patient in considerable danger if they are not administered in a controlled setting. For this reason, along with a short duration of action and low cost-to-benefit ratio in the prehospital setting, colloids are rarely used in prehospital medicine but may be seen in interfacility transports. Examples of colloid solutions include albumin, dextran, Plasmanate, and hetastarch (Hespan).

Isotonic Solutions

As mentioned, IV solutions are also categorized by their tonicity. The three categories related to tonicity are:

- *Isotonic:* 0.9% sodium chloride (normal saline), LR
- *Hypotonic:* 5% dextrose in water (D_5W)
- *Hypertonic:* 9.0% saline, blood products, albumin

The effects of osmotic pressure on a cell are referred to as the tonicity of the solution. Tonicity is the concentration of sodium in a solution and the movement of water in relation to the sodium levels inside and outside the cell:

- An <u>isotonic solution</u> has the same concentration of sodium as does the cell. In this case, water does not shift and no change in cell shape occurs.
- A <u>hypertonic solution</u> has a greater concentration of sodium than does the cell. Water is drawn out of the cell, and the cell may collapse from the increased extracellular osmotic pressure.
- A <u>hypotonic solution</u> has a lower concentration of sodium than does the cell. Water flows into the cell, causing it to swell and possibly burst from the increased intracellular osmotic pressure.

Fluid movement across a cell membrane resulting from hypertonic, isotonic, and hypotonic solutions is illustrated in **Figure 11**. IV fluids introduced into the circulatory system can affect the tonicity of the extracellular fluid, resulting in serious consequences unless care is used.

Isotonic solutions such as <u>normal saline</u> (0.9% sodium chloride) have almost the same <u>osmolarity</u> (concentration of sodium) as serum and other body fluids. As a consequence, isotonic solutions expand the contents of the intravascular compartment without shifting fluid to or from other compartments, or changing cell shape—an important consideration when you are caring for hypotensive or hypovolemic patients. When you are administering isotonic solutions, you must be careful to avoid fluid overloading. Patients with hypertension and congestive heart failure are at greatest risk of this problem. The extra fluid increases preload, which in turn increases the workload of the heart, creating fluid backup in the lungs.

<u>Lactated Ringer's (LR) solution</u> is generally used in the field for patients who have lost large amounts of blood. It contains lactate, which is metabolized in the liver to form bicarbonate—the key buffer that combats the intracellular acidosis associated with severe blood loss. LR solution should not be given to patients with liver problems because they cannot metabolize the lactate. LR has not shown an overwhelming benefit over normal saline for fluid resuscitation and may be potentially detrimental if administered during blood transfusions because the calcium binds to the anticoagulants added to transfused blood, creating a possible blood clot. Whereas some studies suggest that the risk is minimal if the transfusion is performed rapidly, this should not be attempted. LR is also contraindicated for nitroglycerin, nitroprusside, norepinephrine, propranolol, and methylprednisone infusions.

<u>D_5W</u>, 5% dextrose in water, is a unique type of isotonic solution. As long as it remains in the bag, it is considered an isotonic solution. Once it is administered, however, the dextrose is quickly metabolized, and the solution becomes hypotonic. D_5W is rarely administered by itself. It is usually administered when you are preparing medication infusions such as dopamine (Intropin) or amiodarone (Cordorone).

Hypotonic Solutions

A hypotonic solution has a lower concentration of sodium (osmolarity) than the cell's serum. When this fluid is placed in the vascular compartment, it begins diluting the serum. Soon the serum osmolarity is less than that of the interstitial fluid; water is pulled from the vascular compartment into the interstitial fluid compartment and eventually the same process is repeated, pulling water from the interstitial compartment into the cells. Eventually cells swell and possibly burst from the increased intracellular osmotic pressure.

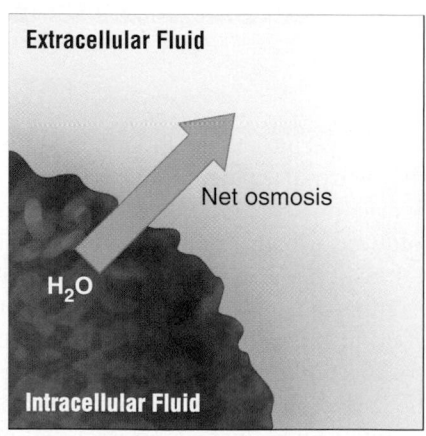

Hypertonic solution

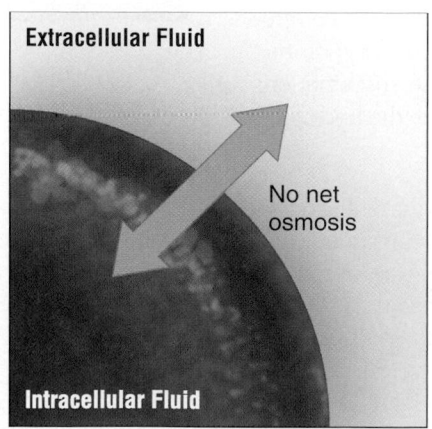

Isotonic solution

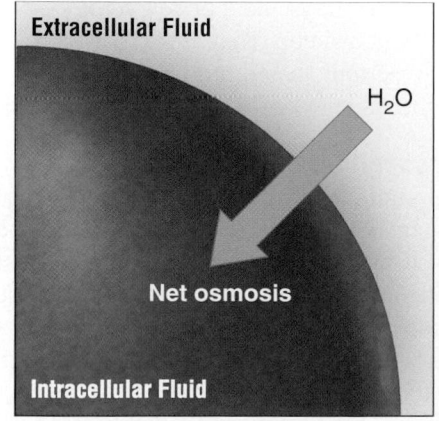

Hypotonic solution

Figure 11 Fluid movement with hypertonic, isotonic, and hypotonic solutions.

Hypotonic solutions hydrate the cells while depleting the vascular compartment. They may be needed for a patient who is receiving dialysis when diuretic therapy dehydrates the cells. Solutions such as hypotonic saline may be used for hyperglycemic conditions such as diabetic ketoacidosis, where high serum glucose levels draw fluid out of the cells and into the vascular and interstitial compartments.

Hypotonic solutions can cause a sudden fluid shift from the intravascular space to the cells, leading to cardiovascular collapse and increased intracranial pressure from shifting fluid into the brain cells. For example, giving D_5W for an extended period can increase intracranial pressure. This makes hypotonic solutions dangerous for patients with stroke or any head trauma. Administering these solutions to patients with burns, trauma, malnutrition, or liver disease is also hazardous because these patients are at risk for developing **third spacing**, an abnormal fluid shift into the serous linings.

Hypertonic Solutions

A hypertonic solution has an osmolarity higher than that of serum, meaning that the solution has more ionic concentration than serum and pulls fluid and electrolytes from the intracellular and interstitial compartments into the intravascular compartment. The danger is that the cells may collapse from the increased extracellular osmotic pressure. Hypertonic solutions shift body fluids into the vascular spaces and help stabilize blood pressure, increase urine output, and reduce edema. These fluids are rarely used in the prehospital setting but may be commonly found during interfacility transports. The high electrolyte concentration of hypertonic solutions may be used for a variety of problems.

Often the term "hypertonic" is used to refer to solutions that contain high concentrations of proteins. These proteins have the same effect on fluid as sodium. Careful monitoring is needed to guard against fluid overloading when you are using hypertonic fluids, especially with patients with impaired heart or kidney function. Also, hypertonic solutions should not be given to patients with diabetic ketoacidosis or others at risk of cellular dehydration.

Oxygen-Carrying Solutions

The best fluid to replace lost blood is whole blood. Unlike the crystalloid and colloid solutions, whole blood contains hemoglobin, which carries oxygen to the body's cells. On occasion (eg, aeromedical transports, multiple-casualty incidents), O-negative blood—a universally compatible blood type—may be used outside a hospital setting. However, because of the refrigeration requirements and other storage issues, general use of whole blood is impractical in the prehospital setting.

Synthetic blood substitutes, which do have the ability to carry oxygen, are being researched and, in some places, field-tested. They show great potential for improving treatment of patients who have lost large amounts of blood. Not only would these synthetic blood substitutes expand circulating volume, but they also would carry and deliver oxygen to the part of the body that needs it the most—the cell.

IV Techniques and Administration

Intravenous means "within a vein." **Intravenous (IV) therapy** involves **cannulation** of a vein with a catheter to access the patient's vascular system. It is one of the most invasive techniques you will perform as a paramedic. **Peripheral vein cannulation** involves cannulating veins of the periphery—that is, veins that can be seen and/or palpated (eg, veins of the hand, arm, or lower extremity and the external jugular vein).

The most important point to remember about IV therapy is to keep the IV equipment sterile. Forethought and attention to detail will help prevent mental and procedural errors while starting the IV line. One way to ensure proper technique is to develop a routine to follow as you assemble the appropriate equipment.

Assembling Your Equipment

To avoid delays and IV site contamination, gather and prepare all your equipment before you attempt to start an IV line. In some cases, the patient's condition may make full preparation difficult, so working as a team becomes critical. The members of your own crew, by anticipating your needs, often can assemble the needed IV equipment. Whereas procedures may vary from service to service, some variation of the following equipment will be available.

- Elastic tourniquet (preferably non-latex)
- Cleaning wipe or solution
- Gauze
- Tape or adhesive bandage
- Appropriate-sized IV catheter
- IV administration set

Choosing an IV Solution

When you are choosing the most appropriate IV solution, you must identify the needs of your patient. Ask yourself the following questions:

- Is the patient's condition critical?
- Is the patient's condition stable?
- Does the patient need fluid replacement?
- Will the patient need medications?

In the prehospital setting, the choice of IV solution is usually limited to two **isotonic crystalloids**, normal saline and LR solution. D_5W is often reserved for administering medication because the presence of dextrose has the potential to alter fluid and electrolyte levels in the body.

Each IV solution bag is wrapped in a protective sterile plastic bag and is guaranteed to remain sterile until the posted expiration date. Once the protective wrap is torn and removed, however, the IV solution must be used within 24 hours. Each IV bag has two ports: an injection port for medication and an **access port** for connecting the administration set. A removable pigtail protects the sterile access port. Once this pigtail is removed, the bag must be used immediately or discarded.

IV solution bags come in different fluid volumes **Figure 12**. Volumes commonly used in hospitals are 1,000 mL, 500 mL, 250 mL, 100 mL, and 50 mL; the more common prehospital volumes are 1,000 mL and 500 mL. The smaller volumes (250 mL and 100 mL) typically contain D_5W or saline and are used for mixing and administering maintenance medication infusions.

Choosing an Administration Set

An **administration set** moves fluid from the IV bag into the patient's vascular system. IV administration sets are sterile as long as they remain in their protective packaging. Each set has a **piercing spike** protected by a plastic cover. Once this spike is exposed and the seal surrounding the cap is broken, the set must be used immediately or discarded.

On most drip sets, a number on the package indicates the number of drops it takes for a milliliter of fluid to pass through the orifice and into the **drip chamber** **Figure 13**. Administration sets come in two primary sizes: microdrip and macrodrip. **Microdrip sets** allow 60 **gtt** (drops) per milliliter (mL) through the needlelike orifice inside the drip chamber. They are ideal for medication administration or pediatric fluid delivery because it is easy to control their fluid flow. **Macrodrip sets** allow 10 or 15 gtt/mL through a large opening between the piercing spike and the drip chamber. They are best used for rapid fluid replacement. Some drip sets allow the provider to dial the desired drip set in; those allow the provider to adjust the drip set to 10, 15, or 60 drops.

Preparing an Administration Set

After choosing the IV administration set and the IV solution bag, verify the expiration date of the solution and check for solution clarity. Prepare to spike the bag with the administration set.

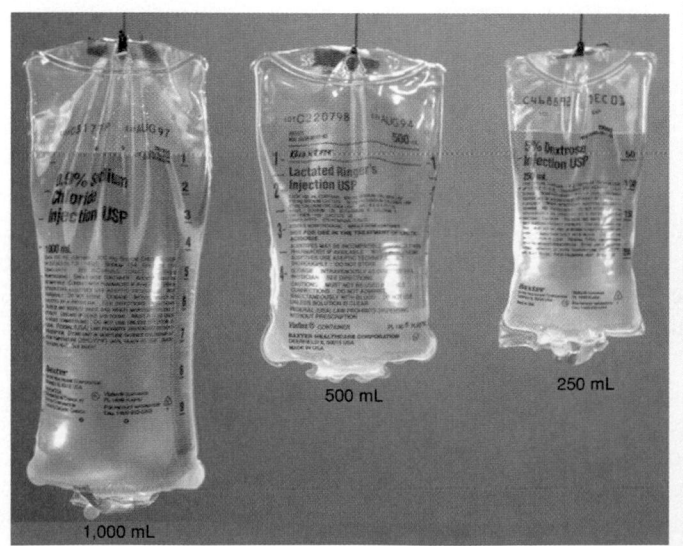

Figure 12 IV solution bags come in different fluid volumes.

1,000 mL

500 mL

250 mL

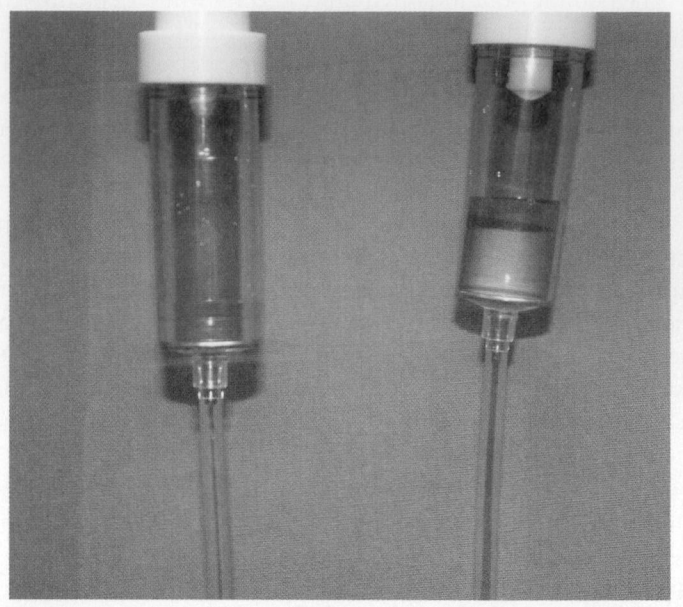

Figure 13 A drip set's packaging contains a number referring to the number of drops it takes for a milliliter of fluid to pass through the orifice into the drip chamber. Two different-sized drip sets are shown here.

The steps for this procedure are shown here and illustrated in **Skill Drill 1**:

Skill Drill 1

1. Remove the protective covering found on the end of the IV bag by pulling on it. The bag is still sealed and will not leak until the piercing spike punctures this port. Remove the protective cover from the piercing spike **Step 1**. (Remember, this spike is sterile!)

2. Move the roller clamp to the off position and slide the spike into the IV bag port until it is seated against the bag **Step 2**.

3. Squeeze the drip chamber to fill to the line marking the chamber, then run fluid into the line to flush the air out of the tubing **Step 3**.

4. Twist the protective cover on the opposite end of the IV tubing to allow air to escape. Do not remove this cover yet because the cover keeps the tubing end sterile until it is needed. Let the fluid flow until air bubbles are removed from the line before turning the roller clamp wheel to stop the flow, or setting the drip rate per the required dose **Step 4**.

5. Next, go back and check the drip chamber; it should be only half-filled. The fluid level must be visible to calculate drip rates. If the fluid level is too low, squeeze the chamber until it fills; if the chamber is too full, invert the bag and the chamber and squeeze the chamber to empty the fluid back into the bag. Hang the bag in an appropriate location with the end of the IV tubing easily accessible **Step 5**.

Skill Drill   1

Spiking the Bag

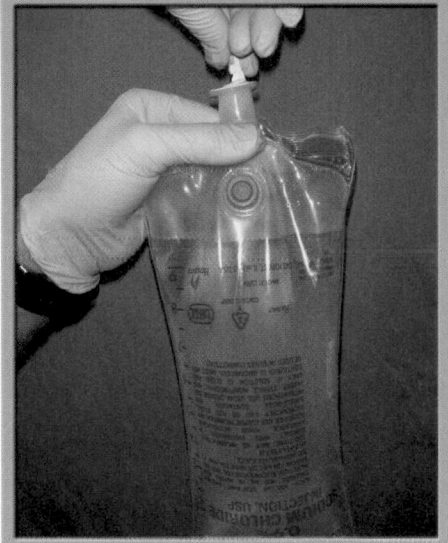

Step 1 Pull on the protective covering on the end of the IV bag to remove it.

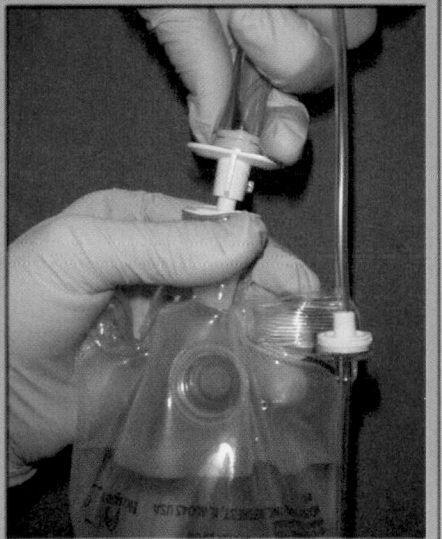

Step 2 Move the roller clamp to the off position and slide the spike into the IV bag until it is seated against the bag.

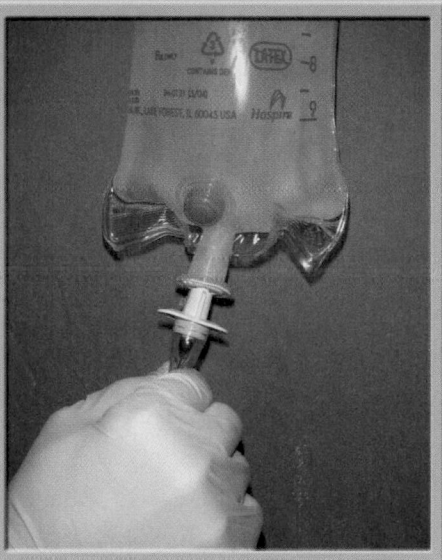

Step 3 Squeeze the drip chamber to fill to the line marking the chamber and then run fluid into the line to flush the air out of the tubing.

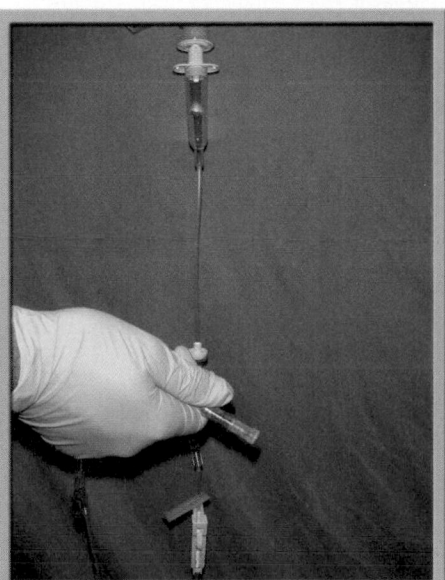

Step 4 Twist the protective cover of the opposite end of the IV tubing to allow air to escape. Do not remove this cover yet. Let the fluid flow until air bubbles are removed from the line before turning the roller clamp wheel to stop the flow, or setting the drip rate per the required dose.

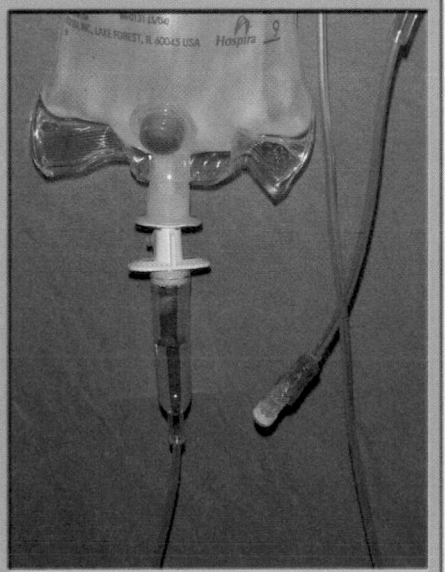

Step 5 Check the drip chamber; it should be only half-filled. If the fluid level is too low, squeeze the chamber until it fills; if the chamber is too full, invert the bag and the chamber and squeeze the chamber to empty the fluid back into the bag. Hang the bag in an appropriate location.

Other Administration Sets

Blood tubing is a macrodrip administration set that is designed to facilitate rapid fluid replacement by manual infusion of multiple IV bags or IV and blood replacement combinations. Most blood tubing administration sets have dual piercing spikes that allow two bags of fluid to be used simultaneously for the same patient **Figure 14**. The central drip chamber has a special filter designed to filter the blood during transfusions.

Fluid control for pediatric patients and certain geriatric patients is important. A microdrip set called a **Volutrol** (also called Buretrol or burette) allows you to fill a 100- or 200-mL calibrated drip chamber with a specific amount of fluid and administer only that amount to avoid inadvertent fluid overload. This type of set is commonly used in pediatric patients. A proximal roller clamp enables you to shut off the Volutrol drip chamber from the IV bag. If the patient needs additional fluids, simply open the proximal roller clamp and fill the Volutrol with more fluid.

■ Choosing an IV Site

It is important for you to select the most appropriate vein for IV catheter insertion. Avoid areas of the vein that contain valves and bifurcations because a catheter will not pass through these areas easily and the needle may cause damage. Valves can be recognized as small bumps located in the vein. Bifurcations are points where one vein may split into two. Use the following criteria to select a vein:

- Locate the vein section with the straightest appearance **Figure 15**.
- Choose a vein that has a firm, round appearance or is springy when palpated.
- Avoid areas where the vein crosses over joints.
- Avoid edematous extremities and any extremity with a dialysis fistula or on the side a mastectomy was done.

If IV therapy is being given for a life-threatening illness or injury, this choice is often limited to the areas that remain open during hypoperfusion. Otherwise, limit IV access to the more distal areas of the extremities: *Start distally; work proximally.* If the most distal site ruptures or infiltrates, you can move up the extremity to the next appropriate site. Because failed cannulation brings the possibility of leakage into the surrounding tissues, any fluid introduced immediately below an open wound has the potential to enter the tissue and cause damage.

Large protruding arm veins can be deceiving in terms of their ease of cannulation. Often these bulging veins can roll from side to side during a cannulation attempt, causing you to

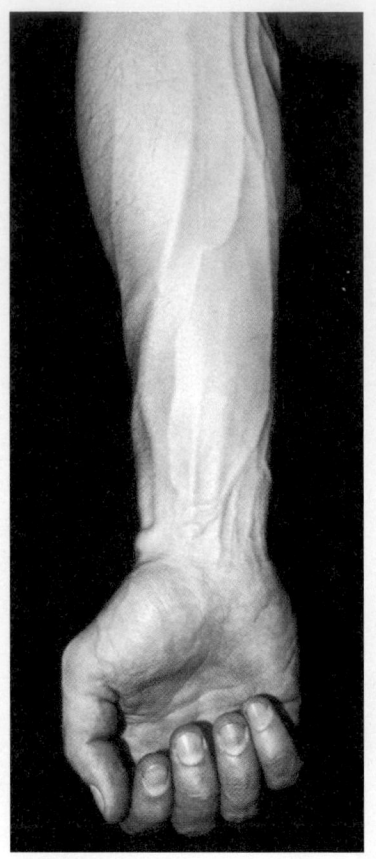

Figure 15 Look for veins that are relatively straight and spring back when palpated.

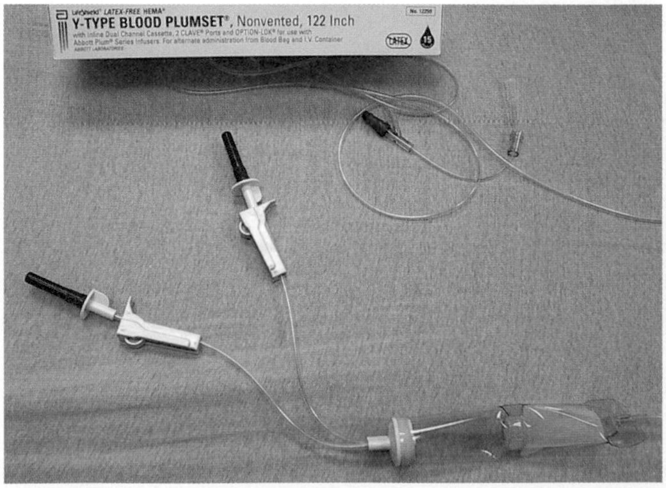

miss the vein. A remedy is to apply manual traction to the vein to lock it into position. Traction techniques differ depending on the location chosen for cannulation. Hold hand veins in place by pulling the skin over the vein taut with the thumb of your free hand as you flex the patient's hand **Figure 16**. Stabilize wrist

Figure 14 Most blood sets have dual piercing spikes that allow two bags of fluid to be used at once for the same patient.

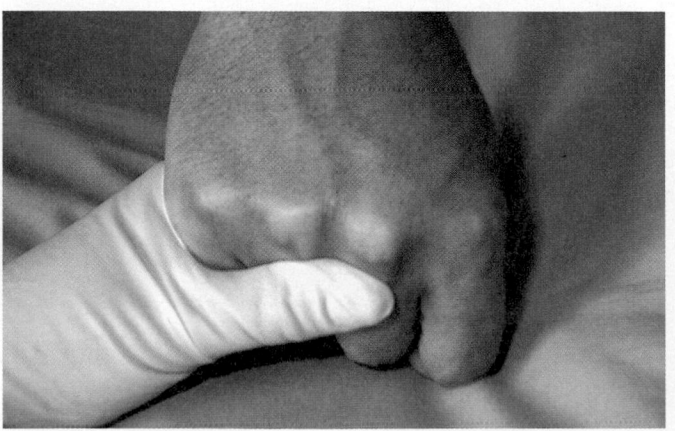

Figure 16 Hold hand veins in place by pulling the skin over the vein taut with the thumb of your free hand as you flex the patient's hand.

veins by flexing the wrist and pulling the skin taut over the vein. Applying lateral traction to the vein with your free hand can stabilize veins in the forearm and <u>antecubital</u> areas. Stabilizing and cannulating the external jugular vein requires a different approach (discussed later in this chapter).

The patient's opinion should also be considered when you are selecting an IV site because he or she may know an IV location that has worked in the past. Avoid attempts to insert an IV in an extremity if it shows signs of trauma, injury, or infection. Also, pay careful attention to areas of the vein that have <u>track marks</u>; they are usually a sign of sclerosis caused by frequent cannulation or puncture of the vein, for example from IV drug abuse.

Hospitals prefer that IV lines be located in nonarticulating areas such as the top of the hand or forearm. This may be taken into consideration if you anticipate long emergency department, ICU, or Med/Surg unit stays. Otherwise, the hospital may reestablish your IV line in a more desirable position. However, in critical situations, you may be unable to take this into consideration.

Some protocols allow IV cannulation of leg veins. Use caution when you are cannulating veins in these areas because they can place the patient at greater risk of <u>venous thrombosis</u> and subsequent <u>pulmonary embolism</u>.

■ Choosing an IV Catheter

Catheter selection should reflect the purpose of the IV line, the age of the patient, and the location for the IV line. The most common types used in the prehospital setting are over-the-needle catheters and butterfly catheters. An <u>over-the-needle catheter</u> **Figure 17** is a Teflon catheter inserted *over* a hollow needle (eg, Angiocath, Terumo, Jelco). A <u>butterfly catheter</u> is a hollow, stainless steel needle with two plastic wings to facilitate its handling **Figure 18**. <u>Through-the-needle catheters</u> (Intracaths)

are plastic catheters inserted *through* a hollow needle; these catheters are rarely used in the prehospital setting.

Table 2 lists the advantages and disadvantages of over-the-needle catheters. These catheters are preferred for use in the prehospital setting for infusing IV fluids or medications in adults and children. They are more readily secured, are less cumbersome than the butterfly catheter, and allow for greater patient movement without the need to immobilize the entire limb.

Table 3 lists the advantages and disadvantages of butterfly catheters. However, these are rarely used, except for on pediatric patients.

Over-the-needle catheters are sized by their diameter, which is referred to as the <u>gauge</u>. The smaller the gauge of the catheter, the larger the diameter. Thus a 14-gauge catheter is of larger diameter than a 22-gauge catheter; 14 gauge is the largest, 27 gauge is the smallest. The larger the diameter, the more fluid that can be delivered through it. The most common lengths are 1¼″ and 2¼″.

Select the largest-diameter catheter that will fit the vein you have chosen or that will be the most appropriate and

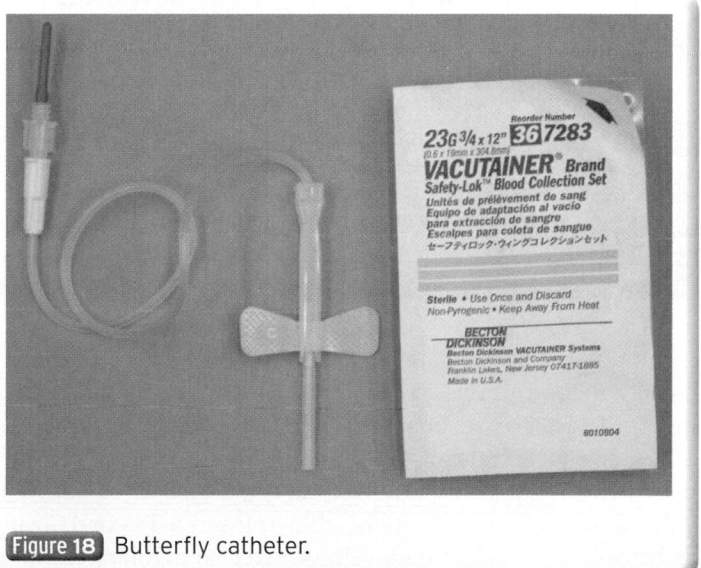

Figure 18 Butterfly catheter.

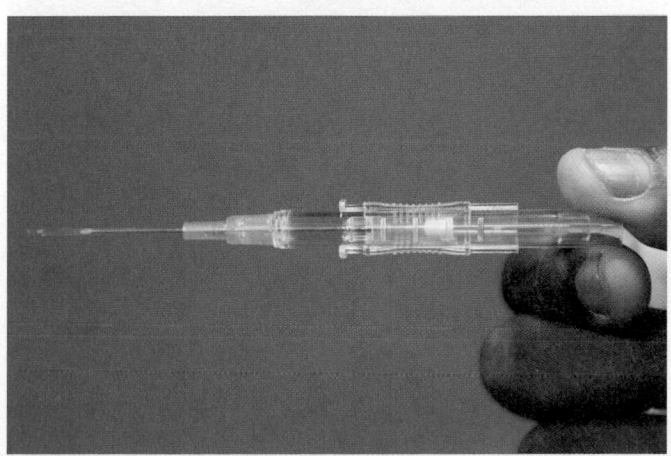

Figure 17 A catheter is a hollow tube that is inserted into a vein in order to keep the vein open, allowing a passageway into the vein. This photo shows an over-the-needle catheter (needle plus catheter).

Table 2 Advantages and Disadvantages of Over-the-Needle Catheters

Advantages	Disadvantages
Less likely to puncture the vein than a butterfly catheter	Risk of sticking the paramedic with contaminated needle as it is withdrawn
More comfortable once in position	More difficult to insert than other devices
Radiopaque for easy identification during x-ray	Possibility of catheter shear

Table 3 Advantages and Disadvantages of Butterfly Catheters

Advantages	Disadvantages
Easiest venipuncture device to insert	May easily cause infiltration. Possible blood cell damage when drawing blood through the butterfly catheter
Useful for scalp veins in infants and in small, difficult veins in geriatric patients for obtaining blood samples	Small-gauge needles limit fluid flow
Small, short needles	

Words of Wisdom

As a general rule, you should start distally and work your way up the patient's extremity when starting an IV line. For patients who need rapid fluid replacement, are in cardiac arrest, or are otherwise in hemodynamically unstable condition, however, you should use a vein that is readily available without a great deal of searching such as the antecubital vein. Unlike other extremity veins (eg, hand, forearm), this vein is usually visible and easier to palpate. A neck vein or an adult IO is another option.

If you think you may be able to establish a larger IV catheter, but are certain you can establish a smaller IV catheter, then choose the smaller IV catheter. Whereas fluid resuscitation may be important, establishing IV access is the priority.

comfortable for the patient. An 18- or 20-gauge catheter is usually a good size for adults who do not need fluid replacement. Metacarpal veins of the hand can usually accommodate 18- or 20-gauge catheters. A 14- or 16-gauge catheter should be used when the patient requires fluid replacement (eg, for hypovolemic shock). You should be able to insert a 14- or 16-gauge catheter into an antecubital vein or external jugular vein in the average adult.

In recent years, an attempt has been made to create over-the-needle catheters that minimize the risk of a **contaminated stick**—when a paramedic punctures his or her skin with the

Special Populations

If you are using an over-the-needle catheter to start an IV line in a pediatric patient, choose among the 20-, 22-, 24-, or 26-gauge catheters, depending on the child's age. Butterfly catheters can be placed in the same locations as over-the-needle catheters and in visible scalp veins in pediatric patients. Scalp veins are best used in young infants.

same catheter that was used to cannulate the vein of a patient. Newer over-the-needle catheters use automatic needle retraction after insertion, usually accomplished with a locking slide mechanism or a spring-loaded slide mechanism.

Inserting the IV Catheter

Each paramedic has a unique technique to insert an IV line, and you should observe many different techniques to determine what works best for you. Two considerations, however, apply to *any* technique:

1. Keep the beveled side of the catheter up when you are inserting the needle in a vein **Figure 19**.
2. Maintain adequate traction on the vein during cannulation.

Apply a constricting band above the site you have chosen for the insertion to allow blood to fill the veins. This creates additional vascular pressure to engorge the veins with blood below the band. It should be snug enough to significantly diminish venous flow but should not hamper arterial flow. The constricting band should be left in place only long enough to complete the IV insertion, obtain blood samples (if needed), and attach the line. *Do not leave the constricting band in place while you assemble IV equipment.*

Constricting bands can be difficult to manage, especially if you are wearing gloves. You should develop a technique that will allow you to release the constricting band with a small tug on one end. Items that can be used as constricting bands include a **Penrose drain**, a blood pressure cuff, or in a pinch, surgical hose.

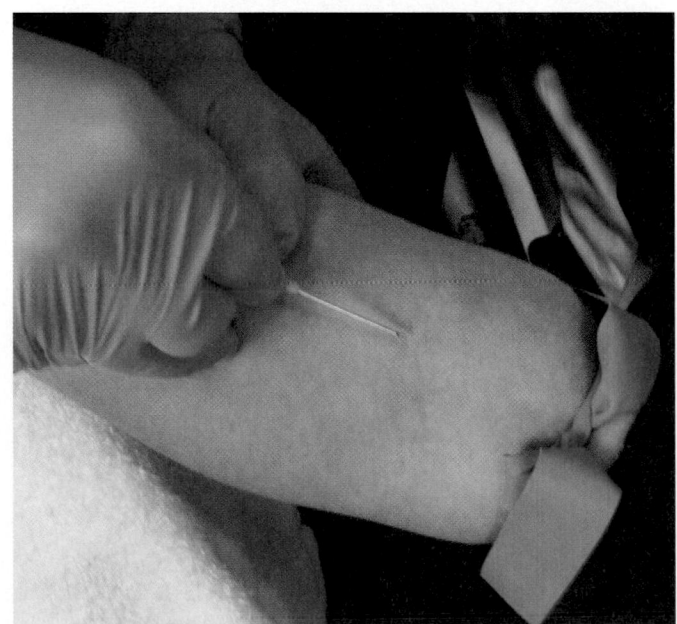

Figure 19 Keep the beveled side of the catheter up when inserting the needle in a vein.

Once you have selected an insertion site, prep it with an alcohol or iodine swab, or chlorhexidine (ChloraPrep). Do not touch the site after it has been prepped. If you contaminate the site, you will need to clean it again **Figure 20**. Apply gentle downward or lateral traction on the vein with your free hand while holding the catheter, bevel side up, in your dominant hand. Take care as you apply traction to avoid collapsing the vein. Begin by establishing an insertion angle of about 45°. Advance the catheter through the skin until the vein is pierced (you should see a flash of blood in the catheter flash

chamber); then immediately drop the angle down to about 15° and advance the catheter a few more centimeters to ensure the catheter sheath is in the vein. Slide the sheath off the needle and into the vein; do not advance the needle too far because it can puncture the other side of the vein. After the catheter is fully advanced, apply pressure to the vein just proximal to the end of the indwelling catheter, remove the needle, and dispose of it in a sharps container, or in the case of other style catheters, trigger the shielding device.

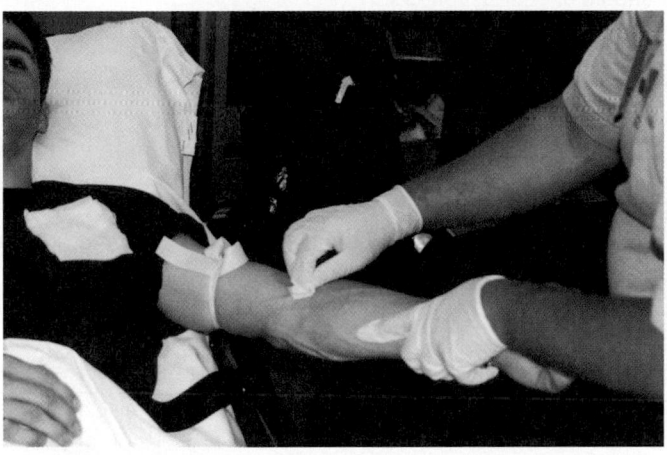

Figure 20 Always use aseptic technique when cleansing the site for IV cannulation. Use the first alcohol pad to clean in a circular motion from the inside out, then use the second to wipe straight down the center.

Words of Wisdom

Iodine helps to make veins more visible in dark-skinned people. As with any patient, make sure the patient is not allergic to iodine.

Securing the Line

Once the catheter is in position and the contents of the IV bag are flowing properly, you must secure the IV line. Tape the area so that the catheter and tubing are securely anchored in case of a sudden pull on the line **Figure 21**. Tear the tape before you start the IV line, because you will need one hand to stabilize the site while you apply the tape. Double back the tubing to create a loop that will act as a shock absorber if the line is pulled accidentally. Cover the insertion site with sterile gauze, and secure it with tape or use a commercially manufactured device (eg, Veniguard, Opsite). Avoid circumferential taping around any extremity because it may impair circulation. If the tubing needs

YOU are the Medic | PART 2

The patient states that the pain level in her left leg is 9 on a scale of 1 to 10 and she is lightheaded and dizzy. Patient states she was running the marathon and suddenly became dizzy, lost her footing, and fell to the ground. She states that when she fell, she heard a snap and felt extreme pain in her leg. She denies any other problem, but states that she did not prehydrate and was not expecting the weather to be this hot.

Recording Time: 1 Minute	
Appearance	Pale and diaphoretic
Level of consciousness	Alert (oriented to person, place, and day)
Airway	Clear and open, maintained by patient
Breathing	28 breaths/min, slightly labored
Circulation	Weak, rapid, thready radial pulse

3. What is the most appropriate treatment for this patient?

4. What type of IV fluid is best for this patient?

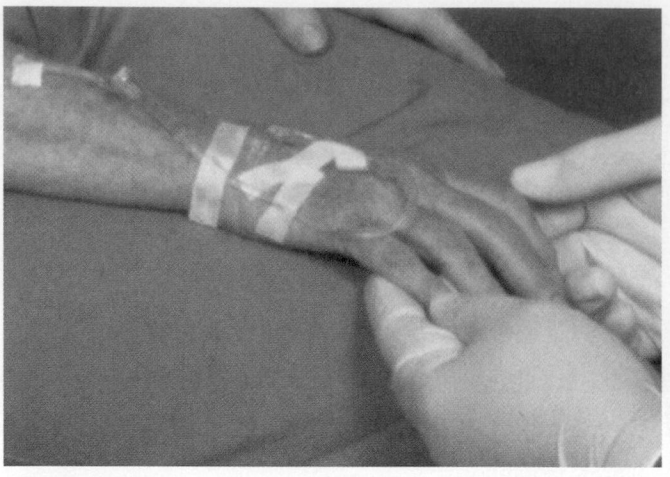

Figure 21 Tape the area so that the catheter and tubing are securely anchored.

Words of Wisdom

Helpful IV Hints

- Allow the patient's arm to hang off the stretcher.
- Pat or rub the area.
- Apply wrapped chemical heat packs for about 60 seconds.
- If you meet resistance from a valve, elevate the extremity.
- After two misses, let your partner try **Figure 22**.
- Try sticking without a constricting band if the IV line keeps infiltrating.
- Never pull the catheter back over the needle.
- The more IV insertions you perform, the more proficient you will become.

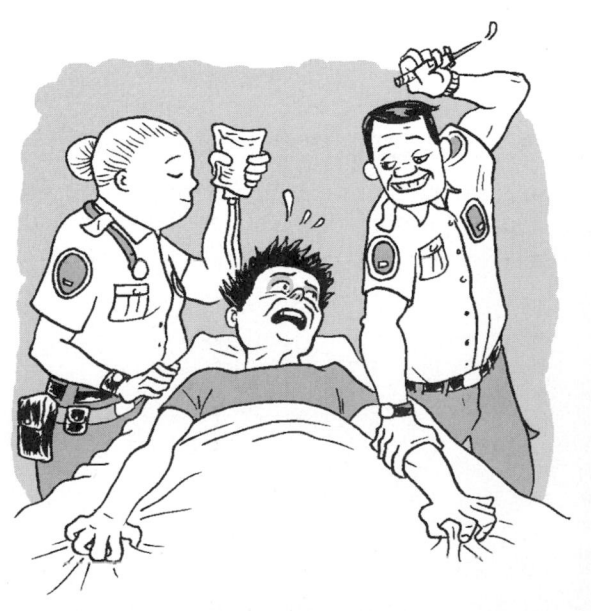

Try seeing it from the patient's point of view.

Figure 22

Documentation and Communication

To document the establishment of an IV line, you need to include five things:

- The gauge of the needle
- The IV attempts versus successes
- The site (for example, left forearm, left external jugular)
- The type of fluid you are administering
- The rate at which the fluid is running

For example, if you initiated an IV line in the left antecubital fossa with an 18-gauge catheter and are infusing normal saline at a rate of 120 mL per hour, the documentation should appear as follows:

18g IV ×1 L ac c̄ NS @ 120 mL/h by Medic 785

to be secured circumferentially because the patient is attempting to pull the line, consider wrapping the extremity and tubing with roller gauze.

To establish vascular access, follow the steps in **Skill Drill 2**:

Skill Drill   2

1. Choose the appropriate fluid, and examine the bag for clarity and expiration date. Make sure that no particles are floating in the fluid and that the fluid is appropriate for the patient's condition and not expired.

2. Choose the appropriate drip set, and attach it to the fluid. A macrodrip set (eg, 10 gtt/mL) should be used for a patient who needs volume replacement; a microdrip set (eg, 60 gtt/mL) should be used for a patient who needs a medication infusion.

3. Fill the drip chamber by squeezing it **Step 1**.

4. Flush or "bleed" the tubing to remove any air bubbles by opening the roller clamp **Step 2**. Make sure no errant bubbles are floating in the tubing.

5. Tear the tape before venipuncture, or have a commercial device available **Step 3**.

6. Apply gloves before making contact with the patient. Palpate a suitable vein **Step 4**. Veins should be "springy" when palpated. Stay away from areas that are hard when palpated.

7. Apply the constricting band above the intended IV site **Step 5**. It should be placed approximately 4″ to 8″ above the intended site.

8. Clean the area using aseptic technique. Use an alcohol pad to cleanse in a circular motion from the inside out. Use a second alcohol pad to wipe straight down the center **Step 6**.

9. Choose the appropriately sized catheter and twist the catheter to break the seal. Do not advance the catheter upward because this may cause the needle to shear the catheter. Examine the catheter and discard it if you discover any imperfections **Step 7**. Occasionally you will find "burrs" on the edge of the catheter.

10. Insert the catheter at an angle of approximately 45° with the bevel up while applying distal traction with the other hand (Step 8). This traction will stabilize the vein and help to keep it from "rolling" as you stick.

11. Observe for "flashback" as blood enters the catheter (Step 9). The clear chamber at the top of the catheter should fill with blood when the catheter enters the vein. If you note only a drop or two, you should gently advance the catheter farther into the vein.

12. Occlude the catheter to prevent blood leaking while removing the stylet. Hold the hub while withdrawing the needle so as not to pull the catheter out of the vein.

13. Immediately dispose of all sharps in the proper container (Step 10).

14. Attach the prepared IV line. Hold the hub of the catheter while connecting the IV line (Step 11).

15. Remove the constricting band (Step 12).

16. Open the IV line to ensure fluid is flowing and the IV is patent. Observe for any swelling or infiltration around the IV site (Step 13). If the fluid does not flow, check whether the constriction band has been released. If infiltration is noted, immediately stop the infusion and remove the catheter while holding pressure over the site with a piece of gauze to prevent bleeding.

17. Secure the catheter with tape or a commercial device (Step 14).

18. Secure IV tubing and adjust the flow rate while monitoring the patient (Step 15).

■ Changing an IV Bag

You may have to change the IV bag for some patients, particularly those who require larger volumes of IV fluid (ie, for hypovolemic shock). Do not allow an IV fluid bag to become *completely* depleted of fluid. Change the bag when about 25 mL of fluid is left.

Like the initial setup of the IV bag and administration set (see Skill Drill 1), replacing the IV bag is a sterile process. If the equipment becomes contaminated, replace it and use new equipment. Always ensure that some fluid remains in the drip chamber and tubing of the set. This simple action will prevent air from entering the patient's vein.

The steps for changing an IV fluid bag are as follows:

1. Stop the flow of fluid from the depleted bag by closing the roller clamp.

2. Prepare the new IV bag by removing the pigtail from the piercing spike port. Inspect the new bag of IV fluid for clarity and discoloration and to ensure that the expiration date has not passed.

3. Remove the piercing spike from the depleted bag and insert it into the port on the new bag. *Do not touch the piercing spike of the administration set.*

4. Ensure that the drip chamber is appropriately filled, and then open the roller clamp and adjust the fluid rate accordingly.

Skill Drill   2

Obtaining Vascular Access

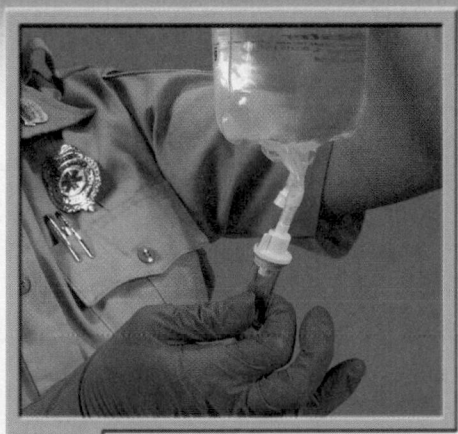

Step **1** Fill the drip chamber by squeezing it.

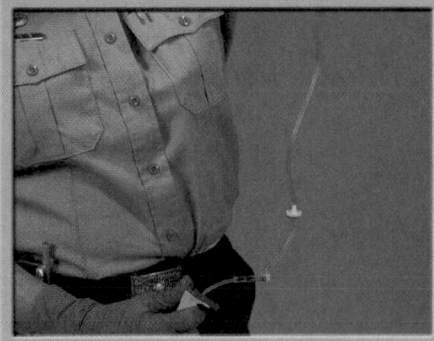

Step **2** Flush or "bleed" the tubing to remove any air bubbles by opening the roller clamp.

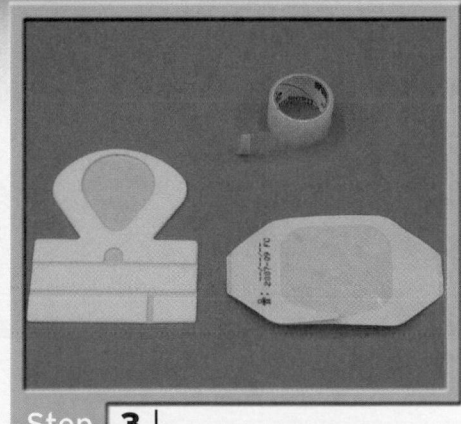

Step **3** Tear the tape before venipuncture, or have a commercial device available.

Continues

Skill Drill   2

Obtaining Vascular Access, continued

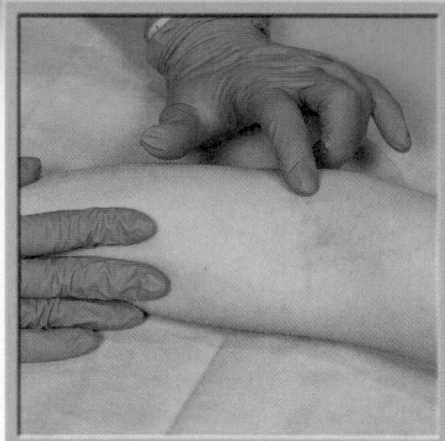

Step 4 Apply gloves before making contact with the patient. Palpate a suitable vein.

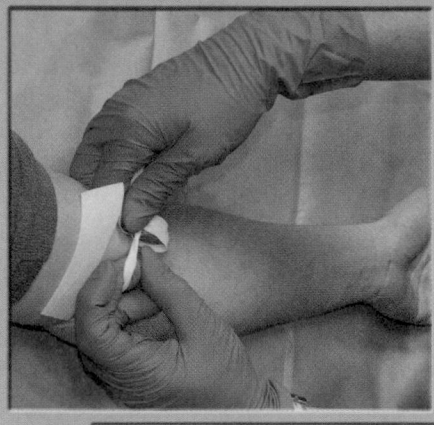

Step 5 Apply the constricting band above the intended IV site.

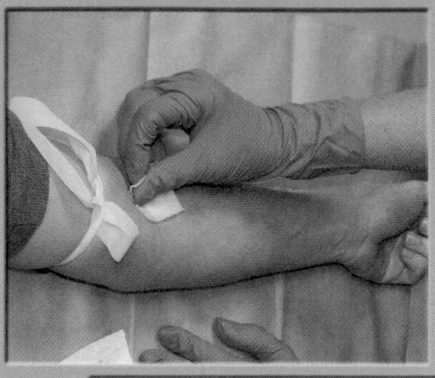

Step 6 Clean the area using aseptic technique. Use an alcohol pad to cleanse in a circular motion from the inside out. Use a second alcohol pad to wipe straight down the center.

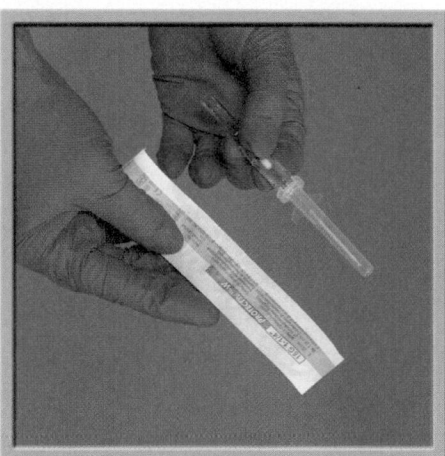

Step 7 Choose the appropriately sized catheter, and examine it for any imperfections.

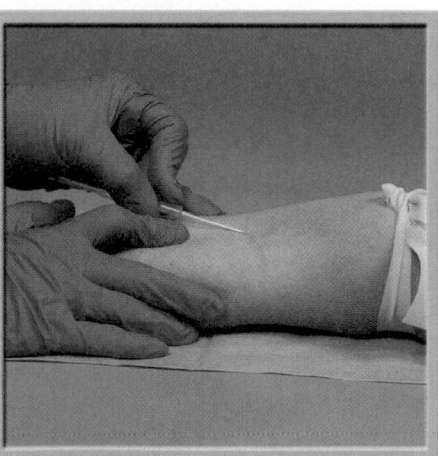

Step 8 Insert the catheter at an angle of approximately 45° with the bevel up while applying distal traction with the other hand.

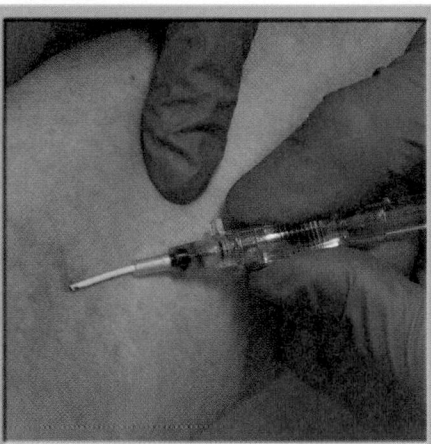

Step 9 Observe for "flashback" as blood enters the catheter. Hold the hub while withdrawing the needle so as not to pull the catheter out of the vein.

Continues

Skill Drill   2

Obtaining Vascular Access, continued

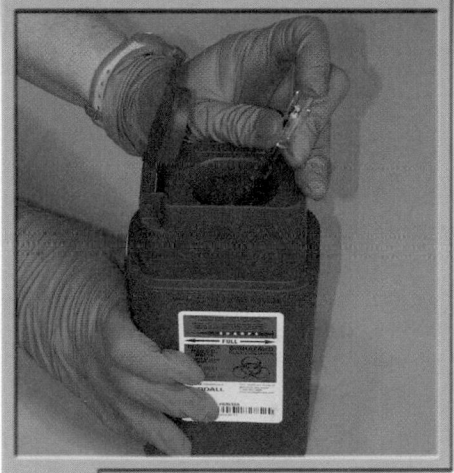

Step 10 Immediately dispose of all sharps in the proper container.

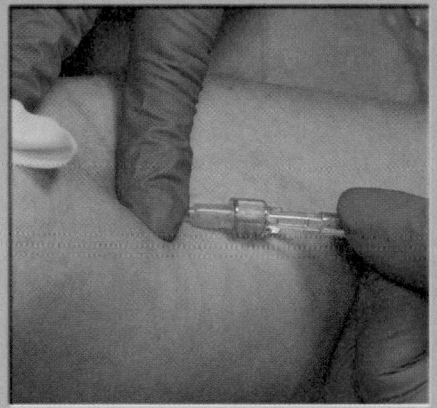

Step 11 Attach the prepared IV line. Hold the hub of the catheter while connecting the IV line.

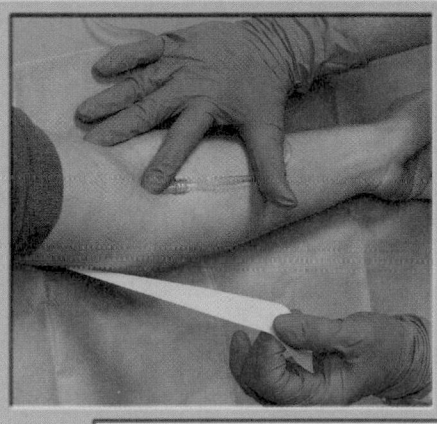

Step 12 Remove the constricting band.

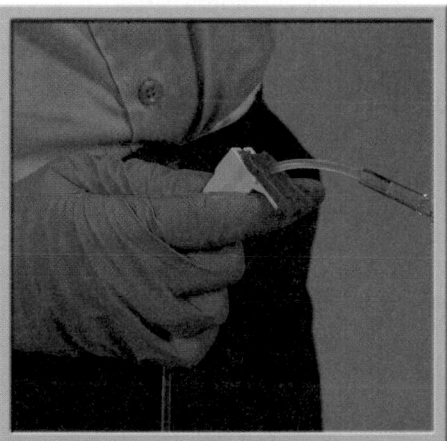

Step 13 Open the IV line to ensure fluid is flowing and the IV is patent. Observe for swelling or infiltration around the IV site.

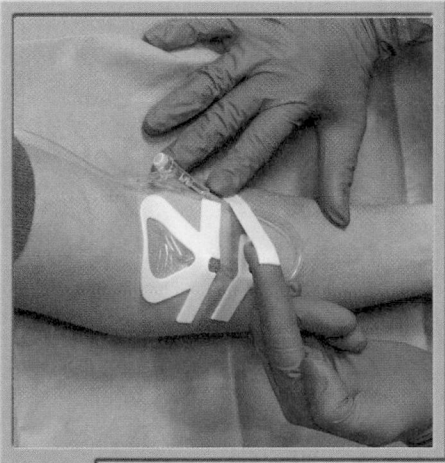

Step 14 Secure the catheter with tape or a commercial device.

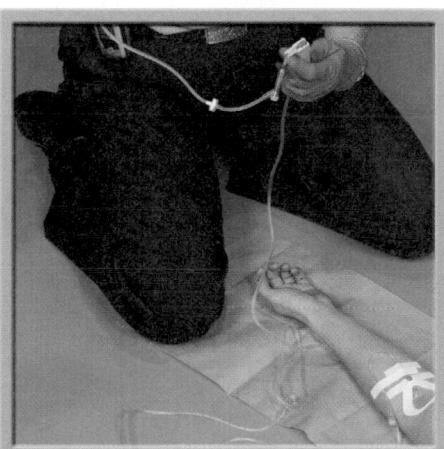

Step 15 Secure the IV tubing and adjust the flow rate while monitoring the patient.

Discontinuing the IV Line

To discontinue the IV line, shut off the flow from the IV with the roller clamp. Gently peel the tape back toward the IV site. As you get closer to the site and the catheter, stabilize the catheter while you loosen the remaining tape holding the catheter in place. Do not remove the IV tubing from the hub of the catheter. Fold a 4″× 4″ piece of gauze and place it over the site, holding it down while you pull back on the hub of the catheter. Gently pull the catheter and the IV line from the patient's vein while applying pressure to control bleeding Figure 23 .

Alternative IV Sites and Techniques

Saline Locks

Saline locks (buff caps) are a way to maintain an active IV site without running fluids through the vein. A saline lock is comprised of a male Luer lock connector, from the standardized Luer taper system created by Hermann Luer, that attaches to the hub of an IV catheter and a female Luer lock connector that can connect to syringes for medication administration or to an IV administration set. Saline locks may have tubing ranging from 1″ to 5″ between the male and female Luer lock connectors. These access ports are used primarily for patients who do not need additional fluids but who may need rapid medication delivery (eg, in case of congestive heart failure or pulmonary edema). A saline lock is attached to the end of an IV catheter and filled with approximately 2 mL of normal saline to keep blood from clotting at the end of the catheter Figure 24 . Because this is a sealed-access site, the saline remains in the port without entering the vein, preventing clotting. These devices are also known as intermittent (INT) sites because they eliminate the need to reestablish an IV each time the patient needs medication or fluid. Some services place a saline lock on every patient to ease the transfer of patient care. This allows the hospital to temporarily disconnect the IV administration without having to reestablish the IV catheter.

External Jugular Vein Cannulation

The external jugular (EJ) vein Figure 25 runs downward and obliquely backward behind the angle of the jaw until it pierces the deep fascia of the neck just above the middle of the clavicle. It ends in the subclavian vein, where valves retard backflow of blood. The EJ vein is fairly large and usually easy to cannulate; however, because the vein lies so near the surface of the skin, it rolls if the vein is not appropriately anchored during cannulation. It is also near other vessels (such as the carotid artery) that may be damaged during cannulation.

You should exhaust all other means of cannulating a peripheral vein (ie, in the arm or hand) before attempting cannulation of the EJ vein. Although it is a "peripheral" vein, more risks are associated with cannulation of this vein— namely, inadvertent puncture of the carotid artery, a *rapidly* expanding hematoma if infiltration occurs, and air embolism.

Follow these steps to cannulate the external jugular vein:

1. Place the patient in a supine, head-down position to fill the jugular vein. Turn the patient's head to the side opposite the intended venipuncture site. *Always* *feel carefully for a pulse before cannulating an external jugular vein. It is imperative not to pierce the carotid artery.*
2. Appropriately cleanse the venipuncture site.
3. Occlude the jugular vein with your finger, distal to the catheter insertion site, to facilitate backflow of blood; this will allow the vein to become more visible.
4. Align the catheter in the direction of the vein, with the point aimed toward the shoulder on the side of the venipuncture Figure 26 .
5. Make the puncture midway between the angle of the jaw and the midclavicular line. Stabilize the vein by placing a finger lightly on top of it just above the clavicle.

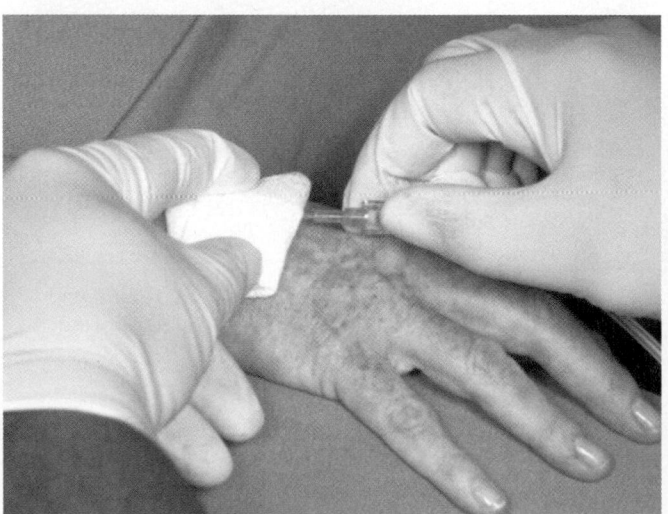

Figure 23 When removing a catheter and IV line, pull gently and apply pressure to control bleeding.

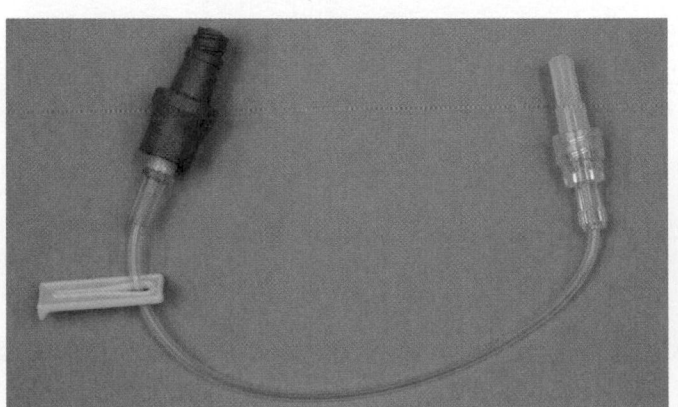

Figure 24 A saline lock is attached to the end of an IV catheter and filled with approximately 2 mL of normal saline in order to keep blood from clotting at the end of the catheter.

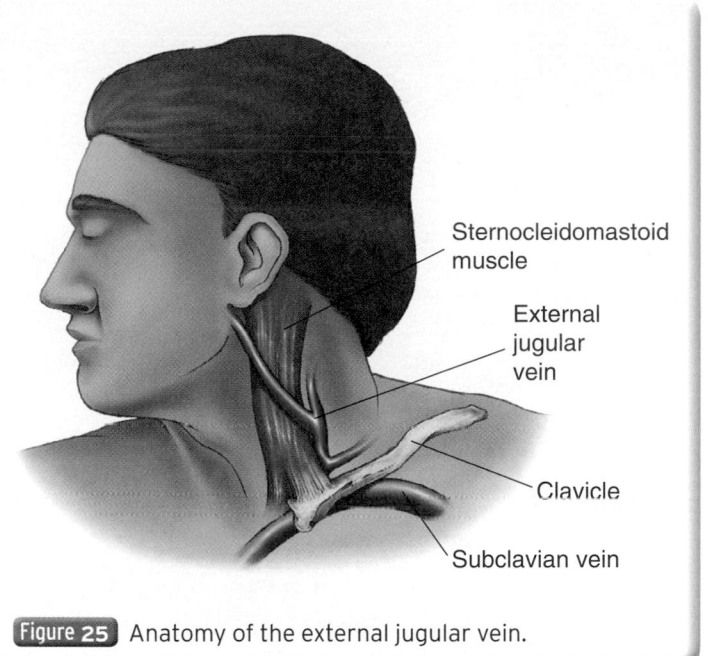

Figure 25 Anatomy of the external jugular vein.

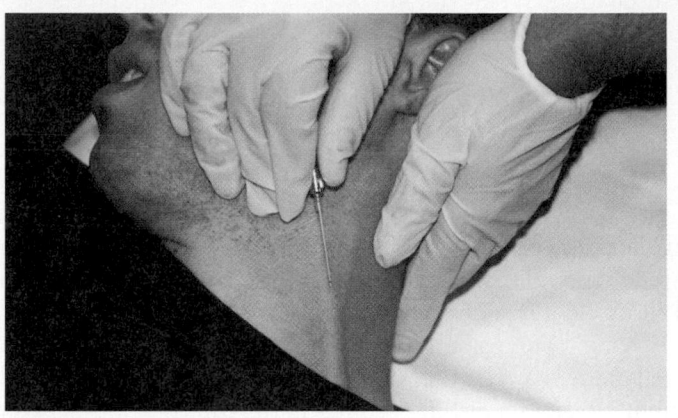

Figure 26 The external jugular vein requires a specific insertion site midway between the angle of the jaw and the midclavicular line with the catheter pointed toward the shoulder on the same side as the venipuncture.

6. Proceed as described for cannulation of a peripheral vein. *Do not let air enter the catheter once it is in the vein.* Patients can draw in as much as 10% of their tidal volume through an open external jugular vein, causing a large air embolism.

7. Tape the line securely but do *not* put circumferential dressings around the neck.

Pediatric IV Therapy Considerations

The same IV solutions and equipment can be used on pediatric patients as on adults, with a few exceptions.

Catheters

If you are using over-the-needle catheters to start a pediatric IV line, the 20-, 22-, 24-, or 26-gauge catheters are best for insertions Figure 27 . Butterfly catheters are ideal for pediatric patients and can be placed in the same locations as over-the-needle catheters and in visible scalp veins. Scalp veins are best used in young infants.

IV Locations

When you are starting an IV line, explain what you are doing to both the child and the parent. A parent can become as stressed as a child, so take time to thoroughly explain the procedure.

The younger the pediatric patient, the fewer choices you have for IV sites. Hand veins are painful and difficult to manage in younger pediatric patients but remain the location of choice for starting peripheral IV lines. Protecting the IV site after it has been established is critical and is sometimes best accomplished by immobilizing the site before cannulation with an arm board.

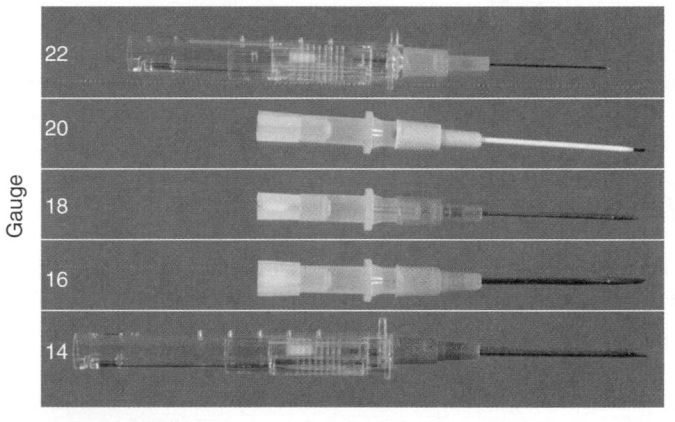

Figure 27 Note the difference in sizes of the catheters.

One of the better techniques for starting pediatric IV lines is to use a penlight to illuminate the veins on the back of the hand. Shine the light through the palm side of the hand to illuminate the veins on the backside of the hand. Be sure not to burn the patient with the penlight, even though this is unlikely. Once a suitable site is located, slightly graze the surface of the hand with your fingernail so you can find the location after you turn off the penlight. Proceed with the IV insertion, using the mark you created as a guide. Sometimes the best choice is an AC (antecubital vein) line with full arm immobilization to avoid dislodging the IV line.

Scalp vein cannulation is often aesthetically unpleasant for both the child and the parents and can produce apprehension in both simply because of the location. In addition, scalp veins can be difficult to cannulate and do not allow for rapid fluid resuscitation. When you are securing a scalp vein, tape a paper cup over the site to avoid applying any direct pressure to the butterfly catheter. Pressure may cause the needle to puncture the other side of the vein and let fluids escape into the tissues (extravasation).

Geriatric IV Therapy Considerations

Smaller catheters may be preferable with elderly patients unless rapid fluid replacement is needed. Some medications commonly used by elderly patients have the tendency to create fragile skin and veins. Often, simply puncturing the vein will cause a massive hematoma. The use of tape can lead to skin damage, so be careful when establishing IV lines in the elderly. Consider using alternative options such as paper tape or commercial devices that reduce the risk of skin damage.

Catheters

Try using the smaller catheters (such as 20, 22, or 24 gauge), because they may be more comfortable for the patient and can reduce the risk of extravasation.

IV Sets

Be careful when you are using macrodrips because they can allow rapid infusion of fluids, which may lead to edema if they are not monitored closely. With both geriatric and pediatric patients, fluid overloading is potentially serious. Always monitor fluid administration carefully.

Locations

In choosing an IV site, you should consider the possibility of poor vein elasticity. One of the consequences of aging is the loss of elasticity in the body tissues. Veins become sclerosed, making them brittle. Certain medications, such as prednisone, can also affect the structure of the vein, making the veins of geriatric patients even more fragile and easily ruptured. Avoid small spidery veins that weave back and forth **Figure 28** because they may rupture easily. Do not use <u>varicose veins</u>; although they often appear to be ideal choices for IV starts, they are almost completely closed off and allow very little circulation.

Factors Affecting IV Flow Rates

Several factors can influence the flow rate of an IV line. For example, if the IV bag is not hung high enough, the flow rate will not be sufficient. Perform the following checks after completing IV administration and whenever a flow problem occurs:

- *Check the IV fluid.* Thick, viscous fluids such as blood products and colloid solutions infuse slowly and may be diluted to help speed delivery. Cold fluids run more slowly than warm fluids. If possible, warm IV fluids before administering them in a cold environment.
- *Check the administration set.* Macrodrips are used for rapid fluid delivery; microdrips deliver a more controlled flow.
- *Check the height of the IV bag.* The IV bag must be hung high enough to overcome gravity. Hang it as high as possible.

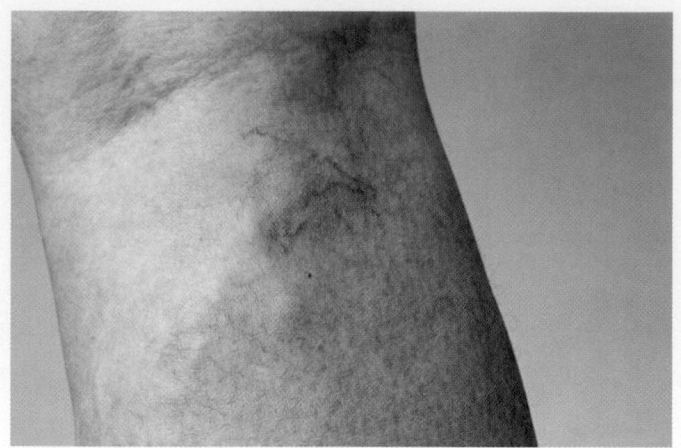

Figure 28 When you are looking for an IV site, avoid small spidery veins and varicose veins.

The closer it is to the patient, the slower it will be. If it falls below the level of the patient, it will begin to draw blood out of the vein.

- *Check the type of catheter used.* The larger the diameter of the catheter (the smaller the number—for example a 14 gauge is of larger diameter than a 20 gauge), the faster fluid can be delivered.
- *Check the constricting band.* Do not leave the constricting band on the patient's arm after completing establishment of the IV line.

Potential Complications of IV Therapy

Problems associated with IV therapy can be categorized as local or systemic reactions. <u>Local reactions</u> include problems such as infiltration and thrombophlebitis. <u>Systemic complications</u> include allergic reactions, circulatory overload, air embolus, vasovagal reactions, and catheter shear.

Local IV Site Reactions and Local Complications

Most local reactions require that you discontinue the IV and reestablish the IV line in the opposite extremity or in a proximal location. Examples of local reactions include infiltration; thrombophlebitis; occlusion; vein irritation; hematoma; nerve, tendon, or ligament damage; and arterial puncture.

Infiltration

<u>Infiltration</u> is the escape of fluid into the surrounding tissue, which causes a localized area of edema. Causes of infiltration include the following problems:

- The IV catheter passes completely through the vein and out the other side.
- The patient moves excessively.

- The tape used to secure the IV line becomes loose or dislodged.
- The catheter is inserted at too shallow an angle and enters only the <u>fascia</u> surrounding the vein (this problem is more common with IV lines in larger veins, such as those in the upper arm and neck).

Signs and symptoms of infiltration include edema at the catheter site, continued IV flow after occlusion of the vein above the insertion site, and patient complaints of tightness, burning, and pain around the IV site.

If infiltration occurs, discontinue the IV line and reestablish it in the opposite extremity or in a more proximal location on the same extremity. Apply direct pressure over the swollen area to reduce further swelling or bleeding into the tissue. Avoid wrapping tape around the extremity because it could create a constricting band.

Occlusion

<u>Occlusion</u> is the physical blockage of a vein or catheter. If the flow rate is not sufficient to keep fluid moving out of the catheter tip such that blood enters the catheter, a clot may form and occlude the flow. The first sign of an occlusion is a decreasing drip rate or the presence of blood in the IV tubing. With a positional IV site, fluid flows at different rates depending on the position of the catheter within the vein; these differences can produce occlusions. Positional IVs may be necessary because of proximity to a valve or because of patient movement that allows the line to become physically blocked, such as the patient resting on the line or crossing his or her arms. Occlusion may also develop if the IV bag nears empty and the patient's blood pressure overcomes the flow, causing fluid backup in the line.

To determine whether an IV line should be reestablished, you may use a syringe prefilled with saline, or you may draw the saline from an IV bag. Once you have the full syringe of clean IV fluid, you will use it to add pressure to the line. Gently apply pressure to the plunger to disrupt the occlusion and reestablish flow **Figure 29**. If flow is reestablished, ensure that the line is free and the rate is sufficient. If the occlusion does not dislodge, discontinue the administration and reestablish the IV line in the opposite extremity or at a proximal location on the same extremity.

Vein Irritation

Occasionally, a patient will experience vein irritation from the IV fluid or medication administration. Patients who have this problem often immediately report that the solution is bothering them (ie, tingling, stinging, itching, and burning). In such cases, observe the patient closely in case an allergic reaction to the fluid develops.

Vein irritation is usually caused by a too-rapid infusion rate. If redness develops at the IV site—a sign suggesting thrombophlebitis—discontinue the IV line and save the equipment for later analysis. Reestablish the IV line in the other extremity with new equipment in case the old equipment contained unseen contaminants.

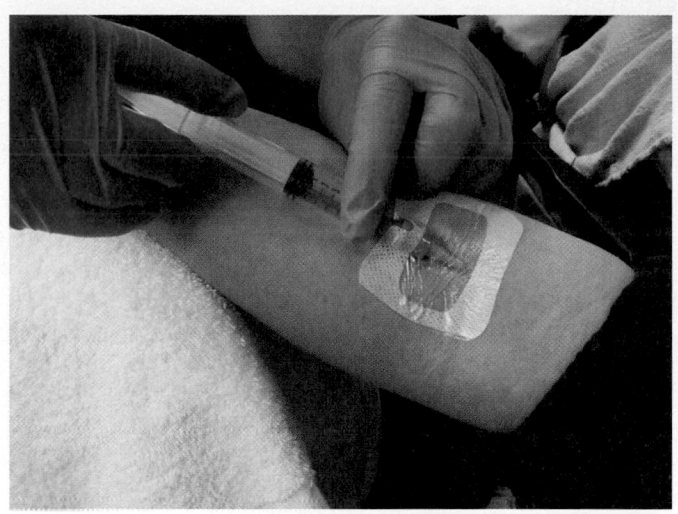

Figure 29 To check if an IV is viable, gently flush the catheter to disrupt the occlusion and reestablish flow. This photo shows a syringe prefilled with saline.

Thrombophlebitis

Infection and <u>thrombophlebitis</u> (inflammation of the vein) may occur in association with venous cannulation; both conditions are most frequently caused by lapses in aseptic technique. Thrombophlebitis is commonly encountered in patients who abuse drugs as well as in patients who are receiving long-term IV therapy in a hospital or hospice setting or with vein-irritating solutions (eg, dextrose solutions, which have a low pH, or hypertonic solutions of any sort). It can also be produced by mechanical factors, such as excessive motion of the IV needle or catheter after it has been placed.

Thrombophlebitis is usually manifested by pain and tenderness along the vein and redness and edema at the venipuncture site. These signs generally do not appear until after several hours of IV therapy, so you are unlikely to see a case of thrombophlebitis in the field setting unless you are conducting an interhospital transport of a patient with an established IV line. In such a case, stop the infusion and discontinue the IV at that site. Warm compresses applied to the site may provide some relief.

It is far better to prevent thrombophlebitis or infection than to treat it afterward. To prevent thrombophlebitis, take the following measures:

- Use a povidone-iodine preparation to scrub and disinfect the skin over the venipuncture site; then do a final wipe with an alcohol swab. Make certain the site is dry before initiating the venipuncture.
- Always wear gloves when you are performing a venipuncture.
- Never touch or otherwise contaminate the site after it has been prepped.
- After inserting the catheter, cover the puncture site with a sterile dressing.
- Anchor the catheter and tubing securely to prevent motion of the catheter within the vein.

Hematoma

A <u>hematoma</u> is an accumulation of blood in the tissues surrounding an IV site, often resulting from vein perforation or improper catheter removal. Blood can be seen rapidly pooling around the IV site, leading to tenderness and pain Figure 30 . Patients with a history of vascular diseases (including diabetes) and patients taking certain medications (eg, corticosteroids or a blood thinner such as warfarin [Coumadin]) or drinking alcohol can have a predisposition to vein rupture or to hematoma development with IV insertion.

If a hematoma develops while you are attempting to insert a catheter, stop and apply direct pressure to help minimize bleeding. If a hematoma develops after a successful catheter insertion, evaluate the IV flow and the hematoma. If the hematoma appears to be controlled and the flow is not affected, monitor the IV site and leave the line in place. If the hematoma develops as a result of discontinuing the IV, apply direct pressure with a 4″ × 4″ gauze pad to the site.

Nerve, Tendon, or Ligament Damage

Improper identification of anatomic structures around the IV site can lead to perforation of tendons, ligaments, and nerves. Selecting an IV site located near joints increases the risk for perforation of these structures. When this type of injury occurs, patients will experience sudden and severe shooting pain. Numbness or tingling in the extremity after the incident is common. Immediately remove the catheter and select another IV site.

Arterial Puncture

You may accidentally puncture the wrong blood vessel if the vein selected for cannulation lies near an artery. The risk of arterial puncture is especially high when cannulating an external jugular vein; therefore, use extreme care. If you insert a catheter into an artery by mistake, bright red blood will spurt back through the catheter. The blood's color and its flow characteristics will alert you to your error. Be aware that patients with

extremely high blood pressures may have a rapid backflow into the bag. Carefully evaluate the incident, the landmarks, and the patient. Immediately withdraw the catheter, and apply direct pressure over the puncture site for at least 5 minutes or until bleeding stops.

To avoid cannulating an artery, always check for a pulse in any vessel you intend to cannulate. Under normal circumstances, veins are near the skin surface and arteries lie much deeper. On occasion, an anatomic anomaly occurs and the vessels become transpositioned, resulting in an artery being superficial.

■ Systemic Complications

Systemic complications can evolve from reactions or complications associated with IV line insertion. They usually involve other body systems and can be life-threatening. If the IV line is established and patent in a patient experiencing a systemic complication, do not remove it because it may be needed for treatment. Potential systemic complications include allergic reactions, pyrogenic reactions, circulatory overload, air embolus, vasovagal reactions, and catheter shear.

Allergic Reactions

Often, allergic reactions associated with IV therapy are minor. However, anaphylaxis—a potentially life-threatening condition—is possible and must be treated aggressively. Allergic reactions can result from a person's unexpected sensitivity to an IV fluid or medication. Such sensitivity could be unknown to the patient, so you must maintain vigilance with any IV for a possible allergic reaction.

The patient presentation depends on the extent of the reaction. Common signs and symptoms of an allergic reaction include itching (pruritus), shortness of breath, edema of the face and hands, urticaria (hives), bronchospasm, and wheezing.

If an allergic reaction occurs, discontinue the IV line and remove the solution. Leave the catheter in place as an emergency medication route. Attach a saline lock, if available. Notify medical control immediately, and maintain an open airway. Monitor the patient's ABCs and vital signs. Keep the solution or medication for evaluation by the hospital (the chapter, *Immunologic Emergencies* covers allergic reactions and anaphylaxis in more detail).

Pyrogenic Reactions

Pyrogens are foreign proteins capable of producing fever. Their presence in the infusion solution or administration set may induce a <u>pyrogenic reaction</u>, which is characterized by an abrupt temperature elevation (as high as 106°F [41.1°C]) with severe chills, backache, headache, weakness, nausea, and vomiting. Occasionally vascular collapse occurs, with all the signs and symptoms of shock. The reaction usually begins within 30 minutes after the IV infusion has been started.

If you observe *any* signs of such a reaction—for example, if the patient reports a headache or backache after you have started running fluids—*stop the infusion immediately!* Start a new

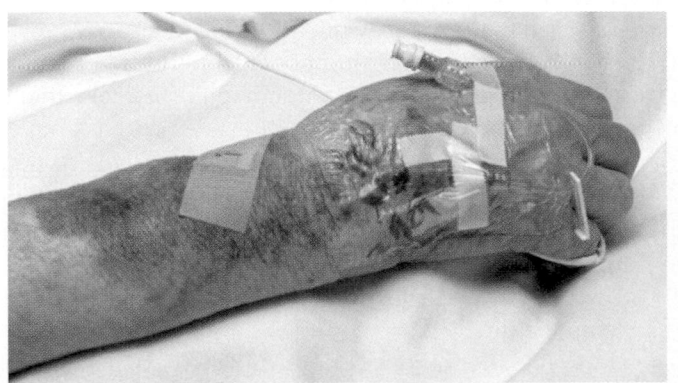

Figure 30 Hematomas can be caused by the improper removal of a catheter, resulting in pooling of blood around the IV site, leading to tenderness and pain.

IV line in the other arm with a *fresh infusion solution*, and remove the first IV. If the patient is showing signs of shock, treat as any other case of shock.

Pyrogenic reactions can be largely avoided by inspecting the IV bag carefully before use. If the bag has any leaks or if the fluid looks cloudy or discolored, select another bag.

Circulatory Overload

Healthy adults can handle as much as 2 to 3 extra liters of fluid without compromise. Problems occur, however, when the patient has cardiac, pulmonary, or renal dysfunction; these types of dysfunction do not tolerate any additional demands from increased circulatory volume. The most common cause of circulatory overload in the prehospital setting is failure to readjust the drip rate after flushing an IV line immediately after insertion. Always monitor the IV line to ensure the proper drip rate. If available, consider using an IV delivery device (eg, Volutrol or Buretrol) for patients who are at risk for circulatory overload.

> ### Special Populations
>
> It is easy to overload elderly patients who need large amounts of IV fluids. Administer small boluses of fluid (200 to 300 mL), and check breath sounds before and after each bolus to ensure that the lungs remain "dry."

Signs and symptoms of circulatory overload include dyspnea, jugular vein distention, and hypertension. Crackles (rales) are often heard when you are evaluating breath sounds. Acute peripheral edema can also be an indication of circulatory overload.

To treat a patient with circulatory overload, slow the IV rate to keep the vein open and raise the patient's head to ease respiratory distress. Administer high-flow oxygen, and monitor vital signs and breathing adequacy. Consider the use of CPAP to push fluid out of the lungs (alveoli).

Air Embolus

Healthy adults can tolerate as much as 200 mL of air introduced into the circulatory system. For patients who are already ill or injured, however, any air introduced into the IV line can present a problem. Properly flushing an IV line will help eliminate the likelihood of an air embolus. Although IV bags are designed to collapse as they empty to help prevent this problem, this collapse does not always occur. Be sure to replace empty IV bags with full ones.

If your patient begins developing respiratory distress with unequal breath sounds, consider the possibility of an air embolus. Other associated signs and symptoms include cyanosis (even in the presence of high-flow oxygen), signs and symptoms of shock, loss of consciousness, and respiratory arrest.

Treat a patient with a suspected air embolus by placing the patient on his or her left side with the head down to trap any air

inside the right atrium or right ventricle, administering 100% oxygen, and rapidly transporting to the closest appropriate facility. Be prepared to assist ventilations if the patient experiences inadequate breathing.

Vasovagal Reactions

Some patients have anxiety concerning needles or the sight of blood. Such anxiety may cause vasculature dilation, leading to a drop in blood pressure and patient collapse. Patients can present with anxiety, diaphoresis, nausea, and <u>syncopal episodes</u>.

> ### Words of Wisdom
>
> Once a catheter has been advanced over a needle, never, never, never pull it back!

Treatment for patients with vasovagal reactions (also known as "vagaling down") centers on treating them for shock:

1. Place patient in the position dictated by protocol for shock management.
2. Apply high-flow oxygen.
3. Monitor vital signs.
4. Establish an IV line in case fluid resuscitation is needed.

Catheter Shear

<u>Catheter shear</u> occurs when part of the catheter is pinched against the needle, and the needle slices through the catheter, creating a free-floating segment. The catheter segment can then travel through the circulatory system and possibly end up in the pulmonary circulation, causing a pulmonary embolus. Treatment involves surgical removal of the sheared tip. If you suspect a catheter shear, place the patient in a left lateral recumbent position with the legs down and the head elevated to try to keep the catheter remnant out of the pulmonary circulation.

Catheter hubs are <u>radiopaque</u> (ie, they appear white on a radiograph) to aid in diagnosing this type of problem. Never rethread a catheter. Dispose of the used one and select a new catheter.

Patients who have experienced catheter shear with pulmonary artery occlusion present with sudden dyspnea, shortness of breath, and possibly diminished breath sounds. Their symptoms mimic the presentation of an air embolus and can be treated the same way. Such patients need continued IV access, and you must try to obtain an IV site in the other extremity.

■ Obtaining Blood Samples

If blood samples are needed—usually at the request of the hospital for laboratory analysis—you should obtain them at the same time you start the IV line. If you have difficulty drawing blood, however, stop and finish establishing the IV line.

To obtain blood samples when you are starting an IV line, you will need the following equipment:

- 15- or 20-mL syringe
- 18- or 20-gauge needle
- **Self-sealing blood tubes**

The blood-tube tops usually come in red, blue, green, and lavender, and should be filled in that order. Use the following mnemonic to help remember the order for filling the tubes: Red Blood Gives Life. The *red*-topped tube contains no additives and is intended to clot if blood typing is needed. The *blue*-topped tube contains the preservative EDTA and is used to help determine a patient's prothrombin time and partial thromboplastin time (values that are used to calculate the patient's blood clotting time). The *green*-topped tube is filled with heparin to prevent clotting and is used to evaluate the patient's electrolyte and glucose levels. *Lavender*-topped tubes are filled with sodium citrate and are often used for a complete blood count, including hematocrit and hemoglobin values.

After the IV catheter is in place, occlude the catheter and remove the constricting band. Attach a 15- or 20-mL syringe to the hub of the IV catheter and draw the necessary amount of blood. Do not pull back on the plunger of the syringe aggressively. Too much pressure can cause hemolysis, which will make the sample useless. *Do not leave the constricting band on while drawing blood with the syringe; doing so may cause waste products to build up in the blood and could skew laboratory test results.* Detach the syringe after the required amount of blood has been obtained, attach the IV tubing, and begin the infusion. Attach an 18- or 20-gauge needle to the syringe, fill the blood tubes with the necessary amount of blood, and immediately dispose of the syringe and needle in a puncture-proof sharps container. *Exercise extreme caution when you are filling blood tubes with this technique; you are handling a "live" needle!*

If IV therapy is not indicated but blood samples are required, you can obtain them by using a cylindrical device that attaches to an 18- or 20-gauge sampling needle (a **Vacutainer**). The blood tubes are inserted into the Vacutainer after the needle it is attached to has entered the vein. To obtain blood using a Vacutainer, follow these steps:

1. Apply a constricting band, and locate a suitable vein—typically, the antecubital vein. Be sure to take standard precautions.
2. Prep the vein as you would when starting an IV line—use an alcohol prep or iodine swab, and cleanse the area in a circular motion, starting from the inside and working your way out.
3. Insert the needle (already attached to the Vacutainer) into the vein.
4. Remove the constricting band, and insert blood tubes into the Vacutainer to obtain the necessary amount of blood **Figure 31**.
5. Remove the needle from the vein, and apply direct pressure.
6. Dispose of the needle in a puncture-proof sharps container.
7. Label all the tubes with the patient's name, the date, the time, and your name as soon as possible to avoid mixing tubes with those of another patient.

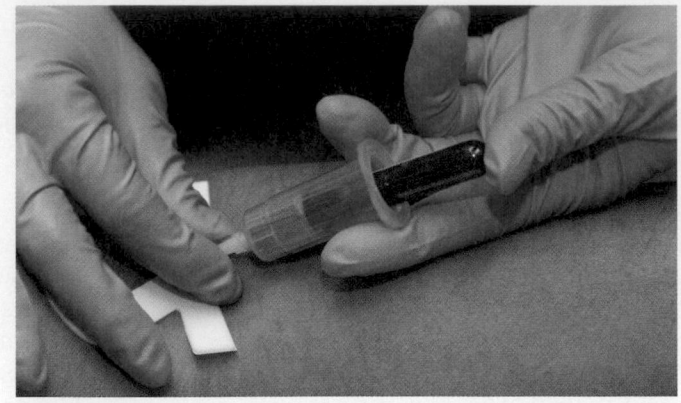

Figure 31 Obtaining blood samples with a Vacutainer.

Once the blood tubes are filled, gently turn them back and forth several times to mix the **anticoagulant** and blood evenly. The exception is the red-topped tube, which is intended to separate the serum from the other blood components. Avoid shaking this tube after the blood has clotted, because the motion may destroy the sample.

For blood tubes to be viable for testing, they must be at least three fourths full. Follow local protocols for the types of blood tubes to fill.

Blood Transfusions

Some states allow paramedics to transport blood and blood products in the interfacility setting. This generally implies that blood infusion was initiated at a transferring facility prior to arrival and that EMS will continue the infusion. Preparation for transports involving blood transfusion can be time consuming because of the amount of data that must be gathered, checked, and rechecked prior to transport.

Blood type is identified by obtaining a type and crossmatch from the patient's bloodwork. After obtaining the patient's blood type, the facility will place a bracelet on the patient that will identify his or her blood type. Any time the bag of blood is changed or care is transferred, the blood being transfused or about to be transfused must be checked against the patient's bracelet and verified by two ALS providers. This can be a paramedic and a nurse, or two paramedics, depending on local, regional, or state regulations.

When blood is being transfused, it is administered through specific blood tubing that has a filter and then mixed with normal saline **Figure 32**. Vital signs should be obtained prior to transport and compared with previous vital signs to identify trends of patient improvement or decline. Vital signs must be assessed every 5 minutes after any additional units of blood are exchanged. When new units are added, you should closely monitor the patient for signs of hemolytic reactions such as tachycardia, hives, airway compromise, wheezing, chest pain, or signs of impending doom. Transfusion reactions are discussed in the chapter, *Hematologic Emergencies*.

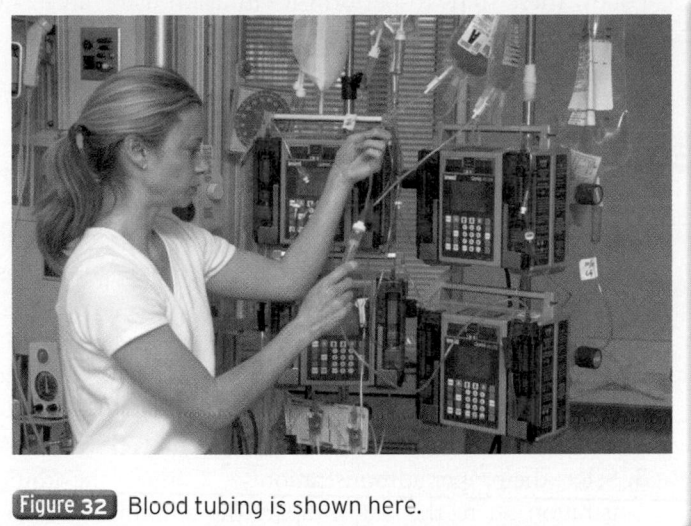

Figure 32 Blood tubing is shown here.

Intraosseous Infusion

<u>Intraosseous</u> means "within the bone." <u>Intraosseous (IO) infusion</u> is a technique of administering fluids, blood and blood products, and medications into the intraosseous space of the proximal tibia, humeral head, or sternum.

Long bones, such as the tibia, consist of a shaft (<u>diaphysis</u>), the ends (<u>epiphyses</u>), and the growth plate (<u>epiphyseal plate</u>) **Figure 33**.

The <u>intraosseous (IO) space</u> collectively comprises the spongy cancellous bone of the epiphyses and the medullary cavity of the diaphysis. Its vasculature drains into the central circulation by a network of venous sinuses and canals.

When a patient is in shock, cardiac arrest, or an otherwise hemodynamically compromised condition, peripheral veins often collapse, making IV access extremely difficult, if not impossible. However, the IO space remains patent, unless the patient has sustained trauma to its bony structure (eg, a fracture). For this reason, the IO space is commonly referred to as a "noncollapsible vein." It quickly absorbs IV fluids and medications and rapidly gets them to the central circulation—as rapidly as is possible with the IV route. Anything that can be given via the IV route—crystalloids, medications, and blood and blood products—can be given via the IO route.

IO infusion is indicated when you are unable to obtain IV access in a critically ill or injured patient (eg, in profound shock, cardiac arrest, or status epilepticus). Historically, IO infusion was reserved for children younger than 6 years when IV access could not be obtained within three attempts or 90 seconds. Although this still holds true, IO infusion has also been approved by the US Food and Drug Administration as an alternative means of establishing vascular access in critically ill or injured adults.

Equipment for IO Infusion

Several products are used for placing an IO needle into the IO space: manually inserted IO needles, the FAST1, the EZ-IO, and the Bone Injection Gun (BIG). Use of these devices requires

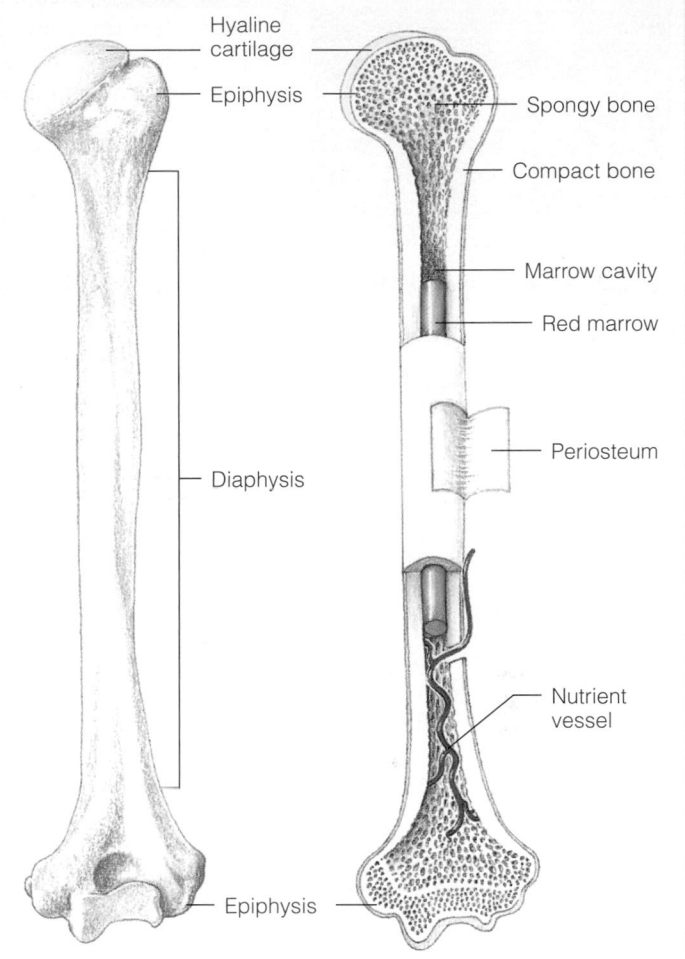

Figure 33 The components of a long bone. **A.** The humerus. Note the long shaft and dilated ends. **B.** Longitudinal section of the humerus showing compact bone, cancellous (spongy) bone, and marrow.

specialized training and thorough familiarity with each device's features, functionality, and clinical application. If your EMS system uses any of these devices, follow local protocols regarding their application.

Manually inserted IO needles (ie, Jamshedi needle, Cook catheter) were the original devices used for establishing IO access in children and are still widely used in the prehospital setting. They consist of a solid boring needle (trocar) inserted through a sharpened hollow needle **Figure 34**. The IO needle is pushed into the bone with a screwing, twisting action. Once the needle pops through the bone, the solid needle is removed, leaving the hollow steel needle in place. The IV tubing is attached to this catheter.

Because manually inserted IO needles are long, rest at a 90° angle to the bone, and are easily dislodged, they require full and careful immobilization. Stabilization is critical for these lines to maintain adequate flow. Stabilize the IO needle in the same manner that you would any impaled object.

The <u>FAST1</u> (First Access for Shock and Trauma) was the first IO device approved for use in adults; *it is not used in children.*

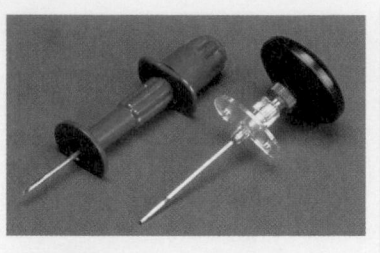

Figure 34 Manually inserted IO needles.

Four design elements allow for this device's IO placement in the sternum: an infusion tube and subcutaneous portal, an introducer, a target/strain relief patch, and a protective dome. The company that developed the FAST1 chose sternum placement based on the ease of locating the manubrium and the easier penetration than other bones.

The **EZ-IO** features a hand-held battery-powered driver, to which a special IO needle is attached **Figure 35**. This device is used to insert an IO needle into the proximal tibia of adults and children and the humeral head in adults when IV access is difficult or impossible to obtain. The battery-powered driver of the EZ-IO is universal, but different sizes of needles are available for adults and children.

The **Bone Injection Gun (BIG)** is a spring-loaded device that is used to insert an IO needle into the proximal tibia of adult and pediatric patients and the humeral head in adults. It comes in an adult size and a pediatric size, though both versions offer the same operational features.

■ Performing IO Infusion

The technique for performing IO infusion requires proper anatomic landmark identification. The flat bone of the proximal tibia—the most commonly used site—is located medial to the tibial tuberosity, the bony protuberance just below the knee. It is necessary to feel the leg to know the difference between the first and second landmarks (these cannot be seen; they must be felt).

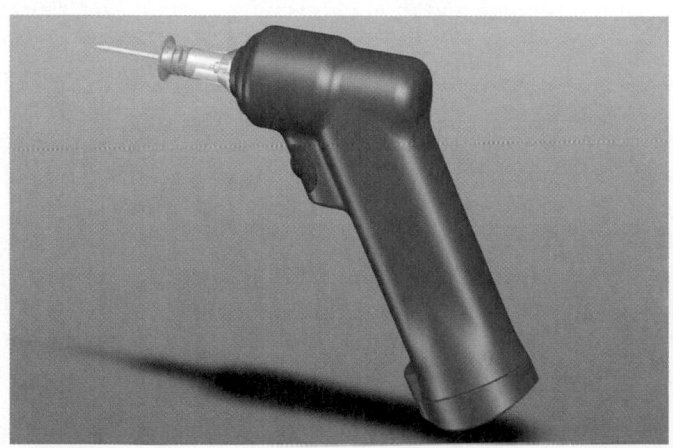

Figure 35 The EZ-IO insertion device features a hand-held battery-powered driver, to which a special intraosseous needle is attached. The battery-powered driver of the EZ-IO is universal, but different sizes of needles are available for adults and children.

Follow these steps to perform IO infusion using an EZ-IO device **Skill Drill 3**.

Skill Drill   3

1. Check the selected IV fluid for proper fluid, clarity, and expiration date. Look for discoloration and for particles floating in the fluid. If found, discard the bag and choose another bag of fluid.

2. Select the appropriate equipment, including an IO needle, syringe, saline, and extension set **Step 1**. A three-way stopcock may also be used to facilitate easier fluid administration.

3. Select the proper administration set. Connect the administration set to the bag. Prepare the administration set. Fill the drip chamber and flush the tubing. Make sure all air bubbles are removed from the tubing.

4. Prepare the syringe and extension tubing.

5. Cut or tear the tape and prepare bulky dressings. This can be done at any time before IO puncture.

6. Take standard precautions **Step 2**. *This must be done before IO puncture.*

7. Identify the proper anatomic site for IO puncture **Step 3**. Palpate the landmarks and then prepare the site.

   - **Tibia placement.** When you are using the BIG in an adult, go 2 cm from the tibial tuberosity toward the inner leg, and then 1 cm up toward the knee. When you are using the EZ-IO (as shown here), go down 2 cm from the patella to the tibial tuberosity, then 1 cm toward the inner leg. It is important to avoid penetrating the epiphyseal (growth) plate in children. When you are using the BIG in a child, go 1 to 2 cm from the tibial tuberosity toward the inner leg, and then 1 cm down toward the foot.

   - **Humerus placement.** Humeral placement is typically reserved for adults. To locate the site, patients should be placed supine with their arm at their side. Identify the midshaft of the humerus and palpate proximally toward the humeral head. Apply pressure to the anterior and inferior parts of the humeral head to locate the greater tubercle. Humerus placement should only be done with an EZ-IO or a BIG. You may need to use the longer needle per protocols.

8. Cleanse the site appropriately **Step 4**. Follow aseptic technique by cleansing in a circular manner from the inside out.

9. Attach the needle to the EZ-IO gun and remove the protective cover **Step 5**.

10. Perform the IO puncture by first stabilizing the tibia, then placing a folded towel under the knee, and finally holding the extremity in a manner to keep your fingers away from the site of puncture. For humeral placement, continue to apply pressure on the anterior and inferior aspects of the humerus.

11. Insert the needle at a 90° angle to the leg. Advance the needle with a twisting motion until a "pop" is felt. Unscrew the cap, and remove the stylet from the needle **Step 6**.

12. Remove the stylet from the catheter **Step 7**.

13. Attach the syringe and extension set to the IO needle **Step 8**. Pull back on the syringe to aspirate blood and particles of bone marrow to ensure proper placement.

14. Slowly inject saline to ensure proper placement of the needle. Responsive patients should receive 1% lidocaine

prior to infusion of fluids. Watch for extravasation, and stop the infusion immediately if it is noted. It is possible to fracture the bone during insertion of the IO. If this happens, you should remove the IO and switch to the other leg.

15. Connect the administration set and adjust the flow rate as appropriate. Fluid does not flow as rapidly through an IO catheter as through an IV line; therefore, crystalloid boluses should be given with a syringe in children and a pressure infuser device in adults.

Skill Drill | 3

Gaining Intraosseous Access With an EZ-IO Device

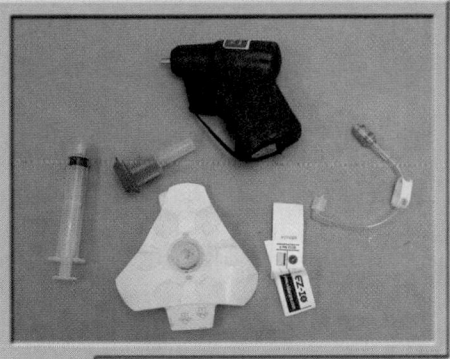

Step 1 Check selected IV fluid for proper fluid, clarity, and expiration date. Select the appropriate equipment, including an IO needle, syringe, saline, and extension tubing. Select the proper administration set. Connect the administration set to the bag. Prepare the administration set, syringe, and extension tubing.

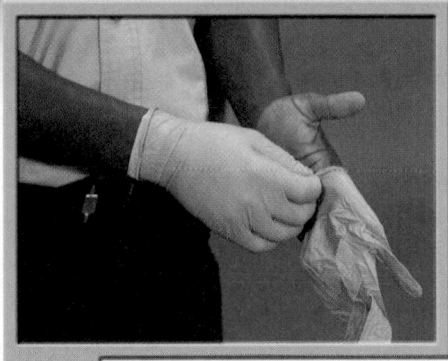

Step 2 Take standard precautions.

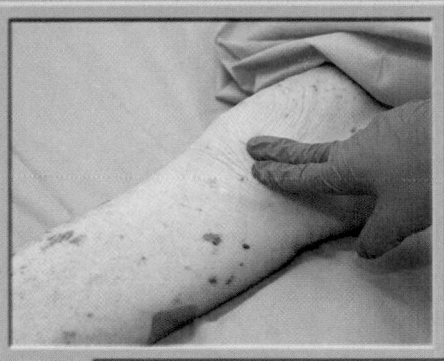

Step 3 Identify the proper anatomic site for IO puncture. Palpate the landmarks and then prepare the site.

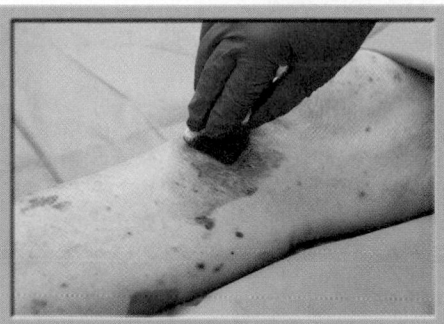

Step 4 Cleanse the site appropriately.

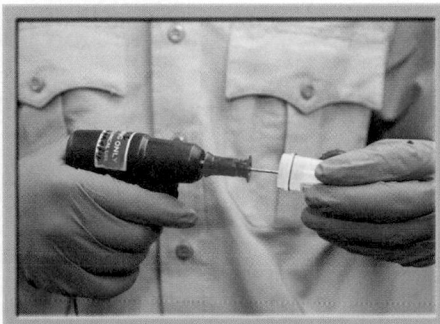

Step 5 Attach the needle to the EZ-IO gun and remove the protective cover.

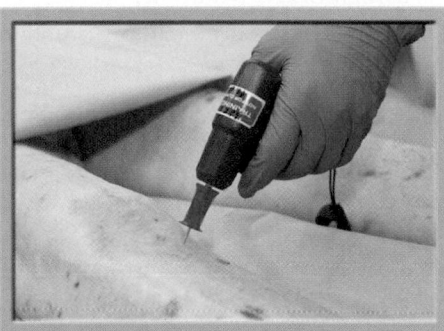

Step 6 Stabilize the tibia, and insert the needle at a 90° angle, advancing it with a twisting motion until a "pop" is felt.

Continues

Skill Drill   3

Gaining Intraosseous Access With an EZ-IO Device, continued

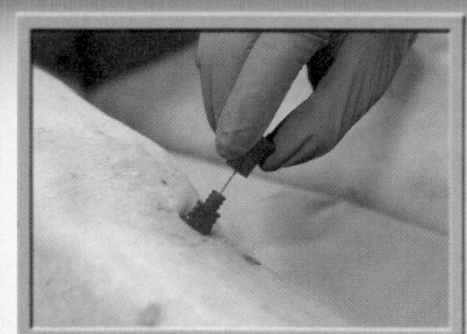

Step 7 Remove the stylet from the catheter.

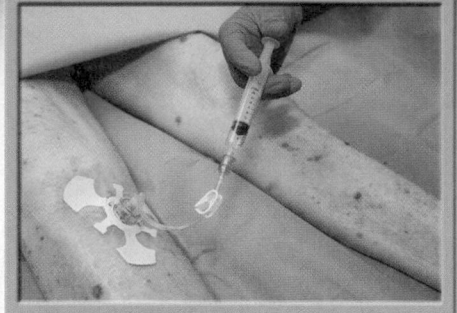

Step 8 Attach the syringe and extension set to the IO needle. Pull back on the syringe to aspirate blood and particles of bone marrow to ensure proper placement. Slowly inject saline to ensure proper placement of the needle. Watch for extravasation, and stop the infusion immediately if it is noted. Connect the administration set, and adjust the flow rate as appropriate. Secure the needle with tape, and support it with a bulky dressing.

16. Secure the needle with tape, and support it with a bulky dressing. Stabilize in place in the same manner that an impaled object is stabilized. Use bulky dressings around the catheter, and tape securely in place. Be careful not to tape around the entire circumference of the leg because this could impair circulation and potentially result in compartment syndrome.

17. Dispose of the needle in the proper container.

▪ Potential Complications of IO Infusion

If proper technique is used (ie, proper anatomic landmark identification, aseptic technique), IO infusion is associated with a relatively low complication rate. The same potential complications associated with IV therapy—thrombophlebitis, local irritation, allergic reaction, circulatory overload, and air embolism—can occur with IO infusion, as well as several others unique to this method of infusion.

Extravasation occurs when the IO needle does not rest in the IO space, but rather rests outside the bone (because the bone was missed completely or is fractured). In such

a case, IV fluid will collect in the soft tissues. The risk of extravasation can be reduced significantly by using the proper insertion technique: *Insert the IO needle at a 90° angle to the bone.* Extravasation should be suspected if the infusion does not run freely or if the site—especially the posterior aspect of the leg—rapidly becomes edematous. If this occurs, discontinue the infusion immediately and reattempt insertion in the opposite leg. Undetected extravasation could result in compartment syndrome.

Osteomyelitis is inflammation of the bone and muscle caused by an infection. According to several studies, osteomyelitis occurs in fewer than 0.6% of IO insertions.

Failure to identify the proper anatomic landmark can damage the growth plate, potentially resulting in long-term bone growth abnormalities in children.

If your insertion technique is too forceful, or if you use an IO needle that is too large for the patient's age or size, fractures can occur.

Through-and-through insertion occurs when the IO needle passes through *both* sides of the bone. To avoid this, stop inserting the needle when you feel a pop. If you feel a "pop, pop," you have likely passed the needle through both sides of the bone. Remove the needle and attempt insertion on the opposite extremity.

Words of Wisdom

With the exception of the FAST1 sternal IO device, all IO devices—manual, spring-loaded, and battery-powered—are primarily used to insert an IO needle into the IO space of the proximal tibia or humeral head. However, other anatomic locations, such as the distal tibia and distal femur, may also be acceptable locations for IO needle insertion.

A pulmonary embolism (PE) can occur if particles of bone, fat, or marrow find their way into the systemic circulation and lodge in a pulmonary artery. You should suspect a PE if the patient experiences acute shortness of breath, pleuritic chest pain, and cyanosis.

Documentation and Communication

When you start an IV line for the purpose of administering a medication, you should set the flow rate just slow enough to keep the vein patent. This slow flow rate can be documented using the acronym KVO, which stands for Keep Vein Open, or TKO, which stands for To Keep Open.

Contraindications to IO Infusion

Cannulation of a peripheral vein remains the preferred route for administering IV fluids and medications. If a functional IV line is available—in a pediatric patient or an adult—IO cannulation is *not* indicated. Other contraindications to IO cannulation and infusion include fracture of the bone intended for IO cannulation, osteoporosis, osteogenesis imperfecta (a congenital disease resulting in fragile bones), and bilateral knee replacements.

Medication Administration

Before administering any medication to a patient, you must have a thorough understanding of how the medication will affect the human body—negatively and positively. This includes familiarity with the medication's mechanism of action, indications, contraindications, side effects, routes of administration, pediatric and adult doses, and antidotes (if available) for adverse reactions.

The first rule of medicine is *primum non nocere*, "The first thing (is) to do no harm." For example, administering the drug atropine to a patient with asymptomatic bradycardia could result in undesirable tachycardia and potential hemodynamic compromise. As a result, you have caused harm to the patient who otherwise did not need the drug. Therefore, it is paramount for you to ensure that a particular drug is clearly indicated to treat the patient's condition.

You must also have an understanding of basic math for pharmacology to calculate the appropriate medication dose. This section begins with a review of basic mathematical principles as they apply to pharmacology and concludes with the various methods of medication administration.

Drug doses and flow rate calculations are often sources of confusion for many prehospital personnel, yet they are skills you will need to use frequently in the field and during your initial training while practicing at skill stations. As a paramedic, you must learn to quickly and accurately calculate medication doses to maximize the chance for a positive patient outcome. Disastrous results, including death, may be the outcome if you administer an inappropriate drug or dose, give it by the wrong route, or give the medication too rapidly or too slowly.

Mathematical Principles Used in Pharmacology

Mathematics Review

This section will discuss the use of fractions, percentages, and decimals. Having basic math skills is imperative for paramedics to appropriately administer medications.

Understanding fractions is important in formula calculation. Fractions represent a portion of a whole number expressed. Fractions are expressed as a numerator (the top number representing the portion available) over the denominator (representing the total quantity). For example, if you have four EMS units available and one of them is dispatched to an emergency, then one fourth (¼) of your units are occupied. Think of fractions as the numerator divided by the denominator. For example, ¼ is the same as $1 \div 4$.

Decimals distinguish numbers that are greater than zero from numbers that are smaller than zero. Whole numbers appear to the left side of the decimal point, and fractions of numbers on the right. Fractions can be easily converted to decimals by dividing the numerator by the denominator. For example, when you are administering atropine to bradycardic adult patients, you administer ½ of a milligram. By dividing 1 by 2, you get 0.5 ($1 \div 2 = 0.5$).

Dividing or multiplying by 10 is simple when you remember the following method. If you are dividing a number by 10, simply move the decimal point to the left. If you are multiplying a number by 10, simply move the decimal point to the right. In other words, if you are dividing the number 20 by 10, moving the decimal point one space to the left results in 2, which is the correct answer. The following examples show this method.

Multiplication problem: 20×10

Step 1: Place the decimal point:

20.0

Step 2: To multiply by 10, move the decimal point one space to the right:

200.0

The answer is 200.

Division problem: $20 \div 10$

Step 1: Place the decimal point:

20.0

Step 2: To divide by 10, move the decimal point one space to the left:

2.00

The answer is 2.

Percentages are a part of 100 and are denoted by the % symbol. Percentages can be represented as a fraction with the denominator being 100; for example, 21% = 21/100. Decimals can also be turned into percentages easily by moving the decimal point over two places (0.21 is equal to 21%).

The Metric System

The metric system is a decimal system based on multiples of ten Figure 36. It is used to measure length, volume, and weight, which are represented as follows:

- Meter (m): The basic unit of length
- Liter (L): The basic unit of volume
- Gram (g): The basic unit of weight

In the metric system, prefixes demonstrate the fraction of the base being used. Commonly used prefixes, from smallest to largest, include the following:

- micro- = 0.000001
- milli- = 0.001
- centi- = 0.01
- kilo- = 1,000.0

Table 4 lists examples of units and abbreviations.

Words of Wisdom

A cubic centimeter (cc) is equal to a milliliter (mL) and may be used interchangeably.

Drugs are supplied in a variety of weights and volumes, and you will be required to convert those weights to volume to administer the appropriate dose of a medication to your patient. Table 5 lists the symbols of weight and volume, with their respective abbreviations, that are used in the metric system. Table 6 lists the metric units of weight and volume and their equivalents.

To administer the appropriate dose of a medication to a patient, you must be able to convert larger units of weight to

smaller ones (for example, g to mg) and larger units of volume to smaller ones (for example, L to mL). Conversely, you must be able to convert smaller units of weight to larger ones (for example, mg to g) and smaller units of volume to larger ones (for example, mL to L).

Drugs are packaged in different units of weight and volume. However, the weight (for example, μg, mg, g) and volume (for example, mL) of the drug to be administered usually comprise only a fraction of the total amount of its packaged form. For example, a physician may order 50 mg of a drug for a patient, but the drug is packaged in grams. Therefore, you must be able to convert grams to milligrams and then determine how much volume is required to achieve the desired dose.

Volume Conversion In the prehospital setting, you will usually be dealing with only two measurements of volume: milliliters and liters. Because 1 L equals 1,000 mL,

Table 4	Units of Measurement				
Volume			**Example**	**Concentration**	
Units	**Abbreviation**			**Units**	**Abbreviations**
kL	Kiloliter		1,000	kg	Kilogram
L	Liter		1	g	Gram
mL	Milliliter		0.001	mg	Milligram
μL or mcL	Microliter		0.000001	μg or mcg	Microgram

Table 5	Symbols Used in the Metric System
Unit	**Symbol**
Weight (smallest to largest)	
microgram	μg (or mcg)
milligram	mg
gram	g (or gm)
kilogram	kg
Volume (smallest to largest)	
milliliter	mL
deciliter	dL
liter	L

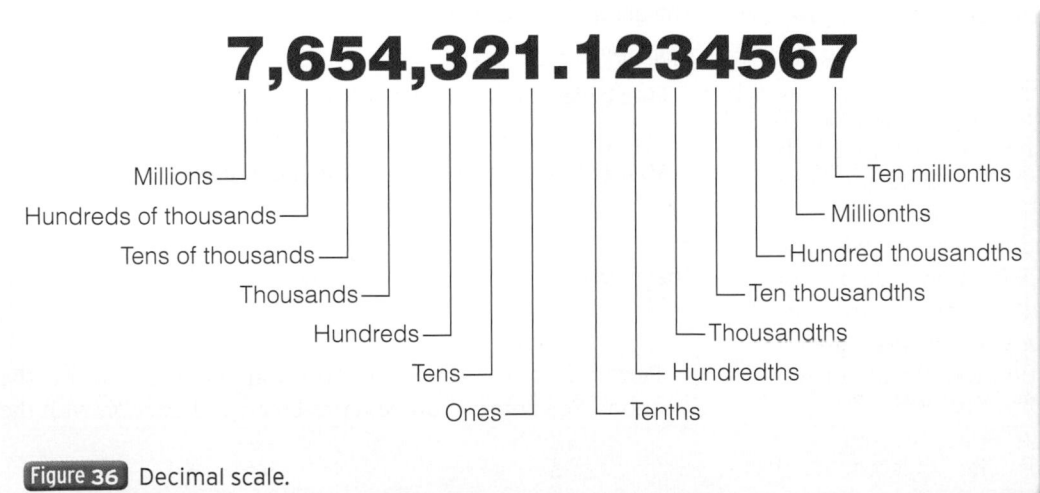

$$7,654,321.1234567$$

Millions
Hundreds of thousands
Tens of thousands
Thousands
Hundreds
Tens
Ones
Tenths
Hundredths
Thousandths
Ten thousandths
Hundred thousandths
Millionths
Ten millionths

Figure 36 Decimal scale.

Table 6 Metric Units and Their Equivalents

Unit	Equivalent
Weight (smallest to largest)	
1 µg	0.001 mg
1 mg	1,000 µg
1 g	1,000 mg
1 kg	1,000 g
Volume (smallest to largest)	
1 mL	1 cc*
100 mL	1 dL
1,000 mL	1 L

*Cubic centimeters (cc) is a unit also used to represent milliliters (mL); therefore, 1 cc is the same as 1 mL (1 cc = 1 mL).

Words of Wisdom

Carry a calculator or EMS field guide, or use a smartphone app to assist you in converting pounds to kilograms or when calculating a drug dosage.

simply divide or multiply by 1,000 or move the decimal point three places to the left or right.

When you are converting mL to L, divide the smaller unit of volume by 1,000 or simply move the decimal point three places to the left, as demonstrated in the following example:

Example 1:
Converting 500 mL of normal saline to L (500 mL = X L)

500 mL ÷ 1,000 = 0.5 L or 500. = 0.5 L normal saline

Conversely, when you are converting L to mL, multiply L by 1,000 or simply move the decimal point three places to the right, as demonstrated in the following example:

Example 1:
Converting 1.5 L of lactated Ringer's to mL (1.5 L = X mL)

1.5 L × 1,000 = 1,500 mL or 1.500 = 1,500 mL

Example 2:
Converting 25 L of lactated Ringer's to mL (25 L = X mL)

25 L × 1,000 = 25,000 mL or 25.000 = 25,000 mL

YOU are the Medic   PART 3

You place the patient on oxygen via a nonrebreathing mask and decide to start an IV line. You choose the left antecubital vein and an 18-gauge catheter. You decide to contact medical control for pain management and fluid rehydration orders. You protect the patient from further exposure to the sun while you prepare to immobilize the leg and then place ice packs under the patient's arms.

Recording Time: 5 Minutes	
Respirations	28 breaths/min
Pulse	140 beats/min, weak and thready
Skin	Flushed and diaphoretic
Blood pressure	86/40 mm Hg
Oxygen saturation (SpO₂)	99%
Pupils	Equal and reactive

5. What type of pain management would be best for this patient? What are the common methods for administration and benefits/problems with each?
6. What are the risks and benefits of using an isotonic solution for fluid replacement?

Weight Conversion

Converting weight is simply a matter of multiplying or dividing by 1,000 *or* moving the decimal point three places to the right or left.

To convert a larger unit of weight to a smaller one, *multiply* the larger unit of weight by 1,000 *or* move the decimal point three places to the *right*, as demonstrated in the following examples:

Example 1:
Converting 25 g of dextrose to mg (25 g = X mg)

$$25 \text{ g} \times 1{,}000 = 25{,}000 \text{ mg } or \text{ } 25.000 \rightarrow = 25{,}000 \text{ mg}$$

Example 2:
Converting 0.15 mg of fentanyl to µg (0.15 mg = X µg)

$$0.15 \text{ mg} \times 1{,}000 = 150 \text{ µg } or \text{ } 0.150 \rightarrow = 150 \text{ µg}$$

Conversely, to convert a smaller unit of weight to a larger unit when the difference is 1,000 (such as mg to g or µg to mg), divide the mg by 1,000 *or* simply move the decimal point three places to the left, as demonstrated in the following examples. Remember that 1 g equals 1,000 mg and 1 mg equals 1,000 µg.

Example 1:
Converting 200 µg of fentanyl to mg (200 µg = X mg)

$$200 \text{ µg} \div 1{,}000 = 0.2 \text{ mg } or \text{ } 200. \leftarrow = 0.2 \text{ mg}$$

Example 2:
Converting 250 mg of dextrose to g (250 mg = X g)

$$250 \text{ mg} \div 1{,}000 = 0.25 \text{ g } or \text{ } 250. \leftarrow = 0.25 \text{ g}$$

Converting Pounds to Kilograms

Most likely your patients will not be able to tell you how much they weigh in kilograms (kg). However, if your patient is able to tell you his or her weight in pounds, you can easily convert that number to kilograms. This information will frequently be available during interfacility transports. For patients who do not know their weight in pounds or who are unresponsive and unable to provide you with this information, you must perform the following steps:

1. Estimate the patient's weight in pounds (lb).
2. Convert pounds to kilograms (kg).

Although many of the drugs given in emergency medicine are administered in a standard dose (eg, 1 mg of epinephrine), others are administered based on the patient's weight in kilograms (eg, 1 to 1.5 mg/kg of lidocaine). In addition, most drugs administered to pediatric patients are based on their weight in kilograms.

Two formulas can be used to convert pounds to kilograms. Use whichever one is easiest for you to remember.

For example, when converting a 170-lb man's weight to kilograms, the formula would be as follows:

Formula 1: Divide the patient's weight in pounds by 2.2 (1 kg = 2.2 lb)

$$170 \text{ lb} \div 2.2 = 77.27 \text{ kg}$$
$$250 \text{ lb} \div 2.2 = 113.64 \text{ kg}$$
$$479.6 \text{ lb} \div 2.2 = 218 \text{ kg}$$
$$6.6 \text{ lb} \div 2.2 = 3 \text{ kg}$$
$$30 \text{ lb} \div 2.2 = 14.09 \text{ kg}$$
$$68 \text{ lb} \div 2.2 = 30.91 \text{ kg}$$

Because the value following the decimal point in this example is less than 0.5, you may round the patient's weight in kilograms to 77. If the value after the decimal point in the first example had been greater than 0.5, you would round the weight in kilograms to 78. Although this may seem negligible, it is good practice to administer the *most* appropriate amount of the drug to the patient.

Formula 2: Divide the patient's weight in pounds by 2 and subtract 10% of that number

For example, when converting a 120-lb woman's weight to kilograms, the formula would be as follows:

$$Step \text{ } 1: 120 \text{ lb} \div 2 = 60$$
$$Step \text{ } 2: 60 \text{ lb} \times 10\% = 6$$
$$Step \text{ } 3: 60 - 6 = 54 \text{ kg}$$

NOTE: This formula provides an approximate weight and is not exact.

Words of Wisdom

A teaspoon is approximately 5 milliliters, and a tablespoon is approximately 15 milliliters. A cup is approximately 240 mL. Drops vary based on the diameter of the dropper. These measurements may be useful to remember if you need to calculate exact amounts of a patient's medication.

Temperature Conversion

The Fahrenheit and Celsius (or centigrade) temperature scales are commonly used to measure temperature. On the **Celsius scale**, water freezes at 0° and boils at 100°. On the **Fahrenheit scale**, water freezes at 32° and boils at 212°. Normal body temperature is 98.6° Fahrenheit (37° Celsius). Values on each of these scales can easily be interconverted by using the following equations:

- To convert Fahrenheit to Celsius: Subtract 32, then multiply by 0.555 (5/9)

$$98.6°\text{F} - 32 \times 0.555 = 36.9 \text{ (37°C)}$$

- To convert Celsius to Fahrenheit: Multiply by 1.8 (9/5), then add 32

$$37°C \times 1.8 + 32 = 98.6°F$$

Fahrenheit → Celsius
$104.2°F - 32 \times 0.555 = 40.1°C$
$100.9°F - 32 \times 0.555 = 38.2°C$
$92.4°F - 32 \times 0.555 = 33.5°C$
Celsius → Fahrenheit
$37.9°C \times 1.8 + 32 = 100.2°F$
$38.6°C \times 1.8 + 32 = 101.4°F$
$32.2°C \times 1.8 + 32 = 90°F$

Calculating Medication Doses

There are multiple formulas for calculating medication doses. This chapter focuses on those formulas that most students find easy to understand. For other calculation formulas, you should consult with your instructor. The method of drug dose calculation demonstrated in this chapter is based on the following three factors:

- Desired dose
- Concentration of the drug available (dose on hand)
- Volume to be administered

Desired Dose

The **desired dose** (ie, the drug order) is the amount of a drug that the physician orders you to give to a patient. It may be expressed as a standard dose (eg, 5 mg of diazepam [Valium], 25 g of 50% dextrose) or as a specific number of micrograms, milligrams, or grams per kilogram of body weight (eg, 1 to 1.5 mg/kg of lidocaine [Xylocaine]).

Drug Concentrations

After you have received a drug order (desired dose), you must determine how much of the drug that you have available. In other words, you must know its **concentration**—the total weight (μg, mg, or g) of the drug contained in a specific amount of volume (mL or L). Sometimes this information is printed on the label of the drug container (eg, Drug X at a concentration of 5 mg/mL); other containers may list the total weight and total volume of the drug separately (eg, 8 mg of morphine sulfate in 2 mL). The following are examples of common prepackaged drug concentrations:

- Lidocaine, 100 mg/10 mL
- Epinephrine, 1 mg/10 mL
- Furosemide, 40 mg/4 mL
- Adenosine, 6 mg/2 mL
- 50% dextrose, 25 g/50 mL
- Fentanyl, 100 μg/1 mL
- Naloxone, 2 mg/5 mL

In the preceding examples, notice that the drugs are contained in different volumes of solution. This is your **volume on hand**. *To administer a drug, you must know the weight of the drug that is present in 1 mL.* This information will tell you the concentration of the drug that you have on hand. The formula for calculating this is as follows:

Total Weight of the Drug ÷ Total Volume in Milliliters = Weight per Milliliter

By using this formula, you can easily calculate how much of the drug is contained in each milliliter.

Example:
Lidocaine, 100 mg/10 mL

100 mg (total weight) ÷ 10 mL (total volume) = 10 mg/mL

Morphine sulfate, 8 mg/2 mL

8 mg ÷ 2 mL = 4 mg/mL

Atropine, 1 mg/10 mL

1 mg ÷ 10 mL = 0.1 mg/mL

Diphenhydramine, 50 mg/2 mL

50 mg ÷ 2 mL = 25 mg/mL

Things become slightly more complex when the label of the drug lists the drug concentration as a percentage—for example, "1% lidocaine (Xylocaine)." What *percentage* means in terms of drug concentration is the number of *grams present in 100 mL*. Thus 1% lidocaine (Xylocaine) contains 1 g of drug in every 100 mL (1 dL). By dividing the numerator and denominator by 100, you will arrive at a concentration of 10 mg/mL:

$$\frac{1\,g}{100\,mL} = \frac{1{,}000\,mg}{100\,mL} = 10\,mg/mL$$

Documentation and Communication

To prevent errors when you are documenting decimals, write 0.2 mg or 2 mg instead of .2 mg or 2.0 mg, which could easily be mistaken for 2 mg or 20 mg, respectively.

Volume To Be Administered

After you have determined the concentration of the drug present in each milliliter, you must calculate how much volume is needed to give the amount of the drug ordered (desired dose). Use the following formula to calculate the volume to be administered:

Desired dose (mg) ÷ concentration of drug on hand (mg/mL) = volume to be administered

Example 1:

Medical control orders you to administer 5 mg of diazepam (Valium) for your patient for sedation. You have a vial of diazepam, which contains 20 mg in 5 mL. How many milliliters of diazepam must you give to achieve the ordered dose of 5 mg?

Step 1: Determine the concentration (in mg/mL).

20 mg ÷ 5 mL = 4 mg/mL (concentration)

Step 2: Determine how much volume to administer.

5 mg (desired dose) ÷ 4 mg/mL (concentration) = 1.25 mL

Example 2:

You are ordered to administer 12.5 g of dextrose to a hypoglycemic patient. You have a prefilled syringe of 50% dextrose containing 25 g in 50 mL. How many milliliters of dextrose will you give?

Step 1: Determine the concentration (in g/mL).

25 g ÷ 50 mL = 0.5 g/mL (concentration)

Step 2: Determine how much volume to administer.

12.5 g (desired dose) ÷ 0.5 g (500 mg)/mL (concentration) = 25 mL

Example 3:

You are treating a patient who has nausea and feels like she is going to vomit. Your protocol says that you can administer 4 mg of ondansetron (Zofran). Ondansetron is packaged in a vial of 4 mg in 2 mL.

Step 1: Determine the concentration (in g/mL).

4 mg ÷ 2 mL = 2 mg/mL (concentration)

Step 2: Determine how much volume to administer.

4 mg (desired dose) ÷ 2 mg/mL (concentration) = 2 mL

Example 4:

During a cardiac arrest your protocols allow you to administer 300 mg of amiodarone (Cordarone) as an antidysrhythmic after epinephrine or vasopressin when ventricular fibrillation or ventricular tachycardia is present. Amiodarone is packaged as 150 mg in 3 mL.

Step 1: Determine the concentration (in g/mL).

150 mg ÷ 3 mL = 50 mg/mL (concentration)

Step 2: Determine how much volume to administer.

300 mg (desired dose) ÷ 50 mg/mL (concentration) = 6 mL

Weight-Based Drug Doses

As mentioned earlier, some medication doses are based on the patient's weight in kilograms. Determining the appropriate dose for the patient requires simply adding one step to the formula that was previously discussed—conversion of the patient's weight in pounds to kilograms. Remember, 1 kg = 2.2 lb.

Example 1:

A 7-year-old girl requires 0.02 mg/kg of atropine to treat symptomatic bradycardia. You have a prefilled syringe of atropine containing 1 mg in 10 mL. The child's mother tells you that she weighs 60 lb. How many milligrams will you give to this child (that is, what is the desired dose)? How much volume will you give to achieve the required dose?

Step 1: Convert the child's weight in pounds to kilograms.

Formula 1: 60 lb ÷ 2.2 = 27.2 kg (round to 27 kg)

Formula 2: 60 lb ÷ 2 − 10% = 27 kg

Step 2: Determine the desired dose.

0.02 mg × 27 kg = 0.54 mg (round to 0.5 mg [desired dose])

Step 3: Determine the concentration.

1 mg ÷ 10 mL = 0.1 mg/mL (concentration)

Step 4: Determine how much volume to administer.

0.5 mg (desired dose) ÷ 0.1 mg/mL (concentration) = 5 mL

Example 2:

You are preparing to intubate a head injury patient who weighs approximately 180 lb. Your protocol calls for lidocaine at 1.5 mg/kg prior to intubation attempts to reduce intracranial pressure. The lidocaine is packaged in a prefilled syringe of 100 mg in 10 mL.

Step 1: Convert the patient's weight in pounds to kilograms.

Formula 1: 180 lb ÷ 2.2 = 81.81 kg (round to 82 kg)

Step 2: Determine the desired dose.

1.5 mg/kg × 82 kg = 123 mg

Step 3: Determine the concentration.

100 mg ÷ 10 mL = 10 mg/mL (concentration)

Step 4: Determine how much volume to administer.

123 mg (desired dose) ÷ 10 mg/mL (concentration) = 12.3 mL

■ Calculating Fluid Infusion Rates

Once the IV or IO catheter is in place, you need to adjust the flow rate according to the patient's clinical condition or as dictated by medical control. To do so, you must know the following information:

- The volume to be infused
- The period over which it is to be infused
- The properties of the administration set you are using—that is, how many drops per milliliter (gtt/mL) it delivers

By knowing in advance the volume to be infused, the period over which it will be infused, and the properties of the administration set, you can calculate the flow rate.

For example, suppose the physician orders an infusion of 1 L (1,000 mL) of normal saline to be infused in 4 hours, and the macrodrip administration set provides 10 gtt/mL:

$$\frac{\text{Volume to be infused} \times \text{gtt/mL of administration set}}{\text{total time of infusion } in\ minutes} = \text{gtt/min}$$

Information:

> Total volume to be infused = 1,000 mL
> gtt/mL of the administration set = 10
> Time of infusion (in minutes) = 4 h × 60 min/h = 240 min

Calculation:

$$\frac{1,000 \text{ mL} \times 10 \text{ gtt/mL}}{240 \text{ minutes}} = \text{approximately 42 gtt/min}$$

Words of Wisdom

If the physician orders a specific number of milliliters to be administered per hour (mL/h), a quick and easy way to calculate the number of drops per minute (gtt/min) with a 60-gtt set is to divide the number of milliliters per hour:

- By 6, if using a macrodrip that provides 10 gtt/mL
- By 4, if using a macrodrip that provides 15 gtt/mL
- By 1, if using a microdrip set that provides 60 gtt/mL

■ Calculating the Dose and Rate for a Medication Infusion

■ Non–Weight-Based Medication Infusions

Following the administration of certain drugs, you may need to begin a continuous infusion to maintain a therapeutic blood level of the drug to prevent a recurrence of the condition. Medication infusions are usually ordered to be administered over a specified period, usually per minute.

To calculate a continuous medication infusion that is not weight-based, you must know the following information in advance:

- The desired dose (μg/min or mg/min)
- The properties of the administration set you are using (eg, microdrip [60 gtt/mL])
- Will you be using an infusion pump? (Mechanical infusion pumps are discussed later in this chapter.)

You will use the same formula to calculate a drug dose as previously discussed. Then, however, you will calculate the desired dose to be administered continuously—usually a certain number of micrograms (μg) or milligrams (mg) per minute.

For example, suppose you have just administered 75 mg of lidocaine to your patient in cardiac arrest, after which time the cardiac rhythm converts to a perfusing rhythm. Medical control then orders you to begin a continuous lidocaine infusion at 2 mg/min. You must determine at how many drops per minute (gtt/min) to set the IV drip rate to deliver the 2 mg/min desired dose. To do so, you will add a certain amount of lidocaine into a bag of IV fluid. In this example, 2 g (2,000 mg) of lidocaine will be added to a 500-mL bag of normal saline, a

common combination. The formula to calculate the continuous infusion rate is as follows:

> *Step 1:* Determine the concentration.
>
> > 2 g (2,000 mg) of lidocaine ÷ 500 mL of normal saline = 4 mg/mL (concentration)
>
> *Step 2:* Determine the amount of volume to infuse per minute (mL/min).
>
> For this calculation, you must recall the desired dose—in this case, 2 mg/min.
>
> To determine the number of mL/min, you perform the following calculation:
>
> > $\frac{2 \text{ mg (desired dose)}}{\text{min}} \times \frac{1 \text{ mL}}{4 \text{ mg}} = 0.5 \text{ mL/min (concentration)}$
>
> *Step 3:* Determine how many drops per minute (gtt/min) at which to set the IV flow rate.

For this calculation, you must know the number of drops per milliliter (gtt/mL) that your IV administration set delivers—a microdrip (60 gtt/mL) or a macrodrip (10 or 15 gtt/mL). For a microdrip administration set (typically used when administering a continuous medication infusion), the number of drops per minute for the IV flow rate would be calculated as follows:

> 0.5 mL/min × 60 gtt/mL ÷ total time in minutes (1) = 30 gtt/min

■ Weight-Based Medication Infusions

Some continuous medication infusions are based on the patient's weight in kilograms. Dopamine (Intropin), for example, is typically administered in a range of 5 to 20 μg/kg/min. By using the previously discussed formula and factoring in the patient's weight in kilograms to determine the desired dose, you will calculate the IV drip rate for a 70-kg patient who requires a continuous dopamine infusion at 5 μg/kg/min. In this example, 800 mg of dopamine will be added to a 500-mL bag of normal saline, a common combination.

Example 1:
> *Step 1:* Determine the desired dose.
>
> > 5 μg/kg/min × 70 kg = 350 μg/min (desired dose)
>
> *Step 2:* Determine the concentration.
>
> > 800 mg (800,000 μg) of dopamine ÷ 500 mL of normal saline = 1.6 mg/mL (concentration)

The caveat here is that dopamine is administered in *micrograms*, not milligrams. Therefore, you must convert the 1.6 mg/mL concentration to μg/mL. Recall that to convert a larger unit of weight to a smaller one, you must multiply by 1,000 *or* move the decimal point three places to the *right*; in other words, 1.6 mg is equal to *1,600 μg*.

Step 3: Determine the amount of volume to infuse per minute (mL/min).

Again, you must recall the desired dose—in this case, 350 μg/min. To determine the number of mL/min, the calculation continues as follows:

$$350 \text{ μg (desired dose)} \div 1,600 \text{ μg/mL}$$
$$\text{(concentration)} = 0.22 \text{ mL/min}$$

Step 4: Determine how many drops per minute (gtt/min) at which to set the IV flow rate.

Again, you must know the properties of the administration set you are using. In this example, you will use the microdrip (60 gtt/mL). The number of drops per minute for the IV flow rate would be calculated as follows:

$$\frac{0.22 \text{ mL}}{\text{min}} \times \frac{60 \text{ gtt}}{\text{mL}} \div \text{Total Time in Minutes (1)} = 13.2 \text{ gtt/min}$$
$$\text{(round to 13 gtt/min)}$$

Dobutamine (Dobutrex) is usually transferred with an IV pump so calculating gtt is rarely needed for this medication. However, paramedics will see this medication in use during interfacility transports, so the following calculation uses dobutamine as an example.

Example 2:
Dobutamine is a common interfacility medication for cardiogenic shock. The dose is generally 2 to 20 μg/kg/min. For this example, you are transferring a 60-kg patient who is on a drip of 10 μg/kg/min. The dobutamine is packaged as 250 mg in a 500-mL bag.

Step 1: Calculate the desired dose.

$$10 \text{ μg/kg/min} \times 60 \text{ kg} = 600 \text{ μg/min (desired dose)}$$

Step 2: Calculate the concentration. The first step in calculating the concentration is to convert the units from mg to μg.

$$250 \text{ mg} \times \frac{1,000 \text{ μg}}{\text{mg}} = 250,000 \text{ μg}$$

$$250,000 \text{ μg} \div 500 \text{ mL} = 500 \text{ μg/mL (concentration)}$$

Step 3: Calculate the amount of volume to infuse per minute (mL/min).

$$600 \text{ μ/min (desired dose)} \div 500 \text{ μg/mL}$$
$$\text{(concentration)} = 1.2 \text{ mL/min}$$

Step 4: Calculate how many drops per minute (gtt/min) at which to set the IV flow rate.

$$1.2 \text{ mL/min} \times 60 \text{ gtt/mL} \div \text{total time in minutes (1)} = 72 \text{ gtt/min}$$

Pediatric Drug Doses

There are numerous methods for determining the appropriate dose of medication for a pediatric patient. Many paramedics use length-based resuscitation tape measures or pediatric wheel charts Figure 37; others carry an EMS field guide with tables or charts specific to pediatric patients. Most drugs used in pediatric emergency medicine are based on the child's weight in kilograms. With the exception of the obviously smaller doses

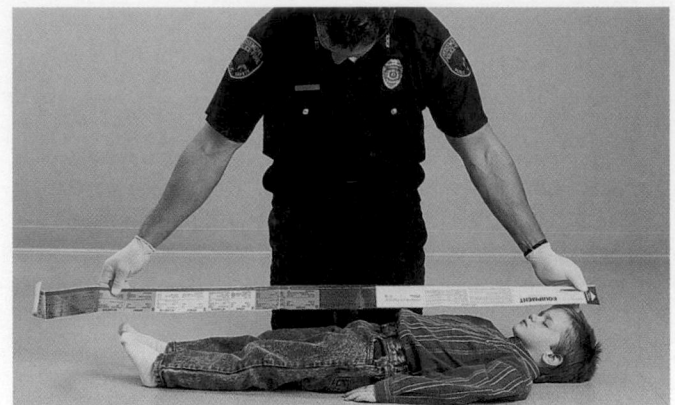

Figure 37 Use of a length-based resuscitation tape measure is one method of calculating pediatric drug doses. The tape measure estimates the child's weight (up to 34 kg) based on his or her length.

Special Populations

The following table lists potentially lethal toddler ingestions:

Medicine	Lethal Dose
Camphor	One teaspoon of oil
Chloroquine	One 500-mg tablet
Clonidine	One 0.3-mg tablet
Glyburide	Two 5-mg tablets
Imipramine	One 150-mg tablet
Lindane	Two teaspoons of 1% lotion
Diphenoxylate/atropine	Two 2.5-mg tablets
Propanolol	One or two 160-mg tablets
Theophylline	One 500-mg tablet
Verapamil	One or two 240-mg tablets

and volumes, the calculations for pediatric drug dosing and medication infusions are the same as they are for adults.

Enteral Medication Administration

<u>Enteral medications</u> are those that are given through some portion of the digestive or intestinal tract. These are also referred to as alimentary medications. This includes medications that are administered orally, through a feeding tube, or rectally.

Oral Medication Administration

Most patients take their daily medications at home by the oral route (PO [per os]). Forms of solid and liquid oral medications include capsules, timed-release capsules, lozenges, pills, tablets, elixirs, emulsions, suspensions, and syrups Figure 38.

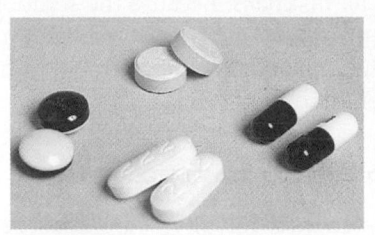

Figure 38 Tablets and capsules, oral medications typically taken by mouth, enter the bloodstream through the digestive system.

Drugs taken by mouth are absorbed at a slow rate from the stomach and intestines—usually somewhere between 30 and 90 minutes. Because absorption is slower, it may be necessary for prehospital providers to initiate PO medications early.

To give oral medications, you may use a small medicine cup, a medicine dropper, a teaspoon, an oral syringe, or a nipple. Gather the appropriate equipment for the form of medication you are administering. Check for indications, contraindications, and precautions, and review the six rights before administering any medication.

Follow these steps when administering an oral medication **Figure 39** .

1. Take standard precautions.
2. Determine the need for the medication based on patient presentation.
3. Obtain a history, including any drug allergies.
4. Follow standing orders, or contact medical control for permission.
5. Check the medication to be sure it is the right medication, it is not cloudy or discolored, and its expiration date has not passed.
6. Determine the appropriate dose. If using a liquid medication, pour the desired amount into a calibrated cup or withdraw the appropriate amount into a syringe or dropper. If administering solid medications, pour the appropriate amount into the lid of the bottle and then place them in the patient's hand.
7. Instruct the patient to swallow the medication with water, if administering a pill or tablet.
8. Monitor the patient's condition, and document the medication given, route, time of administration, and response of the patient.

You may need to calculate the number of pills, capsules, or tablets to give. For PO medications, the concentration is already available on the bottle. For example, during COPD exacerbation, your protocols may call for 60 mg of PO prednisone. The concentration is labeled as 20 mg/tablet.
Calculation:

60 mg (desired dose) ÷ 20-mg tablets (concentration) = 3 tablets

■ Orogastric and Nasogastric Tube Medication Administration

Gastric tubes (orogastric or nasogastric) are occasionally inserted in the prehospital setting to decompress the stomach, perform gastric lavage, or establish a route for enteral medication

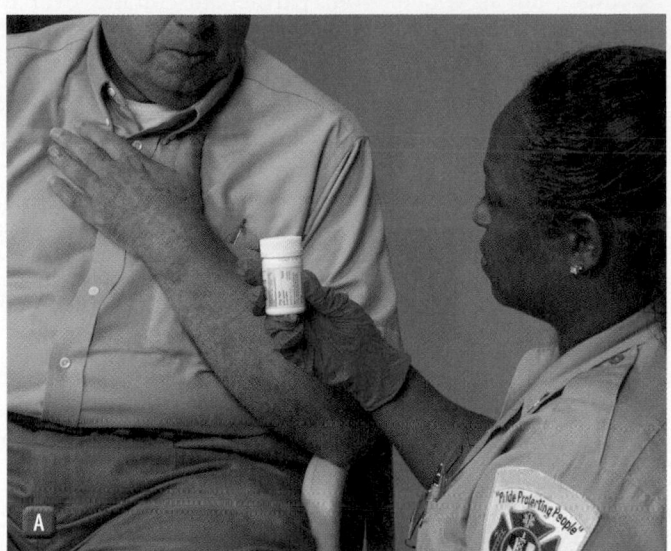

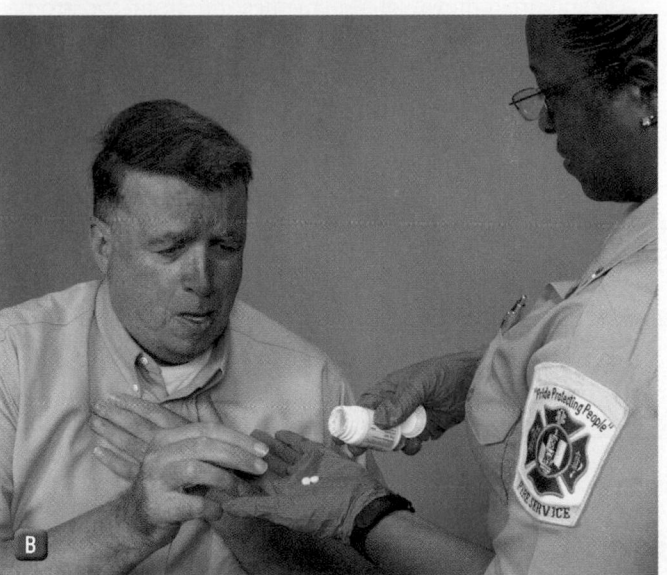

Figure 39 Administering an oral medication. **A.** Check the medication and its expiration date. **B.** Have the patient take the medication. Provide a glass or cup of water if necessary.

administration, though use of this route for medication administration in the field is rare. Some services may allow activated charcoal to be administered by gastric tube for toxic ingestion when PO activated charcoal is contraindicated. Gastric tubes are also commonly present during interfacility transports. The most common solution to be administered through gastric tubes during interfacility transports is tube feeding. The chapter, *Airway Management and Ventilation* describes insertion of orogastric and nasogastric tubes. Follow these steps to administer medications via the gastric tube after the tube has been inserted **Skill Drill 4** :

Skill Drill 4

1. Take standard precautions.
2. Confirm proper gastric tube placement. Attach a 60-mL cone-tipped syringe to the gastric tube and slowly

inject air as you or your partner auscultates over the epigastrium (Step 1).

To further confirm proper placement, withdraw on the plunger of the syringe and observe for the return of gastric contents in the tube. Leave the gastric tube open to air.

3. Draw up 30 to 60 mL of normal saline into the syringe, and irrigate the gastric tube (Step 2). If you meet resistance, ensure that the tube is not kinked.

4. Draw up the appropriate amount of medication, and slowly inject it into the gastric tube (Step 3).

5. Inject 30 to 60 mL of normal saline into the gastric tube following administration of the medication (Step 4). This will ensure that the tube is flushed and that the patient has received the entire dose of the medication.

6. Clamp off the proximal end of the gastric tube (Step 5). Do not attach the gastric tube to suction because this will result in removal of the medication from the stomach. Monitor the patient for adverse reactions. Repeat the medication dose if indicated.

Be sure to use warm saline for injections. Because the solution will be going directly into the digestive tract with a temperature of approximately 98.6°F, a solution at room temperature has the possibility of placing the patient in hypothermia.

■ Rectal Medication Administration

Certain drugs may be administered rectally if you are unable to establish IV or IO access. In the field, diazepam (Valium) can be administered rectally (PR) in patients because IV access can be challenging when the patient is having a seizure. Because the rectal mucosa is highly vascular, medication absorption is rapid and predictable (Figure 40). Because rectal medications are not digested prior to being absorbed by the body's vasculature, they also bypass the first pass metabolism; this is why they have such a rapid onset. Certain antiemetic medications are available in suppository form (eg, promethazine [Phenergan]), and under certain circumstances, you might be asked to administer them. A suppository is a drug mixed in a firm base that melts at body temperature and is shaped to fit the rectum.

Skill Drill   4

Administering Medication via a Nasogastric Tube

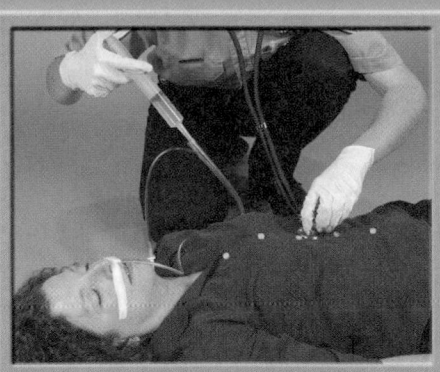

Step 1 Attach a 60-mL syringe to the proximal end of the gastric tube, and slowly inject air into the tube while auscultating over the epigastrium to confirm proper placement. For further confirmation of correct tube placement, aspirate with the syringe and observe for gastric contents.

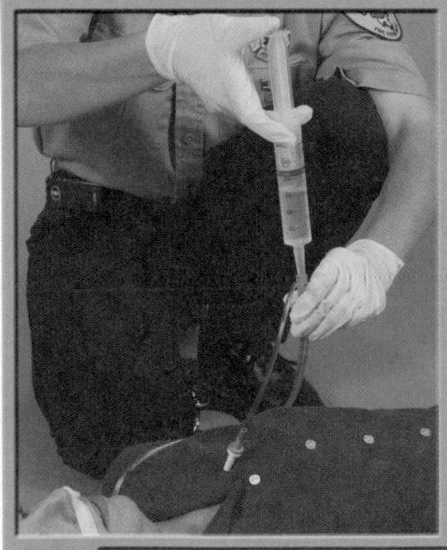

Step 2 Inject 30 to 60 mL of normal saline into the gastric tube to irrigate the tube.

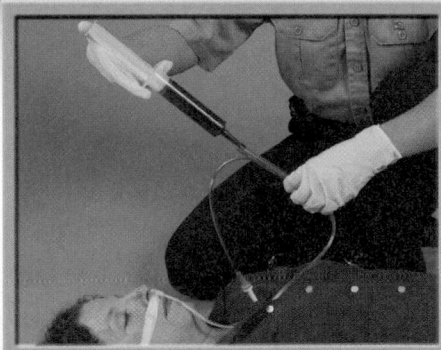

Step 3 Inject the appropriate amount of medication into the gastric tube.

Continues

Skill Drill 4

Administering Medication via a Nasogastric Tube, continued

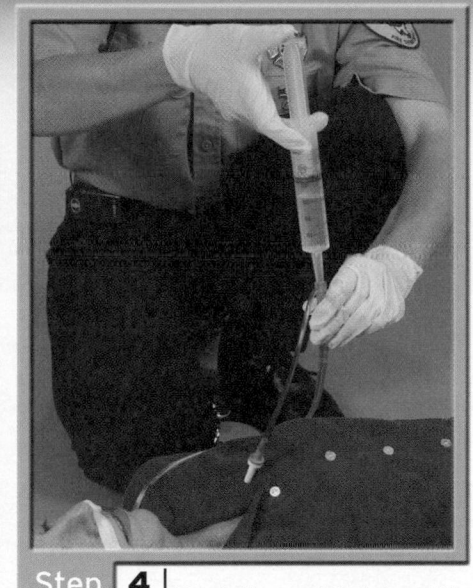

Step 4 Flush the gastric tube with 30 to 60 mL of normal saline to ensure dispersal of the drug into the stomach.

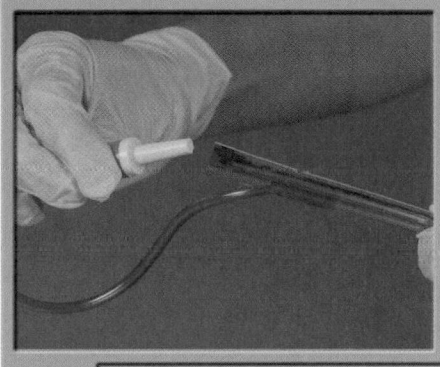

Step 5 Clamp off the proximal end of the gastric tube; do not reattach the tube to suction. Monitor the patient for adverse reactions, and repeat the medication dose if indicated.

approximately $1''$ to $1\frac{1}{2}''$ while instructing the patient to relax and not to bear down.

7. For medications in liquid form, some modifications are needed. You may use a nasopharyngeal airway, a small endotracheal tube, a large-bore IV catheter without a needle, or a commercial device as your delivery device.

  - Lubricate the end of the delivery device with a water-soluble gel, and gently insert it approximately $1''$ to $1\frac{1}{2}''$ into the rectum **Figure 41**.
  - Instruct the patient to relax and not to bear down.
  - With a *needleless* syringe, gently push the medication through the tube.
  - Once the medication has been delivered, remove and dispose of the tube or syringe in an appropriate container.

8. Monitor the patient's condition, and document the medication given, route, time of administration, and response of the patient.

Follow these steps to administer a drug via the rectal route:

1. Take standard precautions.
2. Determine the need for the medication based on patient presentation.
3. Obtain a history, including any drug allergies.
4. Follow standing orders, or contact medical control for permission.
5. Determine the appropriate dose, and check that the medication is the right medication, there is no cloudiness or discoloration, and the expiration date has not passed.
6. When you are inserting a suppository, use a water-soluble gel for lubrication. Insert the suppository into the rectum

Words of Wisdom

Diazepam (Valium) is available in a specially designed container, which is marketed under the name Diastat. The distal end of the container is tapered, which facilitates insertion into the rectum. This feature eliminates the need for syringes or other methods of injecting the medication into the rectum. This is a commonly prescribed medication for children with seizures.

◾ Parenteral Medication Administration

The **parenteral route** refers to any route other than the gastrointestinal tract. Parenteral routes for medication administration include the intradermal, subcutaneous, intramuscular, intravenous, intraosseous, and percutaneous routes. Compared with enterally administered medications (eg, oral, gastric tube), parenterally administered medications are absorbed into the central circulation more quickly and at a more predictable rate, thus achieving their therapeutic effects faster. Of the parenteral drug routes, IV administration is the route most commonly used in the prehospital setting and generally is the quickest route for getting medication into the central circulation.

◾ Syringes and Needles

A variety of needles and syringes are used for administering parenteral medications. Many syringes come prepackaged with a needle already attached. The needles and syringes may also be packaged separately. Syringes consist of a plunger, body or barrel, flange, and tip **Figure 42**. Most syringes are marked with 10 calibrations per milliliter on one side of the barrel, where each small line represents 0.1 mL; the other side of the barrel is marked in minims. Syringes vary from 1 mL to 60 mL; the 3-mL syringe is the one most commonly used for injections. Syringe selection is based on the volume of medication that you will administer **Figure 43**.

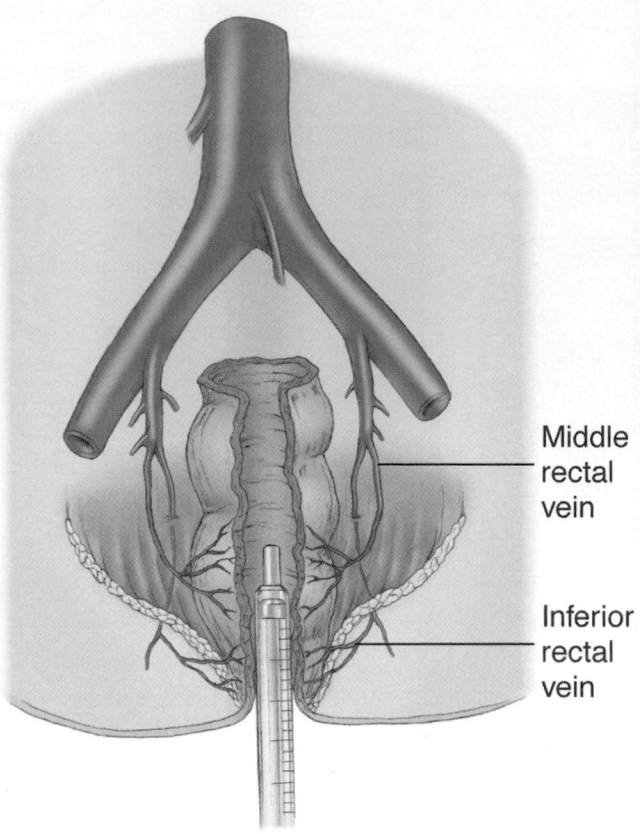

Figure 40 The rectal mucosa is highly vascular. It rapidly and predictably absorbs medications.

Middle
rectal
vein

Inferior
rectal
vein

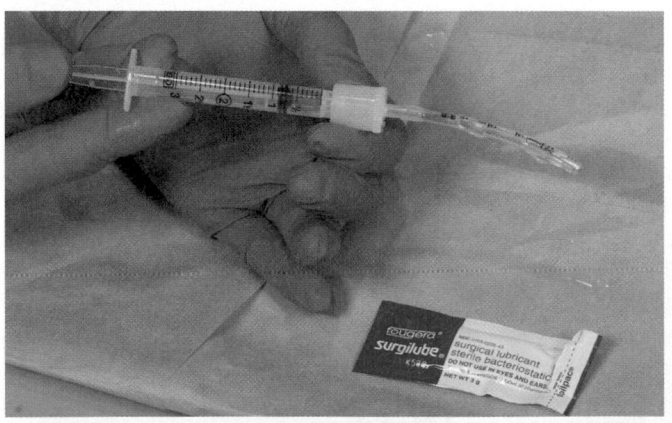

Figure 41 Syringe attached to an endotracheal tube.

Hypodermic needle lengths vary from $\frac{3}{8}''$ to $2''$ for standard injections. As with IV catheters, the gauge of the needle refers to the diameter: The smaller the number, the larger the diameter. Common needle gauges range from 18 to 26. The needle gauge used depends on the route of parenteral medication administration. Smaller-gauge needles, for example, are used for

subcutaneous injections, whereas larger-gauge needles are used for intramuscular and IV injections.

The proximal end of the needle, or hub, attaches to the standard fitting on the syringe. The distal end of the needle is beveled.

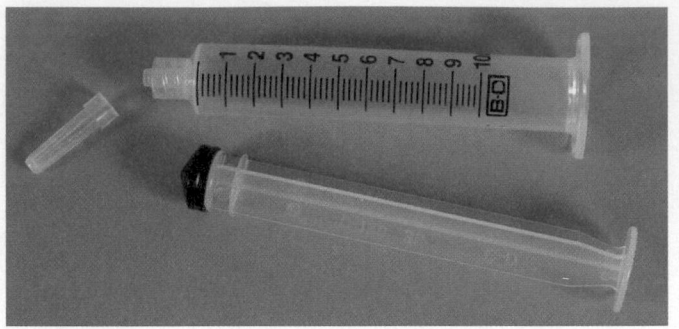

Figure 42 A syringe consists of a plunger, body or barrel, flange, and tip.

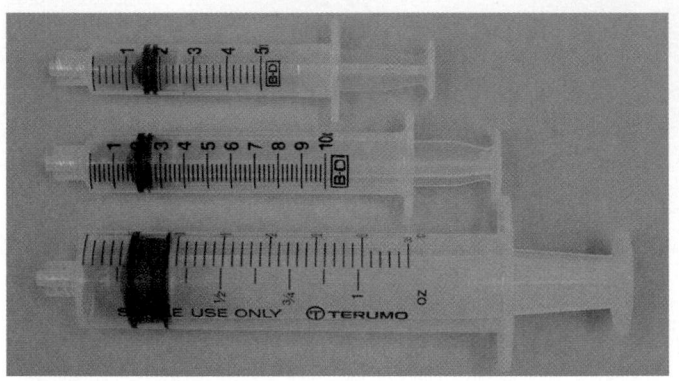

Figure 43 Syringes come in a variety of sizes. Some come with needles already attached, others without needles attached.

Packaging of Parenteral Medications

Ampules

Ampules are breakable sterile glass containers that are designed to carry a single dose of medication **Figure 44**. They may contain as little as 1 mL or as much as 10 mL, depending on the medication.

When you are drawing a medication from an ampule, follow the steps in Skill Drill 5:

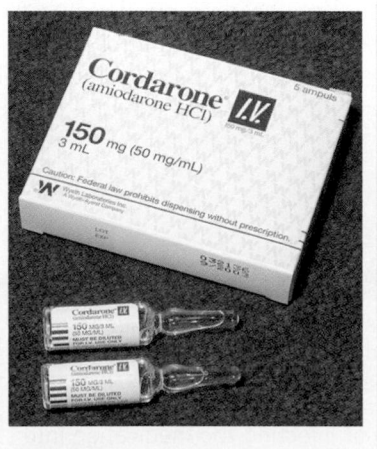

Figure 44 Medication stored in ampules.

Skill Drill 5

1. Check the medication to be sure that the expiration date has not passed and that it is the correct drug and concentration.

2. Shake the medication into the base of the ampule. If some of the drug is stuck in the neck, gently thump or tap the stem (Step 1).

3. Using a 4″ × 4″ gauze pad, an alcohol prep, or an ampule breaker, grip the neck of the ampule and snap it off where the ampule is scored. If the ampule is not scored and an attempt is made to break it, some sharp edges may be present. Drop the stem in the sharps container (Step 2).

4. Insert a filtered needle into the ampule without touching the outer sides of the ampule. Draw the solution into the syringe, and dispose of the ampule in the sharps container (Step 3).

5. Hold the syringe with the needle pointing up, and gently tap the barrel to loosen air trapped inside and cause it to rise (Step 4). Press gently on the plunger to dispel any air bubbles (Step 5).

6. Recap the needle using the one-handed method. Dispose of the needle in the sharps container and attach a standard hypodermic needle to the syringe if necessary to administer the medication.

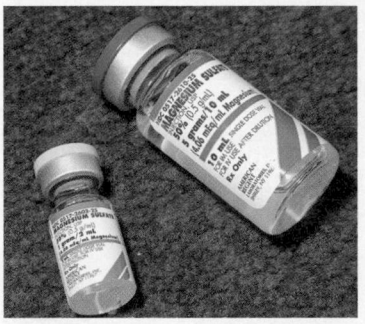

Figure 45 Vials (single-dose and multidose).

Vials

Vials are small glass or plastic bottles with a rubber-stopper top; they may contain single or multiple doses of a medication **Figure 45**. When you are using a vial of medication, you must first determine how much of the drug you will need and how many doses are in the vial.

For a single-dose vial, you may draw up the entire amount in the vial. For multiple-dose vials, you should draw up only the amount needed. Remember that once you remove the cover from a vial, it is no longer sterile. If you need a second dose, clean the top of the vial with alcohol before withdrawing the medication.

Some medications that are stored in vials may need to be reconstituted, such as methylprednisolone sodium succinate (Solu-Medrol) and glucagon. Glucagon is stored in two vials, one with the powdered form of the drug and the other with sterile

Skill Drill 5

Drawing Medication From an Ampule

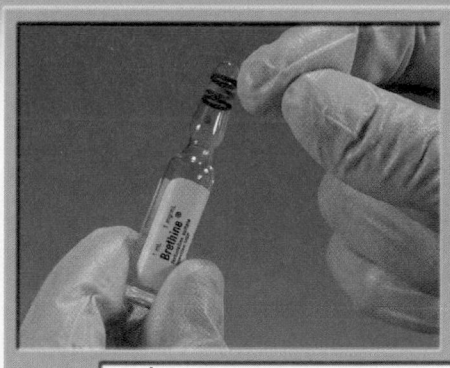

Step 1 Gently tap the stem of the ampule to shake medication into the base.

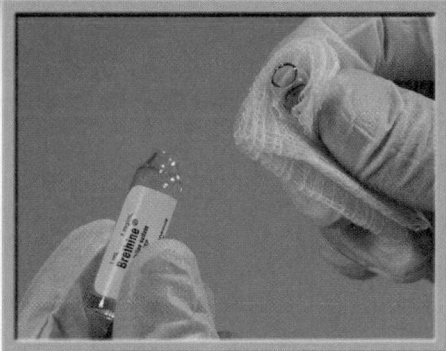

Step 2 Grip the neck of the ampule using a 4″ × 4″ gauze pad, and snap the neck off.

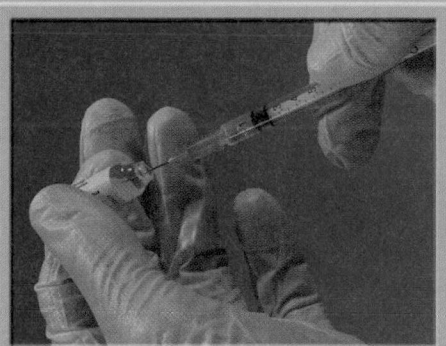

Step 3 Without touching the outer sides of the ampule, insert the needle into the medication in the ampule, and draw the solution into the syringe.

Continues

Skill Drill   5

Drawing Medication From an Ampule, continued

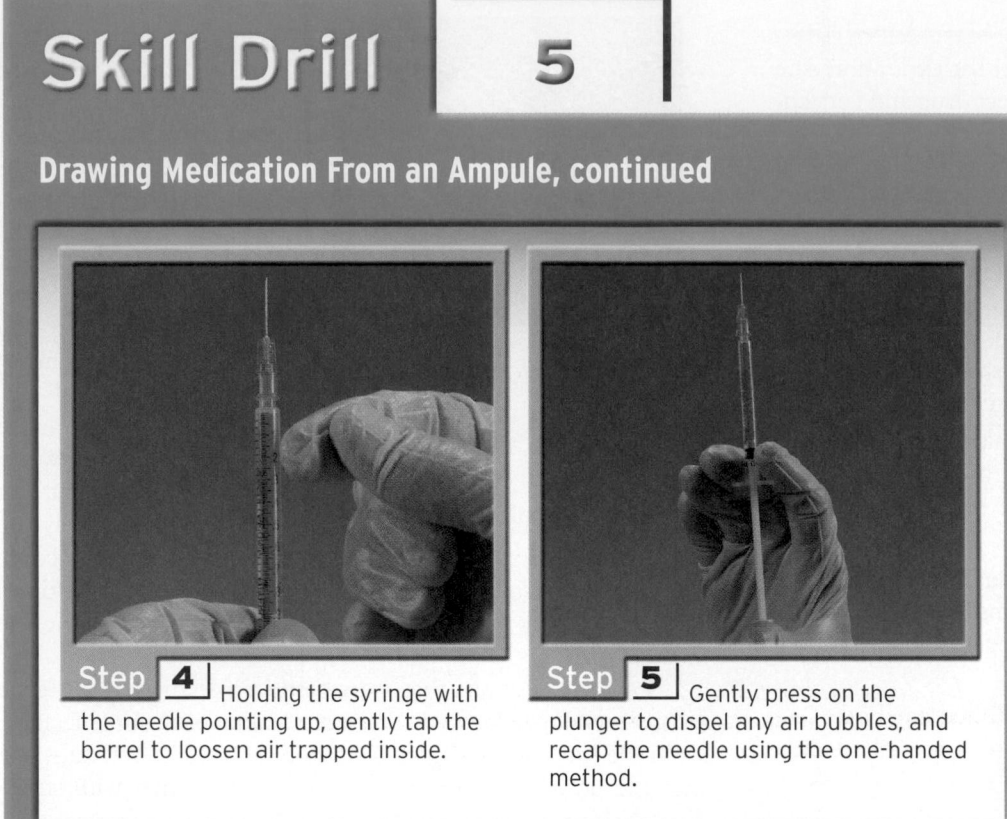

Step 4 Holding the syringe with the needle pointing up, gently tap the barrel to loosen air trapped inside.

Step 5 Gently press on the plunger to dispel any air bubbles, and recap the needle using the one-handed method.

3. Wipe the vial rubber top with an alcohol prep before touching it with the needle. Determine the amount of medication that you will need, and draw that amount of air into the syringe (Step 2). Allow a little extra room to expel some air while removing air bubbles.

4. Invert the vial, clean the rubber stopper with an alcohol prep, and insert the needle through the rubber stopper into the medication. Expel the air in the syringe into the vial and then withdraw the amount of medication needed (Step 3).

5. Once you have the correct amount of medication in the syringe, withdraw the needle from the vial and expel any air in the syringe (Step 4).

6. Recap the needle using the one-handed method (Step 5). Label the syringe if it is not immediately given to the patient.

water. **Drug reconstitution** involves injecting the sterile water (or provided **diluent**) from one vial into the vial that contains the powder, thereby making a solution for injection. To reconstitute the contents of two vials, draw the fluid out of the first vial and inject it into the vial that contains the powder. Shake the vial vigorously to mix the medication before drawing out the contents for administration.

Methylprednisolone sodium succinate is stored in a **Mix-o-Vial**, a single vial divided into two compartments by a rubber stopper (Figure 46). To reconstitute a drug that is contained in a Mix-o-Vial, squeeze the two vials together, which releases the center stopper and allows the contents to mix. Shake vigorously to mix the contents before drawing out the medication.

When you are drawing medication from a vial, follow the steps in Skill Drill 6.

Skill Drill   6

1. Check the medication to be sure that the expiration date has not passed and that it is the correct drug and concentration (Step 1).

2. Remove the sterile cover, or clean the top with alcohol if the vial was previously opened.

Words of Wisdom

Whenever you use a needle to draw up medication from an ampule or vial, to avoid sticking yourself, hold the syringe against your palm with the needle pointing up and draw the ampule or vial down onto the needle using the thumb and forefinger of the palm the syringe is braced against. This especially applies if you are in a moving ambulance.

Prefilled Syringes

Prefilled syringes are packaged in tamper proof boxes. Two types of prefilled syringes exist: those that are separated into a glass drug cartridge and a syringe (Figure 47), and preassembled prefilled syringes (Figure 48). These syringes are designed for ease of use. After all, it is much easier and quicker to use a prefilled syringe when you are treating a patient in cardiac arrest than it is to draw up each individual dose. It is important to remember that with many drug cartridge and syringe systems, both pieces of the assembly may contain sharps and should be disposed of properly. In cases where the medication is too large to fit into a standard sharps container, the medication should be handled with care and disposed of either at the receiving facility's larger sharps container, or at the station in a larger sharps container.

Skill Drill 6

Drawing Medication From a Vial

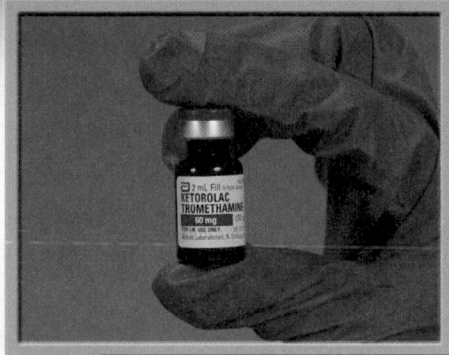

Step 1 Check the medication and its expiration date.

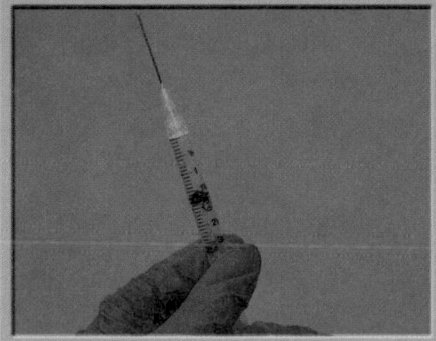

Step 2 Wipe the vial rubber top with an alcohol prep before touching it with the needle. Determine the amount of medication needed, and draw that amount of air into the syringe.

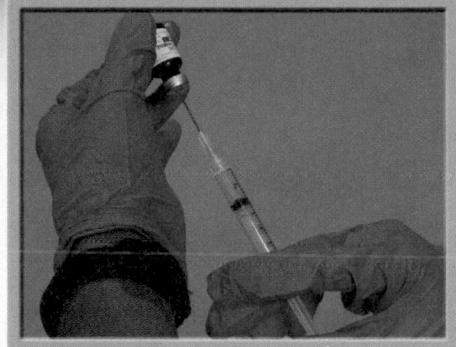

Step 3 Invert the vial, and insert the needle through the rubber stopper. Expel the air in the syringe into the vial, and then withdraw the amount of medication needed.

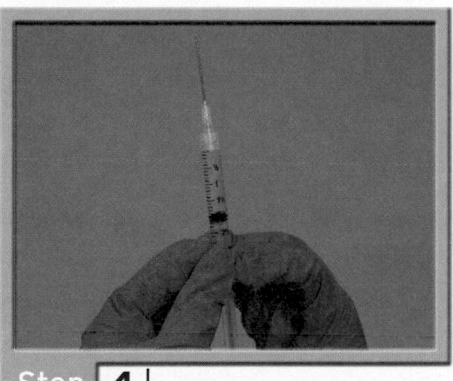

Step 4 Withdraw the needle, and expel any air in the syringe.

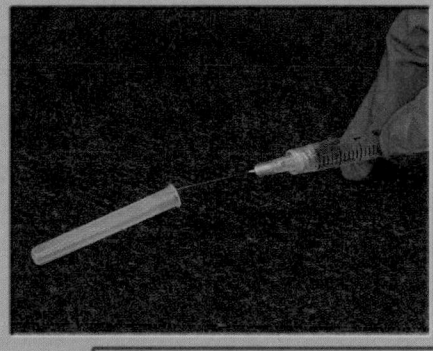

Step 5 Recap the needle using the one-handed method. Label the syringe if the medication is not immediately given to the patient.

To assemble the two-part prefilled syringe, pop the yellow caps off of the syringe and the drug cartridge, insert the drug cartridge into the barrel of the syringe, and screw them together. Remove the needle cover, and expel air in the manner previously described. Follow the steps for the route by which the medication is to be given.

Single-dose disposable medication cartridges that are inserted into a reusable syringe are also available. These syringes are commonly referred to by their brand name of Tubex, Aboject, and Carpuject syringes **Figure 49** .

■ Intradermal Medication Administration

<u>Intradermal</u> injections involve administering a small amount of medication—typically less than 1 mL—into the dermal layer, just beneath the epidermis. The technique involves the use of a 1-mL syringe (for example, a tuberculin syringe) and a 25- to 27-gauge, $\frac{3}{8}''$ to $1''$ needle.

When you are selecting a site for an intradermal injection, you should avoid areas that contain superficial blood vessels to minimize the risk of systemic medication absorption. Because

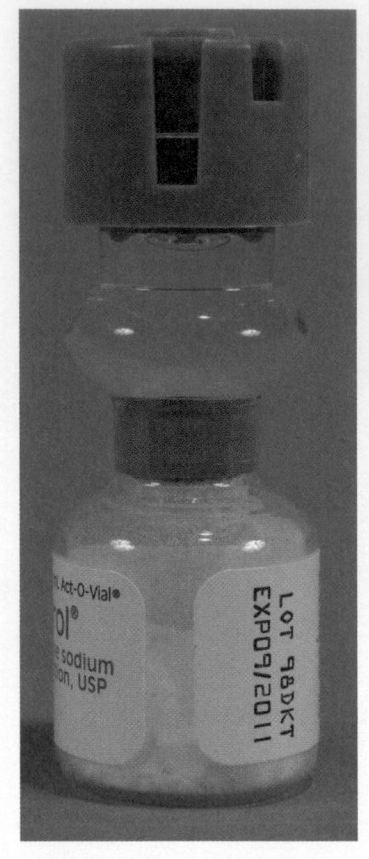

Figure 46 A Mix-o-Vial.

of their high visibility and relative lack of hair, the most common anatomic locations for intradermal injections are the anterior forearm and upper back.

Medications administered intradermally have a slow rate of absorption; there is minimal to no systemic distribution. The medication remains locally collected at the site of the injection. Unless you are anesthetizing the skin before establishing an IV line, you will rarely use the intradermal route to administer medications in the prehospital setting. Instead, these injections are typically given in a physician's office or in the hospital to test a patient for allergies or to perform a PPD (purified protein derivative)—a skin test for tuberculosis.

Follow these steps to administer a medication via the intradermal route:

1. Take standard precautions.
2. Determine the need for the medication based on patient presentation.
3. Obtain a history, including any drug allergies and vital signs.

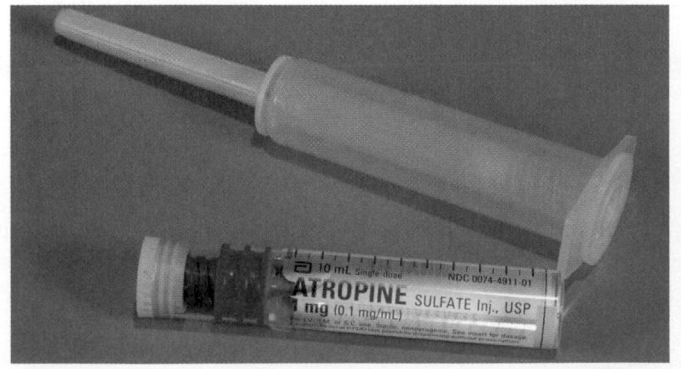

Figure 47 Two-part prefilled syringes are separated into a glass drug cartridge and a syringe (for example, Bristojet).

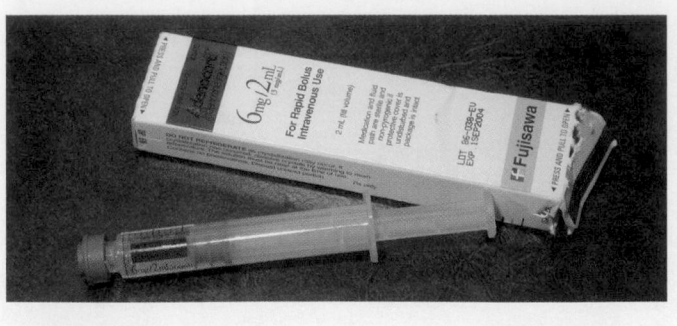

Figure 48 Preassembled prefilled syringe.

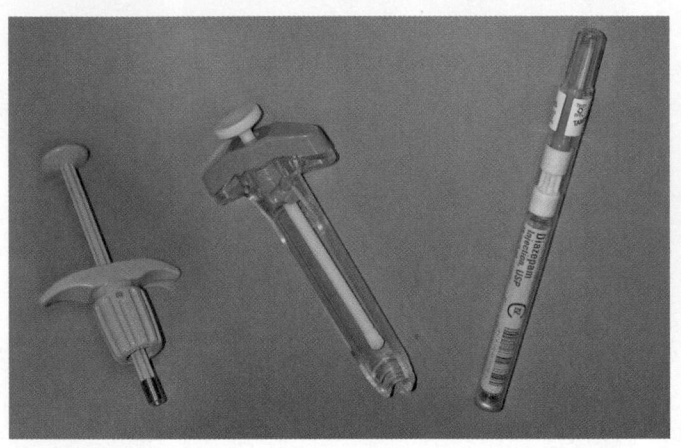

Figure 49 Reusable syringes (left). Disposable medication cartridge (right).

4. Follow standing orders, or contact medical control for permission.
5. Check the medication to ensure that it is the correct one, that it is not cloudy or discolored, and that the expiration date has not passed, and determine the appropriate amount to give for the correct dose.
6. Advise the patient of potential discomfort while explaining the procedure.
7. Assemble and check equipment needed: alcohol preps and a 1-mL syringe with a 25- to 27-gauge, $\frac{3}{8}''$ or $1''$ needle. Draw up the correct dose of medication.
8. Cleanse the area for administration using aseptic technique.
9. Pull the skin taut with your nondominant hand.
10. Insert the needle at a 10° to 15° angle with the bevel up.
11. Slowly inject the medication while observing for the formation of a wheal, or small bump, which indicates that the medication is collecting in the intradermal tissue.
12. Remove the needle. Immediately dispose of the needle and syringe in the sharps container.

13. Monitor the patient's condition, and document the medication given, route, administration time, and response of the patient.

Subcutaneous Medication Administration

Subcutaneous (SC) injections are given into the loose connective tissue between the dermis and the muscle layer Figure 50. Volumes of a drug administered subcutaneously are usually 1 mL or less. The injection is performed using a 24- to 26-gauge 1/2″ to 1″ needle. Common sites for SC injections—in both adults and children—include the upper arms, anterior thighs, and the abdomen Figure 51. Patients who take insulin injections usually vary the sites owing to the multiple (usually daily) injections they require.

Follow the steps in Skill Drill 7 to administer a medication via the subcutaneous route:

Skill Drill 7

1. Take standard precautions.
2. Determine the need for the medication based on patient presentation.
3. Obtain a history, including any drug allergies and vital signs.
4. Follow standing orders, or contact medical control for permission.
5. Check the medication to ensure that it is the correct one, that it is not cloudy or discolored, and that the expiration date has not passed, and determine the appropriate amount and concentration for the correct dose Step 1.

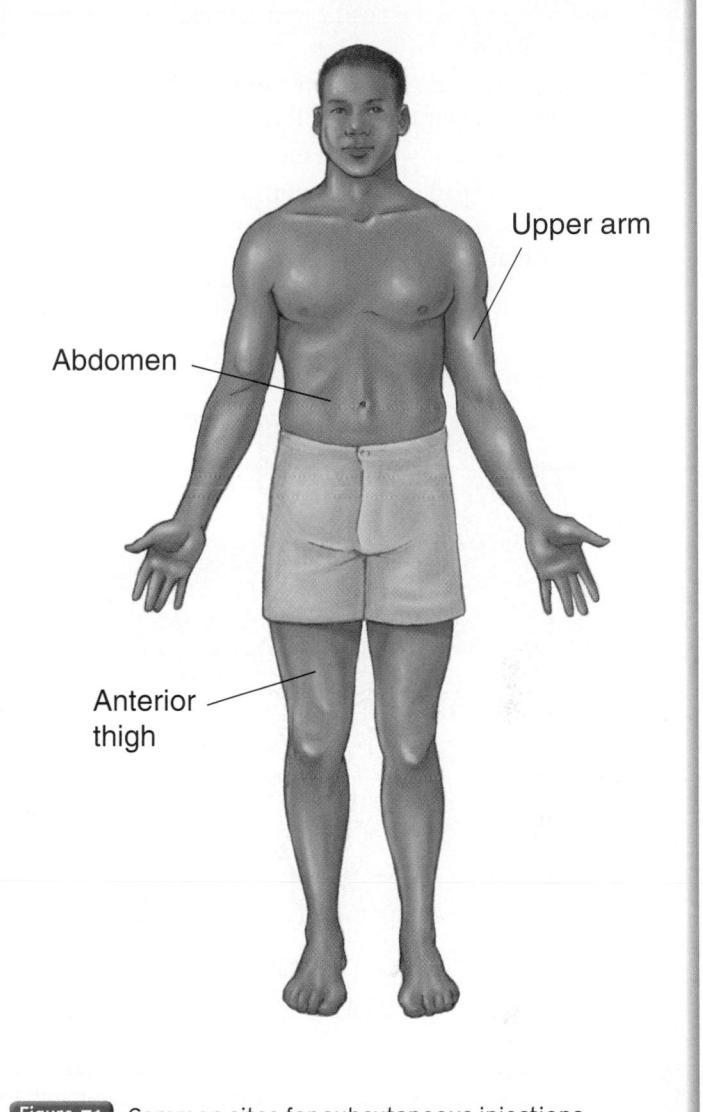

Figure 51 Common sites for subcutaneous injections.

6. Advise the patient of potential discomfort while explaining the procedure.
7. Assemble and check equipment needed: alcohol preps and a 3-mL syringe with a 24- to 26-gauge needle. Draw up the correct dose of medication Step 2.
8. Cleanse the area for the administration (usually the upper arm or thigh) using aseptic technique Step 3.
9. Pinch the skin surrounding the area, advise the patient of a stick, and insert the needle at a 45° angle.

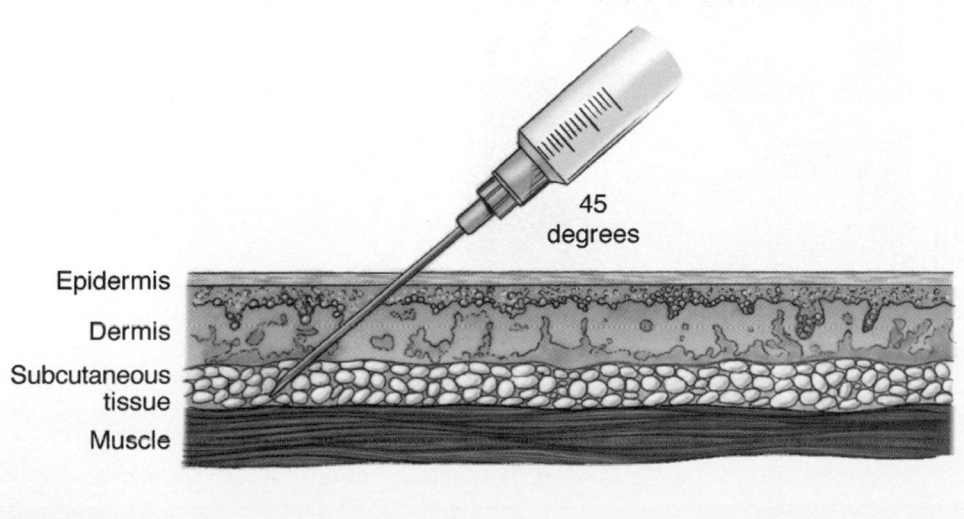

Figure 50 A subcutaneous injection is below the dermis and above the muscle.

10. Inject the medication and remove the needle. Immediately dispose of the needle and syringe in the sharps container (Step 4).

11. To disperse the medication through the tissue, rub the area in a circular motion with your gloved hand.

12. Properly store any unused medication.

13. Monitor the patient's condition, and document the medication given, route, administration time, and response of the patient (Step 5).

■ Intramuscular Medication Administration

Intramuscular (IM) injections are given by penetrating a needle through the dermis and subcutaneous tissue and into the muscle layer (Figure 52). This technique allows administration of a larger volume of medication (up to 5 mL) than the subcutaneous route. Because there is also the potential for damage to nerves due to the depth of the injection, it is important to choose the appropriate site. Common anatomic sites for IM injections for adults and children include the following:

Skill Drill   7

Administering Medication via the Subcutaneous Route

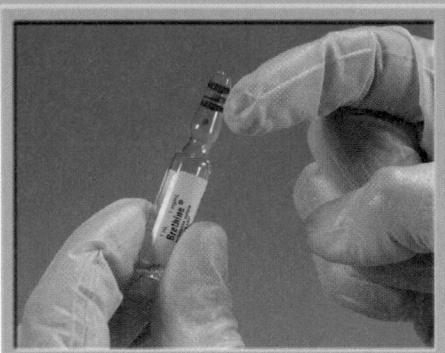

Step 1 Check the medication to ensure that it is the correct one, that it is not discolored, and that the expiration date has not passed.

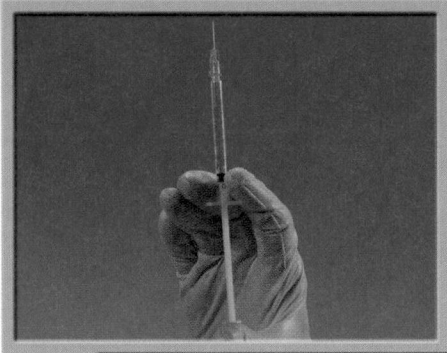

Step 2 Assemble and check the equipment. Draw up the correct dose of medication.

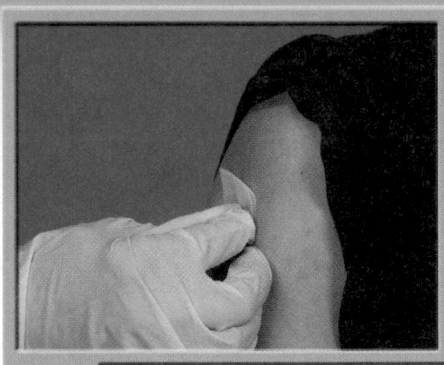

Step 3 Using aseptic technique, cleanse the injection area.

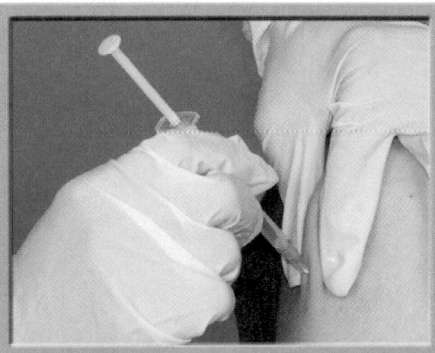

Step 4 Pinch the skin surrounding the area, and insert the needle at a 45° angle. Inject the medication, remove the needle, and hold pressure over the area. Immediately dispose of the needle and syringe in the sharps container.

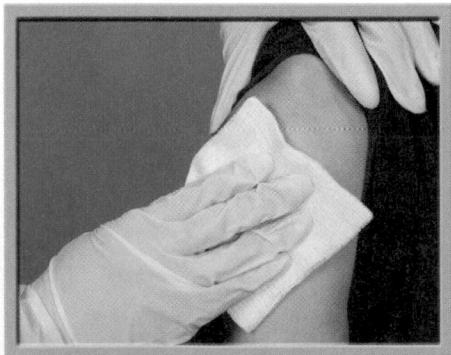

Step 5 To disperse the medication, rub the area in a circular motion. Monitor the patient's condition.

- **Vastus lateralis muscle**—the large muscle on the lateral side of the thigh.
- **Rectus femoris muscle**—the large muscle on the anterior side of the thigh.
- **Gluteal area**—the buttocks, specifically the upper lateral aspect of either side. When injecting into the gluteal area, you should use the upper, outer quadrant to avoid the sciatic nerve.
- **Deltoid muscle**—the muscle of the upper arm that covers the prominence of the shoulder. The site for injection is approximately $1\frac{1}{2}''$ to $2''$ below the acromion process on the lateral side Figure 53.

Follow the steps in Skill Drill 8 to administer a medication via the intramuscular route:

Skill Drill 8

1. Take standard precautions.
2. Determine the need for the medication based on patient presentation.
3. Obtain a history, including any drug allergies and vital signs.
4. Follow standing orders, or contact medical control for permission.
5. Check the medication to ensure that it is the correct one, that it is not cloudy or discolored, and that the expiration date has not passed, and determine the appropriate amount and concentration for the correct dose.
6. Advise the patient of potential discomfort while explaining the procedure.
7. Assemble and check equipment needed: alcohol preps and a 3- to 5-mL syringe with a 21-gauge, $1''$ or $2''$ needle. Draw up the correct dose of medication Step 1.
8. Cleanse the area for administration (usually the upper arm or the hip) using aseptic technique Step 2.
9. Stretch the skin over the cleansed area, advise the patient of a stick, and insert the needle at a 90° angle.
10. Pull back on the plunger to aspirate for blood. The presence of blood in the syringe indicates you may have entered a blood vessel. In such a case, remove the needle, and hold pressure over the site. Discard the syringe and needle in the sharps container. Prepare a new syringe and needle, and select another site.

11. If there is no blood in the syringe, inject the medication and remove the needle Step 3. Immediately dispose of the needle and syringe in the sharps container.
12. Store any unused medication properly.
13. Monitor the patient's condition, and document the medication given, route, administration time, and response of the patient Step 4.

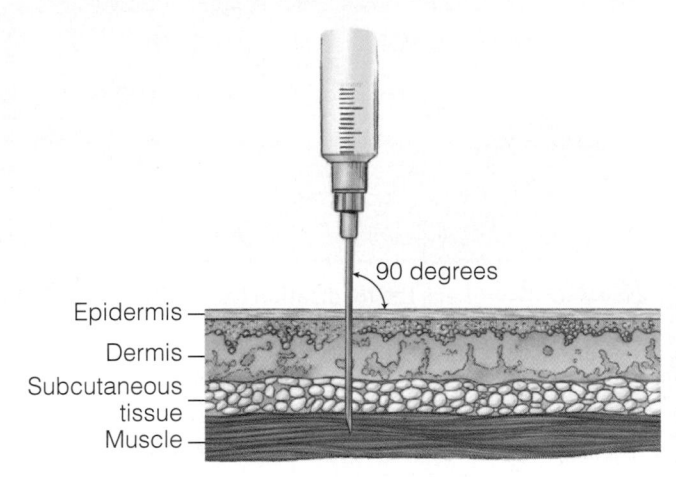

Figure 52 An intramuscular injection is below the dermis and subcutaneous layer and into the muscle.

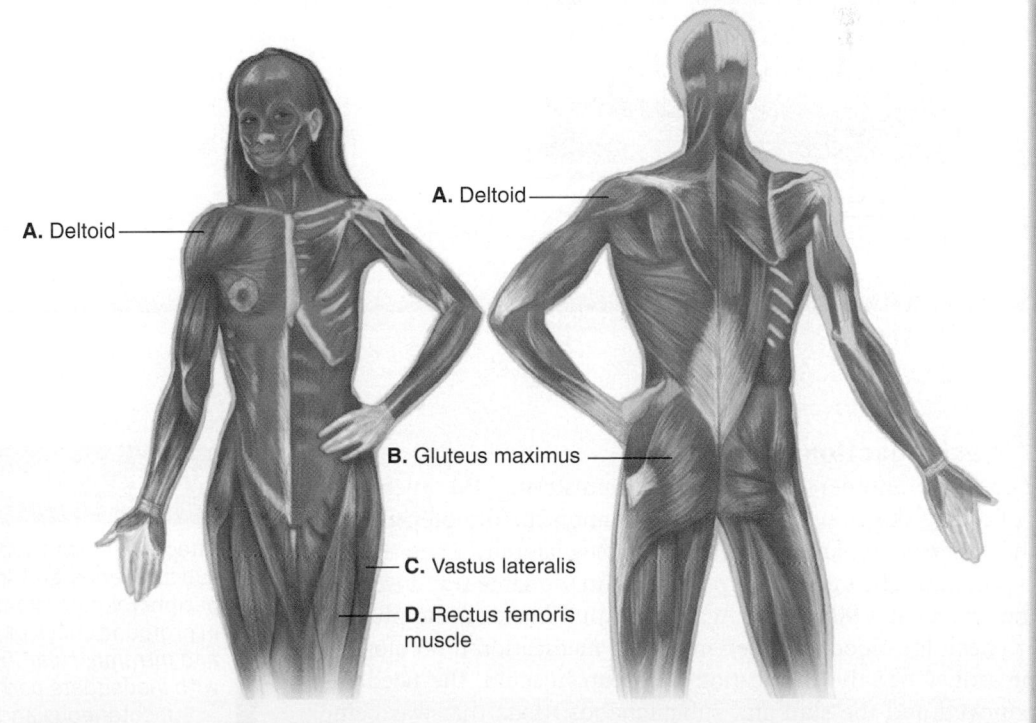

Figure 53 Common sites for intramuscular injections. **A.** Deltoid muscle. **B.** Gluteal area. **C.** Vastus lateralis muscle. **D.** Rectus femoris muscle.

Skill Drill 8

Administering Medication via the Intramuscular Route

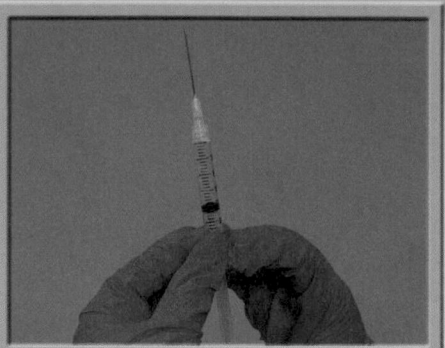

Step 1 Check the medication to ensure that it is the correct one, that it is not discolored, and that its expiration date has not passed. Assemble and check the equipment. Draw up the correct dose of medication.

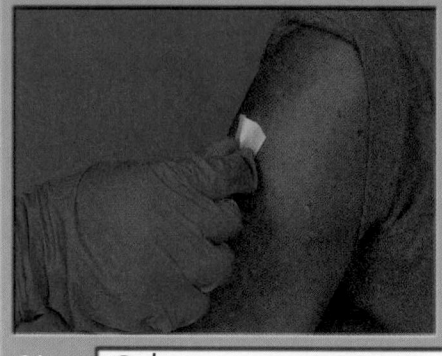

Step 2 Using aseptic technique, cleanse the injection area.

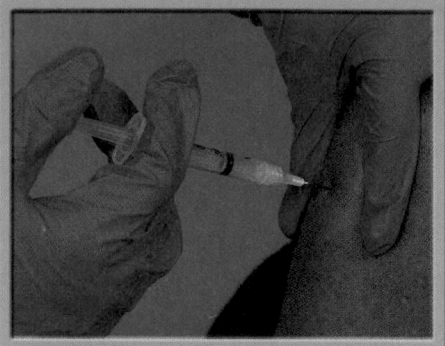

Step 3 Stretch the skin over the area, and insert the needle at a 90° angle. Pull back on the plunger to aspirate for blood. If there is no blood, inject the medication and remove the needle.

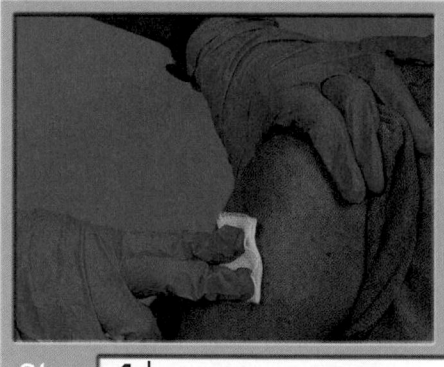

Step 4 Monitor the patient's condition.

Z-Track Injections

Z-track is another method for administering IM injections. Following the steps for IM administration, before Step 8, pull the patient's skin and subcutaneous tissue laterally. Then the site is prepped. The injection is performed in the same way, inserting the needle at a 90° angle. Again, you pull back on the plunger to check for blood and then inject the medication if no blood is present. Once the medication has been injected, the needle is removed and the skin and subcutaneous tissue that was being held is released. By displacing the skin initially and allowing it to come back into place, you allow the skin and subcutaneous tissue to seal in the medication, which minimizes leakage.

Words of Wisdom

Effective absorption of medications administered by the subcutaneous and intramuscular routes requires adequate peripheral perfusion. This is clearly not the case in patients in profound shock or cardiac arrest. Therefore, *subcutaneous and intramuscular injections should not be given to patients with inadequate perfusion* unless no other options exist.

Subcutaneous and intramuscular injections should not be given into skin that is hardened, bruised, red, or otherwise discolored, or stained.

IV Bolus Medication Administration

The IV route places the drug directly into the circulatory system. It is the fastest route of medication administration because it bypasses most barriers to drug absorption. As a result, *there is no room for error with IV administration.* (See "Potential Complications of IV Therapy" earlier in this chapter for details on what can go wrong.) Drugs are administered by direct injection with a needle and syringe into an established peripheral IV line. Many services now use needleless systems to provide protection against needlesticks. When you are using a needleless system, the syringe simply screws into the injection port of the administration set (IV tubing). If a needleless port is punctured with a needle, the system will leak This will require you to switch out the administration set to a new one. If this is a critical situation and time does not warrant you the ability switch out the drip set, you can provide a "temporary patch" on the system by placing a syringe filled with saline on the needleless port.

A **bolus** is a single dose, usually given by the IV route. When given in one mass, it may consist of a small or large quantity of a drug and can be given rapidly or slowly, depending on the drug. Some medications, such as lidocaine and amiodarone, require an initial bolus and then may require a continuous IV infusion to maintain a therapeutic level of the drug. Some medications can have devastating effects if given too fast. For example, promethazine can cause an extreme burning sensation if given too fast. Furosemide may cause tinnitus if given rapidly. Other medications may be ineffective if they are given too slowly. For example, adenosine has a half-life of 10 seconds and will be ineffective if it does not reach the heart in that time frame.

Follow the steps in **Skill Drill 9** when you are administering a medication via the IV bolus route:

Skill Drill   9

1. Take standard precautions.
2. Determine the need for the medication based on patient presentation.
3. Obtain a history, including any drug allergies and vital signs.
4. Follow standing orders, or contact medical control for permission.
5. Check the medication to ensure that it is the correct one, that it is not cloudy or discolored, and that the expiration date has not passed, and determine the appropriate amount and concentration for the correct dose.
6. Explain the procedure to the patient and the need for the medication.
7. Assemble needed equipment, and draw up the medication. Expel any air in the syringe. Draw up 20 mL of normal saline to use as a flush for the medication.

YOU *are the Medic*   PART 4

The physician confirms your order for fentanyl 50-μg IV push and a 500-mL normal saline fluid bolus over 10 minutes. You administer the pain medication and immobilize her leg. You retake her vital signs and carefully load her onto the stretcher and into ambulance. The patient states that her pain is now 6 out of 10, which is a decrease from the original 9.

You begin transport to the hospital and have administered 250 mL of normal saline. You administer another 50 μg of fentanyl and retake her vital signs. The patient states a few minutes later that the pain is 4 out of 10 and her dizziness is starting to resolve. You place the patient on a heart monitor, and a 4-lead ECG reads sinus tachycardia.

Recording Time: 10 Minutes	
Respirations	24 breaths/min
Pulse	120 beats/min
Skin	Flushed and diaphoretic
Blood pressure	90/40 mm Hg
Oxygen saturation (Spo$_2$)	100%
Pupils	PEARRL
ECG	Sinus tachycardia

You arrive at the hospital and have finished administering the 500-mL fluid bolus. The patient reports total relief of light-headedness, and her blood pressure is within normal limits. Her IV line is still patent and in place.

7. You need to administer 50 μg of fentanyl and it comes in an ampule of 100 μg in 2 mL of fluid. How much would you administer?
8. The order was for a 500-mL fluid bolus over 10 minutes. If using a 10-drop set, how many drops per minute would this be?

8. Cleanse the injection port with alcohol, or remove the protective cap if using the needleless system (Step 1).

9. Insert the needle into the port, and pinch off the IV tubing proximal to the administration port. Failure to shut off the line will result in the medication taking the pathway of least resistance and flowing into the bag instead of into the patient.

10. Administer the correct dose of the medication at the appropriate rate. Some medications must be administered quickly, whereas others must be pushed slowly to prevent adverse effects (Step 2).

11. Place the needle and syringe into the sharps container.

12. Unclamp the IV line to flush the medication into the vein. Allow it to run briefly wide open, or flush with a 20-mL bolus of normal saline.

13. Readjust the IV flow rate to the original setting (Step 3).

14. Properly store and label any unused medication.

15. Monitor the patient's condition, and document the medication given, route, time of administration, and response of the patient.

As discussed earlier in this chapter, saline locks are used for patients who are not in need of IV fluid boluses but may need medication therapy. Follow these steps to administer a medication through a saline lock:

1. Take standard precautions.
2. Determine the need for the medication based on patient presentation.
3. Obtain a history, including any drug allergies and vital signs.
4. Follow standing orders, or contact medical control for permission.
5. Check the medication to ensure that it is the correct one, that it is not cloudy or discolored, and that the expiration date has not passed, and determine the appropriate amount and concentration for the correct dose.
6. Explain the procedure to the patient and the need for the medication.
7. Assemble needed equipment, and draw up the medication. Draw up 20 mL of normal saline to use as a flush for the medication.
8. Cleanse the injection port with alcohol, or remove the protective cap if using the needleless system.
9. Insert the needle into the port while holding it carefully, or screw the syringe onto the port. Clamp off the IV tubing proximally to prevent backflow into the IV solution.
10. Pull back slightly on the syringe plunger, and observe for blood return. If blood appears, slowly inject the medication, watching for infiltration. If resistance is felt, or if the patient reports any discomfort, discontinue administration immediately. A new site will need to be established.

Skill Drill 9

Administering Medication via the Intravenous Bolus Route

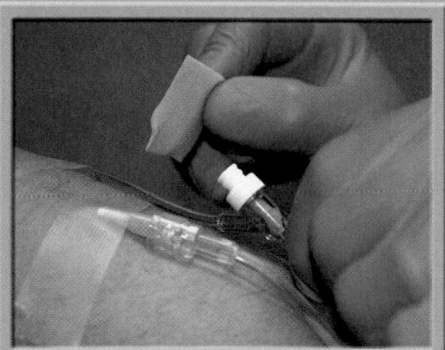

Step 1 Check that the medication is correct, ensure that it is not cloudy or discolored, and check the expiration date. Determine the appropriate dose. Explain the procedure to the patient. Assemble and check the equipment. Cleanse the injection port, or remove the protective cap if using the needleless system.

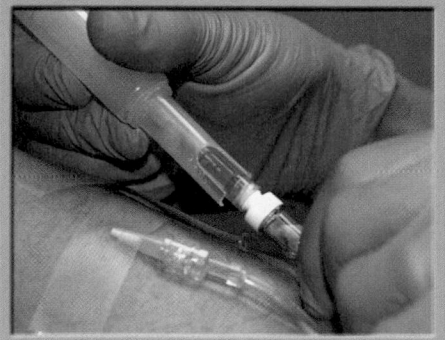

Step 2 Insert the needle into the port, or attach the needleless syringe to the port. Pinch off the IV tubing proximal to the administration port. Administer the correct dose at the appropriate rate.

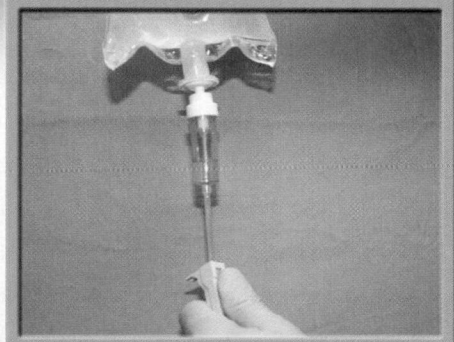

Step 3 Unclamp the IV line to flush the medication into the vein, allowing it to run briefly wide open, or flush with a 20-mL bolus of normal saline. Readjust the IV flow rate to the original setting, and monitor the patient's condition.

11. Place the needle and syringe into the sharps container.

12. Clean the port, and insert the needle with the syringe containing the flush.

13. Flush the saline lock, and place the needle in the sharps container.

14. Store any unused medication properly.

15. Monitor the patient's condition, and document the medication given, route, time of administration, and response of the patient.

Adding Medication to an IV Bag

Certain medications are added to the IV solution itself to be administered as a maintenance infusion—for example, dopamine, lidocaine, and epinephrine. All of these medications require careful titration to achieve the desired effect.

The steps for adding medication to an IV bag are as follows:

1. Check the fluid in the IV bag for clarity or discoloration, and ensure that the expiration date has not passed.

2. Check the drug name on the ampule, vial, or prefilled syringe. Check the concentration of the drug it contains (for example, µg/mL or mg/mL).

3. Compute the volume of the drug to be added to the IV bag. Draw up that amount in a syringe (if a prefilled syringe is used, note the proportion of the volume of the syringe required).

4. Cleanse the medication injection port on the IV bag with an alcohol swab.

5. Inject the desired volume of medication into the IV bag by puncturing the rubber stopper on the medication injection port **Figure 54**.

6. Withdraw the needle, and dispose of the needle and syringe in the sharps container. Agitate the IV bag gently to ensure that the added drug is well mixed in the solution.

7. Label the IV bag with the name of the medication added, the amount added, the concentration of medication in the IV bag (for example, µg/mL or mg/mL), the date and time, and your name.

8. Attach the IV administration set, and prepare the IV bag as discussed earlier in this chapter.

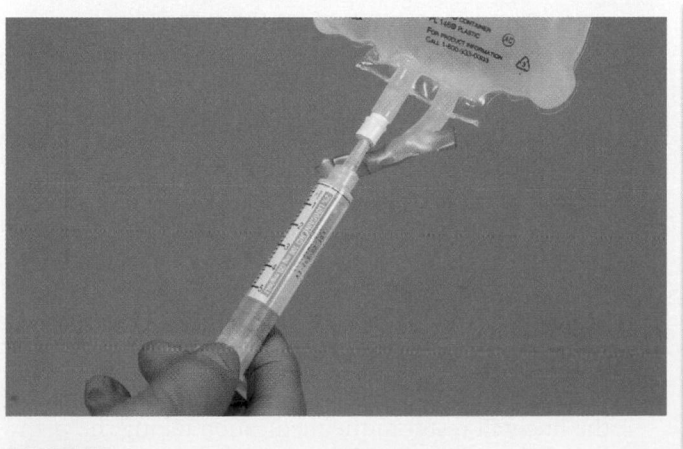

Figure 54 Adding medication to an IV bag.

Words of Wisdom

Medications that are used for maintenance infusions (for example, lidocaine and dopamine) are commonly premixed and prepackaged, which eliminates the need to calculate and draw up the appropriate amount of medication to add to the bag. However, you must still be aware of the concentration (for example, µg/mL or mg/mL) of the drug in the premixed solution and the appropriate maintenance infusion rate.

IV Piggyback

The IV administration set that is connected directly to the hub of the IV catheter is referred to as the primary line. This line is generally used to administer an isotonic solution. Saline is the preferred isotonic solution because it mixes with all medications in the prehospital and interfacility setting. When you are performing a continuous infusion, take the distal end of the drip set that is attached to the mixed medication and connect it to a port on the primary line. The line that is connected to the continuous infusion is referred to as a "piggyback" or secondary line. Multiple lines can be piggybacked onto a primary IV. When multiple lines are present on a patient, it is important to label the lines. This will ensure that when medications are administered en route, there are no medication interactions.

Electromechanical Infusion Pumps

When you are administering a medication maintenance infusion, you should use an electromechanical infusion pump, if available. The infusion pump can also be used to deliver IV fluid maintenance infusions in children and elderly patients to minimize the risk of a "runaway IV" and subsequent circulatory overload.

IV infusion pumps are used heavily in the hospital and during interfacility transports. They are sometimes used in the prehospital setting as well. IV infusion pumps have many advantages as well as several disadvantages. They are beneficial in the aspect that they deliver the rate that is set by the pump without deviating, and they calculate the amount of fluid that has been infused and the amount of fluid remaining. Some problems that can arise include a lack of uniformity among manufacturers. This makes it imperative for you to become familiar with the pumps used by your service. Pumps can also pose problems during transport because of air trapping in the lines that is detected by the pumps. When air is detected, the pump stops the infusion and an alarm sounds. This becomes problematic during transport when the ambulance travels over potholes, makes hard turns, and is exposed to other applied forces.

Electromechanical infusion pumps deliver fluids or medications via positive pressure. Although medications delivered in this manner can result in infiltration of a vein, most infusion pumps are equipped with an alarm that indicates a change in the flow pressure. Other common safety features include alarms that alert you to the presence of occlusion (eg, air in the tubing) or depletion of the medication. Some infusion pumps are designed to accommodate the IV tubing to regulate the flow of IV fluids or medications **Figure 55**, whereas others are designed to accommodate a needleless syringe **Figure 56**.

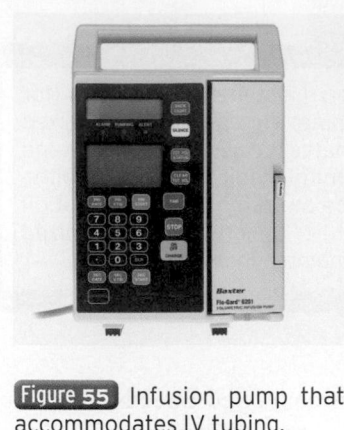

Figure 55 Infusion pump that accommodates IV tubing.

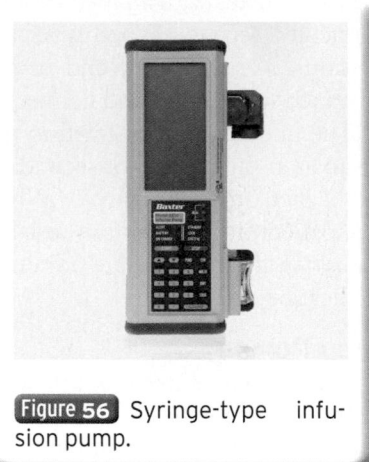

Figure 56 Syringe-type infusion pump.

You should become familiar with some of the terminology related to infusion pumps. Pumps may have multiple chambers for multiple medications. Each chamber can calculate one medication. If the number of medication lines outweighs the available chambers, it may be necessary to transport an isotonic fluid on gravity only. This means that your isotonic line will have the gtt/min set manually as opposed to being set by the pump. The rate is always established in mL/hour. Some IV pumps may have medication databases that will calculate the medication rate by the desired dose and the patient's weight as necessary. The volume to be infused (VTBI) is the amount of solution remaining to be infused. For example, if you were infusing 100 mL of amiodarone and 25 mL has already been infused, then 75 mL is your VTBI. The volume infused (VI) is the amount of solution that has already been administered, 25 mL as stated above. If your infusion pump does not perform medication calculations, this formula will help you determine the rate at which to set the pump:

Example:
Nitroglycerin drips are common interfacility medications for acute coronary syndrome and are being established in the prehospital setting in some areas. The doses range from 5 to 50 μg/min. This calculation will start at 5 μg/min. You have 25 mg in 250 mL.

Step 1: Determine the concentration.

$$25 \text{ mg} \times \frac{1,000 \text{ μg}}{\text{mg}} = 25,000 \text{ μg}$$
$$25,000 \text{ μg} \div 250 \text{ mL} = 100 \text{ μg/mL (concentration)}$$

Step 2: Determine the amount of volume to infuse per minute (mL/min).

For this calculation, you must recall the desired dose–in this case, 5 μg/min. To determine the number of mL/min, you perform the following calculation:

$$5 \text{ μg/min (desired dose)} \div 100 \text{ μg/mL (concentration)}$$
$$= 0.05 \text{ mL/min}$$

Step 3: Determine the rate and VTBI.

The rate can be established by multiplying the mL/min by 60.

$$\frac{0.05 \text{ mL}}{\text{min}} \times \frac{60 \text{ min}}{\text{h}} = 3 \text{ mL/h}$$

The VTBI for nitroglycerin as packaged above is 250 mL unless otherwise requested by medical control. Therefore, infuse this volume at 3 mL/h until it is administered, or until you arrive at the receiving facility.

■ IO Medication Administration

The IO route is used for critically ill or injured children and adults when IV access is difficult or impossible to obtain. Any fluid or medication that may be given through an IV line—bolus or maintenance infusion—can be given by the IO route. Shock, status epilepticus, and cardiac arrest are but a few of the reasons for establishing IO access. Unlike with an IV line, fluid does not flow well into the bone because of resistance; therefore, it is necessary to use a large syringe to infuse the fluid. A **pressure infuser device**— a sleeve placed around the IV bag and inflated to force fluid from the IV bag—should be used when infusing fluids in adults.

Complications of using the IO route are similar to those of the IV route. Along with the complications discussed earlier in this chapter, there is also the potential for compartment syndrome if fluid leaks outside the bone and into the osteofascial compartment.

Follow the steps in Skill Drill 10 to administer a medication via the IO route:

Skill Drill   10

1. Take standard precautions.
2. Determine the need for the medication based on patient presentation.
3. Obtain a history, including any drug allergies and vital signs.
4. Follow standing orders, or contact medical control for permission.
5. Check the medication to ensure that it is the correct one, that it is not cloudy or discolored, and that the expiration date has not passed, and determine the appropriate amount and concentration for the correct dose.
6. Explain the procedure to the patient and/or parent and the need for the medication.
7. Assemble needed equipment, and draw up the medication. Also draw up 20 mL of normal saline for a flush Step 1.
8. Cleanse the injection port of the extension tubing with alcohol, or remove the protective cap if using the needleless system Step 2.
9. Insert the needle into the port, and clamp off the IV tubing proximal to the administration port. This is usually managed with a three-way stopcock. Failure to shut off the line will result in the medication taking the pathway of least resistance and flowing into the bag instead of into the patient.

10. Administer the correct dose of the medication at the proper push rate. Some medications must be administered quickly, whereas others must be pushed slowly to prevent adverse effects (Step 3).

11. Place the needle and syringe into the sharps container.

12. Unclamp the IV line to flush the medication into the site. Flush with at least a 20-mL bolus of normal saline.

13. Readjust the IV flow rate to the original setting.

14. Store any unused medication properly.

15. Monitor the patient's condition, and document the medication given, route, time of administration, and response of the patient (Step 4).

■ Percutaneous Medication Administration

With <u>percutaneous</u> routes of administration, medications are applied to and absorbed through the skin and mucous membranes. Because percutaneously administered medications bypass the gastrointestinal tract, their absorption is more predictable.

Skill Drill | 10

Administering Medication via the Intraosseous Route

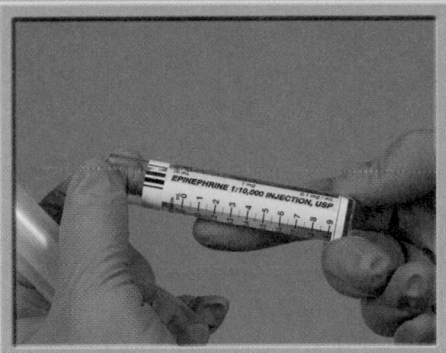

Step 1 Check the medication to ensure that it is the correct one, that it is not discolored, and that the expiration date has not passed. Assemble the equipment, and draw up the medication. Draw up 20 mL of normal saline for a flush.

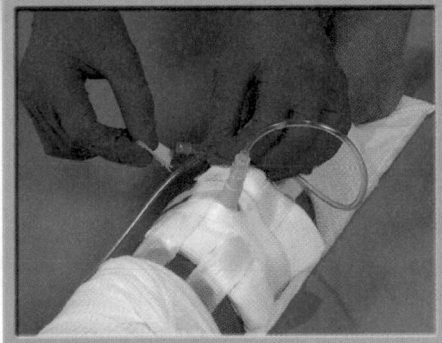

Step 2 Cleanse the injection port, or remove the protective cap if using the needleless system.

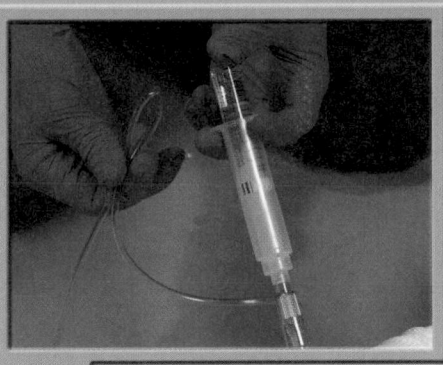

Step 3 Insert the needle into the port, and pinch off the IV tubing proximal to the administration port. Administer the correct dose at the proper push rate.

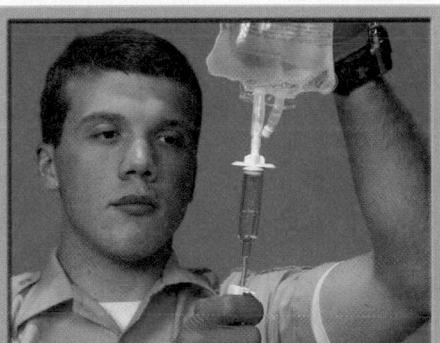

Step 4 Unclamp the IV line to flush the medication into the site, allowing it to run briefly wide open, or flush with a 20-mL bolus of normal saline. Readjust the IV flow rate with a pressure infuser to the original setting, and monitor the patient's condition.

Percutaneous routes of medication administration include the transdermal, sublingual, buccal, ocular, aural, and nasal routes.

Transdermal Medication Administration

Transdermal medications are applied topically—that is, on the surface of the body. Ordinarily, intact skin is an effective barrier to absorption of drugs. However, some drugs have been specially prepared to cross that barrier at a slow steady rate, so the transdermal route is useful for the sustained release of certain medications.

Nitroglycerin, estrogen, nicotine, and analgesic patches, for example, are applied to the skin and release medications over a specified period. Creams, lotions, and pastes (eg, nitroglycerin paste, corticosteroid cream) are also transdermally administered medications.

Factors that can increase the speed of transdermal absorption include administration of too much of the medication (ie, inadvertent or intentional overdose) and thin or nonintact skin. Decreased speed of transdermal absorption can be caused by factors such as thick skin, scar tissue in the area to which the medication is applied, and peripheral vascular disease.

Some medications, such as nitroglycerin paste, may be applied in the prehospital setting. Usually though, providers will be assisting patients with their own transdermal patches. If your service uses nitroglycerin, or another transdermal medication, then you will perform the following steps:

1. Take standard precautions.
2. Determine the need for the medication based on patient presentation.
3. Obtain a history, including any drug allergies and vital signs.
4. Follow standing orders, or contact medical control for permission.
5. Check the medication patch or cream to ensure that it is the correct one and that the expiration date has not passed, and determine the appropriate amount for the correct dose.
6. Explain the procedure to the patient and the need for the medication.
7. Clean and dry the area of the skin where the medication will be applied.
8. Apply the medication to the area in accordance with the manufacturer's specifications.
9. Monitor the patient's condition, and document the medication given, route, time of administration, and response of the patient.

Words of Wisdom

During assessment of your patient, look for transdermal medication patches, especially narcotic and nitroglycerin patches, which can result in hypotension. If the patient is already in a hemodynamically unstable condition, narcotics and nitroglycerin may complicate the clinical picture.

Do not, under any circumstances, administer, assist, or in any other manner come in contact with transdermal medications without taking the proper standard precautions. These medications are designed to go through skin and can easily be absorbed through ungloved hands.

Sublingual Medication Administration

The sublingual (under the tongue) region is highly vascular, so medications given via the sublingual route are rapidly absorbed. Sublingually administered medications, relative to enterally administered medications, get into the circulation much faster. Nitroglycerin—spray or tablet—is a drug that is most commonly administered via the sublingual route **Figure 57** .

Drugs may also be *injected* into the network of veins (venous plexus) under the tongue (basically this is another form of intravenous injection). This technique is especially useful for giving narcotic antagonists to patients who have overdosed on heroin because finding a suitable vein in such patients may be nearly impossible.

To administer a sublingual medication, follow the steps in **Skill Drill 11** .

Skill Drill   11

1. Take standard precautions.
2. Determine the need for the medication based on patient presentation.
3. Obtain a history, including any drug allergies and vital signs.
4. Follow standing orders, or contact medical control for permission.
5. Check the medication to ensure that it is the correct one and that its expiration date has not passed, and determine the appropriate amount for the correct dose **Step 1** .
6. Ask the patient to rinse his or her mouth with a little water if the mucous membranes are dry.
7. Explain the procedure, and ask the patient to lift his or her tongue. Place the tablet or spray the dose under the tongue, or ask the patient to do so.
8. Advise the patient not to chew or swallow the tablet, but to let it dissolve slowly.
9. Monitor the patient's condition, and document the medication given, route, administration time, and patient's response **Step 2** .

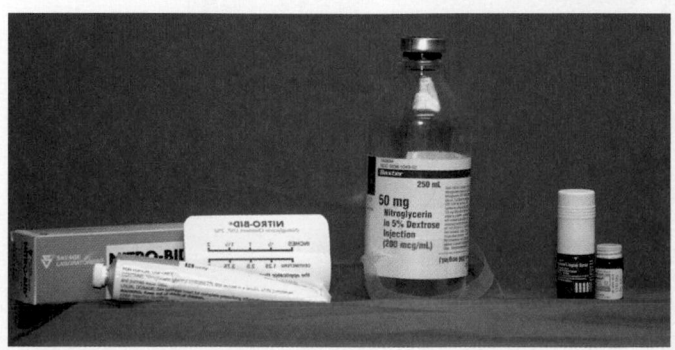

Figure 57 Nitroglycerin is often given sublingually as a spray or a tablet. It is also available as a transdermal patch or paste and can be administered as an IV drip.

Skill Drill   11

Administering Medication via the Sublingual Route

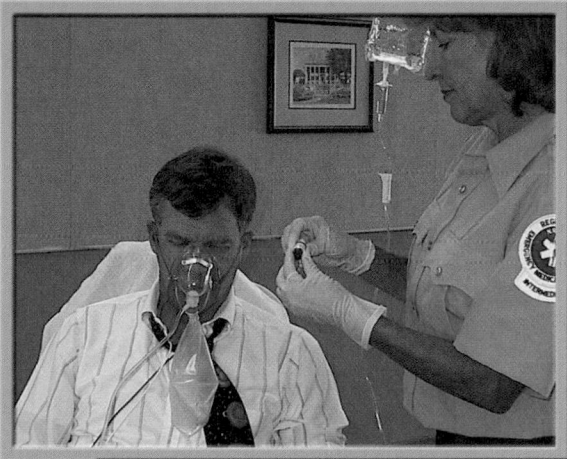

Step 1 Check the medication for drug type and its expiration date, and determine the appropriate amount for the correct dose. Have the patient rinse his or her mouth with a little water if the mucous membranes are dry.

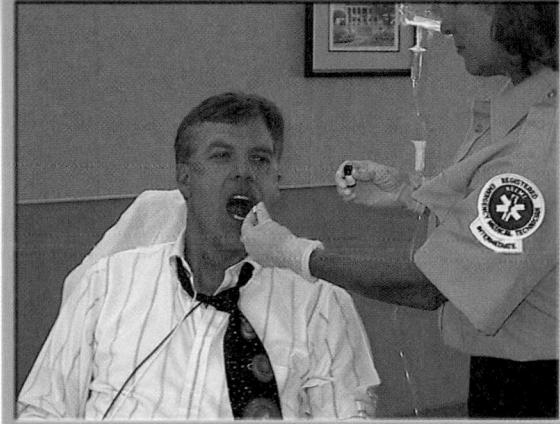

Step 2 Explain the procedure to the patient, and ask the patient to lift his or her tongue. Place the tablet or spray the dose underneath the tongue, or have the patient do so. Advise the patient not to chew or swallow the tablet, but to let it dissolve slowly. Monitor the patient, and document the medication given, route, administration time, and patient's response.

Words of Wisdom

If using a spray medication dispenser, spray it once or twice away from the patient and the crew prior to administration. This will ensure that the dispenser is primed and that the patient will receive the full dose of the medication. Also, as with transdermal medications, use proper standard precautions because nitroglycerin can be absorbed through your hands.

Buccal Medication Administration

The **buccal** region, which is also highly vascular, lies in between the cheek and gums. Most medications administered via the buccal route are in the form of tablets or gels. Glucose is one of the few medications that may be administered buccally in the prehospital setting.

To administer a medication via the buccal route, follow these steps:

1. Take standard precautions.
2. Determine the need for the medication based on patient presentation.
3. Obtain a history, including any drug allergies and vital signs.
4. Follow standing orders, or contact medical control for permission.

5. Check the medication to ensure that it is the correct one and that its expiration date has not passed, and determine the appropriate amount for the correct dose.
6. Explain the procedure to the patient and the need for the medication.
7. Place the medication in between the patient's cheek and gum, or ask the patient to do so.
8. Advise the patient not to chew or swallow the tablet, but to let it dissolve slowly.
9. Monitor the patient's condition, and document the medication given, route, administration time, and response of the patient.

Ocular Medication Administration

Drops or ointments are commonly administered via the **ocular** route. Ocular medications are typically administered for pain relief, allergies, drying of the eyes, or infections. Other than assisting a patient with his or her ocular medication or irrigating a patient's eyes following a toxic exposure, none of the medications used in the prehospital setting are administered via the ocular route.

If a patient asks you to assist him or her with ocular medication administration, follow these steps:

1. Take standard precautions.
2. Confirm that the medication is prescribed to the patient.

3. Place the patient in a supine position, or have the patient place his or her head back and look up.
4. *Without touching the eyeball*, expose the conjunctiva by gently pulling down on the lower eyelid.
5. Administer the required amount of medication on the conjunctival sac by using an eye dropper. Do not apply the medication directly on the eyeball.
6. Advise the patient to close his or her eyes for 1 to 2 minutes.
7. Document the medication name, dose, and administration time.

Aural Medication Administration

Certain medications—mainly antibiotics, analgesics, and ear-wax removal preparations—are administered via the mucous membranes of the <u>aural</u> (ear) canal. As with ocular medications, the aural route is rarely, if ever, used in the prehospital setting.

If you are asked by the patient to assist in administering his or her aural medication, follow these steps:

1. Take standard precautions.
2. Confirm that the medication is prescribed to the patient.
3. Place the patient on his or her side with the affected ear facing up.
4. Expose the ear canal by pulling the ear up and back (adults) or down and back (infants and children).
5. Administer the medication in the appropriate dose with a medicine dropper.
6. Document the medication name, dose, and administration time.

Intranasal Medication Administration

<u>Intranasal</u> (within the nose) medications include nasal spray for congestion or solutions to moisten the nasal mucosa. In recent years, this route of medication administration has become more popular in the prehospital setting. Intranasally administered medications are rapidly absorbed, providing a more rapid onset of action than IM injections. For example, some studies suggest that intranasal fentanyl has an equal onset and duration to IV morphine. Administration of emergency medications via the intranasal route is performed with a <u>mucosal atomizer device (MAD)</u> **Figure 58**. The MAD attaches to a syringe and

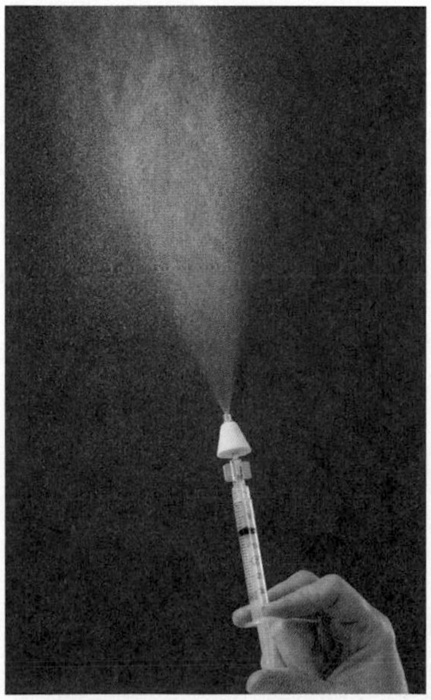

Figure 58 Mucosal atomizer device (MAD).

allows you to spray (atomize) select medications into the nasal mucosa.

Owing to the molecular structure of drugs, only a few emergency medications can be given intranasally, including naloxone (Narcan), midazolam (Versed), glucagon (GlucaGen), ketorlac (Toradol), flumazenil (Romazicon), and fentanyl citrate. Typically, intranasal medications require 2 to 2.5 times the dose of IV medications. Follow local protocol, or consult with medical control about the appropriate doses of these medications and any other medications that may be administered intranasally.

To administer a drug via the intranasal route, follow these steps:

1. Take standard precautions.
2. Determine the need for the medication based on patient presentation.
3. Obtain a history, including any drug allergies and vital signs.
4. Follow standing orders, or contact medical control for permission.
5. Check the medication to ensure that it is the correct one, that it is not cloudy or discolored, and that the expiration date has not passed.
6. Draw up the appropriate dose of medication in the syringe.
7. Attach the mucosal atomizer device to the syringe.
8. Explain the procedure to the patient (or to a relative if the patient is unconscious) and the need for the medication.
9. Spray *half* of the medication dose into each nostril.
10. Dispose of the atomizer device and syringe in the appropriate container.
11. Monitor the patient's condition, and document the medication given, route, time of administration, and response of the patient.

Medications Administered by the Inhalation Route

Nebulizer and Metered-Dose Inhaler

Many medications used in the treatment of respiratory emergencies are administered via the <u>inhalation</u> route. The most common inhaled medication is oxygen. Beta$_2$ agonist bronchodilators (eg, albuterol [Ventolin, Proventil], isoetharine [Bronkosol], metaproterenol [Alupent]) are often administered in the prehospital setting for patients experiencing respiratory distress caused by certain obstructive airway diseases, such as asthma, bronchitis, and emphysema. Other medications, such as ipratropium bromide (Atrovent)—an anticholinergic bronchodilator—are also administered via the inhalation route. Check your drug reference guide or the package insert for the indications, contraindications, and precautions before giving any of these medications.

A patient with a history of respiratory problems will usually have a <u>metered-dose inhaler (MDI)</u> to use on a regular basis or as needed **Figure 59**. MDIs are usually administered by the patient using the patient's own prescribed medications, but paramedics must know how to administer via this route because they may assist the patient with administration. Medications administered by the MDI can be delivered through a mouthpiece held by the patient or by a mask—with or without a spacer device—for young children and patients who are unable to hold the mouthpiece **Figure 60**.

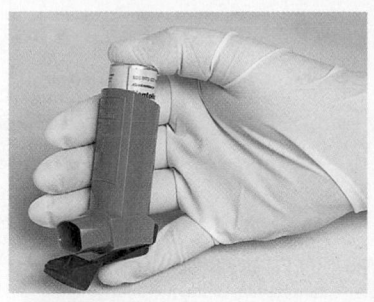

Figure 59 Some medications are inhaled into the lungs with an MDI so that they can be absorbed quickly into the bloodstream.

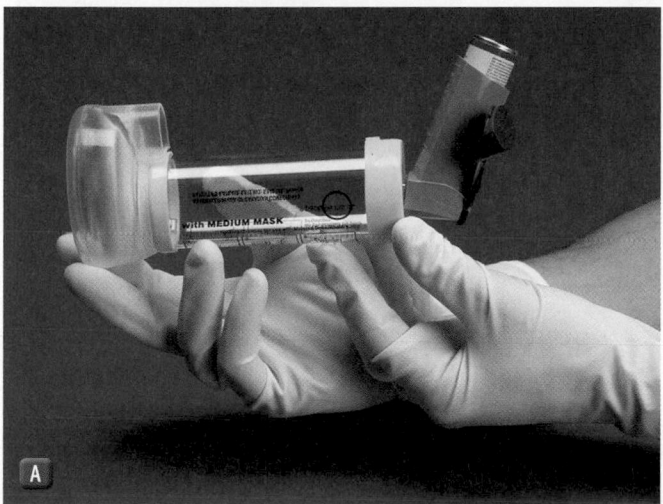

A

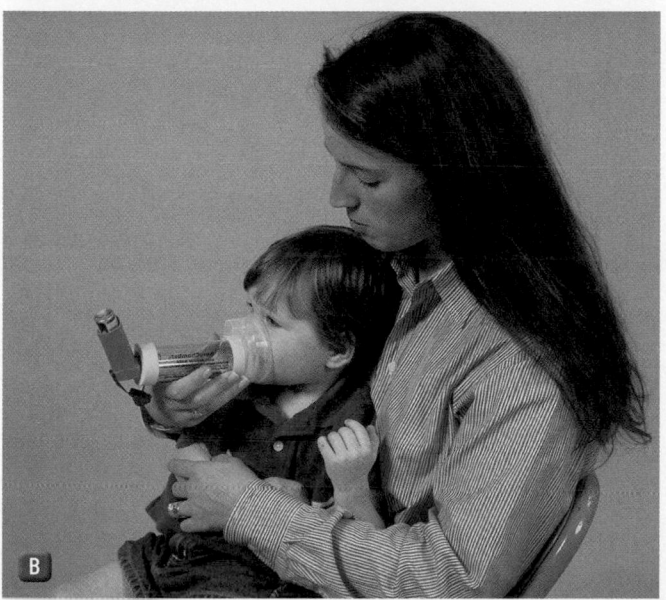

B

Figure 60 **A.** In children, an MDI and spacer can be used with or without a mask. **B.** Children as young as 6 months can use a mask and spacer device.

Follow the steps in **Skill Drill 12** to help a patient self-administer medication from an inhaler:

Skill Drill 12

1. Follow standard precautions.
2. Obtain an order from medical control or follow local protocol.
3. Check that you have the right medication, right patient, right dose, right route, and that the medication is not expired.
4. Make sure that the patient is alert enough to use the inhaler.
5. Check to see whether the patient has already taken any doses.
6. Make sure the inhaler is at room temperature or warmer **Step 1**.
7. Shake the inhaler vigorously several times.
8. Stop administering supplemental oxygen and remove any mask from the patient's face.
9. Ask the patient to exhale deeply and, before inhaling, to put his or her lips around the opening of the inhaler **Step 2**.
10. If the patient has a spacer, attach it to allow more effective use of the medication.
11. Have the patient depress the hand-held inhaler as he or she begins to inhale deeply.
12. Instruct the patient to hold his or her breath for as long as he or she comfortably can to help the lungs absorb the medication **Step 3**.
13. Continue administering supplemental oxygen.
14. Allow the patient to breathe a few times, then give the second dose per direction from medical control or according to local protocol **Step 4**.

Words of Wisdom

Metered-dose inhalers are also called HFAs, after the propellant hydrofluoroalkane that is now used instead of chlorofluorocarbons (CFCs).

For more severe problems, liquid bronchodilators may be aerosolized in a **nebulizer** for inhalation. Small-volume nebulizers (also called updraft or hand-held nebulizers) are the most commonly used method of administration of inhaled medications in the prehospital setting **Figure 61**. Oxygen or a compressed air source is connected to the nebulizer to produce the aerosolized mist.

Some nebulizers have been adapted with child-friendly shapes and images to ease the use with pediatric patients. They may allow for blow-by administration to help the patient tolerate the medication. Other methods used on patients include a nebulized mask that does not require the patient to hold the device. Some adapters have been designed to allow providers

Skill Drill 12

Assisting a Patient With a Metered-Dose Inhaler

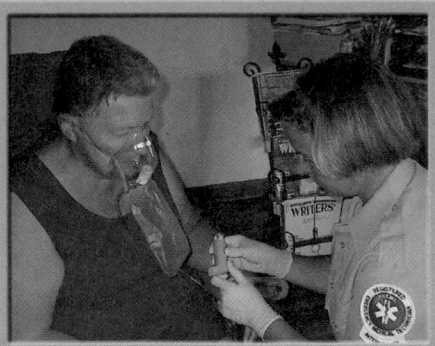

Step 1 Check to make sure you have the correct medication for the correct patient. Check the expiration date. Ensure the inhaler is at room temperature or warmer.

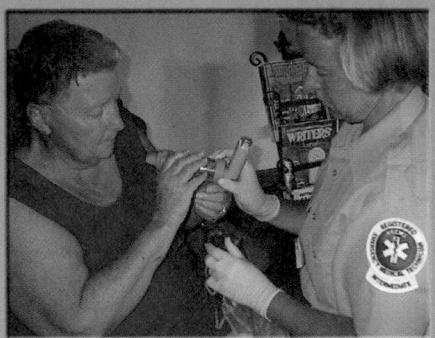

Step 2 Remove any mask. Hand the inhaler to the patient. Instruct about breathing and lip seal. Use a spacer if the patient has one.

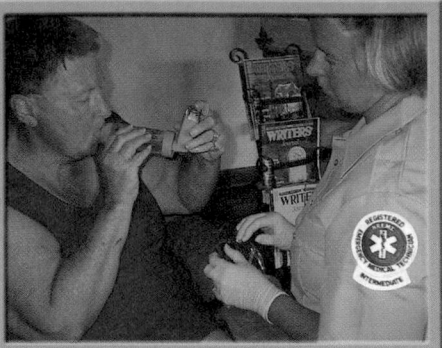

Step 3 Instruct the patient to press the inhaler and inhale one puff. Instruct about breath holding.

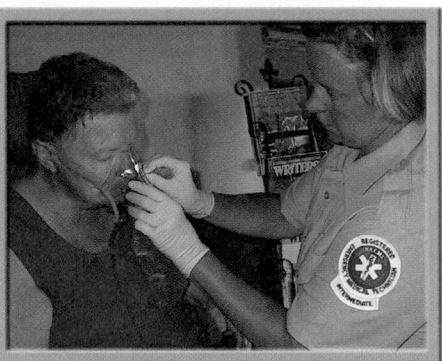

Step 4 Reapply oxygen. After a few breaths, have the patient repeat the dose if medical control or local protocol allows.

to administer nebulized medications to intubated patients with each ventilation. These devices may also be adapted for use with CPAP masks.

Follow the steps in [Skill Drill 13] to administer a medication via a small-volume nebulizer:

Skill Drill 13

1. Take standard precautions.
2. Determine the need for an inhaled bronchodilator based on patient presentation.

3. Obtain a history, including any drug allergies and vital signs.
4. Follow standing orders, or contact medical control for permission.
5. Check the medication and its expiration date. Make sure that you have the right medication and that it is not cloudy or discolored [Step 1].
6. If the medication is in a premixed package, add it to the bowl of the nebulizer. If it is not premixed, add the medication to the bowl and mix it with the specified amount of normal saline, usually 2.5 to 3 mL [Step 2].

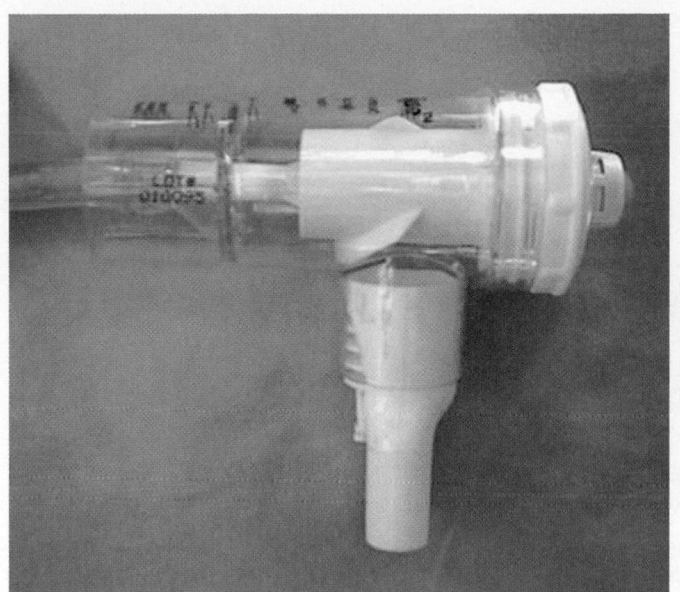

Figure 61 A small-volume nebulizer is used to deliver medications via aerosolized mist.

Controversies

In the past, nebulizers were considered the preferred method of delivering beta-agonist medications for the treatment of asthma attacks. Recent studies, however, have shown that MDIs—especially when used with spacing devices—are at least as effective as nebulizers and have several distinct advantages:

- MDIs are *more convenient* than nebulizers. They do not require any setup time or a source of compressed gas.
- MDIs are *more reliable* than nebulizers. With a nebulizer, one cannot be certain that the patient is getting the full dose of the drug. MDIs deliver a more consistent amount of drug aerosol.
- Because most people with asthma use MDIs at home, using the MDI in an emergency provides an excellent opportunity to *educate the patient* in proper use of the device. Studies have shown that more than half of patients using MDIs at home employ an incorrect and ineffective technique. Showing a patient the correct technique and demonstrating its effectiveness can improve the outcome of subsequent asthma attacks.

7. Connect the T piece with the mouthpiece to the top of the bowl, or the mask to the bowl, and connect it to the oxygen tubing.

8. Set the flowmeter at 6 L/min to produce a steady mist Step 3 .

9. With the MDI or hand-held nebulizer in position, instruct the patient on the proper way to breathe. Have the patient breathe as deeply as possible and hold his or her breath for 3 to 5 seconds before exhaling. Continue to coach the patient as needed.

10. Monitor the patient's condition, and document the medication given, route, time of administration, and response of the patient to the medication Step 4 .

11. Cardiac monitoring is essential when administering a beta agonist. If cardiac dysrhythmias are noted, stop the administration of the medication, administer high-flow oxygen, and contact medical control.

Some patients with respiratory emergencies may be breathing inadequately (ie, inadequate tidal volume, fast or slow respiratory rate) and will not be able to effectively inhale beta-agonist medications into the lungs via a nebulizer or an MDI. In this case, assist with bag-mask ventilation and attach a small-volume nebulizer to the ventilation device. Place a short piece of corrugated tubing—separated by a T piece to connect the nebulizer to—between the bag and mask or endotracheal tube if the patient is intubated.

■ Endotracheal Medication Administration

If IV or IO access is unavailable, certain resuscitative medications can be administered down the endotracheal (ET or ETT for endotracheal tube) tube. For the medication to be adequately dispersed throughout the tracheobronchial tree, you must administer 2 to 2.5 times the standard IV dose. *Only* four medications are accepted nationally to be given down the ET tube; they can easily be remembered by the mnemonic LEAN: Lidocaine, Epinephrine, Atropine, Naloxone (Narcan). While naloxone is accepted to be administered via the ET tube, it is contraindicated for neonates. At the time of print, endotracheal vasopressin has been researched extensively and is showing positive results. As always, check your local protocols prior to administration.

To administer medications via the ET tube, follow these steps:

1. Draw up the appropriate dose of the medication to be administered as your partner ventilates the patient. Dilute the appropriate dose of the medication in 10 mL of normal saline.

2. Disconnect the bag-mask device from the ET tube, and rapidly instill the medication down the ET tube Figure 62 .

3. Immediately reconnect the bag-mask device to the ET tube, and ventilate the patient briskly to facilitate passage of the drug down the trachea and into the lungs.

Long-Term Vascular Access Devices

There may be some situations where IV access is imperative but difficult to obtain. Some of these patients may have a long-term vascular access device inserted. These patients may be receiving an antibiotic regimen, chemotherapy, regular blood draws for chronic disorders, hemodialysis, or other acute or chronic illnesses. These patients will be upfront about their medical device and will generally request that you not insert a peripheral line.

Skill Drill 13

Administering a Medication via Small-Volume Nebulizer

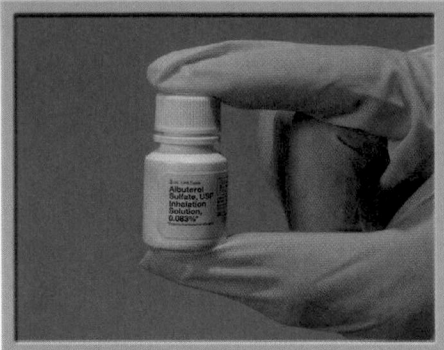

Step 1 Check the medication and the expiration date.

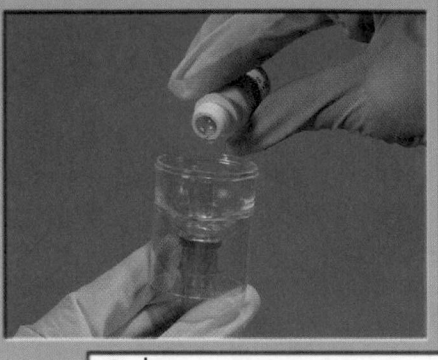

Step 2 Add premixed medication to the bowl of the nebulizer.

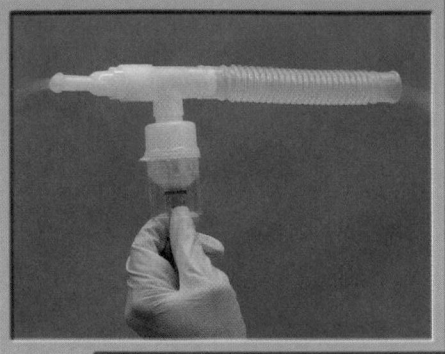

Step 3 Connect the T piece with the mouthpiece to the top of the bowl, connect it to the oxygen tubing, and set the flowmeter at 6 L/min.

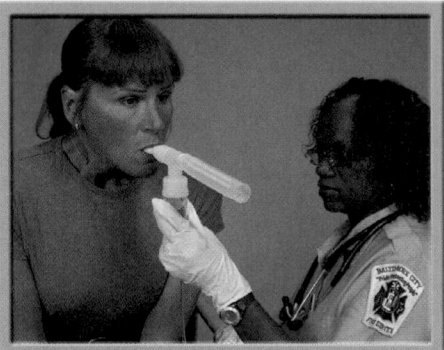

Step 4 Instruct the patient to breathe as deeply as possible and hold his or her breath for 3 to 5 seconds before exhaling. Monitor the patient for effects.

Controversies

Although current practice calls for administering certain resuscitative medications via the ET tube, recent studies have suggested that this route of medication administration may not be particularly effective. Follow local protocols or contact medical control as needed regarding endotracheal drug administration.

If you encounter a patient with a long-term vascular access device, generally there are two types: non-tunneling and implanted. Most protocols only allow the use of these vascular access devices during critical events. These devices are usually preserved with heparin to prevent clotting. Because these devices are not accessed frequently in the prehospital or interfacility setting, it is imperative that you seek out regular training on how to access and use these devices.

Non-tunneling <u>Non-tunneling devices</u> are devices that have been inserted by direct venipuncture through the skin directly into a selected vein. The most common devices that will be encountered in the prehospital and interfacility setting are peripheral inserted central catheters (PICC), midline, and central venous catheters (CVC).

Peripheral inserted central catheters are frequently used for long-term medication administration, chemotherapy, fre-

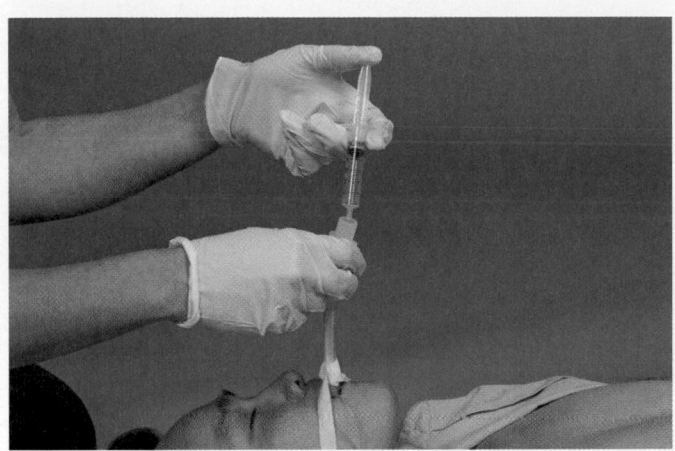

Figure 62 Medication administration via the ET tube is done in some areas but its effectiveness is questionable.

Words of Wisdom

When you are accessing multilumen devices, you should always attempt to access the largest lumen first. If the lumens are the same diameter, then you should access the distal lumen. The lumen that should be used will generally be marked by the number 1.

quent venous sampling, and total parenteral nutrition. PICCs are generally inserted by designated PICC nurses who receive specific training on PICC insertion. The insertion point is usually at the antecubital vein, while the distal end of the PICC usually sits at the superior vena cava and is verified by a radiograph. PICCs may be left in place for 6 to 8 weeks. Some patients may have their PICC accessed by family or home health regularly. The PICC may have a single, double, or triple lumen.

Midlines are also inserted at the antecubital vein. However, unlike a PICC, the distal end of the midline rests at the proximal end of the extremity. Midlines generally can be used for approximately 4 weeks. They also can be used for shorter medication therapies and venous therapies. Central venous catheters are generally inserted in emergent situations by physicians into the subclavian, femoral, or internal jugular, and are used for emergent medication administration, fluid resuscitation, blood administration, or blood sampling. These catheters are generally large-bore and may sit near the vena cava.

The steps for accessing a tunneling device are as follows Skill Drill 14 :

1. Use aseptic technique.
2. Prepare all of the appropriate equipment:
   a. Empty 10- to 20-mL syringe (nothing less than a 10-mL syringe should be used)
   b. 10-mL normal saline flush

   c. Sterile gloves
   d. Alcohol prep
   e. 10-gtt administration set
   f. 500 mL normal saline
3. Ensure that all lumens are clamped. Air embolism is a serious risk with these patients because many of these devices go directly into the vena cava. That is why central lines must be clamped whenever they are not in use.
4. Use an alcohol prep to prepare the lumen that will be used Step 1 .
5. Attach the empty syringe and withdraw a minimum of 10 mL of blood from the lumen Step 2 . Discard this immediately into the sharps container. Do not withdraw too forcefully. If you meet some resistance, gently flush and withdraw. Ask the patient to turn his or her head the opposite direction of the central line.
6. After you have withdrawn the 10 mL of blood, attach the 10-mL syringe filled with normal saline and slowly administer it Step 3 .
7. Attach the prepared IV drip set and set it up for at least 10 mL/h Step 4 . Depending on the size of the catheter, you can infuse at a rate of 125 to 250 mL/h. The line must be running continuously because heparin is not available.
8. Administer IV medications through the attached IV drip set.

Implanted <u>Implanted vascular access devices (VADs)</u> are implanted in surgery, sutured under the skin. These devices are palpable outside the skin but are not exposed to the outside environment. The device consists of a self-sealing core inserted in a stainless steel, titanium, or plastic shell connected to a catheter that runs into the superior vena cava. These devices can only be accessed with a HUBER needle that is non-coring and has a mild angle. These devices can be used for long-term medication administration, total parenteral nutrition, chemotherapy, blood products, or venous blood sampling.

Arterioventricular (AV) fistulas are used for a variety of disorders. They are created by connecting a vein and an artery. For kidney failure, hemodialysis uses AV fistulas to dialyze the blood. Fistulas are also used for plasmapheresis in various disorders such as myasthenia gravis and Guillain-Barré. Fistulas require a unique skill set to access and generally should not be accessed by paramedics.

The steps for accessing an implanted VAD are as follows Skill Drill 15 :

1. Use aseptic technique.
2. Prepare all necessary equipment:
   a. HUBER needle
   b. Empty 10- to 20-mL syringe (nothing less than a 10-mL syringe should be used)
   c. 10-mL normal saline flush
   d. Sterile gloves
   e. Chlorhexidine gluconate (ChloraPrep) or betadine
   f. 10-gtt administration set
   g. 500 mL normal saline

Skill Drill | 14

Accessing a Tunneling Device

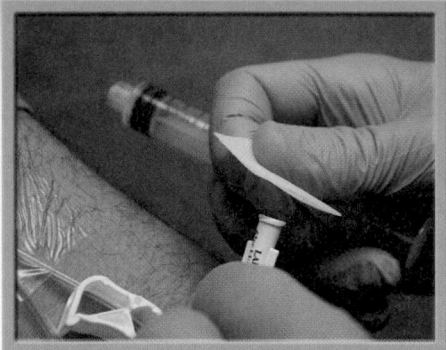

Step 1 Prepare the equipment. Ensure that all lumens are clamped. Use an alcohol prep to prepare the lumen.

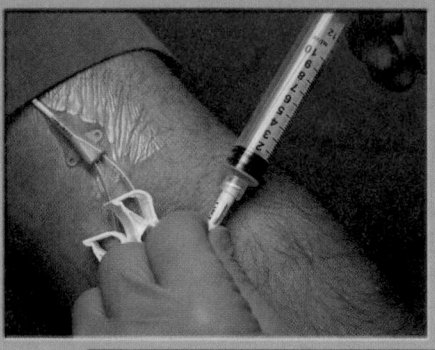

Step 2 Attach the empty syringe and withdraw a minimum of 10 mL of blood. Discard it immediately.

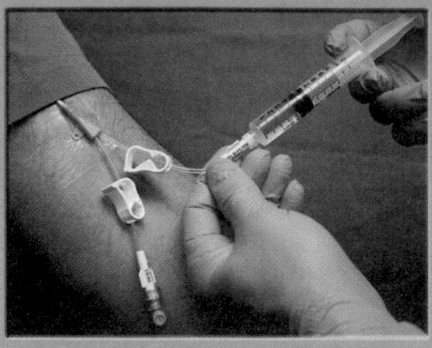

Step 3 Attach the 10-mL syringe filled with normal saline and slowly administer it.

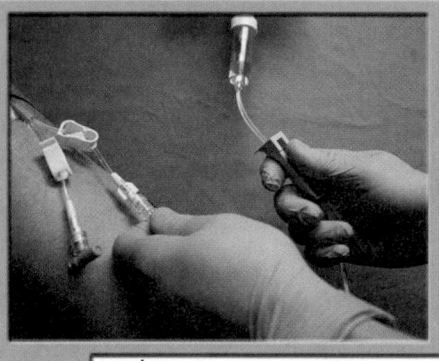

Step 4 Attach the prepared IV drip set and set it up for at least 10 mL/h. Administer the medication.

3. Identify your site in the upper part of the chest. Stabilize it between the thumb and index finger of your nondominant hand.
4. Clean the site with chlorhexidine [Step 1]. If an allergy is present, clean the site with betadine.
5. Apply pressure around the edges of the port to stretch the skin over the injection site [Step 2].
6. While stabilizing the device, insert the HUBER needle at a 90° angle [Step 3].
7. Withdraw at least 10 mL of blood from the needleless extension set [Step 4].
8. Flush the set with the 10-mL normal saline flush.
9. Attach the 10-gtt IV administration set.

10. Administer medications directly into the drop set medication port.

Central lines imply that a patient has a significant medical history that should be investigated and that standard IV access may be difficult to obtain. Accessing these devices is risky and requires proper training. Aseptic technique is imperative considering that many of these devices sit inside the superior vena cava. These devices are all preserved with heparin, which is why providers must withdraw at least 10 mL of blood from the device. Because EMS providers do not routinely carry heparin, EMS providers must keep the IV administration set minimally at KVO/TKO to prevent clots from forming.

Skill Drill 15

Accessing an Implanted Vascular Access Device

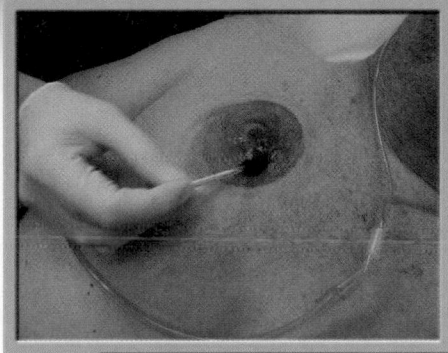

Step 1 Prepare the equipment. Identify and prep the site.

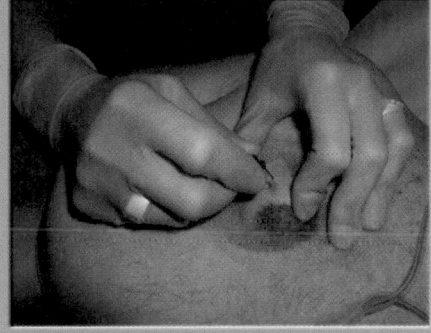

Step 2 Apply pressure around the edges of the port to stretch the skin over the injection site.

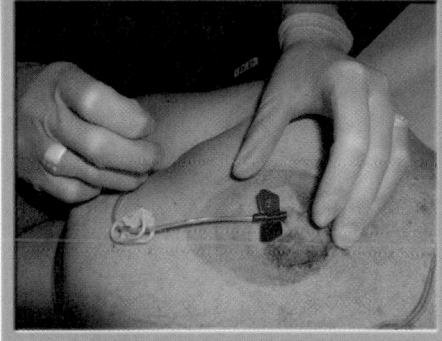

Step 3 Insert the needle at a 90° angle.

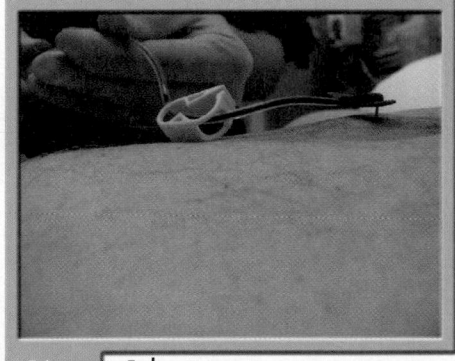

Step 4 Aspirate for blood.

■ Rates of Medication Absorption

The speed at which a drug is absorbed is directly related to the route by which it is given. Obviously, drugs injected directly into the bloodstream (ie, as IV or IO injections) gain access to the central circulation the fastest. Oral medications take longer to achieve their therapeutic effects because they must be absorbed through the gastrointestinal tract first. Table 7 summarizes the various medication routes and their rates of absorption. Table 8 provides examples of medications and their route, onset, peak, and duration. Specific medications are covered in detail in the chapter, *Emergency Medications*.

Words of Wisdom

In rare instances, paramedics may perform peer-assisted medication administration (administering medication to oneself or to one's partner). It may be necessary for the EMS crew to receive medications because they were exposed to a toxic agent. In this case, you would first treat yourself and then your partner.

Table 7 Medication Routes and Rates of Absorption

Route of Administration	Onset of Action*
Intraosseous	30-60 s
Intravenous	30-60 s
Endotracheal	2-3 min[†]
Inhalation	2-3 min
Nasal mucosal atomization (MAD)	3-5 min
Sublingual	3-5 min
Intramuscular injection	10-20 min
Subcutaneous injection	15-30 min
Rectal	5-30 min
Oral	30-90 min
Topical	Minutes to hours

*In a healthy person with adequate perfusion
[†]Recent data suggest that ET drug administration may be less effective than previously thought, especially in poor perfusion states.

Table 8 Examples of Specific Medications

Drug	Route	Onset	Peak	Duration
Metoprolol tartrate (Lopressor)	PO IV	15 minutes Immediate	1 hour 20 minutes	6-12 hours 5-8 hours
Fentanyl citrate (Sublimaze)	Transdermal IV IM Intranasal	6-8 hours Immediate 7-8 minutes 1-2 minutes	12-24 hours 3-5 minutes 20-30 minutes 9-15 minutes	72 hours 20-40 minutes 1-2 hours 20-40 minutes
Naloxone	IV IM ET	0-2 minutes 2-10 minutes 2-10 minutes	0-2 minutes 2-10 minutes 2-10 minutes	20-120 minutes 20-120 minutes 20-120 minutes

YOU *are the Medic*   SUMMARY

1. What are some differential diagnoses for this patient?

The patient is in her early 30s and was running a marathon. Using that line of thinking, you know that the patient may have just tripped and broken her leg. You can also consider that the patient could have experienced a cardiac or respiratory emergency. Using some basic assessments, you will be able to hone in on the primary problem.

2. Is the weather a potential cause for her problem?

Anyone who has worked outside in hot, humid weather knows that no matter what type of physical condition you are in, it will take a toll on your body. A patient who was running a marathon in heat and humidity should be assumed to have a heat-related illness until proven otherwise. The simple treatments for heat exhaustion are BLS and you should recall those steps from your previous EMT training. Remove the patient from the environment, cool the patient, and provide transport to the hospital.

3. What is the most appropriate treatment for this patient?

After BLS care, it is important to rehydrate the patient if dehydration is the working diagnosis that you are making. This patient has a more complex problem because of the broken leg and the pain she is experiencing from the fracture. Therefore, you will need to administer a pain management agent prior to splinting, to help the patient be as comfortable as possible.

4. What type of IV fluid is best for this patient?

An isotonic crystalloid fluid is best for this patient because its chemical makeup is most like the fluids in the body; therefore, it does not cause shifts into or out of intravascular spaces. Lactated Ringer's solution helps for intense blood loss, which is not the situation for this patient. The remaining fluid choices are hypotonic fluids, which hydrate cells while depleting the vascular compartment (common for dialysis patients) or hypertonic fluids, which pull fluid from the cells and into the intravascular compartment (used primarily in the hospital setting).

5. What type of pain management would be best for the patient? What are the common methods for administration and benefits/problems with each?

Because this patient's blood pressure is low and suggests potential shock, the best choice for pain management is fentanyl. The primary benefit of fentanyl is its ability to maintain hemodynamic stability. You have some choices when you are administering fentanyl. The IV route is most likely the best route because this patient needs fluid rehydration. The IV route has the fastest absorption and is the best way of administering medications. You also have the option of administering fentanyl intramuscularly or intranasally. The problem with giving a

medication intramuscularly is the slow absorption rate, whereas the benefit is that the medication can be administered without an IV line. Like intramuscular administration, intranasal administration also has the benefit of not requiring an IV line. The intranasal route is gaining popularity; however, not every agency has a mucosal atomizer in its protocols.

6. What are the risks and benefits of using an isotonic solution for fluid replacement?

The benefit of using an isotonic solution is its rapid ability to increase the patient's blood pressure and increase preload. The risks include the possibility of fluid overload, which is a concern for patients with hypertension and congestive heart failure. The isotonic fluid also cannot carry oxygen, which those patients who are bleeding internally desperately need.

7. You need to administer 50 μg of fentanyl and it comes in an ampule of 100 μg in 2 mL of fluid. How much would you administer?

The desired dose is the amount of a drug that the physician orders you to give to the patient, which is represented by the 50 μg of fentanyl. The drug concentration is how much of the drug you have available, represented here by the 100 μg in 2 mL of fluid. The volume to be administered is the desired dose divided by the concentration of drug on hand:

$$50\ \mu g \div \frac{100\ \mu g}{2\ mL} = 50\ \mu g \times \frac{2\ mL}{\underset{2}{100\ \mu g}} = 1\ mL$$

Because the order is 50 μg and the concentration is 100 μg in 2 mL, there is 50 μg per mL. Therefore, the initial administration of medication is 1 mL of fentanyl.

8. The order was for a 500-mL fluid bolus over 10 minutes. If using a 10-drop set, how many drops per minute would this be?

The formula for fluid administration is to multiply the total volume to be infused by the drops per mL (gtt/mL) of the administration set, divided by the time of infusion in minutes. Therefore:

$$\frac{500\ mL \times 10\ gtt}{10\ min\ mL} = 500\ gtt/min$$

So, your order is to administer 500 mL infused × the drip set ÷ the time in minutes, so the equation looks like 500 × 10 ÷ 10 = 500 drops a minute.

YOU *are the Medic*   **SUMMARY,** *continued*

EMS Patient Care Report (PCR)

Date: 02-23-11	Incident No.: 1232	Nature of Call: Fall		Location: Marathon at mile 16	
Dispatched: 1115	En Route: 1116	At Scene: 1119	Transport: 1137	At Hospital: 1207	In Service: 1237

Patient Information

Age: 34	Allergies: None
Sex: F	Medications: Birth control pills
Weight (in kg [lb]): 60 kg (132 lb)	Past Medical History: None
	Chief Complaint: Dizziness

Vital Signs

Time: 1124	BP: 86/40	Pulse: 140	Respirations: 28	SpO_2: 99%
Time: 1129	BP: 90/40	Pulse: 120	Respirations: 24	SpO_2: 100%
Time:	BP:	Pulse:	Respirations:	SpO_2:
Time: 1139	BP: 96/50	Pulse: 100	Respirations: 22	SpO_2: 100%
Time: 1149	BP: 100/60	Pulse: 80	Respirations: 20	SpO_2: 100%

EMS Treatment
(circle all that apply)

Oxygen @ __12__ L/min via (circle one): NC **NRM** Bag-mask device	Assisted Ventilation	Airway Adjunct	CPR
Defibrillation	Bleeding Control	Bandaging	Splinting	Other

Narrative

EMS arrived on scene to find 34-year-old female marathon runner who states she is dizzy and her left leg hurts. Pt states she was halfway through the marathon when she suddenly became dizzy and tripped, causing her to fall. Pt states when she fell, she heard a snap in her left leg and felt immediate pain. Pt places the pain a 9 on Borg scale. Pt denies any head, neck, or back pain. Pt told EMS she didn't realize it was going to be so hot and did not prehydrate. EMS placed pt on 100% oxygen via NRM. Pt was shaded from sun until treatment could be completed. Vitals were taken and MD 403 contacted for fentanyl pain management orders and a 500-mL fluid bolus for possible dehydration. MD 403 gave orders for 50 μg of fentanyl followed by an additional 50 in 10 minutes if pt still in pain and granted the 500-mL fluid bolus. Pt had IV established by Tech 898 while doctor was being contacted for orders. Tech 898 administered 50 μg fentanyl IVP and began the 500-mL bolus. Pt stated the pain decreased to a 6 and EMS immobilized left tib/fib with frac pak and ice pak. The left leg had some deformity and point tenderness but no open fracture was appreciated. Pt moved to stretcher and then transport begun to St. Mark's Hospital. Pt stated she was still in pain and Tech 898 administered another 50 μg of fentanyl IVP. Pt vitals were monitored throughout and began to improve. Pt states almost complete relief from dizziness and leg pain is now 4 on 10. Pt had no further changes during transport. Pt turned over to Room 5 in the ED with report to the RN. IV was patent and 550 mL infused. Pt states total relief from dizziness.
End of report

Prep Kit

Ready for Review

- The cellular environment contains charged ions, called electrolytes, that are used by the cell for different purposes. These electrolytes include sodium, potassium, calcium, bicarbonate, chloride, and phosphorus. Their electrical charges must remain in balance on either side of the cell membrane.

- There must be a balance of compounds on either side of the cell membrane. If an imbalance occurs, the cell can move chemicals or charges across its membrane by various methods, including osmosis, diffusion, active transport, and filtration.

- Understanding the workings of the intracellular and extracellular chemicals and charges will provide you with a better foundation for understanding why different types of IV solutions are administered for different conditions.

- Techniques for gaining vascular access include cannulation of a peripheral extremity vein, cannulation of the external jugular vein, and cannulation of the IO space. Although the ultimate goal of vascular access is to be able to administer fluids and medications, each of these techniques requires a different approach and must be practiced frequently for initial and ongoing proficiency.

- Several different IV administration sets exist, and you must know which one is most appropriate for a given patient condition. Microdrip sets (60 gtt/mL) are commonly used for medication infusions. Macrodrip sets (10 or 15 gtt/mL) are used when the patient requires IV fluid boluses to treat dehydration, hypovolemic shock, and other states of hemodynamic instability.

- You must consider two factors when choosing an IV catheter: gauge and length. The larger the gauge (the smaller the number), and the shorter the length, the more fluid that can be infused through it. Over-the-needle catheters are the most commonly used IV catheters in the prehospital setting.

- Cannulation of a peripheral extremity vein is the preferred initial means of establishing vascular access. If it is unsuccessful and the patient is critically ill or injured, proceed with IO cannulation without delay. External jugular vein cannulation is usually attempted only after all other techniques of gaining vascular access have failed.

- IO cannulation and infusion are no longer reserved for children only; they can also be used to establish emergency vascular access in adults. The IO space, which acts like a sponge, quickly absorbs fluids and medications and rapidly transports them to the central circulation.

- Although peripheral veins often collapse when a patient is in shock or cardiac arrest, the IO space tends to remain patent. Thus IO cannulation and infusion—in children and adults—may be life-saving measures if peripheral venous access is not possible. Any fluid or medication that can be administered via the IV route can be administered via the IO route and can travel to the central circulation just as rapidly.

- You must be thoroughly familiar with the equipment you are using when performing IO cannulation. Follow local protocols and attend in-service training regarding the specific equipment used for IO cannulation in your EMS system.

- Use aseptic technique when you are performing any invasive procedure to minimize the risk of patient contamination. Always use standard precautions when performing an invasive procedure to maximize your own safety.

- Along with the dispensing of medications comes the responsibility to be thoroughly familiar with each medication carried on your ambulance. Be sure to confirm the drug doses and routes. Remember: *First do no harm.*

- Good math skills and a thorough understanding of the metric system are imperative to providing the right dose of a drug to your patient. The six rights of medication are right patient, right drug, right dose, right route, right time, and right documentation. Administering the wrong drug, using the wrong route, or giving the wrong dose can have disastrous effects.

- All equipment used in the administration of medications must be kept sterile to prevent contamination of the patient. Use proper standard precautions to protect yourself. Needleless systems have made older needle systems increasingly obsolete because the former systems decrease the incidence of needlesticks.

- As a paramedic, you must be familiar with the various routes of medication administration, including the proper use of equipment and proper anatomic locations for administration via each route.

- Enteral medication administration includes the administration of all drugs that may be given through any portion of the gastrointestinal tract. The parenteral route includes any method of drug administration that does not pass through the gastrointestinal tract.

- The IV and IO routes are the fastest routes of medication administration; the oral and transdermal (topical) routes are the slowest.

- When in doubt, always follow local protocols or contact medical control as needed for direction when you are administering a medication. *Never make a hasty critical decision before consulting with a physician!*

Vital Vocabulary

access port A sealed hub on an administration set designed for sterile access to the IV fluid.

acidosis A pathologic condition resulting from the accumulation of acids in the body.

active transport A method used to move compounds across a cell membrane to create or maintain an imbalance of charges.

administration set Tubing that connects to the IV bag access port and the catheter to deliver IV fluid.

alkalosis A pathologic condition resulting from the accumulation of bases in the body.

ampules Small glass containers that are sealed and the contents sterilized.

anion An ion that contains an overall negative charge.

antecubital The anterior aspect of the elbow.

anticoagulant A substance that prevents blood from clotting.

antidiuretic hormone (ADH) A hormone produced by the pituitary gland that signals the kidneys to prevent excretion of water.

antiseptics Chemicals used to cleanse an area before performing an invasive procedure, such as starting an IV line; not toxic to living tissues; examples include isopropyl alcohol and iodine.

aseptic technique A method of cleansing used to prevent contamination of a site when you are performing an invasive procedure, such as starting an IV line.

ataxia A staggered walk or gait.

aural Pertaining to the ear.

bivalent An ion that contains two charges.

blood tubing A special type of macrodrip administration set designed to facilitate rapid fluid replacement by manual infusion of multiple IV bags or IV-blood replacement combinations.

bolus A term used to describe "in one mass"; in medication administration, a single dose given by the IV or IO route; may be a small or large quantity of the drug.

Bone Injection Gun (BIG) A spring-loaded device that is used for inserting an IO needle into the proximal tibia in adult and pediatric patients.

buccal Between the cheek and gums.

butterfly catheter A rigid, hollow, venous cannulation device identified by its plastic "wings" that act as anchoring points for securing the catheter.

cannulation The insertion of a catheter, such as into a vein to allow for fluid flow.

carpopedal spasms Hand or foot spasms; usually the result of hyperventilation or hypocalcemia.

catheter shear Occurs when a needle is reinserted into the catheter, and it slices through the catheter, creating a free-floating segment.

cation An ion that contains an overall positive charge.

Celsius scale A scale for measuring temperature where water freezes at 0° and boils at 100°.

colloid solutions Solutions that contain molecules (usually proteins) that are too large to pass out of the capillary membranes and, therefore, remain in the vascular compartment.

concentration The total weight of a drug contained in a specific volume of liquid.

concentration gradient The natural tendency for substances to flow from an area of higher concentration to an area of lower concentration, within or outside the cell.

contaminated stick The puncturing of an emergency care provider's skin with a needle or catheter that was used on a patient.

crystalloid solutions Solutions of dissolved crystals (for example, salts or sugars) in water; contain compounds that quickly dissociate in solution.

D$_5$W An intravenous solution made up of 5% dextrose in water.

dehydration Depletion of the body's systemic fluid volume.

depolarization The rapid movement of electrolytes across a cell membrane that changes the cell's overall charge. This rapid shifting of electrolytes and cellular charges is the main catalyst for muscle contractions and neural transmissions.

desired dose The amount of a drug that the physician orders for a patient; the drug order.

diaphysis The shaft of a long bone.

diffusion A process where molecules move from an area of higher concentration to an area of lower concentration.

diluent A solution (usually water or normal saline) used for diluting a medication.

disinfectants Chemicals used on nonliving objects to kill organisms; toxic to living tissues.

drip chamber The area of the administration set where fluid accumulates so that the tubing remains filled with fluid.

drug reconstitution Injecting sterile water or saline from one vial into another vial containing a powdered form of the drug.

electrolytes Charged atoms or compounds that result from the loss or gain of an electron. These are ions that the body uses to perform certain critical metabolic functions.

enteral medications Medication administration that involves the medication passing through a portion of the gastrointestinal tract.

epiphyseal plate The growth plate of a bone; a major site of bone development during childhood.

epiphyses The ends of a long bone.

external jugular (EJ) vein Large neck vein that is lateral to the carotid artery.

extracellular fluid (ECF) The water outside the cells; accounts for 15% of body weight.

EZ-IO A hand-held, battery-powered driver to which a special IO needle is attached; used for insertion of the IO needle into the proximal tibia of children and adults.

Fahrenheit scale A scale for measuring temperature where water freezes at 32° and boils at 212°.

fascia The fiberlike connective tissue that covers arteries, veins, tendons, and ligaments.

FAST1 A sternal IO device used in adults; stands for First Access for Shock and Trauma.

flash chamber The area of an IV catheter that fills with blood to help indicate when a vein is cannulated.

gastric tubes Tubes that are commonly inserted in patients in the prehospital setting to decompress the stomach; can also be used to administer certain enteral medications.

gauge The internal diameter of an IV catheter or needle.

gtt A unit of measure that indicates drops.

hematoma An accumulation of blood in the tissues beneath the skin; a potential complication of IV therapy.

hemostasis The body's natural blood-clotting mechanism.

homeostasis The balance of all body systems of the body; also known as homeostatic balance.

hypercalcemia A high serum calcium level.

hyperkalemia A high serum potassium level.

hypertonic solution A solution that has a greater concentration of sodium than does the cell; the increased osmotic pressure can draw water out of the cell and cause it to collapse.

hypocalcemia A low serum calcium level.

hypokalemia A low serum potassium level.

hypotonic solution A solution that has a lower concentration of sodium than does the cell; the increased osmotic pressure lets water flow into the cell, causing it to swell and possibly burst.

implanted vascular access devices (VAD) Devices that are implanted in surgery, sutured under the skin, for the purpose of long-term medication administration, total parenteral nutrition, chemotherapy, blood product administration, and venous blood sampling; an arteriovenous fistula is an example.

infiltration The escape of fluid into the surrounding tissue; the result of vein perforation during IV cannulation.

inhalation Breathing into the lungs; a medication delivery route.

interstitial fluid The water bathing the cells; accounts for about 10.5% of body weight; includes special fluid collections, such as cerebrospinal fluid and intraocular fluid.

intracellular fluid (ICF) The water contained inside the cells; normally accounts for 45% of body weight.

intradermal The layer of the dermis, just beneath the epidermis; a medication delivery route.

intramuscular (IM) Into a muscle; a medication delivery route.

intranasal Within the nose.

intraosseous Within the bone.

intraosseous (IO) infusion A technique of administering fluids, blood and blood products, and medications into the intraosseous space of a long bone, usually the proximal tibia.

intraosseous (IO) space The spongy cancellous bone of the epiphyses and the medullary cavity of the diaphysis, collectively.

intravascular fluid Plasma; the water within the blood vessels, which carries red blood cells, white blood cells, and vital nutrients; normally accounts for about 4.5% of body weight.

intravenous Within a vein.

intravenous (IV) therapy Cannulation of a vein with an IV catheter to access the patient's vascular system.

ionic concentration The amount of charged particles found in a particular area.

ions Charged atoms or compounds that results from the loss or gain of an electron.

isotonic crystalloids Intravenous solutions that do not cause a fluid shift into or out of the cell; examples include normal saline and lactated Ringer's solutions.

isotonic solution A solution that has the same concentration of sodium as does the cell. In this case, water does not shift, and no change in cell shape occurs.

lactated Ringer's (LR) solution A sterile isotonic crystalloid IV solution of specified amounts of calcium chloride, potassium chloride, sodium chloride, and sodium lactate in water.

local reactions Reactions that occur in a localized area; a potential complication of IV therapy.

macrodrip sets Administration sets named for the large orifice between the piercing spike and the drip chamber; allow for rapid fluid flow into the vascular system; allow 10 or 15 gtt/mL, depending on the manufacturer.

medical asepsis A term applied to the practice of preventing contamination of the patient by using aseptic technique.

metabolic Pertaining to the breakdown of ingested foodstuffs into smaller and smaller molecules and atoms that are used as energy sources for cellular function.

metered-dose inhaler (MDI) A pressurized canister that delivers a specific dose of a medication; commonly used for beta-agonist bronchodilators.

metric system A decimal system based on tens for the measurement of length, weight, and volume.

microdrip sets Administration sets named for the small needle-like orifice between the piercing spike and the drip chamber; allow for carefully controlled fluid flow and are ideally suited for medication administration; allow for 60 gtt/mL.

milliequivalent (mEq) Unit of measure for electrolytes.

Mix-o-Vial A single vial divided into two compartments by a rubber stopper; Methylprednisolone sodium succinate (Solu-Medrol) is stored this way.

monovalent An ion that contains one charge.

mucosal atomizer device (MAD) A device that attaches to the end of a syringe that is used to spray (atomize) certain medications via the intranasal route.

nebulizer A device for producing a fine spray or mist that is used to deliver inhaled medications.

non-tunneling devices Devices that have been inserted by direct venipuncture through the skin directly into a selected vein, for the purpose of long-term medication administration, total parenteral nutrition, chemotherapy, and venous blood sampling; peripheral inserted central catheters and central venous catheters are examples.

nonelectrolytes Solutes that have no electrical charge; include glucose and urea; measured in milligrams (mg).

normal saline A solution of 0.9% sodium chloride; an isotonic crystalloid.

occlusion Blockage, usually of a tubular structure such as a blood vessel or IV catheter.

ocular Pertaining to the eye.

online (direct) medical control Type of medical control where the paramedic is in direct contact with a physician, usually via two-way radio or telephone.

osmolarity The ability to influence the movement of water across a semipermeable membrane.

osmosis The movement of water across a semipermeable membrane (for example, the cell wall) from an area of lower to higher concentration of solute molecules.

osteogenesis imperfecta A congenital bone disease that results in fragile bones.

osteomyelitis Inflammation of the bone and muscle caused by infection.

overhydration An increase in the body's systemic fluid volume.

over-the-needle catheter A Teflon (plastic) catheter inserted over a hollow needle.

parenteral route A route of medication administration that involves any route other than the gastrointestinal tract.

Penrose drain A type of surgical drain often used as a constricting band.

percutaneous Through the skin or mucous membrane.

peripheral vein cannulation Cannulating veins of the periphery, that is, those that can be seen and/or palpated. Examples of peripheral veins include those of the hand, arm, and lower extremity and the external jugular vein.

phospholipid bilayer The cell membrane's double layer, consisting of a hydrophilic outer layer composed of phosphate groups, and a hydrophobic inner layer made up of lipids, or fatty acids. It is this structure and composition that allows the cell membrane to have selective permeability.

piercing spike The hard, sharpened plastic spike on the end of the administration set designed to pierce the sterile membrane of the IV bag.

postural hypotension Symptomatic drop in blood pressure related to the patient's body position; detected by measuring pulse and blood pressure while the patient is lying supine, sitting up, and standing. An increase in pulse rate and a decrease in blood pressure in any one of these positions is considered a positive sign for this condition.

prefilled syringes Medication syringes that are prepackaged and prepared with a specific concentration.

pressure infuser device A sleeve that is placed around the IV bag and inflated to force fluid to flow from the IV bag and into the tubing.

pulmonary embolism A blood clot or foreign matter trapped within the pulmonary circulation.

pyrogenic reaction A reaction characterized by an abrupt temperature elevation (as high as 106°F [41°C]) with severe chills, backache, headache, weakness, nausea, and vomiting; a potential complication of IV or IO therapy.

radiopaque Feature of an IV catheter (or any other object) that allows it to appear on a radiograph.

saline locks Special types of IV devices that eliminate the need to hang a bag of IV fluid; also called a buff cap or INT (intermittent); commonly used for patients who do not require fluid boluses but may require medication therapy.

selective permeability The ability of the cell membrane to selectively allow compounds into the cell based on the cell's current needs.

self-sealing blood tubes Glass tubes with self-sealing rubber caps; used to obtain blood samples for laboratory analysis.

sharps Any contaminated item that can cause injury; includes IV needles and catheters, broken ampules or vials, or anything else that can penetrate or lacerate the skin.

sodium-potassium (Na⁺-K⁺) pump The mechanism by which the cell brings in two potassium (K^+) ions and releases three sodium (Na^+) ions.

solute The dissolved particles contained in the solvent.

solution Combination of dissolved elements (solutes) and water (solvent).

solvent The fluid that does the dissolving, or the solution that contains the dissolved components.

standing orders A form of off-line or indirect medical control, where the paramedic performs certain predefined procedures before contacting the physician.

sterile The destruction of all living organisms; achieved by using heat, gas, or chemicals.

subcutaneous (SC) Into the tissue between the skin and muscle; a medication delivery route.

sublingual Under the tongue; a medication delivery route.

syncopal episodes Fainting; brief losses of consciousness caused by transiently inadequate blood flow to the brain.

systemic complications Reactions that affect systems of the body.

third spacing The shifting of fluid into the tissues, creating edema.

thrombophlebitis Inflammation of a vein.

through-the-needle catheters Plastic catheters inserted through a hollow needle; referred to as Intracaths.

tonicity The osmotic pressure of a solution, based on the relationship between sodium and water inside and outside the cell, that takes advantage of their chemical and osmotic properties to move water to areas of higher sodium concentration.

total body water (TBW) Total amount of water in the human body; accounts for approximately 60% of the weight of an average man; divided into various compartments.

track marks The visible scars from repeated cannulation of a vein; commonly associated with illicit drug use.

transdermal Across the skin; a medication delivery route.

Vacutainer A cylindrical device that attaches to an 18- or 20-gauge sampling needle; accommodates self-sealing blood tubes when blood samples are being obtained.

varicose veins Veins on the leg that are large, twisted, and ropelike and can cause pain, swelling, or itching.

venous thrombosis The development of a stationary blood clot in the venous circulation.

vials Small glass or plastic bottles that contain medication; may contain single or multiple doses.

volume on hand The amount of fluid you have on hand, such as the amount of fluid in an IV bag or the amount of fluid in a vial of medication.

Volutrol A special type of microdrip set that features a 100- or 200-mL calibrated drip chamber; used for fluid regulation in patients prone to circulatory overload, such as pediatric and elderly patients; also called a Buretrol.

Assessment
in Action

You and your partner are dispatched to a local diner for a patient with chest pain. You are brought to the patient by staff, where you find a 66-year-old man seated at a table clutching his chest. The patient states he has not been feeling well for the past few days and while he was eating, he began to have some chest pain and trouble breathing. The patient states that he recently went to his doctor, who diagnosed him with pneumonia. The patient states he finished his antibiotics several days ago. You obtain his blood pressure and vital signs and find them all to be within normal limits.

1. What should be your first action with this patient?
   A. Start an IV line.
   B. Administer a nitroglycerin spray.
   C. Attach the patient to the cardiac monitor.
   D. Place the patient on oxygen.

2. You want to administer a nitroglycerin spray to the patient because all his vital signs are normal. How is nitroglycerin spray administered?
   A. Intravenously
   B. Sublingually
   C. Transdermally
   D. Intramuscularly

3. Concerning absorption of the medication in the body for the desired effect, the sublingual administration is absorbed:
   A. very slowly.
   B. slowly.
   C. normally.
   D. rapidly.

4. Another name for a sublingual or transdermal administration of medication is:
   A. inhalation.
   B. parenteral.
   C. enteral.
   D. percutaneous.

5. Aspirin is indicated in this patient. How is aspirin administered and how fast is it absorbed?
   A. Intranasally and quickly, within 5 minutes
   B. Intranasally and slowly, within 1 hour
   C. Orally chewed and quickly, within 15 minutes
   D. Orally swallowed whole and slowly, within 3 hours

6. You have inserted an IV line. All of the following are potential complications except:
   A. infiltration.
   B. flash in the flash chamber.
   C. occlusion.
   D. hematoma.

7. You want to administer a 250-mL fluid bolus over the next 20 minutes using a 10-drop set. At how many drops per minute would you set the rate?
   A. 50 gtt/min
   B. 125 gtt/min
   C. 150 gtt/min
   D. 200 gtt/min

Additional Questions

8. You and your partner are treating an elderly patient who reports shortness of breath. The patient is in rapid atrial fibrillation and the physician orders 10 mg of diltiazem. The medication comes in a vial of 25 mg in 5 mL. How much would you administer?

8. You have just resuscitated a patient who was in cardiac arrest and are initiating the return of spontaneous circulation protocol, which calls for you to administer 2 liters of chilled saline. You have established an intraosseous line to administer medication and you have attached the first liter of chilled saline but cannot get the fluid to flow rapidly. What is the problem?

Emergency Medications

National EMS Education Standard Competencies

Pharmacology

Integrates comprehensive knowledge of pharmacology to formulate a treatment plan intended to mitigate emergencies and improve the overall health of the patient.

Emergency Medications

- Names (pp 546–548)
- Effects (pp 546–548)
- Indications (pp 546–548)
- Routes of administration (pp 546–548)
- Dosages for the medications administered (p 548)
- Actions (p 546)
- Contraindications (p 546)
- Complications (p 546)
- Side effects (p 546)
- Interactions (pp 546–548)

Knowledge Objectives

1. Describe how drugs are classified (p 545).
2. Use appropriate terminology related to pharmacology (pp 546–548).
3. List the components of a drug profile (pp 546–548).

4. Identify airway management medications used by the paramedic, including indications, contraindications, dosages, adverse reactions and side effects, and interactions. (pp 548–579)
5. Identify respiratory medications used by the paramedic, including indications, contraindications, dosages, adverse reactions and side effects, and interactions. (pp 548–579)
6. Identify cardiovascular system medications used by the paramedic, including indications, contraindications, dosages, adverse reactions and side effects, and interactions. (pp 548–579)
7. Identify medications for neurologic conditions that are used by the paramedic, including indications, contraindications, dosages, adverse reactions and side effects, and interactions. (pp 548–579)
8. Identify medications affecting the gastrointestinal system that are used by the paramedic, including indications, contraindications, dosages, adverse reactions and side effects, and interactions. (pp 548–579)
9. Identify any miscellaneous medications that are used by the paramedic, including indications, contraindications, dosages, adverse reactions and side effects, and interactions. (pp 548–579)
10. Give the generic and trade names, actions, indications, contraindications, routes of administration, side effects, interactions, and doses of medications and intravenous fluids that may be administered by the paramedic as dictated by state protocols and local medical direction. (pp 548–579)

Skills Objectives

There are no skills objectives for this chapter.

Introduction

Paramedics are required to know the names, class, mechanism of action, adverse reactions and side effects, interactions, indications, contraindications, complications, routes of administration, dose, and specific administration considerations for all of the following emergency medications and intravenous fluids. Individual states have the authority to include additional medications, which may be taught by your local training agency.

Pharmacology is one of the more difficult subjects to master. As a paramedic, you have to make quick decisions about when to administer medications, what medications to administer, and when administering certain medications would be harmful to the patient. What makes this process even more challenging is that pharmacology is constantly changing; new drugs are released frequently, and paramedics must stay up-to-date on the latest pharmacologic information. A solid understanding of the information in this formulary will help you make the right choices for your patients.

This formulary reflects the most current recommendations and resources, including the 2010 ILCOR Guidelines for emergency cardiac care. It is important to remember that state and regional EMS systems have the right to include medications and indications for these medications that may not be covered in the chapter. Always follow your local protocols.

Medication References

AHA Classification of Recommendations and Level of Evidence

A system of classifying recommendations based on strength of the supporting scientific evidence was used in this chapter:

- **Class I:** This indicates that a treatment should be administered.
- **Class IIa:** This indicates that it is reasonable to administer treatment.
- **Class IIb:** This indicates that treatment may be considered.
- **Class III:** This indicates that treatment should NOT be administered. It is not helpful and may be harmful.

- **Class Indeterminate:** This indicates that either research is beginning on the treatment or that research is continuing on this treatment. There are no recommendations until further research is performed (ie, cannot recommend for or against).

Pregnancy Category Ratings for Drugs

Drugs have been categorized by the Food and Drug Administration (FDA) according to the level of risk to the fetus. These categories are listed for each herein under "Pregnancy Safety" and are interpreted as follows:

- **Category A:** Controlled studies in women fail to demonstrate a risk to the fetus in the first trimester, and there is no evidence of risk in later trimesters; the possibility of fetal harm appears to be remote.
- **Category B:** Either (1) animal reproductive studies have not demonstrated a fetal risk but there are no controlled studies in women or (2) animal reproductive studies have shown an adverse effect (other than decreased fertility) that was not confirmed in controlled studies on women in the first trimester and there is no evidence of risk in later trimesters.
- **Category C:** Either (1) studies in animals have revealed adverse effects on the fetus and there are no controlled studies in women or (2) studies in women and animals are not available. Drugs in this category should be given only if the potential benefit justifies the risk to the fetus.
- **Category D:** There is positive evidence of human fetal risk, but the benefits for pregnant women may be acceptable despite the risk, as in life-threatening diseases for which safer drugs cannot be used or are ineffective. An appropriate statement must appear in the "Warnings" section of the labeling of drugs in this category.
- **Category X:** Studies in animals and humans have demonstrated fetal abnormalities, there is evidence of fetal risk based on human experience, or both; the risk of using the drug in pregnant women clearly outweighs any possible benefit. The drug is contraindicated in women who are or may become pregnant. An appropriate statement must appear in the "Contraindications" section of the labeling of drugs in this category.

YOU are the Medic   PART 1

You are dispatched to a local hotel for a seizure. The dispatcher tells you that you are responding to a 30-year-old woman with a history of seizures. You are also advised that the patient is actively seizing at this time. When you arrive at the room, the patient is lying supine on the bed in a full-body seizure. The patient's husband tells you she has a history of seizures and has not been taking her phenytoin (Dilantin). He adds that she has been seizing actively since he called 9-1-1.

1. What type of seizure is this patient experiencing?
2. What are some of the common causes of seizures?

Federal "Controlled Substance Act of 1970" Schedule Summary

The Controlled Substances Act (CSA), Title II of the Comprehensive Drug Abuse Prevention and Control Act of 1970, is the legal foundation of the government's fight against abuse of drugs and other substances. This law is a consolidation of numerous laws regulating the manufacture and distribution of narcotics, stimulants, depressants, hallucinogens, anabolic steroids, and chemicals used in the illicit production of controlled substances. The Regulatory Agency is the DEA (Drug Enforcement Agency). See the chapter, *Principles of Pharmacology* for more information on drug schedules.

Medical Terminology Related to Pharmacology

Paramedics need to be familiar with terminology related to medications and medication administration, such as common prefixes **Table 1**, common metric conversions **Table 2**, and common medical abbreviations related to pharmacology **Table 3**.

Drug Dosage Calculations

The chapter, *Medication Administration*, discussed drug dosage calculations in detail. The following terms are important to know when performing such calculations:

- **Desired dose**: The quantity of a medication that is to be administered to a patient. This is usually expressed in milligrams, grams, or grains.
- **Concentration** (of the medication on hand): The amount of a medication that is present in the ampule or vial. This is usually expressed in milligrams, grams, or grains.
- **Volume** (of the medication on hand): The amount of a fluid that is present in the ampule or vial in which the medication is dissolved. This is usually expressed in milligrams, grams, or grains.
- **Yield**: The amount of drug in 1 mL.

Table 1 Commonly Used Prefixes

Prefix Name	Prefix Symbol	Prefix Value
micro	μ	1/1,000,000 or 0.000001
milli	m	1/1,000 or 0.001
centi	c	1/100 or 0.01
kilo	k	1,000
mega	M	1 million or 1,000,000

Table 2 Common Metric Conversions

Weight	
1 kilogram (kg)	2.2 pounds (lb)
1 kilogram (kg)	1,000 grams (g or gm)
1 gram (g or gr)	1,000 milligrams (mg)
1 milligram (mg)	1,000 micrograms (μg or mcg)
Volume	
1 liter (L)	1,000 milliliters or cubic centimeters (mL or cc)
Temperature	
37° Celsius (°C)	98.6° Fahrenheit (°F)
Length	
1 centimeter (cm)	10 millimeters (mm)
100 centimeters (cm)	1 meter (m)

Medication Listings

Each entry in this formulary follows a standard format, including the following information:

- Name of medication (other common names)
- **Class**: How the medication is categorized as compared to other medications. This is usually done by grouping those medications with similar characteristics, traits, or primary components.
- **Mechanism of action**: The way in which a medication produces the intended response.
- **Indications**: A circumstance that points to or shows the cause, pathology, treatment, or issue of an attack of disease; that which points out; that which serves as a guide or warning.
- **Contraindications**: Any condition, especially any condition of disease, which renders some particular line of treatment improper or undesirable.
- **Adverse reactions/side effects**: This is an abnormal or harmful effect to an organism caused by exposure to a chemical. It is indicated by some result such as death, a change in food or water consumption, altered body and organ weights, altered enzyme levels, or visible illness. An effect may be classed as adverse if it causes functional or anatomic damage, causes irreversible change in the homeostasis of the organism, or increases the susceptibility of the organism to other chemical or biologic stress. A nonadverse effect will usually be reversed when the organism is no longer being exposed to the chemical.
- **Drug interactions**: This refers to any potential effects that a medication may have when administered in conjunction

Table 3   Common Medical Abbreviations Related to Pharmacology

Abbreviation	Definition	Abbreviation	Definition
ā	before	NKDA	no known diagnosed allergies
α	alpha	NTG	nitroglycerin
amp.	ampule	∅	null or none
APAP	acetaminophen	p̄	after
ASA	aspirin	pc	post cibos (after eating)
β	beta	pedi	pediatric
bid	bis in die (twice a day)	po	per os (by mouth)
c̄	with	pr	per rectus (by rectum)
caps	capsules	prn	per re nata (when necessary)
cc	cubic centimeter	q̄	quisque (every)
D/C	discontinue	qd	quisque die (every day)
dig	digitalis	qh	quisque hora (every hour)
elix	elixir	qid	quarter in die (four times a day)
ET	endotracheal	qod	quaque altera die (every other day)
ETOH	ethyl alcohol	RL	Ringer's lactate
g or gr	gram	s̄	sine (without)
gtt	gutta (drop)	SC	subcutaneous
gtts	guttae (drops)	stat	statim (now or immediately)
HHN	hand-held nebulizer	SVN	small-volume nebulizer
Hs	hora somni (at bedtime)	tid	ter in die (three times a day)
IC	intracardiac	TKO	to keep open
IM	intramuscular	u	unit
IO	intraosseous	ut dict	ut dictum (as directed)
IV	intravenous	®	registered trademark
IVP	intravenous push	♀	female
IVPB	intravenous piggyback	♂	male
kg	kilogram	>	greater than
KO	keep open	<	less than
KVO	keep vein open	≥	greater than or equal to
L or l	liter	≤	less than or equal to
lb	pound	≈	approximately
LR	lactated Ringer's	=	equal to
MAX	maximum	≠	not equal
MDI	Metered-dose inhaler	Δ	change(s)
nitro	nitroglycerin	μ	micro
NKA	no known allergies	μgtt	microdrop

Continues

Table 3 Common Medical Abbreviations Related to Pharmacology, continued

Abbreviation	Definition	Abbreviation	Definition
μg or mcg	microgram	±	plus or minus
mEq	milliequivalent	°	degree(s)
mg	milligram	TM	trademark
min	minute		
mL	milliliter		
MS or MSO$_4$	morphine sulfate		

or in the presence of another medication already in the patient's system, a medication delivery device, or fluid.

- **How supplied:** This is how the manufacturer packages the medication for distribution and sale. Typical methods of packaging are prefilled syringes, vials, or ampules.
- **Dosage and administration:** This is the typical or average volume of the medication that is to be administered to the patient and the route of introduction of the medication to the patient.
- <u>Duration of action</u>: Three values are given: (1) onset: the estimated amount of time it will take for the medication to enter the body/system and begin to take effect, (2) peak effect: the estimated amount of time it will take for the medication to have its greatest effect on the patient/system, and (3) duration: the estimated amount of time that the medication will have any effect on the patient/system.
- **Special considerations:** Additional pertinent information concerning a medication.

Special Populations

Pediatric and geriatric patients often have slower medication absorption and elimination times, necessitating modification of the doses of many drugs administered to these patients. Pregnant patients are limited in the medications they can take because of risk to the fetus.

■ Drug Profiles

■ Activated Charcoal (EZ-Char, Actidose, Liqui-Char)

Class Adsorbent.

Mechanism of action Absorbs toxic substances from the gastrointestinal tract.

Indications Most oral poisonings and medication overdoses; can be used after evacuation of poisons.

Contraindications Oral administration to comatose patients; after ingestion of corrosives, caustics, petroleum distillates (ineffective and may induce vomiting); simultaneous administration with other oral drugs. Use caution in patients experiencing abdominal pain of unknown origin or known GI obstruction.

Adverse reactions/side effects If aspirated, can induce fatal form of pneumonitis; constipation, black stools, diarrhea, vomiting, bowel obstruction.

Drug interactions Bonds with and generally inactivates whatever it is mixed with (eg, syrup of ipecac).

How supplied 25 g (black powder)/125-mL bottle (200 mg/mL); 50 g (black powder)/250-mL bottle (200 mg/mL).

Dosage and administration *Adult:* 1 to 2 g/kg PO or nasogastric tube. *Pediatric:* 1 to 2 g/kg PO or nasogastric tube.

Duration of action *Onset:* Immediate. *Peak effect:* Depends on gastrointestinal function. *Duration:* Will act until excreted.

Special considerations Pregnancy safety: Category C. Often used in conjunction with magnesium citrate. Must be stored in a closed container. Be sure to mix contents well before administration due to separation while being stored. Does not absorb cyanide, lithium, iron, lead, or arsenic.

■ Adenosine (Adenocard)

Class Antidysrhythmic.

Mechanism of action Slows conduction through the AV node; can interrupt re-entrant pathways; slows heart rate by acting directly on the sinus pacemaker cells by slowing impulse formation. The drug of choice for re-entry SVT. Can be used diagnostically for stable, wide-complex tachycardia of unknown origin after two doses of lidocaine.

Indications Conversion of PSVT to sinus rhythm. May convert re-entry SVT due to Wolff-Parkinson-White syndrome. Not effective in converting atrial fibrillation/flutter or V-tach. Most forms of stable narrow-complex SVT.

Contraindications Second- or third-degree AV block (if no pacemaker is present), sick sinus syndrome (if no pacemaker present), bronchoconstrictive or bronchospastic lung disease (asthma, COPD), poison- or drug-induced tachycardia.

Adverse reactions/side effects Generally short duration and mild; headache, dizziness, dyspnea, bronchospasm, dysrhythmias, palpitations, hypotension, chest pain, facial flushing, cardiac arrest, nausea, metallic taste, pain in the head or neck, paresthesia, diaphoresis.

Drug interactions Methylxanthines (theophylline-like drugs) antagonize the effects of adenosine. Dipyridamole (Persantine) potentiates the effect of adenosine. Carbamazepine (Tegretol) may potentiate the AV node blocking effect of adenosine.

How supplied 3 mg/mL in 2-mL and 5-mL flip-top vials.

Dosage and administration *Adult:* 6-mg rapid IV bolus over 1–3 seconds, followed by a 20-mL saline flush and elevate extremity. If no response after 1–2 minutes, administer second dose of 12–mg rapid IV bolus over 1–3 seconds. *Pediatric:* Initial dose 0.1 mg/kg rapid IV/IO push (maximum first dose, 6 mg), followed by a 5- to 10-mL saline flush. Second dose 0.2 mg/kg rapid IV/IO push (maximum second dose, 12 mg), followed by a 5- to 10-mL saline flush.

Duration of action *Onset:* Seconds. *Peak effect:* Seconds. *Duration:* 12 seconds.

Special considerations Pregnancy safety: Category C. May cause bronchoconstriction in asthma patients. Evaluate elderly for signs of dehydration requiring fluid replacement prior to administering adenosine. Short half-life limits side effects in most patients.

Albuterol (Proventil, Ventolin)

Class Sympathomimetic, bronchodilator.

Mechanism of action Selective beta-2 agonist that stimulates adrenergic receptors of the sympathomimetic nervous system. Results in smooth-muscle relaxation in the bronchial tree and peripheral vasculature.

Indications Treatment of bronchospasm in patients with reversible obstructive airway disease (COPD/asthma). Prevention of exercise-induced bronchospasm.

Contraindications Known prior hypersensitivity reactions to albuterol. Tachycardia, dysrhythmias, especially those caused by digitalis. Synergistic with other sympathomimetics.

Adverse reactions/side effects Often dose-related and include headache, fatigue, lightheadedness, irritability, restlessness, aggressive behavior, pulmonary edema, hoarseness, nasal congestion, increased sputum, hypertension, tachycardia, dysrhythmias, chest pain, palpitations, nausea/vomiting, dry mouth, epigastric pain, and tremors.

Drug interactions Tricyclic antidepressants may potentiate vasculature effects. Beta blockers are antagonistic and may block pulmonary effects. May potentiate hypokalemia caused by diuretics.

How supplied Metered-dose inhaler: 90 µg/metered spray. Solution for aerosolization: 0.5% (5 mg/mL), 0.083% (2.5 mg) in 3-mL unit dose nebulizer.

Dosage and administration *Adult:* Administer 2.5 mg. Dilute in 0.5 mL of 0.5% solution for inhalation with 2.5 mL normal saline in nebulizer and administer over 10–15 minutes. Metered-dose inhaler: 1–2 inhalations (90–180 µg); wait 5 minutes between inhalations. *Pediatric:* <20 kg: 1.25 mg/dose via hand-held nebulizer or mask over 20 minutes. >20 kg: 2.5 mg/dose via hand-held nebulizer or mask over 20 minutes. Repeat once in 20 minutes.

Duration of action *Onset:* 5–15 minutes. *Peak effect:* 30 minutes to 2 hours. *Duration:* 3–4 hours.

Special considerations Pregnancy safety: Category C. May precipitate angina pectoris and dysrhythmias. In prehospital emergency care, albuterol should be administered only via inhalation.

Alteplase, Recombinant (tissue plasminogen activator or rTPA, Activase)

Class Fibrinolytic.

Mechanism of action The enzyme binds to the fibrin-bound plasminogen at the clot site, converting plasminogen to plasmin. Plasmin digests the fibrin strands of the clot, restoring perfusion.

Indications Acute myocardial infarction, STEMI, massive pulmonary emboli, acute ischemic cerebrovascular accident.

Contraindications Active internal bleeding, recent surgery (within 2–3 weeks), previous cerebral vascular accident or seizure at onset, prolonged cardiopulmonary resuscitation, intracranial or intraspinal surgery (within 3 months); intracranial neoplasm, arteriovenous malformation, or aneurysm; recent significant trauma, especially head trauma. Uncontrolled hypertension (systolic of greater than 185 mm Hg, diastolic of greater than 110 mm Hg).

Adverse reactions/side effects Intracranial bleeding, headache, reperfusion dysrhythmias, chest pain, hypotension, GI bleeding, nausea, vomiting, abdominal pain.

Drug interactions Acetylsalicylic acid (aspirin) may increase risk of bleeding hemorrhage. Heparin and other anticoagulants may increase risk of hemorrhage.

How supplied 50- and 100-mg powders (requires reconstitution with sterile water to a concentration of 1 mg/mL).

Dosage and administration *Adult:* 15-mg IV bolus over 2 minutes; then 0.75 mg/kg over 30 minutes (not to exceed 50 mg); then 0.50 mg/kg over 60 minutes; maximum total dose of 100 mg (other doses may be prescribed by medical direction). For acute ischemic stroke, 0.9 mg 1kg infused over 60 minutes; administer 10% of total dose in 1 minute and the rest over the next 60 minutes. *Pediatric:* Safety not established.

Duration of action *Onset:* Clot lysis most often within 60–90 minutes. *Peak effect:* Variable. *Duration:* 30 minutes with 80% cleared within 10 minutes.

Special considerations Pregnancy safety: Category C. Closely monitor vital signs. Observe for bleeding. Do not administer IM injections to patients receiving tissue plasminogen activator. Only administer with an infusion pump. Due to severe spontaneous bleeding risk, invasive procedures (eg, IV starts, injections, NG tube, or nasotracheal intubation) should be avoided.

■ Amiodarone (Cordarone, Pacerone)

Class Antidysrhythmic.

Mechanism of action Blocks sodium channels and myocardial potassium channels, delaying repolarization and increasing the duration of action potential.

Indications Ventricular fibrillation, pulseless ventricular tachycardia, unstable ventricular tachycardia in patients refractory to other therapy.

Contraindications Known hypersensitivity to amiodarone or iodine, cardiogenic shock, sinus bradycardia, second- or third-degree AV block (if no pacemaker is present), severe sinus node dysfunction.

Adverse reactions/side effects Dizziness, fatigue, malaise, tremor, ataxia, lack of coordination, adult respiratory distress syndrome, pulmonary edema, cough, progressive dyspnea, congestive heart failure, bradycardia, hypotension, worsening of dysrhythmias, prolonged QT interval, nausea, vomiting, burning at IV site, Stevens-Johnson syndrome.

Drug interactions Use with digoxin may cause digitalis toxicity. Antidysrhythmics may cause increased serum levels. Beta blocker and calcium channel blockers may potentiate bradycardia, sinus arrest, and AV heart blocks.

How supplied 50 mg/mL vials and prefilled syringes. For rapid infusion, add 150 mg/3 mL to a 10-mL D_5W (1.5 mg/mL) run at 600 mL/h on infusion pump.

Dosage and administration *Adult:* Ventricular fibrillation/pulseless ventricular tachycardia unresponsive to CPR, defibrillation, and vasopressors: 300 mg IV/IO push. Initial dose can be followed one time in 3–5 minutes at 150 mg IV/IO push. Recurrent life-threatening ventricular dysrhythmias: Maximum cumulative dose: 2.2 g IV/24 h administered as follows: Rapid infusion: 150 mg IV/IO over 10 minutes (15 mg/minute). May repeat rapid infusion (150 mg IV/IO) every 10 minutes as needed. *Pediatric:* Refractory ventricular fibrillation/pulseless ventricular tachycardia: 5 mg/kg IV/IO bolus. Can repeat the 5 mg/kg IV/IO bolus up to a total dose of 15 mg/kg per 24 h. Maximum single dose: 300 mg. Perfusing supraventricular and ventricular tachycardias: Loading dose 5 mg/kg IV/IO over 20–60 minutes (maximum single dose of 300 mg). Can repeat to maximum dose of 15 mg/kg/day (2.2 g in adolescents). Maximum single dose: 300 mg.

Duration of action *Onset:* Immediate. *Peak effect:* 10–15 minutes. *Duration:* 30–45 minutes.

Special considerations Pregnancy safety: Category D. Monitor patient for hypotension. May worsen or precipitate new dysrhythmias.

■ Amyl Nitrite

Class Antidote, cyanide poisoning adjunct.

Mechanism of action Converts hemoglobin to methemoglobin, which reacts with cyanide and chemically binds with it, preventing any toxic effects.

Indications Cyanide poisoning.

Contraindications None in the emergency setting.

Adverse reactions/side effects Headache, dizziness, weakness, increased ICP, shortness of breath, orthostatic hypotension, tachycardia, syncope, cyanosis of the lips, fingernails, or palms (signs of methemoglobinemia).

YOU *are the Medic*   PART 2

The patient has foam and saliva around her mouth and nose; you hear a gurgling sound coming from behind clenched teeth. The seizure activity is slowing but has not completely stopped. Her husband tells you the long seizure is unusual for her. You and your partner roll the patient onto her side to help clear her airway. Your partner prepares to suction the patient.

Recording Time: 0 Minutes	
Appearance	Tonic-clonic seizures
Level of consciousness	Unresponsive
Airway	Foam and saliva noted around mouth
Breathing	Gurgling
Circulation	Rapid pulse

3. What is the mechanism of action for phenytoin (Dilantin)?

4. Why is it important to know that the patient has not been taking her prescribed medications?

Drug interactions Increased hypotensive effects with antihypertensives, alcohol ingestion, phenothiazines, or beta blockers.

How supplied 0.3-mL ampules for inhalation.

Dosage and administration *Adult:* 1–2 ampules crushed and inhaled for 30 seconds of each minute until sodium nitrite is prepared or administer for 30–60 seconds every 5 minutes until patient is conscious. *Pediatric:* 1 ampule crushed and inhaled for 30 seconds of each minute until sodium nitrite is prepared or administer for 30–60 seconds every 5 minutes until patient is conscious.

Duration of action *Onset:* 30 seconds to 5 minutes. *Peak effect:* Varies. *Duration:* 3 to 5 minutes.

Special considerations Pregnancy safety: Category X. Highly flammable: Avoid exposure to heat or flame. Patient should remain seated or supine during and after administration due to hypotensive effects of this medication. Use caution in administering to patients with cerebral hemorrhage, increased ICP, or hypotension. This is the first step in a three-step treatment for cyanide poisoning followed by sodium nitrite and then sodium thiosulfate.

Aspirin (ASA, Bayer, Ecotrin, St. Joseph, and others)

Class Platelet inhibitor, anti-inflammatory agent.

Mechanism of action Prevents platelets from clumping together, or aggregating, and forming emboli.

Indications New onset chest pain suggestive of acute myocardial infarction.

Contraindications Hypersensitivity. Relatively contraindicated in patients with active ulcer disease or asthma.

Adverse reactions/side effects Bronchospasm, anaphylaxis, wheezing in allergic patients, prolonged bleeding, GI bleeding, epigastric distress, nausea, vomiting, heartburn, Reye syndrome.

Drug interactions Use with caution in patients allergic to NSAIDs.

How supplied 81-mg, 160-mg, and 325-mg tablets. Chewable and standard.

Dosage and administration *Adult:* 160 mg to 325 mg PO. Chewing is preferable to swallowing. *Pediatric:* Not recommended.

Duration of action *Onset:* 30–45 minutes. *Peak effect:* Variable. *Duration:* Variable.

Special considerations Pregnancy safety: Category D. Not recommended in pediatric population.

Atenolol (Tenormin)

Class Beta blocker (beta-1 selective), antidysrhythmic.

Mechanism of action Decreases heart rate, myocardial contractility, and cardiac output. Inhibits dilation of bronchial smooth muscle.

Indications To reduce myocardial ischemia and damage in acute myocardial infarction patients; paroxysmal SVT, atrial flutter, atrial fibrillation, hypertension.

Contraindications Heart failure, cardiogenic shock, bradycardia, lung disease, hypotension, second- or third-degree heart block.

Adverse reactions/side effects Dizziness, bronchospasm, bradycardia, AV conduction delays, hypotension, myocardial infarction, heart failure.

Drug interactions May potentiate antihypertensive effects when given to patients taking calcium channel blockers or MAOIs. Catecholamine-depleting drugs may potentiate hypotension. Sympathomimetic drugs may be antagonized. Signs of hypoglycemia may be masked.

How supplied 5 mg in 10-mL ampules.

Dosage and administration *Adult:* 5 mg slow IV (over 5 minutes). Wait 10 minutes. Give second dose of 5 mg over 5 minutes. *Pediatric:* Not recommended.

Duration of action *Onset:* Within 5 minutes. *Peak effect:* 10 minutes. *Duration:* 2–4 hours.

Special considerations Pregnancy safety: Category D. Atenolol must be given slowly IV over 5 minutes. Concurrent administration with IV calcium channel blockers such as verapamil or diltiazem can cause severe hypotension. Atenolol should be used with caution in patients with liver or renal dysfunction and COPD.

Atropine Sulfate

Class Anticholinergic agent.

Mechanism of action Inhibits the action of acetylcholine at postganglionic parasympathetic neuroeffector sites. Increases heart rate in life-threatening bradydysrhythmias.

Indications Hemodynamically unstable bradycardia, organophosphate poisoning, nerve agent exposure, rapid sequence intubation in pediatrics, beta blocker or calcium channel blocker overdose.

Contraindications Tachycardia, hypersensitivity, unstable cardiovascular status in acute hemorrhage with myocardial ischemia, narrow-angle glaucoma, hypothermic bradycardia.

Adverse reactions/side effects Drowsiness, confusion, headache, tachycardia, palpitations, dysrhythmias, nausea, vomiting, pupil dilation, dry mouth/nose/skin, blurred vision, urinary retention, constipation, flushed, hot, dry skin; paradoxical bradycardia when pushed too slowly or when given at low doses.

Drug interactions Potential adverse effects when administered with digitalis, cholinergics, physostigmine. Effects enhanced by antihistamines, procainamide, quinidine, antipsychotics, benzodiazepines, and antidepressants.

How supplied Prefilled syringes containing 1 mg in 10 mL (0.1 mg/mL). Nebulizer: 0.2% (1 mg in 0.5 mL) and 0.5% (2.5 mg in 0.5 mL).

Dosage and administration *Adult:* Unstable bradycardia: 0.5 mg IV/IO every 3–5 minutes as needed. Not to exceed total dose of 0.04 mg/kg (maximum 3 mg total). Use shorter dosing interval (3 minutes) and higher doses in severe clinical conditions. Organophosphate poisoning: Extremely large doses (2–4 mg or higher) may be needed. *Pediatric:* Unstable bradycardia: 0.02 mg/kg IV/IO (minimum dose: 0.1 mg). May repeat once. Maximum single dose: Child: 0.5 mg. Adolescent: 1 mg. Maximum total dose: Child: 1 mg. Adolescent: 3 mg. ET dose: 0.04–0.06 mg/kg. Rapid sequence intubation: 0.01–0.02 mg/kg IV/IO (minimum: 0.1 mg, maximum: 0.5 mg).

Duration of action *Onset:* Immediate. *Peak effect:* Rapid to 1–2 minutes. *Duration:* 2–6 hours.

Special considerations Pregnancy safety: Category C. Moderate doses may cause pupillary dilation. Paradoxical bradycardia can occur with doses lower than 0.1 mg.

Benzocaine Spray (Hurricane)

Class Topical anesthetic.

Mechanism of action Stabilizes neuronal membrane, which blocks the initiation and conduction of nerve impulses.

Indications Used as a lubricant and topical anesthetic to facilitate passage of diagnostic and treatment devices. Suppresses the pharyngeal and tracheal gag reflex.

Contraindications People with known hypersensitivity to benzocaine.

Adverse reactions/side effects Methemoglobinemia has been reported on extremely rare occasions following the use of benzocaine.

Drug interactions No significant interactions found or known.

How supplied Multi-dose aerosol can of 20% benzocaine.

Dosage and administration *Adult:* 0.5–1 second spray, repeat as needed. *Pediatric:* 0.25–0.5 second spray, repeat as needed.

Duration of action *Onset:* Immediate. *Peak effect:* 30 seconds. *Duration:* 15 minutes.

Special considerations Pregnancy safety: Category C. Topical use only; not for ocular use or injection.

Bumetanide (Bumex)

Class Loop diuretic.

Mechanism of action A potent loop diuretic with a rapid onset and short duration of action. Inhibits the reabsorption of sodium and chloride in the ascending limb of the loop of Henle.

Indications Pulmonary edema, congestive heart failure.

Contraindications Hypersensitivity to bumetanide or sulfonamides, hypovolemia, anuria, electrolyte deficiencies, hepatic coma. Use caution: hepatic cirrhosis, ascites, diabetes, hypersensitivity to furosemide.

Adverse reactions/side effects Dizziness, headache, orthostatic hypotension, ECG changes due to electrolyte depletion, nausea/vomiting, diarrhea, muscle cramps, metabolic alkalosis, hypovolemia, dehydration.

Drug interactions NSAIDs reduce diuretic effect. May increase blood levels of lithium, increasing risk of lithium poisoning.

Antihypertensives and diuretics can cause further hypotension and fluid depletion.

How supplied 0.25 mg/mL vials.

Dosage and administration *Adult:* 0.5 to 1.0 mg IV slowly over 1 to 2 minutes, or IM. *Pediatric:* Safety and effectiveness in pediatric patients is not established.

Duration of action *Onset:* Immediate. *Peak effect:* 15 to 30 minutes. *Duration:* 2 to 4 hours.

Special considerations Pregnancy safety: Category C. Bumetanide does not have the vasodilatory effects of furosemide. 1.0 mg bumetanide = 40 mg furosemide. May precipitate hypokalemic-induced digoxin toxicity.

Calcium Chloride

Class Electrolyte (anion).

Mechanism of action Increases cardiac contractile state (positive inotropic effect). May enhance ventricular automaticity.

Indications Hypocalcemia, hyperkalemia, hypermagnesemia, beta blocker and calcium channel blocker toxicity.

Contraindications Hypercalcemia, ventricular fibrillation, digitalis toxicity.

Adverse reactions/side effects Syncope, cardiac arrest, dysrhythmia, bradycardia, hypotension, asystole, peripheral vasodilation, nausea, vomiting, metallic taste, tissue necrosis at injection site, coronary and cerebral artery spasm.

Drug interactions May worsen dysrhythmias secondary to digitalis toxicity. May antagonize the effects of calcium channel blockers. Do not mix or infuse immediately before or after sodium bicarbonate without intervening flush.

How supplied 10% solution in 10 mL (100 mg/mL) ampules, vials, and prefilled syringes.

Dosage and administration *Adult:* Calcium channel blocker overdose and hyperkalemia: 500 mg to 1,000 mg (5–10 mL of 10% solution) IV push. May repeat as needed. *Pediatric:* Calcium channel blocker overdose and hyperkalemia: 20 mg/kg (0.2 mL/kg) slow IV/IO push. Maximum 1-g dose; may repeat in 10 minutes.

Duration of action *Onset:* 1–3 minutes. *Peak effect:* Variable. *Duration:* 20–30 minutes, but may persist for 4 hours (dose dependent).

Special considerations Pregnancy safety: Category C. Do not use routinely in cardiac arrest. Comparable dose of 10% calcium gluconate is 15–30 mL. Central venous administration is the preferred route in pediatrics if available.

Calcium Gluconate

Class Electrolyte.

Mechanism of action Counteracts the toxicity of hyperkalemia by stabilizing the membranes of the cardiac cells, reducing the likelihood of fibrillation.

Indications Hyperkalemia, hypocalcemia, hypermagnesemia, beta blocker and calcium channel blocker overdose.

Contraindications Ventricular fibrillation, digitalis toxicity, hypercalcemia.

Adverse reactions/side effects Syncope, cardiac arrest, dysrhythmia, bradycardia, hypotension, asystole, peripheral vasodilation, nausea, vomiting, metallic taste, tissue necrosis at injection site, coronary and cerebral artery spasm.

Drug interactions May worsen dysrhythmias secondary to digitalis toxicity. May antagonize the effects of calcium channel blockers. Do not mix or infuse immediately before or after sodium bicarbonate without intervening flush.

How supplied 100 mg/mL of a 10% solution.

Dosage and administration *Adult:* Hyperkalemia: 500–1,000 mg slow IV/IO push (1–1.5 mL/minute) to maximum of 3 grams. Beta blocker and calcium channel blocker overdose: 3–6 grams (30–60 mL) IV/IO followed by a continuous hourly infusion of the same dose. *Pediatric:* Hyperkalemia: 60 to 100 mg/kg IV/IO slowly over a 5–10 minutes to a maximum of 3 grams. Beta blocker and calcium channel blocker overdose: 60 mg/kg (0.6 mL/kg) IV/IO followed by a continuous hourly infusion of the same dose.

Duration of action *Onset:* Immediate. *Peak effect:* Immediate. *Duration:* 30 minutes to 2 hours.

Special considerations Pregnancy safety: Category C. Do not administer by IM or SQ; causes significant tissue necrosis.

Clopidogrel (Plavix)

Class Thienopyridine antiplatelet.

Mechanism of action Inhibits platelet aggregation by blocking activation of the glycoprotein IIb/IIIa complex.

Indications ST elevation MI (STEMI), moderate- to high-risk non-ST elevation MI (NSTEMI), acute coronary syndrome, substitute for aspirin in patients unable to take aspirin.

Contraindications Active GI bleeding, intracranial hemorrhage, known hypersensitivity.

Adverse reactions/side effects Severe neutropenia, thrombotic thrombocytopenic purpura (TTP), GI hemorrhage, cerebral hemorrhage, angioedema, Stevens-Johnson syndrome, rash, flulike symptoms.

Drug interactions Should not to be taken with proton pump inhibitors (omeprazole and similar drugs), use with caution with other anticoagulants (Warfarin, enoxaparin, streptokinase, aspirin).

How supplied 75-mg and 300-mg tablets.

Dosage and administration *Adult:* Loading dose of 300–600 mg PO. *Pediatric:* Not recommended.

Duration of action *Onset:* Rapid. *Peak effect:* 1 hour. *Duration:* 7–10 days.

Special considerations Pregnancy safety: Category B. Often given with other anticoagulants (heparin, eptifibatide) in ACS and MI.

Dexamethasone Sodium Phosphate (Decadron)

Class Corticosteroid, adrenal glucocorticoid.

Mechanism of action Suppresses acute and chronic inflammation; immunosuppressive effects.

Indications Anaphylaxis, asthma, spinal cord injury, croup, elevated intracranial pressure (prevention and treatment), as an adjunct in the treatment of shock.

Contraindications Hypersensitivity, use caution in suspected systemic sepsis.

Adverse reactions/side effects Headache, restlessness, euphoria, psychoses, pulmonary tuberculosis, hypertension, peptic ulcer, nausea, vomiting, GI bleeding, edema, hyperglycemia, immunosuppression, sodium and water retention. None from single dose.

Drug interactions Calcium, metaraminol.

How supplied 100 mg/5 mL vials or 20 mg/1 mL vials.

Dosage and administration *Adult:* 10–100 mg IV (1 mg/kg slow IV bolus). Considerable variance through medical control. *Pediatric:* 0.25–1.0 mg/kg IV/IO/IM. Given one time with maximum dose of 16 mg.

Duration of action *Onset:* Hours. *Peak effect:* 8–12 hours. *Duration:* 24–72 hours.

Special considerations Pregnancy safety: Category C. Protect medication from heat. Toxicity and side effects with long-term use.

Dextrose

Class Carbohydrate, antihypoglycemic.

Mechanism of action Rapidly increases serum glucose levels. Short-term osmotic diuresis.

Indications Hypoglycemia, altered level of consciousness, coma of unknown origin, seizure of unknown origin, status epilepticus.

Contraindications Intracranial hemorrhage.

Adverse reactions/side effects Extravasation leads to tissue necrosis. Cerebral hemorrhage, cerebral ischemia, pulmonary edema, warmth, pain, burning from IV infusion, hyperglycemia.

Drug interactions Sodium bicarbonate, warfarin (Coumadin).

How supplied 500 mg/mL (50%), 250 mg/mL (25%), and 100 mg/mL (10%) prefilled syringes and vials.

Dosage and administration *Adult:* 12.5–25 grams of a 50% solution slow IV push. May be repeated as necessary. *Pediatric:* 1 year and older; 0.5–1 g/kg of a 25% solution slow IV/IO push. May be repeated as necessary. *Neonates and infants:* 200–500 mg/kg of a 10%–25% solution slow IV push (see below). May be repeated as necessary. Maximum concentration of 12.5% (vasculature extremely sensitive to high concentrations).

Duration of action *Onset:* Less than 1 minute. *Peak effect:* Variable. *Duration:* Variable.

Special considerations Pregnancy safety: Category C. Administer thiamine prior to D_{50} in known alcoholic patients. Draw blood

Neonate and Newborn Dosing Chart				
Age	Estimated weight (kg)	Dose	Volume to be infused (mL)	Concentration (%)
Preterm	1.5	0.3 g	3	10
	1.5	0.3 g	2.4	12.50
Birth	3	0.6 g	6	10
	3	0.6 g	4.8	12.50
3 months	5	2.5 g	10	25
6 months	7	3.5 g	14	25
1 year	10	5.0 g	20	25

to determine glucose level before administering. Do not administer to patients with known CVA unless hypoglycemia documented.

How to prepare D_{10}, $D_{12.5}$, and D_{25} from D_{50}:

To make a 10% solution:
- Take 5 mL (2.5 grams) of a 50-mL stock solution of D_{50} and dilute with 20 mL of injectable sterile water:

$$2.5 \text{ g}/25 \text{ mL} = 2{,}500 \text{ mg}/25 \text{ mL} =$$
$$100 \text{ mg}/1 \text{ mL} = 10\% = D_{10}$$

To make a 12.5% solution:
- Take 2.5 mL (1.25 grams) of a 50-mL stock solution of D_{50} and dilute with 7.5 mL of injectable sterile water:

$$1.25 \text{ g}/10 \text{ mL} = 1{,}250 \text{ mg}/10 \text{ mL}$$
$$= 125 \text{ mg}/1 \text{ mL} = 12.5\% = D_{12.5}$$

To make a 25% solution:
- Take 25 mL (12.5 grams) of a 50-mL stock solution of D_{50} and dilute with 25 mL of injectable sterile water:

$$12.5 \text{ g}/50 \text{ mL} = 12{,}500 \text{ mg}/50 \text{ mL}$$
$$= 250 \text{ mg}/1 \text{ mL} = 25\% = D_{25}$$

Diazepam (Valium and others)

Class Benzodiazepine, long-acting; sedative-hypnotic; anticonvulsant; schedule IV drug.

Mechanism of action Potentiates effects of inhibitory neurotransmitters. Raises the seizure threshold. Induces amnesia and sedation.

Indications Acute anxiety states and agitation, acute alcohol withdrawal, muscle relaxant, seizure activity, sedation for medical procedures (eg, intubation, ventilated patients, cardioversion), may be helpful in acute symptomatic cocaine overdose.

Contraindications Hypersensitivity, narrow-angle glaucoma, myasthenia gravis, respiratory insufficiency, coma, head injury.

Adverse reactions/side effects Dizziness, drowsiness, confusion, headache, respiratory depression, hypotension, reflex tachycardia, nausea, vomiting, muscle weakness, tissue necrosis, ataxia, thrombosis, phlebitis.

Drug interactions Incompatible with most drugs, fluids.

How supplied 5 mg/mL prefilled syringes, ampules, vials, and Tubex syringes.

Dosage and administration *Adult:* Seizure activity: 5–10 mg IV q 10–15 minutes PRN (5 mg over 5 minutes) (maximum dose: 30 mg). Premedication for cardioversion: 5–15 mg IV over 5–10 minutes prior to cardioversion. *Pediatric:* Seizure activity: 0.2 mg/kg to 0.5 mg/kg slow IV q 2–5 minutes up to 5 mg (maximum dose 10 mg/kg). Rectal diazepam: 0.5 mg/kg via 2″ rectal catheter and flush with 2–3 mL air after administration.

Duration of action *Onset:* 1–5 minutes. *Peak effect:* 15 minutes. *Duration:* 20–50 minutes.

Special considerations Pregnancy safety: Category D. Short duration for anticonvulsant effect. Reduce dose by 50% in elderly patients.

Digoxin (Lanoxin)

Class Inotropic agent, cardiac glycoside.

Mechanism of action Rapid-acting cardiac glycoside with direct and indirect effects: Increases force of myocardial contraction, increases refractory period of AV node, and increases total peripheral resistance.

Indications Congestive heart failure, re-entry SVTs, ventricular rate control in atrial flutter and atrial fibrillation.

Contraindications Ventricular fibrillation, ventricular tachycardia, digitalis toxicity, hypersensitivity to digoxin.

Adverse reactions/side effects Fatigue, headache, blurred yellow or green vision, seizures, confusion, bradycardia, dysrhythmia, nausea, vomiting, anorexia, skin rash.

Drug interactions Amiodarone, verapamil, and quinidine may increase serum digoxin concentrations by 50%–70%. Concurrent use of digoxin and verapamil may lead to severe heart block. Diuretics may potentiate cardiac toxicity.

How supplied 0.25 mg/mL vials.

Dosage and administration *Adult:* Loading dose 4–6 µg/kg over 5 minutes. Second and third boluses of 2–3 µg/kg to follow at 4- to 8-hour intervals. *Pediatric:* Not recommended in prehospital setting.

Duration of action *Onset:* 5–30 minutes. *Peak effect:* 30–120 minutes. *Duration:* Several days.

Special considerations Pregnancy safety: Category C. Patient receiving IV digoxin must be on a monitor. Patients with known renal failure are prone to developing digitalis toxicity. Hypokalemia, hypomagnesemia, and hypercalcemia potentiate digitalis toxicity. Use carefully in patients with Wolff-Parkinson-White syndrome.

Diltiazem (Cardizem)

Class Calcium channel blocker, antidysrhythmic.

Mechanism of action Slow calcium channel blocker that blocks calcium ion influx during depolarization of cardiac and vascular smooth muscle. Decreases peripheral vascular resistance and causes relaxation of the vascular smooth muscle, resulting in a decrease of both systolic and diastolic blood pressure. Reduces preload and afterload. Reduces myocardial oxygen demand.

Indications Controls rapid ventricular rates due to atrial fibrillation, atrial flutter, and re-entry supraventricular tachycardia.

Contraindications Hypotension, sick sinus syndrome (without functioning pacemaker present), second- or third-degree AV block (without functioning pacemaker present), cardiogenic shock, wide-complex tachycardia (ventricular tachycardia may lead to hemodynamic deterioration and ventricular fibrillation), poison- or drug-induced tachycardia.

Adverse reactions/side effects Dizziness, weakness, headache, dyspnea, cough, dysrhythmias, CHF, peripheral edema, bradycardia, hypotension, AV blocks, syncope, ventricular fibrillation, ventricular tachycardia, cardiac arrest, chest pain, nausea, vomiting, dry mouth.

Drug interactions Caution in patients using medications that affect cardiac contractility. In general, should not be used in patients on beta blockers.

How supplied 5 mg/mL vials (requires refrigeration). 100-mg powder (requires reconstitution with attached fluid) for infusion (1 mg/mL). Add 125 mg/25 mL to a 100-mL bag of D_5W (1 mg/mL).

Dosage and administration *Adult:* Initial dose: 0.25 mg/kg (15–20 mg for the average patient) IV over 2 minutes. If inadequate response, may re-bolus in 15 minutes. Secondary dose: 0.35 mg/kg (20–25 mg for the average patient) IV over 2 minutes.

Maintenance infusion of 5–15 mg/h titrated to physiologically appropriate heart rate. *Pediatric:* Not recommended.

Duration of action *Onset:* 2–5 minutes. *Peak effect:* Variable. *Duration:* 1–3 hours.

Special considerations Pregnancy safety: Category C. Use with caution in patients with renal or hepatic dysfunction. PVCs may be present on conversion of PSVT to sinus rhythm. 500-mg dose of calcium chloride 5 minutes prior to administration of diltiazem can help to block the hypotensive effects in borderline hypotensive patients (blocks baroreceptors in the great vessels).

▇ Diphenhydramine (Benadryl)

Class Antihistamine, anticholinergic.

Mechanism of action Blocks cellular histamine receptors; decreases vasodilation; decreases motion sickness. Reverses extrapyramidal reactions.

Indications Symptomatic relief of allergies, allergic reactions, and anaphylaxis. Blood administration reactions; used for motion sickness and hay fever, relief of acute dystonic reactions caused by phenothiazines; may be useful in phenothiazine overdoses.

Contraindications Asthma, glaucoma, pregnancy, hypertension, narrow-angle glaucoma, infants, patients taking MAOIs.

Adverse reactions/side effects Drowsiness, sedation, seizures, dizziness, headache, blurred vision, paradoxical CNS excitement in children, wheezing, thickening of bronchial secretions, palpitations, hypotension, dysrhythmias, dry mouth, diarrhea, nausea, vomiting.

YOU *are the Medic*   PART 3

Your partner is actively suctioning as much fluid as possible from the patient's airway, resulting in a lessening in the amount of gurgling you hear. Your partner places a nonrebreathing mask on the patient and runs it at 15 L/min while watching her airway carefully. The seizure activity continues to slow but has not completely stopped. You are able to establish an IV line in the patient's left forearm. You call medical control and ask to administer a benzodiazepine to this patient while your partner collects a SAMPLE history.

Recording Time: 5 Minutes	
Respirations	36 breaths/min
Pulse	Rapid
Skin	Pale, warm, clammy
Blood pressure	140 palp
Oxygen saturation (Spo$_2$)	Unable to obtain
Pupils	Equal, reactive

5. What drugs are categorized as benzodiazepines and what are their indications?

6. What dose of diazepam would you administer to this patient?

Drug interactions Potentiates effects of alcohol and other anticholinergics. May inhibit corticosteroid activity. MAOIs prolong anticholinergic effects of diphenhydramine.

How supplied 25- and 50-mg tablets and capsules. 10 mg/mL and 50 mg/mL vials.

Dosage and administration *Adult:* 25–50 mg IM, IV, PO. *Pediatric:* 1–2 mg/kg IV, IO slowly, or IM. If PO: 5 mg/kg/24h.

Duration of action *Onset:* 15–30 minutes. *Peak effect:* 1 hour. *Duration:* 3–12 hours.

Special considerations Pregnancy safety: Category B. Not used in infants. If used in anaphylaxis, must be in conjunction with epinephrine and corticosteroids.

Dobutamine Hydrochloride (Dobutrex)

Class Sympathomimetic, inotropic agent.

Mechanism of action Synthetic catecholamine. Increased myocardial contractility, stroke volume, and increased cardiac output. Minimal chronotropic activity. Increases renal blood flow.

Indications Cardiogenic shock, CHF, left ventricular dysfunction, often used in conjunction with other drugs.

Contraindications Tachydysrhythmias, severe hypotension, idiopathic hypertrophic subaortic stenosis (IHSS), suspected or known poison/drug-induced shock.

Adverse reactions/side effects Headache, dyspnea, tachycardia, hypertension, chest pain, dysrhythmias, PVCs, nausea, vomiting.

Drug interactions Incompatible with sodium bicarbonate and furosemide. Beta blockers may blunt inotropic effects.

How supplied 12.5 mg/mL vials. 250 mg/250 mL D_5W (1,000 µg/mL).

Dosage and administration *Adult:* IV infusion at 2–20 µg/kg/min titrated to desired effect. Max dose 40 µg/kg/min. *Pediatric:* IV infusion at 2–20 µg/kg/min titrated to desired effect (not recommended).

Duration of action *Onset:* 2 minutes. *Peak effect:* 10 minutes. *Duration:* 1–2 minutes after infusion discontinued.

Special Considerations Pregnancy safety: Category B. Monitor blood pressure closely. Titrate dose to maintain a heart rate increase of no greater than 10% of baseline. May increase infarct size in patients with MI. Elderly patients may have a significantly decreased response.

Dolasetron (Anzemet)

Class Serotonin receptor antagonist, antiemetic.

Mechanism of action Selectively blocks the action of serotonin, a natural substance that causes nausea and vomiting.

Indications For the prevention and control of nausea or vomiting. Used in-hospital for patients undergoing chemotherapy or surgical procedures.

Contraindications Known hypersensitivity to dolasetron or other 5-HT3 receptor antagonists; use caution in patients with cardiac dysrhythmias or electrolyte abnormalities.

Adverse reactions/side effects ECG changes (prolonged PR interval and QT interval, widened QRS), dysrhythmias, anaphylactic reaction, headache, hypotension, dyspepsia, fever, dizziness, headache, constipation.

Drug interactions Use with phenothiazines, verapamil, haloperidol, diltiazem, digoxin, beta blockers, and Class III antidysrhythmics can have increased cardiac side effects.

How supplied 20-mg/mL vials and 50–mg and 100–mg tablets.

Dosage and administration *Adult:* 12.5 mg IV one time, 100 mg PO one time. *Pediatric:* 2–16 years old 0.35 mg/kg IV one time to a maximum of 12.5 mg/dose, 1.2 mg/kg PO one time to a maximum of 100 mg/dose. Safety and effectiveness in children younger than 2 years not established.

Duration of action *Onset:* 30 minutes. *Peak effect:* 60 minutes. *Duration:* 4–9 hours.

Special considerations Pregnancy safety: Category B. Injectable form should no longer be used in any patient with chemotherapy-induced nausea and vomiting. Generally has no effect when symptoms are due to motion sickness.

Dopamine Hydrochloride (Intropin)

Class Sympathomimetic, vasopressor, inotropic agent.

Mechanism of action Immediate metabolic precursor to norepinephrine. Produces positive inotropic and chronotropic effects. Dilates renal and splanchnic vasculature. Constricts systemic vasculature, increasing blood pressure and preload. Increases myocardial contractility and stroke volume.

Indications Cardiogenic and septic shock, hypotension with low cardiac output states, distributive shock, second-line drug for symptomatic bradycardia.

Contraindications Hypovolemic shock, pheochromocytoma, tachydysrhythmias, ventricular fibrillation.

Adverse reactions/side effects Extravasation may cause tissue necrosis. Headache, anxiety, dyspnea, dysrhythmias, hypotension, hypertension, palpitations, chest pain, increased myocardial oxygen demand, PVCs, nausea, vomiting.

Drug interactions Incompatible with alkaline solutions (sodium bicarbonate). MAOIs will enhance the effect of dopamine. Bretylium may potentiate effect of dopamine. Beta blockers may antagonize effects of dopamine. When administered with phenytoin, may cause hypotension, bradycardia, and seizures.

How supplied 40 mg/mL and 80 mg/mL prefilled syringes and vials for IV infusion. 400 mg/250 mL D_5W premixed solutions (1,600 µg/mL).

Dosage and administration *Adult:* IV/IO infusion at 2–20 µg/kg/min, slowly titrated to patient response. *Pediatric:* IV/IO infusion at 2–20 µg/kg/min, slowly titrated to patient response.

Duration of action *Onset:* 1–4 minutes. *Peak effect:* 5–10 minutes. *Duration:* Effects cease almost immediately after infusion is discontinued.

Special considerations Pregnancy safety: Category C. Effects are dose-dependent. Dopaminergic response: 2–4 µg/kg/min: dilates vessels in kidneys; increased urine output. Beta-adrenergic response: 4–10 µg/kg/min: positive chronotropic and inotropic effects. Adrenergic response: 10–20 µg/kg/min: primary alpha stimulant/vasoconstriction. Greater than 20 µg/kg/min: reversal of renal effects/override of alpha effects, consider other agents such as epinephrine or norepinephrine infusions. Should be administered by infusion pump.

Epinephrine (Adrenalin)

Class Sympathomimetic.

Mechanism of action Direct-acting alpha and beta agonist. Alpha: vasoconstriction. Beta-1: positive inotropic, chronotropic, and dromotropic effects. Beta-2: bronchial smooth muscle relaxation and dilation of skeletal vasculature. Blocks histamine receptors.

Indications Cardiac arrest (asystole, PEA, ventricular fibrillation and pulseless ventricular tachycardia), symptomatic bradycardia as an alternative infusion to dopamine, severe hypotension secondary to bradycardia when atropine and transcutaneous pacing are unsuccessful, allergic reaction, anaphylaxis, asthma.

Contraindications Hypertension, hypothermia, pulmonary edema, myocardial ischemia, hypovolemic shock.

Adverse reactions/side effects Nervousness, restlessness, headache, tremor, pulmonary edema, dysrhythmias, chest pain, hypertension, tachycardia, nausea, vomiting.

Drug interactions Potentiates other sympathomimetics. Deactivated by alkaline solutions. MAOIs may potentiate effect. Beta blockers may blunt effects.

How supplied 1:1,000 solution: Ampules and vials containing 1 mg/mL. 1:10,000 solution: Prefilled syringes containing 0.1 mg/mL. Auto-injector (EpiPen): 0.5 mg/mL (1:2,000).

Dosage and administration *Adult:* Mild allergic reactions and asthma: 0.3–0.5 mg (0.3–0.5 mL 1:1,000) SC. Anaphylaxis: 1 mg (10 mL of 1:10,000) IV, IO over 5 minutes. Cardiac arrest: IV/IO dose: 1 mg (10 mL, 1:10,000 solution) 3–5 minutes during resuscitation. Follow each dose with a 20-mL flush and elevate arm for 10–20 seconds after dose. Continuous infusion: Add 1 mg (1 mL of a 1:1,000 solution) to 250 mL normal saline or D₅W (4 µg/mL). Initial infusion rate of 1 µg/min titrated to effect (typical dose: 2–10 µg/min). Endotracheal (ET) dose: 2–2.5 mg diluted in 10 mL normal saline. Profound bradycardia or hypotension: 2–10 µg/min; titrate to patient response. Higher dose: Higher doses (up to 0.2 mg/kg) may be used for specific indications: (beta blocker or calcium channel blocker overdose). *Pediatric:* Mild allergic reactions and asthma: 0.01 mg/kg (0.01 mL/kg) of a 1:1,000 solution SC

(maximum of 0.3 mL). Anaphylaxis/severe status asthmaticus: 0.01 mg/kg (0.01 mL/kg) IM of a 1:1,000 solution (maximum single dose: 0.3 mg). Cardiac arrest: IV/IO dose: 0.01 mg/kg (0.1 mL/kg) of a 1:10,000 solution every 3–5 minutes during arrest. All ET doses 0.1 mg/kg (0.1 mL/kg) of a 1:1,000 solution mixed in 3–5 mL of saline until IV/IO access is achieved. Maximum single dose 1 mg. Symptomatic bradycardia: IV/IO dose: 0.01 mg/kg (0.01 mL/kg) of a 1:10,000 solution. All ET doses 0.1 mg/kg (0.1 mL/kg) of a 1:1,000 solution. Continuous IV/IO infusion: Begin with rapid infusion, and then titrate to response. Typical initial infusion: 0.1–1 µg/min. Higher doses may be effective.

Duration of action *Onset:* Immediate. *Peak effect:* Minutes. *Duration:* Several minutes.

Special considerations Pregnancy safety: Category C. May cause syncope in asthmatic children. May increase myocardial oxygen demand. To mix an infusion add 1 mg of epinephrine 1:1,000 to 500 mL D₅W for a yield of 2 mcg/mL. Many states and systems are pulling away from IV/IO/IM administration of 1:1,000 and replacing it with auto-injectors due to the vascular side effects of solo epinephrine 1:1,000 injection.

Epinephrine Racemic (Micronefrin)

Class Sympathomimetic.

Mechanism of action Stimulates beta-2 receptors in lungs: bronchodilation with relaxation of bronchial smooth muscles. Reduces airway resistance. Useful in treating laryngeal edema; inhibits histamine release.

Indications Bronchial asthma, prevention of bronchospasm, croup, laryngotracheobronchitis, laryngeal edema.

Contraindications Hypertension, underlying cardiovascular disease, epiglottitis.

Adverse reactions/side effects Headache, anxiety, fear, nervousness, respiratory weakness, palpitations, tachycardia, dysrhythmias, nausea, vomiting.

Drug interactions MAOIs and bretylium may potentiate effect. Beta blockers may blunt effects.

How supplied Metered-dose inhaler: 0.16–0.25 mg/spray. Solution: 7.5, 15, 30 mL in 1%, 2.25% solution.

Dosage and administration *Adult:* MDI: 2–3 inhalations, repeated every 5 minutes PRN. Solution: dilute 5 mL (1%) in 5 mL saline, administer over 15 minutes. *Pediatric:* Solution: dilute 0.25 mL (0.1%) in 2.5 mL saline (if less than 20 kg); dilute 0.5 mL in 2.5 mL saline (if 20–40 kg); dilute 0.75 mL in 2.5 mL saline (if greater than 40 kg). Administer via hand-held nebulizer.

Duration of action *Onset:* Within 5 minutes. *Peak effect:* 5–15 minutes. *Duration:* 1–3 hours.

Special considerations May cause tachycardia and other dysrhythmias. Monitor vital signs. Excessive use may cause bronchospasm. May have a strong rebound effect after drug wears off.

Eptifibatide (Integrilin)

Class Glycoprotein IIb/IIIa inhibitor, platelet aggregation inhibitor.

Mechanism of action Prevents the aggregation of platelets by binding to the glycoprotein IIb/IIIa receptor, preventing the binding of fibrinogen and von Willebrand factors.

Indications Unstable angina and NSTEMI (ACS) being managed medically. Patients undergoing percutaneous coronary intervention.

Contraindications Any prior intracranial hemorrhage, known malignant intracranial neoplasm, suspected aortic dissection, significant closed head trauma or facial trauma within 3 months, ischemic stroke within 3 months *except* if acute within 3 hours, active internal bleeding or bleeding disorder in past 30 days, surgical procedure or trauma within preceding 6 weeks, platelet count <150,000 × $10^3/\mu L$, hypersensitivity to and concomitant use of another glycoprotein IIb/IIIa inhibitor, severe uncontrolled hypertension (systolic BP >200 mm Hg or diastolic BP >110 mm Hg).

Adverse reactions/side effects Cerebral hemorrhage, pulmonary hemorrhage, hypotension, GI bleeding, internal bleeding, anaphylactic shock.

Drug interactions Thrombolytics, oral anticoagulants, aspirin, NSAIDs, dipyridamole, ticlopidine, and clopidogrel increase effect. Incompatible in the same IV line with furosemide.

How supplied 2 mg/mL vials and 0.75 mg/mL bottles (requires refrigeration).

Dosage and administration *Adult:* Medical management: 180 µg/kg IV bolus over 1–2 minutes, followed by a 2 µg/kg infusion for 72–96 hours. Percutaneous coronary invervention/percutaneous transluminal coronary angioplasty: 180 µg/kg IV bolus over 1–2 minutes followed by a 2 µg/kg infusion, then repeat bolus in 10 minutes. Maximum dose: (based on a 121-kg patient) PCI: 22.6-mg bolus, 15 mg/h infusion, infusion duration 18 to 24 hours after procedure. *Pediatric:* Not recommended.

Duration of action *Onset:* A few minutes. *Peak effect:* 30 minutes to 4 hours. *Duration:* Platelet function recovers within 4 to 8 hours after discontinuation.

Special considerations Pregnancy safety: Category B. Must be administered only with an infusion pump direct from bottle with a vented IV set. Due to severe spontaneous bleeding risk, invasive procedures (eg, IV starts, injections, NG tube, or nasotracheal intubation) should be avoided.

Etomidate (Amidate)

Class Nonbarbiturate hypnotic, anesthesia induction agent.

Mechanism of action Short-acting hypnotic that acts at the level of the reticular activating system.

Indications Premedication for tracheal intubation or cardioversion.

Contraindications Hypersensitivity, labor/delivery.

Adverse reactions/side effects Apnea of short duration, respiratory depression, hypoventilation, hyperventilation, dysrhythmias, hypotension, hypertension, nausea, vomiting, involuntary muscle movement, pain at injection site.

Drug interactions Effects may be enhanced when given with other central nervous system depressants.

How supplied 2 mg/mL vials.

Dosage and administration *Adult:* 0.2–0.6 mg/kg IV over 30–60 seconds (typical adult dose is 20 mg). *Pediatric:* 0.2–0.4 mg/kg IV/IO over 30–60 seconds for rapid sequence intubation (older than 10 years), 1 time only. Maximum dose: 20 mg.

Duration of action *Onset:* <1 minute. *Peak effect:* 1 minute. *Duration:* 5–10 minutes.

Special considerations Pregnancy safety: Category C. Carefully monitor vital signs. Etomidate can suppress adrenal gland production of steroid hormones, which can temporarily cause gland failure. Consider decreasing dose in elderly and patients with cardiac conditions.

Fentanyl Citrate (Sublimaze)

Class Opioid analgesic, schedule II narcotic.

Mechanism of action Binds to opiate receptors, producing analgesia and euphoria.

Indications Pain management, anesthesia adjunct.

Contraindications Known hypersensitivity. Use with caution in traumatic brain injury.

Adverse reactions/side effects Confusion, paradoxical excitation, delirium, drowsiness, CNS depression, sedation, respiratory depression, apnea, dyspnea, dysrhythmias, bradycardia, tachycardia, hypotension, syncope, nausea, vomiting, abdominal pain, dehydration, fatigue.

Drug interactions Increased respiratory effects when given with other CNS depressants.

How supplied 50 µg/mL ampules and Tubex syringes.

Dosage and administration *Adult:* 50 to 100 µg (1µg/kg) IM or IV, IO slow push (over 1–2 minutes) to maximum of 150 µg. *Pediatric:* 1–2 µg/kg IM, IV, or IO slow push (over 1–2 minutes). The safety and efficacy in children younger than 2 years has not been established.

Duration of action *Onset:* 1–3 minutes. *Peak effect:* 3–5 minutes. *Duration:* 30–60 minutes.

Special considerations Pregnancy safety: Category C. Chest wall rigidity possible with a high-dose rapid infusion. A dose of 100 µg of fentanyl citrate is equivalent to 10 mg of morphine or 75 mg of meperidine.

Flumazenil (Romazicon)

Class Benzodiazepine antagonist, antidote.

Mechanism of action Antagonizes the action of benzodiazepines on the central nervous system, reversing the sedative effects.

Indications Reversal of respiratory depression and sedative effects from pure benzodiazepine overdose.

Contraindications Hypersensitivity, tricyclic antidepressant overdose, seizure-prone patients, coma of unknown etiology.

Adverse reactions/side effects Seizures, dizziness, agitation, confusion, headache, visual disturbances, dysrhythmias, chest pain, hypertension, nausea, vomiting, hiccups, rigors, shivering, pain at the injection site.

Drug interactions Toxic effects of mixed drug overdose (especially tricyclics).

How supplied 0.1 mg/mL vials.

Dosage and administration *Adult:* First dose 0.2 mg IV/IO over 15 seconds. Second dose: 0.3 mg may be given over 30 seconds; if no response, give third dose. Third dose: 0.5 mg IV/IO over 30 seconds; if no response, repeat once every minute until adequate response or total of 3 mg is given. *Pediatric:* Not recommended.

Duration of action *Onset:* 1–2 minutes. *Peak effect:* Related to plasma concentration of benzodiazepines. *Duration:* Related to plasma concentration of benzodiazepines.

Special considerations Pregnancy safety: Category C. Be prepared to manage seizures in patients who are physically dependent on benzodiazepines or who have ingested larger doses of other drugs. Flumazenil may precipitate withdrawal syndromes in patients dependent on benzodiazepines. Monitor patients for re-sedation and respiratory depression; be prepared to assist ventilations. Not recommended in combined drug overdoses, especially with TCAs; may result in death. Controversial use in unknown overdose or polysubstance overdose.

▣ Fosphenytoin (Cerebyx)

Class Hydantoin anticonvulsant.

Mechanism of action Modulates voltage-dependent sodium and calcium channels of neurons, inhibits calcium flux across neuronal membranes. Also selectively elevates the excitability threshold of the cell, reducing its response to stimuli.

Indications Status epilepticus, seizure disorder.

Contraindications Bradycardia, Adams-Stokes syndrome, second- or third-degree AV blocks, sinoatrial blocks, known hypersensitivity to fosphenytoin, phenytoin, or other hydantoins.

Adverse reactions/side effects Severe hypotension, bradycardia, dysrhythmias, Stevens-Johnson syndrome, cardiovascular collapse, nystagmus, dizziness, headache, nausea, somnolence, rash, and tremor.

Drug interactions Dopamine may cause severe hypotension. Reacts with many medications, decreasing their effect and increasing the risk of fosphenytoin toxicity. Additive effect with other CNS depressants.

How supplied 75 mg/mL vials.

Dosage and administration *Adult:* loading dose of 10–20 mg PE/kg IM, IV one time to a maximum of 150 mg PE/min IV.

Pediatric: loading dose of 10–20 mg PE/kg IM, IV one time to a maximum of 3 mg PE/kg/min up to 150 mg PE/min IV.

Duration of action *Onset:* 10 minutes. *Peak effect:* 30 minutes. *Duration:* 12 to 28 hours.

Special considerations Pregnancy safety: Category D. Use with caution in patients with hepatic and renal impairment and diabetic, elderly, and debilitated patients. Fosphenytoin dosing is expressed as phenytoin equivalents (PE) to avoid the need for dose conversion between products. Each vial contains 75 mg/mL, which is equivalent to 50 mg/mL of phenytoin.

▣ Furosemide (Lasix)

Class Loop diuretic.

Mechanism of action Blocks the absorption of sodium and chloride at the distal and proximal tubules and the loop of Henle, causing increased urine output.

Indications CHF, pulmonary edema, hypertensive crisis.

Contraindications Hypovolemia, anuria, hypotension (relative contraindication), hypersensitivity, hepatic coma, suspected electrolyte imbalances.

Adverse reactions/side effects Dizziness, headache, ECG changes, weakness, orthostatic hypotension, dysrhythmias, nausea, vomiting, diarrhea, dry mouth, may exacerbate hypovolemia and hypokalemia, hyperglycemia (due to hemoconcentration).

Drug interactions Lithium toxicity may be potentiated because of sodium depletion. Digitalis toxicity may be potentiated by potassium depletion.

How supplied 10 mg/mL vials.

Dosage and administration *Adult:* 0.5–1 mg/kg IV over 1–2 minutes. If no response, double the dose to 2 mg/kg slowly over 1–2 minutes. *Pediatric:* 1 mg/kg IV/IO.

Duration of action *Onset:* 5 minutes. *Peak effect:* 20–60 minutes. *Duration:* 4–6 hours.

Special considerations Pregnancy safety: Category C. Ototoxicity, deafness, and projectile vomiting can occur with rapid administration. Should be protected from light. Vasodilatory effects within 5 minutes; diuretic effects within 30 minutes. Expect a 10–12 mm Hg systolic and a 5–7 mm Hg diastolic drop in blood pressure. Being phased out due to nephrotoxic side effects and greater success rates with CPAP.

▣ Glucagon (GlucaGen)

Class Hyperglycemic agent, pancreatic hormone, insulin antagonist.

Mechanism of action Increases blood glucose level by stimulating glycogenesis. Unknown mechanism of stabilizing cardiac rhythm in beta blocker overdose. Minimal positive inotropic and chronotropic response. Decreases gastrointestinal motility and secretions.

Indications Altered level of consciousness when hypoglycemia is suspected. May be used as a reversal agent in beta blocker and calcium channel blocker overdoses.

Contraindications Hyperglycemia, hypersensitivity.

Adverse reactions/side effects Dizziness, headache, hypertension, tachycardia, nausea, vomiting, rebound hypoglycemia.

Drug interactions Incompatible in solution with most other substances. No significant drug interactions with other emergency medications.

How supplied 1-mg powder in vials (requires reconstitution with diluent provided).

Dosage and administration *Adult:* Hypoglycemia: 0.5–1 mg IM; may repeat in 7–10 minutes. Calcium channel blocker or beta blocker overdose: 3–10 mg IV slowly over 3–5 minutes initially, followed by a 3–5 mg/h infusion as necessary. *Pediatric:* Hypoglycemia: 0.03–0.1 mg/kg IM, IO, SQ, slow IV may repeat in 20 minutes. Maximum dose: 1 mg. Calcium channel blocker or beta blocker toxicity: 0.05–0.15 mg/kg IV/IO over 3–5 minutes initially, followed by a 0.05–0.10 mg/kg/h infusion as necessary.

Duration of action *Onset:* 1 minute. *Peak effect:* 5–20 minutes. *Duration:* 60–90 minutes.

Special considerations Pregnancy safety: Category B. Ineffective if glycogen stores depleted. Should always be used in conjunction with 50% dextrose whenever possible. If patient does not respond to second dose of glucagon, 50% dextrose must be administered.

Haloperidol Lactate (Haldol)

Class Tranquilizer, antipsychotic.

Mechanism of action Inhibits central nervous system catecholamine receptors: strong antidopaminergic and weak anticholinergic. Acts on CNS to depress subcortical areas, mid-brain, and ascending reticular activating system in the brain.

Indications Acute psychotic episodes.

Contraindications Parkinsons disease, depressed mental status, agitation secondary to shock and hypoxia, hypersensitivity.

Adverse reactions/side effects Seizures, sedation, confusion, restlessness, extrapyramidal reactions, dystonia, respiratory depression, hypotension, tachycardia, orthostatic hypotension, QT prolongation, sudden cardiac death, constipation, dry mouth, nausea, vomiting, drooling, blurred vision.

Drug interactions Enhanced central nervous system depression and hypotension in combination with alcohol. Antagonized amphetamines and epinephrine. Other CNS depressants may potentiate effects.

How supplied 5 mg/mL ampules and vials.

Dosage and administration *Adult:* 2–5 mg IM ONLY every 30–60 minutes until sedation is achieved. *Pediatric:* Not recommended.

Duration of action *Onset:* 10 minutes. *Peak effect:* 30–45 minutes. *Duration:* Variable (generally 12–24 hours).

Special considerations Pregnancy safety: Category C. Treat hypotension secondary to haloperidol with fluids and norepinephrine, not epinephrine. Patient may also be taking benztropine mesylate (Cogentin) if on long-term therapy with haloperidol.

Heparin Sodium

Class Anticoagulant.

Mechanism of action Prevents conversion of fibrogen to fibrin. Affects clotting factors IX, XI, XII, plasmin. Does not lyse existing clots.

Indications Acute myocardial infarction, prophylaxis and treatment of thromboembolic disorders (eg, pulmonary emboli and deep venous thrombosis).

Contraindications Hypersensitivity, active bleeding, recent intracranial, intraspinal, or eye surgery, severe hypertension, bleeding tendencies, severe thrombocytopenia.

Adverse reactions/side effects Pain, anaphylaxis, shock, hematuria, GI bleeding, hemorrhage, thrombocytopenia, bruising.

Drug interactions Salicylates, ibuprofen, dipyridamole, and hydroxychloroquine may increase risk of bleeding.

How supplied Common mix: 25,000 units/500 mL (yield 50 units/mL).

Dosage and administration *Adult:* If used with fibrinolytic therapy, always obtain a blood sample for control of partial thromboplastin time before heparin administration. Heparin is given as an IV bolus of 60 U/kg max 4,000 IU (weight adjusted). A continuous infusion is given following the bolus at a rate of 12 IU/kg/h rounded to the nearest 50 (max: 4,000 IU or 1,000 units/h). Follow medical direction and local protocol. *Pediatric:* Not recommended.

Duration of action *Onset:* IV Immediate, (SQ) 20–60 minutes. *Peak effect:* Variable. *Duration:* 4–8 hours.

Special considerations Pregnancy safety: Category C. Heparin dose not lyse existing clots. Heparin along with aspirin is part of the antithrombotic package.

Hydrocortisone Sodium Succinate (Solu-Cortef)

Class Adrenal glucocorticoid.

Mechanism of action Anti-inflammatory; immunosuppressive with salt-retaining actions.

Indications Shock due to acute adrenocortical insufficiency, anaphylaxis, asthma, and COPD.

Contraindications Systemic fungal infections, premature infants (contains benzyl alcohol, which is associated with "fatal gasping syndrome," characterized by CNS depression, metabolic acidosis, and gasping respirations), known hypersensitivity.

Adverse reactions/side effects Headache, vertigo, pulmonary tuberculosis, CHF, hypertension, fluid retention, nausea.

Drugs interactions Incompatible with heparin and metaraminol.

How supplied 100 mg, 250 mg, or 500 mg powder in vials (requires reconstitution with solution provided).

Dosage and administration *Adult:* 4 mg/kg slow IV bolus. *Pediatric:* 2 mg/kg slow IV bolus. Maximum dose: 100 mg.

Duration of action *Onset:* 1 hour. *Peak effect:* Variable. *Duration:* 8–12 hours.

Special consideration Pregnancy safety: Category C. May be used in status asthmaticus as a second-line drug.

Hydroxocobalamin (Cyanokit)

Class Antidote, cyanide poisoning adjunct.

Mechanism of action Binds with cyanide to form nontoxic cyanocobalamin, preventing its toxic effects; excreted renally.

Indications Treatment of known or suspected cyanide poisoning.

Contraindications None in the emergency setting.

Adverse reactions/side effects Hypertension, allergic reactions, GI bleeding, nausea, vomiting, dyspepsia, dyspnea, dizziness, headache, injection site reactions.

Drug interactions Do not administer in the same IV line with diazepam, dobutamine, dopamine, fentanyl, nitroglycerin, propofol, sodium nitrite, and sodium thiosulfate.

How supplied 2.5 g/250-mL glass vials.

Dosage and administration *Adult:* 5 g IV infusion over 15 minutes at a rate of 15 mL/min, one time, may be repeated one time at the same dose to a maximum of 10 g. *Pediatric:* 70 mg/kg IV one time, may be repeated one time at the same dose.

Duration of action *Onset:* Rapid. *Peak effect:* 8–10 min. *Duration:* Varies.

Special considerations Pregnancy safety: Category C. Make sure to reassess the patient's airway, oxygenation, and hydration during administration. The patient may become hypertensive during treatment (greater than 180 mm Hg systolic and 110 mm Hg diastolic are not uncommon) and will return to baseline within 4 hours.

Hydroxyzine (Atarax, Vistaril)

Class Antihistamine, antiemetic, antianxiety agent, anxiolytic.

Mechanism of action Potentiates effects of analgesics. Calming effect without impairing mental alertness. Rapid-acting true ataraxic with probable action of suppressing activity in key locations of the central nervous system's subcortical area. Exerts bronchodilating, antispasmodic, antihistaminic, analgesic, and antiemetic effects.

Indications Potentiates the effects of analgesics. Controls nausea and vomiting in anxiety reactions and motion sickness; preoperative and postoperative sedation.

Contraindications Hypersensitivity, early pregnancy.

Adverse reactions/side effects Drowsiness, agitation, ataxia, dizziness, headache, weakness, wheezing, chest tightness, urinary retention, dry mouth, constipation, pain at injection site.

Drug interactions Potentiates the effects of central nervous system depressants such as narcotics, barbiturates, and alcohol.

How supplied 25, 50 mg/mL vials.

Dosage and administration *Adult:* 25–100 mg IM ONLY. *Pediatric:* 0.5–1 mg/kg/dose IM ONLY.

Duration of action *Onset:* 15–30 minutes. *Peak effect:* 45–90 minutes. *Duration:* 4–6 hours.

Special considerations Pregnancy safety: Category C. Should be administered by IM injection only. Localized burning at the injection site is a common complaint.

Insulin

Class Antidiabetic, hormone.

Mechanism of action Allows glucose transport into cells of all tissues; converts glycogen to fat; produces intracellular shift of potassium and magnesium to reduce elevated serum levels of these electrolytes.

Indications Not used in emergency prehospital setting. Diabetic ketoacidosis or other hyperglycemic state, hyperkalemia (insulin and D_{50} used together to lower hyperkalemic state), nonketotic hyperosmolar coma.

Contraindications Hypoglycemia, hypokalemia.

Adverse reactions/side effects Weakness, fatigue, confusion, headache, seizure, coma, tachycardia, nausea, hypokalemia, hypoglycemia, diaphoresis, itching, swelling, redness.

Drug interactions Incompatible in solution with all other drugs. Corticosteroids, dobutamine, epinephrine, and thiazide diuretics decrease the hypoglycemic effects of insulin. Alcohol and salicylates may potentiate the effects of insulin.

How supplied 30–70 units/mL vials.

Dosage and administration Dosage adjusted relative to blood glucose levels. Standard doses for diabetic coma: *Adult:* 10–25 units SC, IM, or IV, followed by infusion of 0.1 units/kg/h. *Pediatric:* 0.1–0.2 units/kg/h SC, IM, or IV followed by infusion of 50 units/250 mL (0.2 units/mL), at a rate of 0.1–0.2 units/kg/h.

Duration of action *Onset:* Minutes. *Peak effect:* Approximately 1 hour (short-acting); 3–6 hours (intermediate-acting); 5–8 hours (long-acting). *Duration:* Approximately 6–8 hours (short-acting); 24 hours (intermediate-acting); 36 hours (long-acting).

Special considerations Pregnancy safety: Category B. Insulin is the drug of choice for control of diabetes in pregnancy. Usually requires refrigeration. Most rapid absorption if injected in abdominal wall; next most rapid absorption if injected in the arm; slowest absorption if injected into the thigh.

Ipratropium (Atrovent)

Class Anticholinergic, bronchodilator.

Mechanism of action Inhibits interaction of acetylcholine at receptor sites of bronchial smooth muscle, resulting in decreased cyclic guanosine monophosphate and bronchodilation.

Indications Persistent bronchospasm, COPD exacerbation.

Contraindications Hypersensitivity to ipratropium, atropine, alkaloids, peanuts.

Adverse reactions/side effects Headache, dizziness, nervousness, fatigue, tremor, blurred vision, cough, dyspnea, worsening COPD symptoms, tachycardia, palpitations, flushing, MI, dry mouth, nausea, vomiting, GI distress.

Drug interactions None reported.

How supplied Aerosol 18 µg/actuation. 500 µg/mL of a 0.02% solution for nebulized inhalation.

Dosage and administration *Adult:* 250–500 µg via inhalation with hand-held nebulizer every 20 minutes up to 3 times. *Pediatric:* Same as adult.

Duration of action *Onset:* 1–3 minutes. *Peak effect:* 90–120 minutes. *Duration:* 4–6 hours.

Special considerations Pregnancy safety: Category B. *Note: When used in combination with beta-agonists (eg, metaproterenol and albuterol), the beta-agonist is always administered first with a 5-minute wait before administering ipratropium. Shake well before use. Use with caution in patients with urinary retention.*

◼ Isoetharine (Bronchosol, Bronkometer)

Class Sympathomimetic.

Mechanism of action Beta-2 agonist; relaxes smooth muscle of the bronchioles.

Indications Acute bronchial asthma, bronchospasm (especially in COPD patients).

Contraindications Use with caution in patients with diabetes, hyperthyroidism, cardiovascular disease, and cerebrovascular disease.

Adverse reactions/side effects Nervousness, dose-related tachycardia, palpitations, nausea, tremors. Multiple doses can cause paradoxical bronchoconstriction.

Drug interactions Additive adverse effects if given with other beta-2 agonist drugs.

How supplied Multi-dose inhalers and 2-mL unit dose of 1% solution.

Dosage and administration *Adult:* 1–2 inhalations with MDI: COPD: 2.5–5 mg (2.5–0.5 mL) diluted in 3 mL normal saline and nebulized. *Pediatric:* 0.01 mg/kg; maximum dose: 0.5 mL in 3 mL normal saline and nebulized.

Duration of action *Onset:* Immediate. *Peak effect:* 5–15 minutes. *Duration:* 1–4 hours.

Special considerations None.

◼ Ketorolac Tromethamine (Toradol)

Class Nonsteroidal anti-inflammatory (NSAID) analgesic.

Mechanism of action Potent analgesic that does not possess any sedative or anxiolytic activities by inhibiting prostaglandin synthesis.

Indications Short-term management of moderate to severe pain.

Contraindications Allergy to salicylates or other nonsteroidal anti-inflammatory drugs. Patients with history of asthma, bleeding disorders (especially GI related, such as peptic ulcer disease), renal failure.

Adverse reactions/side effects Drowsiness, dizziness, headache, sedation, bronchospasm, dyspnea, edema, vasodilation, hypotension, hypertension, GI bleeding, diarrhea, dyspepsia, nausea.

Drug interactions May increase bleeding time in patients taking anticoagulants.

How supplied 15 mg/mL and 30 mg/mL vials.

Dosage and administration *Adult:* 30–60 mg IM. *Pediatric:* Not recommended.

Duration of action *Onset:* 10 minutes. *Peak effect:* 1–2 hours. *Duration:* 2–6 hours.

Special considerations Pregnancy safety: Category C. Use with caution in elderly patients due to higher risk of renal and fatal GI adverse reactions.

◼ Labetalol (Normodyne, Trandate)

Class Selective alpha and nonselective beta-adrenergic blocker, antihypertensive.

Mechanism of action Blood pressure reduction without reflex tachycardia; total peripheral resistance reduced without significant alteration in cardiac output.

Indications Moderate to severe hypertension.

Contraindications Bronchial asthma, congestive heart failure, cardiogenic shock, second- and third-degree heart block, bradycardia.

Adverse reactions/side effects Fatigue, weakness, depression, headache, dizziness, bronchospasm, wheezing, dyspnea, bradycardia, CHF, pulmonary edema, orthostatic hypotension, ventricular dysrhythmias, nausea, vomiting, diarrhea.

Drug interactions Labetalol may block bronchodilator effects of beta-adrenergic agonists. Nitroglycerin may augment hypotensive effects.

How supplied 5 mg/mL vials.

Dosage and administration *Adult:* 10 mg IV push over 1–2 minutes. May repeat or double every 10 minutes to a maximum dose of 150 mg. Infusion: 2–8 mg/min, titrated to supine blood pressure. *Pediatric:* Not recommended.

Duration of action *Onset:* >5 minutes. *Peak effect:* Variable. *Duration:* 3–6 hours.

Special considerations Pregnancy safety: Category C. Blood pressure, pulse rate, and ECG should be monitored continuously. Observe for signs of congestive heart failure, bradycardia, and bronchospasm. Should only be administered with patient in the supine position.

Levalbuterol (Xopenex)

Class Sympathomimetic, bronchodilator.

Mechanism of action Stimulates beta-2 receptors resulting in smooth muscle relaxation of bronchial tree and peripheral vasculature.

Indications Treatment of acute bronchospasm in patients with reversible obstructive airway disease (COPD/asthma). Bronchospasm prophylaxis in asthma patients.

Contraindications Known hypersensitivity to the drug and other sympathomimetics. Angioedema, tachydysrhythmias, and severe cardiac disease. Avoid use in patients taking phenothiazines; may cause prolonged QT interval and dysrhythmias. Avoid use in patients on sotalol; may decrease bronchodilating effects and cause bronchospasm, prolonged QT interval, and dysrhythmias.

Adverse reactions/side effects Headache, anxiety, dizziness, restlessness, hallucinations, throat irritation, tachycardia, hypertension, hypotension, dysrhythmias, angina, nausea, vomiting, dyspepsia, tremors, hypokalemia, hyperglycemia.

Drug interactions Increased actions of bronchodilators, tricyclic antidepressants, MAOIs, and other adrenergic drugs.

How supplied 0.63 mg, 1.25 mg/3 mL solution for inhalation.

Dosage and administration *Adults:* 1.25 mg to 2.5 mg in 3 mL administered by nebulizer every 20 minutes to a maximum of 3 doses. *Pediatric:* 0.075 mg/kg (minimum of 1.25 mg) administered by nebulizer every 20 minutes to a maximum of 3 doses.

Duration of action *Onset:* 5–15 minutes. *Peak effect:* 60–90 minutes. *Duration:* 6–8 hours.

Special considerations Pregnancy safety: Category C. Use with caution in patients with cardiac dysrhythmias and cardiovascular disorders.

Lidocaine Hydrochloride (Xylocaine)

Class Antidysrhythmic.

Mechanism of action Decreases automaticity by slowing the rate of spontaneous phase 4 depolarization.

Indications Alternative to amiodarone in cardiac arrest from ventricular tachycardia, ventricular fibrillation, stable wide-complex tachycardia (poly- or monomorphic) with normal baseline QT interval, stable monomorphic VT with preserved ventricular function.

Contraindications Hypersensitivity, second- or third-degree AV block in the absence of an artificial pacemaker, Stokes-Adams syndrome, prophylactic use in AMI, wide complex ventricular escape beats with bradycardia.

Adverse reactions/side effects Anxiety, drowsiness, confusion, seizures, slurred speech, respiratory arrest, hypotension, bradycardia, dysrhythmias, cardiac arrest, AV block, nausea, vomiting.

Drug interactions Apnea induced with succinylcholine may be prolonged with high doses of lidocaine. Cardiac depression may occur in conjunction with IV phenytoin. Procainamide may exacerbate CNS effect. Metabolic clearance is decreased in patients with liver disease or in patients taking beta blockers.

How supplied 20 mg/mL of a 2% solution prefilled syringe. 4 mg/mL in D_5W for infusion (1 g/250 mL D_5W).

Dosage and administration *Adult:* Cardiac arrest/pulseless ventricular tachycardia/ventricular fibrillation: Initial dose: 1–1.5 mg/kg IV/IO. Repeat dose: 0.5–0.75 mg/kg IV/IO repeated in 5–10 minutes. Maximum total dose: 3 mg/kg. Stable ventricular tachycardia, wide complex tachycardia of unknown etiology, significant ectopy: Dose range 0.5–0.75 mg/kg and up to 1–1.5 mg/kg. Repeat 0.5–0.75 mg/kg every 5–10 minutes. Maximum total dose: 3 mg/kg. Endotracheal dose: 2–4 mg/kg. Maintenance infusion: 1–4 mg/min (30–50 µg/kg/min); can dilute in D_5W or normal saline. *Pediatric:* IV/IO dose: 1 mg/kg rapid IV/IO push. Maximum dose 100 mg. Continuous IV/IO infusion: 20–50 µg/kg/min. Repeat bolus dose (1 mg/kg) when infusion is initiated if bolus has not been given within previous 15 minutes. Endotracheal dose: 2–3 mg/kg. Rapid sequence intubation: 1–2 mg/kg IV/IO one time only.

Duration of action *Onset:* 1–5 minutes. *Peak effect:* 5–10 minutes. *Duration:* Variable (15 minutes to 2 hours).

Special considerations Pregnancy safety: Category B. Reduce maintenance infusion by 50% if patient is older than 70 years of age, has liver or renal disease, is in CHF, or is in shock. A 75- to 100-mg bolus maintains blood levels for only 20 minutes (if not in shock). Exceedingly high doses of lidocaine can result in death and coma. Avoid lidocaine for reperfusion dysrhythmias after fibrinolytic therapy. Cross-reactivity with other forms of local anesthetics.

Lorazepam (Ativan)

Class Benzodiazepine, short/intermediate acting; sedative, anticonvulsant, schedule IV drug.

Mechanism of action Anxiolytic, anticonvulsant, and sedative effect; suppresses propagation of seizure activity produced by foci in cortex, thalamus, and limbic areas.

Indications Initial control of status epilepticus or severe recurrent seizures, severe anxiety, sedation.

Contraindications Acute narrow-angle glaucoma, coma, shock, suspected drug abuse.

Adverse reactions/side effects Dizziness, drowsiness, CNS depression, headache, sedation, respiratory depression, apnea, hypotension, bradycardia.

Drug interactions May precipitate central nervous system depression if already taking central nervous system depressant medications.

How supplied 2 and 4 mg/mL vials and Tubex syringes.

Dosage and administration Note: When given IV/IO, must be diluted with equal volume of sterile water or sterile saline. When given IM, lorazepam is not diluted. *Adult:* 2–4 mg slow IM/IV at

2 mg/min; may be repeated in 15–20 minutes. Maximum dose of 8 mg. For sedation: 0.05 mg/kg up to 4 mg IM. *Pediatric:* 0.05–0.20 mg/kg slow IV/IO/IM over 2 minutes. May be repeated once in 5–20 minutes. Maximum dose of 0.2 mg/kg.

Duration of action *Onset:* 1–5 minutes. *Peak effect:* Variable. *Duration:* 6–8 hours.

Special considerations Pregnancy safety: Category D. Monitor respiratory rate and blood pressure during administration. Have advanced airway equipment readily available. Inadvertent arterial injection may result in vasospasm and gangrene. Lorazepam expires in 6 weeks when not refrigerated.

Magnesium Sulfate

Class Electrolyte, anti-inflammatory.

Mechanism of action Reduces striated muscle contractions and blocks peripheral neuromuscular transmission by reducing acetylcholine release at the myoneural junction. Manages seizures in toxemia of pregnancy. Induces uterine relaxation. Can cause bronchodilation after beta-agonists and anti-cholinergics have been administered.

Indications Seizures of eclampsia (toxemia of pregnancy), torsades de pointes, hypomagnesaemia, ventricular fibrillation/pulseless ventricular tachycardia that is refractory to amiodarone, life-threatening dysrhythmias due to digitalis toxicity.

Contraindications Heart block, myocardial damage.

Adverse reactions/side effects Drowsiness, CNS depression, respiratory depression, respiratory tract paralysis, abnormal ECG, AV block, hypotension, vasodilation, hyporeflexia.

Drug interactions May enhance effects of other central nervous system depressants. Serious changes in overall cardiac function may occur with cardiac glycosides.

How supplied 50% solution (500 mg/mL) vials (must be diluted to a 10% solution before administering).

Dosage and administration *Adult:* Seizure activity associated with pregnancy: 1–4 g of a 10% solution IV/IO over 3 minutes; maximum dose of 30–40 g/day. Cardiac arrest due to hypomagnesaemia or torsades de pointes: 1–2 g of a 10% solution IV/IO over 5–20 minutes. Torsades de pointes with a pulse: Loading dose of 1–2 g in 50–100 mL of D$_5$W over 5–60 minutes IV. Follow with 0.5–1 g/h IV (titrate dose to control torsades). *Pediatric:* Pulseless ventricular tachycardias with torsades de pointes: 25–50 mg/kg IV/IO bolus of a 10% solution to a maximum dose of 2 grams. Torsades de pointes with pulses/hypomagnesaemia: 25–50 mg/kg IV/IO of a 10% solution over 10–20 minutes to maximum dose of 2 grams. Status asthmaticus: 25–50 mg/kg IV/IO of a 10% solution over 15–30 minutes to a maximum dose of 2 grams.

Duration of action *Onset:* IV/IO: immediate. *Peak effect:* Variable. *Duration:* IV/IO: 30 minutes.

Special considerations Pregnancy safety: Category A. Recommended that the drug not be administered in the 2 hours before delivery, if possible. IV calcium gluconate or calcium chloride should be available as an antagonist to magnesium if needed. Use with caution in patients with renal failure.

Mannitol (Osmitrol)

Class Osmotic diuretic.

Mechanism of action Promotes the movement of fluid from the intracellular space to the extracellular space. Decreases cerebral edema and intracranial pressure. Promotes urinary excretion of toxins.

Indications Cerebral edema, reduce intracranial pressure for certain cause (space-occupying lesions), rhabdomyolysis (myoglobinuria), blood transfusion reactions.

Contraindications Hypotension, pulmonary edema, severe dehydration, intracranial bleeding, CHF.

Adverse reactions/side effects Headache, confusion, seizures, pulmonary edema, tachycardia, chest pain, CHF, hypotension, hypertension, edema, nausea, vomiting, dehydration.

Drug interactions May precipitate digitalis toxicity when given concurrently.

How supplied 250 mL and 500 mL of a 20% solution for IV infusion (200 mg/mL). 25% solution in 50 mL for slow IV push.

Dosage and administration *Adult:* 0.5–1 g/kg IV infusion over 5–10 minutes. Additional doses of 0.25–2 g/kg can be given every 4–6 hours as needed. *Pediatric:* 0.5–1g/kg/dose IV, IO infusion over 30–60 minutes; may repeat after 30 minutes if no effect.

Duration of action *Onset:* 1–3 hours for diuretic effect; 15 minutes for reduction of intracranial pressure. *Peak effect:* Variable. *Duration:* 4–6 hours for diuretic effect; 3–8 hours for reduction of intracranial pressure.

Special considerations Pregnancy safety: Category C. May crystallize at low temperatures; store at room temperature. In-line filter should always be used. Effectiveness depends on large doses and an intact blood-brain barrier. Usage and dosages in emergency care are controversial. Be sure to have ventilatory support available.

Meperidine Hydrochloride (Demerol)

Class Opioid analgesic, schedule II drug.

Mechanism of action Synthetic opioid analgesic whose effects on the central nervous system and smooth muscle organs are similar to morphine, primarily acting as an analgesic and a sedative.

Indications Analgesia for moderate to severe pain.

Contraindications Hypersensitivity to narcotics, diarrhea caused by poisoning, patients taking MAOIs, during labor or delivery of a premature infant, undiagnosed abdominal pain or head injury.

Adverse reactions/side effects Seizures, confusion, sedation, dysphoria, headache, hallucinations, increased ICP, respiratory depression, apnea, hypotension, orthostatic hypotension, syncope, bradycardia, dysrhythmias, nausea, vomiting, constipation, sweating.

Drug interactions Do not give concurrently with MAOIs (even with a dose in the last 14 days). Exacerbates CNS depression when given with other CNS depressants.

How supplied 50 mg/mL and 100 mg/mL prefilled syringes and Tubex syringes.

Dosage and administration *Adult:* 50–100 mg IM, SC. 25–50 mg slowly IV. *Pediatric:* 1–2 mg/kg/dose IV, IO, IM, SC.

Duration of action *Onset:* IM: 10–45 minutes; IV: immediate. *Peak effect:* 30–60 minutes. *Duration:* 2–4 hours.

Special considerations Pregnancy safety: Category C. Use with caution in patients with asthma and COPD. May aggravate seizures in patients with known convulsive disorders. Naloxone should be readily available as antagonist.

Metaproterenol Sulfate (Alupent)

Class Beta-2 adrenergic agonist, bronchodilator.

Mechanism of action Acts directly on bronchial smooth muscle causing relaxation of the bronchial tree and peripheral vasculature.

Indications Bronchial asthma, reversible bronchospasm secondary to bronchitis, COPD.

Contraindications Tachydysrhythmia, hypersensitivity, tachycardia caused by digitalis toxicity.

Adverse reactions/side effects Nervousness, tremor, headache, anxiety, cough, paradoxical bronchospasm, hypertension, chest pain, tachydysrhythmias, palpitations, cardiac arrest, diarrhea, nausea, vomiting, backache, skin reactions, sweating.

Drug interactions Other sympathomimetics may exacerbate cardiovascular effects. MAOIs may potentiate hypotensive effects. Beta blockers may antagonize metaproterenol.

How supplied Metered-dose inhaler: 0.65/mg/spray (15-mL inhaler). Solution: 5% solution in bottles of 10 and 30 mL with calibrated dropper. Alupent inhalation solution unit-dose vial 0.4% or 0.6%.

Dosage and administration *Adult:* Metered-dose inhaler: 2–3 inhalations q 3–4 hours (2 minutes between inhalations). Inhalation solution 5%: Via nebulizer 0.2–0.3 mL of a 5% solution diluted in 2.5 mL saline. *Pediatric:* Metered-dose inhaler: Not recommended. Inhalation solution 5%: Age 6–12 years: 0.1–0.2 mL of a 5% solution diluted in 3 mL saline.

Duration of action *Onset:* 1 minute after inhalation. *Peak effect:* 45 minutes. *Duration:* 3–6 hours.

Special considerations Pregnancy safety: Category C. Monitor for hypotension and tachycardia. Use with caution in patients with coronary artery disease, seizures, hypertension, and diabetes mellitus.

Methylprednisolone Sodium Succinate (Solu-Medrol)

Class Corticosteroid.

Mechanism of action Highly potent synthetic glucocorticoid that suppresses acute and chronic inflammation; potentiates vascular smooth muscle relaxation by beta-adrenergic agonists.

Indications Acute spinal cord trauma, anaphylaxis, bronchodilator for unresponsive asthma.

YOU are the Medic   PART 4

Medical control confirms your request to administer diazepam (Valium) IVP to the patient. You confirm the patient has no medication allergies while you are unlocking your controlled substance container. You confirm the medication, dose, route, and time prior to administering the diazepam. You then slowly administer the diazepam, and the patient's seizure activity stops.

Recording Time: 10 Minutes	
Respirations	24 breaths/min
Pulse	120 beats/min
Skin	Pale, warm, clammy
Blood pressure	142/76 mm Hg
Oxygen saturation (Spo$_2$)	97% on O$_2$
Pupils	Equal and reactive

7. If this patient were more than 20 weeks' pregnant, what medication would you consider?

8. If this patient were diabetic, what medication would you consider?

Contraindications Premature infants, systemic fungal infections, use with caution in patients with gastrointestinal bleeding.

Adverse reactions/side effects Depression, euphoria, headache, restlessness, seizure, increased ICP, pulmonary tuberculosis, hypertension, CHF, nausea, vomiting, peptic ulcer, fluid retention, hypernatremia, hyperkalemia.

Drug interactions Hypoglycemic responses to insulin and hypoglycemic agents may be blunted.

How supplied 40, 125, 500, 1,000 mg powder (requires reconstitution with solution provided).

Dosage and administration *Adult:* Acute spinal cord trauma: 30 mg/kg IV over 30 minutes followed by: Infusion: 5.4 mg/kg/h. Asthma, COPD, anaphylaxis: 1–2 mg/kg IV. *Pediatric:* Acute spinal cord trauma: Same as adult. Status asthmaticus/anaphylaxis: 2 mg/kg/dose IV/IO/IM to a maximum dose of 60 mg.

Duration of action *Onset:* 1–2 hours. *Peak effect:* Variable. *Duration:* 8–24 hours.

Special considerations Pregnancy safety: Category C. Not effective if time of spinal cord injury greater than 8 hours. Crosses the placenta and may cause fetal harm.

Metoprolol Tartrate (Lopressor)

Class Beta blocker, beta-1 selective; antihypertensive, antidysrhythmic.

Mechanism of action Decreases heart rate, conduction velocity, myocardial contractility, and cardiac output. Used to control ventricular response in SVT (PSVT, atrial fibrillation, atrial flutter). Considered second-line agent after adenosine, diltiazem, or digitalis derivative.

Indications PSVT, atrial flutter, atrial fibrillation, reduces myocardial ischemia and damage in patients with AMI.

Contraindications Heart failure, second- or third-degree AV block, first-degree heart block (if PR interval is equal or greater than 0.24 seconds), sick sinus syndrome, cardiogenic shock, bradycardia.

Adverse reactions/side effects Weakness, dizziness, depression, bronchospasm, wheezing, dyspnea, bradycardia, pulmonary edema, CHF, AV blocks, hypotension, heart failure, nausea, indigestion.

Drug interactions Metoprolol may potentiate antihypertensive effects when given to patients taking calcium channel blockers or MAOIs. Catecholamine-depleting drugs may potentiate hypotension. Sympathomimetic effects may be antagonized. Signs of hypoglycemia may be masked.

How supplied 1 mg/mL ampules and vials.

Dosage and administration *Adult:* 5 mg slow IV push at 5-minute intervals to a total of 15 mg. *Pediatric:* Safety not established.

Duration of action *Onset:* 1–2 minutes. *Peak effect:* 5–10 minutes. *Duration:* 3–4 hours.

Special considerations Pregnancy safety: Category C. Metoprolol must be given slow IV over 5 minutes. Concurrent IV administration with IV calcium channel blocker such as verapamil or diltiazem can cause severe hypotension. Metoprolol should be used with caution in patients with liver or renal dysfunction, hypotension, and COPD.

Midazolam Hydrochloride (Versed)

Class Benzodiazepine, short/intermediate acting; schedule IV drug.

Mechanism of action Reversibly interacts with gamma-amino butyric acid (GABA) receptors in the central nervous system causing sedative, anxiolytic, amnesic, and hypnotic effects.

Indications Sedation for medical procedures (eg, intubation, ventilated patients, cardioversion).

Contraindications Acute narrow-angle glaucoma, shock, coma, alcohol intoxication, overdose, depressed vital signs. Concomitant use with barbiturates, alcohol, narcotics, or other central nervous system depressants.

Adverse reactions/side effects Headache, somnolence, respiratory depression, respiratory arrest, apnea, hypotension, cardiac arrest, nausea, vomiting, pain at the injection site.

Drug interactions Should not be used in patients who have taken central nervous system depressants.

How supplied 1 mg/mL and 5 mg/mL vials and Tubex syringes.

Dosage and administration *Adult:* 2–2.5 mg slow IV (over 2–3 minutes). May be repeated to total maximum: 0.1 mg/kg. *Pediatric:* 0.1–0.3 mg/kg IV/IO (maximum single dose: 10 mg).

Duration of action *Onset:* 1–3 minutes, IV and dose dependent. *Peak effect:* Variable. *Duration:* 2–6 hours, dose dependent.

Special considerations Pregnancy safety: Category D. Administer immediately prior to intubation procedure. Requires continuous monitoring of respiratory and cardiac function. Decrease dose by 50% in patients with hepatic and renal dysfunction.

Morphine Sulfate (Roxanol, MS Contin)

Class Opioid analgesic (schedule II narcotic).

Mechanism of action Alleviates pain through CNS action. Suppresses fear and anxiety centers in the brain. Depresses brainstem respiratory centers. Increases peripheral venous capacitance and decreases venous return. Decreases preload and afterload, which decreases myocardial oxygen demand.

Indications Severe CHF, acute cardiogenic pulmonary edema, chest pain associated with acute myocardial infarction, analgesia for moderate to severe acute and chronic pain.

Contraindications Head injury, exacerbated COPD, depressed respiratory drive, hypotension, undiagnosed abdominal pain, decreased level of consciousness, suspected hypovolemia, patients who have taken MAOIs within 14 days.

Adverse reactions/side effects Confusion, sedation, headache, CNS depression, respiratory depression, apnea, bronchospasm, dyspnea, hypotension, orthostatic hypotension, syncope, bradycardia, tachycardia, nausea, vomiting, dry mouth.

Drug interactions Potentiates sedative effects of phenothiazines. CNS depressants may potentiate effects of morphine. MAOIs may cause paradoxical excitation.

How supplied 2 mg/mL, 4 mg/mL, 8 mg/mL, 10 mg/mL ampules, vials, and Tubex syringe.

Dosage and administration *Adult:* STEMI: Initial dose: 2–4 mg slow IV (over 1–5 minutes). Repeat dose: 2–8 mg at 5–15 minute intervals. NSTEMI/Unstable angina. 1–5 mg IV push if symptoms not relieved by nitrates, *use with caution. Pediatric:* 0.1–0.2 mg/kg/dose IV, IO, IM, SC. Maximum dose: 5 mg.

Duration of action *Onset:* Immediate. *Peak effect:* 20 minutes. *Duration:* 2–7 hours.

Special considerations Pregnancy safety: Category C. Morphine rapidly crosses the placenta. Safety in neonates has not been established. Use with caution in the elderly, those with asthma, and in those susceptible to central nervous system depression. Vagotonic effect in patients with acute inferior MI (bradycardia, heart block). Naloxone hydrochloride (Narcan) should be readily available as an antidote.

■ Nalbuphine Hydrochloride (Nubain)

Class Synthetic opioid agonist/antagonist.

Mechanism of action Activates opiate receptor in limbic system of the CNS. Analgesic similar to morphine on a milligram for milligram basis. Agonist and antagonist properties. May be preferred for chest pain in setting of acute MI because it reduces the myocardial oxygen demand without reducing the blood pressure.

Indications Chest pain associated with acute MI, moderate to severe acute pain.

Contraindications Head injury, undiagnosed abdominal pain, diarrhea caused by poison, hypovolemia, hypotension.

Adverse reactions/side effects Headache, dizziness, vertigo, seizure, CNS depression, paradoxical CNS stimulation, respiratory depression, pulmonary edema, hypotension, hypertension, palpitations, bradycardia, nausea, vomiting, dry mouth.

Drug interactions CNS depressants may potentiate effects.

How supplied 10 mg/mL and 20 mg/mL ampules and vials.

Dosage and administration *Adult:* 2–5 mg slowly IV. May repeat 2 mg doses PRN to a maximum dose of 10 mg. *Pediatric:* Not recommended.

Duration of action *Onset:* 2–3 minutes. *Peak effect:* Variable. *Duration:* 3–6 hours.

Special considerations Pregnancy safety: Category B. Use with caution in patients with impaired respiratory function. May precipitate withdrawal syndromes in narcotic-dependent patients. Naloxone should be readily available.

■ Naloxone Hydrochloride (Narcan)

Class Opioid antagonist, antidote.

Mechanism of action Competitive inhibition at narcotic receptor sites. Reverses respiratory depression secondary to opiate drugs. Completely inhibits the effect of morphine.

Indications Opiate overdose, complete or partial reversal of central nervous system and respiratory depression induced by opioids, decreased level of consciousness, coma of unknown origin. Narcotic agonist for the following: morphine sulfate, heroin, hydromorphone (Dilaudid), methadone, meperidine (Demerol), paregoric, fentanyl (Sublimaze), oxycodone (Percodan), codeine, propoxyphene (Darvon). Narcotic agonist and antagonist for the following: butorphanol (Stadol), pentazocine (Talwin), nalbuphine (Nubain).

Contraindications Use with caution in narcotic-dependent patients. Use with caution in neonates of narcotic-addicted mothers.

Adverse reactions/side effects Restlessness, seizures, dyspnea, pulmonary edema, tachycardia, hypertension, dysrhythmias, cardiac arrest, nausea, vomiting, withdrawal symptoms in opioid-addicted patients, diaphoresis.

Drug interactions Incompatible with bisulfite and alkaline solutions.

How supplied 0.4 mg/mL and 1 mg/mL ampules and vials.

Dosage and administration *Adult:* 0.4–2 mg IM/IV/IO/SQ/ET/Intranasal (diluted); minimum single dose recommended: 2 mg. Repeat at 5-minute intervals to a maximum total dose of 10 mg (medical control may request higher amounts). *Pediatric:* 0.1 mg/kg/dose IV/IO/IM/SQ every 2 minutes as needed. Maximum total dose of 2 mg. If no response in 10 minutes, administer an additional 0.1 mg/kg/dose.

Duration of action *Onset:* <2 minutes. *Peak effect:* Variable. *Duration:* 30–60 minutes.

Special considerations Pregnancy safety: Category C. Assist ventilations prior to administration to avoid sympathetic stimulation. Seizures without causal relationship have been reported. May not reverse hypotension. Use caution when administering to narcotic addicts (potential violent behavior). Half-life of naloxone is often shorter than the half-life of narcotics; repeat dosing may be required.

■ Nifedipine (Procardia, Adalat)

Class Calcium channel blocker.

Mechanism of action Inhibits movement of calcium ions across cell membranes; calcium channel blocker; arterial and venous vasodilator; reduces preload and afterload; prevents coronary artery spasm and decreases total peripheral resistance; reduces myocardial oxygen demands; does not prolong AV nodal conduction.

Indications Hypertensive crisis, angina pectoris.

Contraindications Compensatory hypertension, hypotension, cardiogenic shock.

Adverse reactions/side effects Headache, dizziness, nervousness, weakness, mood changes, dyspnea, cough, wheezing, CHF, MI, ventricular dsyrhythmias, hypotension, syncope, nausea, abdominal discomfort, diarrhea.

Drug interactions Beta blockers may potentiate effects. Effects of theophylline may be increased. Antihypertensives may potentiate hypotensive effects.

How supplied 10- and 20-mg liquid-filled capsules.

Dosage and administration *Adult:* 10 mg SL or buccal (puncture end of capsule with needle and squeeze or have patient bite and swallow). May repeat in 30 minutes. *Pediatric:* Not recommended.

Duration of action *Onset:* 15–30 minutes. *Peak effect:* 1–3 hours. *Duration:* 6–8 hours.

Special considerations Pregnancy safety: Category C. Does not slow AV nodal activity. Have beta blocker available for control of reflex tachycardia. Use with caution in geriatric population. Hypotension and angina pectoris may occur.

Special Populations

Almost all medications require lower doses for elderly patients because of diminished renal clearance. Paramedics should be aware of this when administering drugs. Additionally, medications that have a high first-pass metabolism rate through the liver can require additional medication doses to obtain the optimal serum levels. Consult a specific, reliable reference for each medication that is being considered for oral administration, and be sure to rely on medical direction at all times.

Nitroglycerin (Nitrostat, Nitro-Bid, Tridil)

Class Vasodilator.

Mechanism of action Smooth muscle relaxant acting on vasculature, bronchial, uterine, intestinal smooth muscle. Dilation of arterioles and veins in the periphery. Reduces preload and afterload, decreasing workload of the heart and thereby myocardial oxygen demand.

Indications Acute angina pectoris, ischemic chest pain, hypertension, CHF, pulmonary edema.

Contraindications Hypotension, hypovolemia, intracranial bleeding or head injury, pericardial tamponade, severe bradycardia or tachycardia, RV infarction, previous administration in the last 24 hours: tadalafil (Cialis) (48 hours), vardenafil (Levitra), sildenafil (Viagra).

Adverse reactions/side effects Headache, dizziness, weakness, reflex tachycardia, syncope, hypotension, nausea, vomiting, dry mouth, muscle twitching, diaphoresis.

Drug interactions Additive effects with other vasodilators. Incompatible with other drugs IV.

How supplied Tablets: 0.3 mg (1/200 grain). 0.4 mg (1/150 grain). 0.6 mg (1/100 grain). NTG spray: 0.4 mg/actuation. NTG IV (Tridil). 200 μg/mL in D_5W glass vials.

Dosage and administration *Adult:* Tablet: 0.3–0.4 mg sublingually; may repeat in 5 minutes to maximum of 3 doses. NTG spray: 1–2 sprays for 0.5–1 second at 5-minute intervals to a maximum of 3 sprays in 15 minutes. NTG IV infusion: Begin at 10 μg/min; increase by 10 μg/min every 3–5 minutes until desired effect. To a maximum of 200 μg/min. *Pediatric:* Not

recommended. IV infusion: 0.25–0.5 μg/kg/min IV, IO titrated by 1 μg/kg/min (max dose: 5 μg/kg/min).

Duration of action *Onset:* 1–3 minutes. *Peak effect:* 5–10 minutes. *Duration:* SL: 20–30 minutes. IV: 1–10 minutes after discontinuation of infusion.

Special considerations Pregnancy safety: Category C. Hypotension more common in the elderly. If 12-lead ECG shows inferior wall infarct, rule out right ventricular infarct via right-sided 12-lead ECG prior to administering nitroglycerin. Nitroglycerin decomposes when exposed to light or heat, must be kept in airtight containers. Must be administered only with an infusion pump direct from bottle with a vented IV set and non-PVC tubing. Active ingredient may have stinging effect when administered.

Nitropaste (Nitro-Bid Ointment)

Class Vasodilator.

Mechanism of action Smooth muscle relaxant acting on vasculature, bronchial, uterine, intestinal smooth muscle. Dilation of arterioles and veins in the periphery. Reduces preload and afterload, decreasing workload of the heart and thereby myocardial oxygen demand.

Indications Acute angina pectoris, chest pain associated with AMI, hypertension, CHF, pulmonary edema.

Contraindications Hypotension, hypovolemia, intracranial bleeding or head injury, previous administration in the last 24 hours of tadalafil (Cialis) (48 hours), vardenafil (Levitra), sildenafil (Viagra).

Adverse reactions/side effects Headache, dizziness, weakness, reflex tachycardia, syncope, hypotension, nausea, vomiting, dry mouth, muscle twitching, diaphoresis.

Drug interactions Additive effects with other vasodilators.

How supplied 20- to 60-gram tubes of 2% nitroglycerin paste with measuring applicators. Transdermal units of varying doses.

Dosage and administration *Adult:* Paste: Apply ½″ to ¾″ (1–2 cm), 15–30 mg, cover with wrap and secure with tape. Maximum, 5″ (75 mg) per application. Transdermal: Apply unit to intact skin (usually chest wall) in varying doses. *Pediatric:* Not recommended.

Duration of action *Onset:* 30 minutes. *Peak effect:* Variable. *Duration:* 18–24 hours.

Special considerations Pregnancy safety: Category C. Not a great value in prehospital arena. Wear gloves when applying paste. Store paste in a cool place with tube tightly capped. Erratic absorption rates quite common.

Nitrous Oxide 50:50 (Nitronox)

Class Gaseous analgesic and anesthetic.

Mechanism of action Exact mechanism unknown; affects central nervous system phospholipids.

Indications Moderate to severe pain, anxiety, apprehension.

Contraindications Impaired level of consciousness, head injury, inability to follow or comply with instructions, decompression sickness (nitrogen narcosis, air embolism, and air transport), undiagnosed abdominal pain or marked distention, bowel obstruction, hypotension, shock, COPD, cyanosis, chest trauma with pneumothorax.

Adverse reactions/side effects Lightheadedness, drowsiness, respiratory depression, apnea, nausea, vomiting, malignant hyperthermia.

Drug interactions None of significance.

How supplied D and E cylinders (blue and green) of a 50% nitrous oxide and 50% oxygen compressed gas.

Dosage and administration *Adult:* Instruct the patient to inhale deeply through demand valve and mask or mouthpiece. *Pediatric:* Same as above.

Duration of action *Onset:* 2–5 minutes. *Peak effect:* Variable. *Duration:* 2–5 minutes.

Special considerations Pregnancy safety: Category C. Nitrous oxide increases the incidence of spontaneous abortion. Ventilate patient care area during use. Nitrous oxide is nonflammable and nonexplosive. Nitrous oxide is ineffective in 20% of the population.

Norepinephrine Bitartrate (Levophed)

Class Sympathomimetic, vasopressor.

Mechanism of action Potent alpha-agonist resulting in intense peripheral vasoconstriction, positive chronotropic and increased inotropic effect (from 10% beta effect) with increased cardiac output. Alpha-adrenergic activity resulting in peripheral vasoconstriction and beta-adrenergic activity leading to inotropic stimulation of the heart and coronary artery vasodilation.

Indications Cardiogenic shock, unresponsive to fluid resuscitation, significant hypotensive (<70 mm Hg) states.

Contraindications Hypotensive patients with hypovolemia, pregnancy (relative).

Adverse reactions/side effects Headache, anxiety, dizziness, restlessness, dyspnea, bradycardia, hypertension, dysrhythmias, chest pain, peripheral cyanosis, cardiac arrest, nausea, vomiting, urinary retention, renal failure, decreased blood flow to the GI tract, kidneys, skeletal muscle, and skin, tissue necrosis from extravasation.

Drug interactions Can be deactivated by alkaline solutions. Sympathomimetic and phosphodiesterase inhibitors may exacerbate dysrhythmias. Bretylium may potentiate the effects of catecholamines.

How supplied 1 mg/mL vials.

Dosage and administration *Adult:* Dilute 8 mg in 500 mL of D_5W or 4 mg in 250 mL of D_5W (16 µg/mL). Infuse by IV piggyback at 0.1–0.5 µg/kg/min titrated to response (average dose for 70 kg patient 7–35 µg/min). *Pediatric:* Begin at 0.1–2 µg/kg/min IV infusion, adjust rate to achieve desired change in blood pressure and systemic perfusion. Titrated to patient response.

Duration of action *Onset:* 1–3 minutes. *Peak effect:* Variable. *Duration:* 5–10 minutes and lasts only 1 minute after infusion is discontinued.

Special considerations Pregnancy safety: Category C. May cause fetal anoxia when used in pregnancy. Infuse norepinephrine through a large, stable vein to avoid extravasation and tissue necrosis. Often used with low-dose dopamine to spare decreased renal and mesenteric blood flow. Drug or poison-induced hypotension may require higher doses to achieve adequate perfusion.

Ondansetron Hydrochloride (Zofran)

Class Serotonin receptor antagonist; antiemetic.

Mechanism of action Blocks action of serotonin, which is a natural substance that causes nausea and vomiting.

Indications For the prevention and control of nausea or vomiting. Used in hospital for patients undergoing chemotherapy or surgical procedures.

Contraindications Known allergy to ondansetron or other $5-HT_3$ receptor antagonists.

Adverse reactions/side effects Headache, malaise, wheezing, bronchospasm, atrial fibrillation, abnormal ECG, prolonged QT interval, ST segment depression, second-degree AV block, constipation, diarrhea, hives, skin rash.

Drug interactions Not recommended if the patient is taking apomorphine, mesoridazine, pimozide, or thioridazine.

How supplied 2 mg/mL vials.

Dosage and administration *Adult:* 4 mg IV/IM may repeat in 10 minutes. *Pediatric:* 0.1 mg/kg IV/IM.

Duration of action *Onset:* 30 minutes. *Peak effect:* 2 hours. *Duration:* 3–6 hours.

Special considerations Pregnancy safety: Category B.

Oral Glucose (Insta-Glucose)

Class Hyperglycemic, carbohydrate.

Mechanism of action After absorption in the GI tract, glucose is distributed to the tissues providing an increase in circulating blood glucose levels.

Indications Conscious patients with suspected hypoglycemia.

Contraindications Decreased level of consciousness, nausea, vomiting.

Adverse reactions/side effects Nausea, vomiting.

Drug interactions None.

How supplied Paste and gels in various forms.

Dosage and administration *Adult:* 15–45 g PO in patients with an intact gag reflex and the ability to manage their own secretions. *Pediatric:* 5–45 g PO in patients with an intact gag reflex and the ability to manage their own secretions.

Duration of action *Onset:* 10 minutes. *Peak effect:* Variable. *Duration:* Variable

Special considerations Must be swallowed. Glucose is not absorbed sublingually or buccally. Check a glucometer reading before administering oral glucose and repeat at least 10 minutes after.

Oxygen

Class Naturally occurring atmospheric gas.

Mechanism of action Reverses hypoxemia.

Indications Confirmed or expected hypoxemia, ischemic chest pain, respiratory insufficiency, prophylactically during air transport, confirmed or suspected carbon monoxide poisoning, all other causes of decreased tissue oxygenation, decreased level of consciousness.

Contraindications Certain patients with COPD will not tolerate oxygen concentrations over 35%. Hyperventilation.

Adverse reactions/side effects Decreased level of consciousness (COPD patients), decreased respiratory drive in COPD patients, dry mucus membranes.

Drug interactions None.

How supplied Oxygen cylinders (usually green and white) of 100% compressed oxygen gas.

Dosage and administration *Adult:* Cardiac arrest and carbon monoxide poisoning: 100%. Hypoxemia: 10–15 L/min via nonrebreather. COPD: 0–2 L/min via nasal cannula or 28%–35% Venturi mask. Be prepared to provide ventilatory support if higher concentrations of oxygen are needed. *Pediatric:* Same as for adult with exception of premature infant.

Duration of action *Onset:* Immediate. *Peak effect:* Not applicable. *Duration:* Less than 2 minutes.

Special considerations Be familiar with liter flow and each type of delivery device used. Supports combustion.

Oxytocin (Pitocin)

Class Pituitary hormone.

Mechanism of action Increases uterine contractions.

Indications Postpartum hemorrhage after infant and placental delivery.

Contraindications Presence of second fetus, unfavorable fetal position.

Adverse reactions/side effects Coma, seizures, anxiety, subarachnoid hemorrhage, hypotension, tachycardia, dysrhythmias, chest pain, nausea, vomiting, painful uterine contractions, uterine rupture.

Drug interactions Other vasopressors may potentiate hypotension.

How supplied 10 units/mL solution.

Dosage and administration *Adult:* IM administration: 10 units IM following delivery of the placenta. IV administration: Mix 10–40 units in 1,000 mL of nonhydrating diluent: Infused at 20–40 milliunits/min. Titrated to severity of bleeding and uterine response. *Pediatric:* Not applicable.

Duration of action *Onset:* IM: 3–5 minutes; IV: immediate. *Peak effect:* Variable. *Duration:* IM: 30–60 minutes, IV: 20 minutes after infusion is stopped.

Special considerations Pregnancy safety: Category C. Monitor vital signs including fetal heart rate and uterine tone closely.

Pancuronium Bromide (Pavulon)

Class Nondepolarizing neuromuscular blocker/paralytic.

Mechanism of action Binds to the receptor for acetylcholine at the neuromuscular junction.

Indications Induction or maintenance of paralysis after intubation to assist ventilations.

Contraindications Hypersensitivity, inability to control airway and/or support ventilations with oxygen and positive pressure, neuromuscular disease (eg, myasthenia gravis), hepatic or renal failure.

Adverse reactions/side effects Weakness, prolonged neuromuscular block, bronchospasm, apnea, respiratory failure, tachydysrhythmias, transient hypotension, hypertension, PVCs, salivation.

Drug interactions Positive chronotropic drugs may potentiate tachycardia.

How supplied 1 mg/mL and 2 mg/mL ampules and vials.

Dosage and administration *Adult:* 0.06 to 0.1 mg/kg slow IV. Repeat every 30–60 minutes as needed. *Pediatric:* 0.04 to 0.1 mg/kg slow IV/IO.

Duration of action *Onset:* 30 seconds. *Peak effect:* Paralysis in 3–5 minutes. *Duration:* 45–60 minutes.

Special considerations Pregnancy safety: Category C. If patient is conscious, explain the effect of the medication before administration and always sedate the patient before administering pancuronium. Intubation and ventilatory support must be readily available; monitor the patient carefully. Pancuronium has no effect on consciousness or pain. Will not stop neuronal seizure activity. Heart rate and cardiac output will be increased. Decreased doses for patients with renal impairment or myasthenia gravis.

Phenobarbital (Luminal)

Class Barbiturate, long-acting; anticonvulsant; schedule IV drug.

Mechanism of action Generally unknown but believed to reduce neuronal excitability by increasing the motor cortex threshold to electrical stimulation.

Indications Prevention and treatment of seizure activity, status epilepticus.

Contraindications Patients with porphyria, history of sedative or hypnotic addiction, severe liver or respiratory disease.

Adverse reactions/side effects Coma, drowsiness, headache, vertigo, paradoxic excitation, CNS depression, ataxia, bronchospasm, laryngospasm, respiratory depression, hypotension, bradycardia, syncope, nausea, vomiting.

Drug interactions Effects potentiated by other CNS depressants, anticonvulsants, and MAOIs. Incompatible with all other drugs. Flush line before and after use.

How supplied 30 mg/mL, 60 mg/mL, 65 mg/mL, 130 mg/mL ampules and vials and Tubex syringes.

Dosage and administration *Adult:* 100–250 mg slow IV or IM. May repeat as needed in 20–30 minutes. *Pediatric:* 10–20 mg/kg slow IV/IO/IM. Repeat as needed in 20–30 minutes.

Duration of action *Onset:* 3–30 minutes. *Peak effect:* 30 minutes. *Duration:* 4–6 hours

Special considerations Pregnancy safety: Category D. Potential for abuse. Carefully monitor vital signs. Use with caution in patients with pulmonary, cardiovascular, hepatic, or renal insufficiency. Elderly more likely to experience side effects; consider decreasing dose to 75% of the usual dose. Use large, stable vein for injection.

Phenytoin (Dilantin)

Class Anticonvulsant.

Mechanism of action Promotes sodium efflux from neurons, thereby stabilizing the neuron's threshold against the excitability caused by excess stimulation. In similar fashion, decreases abnormal ventricular automaticity and decreases the refractory period in the myocardial conduction system.

Indications Prophylaxis and treatment of major motor seizures, digitalis-induced dysrhythmias.

Contraindications Hypersensitivity, bradycardia, second- and third-degree heart block.

Adverse reactions/side effects Ataxia, agitation, dizziness, headache, drowsiness, CNS depression, respiratory depression, hypotension, tachycardia, vasodilation, heart blocks, dysrhythmias, nausea, vomiting, hepatitis, altered taste, rash, Stevens-Johnson syndrome, nystagmus, pain at injection site.

Drug interactions Serum phenytoin levels increased by anticoagulants, Tagamet, sulfonamides, and salicylates. Metabolism increased by chronic alcohol use. Cardiac depressant effects increased by lidocaine, propranolol, and other beta blockers. Precipitation may occur when mixed with D_5W. Incompatible with many solutions and medications.

How supplied 50 mg/mL vials, prefilled syringes, and Tubex syringes. May be diluted with NS (1–10 mg/mL). Must use inline filter on administration set. IV line should be flushed with 0.9% NS before and after the drug is administered.

Dosage and administration *Adult:* Seizures: 10–20 mg/kg slow IV; not to exceed 1 g or rate of 50 mg/minute. Dysrhythmias: 50–100 mg (diluted) slow IV every 5–15 minutes PRN; maximum 1 g. *Pediatric:* Seizures: 10–20 mg/kg slow IV (1–3 mg/kg/min). Dysrhythmias: 5 mg/kg slow IV; maximum 1 g loading dose.

Duration of action *Onset:* 20–30 minutes. *Peak effect:* 1–3 hours. *Duration:* 18–24 hours but as long as 15 days reported.

Special considerations Pregnancy safety: Category D. Carefully monitor vital signs. Venous irritation may occur (use large stable vein).

Pralidoxime (2-PAM, Protopam)

Class Cholinesterase reactivator, antidote.

Mechanism of action Reactivates cholinesterase to effectively act as an antidote to organophosphate and pesticide poisonings. This action allows for destruction of accumulated acetylcholine at the neuromuscular junction resulting in reversal of respiratory paralysis and paralysis of skeletal muscle.

Indications As an antidote in the treatment of poisoning by organophosphate pesticides and chemicals. Anticholinesterase overdoses.

Contraindications Reduce dose in patients with impaired renal function, patients with myasthenia gravis, inorganic phosphates poisoning.

Adverse reactions/side effects Dizziness, drowsiness, headache, neuromuscular blockade, seizure, laryngospasm, hyperventilation, apnea, tachycardia, cardiac arrest, nausea, muscle rigidity, muscle weakness, rash, pain at injection site.

Drug interactions Avoid use of pralidoxime concurrently with succinylcholine, morphine, aminophylline, theophylline, and other respiratory depressants to include barbiturates, narcotic analgesics, and sedative hypnotics.

How supplied 1 gram powder to be added to solution for infusion. 600 mg/2 mL auto-injector.

Dosage and administration *Adult:* Organophosphate poisoning: Initial dose of 1–2 g as an IV infusion over 30–60 minutes after atropine administration. Dose can be repeated in 1 h if muscle paralysis is still present. 600 mg IM repeat twice more at 15-minute intervals as needed. Anticholinesterase overdose: 1–2 g as an IV infusion over 30–60 minutes. Repeat at 250 mg every 5 minutes as needed. *Pediatric:* 20–40 mg/kg as IV infusion over 15–30 minutes. Dose may be repeated in 1 h if muscle paralysis is still present. If IV administration is not feasible, IM or SC injection may be used.

Duration of action *Onset:* Minutes. *Peak effect:* Variable. *Duration:* Variable.

Special considerations Pregnancy safety: Category C. Slow IV infusion prevents tachycardia, laryngospasm, muscle rigidity. Consider drawing a blood sample prior to administering for hospital to run pretreatment levels. Rapid administration may cause tachycardia, laryngospasm, or muscle rigidity. Treatment will be most effective if given within a few hours after poisoning. Cardiac monitoring should be considered in all cases of severe organophosphate poisoning.

Procainamide Hydrochloride (Pronestyl)

Class Antidysrhythmic.

Mechanism of action Suppresses phase 4 depolarization in normal ventricular muscle and Purkinje fibers, reducing ectopic pacemaker's automaticity; suppresses intraventricular conduction.

Indications Stable monomorphic ventricular tachycardia with normal QT interval, reentry SVT uncontrolled by vagal maneuvers and adenosine, stable wide complex tachycardia of unknown origin, atrial fibrillation with rapid ventricular rate in patients with Wolff-Parkinson-White syndrome.

Contraindications Torsades de pointes, second- and third-degree heart atrioventricular block (without functioning artificial pacemaker), preexisting QT prolongation, digitalis toxicity, tricyclic antidepressant overdose.

Adverse reactions/side effects Confusion, seizures, hypotension, bradycardia, reflex tachycardia, ventricular dysrhythmias, AV blocks, asystole, widening of PR, QRS, and Q-T intervals, nausea, vomiting.

Drug interactions Increases plasma levels of amiodarone and quinidine.

How supplied 100-mg and 500-mg vials.

Dosage and administration *Adult:* Recurrent ventricular fibrillation/pulseless ventricular tachycardia: 20 mg/min slow IV infusion (maximum dose: 17 mg/kg). In urgent situation, up to 50 mg/min may be administered (maximum dose: 17 mg/kg). Other indications: 20 mg/min slow IV infusion until any one of the following occurs: Dysrhythmia suppression, hypotension, QRS widens by >50% of its pretreatment width, or total dose of 17 mg/kg has been given. Maintenance infusion: 1–4 mg/min (diluted in D₅W or normal saline). Reduce dose in presence of renal insufficiency. *Pediatric:* Loading dose 15 mg/kg IV/IO over 30–60 minutes.

Duration of action *Onset:* 10–30 minutes. *Peak effect:* Variable. *Duration:* 3–6 hours.

Special considerations Pregnancy safety: Category C. Potent vasodilation and negative inotropic effects. Hypotension may occur with rapid infusion. Administer cautiously to patients with cardiac, hepatic, or renal insufficiency. Administer cautiously to patients with asthma or digitalis-induced dysrhythmias.

▪ Promethazine Hydrochloride (Phenergan)

Class Phenothiazine, antiemetic, antihistamine.

Mechanism of action H-1 receptor antagonist; blocks action of histamine; possesses sedative, anti-motion, antiemetic, and anticholinergic activity; potentiates the effects of narcotics to induce analgesia.

Indications Nausea/vomiting, motion sickness, sedation for patients in labor, potentiates the analgesic effects of narcotics.

Contraindications Coma, central nervous system depression from alcohol, barbiturates, or narcotics, Reye syndrome, lower respiratory symptoms (eg, asthma).

Adverse reactions/side effects Headache, dizziness, drowsiness, confusion, restlessness, wheezing, chest tightness, thickening of bronchial secretions, palpitations, bradycardia, reflex tachycardia, QT prolongation, postural hypotension, diarrhea, nausea, vomiting.

Drug interactions Additive with other central nervous system depressants. Increased extrapyramidal effects with MAOIs.

How supplied 25 mg/mL, 50 mg/mL ampules and Tubex syringes.

Dosage and administration *Adult:* 12.5–25 mg IV, deep IM, PO, PR. *Pediatric (older than 2 years):* 0.25–0.5 mg/kg dose deep IM.

Duration of action *Onset:* IV: Immediate. *Peak effect:* 30–60 minutes. *Duration:* 4–6 hours.

Special considerations Pregnancy safety: Category C. Convulsions and sudden death when used with children. Use caution in patients with asthma, peptic ulcer, and bone marrow suppression. Do not use in children with vomiting of unknown etiology. Avoid intra-arterial injection. Deep IM injections are the preferred route of administration.

▪ Propofol (Diprivan)

Class Sedative hypnotic, short-acting.

Mechanism of action Produces rapid and brief state of general anesthesia.

Indications Anesthesia induction, anesthesia maintenance, sedation for mechanically ventilated patients.

Contraindications Hypovolemia, known sensitivity including soybean oil, peanuts, and eggs.

Adverse reactions/side effects Seizure, apnea, dysrhythmias, asystole, hypotension, hypertension, nausea, vomiting, involuntary muscle movement, acute renal failure.

Drug interactions No known drug interactions in adults. In pediatric patients when used with fentanyl, propofol can cause profound bradycardia.

How supplied 10 mg/mL intravenous emulsion.

Dosage and administration *Adult:* Induction dose: 1.5–3 mg/kg IV, IO. Maintenance infusion: 25–75 µg/kg/min IV, IO. *Pediatric:* Induction dose: 2.5–3.5 mg/kg IV, IO. Maintenance infusion: 125–300 µg/kg/min IV, IO.

Duration of action *Onset:* <1 minute. *Peak effect:* 1 minute. *Duration:* As long as infusion is running.

Special considerations Pregnancy safety: Category B. Avoid rapid administration in elderly patients to avoid hypotension and airway obstruction. Continue to monitor vital signs and oxygenation. Use large stable vein to avoid injection site pain. Avoid in pregnancy due to neonatal depression.

▪ Propranolol Hydrochloride (Inderal)

Class Beta-adrenergic blocker.

Mechanism of action Nonselective beta-adrenergic blocker that reduces chronotropic, inotropic, and vasodilator response to beta-adrenergic stimulation.

Indications Hypertension, angina pectoris, ventricular tachycardia, ventricular fibrillation refractory to lidocaine, selected supraventricular tachycardia.

Contraindications Sinus bradycardia (if no pacemaker present), second- or third-degree AV block (if no pacemaker present), bronchial asthma, sick sinus syndrome (if no pacemaker present), cardiogenic shock, CHF, and acute pulmonary edema.

Adverse reactions/side effects Weakness, depression, fatigue, anxiety, dizziness, bronchospasm, wheezing, hypotension, bradycardia, CHF, AV blocks, nausea, vomiting, diarrhea, hypoglycemia, hyperglycemia.

Drug interactions Verapamil may worsen atrioventricular conduction abnormalities. Succinylcholine effects may be enhanced. Effects may be reversed by isoproterenol, norepinephrine, dopamine (Intropin).

How supplied 1 mg/mL vials.

Dosage and administration *Adult:* Dilute 1–3 mg in 10–30 mL of D5W. Administer slowly IV at rate of 1 mg/min. Maximum: 5 mg. *Pediatric:* 0.01–0.05 mg/kg/dose slow IV over 10 minutes. Maximum: 3 mg.

Duration of action *Onset:* 15–60 minutes. *Peak effect:* Variable. *Duration:* 6–12 hours.

Special considerations Pregnancy safety: Category C. Closely monitor patient during administration. Use with caution in elderly patients. Atropine should be readily available.

Rocuronium Bromide (Zemuron)

Class Nondepolarizing neuromuscular blocker.

Mechanism of action Antagonizes acetylcholine at the motor end plate producing skeletal muscle paralysis.

Indications Rapid sequence intubation.

Contraindications Known sensitivity to bromides. Use with caution in heart and liver disease.

Adverse reactions/side effects Bronchospasm, wheezing, rhonchi, respiratory depression, apnea, dysrhythmias, tachycardia, transient hypotension and hypertension, nausea, vomiting.

Drug interactions Use of inhalation anesthetics will enhance neuromuscular blockade.

How supplied 10 mg/mL vials.

Dosage and administration *Adult:* 0.6–1.2 mg/kg IV, IO. *Pediatric (older than 3 months):* 0.6–1.2 mg/kg IV, IO.

Duration of action *Onset:* 1–2 minutes. *Peak effect:* Varies. *Duration:* 45–120 minutes.

Special considerations Pregnancy safety: Category B. If patient is conscious, explain the effect of the medication before administration and always sedate the patient before using rocuronium. Intubation and ventilatory support must be readily available. Monitor the patient carefully. Rocuronium has no effect on consciousness or pain. Will not stop neuronal seizure activity. Pulse rate and cardiac output are increased. Decrease doses for patients with renal disease.

Sodium Bicarbonate

Class Systemic hydrogen ion buffer, alkalizing agent.

Mechanism of action Buffers metabolic acidosis and lactic acid buildup in the body caused by anaerobic metabolism secondary to severe hypoxia by reacting with hydrogen ions to form water and carbon dioxide.

Indications Metabolic acidosis during cardiac arrest, tricyclic antidepressant, aspirin, and phenobarbital overdose, hyperkalemia, crush injuries.

Contraindications Metabolic and respiratory alkalosis, hypokalemia, electrolyte imbalance due to severe vomiting or diarrhea.

Adverse reactions/side effects Hypernatremia, metabolic alkalosis, tissue sloughing, cellulitis, or necrosis at injection site. Seizures, fluid retention, hypokalemia, electrolyte imbalance, tetany, sodium retention, peripheral edema.

Drug interactions Increases the effects of amphetamines. Decreases the effects of benzodiazepines, tricyclic antidepressants. May deactivate sympathomimetics (dopamine, epinephrine, norepinephrine).

How supplied 1 mEq/mL of an 8.4% solution in 10- and 50-mL vials and prefilled syringe. 0.5 mEq/mL of a 4.2% solution in 2.5-, 5-, and 10-mL prefilled syringe.

Dosage and administration *Adult:* 1 mEq/kg slow IV, IO push may repeat at 0.5 mEq/kg every 10 minutes. *Pediatric:* 1 mEq/kg slow IV, IO push (dilute in small children to 4.2%).

Duration of action *Onset:* Seconds. *Peak effect:* 1–2 minutes. *Duration:* 10 minutes.

Special considerations Pregnancy safety: Category C. Repeat as needed in tricyclic antidepressant overdose until QRS narrows. Must be used in conjunction with effective ventilation and chest compressions in cardiac arrest. Avoid contact with other medications; may precipitate or inactivate them. Always flush IV line well before and after injecting. Use with caution in patients with CHF and renal disease due to high sodium concentration. Monitor patient closely for signs and symptoms of fluid overload.

Sodium Nitrate

Class Antidote cyanide poisoning adjunct.

Mechanism of action Reacts with hemoglobin to form methemoglobin, which reacts with cyanide and chemically binds with it to prevent toxic effect.

Indications Cyanide poisoning.

Contraindications None in the emergency setting.

Adverse reactions/side effects Hypotension, tachycardia, fainting, nausea, vomiting.

Drug interactions None in the emergency setting.

How supplied 3% solution (30 mg/1 mL) vials.

Dosage and administration *Adult:* 300 mg (10 mL of a 3% solution) slow IV push over 5 minutes or dilute 300 mg in 100 mL of saline and infuse slowly. *Pediatrics:* 10 mg/kg (0.33 mL/kg of a 10% solution) IV/IO over 3–5 minutes.

Duration of action *Onset:* 2–10 minutes. *Peak effect:* Varies. *Duration:* 30 minutes to 2 hours.

Special considerations Pregnancy safety: Category C. Potent vasodilator causes significant hypotension if given too rapidly. Monitor blood pressure closely. Look for signs of methemoglobinemia (eg, cyanosis, vomiting, shock, and coma).

Sodium Thiosulfate

Class Cyanide antidote.

Mechanism of action Converts cyanide to the less toxic thiocyanate, which is then excreted in the urine.

Indications Cyanide poisoning.

Contraindications None in the emergency setting.

Adverse reactions/side effects Diarrhea.

Drug interactions None.

How supplied 12.5 g/50 mL of a 25% solution ampules, vials.

Dosage and administration *Adult:* 12.5 g (50 mL of a 25% solution) IV/IO slow push over 10 minutes. *Pediatrics:* 400 mg/kg (1.65 mL/kg of a 25% solution) IV/IO slow push at a rate of 0.625–1.25 g/min over 10 minutes.

Duration of action *Onset:* 2–10 minutes. *Peak effect:* Varies. *Duration:* 30 minutes to 2 hours.

Special considerations Pregnancy safety: Category C. If response to treatment is inadequate, repeat sodium nitrite and sodium thiosulfate; administer a second dose of each at half the original dose 30 minutes after the first dose. This is the third step in a three-step treatment preceded by amyl nitrite and sodium nitrite.

Streptokinase (Streptase)

Class Thrombolytic.

Mechanism of action Combines with plasminogen to produce an activator complex that converts free plasminogen to the proteolytic enzyme, plasmin. Plasmin degrades fibrin threads and fibrinogen, causing clot lysis.

Indications Acute evolving myocardial infarction, massive pulmonary emboli, arterial thrombosis and embolism, to clear intraventricular cannula.

Contraindications Hypersensitivity, active bleeding, recent cerebral vascular accident, prolonged cardiopulmonary resuscitation, intracranial or intraspinal neoplasm, arteriovenous malformation, recent surgery or significant trauma (particularly head trauma), severe uncontrolled hypertension.

Adverse reactions/side effects Intracranial hemorrhage, bronchospastic hemoptysis, ARDS, reperfusion dysrhythmias, hypotension, MI, GI bleeding, hematuria, abdominal pain, bleeding from other sites, allergic reactions.

Drug interactions Aspirin, heparin, and other anticoagulants may increase risk of bleeding as well as improve outcome.

How supplied 250,000, 750,000, and 1.5 million unit powder (requires reconstitution before administration).

Dosage and administration *Note:* Reconstitute by slowly adding 5 mL of sodium chloride or D_5W, directing stream to side of vial instead of into powder. Gently roll and tilt vial for reconstitution; dilute slowly to 45 mL total. *Adult:* 500,000–1,500,000 IU diluted to 45 mL IV over 1 hour. *Pediatric:* Safety not established.

Duration of action *Onset:* 10–20 minutes (fibrinolysis, 10–20 minutes; clot lysis, 60–90 minutes). *Peak effect:* Variable. *Duration:* 3–4 hours (prolonged bleeding times up to 24 hours).

Special considerations Pregnancy safety: Category C. Thin transparent fibers may occur after reconstitution; they do not interfere with safe use. Do not administer IM injections to patients receiving fibrinolytics. Obtain blood sample for coagulation studies prior to administration. Carefully monitor vital signs. Observe patient for bleeding.

Succinylcholine Chloride (Anectine)

Class Neuromuscular blocker, depolarizing; skeletal muscle relaxant.

Mechanism of action Ultra-short-acting depolarizing skeletal muscle relaxant that mimics acetylcholine as it binds with the cholinergic receptors on the motor end plate, producing a phase 1 block as manifested by fasciculations.

Indications Rapid-sequence intubation.

Contraindications Acute narrow-angle glaucoma, penetrating eye injuries, malignant hyperthermia. Acute injury after multisystem trauma, major burns, or extensive muscle injury. Inability to control airway or support ventilations with oxygen and positive pressure.

Adverse reactions/side effects Apnea, respiratory depression, bradydysrhythmia, tachydysrhythmia, dysrhythmia, cardiac arrest, salivation, prolonged muscle rigidity, rhabdomyolysis, malignant hyperthermia, increased intraocular pressure, hyperkalemia (trauma patients).

Drug interactions Oxytocin, beta blockers, and organophosphates may potentiate effects. Diazepam may reduce duration of action.

How supplied 20 mg/mL vials.

Dosage and administration *Adult:* 1–1.5 mg/kg rapid IV. Repeat once if needed. *Pediatric:* 1–1.5 mg/kg rapid IV/IO. Repeat once if needed. 2 mg/kg in infants.

Duration of action *Onset:* 1 minute. *Peak effect:* 1–3 minutes. *Duration:* 5–10 minutes.

Special considerations Pregnancy safety: Category C. If the patient is conscious, explain the effects of the drug before administration. Consider premedication with atropine, particularly in pediatric age group. Premedication with lidocaine may blunt any increase in intracranial pressure during intubation. Etomidate, diazepam, or midazolam should be used in any conscious patient before undergoing neuromuscular blockade.

Terbutaline Sulfate (Brethine)

Class Beta-2 adrenergic agonist, bronchodilator.

Mechanism of action Selective beta-2 adrenergic receptor activity resulting in relaxation of smooth muscle of the bronchial tree and peripheral vasculature with minimal cardiac effects.

Indications Bronchial asthma, reversible bronchospasm associated with exercise, chronic bronchitis, emphysema.

Contraindications Hypersensitivity, tachydysrhythmias.

Adverse reactions/side effects CNS stimulation, headache, seizure, restlessness, apprehension, wheezing, coughing, bronchospasm, bradycardia, tachycardia, ST wave changes, PVCs, PACs, chest pain.

Drug interactions Cardiovascular effects exacerbated by other sympathomimetics. MAOIs may potentiate dysrhythmias. Beta blockers may antagonize terbutaline.

How supplied 1 mg/mL vials.

Dosage and administration *Adult:* 0.25 mg SC may repeat in 15–30 minutes to maximum dose of 0.5 mg in a 4-hour period. *Pediatric:* Not recommended for children younger than 12 years of age. 0.25 mg SC may repeat in 15–30 minutes to maximum dose of 0.5 mg in a 4-hour period.

Duration of action *Onset:* 5–10 minutes. *Peak effect:* Variable. *Duration:* 1.5–4 hours.

Special considerations Pregnancy safety: Category B. Carefully monitor vital signs. Use with caution in patients with cardiovascular disease, seizure disorder, hypertension, and diabetes. Patient should receive oxygen before and during administration.

Thiamine (Betaxin)

Class Vitamin B.

Mechanism of action Combines with ATP to form thiamine pyrophosphate coenzyme, which is a necessary component for carbohydrate metabolism. The brain is extremely sensitive to thiamine deficiency.

Indications Coma of unknown origin, delirium tremens, beriberi, Wernicke encephalopathy.

Contraindications None.

Adverse reactions/side effects Anxiety, dyspnea, respiratory failure, vasodilation, hypotension, nausea, vomiting.

Drug interactions Give thiamine before glucose under all circumstances.

How supplied 100 mg/mL vials.

Dosage and administration *Adult:* 100 mg slow IV or IM. *Pediatric:* 10–25 mg slow IV or IM.

Duration of action *Onset:* Rapid. *Peak effect:* Variable. *Duration:* Depends on degree of deficiency.

Special considerations Pregnancy safety: Category A. Rapid or large IV doses may cause respiratory difficulties, hypotension, and vasodilation. Anaphylaxis reactions reported.

Tirofiban Hydrochloride (Aggrastat)

Class Glycoprotein IIb/IIIa inhibitor, platelet aggregation inhibitor.

Mechanism of action Inhibits aggregation of platelets by reversibly antagonizing fibrinogen binding to the glycoprotein IIb/IIIa receptor.

Indications Acute coronary syndrome, patients undergoing percutaneous transluminal coronary angioplasty (PTCA) or atherectomy.

Contraindications Trauma or major surgery within the past 30 days, hemorrhagic stroke, intracranial neoplasm. Arteriovenous malformation, aneurysm, or evidence of aortic dissection. Severe uncontrolled hypertension (systolic BP >180 mm Hg, diastolic BP >110 mm Hg), concomitant use of another glycoprotein IIb/IIIa inhibitor, acute pericarditis.

Adverse reactions/side effects Dizziness, pain, sweating, intracranial bleeding, CVA, bradydysrhythmia, dissecting coronary artery aneurysm, GI bleeding, severe bleeding.

Drug interactions Other medications that affect hemostasis: Thrombolytics, oral anticoagulants, aspirin and other nonsteroidal anti-inflammatory agents, dipyridamole, ticlopidine, and clopidogrel.

How supplied 50 µg/mL solution for infusion.

Dose and administration *Adult:* Loading dose: 0.4 µg/kg/min IV for 30 minutes. Infusion: 0.1 µg/kg/min, for 18 to 24 hours post angioplasty. *Pediatric:* Not recommended.

Duration of action *Onset:* A few minutes. *Peak effects:* Early peak in less than 30 minutes, infusion at a steady rate will peak in approximately 6 hours. *Duration:* Platelet function restores 4 to 8 hours after discontinued.

Special considerations Pregnancy safety: Category B. Must be administered only with an infusion pump direct from bottle with a vented IV set. Due to severe spontaneous bleeding risk, invasive procedures (eg, IV starts, injections, NG tube, or nasotracheal intubation) should be avoided.

Vasopressin (Pitressin)

Class Vasopressor

Mechanism of action Stimulation of smooth muscle receptors. Potent vasoconstrictor when given in high doses.

Indications Alternative vasopressor to the first or second dose of epinephrine in cardiac arrest, alternative to epinephrine in asystole, PEA.

Contraindications Use with caution in patients with coronary artery disease, epilepsy, or heart failure.

Adverse reactions/side effects Dizziness, headache, bronchial constriction, MI, chest pain, angina, cardiac dysrhythmia, decreased cardiac output, abdominal cramps, diarrhea, nausea, vomiting, paleness, sweating.

Drug interactions None reported.

How supplied 20 units/mL vials.

Dosage and administration *Adult:* 40 U one-time dose IV/IO to replace the first or second dose of epinephrine in cardiac arrest. 0.02–0.04 U/min continuous. *Pediatric:* 0.4–1 unit/kg IV/IO to a maximum of 40 units to replace the first or second dose of epinephrine in cardiac arrest.

Duration of action *Onset:* Immediate. *Peak effect:* Variable. *Duration:* Variable.

Special considerations Pregnancy safety: Category C. May increase peripheral vascular resistance and provoke cardiac ischemia and angina.

Vecuronium Bromide (Norcuron)

Class Neuromuscular blocker, nondepolarizing.

Mechanism of action Neuromuscular agent with intermediate duration of action that competes with acetylcholine for receptors at the motor end plate, resulting in neuromuscular blockade.

Indications Rapid-sequence intubation.

Contraindications Acute narrow-angle glaucoma, penetrating eye injuries, inability to control airway or support ventilations with oxygen and positive pressure, newborns, myasthenia gravis, hepatic or renal failure.

Adverse reactions/side effects Weakness, prolonged neuromuscular block, bronchospasm, apnea, dysrhythmias, bradycardia, tachycardia, PVCs, transient hypotension, cardiac arrest, excessive salivation.

Drug interactions Use of inhalation anesthetics will enhance neuromuscular blockade.

How supplied 10- and 20-mg powder (requires reconstitution before administration).

Dosage and administration *Adult:* 0.1–0.2 mg/kg IV push. Maintenance dose within 45–60 minutes: 0.8–1.2 mg/kg IV push. *Pediatric:* 0.1–0.3 mg/kg IV/IO. Maintenance dose within 20–35 minutes: 0.01–0.05 mg/kg IV/IO push.

Duration of action *Onset:* 1–3 minutes. *Peak effect:* Varies. *Duration:* 45–90 minutes.

Special Considerations Pregnancy safety: Category C. If patient is conscious, explain the effect of the medication before administration and always sedate the patient before using vecuronium. Intubation and ventilatory support must be readily available. Monitor the patient carefully. Vecuronium has no effect on consciousness or pain. Will not stop neuronal seizure activity. Pulse rate and cardiac output are increased. Decrease doses for patients with renal disease.

■ Verapamil Hydrochloride (Isoptin, Calan)

Class Calcium channel blocker.

Mechanism of action Slow calcium channel blocker that selectively blocks the transmembrane influx of calcium ions into arterial smooth muscles and myocardial cells. Prolongs AV nodal refractory period. Reduces systemic vascular resistance and selective vasodilation of peripheral arteries. Dilates coronary arteries and arterioles.

Indications Paroxysmal supraventricular tachycardia, atrial flutter, and atrial fibrillation with rapid ventricular response, re-entry SVT.

Contraindications Wolff-Parkinson-White syndrome, Lown-Ganong-Levine syndrome, second- or third-degree AV block (without functioning pacemaker), sick sinus syndrome (without functioning pacemaker), hypotension, cardiogenic shock, severe left ventricular dysfunction (ejection fraction less than 30%), wide-complex tachycardias, children younger than 12 months of age, atrial fibrillation.

Adverse reactions/side effects Dizziness, headache, pulmonary edema, sinus arrest, asystole, AV blocks, bradycardia, hypotension, nausea, vomiting, constipation.

Drug interactions Increases the serum concentration of digoxin. Beta-adrenergic blockers may have additive negative

inotropic and chronotropic effects. Antihypertensives may potentiate hypotensive effects.

How supplied 2.5 mg/mL vials.

Dosage and administration *Adult:* 2.5–5 mg IV bolus over 2 minutes (3 minutes in elderly). Repeat dose of 5–10 mg may be given every 15–30 minutes to maximum of 20 mg. *Pediatric:* 0.01–0.02 mg/kg/dose IV, IO push over 2 minutes. Repeat dose in 30 minutes if not effective. *Note:* Not to be used in children younger than 12 months of age.

Duration of action *Onset:* 2–5 minutes. *Peak effect:* Variable. *Duration:* 30–60 minutes.

Special considerations Pregnancy safety: Category C. Closely monitor patient's vital signs. Be prepared to resuscitate. Atrioventricular block or asystole may occur because of slowed atrioventricular conduction.

■ IV Solutions (Colloids and Crystalloids)

Colloids expand plasma volume by colloidal osmotic pressure. Colloids are most often used in hypovolemic shock states. Crystalloids are substances in solution that can diffuse through the intravascular compartment. Crystalloid solutions are used for electrolyte replacement, a route for medication, and short-term intravascular volume expansion.

■ Plasma Protein Fraction (Plasmanate)

Class Natural colloid.

Mechanism of action Plasmanate is a protein-containing colloid that remains in the intravascular compartment. It increases intravascular volume by attracting water from other fluid compartments by virtue of its colloid osmotic pressure.

Indications Hypovolemic shock, especially burn shock; hypoproteinemia (low-protein states)

Contraindications There are no major contraindications to plasma protein fraction when used in the treatment of life-threatening hypovolemic states.

Adverse reactions/side effects Chills, fever, urticaria (hives), nausea, and vomiting have all been reported with plasma protein fraction use.

Drug interactions Solutions should not be mixed with or administered through the same administration sets as other intravenous fluids.

How supplied Plasma protein fraction is supplied in 250- and 500-mL bottles of a 5% solution. An administration set is usually attached.

Dosage and administration The plasma protein fraction infusion rate should be titrated according to the patient's hemodynamic response. In the management of shock secondary to burns, the physician's orders regarding the rate of administration must be closely followed. Standard formulas for IV fluid administration have been developed. The medical control physician will use these in judging the correct rate of intravenous administration.

Duration of action 24–36 hours.

Special considerations Do not use if the solution is cloudy or if you see sedimentation.

Dextran

Class Artificial colloid.

Mechanism of action Dextran is a sugar-containing colloid used as an intravascular volume expander. It remains in the intravascular compartment for approximately 12 hours. It increases intravascular volume by attracting water from other fluid compartments by virtue of its colloid osmotic pressure.

Indications Hypovolemic shock.

Contraindications Dextran should not be administered to patients who have a known hypersensitivity to the drug. It should not be administered to patients with congestive heart failure, renal failure, or known bleeding disorders.

Adverse reactions/side effects Rash, itching, dyspnea, chest tightness, and mild hypotension have all been reported with dextran use. The incidence of these side effects is, however, very low, and reactions are generally mild. Increased bleeding time has also been reported with dextran use due to its interference with platelet function.

Drug interactions Dextran should not be administered to patients who are receiving anticoagulants because it significantly retards blood clotting.

How supplied Dextran 40 and Dextran 70 are supplied in 250- and 500-mL bottles.

Dosage and administration The dosage of dextran is titrated according to the patient's physiologic response.

Duration of action 8–12 hours.

Special considerations In the management of burn shock, it is especially important to follow standard fluid resuscitation regimens to prevent possible circulatory overload.

Hetastarch (Hespan)

Class Artificial colloid.

Mechanism of action Hetastarch is a starch-containing colloid used as an intravascular volume expander. Following administration, the plasma volume is expanded slightly in excess of the volume of hetastarch administered. This effect has been observed for up to 24 to 36 hours. Hetastarch increases intravascular volume by virtue of its colloid osmotic pressure.

Indications Hypovolemic shock, especially burn shock; septic shock.

Contraindications There are no major contraindications to hetastarch when used in the management of life-threatening hypovolemic states.

Adverse reactions/side effects Nausea, vomiting, mild febrile reactions, chills, itching, and urticaria (hives) have been reported with hetastarch administration. Severe anaphylactic reactions have been rarely reported.

Drug interactions Hetastarch should not be administered to patients who are receiving anticoagulants.

How supplied Sterile 6% hetastarch in 0.9% sodium chloride is supplied in 500-mL bottles.

Dosage and administration The dosage of hetastarch is titrated according to the patient's physiologic response.

Duration of action 24–36 hours.

Special considerations Pregnancy safety: Category C. Patients allergic to corn may be allergic to hetastarch.

Lactated Ringer's (Hartmann's Solution)

Class Isotonic crystalloid solution.

Mechanism of action Lactated Ringer's replaces water and electrolytes.

Indications Hypovolemic shock; keep open IV.

Contraindications Lactated Ringer's should not be used in patients with congestive heart failure or renal failure.

Adverse reactions/side effects Rare in therapeutic dosages.

Drug interactions Few in the emergency setting.

How supplied Lactated Ringer's is supplied in 250-, 500-, and 1,000-mL bags, IV infusion.

Dosage and administration Hypovolemic shock; titrate according to patient's physiologic response.

Duration of action Short-term therapy.

Special considerations None.

5% Dextrose in Water (D_5W)

Class Hypotonic dextrose-containing solution.

Mechanism of action D_5W provides nutrients in the form of dextrose as well as free water.

Indications IV access for emergency drugs; for dilution of concentrated drugs for intravenous infusion.

Contraindications D_5W should not be used as a fluid replacement for hypovolemic states.

Adverse reactions/side effects Rare in therapeutic dosages.

Drug interactions D_5W should not be used with phenytoin (Dilantin) or amrinone (Inocor).

How supplied D_5W is supplied in bags of 50, 100, 150, 250, 500, and 1,000 mL.

Dosage and administration D_5W is usually administered through a minidrip (60 drops/mL) set at a rate of "to keep open" (TKO).

Duration of action Short-term therapy.

Special considerations None.

10% Dextrose in Water ($D_{10}W$)

Class Hypertonic dextrose-containing solution.

Mechanism of action $D_{10}W$ provides nutrients in the form of dextrose as well as free water.

Indications Neonatal resuscitation, hypoglycemia.

Contraindications D$_{10}$W should not be used as a fluid replacement for hypovolemic states.

Adverse reactions/side effects Rare in therapeutic dosages.

Drug interactions Should not be used with phenytoin (Dilantin) or amrinone (Inocor).

How supplied D$_{10}$W is supplied in bags of 50, 100, 150, 250, 500, and 1,000 mL.

Dosage and administration The administration rate of D$_{10}$W will usually be dependent on the patient's condition.

Duration of action Short-term therapy.

Special considerations None.

0.9% Sodium Chloride (normal saline)

Class Isotonic crystalloid solution.

Mechanism of action Normal saline replaces water and electrolytes.

Indications Heat-related problems (heat exhaustion, heat stroke), freshwater drowning, hypovolemia, diabetic ketoacidosis, keep open IV.

Contraindications The use of 0.9% sodium chloride should not be considered in patients with congestive heart failure because circulatory overload can be easily induced.

Adverse reactions Rare in therapeutic dosages.

Drug interactions Few in the emergency setting.

How supplied Normal saline is supplied in 250-, 500-, and 1,000-mL bags. Sterile normal saline for irrigation should not be confused with that designed for intravenous administration.

Dosage and administration The specific situation being treated will dictate the rate in which normal saline will be administered. In severe heatstroke, diabetic ketoacidosis, and freshwater drowning, it is likely that you will be called on to administer the fluid quite rapidly. In other cases, it is advisable to administer the fluid at a moderate rate (for example, 100 mL/h).

Duration of action Short-term therapy.

Special considerations None.

0.45% Sodium Chloride (½ normal saline)

Class Hypotonic crystalloid solution.

Mechanism of action One half normal saline replaces free water and electrolytes.

Indications Patients with diminished renal or cardiovascular function for which rapid rehydration is not indicated.

Contraindications Cases in which rapid rehydration is indicated.

Adverse reactions/side effects Rare in therapeutic dosages.

Drug interactions Few in the emergency setting.

How supplied One half normal saline is supplied in 250-, 500-, and 1,000-mL bags.

Dosage and administration The specific situation and patient condition will dictate the rate at which one half normal saline will be administered.

Duration of action Short-term therapy.

Special considerations None.

5% Dextrose in 0.45% Sodium Chloride (D$_5$½NS)

Class Hypertonic dextrose-containing crystalloid solution.

Mechanism of action D$_5$½NS replaces free water and electrolytes and provides nutrients in the form of dextrose.

Indications Heat exhaustion, diabetic disorders; for use as a way to keep open solution in patients with impaired renal or cardiovascular function.

Contraindications D$_5$½NS should not be used when rapid fluid resuscitation is indicated.

Adverse reactions/side effects Rare in therapeutic dosages.

Drug interactions D$_5$½NS should not be used with phenytoin (Dilantin) or amrinone (Inocor).

How supplied D$_5$½NS is supplied in bags containing 250, 500, and 1,000 mL of the fluid.

Dosage and administration The specific situation and patient condition will dictate the rate at which D$_5$½NS should be administered.

Duration of action Short-term therapy.

Special considerations None.

5% Dextrose in 0.9% Sodium Chloride (D$_5$NS)

Class Hypertonic dextrose-containing crystalloid solution.

Mechanism of action D$_5$NS replaces free water and electrolytes and provides nutrients in the form of dextrose.

Indications Heat-related disorders, freshwater drowning, hypovolemia, peritonitis.

Contraindications D$_5$NS should not be administered to patients with impaired cardiac or renal function.

Adverse reactions/side effects Rare in therapeutic dosages.

Drug interactions D$_5$NS should not be used with phenytoin (Dilantin) or amrinone (Inocor).

How supplied D$_5$NS is supplied in bags containing 250, 500, and 1,000 mL of the solution.

Dosage and administration The specific situation and patient condition will dictate the rate at which D$_5$NS is given.

Duration of action Short-term therapy.

Special considerations None.

■ 5% Dextrose in Lactated Ringer's (D$_5$LR)

Class Hypertonic dextrose-containing crystalloid solution.

Mechanism of action D$_5$LR replaces water and electrolytes and provides nutrients in the form of dextrose.

Indications Hypovolemic shock, hemorrhagic shock, certain cases of acidosis.

Contraindications D$_5$LR should not be administered to patients with decreased renal or cardiovascular function.

Adverse reactions/side effects Rare in therapeutic dosages.

Drug interactions D$_5$LR should not be used with phenytoin (Dilantin) or amrinone (Inocor).

How supplied D$_5$LR is supplied in bags containing 250, 500, and 1,000 mL of the fluid.

Dosage and administration In severe hypovolemic shock, D$_5$LR should be infused through a large-bore catheter (14 or 16 gauge). This infusion should be administered "wide open" until a blood pressure of 100 mm Hg is achieved. When the blood pressure is attained, the infusions should be reduced to 100 mL/h. In other cases, the specific situation and patient condition will dictate the rate of administration.

Duration of action Short-term therapy.

Special considerations None.

YOU are the Medic   SUMMARY

1. What type of seizure is this patient experiencing?

A state of continuous seizures or multiple seizures without a return to consciousness is considered status epilepticus. When a patient is experiencing this condition, it is vitally important for you to end the seizure as quickly as possible. The longer the patient seizes, the more hypoxic the patient becomes. The hypoxia will cause brain cells and other tissues to die.

2. What are some of the common causes of seizures?

Seizures can be caused by many things. Some of these causes are hypoglycemia, tumors, head injuries, epilepsy, heat-related emergencies, toxemia, and overdose. It is extremely important to know the medical history of the patient as well as the history of the current event.

3. What is the mechanism of action for phenytoin (Dilantin)?

Phenytoin (Dilantin) promotes sodium efflux from neurons, thereby stabilizing the neuron's threshold against the excitability caused by excess stimulation. Phenytoin (Dilantin) also decreases abnormal ventricular automaticity and decreases the refractory period in the myocardial conduction system.

4. Why is it important to know that the patient has not been taking her prescribed medications?

Most antiseizure medications work by building a constant level of the medication in the patient's system. The goal is to have a sufficient level of the medication to exceed the brain's seizure threshold. If patients who experience seizures have not been compliant with their medication, the level will drop and may fall below the seizure threshold.

5. What drugs are categorized as benzodiazepines and what are their indications?

Diazepam (Valium), lorazepam (Ativan), and midazolam (Versed) are all benzodiazepines, and all three medications are indicated for acute anxiety states and agitation, acute alcohol withdrawal, muscle relaxant, seizure activity, and sedation for medical procedures (eg, intubation, ventilated patients, cardioversion). They may also be helpful in acute symptomatic cocaine overdose.

6. What dose of diazepam would you administer to this patient?

The appropriate dose is 5-10 mg IV q 10-15 minutes PRN (5 mg over 5 minutes) (maximum dose: 30 mg).

7. If this patient were more than 20 weeks' pregnant, what medication would you consider?

In this instance, you would consider magnesium sulfate because of the potential for eclampsia. Magnesium sulfate reduces striated muscle contractions and blocks peripheral neuromuscular transmission by reducing acetylcholine release at the myoneural junction. It also manages seizures in toxemia of pregnancy and induces uterine relaxation.

8. If this patient were diabetic, what medication would you consider?

Dextrose 50% is recommended to correct hypoglycemia. It provides immediate, usable glucose to give insulin something to work on. Dextrose is indicated in hypoglycemia, altered level of consciousness, coma of unknown origin, seizure of unknown origin, and status epilepticus.

YOU are the Medic   SUMMARY, continued

EMS Patient Care Report (PCR)

Date: 07-24-11	Incident No.: 491	Nature of Call: Seizure		Location: 2900 Atlantic, Rm 1065	
Dispatched: 1328	En Route: 1329	At Scene: 1335	Transport: 1352	At Hospital: 1410	In Service: 1425

Patient Information

Age: 30 Sex: F Weight (in kg [lb]): 56 kg (125 lb)	Allergies: No known drug allergies Medications: Phenytoin (Dilantin) Past Medical History: Epilepsy Chief Complaint: Seizures

Vital Signs

Time: 1340	BP: 140 palp	Pulse: Rapid	Respirations: 36	Spo$_2$: Unable to obtain
Time: 1345	BP: 142/76	Pulse: 120	Respirations: 24	Spo$_2$: 97% on O$_2$
Time:	BP:	Pulse:	Respirations:	Spo$_2$:

EMS Treatment
(circle all that apply)

Oxygen @ _15_ L/min via (circle one): NC (NRM) Bag-mask device	Assisted Ventilation	Airway Adjunct:	CPR
Defibrillation	Bleeding Control	Bandaging	Splinting	Other:

Narrative

This unit dispatched to a report of seizures at the Regency Hotel Room 1065. On arrival, we find a 30-year-old woman lying supine on the bed. Pt in full-body tonic/clonic seizures. Husband on scene states the pt has been seizing the entire time from 9-1-1 activation to the current time. Husband states the pt has a history of epilepsy and has not been compliant with taking her phenytoin. Pt rolled to left lateral recumbent to assist with airway control. Suctioning applied, working around clenched teeth. O$_2$ 15 L/min via NRBM applied. IV started of normal saline and medical control contacted for orders. Order confirmed to administer 5 mg diazepam (Valium) IVP to this pt. Pt's seizure activity stopped after administration of the diazepam. Pt moved to unit for transport to university hospital. Report to Sharon RN upon arrival. **End of report**

Prep Kit

Ready for Review

- Paramedics are required to know the names, class, mechanism of action, adverse reactions and side effects, interactions, indications, contraindications, complications, routes of administration, dose, and specific administration considerations for many emergency medications and intravenous fluids.

- Individual states have the authority to include additional medications, which may be taught by your local training agency.

- Because paramedics must make quick decisions about when to administer medications, what medications to administer, and when administering certain medications would be harmful to the patient, it is critically important that they develop a solid understanding of the information in this chapter and stay up-to-date on the latest pharmacologic information.

Vital Vocabulary

<u>adverse reaction/side effect</u> Abnormal or harmful effect to an organism caused by exposure to a chemical. It is indicated by some result such as death, a change in food or water consumption, altered body and organ weights, altered enzyme levels, or visible illness.

<u>class</u> How a medication is categorized as compared to other medications. This is usually done by grouping those medications with similar characteristics, traits, or primary components.

<u>concentration</u> The amount of a medication that is present in the ampule or vial. This is usually expressed in milligrams, grams, or grains.

<u>contraindication</u> Any condition, especially any condition of disease, that renders some particular line of treatment improper or undesirable.

desired dose The quantity of a medication that is to be administered to a patient. This is usually expressed in milligrams, grams, or grains.

drug interactions Any potential effects that a medication may have when administered in conjunction or in the presence of another medication already in the patient's system, a medication delivery device, or fluid.

duration of action Three values are given: (1) onset: the estimated amount of time it will take for the medication to enter the body/system and begin to take effect, (2) peak effect: the estimated amount of time it will take for the medication to have its greatest effect on the patient/system, and (3) duration: the estimated amount of time that the medication will have any effect on the patient/system.

indication A circumstance that points to or shows the cause, pathology, treatment, or issue of an attack of disease; that which points out; that which serves as a guide or warning.

mechanism of action The way in which a medication produces the intended response.

volume The amount of a fluid that is present in the ampule or vial in which the medication is dissolved. This is usually expressed in milligrams, grams, or grains.

yield The amount of drug in 1 mL.

Assessment in Action

Your unit is dispatched to a local playground for a bee sting. The dispatcher advises you the patient is a 7-year-old boy who has a history of allergic reactions to bee stings. When you and your partner arrive on the scene, you find the patient lying on a park bench with his mother screaming at you to hurry. The patient is responsive but has pronounced difficulty breathing and has visible urticaria all over his face and chest.

1. What is the medication classification for diphenhydramine?
   A. Calcium channel blocker
   B. Antihistamine
   C. Antiemetic
   D. Antihypertensive

2. What is the trade name for methylprednisolone sodium succinate?
   A. Streptase
   B. Solu-Medrol
   C. Zofran
   D. Procardia

3. What is the mechanism of action of sympathomimetics?
   A. Blocks the parasympathetic nervous system
   B. Blocks the sympathetic nervous system
   C. Stimulates the parasympathetic nervous system
   D. Stimulates the sympathetic nervous system

4. What is the mechanism of action of beta-2 medications?
   A. Cause bronchial smooth muscle relaxation
   B. Have positive inotropic, chronotropic, and dromotropic effects
   C. Cause bronchial smooth muscle constriction
   D. Cause cholinergic reactions

5. What is the pediatric dose of epinephrine for a child who is experiencing a *mild* allergic reaction and asthma?
   A. 0.01 mg/kg (0.01 mL/kg) of a 1:1,000 solution SQ (maximum of 0.3 mL)
   B. 0.01 mg/kg (0.01 mL/kg) of a 1:10,000 solution SQ (maximum of 0.3 mL)
   C. 0.01 mg/kg (0.1 mL/kg) of a 1:10,000 solution every 3–5 minutes
   D. 0.01 mg/kg (0.1 mL/kg) of a 1:1,000 solution every 3–5 minutes

6. What do adrenergic nerve fibers release?
   A. Corticosteroids
   B. Insulin
   C. Epinephrine
   D. Acetylcholine

Additional Questions

7. Describe the five AHA classifications of recommendations.

8. List the categories of medications regulated under the federal Controlled Substance Act of 1970.

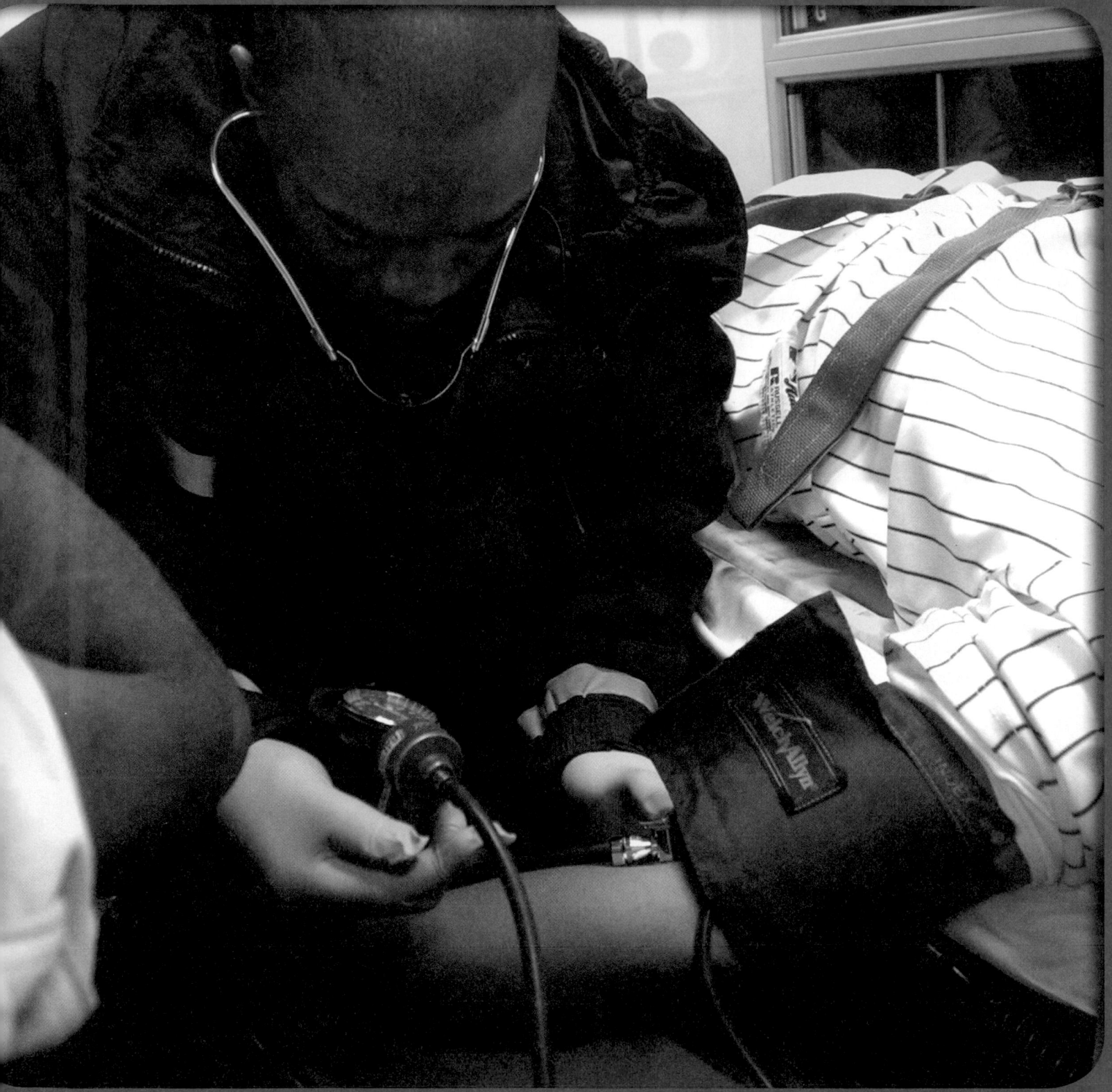

Patient Assessment

National EMS Education Standard Competencies

Assessment

Integrate scene and patient assessment findings with knowledge of epidemiology and pathophysiology to form a field impression. This includes developing a list of differential diagnoses through clinical reasoning to modify the assessment and formulate a treatment plan.

Scene Size-up

- Scene safety (pp 592-594)
- Scene management (pp 592-594)
  - Impact of the environment on patient care (pp 593, 594)
  - Addressing hazards (pp 592-594)
  - Violence (p 593)
  - Need for additional or specialized resources (pp 594-595)
  - Standard precautions (p 595)
  - Multiple patient situations (pp 593, 594)

Primary Assessment

- Primary assessment for all patient situations
  - Initial general impression (p 597)
  - Level of consciousness (p 597)
  - ABCs (pp 597-600)
  - Identifying life threats (p 600)
  - Assessment of vital functions (pp 597-600)
- Begin interventions needed to preserve life (p 600)
- Integration of treatment/procedures needed to preserve life (p 600)

History Taking

- Determining the chief complaint (pp 605, 606-607)
- Investigation of the chief complaint (pp 606-607)
- Mechanism of injury/nature of illness (pp 594, 610-612)
- Past medical history (pp 607-608)
- Associated signs and symptoms (pp 607, 612-614)
- Pertinent negatives (p 612)
- Components of the patient history (pp 606-610)
- Interviewing techniques (pp 605-606)
- How to integrate therapeutic communication techniques and adapt the line of inquiry based on findings and presentation (pp 614-624)

Secondary Assessment

- Performing a rapid full-body exam (p 626)
- Focused assessment of pain (pp 626-627)

- Assessment of vital signs (pp 627-630)
- Techniques of physical examination (pp 626-628, 631-632)
- Respiratory system (pp 648-652)
  - Presence of breath sounds (p 649)
- Cardiovascular system (pp 653-657)
- Neurologic system (pp 672-677)
- Musculoskeletal system (pp 662-667)

Techniques of physical examination for all major

- Body systems (pp 653-657, 662-677)
- Anatomic regions (pp 632-652, 657-662)

Assessment of

- Lung sounds (pp 649-652)

Monitoring Devices

- Obtaining and using information from patient monitoring devices including (but not limited to)
  - Pulse oximetry (p 630)
  - Noninvasive blood pressure (pp 630-631)
  - Blood glucose determination (pp 682-683)
  - Continuous ECG monitoring (pp 680-681)
  - 12-lead ECG interpretation (p 681)
  - Carbon dioxide monitoring (pp 681-682)
  - Basic blood chemistry (pp 682-683)

Reassessment

- How and when to reassess patients (pp 685-686)
- How and when to perform a reassessment for all patient situations (pp 685-686)

Medicine

Integrates assessment findings with principles of epidemiology and pathophysiology to formulate a field impression and implement a comprehensive treatment/disposition plan for a patient with a medical complaint.

Medical Overview

Assessment and management of a

- Medical complaint (pp 590, 597, 601, 603)

Pathophysiology, assessment, and management of medical complaints to include

- Transport mode (pp 594, 597, 601, 603)
- Destination decisions (pp 594, 597, 601, 603)

Knowledge Objectives

1. Identify the components of the patient assessment process and the most important determination made by the paramedic—whether the patient is sick versus not sick. (p 589)

2. Describe how to determine the mechanism of injury (MOI) or nature of illness (NOI) at an emergency and the importance of differentiating trauma patients from medical patients. (pp 590, 594)

3. Discuss some of the possible hazards that may be present at an emergency scene, ways to recognize them, and precautions to protect personal safety. (pp 592-594)

4. List the minimum standard precautions that should be followed and personal protective equipment that should be worn at an emergency scene, including examples of when additional precautions would be appropriate. (p 595)

5. Describe the principal goals of the primary assessment process: to identify and treat life threats and to determine whether immediate transport is required. (p 597)

6. Explain the process of forming a general impression of a patient as part of the primary assessment and the reasons why this step is critical to patient management. (p 597)

7. Describe the assessment of airway status in patients who are responsive and unresponsive, and give examples of possible signs and causes of airway obstruction in each case as well as the appropriate response by the paramedic. (pp 597-598)

8. Describe the assessment of a patient's breathing status, including the key information the paramedic must obtain during this process and the care required for patients who have adequate and inadequate breathing. (p 598)

9. Describe the assessment of a patient's circulatory status, including the different methods for obtaining a pulse and appropriate management depending on the patient's status. (pp 598-600)

10. Describe the assessment of a patient's skin color, temperature, and condition, providing examples of both normal and abnormal findings and the information this provides related to the patient's status. (pp 599-600)

11. Explain the process for determining the priority of patient care and transport at an emergency scene, and give examples of conditions that necessitate immediate transport. (pp 600, 601, 603)

12. Discuss the process of obtaining a history, including its purpose and the initial approach to a patient. (p 605)

13. Describe examples of different techniques a paramedic may use to obtain full and accurate information from patients during the history-taking process. (pp 605-606)

14. Identify the elements of the history to be obtained from responsive medical patients, from family or bystanders in the case of unresponsive medical patients, and with trauma patients. (pp 606-610)

15. Recognize which aspects of the various body systems should be covered during the history-taking process. (pp 612-614)

16. Be able to apply clinical reasoning based on the primary assessment and history-taking results to the patient's unique case. (p 614)

17. Discuss different challenges a paramedic may face when obtaining a patient history, including collection of information on sensitive topics, and strategies a paramedic may use to facilitate each situation. (pp 614-622)

18. Appreciate the unique challenges that arise with history taking with pediatric and geriatric patients. (pp 623-624)

19. Explain the purpose of performing a secondary assessment, the various assessment techniques, and equipment used in the secondary assessment. (pp 626-631)

20. Explain the importance of assessing a patient's mental status, and give examples of different methods used to assess alertness, responsiveness, and orientation. (pp 635-637)

21. Describe normal and abnormal types of lung sounds that may be heard during auscultation. (pp 649-652)

22. Explain general (systemic) conditions considered during the secondary assessment, and then give examples by body system of what the secondary assessment should include based on a patient's chief complaint. (pp 653-657, 662-677)

23. Describe the devices that are used for monitoring a patient's condition during both the secondary assessment and reassessment, including continuous and 12-lead ECG monitoring, carbon dioxide monitoring, and basic blood chemistry. (pp 630-631, 680-683)

24. Explain the importance of performing a reassessment of the patient, including reassessment of the patient's mental status and ABCs as well as re-assessment of any interventions applied and transport priority. (pp 685-686)

Skills Objectives

1. Demonstrate the techniques for assessing a patient's airway, and correctly obtain information related to respiratory rate, rhythm, quality/character of breathing, and depth of breathing. (pp 597-598)

2. Demonstrate how to assess a patient's circulation by evaluating pulses and assessing the skin color and temperature. (pp 598-600)

3. Demonstrate how to perform a rapid exam. (p 601, Skill Drill 1)

4. Demonstrate how to evaluate a patient's orientation and document his or her status correctly. (pp 635-637)

5. Demonstrate how to perform percussion as an assessment technique. (p 627, Skill Drill 2)

6. Demonstrate how to perform a full-body exam for patients with potentially serious—and potentially hidden—injuries. (p 632, Skill Drill 3)

7. Demonstrate how to obtain a patient's orthostatic vital signs to assess the extent of any internal bleeding. (p 658)

8. Demonstrate how to examine a patient's head. (p 640, Skill Drill 4)

9. Demonstrate how to perform a general eye examination. (pp 642-643, Skill Drill 5)

10. Demonstrate how to perform an eye examination with an ophthalmoscope. (p 644, Skill Drill 6)

11. Demonstrate how to perform an ear examination with an otoscope. (p 645, Skill Drill 7)

12. Demonstrate how to examine a patient's neck for injury. (p 647, Skill Drill 8)

13. Demonstrate how to examine a patient's chest, including auscultation of lung fields. (p 649, Skill Drill 9)

14. Demonstrate how to auscultate heart sounds. (pp 654-656, Skill Drill 10)

15. Demonstrate how to examine a patient's abdomen, including use of the techniques of inspection, auscultation, percussion, and palpation. (p 659, Skill Drill 11)

16. Demonstrate how to examine a patient's musculoskeletal system. (p 663, Skill Drill 12)

17. Demonstrate how to examine a patient's peripheral vascular system, including both the upper and lower extremities. (p 668, Skill Drill 13)

18. Demonstrate how to examine a patient's spine for abnormalities, including use of palpation and range-of-motion evaluation. (pp 671-672, Skill Drill 14)

19. Demonstrate how to perform a neurologic examination, including use of the COASTMAP mnemonic and the AVPU scale to test for patient responsiveness. (pp 673-674, Skill Drill 15)

20. Demonstrate how to evaluate deep tendon reflexes and score the patient's responses. (pp 676-677, Skill Drill 16)

Patient Assessment

Scene Size-up

Ensure scene safety

Determine mechanism of injury/nature of illness

Take standard precautions

Determine number of patients

Consider additional/specialized resources

Primary Assessment

Form a general impression

Assess level of consciousness

Assess the airway: identify and treat life threats

Assess breathing: identify and treat life threats

Assess circulation: identify and treat life threats

Perform rapid exam

Determine priority of patient care and transport

History Taking

Investigate the chief complaint (history of present illness)

Obtain SAMPLE history

Secondary Assessment: Medical

Assess vital signs

Use appropriate monitoring devices

Systematically assess the patient
- Full-body exam and/or focused assessment

Secondary Assessment: Trauma

Assess vital signs

Use appropriate monitoring devices

Systematically assess the patient
- Full-body exam and/or focused assessment

Reassessment

Repeat the primary assessment

Reassess vital signs

Reassess the chief complaint

Recheck interventions

Identify and treat changes in the patient's condition

Reassess patient:
- Unstable patients: every 5 minutes
- Stable patients: every 15 minutes

■ Introduction

As a paramedic, one of the most important skills you will develop is the ability to assess a patient. Assessment combines a number of steps—assessing the scene, obtaining a chief complaint and medical history from the patient, and performing a secondary assessment (physical examination). One of the most unique things about your patient assessment skills is that *there is no limit to how good they can be.* In the hospital setting, physicians and nurses are able to use additional resources like x-rays and lab work to aid in their development of a diagnosis. However, most paramedics do not have these resources available and must rely on their ability to effectively obtain an accurate patient history; perform a systematic, organized physical exam; and use diagnostic tools (ie, cardiac monitor, capnography) wisely.

To the patient, the entire assessment process should appear to be a seamless process. To the provider, it is most often a blend of questions and answers with a physical examination. What varies from patient to patient is the number and types of questions that must be asked and the extent to which the patient should be examined before a working diagnosis is reached. Never forget that the entire patient assessment process should be organized and systematic, but, at the same time, be reasonably flexible.

Aside from performing the primary assessment, which focuses on the identification and correction of any life threats to the patient, virtually all of the remaining history-gathering and secondary assessment components come with a lot of latitude as to when each is sequenced into the patient assessment process. In other words, you can perform the majority of your assessment and examination in the order that is in the best interest of patient care, *once the primary assessment and correction of life threats are completed.*

A key part of making your practice of prehospital care successful is for you to develop and cultivate your own style of assessment and an overall strategy for evaluating and providing care for the patients you will encounter in the unique and varied circumstances in the field setting. You will have to work within the parameters of the published standards of care in your system, adding your own personal touches—for example, which gear you take in on a given call or whether you like to kneel, sit, or stand while you interview the patient.

Always remember that your overall job as a paramedic is to quickly identify your patient's problem(s), set your care priorities, develop a patient care plan, and quickly and efficiently execute your plan.

■ Sick Versus Not Sick

The most important assessment skill for you to acquire, and one that comes only from much experience, is that of being able to quickly determine whether the patient is *sick* or *not sick.* This quick, early visual assessment is based on the chief complaint, respirations, pulse, mental status, and skin signs and color. For trauma patients, the mechanism of injury and obvious signs of trauma should be factored in as well. These items together reflect the overall performance of the patient's respiratory, cardiovascular, and neurologic systems and can quickly provide you with a sound medical basis for determining whether a patient is in stable or unstable condition. Abnormalities in any of these areas could indicate a life-threatening condition.

If the patient is sick, the next step is for you to determine "how sick." On one end of the sick scale is a patient with a miserable sinus infection. Is the patient sick? Yes. Is this a life-threatening event? Probably not. On the other end of the scale is a patient whose skin is a dusky gray color, who is struggling to answer your questions, and who is so short of breath that only one- or two-word bursts are possible. Is the patient sick? Yes. Is this a life-threatening event? Based on these signs and symptoms, the answer is yes.

Every time you assess a patient, you have to *qualify* whether your patient is sick or not sick, and then you must *quantify* how sick the patient is. Once this has been accomplished, you are in a position to decide what, if any, care needs to be provided at the scene versus in the ambulance, en route to the hospital.

■ Establishing the Field Impression

More often than not, you will make your <u>field impression</u> based on the patient history and the chief complaint. A field impression is a determination of what you think is the patient's current problem. Your ability to obtain quality information from patients with differing educational, cultural, and ethnic backgrounds; patients with various levels of cognitive ability; and patients impaired by alcohol or drugs is a significant challenge. In addition, you still have to ask the right questions to get the information needed to make the best decisions for your patient.

YOU *are the Medic* | **PART 1**

You are working the night shift and your unit is dispatched for a "man down" in a questionable area of town. The dispatcher informs you that he has no further information because this was from a third-party caller. Your unit is the first on the scene. You see a man lying on his left side on the sidewalk in front of an abandoned strip mall. There appears to be no one around other than the patient. Your partner turns on the scene lights and you see what appears to be blood near the patient.

1. What is your first concern for this scene?
2. How will you address this concern?

Being good at patient assessment can be equated to being a good detective. As you interview your patient, you will sift through the information you obtain, and throughout that process, you will continuously glean clues **Figure 1**. On the basis of these clues, you will ask more questions to seek information relevant to the patient's chief complaint. You may pursue one line of questioning about current medications that yields nothing important, and yet in your next line of questioning about medical history, you discover a wealth of information. Just as a veteran detective methodically collects and analyzes clues to ultimately "solve the case," so must you use a similar process to best meet your patient's needs.

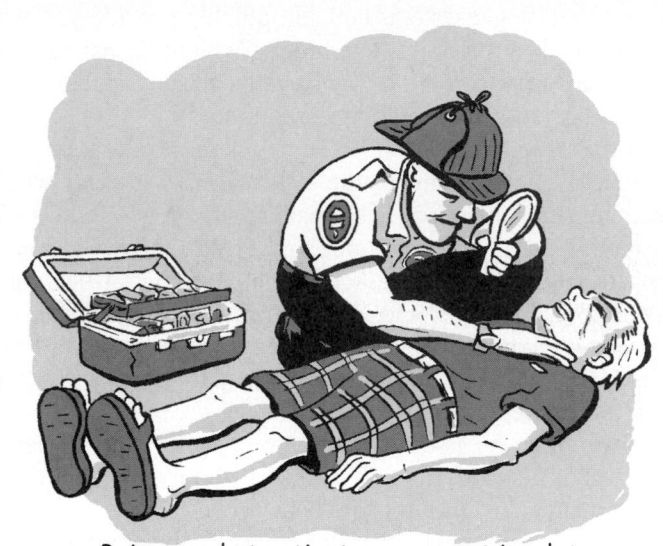

Being good at patient assessment is a lot like being a good detective

Figure 1

In time, every paramedic develops his or her own *style* of patient assessment. As you work at developing this most important job skill, it is critical that you think of patient assessment as a "fluid" process. The overall assessment process must be organized and systematic but still flexible enough to allow you to maximize your information gathering. As the patient interview unfolds, you need be able to change the sequence of your questioning as the situation or patient's condition dictates. You must know when to expand your questioning to elicit more information and when to focus your questioning to ascertain the most relevant facts.

Medical Versus Trauma

There are two basic categories of patient problems: medical and trauma. For patients with medical problems, identifying their chief complaint and sifting carefully through their medical history will allow you to provide the quality care the patients need. In contrast to medical emergencies, trauma calls are generally the result of unexpected events. When trauma is the primary culprit, the patient's medical history may have less impact on your care plan. For that reason, trauma cases require a modified approach to assessment, which is covered in more detail in the chapter, *Trauma Systems and Mechanism of Injury*.

That said, it is important to never forget that medical events can cause trauma. For example, a person with diabetes who takes insulin may forget to eat breakfast; the patient's blood glucose level then drops and, as a result, the patient falls down the steps. By comparison, traumatic events can produce medical problems. For example, a person with asthma might be involved in a motor vehicle crash, and the stress of the event then results in an asthma attack. Keep your mind open to the varied patient care scenarios you may encounter in your practice so you are mentally ready to respond to your patient's needs. Remember: any given call may be 100% trauma, 100% medical, or any combination of the two.

Patient Assessment

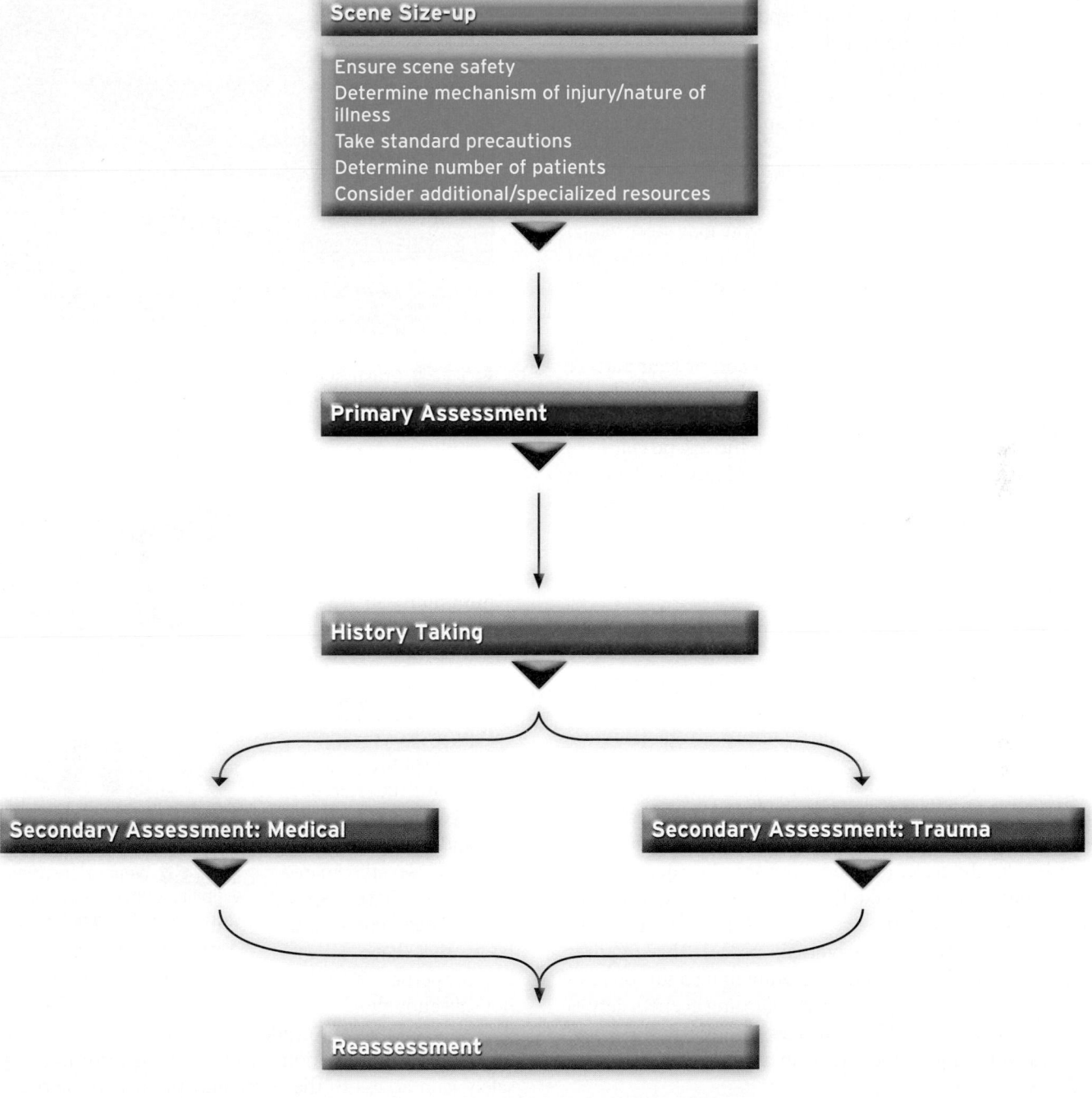

Scene Size-up

Ensure scene safety
Determine mechanism of injury/nature of illness
Take standard precautions
Determine number of patients
Consider additional/specialized resources

Primary Assessment

History Taking

Secondary Assessment: Medical

Secondary Assessment: Trauma

Reassessment

Scene Size-up

Determining the dynamics of scene management begins by assessing the scene itself, a process known as <u>scene size-up</u>. Regardless of when and where you respond to an emergency call, the first step—before any patient care is initiated—is to take a look around and evaluate the overall safety and stability of the emergency scene for any risks to you or any other member of the rescue team, the patient, and any friends, family, and bystanders. Additionally, you need to make sure that you have safe and secure access into the scene for your team and their equipment, and ready egress out of the scene as well. Lastly, you need to consider any specialty resources you may need, such as a hazmat team or police support, and get them en route and heading in your direction. Remember, the sooner you call for help, the sooner help arrives.

If you do not take a few moments to evaluate the scene and address safety issues, you may find that you and/or your partner have joined the list of casualties. An injured paramedic simply adds to the list of injured and subtracts from the list of rescue resources, making more work for the rest of the rescue team.

The success of the overall coordination of any incident can be impacted greatly by your ability to perform an adequate scene size-up. This step sets the tone for the remainder of the incident. Without this early assessment, the scene is likely to be chaotic and patient care will suffer.

Scene Safety

In the size-up of the emergency scene, your main focus is to ensure the safety and well-being of your EMS team and any other emergency responders. Ask yourself, "Is it safe for me and my team to enter this scene and to approach the patient?" To answer that question, you need to use a "wide-angle lens" thought process when you assess and evaluate the scene. If the answer to the question is "Yes, the scene is safe," then establish patient contact and proceed with your assessment. However, if the answer is "No, the scene does not appear to be safe," then do what is necessary to either make the scene safe or request additional resources to secure the scene before beginning patient care. Ensuring scene safety is a dynamic process that requires constant reassessment. Scene and environmental conditions can change rapidly; maintaining vigilance regarding scene safety is an important concept for EMS providers to understand. Some of the issues you might encounter in particular scenes are described next.

Crash and rescue scenes often include multiple risks and extrication hazards, such as unstable vehicles, moving traffic, leaking fuel, jagged metal and broken glass, fire or explosion hazards, downed power lines, and, possibly, hazardous materials **Figure 2**. In addition, just conducting EMS and rescue operations in an active roadway poses a hazard. Many motorists are more interested in viewing the incident scene as they pass, commonly referred to as "rubbernecking," rather than watching for EMS workers in the roadway. Therefore, even at incidents in which there appear to be limited dangers involved in the extrication process, the threat of another motorist disrupting

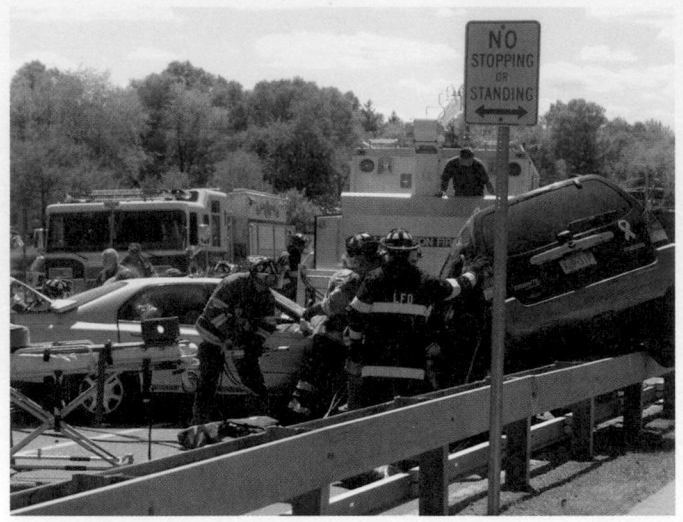

Figure 2 Crash scenes have many risks to you, your partners, and the patient.

your scene is always a possibility. When you are working next to a public roadway, wear, at a minimum, an American National Standards Institute 207 certified high-visibility public safety vest **Figure 3**. The vest provides you appropriate visibility while minimizing interference with your other clothing and equipment. In addition, several manufacturers have specialty gloves, coats, and boots that have reflective properties. It is always better to be overly safe rather than not safe enough.

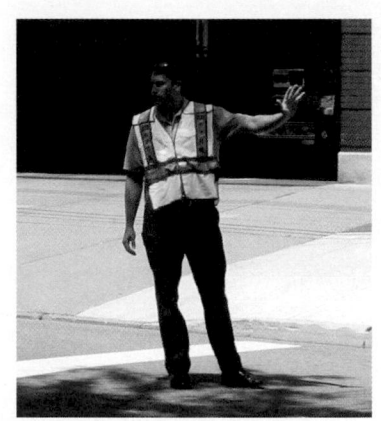

Figure 3 Wear a certified high-visibility public safety vest when working next to a public roadway.

Another major consideration is that of access and egress. When all is said and done, you and your team must be able to safely gain access to the scene and the patient, and then safely exit with the patient. If the scene cannot be stabilized to your liking, you need to consider the possibility of making a snatch and grab—ie, a quick entry to find the patient, doing the *absolute* least you have to that will allow the patient to be moved safely, and a quick exit with your patient to a more secure, stable location. In many cases, that will be the confines of your ambulance.

In all cases, you need to establish a safe perimeter to keep bystanders out of harm's way. At some point scene tape or barricades may be required, but initially, scene security is usually established simply with personnel assigned that task. Without that perimeter, allowing bystanders uncontrolled entry into the emergency scene can quickly cause chaos, greatly complicating the call, negatively impacting patient care, and increasing the likelihood of injury to patients, bystanders, and members of the EMS team.

Arriving at a scene with hazards and multiple patients can easily become overwhelming to your EMS team. Formulating a basic plan with your team and visually scanning the scene should take place before exiting the vehicle. This allows for coordination in your patient care and the opportunity to request additional resources earlier. For example, when you arrive at the scene of a motor vehicle crash, you may notice multiple patients in potentially unstable vehicles. In addition, the incident may be located at a busy intersection with multiple motor vehicles driving past the scene. At this point, it becomes apparent that resources such as the fire department (and possibly specialized rescue resources) and police will be needed at the scene. The fire department and rescue can aid with vehicle stabilization and patient extrication, and the police department can aid with traffic control. In addition, with multiple patients involved, this would be a good time to request additional ambulances if necessary.

Toxic substances are found at many scenes. From the lawn and garden chemicals found in almost every home to the countless chemicals used in industry and manufacturing, you should always be alert for the presence of toxic substances. You should also be wary of working in toxic environments—that is, where the atmosphere itself is toxic. Smoke is the by-product of incomplete combustion and can contain many toxins, pathogens, and carcinogens. In these cases, having proper body and respiratory protection is a must before entering the scene and initiating patient care Figure 4 .

Do not just think of crime scenes in the past tense because there is always the possibility that more violence may occur. Under ideal circumstances, when EMS personnel are dispatched to a potential crime scene, law enforcement personnel should enter and secure the scene first. All too frequently, however, the EMS team arrives first and unknowingly enters a crime scene. For example, dispatch might receive a call for an injured person; on arrival, the EMS team might discover that the patient has received a gunshot wound. Law enforcement personnel should be requested immediately in such cases because it is nearly impossible for you and your partner

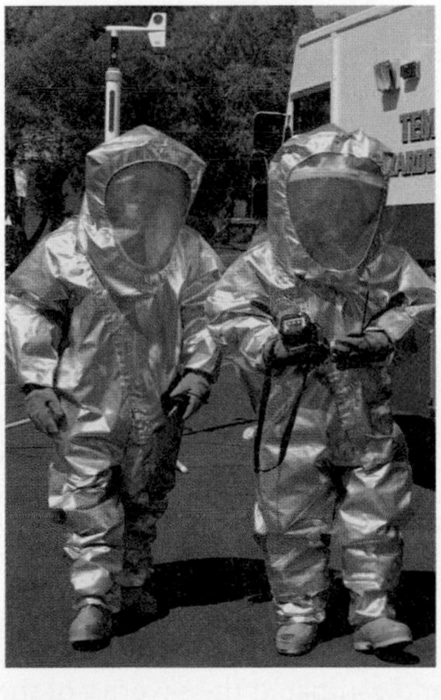

Figure 4 Scenes involving toxic substances may require specially trained rescuers with extra protective equipment.

to control the scene and care for the patient at the same time Figure 5 —and because the perpetrator could return.

When you are faced with a currently unstable scene or one that begins deteriorating and destabilizing (for example, people become progressively louder or more unruly or make aggressive gestures or threats), consider retreating to your rig until the scene is secured and deemed safe. If you believe that you can maneuver safely and remove the patient from the scene with you, do so but remember that making such an attempt is clearly a judgment call on your part. When you are dispatched to a scene in which there is a high potential for violence, you and your partner should formulate a plan of escape should the scene become unsafe. When you arrive at the scene, park your vehicle away from the scene and refrain from entering the scene until law enforcement personnel have secured the area.

In addition to the threat of potential violence from bystanders, the risk of patients becoming violent toward EMS providers is always present, particularly when cocaine or methamphetamines are involved. You should carefully and thoroughly survey the scene to provide you with clues regarding potentially violent patients. Behavioral emergencies are common and challenging calls, and they always present with the possibility of some sort of violent outbreak occurring.

With the trend toward increased manufacture and abuse of methamphetamines, EMS personnel are seeing a growing number of patients who are on the tail end of multiple sleepless days fueled by methamphetamine. These people are often paranoid, emotionally unstable, and almost always armed, making them far more a threat than an average patient with a non–drug-induced behavioral emergency. In addition, methamphetamine and crack users are at high risk of experiencing excited or agitated delirium, such that they may present in a blind rage and are almost uncontrollable. Never hesitate to call for law enforcement assistance when you are managing any patient who has the potential to become violent. Further

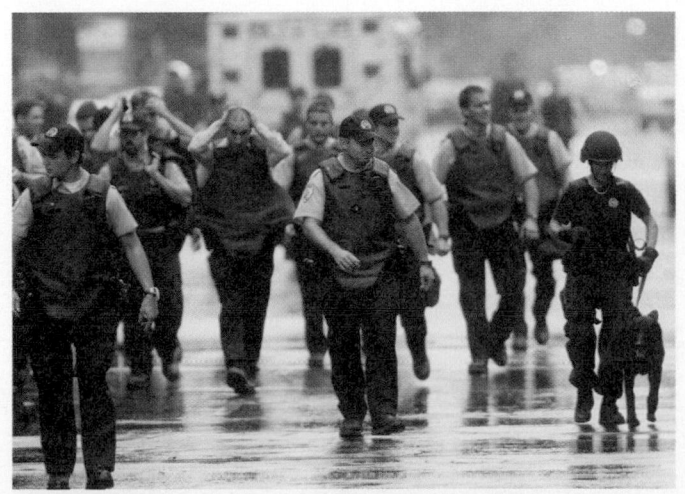

Figure 5 If the scene is unsafe, request law enforcement support, and wait in your vehicle at a safe distance.

information regarding violent patients is provided in the chapter, *Psychiatric Emergencies*.

Other risks at the scene relate to the physical environment, rather than the people who populate that environment. Unstable surfaces are everyday occurrences in the field. In some parts of the United States, snow- or ice-covered surfaces can persist for 3 or 4 months out of the year. Rain occurs most everywhere. Most of the United States has terrain issues ranging from minor hills to mountains to sandy beaches. Thus, working on unstable surfaces is an inevitable part of prehospital medicine **Figure 6**. Take the time to make all of your patient lifts and moves as safe and controlled as possible. Making a commitment to focus on this aspect of your practice will go a long way toward helping prevent a fall and a possible injury.

You should also consider the stability of the structures around you and the threat of a possible secondary collapse. If you have any doubts about the structural integrity of any scene, leave the area, establish a safe perimeter, and request additional resources to ensure a safe scene.

Whereas protecting the emergency response team is clearly a priority, so is protecting the patient and bystanders. Once safety for the EMS team has been established, the safety of the patient is the next priority. As discussed earlier, if the scene at any time becomes unsafe for EMS providers, it also becomes unsafe for the patient. The first step is to take action to minimize hazards posed to the EMS team and patient. If you are unable to minimize the hazard, you must move the patient to a safe area, as long as doing so does not place the paramedic's safety at risk. After the safety of the patient is taken into consideration, the paramedic must consider the safety of bystanders. Many bystanders attempt to help during an emergency; always remember that they are not trained to handle EMS equipment, illnesses, or injuries. An exception to that is if a bystander is a health care provider by profession; in that case, it is best to contact medical control regarding whether this person should play a role, and determine what that role should be. You should make

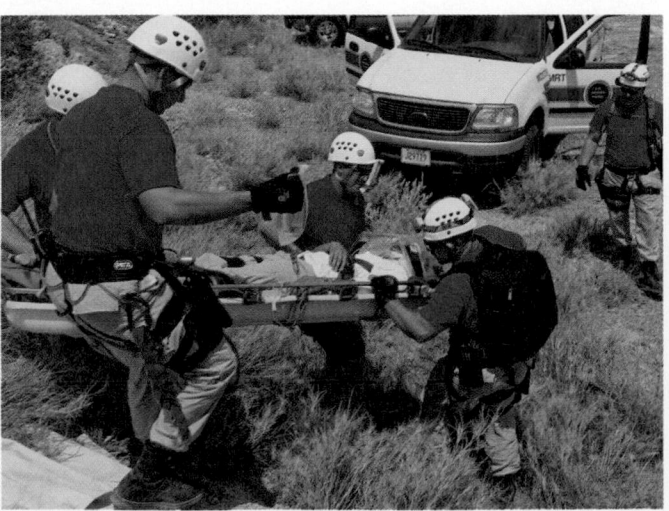

Figure 6 At times you may need a team to carry patients out of areas with unstable terrain.

every attempt to protect bystanders from becoming patients as well. This can be accomplished by establishing a perimeter or barrier around an emergency scene to prevent bystanders or the media from entering and potentially becoming patients. There are times when it is best to isolate the patient or bystanders in order to facilitate appropriate patient care or to establish a safer environment. If at any time the scene becomes unsafe for bystanders, EMS providers should have the bystanders immediately removed from the scene with the help of law enforcement.

Environmental issues can also influence scene safety and the patient care process. The longer a patient is exposed to wind and rain, the more likely it is that hypothermia will become a factor. Conversely, a hot asphalt highway is not a good place for a patient either. When the environment is unfriendly, perform the primary assessment, address life threats, and move the patient into the controlled environment of the ambulance as quickly as possible.

Mechanism of Injury or Nature of Illness

Most calls to 9-1-1 will be for a medical emergency or some form of trauma. Remember, a call for a sick man could be for a hypoglycemic patient who fell and injured himself as a result of a low blood glucose level. Similarly, a trauma patient may have crashed her car when she passed out because of an abnormal heart rhythm. Prudent paramedics keep their minds open to multiple possibilities when trying to figure out what is going on with patients. Failure to keep an open mind leads to "tunnel vision" and poor patient care.

The **mechanism of injury (MOI)** is the way in which traumatic injuries occur—the forces that act on the body to cause damage. Assessing and evaluating the MOI can help you predict the likelihood of certain injuries having occurred and estimate their severity. (The patterns of injuries sustained in traumatic events are discussed in detail in the chapter, *Trauma Systems and Mechanism of Injury*.)

On medical calls, you should quickly determine from the patient (or family, friends, or bystanders) why EMS services were requested. The **nature of illness (NOI)** is the general type of illness a patient is experiencing.

At this point of the call, if there is more than one patient or if the patient is obese (so that multiple responders will be needed to remove the person from the scene), you may need to request additional resources. On a medical call, if multiple patients are present and have similar symptoms or complaints, consider carbon monoxide poisoning (or contact with some other noxious agent) or food poisoning as prime candidates. Irrespective of the cause of the problem, the presence of multiple patients means that they must be triaged to determine which additional resources you need and how you will allocate your resources.

Likewise, when multiple patients require care at a trauma scene, you must triage all patients. Once you have identified the total number of patients and estimated the severity of their injuries, make certain that you have requested enough additional resources to support the efforts of emergency medical responders already on the scene—for example, additional EMS, fire, police, rescue, public utilities, or hazardous materials personnel. Listen for clues in the dispatch information, such as the number of patients, potential hazards, and bystanders; this information might lead you to make a request for additional resources earlier. Consider activating law enforcement early when protection of the patient or securing the scene from bystanders may be necessary. Depending on the number of patients and the amount of resources needed, activation of the incident command system (ICS) may be necessary.

While not all available resources may be needed at a scene, you should be familiar with the various specialized resources available to you. These specialized resources use specific equipment when carrying out their operations to ensure their own safety. Chemical and biological suits, specialized extrication equipment, and ascent or descent gear may be needed at a given scene. It is important to note that only specially trained responders should participate in these rescue operations.

The process of scene size-up needs to be completed in a short amount of time. Once you have digested the dispatch information, evaluated the overall scene and safety, determined the MOI or NOI, and summoned additional help, you are ready to manage patient care. By contrast, if the responding crew can manage the situation without further assistance, you should assess the need for spinal motion restriction and continue with patient care. Based on the scene size-up and MOI, EMS providers must ensure that spinal motion restriction takes place on reaching the patient. Indications for spinal motion restriction are covered further in the chapter, *Head and Spine Trauma*.

Standard Precautions

To reemphasize the point made earlier, your first and foremost concern on any call is ensuring your own safety and the safety of the other EMS team members **Figure 7**. After all, you cannot help the patient if you become injured and cannot provide care. Suppose you contract an infectious disease because you neglected to follow standard precautions; you may then miss time from work because you are sick. In the worst-case scenario, you might contract a career-ending or life-threatening disease.

Any patient with whom you come into contact should be treated as potentially infectious. Diseases such as human immunodeficiency virus (HIV) and hepatitis B and C do not discriminate: They can be found in suburban children and urban children, elderly in residential homes and elderly in nursing homes, and business professionals and homeless persons. Standard precautions were developed to ensure that health care workers would treat all patients the same way— that is, as potentially infectious.

You should wear properly sized gloves on every call. If blood or other fluids could potentially splash or spray, wear

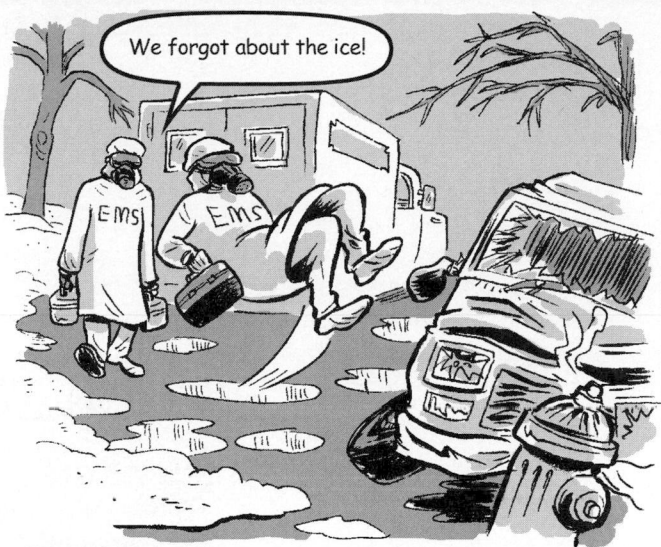

We forgot about the ice!

EMS

EMS

The size-up of the emergency scene is a critical process. . .

Figure 7

eye protection. When inhaled particles are a risk factor, wear a properly sized and fitted mask (HEPA or N95). In rare cases, a gown is also indicated. Always take the steps necessary to protect yourself on calls. When you are in doubt about the nature of the threat, it is always better to err on the side of caution and protect yourself too much rather than too little. Infection control is covered in depth in the chapter, *Workforce Safety and Wellness*. Remember to change your gloves in between patients to prevent any possible contamination and to immediately wash your hands or use an alcohol-based hand sanitizer every time you remove or change your gloves. Handwashing is the number one way to prevent the transmission of disease.

Whereas using standard precautions and protecting yourself from bodily fluids is important, you also need to consider the other hazards involved with patient care and take the necessary precautions to protect yourself. Personal protective equipment (PPE) includes clothing or specialized equipment that provides some protection to the wearer from substances that may pose a health or safety risk. It includes items like steel-toe boots to protect your feet and toes, helmets, heat-resistant outerwear, a self-contained breathing apparatus, and leather gloves. While these items will not necessarily protect you from bodily fluids, they will provide protection from the other environmental hazards present at many EMS incidents.

Patient Assessment

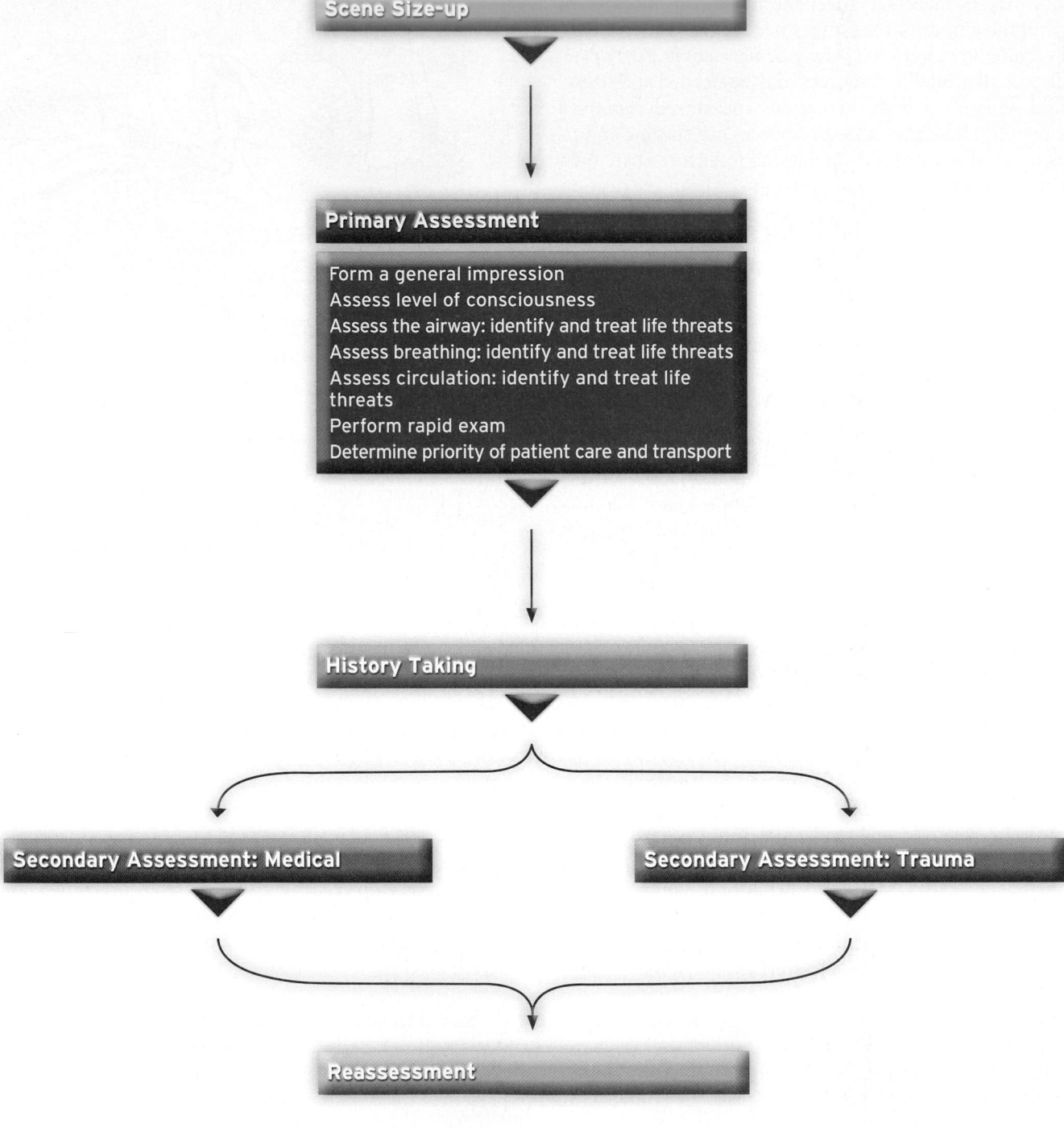

Scene Size-up

Primary Assessment

Form a general impression
Assess level of consciousness
Assess the airway: identify and treat life threats
Assess breathing: identify and treat life threats
Assess circulation: identify and treat life threats
Perform rapid exam
Determine priority of patient care and transport

History Taking

Secondary Assessment: Medical

Secondary Assessment: Trauma

Reassessment

Primary Assessment

Form a General Impression

The <u>primary assessment</u> is the most time-intensive portion of the assessment process because it focuses on the identification and management of life-threatening problems. In the first 60 to 90 seconds, as you look at, talk with, and touch your patient, you should be able to identify threats to the ABCs (airway, breathing, and circulation). More often than not, you will form the <u>general impression</u> of your patient based almost solely on the initial patient presentation and chief complaint. As additional information becomes available, always try to remain objective, and avoid an early case of tunnel vision, ie, making a field diagnosis with limited clinical information.

Each of us, without even trying or being conscious of doing so, makes dozens of observations about the appearance of another person during the first few seconds of an encounter—for example, whether the other person is sitting or standing, overweight or thin, smiling or frowning, dressed neatly or ill-kempt. When assessing a patient, you must make similar observations, but in a much more conscious, objective, and systematic manner, looking for specific clues to give you an immediate sense of the seriousness of the situation. A complaint of "I just can't catch my breath" that comes to you in one- or two-word bursts clearly points to an extremely sick patient. A patient reporting "chest pain" after being stabbed in the chest is an even more obvious example of a priority.

The focus here is trying to answer two questions. First, is my patient in stable or unstable condition? If in stable condition, might he or she potentially become unstable? These questions can be simplified by rephrasing them as a single question. Second, is my patient sick or not sick? In the case of trauma, the questions take a slightly different form: Is my patient hurt? If so, how badly hurt is he or she?

Whether the call is for a medical or trauma case, the first question is a qualification and the second is a quantification. "Is my patient sick?" has a yes or no answer, whereas "How sick is my patient?" attempts to rate the event's severity. With time and experience, you should be able to answer both questions in that 60- to 90-second window, forming your general impression.

The patient's mental status is often one of the prime indicators of how sick the patient really is. Changes in the state of consciousness may provide the first clue to an alteration in the patient's condition, so you should establish a baseline as soon as you encounter the patient. At the same time you are assessing mental status, if trauma is involved, you need to decide whether you will implement spinal motion restriction procedures.

Once the questions about the severity of the patient's complaint are answered, you can move forward with determining your priorities of care, developing a care plan, and putting the care plan into action. If the primary problem seems to be a traumatic injury, identify and evaluate the MOI. If the primary problem seems to be medical, identify the NOI. As you mentally move through this process, keep in mind that an injured patient might have a medical component to his or her problem, just as a patient with a medical emergency might have a trauma component to his or her problem.

You will also need to identify the age and sex of your patient because each of these factors may change how your patient presents. For example, an older woman having a heart attack might have no chest pain, whereas an older man with the same condition may have severe chest pain. Likewise, a girl of middle school age will often be more emotionally mature than a boy of the same age, changing how each child answers your questions and reacts to the emergency itself.

The information gleaned from the primary assessment is crucial to the overall outcome for your patient. Treat life threats as you find them, but also decide what additional care is needed, what needs to be done on scene versus en route, when to initiate transport, and which facility is most appropriate given your patient's unique needs.

The quickest and simplest way to assess the patient's mental status or level of consciousness (LOC) is to use the <u>AVPU</u> process:

A *Alert* to person, place, and day
V Responsive to *verbal* stimuli
P Responsive to *pain*
U *Unresponsive*

When you are classifying the response to stimuli, grade the patient according to the best response you can elicit. For example, a patient passed out on the street who moans in response to a loud shout from the paramedic would score a V on the AVPU scale. Response to tactile stimuli (eg, pinching the nail bed, twisting the skin of the forearm) would earn a P. No response to verbal or tactile stimuli would be classified as U.

Assess the Airway

Assessment of the patient's airway status focuses on two questions: Is the airway open and patent? If it is open, is it likely to remain so? For air to be drawn into the lungs, the airway has to be properly positioned and not obstructed (open from an anatomic perspective). If you hear sonorous (snoring respirations), think "position problem"—the sounds you are hearing are most likely from the tongue partially obstructing the airway. If you hear gurgling or bubbling sounds, think "suction"—there are most likely fluids such as blood, mucus, or vomit in the mouth or posterior pharynx.

When you are considering airway management options, move your thinking along a line from simple to complex. The easiest problem to solve is one of position. Its resolution requires no equipment and can be done quickly. The possibility of a spine injury (or lack thereof) drives the decision of which technique to use to open the airway (head tilt–chin lift or, for trauma, the jaw-thrust maneuver). In the case of obstruction, such as by food, BLS procedures to clear the obstruction require no equipment and can be done quickly.

Assessment of a patient's airway is completed in the same way regardless of the patient's age. In responsive patients of any age, talking or crying will give clues about the adequacy of the airway. For all unresponsive patients, you must establish responsiveness and assess breathing. If breathing is ineffective or absent, you must open the airway with a head tilt–chin lift (in nontrauma patients) or jaw-thrust maneuver (in trauma patients).

When you are performing the head tilt–chin lift maneuver, remember the anatomic differences in the various age groups and make sure that you do not create an airway obstruction with improper positioning of the head. Infants and young children do not have the developed tracheal rings that provide support for this structure in adults, which means their trachea is easily collapsed or occluded when the head position changes.

Suctioning takes longer (because of the need to set up and use the equipment) and is a more complicated procedure than positioning. If you suction the patient for too long, you may create new problems—hypoxia and bradycardia secondary to vagal stimulation.

If a mechanical means is required to keep the airway open and patent, you must choose an airway adjunct. If you opt to place an oropharyngeal or nasopharyngeal airway, you must retrieve the equipment, choose the right size for the specific patient, and then place the airway. This procedure takes considerable time.

If you determine that the patient cannot maintain his or her airway and you cannot maintain it by any other means, you need to use a more invasive technique, such as endotracheal intubation. This invasive procedure involves several pieces of equipment: a laryngoscope handle, a laryngoscope blade, a properly sized endotracheal tube, a syringe, a stylet, an oropharyngeal airway, a waveform end-tidal carbon dioxide capnography device, a 10-mL syringe, a bag-mask device, and a method to secure the tube once it is placed. Obviously, gathering the equipment, preparing the patient, and performing the intubation procedure are more time intensive than the previously mentioned interventions.

Other advanced airway management options include use of a multilumen airway (Combitube), King LT airway, laryngeal mask airway, or surgical airway (discussed in the chapter, *Airway Management and Ventilation*).

Assess Breathing

As with the assessment of the airway, the assessment of breathing likewise focuses on two questions: First, is the patient breathing? If not, then you have to breathe for the patient. Second, if the patient is breathing, is breathing adequate?

As discussed in detail in the chapter, *Airway Management and Ventilation*, the minute volume equals the respiratory rate multiplied by the tidal volume inspired with each breath. For example, a patient breathing slowly and deeply at 10 breaths/min and 500 mL/breath has a minute volume of 5,000 mL. By comparison, a patient breathing faster and shallower at a rate of 24 breaths/min and 200 mL/breath would have a minute volume of 4,800 mL. On a per-minute basis, the volumes of the two patients are virtually identical, even though the second patient is breathing more than twice as fast as the first patient. Always keep in mind that the amount of air actually moved in and out of the lungs each minute is the best measure of breathing adequacy.

Besides the assessment of tidal volume, note the patient's breathing rate, the work of breathing (accessory muscle use, retractions, effort of breathing), breath sounds, skin color, and LOC or mental status as part of the breathing assessment. As a general rule, a breathing rate of greater than 24 breaths/min is considered too fast. Likewise, a breathing rate of 8 breaths/min is considered too slow. In both cases, though more so with the patient breathing at 8 breaths/min versus 24 breaths/min, prompt treatment needs to be initiated.

The techniques used to assess a patient's breathing status consist of assessing for chest rise and fall, noting symmetry of the chest wall and the depth of respirations. Assess for breath sounds by using your sense of hearing or by auscultation with a stethoscope. Finally, assess for air movement by placing your cheek or the palm of your hand near the patient's mouth.

Assess Circulation

Assessing the pulse gives a rapid check of the patient's cardiovascular status and provides information about the rate, strength, and regularity of the heartbeat. In adults and children, the pulse is best palpated over the radial artery (in responsive patients) and the carotid artery (in unresponsive patients) by using the tips of your index and middle fingers. If a pulse cannot be found, begin chest compressions. In responsive or unresponsive infants, palpate the pulse over the brachial artery. First measure the pulse rate by counting the number of beats during 15 seconds; then multiply by 4. If the pulse is irregular or slow, it is best to count for a full minute. If for some reason you are unable to palpate a radial pulse, reassess for a pulse using the carotid artery. The normal pulse rate for adults is between 60 and 100 beats/min, though well-conditioned people may have resting rates in the 40s, whereby people who are out of condition might have a resting heart rate of 112 beats/min. In general, a heart rate of less than 60 beats/min is considered slow and is referred to as bradycardia. Rates of higher than 100 beats/min are considered fast and are referred to as tachycardia.

As you count the pulse rate, note the force of the pulse. A normal pulse feels "full," as if a strong wave has passed beneath your fingertips. With severe vasoconstriction or in the case of hypotension with a fast pulse, the pulse may feel weak or "thready, meaning it is just tapping along." By comparison, a patient who is hypertensive will produce a pulse that is more forceful than usual—a "bounding" pulse.

Finally, note the rhythm of the pulse. A normal rhythm is regular, like the ticking of a clock. If some beats come early or late or are skipped, the pulse is considered irregular. Although many cardiac dysrhythmias are not life threatening, in the case of heart blocks, an irregular pulse can indicate a serious condition. As such, consider all patients with an irregular pulse to be at risk of deterioration until proven otherwise.

Report your findings by describing the rate, force, and rhythm of the pulse. For example, state that "The patient's pulse was 72, full, and regular," or "The pulse was 138, thready, and regular."

Once the pulse location, quality, and rate have been assessed, a quick overall visual inspection of the skin is necessary to assess for any active bleeding that needs to be addressed. If a source of bleeding is found, every effort should be made to control it.

Capillary refill is evaluated to assess the ability of the circulatory system to restore blood to the capillary system. When evaluated in an uninjured limb, capillary refill time may provide an indication of the patient's level of perfusion. Capillary refill, however, can be affected by the patient's body temperature, position, preexisting medical conditions, and medication. Other conditions not related to the body's circulation may also slow capillary refill. These conditions include, but are not limited to, the patient's age, exposure to a cold environment, frozen tissue (frostbite), and vasoconstriction. Injuries to bones and muscles of the extremities may cause local circulatory compromise, resulting in hypoperfusion.

Assessment of capillary refill is most often used in pediatric patients. To test capillary refill, place your thumb on the patient's finger and gently compress **Figure 8A**. Blood will be forced from the capillaries in the nail bed. Remove the pressure applied against the tip of the patient's finger. The nail bed will remain blanched for a brief period. As the underlying capillaries refill with blood, the nail bed will be restored to its normal pink color.

Capillary refill should be prompt. With adequate perfusion, the color in the nail bed should be restored within 2 seconds, or about the time it takes to say "capillary refill" at a normal rate of speech **Figure 8B**. You should suspect poor peripheral circulation when the capillary refill takes more than 2 seconds or the nail bed remains blanched. It is important to note that capillary refill is a more accurate test of perfusion in pediatric patients than in adults. With the underlying comorbidities found in adult patients, capillary refill time can be a less reliable indicator of perfusion.

A bluish nail bed may indicate that the capillaries are refilling with blood drawn from the veins rather than with oxygenated blood from the arteries, making the test invalid. You should also consider the capillary refill test invalid if the patient is in or has been exposed to a cold environment or if the patient is older. In both situations, delayed capillary refill may be normal.

To assess capillary refill in older infants and children younger than 6 years, press the skin or nail bed and determine how long it takes for the color to return. In newborns and young infants, press the forehead, chin, or sternum to determine capillary refill time. As with adults, normal capillary refill takes 2 seconds or less. However, it is a much more reliable indicator of cardiovascular status in children than it is in adults and should be recorded for all your pediatric patients.

As part of this phase of the primary assessment, assess the patient's skin for color, temperature, and moisture. Collectively, these criteria provide insight into the patient's overall

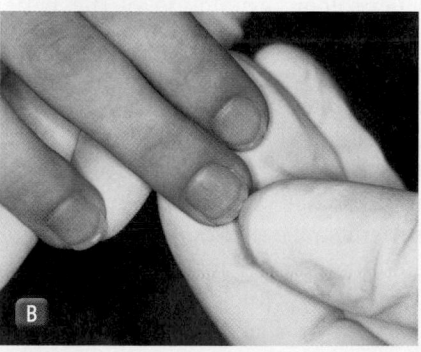

Figure 8 **A.** To test capillary refill, gently compress the fingertip until it blanches. **B.** Release the fingertip, and count until it returns to its normal pink color.

perfusion. Use the back of your hand to assess the warmth and moisture of the patient's skin because it tends be more sensitive than your palm **Figure 9**.

The color of the skin **Table 1**, especially in light-skinned patients, reflects the status of the circulation immediately underlying the skin, including the oxygen saturation of the blood. In people of color, changes may not be readily evident in the skin but may be assessed by examining the mucous membranes (such as the lips or conjunctivae). When the blood vessels supplying the skin are fully dilated, the skin becomes warm and pink. When the blood vessels supplying the skin constrict or the cardiac output drops, the skin becomes pale or mottled and cool. If the patient does not get enough oxygen—for example, in a narcotic overdose in which the patient is breathing four times per minute—the blood will desaturate as the oxygen level drops; the skin will then turn a dusky gray or blue (cyanosis). Pallor occurs if arterial blood flow ceases to part of the body, as in the case of a blood clot or massive bleeding. Hypothermia will also result in pallor as the body shunts blood to the core and away from the extremities.

Skin temperature rises as peripheral blood vessels dilate; it falls as blood vessels constrict. Fever and high environmental

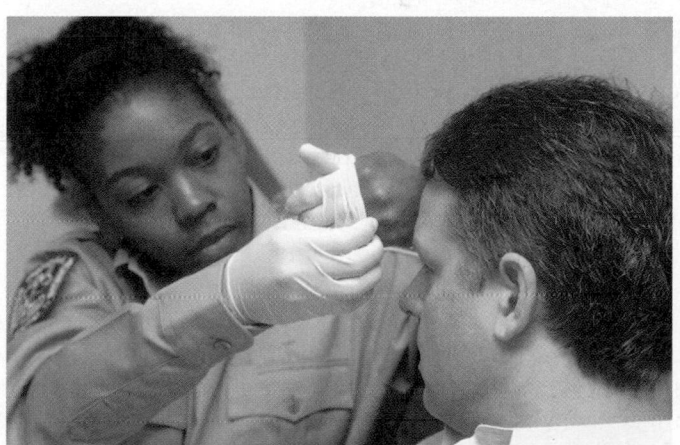

Figure 9 Assessing the skin condition. Use the back of the hand to assess the temperature and moisture of the skin.

Table 1 **Inspection of the Skin**

Skin Color	Possible Cause
Red	Fever Hypertension Allergic reactions Carbon monoxide poisoning (late sign)
White (pallor)	Excessive blood loss Fright
Blue (cyanosis)	Hypoxemia, oxygen desaturation
Mottled	Cardiovascular embarrassment (as in shock), disseminated intravascular coagulopathy

temperatures usually stimulate vasodilation, whereas shock elicits vasoconstriction. Normal skin is moderately warm and dry. The dryness or moisture of the skin is largely determined by the sympathetic nervous system. Stimulation of the sympathetic nervous system, as in shock or any other severe stress or pain, causes sweating. Depression of the sympathetic nervous system, as in an injury to the thoracic or lumbar spine, can cause the skin in the affected area to become abnormally dry and cool **Table 2**.

Restoring Circulation

If a patient has inadequate circulation, you must take immediate action to restore or improve circulation, control severe bleeding, and improve oxygen delivery to the tissues. The apparent absence of a palpable pulse in a responsive patient is indicative of a low cardiac output state—not cardiac arrest. However, if you cannot feel a pulse in an unresponsive adult, you should begin CPR if an automated external defibrillator (AED) or manual defibrillator is not readily available. Once an AED or manual defibrillator is available, immediately assess the need for defibrillation. Remember to follow standard precautions, which may include use of a barrier device for ventilation, gloves, and protective eyewear. Performing CPR and using an AED on a patient who has no pulse and is unresponsive is discussed in the chapter, *Cardiovascular Emergencies*.

Although the AED is not indicated for patients with traumatic cardiac arrest or for patients younger than 1 year, you must evaluate the cardiac rhythm of any patient in cardiac arrest with a manual cardiac monitor/defibrillator, trauma and age notwithstanding. Identifying the patient's cardiac rhythm will enable you to administer the most appropriate medication therapy. Although patients with traumatic cardiac arrest will likely require intravenous fluid therapy for blood loss, certain medications will be needed to treat the cardiac arrest itself.

Continued impaired circulation is devastating to the body's cells because it deprives the cells of vital oxygen, which is necessary for cell function. CPR and bleeding control are intended to maintain circulation. Oxygen delivery is improved through the administration of 100% supplemental oxygen. Any patient with impaired circulation should receive high-flow oxygen via a nonrebreathing mask or assisted ventilation to improve oxygen delivery at the cellular level.

Assess and Control External Bleeding

Perform a __rapid exam__ of the patient to identify any major external bleeding. In some cases, blood loss can be very rapid and can quickly result in shock or even death. Therefore, this step demands your immediate attention. Signs of blood loss include active bleeding from wounds and/or evidence of bleeding such as blood on the clothes or near the patient. Serious bleeding from a large vein may be characterized by steady blood flow. Bleeding from an artery is characterized by a spurting flow of blood. When you evaluate an unresponsive patient, do a sweep for blood quickly and lightly by running your gloved hands from head to toe, pausing periodically to see if your gloves are bloody.

Immediately control all life-threatening external bleeding. More information about controlling bleeding and applying a tourniquet is found in the chapter, *Bleeding*.

Identify and Treat Life Threats

Many conditions present an immediate threat to life, and one of your key roles is to determine if a life threat is present and, if so, to quickly address it. In many situations, there is a process the body takes when reacting to a life threat.

The first observation that you will most likely make is that there will be a loss of meaningful communication between you and the patient. A dying person becomes less aware of his or her surroundings and stops making attempts to communicate. After a variable period, loss of consciousness occurs. The patient becomes totally unresponsive to external stimuli. The muscles become slack, among them the muscles of the jaw, thus permitting the tongue to sag against the posterior part of the throat. This in turn leads very quickly to airway obstruction. Air can no longer enter the lungs, and within a few minutes the patient stops breathing. The heart cannot continue to function without oxygen, and it stops beating. Within a few minutes, a number of brain cells begin to die, leading to irreversible brain damage. There are only a few conditions that cause sudden death: airway obstruction, respiratory arrest, cardiac arrest, and severe bleeding. Often these conditions are reversible, but to reverse them, you have to be able to recognize them quickly and take immediate steps to correct them. This is the purpose of the primary assessment.

Assess the Patient for Disability
Perform a Neurologic Evaluation

Once you have examined the patient's airway, breathing, and circulation and addressed any life-threatening issues, you should perform a brief neurologic evaluation of the patient. Assess the patient for any gross neurologic deficits. This can be easily accomplished by having the patient carefully move all extremities to assess for any motor deficits. During this exam, assess for motor strength and weakness bilaterally by adding resistance to each extremity and asking the patient to move the extremity against the resistance of your hands. Assess grip strength by having the patient squeeze two of your fingers; this is done bilaterally and simultaneously to assess for any unilateral neurologic deficits. Finally, quickly assess for any loss of sensation by using a blunt or sharp object and touching the distal portions of the extremities to assess for any gross sensory loss.

Be Mindful of Exposure Concerns

When you are performing a physical exam on any patient, you need to visually inspect each area being examined to make an accurate and thorough assessment of the patient. Whereas not

Table 2 Palpation of the Skin	
Skin Condition	**Possible Cause**
Hot, dry	Excessive body heat (heatstroke)
Hot, wet	Reaction to increased internal or external temperature
Cool, dry	Exposure to cold
Cool, wet	Shock

every patient needs to be completely exposed for appropriate assessment to occur, it is very important to keep in mind that you cannot assess what you cannot see. Therefore, proper exposure of each area being examined is essential to the physical exam process.

Perform a Rapid Exam

The rapid exam is a quick and thorough palpation of the body. You will need to take 60 to 90 seconds and perform a rapid exam of the patient's body to identify injuries that must be managed and/or protected immediately. This is an abbreviated exam as opposed to the more focused physical examination that will be performed during the secondary assessment. The rapid exam is used to identify injuries that must be managed and/or protected before and during packaging and loading the patient for transport.

An example of how to perform a rapid exam on a patient who is ambulatory after a motor vehicle crash follows:

1. Face the patient and observe for any asymmetry (face, shoulder droop, foot rotation) or any obvious defects to the head, chest, abdomen, or extremities. Look for work of breathing.
2. Start with the scalp, and palpate the entire surface of the skull, then down to C7 of the cervical spine, while asking "Does anything on your head or neck hurt?"
3. Squeeze and roll the shoulder girdles, compress the sternum for stability while asking, "Did any of that hurt? Does it hurt to breathe?"
4. Gently palpate the abdomen, and gently rock the pelvis while asking, "Does anything in your belly or your hips hurt?"
5. Circumferentially grasp each arm at the shoulder girdle and slide your hands down to the wrist. Palpate the legs from the thighs to the ankle, while asking, "Does anything on your arms or legs hurt?"
6. Ask, "Can you gently wiggle your fingers and toes? Do they feel basically the same, equal from side to side?"
7. Ask, "Do you feel like you could be bleeding from anywhere?"

The physical examination you perform is based on the needs of your patient. The following are guidelines on how and what to assess during a physical examination:

- **Inspection.** Inspection is simply looking at your patient for abnormalities and asymmetry. This is done by looking for anything that may indicate a problem. For example, swelling in a lower extremity may indicate an acute injury or a chronic illness.
- **Palpation.** Palpation is the process of touching or feeling the patient for abnormalities, such as swelling or structures that are anatomically out of place, ie, a dislocated elbow. At times palpation is gentle, and at other times it is firmer and will help you to identify where the patient has pain. Your fingertips are best suited for detecting texture and consistency, while the back of your hand is best suited for noting temperature.
- **Auscultation.** Auscultation is the process of listening to sounds the body makes by using a stethoscope. For example, when you are measuring a patient's blood pressure,

you listen to the flow of blood against the brachial artery with the head of the stethoscope. This is auscultation of a blood pressure.

The mnemonic **DCAP-BTLS** will help remind you what to look for any time you are inspecting and palpating various body regions. Each area of the body is evaluated for the following:

- Deformities
- Contusions
- Abrasions
- Punctures/penetrations/paradoxical movement
- Burns
- Tenderness
- Lacerations
- Swelling

To perform a rapid exam of the patient, follow the steps in **Skill Drill 1**. Remember, this should take no longer than 60 to 90 seconds!

Skill Drill   1

1. Assess the head, looking and feeling for DCAP-BTLS and **crepitus** (a grating or grinding sensation or sound made when two pieces of broken bone are rubbed together) **Step 1**.
2. Assess the neck, looking and feeling for DCAP-BTLS, jugular venous distention, tracheal deviation, and crepitus **Step 2**. In trauma patients, you should now apply a cervical spinal immobilization device **Step 3**. It is particularly important to assess the neck before covering it with a cervical collar.
3. Assess the chest, looking and feeling for DCAP-BTLS, paradoxical motion, and crepitus. You should also listen to breath sounds on both sides of the patient's chest **Step 4**.
4. Assess the abdomen, looking and feeling for DCAP-BTLS, rigidity (firm or soft), and distention **Step 5**.
5. Assess the pelvis, looking for DCAP-BTLS. If there is no pain, gently compress the pelvis downward and inward to look for tenderness and instability **Step 6**.
6. Assess all four extremities, looking and feeling for DCAP-BTLS. Also assess bilaterally for distal pulses and the motor and sensory function **Step 7**.
7. Assess the back and buttocks, looking and feeling for DCAP-BTLS. In all trauma patients, you should maintain in-line stabilization of the spine while rolling the patient on his or her uninjured side in one motion **Step 8**. If you are placing the patient on a backboard, ideally you should check the back before you finish log rolling the patient onto a backboard. If you use a scoop stretcher, you will not be able to inspect or palpate the lower thoracic and lumbar spine.

Make a Transport Decision

As noted previously, early in the assessment process, you need to identify priority patients who will benefit from limited time at the scene and rapid transport, as in the case of a patient with

Primary Assessment

Skill Drill   1

Performing a Rapid Exam

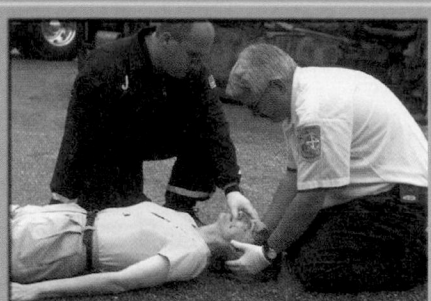

Step 1 Assess the head. Have your partner maintain in-line stabilization of the head and neck if trauma is suspected.

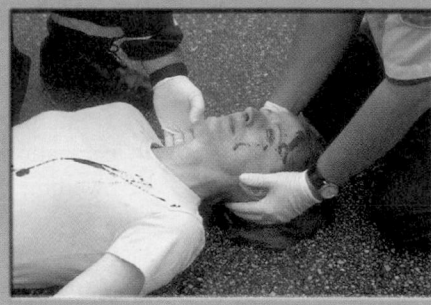

Step 2 Assess the neck.

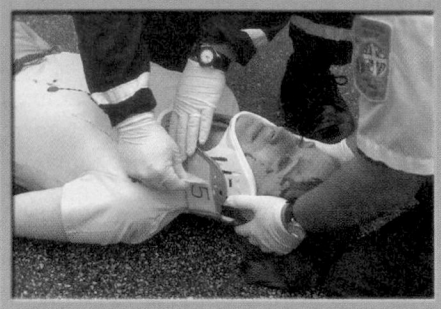

Step 3 Apply a properly-sized cervical spinal immobilization device on trauma patients.

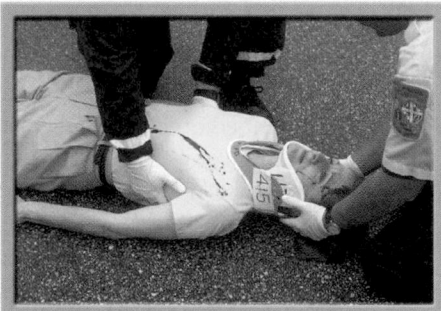

Step 4 Palpate both sides of the chest.

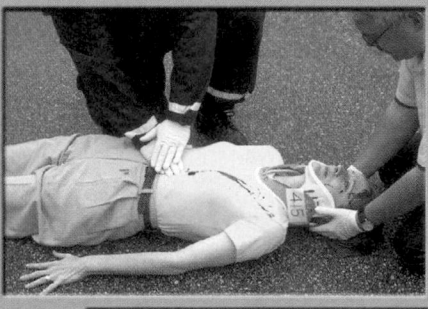

Step 5 Assess the abdomen.

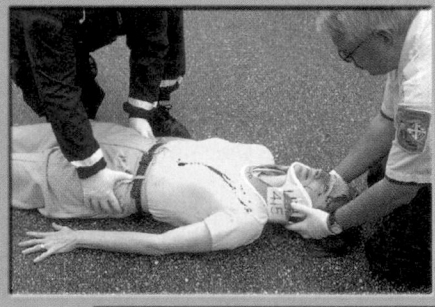

Step 6 Assess the pelvis. If there is no pain, gently compress the pelvis downward and inward to look for tenderness and instability.

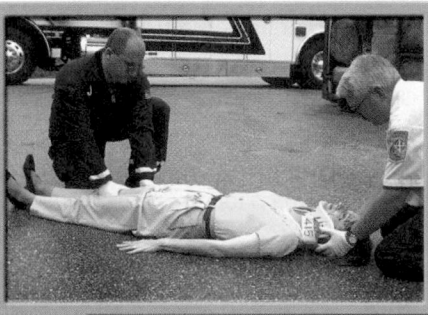

Step 7 Assess all four extremities. Assess pulse and the motor and sensory function.

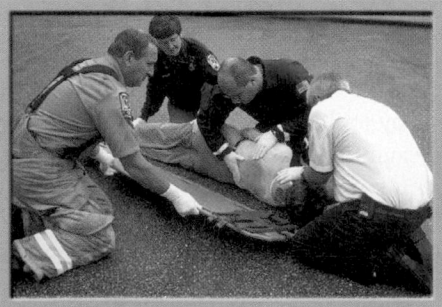

Step 8 Assess the back. In trauma patients, roll the patient in one motion.

internal bleeding from trauma. These patients are typically deemed to be in either unstable or potentially unstable condition. Such patients usually need surgery and blood replacement, neither of which can be accomplished in the field setting.

Patients deemed not to be high-priority cases are generally in stable condition. These patients, while injured, are not necessarily in critical condition (unstable) and, therefore, do not require expedient transport.

Transporting patients to the hospital is not without risk. When you are transporting patients in unstable and potentially unstable condition to the hospital, you need to ensure that it is accomplished in a fast and efficient manner, but keep in mind that safety should always be your top priority.

With a priority patient, you need to expedite transport, doing only what is absolutely necessary at the scene and handling everything else en route, including the appropriate history taking, secondary assessment, and reassessment. The following is a list of priority patients:

- **Poor general impression.** The patient is in obvious distress and does not "look well."
- **Unresponsive patients.** Unresponsiveness is never a good sign and typically points to a patient in serious or critical condition who may not be able to protect his or her airway.
- **Responsive but does not or cannot follow commands.** Altered mentation is another bad sign; the question you

need to answer is "How bad?", especially if there is a possible traumatic brain injury.

- **Difficulty breathing.** Breathing problems are one of the most common chief complaints in prehospital care. Patients who have difficulty breathing are in trouble; those who are "working to breathe" are in much bigger trouble.
- **Hypoperfusion or shock.** Without question, hypoperfusion or shock is an obvious sign of a high-risk patient. A weak or absent peripheral pulse, sustained tachycardia, and pale, cool, wet skin all point to a very ill patient.
- **Complicated childbirth.** Anything that presents from the birth canal other than the newborn's head represents a situation not likely to be managed in the field setting.
- **Chest pain with a systolic blood pressure of less than 100 mm Hg.** Especially in the context of tachycardia, this sign indicates potential signs of shock or cardiac compromise and a high-risk patient in unstable condition.
- **Uncontrolled bleeding.** Whether internal or external, such bleeding is a serious life threat.
- **Severe pain anywhere.** Any person with severe pain, especially enough to wake the person up in the middle of the night, should be considered a priority patient.
- **Multiple injuries.** Whereas a patient may have multiple minor injuries that by themselves are not serious, several small problems can add up to one large problem.

YOU are the Medic   PART 2

You immediately request law enforcement personnel to respond to the scene and advise the dispatcher of what you see. You use the PA system to say to the patient, "If you can hear me, wave at me." The patient raises his hand to your direction. Law enforcement personnel arrive with two patrol cars as the patient signals you. The officers approach the patient, and then gesture for you to come to the patient. The first officer tells you the patient has been stabbed in the chest. The patient's shirt is bloody and you cannot see a knife or other implement that may have been used to stab the chest. The patient looks up at you but says nothing when you ask him what happened.

Recording Time: 3 Minutes	
Appearance	Awake
Level of consciousness	Follows command
Airway	Open
Breathing	Adequate
Circulation	Adequate

3. What is your general impression of this patient?

4. What is your next step in the assessment of this patient?

History Taking

Patient Assessment

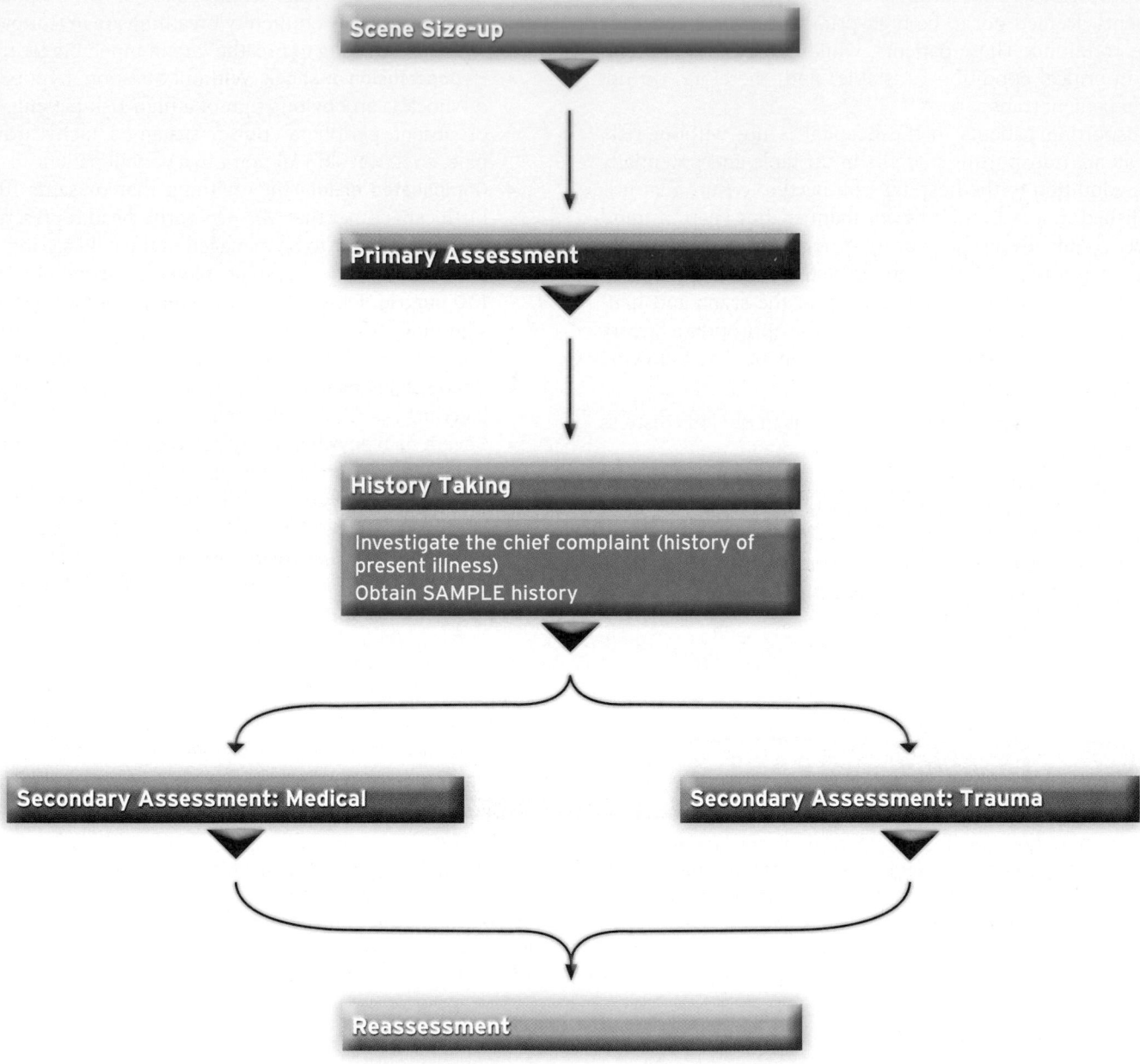

Scene Size-up

Primary Assessment

History Taking

Investigate the chief complaint (history of present illness)
Obtain SAMPLE history

Secondary Assessment: Medical

Secondary Assessment: Trauma

Reassessment

History Taking

Purpose

The purpose of obtaining a <u>patient history</u> is to gain information about the patient and learn about the events surrounding the incident. You are seeking to obtain a clear and accurate history of the immediate event and the pertinent past medical history, noting details that will assist you in distinguishing potential life threats from nonemergency complaints. When appropriate, expanded details about the patient history may be appropriate.

As a general rule, ask open-ended questions; they typically yield more information. Close-ended questions (those that can be answered yes or no) are still useful and can yield valuable information; just not much in the way of detail. Avoid asking leading questions, because they may serve to take the patient down an information pathway they never intended to go down. There are times that you will need to ask very direct questions, such as with a depressed patient, "Have you had thoughts about hurting yourself or committing suicide?"

Ensure that the questions you ask are age-appropriate and education-appropriate for your patient. Also, be patient. Ask a question and then wait for the answer. Rushing your patient along almost ensures you will not capture the information you want and need.

During the assessment process, you may find time to do some patient teaching, for example, "You may want to consider using a week-at-a-time pill box to help you stay compliant with your medications."

Patient Information

A number of components collectively make up the patient history. On most runs, the two most important pieces of patient history information that you need to obtain are the patient's name and the chief complaint. After that, you can obtain the rest of the patient history in whatever order is most conducive to good patient care and most convenient.

Your first step in approaching your patient is to introduce yourself and to explain that you are a paramedic. Then you can ask your patient his or her name and why he or she asked for your help (the chief complaint). Along with the patient's *name*, you need to ask about the *day of the week, time, location,* and *events* surrounding the current situation. This is important information and gives you the chance to quickly determine whether the patient is alert to person, place, time, and events. Your EMS system may require you to collect some additional identifying data such as age, sex, race, address, and occupation. You will also want to know who called 9-1-1: Did the patient place the call for help, or was it a friend, family member, or bystander who made the call? As you look at the patient, note any medical jewelry that may offer valuable information.

If emergency medical responders are already on the scene, find out the information they have already obtained and the results of any care they provided, such as: If the patient was bleeding, is it now controlled? Was oxygen administered? Have the patient's medications been tracked down (including prescriptions, over-the-counter medications, and supplements)? This information saves time by avoiding your having to ask the same questions again.

Techniques for History Taking

Every time you care for a patient, you must first establish a professional relationship. In most cases, this is a short-term relationship, often less than 2 hours' duration, until you provide your hand-off report and turn the patient over to the emergency department staff.

Your Appearance and Demeanor

Although time is short, you will want to have a positive patient outcome in the care you provide and the communication you establish with all involved. When you first meet your patients, they should be looking at a clean, neat, health care provider. You should have good personal hygiene and grooming and attire that is professional, clean, and pressed Figure 10 . If you look professional, your patients will likely form a good first impression of you. By comparison, if you don't look professional, it may be difficult for your patient to trust that you are indeed a professional. Gaining the trust of your patient is an important aspect of care.

Along with your appearance, there is the matter of your demeanor. On every call, your attitude is always on display. If you are unhappy, a look of unhappiness may appear on your face. Remember that your facial expressions and body language send powerful messages. If you have come to believe that calls to 9-1-1 need to meet *your* expectations, *you are wrong.* If patients think a problem is serious enough to merit a call to 9-1-1, you have an obligation to treat patients and their complaints accordingly—professionally and to the best of your ability.

Introduce yourself to your patient and tell him or her the name of your service and your certification level. Introduce your partner as well.

Try to interview the patient in a private setting. Most people do not want to admit to having some bad habits (for example, cigarettes) that have a negative impact on their health, but if it is information you need, then obtain it. Do not hesitate to ask any nonessential personnel to leave the room or to at least step back, because you will frequently find yourself asking your patients personal or intimate questions, requesting information that you need to know. If the setting makes the patient feel threatened or uncomfortable, the patient may choose to not answer

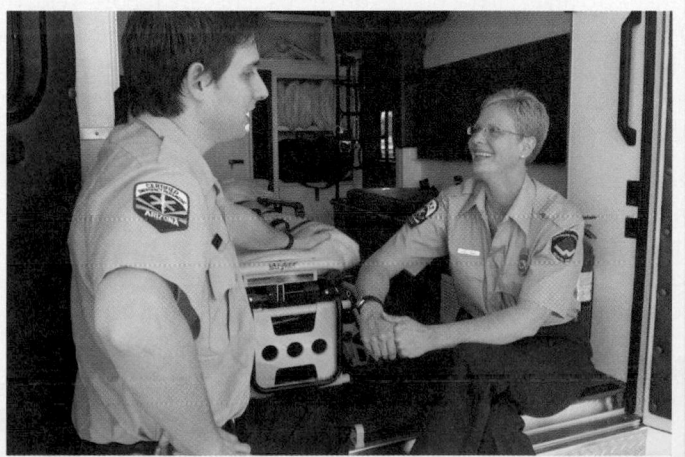

Figure 10 Your appearance should be professional and your demeanor positive and friendly.

your questions or to answer inaccurately. Working to ensure the patient's privacy, confidentiality, and comfort level goes a long way toward establishing positive patient rapport and encourages more honest, open communication.

Confidentiality

As discussed in the chapter, *Medical, Legal, and Ethical Issues*, it is your duty to maintain confidentiality of the patient's information. The Health Information Portability and Accountability Act (HIPAA) and state laws govern the disclosure of patient information. You need to be familiar with the relevant laws. Also, showing the patient that you respect the confidentiality of his or her medical information helps build rapport and contributes to the overall patient care experience.

How to Address the Patient

After introducing yourself, ask the patient his or her name and how he or she would like to be addressed. Err on the side of formality, using Mr., Miss, Mrs., or Ms. There is a world of difference in Mr. John Markham (formal), John (more casual), or Johnnie (really casual). Your patient will say, "Call me John" if that is what he prefers. Calling patients by the name of their choosing is professional, but assuming formality will help establish better rapport than being too familiar.

Avoid "catch-all names" or "pet names" like pal, buddy, sport, dude, friend, honey, sweetie, cutie, and darling. You can bog down the process of obtaining a history by demeaning the patient and treating the patient unprofessionally. Using casual nicknames also can be problematic when there are cultural differences. Some terms have negative connotation in some cultures. You need to be familiar with the cultural groups in your area and with issues that could lead to misunderstanding.

Note Taking

As you get ready to start the assessment process, let the patient know that you are going to be asking a number of questions and that while he or she is answering, you or your partner will be taking notes. This lets patients know they are not being ignored and that the information being provided is important enough to write down **Figure 11**.

Too often, EMS providers read off a list of questions to patients to fill in all the blanks on the patient care report. With this approach comes the problem of making little to no eye contact with the patient. Do not bury your nose in the tablet computer or clipboard! If possible, position yourself at the eye level of your patient. Maintain good eye contact and pay attention.

Reviewing the Medical History and Information Reliability

Frequently, you will obtain information not just from your patient but also from other sources. It is important that you document the source of this information in your record. Family

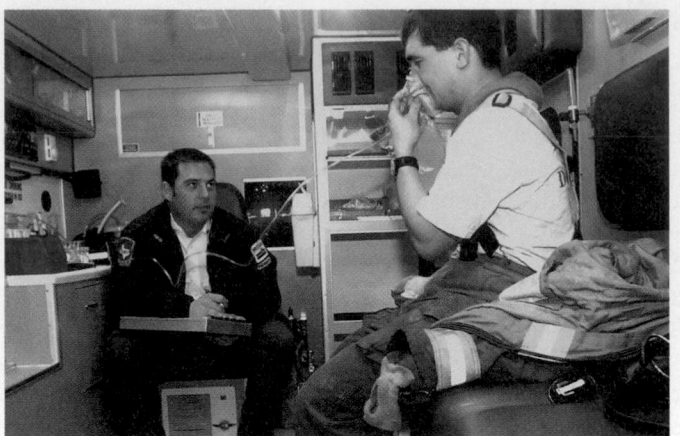

Figure 11 You may want to take notes on an assessment card during the patient history.

members are commonly involved at emergency scenes, as are friends. Law enforcement personnel and bystanders also can be valuable sources of information. Never forget that the best source of information is your patient. Answers provided by others may be less accurate, and therefore, less helpful.

A large number of the patient contacts in day-to-day EMS are routine patient transfers from assisted living or extended care facilities to the hospital and back. Take a few moments to review the transfer paperwork. You need to know the medical history of the patient so that you will be prepared to provide care should your planned routine transfer suddenly turn unroutine.

Again, always keep in mind the importance of evaluating your sources of information for reliability. Although the medical records in the transfer packet from an extended care or other health care facility should be assumed to be reasonably accurate, individual performances of caregivers inevitably vary. When all is said and done, you are responsible for patient care decisions, so make sure you work with information that is as accurate as possible.

Responsive Medical Patients

For a responsive patient with a medical problem, you will usually form your working field impression based on information gathered during the history-taking process. The secondary assessment and any diagnostic tests you perform after obtaining the history will help you further pinpoint the problem.

After the introductions are over, start gathering information. Take a moment to make sure the patient is as comfortable as possible before you start—warm or cool enough, privacy ensured—and that you have gained the patient's confidence and trust.

Chief Complaint

The patient's **chief complaint** is the most serious thing that the patient is concerned about. This is the reason the patient or someone else called 9-1-1. Ideally, the chief complaint should be recorded in the patient's own words. For example, if the patient says, "My feet hurt," then you write "My feet hurt" in quotation marks for the chief complaint in your documentation. For patients who are unable to speak or who are unresponsive, writing their primary medical condition or simply "unresponsive" is generally considered acceptable. The chief complaint should include what is wrong and why treatment is being sought.

With a responsive medical patient, you must first identify the chief complaint. In most cases, some type of pain, discomfort, or body dysfunction (such as "hasn't had a bowel movement in 4 days") prompts the call for help. In some cases, the complaint may be vague (such as "I just don't feel right today"). Vague complaints are common in older people, especially postmenopausal women. Vague complaints also challenge you to ask the right questions and be a patient listener as you work to obtain the information you need to make good care decisions Figure 12 .

History of the Present Illness

After determining the chief complaint, you should obtain the <u>history of the present illness</u>. To obtain a full, clear, chronologic account of the symptoms the patient is experiencing, the mnemonic OPQRST offers an easy-to-remember approach to analyzing a patient's chief complaint that is simple and effective. For example, when exploring a complaint of pain:

- **Onset.** What were you doing when the pain started?
- **Provocation.**
  - Did the pain start all of a sudden or come on over a period of time?
  - Does anything make the pain go away or feel better or feel worse?
- **Quality.** If you were trying to make me feel the way you do, what would you do to me to give me that same feeling?
- **Region/Radiation/Referral.**
  - Can you point to the place where it hurts?
  - Does the pain stay there, or does it go somewhere else?
- **Severity.** On a scale of 1 to 10, with 1 being very minor and 10 the worst pain you have ever felt, how would you rank this?
- **Time.** How long have you felt this way?

Documentation and Communication

Documenting pain severity ratings is important. Also note how distressed the patient appears: mild, moderate, or severe.

The SAMPLE mnemonic can also be useful in the interviewing process: Signs and symptoms of current complaint; Allergies; Medications; Pertinent past history; Last oral intake; and Events that led to the current injury or illness.

The history of the present illness starts with one of the most open-ended of all medical questions: "What is going on today that made you call 9-1-1?" An open-ended question cannot be answered with a "yes" or "no." This or a similar question will get the conversation moving. More often than not, the answer you get involves some problem(s) with the person being in pain or discomfort. If your patient's behavior is inappropriate, consider the possibility that it might be a psychiatric emergency or the patient may have altered mentation secondary to drug or alcohol ingestion.

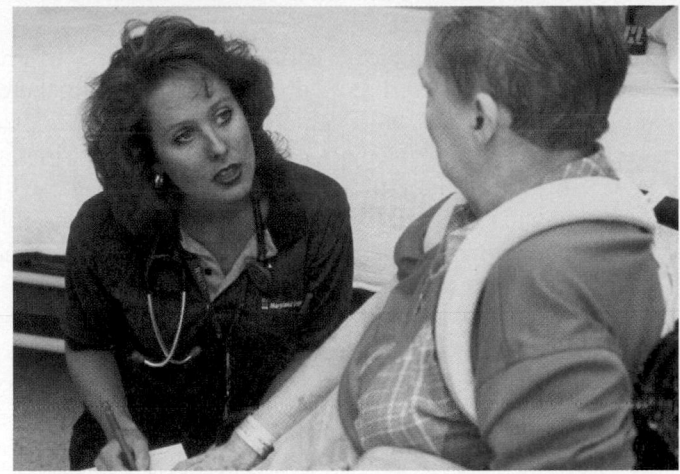

Figure 12 Be especially patient when obtaining information about a vague complaint.

Sometimes patients will have multiple complaints. Suppose a 64-year-old man tells you, "I'm really weak, and it feels like there are butterflies in my chest." You will need to determine whether these symptoms are related. If you believe that they are related, to provide appropriate care, you need to identify the *origin of the problem*. In this case, you may want to ask, "Have you had this problem before?" to see if the patient has issues with tachycardias and weakness in the past.

Now suppose the patient is complaining of "being dizzy and having pain in her left ankle." You might then ask questions and determine, for example, that the two complaints are not related. You must then decide which of the two conditions is your priority.

Once you have established the chief complaint(s), you will want to flesh out the history of the present illness. This information should provide you with a clear sequence and chronologic account of the patient's <u>signs</u> and <u>symptoms</u>—that is, *what happened* and *when*. Signs are objective observations or measurements that you make, and symptoms are subjective information that the patient tells you.

While you are taking the history, always look for a medical information tag or card. Medical identification devices may take the form of a bracelet, necklace, or wallet card. Such a device is used to identify patients with a history of allergies, certain medical conditions (such as diabetes, cardiac conditions, AICD/pacemaker, hypertension, renal disease), and other conditions that may need to be addressed in the treatment of the patient.

Past Medical History

The <u>past medical history</u> gives you an opportunity to learn about any pertinent or chronic underlying medical conditions the patient may have. Whereas not all aspects of the past history may seem important at the present time, a careful and thorough history will help paint a clear picture of the patient's overall health status. Not only will this potentially help you in your assessment, but it will help with the overall continuity of care from other health care providers who may be caring for the patient once at the hospital.

The past medical history is frequently linked to the patient's current problem. For example, people with diabetes who do not manage their blood glucose levels experience progressively worsening problems with their peripheral circulation, eyesight, and kidney function. Also, most patients with stable angina will eventually make the transition into unstable angina; at some point, the patient's condition may worsen and the patient may have a heart attack.

The past medical history should include current medication and dosages. Once again, while this information may not seem important at the time, this information may be quite helpful later on in the patient care process. Not only should information about prescription medications be obtained, but any over-the-counter medications and herbal/alternative medication therapies or dietary supplements should be identified as well. In addition, any allergies the patient may have should be documented. This includes not only allergies to medications, but also allergies to other substances (ie, food, detergents, animals). When you are recording this information, ask the patient what their reaction is to each specific allergy. This will provide valuable information later on in the patient care process.

A brief assessment of childhood illnesses along with immunizations should be assessed if time allows. This will help to rule in or rule out disease processes when you are taking a history and performing a secondary assessment.

Ask the patient about adult illnesses or any condition that he or she has that is currently being treated by a physician. This information will provide insight and details that may pertain to the current emergent medical problem. For example, if the patient is reporting chest pain, a past medical history of hypertension, hyperlipidemia, and diabetes are important elements that may pertain to the patient's chest pain because all of those conditions are considered independent risk factors for an acute myocardial infarction. You will need to assist some patients in filtering this information so it can be helpful to you. Some patients may want to tell you about every cold and splinter they have ever had in their life. Other patients will offer little information or take you so literally that it may obscure your assessment. For example, if you ask a patient, "Do you have any heart problems," such a patient might say, "No." When you open the patient's shirt, however, you find a scar running down the middle of the chest from open-heart surgery. You reply, "I thought you said you didn't have any heart problems," The patient's response: "I don't have any heart problems. I did a few years ago, but they fixed it."

Ask the patient about past surgeries. A great way to approach this is if you notice any surgical scars in your primary assessment, you could ask the patient how they got that scar. However, not all surgical scars are noticeable, and some procedures do not leave a scar at all. Therefore, you will need to ask each patient about past surgeries, including when they occurred.

A history describing past hospitalizations and any disabilities from previous illnesses will help to fine-tune your assessment. A patient with a previous history of hospitalization for chronic obstructive pulmonary disease, for example, should

be able to give you clues as to how advanced the disease might be or to the severity of the disease. A neurologic deficit from a previous traumatic event might obscure the physical exam findings in a potential stroke patient; therefore, asking about previous disabilities is important.

The emotional affect of the patient provides insight into the overall mental health of the patient. In addition, it helps you assess the mental status of the patient. A patient just involved in a motor vehicle crash is likely to be emotionally upset. When a patient appears to have an emotional response that is not typical or appropriate for the current event, you must consider the notion of a possible altered mental status in the patient. Ask about any mental health problems the patient might be having and whether he or she has ever been hospitalized for a mental health problem. Although it is often difficult for patients and families to admit to mental health problems, if you are matter-of-fact and dignified in asking the question, you can get an honest answer.

As you inquire about the patient's past medical history, take the time to explore how some of his or her problems were solved (eg, "It took a couple of breathing treatments before I felt better" or "After my last asthma attack, I had to be intubated and was in the hospital on a ventilator for a week").

Equally important is the situation in which the patient presents with a problem he or she has never experienced. An acute presentation of a new problem or condition is best considered serious until proven otherwise.

Current Health Status

One of the more challenging aspects of the history-taking process is that of pulling together the patient's **current health status**, because it is made up of many unrelated pieces of information. However, it often ties together some of the past history with the history of the current event, so it has definite value to the assessment process. The patient's current health status is a composite picture that includes numerous factors in the patient's life. To some degree, each of these items may have contributed to the problem you are confronted with today.

Questions that will be most helpful in obtaining a useful history of the patient's current health status include the following:

- What prescription medicines are you currently taking? How much and how often? (Patients can and do confuse when and how to take their medications—and if your patient has, you could be witnessing a drug reaction. Also, as you gain experience as a paramedic, your familiarity with the drugs will give you an idea of the patient's illness. Medications will also give you a clue about mental health problems or dementia without your needlessly antagonizing a reluctant patient.)
- Do you take any over-the-counter medications such as aspirin, or supplements such as herbs or vitamins?
- Are you allergic to anything?
- Do you smoke? How much? Do you drink beer, wine, or cocktails? How often?
- Have you been smoking or taking drugs (licit or illicit) other than cigarettes? (Assure your patient of confidentiality when you are making such inquiries.)

- What did you have to eat yesterday and today?
- Ask about screening tests that are appropriate. For example, for difficulty breathing, ask, "Have you had a chest x-ray lately?"
- Are your immunizations up-to-date? Have you had a flu shot or pneumococcal vaccine? Ask about children's immunizations, too.
- Have you been getting a good night's sleep? Look for maladaptive sleep patterns.
- Do you like to exercise? How much?
- What kinds of chemical cleaners do you have in your house? Do you have any strong chemicals where you work? You might need to probe for environmental hazards.
- Does the family use seat belts and car seats for the children? Do you have baby gates? Are medicines locked away (if it seems necessary)?
- Do you have a history of any specific diseases in your family?
- Where do you live? What do you like to do at home? Is there anyone in your life whom you might be afraid of? (You might need to assess a difficult home situation, ie, failure to thrive.)
- How do you spend your time during the day?
- Do you have anything in your religion that would prevent me from administering treatment?
- Are you an optimistic person? (You might feel it important to get your patient's overall outlook on life.)

Of course, you do not have to obtain each and every piece of information on this list for every patient. It takes time and practice and a certain amount of common sense for you to know the right questions to ask each patient. You have to decide which of the listed items you want to explore and which you do not. For a really sick patient with immediate life threats, you may have no time to explore any of them. For a patient in stable condition who appears to be in no apparent distress, you may have time and decide to explore all relevant topics.

Family History

A brief family history helps to establish patterned and risk factors for potential diseases. If a 35-year-old man with chest pain tells you that his father died of a heart attack at age 39, you should be concerned this patient could be experiencing a massive heart attack as well. Remember that not every aspect of the family history is necessarily important in the immediate emergent setting. Your information should be pertinent information related to the patient's current medical condition.

Social History

The social history is not typically gathered in the prehospital area. However, it provides valuable information regarding the

overall health status of the patient and helps to identify risk factors for various disease processes. Ask the patient about any smoking habits. If the patient has a smoking history or currently smokes, information about the quantity of smoking along with the length of time is essential. This is typically recorded in what is known as "pack-years." A patient who smokes one pack of cigarettes per day for 15 years is charted as a "15 pack-year history." A patient who smokes ½ pack of cigarettes per day for 15 years is charted as a "7 ½ pack-year history."

In addition to smoking, you should gather information regarding alcohol consumption (How much? How often? What drink?) and recreational/prescription drug use and abuse. Some patients may be reluctant to divulge such information freely out of fear of prosecution. While all paramedics understand that some patients may have broken the law, it is important to remind them that your primary responsibility is to provide medical care and that certain information is necessary for you to treat them appropriately.

The social history may include information regarding sexual habits. Discussing sexual habits is an uncomfortable topic, even for the most seasoned paramedics. Use caution and tact when you are ascertaining this information; few patient encounters require a detailed sexual history. However, in some patients, obtaining a sexual history is important. For instance, a woman in her 20s with left lower quadrant pain and a missed menstrual cycle could have an ectopic pregnancy, a potentially life-threatening emergency. A sexual history of this patient will be an important aspect of the overall patient assessment.

Questions regarding the patient's diet are also part of the patient's social history. Your patient's typical daily food intake is important information when you are determining patient

> ### Special Populations
>
> Without question, two of the most difficult groups of patients are pediatrics and geriatrics. With pediatric patients, patient history gathering from the patient usually does not work well until they are 2 or 3 years of age. Most of the problems encountered in the field for pediatric patients are respiratory related or fluid related. Just a day or two of vomiting or diarrhea can put a small child at high risk. With trauma, pediatric patients have to deal with being top-heavy (more likely to fall and strike their heads, especially in car versus pedestrian incidents).
>
> By comparison, geriatrics have certain unique characteristics. With aging often comes decreased sensorium, so complaints of pain are less frequent. Diabetes will add the problems of peripheral neuropathies, further diminishing sensitivity to pain, as well as eyesight and kidney problems. Compliance with medications is a challenge for any patient, but much more so for the elderly.
>
> Balance and equilibrium issues increase the likelihood of falls. Many of the elderly are on blood thinners as part of the regimen for treating atrial fibrillation, and even a minor fall can be deadly if blood cannot clot in a timely fashion. A fall can be lethal for the elderly as evidenced by hip fracture data; roughly 50% of the elderly who fall and break a hip will not survive the event.

> ### Special Populations
>
> In some cases, a patient's religious beliefs may be relevant—for example, if the beliefs pertain directly to medical care. If your patient indicates that such beliefs are important, this information should be passed along to emergency department staff.

History Taking

care. Questions regarding the timing and quantity of food consumption are appropriate to ask and may help to narrow down the list of possible differential diagnoses. For example, patients who do not eat certain foods because of personal, cultural, or religious reasons may experience nutritional deficiencies that are reflected in their symptoms.

A patient's occupation, environment, and travel history may need to be questioned to complete the social history. Occupation identification provides information about possible exposures to toxic substances and gives details regarding physical health. The environment in which the patient resides provides details regarding lifestyle and chronic exposures. A travel history may or may not be an important detail when you are obtaining a history. There are illnesses not common in the United States that people may potentially contract while traveling and bring back to this country. In addition, many of those illnesses are communicable and place EMS providers at potential risk. A travel history is also useful when pulmonary embolism is suspected. People who are on long airplane rides are prone to developing blood clots from not moving their lower extremities for extended periods of time. Any time a patient may present with an abnormal illness, a travel history should be obtained.

Unresponsive Patients

With an unresponsive patient, you start at a disadvantage in your assessment because your most reliable source of information—the patient—cannot answer your questions. Owing to this serious limitation, history taking and secondary assessment of an unresponsive patient is much like a trauma assessment. You must rely on a thorough head-to-toe physical examination plus the normal diagnostic tools (pulse oximetry, capnography, cardiac monitor, and glucometer) to acquire the information needed to care for your patient (discussed later in the section, Secondary Assessment of Unresponsive Patients). If family or friends are present, they may be able to provide you information about the patient's chief complaint, history of the present illness, past medical history, and possibly current health status. Nevertheless, the information they offer is almost never as good as that provided directly by the patient. Look for items that may assist you in learning more about the patient's condition. Items such as pill containers and medical jewelry can provide invaluable insight into a patient's underlying conditions.

Trauma Patients

As you move into the history taking for a trauma patient, quickly revisit all of the information from the primary assessment, including reconsidering the MOI. Collectively, these data may help you identify patients who need to be priority transports to the trauma center.

A number of mechanisms have the potential to produce life-threatening injuries Figure 13 :

- Ejection from *any* vehicle (car, motorcycle, or all-terrain vehicle)
- Death of another patient in the same vehicle

- Falls of greater than 15′ to 20′ or three times the patient's height
- Vehicle rollover
- High-speed vehicle crash (35 miles per hour or greater)
- Vehicle-pedestrian collision
- Motorcycle crash
- Penetrating wounds to the head, chest, or abdomen

Note that unresponsiveness or altered mental status following trauma suggests potential injury, usually a traumatic brain injury, even if the MOI does not seem significant.

If the patient is an infant or a child, MOIs that would indicate a high-priority patient include the following Figure 14 :

- Falls from more than 10′ or two to three times the child's height
- Fall of less than 10′ with loss of consciousness
- Medium- to high-speed vehicle crash (25 miles per hour or greater)
- Bicycle collision

In many cases, multiple MOIs come into play during a traumatic event—for example, a lateral collision that leaves the patient with a crushed upper arm and pelvic girdle and also penetrating trauma from the piece of door trim impaled in the chest. A patient with any of the previously mentioned mechanisms should immediately raise your index of suspicion. Two or more serious MOIs markedly increase the chance of a patient sustaining a serious or fatal injury.

Seat belts and air bags have significantly reduced the death and disability associated with motor vehicle crashes (MVCs). However, you should be aware that seat belts and air bags can also cause injuries. When you are evaluating a patient who was involved in an MVC, you should look for and ask questions to determine whether seat belts and/or air bags were involved. Check the clavicles where the shoulder strap crosses. The clavicles are small bones, and the subclavian vein and arteries run directly underneath them. In shorter patients, the shoulder strap mounted on the B column in a car can ride up across the neck, increasing the risk of soft-tissue and cervical spine injury. Examine the area where the lap belt crosses the pelvic girdle. If the belt is not across the iliac spine but has ridden up over the lower abdomen, the patient has an increased risk of organ damage and thoracic or lumbar spine injury. Passengers who tuck the shoulder harness under their arms for comfort and are then involved in rollover crashes are at high risk of death from liver injuries caused by the improperly positioned belt.

Air bags have saved countless lives, but many people do not realize that an air bag is a secondary restraint system, designed to work with seat belts to reduce injuries. When the seat belt is not used and a crash occurs, the air bag deploys, momentarily catching the patient. As the air bag deflates, it releases the driver or passenger, who continues moving forward and may go down-and-under (into the dashboard) or up-and-over (into the steering wheel and/or windshield). When you are at the scene of any crash with air bag deployment, lift the bag and look underneath for a bent steering wheel—another potential source of life-threatening internal injuries. During your hand-off report at

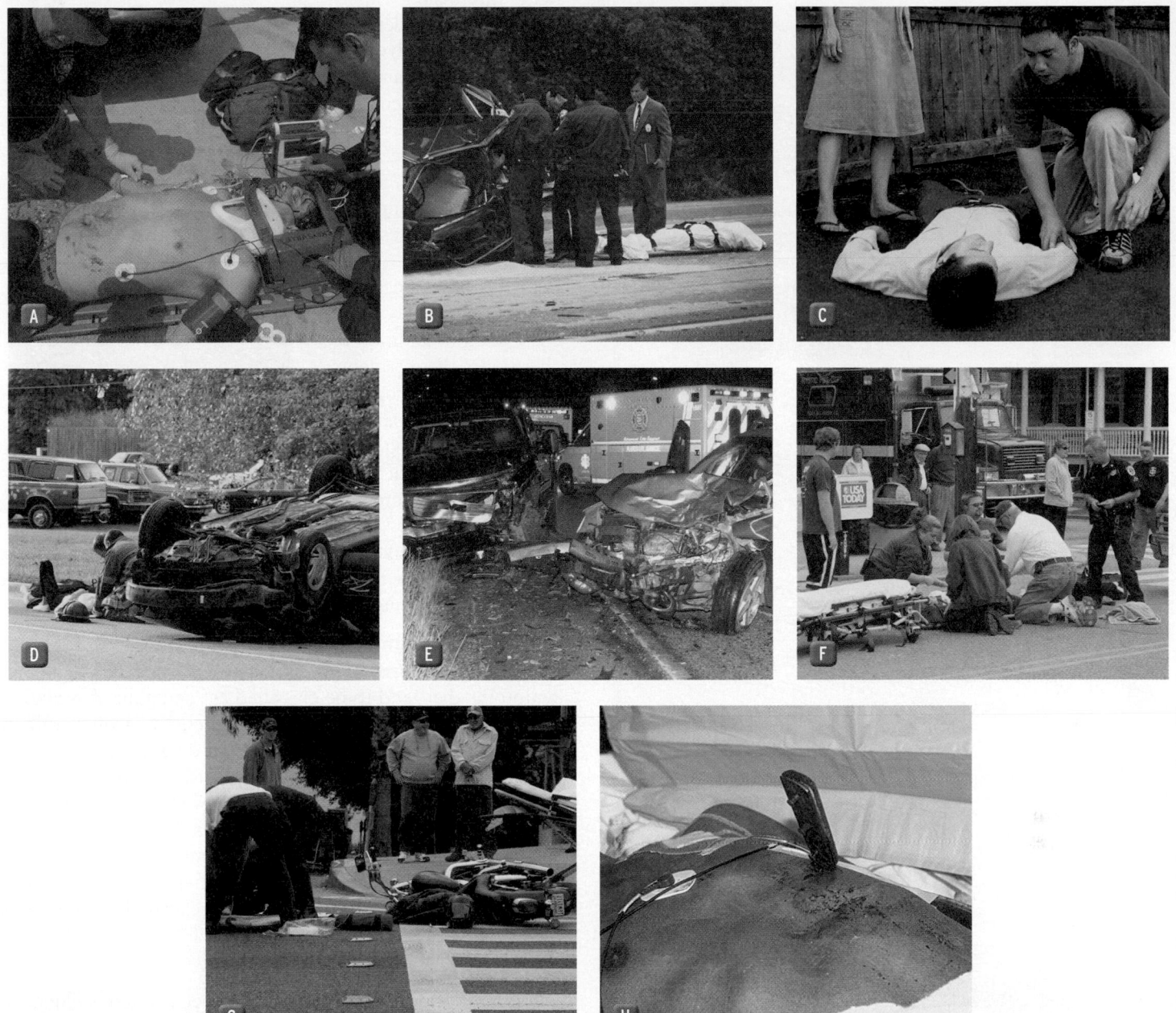

Figure 13 Significant mechanisms of injury. **A.** Ejection from *any* vehicle (car, motorcycle, ATV). **B.** Death of another patient in the same passenger compartment. **C.** Falls from more than 20′. **D.** Vehicle rollover. **E.** High-speed motor vehicle crash. **F.** Vehicle-pedestrian collision. **G.** Motorcycle crashes. **H.** Penetrating wounds to the head, chest, or abdomen.

the hospital, make sure that you tell hospital personnel whether seat belts were worn, properly positioned, and whether the air bag deployed.

Child safety seats have also saved countless lives **Figure 15**. If they are improperly installed or positioned in the vehicle, however, they can be rendered useless as a safety device. If the car seat comes loose during a crash, the risk of face, head, neck, and spine trauma to the child increases markedly. Similarly, if the child is too large or too small for the seat, the seat will not provide the intended level of protection.

Patients With Minor Injuries or No Significant Mechanism of Injury

Most trauma calls involve patients with a single, isolated injury or, on occasion, several minor injuries. In almost all of these cases, the lack of serious or critical injuries is consistent with the lack of a significant MOI: A collision on the basketball court results in a sprained ankle; a skater crashes and ends up with a Colles fracture; a loose piece of metal spins off a lathe in the machine shop, lacerating the machinist's forearm. Patients should not show any signs of systemic involvement

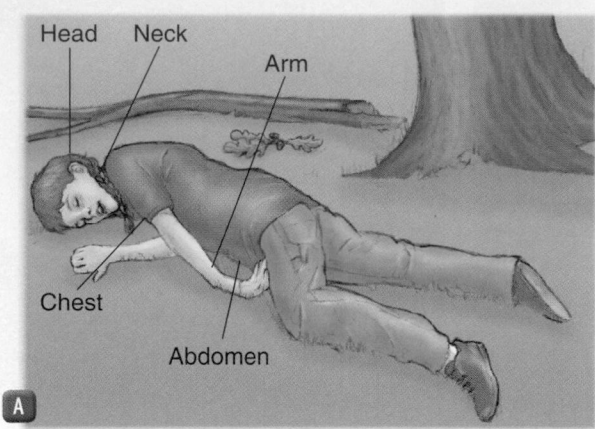

A — Head, Neck, Arm, Chest, Abdomen

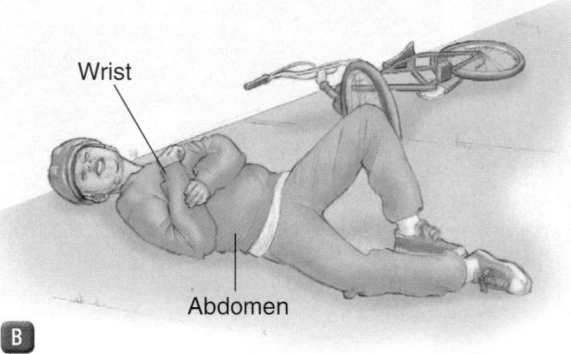

B — Wrist, Abdomen

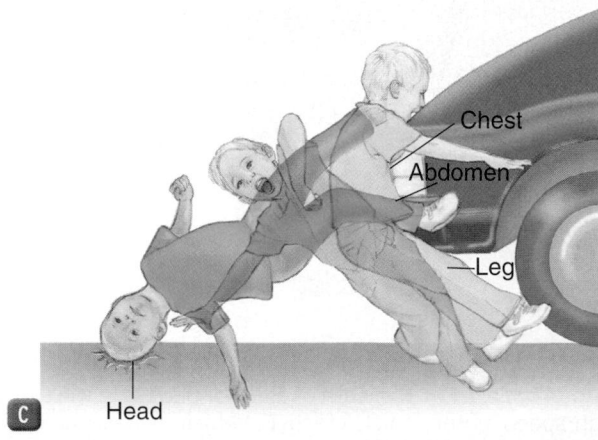

C — Chest, Abdomen, Leg, Head

Figure 14 Significant mechanisms of injury for an infant or child. **A.** Falls from more than 10′. **B.** Bicycle collision. **C.** Vehicle-pedestrian collision.

(hypotension). If they do, there is more going on than an isolated injury. You need to continue with your assessment with the goal of finding the more serious problem and correcting it.

Review of Body Systems
The review of body systems during history taking is a way to gain additional information that could help determine a

field impression. Many prehospital providers use **pertinent negatives** as a way to help gain this information. When you are determining pertinent negatives, you are looking for a lack of certain signs and symptoms specific to illnesses. For instance, people experiencing a myocardial infarction typically have chest pain. In addition to chest pain, these patients often report shortness of breath, nausea and vomiting, sweating, and syncope. A lack of these additional symptoms or the presence of them could help you make a more accurate field impression. Another example would be the patient who struck his head but denies any loss of consciousness.

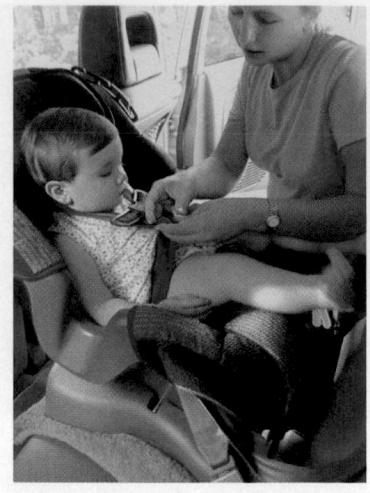

Figure 15 A child should be properly positioned in a car seat in the rear seats of the vehicle.

General Symptoms
Many patients present with vague, nonspecific signs and symptoms that tend to be classified as "generalized weakness" and "flu-like symptoms." In these patients it is often difficult to differentiate between potential field diagnoses; therefore, it is helpful for you to ask questions regarding fever, chills, malaise, fatigue, night sweats, and weight variations. While there is an endless of list of potential diseases in which any of these symptoms can be found, it is important for you to ascertain this information to help establish the field impression and in turn, to aid the hospital personnel in treating the patient once they assume care.

Skin, Hair, and Nails
Questions in this body system should focus on items like rashes (particularly in the pediatric population), itching or hives, and sweating. This system tends to be one of the most forgotten systems when performing the physical exam, and yet it is one of the most important. Remember that symptoms vary because they are subjective, but signs such as sweating and pallor have significance that should not be downplayed. It is important for you to look for and ask about these conditions because many patients will dismiss many of these subtle signs and symptoms or neglect to communicate them to you.

Musculoskeletal
The musculoskeletal system is affected by many illnesses. Whereas issues with the musculoskeletal system tend to be attributed to trauma, many medical conditions affect this system as well. For patients reporting signs and symptoms that could be associated with the musculoskeletal system, you should ask questions about joint pain, loss of range of motion, and any swelling, redness, erythema, and localized heat or deformity.

Head and Neck

There are multiple structures within the head and neck that could affect the overall health status of a patient. Particular attention should be given to patients experiencing a severe headache or loss of consciousness because these could be resulting from potentially life-threatening conditions.

Eyes

When you are asking questions regarding the eyes and vision, ask about visual acuity, blurred vision, diplopia (double vision), photophobia (sensitivity to light), pain, changes in vision, and flashes of light seen in the field of vision.

Ears

Questions should focus on hearing loss, pain, discharge, tinnitus (ringing in the ears), and vertigo (sensation of the room spinning).

Nose

Ask about sense of smell, rhinorrhea (runny nose), obstruction, epistaxis, postnasal discharge, and sinus pain.

Throat and Mouth

Questions should focus on complaints such as sore throat, bleeding, pain, dental issues, ulcers, and changes to taste sensation.

Endocrine

The endocrine system is a complicated network of hormone-secreting glands that help to regulate various functions in the human body. Many diseases of the endocrine system are seen in the EMS environment and should be included in your review of systems. Because multiple glands and organs are part of the endocrine system, there is a broad range of questions to ask patients. Ask your patient if he or she has ever been told that he or she has enlargement to the thyroid gland. While subtle enlargement is typically only noticed with palpation, excessive enlargement is generally noticed by the patient.

Additional questions about the endocrine system pertain to temperature intolerance, skin changes, swelling of hands and feet, any weight changes, polyuria (increased frequency of urination), polydipsia (increased thirst), polyphagia (increased appetite), and any changes in body and facial hair.

Chest and Lungs

Complaints regarding the heart and lungs are common reasons for requesting EMS assistance. A review of systems would not be complete without screening for possible cardiac and respiratory conditions. Patients should always been screened for dyspnea and chest pain. Other respiratory questions should be focused toward coughing, wheezing, hemoptysis (coughing up blood), and tuberculosis status. With regarding to coughing, a description of the cough, including production of mucus or phlegm, should be noted. When you are questioning a patient about cardiac complaints, the initial focus is on whether this is a first-time or recurring event, followed by questions about pain or discomfort. As described earlier, attention to the onset of pain, its duration, quality, provocation, and palliation should be explored. Other questions related to the heart and blood vessels are regarding orthopnea, edema, and past cardiac evaluation and tests.

Hematology

Ask your patients about any history of anemia, bruising, and fatigue. Anemia may exacerbate multiple conditions that could be seen during EMS calls. Bruising should be noted, especially when it is atraumatic. This could suggest a clotting disorder that may affect traumatic injuries as well as other medical conditions. Note any bruising that may point toward a possible physical abuse scenario, keeping in mind that paramedics are mandatory reporters.

Lymph Nodes

Tender and enlarged lymph nodes can be seen with conditions ranging from infections to cancers. Notably, many patients encountered in the EMS environment will be experiencing infections. Questioning about tender and enlarged lymph nodes can point towards a possible field impression.

Gastrointestinal

Gastrointestinal (GI) complaints can be common in EMS patients. Paramedics need to have an understanding of GI ailments and ask appropriate questions in the review of systems to help distinguish the various illnesses. Patients should be asked about appetite, general digestion, food allergies and intolerances, heartburn, any nausea and vomiting, diarrhea, hematemesis (blood in vomit), bowel regularity, changes in stool (size, shape, smell, and color), flatulence, jaundice, and any past GI evaluations and tests. Pay particular attention to signs and symptoms that point toward active GI bleeding, a potentially life-threatening condition.

Genitourinary

Many patients fail to freely offer information regarding urination. Some people attribute changes in urinary habits to aging, but in fact many times this is a new finding that needs to be addressed. It is important for you to ask questions regarding urinary habits or changes in urinary habits. Many times changes in these habits could be indicative of an underlying infection. You should question patients about any dysuria (painful urination), increased frequency of urination, urgency (sudden need to urinate), nocturia (waking up in the middle of the night to urinate), hematuria (blood in urine), polyuria (excessive urination), and pain to the flank and suprapubic region when you suspect that an underlying urinary problem could be related to the chief complaint.

The genitourinary system also includes the genitals. As mentioned earlier, discussing one's genitals with a complete stranger is not easy for most people. However, conditions such as sexually transmitted diseases are serious issues. Even though this may be an embarrassing topic for both patients and paramedics, questions regarding any current or history of sexually transmitted diseases should be asked.

Some questions are specific to the male and female genders. Recall that both the male and the female sex organs secrete hormones belonging to the endocrine system. When you are questioning male patients, ask about erectile dysfunction, any fluid discharge, and testicular pain. It may seem trivial to the patient, but issues with erectile dysfunction are frequently related to systemic diseases like hypertension or diabetes. In addition, the medications used to treat many of these conditions can affect the care provided by paramedics, ie, do not give nitroglycerin to a patient taking erectile dysfunction drugs like Viagra or Cialis. Females should be questioned about menstrual regularity, last menstrual period, dysmenorrhea, vaginal discharge, abnormal bleeding, pregnancies, and contraception use. Further discussion of female gynecologic and obstetric issues appears in the chapter, *Gynecologic Emergencies*.

Neurologic

The nervous system is intricate and often difficult to understand. When patients summon EMS for a neurologic complaint, you need to understand the importance for assessing possible neurologic pathology and ask certain questions when performing the review of systems that cover or involve the nervous system. Patients should be asked about a history of seizures or syncope, and loss of sensation, weakness in extremities, paralysis, loss of coordination or memory, and muscle twitches or tremors. Be alert for signs of facial asymmetry, especially when the chief complaint is headache. If you suspect stroke or a transient event, run the patient through the Cincinnati Stroke Scale. The Cincinnati Stroke Scale is discussed in detail in the chapter, *Neurologic Emergencies*. Neurologic complaints are relatively common in EMS; therefore, it is essential that you consider these questions when performing a patient history.

Psychiatric

Many times, paramedics are called to the scene to deal with a behavioral health emergency. Considering the breadth of behavioral health issues, you need to question patients appropriately to differentiate between the various mental illnesses. This step is important not only to deliver appropriate patient care, but also to ensure the safety of yourself, the crew, and the patient. Patients should be asked about a history or any current depression, mood changes, difficulty concentrating, any anxiety, irritability, sleep disturbances, fatigue during the day, and suicidal or homicidal ideations.

Clinical Reasoning

Clinical reasoning combines knowledge of anatomy, physiology, pathophysiology, and the patient's complaints to help direct questioning when you are obtaining a history. Note any abnormal symptoms or physical findings, as well as their anatomic location. Pay careful attention to any signs or symptoms that are inconsistent with your working diagnosis, because they may point you in a different direction. As the interview questions are answered, you begin to analyze the answers based on your underlying medical knowledge. Once the history of the chief complaint, history of the present illness, past medical history, and review of systems have been completed, you can begin to develop the **differential diagnosis**—a working hypothesis of the nature of the problem.

Just like a scientist, you can then begin to test this hypothesis to determine whether it holds true. This is accomplished through further assessment and testing. The process evolves as different questions are asked based on the patient's answers. This exploration, in turn, will help to focus your physical assessment and narrow down your potential field diagnoses. You may use various methods to test theories (ie, 12-lead ECG, glucose check). This additional information is combined with the existing knowledge, and a differential is narrowed even further.

When you are developing differential diagnoses, start with broad possibilities—that is, which body systems might be contributing to the patient's complaint. For instance, chest pain could involve the cardiac, respiratory, or gastrointestinal systems. This approach will help you to avoid "tunnel vision," which is defined as locking into a diagnosis early before considering all the possibilities. Because chest pain could involve multiple systems, it is important for paramedics to consider all the possible diagnoses and rule each one out systematically in order to determine a diagnosis.

You should first begin by considering the patient's chief complaint. A significant number of illnesses or conditions can be ruled out quickly by just determining the chief complaint. Suppose, for instance, a patient reports chest pain. Your knowledge gives you insight into the potential problems that can cause chest pain. Your differentials might include a heart attack, gastroesophageal reflux, a pulmonary embolism, or an aortic dissection. A patient reporting chest pain is not likely to have gastrointestinal bleeding; therefore, you can use the chief complaint to immediately narrow the diagnosis. In addition to the chief complaint, the associated signs and symptoms along with the history will narrow the possible choices even further.

The physical exam (discussed later in this chapter) is another important aspect of clinical reasoning. Tenderness or other specific exam findings help to point you toward specific anatomic locations can help tighten up your diagnostic possibilities. Once you are able to identify the possible organ systems involved, you can use your knowledge of pathophysiology to determine the most likely diagnosis.

Once you have determined your working diagnosis, be sure to continue your questioning of the patient to help confirm your diagnosis. In addition, make sure you reevaluate the overall situation and complaint to make sure all of the patient issues have been addressed.

Communication Techniques
Encourage Dialogue

On the basis of the questions asked and answers received, and data from your diagnostics, you will make patient care decisions. A number of approaches and conversation techniques can help to improve the volume and quality of information you obtain during the patient interview. Techniques were discussed in the chapter, *EMS Communications* and are summarized in **Table 3**.

Remember that patients of all ages are hesitant to share private or embarrassing information. You need to make your patients feel so secure with you so that they will give you the information you need. Remember the importance of speaking in layperson terminology, not in the language of medicine. Patients with no background in medicine will generally use nonmedical terms to answer your assessment questions **Figure 16**.

Empathetic Response

Empathy is often described as one step further than sympathy; empathy is a psychological gift that allows you to feel what your patient is feeling—putting yourself into his or her shoes.

Table 3   Communication Techniques

Technique	Definition	Examples
Facilitation	Using techniques that encourage your patient to feel open to giving you any information you need.	Pay attention. Make eye contact. Repeat key information from the patient's answers. Nod your head. Use phrases such as: ■ "That's helpful." ■ "Anything else you can think of?" ■ "Please go on."
Reflection	Pausing to consider something significant that you've just been told.	Your patient says: "I couldn't catch my breath." You respond: "That's very helpful. Hold on a second, and let me think about that for a moment."
Clarification	The technique of asking your patients for more information when some aspect of the history is vague or unclear to you.	Paramedic: "What's going on today, Mrs. Hendrickson?" Patient: "Oh I don't know. I'm just . . . well I'm just not feeling like myself." Paramedic: "I'm sorry. Could you try to be a little more specific? If you could do that, it will help me figure out what's going on with you today." Patient: "I'm always full of energy first thing in the morning, but I'm so weak right now that I couldn't even take Princess outside."
Confrontation	Making your patient aware that you perceive something that is not consistent with his or her behavior, the actual scene, or the information the patient is giving you.	Use a direct approach; for example, with a chronically depressed patient, ask about whether he or she is contemplating suicide and if so, if he or she has a plan. Remain professional and nonjudgmental, but direct.
Interpretation	Inferring the cause of the patient's distress, then asking the patient if you are right.	Maintain a diplomatic approach. Use the phrase: "So, if I understand you correctly . . ."

History Taking

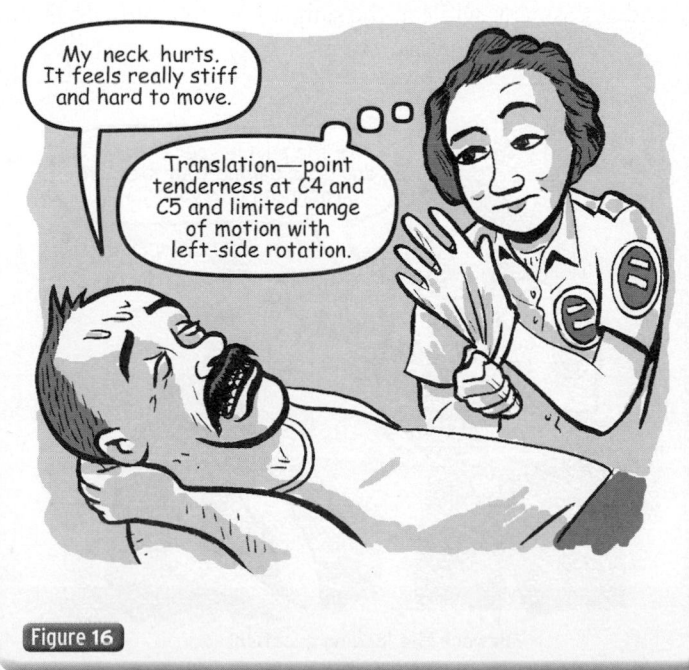

Figure 16

At times, you will hear sad and tragic information from your patients. Do not hesitate to communicate your feelings and address the emotional impact of what has been said Figure 17 .

Documentation and Communication

Do not put words into the patient's mouth, or ideas into the patient's head, such as, "Is the pain in your chest a dull ache? Does it radiate behind your sternum and into your jaw?"

When a patient may not have an overt medical problem, you should consider the possibility that he or she might be depressed and that a mental health referral is needed.

Paramedics, unlike most other health care providers, see people when the illness or trauma just occurred. Your patients are uniquely vulnerable and uniquely demanding. Try your best to develop empathy for your patients.

Earlier chapters discussed ways of being knowledgable of the various resources that may be of help for your patients. Empathy can help you set your patient on a path to healing—no matter what the diagnosis.

Asking About Feelings

Asking about feelings is one of the most difficult roles of a paramedic. But as part of a good health history, you will need to ask if a patient is tired, depressed, or any number of feelings that are most easily dealt with by denial. (You will even need

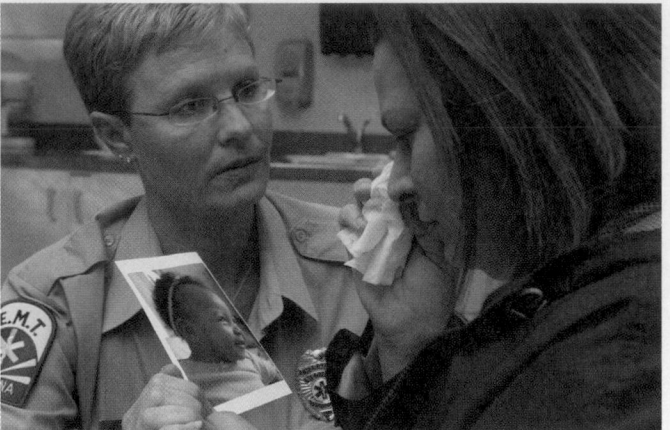

Figure 17 Be as empathetic as possible when the patient conveys sad or tragic information.

to ask these questions of a colleague if you see the symptoms in him or her.)

Try to keep possible unpleasant sights, sounds, and smells from your patient who is feeling badly. You can also validate feelings: "This is a tough situation." That is empathy in action. Do your best to attend to psychological needs continuously throughout a call. It is a challenging part of the paramedic's job, but these needs profoundly affect a person's physical health.

While being empathetic with your questioning, it is important to be effective. Do not ask, "Are you okay?" This is the most tempting of all questions (and it *can* be answered with a yes or no!). Instead, ask for facts first, and then follow up. When asked, most people would deny that they are exhausted, frazzled, scared, or depressed. Your patients met you only a few minutes ago. Establish that you are a caring health professional by asking a series of "safe" questions about physical health before you ask about mental health issues.

Getting More Information
You may have obtained much information from your patient, but in many cases, you need to refine your thinking to come up with the most probable diagnosis. Suppose you were exploring a particular symptom such as "abdominal pain" with your patient. (As you will soon learn, abdominal pain can suggest a startlingly large number of diagnoses.) Some possible questions you might ask the patient about the *region* or location of the pain include the following:

- Where exactly does it hurt?
- Can you point to where it hurts with one finger, or is it in a more specific area?
- Does the pain stay right there, or does it move or radiate anywhere else?
- If your pain does move or radiate, where does it go?

Questions you may ask about the *quality* of the abdominal pain include the following:

- How would you describe the quality of your pain?
- Does the pain come and go, or is it constant?

- If you wanted me to feel the same feeling that you do, what would you do to me to make me feel that way?

Questions you may ask about the *severity* of the abdominal pain include the following:

- In your opinion, how bad is this pain?
- Is it more of an uncomfortable feeling or a feeling of hurt?
- Would you say the pain is similar to or worse than previous episodes?
- On a scale of 1 to 10, with 10 being the *worst* pain you have ever felt and 1 being very minor, how would you rate your pain?

The questions in these lists are not exhaustive or all-inclusive. Add, delete, and modify questions as necessary. Use open-ended questions whenever you can **Figure 18**. If possible, do not ask questions that can be answered with a "yes" or "no"—but ask your patient a close-ended question if that is what the situation requires. Avoid leading questions, which are phrased in a way that suggests the paramedic's opinion, rather than directing the patient to give an answer based on his or her own observations. An example of a leading question is, "Do you think this is a cardiac emergency?" Many patients, particularly the elderly, are eager to please and will give an answer in order to please the interviewer. Asking leading questions may lead to the wrong diagnosis and hinder patient care.

Try to be *orderly* and *systematic* in your information gathering and assessment, while at the same time remaining *flexible* in

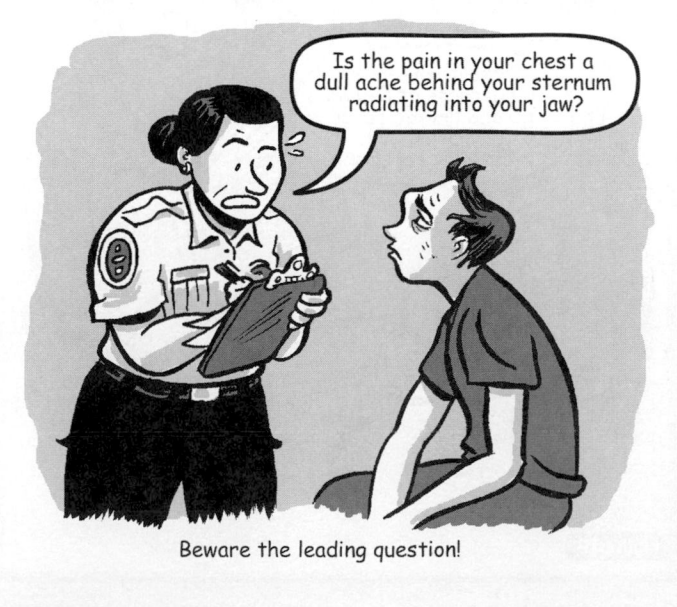

Beware the leading question!

Figure 18

your approach. Being flexible in an emergency is more difficult than it sounds, but it is attainable with practice—lots and lots of practice.

Asking Direct Questions

To complete the history, direct questions could be required. If a patient is not giving you usable facts about himself or herself, and if you need a date, time, or other specific information, you should ask for it.

Applying Clinical Reasoning

When all is said and done, the result of your assessment should be to figure out the most likely reason for your patients' chief complaint and how best to address it. In the chapter, *Critical Thinking and Clinical Decision Making*, you will learn the details of critical thinking. For now, recognize that critical thinking consists of (1) concept formation, (2) data interpretation, (3) application of principles (guidelines or algorithms), (4) reflection in action (being willing to change course as you interpret your patient's condition), and (5) reflection on action (doing honest and thorough postrun critiques to benefit learning).

Being able to think and perform well under pressure is a big part of being able to be a good paramedic. In many ways, critical thinking and decision making are just two more skills you will need to work on, not just while you are a student, but for the rest of your career as a practicing paramedic.

One of the most important elements of the interview process is for you to be a *great listener,* and a big part of being a great listener is also being a *patient listener.* For a number of reasons, patients can be slow to respond. Maybe they did not hear your question, or maybe they did not understand you. Maybe they are afraid to answer. Ask, then wait, and give your patients time to gather their thoughts so they can answer you.

Communicate with your patients by using terminology matched to their knowledge and understanding. On the one hand, a patient who is an emergency department nurse or a retired surgeon will understand medical terminology. On the other hand, a patient who speaks little English needs simple and focused communication.

Throughout the assessment process, look for nonverbal communication, such as changes in facial expression, heavy sighs, or aggressive gestures (finger pointing), any of which can impact your information processing.

Getting a History on Sensitive Topics

As a paramedic, you will be privileged to care for people who depend on you during some of the worst moments of their lives. You represent hope and comfort no matter how difficult, even horrific, your patient's situation might be.

Some sensitive factors like drug and alcohol abuse can stand in the way of your best efforts for the health of your patients. Here are some ways that can help you be the paramedic you want to be, no matter how sensitive the situation.

Alcohol and Drug Abuse

People who regularly abuse drugs or alcohol become adept at hiding the signs and symptoms from their friends, family, and workplace associates and denying there is a problem. Such denial can go on for years, and the signs and symptoms can be hidden even from people closest to the patient.

If asked how much alcohol or drug has been consumed, the amount is routinely understated. Some experienced paramedics say the standard answer to the question about how many drinks is "two," when the behavior and physical signs indicate many more. According to the National Highway Traffic Safety Administration (NHTSA), a significant number of fatalities from motor vehicle crashes in the United States involve alcohol **Figure 19** .

It is probable that an alcohol-impaired patient will give an unreliable history, especially regarding pain. Do not assume that all information you are told is completely accurate. Keep in mind that alcohol can mask any number of signs and symptoms. When a patient who experienced a significant traumatic event denies neck or back pain, if you smell what you believe to be alcohol on the patient's breath or the patient's behavior raises your suspicion of alcohol or drug use, take precautions to restrict spinal motion.

Alcohol is a legal drug. If your patient is using other substances to "get high," using them is most likely illegal. The fear of punishment for illegal use of drugs might lead patients to deny their use. Let your patient know that you are a medical provider and that anything that he or she tells you will be kept in confidence. Do your best to win your patient's trust because you need accurate information to provide proper treatment.

Keep your best professional attitude as you work with patients whom you suspect of using drugs or alcohol. You should never judge your patients by appearances or behavior. An unkempt homeless person might be in desperate need of assessment and immediate care for head trauma, not alcoholism.

Physical Abuse, Domestic Violence, and Sexual Assault

As a paramedic, you are required to report a case if you have reason to suspect physical abuse or domestic violence. Although it is inappropriate for you to accuse someone of abuse at the scene, never hesitate to call for law enforcement personnel if you have reason to believe that abuse has occurred. Police can help stabilize the scene, provide another set of professional eyes, and, if necessary, take someone into custody.

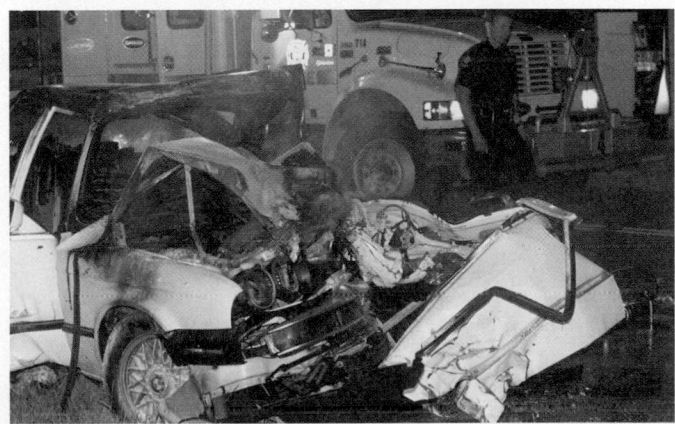

Figure 19 Many crashes involve alcohol. In these cases, the patient history may not be reliable.

A number of clues may lead you to suspect domestic violence. Injuries inconsistent with the information you are being given are common, as are multiple injuries in various stages of healing. Unspoken messages may be given by the family's behavior. You may notice the cowering posture of the woman at the kitchen table as her husband or significant other towers over her and answers your questions for her. If the injured family member does not give you the information but waits for someone else to speak up, that is a clue that the injured family member is being repressed. You can suggest that the significant other who is doing all the talking go to the ambulance to help with the stretcher. The moment the door shuts, you may receive valuable information, such as "My husband is beating me and I'm scared to death. You have got to get me out of here before he kills me or one of the kids." *Immediately* request law enforcement personnel if this or if anything close to this type of situation happens.

Words of Wisdom

If you find yourself suddenly in a potentially dangerous position and your partners are not aware of it, use a predetermined code word to alert them. One inconspicuous code is to use the trade name of something in your ambulance—"Could you get the Ferno cot?" Your partners should know that it means there is danger and that they should summon law enforcement personnel.

Emergency scenes involving domestic violence are some of the most dangerous for EMS and law enforcement professionals alike Figure 20 . Do not even think of handling them without law enforcement personnel on hand.

In cases of sexual assault or rape, handle all clothing per local protocol and bag it with any other evidence (use paper bags rather than plastic). Sexual assault and rape have a significant psychological impact. Be supportive, caring, and nonjudgmental during your care. It is ideal to have an EMS provider who is the same sex as the victim.

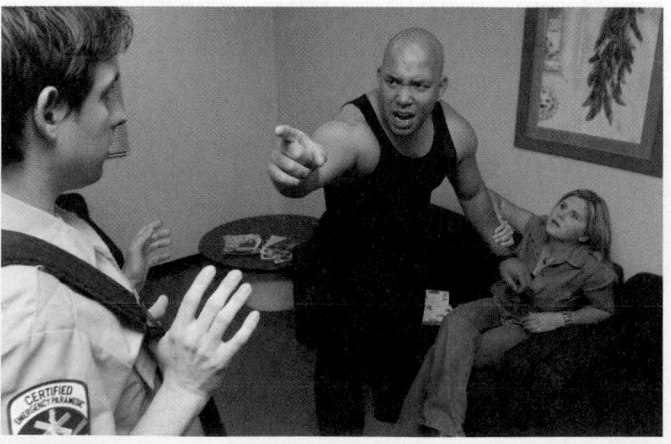

Figure 20 Do not handle potentially violent calls alone. Summon law enforcement personnel.

Sexual History

A number of factors may influence a patient to be less than forthcoming about sexual history. Religious upbringing, cultural or societal mores, and exotic or bizarre sexual tastes may inhibit a patient from sharing his or her sexual history. When you obtain a patient's sexual history, talk to the patient in a setting that is as private as possible.

Keep your questions focused. For a woman reporting acute abdominal pain, foul-smelling vaginal discharge, pain on urination, or genital lesions, you will need to know when your patient last had her period and when she last had sexual intercourse. You will also need to find out if there is vaginal bleeding, whether she has had multiple sex partners, the characteristics of the vaginal discharge, and whether she uses a birth control method.

Special Populations

Some younger teens may be confused when asked about sexual issues. Be direct and avoid using questions like "Are you sexually active?" Some young people may think "active" means "often."

Men who report pain on urination, discharge from the penis, or genital lesions need to be asked about their most recent sexual encounter, whether they use condoms, and the characteristics of their discharge and lesions.

You may need to ask female and male patients if they have ever been tested for HIV, AIDS, or hepatitis. Do not interject any opinions or biases about sexual choices or behavior. Their choices are not your choices, just as your choices are not theirs. Every patient you care for deserves to be treated with compassion and respect.

Cultural Competence

To effectively communicate to save lives, you must strive to understand the differences inherent in all people. Only then can you adjust your efforts to accommodate and overcome cultural barriers. The most common barriers to communication include those related to race, ethnicity, age, gender, language, education, religion, geography, and economic status. The collection of all these characteristics can be termed "culture." You cannot treat your patients effectively if you use your own culture as your only reference—EMS providers cannot impose their own morality on patients. Understanding other cultures is important, especially the cultures in your region. This knowledge will help you communicate effectively when you care for patients who have different cultural backgrounds than yours.

Culture and ethnicity are not the same thing, though a person's culture may be affected by his or her ethnicity. Cultural beliefs may relate to a person's age as well as his or her ethnicity, among other factors.

Culture has an impact on our modern society in a number of ways. Cultural beliefs can affect many medical decisions and treatment plans. It is your responsibility to respect a person's ideas and beliefs, even when yours are not the same. For example, some cultures believe that illness may be caused by evil spirits. When you are treating a patient who believes that an evil spirit is the cause of an illness, do not dismiss the belief and fear. Be compassionate. Your approach will ensure that communication is kept open to maintain continuity of care.

Dietary practices and family relationships need to be considered during patient care. As a part of a culture, people consume certain foods in their diet that may not be healthy. For this reason, certain cultural groups are more prone to diabetes and heart disease. When you have the opportunity, making recommendations regarding healthy eating choices can positively affect the entire family. In cultures that have an identified leader in the household who makes all the decisions regarding diet and medical care, it is important for you to establish a good relationship with that person in order to facilitate patient care. With regard to health care, certain cultures and religions do not believe in administering vaccinations and medications for disease prevention and treatment. Some of these groups object to the transfusion of blood products, regardless of the illness. For this reason, paramedics should always gain consent before administering any medication to a patient. Understand that as long as the patient is mentally competent, he or she has the right to refuse treatment of any kind.

A person's socioeconomic status may relate to overall physical health. Persons with lower socioeconomic status have fewer financial resources to maintain good health. It is your responsibility to provide the best possible care for all patients regardless of their socioeconomic status.

Classes and seminars are available that focus on dealing with cultural differences. What do all of these classes and seminars actually teach? In a word, "respect." EMS providers need to be sensitive to how their behavior affects patients of other cultures.

Because the social practices, mannerisms, etiquette, and idiosyncrasies of cultures are numerous, it is critical that you are open to educating yourself. Research the cultural groups, ethnic groups, or religious groups that are prevalent in your area of practice and learn the best ways to communicate and facilitate optimal patient care. You may not get everything right when you encounter a person from another culture, but your efforts at communicating will reflect your respect, which makes a positive impression. Remember the importance of manners. Use phrases such as "Yes, sir," "No, ma'am," "Thank you," "Please," "Would you . . .," "Could you . . .," and "May I . . .." Regardless of culture, these phrases help instill confidence and help establish a professional relationship with your patient. If at any time you note that the patient becomes embarrassed or uncomfortable, adjust your approach, if possible, to help maintain the patient's dignity.

Finally, remember that manners, hand gestures, and body language have different meanings in different cultures. Try to develop a communication style that is free of mannerisms or gestures that can be misinterpreted or that have culture-specific meanings.

Special Challenges in History Taking

It is impossible to address every scenario you may encounter in your work as a paramedic. Nevertheless, certain challenges recur in history taking.

Silence

When you are obtaining your patient's history, do not let a period of silence from your patient make you uneasy. Your patient may be simply trying to gather his or her thoughts, trying to recall possibly distant details relative to the questions(s) you just asked, or trying to decide if he or she trusts you enough to answer your question(s) truthfully or at all.

Learn how to time your questions; ask, and then *wait*. What seems like an eternity to you is only 1 or 2 seconds to your patient.

Finally, patients may become silent when a paramedic displays a lack of sensitivity. If you cannot seem to determine the cause of your patient's silence, consider whether your manner could be silencing the patient, and adjust your approach.

Remain alert for nonverbal signs of distress. Pain, psychological distress, or fear often registers in body movements and facial expression. As you work in the field while you are a student, you will learn how to read the many nonverbal cues that patients give. The paramedics you work with will help, as will working with experienced caregivers in the emergency department and the hospital.

Overly Talkative Patients

Another challenge you will face will be patients who are overly talkative. Some people learn to talk endlessly as a way of socializing, but you must consider possible clinical reasons for the chattiness. Recovering from a fight-or-flight situation, consuming a triple espresso 15 minutes ago, or taking an illegal drug—cocaine, crack, or methamphetamine—might be the reason. Whatever the cause, the first requirement of dealing with a talkative patient is to again keep your patience. Try giving the patient free reign for the first few minutes. You might not be able to get as comprehensive a history as you would like with such a patient.

After a few minutes, try interrupting the patient to ask for clarification of a piece of information. This gives you an opportunity to quickly summarize what you have just heard.

Remember that there is a positive side to an overly talkative patient—you are better off with too much information than with too little or no information.

Patients With Multiple Symptoms

Although your calls would be much simpler if each of your patients had only a single complaint, that is not reality. Sometimes you will be presented with "linked" complaints such as "It feels like my heart is just fluttering, and I'm really dizzy." In this case, both symptoms can be tied to the patient having a high pulse rate and a falling blood pressure as a result.

On other occasions, especially with older patients, you may be dealing with multiple causes. A patient with diabetes who is having a cardiac crisis may easily forget that he or she has taken insulin and, therefore, take it again. One of the classic musts in EMS is to *always check the blood glucose level* on patients with *altered mentation*, whether they have a history of diabetes or not.

You need to learn to prioritize your patient's complaints. Only when that is accomplished can you develop an appropriate care plan as you decide which of your patient's problems you need to address and in which order you need to address them.

No matter how sure you are about your working diagnosis, *always* remain open to the possibility that something else is going on with your patient that you may need to address.

Anxious Patients

Although you may not want to believe it, you may be a cause of many of your patients being overly anxious. No matter how much the public loves to watch emergencies on television, it is frightening to see an ambulance, fire engine, or squad car pull up and stop in front of the house. You should expect your patient to initially be somewhat anxious, but he or she should start to calm down shortly after your arrival. If not, you'll need to consider other possibilities. High anxiety is an early sign of physiologic shock, which must be treated immediately. Alternatively, your patient could be hiding something, such as physical abuse or the use of illegal drugs.

Words of Wisdom

A common cause of anxiety is hypoxia, or low levels of oxygen in the blood. The patient may be sweaty and restless and become agitated easily. Hypoxia is often misinterpreted as panic.

Be sensitive to verbal and nonverbal clues, always keeping in mind that any information you fail to obtain could be the information you need to treat your patient.

Reassurance

When you are communicating with patients, you should be poised and confident, with a positive demeanor. With that positive demeanor also comes the temptation to reassure your patients, sometimes inappropriately. Be cautious about what you tell your patients so that you do not make promises you cannot deliver.

For example, you may be tempted to reassure a metal worker who caught his wedding ring on a piece of metal that a few stitches will be all that is needed in terms of treatment. In reality, many circumferential finger cuts can result in an amputation. Imagine how much distress you will cause your patient when he arrives at the hospital and receives news that is not so positive.

In addition, if your reassurance is inappropriate, your patient could choose not to share quite as much information as he or she might have under other circumstances, leaving you with less information rather than more.

Anger and Hostility

Frequently you will find yourself the target of patients' and family members' frustrations, which may manifest as anger or hostility. Anger and hostility at unfairness and harsh realities are normal. Remember, do not take these situations personally—take them professionally.

A valuable coping skill that you can use is not to get angry yourself. When you are in control of your own anger, you can work to calm the situation. Be attentive to changes in body language, such as threatening gestures or an escalating volume of the conversation or, worse yet, having a heated dialog melt down into an outright yelling match. When people are angry or hostile, the worst thing you can do is get angry yourself.

On any call, establishing a safe and secure scene is your first order of business. If you cannot calm the patient or family members, it is time to consider calling for law enforcement personnel. If the patient or a family member is hostile, you might need to tell the person directly that if he or she continues to shout, you will not feel safe enough to provide care to them and will need to seek the assistance of law enforcement personnel. However, if the patient and/or the family members are already angry, telling them that the police are on the way will not make them any happier. In worst case scenarios, you may have to withdraw to the safety of your ambulance to wait for the police to arrive.

Special Populations

Most patients are older than the paramedics taking care of them. They can feel threatened by strange "youngsters" telling them what is best for them. Listen and be respectful to your older patients. They often do know what is best for themselves.

If the hostile person suddenly leaves the room, especially in the middle of the conversation, you or your partner should follow the person, while working to calm him or her and defuse the situation. What you are also doing is making certain that the person does not go to another room, get a handgun or other weapon, and come back and shoot you, your partner, and maybe even the patient.

Intoxication

When your patient is intoxicated, whether from alcohol or drugs, obtaining a good medical history becomes difficult. Intoxication may mask symptoms, such as pain. With intoxication also comes a decrease in patience; while the patient is trying to explain things to you, his or her hostility or anger can escalate faster than if he or she were not intoxicated. A common scenario for this type of situation occurs at minor vehicle accidents, where the intoxicated person wants to get back in the car and continue on his or her way. The patient's behavior can become explosive. In such cases, do not aggravate the patient. Your ability to be patient and diplomatic is paramount in such potentially dangerous situations.

Dealing with intoxicated people can be frustrating for you; however, remain objective and nonjudgmental. Remember, you are there to provide help.

Crying

Sometimes people cry because they are happy or sad. Although these are certainly common reasons for crying, other possibilities exist.

When an unexpected event occurs, it can overwhelm people emotionally. Patients and their family members, along with their friends and neighbors, can suddenly find themselves under extreme levels of stress as a result of the emergency situation at hand. Just as some people react with anger and hostility to a stressful situation, others cry.

Once again, patience goes a long way. You cannot expect a person who is crying to immediately stop.

Fortunately, the presence of EMS arriving on the scene often exerts a calming effect. During the course of your career, you will be surprised at how often you hear someone say, usually the moment you walk in the door, "Thank goodness, the paramedics are here!" Collectively, your calm demeanor and patient approach; appropriate touch, such as a hand on the shoulder; and a quiet, "I'm in control now" tone of voice will help a person stop crying and allow you to begin your assessment and care.

Depression

Depression is a common reason for seeking medical attention. If a patient seems sad, hopeless, restless, and irritable; has sleep or eating disruptions; says that he or she feels his or her energy is low; or has pain for which you cannot find a source, consider that your patient might be depressed.

There are two basic types of depression: situational and chronic. Situational depression describes a reaction to a stressful event in a patient's life. Chronic depression is ongoing and does not seem to have an apparent cause.

Depression is a normal human response. In the case of situational depression, many people accept what has happened and begin to get on with their life again. However, sometimes this does not happen and they fall victim to chronic depression. Both forms of depression can lead to harmful behavior, including suicide.

You must ask about your patient's feelings to assess for risk of suicide. If the patient indicates that he or she could commit suicide, follow your protocol to ensure that this patient is connected to a mental health professional.

Sexually Attractive or Seductive Patients

It is not abnormal for clinicians and patients to be sexually attracted to each other. Although these feelings are normal, it is *never* appropriate for a clinician to act on them. If a patient becomes seductive or makes sexual advances, frankly but firmly make clear that your relationship is professional, rather than personal. Should this occur, try to keep your partner, a member of the law enforcement community, or a family member in the room with you at all times as a witness to any events that occur and a support person to help the patient recognize that the behavior is inappropriate.

Make absolutely certain that you do not cross the line that separates personal from professional behavior, and do not allow the patient to cross that line either.

Confusing Behaviors or Histories

Paramedics sometimes find that the patient's history given at the scene is different from the history the patient gives to the physician in the hospital emergency department. Sometimes the information is so different that it seems as if this is an entirely different patient. Patients may be too frightened or embarrassed to give particular information to a paramedic but will give a physician the vital information.

There are many other possibilities that can account for confusing behavior on the part of your patients, such as hypoxia, a toxic environment, a cerebrovascular accident (stroke), or transient ischemic attack. You will need to consider the possibility of mental illness or drug-induced delirium. In addition, organic causes such as Alzheimer disease, dementia, or a brain tumor can contribute to any discrepancies. The human brain is an impressive organ, but it may malfunction for any number of reasons. More often than not, the problem is related to glucose or oxygen, two fuels that are essential to the brain, though it can store neither of them.

Limited Education or Intelligence

Never, ever presume that you will not be able to obtain a history from a patient—any patient. Some patients will not have much knowledge of the health care system or its specialized vocabulary. Other patients will be developmentally challenged. Assume that you can get at least some worthwhile history from all patients. Assume that it is your job to keep asking questions in different ways until you get the answers you need.

Do not try to impress patients with medical terminology. Simple phrases will be much more readily understood. On the one hand, asking someone, "Do you think you are having an attack of unstable angina?" may get you little more than a blank stare in return. On the other hand, asking, "Are you having chest pain?" may get you just the information you need to proceed with caring for your patient.

With a skillful question and answer approach (and patience), you can frequently obtain adequate information from patients with limited education or intellectual capabilities. Be alert for partial answers to your questions or omissions. These are patients who commonly may not know or be able to recall the information you are requesting. For patients who are severely mentally challenged, you may need to get information from family members, friends, or another caregiver.

Language Barriers

The world has many groups of people who do not speak the primary language of the countries in which they live. But when they are sick, you will want to give them the best possible care **Figure 21**.

The first person to look to for help is someone who speaks your language and your patient's language—an interpreter.

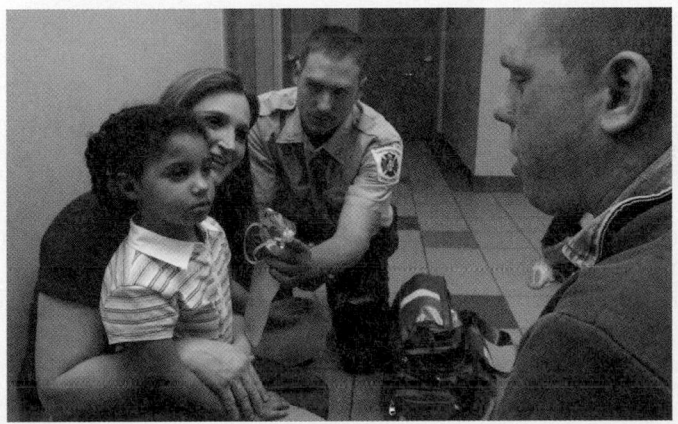

Figure 21 You will work with people of other cultures, which may require using an interpreter.

History Taking

(If there are large groups of people who speak one language in your service area, it would be wise to learn how to ask for an interpreter in that other language.) You must understand that using an interpreter comes with inherent risks, because ultimately, the interpreter acts as a filter. How a question is phrased can make a world of difference; therefore, it is best to ask closed questions that yield short answers. For example, "Are you having trouble breathing?" The tradeoff is that these types of questions do not yield large volumes of information; however, if you are thoughtful with your questions, and wait for the patient's reply, you should be able to extract what you need to provide care. Lastly, take a moment and remind the interpreter that he or she should not share this private information about the patient with anyone else.

Often, the only person available to interpret will be your patient's child—children absorb a new language quickly in their schools. However, if you can find someone older and not so intimately attached to your patient, it would be better for getting a good history. Keep your questions as straightforward as possible, and do your best not to scare a child.

Documentation and Communication

Be aware that medical terms and jargon often do not translate well, such as "ECG leads," "CAT scan," "JAWS," and "stool."

Maintaining patient confidentiality should be considered when selecting an appropriate interpreter. For this reason, using a certified medical interpreter is the preferred choice. Not only are certified interpreters trained in understanding medical terminology, they are also aware of patient confidentiality issues. Confidentiality may become a potential problem when choosing a family member or a bystander to interpret. The patient may not want certain medical information divulged through an interpreter. Therefore, every attempt should be made to find a qualified medical interpreter to make sure the patient's rights are not violated. Realistically, finding a medical interpreter in the EMS environment may not be practical, but it should be considered.

You must not, however, let a few broken words of yours be a substitute for an interpreter. Also understand that simply speaking louder during your questioning will not overcome a language barrier.

Hearing Problems

Another interesting challenge relates to working with patients with hearing problems. Hearing problems can range from a slight impairment to total deafness. For patients such as older people who may have only minimal impairment, speaking slowly and slightly louder may be all that is necessary. For people with a more severe problem, you may want to let them wear your stethoscope as you hold the bell and speak to them. If you do this, make sure to clean the earpieces before you offer them to the patient and before you put them back on.

When you are addressing patients who are totally deaf but who can read lips, address them face-to-face, slowing your speech slightly so that you are speaking clearly. With medical communications, however, you should find an interpreter who knows American Sign Language. Writing out medical communications is also a way of getting a patient history, but is very time-consuming.

On your successful completion of a paramedic program, two of the best investments in continuing education you can make for your future are learning conversational Spanish and learning sign language.

Visual Impairment or Blindness

Many patients with varying degrees of visual impairment are self-sufficient and live independent, productive lives. People who are blind have the greatest challenge. When you are interacting with a visually impaired or blind patient, first and foremost, be careful to announce yourself, giving your patient your identity and your reason for being there. If you pull up a chair to sit next to a blind patient, remember to put it back exactly where you found it; the same is true if furniture has to be moved to provide access or egress. Blind people who have their living environments situated the way they want it can get around with remarkable ease. Make sure you leave things the way you found them.

Words of Wisdom

Patients' medication(s), their living quarters, and the name of their doctor can often give clues about medical history. For example, insulin means the patient has diabetes; oxygen tanks and nebulizers in the house probably denote chronic lung disease; and the physician's name can be that of a specialist, like an oncologist or psychiatrist.

Once you move the visually impaired or blind patient to the ambulance, he or she is in a foreign environment and dependent on the EMS team for transport and assistance with an orderly transition into the emergency department. Be sure to tell the person what you are doing and the location of the transport vehicle at all times (for example, "We'll be at the hospital in about 10 minutes" or "We're at the hospital and will be wheeling you off the ambulance and into the emergency department in just a minute").

Family and Friends

Some patients might not be able to give you any or much information, and you will need to turn to their family and friends for assistance. Although you need the information to help your patient, be aware that the farther you go from the primary source, the greater the chance the information will contain inaccuracies. Like working with interpreters, family and friends often function as filters for information. Try to obtain accurate data when possible because it will then be easier for you to form an accurate working diagnosis and provide the best care possible.

Also, remember that you cannot reveal medical information about your patient to the family, so forming your questions will be difficult. However, obtaining information about your patient is critical, so work with people who can help your patients.

Age-Related Considerations
Pediatric Patients

The initial approach to any pediatric patient should be similar to that of an adult—with a few exceptions. You always begin with a scene size-up; assessment and treatment of life-threatening conditions affecting airway, breathing, and circulation; and forming a general impression and treatment strategy. There are differences, however, in the overall interaction you have with the patient and the parents.

Obtaining an accurate history of the present illness can be difficult in the pediatric population. Whereas every effort should be taken to include the child in the history-taking process, the most accurate and complete history will come from the parents or a responsible caregiver. Typically the parents are familiar with their children's habits and demeanor and know when something is wrong. Therefore, when a parent is showing signs of concern and tells you the child is not acting appropriately, you should listen.

Many times parents call for EMS out of fear for the welfare of their child. It is important for you as the health care provider to not only understand the fears the parents might have, but also continue to ascertain and investigate those fears in more detail. For instance, a febrile seizure in a pediatric patient is a fairly common entity encountered in EMS work and a relatively benign condition; however, for a new parent, it can be an emotionally traumatic event that creates all kinds of fears. Parents want to know what is wrong with their child and will typically go to sources like the Internet for answers. The problem with this approach is that it leaves a great deal to the imagination, and Internet sources are not always credible. Therefore, a parent of a child experiencing a febrile seizure is likely not just thinking about the immediate event, but is also worried about all of the possible causes of a seizure (eg, bleeding into the brain, brain tumors, cancer), when in reality it may be a benign condition. You need to be aware of these fears and take them into consideration when dealing with parents.

When you are obtaining information from the parent or caregiver, first begin by paying attention to the relationship between this person and the child. Typically, sick children cling to the parent or caregiver and are reluctant to allow a paramedic to examine them or remove them from the arms of the parent or caregiver. A child who readily allows you to remove him or her from the parent for examination should raise your concern about how sick the child actually is and should bring into consideration the possibility of neglect and/or abuse.

When you are obtaining a past medical history, your questions should be tailored to the age of the child. In neonates and infants, a maternal health history is important. You should ask questions about the mother's health status during pregnancy, the type of prenatal care provided, use of medications, hormones, and vitamins, and illicit drug or alcohol use during pregnancy. A birth history should also be obtained. You want to know about the duration of pregnancy, the location of the birth, labor conditions, any delivery complications, whether it was a vaginal or cesarean delivery, the condition of the infant at birth, and the birth weight.

History Taking

YOU *are the Medic*   PART 3

You immediately determine that the patient has the potential to deteriorate quickly. Your partner assembles the equipment necessary to stabilize the patient's spine. You determine that the patient is responsive, disoriented, and nonverbal. You cut the patient's shirt off and find an approximate 1" penetration on the left side of the chest just inferior to the center of the clavicle. The wound has stopped bleeding. You apply an occlusive dressing. The patient is breathing rapidly and appears to be very restless.

Recording Time: 5 Minutes

Respirations	28 breaths/min, shallow
Pulse	122 beats/min, weak
Skin	Cool, pale, dry
Blood pressure	90/64 mm Hg
Oxygen saturation (Spo$_2$)	93% on room air
Pupils	Equal and reactive

5. On the basis of your assessment of the ABCs, what is your first priority in the care of this patient?

6. Can you determine the priority of this patient at this point?

The first month following birth, otherwise known as the neonatal period, is also an important part of the pediatric history. Questions should be asked about congenital anomalies, feeding issues, the presence of jaundice, evidence of any illness, and developmental landmarks.

Around the age of 3 to 5 years, children become very capable of providing history of the current problem. Once in school, the focus of questioning should change based on the age of the child. Asking about the child's performance in school helps to determine whether there are any developmental problems or learning disabilities. Questioning should also focus on the child's dentition, growth, sexual development, illnesses, and immunizations.

Once the child moves into the adolescent phase of development, you should now focus more on the adolescent in the history taking, and less on the parent. Adolescents struggle for independence and understand they are in charge of their bodies. Gathering your history from the adolescent helps to establish trust and a good rapport. As the line of questioning for an adolescent becomes more private, consider interviewing the patient in a more private location. Questioning should focus on risk-taking behaviors, self-esteem issues, rebelliousness, drug and alcohol use, and sexual activity. Some of these patients may be reluctant to discuss these issues with you, which is why establishing trust and rapport is so important.

In addition to gathering information about the child, make sure you gather an accurate family history. Specifically ask questions about maternal gestational history and any deceased siblings. Ask about the personal social status of the family and the conditions of the home.

A review of systems should also be included in the pediatric history. While every system should be covered, attention should be made toward the skin for any lesions; the ears for any history of otitis media (inner ear infections); the nose for any snoring, mouth breathing, and environmental allergies; and the teeth for dental issues.

Geriatric Patients

Geriatric patients can pose a rather different challenge for paramedics. This patient population is growing and frequently represents the primary customer for EMS. It brings with it a variety of medical and traumatic issues not seen in other patients. You need to have a fundamental knowledge of geriatric patients and be prepared to deal with this population on a daily basis.

As people begin to age, the senses become dull, particularly hearing and vision. Thus an elderly patient may have difficulty hearing your questions during the patient assessment. If the patient has eyeglasses or a hearing aid, make sure these aids are available during the interview. You may need to speak a little more slowly and louder when you are treating these patients; however, do not assume that all elderly patients have difficulty hearing. In addition, it may be helpful to face your patient when asking questions in case the patient reads lips to help with communication. Accommodating these sensory losses can improve the information gathered during the patient assessment.

Geriatric patients tend to have multiple chronic medical problems that can occasionally complicate the history-taking process. Multiple chief complaints can make it difficult for you to decipher between what is an acute complaint versus a chronic complaint. In addition, these patients often take a multitude of prescription and nonprescription medications that may contribute to their various complaints. It is a recognized pharmacologic phenomenon that any patient taking five or more drugs likely has some form of drug interaction. These **iatrogenic** illnesses caused by medications can mask other conditions that may need immediate medical attention. Accidental overdoses and adverse drug reactions are also a common issue in the geriatric population. You need to gather an accurate medication history along with current dosages to assist other health care providers with continued care of the patient.

Disease symptoms may become less dramatic in the older patient. As the body ages, responses to things like shock and pain are often dulled. This can complicate the assessment process because these patients frequently do not exhibit the "textbook" response to some illnesses. Their symptoms may be vague and nonspecific, especially in postmenopausal women having myocardial infarction. You should always have a high clinical index of suspicion when treating the elderly and must always consider the worst-case scenario.

You should consider including a functional assessment during the systems review in the elderly patient with an apparent disability. This typically includes assessment of mobility at home and in the community, upper extremity function and limitations, and activities of daily living. Physicians will typically assess instrumental activities of daily living (IADLs) when examining an elderly patient. This includes assessment of items like getting dressed, bathing, and cooking, and may even extend to areas like financial management and shopping. You can assist in this process by assessing some of these functions in the field; this evaluation should be part of the assessment of patients in both stable and unstable condition as time allows.

Patient Assessment

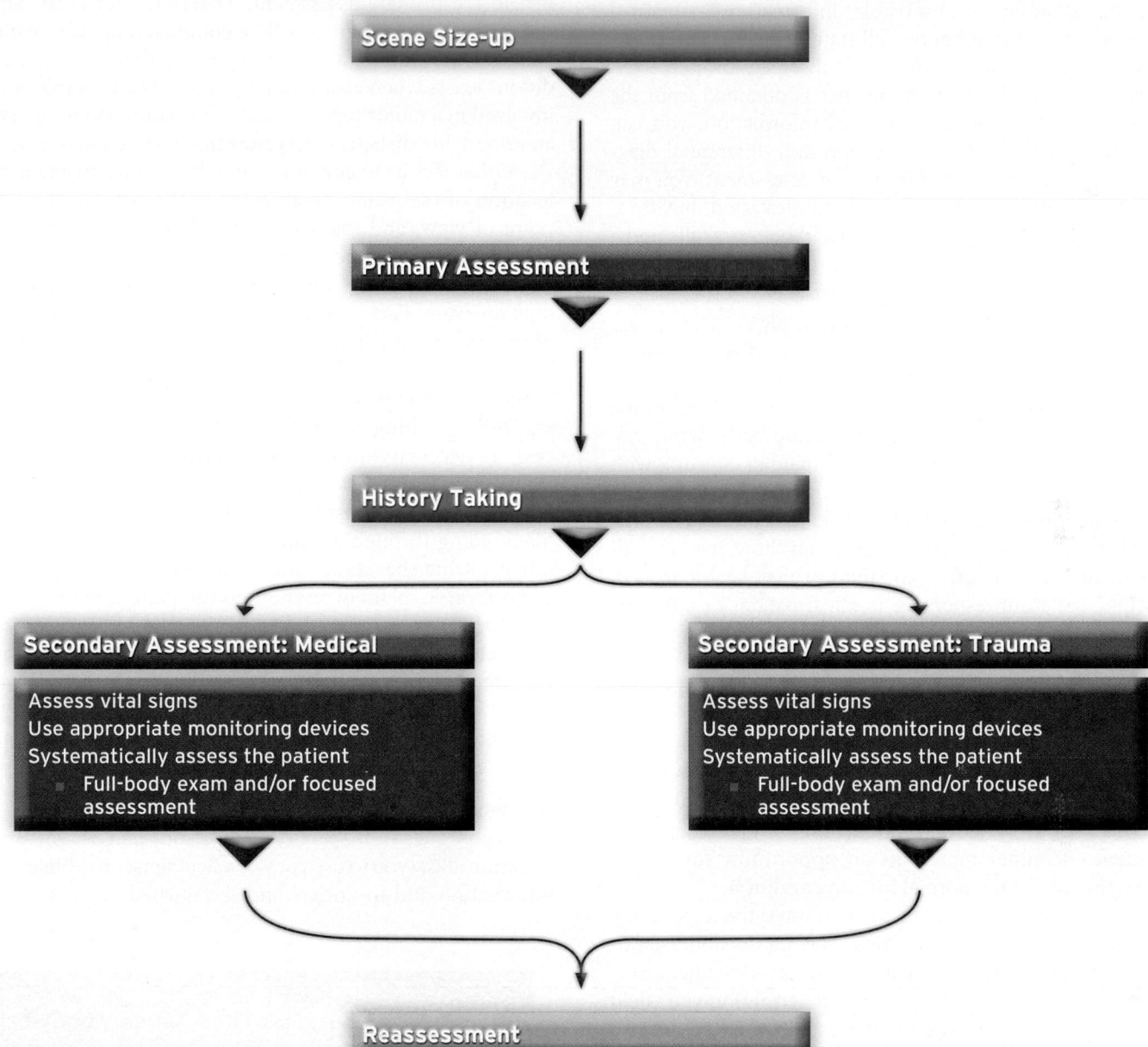

Scene Size-up

Primary Assessment

History Taking

Secondary Assessment: Medical

Assess vital signs
Use appropriate monitoring devices
Systematically assess the patient
  - Full-body exam and/or focused
    assessment

Secondary Assessment: Trauma

Assess vital signs
Use appropriate monitoring devices
Systematically assess the patient
  - Full-body exam and/or focused
    assessment

Reassessment

■ Secondary Assessment

Secondary assessment is the process by which quantifiable, objective (based on fact or observable) information is obtained from a patient about his or her overall state of health. This information is compared with subjective (observed or perceived by the patient), historic information that is obtained from the patient. Armed with these two types of information, you can obtain a comprehensive field impression and differential diagnosis of the patient. While performing an assessment, you may see the patient's condition as a clinical manifestation; however, a caring and empathetic approach will yield better results and a more accurate evaluation. Likewise, putting forth a professional appearance and demeanor will instill trust and confidence in your patient as to your abilities as a care provider.

The secondary assessment (also known as physical examination) consists of two elements—obtaining vital signs that measure overall body function and performing a head-to-toe survey that evaluates the workings of specific body organ systems. This survey is done in a sequential manner, starting with the head, moving down to the toes, ensuring that every aspect of the body's function is evaluated. Of course, the conditions in the prehospital setting may determine precisely how the secondary assessment is performed. Sometimes, it may be condensed. For example, for an unresponsive medical patient or a trauma patient with a significant MOI, there may only be time to perform a rapid exam.

The overall patient assessment is intended to determine whether a problem exists, so that actions can be taken to manage that problem. Before you can appreciate abnormalities on examination, you must understand the wide variety of normal presentations. This is something that can be learned only through direct hands-on experience and interaction with patients. Thus every patient encounter represents an opportunity for you to gain experience about the normal human condition.

As you approach your patient, keep in mind the major body systems and their anatomic locations. Having an understanding of anatomy and physiology will be a tremendous help during the assessment and will help you in determining your field impression. For example, when you are palpating the chest it is important to remember the heart, lungs, great vessels, and the esophagus are located in that anatomic region and should be considered when a patient complains of pain to that area. In addition, an understanding of the gastrointestinal system and the location of specific organs in the abdominal cavity can help narrow down a differential diagnosis.

As stated earlier, the general approach to examining a patient should be completed systematically. However, the actual start of your examination is determined by several factors, such as the stability of the patient, the chief complaint, the history, and the communication ability of the patient. A patient who complains of isolated ankle pain does not necessarily warrant an exam that begins with assessment of the head. With that said, a multisystem trauma patient may require an examination that includes a rapid exam from head-to-toe from the beginning of the assessment. Some patients, depending on their level of stability, may never get a complete assessment because you will be too busy managing the life-threatening injuries identified in the primary assessment. Therefore, not every aspect of the secondary assessment will be completed in every patient. In addition, the additional challenge of underlying co-medical conditions exists when examining a patient. For example, a patient involved in a motor vehicle crash who is unresponsive may have an underlying diabetic emergency that resulted in the crash.

Other factors to consider when beginning an exam include location of the exam, positioning of the patient, the patient's point of view, and maintaining professionalism. Always consider your environment when examining a patient and ask yourself if this is the most appropriate environment to conduct an exam. Factors such as noise, lighting, and the position of the patient might hinder your assessment. In addition, the patient's privacy should always be considered, not only because of the need to expose your patient, but also to inhibit bystanders from watching and listening during the examination process. If necessary and feasible, move the patient to a more private location, such as the ambulance, before conducting an in-depth secondary assessment. Remember that the patient is likely going through an emotional and traumatic event. Your touch during the examination will contribute to the patient's stress level. Explain everything to the patient before you actually perform the exam to help alleviate the patient's stress. This will help to establish a level of professionalism and show that you are attentive to the patient's needs. Keep in mind that most people do not care for physical examinations, so being kind, professional, and compassionate will go a long way toward calming their anxiety and fears.

Assessment Techniques

The techniques of inspection, palpation, percussion, and auscultation allow you to use your physical senses to obtain physical information and to understand the normal (versus abnormal)

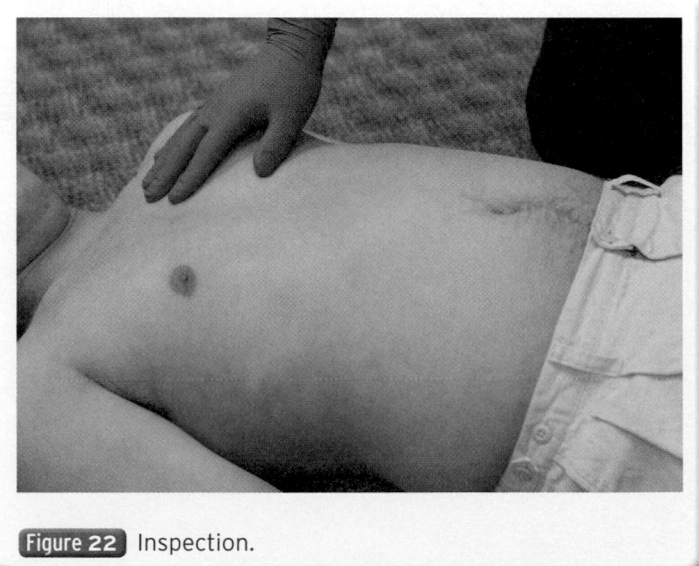

Figure 22   Inspection.

functions of a patient's body. __Inspection__ involves looking at the patient, either in general or at a specific area (ie, a patient's overall appearance from the doorway versus looking specifically at the chest wall for abnormalities/deformities) **Figure 22**. __Palpation__ is physical touching for the purpose of obtaining information—for example, tenderness (elicited pain), deformity, crepitance, masses, pulse quality, and abnormal organ enlargement **Figure 23**. You will typically use your fingertips to check pulses, but will use your palms to sweep across and around the skull to assess structural integrity as well as to assess for defects, ie, knots or dents. Use the back of your hand to touch a patient's skin for fever assessment, because it is more sensitive than your palm.

Various techniques of palpation are used to examine specific areas. Palpation with the hands and fingertips is typically performed on the chest, abdomen, and extremities. This can be accomplished by keeping your hand and forearm on a horizontal plane, with fingers together and flat on the patient, and palpating with a sliding or dipping motion depending on the area being examined. Palpation with fingertips may be reserved for examining the distal extremities, the head, and the neck. The ulnar surface of the hand is commonly used when examining the abdomen. Some patients will immediately tense their abdominal muscles during the exam, regardless of whether there is pain. When you use only the ulnar surface of one hand, the exam seems less intrusive to the patient and the results are more likely to be accurate. Palpation with the dorsal aspect of the hand can be used in the same manner as the ulnar surface. This technique is also used when assessing skin temperature.

__Percussion__ entails gently striking the surface of the body, typically where it overlies various body cavities. This technique allows you to detect changes in the densities of the underlying structures. For example, percussion of a normal lung will yield medium to loud, low-pitched, resonant sounds. Percussion sounds over muscle and bone should be soft, high-pitched, and flat. Percussion sounds over hollow organs such as the intestines are often described as loud, high-pitched, and tympanic (like a drum).

Percussion is a skill that requires a lot of practice to perfect. An internist who performs this skill a dozen times a day becomes competent quickly. By comparison, percussion is rarely done in the field and as such, is a minimally developed skill for most providers. Follow the steps in **Skill Drill 2**:

Skill Drill   2

1. Place your nondominant hand lightly against the surface to be examined (Step 1).
2. Hyperextend the middle finger and apply firm pressure to the surface to be percussed (Step 2).
3. Directly strike the middle phalanx of the middle finger with one or two fingertips of the other hand (Step 3).
4. Apply the same force over each area of the body to accurately compare the sounds produced by percussion.

__Auscultation__ involves listening with a stethoscope. The body generates a variety of high- and low-frequency sounds—both normal and abnormal—that can be detected via auscultation. Bowel sounds can be assessed via auscultation, as can lung sounds. Appreciating the presence of and differences in auscultated sounds requires keen attention, a thorough understanding of what "normal" sounds like, and lots of practice.

Vital Signs

Vital signs consist of a measurement of pulse rate, rhythm, and quality; respiratory rate, rhythm, and quality; blood pressure; temperature; and pulse oximetry. Other than overall patient appearance, vital signs provide the most objective data for determining patient status. Their measurement requires you to use the techniques of auscultation, palpation, and inspection.

Words of Wisdom

When done properly, palpation should never cause harm. Deep palpation is rarely done in EMS, and requires practice and knowing when to stop.

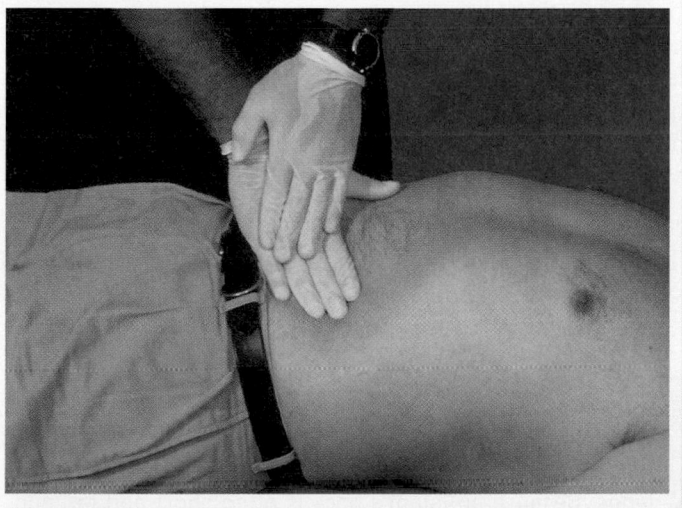

Figure 23 Palpation.

Words of Wisdom

There are important differences between the bell and diaphragm of the stethoscope. The bell is cup-shaped and is used to listen for deep and low-pitched sounds (heart sounds). It is placed lightly on the skin, just enough to make a seal. The diaphragm is flat-shaped and is used to listen for high-pitched sounds (breath, bowel, and normal heart sounds); it is placed firmly on the skin.

Secondary Assessment

Skill Drill   2

Performing Percussion

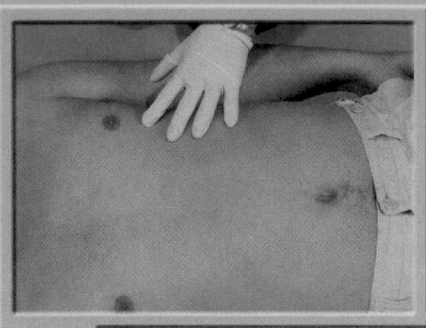

Step 1 Place your hand lightly against the surface to be examined.

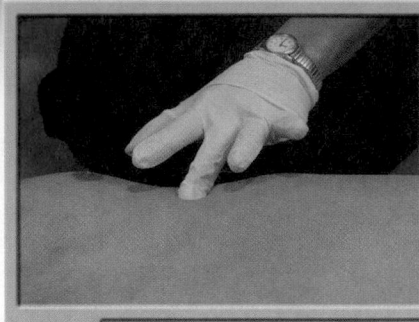

Step 2 Hyperextend the middle finger and apply firm pressure.

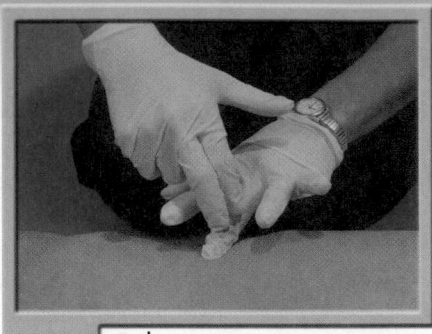

Step 3 Strike the middle finger with one or two fingertips of the other hand.

Words of Wisdom

Be aware that the patient's age, underlying physical and mental conditions, and current medications can affect the patient's vital signs. Like any other assessment tool, consider the vital signs but devote your attention to the patient's presentation.

Vital signs are aptly named; strict attention should be paid to the assessment of these critically important parameters. Normal limits can vary depending on several factors, including age and medication use, and vital signs should be interpreted with those factors in mind. Vital signs should be obtained both accurately and serially to help determine overall stability of the patient. Because vital signs can change dramatically over relatively short time periods, failing to check them frequently, especially in the context of a significantly ill or injured patient, can lead to poor patient care.

Pulse

<u>Pulse</u> measurements should assess the rate, presence, location, quality, and regularity of the pulses. To palpate the pulse,

gently compress an artery against a bony prominence, which allows you to feel the pressure wave generated by the heart's contraction. Pulses can be obtained at several points in the body, including the radial, brachial, femoral, and carotid arteries **Figure 24**. When you are formally counting the pulse rate, time the pulses for a minimum of 15 seconds and then multiply by 4 to obtain the rate per minute. Palpating a pulse is a basic way to evaluate cardiac output. EMS providers should compare proximal and distal pulses during patient evaluations.

Although it is appropriate to check for the presence of a central pulse in an unresponsive patient, the actual pulse rate should be counted in the most peripheral location that can be palpated. In the responsive patient, you may want to determine the respiratory rate while you appear to be checking the pulse; this may decrease the tendency of patients to inadvertently alter their breathing pattern or rate when they become aware of being evaluated.

Respiration

The respiratory rate is typically measured by inspection of the patient's chest, but overall respiratory effort can be assessed

Words of Wisdom

Whenever possible, avoid taking a blood pressure on a painful/injured extremity, on an arm with an arteriovenous shunt or fistula, or on a postmastectomy side. This can cause pain and/or result in inaccurate readings.

Special Populations

Palpating the pulse in an infant often presents a real challenge. Because an infant's neck is often short and fat, and the pulse is quite fast, you may have a hard time finding the carotid pulse. Therefore, in infants younger than 1 year, you should palpate the brachial artery to assess the pulse.

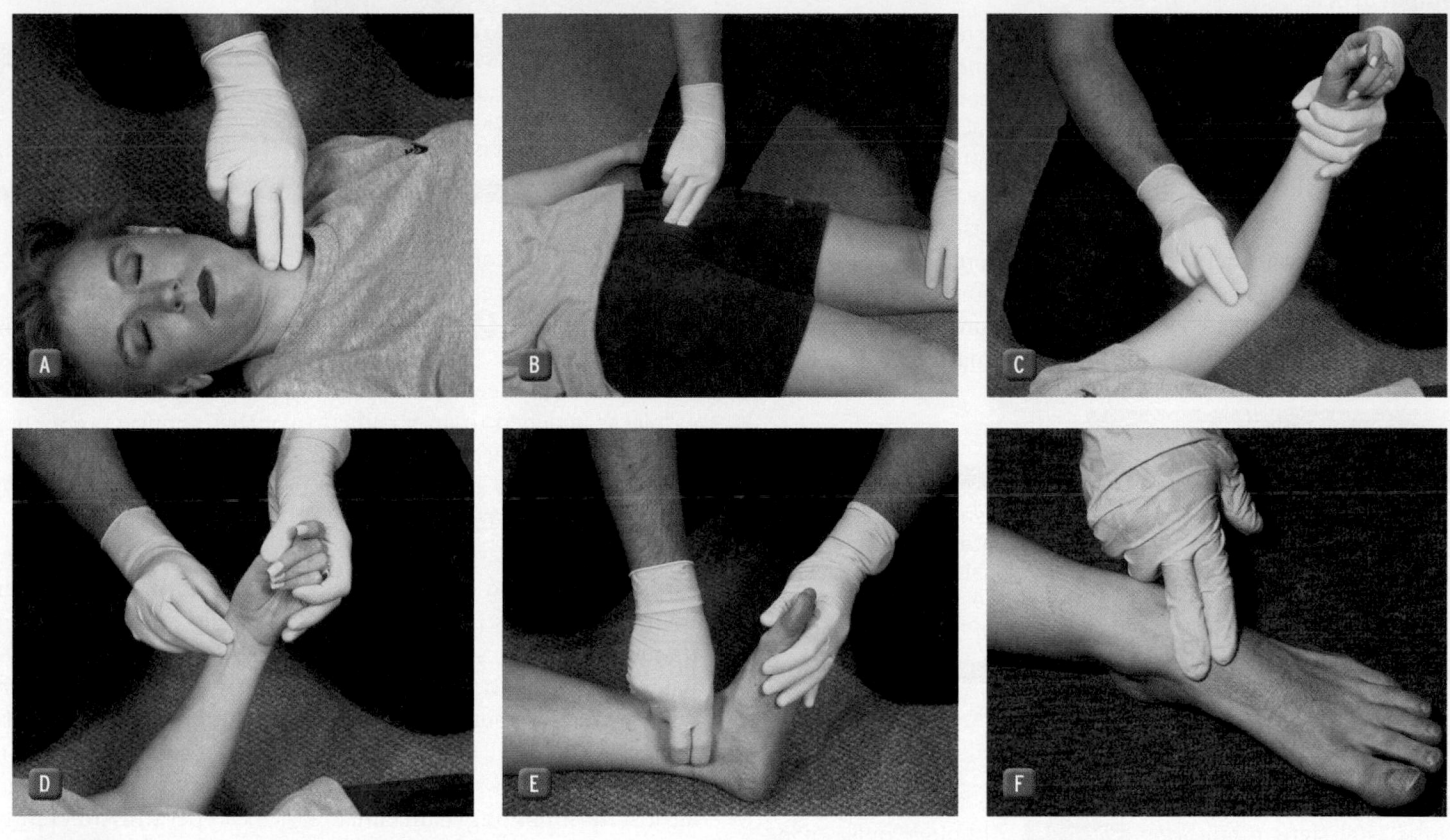

Figure 24 Common pulse points. **A.** Carotid pulse. **B.** Femoral pulse. **C.** Brachial pulse. **D.** Radial pulse. **E.** Posterior tibial pulse. **F.** Dorsalis pedis pulse.

by visualizing portions of the abdominal wall, neck, face, and accessory muscle use. Although the absolute respiratory rate is important, the quality of the respiratory effort should be evaluated as well. You should also learn to recognize pathologic respiratory patterns or rhythms (eg, tachypnea, Kussmaul, Cheyne-Stokes, and Biot breathing). Similarly, you should recognize when patients exhibit tripod positioning, accessory muscle use, or retractions. This information is especially critical in the assessment of pediatric patients. The respiratory rate should be measured for a minimum of 30 seconds, and then multiplied by 2 to obtain the rate per minute for pediatric patients. Assessment of work of breathing in a pediatric patient is one of the single most predictive signs available; therefore, when you see a child with excessive work of breathing who begins to show the signs of ventilator fatigue, a physiologic collapse is usually moments away.

Blood Pressure

<u>Blood pressure</u> is the measurement of the force exerted against the walls of the blood vessels. It is commonly measured in a peripheral artery, although it can be obtained essentially anywhere in the circulatory system. Blood pressure is the product of cardiac output and peripheral vascular resistance, so it includes two components: systolic pressure and diastolic pressure. <u>Systolic pressure</u> is created by the left ventricle while it is contracting (ie, in systole). <u>Diastolic pressure</u> is the result of

residual pressure in the system while the left ventricle is relaxing (ie, in diastole). Normally, diastolic pressure should not go to zero, because peripheral vascular resistance in the arteriolar side of the circulatory system should continually provide for a diastolic pressure. The coronary arteries receive blood flow by this mechanism, so lower diastolic pressure means less myocardial perfusion.

Words of Wisdom

Many patients exhibit an increase in blood pressure due to anxiety and the stress of an acute injury or illness. Look at your patient as well as trends in vital signs before concluding that the blood pressure is truly abnormal.

Blood pressure must be measured using a cuff that is appropriate to the patient's size and habitus (physique or body build). Too small or tight a cuff will yield an artificially high pressure; too large or loose a cuff will give inappropriately low results. Although blood pressure ideally should be auscultated, it can be palpated to estimate the systolic pressure but this introduces more margin of error. Periodic inspection of the blood pressure cuff's gauge is important because it can lose accuracy and require recalibration.

Secondary Assessment

Temperature

Many methods can be used to evaluate body temperature. If you use a device for measuring the tympanic membrane temperature in order to obtain a patient's body temperature, be aware of extrinsic factors that may increase or decrease the temperature reading. Make sure the external auditory canal is free of cerumen (ear wax), which can lower the temperature reading. Position the probe in the canal so that the infrared beam is aimed at the tympanic membrane (otherwise the measurement will be invalid). Wait 2 to 3 seconds until the digital temperature reading appears. This method measures core body temperature, which is higher than the normal oral temperature by approximately 1.4°F (0.8°C).

Words of Wisdom

The accuracy of tympanic membrane temperatures has been called into question by some data, especially in patients with severe infections. If your patient looks sick, feels warm, and the tympanic membrane temperature is "normal," consider using a different type of thermometer.

Pulse Oximetry

Arterial oxygen saturation determination made via **pulse oximetry** has earned a place in emergency health care as part of regular vital signs monitoring **Figure 25**. Although pulse oximetry is a valuable tool, it should never be used as an absolute indicator of the need for oxygen therapies. Pulse oximetry measures the percentage of hemoglobin saturation and can provide inaccurate information in certain situations. You need to understand potential limitations with pulse oximetry to appropriately process the information it provides. Inaccurate readings may be obtained for a variety of reasons—for example, a hypotensive or hypothermic patient, carbon monoxide poisoning, abnormal hemoglobin (ie, sickle cell disease or anemia), vascular dyes, patient motion, incorrect placement, and even certain types of nail polish.

Equipment Used in the Secondary Assessment

Equipment used to perform the secondary assessment includes a stethoscope, blood pressure cuff (sphygmomanometer),

Words of Wisdom

Remember to look at your patient, not the "number." If the patient looks sick but the pulse oximetry reading is "normal," then the patient is still sick.

capnography, glucometry, ophthalmoscope, otoscope, scissors, a reliable light source, gloves, and a sheet or blanket.

Stethoscopes **Figure 26** are available in two forms: acoustic and electronic. Today's acoustic stethoscope, which is the most commonly seen in the prehospital setting, consists of two earpieces attached to an air-filled tube that connects to a chest piece. The chest piece has two sides—a diaphragm (plastic disk) and a bell (hollow cup)—that can be placed against the patient to sense sounds. The diaphragm is vibrated by the sounds of the body, which are then transmitted up to the stethoscope's earpieces; thus the diaphragm side is used to pick up higher-frequency sounds. The bell, which usually transmits lower-frequency sounds, senses the sounds directly off the skin of the patient. Some stethoscopes have attenuated diaphragms, meaning they have an outer metal ring and another ring closer to the center of the head. Pushing lightly on the head allows you to listen to one set of sounds. Pressing firmly seats the diaphragm against the inner ring, which makes the head perform differently.

The acoustic stethoscope does not amplify sounds; rather, it simply blocks out ambient noises, allowing you to hear and appreciate the sounds of the body. In contrast, the electronic stethoscope converts the acoustic sound waves into an electronic signal that is then amplified.

The **sphygmomanometer**, or blood pressure cuff, is used in the measurement of the patient's blood pressure **Figure 27**. The traditional device consists of an inflatable cuff, which occludes blood flow, and a manometer (pressure meter), which is used to determine the pressure in the artery at various points in the secondary assessment. These two components are connected via tubing. In manual cuffs, a separate tube connects to an inflation bulb.

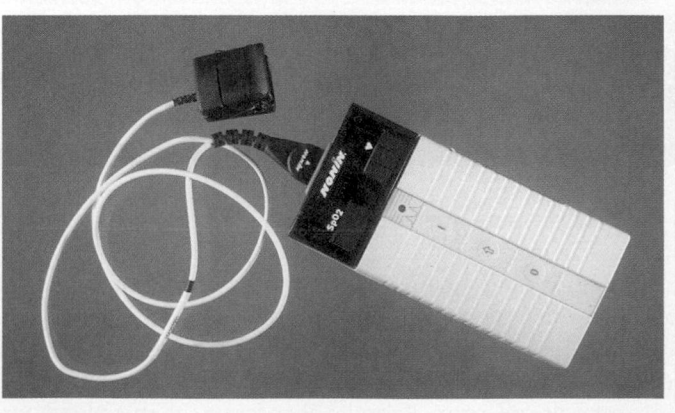

Figure 25 A pulse oximeter.

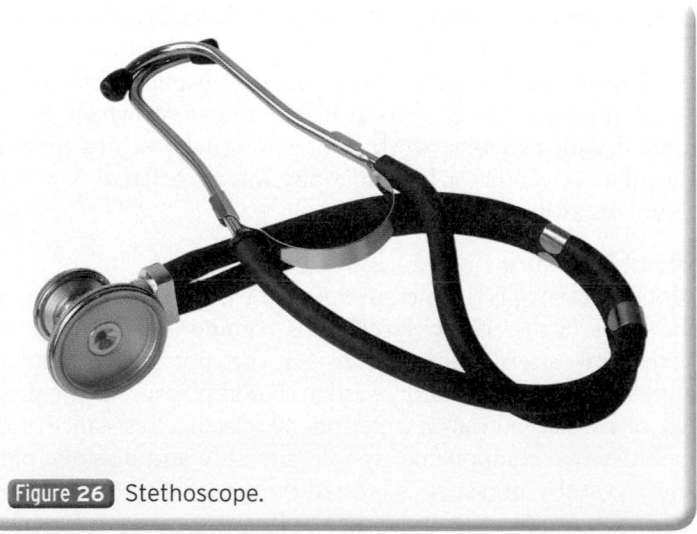

Figure 26 Stethoscope.

There are also bladderless blood pressure cuffs on the market as well, though they can be uncomfortable against bare skin.

Many sizes of blood pressure cuffs are available, and using the appropriate size for the patient is essential to obtain an accurate reading. The cuff should be one half to two thirds the size of the upper arm. The blood pressure measurement is separated into systolic and diastolic pressures and is reported in millimeters of mercury (mm Hg).

The <u>ophthalmoscope</u> allows you to look into a patient's eyes and view the retina and aqueous fluid. This tool consists of a concave mirror and a battery-powered light, which is usually contained in the device's handle **Figure 28**. You look through a monocular eyepiece that is usually equipped with a rotating disk of lenses; selection of a lens allows for adjustment of the depth and magnification. Use of the ophthalmoscope is usually reserved for hospital and physician's office examination because effective evaluation requires dilation of the patient's pupils with medication and a lot of diagnostic expertise to be able to accurately determine what you are looking at and what it means clinically.

The <u>otoscope</u> is used to evaluate the ears of a patient. This instrument consists of a head and a handle. The head contains an electric light source and a low-power magnifying lens. The front of the headpiece has an attachment for a disposable plastic earpiece (speculum). The examiner inserts the speculum into the ear and looks through a lens on the rear of the headpiece. Some otoscopes include a sliding rear window that allows for the insertion of an additional instrument (eg, to remove ear wax). Most have an insertion point for a bulb that is used to push air into the ear canal, allowing the examiner to visualize the movement of the tympanic membrane. The rechargable batteries are located in the handle unless it is a wall-mounted unit, such as those found in a physician's office.

The Physical Examination

Remember that as soon as you approach the scene, you will already begin to gain information regarding the patient's overall presentation **Figure 29**. A patient lying on the ground on a rainy, cool evening should be considered hypothermic until proven otherwise. A quick look at the environment in which the patient is found and the general appearance of the patient provides a substantial amount of information before you begin to speak.

Look for signs of significant distress such as mental status changes, anxiousness, labored breathing, difficulty speaking, diaphoresis, obvious pain, obvious deformity, and guarding or splinting of a painful area. It is not uncommon for persons experiencing substantial and incapacitating pain to present with a quiet and still affect.

Other aspects that may be readily apparent and worth noting include dress, hygiene, expression, overall size, posture, untoward odors, and overall state of health. When you are characterizing the overall state of the patient, be sure to use appropriate terms to describe the degree of distress: no apparent distress, mild (slight or not harsh), moderate (small or average), acute (very great or bad), and severe (dangerous or difficult to endure). Other acceptable terms to describe the general state of a patient's health include chronically ill, frail, feeble, robust, and vigorous.

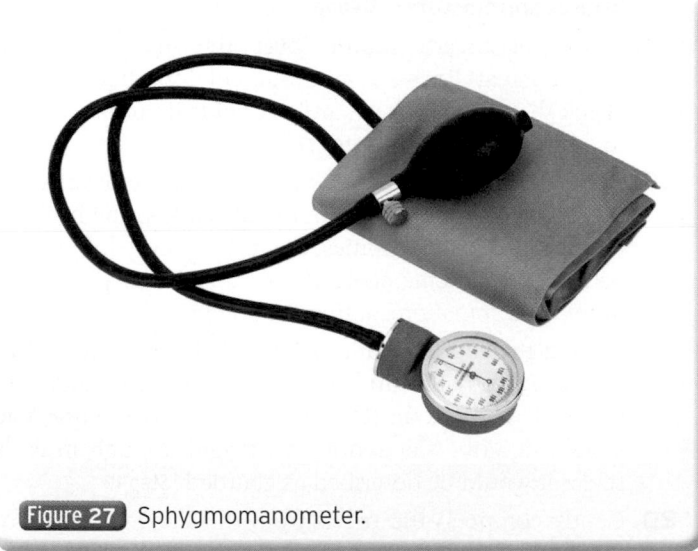

Figure 27 Sphygmomanometer.

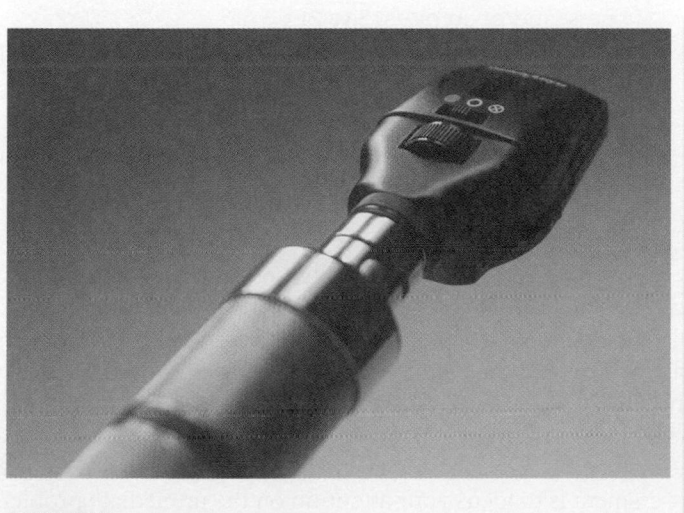

Figure 28 Ophthalmoscope.

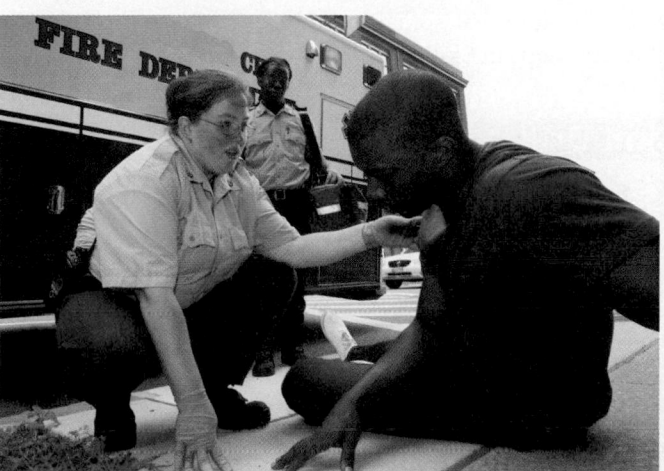

Figure 29 Get a general impression of the overall situation as you approach the patient.

The physical examination of a patient in the prehospital setting is the most important skill a health care provider can master. This ability is first developed as an EMT and should be refined as an advanced practitioner. Establishing vascular access, administering medications, and performing endotracheal intubation are mechanical skills that require extensive practice to achieve proficiency. By comparison, the skills of patient assessment and interpreting the findings of a physical examination truly separate the accomplished paramedic from the basic provider. The physical examination consists of a comprehensive review of systems to determine the nature and extent of the patient's illness or injury.

The secondary assessment should be driven by the information you gathered during the primary assessment and the history-taking phase. For a patient who tells you, "I just can't catch my breath," assessment of breath sounds early on is a must. If the patient tells you, "My leg feels numb," assessment of pulse, motor function, and sensation in the affected and unaffected extremities is indicated. You need to exercise good judgment to make the best use of your time. Do not waste time palpating a patient's abdomen or auscultating heart sounds if the person reports knee pain. In general, the care you provide for a responsive medical patient will be driven by your local protocols in conjunction with your consultation with the base station physician.

The Full-Body Exam

The **full-body exam** is a systematic head-to-toe examination. Like the rapid exam, the full-body exam includes both looking and palpating. The goal of this process is to identify hidden injuries or identify causes that may not have been found during the 60- to 90-second rapid exam that took place during the primary assessment. Any patient who has sustained a significant MOI, is unresponsive, or is in critical condition should receive this type of examination. An unresponsive patient is unable to tell you what is wrong; therefore, this type of examination may give you clues to identify the problem.

To perform a full-body exam of a patient with no suspected spinal injuries, follow the steps in `Skill Drill 3`. To perform a full-body exam in which the patient has sustained significant trauma, be sure that spinal immobilization is still in place and follow the steps in Skill Drill 3:

Skill Drill   3

1. Look at the face for obvious lacerations, bruises, fluids, and deformities `Step 1`.
2. Inspect the area around the eyes and eyelids `Step 2`.
3. Examine the eyes for redness and for contact lenses. Assess the pupils using a penlight `Step 3`.
4. Look behind the patient's ears to assess for bruising (the Battle sign) `Step 4`.
5. Use the penlight to look for drainage of spinal fluid or blood in the ears `Step 5`.
6. Look for bruising and lacerations about the head. Palpate for tenderness, depressions of the skull, and deformities `Step 6`.

7. Palpate the zygomas for tenderness, symmetry, and instability `Step 7`.
8. Palpate the maxillae `Step 8`.
9. Check the nose for blood and drainage `Step 9`.
10. Palpate the mandible `Step 10`.
11. Assess the mouth and nose for cyanosis, foreign bodies (including loose or broken teeth or dentures), bleeding, lacerations, and deformities `Step 11`.
12. Check for unusual odors on the patient's breath `Step 12`.
13. Look at the neck for obvious lacerations, bruises, and deformities. Observe for jugular venous distention and/or tracheal deviation `Step 13`.
14. Palpate the front and the back of the neck for tenderness and deformity `Step 14`.
15. Look at the chest for obvious signs of injury before you begin palpation. Be sure to watch for movement of the chest with respirations `Step 15`. Assess the work of breathing.
16. Gently palpate over the ribs to assess structural integrity and elicit tenderness. Avoid pressing over obvious bruises and fractures `Step 16`.
17. Listen for breath sounds over the midaxillary and midclavicular lines—a minimum of four fields if you check the anterior chest, and six fields if you are assessing the posterior chest `Step 17`.
18. Lung assessment must include the bases and apices of the lungs `Step 18`. At this point, also assess the back for tenderness and deformities, so that you only log roll the patient once. Remember, if you suspect a spinal cord injury, use spinal precautions as you log roll the patient.
19. Look at the abdomen and pelvis for obvious lacerations, bruises, and deformities. Gently palpate the abdomen for tenderness. If the abdomen is unusually tense, you should describe the abdomen as rigid, though in early stages it would be described as guarded `Step 19`.
20. Gently compress the pelvis from the sides to assess for tenderness `Step 20`.
21. Gently press the iliac crests to elicit instability, tenderness, and/or crepitus `Step 21`.
22. Inspect all four extremities for lacerations, bruises, swelling, deformities, and medical alert anklets or bracelets. Also assess distal pulses and motor and sensory function in all extremities `Step 22`. Compare right and left sides whenever possible.

The Focused Assessment

A **focused assessment** is generally performed on patients who have sustained nonsignificant MOIs and on responsive medical patients. This type of examination is based on the chief complaint. For example, in a person reporting a headache, you should carefully and systematically assess the head and/or the neurologic system. A person with a laceration on the arm may need to only have that arm evaluated. The goal of a focused assessment is to focus your attention on the immediate problem. `Table 4` gives examples of common chief complaints and their corresponding focused assessment.

Skill Drill | 3

Performing the Full-Body Exam

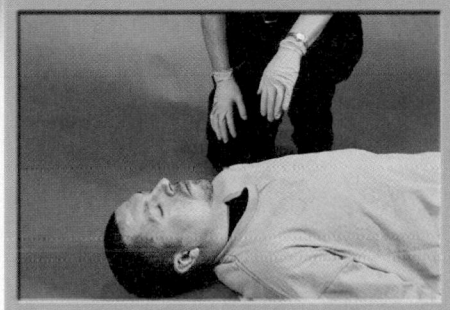

Step 1 Observe the face.

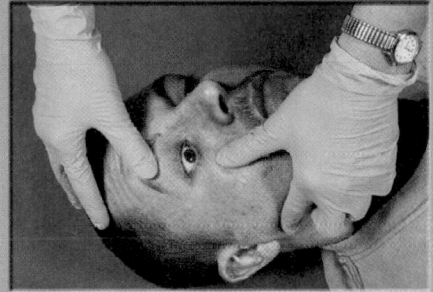

Step 2 Inspect the area around the eyes and eyelids.

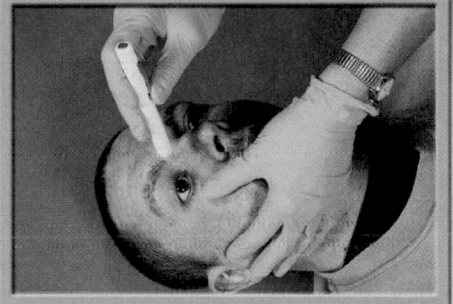

Step 3 Examine the eyes for redness and contact lenses. Check pupil function.

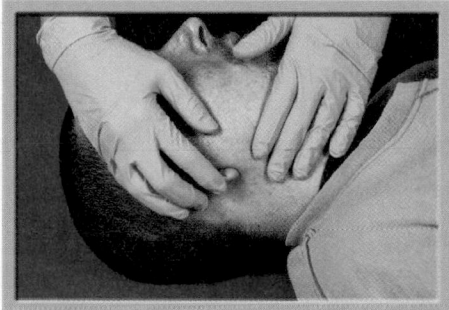

Step 4 Look behind the ears for the Battle sign.

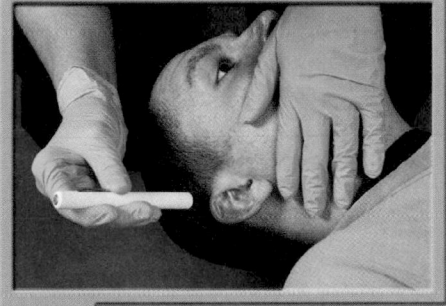

Step 5 Check the ears for drainage or blood.

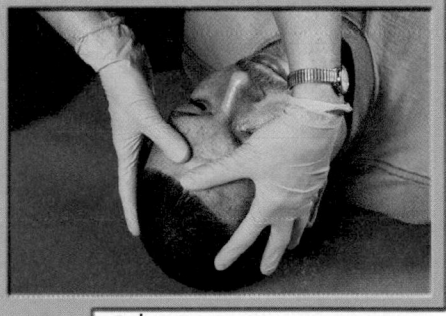

Step 6 Observe and palpate the entire surface of head.

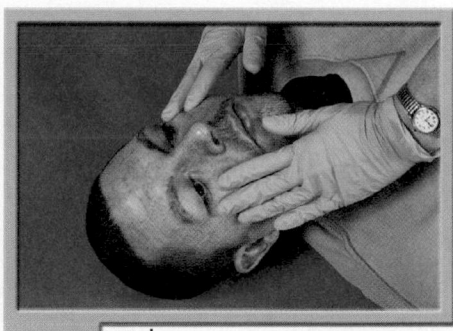

Step 7 Palpate the zygomas.

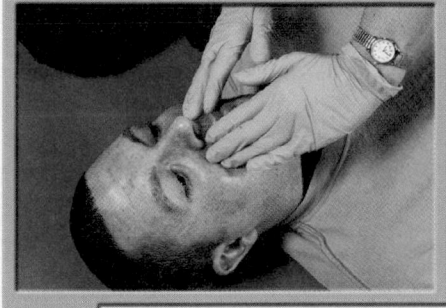

Step 8 Palpate the maxillae.

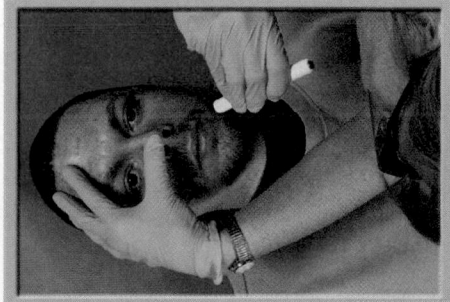

Step 9 Check the nose for blood and drainage.

Secondary Assessment

Continues

Skill Drill 3

Performing the Full-Body Exam, continued

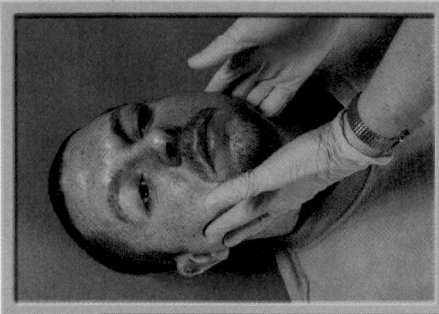

Step 10 Palpate the mandible.

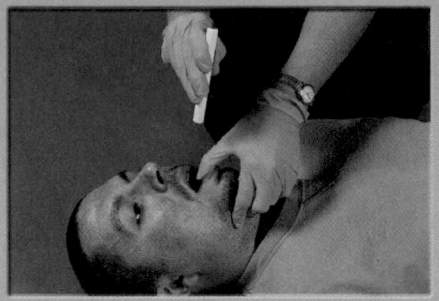

Step 11 Assess the mouth and nose.

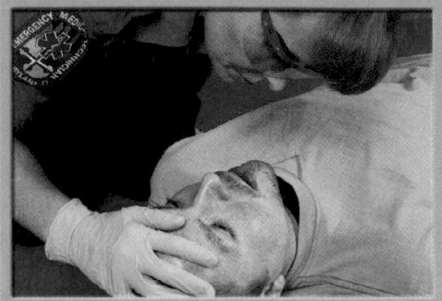

Step 12 Check for unusual breath odors.

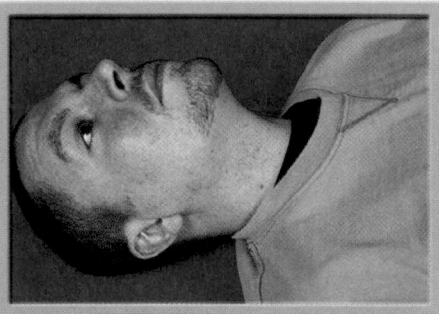

Step 13 Inspect the neck. Observe for jugular venous distention and/or tracheal deviation.

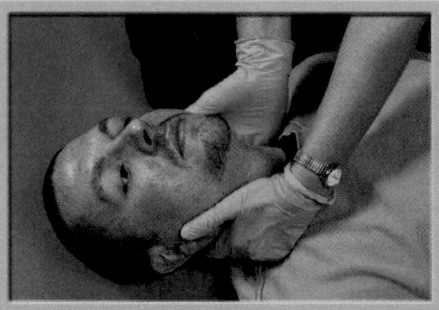

Step 14 Palpate the front and back of the neck.

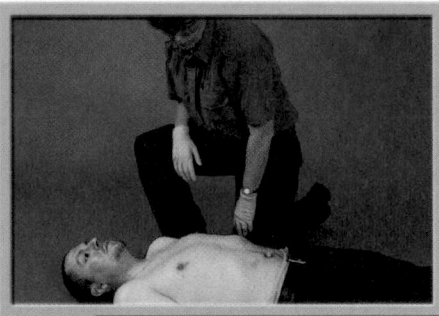

Step 15 Inspect the chest, and observe breathing motion.

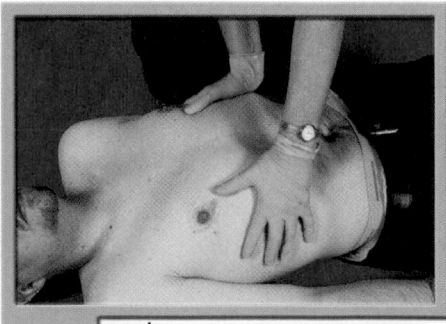

Step 16 Gently palpate over the ribs.

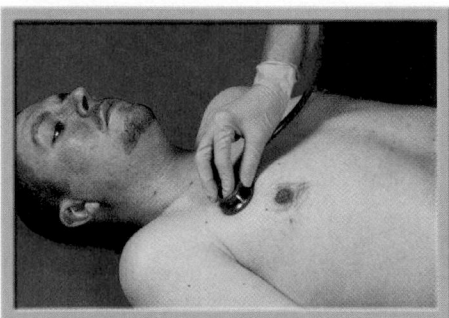

Step 17 Listen to anterior breath sounds (midaxillary, midclavicular).

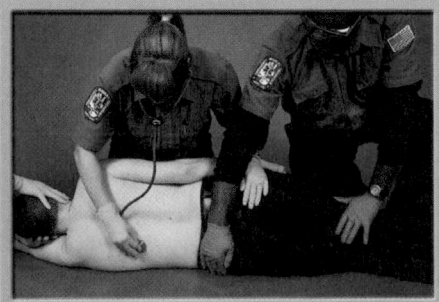

Step 18 Listen to posterior breath sounds (bases, apices). At this point, also inspect the back.

Secondary Assessment

Continues

Skill Drill | 3

Performing the Full-Body Exam, continued

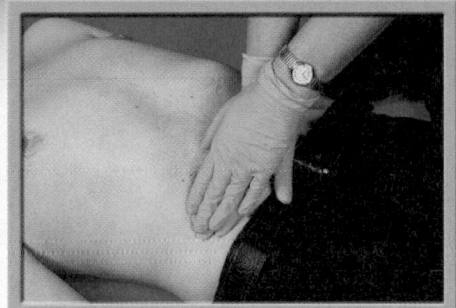

Step 19 Observe and then palpate the abdomen and pelvis.

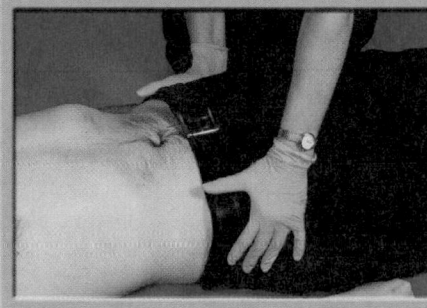

Step 20 Gently compress the pelvis from the sides.

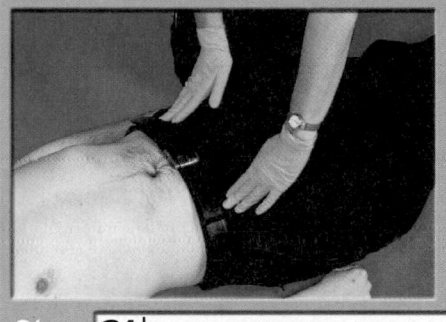

Step 21 Gently press the iliac crests.

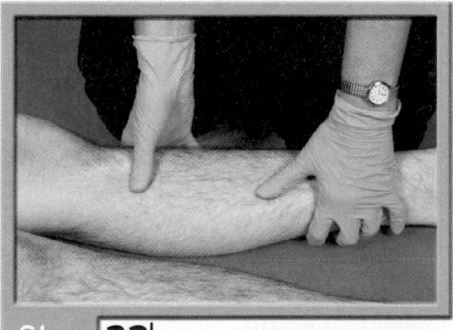

Step 22 Inspect the extremities; assess distal circulation and motor and sensory function.

The most common complaints from a responsive medical patient will involve the head, heart, lungs, or abdomen, individually or in combination.

Words of Wisdom

Many technologic devices are available to EMS personnel to aid in patient assessment. Whereas they are considered excellent equipment, always remember that you are assessing a patient—not a machine. Take the time to explain what your tools are and why you are using them. This simple action may help lessen patient anxiety.

Mental Status

For patients with a "head" problem (confusion, headache, altered mentation), you should assess and palpate the head looking for signs of trauma. Check for facial asymmetry, such as facial droop or other signs of a suspected stroke. Dilated or constricted pupils may point to recreational drug use, whereas red conjunctiva may suggest drug or alcohol use. Elevated blood pressure often accompanies a headache, possibly secondary to hypertension.

Evaluation of a patient's mental status involves assessing cognitive function (ie, ability to use reasoning). At a minimum, evaluate the patient's degree of alertness. Use the AVPU mnemonic as described in the section, Primary Assessment, to help identify the patient's level of consciousness.

You can further assess mental status by considering whether the patient is <u>alert and oriented (A × O)</u> in four areas: person, place, day of the week, and the event itself. Assessing whether the patient can recall his or her name tests long-term memory, whereas assessing whether the patient knows where he or she is and what happened tests short-term memory.

The most reliable and consistent method of assessing mental status and neurologic function is the <u>Glasgow Coma Scale (GCS)</u>, which assigns a point value (score) for eye opening, verbal response, and motor response; these values are added

Table 4   Common Chief Complaints and Focused Assessments

Chief Complaint	Focused Assessment
Chest pain	Evaluate skin, pulse, and blood pressure. Look for trauma to the chest, assess the external jugular veins, and listen to breath sounds. Assess for pedal/dependent edema.
Abdominal pain	Evaluate skin, pulse, and blood pressure. Look for trauma to the abdomen, and palpate the abdomen for tenderness or rigidity.
Shortness of breath	Evaluate skin, pulse, blood pressure, and rate and depth of respirations. Assess for airway obstruction. Listen carefully to breath sounds, and assess for hypoxemia (that is, use pulse oximetry). Assess for pedal/dependent edema.
Dizziness	Evaluate skin, pulse, blood pressure, and adequacy of respirations. Monitor the level of consciousness and orientation carefully. Check the head for signs of trauma. Evaluate for signs of stroke, including facial droop, slurred speech, and one-sided weakness. Check for a history of inner ear problems.
Any pain associated with bones or joints	Evaluate skin, pulse, movement, and sensation adjacent and distal to the affected area.

Table 5   Glasgow Coma Scale

Eye Opening		Best Verbal Response		Best Motor Response	
Spontaneous	4	Oriented and converses	5	Follows commands	6
To verbal command	3	Disoriented conversation	4	Localizes pain	5
To pain	2	Speaking but nonsensical	3	Withdraws to pain	4
No response	1	Moans or makes unintelligible sounds	2	Decorticate flexion	3
		No response	1	Decerebrate extension	2
				No response	1

Scores:
15: Indicates no neurologic disabilities
13–14: Mild dysfunction
9–12: Moderate to severe dysfunction
8 or less: Severe dysfunction (The lowest possible score is 3.)

Special Populations

Mental status may be difficult to evaluate in children. First, determine whether the child is alert. Even infants should be alert to your presence and should follow you with their eyes (a process called "tracking"). Ask the parent whether the child is behaving normally, particularly in regard to alertness. Most children older than 2 years should know their own name and the names of their parents and siblings. Evaluate mental status in school-age children by asking about holidays, recent school activities, or teachers' names.

for a total score (**Table 5**). While it may take slightly longer to perform than the AVPU, calculating a GCS score provides much greater insight into the patient's overall neurologic function.

Here is a sample scenario for you to work through. You encounter an older man who tracks you with his eyes as you enter his room. As you speak with the man, you note that his verbal response is disoriented, even though he follows your commands. His GCS values would be 4, 4, and 6, for a total score of 14. By comparison, if the patient opened his eyes only to pain, moaned as the only verbal response, and withdrew to pain, he would be assigned GCS values of 2, 2, and 4, for a total score of 8. Clearly, a child or infant will respond differently than an adult. A modified assessment should be used for these patients. This issue is addressed in the chapter, *Pediatric Emergencies.*

Once the basic mental status has been assessed, you should conduct a thorough mental status examination, especially in patients experiencing a behavioral emergency. This examination begins by assessing the patient's general appearance, including posture and facial expression. Note the patient's posture and ability to relax. Does the posture change with topics of discussion, with activities, or with certain people around the patient? A tense posture, restlessness, and fidgeting suggest the patient may be experiencing anxiety, while a slumped posture with slow movement might indicate an underlying depression. Observe the patient's face, both at rest and when the patient

interacts with others. Watch for variations in expression with topics of discussion. Ask yourself if the facial expressions are appropriate. A face that is relatively immobile (for example, a patient who does not blink, or whose face appears to be frozen in a stare) throughout the exam may indicate an underlying Parkinson disease.

Note the patient's speech and language patterns. Pay attention to the quantity, rate, volume, articulation, and fluency of speech. Alterations in language suggest an underlying psychiatric or central nervous system disease.

Ask the patient about his or her mood. This is an objective statement similar to the chief complaint. Simply asking "how do you feel" may give you an appropriate response; however, more direct questioning regarding mood might be needed. All patients should be asked about suicidal ideations. Any patient who expresses thoughts of suicide should be evaluated at an appropriate facility.

Assessment of the patient's thoughts and perceptions is an important part of the complete mental status exam. Here you will assess the logic, relevance, organization, and coherence of the patient's thoughts. This is done simply by listening to the patient's conversation. Watch for occurrences such as abrupt shifting of the conversation from one subject to another, invented or distorted words, and speech that is largely incomprehensible, which may indicate an underlying disorder such as schizophrenia. The patient's perceptions deal with senses. Ask your patient if he or she sometimes hears or sees things that others do not. In addition, ask patients if they feel things even when there is nothing touching them. Patients who answer "yes" to any of these questions may be experiencing hallucinations that are related to an underlying psychiatric illness or an illness affecting the central nervous system.

You should assess information relevant to thought content during the exam. This is also assessed by listening. Listen for content that suggest phobias, obsessions, anxieties, and delusions. Delusions are false, fixed, personal beliefs that are not shared by other members of the patient's culture. It is important that any observations made regarding the patient's thought content be relayed to the hospital.

Assess the patient's insight and judgment. Insight shows the patient's awareness of his or her illness and need for treatment. You can simply ask, "What do you think is wrong?" Some patients may respond by saying, "I'm depressed and I know I need to get help." This demonstrates positive insight into his or her illness. However, some patients may tell you that it is normal to hear voices and feel they do not need treatment. These patients are considered to be lacking insight. You can usually assess judgment by noting the patient's response to family situations, jobs, use of money, and interpersonal conflicts. You can ask, "Who is going to look after your home while you are in the hospital?" Any inappropriate response may indicate an underlying delirium, dementia, developmental delay, or psychotic state.

Finally, the complete mental status examination includes an assessment of the patient's cognitive function. This can be accomplished by assessing the patient's attention, memory, and ability to learn new items. There are several ways to assess the patient's attention. Two common methods of assessing attention include *serial 7s* and *spelling backwards*. Serial 7s is conducted by having the patient start at 100, subtract 7, and continue subtracting 7. Note the patient's effort, speed, and accuracy of responses. Spelling backwards is another way to assess attention. Ask the patient to spell a five-letter word, such as W-O-R-L-D forward, and then backward. Once again, note the patient's effort, speech, and accuracy. When you are assessing memory, begin by assessing remote memory such as birthdays, anniversaries, schools attended, and jobs held. It can be difficult to assess accuracy of remote memory if there is no one available to confirm the patient's answers, and thus it is not always the most accurate assessment tool. After the remote memory is assessed, inquire about the patient's recent memory. This could involve the events of the day. Ask the patient what medications he or she took today. You could even ask what the patient ate for breakfast, but like remote memory, someone will need to be available to confirm the answer. Finally, assess the patient's ability to learn new things. This can be assessed by giving the patient three or four objects (eg, ball, key, lawnmower) to remember and asking the patient to recite them 3 to 5 minutes later.

Skin, Hair, and Nails
Skin
The skin, which is the largest organ system in the body, serves three major functions: It regulates the temperature of the body, it transmits information from the environment to the brain, and it protects the body in the environment.

The skin is the major organ governing the body's thermoregulation. In a cold environment, constriction of the blood vessels shunts blood away from the skin to decrease the amount of heat being lost through radiation from the body surface (observed as pale skin). When the outside environment is hot, the vessels in the skin dilate, the skin becomes flushed or red, and heat is lost as it radiates from the body surface. Also, in a hot environment, sweat is secreted to the skin surface from the sweat glands. Energy, in the form of body heat, is lost during the evaporation process, which causes body temperature to fall. It is worth noting that at a humidity level of more than 85%, evaporation does not work.

Information from the environment is carried to the brain through a rich supply of sensory nerves that originate in the skin. Nerve endings that lie in the skin are adapted to perceive and transmit information about heat, cold, external pressure, pain, and the position of the body in space. In this way, the skin recognizes changes in the environment. It also reacts to pressure, pain, and pleasurable stimuli.

The skin is composed of two layers: the epidermis and the dermis **Figure 30**. The **epidermis**, or outermost layer, is the body's first line of defense. It serves as the principal barrier

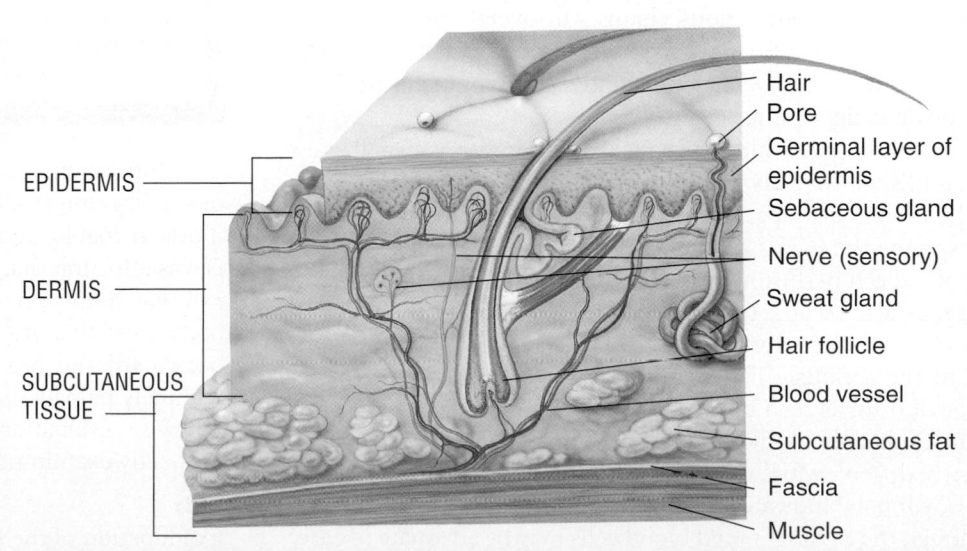

EPIDERMIS

DERMIS

SUBCUTANEOUS TISSUE

Hair
Pore
Germinal layer of epidermis
Sebaceous gland
Nerve (sensory)
Sweat gland
Hair follicle
Blood vessel
Subcutaneous fat
Fascia
Muscle

Figure 30 The skin is composed of a tough external layer (the epidermis) and a vascular inner layer (the dermis).

against water, dust, microorganisms, and mechanical stress. Underlying the epidermis is the <u>dermis</u>—a tough, highly elastic layer of connective tissues. This complex material is composed chiefly of collagen fibers, elastic fibers, and a mucopolysaccharide gel. Numerous <u>fibroblasts</u> (cells that secrete collagen, elastin, and ground substance) are found within the dermis as well.

The dermis is subdivided into the papillary dermis and a reticular layer. The vasculature inside the papillary dermis serves two functions—it provides nutrients to the epidermis and it aids in thermoregulation. Dilation of these vessels increases blood flow to the skin, allowing heat to dissipate. Conversely, blood vessel constriction results in retention of heat. The reticular layer consists of dense, irregular connective tissue, which provides both strength and elasticity. With age, the skin undergoes significant changes, including loss of the collagen connective tissues and diminished capillary supply.

Examination of the skin involves both inspection and palpation. Pay careful attention to the skin color, moisture, temperature, texture, <u>turgor</u>, and any significant lesions. Look for evidence of diminished perfusion, evaluate for pallor and cyanosis, and be wary of <u>diaphoresis</u>. Reddened or pink skin can be seen in a variety of normal states, but it is also evident in states of relative <u>vasodilation</u> (flushing). Flushed skin is usually apparent in patients with fever, and it may be seen in patients experiencing an allergic process. Reddened skin should also be considered in the context of superficial burns.

Special Populations

When assessing skin turgor in an older patient, use the skin of the upper chest. This is a much more reliable indicator than the extremities.

Perhaps the quickest and most reliable initial way to evaluate a patient's overall degree of distress is to look at the skin. Relatively subtle but serious changes in overall circulation are usually manifested early on in the skin's appearance. Evaluate the skin's color, relative moisture, and relative temperature. Note any obvious deformities.

Examining the skin for changes in perfusion is usually best accomplished in areas in which the epidermis is thinnest, such as the fingernails, lips, and conjunctivae. It is sometimes useful to examine the palms and soles as well. <u>Pallor</u> is present when red blood cell perfusion to the capillary beds of the skin is poor. You may also be able to detect pallor by looking at the patient's lips or eye conjunctiva. Pale skin is a relatively common finding in the seriously ill patient and may indicate severe <u>vasoconstriction</u>, as seen in profound anemia, acute cardiovascular events, other shock-like states, and hypothermia. Local areas of blanched, cool, white skin are typical of frostbite.

<u>Cyanosis</u> indicates a relative lack of oxygen perfusion, although the number of red blood cells may be adequate to carry any available oxygen. Cyanosis correlates extremely well with low arterial oxygen saturation. It can be visualized generally in the skin, but more specifically in the fingernail beds, face,

and lips. Although cyanotic skin is commonly seen in states of oxygen desaturation, it can also be a function of hypothermia, especially in young patients. <u>Mottling</u> is a typical finding in states of severe protracted hypoperfusion and shock and is easily recognized in seriously ill or injured pediatric patients. However, when mottling is seen in a pediatric patient, do not immediately consider the finding "normal." It is important to consider all aspects of the history and physical exam in order to make sure there is no evidence of hypoperfusion.

<u>Ecchymosis</u> is localized bruising or blood collection within or under the skin. Evaluate large ecchymoses for the possibility of serious underlying soft-tissue, bony, or organ injury. Serious wounds to the head, neck, and torso should also be noted, as well as any evidence of a potential hemorrhage.

It takes practice to accurately gauge patients' relative perfusion and hydration status. Becoming familiar with the abnormal findings of the skin and mucous membranes is an excellent aid in judging both. Turgor relates directly to hydration. Poor skin turgidity is an expression of poorly hydrated skin, with associated <u>tenting</u> evident in extreme cases, particularly in young children. Just a few hours of profuse vomiting and diarrhea can leave an infant seriously dehydrated. Because of normal changes in elastin and connective tissues with advanced age, skin turgor is an insignificant indicator in geriatric patients, as is skin that is abnormally dry to the touch. Paying attention to skin temperature can sometimes prove useful when you are trying to determine the etiologies of different problems (eg, respiratory distress). Sometimes making a clinical distinction between congestive heart failure with pulmonary edema versus pneumonia is a function of the patient's temperature, which may be readily apparent from tactile examination of the skin.

Words of Wisdom

When you are inspecting the skin, always be alert for signs of possible abuse or maltreatment. Multiple bruises at different stages of healing or even pressure sores may raise concerns about possible physical abuse and should be reported. Fingerprint bruises, ie, from being grabbed, lifted, or dragged, should always make you suspicious.

Skin lesions may sometimes be the only external evidence of a serious internal injury. Take note of any large areas of ecchymosis, palpable crepitus (palpable fractures), and open wounds. Devastating internal injuries can result from wounds whose only external signs appear to be relatively benign. Be aware of any body areas that are hidden by clothing or by devices such as a backboard and head immobilizer. Always visually inspect and manually palpate the patient's back and expose the entire body. Likewise, evaluation for rashes is usually best accomplished by discreetly examining areas of skin otherwise hidden by clothing.

Hair

Examination of the hair is done by inspection and palpation. In this survey, note the quantity, distribution, and texture of the hair. Recent changes in the growth or loss of hair can indicate an underlying endocrine disorder, such as diabetes, or may result from treatment modalities for disease processes (eg, chemotherapy or radiation treatment of cancer). Although the recent loss of hair may be related to a disease process, the thinning and loss of hair can also be a normal finding in the older patient. Hair that has been forcibly ripped often points to an abuse scenario.

Nails

The examination of the fingernails and toenails can reveal many subtle findings [Table 6]. The color, shape, texture, and presence or absence of lesions should all be assessed. The normal nail should be firm and smooth on palpation. Normal changes to the nails with aging include the development of striations and a change in color (yellowish tint) related to the reduction in body calcium. Overly thick nails or nails that have lines running parallel to the finger often suggests a fungal infection.

Head, Eyes, Ears, Nose, and Throat

The head, eyes, ears, nose, and throat (HEENT) exam consists of a comprehensive evaluation of the head and related structures. It is crucial because the head contains the brain, numerous important sensory organs, and all of the upper airway anatomy. The eyes are a nervous system structure that involves both motor pathways (lids, extraocular muscles, pupillary constrictors, corneal blink reflex) and sensory pathways. The ears provide for both hearing and balance control. The nose is a sensory organ involved with the senses of smell and taste; it also plays an important role in assisting with breathing. The throat consists of the mouth and posterior pharynx, and all the structures intrinsic to them. This complicated organ simultaneously coordinates many motor and sensory functions, while also coordinating the initial activities of both the respiratory and digestive systems.

Head

The head is divided into two parts: the cranium and the face. The cranium, or skull, contains the brain. The brain connects to

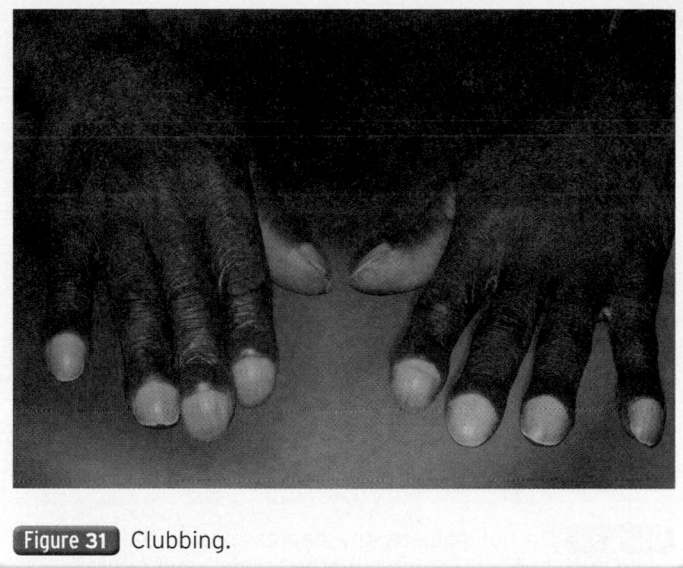

Figure 31 Clubbing.

the spinal cord through the foramen magnum, a large opening at the base of the skull. The most posterior portion of the cranium is the occiput. On each side of the cranium, the lateral portions are called the temples or temporal regions. Between the temporal regions and the occiput lie the parietal regions. The forehead is called the frontal region. Just anterior to the ear, in the temporal region, you can feel the pulse of the superficial temporal artery. A layer of muscle fascia covers the skull. The thick skin covering the cranium, which usually bears hair, is called the scalp.

Within the skull lie the meninges, three distinct layers of tissue that suspend the brain and the spinal cord within the skull and the spinal canal. The dura mater is the tough, fibrous, outer layer that resembles leather. It forms a sac that contains the central nervous system (CNS), with small openings through which the peripheral nerves exit. The inner two layers of the meninges, called the arachnoid and the pia mater, are much thinner than the dura mater. They contain the blood vessels that nourish the brain and spinal cord. Cerebrospinal fluid (CSF) is produced in a chamber inside the brain, called the third ventricle. CSF fills the space between the meninges and acts as a shock absorber.

When you are examining the head, you should both feel it and inspect it visually. This step is important in the management of potential trauma patients and with patients who have altered mental status or are unresponsive. Inspect and feel the entire cranium for signs of deformity or asymmetry, being careful not to palpate any depressions because you do not want to push bone fragments into the cranial vault or the brain [Figure 32]. Note any warm, wet areas; they usually represent blood, CSF, or a combination of the two. If you find evidence of external bleeding, attempt to separate the hair manually and irrigate the clot; this should allow you to identify the source of bleeding. Evaluate the skull for any deformity, step-off, or tenderness. Observe the general shape and contour of the skull. Look for scars or shunts that suggest a history of trauma or problems with the CNS. If you suspect the presence of a cerebral shunt, inquire from the patient where the shunt was placed and where it drains in the body.

Table 6	Abnormal Findings in the Nails	
Condition	Findings	Possible Cause
Beau lines	Transverse depressions in the nail inhibiting growth	Systemic illness, severe infection, or nail injury
Clubbing	The angle between the nail and the nail base approaches or exceeds 180°	Flattening and enlargement of the fingertips is associated with chronic respiratory disease [Figure 31]
Psoriasis	Pitting, discoloration, and subungual thickening of the nail	Autoimmune disease
Splinter hemorrhages	Red or brown linear streaks in the nail bed	Bacterial endocarditis or trichinosis
Terry nails	Transverse white bands that cover the nail except for the distal tip	Cirrhosis

Secondary Assessment

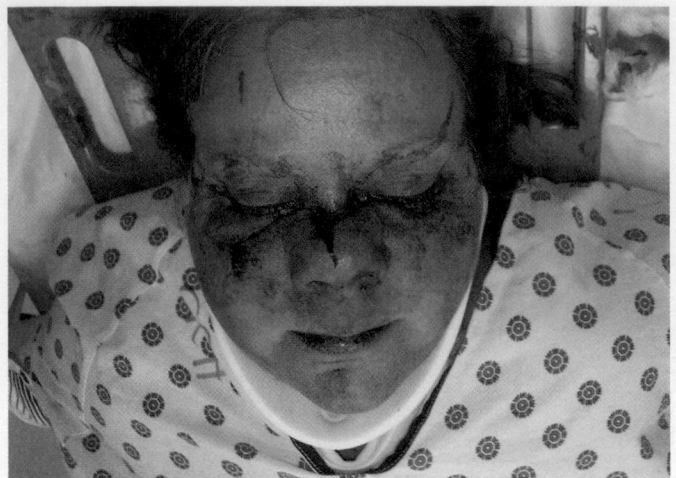

Figure 32 Do not palpate any depressions in the skin; you could push bone fragments into the cranial vault or brain.

Special Populations

Always inspect the fontanelle in infants.
- Bulging = Increased intracranial pressure in a quiet child
- Sunken = Dehydration

In children younger than 18 months, routinely palpate the anterior fontanelle (the "soft spot"). Prior to its normal physiologic closure, it can serve as an excellent relative indicator of hydration and intracranial pressure. The fontanelle is usually characterized as open and flat (the normal state), bulging (common while crying, pathologic when observed in a quiet child), and sunken (in severe dehydration).

When you are evaluating the face, observe the color and moisture of the skin, as well as expression, symmetry, and contour of the face itself. Asymmetry of the face could suggest an underlying nerve system problem such as a stroke or facial nerve palsy. Also pay attention to any swelling or apparent areas of injury, and note any signs of respiratory distress. Use the mnemonic DCAP-BTLS—Deformities, Contusions, Abrasions, Punctures/penetrations, Burns, Tenderness, Lacerations, and Swelling—to assist you during the secondary assessment. Follow the steps in **Skill Drill 4** to assess the head:

Words of Wisdom

Protecting fragile CNS structures from further damage is vital to the patient's prospects for living a normal life. Lean toward caution and overprotection in assessing and treating possible brain and spinal cord injuries.

Skill Drill 4

1. Visually inspect the head, looking for any obvious DCAP-BTLS **Step 1**.
2. Palpate the top and back of the head to locate any subtle abnormalities **Step 2**. Use a systematic approach, going from front to back, to ensure that nothing is missed.
3. Part the hair in several places to examine the condition of the scalp. Identify any lesions under the hair **Step 3**.
4. Note any pain during the process (this exam should not cause the patient any pain).
5. Palpate the structure of the face noting any DCAP-BTLS. Pay attention to the condition of the skin, hair distribution, and shape of the face **Step 4**.

Eyes

The eyes are a tremendously complex sensory organ **Figure 33**. They process light stimuli for the brain, so that the brain is able to decode light impulses presenting to the eyes and form a visual image. The eyes are a critical link to the CNS, and as such they allow the examiner to more precisely assess the functions of the CNS.

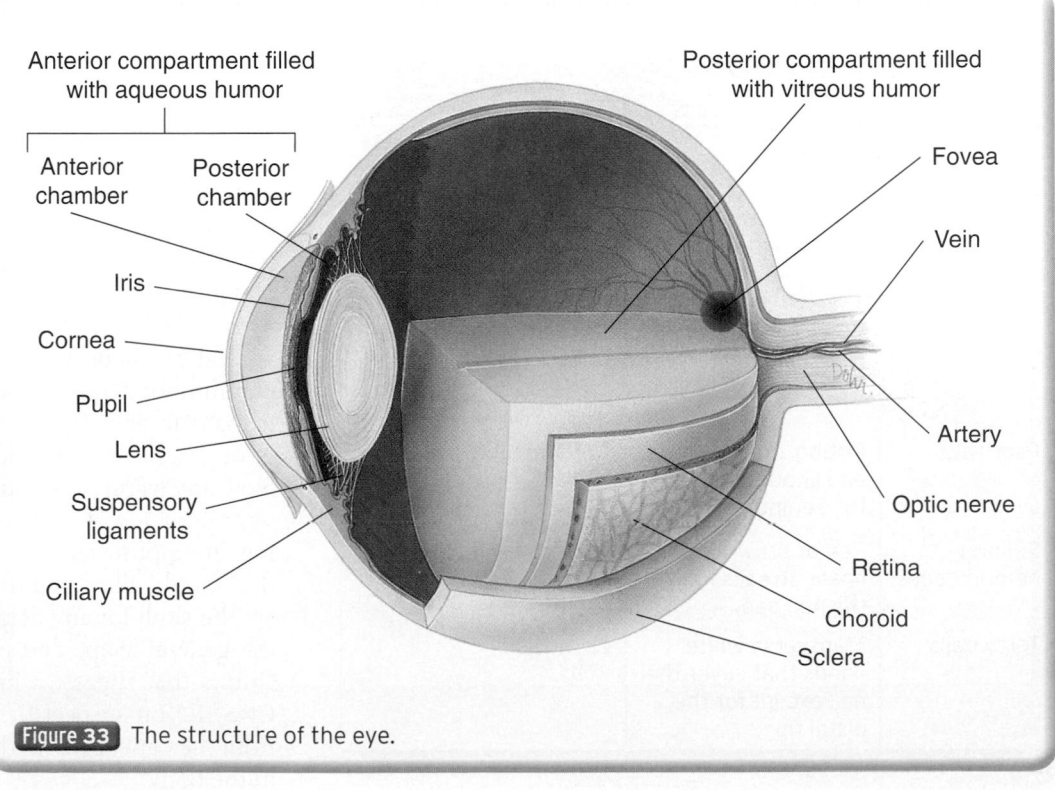

Figure 33 The structure of the eye.

Secondary Assessment

Skill Drill 4

Assessing the Head

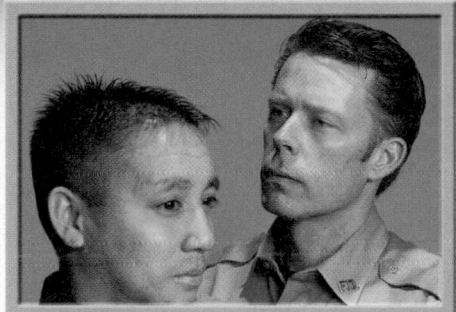

Step 1 Visually inspect the head, looking for any obvious DCAP-BTLS.

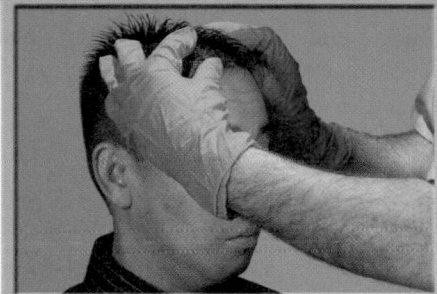

Step 2 Palpate the top and back of the head to locate any subtle abnormalities.

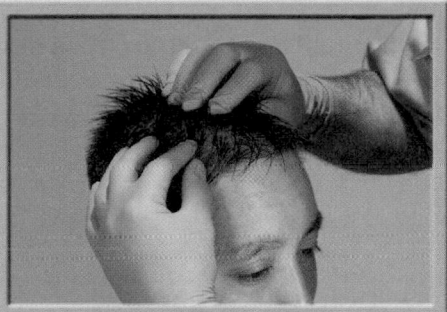

Step 3 Part the hair in several places to examine the condition of the scalp.

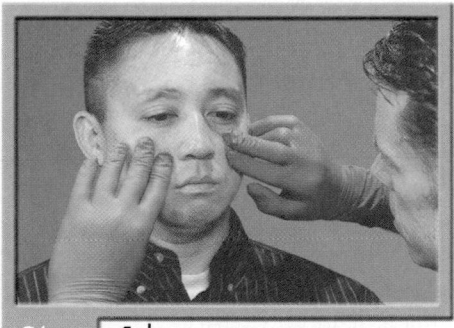

Step 4 Palpate the structure of the face, noting any DCAP-BTLS.

Each eye consists of an anterior chamber and a posterior chamber, which are always assessed in a standardized fashion (ie, from "front to back"). The outer aspects of the eye are checked first, with deeper structures subsequently evaluated. Carefully inspect and palpate the upper and lower orbits, starting at the nose and working toward the lateral edge. General issues to ask about include any pain or redness, loss of vision, **diplopia** (double vision), photophobia, blurring, discharge, and corrective lens use. Note periorbital ecchymosis (raccoon eyes).

After you address these general questions, assess the patient for **visual acuity** — that is, the ability or inability to see, and how well the patient can see. Check visual acuity by examining each eye in isolation. If corrective lenses are normally worn, check visual acuity with the correction in place. The standard device for checking visual acuity is the Snellen ("E") chart Figure 34 , although it is not an appropriate tool in the prehospital setting. More appropriate tools in this environment include simple tests such as light/dark discrimination and finger counting. Finger counting should be done from a noted distance,

typically 6′, 3′, and 1′. Reporting on visual acuity must include the distance from which finger counting was measured.

The pupil is a circular opening in the center of the pigmented iris of the eye. The diameter and reactivity of the patient's pupil to light reflect the status of the brain's perfusion, oxygenation, and condition. The pupils are normally round and of approximately equal size; they serve as optical diaphragms, adjusting their size depending on the available light. In normal room light, the pupils appear to be midsized. With less light, they dilate to allow more light to enter the eye, in an attempt to improve visibility in dim light. With high light levels or when a bright light is suddenly introduced, the pupils instantly constrict, allowing less light to enter and protecting the sensitive receptors in the inner eye from damage. When a brighter light is introduced into one eye (or higher levels of light enter one eye only), both pupils should constrict equally to the appropriate size for the pupil receiving the most light.

In the absence of any light, the pupils will become fully relaxed and dilated. When light is introduced, each eye

Secondary Assessment

sends sensory signals to the brain, indicating the level of light received. Pupil size is regulated by a series of continuous motor commands that the brain automatically sends through the oculomotor nerves (third cranial nerve) to each eye. Normally, pupil size changes instantly to any change in light level.

When you are assessing the pupils, check for size (in millimeters), shape, and symmetry. Also check for a reaction to light shined on them, performing this assessment in as darkened an environment as possible. Asymmetric pupils (anisocoria, which can be found in 20% of the population) may indicate significant ocular or neurologic pathology, but must be correlated with the patient's overall presentation Figure 35 . Topical applications of certain medicines and substances can also provoke pupillary changes.

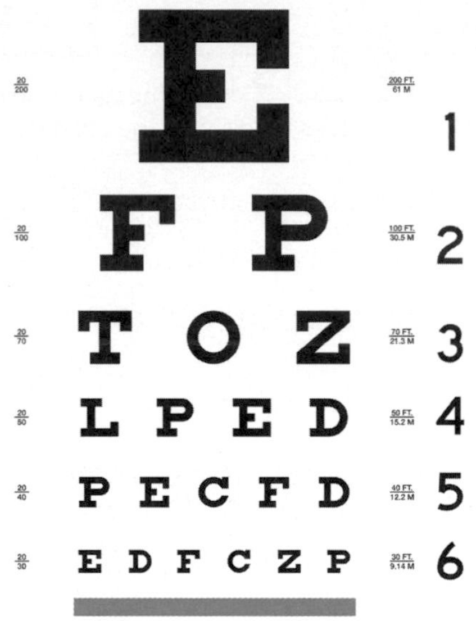

Muscles are responsible for physically moving the eyes from side to side and up and down, which allows for seamless binocular vision. When a patient is asked to use his or her eyes to follow your finger, which you are moving in a "Z" or "H" pattern, the eyes should move smoothly and symmetrically with the finger movement. Evaluate whether the eyes move in harmony (conjugate gaze) and whether they can track in all fields (up, down, left, right, across). Visual field examination assesses the retina's (and therefore the optic nerve's) ability to perceive light. This is done by checking the patient's peripheral vision, examining each eye separately.

Following the general eye exam, a more precise penlight exam is typically undertaken Figure 36 . Check the lids, lashes, and tear ducts. Look for foreign bodies, evidence of wounds and trauma, and discharge. Turn up the lids to look for foreign bodies, and inspect the conjunctivae and sclera. The sclera ought to be white, not jaundiced or injected (red). Painless subconjunctival hemorrhage is a common but benign presentation. The conjunctivae should be pink—not cyanotic, pale, or overly reddened. The cornea and lens will be difficult to examine without additional assessment tools—although in a trauma situation, you should note whether the globe is patent. Next, examine the anterior chamber and iris for clarity, noting any cloudiness or bleeding. Finally, examine the posterior chamber and retina; however, this exam is more useful after chemical dilation of the pupil and appropriate use of an ophthalmoscope.

To examine the eye, follow the steps in Skill Drill 5 :

Skill Drill 5

1. Examine the exterior portion of the eye. Look for any obvious trauma or deformity Step 1 .
2. Ask the patient about any pain, altered vision (eg, blurred or double vision), discharge, or sensitivity to light.

Figure 34 Due to its size and complexity, the Snellen chart is not a good prehospital tool.

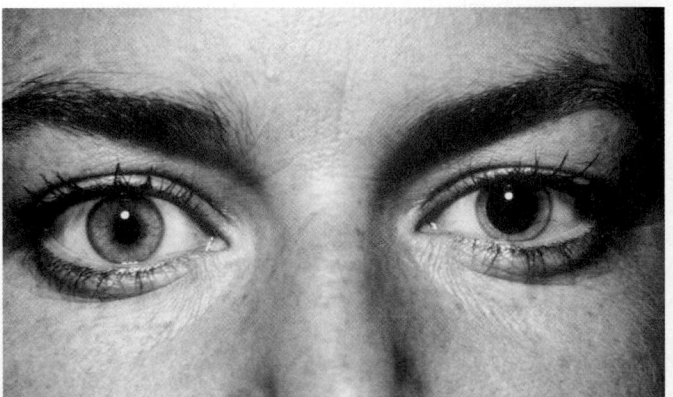

Figure 35 Asymmetric pupils may be normal or may signify a severe brain injury.

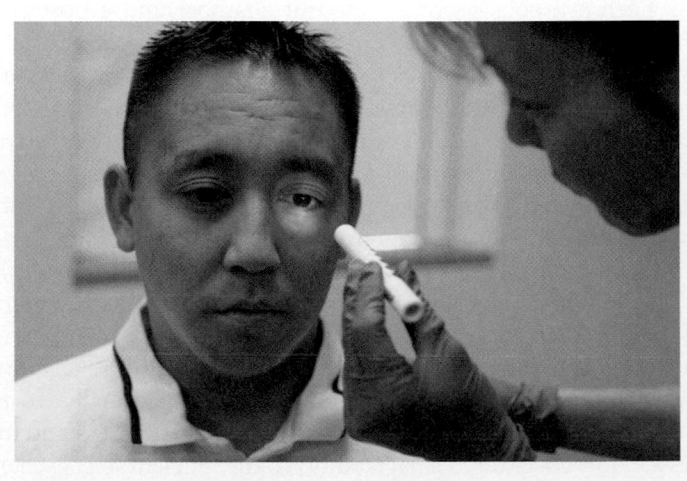

Figure 36 Penlight exam of the eye.

Secondary Assessment

Skill Drill 5

Examining the Eye

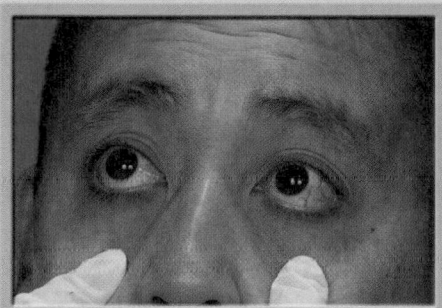

Step 1 Examine the exterior portion of the eye.

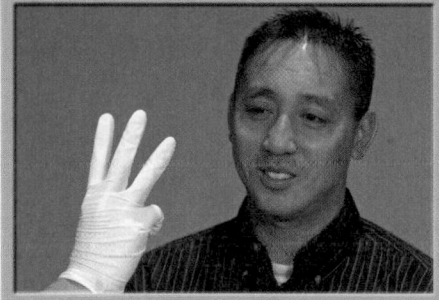

Step 2 Measure visual acuity by having the patient count the number of fingers you are holding up at varying distances.

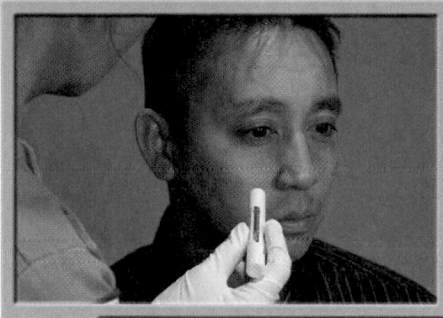

Step 3 Test the pupils for their reaction to light.

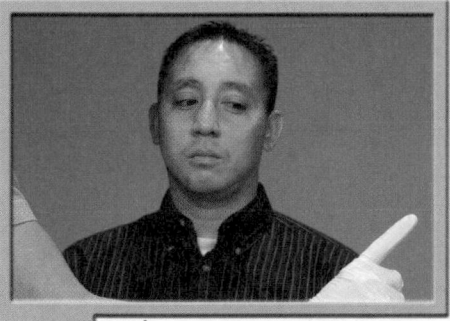

Step 4 Test for cranial nerve function by asking the patient to follow your fingers in a "Z" or "H" pattern.

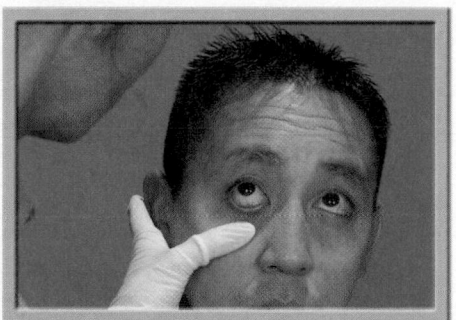

Step 5 Inspect the eyelids, lashes, and tear ducts.

3. Measure visual acuity by having the patient count the number of fingers you are holding up at varying distances (usually 6′, 3′, and 1′ away from the patient). Perform this exam on each eye independently of the other **Step 2**.

4. Examine the pupils for size, shape, and symmetry. They should be equal.

5. Test the pupils for their reaction to light. Both pupils should constrict when exposed to light, and they should be equal in their response **Step 3**.

6. Test for cranial nerve function by asking the patient to follow your fingers in a "Z" or "H" pattern. Note any abnormal movement of the eyes **Step 4**.

7. Inspect the eyelids, lashes, and tear ducts for evidence of trauma, foreign bodies, or discharge **Step 5**.

Words of Wisdom

Test for cranial nerve function by asking the patient to follow your fingers in a "Z" or "H" pattern. Failure to follow in a certain direction indicates weakness of an extraocular muscle or dysfunction of a cranial nerve innervating it.

Words of Wisdom

Cataracts appear as opaque black areas against the red reflex.

Secondary Assessment

To examine the eye with an ophthalmoscope, follow the steps in Skill Drill 6:

Skill Drill 6

1. Darken the environment as much as possible.
2. Ask the patient to look straight ahead and focus on a distant object Step 1.
3. Set the light on the ophthalmoscope to a setting no brighter than necessary and the lens to 0 unless another setting works better for your eyes.
4. Use your right hand and eye to examine the patient's right eye; use your left hand and eye to examine the patient's left eye Step 2.
5. Place the scope to your eye and look into the patient's pupil from 10″ to 20″ away at a 45° angle to the eye. You should see the retina as a "red reflex" or a bright orange glow Step 3.
6. Slowly move toward the patient to appreciate the structures of the fundus. Adjust the lens as needed to improve the focus. Locate a blood vessel and follow it back to the disk. Use this blood vessel as a point of reference.
7. Inspect for the size, color, and clarity of the disk. Note the integrity of the blood vessels and any lesions present on the retina. Move nasally to observe the macula Step 4.
8. Repeat the process with the other eye.

Words of Wisdom

Use of the ophthalmoscope requires frequent practice. It is rarely used in prehospital care.

Skill Drill 6

Eye Examination With an Ophthalmoscope

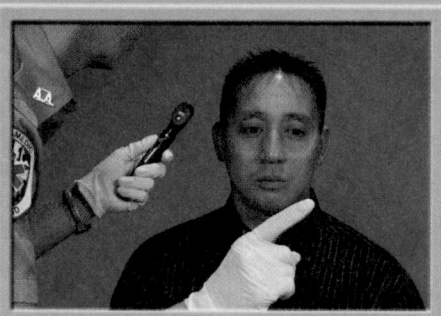

Step 1 Ask the patient to look straight ahead and focus on a distant object.

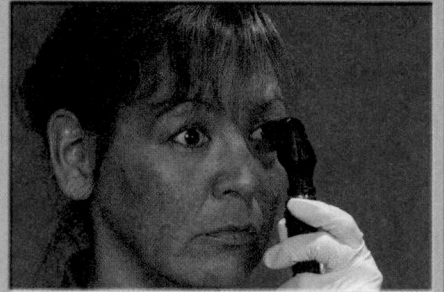

Step 2 Use your right hand and eye to examine the patient's right eye; use your left hand and eye to examine the patient's left eye.

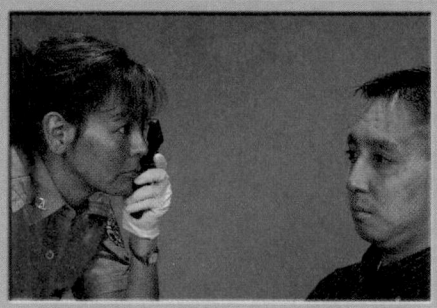

Step 3 Place the scope to your eye and look into the patient's pupil from 10″ to 20″ away at a 45° angle to the eye.

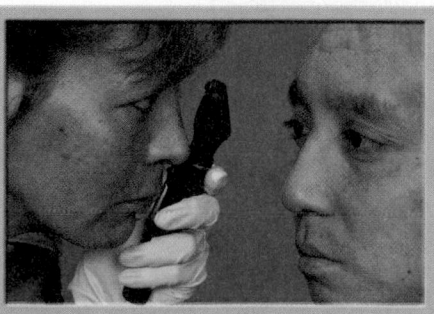

Step 4 Inspect for the size, color, and clarity of the disk.

Ears

The ear is a sensory organ that is chiefly involved with hearing and sound perception but is also intimately involved with balance control. The ear consists of an outer portion, a middle portion, and an inner portion Figure 37 .

The external ear consists of the pinna, or auricle (the part lying outside of the head), and the external auditory canal, which leads in toward the tympanic membrane, or eardrum.

The middle ear contains three small bones (hammer, anvil, and stirrup) that move in response to sound waves hitting the tympanic membrane. This mechanism controls how a person hears and differentiates sounds. The middle ear is connected to the nasal cavity by the eustachian tube, or internal auditory canal. This connection permits equalization of pressure in the middle ear when external atmospheric pressure changes.

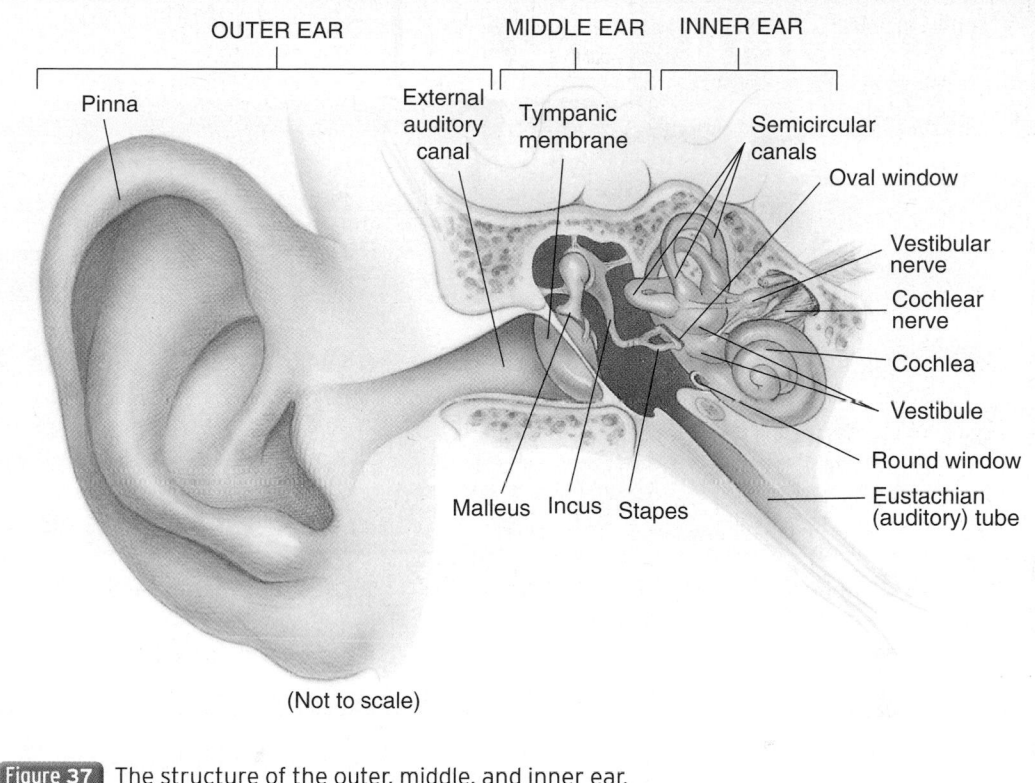

OUTER EAR   MIDDLE EAR   INNER EAR

Pinna

External auditory canal

Tympanic membrane

Semicircular canals

Oval window

Vestibular nerve

Cochlear nerve

Cochlea

Vestibule

Round window

Eustachian (auditory) tube

Malleus Incus Stapes

(Not to scale)

Figure 37 The structure of the outer, middle, and inner ear.

The inner ear consists of bony chambers filled with fluid. As the head moves, so does the fluid. In response, fine nerve endings within the fluid send impulses to the brain, indicating the position of the head and the rate of change of position.

Assessing the ears essentially involves checking for new aberrations in hearing perception plus inspecting and palpating for wounds, swelling, or drainage (pus, blood, CSF). Often the mastoid process of the skull, which is palpated immediately posterior to the auricle, is assessed for discoloration and tenderness (Battle sign). Abnormalities of the external canal and tympanic membrane are visualized by use of an otoscope. Follow the steps in Skill Drill 7 :

Skill Drill   7

1. Select an appropriately sized speculum. Dim the lights as much as possible.
2. Ensure that the ear is free of foreign bodies.
3. Place your hand firmly against the patient's head and gently grasp the patient's auricle. Move the ear to best visualize the canal, usually upward and back in the adult patient Step 1 .
4. Instruct the patient not to move during the exam to avoid damaging the ear.
5. Turn on the otoscope and insert the speculum into the ear Step 2 . Insertion toward the patient's nose usually

Words of Wisdom

When looking for a foreign body, do not advance an otoscope tip blindly; you may accidentally push the foreign body in further.

provides the best view. Do not insert the speculum deeply into the canal.

6. Inspect the canal for any lesions or discharge. A small amount of cerumen (ear wax) is normal Step 3 .
7. Visualize the tympanic membrane (eardrum), and inspect it for integrity and color. It should be translucent or a pearly gray color. Note any signs of inflammation, including swelling or discoloration (pink or redness in the canal or tympanic membrane).

Nose

The nose is a sensory organ involved with smell and taste; it is also part of the respiratory system. When you are assessing injuries involving the nose, it helps to picture the inside of the nose itself Figure 38 . The nasal cavity is divided into two sections or chambers by the nasal septum, which is made of cartilage. Each nasal chamber contains three layers of bone (the turbinates) that are covered with a moist lining. Both chambers have superior, middle, and inferior turbinates. During nasal breathing, the air moves through the nasal chambers and is filtered and humidified as it passes over the turbinates.

Skill Drill 7

Examining the Ear With an Otoscope

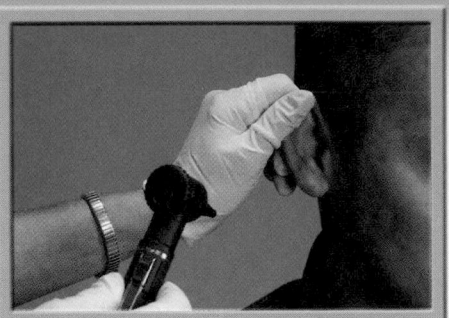

Step 1 Place your hand firmly against the patient's head and gently grasp the patient's auricle.

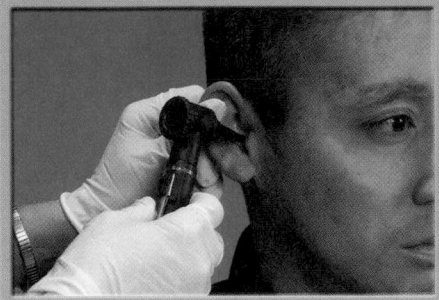

Step 2 Turn on the otoscope and insert the speculum into the ear.

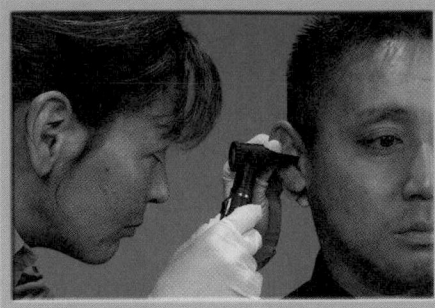

Step 3 Inspect the canal for any lesions or discharge.

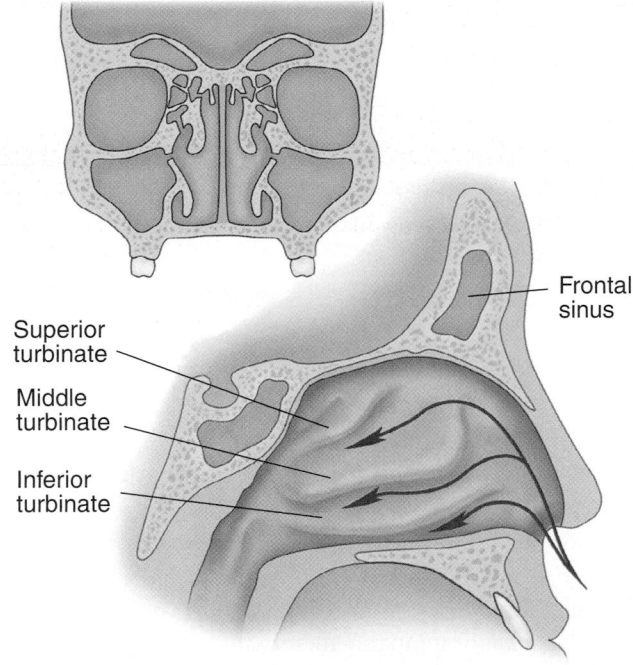

Figure 38 The nose has two chambers, divided by the septum. Each chamber is composed of layers of bone called turbinates. Above the nose are the frontal sinuses. On either side of the nose are the orbits of the eyes.

Frontal sinus

Superior turbinate

Middle turbinate

Inferior turbinate

When you are checking the nose, assess it both anteriorly and inferiorly. Look for evidence of asymmetry, deformity, wounds, foreign bodies, discharge or bleeding, and tenderness. Note any evidence of respiratory distress, such as flaring of the nostrils. Inspect the exterior of the nose, looking for color changes, symmetry, and structural abnormalities. The nose should be firm and the nares clear of obstruction. Examine the column of the nose; it should be midline with the face. Inspect the septum for any deviation from midline. The nares should be symmetric. Slight deviation or asymmetry of the nares, septum, and column are normal findings; however, gross abnormalities should be noted. Note any drainage or discharge. Small amounts of mucosal discharge are normal, but large amounts of mucus and any blood or CSF fluid are serious findings.

Throat

Assessment of the throat should include an evaluation of the mouth, the pharynx, and sometimes the neck. The throat is a conduit for both respiration and digestion, and it is in close proximity to numerous vital neurovascular structures.

> ### Words of Wisdom
>
> Frank blood or clear, watery drainage (CSF) from the ears or nose following trauma suggests a basilar skull fracture.

As part of the assessment of overall hydration status, pay close attention to the lips, teeth, oral mucosa, and tongue. In patients who present with markedly altered mental status, you will need to rapidly determine upper airway status; prompt assessment of the throat and upper airway structures is mandatory. Depending on the situation, assess for the presence of a foreign body or aspiration in either the throat or lower airway structures. Situations requiring removal of foreign bodies, secretions, or blood can manifest in many types of emergency cases. Always be prepared to assist with clearing the pharynx using manual techniques and suction.

Secondary Assessment

The examination of the mouth begins with the lips, which should be pink and free of edema or surface irregularities. Confirm that the mouth is symmetric. The gums should be pink, with no lesions or edema. Cyanosis often presents early around the lips. Be alert for this sign!

Inspect the airway to ensure that it is free of obstructions. Visualize the tongue, noting its color, size, and moisture. The tongue should be located at midline, without swelling, and moist.

Inspect and palpate the maxilla and the mandible, assessing the integrity and symmetry of both structures. Open the mouth, and look for signs of trauma (such as cracked or missing teeth, or missing crowns or onlays). Check the bite for fit.

Examine the oropharynx, identifying any discoloration or pustules that might indicate an infection. Be alert for any unusual odors on the patient's breath (such as alcohol or ketones). Check the posterior pharynx for fluids that may need to be suctioned. Inspect the uvula for edema and redness.

The neck is an extraordinarily muscular region, through which many vital structures pass. External anatomy includes the jaw, cricothyroid membrane, external jugular veins, thyroid cartilage, suprasternal notch, and cervical spinous processes. When you are assessing the neck, take the time to look for any abnormalities, including those related to symmetry, masses, and venous distention. When you are noting venous distention, consider the patient's body position relative to lying flat (0°). Describe how far up the neck the distention tracks (from the base of the neck to the angle of the jaw), either by approximation or using a centimeter scale. Palpate the carotid pulses and note relative strength of impulse. Look for any pulsating or expanding mass near the carotid pulse point. Palpate the suprasternal notch in an effort to identify any tracheal deviation. Look for the presence of a tracheal stoma. These are present in patients who have had a laryngectomy, and the stoma serves as their only means of a patent airway. Therefore, assess the stoma to make sure it is free of any obstruction. In these patients, all airway management should focus around the stoma. Have the patient open and close the jaws while you palpate over the temporomandibular joint during your examination of the jaw. To examine the neck, follow the steps in Skill Drill 8 :

Skill Drill 8

1. If trauma is suspected, take precautions to protect the cervical spine Step 1 .
2. Assess for the usage of accessory muscles during respiration.
3. Palpate the neck to find any structural abnormalities or subcutaneous air, and to ensure the trachea is midline. Begin at the suprasternal notch and work your way toward the head Step 2 . Be careful about applying pressure to the area of the carotid arteries because it may stimulate a vagal response.
4. Assess the lymph nodes and note any swelling, which may indicate infection Step 3 .
5. Assess the jugular veins for distention; it may indicate a problem with blood returning to the heart Step 4 .

Cervical Spine

The cervical spine is the pathway by which the spinal cord makes its way out of the brain and into the torso, enabling the spinal nerves to emanate to and innervate the rest of the body Figure 39 . It is also the point at which the head connects to the body. The spine is supported by a large mass of muscle, as well as multiple tendinous and ligamentous supports. Cervical injury can present in a variety of ways, and the assessment for such injury must be conducted in a careful manner.

Evaluate the patient first for the MOI and then for the presence of pain. Does the patient have an altered mental status, or did a loss of consciousness occur at the time of the event? Is there a significant MOI, or do multiple or serious distracting injuries make assessment of the cervical spine difficult? Is the patient under the influence of any intoxicating substances? Being able to confidently answer all of those questions will allow you to decide which patients may (or may not) require further treatment of a potential cervical spine injury.

When you are examining the cervical spine, inspect and palpate it, looking for evidence of tenderness and deformity. Pain is the single most reliable indicator of a spine injury or spinal cord injury. Midline posterior tenderness involving the bony spinous processes should always raise concerns. Palpable discomfort over the lateral aspects of the neck usually signals a muscular or ligamentous problem, not an injury to the bony spinal column itself. Any manipulations that result in pain, tenderness, or tingling should prompt you to stop the exam *immediately* and place the patient into a properly sized collar. With any complaints of neck pain in patients who have sustained a significant MOI, immediate stabilization of the head, neck, and complete spine is essential. Continued assessment of a patient's range of motion should take place only when there is no potential for serious injury.

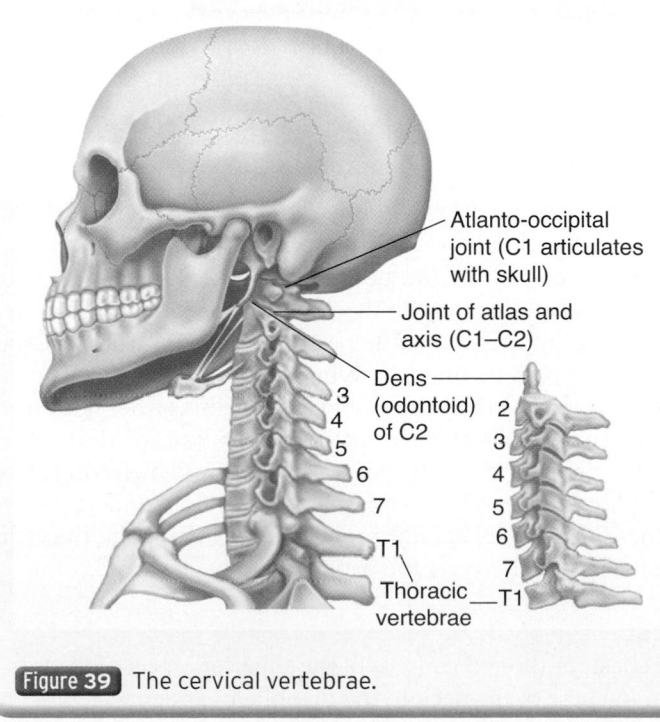

Figure 39 The cervical vertebrae.

Skill Drill   8

Examining the Neck

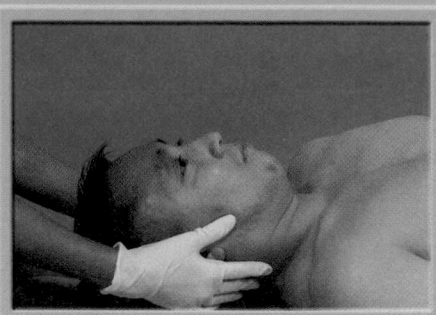

Step 1 If trauma is suspected, take precautions to protect the cervical spine.

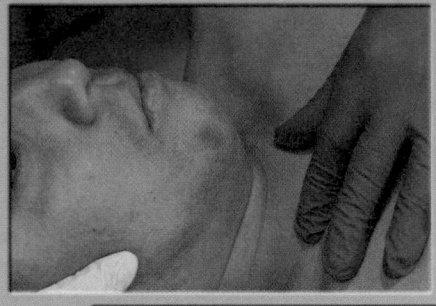

Step 2 Palpate the neck to find any structural abnormalities or subcutaneous air, and to ensure the trachea is midline. Begin at the suprasternal notch and work your way toward the head.

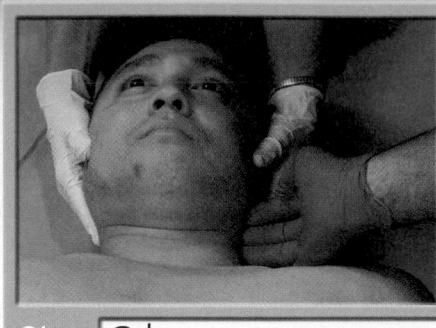

Step 3 Assess the lymph nodes.

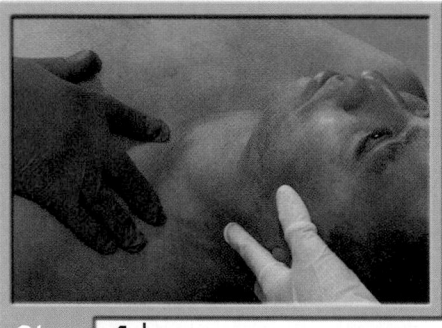

Step 4 Assess the jugular veins for distention.

When you are ranging the neck to assess for an underlying injury, first perform the activity in a passive manner, in which you are in control of the head and neck. Next, conduct the exam actively—that is, with the patient performing the directed maneuvers but cautioning the patient to stop if he or she experiences any pain or tingling. When you are checking range of motion, first have the patient slowly rotate his or her head from shoulder to shoulder. Then, if there is no pain or discomfort, have the patient extend the head back, followed by flexing of the head and neck, touching chin to chest. Any discomfort elicited by these maneuvers should prompt you to terminate the exam immediately and protect the patient's spine.

Chest

The chest (or thorax) consists of the superior aspect of the torso, from the base of the neck to the diaphragm as delineated by the costal arch **Figure 40**. The chest wall is divided into anterior and posterior portions—literally, the patient's front and back. The back of the chest extends down the patient's back, to the level of the diaphragm posteriorly, which tends to move up and down with breathing. The chest contains many vital structures, including the lungs and mediastinal elements (heart, great vessels). The chest wall serves as a protective covering for the internal components. It consists of numerous musculoskeletal, vascular, nervous, connective, and lining structures.

Typically, the chest exam proceeds in three phases. The chest wall is checked, a pulmonary evaluation is conducted, and finally the cardiovascular assessment is performed. The chest must be inspected to assess for deformities in wall patency as well as to look for external clues of respiratory distress. Expose the chest and then begin its assessment, using the techniques of inspection, palpation, percussion, and auscultation.

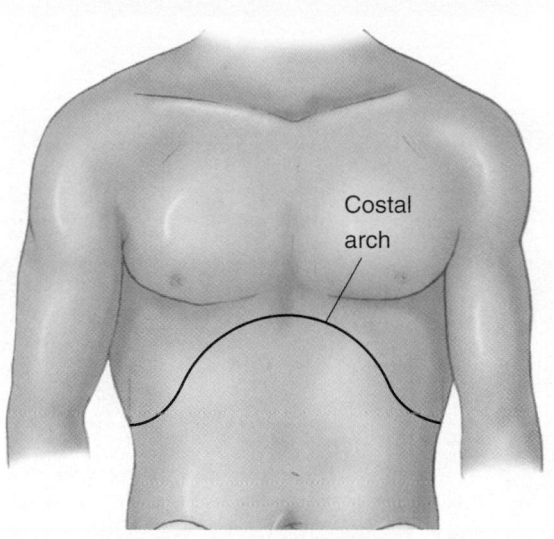

Figure 40 The chest (thorax) consists of the superior aspect of the torso, from the base of the neck to the diaphragm as delineated by the costal arch.

The examination of the posterior chest is the same as the examination of the anterior chest. Follow the steps in Skill Drill 9 :

Skill Drill 9

1. Ensure the patient's privacy as best you can.
2. Inspect the chest for any obvious DCAP-BTLS Step 1 .
3. If you find any open wounds, dress them appropriately.
4. Note the shape of the patient's chest—it can give you clues to many underlying medical conditions (eg, emphysema) Step 2 .
5. Look for any surgical scars that may be a result of pacer implantation or a midline scar (a "zipper") that indicates previous cardiac surgery. Palpation of the chest may also reveal air under the skin (ie, subcutaneous emphysema).
6. Auscultate the lung fields, noting any abnormal lung sounds Step 3 .
7. Use percussion to detect any abnormalities Step 4 .
8. Auscultate for heart tones.
9. Repeat the appropriate portions of the examination for the posterior aspect of the thorax.

Compare the two sides of the chest for symmetry. Observe the chest wall for respiratory effort, and document the respiratory rate, depth, and rhythm. Listen to the patient's breathing, look for signs of obstruction, and note the general shape of the chest wall. Pay close attention to any signs of abnormal breathing movements (paradox, accessory muscle use, impaired or diminished breathing movement) and retractions (suprasternal, sternal, intercostal, and subcostal). The presence of retractions is an important indicator of pulmonary issues, especially in children. Note any chest deformities, such as barrel chest (chronic obstructive pulmonary disease [COPD]), flail segments/subcutaneous

air (trauma), kyphoscoliosis of the spine (compression fractures, COPD), significant bruising, and any suspicious wounds. Remember—flail segments may not have paradoxical movement early on due to the splinting effect of muscle spasms.

When you are palpating the chest wall, note any tenderness or crepitance/crepitus. Be sure to palpate areas that were initially noted to be abnormal on inspection. Palpation will also enable you to better appreciate respiratory symmetry and expansion, and the overall work of breathing. Although often impractical in the prehospital environment, percussion of the chest wall can allow for enhanced evaluation of the underlying chest cavity by distinguishing either dullness or hyperresonance versus normal resonance.

Auscultate the breath sounds Figure 41 . Remember to always auscultate directly to the patient's skin, not through his or her shirt. Listening over the fabric will result in breath sounds being muted by the clothing. The lungs consist of five discrete lobes: The right side contains the right upper, right middle, and right lower lobes; the left side contains the left upper and left lower lobes, as well as the lingual Figure 42 . During your examination, listen over each lobe, both anteriorly and posteriorly. Have the patient take as deep a breath as he or she can via an

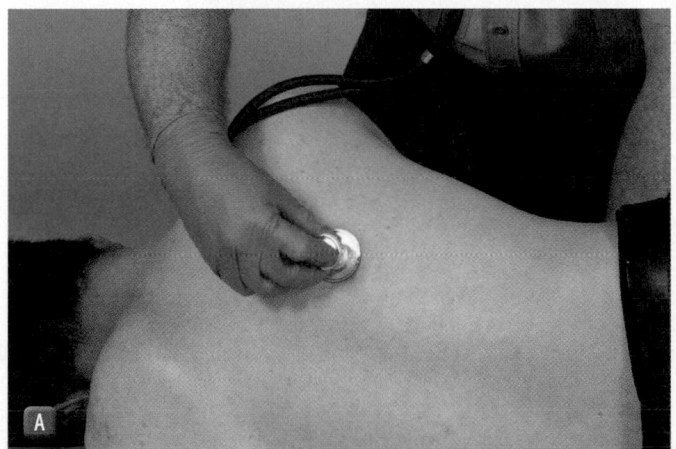

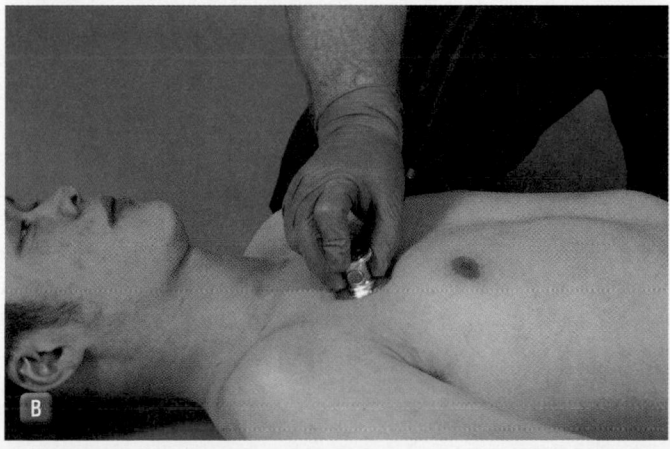

Figure 41 Auscultate the breath sounds on both sides of the chest.

Secondary Assessment

Skill Drill 9

Examining the Chest

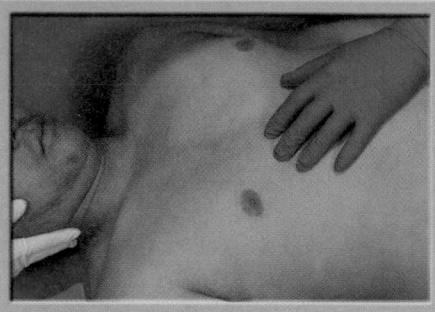

Step 1 Inspect the chest for any obvious DCAP-BTLS.

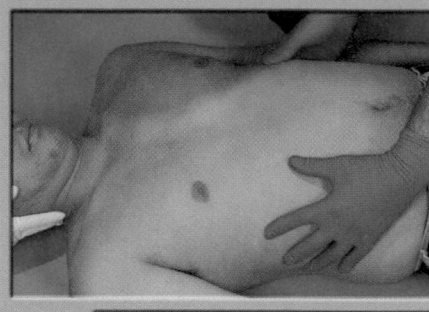

Step 2 Note the shape of the chest and symmetry of movement.

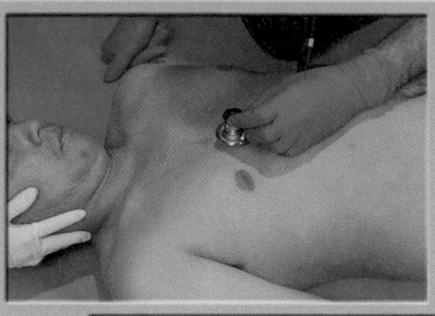

Step 3 Auscultate the lung fields, noting any abnormal lung sounds.

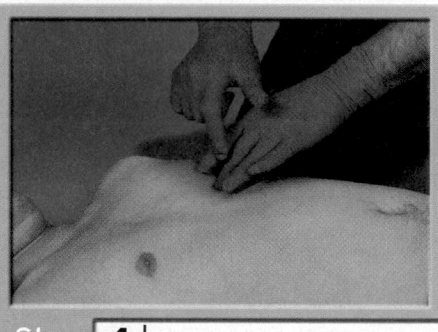

Step 4 Percuss the chest to detect any abnormalities.

Secondary Assessment

open mouth to facilitate your auscultatory assessment. Listen to as many portions of the lungs as possible, preferably avoiding any bony prominences, attached medical equipment, and, as mentioned, clothing. You can almost always hear a patient's breath sounds better from the patient's back; therefore, if the patient's back is accessible, listen there and assess six fields. If you have stabilized the patient or if the patient is in a supine position, listen from the front and sides and assess four fields. Always use the best stethoscope available.

Normal breath sounds are clear and quiet during inspiration and expiration. Tracheal sounds (noted over the trachea) are loud and harsh. The loud, high-pitched, and hollow sounds noted over the manubrium (over the mainstem bronchus) are known as bronchial sounds. The soft, breezy, and lower pitched sounds found at the midclavicular line are known as <u>bronchovesicular sounds</u>. The finer and somewhat fainter breath sounds noted in the lateral wall of the chest are from the smaller bronchioles and alveoli and are known as <u>vesicular sounds</u>.

Pathologic or <u>adventitious breath sounds</u> include the following:

- **Wheezing breath sounds.** These sounds suggest an obstruction of the lower airways. <u>Wheezing</u> is a high-pitched whistling sound that is most prominent on expiration but can be heard on inspiration in sicker patients.

    If wheezing is unilateral, an aspirated foreign body or infection should be suspected. If wheezing is bilateral, suspect asthma. Other causes include an inhaled irritant such as chlorine or other less common lung diseases such as asbestosis may be the problem.

- <u>Rales</u>. Wet breath sounds may indicate cardiac failure or infection, especially in a young child. Rales are

Words of Wisdom

The lungs are hyperinflated in patients with chronic emphysema, resulting in hyperresonance where you would expect to hear cardiac dullness.

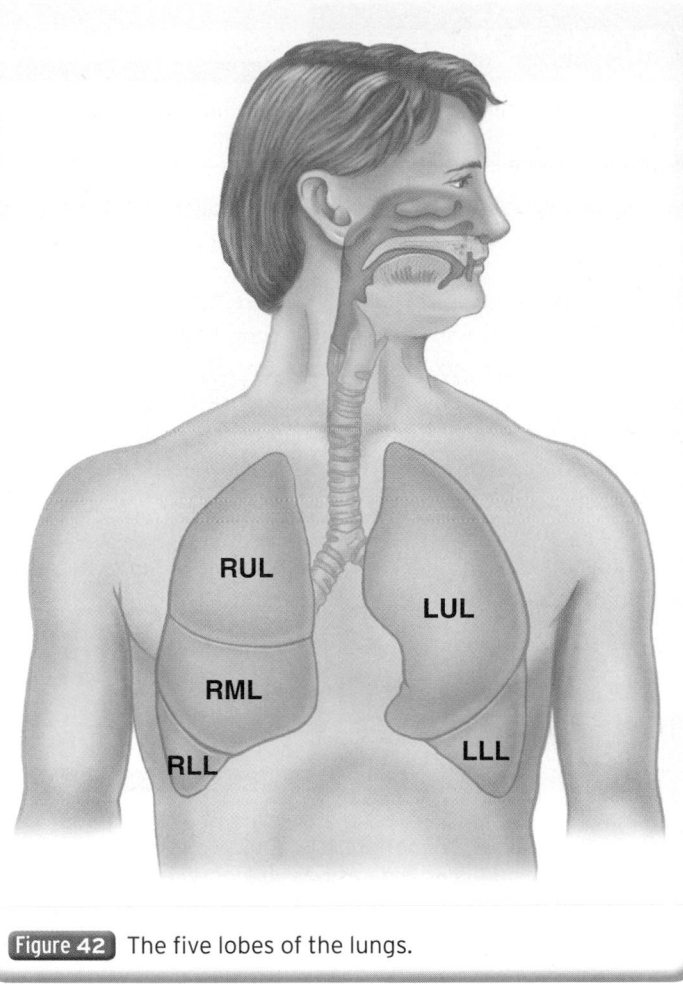

Figure 42 The five lobes of the lungs.

often difficult to hear, especially in the back of a moving ambulance. A moist crackling, usually on inspiration and expiration, is called crackles. Rales and crackles are produced by oxygen passing through moisture in the bronchoalveolar system or by closed alveoli opening abruptly.

- Rhonchi. Rhonchi, or congested breath sounds, are continuous sounds with a lower pitch and a rattling quality and are indicative of fluid in the larger airways in the lungs. They may indicate the presence of mucus in the lungs, for example from the presence of an infection (such as pneumonia) or inflammation (such as bronchitis). Expect to hear low-pitched, noisy sounds that are most prominent on expiration. The patient often reports a productive cough associated with these sounds. Aspiration of fluid may also result in rhonchi.

- Stridor. Stridor is a brassy, crowing sound often heard without a stethoscope. It is caused by the narrowing, swelling, or obstruction of the upper airway and may indicate that the patient has an airway obstruction in the neck or upper part of the chest. It is most prominent on inspiration. Stridor may be caused by bacterial epiglottitis, viral croup, swelling from upper airway burns, or a partial foreign body airway obstruction. Stridor often indicates a life-threatening problem, because stridor equates to an 85% reduction in airway size. The onset of crowing or stridor in

the presence of fever or upper respiratory infection should be recognized as a potential threat to life.

- Pleural friction rubs. These sounds are squeaking or grating sounds that occur when the pleural linings rub together. If this occurs, the pleural layers have lost their lubrication, most commonly due to inflammation of the pleura. This condition is usually associated with pain on inspiration. The sounds may be heard any time the chest wall moves; therefore, they can be heard on inspiration, expiration, or both.

Words of Wisdom

Percussion of the chest produces hyperresonance when the thorax is full of air and hyporesonance, or dullness, when it is full of blood.

While having a true appreciation for these adventitious sounds takes a great deal of practice, at times even the most experienced provider has difficulty deciphering the various pathologic lung sounds. In these instances, it might be helpful to describe the sounds rather than attempt to immediately classify them. Ask yourself if the sounds appear to be dry or moist. Moist sounds might suggest pneumonia or pulmonary edema. Are the sounds continuous or intermittent? Continuous sounds suggest a pathologic process, whereas intermittent sounds could be from a partial foreign body obstruction or a reversible process such as bronchospasm. Define the sounds as course or fine. Course sounds are louder and harsher and suggest a possible problem in the bronchial tree, whereas fine sounds are quieter and sometimes associated with a lower airway problem.

One of the most important—and perhaps most often overlooked—aspects of pulmonary assessment is appreciating when breath sounds are diminished or absent. You cannot be aware of this phenomenon without first developing an appreciation of the wide spectrum of normal presentations that exist. Before going out into the field, you should spend many hours listening to normal breath sounds so that you develop an understanding of what constitutes the many variations of normal breathing. After that, you will spend time listening to patients with respiratory difficulty, preferably alongside an experienced person who can point out the significant variations in the presenting abnormalities.

Decreased breath sounds can be localized to a portion of one lung, or they can encompass the entire chest. When hypoventilation is suspected, you must take immediate action. Decreased breath sounds typically signal a lack of respiratory excursion or decreased tidal volume. Numerous problems can cause decreased breath sounds, including pneumothorax, hemothorax, pleural effusion, pulmonary edema, atelectasis/consolidation, exacerbated COPD, status asthmaticus, opiate intoxication, pneumonia, bronchitis, and altered mental status.

If decreased breath sounds are localized to a specific area, assess transmitted voice sounds to see if there is any increased vocal resonance, which is a sign of consolidation in the lung, suggesting possible pneumonia. Further assessment of increased

Secondary Assessment

vocal resonance can be made by testing for **bronchophony**. This is accomplished by placing the diaphragm of the stethoscope over the area of potential consolidation and asking the patient to say the words "ninety-nine." In healthy lung tissue, the term should sound muffled and indistinct; however, if the sound is louder and clear, this is considered bronchophony and suggests an area of consolidation. A similar test, called **whispered pectoriloquy**, is performed in the same manner but with the patient whispering the words "ninety-nine." Once again, a normal response should be muffled and indistinct. A louder and clearer whisper is considered a positive test of whispered pectoriloquy. Another test for consolidation is **egophony**. Here you place the diaphragm over the area of decreased breath sounds and ask the patient to say "ee." A normal response will elicit a muffled long E sound. However, if there is any consolidation in the area, the sound will sound like "ay." Keep in mind that these tests require an optimal listening environment; something that is hard to find at an emergency scene.

During the respiratory assessment, pay attention to the respiratory rate, depth, and effort, as these will help to determine the level of distress a patient might be experiencing. For patients with respiratory complaints, assess breath sounds early and often. Possible findings or problems include the following:

- Lung fields with absent breath sounds: pneumothorax, hemothorax
- Silent breath sounds: status asthmaticus
- Lung fields with areas of consolidation: pneumonia, lung contusion
- Wheezing (localized or diffuse): asthma or bronchoconstriction
- Rales (wet lung sounds): pulmonary edema, heart failure, toxic inhalation, submersion

Words of Wisdom

Normal breathing should be quiet and not grossly evident to you. If you can see or hear the patient working hard to breathe, there is a problem.

For any patient with a respiratory complaint, you should be alert for the appearance of accessory muscle use or retractions, both of which are signs of increased work of breathing. Also, look for the signs of ventilatory fatigue, such as decreased mentation or a tired, worn-out appearance that often precedes ventilatory failure and, frequently, respiratory or cardiac arrest. This is especially true for children. Watch for the appearance of jugular venous distention (JVD) with respiratory patients because it may point to pneumothorax or heart failure.

Words of Wisdom

It may be difficult to assess the stability of a large patient's chest for paradoxical motion. Try fanning out the fingers of both of your hands as wide as possible; then assess the up-and-down motion of the patient's breathing. This will give you a better assessment of equality and movement of the chest with respiration.

Secondary Assessment

YOU *are the Medic*   PART 4

Your crew has finished securing the patient into full spinal precautions and you have started an IV line. You move the patient to the ambulance for transport to the trauma center.

Recording Time: 10 Minutes	
Respirations	28 breaths/min, shallow
Pulse	120 beats/min, weak
Skin	Cool, pale, dry
Blood pressure	92/62 mm Hg
Oxygen saturation (Spo$_2$)	96% on 15 L/min O$_2$ via nonrebreathing mask
Pupils	Equal and reactive

7. How can you determine the level of internal damage if you do not have the implement used in the stabbing?

8. Is past medical history relevant in this case?

Cardiovascular System

The cardiovascular system circulates blood throughout the body, an activity that maintains perfusion of the body's tissues **Figure 43**. The cardiovascular system comprises a pump (the heart), a set of pipes (the blood vessels), and a liquid transported within those pipes (blood).

Blood consists of plasma, red blood cells, white blood cells, and platelets. Plasma is essentially a mild saline solution, but it also contains blood-clotting factors and particles that play important roles in the body's immune response.

The complex arrangement of connected tubes in the circulatory system includes the arteries, arterioles, capillaries, venules, and veins. This system is entirely closed, with capillaries connecting the arterioles and the venules.

Blood flows through two circuits in this system: the systemic circulation in the body and the pulmonary circulation in the lungs. The systemic circulation carries oxygen-rich blood from the left ventricle through the body and back to the right atrium. As this blood passes through the tissues and organs, it gives up oxygen and nutrients and absorbs cellular wastes and carbon dioxide. The cellular wastes are, in turn, eliminated as the blood flows through the liver and the kidneys. The pulmonary circulation carries oxygen-poor blood from the right ventricle through the lungs and back into the left atrium.

The cardiac cycle involves the events of cardiac relaxation (diastole), filling, and contraction (systole). These mechanical events are coordinated electrically with the heart's pacing and conduction system. The heart consists of four chambers: two atria (upper chambers) and two ventricles (lower chambers). Each side of the heart contains one atrium and one ventricle. The interatrial septum (membrane) separates the two atria; a thicker wall, the interventricular septum, separates the right and left ventricles. Each atrium receives blood that is returned to the heart from other parts of the body; each ventricle pumps blood out of the heart. The upper and lower portions of the heart are separated by the atrioventricular valves, which prevent backward flow of blood. The semilunar valves, which are located between the ventricles and the arteries into which they pump blood, serve a similar function **Figure 44**.

Blood enters the right atrium via the superior and inferior vena cavae and the coronary sinus, which consists of veins that collect blood returning from the walls of the heart. Blood from four pulmonary veins enters the left atrium. Between the right and left atria is the fossa ovalis, a depression that represents the former location of the foramen ovale, an opening between the two atria that is present in the fetus.

The cardiac cycle coordinates the movement of blood between the chambers of the heart. The atria always relax and contract together, as do the ventricles. While the atria are contracting (and filling the ventricles), the ventricles are relaxing. Conversely, when the ventricles are contracting, the atria are relaxing, being filled by either the vena cava or the pulmonary veins.

The contraction and relaxation of the heart, combined with the flow of blood, generates characteristic heart sounds during auscultation with a stethoscope. The normal pattern sounds much like this: "lub-DUB lub-DUB, lub-DUB ..." The "lub" is referred to as the first heart sound or S_1, and the "DUB" (emphasized because it is often louder) as the second heart sound or S_2. Pathologic heart sounds include S_3 and S_4 **Figure 45**. The S_3 or third heart sound is a soft, low-pitched heart sound that occurs about one third of the way through diastole. Although S_3 is sometimes present in healthy young people, it most commonly is associated with abnormally increased filling pressures in the atria secondary to moderate to severe heart failure. S_4, which is considered a "gallop" rhythm, is a moderately pitched sound that occurs immediately before the normal S_1 sound; it is always abnormal. The S_4 sound represents either decreased stretching (compliance) of the left ventricle or increased pressure in the atria. Events on

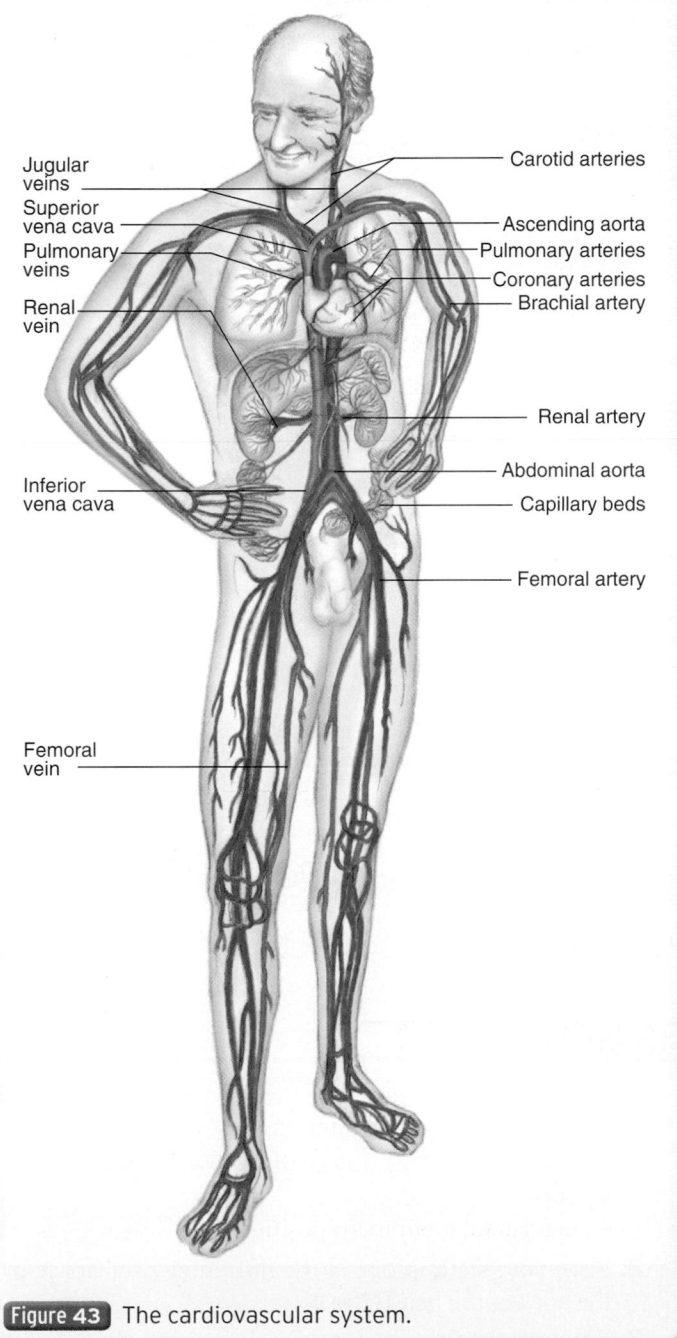

Jugular veins
Superior vena cava
Pulmonary veins
Renal vein
Inferior vena cava
Femoral vein

Carotid arteries
Ascending aorta
Pulmonary arteries
Coronary arteries
Brachial artery
Renal artery
Abdominal aorta
Capillary beds
Femoral artery

Figure 43 The cardiovascular system.

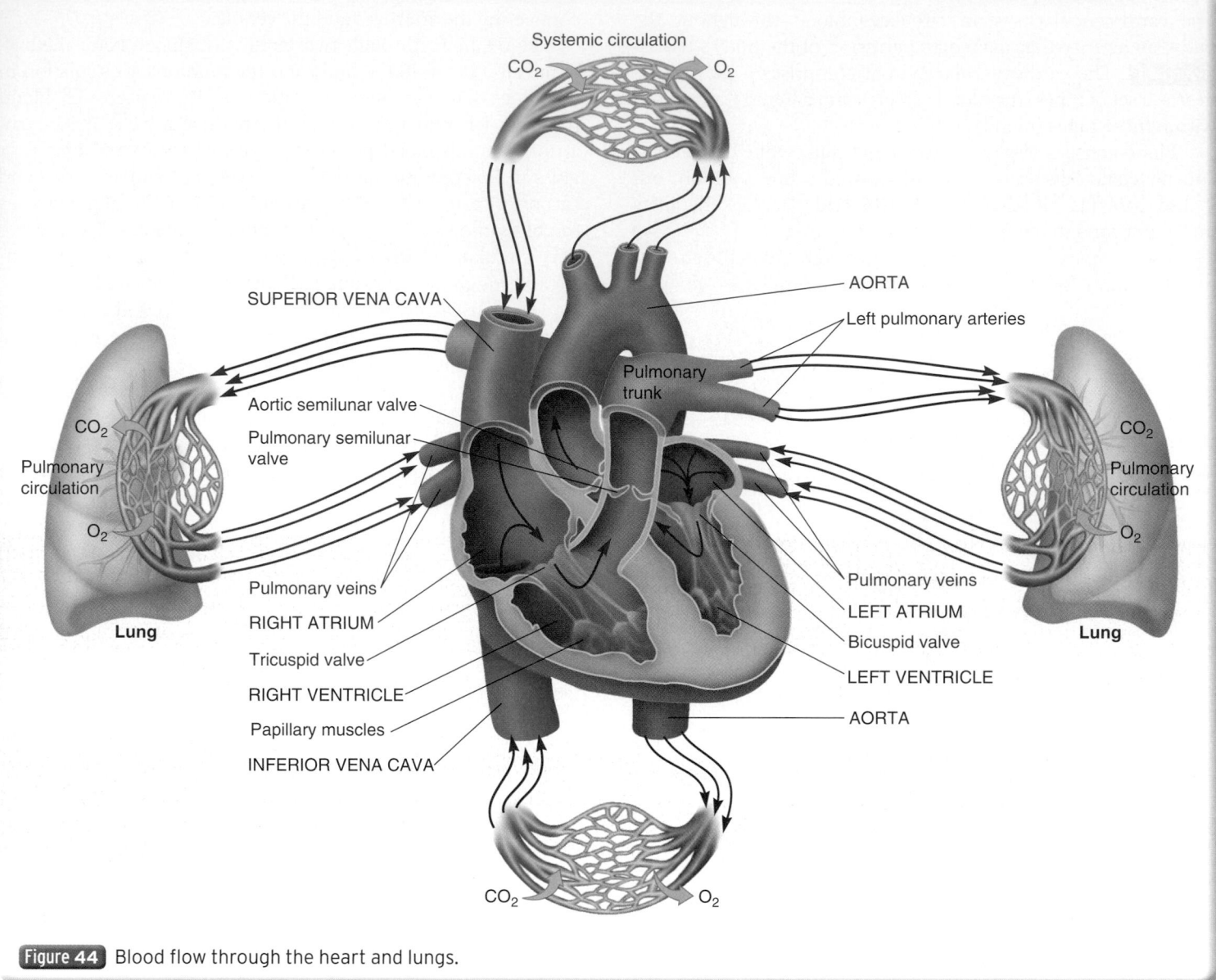

Systemic circulation

CO_2 O_2

AORTA

SUPERIOR VENA CAVA

Left pulmonary arteries

Pulmonary trunk

Aortic semilunar valve

Pulmonary semilunar valve

CO_2

Pulmonary circulation

O_2

CO_2

Pulmonary circulation

O_2

Pulmonary veins

RIGHT ATRIUM

LEFT ATRIUM

Tricuspid valve

Bicuspid valve

RIGHT VENTRICLE

LEFT VENTRICLE

Papillary muscles

AORTA

INFERIOR VENA CAVA

Lung

Lung

CO_2 O_2

Figure 44 Blood flow through the heart and lungs.

the right side of heart usually occur slightly later than those on the left side, creating two discernible sounds rather than one heart sound. This is known as **splitting**. This most commonly occurs with S_2 and is typically associated with respiratory patterns (physiologic split). However, a split S_2 that is fixed and does not change with respirations is indicative of a potentially serious heart problem and warrants further evaluation.

Heart sounds can be appreciated by listening to the chest wall in the parasternal areas superiorly and inferiorly as well

as in the region superior to the left nipple. Follow the steps in Skill Drill 10:

Words of Wisdom

The S_3 sound is associated with heart failure and is always abnormal in patients older than 35 years.

Skill Drill   10

1. Place the patient in one of these positions, to bring the heart closer to the left anterior chest wall:
   - Sitting up and leaning slightly forward Step 1
   - Supine
   - Left lateral recumbent position

2. Place your stethoscope at the fifth intercostal space over the apex of the heart Step 2.

3. To appreciate the S_1 sound, ask the patient to breathe normally and hold the breath on expiration.

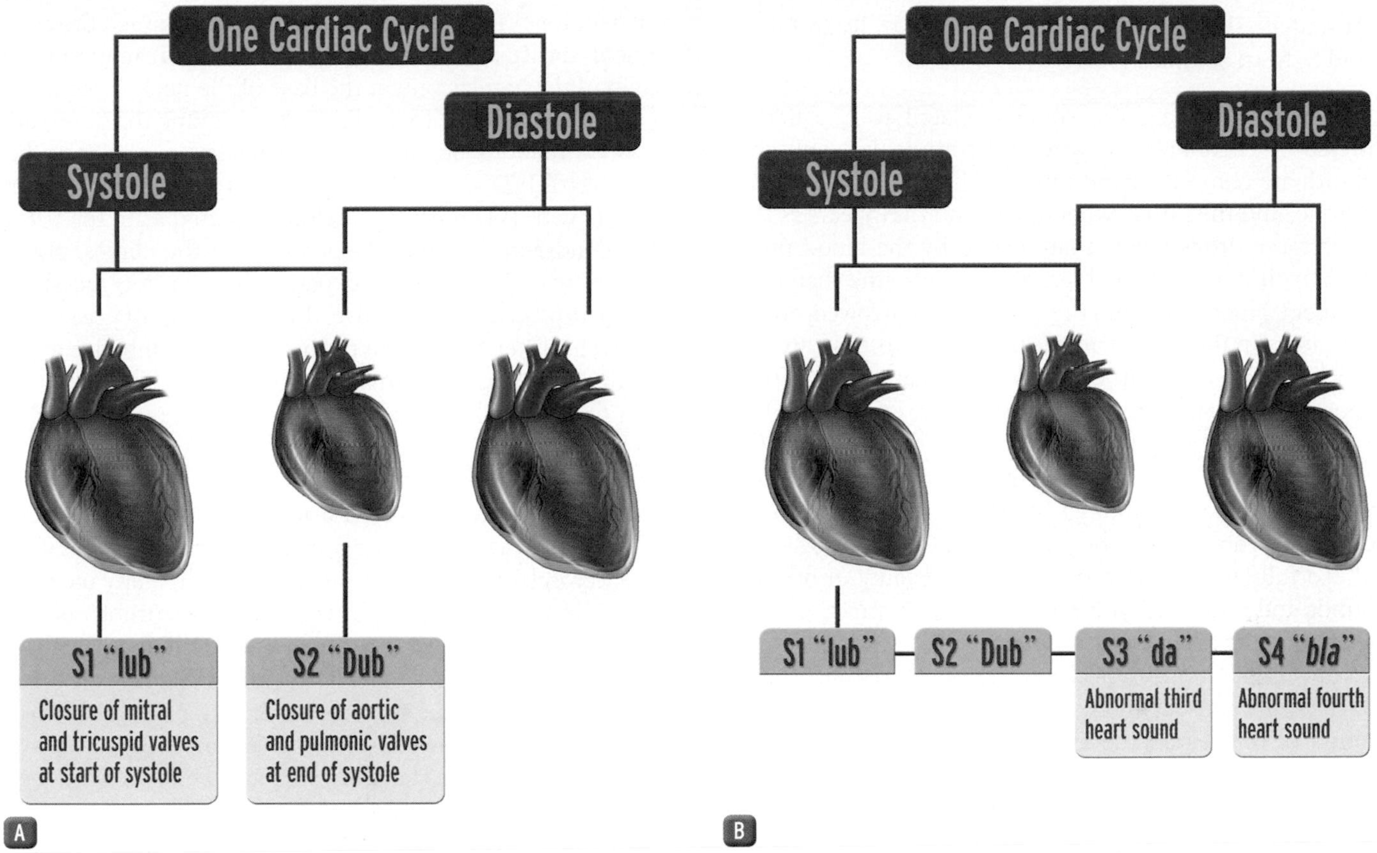

One Cardiac Cycle

Diastole

Systole

S1 "lub"	**S2 "Dub"**
Closure of mitral and tricuspid valves at start of systole	Closure of aortic and pulmonic valves at end of systole

A

One Cardiac Cycle

Diastole

Systole

S1 "lub"	**S2 "Dub"**	**S3 "da"**	**S4 "bla"**
		Abnormal third heart sound	Abnormal fourth heart sound

B

Figure 45 Heart sounds. **A.** The normal S$_1$ and S$_2$ heart sounds. **B.** The abnormal S$_3$ and S$_4$ heart sounds.

Skill Drill   10

Auscultating Heart Sounds

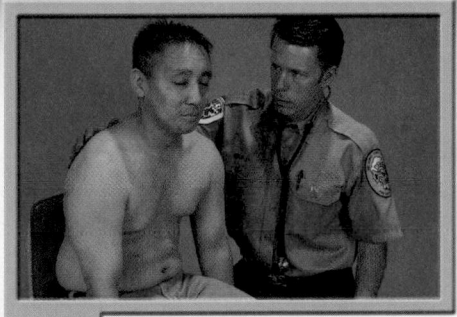

Step 1 Place the patient in a position that will bring the heart closer to the left anterior chest wall, such as sitting up and leaning slightly forward.

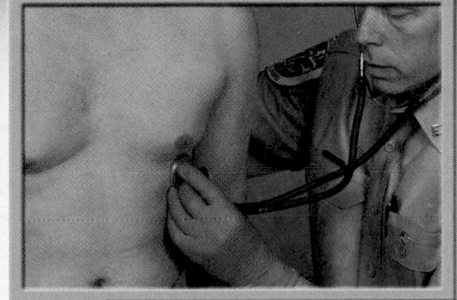

Step 2 Place your stethoscope at the fifth intercostal space over the apex of the heart.

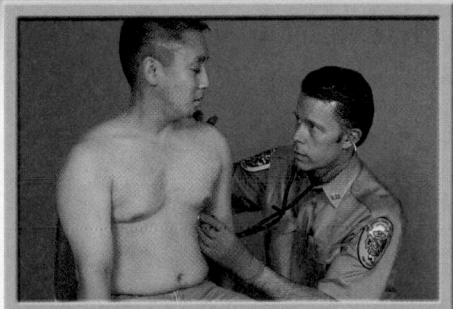

Step 3 Ask the patient to breathe normally and hold the breath on inhalation.

Secondary Assessment

4. To appreciate the S₂ sound, ask the patient to breathe normally and hold the breath on inhalation `Step 3`.

5. Auscultate the area above the left nipple to listen for S₃ and S₄ heart sounds.

<u>Korotkoff sounds</u> are the sounds related to a patient's blood pressure. There are five Korotkoff sounds, but only the first and fifth are clinically significant: the first is the thumping of the systolic, and the fifth is when the sound disappears as the diastolic pressure drops below that created by the blood pressure cuff. A <u>bruit</u> is an abnormal "whoosh"-like sound that indicates turbulent blood flow moving through a narrowed artery (most significant in the carotid arteries). A <u>murmur</u> is an abnormal whoosh-like sound heard over the heart that indicates turbulent blood flow around a cardiac valve. Murmurs are graded as a range of intensity from 1 (softest) to 6 (loudest). Many people have normal, physiologic murmurs. In some patients, they can represent a degree of pathology, depending on the nature of the underlying problem and the specific anatomy of the valve involved. To fully appreciate the nature and quality of normal heart sounds and murmurs, you must thoroughly practice your listening skills using excellent equipment.

Arterial pulses are a physical expression of systolic blood pressure. They are caused when contraction of the left ventricle and ejection of blood into the systemic circulation generate a pressure wave, which then travels throughout the arterial system. Arterial pulses are palpable wherever an artery crosses a bony prominence.

Venous pressure tends to be low. In fact, in the normal setting, the pressure in the vena cava just before blood is received into the right atrium is close to zero. Veins are relatively non-muscular, thin-walled vessels that have no effect on systemic vascular resistance and do not assist in promoting systemic blood pressure. Blood flows through the venous system and returns to the heart in part because it is propelled from behind in a continuous fashion, draining the capillary network. Most venous return of blood is a function of the respiratory cycle, generated by negative intrathoracic pressure that is developed at inspiration during normal breathing.

Assess the extremities, particularly the lower extremities, for any signs of venous obstruction or insufficiency. Signs include venous engorgement, palpable varicosities, edema, swelling, hyperpigmentation, and mild erythema. Patients may complain of swelling, painful superficial veins, heaviness in the extremities, and changes in skin color.

Occasionally, you can estimate the capacity of the venous system by observing a patient's jugular venous pressure, also known as <u>jugular venous distention (JVD)</u>. Any time you see JVD, ask yourself where is the venous obstruction that is impeding blood return to the heart? If the patient has penetrating left chest trauma, JVD may indicate cardiac tamponade. If the patient has pedal edema, consider heart failure. Specifically, in right-sided heart failure, blood tends not to be readily accepted into the right atrium. Venous capacitance increases in an effort to compensate for this failure, which in turn results in elevated pressures and corresponding JVD. JVD can be most readily observed by evaluating the anterolateral aspects of the

neck; it can also be provoked in a normal person by having the person lie supine and elevate the legs. While you are examining a patient for JVD, it is important to note how much distention is present, measured in terms of centimeters of distention from the origin of the jugular vein at the base of the neck. Note the angle of the patient relative to 0° (flat) while making the observation.

In situations involving hypotension, there may be no evidence of JVD, even while the patient is supine. Hypotensive patients with JVD must be carefully assessed as to the nature of their condition, however. Depending on the clinical situation, patients with JVD may be experiencing cardiogenic shock or have a ruptured cardiac valve. In the setting of chest trauma, neck vein distention and hypotension may symbolize a tension pneumothorax or pericardial tamponade.

The ability of the circulatory system to constrict and dilate can diminish markedly as a person ages. Although this limitation may vary considerably from patient to patient, an older patient's ability to compensate for cardiovascular insults may be profoundly curtailed by age-related changes, especially arterial atherosclerosis and diabetes. In addition, many medications that older persons routinely use to manage problems such as high blood pressure can negatively affect the body's ability to handle sudden changes in the demand for blood supply (ie, the body wants to increase the pulse rate, but a beta blocker medication will not let the pulse rate accelerate). By contrast, children and young adults have an enhanced ability to vasoconstrict and increase the pulse rate to compensate for a vascular insult; this compensation mechanism can fool you into believing that young patients are "less sick" than they actually are.

When you are examining a patient's cardiovascular system, pay attention to arterial pulses, noting their location, rate, rhythm, and quality. In addition, note the amplitude of the pulses (eg, weak and thready vs strong and bounding). Obtain an accurate blood pressure, and repeat this measurement periodically to assess the patient's hemodynamic stability. Note if the patient has a history of hypertension, and if so, note which class of hypertension the patient falls into `Table 7`. Palpate the carotid arteries and listen to them with the bell of the stethoscope to assess for any bruits. While inspecting and palpating the chest, listen for heart sounds. Feel the chest wall to locate the point of maximum impulse (PMI) and appreciate the apical pulse. Palpate for any <u>lifts</u> or <u>heaves</u> in the chest wall, suggesting hypertrophy, or for

Table 7 Hypertension Classifications		
Hypertension Classification	**Systolic Blood Pressure (mm Hg)**	**Diastolic Blood Pressure (mm Hg)**
Normal	< 120	and < 80
Prehypertension	120–139	or 80–89
Stage 1 hypertension	140–159	or 90–99
Stage 2 hypertension	> 160	or > 100

any thrills (humming vibration). A palpable thrill suggests an underlying bruit or murmur and warrants further investigation. Listen over the areas where the cardiac valves are located. The aortic valve is found near the second intercostal space, to the right of the sternum. The pulmonic valve lies near the second intercostal space, to the left of the sternum. The tricuspid valve is auscultated over the lower left sternal border. The mitral valve can be assessed over the cardiac apex, lateral to the lower left sternal border near the midclavicular line. Note the intensity of the heart sounds, and listen for S_1, S_2, and any extra sounds and murmurs.

For a suspected heart problem, assess the pulse for regularity and strength, and examine the skin for signs of hypoperfusion (pallor, cool, wet) or oxygen desaturation (cyanosis). If the pulse feels irregular, assess it over 1 minute, rather than 30 seconds, in order to obtain a more accurate rate. Listen to breath sounds—many cardiac problems are associated with respiratory problems (such as rales secondary to pulmonary edema). Obtain baseline vital signs. Serious hypotension with sustained or progressive tachycardia is common in cardiogenic shock; stay alert for this condition because its mortality rate is more than 80%. Check for JVD because it can indicate heart failure, cardiac tamponade, or pneumothorax. Examine the extremities for signs of peripheral edema that may result from right-sided heart failure.

When you are performing a cardiac exam in a neonate or infant, the definition of normal and abnormal findings differs from that of an adult. Paramedics should always assess for signs of cardiac compromise and insufficiency. When you are performing a visual inspection, be alert for cyanosis. Immediately following birth it is common for neonates to have acrocyanosis (cyanosis in the extremities). While in the adult population cyanosis in the extremities is an indication of severe hypoxia, in the neonate population acrocyanosis may be a normal variant following birth. Many times this is related to the ambient temperature in the room. When listening for heart sounds, you may notice some abnormal sounds that are considered normal variants in the pediatric population. For example, the presence of an S_3 in the pediatric population is considered a benign finding as long as the patient does not display any other signs of cardiac compromise. The presence of a split S_2 is relatively common in young children and is considered a benign finding when the split is associated with respiratory patterns. If the split S_2 is fixed regardless of the respiratory pattern, this warrants further evaluation because it is typically associated with a defect in the septum. The point of maximum impulse is not always palpable in infants and is affected by respiratory patterns, a full stomach, and the infant's positioning.

Abdomen

Because of the large number of organs within the abdomen, the location of organs and their related medical complaints are most easily described by dividing the abdomen into imaginary quadrants. The umbilicus (navel) serves as the central reference point. The diaphragm, the large dome-shaped muscle used for respiration, is at the top of the abdominal cavity, and the pelvis is at the bottom. The quadrants are divided by a set of imaginary perpendicular lines intersecting at the umbilicus **Figure 46**.

The abdomen contains almost all of the organs of digestion, the organs of the urogenital system, and significant

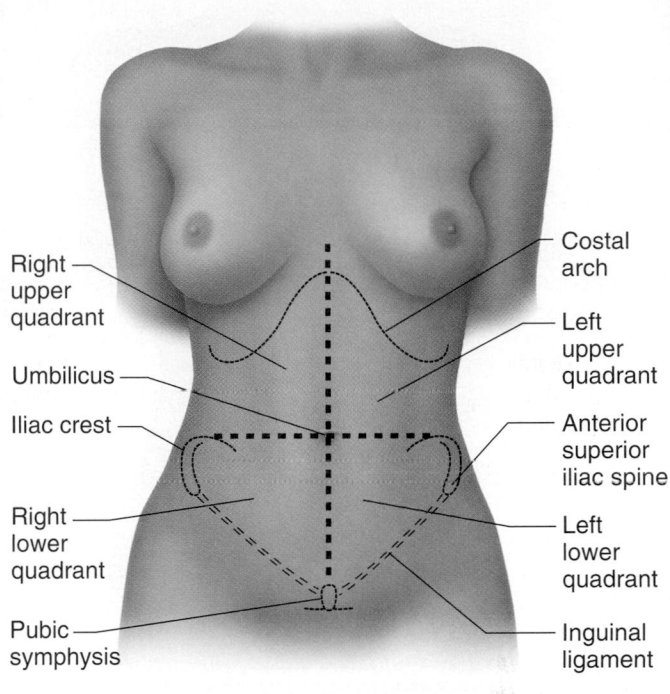

Figure 46 The abdomen is divided into four quadrants by imaginary vertical and horizontal lines.

neurovascular structures. The abdominal wall is a relatively thick muscular organ that overlies the peritoneum. The peritoneum is itself a well-defined layer of fascia made up of the parietal and visceral peritoneum. Abdominal organs are often characterized as being either intraperitoneal or extraperitoneal, depending on where they reside in relation to this layer. Intraperitoneal organs include the stomach, proximal duodenum of the small intestine, pancreas, jejunum, ileum, appendix, cecum, transverse colon, sigmoid colon, proximal rectum, liver, gallbladder, spleen, omentum, and female internal genitalia. Extraperitoneal organs include the mid- and distal duodenum, abdominal aorta, mid- and lower rectum, kidneys, pancreatic tail, adrenal glands, ureters, renal blood vessels, gonadal blood vessels, ascending colon, descending colon, and urinary bladder.

The abdominal organs can be topographically organized and sequentially assessed by viewing the overlying abdominal wall in a subdivided fashion. This is typically done in quadrants—left upper quadrant (LUQ), right upper quadrant (RUQ), left lower quadrant (LLQ), right lower quadrant (RLQ)—or ninths: right hypochondrial, RH; epigastric, E; left hypochondrial, LH; right lumbar, RL; umbilical, U; left lumbar, LL; right iliac, RI; hypogastric, II; left iliac, LI **Figure 47**.

One of the most challenging complaints for you to assess in the field setting is that of abdominal pain because it can result from multiple causes and often presents with little or no external signs. The following three basic mechanisms produce abdominal pain:

- *Visceral pain* results when hollow organs are obstructed, thereby stretching the smooth muscle wall, which in turn produces cramping and more diffuse, widespread pain.

Image labels: Right upper quadrant, Umbilicus, Iliac crest, Right lower quadrant, Pubic symphysis, Costal arch, Left upper quadrant, Anterior superior iliac spine, Left lower quadrant, Inguinal ligament

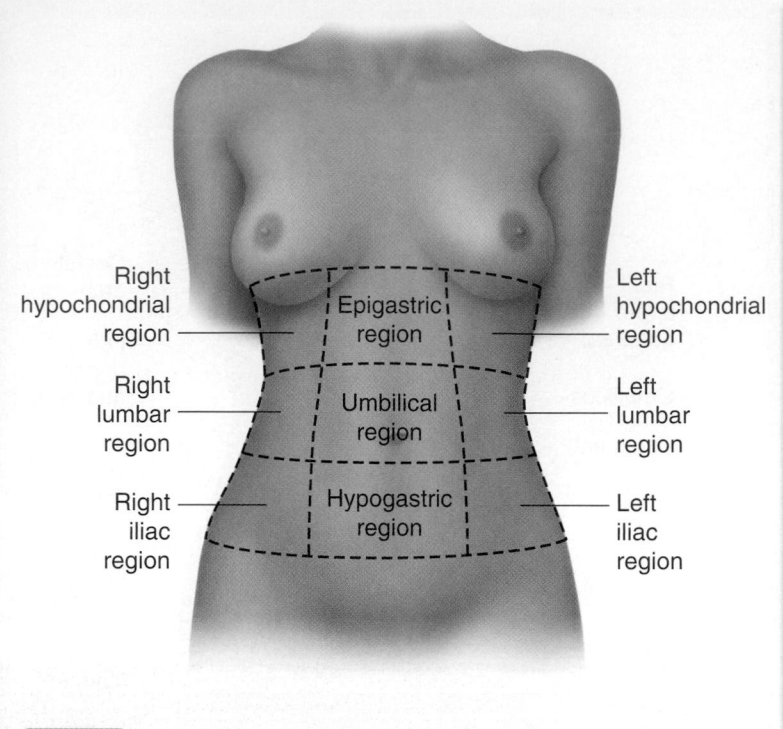

Right hypochondrial region

Epigastric region

Left hypochondrial region

Right lumbar region

Umbilical region

Left lumbar region

Right iliac region

Hypogastric region

Left iliac region

Figure 47 The abdomen can also be divided into nine regions.

- *Inflammation* or irritation of the somatic pain fibers located in the skin, the abdominal wall, and the musculature may produce sharp, localized pain, as in the case of pelvic inflammatory disease or appendicitis. If gastric contents, blood, or urine enters the peritoneum, it will also produce somatic pain, albeit usually much less localized and more diffuse.
- *Referred pain* has its origin in a particular organ but is described by the patient as pain in a different location. Examples include flank pain associated with kidney stones, inner thigh pain from appendicitis or pelvic inflammatory disease, scapular pain from cholecystitis, and groin pain (waves of pain) from renal colic.

Obtaining any appropriate history relevant to the situation is critical to help you determine the nature of an abdominal problem. Historic information should include the location, quality, and severity of the discomfort; time of onset and duration of symptoms; significant activities at the onset of distress; any aggravating or alleviating factors; and any associated symptoms, including nausea, vomiting, febrile symptoms, or changes in dietary, bowel, or bladder habits.

Inspection and palpation of the abdomen can provide valuable information, although it is often general. Tightness or guarding can result from internal bleeding, an inflamed organ, and many other causes. With upper left quadrant pain, possible sources include a ruptured spleen from a sickle cell crisis and mononucleosis. Patients with lower left abdominal pain, especially if they have a history of constipation, nausea, vomiting, and fever, should be suspected of having diverticulitis. With lower right abdominal pain, appendicitis is a likely culprit. Generalized abdominal pain in women of childbearing age can be the result of an ectopic pregnancy, a ruptured ovarian cyst, or

some other obstetric or gynecologic problem, some of which can be life threatening.

Obtaining baseline vital signs is an integral part of any secondary assessment. Clues provided will help you determine the seriousness of the patient's condition and the function of internal organs. Remember that shock, whether medical or trauma-related, is seen in different stages. Changes in a patient's blood pressure may be the last piece of evidence you see when shock changes from one level to the next. Keep in mind that blood pressure must be sufficient to maintain adequate end-organ perfusion.

<u>Orthostatic vital signs</u>, also called the tilt test, are measurements of a patient's blood pressure and pulse that are taken in the supine and sitting or standing positions. The results of such a test can help you determine the extent of volume depletion. The tilt test is generally used for patients with complaints of nausea, vomiting, diarrhea, syncope, and potential gastrointestinal problems; it indicates whether the patient needs fluid replacement. Normally, baroreceptors in the body sense changes in the blood pressure and volume and stimulate a catecholamine and renin-aldosterone response. This, in turn, causes peripheral vasoconstriction, increased pulse rate, and fluid retention, which puts more blood into core circulation and increases volume and blood pressure. In patients who are volume-depleted, there is not enough circulating blood to push into the core circulation, especially when they move from a supine position to sitting or standing.

Words of Wisdom

If a patient becomes dizzy when moving from a supine position to sitting up, do not have him or her stand up because he or she will likely pass out.

In some studies, a tilt test or orthostatic change is considered positive when the patient's blood pressure shows a decrease in systolic pressure (up to 20 mm Hg), an increase in diastolic pressure of 10 mm Hg (a narrowing pulse pressure), and an increase in the pulse rate by 20 beats/min. Vital signs should be taken at 1-minute intervals between moving a patient to a new position, and the cuff should be placed on the same arm in the same location. Documentation should include whether the pulse was regular, if the patient is being monitored and there is an attached strip, and whether the patient is experiencing other symptoms. If a fluid bolus for volume replacement is

Words of Wisdom

Assess the abdomen for the following:
- Tenderness
- Rigidity
- Swelling
- Guarding
- Distention

given, providers should repeat the orthostatic assessment after assessing lung sounds.

When you are examining a patient's abdomen, generally it is best to make the patient as comfortable as possible. Sometimes this requires administering some pain medication first; this usually allows the patient to be more cooperative and better able to focus with less discomfort. To assess the abdomen, the patient must be in a supine position. To examine and palpate/percuss over the posterior aspects of the abdomen, however, you should either have the patient sit up or log roll him or her at some point.

Prior to palpating the abdomen, have the patient point to the area of greatest discomfort. Avoid touching that area until last. Work slowly and avoid quick movements. When appropriate, speak with the patient about the nature of the illness while palpating the abdomen. Once an area of tenderness has been localized, attempt to visualize which structures may underlie it and think about what might potentially be causing the problem. In situations of penetrating trauma, this step is less of a priority: It is difficult to localize which areas may be damaged with a high-velocity wound by visualizing and palpating the

abdominal wall. Always proceed with abdominal assessment in a systematic fashion, routinely performing inspection, auscultation, percussion, and palpation, in that order quadrant by quadrant. Follow the steps in Skill Drill 11:

Skill Drill 11

1. Inspect the abdomen for any DCAP-BTLS Step 1.
2. Note any surgical scars because they may be clues to an underlying illness.
3. Look for symmetry and the presence of any distention.
4. Auscultate the abdomen for bowel sounds Step 2.
5. Perform percussion.
6. Palpate the four quadrants of the abdomen in a systematic pattern, beginning with the quadrant farthest from the patient's complaint of pain Step 3.
7. Note any tenderness or rigidity, and pay special attention to the patient's expressions because they may yield valuable information Step 4.

Skill Drill 11

Examining the Abdomen

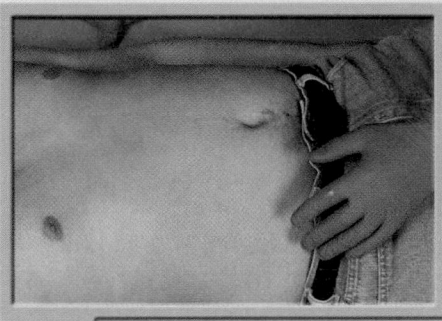

Step 1 Inspect the abdomen for any DCAP-BTLS.

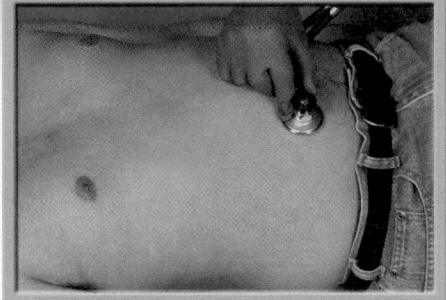

Step 2 Auscultate the abdomen for bowel sounds (if time and quiet environment permit).

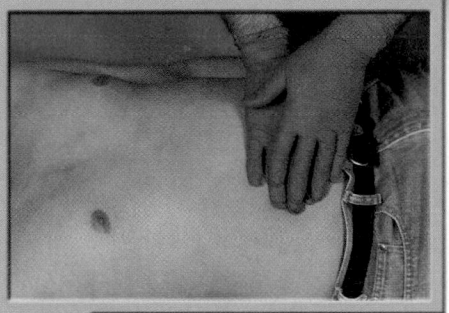

Step 3 Palpate the four quadrants of the abdomen in a systematic pattern, beginning with the quadrant farthest from the patient's complaint.

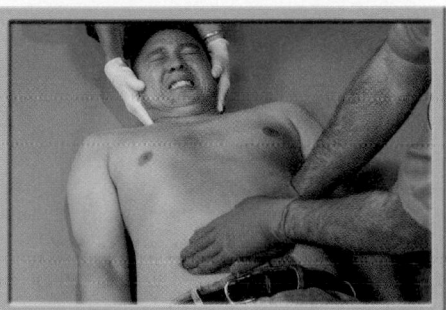

Step 4 Note any tenderness or rigidity.

Words of Wisdom

When you are palpating the abdomen, always begin on the side opposite the site of pain.

Start your assessment of the abdomen by looking at the skin as well as the contour and overall appearance of the abdominal wall. Note whether the abdomen is symmetric. Inspect the entire area for signs of swelling or bruising. Bluish discoloration in the periumbilical area (Cullen sign) or along the flanks (Grey Turner sign) is indicative of intraperitoneal hemorrhage, with two of the more common causes being ruptured ectopic pregnancy and acute pancreatitis. Look for a rash or other signs of an allergic reaction. Take note of scars from previous trauma or surgeries. Finally, note any wounds, striae, dilated veins, or generalized distention or localized masses.

Words of Wisdom

Patient restlessness and constant repositioning occur with the colicky pain of gastroenteritis or bowel obstruction. Absolute stillness, resisting any movement, is demonstrated with the pain of peritonitis (inflammation of the peritoneum). Knees flexed, facial grimacing, and rapid/uneven respirations also indicate signs of pain.

The abdomen can be described as flat, rounded, protuberant (bulging out), scaphoid, or pulsatile. Any abdominal distention needs to be distinguished from obesity. An obese abdomen tends to be more protuberant than distended, and is typically exceptionally pliable. A patient with intra-abdominal pathology who also happens to have significant obesity will present a challenge in this regard.

Some patients may have **ascites**, a collection of fluid within the peritoneal cavity. Ascites is consistent with an underlying edema, but instead of affecting the interstitial tissues of the legs, it involves the abdomen. The patient's abdomen may appear markedly distended, and a visible or palpable fluid wave may be evident during examination, with shifting dullness noted to percussion. Ascites is most typically seen in patients with liver disease, but it can also be appreciated with underlying malignancy and, to a certain extent, with renal and cardiac insufficiency.

Auscultation of the abdomen is commonly performed as part of the routine abdominal examination, although it may have limited utility in the prehospital setting. To hear bowel sounds, the setting must be fairly quiet and the patient must remain still. Make sure you take enough time to ensure an adequate assessment. Differentiating normal from abnormal can sometimes be challenging, so you should practice this skill on many healthy people to get a full appreciation for the abnormal situations you are likely to encounter.

When you are assessing bowel sounds, make note of their presence or absence. Sometimes the abnormality is characterized

Words of Wisdom

Hyperactive sounds are loud, high-pitched, rushing, or tinkling sounds that signal increased motility. Hypoactive or absent sounds follow recent abdominal surgery or are a sign of inflammation of the peritoneum.

by hyperactivity or hypoactivity, rather than a total lack of sounds. Bowel sounds can also be described as increased, decreased, or absent. In the case of hyperactive sounds, note their frequency and character. With an obstruction, the sounds are often referred to as high-pitched and tinkling.

In addition to bowel sounds, use the bell of the stethoscope to listen for any bruits in the abdomen. Recall that bruits are sounds made from turbulent blood flow through arteries. In the abdominal cavity, you should listen for bruits over the aorta, the right and left renal arteries, and the common iliac arteries. Bruits in these areas suggest stenosis or blockages of the arteries.

Palpation yields perhaps the most significant diagnostic information during the abdominal examination—that is, tenderness (elicited pain). You may then be able to correlate historic information related to the patient's current illness or situation and the findings from the examination, and determine what is wrong. Pain from the upper left quadrant should always be assumed to be the spleen, unless that can be ruled out. Misdiagnosing a ruptured spleen can result in a fatality. If you palpate the liver and see significant JVD, this suggests liver disease or inflammation secondary to hepatitis.

Palpate each quadrant gently but firmly, and recognize that the patient may respond in many ways. In a normal abdomen, the cavity should appear soft without any tenderness or masses. A moan, a guarding posture or withdrawing, or a facial grimace all send the same message: You have touched something or somewhere that causes pain or discomfort. That key information is worth pursuing with your assessment. Consider any signs or symptoms of abdominal injury as serious and indicative of a high-priority patient in unstable condition.

A patient who contracts his or her abdominal muscles shows the sign called **guarding**. Guarding can be either a voluntary or involuntary act, and is typically encountered when the patient has peritoneal irritation.

Rebound tenderness checks are rarely done in the field setting primarily because they can be painful for the patient as you slowly push down and then rapidly release sections of the abdomen. A positive sign (the patient cries out or withdraws) indicates peritoneal irritation. Such irritation may arise when an organ underlying the peritoneum becomes inflamed, or when a hollow organ ruptures and empties its contents into the peritoneal cavity. In trauma cases, however, solid-organ bleeding does not always result in peritoneal irritation and guarding. Large-volume bleeding with peritoneal distention will result in this phenomenon, for example. Marked peritoneal irritation and guarding is referred to as abdominal rigidity. This clinically important feature often results in urgent surgical evaluation and intervention. Guarding and rigidity are often encountered in trauma patients, but may also be seen in patients with appendicitis, cholecystitis, hollow-organ perforation, pancreatitis, and diverticulitis.

Patients with less discrete guarded tenderness to palpation may have a more visceral problem. Although this may represent an early manifestation of a serious condition, it can also be associated with various degrees of bowel obstruction, renal colic, biliary colic, or urinary tract infection. Often the pain is less localized on palpation, and is deep-seated and poorly described by the patient. Cases of colic typically involve a problem with peristalsis, the wave-like contraction motion of a hollow tubular structure (eg, small and large intestine, common bile duct, or ureter). A stone may obstruct the tube, for example, or an adhesion or hernia may prevent proper intestinal peristalsis. Some patients will describe the pain as "wave-like," or waxing and waning in nature. Other lower abdominal sources of pain and tenderness include genitourinary processes.

When you are palpating the abdominal cavity, you may attempt to palpate organs such as the liver, gallbladder, and spleen. To palpate the liver, place your left hand behind the patient, parallel to and supporting the right 11th and 12th ribs and adjacent soft tissues below. Place your right hand on the patient's right abdomen just below the rib cage. Ask the patient to take a deep breath. Try to feel the liver edge as it comes down to meet your fingertips. If you feel it, lighten the pressure of your palpating hand slightly so that the liver can slip under your finger pads and you can feel its anterior surface. The same technique can be used when assessing the gallbladder. While the gallbladder is typically not palpable, pain elicited or a sudden gasp from the patient indicates possible inflammation of the gallbladder. The only difference in the technique is when the patient takes a deep breath, attempt to move your fingertips under the liver edge, rather than palpating the anterior surface. This will bring your fingertips closer to the gallbladder. The spleen is a very difficult organ to palpate, and it is likely you will only be able to actually palpate the spleen when it is inflamed. With your left hand, reach over and around the patient to support and press forward the lower left rib cage and adjacent soft tissue. With your right hand below the left costal margin, press in toward the spleen. Begin palpation low enough so that you are below a possible enlarged spleen. Ask the patient to take a deep breath and try to feel the tip or edge of the spleen as it comes down to meet your fingertips.

Vascular sources can cause significant abdominal pain, most notably aortic aneurysm. Occasionally a markedly dilated aorta can be seen pulsating in the upper midline abdomen. If the patient has an obvious pulsatile mass, do not palpate it. However, if no pulsatile mass is seen, proceed with palpation of the abdomen. A ruptured aortic aneurysm also tends to be tender to palpation. Once you suspect an aortic aneurysm,

care should be taken to minimize manipulation. The aorta is a retroperitoneal structure, so a lack of obvious findings while assessing the anterior abdomen does not rule out this diagnosis in an otherwise proper clinical setting. Other notable palpable abdominal wall masses include **hernia**, a localized weakening of the abdominal wall musculature. Occasionally you might find a hernia in the ventral wall of the abdomen. This is different from a hernia that might be found in the groin. Many of these types of hernias, such as umbilical hernias, are congenital, whereas others may be acquired through previous abdominal surgeries. Hernias in the ventral wall are not always visible. If you suspect but do not see an umbilical or incisional hernia, place the patient in the supine position and ask the patient to raise his or her head and shoulders off the table. The bulge of a hernia will usually appear with this action. Most of the time, these findings are considered benign in the EMS environment. However, it is a true medical emergency if a section of bowel becomes entrapped and strangled in the hernia. In these cases the patient will have symptoms that include pain, fever, and possibly shock.

Female Genitalia

The female genitalia consist of the ovaries, fallopian tubes, uterus, vagina, and external genitalia **Figure 48**. The ovaries lie in the lowermost abdomen, in the inguinal regions, just superior to the inguinal creases. During a woman's reproductive years, the ovaries produce specialized hormones and ova. Hormonal regulation results in the maturation and release of an ovum roughly once a month as part of the menstrual cycle during that time.

After its release by the ovary, the ovum enters the fallopian tube and travels to the uterus. In the nonpregnant state, the uterus is a small structure that is not palpable on external examination. This hollow, muscular organ opens via the cervix into the vagina. Its inner lining thickens in response to hormonal stimulation, corresponding with the ripening and release of an ovum from the ovary.

The uterus receives sperm via the vagina and cervix. Pregnancy can result if sperm and ova successfully combine and become implanted in the lining of the uterine wall. If such fertilization does not occur, the uterine lining will slough and pass from the body with the menstrual flow.

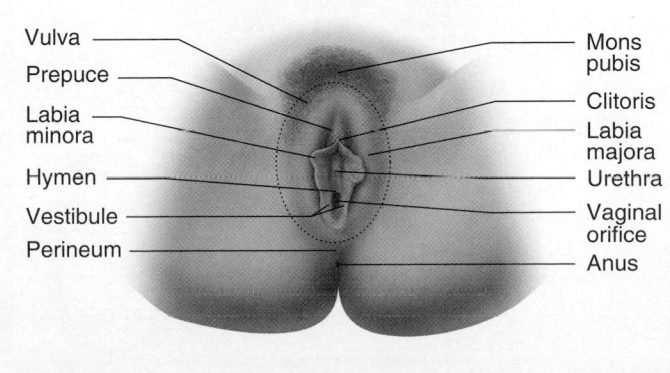

Figure 48 The female external genitalia.

In general, assessment of female genitalia is performed in a limited and discreet fashion. Always keep the patient appropriately draped during the course of the examination. Male paramedics should be assisted by a woman. Reasons to examine the genitalia include concern over life-threatening hemorrhage or imminent delivery in childbirth (checking for crowning).

While you are assessing the abdomen, palpate both the bilateral inguinal regions and the hypogastric region. If the decision is made to examine the genitalia specifically, limit the examination to inspection only. Pain and tenderness in the fallopian tubes and ovaries can be elicited during patient assessment. Clinically significant causes of this pain include ectopic pregnancy, complications of third-trimester pregnancy, and nonpregnant ovarian problems or pelvic infections. In the trauma patient where pelvic fracture is a concern, genital bleeding is a possibility, albeit an unlikely one. In the case of injury involving intentional trauma, significant bleeding is possible; if you must intervene in this kind of situation, be sure to preserve any garments and give them to the police as soon as possible. In general, make note of the amount and quality of any bleeding, as well as any inflammation, discharge, swelling, or lesions of the genitalia.

Male Genitalia

The male reproductive system consists of the testes, reproductive ducts, prostate, penis, and urethra **Figure 49**. The testes are analogous to the ovaries, in that they are the principal organs of reproduction and are responsible for manufacturing sperm. The testes, which lie outside the torso in a sac called the scrotum, produce hormones, seminal fluid (semen), and reproductive cells (sperm). The sperm and seminal fluid are transported

from the testes to the lower abdomen, where they are stored in the seminal vesicles.

During sexual intercourse, semen is ejaculated through the urethra. During its passage through the urethra, the prostate gland adds fluids to the semen. The urethra passes through the penis, which is a highly vascular structure. Reflexive arteriolar dilation within the penis results in penile engorgement and subsequent erection.

When you are examining male genitalia, make certain that your partner is present and perform the exam in a limited and discreet fashion. In the prehospital setting, situations requiring assessment of the male genitalia are limited. Always assess the entire abdomen and note any pertinent findings because occasionally lower abdominal problems are referred from the genitalia. Situations of testicular torsion or inguinal hernia sometimes present with a complaint of lower abdominal pain but minimal abdominal tenderness. In the case of a trauma patient, assess for the possibility of significant genital bleeding and injury, or underlying fracture. Note any inflammation, discharge, swelling, or lesions. Also, take note of priapism in male patients; a prolonged erection is usually the result of a spinal cord injury. In addition, look for evidence of urinary incontinence, especially in an unresponsive patient. Incontinence in an unresponsive patient could suggest a possible spinal cord injury or seizure.

Anus

The anus—the distal orifice of the alimentary canal—is often evaluated at the same time as the genitalia. It is examined in only a limited number of circumstances, and is always done with the patient appropriately draped and your partner present. With a positive history or signs or symptoms of trauma, examine the area to assess for the need of bleeding control or another intervention (such as treatment for shock, care of eviscerated parts). Examination usually occurs with the patient lying in a laterally recumbent position, and involves inspection only. Examine the sacrococcygeal and perineal areas, noting obvious bleeding, trauma, lumps, ulcers, inflammation, rash, abrasions, or evidence of fecal incontinence.

Musculoskeletal System

The extremities consist of both soft tissues and bones. Joints are areas where bone ends abut each other and form a kind of hinge, creating a jointed appendage. Joints are filled with shock-absorbing linings and fluid (synovium), and are held together by ligaments. They allow the body to perform mechanical work. Indeed, the mechanical process of motion becomes possible when the joints are flexed and extended by skeletal (or striated) muscles that traverse the joints. Skeletal muscles are anchored to bone via tendons, with each muscle being named according to its location and function.

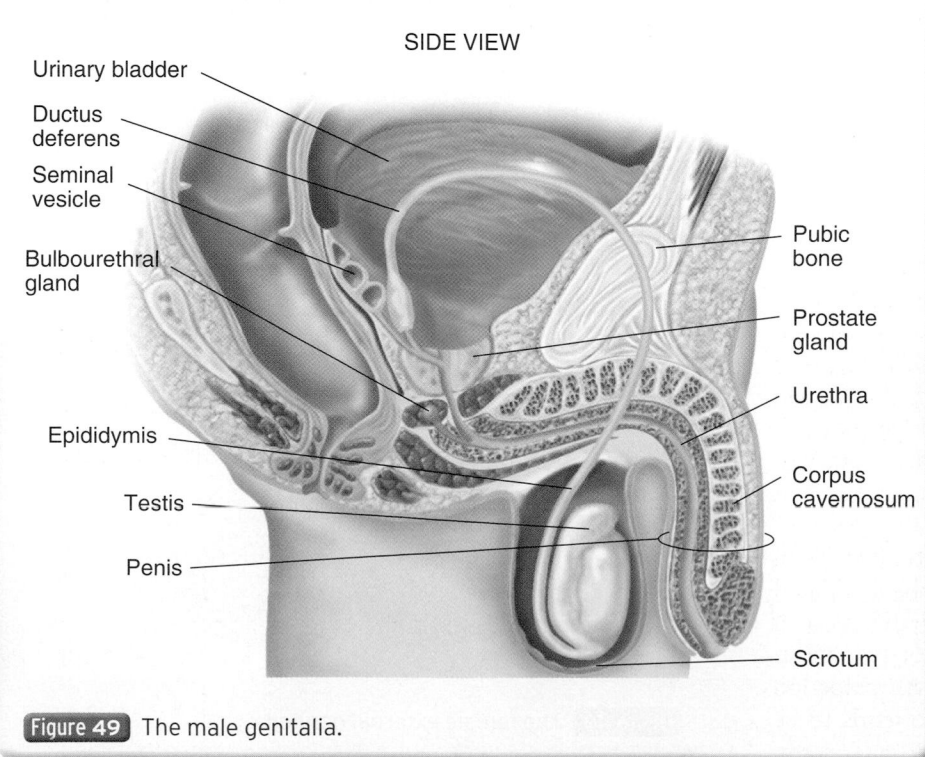

SIDE VIEW

- Urinary bladder
- Ductus deferens
- Seminal vesicle
- Bulbourethral gland
- Epididymis
- Testis
- Penis
- Pubic bone
- Prostate gland
- Urethra
- Corpus cavernosum
- Scrotum

Figure 49 The male genitalia.

The principal joints of the upper extremities include the shoulder (acromioclavicular and glenohumeral joints), elbow (olecranon), and wrist (radiocarpal). The principal joints of the lower extremities include the hip (acetabulum), knee (patellar), and ankle (tibiotalar).

As joints age, they become more vulnerable to repetitive motion stress and trauma, and they lose much of their articular abilities due to inflammation and breakdown of the synovium, leading to osteoarthritis in older adults. Disruption of the bones, joints, and soft tissues can take a variety of forms, and discomfort or disability may be a manifestation of an acute problem, a chronic problem, or a combination of the two. In older patients, musculoskeletal complaints are common. As the joints and muscles change with age, so does their ability to move around. Older patients are likely to have decreased mobility and range of motion secondary to joint and muscle changes. In addition to the joint changes mentioned earlier, the muscle mass in adults begins to decrease with age and with lack of use. Older adults tend to live a more sedentary lifestyle, which contributes to arthritis and loss of muscle mass. A common finding when assessing joints is crepitus with movement. Whereas this would be considered an abnormal finding in the younger population, this is considered a normal variant of aging and is typically associated with advanced arthritis.

Common types of musculoskeletal and soft-tissue injuries include fractures, sprains, strains, dislocations, contusions, hematomas, and open wounds. Fractures may be characterized in a number of ways. For example, an open fracture is essentially a fracture with direct communication to the exterior surface of the body, or simply an open wound in close proximity to the site of a presumed fracture.

Although fractures always involve a pathologic process, it is important to distinguish a <u>pathologic fracture</u> from a <u>physiologic fracture</u>. A physiologic fracture occurs when abnormal forces are applied to normal bone structures, producing a fracture. A pathologic fracture occurs when normal forces are applied to abnormal bone structures, producing a fracture. Physiologic fractures usually occur in the setting of high-force blunt injury. Pathologic fractures often occur as a result of decreased bone density, such as osteopenia or occult malignancy.

When you are examining the skeleton and joints, pay attention to their structure and function. Consider how the joint and associated extremity look and how well they work. Does the extremity look normal, and does it move easily? In particular, note any limitation in range of motion, pain with range of motion, or bony crepitance. When assessing the joints and extremities, look for evidence of inflammation or injury, such as swelling, tenderness, increased heat, redness, ecchymosis, or decreased function. Also evaluate the joint or extremity for obvious deformity, diminished strength, atrophy, or asymmetry from one side to the other. The examination of the musculoskeletal system should not cause the patient any pain; if any occurs, it should be considered an abnormal finding. Follow the steps in Skill Drill 12 :

Skill Drill 12

1. Beginning with upper extremities, inspect the skin overlying the muscles, bones, and joints for soft-tissue damage Step 1 .

2. Note any deformities or abnormal structure.

3. Check for adequate distal pulse, motor, and sensation to each extremity Step 2 .

4. Inspect and palpate the hands and the wrists, noting any DCAP-BTLS.

5. Ask the patient to flex and extend the joints of the fingers, hands, and wrist, noting any abnormalities in the range of motion. If the patient experiences any discomfort, stop that portion of the exam immediately Step 3 .

6. Inspect and palpate the elbows, noting any abnormalities. Ask the patient to flex and extend the elbow to determine the range of motion.

7. Ask the patient to turn the hand from the palm-down position to the palm-up position and back again, noting any pain or abnormalities Step 4 .

8. Inspect and palpate the shoulders. Ask the patient to shrug the shoulders and raise and extend both arms Step 5 .

9. Inspect the skin overlying the lower extremities.

10. Ask the patient to point and bend the toes to establish the range of motion Step 6 .

11. Ask the patient to rotate the ankle, checking for pain or restricted range of motion Step 7 .

12. Inspect and palpate the knee joints and patella. Ask the patient to bend and straighten both to establish the range of motion Step 8 .

13. Check for structural integrity of the pelvis by applying gentle pressure to the iliac crests and pushing in and then down Step 9 .

14. Ask the patient to lift both legs by bending at the hip and then turning the legs inward and outward. Note any abnormalities Step 10 .

Words of Wisdom

Point tenderness is the most reliable indicator of an underlying closed fracture.

Often the diagnosis of a problem involving the shoulders and related structures can be made simply by noting the patient's posture at the time of first contact with paramedics Figure 50 . For example, a glenohumeral joint dislocation may

Secondary Assessment

Skill Drill | 12

Examining the Musculoskeletal System

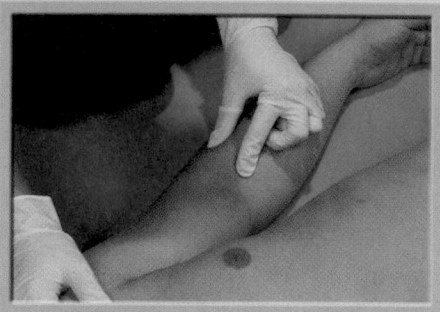

Step 1 Inspect the skin overlying the muscles, bones, and joints for soft-tissue damage.

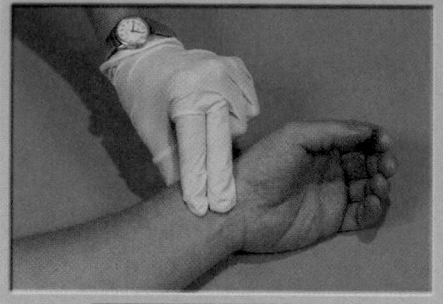

Step 2 Check for adequate distal pulse, motor, and sensation to each extremity.

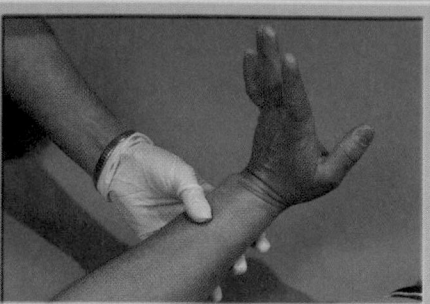

Step 3 Ask the patient to flex and extend the joints of the fingers, hands, and wrist to establish range of motion.

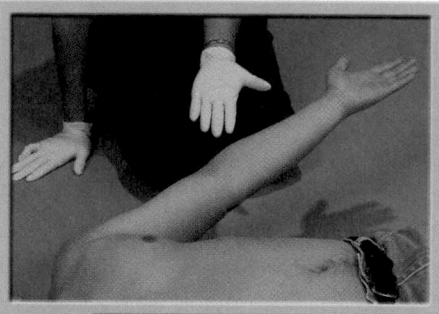

Step 4 Ask the patient to turn the hand from the palm-down position to the palm-up position and back again.

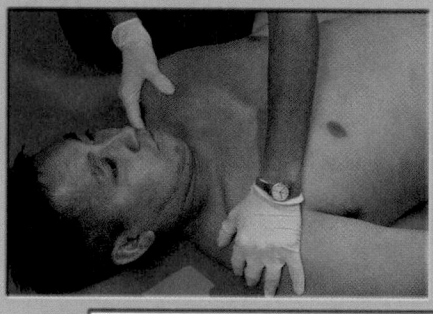

Step 5 Inspect and palpate the shoulders.

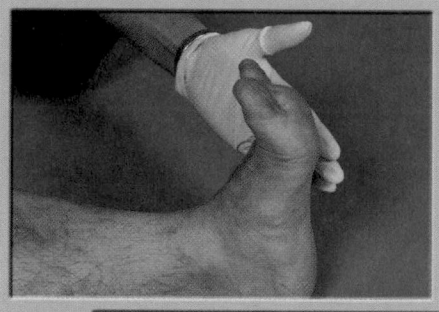

Step 6 Inspect and palpate the bony structures. Ask the patient to point and bend the toes to establish range of motion.

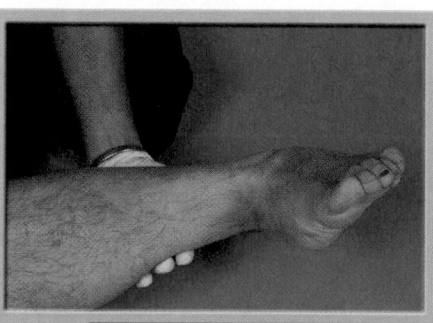

Step 7 Ask the patient to rotate the ankle, checking for pain or restricted range of motion.

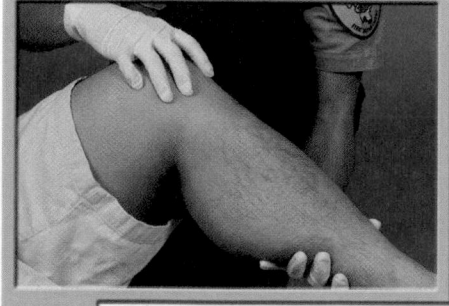

Step 8 Inspect and palpate the knee joints and patella. Ask the patient to bend and straighten both to establish range of motion.

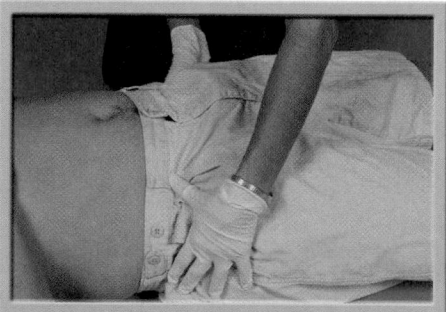

Step 9 Check for structural integrity of the pelvis by applying gentle pressure to the iliac crests and pushing in and then down.

Secondary Assessment

Continues

Skill Drill 12

Examining the Musculoskeletal System, continued

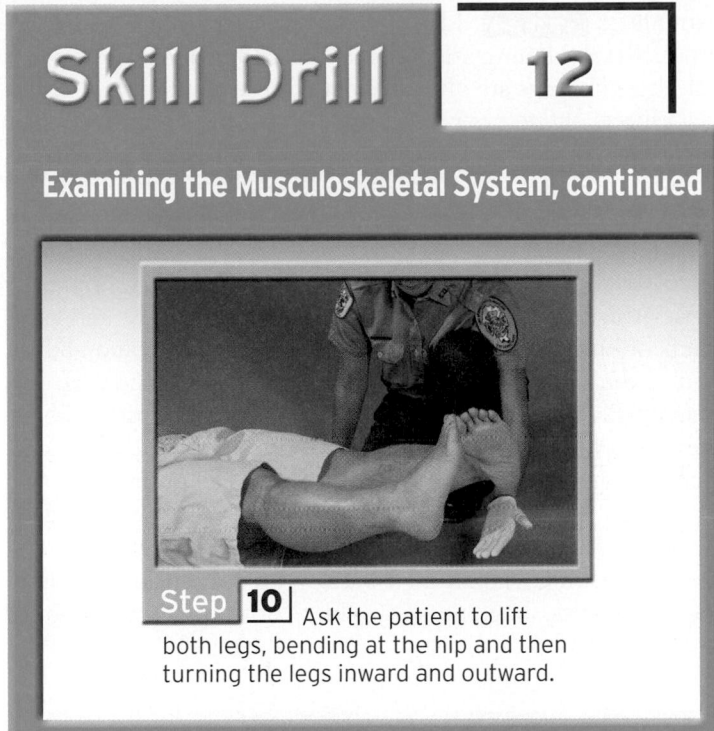

Step 10 Ask the patient to lift both legs, bending at the hip and then turning the legs inward and outward.

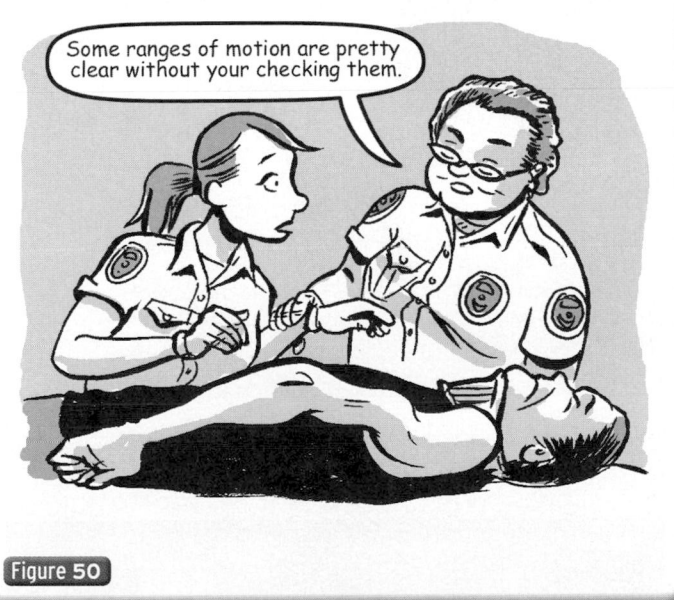

Some ranges of motion are pretty clear without your checking them.

Figure 50

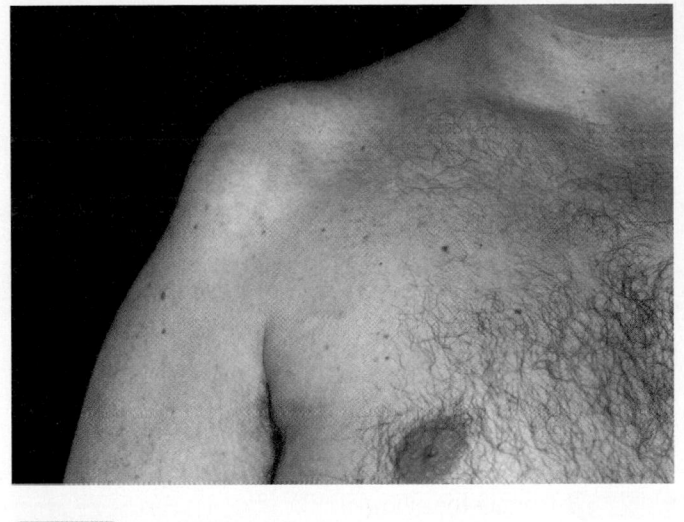

Figure 51 Abnormal squaring of the shoulder.

Words of Wisdom

When you are assessing a patient with a possible shoulder dislocation, position yourself behind the patient and compare the shoulders. The dislocated side is usually lower than the uninjured side.

be manifested as the loss of normal contour of the shoulder, with abnormal squaring of the lateral aspect of the shoulder and the humeral head visible and/or palpable in the soft tissues of the chest wall, in the subacromial region **Figure 51**.

When you are palpating the proximal upper extremity and shoulder, be sure to assess the sternoclavicular joint, acromioclavicular joint, subacromial area, and bicipital groove (origin of the biceps, just distal to the anterior aspect of the humeral head). Note any tenderness, swelling, crepitance, deformity, rotation, or ecchymosis in these areas.

When possible, check the patient's range of motion by asking the patient to raise the arms to the vertical position, above the head. Next, have the patient demonstrate external rotation and abduction by placing both hands behind the neck with the elbows out to the sides. Finally, perform internal rotation by having the patient place both hands behind the lower back.

Evaluation of the elbows should start with an overall inspection for gross deformity or abnormal rotation. Palpate the elbow between the epicondyles and olecranon, and palpate the epicondyles and olecranon themselves **Figure 52**. Note any tenderness, crepitance, swelling, or thickening. Range-of-motion testing should be performed last because suspicion of significant pathology or fracture of the elbow mandates appropriate immobilization as soon as possible. When ranging the elbows, flex and extend them both passively and actively. Then have the patient supinate and pronate the forearms while the elbows are flexed at the patient's sides.

When you are checking the hands and wrists, inspect them for any abnormalities, including swelling, redness, contusions, wounds, nodules, deformities, or atrophy. Palpate the hands, feeling the medial and lateral aspects of each interphalangeal joint on each finger **Figure 53**. Squeeze the hands, compressing the metacarpophalangeal joints. Palpate the carpal bones of the

Secondary Assessment

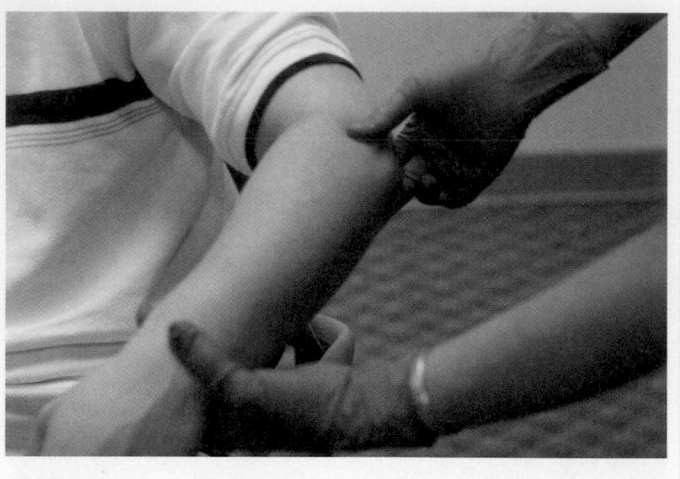

Figure 52 Palpate the elbow.

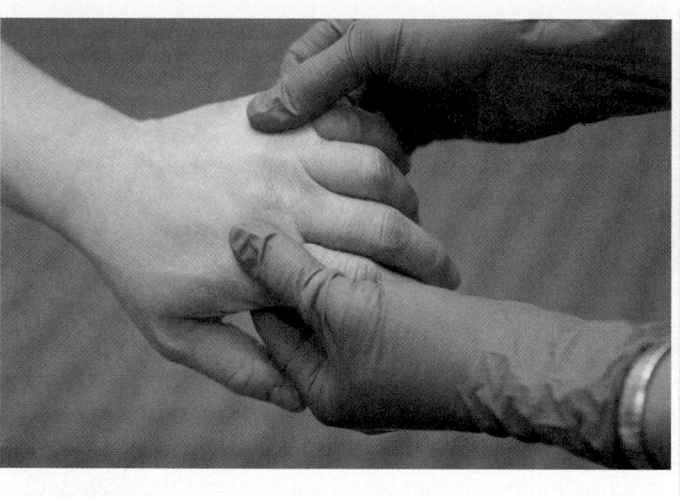

Figure 53 Palpate the hand and fingers.

wrists, noting any areas of swelling, tenderness, or bogginess. Perform range-of-motion evaluations by asking the patient to make fists with both hands, then extend and spread the fingers, then flex and extend the wrists, and finally move the hands laterally and medially with the palms facing down. Check capillary refill, symmetry of radial pulses, and overall limb temperature at this point.

A rapid appreciation of injury or disability involving the lower extremities can be made by evaluating the patient's ability to walk. Of course, this may not be a practical first approach to assessment in many prehospital cases.

Examination of the knees and hips begins with inspection of overall alignment and symmetry of the lower

Words of Wisdom

Heberden and Bouchard nodules are hard and nontender and occur with osteoarthritis.

extremities **Figure 54**. Identify any lower extremity deformity, especially shortening and/or rotation, either internal or external; these findings are often evident with an injury to the proximal aspects of the lower extremity or hip joint. In particular, an open book pelvic fracture, which presents with both feet rotated outward, is a life-threatening injury. Look for evidence of thickening, swelling, or bruising of the thigh. Note any crepitance or palpable tenderness. If possible, range the knees and hips in an effort to determine the presence of underlying injury to those structures. Ask the patient to bend each knee and raise the bent knee toward the chest. Assess for rotation and abduction of the hips, both passively and actively. Palpate each hip individually—specifically, distal to the inguinal crease and over the anterior, lateral, and posterior aspects. Finally, palpate and gently compress the pelvis downward and then inward.

When you are examining the ankles and feet, observe all surfaces. Note any wounds, deformities, discolorations, nodules, or swelling. Palpate all aspects of the feet and ankles, noting tenderness, bogginess, swelling, or crepitance. Measure

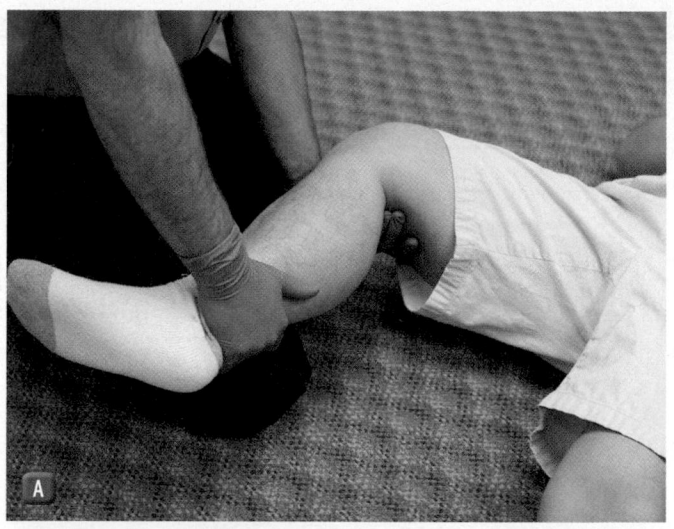

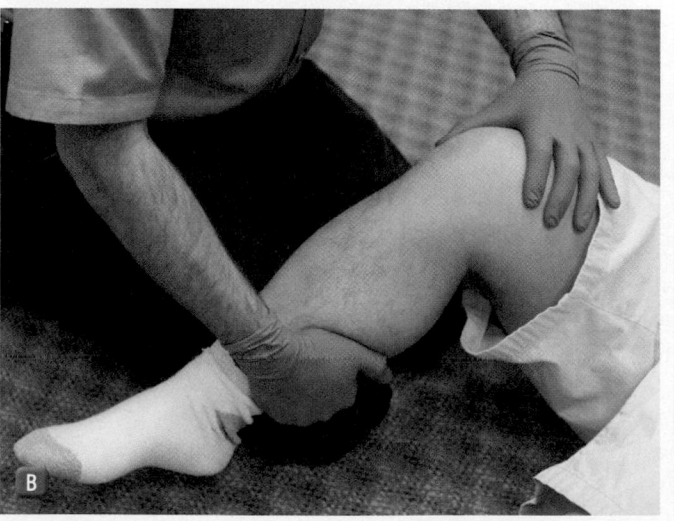

Figure 54 Examination of the lower extremities. **A.** Hip. **B.** Knee.

distal pulses over the dorsalis pedis and posterior tibialis, and assess the overall limb temperature at this point. A decrease in pulses might be noted in older patients, especially those with a history of moderate edema and peripheral vascular disease. Due to the sheer size of anatomy in young pediatric patients, pulses may be difficult to palpate. In this situation, capillary refill will be a more reliable indicator of perfusion. Assess range of motion by having the patient plantar flex, dorsiflex, and invert and evert the ankles and feet. Be sure to check the forefoot and toes by inspection, palpation, and range-of-motion testing **Figure 55**.

Peripheral Vascular System

The peripheral vascular system comprises all aspects of the circulatory system, except for the heart, the great vessels immediately involved with the mediastinum, and the coronary circulation. Thus it includes all of the body's arteries, veins, arterioles, venules, capillaries, lymphatics, and the respective fluids that fill these structures.

The lymphatic system is an intricate network of nodes and ducts of various sizes that are dispersed throughout the body **Figure 56**. Lymph nodes are larger accumulations of lymphatic tissue, and smaller amounts of lymph are distributed by tissue throughout the body. All lymphatic tissue contains large numbers of immunologically active cells; thus the lymphatics manage a key function in the body's immune system. The ducts contain a fat-rich fluid known as lymph, which transports materials from the lymph tissue into the central venous circulation via the thoracic ducts.

Perfusion occurs in the peripheral circulation via the network of capillary beds. Blood cells and plasma in close proximity to tissue offload substances required by the cells for proper metabolic functioning, and simultaneously pick up metabolic wastes for transport out of the tissues, ultimately for elimination from the body. Impaired functioning of the peripheral vascular system means that the capillary beds cannot provide for adequate tissue and organ perfusion—this is a significant source of morbidity and mortality. Diseases of the peripheral vascular system are often seen in patients with other

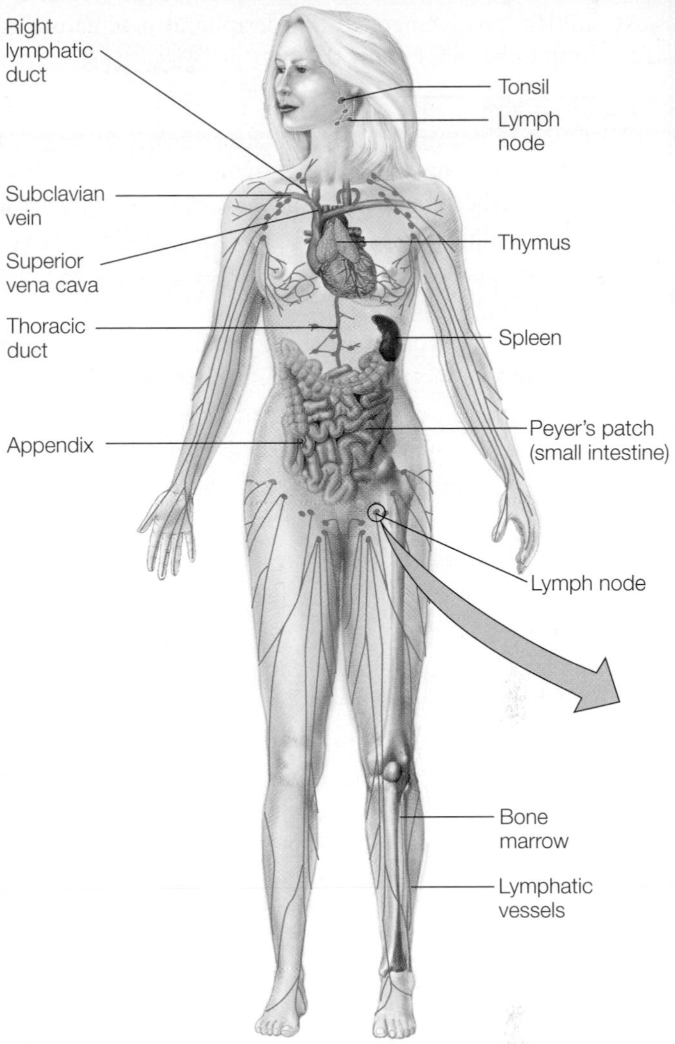

Figure 56 Lymphatic system.

underlying medical conditions, such as diabetes, hypertension, dyslipidemia, obesity, and tobacco use. These disease processes typically target and cause malfunctioning of the smaller-diameter vessels of the peripheral vascular system, resulting in disease states of the tissues and organs that depend on those vessels for proper functioning. With age and the occurrence of these various disease processes, the vasculature becomes less able to rapidly manage changes in perfusion requirements, so it can itself become a source of illness.

When you are assessing the peripheral vascular system, pay attention to both the upper and lower extremities. Look for signs indicative of either acute or chronic vascular problems. A wide range of disorders can affect the peripheral vascular system—from chronic venous stasis and lymphedema to intermittent claudication (cramp-like pain in the lower legs due to poor circulation or low potassium levels) and acute arterial occlusion. Peripheral vascular disease can manifest in many forms, depending on the point in the vasculature where the abnormality is located. Carotid artery disease can manifest as a stroke, for example, while arterial embolization involving the

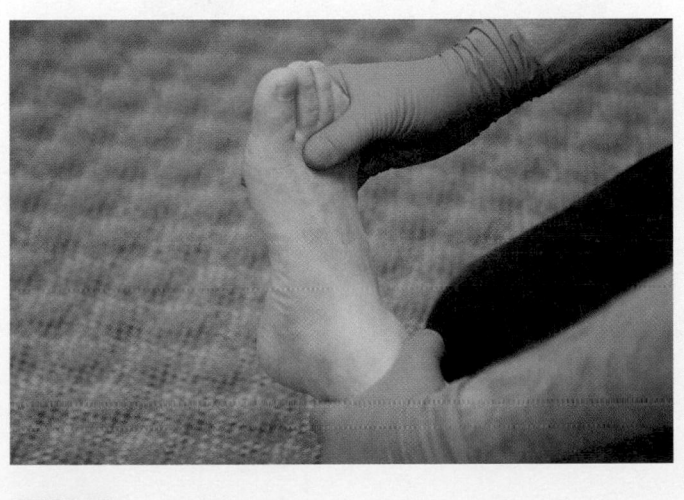

Figure 55 Inspect the feet.

mesenteric vessels can result in bowel ischemia and necrosis. In the extremities, involvement of the peripheral vasculature can result in limb ischemia. Follow the steps in Skill Drill 13:

Skill Drill   13

1. While examining the upper extremities, note any abnormalities in the radial pulse, skin color, or condition Step 1.

2. If abnormalities are noted in the distal pulse, work your way proximally, checking these pulse points and noting your findings Step 2.

3. Palpate the epitrochlear and brachial nodes of the lymphatic system, noting any swelling or tenderness Step 3.

4. Examine the lower extremities, noting any abnormalities in the size and symmetry of the legs Step 4.

5. Inspect the skin color and condition, noting any abnormal venous patterns or enlargement Step 5.

6. Check distal pulses, noting any abnormalities Step 6.

7. Palpate the inguinal nodes for swelling or tenderness Step 7.

8. Evaluate the temperature of each leg relative to the rest of the body and to each other.

9. Evaluate for pitting edema in the legs and feet Step 8.

When you are checking the upper extremities, inspect them from fingertips to shoulders. Note the extremity's relative size, and evaluate it for symmetry by comparing one side with the other. Pay attention to any obvious swelling, unusual venous patterns, the color and texture of the skin, and the color of the nail beds. Palpate the radial pulses simultaneously, and compare each side with the other. In situations of unilaterally absent pulses, check proximally over the brachial pulse sites. When you are evaluating a limb for ischemia, consider the five Ps of acute arterial insufficiency: Pain, Pallor, Parasthesias/Paresis, Poikilothermia (inability to maintain a constant core body temperature independent of ambient temperature), and Pulselessness. The loss of a palpable pulse is probably the worst indicator of such a problem because it is considered a late finding. If indicated, palpate the epitrochlear and axillary lymph nodes, noting their size, tenderness, overlying redness, and mobility.

Proper evaluation of the vascular status of the lower extremities requires the patient to be lying down and draped appropriately. Remove the patient's socks, stockings, and shoes before proceeding with the exam. Inspect the lower extremities from the groin and buttocks to the feet. Always examine the lower extremities by comparing the right side with the left side. Look at the size and symmetry of the legs, noting any localized versus generalized swelling. Pay attention to any remarkable superficial venous patterns or venous enlargement. Observe the skin pigmentation, as

Words of Wisdom

Bilateral, dependent, pitting edema occurs with systemic conditions such as heart failure and hepatic cirrhosis. Unilateral edema occurs with local conditions such as occlusion of a deep vein.

well as the skin color and texture. Rubor, ecchymosis, or pallor may all be encountered in patients with significant vascular insufficiency. Also note the presence of any rashes, scars, and ulcers, and determine whether they are shallow or deep.

Palpate pulses in the lower extremities to assess the arterial circulation. In particular, palpate pulses over the dorsalis pedis, the posterior tibialis, and the femoral regions. The popliteal pulse can also occasionally be appreciated. Note the temperature of the feet and legs, and attempt to palpate edema in the legs. To do so, press your thumb over the dorsum of the foot and anteriorly over the tibias, holding the thumb with firm, gentle pressure for at least 5 seconds. If indicated, palpate the superficial inguinal lymph nodes, noting their size, tenderness, any overlying redness, and mobility.

Words of Wisdom

Pitting edema 4-point scale:

+1 = 0″ – 1/4″

+2 = 1/4″ – 1/2″

+3 = 1/2″ – 1″

+4 = >1″

Spine

Earlier, assessment of the cervical spine was introduced in the section, Neck. This section covers complete assessment of the spine. The spine represents the core of the axillary skeleton. It consists of 33 individual vertebrae, the lower nine of which are fused Figure 57. The vertebrae are irregularly shaped bones that articulate with each other in a complex fashion. The spine provides anchoring points for the skull, shoulders, ribs,

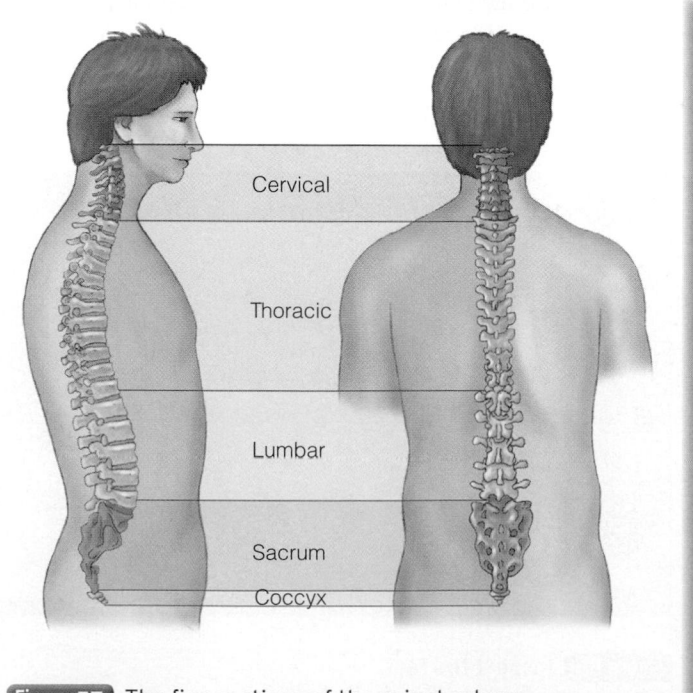

Figure 57   The five sections of the spinal column.

Skill Drill | 13

Examining the Peripheral Vascular System

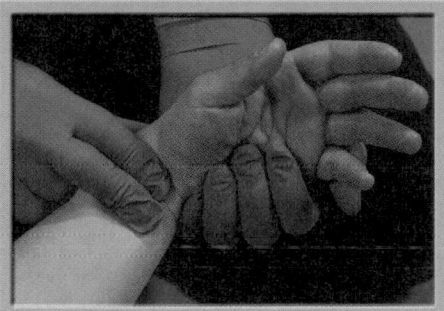

Step 1 Note any abnormalities in the radial pulse, skin color, or condition.

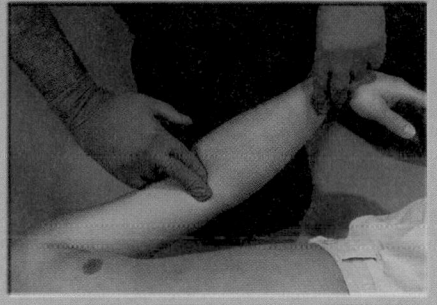

Step 2 If abnormalities are noted in the distal pulse, work your way proximally, checking these pulse points and noting your findings.

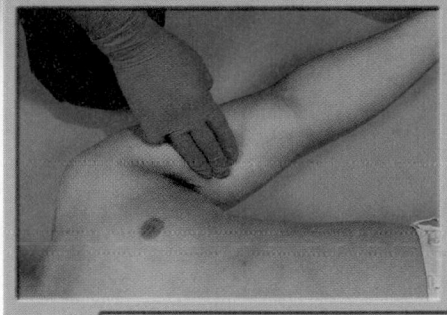

Step 3 Palpate the epitrochlear and brachial nodes of the lymphatic system, noting any swelling or tenderness.

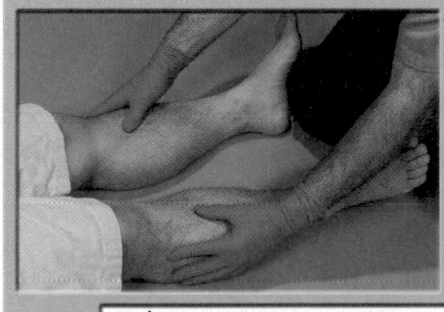

Step 4 Examine the lower extremities, noting any abnormalities in the size and symmetry of the legs.

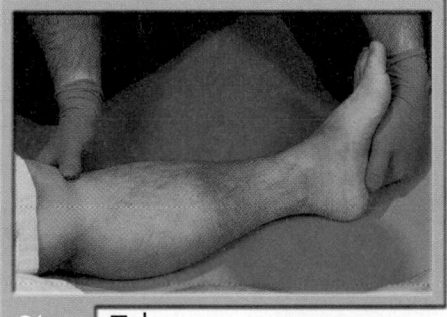

Step 5 Inspect the skin color and condition, noting any abnormal venous patterns or enlargement.

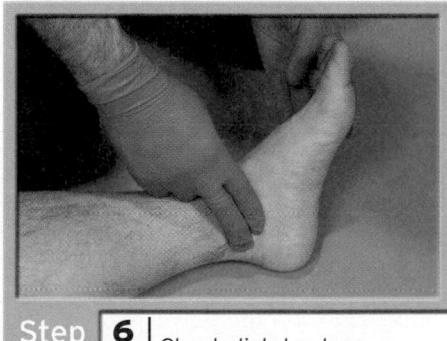

Step 6 Check distal pulses.

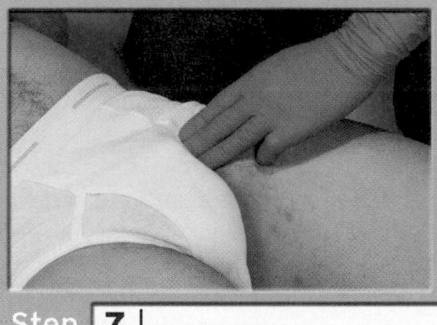

Step 7 Palpate the inguinal nodes for swelling or tenderness.

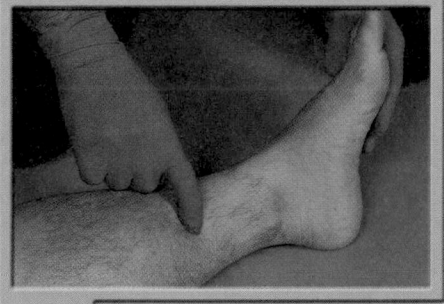

Step 8 Evaluate for pitting edema in the legs and feet.

and pelvis. It also protects the spinal cord and provides the passageway through which spinal nerves travel to and from the peripheral nervous system.

When you are assessing the spine, begin by inspecting the back from both the posterior and lateral aspects. The spine features several curves, representing the cervical, thoracic, and lumbar regions. <u>Lordosis</u> refers to the inward curve of the lumbar spine just above the buttocks. An exaggerated form of lordosis results in swayback **Figure 58**. <u>Kyphosis</u> refers to the outward curve of the thoracic spine **Figure 59**. It is frequently

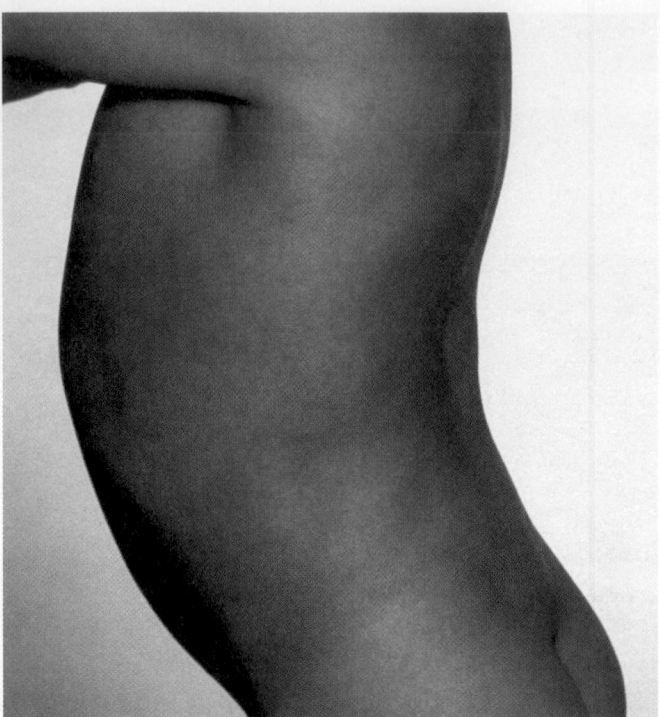

Figure 58 Lordosis is inward curvature of the lumbar spine just above the buttocks.

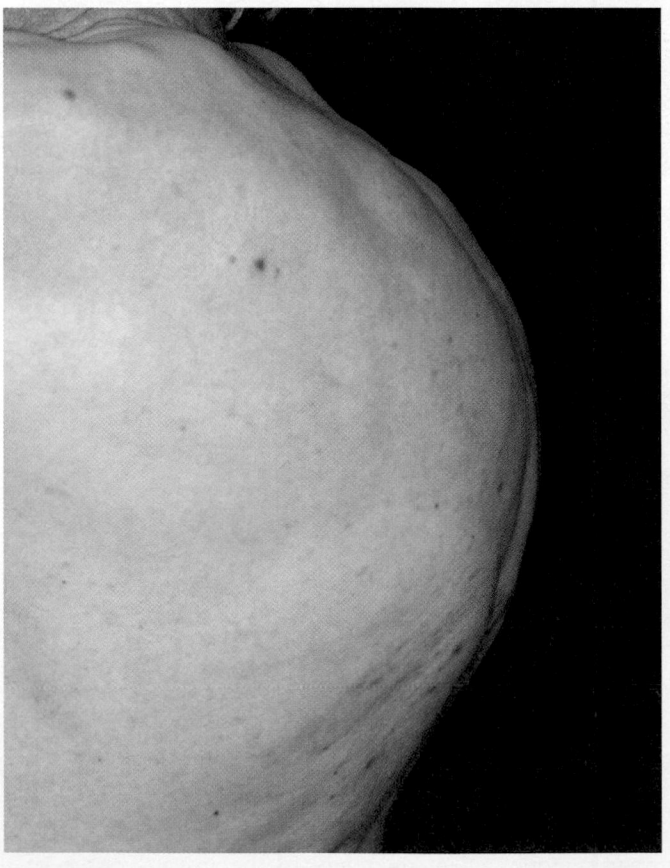

Figure 59 Kyphosis is outward curvature of the spine; it can be exaggerated in elderly patients.

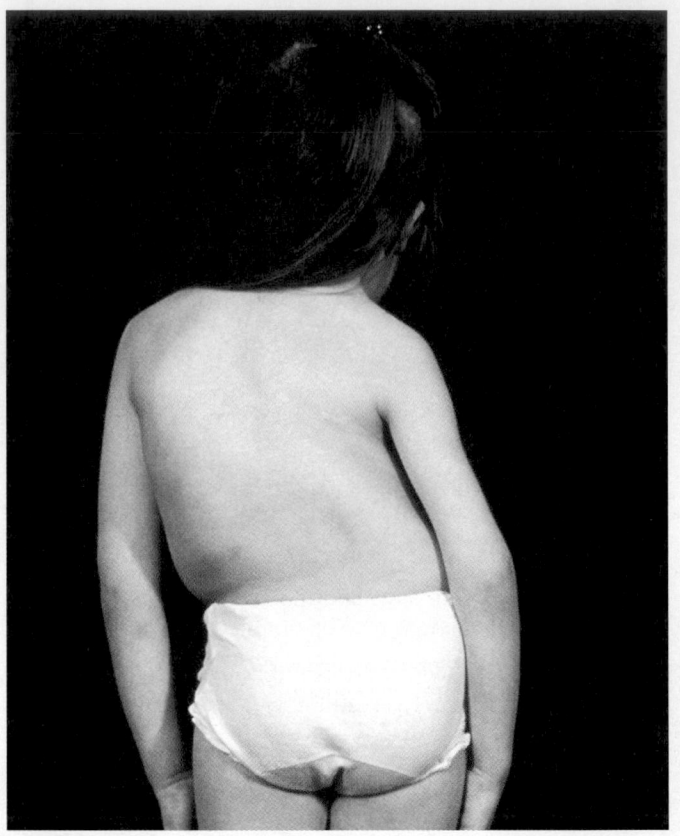

Figure 60 Scoliosis is sideways curvature of the spine.

exaggerated in elderly persons due to degenerative joint disease, osteoporosis, and vertebral compression fractures. At its worst, kyphosis can become a source of restrictive lung disease, a form of COPD. <u>Scoliosis</u> is a sideways curvature of the spine, and is always abnormal Figure 60 . When you are examining the spine, look for differences in the height of the shoulders as well as differences in the heights of the iliac crests of the pelvis. Be sure to take a moment and look at the entire back at this point, noting any wounds or ecchymosis.

Palpation of the spine is typically done while the patient is supine, often when he or she has been log rolled onto one side to facilitate access to the back and placement of a spinal immobilization device. When you are palpating the spine, use the thumb to touch each spinous process. This allows you to identify any tenderness, step-off, or crepitance. Identification of an abnormality should prompt you to institute proper splinting and protective measures.

While you are examining the spine, it is also appropriate to check the rest of the back for any other significant findings on palpation. Tap over the costovertebral angles, and palpate the scapulae, paraspinal areas, and base of the neck. Also check the buttocks.

Finally, perform a range-of-motion evaluation. Although this evaluation may be of limited utility in the prehospital setting, in areas that practice selective spinal immobilization, it may prove quite helpful. Range of motion should always be checked passively first, with you controlling the range. It is then done actively, with the patient controlling the range. If at any time during ranging you elicit pain in the spine or tingling

Words of Wisdom

Log rolling the patient onto a backboard is always a valuable opportunity to examine the back for signs of injury. Instruct and position assistants to ensure your ability to inspect and palpate the back briefly while the patient is rolled onto the side.

in the extremities, stop that phase of assessment immediately and immobilize the spine. Ranging the cervical spine should require rather limited movements. In contrast, ranging the remainder of the spine may include somewhat exaggerated motions, including flexion and extension, with the patient front- and back-bending. Lateral bending can also be appreciated, as can leftward and rightward rotation. Pay attention to the smoothness and symmetry of the patient's movements, along with the actual degree of motion elicited. Follow the steps in Skill Drill 14:

Skill Drill 14

1. Inspect the cervical, thoracic, and lumbar curves for any abnormalities [Step 1].
2. Evaluate the heights of the shoulders and the iliac crests [Step 2]. Differences from one side to the other may indicate abnormal curvature of the spine.
3. Palpate the posterior portion of the cervical spine, noting any point tenderness or structural abnormalities [Step 3].
4. In the nontrauma patient, and in the absence of reported pain, ask the patient to move the head forward, backward, and from side to side [Step 4].

Skill Drill | 14

Examining the Spine

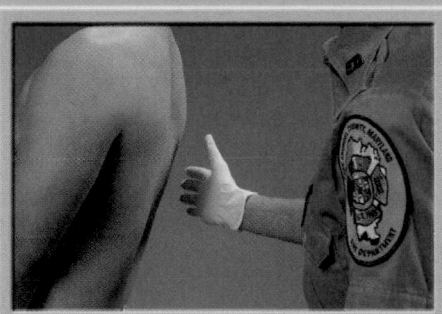

Step 1 Inspect the cervical, thoracic, and lumbar curves for any abnormalities.

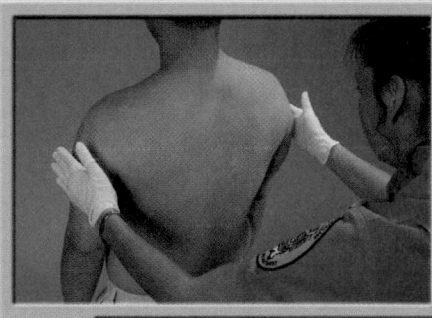

Step 2 Evaluate the heights of the shoulders and the iliac crests.

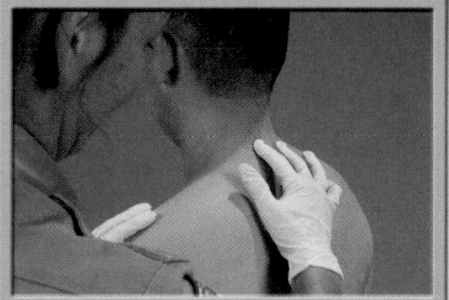

Step 3 Palpate the posterior portion of the cervical spine, noting any point tenderness or structural abnormalities.

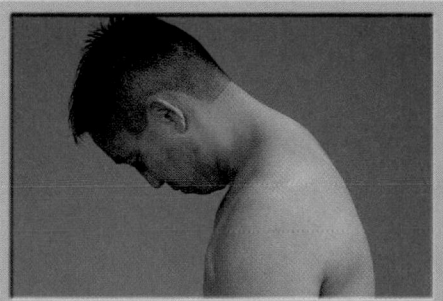

Step 4 In the nontrauma patient, and in the absence of reported pain, ask the patient to move the head forward, backward, and from side to side.

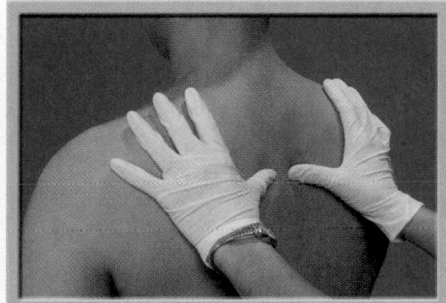

Step 5 Palpate each vertebra with the thumbs.

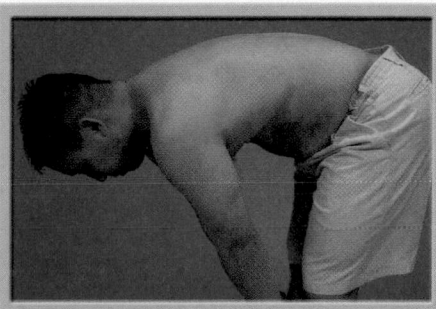

Step 6 In the absence of pain or trauma, ask the patient to bend at the waist in each direction to establish the range of motion.

5. Move down the spine, palpating each vertebra with the thumbs to note any tenderness or instability (Step 5).

6. In the absence of pain or trauma, ask the patient to bend at the waist in each direction to establish the range of motion (Step 6).

Nervous System

Structure and Function of the Nervous System

The nervous system is the body's master control system. It constantly receives information about the body's internal and external environments, and it continuously readjusts the body's systems in response to changes in those environments. The nervous system includes two portions: the central nervous system (CNS), which consists of the brain and spinal cord, and the peripheral nervous system (PNS), which includes the remaining motor and sensory nerves.

The brain is an extraordinarily complex structure, with an enormous perfusion requirement. It is constantly active at both conscious and unconscious levels. The brain comprises the cerebrum, cerebellum, and medulla (brainstem). The cerebrum takes charge of all of the brain's conscious processes; it is divided into four discrete lobes (frontal, temporal, parietal, and occipital). The cerebellum is responsible for coordinating balance. The brainstem handles all of the unconscious deeper processes.

With the exception of the cranial nerves, all nerves are ultimately channeled to the brain via the spinal cord. The spinal cord plays the role of a large conduit, passing information back and forth along itself. The peripheral nerves that emanate from the spinal cord, which are known as spinal nerves, have both motor and sensory pathways. Motor nerves control some aspect of motion or movement, whereas sensory nerves receive external signals and send them to the brain for processing and motor response. Motor tracts run from the spinal cord to the body outwardly; sensory nerves run from the body to the cord inwardly.

Cranial nerves are not mediated by the spinal cord but rather go directly to and from the brain, originating at the medulla. They innervate the face, head, and parts of the neck, with the exception of the vagus nerve, which runs down the neck and into the chest and abdomen. There are 12 cranial nerves in total. They play roles in a wide variety of motor and sensory functions (Table 8) that involve both the voluntary and autonomic nervous systems (discussed later in this section).

The peripheral nerves are covered with a sheet-like material called myelin. Myelin promotes rapid transmission of impulses along the nerve. In the newborn, several of the major motor pathways (or long tracts) are not fully myelinated. Over time, however, myelin is completely deposited and the motor pathways become fully functional. Conversely, with advancing age and the occurrence of various disease states, neurologic functions can deteriorate. This failure may take the form of a cognitive problem (eg, dementia), or it may lead to a physical disability (eg, the problems seen with parkinsonism and cerebrovascular disease).

In addition to the central/peripheral distinctions, the nervous system may be divided into involuntary (autonomic) and voluntary portions, with the autonomic nervous system being further subdivided into the sympathetic and parasympathetic systems. **Reflexes** are involuntary motor responses to specific sensory stimuli, such as a tap on the knee or stroking the eyelash. The location of what is stimulated determines which muscle will contract to produce a reflexive response. Spinal reflexes occur when sensory input comes from receptors in the muscles, joints, and skin. The motor response to this stimulation occurs entirely within the spinal cord; no brain processing is required. Other reflexes include the deep tendon reflexes

Table 8 Cranial Nerves

Number	Name	Motor vs Sensory	Functions
I	Olfactory	Sensory	Smell
II	Optic	Sensory	Light perception and vision
III	Oculomotor	Motor	Pupil constriction, eye movements
IV	Trochlear	Motor	Eye movements
V	Trigeminal	Motor and sensory	Motor: chewing Sensory: face, sinuses, teeth
VI	Abducens	Motor	Eye movements
VII	Facial	Motor	Facial movements
VIII	Vestibulocochlear	Sensory	Hearing, balance perception
IX	Glossopharyngeal	Motor and sensory	Motor: throat and swallowing, gland secretion Sensory: tongue, throat, ear
X	Vagus	Motor and sensory	Heart, lungs, palate, pharynx, larynx, trachea, bronchi, GI tract, external ear
XI	Spinal accessory	Motor	Shoulder and neck movements
XII	Hypoglossal	Motor	Tongue, throat, and neck movements

Words of Wisdom

A Babinski test may be used to check for neurologic function. It is accomplished by stimulating the sole of the foot by rubbing with your thumb or running a pen or other pointed object along the sole of the foot. In a normal reaction, the great toe will flex. However, you should *not* perform a Babinski test on a patient who has injuries to the lower extremities. This test could cause the patient to pull the leg back, causing pain.

and the superficial and brainstem reflexes. <u>Primitive reflexes</u>—including the Babinski, grasping, and sucking signs—are normal findings in infants. In older people, once the long motor pathways of the PNS have become fully myelinated, the primitive reflexes represent abnormal findings, typical of injury or disconnection between the cerebral cortex and the brainstem.

The Neurologic Exam

The check of the nervous system is one of the most time-consuming elements of the physical exam. There will be times when a complete and thorough neurologic exam will not be possible in the field; however, if the patient is displaying signs and symptoms of a neurologic problem, every attempt should be made to perform a complete neurologic exam. At a minimum, the neurologic exam should determine the patient's baseline mental status (AVPU), cranial nerve function (pupils, eyes, smile, speech, swallow, shoulder shrug), distal motor function (ability to move), and distal sensory function (ability to feel). It may also test the deep tendon reflexes if necessary.

First, assess the patient's overall mental status. Is the patient awake? If so, is the patient alert, and to what degree? If a change in level of consciousness has occurred, what kind of stimulus does it take to get a response, and to what degree does the patient's mental status improve? In the case of an altered mental status, do you observe any unusual postures? Is there any alteration in physical status (eg, is the ability to move successfully and symmetrically preserved)? A detailed explanation of the mental status examination was covered earlier in the chapter. Here is a quick review using the mnemonic (COASTMAP):

- **Consciousness.** Along with level of consciousness, note the patient's ability to pay attention and concentrate. Is the patient easily distracted?
- **Orientation.** Ask about the year, season, month, day, and date. Have the patient identify the present location—that is, state, town, and specific location. Can the patient recall and describe the event(s) currently going on?
- **Activity.** Does the patient appear anxious or restless? Is he or she sitting still, scarcely moving at all? Is he or she making any strange or repetitive motions (possibly because of methamphetamine use)?
- **Speech.** Note the rate, volume, articulation, and intonation of the patient's speech. Does it sound pressured? Does the speech have a flat, monotone delivery consistent with depression? Is the speech garbled or slurred (dysarthria)? Garbled or slurred speech may have many

causes, including alcohol or drug impairment, stroke, and traumatic brain injury.

- **Thought.** Listen to the patient's story. What is on his or her mind? Is the patient making sense? Is there anything unusual about his or her reasoning? Is the patient expressing apparently false ideas (delusions)? Are voices telling the patient what to do or think (psychotic)? Does the patient report that people are "out to get me" (paranoia)?
- **Memory.** You can usually form an impression of the patient's memory by listening to his or her reconstruction of events. A more precise assessment requires asking a few questions. Ask the patient if you may test his or her memory. If the patient assents, slowly say the names of three unrelated subjects (such as apple, bicycle, sewing machine). Now ask the patient to repeat those words; that will test registration. A few minutes later, ask the patient if he or she can remember the three words you named before; that tests retention and memory.
- **Affect.** The patient's affect (mood) may be most apparent in his or her body language. The patient sitting with shoulders drooping and head bent, for example, conveys depression. Note whether the affect—the expression of inner feelings—seems appropriate to the situation.
- **Perception.** Detecting disorders of perception may be difficult because patients are often hesitant to answer questions about hallucinations. Sometimes it is helpful to ask the patient, "Do you ever hear things that other people can't hear?"

It is also helpful to assess the Glasgow Coma Scale (discussed earlier in this chapter), which was designed as a tool to assist in better assessing people with significant alterations in mental status, and was originally intended for use in the trauma setting. It simultaneously scores several parameters, including eye opening, verbal acuity, and motor activity, and attempts to provide a numeric score as a rapid means of defining severity of brain dysfunction and potential prognosis. Follow the steps in **Skill Drill 15** :

Skill Drill 15

1. Assess the patient's mental status by using the AVPU mnemonic.
2. Note the patient's posture.
3. Evaluate cranial nerve function **Step 1**.
4. Evaluate the patient's neuromuscular status by checking muscle strength against resistance **Step 2**. Use the grading system described later in this chapter to grade all extremities.
5. Evaluate the patient's coordination by performing the finger-to-nose test using alternating hands **Step 3**.
6. If appropriate, test the patient's gait and balance by having the patient walk heel-to-toe or perform the heel-to-shin stance **Step 4**.
7. Perform the pronator drift test by asking the patient to close his or her eyes and hold both arms out in front of the body **Step 5**. There should be no difference in movement on either side.

Skill Drill 15

Examining the Nervous System

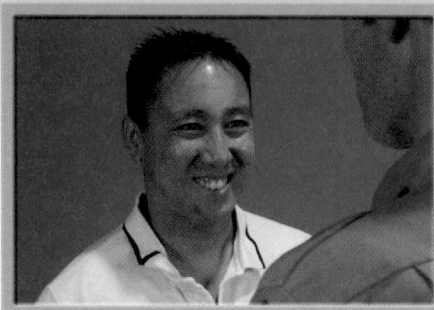

Step 1 Evaluate cranial nerve function.

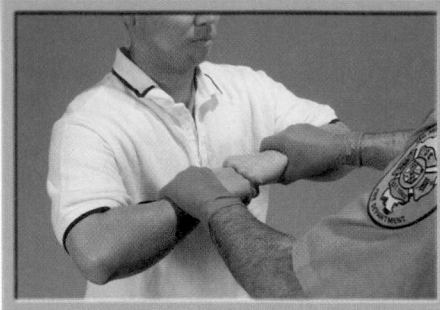

Step 2 Evaluate the patient's neuromuscular status by checking muscle strength against resistance.

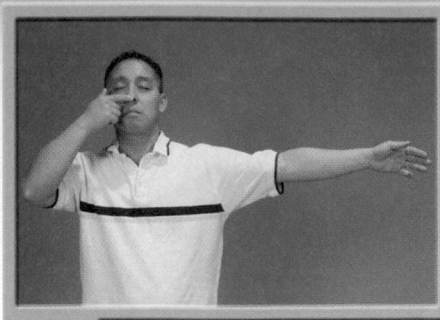

Step 3 Evaluate the patient's coordination by performing the finger-to-nose test using alternating hands.

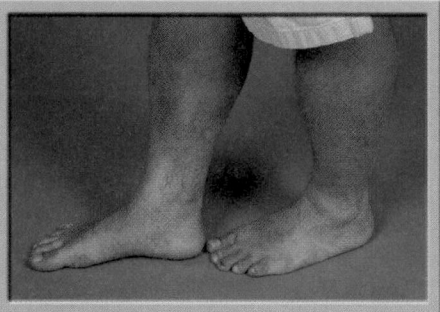

Step 4 If appropriate, test the patient's gait and balance by having the patient walk heel-to-toe or perform the heel-to-shin stance.

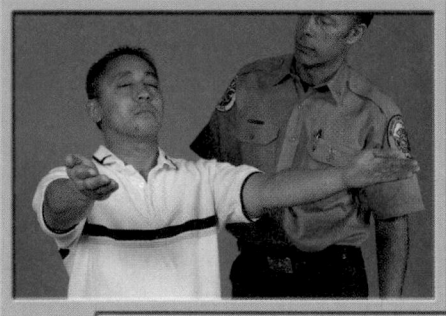

Step 5 Perform the pronator drift test by asking the patient to close his or her eyes and hold both arms out in front of the body.

8. Evaluate the patient's sensory function by checking his or her responses to both gross and light touch.
9. If appropriate, check for deep tendon reflexes.

Words of Wisdom

Restlessness is a danger signal!

After assessment of the patient's overall mental status, you should begin the comprehensive neurologic exam. Of course, such an exam is not needed in every case. Its details may vary greatly, depending on the nature of the patient's problem. Also, many portions of the neurologic exam may have been completed earlier, during other aspects of the patient assessment. Keep track of these initial findings so that you can report them, they are not needlessly repeated, and any subsequent changes in status can

be noted. Are left- and right-sided motor and sensory findings symmetric? If not, how do they differ? Does the presenting problem appear to be more of a CNS or a PNS malfunction, or is it secondary to swelling or bone displacement from trauma?

When testing the cranial nerves, a number of simple maneuvers can be employed to determine the presence and degree of disability Table 9 . With practice, the entire cranial nerve examination can be performed in less than 3 minutes. That said, do not waste time performing this examination if the patient has more pressing needs.

Adequate evaluation of the motor system involves assessment of several distinct areas. Although motor activity may represent the localized workings of the musculoskeletal system, the nervous system has an overriding influence on motor activity. Observe the patient's initial posture and body position Figure 61 as well as the body position both at rest and with movement, if appropriate. Watch for any apparent involuntary movements, and document their quality, rate, rhythm,

Secondary Assessment

Table 9 Tests for Disability in Cranial Nerves

Cranial Nerve	Test
I	Check smell
II	Check visual acuity
III	Check pupil size, shape, symmetry, response to light, eye movements
IV	Check eye movements
V	Check jaw clench; touch both sides of face at forehead, cheeks, and jaw
VI	Check eye movements
VII	Check facial symmetry; look for abnormal movements; raise eyebrows, grin broadly, frown, shut eyes tightly, puff out cheeks; note any asymmetry
VIII	Check hearing and balance
IX, X	Check swallowing; perform general physical exam
XI	Check shoulder shrug; turn head from left to right and back
XII	Check swallowing; turn head from left to right and back

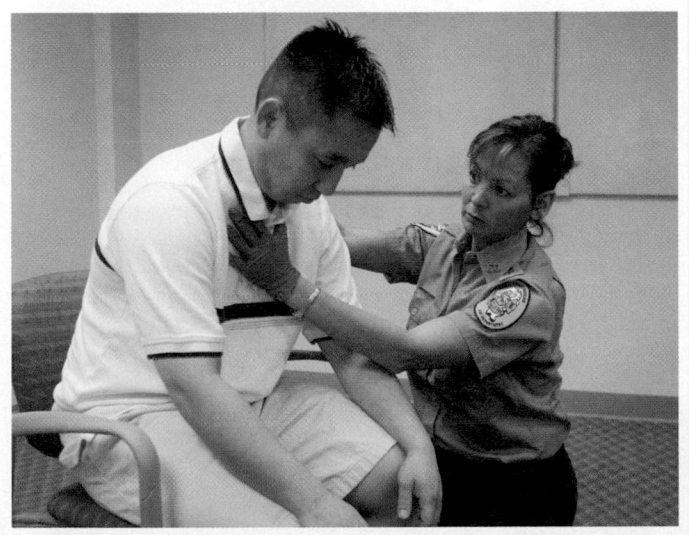

Figure 61 Note the patient's posture and body position.

and amplitude. Try to determine whether these involuntary movements are related to the patient's posture or activity, and think about whether their presentation includes a component of fatigue or emotion. Make a general assessment of the bulk of the patient's major muscle groups. Compare these muscles' sizes and contours. Note associated muscle tone by checking for resistance to passive movement.

An important part of the motor exam is the evaluation of overall muscle strength. To perform this assessment, have the patient actively move against the examiner's resistance. Strength is graded on a scale of 1 to 5:

1: No muscle contraction or twitch detectable
2: Only active movement with gravity eliminated
3: Active movement against gravity obtained
4: Active movement against some resistance or with fatigue evident
5: Active movement against full resistance without evident fatigue

Strength is expressed as a ratio—for example, "strength is 4 over 5 (4/5) in the bilateral upper and lower extremities"; 5/5 is a state of normal muscle tone. When checking strength, and depending on the location of the muscle groups involved, be prepared to test for flexion, extension, grip, abduction, adduction, and opposition.

Checking coordination is an important part of the neurologic exam because it tests a variety of nervous system functions, especially those involving cerebellar functioning. Coordination is assessed by evaluating a patient's ability to perform rapid alternating movements, point-to-point movements (including finger-to-nose and heel-to-shin testing), stance, and gait. Gait and stance should be evaluated only in those subjects whose status allows them to be safely placed in a standing position. Note any upper extremity tremors, flaps, or pronator drift at this point as well.

Coordination is not the only cerebellar function that the paramedic should be testing. <u>Proprioception</u> involves the patient's understanding and interpretation of the positioning of an extremity and is a function of the cerebellum. Loss of proprioception can be seen in conditions such as trauma, multiple sclerosis, vitamin B_{12} deficiency, and peripheral neuropathy. Test for proprioception by grasping the patient's big toe, holding it by its sides between your thumb and index finger, and then pulling it away from the other toes. Demonstrate for the patient "up" and "down" as you move the patient's toe clearly upward and downward. Then, with the patient's eyes closed, ask for a response of "up" or "down" when you are moving the large toe.

Just as evaluation of motor function tests the workings of the nervous system from the brain outward to the body, so testing sensory function checks the workings of the nervous system from the body inward to the brain. In general, sensory processes are tested bilaterally, looking for changes in symmetry from one side to the other, as well as comparing proximal to distal processes. When performing the primary assessment on a patient appearing severely ill, a sensory exam is typically the first evaluation done. In this exam, both primary and cortical sensory functions should be assessed. Initial "shake and shout" maneuvers represent an attempt to find evidence of preserved higher cerebral functioning. This testing determines whether the patient's primary sensory function is intact. Typically these tests look for any response to gross stimuli (eg, a loud shout in the face) or implementation of more noxious forms of stimuli (eg, squeezing the nail bed, twisting the skin of the forearm). Once primary sensory function is determined to be intact, minimal perception of gross versus light touch should be tested (no equipment is required). This testing evaluates areas of cortical sensory function. More involved sensory evaluation involves checking sharp versus dull perception and two-point discrimination. In order to appropriately assess cortical function, the primary function must be intact. The primary sensory cortex in the brain uses sensory information gathered in order to perform the more distinct cortical functions. Therefore, if there is disruption in the primary function, examination of cortical function will not be reliable. Sensation is commonly reported in relation to dermatomal location on the body's surface. **Dermatomes** are distinct areas of skin that correspond to specific spinal or cranial nerve levels where sensory nerves enter the CNS.

Follow the steps in [Skill Drill 16] to evaluate deep tendon reflexes. Scoring of deep tendon reflexes is covered in [Table 10].

Skill Drill 16

1. Place the patient in the sitting position [Step 1].
2. Flex the patient's arm to 45° at the elbow. Locate the biceps tendon in the antecubital fossa. Place your thumb over the tendon, with your fingers behind the elbow. Strike your thumb with the reflex hammer, noting the flexion of the elbow [Step 2].
3. With the patient's arm remaining at a 45° angle, rest the patient's forearm on your arm with the hand slightly pronated. Strike the patient's brachioradial tendon proximal to the wrist, noting the flexion of the elbow [Step 3].

Skill Drill 16

Evaluating Deep Tendon Reflexes

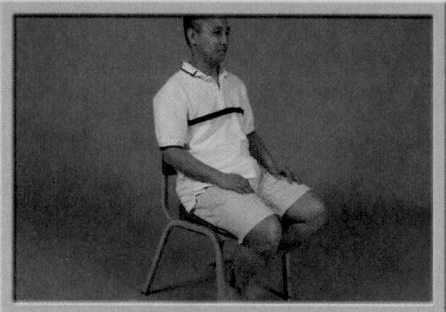

Step 1 Place the patient in the sitting position.

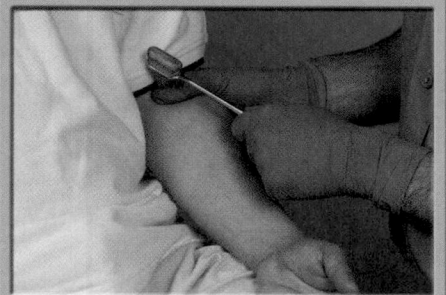

Step 2 Flex the patient's arm to 45° at the elbow. Locate the biceps tendon in the antecubital fossa. Place your thumb over the tendon, with your fingers behind the elbow. Strike your thumb with the reflex hammer, noting the flexion of the elbow.

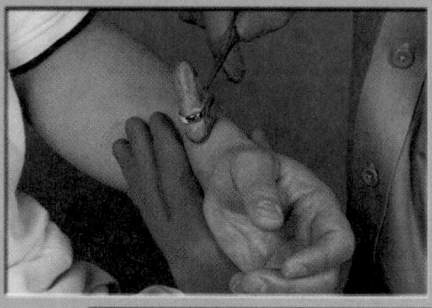

Step 3 With the patient's arm remaining at a 45° angle, rest the patient's forearm on your arm with the hand slightly pronated. Strike the patient's brachioradialis tendon proximal to the wrist, noting the flexion of the elbow.

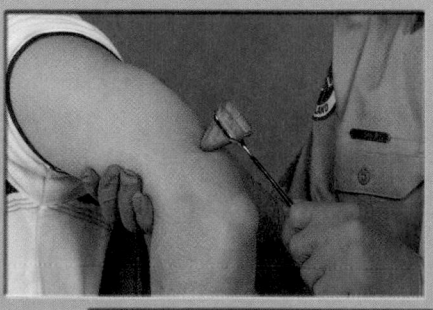

Step 4 Flex the patient's arm at the elbow 90° and rest his or her hand against the body. Locate and strike the triceps tendon, noting contraction of the triceps or extension of the elbow.

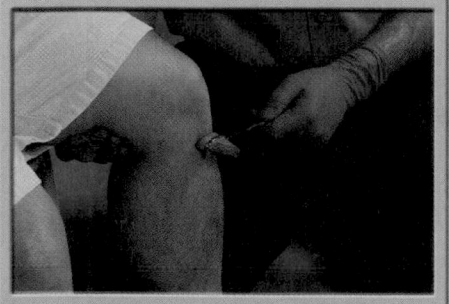

Step 5 Flex the patient's knee to 90°, allowing the leg to dangle. Support the upper leg with your hand, and strike the patellar tendon just below the patella.

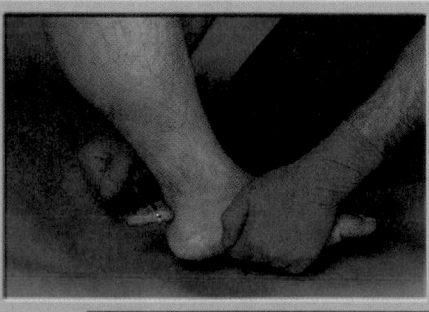

Step 6 With the patient's leg in the same position, hold the heel of the patient's foot in your hand. Strike the Achilles tendon.

Table 10	Scoring of Deep Tendon Reflexes
Grade	**Deep Tendon Reflex Response**
0	No response
1+	Sluggish
2+	Active (expected response)
3+	Slightly hyperactive
4+	Hyperactive

4. Flex the patient's arm at the elbow 90° and rest his or her hand against the body. Locate and strike the triceps tendon, noting contraction of the triceps or extension of the elbow [Step 4].

5. Flex the patient's knee to 90°, allowing the leg to dangle. Support the upper leg with your hand, and strike the patellar tendon just below the patella. Note the contraction of the quadriceps and the extension of the lower leg [Step 5].

6. With the patient's leg in the same position, hold the heel of the patient's foot in your hand. Strike the Achilles tendon, noting the plantar flexion of the foot [Step 6].

Results of the Neurologic Exam

Abnormal findings on the neurologic exam can take a wide variety of forms. Most common are mental status changes that can represent any number of acute and chronic processes, many of which have a non-neurologic origin. Oftentimes, mental status changes represent changes in perfusion or are encountered as a subtle indicator of early sepsis (which is common in the elderly population).

Distinguishing between delirium and dementia, when dealing with a patient with abnormal mental status, is also important. **Delirium** is more consistent with an acute sudden change in mental status, secondary to some significant underlying aberration. **Dementia** is representative of a gradual and pervasive deterioration of cognitive cortical functions, typically secondary to the slow progression of some disease state, ie, Alzheimer disease.

Commonly encountered motor abnormalities include facial and extremity strength asymmetry along with difficulty in speaking (expressive **aphasia**). These signs are typical of cerebrovascular disease. Other commonly encountered abnormalities include ataxia, dystonia, seizures, vertigo, visual changes, tinnitus, and tremor. In the setting of trauma, global changes in mental status are more indicative of intracranial mass lesions, whereas decreased extremity motor function may present with proximal versus distal asymmetry and objective **parasthesias** (tingling or sensory changes), which is more consistent with a spinal lesion.

Secondary Assessment of Unresponsive Patients

After completing the primary assessment and assuming you have ruled out trauma, position unresponsive patients in the recovery position (left lateral recumbent position) to facilitate drainage of vomit, blood, or other fluids and to help prevent aspiration. If trauma is a factor, position the patient in neutral alignment, place a properly sized and fitted rigid cervical collar, and implement spinal motion restriction procedures as per the local protocol.

Perform a thorough assessment of the head, neck, chest, abdomen, pelvis, posterior body, and extremities, looking for signs of illness such as rash or urticaria, fever, unusual or excessive bruising, pulmonary or peripheral edema, and irregular pulse. Follow up your examination with at least two sets of vital signs—one taken now and another obtained a few minutes after you have started your initial interventions (such as supplemental oxygen and IV therapy). The first set establishes a baseline (baseline vital signs); the second and additional sets (serial vital signs) provide comparative data to help you evaluate whether the patient's condition is improving, status quo, or worsening. If time allows, additional sets of vital signs add further data, allowing you to map trends (such as a progressively increasing pulse rate). Make sure the vital signs include an auscultated blood pressure, accurate pulse and respiratory rates, and the patient's temperature. A recheck of breath sounds is always a prudent choice as well. All unresponsive patients should have their posture assessed. If there is no spontaneous movement, you may need to apply a painful stimulus. A normal response should involve the patient pushing the stimulus away or withdrawing from it. Abnormal postural responses of the trunk and extremities include decorticate and decerebrate posturing. More information on postural presentations can be found in the chapter, *Neurologic Emergencies*.

Unresponsive patients should always be considered in unstable condition and at high risk, so rapid transport to the appropriate facility is indicated. Throughout transport, perform reassessment, which includes rechecking the ABCs and reassessing anything associated with the patient's chief complaint.

Secondary Assessment of Trauma Patients

Trauma patients may be classified into two major groups: patients with an isolated injury and patients with multisystem trauma. The biggest difference from a secondary assessment perspective is that an isolated injury allows you to immediately focus on the main problem. In contrast, with multisystem trauma, you must first find all (or as many as you can reasonably find) of the various problems (for example, a hematoma on the forehead, a fractured arm, and neck and lower back pain). Then you need to prioritize the injuries by severity and the order in which you plan to address them. During the assessment, you must continually think about how each injury or condition relates to the others. For example, the mortality rate doubles for a patient with a serious traumatic brain injury who has just a single episode of hypotension. In such a case, you not recognizing and addressing the hypotension and the lack of adequate perfusion pressure has a huge impact—in some cases, a fatal impact.

Another important consideration is the "high visibility factor" of many injuries, which sometimes creates a visual distraction.

Words of Wisdom

The salvage of lives takes precedence over the salvage of limbs.

A compound fracture of the lower leg and ankle, with the foot twisted sideways and jammed under the brake pedal in a car, is not a pretty sight events—but it is not a life-threatening injury. Because of the visual distraction, you might focus on the grossly deformed ankle and miss the early signs and symptoms of shock caused by the internal injuries and bleeding that you cannot see.

Any trauma patient who is unresponsive or has altered mentation should be considered a high-risk, priority patient and requires immediate transport to a trauma center. An unresponsive patient may have a traumatic brain injury, stroke, hypoglycemia, or alcohol or drug intoxication. All are serious events—even potentially lethal—with some (such as traumatic brain injury) being devastating injuries.

Recall that you will perform the rapid exam on trauma patients to obtain a quick 60- to 90-second impression of a patient's injuries before he or she is immobilized. Though there may not always be time for further physical examinations of trauma patients, when time and patient condition do allow for it, perform further physical examinations.

Keep in mind that the most visible injury you may be looking at (the scalp laceration) or the most painful injury the patient reports (the fractured and dislocated ankle) may not be nearly as serious as the most lethal injury the patient has (the ruptured spleen). A splenic injury, for example, is not visible and less painful than the other two injuries.

Before you physically examine a trauma patient, make sure that the patient's cervical spine is manually immobilized in the neutral position. Quickly reassess the patient's current mental status, comparing it with the baseline you established when you first encountered the patient. Last, revisit your transport decision. If you decide that the patient needs immediate transport, perform the rapid exam and do not delay transport in order to perform more thorough examinations.

If you do perform additional physical examinations of the trauma patient beyond the rapid exam, note that it is a good idea to check your gloves for blood after each area of the body is assessed. This will help you note any areas that have active bleeding. If you do not check your gloves frequently, you may be unsure which part of the body the blood came from, and will have to redo the entire process.

Also, mentally piece together all that you now know about your patient, including the chief complaint, the history of the present event, the medical history, and any information about the patient's current health status. Combine that knowledge with the other information and insights you have gained from your various assessments, along with the information obtained from your diagnostics, and you should have more than enough information to make good clinical choices for your patient.

Additional physical examinations of the trauma patient will help you find any life threats you may have missed in the primary assessment, but need to be done quickly. Remember that examining a trauma patient *takes lots and lots of practice*.

Secondary Assessment of Infants and Children

When you are caring for infants and children, you will need to alter your approach to patient assessment in general. Because a young child might not be able to speak, your assessment of his

or her condition must be based in large part on what you can see and hear yourself, and what you can learn from parents or caregivers.

Examining a child requires understanding that you may have to deal with several sources of information. Remember that families may be helpful in providing vital information about the injury or illness. If possible, and if the patient is of an adequate age and developmental status, you should also attempt to elicit some information from the patient first before moving on to parents or others.

In the secondary assessment, the goals of assessment in children are the same as those for adult patients. If possible, obtain the permission of the parent or guardian before conducting a physical examination. Explain to the child that you are going to check him or her because you are a paramedic, and that you are here to help. In a situation of acute life-threatening illness or injury, rapidly conduct the primary assessment and manage life-threatening conditions as with an adult patient.

When time permits, consider certain age-related strategies for attempting to facilitate the examination. Overall, children tend to do better being examined from toe to head, as opposed to the reverse method commonly used with adults. This strategy tends to gain trust and decreases the child's fear. Infants are usually not overly distressed by being manipulated by adults, so the basic approach to assessment is reasonable with them. Pay close attention to vital signs and physical findings because the ability to obtain a helpful history is limited.

When you are examining a newborn or neonate, be aware of normal and abnormal presentations on the physical exam. Inspect the skin for any abnormalities. Common findings such as vernix (a white cheesy material), edema, and Mongolian spots (dark or bluish pigmentation over the buttocks and lower lumbar regions in African, Asian, and Mediterranean patients) are considered to be normal variants. Jaundice can appear in healthy babies 2 to 5 days after birth and typically disappears after about a week. Jaundice that progresses beyond 2 to 3 weeks should raise suspicion for biliary obstruction or liver disease. Examine the head for symmetry and abnormalities. Because the sutures in the skull are not fused at birth, it is common for the head to appear asymmetric immediately after birth. This normal variation allows the head to fit through the birth canal. In these cases, provide the parents with reassurance and explain that the head will typically appear more symmetric within the next few days. Be aware that most young infants lack muscle strength in the neck and are unable to control motion of the head. It is important to provide support of the head and neck at all times when examining young infants. Examine the eyes of the neonate and look for irregularities. A newborn who truly cannot open an eye may have a congenital defect. Watch for abnormal eye movement such as nystagmus (wandering or shaking eye movements) and strabismus (alternating convergence for divergence creating a crossed-eye appearance). Look for abnormalities in the sclera and pupils. Subconjunctival hemorrhages are common in newborns. Examine for any drainage or ocular discharge because this may be associated with a blocked tear duct. Inspect the newborn's umbilical cord to detect abnormalities. Normally, there are two thick-walled umbilical arteries and one larger but thin-walled umbilical vein, which is usually located in the 12-o'clock position. Note the presence of any abnormal abdominal findings, such as hernias.

Children are prone to dehydration and infection (eg, sepsis), and assessment for trauma should always be a consideration as well. In infants, the fontanelles play a key role in the assessment of fevers and dehydration. A depressed anterior fontanelle may be a sign of dehydration in an infant and warrants further evaluation. Bulging fontanelles are associated with increased intracranial pressure and are typically seen when the baby cries, vomits, or has an underlying pathologic condition.

Children from ages 1 to 3 years can be challenging to work with, and as a rule will strenuously object to being touched or manipulated by a stranger. The toe-to-head approach is a good strategy in this age group. Decide which aspects of the exam must be performed, set some reasonable ground rules for the exam, and then examine the patient accordingly. Practice ways to safely and adequately hold young patients to facilitate the assessment. If possible, have family members assist with this task.

Children from ages 4 to 5 years are typically much less of a management challenge for you. They are usually cooperative and helpful with the exam, and the standard head-to-toe approach can usually be employed. School-age children tend to be cooperative as well, and should be actively engaged in the examination process. Be sure to take the time to explain what you are doing while you are examining them.

Adolescent evaluation can be a bit more demanding because these patients tend to have feelings more directed at preserving their autonomy, and they can be concerned about how a given situation may involve either parents or peers. They also tend to be concerned with bodily integrity, so be prepared to reassure them that things are okay if a physical finding is not concerning.

When you are dealing with the assessment of children, some general principles apply. No matter how stressful or disturbing the situation, remain calm, patient, and gentle. Be honest with children; if something is likely to hurt, say so—but you do not need to elaborate. If at all possible, attempt to keep children and parents together. Many children normally harbor fears over separation; in the setting of acute illness or injury, these anxieties will only be worsened. Remember that pediatric patients presenting in the prehospital setting are often victims of trauma. Be sure to appropriately assess for injury, and treat appropriately. Do not neglect a child's pain.

Physical exam techniques vary slightly in the pediatric population depending on the patient's age. While inspection remains the same, auscultation may vary. Specific findings regarding heart auscultation were discussed earlier. Auscultation of a quiet infant's abdomen is simple. A common finding is an array of active tinkling bowel sounds when the stethoscope is placed on the belly. Because children are reactive to cold stimuli, warming the diaphragm of your stethoscope before placing it on the skin might help yield a more accurate result. You can percuss an infant's abdomen as you would an adult's; however, a more tympanic sound might be noted. Palpation techniques in pediatric patients will vary with age. In most infants, palpation is straightforward because infants like to be touched. However, as children age and "stranger anxiety" progresses, patients may be more likely to resist palpation. Palpation is intrusive, especially in the abdominal area. For this reason, exam techniques that are more likely to be resisted by a child should be performed near the end of your examination. More information on the assessment of pediatric patients can be found in the chapter, *Pediatric Emergencies.*

Recording Secondary Assessment Findings

Medical information may be presented in both verbal and written forms. Recording of information should always be done in an orderly and concise manner, without omitting important information. The obtained information may then be practically and accurately relayed to the receiving medical staff. In addition, documentation ensures that an accurate historic accounting of the patient's problems prior to entering the hospital will legally exist in the formal medical record. A number of acceptable formats are currently in use. You must use the forms that are recommended by your medical director. Modification of a format is acceptable as long as it preserves the basic requirements for medical documentation.

A secondary assessment requires a physical interaction between you and the patient, and it can be successfully performed on a patient who cannot communicate. When you are recording examination findings, note objective signs, pertinent negatives, and other similar relevant information. Objective information is commonly recorded in a standard format, in the same order as used for the verbal or written report.

Words of Wisdom

Remember the legal and ethical components to the secondary assessment:

1. Respect the patient's autonomy in decision making.
2. Be accountable to the patient.
3. Respect the patient's confidentiality and privacy.
4. Obtain consent.
5. Recognize assault and battery.
6. Understand and respect advance directives.
7. Document facts accurately and nonjudgmentally.

Limits of the Secondary Assessment

The ability to competently perform a secondary assessment is one of the most valuable skills you can possess. This assessment can, for example, uncover information that the patient is unable or unwilling to share. An accomplished clinician will use this skill in conjunction with the history taking and other diagnostic tools to form an impression and formulate a treatment plan.

Nevertheless, despite the emphasis placed on a comprehensive physical examination, the secondary assessment has limitations. Even the most experienced physician understands that not everything can be discovered in such an assessment. In the prehospital setting, it is important to remember that evaluation by a trained physician coupled with laboratory and radiographic studies may be needed for a definitive diagnosis.

Monitoring Devices

Whereas the history-taking and secondary assessment process is the best method for determining a differential diagnosis in your patient, the use of certain diagnostic and monitoring devices, and laboratory tests are typically used by paramedics to aid in the assessment process. These devices are designed to assist the paramedic with diagnostic assessment and monitoring of patients. Keep in mind that while these devices are helpful, they cannot replace a good history and secondary assessment. Too often paramedics are found relying on monitoring devices and not on the physical exam and patient presentation. This is a pitfall you must avoid. Always remember to treat your patient—not the monitor.

Continuous ECG Monitoring

The purpose of continuous ECG monitoring in the prehospital environment is to establish a baseline of ECG rhythm and to monitor for dynamic changes in cardiac electrical activity while the patient is in your care.

Patients who present with any cardiac-related signs and symptoms or potential signs and symptoms of illnesses with cardiac impact should be on continuous cardiac monitoring. Coincidentally, this indication is quite common in EMS calls, which is why paramedics frequently place patients on cardiac monitors as part of their routine ALS care.

Most ECG monitors designed for the prehospital environment typically work in the same fashion. To monitor the cardiac rhythm appropriately, the electrodes must be placed on the patient accurately **Figure 62**. Cardiac monitoring devices typically use anywhere from three to five leads for rhythm monitoring. The leads are usually colored and labeled to help with placement. The lead wires are attached to electrodes, which are adhesive disks with a gel center to aid in skin contact. Some manufacturers offer a "diaphoretic" electrode that sticks to a sweating patient more effectively.

Bipolar leads are used for monitoring purposes—that is, lead I, II, or III. These leads, also called limb leads, consist of two electrodes, one positive and one negative, that are placed on two different limbs. When using bipolar leads, any impulse in the body moving to a positive electrode will cause a positive deflection on the ECG. Conversely, if an impulse is moving toward a negative electrode, it will result in negative deflection on the ECG tracing. A lack of electrical impulse will produce an isoelectric or flat line. If the impulse moves perpendicular to the lead, the result will be a "biphasic" waveform, which is above and below the isoelectric baseline.

When positioned on the chest, these leads form a triangle around the heart, called the Einthoven triangle **Figure 63**. ECG monitors have the ability to change the polarity of the leads so that you can view leads I, II, and III by turning a knob or pressing a shift key. Many of the newer ECG monitors allow you to see all three of these leads at the same time.

Whereas continuous ECG monitoring provides real-time visibility of the cardiac electrical activity, it only shows you one aspect of the heart's electrical activity. An ECG tracing will not give you any information regarding the muscular function of the heart, nor will it always provide you with an accurate assessment of the blood supply to the cardiac muscle via the coronary vessels. The heart is like a light bulb in a socket—the light bulb contains everything it needs inside it in order to function; however, it needs electricity. When a light bulb burns out

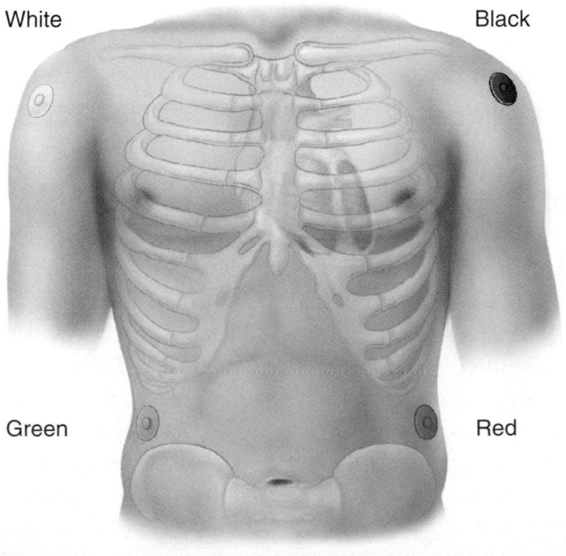

White

Black

Green

Red

Figure 62 4-lead electrode placement.

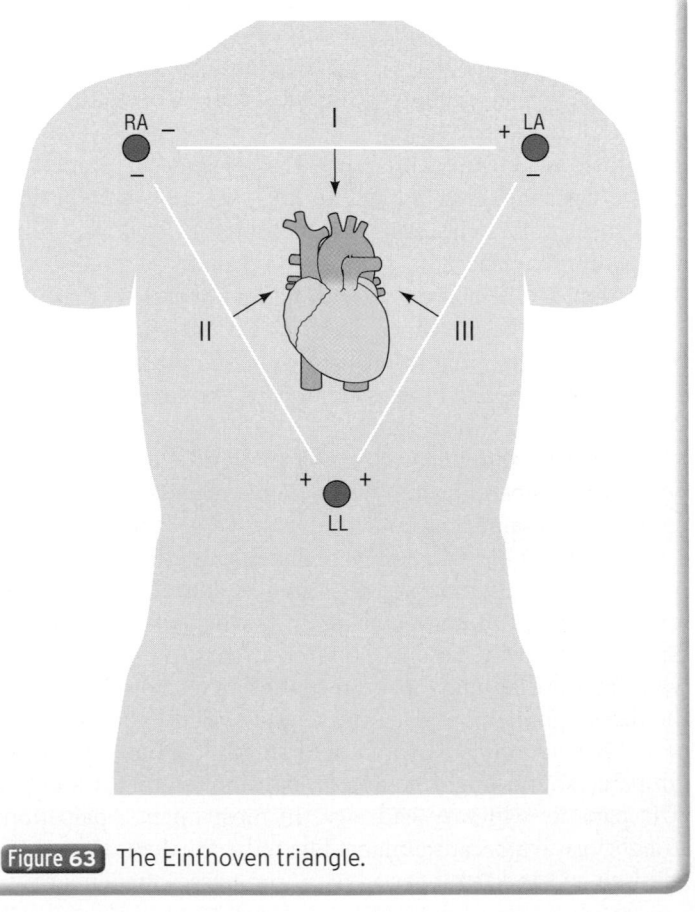

Figure 63 The Einthoven triangle.

and stops working, it does not mean that the electricity flowing to the bulb in the socket has stopped. You would not stick your wet fingers in the socket of a burned-out light bulb to see if there is electrical current present because if the switch remains on, the electricity is there. The same principle works here. There are times when the ECG looks normal, but the heart is still not functioning properly. More information regarding interpretation of ECGs can be found in the chapter, *Cardiovascular Emergencies*.

12-Lead ECG Monitoring

For the purposes of rhythm interpretation, a single lead (usually lead II) is usually sufficient. To localize the site of injury to the heart muscle, however, you must be able to look at the heart from several angles. That is precisely the purpose of a 12-lead ECG.

A 12-lead ECG analysis is indicated in any patient who might have a cardiac-related condition. Any patient with chest pain should undergo ECG analysis, but this monitoring should also be instituted for any patient with a history of heart problems. Given that age is a contributing factor to heart disease, ECG analysis is appropriate for elderly patients in many situations. Indeed, the ECG should be thought of as another vital sign, similar to blood pressure or pulse oximetry.

The addition of the 12-lead ECG to the paramedic's "tool box" has opened the door for more advanced patient care in the field. Paramedics are now able to diagnose ST elevation myocardial infarction (STEMI) in the patient's home. This early recognition of a myocardial infarction allows hospitals to prepare before patient arrivals, thus decreasing time to definitive care. In addition, paramedics in some areas of the United States are performing early intervention in the field by administering fibrinolytics to STEMI patients or diverting them to cardiac centers with catheterization labs.

The only way to learn how to take a 12-lead ECG is to practice with the equipment itself. Here are some guidelines to help ensure that the ECGs you obtain are of the highest quality possible.

- The patient should be supine. If the patient feels short of breath in that position, you may elevate the back of the stretcher about 30°.
- Make sure the patient does not become chilled because shivering will produce artifact in the ECG tracing. Note that 12-lead ECGs are more sensitive to artifact than 3-lead monitoring ECGs.
- Prepare the patient's skin as you would for placing monitoring electrodes.
- Connect the four limb electrodes. Double-check that the correct electrode is on each limb (the "LA" electrode is on the left arm, the "RA" electrode is on the right arm, and so on). Confirm that the limb electrodes are on the same arms and legs and not on the trunk of the body.
- Connect and apply the precordial leads as indicated in **Figure 64**.
- Record the ECG.

Interpretation of 12-lead ECGs is discussed in detail in the chapter, *Cardiovascular Emergencies*.

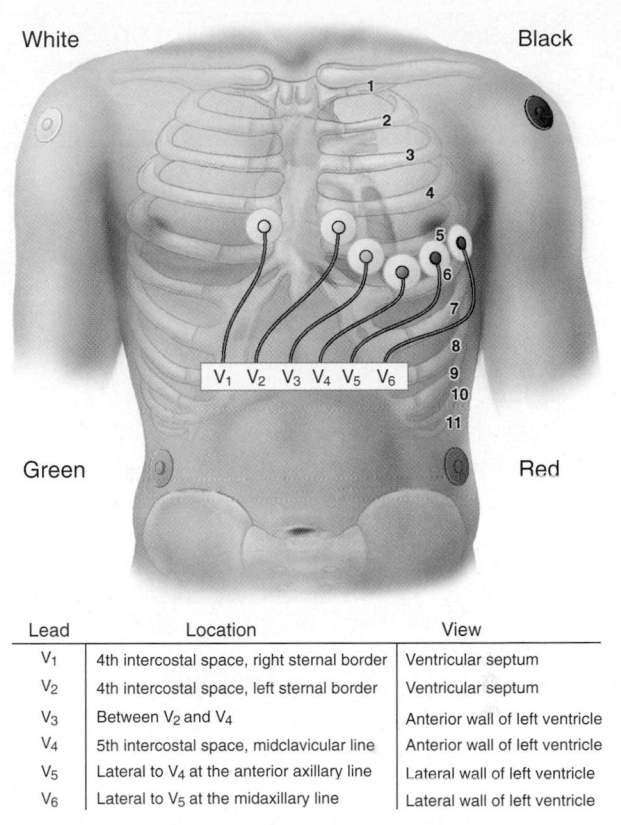

Lead	Location	View
V_1	4th intercostal space, right sternal border	Ventricular septum
V_2	4th intercostal space, left sternal border	Ventricular septum
V_3	Between V_2 and V_4	Anterior wall of left ventricle
V_4	5th intercostal space, midclavicular line	Anterior wall of left ventricle
V_5	Lateral to V_4 at the anterior axillary line	Lateral wall of left ventricle
V_6	Lateral to V_5 at the midaxillary line	Lateral wall of left ventricle

Figure 64 12-lead electrode placement.

Carbon Dioxide Monitoring

As you learned in the chapter, *Anatomy and Physiology*, carbon dioxide is a naturally occurring by-product of cellular metabolism in the human body. As the metabolism in a patient's body changes to counteract stressors, change in the output of carbon dioxide can be seen and measured. You must be able to recognize carbon dioxide output in a patient and use that information to determine treatment strategies.

There are two ways in which carbon dioxide is monitored in the field: capnometry and capnography. **Capnometry** typically consists of a disposable or electronic device that provides you with a means of showing carbon dioxide output. **Capnography** not only includes a measurement of carbon dioxide output but also provides a wave form that gives you further insight into the overall ventilatory status of your patient.

A capnographer is a practical and easy-to-use device in the prehospital environment. Whereas the older models were heavy and sometimes difficult to operate, the new devices are user-friendly and easy to interpret. While these devices can be used to confirm endotracheal tube placement, they can also be used in your conscious and breathing patients. The value of this device is in the waveform provided **Figure 65**. Consider this to be the ECG of ventilation. This will give you insight into bronchospasm, shock, and acidosis. When used for intubated patients, the device is placed on the proximal end of the endotracheal tube and then is connected into your portable ECG monitor or a separate monitoring device. For breathing patients, a special nasal cannula adapted for collecting CO_2 while

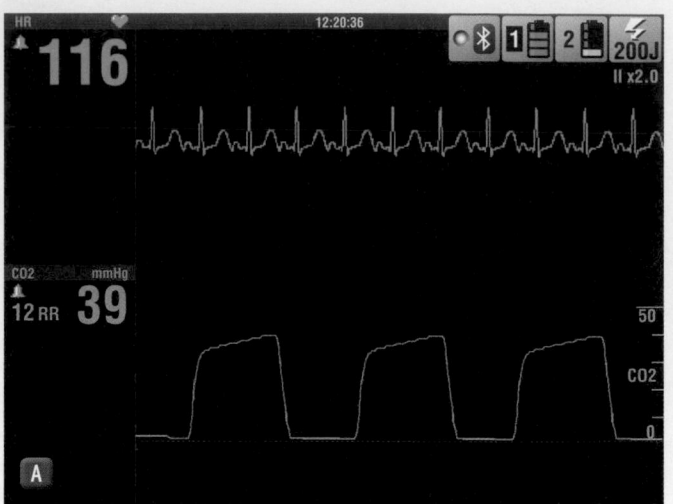

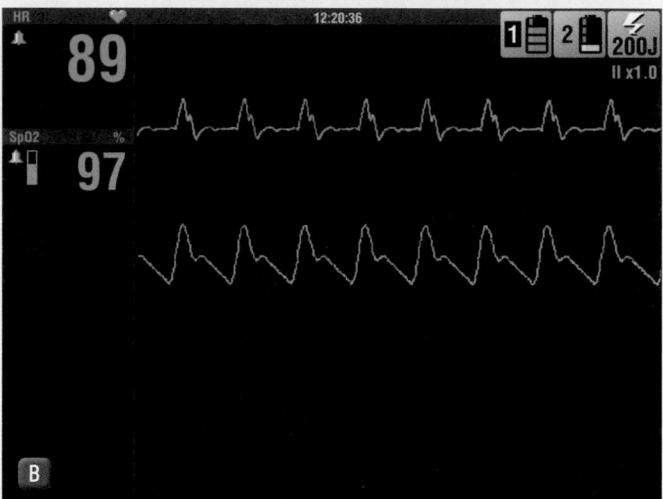

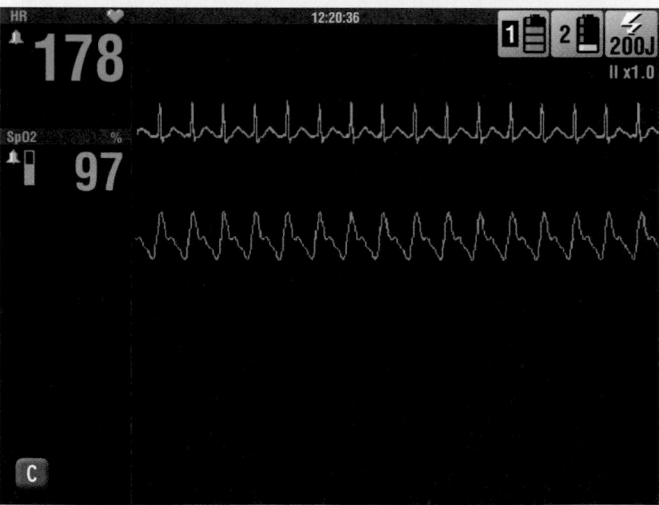

Figure 65 Waveform capnography is the preferred method for carbon dioxide monitoring. These screens also show the patient's ECG. **A.** Tachycardia. **B.** Ventricular tachycardia. **C.** Supraventricular tachycardia.

administering oxygen is used. Whereas this device is superior in monitoring quality to the capnometer, it too has limitations. These devices typically require a minimal airflow in order to calculate a reading, require calibration, and are sometimes affected from secretions getting into the tubing.

Conversely, the purpose of capnometry is to provide verification of correct endotracheal tube placement. The idea is that the capnometer is placed on the proximal end of an endotracheal tube. If the tube is in the trachea, exhaled CO_2 should pass by the sensor and provide information about tube placement. This sounds easy enough; however, it is not without limitations.

Capnometry and capnography are discussed in more detail in the chapter, *Airway Management and Ventilation*.

Basic Blood Chemistry

There are a variety of elements found in blood that aid you in determining a differential diagnosis. Whereas results from the history taking and secondary assessment are paramount in determining the differential diagnosis, sometimes a laboratory result helps to confirm the diagnosis. You can use some of these basic blood chemistry tests in the field to aid in determining a differential diagnosis.

Blood Glucometer

Measuring the blood glucose level of every patient who has altered mentation as part of his or her clinical presentation is a must in EMS. It is a relatively easy test to perform and provides you with rapid information regarding the level of available glucose in the patient's bloodstream. If the glucose level is low, this can help you in determining the differential diagnosis for an unresponsive patient. On the same note, if the level is high in a patient with nausea, vomiting, and abdominal pain with a change in mental status, it may help you to determine a diagnosis of diabetic ketoacidosis.

Blood glucose should be assessed in all known diabetic patients, all patients who are unresponsive for unknown reasons, and for patients with generalized malaise/weakness. In addition, a blood glucose level can be assessed on any patient whom you feel has a poor general impression.

There are generally two ways to obtain a rapid blood glucose reading in the field: from the hub of an IV catheter and from a finger stick. When obtaining a blood sample from an IV catheter, establish IV access as usual, place the test strip against the hub of the catheter before you connect the IV tubing, and allow a drop of blood to touch the test strip while being careful not to contaminate yourself with the patient's blood. For those patients with an already infusing IV, you will need to use a lancet needle to obtain a drop of blood. Cleanse the site (finger) with antiseptic and puncture the site with the lancet needle. Immediately dispose of the needle in a sharps container and obtain a drop of blood on the test strip. When finished, place a bandage over the puncture site.

Most newer glucometers take only a few seconds to give you a reading. Keep in mind that while this is convenient for you, there are some accuracy issues to consider. Rapid does not always equal accurate. Glucometers should be calibrated on a regular basis in order to maintain accuracy. In addition, you should verify that the test strips are correct for the glucometer you are using and that they have not expired. You must also make sure you have prepped the site adequately, and that the finger is clean.

Cardiac Biomarkers

Cardiac biomarkers are used to assess for the presence of damage to cardiac muscle. Typically, such blood tests are performed to determine whether a myocardial infarction has taken place. Earlier discussion in this chapter covered the use of 12-lead ECGs in the field to help determine the presence of STEMI; however, most heart attacks are known as non-ST myocardial infarctions (NSTE-MIs). These are typically diagnosed using cardiac biomarkers. Although these blood tests are usually done in a lab, several field versions are now available to measure these markers quickly.

In the EMS environment, these markers should be assessed in all cardiac patients, depending on local protocol, as well as in patients who are presenting with signs and symptoms of a stroke. The procedure is similar to that of obtaining a blood glucose level.

The accuracy of this method of testing reflects the effectiveness of the calibration process, use of appropriate testing medium (ie, strips), and use of non-expired items. In addition, when assessing for a myocardial infarction, you must understand that elevation of cardiac biomarkers can take several hours before it is present in a patient's blood. Therefore, just because elevated levels may not be seen in the field, you cannot rule out that a myocardial infarction is not taking place. Myocardial infarction is discussed in more depth in the chapter, *Cardiovascular Emergencies*.

Other Blood Tests

With the invention of rapid laboratory testing devices, more EMS systems are beginning to perform basic laboratory tests in the field. Whereas many of these tests may not be used in the emergency setting, they are being used quite often for specialty care transports.

Tests such as a basic and complete metabolic profile (CHEM 7 and CHEM 12) give you insight into the electrolyte status of the patient, along with his or her renal and, sometimes, liver function. The brain natriuretic peptide (BNP) level is typically elevated in a patient experiencing an exacerbation of chronic heart failure. A BNP test helps you to differentiate cardiac versus pulmonary causes of respiratory distress.

Arterial blood gases are an invasive test requiring the puncture of an artery to obtain a sample for testing. This test is valuable for patients experiencing respiratory distress/failure, for ventilated patients, and for the assessment of respiratory and metabolic acidosis. While this test is not typically performed in the prehospital environment, it may prove to be quite helpful in the specialty care transport arena.

Secondary Assessment

Patient Assessment

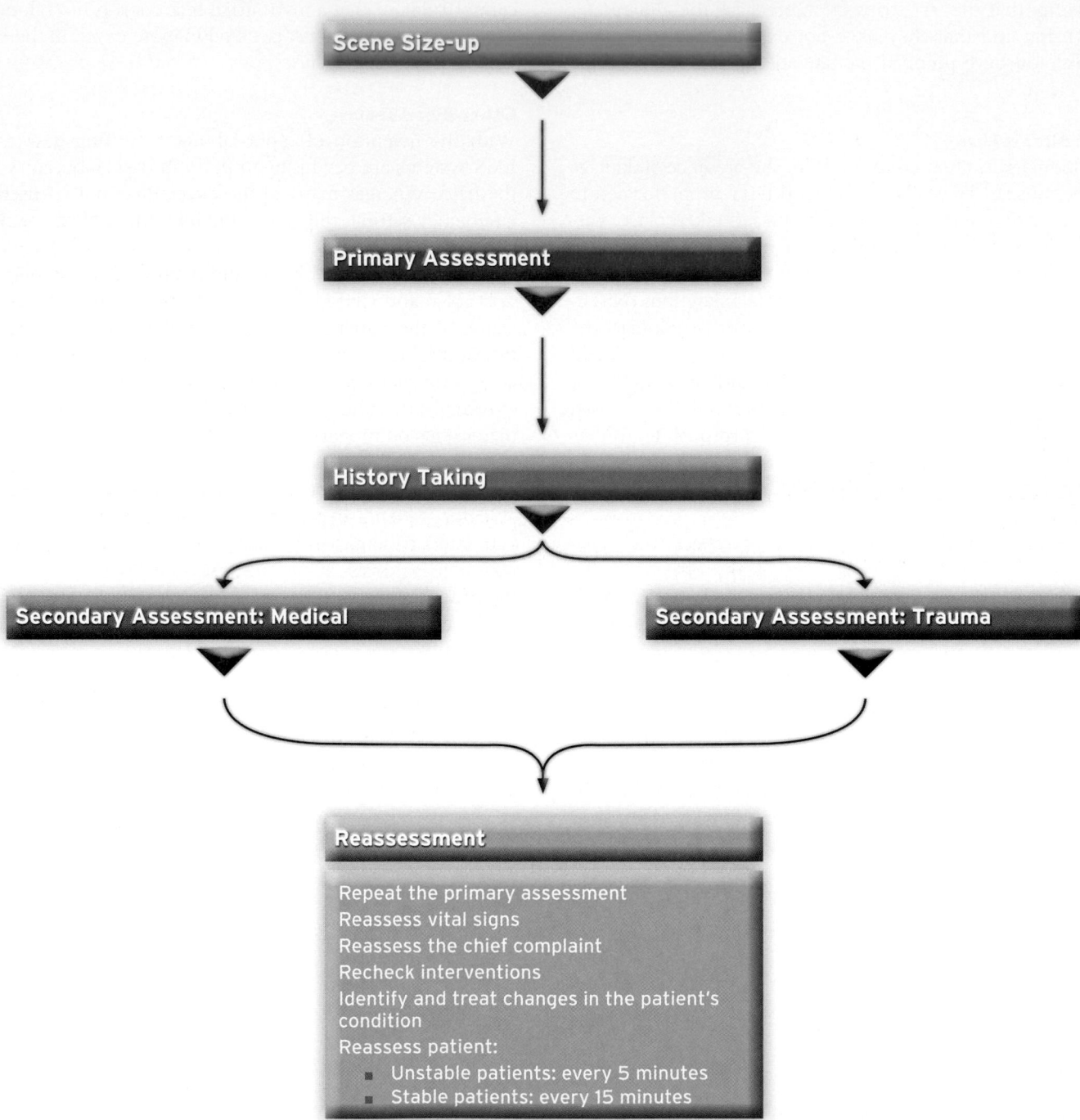

Scene Size-up

Primary Assessment

History Taking

Secondary Assessment: Medical

Secondary Assessment: Trauma

Reassessment

Repeat the primary assessment
Reassess vital signs
Reassess the chief complaint
Recheck interventions
Identify and treat changes in the patient's condition
Reassess patient:
- Unstable patients: every 5 minutes
- Stable patients: every 15 minutes

Reassessment

After the primary assessment, <u>reassessment</u> is the single most important assessment process you will perform. When performing reassessment, you must reassess the ABCs, make certain you have adequately addressed the chief complaint, obtain another set of vital signs, and close any other patient care loops, such as dressing small wounds and placing ice packs. Reassessment represents a continuous, yet cyclical, process that you perform throughout transport, right up to the time you turn patient care over to the emergency department staff. For patients in stable condition, you should do a reassessment every 15 minutes or so. For patients in unstable condition, you need to make a concerted effort to repeat the reassessment every 5 minutes.

Reassessment of Mental Status and the ABCs

Reassessment combines repetition of the primary assessment, reassessment of vital signs and breath sounds, and repetition of the secondary assessment. During the reassessment, you continue to evaluate and reevaluate the patient's status and any treatments already administered. Trends in the patient's current condition may give clues about the effectiveness of treatments. Compare vital signs. Have interventions improved the patient's condition? Are identified problems better or worse? This information indicates which changes have occurred and which critical conditions have been addressed and corrected.

First, compare the patient's LOC with your baseline assessment. Is the LOC changing? If so, how? If mentation is decreasing, can the patient still protect the airway? If you have doubts, consider inserting an advanced airway.

Second, review the patient's airway. Is it patent? Swelling, bleeding, or just a change of position can quickly obstruct the airway, so make certain that the airway is properly positioned and dry. Always be prepared to suction, and do not delay if you hear gurgling in the upper airway. It is far better to prevent aspiration than to treat it later. If the airway needs to be secured, prepare the patient for intubation and perform the procedure immediately. Once intubation is accomplished, recheck lung sounds and perform oximetry and capnography periodically to confirm that the tube is properly placed.

Third, reassess breathing. Is the patient breathing adequately? If not, figure out why and correct the problem. For hypoventilation, assist breathing with oxygen and a bag-mask device. Correct hypoxia with high-concentration oxygen therapy. For patients with diminished or absent breath sounds, JVD, and progressive dyspnea (signs of pneumothorax), decompress the chest.

Stay alert for signs that the patient is experiencing ventilatory fatigue (for example, decreasing pulse oximetry reading, patient looks increasingly tired). Be especially alert for this possibility in children because it is a classic sign that precedes disaster for the patient. Patients of any age who are going into ventilatory fatigue need to have their airway aggressively managed for them.

Finally, reassess the patient's circulation. Assess overall skin color as an initial measure of cardiovascular function and hemodynamic status. With pale, cool, wet skin, think shock; with cyanosis, think oxygen desaturation; with mottling, think end-stage shock.

Make certain that all bleeding is controlled. If you find blood-soaked dressings, add more fresh dressings to the stack and rebandage in place. Reassess the blood pressure, watching closely for signs that the patient is beginning to decompensate.

Reassess the pulse, including its rate, strength, and regularity. Progressive tachycardia may indicate that the patient's problem is uncorrected (he or she is still bleeding, is hypoxic, or is developing cardiogenic shock). In contrast, sustained or progressively worsening bradycardia may reflect rising intracranial pressure (from trauma or a stroke) or end-stage shock.

The physiologic response of pediatric and geriatric patients during a crisis may differ and therefore may require a different approach to reassessment. Adult patients have a tendency to show signs of deterioration as their conditions begin to become unstable. The condition of a pediatric patient, however, will decompensate much more quickly; therefore, it is imperative that you frequently reassess pediatric patients. Any indication of a decrease in mental status or changes to airway, breathing, and circulation should prompt immediate intervention. Geriatric patients differ from adult and pediatric patients in that many of them lack appropriate compensatory mechanisms and therefore may not show signs of deterioration as their conditions become unstable. In addition, many of these patients have underlying diseases or take medications that mask the true assessment findings. For example, a patient who is going into shock would typically demonstrate an increase in pulse rate. However, many geriatric patients either lack the ability to increase their pulse rate or take medications that block the pulse rate from increasing. Reassessment of mental status may also prove challenging in this population. For some patients, an altered mental status is their baseline behavior; therefore, it becomes difficult to assess whether the patient is showing signs of improvement. Frequent reassessment of this population is necessary in order to determine and monitor a patient's overall progress and stability.

Reassessment of Patient Care and Transport Priorities

After reassessing the patient, think about your present care plan. Have you addressed all life threats? Based on what you now know, do you need to revise your priority list? If so, make the change and get on with patient care. In contrast, if your plan is working well and you have addressed most or all of the patient's complaints, there is no need to revise the care plan.

While you are reevaluating your patient care priorities, you should reassess the transport plan as well. Should routine transport be stepped up to priority? Is the patient's condition worsening to the point that you need to consider diverting to a closer facility? Do you need to set up a rendezvous with an air ambulance and fly the patient to the health care facility? If your patient's condition has improved and stabilized, you should step down from priority and transport the patient as a routine case, the clearly safer choice.

Get another complete set of vital signs, and compare them with the expected outcomes from your therapies. For example, if you administered a 500-mL bolus of normal saline to a patient with gastrointestinal bleeding, you usually would expect a rise in blood pressure and a decrease in pulse rate.

With any priority patient, you should have, at a minimum, three sets of vital signs—and that would be if you had a short transport. With most priority patients, you will have four or five sets of vital signs. Thus, you can look for trends or patterns such as a slowing pulse, rising blood pressure, and erratic respiratory patterns that represent the **Cushing reflex**, a grave sign for patients with head trauma. Alternatively, narrowed

pulse pressure, muffled heart tones, and JVD are associated with cardiac tamponade (**Beck triad**), usually secondary to penetrating chest trauma.

The last element of the reassessment is to revisit the patient's complaints (from the history taking), along with your interventions. Have any complaints improved or resolved? Has the 9 over 10 chest pain improved with the nitroglycerin you administered? Did the second albuterol treatment ease the patient's breathing? Which situations remain unresolved? Situations that are worsening are especially concerning because they could mean an unseen problem or ineffective interventions. If you have not reached the receiving facility, get ready to do the reassessment process again—that is why it is called the reassessment. Finally, document all of your findings with each reassessment so that your medical record is accurate and complete.

Words of Wisdom

Understand that you cannot hear narrowing pulse pressures until you've taken two or three blood pressures. Multiple checks provide the comparative data you need.

YOU are the Medic SUMMARY

1. What is your first concern for this scene?

You do not know at this point what happened to this patient. This may or may not be a crime scene. Either way, the main focus is to ensure the safety and well-being of you and your partner. Ask yourself, "Is it safe for me and my team to enter this scene and to approach the patient?" To answer that question, you need to use a "wide-angle lens" thought process when you assess and evaluate the scene. If the answer to the question is "Yes, the scene is safe," then establish patient contact and proceed with your assessment. However, if the answer is "No, the scene does not appear to be safe," then either perform whatever may be necessary to make the scene safe or request additional resources before entering the scene.

2. How will you address this concern?

Frequently the EMS team arrives first and unknowingly enters a crime scene. In this case, the dispatcher received the call from a third-party caller, which usually means someone who is not with the patient. Law enforcement personnel should be requested immediately in such cases because it is nearly impossible for you and your partner to control the scene and care for the patient at the same time, and because the perpetrator could return with additional weapons. If you are in doubt about what to do, protect yourself and your crew before anything else. This may equate to staying in the ambulance until law enforcement personnel arrive to secure the scene.

3. What is your general impression of this patient?

In the first 60 to 90 seconds, as you look at, talk with, and touch your patient, you should be able to identify obvious threats to the ABCs. More often than not, you will form the general impression of your patient based almost solely on the initial presentation and chief complaint. In the case of trauma ask, "Is my patient hurt? If so, how badly?" In this case, you know the patient is responsive and bleeding from a wound to the chest. Once these questions are answered, you can move forward with determining your priorities of care, developing a care plan, and putting the care plan into action.

4. What is your next step in the assessment of this patient?

Changes in the state of consciousness may provide the first clue to an alteration in the patient's condition, so establish a baseline as soon as you encounter the patient. At the same time you are assessing mental status, if trauma is involved, you need to decide whether you will implement spinal motion restriction procedures. The quickest and simplest way to assess the patient's mental status or level of consciousness (LOC) is to use the AVPU process:

A Alert to person, place, and day

V Responsive to Verbal stimuli

P Responsive to Pain

U Unresponsive

5. On the basis of your assessment of the ABCs, what is your first priority in the care of this patient?

Assessment of the patient's airway status focuses on two questions: Is the airway open and patent? Is it likely to remain so? If you determine that the patient cannot maintain his or her airway, an oral or nasal airway may resolve the problem. However, if you cannot maintain it by any other means, you need to use a more invasive technique, such as endotracheal intubation. Breathing is proportional and related to airway adequacy. The assessment of breathing likewise focuses on two questions: First, is the patient breathing? If not, then you have to breathe for the patient. Second, if the patient is breathing, is breathing adequate? Again, if breathing is not adequate, do what is necessary to support the patient's breathing or consider performing rapid sequence intubation.

6. Can you determine the priority of this patient at this point?

When you have a priority patient, you need to expedite transport, doing only what is absolutely necessary at the scene and handling everything else en route, including the appropriate history taking and physical examination. This patient presents with a poor general impression, is responsive but does not or cannot follow commands, and has difficulty breathing. Based solely on these three criteria, this patient is a priority.

YOU *are the Medic*   SUMMARY, *continued*

7. How can you determine the level of internal damage if you do not have the implement used in the stabbing?

The chest contains many structures that are vital to life; any injury to the chest, regardless of the object used, has the potential to cause significant internal damage. The chest (or thorax) consists of the superior aspect of the torso, from the base of the neck to the diaphragm as delineated by the costal arch. The chest wall is divided into anterior and posterior portions–literally, the patient's front and back. The back of the chest extends down the patient's back, to the level of the diaphragm posteriorly, which tends to move up and down with breathing. The chest contains many vital structures, including the lungs and mediastinal elements (heart, great vessels). The chest wall serves as a protective covering for the internal components. It consists of numerous musculoskeletal, vascular, nervous, connective, and lining structures.

8. Is past medical history relevant in this case?

The past medical history gives you an opportunity to learn about any pertinent or chronic underlying medical conditions the patient may have. Whereas not all aspects of the past history may seem important with this patient, a careful and thorough history will help paint a clear picture of the overall health status of the patient. In this case, the patient may not be willing or able to provide this information to you. Use the information you obtained from your assessment and inspection of the patient as much as possible. Always stay alert for any medical alert bracelets or devices and take note of any scars possibly indicating that the patient has had open heart surgery or had a pacemaker or automated internal cardioverter-defibrillator implanted in the chest wall.

EMS Patient Care Report (PCR)

Date: 04-28-11	Incident No.: 902	Nature of Call: Stabbing		Location: 4th Ave/Main St	
Dispatched: 0200	En Route: 0201	At Scene: 0205	Transport: 0215	At Hospital: 0225	In Service: 0240

Patient Information

Age: Approx 30 Sex: M Weight (in kg [lb]): 75 kg (165 lb)	Allergies: Unknown Medications: Unknown Past Medical History: Unknown Chief Complaint: 1″ penetrating to upper left chest

Vital Signs

Time: 0209	BP: 90/64	Pulse: 122	Respirations: 28	Spo$_2$: 93% on room air
Time: 0214	BP: 92/62	Pulse: 120	Respirations: 28	Spo$_2$: 96% on 15 L/min
Time:	BP:	Pulse:	Respirations:	Spo$_2$:

EMS Treatment
(circle all that apply)

Oxygen @ __15__ L/min via (circle one): NC (NRM) Bag-mask device	Assisted Ventilation	Airway Adjunct:	CPR
Defibrillation	Bleeding Control	Bandaging	Splinting	Other:

Narrative

Unit 84 dispatched for a man down in front of the strip mall at 4th Avenue & Main Street. This unit arrived on scene prior to all other responders to find this pt lying left lateral recumbent on the sidewalk. There appears to be no one else present on the scene. Prior to exiting the vehicle, scene lights reveal what appears to be blood on the sidewalk near the pt's chest. Using the PA system assessment was made of the level of consciousness due to scene safety concerns. Pt demonstrated following commands at that time. PD on scene approximately 1 minute after our arrival. Scene secured for pt assessment and treatment. Pt is approx. 30-year-old man with a penetrating wound, approx 1″ in length just inferior to the center of the left clavicle. Bleeding has stopped. Occlusive dressing applied. Pt is responsive, responds to commands, but is not verbal. Pt placed in full spinal precautions. VS as noted and 15 L/min O$_2$ via NRM applied. IV NS established with 16ga, right AC. Pt able to maintain own airway but having increased difficulty breathing upon lying supine on the backboard. Pt moved to ambulance for emergency transport to the trauma center. Head of the backboard raised 15%, which provided some relief to breathing effort. Pt report given to Dr. Solomon upon arrival. **End of report**

Prep Kit

- Patient assessment is the platform on which quality prehospital care is built and the single most important skill you bring to bear on patient care.

- Patient assessment is a process composed of five main components: scene size-up, primary assessment, history taking, secondary assessment, and reassessment.

- The first step of the patient assessment process is the scene size-up because your first and foremost concern on any call is ensuring your own safety and the safety of the other EMS team members.

- During the size-up, you also make a determination of the mechanism of injury or nature of the patient's illness.

- Another important step in protecting yourself is to take standard precautions. Be sure to don all necessary personal protective equipment before approaching the patient.

- The first step in the primary assessment is to form a general impression of the patient's condition. While walking up to the patient, note whether the patient appears to be in stable or unstable condition, and observe the environment for clues.

- During the primary assessment, you should be able to identify threats to the ABCs; these life threats should be addressed immediately.

- After assessing the patient for disability, you must make a transport decision and, if the patient has sustained trauma, perform a rapid exam to identify injuries that require care prior to immobilizing the patient.

- Once the primary assessment is complete and all life threats have been addressed, you can move into the history-taking phase of patient assessment.

- Patient history is a primary means of diagnosing the chief complaint in the field; its value depends on the your ability to skillfully elicit full and accurate information. For responsive medical patients, you should ask questions about each body system to obtain a thorough picture of the patient's health.

- The first part of a patient's history also serves as a good mental status examination: ask for the patient's name; the date, time, and location; the chief complaint; and the events leading up to the request for EMS assistance.

- After clarifying the history of the present illness, ask the patient about his or her past medical history, the general state of his or her health, and any pertinent family history. As part of this questioning, write down a list of medications your patient is taking, and allergies.

- For responsive medical patients, the history may generally be obtained directly from the patient, although assistance may be needed with certain patients (eg, pediatric patients); for unresponsive medical patients and trauma patients, it may be necessary to obtain the history from family members or bystanders.

- Use constructive communications skills as you talk with patients: facilitation, reflection, clarification, empathy, confrontation, interpretation, and asking directly about feelings.

- At times you will need to ask patients about sensitive topics, such as alcohol or drug abuse, physical abuse or violence, or sexual history. Be familiar with techniques for successfully asking patients about these topics.

- Obtaining a history from a geriatric patient may involve challenges. Older patients may have multiple medical problems, may be taking numerous medications, and may present differently than adults, making their emergencies potentially more complex. They may have sensory losses that may require that you adjust your approach in order to gain the needed information.

- Work on strategies within your service and with your partner for positive communications with patients who are silent, overly talkative, seductive, having multiple symptoms, anxious, needing reassurance, angry or hostile, intoxicated, crying, or depressed.

- Secondary assessment (also known as the head-to-toe physical examination) is the process by which quantifiable, objective information is obtained from a patient about his or her overall state of health.

- There are times when you may not have time to perform a secondary assessment at all if the patient has serious life threats. Or, you may focus on the area of the chief complaint first, then move on to assessing all other body systems if time permits. The two types of physical examinations are the full-body exam and the focused assessment.

- The secondary assessment includes obtaining vital signs that measure overall body function, and performing a head-to-toe survey that evaluates the workings of specific body organ systems. This survey is done in a sequential manner, ensuring that every aspect of the body's function is evaluated.

- The techniques of inspection, palpation, percussion, and auscultation allow you to use your physical senses to obtain physical information and to understand the normal (versus abnormal) functions of a patient's body.

- Vital signs consist of a measurement of blood pressure; pulse rate, rhythm, and quality; respiratory rate, rhythm, and quality; temperature; and, if indicated, pulse oximetry. Other than overall patient appearance, vital signs are some of the most valuable objective data for determining patient status.

- Monitoring devices used by the paramedic include continuous ECG monitoring, 12-lead ECG, carbon dioxide monitoring (capnography and capnometry), blood chemistry analyses, and cardiac biomarkers, among others.

- You need to alter your approach to patient assessment when dealing with infants and children. Because a young child might not be able to speak, your assessment of his or her condition must be based in large part on what you can see and hear yourself. Family members or caregivers may also be able to provide useful information.

- After the primary assessment, the reassessment is the single most important assessment process you will perform.

- The reassessment is performed on all patients. It gives you an opportunity to reevaluate the chief complaint and to reassess interventions to ensure that they are still effective. Information from the reassessment may be used to identify and treat changes in the patient's condition.

- A patient in stable condition should be reassessed every 15 minutes, whereas a patient in unstable condition should be reassessed every 5 minutes. A critical patient needs to be evaluated continuously.

■ Vital Vocabulary

adventitious breath sounds Abnormal breath sounds such as wheezes, rhonchi, rales, stridor, and pleural friction rubs.

alert and oriented (A × O) A determination made when assessing mental status by looking at whether the patient is oriented to four elements: person, place, time, and the event itself. Each element provides information about different aspects of the patient's memory.

aphasia The impairment of language that affects the production or understanding of speech and the ability to read or write.

ascites Abnormal accumulation of fluid in the peritoneal cavity.

aspiration The introduction of vomit or other foreign material into the lungs.

auscultation The method of listening to sounds within the body with a stethoscope.

AVPU A method of assessing mental status by determining whether a patient is Awake and alert, responsive to Verbal stimuli or Pain, or Unresponsive; used principally in the primary assessment.

Battle sign Bruising over the mastoid process, which may be indicative of a skull fracture; also known as raccoon eyes.

Beck triad The combination of a narrowed pulse pressure, muffled heart tones, and jugular venous distention associated with cardiac tamponade; usually resulting from penetrating chest trauma.

blood pressure The measurement of the force exerted against the walls of the blood vessels as the heart contracts and relaxes; it is calculated as the product of cardiac output and peripheral vascular resistance.

bronchophony A test of decreased breath sounds performed by placing the diaphragm of the stethoscope over the area in question while the patient says "ninety-nine"; a loud, clear sound indicates lung consolidation.

bronchovesicular sounds Pertaining to the bronchial tubes and the alveoli with special reference to sounds intermediate between bronchial or tracheal sounds and alveolar sounds.

bruit An abnormal "whoosh"-like sound of turbulent blood flow moving through a narrowed artery, usually heard in the carotid arteries.

capnography A noninvasive diagnostic tool that can quickly and efficiently provide information on a patient's ventilatory and circulatory status.

capnometry The use of a capnometer, a device that measures the amount of expired carbon dioxide.

cerumen Ear wax.

chief complaint The problem for which the patient is seeking help.

crepitus Crackling, grating, or grinding that is often felt or heard when two ends of bone rub together.

current health status A composite picture of a number of factors in a patient's life, such as dietary habits, current medications, allergies, exercise, alcohol or tobacco use, recreational drug use, sleep patterns and disorders, and immunizations.

Cushing reflex The combination of a slowing pulse, rising blood pressure, and erratic respiratory patterns; a grave sign for patients with head trauma or cerebrovascular accident.

cyanosis A bluish-gray skin color that is caused by reduced levels of oxygen in the blood.

DCAP-BTLS A mnemonic for assessment in which each area of the body is evaluated for Deformities, Contusions, Abrasions, Punctures/penetrations, Burns, Tenderness, Lacerations, and Swelling.

delirium Change in mental status that is marked by the inability to focus, think logically, and maintain attention.

dementia The slow onset of progressive disorientation, shortened attention span, and loss of cognitive function.

dermatomes Distinct areas of skin that correspond to specific spinal or cranial nerve levels where sensory nerves enter the central nervous system.

dermis The tough, highly elastic layer of connective tissues underlying the dermis.

diaphoresis Excessive sweating; it is often associated with shock.

diastolic pressure The result of residual pressure in the circulatory system while the left ventricle is relaxing (ie, in diastole).

differential diagnosis The process of weighing the probability of one disease versus other diseases by comparing clinical findings that could account for a patient's illness.

diplopia Double vision.

ecchymosis Localized bruising or blood collection within or under the skin.

egophony A test of decreased breath sounds performed by placing the diaphragm of the stethoscope over the area in question while the patient says "ee"; an "ay" sound indicates lung consolidation.

epidermis The outermost layer of the skin that acts as the body's first line of defense.

fibroblasts Cells that secrete collagen, elastin, and ground substance.

field impression A determination of what you think is the patient's current problem, usually based on the patient history and the chief complaint.

focused assessment A type of physical assessment that is typically performed on patients who have sustained an isolated injury or on responsive medical patients. This type of examination is based on the chief complaint and focuses on one body system or part.

full-body exam A systematic head-to-toe examination that is performed during the secondary assessment of a patient who has sustained a significant mechanism of injury, is unresponsive, or is in critical condition.

general impression The overall initial impression that determines the priority for patient care; based on the patient's surroundings, the mechanism of injury, signs and symptoms, and the chief complaint.

Glasgow Coma Scale (GCS) An evaluation tool used to determine level of consciousness, which evaluates and assigns point values (scores) for eye opening, verbal response, and motor response, which are then totaled; effective in helping predict patient outcomes.

guarding Contraction of the abdominal muscles in patients.

heave A sensation felt upon palpation of the chest wall, in which the heart beats extremely strongly; suggests hypertrophy; also called a lift.

hernia Protrusion of any organ through an opening into a body cavity where it does not belong.

history of the present illness Information about the chief complaint, obtained using the OPQRST mnemonic.

iatrogenic Related to a side effect or complication of treatment.

inspection Looking at the patient, either in general or at a specific area (ie, a patient's overall appearance from the doorway, versus looking specifically at the chest wall for abnormalities/deformities).

jugular venous distention (JVD) Distention of the veins in the neck indicating decreased venous return to the heart.

Korotkoff sounds Sounds related to blood pressure measurement that are heard by stethoscope.

kyphosis Outward curve of the thoracic spine.

lift A sensation felt upon palpation of the chest wall, in which the heart beats extremely strongly; suggests hypertrophy; also called a heave.

lordosis Inward curve of the lumbar spine just above the buttocks. An exaggerated form of lordosis results in the condition known as swayback.

mechanism of injury (MOI) The series of events that result in traumatic injuries; the forces that act on the body to cause damage.

mottling A blotchy pattern on the skin; a typical finding in states of severe protracted hypoperfusion and shock.

murmur An abnormal "whoosh"-like sound heard over the heart that indicates turbulent blood flow around a cardiac valve.

nature of illness (NOI) The general type of illness a patient is experiencing.

ophthalmoscope An instrument used to look into a patient's eyes and view the retina and aqueous fluid; consists of a concave mirror and a battery-powered light that is usually contained in the handle.

orthostatic vital signs Assessing vital signs in two different patient positions (for example, from a lying to a sitting position) to determine the degree of hypovolemia; also called a tilt test.

otoscope A tool used to examine the ears of a patient; consists of a head and a handle. The head contains an electric light source and a low-power magnifying lens.

pallor Paleness.

palpation Physical touching for the purpose of obtaining information.

parasthesias Tingling feeling or sensory change.

past medical history Information obtained during the history-taking process, such as the patient's general state of health, childhood and adult diseases, surgeries and hospitalizations, psychiatric and mental illnesses, or traumatic injuries, which may relate to the patient's current problem.

pathologic fracture A fracture that occurs when normal forces are applied to abnormal bone structures.

patient history Information about the patient's chief complaint, present symptoms, and previous illnesses.

percussion Gently striking the surface of the body, typically overlying various body cavities, to detect changes in the densities of the underlying structures.

perfusion The body's ability to deliver oxygen and nutrients at the cellular level and to remove the waste products of metabolism for elimination.

pertinent negatives A lack of certain signs and symptoms one would normally expect to see specific to illnesses or conditions.

physiologic fracture A fracture that occurs when abnormal forces are applied to normal bone structures.

pleural friction rubs Squeaking or grating sounds that occur when the pleural linings rub together, which may be heard on inspiration, expiration, or both; commonly caused by inflammation of the pleura.

primary assessment The part of the assessment process that focuses on identifying immediately or potentially life-threatening conditions so that you can initiate lifesaving care.

primitive reflexes Reflex reactions such as Babinski, grasping, and sucking signs normally found in young patients.

proprioception The ability to perceive the position and movement of one's body or limbs.

pulse The palpation of the heartbeat by using the fingers at a point where an artery passes close to a bone.

pulse oximetry An assessment tool that measures oxygen saturation of hemoglobin in the capillary beds.

rales Rattling, bubbling, or crackling lung sounds indicative of fluid in the small airways; also known as crackles.

rapid exam A 60- to 90-second nonsystematic review and palpation of the patient's body to identify injuries that must be managed or protected immediately; conducted during the primary assessment and includes the mnemonic DCAP-BTLS.

reassessment The part of the assessment process in which problems are reevaluated and responses to treatment are assessed.

reflexes Involuntary motor responses to specific sensory stimuli, such as a tap on the knee or stroking the eyelash.

rhonchi Lung sounds that resemble snoring.

rubor Redness; one of the classic signs of inflammation.

scene size-up A quick assessment of the scene and its surroundings made to provide information about scene safety and the mechanism of injury or nature of illness, before you enter and begin patient care.

scoliosis Sideways curvature of the spine.

secondary assessment The process by which more detailed, quantifiable, objective information is obtained from a patient about his or her overall state of health.

signs Indications of illness or injury that the examiner can see, hear, feel, smell, and so on.

sphygmomanometer A blood pressure cuff.

splitting In the context of heart sounds, the situation in which events on the right side of heart occur slightly later than those on the left side, and create two discernible sounds rather than one heart sound.

stridor A harsh, high-pitched, crowing inspiratory sound, such as the sound often heard in acute laryngeal obstruction.

symptoms The pain, discomfort, or other abnormality that the patient feels.

systolic pressure Blood pressure created by the left ventricle while it is contracting (ie, in systole).

tenting A condition in which the skin slowly retracts after being pinched and pulled away slightly from the body; a sign of dehydration.

thrill A humming vibration that can be palpated through the chest wall; suggests an underlying bruit or murmur.

turgor Loss of elasticity in the skin.

vasoconstriction Narrowing of a blood vessel, such as with hypoperfusion or cold extremities.

vasodilation Widening of a blood vessel.

vesicular sounds Normal breath sounds made by air moving in and out of the alveoli; heard over a normal lung.

visual acuity The ability or inability to see, and how well one can see.

wheezing A high-pitched, whistling breath sound caused by air traveling through narrowed air passages within the bronchioles; a sign of lower airway obstruction.

whispered pectoriloquy A test of decreased breath sounds performed by placing the diaphragm of the stethoscope over the area in question while the patient whispers "ninety-nine"; a loud, clear sound indicates lung consolidation.

Assessment in Action

You and your partner are on scene with a patient who is having chest pain. You have already completed your primary assessment and have administered high-flow oxygen to the patient by a nonrebreathing mask. The patient rates his pain a 12 on a scale of 1 to 10 and describes it as a squeezing sensation. The patient has no prior history of cardiac problems.

1. What is the best method for determining a differential diagnosis for your patient?
   A. The capnography reading
   B. The vital signs
   C. The cardiac monitor
   D. The history and physical examination

2. Placing electrodes on the patient's chest to form a triangle around the heart is called:
   A. Einthoven triangle.
   B. Starling's law.
   C. Beck triad.
   D. Cushing triad.

3. Who is a candidate for 12-lead ECG monitoring?
   A. Patients with general complaints
   B. Patients who only have no cardiac history
   C. Patients who may have a cardiac condition
   D. Patients with pacemakers

4. What does capnography measure?
   A. Oxygen
   B. Carbon dioxide
   C. STEMI criteria
   D. Level of consciousness

5. Cardiac biomarkers are used to determine:
   A. the presence of damage to the heart muscle.
   B. the presence of carbon dioxide.
   C. the presence of cholesterol.
   D. the presence of oxygen.

6. Elevation in cardiac biomarker readings in the presence of a myocardial infarction may take:
   A. seconds.
   B. minutes.
   C. hours.
   D. days.

Additional Questions

7. Why is the statement, "mind your manners" important in EMS?

8. What is clinical reasoning?

Critical Thinking and Clinical Decision Making

National EMS Education Standard Competencies

Assessment

Integrate scene and patient assessment findings with knowledge of epidemiology and pathophysiology to form a field impression. This includes developing a list of differential diagnoses through clinical reasoning to modify the assessment and formulate a treatment plan.

Knowledge Objectives

1. List and explain the four cornerstones of effective paramedic practice: (1) gathering, evaluating, and synthesizing; (2) developing and implementing a patient care plan; (3) using judgment and independent decision making; and (4) thinking and working under pressure. (pp 695-698)

2. Explain the benefits and drawbacks of patient protocols or standing orders and patient care algorithms in the EMS system in which you work. (p 696)

3. Explain how to distinguish patients with critical life threats from those in serious condition and those with minimal non-life-threatening injuries. (p 698)

4. Describe the stages of critical thinking and thought processing in the prehospital setting: concept formation, data interpretation, application of principle, reflection in action, and reflection on action. (pp 698-701)

5. List and explain the *Six Rs* of critical thinking: (1) Read the scene; (2) Read the patient; (3) React; (4) Reevaluate; (5) Revise the plan; (6) Review your performance. (pp 702-704)

Skills Objectives

There are no skills objectives for this chapter.

Introduction

The most fundamental description of what a paramedic does on a day-to-day basis is as follows: identify problems, set patient care priorities, develop a care plan, and, finally, execute that plan. While these steps are crucial, **cookbook medicine**—the practice of following steps without thinking about what you are doing or whether it is working—is not an effective way to practice these steps. Effective medicine requires that the provider be a *thinking cook* because many patients present atypically when compared with textbook descriptions. To further complicate matters, the prehospital environment is dynamic, which can affect the stability of any scene Figure 1 . Some paramedics who have worked in hospital emergency departments say that the chaos of the emergency department cannot be compared with the setting of the streets. Still, a paramedic working in the prehospital setting is expected to provide *quality* patient care.

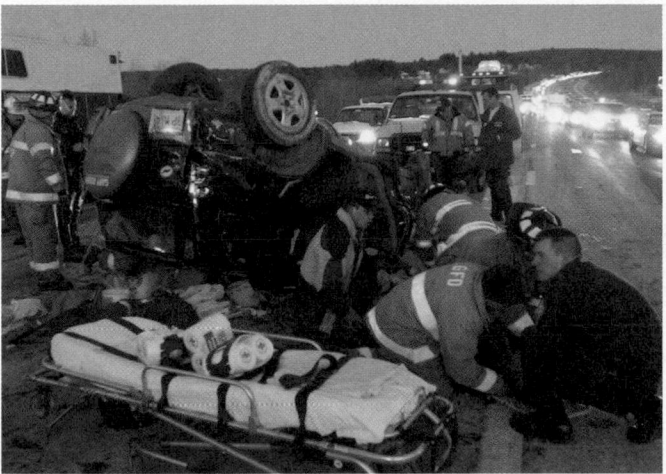

Figure 1 Your work as a paramedic is rarely done in a quiet, stress-free setting. Learn the skill of making decisions in a chaotic environment.

This chapter is divided into two parts: first, an explanation of critical thinking, and second, a discussion about how you can apply critical thinking skills in the streets. Initially, you will learn about *the science of thinking*. This topic will then be followed by the practical subject matter: how to use this knowledge and *take it to the streets*. To become a master at critical thinking and clinical decision making, you will need to know the cornerstones of the thinking processes and the terms that describe them.

The Cornerstones of Effective Paramedic Practice

Gathering, Evaluating, and Synthesizing

The first cornerstone of your practice involves *gathering, evaluating,* and *synthesizing* information. Every day, call by call, you will find yourself challenged as you try to obtain information from patients of different age groups and educational backgrounds, with varying abilities to communicate. At times, alcohol or other drug use will impair a patient's ability to respond to your questions, which will further complicate the patient assessment process.

Once you have gathered the information, you must assess and evaluate it to formulate a treatment plan. You must check the validity of the information—often relying on your own judgment and communication skills. For example, you may encounter a patient with a minor sprained ankle who asks you for morphine for pain. You may initially think that this person is an illicit drug user. Another consideration, however, is that your patient may be a health care professional or is knowledgeable about medications and has a low tolerance for pain. Because morphine is not a first-line drug for a sprained ankle, however, you will need to explain to your patient why the drug cannot be administered. The thinking paramedic must be as objective as possible in the decision-making process.

Once you have evaluated the information you obtained from the scene, the patient, or a bystander, and determined which information is valid or invalid, you need to process—or *synthesize*—this information.

YOU *are the Medic* | PART 1

You and your partner are dispatched to Cheers Cheerleading gym for a 12-year-old girl who injured her shoulder during cheerleading practice. On arrival, you ascend to the 3rd floor and see a girl surrounded by people holding her left arm. One staff member tells you that the patient was practicing a pyramid maneuver and was not caught upon dismount. The patient fell approximately 8′ onto a spring floor with her arms outstretched.

1. What is your concept formation of the call based on the information you have been provided?
2. What is included in your primary assessment of this patient?

Words of Wisdom

Remember, your professional ethics demand that you consider all the possibilities when communicating with a patient. Do not be judgmental. You must focus on how you can best meet your patient's needs.

For example, consider a patient, a 64-year-old man having chest pains, who has had type 1 diabetes since childhood, started smoking in high school, and has had chronic obstructive pulmonary disease (COPD) since his 50s. Synthesis requires that you consider how each element interacts with the others, and ultimately how they impact your patient's current condition Figure 2 .

Words of Wisdom

After you have established a working diagnosis, your treatment plan will be determined by the patient care protocols or standing orders in the EMS system where you work.

In this scenario the patient has diabetes. Diabetes, a metabolic dysfunction, is related to circulatory complications. It often leads to the development of vascular disease. In addition, in the context of shock, a high blood glucose level can make progressively thickening blood stickier, further worsening the situation. Also, whereas an extremely low blood glucose level may kill someone or result in brain damage quickly, a chronic, higher-than-normal blood glucose level takes its toll on every organ and every body system. Think about how many long-term diabetics you encounter with vision problems or amputated fingers or toes. The patient's COPD, which is primarily a disease of gas exchange, frequently results in a combination of hypoxia (low levels of oxygen in the blood) and hypercarbia (high levels of carbon dioxide in the blood). You need to assess the new onset of chest pain. It is likely that coronary artery disease has caused one or more of the vessels of the heart muscle to become blocked, in turn causing this part of the heart to begin to necrose, or die. Taking all the information you have gathered and synthesizing it would basically work something like this: "I have a patient with diseases of both circulation and gas exchange. There is a possibility that part of the patient's heart is dying because vessels are unable to deliver oxygenated blood to a portion of the heart muscle." You must treat the combined effect of your patient's disease processes to prevent the unperfused section of the heart from dying, which may cause the death of your patient. This is the synthesis part—taking individual conditions and mentally gluing them together to determine their potential for having a life-threatening impact. In the scenario described above, the patient should be considered to be having acute coronary syndrome (ACS), a potentially life-threatening condition.

Developing and Implementing a Patient Care Plan

The second cornerstone of your practice is the *development and implementation of a patient care plan*. This is actually much simpler than analyzing the validity of the information you have gathered. Once you have determined the patient's primary problem by identifying the chief complaint and establishing your working diagnosis, your treatment plan is defined and guided by the patient care protocols or standing orders in the EMS system where you work.

Protocols or standing orders define the essential standard of care for patients with certain injuries, illnesses, or behavioral conditions. They further specify performance parameters, ie, what you can or cannot do without direct medical control, as well as when you need to contact medical control before providing care. Collectively, protocols promote both a standard approach and a standard of quality care as defined by regional, state, or national standards.

Unfortunately, protocols, standing orders, and patient care algorithms only address classic patient care presentations. As a rule, they do not address vague patient complaints that do not fit into a neat clinical description—nor do they address patients with multiple disease etiologies (remember synthesis?). Those patients will require multiple treatment modalities as part of the care plan.

Therefore, your next step is to decide what you should do to best meet your patient's needs.

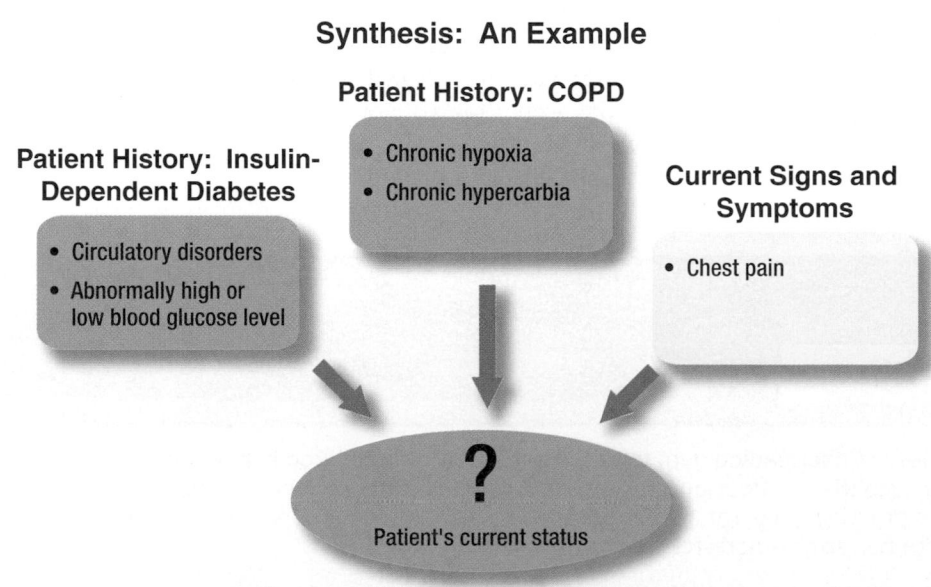

Synthesis: An Example

Patient History: COPD
- Chronic hypoxia
- Chronic hypercarbia

Patient History: Insulin-Dependent Diabetes
- Circulatory disorders
- Abnormally high or low blood glucose level

Current Signs and Symptoms
- Chest pain

?
Patient's current status

Figure 2 When you synthesize the patient information you have gathered, assess the relative importance of the patient's medical history (blue boxes) and his or her current signs and symptoms (yellow box). These factors usually affect each other.

Using Judgment and Independent Decision Making

The third cornerstone is *using judgment and independent decision making* Figure 3 . For example, you have been called to a factory where a machinist has been injured on the job and has a serious gash to the upper part of his leg. You see a significant amount of blood gushing from the area of his femoral artery with every contraction of his heart. In such a situation, it is in the patient's best interest to delay any contact with medical control until the bleeding is resolved and you are en route. You must take action or the patient may die. Even under the best circumstances, your patient

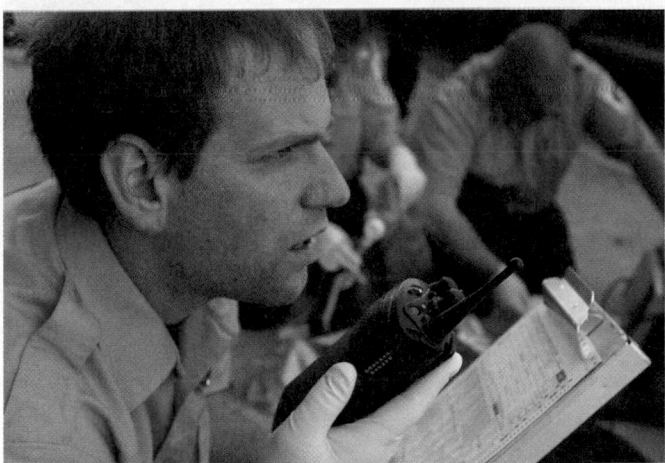

Figure 3 Every call has its own unique circumstances and challenges. Much of your patient care rests with the use of careful, nonjudgmental decision making.

may have died well before you completed a call with medical control. To save the patient, you immediately recognize the severed artery as an immediate life threat and apply continuous direct pressure, and, ideally, a tourniquet to ensure bleeding control.

In another scenario you may encounter, you have a patient who is in cardiac arrest on her front porch. In such a situation, you would immediately perform high-quality CPR on scene, including defibrillation if indicated. Then, once en route, you would perform ALS care, such as securing the airway and obtaining vascular access. If that same patient were in a third-story attic apartment with a small, treacherous exterior stairway access, there may be a different range of outcomes—from the patient being fully resuscitated and viable to being pronounced dead at the scene. Because of the physical environment, you realize it is impossible to quickly and efficiently remove the patient from the apartment for transport to the receiving facility. As such, you have a decision to make. Either the resuscitation is ended, or you resuscitate and stabilize the patient before packaging and transport. As circumstances change, so may your treatment plan. However, necessary treatment changes will only happen if you are using your critical thinking and decision-making skills to the best of your abilities.

Thinking and Working Under Pressure

The fourth and final cornerstone of your practice is your ability to *think and work under pressure*. Imagine ringing the doorbell at the address to which you have been dispatched and having the door open and a hysterical mother hands you a cyanotic, apneic 18-month-old child who has been submerged in a bathtub. Critical thinking tells you that the child must start breathing within the

---

YOU *are the Medic* PART 2

As you talk with the staff member, he tells you that they watched her fall, and reports that only her arm was injured. There was no trauma to the head or neck. You examine the patient and find that her left arm has an angular deformity in the region of the humerus. It is obvious that there is abnormal motion there every time she tries to move, and she is unable to move it without significant pain. The patient rates her level of pain as 9 on a scale of 1 to 10, but denies having any head, neck, or back pain. You obtain her vital signs while a staff member continues holding her arm. The patient's parents are not on scene, but the staff member tells you that they are being contacted. Although the patient is visibly shaken, she is not crying and is answering questions appropriately.

Recording Time: 0 Minutes	
Appearance	Visibly upset
Level of consciousness	Alert and oriented
Airway	Open and patent
Breathing	Normal, 22 breaths/min
Circulation	Radial pulse, tachycardic

3. Have you gathered enough data to turn your field impression into patient care?

4. Should you administer pain medication?

next few seconds or cardiac arrest will occur, further decreasing the likelihood of saving the child's life. Only a combination of knowledge coupled with excellent psychomotor clinical skills will allow you to avert a patient care disaster: the death of the child. You must be able to work under extreme pressure and be able to think and perform quickly and effectively.

■ The Range of Patient Conditions

One of the key elements of your practice is to be able to quickly determine if your patient is *sick or not sick.* For patients who are sick, you must be able to quantify *how sick they are,* which in turn allows you to make the best choices as to the care you must provide at the scene and the care you should provide in the ambulance while en route.

Special Populations

To improve your ability to recognize whether an infant or child is sick or not sick, take every continuing education pediatrics course and read every pediatric-related article you can.

Clear thinking in a chaotic emergency starts with a triage process. Critical patients need immediate care to survive. Serious patients need care within the next few minutes to possibly the next half hour (or they become critical patients) to have a positive outcome **Figure 4** . The two groups of patients who are left are the mortally wounded or dead, and those often termed the walking wounded or minimally injured. For the sake of discussion, the walking wounded will be referred to as non-life threats.

Examples of patients with *critical life threats* would include those with the following injuries/illnesses:

- Major multisystem trauma
- Devastating single-system trauma
- End-stage disease presentations
- Acute presentations of chronic conditions

Examples of patients in *serious condition* would include those with the following injuries/illnesses:

- Serious multisystem trauma
- Acute presentations of "first-time" medical events
- Multiple disease etiologies

Examples of patients who are "walking wounded" or have *minimal, non-life-threatening injuries* would include those with the following injuries/illnesses:

- Simple abrasions
- Partial-thickness burns of an extremity of less than 5% body surface area
- Small lacerations with only capillary bleeding

■ Critical Thinking and Clinical Decision Making

It is important for you to understand the processes of *thinking* and *decision making.* By having a better understanding of how

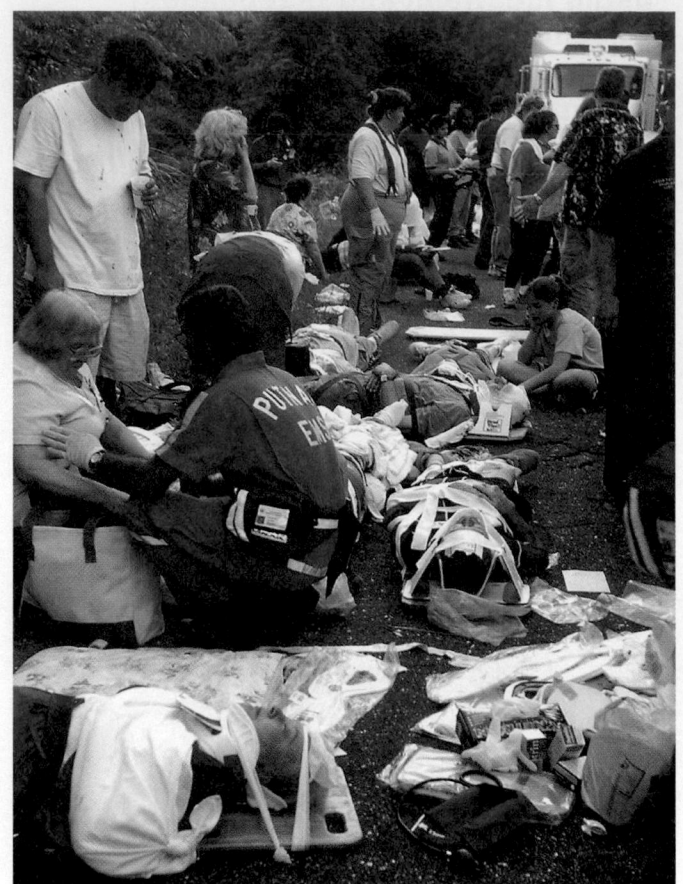

Figure 4 With multiple patients, you must quickly assess and prioritize the urgency of each patient's condition.

your thoughts are formed and processed, you can learn to think more effectively.

■ Concept Formation

The first stage of the thought process in prehospital care is that of gathering information—things you see, hear, smell, or feel and that which you gather from your diagnostic tools. This process is called **concept formation**.

The process starts as you arrive at the scene and evaluate it from a safety perspective for both the EMS team and your patient. You need to evaluate the mechanism of injury for trauma, or in the case of medical calls, the nature of the present illness. How does your patient present? Does the patient appear uncomfortable, frightened, or deathly ill? You need to assess the patient's level of consciousness (LOC), in part to determine whether the patient can provide you with reliable information to act on. This initial evaluation of his or her LOC will also establish baselines to refer to later as the call progresses and the patient's condition changes.

You move further into the information-gathering process as you perform your primary assessment, focusing on the identification of any serious threats to your patient's life that you need to immediately address. You continue on as you perform an appropriate physical examination, ie, the secondary assessment.

After you identify the patient's chief complaint, you need to obtain a pertinent medical history, including any medications the patient is taking: prescription, over-the-counter, illicit, or possibly herbal.

One of the most important observations you need to judge is your patient's affect, ie, the emotional state reflected in physical behavior **Figure 5**. The affect might not tally with what the patient tells you. For example, you may treat a patient who presents with manic behavior that can be associated with amphetamine abuse, yet the patient denies any drug use. You might even see drug paraphernalia. You must assess the accuracy of the information you are receiving if it does not match what you are seeing and hearing.

Last, you need to obtain the patient's vital signs by using your primary diagnostic tools: the glucometer, pulse oximeter, capnometer, cardiac monitor, blood pressure cuff, and stethoscope.

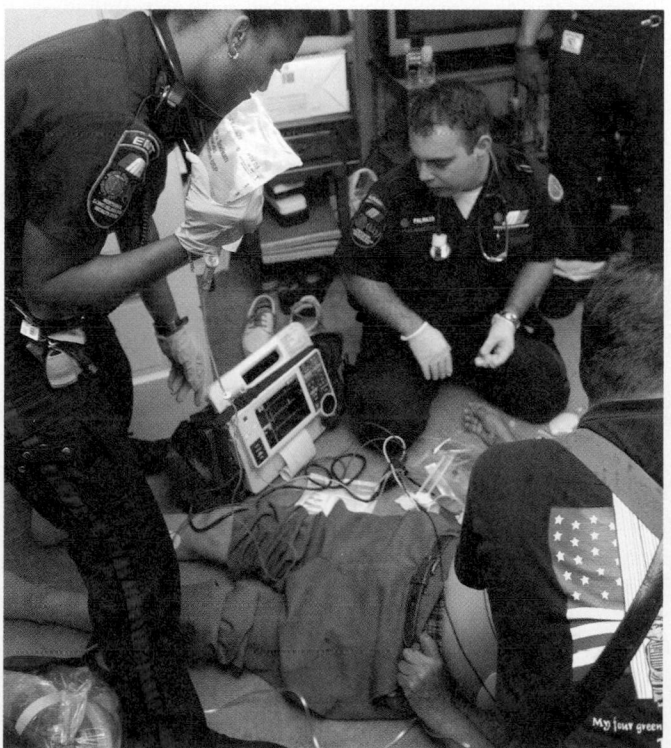

Figure 5 Take in clues not only from your patient's status, but also from his or her surroundings. Assess the entire environment to make sure that you fully understand its impact on your patient's condition.

Data Interpretation

During the second stage of the critical thinking process, you must evaluate all the information you have gathered, which is called <u>data interpretation</u>. You will need a solid background in anatomy and physiology and pathophysiology to understand how the body works and how it responds when problems arise. Another key element is your base of experience. If you have come to the paramedic program with significant experience as an EMT, you will have an excellent platform to build on. However, even without that background, applying yourself in your studies will help you to meet the challenges of working in EMS.

How you think and form conclusions is affected not only by the attitudes of your patients but also by your attitude as a provider. This means, for example, you should never consider a call a waste of your time or talent. Furthermore, unprofessional comments such as, "I can't believe you called us for THIS!" show a lack of compassion and interest in providing quality patient care. Having a negative attitude about any patient or patient care situation will almost guarantee that the care you provide will be suboptimal. To maintain the standards of care set by your profession, you must provide the best care you can for every patient you encounter.

Application of Principle

The third stage of the critical thinking process comes when your initial field impression becomes your working diagnosis. The key word here is "working." Think of it as being "tentative." It is what you believe to be the problem and the focus of your treatment.

From this point on, your treatment plan is driven by the patient care protocols, or standing orders, in the system where you work. Protocols represent the standard of care and describe the treatments and interventions you are expected to provide. In addition, the protocols further define what you as a paramedic *can do* without contacting medical control, as well as what therapies or interventions you *cannot do* without obtaining orders from medical control.

Reflection in Action

You are now actively treating your patient while monitoring the effects of your interventions. Think of *reflection in action* as simply *thinking while doing*.

If your patient is having difficulty breathing, for example, you would apply a nonrebreathing mask with oxygen flowing at 15 L/min. After a few minutes you should ask the patient, "Is it getting any easier for you to breathe?" It is important to periodically check your interventions to see whether they are making the patient feel better. If you ask your patient how your treatment is working, you will also be reassuring your patient that you are

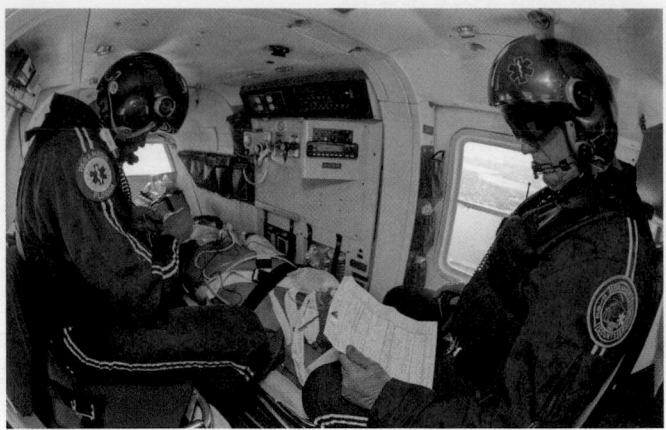

Figure 6 A patient's condition can change rapidly—especially when critically ill or injured. Continually monitor any changes to a patient's condition.

severe. This is key information, because you know that the pain associated with a heart attack is not relieved by simply sitting still and not moving. You now *revise your impression* and focus your assessment on the possibility of a musculoskeletal injury, and your treatment plan and interventions change accordingly.

Instead of giving the patient aspirin, nitroglycerin, and high-flow oxygen to improve delivery of oxygen to a potentially infarcting heart, you now provide nitrous oxide, fentanyl, or morphine sulfate for pain relief for an isolated musculoskeletal injury.

One of the key elements of this stage of the critical thinking process is to avoid *tunnel vision*; you need to keep your mind open to all the possible causes of your patient's current condition. Keep in mind that your patient might be having a heart attack that presents in a way that differs from the typical signs and symptoms, so reassess constantly.

concerned and on top of the situation **Figure 6**. Reassessment is an important and ongoing part of your patient care.

In another scenario, a 58-year-old man has experienced chest pain while moving rocks to landscape his yard. Although he has no history of cardiac disease, he is in the right age group for you to suspect a heart problem. When you ask him if he can pinpoint where the pain seems to be, he points to a spot on his chest directly over his heart. His heart could still be the problem, so you continue with the same care plan.

Then you ask if anything makes the pain better or worse and the patient explains that if he holds his left arm still, the pain goes away. However, with arm movement the pain is

Words of Wisdom

To provide optimal patient care, paramedics need to avoid tunnel vision, or narrow-mindedness, when it comes to determining the cause of a patient's condition. Do not focus only on your initial impression. As you gather information, modify your treatment plan according to the patient's needs.

■ Reflection on Action

The last stage in the critical thinking process occurs after the call is over and is commonly associated with run review or run critiques. This is the time when you look back at the call and reflect on how you gathered and processed information and

YOU *are the Medic* | PART 3

The patient is in visible pain and you ask her to describe it. She states that the pain is "really bad" in her left shoulder. The staff member tells you that she has tried calling the parents twice but has not reached them yet. She says she will continue to try. You decide to call medical control regarding pain medication. You give the physician a report, including her size and weight (5′ tall, 100 lb), and he advises you to administer 2 mg of morphine followed by another dose of 2 mg 10 minutes later. You start an IV line and administer 2 mg of morphine.

Recording Time: 5 Minutes	
Respirations	26 breaths/min
Pulse	110 beats/min
Skin	Warm and dry
Blood pressure	110/80 mm Hg before morphine Two minutes after morphine administration: 100/50 mm Hg
Oxygen saturation (Spo$_2$)	100%
Pupils	PEARRL

5. What is your working diagnosis?

6. What effects can be expected from the administration of morphine?

reached the decisions that you did. One of the most difficult aspects of this stage is learning to accept that something went wrong or that better treatment choices could have been made. It is important to establish an attitude that there is always room for personal and professional improvement. A review of the run is an excellent opportunity to evaluate what might have gone wrong and to improve your skills as a paramedic.

You will periodically encounter patients with atypical presentations, meaning that some patients just do not follow the classic textbook signs and symptoms. For example, you may see a patient with a neck fracture who has no pain. Even though pain is the single best predictor of a possible spine injury, it is not an absolute predictor. To make an accurate diagnosis, you must also use all that you have learned about communication with patients—your patient might come from a culture that minimizes the presence of pain.

Reflection gives you the chance to continuously improve your thinking and decision making, and, in turn, your patient care as you become more experienced. Always having an attitude that is open to learning makes every run you go on, every class you take, and every run review you attend another opportunity to improve your skills **Figure 7**. Growth will not happen if you cannot admit mistakes or if you are unwilling to continue to learn. The successful completion of the paramedic class is only the starting point in your career as an ALS provider. To provide the best possible care requires that you make a commitment to a *lifetime of learning*. The most important trait for a successful lifetime career in EMS is a true desire to continuously improve as a paramedic.

In review, the fundamental elements that contribute to the critical thinking and clinical decision-making process are listed below. As you look over each item on the following list, ask yourself, *"Do I have this quality already, or do I need to develop it?"*

- Adequate fund of knowledge in anatomy and pathophysiology
- Ability to gather and organize data and form concepts
- Ability to focus on specific and multiple elements of data
- Ability to identify and deal with **medical ambiguity**—the uncertainty regarding the specific cause of the patient's condition; few calls follow the scripts in your protocols to the letter.

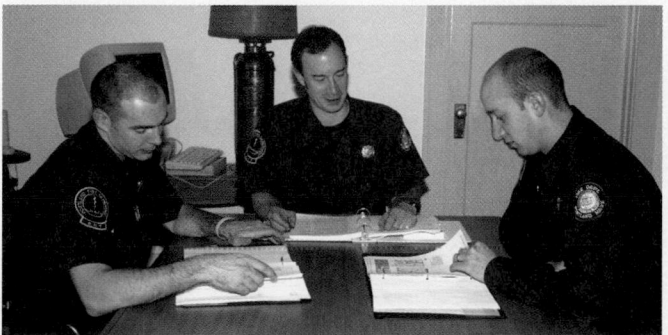

Figure 7 A formal review, or audit, of your performance can seem intimidating. However, it is also an opportunity for you to gain important feedback and improve as a paramedic.

- Skill in differentiating between relevant and irrelevant data
- Capability to analyze and compare similar situations
- Capability to analyze and compare contrary situations
- Ability to articulate your reasoning and construct arguments

From Theory to Practical Application

A number of unique factors come into play with every call. Consider the following scenario:

You are dispatched to a "car off the road" involving a single car with four passengers that has spun off into a ditch at an estimated speed of 35 miles per hour. Think about how each of the following variables might change how you respond to and manage the call.

- The passengers were not wearing seat belts.
- The car was traveling at 65 miles per hour.
- The vehicle flipped over and is on its roof.
- It is 20°F outside and the crash was not discovered for at least an hour.

As you can see from the list, changes in variables create many possible new outcomes for patients, and therefore your ability to manage the call and patient care properly also becomes more challenging.

Even if only a few of the calls you respond to on a day-to-day basis represent life-threatening emergencies, it is important that you handle every call in the same professional manner and provide the best care possible.

Words of Wisdom

Never be fooled by patients who initially appear uninjured or healthy. Never hesitate to take a thorough history and perform a complete physical examination.

Remember that you have to learn to cope with your own reactions, such as the impact of the "fight-or-flight" response, when you are confronted with extreme cases. This response can impair your critical thinking skills and diminish your concentration and assessment abilities. One way to counter these negative effects is to improve your mental conditioning and your skill performance. Practice your skills until you can do them instinctively and can perform them on command in the skills lab setting. Once you reach that level of skill performance, you can quickly draw on them in a real-life setting, allowing you to better focus on patient assessment or other decision-making areas.

Facilitate better thinking under pressure by memorizing the following mental checklist for all calls:

1. Take a moment to *scan the situation*.
2. Take another moment to *stop and think*.

3. *Move forward and make decisions and act* on behalf of your patient.
4. *Stay calm*, and maintain clear, concise *mental control*.
5. Regularly and continually *reevaluate your patient*.

■ Taking It to the Streets

When you are out on a call, critical thinking can be summed up with the *Six Rs*.

■ 1. Read the Scene

An emergency scene is filled with information readily available to you. Equally important to consider is that this information is *only* available at the scene and becomes unavailable the moment you initiate transport to the hospital. Some of the primary elements involved in reading the scene are evaluating the overall safety of the situation, the environmental conditions, the immediate surroundings, access and egress issues, and finally, in the case of trauma, evaluating the mechanism of injury **Figure 8**. In particular, when you are looking at the mechanism of injury, take time to evaluate all aspects of the incident. For example, with a car crash, look at the length of the skid marks or note whether there are none, what the vehicle struck, how much intrusion there is into the passenger compartment, and whether seat belts were worn and the headrest is properly positioned. In another example, involving a patient who fell, you would look for the height of the fall, how the patient landed, and what the patient landed on.

Other issues to consider when you interpret the scene include assessing the environment. Was it hot, cold, or wet?

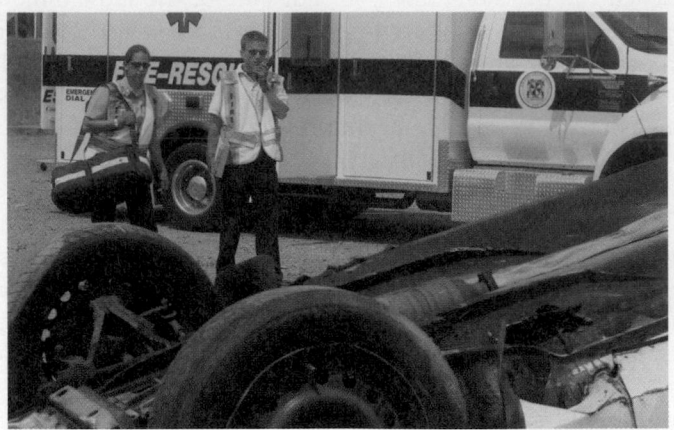

Figure 8 Although you need to focus on treating patients as soon as possible, always take a moment to register important information about the scene. What has happened that will help you remain safe and provide quality patient care?

Also, are there eyewitnesses or friends or family to provide additional information?

■ 2. Read the Patient

One of the greatest skills you can develop is learning to read a patient quickly. As you approach the patient, does the patient see you and track you with his or her eyes? Offer the patient your hand to shake, introduce yourself, and ask why 9-1-1 was called. If the patient takes your hand and answers you appropriately, you have just determined that the patient has a Glasgow

YOU *are the Medic* | PART 4 |

On reassessment, the patient feels less pain and rates it as 5 on a scale of 1 to 10. You proceed to immobilize the arm. While you are moving the patient onto a stretcher the patient's aunt arrives on the scene. You give the aunt a complete report and tell her you will be transporting her niece to the local hospital for treatment. You advise the aunt that you are administering a second dose of morphine. The aunt tells you "No!" and says you should not have given pain medication to her niece.

Recording Time: 10 Minutes	
Respirations	18 breaths/min
Pulse	70 beats/min
Skin	Warm and dry
Blood pressure	100/60 mm Hg
Oxygen saturation (Spo$_2$)	100%
Pupils	Equal
ECG	Sinus without ectopy

7. How should you respond to the aunt's statement that pain medication should not have been administered?

8. Did you have the right to give the patient pain medication without a parent present?

Coma Scale score of 15 (spontaneous eye opening, follows commands, appropriate verbal response). Other components of effectively reading a patient include the following:

- **Observe the patient.** What is the patient's LOC and level of comfort or discomfort? Skin color? Position? Work of breathing? Any obvious deformity or asymmetry?
- **Talk to the patient.** Determine the chief complaint. Is this a new problem or the worsening of a preexisting condition? Obtain the medical history and the history of the present problem.
- **Touch the patient.** Assess the skin temperature and moisture level. Assess the pulse rate, regularity, and strength.
- **Auscultate lung sounds.** Confirm the adequacy or inadequacy of breathing and assess the patency of the airway.
- **Identify life threats.** Correct any life threats relative to airway, breathing, and circulation in the order you find them.
- **Obtain complete and accurate vital signs** Figure 9 . For every patient, even for routine BLS transfer patients, you must obtain a baseline set of vital signs. For patients with serious problems, two sets of vital signs provide comparative data. With critical patients, three or more sets of vital signs allow you to assess trends and to reassess whether the patient's condition is stabilizing, improving, or getting worse. If your patient's condition is deteriorating, multiple sets of vital signs will track the progression.

3. React

Your first priority in patient care is to treat any life threats. Next, consider possible causes of your patient's symptoms and either rule certain conditions in or out as you gather more information and develop a working diagnosis.

If at the end of your assessment you have not been able to develop a working diagnosis, provide care based on the presenting signs and symptoms. If your patient is having difficulty breathing, administer high-flow oxygen and place

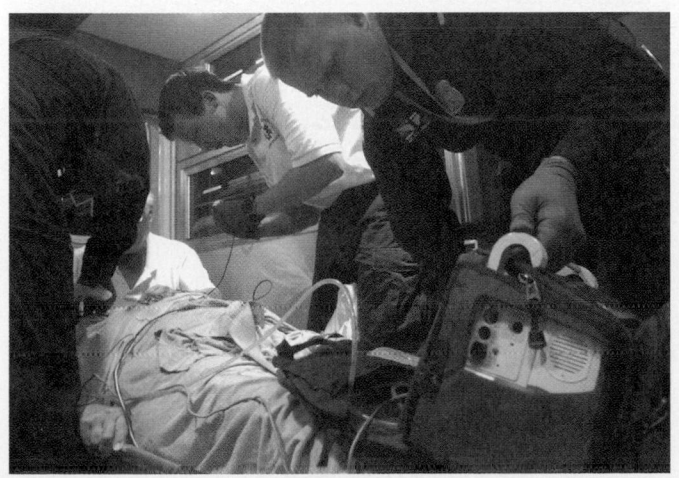

Figure 9 The more accurate your patient information, the more reliable your diagnosis. Take the time to obtain a set of baseline vital signs for every patient.

the patient in a position of comfort. For signs and symptoms of shock, keep the patient warm, administer high-flow oxygen, and establish one or two large-bore IV lines en route while you continue to try to search for the cause of the condition. You will often care for patients whose conditions cannot be diagnosed until they reach the hospital.

4. Reevaluate

As patient care is continuing, make certain that you follow up on any interventions. See whether the splint you applied has eased the pain in your patient's injured leg. If you are treating frequent premature ventricular contractions (PVCs) and salvos with an anti-dysrhythmic medication, check the monitor to see if the PVCs have resolved. On challenging calls it is easy to get into "treatment mode" and just focus on *doing things* and forgetting to follow up on whether what you are doing is actually improving the patient's condition.

As you reassess your patient, take the time to add any information you may have gathered from the secondary assessment to the primary assessment. For example, you find that your patient has no breath sounds in the upper right lobes secondary to a fractured rib that caused a small pneumothorax. By itself, the small pneumothorax is not an immediate life threat to a relatively healthy person. The patient, however, also has bilateral fractured femurs, significant blood loss, and a minor head injury. Under those circumstances, a small pneumothorax may complicate matters far more than if it were a single, isolated condition. When you care for patients, especially trauma patients with multiple injuries, it is up to you to assess their cumulative impact as you develop your treatment plan to make sure nothing is overlooked that can be addressed in the field.

5. Revise the Plan

As you continue to care for your patient, you may get indications that what you once thought was a head injury is a problem secondary to glue sniffing—two very different causes. The thinking paramedic, no matter how sure he or she is of the working diagnosis, always keeps part of the thought process open to other possibilities. As the call unfolds and other information becomes available, you should always be prepared to change your treatment direction as necessary. By remaining mentally "light on your feet," you position yourself to be receptive to changing presentations or circumstances, which, in turn, helps you avoid tunnel vision.

■ 6. Review Your Performance

Again, once a call is over, you as a provider have the opportunity to look back and reexamine your work **Figure 10**. Whether this review is in the formal setting of a continuous quality improvement (CQI) meeting or just back at the station reviewing the call with your partner, taking the time to critically look at your work allows for real growth opportunities. This is particularly true when you have made a mistake. Whereas success is satisfying and certainly feels good, there is little growth opportunity to be achieved. However, when you make a mistake, take the time to analyze the call so that you can avoid repeating your behavior and making the same mistake. Mistakes will only change if you want to find out what they were and why they recurred. Excellence in prehospital care is the gradual result of you as a provider constantly striving to improve your practice, which requires that you *always* have an attitude that is open to learning.

Being a thinking paramedic will only happen if you choose to work on your critical thinking skills day by day, call by call, throughout your career. If you continue to improve the way you think and make decisions, your patient care will improve as well. Your reward will be excellence in your practice—the ultimate job satisfaction.

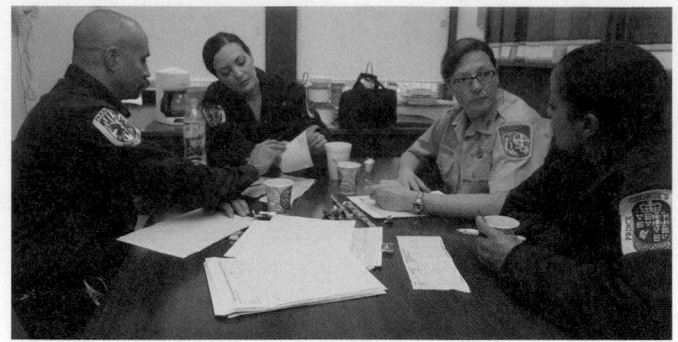

Figure 10 You can learn something new with every call you run. One of the best ways to review your performance–and to continually learn and improve–is to talk it over with peers.

YOU are the Medic   SUMMARY

1. What is your concept formation of the call based on the information you have been provided?

Concept formation takes into consideration everything that you see, hear, and feel. The call was for a child who injured her shoulder during cheerleading practice. On scene, you are told by a staff member that the patient fell 8' onto a spring floor with her arms outstretched. You realize that you will be caring for a pediatric patient with injuries that may be severe.

2. What is included in your primary assessment of this patient?

You need to immediately rule out any injury to the patient's cervical spine, back, or head. Assess the patient's vital signs, including her level of consciousness and the ABCs. Monitor the patient's respiratory status and place the patient on oxygen if there are any signs of difficulty breathing. Also, ask the patient whether pain medication would be helpful to her prior to immobilizing her arm in a sling. Remember that parental consent must be obtained, if possible, before providing emergency treatment to a minor.

3. Have you gathered enough data to turn your field impression into patient care?

You have enough information to make a working treatment plan. The patient has sustained an isolated trauma to her arm. Critical actions that must be completed are immobilization of the arm, making the patient comfortable, and transporting the patient to a hospital for further treatment.

4. Should you administer pain medication?

You are ethically responsible for making your patient as comfortable as possible. Recent studies have shown, however, that prehospital providers are less likely to give pain medication

to pediatric patients than to adults. Pediatric patients may be administered medication to help relieve pain. If a parent or guardian is not available, emergency treatment to sustain life may be undertaken without consent under the doctrine of implied consent. Emergency treatment to relieve pain may frequently be provided also in the absence of available parental consent, but this is more variable from jurisdiction to jurisdiction. When in doubt, obtain online guidance from medical control. Know your state laws and local protocols concerning the treatment of minors.

5. What is your working diagnosis?

You have ruled out multisystem trauma and determined that the patient has an isolated extremity trauma. There is no medical condition associated with the emergency, and the patient denies having any significant medical history or medication allergies. Your treatment includes immobilization of the injury and providing the patient comfort care while en route to the hospital.

6. What effects can be expected from the administration of morphine?

Morphine is a common narcotic analgesic that is carried by many EMS agencies. The effect of morphine is different for each patient. Although pain medication may not eliminate the patient's pain, it will reduce the level of pain. Some benefits to giving pain medication are a more relaxed patient, which will result in positive changes in vital signs and a decreased level of anxiety. Some patients may be allergic to pain medications; any allergies should be established prior to medication administration. Pain medications sometimes cause adverse effects, such as nausea and/or vomiting. Those effects should be anticipated and can be treated with an antiemetic medication such as ondansetron.

YOU *are the Medic* | **SUMMARY,** *continued*

7. How should you respond to the aunt's statement that pain medication should not have been administered?

Minors present special issues for the paramedic. Usually a parent is the legal decision maker for a child; a relative is not a legal decision maker unless there is documentation signed by the mother or father stating otherwise. Recognizing that the relative may have a valid concern, explain that your treatment was authorized by a physician and is standard care. Advise the aunt to contact the patient's parents to discuss her concerns.

8. Did you have the right to give the patient pain medication without a parent present?

Under certain circumstances you do have the right to treat a minor without a parent present. In this situation, you have been given the authority by medical control to treat the patient. Often, obtaining consent to treat a child may be difficult. At times, a parent or guardian of a child may not want you to treat the child for a variety of reasons. In such cases, you must respect the parent's (or guardian's) wishes and discuss the medical consequences of that decision with him or her. However, you may not withhold care from the patient when the person requesting this is not the parent or guardian. Remember that as a patient advocate, you need to be aware of the problems associated with obtaining permission and be prepared to discuss the need for care.

EMS Patient Care Report (PCR)

Date: 04-24-11	**Incident No.:** 110435	**Nature of Call:** Child injured		**Location:** Cheers Cheerleading gym	
Dispatched: 1102	**En Route:** 1103	**At Scene:** 1105	**Transport:** 1130	**At Hospital:** 1145	**In Service:** 1200

Patient Information

Age: 12 **Sex:** F **Weight (in kg [lb]):** 45 kg (100 lb)	**Allergies:** None **Medications:** None **Past Medical History:** None **Chief Complaint:** Upper arm pain

Vital Signs

Time: 1110	**BP:** 110/80; two min after morphine admin, 100/50	**Pulse:** 110	**Respirations:** 26	**Spo$_2$:** 100%
Time: 1115	**BP:** 100/60	**Pulse:** 70	**Respirations:** 18	**Spo$_2$:** 100%
Time:	**BP:**	**Pulse:**	**Respirations:**	**Spo$_2$:**

EMS Treatment
(circle all that apply)

Oxygen @ _____ L/min via (circle one): NC NRM Bag-mask device	**Assisted Ventilation**	**Airway Adjunct**	**CPR**
Defibrillation	**Bleeding Control**	**Bandaging**	~~**Splinting**~~	**Other**

Narrative

Arrived on scene to find 12-year-old girl in care of coaching staff. Staff states pt was on top of a pyramid performing a cheerleading maneuver and was not caught upon dismount. Pt states she fell about 8' onto her left arm and right arm, with most of the force absorbed by the left arm. The floor at gym was on springs and was able to absorb most of the energy of the fall. Pt states she has "really bad" pain in her left upper arm. Pt denies any head, neck, or back pain. Pt denies any other injury, problem, or pain other than in her left arm. Assessment of the pt's arm reveals extreme pain with arm movement. Pt agreed to receive medication treatment for pain. Medical control at Memorial Hospital authorized 2 mg of morphine initially and another 2 mg after 10 minutes if pain is still severe. Hospital staff will be awaiting our arrival. IV line established in right AC vein with 20-gauge needle, saline well attached, and saline drip started at KVO rate. 2 mg of morphine administered at 1115 followed by 10-mL flush. Minutes later the pt stated the pain level changed from 9 to 5, and pt's arm was immobilized with a sling. Pt moved to ambulance and reassessed; vital signs taken and noted above. Pt stated pain level was still at 5 after 10 minutes. Pt was given second dose of 2 mg of morphine. Pt's aunt met us prior to leaving for hospital and expressed displeasure with EMS giving her niece morphine. EMS reassured aunt that pt treatment was authorized by medical control physician and stated that pt was feeling much better and in less pain. Pt transported without further incident. Vital signs monitored and pt's pain decreased from 5 to 4. Pt released to nurse in ED room 4 with report. IV patent and less than 200-mL infused. RN witnessed waste of 6 mg of morphine. Waste form attached to PCR. **End of report**

Prep Kit

- The first cornerstone of your practice as a paramedic is having the ability to *gather*, *evaluate*, and *synthesize* information.

- Once you have gathered information, assess and evaluate its validity and the impact it may have on the patient care plan you are developing.

- Once you have evaluated the information you obtained from the scene, the patient, or any bystanders and determined what information is valid, then you need to process—or *synthesize*—that information.

- The second cornerstone of your practice is the *development and implementation of a patient care plan*.

- Your care plan is almost always defined by the patient care protocols or standing orders in the EMS system where you work.

- The third cornerstone is *judgment and making independent decisions*.

- The fourth and final cornerstone of your practice is your ability to *think and work under pressure*.

- The first stage of the thought process in prehospital care is gathering information—things you see, hear, smell, or feel or obtain with your diagnostics. This is *concept formation*.

- The second stage of the critical thinking process is *data interpretation*—evaluating the information you have gathered.

- The last stage in the critical thinking process occurs after the call is over and is commonly associated with run review or run critiques. Look back at the total call and reflect on how you processed all the information you gathered and reached the decisions that you did.

- The *Six Rs* can be used to summarize what must be done on a call:
  - Read the scene
  - Read the patient
  - React
  - Reevaluate
  - Revise the plan
  - Review your performance

- Excellence in prehospital care results from a constant effort to improve your practice, which requires that you *always* have an attitude that is open to learning.

Vital Vocabulary

__concept formation__ Pattern of understanding based on initially obtained information.

__cookbook medicine__ Blindly following a protocol or algorithm without thinking about what you are doing and whether or not it is working.

__data interpretation__ The process of reaching conclusions based on comparing the patient's presentation with information from your training, education, and past experiences.

__medical ambiguity__ Vague or unclear aspects of medicine.

Assessment
in Action

You are dispatched to a domestic dispute between brothers. The police are on the scene and state there were two patients involved in a street brawl. You arrive on the scene and find a 16-year-old boy with a swollen, bruised eye with a laceration (bleeding is controlled) and a 7-year-old boy with a bruise to his right arm. The mother is on the scene.

1. Which of the following elements is not involved in reading the scene?
   A. Evaluating the scene safety
   B. Evaluating environmental conditions
   C. Evaluating the location of the ambulance
   D. Evaluating access and egress issues

2. After reading the scene, the next step in the *Six Rs* of critical thinking is:
   A. relieving the patient of worry.
   B. readying the ambulance for transport.
   C. requesting ALS.
   D. reading the patient.

3. The third step of critical thinking, called *React*, involves which of the following as your first priority in patient care?
   A. Correct life threats.
   B. Consider the worst-case scenario.
   C. Complete a head-to-toe assessment.
   D. Establish command.

4. The patients are both alert and have calmed down. Initially you and your partner apply ice packs to each patient while you continue your assessments and begin treatment, including splinting the injured arm and providing pressure to maintain bleeding control for the laceration. You each inquire as to how your patient is feeling. Which step is this in the *Six Rs*?
   A. Request
   B. Reevaluate
   C. React
   D. Review

5. You and your partner decide that both patients should be transported to the hospital for evaluation. With the process of concept formation, including the primary assessment of each patient, you determine that the 7-year-old requires a radiograph to ascertain if there is a broken bone, and the 16-year-old needs stitches for the laceration. Evaluating all the information you have gathered is called:
   A. data interpretation.
   B. working diagnosis.
   C. reflection in action.
   D. read the scene.

6. A few days after the call, you receive a message from your QI supervisor saying that your documentation and care were exceptional. This feedback helps you:
   A. realize you are an exceptional provider.
   B. review your performance.
   C. understand that you cannot make mistakes.
   D. revise your patient care plan for future runs.

7. If you arrived on the scene and found the fight still occurring and no police presence, using your best judgment and independent decision making, what would you do?
   A. Stop your vehicle and remain inside.
   B. Get out of your vehicle and stop the fight.
   C. Stop your vehicle and yell for them to stop.
   D. Leave the scene until police arrive and secure it.

Additional Questions

8. You are in your station doing chores and a 16-year-old walks in complaining of chest pain. How do you treat the patient?

Airway Management

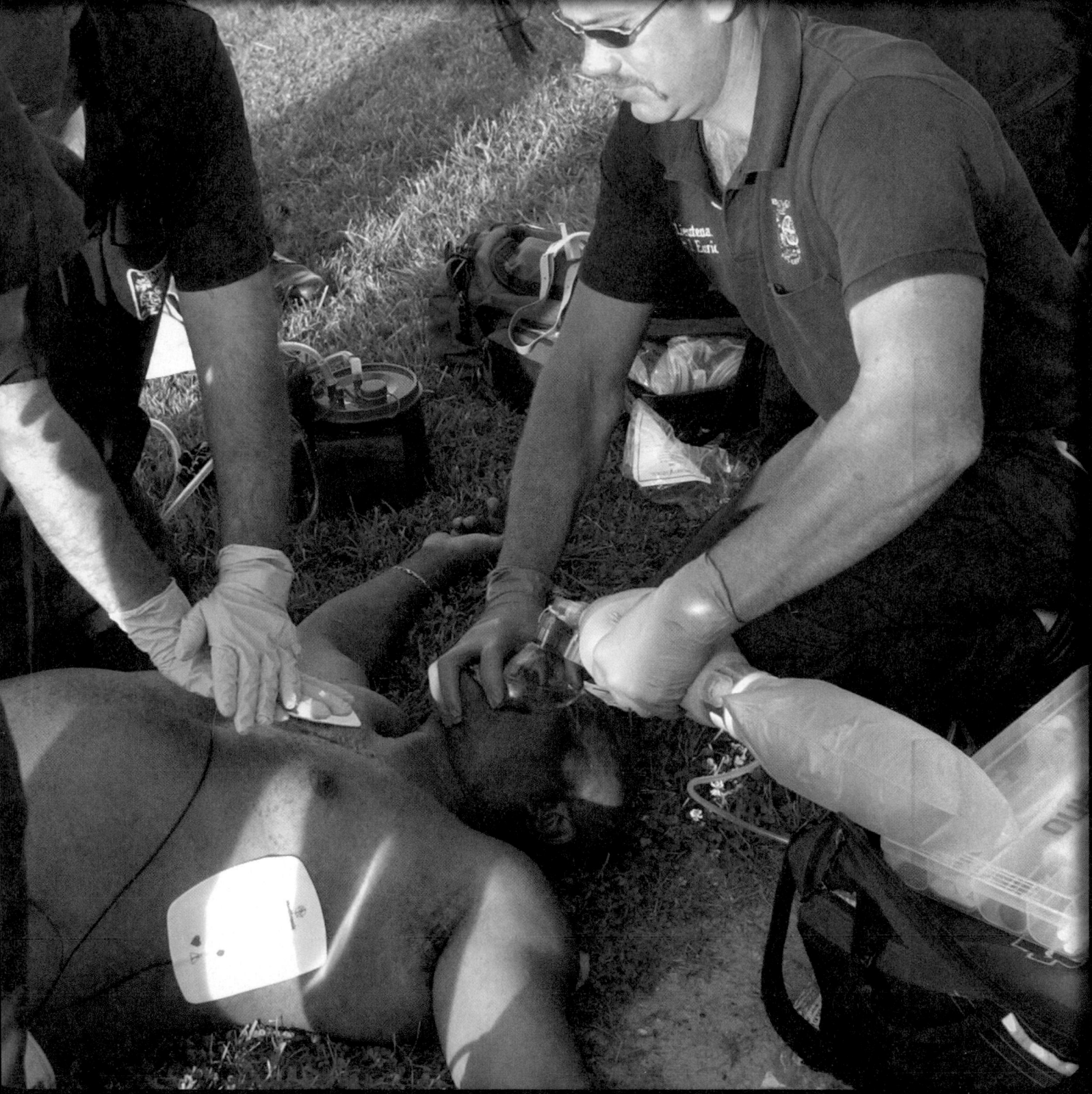

15 Airway Management and Ventilation

Airway Management and Ventilation

National EMS Education Standard Competencies

Airway Management, Respiration, and Artificial Ventilation

Integrates complex knowledge of anatomy, physiology, and pathophysiology into the assessment to develop and implement a treatment plan with the goal of ensuring a patent airway, adequate mechanical ventilation, and respiration for patients of all ages.

Airway Management

- Airway anatomy (pp 712-717)
- Airway assessment (pp 728-732)
- Techniques of ensuring a patent airway (pp 736-737)

Respiration

- Anatomy of the respiratory system (pp 712-717)
- Physiology and pathophysiology of respiration (pp 717-728)
  - Pulmonary ventilation (p 717)
  - Oxygenation (pp 722-723)
  - Respiration (p 723)
    - External (p 723)
    - Internal (p 724)
    - Cellular (p 724)
- Assessment and management of adequate and inadequate respiration (pp 725-732)
- Supplemental oxygen therapy (pp 750-756)

Artificial Ventilation

Assessment and management of adequate and inadequate ventilation

- Artificial ventilation (pp 758-761)
- Minute ventilation (pp 720, 726)
- Alveolar ventilation (p 720)
- Effect of artificial ventilation on cardiac output (p 728)

Knowledge Objectives

1. Describe the major structures of the respiratory system, including the upper and lower airway. (pp 712-717)
2. Discuss the physiology of breathing, including ventilation, oxygenation, and respiration. (p 717)
3. Discuss important concepts related to ventilation, including partial pressure, volumes, and neural and chemical control of ventilation. (pp 717-725)
4. Explain positive-pressure ventilation versus negative-pressure ventilation. (pp 756-757)
5. Discuss respiratory drive versus hypoxic drive. (pp 721-722)

6. Describe factors related to pathophysiology of respiration, including ventilation/perfusion ratio mismatch, hypoventilation, hyperventilation, and circulatory compromise. (pp 726-727)
7. Discuss acid/base imbalance, specifically respiratory acidosis and respiratory alkalosis. (p 728)
8. List the signs of adequate breathing. (p 729)
9. List the signs of inadequate breathing. (pp 729-730)
10. List abnormal breathing patterns to recognize when assessing a patient's breathing. (p 731)
11. Discuss how to assess a patient's breath sounds. (pp 730-732)
12. List methods for end-tidal carbon dioxide assessment, and discuss its importance. (pp 735-736)
13. Describe the assessment and care of a patient with apnea. (pp 758-761)
14. Understand how to assess for adequate and inadequate respiration, including the use of pulse oximetry. (pp 729-730, 733-734)
15. Understand how to assess for a patent airway. (pp 728-732)
16. Describe how to perform the head tilt-chin lift maneuver. (p 738)
17. Describe how to perform the jaw-thrust maneuver. (p 738)
18. Describe how to perform the tongue-jaw lift. (p 738)
19. Understand the importance and techniques of suctioning. (pp 739-742)
20. Explain how to measure and insert an oropharyngeal (oral) airway. (p 744)
21. Describe how to measure and insert a nasopharyngeal (nasal) airway. (p 746)
22. Explain the use of the recovery position to maintain a clear airway. (p 737)
23. Describe the importance of giving supplemental oxygen to patients who are hypoxic. (p 750)
24. Understand the basics of how oxygen is stored and the various hazards associated with its use. (pp 750-752)
25. Describe the use of a nonrebreathing mask, and state the oxygen flow requirements for its use. (p 754)
26. Understand the indications for using a nasal cannula rather than a nonrebreathing face mask. (pp 754-755)
27. Describe the indications for use of a humidifier during supplemental oxygen therapy. (pp 754, 756)
28. Explain the steps to take to perform mouth-to-mouth, mouth-to-nose, and mouth-to-mask ventilation. (p 758)
29. Describe the use of a one-, two-, or three-person bag-mask device and a manually triggered ventilation (MTV) device. (pp 758-762)
30. Discuss automatic transport ventilators and how to use them. (p 762)
31. Describe the signs associated with adequate and inadequate artificial ventilation. (p 761)
32. Describe the indications, contraindications, and complications of use of continuous positive airway pressure (CPAP). (pp 763-764)
33. Explain considerations surrounding gastric distention and how to perform nasogastric and orogastric decompression. (pp 765-766)
34. Discuss airway management considerations for patients with a laryngectomy, tracheostomy, or stoma. (pp 769-772)

35. List the advanced airway devices and techniques available to the paramedic. (pp 774-775)

36. Discuss methods used to predict the difficult airway. (pp 775-776)

37. Describe the advantages, disadvantages, and equipment used when performing endotracheal intubation. (pp 776-780)

38. Explain how to determine correct endotracheal tube size. (pp 776-777)

39. List factors to consider when determining correct laryngoscope blade size. (pp 777-778)

40. Discuss the indications, contraindications, advantages, disadvantages, and complications of orotracheal intubation. (pp 778-786)

41. List the methods available for confirming correct endotracheal tube placement and the advantages and disadvantages of each method. (pp 784-785)

42. Describe how to secure an endotracheal tube. (p 786)

43. Discuss the indications, contraindications, advantages, disadvantages, and complications of nasotracheal intubation. (pp 786-790)

44. Discuss the indications, contraindications, advantages, disadvantages, and complications of digital intubation. (pp 790-794)

45. Discuss the indications, contraindications, advantages, disadvantages, and complications of transillumination intubation. (pp 794-798)

46. Discuss the indications, contraindications, advantages, disadvantages, and complications of retrograde intubation. (pp 798-802)

47. Explain what to do when intubation fails. (pp 802-803)

48. Explain how to perform tracheobronchial suctioning. (p 803)

49. Discuss considerations related to field extubation. (pp 803-804)

50. Discuss the indications, contraindications, advantages, disadvantages, and complications of endotracheal intubation in the pediatric patient. (pp 805-810)

51. Explain how to determine correct endotracheal tube size for a pediatric patient. (pp 805-806)

52. List factors to consider when determining correct laryngoscope blade size for a pediatric patient. (p 805)

53. List possible pharmacologic adjuncts to airway management and ventilation, including both sedatives and neuromuscular blocking agents used for emergency intubation. (pp 810-812)

54. Discuss the procedure for performing rapid-sequence intubation (RSI). (pp 812-813)

55. Discuss the esophageal tracheal Combitube (ETC), including how it works, its indications, contraindications, and complications, and the procedure for inserting it. (pp 814-815)

56. Discuss the laryngeal mask airway (LMA), including how it works, its indications, contraindications, and complications, and the procedure for inserting it. (pp 815, 817-819)

57. Discuss King LT airway devices, including how they work, their indications, contraindications, and complications, and the procedure for inserting them. (pp 818, 820-821)

58. Discuss the Cobra perilaryngeal airway (CobraPLA), including how it works, its indications, contraindications, and complications, and the procedure for inserting it. (pp 821-823)

59. Discuss the indications, contraindications, advantages, disadvantages, and complications of performing open cricothyrotomy. (pp 824-827)

60. Discuss the indications, contraindications, advantages, disadvantages, and complications of performing needle cricothyrotomy. (pp 828-831)

61. Understand the causes of foreign body airway obstruction. (pp 746-748)

62. Describe the management of mild and severe foreign body airway obstruction in an adult, a child, and an infant. (pp 749-750)

Skills Objectives

1. Demonstrate use of pulse oximetry. (pp 733-734)

2. Demonstrate how to position the unresponsive patient. (p 737)

3. Demonstrate the steps in performing the head tilt-chin lift maneuver. (p 738, Skill Drill 1)

4. Demonstrate the steps in performing the jaw-thrust maneuver. (p 738, Skill Drill 2)

5. Demonstrate the steps in performing the tongue-jaw lift maneuver. (p 738, Skill Drill 3)

6. Demonstrate how to place a patient in the recovery position. (p 737)

7. Demonstrate how to operate a suction unit. (pp 739-742)

8. Demonstrate how to suction a patient's airway. (pp 741-742, Skill Drill 4)

9. Demonstrate the insertion of an oral airway. (p 744, Skill Drill 5)

10. Demonstrate the insertion of an oral airway with a 90° rotation. (p 744, Skill Drill 6)

11. Demonstrate the insertion of a nasal airway. (p 746, Skill Drill 7)

12. Demonstrate how to use Magill forceps to remove an object that is in the airway. (p 750, Skill Drill 8)

13. Demonstrate how to place an oxygen cylinder into service. (pp 753-754, Skill Drill 9)

14. Demonstrate the use of a partial rebreathing mask in providing supplemental oxygen therapy to patients. (p 755)

15. Demonstrate the use of a Venturi mask in providing supplemental oxygen therapy to patients. (p 755)

16. Demonstrate the use of a humidifier in providing supplemental oxygen therapy to patients. (p 756)

17. Demonstrate how to assist a patient with ventilations using the bag-mask device for one and two rescuers. (pp 760-761)

18. Demonstrate mouth-to-mask ventilation. (p 758, Skill Drill 10)

19. Demonstrate the use of a manually triggered ventilation device to assist in delivering artificial ventilation to the patient. (pp 761-762)

20. Demonstrate the use of an automatic transport ventilator to assist in delivering artificial ventilation to the patient. (p 762)

21. Demonstrate the use of CPAP. (p 764, Skill Drill 11)

22. Demonstrate insertion of a nasogastric tube. (pp 766-768, Skill Drill 12)

23. Demonstrate insertion of an orogastric tube. (pp 768-769, Skill Drill 13)

24. Demonstrate how to suction a stoma. (p 770, Skill Drill 14)

25. Demonstrate mouth-to-stoma ventilation using a resuscitation mask. (p 770, Skill Drill 15)

26. Demonstrate bag-mask device-to-stoma ventilation. (p 770, Skill Drill 16)

27. Demonstrate how to replace a dislodged tracheostomy tube. (pp 771-772, Skill Drill 17)

28. Demonstrate how to secure an endotracheal tube. (p 786)

29. Demonstrate the entire procedure for orotracheal intubation using direct laryngoscopy. (p 786, Skill Drill 18)

30. Demonstrate how to perform blind nasotracheal intubation. (p 790, Skill Drill 19)

31. Demonstrate how to perform digital intubation. (p 794, Skill Drill 20)

32. Demonstrate how to perform transillumination intubation. (p 798, Skill Drill 21)

33. Demonstrate how to perform retrograde intubation. (pp 800-802, Skill Drill 22)

34. Discuss how to perform face-to-face intubation. (pp 801-802)

35. Demonstrate how to perform tracheobronchial suctioning. (p 803, Skill Drill 23)

36. Demonstrate how to perform endotracheal intubation in the pediatric patient. (p 807, Skill Drill 24)

37. Demonstrate how to perform rapid-sequence intubation (RSI). (pp 812-813)

38. Demonstrate insertion of the Combitube. (p 815, Skill Drill 25)

39. Demonstrate insertion of the laryngeal mask airway. (pp 818-819, Skill Drill 26)

40. Demonstrate insertion of the King LT airway. (p 821, Skill Drill 27)

41. Demonstrate insertion of the Cobra perilaryngeal airway. (pp 822-823, Skill Drill 28)

42. Demonstrate how to perform open cricothyrotomy. (pp 826-828, Skill Drill 29)

43. Demonstrate how to perform needle cricothyrotomy and translaryngeal catheter ventilation. (pp 830-831, Skill Drill 30)

Introduction

Establishing and maintaining a <u>patent</u> (open) airway and ensuring effective oxygenation and ventilation are vital aspects of effective patient care. Attempting to stabilize the condition of a patient whose airway is compromised is futile. The human body needs a constant supply of oxygen to carry out the physiologic processes necessary to sustain life; the airway is where it all begins. Few situations will cause such acute deterioration and death more rapidly than airway or ventilation compromise. To preserve life, the airway must remain patent at all times—regardless of the situation.

The function of the respiratory system is simple: It brings in oxygen and eliminates carbon dioxide (the primary waste product of oxygen metabolism). If this process is interrupted, vital organs of the body will not function properly. For example, the brain can survive for only 6 minutes or so without oxygen before permanent death of brain cells occurs.

Failure to manage the airway or inappropriate management of the airway is a major cause of preventable death in the prehospital setting. *The basic airway management techniques learned in initial EMT education are among the most crucial skills for a paramedic.* The failure to use basic airway techniques, improper performance of the techniques (such as improper bag-mask seal or improper airway positioning), a rush to use advanced interventions, and failure to reassess the patient's condition increase mortality and morbidity. Therefore, a large portion of this chapter is dedicated to reinforcement of basic airway management skills.

Paramedics must understand the importance of early detection of airway problems, rapid and effective intervention, and continual reassessment of a patient with airway or breathing compromise.

This chapter describes the airway in detail, beginning with a review of the anatomy and physiology of the respiratory system and the processes of ventilation, oxygenation, and respiration.

A "basic-to-advanced" approach—just as airway management should be performed in the field—is followed to emphasize the criticality of securing a patent airway and ensuring adequate ventilation, oxygenation, and respiration. The chapter then describes the various techniques in the order in which they should be performed: opening and maintaining a patent airway, recognizing and treating airway obstructions, assessing a patient's ventilation and oxygenation status, administering supplemental oxygen, and providing ventilatory assistance. Although a responsive patient may not need to have his or her airway manually opened by the paramedic and may need only supplemental oxygen, paramedics must remember the order in which steps should be performed, bypassing steps that do not apply to the particular situation. Finally, advanced techniques, including advanced airway devices and procedures, are then discussed in detail.

Anatomy of the Respiratory System

The respiratory system consists of all the structures in the body that make up the airway and help us breathe, or ventilate **Figure 1**. The airway is divided into the upper and lower airways. Structures that help us breathe include the diaphragm, the intercostal muscles, accessory muscles of breathing, and the nerves from the brain and spinal cord to those muscles. Ventilation is the movement of air into and out of the lungs. The diaphragm and intercostal muscles are responsible for the regular rise and fall of the chest that accompany normal breathing.

Anatomy of the Upper Airway

The <u>upper airway</u> consists of all anatomic airway structures above the level of the vocal cords—the nose, mouth, jaw, oral cavity, and pharynx (throat). The larynx is considered the point of division between the upper and lower airways. The major functions of the upper airway are to warm, filter, and humidify

YOU *are the Medic* PART 1

At 4:20 PM, your alert tones sound, "Medic 81, respond to 201 East Grayson Street for a 56-year-old man with breathing problems." You and your partner proceed to the scene with a response time of approximately 6 minutes. An engine company is dispatched to provide assistance.

1. What should you anticipate as being your first priority on making contact with this patient?

2. What is the difference between managing a patient's airway and ensuring adequate ventilation and oxygenation?

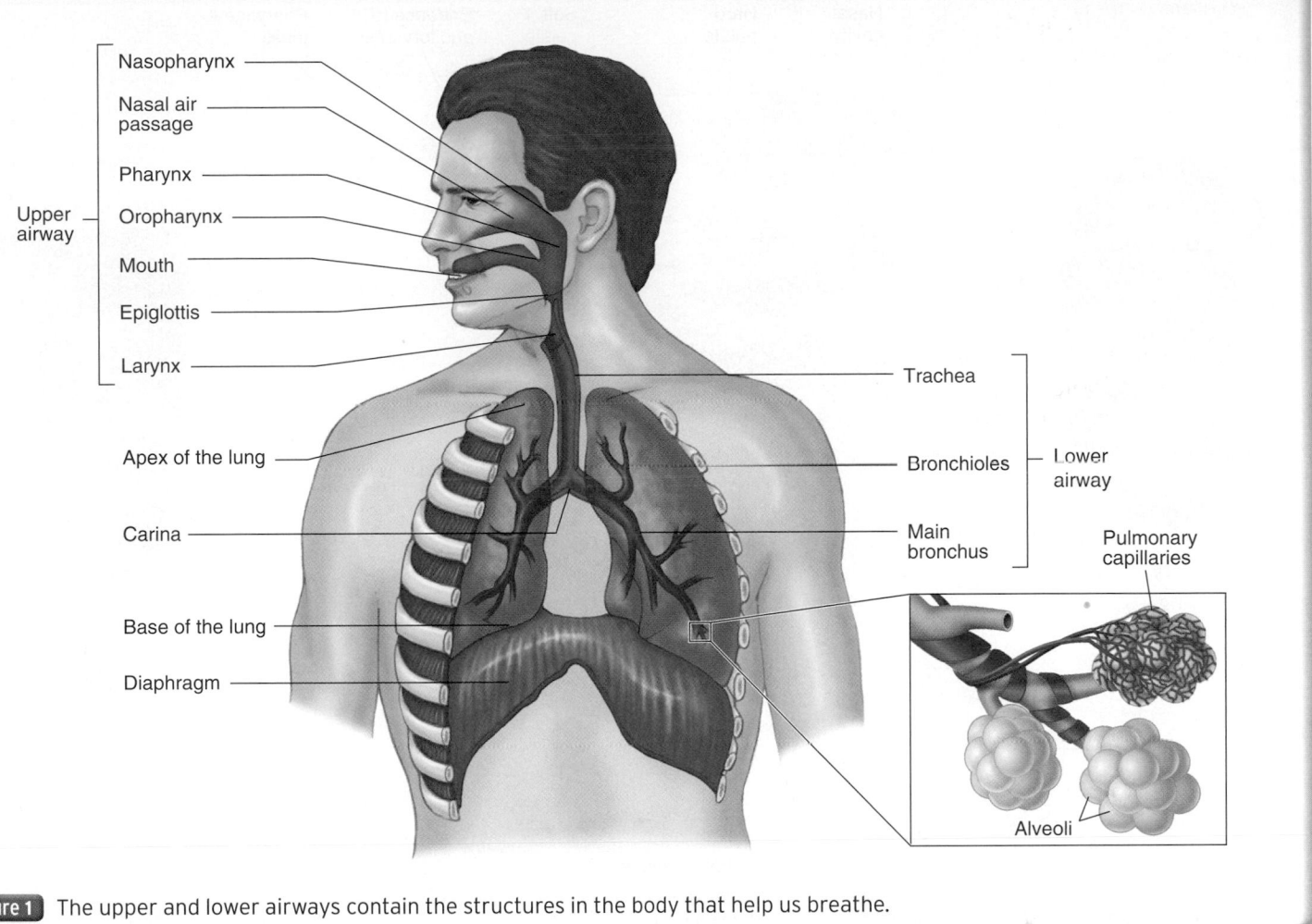

Upper airway
- Nasopharynx
- Nasal air passage
- Pharynx
- Oropharynx
- Mouth
- Epiglottis
- Larynx

Apex of the lung
Carina
Base of the lung
Diaphragm

Trachea
Bronchioles
Main bronchus

Lower airway

Pulmonary capillaries
Alveoli

Figure 1   The upper and lower airways contain the structures in the body that help us breathe.

air as it enters the body through the nose and mouth. Warming helps protect a person from hypothermia. Humidification is accomplished as the air picks up moisture from the soft tissues of the airway. The **pharynx** is a muscular tube that extends from the nose and mouth to the level of the esophagus and trachea. The pharynx is composed of the nasopharynx, oropharynx, and the laryngopharynx (also called the hypopharynx). The laryngopharynx is the lowest portion of the pharynx; it opens into the larynx anteriorly and the esophagus posteriorly **Figure 2A**.

Nasopharynx

On inhalation, air normally enters the body through the nose and passes into the **nasopharynx**, which is formed by the union of the facial bones.

The entire nasal cavity is lined with a ciliated mucous membrane that keeps contaminants such as dust and other small particles out of the respiratory tract. In illness, the body produces additional mucus to trap potentially infectious agents. This mucous membrane is extremely delicate and has a rich blood supply. Any trauma to the nasal passages, such as improper or overly aggressive placement of airway devices, may result in profuse bleeding from the posterior nasal cavity. Bleeding from this area cannot be controlled by direct pressure. Extrinsic

factors (such as cocaine use) can also damage the delicate nasal passages or the septum, which separates the two nares.

Three bony shelves, called **turbinates**, protrude from the lateral walls of the nasal cavity and extend into the nasal passageway, parallel to the nasal floor. The turbinates increase the surface area of the nasal mucosa, thereby improving the processes of warming, filtering, and humidification of inhaled air.

The nasopharynx is divided into two passages by the **nasal septum**, a rigid partition composed of the ethmoid and vomer bones and cartilage. Normally, the nasal septum is in the midline of the nose. In some people, the septum may be deviated to one side or the other—a condition that becomes important when contemplating insertion of a nasal airway device.

Along the lateral walls of the nasal passageway are numerous openings that extend into the frontal and maxillary **sinuses**. Because of their proximity to and direct communication with the nasal passage, the frontal and maxillary sinuses are referred to as the **paranasal sinuses** **Figure 3**. The sinuses prevent contaminants from entering the respiratory tract and act as tributaries for fluid to and from the eustachian tubes and tear ducts. Fractures of the bones that comprise the sinuses may cause cerebrospinal fluid (CSF) to leak from the nose (**cerebrospinal rhinorrhea**) or the ears (**cerebrospinal otorrhea**). In some

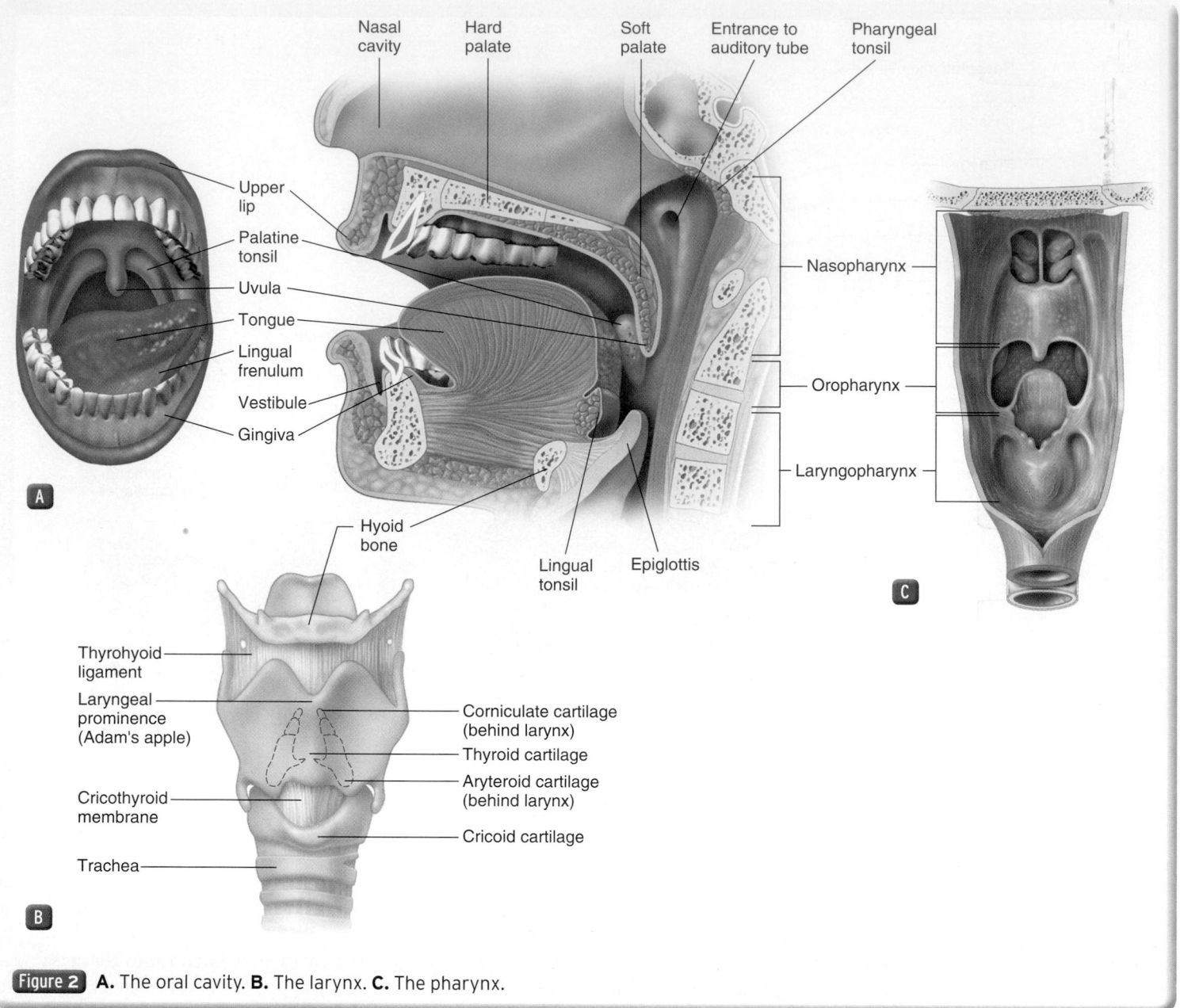

Figure 2 **A.** The oral cavity. **B.** The larynx. **C.** The pharynx.

cases, CSF may drain from the posterior nasopharynx down the patient's throat, causing a salty taste in the mouth.

Oropharynx

The **oropharynx** forms the posterior portion of the oral cavity, which is bordered superiorly by the hard and soft palates, laterally by the cheeks, and inferiorly by the tongue **Figure 2B**. The 32 adult teeth are embedded in the gums in such a manner that significant force is required to dislodge them. However, trauma of lesser severity may result in fracture or avulsion of the teeth, potentially obstructing the upper airway or causing **aspiration** of tooth fragments into the lungs.

The tongue is a large muscle attached to the mandible and the **hyoid bone**—a small, horseshoe-shaped bone to which the jaw, epiglottis, and thyroid cartilage attach as well. From an airway perspective, the most important anatomic consideration regarding the tongue is its tendency to fall back and occlude the posterior pharynx when the mandible relaxes. In fact, the tongue is the most common cause of anatomic upper airway obstruction, especially in patients with a decreased level of consciousness (LOC).

The **palate** forms the roof of the mouth and separates the oropharynx and nasopharynx. Its anterior portion, which is formed by the maxilla and palatine bones, is called the hard palate. The soft palate is posterior to the hard palate. The **palatoglossal arch**, the posterior border of the oral cavity, is an extension of the soft palate.

The **uvula**, a soft-tissue structure that resembles a punching bag, extends into the palatoglossal arch at the base of the tongue in the posterior aspect of the oral cavity.

The **palatopharyngeal arch** is the entrance to the throat, or pharynx. The tonsils, which are composed of lymphatic tissue, trap bacteria and help fight infection. The <u>palatine tonsils</u> are paired structures that lie just behind the walls of the palatoglossal arch, anterior to the palatopharyngeal arch. The pharyngeal tonsil, also known as the <u>adenoid</u>, is located on the posterior nasopharyngeal wall. The lingual tonsils are at the base of the tongue Figure 4 . The adenoids and tonsils often become swollen and infected. Severe swelling of the tonsils can potentially cause obstruction of the upper airway.

■ Anatomy of the Lower Airway

The function of the lower airway is to exchange oxygen and carbon dioxide. Externally, it extends from the fourth cervical vertebra to the xiphoid process. Internally, it spans the glottis to the pulmonary capillary membrane Figure 5 .

Larynx

The <u>larynx</u> is a complex structure formed by many independent cartilaginous structures Figure 2C . It marks where the upper airway ends and the lower airway begins.

The <u>thyroid cartilage</u> is a shield-shaped structure formed by two plates that join in a "V" shape anteriorly to form the laryngeal prominence known as the Adam's apple. The laryngeal prominence is more pronounced in men than in women; it can also be difficult to locate in obese or short-necked patients. The thyroid cartilage is suspended from the hyoid bone by the thyroid ligament and is directly anterior to the glottic opening.

The <u>cricoid cartilage</u>, or cricoid ring, lies inferiorly to the thyroid cartilage; it forms the lowest portion of the larynx. The cricoid cartilage is the first ring of the trachea and the only upper airway structure that forms a complete ring.

Between the thyroid and cricoid cartilage is a ligament called the <u>cricothyroid membrane</u>, which is a site for emergency surgical and nonsurgical access to the airway (cricothyrotomy). Because it is bordered laterally and inferiorly by the highly vascular thyroid gland, the paramedic must locate the anatomic landmarks carefully when accessing the airway via this site.

Glottis

The <u>glottis</u>, also called the glottic opening, is the space between the vocal cords and the narrowest portion of the adult airway Figure 6 . Airway patency in this area is heavily dependent on adequate muscle tone. The lateral borders of the glottis are the <u>vocal cords</u>. At rest, these white bands of tough tissue are partially separated (that is, the glottis is partially open). During forceful inhalation, the vocal cords open widely to provide minimum resistance to air flow.

The superior border of the glottis is the <u>epiglottis</u>. This leaf-shaped cartilaginous flap prevents food and liquid from entering the glottis during swallowing. The epiglottis is attached to the thyroid chartilage by the <u>thyroepiglottic ligament</u>, to the base of the tongue by the <u>glossoepiglottic ligament</u>, and to the hyoid bone by the <u>hyoepiglottic ligament</u>. Because of the ligamentous

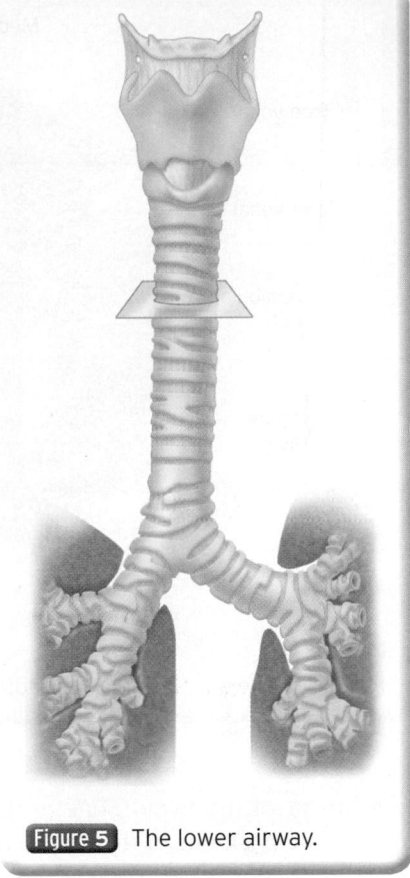

Figure 5 The lower airway.

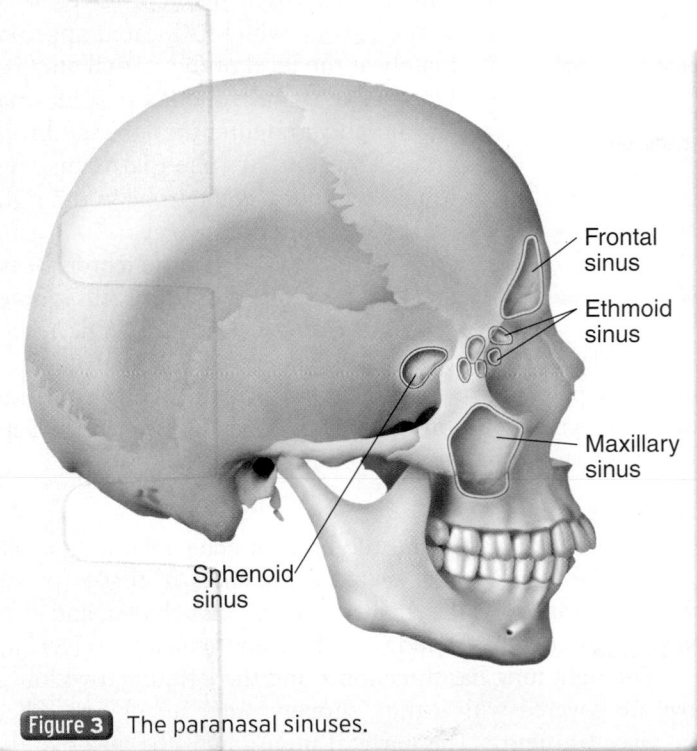

Figure 3 The paranasal sinuses.

Frontal sinus
Ethmoid sinus
Maxillary sinus
Sphenoid sinus

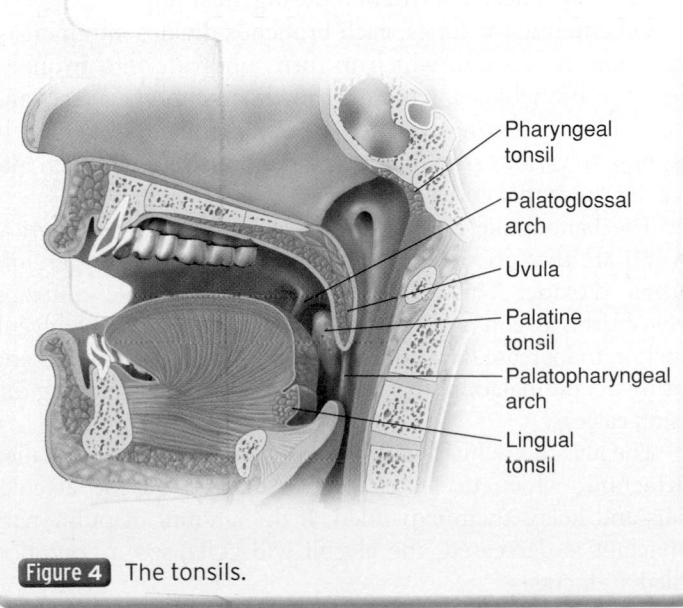

Figure 4 The tonsils.

Pharyngeal tonsil
Palatoglossal arch
Uvula
Palatine tonsil
Palatopharyngeal arch
Lingual tonsil

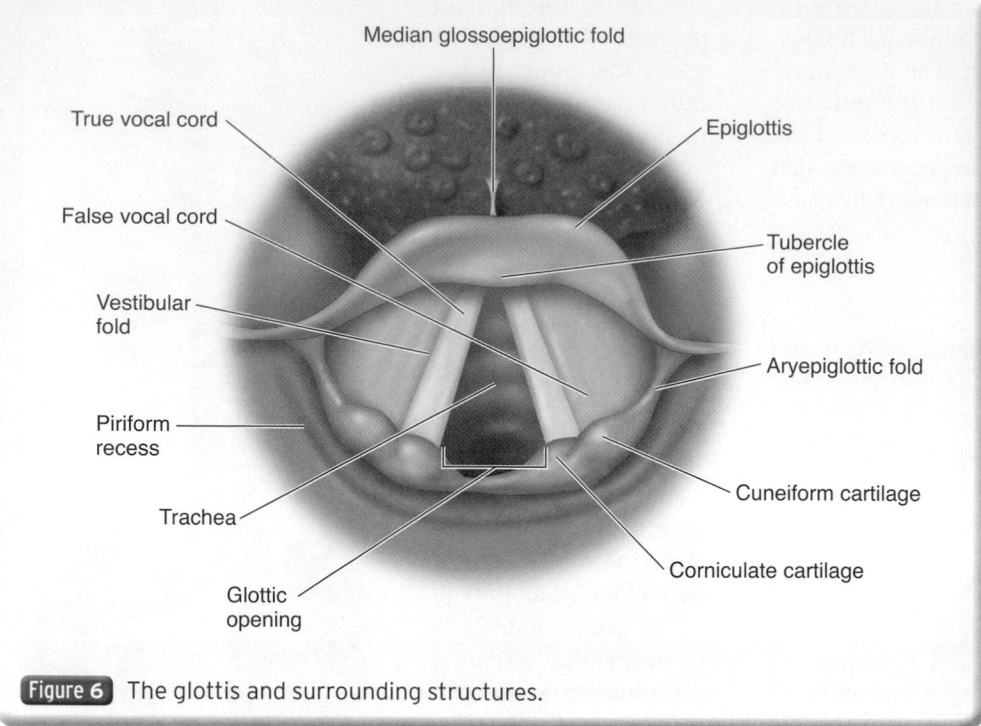

True vocal cord

Median glossoepiglottic fold

Epiglottis

False vocal cord

Tubercle
of epiglottis

Vestibular
fold

Aryepiglottic fold

Piriform
recess

Cuneiform cartilage

Trachea

Corniculate cartilage

Glottic
opening

Figure 6 The glottis and surrounding structures.

attachment of the hyoid bone to the soft tissues of the upper airway, the positions of the tongue and epiglottis change as the hyoid bone is moved. This movement occurs during the head tilt–chin lift maneuver and by direct forward displacement of the base of the tongue, as is often done during intubation. The **vallecula** is the anatomic space, or "pocket," located between the base of the tongue and the epiglottis. It is an important landmark for endotracheal (ET) intubation.

At the inferior border of the glottic opening are the corniculate and cuneiform cartilages, which appear as bumps just below the glottis. The **arytenoid cartilages** are pyramidlike cartilaginous structures that form the posterior attachment of the vocal cords; they are valuable guides for ET intubation. As the arytenoid cartilages pivot, the vocal cords open and close, which regulates the passage of air through the larynx and controls the production of sound; hence, the larynx is sometimes called the "voice box."

The **piriform fossae** are two pockets of tissue on the lateral borders of the larynx. Airway devices are occasionally inadvertently inserted into these pockets, resulting in a tenting of the skin under the jaw.

When the airway is stimulated (such as during aspiration of foreign material or submersion incident), defensive reflexes cause a **laryngospasm**—spasmodic closure of the vocal cords, which seals off the airway. This reflex normally lasts a few seconds. Persistent laryngospasm, however, can threaten airway patency by preventing ventilation altogether.

Trachea

The **trachea**, or windpipe, is the conduit for air entry into the lungs. This tubular structure is approximately 10 to 12 cm long and consists of a series of C-shaped cartilaginous rings. The

trachea begins immediately below the cricoid cartilage and descends anteriorly down the midline of the neck and chest to the level of the fifth or sixth thoracic vertebra in the mediastinum—the space between the lungs that contains, in addition to the trachea, the heart, great vessels, and a portion of the esophagus. The shape of the tracheal rings enables food to pass down the esophagus easily during swallowing. Anatomically, the esophagus lies posterior to the trachea.

The trachea divides into the right and left mainstem **bronchi** at the level of the **carina**, which is located approximately at the level of the sternal angle of Louis. The right bronchus is somewhat shorter and straighter than the left bronchus. Thus, an ET tube that is inserted too far will often come to lie in the right mainstem bronchus.

The trachea and mainstem bronchi are lined with mucous-producing cells (**goblet cells**), cilia, and beta-2 adrenergic receptors. Goblet cells secrete a sticky lining that traps small particles and other potential contaminants. Cilia move back and forth to sweep foreign material out of the airway. Beta-2 adrenergic receptors, when stimulated, result in bronchodilation.

Lungs

All of the blood vessels and the bronchi enter each lung at the **hilum**. The lungs consist of the entire mass of tissue (parenchyma) that includes the smaller bronchi, bronchioles, and alveoli **Figure 7**. In total, the lungs can hold approximately 6 L of air.

The right lung has three lobes and the left lung, two lobes, that are covered with a thin, slippery outer membrane called the **visceral pleura**. The **parietal pleura** lines the inside of the thoracic cavity. A small amount of fluid is found between the pleurae, which decreases friction during breathing.

On entering the lungs, each bronchus divides into increasingly smaller bronchi, which in turn subdivide into **bronchioles**. The bronchioles, which are made of smooth muscle and lined with beta-2 adrenergic receptors, can dilate or constrict in response to various stimuli. The smaller bronchioles branch into alveolar ducts that end at the alveolar sacs.

The balloonlike clusters of single-layer air sacs known as **alveoli** are the functional site for the exchange of oxygen and carbon dioxide. This exchange occurs by simple diffusion between the alveoli and the pulmonary capillaries. The alveoli function to increase the surface area of the lungs; as they expand during deep inhalation, they become even thinner, making diffusion easier.

The alveoli are lined with a phospholipid compound called **surfactant**, which decreases surface tension on the alveolar walls and keeps them expanded. If the amount of pulmonary surfactant is decreased, the alveoli will collapse—a condition called **atelectasis**.

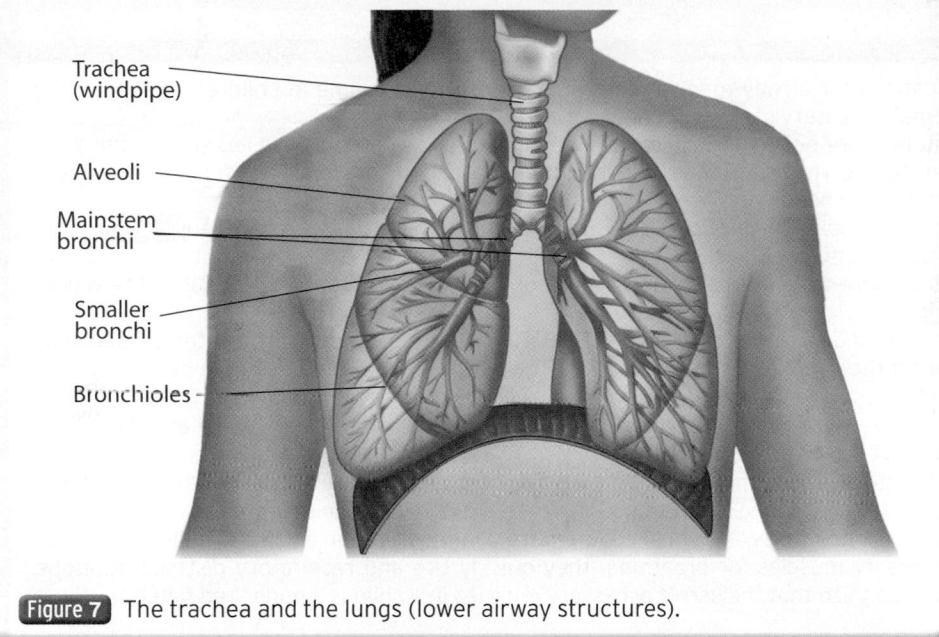

Figure 7 The trachea and the lungs (lower airway structures).

Finally, it is useful to be familiar with the landmarks shown in **Figure 8** when assessing and managing the airway.

Physiology of Breathing

The respiratory and cardiovascular systems work together to ensure that a constant supply of oxygen and nutrients is delivered to every cell in the body and that carbon dioxide and other waste products are removed from every cell **Table 1**. If one of these systems is compromised, oxygen delivery is not effective and cellular death may occur. The following sections describe the processes of ventilation, oxygenation, and respiration.

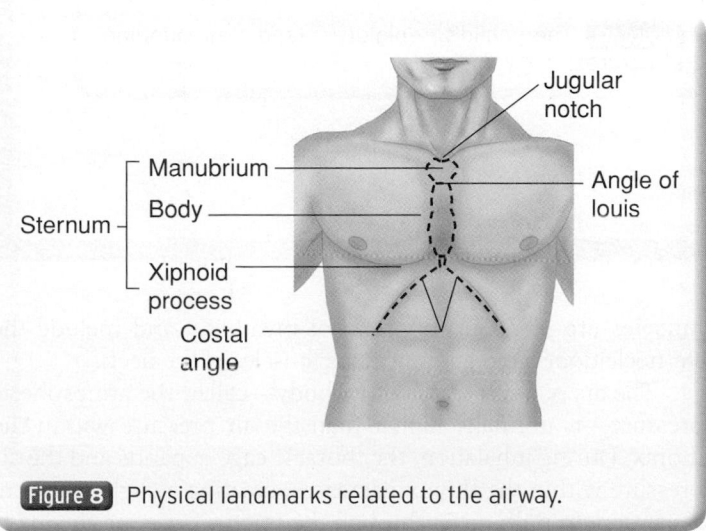

Figure 8 Physical landmarks related to the airway.

Ventilation

Pulmonary **ventilation**—the process of moving air into and out of the lungs—is necessary for oxygenation and respiration. Ventilation consists of two phases: inhalation (inspiration) and exhalation (expiration). Adequate, continuous ventilation is essential for life and, therefore, is one of the highest priorities in treating any patient. If a patient is not breathing or is breathing inadequately, you must immediately intervene to ensure adequate ventilation.

Inhalation

The Role of Muscles

The active, muscular part of breathing is called **inhalation**. It is governed by **Boyle's law**, which states that the pressure of a gas is inversely proportional to its volume. When a person inhales, air enters the body through the mouth and nose and moves to the trachea. This air travels to and from the lungs, filling and emptying the alveoli. During inhalation, the diaphragm and intercostal muscles contract. When the diaphragm contracts, it descends and enlarges the thoracic cage from top to bottom, and when the intercostal muscles contract, they lift the ribs up and out. The combined actions of these structures enlarge the thorax in all directions. Maximum inhalation occurs when the diaphragm and intercostal muscles are contracted and the lungs fill with air.

The diaphragm is a specialized skeletal muscle. Innervated by the phrenic nerve, the diaphragm functions as a voluntary and an involuntary muscle. It acts as a voluntary muscle when a person takes a deep breath, coughs, or holds his or her breath—all actions that are under voluntary (somatic) control. However, unlike other skeletal muscles, the diaphragm functions as an involuntary muscle whenever voluntary function ceases, such as when coughing stops and during sleep. Voluntary use of the diaphragm cannot continue indefinitely. When the concentration of carbon dioxide rises in the blood, the autonomic regulation of breathing resumes under control of the brainstem.

Table 1 Ventilation, Oxygenation, and Respiration	
Function	**Definition**
Ventilation	The physical act of moving air into and out of the lungs
Oxygenation	The process of loading oxygen molecules onto hemoglobin molecules in the bloodstream
Respiration	The actual exchange of oxygen and carbon dioxide in the alveoli and the tissues of the body

Special Populations

Although the maneuvers, techniques, and indications for airway management are essentially the same in children as they are in adults, several anatomic differences in children make mastery of these techniques critical.

Infants and small children have a proportionately larger occiput, which causes the head to flex when the child lies supine; this position itself can cause an airway obstruction. When positioning the airway of an infant or a child, you should place a folded towel under his or her shoulders to maintain a neutral position of the head.

Compared with adults, children have a proportionately smaller mandible and a proportionately larger tongue **Figure 9**. Both factors increase the incidence of airway obstruction in children.

The child's epiglottis is more floppy and omega-shaped (Ω) than an adult's. As a consequence, it must be lifted out of the way to visualize the vocal cords for intubation **Figure 10**.

In general, the infant's and child's airway is smaller and narrower at all levels. The larynx lies more superior and anterior than in an adult—an important consideration when visualizing the vocal cords for intubation. The larynx is also funnel-shaped because of the narrow, underdeveloped cricoid cartilage. In children younger than 10 years, the narrowest portion of the airway is at the cricoid ring. Further narrowing of the child's inherently narrow airway, such as that caused by soft-tissue swelling or foreign body aspiration, can result in a major increase in airway resistance and breathing inadequacy.

Children do not have well-developed chest musculature, and their ribs and cartilage are softer and more pliable than an adult's. As a result, the thoracic cavity cannot optimally contribute to lung expansion. Children rely heavily on their diaphragm for breathing, which moves their abdomen in and out. For this reason, infants and small children are commonly referred to as "belly breathers." When infants and children need to use the accessory muscles for breathing, they quickly tire and respiratory distress develops, followed by respiratory arrest. Paramedics must recognize that the use of accessory muscles in a child is a huge "red flag."

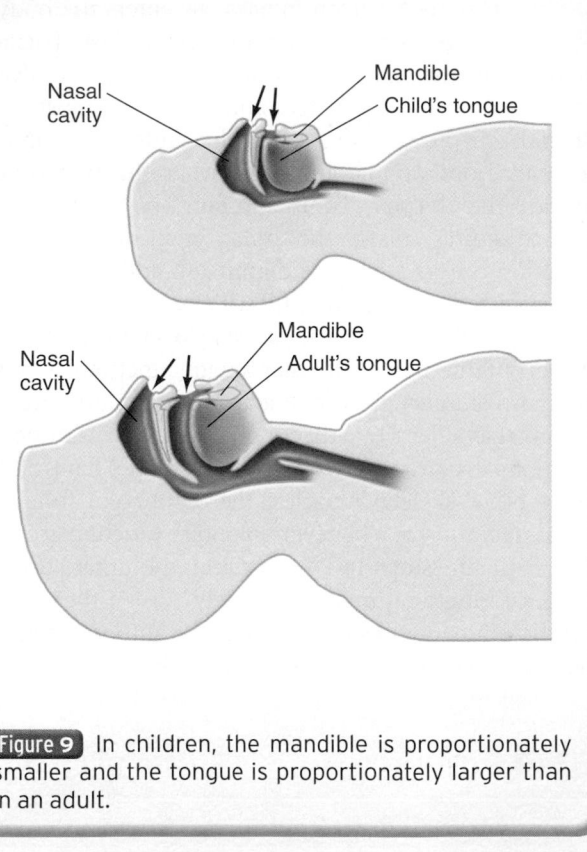

Figure 9 In children, the mandible is proportionately smaller and the tongue is proportionately larger than in an adult.

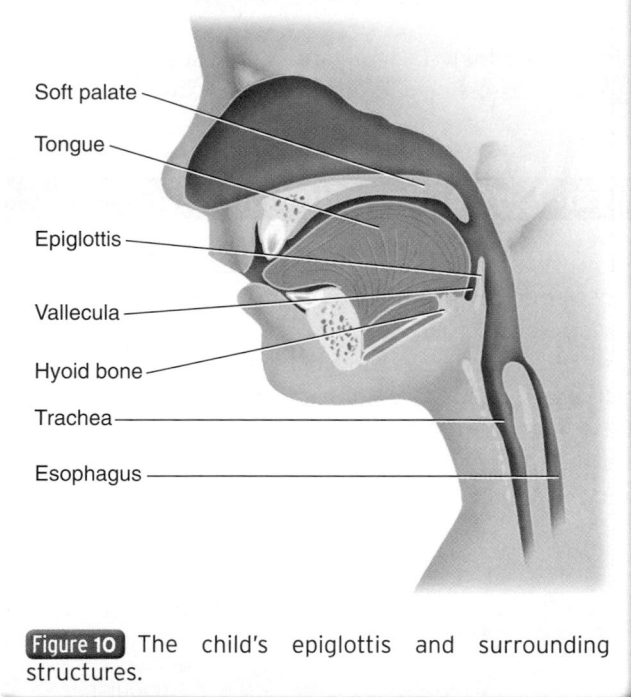

Figure 10 The child's epiglottis and surrounding structures.

The lungs have no muscle tissue; therefore, they cannot move on their own. They need the help of other structures to be able to expand and contract during inhalation. Therefore, the ability of the lungs to function properly is dependent on the movement of the chest and supporting structures. These structures include the thorax, the thoracic cage (chest cage), the diaphragm, the intercostal muscles, and the accessory muscles. **Accessory muscles** are secondary muscles of breathing, and include the sternocleidomastoid and trapezius muscles of the neck.

The air pressure outside the body—called the atmospheric pressure—is normally higher than the air pressure within the thorax. During inhalation, the thoracic cage expands and the air pressure within the thorax decreases, creating a slight vacuum. This vacuum pulls air in through the trachea, causing the lungs

Words of Wisdom

Normal breathing involves negative intrathoracic pressure and the pulling of air into the lungs (negative-pressure ventilation). With ineffective chest movement (such as with reduced tidal volume) or no chest movement (as in apnea), negative intrathoracic pressure cannot be created. When this occurs, the only way to move air into the lungs is by **positive-pressure ventilation**, the forcing of air into the lungs. Positive pressure can be created with a bag-mask device, pocket face mask, or mechanical ventilation device.

to fill—a process called **negative-pressure ventilation**. When the air pressure inside the thorax equals the air pressure outside the body, air stops moving. Gases, such as oxygen and carbon dioxide, move from an area of higher pressure to an area of lower pressure (diffusion) until the pressures are equal. At this point, the air stops moving and inhalation stops.

It may help you to understand this if you think of the thoracic cage as a bell jar in which balloons are suspended.

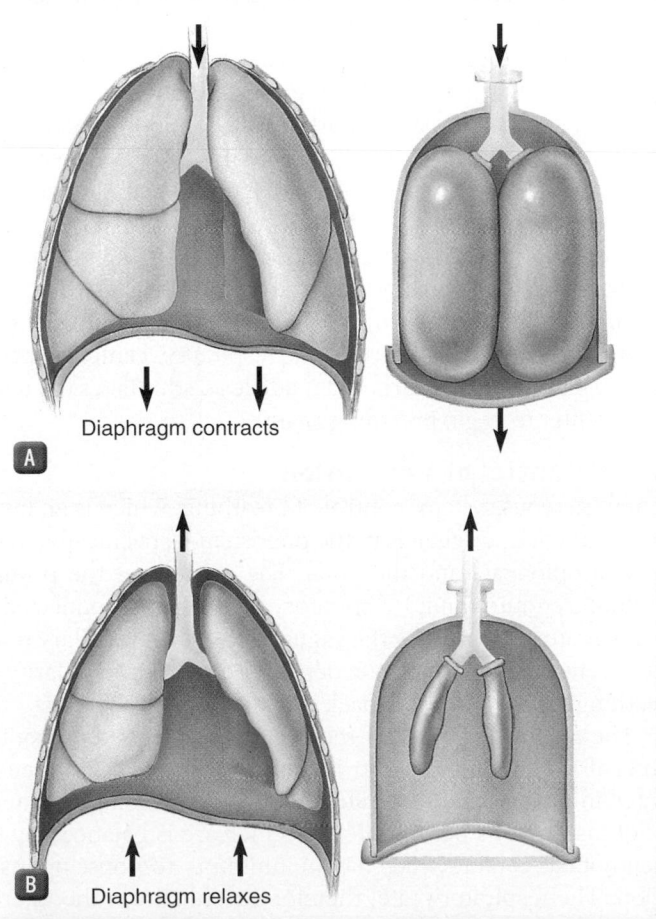

A. Diaphragm contracts

B. Diaphragm relaxes

Figure 11 The mechanism of ventilation can be illustrated by a bell jar. **A.** Inhalation and chest expansion, anatomic (left) and bell jar (right). **B.** Exhalation and chest contraction, anatomic (left) and bell jar (right).

In this example, the balloons are the lungs. The base of the jar is the diaphragm, which moves up and down slightly with each breath. The ribs, which are the sides of the jar, maintain the shape of the chest. The only opening into the jar is a small tube at the top, similar to the trachea. During inhalation, the bottom of the jar moves down slightly, causing a decrease in pressure in the jar and creating a slight vacuum. As a result, the balloons fill with air **Figure 11**.

The Role of Diffusion

The process of oxygen transfer from air into the capillaries in the alveoli involves diffusion. Several concepts are useful in understanding this process.

Partial pressure is a term used to describe the amount of gas in air or dissolved in liquid, such as the blood, and is governed by **Henry's law**, which states that the amount of a gas in a solution varies directly with the partial pressure of a gas over a solution. In other words, as the pressure of a gas over a liquid decreases, the amount of gas dissolved in the liquid will also decrease. As more pressure is applied over the liquid, more gas can be dissolved in the liquid. In practical terms, this law states that molecules of a gas can be dissolved in a liquid and remain in the liquid as long as the liquid is in a pressurized, closed container (eg, the circulatory system).

Partial pressure is measured in millimeters of mercury (mm Hg), or torr. The partial pressure of oxygen in air residing in the alveoli is 104 mm Hg. Carbon dioxide enters the alveoli from the blood and causes a partial pressure of 40 mm Hg.

Deoxygenated arterial blood from the heart has a partial pressure of oxygen (PaO_2) that is lower than the partial pressure of oxygen in the alveoli. The body attempts to equalize the partial pressure, which results in oxygen diffusion across the alveolar-capillary membrane into the blood; carbon dioxide diffuses into the alveoli and is eliminated as waste during exhalation. Oxygen and carbon dioxide both diffuse until the partial pressure in the air and the blood is equal. This process occurs in reverse when the arterial blood reaches the tissues. Oxygen diffuses into the tissue fluid and then into the cells, and carbon dioxide diffuses out of the cells and into the fluid and blood.

Lung Volumes

The entire process of inhalation is focused on delivering oxygen to the alveoli. Breathing becomes deeper as the tidal volume responds to the increased metabolic demand for oxygen. However, not all of the inhaled air reaches the alveoli. The volume of air that reaches the alveoli is called alveolar volume (also referred to as alveolar ventilation). **Alveolar volume** is determined by subtracting the amount of *dead space volume* from the *tidal volume*. **Tidal volume (V_T)**, a measure of the depth of breathing, is the amount of air (in milliliters ([mL]) that is moved into or out of the respiratory tract during one breath. The normal tidal volume for a healthy adult is 5 to 7 mL/kg (about 500 mL). In infants and children, the normal tidal volume is approximately 6 to 8 mL/kg.

Dead space volume (V_D) is the portion of the tidal volume that does not reach the alveoli and, therefore, does not participate in gas exchange. Anatomic dead space contains air that remains in the mouth, nose, trachea, bronchi, and larger bronchioles, which can add up to approximately 150 mL in a healthy man. Certain respiratory diseases increase dead space volume by creating intrapulmonary obstructions or atelectasis (alveolar collapse); these areas are called **physiologic dead space**.

Minute ventilation, also referred to as **minute volume** (V_M), is the amount of air moved through the respiratory tract—including the anatomic dead space—in 1 minute, and is calculated by multiplying the tidal volume and respiratory rate. **Alveolar minute volume (V_A)**—also referred to as minute alveolar ventilation—is a more precise measurement. It represents the *actual* volume of air that reaches the alveoli and participates in pulmonary gas exchange each minute. Alveolar minute volume can be calculated by subtracting the dead space volume from the tidal volume, then multiplying that number by the **respiratory rate** (the number of times a person breathes in 1 minute). Therefore, if a patient has a respiratory rate of 12 breaths/min, a tidal volume of 500 mL, and a dead space volume of 150 mL, his or her alveolar minute volume would be 4,200 mL (4.2 L), as follows:

$$500\,mL\,(V_T) - 150\,mL\,(V_D) \times 12\,breaths/min = 4,200\,mL\,(V_M)$$

Variations in tidal volume, respiratory rate, or both affect alveolar minute volume. For example, if a patient is breathing at a rate of 12 breaths/min, but the tidal volume is reduced (shallow breathing), the alveolar minute volume will decrease. Conversely, if a patient is breathing at a rate of 12 breaths/min and the tidal volume increases (deep breathing), the alveolar minute volume will increase. Conversely, alveolar minute volume will decrease if the tidal volume or the respiratory rate (or both) decreases. It is important to note that as respirations become faster, they often become more shallow (reduced tidal volume). When respirations are too rapid *and* too shallow, much of the inhaled air may reach only the anatomic dead space before it is promptly exhaled, resulting in smaller volumes of air reaching the alveoli. As a result, the alveolar minute volume would decrease.

A final term related to inspiration is **inspiratory reserve volume**, which is the amount of air that can be inhaled in addition to the normal tidal volume; it is normally about 3,000 mL in a healthy adult.

Following an optimal inspiration, the amount of air that can be forced from the lungs in one exhalation is called the **functional reserve capacity**. The amount of air that can be exhaled following normal (relaxed) exhalation is called the **expiratory reserve volume**; this amount is about 1,200 mL. Even forceful exhalation, however, cannot completely empty the lungs of air. **Residual volume** is the air that remains in the lungs after maximal exhalation; it is also about 1,200 mL in a healthy man. The **vital capacity** is the amount of air that can be forcefully exhaled after a full inhalation; in a healthy man, this amount is approximately 4,800 mL. The **total lung capacity**, or maximum amount of air the lungs can hold, is the vital capacity plus the residual volume. In a healthy man, this amount is about 6,000 mL (6 L). Various respiratory and cardiac diseases affect the various lung volumes.

Exhalation

Unlike inhalation, **exhalation** does not normally require muscular effort; therefore, it is a passive process. As the chest expands, mechanical receptors, known as stretch receptors, in the chest wall and bronchioles send a signal to the apneustic center via the vagus nerve to inhibit the respiratory center, and exhalation occurs. This feedback loop, a combination of mechanical and neural control, is called the **Hering-Breuer reflex** and terminates inhalation to prevent overexpansion of the lungs. The diaphragm and intercostal muscles relax, which increases intrapulmonary pressure. The natural elasticity, or recoil, of the lungs passively removes the air. When the size of the thoracic cage decreases, air in the lungs is compressed into a smaller space. The air pressure within the thorax then becomes higher than the outside pressure, and the air is pushed out through the trachea.

Regulation of Ventilation

The body's need for oxygen is dynamic; it is constantly changing. The respiratory system must be able to accommodate the changes in oxygen demand by altering the rate and depth of ventilation. These changes are regulated primarily by the pH of the CSF, which is directly related to the amount of carbon dioxide dissolved in the plasma portion of the blood (Pa_{CO_2}). The regulation of ventilation involves a complex series of receptors and feedback loops that sense gas concentrations in the body fluids and send messages to the respiratory center in the brain to adjust the rate and depth of ventilation accordingly. For most people, the drive to breathe is based on pH changes (related to the carbon dioxide level) in the blood and CSF. In healthy people, when the oxygen level rises, the respiratory center suspends breathing until a rising carbon dioxide level stimulates the respiratory center to begin breathing again.

Neural Control of Ventilation

Neural (nervous system) control of breathing, which is an involuntary function, originates in the brainstem—specifically, in the medulla oblongata and the pons. The medulla is the primary involuntary (autonomic) respiratory center. It is connected to the respiratory muscles by the vagus nerve. The medullary respiratory centers control the rate, depth, and rhythm (regularity) of breathing in a negative feedback interaction with the pons.

The apneustic center of the pons is the secondary control center if the medulla fails to initiate breathing. The apneustic center influences the respiratory rate by increasing the number of inspirations per minute. This increase is balanced by the pneumotaxic center, which has an inhibitory response on inspiration. The respiratory rate, therefore, results from the interaction between these two centers.

Chemical Control of Ventilation

The goal of the respiratory system is to keep the blood concentrations of oxygen and carbon dioxide and its acid-base balance within very narrow ranges. The body has a number of receptors that monitor variables and provide feedback to the respiratory centers to adjust the rate and depth of respiration based on the body's needs. These **chemoreceptors** have important effects on respiratory rate and depth.

Chemoreceptors that constantly monitor the chemical composition of body fluids are located throughout the body to provide feedback on many metabolic processes. Three sets of chemoreceptors affect respiratory function: those located in the carotid bodies, those in the aortic arch, and the central chemoreceptors.

The chemoreceptors that measure the amount of carbon dioxide in arterial blood are located in the carotid bodies and the aortic arch Figure 12 . These receptors sense tiny changes in the carbon dioxide level and send signals to the respiratory center via the glossopharyngeal nerve (9th cranial nerve) and the vagus nerve (10th cranial nerve).

Central chemoreceptors, which monitor the pH of the CSF, are located adjacent to the respiratory centers in the medulla. The acidity of the CSF is an indirect measure of the amount of carbon dioxide in arterial blood because the carbon dioxide in the blood readily diffuses across the blood-brain barrier and combines with water to form carbonic acid (H_2CO_3). The carbonic acid dissociates, and the pH drops as the hydrogen ion (H^+) concentration increases. An increase in the acidity of the CSF triggers the central chemoreceptors to increase the rate and depth of breathing. These central chemoreceptors are very sensitive to small changes in pH and provide for "fine-tuning" of the body's acid-base balance.

While the primary control of ventilation is the pH of the CSF, the amount of oxygen dissolved in the blood plasma (Pao_2) has a secondary and protective role. The chemoreceptors located in the aortic arch and carotid bodies also respond to decreases in Pao_2 by sending messages to the respiratory centers to increase breathing. Under normal conditions, these chemoreceptors serve as a backup to the primary control of ventilation, which is based on the level of carbon dioxide in the blood and the pH of the CSF.

When serum carbon dioxide or hydrogen ion levels increase because of a medical condition or traumatic injury involving the respiratory system, chemoreceptors stimulate the dorsal and ventral respiratory groups in the medulla to increase the respiratory rate, thus removing more carbon dioxide or acid from the body. The **dorsal respiratory group** is responsible for initiating inspiration based on the information received from the chemoreceptors. The **ventral respiratory group** is primarily responsible for motor control of the inspiratory and expiratory muscles.

Hypoxic Drive Patients with chronic obstructive pulmonary disease (COPD), such as emphysema and chronic bronchitis, have difficulty eliminating carbon dioxide through exhalation; therefore, they always have higher blood levels of carbon dioxide. The high level can potentially alter their **primary respiratory drive** (which is based on increased arterial CO_2 levels and the pH of the CSF). The theory is that the respiratory centers in the brain gradually accommodate elevated carbon dioxide levels. In patients with end-stage COPD, the body uses a "backup system" to control breathing. This theory of secondary control, called the **hypoxic drive**, stimulates breathing when the arterial oxygen level falls. However, the nerves in the brain, the walls of the aorta, and the carotid arteries that act as oxygen sensors (chemoreceptors)

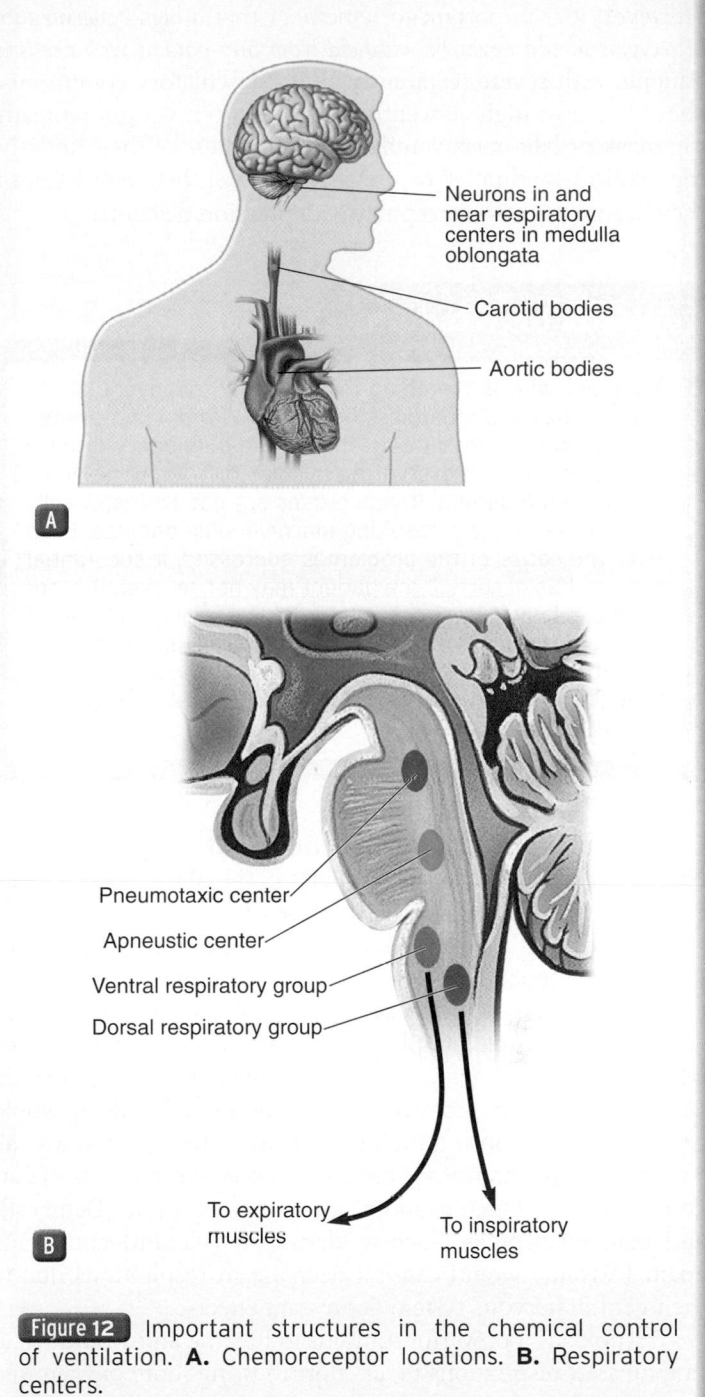

A

B

 Figure 12 Important structures in the chemical control of ventilation. **A.** Chemoreceptor locations. **B.** Respiratory centers.

Labels in figure:
- Neurons in and near respiratory centers in medulla oblongata
- Carotid bodies
- Aortic bodies
- Pneumotaxic center
- Apneustic center
- Ventral respiratory group
- Dorsal respiratory group
- To expiratory muscles
- To inspiratory muscles

are easily satisfied with a minimal level of oxygen. Therefore, the hypoxic drive is much less sensitive and less powerful than the carbon dioxide sensors in the brainstem. Hypoxic drive is typically found in end-stage COPD and not in patients with a recent diagnosis of COPD. Providing high concentrations of oxygen over time will increase the amount of oxygen dissolved in the blood plasma (Pao_2). However, many physicians believe this could negatively affect the body's drive to breathe.

Regardless of the current research, it remains that a certain amount of caution should be taken when administering high concentrations of oxygen to patients with end-stage COPD. However, it is important to remember that *a high concentration of oxygen should never be withheld from any patient who needs it.* Patients with severe respiratory and/or circulatory compromise should receive high concentrations of oxygen via nonrebreathing mask or bag-mask ventilation—regardless of their underlying medical conditions. Be prepared to assist their ventilations if they become sleepy or respiratory depression develops.

Words of Wisdom

A patient who is breathing inadequately (hypoventilation) requires oxygen, regardless of history. Withholding oxygen from a patient with chronic obstructive pulmonary disease in an attempt to preserve the hypoxic drive may be detrimental to the patient. If vital organs are not perfused, cells and tissues may die, resulting in irreversible damage. Even after the cause of the problem is addressed, if substantial damage has occurred, the patient may not recover. By ventilating a hypoxic patient, vital organs remain perfused. If the hypoxic drive is eliminated, organs are still oxygenated. Once the cause of the original problem is corrected, the patient is weaned off the ventilator and could return to a normal, productive life.

Control of Ventilation by Other Factors

Numerous factors other than changes in the pH, $Paco_2$, and Pao_2 can influence ventilation. As the body temperature rises (that is, in the case of fever), respirations increase in response to the increased metabolic activity. Certain medications cause respirations to increase or decrease, depending on their physiologic action. For example, amphetamines (such as methylphenidate [Ritalin] and dextroamphetamine-amphetamine combination [Adderall]), which produce a sympathomimetic effect, would cause an increase in respirations. Pain and strong emotions can also increase respirations. Conversely, excessive amounts of narcotic analgesics (such as morphine and meperidine [Demerol]) and benzodiazepines (such as diazepam [Valium] and lorazepam [Ativan]) would cause a decrease in respirations due to their central nervous system depressant effects.

Hypoxia is a powerful stimulus to breathe and would result in increased respirations in an effort to bring more oxygen into the body. Conversely, acidosis increases respirations as a compensatory response to promote the elimination of excess acids produced by the body.

A person's metabolic rate also influences the rate of breathing. When the metabolic rate is high (such as during exercise), respirations increase to eliminate the excess carbon dioxide produced. Conversely, when the metabolic rate is low (such as during sleep), respirations slow.

■ Oxygenation

Oxygenation is the process of loading oxygen molecules onto hemoglobin molecules in the bloodstream. Adequate oxygenation is required for internal respiration; however, it does not guarantee that internal respiration is taking place. Oxygenation requires that the air used for ventilation contains an adequate percentage of oxygen. While oxygenation cannot occur without ventilation, ventilation is possible without oxygenation. Ventilation without oxygenation may occur in places where the oxygen level in the air has been depleted, such as in mines and confined places. Oxygenation can also be impeded when other gases—for example, carbon monoxide (CO)—prevent oxygen from binding to hemoglobin.

Ventilation without adequate oxygenation also occurs in climbers who ascend too quickly to an altitude with inadequate atmospheric pressure. At high altitudes, the percentage of oxygen remains the same (20.8%), but the atmospheric pressure makes it difficult to adequately bring sufficient amounts of oxygen into the body.

The **fraction of inspired oxygen (Fio_2)** is the percentage of oxygen in inhaled air. The Fio_2 increases when supplemental oxygen is given to a patient and is commonly documented as a decimal number. A person breathing room air, which contains about 21% oxygen, would be documented as having an Fio_2 of 0.21. A nonrebreathing mask, which delivers about 90% oxygen, would be documented as delivering an Fio_2 of 0.90 to an adequately breathing patient.

The Oxyhemoglobin Dissociation Curve

Hemoglobin, a protein that is necessary for life, is an iron-containing molecule that has a great affinity for oxygen molecules. Approximately 95% of the protein in a red blood cell is hemoglobin. Common laboratory tests performed to quantify a person's hemoglobin level and to determine the ratio of red blood cells to plasma are hemoglobin and hematocrit measurements (sometimes abbreviated H and H). Hemoglobin levels are reported in grams per deciliter (dL); normal values are 14 to 16 g/dL for men and 12 to 14 g/dL for women. Hematocrit values indicate the percentage of red blood cells in whole blood. Normal hematocrit values are 45% to 52% for men and 37% to 48% for women.

One hemoglobin molecule reversibly binds with four oxygen molecules. Oxygen saturation (expressed as Spo_2 if measured by pulse oximetry and as Sao_2 if measured in the arterial blood gases [ABGs]) is proportional to the amount of oxygen dissolved in the plasma component of the blood (Pao_2). The relationship between the Pao_2 and Sao_2/Spo_2 is represented by the oxyhemoglobin dissociation curve **Figure 13**. Note that under normal conditions ($Pao_2 = 105$ mm Hg), the Spo_2/Sao_2 is approximately 98%.

While deoxygenated is often the term used to describe the venous blood returning to the heart during circulation, the blood is not completely devoid of oxygen. Some oxygen is still bound to the hemoglobin because the ability of the respiratory system to supply oxygen to the rest of the body exceeds the demand in normal resting conditions. When metabolism increases, however, the demand for oxygen increases and venous blood contains less oxygen. As blood is circulated to the tissue level, the Pao_2 begins to drop. At this point, the hemoglobin releases its oxygen molecules to make them available for cellular respiration.

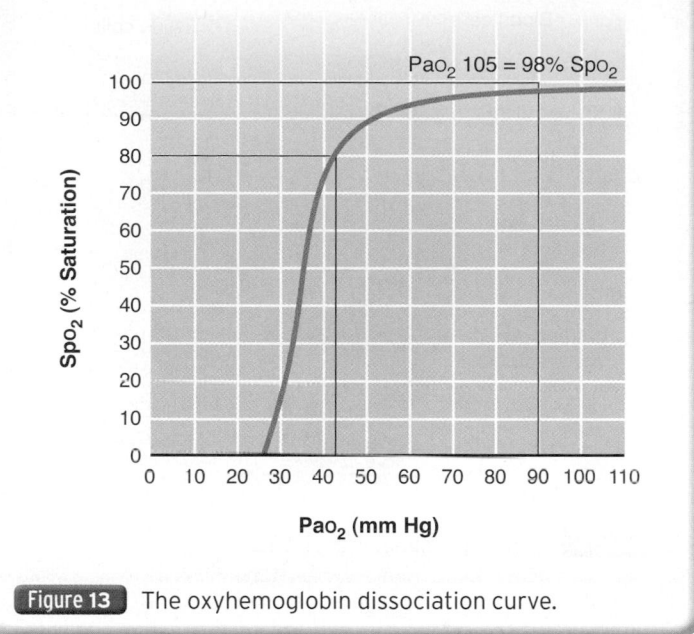

Figure 13 The oxyhemoglobin dissociation curve.

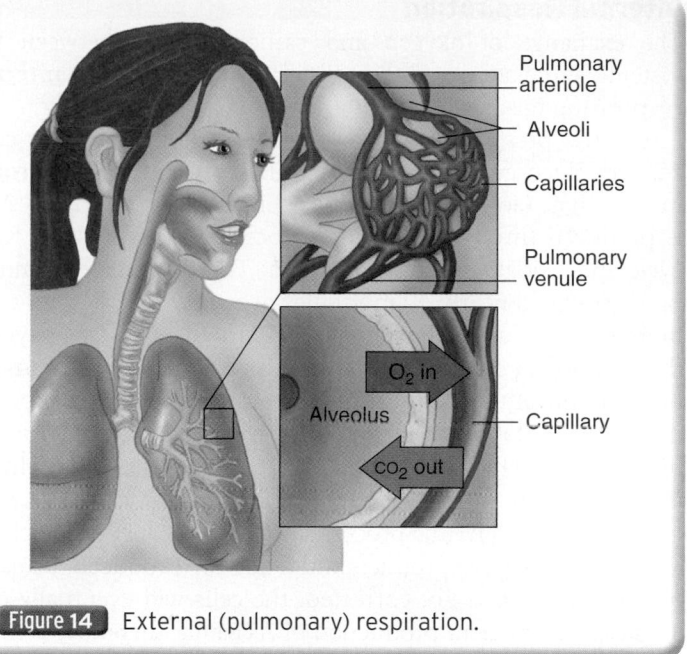

Figure 14 External (pulmonary) respiration.

Hemoglobin has the ability to change how tightly it holds onto oxygen in response to changes in metabolism. More oxygen molecules are released as the acidity of the blood increases (when the pH decreases). This change results in a shift in position of the oxyhemoglobin dissociation curve. Various other conditions can also shift the entire curve to the left or right. A shift to the right causes the hemoglobin to give up its oxygen faster and earlier. A shift to the left has the opposite effect. Acidosis (decreased pH) and increased carbon dioxide levels cause the curve to shift to the right. Alkalosis (increased pH) and a decrease in carbon dioxide levels cause the curve to shift to the left, causing the hemoglobin to hold on to more oxygen.

■ Respiration

All living cells perform a specific function and need energy to survive. Cells take energy from nutrients through a series of chemical processes. The name given to these processes is **metabolism**. During metabolism, each cell combines nutrients (such as glucose) and oxygen and produces energy in the form of adenosine triphosphate (ATP) and waste products, primarily carbon dioxide and water. **Respiration**, the process of exchanging oxygen and carbon dioxide, allows the body a regular means of providing the cells with oxygen and disposing of waste (carbon dioxide). Respiration involves ventilation, diffusion of oxygen and carbon dioxide between the blood and the pulmonary alveoli, and the transport of oxygen and carbon dioxide throughout the body.

External Respiration

External respiration (pulmonary respiration) is the process of exchanging oxygen and carbon dioxide between the alveoli and the blood in the pulmonary capillaries **Figure 14**.

Fresh air that is inspired into the lungs contains about 21% oxygen, 78% nitrogen, and 0.3% carbon dioxide. As this air reaches the alveoli, it comes into contact with a combination of phospholipids called surfactant, which, as previously discussed, reduces surface tension within the alveoli and keeps them expanded; this expansion facilitates the exchange of oxygen and carbon dioxide. It is important to remember that although adequate ventilation is necessary for external respiration to take place, it does not guarantee that external respiration is being achieved.

Once the oxygen crosses the alveolar membrane, it is bound to hemoglobin. Hemoglobin molecules that are low in oxygen concentration are pumped from the right side of the heart into the capillaries of the pulmonary circulation. The capillaries surround the alveoli containing high concentrations of oxygen (from inspired air). The hemoglobin molecules pick up fresh oxygen as it crosses the alveolar membrane and transport it back to the left side of the heart, where it is pumped out to the rest of the body. Under normal conditions, 96% to 100% of the hemoglobin receptors contain oxygen.

Words of Wisdom

The blood does not use all the inhaled oxygen as it passes through the body. Exhaled air contains approximately 16% oxygen and 3% to 5% carbon dioxide; the rest is nitrogen. Therefore, when mouth-to-mouth (or mask) ventilation is provided to a patient who is not breathing, the patient is receiving a 16% concentration of oxygen with each of the rescuer's exhaled breaths.

Internal Respiration

The exchange of oxygen and carbon dioxide between the systemic circulation and the cells of the body is called <u>internal respiration</u> (also called <u>cellular respiration</u>) Figure 15 .

In the presence of oxygen, the mitochondria of the cells convert glucose into energy through a process called **aerobic metabolism** (aerobic respiration). Energy in the form of ATP is produced through a series of processes known as the Kreb cycle and oxidative phosphorylation. Together, these chemical processes yield nearly 40 molecules of energy-rich ATP for each molecule of glucose metabolized. Without adequate oxygen, the cells do not completely convert glucose into energy, and lactic acid and other toxins accumulate in the cell. This process, **anaerobic metabolism** (anaerobic respiration), cannot meet the metabolic demands of the cell. Although another intracellular process, glycolysis, also contributes to ATP production and does not require oxygen, this process results in less ATP production, and lactic acid waste products and toxins are produced. If anaerobic metabolism is not corrected, the cells will eventually die. To support sufficient production of ATP and, therefore, aerobic internal respiration, adequate perfusion (circulation of blood within an organ or tissue) and ventilation must be present. Although perfusion and ventilation are necessary for internal respiration, they do not guarantee that aerobic internal respiration will occur.

When the mitochondria within each cell use oxygen to convert glucose to energy, carbon dioxide—the main waste product—accumulates in the cell. Carbon dioxide is then transported through the circulatory system and back to the lungs for exhalation.

Without oxygen, anaerobic metabolism creates a series of events that will eventually lead to cellular death. Initially, cells become hypoxic, and as stores of glucose are depleted, lactic acid, which is the by-product of glycolysis, remains. The increased acidic environment destroys the cellular proteins, in turn leading to cellular death and infarction of tissue as more cells become ischemic and then necrotic.

Understanding the processes of ventilation, oxygenation, and respiration is important for paramedics. The overall goal of these mechanisms is to provide an adequate supply of oxygen to the cells of the body. When one of these processes fails or becomes disrupted, cells will die. Figure 16 summarizes barriers to proper ventilation, oxygenation, and respiration, which will be helpful to remember when assessing and treating patients. By recognizing the signs and symptoms of inadequate tissue perfusion and oxygenation, you can immediately intervene and correct a potentially life-threatening condition.

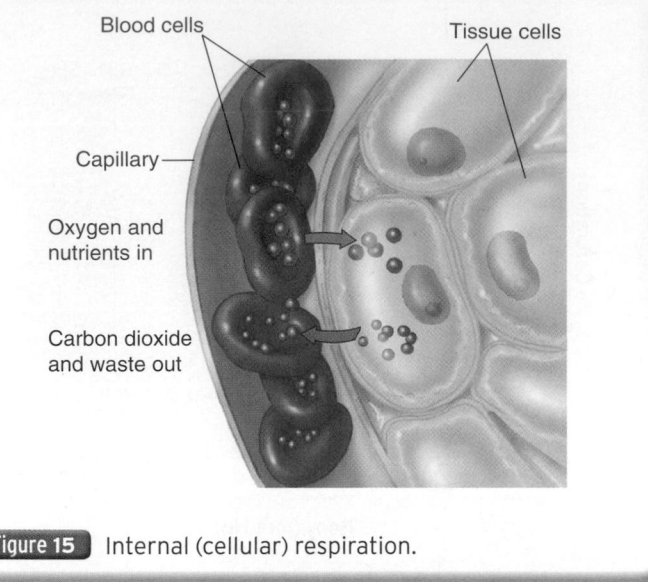

Figure 15 Internal (cellular) respiration.

YOU are the Medic   PART 2

You arrive at the scene and determine that it is safe to enter the residence. You find the patient sitting on the couch, leaning forward, in obvious distress. He is conscious and alert, but anxious, and speaks to you in broken sentences. His skin is notably pale and diaphoretic. His wife tells you that he suddenly began experiencing breathing difficulty about 20 minutes ago and that he had been fine all day. As you complete your primary assessment, your partner gives the patient high-flow oxygen via a nonrebreathing mask.

Recording Time: 1 Minute	
Appearance	Anxious, diaphoretic
Level of consciousness	Alert (oriented to person, place, and day)
Airway	Open; clear of secretions or foreign bodies
Breathing	Rapid and labored; accessory muscle use; preferential positioning
Circulation	Radial pulses, rapid and weak; skin, pale and diaphoretic

3. Is this patient maintaining his own airway spontaneously?

4. How should you proceed with your assessment of this patient?

Definition	Barriers
Ventilation	
• The physical act of moving air into and out of the lungs	• Chest trauma (impaired muscles: diaphragm, intercostal muscles, or accessory muscles; damage to airway structures) • Burns (impaired airflow into trachea) • Head or spine trauma (damage to respiratory centers) • Neck trauma (physical damage to airway structures) • Medications that depress the central nervous system • Airway obstruction (physical blockage of airway by any substance—foreign body; tongue; fluid; tissue; swelling from allergic reaction, infection, or asthma) • Bronchoconstriction (from allergic reaction, infection, asthma) • Respiratory disease • Cardiac disease • Neuromuscular disorders • Hypoventilation • Hyperventilation
Oxygenation	
• The process of loading oxygen molecules onto hemoglobin molecules in the bloodstream	• Carbon monoxide (prevents oxygen from binding to hemoglobin) • High altitude (insufficient oxygen in the environment) • Confined space (insufficient oxygen in the environment) • Mine (insufficient oxygen in the environment)
Respiration	
• The exchange of oxygen and carbon dioxide in the alveoli and the tissues of the body	• Anaerobic metabolism • Hypoglycemia • Circulatory compromise (blood loss, pulmonary embolism, pneumothorax, hemothorax, hemopneumothorax) • Anemia

Figure 16 Ventilation, oxygenation, and respiration are required for oxygen to reach the tissues. If any of these functions does not occur, the patient will receive insufficient oxygen. Barriers to each of these functions are listed in this figure.

Pathophysiology of Respiration

Multiple conditions can inhibit the body's ability to effectively provide oxygen to the cells. Disruption of pulmonary ventilation, oxygenation, and respiration will cause immediate effects on the body. As a paramedic, you must recognize these conditions and correct them immediately. It is important to be able to distinguish a primary ventilation problem from a primary oxygenation or respiration problem. For example, overdose of a CNS depressant drug (ie, narcotic/opiate, barbiturate) has a negative effect on respiratory rate and depth (tidal volume), and causes, at least initially, a ventilation problem. If ventilation is impaired, adequate oxygen will not be taken into the lungs and distributed to the cells and tissues of the body. By contrast, a person trapped in a place that is devoid of oxygen may develop an oxygenation problem first; he or she is ventilating adequately,

but is not breathing in adequate amounts of oxygen. As a result, oxygen delivery to the cells and tissues will be compromised, resulting in a respiration problem.

Every cell in the body needs a constant supply of oxygen to survive. Whereas some tissues are more resilient than others, eventually all cells will die if deprived of oxygen **Figure 17**. To provide adequate amounts of oxygen to the tissues of the body, sufficient levels of external respiration and perfusion—circulation of blood within an organ or tissue in adequate amounts to meet the cells' current needs—must take place.

Hypoxia

Failure to meet the body's needs for oxygen may result in hypoxia. <u>Hypoxia</u> is a dangerous condition in which the tissues and cells do not receive enough oxygen. If hypoxia is uncorrected, death may occur quickly.

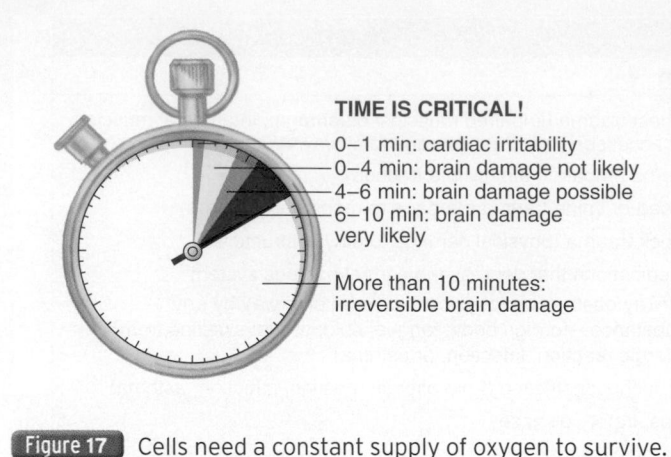

TIME IS CRITICAL!

0–1 min: cardiac irritability

0–4 min: brain damage not likely

4–6 min: brain damage possible

6–10 min: brain damage very likely

More than 10 minutes: irreversible brain damage

Figure 17 Cells need a constant supply of oxygen to survive. Some cells may be severely or permanently damaged after 4 to 6 minutes without oxygen.

Patients who are breathing inadequately will show varying signs and symptoms of hypoxia. The onset and degree of tissue damage caused by hypoxia often depend on the quality of ventilations. Early signs of hypoxia include restlessness, irritability, apprehension, tachycardia, and anxiety. Late signs of hypoxia include mental status changes, a weak (thready) pulse, and cyanosis. Responsive patients often report a feeling of shortness of breath (**dyspnea**) and may not be able to speak in complete sentences. The best time to give a patient oxygen is before the signs and symptoms of hypoxia appear.

Ventilation-Perfusion Ratio and Mismatch

The lungs have a functional role in placing ambient (room) air in proximity to circulating blood to permit gas exchange by simple diffusion. To accomplish this, air and blood flow must be directed to the same place at the same time. In other words, ventilation and perfusion must be matched. A failure to match ventilation and perfusion, or **V̇/Q̇ mismatch**, lies behind most abnormalities in oxygen and carbon dioxide exchange.

In most people, the normal resting minute ventilation is approximately 6 L/min. About one third of this volume fills dead space; therefore, resting alveolar volume is approximately 4 L/min. However, pulmonary artery blood flow is approximately 5 L/min, yielding an overall ratio of ventilation to perfusion of 4:5 L/min, or 0.8 L/min. Because neither ventilation nor perfusion is distributed equally, both are distributed to dependent regions of the lungs at rest. However, an increase in gravity-dependent flow is more marked with perfusion (blood) than with ventilation (air). Hence, the ratio of ventilation to perfusion is highest at the apex of the lung and lowest at the base.

When ventilation is compromised but perfusion continues, blood passes over some alveolar membranes without gas exchange taking place; therefore, not all alveoli are enriched with oxygen. The result is a lack of oxygen diffusing across the membrane and into the circulatory system. Along the same lines, carbon dioxide is also unable to diffuse across the membrane and is recirculated into the bloodstream. This condition results in a V̇/Q̇ mismatch and could lead to severe hypoxemia if the problem is not recognized and treated.

Similar problems can occur when perfusion across the alveolar membrane is disrupted. Even though the alveoli are filled with fresh oxygen, disruption in blood flow does not allow for optimal exchange of gases across the membrane. The result of inadequate perfusion is less oxygen absorption in the bloodstream and less carbon dioxide removal. This V̇/Q̇ mismatch can also lead to hypoxemia, and the patient needs immediate intervention to prevent further damage or death.

Factors Affecting Ventilation

Maintaining a patent airway is critical for the provision of oxygen to the tissues of the body. There are many intrinsic (internal) and extrinsic (external) factors that can cause airway obstruction. Intrinsic conditions such as infection, allergic reactions, and unresponsiveness (possibly leading to airway obstruction by the tongue) can significantly restrict the ability to maintain a patent airway. Swelling from infections and allergic reactions can be fatal if not aggressively managed with medications and, possibly, advanced airway management techniques. The tongue is the most common airway obstruction in an unresponsive patient. This airway obstruction, while easily corrected, can result in hypoxia and hinder adequate tissue perfusion. Snoring respirations and an improper position of the head and/or neck are good indicators that the tongue may be obstructing the airway. Prompt correction of this obstruction is necessary for adequate ventilation and oxygenation.

Some factors affecting pulmonary ventilation are not necessarily directly part of the respiratory system. The central and peripheral nervous systems have key roles in the regulation of breathing. Interruptions in these systems can have a drastic effect on the ability to breathe effectively. Medications that depress the central nervous system (such as opiates or opioids and benzodiazepines), if taken in excess, lower the respiratory rate and reduce the tidal volume. This lower rate and tidal volume will decrease alveolar volume and overall minute volume. As a result, the amount of carbon dioxide in the respiratory and circulatory systems is increased, resulting in an overall increase of the carbon dioxide content of the blood. Trauma to the head and spinal cord can also interrupt nervous control of ventilation, resulting in decreased respiratory function and even failure. Neuromuscular disorders, such as muscular dystrophy and poliomyelitis, can also affect the nervous system's control of breathing. Muscular dystrophy causes degeneration of muscle fibers, slowing motor development, and loss of muscle contractility. Curvature of the spine is also likely in patients with muscular dystrophy and can impair pulmonary function. Poliomyelitis is a viral neuromuscular disorder that can affect the nerves, including those that regulate ventilation, and result in paralysis. Neuromuscular blocking agents (paralytics), such as those used to facilitate intubation, effectively paralyze a patient and induce apnea.

Patients with allergic reactions might have not only a potential airway obstruction due to swelling (angioedema), but also a decrease in pulmonary ventilation from bronchoconstriction.

As the bronchioles constrict, air is forced through smaller lumens, resulting in decreased ventilation. Bronchoconstriction is also associated with conditions such as COPD and asthma.

Extrinsic factors affecting pulmonary ventilation can include trauma and foreign body airway obstruction. Trauma to the airway or chest requires immediate evaluation and intervention. Blunt or penetrating trauma and burns can disrupt airflow through the trachea and into the lungs, quickly resulting in oxygenation deficiencies. In addition, trauma to the chest wall can result in structural damage to the thorax, leading to inadequate pulmonary ventilation. For example, a patient with numerous rib fractures or a flail chest may purposely breathe shallowly in an attempt to alleviate the pain caused by the injury; this is called respiratory splinting and can result in decreased pulmonary ventilation. Proper ventilatory support is crucial to the outcome of patients with such injuries or conditions.

If carbon dioxide production exceeds the body's ability to eliminate it by ventilation, the partial pressure of carbon dioxide ($Paco_2$) rises, resulting in **hypoventilation**. Theoretically, hypoventilation can occur in two ways: carbon dioxide production can exceed the body's ability to eliminate it, or carbon dioxide elimination can be depressed to the extent that it no longer keeps up with normal metabolism.

At the other extreme is **hyperventilation**, which occurs when carbon dioxide elimination exceeds carbon dioxide production. For example, patients experiencing an anxiety attack tend to breathe very deeply and rapidly, so they eliminate carbon dioxide at a rate faster than their body produces it. The level of carbon dioxide in their blood then falls below normal, and they experience symptoms such as dizziness and numbness or tingling in the face and extremities.

In addition to factors discussed thus far, decreases or increases in minute volume can lead to problems with carbon dioxide levels in the blood (Table 2). A decrease in the minute volume decreases carbon dioxide elimination, resulting in a buildup of carbon dioxide in the blood (**hypercarbia**). An increase in the minute volume increases carbon dioxide elimination, which lowers the carbon dioxide content of the blood (**hypocarbia**).

■ Factors Affecting Oxygenation and Respiration

External elements in the environment can affect the overall process of respiration. For proper respiration to occur at the cellular level, oxygenation and perfusion must function efficiently.

External Factors

Adequate respiration requires proper ventilation and oxygenation. External factors such as atmospheric pressure and the partial pressure of oxygen in the ambient air have a key role in the overall process of respiration. At high altitudes, the percentage of oxygen remains the same, but the partial pressure decreases because the total atmospheric pressure decreases. The low partial pressure of oxygen can make it difficult—or impossible—to adequately oxygenate the tissues, thus interrupting internal respiration. In addition, closed environments, such as mines and trenches, may also have decreases in ambient oxygen, resulting in poor oxygenation and respiration.

Carbon monoxide, along with other toxic gases, displaces oxygen in the environment and makes proper oxygenation and respiration difficult. In particular, CO has a much greater affinity for hemoglobin than does oxygen (250 times more). The attachment of CO molecules to the hemoglobin molecules, which forms carboxyhemoglobin (COHb), inhibits the proper transport of oxygen to the tissues and can cause false pulse oximetry readings.

Internal Factors

Conditions that reduce the surface area for gas exchange also decrease the body's oxygen supply, leading to inadequate tissue perfusion. Medical conditions such as pneumonia, pulmonary edema, and COPD may also result in a disturbance of cellular metabolism. These conditions decrease the surface area of the alveoli by damaging the alveoli or by leading to an accumulation of fluid in the lungs.

Nonfunctional alveoli inhibit the diffusion of oxygen and carbon dioxide. As a result, blood entering the lungs from the right side of the heart bypasses the alveoli and returns to the left side of the heart in an unoxygenated state—a condition called **intrapulmonary shunting**.

Submersion (previously called near drowning) victims and patients with pulmonary edema have fluid in the alveoli. This accumulation of fluid inhibits adequate gas exchange at the alveolar membrane and results in decreased oxygenation and respiration. In addition, exposure to certain environmental conditions (such as high altitudes) or occupational hazards (such as epoxy resins) can result in fluid accumulation in the alveoli over time, resulting in an overall decrease in respiration. These conditions can result in anaerobic respiration and an increase in lactic acid accumulation. Excess lactic acid in the blood lowers the pH and can result in numerous life-threatening conditions, such as cardiac dysrhythmias, coma, and shock.

Other conditions that affect the cells of the body include hypoglycemia, hormonal imbalances, and infection. As oxygen and glucose levels decrease, the body is unable to maintain a homeostatic balance with regard to energy production. If the metabolic needs of the body cannot be met, cellular death is likely. Infection also increases the metabolic needs of the body and disrupts homeostasis. If the disruption in homeostasis is not corrected, the cells will die as well. If the levels of the hormone insulin decrease in the body, the cellular uptake of glucose will decrease. Without sufficient glucose, the cells will metabolize fatty acids, resulting in ketoacidosis—a form of metabolic acidosis.

Table 2 Carbon Dioxide Balance

	Hypoventilation	Hyperventilation
Minute volume	↓	↑
CO_2 elimination	↓	↑
$Paco_2$	↑ (hypercarbia)	↓ (hypocarbia)

Circulatory Compromise

As mentioned, the circulatory system must function efficiently for respiration to occur. When the circulatory system is compromised, perfusion becomes inadequate and the body's oxygen demands will not be met.

Obstruction of blood flow to individual cells and tissues is typically related to trauma emergencies that paramedics may encounter. These conditions include simple or tension pneumothorax, open pneumothorax (sucking chest wound), hemothorax, hemopneumothorax, and pulmonary embolism. All of these conditions inhibit gas exchange at the tissue level as a result of their effects on the respiratory and circulatory systems. In addition, conditions such as heart failure and cardiac tamponade inhibit the ability of the heart to effectively pump oxygenated blood to the tissues.

Blood loss and anemia—a deficiency of red blood cells—reduce the oxygen-carrying ability of the blood. Without sufficient circulating red blood cells, there are not enough hemoglobin molecules available to bind with oxygen.

When the body is in a state of shock, oxygen is not delivered to the cells efficiently. Hemorrhagic shock (a form of hypovolemic shock) is an abnormal decrease in blood volume, because of bleeding, that causes inadequate oxygen delivery to the body. In contrast, vasodilatory shock is not caused by a decrease in blood volume, but by an increase in the size of the blood vessels. As the diameter of the blood vessels increases, the blood pressure decreases and blood flow diminishes; oxygen is not delivered to the tissues in an effective manner. Both forms of shock result in poor tissue perfusion that leads to anaerobic metabolism. Any patient suspected of being in shock should be treated aggressively to prevent further interruptions in tissue perfusion.

■ Acid-Base Balance

Hypoventilation and hyperventilation, along with hypoxia, can cause disruptions in the acid-base balance in the body that may lead to rapid deterioration in a patient's condition and death. The respiratory system and the renal system have roles in maintaining homeostasis. Homeostasis is the tendency toward stability in the body's internal environment and requires a balance between the acids and bases. When there is an excess of acid in the body, the fastest way to eliminate it is through the respiratory system. Excess acid can be expelled as carbon dioxide from the lungs. Conversely, slowing respirations will increase the level of carbon dioxide. The renal system regulates pH by filtering out more hydrogen and retaining bicarbonate when needed, or doing the reverse. The fastest way the body can eliminate excess H^+ ions is to create water and carbon dioxide, which can be expelled as gases from the lungs.

Anything that inhibits respiratory function can lead to acid retention and acidosis. Any time a patient is in respiratory distress or is unable to breathe, acidosis quickly develops. Acidosis can develop as a result of abnormal respiratory function (as with bradypnea, tachypnea, labored breathing, or shallow breathing [reduced tidal volume]). Alkalosis can also develop if the respiratory rate is too high (or the volume too much).

There are four main clinical presentations of acid-base disorders:

- Respiratory acidosis
- Respiratory alkalosis
- Metabolic acidosis
- Metabolic alkalosis

Fluctuations in pH due to the available bicarbonate in the body result in metabolic acidosis or alkalosis, whereas fluctuations in pH due to respiratory disorders result in respiratory acidosis or alkalosis. The focus here is on respiratory acidosis and respiratory alkalosis.

Acid-base disorders that are not immediately correctable by the body's buffering systems cause the body to initiate compensatory mechanisms to help return levels to normal. For example, metabolic acidosis may create respiratory alkalosis as a compensatory response. Patient management often involves treating more than one form of acid-base imbalance.

Words of Wisdom

The Effects of Ventilation on Cardiac Output

During normal breathing, the negative pressure created by each breath increases venous return of blood to the heart. Just as negative intrathoracic pressure draws air into the chest cavity through the airway, the same pressure also draws venous blood back to the heart from the head (via the superior vena cava) and abdomen (via the inferior vena cava).

When patients transition from negative-pressure ventilation to positive-pressure ventilation (such as when they are being ventilated with a bag-mask device), they lose this stimulus for venous return, and some patients may experience decreased cardiac output and hypotension as a result. The increased intrathoracic pressure caused by positive-pressure ventilation creates a pressure gradient against which the heart must pump. This increases the afterload (the amount of resistance against which the ventricle must contract), which can further decrease cardiac output. The greater the pressure used to ventilate an apneic or a hypoventilating patient, the greater the decrease in preload (the volume of blood that returns to the heart), which occurs when the heart is literally squeezed by increased intrathoracic pressure.

Patients who are hypotensive, in shock, or otherwise in hemodynamically unstable condition may experience profound changes in blood pressure as a result of the hemodynamic effects of positive-pressure ventilation. The best way to minimize this complication is to ventilate the patient for a period of 1 second–just enough to cause visible chest rise–and avoid ventilating the patient too fast.

■ Patient Assessment: Airway Evaluation

The importance of carefully assessing a patient's airway and ventilatory status cannot be overemphasized. In the field, you will encounter patients with a variety of airway problems—some of these problems are easily corrected; others require aggressive management. *The care you provide to a patient with an airway or ventilation problem is only as good as the assessment you perform.*

Recognizing Adequate Breathing

An adult who is responsive, alert, and able to speak in complete sentences with a normal voice has no *immediate* airway or breathing problems. Normal breathing in an adult at rest is characterized by a rate between 12 and 20 breaths/min Table 3 with adequate depth (tidal volume), a regular pattern of inhalation and exhalation, and clear and equal breath sounds bilaterally. Breathing at rest should appear effortless, and changes in rate and regularity should be *subtle*—not obvious.

Recognizing Inadequate Breathing

Any patient you encounter—especially one with a respiratory complaint—should be assessed for breathing adequacy. Just because a patient is breathing does not indicate that he or she is breathing *adequately*. Generally speaking, if you can see or hear a patient breathe, there is a problem.

An adult patient who presents with respiratory distress and is breathing at a rate of less than 12 breaths/min or more than 20 breaths/min must be evaluated for other signs of inadequate ventilation, such as shallow breathing (reduced tidal volume), an irregular pattern of breathing, altered mentation, and **adventitious** (abnormal) airway sounds. **Cyanosis**—a blue or purple skin color—is a clear indicator of a low blood oxygen content.

Patients with respiratory distress often compensate with preferential positioning, such as an upright sniffing (tripod) position, or a semi-Fowler (semisitting) position. Patients experiencing respiratory distress will avoid a supine position because it will worsen their breathing difficulty.

The potential causes of respiratory distress and inadequate ventilation are numerous and include severe infection (sepsis), trauma, brainstem insult, a noxious or oxygen-poor environment, and renal failure. Respiratory distress may be the result of an upper and/or lower airway obstruction, respiratory muscle impairment (as in spinal cord injury), or central nervous system impairment (as in head injury and drug overdose).

Words of Wisdom

Hypoxemia is defined as a low level of oxygen in arterial blood. Hypoxia, as discussed earlier, is a deficiency of oxygen at the tissue and cellular levels. Although these terms are often used interchangeably, *they are different processes*. Hypoxemia can be reversed by administering supplemental oxygen, whereas hypoxia requires more aggressive oxygenation and, in some cases, ventilatory support. Left untreated, hypoxia will lead to **anoxia**—a lack of oxygen that results in tissue and cellular death.

Table 3 Normal Respiratory Rate Ranges

Adults	12 to 20 breaths/min
Children	15 to 30 breaths/min
Infants	25 to 50 breaths/min

If a patient's airway is not patent, or if breathing is absent or inadequate, all therapies that you may attempt will prove futile. Proper airway management involves opening the airway, clearing the airway, assessing breathing, and providing the appropriate intervention(s)—in that order.

Evaluation of a patient with a respiratory complaint includes visual observations, palpation, and auscultation. Visual techniques should be used at first sight of the patient—literally from the door as you enter the room. The following questions should be answered when assessing a patient with respiratory distress:

- How is the patient positioned? Is he or she in a tripod position (elbows out)?
- Is the patient experiencing **orthopnea** (positional dyspnea)?
- Is rise and fall of the chest adequate (adequate tidal volume)?
- Is the patient gasping for air (air hunger)?
- What is the skin color? Is the skin moist or clammy (diaphoretic)?
- Is there flaring of the nostrils?
- Is the patient breathing through pursed lips?
- Do you note any **retractions** (skin pulling between and around the ribs during inhalation):
  - Intercostal?
  - At the suprasternal notch?
  - At the supraclavicular fossa?
  - Subcostal?
- Is the patient using accessory muscles to breathe?
- Is the patient's chest wall moving symmetrically? (**Asymmetric chest wall movement**, when one side of the chest moves less than the other, indicates that airflow into one lung is decreased.)
- Is the patient taking a series of quick breaths, followed by a prolonged exhalation phase?

A patient with inadequate ventilation may appear to be working hard to breathe (labored breathing). Labored breathing requires effort and may involve the use of accessory muscles. Accessory muscles include the sternocleidomastoid muscles (neck muscles), the chest pectoralis major muscles, and the abdominal muscles.

Accessory muscles are not used during normal breathing. Signs of inadequate ventilation in adults include the following:

- Respiratory rate of fewer than 12 breaths/min or more than 20 breaths/min in the presence of dyspnea
- Irregular rhythm, such as taking a series of deep breaths followed by periods of apnea
- Diminished, absent, or noisy auscultated breath sounds
- Abdominal breathing
- Reduced flow of exhaled air at the nose and mouth
- Unequal or inadequate chest expansion, resulting in reduced tidal volume
- Increased effort of breathing—use of accessory muscles
- Shallow depth of breathing (reduced tidal volume)
- Skin that is pale, cyanotic, cool, moist (clammy), or mottled
- Retractions
- Staccato speech patterns (one- or two-word dyspnea)

When you are assessing a patient with respiratory distress, consider the external environment, such as high altitude and enclosed spaces, which can be associated with impaired oxygenation. Do not forget personal safety if the environment is unsafe.

Feel for air movement at the nose and mouth. Observe the chest for symmetry, and note any **paradoxical motion**—the inward movement of a segment of the chest during inhalation and outward movement of the chest during exhalation, opposite normal chest movement and an indication of a flail chest. Assess for **pulsus paradoxus**. Pulsus paradoxus is a clinical finding in which the systolic blood pressure drops more than 10 mm Hg during inhalation. A change in pulse quality, or even the disappearance of a pulse during inhalation, may also be detected. Pulsus paradoxus is generally seen in patients with decompensating COPD, severe pericardial tamponade, or other conditions that cause an increase in intrathoracic pressure (such as tension pneumothorax and a severe asthma attack).

A history of the present illness is a vital part of your assessment of a patient with respiratory distress. You should ask questions to determine the evolution of the current problem:

- Was the onset of the problem sudden or gradual?
  - Some people may perceive respiratory distress that occurred 2 days earlier as arising gradually, when, in fact, the onset was sudden; the patient may have waited 2 days before calling for help.
- Is there any known cause or "trigger" of the event?
  - Asthma is commonly exacerbated by stress or cold weather. A foreign body airway obstruction is commonly preceded by a sudden onset of difficulty in breathing during a meal or, in children, while playing with small toys or other objects.
- What is the duration (is it constant or recurrent)?
- Does anything alleviate or exacerbate the problem?
- Are there any other associated symptoms, such as a productive cough (if yes, what color is the sputum?), chest pain or pressure, or fever?
- Were any interventions attempted before EMS arrival?
- Has the patient been evaluated by a physician or admitted to the hospital for this condition in the past?
  - Determine specifically whether the patient was hospitalized or seen in the emergency department and then released. If the patient was hospitalized, ask whether he or she was admitted to an intensive care unit or a regular, unmonitored floor. A condition that warranted an intensive care unit admission is clinically significant.
- Is the patient currently taking any medications?
  - Do not simply ask which medications were taken today. Instead, determine the *overall* compliance by asking whether the patient has been taking the medications as prescribed. Ask "Have you been able to take all of your pills as directed?" "Is there anything that has stopped you from taking your pills as directed, such as running out of some of the pills?" "Is there something that bothers you about taking a certain pill?" Verify this information by looking at the prescription date on the medication bottle(s) and by reading the prescription directions.

- Ask whether the patient has had any changes in his or her current prescription, such as a new medication or changes in the prescribing directions of an existing medication.
- Does the patient have any risk factors that could cause or exacerbate his or her condition, such as alcohol or illicit drug use, cigarette smoking, or an inadequate diet?

Evaluate the patient for protective reflexes of the airway. These include coughing, sneezing, and gagging. A patient whose cough mechanism is suppressed—whether by drugs, by pain, by trauma, or by any other cause—is at serious risk of aspirating foreign material. Sneezing is usually elicited by irritation of the nose.

The **gag reflex** is a spastic pharyngeal and esophageal reflex caused by stimulation of the posterior pharynx to prevent foreign bodies from entering the trachea. The **eyelash reflex** is a fairly reliable indicator of the presence or absence of an intact gag reflex in an unresponsive patient **Figure 18**. If the patient's lower eyelid contracts when you gently stroke the upper eyelashes, he or she probably has an intact gag reflex.

Sighing is a slow, deep inhalation followed by a prolonged and sometimes quite audible exhalation. Sighing periodically hyperinflates the lungs, thereby reexpanding atelectatic (collapsed) alveoli. The average person sighs about once per minute. Hiccuping is a sudden inhalation, due to spasmodic contraction of the diaphragm, cut short by closure of the glottis. Hiccuping serves no physiologic purpose, although persistent hiccups may be clinically significant.

Patients with serious injuries or illness may present with changes in their respiratory pattern. **Table 4** shows various abnormal respiratory patterns and their causes.

■ Assessment of Breath Sounds

While you are assessing breathing, auscultate breath sounds with a stethoscope. They should be clear and equal on both sides of the chest (bilaterally), anteriorly, and posteriorly. Compare

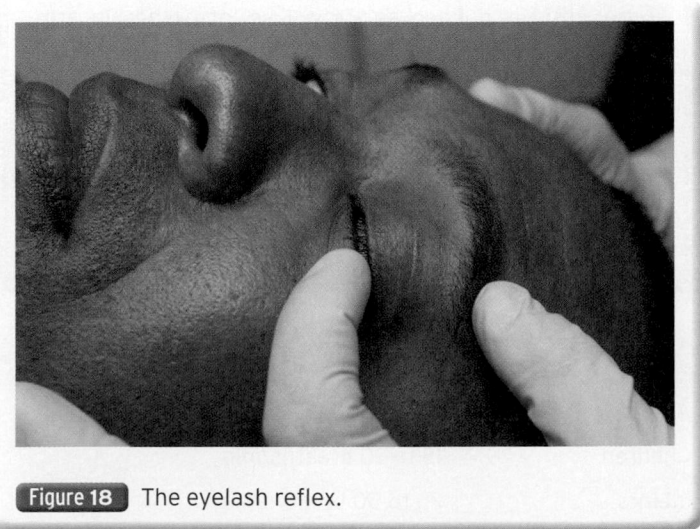

Figure 18 The eyelash reflex.

each apex (top) of the lung with the opposite apex and each base (bottom) of the lung with the opposite base.

Breath sounds are created as air moves through the tracheobronchial tree. The size of the airway determines the type

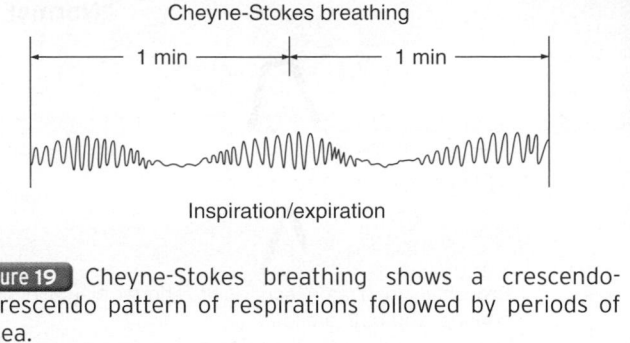

Figure 19 Cheyne-Stokes breathing shows a crescendo-decrescendo pattern of respirations followed by periods of apnea.

Table 4	Abnormal Respiratory Patterns
Cheyne-Stokes respirations	Gradually increasing rate and depth of respirations followed by a gradual decrease of respirations with intermittent periods of apnea; associated with brainstem insult **Figure 19**.
Kussmaul respirations	Deep, rapid respirations; seen in patients with diabetic ketoacidosis.
Biot (ataxic) respirations	Irregular pattern, rate, and depth of breathing with intermittent periods of apnea; results from increased intracranial pressure.
Apneustic respirations	Prolonged, gasping inhalation followed by extremely short, ineffective exhalation; associated with brainstem insult.
Agonal gasps	Slow, shallow, irregular, or occasional gasping breaths; results from cerebral anoxia. Agonal gasps may be seen when the heart has stopped but the brain continues to send signals to the muscles of respiration. This is not considered a form of respiration.

of sound that will be produced. There are significant differences in adult, child, and infant airways, resulting in differences in breath sounds. The trachea and bronchi have large diameters; therefore, the sound produced is higher pitched and is heard during inspiration and expiration. Breath sounds are heard over the majority of the chest, representing airflow into the alveoli. **Tracheal breath sounds**, also called bronchial breath sounds, are heard by placing the stethoscope diaphragm over the trachea or over the sternum. Assess breath sounds for duration, pitch, and intensity. **Vesicular breath sounds** are softer, muffled sounds and have been described as wind blowing through the trees. The expiratory phase is barely audible. **Bronchovesicular sounds** are a combination of the two and are heard in places where airways and alveoli are found—the upper part of the sternum and between the scapulae. Locations for these sounds are shown in **Figure 20**. **Figure 21** describes the normal breath sounds. Bronchovesicular sounds should be assessed for duration, pitch, and intensity.

Duration refers to the length of time for the inspiratory and expiratory phase of the breath. Normally, expiration is at least twice as long as inspiration. This relationship is expressed by the **I/E ratio** (inspiratory/expiratory ratio); a normal I/E ratio is 1:2. When a patient's lower airway is obstructed and he or she has difficulty getting air out (as in asthma, for example), the expiratory phase is prolonged and may be four to five times as long as

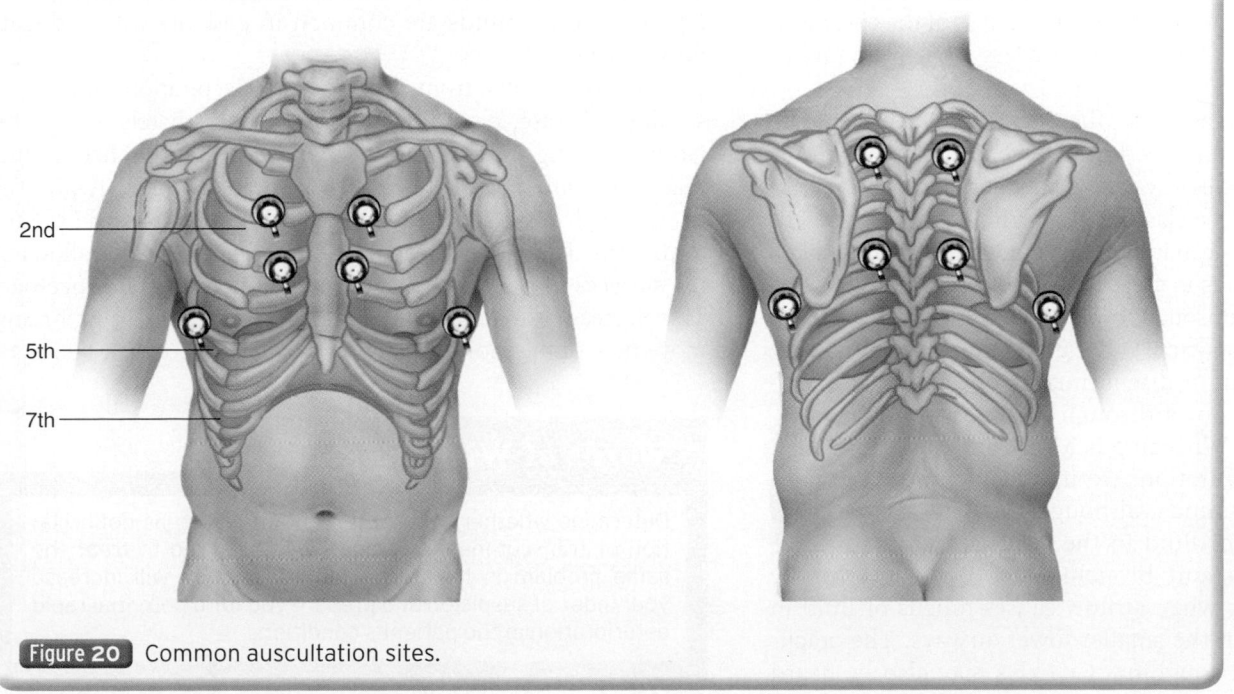

Figure 20 Common auscultation sites.

2nd
5th
7th

"Normal" Breath Sounds

Tracheal. Inspiratory and expiratory sounds are both loud.

Bronchial. Inspiratory sounds are shorter than expiratory sounds, and both are loud.

Bronchovesicular. Inspiratory and expiratory sounds are about the same, and of medium intensity.

Vesicular. Inspiratory sounds last longer than expiratory sounds, and both are faint.

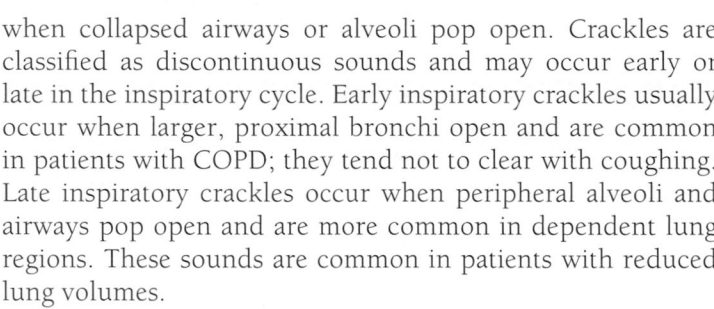

The thickness of the bars shows intensity (loudness) of the breath, and slope correlates with pitch (steeper slope, higher pitch).

Figure 21 Normal breath sounds are heard over different parts of the chest. Breath sounds become softer away from the largest airways. The character during inspiration versus expiration also changes.

inspiration; in this case, the I/E ratio would be 1:4 or 1:5. In patients who are tachypneic, the expiratory phase is short and approaches that of inspiration; in this case, the I/E ratio may be 1:1.

Pitch is described as higher or lower than normal, as in stridor or wheezing. The intensity of sound depends on airflow rate, constancy of flow throughout inspiration, patient position, and the site selected for auscultation. Thickness of the chest wall may affect the intensity. Sounds that are less intense are said to be diminished.

A common error in assessing the intensity of breath sounds occurs when auscultation is performed over the patient's clothing. Always auscultate directly on the patient's skin.

Sounds that might be classified as normal—but are present in an unexpected area—can indicate an abnormal condition. For example, tracheal sounds in areas that should produce vesicular sounds may indicate consolidation or pneumonia.

Adventitious (abnormal) breath sounds are usually classified as continuous or discontinuous. **Wheezing** is a continuous sound as air flows through a constricted lower airway, as with asthma. Wheezing is a high-pitched sound that may be heard on inspiration, expiration, or both. **Rhonchi** are also continuous sounds, although they are low-pitched; they indicate mucus or fluid in the larger lower airways (as in pulmonary edema and bronchitis). **Crackles** (formerly known as rales) occur when airflow causes mucus or fluid in the airways to move in the smaller lower airways. The crackles tend to clear with coughing. Crackles may also be heard

when collapsed airways or alveoli pop open. Crackles are classified as discontinuous sounds and may occur early or late in the inspiratory cycle. Early inspiratory crackles usually occur when larger, proximal bronchi open and are common in patients with COPD; they tend not to clear with coughing. Late inspiratory crackles occur when peripheral alveoli and airways pop open and are more common in dependent lung regions. These sounds are common in patients with reduced lung volumes.

Stridor results from foreign body aspiration, infection, swelling, disease, or trauma within or immediately above the glottic opening. Stridor produces a loud, high-pitched sound that is typically heard during the inspiration phase. A **pleural friction rub** results from inflammation that causes the pleura to thicken. The pleural space can decrease as a result, allowing the surfaces of the visceral and parietal pleura to rub together. This decrease often creates stabbing pain with breathing or any movement of the thorax.

Words of Wisdom

Determine whether other interventions (such as defibrillation or transcutaneous pacing) were required to treat the same problem in the past. This information will increase your index of suspicion and prepare you for a potential rapid deterioration in the patient's condition.

Quantifying Ventilation and Oxygenation

In addition to your hands-on assessment of the patient with an airway or breathing problem, several methods and devices are used to quantify—that is, assign a numeric value to—ventilation and oxygenation.

Pulse Oximetry

Pulse oximetry is a simple, rapid, safe, and noninvasive method of measuring—minute by minute—how well a person's hemoglobin is saturated.

A **pulse oximeter** measures the percentage of **hemoglobin (Hb)** in the arterial blood that is saturated with oxygen Figure 22 . Under normal circumstances, hemoglobin is saturated with oxygen (Sp_{O_2}). A sensor probe, clipped to the patient's finger or earlobe, uses a light-emitting diode (LED) to transmit light through the vascular bed to a light-sensing detector. The amount of light transmitted across the vascular bed depends on the proportion of hemoglobin that is saturated with oxygen. To ensure that the instrument is measuring arterial and not venous oxygen saturation, pulse oximeters are designed to assess only pulsating blood vessels. As a consequence, they also measure the patient's pulse. One way to check the functioning of a pulse oximeter is to compare the pulse reading it provides with your own measurement of the patient's pulse by palpation. Refer to the manufacturer's instructions for the device being used.

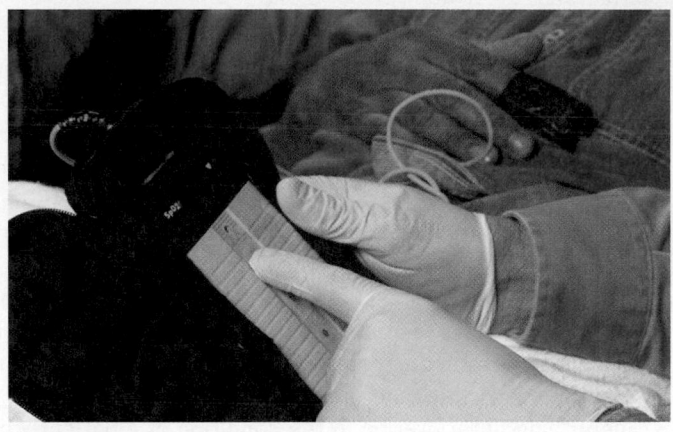

Figure 22   Pulse oximetry is a noninvasive method of assessing arterial oxygen saturation (Sp_{O_2}).

A normally oxygenated, normally perfused person should have an Sp_{O_2} of greater than 95% while breathing room air. A reading of less than 95% in a nonsmoker suggests hypoxemia; a reading of less than 90% signals a need for aggressive oxygen therapy.

YOU *are the Medic*   PART 3

The patient's breath sounds are diminished bilaterally, but otherwise equal. Your partner obtains the patient's vital signs and attaches the cardiac monitor, which reveals sinus tachycardia. Your partner removes the nonrebreathing mask, applies an $ETCO_2$ nasal cannula, and reapplies the nonrebreathing mask. An $ETCO_2$ of 49 mm Hg is noted and documented.

The patient's wife tells you that her husband has congestive heart failure and high blood pressure and has experienced two heart attacks in the past. He also has esophageal cancer and just completed his last round of chemotherapy and radiation therapy 2 days ago. She hands your partner a list of the patient's medications. The patient remains conscious and alert but is still experiencing significant respiratory distress. His oral temperature reads 97.9°F.

Recording Time: 5 Minutes	
Respirations	26 breaths/min; labored
Pulse	120 beats/min; weak
Skin	Pale and diaphoretic
Blood pressure	128/70 mm Hg
Sp_{O_2}	90% (on oxygen)
$ETCO_2$	49 mm Hg
ECG	Sinus tachycardia

5. What information have you learned from the patient's $ETCO_2$ and pulse oximetry readings?

6. Is there a correlation between $ETCO_2$ and Pa_{CO_2}? If so, what is it?

Situations in which pulse oximeters may be useful in prehospital emergency care include the following:

- **Monitoring the oxygenation status of a patient during an intubation attempt or during suctioning.** The low-saturation alarm on the pulse oximeter can signal that the paramedic should abort the intubation attempt and ventilate the patient.
- **Identifying deterioration in the condition of a trauma victim.** In a patient with multiple trauma, the signs of a developing tension pneumothorax, for example, may not be evident until the problem is quite advanced. A declining SpO_2 level can alert a paramedic that something bad is happening and prompt a search for the cause of the problem.
- **Identifying deterioration in the condition of a patient with cardiac disease.** Pulse oximetry may enable early identification of patients who are experiencing congestive heart failure in the wake of a myocardial infarction.
- **Identifying high-risk patients with respiratory problems.** For example, pulse oximetry may identify patients with asthma who are having serious attacks or patients with emphysema who are in severe decompensation.
- **Assessing vascular status in orthopaedic trauma.** Pulse oximetry is routine practice in assessing a fractured extremity to evaluate the pulse distal to the fracture. Loss of a pulse means that the limb is in jeopardy and may require urgent action in the field if transport time is long. A pulse oximeter clipped to a finger or toe on a broken limb might provide critical information about the ongoing circulation to the limb.

The usefulness of a pulse oximeter depends on its ability to provide accurate information. A pulse oximeter that gives a reading of 99% when the patient is actually severely hypoxemic will not provide helpful information and could lead to inadequate or erroneous interventions. Be aware of circumstances that might produce erroneous readings:

- **Bright ambient light** may enter the spectrophotometer of the pulse oximeter and create an incorrect reading. Protect the sensor clip by covering it with a towel or aluminum foil.
- **Patient motion** can confuse the pulse oximeter because it may mistake motion for arterial pulsation and read the oxygen saturation from a vein rather than an artery.
- **Poor perfusion** makes it difficult for the oximeter to sense a pulse and therefore to generate a reading. Poor perfusion occurs in states such as shock, cardiac arrest, and cold exposure. If the vessels in a patient's limbs are constricted and the limbs are cold, it may be necessary to place the pulse oximeter clip on the earlobe or nose.
- **Nail polish** will prevent the sensor from working properly. Carry disposable acetone (nail polish remover) swabs to quickly remove nail polish.
- **Venous pulsations** may occur in some patients with right-sided heart failure due to the systemic backup of blood. If a vein is pulsating, the oximeter may regard it as an artery and measure venous oxygen saturation.
- **Abnormal hemoglobin** may produce a falsely normal SpO_2.

The two types of hemoglobin normally found are **oxyhemoglobin (HbO_2)**, hemoglobin that is occupied by oxygen, and **reduced hemoglobin**, the hemoglobin after the oxygen has been released to the cells. However, in the presence of **methemoglobin (metHb)** (a compound formed by oxidation of the iron on the hemoglobin), and **carboxyhemoglobin (COHb)** (hemoglobin loaded with CO), normal SpO_2 values may be observed, even though the body is not receiving sufficient oxygen. Carbon monoxide binds to hemoglobin 250 times more readily than oxygen. A **CO-oximeter**, sometimes called a CO monitor, is a device that measures absorption at several wavelengths to distinguish HbO_2 from COHb and determines the HbO_2 saturation—the percentage of oxygenated Hb compared with the total amount of hemoglobin—including COHb, metHb, HbO_2, and reduced Hb **Figure 23**. When a patient presents with CO poisoning, the CO-oximeter will detect this Hb—expressed as SpCO—and will report a markedly reduced HbO_2 saturation. Remember to not depend solely on pulse oximetry, and be aware of its limitations.

Peak Expiratory Flow Measurement

In patients with certain reactive airway diseases (such as asthma), bronchoconstriction can be evaluated by measuring the peak rate of a forceful exhalation with a peak expiratory flowmeter **Figure 24**. An increasing **peak expiratory flow** suggests that the patient is responding to treatment (such as inhaled bronchodilators). A decreasing peak expiratory flow may be an early indication that the patient's condition is deteriorating.

Words of Wisdom

When in Doubt, Look at the Patient!
Always weigh the information provided by pulse oximetry (or any other device) against clinical observations. If the patient is turning blue and struggling to breathe, ignore the pulse oximeter reading that suggests the patient is adequately oxygenated.

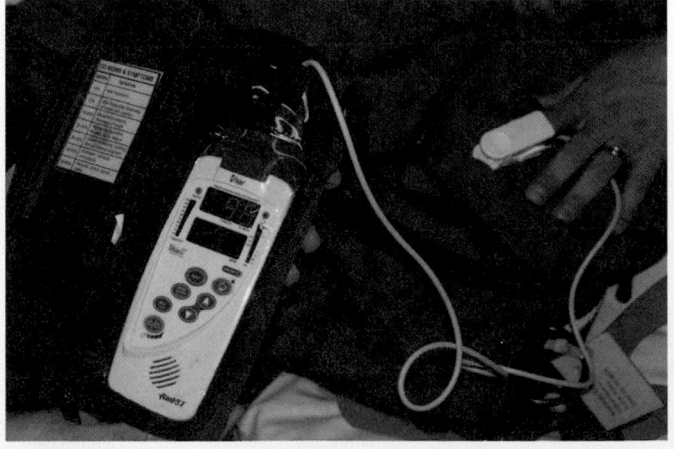

Figure 23 A carbon monoxide oximeter has the ability to distinguish oxyhemoglobin from carboxyhemoglobin.

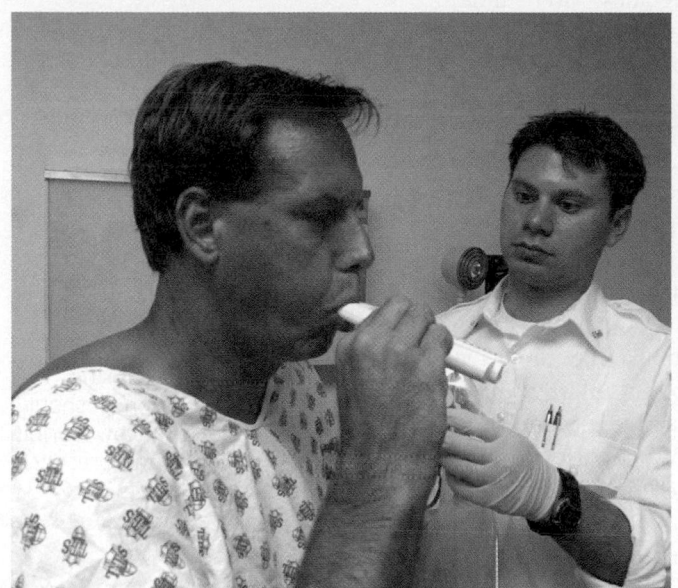

Figure 24 Peak expiratory flowmeters are used to quantify the degree of bronchoconstriction.

Peak expiratory flow varies based on gender, height, and age. Healthy adults have a peak expiratory flow rate of 350 to 750 mL. To assess peak expiratory flow, place the patient in a seated position with legs dangling. Assemble the flowmeter, and ensure that it reads zero. Ask the patient to take a deep breath, place the mouthpiece in his or her mouth, and exhale as forcefully as possible (make sure no air leaks around the device or comes from the patient's nose). Perform the test three times, and take the best peak flow rate of the three readings.

Arterial Blood Gas Analysis

Analysis of ABGs provides the most comprehensive quantitative information about the respiratory system. In this procedure, blood is obtained from a superficial artery, such as the radial or femoral artery. The blood is then analyzed for pH, $Paco_2$, Pao_2, Hco_3^- (concentration of bicarbonate ions), base excess (indicating acidosis or alkalosis), and Sao_2. Normal ABG values are summarized in Table 5.

With ABG measurements, the values of pH and Hco_3^- are used to evaluate the acid-base status of the patient. The $Paco_2$

Table 5 Normal Arterial Blood Gas Values	
pH	7.35 to 7.45
Pao_2	80 to 100 mm Hg
$Paco_2$	35 to 45 mm Hg
Hco_3^-	22 to 26 mEq/L
Base (excess or deficit)	±2 to ±3 mEq/L
Sao_2	>95%

is an indicator of the effectiveness of ventilation. The values of Pao_2 and Sao_2 are indicators of oxygenation. To maintain normal ABG values, a balance between alveolar volume and perfusion of the alveolar capillaries must be maintained.

Because paramedics are typically not trained to obtain arterial blood specimens and do not carry the equipment needed to analyze the patient's blood, they rely on noninvasive methods of assessing ventilation and oxygenation (such as pulse oximetry and capnography/capnometry).

End-tidal Carbon Dioxide ($ETCO_2$) Assessment

End-tidal CO_2 ($ETCO_2$) monitors detect the presence of carbon dioxide in exhaled air and are important adjuncts for determining ventilation adequacy. These devices work by analyzing air samples through a special $ETCO_2$ nasal cannula in a spontaneously breathing patient with an adequate airway. They can also be used to assess ventilation adequacy in patients in whom an advanced airway (such as an ET tube, a King LT, a laryngeal mask airway [LMA], or a tracheostomy tube) has been inserted.

Because carbon dioxide rapidly equilibrates in the alveolar gases, the carbon dioxide concentration in exhaled gases—particularly the gases present near the end of exhalation—closely approximate arterial $Paco_2$ levels, which normally range between 35 and 45 mm Hg. Typically, $ETCO_2$ is approximately 2 to 5 mm Hg lower than the arterial $Paco_2$. Because carbon dioxide is not present in the esophagus, use of an $ETCO_2$ detector is a reliable (and *essential*) method for confirming and monitoring advanced airway placement.

The $ETCO_2$ detectors may be digital, waveform, digital/waveform, or colorimetric. A **capnometer** provides quantitative information, in real time, by displaying a numeric reading of exhaled carbon dioxide. It uses a special adapter, which attaches between the advanced airway device and bag-mask device. Tubing from the adapter then connects to a capnometry machine Figure 25. Many portable cardiac monitor/defibrillators used in the prehospital setting have capnometry capability, as well as the capability for pulse oximetry.

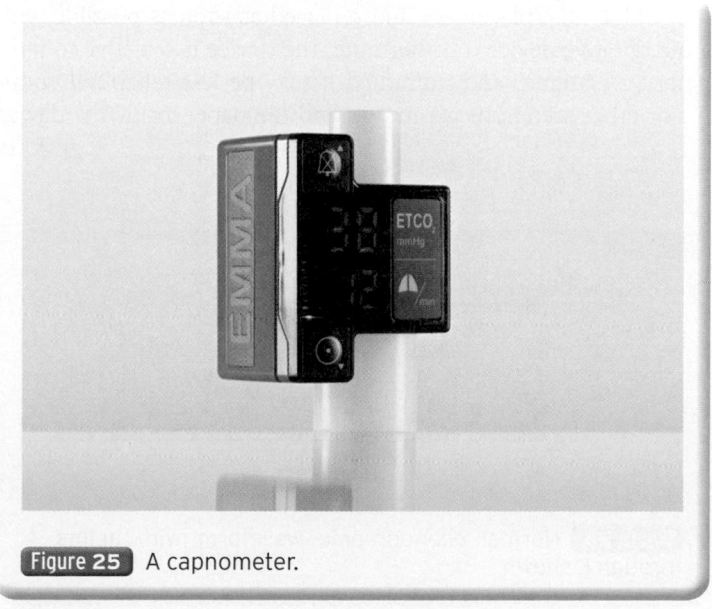

Figure 25 A capnometer.

A **capnographer** performs the same function and attaches in the same way as the capnometer, but it provides a graphic representation of exhaled carbon dioxide. There are three types of capnographers—waveform, digital/waveform, and colorimetric.

Waveform capnography provides quantitative, real-time information regarding the patient's exhaled carbon dioxide level. Unlike capnometry, however, waveform capnography displays a graphic waveform on the portable cardiac monitor/defibrillator. In many cases, portable cardiac monitor/defibrillators provide a numeric reading *and* a waveform (digital/waveform capnography). Capnography is used in cardiac arrest as an early indicator of the return of spontaneous circulation, discussed further in the chapter, *Cardiovascular Emergencies*.

It is important to understand the features of the capnographic waveform, including contour, baseline level, and rate and rise of the carbon dioxide level. There are four distinct phases **Figure 26** . The first phase (A-B), also known as the respiratory baseline, is the initial stage of exhalation; the gas sample is dead space gas, free of carbon dioxide. At point B, there is a mixture of alveolar gas with dead space gas, resulting in an abrupt rise in carbon dioxide levels; phase B-C is called the expiratory upslope. The expiratory or alveolar plateau is represented by phase C-D, and the gas sampled is essentially alveolar. Point D is the maximal $ETCO_2$ level—the best reflection of the alveolar carbon dioxide level. Fresh gas is introduced during the inspiratory downstroke (phase D-E), and the waveform returns to the baseline level of carbon dioxide—approximately 0.

A **colorimetric capnographer** provides qualitative (that is, it does not assign a numeric value) information regarding the presence of carbon dioxide in the patient's exhaled breath. The device is attached between the advanced airway and bag-mask device. After 6 to 8 positive-pressure breaths—the amount of time it takes for carbon dioxide to accumulate in the device—the specially treated paper inside the detector should turn from purple to yellow during exhalation, indicating the presence of exhaled carbon dioxide **Figure 27** .

It should be noted that the colorimetric capnographer is a "spot-check" device and should be used during *initial* confirmation of ET tube placement and replaced as soon as possible with a quantitative device. Furthermore, the device is sensitive to temperature extremes and humidity; it may be less reliable if vomitus or other secretions get into it; and the paper inside the device

degrades over time, resulting in a less reliable reading—despite the presence of exhaled carbon dioxide.

Capnography can also serve as an indicator of chest compression effectiveness and to detect return of spontaneous circulation. The provision of this information is possible because blood must circulate through the lungs for carbon dioxide to be exhaled and measured.

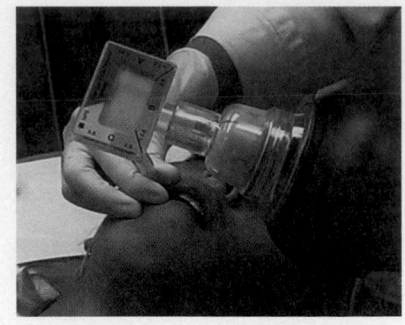

Figure 27 The paper inside the colorimetric capnographer should turn from purple to yellow during exhalation, indicating the presence of exhaled carbon dioxide.

Use of $ETCO_2$ monitoring is limited in the face of cardiac arrest. In a patient with a short arrest interval, exhaled carbon dioxide may be detected despite a lack of perfusion. Patients with prolonged cardiac arrest, however, will have minimal to no exhaled carbon dioxide because of severe acidosis and minimal or no carbon dioxide return to the lungs.

When assessing the ventilation status of any patient, whether he or she is spontaneously breathing, apneic with a pulse, or pulseless and apneic, it is critical to understand and recognize the causes of increased and decreased $ETCO_2$ levels to make necessary adjustments to your treatment **Table 6** .

◼ Airway Management

Air will reach the lungs only if it travels through the trachea. Therefore, a patent airway is essential. Patency is obvious in a responsive patient who is able to talk. In a patient with an

Normal

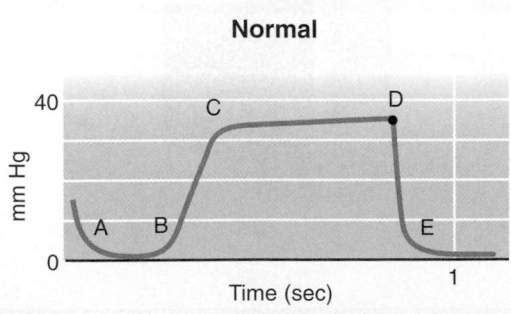

Figure 26 Normal capnographic waveform with points A through E shown.

Table 6   Causes of Increased and Decreased $ETCO_2$

	↑ $ETCO_2$	↓ $ETCO_2$
Spontaneously breathing	Hypoventilation	Hyperventilation
Apneic with a pulse	Ventilating too slowly	Ventilating too rapidly
Apneic and pulseless	Ventilating too slowly Could indicate ROSC†	Misplaced endotracheal tube* Decreased CO_2 return to the lungs (prolonged arrest) Ventilating too rapidly‡

*$ETCO_2$ LED reads 0, and capnographic waveform is flat.
†ROSC indicates return of spontaneous circulation. There is an abrupt increase in $ETCO_2$ (typically > 40 mm Hg).
‡In an arrest of short interval.

altered LOC, however, the airway is often not patent and manual maneuvers will be required to open it. In addition, artificial airway adjuncts may be needed to assist in maintaining the airway. In a compromised airway, clearing the airway and maintaining patency are vital. Clearing the airway means removing obstructing material, tissue, or fluids from the nose, mouth, and throat. Maintaining the airway means keeping the airway patent so that air can enter and leave the lungs freely Figure 28 .

Positioning the Patient

In a perfect world, all patients would present in a supine position, so that you could quickly assess them and intervene without moving them. If an unresponsive patient is found in a prone position, however, you must position him or her properly so that you can assess the need for ventilations or cardiopulmonary resuscitation (CPR).

To move a patient to a supine position, log roll the person as a unit. Once the patient is in a supine position, quickly assess for breathing by visualizing the chest for visible movement. If the patient is breathing adequately and is not injured, position him or her in the recovery position. The **recovery position**, which involves placing the patient in a left lateral recumbent position, should be used in all nontrauma patients

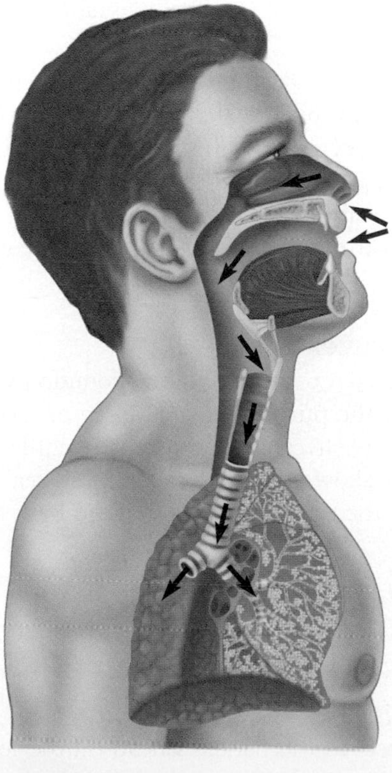

Figure 28 Air reaches the lungs only if it travels through the trachea. Maintaining the airway means keeping the airway patent so that air can enter and exit the lungs freely.

with a decreased LOC who are able to maintain their own airway spontaneously and are breathing adequately Figure 29 .

Manual Airway Maneuvers

If an unresponsive patient has a pulse, but is not breathing (or has only agonal gasps), you must open the airway manually to provide rescue breathing. The most common cause of airway obstruction in an unresponsive patient is the tongue Figure 30 . To correct this problem, manually maneuver the patient's head

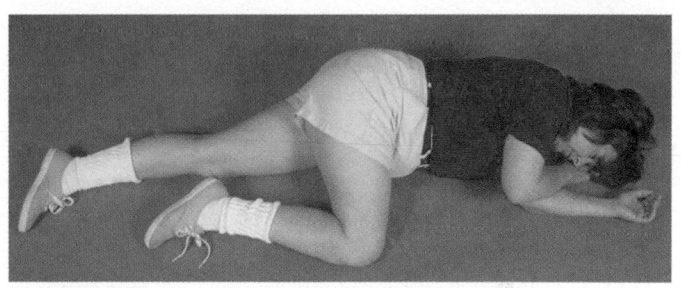

Figure 29 The recovery position.

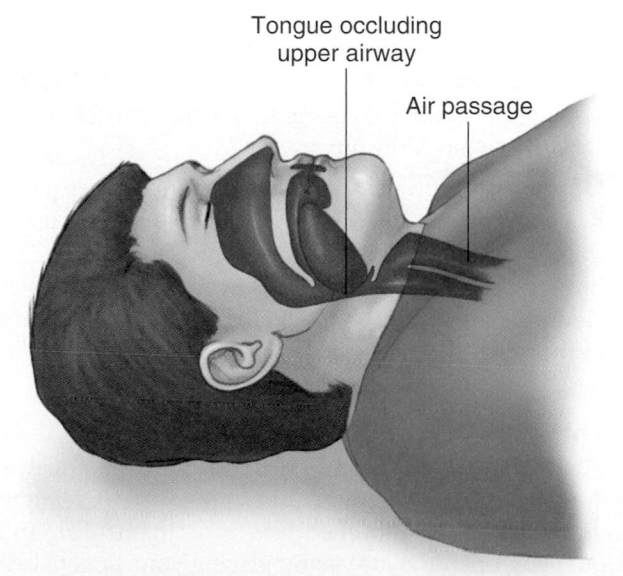

Tongue occluding upper airway

Air passage

Figure 30 When the tongue falls back and occludes the posterior pharynx, it may obstruct the airway.

to propel the tongue forward and open the airway by using the head tilt–chin lift maneuver or the jaw-thrust maneuver (with or without head tilt).

Head Tilt–Chin Lift Maneuver

Opening the airway can often be done quickly and easily by simply tilting the patient's head back and lifting the chin. This **head tilt–chin lift maneuver** is the preferred technique for opening the airway of a patient who has not sustained trauma. Occasionally, this simple maneuver is all that is required for the patient to resume breathing. The following are some considerations when using the head tilt–chin lift maneuver:

- **Indications.** An unresponsive patient, no mechanism for cervical spine injury, or a patient who is unable to protect his or her own airway
- **Contraindications.** A responsive patient or a possible cervical spine injury
- **Advantages.** No equipment required and simple, safe, and noninvasive
- **Disadvantages.** May be hazardous to patients with spinal injury and no protection from aspiration

Perform the head tilt–chin lift maneuver as listed here and shown in **Skill Drill 1**:

Skill Drill 1

1. With the patient in a supine position, position yourself beside the patient's head **Step 1**.
2. Place one hand on the patient's forehead, and apply firm backward pressure with your palm to tilt the patient's head back **Step 2**. This extension of the neck will propel the tongue forward, away from the posterior pharynx and clear the airway.
3. Place the tips of your fingers of your other hand under the lower jaw near the bony part of the chin **Step 3**. Do not compress the soft tissue under the chin because this action may block the airway.
4. Lift the chin upward, bringing the entire lower jaw with it, helping to tilt the head back **Step 4**. Do not use your thumb to lift the chin. Lift so that the teeth are nearly brought together, but avoid closing the mouth completely. Continue to hold the forehead to maintain a backward tilt of the head.

Jaw-Thrust Maneuver

If you suspect that the patient has experienced a cervical spine injury, open his or her airway with the **jaw-thrust maneuver**, also referred to as the modified jaw-thrust maneuver. In this technique, you open the airway by placing your fingers behind the angle of the jaw and lifting the jaw forward. The jaw is displaced forward at the mandibular angle. Following are some considerations when using the jaw-thrust maneuver:

- **Indications.** An unresponsive patient, possible cervical spine injury, or a patient who is unable to protect his or her own airway
- **Contraindications.** A responsive patient with resistance to opening the mouth. The jaw-thrust maneuver may be needed in a responsive patient who has sustained a jaw fracture to keep the tongue away from the back of the throat
- **Advantages.** May be used in patients with cervical spine injury, may use with cervical collar in place, and no special equipment required
- **Disadvantages.** Cannot maintain if patient becomes responsive or combative, difficult to maintain for an extended time, very difficult to use in conjunction with bag-mask ventilation, thumb must remain in place to maintain jaw displacement, requires second rescuer for bag-mask ventilation, and no protection against aspiration

Perform the jaw-thrust maneuver as listed here and shown in **Skill Drill 2**:

Skill Drill 2

1. Position yourself at the top of the supine patient's head **Step 1**.
2. Place the meaty portion of the base of your thumbs on the zygomatic arches, and hook the tips of your index fingers under the angle of the mandible, in the indentation below each ear **Step 2**.
3. While holding the patient's head in a neutral in-line position, displace the jaw upward and open the patient's mouth with the tips of your thumbs **Step 3**. Because opening and maintaining a patent airway is so critical, you should *carefully* perform the head tilt–chin lift maneuver if the jaw-thrust maneuver fails to adequately open the airway.

Tongue-Jaw Lift Maneuver

The **tongue-jaw lift maneuver** is used more commonly to open a patient's airway for the purpose of suctioning or inserting an oropharyngeal airway. It cannot be used to ventilate a patient because it will not allow for an adequate mask seal on the patient's face. Perform the tongue-jaw lift as listed here and shown in **Skill Drill 3**:

Skill Drill 3

1. Position yourself at the side of the patient **Step 1**.
2. Place the hand closest to the patient's head on the forehead **Step 2**.
3. With the other hand, reach into the patient's mouth and hook your first knuckle under the incisors or gum line. While holding the patient's head and maintaining the hand on the forehead, lift the jaw straight up **Step 3**.

Skill Drill   1

Head Tilt-Chin Lift Maneuver

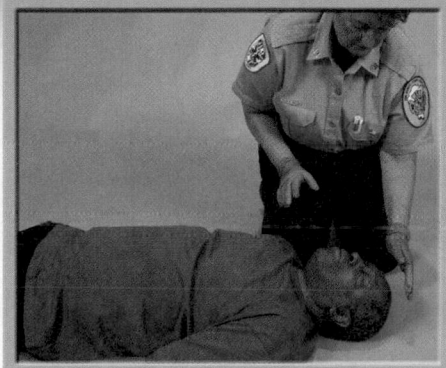

Step 1 Position yourself at the patient's side.

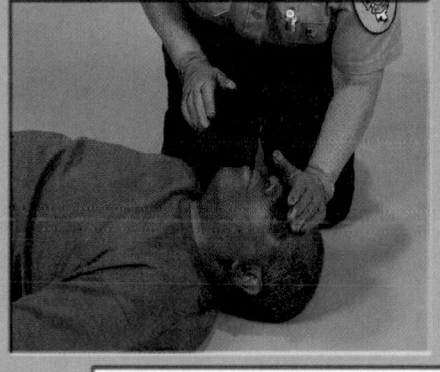

Step 2 Place the hand closest to the patient's head on the forehead.

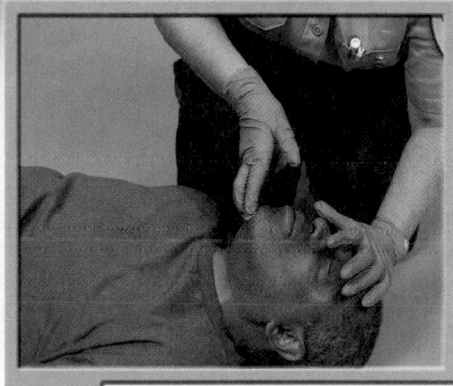

Step 3 With your other hand, place two fingers on the underside of the patient's chin.

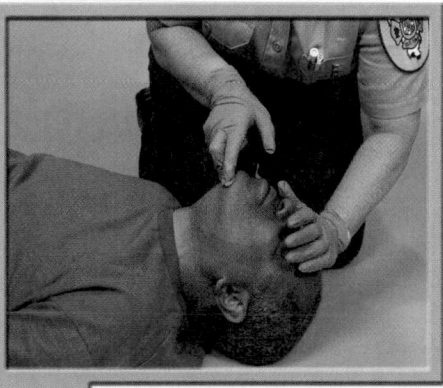

Step 4 Simultaneously apply backward and downward pressure to the patient's forehead and lift the jaw straight up. Do not depress the soft tissue below the chin.

■ Suctioning

When the patient's mouth or throat becomes filled with vomitus, blood, or secretions, a suction apparatus enables you to remove material quickly and efficiently, thereby allowing you to ventilate the patient. Ventilating a patient with secretions in his or her mouth will force material into the lungs, resulting in an upper airway obstruction or aspiration. Therefore, clearing the patient's airway with suction, if needed, is your next priority after opening the patient's airway with the manual maneuvers previously discussed. *If you hear gurgling, the patient needs suctioning.*

■ Suctioning Equipment

Ambulances should carry a fixed suction unit (which operates off a vacuum from the engine) and a portable suction unit (battery-operated or hand-powered) **Figure 31**. Regardless of

Skill Drill 2

Jaw-Thrust Maneuver

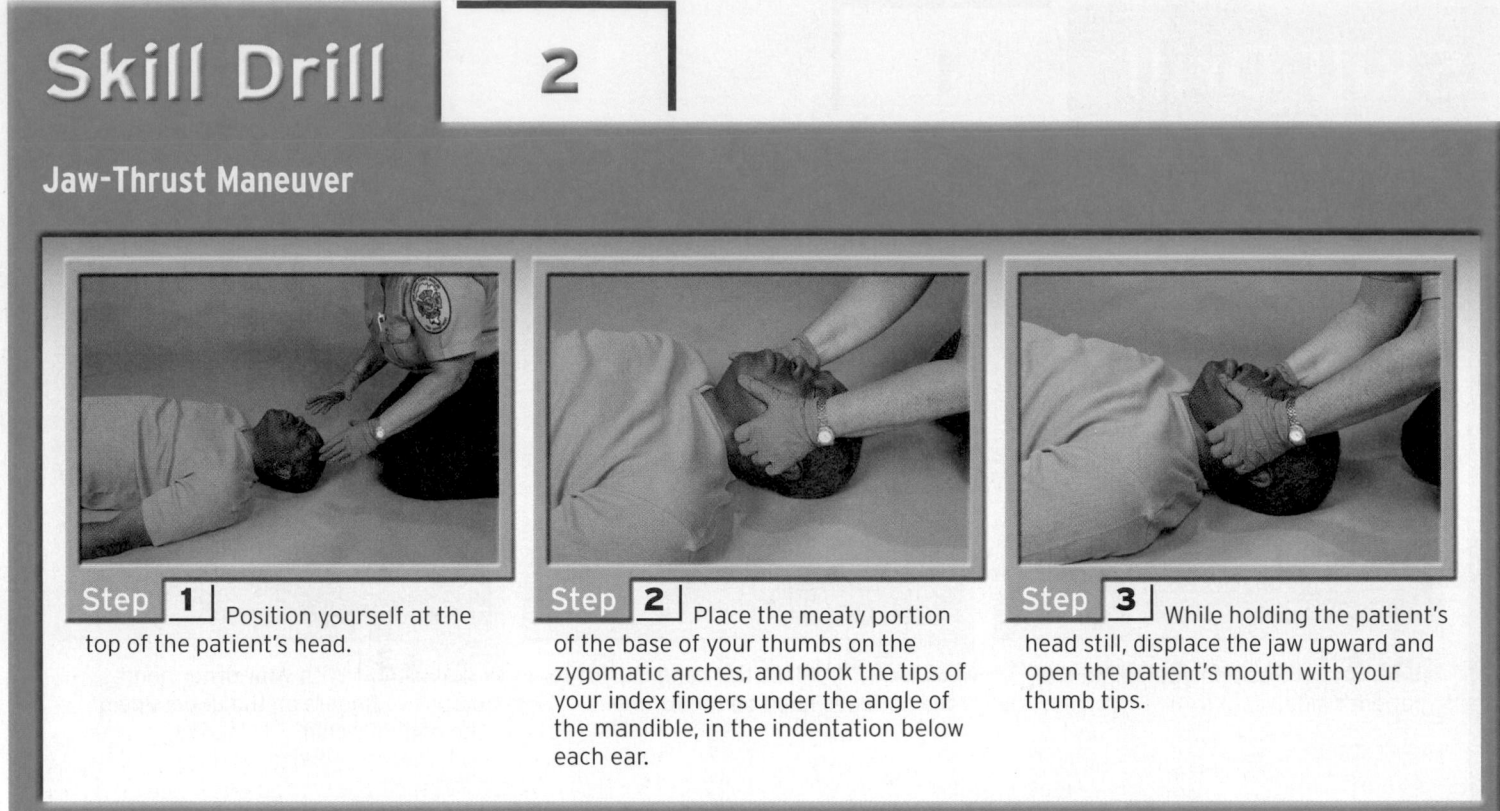

Step 1 Position yourself at the top of the patient's head.

Step 2 Place the meaty portion of the base of your thumbs on the zygomatic arches, and hook the tips of your index fingers under the angle of the mandible, in the indentation below each ear.

Step 3 While holding the patient's head still, displace the jaw upward and open the patient's mouth with your thumb tips.

your location—in the patient's residence, the middle of a field, or the back of the ambulance—you must have quick access to suction. It is essential for resuscitation.

Hand-operated suctioning units with disposable canisters are reliable, effective, and relatively inexpensive; they can easily fit into your first in bag. Mechanical or vacuum-powered suction units should be capable of generating a vacuum of 300 mm Hg within 4 seconds of clamping off the tubing. The amount of suction should be adjustable for use in children and intubated patients. Check the vacuum on the mechanical suction unit at the beginning of every shift by turning on the device, clamping the tubing, and making sure the pressure gauge registers 300 mm Hg. Ensure that all battery-charged units have fully charged batteries. **Table 7** lists the advantages and disadvantages of the most common types of suction devices.

Regardless of which type of suction unit you are using, the device must generate enough vacuum pressure to adequately suction the patient's mouth and oropharynx. In addition to the suctioning unit, the following supplies should be readily accessible at the patient's head:

- Wide-bore, thick-walled, nonkinking tubing
- Soft and rigid suction catheters
- A nonbreakable, disposable collection bottle
- A supply of water for rinsing the catheters

A suction catheter is a hollow, cylindrical device that is used to remove fluids and secretions from the patient's airway.

A Yankauer catheter (**tonsil-tip catheter**) is a good option for suctioning the pharynx in adults and the preferred device for infants and children. These plastic-tip catheters have a large diameter and are rigid, so they do not collapse. Rigid catheters are capable of suctioning large volumes of fluid rapidly. Tips with a curved contour allow for easy, rapid placement in the oropharynx **Figure 32**.

Soft plastic, nonrigid catheters, sometimes called French or **whistle-tip catheters**, can be placed in the oropharynx or nasopharynx or down an ET tube. They come in various sizes and have a smaller diameter than rigid catheters. Soft catheters are used to suction the nose and liquid secretions in the back of the mouth and in situations in which a rigid catheter cannot be used, such as for a patient with a stoma **Figure 33**. For example, a rigid catheter could break a tooth in a patient with clenched teeth, whereas a flexible catheter may be worked along the cheeks without causing injury. Suction tubing without the attached catheter facilitates suctioning of large debris in the oropharynx and allows access to the back of the pharynx in a patient with clenched teeth.

■ Suctioning Techniques

Mortality increases significantly if a patient aspirates; therefore, suctioning the upper airway is critical to avoid this potentially fatal event. Suctioning removes not only liquids from the airway, but also oxygen. For that reason, any patient who is to be

Skill Drill 3

Tongue-Jaw Lift Maneuver

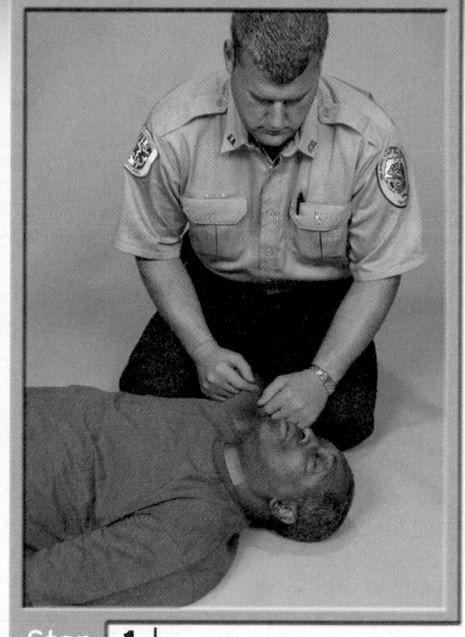

Step 1 Position yourself at the patient's side.

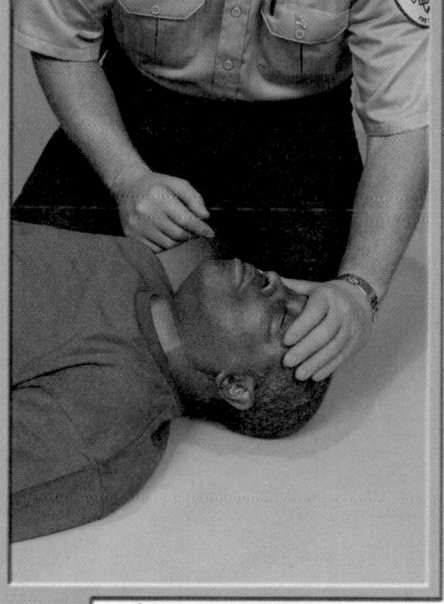

Step 2 Place the hand closest to the patient's head on the forehead.

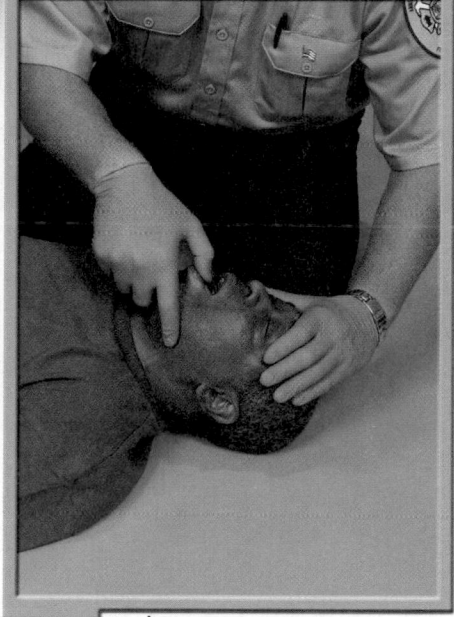

Step 3 With your other hand, reach into the patient's mouth and hook your first knuckle under the incisors or gum line. While holding the patient's head and maintaining the hand on the forehead, lift the jaw straight up.

suctioned should be adequately preoxygenated; this step will provide a small oxygen reserve that can be drawn upon while you are suctioning. Even so, each suctioning attempt must be limited to a maximum of 15 seconds in an adult (10 seconds in children; 5 seconds in infants). Be careful not to stimulate the back of the throat, especially in a young child or an infant because the vagal stimulus can cause the pulse rate to drop. After the patient has been suctioned, continue ventilation and oxygenation.

Soft-tip catheters must be lubricated when suctioning the nasopharynx and are best used when passed through an ET tube. The catheter is inserted, and suction is applied during extraction of the catheter to clear the airway. After the patient has been suctioned, reevaluate the patency of his or her airway, and continue to ventilate and oxygenate as needed.

Before inserting any suction catheter into a patient, make sure you measure for the proper size, from the corner of the mouth to the earlobe. Never insert a catheter past the base of the tongue because it may cause the patient to gag or vomit.

The steps for properly suctioning a patient's airway are listed here and shown in Skill Drill 4 :

Skill Drill 4

1. Turn on the assembled suction unit Step 1 .
2. Measure the catheter from the corner of the mouth to the earlobe Step 2 .
3. Before applying suction, turn the patient's head to the side (unless you suspect cervical spine injury), open the patient's mouth by using the cross-finger technique or

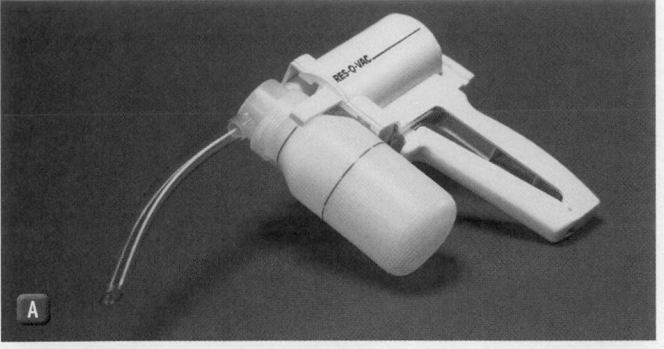

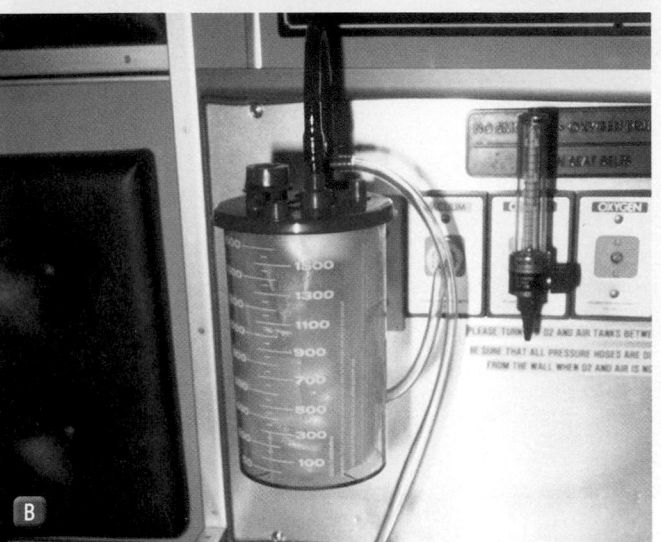

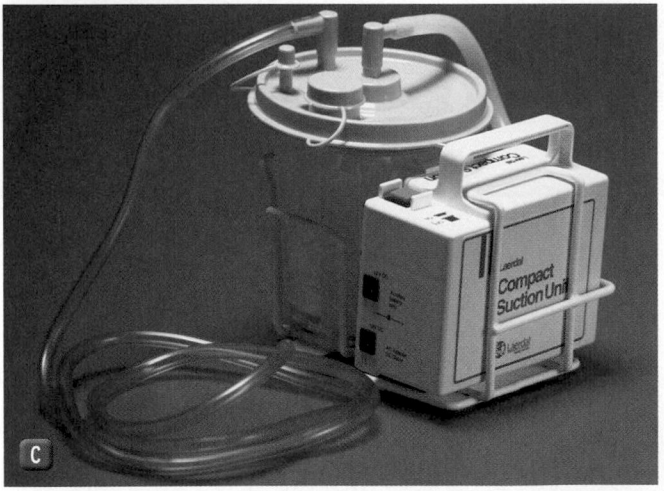

Figure 31 Effective suctioning equipment is essential for good airway management. **A.** Hand-operated device. **B.** Fixed unit. **C.** Portable unit.

Table 7 Suction Devices

Suction Device	Advantages	Disadvantages
Hand-powered portable	■ Lightweight ■ Portable ■ Mechanically simple ■ Inexpensive	■ Limited volume ■ Manually powered ■ Fluid contact ■ Components not disposable
Oxygen-powered portable	■ Lightweight ■ Small	■ Limited suction power ■ Uses a lot of oxygen for limited suctioning power
Battery-operated portable	■ Lightweight ■ Portable ■ Excellent suction power ■ Most problems can be identified and fixed in the field	■ More complicated mechanics ■ May lose battery integrity over time ■ Some fluid contact ■ Components not disposable
Mounted vacuum-powered	■ Extremely strong vacuum ■ Adjustable vacuum power ■ Components disposable	■ Not portable ■ Fluid contact ■ Cannot "field service" or substitute power source

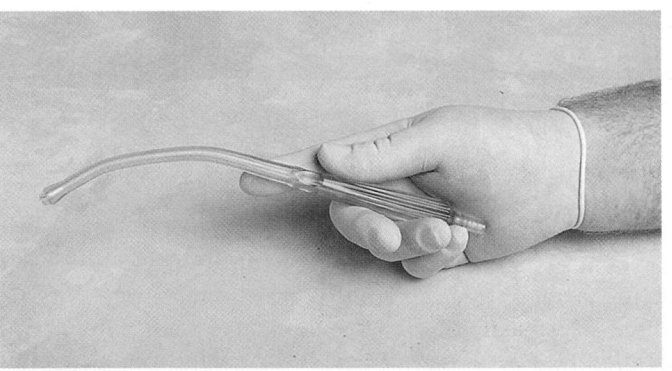

Figure 32 Tonsil-tip catheters are a good choice for suctioning the oropharynx because they have wide-diameter tips and are rigid.

tongue-jaw lift, and insert the tip of the catheter to the predetermined depth. Do not suction while inserting the catheter [Step 3].

4. Apply suction in a circular motion as you withdraw the catheter. Do not suction an adult for more than 15 seconds [Step 4].

■ Airway Adjuncts

After manually opening the airway of an unresponsive patient and using suction as needed to clear away any blood or other secretions, an artificial airway adjunct may be needed to help maintain airway patency. *An artificial airway is not a substitute for proper head*

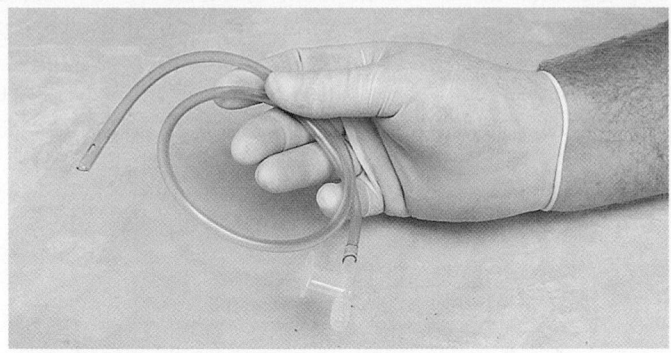

Figure 33 French (whistle-tip) catheters are used in situations in which rigid catheters cannot be used, such as when a patient has a stoma or if the patient's teeth are clenched. Flexible catheters can also be passed down a tube.

Words of Wisdom

Suctioning Time Limits	
Adult	15 seconds
Child	10 seconds
Infant	5 seconds

positioning. Even after an airway adjunct has been inserted, the appropriate manual position of the head must be maintained.

■ Oropharyngeal Airway

The oropharyngeal (oral) airway is a curved, hard plastic device that fits over the back of the tongue with the tip in the

Skill Drill 4

Suctioning a Patient's Airway

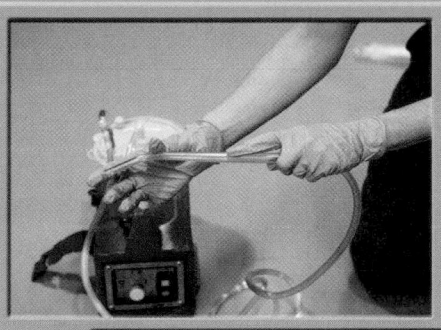

Step 1 Make sure the suctioning unit is properly assembled, and turn on the suction unit.

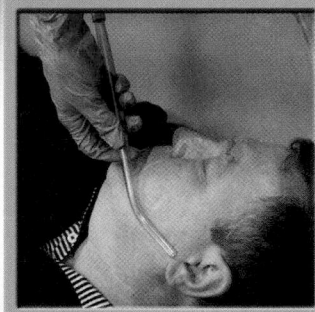

Step 2 Measure the catheter from the corner of the mouth to the earlobe.

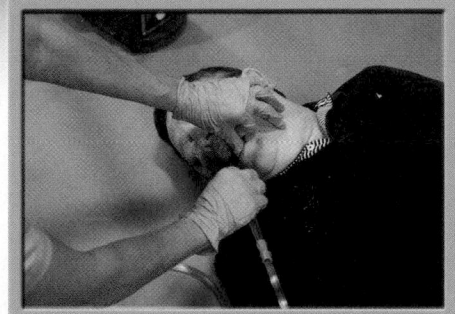

Step 3 Turn the patient's head to the side (unless you suspect cervical spine injury), open the mouth using the cross-finger technique if necessary, and insert the catheter to the predetermined depth without suctioning.

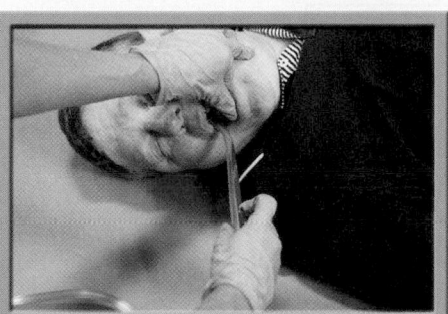

Step 4 Apply suction in a circular motion as you withdraw the catheter. Do not suction an adult for more than 15 seconds.

posterior pharynx **Figure 34**. It is designed to hold the tongue away from the posterior pharyngeal wall, and its use makes it much easier to ventilate patients with a bag-mask device. The oral airway can also serve as an effective bite-block, preventing an intubated patient from biting down on the ET tube.

An oral airway should be inserted promptly in unresponsive patients—breathing or not—who have no gag reflex. Because its distal end sits in the back of the throat, this device will stimulate gagging and retching in a responsive patient. For that reason, the oropharyngeal airway should be used only in unresponsive patients without a gag reflex. To assess a patient's gag reflex, use the eyelash reflex (discussed earlier in this chapter). *If the patient gags during insertion of the oral airway, remove the device immediately and be prepared to suction the oropharynx.* Following are some considerations when using an oropharyngeal airway:

- **Indications.** Unresponsive patients and absent gag reflex
- **Contraindications.** Responsive patients and patients with a gag reflex
- **Advantages.** Noninvasive, easily placed, and prevents blockage of the glottis by the tongue
- **Disadvantages.** No prevention of aspiration
- **Complications.** Unexpected gag may cause vomiting, or improper technique may cause pharyngeal or dental trauma.

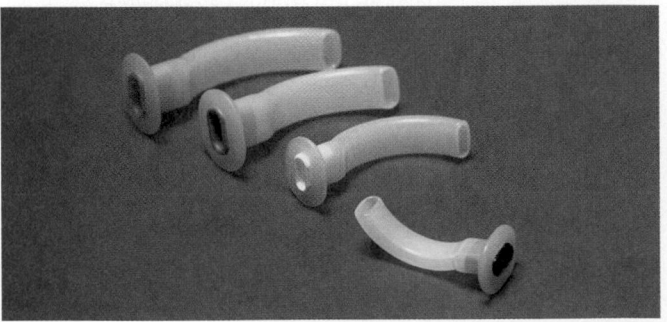

Figure 34 An oral airway is used for unresponsive patients who have no gag reflex. It helps to keep the tongue from blocking the airway.

If the oral airway is improperly sized or is inserted incorrectly, it could push the tongue back into the pharynx, creating an airway obstruction. Rough insertion of the airway can injure the hard palate, resulting in oral bleeding and creating a risk of vomiting and aspiration. Before inserting an oral airway, suction the oropharynx as needed to ensure that the mouth is clear of blood or other fluids. The steps for inserting an oral airway are listed here and shown in **Skill Drill 5**:

Skill Drill   5

1. To select the proper size, measure the distance from the patient's earlobe to the corner of the mouth **Step 1**.
2. Open the patient's mouth with the cross-finger technique or tongue-jaw lift. Hold the airway upside down with your other hand. Insert the airway with the tip facing the roof of the mouth **Step 2**.
3. Rotate the airway 180°, flipping it over the tongue. When inserted properly, the airway will rest in the mouth, with the curvature of the airway following the contour of the tongue. The flange should rest against the lips, with the distal end in the posterior pharynx **Step 3**.

If you encounter difficulty while inserting the oral airway, try this alternative technique listed here and shown in **Skill Drill 6**:

Skill Drill   6

1. Use a tongue blade to depress the tongue, ensuring that the tongue remains forward **Step 1**.
2. Insert the oral airway sideways from the corner of the mouth, until the flange reaches the lips **Step 2**.
3. Rotate the oral airway 90°, removing the tongue blade as you exert gentle backward pressure on the oral airway, until the flange rests securely in place against the lips **Step 3**.

Nasopharyngeal Airway

The **nasopharyngeal (nasal) airway** is a soft, rubber tube that is inserted through the nose into the posterior pharynx behind

Skill Drill   5

Inserting an Oral Airway

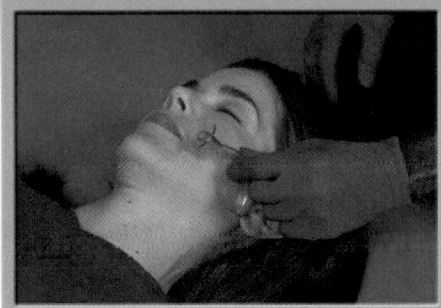

Step 1 Size the airway by measuring the distance from the patient's earlobe to the corner of the mouth.

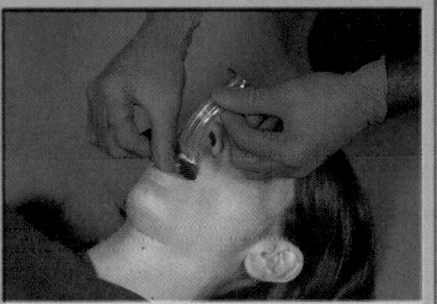

Step 2 Open the patient's mouth with the cross-finger technique or tongue-jaw lift. Hold the airway upside down with your other hand. Insert the airway with the tip facing the roof of the mouth, and slide it in until it touches the roof of the mouth.

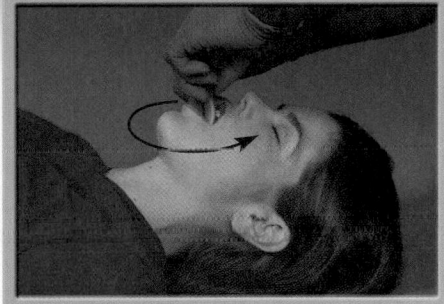

Step 3 Rotate the airway 180° after it passes the soft palate. Insert the airway until the flange rests on the patient's lips and teeth. In this position, the airway will hold the tongue forward.

Skill Drill   6

Inserting an Oral Airway With a 90° Rotation

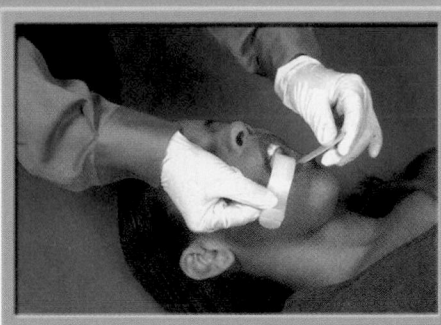

Step 1 Depress the tongue with a tongue blade so the tongue remains forward.

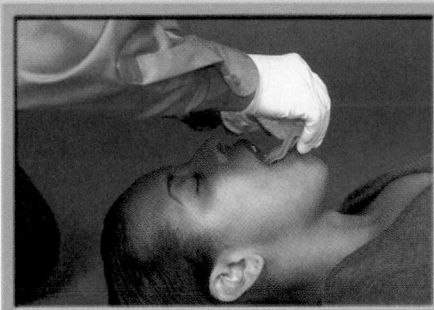

Step 2 Insert the oral airway sideways from the corner of the mouth, until the flange reaches the lips.

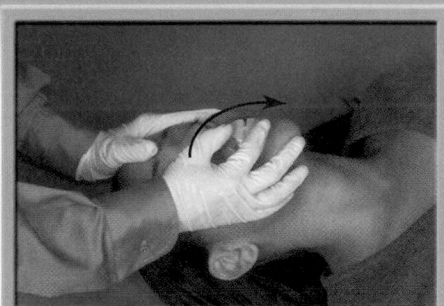

Step 3 Rotate the oral airway 90°, and remove the tongue blade as you exert gentle backward pressure on the oral airway until the flange rests securely in place against the lips.

Special Populations

In children, using a tongue blade to hold the tongue down while inserting an oral airway is the preferred method. Because the airways of children are less developed than those of adults, rotating the oral airway in the posterior pharynx may cause damage.

the tongue, thereby allowing passage of air from the nose to the lower airway. Nasal airways range in size from 12 French to 32 French; the length of the nasal airway depends on its size. A nasal airway is much better tolerated than an oral airway in patients who have an intact gag reflex but an altered LOC Figure 35 . Do not use this device if the patient has experienced trauma to the nose or you have reason to suspect a skull fracture (for example, CSF leakage from the nose). Inserting the airway in such cases may cause it to enter the brain through the hole caused by the fracture.

The nasopharyngeal airway must be inserted gently to avoid precipitating epistaxis (nosebleed). Lubricate the airway generously with a water-soluble gel, preferably one that contains a local anesthetic, and slide it gently, tip downward, into one nostril. *Do not try to force it.* If you meet resistance, try to pass the airway down the other nostril. Following are considerations when using a nasopharyngeal airway:

- **Indications.** Unresponsive patients and patients with an altered mental status who have an intact gag reflex
- **Contraindications.** Patient intolerance; presence of facial (specifically, the nose) fracture or skull fracture
- **Advantages.** Can be suctioned through, provides a patent airway, can be tolerated by responsive patients, can be safely placed "blindly," no requirement for the mouth to be open
- **Disadvantages.** Improper technique may result in severe bleeding (resulting epistaxis may be extremely difficult to control), and does not protect from aspiration.

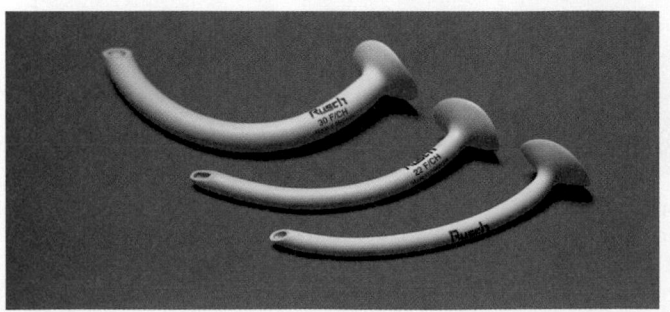

Figure 35 A nasal airway is better tolerated by patients who have an intact gag reflex.

The steps for inserting a nasal airway are listed here and shown in Skill Drill 7 :

Skill Drill 7

1. Before inserting the airway, make sure you have selected the proper size. Measure the distance from the tip of the nostril to the earlobe. In almost all people, one nostril is larger than the other. The diameter should be roughly equal to the patient's little finger Step 1 .
2. After lubricating the nasal airway with a water-soluble gel, place the airway in the larger nostril, with the curvature of the device following the curve of the floor of the nose and the bevel facing the septum Step 2 .
3. Place the bevel toward the septum, and insert it gently along the nasal floor, parallel to the mouth. *Do not force the airway* Step 3 .
4. When completely inserted, the flange should rest against the nostril. The distal end of the airway will open into the posterior pharynx Step 4 .

As an alternative, the proper size of nasal airway can be determined by measuring from the tip of the nostril to the angle of the jaw rather than the earlobe. If the nasal airway is too long, it may obstruct the patient's airway. If the patient becomes intolerant of the nasal airway, gently remove it from the nasal passage. Although a nasal airway is not as likely to cause vomiting as an oral airway, you should still have suction readily available.

Airway Obstructions

The airway connects the body to the life-giving oxygen in the atmosphere. If it becomes obstructed, this lifeline is cut and the patient dies—often within minutes. Paramedics must recognize the signs of an obstructed airway and immediately take corrective action.

Causes of Airway Obstruction

In an adult, sudden foreign body airway obstruction usually occurs during a meal. In children, it typically occurs while eating or playing with small toys. An otherwise healthy child who presents with a sudden onset of difficulty breathing—especially in the absence of fever—should be suspected of having a foreign body airway obstruction. Airway obstruction, however, has a multitude of other causes, including the tongue, laryngeal edema, laryngeal spasm (laryngospasm), trauma, and aspiration.

When the airway is obstructed because of an infectious process or a severe allergic reaction, repeated attempts to clear the airway as if it were obstructed by a foreign body will be unsuccessful and potentially harmful. These conditions require specific management (discussed in the appropriate chapters of this book) and prompt transport to an appropriate medical facility.

Skill Drill   7

Inserting a Nasal Airway

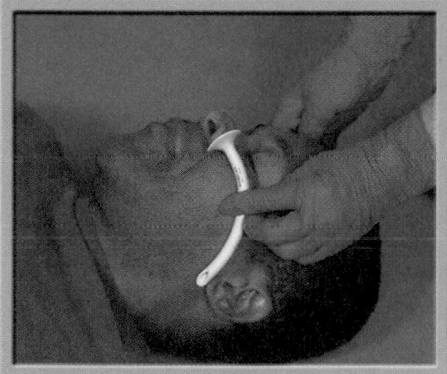

Step 1 Determine the size of the airway by measuring the distance from the tip of the nostril to the patient's earlobe. Coat the tip with a water-soluble lubricant.

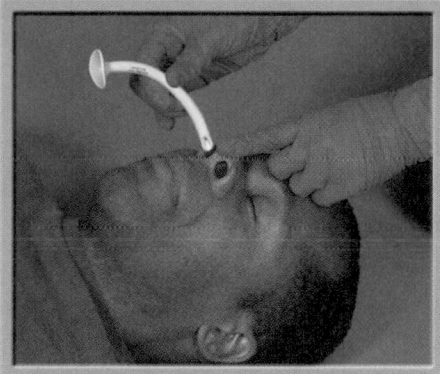

Step 2 Insert the lubricated airway into the larger nostril, with the curvature following the floor of the nose and the bevel facing the septum.

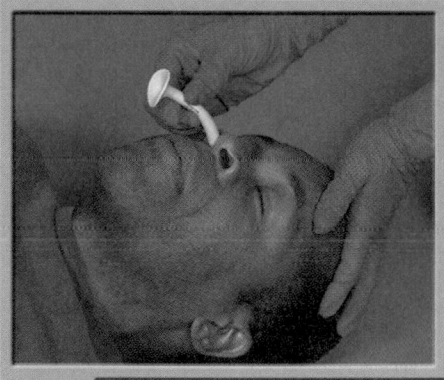

Step 3 Gently advance the airway. If using the left nostril, insert the nasal airway until it meets with resistance, then rotate the airway 180° into position. *This rotation is not required if you are using the right nostril.*

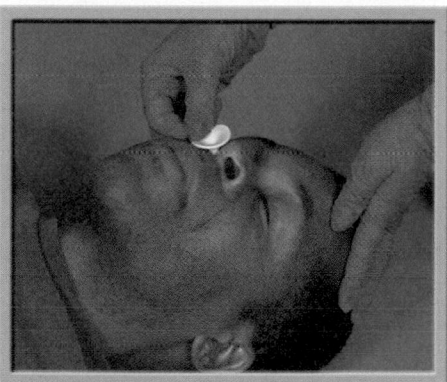

Step 4 Continue until the flange rests against the nostril. If you feel any resistance or obstruction, remove the airway and insert it into the other nostril.

Tongue

In a patient with an altered LOC, the jaw relaxes and the tongue tends to fall back against the posterior wall of the pharynx, closing off the airway. A patient with partial obstruction from the tongue will have snoring respirations; a patient whose airway is completely obstructed will have no respirations. Fortunately, obstruction of the airway by the tongue is simple to correct using a manual maneuver (such as head tilt–chin lift or jaw-thrust).

Foreign Body

A significant number of people die of foreign body airway obstructions each year, often as the result of choking on a piece of food. The typical victim is middle-aged or older and wears dentures. The person has usually consumed alcohol, which depresses protective reflexes and adversely affects judgment about how large a piece of food can be prudently placed in the mouth. In addition, people with conditions that decrease their airway reflexes (such as stroke) are at an increased risk for a foreign body airway obstruction. A foreign body may cause a mild or severe airway obstruction, depending on the size of the object and its location in the airway.

Signs may include choking, gagging, stridor, dyspnea, **aphonia** (inability to speak), and **dysphonia** (difficulty speaking). Treatment depends on whether the patient is effectively moving air. Techniques for foreign body airway obstruction removal are discussed later in this chapter.

Laryngeal Spasm and Edema

A laryngeal spasm (laryngospasm) results in spasmodic closure of the vocal cords, completely occluding the airway. It is often caused by trauma during an overly aggressive intubation attempt or occurs immediately on extubation, especially when the patient has an altered LOC.

Laryngeal edema causes the glottic opening to become extremely narrow or totally closed. Conditions that commonly cause this problem include epiglottitis, anaphylaxis, or inhalation injury (such as burns to the upper airway).

Airway obstructions caused by laryngeal spasm or edema may be relieved by aggressive ventilation to force air past the narrowed airway or a forceful upward pull of the jaw in an attempt to reposition the airway. In certain cases, muscle relaxant medications may be effective in relieving laryngeal spasm. Do not let your guard down after the laryngospasm has appeared to have resolved; resolution of the crisis does not mean that laryngospasm will not recur. The patient should be transported to the hospital for evaluation.

Laryngeal Injury

Airway patency depends on good muscle tone to keep the trachea open. Fracture of the larynx increases airway resistance by decreasing airway size due to decreased muscle tone, laryngeal edema, and ventilatory effort. An advanced airway may be required to maintain a patent airway. Penetrating and crush injuries to the larynx can compromise the airway secondary to swelling and bleeding. As with laryngeal fractures, advanced airway management may be required.

Aspiration

Aspiration of blood or other fluid significantly increases mortality. In addition to potentially obstructing the airway, aspiration destroys delicate bronchiolar tissue, introduces pathogens into the lungs, and decreases the patient's ability to ventilate (or be ventilated).

Suction should be readily available for any patient who is unable to maintain his or her own airway. Patients requiring emergency care should always be assumed to have a full stomach.

■ Recognition of an Airway Obstruction

A foreign body lodged in the upper airway can cause a mild (partial) or severe (complete) airway obstruction. A rapid but careful assessment is required to determine the seriousness of the obstruction because the differences in managing mild versus severe cases are significant.

A patient with a mild airway obstruction is responsive and able to exchange air but may show varying degrees of respiratory

---

YOU are the Medic   PART 4

The engine company arrives with two EMTs. Shortly after completing your assessment, you note that the patient's level of consciousness has deteriorated; he is now only responsive to painful stimuli. His face and neck have become cyanotic, his Spo_2 has decreased to 80%, and his $ETCO_2$ has increased to 58 mm Hg.

Recording Time: 8 Minutes	
Level of consciousness	P (responds to painful stimuli [trapezius pinch])
Respirations	8 breaths/min; labored and shallow
Pulse	130 beats/min; weak and regular
Skin	Diaphoretic and cyanotic
Blood pressure	116/60 mm Hg
Spo_2	80% (on oxygen)
$ETCO_2$	58 mm Hg
ECG	Sinus tachycardia, no ectopy

7. Why is this patient's condition deteriorating despite high-flow oxygen?

8. How must you adjust your current treatment?

distress. The patient will usually have noisy respirations and may be coughing. He or she may wheeze between coughs but does not become cyanotic. *Patients with a mild airway obstruction should be left alone. A forceful cough is the most effective means of dislodging the obstruction.* Attempts to manually remove the object could force it farther down into the airway and cause a severe obstruction. Closely monitor the patient's condition, and be prepared to intervene if you see signs of severe airway obstruction.

A patient with a severe airway obstruction typically experiences a sudden inability to breathe, talk, or cough—classically during a meal. The patient may grasp at his or her throat (universal sign of choking), begin to turn cyanotic, and make frantic, exaggerated attempts to move air Figure 36 . Patients with a severe airway obstruction have a weak, ineffective, or absent cough and are in marked respiratory distress; weak inspiratory stridor and cyanosis are often present.

Emergency Medical Care for Foreign Body Airway Obstruction

If a patient with a suspected airway obstruction is responsive, ask, "Are you choking?" If the patient nods "yes" and cannot speak, begin treatment immediately. If the obstruction is not promptly cleared, the amount of oxygen in the blood will decrease dramatically, resulting in severe hypoxia and death.

Words of Wisdom

Causes of Airway Obstruction
- Relaxation of the tongue in an unresponsive patient
- Foreign objects—food, small toys, balloons, dentures
- Blood clots, broken teeth, or damaged oral tissue following trauma
- Airway tissue swelling—infection, allergic reaction
- Aspirated vomitus (stomach contents)

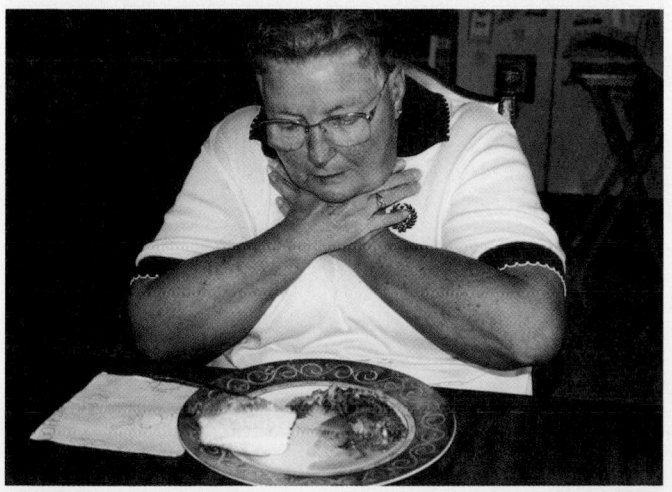

Figure 36 The universal sign of choking.

If, after opening the airway, you are unable to ventilate the patient (no visible chest rise) or you feel resistance when ventilating (poor lung compliance), reopen the airway and again attempt to ventilate the patient. **Lung compliance** is the ability of the alveoli to expand when air is drawn into the lungs during negative-pressure ventilation or pushed into the lungs during positive-pressure ventilation. Poor lung compliance is characterized by increased resistance during ventilation attempts.

If large pieces of vomitus, mucus, loose dentures, or blood clots are found in the airway, sweep them forward and out of the mouth with your gloved index finger. *Blind finger sweeps of the mouth—regardless of the patient's age—are not recommended and may cause further harm; attempt to remove only foreign bodies that you can see and easily retrieve.* After the patient's airway is open, insert your index finger down along the inside of the patient's cheek and into his or her throat at the base of the tongue, then try to hook the foreign body to dislodge it and maneuver it into the mouth. Take care not to force the foreign body deeper into the airway. Do *not* blindly insert any object other than your finger into the patient's mouth to remove a foreign body because an instrument jammed into the throat can damage the delicate structures of the pharynx and compound the obstruction with hemorrhage. Suctioning should be used to clear the airway of secretions as needed.

Words of Wisdom

Blind insertion of any instrument, whether improvised or specially designed, into a patient's pharynx is extremely dangerous. Do not do it!

The **abdominal thrust maneuver** (also called the Heimlich maneuver) is the most effective method of dislodging and forcing an object out of the airway of a responsive adult or child. It aims to create an artificial cough by forcing residual air out of the victim's lungs, thereby expelling the object. You should perform the Heimlich maneuver on any responsive child or adult with a severe airway obstruction until the obstructing object is expelled or until the patient becomes unresponsive. If a responsive patient with a severe airway obstruction is in the advanced stages of pregnancy or is morbidly obese, perform chest thrusts instead of abdominal thrusts.

If the responsive patient with a severe airway obstruction becomes unresponsive, carefully position him or her supine on the ground and begin chest compressions. Perform 30 chest compressions (15 compressions if two rescuers are present and the patient is an infant or a child), and then open the airway and

---

Special Populations

According to 2010 guidelines for CPR and emergency cardiovascular care, a child is a person from about 1 year of age until the onset of puberty (12 to 14 years of age).

look in the mouth. *Attempt to remove the foreign body only if you can see it.* After looking in the mouth, attempt to deliver a rescue breath. If the first breath does not produce visible chest rise, reopen the airway and reattempt to ventilate. If both breaths fail to produce visible chest rise, continue chest compressions.

If you are unable to relieve a severe airway obstruction in an unresponsive patient with the basic techniques previously discussed, you should proceed with **direct laryngoscopy** (visualization of the airway with a laryngoscope) for the removal of the foreign body. Insert the laryngoscope blade into the patient's mouth. If you see the foreign body, carefully remove it from the upper airway with **Magill forceps**, a special type of curved forcep **Figure 37**.

The steps for removal of an upper airway obstruction with Magill forceps are listed here and shown in **Skill Drill 8**:

Skill Drill 8

1. With the patient's head in the sniffing position, open the patient's mouth and insert the laryngoscope blade **Step 1**.
2. Visualize the obstruction, and retrieve the object with the Magill forceps **Step 2**.
3. Remove the object with the Magill forceps **Step 3**.
4. Attempt to ventilate the patient **Step 4**.

Words of Wisdom

A patient with a severe upper airway obstruction has very little time before severe hypoxia develops. If several attempts to relieve the obstruction with conventional BLS methods fail, you should proceed with direct laryngoscopy without delay. As you are performing BLS maneuvers, your partner should be preparing the laryngoscope handle and blade.

Supplemental Oxygen Therapy

Supplemental oxygen should be administered to any patient with potential hypoxia, regardless of his or her clinical appearance. In some conditions, a part of the patient's body does not receive enough oxygen, *even though the oxygen supply to the body*

as a whole is adequate. For example, when a patient experiences an acute myocardial infarction (heart attack), a portion of the myocardium is hypoxic, *even though the rest of the body is well oxygenated.* Increasing the available oxygen supply also enhances the body's compensatory mechanisms during shock and other distressed states.

The oxygen-delivery method must be appropriate for the patient's ventilatory status and should be reassessed frequently and adjusted accordingly based on the patient's clinical condition and breathing adequacy.

Oxygen Sources

Oxygen Cylinders

Pure (100%) oxygen is stored in seamless steel or aluminum cylinders, whose colors may vary from silver, to chrome, to green, or some combination thereof. Make sure that the cylinder is labeled "medical oxygen." Also, look for letters and numbers stamped on the collar of the cylinder **Figure 38**. Of particular importance are the month and year stamps, which indicate when the cylinder was last hydrostatically tested.

Oxygen cylinders are available in various sizes. You will most often use the D cylinder, which contains 350 L of oxygen and is typically carried from the ambulance to the patient, and the M cylinder, which contains 3,000 L of oxygen and remains on board the ambulance as a main supply tank.

Oxygen delivery is measured in terms of liters per minute (L/min). As a precaution against running out at an inconvenient moment, you should replace an oxygen cylinder with a full one when the pressure falls to 200 psi or lower. That level is called the **safe residual pressure**, indicating that it is *unsafe* to continue using the oxygen cylinder. In some EMS systems, the safe

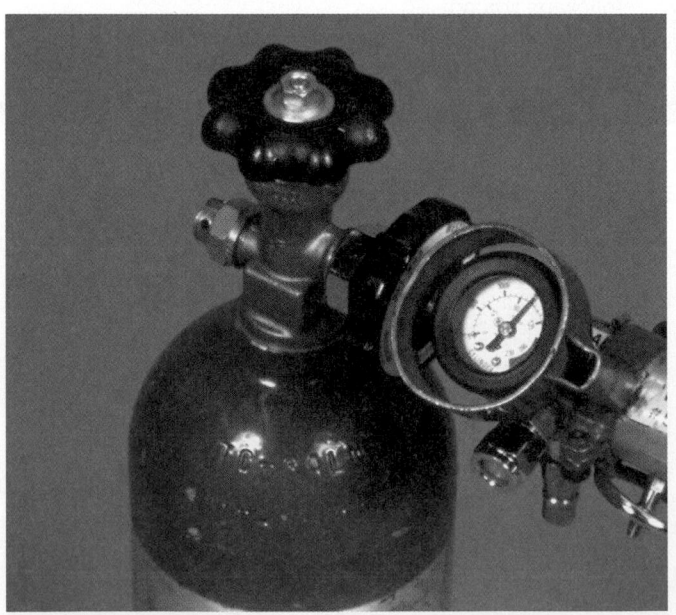

Figure 38 Oxygen cylinders for medical use have a series of letters and numbers stamped into the metal on the collar of the cylinder.

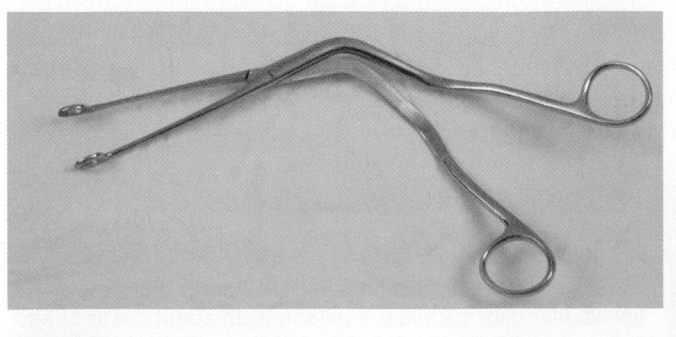

Figure 37 Magill forceps.

Skill Drill 8

Removal of an Upper Airway Obstruction With Magill Forceps

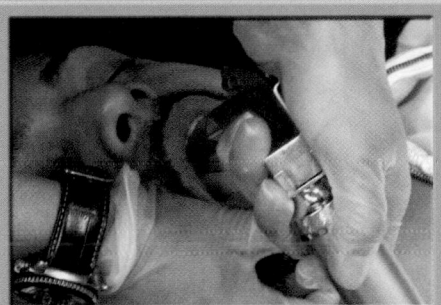

Step 1 With the patient's head in the sniffing position, open the patient's mouth and insert the laryngoscope blade.

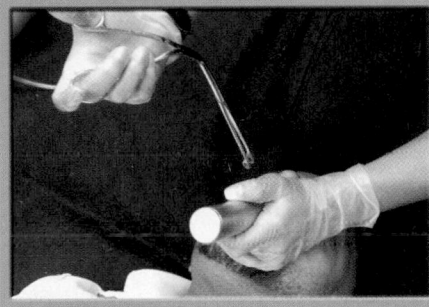

Step 2 Visualize the obstruction, and retrieve the object with the Magill forceps.

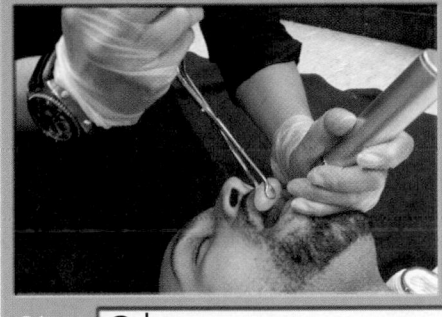

Step 3 Remove the object with the Magill forceps.

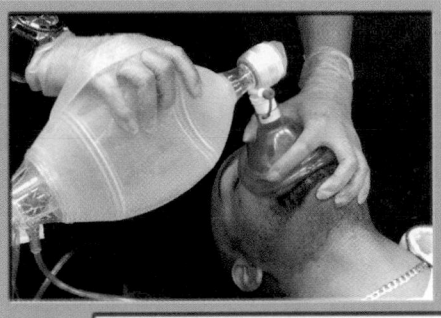

Step 4 Attempt to ventilate the patient.

residual pressure for an oxygen cylinder is 500 psi. On the basis of the pressure in the oxygen cylinder and the flow rate of oxygen delivery, you can calculate how long the supply of oxygen in the cylinder will last—that is, the tank life Table 8 .

Liquid Oxygen

Liquid oxygen is oxygen that is cooled to its aqueous state. It converts to a gaseous state when warmed. Although much larger volumes of gaseous oxygen can be stored in the aqueous state, units for liquid oxygen generally require upright storage Figure 39 . In addition, there are special requirements for large-volume storage and cylinder transfer.

■ Safety Reminders

Any cylinder containing compressed gas under high pressure has the potential, under specific conditions, to assume the properties of a rocket. Furthermore, oxygen presents the additional hazard of fire because it supports the combustion process. For

Table 8 Oxygen Cylinders: Duration of Flow
Formula
(Tank Pressure in psi* − 200 psi [the safe residual pressure]) × Cylinder Constant/Flow Rate in L/min = Duration of Flow in min
Cylinder Constant
D = 0.16   G = 2.41 E = 0.28   H = 3.14 M = 1.56   K = 3.14
Steps
Determine the life of an M cylinder that has a pressure of 2,000 psi and a flow rate of 10 L/min. $$\frac{(2{,}000 - 200) \times 1.56}{10} = \frac{2{,}808}{10} = 281\,\text{min, or 4 h 41 min}$$
*Note: psi indicates pounds per square inch.

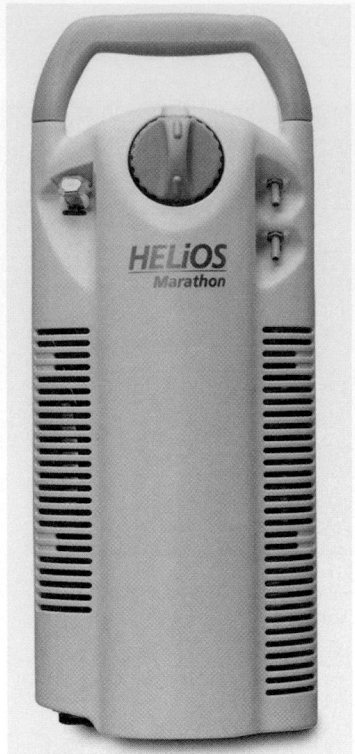

Figure 39 Liquid oxygen converts to a gas when warmed. It must be stored upright.

these reasons, safety precautions are necessary when you are handling oxygen cylinders:

- Keep combustible materials, such as oil and grease, away from contact with the cylinder itself, the regulators, fittings, valves, and tubing.
- Do not permit smoking in any area where oxygen cylinders are in use or on standby.
- Store oxygen cylinders in a cool, well-ventilated area. Do not subject the cylinders to temperatures above 125°F (approximately 50°C).
- Use an oxygen cylinder only with a safe, properly fitting regulator valve.

Regulator valves for one gas should never be modified for use with another gas.

- Close all valves when the cylinder is not in use, even if the tank is empty.
- Secure cylinders so that they will not topple over. In transit, keep them in a proper carrier or rack, or strap them onto the stretcher with the patient.
- When working with an oxygen cylinder, always position yourself to its side. Never place any part of your body over the cylinder valve. A loosely fitting regulator can be blown off the cylinder with sufficient force to demolish any object in its path.
- Have the cylinder hydrostat tested every 10 years to make sure it can still sustain the high pressures required. The original test date is stamped onto the cylinder together with its serial number.

Oxygen Regulators and Flowmeters

High-pressure regulators are attached to the cylinder stem to deliver cylinder gas under high pressure. These regulators are used to transfer cylinder gas from tank to tank, such as when you are refilling a portable oxygen cylinder.

The pressure of gas in a full oxygen cylinder is approximately 2,000 psi. Clearly, this is far too much pressure to deliver directly into a patient's airway. Instead, gas flow from an oxygen cylinder to the patient is controlled by a **therapy regulator**, which attaches to the stem of the oxygen cylinder and reduces the high pressure of gas to a safe range (about 50 psi).

Flowmeters, which are usually permanently attached to the therapy regulator, allow the oxygen delivered to the patient to be adjusted within a range of 1 to 25 L/min. The two types of flowmeters most commonly used are the pressure-compensated flowmeter and the Bourdon-gauge flowmeter.

A **pressure-compensated flowmeter** incorporates a float ball within a tapered calibrated tube; this float rises or falls based on the gas flow in the tube. The gas flow is controlled by a needle valve located downstream from the float ball. Because this type of flowmeter is affected by gravity, it must remain in an upright position to obtain an accurate flow reading **Figure 40**.

By contrast, the **Bourdon-gauge flowmeter** is not affected by gravity and can be placed in any position. This pressure gauge is calibrated to record the flow rate **Figure 41**. The major disadvantage of this type of flowmeter is that it does not compensate for backpressure. As a result, it will usually record a higher flow rate when there is any obstruction to gas flow downstream.

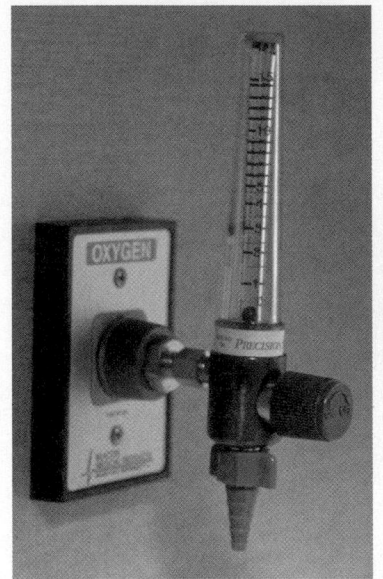

Figure 40 Pressure-compensated flowmeters contain a float ball that rises or falls based on the gas flow in the tube. It must remain in an upright position for an accurate flow reading.

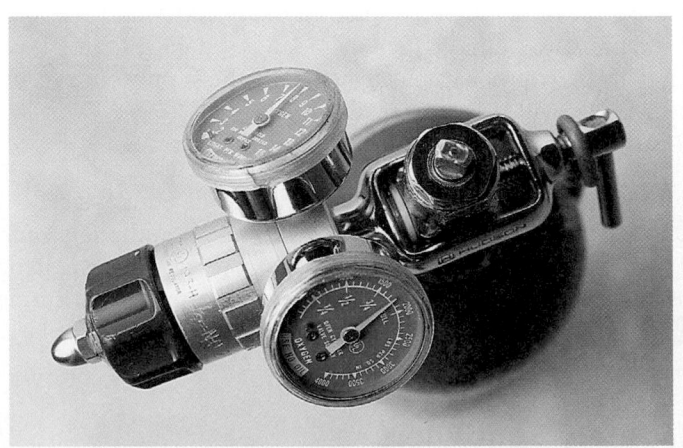

Figure 41 The Bourdon-gauge flowmeter is not affected by gravity and can be placed in any position.

Preparing an Oxygen Cylinder for Use

Before administering supplemental oxygen, you must prepare the oxygen cylinder and therapy regulator. To place an oxygen cylinder into service, follow the steps listed here and shown in **Skill Drill 9**:

Skill Drill   9

1. Inspect the cylinder and its markings. Remove the plastic seal covering the valve stem opening (if commercially filled). Inspect the opening to ensure that it is free of dirt and other debris. With the tank facing away from

yourself and others, use an oxygen wrench to "crack" the cylinder—quickly opening and closing the valve to ensure that dirt particles and other contaminants do not enter the oxygen flow **Step 1**.

2. Attach the regulator/flowmeter to the valve stem, ensuring that the pin-index system is correctly aligned. A metal or plastic O-ring is placed around the oxygen port to optimize the airtight seal between the collar of the regulator and the valve stem **Step 2**.

3. Place the regulator collar over the cylinder valve, with the oxygen port and indexing pins on the side of the valve stem that has three holes. Align the regulator so that the

Skill Drill   9

Placing an Oxygen Cylinder Into Service

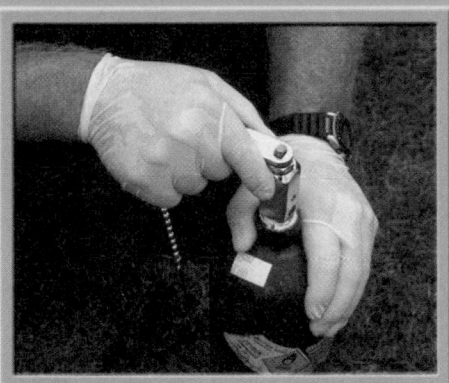

Step 1 Using an oxygen wrench, turn the valve counterclockwise to "crack" the cylinder.

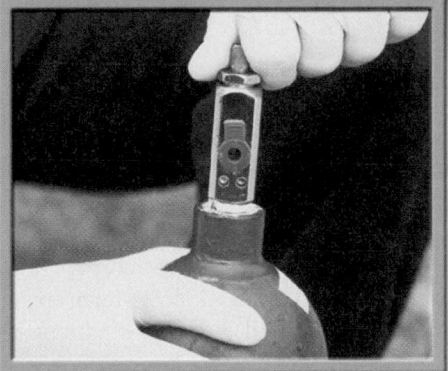

Step 2 Attach the regulator/ flowmeter to the valve stem using the two pin-indexing holes, and make sure that the O-ring is in place over the larger hole.

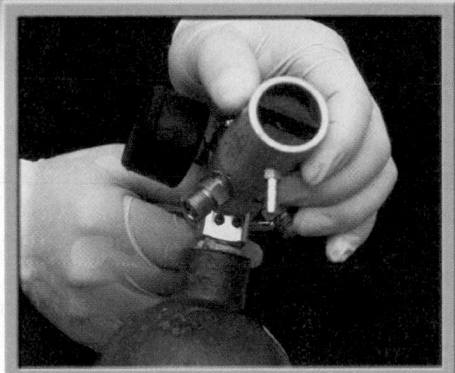

Step 3 Align the regulator so that the pins fit snugly into the correct holes on the valve stem and hand-tighten the regulator.

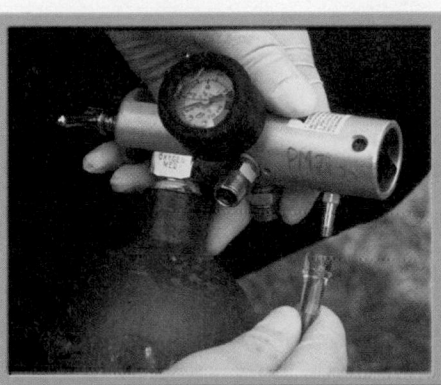

Step 4 Attach the oxygen connective tubing to the flowmeter.

oxygen port and the pins fit into the correct holes on the valve stem; align the screw bolt on the opposite side with the dimpled depression. Tighten the screw bolt until the regulator is firmly attached to the cylinder. At this point, you should not see any space between the sides of the valve stem and the interior walls of the collar Step 3.

4. With the regulator firmly attached, open the cylinder and read the pressure level on the regulator gauge. Follow your local protocols regarding minimum cylinder pressures.

5. A second gauge or a selector dial on the flowmeter indicates the oxygen flow rate. Attach the oxygen connective tubing to the "Christmas tree" nipple on the flowmeter and select the oxygen flow rate that is appropriate for your patient's condition Step 4.

Supplemental Oxygen-Delivery Devices

In general, the oxygen-delivery equipment that is used in the prehospital setting is limited to nonrebreathing masks, bag-mask devices, and nasal cannulas, depending on local protocol. However, you may encounter other devices during transports between medical facilities.

Nonrebreathing Mask

The **nonrebreathing mask** is the preferred device for providing supplemental oxygen to spontaneously breathing patients in the prehospital setting. With a good mask-to-face seal and a flow rate of 15 L/min, it is capable of providing between 90% and 100% inspired oxygen (Fio_2).

The nonrebreathing mask is a combination mask and reservoir bag system. Oxygen fills a reservoir bag that is attached to the mask by a one-way valve, permitting the patient to inhale from the reservoir bag but not to exhale back into it. The only gas that can enter the reservoir, therefore, is 100% oxygen piped in from the oxygen cylinder. Exhaled gas escapes through one-way flapper valves located on the side of the mask Figure 42.

Before administering oxygen to a patient with a nonrebreathing mask, you must ensure that the reservoir bag is completely filled. The oxygen flow rate is adjusted from 12 to 15 L/min to prevent collapse of the bag during inhalation. Use a pediatric nonrebreathing mask, which has a smaller reservoir bag, for infants and small children; they inhale smaller volumes of air.

The nonrebreathing mask is indicated for spontaneously breathing patients who require high-flow oxygen concentrations (such as in shock or with hypoxia from any cause) and are breathing adequately (that is, adequate tidal volume, normal rate and regularity). Contraindications include apnea and poor respiratory effort. Because the nonrebreathing mask delivers oxygen passively, the patient's respirations must be of adequate depth to open the one-way valve and draw air from the reservoir bag into the lungs. A patient with a marked reduction in tidal volume (shallow breathing) will benefit little, if at all, from a nonrebreathing mask.

Nasal Cannula

The **nasal cannula** delivers oxygen via two small prongs that fit into the patient's nostrils Figure 43. With an oxygen flow rate of 1 to 6 L/min, the nasal cannula can provide an oxygen concentration of 24% to 44%. Higher flow rates will merely irritate the nasal mucosa without increasing the delivered oxygen concentration. An oxygen humidifier should be used when giving oxygen via nasal cannula for a prolonged period because it will help prevent mucosal drying and irritation.

The nasal cannula provides low to moderate oxygen enrichment and is most beneficial for patients who require long-term oxygen therapy (such as for COPD). It is ineffective if the patient is apneic, has poor respiratory effort, is severely hypoxic, or is a mouth-breather. In the prehospital setting, the nasal cannula is primarily used when patients who need oxygen cannot tolerate a nonrebreathing mask or if they require only low concentrations of oxygen to maintain an oxygen saturation greater than 94%.

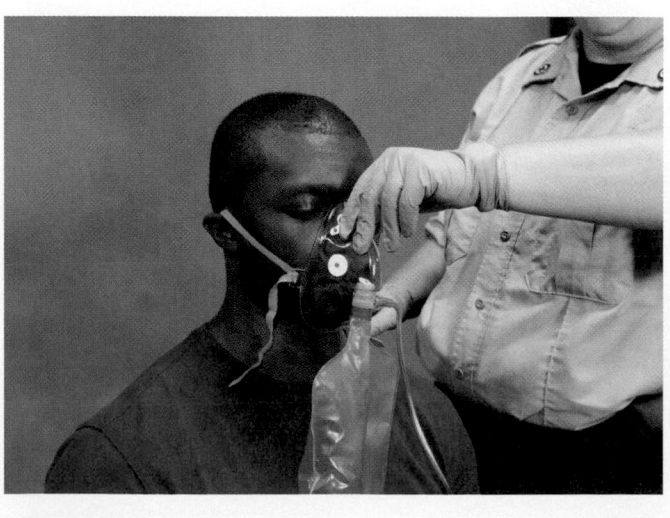

Figure 42 Nonrebreathing mask.

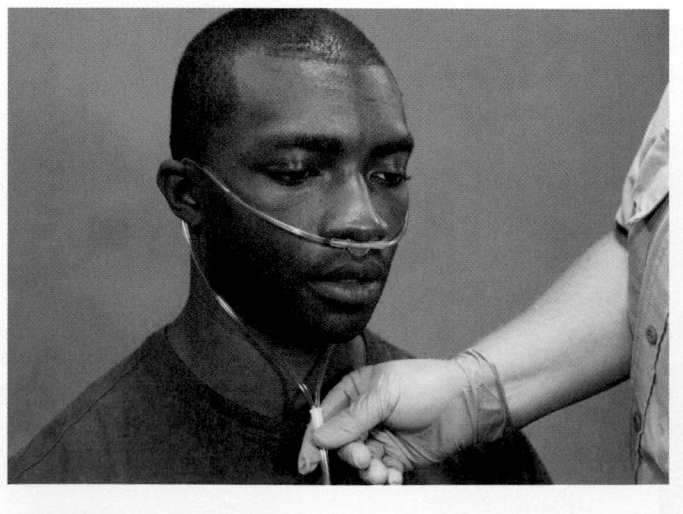

Figure 43 Nasal cannula.

The nasal cannula is generally well tolerated, especially by patients who are claustrophobic and intolerant of an oxygen mask over their face. However, it does not provide high volumes or concentrations of oxygen.

Partial Rebreathing Mask

A **partial rebreathing mask** is similar to the nonrebreathing mask except that it lacks a one-way valve between the mask and the reservoir **Figure 44**. Room air is not drawn in with inhalation, but residual exhaled air is mixed in the mask and rebreathed.

Contraindications are the same as for the nonrebreathing mask—any patient with apnea or inadequate tidal volume. Because inhaled gas is not mixed with room air, higher oxygen concentrations are attainable—at flow rates of 6 to 10 L/min, an oxygen concentration of 35% to 60% becomes possible. Increasing the oxygen flow rate beyond 10 L/min will not enhance the oxygen concentration, and leakage from the mask around the face decreases the amount of oxygen inhaled by the patient.

Venturi Mask

The **Venturi mask** draws room air into the mask along with the oxygen flow, allowing for the administration of highly specific oxygen concentrations **Figure 45**. Depending on the adapter used, the Venturi mask can deliver 24%, 28%, 35%, or 40% oxygen. Venturi masks are especially useful in the hospital management of patients with COPD and other chronic respiratory diseases. They offer little advantage in prehospital care, except in the long-range transport of patients with such conditions.

Tracheostomy Masks

Patients with tracheostomies do not breathe through their nose and mouth; therefore, a face mask or nasal cannula would be ineffective for providing oxygen. Masks designed specifically for patients with tracheostomies cover the tracheostomy hole (stoma) and have a strap that goes around the neck. These masks are usually available in intensive care units, where many patients have tracheostomies, and may not be available in the emergency setting. If you do not have a tracheostomy mask, you can improvise by placing a face mask over the stoma. Even though the

mask is shaped to fit the face, you can usually get an adequate fit over the patient's neck by adjusting the strap **Figure 46**.

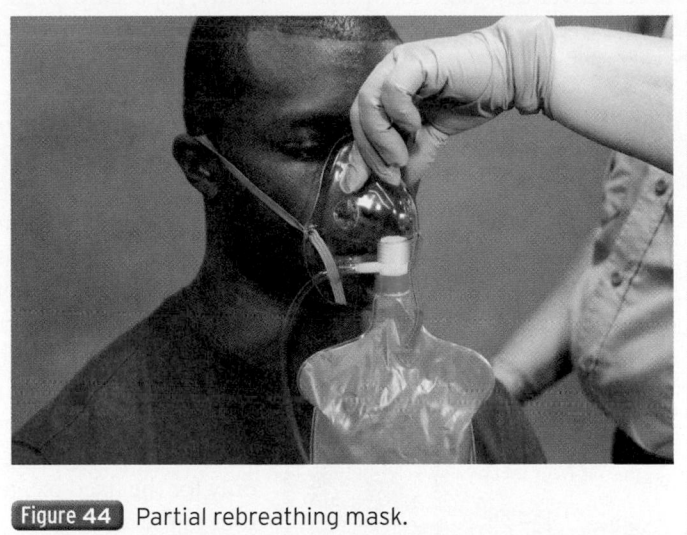

Figure 44 Partial rebreathing mask.

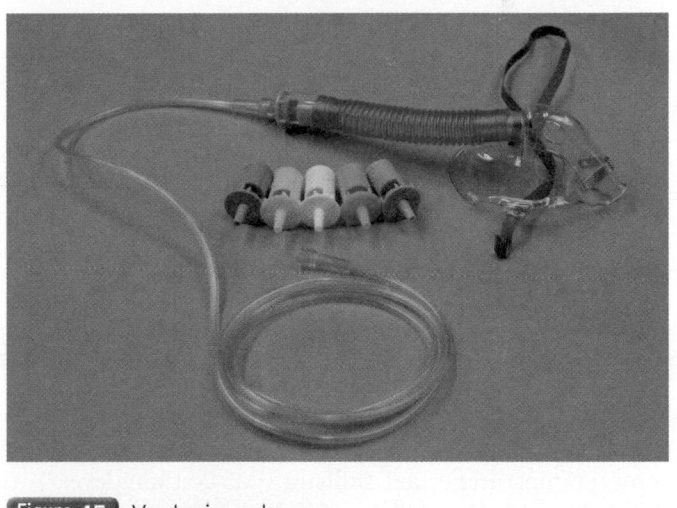

Figure 45 Venturi mask.

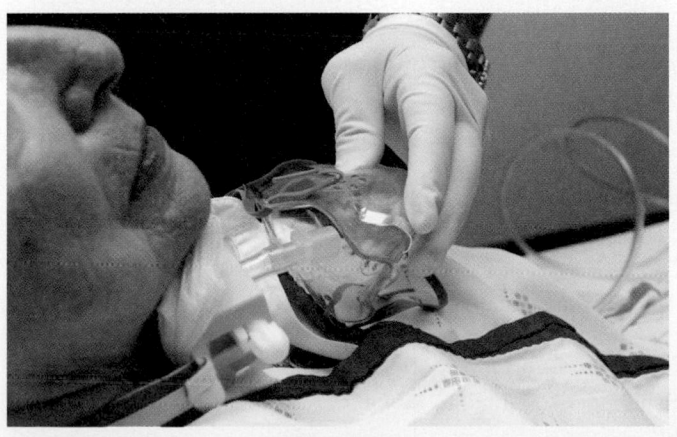

Figure 46 If a tracheostomy mask is not available, a face mask can be used instead.

Oxygen Humidifier

Oxygen stored in cylinders has zero humidity, and it is not a good idea to deliver dry gases to a patient's airway, especially for long periods. In fact, oxygen that is entirely devoid of moisture will rapidly dry the patient's mucous membranes. An <u>oxygen humidifier</u> consists of small bottle of sterile water through which the oxygen leaving the cylinder becomes moisturized before it reaches the patient Figure 47 . Because the humidifier must be kept in an upright position, however, it is practical only for the fixed oxygen unit in the ambulance.

Oxygen humidifiers can be a source of infection for the patient. For this reason, you should either fill the nondisposable bottle halfway with sterile water and clean the bottle in between patients, or use a disposable bottle.

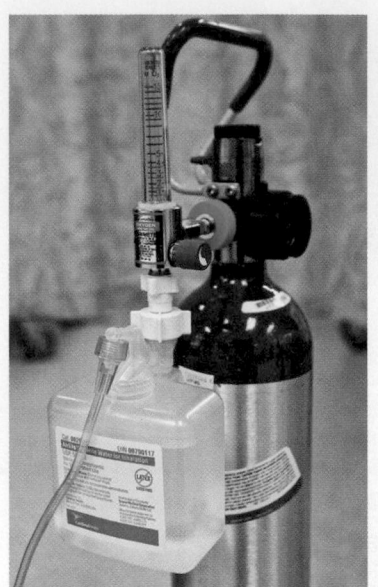

Figure 47 Administering humidified oxygen is preferred for long-range transports to avoid drying the patient's mucous membranes.

Ventilatory Support

Obviously, a patient who is not breathing needs artificial ventilation and 100% supplemental oxygen. Artificial ventilation is among the most important skills in EMS—at any level. Artificial ventilation is the skill of providing assisted ventilation to a patient who is breathing spontaneously, or by ventilating a patient who is not breathing at all. Artificial ventilation techniques are extremely effective when performed properly. Mastery of these techniques is imperative.

Patients who are breathing inadequately, such as too fast or too slowly with reduced tidal volume (shallow breathing), are typically unable to speak in complete sentences. An irregular breathing pattern may also require artificial ventilation to assist in maintaining adequate minute volume. Fast, shallow breathing can be just as dangerous as very slow breathing. Fast, shallow breathing moves air primarily in the larger airway passages (dead space) and does not allow for adequate exchange of oxygen and carbon dioxide in the alveoli. Signs of altered mental status and inadequate minute volume are indications for assisted ventilation. In addition, excessive accessory muscle use and fatigue from labored breathing are signs of potential respiratory failure. Patients with these signs need immediate treatment. Two treatment options are available for patients with severe respiratory distress or respiratory failure: assisted ventilation with a bag-mask device or continuous positive airway pressure (CPAP). The purpose of assisted ventilation is to improve the overall oxygenation and ventilatory status of the patient. CPAP is discussed later in this chapter; the focus of this section is assisted ventilation with a bag-mask device.

Normal Ventilation Versus Positive-Pressure Ventilation

As discussed earlier, the act of moving air into and out of the lungs is based on pressure changes within the thoracic cavity. During normal ventilation, the diaphragm contracts and negative pressure is generated in the chest cavity. This negative pressure draws air into the chest through the trachea in an attempt to equalize the pressure in the chest with the pressure of the external atmosphere (negative-pressure ventilation). However, positive-pressure ventilation generated by a device, such as a bag-mask device, forces air into the chest cavity from the external environment. The difference between normal ventilation and positive-pressure ventilation can create challenges for paramedics Table 9 .

Table 9 Normal Ventilation Versus Positive-Pressure Ventilation		
	Normal Ventilation	**Positive-Pressure Ventilation**
Air movement	Air is sucked into the lungs due to the negative intrathoracic pressure created when the diaphragm contracts.	Air is forced into the lungs by means of mechanical ventilation.
Blood movement	Normal breathing allows blood to naturally be pulled back to the heart.	Intrathoracic pressure is increased, not allowing blood to be adequately pulled back to the heart and resulting in reduction of the amount of blood pumped by the heart.
Airway wall pressure	Not affected during normal breathing	More volume is required to have the same effects as normal breathing. As a result, the walls are pushed out of their normal anatomic shape.
Esophageal opening pressure	Not affected during normal breathing	Air is forced into the stomach, causing gastric distention that could result in vomiting and aspiration.
Overventilation	Not typical of normal breathing	Forcing volume and rate results in increased intrathoracic pressure, gastric distention, and decreased cardiac output (hypotension).

The physical act of the chest wall expanding and recoiling during breathing aids the circulatory system in returning blood to the heart. During normal ventilation, the chest wall movement works similar to a pump. The pressure changes in the thoracic cavity help draw venous blood back to the heart, which improves preload. However, when positive-pressure ventilation is initiated, more air is needed to achieve the same oxygenation and ventilatory effects of normal breathing. This increase in airway wall pressure causes the walls of the chest cavity to push out of their normal anatomic shape. As a result, there is an increase in the overall intrathoracic pressure within the chest cavity. Positive pressure affects venous return to the heart (reduced preload). The blood flow is decreased due to the increased pressure in the chest. This decreased blood flow results in insufficient venous return to the heart, and as a result, the amount of blood pumped out of the heart is reduced. Therefore, it is imperative that paramedics regulate the rate and volume of artificial ventilations to help prevent this drop in cardiac output. Cardiac output is a function of stroke volume multiplied by the pulse rate. Stroke volume is the amount of blood ejected by the ventricle in one cardiac cycle. The pulse rate is assessed by palpating the pulse for 1 minute. The cardiac output is the amount of blood ejected by the left ventricle in 1 minute.

Another difference between normal ventilation and positive-pressure ventilation is the control of airflow. When a person breathes, air enters the trachea and, generally, not the esophagus. However, the force generated from positive-pressure ventilation allows air to enter not only the trachea, but also the esophagus. Ventilations that are too forceful can open the esophagus—normally a flat tube—and instill air in the stomach. This potential complication—called gastric distention—is discussed later in this chapter.

Assisted Ventilation

Follow these steps to assist a patient's ventilations using a bag-mask device. Remember to follow standard precautions as needed when managing the patient's airway.

1. Explain the procedure to the patient.
2. Place the mask over the patient's nose and mouth.
3. Squeeze the bag each time the patient inhales, maintaining the same rate as the patient, coaching the patient as needed.
4. After the initial 5 to 10 breaths, slowly adjust the rate and deliver the appropriate tidal volume.
5. Adjust the rate and tidal volume to maintain adequate minute volume.

Words of Wisdom

Methods of positive-pressure ventilation (listed in order of preference):
- Two-person bag-mask device with reservoir and supplemental oxygen
- Mouth-to-mask with one-way valve and supplemental oxygen attached
- Manually triggered ventilation device (flow-restricted, oxygen-powered ventilation device)
- One-person bag-mask device with oxygen reservoir and supplemental oxygen

Note: This order of preference has been stated because research has demonstrated that personnel who infrequently ventilate patients have great difficulty maintaining an adequate seal between the mask and the patient's face.

YOU are the Medic | PART 5

The patient's head is appropriately positioned, a nasopharyngeal airway is inserted, and your partner begins assisting the patient's breathing with a bag-mask device attached to high-flow oxygen. As the EMTs from the engine company bring in the stretcher, you quickly reassess the patient and prepare him for transport.

Recording Time: 11 Minutes	
Level of consciousness	U (unresponsive)
Respirations	8 breaths/min (baseline); ventilations being assisted
Pulse	128 beats/min; weak and regular
Skin	Cyanotic and diaphoretic
Blood pressure	110/58 mm Hg
Spo$_2$	84% (with assisted ventilation and oxygen)
ETCO$_2$	56 mm Hg
ECG	Sinus tachycardia

9. Why must you use caution when providing positive-pressure ventilation?

10. Is it necessary to adjust your current treatment? If so, how?

Artificial Ventilation

Without immediate treatment, patients who are in respiratory arrest will die. However, the act of breathing for a patient, or artificial ventilation, is not a skill you should take lightly. Once you determine that a patient is not breathing, you must begin artificial ventilation immediately. The methods that you may use to provide artificial ventilation include the mouth-to-mask technique; a one-, two-, or three-person bag-mask device technique; and the manually triggered ventilation device.

Mouth-to-Mouth, Mouth-to-Nose, and Mouth-to-Mask Ventilation

As you learned in your CPR course, mouth-to-mouth ventilation is routinely performed with a barrier device, such as a mask with a one-way valve or a plastic face shield **Figure 48**. A barrier device is a protective item that features a plastic barrier placed on a patient's face with a one-way valve to prevent the backflow of secretions, vomitus, and gases. Barrier devices provide adequate protection for paramedics.

Mouth-to-mouth is the most basic form of ventilation. Mouth-to-nose is simply ventilating through the nose rather than the mouth. Indications for this type of ventilation include apnea and the lack of availability of other ventilation devices.

Although mouth-to-mouth and mouth-to-nose ventilation require no special equipment and can provide adequate tidal volume, there are other methods of providing artificial ventilation that are safer for paramedics. The disadvantages of the mouth-to-mouth and mouth-to-nose techniques include the risk of unknown communicable diseases and psychological barriers associated with these methods.

Mouth-to-mask ventilation is preferred over the mouth-to-mouth and mouth-to-nose techniques. Advantages of using a mask include placing a physical barrier between your mouth and the patient's mouth. Most masks feature a one-way valve to prevent exposure to blood and other body fluids. It is also easier to secure an effective seal with a mask because you can use both hands, which enables the provision of adequate tidal volume to the patient.

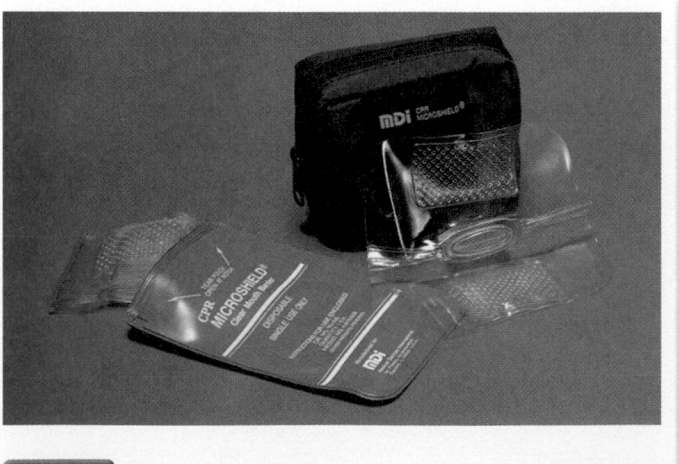

Figure 48 Plastic face shield.

A mask with an oxygen inlet provides oxygen during mouth-to-mask ventilation to supplement the air from your own lungs. Remember that the gas you exhale contains 16% oxygen, which is adequate to sustain a patient's life for a limited period. With the mouth-to-mask system, however, the patient receives the additional benefit of significant oxygen enrichment with inspired air—up to 55%.

The mask may be shaped like a triangle or a doughnut, with the apex (top) placed across the bridge of the nose. The base (bottom) of the mask is placed in the groove between the lower lip and the chin. In the center of the mask is a chimney with a 15-mm connector.

To perform mouth-to-mask ventilation, follow the steps listed here and shown in **Skill Drill 10**:

Skill Drill 10

1. Kneel at the patient's head. Open the airway by using the head tilt–chin lift or the jaw-thrust maneuver if trauma is suspected. Insert an oral or nasal airway to help maintain airway patency. Connect the one-way valve to the face mask, and place the mask on the patient's face. Make sure the top is over the bridge of the nose and the bottom is between the lower lip and chin. Hold the mask in position by placing your thumbs over the top part of the mask and your index fingers over the bottom half. Grasp the patient's lower jaw with the next three fingers on each hand. Place your thumbs on the dome of the mask, making an airtight seal by applying firm pressure between the thumbs and fingers. Maintain an upward and forward pull on the lower jaw with your fingers to keep the airway open **Step 1**.

2. Take a deep breath, and exhale through the open port of the one-way valve. Deliver the breath over a period of 1 second as you observe for visible chest rise **Step 2**.

3. Remove your mouth, and watch for the patient's chest to fall during passive exhalation **Step 3**.

Ventilation effectiveness is best determined by watching the patient's chest rise and fall and feeling for resistance of the patient's lungs as they expand. You should also hear and feel air escape as the patient passively exhales. Make sure you provide the correct number of breaths per minute for the patient's age **Table 10**.

The Bag-Mask Device

With an oxygen flow rate of 15 L/min and an adequate seal, a **bag-mask device** with an oxygen reservoir can deliver nearly 100% oxygen. Most bag-mask devices on the market include modifications or accessories (reservoirs) that permit the delivery of oxygen concentrations approaching 100%. However, the device can deliver only as much volume as can be squeezed out of the bag by hand. The bag-mask device provides less tidal volume than mouth-to-mask ventilation; however, it delivers a much higher oxygen concentration.

Skill Drill 10

Mouth-to-Mask Ventilation

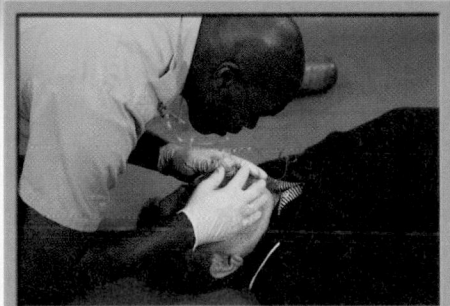

Step 1 Once the patient's head is properly positioned and an airway adjunct is inserted, place the mask on the patient's face. Seal the mask to the face using both hands.

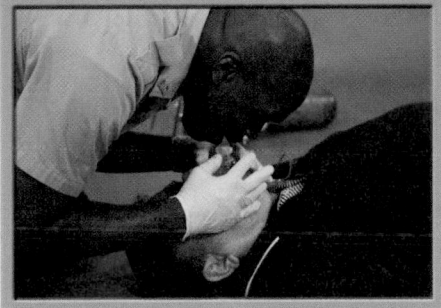

Step 2 Exhale slowly into the open port of the one-way valve until you notice visible chest rise.

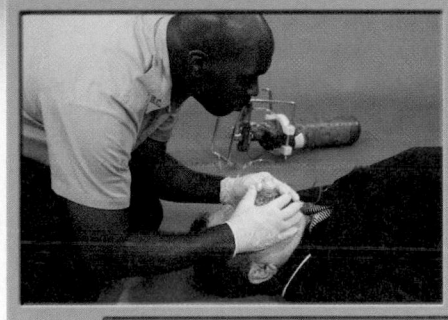

Step 3 Remove your mouth, and watch the patient's chest fall during exhalation.

Table 10 Ventilation Rates	
Adult*	Apneic with a pulse: 10 to 12 breaths/min ■ With or without an advanced airway in place (eg, ET tube, LMA) Apneic and pulseless: 8 to 10 breaths/min ■ After an advanced airway has been inserted
Infant and Child*	Apneic with a pulse: 12 to 20 breaths/min ■ With or without an advanced airway in place (eg, ET tube, LMA) Apneic and pulseless: 8 to 10 breaths/min ■ After an advanced airway has been inserted

Abbreviations: ET indicates endotracheal; and LMA, laryngeal mask airway.
*Avoid hyperventilating any patient; hyperventilated lungs may "squeeze" the heart, thus impeding venous return and subsequent cardiac output. Hyperventilation also increases the risk of regurgitation and aspiration.

Words of Wisdom

Airway management and ventilation procedures often expose you to blood, vomitus, and oral secretions. While blood is the most potentially infectious body fluid, you should exercise great caution to avoid contact with *all* body fluids. Wear gloves for all airway and ventilation procedures and when handling airway equipment that might have been contaminated with body fluids. To mitigate the risk of splashing or droplets of body fluid coming in contact with your mouth, nose, and eyes, wear a mask and protective eyewear or a face shield, especially when inserting an advanced airway. In cases of significant blood splashing, such as in trauma, you should also wear a protective gown, if possible.

The bag-mask device is the most common device used to ventilate patients in the prehospital setting. An experienced paramedic will be able to provide adequate tidal volume with the bag-mask device. Use of the device, however, is a difficult skill to master. Mask seal on a medical patient may be difficult to maintain with only one rescuer. Because it takes two hands to perform a jaw-thrust maneuver, it takes two rescuers to use the bag-mask device on a trauma patient unless an advanced airway has already been inserted. The amount of tidal volume and the concentration of oxygen delivered to the patient are dependent on mask seal integrity. Paramedics should practice frequently by ventilating a manikin with the bag-mask device.

Bag-Mask Device Components

All adult bag-mask devices should have the following components and characteristics:

- A disposable, self-inflating bag
- No pop-off valve or, if one is present, the capability of disabling the pop-off valve
- An outlet valve that is a true nonrebreathing valve

- An oxygen reservoir that permits delivery of a high concentration of oxygen
- A one-way, no-jam inlet valve system that provides an oxygen inlet flow at a maximum of 15 L/min with a standard 15/22-mm fitting for a face mask and an advanced airway (that is, ET tube, LMA, King LT, Combitube)
- A transparent face mask
- The ability to perform under extreme environmental conditions, including extreme heat and cold

The total amount of gas in the reservoir bag of an adult bag-mask device is usually 1,200 to 1,600 mL. The pediatric bag contains 500 to 700 mL, and the infant bag holds 150 to 240 mL.

The volume of air (oxygen) to deliver to the patient is based on one key observation—visible chest rise. A delivered tidal volume of 500 to 600 mL (6–7 mL/kg) per breath will produce visible chest rise in most adults. When using a bag-mask device, whether supplemental oxygen is attached or not, you should deliver each breath over a period of 1 second—just enough to produce visible chest rise—at the appropriate rate. Breaths that are given too forcefully or too fast can result in two negative effects: gastric distention (and the associated risks of vomiting and aspiration) and decreased venous return to the heart (preload) due to increased intrathoracic pressure.

Inadequate tidal volume and oxygen may be delivered because of improper technique, an ineffective mask-to-face seal, or the presence of gastric distention. Training and practice are key to the proper use of the bag-mask device.

Bag-Mask Device Technique

Whenever possible, you and your partner should work together to provide ventilation with the bag-mask device. One paramedic can maintain a good mask seal by securing the mask to the patient's face with two hands while the other paramedic squeezes the bag. Ventilation using a bag-mask device is a challenging skill; it may be very difficult for one EMS provider to maintain a proper seal between the mask and the face with one hand while squeezing the bag well enough to deliver an adequate volume of air to the patient. This skill can be difficult to maintain if you do not have many opportunities to practice. Effective one-person bag-mask ventilation requires considerable experience. Also, performance of this skill depends on having enough personnel to carry out other actions that need to be done at the same time, such as chest compressions, putting the stretcher in place, or helping lift the patient onto the stretcher.

Follow these steps to use the two-person bag-mask device technique:

1. Kneel above the patient's head. If possible, your partner should be at the side of the head. Select the proper size mask.
2. Maintain the patient's neck in a hyperextended position unless you suspect a cervical spine injury, in which case you should stabilize the patient's head and neck in a neutral position and use the jaw-thrust maneuver. Open the patient's mouth, and suction as needed. Insert an oral or nasal airway to help maintain airway patency.

3. Place the mask on the patient's face. Make sure the top is over the bridge of the nose and the bottom is in the groove between the lower lip and the chin. If the mask has a large, round cuff around the ventilation port, center the port over the patient's mouth. Inflate the collar to obtain a better fit and seal to the face if necessary.
4. Bring the lower jaw up to the mask with your last three fingers. This step will help to maintain an open airway. Make sure you do not grab the fleshy part of the neck because you may compress structures and create an airway obstruction. If you think the patient may have a spinal injury, make sure your partner manually stabilizes the cervical spine as you move the lower jaw.
5. Connect the bag to the mask if you have not already done so.
6. Hold the mask in place while your partner squeezes the bag with two hands until the patient's chest visibly rises **Figure 49**. If a spinal injury is suspected, stabilize the patient's head and neck with your forearms while maintaining an adequate mask-to-face seal with your hands. Continue squeezing the bag once every 5 to 6 seconds for adults and once every 3 to 5 seconds for infants and children.
7. If you are alone, hold your index finger over the lower part of the mask and your thumb over the upper part of the mask, and then use your remaining fingers to pull the lower jaw into the mask. This is called the EC-clamp method and will maintain an effective mask-to-face seal **Figure 50**. Use the head tilt–chin lift maneuver to make sure the neck is extended. Squeeze the bag with your other hand in a rhythmic manner once every 5 to 6 seconds for adults and once every 3 to 5 seconds for infants and children.
8. Observe for gastric distention, changes in compliance of the bag with ventilations, and improvement or deterioration of the patient's clinical status.

When using the bag-mask device to assist ventilation, you should squeeze the bag as the patient inhales. Then, for the next

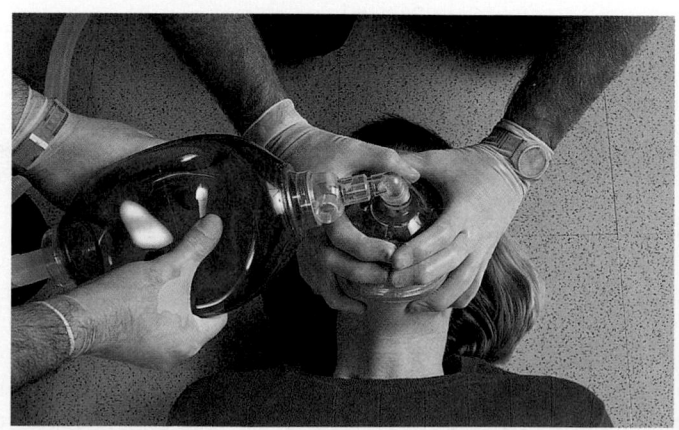

Figure 49 With two-person bag-mask ventilation, you should hold the mask in place while your partner squeezes the bag with two hands until the patient's chest visibly rises.

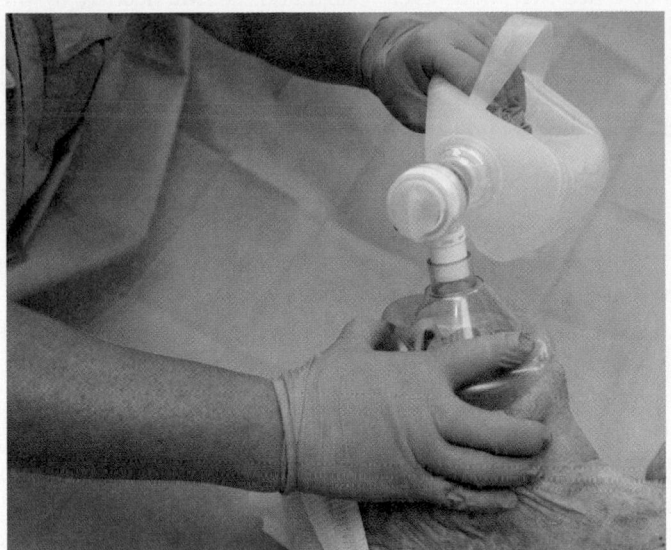

Figure 50 Maintain the seal of the mask to the face using the EC-clamp technique if you must ventilate alone.

5 to 10 breaths, slowly adjust the rate and tidal volume until an adequate minute volume is achieved.

To assist ventilations of a patient who is breathing too fast (hyperventilation) with reduced tidal volume, you must first explain the procedure to the patient if he or she is coherent. Initially assist ventilations at the rate at which the patient has been breathing, squeezing the bag each time the patient inhales. Then, for the next 5 to 10 breaths, slowly adjust the rate and tidal volume until an adequate minute volume is achieved.

As you are assisting ventilations with a bag-mask device, you should evaluate the effectiveness of your ventilations. Artificial ventilations are not adequate if the patient's chest does not rise and fall with each ventilation, the rate of ventilation is too slow or too fast for the patient's age, or the pulse rate does not improve. If the patient's chest does not rise and fall, you may need to reposition the head or insert an oral or nasal airway.

If the patient's stomach, rather than the chest, seems to be rising and falling, you should reposition the head. In a patient with a possible spinal injury, you should reposition the jaw rather than the head. If too much air is escaping from under the mask, reposition the mask for a better seal. If the patient's chest still does not rise and fall after you have made these corrections, check for an airway obstruction. If an obstruction is not present, you should attempt ventilation with another airway device.

Advanced airway techniques are beneficial when ventilation with basic means is not effective, the patient has a cervical spine injury, or the patient's condition otherwise warrants.

■ Manually Triggered Ventilation Devices

Another method of providing artificial ventilation is with the manually triggered ventilation device, also known as the flow-restricted, oxygen-powered ventilation device. This type of device is mainly used to ventilate apneic or hypoventilating patients, although it can also be used to provide supplemental oxygen to breathing patients. Manually triggered ventilation devices have a "demand valve" that is triggered by the negative pressure generated by inhalation. This valve automatically delivers 100% oxygen as the patient begins to inhale and stops the flow of gas at the end of the inhalation phase of the respiratory cycle. Because the manually triggered ventilation device makes an airtight seal with the patient's face, the gas that the patient inspires is nearly 100% oxygen.

The major advantage to this device is that it allows one rescuer to use both hands to maintain a mask-to-face seal while providing positive-pressure ventilation to a spontaneously breathing patient. It also reduces rescuer fatigue associated with using a bag-mask device on extended transports. However, recent findings suggest that manually triggered ventilation devices are associated with difficulty in maintaining adequate ventilation without assistance and should not be used routinely because of the high incidence of gastric distention and possible damage to structures within the chest cavity due to excessive pressure (barotrauma). *This device should not be used for ventilating infants or children or for patients with COPD or possible cervical spine or chest injury.*

Because the rescuer is not squeezing a bag, it is virtually impossible to assess for lung compliance when using the manually triggered ventilation device. As a result, the rescuer should be especially cautious when ventilating; the high ventilatory pressures generated by the device may damage the lung tissue if not carefully monitored. An adult normally consumes 5 L/min of oxygen during ventilation, versus 15 to 25 L/min with the manually triggered device.

Generally, patients find it most comfortable if they hold the mask to their face themselves. The manually triggered ventilation device is an efficient way to conserve oxygen because it delivers only the volume needed by the patient during inhalation, rather than wasting oxygen with a constant flow. These masks, however, are relatively expensive and typically not disposable. The entire unit must be properly disinfected after each use.

The plastic housing of the manually triggered ventilation device has a 22-mm adapter designed to fit into standard ventilation masks. When the button on the top of the regulator is pressed, oxygen flows at a constant rate. Although the manually triggered device solves the pressure and flow rate problems of bag-mask ventilation, one hand is still needed to press the button to ventilate, leaving only one hand to maintain the mask seal and the airway.

Components of Manually Triggered Ventilation Devices

Manually triggered ventilation devices should have the following components and characteristics **Figure 51**:

- A peak flow rate of 100% oxygen of up to 40 L/min
- An inspiratory pressure safety release valve that opens at approximately 30 cm of water and vents any remaining volume to the atmosphere or stops the flow of oxygen
- An audible alarm that sounds whenever the relief valve pressure is exceeded
- The ability to operate satisfactorily under normal and varying environmental conditions
- A trigger (or lever) positioned so that both of the rescuer's hands can remain on the mask to provide an airtight seal while supporting and tilting the patient's head and keeping the jaw elevated

Learning how to use these devices correctly requires proper training and considerable practice. As with bag-mask devices, you must make sure there is an airtight fit between the mask and the patient's face. The amount of pressure that is necessary to ventilate a patient adequately varies according to the size of the patient, the patient's lung volume, and the condition of the lungs. Pressures that are too great can cause a pneumothorax. It is critical for the paramedic to keep his or her eyes on the patient's chest at all times in order to avoid hyperinflation of the lungs. *Always follow local protocol when using these devices.*

■ Automatic Transport Ventilators

The main advantage of manually triggered ventilation devices is the constant flow rate that subsequently controls the upper airway pressure. However, one hand is still needed to press the button and ventilate the patient. Variations in the rate and duration of ventilation are also possible. The **automatic transport ventilator (ATV)** solves these problems. The steps for using the ATV are as follows:

1. Attach the ATV to the wall-mounted oxygen source.
2. Set the tidal volume and ventilatory rate on the ATV as appropriate for the patient's age and condition.
3. Connect the ATV to the 15/22-mm fitting on the ET tube or other advanced airway device.
4. Auscultate the patient's breath sounds, and observe for equal chest rise to ensure adequate ventilation.

The ATV is essentially a manually triggered ventilation device attached to a control box that allows the variables of ventilation—rate and tidal volume—to be set **Figure 52**. Although the ATV lacks the sophisticated controls of a hospital ventilator, it frees your hands to perform other non–airway-related tasks. However, even though the ATV is helpful to paramedics, a bag-mask device should always be readily available should the ATV malfunction.

Most models have adjustments for respiratory rate and tidal volume. In most cases, the respiratory rate is set at the midpoint or average for the patient's age. The paramedic can estimate tidal volume using a formula based on 6 to 7 mL/kg, which can be adjusted based on chest rise and the patient's physiologic response. Automatic transport ventilators are considered volume-cycled, rate-controlled ventilators, which means that they deliver a preset volume at a preset ventilatory rate, although this does not guarantee that all of the volume is being delivered to the lungs, unless the patient is intubated. When using the ATV in the intubated patient who is in cardiac arrest, it is critical to set the rate and tidal volume accordingly in order to reduce the risk of hyperventilation.

Like manually triggered ventilation devices, the ATV is generally oxygen-powered, although some models may require an external power source. Whereas this device requires oxygen, it generally consumes 5 L/min of oxygen, unlike a bag-mask device that uses 15 to 25 L/min. In addition, just like the manually triggered ventilation device, the ATV has a pressure-relief valve, which can lead to hypoventilation in patients with inadequate lung compliance, increased airway resistance, or airway obstruction. There is the possibility of barotrauma if the relief valve fails or if ventilation is overzealous.

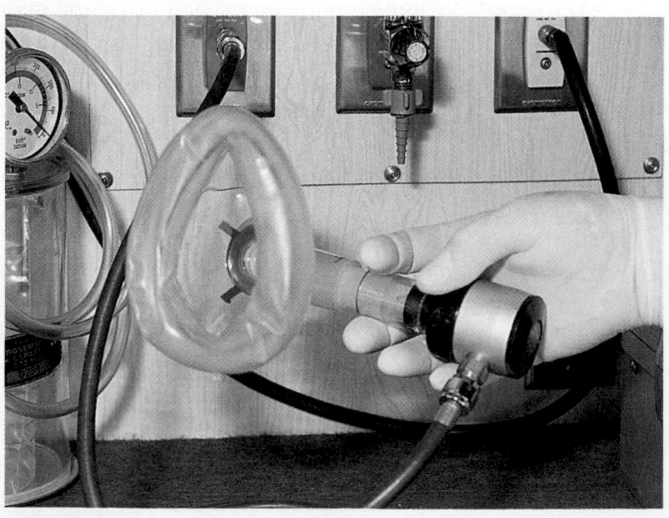

Figure 51 A manually triggered ventilation device can deliver up to 100% oxygen.

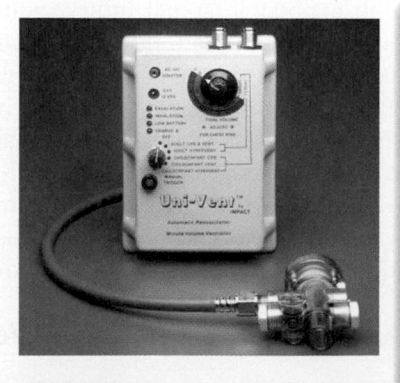

Figure 52 Automatic transport ventilator.

Special Populations

Artificial Ventilation of Pediatric Patients

The flat nasal bridge of pediatric patients makes achieving an effective mask-to-face seal more difficult. Compressing the mask against the face to improve mask seal may result in obstruction. The best mask seal is achieved by the two-person bag-mask ventilation technique with jaw displacement.

A pediatric bag-mask device with a minimum tidal volume of 450 mL should be used for full-term neonates and infants. In children (1 year old to the onset of puberty [12 to 14 years old]), consider the size of the child when determining bag size. An adult bag with a 1,500-mL volume may be used, but a pediatric bag-mask device is preferred. Children older than 12 to 14 years require an adult-sized bag-mask device for adequate ventilation. Choose a size to ensure a proper mask fit. The mask should reach from the bridge of the nose to the cleft of the chin. A length-based resuscitation tape may also be used to determine the most appropriately sized bag-mask device for pediatric patients who weigh up to 75 lb (~34 kg).

When you are ventilating a pediatric patient, ensure that there is a proper mask seal by using the EC-clamp technique. Place the mask over the mouth and nose, avoiding compression of the eyes. With one hand, place your thumb on the mask at the apex (over the nose) and your index finger on the mask at the chin to form a "C." With gentle pressure, push down on the mask to establish an adequate seal. Maintain the airway by lifting the bony prominence of the chin with your remaining fingers, forming an "E." Avoid placing pressure on the soft area under the chin because this pressure may cause an airway obstruction.

Deliver each ventilation over 1 second—just enough to produce visible chest rise. *Do not overinflate.* Deliver one breath every 3 to 5 seconds (12 to 20 breaths/min), allowing adequate time for exhalation. While ventilating, look for adequate chest rise. Auscultate lung sounds at the third intercostal space on the midaxillary line bilaterally. Also assess for improvement in skin color and pulse rate.

◣ Continuous Positive Airway Pressure

Continuous positive airway pressure (CPAP) is a noninvasive means of providing ventilatory support for patients experiencing respiratory distress. Many people with obstructive sleep apnea wear a CPAP unit at night to maintain their airway while they sleep. During the past several years, the use of CPAP in the prehospital setting has proven to be an excellent adjunct in the treatment of respiratory distress caused by acute pulmonary edema, obstructive lung disease, and acute bronchospasm (as in asthma)—especially when used in conjunction with beta-2 agonists. Typically, many patients with these conditions would be managed with advanced airway techniques, such as ET intubation. Research has shown a significant increase in morbidity and mortality when patients with these conditions are intubated for the condition in the prehospital setting. Early intervention with CPAP is an alternative means of providing ventilatory assistance and can prevent the need for intubation. Because of the simplicity of the device and its great benefit to patients, CPAP is becoming widely used by paramedics.

Continuous positive airway pressure increases pressure in the lungs, opens collapsed alveoli and prevents further alveolar collapse (atelectasis), pushes more oxygen across the alveolar membrane, and forces interstitial fluid back into the pulmonary circulation. The desired effect of CPAP is to improve pulmonary compliance and make spontaneous ventilation easier. The therapy is typically delivered through a face mask that is secured to the head with a strapping system. A good seal with minimal leakage between the face and mask is essential.

The face mask is fitted with a pressure relief valve that determines the amount of pressure delivered to the patient (such as 5 cm of water [cm H_2O]). This pressure results in a high inspiratory flow and the need to push a pressure valve open with exhalation. While a great deal of effort on the part of a patient who is already in distress may seem necessary, many patients make a dramatic turnaround when CPAP is applied.

◼ Indications for CPAP

Continuous positive airway pressure is indicated for patients experiencing respiratory distress in which their own compensatory mechanisms cannot keep up with their oxygen demand. Whereas the condition of most patients improves after the application of CPAP, it is important to remember that CPAP is merely treating the symptoms and not necessarily the underlying pathology.

The following are some general guidelines for using CPAP:

- Patient alert and able to follow commands
- Obvious signs of moderate to severe respiratory distress (such as accessory muscle use, tripod position, retractions) from an underlying disease such as congestive heart failure with pulmonary edema, obstructive lung disease (such as COPD), and acute bronchospasm (as in acute asthma)
- Respiratory distress after submersion
- Rapid breathing (more than 26 breaths/min), such that it affects overall minute volume
- Pulse oximetry reading of less than 90%

Whereas these guidelines should be considered when assessing the need for CPAP, it is important that you follow your local guidelines and protocols.

◼ Contraindications to CPAP

Continuous positive airway pressure has proven to be immensely beneficial to patients experiencing respiratory distress from acute pulmonary edema, acute bronchospasm, and obstructive lung disease; however, there are times when CPAP is not appropriate.

The following are general contraindications for CPAP use:

- Respiratory arrest
- Hypoventilation (slow respiratory rate and/or reduced tidal volume)

- Signs and symptoms of a pneumothorax or chest trauma
- Tracheostomy
- Active gastrointestinal bleeding or vomiting
- Patient unable to follow verbal commands
- Inability to properly fit the CPAP system mask and strap
  - Excessive facial hair or dysmorphic facial features can impede your ability to ensure a proper-fitting mask
- Inability to tolerate the mask

In addition, you should always reassess the patient for signs of clinical deterioration and/or respiratory failure. Although CPAP is an excellent tool to assist with ventilation, not all patients will experience improvement in their condition with this device. Once signs of respiratory failure become apparent or the patient is no longer able to follow commands, CPAP should be removed, and positive-pressure ventilation with a bag-mask device attached to high-flow oxygen should be initiated. In some cases, intubation will be required.

■ Application of CPAP

Several varieties of CPAP units are available to EMS services; however, most follow the same general guidelines for use and setup. The CPAP units are generally composed of a generator, a mask, a circuit that contains corrugated tubing, a bacteria filter, and a one-way valve. During the expiratory phase, the patient exhales against a resistance called **positive end-expiratory pressure (PEEP)**. Within the CPAP generator is a valve that determines the amount of PEEP; however, some CPAP models have PEEP valves that connect separately. Depending on the device, the PEEP is controlled by manually adjusting the PEEP using a manometer or predetermined by a fixed setting on the PEEP valve. A PEEP of 5 to 10 cm H_2O is generally an acceptable therapeutic range for a patient using CPAP. Always consult the operations manual of a particular CPAP device for proper assembly instructions.

Because most CPAP units are powered by oxygen, it is important to have a full cylinder of oxygen when using CPAP and a backup cylinder. Some CPAP units use a continuous flow of oxygen, whereas others use oxygen on more of a demand basis. Continuously monitor the amount of available oxygen in the cylinder. Some CPAP units will empty a D cylinder in as little as 5 to 10 minutes. Therefore, proper planning for oxygen consumption is necessary when considering applying CPAP. In addition, some of the newer CPAP devices allow the provider to adjust the F_{IO_2}. Most CPAP devices are set to deliver a fixed F_{IO_2} of 30% to 35%; however, some can deliver as high as 80%.

Follow the steps listed here and shown in **Skill Drill 11** to use CPAP:

Skill Drill   11

1. Check your equipment, then connect the circuit to the CPAP device. **Step 1**.
2. Connect the face mask to the circuit tubing **Step 2**. Once the system is connected, check to see if there is an on/off button or switch. Some of the newer models have this feature. Make sure the device is set in the "on" position before you apply CPAP to the patient.
3. Connect the tubing to the oxygen tank **Step 3**.
4. Confirm that the device is working, and place the mask over the patient's mouth and nose, creating as much of an airtight seal as possible. This task can be rather difficult depending on the patient. Many patients resist the application of the mask to their face while in severe respiratory distress. Explain the application to the patient, and coach him or her through the initial application of the mask. Allowing the patient to hold the mask to his or her face initially may be beneficial in alleviating some of the stress and anxiety associated with CPAP application **Step 4**.
5. Once the mask is on the face, use the strapping mechanism to secure it to the patient's head, making sure the seal between the mask and face remains intact. Consult the manufacturer's guidelines for specific strapping instructions **Step 5**.
6. Adjust the PEEP valve and F_{IO_2} according to the manufacturer's recommendations to maintain adequate oxygenation and ventilation. With CPAP in place, the patient's oxygenation status should improve, the work of breathing should decrease, and the ease of speaking should increase. Constant reassessment of patients for signs of clinical deterioration is essential **Step 6**.

■ Complications of CPAP

The application and administration of CPAP is a relatively easy process. However, some patients may find CPAP claustrophobic and will resist the application. As patients become more hypoxic, the application of the mask to their face is sometimes perceived as suffocation, rather than an attempt to them breathe. In any event, it is important to explain the application to patients and coach them through the process. Do not force the mask on any patient. Forceful application will create a higher level of anxiety and increase oxygen demand. Coach patients through the application of CPAP, allowing them to adjust to the situation. Coaching patients is not always easy; it takes practice and a willingness to work closely with your patient during a rather difficult time.

Because of the high volume of pressure generated by CPAP, causing a pneumothorax due to barotrauma is possible. Whereas some literature suggests a pneumothorax is unlikely, you should be aware of this risk and continually assess your patient for signs and symptoms of a pneumothorax.

In addition to pneumothoraces, increased pressure in the chest cavity can result in hypotension. As the intrathoracic pressure increases, venous blood returning to the heart (preload) meets resistance from the increased pressure in the chest, which can result in a sudden drop in blood pressure. While hypotension is not common with lower levels of CPAP, continuous monitoring of blood pressure is essential.

As with any form of positive-pressure ventilation in the unprotected airway, air may enter the stomach, which increases the risk of aspiration if vomiting occurs.

Skill Drill 11

Using CPAP

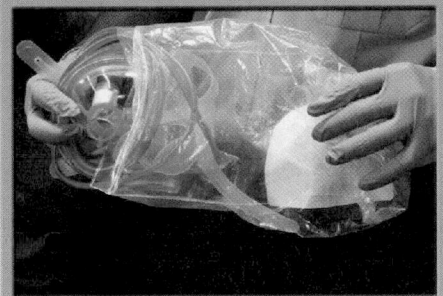

Step 1 Check your equipment, then connect the circuit to the CPAP device.

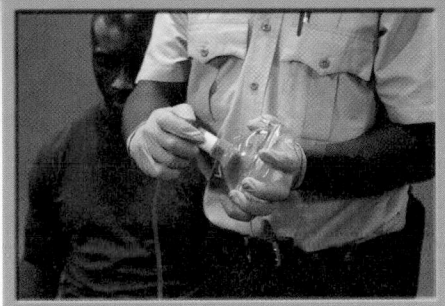

Step 2 Connect the face mask to the circuit tubing.

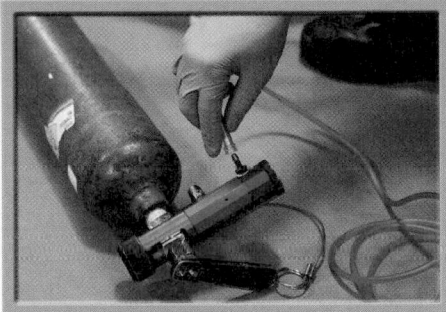

Step 3 Connect the tubing to the oxygen tank.

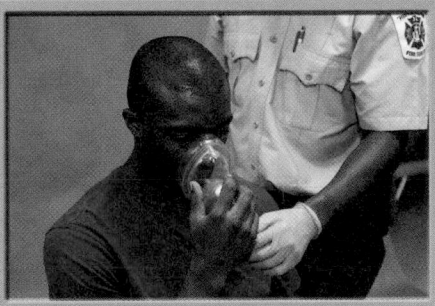

Step 4 Confirm that the device is on before you apply it to the patient's face. Place the mask over the patient's mouth and nose, or allow the patient to hold it to his or her mouth and nose. Allow the patient to get used to the mask.

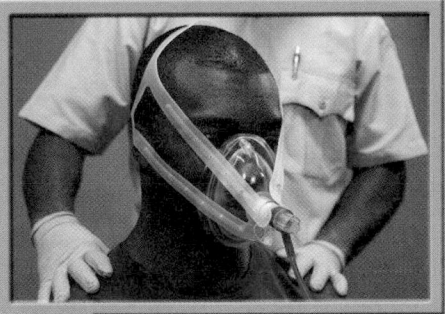

Step 5 Use the strapping mechanism to secure the CPAP to the patient's head. Make sure there is a tight seal.

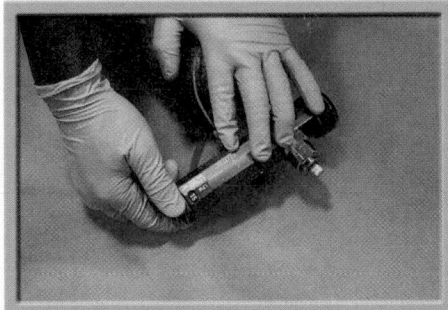

Step 6 Adjust the PEEP valve and the F_{IO_2} according to the manufacturer's recommendations to maintain adequate oxygenation and ventilation. Reassess the patient.

Words of Wisdom

Bilevel positive airway pressure (BiPAP), another form of noninvasive positive-pressure ventilation, is also used to treat patients with obstructive lung disease, acute bronchospasm, and acute pulmonary edema. Whereas CPAP delivers a single pressure (which is most beneficial to the patient during exhalation), BiPAP delivers two pressures—a higher inspiratory positive airway pressure (IPAP), which opens the lower airways, and a lower expiratory positive airway pressure (EPAP), which helps keep the lower airways open. Common BiPAP settings deliver 10 cm H_2O during inhalation and 5 cm H_2O during exhalation. The indications, contraindications, and precautions for BiPAP are the same as they are for CPAP. Follow your EMS system protocols regarding the use of BiPAP and the desired IPAP and EPAP settings.

■ Gastric Distention

Any form of artificial ventilation that blows air into the patient's mouth—as opposed to blowing air directly into the trachea via an ET tube—may lead to inflation of the patient's stomach with air. **Gastric distention**—inflation of the patient's stomach with air—is especially likely to occur when excessive pressure is used to inflate the lungs, when ventilations are performed too fast or too forcefully, or when the airway is partially obstructed during ventilation attempts. The pressure in the airway forces open the esophagus, and air flows into the stomach. Gastric distention occurs most often in children but is common in adults as well.

A distended stomach is harmful for at least two reasons. First, it promotes regurgitation of stomach contents, which can lead to aspiration of the stomach contents. Second, a distended stomach pushes the diaphragm upward into the chest, reducing the amount of space in which the lungs can expand.

Signs of gastric distention include an increase in the diameter of the stomach, an increasingly distended abdomen, and increased resistance to bag-mask ventilations. If these signs are noted, you should reassess and reposition the airway as needed and observe the chest for adequate rise and fall as you continue ventilating. In addition, limit ventilation times to 1 second or the time needed to produce adequate chest rise.

■ Invasive Gastric Decompression

Invasive gastric decompression involves inserting a <u>gastric tube</u> into the stomach and removing the contents with suction. The gastric tube is an effective tool for removing air and liquid from the stomach because removal of the stomach contents decreases the pressure on the diaphragm and virtually eliminates the risks of regurgitation and aspiration. In certain cases of poisoning, activated charcoal can be instilled via a gastric tube.

The gastric tube can be inserted into the stomach through the mouth (<u>orogastric [OG] tube</u>) or through the nose (<u>nasogastric [NG] tube</u>). Use of a gastric tube should be considered for any patient who will need positive-pressure ventilation for an extended period, especially if the patient is not intubated. An NG or OG tube should also be inserted when gastric distention interferes with ventilations—for example, when children are receiving positive-pressure ventilation or have swallowed large volumes of air because of increased work of breathing.

The NG and OG tubes must be used with extreme caution in any patient with known esophageal disease (such as tumors or varices). They should never be used in a patient whose esophagus is not patent. After insertion, make sure that the tube has been placed into the stomach. Occasionally, it may remain in the esophagus without actually entering the stomach (supragastric placement) or may have been placed into the trachea.

Nasogastric Tube
An NG tube is inserted through the nose, into the nasopharynx, through the esophagus, and into the stomach **Figure 53**. In airway management and ventilation, it decompresses the stomach, thereby decreasing pressure on the diaphragm and limiting the risk of regurgitation. The NG tube is also used to perform gastric lavage—a procedure in which the stomach is decontaminated following a toxic ingestion.

The NG tube is relatively well tolerated, even by patients who are responsive. Patients can still talk with an NG tube in place, and, after a few hours, most patients get used to it. For these reasons, the NG route of insertion is generally preferred for responsive patients.

During the insertion of an NG tube, most patients who are responsive will gag and may vomit, even if their gag reflex is suppressed. In a patient with a decreased LOC, vomiting can seriously threaten the airway.

Insertion of an NG tube in patients with severe facial injuries, particularly midface fractures and skull fractures, is contraindicated because the NG tube may be inadvertently inserted through the fracture and into the cranial vault. For patients with these conditions, use the OG route of insertion.

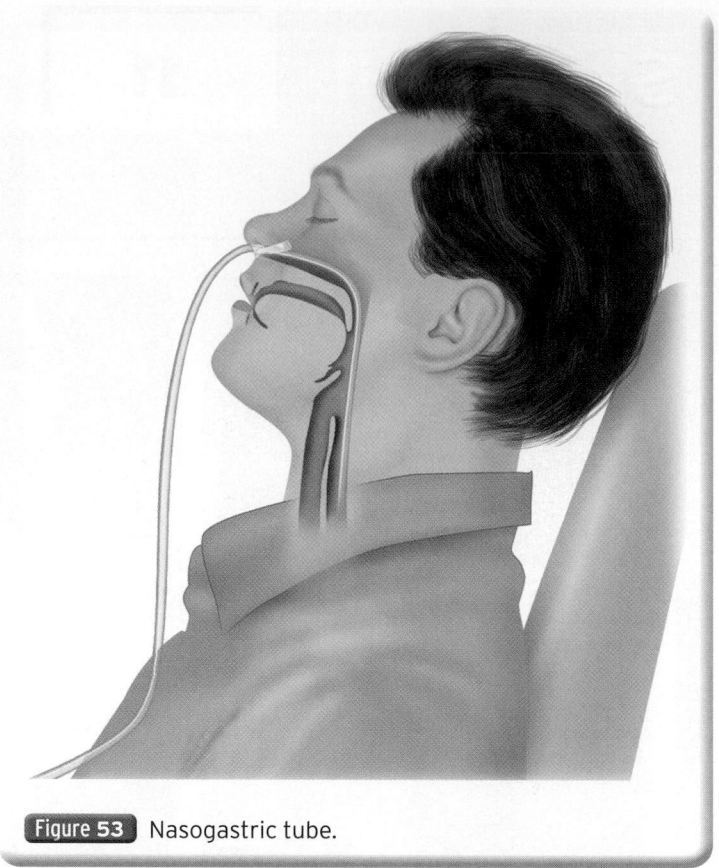

Figure 53 Nasogastric tube.

Improper technique during NG tube insertion can cause trauma to the nasal passageways, esophagus, or gastric lining; therefore, you must use caution and be gentle when inserting the tube.

Use of the NG tube in patients who are not intubated may interfere with the mask seal of the bag-mask device. If you cannot effectively ventilate a patient because of severe gastric distention, however, you must balance the benefit of gastric decompression against the risk of a poor mask seal and determine which has a higher priority. Of course, if the patient is unresponsive and requires ET intubation, you can easily pass an ET tube around the NG tube.

The steps of NG tube insertion are listed here and shown in **Skill Drill 12**:

Skill Drill   12

1. Explain the procedure to the patient, and oxygenate him or her, if necessary and possible. Ensure that the patient's head is in a neutral or slightly flexed position. Suppress the gag reflex with a topical anesthetic spray **Step 1**.

2. Constrict the blood vessels in the nares with a topical alpha-agonist if available **Step 2**.

3. Measure the tube for the correct depth of insertion (nose to ear to xiphoid process) **Step 3**.

4. Lubricate the tube with a water-soluble gel **Step 4**.

5. Advance the tube gently along the nasal floor **Step 5**.

6. Encourage the patient to swallow or drink to facilitate passage of the tube into the esophagus **Step 6**.

Skill Drill 12

Nasogastric Tube Insertion in a Responsive Patient

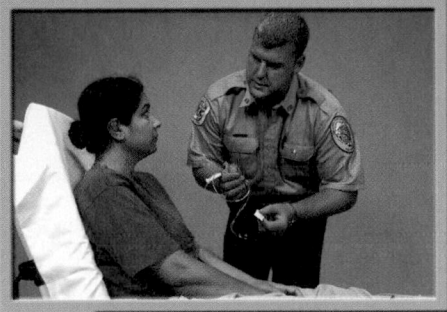

Step 1 Explain the procedure to the patient, and oxygenate the patient if necessary. Ensure the patient's head is in a neutral position, and suppress the gag reflex with a topical anesthetic spray.

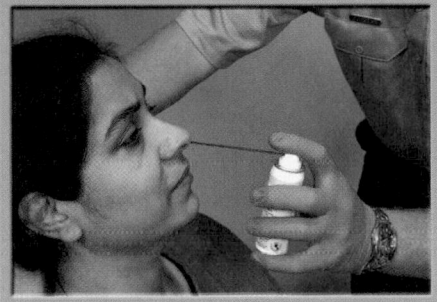

Step 2 Constrict the blood vessels in the nares with a topical alpha-agonist if available.

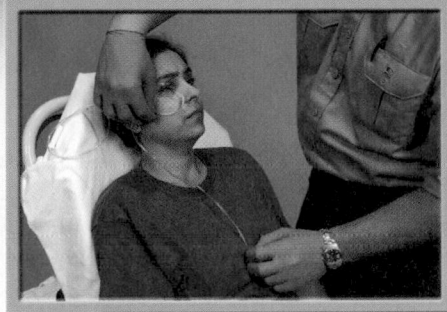

Step 3 Measure the tube for the correct depth of insertion (nose to ear to xiphoid process).

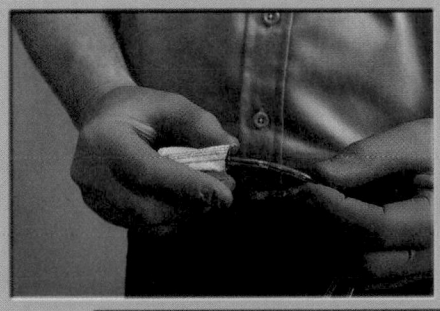

Step 4 Lubricate the tube with a water-soluble gel.

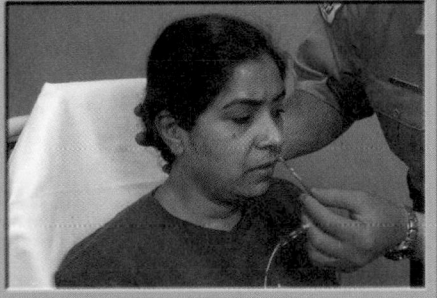

Step 5 Advance the tube gently along the nasal floor.

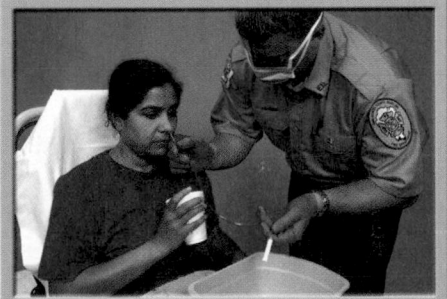

Step 6 Encourage the patient to swallow or drink to facilitate passage of the tube.

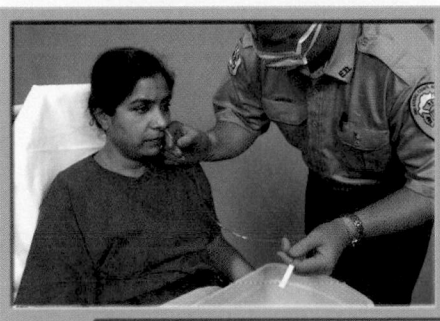

Step 7 Advance the tube into the stomach.

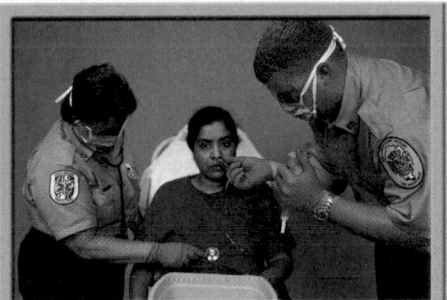

Step 8 Confirm placement: Auscultate over the epigastrium while injecting 30 to 50 mL of air, and/or observe for gastric contents in the tube. There should be no reflux around the tube.

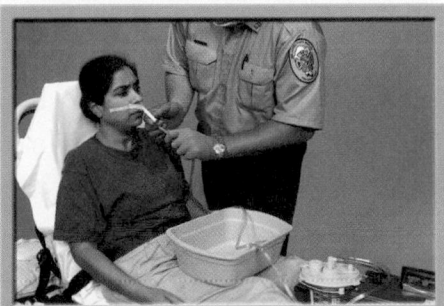

Step 9 Apply suction to the tube to aspirate the gastric contents, and secure the tube in place.

7. Advance the tube into the stomach Step 7.

8. Confirm proper placement: Auscultate over the epigastrium while injecting 30 to 50 mL of air into the tube, and/or observe for gastric contents in the tube Step 8.

9. Apply suction to the tube to aspirate the stomach contents, and secure the tube in place Step 9.

Orogastric Tube

An OG tube serves the same purpose as an NG tube but is inserted through the mouth instead of the nose Figure 54. The advantages and disadvantages of the OG tube are essentially the same as they are for the NG tube. The major differences are that the OG tube carries no risk of nasal bleeding and is safer in patients with severe facial trauma. In addition, you can use larger tubes, which is helpful if the patient requires aggressive gastric lavage.

The OG tube, however, is less comfortable for responsive patients, causing gagging much more often, and increases the possibility of vomiting. Responsive patients also tend to bite the tube as it is passed orally.

The OG route is generally preferred for patients who are unresponsive without a gag reflex. Because they need aggressive airway management, the OG tube is almost always inserted *after* the patient's airway is protected with an ET tube; insertion of the OG tube before intubating the patient may obscure your view of the vocal cords.

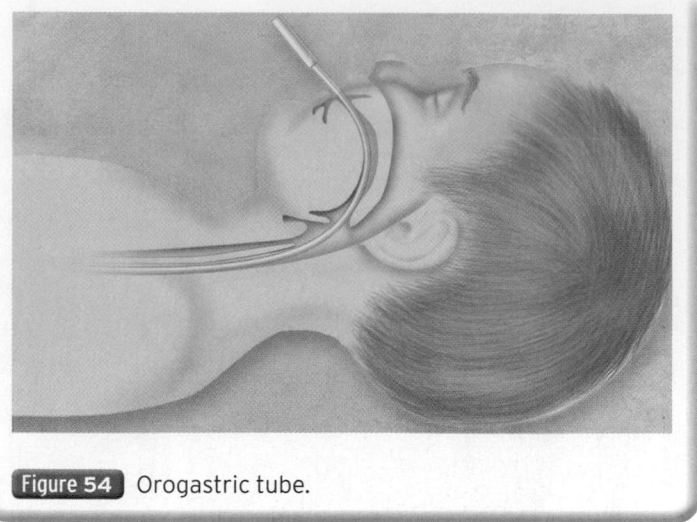

Figure 54 Orogastric tube.

The steps of OG tube insertion are listed here and shown in Skill Drill 13:

Skill Drill 13

1. Position the patient's head in a neutral or slightly flexed position.

2. Measure the tube for the correct depth of insertion (mouth to ear to xiphoid process) Step 1.

YOU are the Medic   PART 6

After adequate preoxygenation, a 7.5-mm ET tube is inserted and confirmed by auscultation of the epigastrium and lung fields and quantitative waveform capnography, which is connected to the cardiac monitor. After noting and documenting the centimeter marking on the ET tube at the patient's teeth, you secure the tube in place, secure the patient to the stretcher, and load him into the ambulance. An engine company EMT drives the ambulance to the hospital, which is located 25 miles away, so your partner can assist you in the back with the patient.

En route to the hospital, the patient starts moving his head and is becoming slightly combative. You reassess him and note that his vital signs have improved. Your estimated time of arrival at the hospital is 18 minutes.

Recording Time: 15 Minutes	
Level of consciousness	U (unresponsive)
Respirations	8 breaths/min (baseline); intubated and ventilations being assisted
Pulse	112 beats/min; weak and regular
Skin	Cyanosis resolving; skin remains diaphoretic
Blood pressure	116/60 mm Hg
SpO_2	94% (with assisted ventilation and oxygen)
$ETCO_2$	47 mm Hg
ECG	Sinus tachycardia

11. Should you extubate this patient? Why or why not?

Skill Drill | 13

Orogastric Tube Insertion

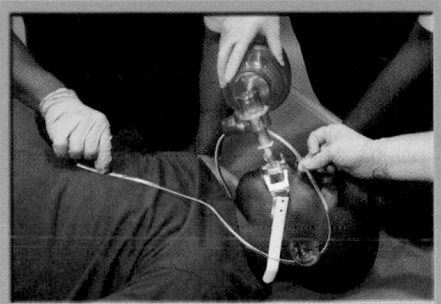

Step 1 Position the patient's head in a neutral or slightly flexed position. Measure the tube for the correct depth of insertion (mouth to ear to xiphoid process).

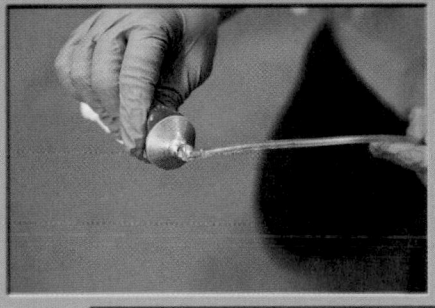

Step 2 Lubricate the tube with a water-soluble gel.

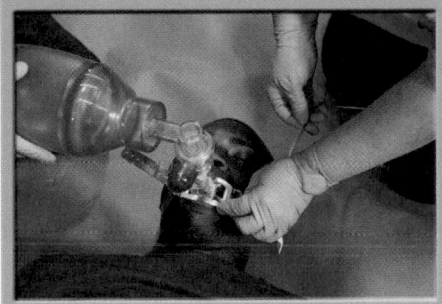

Step 3 Introduce the tube at the midline, and advance it gently into the oropharynx. Advance the tube into the stomach.

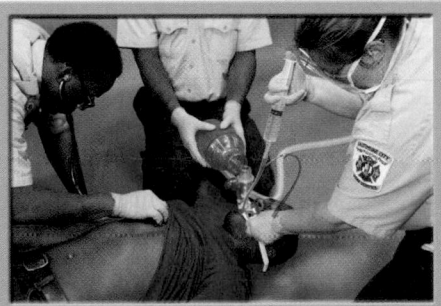

Step 4 Auscultate over the epigastrium to confirm correct placement. Afterwards, auscultate over the lung fields to confirm that the endotracheal tube has not been dislodged.

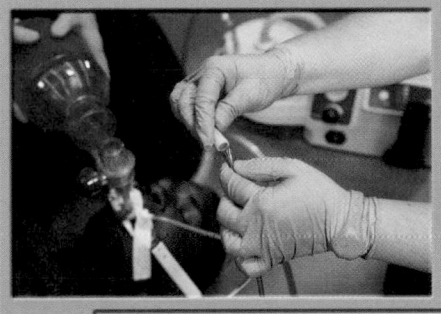

Step 5 Apply suction to the tube to aspirate the stomach contents.

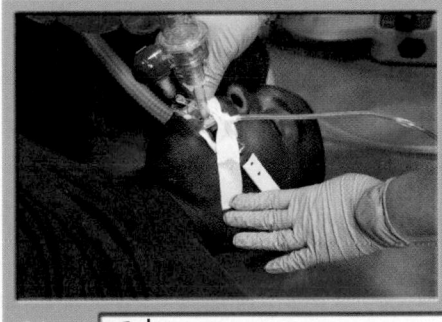

Step 6 Secure the tube in place.

3. Lubricate the tube with a water-soluble gel (Step 2).

4. Introduce the tube at the midline, and advance it gently into the oropharynx.

5. Advance the tube into the stomach (Step 3).

6. Confirm proper placement: Auscultate over the epigastrium while injecting 30 to 50 mL of air and/or observe for gastric contents in the tube. There should be no reflux around the tube. Afterwards, auscultate over the lung fields to confirm that the endotracheal tube has not been dislodged (Step 4).

7. Apply suction to the tube to aspirate the stomach contents (Step 5).

8. Secure the tube in place (Step 6).

■ Special Patient Considerations

■ Laryngectomy, Tracheostomy, Stoma, and Tracheostomy Tubes

A **laryngectomy** is a surgical procedure in which the larynx is removed. This procedure is performed by making a **tracheostomy** (surgical opening into the trachea), thus creating a **stoma**, an orifice that connects the trachea to the outside air. The tracheal stoma is located in the midline of the anterior part of the neck. Surgical removal of the entire larynx is called **total laryngectomy**. A person who has had this procedure is sometimes known as a laryngectomee, or "neck breather"—he or she breathes through the stoma in his or her neck. Because there is no longer any connection between the patient's pharynx and lower airway, you cannot ventilate the patient by the mouth-to-mask technique. The air blown into the mouth or nose can only go down the esophagus into the stomach; it will not reach the lower airway.

A **partial laryngectomy** entails surgical removal of a portion of the larynx. People who have had this procedure are called "partial neck breathers"—they breathe through the stoma *and* the nose or mouth. In practice, you may not be able to tell whether a person has had a total or partial laryngectomy until you attempt artificial ventilation.

Suctioning of a Stoma

You may encounter patients who require suctioning of thick secretions from the stoma. Failure to recognize and identify this need could result in hypoxia. It is not uncommon for a patient's stoma to become occluded with mucous plugs. Patients with a laryngectomy have a less efficient cough and, therefore, difficulty spontaneously clearing the stoma.

Suctioning of the patient's stoma must be performed with extreme care, especially if laryngeal swelling is suspected. Even the slightest irritation of the tracheal wall can result in a violent laryngospasm and complete airway closure. Limit suctioning of the stoma to 10 seconds.

The steps for suctioning a stoma are listed here and shown in Skill Drill 14 :

Skill Drill 14

1. Take standard precautions (gloves and face shield) Step 1 .
2. Preoxygenate the patient with a bag-mask device and 100% oxygen Step 2 .
3. Inject 3 mL of sterile saline through the stoma and into the trachea Step 3 .
4. Instruct the patient to exhale (if he or she is responsive), and insert the catheter (without providing suction) until resistance is felt (no more than 12 cm) Step 4 .
5. Suction while withdrawing the catheter Step 5 .
6. Resume oxygenating the patient with a bag-mask device and 100% oxygen Step 6 .

Ventilation of Stoma Patients

Neither the head tilt–chin lift nor the jaw-thrust maneuver is required for ventilating a patient with a stoma. If the patient has a stoma and no tracheostomy tube in place, ventilations can be performed using the mouth-to-stoma (with a resuscitation mask) technique or with a bag-mask device. Regardless of the technique used, you should use an infant- or child-sized mask to make an adequate seal over the stoma. Seal the patient's nose and mouth with one hand to prevent the leakage of air up the trachea. Release the seal of the patient's mouth and nose following each ventilation, allowing exhalation to occur through the upper airway. Two rescuers are needed to perform bag-mask device-to-stoma ventilations: one to seal the nose and mouth and the other to squeeze the bag-mask device. If you are unable to ventilate a patient who has a stoma, try suctioning the stoma and mouth with a French or soft-tip catheter before providing artificial ventilation through the nose and mouth. Note that this would

only work if the patient had a partial laryngectomy, not if he or she had a total laryngectomy. If you seal the stoma during ventilation, the ability to artificially ventilate the patient in this way may be improved, or it may help to clear any obstructions.

The steps for performing mouth-to-stoma ventilation with a resuscitation mask are listed here and shown in Skill Drill 15 :

Skill Drill 15

1. Position the patient's head in a neutral position with the shoulders slightly elevated Step 1 .
2. Locate and expose the stoma site Step 2 .
3. Place the resuscitation mask (pediatric mask preferred) over the stoma, and ensure an adequate seal Step 3 .
4. Maintain the patient's neutral head position, and ventilate the patient by exhaling directly into the resuscitation mask.
5. Assess the patient for adequate ventilation by observing his or her chest rise and feeling for air leaks around the mask Step 4 .
6. If air leakage is evident, seal the patient's mouth and nose and ventilate Step 5 . For best results, use a pediatric mask on the stoma.

The steps for performing bag-mask device-to-stoma ventilation are listed here and shown in Skill Drill 16 :

Skill Drill 16

1. With the patient's head in a neutral position, locate and expose the stoma Step 1 .
2. Place the bag-mask device over the stoma, and ensure an adequate seal.
3. Ventilate the patient by squeezing the bag-mask device, and assess for adequate ventilation by observing chest rise and feeling for air leaks when using a mask. Seal the mouth and nose if an air leak is evident from the upper airway Step 2 .
4. Auscultate over the lungs to confirm adequate ventilation Step 3 .

Tracheostomy Tubes

A **tracheostomy tube** is a plastic tube placed within the tracheostomy site (stoma) Figure 55 . It requires a 15/22-mm adapter to be compatible with ventilatory devices, such as a mechanical ventilator or bag-mask device. Patients with a tracheostomy tube may receive supplemental oxygen via tubing designed to fit over the tube or by placing an oxygen mask over the tube. Ventilation is accomplished by simply attaching the bag-mask device to the tracheostomy tube.

Patients with a tracheostomy tube who experience sudden dyspnea often have thick secretions in the tube. In this case, perform suctioning through the tracheostomy tube as you would through a stoma.

When a tracheostomy tube becomes dislodged, **stenosis** (narrowing) of the stoma may occur. Stenosis is potentially

Skill Drill | 14

Suctioning of a Stoma

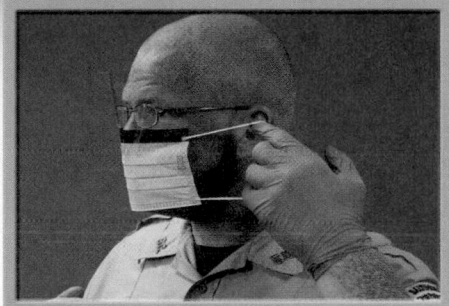

Step 1 Take standard precautions (gloves and face shield).

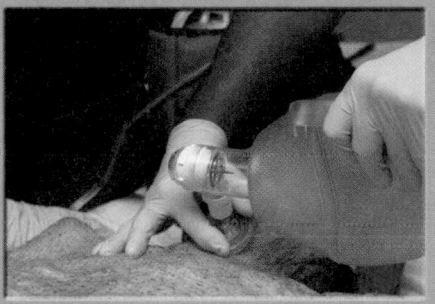

Step 2 Preoxygenate the patient with a bag-mask device and 100% oxygen.

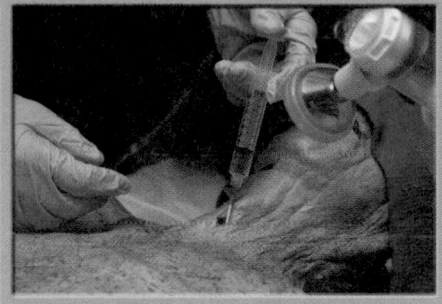

Step 3 Inject 3 mL of saline through the stoma and into the trachea.

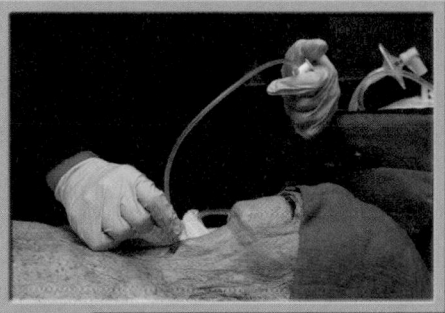

Step 4 Instruct the patient to exhale, and insert the catheter (without providing suction) until resistance is felt (no more than 12 cm).

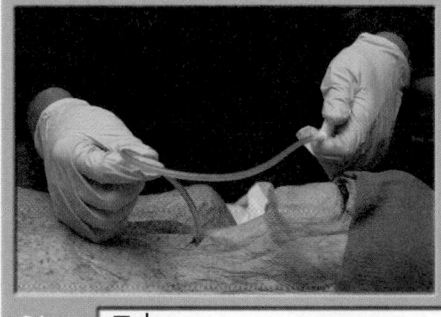

Step 5 Suction while withdrawing the catheter.

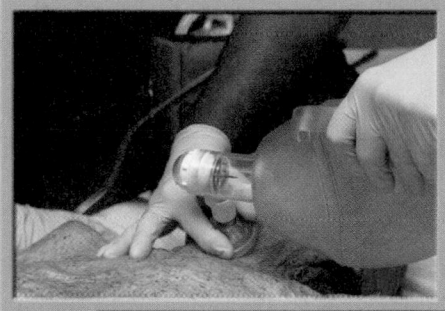

Step 6 Resume oxygenating the patient with a bag-mask device and 100% oxygen.

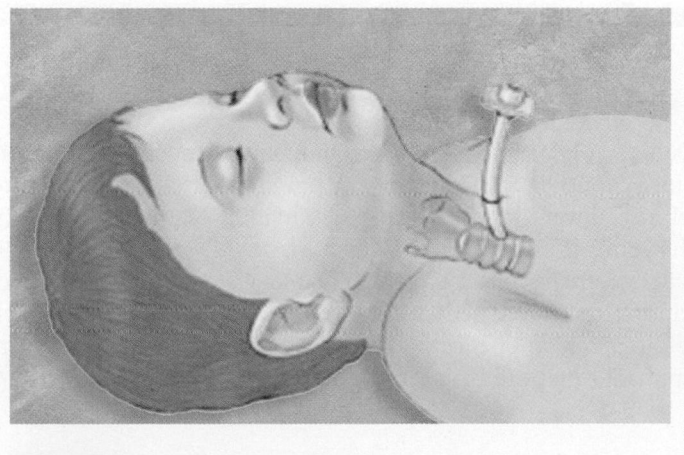

Figure 55 A tracheostomy tube.

life-threatening because soft-tissue swelling decreases the stoma's diameter and impairs the patient's ventilatory ability. In such cases, you may not be able to replace the tracheostomy tube itself and may have to insert an ET tube into the stoma before it becomes totally occluded. Because a patient with a stoma already has a significant medical problem (such as brain injury, chronic respiratory insufficiency), he or she may be less tolerant of even brief periods of hypoxia.

The steps for replacing a dislodged tracheostomy tube are listed here and shown in **Skill Drill 17**:

Skill Drill | 17

1. Take standard precautions (gloves and face shield). Assemble the equipment. **Step 1**.

2. Lubricate the same-sized tracheostomy tube or an ET tube (at least 5.0 mm) **Step 2**.

Skill Drill | 15

Mouth-to-Stoma Ventilation Using a Resuscitation Mask

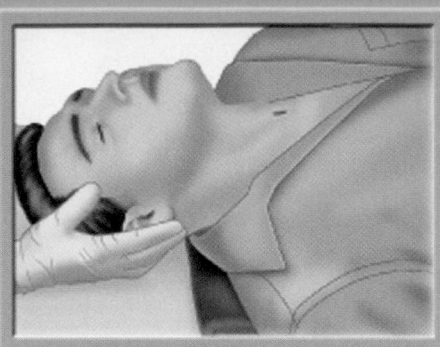

Step 1 Position the patient's head in a neutral position with the shoulders slightly elevated.

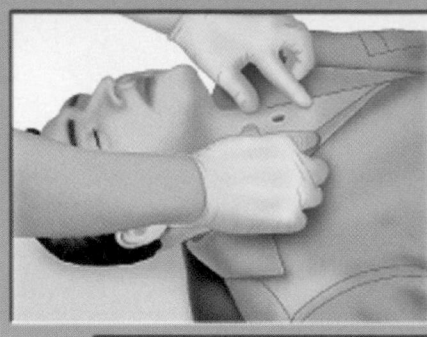

Step 2 Locate and expose the stoma site.

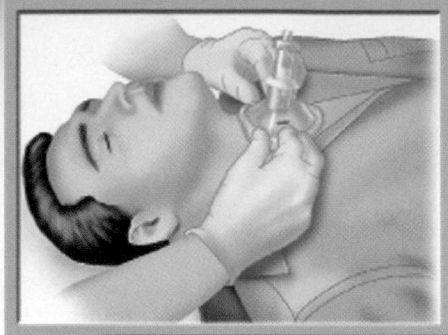

Step 3 Place the resuscitation mask (pediatric mask preferred) over the stoma, and ensure an adequate seal.

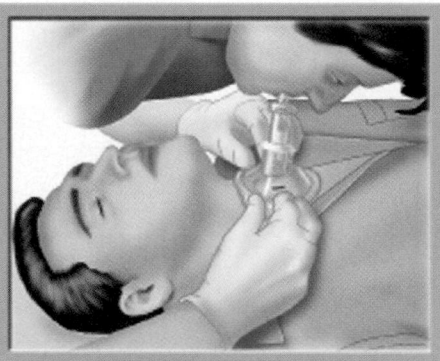

Step 4 Maintain the patient's neutral head position, and ventilate the patient by exhaling directly into the resuscitation mask. Assess the patient for adequate ventilation by observing his or her chest rise and feeling for air leaks around the mask.

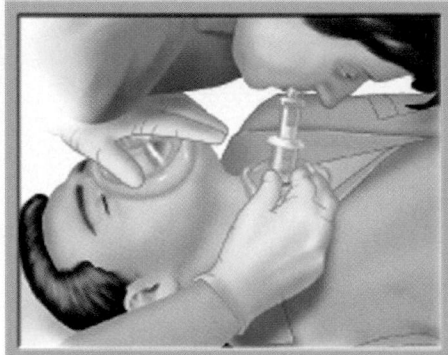

Step 5 If air leakage is evident, seal the patient's mouth and nose and ventilate. For best results use a pediatric mask on the stoma.

3. Instruct the patient to exhale, and gently insert the tube approximately 1 to 2 cm beyond the balloon cuff (**Step 3**).

4. Inflate the balloon cuff (**Step 4**).

5. Ensure that the patient is comfortable, and confirm patency and proper placement of the tube by listening for air movement from the tube and noting the patient's clinical status. Ensure that a false lumen was not created (**Step 5**).

6. Auscultate the lungs to confirm correct tube placement (**Step 6**).

■ Dental Appliances

Dental appliances, which are frequently encountered in the elderly population, can take many different forms: dentures (upper, lower, or both), bridges, individual teeth, and braces (in the younger population). When assessing the airway of a patient with a dental appliance, especially one who is unresponsive, you must determine whether the appliance is loose or fitting well. If the dental appliance fits well, leave it in place. A well-fitting appliance helps to maintain the structure of the face, facilitating

Skill Drill | 16

Bag-Mask Device-to-Stoma Ventilation

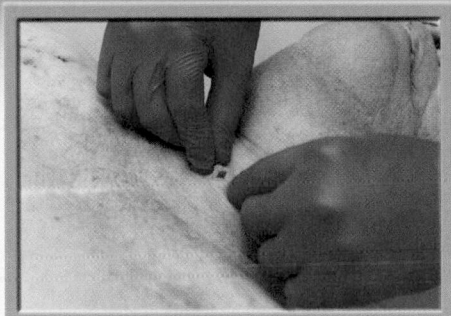

Step 1 With the patient's head in a neutral position, locate and expose the stoma.

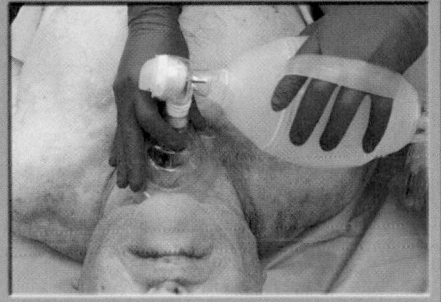

Step 2 Place the bag-mask device over the stoma, and ensure an adequate seal. Ventilate the patient by squeezing the bag-mask device, and assess for adequate ventilation by observing chest rise.

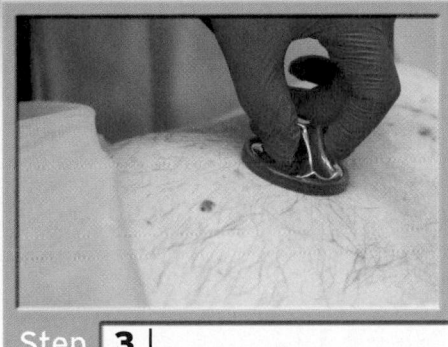

Step 3 Auscultate over the lungs to confirm adequate ventilation.

an effective mask-to-face seal if the patient requires mouth-to-mask or bag-mask ventilation. If the appliance is loose, however, it could easily become an airway obstruction and should be removed.

If an unresponsive patient has an airway obstruction caused by a dental appliance, perform the usual steps in clearing an obstruction, such as chest compressions, direct laryngoscopy, and use of the Magill forceps. Great care must be taken if the obstruction is caused by a bridge; these devices often contain sharp metal ends that can easily lacerate the posterior pharynx or larynx.

Often it is not the dental appliance itself that hinders a paramedic's ability to manage a patient's airway, but rather attempts to identify and remove the device. A paramedic may become overly concerned with the presence of the dental appliance rather than concentrating on managing the airway. In addition, the oropharyngeal anatomy may be somewhat distorted by the presence of a dental appliance.

In general, it is best to remove dental appliances before intubating a patient. Once the ET tube is in place and has been secured, removal of the dental appliance will be extremely difficult and dangerous because it may cause dislodgement of the tube or inflict unnecessary oropharyngeal trauma.

Facial Trauma

It can be especially challenging to effectively manage the airway of a patient with facial injuries **Figure 56**. Because the face is highly vascular, facial trauma can result in severe tissue swelling and bleeding into the airway. Control bleeding with direct pressure, and suction the airway as needed. You may encounter a patient with severe facial trauma who is breathing inadequately *and* has severe oropharyngeal bleeding—both problems are life-threatening. This situation is most effectively managed by suctioning the patient's airway for 15 seconds (less in infants and children) and then providing positive-pressure ventilation for 2 minutes. This alternating pattern of suctioning and ventilating should continue until the oral secretions have been cleared or the patient's airway has been secured with an ET tube.

Facial injuries should also increase your index of suspicion for a cervical spine injury. Therefore, when managing the airway, use the jaw-thrust maneuver and keep the patient's head in a neutral in-line position. Endotracheal intubation of a trauma patient is most effectively performed by two paramedics—one who maintains neutral in-line stabilization of the patient's head and the other who performs the intubation. An alternative technique, especially if you are the only paramedic

Skill Drill 17

Replacing a Dislodged Tracheostomy Tube With a Temporary Endotracheal Tube

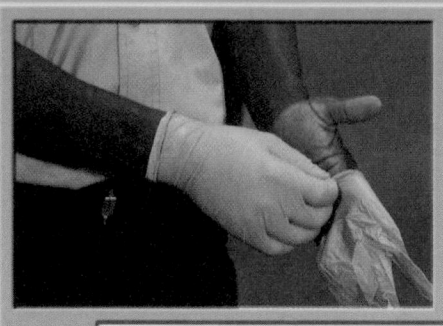

Step 1 Take standard precautions (gloves and face shield). Assemble the equipment.

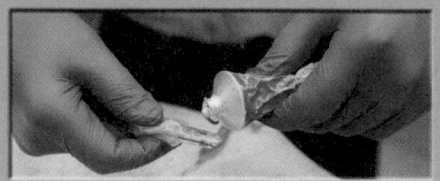

Step 2 Lubricate the same-sized tracheostomy tube or an ET tube (at least 5.0 mm).

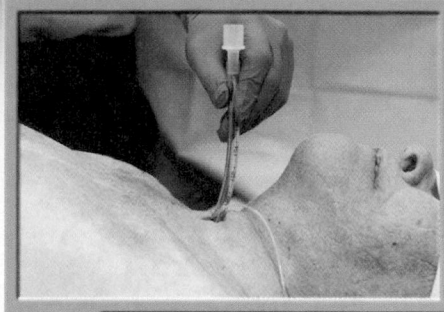

Step 3 Instruct the patient to exhale, and gently insert the tube approximately 1 to 2 cm beyond the balloon cuff.

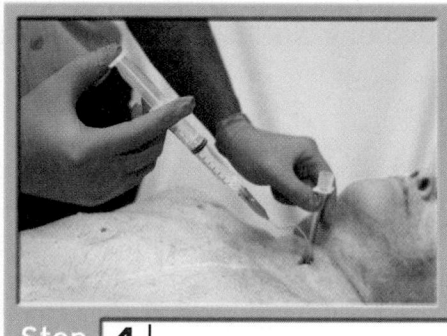

Step 4 Inflate the balloon cuff.

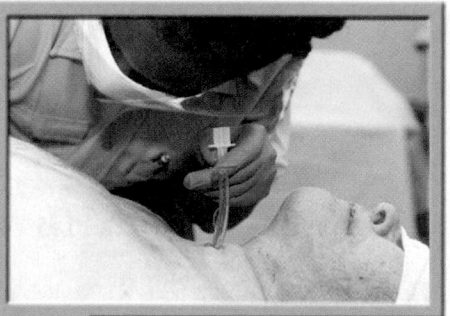

Step 5 Ensure that the patient is comfortable, and confirm patency and proper placement of the tube by listening for air movement from the tube and noting the patient's clinical status. Ensure that a false lumen was not created.

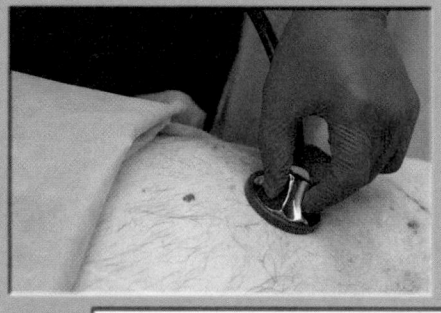

Step 6 Auscultate the lungs to confirm correct tube placement.

managing the patient's airway, is to stabilize the patient's head in a neutral in-line position with your thighs and then perform the intubation.

When you are ventilating a patient with facial injuries, stay alert for changes in ventilation compliance or sounds that may indicate laryngeal edema (such as stridor). If you are unable to effectively ventilate or orally intubate a patient with severe facial injuries, perform a cricothyrotomy (surgical or needle). Advanced airway management, including ET intubation, multi-lumen and supraglottic airway devices, and needle and surgical cricothyrotomy are discussed next.

■ Advanced Airway Management

One of the most common mistakes in the situation of respiratory or cardiac arrest is to proceed with advanced airway management too early, forsaking the basic techniques of establishing and maintaining a patent airway in a patient who is already hypoxic. *Never abandon the basics of airway management—do not immediately proceed with advanced techniques simply because you can.*

After establishing and maintaining a patent airway with basic techniques and maneuvers, you should consider advanced airway management. Patients primarily require advanced airway management for two reasons: failure to maintain a patent airway and/or failure to adequately oxygenate and ventilate. Advanced airway management involves the insertion of a number of advanced airway devices that are designed to facilitate adequate oxygenation and ventilation. The remainder of the chapter discusses and illustrates the following advanced airway devices and techniques:

- ET tube
  - Orotracheal intubation
  - Blind nasotracheal intubation
  - Digital intubation
  - Intubation via transillumination
  - Face-to-face intubation
  - Retrograde intubation
- King LT airway
- Laryngeal mask airway (LMA)
- Cobra perilaryngeal airway (CobraPLA)
- Esophageal tracheal Combitube (ETC)
- Surgical and needle cricothyrotomy

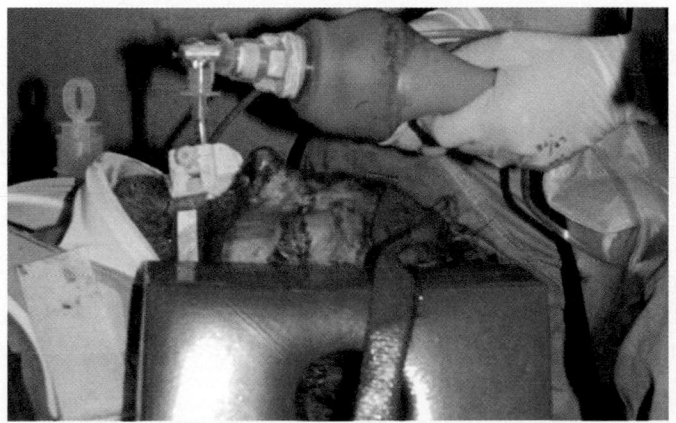

Figure 56 Airway management can be especially challenging in patients with facial injuries.

Predicting the Difficult Airway

In the prehospital setting, it is estimated that 20% of all intubations are classified as "difficult." Paramedics must decide how to accomplish airway management. Can I manage this airway with BLS techniques? Can I intubate this patient's trachea? There are several factors to consider when caring for a patient who has a difficult airway.

History is one factor. Anatomic findings suggestive of a difficult airway may include congenital abnormalities (ie, dysmorphic face), recent surgery, trauma, infection, or neoplastic diseases (such as cancer).

A commonly used mnemonic to guide assessment of the difficult airway is LEMON, which stands for:

Look externally
Evaluate 3-3-2
Mallampati
Obstruction
Neck mobility

As indicated by the "L" in the mnemonic, simply looking at the patient may indicate the relative difficulty that may be encountered in airway management. Patients with short, thick necks may be difficult to intubate. Morbid obesity significantly complicates intubation. Dental conditions, such as an overbite or "buck" teeth, may make intubation difficult.

The "E" stands for Evaluate 3-3-2. Three anatomic measurements are assessed using the **3-3-2 rule** **Figure 57**. The first "3" refers to mouth opening. Ideally, a patient's mouth should open at least three fingerwidths (approximately 5 cm). A width of less than three fingers indicates a potentially difficult airway. The second "3" refers to the length of the mandible. At least three fingerwidths is optimal. This length is measured from the tip of the chin to the hyoid bone. Smaller mandibles have less room for displacement of the tongue and epiglottis and can make airway management more difficult. The "2" part of this rule refers to the distance from the hyoid bone to the thyroid notch; it should be at least two fingers wide.

The "M" stands for Mallampati. An anesthesiologist, Mallampati, developed the **Mallampati classification** to predict

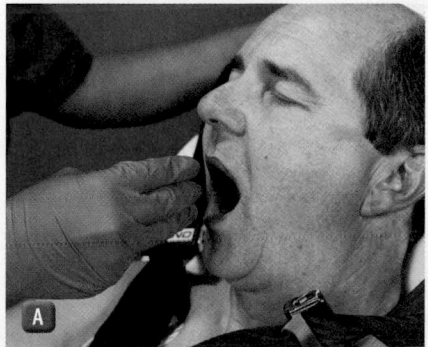
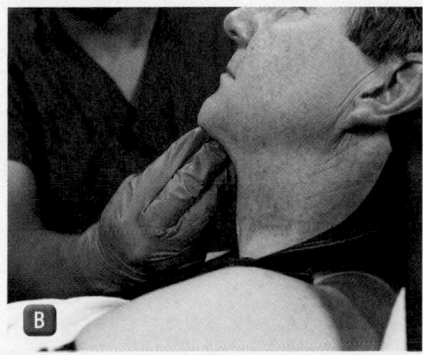
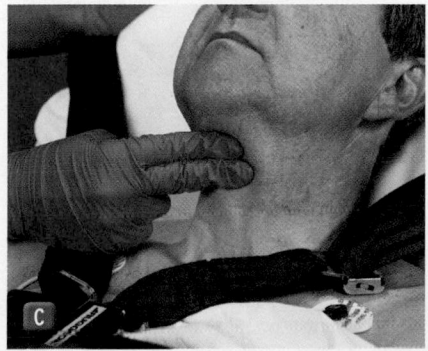

Figure 57 The 3-3-2 rule. **A.** The mouth should be at least three fingers wide when open. **B.** The space from the chin to the hyoid bone should be at least three fingers wide. **C.** The distance from the hyoid bone to the thyroid notch should be at least two fingers wide.

the relative difficulty of intubation Figure 58 . This classification notes the oropharyngeal structures visible in an upright, seated patient who is fully able to open his or her mouth. Although this is an accurate predictor of intubation difficulty, it is of limited value in unresponsive patients and in patients who cannot follow commands. If a patient is cooperative and able to comply with this evaluation, emergency prehospital intubation is probably not indicated. However, the evaluation is important because it can provide useful information should intubation become necessary.

The "O" stands for obstruction. Anything that might interfere with visualization or ET tube placement should be noted. Foreign body, obesity, hematoma, and masses are all examples of situations that can create a difficult airway.

The "N" stands for neck mobility. The ideal position for visualization and intubation is the "sniffing position" with the adult head slightly elevated and extended. Neck mobility problems are most commonly associated with trauma patients (due to cervical collars or injury) and elderly patients (due to osteoporosis or arthritis). The inability to place the patient in the sniffing position can significantly reduce your ability to visualize the airway.

Endotracheal Intubation

Endotracheal intubation is defined as passing an ET tube through the glottic opening and sealing the tube with a cuff inflated against the tracheal wall. When the tube is passed into the trachea through the mouth, the procedure is called orotracheal intubation. When the tube is passed into the trachea through the nose, the procedure is called nasotracheal intubation.

Intubation of the trachea is the *most* definitive means of achieving complete control of the airway. A solid understanding of the basics of this technique is needed when making urgent decisions about when to intubate a patient. Following are considerations when performing ET intubation:

- **Advantages.** Provision of a secure airway, protection against aspiration, and provision of an alternative route to the IV or intraosseous (IO) route for certain medications (*as a last resort*)
- **Disadvantages.** Special equipment required and physiologic functions of the upper airway (warming, filtering, humidifying) bypassed
- **Complications.** Bleeding, hypoxia, laryngeal swelling, laryngospasm, vocal cord damage, mucosal necrosis, and barotrauma

Endotracheal Tubes

The basic structure of an endotracheal (ET) tube Figure 59 includes the proximal end, the tube itself, the cuff and pilot balloon, and the distal tip. The proximal end is equipped with a standard 15/22-mm adapter that allows it to be attached to any ventilation device. It also includes an inflation port with a pilot balloon; the distal cuff is inflated with a syringe attached to the inflation port, which has a one-way valve. The pilot balloon indicates whether the distal cuff is inflated or deflated once the tube has been inserted into the mouth.

Centimeter markings along the length of the ET tube provide a measurement of its depth. The distal end of the tube has a beveled tip to facilitate insertion and an opening on the side called Murphy's eye, which enables ventilation to occur even if the tip becomes occluded by blood, mucus, or the tracheal wall.

Endotracheal tubes range in size from 2.5 to 9.0 mm in inside diameter, and their length ranges from 12 to 32 cm Figure 60 . Sizes ranging from 5.0 to 9.0 mm are equipped with a distal cuff that, when inflated, makes an airtight seal with the tracheal wall.

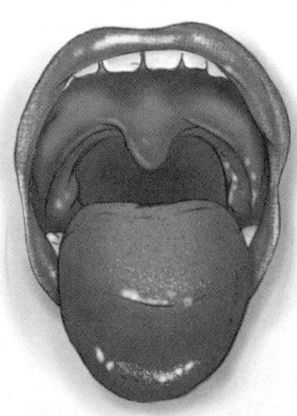
Class I
Entire posterior pharynx is fully exposed

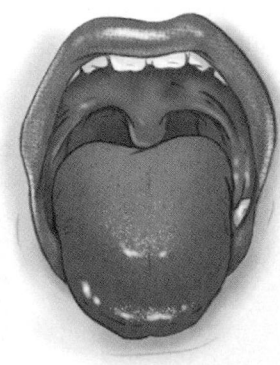
Class II
Posterior pharynx is partially exposed

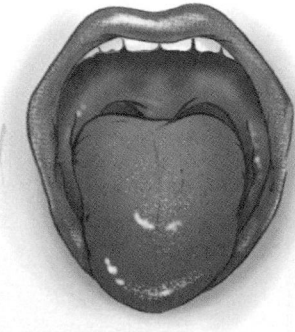
Class III
Posterior pharynx cannot be seen; base of the uvula is exposed

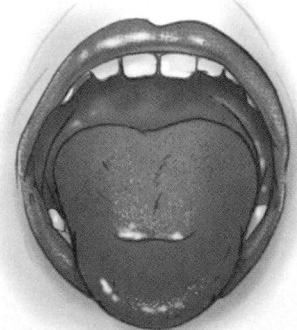
Class IV
No posterior pharyngeal structures can be seen

Figure 58 Mallampati classification.

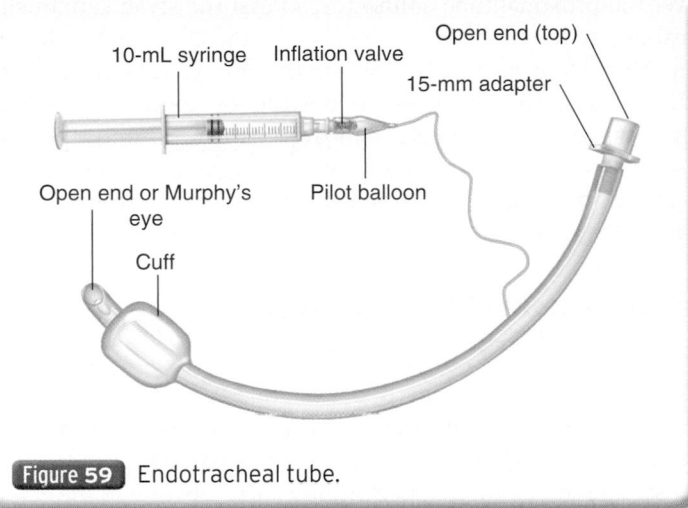

Figure 59 Endotracheal tube.

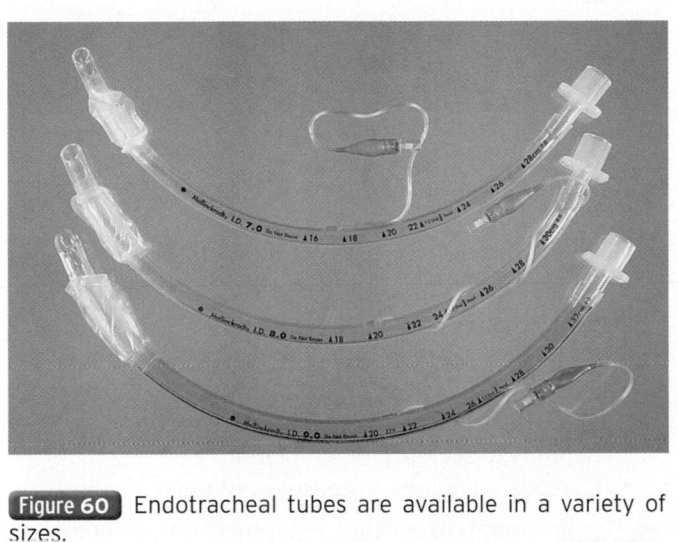

Figure 60 Endotracheal tubes are available in a variety of sizes.

A tube that is too small for the patient will lead to increased resistance to airflow and difficulty in ventilating. A tube that is too large can be difficult to insert and may cause trauma. Usually, a woman will require a 7.0- to 8.0-mm tube, and a man will require a 7.5- to 8.5-mm tube.

In pediatric patients, ET tubes ranging from 2.5 to 4.5 mm are used. In children, the funnel-shaped cricoid ring (the narrowest portion of the pediatric airway) forms an anatomic seal with the ET tube, eliminating the need for a distal cuff in most cases. The proximal end of the tube still has a 15/22-mm adapter for use with standard ventilation devices, and the distal end has a beveled tip with distal end markings. However, because it lacks a balloon cuff, there is no pilot balloon.

A number of anatomic clues can help determine the proper size of ET tube for adults and children. The internal diameter of the nostril is a good approximation of the diameter of the glottic opening. The diameter of the little finger or the size of the thumbnail is also a good approximation of airway size. Because all attempts to predict the tube size required for a given patient

are estimates, however, you should always have *three* ET tubes ready: one tube of the size you *think* will be appropriate, one a size larger, and one a size smaller.

Laryngoscopes and Blades

A laryngoscope is required to perform orotracheal intubation by direct laryngoscopy—a procedure in which the vocal cords are directly visualized for placement of the ET tube. The <u>laryngoscope</u> consists of a handle and interchangeable blades Figure 61 . The handle contains the power source for the light on the laryngoscope blade. Most laryngoscopes run on disposable batteries, but some are rechargeable. The handle has a bar designed to connect with a notch on the blade Figure 62 . When the blade is moved into the perpendicular position, the bright light shines near the tip of the blade.

The two most common types of laryngoscope blades are the straight (Miller and Wisconsin) blade and the curved (Macintosh) blade. The <u>straight laryngoscope blade</u> is designed so that its tip will extend beneath the epiglottis and lift it up

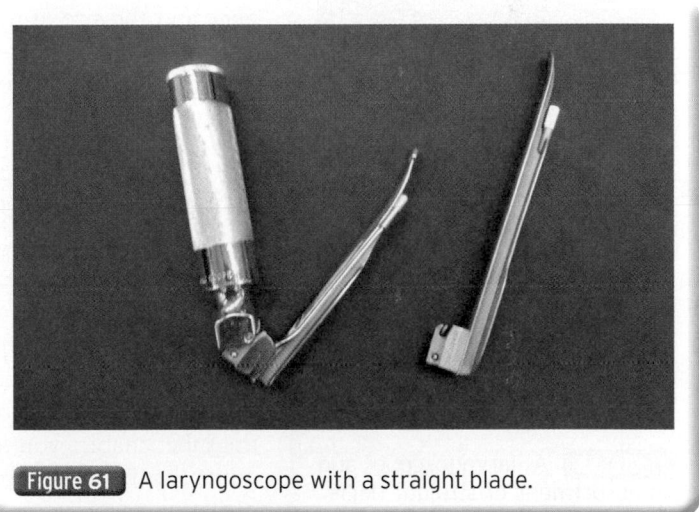

Figure 61 A laryngoscope with a straight blade.

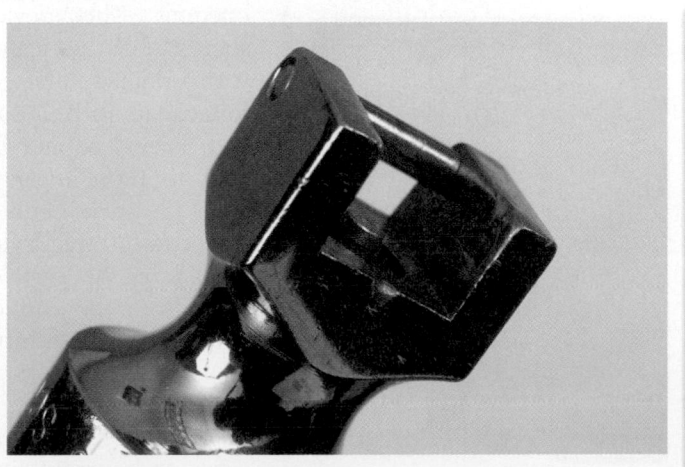

Figure 62 The laryngoscope's handle has a bar designed to connect with a notch on the blade.

Figure 63—a particularly useful feature in infants and small children, who often have a long, floppy epiglottis that is difficult to elevate out of the way with a curved blade. In an adult, use of a straight blade requires great care; if used improperly and levered across the upper jaw, the straight blade is more likely to damage the patient's teeth. The **curved laryngoscope blade** is less likely to be levered against the teeth by an inexperienced paramedic **Figure 64**. The direction of the curve conforms to that of the tongue and pharynx, so the blade follows the outline of the pharynx with relative ease. The tip of the curved blade is placed in the vallecula (the space between the epiglottis and the base of the tongue) rather than beneath the epiglottis; it indirectly lifts the epiglottis to expose the vocal cords. You should have curved *and* straight blades readily available during an orotracheal intubation attempt.

Blade sizes range from 0 to 4. Sizes 0, 1, and 2 are appropriate for infants and children, whereas 3 and 4 are considered adult sizes. For pediatric patients, blade sizes are often recommended based on the child's age or height. Most paramedics choose the blade for adults based on experience and the size of the patient (3 for average-sized adults and 4 for larger persons).

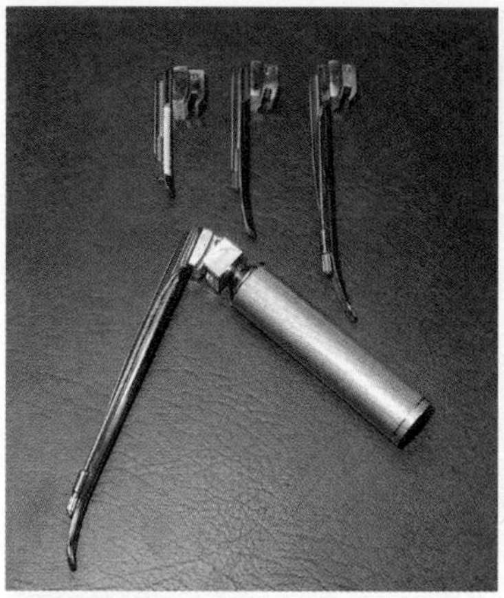

It is common, especially in emergency situations, to be unable to obtain a full view of the glottic opening. The **stylet**, a semirigid wire that is inserted into the ET tube to mold and maintain the shape of the tube, enables you to guide the tip of the tube over the arytenoid cartilage, even if you cannot see the entire glottic opening. This device should be lubricated with a water-soluble gel to facilitate its removal, and its end should be bent to form a gentle "hockey stick" curve. The end of the stylet should rest at least ½″ back from the end of the ET tube; if the stylet protrudes beyond the end of the tube, it may damage the vocal cords and surrounding structures. Bend the other end of the stylet

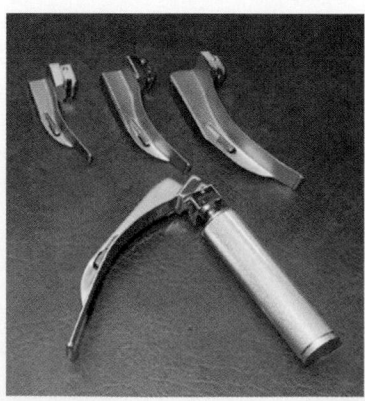

Figure 63 A laryngoscope and an assortment of straight (Miller or Wisconsin) blades.

Figure 64 A laryngoscope and an assortment of curved (Macintosh) blades.

over the proximal tube connector, so that the stylet cannot slip farther into the tube.

Magill forceps have two uses in the emergency setting. First, they are used to remove airway obstructions under direct visualization, as discussed earlier in this chapter. Second, they are used to guide the tip of the ET tube through the glottic opening if the proper angle cannot be achieved with simple manipulation of the tube.

Orotracheal Intubation by Direct Laryngoscopy

Orotracheal intubation by direct laryngoscopy involves inserting an ET tube through the mouth and into the trachea while visualizing the glottic opening with a laryngoscope; it is the most common method of performing ET intubation in the emergency setting. The indications and contraindications for orotracheal intubation include the following:

- Indications
  - Airway control needed as a result of coma, respiratory arrest, and/or cardiac arrest
  - Ventilatory support before impending respiratory failure
  - Prolonged ventilatory support required
  - Absence of a gag reflex
  - Traumatic brain injury
  - Unresponsiveness
  - Impending airway compromise (as in burns or trauma)
  - Medication administration (as a *last* resort)
- Contraindications
  - An intact gag reflex
  - Inability to open the patient's mouth because of trauma, dislocation of the jaw, or a pathologic condition
  - Inability to see the glottic opening
  - Copious secretions, vomitus, or blood in the airway

Table 11 summarizes the equipment and preparation required before performing orotracheal intubation. Make a copy of this table, and affix it to your intubation kit, so that you can check the kit systematically at the beginning of every shift.

Standard Precautions

Intubation may expose you to blood or other body fluids, so take proper precautions when performing this procedure. In addition to gloves, wear a mask that covers your entire face, which will be relatively close to the patient's mouth and nose, and that will protect you if the patient vomits or coughs during intubation.

Words of Wisdom

Perform ventilations with a bag-mask device and 100% oxygen for at least 2 to 3 minutes before attempting intubation. The patient needs an oxygen reserve to tolerate the period without ventilation that will occur during insertion of an advanced airway. You also need the time to check your equipment properly.

Words of Wisdom

Video Laryngoscopy

A number of video laryngoscopes are on the market—some with a laryngoscope and separate video monitor, and others with the video monitor attached to the laryngoscope itself. Video laryngoscopy is becoming popular in the hospital and prehospital settings because it facilitates visualization of the vocal cords—even in patients with the most difficult airways. Instead of trying to visualize the vocal cords around the laryngoscope, the intubator can guide placement of the ET tube with the use of a video monitor.

The GlideScope Ranger features a reusable video baton laryngoscope to which sterile, single-use blades of various sizes are attached Figure 65 . The video baton is attached to an 8.9-cm high-resolution video monitor that allows a paramedic to visualize the vocal cords and see the ET tube passing between them Figure 66 .

The McGrath features a 1.7″ LED video monitor that is attached to the laryngoscope itself Figure 67 . The video monitor can be tilted and/or rotated as needed for optimal view, thus reducing glare in bright environments. Sterile, disposable blades—ranging in size from infant to adult—slide into the laryngoscope, which can be adjusted in size to accommodate large and small patients.

Video laryngoscopy can be beneficial in a variety of environments and can enhance paramedics' ability to visualize the glottic opening and vocal cords. Consult the manufacturer's guidelines regarding the use of video laryngoscopes.

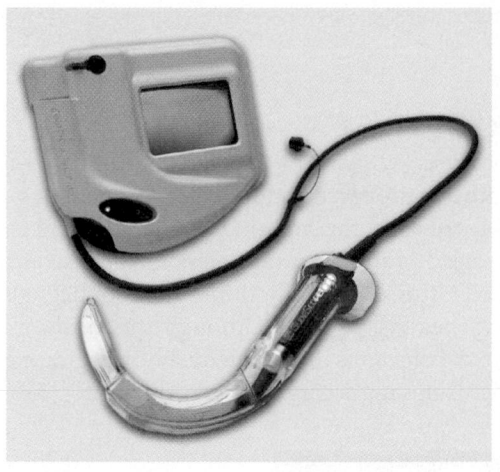

Figure 65 GlideScope Ranger® video laryngoscope.

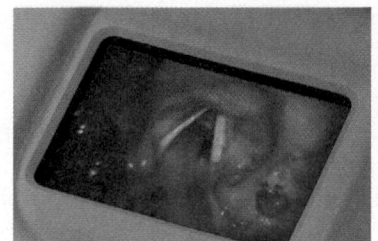

Figure 66 A high-resolution video monitor facilitates a paramedic's view of the vocal cords.

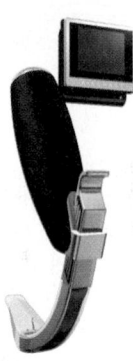

Figure 67 The McGrath® video laryngoscope.

Table 11 Preparing Equipment for Intubation

Equipment	What to Check, Prepare, and Assemble
Ventilation equipment	Have your partner ventilate the patient while you are assembling, checking, and preparing your equipment. Ensure that the patient is being ventilated with 100% oxygen and that the pulse oximeter reading is as close to 100% as possible (minimum of > 95%).
ET tube	Select the proper size tube (7.0-7.5 for women; 7.5-8.5 for men). Inject 10 mL of air into the cuff, and ensure that the cuff holds air. Confirm that the 15/22-mm adapter is firmly inserted into the tube. Insert the stylet, and ensure that the tip is proximal to the Murphy's eye. Bend the tube/stylet into a "hockey stick" configuration. Increase the angle of the bend if you anticipate a difficult intubation.
Laryngoscope and blades	You should have an assortment of blades (straight and curved) available because some patients are easier to intubate with one than with the other. Confirm that the blade you select is free of nicks, which could easily cause soft-tissue trauma to the upper airway. Check the bulb to ensure that the light is "bright, white, steady, and tight." The light should be bright enough so that it is uncomfortable to look at directly. It should be white, not yellow or dim. The light should not flicker, especially as the blade is moved on the handle. Most important, the bulb must be tightly screwed into the blade to prevent it from being aspirated into the lungs.

Continues

Table 11 **Preparing Equipment for Intubation,** continued

Equipment	What to Check, Prepare, and Assemble
Towels	Towels may be needed to properly position the patient's head.
Suction	Suction may be needed to clear the airway of blood or other secretions to obtain an adequate laryngoscopic view of the glottic opening and vocal cords.
Magill forceps	Have Magill forceps available should you need to guide the ET tube between the vocal cords or if you encounter a foreign body obstruction during laryngoscopy.
Confirmation devices	Stethoscope and an end-tidal CO_2 ($ETCO_2$) detector (*quantitative capnography should be used to confirm initial and ongoing ET tube placement*). Other devices include the colorimetric $ETCO_2$ detector and esophageal detector device bulb or syringe.
ET tube-securing device	Have the appropriate device readily available to secure the ET tube. A commercial device specifically designed to secure the ET tube is recommended.

Abbreviation: ET indicates endotracheal.

Preoxygenation

Adequate preoxygenation with a bag-mask device and 100% oxygen is a critical step before intubating a patient. You should preoxygenate an apneic or hypoventilating patient for 2 to 3 minutes. During the intubation attempt, the patient will undergo a period of "forced apnea," during which time he or she will not be ventilated. The goal of preoxygenation is to prevent hypoxia from occurring during this time. Unfortunately, you will be unable to perform an extensive preintubation evaluation of the patient (such as obtaining hemoglobin and hematocrit values), and patients who are intubated in the prehospital setting are usually in physiologically unstable condition.

You should monitor the patient's SpO_2 and achieve as close to 100% saturation as possible during the 2- to 3-minute period of preoxygenation. During the intubation attempt, you must continually monitor the SpO_2 and maintain it at greater than 95%.

Words of Wisdom

Ideally, a patient should have an SpO_2 of 100% (or as close to it as possible) before an intubation attempt. Preoxygenate the patient for 2 to 3 minutes, while monitoring his or her SpO_2 reading. If you are attempting to preoxygenate the patient, and the SpO_2 continues to drop despite your best efforts at basic airway management and ventilation, it is best to proceed with intubation without delay.

The consequences of even brief periods of hypoxia can be disastrous. Do not rely solely on pulse oximetry to quantify a patient's oxygenation status; it can produce falsely high readings, even if the patient is severely hypoxic. Although some sequelae of hypoxia are dramatic and occur immediately, most are subtle and occur gradually. Some of the poor neurologic outcomes following aggressive airway management result from intubation-induced hypoxia.

Positioning the Patient

Successful laryngoscopy will be extremely difficult—if not impossible—without proper positioning of the patient's head. The airway has three axes: the mouth, the pharynx, and the larynx. When the head is in a neutral position, these axes are at acute angles, facilitating entry of food into the esophagus rather than into the trachea **Figure 68A**. Although this positioning is advantageous to a conscious, spontaneously breathing person, the angles of these axes make laryngoscopy difficult.

Words of Wisdom

If the patient has experienced a possible neck injury, his or her head must be placed in a neutral in-line position. Do not use the sniffing position or extend the patient's head in any way. Intubation of a trauma patient is *most* effectively performed by two paramedics.

To facilitate visualization of the airway, the three axes must be aligned to the greatest extent possible. This alignment is most effectively achieved by placing the patient in the "sniffing" position (the position of the head when intentionally sniffing). The position involves approximately a 20° extension of the **atlanto-occipital joint** and a 30° flexion of the neck at C6 and C7 for a patient with a short neck and/or "no chin." In such situations, increasing the angle even further will help improve visualization **Figure 68B**.

In most supine patients, the sniffing position can be achieved by extending the head and elevating the occiput 2.5 to 5 cm. Elevate the head and/or neck with folded towels until the ear is at the level of the sternum **Figure 69**. When you are using towels, their thickness can easily be adjusted by changing the number of folds. With obese patients, padding under the head alone may not result in the sniffing position; you may need to add padding under the shoulders and neck as well. To determine whether the patient is in a true sniffing position, view the person from the side to evaluate the adequacy of his or her head position.

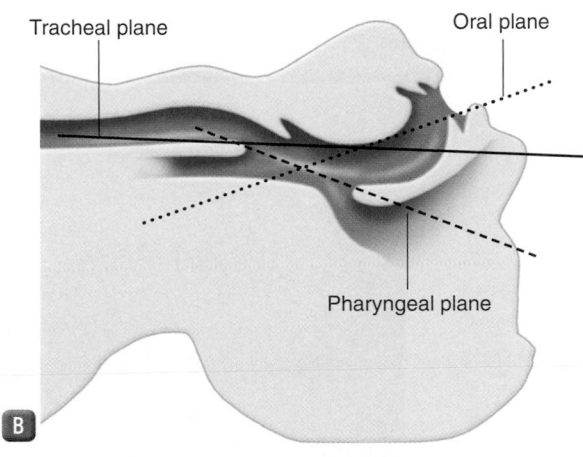

Figure 68 Three axes of the airway: oral, pharyngeal, and tracheal. **A.** Neutral position. **B.** Sniffing position.

Blade Insertion

After you have properly positioned the patient's head and provided preoxygenation, direct your partner to stop ventilating. Position yourself at the top of the patient's head. If the patient is on a stretcher, you can squat to put your head at the level of the patient's face. If the patient is on the floor or ground, you may need to kneel and lean forward or lie down to get into the proper position Figure 70 .

Grasp the laryngoscope with your left hand, and hold it as far down on the handle as possible. If the patient's mouth is not open, place the side of your right-hand thumb just below the bottom lip and push the mouth open, or "scissor" your thumb and index finger between the molars. As an alternative, you can open the mouth with the tongue-jaw lift maneuver.

Insert the blade into the *right* side of the patient's mouth. Use the flange of the blade to sweep the tongue gently to the left side of the mouth while moving the blade into the midline. Take care not to catch the patient's lips between the laryngoscope blade and the teeth. Moving the tongue from right to left is a critical step. If you simply insert the blade in the midline, the tongue will hang over both sides of the blade and all you will see is the tongue Figure 71 .

Slowly advance the blade—the curved blade into the vallecula or the straight blade beneath the epiglottis—while sweeping the tongue to the left. Exert *gentle* traction at a 45° angle to the floor as you lift the patient's jaw. *Do not "pry" back on the laryngoscope;* prying will cause you to use the patient's upper teeth as a fulcrum, resulting in breaking and potential aspiration of teeth Figure 72 . Keeping your back and your left arm straight as you pull upward allows you to use the strength of your shoulders to lift the patient's jaw and decreases the likelihood of levering the laryngoscope blade against the patient's teeth Figure 73 . The correct motion is similar to holding a glass and offering a toast.

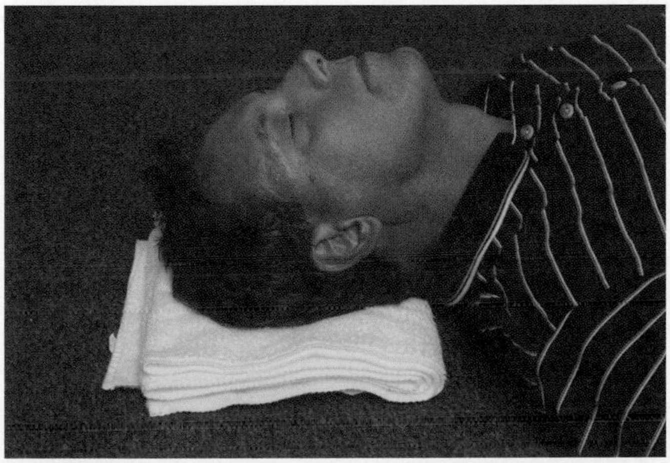

Figure 69 Head elevation is best achieved with folded towels positioned under the head.

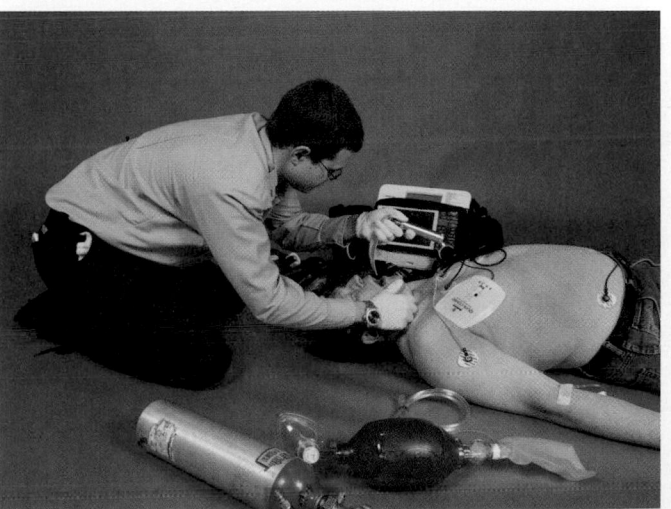

Figure 70 If the patient is on the floor or ground, you may need to kneel and lean forward or lie on the floor to get into the proper position.

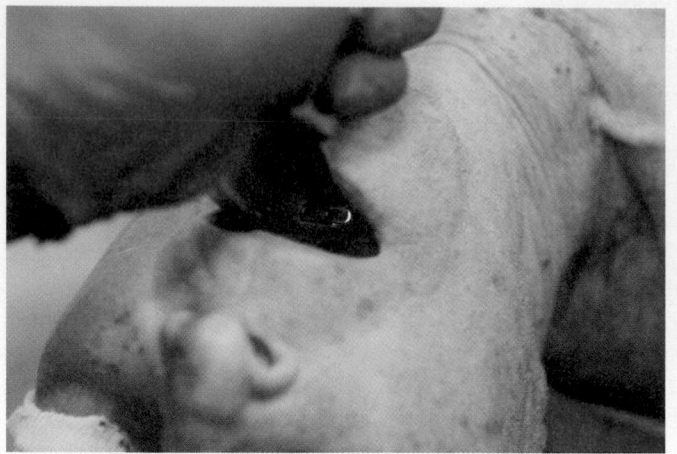

Figure 71 The tongue is a sticky, amorphous structure that can be a major hindrance to visualizing the airway. Proper manipulation of the blade in the mouth is critical to controlling the tongue.

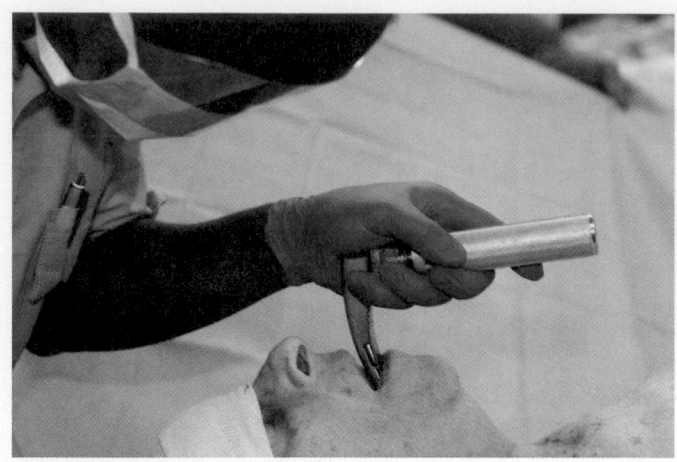

Figure 73 Keep your back and your left arm straight as you pull upward so that you use the strength of your shoulders to lift the patient's jaw.

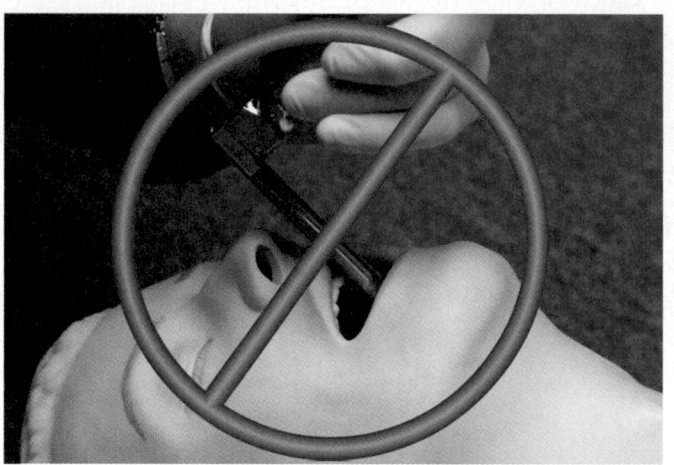

Figure 72 Prying against the upper teeth with the laryngoscope can result in breaking and potential aspiration of the teeth and, therefore, must be avoided.

view. The vocal cords are the white fibrous bands that lie vertically within the glottic opening; they should be slightly open **Figure 74**.

The **gum elastic bougie** is a flexible device that is approximately 1 cm in diameter and 60 cm long.

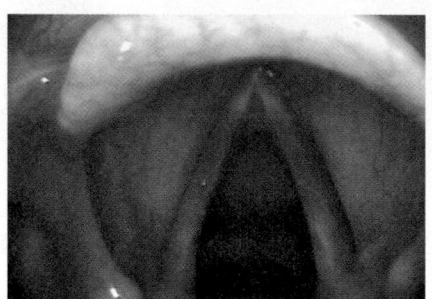

Figure 74 Laryngoscopic view of the vocal cords (white fibrous bands).

A 1-cm, 30° bend is found at the distal tip **Figure 75**. Reusable and disposable versions are available in adult and pediatric sizes. The gum elastic bougie is used in epiglottis-only views to facilitate intubation. It can make intubation possible in some difficult situations, especially when your view of the glottic opening is limited. The gum bougie is rigid enough that it can be easily directed through the glottic opening, yet flexible enough that it does not cause damage to the tracheal walls.

The gum bougie is inserted through the glottic opening under direct laryngoscopy. The angle at its distal tip facilitates entry into the glottic opening and enables you to "feel" the ridges of the tracheal wall **Figure 76**. Once the gum bougie is placed deeply into the trachea, it becomes a guide for the ET tube. Simply slide the tube over the gum bougie and into the trachea. Remove the gum bougie, ventilate, and confirm proper ET tube placement.

Tube Insertion

Once you have visualized the glottic opening, pick up the preselected ET tube in your right hand, holding it near the connector as you would hold a pencil. Under direct vision, insert the tube

Visualization of the Glottic Opening

Continue *lifting* the laryngoscope as you look down the blade. You should see some familiar anatomic landmarks—the epiglottis or the arytenoid cartilage. Identifying these structures enables to you make small adjustments in the position of the blade to aid in visualization of the glottic opening.

With the curved blade, "walk" the blade down the tongue because the vallecula and the epiglottis lie at the base of the tongue. With the straight blade, insert the blade straight back until the tip touches the posterior pharyngeal wall.

As you continue to work the tip of the blade into position (lifting the epiglottis with the straight blade or the vallecula with the curved blade), the glottic opening should come into full

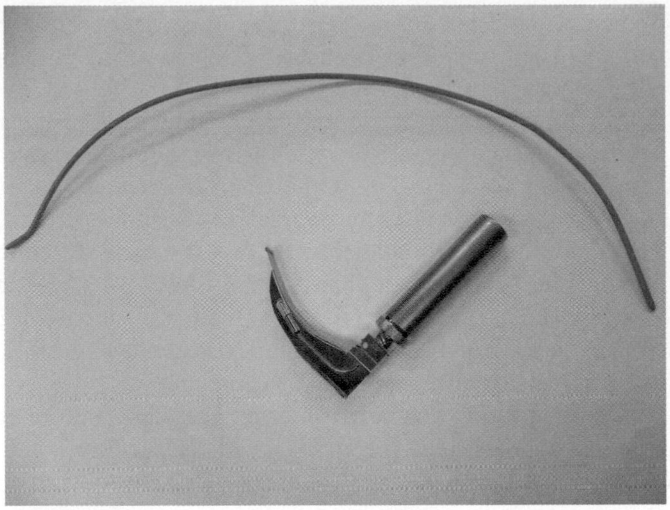

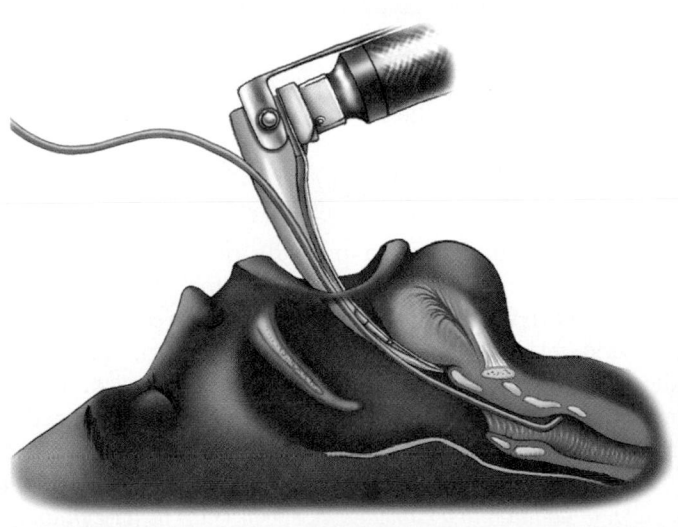

Figure 75 A gum elastic bougie shown next to a laryngoscope.

Figure 76 The angle at the distal tip of the gum elastic bougie facilitates entry into the glottic opening and enables you to feel the ridges of the tracheal wall.

from the right corner of the patient's mouth through the vocal cords. Continue to insert the tube until the proximal end of the cuff is 1 to 2 cm past the vocal cords. *You must see the tip of the ET tube pass through the vocal cords. If you cannot see the vocal cords, do not insert the tube.* An ET tube shoved blindly down the throat will almost always come to rest in the esophagus, not in the trachea; the only way to be certain that the tube has passed through the vocal cords is to *see* it pass through the vocal cords. If you take your eye off the tip of the tube (and the vocal cords), even for a second, you significantly increase the likelihood of allowing the tube to slip into the esophagus.

A major mistake of beginners is to try to pass the tube down the barrel of the laryngoscope blade—especially when using a

Words of Wisdom

Improving Your Laryngoscopic View
If you are having difficulty seeing the glottic opening, consider having your assistant perform the **BURP maneuver**: backward/upward/rightward pressure. The BURP maneuver—also known as external laryngeal manipulation—is performed by locating the lower third of the thyroid cartilage and applying pressure back, up, and to the right. If performed correctly, the BURP maneuver can improve your laryngoscopic view of the glottic opening and vocal cords **Figure 77**.

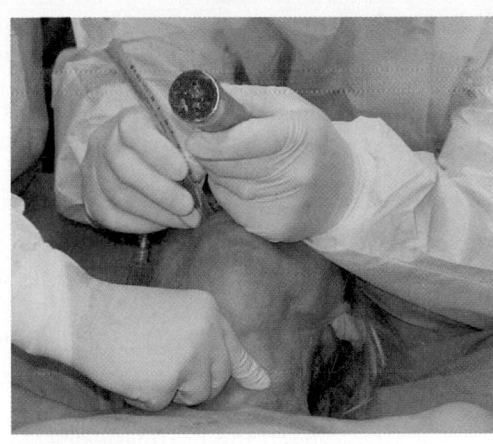

Figure 77 The BURP maneuver—displacing the larynx back, up, and to the right—may help visualize the vocal cords.

straight blade. The laryngoscope blade is not designed as a guide for the tube; it is a tool used only to visualize the glottic opening. Placing the tube down the barrel of the blade will obscure your view of the glottic opening and should be avoided **Figure 78**.

Ventilation

After you have seen the cuff of the ET tube pass roughly ½″ beyond the vocal cords, gently remove the blade, hold the tube securely in place with your right hand, and remove the stylet from the tube. Inflate the distal cuff with 5 to 10 mL of air, and

Words of Wisdom

An intubation attempt should not take more than 30 seconds. Thirty seconds begins when you stop ventilating with the bag-mask device and resume ventilations with the bag-mask device attached to the ET tube. If you are unable to intubate the patient within 30 seconds, abort the attempt and reoxygenate the patient for at least 30 seconds to 1 minute with 100% oxygen before attempting intubation again. *If the patient is in cardiac arrest, do not interrupt chest compressions to insert an ET tube.*

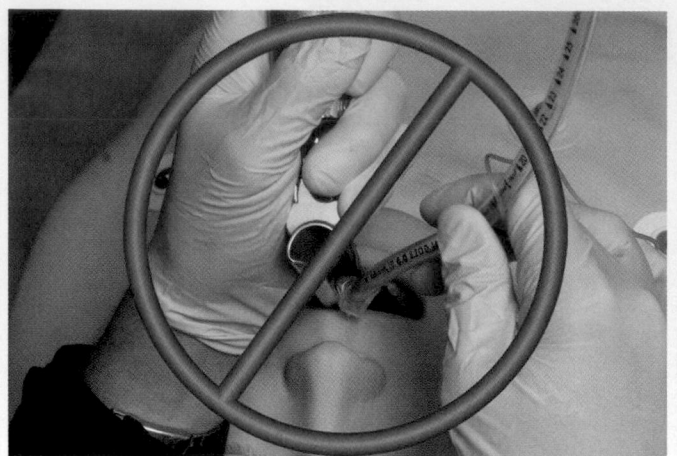

Figure 78 Placing a tube down the barrel of the blade obscures your view of the glottic opening and should be avoided.

then detach the syringe from the inflation port. If the syringe is not removed *immediately* following inflation of the distal cuff, air from the cuff may leak back into the syringe, resulting in a loss of an adequate seal between the cuff and the tracheal wall. Avoid inflating the distal cuff with excess pressure, which may cause tissue necrosis of the tracheal wall.

Have your assistant attach the bag-mask device to the ET tube and continue ventilation. An in-line T-piece capnography monitor, which is attached to the cardiac monitor/defibrillator, should be placed between the bag-mask device and ET tube. As the first ventilations are delivered, look at the patient's chest to ensure that it rises with each ventilation. At the same time, listen with a stethoscope to both lungs at the apices and bases and to the stomach over the epigastrium. If the tube is properly positioned, you will hear equal breath sounds bilaterally and a quiet epigastrium. Epigastric sounds may be transmitted to the lungs in obese patients or patients with significant gastric distention, however, leading you to believe that you have inadvertently intubated the esophagus.

Ventilation should continue as dictated by the patient's age. An apneic adult with a pulse should be ventilated at a rate of 10 to 12 breaths/min (one breath every 5 to 6 seconds), and an apneic infant or child with a pulse should be ventilated at a rate of 12 to 20 breaths/min (one breath every 3 to 5 seconds). If the patient (adult, child, or infant) is in cardiac arrest, ventilate him or her at a rate of 8 to 10 breaths/min (one breath every 6 to 8 seconds); do not stop chest compressions to deliver ventilations (asynchronous CPR).

Confirmation of Tube Placement

Visualizing the ET tube passing between the vocal cords is your first—and most reliable—method of confirming that the tube has entered the trachea; however, you must continue gathering information to assess the location of the tube. A misplaced tube that goes undetected is a fatal error. You must incorporate multiple assessment findings into the determination of where the tube is located.

Auscultation is the next step in confirming proper tube placement. Unequal or absent breath sounds suggest esophageal placement, right mainstem bronchus placement, pneumothorax, or bronchial obstruction.

Bilaterally absent breath sounds or gurgling over the epigastrium when auscultating during ventilation indicates that you have intubated the esophagus rather than the trachea. In that case, you must *immediately* remove the ET tube and be prepared to vigorously suction the patient's airway. If gastric distention is present, the likelihood of emesis is increased. After clearing the airway with suction (if needed), ventilate the patient with a bag-mask device and 100% oxygen for 30 seconds to 1 minute before you make another attempt at intubation.

If breath sounds are heard only on the right side of the chest, the tube has likely been advanced too far and entered the right mainstem bronchus. Follow these steps to reposition the tube:

1. Loosen or remove the tube-securing device.
2. Deflate the distal cuff.
3. Place your stethoscope over the left side of the chest.
4. While ventilation continues, *slowly* retract the tube while simultaneously listening for breath sounds over the left side of the chest.
5. Stop as soon as bilaterally equal breath sounds are heard.
6. Note the depth of the tube (in cm) at the patient's teeth.
7. Reinflate the distal cuff.
8. Secure the tube.
9. Resume ventilations.

If the ET tube has been properly positioned in the trachea, the bag-mask device should be easy to compress and you should see corresponding chest expansion. Increased resistance (decreased ventilation compliance) during ventilations may indicate gastric distention, esophageal intubation, or tension pneumothorax. Each of these conditions warrants immediate reassessment and corrective action.

Continuous waveform capnography (discussed earlier in this chapter), in addition to a clinical assessment (such as auscultation of breath sounds and over the epigastrium and assessing for visible chest rise), is regarded as the most reliable method of confirming and monitoring correct placement of the ET tube. The ideal time to attach the capnography T-piece is when the bag-mask device is attached to the ET tube. If waveform capnography is not available, a colorimetric $ETCO_2$ detector (also discussed earlier in this chapter) or an esophageal detector device—along with a clinical assessment of the patient—can be used.

The **esophageal detector device** is a bulb or syringe with a 15/22-mm adapter. With the syringe model, the syringe is attached to the end of the ET tube and the plunger is withdrawn, creating negative pressure **Figure 79**. If the tube is in the trachea (which has rigid, noncollapsible walls), air is easily drawn into the syringe and the plunger does not move when released. Unlike the trachea, however, the esophagus is a flaccid, easily collapsible tube. Thus, if the tube is in the esophagus, a vacuum is created as the plunger of the esophageal detector device is withdrawn and the plunger moves back toward zero when released.

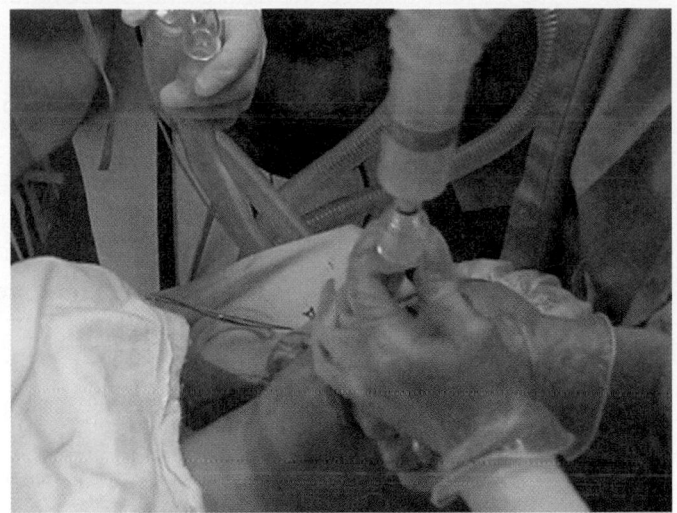

Figure 79 With the esophageal detector device syringe, the ability to freely withdraw air indicates placement of the tube in the trachea.

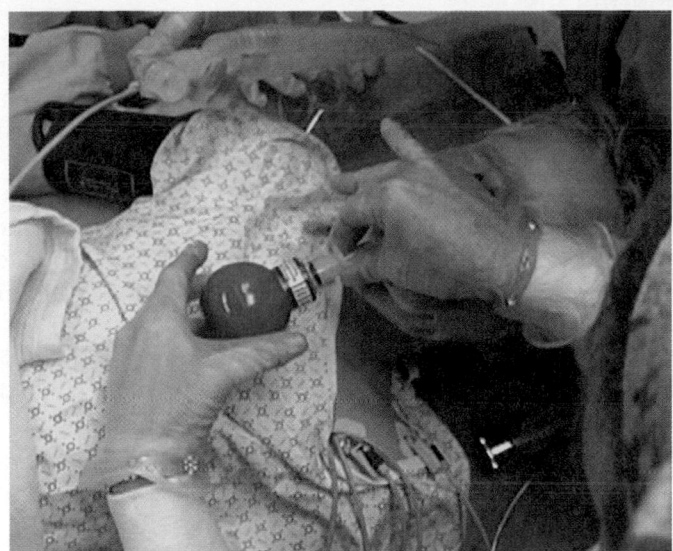

Figure 80 If the endotracheal tube is in the trachea, the bulb of the esophageal detector device should briskly fill with air.

With the bulb model, the bulb is squeezed and then attached to the end of the ET tube. If it remains collapsed or inflates slowly, the esophageal wall has occluded the distal tip of the tube, indicating that esophageal intubation has likely occurred. If the bulb briskly expands, the tube is properly positioned in the trachea **Figure 80**.

After confirming proper tube placement, note and mark the ET tube with ink or piece of tape at the point where it emerges from the patient's mouth; this mark will enable health care personnel involved in the subsequent care of the patient to determine whether the tube has slipped in or out. The average depth for adults is 21 to 25 cm.

YOU *are the Medic*   PART 7

After establishing IV access and obtaining a 12-lead ECG, which reveals no gross evidence of myocardial ischemia or injury, you call in your radio report to the receiving hospital and reassess the patient. The patient is responsive to painful stimuli but is tolerating the ET tube after the administration of 5 mg of midazolam (Versed). Your partner continues to assist ventilations.

Recording Time: 20 Minutes	
Level of consciousness	P (sedated with midazolam [Versed])
Respirations	10 breaths/min (baseline); intubated and ventilations being assisted
Pulse	104 beats/min; regular and strong
Skin	Less diaphoretic; cyanosis continues to resolve
Blood pressure	122/64 mm Hg
Spo$_2$	99% (with assisted ventilation and oxygen)
ETCO$_2$	28 mm Hg; decreased waveform height
ECG	Sinus tachycardia in lead II; 12-lead ECG reveals the same

12. What are some possible causes of the patient's decreasing ETCO$_2$ and waveform height? What must you do to determine the cause?

13. What would you expect the patient's ETCO$_2$ reading and waveform to do if he were not being adequately ventilated?

Securing the Tube

The last, and very important step, is to secure the ET tube. Inadvertent extubation is relatively common and can be traumatic to the patient. There are few things more discouraging than accomplishing a difficult intubation and having the tube slip out of the trachea. Reintubation will almost certainly be even more difficult. *Never take your hand off the ET tube before it has been secured with an appropriate device.* Even then, it is a good idea to support the tube manually while you ventilate the patient to avoid a sudden jolt from the bag-mask device that pulls the tube from the trachea.

Many commercial tube-securing devices are available. You should be familiar with the specific device used by your EMS system. The steps for securing an ET tube are reviewed here:

1. Note the centimeter marking on the ET tube at the level of the patient's teeth.
2. Remove the bag-mask device from the ET tube.
3. Position the ET tube in the center of the patient's mouth.
4. Place the securing device over the ET tube. Tighten the screw to secure it in place. Fasten the strap.
5. Reattach the bag-mask device, auscultate again over the apices and bases of the lungs and over the epigastrium, and note the capnography reading and waveform.

Many commercially manufactured ET tube–securing devices feature a built-in bite block to prevent the patient from occluding the tube if he or she bites down or experiences a seizure. If you do not have a commercially manufactured ET tube–securing device, you can secure the tube in place with tape and insert a bite block or oral airway between the patient's molars to prevent him or her from biting the tube.

It is also important to minimize head movement in an intubated patient. With a firmly secured tube, the tip can move as much as 5 cm during head flexion and extension. Consider applying a cervical collar, placing the patient on a long backboard, and stabilizing the patient's head with lateral immobilization blocks to reduce the likelihood of tube dislodgement during transport.

The steps for orotracheal intubation by direct laryngoscopy are summarized here and shown in **Skill Drill 18**:

Skill Drill   18

1. Take standard precautions (gloves and face shield) **Step 1**.
2. Measure and insert an oropharyngeal airway using one of the techniques described in Skill Drills 5 and 6 **Step 2**.
3. Preoxygenate the patient for 2 to 3 minutes with a bag-mask device and 100% oxygen **Step 3**.
4. Check, prepare, and assemble your equipment **Step 4**.
5. Place the patient's head in the sniffing position **Step 5**.
6. Remove the oropharyngeal airway, then insert the blade into the right side of the patient's mouth, and displace the tongue to the left **Step 6**.
7. Gently lift the long axis of the laryngoscope handle until you can visualize the glottic opening and the vocal cords **Step 7**.
8. Insert the ET tube through the right corner of the mouth **Step 8**.
9. Visualize its entry between the vocal cords **Step 9**.
10. Remove the laryngoscope from the patient's mouth **Step 10**.
11. Remove the stylet from the ET tube **Step 11**.
12. Inflate the distal cuff of the ET tube with 5 to 10 mL of air, and *immediately* detach the syringe from the inflation port **Step 12**.
13. Attach an ETCO$_2$ detector (waveform capnography preferred) to the ET tube **Step 13**.
14. Attach the detector to the monitor **Step 14**.
15. Attach the bag-mask device and ventilate. Listen over both lungs and over the stomach for ventilations **Step 15**.
16. Secure the ET tube with a commercial device or tape. Continue to reassess the patient **Step 16**.

Documentation and Communication

On the patient care report, document the means of assessing placement of the ET tube, such as breath sounds, visualization, and waveform capnography findings. The depth of the tube, as noted by the centimeter marking at the patient's teeth, should also be documented. In addition, indicate when correct placement was confirmed: at the time the ET tube was placed, any time the patient was moved (ie, from the floor to the stretcher, loaded into the ambulance), and on arrival at the hospital.

Nasotracheal Intubation

Nasotracheal intubation is the insertion of a tube into the trachea through the nose. In the prehospital setting, it is usually performed without directly visualizing the vocal cords—hence the term "blind" nasotracheal intubation.

Blind nasotracheal intubation is an excellent technique for establishing control over the airway in situations when it is difficult or hazardous to perform laryngoscopy. Because the procedure must be performed on patients with spontaneous breathing, it is less likely to result in hypoxia.

Indications and Contraindications

Nasotracheal intubation is indicated for patients who are breathing spontaneously but require definitive airway management to prevent further deterioration of their condition. Responsive patients and patients with an altered mental status and an intact gag reflex who are in respiratory failure because of conditions such as COPD, asthma, or pulmonary edema are excellent candidates for nasotracheal intubation.

Nasotracheal intubation is contraindicated in apneic patients (that is, in respiratory or cardiac arrest), who should be orotracheally intubated. This procedure is also contraindicated in patients with head trauma and possible midface fractures, as evidenced by CSF drainage from the nose following a head injury. In patients with these injuries, a nasally inserted

ET tube may enter the cranial vault and penetrate the brain. Other contraindications to nasotracheal intubation include anatomic abnormalities, such as a deviated septum or nasal polyps, and frequent cocaine use. Nasal insertion of an ET tube in patients with these contraindications may result in severe epistaxis.

Skill Drill | 18

Intubation of the Trachea Using Direct Laryngoscopy

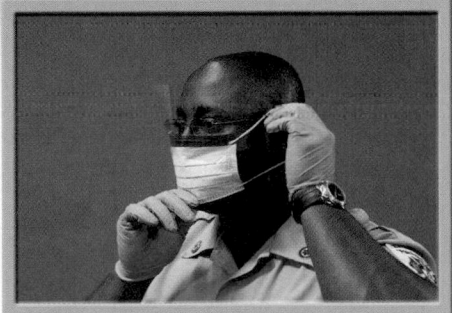

Step 1 Take standard precautions (gloves and face shield).

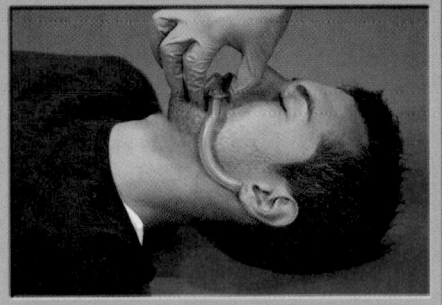

Step 2 Measure and inspect an oropharyngeal airway using one of the techniques described in Skill Drills 5 and 6.

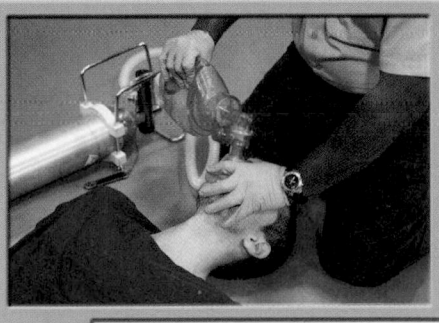

Step 3 Preoxygenate the patient for 2 to 3 minutes with a bag-mask device and 100% oxygen.

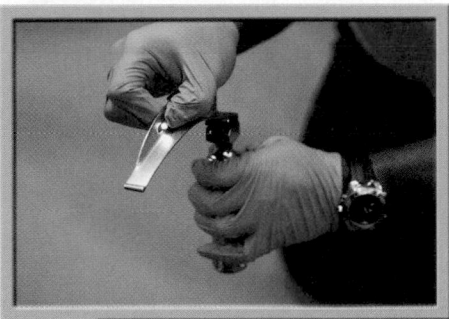

Step 4 Check, prepare, and assemble your equipment.

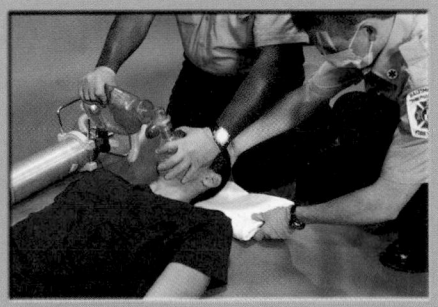

Step 5 Place the patient's head in the sniffing position.

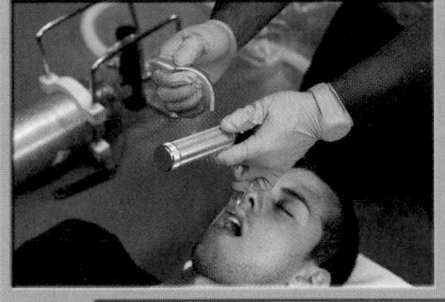

Step 6 Remove the oropharyngeal airway, then insert the blade into the right side of the patient's mouth, and displace the tongue to the left.

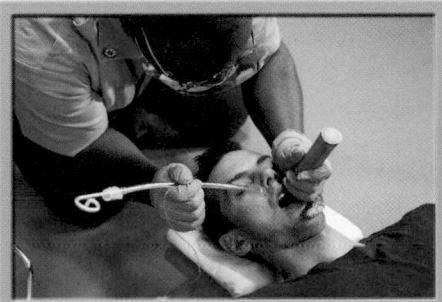

Step 7 Gently lift the long axis of the laryngoscope handle until you can visualize the glottic opening and the vocal cords.

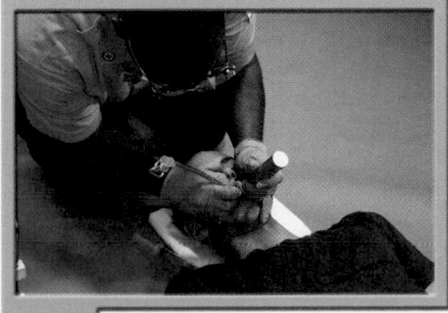

Step 8 Insert the ET tube through the right corner of the mouth.

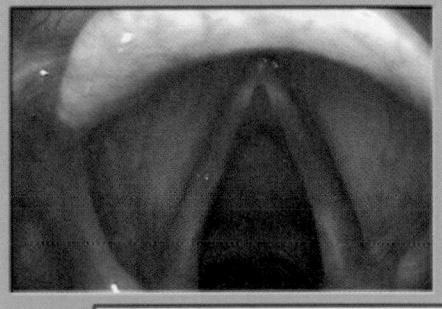

Step 9 Visualize its entry between the vocal cords.

Continues

Skill Drill | 18

Intubation of the Trachea Using Direct Laryngoscopy, continued

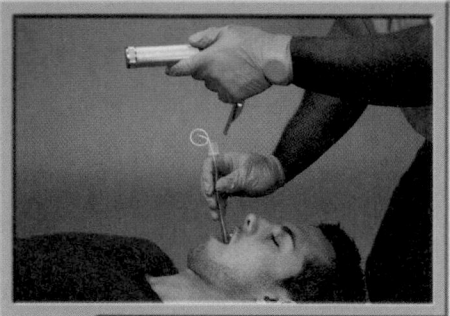

Step 10 Remove the laryngoscope from the patient's mouth.

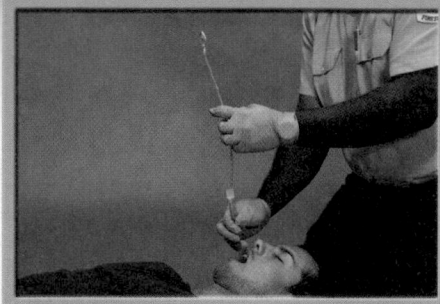

Step 11 Remove the stylet from the ET tube.

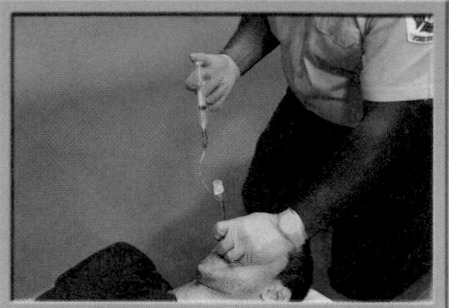

Step 12 Inflate the distal cuff of the ET tube with 5 to 10 mL of air, and detach the syringe from the inflation port.

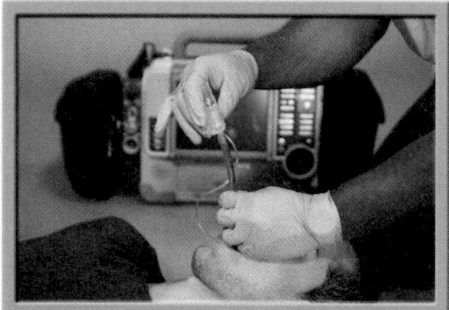

Step 13 Attach the end-tidal carbon dioxide detector to the ET tube.

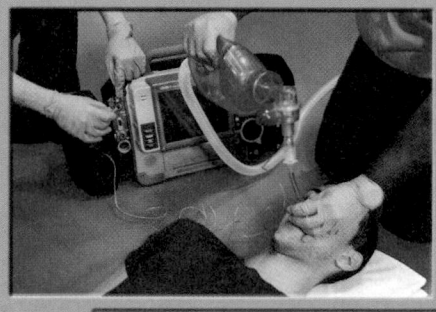

Step 14 Attach the detector to the monitor.

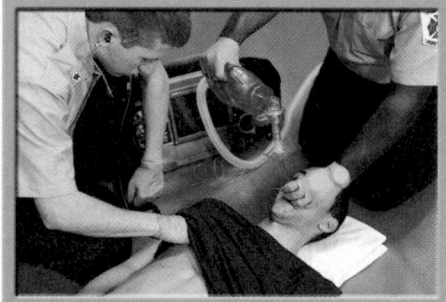

Step 15 Attach the bag-mask device and ventilate. Listen over both lungs and over the epigastrium for ventilations.

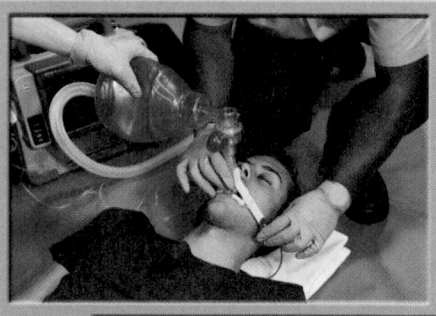

Step 16 Confirm placement, and then secure the ET tube. Continue to reassess the patient.

Avoid nasotracheal intubation, if possible, in patients with blood-clotting abnormalities and in patients who take anticoagulation medications (such as warfarin [Coumadin]). These situations also increase the likelihood and severity of epistaxis following insertion of anything in the nose.

Advantages and Disadvantages

The primary advantage of blind nasotracheal intubation is that it can be performed on patients who are responsive and breathing. This procedure does not require placement of anything in the mouth (such as a laryngoscope), so the nasotracheal route is associated with much less retching and a lower risk of vomiting in patients with an intact gag reflex.

Another major advantage of nasotracheal intubation is that there is no need for a laryngoscope, which eliminates the risk of trauma to the teeth or soft tissues of the mouth. Because the patient's mouth does not need to be opened, this technique is better suited to patients with limited temporomandibular joint mobility, such as patients with mandibular wiring, mandibular fractures, seizures, or clenched teeth (**trismus**).

Nasotracheal intubation does not require the patient to be placed in a sniffing position, which makes it an ideal technique for intubating patients with a possible spinal injury, unless a midface fracture is suspected. Finally, because the tube is inserted through the nose, the patient cannot bite the tube. Furthermore, it can be secured more easily than a tube that is inserted orally because the nose generally has less secretions than the mouth.

On the downside, because nasotracheal intubation is a blind technique, one of the major tube confirmation methods—visualizing the tube passing through the vocal cords—cannot be used. Confirming proper tube position is critical, regardless of the intubation method used; however, paramedics should be even more diligent when confirming tube placement following nasotracheal intubation.

Complications

Bleeding is the most common complication associated with nasotracheal intubation. If intubation is successful, the airway is protected and the risk of aspiration is eliminated. However, severe bleeding can occur, especially with rough technique, posing an additional threat to an already compromised airway as the swallowing of blood greatly increases the likelihood of vomiting and subsequent aspiration.

The incidence of bleeding associated with nasotracheal intubation can be reduced by gentle insertion of the tube into the nostril and lubrication of the tip with a water-soluble gel. If available, an anesthetic lubricant containing a vasoconstrictive agent (such as phenylephrine hydrochloride [Neo-Synephrine]) will reduce the amount of patient discomfort and the likelihood and severity of nasal bleeding.

Equipment

The same equipment used for orotracheal intubation—minus the laryngoscope and stylet—is used for blind nasotracheal intubation. Standard ET tubes can be used for orotracheal and nasotracheal intubation, although they should be 1.0 to 1.5 mm smaller when inserted nasally. When choosing the size of tube, select one that is slightly smaller than the nostril in which it will be inserted.

Some ET tubes have been designed specifically for blind nasotracheal intubation. For example, the Endotrol tube **Figure 81** is slightly more flexible than a standard ET tube and is equipped with a "trigger" that is attached to a piece of line, which is itself attached to the tip of the tube. Pulling the trigger moves the tip of the tube anteriorly and increases the tube's overall curvature. This feature replaces the function of the stylet.

The movement of air through the ET tube helps determine proper tube placement following nasotracheal intubation.

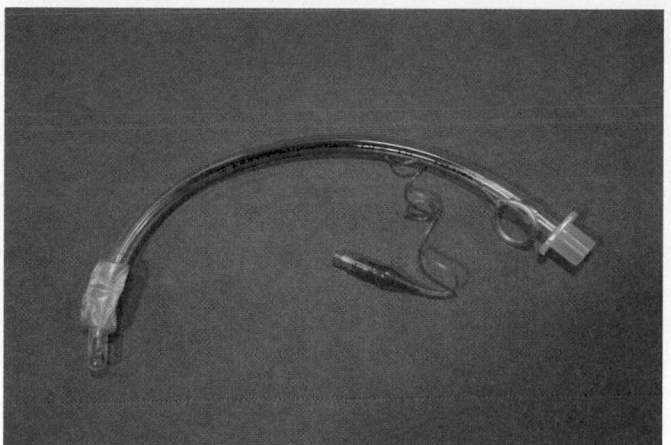

Figure 81 The Endotrol tube makes nasotracheal intubation safer, easier, and more efficient.

Table 12	**Devices Used to Determine Maximum Airflow Through the Tube During Nasotracheal Intubation**
Humid-Vent 1	A device that attaches to the 15/22-mm adapter at the end of the ET tube to prevent secretions from being expelled from the tube.
BAAM (Beck Airway Airflow Monitor)	A small whistle that attaches to the 15/22-mm adapter and emits a high-pitched sound as air moves in and out of the tube.
Stethoscope with head removed	Stethoscope tubing placed in the proximal 2 to 3 cm of the ET tube enables a paramedic to hear air movement without placing his or her face next to the tube.
IV tubing attached to an earpiece	The tubing in the proximal 2 to 3 cm of the ET tube enables the intubator to hear air movement without placing his or her face next to the tube.
Abbreviation: ET indicates endotracheal.	

A number of devices have been developed to allow a paramedic to confirm successful nasotracheal intubation without the need to place his or her face next to the tube, thus risking contact with contaminants in the patient's exhaled breath **Table 12**.

■ Technique for Nasotracheal Intubation

When you perform blind nasotracheal intubation, you use the patient's spontaneous respirations to guide a nasotracheal tube into the trachea and confirm proper placement. The tube is advanced as the patient inhales, at which point the vocal cords are open at their widest, which facilitates placement of the tube into the trachea.

After preparing your equipment and preoxygenating the patient, insert the tube into the nostril with the bevel facing toward the nasal septum. The right nostril is typically used because the curvature of the tube is in the correct orientation in relation to the bevel. If the right nostril is obstructed or if significant resistance is met, insert the tube into the left nostril, but rotate the tube 180° as its tip enters the nasopharynx.

The angle of insertion is critical when performing nasotracheal intubation. Aim the tip of the tube straight back toward the ear Figure 82. The goal is to follow the floor of the nasal cavity until the tube enters the nasopharynx. *Do not* insert the tube with the tip aimed upward toward the eye; doing so can damage the turbinates and cause significant bleeding.

As the tube is advanced into the nasopharynx, you will begin to hear air rushing in and out of the tube as the patient breathes. Your goal is to position the tube just above the glottic opening so that the patient will draw the tube into the trachea when he or she inhales deeply. Manipulate the patient's head to control the position of the tip of the tube. Cup your left hand (if the tube is inserted in the right nostril) under the patient's occiput. Move the patient's head until you find the position that offers the maximum amount of air moving through the tube. At this point, the tube should be positioned just above the glottic opening.

As the patient inhales, the negative pressure created by inhalation facilitates movement of the tube through the glottic opening. Instruct the patient to take a deep breath, and *gently* advance the tube with the inhalation. Placement of the tube in the trachea will be evidenced by an increase in air movement through the tube.

If you see a soft-tissue bulge on either side of the airway, the tube has probably been inserted into the piriform fossa. Hold the patient's head still and slightly withdraw the tube. Once maximum airflow is detected, advance the tube on inhalation. If you do not see a soft-tissue bulge and no air is moving through the tube, the tube has entered the esophagus. Withdraw the tube until you detect airflow, and then extend the head.

Once the tube has been properly positioned, inflate the distal cuff with the minimum amount of air necessary to achieve an airtight seal. Attach a bag-mask device to the tube, and ventilate the patient according to his or her clinical condition. Because you do not have the benefit of visualizing the tube passing between the vocal cords, confirmation (by multiple techniques) and continuous monitoring of proper tube position are more important following blind nasotracheal intubation than with any other intubation technique. Although the movement of air in and out of the tube during breathing is a good indicator that the tube is in the trachea, it is not foolproof. In many cases, only the tip of the nasotracheal tube has passed through the glottic opening; even slight patient movement may dislodge the tube into the esophagus, which might not be recognized. Movement of the tube can also result in right mainstem placement.

Clean up any secretions or excess lubricant, and secure the tube with tape. Document the depth of insertion at the nostril, and monitor it frequently to detect movement of the tube. The steps for performing blind nasotracheal intubation are listed here and shown in Skill Drill 19:

Skill Drill 19

1. Take standard precautions (gloves and face shield) Step 1.
2. Preoxygenate the patient whenever possible with a bag-mask device and 100% oxygen Step 2.
3. Check, prepare, and assemble your equipment Step 3.
4. Place the patient's head in a neutral position Step 4.
5. Preform the nasotracheal tube by bending it in a circle Step 5.
6. Administer a nasal spray to the patient for comfort Step 6.
7. Lubricate the tip of the tube with a water-soluble gel Step 7.
8. Gently insert the nasotracheal tube into the more compliant nostril, with the bevel facing toward the nasal septum, and advance the tube along the nasal floor Step 8.
9. Advance the nasotracheal tube through the vocal cords as the patient inhales Step 9.
10. Inflate the distal cuff with 5 to 10 mL of air, and detach the syringe Step 10.
11. Attach an ETCO$_2$ detector (waveform capnography preferred) to the nasotracheal tube Step 11.
12. Attach the detector to the monitor Step 12.
13. Attach the bag-mask device, ventilate, and auscultate over the apices and bases of both lungs and over the epigastrium. Secure the nasotracheal tube Step 13.

Words of Wisdom

Keep a laryngoscope and Magill forceps within easy reach in case the patient becomes apneic during the procedure or you are unable to thread the tip of the tube through the glottic opening blindly. In these cases, you will need to complete the procedure under direct laryngoscopy.

■ Digital Intubation

Suppose you are in the midst of attempting to intubate your patient and suddenly the light on your laryngoscope sputters

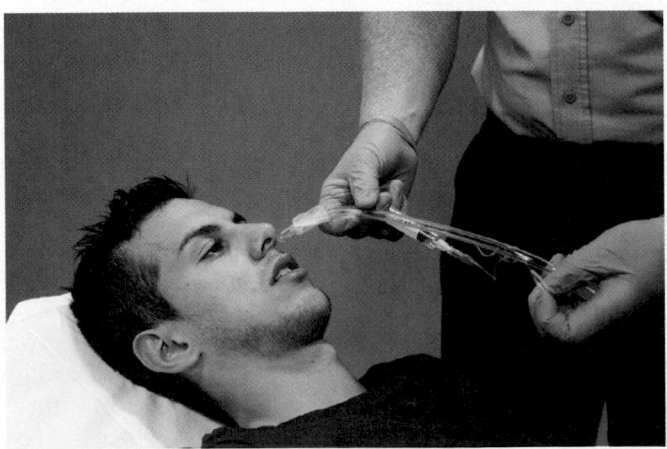
Figure 82 Aim the tip of the tube straight back toward the ear.

out. You must have a contingency plan for these kinds of unexpected events, including a set of fresh batteries and a backup laryngoscope handle.

Fortunately, there *is* a way to intubate the trachea without a laryngoscope. <u>**Digital intubation**</u> (also referred to as "blind"

or "tactile" intubation) involves directly palpating the glottic structures and elevating the epiglottis with your middle finger while guiding the ET tube into the trachea by using the sense of touch. Being adept at digital intubation provides you with an option in some extreme circumstances, such as equipment

Skill Drill | 19

Performing Blind Nasotracheal Intubation

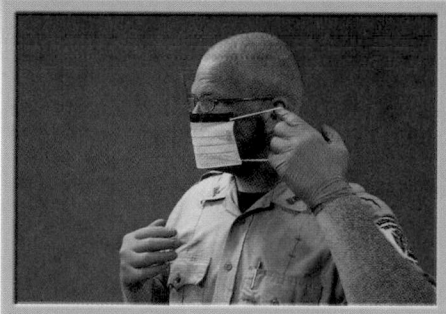

Step 1 Take standard precautions (gloves and face shield).

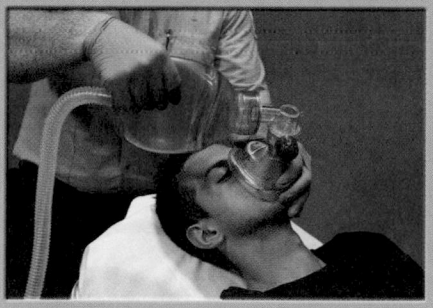

Step 2 Preoxygenate the patient whenever possible with a bag-mask device and 100% oxygen.

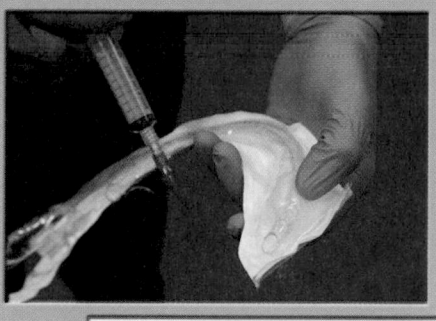

Step 3 Check, prepare, and assemble your equipment.

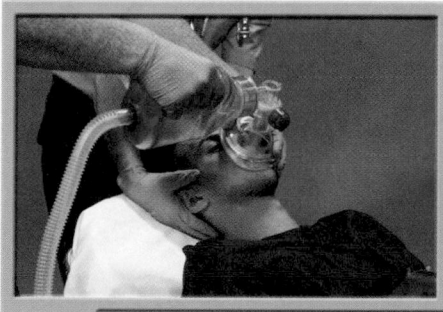

Step 4 Place the patient's head in a neutral position.

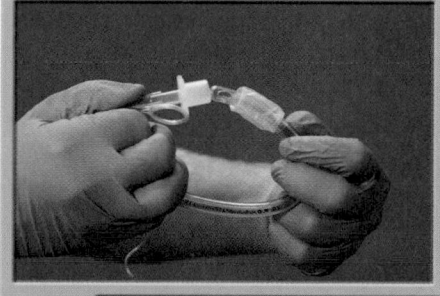

Step 5 Preform the nasotracheal tube by bending it in a circle.

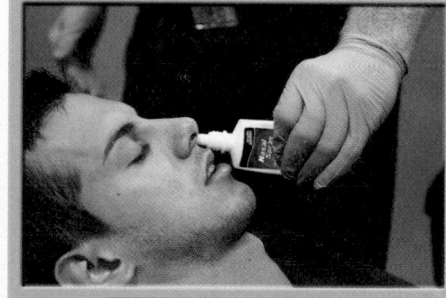

Step 6 Administer a nasal spray to the patient for comfort.

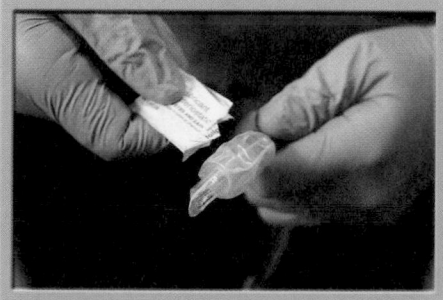

Step 7 Lubricate the tip of the tube with a water-soluble gel.

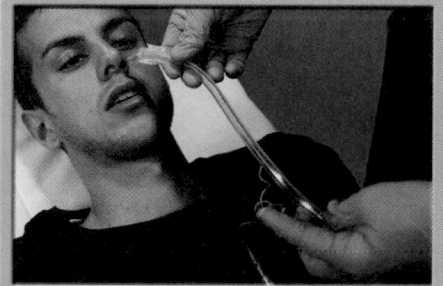

Step 8 Gently insert the nasotracheal tube into the more compliant nostril, with the bevel facing toward the nasal septum, and advance the tube along the nasal floor.

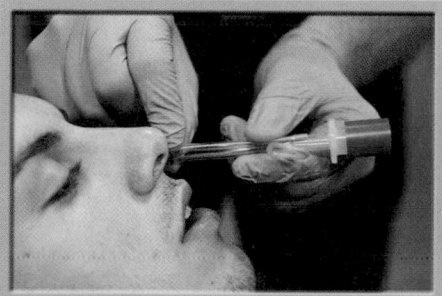

Step 9 Advance the nasotracheal tube through the vocal cords as the patient inhales. The BAAM® device can be helpful in this step.

Continues

Skill Drill   19

Performing Blind Nasotracheal Intubation, continued

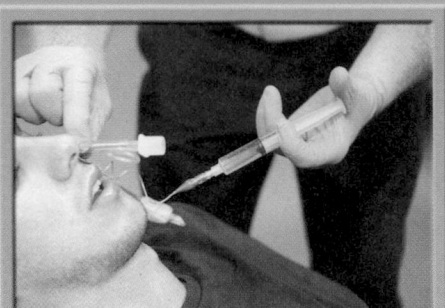

Step 10 Inflate the distal cuff with 5 to 10 mL of air, and detach the syringe.

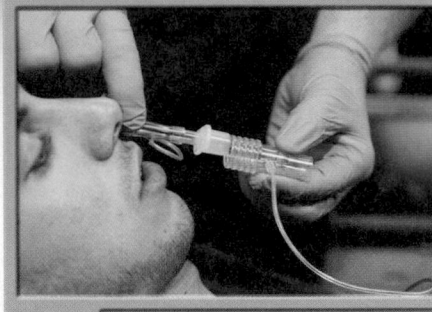

Step 11 Attach an end-tidal carbon dioxide detector to the nasotracheal tube.

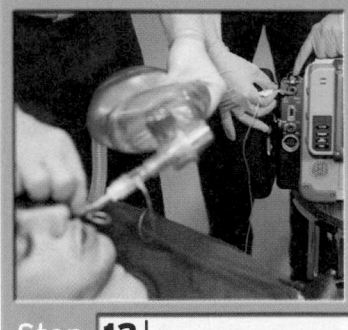

Step 12 Attach the detector to the monitor.

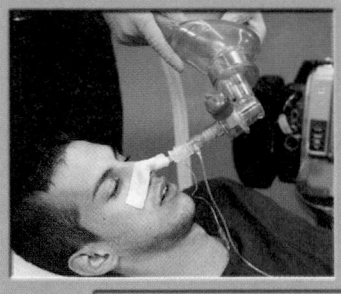

Step 13 Attach the bag-mask device, ventilate, and auscultate over the apices and bases of both lungs and over the epigastrium. Ensure proper tube placement with waveform capnography. Secure the nasotracheal tube.

failure when attempting to intubate an apneic patient, who, because of his or her apnea, is not a candidate for blind nasotracheal intubation.

Indications and Contraindications

Digital intubation may be used in the following exceptional circumstances:

- A laryngoscope is not available or has malfunctioned.
- Other techniques to intubate the patient have failed.
- The patient is in a confined space.
- The patient is extremely obese or has a short neck.
- Copious secretions obscure your view of the airway.
- The head cannot be moved owing to trauma, or immobilization equipment interferes with direct laryngoscopy.
- Massive airway trauma has made visualization of the intubation landmarks impossible.

Although digital intubation can be performed in pediatric patients, the size of an adult's fingers (it takes two fingers) relative to the size of the child's mouth usually makes the technique impossible. Also, digital intubation is absolutely contraindicated if the patient is breathing, is not deeply unresponsive, or has an intact gag reflex.

Advantages and Disadvantages

Because digital intubation does not require a laryngoscope, this technique is most advantageous in case of equipment failure. It is also ideal in situations in which your view of the vocal cords is obscured by copious, uncontrollable oral secretions. Because digital intubation does not require the patient's head to be in a sniffing position, it can be performed on trauma patients and patients whose heads cannot be placed in a sniffing position (such as obese or short-necked patients).

The major disadvantage of digital intubation is that it requires placing your fingers in the patient's mouth, posing a risk of being bitten. Digital intubation should therefore be performed only in patients who are deeply unresponsive and apneic *and* who have a bite block in their mouth to prevent closure. There is also a potential risk of exposure to an infectious disease. The patient's teeth could easily tear through gloves, especially if the teeth are sharp or broken.

Successful placement of an ET tube via digital intubation depends on frequency of practice, experience, manual dexterity, and the size and length of the paramedic's fingers. Paramedics with short fingers or fingers with large diameter will have greater difficulty performing digital intubation.

Complications

Misplacement of the ET tube is the major complication of digital intubation. Although the intubation is tactilely guided, it is easy to misdirect the tip of the tube during insertion. Therefore, diligent attention to tube confirmation is absolutely essential.

Because it does not require the use of a laryngoscope, digital intubation is associated with a much lower incidence of dental trauma; however, the insertion of a bite block or dental prod can cause lip trauma and tooth damage. In addition, vigorous attempts at insertion or improper technique can cause airway trauma or swelling.

Any intubation attempt, regardless of the technique used, can result in hypoxia. Therefore, you must carefully monitor the patient's clinical condition (such as pulse oximetry readings, skin color, and pulse rate) during the technique, limit intubation attempts to 30 seconds, and ventilate the patient appropriately between attempts.

Equipment

Less equipment is needed for digital intubation. In fact, you will usually attempt the digital technique because you have limited (or malfunctioning) equipment. Except for the laryngoscope, you will essentially use the same equipment as required for orotracheal intubation, plus your fingers. That is, you will need traditional intubation equipment and supplies—a stylet, $ETCO_2$ detector (waveform capnography preferred) or esophageal detector device, and an appropriate device to adequately secure the tube.

Technique for Digital Intubation

Because of the variety of alternative airway devices available (such as Combitube, King LT, and LMA), digital intubation is rarely performed. Nevertheless, you should work, through frequent practice, to become just as skilled and competent with digital intubation as you are with more common advanced airway management techniques.

Prepare your equipment for the digital intubation as your assistant ventilates the patient with a bag-mask device and 100% oxygen. Select an ET tube that is one half to a full size smaller than that used for intubation with direct laryngoscopy. In this technique, the tip of the tube is guided into the trachea while using your index finger as a leverage point. A stylet provides the tube with the rigidity necessary to make the bend in the tube. Two configurations are recommended; you should practice with both to determine your preference.

- In an "open J" configuration, the stylet is inserted and a large J shape is made in the distal end of the tube.
- In the "U-handle" configuration, the tube is bent into a U shape and the proximal half of the tube is bent into a 90° handle toward your dominant hand **Figure 83**.

Because a sniffing position is not required to perform digital intubation, you can be positioned at the patient's left side facing toward the head. This position facilitates digital intubation if the patient is trapped in a seated or standing position **Figure 84**.

Before considering placing your fingers in the patient's mouth, insert a bite block or the flange of an oral airway, turned

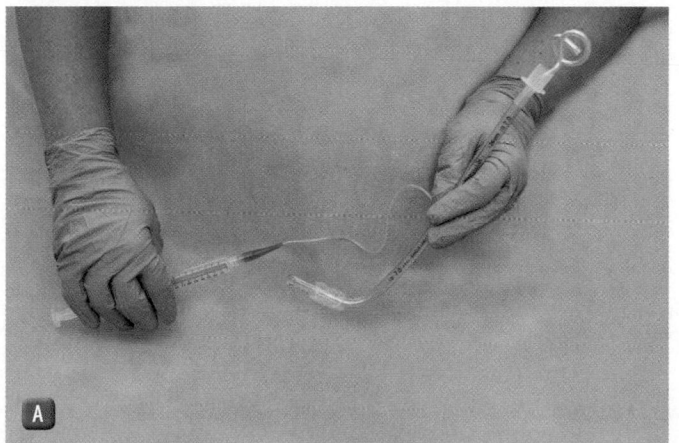

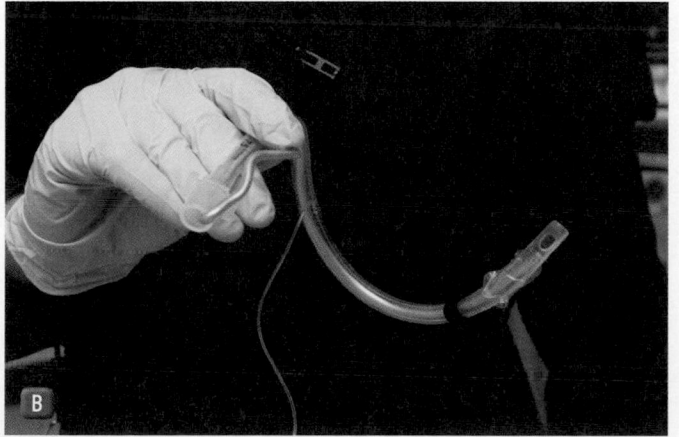

Figure 83 **A.** Open J configuration. **B.** The U-handle configuration.

sideways, between the patient's molars Figure 85 . This action will prevent complete closure of the patient's mouth, providing protection for your fingers in the event of a sudden change in consciousness or seizure.

Insert the index and middle fingers of your left hand into the right side of the patient's mouth. Press down against the tongue as you slide your fingers along the midline of the tongue until you can feel the epiglottis. Then pull the epiglottis forward with your middle finger.

Hold the ET tube in your right hand, as you would hold a pencil, and insert it into the left side of the patient's mouth. Advance the tube along the outer surface of your left index finger or between your middle and index fingers, and guide its tip toward the glottis. Once you feel the cuff of the tube pass about 2″ beyond the tip of your finger, stabilize the tube with your right hand while you gently withdraw your two left fingers from the patient's mouth.

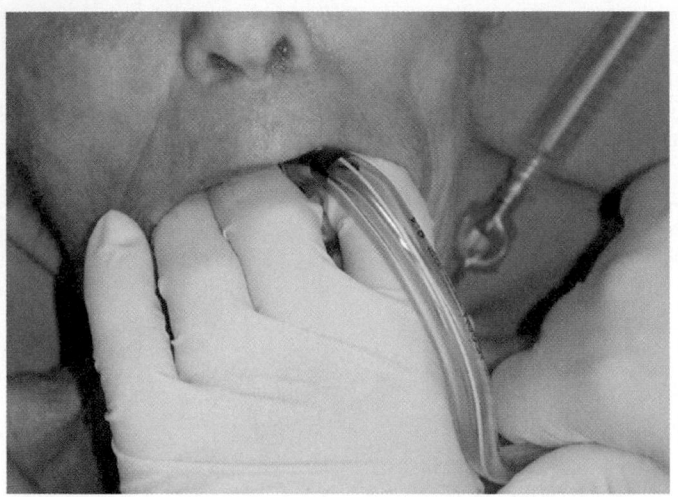

Figure 84 If the patient is trapped in a seated or standing position, digital intubation can be performed from a position facing the patient.

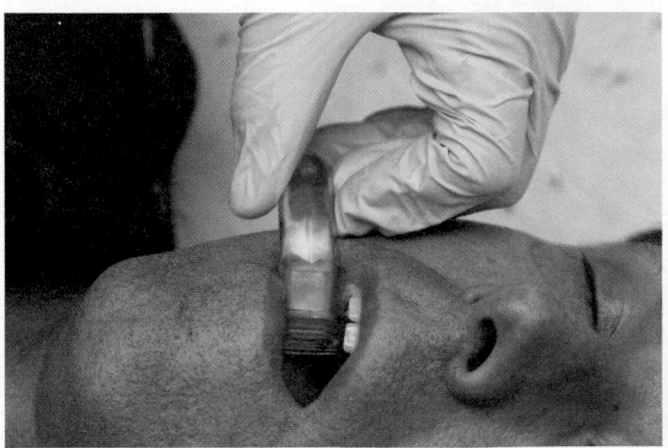

Figure 85 The flange of an oral airway should be inserted into the mouth and turned sideways to act as a bite block.

After the tube has been positioned and stabilized manually, carefully remove the stylet and inflate the distal cuff with 5 to 10 mL of air. (Do not forget to detach the syringe from the inflation port.) Attach the bag-mask device to the ET tube—with an ETCO$_2$ detector between the bag and tube—and ventilate the patient while observing for visible chest rise.

Because digital intubation is a blind technique, rigorous protocol for confirmation of tube placement must be followed. Auscultate both lungs and over the epigastrium, monitor the ETCO$_2$, and properly secure the tube in place. Continue ventilations according to the patient's clinical condition.

The steps for performing digital intubation are listed here and shown in Skill Drill 20 :

Skill Drill   20

1. Take standard precautions (gloves and face shield) Step 1 .
2. Insert an airway adjunct if needed Step 2 .
3. Preoxygenate the patient for 2 to 3 minutes with a bag-mask device and 100% oxygen Step 3 .
4. Check, prepare, and assemble your equipment Step 4 .
5. Bend the ET tube by placing a slight curve at its distal end (like a hockey stick) Step 5 .
6. Have a second provider hold the patient's head in neutral position while one provider continues to preoxygenate the patient. If you did not insert an airway adjunct earlier, at this point, place a bite block in between the patient's molars to prevent the patient from biting your fingers Step 6 .
7. Insert the middle and index fingers of one hand into the patient's mouth, and shift the patient's tongue forward as you advance your fingers toward the patient's larynx. Palpate and lift the epiglottis with your middle finger Step 7 .
8. Advance the tube with your other hand and guide it between the vocal cords with your index finger Step 8 .
9. Remove the stylet from the ET tube Step 9 .
10. Inflate the distal cuff of the ET tube with 5 to 10 mL of air, and detach the syringe Step 10 .
11. Attach the ETCO$_2$ detector (waveform capnography preferred) to the ET tube Step 11 .
12. Attach the bag-mask device and ventilate. Auscultate over the apices and bases of both lungs and over the epigastrium Step 12 .
13. Secure the ET tube Step 13 .

■ Transillumination Techniques for Intubation

Transillumination intubation, like digital intubation, is rarely considered a first-line technique to definitively secure the airway, but it may prove valuable in some situations. The tissue that overlies the trachea is relatively thin. Therefore, a bright light source placed inside the trachea emits a bright, well-circumscribed light that is visible on the outside of the trachea and the external soft tissue that overlies it.

Skill Drill 20

Performing Digital Intubation

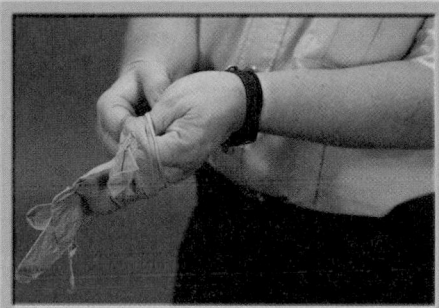

Step 1 Take standard precautions (gloves and face shield).

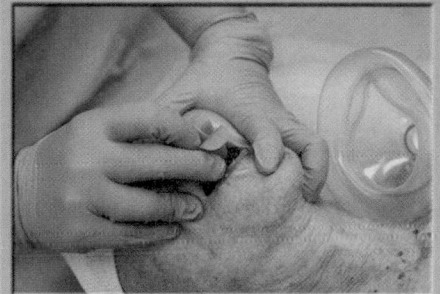

Step 2 Insert an airway adjunct if needed.

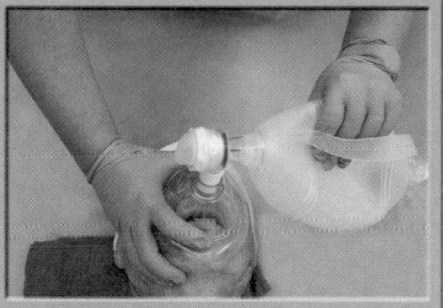

Step 3 Preoxygenate the patient for 2 to 3 minutes with a bag-mask device and 100% oxygen.

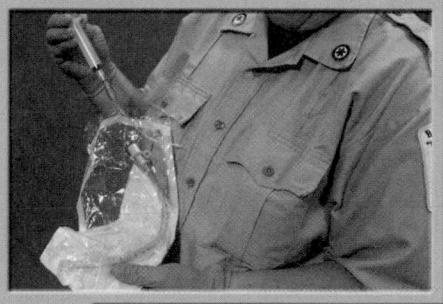

Step 4 Check, prepare, and assemble your equipment.

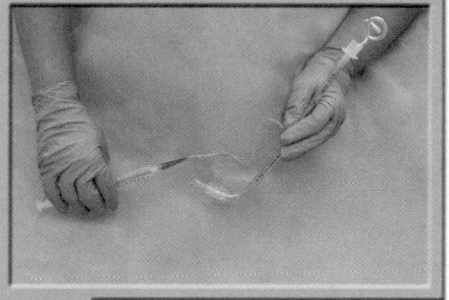

Step 5 Bend the ET tube by placing a slight curve at its distal end (like a hockey stick).

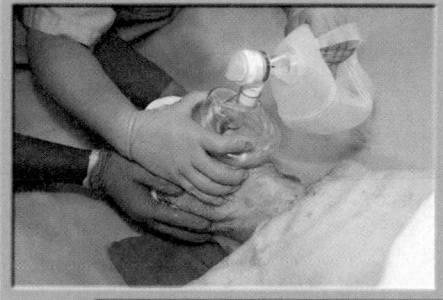

Step 6 Have a second provider hold the patient's head in neutral position while one provider continues to preoxygenate the patient. If you did not insert an airway adjunct earlier, at this point, place a bite block in between the patient's molars to prevent the patient from biting your fingers.

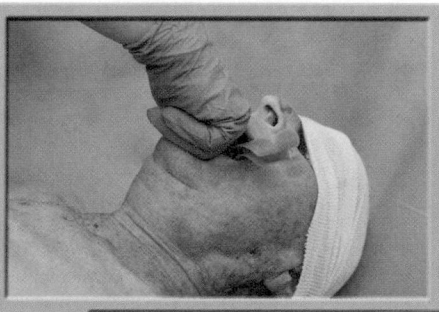

Step 7 Insert the middle and index fingers of one hand into the patient's mouth and shift the patient's tongue forward as you advance your fingers toward the larynx. Palpate and lift the epiglottis with your middle finger.

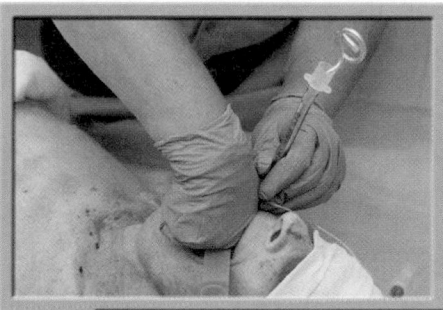

Step 8 Advance the tube with your other hand and guide it between the vocal cords with your index finger.

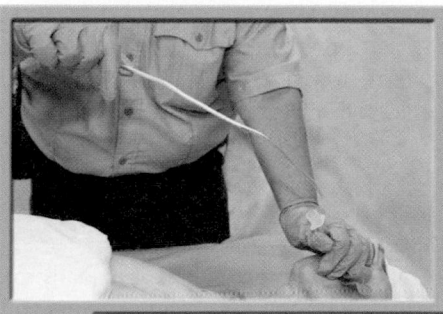

Step 9 Remove the stylet from the ET tube.

Continues

Skill Drill 20

Performing Digital Intubation, continued

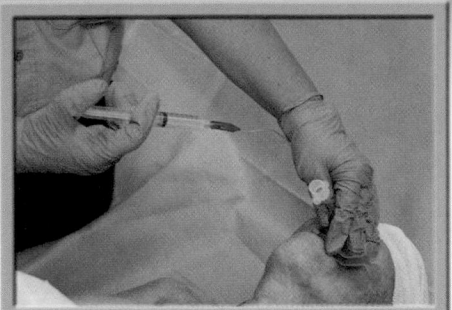

Step 10 Inflate the distal cuff of the ET tube with 5 to 10 mL of air, and detach the syringe.

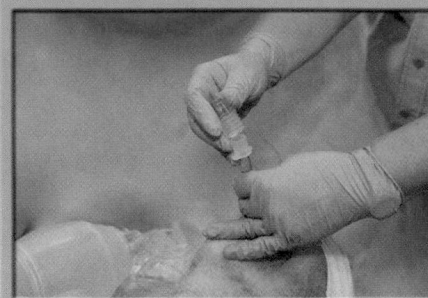

Step 11 Attach the end-tidal carbon dioxide detector to the ET tube.

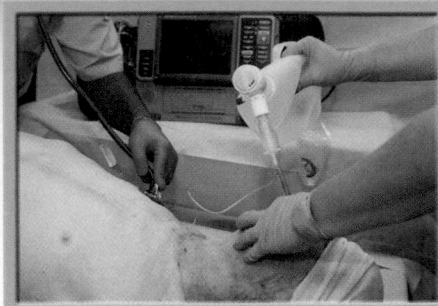

Step 12 Attach the bag-mask device and ventilate. Auscultate over the apices and bases of both lungs and over the epigastrium. Ensure proper tube placement with waveform capnography.

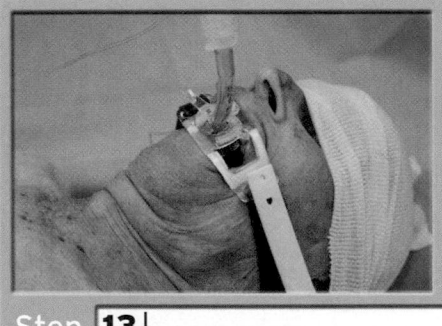

Step 13 Secure the ET tube.

A number of devices can be used to intubate the trachea with the transillumination technique Figure 86. You should be familiar with your specific equipment and consult the product documentation for instructions in its use. In this section, the term "lighted stylet" will be used generically to describe any malleable stylet with a bright light source at its distal end that can be used to guide intubation.

Indications and Contraindications

Transillumination intubation can be used whenever a patient needs to be intubated, but it is usually performed after other intubation techniques have failed. This technique is absolutely contraindicated in patients with an intact gag reflex and in patients with an airway obstruction. When determining whether transillumination should be attempted, consider the amount of soft tissue overlying the trachea. Transillumination may be difficult in obese patients and patients with short, muscular necks.

Theoretically, it is possible to perform transillumination in pediatric patients; however, the stylet *must* fit inside the ET tube. Most lighted stylets will not fit in tubes smaller than 6.0 mm.

Advantages and Disadvantages

Because transillumination does not involve the use of a laryngoscope, it largely avoids the problems associated with laryngoscopy (such as dental and soft-tissue trauma). In contrast with other blind intubation techniques (such as digital and nasotracheal), transillumination adds a visual parameter—a light at the midline of the neck—that increases the chance for successful tube placement. Furthermore, this technique does not require visualization of the glottic opening, so the tube can be inserted through copious secretions. Finally, because the patient's head does not need to be in a sniffing position, transillumination can be safely performed in patients with a possible spinal injury.

The major disadvantages of transillumination are the requirements for special equipment—namely, a bright light source at the tip of the malleable stylet—and proficiency with its use. As a consequence of the requirement for a bright light source, transillumination can be difficult or impossible in brightly lit areas. If you are inside, you may be able to dim the lights to perform this procedure.

esophagus is the main complication. Strict attention to tube confirmation techniques is needed following transillumination-guided intubation.

Equipment

Whether specifically designed or modified, the single most important piece of equipment required for transillumination-guided intubation is a device with a rigid stylet and a bright light source at the end. Because the light may not always be aimed directly at the skin surface, it should shine laterally and forward. The lighted stylet must be long enough to accommodate a standard-length ET tube, and there should be some method of adequately securing the stylet within the tube.

Technique for Transillumination-Guided Intubation

As with any intubation technique, the patient must be preoxygenated for at least 2 to 3 minutes with a bag-mask device and 100% oxygen. Your assistant can perform this task as you prepare your equipment.

Select the appropriately sized ET tube, and check the cuff to ensure that it holds air. Lubricate and insert the lighted stylet so that the light is positioned immediately at (but not beyond) the tip of the tube. Ensure that the stylet is firmly seated into the tube.

Prepare the tube by bending it into the proper shape to facilitate entry of the tube into the trachea and to ensure that the light will be visible at the anterior part of the neck. The stylet should be straight, with a sharp 90° angle in the tube-stylet assembly just proximal to the cuff. This bend in the tube must be sharp because it will act as the pivot point when you direct the

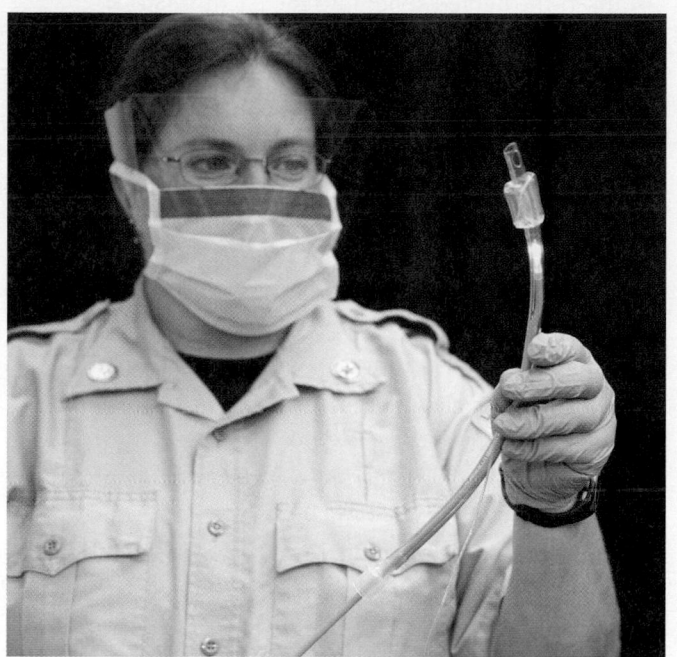

Figure 86 In transillumination intubation, a lighted stylet is inserted into the ET tube.

Complications

Although transillumination is not an entirely blind technique, the intubator cannot directly visualize the tube passing between the vocal cords. Therefore, misplacement of the tube in the

YOU *are the Medic* | PART 8

The rate at which your partner is assisting the patient's ventilations is adjusted accordingly, and your reassessment reveals that his clinical condition has improved. You note spontaneous movement of the patient's eyes, but he remains tolerant of the ET tube.

Recording Time: 25 Minutes	
Level of consciousness	P (responds to painful stimuli; eye movement noted; sedated with midazolam [Versed])
Respirations	10 breaths/min (baseline); intubated and ventilations being assisted
Pulse	90 beats/min; regular and strong
Skin	Pink, warm, and dry
Blood pressure	118/62 mm Hg
Spo$_2$	99% (with assisted ventilation and oxygen)
ETCO$_2$	38 mm Hg; normal waveform
ECG	Normal sinus rhythm

14. What impact does inadequate or absent ventilation have on respiration?

15. Is further treatment required for this patient at this time?

stylet into the trachea; it will also place the light in the proper position to illuminate the anterior part of the neck.

Place the patient's head in a neutral or slightly extended position. This position will move the epiglottis off the posterior pharyngeal wall and facilitate entry of the ET tube into the glottic opening. Extension of the patient's head will also provide maximum exposure of the anterior part of the neck, enhancing visualization of the lighted stylet under the soft tissue as it moves down the airway. The intubator is typically positioned at the patient's head.

While holding the lighted stylet in your dominant hand, displace the patient's jaw forwardly by grasping it with your thumb and forefinger. This step will ensure that the epiglottis is not covering the glottic opening. Turn on the lighted stylet, and insert the device in the midline of the patient's mouth, with the tip directed toward the laryngeal prominence. The goal is to lift the epiglottis with the ET tube–stylet combination.

As you continue to insert the tube-stylet assembly, draw your wrist toward you. The light should become visible at the midline of the neck. A tightly circumscribed light slightly below the thyroid cartilage indicates that the tip of the tube has entered the trachea. A faintly glowing light and bulging of the soft tissue above the thyroid cartilage indicates that the tip of the tube is in the vallecular space. If the tip is in this space, withdraw the tube slightly, displace the jaw forward, and readvance the tube-stylet assembly. A dim, diffuse light at the anterior part of the neck typically indicates esophageal placement. In this case, slightly withdraw the tube-stylet assembly and slightly extend the patient's head. You may also consider increasing the angle of the bend in the tube. These actions should reposition the tube-stylet assembly at the glottic opening. If you continue to encounter difficulty, abort the procedure and ventilate the patient with a bag-mask device and 100% oxygen before reattempting insertion of the tube-stylet assembly.

Once a bright, tightly circumscribed light is visible at the midline and just below the thyroid cartilage, hold the stylet in place and advance the tube approximately 2 to 4 cm into the trachea. When the tube is securely in the trachea, manually stabilize it in place with your nondominant hand and carefully withdraw the lighted stylet.

Inflate the distal cuff of the ET tube with 5 to 10 mL of air, detach the syringe from the inflation port, and attach the bag-mask device to the ET tube. Ventilate the patient while auscultating over the apices and bases of both lungs and over the epigastrium. Following subjective and objective confirmation of proper tube placement, secure the tube in place with the appropriate device and continue ventilations according to the patient's clinical condition.

The steps for performing intubation with the transillumination technique are listed here and shown in **Skill Drill 21**:

Skill Drill 21

1. Take standard precautions (gloves and face shield) **Step 1**.
2. Preoxygenate the patient for 2 to 3 minutes with a bag-mask device and 100% oxygen **Step 2**.
3. Check, prepare, and assemble your equipment **Step 3**.
4. Insert the lighted stylet into the ET tube **Step 4**.
5. Bend the ET tube by placing a slight curve at its distal end (like a hockey stick), and turn on the lighted stylet **Step 5**.
6. Lift the patient's tongue and mandible anteriorly **Step 6**.
7. Insert the ET tube into the midline of the patient's mouth and slowly advance toward the larynx, but stop before passing through the vocal cords **Step 7**.
8. Observe for a tightly circumscribed light at the midline of the neck, and advance the ET tube 2 to 4 cm farther **Step 8**.
9. Remove the stylet from the ET tube **Step 9**.
10. Inflate the distal cuff of the ET tube with 5 to 10 mL of air, and detach the syringe **Step 10**.
11. Attach the ETCO$_2$ detector (waveform capnography preferred) to the ET tube **Step 11**.
12. Attach the bag-mask device, ventilate, and auscultate over the apices and bases of both lungs and over the epigastrium **Step 12**.
13. Secure the ET tube **Step 13**.

Retrograde Intubation

When intubation is unsuccessful by standard methods, the technique of <u>retrograde intubation</u> may be used. This technique is rarely performed in the prehospital environment and is only relevant in EMS systems where local protocols indicate this as a paramedic skill. In retrograde intubation, a needle is placed percutaneously within the trachea via the cricothyroid membrane. A wire is placed toward the head through the needle upward through the trachea and into the mouth. The wire is then visualized and secured, and the ET tube is placed over the wire and guided into the trachea. The wire is subsequently removed, and the ET tube is advanced and secured.

Indications for retrograde intubation include the following:

- Upper airway obstruction
- Copious secretions in the airway
- Failure to intubate the trachea by less invasive methods

Contraindications to retrograde intubation include the following:

- Lack of familiarity with the procedure
- Laryngeal trauma
- Unrecognizable or distorted landmarks
- Coagulopathy (relative contraindication)
- Severe hypoxia (due to inability to ventilate during the procedure and time to perform the procedure)

Complications of retrograde intubation include the following:

- Hypoxia
- Cardiac dysrhythmias
- Mechanical trauma
- Infection
- Increased intracranial pressure

The assessment findings and transport complications with retrograde intubation are the same as with standard intubation.

Skill Drill 21

Performing Transillumination Intubation

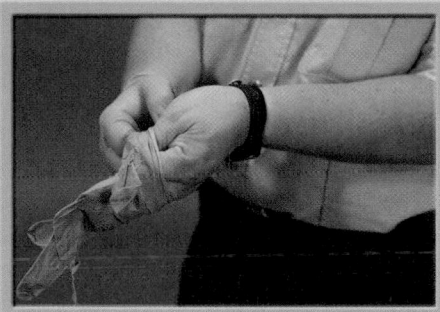

Step 1 Take standard precautions (gloves and face shield).

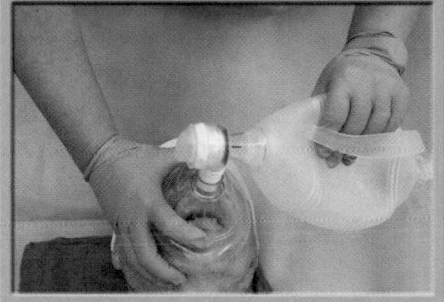

Step 2 Preoxygenate the patient for 2 to 3 minutes with a bag-mask device and 100% oxygen.

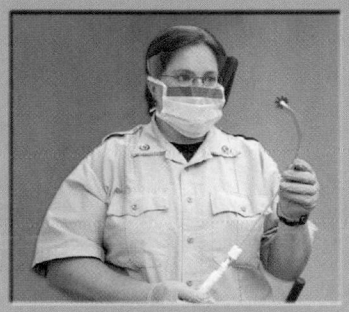

Step 3 Check, prepare, and assemble your equipment.

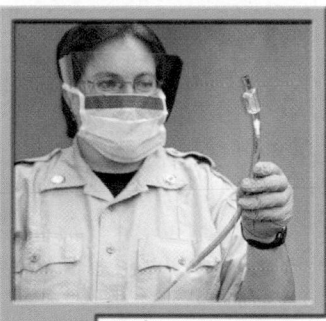

Step 4 Insert the lighted stylet into the ET tube.

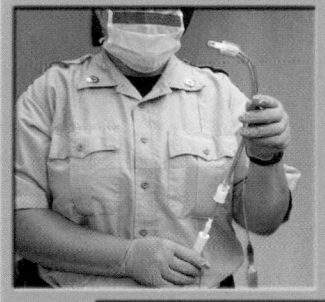

Step 5 Bend the ET tube by placing a slight curve at its distal end (like a hockey stick), and turn on the lighted stylet.

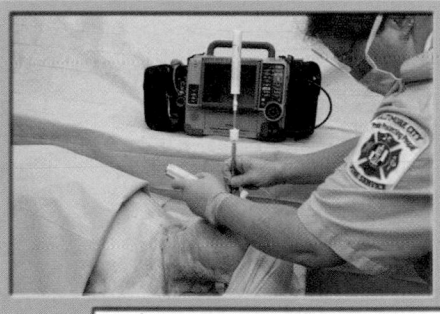

Step 6 Lift the patient's tongue and mandible anteriorly.

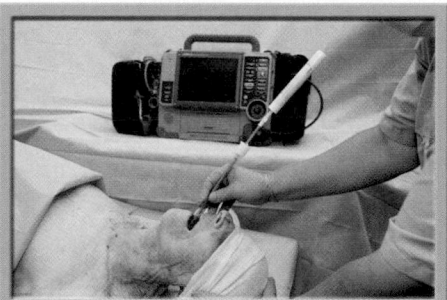

Step 7 Insert the ET tube into the midline of the patient's mouth and slowly advance toward the larynx, but stop before passing through the vocal cords.

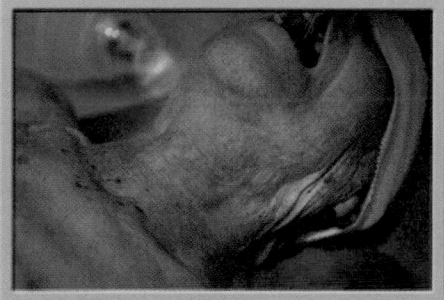

Step 8 Observe for a tightly circumscribed light at the midline of the neck, and advance the ET tube 2 to 4 cm farther.

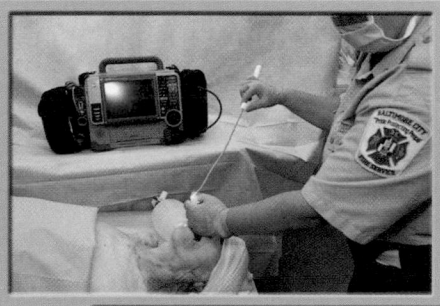

Step 9 Remove the stylet from the ET tube.

Continues

Skill Drill   21

Performing Transillumination Intubation, continued

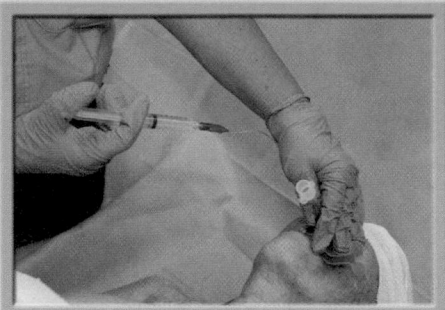

Step 10 Inflate the distal cuff of the ET tube with 5 to 10 mL of air, and detach the syringe.

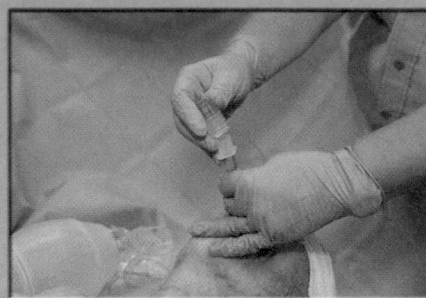

Step 11 Attach the end-tidal carbon dioxide detector to the ET tube.

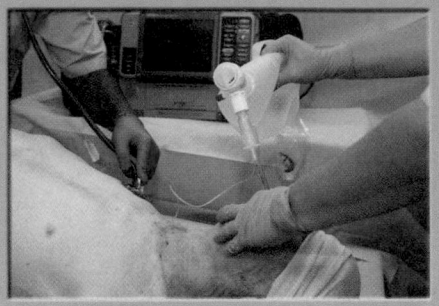

Step 12 Attach the bag-mask device, ventilate, and auscultate over the apices and bases of both lungs and over the epigastrium. Ensure proper tube placement with waveform capnography.

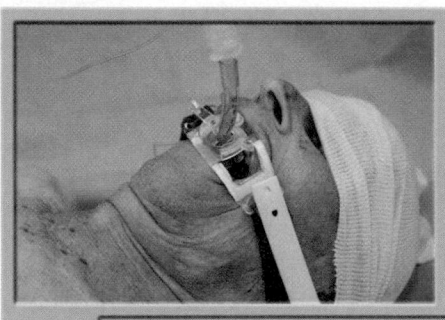

Step 13 Secure the ET tube, and recheck breath sounds.

The steps for performing retrograde intubation are listed here and shown in Skill Drill 22:

Skill Drill   22

1. Take standard precautions (gloves and face shield).
2. Place the patient supine.
3. Ventilate the patient with 100% oxygen via the appropriate device while preparing the equipment and the patient.
4. Cleanse the anterior part of the neck from the laryngeal prominence to just below the cricoid ring, and position a fenestrated drape **Step 1**.
5. If the patient is responsive, consider numbing the area over the cricothyroid membrane using a local anesthetic **Step 2**.
6. Puncture the cricothyroid membrane using a large needle aligned with the airway and pointed approximately 30°

cephalad (toward the head), perpendicular at the level of the cricothyroid membrane **Step 3**.

7. Identify the tracheal lumen by aspiration of air into the syringe attached to the needle **Step 4**.
8. Pass the 70-cm guide wire through the catheter until it appears in the oropharynx, mouth, or one of the nares **Step 5**.
9. If the guide wire is in the oropharynx, grasp it with a clamp or Magill forceps, and pull the wire partially out of the mouth, ensuring that the distal end is still emerging from the neck and the wire is pulled taut **Step 6**.
10. Insert the guide wire coming from the mouth, through the lumen of the ET tube **Step 7**.
11. Advance the ET tube into the trachea **Step 8**.
12. Verify tube placement by auscultating the lungs bilaterally and over the epigastrium, and attach an ETCO$_2$ detector (waveform capnography preferred) **Step 9**.

13. Once tube placement is confirmed, remove the guide wire by pulling on the distal end emerging from the neck, then advance the tube 2 to 3 cm further (Step 10).

14. If tube placement is incorrect, remove and attempt to ventilate. If ventilating adequately, continue to ventilate with high-flow oxygen and reassess. Determine if additional attempts at retrograde intubation are warranted or if another means of securing the airway is necessary (such as cricothyrotomy) (Step 11).

15. Secure the ET tube in place, and continue to ventilate (Step 12).

Face-to-Face Intubation

Intubation may be performed with the paramedic's face at the same level as the patient's face when other positions are not possible—for example, in a motor vehicle crash in which the patient is seated in a tight space and the space above the head cannot be accessed. This technique is called <u>face-to-face intubation</u>, or the "Tomahawk" method. The procedure is essentially the same as orotracheal intubation using direct laryngoscopy, with the following exceptions:

- The patient's head cannot be placed in the sniffing position. It is manually stabilized by a second paramedic during the entire procedure.

Skill Drill | 22

Performing Retrograde Intubation

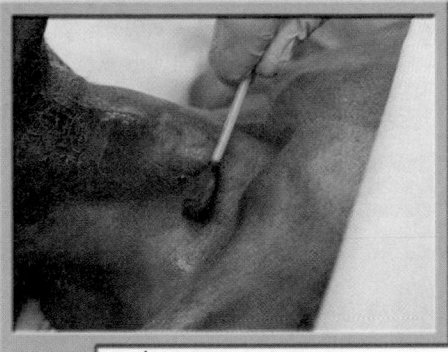

Step 1 Take standard precautions (gloves and face shield). Place the patient supine. Ventilate the patient while preparing the equipment and the patient. Cleanse the anterior part of the neck from the laryngeal prominence to just below the cricoid ring, and position a fenestrated drape.

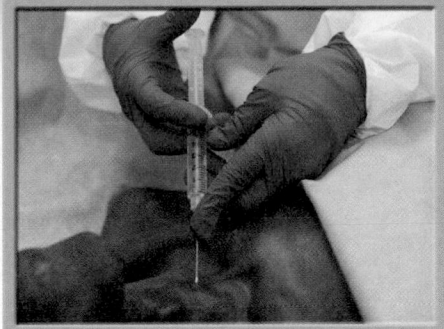

Step 2 Numb the area over the cricothyroid membrane using a local anesthetic if the patient is responsive.

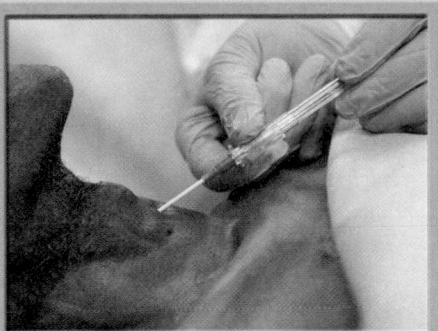

Step 3 Puncture the cricothyroid membrane using a large needle aligned with the airway and pointed approximately 30° cephalad, perpendicular at the level of the cricothyroid membrane.

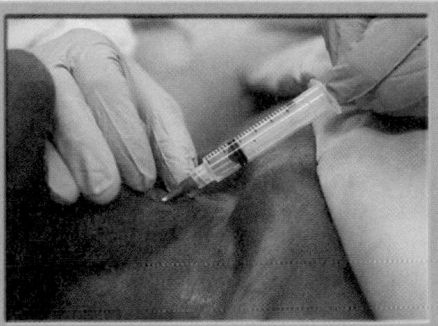

Step 4 Identify the tracheal lumen by aspirating the syringe attached to the needle.

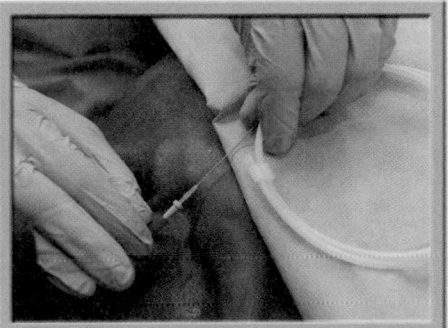

Step 5 Pass the 70-cm guide wire through the catheter until it appears in the oropharynx, mouth, or one of the nares.

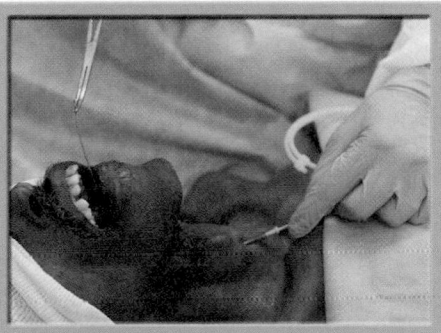

Step 6 If the guide wire is in the oropharynx, grasp it with a clamp and pull the wire partially out of the mouth, ensuring that the distal end is still emerging from the neck and the wire is pulled taut.

Continues

Skill Drill | 22

Performing Retrograde Intubation, continued

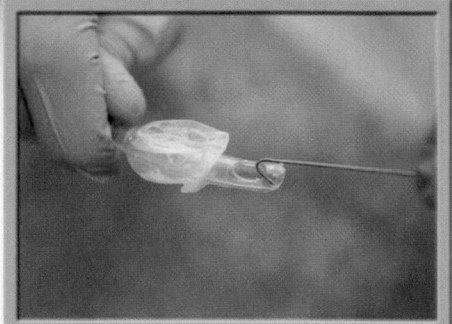

Step 7 Insert the guide wire emerging from the mouth, through the lumen of the ET tube.

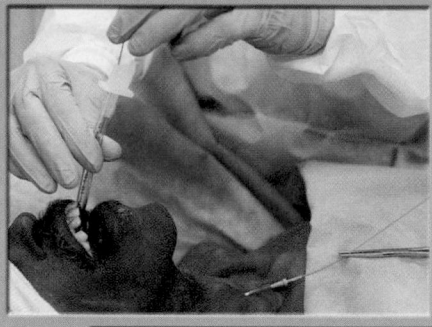

Step 8 Advance the ET tube into the trachea.

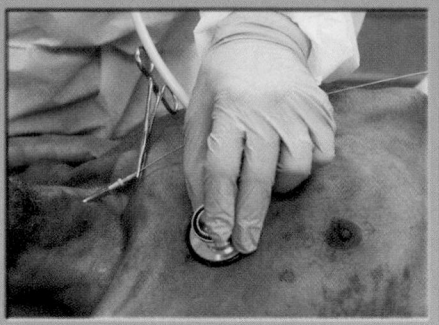

Step 9 Auscultate the chest bilaterally and over the epigastrium. Ensure proper tube placement with waveform capnography.

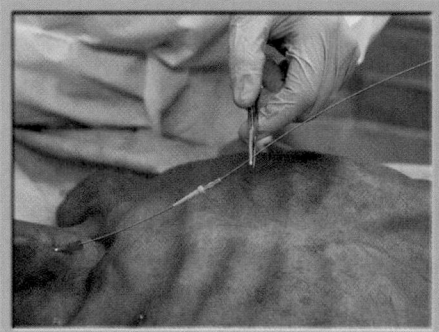

Step 10 Once tube placement is confirmed, remove the guide wire by pulling on the distal end emerging from the neck.

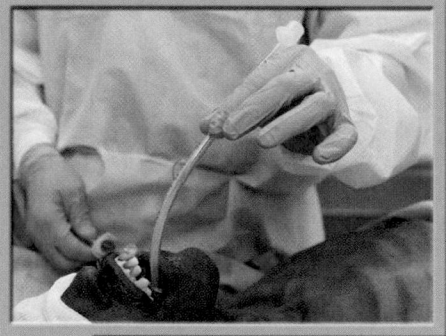

Step 11 If tube placement is incorrect, remove the tube and start over or switch to a different technique.

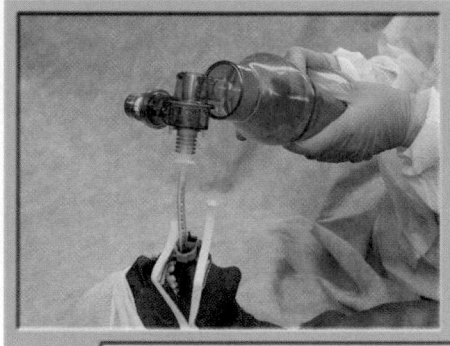

Step 12 Secure the ET tube in place and ventilate.

- The laryngoscope (with a curved [Macintosh] blade) is held in the right hand with the blade facing downward like a hatchet, and the ET tube is held in the left hand. The laryngoscope blade is inserted into the right side of the patient's mouth, the tongue is swept to the patient's left, and the vocal cords are visualized.
- Once the laryngoscope blade has been placed, the paramedic who is intubating may slightly adjust the patient's head for better visualization by pulling the mandible forward while pressing down.

■ Failed Intubation

It is estimated that the failed intubation rates are around 5%, but this is currently a controversial area and being closely studied, since some studies have demonstrated higher failed intubation rates when multiple attempts are taken into consideration. At the service and regional level this is an extremely important procedure to be closely monitored by physician-led quality-assurance efforts, since the implications for failed intubation and, more importantly, an unrecognized misplaced ET tube (in the esophagus) is significant for the paramedic, the service's medical director, and the regional system, as well as potentially fatal for the patient.

A failed airway attempt is defined as the failure to maintain acceptable oxygen saturation during or after one or more failed intubation attempts or a total of three failed intubation attempts by an experienced intubator—even when the oxygen saturation can be maintained. Ways to minimize complications of airway management have been discussed. However, you frequently do

Words of Wisdom

Endotracheal Intubation: Points to Remember
- Never attempt endotracheal (ET) intubation before the patient has been adequately preoxygenated.
- Assemble and check all equipment before you begin.
- Position is everything! Ensure that the patient's head is in the proper position to align the airway axes.
- Do not rush. Work with deliberate speed.
- Get it right the first time. The second attempt will likely be more difficult. Remember that a patent BLS airway is acceptable until a more experienced provider has time to insert an advanced airway.
- Confirm that the ET tube is in the right place. Take nothing for granted.
- Secure the ET tube appropriately. Otherwise, you might soon be trying to reinsert it.
- Even when the tube is properly secured, stabilize it with your hand as you ventilate the patient.
- Consider applying a cervical collar and lateral head immobilization after intubating a patient. Doing so will minimize the amount of head movement and the risk of inadvertent extubation.
- Reconfirm proper ET tube placement after *any* major patient move (ie, from the ground to the stretcher, after loading into the ambulance, transferring the patient to the hospital stretcher).

not have a choice of methods in the prehospital setting. So, what do you do? Many rescue airway techniques are available.

- Perform simple BLS airway maneuvers with an oral airway and/or a nasal airway and a bag-mask device. With good technique, adequate oxygenation and ventilation can be provided. The objective is to ventilate and oxygenate—not intubate.
- Consider using a rescue airway device, such as the King LT, LMA, or Combitube, all of which are discussed later in this chapter.

Tracheobronchial Suctioning

Tracheobronchial suctioning involves passing a suction catheter into the ET tube to remove pulmonary secretions. The first rule to remember about performing tracheobronchial suctioning is this: Do not do it if you do not have to! This kind of suctioning requires strict attention to sterile technique, which is nearly impossible to maintain in the prehospital environment. Suctioning the trachea can also cause cardiac dysrhythmias; cardiac arrest has been reported during tracheobronchial suctioning. For these reasons, you should avoid suctioning through an ET tube *unless secretions are so massive that they interfere with ventilation.* If tracheobronchial suctioning must be performed, use sterile technique (if possible), and monitor the patient's cardiac rhythm and oxygen saturation during the procedure.

Preoxygenation of the patient is essential before performing tracheobronchial suctioning. Lubricate a soft-tip (whistle-tip) catheter, and preoxygenate the patient for at least 2 to 3 minutes. It may be necessary to inject 3 to 5 mL of sterile water down the ET tube to loosen thick pulmonary secretions.

Gently insert the suction catheter down the ET tube until resistance is felt. Apply suction as the catheter is extracted, taking care not to exceed 10 seconds in an adult. After tracheobronchial suctioning is complete, reattach the bag-mask device, continue ventilations, and reassess the patient.

The steps for performing tracheobronchial suctioning are listed here and shown in Skill Drill 23 :

Skill Drill 23

1. Check, prepare, and assemble your equipment Step 1 .
2. Lubricate the suction catheter Step 2 .
3. Preoxygenate the patient Step 3 .
4. Detach the bag-mask device, and inject 3 to 5 mL of sterile water down the ET tube Step 4 .
5. Gently insert the catheter into the ET tube until resistance is felt Step 5 .
6. Suction in a rotating motion while withdrawing the catheter. Monitor the patient's cardiac rhythm and oxygen saturation during the procedure Step 6 .
7. Reattach the bag-mask device, and resume ventilation and oxygenation Step 7 .

Field Extubation

Extubation is the process of removing the tube from an intubated patient. Patients are rarely extubated in the prehospital setting. Generally, the only reason to consider performing extubation in the field is a patient who is *unreasonably* intolerant of the ET tube (for example, extremely combative, gagging, or retching). In general, it is better to sedate the patient rather than remove the ET tube, but sedation may not be an option in all EMS systems or for patients in hemodynamically unstable condition. Before performing field extubation, you should contact medical control or follow locally established protocols.

The most obvious risk associated with extubation is overestimation of the patient's ability to protect his or her own airway. In addition, when extubation is performed on responsive patients, there is a high risk of laryngospasm, and most patients experience some degree of upper airway swelling because of the trauma of having the tube in the trachea. These two facts, along with the ever-present potential for vomiting, make successful reintubation challenging, if not impossible. If you are not *absolutely* sure that you can reintubate the patient, do not remove the ET tube. Instead, sedate the patient with a benzodiazepine. If a paralytic drug was used to facilitate intubation, consider administering additional doses in conjunction with a benzodiazepine. Field extubation is absolutely contraindicated if there is *any* risk of recurrent respiratory failure or uncertainty about a patient's ability to maintain his or her own airway spontaneously.

If field extubation is indicated, you must first ensure that the patient is adequately oxygenated. Discuss the procedure with the patient, and explain what you plan to do. If possible, have the patient sit up or lean slightly forward so that he or she is in a safe position should vomiting occur after extubation. Assemble and

Skill Drill 23

Performing Tracheobronchial Suctioning

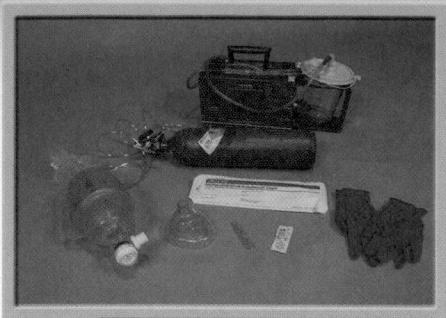

Step 1 Check, prepare, and assemble your equipment.

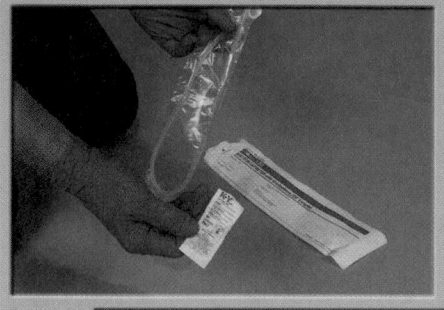

Step 2 Lubricate the suction catheter.

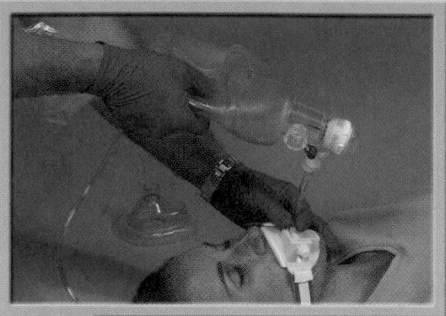

Step 3 Preoxygenate the patient.

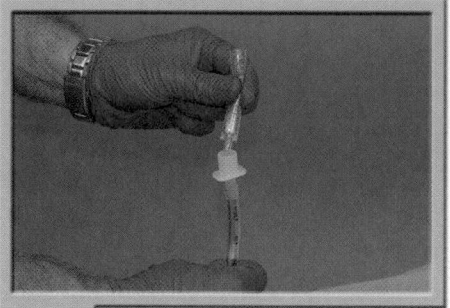

Step 4 Detach the bag-mask device, and inject 3 to 5 mL of sterile water down the ET tube.

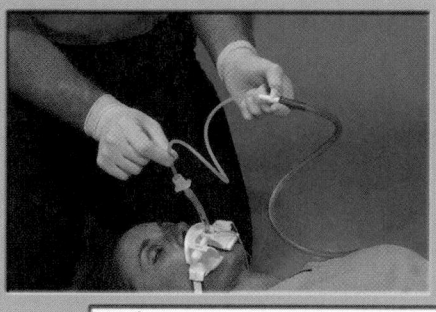

Step 5 Gently insert the catheter into the ET tube until resistance is felt.

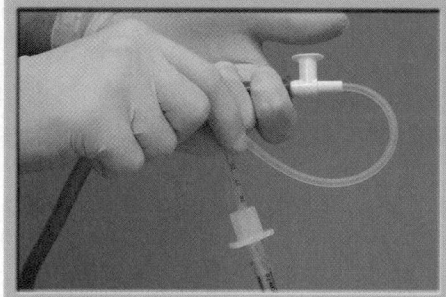

Step 6 Suction in a rotating motion while withdrawing the catheter. Monitor the patient's cardiac rhythm and oxygen saturation during the procedure.

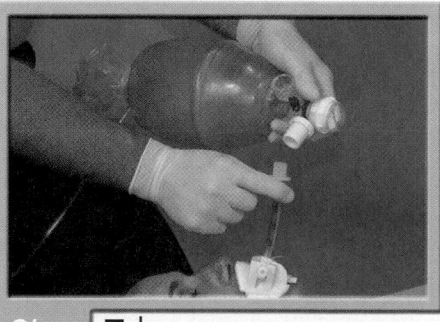

Step 7 Reattach the bag-mask device, and resume ventilation and oxygenation.

have available all equipment to suction, ventilate, and reintubate, if necessary. After confirming that the patient remains responsive enough to protect his or her own airway, suction the oropharynx to remove any secretions or debris that may threaten the airway once the tube has been removed. Deflate the distal cuff on the ET tube as the patient begins to exhale so that any accumulated secretions proximal to the cuff are not aspirated into the lungs. On the next exhalation, *remove the tube in one steady motion*, following the curvature of the airway. Place a towel or emesis basin in front of the patient's mouth in case vomiting occurs.

Pediatric Endotracheal Intubation

Although ET intubation has been considered the means for definitive prehospital airway management in adults, recent studies suggest that effective bag-mask ventilations in pediatric patients can be as effective as intubation when transport times are short. However, if bag-mask ventilations are not producing adequate ventilation and oxygenation, the infant or child should be intubated. Indications for ET intubation in pediatric patients are the same as those in adults:

- Cardiopulmonary arrest
- Respiratory failure or arrest
- Traumatic brain injury
- Unresponsiveness
- Inability to maintain a patent airway
- Need for prolonged ventilation
- Need for ET administration of resuscitative medications (if no IV or IO access available)

Certain anatomic differences between children and adults have a key role in a successful intubation because proper airway positioning is critical Table 13 .

Laryngoscope and Blades

Although any laryngoscope handle can be used to intubate a child, most paramedics prefer the thinner pediatric handles. Straight blades facilitate lifting of the floppy epiglottis. If a curved blade is used, the tip of the blade is positioned in the vallecula to lift the jaw and epiglottis to visualize the vocal cords.

The blade should extend from the child's mouth to the tragus of the ear. Acceptable means of measuring this length include use of a length-based resuscitation tape measure or using the following general age group–based guidelines:

- Premature newborn: size 0 straight blade
- Full-term newborn to 1 year: size 1 straight blade
- 2 years to adolescent: size 2 straight blade
- Adolescent and older: size 3 straight or curved blade

Table 13 Differences in the Pediatric Airway
Infants and small children (up to 5 or 6 years of age) have a larger, rounder occiput, which causes the head of an infant or small child who lies supine to be in a flexed position.
In children, the tongue is proportionately larger and the mandible is proportionately smaller—differences that increase children's propensity for airway obstruction.
The epiglottis in a child is more floppy and omega-shaped, so it must be lifted, or positioned, out of the way to visualize the vocal cords.
The trachea in a child is smaller, shorter, and narrower than an adult's, and it is positioned more anteriorly and superiorly.
The narrowest portion of the child's airway is the cricoid ring, which is below the vocal cords (subglottic), and the anatomy below the vocal cords is funnel-shaped. This difference makes a cuff less necessary for occluding the trachea; the developing cartilage of the cricoid ring could be injured by inflation of a cuffed ET tube.

Endotracheal Tubes

In infants and children, there are many methods to estimate the appropriate size of ET tube to be used. Because length has been shown to be a better estimator of weight than age, a length-based resuscitation tape measure should be used if one is available Figure 87A . The tape measure will provide information not only about the proper size ET tube, but also about the proper size of basic airway adjuncts, drug doses, defibrillation and cardioversion settings, and other care. If a resuscitation tape measure is not available, either of the following formulas can be used for children older than 1 year. To obtain the correct answer, calculate the items in brackets first.

- [Age (in years) + 16] ÷ 4
  - A 4-year-old child would need a 5.0-mm tube ([4 + 16] ÷ 4 = 5.0)
- [Age (in years) ÷ 4] + 4
  - A 2-year-old child would need a 4.5-mm tube ([2 ÷ 4] + 4 = 4.5)

Certain anatomic clues, such as the nares or the width of the nail on the little finger Figure 87B , can be used to estimate tube size, or general guidelines based on the child's age group can be followed Table 14 .

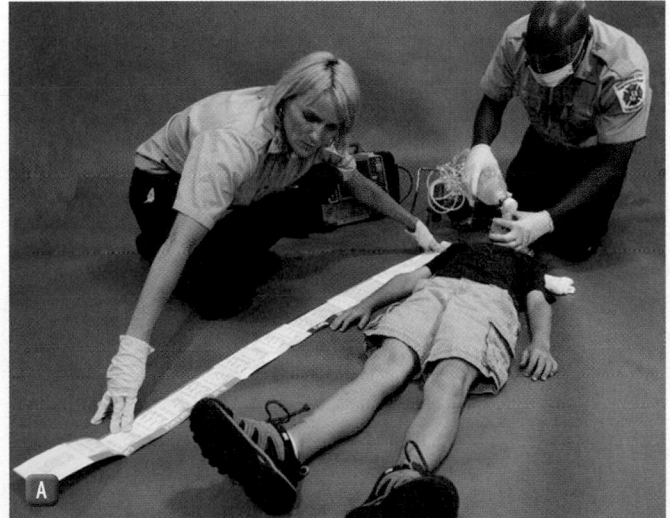

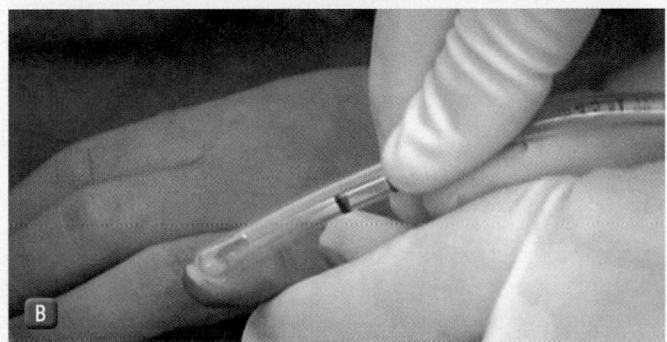

Figure 87 **A.** A length-based resuscitation tape measure can help estimate a child's endotracheal (ET) tube size. **B.** The width of the child's smallest fingernail (or the external diameter of one of the nares) can be used to estimate ET tube size.

Table 14 Guidelines for Selecting Pediatric Endotracheal Tubes

Age Group	Endotracheal Tube (mm)	Insertion Depth (cm)
Premature infant	2.5-3.0 uncuffed	8.0
Full-term infant	3.0-3.5 uncuffed	8.0-9.5
Infant to 1 year	3.5-4.0 uncuffed	9.5-11.0
Toddler	4.0-5.0 uncuffed	11.0-12.5
Preschool	5.0-5.5 uncuffed	12.5-14.0
School age	5.5-6.5 uncuffed	14.0-20.0
Adolescent	7.0-8.0 cuffed	20.0-23.0

Cuffed ET tubes are generally not used in the field until the child is 8 to 10 years old, unless otherwise specified by your medical director or local protocols. A cuff at the cricoid ring is unnecessary to obtain a seal in children in this age range. Furthermore, a cuff can cause ischemia and damage the tracheal mucosa at the level of the cricoid ring. Endotracheal tubes smaller than 5.0 mm generally do not have a cuff. When selecting the appropriate size of ET tube, you should have tubes one size smaller and one size larger than expected for situations in which there is variability in the child's upper airway diameter.

The appropriate depth of insertion of the ET tube is 2 to 3 cm beyond the vocal cords. After the tube has been inserted, the depth at the corner of the child's mouth should be recorded and monitored. For uncuffed tubes, a black band—the vocal cord guide—often encircles the tube at the distal end. When you see this band at the level of the vocal cords, stop. Cuffed tubes should be inserted until the cuff is just below the level of the vocal cords. Another guideline is to insert the tube to a depth equal to three times the inside diameter (mm) of the ET tube. For example, a 4.0-mm tube should be inserted to a depth of 12.0 cm ($12.0 = 3 \times 4$ mm).

Pediatric Stylet

The use of a stylet, for the most part, is a matter of personal preference when intubating pediatric patients. If a stylet is used, insert it into the ET tube, stopping at least 1 cm from the end of the tube. Pediatric stylets will fit into tube sizes 3.0 to 6.0 mm, whereas adult stylets are used for tube sizes 6.0 mm or larger. After inserting the stylet into the ET tube, bend the tube into a gentle upward curve. In some cases, bending the tube into the shape of a hockey stick is beneficial.

Preoxygenation

Adequate preoxygenation with a bag-mask device and 100% oxygen for at least 2 to 3 minutes before attempting intubation cannot be overemphasized—respiratory failure or arrest is the most common cause of cardiac arrest in the pediatric population. While preoxygenating a child, you must also ensure that the child's head is in the proper position: the sniffing position or the neutral position for patients with suspected trauma. If needed, insert an airway adjunct; in conjunction with proper manual positioning of the head, it will maintain airway patency and facilitate effective ventilation.

Additional Preparation

Stimulation of the parasympathetic nervous system with resultant bradycardia can occur during intubation in children; therefore, you should monitor the child's cardiac rhythm. A pulse oximeter should be used throughout the intubation attempt to monitor the child's pulse rate and oxygen saturation. In addition, suction should be readily available to clear oral secretions from the child's airway. In some situations, atropine sulfate in a dose of 0.02 mg/kg may be administered to prevent vagal nerve–induced bradycardia due to parasympathetic stimulation.

Intubation Technique

With the child's head in a sniffing position, open his or her mouth by applying thumb pressure on the chin. Some children may require use of the cross-finger technique: use your thumb and index finger or thumb and middle finger to push the upper and lower teeth apart. If an oral airway has been inserted, remove it. If needed, suction the child's mouth and pharynx to remove any secretions.

Hold the laryngoscope handle in your left hand, using your thumb, index finger, and middle finger to hold the handle (the "trigger finger" position). Insert the laryngoscope blade in the right side of the child's mouth, sweeping the tongue to the left side and keeping it under the blade. Advance the blade straight along the tongue, while applying gentle traction upward along the axis of the laryngoscope handle at a 45° angle. *Never use the teeth or gums as a fulcrum for the blade.* A child's teeth could easily be loosened or cracked during a traumatic intubation attempt.

When the blade passes the epiglottis, gently lift the epiglottis if you are using a straight blade. If you are using a curved blade, place the tip of the blade in the vallecula, and lift the jaw, tongue, and blade gently at a 45° angle.

Identify the vocal cords and other normal anatomic landmarks. If they are not visible, consider the BURP maneuver, although this may be more difficult in children than in adults. Additional gentle suctioning may be needed to facilitate your view of the vocal cords.

Hold the ET tube in your right hand, and insert the tube from the right-side corner of the child's mouth. Do not pass the tube through the channel of the laryngoscope blade because you will lose sight of the vocal cords. Guide the tube through the vocal cords, and advance the tube until the glottic or vocal cord mark (black band) is positioned just beyond the vocal cords (approximately 2 to 3 cm). Record the depth of the tube as measured at the right-side corner of the child's mouth, and remove the laryngoscope blade.

Carefully remove the stylet if one was used, while holding the tube securely in place. Next, recheck the tube depth to ensure that it did not become displaced during removal of the stylet. If you are using a cuffed ET tube, inflate the cuff with just enough air to form a seal between the tube and tracheal wall. Attach the tube to a bag-mask device and 100% oxygen, with an ETCO$_2$ detector (waveform capnography preferred) between the bag and tube.

Confirm proper ET tube placement by using several techniques. Observe the patient for bilateral chest rise during ventilation. Auscultate the lungs bilaterally at the midaxillary line at the third intercostal space, listening for two breaths in each location. If breath sounds are decreased on the left side, the tube may be positioned too deep and aimed toward or in the right mainstem bronchus. To correct this problem, listen to the left side of the chest while ventilating and *carefully* withdrawing the tube, until breath sounds are equal on both sides of the chest. Rerecord the depth of the tube.

Breath sounds travel easily in a child because of the small chest. Auscultate over the epigastrium to ensure that no bubbling or gurgling sounds are present. These sounds indicate esophageal intubation, mandating *immediate* removal of the tube, suctioning as needed, and ventilation with a bag-mask device and 100% oxygen before reattempting intubation.

Additional clinical methods to confirm proper ET tube placement include improvement in the child's skin color, pulse rate, and oxygen saturation and the use of waveform capnography. If you must use the colorimetric ETCO$_2$ detector or EDD, which are less reliable than waveform capnography, remember two important points: (1) The adult colorimetric ETCO$_2$ detector cannot be used in children weighing less than 15 kg and (2) The esophageal bulb or syringe cannot be used in children weighing less than 20 kg.

After you confirm proper tube placement, hold the ET tube firmly in place and secure it with an appropriate device. Although several methods for securing an ET tube exist, no single method is foolproof. One person should always hold the tube in place while another properly secures it.

It is important to reconfirm tube placement not only after securing the tube, but also following any patient movement (such as onto the stretcher or into the ambulance), because tubes can easily become dislodged. To do so, auscultate for bilateral breath sounds and epigastric sounds. Once tube position has been confirmed, resume ventilations with 100% oxygen at the appropriate rate.

If you realize the tube is too large or you cannot identify the vocal cords and glottic landmarks, abort the intubation attempt and ventilate the child with the bag-mask device and 100% oxygen. Modify your equipment selection accordingly, and start the procedure from the beginning. If intubation cannot be accomplished after two attempts, discontinue attempts, and resume bag-mask ventilation for the remainder of the transport.

The steps for performing pediatric ET intubation are listed here and shown in Skill Drill 24 :

Skill Drill 24

1. Take standard precautions (gloves and face shield) Step 1 .
2. Check, prepare, and assemble your equipment Step 2 .
3. Measure an adjunct if needed Step 3 .
4. Manually open the child's airway, and insert an adjunct, if needed Step 4 .
5. Preoxygenate the child with a bag-mask device and 100% oxygen for at least 2 to 3 minutes Step 5 .
6. Measure the length of the child using a length-based resuscitation tape Step 6 .
7. Remove the airway adjunct if one was placed. Insert the laryngoscope in the right side of the mouth, and sweep the tongue to the left. Lift the tongue with firm, gentle pressure. Avoid using the teeth or gums as a fulcrum Step 7 .
8. Identify the vocal cords. If the cords are not yet visible, instruct your partner to perform the BURP maneuver, if possible Step 8 .

9. Introduce the ET tube in the right corner of the child's mouth Step 9 .
10. Pass the ET tube through the vocal cords to approximately 2 to 3 cm below the vocal cords. Inflate the cuff if a cuffed tube is used Step 10 .
11. Attach an ETCO$_2$ detector (waveform capnography preferred).
12. Attach the bag-mask device, and auscultate for equal breath sounds over each lateral chest wall high in the axillae. Ensure absence of breath sounds over the epigastrium Step 11 .
13. Secure the ET tube, noting the placement of the distance marker at the child's teeth or gums, and reconfirm tube placement Step 12 .

If an intubated child's condition acutely deteriorates, you must take immediate action to identify and correct the underlying problem. The DOPE mnemonic (**D**isplacement, **O**bstruction, **P**neumothorax, and **E**quipment failure) can be used to recall the common causes of acute deterioration in an intubated child Table 15 .

Table 15	**Troubleshooting Acute Deterioration With the DOPE Mnemonic in an Intubated Child**
Displacement	■ Reauscultate breath sounds and any sounds over the epigastrium. ■ If breath sounds are stronger on the right, slowly withdraw the tube until they are equal bilaterally. ■ If breath sounds are absent and you hear epigastric gurgling, immediately remove the endotracheal tube, suction as needed, and ventilate with a bag-mask device and 100% oxygen.
Obstruction	■ If thick pulmonary secretions are interfering with your ability to effectively ventilate an intubated child, perform tracheobronchial suctioning. ■ Consider tube obstruction if ventilation compliance is decreased (that is, it is difficult to squeeze the bag).
Pneumothorax	■ Suspect a pneumothorax if breath sounds are stronger on the *left* and decreased or absent on the right; such findings are not consistent with right mainstem bronchus intubation. ■ Ventilation compliance may also be decreased in a child with a pneumothorax. ■ Prepare to perform needle decompression.
Equipment failure	■ Ensure that you are giving 100% oxygen. ■ Check the reservoir bag on the bag-mask device for tears, ensure that the device is attached to a 100% oxygen source, and check the bag itself for tears. ■ Immediately replace defective or damaged equipment.

Complications of Endotracheal Intubation

Complications associated with ET intubation in pediatric patients are essentially the same as those for adult patients:

- **Unrecognized esophageal intubation.** *Frequently* monitor the position of the tube, especially after *any* major patient move. Use continuous waveform capnography.

Skill Drill | 24

Performing Pediatric Endotracheal Intubation

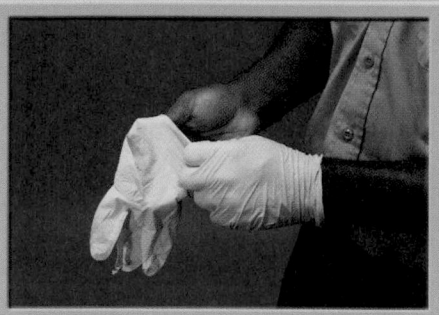

Step 1 Take standard precautions (gloves and face shield).

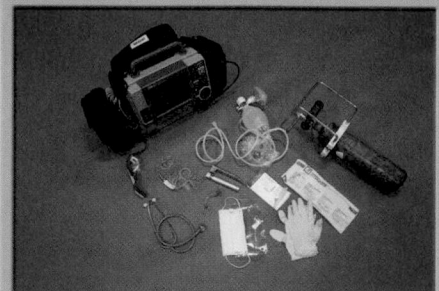

Step 2 Check, prepare, and assemble your equipment.

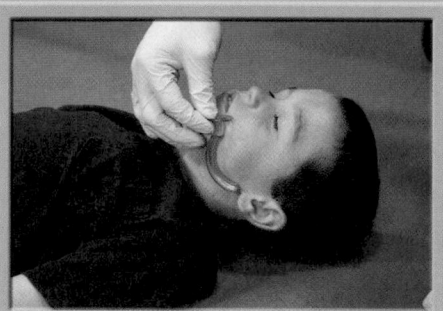

Step 3 Measure an adjunct if needed.

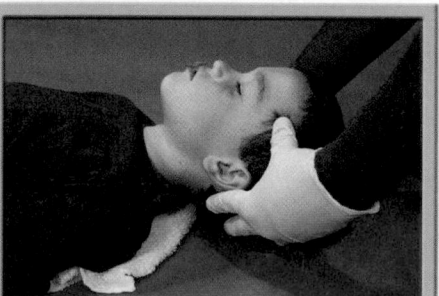

Step 4 Manually open the child's airway and insert an adjunct if needed.

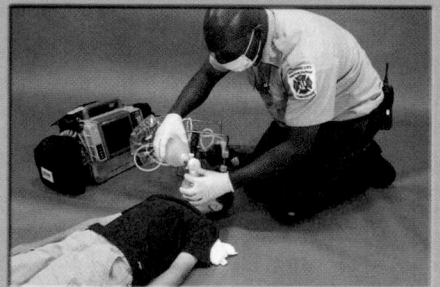

Step 5 Preoxygenate the child with a bag-mask device and 100% oxygen for at least 2 to 3 minutes.

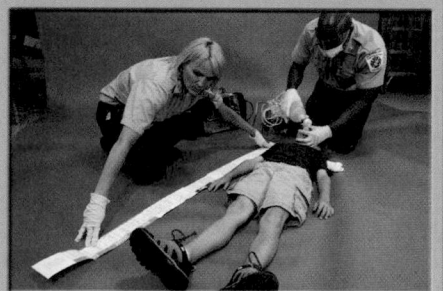

Step 6 Measure the length of the child using a length-based resuscitation tape.

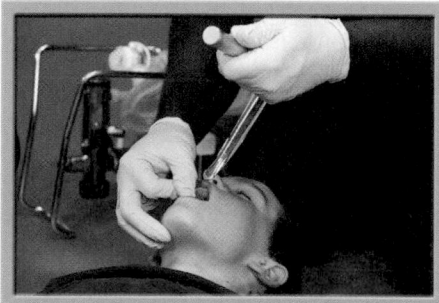

Step 7 Remove the airway adjunct if one was placed. Insert the laryngoscope in the right side of the mouth and sweep the tongue to the left. Lift the tongue with firm, gentle pressure. Avoid using the teeth or gums as a fulcrum.

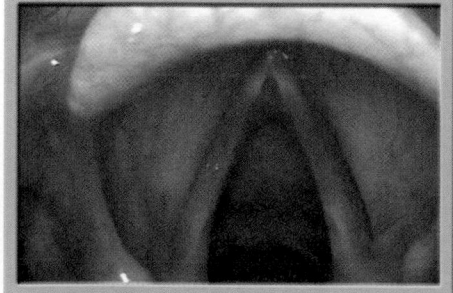

Step 8 Identify the vocal cords. If the cords are not yet visible, instruct your partner to perform the BURP maneuver, if possible.

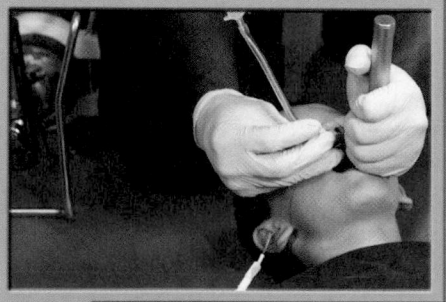

Step 9 Introduce the ET tube in the right corner of the child's mouth.

Continues

Skill Drill | 24

Performing Pediatric Endotracheal Intubation, continued

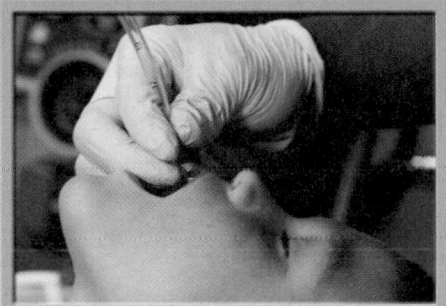

Step 10 Pass the ET tube through the vocal cords to approximately 2 to 3 cm below the vocal cords. Inflate the cuff if a cuffed tube is used.

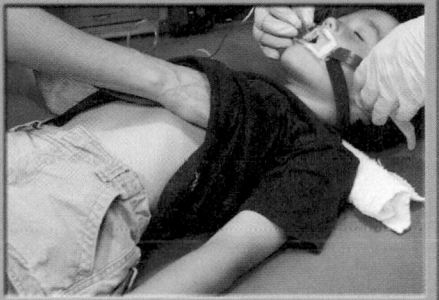

Step 11 Attach an ETCO$_2$ detector. Attach the bag-mask device, and auscultate for equal breath sounds over each lateral chest wall high in the axillae. Ensure absence of breath sounds over the epigastrium. Ensure proper tube placement with waveform capnography.

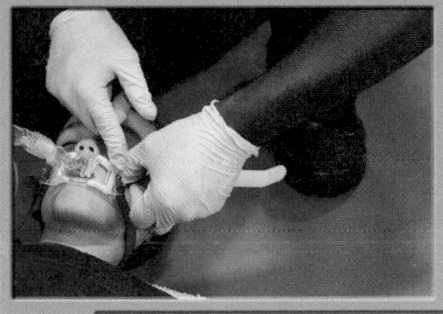

Step 12 Secure the ET tube.

YOU *are the Medic* | PART 9

You continue to monitor the patient throughout the duration of the transport. Additional midazolam (Versed) is administered to facilitate the patient's tolerance of the ET tube. His vital signs are reassessed, and a second 12-lead ECG reveals a normal sinus rhythm without gross evidence of myocardial ischemia or injury.

The patient's condition remains unchanged for the duration of the transport. You continue to monitor him for signs of further improvement or deterioration in his condition. The patient is delivered to the emergency department staff. You give your verbal report to the receiving physician, who reconfirms correct ET tube placement, and then return your unit to service.

Recording Time: 30 Minutes	
Level of consciousness	P (responds to painful stimuli; eye movement noted; sedated with midazolam [Versed])
Respirations	10 breaths/min (baseline); intubated and ventilations being assisted
Pulse	84 beats/min; regular and strong
Skin	Pink, warm, and dry
Blood pressure	126/70 mm Hg
Spo$_2$	100% (with assisted ventilation and oxygen)
ETCO$_2$	40 mm Hg; normal waveform
ECG	Normal sinus rhythm in lead II; 12-lead ECG reveals the same

16. What actions should you take to troubleshoot acute deterioration of the condition of an intubated patient?

- Induction of emesis and possible aspiration. *Always* have a suctioning device immediately available.
- **Hypoxia resulting from prolonged intubation attempts.** Limit pediatric intubation attempts to *20 seconds*. Monitor the child's cardiac rhythm and oxygen saturation during intubation.
- **Damage to teeth, soft tissues, and intraoral structures.** Technique, technique, technique!

Words of Wisdom

A single pediatric intubation attempt should not exceed 20 seconds. If intubation cannot be performed within this time, abort the attempt and resume bag-mask ventilations with 100% oxygen.

Pharmacologic Adjuncts to Airway Management and Ventilation

Pharmacologic agents in airway management are used to decrease the discomfort of intubation, decrease the incidence of complications associated with laryngoscopy and intubation, and make aggressive airway management possible for patients who need it but are unable to cooperate.

Sedation in Emergency Intubation

Sedation is used in airway management to reduce a patient's anxiety, induce amnesia, and decrease the gag reflex. It is useful for anxious, combative, or agitated patients and for patients who need aggressive airway management but who are too responsive to tolerate intubation. If used properly and under the correct circumstances, sedation effectively increases patient compliance and comfort, making definitive airway management easier and safer to perform. If used improperly, however, it can cause further harm.

The complications associated with sedation in airway management are related primarily to undersedation and oversedation. Undersedation can result in inadequate patient cooperation, the complications of gagging (such as trauma, tachycardia, hypertension, vomiting, and aspiration), and incomplete amnesia of the event. Oversedation can result in uncontrolled general anesthesia, loss of protective airway reflexes, respiratory depression, complete airway collapse, and hypotension.

Words of Wisdom

Hypersensitivity to sedative medications is the primary contraindication to the use of these drugs. Obtain an accurate, thorough medical history, to the extent possible, before giving any drug to any patient.

The level of sedation desired dictates the amount of medication administered. A patient's response to sedatives is dose-dependent. Paramedics should follow local protocol or

Table 16   Sedatives Used in Airway Management

Drug Type	Examples
Butyrophenones: sedative	Haloperidol (Haldol) Droperidol (Inapsine)
Benzodiazepines: sedative-hypnotic	Diazepam (Valium) Midazolam (Versed)
Barbiturates: sedative-hypnotic	Thiopental (Pentothal, Trapanal) Methohexital (Brevital)
Narcotics (opioids): sedative-analgesic	Fentanyl (Sublimaze) Alfentanil (Alfenta)
Nonnarcotic/nonbarbiturate: sedative-hypnotic	Etomidate (Amidate)

contact medical control regarding the appropriate dose for a given patient.

Two major classes of sedatives are commonly used in airway management: analgesics and sedative-hypnotics **Table 16**. Analgesics decrease the perception of pain. Sedative-hypnotics induce sleep and decrease anxiety; they do not reduce pain.

Butyrophenones

Butyrophenones are potent, effective sedatives. Two of these drugs, haloperidol (Haldol) and droperidol (Inapsine), are frequently used in emergency situations for anxiolysis, the relief of anxiety. These medications are effective for calming agitated patients, trauma patients who are combative, patients who are experiencing alcohol withdrawal, and patients with acute psychoses. They do not produce apnea and have little effect on the cardiovascular system. Droperidol is faster acting than haloperidol and is generally preferred in emergency situations. Butyrophenones are not recommended for induction of anesthesia.

Benzodiazepines

Benzodiazepines are sedative-hypnotic drugs. Diazepam (Valium) and midazolam (Versed) provide muscle relaxation and mild sedation and are used extensively as anxiolytic and antiseizure medications. They also provide anterograde amnesia, which is beneficial for invasive or uncomfortable procedures; the patient likely will not recall the event.

Midazolam is two to four times as potent as diazepam, is faster acting, and has a shorter duration of action. Because large doses of midazolam are necessary to achieve the desired effect, it should not be used as an induction agent. Some clinicians use midazolam to induce general anesthesia before intubation; however, the likelihood of complications increases because of the large dose necessary to induce muscle relaxation. In general, the use of neuromuscular blockers (paralytics) to achieve muscle relaxation is preferred because they require smaller doses to achieve the desired effect.

Respiratory depression and slight hypotension are potential side effects of benzodiazepine administration. Flumazenil (Romazicon) is a benzodiazepine antagonist that can reverse the effects of diazepam and midazolam.

Barbiturates

Barbiturates are sedative-hypnotic medications that have a long history of use. Thiopental (Pentothal, Trapanal) is short acting and causes a rapid onset of profound sedation; however, the brand-name Pentothal is no longer available in the United States. Methohexital (Brevital) is ultra-short acting and twice as potent as thiopental. Barbiturates can cause significant respiratory depression and a drop in blood pressure of approximately 10% in normovolemic patients. This drop in blood pressure can be profound and potentially irreversible in hypovolemic patients.

Opioids/Narcotics

Opioids are potent analgesics with sedative properties. Narcotics are used in emergency airway management as a premedication, during induction, and in maintenance of sedation or amnesia. The two most commonly used narcotics for airway management are fentanyl (Sublimaze) and alfentanil (Alfenta). Fentanyl is 70 to 150 times more potent than morphine. It has a rapid onset of action and a relatively short duration of action. Alfentanil is less potent than fentanyl but has a faster onset of action and a shorter duration of action. It is also eliminated from the body faster.

Opioids can cause profound respiratory and central nervous system depression and produce severe hypotension and bradycardia, especially in hemodynamically unstable patients. These negative effects can be reversed with naloxone (Narcan), a narcotic antagonist.

Nonnarcotic/Nonbarbiturate

Etomidate (Amidate) is a nonnarcotic, nonbarbiturate hypnotic-sedative drug often used in the induction of general anesthesia. It is a fast-acting agent of short duration. This drug has little effect on pulse rate, blood pressure, and intracranial pressure (ICP) and does not cause the histamine release and bronchoconstriction that may occur with other agents. However, a high incidence of uncomfortable myoclonic muscle movement is associated with its use. Etomidate is a useful induction agent in patients with coronary artery disease, increased ICP, or borderline hypotension/hypovolemia.

Words of Wisdom

Combativeness, aggressiveness, and belligerence should be considered signs of cerebral hypoxia until proven otherwise. You must be firm and direct but still treat your patients with respect and empathy. Keep in mind that they are fighting for their lives, not with you.

Neuromuscular Blockade in Emergency Intubation

Cerebral hypoxia can make an ordinarily docile person combative, aggressive, belligerent, and uncooperative, resulting in a difficult and potentially dangerous situation—for the patient and paramedics. A patient with cerebral hypoxia must be treated with aggressive oxygenation and ventilation, but combativeness or other resistive behavior often makes this task difficult, if not impossible. Clenching of the patient's teeth due to spasm of the jaw muscles (trismus) and laryngospasm can also hamper your efforts to obtain a definitive airway.

In the past, physical restraint of a combative patient was common to enable obtaining a definitive airway. A safer, more effective approach is "chemical paralysis" with neuromuscular blocking agents (paralytics). With the patient chemically sedated and paralyzed, his or her protective airway reflexes are lost; you can effectively perform oxygenation and ventilation, and the patient will not gag during insertion of an ET tube.

Neuromuscular Blocking Agents

Although sedatives alone can be used to facilitate intubation, the incidence of complications and side effects is unacceptably high. It is much more effective to administer a drug specifically designed to induce paralysis. Paralytic drugs affect every skeletal muscle in the body, including the diaphragm and the intercostal muscles. Within about 1 minute of receiving an IV dose of a paralytic, a patient will become totally paralyzed. That is, the patient will stop breathing; his or her jaw muscles will go slack, and the base of the tongue will fall back against the posterior pharynx and obstruct the airway. Put bluntly, paralytics convert a breathing patient with a marginal airway into an apneic patient with no airway. Before you bring about such a change, you must be absolutely sure that you can secure his or her airway with an ET tube or other advanced airway device. Once a patient is paralyzed, you are completely responsible for the patient's breathing and well-being. Fortunately, paralytic agents do not affect cardiac or smooth muscle.

A paralyzed patient *appears* to be asleep or unresponsive, but is not! Paralytic agents, unlike sedatives, have no effect on LOC. The patient is fully aware and can hear, feel, and think.

Pharmacology of Neuromuscular Blocking Agents

To understand how medications induce paralysis, recall how skeletal muscles contract. All skeletal (striated) muscles are voluntary and require input from the somatic nervous system to initiate contraction. As an impulse to contract reaches the terminal end of a motor nerve, acetylcholine (ACh) is released into the synaptic cleft (the junction between the nerve cell and the muscle cell). This neurotransmitter diffuses across the short distance of the synaptic cleft and binds to receptor sites on the motor end plate. Acetylcholine occupying the receptor sites triggers changes in electrical properties of the muscle fiber, a process called depolarization. When enough motor end plates have been depolarized, a threshold is reached and the muscle fiber contracts. Depolarization lasts for only a few milliseconds because of the presence of acetylcholinesterase, an enzyme that quickly removes ACh from the synaptic cleft and from the receptors on the motor end plate.

Paralytic medications function at the neuromuscular junction and relax the muscle by impeding the action of ACh. Collectively, paralytics are referred to as neuromuscular blocking agents. They are classified into two categories: depolarizing and nondepolarizing agents. **Table 17** lists the standard doses for these agents used in the prehospital setting.

Table 17 Neuromuscular Blocking Drug Doses

Drug	Dose
Succinylcholine (depolarizing)	1-1.5 mg/kg via IV push (initial dose); repeated doses can be given based on the patient's clinical response
Vecuronium bromide* (nondepolarizing)	0.1-0.2 mg/kg via IV push (initial dose for adults and children older than 10 years); 0.01-0.015 mg/kg can be given 20-40 min after initial dose
Pancuronium bromide* (nondepolarizing)	0.06-0.1 mg/kg via IV push (initial dose for adults and children older than 1 month); can repeat at 0.01 mg/kg every 20-60 min, as needed
Rocuronium bromide* (nondepolarizing)	0.6-1.2 mg/kg

*Administer 10% of the initial dose (defasciculating dose) before administering succinylcholine.

Words of Wisdom

Paralysis Versus Sedation
Imagine what it must be like to be completely paralyzed. You cannot blink, talk, move, or, most important, breathe! You are completely dependent on others to keep you alive. *Paralytic agents do not induce sedation or amnesia.* If you administer only a paralytic agent, the patient will be fully responsive and remember the entire event. Therefore, unless contraindicated, you must sedate a patient *before* administering a paralytic. *Paralysis without sedation is a form of patient abuse!*

Depolarizing Neuromuscular Blocking Agent

A <u>depolarizing neuromuscular blocker</u> competitively binds with the ACh receptor sites but is not affected as quickly by acetylcholinesterase. Therefore, it causes depolarization of the muscle and prevents future signals for depolarization from having an effect because all of the ACh receptor sites are already occupied.

<u>Succinylcholine chloride</u> (Anectine) is the only depolarizing neuromuscular blocking agent. Because succinylcholine causes depolarization, <u>fasciculations</u>—characterized by brief, uncoordinated twitching of small muscle groups in the face, neck, trunk, and extremities—can be observed during its administration. These fasciculations tend to cause generalized muscle pain at the termination of paralysis (when the succinylcholine wears off).

Depolarizing neuromuscular blockers are characterized by a very rapid onset (60–90 seconds) of total paralysis and a relatively short duration of action (5–10 minutes). For this reason, succinylcholine is often used as an initial paralytic. With this drug, if you are unable to secure the patient's airway, you have to support ventilation for only a short period before the patient can breathe again on his or her own.

Succinylcholine should be used with caution in patients with burns, crush injuries, and blunt trauma—that is, conditions that can result in hyperkalemia. In addition, because its chemical structure is similar to that of ACh, succinylcholine can cause bradycardia, especially in pediatric patients. Administration of atropine sulfate, which prevents succinylcholine-induced bradycardia, should precede the administration of succinylcholine in pediatric patients, if possible.

Words of Wisdom

If you administer only a short-acting paralytic (namely, succinylcholine) to your patient without administering a long-acting paralytic (eg, vecuronium, rocuronium) after the patient has been intubated, you will have to give the medication by continuous infusion or administer a bolus every 5 minutes. This approach significantly increases the risk of complications.

Nondepolarizing Neuromuscular Blocking Agents

<u>Nondepolarizing neuromuscular blockers</u> also bind to ACh receptor sites; however, unlike depolarizing neuromuscular blockers, they do not cause depolarization of the muscle fiber. When given in sufficient quantity, the amount of nondepolarizing medication exceeds the amount of ACh in the synaptic cleft, and the critical threshold of depolarization cannot be achieved. Thus, when nondepolarizing paralytics are administered in small quantities before administering a depolarizing paralytic, they prevent fasciculations. The defasciculating dose is typically 10% of the normal dose; it does not induce paralysis, but causes weakness.

The most commonly used nondepolarizing neuromuscular blockers are vecuronium bromide (Norcuron), pancuronium bromide (Pavulon), and rocuronium bromide (Zemuron). All three agents have a duration of action longer than that of succinylcholine. <u>Vecuronium</u> has a rapid onset of action (2 minutes) and a duration of action of about 45 minutes. <u>Rocuronium</u> has a rapid onset of action (< 2 minutes) and a duration of action of 45 to 60 minutes. <u>Pancuronium</u> also has a rapid onset of action (3–5 minutes) and a duration of action of 1 hour.

Nondepolarizing neuromuscular blockers, because of their longer duration of action, are ideal when a patient requires extended periods of paralysis, such as when there is a prolonged transport time or when the patient's airway has been secured and you need to manage other injuries or conditions. However, these agents should not be given before the patient's airway has been secured.

Rapid-Sequence Intubation

<u>Rapid-sequence intubation (RSI)</u>, also referred to as pharmacologically assisted intubation, represents a culmination and integration of all of your airway, problem-solving, and decision-making skills into one procedure. It includes the safe, smooth, and rapid induction of sedation and paralysis followed immediately by intubation. Although RSI has been successfully performed in the operating room for years, its use in the prehospital setting is relatively new. It is generally used for responsive or combative patients who need to be intubated but who are unable to cooperate.

Preparation of the Patient and Equipment

The experience of being intubated is frightening for patients, so you must explain what you are going to do and reassure the patient that he or she will be asleep during the procedure and will not feel or remember anything. Apply a cardiac monitor and pulse oximeter. Check, prepare, and assemble your equipment, and ensure that it is in good working order. In particular, have suction immediately available.

Preoxygenation

All patients undergoing RSI should be adequately preoxygenated before the procedure is begun. If the patient is breathing spontaneously and has adequate tidal volume, apply high-flow oxygen via nonrebreathing mask. However, if the patient is hypoventilating, assisted ventilations with a bag-mask device and high-flow oxygen may be necessary. Bag-mask ventilation before RSI should be avoided whenever possible to avoid gastric distention and the associated risks of regurgitation and aspiration.

Premedication

Stimulation of the glottis associated with intubation can cause dysrhythmias and a substantial increase in ICP—a particularly problematic issue for patients with closed head injuries or other conditions associated with increased ICP. If you are performing RSI on a patient with closed head trauma, your protocols may call for the administration of 1 to 1.5 mg/kg of lidocaine. Lidocaine has been shown to have mixed results regarding its ability to blunt the sympathetic response to intubation, although it has been shown to blunt the increase in ICP associated with suctioning and laryngeal stimulation.

If your initial paralytic of choice is succinylcholine, you should administer a defasciculating dose—typically 10% of the normal dose—of a nondepolarizing paralytic, if time permits. Atropine sulfate should also be administered to decrease the incidence of bradycardia associated with the administration of succinylcholine. The usual dose for an adult is 0.5 mg and for infants and children is 0.02 mg/kg.

Sedation and Paralysis

As long as the patient is in hemodynamically stable condition (systolic blood pressure of > 90 mm Hg), administer a sedative agent to induce sedation and amnesia. As soon as the patient is adequately sedated, administer the paralytic agent. The onset of paralysis will be quick and should be complete within 2 minutes. Observe for apnea, check for laxity of the mandible, and assess for the loss of the eyelash reflex; these are signs of adequate paralysis.

Intubation

Intubate the trachea as carefully as possible. If you cannot accomplish the intubation within 30 seconds, stop and ventilate the patient for 30 to 60 seconds with a bag-mask device and 100% oxygen before trying again. *If you must ventilate the patient with a bag-mask device, do so slowly (1 second per breath [enough to produce visible chest rise]).*

Once the tube is in the trachea, inflate the cuff, remove the stylet, verify correct position of the ET tube (by auscultation and continuous waveform capnography). Secure the tube in place as usual, and continue ventilations at the appropriate rate.

Words of Wisdom

Rapid-sequence intubation should be attempted only if you have confidence that you will be able to intubate and ventilate the patient or ventilate the patient without intubation, if necessary. Otherwise, a patient who has been sedated and paralyzed will die. Above all, do no harm!

Maintenance of Paralysis and Sedation

When you are absolutely sure that you have successfully intubated the trachea, depending on your transport time, additional paralytic administration may be necessary. If you administered succinylcholine initially (with a short duration of action), administer a nondepolarizing agent (such as vecuronium or rocuronium) to maintain long-term paralysis. If you administered a long-acting paralytic initially, additional dosing is usually not necessary for short transport times. Administer additional sedation as needed if the patient's blood pressure is adequate.

While the general steps of RSI are the same for all patients, some modification is necessary for patients in unstable condition. If the patient's oxygen saturation drops, you have no choice except to ventilate (*slowly*). If the patient is in hemodynamically unstable condition, you must judge whether sedation is appropriate or whether the risk of profound hypotension is too great to sedate the patient before inducing paralysis. **Table 18** lists sample protocols for RSI in patients in hemodynamically stable or unstable condition.

Table 18 Sample Protocols for Rapid-Sequence Intubation

For patients in hemodynamically stable condition:
1. Prepare patient and equipment.
2. Preoxygenate with 100% oxygen for at least 2 to 3 minutes.
3. Administer a defasciculating dose of a nondepolarizing paralytic, lidocaine, or atropine.
4. Sedate.
5. Administer succinylcholine.
6. Intubate and verify correct tube placement.
7. Properly secure the ET tube.
8. Administer a nondepolarizing paralytic (standard dose), as needed, and maintain adequate sedation.

For patients in hemodynamically unstable condition:
1. Prepare patient and equipment.
2. Preoxygenate and ventilate as necessary.
3. Consider sedation.
4. Administer succinylcholine.
5. Intubate and confirm correct tube placement.
6. Properly secure the ET tube.
7. Administer a nondepolarizing paralytic.

Alternative Advanced Airway Devices

Multilumen Airways

Multilumen airway devices are inserted blindly and have been clinically proven to secure the airway and allow for better ventilation than a bag-mask device and simple airway adjunct in most cases. Two such devices, called **multilumen airways**, are the **Combitube** Figure 88 and the pharyngotracheal lumen airway. The pharyngotracheal lumen airway is the predecessor to the Combitube; because it is now rarely used, the focus will be on the Combitube.

The Combitube has a long tube that is blindly inserted into the airway. In contrast with single-lumen airways, the tube can be used for ventilation whether it is inserted into the esophagus or trachea Figure 89 . Although these devices almost always come to rest in the esophagus, they can function as an ET tube if inserted into the trachea. Multilumen airways contain two

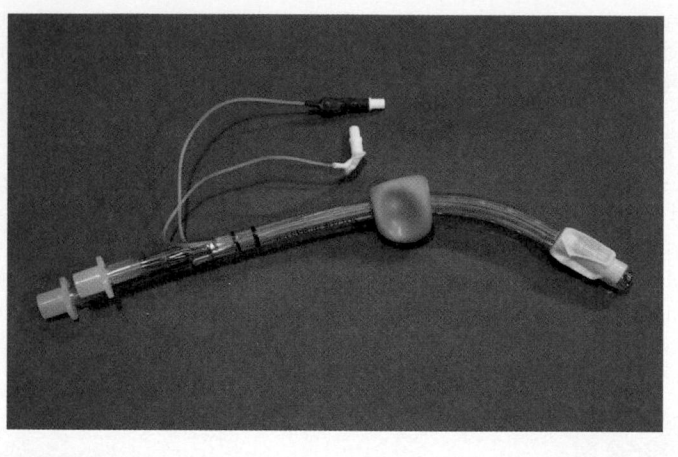

Figure 88 Combitube.

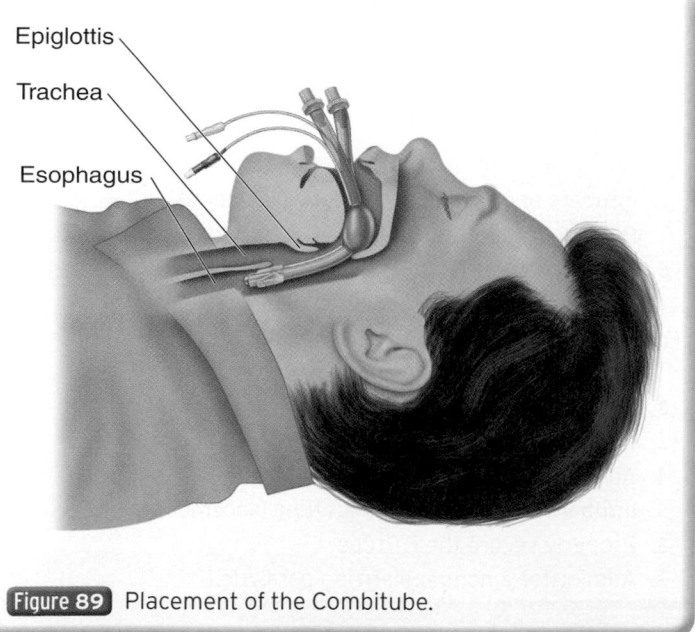

Epiglottis

Trachea

Esophagus

Figure 89 Placement of the Combitube.

lumens, which function appropriately based on tube position and ventilating through the correct lumen. Each lumen has a standard 15/22-mm ventilation adapter, which accommodates any ventilation device (such as a bag-mask device or manually triggered ventilator). The proper port for ventilation depends on where the tube is located. They also contain an oropharyngeal balloon, which eliminates the need for a mask seal.

Indications and Contraindications for Multilumen Airways

Multilumen airways are indicated for airway management of deeply unresponsive, apneic patients with no gag reflex in whom ET intubation is not possible or has failed. If the patient regains consciousness, the device must be removed.

Neither of the multilumen airways can be used in children younger than 16 years, and they should be used only for patients between 5' and 7' tall. A smaller version of the Combitube—called the Combitube SA (small adult)—can be used for patients more than 4' tall. Because the device is inserted into the esophagus most of the time, use is contraindicated in patients with esophageal trauma, patients with a known pathologic condition of the esophagus (such as esophageal varices or cancer), patients who have ingested a caustic substance, or patients who have a history of alcoholism.

Advantages and Disadvantages of Multilumen Airways

The major advantage of the multilumen airway is that, in effect, it cannot be improperly placed; effective ventilation is possible whether the tube enters the esophagus or the trachea. Insertion of the multilumen airway is also technically easier than ET intubation. Furthermore, because insertion of the airway is performed with the patient's head in the neutral position, cervical spine movement is kept to a minimum. In addition, no mask seal is required to ventilate with the Combitube.

Multilumen airways also provide some patency to the airway. If the tube is placed in the trachea, it functions exactly like an ET tube, and no upper airway positioning is required. If the tube is placed in the esophagus, the pharyngeal balloon creates an airtight seal in the oropharynx, making the tongue position less of a factor in the maintenance of a patent airway. A jaw-thrust maneuver should easily alleviate any ventilatory difficulty if the epiglottis partially obstructs the airway.

Use of a multilumen airway requires strict attention and good assessment skills because *ventilation in the wrong port results in no pulmonary ventilation*. These devices are usually considered temporary airways and should be replaced as soon as possible. The pharyngeal balloon reduces but does not completely eliminate the risk of aspiration. In addition, intubating the trachea via direct laryngoscopy with a multilumen airway in place, although possible, can be extremely challenging.

Complications of Multilumen Airways

The most significant complication associated with the use of multilumen airways is *unrecognized* displacement of the tube into the esophagus. (It is okay if the tube is placed in the esophagus, but the paramedic must realize this in order to effectively ventilate.) Therefore, good assessment skills are essential to properly confirm tube placement, and multiple confirmation techniques should be used following insertion of the device.

Laryngospasm, vomiting, and possible hypoventilation may occur during insertion of a multilumen airway. In addition, pharyngeal or esophageal trauma may result from improper technique.

Ventilation may be difficult if the pharyngeal balloon pushes the epiglottis over the glottic opening. A few cases of difficult ventilation have occurred with multilumen airways. However, in all cases, ventilation became easier when the device was withdrawn 2 to 4 cm.

Insertion Techniques

The Combitube consists of a single tube with two lumens, two balloons, and two ventilation attachments. One of the lumens is open at its distal end, and the other is closed. The closed lumen has side holes to the pharyngeal balloon. The proximal balloon is designed to be inflated with 100 mL of air and provide a pharyngeal seal. The distal balloon is inflated with 15 mL of air and makes an airtight seal with the walls of the trachea (in case of tracheal placement) or provides esophageal obturation (in case of esophageal placement) **Figure 90**.

Before inserting a multilumen airway, check and prepare your equipment. Check both cuffs, and ensure that they hold air. The patient should be preoxygenated before insertion. Ventilation should not be interrupted for longer than 30 seconds to insert the airway. For insertion, the patient's head should be placed in a neutral position.

- **Forwardly displace the jaw.** With the patient's head in a neutral position, insert the thumb of your gloved nondominant hand into the patient's mouth and lift the jaw. This action lifts the hyoid bone and pulls the base of the tongue off the posterior pharyngeal wall.
- **Insert the device.** Following the curvature of the tube, insert the device blindly into the posterior pharynx. The Combitube is inserted until the incisors are between the two black lines printed on the tube. Be gentle, and stop advancing the tube if you meet resistance.

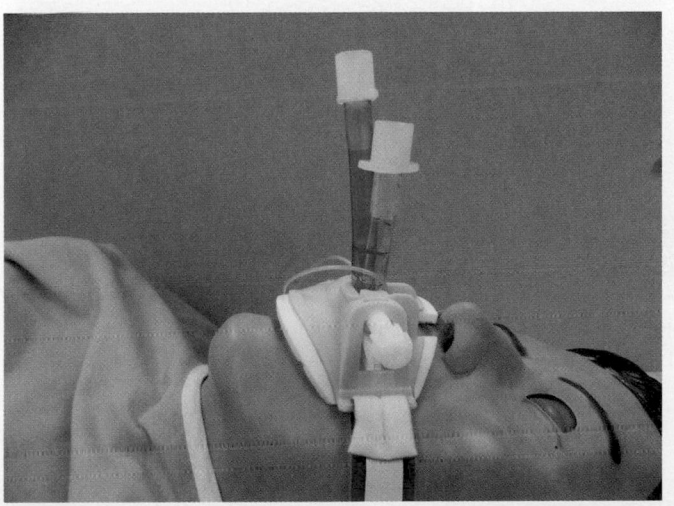

Figure 90 Ventilation with a Combitube in place.

- The Combitube has two independent inflation valves that must be inflated sequentially. The first inflation valve goes to the balloon on the pharyngeal tube (blue [No. 1] tube) and is inflated with 100 mL of air. The second inflation valve inflates the distal balloon of the tracheal tube (clear [No. 2] tube) and is filled with 15 mL of air.

When inserting a multilumen airway, confirmation of ventilation is critical. If you ventilate through the wrong tube, the patient will receive no pulmonary ventilation and you could actually be instilling air directly into the stomach. The steps for insertion of a Combitube are listed here and shown in **Skill Drill 25**:

Skill Drill 25

1. Take standard precautions (gloves and face shield) **Step 1**.
2. Preoxygenate the patient whenever possible with a bag-mask device and 100% oxygen **Step 2**.
3. Gather your equipment **Step 3**.
4. Place the patient's head in a neutral position **Step 4**.
5. Open the patient's mouth with the tongue-jaw lift maneuver, and insert the Combitube in the midline of the patient's mouth. Insert the tube until the incisors or alveolar ridge lies between the two reference marks **Step 5**.
6. Inflate the pharyngeal cuff with 100 mL of air **Step 6**.
7. Inflate the distal cuff with 15 mL of air **Step 7**.
8. Ventilate the patient through the longest tube (blue tube) first. Chest rise indicates esophageal placement of the distal tip; continue to ventilate **Step 8**.
9. No chest rise indicates tracheal placement (switch ports and ventilate) **Step 9**.
10. Confirm placement by auscultating breath sounds and epigastric sounds, and attach a capnography monitor.

Following inflation of the balloons, begin to ventilate the patient. With the Combitube, ventilate through the longer (blue) tube first. Observe for chest rise and auscultate breath and epigastric sounds. If there are no breath sounds (or epigastric sounds are present) and the chest does not rise and fall with ventilation, switch immediately to the shorter (clear) tube. Be sure to continuously monitor ventilation. Both multilumen airways are generally secure in the airway owing to the large pharyngeal balloons. However, it is still important to secure the device in place once ventilations are confirmed. Continuous waveform capnography should be used to confirm the presence of exhaled carbon dioxide, which further confirms proper ventilation.

■ Supraglottic Airway Devices

Laryngeal Mask Airway

The **laryngeal mask airway (LMA)** **Figure 91** was originally developed for use in the operating room. It provides a viable option for patients who require more airway and ventilatory support than bag-mask ventilation can provide but do not require ET intubation.

Skill Drill 25

Inserting a Combitube

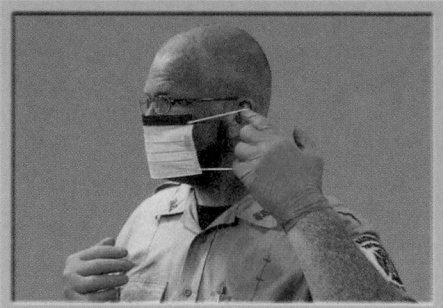

Step 1 Take standard precautions (gloves and face shield).

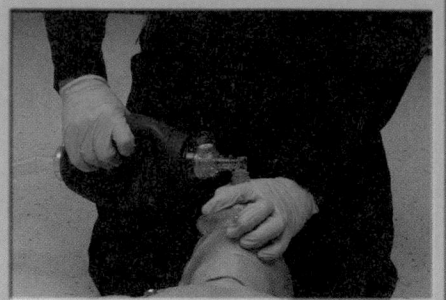

Step 2 Preoxygenate the patient with a bag-mask device and 100% oxygen.

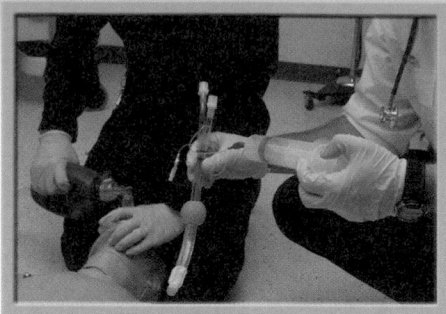

Step 3 Gather your equipment.

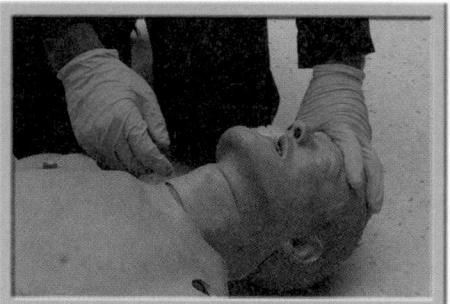

Step 4 Place the patient's head in a neutral position.

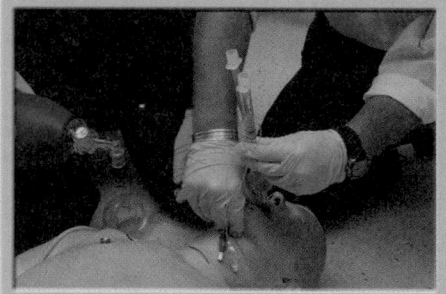

Step 5 Open the patient's mouth with the tongue-jaw lift maneuver, and insert the Combitube in the midline of the patient's mouth. Insert the tube until the incisors lie between the two reference marks.

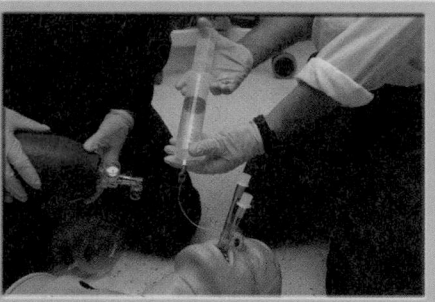

Step 6 Inflate the pharyngeal cuff with 100 mL of air.

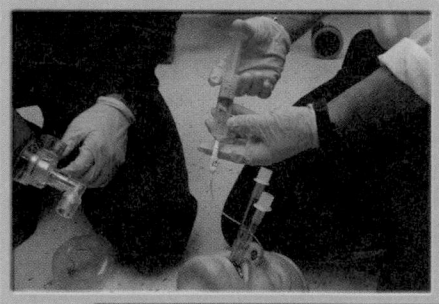

Step 7 Inflate the distal cuff with 15 mL of air.

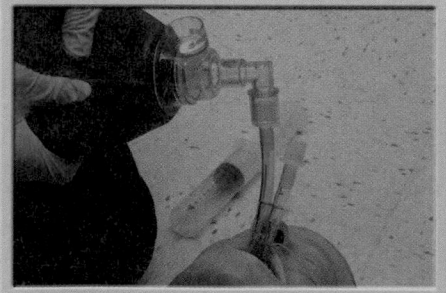

Step 8 Ventilate the patient through the pharyngeal (blue) tube first. Chest rise indicates esophageal placement of the distal tip; continue to ventilate.

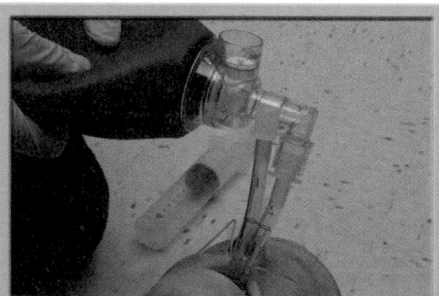

Step 9 No chest rise indicates tracheal placement; switch ports and ventilate. Ensure proper tube placement with waveform capnography.

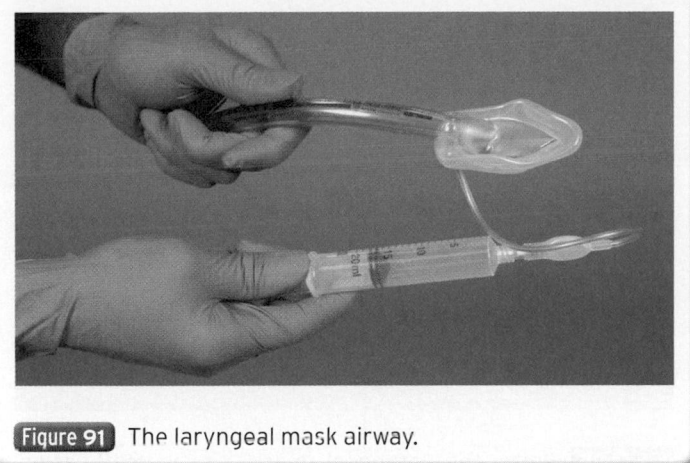

Figure 91 The laryngeal mask airway.

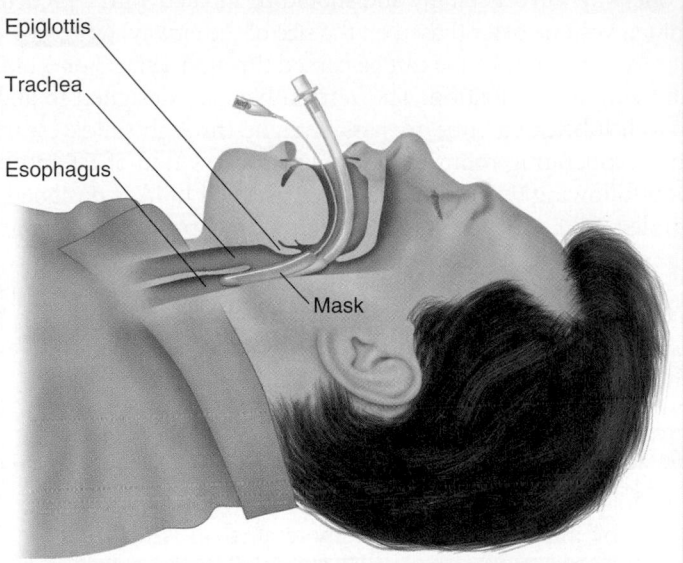

Epiglottis

Trachea

Esophagus

Mask

Figure 92 When properly positioned, the opening of the laryngeal mask airway is at the glottic opening, the tip is at the entrance of the esophagus, the lateral portions in the piriform fossae, and the upper border at the base of the tongue.

The LMA is designed to provide a conduit from the glottic opening to the ventilation device. It surrounds the opening of the larynx with an inflatable silicone cuff positioned in the hypopharynx. When properly inserted, the opening of the LMA is positioned at the glottic opening, and the tip is inserted into the proximal esophagus, the lateral portions in the piriform fossae, and the upper border at the base of the tongue. The inflatable cuff conforms to the contours of the airway and forms a relatively airtight seal **Figure 92**.

Indications and Contraindications for the LMA The LMA should be considered as one possible alternative to bag-mask ventilation when the patient cannot be intubated.

The LMA is less effective in obese patients and should not be used in morbidly obese patients. Pregnant patients and patients with a hiatal hernia are at an increased risk for regurgitation and must be evaluated carefully if LMA use is considered. The LMA is ineffective for the ventilation of patients requiring high pulmonary pressures (such as patients with COPD or congestive heart failure).

Advantages and Disadvantages of the LMA The LMA has many advantages compared with ventilating an unprotected airway with a mask. The LMA has been shown to provide better ventilation than a bag-mask device and an oral and/or nasal airway, and ventilation with an LMA does not require the continual maintenance of a mask seal. Compared with ET intubation, LMA insertion is easier because it does not require laryngoscopy. There is significantly less risk of soft-tissue, vocal cord, tracheal wall, and dental trauma than with ET intubation and other forms of intubation that rely on blocking the esophagus. The LMA provides protection from upper airway secretions, and the tip of the LMA wedged into the proximal esophagus most likely provides some obturation.

The main disadvantage of the LMA—especially in emergency situations—is that it does not provide protection against aspiration. In fact, the LMA actually increases the risk of aspiration if the patient regurgitates because the stomach contents would most likely be directed into the trachea.

During prolonged LMA ventilation, some air may be insufflated into the stomach because the seal made in the airway is not airtight. Because of the risk of aspiration, it is unlikely that the LMA will ever replace ET intubation in prehospital emergency care. *The LMA should not be considered a primary airway in emergency situations.* It should, however, be considered superior to bag-mask ventilation in patients who cannot be endotracheally intubated.

Complications of Using the LMA The most significant complications associated with use of the LMA involve regurgitation and subsequent aspiration. The product literature states that the LMA should be used only in patients who are fasting. Unfortunately, this would eliminate all patients in emergency situations, who should always be presumed to have full stomachs. You must weigh the risk of aspiration against the risk of hypoventilation with bag-mask ventilation in the context of the clinical scenario.

You should observe the patient for clinical indications of adequate ventilation (that is, chest rise and breath sounds) during LMA ventilation. Hypoventilation of patients who require high ventilatory pressures can also occur, and a few cases of upper airway swelling have been reported.

Equipment for the LMA The LMA comes in seven sizes and is sized based on the patient's weight. The device consists of a tube and an inflatable mask cuff. The cuff provides a collar that positions the opening of the tube at the glottic opening when inflated. Two vertical bars at the opening of the tube prevent occlusion. The proximal end of the tube is fitted with a standard 15/22-mm adapter that is compatible with any ventilation device. The cuff has a one-way valve assembly and should be inflated with a predetermined volume of air (based on the size of the airway) Figure 93 .

A 6.0-mm ET tube can be passed through a size 3 or 4 LMA, allowing for intubation. The vertical bars are designed to allow a well-lubricated tube to pass straight through, and research in the operating room found a high success rate of ET intubation following this technique. The Fasttrach LMA is designed to guide an ET tube into the trachea and may prove to be a viable alternative to direct laryngoscopy Figure 94 .

Insertion Technique Before insertion, check and prepare all equipment. The steps for inserting an LMA are listed here and shown in Skill Drill 26 :

Skill Drill 26

1. Take standard precautions. Check the cuff of the LMA by inflating it with 50% more air than is required for the size of airway to be used. Then deflate the cuff completely Step 1 . The cuff should be completely deflated so that no folds appear near the tip. Deflation is best accomplished by pressing the device, cuff down, on a flat surface Figure 95 .

2. Lubricate the outer rim of the device Step 2 .

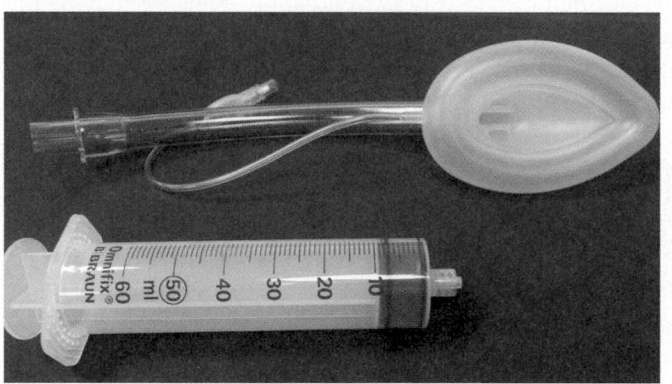

Figure 93 The laryngeal mask airway with the cuff inflated.

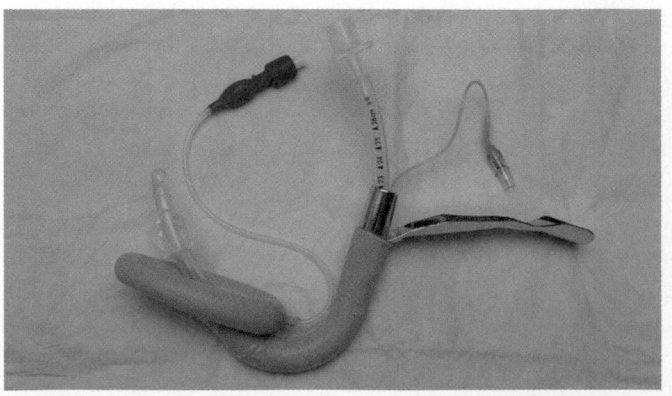

Figure 94 The Fasttrach laryngeal mask airway with a 6.0-mm endotracheal tube.

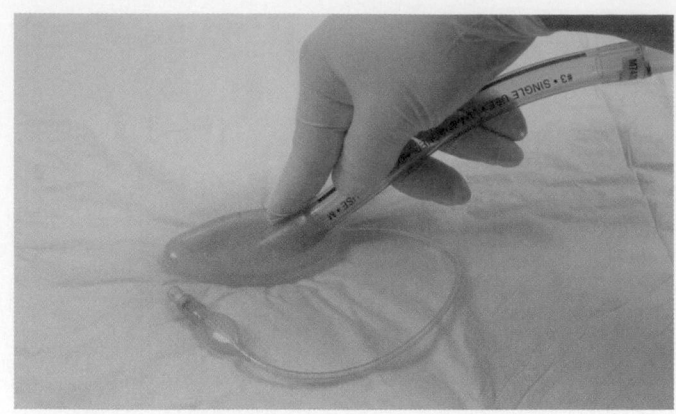

Figure 95 Press the laryngeal mask airway, cuff down, against a flat surface to remove all wrinkles from the cuff.

3. Preoxygenate the patient before insertion. Ventilation should not be interrupted for more than 30 seconds to accomplish airway placement. Place the patient in the sniffing position Step 3 .

4. Insert your finger between the cuff and the tube. Proper insertion of the LMA depends on holding the device properly. Place the index finger of your dominant hand in the notch between the tube and the cuff. Open the patient's mouth Step 4 .

5. Insert the LMA along the roof of the mouth. The key to proper insertion is to slide the convex surface of the airway along the roof of the mouth. Use your finger to push the airway against the hard palate Step 5 . Once it slides past the tongue, the LMA will move easily into position.

6. Inflate the cuff with the amount of air indicated for the size of airway being used Step 6 . If the LMA is properly positioned, it will move out of the airway slightly (1–2 cm) as it moves into position. This is a good indication that the LMA is in the correct position.

7. Begin to ventilate the patient. Confirm chest rise and the presence of breath sounds. Continuously and carefully monitor the patient's condition Step 7 .

Documentation and Communication

If adverse events occur with the use of advanced airway devices, such as bleeding or trauma, be sure to document these occurrences on the patient care report form.

King LT Airway

The **King LT airway** is a latex-free, single-use, single-lumen airway that is blindly inserted into the esophagus Figure 96 and can be used to provide positive-pressure ventilation to apneic patients and maintain a patent airway in spontaneously

Skill Drill | 26

LMA Insertion

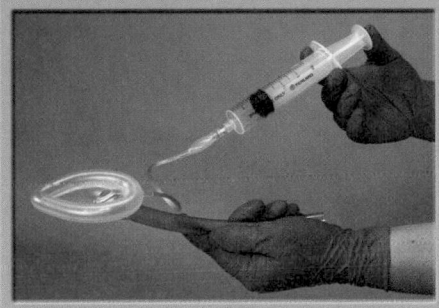

Step 1 Take standard precautions. Check the cuff of the LMA by inflating it with 50% more air than is required for the size of airway to be used. Then deflate the cuff completely.

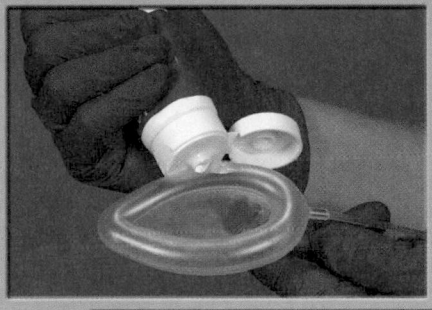

Step 2 Lubricate the outer rim of the device.

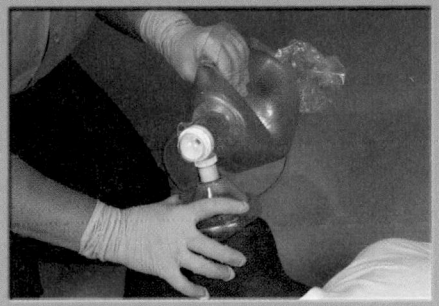

Step 3 Preoxygenate the patient before insertion. Ventilation should not be interrupted for more than 30 seconds to accomplish airway placement. Place the patient in the sniffing position.

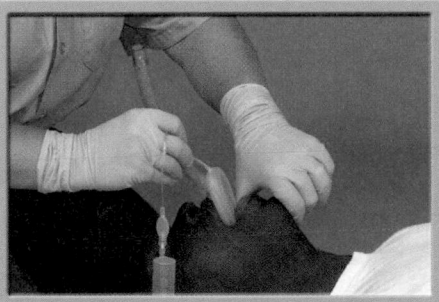

Step 4 Lift the jaw with one hand, and begin to insert the device with the other hand.

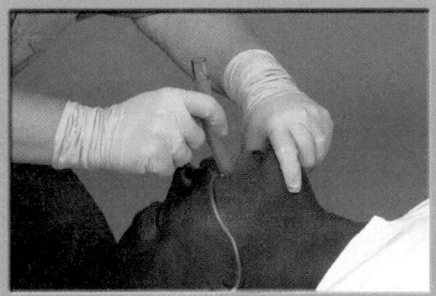

Step 5 Insert the LMA along the roof of the mouth. Use your finger to push the airway against the hard palate.

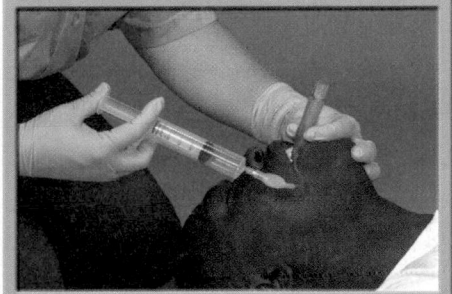

Step 6 Inflate the cuff with the amount of air indicated for the airway being used.

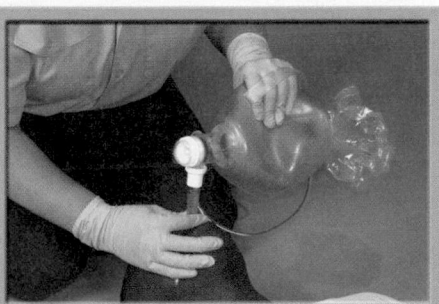

Step 7 Begin to ventilate the patient. Confirm chest rise and the presence of breath sounds. Ensure proper tube placement with waveform capnography. Continuously and carefully monitor the patient's condition.

breathing patients who require advanced airway management. The King LT is available in adult and pediatric sizes.

The device consists of a curved tube with ventilation ports located between two inflatable cuffs. Both cuffs are inflated simultaneously using a single valve. When the airway is properly placed, in the esophagus, the distal cuff seals the esophagus, and the proximal cuff seals the oropharynx **Figure 97**. Openings located between these two cuffs provide ventilation of the lungs once positioning is confirmed. Studies have shown that the King LT can be inserted more easily and quickly than the Combitube and can be used successfully as a rescue airway device.

Two types of King LT airway are available: the King LT-D and the King LTS-D. The King LT-D can be used in adults and children in the prehospital setting, whereas the King LTS-D is used only in adults. Five sizes of each type are available, and sizes are based on the patient's height and or weight. Each size

Table 19 King LT-D and LTS-D Sizes, Patient Criteria, and Cuff Volumes			
Size	Connector Color	Height and Weight Criteria	Cuff Volume
2	Green	35″–45″ or 12-25 kg	25-35 mL*
2.5	Orange	41″–51″ or 25-35 kg	30-40 mL*
3	Yellow	4′-5′	LT-D (45-60 mL) LTS-D (40-55 mL)
4	Red	5′-6′	LT-D (60-80 mL) LTS-D (50-70 mL)
5	Purple	> 6′	LT-D (70-90 mL) LTS-D (60-80 mL)

*Sizes 2 and 2.5 are available only in the King LT-D.

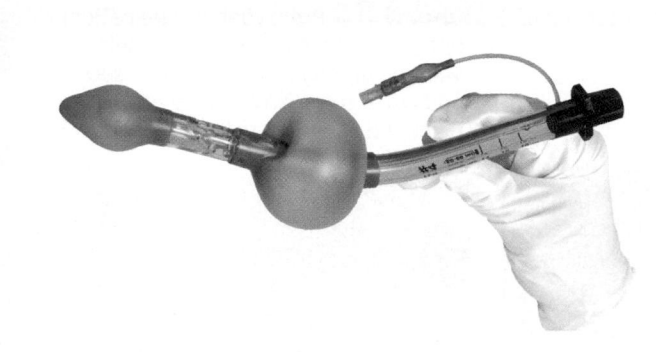

Figure 96 The King LT is a single-lumen airway that is blindly inserted into the esophagus.

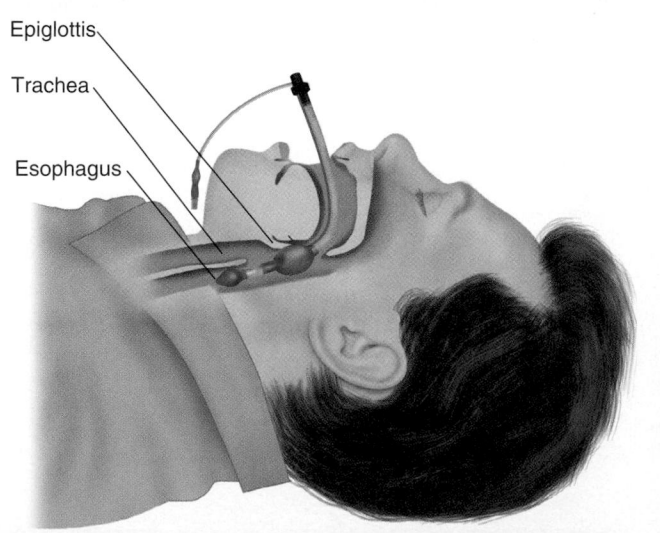

Epiglottis

Trachea

Esophagus

Figure 97 Placement of the King LT airway. When properly placed, the distal cuff seals the esophagus, and the proximal cuff seals the oropharynx.

has a different color of proximal connector and requires different cuff inflation pressures **Table 19**. EMS kits are not sterile and contain a single King LT-D or LTS-D, a syringe for cuff inflation, water-soluble lubricant, and instructions for use.

The King LT-D (see Figure 96) and the King LTS-D share most of the same features. Both have a proximal pharyngeal cuff and a distal cuff and several ventilation outlets at the distal part of the tube. In both, an ET tube introducer (a gum elastic bougie) can be inserted through the tube, where it exits at a "ramp" between the pharyngeal and distal cuffs. If an ET tube needs to be inserted, the tube introducer is simply inserted through the King airway and into the trachea. The King is then removed, and an ET tube is directed into the trachea by placing it over the tube introducer.

The distal end of the LT-D is closed, whereas the distal end of the LTS-D is open. This opening permits insertion of a suction catheter (up to 18F) through a gastric access lumen on the proximal end of the LTS-D for gastric decompression **Figure 98**.

Indications for the King LT Airway The King LT airway is an alternative to bag-mask ventilation when a rescue airway device is required for a failed intubation attempt. The King LT airway has the same advantages, disadvantages, complications, and special considerations as the Combitube.

Contraindications to the King LT Airway The King LT airway does not eliminate the risk of vomiting and aspiration. High airway pressures can cause air to leak into the stomach or out of the mouth. The King LT airway should not be used in patients with an intact gag reflex, patients with known esophageal disease, or patients who have ingested a caustic substance. As with other advanced airway devices, proper placement is confirmed by observing chest rise, auscultating the lungs and epigastrium, and using waveform capnography.

Complications of the King LT Airway As with multilumen airway devices, it is reasonable to assume that laryngospasm, vomiting,

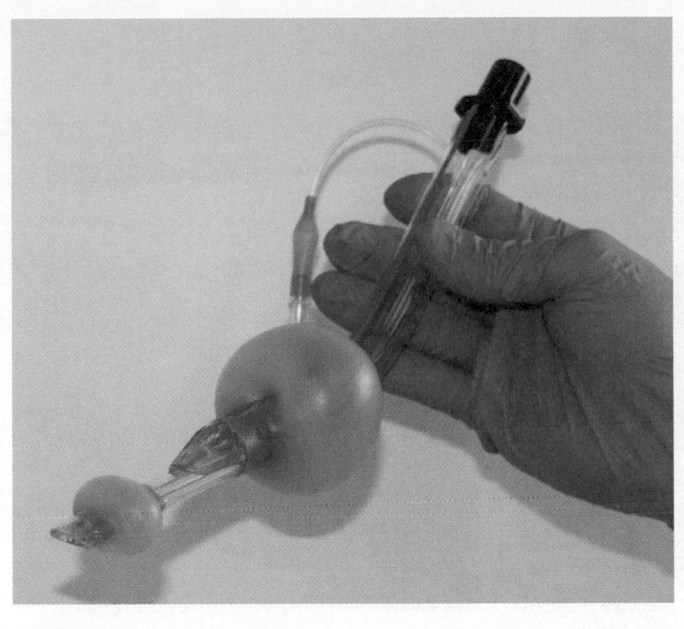

Figure 98 The King LTS-D.

and possible hypoventilation may occur. Trauma may also result from improper insertion technique. Ventilation may be difficult if the pharyngeal balloon pushes the epiglottis over the glottic opening. If this problem occurs, gently withdraw the device—without deflating either of the cuffs—until ventilation becomes easier.

Insertion Technique As previously discussed, the King LT airway comes in five sizes; the patient's height and weight determine the size that should be used. The steps for inserting the King LT airway are listed here and shown in Skill Drill 27 :

Skill Drill 27

1. Take standard precautions (gloves and face shield) Step 1 .

2. Preoxygenate the patient with a bag-mask device and 100% oxygen Step 2 .

3. Gather your equipment Step 3 .

4. Choose the proper size of King LT airway for the patient. Test the cuffs for proper inflation. Ensure that all air is removed from the cuffs before insertion. Lubricate the tip of the device with a water-soluble lubricant for easy insertion and minimal airway damage.

5. Place the patient's head in a neutral position, unless contraindicated (use the jaw-thrust maneuver if trauma is suspected). In your dominant hand, hold the King LT at the connector. With your other hand, hold the patient's mouth open while positioning the head Step 4 .

6. Insert the tip of the device into the corner of the mouth, and continue to advance it behind the base of the tongue while rotating the device. When rotation is complete, the blue line on the device should face the patient's chin.

7. Continue to gently advance the device until the base of the connector is aligned with the patient's teeth or gums. Do not use excessive force.

8. Inflate the cuffs with the recommended amount of air or enough to just seal the device Step 5 .

9. Attach the tube to the bag-mask device, and confirm tube placement by auscultating the lungs and epigastrium and attaching waveform capnography Step 6 . Add additional air to the cuffs to maximize airway seal, if needed.

10. Once placement is confirmed, secure the tube and begin ventilating the patient.

Cobra Perilaryngeal Airway

The <u>Cobra perilaryngeal airway (CobraPLA)</u> was first introduced as a device to ventilate patients with difficult airways. It is so named because of the "cobra" shape of the distal part of the airway Figure 99 . The shape allows the device to slide easily along the hard palate and to hold the soft tissue of the airway away from the laryngeal inlet (hence, "perilaryngeal") once in place. It is a supraglottic device with a tube for ventilation and a circumferential cuff (that sits in the hypopharynx at the base of the tongue) proximal to the distal end, which is the ventilation outlet. It also has a 15/22-mm standard adapter and the distal widened end that holds soft tissue apart and allows for ventilation of the trachea. The distal tip is proximal to the esophagus and seals the hypopharynx. When the cuff is inflated, it raises the tongue and creates an airway seal allowing for ventilation. Because the insertion technique is simple, personnel with little or no experience often are successful.

The CobraPLA is available in eight sizes. Proper size is determined by the one that comfortably fits through the patient's mouth.

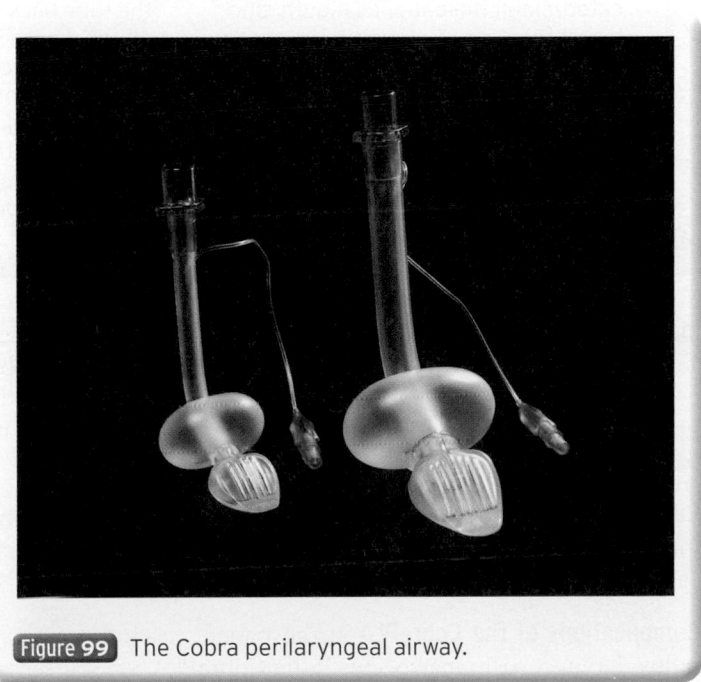

Figure 99 The Cobra perilaryngeal airway.

Skill Drill | 27

Inserting a King LT Airway

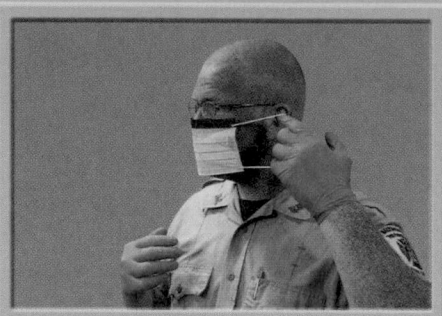

Step 1 Take standard precautions (gloves and face shield).

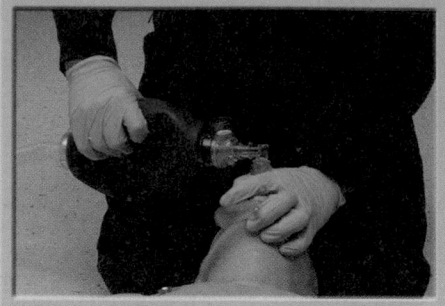

Step 2 Preoxygenate the patient with a bag-mask device and 100% oxygen.

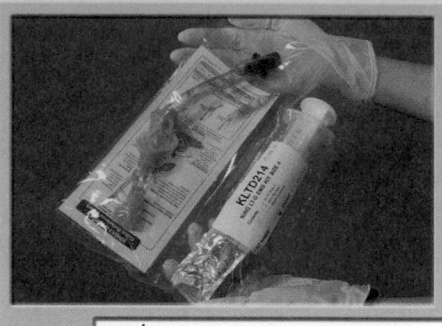

Step 3 Gather your equipment.

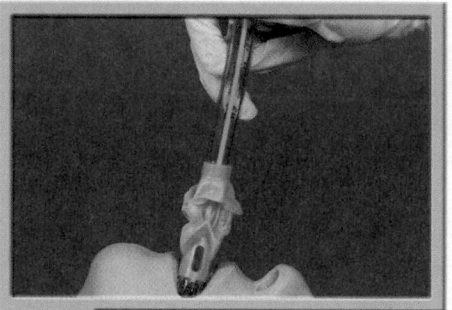

Step 4 Place the patient's head in a neutral position unless contraindicated. Open the patient's mouth, and insert the King LT airway in the corner of the mouth.

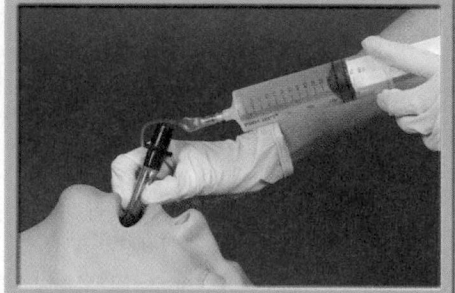

Step 5 Advance the tip behind the base of the tongue while rotating the tube back to midline so the blue line on the device faces the patient's chin. Gently advance the device until the base of the connector is aligned with the teeth or gums. Do not use excessive force. Inflate the cuffs with the recommended amount of air or enough to just seal the device.

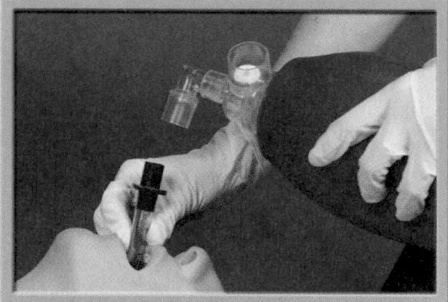

Step 6 Attach the tube to the bag-mask device, and confirm tube placement. Ensure proper tube placement with waveform capnography. Once placement is confirmed, secure the tube and begin ventilating the patient.

Indications for the CobraPLA The CobraPLA is used in a manner similar to that for other supraglottic airway devices and can be used in pediatric patients. Because the device does not provide protection against aspiration, it is recommended for use only in patients who are not at risk for vomiting.

Contraindications to Use of the CobraPLA Contraindications include the risk for aspiration and massive trauma to the oral cavity.

Complications of the CobraPLA If the patient has an intact gag reflex, laryngospasm may occur. If the CobraPLA is not inserted far enough, inflation of the cuff may cause the tongue to protrude from the mouth, disrupting an adequate seal. Using the proper size is vital because the patient cannot be ventilated if the device is too small and passes into the laryngeal inlet. However, in such cases, it can be removed and another size inserted with minimal trauma to the oropharynx.

Insertion Technique The steps for inserting a CobraPLA are listed here and shown in Skill Drill 28 :

Skill Drill | 28

1. Take standard precautions (gloves and face shield).
2. Preoxygenate the patient whenever possible with a bag-mask device and 100% oxygen.

3. Gather and inspect your equipment.

4. Fully deflate the cuff of the CobraPLA, and fold it back against the breathing tube.

5. Apply a water-soluble lubricant liberally to the front and back of the CobraPLA head and to the cuff.

6. Place the patient's head in the sniffing position.

7. Open the patient's mouth with a scissor maneuver with your nondominant hand, gently pulling the mandible upward (Step 1).

8. Direct the distal end straight back between the tongue and hard palate with your dominant hand while lifting the jaw with your nondominant hand. Do not direct the CobraPLA tip against the hard palate.

9. Continue advancing the CobraPLA until modest resistance is encountered as the device tip reaches the glottis (Step 2).

10. Inflate the cuff with only enough air to achieve a good seal (Step 3). Never overinflate the cuff. Inflate with less than the maximum volume recommended until there is no leak obtained with positive-pressure ventilation.

11. Ventilate the patient to confirm correct placement and to measure the pressure at which an audible leak occurs. Confirm placement by observing for chest rise and auscultating over the neck, chest, and epigastric region. Attach waveform capnography.

12. Secure the tube in place.

Skill Drill | 28

Inserting a Cobra Perilaryngeal Airway (CobraPLA)

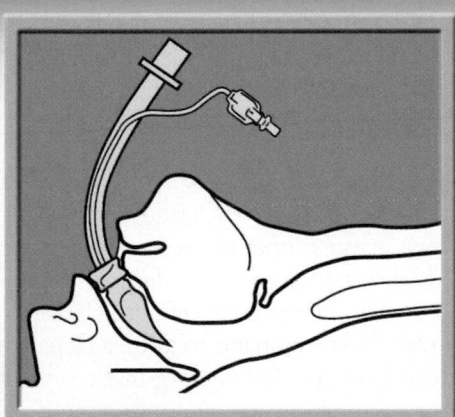

Step 1 Take standard precautions. Preoxygenate the patient. Gather, inspect, and prepare your equipment. Fully deflate the cuff of the CobraPLA, and fold back against the breathing tube. Apply a water-soluble lubricant liberally to the front and back of the CobraPLA head and to the cuff. Place the patient's head and neck in the sniffing position. Open the patient's mouth with a scissor maneuver with your nondominant hand, gently pulling the mandible upward. Direct the distal end of the CobraPLA straight back between the tongue and hard palate while lifting the jaw with your other hand.

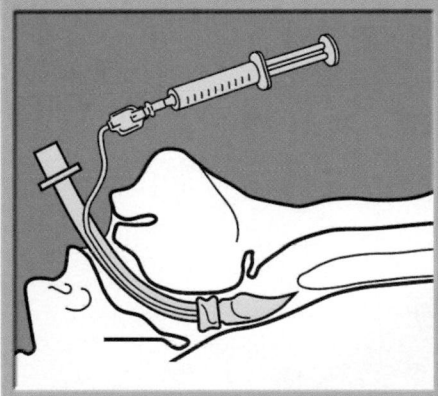

Step 2 Continue advancing the CobraPLA until modest resistance is encountered.

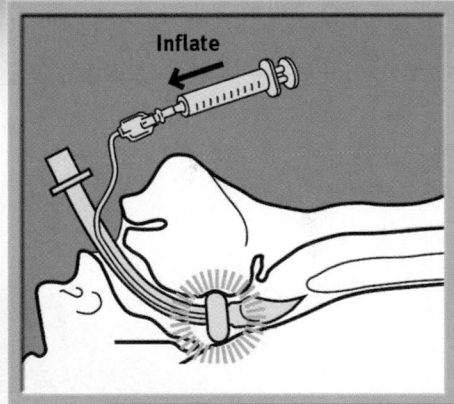

Step 3 Inflate the cuff with only enough air to achieve a good seal. Never overinflate the cuff. Ventilate the patient to confirm correct placement and to measure the pressure at which an audible leak occurs. Confirm placement by observing for chest rise and auscultating over the neck, chest, and epigastric region. Ensure proper tube placement with waveform capnography. Secure the tube in place.

Surgical and Nonsurgical Cricothyrotomy

In most cases, a paramedic is able to secure a patent airway with relative ease using basic (bag-mask device with oral airway) or advanced (ET intubation) methods. In some situations, however, the patient's condition or other factors preclude the use of conventional airway techniques, and a more aggressive and invasive approach must be taken to secure the airway and maximize survival.

Two methods of securing a patent airway can be used when conventional techniques and methods fail: the open (surgical) cricothyrotomy and translaryngeal catheter ventilation (nonsurgical or needle cricothyrotomy). To perform these procedures, you must be familiar with the key anatomic landmarks that lie in the anterior aspect of the neck Figure 100 .

In addition, you must be familiar with the important blood vessels in this area. The superior cricothyroid vessels run at a transverse angle across the upper third of the cricothyroid membrane. The external jugular veins run vertically and are located lateral to the cricothyroid membrane. Therefore, the paramedic must use great care when incising the cricothyroid membrane.

When performing cricothyrotomy, you should expect to encounter some minor bleeding from the subcutaneous and small skin vessels as you incise the cricothyroid membrane. This bleeding should be easily controlled with light pressure after the tube has been inserted into the trachea.

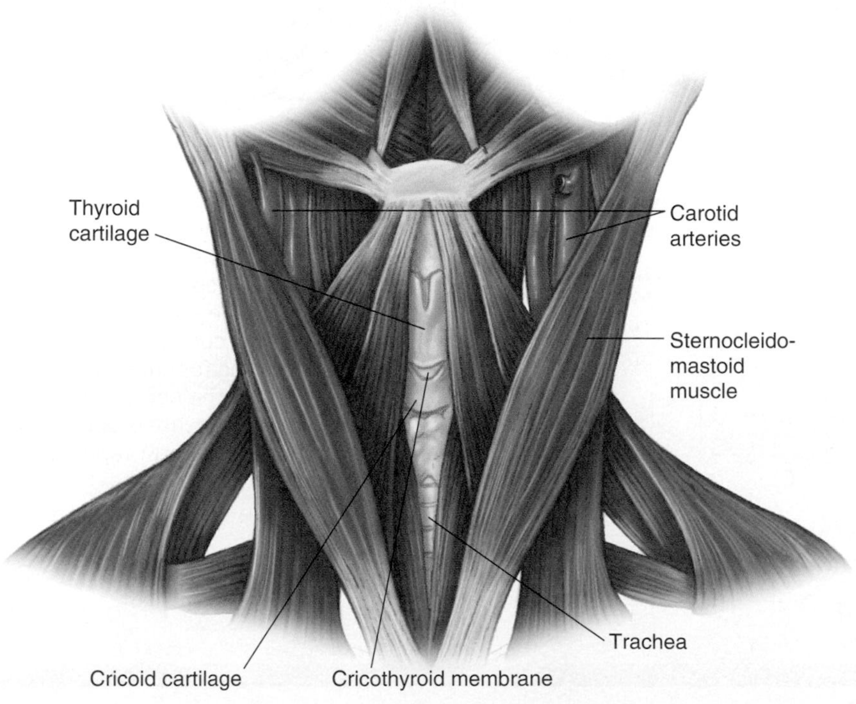

Open Cricothyrotomy

Open cricothyrotomy (surgical cricothyrotomy) involves incising the cricothyroid membrane with a scalpel and inserting an ET or tracheostomy tube directly into the subglottic area (below the vocal cords) of the trachea. The cricothyroid membrane is the ideal site for making a surgical opening into the trachea because no important structures lie between the skin and the airway. The airway at this level lies relatively close to the skin and is easy to enter through the thin cricothyroid membrane. The posterior wall of the airway at this level is formed by the tough cricoid cartilage, which helps prevent accidental perforation through the back of the airway into the esophagus.

There are several types of surgical cricothyrotomies. As previously discussed, open (surgical) cricothyrotomy involves incising the patient's skin and cricothyroid membrane and inserting an ET tube or tracheostomy tube. A modified cricothyrotomy is another type of cricothyrotomy. Several commercial modified cricothyrotomy kits are available, many of which use a modification of the **Seldinger technique** to enable placement of the airway. The Seldinger technique uses a needle and guide wire or guide catheter for tube placement in blood vessels or other hollow organs Figure 101 . Other devices for performing a cricothyrotomy, such as the Nu-Trake and Pertrach, are commercially manufactured airway placement devices that may be used in the prehospital setting. These devices do not use the Seldinger technique, but instead use a device that functions as an introducer and an airway Figure 102 .

Indications and Contraindications

Open cricothyrotomy is indicated when a patent airway cannot be secured with more conventional means. *It is not the preferred means of initially securing a patient's airway.* For example, if you are unable to intubate a patient but can provide effective bag-mask ventilations, cricothyrotomy would not be appropriate.

Situations that may preclude conventional airway management include severe foreign body obstructions of the upper airway that cannot be extracted with Magill forceps and direct laryngoscopy, airway obstructions from swelling (such as epiglottitis, anaphylaxis, and upper airway burns), massive maxillofacial trauma, and the inability to open the patient's mouth. Patients with massive maxillofacial trauma Figure 103 often have associated mandibular fractures, which makes it extremely difficult to maintain an effective mask-to-face seal with a bag-mask device. Intubation in patients with these injuries would also be extremely difficult because of posterior tongue lacerations with profuse bleeding. In such cases, frequent suctioning to prevent aspiration would delay intubation and increase hypoxia.

Figure 100 Anatomy of the anterior aspect of the neck.

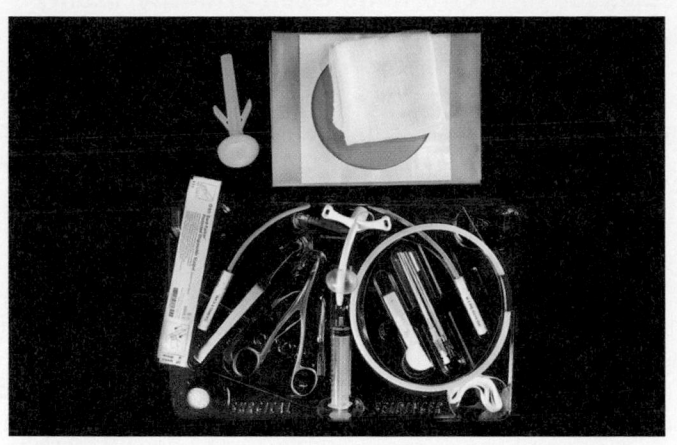

Figure 101   The Cook critical care Melker cricothyrotomy catheter kit.

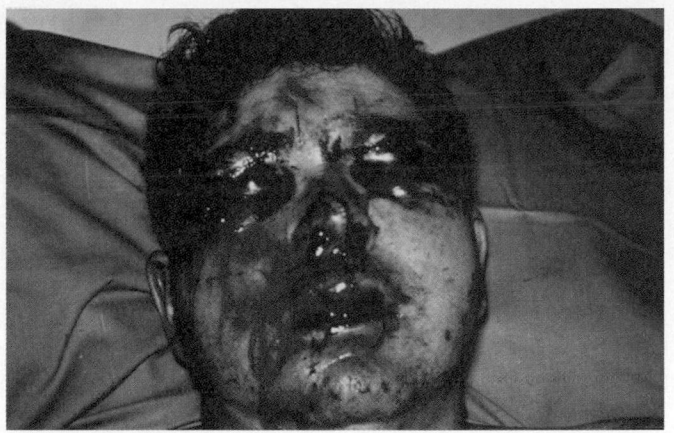

Figure 103   Patients with massive maxillofacial trauma often have mandibular fractures or profuse bleeding in the oropharynx, both of which can make bag-mask ventilations and intubation extremely difficult, if not impossible.

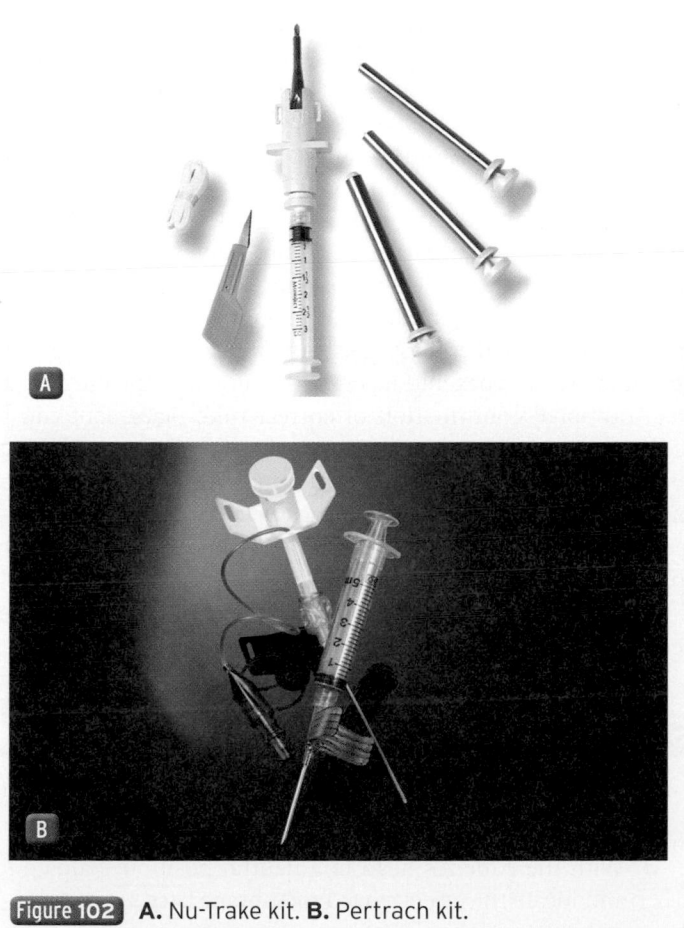

Figure 102   **A.** Nu-Trake kit. **B.** Pertrach kit.

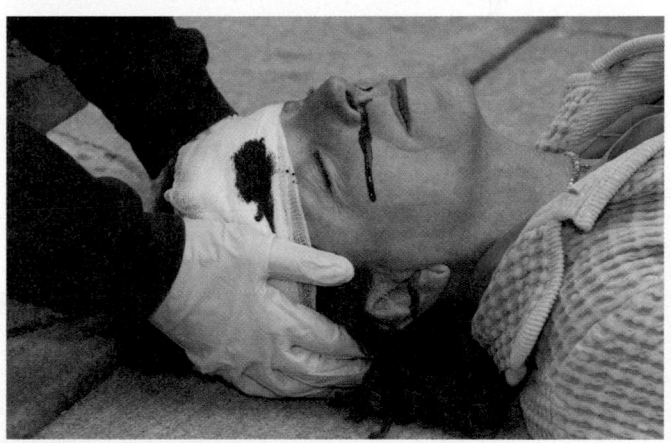

Figure 104   Endotracheal intubation may not be possible in patients with a head injury and trismus. Nasotracheal intubation is contraindicated in patients with head injury and fluid drainage from the ears or nose.

skull fracture or a fracture of the cribriform plate likely is present. If nasotracheal intubation is attempted, the ET tube or nasal airway may be placed into the cranial vault.

As noted earlier, the main contraindication for open cricothyrotomy is the ability to secure a patent airway by less invasive means. Other contraindications include the inability to identify the correct anatomic landmarks (cricothyroid membrane), crushing injuries to the larynx and tracheal transection, underlying anatomic abnormalities (such as trauma, tumors, or subglottic stenosis), and age younger than 8 years. The larynx of a small child is generally unable to support a tube large enough to produce effective ventilation without causing damage to the larynx; a needle cricothyrotomy (discussed later in this chapter) would be safer for young children.

In situations in which cricothyrotomy is contraindicated, the patient must be rapidly transported to the closest appropriate facility, where an emergency tracheostomy can be performed.

Patients with head injuries and trismus (clenched teeth) may require cricothyrotomy, especially if you do not have the resources or protocols to perform RSI. Furthermore, head injury, which is commonly accompanied by facial trauma, is a contraindication for nasotracheal intubation and placement of a nasopharyngeal airway, especially if fluid is draining from the patient's ears or nose Figure 104 . If this fluid is CSF, a basilar

Advantages and Disadvantages

Open cricothyrotomy can be performed quickly, and without manipulating the cervical spine. The latter characteristic is especially advantageous because many cricothyrotomies involve patients with massive facial trauma.

Disadvantages of cricothyrotomy include the difficulty encountered in performing the procedure in children, which is why it is contraindicated in children younger than 8 years of age, and in patients with short, muscular, or fat necks. In contrast with needle cricothyrotomy, an open cricothyrotomy is more difficult to perform; however, inserting a large-bore tube (such as an ET tube or a tracheostomy tube) permits achieving greater tidal volume, which facilitates more effective oxygenation and ventilation.

Complications

Some minor bleeding should be expected when an open cricothyrotomy is performed. More severe bleeding is usually the result of laceration of the external jugular vein. Incising the cricothyroid membrane vertically, instead of horizontally, will minimize the risk of this potential complication. It will also minimize the risk of damaging the highly vascular thyroid gland. After the incision has been made, gently inserting the tube will minimize the risks of perforating the esophagus and damaging the laryngeal nerves.

An open cricothyrotomy must be performed quickly. Taking too long to complete a cricothyrotomy will result in unnecessary hypoxia, which may result in cardiac dysrhythmias, permanent brain injury, and/or cardiac arrest.

> ### Words of Wisdom
>
> Frequent practice on a cadaver, if available, or a special cricothyrotomy manikin, will maximize your ability to perform cricothyrotomy quickly. In general, skills that are not frequently performed in the field should be routinely practiced to maintain proficiency and competence.

Tube misplacement should be suspected when subcutaneous emphysema is encountered after performing a cricothyrotomy. Subcutaneous emphysema occurs when air infiltrates the subcutaneous (fatty) layers of the skin and is characterized by a "crackling" sensation when palpated.

Any invasive procedure performed in the prehospital setting has the risk of infection to patients. Therefore, you should maintain aseptic technique to the extent possible when performing an open cricothyrotomy.

Equipment

If a commercially manufactured cricothyrotomy kit is not available, you must prepare the following equipment and supplies:

- Scalpel
- ET or tracheostomy tube (6.0 mm minimum)
- Commercial device (or tape) for securing the tube
- Curved hemostats
- Suction apparatus
- Sterile gauze pads for bleeding control
- Bag-mask device attached to 100% oxygen

Technique for Performing Open Cricothyrotomy

Once you determine that an open cricothyrotomy is needed, you must proceed rapidly, yet cautiously. Identify the cricothyroid membrane by palpating for the V notch of the thyroid cartilage, which feels like a high, sharp bump. Stabilize the larynx between your thumb and middle fingers while you palpate with your index finger. When you have located the V notch, slide your index finger down into the depression between the thyroid and cricoid cartilage; that is the cricothyroid membrane.

While you are locating and preparing the site, your partner should be preparing your equipment and ensuring that the cardiac monitor and pulse oximeter are attached to the patient.

Maintain aseptic technique as you cleanse the area with iodine; avoid touching the area once cleansed. While stabilizing the larynx with one hand, make a 1- to 2-cm vertical incision over the cricothyroid membrane. Some advocate making an additional 1-cm incision horizontally across the membrane to facilitate easier placement of the tube. If you do so, remember that the thyroid gland and external jugular veins are lateral to the area and can be damaged if the horizontal incision is too long. Once the incision has been made, insert the curved hemostats into the opening and spread it apart. Your partner should be readily available to control any bleeding that might occur.

With the trachea exposed, gently insert a 6.0-mm cuffed ET tube or a 6.0 tracheostomy (**Shiley**) tube and direct it into the trachea. Once the tube is in place, inflate the distal cuff with the appropriate volume of air—typically 5 to 10 mL. Attach the bag-mask device to the standard 15/22-mm adapter on the tube, and ventilate the patient while your partner auscultates to ensure the presence of bilaterally clear breath sounds and the absence of epigastric sounds. If epigastric sounds are heard, you have likely perforated the trachea and inserted the tube into the esophagus.

Additional confirmation of correct tube placement can be accomplished by attaching an ETCO$_2$ detector between the tube and bag-mask device. After confirming proper tube placement, ensure that any minor bleeding has been controlled, properly secure the tube, and continue to ventilate the patient at the appropriate rate.

The steps for performing an open cricothyrotomy are listed here and shown in Skill Drill 29 :

Skill Drill 29

1. Take standard precautions (gloves and face shield) Step 1 .
2. Check, assemble, and prepare the equipment Step 2 .
3. With the patient's head in a neutral position, palpate for and locate the cricothyroid membrane Step 3 .
4. Cleanse the area with an iodine-containing solution Step 4 .
5. Stabilize the larynx, and make a 1- to 2-cm vertical incision over the cricothyroid membrane Step 5 .
6. Puncture the cricothyroid membrane Step 6 .
7. Make a horizontal cut 1 cm in each direction from the midline. Spread the edges of the incision apart with curved hemostats Step 7 .
8. Insert the tube into the trachea Step 8 .

9. Attach an ETCO₂ detector between the tube and the bag-mask device (Step 9).

10. Ensure proper tube placement with waveform capnography. Attach the ETCO₂ detector to the monitor (Step 10).

11. Ventilate the patient (Step 11).

12. Confirm correct tube placement by auscultating the apices and bases of both lungs and over the epigastrium (Step 12).

13. Secure the tube with a commercial device or tape. Reconfirm correct tube placement, and resume ventilations at the appropriate rate (Step 13).

Skill Drill | 29

Performing an Open Cricothyrotomy

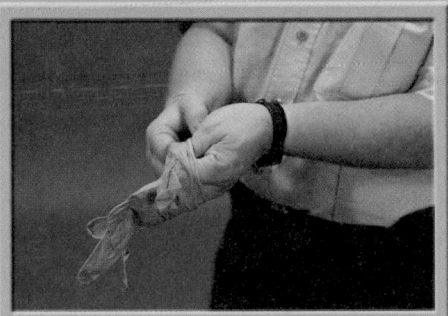

Step 1 Take standard precautions (gloves and face shield).

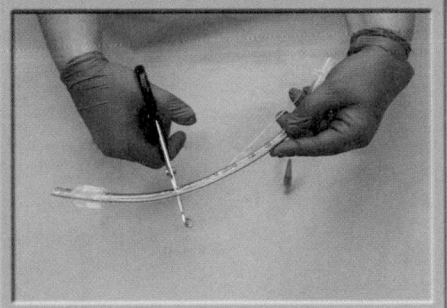

Step 2 Check, assemble, and prepare the equipment. Cutting the tube is shown here.

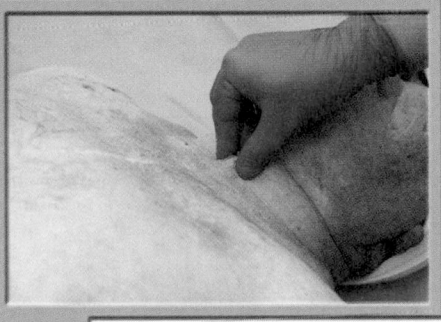

Step 3 With the patient's head in a neutral position, palpate for and locate the cricothyroid membrane.

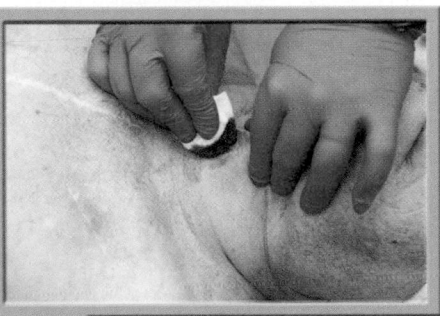

Step 4 Cleanse the area with an iodine-containing solution.

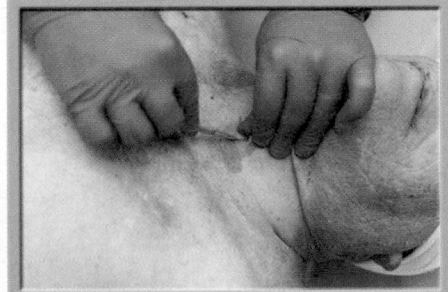

Step 5 Stabilize the larynx, and make a 1- to 2-cm vertical incision over the cricothyroid membrane.

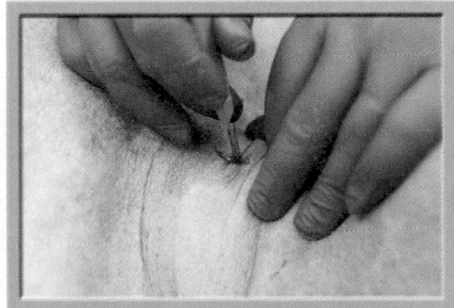

Step 6 Puncture the cricothyroid membrane.

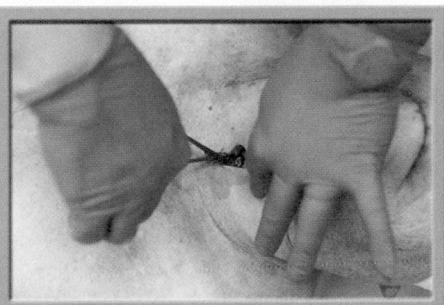

Step 7 Make a horizontal cut 1 cm in each direction from the midline. Spread the incision apart with curved hemostats.

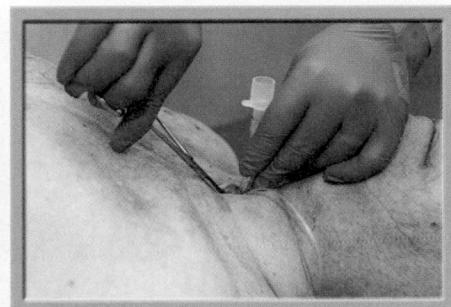

Step 8 Insert the tube into the trachea.

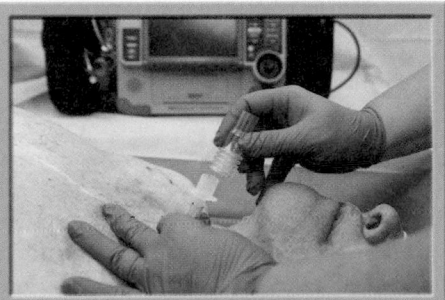

Step 9 Attach an ETCO₂ detector between the tube and the bag-mask device.

Continues

Skill Drill   29

Performing an Open Cricothyrotomy, continued

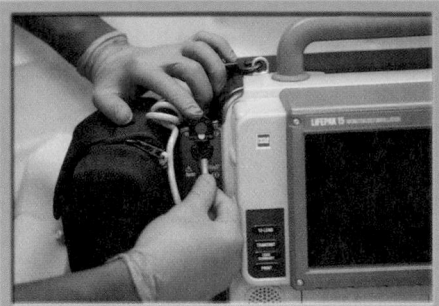

Step 10 Ensure proper tube placement with waveform capnography. Attach the ETCO₂ detector to the monitor.

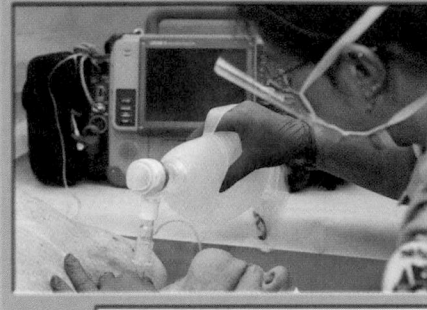

Step 11 Ventilate the patient.

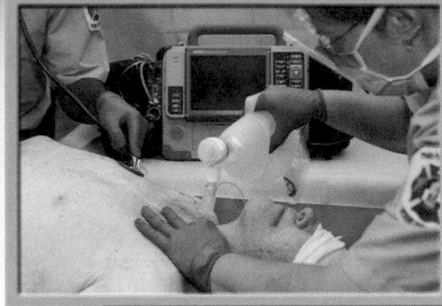

Step 12 Confirm correct tube placement by auscultating the apices and bases of both lungs and over the epigastrium.

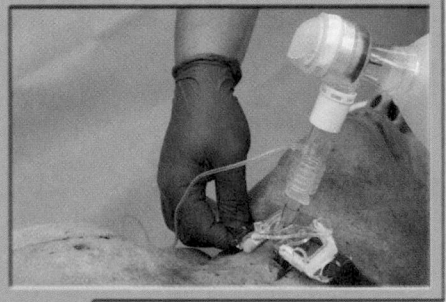

Step 13 Secure the tube with a commercial device or tape. Reconfirm correct tube placement, and resume ventilations at the appropriate rate.

■ Needle Cricothyrotomy

Needle cricothyrotomy also uses the cricothyroid membrane as an entry point into the airway. In this procedure, a 14- to 16-gauge over-the-needle IV catheter is inserted through the cricothyroid membrane and into the trachea. Adequate oxygenation and ventilation are then achieved by attaching a high-pressure jet ventilator (**Figure 105**) to the hub of the catheter. Known as **translaryngeal catheter ventilation**, this procedure is commonly used as a temporary measure until a more definitive airway can be obtained (such as open cricothyrotomy or tracheostomy).

Indications and Contraindications

The indications for needle cricothyrotomy and translaryngeal catheter ventilation are essentially the same as for the open cricothyrotomy—the inability to ventilate the patient by other, less invasive techniques; massive maxillofacial trauma; inability to open the patient's mouth; and uncontrolled oropharyngeal bleeding.

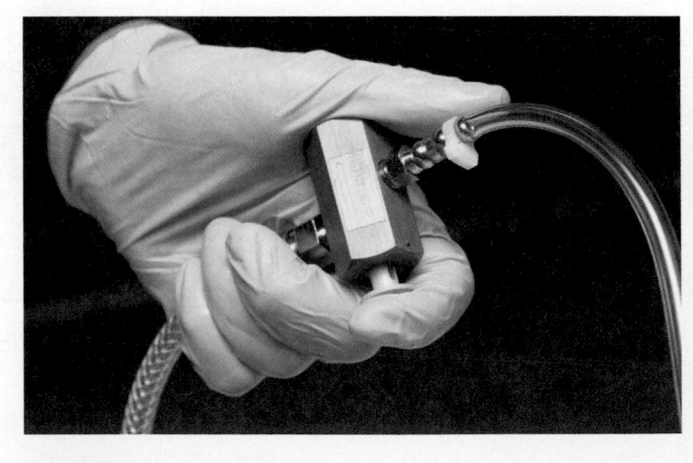

Figure 105 High-pressure jet ventilator.

Needle cricothyrotomy is contraindicated in patients who have a severe airway obstruction above the site of catheter insertion. Exhalation is not as effective with a small-bore catheter as with a large-bore tube (namely, an ET tube or a tracheostomy tube). In addition, exhalation via the glottic opening is not possible because the airway is completely obstructed above the catheter insertion site. As the result of minimal and ineffective exhalation, hypercarbia and hypoxia may occur. The high-pressure ventilator used with needle cricothyrotomy would cause an increase in intrathoracic pressure, resulting in **barotrauma** and a potential pneumothorax. Barotrauma can also be caused by overinflation of the lungs with the jet ventilator, so take care to open the release valve only until the patient's chest adequately rises.

If the equipment necessary to perform translaryngeal catheter ventilation is not immediately available, you should perform an open cricothyrotomy.

Advantages and Disadvantages

Compared with an open cricothyrotomy, needle cricothyrotomy is faster and technically easier to perform. In particular, it is associated with a lower risk of causing damage to adjacent structures because you are puncturing the cricothyroid membrane with an IV catheter—not incising it with a scalpel. Needle cricothyrotomy also allows for subsequent intubation attempts because it uses a small-bore catheter, thus allowing an ET tube to easily pass beside it. This advantage could be particularly beneficial if you do not have the equipment or protocols to perform an open cricothyrotomy. In addition, this procedure does not require manipulation of the patient's cervical spine.

Words of Wisdom

If you do not have the protocols to perform an open crico-thyrotomy and/or you do not have a jet ventilator on your ambulance, there is an alternative—albeit less effective—method of ventilating the patient via needle cricothyrotomy. Attach a 7- to 7.5-mm endotracheal (ET) tube adapter into the barrel of a 10-mL syringe. Next, connect the syringe to the intravenous catheter that has been inserted into the cricothyroid membrane. Connect the bag-mask device to the ET tube adapter, and begin ventilations. Although you will not be able to deliver nearly the tidal volume as would be possible with a jet ventilator, this approach may be your only alternative to provide some oxygenation and ventilation until a more definitive airway can be achieved at the emergency department.

There are, however, disadvantages to performing a needle cricothyrotomy. Using a smaller-bore tube (such as an over-the-needle IV catheter) to ventilate the patient does not provide protection from aspiration as an ET tube or tracheostomy tube would during an open cricothyrotomy (a larger-bore tube, combined with the distal cuff, would fill the diameter of the trachea, protecting it from esophageal regurgitation). Also, this technique requires a specialized, high-pressure jet ventilator to provide adequate tidal volume. This jet ventilator will expend high volumes of oxygen rapidly.

Complications

Improper catheter placement can result in severe bleeding caused by damage to adjacent structures. Even if the catheter is correctly placed, excessive air leakage around the insertion site can cause subcutaneous emphysema, especially if the patient has undetected laryngeal trauma. If too much air infiltrates into the subcutaneous space, compression of the trachea and subsequent obstruction may occur.

Extreme care must be exercised when ventilating a patient by using a jet ventilator. The release valve should be opened just long enough for adequate chest rise to occur. Overinflation of the lungs can result in barotrauma, which involves a risk of pneumothorax. Conversely, opening the release valve for too short a period could cause hypoventilation, resulting in inadequate oxygenation and ventilation.

Equipment

The following equipment is needed to perform needle cricothyrotomy and translaryngeal catheter ventilation:

- Large-bore IV catheter (14–16 gauge)
- 10-mL syringe
- 3 mL of sterile water or saline
- Oxygen source (50 psi)
- High-pressure jet ventilator device and oxygen tubing

Technique for Performing Needle Cricothyrotomy

When preparing your equipment, draw up approximately 3 mL of sterile water or saline into a 10-mL syringe and attach the syringe to the IV catheter. Next, place the patient's head in a neutral position, and locate the cricothyroid membrane. If time permits, cleanse the area with an iodine-containing solution.

While you are stabilizing the patient's larynx, carefully insert the needle into the midline of the cricothyroid membrane at a 45° angle toward the feet (caudally). You should feel a pop as the needle penetrates the membrane. After the pop is felt, insert the needle approximately 1 cm farther, and then aspirate with the syringe. If the catheter has been correctly placed, you should be able to easily aspirate air and see the saline or water bubbling within the syringe. If blood is aspirated or if you meet resistance, you should reevaluate catheter placement because it is likely outside the trachea.

After confirming correct placement, advance the catheter over the needle until the catheter hub is flush with the skin, then withdraw the needle and place it in a puncture-proof biohazard container. Next, attach one end of the oxygen tubing to the catheter and the other end to the jet ventilator.

Begin ventilations by opening the release valve on the jet ventilator and observing for adequate chest rise. Auscultation of breath and epigastric sounds will further confirm correct catheter placement. To prevent overexpansion of the lungs and subsequent barotrauma, turn the release valve off as soon as you see the chest rise. Exhalation will occur passively via the glottis. Ventilate the patient as dictated by his or her clinical condition.

Secure the catheter by placing a folded 4″ × 4″ gauze pad under the catheter and taping it in place. Continue ventilations while frequently reassessing the patient for adequacy of ventilations and for potential complications (such as subcutaneous emphysema from incorrect placement).

The steps for performing needle cricothyrotomy with translaryngeal catheter ventilation are listed here and shown in Skill Drill 30 :

Skill Drill 30

1. Take standard precautions (gloves and face shield) Step 1 .
2. Attach a 14- to 16-gauge IV catheter to a 10-mL syringe containing approximately 3 mL of sterile saline or water Step 2 .

3. With the patient's head in a neutral position, palpate for and locate the cricothyroid membrane Step 3 .
4. Cleanse the area with an iodine-containing solution Step 4 .
5. Stabilize the larynx, and insert the needle into the cricothyroid membrane at a 45° angle toward the feet Step 5 .
6. Aspirate with the syringe to determine correct catheter placement Step 6 .
7. Slide the catheter off of the needle until the hub of the catheter is flush with the patient's skin Step 7 .

Skill Drill 30

Performing Needle Cricothyrotomy and Translaryngeal Catheter Ventilation

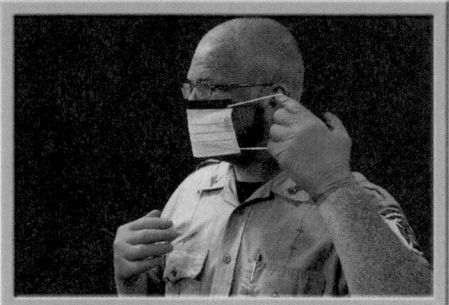

Step 1 Take standard precautions (gloves and face shield).

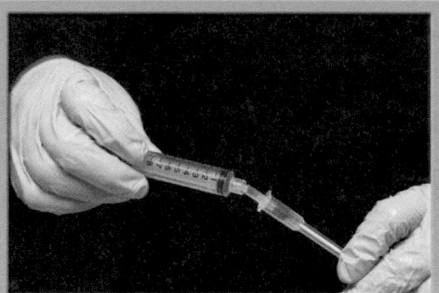

Step 2 Attach a 14- to 16-gauge IV catheter to a 10-mL syringe containing approximately 3 mL of sterile saline or water.

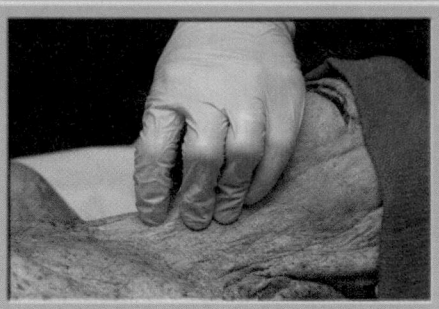

Step 3 With the patient's head in a neutral position, palpate for and locate the cricothyroid membrane.

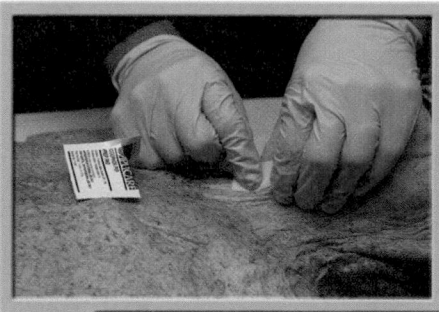

Step 4 Cleanse the area with an iodine-containing solution.

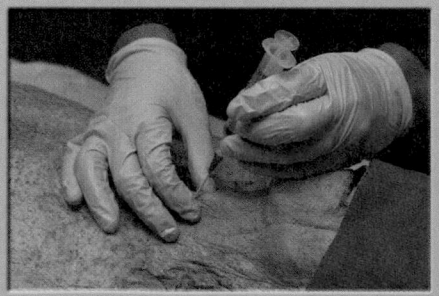

Step 5 Stabilize the larynx, and insert the needle into the cricothyroid membrane at a 45° angle toward the feet.

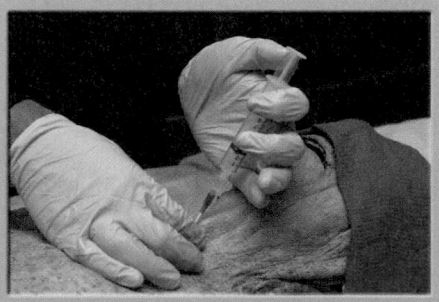

Step 6 Aspirate with the syringe to determine correct catheter placement.

Continues

Skill Drill 30

Performing Needle Cricothyrotomy and Translaryngeal Catheter Ventilation, continued

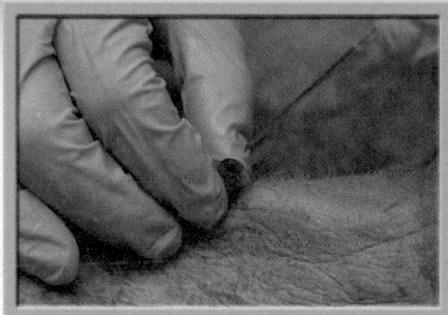

Step 7 Slide the catheter off of the needle until the hub of the catheter is flush with the patient's skin.

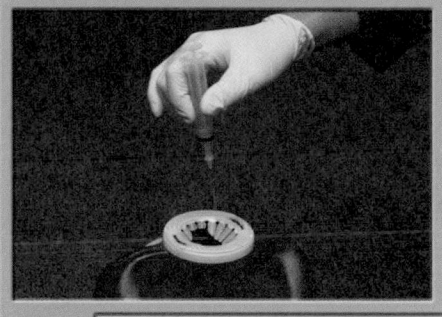

Step 8 Place the syringe and needle in a puncture-proof container.

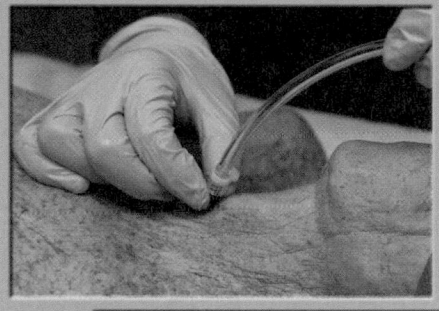

Step 9 Connect one end of the oxygen tubing to the catheter and the other end to the jet ventilator. Maintain manual stabilization of the catheter until it has been secured in place to avoid dislodgment with jet ventilation.

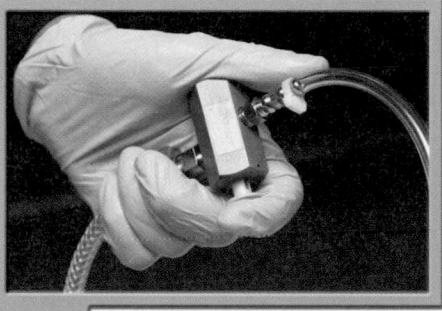

Step 10 Open the release valve on the jet ventilator, and adjust the pressure accordingly to provide adequate chest rise.

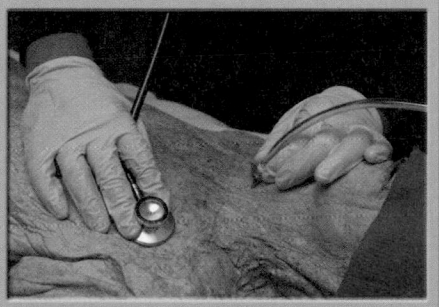

Step 11 Auscultate the apices and bases of both lungs and over the epigastrium to confirm correct catheter placement.

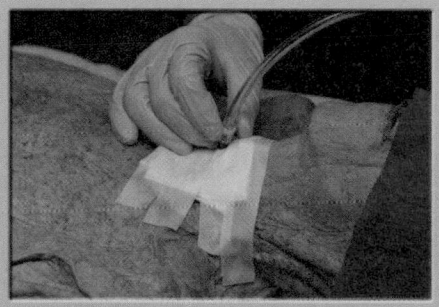

Step 12 Secure the catheter with a 4" × 4" gauze pad and tape. Continue ventilations while frequently reassessing for adequate ventilations and potential complications.

8. Place the syringe and needle in a puncture-proof container **Step 8**.

9. Connect one end of the oxygen tubing to the catheter and the other end to the jet ventilator **Step 9**.

10. Open the release valve on the jet ventilator, and adjust the pressure accordingly to provide adequate chest rise **Step 10**.

11. Auscultate the apices and bases of both lungs and over the epigastrium to confirm correct catheter placement **Step 11**.

12. Secure the catheter with a 4" × 4" gauze pad and tape. Continue ventilations while frequently reassessing for adequate ventilations and potential complications **Step 12**.

YOU *are the Medic*   SUMMARY

1. What should you anticipate as being your first priority on making contact with this patient?

After ensuring the safety of you and your partner and taking the appropriate standard precautions, your first priority when caring for any patient—especially one with a respiratory problem—is to obtain and maintain a patent airway. Patients who are conscious, alert, and talking obviously have a patent airway. However, patients with a decreased level of consciousness (LOC) have less than complete control over their own airway and often need some form of airway management.

Some patients only require manual positioning of the head to maintain the airway; others require manual positioning and a simple airway adjunct (namely, oral or nasal airway). If there are secretions in the patient's mouth, they must be immediately removed with suction. Depending on your ability to maintain the patient's airway with simple maneuvers, as well as factors such as your transport time to the hospital and the patient's clinical status, an advanced airway device (such as a King, LMA, Combitube, or ET tube) may be needed to maintain airway patency.

Without a patent airway, you cannot assess the patient's breathing adequacy or take steps to ensure adequate ventilation and oxygenation.

2. What is the difference between managing a patient's airway and ensuring adequate ventilation and oxygenation?

Airway management involves mechanical interventions aimed at ensuring that a patient's airway remains open (patent) and clear of secretions or foreign bodies. For example, the head tilt–chin lift and jaw-thrust maneuvers—both of which involve mechanical manipulation—are used to lift the tongue off of the posterior pharynx and align the airway structures, thereby providing a clear path for air to enter and exit the lungs. In some cases, simply opening the patient's airway with a manual maneuver will allow him or her to resume adequate breathing. Insertion of a simple airway adjunct (namely, oral or nasal airway) is another example of airway management. In conjunction with manual positioning, simple adjuncts maintain an open airway by preventing the tongue from occluding the glottic opening. Some patients have secretions, blood, or foreign bodies in the airway; this is an *immediate* threat to life and must be treated rapidly with suction or airway obstruction removal techniques (such as abdominal thrusts, laryngoscopy and foreign body removal with Magill forceps). In many cases, basic techniques of opening and maintaining a patent airway will enable you to adequately ventilate and oxygenate the patient. However, if basic interventions are not effective, an advanced airway device (such as the King, LMA, Combitube, or ET tube) should be inserted. These devices are designed to bypass the structures of the upper airway, thereby directly or indirectly isolating the trachea and allowing you to ventilate and oxygenate the patient. If a patient's airway is not properly managed, the processes of adequate ventilation and oxygenation cannot occur. *You must first provide a clear path for air to enter the lungs!*

Adequate ventilation means that the patient can move enough air into and out of his or her lungs spontaneously (without assistance) or that a paramedic can do so by providing

positive-pressure ventilation with a bag-mask device or pocket face mask or through an advanced airway device. To adequately oxygenate a patient, adequate ventilation must be established *first*. Oxygenation involves the delivery of sufficient oxygen to the circulatory system via the lungs and its subsequent binding to the hemoglobin molecules on the red blood cells for delivery to the body's tissues and cells.

Ventilation is the simple act of moving air into and out of the lungs; therefore, it is possible to ventilate but not oxygenate. An example of this is a pulmonary embolism; the patient is ventilating, but a pulmonary arterial blockage is impeding blood flow from the right side of the heart to the lungs where it can be reoxygenated. It is not possible, however, to oxygenate without adequate ventilation; if a patient cannot ventilate, how can he or she get air into the lungs to be oxygenated?

If the patient is breathing adequately, administer supplemental oxygen with a nonrebreathing mask or nasal cannula. However, if the patient is not breathing or is breathing inadequately (such as shallow breathing [reduced tidal volume], respirations that are too fast or too slow, or grossly irregular breathing pattern), you must provide some form of positive-pressure ventilation and ensure that supplemental oxygen is attached to the device used to ventilate the patient.

3. Is this patient maintaining his own airway spontaneously?

There is a difference between an "airway problem" and a "breathing problem." A critical part of the assessment process is to determine if the patient is able to maintain his or her own airway spontaneously or if you must intervene to maintain the airway. If a patient is conscious and alert, is able to speak, is not making abnormal airway sounds (such as snoring or gurgling), and is able to expel any secretions from his or her mouth, his or her airway is patent and self-maintained.

The patient appears to be maintaining his own airway at present, although this is no indication that he will be able to do this for the duration of your contact with him. He clearly has a breathing problem, as evidenced by his respiratory distress, accessory muscle use, preferential positioning, and inability to speak in complete sentences.

Never assume that a self-maintained airway will remain so—especially in a patient with a breathing problem. You must perform *frequent* assessments and be prepared to rapidly intervene. For example, if the patient's LOC begins to deteriorate, manual positioning (such as with the head tilt–chin lift maneuver) and a simple adjunct may be needed to help maintain the airway. If this approach is not effective, advanced airway management will be necessary. Remember, a compromised airway will not allow for adequate ventilation and oxygenation; watch your patient!

4. How should you proceed with your assessment of this patient?

After identifying and correcting any immediate threats to life (primary assessment), your next step in the assessment of a patient with respiratory distress should be to perform a rapid scan of the body to detect any other abnormalities and then obtain additional information that may help lead you to a field impression and treatment specific to the patient's condition (secondary assessment).

Use of the OPQRST (**O**nset, **P**rovocation/palliation, **Q**uality, **R**adiation, **S**everity, **T**ime of onset) mnemonic will help you obtain further information about the patient's breathing problem. For example, it is clinically significant that his respiratory distress was of an acute onset. This knowledge makes conditions such as pneumonia less likely, although not impossible, and conditions such as spontaneous pneumothorax or pulmonary embolism—both of which present acutely—more likely.

Further assessment of the patient with respiratory distress includes assessing oxygen saturation (Spo$_2$) and end-tidal CO_2 (ETCO$_2$); this quantitative information will enable you to assess the degrees of hypoxemia and hypercarbia, respectively. It is important to remember that oxygen is indicated for *any* patient with respiratory distress—regardless of pulse oximetry and capnometry/capnography readings.

When assessing a patient with respiratory distress, it is important to determine if the patient's problem stems from the upper airway or lower airway. Auscultating the patient's breath sounds will help differentiate an upper airway problem from a lower airway problem. Adventitious sounds such as wheezing, crackles, or rhonchi indicate a lower airway problem, while stridor indicates an upper airway problem.

Cardiac monitoring is also essential for any patient with a breathing problem. Hypoxemia can cause potentially life-threatening dysrhythmias, especially in patients with a history of cardiac disease. A 12-lead ECG is also indicated; in some patients, acute respiratory distress is the only presenting symptom of an acute coronary syndrome.

---

5. What information have you learned from the patient's ETCO$_2$ and pulse oximetry readings?

Oxygen saturation (Spo$_2$) reflects the percentage of oxygen that is bound to the hemoglobin in the blood. Spo$_2$ in a healthy adult who does not smoke should be greater than 95% while breathing room air. An Spo$_2$ of less than 95% indicates hypoxemia, while an Spo$_2$ of less than 90% indicates significant hypoxemia and the need for aggressive oxygenation. In addition to his low Spo$_2$ reading (90% with supplemental oxygen), the patient is anxious and tachycardic; these are also important clinical indicators of hypoxemia. It is important to note that hypoxemia and hypoxia are not the same. Hypoxemia is a decreased amount of oxygen in arterial blood. Hypoxia is a dangerous condition in which there is an inadequate supply of oxygen at the cellular level. Hypoxemia can often be reversed by simply administering supplemental oxygen; hypoxia may not be so easily reversed with supplemental oxygen and often requires more aggressive treatment, such as assisted ventilation. Pulse oximetry is a useful tool in your overall assessment of a patient with respiratory distress but should not replace a hands-on physical examination.

End-tidal carbon dioxide (ETCO$_2$) represents the amount of CO_2 (in mm Hg) that is eliminated from the body via the lungs. In a healthy adult, ETCO$_2$ should range between 35 and 45 mm Hg. A reading of less than 35 mm Hg indicates that the patient is eliminating too much CO_2 (hypocarbia). Low ETCO$_2$ readings

in a spontaneously breathing patient are often seen with hyperventilation and as a response of the respiratory buffer system to metabolic acidosis (such as in diabetic ketoacidosis and aspirin overdose). An ETCO$_2$ of more than 45 mm Hg, however, indicates that the patient is retaining CO_2 (hypercarbia) because of compromised ventilation.

Like pulse oximetry, capnometry and capnography are adjuncts to a comprehensive hands-on assessment of a patient with respiratory distress. Based on his current readings (↓ Spo$_2$ and ↑ ETCO$_2$), along with the findings of your physical exam, you should conclude that your patient is hypoxemic and hypercarbic. Therefore, you must carefully monitor his condition; if his LOC begins to deteriorate, it will likely be necessary to assist his ventilations with supplemental oxygen.

---

6. Is there a correlation between ETCO$_2$ and Paco$_2$? If so, what is it?

The partial pressure of carbon dioxide in arterial blood (Paco$_2$) is derived from the amount of carbon dioxide dissolved in the blood plasma and can be measured only by arterial blood gas (ABG) measurement. In a healthy person, the arterial Paco$_2$ should range between 35 and 45 mm Hg.

Although ETCO$_2$ and arterial Paco$_2$ both assess for hypercarbia, they measure the carbon dioxide level differently. Paco$_2$ is assessed by analyzing arterial blood, while ETCO$_2$ is assessed by noting the reading during breathing, specifically, exhalation. ETCO$_2$ can serve as an *approximate measurement* of a patient's arterial Paco$_2$. ETCO$_2$ is typically about 2 to 5 mm Hg lower than the Paco$_2$.

---

7. Why is this patient's condition deteriorating despite high-flow oxygen?

Despite high-flow oxygen via a nonrebreathing mask, your patient's condition has deteriorated significantly. His mental status indicates that he is no longer able to bring in enough oxygen to maintain adequate cerebral perfusion. During your initial contact with the patient, you found that he was experiencing respiratory distress, and although his Spo$_2$ and ETCO$_2$ indicated hypoxemia and hypercarbia, the fact that he was conscious and alert indicated that he was still able to compensate—through increased work of breathing—to maintain adequate cerebral perfusion.

Your patient's condition has deteriorated because he is no longer breathing adequately on his own. His respirations, in addition to being labored, are now shallow, and his respiratory rate has decreased *significantly* (from 26 breaths/min to 8 breaths/min); these are indicators that he has become fatigued because of hypoxia and worsened hypercarbia. Shallow breathing (reduced tidal volume [V_T]) and a marked decrease in respiratory rate will result in a reduction in minute alveolar volume (MV_A), which is affected by V_T, respiratory rate, or both.

Oxygen that is delivered passively, such as through a nonrebreathing mask or nasal cannula, can adequately oxygenate a patient provided that he or she has adequate ventilation—that is, adequate tidal volume and rate. It takes a certain volume to breathe oxygen from the delivery device into the lungs. When ventilation becomes compromised, passive oxygenation will be of little to no benefit.

YOU *are the Medic* | SUMMARY, *continued*

8. How must you adjust your current treatment?

When any patient's condition deteriorates, your first priority is to repeat the primary assessment and rapidly correct any problems with the ABCs. If a patient's LOC decreases, you must assume that he or she can no longer maintain his or her own airway. Manually open the patient's airway, assess the oropharynx for secretions (use suction as needed), and insert a simple airway adjunct. Because the patient is not completely unconscious and likely has a gag reflex, a nasopharyngeal airway would be appropriate. *Remember, you must correct an airway problem before you can treat a breathing problem.*

After ensuring a patent airway, you must quickly turn your attention to his breathing. His own respiratory effort is no longer adequate; therefore, he requires some form of positive-pressure ventilation assistance. Initially, this should be performed with a bag-mask device attached to supplemental oxygen, with the goal to restore tidal volume *and* adequate oxygenation.

Ventilate the patient at a rate of 10 to 12 breaths/min, and give each breath over 1 second–just enough to produce visible chest rise. Monitor the patient's Spo_2, $ETco_2$, pulse rate, and skin color while you are ventilating him. If your ventilations are effective, you should see an increase in his Spo_2, decreases in his $ETco_2$ and pulse rate, and improvement in his skin color. If these clinical signs are not observed or if you are experiencing difficulty ventilating him with a bag-mask device, you should proceed to advanced airway management.

9. Why must you use caution when providing positive-pressure ventilation?

When providing positive-pressure ventilation to a patient whose airway is not secured with an advanced device, you must use caution to minimize the incidence of gastric distention and the associated risks of regurgitation and aspiration. Ventilating the patient at an age-appropriate rate (10 to 12 breaths/min [one breath every 5 to 6 seconds] in an adult) and by delivering each breath over a period of 1 second while observing for visible chest rise is most effective.

If gastric distention impairs your ability to effectively ventilate the patient, invasive gastric decompression should be performed by inserting a nasogastric (NG) tube. An NG tube is often inserted after the airway has been secured with an advanced device. Even though the airway has been secured, gastric distention that occurred during bag-mask ventilation may make it difficult to adequately ventilate the patient after intubation has been performed.

Positive-pressure ventilation also affects cardiac output. Unlike normal breathing, which facilitates venous return to the heart (preload) through negative-pressure ventilation (the drawing of air into the lungs), positive-pressure ventilation (pushing air into the lungs) causes an increase in intrathoracic pressure, which increases the pressure against which the heart must pump (afterload). Increased intrathoracic pressure can also impair preload by literally squeezing the heart. As a result, positive-pressure ventilation can reduce a patient's cardiac output and cause hypotension.

For the reasons explained, you must carefully monitor the hemodynamic status (that is, blood pressure and pulse rate) of any patient who is receiving positive pressure ventilation. *Do not hyperventilate the patient*; doing so will increase the risk of hemodynamic compromise, whether the patient's airway is secured with an advanced device or not.

10. Is it necessary to adjust your current treatment? If so, how?

Despite assisted ventilation with high-flow oxygen, the patient's condition has not improved; in fact, it has deteriorated further. He is now unresponsive, he is still cyanotic and tachycardic, and his Spo_2 and $ETco_2$ readings have not improved.

Before proceeding to advanced airway management, you should troubleshoot what you are currently doing. This must be done quickly, however, or the patient's condition may deteriorate further and cardiopulmonary arrest may occur.

A common complication of using the bag-mask device is the inability to maintain an effective mask-to-face seal, especially if one rescuer is ventilating the patient, in which case he or she must maintain a mask-to-face seal with one hand and squeeze the bag with the other. If another rescuer is available, two-person bag-mask ventilation should be performed. Reevaluate the position of the patient's head; is it properly positioned? Does his chest visibly rise with each ventilation? Are you ventilating him at the appropriate rate? Does he have secretions in his airway that need to be removed with suction? Are you ventilating him with high-flow oxygen? In many cases, basic troubleshooting can identify why a patient's condition is not improving or is continuing to deteriorate.

If it is determined that you are ventilating the patient adequately, and the patient's condition is still deteriorating, it will be necessary to secure his airway with an advanced device.

There are several devices that would be suitable for this patient, such as a perilaryngeal airway (such as the Cobra-PLA), a supraglottic airway (such as the laryngeal mask airway [LMA]), or an ET tube. Devices that are inserted into the esophagus, such as the King LT and Combitube, however, are contraindicated for this patient because of his history of esophageal cancer.

In some cases, the advanced airway device you choose will be based on locally established protocol; it is not uncommon for medical directors to instruct paramedics to insert a CobraPLA or an LMA before attempting ET intubation. Either way, you must act quickly to secure the patient's airway and restore ventilation and oxygenation.

11. Should you extubate this patient? Why or why not?

No! Extubation–the process of removing the tube from an intubated patient–is rarely performed in the prehospital setting. Generally, the only reason to consider extubation in the field is if the patient is *unreasonably* intolerant of the ET tube (such as extremely combative, gagging, or retching). Your patient is moving his head and is *slightly* combative, which would not constitute unreasonable intolerance.

The most obvious risk associated with extubation is overestimating a patient's ability to protect his or her own airway. Furthermore, when extubation is performed on conscious or semiconscious patients, there is a high risk of laryngospasm, and most patients experience some degree of upper airway swelling due to the trauma associated with having a tube in the trachea. These two facts, along with the ever-present risk of vomiting, make successful reintubation challenging, if not impossible.

If you are not *absolutely* sure that you can reintubate the patient, do not remove the tube. Field extubation is absolutely contraindicated if there is *any* risk of recurrent respiratory failure or if you are uncertain that the patient can maintain his or her own airway spontaneously.

Because your patient is not unreasonably intolerant of the tube, it would be far more prudent to sedate him. Benzodiazepines, such as midazolam (Versed), lorazepam (Ativan), and diazepam (Valium) are commonly used to sedate intubated patients who are "fighting the tube." In addition to the sedative effects of benzodiazepines, they also induce amnesia, meaning that the patient will likely not remember being intubated. Depending on your local protocol, a neuromuscular blocking agent (paralytic) may also be considered, although this intervention largely depends on your transport time.

12. What are some possible causes of the patient's decreasing $ETCO_2$ and waveform height? What must you do to determine the cause?

Any change—especially an acute change—in $ETCO_2$ should prompt an *immediate* reassessment of ET tube placement. If the ET tube slips out of the trachea and into the esophagus, you will note an *acute and profound decrease* in $ETCO_2$ (leading to a complete loss of $ETCO_2$) and a rapidly decreasing waveform amplitude, which will eventually become flat. Remember, there is no carbon dioxide in the stomach, which explains the sudden loss of $ETCO_2$; there is no carbon dioxide to measure, so the capnographer will simply not display a number. Of course, disconnection of the capnography tubing from the cardiac monitor will also cause a sudden loss of $ETCO_2$ and a capnographic waveform; check your equipment.

If waveform capnography suggests ET tube dislodgement, immediately observe the chest for symmetric rise and fall and reauscultate the epigastrium and lungs fields. If breath sounds are heard and there are no sounds over the epigastrium, use another intubation confirmation device, such as a colorimetric capnographer or an esophageal detector device. It is important to remember that no one method of ET tube placement confirmation is infallible; several assessment techniques should be used. If breath sounds are not heard and gurgling is heard over the epigastrium, remove the ET tube immediately, insert a basic airway adjunct, and resume ventilations with a bag-mask device.

If you confirm that the patient is still correctly intubated, you should turn your attention to the rate at which the patient's ventilations are being assisted. A ventilation rate that is too fast (hyperventilation) will drive the patient's $ETCO_2$ reading down (and produce a smaller waveform) because too much carbon dioxide is being eliminated from the lungs. To correct this problem, ensure that the patient is being ventilated at the appropriate rate of 10

to 12 breaths/min. The rate of ventilation in an intubated patient is best guided by capnography, with the goal to maintain an $ETCO_2$ between 35 and 45 mm Hg. In most patients, you can maintain a therapeutic $ETCO_2$ with only slight variations in ventilatory rate.

Other causes of decreased $ETCO_2$ include decreased carbon dioxide production (such as in hypothermia, sedation, paralysis, and acidosis) and decreased carbon dioxide delivery to the lungs because of decreased cardiac output (such as in blood loss and cardiogenic shock). Hyperventilation can impair preload and cause a decrease in cardiac output as well.

13. What would you expect the patient's $ETCO_2$ reading and waveform to do if he was not being adequately ventilated?

If an intubated patient with spontaneous perfusion (that is, he or she has a pulse), is not being adequately ventilated, you should expect to see an increase in his or her $ETCO_2$ and an increase in the height of the capnographic waveform. This is typically an indication that the patient is not being ventilated fast enough (hypoventilation), resulting in pulmonary carbon dioxide retention. Remember that *any* change in $ETCO_2$ should prompt an *immediate* reassessment of ET tube placement using the methods previously described.

After confirming correct ET tube placement, reassess the rate at which the patient is being ventilated. Provided the patient has a pulse and the ET tube is still in the trachea, you should be able to restore a therapeutic $ETCO_2$ by increasing the rate of ventilation accordingly.

14. What impact does inadequate or absent ventilation have on respiration?

As previously discussed, ventilation is the movement of air into and out of the lungs. During normal (unassisted) breathing, ventilation occurs when the diaphragm and intercostal muscles contract, which causes an increase in the vertical and horizontal dimensions of the thoracic cavity. As a result, intrathoracic pressure falls below that of atmospheric pressure and air is drawn into the lungs (negative-pressure ventilation). By contrast, positive-pressure ventilation—the pushing or forcing of air into the lungs—is provided by the rescuer with a bag-mask or other ventilation device.

Respiration is the exchange of gases (oxygen and carbon dioxide) between the body and its environment. Pulmonary (external) respiration is the exchange of oxygen and carbon dioxide in the lungs, whereas cellular (internal) respiration is the exchange of oxygen and carbon dioxide at the cellular level. Both forms of respiration rely on the critical processes of ventilation *and* oxygenation.

If ventilation is inadequate or absent, oxygenation will be as well. Remember, oxygenation is not possible without ventilation. During ventilation (positive and negative pressure), oxygen is delivered to the lungs, where it diffuses across the pulmonary-capillary membrane and into the alveoli. At the same time, carbon dioxide, returning from the right side of the heart, diffuses out of the alveoli and is eliminated from the body during exhalation. After the exchange of oxygen and carbon dioxide in the lungs (pulmonary

YOU *are the Medic* | SUMMARY, *continued* |

[external] respiration), oxygen binds to the hemoglobin, is returned to the left side of the heart, and is distributed to the tissues and cells. If there is no mechanism to bring oxygen into the lungs (namely, ventilation), there is nothing to load onto the hemoglobin molecules of the red blood cells in the circulatory system *and* the body will retain carbon dioxide. Cellular (internal) respiration is not possible without pulmonary (external) respiration. In the absence of oxygen, the cells will transition from aerobic (with oxygen) to anaerobic (without oxygen) metabolism. The by-products of aerobic metabolism are carbon dioxide and water; the by-products of anaerobic metabolism are lactic and pyruvic acid. Acidosis impairs the body's ability to be oxygenated and *must* be treated as early as possible. Acidosis can be prevented by ensuring adequate ventilation *and* oxygenation. If ventilation *and* oxygenation are not quickly restored, the cells and, ultimately, the organism—that is, the patient—will die.

15. Is further treatment required for this patient at this time?

Compared with previous assessments, your patient's clinical status has markedly improved. However, the underlying cause of his respiratory problem has not been identified, and his condition will likely deteriorate without the treatment you are providing. Therefore, simply keep doing what you are doing and *closely* monitor his mental status, vital signs, ECG, Spo_2, and $ETCO_2$.

16. What actions should you take to troubleshoot acute deterioration of the condition of an intubated patient?

The importance of *frequently* reassessing an intubated patient cannot be overemphasized. Do not let your guard down when the patient's clinical status appears to be improving; it can deteriorate very quickly, and you must be able to rapidly identify and correct the problem.

Without doubt, the most lethal complication that can occur in an intubated patient is unrecognized dislodgement of the ET tube. In the back of a moving ambulance, breath sounds may be difficult to hear, and factors such as obesity and certain respiratory diseases that cause "stiff lungs" (such as COPD) can make chest rise less obvious—even if the patient is correctly intubated. Therefore, quantitative waveform capnography is absolutely critical and is the recommended method for ongoing confirming and monitoring of the placement of the ET tube. If you note the sudden loss of a numeric $ETCO_2$ reading and the capnographic waveform becomes flat, make sure that the tubing from the

in-line capnographer has not been disconnected from the cardiac monitor. If it has, simply reconnecting it should restore a numeric $ETCO_2$ value and waveform.

If an intubated patient's clinical status acutely deteriorates (such as cyanosis, increasing pulse rate, or decreasing Spo_2), immediately look at the numeric $ETCO_2$ reading and capnographic waveform. If a loss of a numeric $ETCO_2$ reading and waveform is noted, you should immediately remove the ET tube, insert a simple airway adjunct, and resume ventilations with a bag-mask device. Continuing to ventilate the patient through the ET tube and auscultating breath sounds—which may be difficult to hear over the drone of the ambulance engine—wastes time and deprives the patient of oxygen. If you observe stomach contents in the tube, extubation must occur immediately. If you are at the scene and it is reasonably quiet, reauscultating the lung fields and epigastrium would not be unreasonable. Use of qualitative devices, such as the esophageal detector device and colorimetric capnographer, has been shown to be of limited value; follow your local protocols regarding the use of these devices.

The mnemonic "DOPE" is an excellent tool for troubleshooting acute deterioration of the condition of an intubated patient. It stands for Displacement/dislodgement, Obstruction, Pneumothorax, and Equipment.

Assessing for tube dislodgement has already been discussed. If there are thick pulmonary secretions in the ET tube, you may note decreased compliance (increased resistance) while ventilating and can often hear gurgling in the tube. If this occurs, instill 3 to 5 mL of sterile saline down the ET tube and pass a flexible suction catheter down the tube to clear the secretions. If the suction catheter passes easily and you do not retrieve any secretions, look at the symmetry of the chest and reauscultate breath sounds. Asymmetrical chest movement and decreased or absent breath sounds on one side of the chest should alert you to the possibility of a pneumothorax. Other signs of a pneumothorax include decreased ventilation compliance, hypotension, tachycardia, and cyanosis. Treatment for a pneumothorax involves needle decompression on the affected side of the chest.

Finally, check the status of your equipment. Are high-flow oxygen and an oxygen reservoir attached to the bag-mask device? Is the bag-mask device defective? Have you depleted your oxygen source? Check from "patient to tank" to ensure that the cause of the patient's deteriorating status is not equipment malfunction.

EMS Patient Care Report (PCR)

Date: 11-02-11	**Incident No.:** 10111501	**Nature of Call:** Respiratory distress		**Location:** 201 East Grayson St	
Dispatched: 1620	**En Route:** 1621	**At Scene:** 1626	**Transport:** 1645	**At Hospital:** 1702	**In Service:** 1720

Patient Information

Age: 56 **Sex:** M **Weight (in kg [lb]):** 77 kg (171 lb)	**Allergies:** Codeine, contrast dye **Medications:** Lisinopril, furosemide, potassium chloride, digoxin, clopidogrel **Past Medical History:** CHF, HTN, AMI, esophageal CA **Chief Complaint:** "I can't breathe"

YOU *are the Medic*   SUMMARY, *continued*

Vital Signs

Time: 1631	BP: 128/70	Pulse: 120	Respirations: 26	Spo$_2$: 90%	ETCO$_2$: 49	ECG: Sinus tachycardia
Time: 1634	BP: 116/60	Pulse: 130	Respirations: 8	Spo$_2$: 80%	ETCO$_2$: 58	ECG: Sinus tachycardia
Time: 1637	BP: 110/58	Pulse: 128	Respirations: 8	Spo$_2$: 84%	ETCO$_2$: 56	ECG: Sinus tachycardia
Time: 1641	BP: 116/60	Pulse: 112	Respirations: 8	Spo$_2$: 94%	ETCO$_2$: 47	ECG: Sinus tachycardia
Time: 1646	BP: 122/64	Pulse: 104	Respirations: 10	Spo$_2$: 99%	ETCO$_2$: 28	ECG: Sinus tachycardia
Time: 1651	BP: 118/62	Pulse: 90	Respirations: 10	Spo$_2$: 99%	ETCO$_2$: 38	ECG: Normal sinus rhythm
Time: 1656	BP: 126/70	Pulse: 84	Respirations: 10	Spo$_2$: 100%	ETCO$_2$: 40	ECG: Normal sinus rhythm
Time: 1701	BP: 124/68	Pulse: 80	Respirations: 10	Spo$_2$: 100%	ETCO$_2$: 39	ECG: Normal sinus rhythm

EMS Treatment
(circle all that apply)

Oxygen @ __15__ L/min via (circle one): NC **(NRM)** Bag-mask device		**Assisted Ventilation**	**Airway Adjunct** NPA	CPR
Defibrillation	Bleeding Control	Bandaging	Splinting	**Other:** ET (tube size 7.5 mm) by direct visualization, cardiac monitoring, 12-lead ECG **Medication:** Midazolam Time: 1647 Dose: 5 mg Route: IV push **Medication:** Midazolam Time: 1655 Dose: 5 mg Route: IV push

Narrative

9-1-1 dispatch for a pt with "breathing problems." Arrived on scene and found the pt, a 56-year-old man, sitting on the couch leaning forward to breathe. He was conscious and alert. His airway was clear of secretions and foreign bodies; however, his breathing was obviously labored, he could speak only in minimal-word sentences, and he was using accessory muscles to breathe. His skin was notably pale and diaphoretic, and his radial pulses were rapid and weak. Administered high-flow oxygen via nonrebreathing mask and continued assessment. Breath sounds were diminished bilaterally, but equal, and chest wall movement was symmetric. Obtained initial vital signs and assessed pt's ETCO$_2$ (per capnography), which read 49 mm Hg. Cardiac monitor was applied and revealed sinus tachycardia without ectopy; 12-lead ECG revealed the same. The pt's wife states that his medical history includes congestive heart failure (CHF), hypertension, acute myocardial infarction × 2, and esophageal cancer. She further stated that he just completed his last round of chemotherapy and radiation 2 days ago and had been fine all day when he suddenly began experiencing difficulty breathing. His oral temperature was 97.9°F. The pt does not have any known history of respiratory problems and has never experienced acute exacerbation of his CHF. During the course of the assessment, the pt's condition markedly deteriorated; his mental status decreased, his Spo$_2$ decreased, his ETCO$_2$ reading increased, and cyanosis developed. Manually positioned pt's head, inserted nasopharyngeal airway, and began assisting pt's ventilations at 12 breaths/min with bag-mask device. Reassessment revealed no improvement and pt was now unresponsive; therefore, the decision to perform endotracheal intubation was made. Pt was successfully intubated and ET tube placement was confirmed by waveform capnography (ETCO$_2$ reading: 40 mm Hg), the presence of clear and equal breath sounds (auscultation time: 1638), and absent epigastric sounds. Began transport to the hospital and continued to monitor the pt's condition en route. His clinical status improved, and he became somewhat intolerant of the ET tube. Established vascular access and administered 5 mg of midazolam, with positive effect. Obtained second 12-lead ECG, which remained unchanged from previous tracing. Throughout remainder of transport, pt's condition continued to improve; his Spo$_2$, ETCO$_2$, and heart rate indicated hemodynamic stability, and spontaneous eye movement was noted. Additional midazolam was administered as needed for sedation. Cardiac monitoring revealed normal sinus rhythm without ectopy, and pt's vital signs remained stable. Delivered pt to emergency department staff and gave verbal report to receiving physician. ET tube placement was reconfirmed by waveform capnography (40 mm Hg) and auscultation of breath sounds, which were clear and equal bilaterally, and absent epigastric sounds. IV line was patent at time of pt care transfer. Medic 81 cleared the hospital and returned to service at 1716. **End of report**

Prep Kit

- The upper airway consists of all structures above the vocal cords—the larynx, oropharynx, nasopharynx, and tongue. Its functions include warming, filtering, and humidification of inhaled air.

- The lower airway consists of all structures below the vocal cords—the trachea, mainstem bronchi, bronchioles, pulmonary capillaries, and alveoli. Pulmonary gas exchange takes place at the alveolar level in the lungs.

- The diaphragm is the major muscle of breathing; it is innervated by the phrenic nerves. The intercostal muscles, the muscles between the ribs, are innervated by the intercostal nerves. Accessory muscles, which are used during times of respiratory distress, include the sternocleidomastoid muscles of the neck.

- The respiratory and cardiovascular systems work together to ensure that constant supplies of oxygen and nutrients are delivered to every cell in the body and that carbon dioxide and other waste products are removed from every cell.

- Ventilation, oxygenation, and respiration are crucial for the tissues to receive the needed nutrients.

- Ventilation is the act of moving air into and out of the lungs. For ventilation to occur, the diaphragm and intercostal muscles must function properly. Diffusion allows oxygen to transfer from the air into the capillaries.

- Changes in oxygen demand are regulated primarily by the pH of the cerebrospinal fluid (CSF), which is directly related to the amount of carbon dioxide dissolved in the plasma portion of the blood ($Paco_2$). The medullary respiratory centers in the brainstem control the rate, depth, and rhythm of breathing. Chemoreceptors monitor the chemical composition of the blood and provide feedback to the respiratory centers.

- Negative-pressure ventilation is the drawing of air into the lungs due to changes in intrathoracic pressure. Positive-pressure ventilation is the forcing of air into the lungs and is provided via bag-mask device, pocket mask, or mechanical ventilation device to patients who are not breathing (apneic) or are breathing inadequately.

- Oxygenation is the process of loading oxygen molecules onto hemoglobin in the bloodstream. Oxygenation may not occur if the environment is depleted of oxygen or if the environment contains carbon monoxide, which prevents oxygen from binding to hemoglobin.

- Respiration is the exchange of oxygen and carbon dioxide in the alveoli and tissues of the body. Cells normally perform aerobic respiration, which converts glucose into energy. Without oxygen, cells perform anaerobic metabolism, which cannot meet the metabolic demands of the cell. Ultimately, anaerobic metabolism will lead to cell death if the lack of oxygen not corrected.

- The primary breathing stimulus in a healthy person is based on increasing arterial carbon dioxide levels. The hypoxic drive—a backup system to breathe—is based on decreasing arterial oxygen levels.

- Conditions that can inhibit the body's ability to effectively deliver oxygen to the cells are many. With ventilation/perfusion ratio mismatch, ventilation may be compromised but perfusion continues, leading to a lack of oxygen diffusing into the bloodstream, which can lead to severe hypoxemia.

- Other factors that impede delivery of oxygen to cells include airway swelling, airway obstruction, medications that depress the central nervous system, neuromuscular disorders, respiratory and cardiac diseases, hypoglycemia, circulatory compromise, submersion, and trauma to the head, neck, spine, or chest.

- Hypoventilation and hyperventilation, along with hypoxia, can cause disruptions in the acid-base balance in the body that may lead to rapid deterioration in a patient's condition and death. When there is an excess of acid in the body, the fastest way to eliminate it is through the respiratory system. Excess acid can be expelled as carbon dioxide from the lungs. Conversely, slowing respirations will increase the level of carbon dioxide. Respiratory acidosis and respiratory alkalosis can result from a number of conditions and can be life threatening.

- Adequate breathing in the adult features a respiratory rate between 12 and 20 breaths/min, adequate depth (tidal volume), a regular pattern of inhalation and exhalation, symmetric chest rise, and bilaterally clear and equal breath sounds.

- Inadequate breathing features a rate that is too slow (< 12 breaths/min) or too fast (> 20 breaths/min), a shallow depth of breathing (reduced tidal volume), an irregular pattern of inhalation and exhalation, asymmetric chest movement, adventitious airway sounds, cyanosis, and an altered mental status.

- It is important to be able to recognize abnormal breathing patterns when assessing a patient. These include Cheyne-Stokes respirations, Kussmaul respirations, Biot (ataxic) respirations, apneustic respirations, and agonal gasps.

- While assessing breathing, auscultate breath sounds with a stethoscope. Breath sounds represent airflow into the alveoli. They should be clear and equal on both sides of the chest (bilaterally), anteriorly, and posteriorly. Abnormal breath sounds include wheezing, rhonchi, crackles, stridor, and pleural friction rub.

- The pulse oximeter measures the percentage of blood that is saturated with oxygen (Spo_2). This type of measurement depends on adequate perfusion to the capillary beds and can be inaccurate when the patient is cold, is in shock, or has been exposed to carbon monoxide.

- Peak expiratory flow is a fairly reliable assessment of the severity of bronchoconstriction. It is also used to gauge the effectiveness of treatment, such as inhaled beta-2 agonists (such as albuterol).

- End-tidal CO_2 ($ETCO_2$) monitors detect the presence of carbon dioxide in exhaled air and are important adjuncts for determining ventilation adequacy. These monitors can analyze air samples of a spontaneously breathing patient or can be used when an advanced airway has been inserted. Quantitative waveform capnography is the "standard" and is the most accurate method for monitoring $ETCO_2$.

- Patients with inadequate breathing require some form of positive-pressure ventilation; patients with adequate breathing who are suspected of being hypoxemic require 100% supplemental oxygen via a nonrebreathing mask. Never withhold oxygen from any patient suspected of being hypoxemic.

- Unrecognized inadequate breathing will lead to hypoxia, a dangerous condition in which the body's cells and tissues do not receive adequate oxygen.

- Regardless of the patient's condition, his or her airway must remain patent at all times. The first step in airway management is to position the patient. The recovery position involves placing the patient in a left lateral recumbent position. It is the preferred position to maintain the airway of unresponsive patients without traumatic injuries who are breathing adequately.

- The patient's head must be properly positioned. Manual airway maneuvers include the head tilt–chin lift, jaw-thrust (with and without head tilt), and the tongue-jaw lift.

- Clearing the airway means removing obstructing material; maintaining the airway means keeping it open, manually or with adjunctive devices.

- Oropharyngeal suctioning may be required after opening a patient's airway. Rigid (tonsil-tip) catheters are preferred when suctioning the pharynx. Soft, plastic (whistle-tip) catheters are used to suction secretions from the nose and can be passed down an endotracheal tube to suction pulmonary secretions.

- Oropharyngeal suction should be limited to 15 seconds in an adult, 10 seconds in a child, and 5 seconds in an infant.

- Airway obstruction can be caused by choking on food (or, in children, on toys), epiglottitis, inhalation injuries, airway trauma with swelling, and anaphylaxis. It is critical to differentiate between a mild (partial) airway obstruction and a severe (complete) airway obstruction.

- Chest compressions, finger sweeps (only if the object can be seen and easily retrieved), manual removal of the object, and attempts to ventilate is the recommended sequence of events to attempt to remove a foreign body airway obstruction in an unresponsive adult. Abdominal thrusts should be performed continuously in a responsive adult or child with an airway obstruction until the obstruction is relieved or he or she becomes unresponsive.

- Basic airway adjuncts include the oropharyngeal (oral) airway and the nasopharyngeal (nasal) airway. The oral airway keeps the tongue off of the posterior pharynx; it is used only in unresponsive patients without a gag reflex. The nasal airway is better tolerated in patients with altered mental status who have an intact gag reflex.

- Supplemental oxygen should be administered to any patient with potential hypoxia, regardless of his or her clinical appearance. Be familiar with oxygen cylinder sizes and their duration of flow, and always practice safety precautions when using oxygen.

- The nonrebreathing mask is the preferred device for providing oxygen to adequately breathing patients in the prehospital setting; it can deliver up to 90% oxygen when the flow rate is set at 15 L/min. The nasal cannula should be used if the patient cannot tolerate the nonrebreathing mask; it can deliver oxygen concentrations of 24% to 44% when the flowmeter is set at 1 to 6 L/min. Other types of oxygen-delivery devices include the partial rebreathing mask and Venturi mask.

- The methods of providing artificial ventilation—in order of preference—include the two-person bag-mask technique, mouth-to-mask with one-way valve and supplemental oxygen attached, manually triggered ventilation device, and the one-person bag-mask technique. Use extreme caution with the manually triggered ventilation, and never use this device in children and patients with thoracic injuries.

- Continuous positive airway pressure (CPAP) has been clinically proven to improve a patient's breathing by forcing fluid from the alveoli (in pulmonary edema) or dilating the bronchioles (in obstructive lung diseases and asthma). It involves the patient breathing against a certain amount of positive pressure during exhalation. CPAP has also been shown to reduce the need for intubation.

- Check for loose dental appliances in a patient before providing artificial ventilation. Loose dental appliances should be removed to prevent them from obstructing the airway; tight-fitting dental appliances should be left in place during artificial ventilation.

- Dental appliances should be removed before intubating a patient. Removing them after the patient has been intubated may result in inadvertent extubation.

- Patients with massive maxillofacial trauma are at high risk for airway compromise due to oral bleeding. Assist ventilations, and provide oral suctioning, as needed.

- Ventilating too forcefully or too fast can cause gastric distention, which can cause regurgitation and aspiration. Administering ventilations over 1 second—just enough to produce visible chest rise—will reduce the incidence of gastric distention and the associated risks of regurgitation and aspiration.

- Invasive gastric decompression involves the insertion of a gastric tube into the stomach. A nasogastric tube is inserted into the stomach via the nose; an orogastric tube is inserted into the stomach via the mouth.

- Patients with a tracheal stoma or tracheostomy tube may require ventilation, suctioning, or tube replacement. Ventilation through a tracheostomy tube involves attaching the bag-mask device to the 15/22-mm adapter on the tube; ventilation of a patient with a stoma and no tracheostomy tube can be performed with a pocket mask or bag-mask device. Use pediatric-size masks when ventilating a patient through a stoma.

Prep Kit, continued

- Unresponsive patients or patients who cannot maintain their own airway should be considered candidates for endotracheal (ET) intubation, the insertion of an ET tube into the trachea. In orotracheal intubation, the ET tube is inserted into the trachea via the mouth; in nasotracheal intubation (a blind technique), the ET tube is inserted into the trachea via the nose. Other methods of ET intubation include digital (or tactile) intubation, retrograde intubation, face-to-face intubation, and intubation with the use of a lighted stylet (transillumination).

- An important step in intubation is confirmation of tube placement. Continuous waveform capnography, in addition to a clinical assessment (such as auscultation of breath sounds and over the epigastrium and assessing for visible chest rise), is regarded as the most reliable method of confirming and monitoring correct placement of the ET tube.

- If an attempted intubation does not result in acceptable oxygen saturations, perform simple BLS maneuvers with an oral airway and/or nasal airway and a bag-mask device, and consider using another airway device.

- Tracheobronchial suctioning is indicated if the condition of an intubated patient deteriorates because of pulmonary secretions in the ET tube.

- Extubation should not be performed in the prehospital setting unless the patient is unreasonably intolerant of the tube. It is generally best to sedate an intubated patient who is becoming intolerant of the ET tube.

- Pediatric ET intubation involves the same technique as for adult patients, but with smaller equipment.

- Rapid-sequence intubation (RSI) involves using pharmacologic agents to sedate and paralyze a patient to facilitate placement of an ET tube. It should be considered when a responsive or combative patient requires intubation but cannot tolerate laryngoscopy.

- Drugs used for RSI include sedatives, such as diazepam (Valium) and midazolam (Versed), and neuromuscular blocking agents (paralytics) to induce complete paralysis. The latter agents are classified into depolarizing (succinylcholine) and nondepolarizing (such as vecuronium, pancuronium, and rocuronium) paralytics.

- Alternative airway devices, which may be used if ET intubation is not possible or is unsuccessful, include the Combitube, laryngeal mask airway, King LT airway, and Cobra perilaryngeal airway.

- Open (surgical) cricothyrotomy involves incising the cricothyroid membrane, inserting a tracheostomy tube or ET tube into the trachea, and ventilating the patient with a bag-mask device. Needle cricothyrotomy involves inserting a 14- to 16-gauge over-the-needle catheter through the cricothyroid membrane and ventilating the patient with a high-pressure jet ventilation device.

■ Vital Vocabulary

3-3-2 rule A method used to predict difficult intubation. A mouth opening of less than three fingers wide, a mandible length of less than three fingers wide, and a distance from hyoid bone to thyroid notch of less than two fingers wide indicate a possibly difficult airway.

abdominal thrust maneuver Abdominal thrusts performed to relieve a foreign body airway obstruction.

accessory muscles The muscles not normally used during normal breathing; include the sternocleidomastoid muscles of the neck, the chest pectoralis major muscles, and the abdominal muscles.

acetylcholine (ACh) A chemical neurotransmitter of the parasympathetic nervous system.

adenoid The pharyngeal tonsil; located on the posterior nasopharyngeal wall.

adventitious Abnormal.

aerobic metabolism The metabolism that can proceed only in the presence of oxygen.

afterload The pressure gradient against which the heart must pump. Increasing the afterload can decrease cardiac output.

agonal gasps Slow, shallow, irregular respirations or occasional gasping breaths; result from cerebral anoxia.

alveolar minute volume (V_A) The amount of air that actually reaches the alveoli per minute and participates in gas exchange.

alveolar volume Volume of inhaled air that reaches the alveoli and participates in gas exchange; equal to tidal volume minus dead space volume and is approximately 350 mL in an average adult; also called alveolar ventilation.

alveoli Balloonlike clusters of single-layer air sacs that are the functional site for the exchange of oxygen and carbon dioxide in the lungs.

anaerobic metabolism The metabolism that takes place in the absence of oxygen; the principal by-product is lactic acid.

anoxia An absence of oxygen.

anterograde amnesia An inability to remember events after the onset of amnesia.

anxiolysis The relief of anxiety.

aphonia The inability to speak.

apneustic respirations Prolonged gasping inspirations followed by extremely short, ineffective expirations; associated with brainstem insult.

arytenoid cartilages Pyramid-like cartilaginous structures that form the posterior attachment of the vocal cords.

aspiration The entry of fluids or solids into the trachea, bronchi, and lungs.

asymmetric chest wall movement Unequal movement of the two sides of the chest; indicates decreased airflow into one lung.

atelectasis Collapse of the alveoli.

atlanto-occipital joint The joint formed at the articulation of the atlas of the vertebral column and the occipital bone of the skull.

automatic transport ventilator (ATV) A portable mechanical ventilator attached to a control box that allows the variables of ventilation (such as rate and tidal volume) to be set.

bag-mask device A manual ventilation device that consists of a bag, mask, reservoir, and oxygen inlet; capable of delivering up to 100% oxygen.

barbiturates Sedative-hypnotic medications; include drugs such as thiopental (Pentothal, Trapanal) and methohexital (Brevital).

barotrauma Trauma resulting from excessive pressure.

benzodiazepines Sedative-hypnotic drugs that provide muscle relaxation and mild sedation; include drugs such as diazepam (Valium) and midazolam (Versed).

Biot (ataxic) respirations Irregular pattern, rate, and depth of respirations with intermittent periods of apnea; result from increased intracranial pressure.

Bourdon-gauge flowmeter An oxygen flowmeter that is commonly used because it is not affected by gravity and can be placed in any position.

Boyle's law States that the pressure of a gas is inversely proportional to its volume.

bronchi The main branches of the trachea; subdivide into smaller bronchi and bronchioles that conduct air into and out of the lungs.

bronchioles The subdivision of smaller bronchi in the lungs; made of smooth muscle and dilate or constrict in response to various stimuli.

bronchovesicular sounds A combination of the tracheal and vesicular breath sounds; heard where airways and alveoli are found, the upper part of the sternum and between the scapulas.

BURP maneuver The backward, upward, rightward pressure used during intubation to improve the laryngoscopic view of the glottic opening and vocal cords; also called external laryngeal manipulation.

butyrophenones Potent, effective sedatives; include drugs such as haloperidol (Haldol) and droperidol (Inapsine).

capnographer A device that attaches between the endotracheal tube and bag-mask device; provides graphic information about the presence of exhaled CO_2.

capnometer A device that performs the same function and attaches in the same way as a capnographer but provides a digital reading of the exhaled CO_2.

carboxyhemoglobin (COHb) Hemoglobin loaded with carbon monoxide (CO).

carina A ridgelike projection of tracheal cartilage located where the trachea bifurcates into the right and left mainstem bronchi.

cellular respiration A biochemical process resulting in the production of energy in the form of adenosine triphosphate; also called metabolism.

cerebrospinal otorrhea Cerebrospinal fluid drainage from the ears.

cerebrospinal rhinorrhea Cerebrospinal fluid drainage from the nose.

chemoreceptors Sense organs that monitor the levels of oxygen and carbon dioxide and the pH of the CSF and blood and provide feedback to the respiratory centers to modify the rate and depth of breathing based on the body's needs at any given time.

Cheyne-Stokes respirations A gradually increasing rate and depth of respirations followed by a gradual decrease with intermittent periods of apnea; associated with brainstem insult.

Cobra perilaryngeal airway (CobraPLA) A supraglottic airway device with a shape that allows the device to slide easily along the hard palate and to hold the soft tissue away from the laryngeal inlet.

colorimetric capnographer A device that attaches between the endotracheal tube and bag-mask device; uses special paper that should turn from purple to yellow during exhalation, indicating the presence of exhaled CO_2.

Combitube A multilumen airway device that consists of a single tube with two lumens, two balloons, and two ventilation ports; an alternative device if endotracheal intubation is not possible or has failed.

continuous positive airway pressure (CPAP) A method of ventilation used primarily in the treatment of critically ill patients with respiratory distress; can prevent the need for endotracheal intubation.

CO-oximeter A device that measures absorption at several wavelengths to distinguish oxyhemoglobin from carboxyhemoglobin.

crackles The breath sounds produced as fluid-filled alveoli pop open under increasing inspiratory pressure; can be fine or coarse; formerly called rales.

cricoid cartilage Forms the lowest portion of the larynx; also called the cricoid ring; the first ring of the trachea and the only upper airway structure that forms a complete ring.

cricothyroid membrane A thin, superficial membrane located between the thyroid and cricoid cartilage that is relatively avascular and contains few nerves; the site for emergency surgical and nonsurgical access to the airway.

curved laryngoscope blade A blade designed to fit into the vallecula, indirectly lifting the epiglottis and exposing the vocal cords; also called the Macintosh blade.

cyanosis Blue or purple skin; indicates inadequate oxygen in the blood.

dead space volume (V_D) Any portion of the airway that does not contain air and cannot participate in gas exchange.

depolarizing neuromuscular blocker A drug that competitively binds with the acetylcholine receptor sites but is not affected as quickly by acetylcholinesterase; succinylcholine is the only one.

digital intubation A method of intubation that involves directly palpating the glottic structures and elevating the epiglottis with the middle finger while guiding the endotracheal tube into the trachea by using the sense of touch.

direct laryngoscopy Visualization of the airway with a laryngoscope.

dorsal respiratory group A portion of the medulla oblongata where the primary respiratory pacemaker is located.

dysphonia Difficulty speaking.

dyspnea Difficult or labored breathing.

endotracheal (ET) tube A tube that is inserted into the trachea for definitive airway maintenance; equipped with a distal cuff, proximal inflation port, a 15/22-mm adapter, and centimeter markings on the side.

endotracheal intubation Inserting an endotracheal tube through the glottic opening and sealing the tube with a cuff inflated against the tracheal wall.

end-tidal CO_2 ($ETCO_2$) monitors Devices that detect the presence of carbon dioxide in exhaled air.

epiglottis A leaf-shaped cartilaginous structure that closes over the trachea during swallowing.

esophageal detector device A bulb or syringe that is attached to the proximal end of the endotracheal (ET) tube; a device used to confirm proper ET tube placement.

etomidate A nonnarcotic, nonbarbiturate hypnotic-sedative drug; also called Amidate.

exhalation Passive movement of air out of the lungs; also called expiration.

expiratory reserve volume The amount of air that can be exhaled following a normal exhalation; average volume is about 1,200 mL.

external respiration The exchange of gases between the lungs and the blood cells in the pulmonary capillaries; also called pulmonary respiration.

extubation The process of removing the tube from an intubated patient.

eyelash reflex Contraction of a patient's lower eyelid when the upper eyelashes are gently stroked; a fairly reliable indicator of the presence or absence of an intact gag reflex.

face-to-face intubation Performing intubation at the same level as the patient's face; used when the standard position is not possible. In this position, the laryngoscope is held in the provider's right hand and the endotracheal tube in the left.

fasciculations Brief, uncoordinated twitching of small muscle groups in the face, neck, trunk, and extremities; may be seen after the administration of a depolarizing neuromuscular blocking agent (succinylcholine).

fraction of inspired oxygen (FIO_2) The percentage of oxygen in inhaled air.

functional reserve capacity The amount of air that can be forced from the lungs in a single exhalation.

gag reflex An automatic reaction when something touches an area deep in the oral cavity that helps protect the lower airway from aspiration.

gastric distention The enlargement or expansion of the stomach, often with air; can be a complication of ventilating the esophagus instead of the trachea.

gastric tube A tube that is inserted into the stomach to remove its contents.

glossoepiglottic ligament The ligament between the tongue and the epiglottis.

glottis The vocal cords and the opening between them.

goblet cells Mucus-producing cells found mainly in the respiratory and intestinal tracts.

gum elastic bougie A flexible device that is inserted between the glottis under direct laryngoscopy; the endotracheal tube is threaded over the device, facilitating its entry into the trachea.

head tilt–chin lift maneuver Manual airway maneuver that involves tilting the head back while lifting up on the chin; used to open the airway of an unresponsive nontrauma patient.

hemoglobin (Hb) An iron-containing protein within red blood cells that has the ability to combine with oxygen.

Henry's law A law of gas that states that the amount of a gas in a solution varies directly with the partial pressure of a gas over the solution.

Hering-Breuer reflex A protective mechanism that terminates inhalation, thus preventing overexpansion of the lungs.

hilum The point of entry of blood vessels, nerves, and bronchi into each lung.

hyoepiglottic ligament The ligament between the hyoid bone and the epiglottis.

hyoid bone A small, horseshoe-shaped bone to which the jaw, tongue, epiglottis, and thyroid cartilage attach.

hypercarbia Increased carbon dioxide content in arterial blood.

hyperventilation A condition in which an increased amount of air enters the alveoli; carbon dioxide elimination exceeds carbon dioxide production.

hypocarbia Decreased carbon dioxide content in arterial blood.

hypoventilation A condition in which a decreased amount of air enters the alveoli; carbon dioxide production exceeds the body's ability to eliminate it by ventilation.

hypoxemia A decrease in arterial oxygen level.

hypoxia A lack of oxygen to cells and tissues.

hypoxic drive Secondary control of breathing that stimulates breathing based on decreased PaO_2 levels.

I/E ratio Inspiratory/expiratory ratio; an expression for comparing the length of inspiration with that of expiration, normally 1:2, meaning that expiration is twice as long as inspiration (not measured in seconds).

inhalation The active process of moving air into the lungs; also called inspiration.

inspiratory reserve volume The amount of air that can be inhaled in addition to the normal tidal volume.

internal respiration The exchange of gases between the blood cells and the tissues.

intrapulmonary shunting Bypassing of oxygen-poor blood past nonfunctional alveoli.

jaw-thrust maneuver A technique to open the airway by placing the fingers behind the angle of the jaw and bringing the jaw forward; used when a patient may have a cervical spine injury.

King LT airway A single-lumen airway that is blindly inserted into the esophagus; when properly placed in the esophagus, one cuff seals the esophagus, and the other seals the oropharynx.

Kussmaul respirations Deep, gasping respirations; common in diabetic ketoacidosis.

laryngeal mask airway (LMA) A device that surrounds the opening of the larynx with an inflatable silicone cuff positioned in the hypopharynx; an alternative device to bag-mask ventilation.

laryngectomy A surgical procedure in which the larynx is removed.

laryngoscope A device that is used in conjunction with a laryngoscope blade to perform direct laryngoscopy.

laryngospasm Spasmodic closure of the vocal cords.

larynx A complex structure formed by many independent cartilaginous structures that all work together; where the upper airway ends and the lower airway begins.

lung compliance The ability of the alveoli to expand when air is drawn into the lungs during negative-pressure ventilation or positive-pressure ventilation.

Magill forceps A special type of forceps that is curved, thus allowing paramedics to maneuver it in the airway.

Mallampati classification A system for predicting the relative difficulty of intubation based on the amount of oropharyngeal structures visible in an upright, seated patient who is fully able to open his or her mouth.

metabolism The chemical processes that provide the cells with energy from nutrients.

methemoglobin (metHb) A compound formed by oxidation of the iron on hemoglobin.

minute volume (V_M) The amount of air that moves in and out of the respiratory tract per minute.

multilumen airways Airway devices with a single long tube that can be used for esophageal obturation or endotracheal tube ventilation, depending on where the device comes to rest following blind positioning.

Murphy's eye An opening on the side of an endotracheal tube at its distal tip that permits ventilation to occur even if the tip becomes occluded by blood, mucus, or the tracheal wall.

nasal cannula A device that delivers oxygen via two small prongs that fit into the patient's nostrils; with an oxygen flow rate of 1 to 6 L/min, an oxygen concentration of 24% to 44% can be delivered.

nasal septum A rigid partition composed of bone and cartilage; divides the nasopharynx into two passages.

nasogastric (NG) tube A gastric tube is inserted into the stomach through the nose.

nasopharyngeal (nasal) airway A soft rubber tube about 6″ long that is inserted through the nose into the posterior pharynx behind the tongue, thereby allowing passage of air from the nose to the lower airway.

nasopharynx The nasal cavity; formed by the union of the facial bones.

nasotracheal intubation Insertion of an endotracheal tube into the trachea through the nose.

needle cricothyrotomy Insertion of a 14- to 16-gauge over-the-needle IV catheter (such as an Angiocath) through the cricothyroid membrane and into the trachea.

negative-pressure ventilation Drawing of air into the lungs; airflow from a region of higher pressure (outside the body) to a region of lower pressure (the lungs); occurs during normal (unassisted breathing).

nondepolarizing neuromuscular blockers Drugs that bind to acetylcholine receptor sites; they do not cause depolarization of the muscle fiber; examples are vecuronium (Norcuron) and pancuronium (Pavulon).

nonrebreathing mask A combination mask and reservoir bag system in which oxygen fills a reservoir bag attached to the mask by a one-way valve permitting a patient to inhale from the reservoir bag but not to exhale into it; at a flow rate of 15 L/min, it can deliver 90% to 100% inspired oxygen.

open cricothyrotomy An emergency incision of the cricothyroid membrane with a scalpel and insertion of an endotracheal or a tracheostomy tube directly into the subglottic area of the trachea; also called surgical cricothyrotomy.

opioids Potent analgesics with sedative properties; examples are fentanyl (Sublimaze) and alfentanil (Alfenta); also called narcotics.

orogastric (OG) tube A gastric tube inserted into the stomach through the mouth.

oropharyngeal (oral) airway A hard plastic device that is curved so that it fits over the back of the tongue with the tip in the posterior pharynx.

oropharynx Forms the posterior portion of the oral cavity, which is bordered superiorly by the hard and soft palates, laterally by the cheeks, and inferiorly by the tongue.

orotracheal intubation Insertion of an endotracheal tube into the trachea through the mouth.

orthopnea Positional dyspnea.

oxygen humidifier A small bottle of water through which the oxygen leaving the cylinder is moisturized before it reaches the patient.

oxygenation The process of adding oxygen, such as for delivery to the cells.

oxyhemoglobin (HbO_2) Hemoglobin that is occupied by oxygen.

palate The structure that forms the roof of the mouth and separates the oropharynx and nasopharynx.

palatine tonsils Paired lymphatic tissues that lie on the lateral walls of the palatoglossal arch and anterior to the palatopharyngeal arch.

palatoglossal arch The posterior border of the oral cavity.

palatopharyngeal arch The entrance from the oral cavity into the throat.

pancuronium A nondepolarizing neuromuscular blocking agent; used to maintain paralysis following succinylcholine-facilitated intubation; also called Pavulon.

paradoxical motion The inward movement of the chest during inhalation and outward movement during exhalation; the opposite of normal chest wall movement during breathing.

paralytics Drugs that paralyze skeletal muscles; used in emergency situations to facilitate intubation; also called neuromuscular blocking agents.

paranasal sinuses The frontal and maxillary sinuses.

parietal pleura Thin membrane that lines the chest cavity.

partial laryngectomy Surgical removal of a portion of the larynx.

partial pressure The amount of gas in air or dissolved in fluid, such as the blood; measured in millimeters of mercury (mm Hg) or torr.

partial rebreathing mask A mask similar to the nonrebreathing mask but without a one-way valve between the mask and the reservoir; room air is not drawn in with inspiration; residual expired air is mixed in the mask and rebreathed.

patent Open.

peak expiratory flow An approximation of the extent of bronchoconstriction; used to determine whether therapy (such as with inhaled bronchodilators) is effective.

pharynx The throat.

physiologic dead space Additional dead space created by intrapulmonary obstructions or atelectasis.

piriform fossae Two pockets of tissue on the lateral borders of the larynx.

pleural friction rub The result of an inflammation that causes the pleura to thicken, decreasing the pleural space and allowing the pleurae to rub together.

positive end-expiratory pressure (PEEP) Mechanical maintenance of pressure in the airway at the end of expiration to increase the volume of gas remaining in the lungs.

positive-pressure ventilation Forcing of air into the lungs.

preload The pressure of blood that is returned to the heart (venous return).

pressure-compensated flowmeter An oxygen flowmeter that incorporates a float ball in a tapered calibrated tube; the float rises or falls according to the gas flow in the tube; is affected by gravity and must remain in an upright position for an accurate reading.

primary respiratory drive The normal stimulus to breathe; based on fluctuations in Pa_{CO_2} and pH of the cerebrospinal fluid.

pulse oximeter A device that measures oxygen saturation (Sp_{O_2}).

pulsus paradoxus A drop in the systolic blood pressure of 10 mm Hg or more; commonly seen in patients with pericardial tamponade or severe asthma.

rapid-sequence intubation (RSI) A specific set of procedures, combined in rapid succession, to induce sedation and paralysis and intubate a patient quickly.

recovery position Left-lateral recumbent position; used in all unresponsive nontrauma patients who are able to maintain their own airway spontaneously and are breathing adequately.

reduced hemoglobin The hemoglobin after the oxygen has been released to the cells.

residual volume The air that remains in the lungs after maximal exhalation.

respiration The process of exchanging oxygen and carbon dioxide.

respiratory acidosis A pathologic condition characterized by a blood pH of less than 7.35 and caused by the accumulation of acids in the body from a respiratory cause.

respiratory alkalosis A pathologic condition characterized by a blood pH of greater than 7.45 and resulting from the accumulation of bases in the body from a respiratory cause.

respiratory rate The number of times a person breathes in 1 minute.

retractions Skin pulling between and around the ribs during inhalation; a sign of respiratory distress.

retrograde intubation A technique in which a wire is placed through the trachea and into the mouth with a needle via the cricoid membrane; the endotracheal tube is then placed over the wire and guided into the trachea.

rhonchi A continuous, low-pitched sound; indicates mucus or fluid in the larger lower airways.

rocuronium A nondepolarizing neuromuscular blocking agent; used to maintain paralysis following succinylcholine-facilitated intubation; also called Zemuron.

safe residual pressure The pressure at which an oxygen cylinder should be replaced with a full one; often is 200 psi.

sedation The reduction of a patient's anxiety, induction of amnesia, and suppression of the gag reflex, usually by pharmacologic means.

Seldinger technique A technique that involves inserting a needle with a syringe, then inserting a guide wire into the needle, removing the needle, making an incision, and inserting a catheter over the guide wire; the guide wire is then removed.

Shiley A type of tracheostomy tube.

sinuses Cavities formed by the cranial bones that trap contaminants from entering the respiratory tract and act as tributaries for fluid to and from the eustachian tubes and tear ducts.

stenosis A narrowing, such as of a blood vessel or stoma.

stoma In the context of the airway, the resultant orifice of a tracheostomy that connects the trachea to the outside air; located in the midline of the anterior part of the neck.

straight laryngoscope blade A blade designed to lift the epiglottis and expose the vocal cords; also called the Miller blade.

stridor A high-pitched inspiratory sound representing air moving past an obstruction within or immediately above the glottic opening.

stylet In the context of intubation, a semirigid wire inserted into an endotracheal tube to mold and maintain the shape of the tube.

succinylcholine chloride A depolarizing neuromuscular blocker frequently used as the initial paralytic during rapid-sequence intubation; causes muscle fasciculations; also called Anectine.

surfactant A proteinaceous substance that lines the alveoli; decreases alveolar surface tension and keeps the alveoli expanded.

therapy regulator A device that attaches to the stem of the oxygen cylinder and reduces the high pressure of gas to a safe range (about 50 psi).

thyroepiglottic ligament The attachment of the thyroid cartilage to the epiglottis.

thyroid cartilage The main supporting cartilage of the larynx; a shield-shaped structure formed by two plates that join in a "V" shape anteriorly to form the laryngeal prominence known as the Adam's apple.

tidal volume (V_T) A measure of the depth of breathing; the volume of air that is inhaled or exhaled during a single respiratory cycle.

tongue-jaw lift maneuver A manual maneuver that involves grasping the tongue and jaw and lifting; commonly used to suction the airway and to place certain airway devices.

tonsil-tip catheter A hard or rigid suction catheter; also called a Yankauer catheter.

total laryngectomy Surgical removal of the entire larynx.

total lung capacity The total volume of air that the lungs can hold; approximately 6 L in an average man.

trachea The conduit for all entry into the lungs; a tubular structure that is approximately 10 to 12 cm long and composed of a series of C-shaped cartilaginous rings; also called the windpipe.

tracheal breath sounds Breath sounds heard by placing the stethoscope diaphragm over the trachea or sternum; also called bronchial breath sounds.

tracheobronchial suctioning Inserting a suction catheter into the endotracheal tube to remove pulmonary secretions.

tracheostomy A surgical opening into the trachea.

tracheostomy tube A plastic tube placed within the tracheostomy site (stoma).

transillumination intubation A method of intubation that uses a lighted stylet to guide the endotracheal tube into the trachea.

translaryngeal catheter ventilation A method used in conjunction with needle cricothyrotomy to ventilate a patient; requires a high-pressure jet ventilator.

trismus Clenched teeth caused by spasms of the jaw muscles.

turbinates Three bony shelves that protrude from the lateral walls of the nasal cavity and extend into the nasal passageway, parallel to the nasal floor; they increase the surface area of the nasal mucosa, thereby improving warming, filtering, and humidification of inhaled air.

upper airway Consists of all anatomic airway structures above the level of the vocal cords.

uvula A soft-tissue structure that resembles a punching bag; located in the posterior aspect of the oral cavity, at the base of the tongue.

vallecula An anatomic space, or "pocket," located between the base of the tongue and the epiglottis; an important anatomic landmark for endotracheal intubation.

vecuronium A nondepolarizing neuromuscular blocking agent; used to maintain paralysis following succinylcholine-facilitated intubation; also called Norcuron.

ventilation The process of moving air into and out of the lungs.

ventral respiratory group A portion of the medulla oblongata that is responsible for modulating breathing during speech.

Venturi mask A mask with a number of interchangeable adapters that draws room air into the mask along with the oxygen flow; allows for the administration of highly specific oxygen concentrations.

vesicular breath sounds Soft, muffled breath sounds in which the expiratory phase is barely audible.

visceral pleura The thin membrane that covers the lungs.

vital capacity The amount of air that can be forcefully exhaled after a full inhalation; approximately 4,800 mL in an average man.

vocal cords White bands of tough tissue that are the lateral borders of the glottis.

V̇/Q̇ mismatch An imbalance in the amount of oxygen received in the alveoli and the amount of blood flowing through the alveolar capillaries.

waveform capnography A waveform display of exhaled carbon dioxide shown on a portable cardiac monitor/defibrillator.

wheezing A high-pitched whistling sound that may be heard on inspiration, expiration, or both; indicates air movement through a constricted lower airway, as with asthma.

whistle-tip catheters Soft plastic, nonrigid catheters; also called French catheters.

Assessment in Action

You and your paramedic partner are dispatched to a residence for a woman with "breathing problems." You arrive at the scene 4 minutes after being dispatched and are greeted at the door by the patient's husband, who tells you that his wife, who has congestive heart failure, "can't get enough air."

Your primary assessment reveals that the woman is conscious and alert but is experiencing obvious breathing difficulty. Her respirations are rapid and labored, her pulse is rapid and weak, and you notice dried blood around her mouth. Your partner applies high-flow oxygen as you continue your assessment.

1. Which of the following conditions would *not* impair pulmonary respiration?
   A. Increased surfactant
   B. Widespread atelectasis
   C. Fluid within the alveoli
   D. Increased alveolar surface tension

2. What would occur if an adult were breathing at a rate of 50 breaths/min?
   A. Increased tidal volume and increased minute volume
   B. Increased tidal volume and decreased minute volume
   C. Decreased tidal volume and increased minute volume
   D. Decreased tidal volume and decreased minute volume

3. In contrast with hypoxemia, hypoxia:
   A. is easily treated by administering supplemental oxygen.
   B. is defined as a deficiency of oxygen at the cellular level.
   C. can be ruled out in the prehospital setting with pulse oximetry.
   D. is defined as an absence of oxygen to the brain and vital organs.

4. As you are auscultating the patient's breath sounds, you hear diffuse crackles to the apices and bases of her lungs bilaterally. This finding indicates:
   A. widespread collapsing of the alveoli.
   B. fluid accumulation in the larger airways.
   C. air moving through narrowed air passages.
   D. mucus or fluid in the smaller lower airways.

5. One of the purposes of continuous positive airway pressure (CPAP) is to:
   A. increase tidal volume.
   B. improve cardiac preload.
   C. force fluid from the alveoli.
   D. reduce hypoxia during apnea.

6. You ultimately decide to administer CPAP to this patient. Her clinical status does not seem to be improving, so you consider whether you will need to perform rapid-sequence intubation. Which of the following findings is consistent with a "2" on the Mallampati airway classification scale?
   A. Entire posterior pharynx is fully exposed
   B. No posterior pharyngeal structures seen
   C. Posterior pharynx is partially exposed
   D. Posterior pharynx cannot be seen; base of the uvula visible

7. Medications used for the express purpose of facilitating endotracheal intubation include:
   A. rocuronium bromide.
   B. atropine sulfate.
   C. midazolam hydrochloride.
   D. lidocaine hydrochloride.

8. Any airway device that is designed to enter the esophagus is contraindicated in patients who:

    A. are in cardiopulmonary arrest.

    B. have ingested a caustic substance.

    C. require short-term ventilatory support.

    D. are in need of definitive airway care.

Additional Questions

You and your paramedic partner are treating a 55-year-old woman who presented with acute shortness of breath. She has a history of congestive heart failure, hypertension, and coronary artery disease. She is extremely restless and agitated and is experiencing marked respiratory distress. Your partner applies oxygen via nonrebreathing mask, which she quickly pulls away from her face. Auscultation of her lungs reveals diffuse rhonchi bilaterally. You apply CPAP to the patient, but again, she will not allow a mask to be placed on her face. She is showing signs of physical exhaustion, her heart rate is rapid and weak, and facial cyanosis is developing. Her SpO_2 reads 79% and her $ETCO_2$, per nasal/oral cannula, reads 60 mm Hg. You are approximately 25 miles away from the closest appropriate medical facility.

9. What action(s) must you take to prevent the development of respiratory arrest and subsequent cardiac arrest?

10. What $ETCO_2$ readings would you expect to see in a patient with persistent cardiac arrest versus a patient with return of spontaneous circulation?

11. How does external respiration differ from internal respiration?

12. In contrast to negative-pressure ventilation, what are the effects of positive-pressure ventilation on cardiac output?

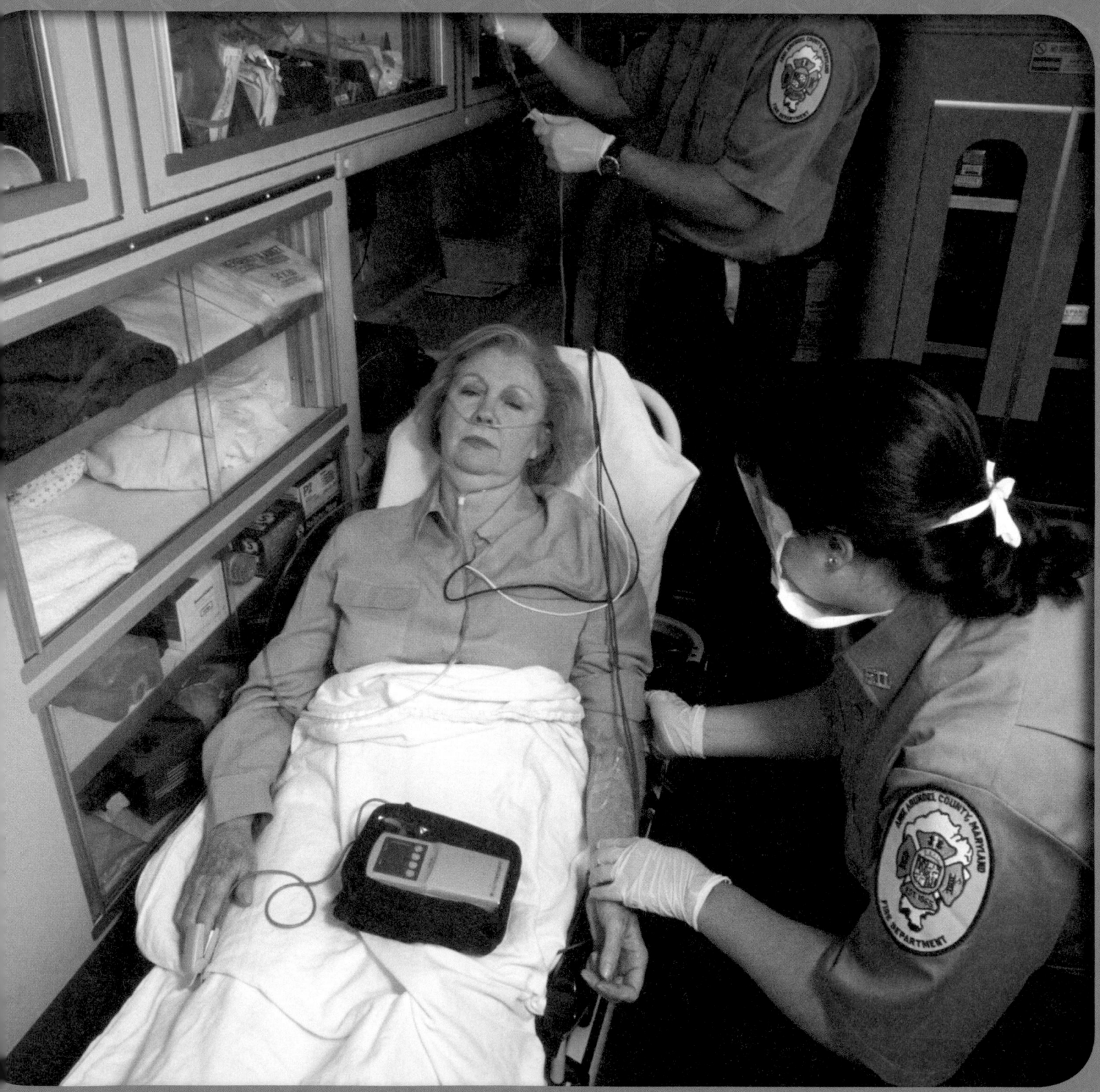

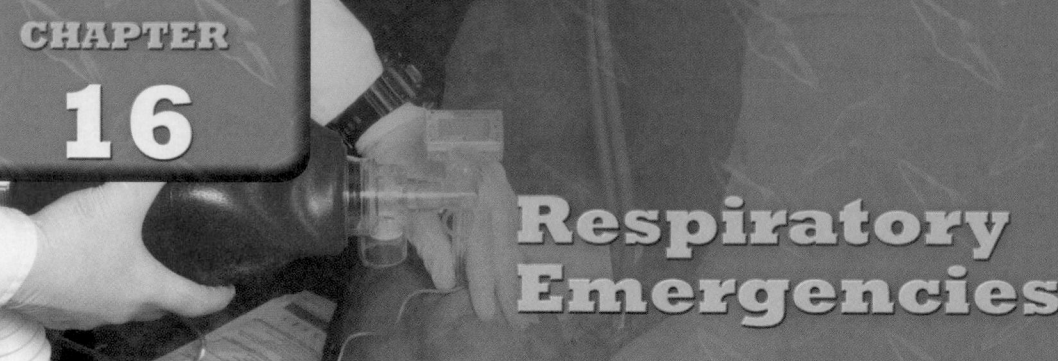

Respiratory Emergencies

National EMS Education Standard Competencies

Medicine

Integrates assessment findings with principles of epidemiology and pathophysiology to formulate a field impression and implement a comprehensive treatment/disposition plan for a patient with a medical complaint.

Respiratory

Anatomy, signs, symptoms, and management of respiratory emergencies including those that affect the

- Upper airway (pp 854-856)
- Lower airway (p 856)

Anatomy, physiology, pathophysiology, assessment, and management of

- Epiglottitis (pp 886, 887)
- Spontaneous pneumothorax (p 896)
- Pulmonary edema (p 895)
- Asthma (pp 888-890)
- Chronic obstructive pulmonary disease (pp 890-892)
- Environmental/industrial exposure (pp 894, 895)
- Toxic gas (pp 894, 895)
- Pertussis (p 898)
- Cystic fibrosis (p 898)
- Pulmonary embolism (pp 896, 897)
- Pneumonia (p 893)
- Viral respiratory infections (pp 892, 893)
- Obstructive/restrictive disease (pp 890-892)

Anatomy, physiology, epidemiology, pathophysiology, psychosocial impact, presentations, prognosis, and management of

- Acute upper airway infections (p 886)
- Spontaneous pneumothorax (p 896)
- Obstructive/restrictive lung diseases (pp 890-892)
- Pulmonary infections (pp 892, 893, 895)
- Neoplasm (p 894)
- Pertussis (p 898)
- Cystic fibrosis (p 898)

Shock and Resuscitation

Integrates comprehensive knowledge of causes and pathophysiology into the management of cardiac arrest and pre-arrest states.

Integrates a comprehensive knowledge of the causes and pathophysiology into the management of shock, respiratory failure, or arrest, with an emphasis on early intervention to prevent arrest.

Knowledge Objectives

1. Discuss the epidemiology, morbidity, and mortality of respiratory illness in the United States. (p 852)
2. Define hypoventilation and hyperventilation, and outline the conditions with which they are often associated. (pp 852-854)
3. List the structures of the upper and lower airways and accessory structures of the respiratory system. (pp 854-856)
4. List the three primary functions of the respiratory system. (p 861)
5. Explain how gas exchange occurs at the interface of the alveoli and the pulmonary capillary bed. (pp 858, 859)
6. Analyze the neurologic, cardiovascular, muscular, and renal mechanisms of respiratory control. (pp 861-863)
7. Analyze proper measures for ensuring scene safety when called to care for a patient with dyspnea. (p 863)
8. Describe the factors that contribute to a general impression of the patient's condition and an accurate estimation of his or her degree of respiratory distress. (pp 863, 864)
9. Discuss the typical presentation of a patient with dyspnea, and list the signs and symptoms that indicate a high level of respiratory distress. (p 864)
10. Explain the special patient assessment and care considerations for older adult patients with respiratory distress. (p 864)
11. Identify breathing alterations that may indicate respiratory distress, and become familiar with the signs of increased work of breathing. (p 864)
12. Describe the abnormal breathing patterns associated with neurologic insults that depress the respiratory center in the brain. (p 868)
13. Become familiar with the signs of lung consolidation, including abnormal breath sounds associated with excessive fluid in the lungs. (pp 865-868)
14. Explain how to assess the adequacy of the circulation of a patient with dyspnea. (p 869)
15. Discuss how transport decisions are made for patients with respiratory distress. (p 870)
16. Describe how to investigate the chief complaint of a patient who is having trouble breathing. (p 870)
17. Identify each component of the SAMPLE history as it applies to patients with dyspnea. (pp 871, 872)
18. List the over-the-counter medications likely to be used by patients with respiratory conditions, and explain what each is used for. (p 872)
19. Describe the components of the physical examination of a patient with dyspnea. (pp 873, 874)
20. Survey the devices used to monitor patients with respiratory complaints. (pp 874-877)
21. Describe interventions available for treating patients with dyspnea. (pp 880-886)

22. Discuss the pathophysiology, assessment, and management of a patient whose upper airway has an anatomic or foreign body obstruction. (p 886)

23. Discuss the pathophysiology, assessment, and management of a patient who has upper airway inflammation caused by infection. (pp 886-887)

24. Discuss the pathophysiology, assessment, and management of a patient who has aspirated food, liquid (including blood), or a foreign body. (pp 887, 888)

25. Discuss the pathophysiology, assessment, and management of a patient with an obstructive lower airway disease. (p 888)

26. List and explain the three features that characterize asthma and how each is treated. (pp 888-890)

27. Compare the signs and symptoms of asthma, emphysema, and chronic bronchitis. (pp 890, 891)

28. Discuss complications that can cause a patient with COPD to decompensate. (pp 891-892)

29. Explain the concepts of hypoxic drive and auto-PEEP as they relate to COPD. (p 892)

30. Discuss the pathophysiology, assessment, and management of patients with pulmonary infections, atelectasis, cancer, toxic inhalations, pulmonary edema, and acute respiratory distress syndrome. (pp 892-895)

31. Discuss the pathophysiology, assessment, and management of patients with pneumothorax, pleural effusion, and pulmonary embolism. (pp 896, 897)

32. Describe age-related variations in respiratory anatomy and the pathophysiology of respiratory disease. (pp 897, 898)

Skills Objectives

1. Demonstrate the process of history taking for a patient with dyspnea. (pp 870-872)

2. Demonstrate how to help a patient use a metered-dose inhaler. (pp 879, 880)

3. Demonstrate how to teach a patient to use a small-volume nebulizer. (p 879)

4. Demonstrate the application of a CPAP/BiPAP unit. (pp 883-885)

Introduction

Few reasons for dialing 9-1-1 are more compelling than the feeling of being unable to breathe (dyspnea). In most cases, respiratory distress is caused by a problem that originates in the respiratory system itself. This chapter examines some of those problems. The discussion begins with a survey of the anatomy and physiology of the respiratory system. The next topic is the assessment of a patient whose chief complaint is dyspnea—namely, which aspects to emphasize in obtaining the history and carrying out the physical examination. The chapter concludes with an in-depth look at some of the problems that may assault each component of the respiratory system—from the respiratory control centers in the brain to the alveolus, the smallest functional unit of respiration in the lung.

Epidemiology

Respiratory disease is one of the most common pathologic conditions, making respiratory distress one of the most common EMS dispatches. Asthma and chronic obstructive pulmonary disease (COPD) are among the top 10 chronic conditions that cause restricted activity. About 10% of people older than 65 years have COPD. Of all Americans, 15 million have asthma, resulting in a half million hospitalizations and 5,000 deaths annually. Pneumonia, described by Hippocrates in 400 BC, remains one of the most common fatal illnesses in developing countries, and it accounts for 6% of in-hospital deaths in the United States.

Some respiratory diseases, such as cystic fibrosis, are genetic (or intrinsic), while others, such as the occupational lung diseases, are caused by external (or extrinsic) factors. The cause of many respiratory diseases is a complex combination of factors that researchers have yet to fully decipher. In 80% to 90% of cases, COPD is related to cigarette smoking, for example, but 5% can be attributed to the genetic absence of a critical enzyme (alpha-1 antitrypsin). The cause of asthma is even more complex and may be affected by genetics, race, geographic location, diet, allergies, childhood illnesses, or some combination of these factors. Intrinsic factors such as genetics, cardiac disease, and even stress are often combined with extrinsic factors such as smoking and environmental pollutants, creating a multifactorial mechanism for respiratory illness.

Hypoventilation

When the lungs fail to work properly, carbon dioxide is not efficiently disposed of and accumulates in the blood. The carbon dioxide combines with water to form bicarbonate ions and hydrogen (H^+) ions, also known as acid (pH is an expression of how many free H^+ ions are in a solution). The result is acidosis.

Acidosis can occur if hypoventilation is not recognized. Impaired **ventilation** can be attributed to a variety of factors, as shown in Table 1. Each of these factors is examined in detail later in the chapter.

Table 1 Selected Causes of Impaired Ventilation	
Category of Impairment	**Conditions**
Upper airway obstruction	Foreign body obstruction Infection Trauma
Lower airway obstruction	Trauma Obstructive disease Increased mucus production Airway swelling (edema)
Chest wall impairment	Pneumothorax Flail chest Pleural effusion Restrictive disease (scoliosis, kyphosis)
Neuromuscular impairment	Overdose Lou Gehrig disease (amyotrophic lateral sclerosis) Carbon dioxide narcosis

YOU are the Medic   PART 1

You are dispatched to a medical alarm at a large, rent-assisted building complex. When you arrive, you and your partner grab your gear and head to the closest entrance to the building. You enter the apartment on the fifth floor and find a 74-year-old man with ashen gray skin who is diaphoretic and struggling to breathe. The patient lives alone and is speaking in 1- to 2-word sentences.

1. What initial "from the door" findings make you concerned for this patient?
2. What are your priorities for this patient?

The carbon dioxide level is also directly related to pH (acid-base balance). Patients who are hyperventilating usually have respiratory alkalosis. As their carbon dioxide level dips, their pH level rises. Patients who are hypoventilating usually have respiratory acidosis. As their carbon dioxide level goes up, their pH level drops.

Many types of problems can cause patients to **hypoventilate**:

- **Conditions that impair lung function.** When a patient is breathing but gas exchange is impaired, the carbon dioxide level rises. This situation can happen in severe cases of atelectasis, pneumonia, pulmonary edema, asthma, and COPD.
- **Conditions that impair the mechanics of breathing.** Gas flow can be suppressed by a high cervical fracture, flail chest, diaphragmatic rupture, severe **retractions**, an abdomen full of air or blood, abdominal or chest binding (using a pneumatic antishock garment or immobilization straps), and anything else that restricts the pressure changes that facilitate respiration.

  Obesity hypoventilation syndrome (also known as pickwickian syndrome) is respiratory compromise related to morbid obesity. One of the earliest descriptions of the combination of obesity, respiratory compromise, and sleep apnea is found in the character of Joe the "fat boy" in Charles Dickens's *Pickwick Papers*. Joe would fall asleep in midsentence, snore loudly, and generally have signs of hypercapnia. This syndrome is not on the decline, given the nationwide increase in obesity.

- **Conditions that impair the neuromuscular apparatus.** Patients who have had head trauma, intracranial infections, or brain tumors may have damage to the respiratory centers of the brain, which in turn may compromise ventilation. Serious injury to the spinal cord (above the level of the fifth cervical vertebra [C5]) may block the nerve impulses that stimulate breathing. **Guillain-Barré syndrome**, in which progressive muscle weakness and paralysis that move up the body from the feet, can result in ineffective breathing if the paralysis reaches the diaphragm. Amyotrophic lateral sclerosis (also known as Lou Gehrig disease) also causes progressive muscle weakness. This disease is fatal, with death usually attributable to respiratory failure as the muscles of respiration become unable to maintain adequate ventilation.

  Botulism is caused by the bacterium *Clostridium botulinum*. Although somewhat rare, it is usually caused by food poisoning or by giving infants raw (unpasteurized) honey, which may be contaminated with spores of the bacterium. Botulism can cause muscle paralysis and is usually fatal when it reaches the muscles of respiration.

- **Conditions that reduce respiratory drive.** Perhaps the most common hypoventilation crisis paramedics see is acute heroin overdose. Intoxication with alcohol, narcotics, and a host of other drugs and toxins can reduce the respiratory drive. Head injury, hypoxic drive, and asphyxia are all associated with grossly low respiratory rates and volumes.

The ultimate expression of hypoventilation is respiratory arrest followed by cardiac arrest.

In these circumstances, aggressive treatment must be initiated to assist the patient's respiratory efforts.

■ Hyperventilation

Hyperventilation occurs when people breathe in excess of metabolic need by increasing the rate or depth of respiration or both, releasing more carbon dioxide than normal. The result is alkalosis. When this cycle is triggered by emotional distress or a panic attack, it may be called hysterical hyperventilation or hyperventilation syndrome. The falling carbon dioxide level may make the person feel short of breath, so the person tends to become even more anxious and breathe even more rapidly and deeply. In acute hyperventilation syndrome, patients usually feel as if they cannot breathe at all. Hyperventilation that is not caused by some metabolic crisis is usually self-limiting.

Respiratory alkalosis causes numbness or tingling in the hands and feet and around the mouth. If it continues, patients may complain of chest pain and will ultimately experience **carpopedal spasm**, during which the hands and feet are clenched into a clawlike position. These symptoms frighten the patient even further and usually make him or her hyperventilate even more. A hysterical patient may eventually lose consciousness, but not before experiencing extreme distress. If the patient does not calm down and stop hyperventilating on awakening, the process could repeat itself.

The traditional therapy for hyperventilation called for patients to rebreathe their own carbon dioxide from a paper bag or from a partial rebreathing mask set at 21% oxygen (in other words, not attached to supplemental oxygen). This practice can be dangerous for two important reasons:

1. Patients quickly exhaust the oxygen in the gas they are breathing (and rebreathing). Hyperventilation does not mean that the patient has too much oxygen, but rather that he or she is releasing too much carbon dioxide. Rebreathing carbon dioxide can cause hypoxia, which is counterproductive when trying to stop a relatively benign hyperventilation episode.
2. Hyperventilation in a patient with acidosis might represent the body's attempt to drive the pH level back up to normal. In a patient with diabetic ketoacidosis, for example, too much acid is produced because of inadequate glucose metabolism, so the body attempts to compensate for the acidosis by hyperventilation (**Kussmaul respirations**). A variety of overdoses, toxic exposures, and metabolic abnormalities can also produce acidosis and compensatory hyperventilation, and *none should be treated by rebreathing carbon dioxide*. Never conclude that a patient is "just hyperventilating" until all possible causes of the presentation have been ruled out, which is difficult or perhaps impossible in the field.

Ultimately, treatment may include sedating a person who is truly hysterical and is hyperventilating, but that rarely occurs in the field. Frequently, hyperventilation is triggered by an emotional stressor, such as a family fight or receiving distressing news. More often than not, a variety of psychological support techniques will help. An important part of patient care is to help the patient understand that if the behavior that precipitated the hyperventilation is repeated, the hyperventilation will likely recur.

Other psychological support techniques include breathing with the patient, having the patient count to two between breaths (gradually increasing to higher numbers), and various distraction techniques (such as asking the patient to recount his or her life story). Sometimes singing a song with the patient will require him or her to use some breathing control and will terminate the episode. Help the patient not feed into the anxieties by using the aforementioned techniques.

■ Anatomy and Physiology

The primary structures of the respiratory system are often compared with an inverted tree, with the trachea representing the trunk and the <u>alveoli</u> resembling the leaves. That is a useful analogy, but in reality, a tree would have to branch 24 times and have nearly a billion leaves to match the intricacy of the respiratory system **Figure 1**. Imagine attempting to pull fluid from the ground into the leaves by exerting negative pressure at the leaf ends, and the complexities of breathing become apparent.

■ Structures of the Upper Airway

Nostrils and Nose
Air enters the upper airway primarily through the nares (nostrils) of the nose. Nares are lined with nasal hairs, which serve as filters to catch particulate matter. The external nares are separated by the nasal septum. Quiet breathing usually allows air to flow through the nose. Even people who breathe through their mouths usually have some nasal airflow.

Turbinates
After passing through the nares, air is pulled across the <u>turbinates</u> (sometimes called conchae). These highly vascular ridges of tissue are covered with a mucous membrane that traps particulate matter. The large surface area of the turbinates allows air to be warmed and humidified as it passes through **Figure 2**. Processes such as intubation and <u>tracheotomy</u> force inhaled air to bypass the nose, therefore bypassing the humidification and filtering. Because the turbinates contain many blood vessels, they swell easily, causing a stuffy nose, and are prone to bleeding (<u>epistaxis</u>).

Mouth and Oropharynx
The mouth and <u>oropharynx</u> also contain many blood vessels and are covered by a mucous membrane. <u>Edema</u> (swelling) of these structures can be extreme and dangerous. Bee stings to the lips or tongue can cause profound swelling. <u>Angioedema</u> **Figure 3** is a vascular reaction characterized by severe swelling, often around the eyes and lips. Swelling may involve the tongue and mouth. The reaction may be caused by an allergy and other factors, such as exposure to sunlight or water, but the cause may be unknown. Always ask a patient who may be experiencing an allergic reaction if his or her tongue feels thick. Monitor the patient's speech for symptoms of oral or laryngeal swelling, such as low volume or a raspy voice.

Hypopharynx
The oropharynx and nasopharynx meet in the back of the throat at the hypopharynx (sometimes called the *posterior pharynx*). The gag reflex is most profound in this area. Triggering the gag reflex, on purpose or by accident, can cause vagal bradycardia (a slow heartbeat caused by stimulation of the vagus nerve), vomiting, and increased intracranial pressure. A strong gag reflex may make the use of airway devices difficult or inappropriate. Conversely, patients with a diminished or absent gag reflex may require endotracheal (ET) intubation to help isolate and protect the airway from foreign materials and secretions.

Larynx and Glottis
The <u>larynx</u> (voice box) **Figure 4** and <u>glottis</u> (the vocal cords and the opening between them, at the top of the trachea) are typically considered the dividing line between the upper airway and the sterile lower airway. The thyroid cartilage is the most obvious external landmark of the larynx. The glottis and vocal cords are situated in the middle of the cartilaginous structure of the thyroid.

Several cartilages, sometimes visible during intubation, support the vocal cords. The

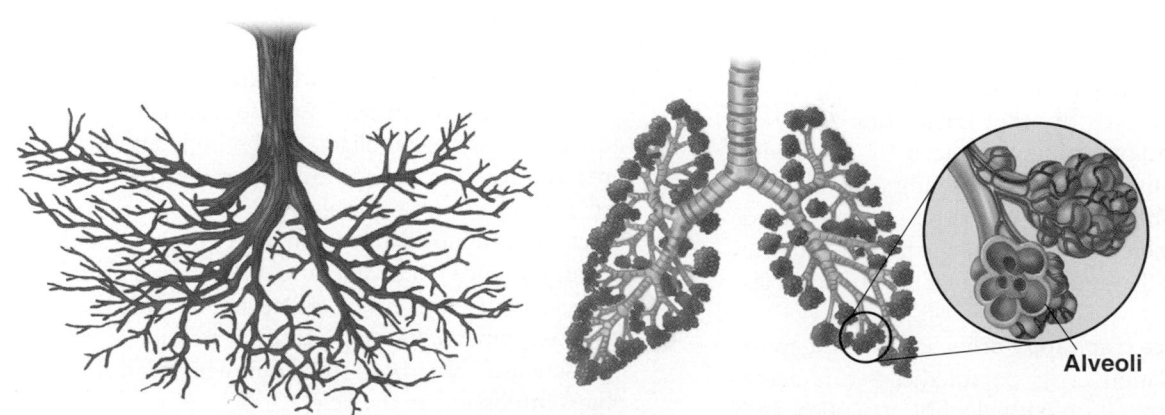

Alveoli

Figure 1 The tracheobronchial tree branches in much the same way as a real tree, except that even the most magnificent tree has only a small fraction of the branches as are in a lung.

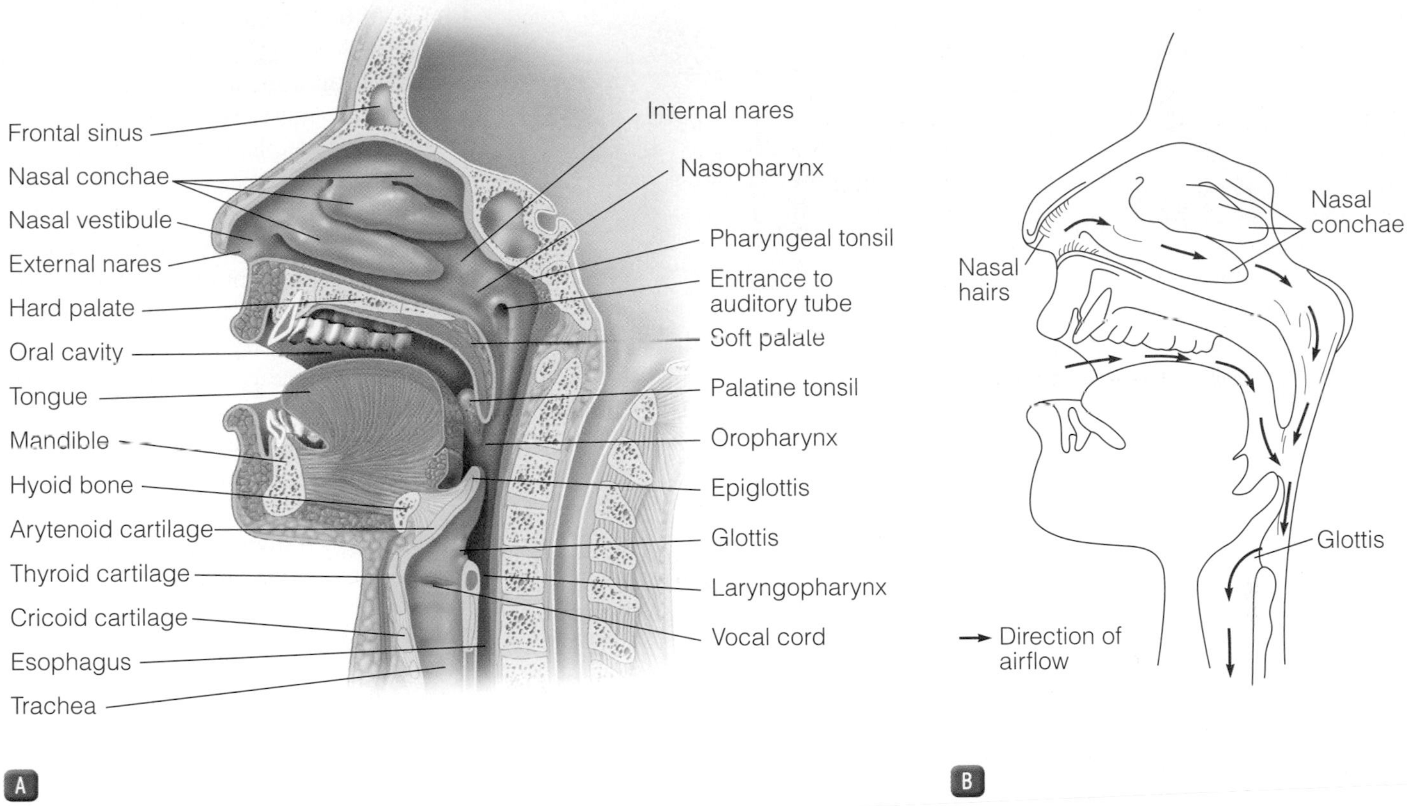

Frontal sinus

Nasal conchae

Nasal vestibule

External nares

Hard palate

Oral cavity

Tongue

Mandible

Hyoid bone

Arytenoid cartilage

Thyroid cartilage

Cricoid cartilage

Esophagus

Trachea

Internal nares

Nasopharynx

Pharyngeal tonsil

Entrance to auditory tube

Soft palate

Palatine tonsil

Oropharynx

Epiglottis

Glottis

Laryngopharynx

Vocal cord

Nasal conchae

Nasal hairs

Glottis

→ Direction of airflow

A

B

Figure 2 **A.** The upper airway serves to heat and humidify the air that passes through it. **B.** Direction of airflow. An important filter is lost when the upper airway is bypassed during intubation.

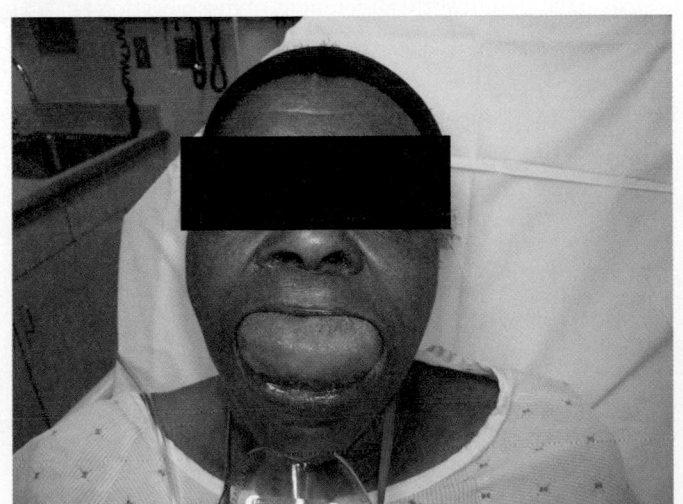

Figure 3 Angioedema is an acute swelling, sometimes of the lips and tongue, which may be caused by an allergic reaction. Some medications cause angioedema after the first or second dose.

arytenoid cartilages appear as two pearly white lumps at the distal end of each vocal cord. These lumps are individually named the *cuneiform* and *corniculate cartilages*. They may be visible during laryngoscopy. On either side of the glottis are pockets of tissue called the **piriform fossae** (singular *fossa*, from a Latin word meaning "trench") **Figure 5**.

The epiglottis covers the glottis like a trapdoor during swallowing, keeping food and liquid from entering the trachea. Many people aspirate food or liquids from the perimeter of the epiglottis, whereas others have no trouble swallowing even after the epiglottis has been surgically removed.

The **cricoid cartilage** can be palpated just below the thyroid cartilage in the neck. It forms a complete ring and helps hold the trachea in an open position. The small space between the thyroid and cricoid cartilages is the **cricothyroid membrane**. The membrane does not contain many blood vessels and is covered only by skin and minimal subcutaneous tissue. It is a potential site for performing a cricothyrotomy (an incision through the skin and cricothyroid membrane to relieve difficulty breathing caused by an airway obstruction) if the airway cannot be secured with an advanced airway device. The rest of the neck contains large blood vessels, important nerves, and other critical

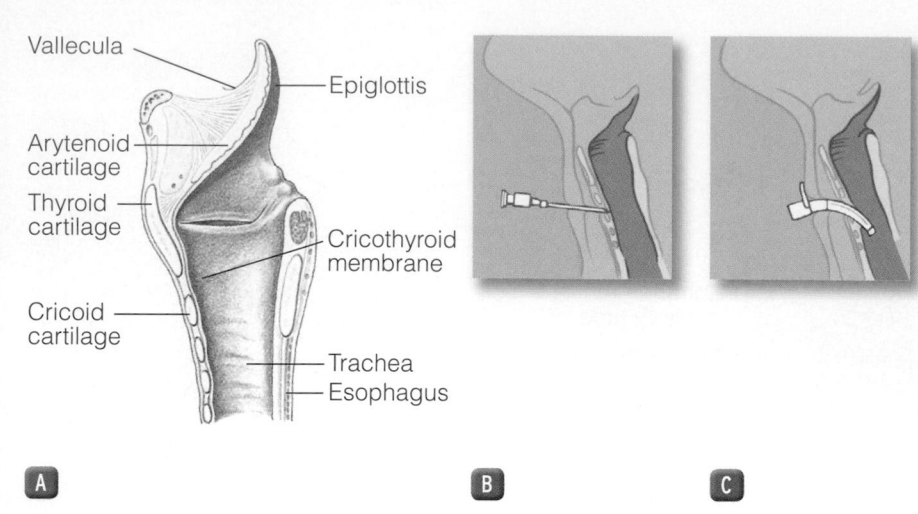

A   B   C

Figure 4 To perform a number of airway management skills, a thorough understanding of the anatomy of the larynx is imperative. **A.** Anatomy of the larynx. **B.** An IV cannula is inserted into the cricothyroid membrane. **C.** A tracheostomy tube is inserted below the cricoid cartilage.

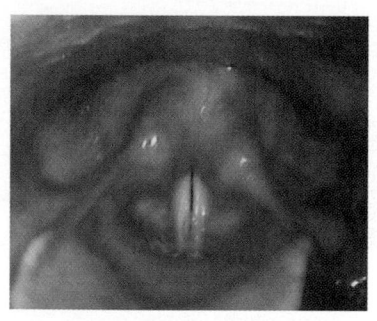

Figure 5 The arytenoid cartilages and piriform fossae are sometimes the only landmarks visible during a difficult intubation. The arytenoid cartilages are a pair of small, pyramid-shaped cartilages to which the vocal cords are attached.

anatomic structures that must be avoided when performing a cricothyrotomy.

Trauma or swelling of any of the laryngeal structures can create a life-threatening airway obstruction **Figure 6** . In the worst-case scenario, this entire anatomic region may be bypassed by a **tracheostomy** (a surgical opening into the trachea). By their very nature, traumatic injuries may alter the typical anatomy of the upper airway. Procedures such as a cricothyrotomy can prove highly challenging when the airway is choked with blood and vomitus and the anatomic landmarks are obscured by swelling or subcutaneous air.

Structures of the Lower Airway

The alveoli and terminal bronchioles comprise most of the lung mass. The connective tissue, small airways, and alveoli are collectively referred to as the lung parenchyma.

Tracheobronchial Tree

The trunk of the tracheobronchial tree is the trachea, or windpipe, which carries air to the lungs. The trachea extends about 10 to 13 cm, from the larynx to the left and right mainstem bronchi. This point of bifurcation, at the **carina**, is at roughly the level of the fifth thoracic vertebra (approximately nipple level) **Figure 7** . In adults, the right mainstem bronchus typically branches at a less acute angle than the left. This anatomic peculiarity explains why an ET tube that is advanced too far almost always goes into the right mainstem bronchus in an adult. Similarly, aspirated foreign bodies often end up in the right mainstem bronchus.

The mainstem bronchi branch into lobar bronchi, segmental bronchi, subsegmental bronchi, and bronchioles. These structures account for about 15 branches of the airway. They are lined with ciliated epithelium. **Cilia** are small hairlike structures that rhythmically wave in a pattern that helps move particulate matter up and out of the airway **Figure 8** .

Bronchioles

Gas transfer is most efficient in the alveoli, but a significant amount of gas is also exchanged across the respiratory bronchioles **Figure 9** . The terminal bronchioles are thin and have little cellular structure, which is helpful for gas exchange, but also means that the bronchioles lack cilia, have no protective blanket of mucus, and are not shielded by smooth muscle or a more rigid structure. Once foreign material reaches the terminal bronchioles and alveoli (parts of the lung collectively known as the lung **parenchyma**), it never comes out. Most people have black spots on their lungs from simply living in an industrialized society. Smokers and people who work around coal dust or other particulates may have significantly larger areas of discoloration **Figure 10** .

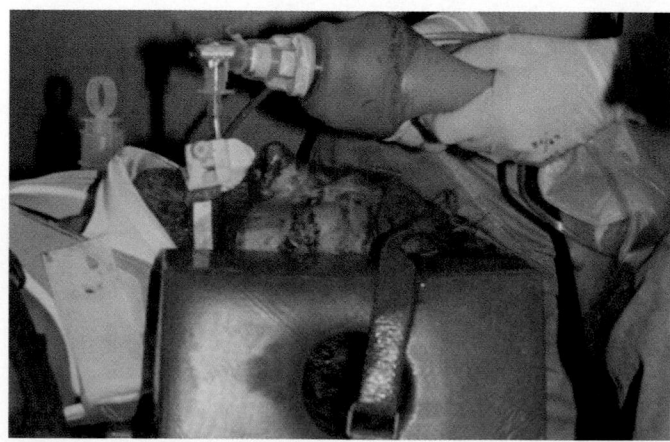

Figure 6 Trauma to the head and neck can completely obscure the anatomy of the airway. It is important to be comfortable enough with airway anatomy to manage the airway even when it has been significantly altered.

Goblet cells also line the airways. These cells produce mucus that blankets the entire lining of the conducting airways. The mucus covers the cilia, forming a two-layered blanket that is thick on the surface (gel layer) and thin and watery next to the cilia (sol layer). The gel layer is thick and floats over the sol layer. In a healthy person, cilia constantly push the gel layer up and out of the airway. As the cilia beat, they reach out into the gel layer, pushing it up and toward the glottis. On the return stroke, the cilia collapse into the sol layer, so that they do not pull the gel layer back down. In this manner, the cilia slowly move the entire gel layer up and out of the tracheobronchial tree, where it is swallowed or expectorated.

If a person is dehydrated or has taken medications such as antihistamines that dry the normal secretions, the sol layer will begin to dry up, and the cilia will not be able to move secretions effectively. The same is true if the patient is overhydrated: the cilia will wave meaninglessly in a deep watery layer without ever affecting the thick gel layer.

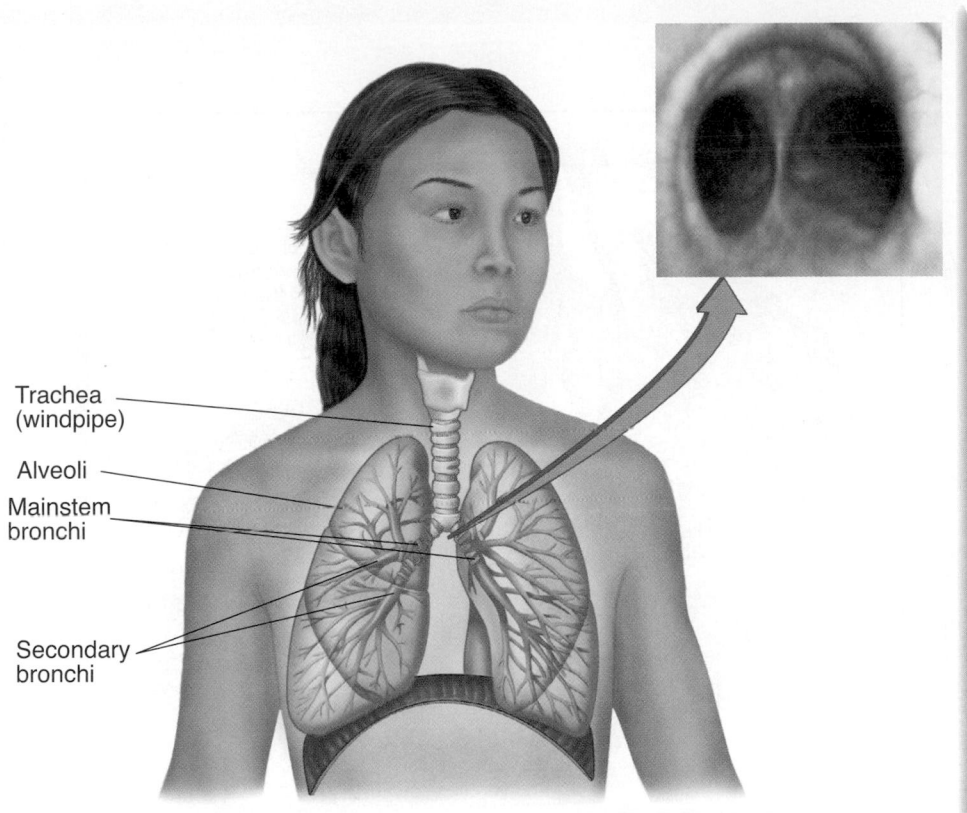

Figure 7 The point of bifurcation of the right and left mainstem bronchi is at the carina. In an adult, this location is at roughly the fifth intercostal space.

Trachea (windpipe)
Alveoli
Mainstem bronchi
Secondary bronchi

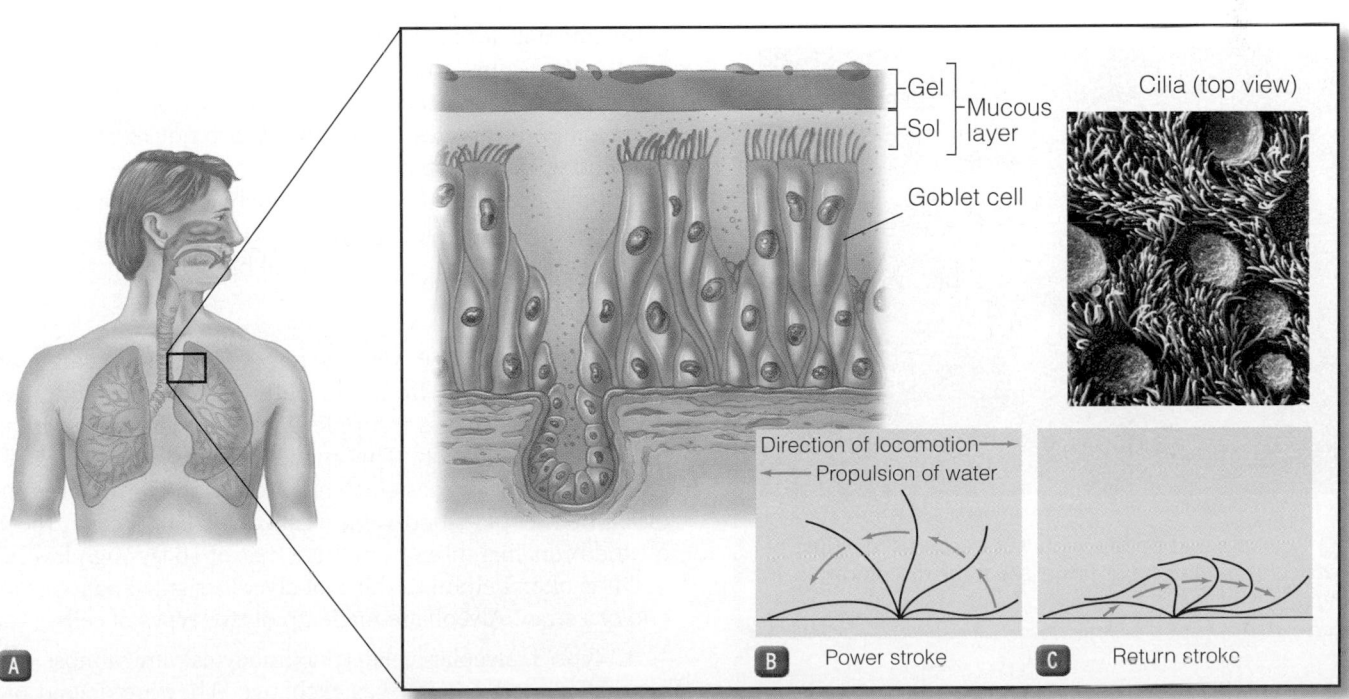

Figure 8 Cilia line the larger airways of the respiratory tract **(A)**. Their regular pattern of movement between the gel and sol layers of mucus helps move foreign material out of the tracheobronchial tree **(B and C)**.

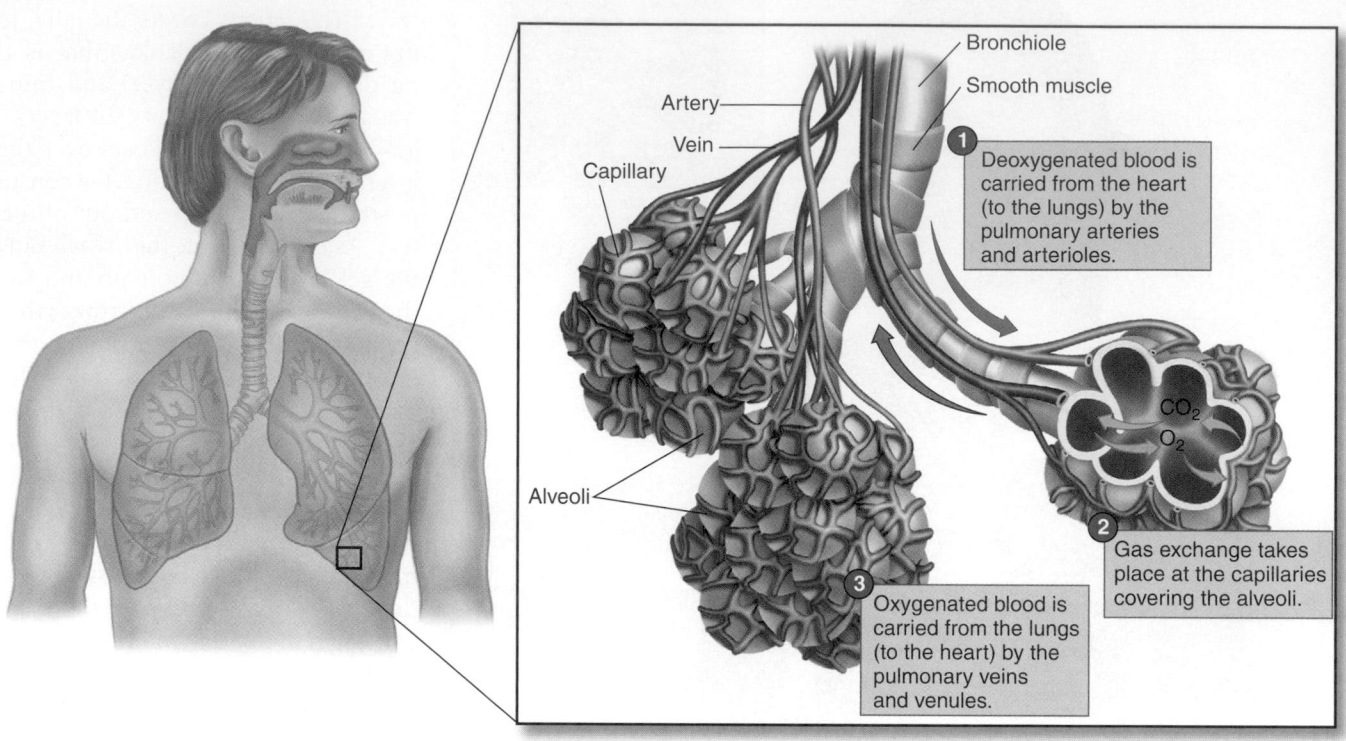

Figure 9 The respiratory bronchioles, sometimes called terminal bronchioles, include the alveoli and the last several branches of the tracheobronchial tree. Gas exchange occurs over this entire area, not just the alveoli.

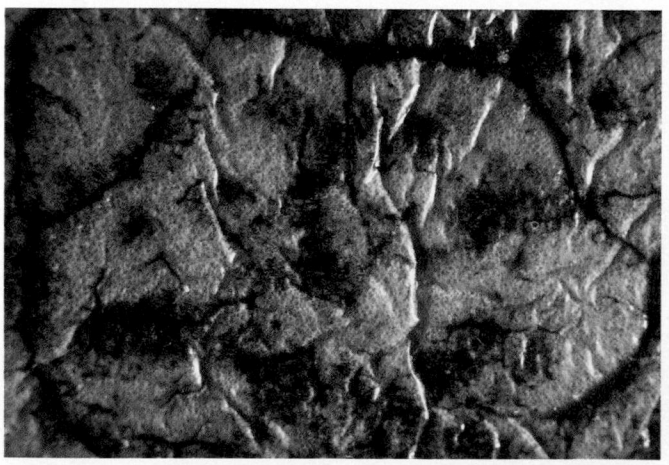

Figure 10 Smokers and people who work around coal dust or other particulates may have large areas of discoloration in their lungs.

<u>Smooth muscle</u> surrounds the conducting airways down to the subsegmental level. Bronchoconstriction occurs when the smooth muscle narrows these larger airways. Below the

subsegmental level, bronchodilator medications have little effect. Wheezing that is resolved with administration of bronchodilator medication was probably caused by constriction of the smooth muscles. Wheezing that is not resolved by these medications may have been caused by any of several pathologic conditions deeper in the tracheobronchial tree. The terminal airways and alveoli include branches 16 through 24 of the tracheobronchial tree, the so-called terminal bronchioles.

Alveoli

Gas Exchange Interface <u>Gas exchange</u> is the process by which deoxygenated blood from the pulmonary circulation releases carbon dioxide and is resupplied with oxygen before it enters the cardiac circulation. This process occurs at the level of the alveoli, the tiny air sacs clustered around the terminal bronchioles. Microscopic blood vessels called *capillaries* cover the alveoli and bronchial tubes from branch level 16 through level 24.

It is often helpful to think of alveoli as small balloons at the end of a straw. Alveoli are made up of two types of cells:

1. Type I alveolar cells (pneumocytes) are almost empty, allowing for better gas exchange. They are devoid of cellular components that would permit them to reproduce.

2. Each alveolus has several type II pneumocytes, which can make new type I cells and also produce a substance

known as **surfactant**, which reduces surface tension and helps keep the alveoli expanded. When alveoli are damaged by infection, cigarette smoking, or other trauma, their ability to repair themselves correlates directly to the number of type II cells that remain. Once all of the type II cells in an alveolus have been destroyed, the alveolus cannot make new cells or surfactant and is essentially dead.

Alveoli function best when they are kept partially inflated. Blowing up a balloon takes a lot of pressure. Once the balloon is partially inflated, however, it is much easier to inflate it the rest of the way. The same is true of alveoli. By reducing the surface tension of the alveoli, surfactant makes it easier for them to expand. When surfactant is washed out of the alveoli, as may occur in pulmonary edema, near-drowning, or severe shock, they are much more likely to collapse.

Collapsed, fluid-filled, or pus-filled alveoli do not participate in gas exchange. Instead, these alveoli contribute to a **shunt**, in which blood from the right side of the heart bypasses the alveoli and returns to the left side of the heart in an unoxygenated state, perhaps resulting in hypoxemia. Problems with ventilation, perfusion, or both can prevent oxygen from reaching the bloodstream Table 2 .

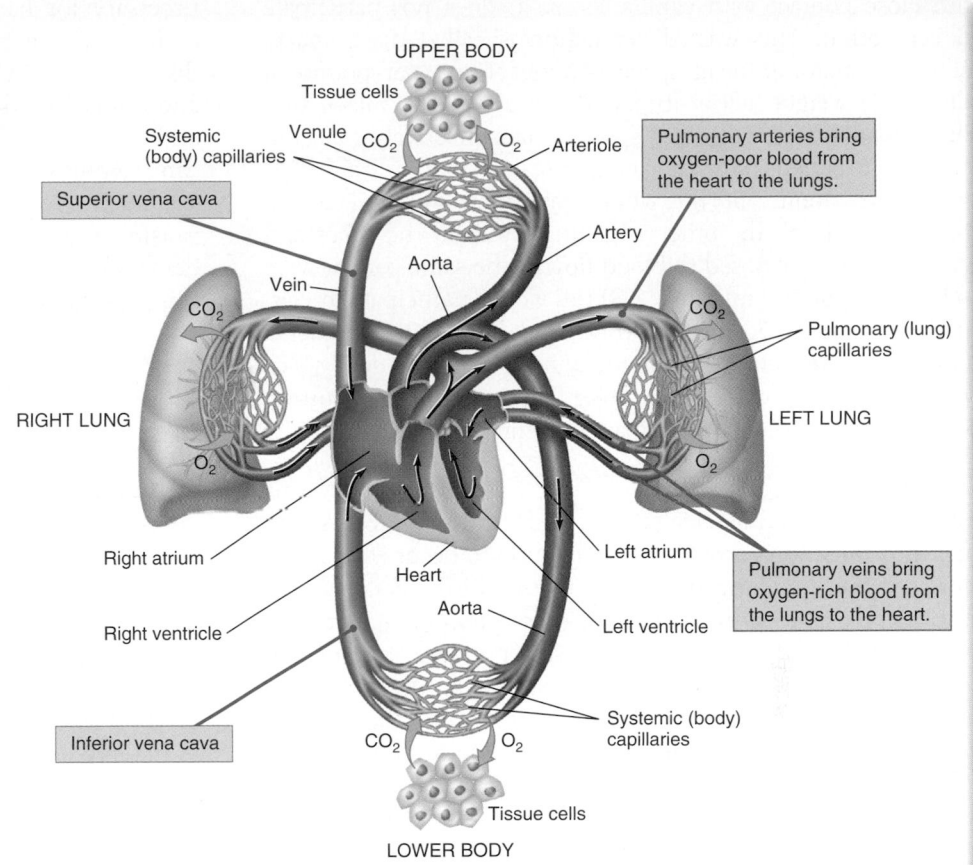

Figure 11 Pulmonary circulation begins as blood leaves the right ventricle via the pulmonary artery. The pulmonary capillary bed brings red blood cells close to the terminal bronchioles. After picking up oxygen, the blood returns to the left atrium via the pulmonary veins.

Pulmonary Capillary Bed The pulmonary circulation begins at the right ventricle, where the pulmonary artery (the only artery that usually carries deoxygenated blood) branches into increasingly smaller vessels until the pulmonary capillary bed surrounds the alveoli and terminal bronchioles Figure 11 . There is significantly more circulation to the lung bases than there is to the lung apices. Because humans are upright, gravity-dependent creatures, most infections and pathologic conditions occur at the base of the lung.

Like all capillaries in the body, the pulmonary capillaries are narrow and normally allow red blood cells to pass through only in single file. People with chronic lung disease and chronic **hypoxia** often generate a surplus of red blood cells over time, which makes their blood thick (**polycythemia**). Viscous blood that is pushed through the tiny pulmonary capillaries can place a significant strain on the right side of the heart. When the alveoli are distended by COPD, they push against the capillary bed, further narrowing the capillaries and straining the right side of the heart. Right-sided heart failure because of chronic lung disease is known as **cor pulmonale**.

Interstitial Space The network of gaps between the air-filled alveoli and the capillaries, which supply deoxygenated blood, is called the *interstitial space*. The interstitial space is filled with interstitial (inter-cellular) fluid, but it can expand with excess fluid or white blood cells and other cellular debris from infection, making gas exchange more difficult.

Inspired gas is distributed to the millions of alveoli by a network of conducting airways. Gas in these tubes does not come

Table 2	Alveoli and Capillary Supply Problems		
	Ventilation	**Perfusion**	**Examples**
Dead space	Good	Poor	Pulmonary embolus or shock
Shunt	Poor	Good	Pneumonia or atelectasis
Silent	Poor	Poor	Cardiac arrest

into close contact with capillaries, so it does not participate in ventilation. This wasted ventilation is called <u>dead space</u>. Typically, anatomic dead space is about 1 mL per pound of ideal body weight (a 150-lb person has about 150 mL of anatomic dead space). This dead space remains relatively constant. If a 150-lb patient took an average breath (<u>tidal volume</u> [V_T]) of 700 mL, about 550 mL would participate in ventilation at the alveolar level; the other 150 mL would fill the tubes and would never be exposed to blood flow. If the same patient were to have a V_T of 500 mL, only 350 mL would participate in ventilation, because 150 mL would be stuck in the tubes. Patients with chronic respiratory disease may have increased dead space (physiologic dead space), indicating that an even larger portion of each breath does not participate in respiration.

Chest Wall

The chest wall and associated muscles form a bellows system that must function correctly for ventilation to occur. The spine, sternum, and ribs form the basic structure of the bellows. The diaphragm is the primary muscle of respiration. It stretches across the bottom of the thorax, causing pressure changes that move air in and out of the top of the bellows at the glottis. The muscles and connective tissues of the ribs make the thoracic cavity airtight to maintain the pressure. The shiny, slippery pleural membranes line the inside of the thorax (the parietal pleura) and the outside of the lungs (the visceral pleura), allowing the organs to move smoothly within the chest. If air, blood, or pus leaks or seeps into the space between the visceral and parietal pleura (the pleural space), the result is pain, decreased lung motion, and, ultimately, lung collapse if the buildup continues unchecked.

When the body is healthy, this bellows system works efficiently, allowing movement of the tremendous amounts of air necessary for hard work and play. Trauma and diseases of the bones and muscles (kyphosis and scoliosis Figure 12) can significantly impair the ability to move air, causing a group of disorders known as <u>restrictive lung diseases</u>.

Mediastinum The heart and large blood vessels take up space in the middle of the chest between the lungs. The large conducting airways (trachea and mainstem bronchi) and some other organs (the thymus in children) also reside in this space, and they collectively show up on a chest radiograph as the large white area in the middle. This "middle ground" is referred to as the mediastinum. The mediastinum might widen if the patient is bleeding from a ruptured aorta, or it might trap air from a traumatic injury (pneumomediastinum).

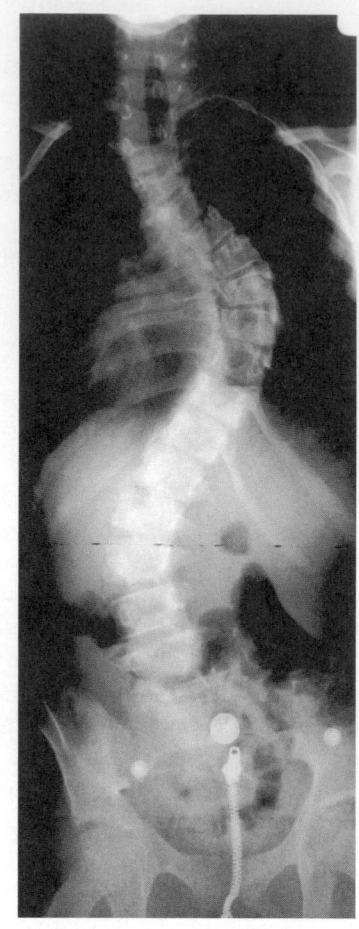

Figure 12 Diseases of the bones, such as scoliosis, can impair the patient's ability to move air because of chest compression.

YOU are the Medic   PART 2

It is evident to you that this patient is struggling to breathe. The patient tells you that he woke up suddenly with difficulty breathing and weakness. Your partner prepares to administer 100% oxygen via nonrebreathing mask and obtain vital signs. When you initially listen for lung sounds, you hear rales in the apices and diminished lung sounds in the bases. No medication bottles are in obvious view.

Recording Time: 1 Minute	
Appearance	Ashen gray, poor
Level of consciousness	Alert (oriented to person, place, and day)
Airway	Open; patent
Breathing	Rapid and shallow with crackles (rales)
Circulation	Weak and rapid radial pulse

3. What is your working diagnosis at this time?

4. What assessment and treatment steps will you want to accomplish on scene?

Functions of the Respiratory System

Respiration is the process by which oxygen is taken into the body, distributed to the cells, and used by the cells to make energy. The oxygen must be supplied by the lungs and circulatory systems. The primary by-product of this process is carbon dioxide. Under normal circumstances, the carbon dioxide generated during cellular respiration is returned to the lungs by the circulatory system, where it is exhaled during ventilation.

A sound understanding of normal ventilation, diffusion, and perfusion and the common problems associated with each will allow paramedics to think critically and understand which treatments are likely to help.

Ventilation

Ventilation is the movement of air in and out the lungs. With the use of supplemental oxygen, reasonable and even high oxygen levels are easy to maintain in patients who have healthy lungs, even if ventilation is severely compromised. The best measurement of ventilation, however, is the carbon dioxide level. Normal breathing removes just enough carbon dioxide to keep the acid-base status balanced. In fact, the volume of ventilation (minute volume) is controlled to a large extent by the acid-base balance of the blood. The body must maintain the $Paco_2$ in the range of 35 to 45 mm Hg. An acidic pH will stimulate breathing, and an alkaline pH slows breathing. In a person at rest, that goal is usually accomplished by breathing a tidal volume of around 500 mL at a rate of 12 to 16 breaths/min—that is, with a minute volume in the range of 6 to 8 L. During deep sleep, a smaller minute volume may suffice, whereas muscular exertion associated with exercise may require a larger minute volume. As long as the $Paco_2$ remains in the normal range, ventilation is considered normal.

Diffusion

For a molecule of oxygen to travel from an alveolus to a red blood cell, it must first diffuse (pass through) one side of the alveolar cell, across the membrane, and out the other side. It must then traverse the interstitial space and diffuse into the capillary wall, across *that* cell membrane, and out the other side. This trip happens billions of times, breath after breath, in all air-breathing creatures.

Some lung diseases cause thickening of the alveoli, or the buildup of fluid between the alveoli and the capillaries, making it difficult for oxygen to diffuse into the blood. In these cases, a patient may be ventilating just fine but has difficulty oxygenating.

Effective diffusion is driven by having a higher concentration of oxygen in the alveoli than there is in the bloodstream. If an oxygen-poor gas is inhaled, diffusion might stop or even go in the wrong direction. We give patients supplemental oxygen in an attempt to drive the diffusion of larger amounts of oxygen into the blood, but if other factors (such as bronchospasm or swelling or fluid in the airspaces) prevent the oxygen from reaching the alveoli, the supplemental oxygen will be of little value. If the hemoglobin molecules are already saturated with oxygen, additional supplemental oxygen is of little value, making the potential for the damage to tissues by oxygen a greater concern.

Perfusion

Perfusion refers to the circulatory component of the respiratory system. If blood does not consistently flow through the pulmonary vessels, good ventilation and diffusion are wasted because adequate oxygen cannot come into contact with the blood. A large pulmonary embolus can block blood flow to an entire lung. Patients who are anemic (low <u>hemoglobin</u> level) or hypovolemic (low blood volume) also have an impaired ability to transport oxygen and carbon dioxide.

Mechanisms of Respiratory Control

Neurologic Control

The neurologic control of respiration is centered in the medulla, but at least four parts of the brainstem are responsible for the smooth, rhythmic breathing that occurs without conscious effort. One area of the brain helps control respiratory rate, another depth, another inspiratory pause, and yet another rhythmicity. Another mechanism of neurologic control of breathing is a set of stretch receptors in the lungs that cause a person to cough if he or she takes too deep a breath. This response, called the <u>Hering-Breuer reflex</u>, helps regulate the depth of respiration and keeps the lungs from overinflating. This reflex is of little help to an unresponsive patient, but it explains why a conscious patient will cough violently if ventilated with too large a tidal volume.

The phrenic nerve, which innervates the diaphragm, and the thoracic spinal nerves that innervate the intercostal muscles are other mechanisms of neurologic control.

Cardiovascular Regulation

The lungs are closely linked to cardiac function. Some whimsically describe the lungs as an organ that lies between the right and left sides of the heart. While this description is not anatomically correct, changes in the right or left side of the heart can have dramatic pulmonary consequences. When the prevalence of acute cardiac disorders is considered along with the total number of patients with respiratory disorders, it is easy to see how "shortness of breath" is a common, diagnostically challenging dispatch.

Left-sided heart failure typically progresses much faster than right-sided heart failure. Right-sided heart failure may slowly worsen over many days, whereas left-sided heart failure resulting from a massive acute myocardial infarction can kill a person in a matter of minutes. Thinking of the lungs as lying between the right and left sides of the heart (in terms of function) provides an accurate conceptualization: The right side of the heart pumps blood to the lungs, and the left side of the heart receives blood from the lungs and then pumps it around the body. Any major change in the function of the lungs, the right side of the heart, or the left side of the heart almost always affects the other components.

The body's immediate response to mild hypoxemia is to increase the heart rate (possibly to a rate of more than 130 beats/min, or tachycardia). Severe hypoxia often causes bradycardia. Any uncorrected hypoxic insult may trigger a lethal cardiac arrhythmia, such as ventricular fibrillation or ventricular tachycardia. Changes in fluid balance, right-sided heart pumping pressure, or left-sided heart pumping pressure can cause various forms of congestive heart failure (CHF). Thorough evaluation of the cardiovascular system is essential to proper evaluation of a patient with a respiratory problem.

Muscular Control

The body is designed to take in air by means of negative pressure. Think about a vacuum cleaner at the base of the lungs sucking in air during inhalation. This air is pulled in through the mouth and the nose, over the turbinates, and around the complex terrain of the epiglottis and glottis. Air typically does not enter the esophagus and stomach because it is preferentially sucked into the trachea **Figure 13**.

This negative-pressure vacuum effect occurs because the thorax is essentially an airtight box with the flexible diaphragm at the bottom and an open tube (the trachea) at the top. The diaphragm is innervated by the phrenic nerves, which arise from the third through fifth cervical nerve roots (hence the phrase "C3 to C5 keep the diaphragm alive"). During quiet breathing, when the diaphragm flattens, the overall size of the container increases, and air is sucked in through the tube at the top to fill the increasing space inside the thorax. The amount of

air moved each minute (minute ventilation) can be increased by dropping the diaphragm more aggressively (deep breathing) or by breathing more rapidly (tachypnea).

When greater amounts of air must be moved, such as during exercise or illness, accessory muscles, some of which are innervated by cranial nerves, can be recruited to cause more dramatic pressure changes. The intercostal muscles attach each rib to the ribs above it. These muscles allow the ribs to be pulled up and out, expanding the thoracic cavity and allowing more air to be taken in. Accessory muscles of the neck and back and elsewhere, such as the shoulder girdle, can also help open up the thorax.

Any traumatic opening of the thorax provides an alternative route for air to be sucked in. This air ends up in the pleural space, resulting in a sucking chest wound **Figure 14**. When multiple ribs are broken in more than one place (flail chest), free-floating sections of the thorax are pulled in as the patient breathes, limiting the amount of air that can be sucked in through the trachea.

Exhalation is usually a passive process. After the size of the thorax has increased during inhalation, the components of the respiratory system return to their original places, and air is pushed out of the trachea under positive pressure.

Renal Status

Fluid balance, acid-base balance, and blood pressure are controlled, in part, by the kidneys. Each of these factors also affects the pulmonary mechanics and, hence, the delivery of

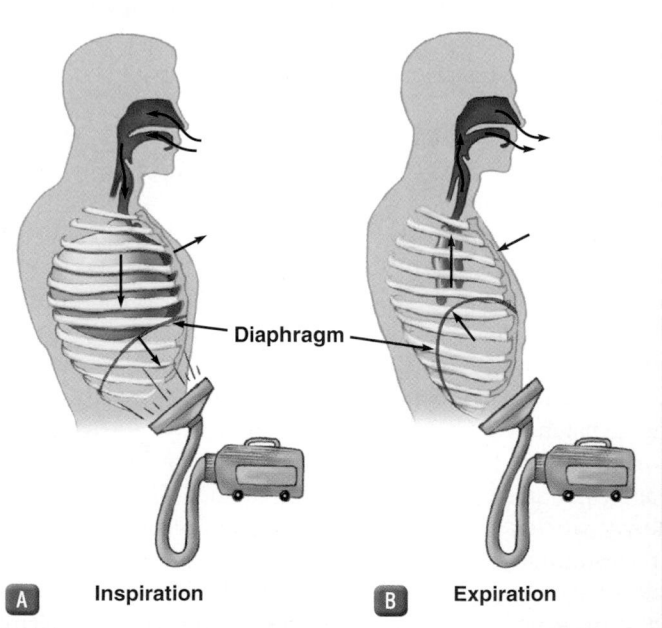

A   Inspiration   **B**   Expiration

Figure 13 Normal ventilation is negative pressure ventilation, meaning that air is sucked into the lungs, much as a vacuum cleaner sucks in air. The negative pressure pulls down the diaphragm, causing the lungs to fill **(A)**. When the pressure is released, the diaphragm relaxes and the lungs empty **(B)**. Compare with positive pressure ventilation, shown in Figure 34.

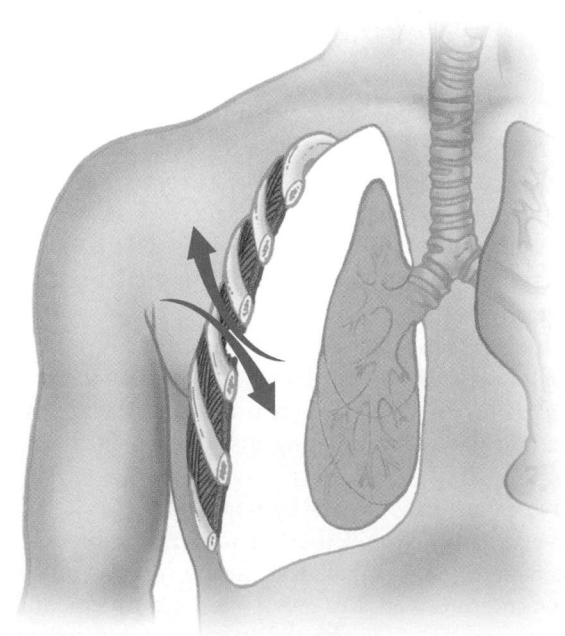

Figure 14 A sucking chest wound reduces ventilation by allowing air to enter the thorax during the inspiratory or negative pressure phase of ventilation.

oxygen to the tissues. Patients with severe renal disease often present with respiratory signs and symptoms, so paramedics should always note signs of severe renal disease when evaluating their condition. The condition of patients who have CHF because of renal disease can be difficult to manage because **diuresis** may be difficult or impossible. Patients who have renal disease may also have acid-base disturbances that cause them to hyperventilate and that are sometimes mistaken for respiratory disorders. Often, a patient's need for emergency dialysis may have an influence on transport decisions and options.

Assessment of a Patient With Dyspnea

Evaluation of the respiratory organs is clearly an important component of assessing respiratory emergencies. However, the job performed by the respiratory system so dramatically affects other body systems that a thorough respiratory assessment includes much more than listening to the patient's lungs.

As always, remember that recognizing and treating life threats is the priority in the primary assessment and throughout care. Because many respiratory ailments are life threatening, the respiratory assessment is always an early step in patient assessment.

Scene Size-up

Paramedics should always think first of observing standard precautions and using proper personal protective equipment, which is vital whenever exposure to blood, body fluids, or respiratory secretions is possible. In addition, the patient may have a respiratory infection that could be communicable by sputum, respiratory droplets, or airborne particles (see the chapter, *Infectious Diseases*). The minimum personal protective equipment when treating a patient with respiratory distress should be examination gloves, eye protection, and a HEPA (high-efficiency particulate air) respirator. A face shield and gown may also be used if the patient is suspected of having a respiratory infection.

Pulmonary complaints are associated with a broad range of situations and toxins, including atmospheres with decreased oxygen concentrations (enclosed, improperly ventilated spaces, such as methamphetamine laboratories), silos, carbon monoxide, and irritant gases. Some respiratory illnesses are highly contagious. It is therefore essential to evaluate scene safety on every call, even a "routine" dispatch for shortness of breath.

Respiratory diseases can cause trouble in a variety of ways. Respiratory disease can impair ventilation, diffusion, perfusion, or a combination of the three.

Rapid-onset dyspnea may be caused by acute bronchospasm, anaphylaxis, pulmonary embolism, or pneumothorax. **Paroxysmal nocturnal dyspnea** is dyspnea that comes on suddenly in the middle of the night and may be an ominous sign as it may signal left-sided heart failure.

Factors that limit the ability of the diaphragm to move (such as advanced pregnancy, obesity, and air or blood in the abdomen), conditions that restrict chest wall movement (such as crush injuries, tightly applied immobilization devices, and an abnormal spinal curvature like scoliosis or kyphosis), and injuries that disrupt the integrity of the thoracic cage (such as flail chest) hinder a patient's ability to move air.

Primary Assessment

The following pages discuss signs associated with life-threatening respiratory distress. A multitude of obvious and subtle signs must be assessed during the first few moments of every patient encounter.

Form a General Impression

One glance at a patient may suggest a body type associated with a particular pathologic condition. The classic presentation of a patient with emphysema includes a barrel chest (a chest that is larger in the front-to-back dimension than in the side-to-side dimension from years of having air trapped in the thorax), muscle wasting (because of using body mass for energy), and pursed-lip breathing (because of the obstructive disease). Patients with emphysema are often tachypneic and do not typically present with profound hypoxia and cyanosis.

Patients who have chronic bronchitis tend to be more sedentary and, thus, may be obese. They are often encountered in a chair or recliner, where they sleep in an upright position. A wastebasket may overflow with tissues, and a cup into which they spit their copious secretions and a full ashtray may be nearby. Men with chronic bronchitis might keep a urinal near the chair to avoid frequent trips to the bathroom. A table next to the chair may have several medications, inhalers, or an aerosol nebulizer. Such a scene can disclose volumes of information about the patient and his or her history long before a paramedic places a stethoscope on the chest.

Oxygen demand increases with any kind of exertion. If a patient's condition is stable at rest, observe his or her condition during typical exertion. Does the patient become dyspneic when moving from the chair to the stretcher, when going to the bathroom, or while eating? Note the patient's oxygen saturation while at rest and during any simple exertion. Check infants while they are eating or after they cry.

Increased work of breathing, anxiety, hypoxia, or fever can all trigger a sympathetic nervous system response resulting in tachycardia, diaphoresis, and pallor. It is interesting to note that the heart rate often decreases as patients respond to treatment even though that treatment often involves the use of sympathetic stimulators that may increase the heart rate.

Severely ill patients with end-stage diseases, cancer, or immune system disorders are often easy to identify, as are the sickly appearance, rigors, and chills of a patient with pneumonia. Tall, thin young adults are predisposed to spontaneous pneumothorax, and women who smoke and take birth-control pills are predisposed to pulmonary embolus.

Clues to a variety of pathologic conditions may be evident immediately, but keep in mind that they are only clues. Avoid making a hasty field impression based on minimal information. The patient's presentation may suggest a particular condition, but these suspicions must be confirmed by a thorough assessment.

Airway and Breathing
Position and Degree of Distress
Patients in respiratory distress tend to seek the sitting position. The tripod position involves leaning forward and rotating the scapulae outward by placing the arms on a table with elbows out, or placing the hands on the knees **Figure 15**. This position opens up a little more space in the lung apices for airflow and drops the abdominal structures away from the diaphragm. Because there is considerably more perfusion to the lung bases than to the apices, this maneuver may use more energy than it gains in oxygenation. Beware of a patient in respiratory distress who is willing to lie flat; this could be a sign of sudden deterioration in the patient's condition.

Purposeful hyperextension occurs when a patient maximizes airflow through the upper airway by holding his or her head in the head tilt–chin lift position, or "sniffing" position. This position may indicate upper airway swelling, but it is also commonly seen in patients who are trying to maximize airflow. Maintaining this position uses up valuable energy. A patient with severe respiratory disease who begins to feel fatigued may hold his or her head up in this position only during inhalation, letting it fall into flexion during exhalation. This head bobbing is an ominous sign of imminent decompensation and is frequently preterminal behavior.

Breathing Alterations
Breathing alterations can be much more complex. They can involve problems with the conducting airways (branches), such as asthma or bronchitis; difficulties at the alveolar level, such as pneumonia or emphysema; problems with the muscles and nerves that make breathing work, as in Guillain-Barré syndrome or spinal cord injury; and problems with the rigid structure of the thorax, such as flail chest, that hamper the pressure changes that make breathing work.

Words of Wisdom

Maintaining the airway and breathing for a patient are not the same. Many patients need assistance to establish a patent airway. An open airway, however, does not ensure that an adequate volume of gas is moving in and out of the lungs. Proper ventilation is necessary to oxygenate the blood and to remove carbon dioxide. Increasing the amount of available oxygen ensures that even a patient who is not moving adequate volumes of gas (that is, hypoventilating) can maintain adequate oxygen saturation. If ventilation remains inadequate, a hypoventilating patient will become hypercapnic (too much carbon dioxide in the blood) and acidotic (pH of arterial blood is too low). These conditions interrupt important body systems and are fatal if uncorrected.

Increased Work of Breathing
Patients using accessory muscles to breathe are in danger of tiring out, so noting such muscle use is important. Is the patient using the muscles of the abdomen to push air out (as in asthma or COPD), or is the patient using muscles in the chest and neck to pull air in **Figure 16**? Infants and small children have substantial elasticity in the chest wall; when they use accessory muscles to breathe, the flexible cartilage of the sternum or ribs often collapses, causing bony retractions. In adults and children, profound intrathoracic pressure changes can cause the peripheral pulses to weaken (or disappear) during inspiration (pulsus paradoxus), and pulses are easier to palpate during exhalation. Patients using accessory muscles to breathe may have dramatic pressure changes within the thorax and exhibit these and other signs of increased work of breathing, summarized in **Table 3**. These signs may indicate life-threatening respiratory distress.

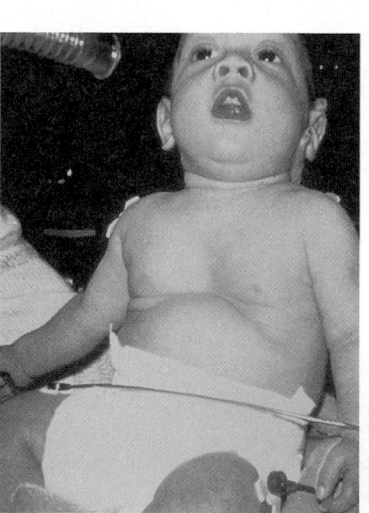

Figure 16 Bony retraction not only is a sign of severe distress and increased work of breathing, but also contributes to respiratory failure. With inhalation, the lower sternum is pulled into the lungs. Every cubic centimeter of space displaced by the retraction is a cubic centimeter of air that cannot reach the airways.

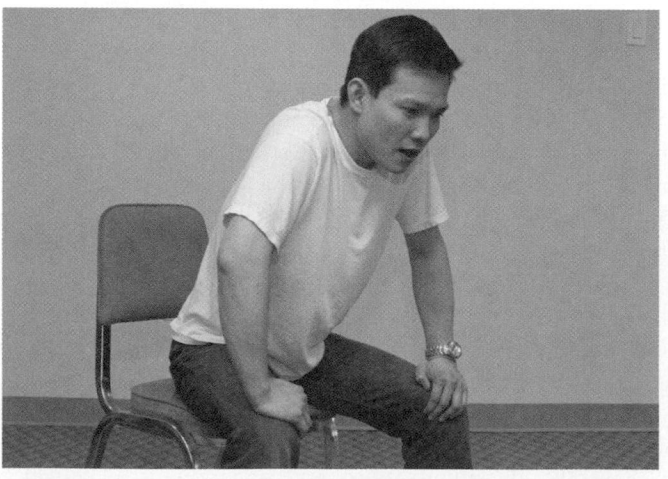

Figure 15 The tripod position (elbows out) allows better diaphragmatic movement by getting the abdomen out of the way and allows somewhat more airflow to the apices by rotating the scapulae laterally. This takes work, which requires more oxygen.

Altered Rate and Depth of Respiration

Assessing the rate and depth of breathing is an obvious component of respiratory assessment, but rate and depth are often not accurately determined. The rate may be a commonly "guessed" vital sign, but respiratory depth is even more commonly misjudged. A patient with an adequate rate but a low volume will still have an inadequate minute volume (respiratory rate × tidal volume = minute volume). The respiratory rate can vary significantly from minute to minute. Be sure to monitor trends in respiratory rate (increasing, decreasing) rather than concentrating on a specific rate from the beginning of the assessment. While assessing the patient's respiration, note the pattern (see Table 6) and the inspiratory-to-expiratory (I/E) ratio. Is the patient working hard to inhale, exhale, or both? Does the breath have a peculiar odor (such as the acetone odor associated with diabetic ketoacidosis)? Are there any audible abnormal respiratory noises? As a general rule, *any* respiratory noises that are audible without a stethoscope are abnormal.

Abnormal Breath Sounds

Whenever possible, auscultate the lungs systematically. Although examiners tend to compare the left and right sides, the lungs are not symmetric. The right lung has three lobes: the upper, middle, and lower. The left lung has only two lobes: the upper and lower. It is important to understand where to listen to hear each lobe **Figure 17**.

Some pathologic conditions are gravity-dependent, meaning that most types of pneumonia and CHF are found in the lung bases. Wheezing may be diffuse and spread throughout the lung fields. The bases are almost exclusively heard by listening on the patient's back.

The upper lobes, which rarely have abnormalities, are heard by listening on the anterior part of the chest. The right

Table 3	Signs of Increased Work of Breathing
Sign	**Description**
Bony retractions	During inhalation, the sternum or ribs pull back or recede (retract) into the chest, creating a visible deformity with each breath.
Soft-tissue retractions	Soft tissue is drawn in around the bones during inhalation. Dramatic retractions can be seen in the supraclavicular, intercostal, and subxiphoid areas.
Nasal flaring	The nostrils are pulled wide open during inhalation.
Tracheal tugging	During inhalation, the thyroid cartilage is pulled upward and the area just above the sternal notch is drawn in.
Paradoxical respiratory movement	During inhalation, the epigastrium is pulled in as the abdomen is pushed out, creating a seesaw effect as the two move in opposite directions.
Pulsus paradoxus	The weak or absent peripheral pulses on inhalation are caused by extreme pressure changes in the thorax.
Pursed-lip breathing	Patients with obstructive diseases (such as chronic obstructive pulmonary disease and acute asthma) have trouble pushing air out. It is more effective to exhale slowly over a longer period than to try to push the air out forcefully. Many patients learn to purse their lips (like a kiss) and exhale slowly through this restricted orifice. This technique allows them to exhale more efficiently and provides a clue to the disease.
Grunting	In infants and young children with lower airway illness, the glottis closes at the end of exhalation, so there is grunting at the end of each breath. This maneuver provides a small amount of pressure that helps keep the alveoli open (as with positive end-expiratory pressure). The grunts may be audible, or a stethoscope may be required to hear them, but grunting is a classic sign of respiratory distress in infants.

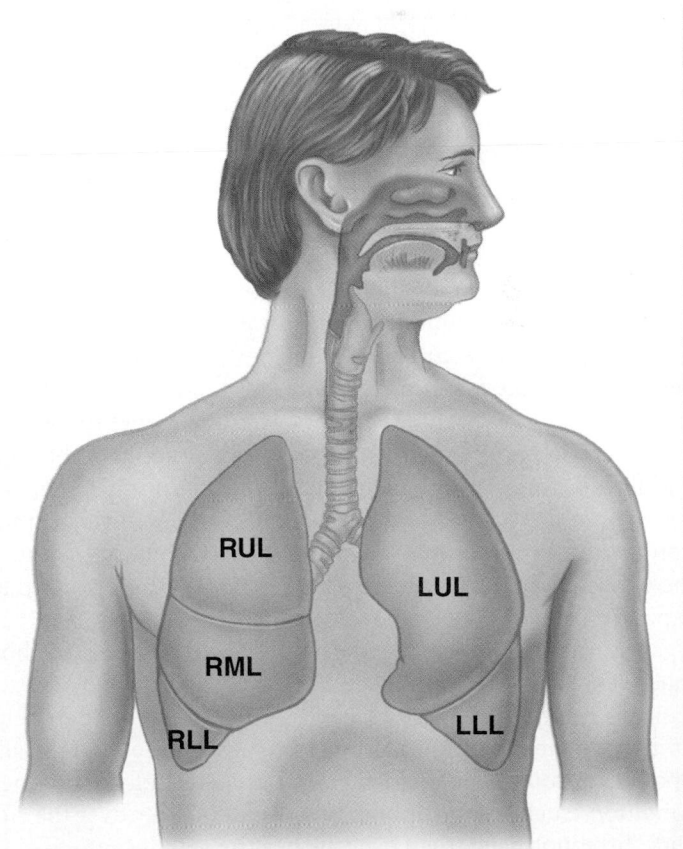

Figure 17 The lungs are not symmetric. Most acute pathologic conditions are best heard in the lung bases, requiring that the stethoscope be placed on the patient's back. The right middle lobe is best heard beneath the right breast or just lateral to it. LUL, left upper lobe; LLL, left lower lobe; RUL, right upper lobe; RML, right middle lobe; RLL, right lower lobe.

middle lobe can best be heard by listening just beneath or lateral to the right breast. The best left-right differentiation can be noted in the midaxillary line; this is the best place to listen to confirm ET tube placement. Listening to the anterior part of the chest allows the examiner to hear the noisemaker (the ET tube), whether it is in the trachea or the esophagus.

The breath sounds are made by turbulent flow in the large airways as they are transmitted through the chest to the stethoscope. Tracheal breath sounds are not commonly auscultated, but note how harsh and tubular they sound. Bronchial breath sounds are also quite loud, but note that exhalation predominates. Farther toward the periphery, bronchovesicular sounds are softer and sound the same during inspiration and expiration. The most commonly heard breath sounds are the soft, breezy vesicular sounds heard in the periphery. They have a much more obvious inspiratory component. Listen to a large number of healthy lungs to become familiar with the four different sounds **Figure 18**. Some pathologic conditions cause normal breath sounds to be heard in abnormal places.

Sound moves better through fluid than it does through air. Thus, the more air in a patient's chest (as in COPD or asthma), the more distant or diminished the breath sounds will be at the periphery, if they are audible at all. Conversely, the "wetter" the patient's lungs are (as in pneumonia; consolidation, when fluid causes the lungs to become firm; or CHF), the louder the sounds will be at the periphery. If a patient has pneumonia in the right middle lobe, bronchovesicular sounds (equal during inspiration and expiration) or even bronchial sounds (louder during expiration than inspiration) may be heard in the periphery, instead of the expected vesicular sounds (louder during inspiration than expiration).

The quality of the breath sounds also depends on how much extra tissue comes between the stethoscope and the patient's respiratory structures. For this reason, it is often helpful to compare breath sounds on the right with those on the left. The breath sounds of a patient who has a one-sided pathologic condition (such as pneumonia) may sound *louder* over the side with the abnormality than over the healthy side.

Breath sounds and vocalizations travel more efficiently through a firm, fluid-filled lung than through a healthy lung, but they travel poorly through a hyperinflated lung. If a patient speaks during chest auscultation, the examiner cannot usually understand what he or she is saying through the stethoscope. If the patient's words are audible, it may mean that the patient has consolidation from pneumonia or atelectasis. These sounds

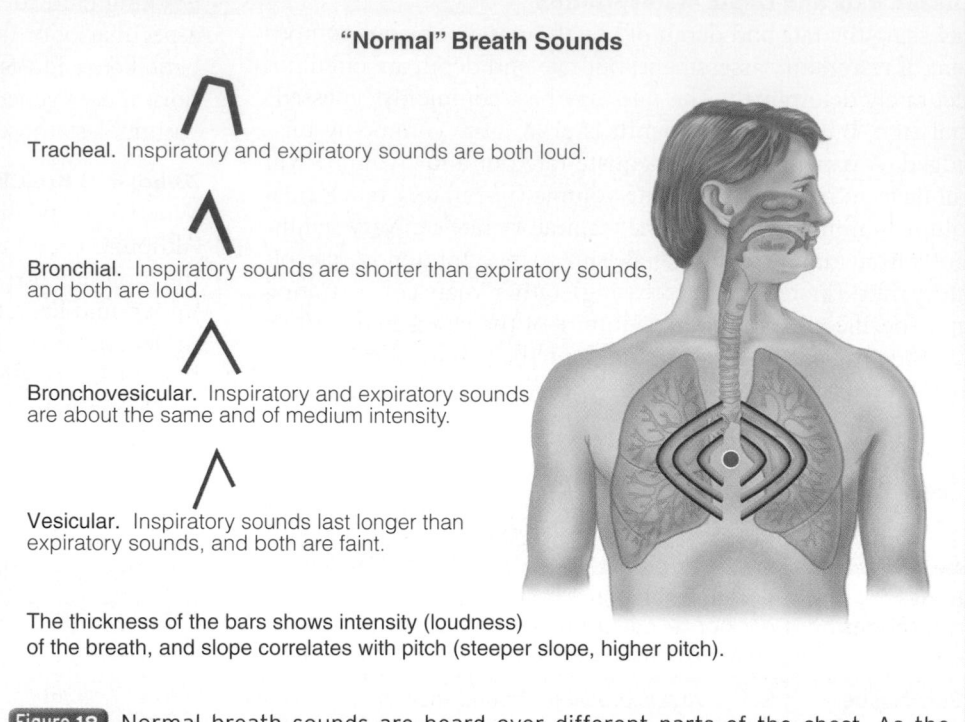

"Normal" Breath Sounds

Tracheal. Inspiratory and expiratory sounds are both loud.

Bronchial. Inspiratory sounds are shorter than expiratory sounds, and both are loud.

Bronchovesicular. Inspiratory and expiratory sounds are about the same and of medium intensity.

Vesicular. Inspiratory sounds last longer than expiratory sounds, and both are faint.

The thickness of the bars shows intensity (loudness) of the breath, and slope correlates with pitch (steeper slope, higher pitch).

Figure 18 Normal breath sounds are heard over different parts of the chest. As the stethoscope moves away from the largest airways, breath sounds become softer. The character of sounds during inspiration versus exhalation also changes.

will be clearest directly over the consolidated lobe. **Table 4** lists signs of consolidation.

__Adventitious__ (abnormal) breath sounds are the extra noises that can be heard on top of the breath sounds described previously. Continuous sounds (for example, a wheeze) can be heard across some portion of each breath. Discontinuous sounds are the instantaneous pops, snaps, and clicks known as __crackles__ **Figure 19**.

Wheezes are high-pitched, whistling sounds made by air being forced through narrowed airways, which makes them vibrate, much like the reed in a musical instrument. Wheezing

Table 4   Signs of Consolidation

Sign	Test
Bronchophony	When a patient says "99" repeatedly, it sounds like a hum through a normal lung. Through a consolidated lung, you can understand the words "99."
Egophony	The patient says "eeeeee" while you are auscultating, and you hear "aaaaaa." The sound may be heard particularly well over a pleural effusion.
Whispered pectoriloquy	The patient whispers while you are auscultating, and you can understand what is said.

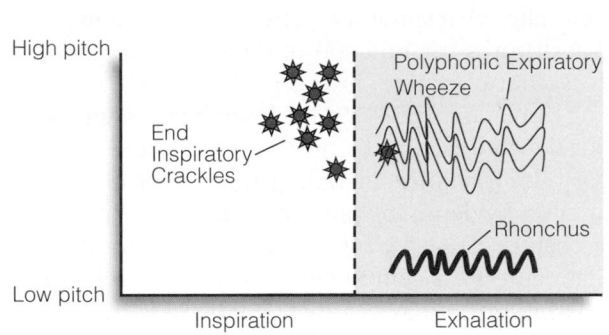

Figure 19 Adventitious sounds can be described as continuous (wheezes and rhonchi) or discontinuous (crackles). They can also be characterized by their pitch (such as high or low), by where they are in the respiratory cycle (end inspiration or forced exhalation), and by their complexity (monophonic versus polyphonic).

(**monophonic**); if many bronchi are vibrating, the wheeze may have many notes, like a bagpipe (**polyphonic**). Note when the sound is heard in the respiratory cycle. Does the wheeze occur during inspiration and exhalation? Just during exhalation? Or just at the end of exhalation?

Crackles are any discontinuous noises heard during auscultation of the lungs and are caused by the popping open of air spaces (fine crackles) or the movement of fluid or secretions in the larger airways (coarse crackles). They are usually associated with increased fluid in the lungs. These sounds are often referred to as *crackles*. In some parts of the country, the terms *rales* and *rhonchi* persist. **Rales** usually refers to the high-pitched crackles heard in the lung bases at the end of inspiration. Rales are consistent with pulmonary edema. **Rhonchi** is a nonspecific term that usually refers to low-pitched crackles caused by secretions in the larger airways. A pleural friction rub sounds like two pieces of wet rubber being drawn over each other and is heard when the patient has pleurisy (infection or edema of the pleural membranes).

Audible sounds—stridor from upper airway obstruction and grunting from lower airway obstruction—are often audible. A low-pitched gurgling sound is sometimes heard as patients become unable to clear their own secretions (sometimes called a "death rattle"). Wheezes and crackles that are audible when entering a room are obviously more impressive than sounds that require a stethoscope to hear. As patients become more sick, the various "musical" emissions become louder. As respiratory distress worsens, the noises may again diminish. The most ominous breath sounds are no breath sounds at all. An absence of

may be diffuse, as in asthma and CHF, or localized, as when a foreign body obstructs a bronchus. Pathologic conditions such as asthma rarely cause one-sided wheezing. Have the patient cough, and listen again. If the sound emanates from only one side; it could be caused by the movement of secretions. If a single bronchus is vibrating, the wheeze will be a single note

---

YOU *are the Medic* | **PART 3** |

Your patient has been given oxygen via nonrebreathing mask, although this intervention does not seem to be improving the patient's condition. His oxygen saturation level is still in the low 80s, so you decide to apply continuous positive airway pressure (CPAP). The patient is becoming hypoxic and is no longer following your commands. He is visibly anxious and asking you to help him. Your partner helps assemble the CPAP equipment while you begin continuous 4-lead monitoring and you monitor his ECG. The 12-lead shows ST elevations in leads 2 and 3. You inquire again if the patient is experiencing any chest pain, which he denies.

Recording Time: 5 Minutes	
Respirations	34 breaths/min; shallow and rapid
Pulse	110 beats/min; weak
Skin	Gray and clammy
Blood pressure	140/100 mm Hg
Oxygen saturation (Spo$_2$)	80% with oxygen by nonrebreathing mask
Pupils	Equal

5. Is this patient experiencing an airway problem or a breathing problem?

6. Does the absence of chest pain mean the patient is not having a heart attack?

breath sounds indicates that the patient is not moving enough air to ventilate the lungs. *Silence means danger*.

Noisy breathing is obstructed breathing. **Snoring** indicates partial obstruction of the upper airway by the tongue—a form of obstruction that is easily corrected by head-tilt maneuvers. Gurgling signals the presence of fluid in the upper airway. **Stridor**, a harsh, high-pitched sound heard during inhalation, indicates narrowing, usually as a result of swelling (laryngeal edema).

Quiet breathing can also be revealing. A patient with tachypnea who has crystal clear breath sounds may have hyperventilation syndrome but may also be breathing rapidly because of acidosis. Quiet tachypnea suggests possible shock. Paramedics occasionally assume that tachypnea caused by pain, anxiety, or metabolic disorders is the patient's primary problem and mistakenly administer aerosol treatments when the real problem is diabetic crisis or sepsis.

Sputum

It is probably not necessary to discuss the pathologic conditions suggested by various sputum colors, but it is appropriate to note whether the patient is coughing up discolored sputum Table 5 . Many smokers and people with chronic respiratory diseases cough up sputum every day (especially first thing in the morning), so determine if the color or amount of this sputum has changed. Some people keep a cup or emesis basin nearby to spit in. Others do not spit out the sputum.

Increased sputum production coupled with fever and chills is a classic presentation of an infection such as pneumonia. Blood-tinged sputum may be a warning sign of **tuberculosis**, or it may mean the patient has been coughing forcefully and small blood vessels in the airway have broken. When air is forced through airways filled with pulmonary edema fluid, the pink foam or froth commonly associated with CHF is created. It is important to note whether the mucus is **purulent** (puslike). Ask the patient about the color of mucus coughed up and whether the color or any other characteristic is a change from the usual for the patient.

Abnormal Breathing Patterns

Major neurologic insults may also manifest themselves with some altered respiratory pattern. Brain trauma or any event that disturbs the function of the brain may depress the respiratory control centers in the medulla. For example, the increasing intracranial pressure in closed head trauma may literally put the squeeze on the medulla to produce a variety of respiratory abnormalities, including apnea. A stroke may have a similar effect by depriving portions of the brain of circulation (see the chapter, *Cardiovascular Emergencies*). Overdoses with drugs that depress the central nervous system (such as narcotics and barbiturates) may also severely depress the activity of the respiratory center.

Severe traumatic brain injuries result in bizarre respiratory patterns when one or more of these respiratory centers are damaged or deprived of adequate blood flow. Table 6 summarizes various breathing patterns.

Table 5 Classic Sputum Types

Type of Sputum	Causes
Frothy, sometimes with a pink tinge	Congestive heart failure
Thick	Dehydration or antihistamine use
Purulent	Infectious process (because the pus contains dead white blood cells)
Yellow, green, brown	Older secretions in various stages of decomposition
Clear or white	Bronchitis
Blood-streaked	Tumor, tuberculosis, pulmonary edema, or trauma from coughing

Table 6 Breathing Patterns

Pattern	Comments
Agonal	Irregular gasps that are widely spaced; usually represent stray neurologic impulses in a dying patient; occasional agonal gasp not unusual in patients with no pulse; not actually considered a form of breathing
Apneustic	Characterized by a prolonged inspiratory hold (sometimes called "fish breathing"); follows damage to the pneumotaxic center in the brain; an ominous sign of severe brain injury
Ataxic	Chaotically irregular respirations that indicate severe brain injury or brainstem herniation
Biot respirations	Irregular pattern, rate, and depth of respirations, characterized by intermittent patterns of apnea; indicates severe brain injury or brainstem herniation
Bradypnea	Unusually slow respiration
Central neurogenic hyper-ventilation	Tachypneic hyperpnea; rapid and deep respirations caused by increased intracranial pressure or direct brain injury; drives carbon dioxide level down and pH up, resulting in respiratory alkalosis
Cheyne-Stokes respirations	Crescendo-decrescendo breathing with a period of apnea between cycles; not considered ominous unless grossly exaggerated or occurs in a patient with brain trauma
Cough	Forced exhalation against a closed glottis; an airway-clearing maneuver; also seen when foreign substances irritate the airways; controlled by the cough center in the brain (Antitussive medications work on the cough center to reduce this sometimes annoying physiologic response.)

Continues

Table 6 Breathing Patterns, continued

Pattern	Comments
Eupnea	Normal breathing
Hiccup	Spasmodic contraction of the diaphragm, causing short exhalations with a characteristic sound; sometimes seen in cases of diaphragmatic (or phrenic) nerve irritation from acute myocardial infarction, ulcer disease, or endotracheal intubation
Hyperpnea	Abnormally increased rate and depth of breathing; seen in various neurologic and chemical disorders, including overdose with certain drugs
Hypopnea	Abnormally decreased rate and depth of breathing
Kussmaul respirations	The same pattern as in central neurogenic hyperventilation but caused by the body's response to metabolic acidosis, attempting to rid itself of blood acetone via the lungs; seen in diabetic ketoacidosis; accompanied by a fruity (acetone) breath odor and, usually, cracked and dry mouth and lips
Sighing	Periodically taking a deep breath of about twice the normal volume; forces open alveoli that routinely close from time to time.
Tachypnea	Unusually rapid breathing; does not reflect depth of respiration and does not mean a patient is hyperventilating (breathing too rapidly and deeply, resulting in a lowered carbon dioxide level); often involves moving only small volumes of air, or *hypo*ventilation (much like a panting dog)
Yawning	Seems beneficial in the same manner as sighing

Most of the respiratory centers are in and around the brainstem Figure 20 . Patients who have serious trauma to the upper cerebral hemispheres (such as from a gunshot wound) are often still breathing despite mortal wounds. Apneustic breathing results from damage to the pneumotaxic center in the brain, which regulates inspiratory pause. A patient with apneustic respirations will have a short, brisk inhalation with a long pause before exhalation. This pattern indicates severe pressure within the cranium or direct trauma to the brain. Similarly, Biot's respirations are seen when the center that controls breathing rhythm is damaged. This respiratory pattern is grossly irregular, sometimes with lengthy apneic periods.

Cheyne-Stokes respirations are more of a high-brain function. Many deep sleepers or intoxicated people will have this type of respiratory pattern. The depth of breathing (or volume of snoring) gradually increases and then decreases (crescendo-decrescendo), followed by an apneic period. The apneic period is usually brief in a relatively healthy person.

Exaggerated Cheyne-Stokes respirations, in which the crescendo-decrescendo is much more prominent, may be seen in patients who have a severe brain injury. The apneic period may last 30 to 60 seconds.

Injury high in the spinal cord may paralyze the intercostal muscles and even the diaphragm. Polio attacks the nerves that supply the respiratory muscles, but certain chronic illnesses, such as myasthenia gravis, weaken the respiratory muscles themselves. The net effect of these conditions is the inability of the respiratory muscles to function normally in response to the respiratory drive. As a consequence, the tidal volume is shallow and the minute volume is correspondingly decreased. Patients with such conditions often need assisted ventilation to increase the tidal volume and, thus, minute volume.

Circulation

Assessing skin color is a fast way to begin forming an early impression of the patient's circulation Figure 21 . Although it is important to note the generalized cyanosis of oxygen desaturation or the profound pallor of shock, more subtle information can be gained by assessing the mucous membranes. The tissue inside the mouth, under the eyelids, and even under the nail beds is usually the same pink color in all healthy patients. A few notable variations are as follows:

- **Cyanosis.** Healthy adults have a hemoglobin level of 12 to 14 g/dL. With a hemoglobin level in this range, a person will begin to exhibit the blue discoloration of cyanosis when about 5 g/dL is desaturated (does not have oxygen attached). That means the oxygen saturation would be roughly 65%! If a person's hemoglobin level were only 10 g/dL, 50% of it (5 of the 10 g/dL) would have to be desaturated before the patient would look cyanotic. Some patients in cardiac arrest have deep blue skin, whereas others are pale. Similarly, in patients with high hemoglobin levels (patients with chronic respiratory disease), cyanosis may develop earlier than in patients with normal hemoglobin levels. Of course, there are slight variations in what is considered normal. Also, some patients with chronic respiratory conditions who have an artificially low oxygen saturation may also have a low level of chronic cyanosis. Patients with chronic bronchitis often have chronically low oxygen levels and relatively high hemoglobin levels, resulting in chronic peripheral cyanosis.
- **Chocolate brown skin.** High levels of methemoglobin derived from nitrates and some toxic exposures may turn the mucous membranes brown. This transformation is typically more evident in the patient's venous blood than in the skin and mucous membranes.
- **Pale skin.** Pale skin and mucous membranes are caused by a reduction of blood flow to the small vessels near the surface of the skin. The source of this condition could be hypoxia; shock; catecholamine release, such as from epinephrine or norepinephrine; or a cold environment.

Note whether the patient's mucous membranes are moist. Dehydration can be seen in the mucous membranes of the mouth and eyes. Dry, cracked lips; a dry, furrowed tongue; and

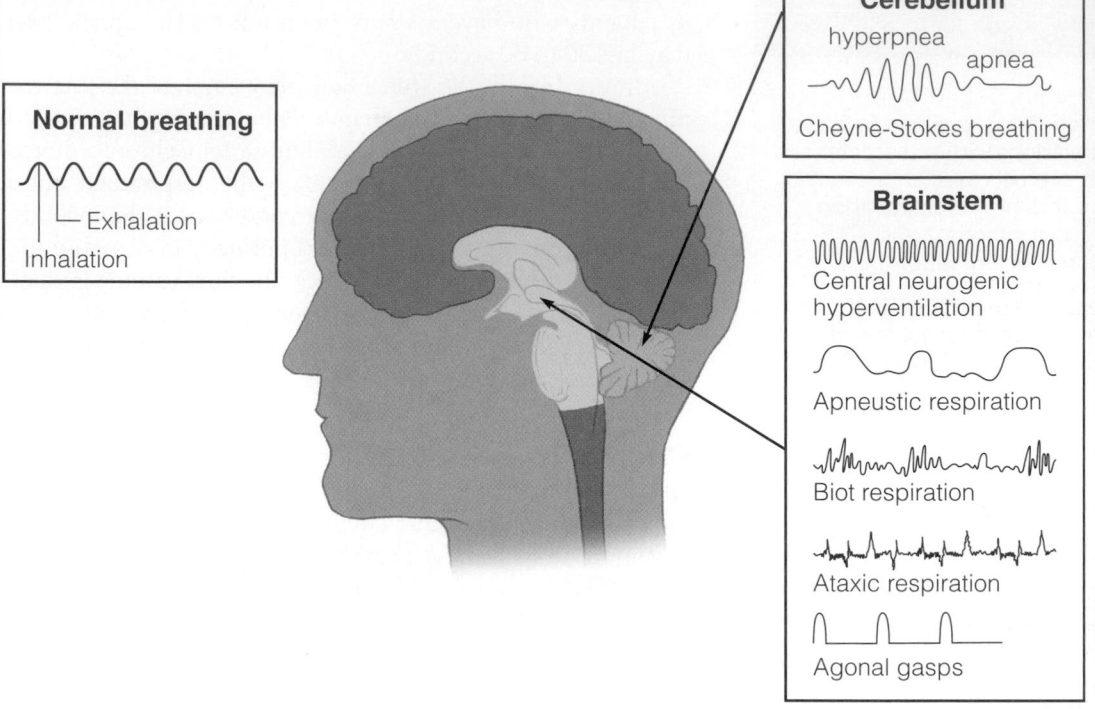

Normal breathing

Exhalation
Inhalation

Cerebellum

hyperpnea   apnea

Cheyne-Stokes breathing

Brainstem

Central neurogenic hyperventilation

Apneustic respiration

Biot respiration

Ataxic respiration

Agonal gasps

Figure 20 The neurologic control of respiration is complex, and many variations in the respiratory pattern may be noted in the scenario of brain injury. The respiratory patterns shown—each recorded for 1 minute—have been documented using an end-tidal carbon dioxide ($ETCO_2$) detector. Note that most irregular breathing patterns are controlled by the brainstem.

Transport Decisions

The treatment of acute cardiac and respiratory disorders is foundational in virtually all emergency departments. Patients with respiratory problems are usually transported to the closest hospital. In some settings, specialty pediatric centers are an option for children, particularly children with tracheostomies, home ventilators, or other sophisticated ventilatory supports.

Patients whose respiratory distress is related to renal failure would benefit from being taken to a facility that can provide emergency dialysis. (Not all centers that provide routine dialysis offer it on weekends or during the evening or night.)

When multiple emergency departments are available, paramedics should weigh the benefits of taking a patient to his or her preferred facility, where their previous laboratory and x-ray results and their own physician may be available, versus the closest facility if only a few minutes of travel time separate the options. Patients with acute decompensation should usually go to the closest facility, but the majority of patients with respiratory problems can tolerate a few extra minutes if it facilitates their care after they arrive.

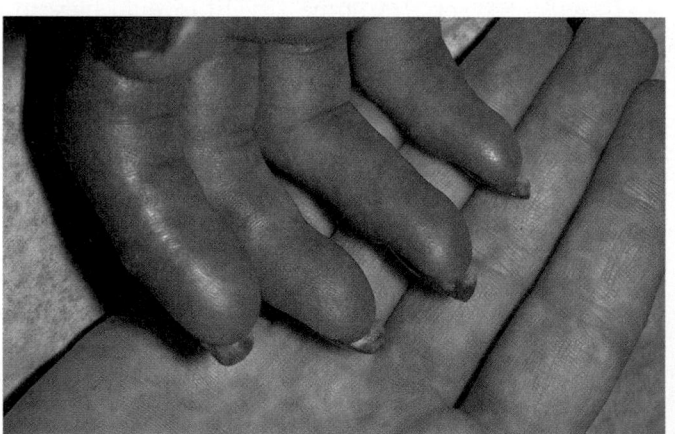

Figure 21 Skin color can provide an early, fast indication of several disease processes. Cyanosis (shown here) presents as bluish skin and indicates at least 5 g/dL of unoxygenated hemoglobin. Carbon monoxide intoxication can present as cherry-red skin, although this is a late sign. When making any preliminary diagnosis, allow for wide variation in the skin color and tone in patients.

History Taking

Investigate the Chief Complaint

Ask patients to explain in their own words what they are feeling. Many patients will identify their problem and explain the best way to treat it without the need to dig for the information. Patients with chronic respiratory conditions are often knowledgeable about the disease or disorder and may have tried several treatment options already. They might reveal that have been intubated and treated with a ventilator before. Many patients with chronic respiratory disease have some symptoms all of the time. The pertinent question for them is "What changed that made you call for an ambulance today?" Increased cough, a change in the amount or color of sputum, fever, or wheezing may be some of the chief complaints, in addition to the usual dyspnea. Chest pain is also a common chief complaint, whether from myocardial ischemia that caused acute left-sided heart failure or pneumonia and pleural infection resulting in chest pain with each breath.

dry, sunken eyes point to obvious dehydration. The skin of an older patient may always look dry with poor turgor, so skin assessment may be of less value in some older people.

One challenge in assessing patients with respiratory problems is that they may not be able to talk because of the difficulty breathing. Although it is usually best to ask open-ended questions and permit patients to tell their own stories, dyspneic patients may be able to speak only in short sentences or may be able to only nod in response to a series of yes-or-no questions. In some cases, the bulk of the history taking may have to be hastily obtained from a family member or gleaned from the few clues (such as medications) immediately available. Basic therapy (such as oxygen or aerosol therapy) often must be instituted before getting the complete story from a patient. Sometimes, a patient must immediately be intubated, which will eliminate the ability to get a direct history from that point on.

When patients are able to discuss their chief complaint with you, they may often be able to tell you exactly what the problem is. If they have one of the common respiratory illnesses (such as asthma, COPD, or CHF), they may be having an acute flare-up (called an exacerbation), or they might have one of the following common problems.

- **Asthma With Fever.** When patients with reactive airways begin wheezing, their inhalers usually will help for only a little while before symptoms return. The typical asthma attack that responds to treatment but occurs again in a few hours is sometimes caused by an underlying infection (such as pneumonia or bronchitis) that continually triggers the asthmalike symptoms. The asthma attack will not subside until the trigger is treated. Does the patient have a fever or chills? Is he or she coughing up sputum? What is the color of the sputum?

- **Failure of a Metered-Dose Inhaler.** Metered-dose inhalers indicate how many actuations (puffs) they are designed to deliver, but most patients do not keep close track of their use. Often the medication may be exhausted even though some propellant remains in the canister. A patient may have been inhaling nothing but propellant for days, which explains why the wheezing is not getting better. Similar problems can occur when patients use outdated medications or medications that have been overheated or improperly stored (left in a hot automobile or similar environment). In these cases, the bronchodilator from your ambulance may be effective, even though the patient's has failed. Another possible problem is that patients who do not fully understand how to use the device do not inhale at an appropriate point and then spray the medicine on the inside of the mouth. This is one reason that physicians often prescribe a spacer device to be used with the metered-dose inhaler.

- **Travel-Related Problems.** Some patients present with significant pulmonary edema after a lengthy journey. The culprit: not wanting to take diuretics while traveling. Remember to ask the obvious: "What medications do you use?" Which should always be followed by: "Did you take them during your travels?"

- **Dyspnea Triggers.** Just because a person knows the triggers for his or her reactive airways, such as pets, perfume, cigarette smoke, cold, or pollen, does not mean the triggers can always be avoided. A social or family situation may be important enough to risk having an episode of dyspnea, and no one can always prevent contact with all triggers (many of which are present in public places).

- **Seasonal Issues.** Bacteria, molds, and fungi can grow in heating ducts and air conditioners during the off-seasons. When the weather suddenly changes, and use of heating systems or air conditioners begins, an increase in calls from people with chronic respiratory diseases can be expected. Excessive heat, humidity, cold, pollen, dust, and smog can cause a flare-up of respiratory disease.

- **Noncompliance With Therapy.** Some people with chronic respiratory disease rebel against therapy as an attempt to regain control over their lives. Sometimes, the long-term nature of the therapy is not fully understood, and they attempt to wean themselves off their medications, oxygen, or respiratory support devices. Unfortunately, a crisis may result.

  Some patients have been prescribed home oxygen, aerosol therapy, continuous positive airway pressure (CPAP), bilevel positive airway pressure (BiPAP), or a variety of medications that they do not use or use only sporadically. Some medications, such as oral corticosteroids, can cause dangerous complications if use is stopped abruptly.

- **Failure of Technology or Running Out of Medicine.** Advances in technology have allowed patients who have chronic respiratory disease much more freedom to leave the house and to travel. Therefore, paramedics may be called to assist someone whose oxygen tank has run dry, whose portable ventilator has suddenly malfunctioned, or whose medications were left behind or lost with the luggage.

  When it is possible to discuss the history of the present illness with patients, several lines of discussion can provide important data.

SAMPLE History

The mnemonic SAMPLE (signs and symptoms, allergies, medications, pertinent past medical history, last oral intake, events preceding the onset of the complaint) helps paramedics systematically obtain information about the history of present illness and the medical history.

- **Signs and symptoms.** Respiratory difficulty must always be evaluated in light of the patient's cardiovascular and renal status. Many acute myocardial infarctions present as CHF, as do renal crises. Tachypnea can signal anxiety, diabetes, or shock. In addition, the vast majority of chronically ill patients have a respiratory component to their disease. A whole host of pathologic conditions can masquerade as respiratory distress, especially in patients who have underlying respiratory disease. Do not be too quick to conclude that the patient's *only* problem is a relatively straightforward respiratory issue. Always dig deeper to determine what else may be triggering or worsening the patient's respiratory distress.

- **Allergies.** A person's knowledge of the triggers for his or her respiratory difficulties does not mean that the person can always avoid the triggers. In your assessment, ask whether the person has been exposed to a known trigger.

- **Medications.** Part of a thorough history includes reviewing the patient's prescribed and over-the-counter medications. Many patients take multiple medications. A common combination might include a rapid-acting **beta-2 agonist** (rescue inhaler), a corticosteroid, and a slow-acting bronchodilator.

Dyspneic patients might resort to using—and sometimes misusing—over-the-counter medications in addition to their prescribed medications. The following is a list of over-the-counter medications that a patient may be using in conjunction with his or her prescribed medications:

- *Antihistamines* dry secretions and should not be taken by people who have asthma. Antihistamines are a common ingredient in many over-the-counter cough and cold medications.
- *Antitussives* are used to suppress coughs. Because coughing helps clear secretions from the airways, suppressing a cough might not be helpful. Coughs can be annoying, particularly if they interrupt sleep. However, the need for comfort must be weighed against the need to rid the airway of excess secretions. Overuse of antitussives can cause sedation, reduce respiratory drive, and cause excessive plugging of the airway with secretions. Many over-the-counter cough syrups also contain antihistamines that can cause problems if not used appropriately.
- *Bronchodilators* are available in some over-the-counter preparations. They often produce a nonspecific response, meaning that the medication may also have a significant effect on the heart and blood vessels, particularly when taken in addition to prescription bronchodilators. The most common over-the-counter bronchodilators are simply attenuated (diluted) forms of epinephrine.
- *Diuretics* can be found in diet pills and caffeine-containing products. However, the most common diuretics overused by people are the beverages that they drink. People are often told to drink plenty of fluids to maintain hydration, but drinking beverages that contain alcohol or caffeine, except in moderation, will have the opposite effect.
- *Expectorants* thin pulmonary secretions so that they can be coughed up. Most common expectorants can be purchased in over-the-counter products. Many products combine expectorants with antitussives or antihistamines. These combinations are often at odds with each other. People with increased mucus production should avoid antihistamine products, taking only products that contain guaifenesin (a type of expectorant).

By following a simple pattern of interviewing, it is possible to determine which medications the patient is supposed to take (which often gives valuable clues to other problems), whether the patient is taking the medications correctly, and whether the patient has any medication allergies.

- **Pertinent past medical history.** An asthma attack, CHF, pneumonia in immunocompromised patients, and even spontaneous pneumothorax are often repeating pathologic conditions. A patient's experience with these types of events can serve as a baseline to assess the current condition. Ask these questions: Do you feel better or worse than last time? How often does this happen to you? What did the doctor tell you it was? What helped you or what happened last time?

In addition, ask patients about tobacco use, exposure to secondhand smoke, and other possible toxic exposures.

- **Last oral intake.** The typical reason to ascertain the patient's last oral intake is concern about a full stomach should ET intubation be required. Patients with chronic respiratory disease also tend to eat and drink less when they become acutely ill, which adds dehydration and hypoglycemia or malnutrition to their already complex physiologic needs.

- **Events preceding the onset of the complaint.** It is important to determine what was happening just before or when the problem began. In addition, the speed with which the patient's distress has worsened is an important consideration in determining the underlying cause. Did this problem arise suddenly, or did it get worse over time? How long has it been this bad? The position of comfort and difficulty speaking may also indicate the degree of distress. A patient who is comfortable while lying flat and speaking in full sentences can be deemed to be in little distress. A patient who is sitting in a **Fowler's position** and speaking only in two- or three-word statements is probably in considerable distress, possibly even life-threatening distress. The patient might be described as having "three-word dyspnea."

Documentation and Communication

Remember to consult medical control. Report all pulmonary medications the patient is taking, and note whether they are oral, inhaled, or parenteral. If the patient uses an inhaler, report when the patient last used it, how many puffs were used at that time, and what the label instructs about dosage.

When respiratory disorders are chronic or recurring, patients may already have strategies to manage their crises. Determine what the patient may have already tried and whether it had any effect (positive or negative). Ask what the patient was doing when the episode of dyspnea began. Patients also often know exactly what caused their problems.

■ Secondary Assessment

Physical Examination

By the time a patient's history has been elicited, some important information should be known about his or her physical signs, such as level of consciousness, position, and degree of distress. This section presents the components of the physical exam in sequence, noting at each step the points of particular relevance to a patient with dyspnea.

Neurologic Assessment

Assessing the level of consciousness is imperative in patients with dyspnea. Although the patient's arterial blood gases cannot be measured in the field, the patient's brain is constantly doing precisely that. Any decline in Pao_2 (hypoxemia) will manifest initially as restlessness, confusion, and, in worst-case scenarios, as combative behavior. An increase in $Paco_2$, by contrast, usually has sedative effects, making the patient sleepy and difficult to rouse.

The respiratory system is involved in the delivery of oxygen to the bloodstream and the removal of carbon dioxide from the body. If the lungs are not functioning appropriately, both of these vital functions may be impaired. Failure to deliver oxygen efficiently results in cellular hypoxia. Hypoxia kills cells by making it impossible for them to make enough energy to do their work; it also causes acidosis. The brain is sensitive to reduced levels of oxygen. For this reason, any alteration in level of consciousness could represent a degree of respiratory compromise. Anxiety can be an early sign of hypoxia, while confusion, lethargy, and coma are typically later signs. A brief seizure often accompanies a hypoxic event or cardiac arrest. Dizziness and tingling extremities could signify hyperventilation.

Neck Exam

In the neck, look for __jugular venous distention__ when a patient is in a semisitting position. Jugular venous distention is a condition in which the jugular veins are engorged with blood. It is common in patients who have an obstructive lung disease such as asthma or COPD. Healthy young adults often have jugular venous distention when they are supine, and it is common to see gross jugular venous distention when people are laughing or singing **Figure 22**.

When jugular venous distention is present in patients who are sitting upright, it can provide a rough measure of the pressure in the right atrium of the heart. Distended neck veins may implicate cardiac failure as the source of dyspnea. Jugular venous distention may also indicate high pressure in the thorax, which keeps the blood from draining out of the head and neck. Cardiac tamponade, pneumothorax, heart failure, and COPD can all cause jugular venous distention. Hepatojugular reflux occurs when mild pressure on the patient's liver causes the jugular veins to engorge further. This is a specific sign of right-sided heart failure.

Jugular venous distention must be interpreted in the light of the patient's position and other vital signs. Grossly distended jugular veins despite a blood pressure of 80/40 mm Hg in a

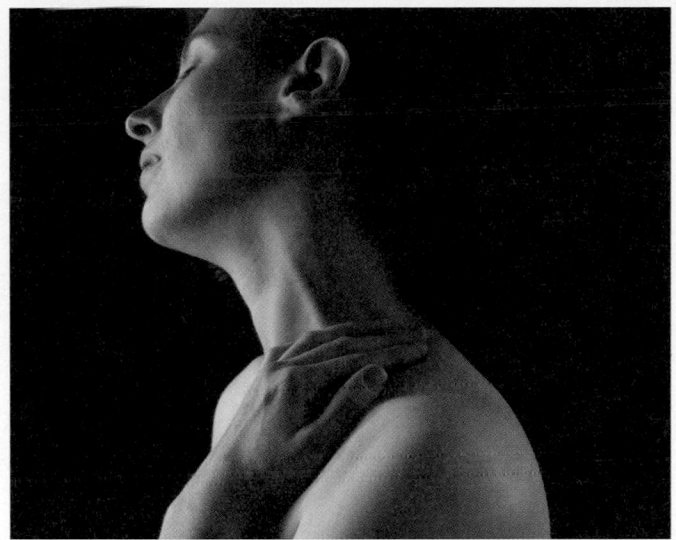

Figure 22   Jugular venous distention may be a normal finding in a healthy young adult who is supine or laughing. In an adult who is sitting upright, however, distention may indicate that blood is backing up as it tries to enter the thorax or the right atrium.

trauma patient should cause considerable concern; however, jugular venous distention in a healthy 20-year-old person who is lying flat (but not while sitting) is of little concern.

While you are looking at the neck, note the trachea. Tracheal deviation is a classic—albeit late—sign of a tension pneumothorax **Figure 23**. Tension pneumothorax is difficult to see except in extreme cases. On a radiograph, the trachea can clearly be seen deviating because of a tension pneumothorax. The deviation occurs behind the sternum, so it may not be seen or felt. Consider palpating the trachea at the suprasternal notch.

Chest and Abdominal Exam

Hepatojugular reflux is specific to right-sided heart failure. When the right ventricle is not pumping effectively, blood backs up, making it difficult for the jugular veins and the large reservoir of blood in the liver to drain into the thorax. As a result, the combination of jugular venous distention and hepatomegaly (distended liver) may present in right-sided heart failure. Pressing gently on the liver will further engorge the jugular veins (hepatojugular reflux). You can elicit this sign of right-sided heart failure when a patient in respiratory distress is sitting up in a semi-Fowler's (45°) position.

Feel the chest for vibrations as the patient breathes (__tactile fremitus__); secretions in the large airways are usually easy to feel and to hear. Some recommend percussion of the chest. With experience, it is possible to distinguish between the sounds of a normal chest and the sounds of a large pneumothorax, but percussion remains a difficult procedure to use in the field because of ambient noise.

Trauma to the chest or abdomen can cause respiratory distress by a variety of mechanisms (see the chapters, *Chest Trauma* and *Abdominal and Genitourinary Trauma*).

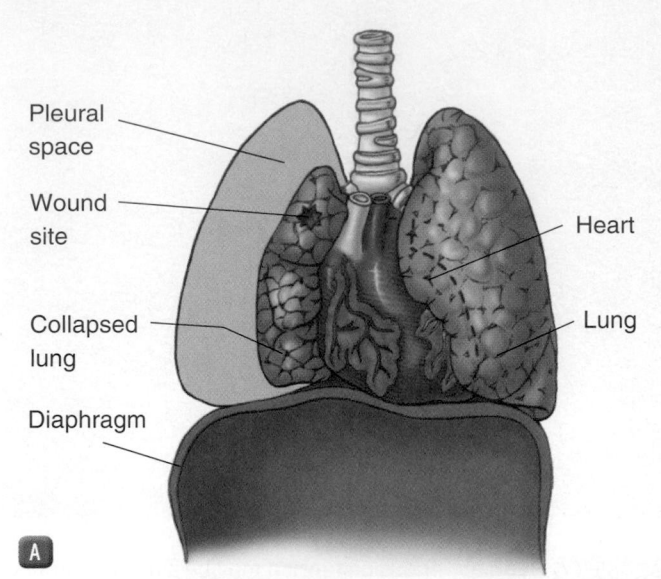

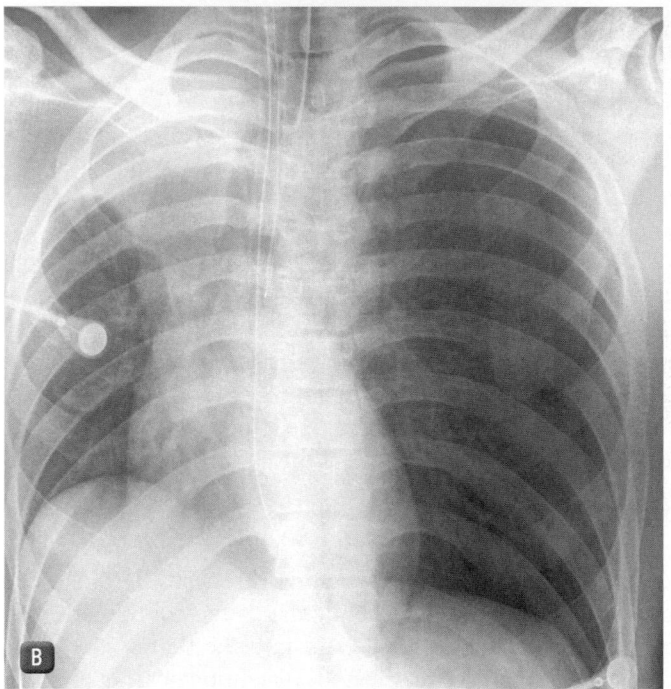

Figure 23 A pneumothorax occurs when air leaks into the pleural space between the lung and the chest wall **(A)**. The radiograph **(B)** shows a collapsed lung on the right, which appears darker.

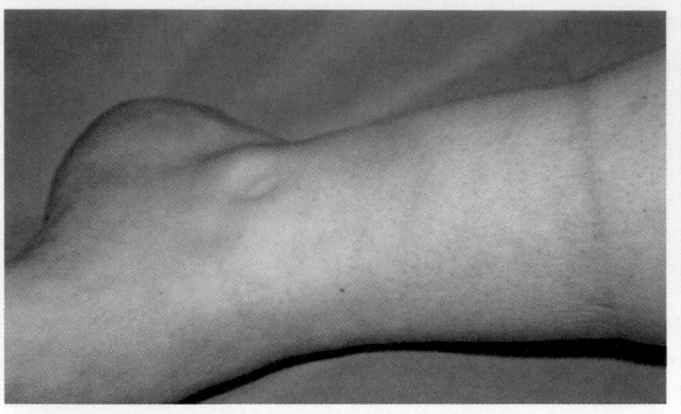

Figure 24 Pitting edema is present when the fingers leave a temporary depression in the tissue.

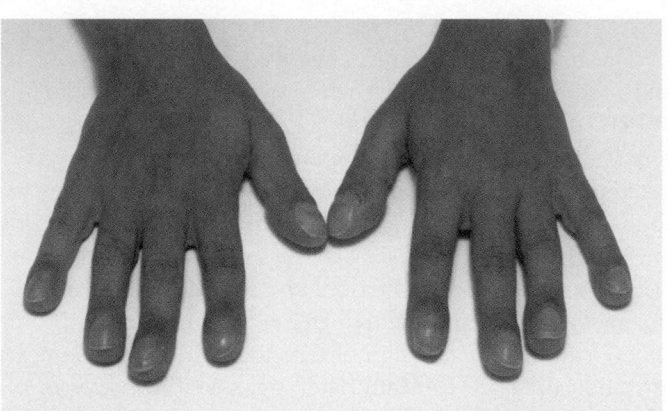

Figure 25 Digital clubbing is a sign of chronic hypoxia. It is seen in young people who have congenital heart disease and in older people who have severe chronic lung disease.

Examination of the Extremities

Does the patient have edema of the ankles or lower back? If so, does it pit when a finger is pushed into the edematous tissue **Figure 24**? Is there peripheral cyanosis? Check the pulse. Does the patient have profound tachycardia (from exertion or hypoxia)? Is there **pulsus paradoxus**? Also note the patient's skin temperature. Does the patient have an obvious fever, or is the patient's skin cool and clammy from shock? Is there distal clubbing (from chronic hypoxia) **Figure 25**?

Vital Signs

Vital signs besides the respiratory rate and quality of respirations will provide obvious clues to the respiratory workload. Patients under stress can be expected to have tachycardia (because of hypoxemia, the use of sympathomimetic drugs, and the stress of dyspnea) and hypertension (for the same reasons). Bradycardia, hypotension, and falling respiratory rates are ominous signs of impending arrest in patients with respiratory diseases.

Monitoring Devices

As appropriate to the patient care plan, apply any monitors that are immediately available. Repeated vital signs, ECG, and pulse oximetry readings are the data most commonly collected. In some situations, depending on available equipment, peak expiratory flow, $ETCO_2$, and transcutaneous carbon monoxide levels might be recorded.

Stethoscope

Practically speaking, the stethoscope is the single most important investment a paramedic will make. A paramedic should buy the best he or she can afford and take good care of it. Periodically check to make sure the earpieces are clean and clear of earwax. Regularly wipe the length of the main tubing with an all-purpose cleaner. This cleaning helps slow the breakdown of the tube from the oils picked up when it is placed around the neck.

The diaphragm of the stethoscope is for high-pitched sounds (breath sounds); the bell (if present) is for low-pitched sounds (some heart tones). Pressing the bell firmly against the skin stretches the skin beneath it and makes it act like a diaphragm. Therefore, the bell should be placed lightly against the skin to hear the lower pitched sounds. Some newer stethoscopes take advantage of this principle, allowing a single head to help transmit high and low-pitched sounds based on the pressure exerted by the operator. In older style stethoscopes, the bell rotates to allow the examiner to hear the sounds better.

The ear canals tend to point anteriorly in your skull (toward your eyes). The earpieces on the scope can be tilted farther forward for a better fit. But be careful: accidentally placing the scope in the ears backward causes the earpieces to hit the sides of the ear canal, obscuring nearly all sound.

The following guideline applies to stethoscopes: the longer the tubing, the more extraneous noise will be heard. Avoid overly long stethoscopes. Higher quality stethoscopes have a tubing-within-the-tubing design that limits external noise interference. Although the Sprague-Rappaport design is popular, its two parallel tubes often bang against each other while moving, which can create extra noise.

Pulse Oximeter

Under normal circumstances, a pulse oximeter is a noninvasive device that measures the percentage of a patient's hemoglobin that has oxygen attached to it **Figure 26**. For example, an oxygen saturation of 97% indicates that 97% of the patient's hemoglobin has oxygen attached to it. Oxygen saturation greater than 95% is considered normal. Most healthy people would feel short of breath at a saturation rate of less than 90%.

A pulse oximeter must "see" a pulsatile capillary bed to read properly. Nail polish may need to be removed with an acetone nail polish remover before a reading can be obtained (although some research indicates that if a consistent reading is being taken through nail polish, the reading is probably accurate). Inadequate peripheral perfusion, cold extremities, or patient movement (tremors or shivering) can make the reading inaccurate. Most pulse oximeters also display the patient's pulse rate; this reading should match the patient's palpated heart rate.

If the patient's hemoglobin level is low (as a consequence of trauma or hemorrhage, for example), the pulse oximetry result will be correspondingly high. If the reading shows only 6 g/dL of hemoglobin (normal, 14 g/dL), ideally all of the hemoglobin will have oxygen attached to it (100% saturation).

A patient with an abnormally high hemoglobin level, as is common in chronic hypoxia such as in cases of COPD, or a patient who lives at a high altitude, such as in Denver, Colorado, will have a correspondingly low oxygen

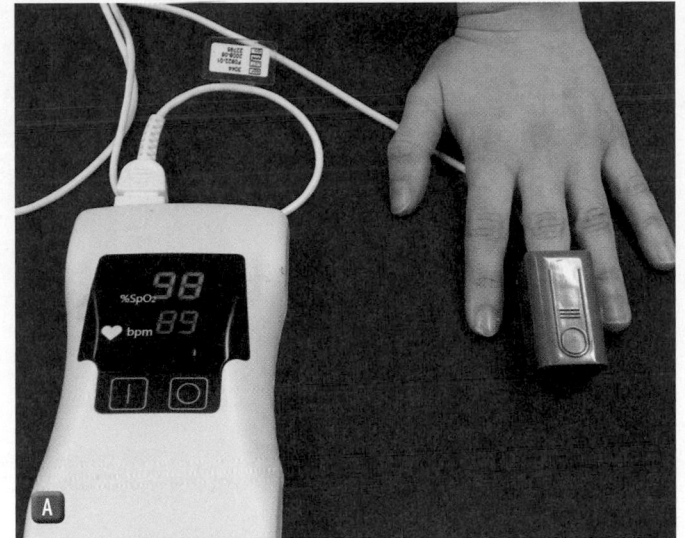

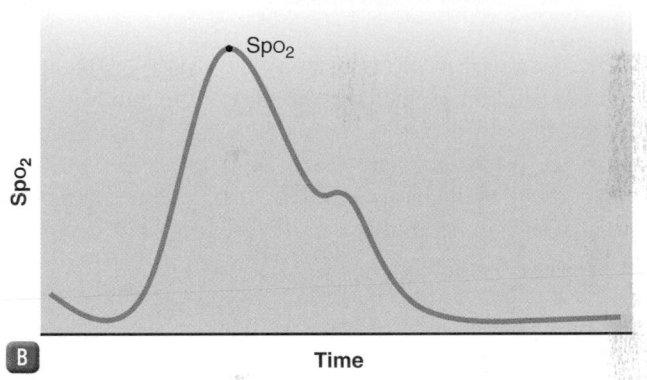

Figure 26 Pulse oximeters come in many sizes and, increasingly, are built into cardiac monitors **(A)**. Some oximeters provide a waveform **(B)**, which should demonstrate this characteristic shape when the oximeter is properly sensing.

saturation. For example, a patient with a combination of moderate hypoxia and polycythemia (excess red blood cell production) may have a normal oxygen saturation level as low as 89% to 90%.

While it is relatively easy to measure oxygenation, a favorable oxygen saturation result does not necessarily mean that all is well. A pulse oximeter cannot differentiate between an oxygen molecule attached to hemoglobin and a carbon monoxide molecule attached to hemoglobin. Most people who live in an industrialized society have a 1% to 2% carbon monoxide level all the time. Smokers may have a level as high as 3% to 4%. Thus, a 97% pulse oximetry reading may actually comprise 95% oxygen saturation and 2% carbon monoxide saturation. A patient whose hemoglobin has a toxic or even fatal level of carbon monoxide attachment may nevertheless show a normal or high pulse oximetry value. Fortunately, portable devices that specifically measure carbon monoxide levels are poised to become important tools, enabling paramedics to readily assess for carbon monoxide poisoning in the field **Figure 27**.

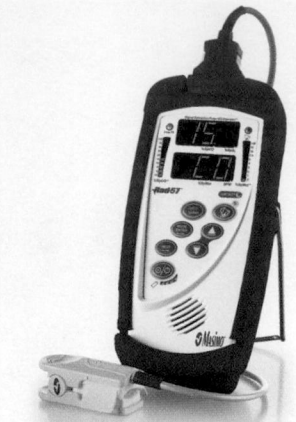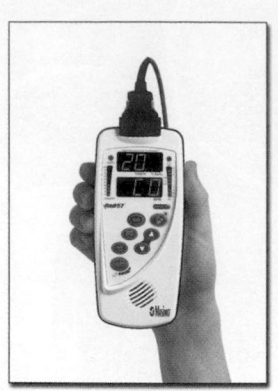

Figure 27 Devices are available that can measure oxygen saturation and carbon monoxide levels.

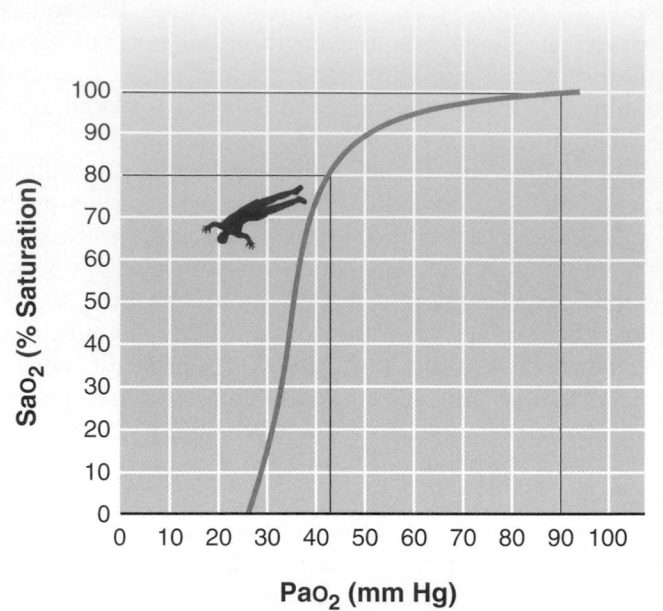

Figure 28 The oxyhemoglobin dissociation curve. As patients become increasingly hypoxemic (lower Pao_2), they may "fall off" the curve as their saturation drops rapidly.

The oxyhemoglobin dissociation curve **Figure 28** illustrates the relationship between oxygen saturation and the amount of oxygen dissolved in the plasma (Pao_2). It demonstrates that when oxygen molecules are scarce, they bind easily to hemoglobin, so that small changes in Pao_2 bring about relatively large changes in oxygen saturation. As the hemoglobin begins to fill up with oxygen molecules, larger changes in Pao_2 (shown on the horizontal axis) are required to produce changes in oxygen saturation.

Using a nonrebreathing mask for a healthy patient may increase the saturation level from 96% to 99%, whereas giving oxygen by a nasal cannula at 2 L/min to a hypoxic patient may increase the oxygen saturation from 80% to 92% (a more significant change). Conversely, the more hypoxic patients become, the faster they will "desaturate" as they "fall off" the steep part of the oxyhemoglobin dissociation curve. Other factors, such as acid-base balance, body temperature, and amount of hemoglobin, can also affect the entire system and shift the entire curve to the left or the right.

End-Tidal Carbon Dioxide Detector

Carbon dioxide is returned to the lungs in the venous blood, where it is exhaled during ventilation. This exhaled carbon dioxide can be measured by various means. *Capnometry* is the term that refers to the detection of $ETCO_2$ (a colorimetric detector is a capnometer) to confirm correct placement of an ET tube. Wave capnography is $ETCO_2$ monitoring by means of a device that measures the actual amount of carbon dioxide during a time (minutes or hours) and plots the resulting values graphically as a waveform. In other words, capnography provides numeric data, whereas capnometry simply confirms the presence of carbon dioxide.

Colorimetric **end-tidal carbon dioxide** ($ETCO_2$) detecting does not measure the exact amount of carbon dioxide exhaled, but it indicates whether carbon dioxide is present in *reasonable* amounts in the exhaled breath of a patient **Figure 29**. This type

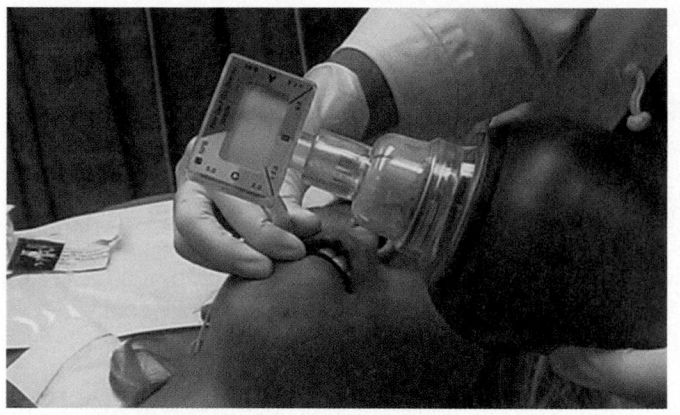

Figure 29 Colorimetric CO_2 detectors used to be popular prior to the availability of waveform capnography in the field.

of monitoring helps in identifying placement of an ET tube. Air exhaled through an ET tube that has been properly placed in the trachea of a patient with normal perfusion should contain 4% to 5% carbon dioxide (a yellow reading on the colorimetric device). If the tube has been mistakenly placed in the esophagus, less than 0.5% carbon dioxide will be present in the exhaled gas (a purple reading). Note that the monitor might be incorrect (or fooled) if the patient has carbon dioxide trapped in the stomach from the ingestion of carbonated beverages, so confirm the reading over at least six breaths to be certain it is not a false-positive.

The exact percentage of carbon dioxide contained in the last few milliliters of the patient's exhaled air can be measured by a special sensor. For example, some electronic ETCO$_2$ detectors use a photoelectric sensor that relies on absorption of infrared light by carbon dioxide to provide this measurement. The sensor can evaluate ETCO$_2$ in a spontaneously breathing patient via a specialized nasal cannula–type device, or it can be attached to the end of an ET tube. These devices typically display a waveform Figure 30 that can give additional data about the patient's respiratory status. In addition, such monitors serve as alarms that can alert paramedics to changes in respiratory rate or depth. This kind of monitoring is called **waveform capnography**.

The recent realization that the amount of ETCO$_2$ in the exhaled breath of a patient in cardiac arrest is an important indicator of the effectiveness of cardiopulmonary resuscitation (CPR) has led to a significantly increased awareness of this important value. In cardiac arrest, an ETCO$_2$ of less than 10 torr (torr = mm Hg) may indicate less-than-optimal CPR compressions. A sudden increase in ETCO$_2$ (from 10 to 35 mm Hg, for example) may be the earliest indicator of the return of spontaneous circulation. Keep in mind that the ETCO$_2$ value can be dramatically affected by the rate and depth of ventilation. The ultimate value of this parameter depends on a provider's ability to maintain ventilation at recommended levels (8 to 10 breaths/min at 6 to 7 mL/kg in an adult in cardiac arrest).

Peak Expiratory Flow

The peak flow is the maximum flow rate at which a patient can expel air from the lungs. (The chapter, *Airway Management and Ventilation* describes the use of a peak expiratory flowmeter.) A lower value indicates that the patient's larger airways are narrowed by bronchial constriction or bronchial edema. Many patients who have pulmonary disease check their peak flow twice a day and chart the results. They may present this chart when EMS personnel arrive. Normal peak flow values vary by age, sex, and height, but generally run from about 350 to 700 L/min; a peak flow less than 150 L/min is considered inadequate and signals significant distress. Some people with chronic asthma have a peak flow that never exceeds 100 L/min.

Reassessment

Interventions

Before administering the medications discussed in the following sections, a variety of other standard interventions should have already been implemented. Oxygen to keep the saturation above 93% and an intravenous line are typical interventions for any patient who needs advanced life support. Psychological support is also an important consideration for a patient with dyspnea. Your efforts to reduce that patient's anxiety with a calm, professional, and caring demeanor can help reduce the patient's heart rate and blood pressure and allow the patient to maximize breathing effectiveness.

In general, the sympathetic and parasympathetic nervous systems act as opposites. In terms of heart rate and bronchodilation, it is reasonable to think of them as the gas (sympathetic stimulation speeds the heart rate [beta-1] and produces bronchodilation [beta-2]) and the brake (parasympathetic stimulation slows the heart rate and causes bronchoconstriction). Anticholinergic medications block the parasympathetic response, so they are like taking the foot off the brake. It would be difficult to drive a car if someone were placing constant pressure on the brake pedal. Likewise, bronchodilation can be enhanced by specifically blocking the bronchoconstriction mechanism Figure 31.

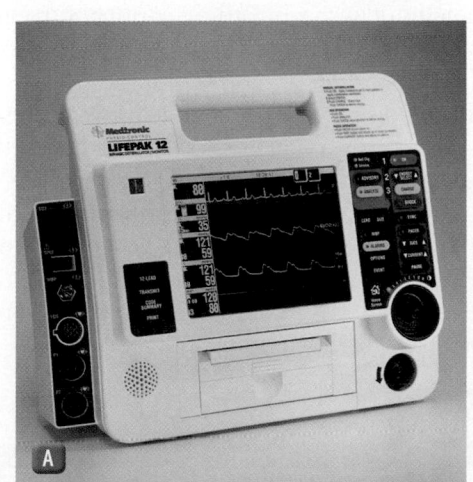

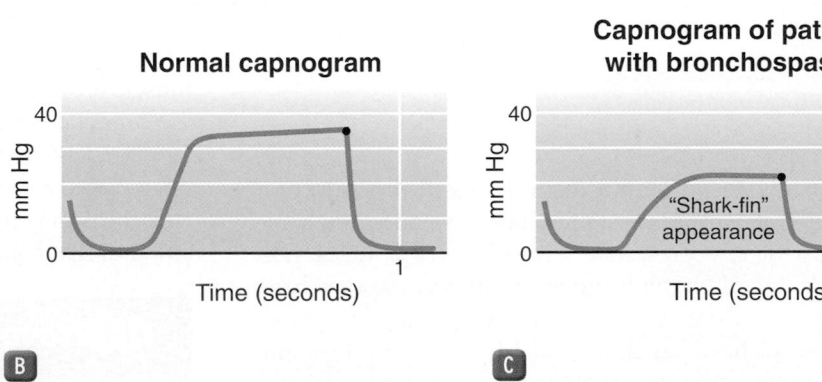

Normal capnogram

Capnogram of patient with bronchospasm

"Shark-fin" appearance

Time (seconds)

Time (seconds)

Figure 30 The waveform supplied by end-tidal carbon dioxide (ETCO$_2$) detectors **(A)** provides important data in addition to the ETCO$_2$ value. Variations in waveform shape—normal is shown in graph **(B)**—may help identify air-trapping disorders such as asthma **(C)** and chronic obstructive pulmonary disease. It may also document altered respiratory patterns and serve as an alarm for apnea, bradypnea, and tachypnea.

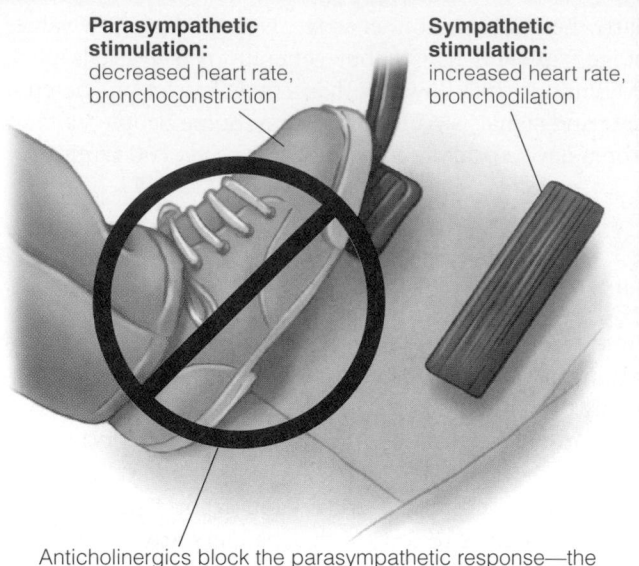

Parasympathetic stimulation: decreased heart rate, bronchoconstriction

Sympathetic stimulation: increased heart rate, bronchodilation

Anticholinergics block the parasympathetic response—the equivalent to taking the foot off of the brake pedal.

Figure 31 Blocking the parasympathetic nervous system (the anticholinergic effect) is like pulling the foot off the brake pedal, whereas giving sympathetic nervous system stimulators is like stepping on the gas.

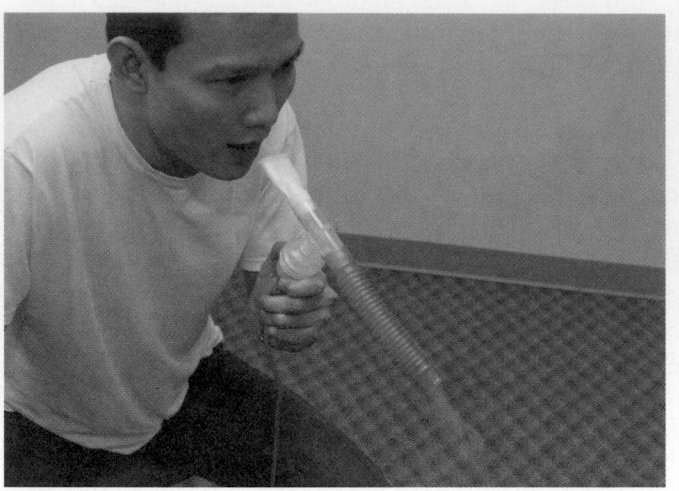

Figure 32 Aerosol nebulizers are often used to deliver medications directly to the respiratory tract. Unfortunately, they may give only 35% oxygen during a treatment. Flow rate is an important factor in how much medication reaches the lungs.

In the past, the strategy was to disperse atropine (the most common parasympathetic blocker) through an aerosol. Today, a medication specifically designed for aerosol use, ipratropium, is available. It is also available in a metered-dose inhaler. The combination of albuterol (a beta-2 agonist) and ipratropium (an anticholinergic) is also available as a premixed "cocktail," as an aerosol or a metered-dose inhaler.

Anticholinergics have emerged as a central component in the management of COPD. Tiotropium (Spiriva), a once-a-day anticholinergic for this indication, is taken via a type of dry powder inhaler. Patients taking tiotropium would not typically also use aerosol ipratropium.

Some of these medications are administered in the home by using an aerosol nebulizer, a metered-dose inhaler, or a dry powder inhaler.

Aerosol Therapy

Aerosol nebulizers deliver liquid medications in the form of a fine mist **Figure 32**. Particles that are 5 μm or smaller ride laminar airflow into the lower respiratory tract. Larger particles "rain out" in the mouth and pharynx and are swallowed, so they have little ultimate effect. To generate the optimal particle size, most nebulizers need to have gas flow of at least 6 L/min. Running the gas more slowly generates particles that are too large; running it significantly faster makes the treatment go faster, with the potential of less medication delivery.

In the home, most people run their aerosol treatments off of a small air compressor; in the ambulance, this therapy usually runs off of tanked oxygen or a wall unit attached to the main oxygen supply. As a result, the patient might receive only 35% to 40% oxygen via an aerosol treatment, which is still more than

the 21% oxygen contained in room air but may be less needed by patient with significant hypoxia. The relative drop in the fraction of inspired oxygen when removing a patient's nonrebreathing mask to give an aerosol treatment may be a contraindication to the procedure, particularly if the aerosol treatment has a minimal potential to improve the patient's condition.

A nebulizer can be attached to a mouthpiece (pipe), a face mask, or a tracheostomy collar, or it can simply be held in front of the patient's face (the so-called blow-by technique). The smaller the amount of mist the patient inhales, however, the less medication he or she receives. Blow-by and mouthpiece treatments are ineffectual if patients continually turn their heads or remove the mouthpiece to answer questions. As such, once the decision has been made to deliver a breathing treatment, try to stop the conversation and let the patient focus on inhaling the medication.

An aerosol treatment is a simple method of delivering drugs, such as bronchodilators. Bronchodilators relax the smooth muscle around the larger bronchi and are a significant therapy for bronchoconstriction. Strictly speaking, aerosol bronchodilators do not reduce swelling, push fluid out of the lungs, or open closed alveoli. However, patients with pneumonia, CHF, or atelectasis may have a small amount of secondary bronchoconstriction that could be reversed with a bronchodilator.

Controversies

In some systems, aerosol treatments are given to anyone who is dyspneic under the belief that "it might help, and it usually does not hurt"; in other systems, the use of aerosol bronchodilators is restricted to situations in which they are clearly indicated. Be sure to consult medical direction and your local protocols to keep abreast of how this class of medications is used in your region.

Although bronchodilators are the drugs most commonly delivered by this method, corticosteroids, anesthetic agents, antitussives, and mucolytics can be dispersed through an aerosol. Aerosol lidocaine is extremely effective for numbing the upper airway before procedures, and aerosol fentanyl is used to reduce chronic coughing in patients who are terminally ill with lung cancer.

Aerosols also deliver significant humidity to the airway. A quick way to provide a cooling mist to the swollen upper airway of a patient with burns or a child with croup is to give an aerosol treatment of saline solution. The chapter, *Burns* describes burns of the upper airway in more detail. Check with medical control or follow local protocols to learn more about these less common uses of aerosol therapy.

The newer aerosol bronchodilators cause far less tachycardia than the older, less beta-2–specific ones. As a result, it has become possible to give repeated treatments to patients with bronchospasm. Continuous nebulizers are available that hold up to 10 times the usual medication dosages and run for an hour or more. However, the potential for some beta-1 stimulation (causing tachycardia) remains, and some physicians are concerned that aerosol bronchodilators could worsen tachycardia in a patient with underlying cardiac disease. Tachycardia is almost always already present in patients with dyspnea, so be sure to consult medical control or local protocols for guidance. The steps for administering medications via small-volume nebulizer are shown in the chapter, *Medication Administration*.

Metered-Dose Inhalers

When properly used, a metered-dose inhaler should deliver the same amount of medication as an aerosol treatment. This device is small, easy for patients to carry and use, and convenient. Because it does not require additional equipment (such as a nebulizer or air compressor), it is usually the delivery method of choice for bronchodilators and corticosteroids in the home setting **Figure 33**. Because patients use (and may misuse) their own inhalers in the home, be sure to document how often the patient has been "taking an extra puff." Do not forget to consult

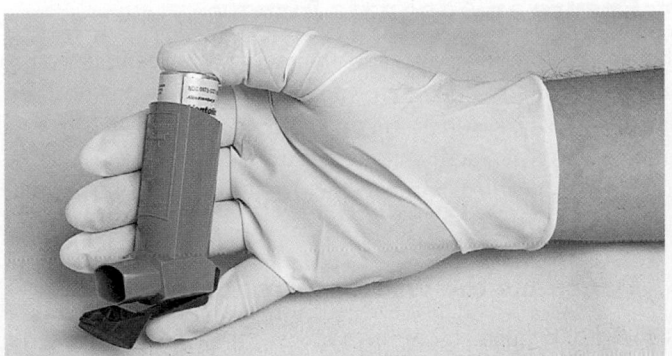

Figure 33 Metered-dose inhalers are a common delivery platform for respiratory medications. Their effectiveness is greatly increased by the use of a spacer device (not shown), which regulates the release of medication into the inhaler.

medical control before administering additional doses if this is required in your system.

The metered-dose inhalers on the ambulance should ideally be equipped with **spacers**. A spacer is a device that collects the medication as it is released from the canister, allowing more to be delivered to the lungs and less to be lost to the environment. Remember, the mist coming out of the inhaler is not what reaches the patient's alveoli; rather, the 5-μm particles, which stay suspended in the spacer for several minutes, are pulled deep into the lungs by smooth laminar flow. When a spacer is used, the patient does not have to worry about timing the inhalation to coincide with the discharge of the inhaler. Spacers also reduce deposition of the drug into the mouth and oropharynx, which is a problem with inexperienced users.

In addition to improving the delivery of the medication to patients, the spacer also allows paramedics to use the same expensive inhaler for multiple patients. Each patient gets a new spacer, but the inhaler can be used over and over. Be sure to use a system to keep track of how many times an inhaler has been used so that patients receive the proper amount of medication and not just propellant.

Achieving the proper technique when using a metered-dose inhaler is not difficult, but it requires constant reinforcement. The steps for administering medication with a metered-dose inhaler are shown in the chapter, *Medication Administration*.

The following are some tips on how to avoid common errors when using or administering a metered-dose inhaler:

- The mist from a metered-dose inhaler is not breath spray. Patients need to deeply inhale as they discharge the inhaler to draw the medication deep into their lungs. Placing the inhaler directly into the mouth (without a spacer) often causes much of the medication to fall on the posterior pharynx, and it is swallowed and digested, thus negating its intended effect.
- Some patients mistakenly blow into the spacer. Tell them to think of the spacer as a big straw, and they should try to suck the medication out of the bottom.
- Many spacers make a harmonica-like sound if the patient sucks too hard. The best particle deposition comes from smooth, low-pressure, laminar flow. Sucking too hard causes turbulent flow, which makes many of the particles stick to the trachea and large bronchi, where they are not as effective.
- Patients should try to inhale the medication deeply and then hold their breath for a few seconds. This is a lot to ask of someone who is dyspneic, and it is not always possible. Sometimes the inhalation causes the patient to cough immediately after inhaling the medication, which precludes delivery of a full dose but may be unavoidable.
- Make sure the inhaler contains medication. Most inhalers list the number of puffs of medication in the canister on the label. Patients should be encouraged to keep track of how many times they have used the inhaler and to discard it when they reach the recommended number of uses. Just because fluid is sloshing around in the canister when it is shaken does not mean that there is any medication left.

- Keep the spacer and canister holder clean. The spacer and canister holder should occasionally be rinsed off to avoid inhaling dust and other particles. In addition, respiratory devices should be dried after they are cleaned to avoid the growth of microorganisms.
- After using a corticosteroid inhaler, patients are encouraged to rinse out their mouth with water or mouthwash. Residual corticosteroid in the pharynx can predispose to thrush, an annoying fungal infection in the pharynx or mouth.

Special Populations

In asthma camp, children learn to take a puff of their bronchodilator inhaler, turn over an hourglass egg timer, and wait 1 or 2 minutes before taking the next puff. This strategy lets the first puff open up the airways a little so the second puff gets in deeper.

Failure of a Metered-Dose Inhaler

Metered-dose inhalers have some drawbacks. Using such a device requires a cooperative patient who is willing and able to perform the maneuver correctly. Because the entire dose is delivered in one or two breaths, little or no medication will reach the lungs if improper technique is used to administer the dose. An inhaler may be contraindicated for a patient who is not moving enough air to effectively draw the medication into the lungs. In addition, the patient may not realize when he or she is using an empty inhaler—in other words, the canister contains some propellant, but no medication.

A patient who does not fully understand how to use the device may inhale at an inappropriate point and end up spraying the medicine on the inside of the mouth. This is one reason that physicians often prescribe a spacer device to be used with the metered-dose inhaler.

Dry Powder Inhalers

Some respiratory medications are most stable in the form of a fine powder. Several common corticosteroids and slow-acting bronchodilators are often dispensed by means of a plastic disk that holds about 1 month's worth of medication. Each time the device is opened, the small plastic blister that holds a dose is rotated into position. The patient then pushes a small lever to puncture the blister, presses the disk to his or her lips over the opening, and inhales deeply to suck the powder out of the device. These devices are reasonably convenient and easy to use, but they are rarely used during emergency care.

Documentation and Communication

Teach patients to use their rescue inhalers before taking corticosteroids, slow-acting bronchodilators, and other medications. A rescue inhaler dilates the bronchi so that subsequent medications are more effective.

This device is used to deliver reasonably expensive medications, so do not to open and close it repeatedly; it is possible to waste several days' worth of medication as the blisters rotate into and then past their position to be punctured.

Other devices require the patient to insert a capsule of powdered medication, which is then pierced when the patient compresses a button or lever on the device. The patient sucks the powder out using a technique similar to that previously described.

Communication and Documentation

Contact medical control to report any change in level of consciousness or any increased difficulty breathing. Consistent with local protocol, contact medical control before assisting with administration of any prescribed medications. Document any changes, noting what time they occurred, and document any orders given by medical control.

■ Emergency Medical Care

This section discusses management of a patient with dyspnea. Management of specific diseases and conditions is discussed later in the chapter.

Paramedics have a relatively short list of tools to treat respiratory compromise. At the most basic level, the goal is to provide supportive care, administer supplemental oxygen therapy, and provide monitoring and transport. In actuality, little can be done in the field to alter the course of the pathologic condition (such as COPD, pneumonia, or pulmonary contusion).

The primary exception is the treatment of bronchoconstriction. A host of bronchodilators are available to help relax bronchial smooth muscle. This therapy can be extremely helpful if the patient's primary problem is bronchial muscle spasm resulting from anaphylaxis or asthma. Bronchodilator therapy may be somewhat helpful to many other patients as well.

At the other end of the spectrum of care are patients with overt respiratory failure. The primary approach is to take over the work of breathing completely by intubating and manually ventilating the patient.

■ Ensure an Adequate Airway

The first part of assessing and managing any respiratory problem is to ensure an open and maintainable airway. Food, gum, chewing tobacco, and like items should be removed from the patient's mouth. Suction if necessary, and keep the airway in the optimal position, which typically is the position that makes the patient most comfortable.

■ Decrease the Work of Breathing

Even under normal circumstances, muscles must work to allow breathing, and they must work much harder during respiratory distress. This extra work comes at a cost. People who have asthma, for example, can often compensate for respiratory distress by devoting substantial energy to breathing. They can maintain their oxygen and carbon dioxide levels in an acceptable range as long as they continue to apply their muscles to this effort. The tremendous workload uses large amounts of energy, which requires even more oxygen and ventilation. Patients in such a condition typically are not in a position to eat and drink normally, so they become progressively more dehydrated, malnourished, and fatigued. At some point, they will tire and be unable to continue the necessary work of breathing; they will look sleepy, the rate and depth of respirations will slowly drop, and they will experience decompensation (respiratory failure).

The Trendelenburg and supine positions, especially for an overweight patient, cause the abdominal organs to compress the diaphragm. With each breath, the patient must move the abdominal contents out of the way to expand the thorax and breathe. Abdominal distention with air or blood compounds the situation. Shortness of breath induced by lying flat is called __orthopnea__. It explains why most people maintain a sitting position when they are short of breath. To decrease the work of breathing, help the patient sit up if he or she is more comfortable in that position. Remove constricting clothing, such as belts and tight collars. *Do not make the person walk.* Relieve gastric distention, perhaps with a nasogastric tube. Do not bind the chest or make the patient lie on the side of the unaffected lung.

◼ Provide Supplemental Oxygen

It is essential to provide supplemental oxygen to any patient who needs it. Like any other drug, administer oxygen in the concentrations necessary to be effective. Patients who are not breathing adequately should receive bag-mask ventilation with supplemental oxygen. Closely reassess the patient's breathing status, and adjust treatment accordingly. Pulse oximetry is a useful guide to oxygenation if it is accurate (the pulse rate on the oximeter matches the palpated pulse) and if the patient's hemoglobin level is relatively normal.

It is safe to administer oxygen in concentrations less than 50% to almost anyone, and it is appropriate to do so when there is a reasonable chance the patient would benefit from it. Oxygen concentrations higher than 50% should be reserved for patients who have hypoxia that does not respond to lower concentrations, and the use of 100% oxygen should be limited to the shortest period necessary.

Of the oxygen in the body, 97% is bound to hemoglobin. The other 3% is dissolved in the plasma. Once all of the hemoglobin in the blood has been saturated with oxygen, further exposure to high concentrations of oxygen begins to damage the lung tissue in as little as 3 hours.

In the past, the inability to accurately measure oxygenation in the field, coupled with a lack of understanding of the hazards of high-concentration oxygen therapy, led to the common practice of giving 100% oxygen to any patient with dyspnea or any degree of hypoxia. That practice may warrant reconsideration, particularly in EMS systems where transport times may be prolonged. High concentrations of oxygen should be maintained for long periods (longer than 3 hours) only when the risk of long-term lung damage is outweighed by the need to save the patient's life. However, there is no evidence that short periods of high-dose oxygen administration (100% for up to 2 hours) is in any way dangerous.

YOU are the Medic   PART 4

While your partner prepares the patient for transport, you transmit the 12-lead ECG to the hospital and administer a dose of nitroglycerin paste. The patient's condition is still deteriorating. You have your partner begin positive pressure ventilation with a bag-valve mask device, and you establish an IV line. The patient initially resists but eventually becomes more comfortable and tolerates the treatment. You administer 40 mg of furosemide (Lasix) after confirming that the IV line is patent. As soon as the patient is in the ambulance, you begin priority 1 transport to the hospital. You contact medical control and request the use of additional nitroglycerin paste and additional furosemide. The physician grants the requests and also gives an order to administer 162 to 325 mg of aspirin to the patient. During transport, the patient's oxygen saturation progressively increases with treatment.

Recording Time: 10 Minutes	
Respirations	28 breaths/min; assisted
Pulse	100 beats/min
Skin	Pale and diaphoretic
Blood pressure	130/100 mm Hg
Oxygen saturation (Spo$_2$)	85% with oxygen by mask at 15 L/min and increasing
Pupils	Equal and reactive

7. What is the rationale for administering nitroglycerin if the patient is not experiencing chest pain?

■ Administer a Bronchodilator

Many patients who have respiratory distress can receive some benefit from bronchodilation, and some patients receive substantial benefit. Today's aerosol bronchodilators rarely hurt patients, so paramedics tend to use them aggressively in the field. Patients who do not have bronchospasm will probably benefit only slightly from aerosol bronchodilators, and the oxygen concentration that is delivered might need to be reduced during a typical aerosol treatment. In these circumstances, use of a nonrebreathing mask is a better choice than the aerosol treatment. Follow local protocol, but remember that bronchodilators are ineffective in conditions such as pneumonia, pulmonary edema, and heart disease.

Fast-Acting Bronchodilators

The most commonly used and fastest-acting bronchodilators work by stimulating the beta-2 receptors in the lungs—part of the sympathetic nervous system. These so-called rescue inhalers provide almost instant relief, a property that sometimes leads to their misuse. Present-day bronchodilators are beta-2–specific,

meaning that they stimulate only beta-2 receptors, without acting on other parts of the body. Many patients, however, still use older, less specific medications. Albuterol (Proventil, Ventolin), which is currently the most common beta-2 agonist, is routinely given every 4 hours, but more frequent treatments and even continuous therapy for hours at a time are often used without the occurrence of tachycardia.

Slow-Acting Bronchodilators

A variety of bronchodilators work by mechanisms other than beta-2 stimulation. Although most of these medications do not provide immediate relief of symptoms, if taken daily, they can reduce the frequency and severity of asthma attacks. Patients who are accustomed to the immediate change in their symptoms after using beta-2 agonists often complain that these agents do not work and need encouragement to take them as prescribed until the long-term benefits become evident.

Popular long-acting bronchodilators include salmeterol (Serevent) and cromolyn (Intal, NasalCrom). Such agents have dramatically improved the quality of life for many patients who have respiratory illness and who use the drugs correctly.

Leukotriene Modifiers

In some patients, bronchoconstricting chemicals called leukotrienes are released, particularly during an allergic response. A leukotriene blocker, such as montelukast (Singulair), which is usually taken orally, may be effective.

Methylxanthines

Methylxanthines, which include aminophylline and theophylline, were once the mainstay of therapy for asthma and COPD. Their popularity has declined in recent years because their adverse effects (particularly cardiac effects) are more onerous compared with those of the new drugs available. Some patients who have long-term COPD, however, still take aminophylline or theophylline. These drugs can be administered orally (in tablet form or in sprinkles placed on food); they can also be given intravenously. Overdose with these agents may cause cardiac dysrhythmias and hypotension, and the level of the drugs in the bloodstream must be closely monitored.

Electrolytes

Some studies indicate that magnesium has a role in bronchodilation, although this link remains controversial. In devastating asthma attacks, some physicians give 0.5 to 2 g of magnesium sulfate intravenously as a last-ditch effort before intubating. Consult with medical control, or follow local protocols regarding this therapy.

Corticosteroids

Corticosteroids are used to reduce bronchial swelling (edema). These corticosteroids are different from the anabolic corticosteroids that may be abused by athletes. The corticosteroids used in respiratory medicine have a variety of adverse effects. Long-term corticosteroid use can cause Cushing syndrome, which is characterized by the classic moon face and generalized edema. Corticosteroids cause rapidly changing blood glucose levels and can blunt the immune system, allowing an infection to flourish.

Discontinuing the use of corticosteroids such as prednisone must be done gradually. Because of the long-term adverse effects, a course of corticosteroid therapy is usually prescribed that lasts 1 or 2 weeks, with a particular end date in an attempt to avoid long-term use.

Inhaled Corticosteroids Inhaled corticosteroids do not seem to have the same adverse effects as their oral counterparts. For that reason, inhaled corticosteroids are becoming standard adjuncts to the treatment of asthma and COPD. Two of the components in the asthma triad can be addressed by a slow-acting bronchodilator to reduce bronchospasm and an inhaled corticosteroid to reduce airway edema. (The third component of the triad is increased mucus production. Asthma is discussed in more detail later in the chapter.)

Intravenous Corticosteroids In an emergency, it is common to give corticosteroids intravenously. A single bolus of IV corticosteroids does not seem to cause negative long-term consequences and is reasonably safe. Methylprednisolone and hydrocortisone are IV corticosteroid preparations given as an IV bolus, usually for acute exacerbations of COPD or acute asthma attacks. Their onset of action takes hours, so no results will be seen in the field. As always, consult local protocols and medical control before administering these agents.

■ Administer a Vasodilator

A variety of strategies that cause vasodilation, thereby sequestering more fluid in the venous circulation and decreasing preload, are potential treatments for pulmonary edema. Nitrates, from sublingual nitroglycerin tablets to nitroglycerin drips, can be used as long as the patient has adequate blood pressure and does not take a phosphodiesterase inhibitor such as sildenafil (Viagra) or tadalafil (Cialis). Morphine sulfate decreases anxiety but probably does not increase venous capacitance as much as once thought. Its use in pulmonary edema is not as common as it once was.

■ Restore Fluid Balance

Rehydration is supplemental therapy for patients with respiratory problems who are dehydrated (for example, some patients who have pneumonia or asthma). It is common to give a fluid bolus to younger patients who are dehydrated. In any elderly patient or patient who has cardiac dysfunction, pulmonary edema could be caused by the administration of too much fluid. Always assess breath sounds before and after giving a fluid bolus to be certain that the patient does not become overhydrated. Because the condition of a patient with respiratory problems can deteriorate precipitously, having an IV line in place is a wise precaution.

■ Administer a Diuretic

Not every patient who has crackles has pulmonary edema. Giving diuretics to patients who have pneumonia or asthma may worsen their overall condition by dehydrating them and causing secretions to further plug smaller airways.

Diuretics are used to help reduce blood pressure and to maintain fluid balance in patients who have heart failure. Patients with pulmonary edema may benefit from a diuretic to remove excess fluid from the circulation, which ultimately keeps it out of the lungs. Loop diuretics (bumetanide [Bumex] and furosemide) are the most commonly used agents in emergency situations. Thiazide diuretics are commonly taken orally to treat high blood pressure and heart failure.

Many diuretics cause the loss of not only fluid, but also potassium. Patients who do not take potassium supplements may have low potassium levels and a resulting predisposition to cardiac dysrhythmias and chronic muscle cramping.

Do not give diuretics to patients who have pneumonia or to patients who are already dehydrated—reserve their use for patients who clearly have pulmonary edema. Some EMS systems reserve furosemide in standing orders only for patients with "wet" lungs and peripheral edema, and others have removed it from their prehospital formulary because it has been overused.

Patients who have some degree of renal failure may require sizable doses of diuretics or may have no response to them. If a patient requires dialysis for renal failure, trying to induce diuresis is unlikely to be effective. While the management of respiratory distress is routine in virtually all emergency departments, a dialysis patient in pulmonary edema may be best served in a hospital with the ability to provide emergency dialysis. This may be one of the few circumstances in which a paramedic must make a decision to transport a patient with respiratory problems to a specialty center instead of the local emergency department.

■ Support or Assist Ventilation

If the patient becomes fatigued, breathing might need to be supported in a more aggressive manner. Therapy with CPAP and BiPAP is becoming increasingly common and can preclude the need for intubation in many patients. Some patients may simply require bag-mask ventilation for a short period to reoxygenate, improve hemoglobin saturation, and reduce the Pa_{CO_2} level.

It is important for paramedics to be confident in bag-mask ventilation technique to avoid worsening a patient's condition. Trying to assist breathing for a patient who is *already breathing on his or her own* is one of the most difficult interventions. Gastric distention and vomiting from overaggressive ventilation can complicate an already worsening situation. As always, *do no harm*. The same is true when providing sedation to anxious and possibly combative patients. The need to control a patient's behavior must be balanced against the possibility of depressing respirations further. It is almost always counterproductive to sedate patients in the field to treat erratic behavior that results from dyspnea.

Continuous Positive Airway Pressure

Continuous positive airway pressure is used in two distinctly different ways: to treat obstructive sleep apnea and to treat respiratory failure.

Many people with obstructive sleep apnea wear a CPAP unit at night to maintain their airways during sleep. This type of CPAP may be applied via nasal pillows, a nasal mask, a face mask that resembles a typical mask used for bag-mask ventilation, or a mask that covers the entire face. This is *not* the type of CPAP used for critically ill patients. The positive pressure delivered maintains the stability of the posterior pharynx, thereby preventing obstruction of the upper airway when the person sleeps. This pressure limits hypoxic episodes and snoring.

The CPAP used as therapy for respiratory failure is almost always delivered through a mask that is secured to the face by some type of strapping system. When positive pressure ventilation (that is, with a pocket mask or bag-mask ventilation) is given, air is forced into the upper airway and flows into the trachea and esophagus unless steps are taken to help direct it into the trachea Figure 34. Indeed, positive pressure ventilation with bag-mask ventilation or a pocket mask is physiologically the opposite of normal (negative pressure) ventilation.

When a bag-mask device is used for ventilation, positive pressure is created in the chest. The more forcefully the bag is squeezed, the higher the positive pressure. A pressure that is too high can cause several problems. Simple pneumothorax can evolve into tension pneumothorax, air leaks can produce huge amounts of subcutaneous air, and high intrathoracic pressure can retard, or even completely block, venous return. In recent years, prehospital providers have begun to understand the ramifications of positive pressure ventilation during low-flow states such as shock and cardiac arrest. This understanding has led to CPR guidelines that stress lower ventilation rates, smaller volumes, and lower pressures. CPR is based on principles of hemodynamics, and the rate, volume, and pressure of delivered breaths can quickly do more harm than good during resuscitation.

Administering CPAP increases pressure in the chest. If the patient's blood pressure is already low, too much CPAP can stop venous return to the heart and cause a sudden drop in blood pressure. This problem is uncommon with lower levels of CPAP, but blood pressure should be carefully monitored whenever CPAP is used (especially at levels more than 10 cm H_2O). Keep in mind that CPAP can turn a simple pneumothorax into a tension pneumothorax in only a few breaths.

Ensure a good seal with minimal leakage Figure 35. In the field, 100% supplemental oxygen is the most common driving gas for the positive pressure. Be vigilant about monitoring the gas supply—depending on the flow and the patient's respiratory rate, some CPAP units may empty a D cylinder in as little as 5 or 10 minutes. The mask is fitted with a pressure-relief valve that determines the amount of pressure delivered (such as 5 cm H_2O). The effect is similar to being in a gale-force wind (high inspiratory flow) and having to push a pressure valve open with exhalation. This would seem to require a great deal of effort and tire out a patient in decompensating respiratory failure, but many patients in critical condition make a dramatic turnaround when CPAP is applied.

Some patients find the CPAP mask claustrophobic and will fight its application. Some patients can be talked through the process with good results, but other patients simply cannot tolerate the mask. Do not fight with a patient who is unwilling to use the mask; doing so will increase the patient's anxiety, cardiac workload, and cardiac oxygen consumption. When CPAP works as intended, it can provide dramatic relief and avoid intubation. When it fails, it is critical to recognize a deteriorating condition and be prepared to move to the next step (usually intubation). Within several minutes of application, the patient's oxygen saturation should increase and the respiratory rate should decrease. The success of CPAP is inversely related to the patient's respiratory rate soon after its application. If this rate *increases*, the therapy is likely to fail; if this rate *decreases*, the therapy is likely to succeed.

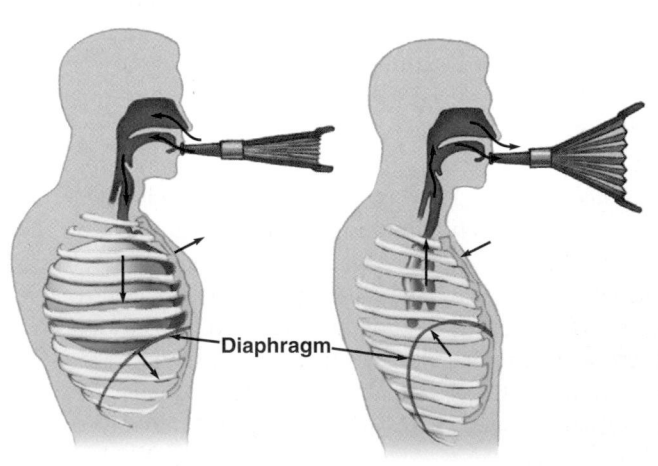

Ventilation   **Exhalation**

Figure 34 Positive pressure ventilation is physiologically the opposite of normal ventilation. Air is pushed into the respiratory tract with bag-mask ventilation and can enter the esophagus and stomach unless careful technique is used. Compare with negative pressure ventilation, shown in Figure 13.

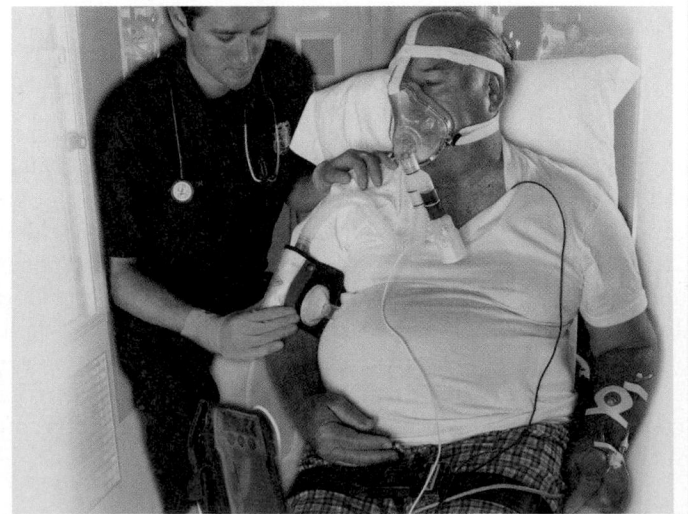

Figure 35 The continuous positive airway pressure used in the acute setting is usually administered via face mask, which must make a tight seal to function properly.

Bilevel Positive Airway Pressure

In BiPAP, one pressure can be delivered during inspiration (inspiratory positive airway pressure) and a different pressure can be delivered during exhalation (expiratory positive airway pressure). Instead of delivering 20 cm H_2O as in CPAP, BiPAP set at 20/8 gives 20 cm H_2O pressure during inhalation and 8 cm H_2O pressure during exhalation. Because this type of positive airway pressure is more like normal breathing, it is often more comfortable for patients. It causes a pressure variation in the chest, which allows for more normal blood flow. The BiPAP device is also more complex and expensive, and it is not commonly used in the field.

Automated Transport Ventilators

Automated transport ventilators are essentially flow-restricted oxygen-powered ventilation devices with built-in timers. They can be set to deliver a particular volume of oxygen at a particular rate, which can be helpful when an extra pair of hands is needed Figure 36 . They are a particularly good substitute for bag-mask ventilation for patient in cardiac or respiratory arrest. Basic automated transport ventilators may not offer advanced features, such as alarms, flow rate controls, and a selection of ventilatory modes. They are *not* little ventilators and are *not* intended to ventilate patients without direct observation and attention by a skilled paramedic.

Conscious patients require up to 150 L/min of flow to breathe comfortably. Most automated transport ventilators are permanently set to deliver 40 L/min, which would be extremely uncomfortable for a spontaneously breathing patient. Flow-restricted oxygen-powered ventilation devices and automated transport ventilators are preset to 40 L/min, which is the optimal flow for ventilating a patient in cardiac arrest—via face mask and without causing gastric distention.

■ Intubate the Patient

Ultimately, patients who are in respiratory failure may need to be intubated and ventilated. Intubation can be lifesaving, and

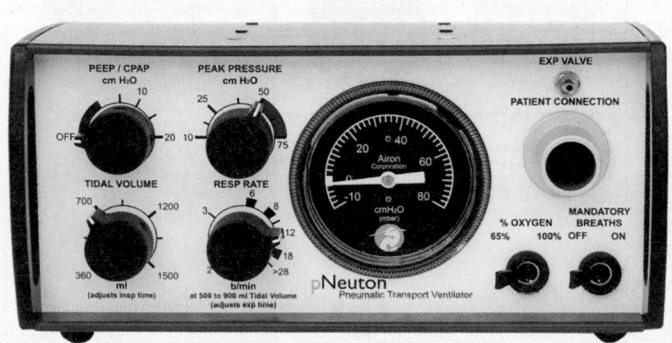

Figure 36 Portable versions of this automatic transport ventilator can be used in the field to dial in specific ventilation rates and volumes. This can be useful in cardiac arrest once the patient has an advanced airway inserted to assure proper ventilation.

many patients can be extubated within a day or two and have an excellent outcome. However, there are some issues to consider when intubating a patient. Paramedics must weigh these issues along with the protocols, medical direction, and any expression of the patient's wishes. Keep these issues in mind:

- Intubation should be the last option for patients who have severe asthma. Patients with asthma are extremely difficult to ventilate and are prone to pneumothoraces.
- Be proactive; ventilate patients *before* cardiac arrest occurs. When in doubt, attempt to ventilate. A patient who is combative may not be ready for intubation. If a patient allows intubation, it was probably necessary. Patients who are conscious, yet still in respiratory distress will require sedation and neuromuscular blocking medications (through rapid-sequence intubation) to facilitate intubation.
- Patients who have had a stroke or who are severely intoxicated may have little or no gag reflex, the lack of which poses a grave danger if the patient vomits. Consider intubating patients in these situations to protect the airway even if ventilation is adequate.
- Some patients who have diabetes or have overdosed present with an obvious need for intubation. However, if an ampule of 50% dextrose or naloxone (Narcan) is likely to completely change that picture, it might be better to use bag-mask ventilation for a few minutes to monitor the effect of the initial therapy, assuming ventilation can be done without causing gastric distention and vomiting. Ventilate slowly (over 1 second), and use only enough ventilation to produce visible chest rise.

■ Inject a Beta-Adrenergic Receptor Agonist Subcutaneously

Drug administration methods that require the patient to inhale the medication may be unreliable or ineffective when the patient's breathing effort is inadequate (reduced tidal volume). In some circumstances, it may be beneficial to attempt beta-2 stimulation the old way—that is, by administering subcutaneous or intramuscular terbutaline or epinephrine. These medications are not as beta-2-specific as their aerosol cousins, so they will also cause more tachycardia (beta-1 stimulation) and hypertension (alpha stimulation), but when a patient's airways are severely closed, they are sometimes the more effective approach. Be particularly careful using these agents in elderly patients who may not tolerate the additional cardiac stimulation well.

■ Instill Medication Directly Through an Endotracheal Tube

Under certain circumstances, such as cardiac arrest when prompt vascular access is delayed, the administration of select drugs (such as epinephrine or atropine) via the ET tube is an option. The dose of epinephrine is usually 2 to 2.5 times the usual dose because much of the drug does not reach the terminal bronchioles for absorption into the bloodstream. Newer devices "mist" the drug into the tube, which can be done without interrupting CPR. Although American Heart Association guidelines discourage endotracheal drug delivery, it is an option if all else fails.

Pathophysiology, Assessment, and Management of Obstructive Upper Airway Diseases

Anatomic Obstruction

Pathophysiology

The most common cause of upper airway obstruction in a semiconscious or an unconscious patient is the tongue. Every year, obstruction caused by the tongue results in the death of some trauma patients, patients in insulin shock, patients who have had a seizure, or patients who are intoxicated.

Assessment

Assessment of the airway is among the most foundational skills of paramedics. Anyone with a decreased level of consciousness, particularly if in a supine position, is at risk for some upper airway obstruction. Sonorous (snoring) respirations are an obvious sign that breathing is at least partially obstructed. Other signs include gurgling, squeaking, and bubbling sounds during breathing. Stridor may be associated with accessory muscle use or retractions if the patient is attempting to breathe through an obstructed airway.

Management

Many times, bystanders place a pillow behind the head of an unresponsive person, which exacerbates this problem. If the patient is snoring, remove the pillow and reposition the patient's airway.

Excess soft tissue in the airway is one cause of obstructive sleep apnea, and some people go so far as to have tissue surgically removed from their pharynx to limit this anatomic obstruction. Fortunately, the soft tissue of the upper airway can be manually displaced with a variety of basic maneuvers, which were discussed in the chapter, *Airway Management and Ventilation*. If restriction of spinal motion is not needed, an unconscious patient may be positioned in the recovery position to avoid blocking the airway. The recovery position is the safest position for many patients who have had a seizure or are hypoglycemic or intoxicated. It also reduces the risk of aspiration if the patient vomits.

Inflammation Caused by Infection

Pathophysiology

A variety of infections can cause swelling in the upper airway. Infections can lead to <u>laryngotracheobronchitis</u>, which is inflammation of the larynx, trachea, and bronchi. An acute form of laryngotracheobronchitis is a common cause of <u>croup</u>, a condition characterized by stridor, hoarseness, and a barking cough that most commonly occurs in infants and small children. (Some authors consider laryngotracheobronchitis and croup to be the same.) Poiseuille's law holds that as the diameter of a tube decreases, resistance to flow increases exponentially. This law explains why children—who have narrow airways—have croup when an infection causes upper airway swelling, whereas adults with the same infection do not **Figure 37** . Viral infections are more common than bacterial infections as an underlying cause of croup. Croup may also be caused by allergies that result in airway swelling and obstruction and obstruction with a foreign body.

The palatine tonsils can also become impressively inflamed in children, but this condition is rarely life threatening. When a child is properly positioned for intubation, inflamed tonsils do not typically obstruct a clear view of the glottis, but take care to avoid injuring them with the laryngoscope because the tonsils can swell and bleed if traumatized.

Assessment

In recent decades, many deadly upper airway conditions, such as epiglottitis, have become rare as a result of widespread immunization efforts. Unfortunately, the rate of childhood

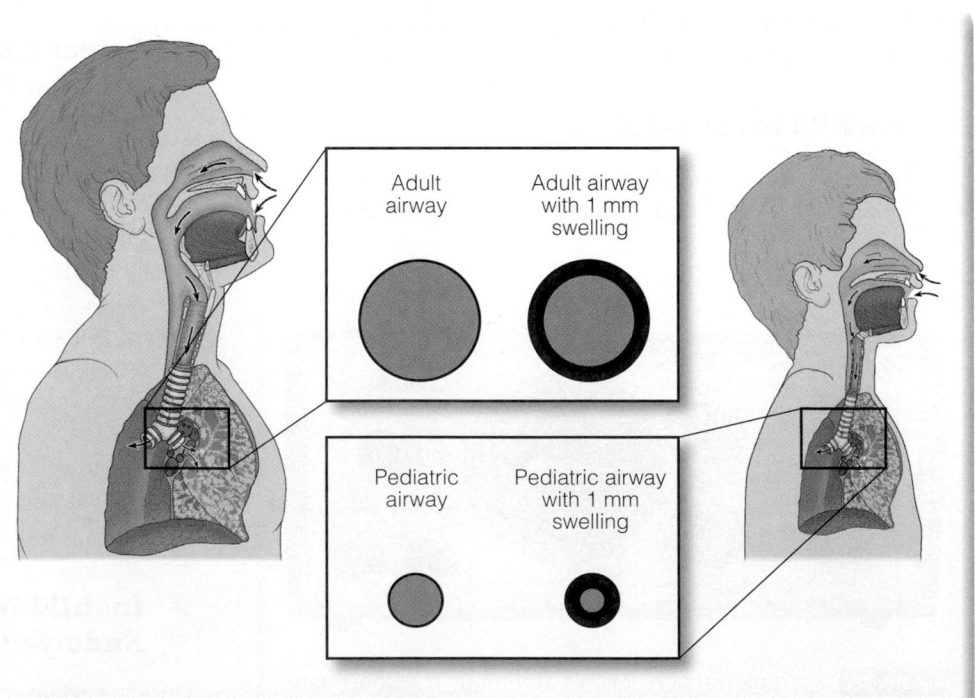

Figure 37 Any constriction of the airway (caused by a condition such as asthma) can severely reduce the volume of airflow, especially in children. Poiseuille's law states that as the diameter of a tube decreases, resistance to flow increases exponentially.

immunizations has begun to decline as the general public becomes complacent about these diseases, so paramedics must remain vigilant for these pathologic conditions. Table 7 lists inflammatory conditions that can impair the upper airway, with some of the signs and symptoms that may accompany each.

Table 7 Inflammatory Conditions That Can Impair the Upper Airway

Condition	Comments
Croup	A condition most commonly found in children between 6 months and 3 years old, but can occur at any age; in northern areas, most common between October and March; characterized by stridor, hoarseness, and a barking cough; distressing but not typically fatal; may be a result of laryngotracheobronchitis with a viral or bacterial infection as the underlying cause. Do not manipulate the airway.
Epiglottitis	Severe, rapidly progressive inflammation of the epiglottis and surrounding tissues, usually due to an infection (most commonly with *Haemophilus influenzae* type b), that may be fatal because of sudden respiratory obstruction; a life-threatening emergency; signs and symptoms include sore throat, fever, drooling, hoarseness, and purposeful hyperextension of the neck; once more common in children, it is now rare due to widespread immunization against H flu, leaving unimmunized adults as the most common susceptible group. Fortunately, the pathology is less life threatening in adults.
Peritonsillar abscess	Uncommon in children, more common in young adults; **abscess** forms near one pharyngeal tonsil; symptoms include fever and sore throat; may be mistaken for epiglottitis until a lateral abscess (instead of enlarged epiglottis) is seen in the throat. Do not manipulate the airway.
Retropharyngeal abscess	Most common in children; caused by infection in retropharyngeal lymph nodes and by direct trauma to pharynx; signs and symptoms include fever and sudden stridor; may be mistaken for epiglottitis until laryngoscopic examination reveals retropharyngeal abscess (instead of cherry-red epiglottis). Do not manipulate the airway.
Diphtheria	Causative bacterium attacks and kills layer of epithelial tissue, creating **pseudomembrane**, often in tonsillar area; membrane (and swelling of upper airway caused by disease) can obstruct upper airway; no longer common because of diphtheria, tetanus, and pertussis (DTP) immunization. Do not manipulate the airway.
Enlarged tonsils	**Palatine tonsils** can swell excessively, sometimes to golf ball size; associated with fever, difficulty swallowing, and throat pain; rarely obstruct the airway but can cause snoring and stridor. Do not manipulate the airway.

Words of Wisdom

Immunizations have significantly reduced the incidence of many infectious diseases, such as diphtheria; however, an increasing number of people in the United States do not receive immunizations (because of poverty, lack of access to health care, geographical isolation) or refuse to be immunized (because of fears that immunizations cause other diseases or beliefs that immunizations are unnecessary), causing the resurgence of some diseases. In addition, because the effects of immunizations do not last forever, conditions such as epiglottitis may be seen in adults in their 20s and 30s, albeit rarely.

Croup and tonsillitis are common, especially in children, but the other conditions mentioned are rare. When these pathologic conditions occur, they are critical emergencies, because swelling can rapidly obstruct the airway, making orotracheal intubation extremely difficult or impossible. *Avoid manipulating the airway* unless absolutely necessary. Ventilation is usually possible with careful bag-mask technique.

Management

If intubation is essential because of an inability to effectively ventilate the patient with bag-mask ventilation, the airway may prove to be entirely obscured by the swelling and attempts at laryngoscopy may worsen the swelling. Ask a partner to press on the patient's chest while you look for a stream of bubbles coming from the airway (use an ET tube at least two full sizes smaller than the size that would typically be appropriate for that patient). If this effort fails after a single attempt, a needle or surgical cricothyrotomy will be necessary. It is better to defer surgical attempts to the staff at the closest hospital, but time may force you to use an invasive airway approach if permitted in your system.

▮ Aspiration

The inhalation of anything other than breathable gases is called aspiration. Patients can aspirate fresh or salt water, blood, vomitus, or food. Patients who receive tube feedings are at particular risk for aspiration if they are placed supine immediately after receiving a large feeding. A large percentage of geriatric patients have impaired swallowing from strokes or other neurologic impairments. Unresponsive patients are at risk for the aspiration of vomitus. The aspiration of stomach contents carries the additional risk of aspiration **pneumonitis**, in which the gastric acid irritates lung tissue. This risk is in addition to the risk of pneumonia from any bacteria in the aspirated material.

Pathophysiology

Aspiration of stomach contents into the lungs has a significantly high mortality rate. It is a common but profoundly dangerous complication in patients who have had a cardiac arrest and in unresponsive patients who have had trauma or who have overdosed.

Aspiration of foreign bodies, such as nuts or broken teeth, may also occur. Most adults choke only when they are intoxicated or traumatized or have a reduced gag reflex from a stroke or aging. Chronic aspiration of food is also a common cause of <u>pneumonia</u> in older patients.

Assessment

What is the scenario surrounding your patient's sudden onset of dyspnea? Did it occur immediately after eating? Does the patient have a gastric feeding tube, and if so, when was the last feeding and how large was it? Is the material suctioned from the patient's airway the same color as the tube feeding? Is there particulate matter in the suctioned material? A fever and cough may present several hours after an aspiration-prone event, like a seizure or episode of unresponsiveness. Some patients aspirate chronically and may have a history of aspiration pneumonia.

Management

Follow these guidelines when treating patients at risk for aspiration or who have aspirated:

1. Aggressively reduce the risk of aspiration by avoiding gastric distention when ventilating and by decompressing the stomach with a nasogastric tube whenever appropriate.
2. Aggressively monitor the patient's ability to protect his or her own airway, and protect the patient's airway with an advanced airway when needed.
3. Aggressively treat aspiration with suction and airway control if steps 1 and 2 fail.

Patients at risk for aspiration should not eat when they are having difficulty breathing. If basic life-support maneuvers fail to clear an obstructed airway, use laryngoscopy and Magill forceps, and, if necessary, perform a needle or surgical cricothyrotomy, if allowed by local protocol.

■ Pathophysiology, Assessment, and Management of Obstructive Lower Airway Diseases

Obstructive lower airway diseases are characterized by diffuse obstruction to airflow within the lungs. The most common obstructive airway diseases are emphysema and chronic bronchitis (chronic diseases) and asthma (an acutely episodic syndrome); these three conditions collectively affect as many as 10% to 20% of adults in the United States. Emphysema and chronic bronchitis are collectively classified as COPD because the changes in pulmonary structure and function are chronic, progressive, and irreversible. Asthma is considered a separate entity because—at least in its early stages—it is a condition of *reversible* airway narrowing.

Obstructive disease occurs when the positive pressure of exhalation causes the small airways to pinch shut, trapping gas in the alveoli. The harder the patient tries to push air out, the more it is trapped in the alveoli Figure 38. Hence, patients with obstructive disease have large amounts of gas trapped in their lungs that they cannot effectively expel. Patients with obstructive disease learn that exhaling slowly at a low pressure is more effective than exhaling rapidly at high pressure.

Patients with obstructive airway disease may have a variety of physical findings that can indicate the nature of their disease:

- **Pursed-lip breathing.** Breathing in this way allows patients to exhale slowly under controlled pressure.
- **Increased I/E ratio.** The I/E ratio is typically 1:2 in healthy people breathing quietly. In other words, it takes about twice as long to exhale as it does to inhale. Patients who are gravely ill with obstructive disease may have an I/E ratio as high as 1:6 or 1:8.
- **Abdominal muscle use.** Abdominal muscles help to push air out (during exhalation). Patients with obstructive disease must work to push air out with every breath. People with asthma may complain of abdominal pain after an attack because they do the equivalent of hundreds of sit-ups with each forced exhalation.
- **Jugular venous distention.** The trapped air creates a higher pressure in the thorax. Blood draining into the superior vena cava from the head and neck can back up in the jugular veins, causing jugular venous distention.

■ Asthma

Pathophysiology

The name asthma (from a Greek word meaning "panting") was first given to this disease by the second-century Greek physician Areatus "because in the paroxysms, the patients also pant for breath." Bronchial asthma is characterized by an increased reactivity of the trachea and bronchi to a variety of stimuli. The hyperreactivity results in widespread, reversible narrowing of the airways, or bronchospasm Figure 39. Asthma makes it difficult to exhale. Air is trapped in the distal portions of the lung and does not allow air from the next inhalation to enter the alveoli.

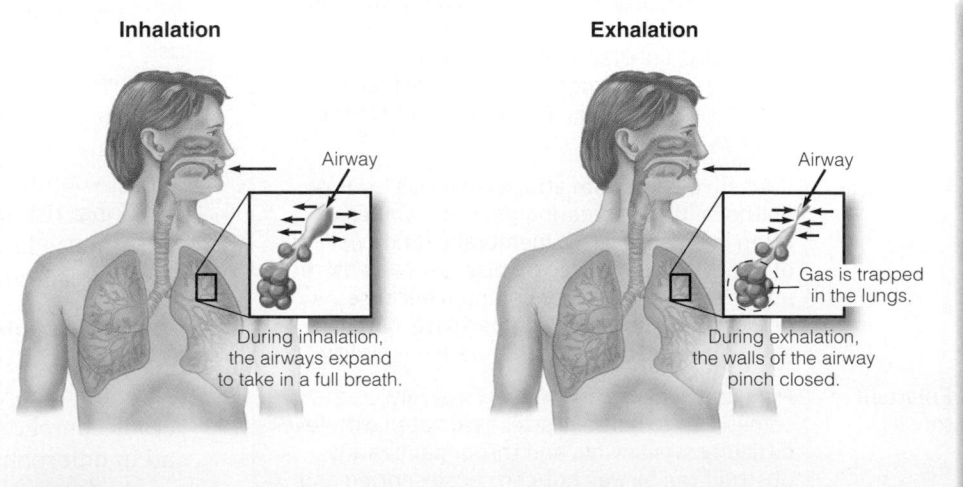

Figure 38 Obstructive disease involves changes in the smaller airways that cause them to pinch closed during exhalation, trapping air inside the lungs. Healthy airways narrow during exhalation but not to the extent that causes obstruction or air trapping.

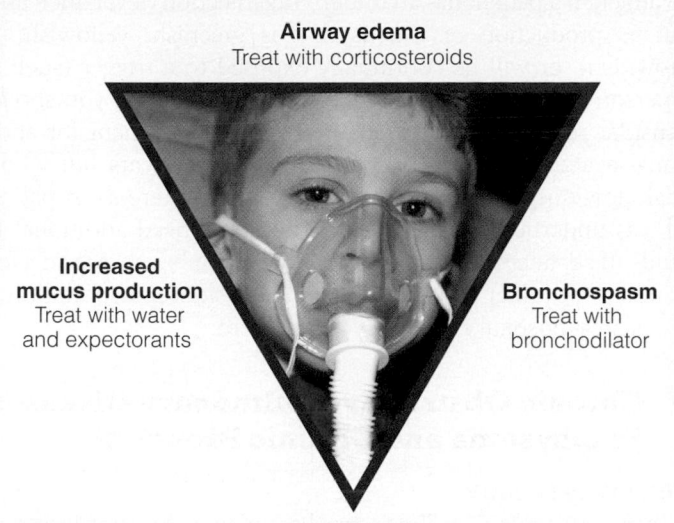

Airway edema
Treat with corticosteroids

Increased mucus production
Treat with water and expectorants

Bronchospasm
Treat with bronchodilator

Figure 39 The asthma triad demonstrates the three primary components of asthma and the corresponding treatments for each component. Asthma presents differently in different people, so individual treatments need to vary as well.

Words of Wisdom

The term *asthma* describes a triad of airway problems: bronchospasm, increased mucus production, and peripheral airway edema. It may present differently in different people, but it is a common pathologic condition.

More than 24 million people in the United States reported having asthma in 2009, and the incidence seems to be increasing. Each year, 2 million people visit an emergency department because of asthma, and one quarter of them will be admitted to the hospital.

The fastest-growing asthma rates are observed in children younger than 5 years. Overall death rates from asthma are also higher in people younger than 35 years. Asthma is more common in males but tends to be more severe in females. African Americans, especially if living in large urban centers, are three times more likely to be diagnosed with asthma and have death rates that are five times higher than those observed in other racial groups.

Patients who have potentially fatal asthma often have severely compromised ventilation all of the time. They are at serious risk if acute bronchospasm is triggered or if they have an infection. A patient who has asthma is at high risk of respiratory arrest if he or she has a history that includes any of the factors in Table 8. Not following the medication regimen and severe psychiatric disorders also predispose a patient with asthma to a fatal attack.

Death rates from asthma are increasing across the United States, although not equally across all populations. Approximately 5,000 people (1 in 100 admissions) will die of asthma annually. The overall mortality rate for this disease is 5%.

Table 8 Factors That Indicate an Increased Risk of Asthma-Related Death
■ Previous intubation for respiratory failure or respiratory arrest
■ Respiratory acidosis
■ Two or more admissions to the hospital despite oral corticosteroid use
■ Two or more episodes of pneumothorax

When patients begin wheezing, their inhalers usually will help for only a short time before symptoms return. The typical asthma attack that responds to treatment but occurs again in a few hours is sometimes caused by an underlying infection (such as pneumonia or bronchitis) that continually triggers the asthmalike symptoms. The asthma attack will not subside until the patient receives treatment of the trigger. Does your patient have a fever or chills? Is he or she coughing up colored sputum?

Status asthmaticus is a severe, prolonged asthmatic attack that cannot be stopped with conventional treatment. **It is a dire medical emergency**. Just as a person with COPD ordinarily does not call for an ambulance unless his or her condition has markedly changed, a person with asthma does not usually dial 9-1-1 unless the attack is much worse than usual. It is reasonable to assume that **any person with asthma who feels sick enough to call an ambulance may be in status asthmaticus until proved otherwise**.

On examination, a patient in status asthmaticus will be desperately struggling to move air through obstructed airways, with prominent use of the accessory muscles of breathing. The chest will be maximally hyperinflated. Breath sounds and wheezes may be entirely inaudible because air movement is negligible, and the patient will usually be exhausted, severely acidotic, and dehydrated.

Assessment

Sometimes asthma is referred to as reactive airway disease to indicate that the patient experiences bronchospasm when exposed to certain triggers, such as dust, cold, or smoke. In addition, edema and inflammation of the airways and increased mucus production can cause significant airway obstruction. Asthma characteristically occurs in acute attacks of variable duration. Between attacks, the person may be relatively asymptomatic.

Bronchospasm Bronchospasm is caused by the constriction of smooth muscle that surrounds the larger bronchi in the lungs Figure 40. Bronchospasm may occur because of stimulation by an allergen or irritants such as dust, perfume, animal dander, or cold temperatures or by other stimuli such as exercise or stress. When air is forced through the constricted airways, it causes them to vibrate, which creates wheezing. Bronchospasm can also reduce the peak expiratory flow by causing turbulent airflow. The primary treatment of bronchospasm is nebulized bronchodilator medication.

Bronchial Edema Swelling of the bronchi and bronchioles also creates turbulent airflow, wheezing, and air trapping.

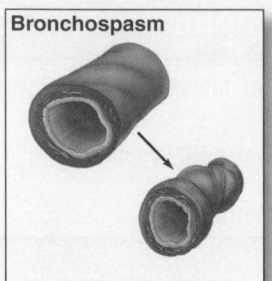
With bronchospasm, the muscle contracts, causing the entire tube to narrow.

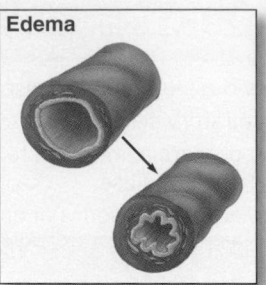
With edema, the wall of the tube swells, causing only the lumen to narrow.

Figure 40 Bronchospasm is a constriction (narrowing) of both the inside and outside diameters of the airway, whereas with bronchial edema only the inside diameter (bronchial lumen) is constricted. Both reduce the functional diameter of airways.

Bronchodilator medications do little to reduce bronchial edema. If a patient takes such a medication and the peak flow does not dramatically improve, some degree of bronchial edema is likely.

Increased Mucus Production Thick secretions may plug the distal airways and contribute to air trapping. People who have asthma may be significantly dehydrated because of their increased fluid loss from tachypnea and their often-poor fluid intake. Dehydration makes secretions even thicker, further worsening the air trapping. Taking antihistamine medications may further thicken secretions.

Management
Most people who have asthma have a combination of these three pathologic conditions, although their predominance varies in individual patients.

- **Bronchospasm.** The condition of a person with asthma characterized primarily by bronchoconstriction would respond well to aerosol bronchodilators.
- **Bronchial edema.** The condition of a person with asthma characterized primarily by bronchial edema would respond much less to aerosol bronchodilators and probably would not show significant improvement until administered corticosteroids have taken effect. Corticosteroids may or may not be given in the field setting because, unlike bronchodilators, which can improve breathing immediately, corticosteroids take a few hours to reduce inflammation.
- **Excessive mucus secretion.** The primary approach to dealing with secretions in a person with asthma is to improve hydration. Mucolytics, which break down thick mucus, and expectorants, which loosen thick secretions so that they can be coughed out, are also sometimes used, most often in the hospital setting.

Transport Considerations Many patients routinely manage their asthma at home and may resist transport to the hospital once their most acute symptoms have been relieved. Important transport decisions include attempting to determine the trigger for an attack. If a patient has an underlying infection (fever, increased mucus production or mucus that is greenish, yellowish, or brownish), or will be continually exposed to a trigger (such as a person who wears a strong fragrance or smokes), you should consider removing the patient from the environment for additional evaluation. A patient whose wheezing clears but whose peak flow does not improve may need corticosteroids. A patient who is undernourished or dehydrated may need additional IV fluids. If advanced life support assistance will be more than a few minutes away after you leave, strongly consider transportation to the nearest hospital emergency department.

Chronic Obstructive Pulmonary Disease: Emphysema and Chronic Bronchitis

Pathophysiology
Chronic obstructive pulmonary disease comprises at least two distinct clinical entities: emphysema and chronic bronchitis. Emphysema is thought to damage or destroy the fragile structure of the terminal bronchioles. Groups of alveoli merge into large blebs, or bullae, which are far less efficient than normal lung tissue because they have less surface area for gas exchange. This part of the tracheobronchial tree becomes so weak that its branches collapse during exhalation, trapping air in the alveoli.

Chronic bronchitis is defined as sputum production most days of the month for 3 or more months out of the year for more than 2 years. The hallmark of this disease is excessive mucus production in the bronchial tree, which is nearly always accompanied by a chronic or recurrent productive cough (a cough that produces phlegm). A typical patient who has chronic bronchitis is almost invariably a heavy cigarette smoker. He or she is usually overweight and congested and sometimes has a bluish complexion. Blood gas levels tend to be abnormal, with elevated Pa_{CO_2} (hypercapnia) and decreased Pa_{O_2} (hypoxemia) levels. Often, the patient has associated heart disease and right-sided heart failure (cor pulmonale).

Words of Wisdom

Over the years, people with chronic obstructive pulmonary disease (COPD) learn how much exertion they can tolerate, in what position sleep is possible, and so forth. So when a person with COPD calls for an ambulance, it nearly always means that something has changed for the worse.

Assessment
Emphysema and chronic bronchitis represent two extremes of the COPD spectrum. In reality, as the disease progresses, most patients with COPD fall somewhere between these two clinical extremes, showing signs and symptoms of both disease processes.

Many patients who have emphysema have a barrel chest caused by chronic lung hyperinflation. The patients are often tachypneic because they attempt to maintain a normal carbon dioxide level despite their dysfunctional lungs. They often use extreme amounts of energy attempting to breathe, using their own muscle mass for energy in the process.

Among the causes of diffuse wheezing are acute left-sided heart failure ("cardiac asthma"), smoke inhalation, chronic bronchitis, and acute pulmonary embolism. Localized wheezing reflects an obstruction, by foreign body or tumor, in a specific area. Only a careful history and physical examination will reveal the correct diagnosis.

Words of Wisdom

It is particularly important to distinguish the wheezing of asthma from that caused by left-sided heart failure because the treatments of the two conditions are markedly different.

The following are some common issues that cause decompensation in a patient who has COPD.

Chronic Obstructive Pulmonary Disease With Pneumonia Because these patients are chronically ill, have poor secretion clearance, and sometimes have excessive mucus production (which acts like a culture medium for pathogenic microorganisms), they often have lung infections. Assessment should ascertain the presence of a fever, whether the color or amount of their sputum production changed, the presence of other signs of infection (such as body aches, general malaise, or pain when breathing), and whether auscultated breath sounds are consistent with pneumonia (such as localized or one-sided crackles). A patient who obviously has COPD might also have another condition, including other respiratory conditions.

Chronic Obstructive Pulmonary Disease With Right-sided Heart Failure It is a laborious task for the right side of the heart to push thick blood—thick because of polycythemia—through capillaries compressed by hyperinflated alveoli. This situation commonly causes right-sided heart failure because of lung disease (cor pulmonale). If patients take in too much salt or fluid or do not excrete sufficient fluid (because of renal failure or not using diuretics as prescribed), they may have an episode of CHF. Assessment should look for peripheral edema, jugular venous distention with hepatojugular reflux, end inspiratory crackles (sometimes difficult to differentiate crackles of CHF from crackles always present because of COPD), a progressive increase in dyspnea over several days, a greater-than-usual fluid intake, and improper use of diuretics.

Chronic Obstructive Pulmonary Disease With Left-sided Heart Failure Patients with COPD are at high risk of sudden cardiac arrest. Any abrupt left ventricular dysfunction, such as an acute myocardial infarction or a cardiac rhythm disturbance (dysrhythmia), can cause rapid-onset, left-sided heart failure. Do not allow an initial impression of COPD preclude swift identification of an acute myocardial infarction.

Acute Exacerbation of Chronic Obstructive Pulmonary Disease In an acute exacerbation, no copathologic condition such as CHF or pneumonia clearly accounts for the sudden decompensation.

Documentation and Communication

Seek guidance from the medical director and observe local protocols when treating a patient with severe COPD or asthma who is in cardiac arrest or near-arrest.

Instead, the patient's condition suddenly becomes worse, often because of some environmental change such as weather, humidity, or recent activation of the heating or cooling system. An acute exacerbation can also be prompted by the inhalation of trigger substances, such as dust, mold, animal dander, or fresh paint.

Advances in technology have allowed people with chronic respiratory disease much more freedom to get out of the house and to travel. Paramedics may be called to assist a person who has an acute exacerbation of COPD when an oxygen tank runs dry or a portable ventilator malfunctions, medications are left at home or packed in checked baggage that is misdirected, or therapy is deliberately discontinued because the person wants to regain some control over his or her life or does not understand the importance of the therapy.

End-Stage Chronic Obstructive Pulmonary Disease Patients with severe COPD eventually reach a point at which their lungs can no longer support oxygenation and ventilation. Their calls to 9-1-1 become more frequent as their condition deteriorates. Some will be in hospice care. In the end stages of the disease, it can be difficult to determine whether a patient has an exacerbation that can be resolved or has reached the end of the disease process. Endotracheal intubation may make it impossible for a patient to make his or her wishes known. In addition, the more frequently a patient requires intubation and mechanical ventilation, the more difficult ventilator weaning becomes. Apprehension about these bleak prospects heightens the patient's anxiety, thus escalating cardiac workload and cardiac oxygen consumption—a potentially lethal combination for a patient with end-stage COPD.

Each EMS system has its own ways of dealing with do-not-resuscitate orders. It is important to secure documentation of the patient's wishes as the terminal phase of the disease begins. Follow local protocol or contact medical control as needed regarding such issues.

Chronic Obstructive Pulmonary Disease and Trauma People with COPD are as susceptible to trauma as the rest of the population. However, COPD lessens a person's ability to tolerate trauma. Many patients with COPD must sit up to breathe, so the common act of strapping them to a long board can lead to decompensation. Anyone who has performed CPR compressions on a patient with chronic emphysema knows how poorly the chest wall tolerates trauma. Even when patients with COPD survive the initial trauma, they are susceptible to pulmonary emboli and infections during recovery. Monitor patients with chronic lung disease closely because they typically have a much smaller reserve and decreased ability to compensate. Patients with

COPD rarely have a "normal" oxygen saturation; their normal might be less than 90%. Providing oxygen to achieve a saturation of 98% is unrealistic and might be harmful.

Management

Although little can be done in the field to provide long-term relief for patients with COPD, the associated bronchospasm, edema, fluid, or hypoxia can often be relieved, helping improve the patient's immediate situation.

Patients with COPD are often debilitated by the disease and have little or no respiratory reserve to help them deal with additional respiratory insults. Paramedics must actively try to determine the circumstances that tipped the precarious balance from relative stability to a state of respiratory insufficiency that prompted a call to 9-1-1. Effective management of COPD requires an understanding of the concepts of hypoxic drive and auto-PEEP (positive end-expiratory pressure).

Hypoxic Drive Hypoxic drive is a situation in which a person's stimulus to breathe comes from a decrease in Pao_2 rather than the normal stimulus, an increase in $Paco_2$. When a patient has chronic hypoventilation, bicarbonate (Hco_3) ions migrate into the cerebrospinal fluid, fooling the brain into thinking that acid and base are in balance. The patient's respiratory center might then switch to a hypoxic drive, meaning that the primary stimulus to breathe comes from decreased levels of oxygen, rather than from increased levels of carbon dioxide.

This phenomenon affects only a small percentage of patients who have the most relentless forms of pulmonary disease. It occurs during the end stage of the disease process. Paramedics must decide whether the administration of oxygen is appropriate for any given patient. In making this decision, consider the following points:

1. Only a small subset of patients with COPD breathe because of hypoxic drive, but it is impossible to know who they are by just looking at them.
2. Patients who breathe because of hypoxic drive do not suddenly become apneic after breathing oxygen. High levels of oxygen slowly depress the respiratory drive, and the respiratory rate slowly declines into the single digits before a patient becomes apneic. A paramedic is likely to recognize this phenomenon during a transport; the real concern is for a patient in a hospital or an extended care facility who is given 100% supplemental oxygen and left alone for a prolonged period.
3. Verbal and physical stimulation can encourage breathing. If the respiratory rate begins to drop, gently shake the patient and yell "Breathe!" This technique works well in the early stages.
4. If a patient becomes apneic because of increased oxygenation, his or her skin may still appear perfused.
5. If the patient becomes apneic, provide artificial ventilation and consider intubation.
6. The decision to intubate a patient with hypoxic drive is often complex. Once intubated, the patient may have to live what is left of his or her life on a ventilator, which is counter to many patients' wishes.

7. Although oxygen saturation (Spo_2) readings may be a valuable adjunct in deciding whether to intubate, Spo_2 values are less useful in cases of COPD because they fail to shed light on the carbon dioxide level.

Words of Wisdom

Never withhold oxygen therapy from any patient in respiratory distress, even (or especially) a patient with chronic obstructive pulmonary disease.

Supplemental oxygen is integral to therapy for many patients, so it does not make sense to withhold oxygen from someone who needs it for fear of decreasing the respiratory drive in the few patients who might have this complication. Keep in mind that oxygen saturations of 93% are acceptable, and many patients with COPD routinely have even lower values. It is not necessary or desirable to oxygenate these patients to oxygen saturation levels of 99% or 100%

Auto-PEEP Not everyone should be ventilated the same way. When ventilating a patient who has severe obstructive disease, such as patients with decompensated asthma or COPD, remember the difficulty exhaling. Complete exhalation must be allowed before the next breath is delivered or pressure in the thorax will continue to rise. This phenomenon, which is called auto-PEEP, can eventually cause a pneumothorax or cardiac arrest. If the pressure in the chest exceeds the pressure of blood returning to the heart, limiting venous return, cardiac arrest may occur.

Patients in whom auto-PEEP is a concern should be ventilated at a rate of as little as 4 to 6 breaths/min. Such restraint is difficult, but it is an absolute necessity to avoid the dire consequences of raising the thoracic pressure with each breath. Remember that the standard ventilation rate for adults in cardiac arrest is only 8 to 10 breaths/min in patients without COPD.

■ Pathophysiology, Assessment, and Management of Common Respiratory Problems

■ Pulmonary Infections

Pathophysiology

Bacteria, viruses, fungi, and protozoa cause infections. The respiratory tract is particularly vulnerable to a variety of airborne agents and to agents that reside in the nose or throat and may migrate into the lungs.

In general, infectious diseases cause swelling of the respiratory tissues, an increase in mucus production, and the production of pus. Swelling in well-perfused respiratory tissues can be dramatic, particularly in the upper airway. This is problematic because the resistance to airflow increases exponentially when the airway diameter is narrowed (Poiseuille's law). Alveoli can also become nonfunctional if they fill with pus, as occurs in pneumonia.

Pneumonia may be caused by any of a variety of bacterial, viral, and fungal agents. Bacterial pneumonia is most often caused by the *Streptococcus pneumoniae* bacterium, for which an effective vaccine is now available. This type of pneumonia is responsible for about 10% of hospital admissions in the United States and, despite the use of antibiotics, has a mortality rate of 5% to 10%. In many other countries, pneumonia is the leading cause of death.

Older people, people with chronic illnesses, and people who smoke are at greater risk of pneumonia. Anyone who is not ventilating effectively, who has excessive secretions (such as in COPD or asthma, postoperatively, or bedridden or sedentary status), or who is immunocompromised (from human immunodeficiency virus, other illnesses, posttransplantation immunosuppression, or chemotherapy) is at risk for the development of pneumonia. Patients with acquired immunodeficiency syndrome are particularly susceptible to *Pneumocystis jiroveci* pneumonia; it is a primary cause of morbidity and mortality. All high-risk patients are strongly encouraged to receive the pneumonia vaccine annually.

Another important consideration is that antibiotic-resistant organisms (such as methicillin-resistant *Staphylococcus aureus* and vancomycin-resistant enterococci, discussed in the chapter, *Infectious Diseases*) can colonize the respiratory tract. The aerosolization of these organisms when a patient coughs or during advanced airway procedures is potentially more dangerous to paramedics than when infections caused by these organisms exist in a decubitus ulcer covered with a dressing. When presented with a patient in isolation because of an infection with methicillin-resistant *S aureus* (or a similar organism), always ask *where* the organism was found and wear proper respiratory protection if the organism is in the respiratory tract.

Assessment

A patient with pneumonia usually reports several hours to days of weakness, productive cough, fever, and sometimes chest pain worsened by coughing. The illness may have started abruptly, with shaking chills (rigors), or it might have come on more gradually, with progressive weakness. As the patient's history of recent illness is obtained, be particularly attuned to comments such as "…and I just got over the flu about a week ago." Pneumonia is often a secondary infection that follows a bout of influenza and is one of the leading causes of death under those circumstances.

Physical examination of a patient with pneumonia often reveals a grievously ill or toxic appearance. The patient may or may not be coughing. Crackles may be heard on auscultation of the chest, and the patient may have increased tactile fremitus and sputum production. In advanced cases, diminished or absent breath sounds are noted in areas of consolidation. Sputum may be thick (because of dehydration) or purulent. If the infection also causes swelling of the pleural membranes, the patient may experience significant pain when breathing, especially when taking a deep breath or coughing. A pleural friction rub may be heard over the involved area.

Pneumonia often occurs in the lung bases, typically on only one side. Patients may therefore have a "coughing fit" when turning from one side to the other. Sometimes patients' oxygen saturation will be significantly lower when they lie on one side versus the other. When the "good lung" is up, respiratory status may seem much better than when the good lung is compressed by body weight.

Patients with pneumonia are often dehydrated. Rehydration may temporarily worsen their condition as the thick secretions liquefy and expand in the chest. Supportive care includes oxygenation, secretion management (suctioning), and transport to the closest receiving facility. Bronchodilators will not help pneumonia, but they may slightly improve the patient's ability to ventilate.

Management

Infections of the upper airway may require aggressive airway management approaches. Infections in the lower airway are usually treated with supportive care and by transport to the hospital.

■ Atelectasis

Pathophysiology

The alveoli are vulnerable to a number of disorders. They may collapse from obstruction somewhere in the proximal airways or from external pressures produced, for example, by pneumothorax or hemothorax. They may fill with pus in pneumonia, with blood in pulmonary contusion, or with fluid in near-drowning or CHF. In addition, smoke or toxic gases may displace the fresh air that should be present in the alveoli.

Under normal conditions, most of the air that moves in and out of the lungs (about 79%) is the relatively inert gas nitrogen, which keeps the alveoli open. If a patient is given 100% oxygen, any alveolus that plugs will collapse once all of the oxygen diffuses out. Patients receiving high concentrations of oxygen have this type of atelectasis.

The human body has billions of alveoli, and it is common for some of them to collapse from time to time. Humans (and most mammals) periodically sigh, cough, sneeze, and change positions, all actions that are thought to help open closed alveoli and avoid decreased ventilation to any one part of the lung. When people do not use these actions, for example, because they are sedated or in a coma or deep breathing or moving causes pain, increasing numbers of alveoli in sections of the lung may collapse and not reopen. Like balloons, alveoli are more difficult to blow open once they have completely collapsed; eventually, entire lung segments collapse. This condition is called <u>atelectasis</u>, and it increases the chance of pneumonia developing in the affected areas.

Assessment

Although atelectasis can be a significant disease by itself, the larger concern is that the affected areas become breeding grounds for pathogens, resulting in pneumonia. This is a concern in any patient who has a fever in the days following chest or abdominal surgery, particularly if breath sounds are decreased or abnormally colored sputum is coughed up.

Management

Postsurgical patients are encouraged to cough, deep breathe, and get out of bed, even though it is painful. People who cannot get out of bed may get atelectasis, which can lead to hypoxia or predispose a patient to lung infections and pneumonia.

In the hospital, patients are constantly encouraged to take deep breaths. A device called an incentive spirometer helps patients quantify the depth of their breaths **Figure 41**. These devices are often sent home with patients for continued use after discharge from the hospital (such as after rib fracture or chest surgery). Paramedics can reinforce deep breathing in patients who would benefit from it and can be watchful for atelectasis in patients who are sedentary or who take medications with sedative effects, including some analgesics.

■ Cancer

Pathophysiology

Lung cancer is one of the most common forms of cancer, especially among people who smoke cigarettes and people exposed to occupational lung hazards, such as asbestos, coal dust, and secondhand smoke. Although lung cancer was traditionally considered predominantly a disease of men, today 45% of new cases of lung cancer occur in women, most likely because of the increase in smoking among women.

Assessment

Lung cancer often is identified when tumors in the large airways bleed, causing <u>hemoptysis</u> (coughing up blood in the sputum) and uncontrollable coughing. It is frequently accompanied by COPD and impaired lung function. The lung is also a common site for the <u>metastasis</u> of cancer from other body sites.

Other cancer may invade the lymph nodes in the neck, producing tumors that threaten to occlude the upper airway.

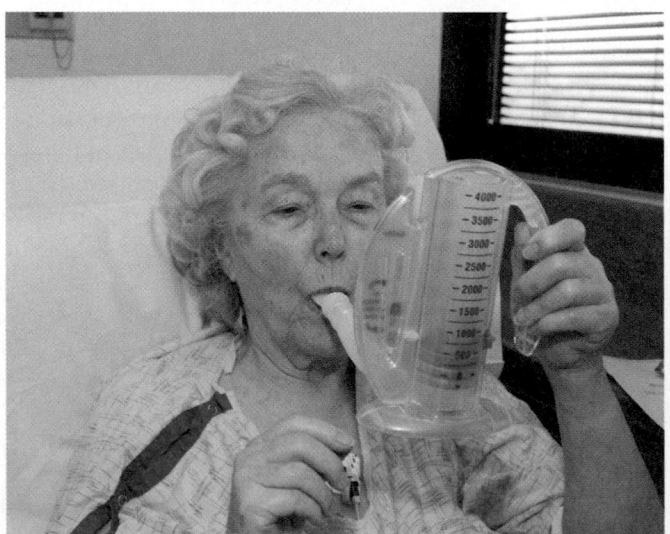

Figure 41 An incentive spirometer helps patients quantify how deep their breathing is. It helps them take deep breaths to avoid atelectasis.

Patients with various types of cancer may have pulmonary complications from chemotherapy or radiation therapy. Lung irradiation, for example, may be associated with some degree of pulmonary edema. Tumors or treatment may also cause <u>pleural effusion</u>, which can present with rapidly progressing dyspnea.

Management

Paramedics can support oxygenation and ventilation and provide some amount of pain management, but there is little prehospital treatment specific to pleural effusions or hemoptysis other than transport to the hospital. Paramedics are sometimes called to assist with end-of-life issues for patients with cancer. Patients in hospice care, for example, may present with depressed respiration caused by the large amounts of narcotics used to relieve pain, anxiety, or other symptoms. In this type of narcotics overdose, titrate naloxone (Narcan) *only* to improve respiration—do not completely reverse the patient's primary pain control, or the patient may be plunged abruptly into complete misery. In the past, the respiratory depressant effects of narcotics and antianxiety agents may have been overemphasized, but now these agents are gaining increased popularity in the management of chronic pain, chronic cough, and anxiety in end-of-life scenarios. For example, fentanyl citrate (Sublimaze), a strong narcotic, is sometimes dispensed through an aerosol device to suppress chronic coughing in patients who have end-stage lung cancer.

■ Toxic Inhalations

Pathophysiology

Many potentially toxic substances can be inhaled into the lungs. The type of damage depends largely on the water solubility of the toxic gas. **Table 9** shows how toxic gases are categorized.

Assessment

Highly water-soluble gases like ammonia will react with the moist mucous membranes of the upper airway and cause swelling and irritation. If the substance gets in the patient's eyes, they will also burn and feel inflamed and irritated.

Less water-soluble gases may get deep into the lower airway, where they may do damage over time. Such toxic gases have

Table 9   Categorization of Toxic Gases

Category	Example	Effects
Highly water soluble	Ammonia	Acute upper airway irritation
Moderately water soluble	Chlorine	Depends on concentration and amount of exposure; range from coughing, wheezing, rales, and pulmonary edema to chemical burns
Minimally water soluble	Phosgene	Delayed onset of pulmonary edema

been used in war to disable the enemy, because they do not cause immediate distress, but rather cause pulmonary edema up to 24 hours later. The gases phosgene and nitrogen dioxide behave in this manner.

Some common gases, for example chlorine, are moderately water soluble and cause problems somewhere between the extremes of irritation and pulmonary edema. Severe exposure may present with upper airway swelling, whereas lower-level exposure may present with the classic delayed-onset, lower airway damage. A common household error is pouring drain cleaner and chlorine bleach into a drain in an attempt to clear a clog, which may produce an irritant chlorine gas that can sicken the person and everyone in the home or building. Industrial settings often use irritant gas–forming chemicals in large quantities and in higher concentrations than available for home use, creating the possibility for incidents that expose a larger number of people or a more toxic gas. Paramedics should note industrial settings in their area that are high risk for this type of incident.

Management

A patient who has been exposed to such a substance must be removed from contact with the toxic gas immediately and provided with 100% supplemental oxygen or assisted ventilation if breathing is impaired (if there is reduced tidal volume). If the upper airway is compromised, aggressive airway management (such as intubation or a cricothyrotomy) may be required.

Patients who have been exposed to slightly water-soluble gases may feel fine initially but have acute dyspnea many hours later. When such an exposure is suspected, patients should strongly consider transport to the closest emergency department for observation and further assessment.

■ Pulmonary Edema

Pathophysiology

Fluid buildup in lung tissue and air spaces occurs when fluid from the blood plasma migrates into the lung parenchyma. This pulmonary edema compromises gas exchange long before overt signs are present.

Pulmonary edema can be classified as high pressure (cardiogenic) or high permeability (noncardiogenic). Cardiogenic pulmonary edema is often called CHF and can result from dysfunction of the right or the left ventricle, chronic hypertension, or cardiac diseases such as myocarditis. (These problems are discussed in greater detail in the chapter, *Cardiovascular Emergencies*.)

Noncardiogenic pulmonary edema occurs in cases of acute hypoxemia, such as when inhaled toxins or near-drowning damage alveolar tissue, causing fluid to seep into the lungs. Toxins or drugs in the bloodstream (such as toxins when a patient is in shock or using heroin) can damage the pulmonary capillaries and have the same effect. Sometimes trauma, severe shock, cardiac arrest, or even altitude changes can damage the alveoli and capillaries, causing acute respiratory distress syndrome or high-altitude pulmonary edema.

Assessment

Some patients present with significant pulmonary edema after a lengthy journey, because they did not take diuretics while traveling. If a patient has been traveling, ask about medications prescribed and whether they have been taken regularly.

Early in pulmonary edema, few signs are apparent. By the time fine crackles in the bases of the lungs become audible at the end of inspiration, fluid has leaked out of the capillaries, increased the diffusion space between the alveoli and capillaries, swollen the alveolar walls, and begun to seep into the alveoli. This sound is caused by fields of "wet" alveoli popping open as the lungs reach maximal inflation. Always listen to the lower lobes of the lungs through the patient's back (but never through clothing).

As pulmonary edema worsens, crackles may originate higher in the patient's lung fields—often described as "crackles up to the subscapular level" or "crackles up to the apices." As fluid migrates into the larger airways and mixes with mucus, coarse crackles will become audible during inspiration and exhalation and tactile fremitus may be identified. Ultimately, the patient will begin to cough up watery sputum that often has a pink tinge (from red blood cells). As air is forced in and out of the fluid-filled lungs, the fluid may bubble and foam. Coughing up pink, foamy, or blood-tinged sputum is a classic sign of severe pulmonary edema.

■ Acute Respiratory Distress Syndrome

Pathophysiology

Acute respiratory distress syndrome (also known as ARDS, shock lung, Da Nang lung, and, in neonates, hyaline membrane disease) is seldom seen in the field, but paramedics may have a vital role in preventing this devastating pathologic condition. This syndrome is caused by diffuse damage to the alveoli, perhaps as a result of shock, aspiration of gastric contents, pulmonary edema, or a hypoxic event. It seems to be worse when there is some direct damage to the lungs, as in trauma patients who have severe pulmonary contusions.

Picture the alveoli as a beach surrounded by the sea of the bloodstream. During a near-death crisis, changes in permeability allow the tide to come in and wash over the beach. When the tide goes out, it washes away the surfactant in the alveoli and leaves remains (such as dead cells and bacteria) behind on the shore. The alveoli become stiff (noncompliant) and difficult to ventilate. They ultimately require mechanical ventilation under extraordinarily high pressure, which causes even more damage. The delivery of high oxygen concentrations for prolonged periods causes an additional layer of destruction.

Assessment

Typically, ARDS is not seen in the field, but paramedics might be asked to transport a patient with ARDS between facilities. Assessment is similar to that for any patient with a respiratory problem. Document oxygen saturation, breath sounds, and any sudden changes in condition. Patients with ARDS typically have "stiff" lungs (that is, low compliance). During manual ventilation, ventilation pressures should be monitored and care taken to not overventilate and cause further damage.

Pathophysiology, Assessment, and Management of Problems Outside the Lung Parenchyma

■ Pneumothorax

Pathophysiology

When a patient has a pneumothorax, air typically collects between the visceral and parietal pleura lining the inside of the chest cavity. Some people have blebs in the lung parenchyma that are congenital or that are caused by COPD and that predispose them to this condition. Blebs are weak spots that can rupture under stress, causing a spontaneous pneumothorax. The stress that ruptures the bleb may be as simple as coughing or as severe as aggressive bag-mask ventilation. People who have severe asthma are prone to blebs, as are tall, thin people, especially people who smoke.

Assessment

Some patients have had multiple simple pneumothoraces in their life and may actually say: "I'm having another pneumothorax." Patients may describe feeling a sharp pain after coughing, followed by increasing dyspnea during the subsequent minutes or hours.

Management

Most patients will not require acute intervention, such as needle chest decompression, but they must at least receive oxygen and have their respiratory status closely monitored en route to the hospital.

■ Pleural Effusion

Pathophysiology

When fluid collects between the visceral and parietal pleura, it produces a pleural effusion **Figure 42**. The sac of fluid formed is similar to a blister, in which repeated trauma to the tissues causes more fluid to collect. Effusions can be caused by infections, tumors, or trauma.

To visualize how this condition arises, imagine a blister forming at the base of the lung. The tissues rub against each other breath after breath, causing inflammation and fluid to accumulate in the space. Some pleural effusions can contain several liters of fluid. A large effusion decreases lung capacity and causes dyspnea.

Assessment

It may be difficult to hear any breath sounds through the effusion. Because the effusion is filled with fluid, the patient's position will affect his or her ability to breathe.

Management

Shifting positions may cause significantly more dyspnea, and patients usually will resist being placed into anything other than the Fowler's position. Supportive care, including proper

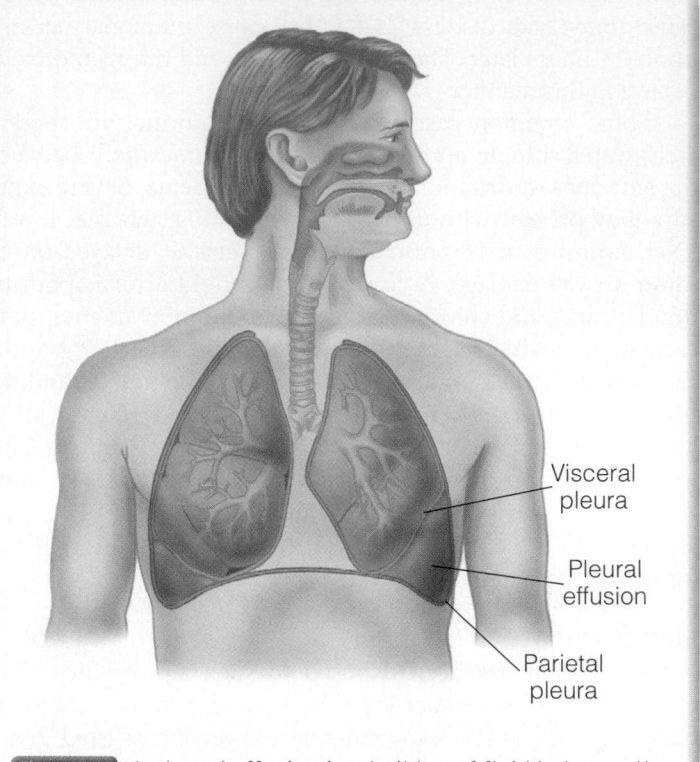

Figure 42 A pleural effusion is a buildup of fluid between the visceral and parietal pleura.

Visceral pleura

Pleural effusion

Parietal pleura

positioning and aggressive supplemental oxygen administration, should be used until the patient can be transported to a facility at which the effusion can be definitively treated.

■ Pulmonary Embolism

Pathophysiology

The pulmonary circulation may be compromised by a blood clot (embolism), a fat embolism from a broken bone, an amniotic fluid embolism from leakage of amniotic fluid during pregnancy, or an air embolism resulting from air entering the circulation from a laceration in the neck or an IV administration set that was improperly flushed or not flushed. A large embolism, of whatever type, will usually lodge in a major branch of the pulmonary artery and prevent blood flow through that branch. Adequate gas exchange in the lungs requires functional alveoli to provide oxygen and take up carbon dioxide and intact pulmonary vessels to convey oxygen-poor blood to the alveoli. Normal alveoli will be of little use if the venous blood cannot reach them, as is the situation in pulmonary embolism.

Assessment

Pulmonary embolism is one of the most frequently misdiagnosed conditions in emergency medicine because of its confusing presentation. The early presentation may reveal normal breath sounds with good peripheral aeration, diverting attention away from a pulmonary pathology. The classic presentation is sudden dyspnea and cyanosis and, perhaps, a sharp pain in the chest. A hallmark of pulmonary embolism is that the cyanosis does not resolve with oxygen therapy.

Pulmonary emboli often originate in the large veins of the leg, particularly the greater saphenous vein, where a clot can form and migrate through the venous circulation, passing through the right side of the heart and into the pulmonary circulation **Figure 43**. Patients with thrombophlebitis (inflammation of the veins in the legs) are at high risk for pulmonary embolism. They may have the Homan sign (calf pain during dorsiflexion of the foot caused by thrombophlebitis in the leg).

Clots also tend to form when a person is immobile for a prolonged period, such as during a long car trip or lengthy airplane flight.

Management

Bedridden patients are often prescribed anticoagulants or wear special stockings or other devices to reduce the formation of blood clots in the legs. Especially for patients with a history of deep venous thrombosis, a **Greenfield filter** may be inserted by a physician. This device, which opens like a mesh umbrella in the main vein that returns blood to the heart, is intended to catch clots that break loose and travel from the legs.

An exceptionally large pulmonary embolus that lodges at the bifurcation of the right and left pulmonary arteries is called a *saddle embolus*, and it may be immediately fatal. Cardiac arrest caused by a large pulmonary embolus is a perilous situation

that few patients survive. Patients with such an embolus often have **cape cyanosis**—deep cyanosis of the face, neck, chest, and back—despite good-quality CPR and ventilation with 100% supplemental oxygen. One hallmark of pulmonary embolus is cyanosis that does not respond to oxygen. Patients who do not respond to oxygen, or who complain of chest pain, must be transported to the nearest emergency facility.

■ Age-Related Variations

Most patients with COPD, pulmonary edema, and other common respiratory ailments are in the second half of their lives. Asthma is often seen in younger patients but can flare at any time. As with most systems, there are anatomic and physiologic differences related to respiratory ailments in children.

■ Anatomy

In children, the upper airway has several important anatomic considerations (see the chapter, *Airway Management and Ventilation*). Children have large heads relative to the size of their bodies.

■ Pathophysiology

Infants have a limited ability to compensate for respiratory insults and often expend huge amounts of energy to breathe. At times, infants are intubated to take over the work of breathing even though adequate physiologic parameters are maintained. In older children, increasing compensatory skills develop, and juvenile patients with asthma can sometimes compensate for days, with adequate oxygen saturation, before literally tiring out and dying of fatigue.

Many infants and children with respiratory problems have respiratory distress (difficulty breathing), some have respiratory failure (which invariably leads to decompensation), and a few are in respiratory arrest. If the child in respiratory arrest can be resuscitated before cardiac arrest occurs, survival with a return to full function is likely. Any respiratory compromise in children must be monitored closely and the child transported to the closest emergency department. If a pediatric-specific emergency department is available, consult medical direction or your local transport protocols for advice. Some of the respiratory diseases common among pediatric patients include the following:

- **Foreign body obstruction of the upper airway.** Toddlers explore the world with their mouths, and small items like peanuts and coins can lodge in the upper airway. The soft latex of a balloon that has deflated or popped can be sucked into a child's airway past the cricoid ring, where a paramedic is unlikely to be able to remove it. Because of this hazard, avoid blowing up a glove and giving it to children as a toy.

  Pencil erasers, candy, and beans frequently obstruct a nostril. These items are often in the nose for a day or two before the child has pain and a foul-smelling nasal discharge. Paramedics should not try to remove the obstruction. Emergency department personnel are skilled in removing such objects.

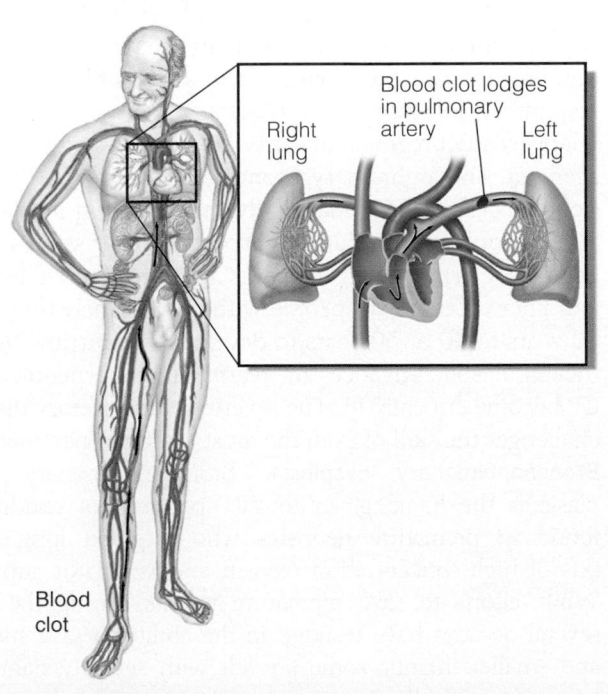

Figure 43 Pulmonary emboli are most common in sedentary people, in whom an embolus typically forms in the legs or pelvis. The embolus passes through the right side of the heart and lodges in the pulmonary artery, blocking blood flow to a portion of the lung.

- **Infection.** Several infections can cause dangerous inflammation and swelling of the upper airway. The diseases include croup, laryngotracheobronchitis (a cause of croup), epiglottitis, bacterial tracheitis, and retropharyngeal abscesses. Be wary of children with high fevers and stridor.

- **Lower airway disease.** Diseases of the lower airway are common in children. Even relatively minor viral infections can cause significant respiratory distress in small children. One millimeter of swelling in an adult airway might be annoying and cause a scratchy throat. The same amount of swelling in a young child's airway can cause respiratory distress.

- **Asthma.** Asthma often presents during childhood, and it may take a while to figure out a particular child's triggers. Asthma usually includes a component of bronchospasm that causes wheezing. While it has long been believed that "infants do not get asthma," it is increasingly recognized that even infants can have reactive airway disease caused by specific triggers.

- **Bronchiolitis.** Some children have bronchiolitis, or inflammation of the bronchioles. This condition is caused by swelling, not bronchospasm. In fact, the bronchioles are usually too deep in the airway to be surrounded by any smooth muscle, so aerosol bronchodilators will rarely help. One definition of bronchiolitis is wheezing that is unresponsive to bronchodilators. (Adults sometimes have inflammation and plugging of the bronchioles that results in pneumonia distal to the blockages. This bronchiolitis obliterans with organizing pneumonia is referred to as BOOP.)

- **Pneumonia.** Children are susceptible to pneumonia because their immune system may not be as strong as in a typical adult. Common infectious diseases like the seasonal flu and upper respiratory infections sometimes progress to a far more dangerous pneumonia. Maintain a high index of suspicion when called for children with any drop in oxygen saturation, particularly if they have a fever or abnormal breath sounds.

- **Pertussis.** Pertussis, also known as whooping cough, is a good example of a highly contagious bacterial disease. Children are typically vaccinated against pertussis as a part of their routine childhood immunizations, and pertussis had become a rare disease in the United States. Unfortunately, immunizations rates have fallen because of apathy, lack of access to medical care, and the growing fear of some parents that immunizations have negative consequences. Once-rare diseases like pertussis are making a comeback. Pertussis begins with mild symptoms, like any other upper respiratory tract infection, but progresses in 1 or 2 weeks to paroxysms of coughing that often produce a characteristic whoop when the child attempts to inhale after a coughing fit. The cough can last as long as 6 weeks, earning pertussis the title "the 100-day cough." The cough can be so severe that it can cause postcough vomiting, conjunctival hemorrhage, and cyanotic hypoxia. Elderly patients occasionally have pertussis, presumably because their childhood immunizations have lost their effectiveness.

Special Populations

Many children with high-tech medical devices live at home. Tracheotomies are not uncommon. The pediatric tracheostomy tube is often too small to have an inner cannula that can be removed if it becomes clogged with secretions (see the chapter, *Airway Management and Ventilation*). As a result, the tube sometimes is coughed out, and a well-meaning caregiver sometimes causes trauma trying to reinsert it. Multiple options are available for dealing with tracheostomy emergencies in children. A small endotracheal tube can be inserted through the tracheostomy. A standard oral endotracheal intubation can usually be performed. Make sure the endotracheal tube comes to rest below the level of the tracheostomy, or cover the tracheostomy and ventilate the patient with a bag-mask device.

The pertussis immunization lasts for 5 to 10 years, so adults can contract the disease even if they were vaccinated as children. An infected adult can transmit the infection to a child. It is important for paramedics to pay attention to their own health, vaccinations, and immune system. They will probably be exposed to tuberculosis, pertussis, hepatitis B, and a variety of other pathogenic organisms and contagious diseases during their careers (see the chapter, *Infectious Diseases*).

- **Cystic fibrosis.** Cystic fibrosis (CF) is a hereditary disease that affects the respiratory and digestive systems. It is the most common life-shortening hereditary disease among people of European descent. People with CF produce copious amounts of thick mucus in their respiratory and digestive tracts, which makes them susceptible to chronic respiratory infections and requires them to maintain a relatively strict regimen of aerosol treatments, mucus management, and pulmonary exercise. People with CF have frequent respiratory illnesses that require hospitalization. Some people require lung transplants. Great strides have been made in the management of CF during the last decade, and life expectancy of people with CF has increased from 20 years to 40 or 50 years in developed countries. Nevertheless, despite advances in treatment, some people with CP become critically ill. The severity of respiratory disease challenges the skill of even the most seasoned paramedics.

- **Bronchopulmonary dysplasia.** Bronchopulmonary dysplasia is the name given to the spectrum of conditions found in premature neonates who required long periods of high-concentration oxygen and ventilator support. While efforts to save premature infants during the past several decades have resulted in the ability to save smaller and smaller infants, some are left with severely damaged lungs, occasionally requiring long-term ventilator support. Researchers in this area initially thought that barotrauma from ventilators was the primary cause, but studies have increasingly pointed to the role of high-concentration oxygen in damaging the lungs. Children with bronchopulmonary dysplasia may use home ventilators, have tracheostomies, or have fragile lungs and many pulmonary complications.

YOU *are the Medic* | SUMMARY |

1. What initial "from the door" findings make you concerned for this patient?

The patient's initial appearance should raise red flags for you because his ashen gray skin signals hypoxia. The patient speaking in only 1- or 2-word sentences indicates that his oxygen saturation is low and he is struggling for enough oxygen. An initial impression of this patient should tell you that he is in serious distress and needs rapid, decisive care.

2. What are your priorities for this patient?

Oxygen is your priority. Through proper assessment and interviewing techniques, you need to ascertain why this patient is not getting enough oxygen and treat the cause. Aggressive airway and breathing care are paramount for this patient.

3. What is your working diagnosis at this time?

Pulmonary edema is the most accurate working diagnosis based on the information you have so far, although it is not clear why this patient is experiencing the edema. Although no medications are found on the scene, it is possible that the patient has prescriptions for medications that should be taken. You also need to rule out a heart attack in this patient; heart failure can also cause pulmonary edema.

4. What assessment and treatment steps will you want to accomplish on scene?

This patient's condition is serious, so you do not want to spend a lot of time on the scene; however, certain skills that are difficult to accomplish en route should be completed at the scene. Obtaining a 12-lead ECG, for example, needs to be done before you begin transport because doing so while moving can be a challenge and often results in too much artifact to allow an accurate interpretation. Vital signs can also be difficult to accomplish while driving to the hospital because of road noise, so getting a baseline set makes good clinical sense.

5. Is this an airway problem or a breathing problem?

This is a breathing problem. The patient is able to speak and move air, although with some difficulty. The problem is that the patient's lungs are not properly exchanging air because they are full of fluid—diminishing the amount of fluid in the lungs will help gas exchange and allow the needed oxygen to reach all of the cells.

6. Does the absence of chest pain mean the patient is not having a heart attack?

Not necessarily. Patients can be having a heart attack even though they are not experiencing any chest pain. Never rule out the possibility of a heart attack in the presence of pulmonary edema. A number of diagnostic tests will need to be given in the hospital to determine if the patient is having a heart attack. At this point, you should contact medical control with a report and request permission to give aspirin.

7. What is the rationale for administering nitroglycerin if the patient is not experiencing chest pain?

Nitroglycerin has some vasodilatory effects, which aid in eliminating the fluid from the patient's lungs and help free the surfaces needed for gas exchange, which, in turn, allows oxygen to reach the cells and tissue. However, expanding the vasculature also lowers the patient's blood pressure and possibly lowers the preload to the heart.

EMS Patient Care Report (PCR)

Date: 5-05-11	Incident No.: 550	Nature of Call: Medical alarm		Location: 222 Fifth Street	
Dispatched: 0900	En Route: 0901	At Scene: 0903	Transport: 0915	At Hospital: 0922	In Service: 0939

Patient Information

Age: 74 Sex: M Weight (in kg [lb]): 100 kg (220 lb)	Allergies: None Medications: Unknown Past Medical History: Unknown Chief Complaint: Difficulty breathing

Vital Signs

Time: 0908	BP: 140/100	Pulse: 110	Respirations: 34	Spo$_2$: 80%
Time: 0913	BP: 130/100	Pulse: 100	Respirations: 28	Spo$_2$: 85%
Time:	BP:	Pulse:	Respirations:	Spo$_2$:

YOU are the Medic   SUMMARY, continued

EMS Treatment (circle all that apply)				
Oxygen @ __15__ L/min via (circle one): NC NRM **Bag-mask device**		Assisted Ventilation	Airway Adjunct:	CPR
Defibrillation	Bleeding Control	Bandaging	Splinting	Other:
Narrative				

Arrived to find a 74-year-old man in severe breathing distress. Pt states in 1- to 2-word sentences that he awoke this way and thinks he is going to die. Pt is not able to provide a history owing to severe breathing distress. Pt is in tripod position, skin color is ashen gray, and Pt is diaphoretic. Pt given 100% oxygen while breath sounds were obtained. Breath sounds reveal rales in apices and diminished sounds in bases. Pt denies history of fluid in lungs. Oxygen administration changed to CPAP. Pt becoming more anxious and is not following instructions. Monitor showed sinus tachycardia while vital signs were being obtained. Pt not tolerating CPAP and oxygen saturation falling; decision made to assist ventilations with positive pressure bag-mask ventilation. Decision made not to intubate on scene given short transport time to hospital. My partner performed ventilations while 12-lead ECG was obtained. 12-lead ECG shows some ST elevation in chest leads V2 and V3 and Pt was transmitted to destination hospital. Pt moved onto stretcher and placed in upright position. Pt given 1 inch of nitroglycerin paste and was tolerating assisted ventilation well. Pt moved into ambulance, vital signs obtained again, and transport begun to hospital. Pt had IV established and was given 40 mg of furosemide at 0928. MD 413 contacted at Mercy Hospital; full report given; requested permission to give additional nitroglycerin paste and additional furosemide. MD 413 granted both requests and stated to give Pt 324 mg of aspirin. Orders confirmed; furosemide administered and 1 inch of nitroglycerin paste applied at 0930. Shortly afterward, Pt began to feel better and did not need further assistance with ventilation. CPAP resumed and Pt able to answer questions appropriately. Oxygen saturation progressively increased with treatment during transport. Arrival at Mercy Hospital at 0933 and Pt admitted to room 5 with report to RN. CPAP maintained until respiratory therapist arrived with device. Pt had significant improvement at time of turnover. IV remained patent; less than 150 mL infused. **End of report**

Prep Kit

www.Paramedic.EMSzone.com

◼ Ready for Review

- Respiratory disease is one of the most common pathologic conditions, and, as a result, respiratory distress is one of the most common reasons for EMS dispatches.

- Impaired ventilation may be caused by upper airway obstruction, lower airway obstructive disease, chest wall impairment, or neuromuscular impairment.

- Respiratory failure, or hypoventilation, can occur from a multitude of pathologic conditions, from injuries to the lungs, heart, and neurologic system to overdoses. Care includes providing supplemental oxygen.

- In hyperventilation syndrome, ventilation is excessive. If it continues, the patient may experience chest pain, carpopedal spasm, and alkalosis.

- The nasal hairs in the nares (nostrils) filter particulates from the air, which flows through the nose and is warmed, humidified, and additionally filtered by the turbinates.

- The mouth and oropharynx are highly vascular structures covered by a mucous membrane. The hypopharynx is the junction of the oropharynx and nasopharynx.

- The larynx and glottis are typically considered the dividing line between the upper airway and the lower airway. The thyroid cartilage is the most obvious external landmark of the larynx. The glottis and vocal cords are found in the middle of the thyroid cartilage.

- The cricoid cartilage can be palpated just below the thyroid cartilage in the neck. It forms a complete ring and maintains the trachea in an open position. Applying cricoid pressure, known as the Sellick maneuver, is no longer recommended.

- The small space between the thyroid and cricoid cartilages is the cricothyroid membrane. Because it contains few blood vessels and is covered only by skin and minimal subcutaneous tissue, it is a preferred area for inserting a large IV catheter or a small breathing tube.

- The primary components of the respiratory system are like an inverted tree, with the trachea representing the trunk and the alveoli resembling the leaves.

- The trachea bifurcates into the left and right mainstem bronchi of the lungs at a ridgelike projection of tracheal cartilage called the *carina*.

- Cilia line the larger airways and help move foreign material out of the tracheobronchial tree. If a patient is dehydrated or has taken medications that dry secretions (such as antihistamines), the cilia will not be able to effectively move secretions. The same is true if the patient is overhydrated.

- Pulmonary circulation begins at the right ventricle, where the pulmonary artery branches into increasingly smaller vessels until it reaches the pulmonary capillary bed, which surrounds the alveoli and terminal bronchioles. Gas exchange occurs at the interface of the alveoli and the pulmonary capillaries.

- The interstitial space can fill with blood, pus, or air, causing pain, stiff lungs, and lung collapse.

- The primary functions of the respiratory system are ventilation, perfusion, and diffusion.

- Mechanisms of respiratory control are neurologic, cardiovascular, muscular, and renal.

- Patients who have traumatic brain injuries may exhibit abnormal respiratory patterns, including agonal gasps; apneustic and ataxic patterns; Biot, Cheyne-Stokes, and Kussmaul respirations; and central neurogenic hyperventilation, bradypnea, hyperpnea, hypopnea, and tachypnea.

- The brain is sensitive to reduced levels of oxygen. It requires a regular supply of oxygen and glucose to function but can store neither. An altered level of consciousness could represent respiratory compromise.

- Respiratory disease can cause impairment in ventilation, diffusion, perfusion, or combination of the three.

- Certain respiratory diseases have classic presentations that might help with the primary assessment.

- It is critical to evaluate how hard a patient is working to breathe. Patients in respiratory distress may be able to compensate at first, but will eventually become sleepy, have a decreased respiratory rate and depth, and then experience decompensation.

- Assessing a patient's position of comfort and level of difficulty speaking may help in determining the patient's degree of distress. A patient sitting in a Fowler's position and speaking only in two- or three-word statements, for example, is probably in considerable distress.

- Patients in respiratory distress tend to seek the tripod position. The condition of a patient in respiratory distress who is willing to lie flat may be quickly deteriorating. Head bobbing is also an ominous sign.

- Other signs of life-threatening respiratory distress include bony retractions, soft tissue retractions, nasal flaring, tracheal tugging, paradoxical respiratory movement, pulsus paradoxus, pursed-lip breathing, and grunting.

- Note any audible abnormal respiratory noises. Noisy breathing is obstructed breathing.

- Snoring indicates partial obstruction of the upper airway by the tongue. Stridor indicates narrowing of the upper airway, usually as a result of swelling (laryngeal edema).

- Auscultate the lungs whenever possible. Adventitious breath sounds are the extra noises audible during auscultation; they include wheezing and crackles.

- Crackles are any discontinuous noises heard during auscultation of the lungs. They are caused by the popping open of air spaces and are usually associated with increased fluid in the lungs.

- Wheezes are high-pitched, whistling sounds made by air being forced through narrowed airways, which makes them vibrate. Wheezing may be diffuse in conditions such as asthma and congestive heart failure or localized when caused by a foreign body obstructing a bronchus.

- *Silence means danger!* If breath sounds are inaudible with a stethoscope, the patient is not moving enough air to ventilate the lungs.

- The respiratory system delivers oxygen to the body and removes the primary waste product of metabolism, carbon dioxide. If the lungs are not functioning properly, both of these vital functions may be impaired. Hypoxia, cell death, and acidosis can then occur.

- Patients with dyspnea are usually transported to the nearest facility.

- Patients who have chronic respiratory disease are often knowledgeable about their disease and may have tried several treatment options already. Ask them about these efforts and what results, if any, they produced.

- Onset and duration of distress are important considerations in determining the underlying cause. Find out if the problem happened suddenly or gradually worsened over time.

- Find out if the patient's condition is a recurrence of a past condition. If so, compare the current situation with other episodes.

- A patient who has respiratory disease may not be able to talk because he or she is having difficulty breathing. The history may have to be obtained from a family member or from only a few clues.

- Assess the patient's mucous membranes for cyanosis (a bluish or dusky color), pallor, and moisture.

- Assessing the level of consciousness is extremely important in dyspneic patients.

- Look for jugular venous distention in the neck, with the patient in a semisitting position. Distended neck veins may be caused by cardiac failure.

- Feel the chest for vibrations as the patient breathes. Check for edema of the ankles and lower back. Check for peripheral cyanosis. Check the pulse, and note the patient's skin temperature. Apply any available monitors.

- A pulse oximeter indicates the percentage of the patient's hemoglobin that has oxygen attached. An oxygen saturation level greater than 95% is considered normal.

- Exhaled carbon dioxide can be monitored with colorimetric end-tidal carbon dioxide devices or with wave capnography.

- The peak flow is the maximum flow rate at which the patient can expel air from the lungs. Normal peak flow ranges from about 350 to 700 L/min. A peak flow of less than 150 L/min is insufficient and signals that the patient is in significant respiratory distress.

- Metered-dose inhalers deliver bronchodilators and corticosteroids as an aerosol treatment. Dry powder inhalers deliver a measured dose of medication in the form of a fine powder. Little or no medication may reach the lungs if improper technique is used.

- Aerosol nebulizers deliver liquid medications in the form of a fine mist to the respiratory tract. Weigh the potential benefits of aerosol therapy against the lower fraction of inspired oxygen delivered during the treatment.

- Emergency medical care for patients with dyspnea may include securing the airway; decreasing the work of breathing; administering supplemental oxygen, bronchodilators, leukotriene modifiers, methylxanthines, electrolytes, inhaled corticosteroids, vasodilators, or diuretics; supporting or assisting ventilation; intubating the patient; injecting a beta-adrenergic receptor agonist subcutaneously; and/or instilling medication directly through an endotracheal tube.

- In managing the condition of a patient who is in respiratory distress, begin by ensuring that there is an open and maintainable airway. Suction if necessary, and keep the airway optimally positioned. Remove constricting clothing. Reduce the patient's effort to breathe.

- Drug administration methods that require the patient to inhale the medication may become unreliable or ineffective when the patient's airways are severely compromised. Some cases may warrant administering medications subcutaneously.

- Medications can be instilled directly into the tracheobronchial tree when patients are intubated or have a tracheostomy. Stop CPR compressions for a moment while instilling the medication.

- Continuous positive airway pressure (CPAP) is used as therapy for respiratory failure. Within several minutes of application, the patient's oxygen saturation should increase, and the respiratory rate should decrease.

- Bilevel positive airway pressure (BiPAP) is CPAP that delivers one pressure during inspiration and a different pressure during exhalation. It is more like normal breathing and is often more comfortable for patients.

- Automated transport ventilators are essentially flow-restricted oxygen-powered breathing devices with timers. They are particularly good choices for filling the role of the bag-mask ventilator when the patient is in cardiac or respiratory arrest but are not intended to ventilate patients without direct observation and attention from a skilled practitioner.

- Patients in respiratory failure may ultimately need to be intubated. There are major drawbacks and risks to intubating in the field, but it can also be lifesaving. Weigh these issues along with protocols, medical direction, and the patient's wishes.

- Anatomic or foreign body obstructions of the upper airway, including aspiration of stomach contents, can cause seizures and death. Avoid causing gastric distention when administering bag-mask ventilation, and monitor the patient's ability to protect his or her airway. If the patient cannot protect his or her airway, the patient must be intubated.

- Infections can cause swelling in the upper airway. Croup is one of the most common conditions causing airway swelling, although it usually occurs only in small children.

- Common obstructive airway diseases include emphysema, chronic bronchitis, and asthma. Emphysema and chronic bronchitis are collectively classified as COPD.

- Asthma is caused by allergens or irritants and is characterized by widespread, reversible narrowing of the airways (bronchospasm), edema of the airways, and increased mucus production. It can cause significant airway obstruction.

- Primary treatment of bronchospasm is bronchodilator medication. Primary treatment of bronchial edema is corticosteroids, which may or may not be administered in the field setting.

- Status asthmaticus is a severe, prolonged asthmatic attack that cannot be stopped with conventional treatment. It is a dire medical emergency. Any person with asthma who feels sick enough to call an ambulance is in status asthmaticus until proved otherwise.

- When a patient has recurring asthma attacks, his or her inhaler could be empty or the medication could no longer be effective. Try administering a new bronchodilator.

- Noncompliance with the prescribed medication regimen could trigger an asthma attack. Ask what the patient was doing when the asthma attack began. Ask if the patient took his or her medications today. Ask if movement worsens the dyspnea.

- Emphysema is a chronic weakening and destruction of the walls of the terminal bronchioles and alveoli. A patient with emphysema classically has a barrel chest, muscle wasting, and pursed-lip breathing. Tachypnea is often present.

- Chronic bronchitis is characterized by excessive mucus production in the bronchial tree, nearly always accompanied by a chronic or recurrent productive cough. A patient with chronic bronchitis tends to be sedentary and obese, sleep in an upright position, use many tissues, have copious secretions, and be cyanotic.

- In assessing patients who have COPD, search for the cause of a worsened condition that prompted the call for help. Look for signs of infection, peripheral edema, jugular venous distention with hepatojugular reflux, and crackles. Find out if the onset of dyspnea was sudden or gradual.

- Hypoxic drive is a phenomenon in which high levels of oxygen decrease the patient's respiratory drive. Nevertheless, supplemental oxygen should not be withheld.

- Not every patient should be ventilated the same way. Allow the patient to exhale completely before the next breath is delivered. If the patient is not allowed to do so, pressure in the thorax will rise, eventually causing pneumothorax or cardiac arrest. This phenomenon is called auto-PEEP. If auto-PEEP is a risk, ventilation should be at a rate of 4 to 6 breaths/min. The standard ventilation rate for adults without COPD is 8 to 10 breaths/min.

- Pneumonia may be caused by a variety of bacterial, viral, and fungal agents. A patient with pneumonia usually reports weakness, productive cough, fever, and sometimes chest pain that worsens with coughing. Supportive care includes oxygenation, suctioning, and transport to an appropriate facility.

- Atelectasis is alveolar collapse as a result of proximal airway obstruction, pneumothorax, hemothorax, toxic inhalation, or other causes. Incentive spirometry can help prevent atelectasis in postsurgical patients and others.

- Lung cancer is often characterized by hemoptysis and is increasing among women.

- Damage caused by inhalation of a toxic gas depends on the water solubility of the gas.

- Pulmonary edema occurs when fluid migrates into the lungs. A patient expectorating foamy pink secretions probably has severe pulmonary edema.

- Acute respiratory distress syndrome is caused by diffuse alveolar damage as a result of aspiration, pulmonary edema, or some other alveolar insult.

- When a patient has a pneumothorax, air collects between the visceral pleura and the parietal pleura. Administer supplemental oxygen, and monitor the patient's respiratory status closely.

- Pleural effusion will cause dyspnea. Supportive care, including proper positioning and aggressive oxygen administration, should be given.

- A pulmonary embolism occurs when a blood clot breaks off in the circulation and travels to the lungs, blocking blood flow and nutrient exchange. Bedridden patients and people with thrombophlebitis are at risk of pulmonary embolism. The hallmark of a pulmonary embolus is cyanosis that does not resolve with oxygen therapy.

- Infants are less able than older children to compensate for respiratory insults.

- Infants and children with respiratory problems may be in respiratory distress (difficulty breathing), respiratory failure (a condition that invariably leads to decompensation), or respiratory arrest. It is important to resuscitate a child before cardiac arrest occurs.

◼ Vital Vocabulary

__abscess__ A collection of pus in a sac, formed by necrotic tissues and an accumulation of white blood cells.

__adventitious__ A type of breath sound that occurs in addition to the normal breath sounds; examples are crackles and wheezes.

__alveoli__ The saclike units at the end of the bronchioles where gas exchange takes place (singular, alveolus).

__angioedema__ A vascular reaction that may have an allergic cause and may result in profound swelling of the tongue and lips.

__arytenoid cartilages__ One of the paired, pitcher-shaped cartilages at the back of the larynx, at the upper border of the cricoid cartilage.

__aspiration__ The drawing in or out by suction. In the lungs, aspiration of food, liquids, blood, or foreign objects can occur when a patient is unable to protect his or her own airway.

__atelectasis__ The collapse of the alveolar air spaces of the lungs.

__beta-2 agonist__ A pharmacologic agent that stimulates the beta-2 receptor sites found in smooth muscle; includes common bronchodilators such as albuterol and levalbuterol.

__botulism__ Poisoning from eating food containing botulinum toxin.

__bronchospasm__ Severe constriction of the bronchial tree.

__cape cyanosis__ Deep cyanosis of the face and neck and across the chest and back; associated with little or no blood flow; a particularly ominous sign.

__carina__ A ridgelike projection of tracheal cartilage located where the trachea bifurcates into the right and left mainstem bronchi.

__carpopedal spasm__ Contorted position of the hand or foot in which the fingers or toes flex in a clawlike manner; may result from hyperventilation.

__chronic bronchitis__ A chronic inflammatory condition affecting the bronchi that is characterized by excessive mucus production as a result of overgrowth of the mucous glands in the airways.

__cilia__ The hairlike microtubule projections on the surface of a cell that can move materials over the cell surface.

__cor pulmonale__ Heart disease that develops because of chronic lung disease, affecting primarily the right side of the heart.

__crackles__ The abnormal breath sounds that have a fine, crackling quality; previously called rales.

__cricoid cartilage__ The ringlike cartilage forming the lower and back part of the larynx.

__cricothyroid membrane__ The membrane between the cricoid and thyroid cartilages of the larynx.

croup A common disease of childhood due to upper airway obstruction and characterized by stridor, hoarseness, and a barking cough.

dead space The portion of the tidal volume that does not reach the alveoli and, thus, does not participate in gas exchange.

diuresis The production of large amounts of urine by the kidney.

emphysema The infiltration of any tissue by air or gas; a chronic obstructive pulmonary disease characterized by distention of the alveoli and destructive changes in the lung parenchyma.

end-tidal carbon dioxide The carbon dioxide contained in the last few milliliters of exhaled air; the unit of measure is a percentage.

epistaxis Nosebleed.

Fowler's position A sitting position with the head elevated to 90° (sitting straight upright).

gas exchange The process by which oxygen-depleted blood from the pulmonary circulation releases carbon dioxide and is enriched with oxygen; occurs by diffusion at the interface of the alveoli and the pulmonary capillary bed; newly oxygen-enriched blood enters the cardiac circulation for distribution to the body's tissues.

glottis The vocal cords and the opening between them.

goblet cells The mucus-producing cells found mainly in the respiratory and intestinal tracts.

Greenfield filter A mesh filter placed in the inferior vena cava to catch blood clots in patients who are at high risk of pulmonary embolus.

Guillain-Barré syndrome A disease of unknown cause that involves progressive paralysis that moves from the feet to the head (ascending paralysis); if paralysis reaches the diaphragm, the patient may require respiratory support.

hemoglobin The oxygen-carrying pigment of red blood cells; when it has absorbed oxygen in the lungs, it is bright red and called oxyhemoglobin; after oxygen has been given up in the tissues, hemoglobin is purple and called reduced hemoglobin.

hemoptysis Coughing up blood.

Hering-Breuer reflex The nervous system mechanism that terminates inhalation and prevents lung overexpansion.

hypoventilate To move inadequate volumes of air into the lungs.

hypoxia A dangerous condition in which the supply of oxygen to the tissues is reduced.

hypoxic drive A situation in which a person's stimulus to breathe comes from a decrease in Pao_2 rather than the normal stimulus, an increase in $Paco_2$.

jugular venous distention The visible bulging of the jugular veins when a patient is in semi-Fowler's or full Fowler's position; indicates inadequate blood movement through the heart and/or lungs.

Kussmaul respirations A respiratory pattern characteristic of diabetic ketoacidosis, with marked hyperpnea and tachypnea.

laryngotracheobronchitis Inflammation of the larynx, trachea, and bronchi.

larynx The organ of voice production.

metastasis The transfer of a disease from one organ or part of the body to another that is not directly connected to the original site; often used to describe a cancer that has spread to other parts of the body.

monophonic The sound of one note during wheezing, caused by the vibration of a single bronchus.

orthopnea Severe dyspnea experienced when recumbent and relieved by sitting or standing up.

palatine tonsils One of three sets of lymphatic organs that constitute the tonsils; located in the back of the throat, on each side of the posterior opening of the oral cavity; help protect the body from bacteria introduced into the mouth and nose.

parenchyma The functional portions of a gland or solid organ.

paroxysmal nocturnal dyspnea Severe shortness of breath occurring at night after several hours of recumbency, during which fluid pools in the lungs.

piriform fossae Hollow pockets on the lateral portions of the glottic opening.

pleural effusion Excessive accumulation of fluid in the pleural space.

pneumonia Inflammation of the lung caused by an infectious agent.

pneumonitis Inflammation of the lung; implies lung inflammation from an irritant such as a chemical, dust, or radiation, or from aspiration.

polycythemia The production of more red blood cells over time, making the blood "thick"; a characteristic of people who have chronic lung disease and chronic hypoxia.

polyphonic The sound of multiple notes during wheezing; caused by the vibrations of many bronchi.

pseudomembrane A false membrane formed by a dead tissue layer; seen in the posterior pharynx of patients with diphtheria.

pulsus paradoxus Weakening or loss of a palpable pulse during inhalation; characteristic of cardiac tamponade and severe asthma.

purulent Full of pus; having the character of pus.

rales Old term for abnormal breath sounds that have a fine, crackling quality; now called *crackles*.

reactive airway disease A term used to describe any condition that causes hyperreactive bronchioles and bronchospasm.

restrictive lung diseases Diseases that limit the ability of the lungs to expand appropriately. Skeletal abnormalities (kyphosis and scoliosis) are a common example of restrictive lung disease.

retractions The drawing in of the intercostal muscles and the muscles above the clavicles in respiratory distress.

rhonchi Coarse, low-pitched breath sounds heard in patients who chronically have mucus in the airways (singular, rhonchus).

shunt A situation in which a portion of the output of the right side of the heart reaches the left side of the heart without being oxygenated in the lungs; may be caused by atelectasis, pulmonary edema, or a variety of other conditions. In hemodialysis, an anastomosis between a peripheral artery and vein.

smooth muscle The nonstriated involuntary muscle found in vessel walls, glands, and the gastrointestinal tract.

snoring A noise made during inhalation when the upper airway is partially obstructed by the tongue.

spacers The devices that collect medication as it is released from the canister of a metered-dose inhaler, allowing more medication to be delivered to the lungs and less to be lost to the environment.

status asthmaticus A severe, prolonged asthma attack that cannot be stopped with conventional treatment, such as the administration of epinephrine.

stridor The harsh, high-pitched sound associated with severe upper airway obstruction, such as that caused by laryngeal edema.

surfactant A liquid protein substance that coats the alveoli in the lungs; it reduces the surface tension and helps keep the alveoli expanded.

tactile fremitus Vibrations in the chest that can be felt with a hand on the chest as the patient breathes.

tidal volume The amount of air inhaled or exhaled during one breath.

tracheostomy The opening created during a tracheotomy procedure.

tracheotomy Surgically opening the trachea to create an airway.

tuberculosis A chronic bacterial disease caused by *Mycobacterium tuberculosis* that usually affects the lungs but can also affect other organs such as the brain and kidneys.

turbinates A set of bony convolutions in the nasopharynx that help to maintain smooth airflow and warm, humidify, and filter the air as it is inhaled.

waveform capnography A monitoring method that measures the exhaled carbon dioxide level and displays the value numerically and as a waveform tracing.

ventilation The process of exchanging air between the lungs and the environment; includes inhalation and exhalation.

Assessment in Action

You are dispatched to a medical clinic for an 18-year-old woman complaining of difficulty breathing. According to the nurse on scene, the patient has a history of asthma as a child but has not had a problem during the last couple of years. You listen to the lungs and hear wheezes in all fields. The patient's vital signs are stable, so you decide to administer a nebulizer with albuterol and ipratropium (Atrovent). The patient states she was mowing her lawn when the breathing difficulty started.

1. Why is asthma considered a reactive airway disease?
   A. The patient reacts poorly with asthma.
   B. The asthma attack occurs most often when exposed to a trigger.
   C. Asthma interacts with other diseases the patient has.
   D. Patients experience asthma only in response to environmental triggers.

2. Is the number of people reported to have asthma in the United States increasing or decreasing?

3. Status asthmaticus is a:
   A. short asthma attack that ends spontaneously.
   B. long asthma attack the ends spontaneously.
   C. pseudoasthma attack.
   D. severe, prolonged asthma attack that cannot be stopped with conventional treatment.

4. The breathing treatment you administer is primarily to help with:
   A. reduction of mucus production.
   B. elimination of the response to a trigger.
   C. reduction of bronchospasm.
   D. reduction of anxiety.

5. The wheezing you hear is primarily caused by:
   A. air trapped in the lungs.
   B. air forced through constricted tubes, which causes them to vibrate.
   C. air moving normally in lungs.
   D. air moving through mucus in the lungs.

6. Because the patient is a woman, you know that:
   A. her asthma attacks are normally self-limiting.
   B. she is more likely to have asthma than a man.
   C. she is at less risk of having a severe attack than a man.
   D. she has a greater risk of having a severe attack than a man.

7. What other medications may help the patient during the next few hours?
   A. Antibiotics
   B. Corticosteroids
   C. Epinephrine
   D. Oxygen only

Additional Questions

8. What are some signs that a pediatric patient is in respiratory distress?

9. Will administering 100% oxygen to a patient who has had COPD for a long time cause respiratory arrest?

Cardiovascular Emergencies

National EMS Education Standard Competencies

Medicine
Integrates assessment findings with principles of epidemiology and pathophysiology to formulate a field impression and implement a comprehensive treatment/disposition plan for a patient with a medical complaint.

Cardiovascular
Anatomy, signs, symptoms, and management of

- Chest pain (pp 928-930)
- Cardiac arrest (pp 1003-1011)

Anatomy, physiology, epidemiology, pathophysiology, psychosocial impact, presentations, prognosis, and management of

- Acute coronary syndrome (p 1013)
  - Angina pectoris (pp 1012-1013)
  - Myocardial infarction (pp 1013-1018)
- Heart failure (pp 1018-1021)
- Nontraumatic cardiac tamponade (p 1021)
- Hypertensive emergencies (pp 1024-1025)
- Cardiogenic shock (pp 1021-1022)
- Vascular disorders (pp 1011-1012)
  - Abdominal aortic aneurysm (p 1024)
  - Arterial occlusion (pp 1011-1012)
  - Venous thrombosis (p 1012)
- Aortic aneurysm/dissection (pp 1022-1024)
- Thromboembolism (p 1012)
- Cardiac rhythm disturbances (pp 936, 937)
- Infectious diseases of the heart (p 1025)
  - Endocarditis (p 1025)
  - Pericarditis (p 1025)
- Congenital abnormalities (p 1026)

Shock and Resuscitation
Integrates comprehensive knowledge of causes and pathophysiology into the management of cardiac arrest and pre-arrest states.

Integrates a comprehensive knowledge of the causes and pathophysiology into the management of shock, respiratory failure or arrest with an emphasis on early intervention to prevent arrest.

Knowledge Objectives
1. Describe risk factors related to cardiovascular disease. (p 910)
2. Understand the basic structure and function of the cardiovascular system. (pp 910-912)
3. Identify the major normal and abnormal heart sounds. (pp 934-935)
4. Describe the cardiac cycle, including diastole and systole. (p 912)
5. Identify the various types of blood vessels. (p 914)
6. Explain how the heart functions as a pump, including the concepts of cardiac output, stroke volume, heart rate, and ejection fraction. (pp 915, 917-918)
7. Understand how electrical conduction activity occurs within the heart. (pp 918-921)
8. Understand how the autonomic nervous system controls the functioning of the heart. (pp 921-923)
9. Identify the various classes of drugs that influence the sympathetic nervous system. (pp 923-927)
10. Understand how the sympathetic nervous system regulates blood pressure. (pp 927-928)
11. Explain patient assessment procedures for cardiovascular problems, including scene size-up, primary assessment, history taking, secondary assessment, and reassessment. (pp 928-936)
12. Recognize the medications commonly prescribed to patients with cardiovascular diseases. (pp 930-933)
13. Describe the placement of leads and electrodes in 3-lead ECG monitoring. (pp 937-938)
14. Identify the components of an ECG rhythm strip. (pp 942-944)
15. Understand how to determine heart rate. (pp 945-947)
16. Describe the placement of 12-lead ECG leads. (pp 939, 941)
17. Describe the placement of 15- and 18-lead ECG leads. (pp 940-941)
18. Understand how to interpret 12-lead ECG findings, including atrial, junctional, and ventricular rhythms. (pp 944-947, 968-990)
19. Recognize normal sinus rhythm, and list the various types of cardiac dysrhythmias. (pp 947-964)
20. Discuss manual defibrillation, cardioversion, and transcutaneous pacing as techniques for managing cardiac emergencies. (pp 990-1000)
21. Understand the indications and procedure for operating an automated external defibrillator (AED). (pp 994-995)
22. Describe emergency medical care for the symptomatic patient with bradycardia. (pp 999, 1001-1002)
23. Describe emergency medical care for the symptomatic patient with tachycardia. (pp 1001, 1003, 1005)
24. Describe emergency medical care for the patient with cardiac arrest, including the elements of basic life support (BLS) and advanced cardiac life support (ACLS). (pp 1003-1010)
25. Describe the components of care following resuscitation, including how to determine return of spontaneous circulation. (p 1010)
26. Describe the pathophysiology of atherosclerosis, peripheral vascular disorders, acute coronary syndrome, and angina pectoris. (pp 1011-1013)
27. Discuss the assessment and management of coronary disease and angina. (pp 1012-1013)
28. List the signs and symptoms of acute myocardial infarction (AMI). (pp 1014-1015)

29. Explain the procedure for managing AMI and suspected AMI in the field, including STEMI and non-STEMI presentations. (pp 1015-1017)

30. Understand the benefits of reperfusion techniques (fibrinolysis and percutaneous intervention) in patients with AMI or suspected AMI. (pp 1017-1018)

31. Discuss the pathophysiology of congestive heart failure and its signs, symptoms, and treatment. (pp 1018-1021)

32. Discuss the pathophysiology of cardiac tamponade and its signs, symptoms, and treatment. (p 1021)

33. Discuss the pathophysiology of cardiogenic shock and its signs, symptoms, and treatment. (pp 1021-1022)

34. Describe the pathophysiology, assessment, and management of aortic aneurysms, including both acute dissecting aneurysm of the aorta and expanding and ruptured abdominal aortic aneurysms. (pp 1022-1024)

35. Discuss the pathophysiology of hypertensive emergencies and their signs, symptoms, and treatment. (pp 1024-1025)

36. Describe the risks posed by thromboembolism. (p 1012)

37. Identify types of congenital heart disease. (p 1026)

38. Describe the pathophysiology of hypertrophic cardiomyopathy. (p 985)

39. Describe the pathophysiology of other cardiovascular anomalies: coarctation of the aorta, truncus arteriosus, tricuspid atresia, hypoplastic left heart syndrome, tetralogy of Fallot, transposition of the great arteries, and total anomalous pulmonary venous return. (see chapter, *Neonatal Emergencies*)

40. Describe how infections—endocarditis, pericarditis, and rheumatic fever—can damage the heart. (pp 1025-1026)

Skills Objectives

1. Demonstrate how to assess and provide emergency medical care for a patient with chest pain or discomfort. (pp 928-936, 1013-1016)

2. Demonstrate how to perform cardiac monitoring. (p 938, Skill Drill 1)

3. Demonstrate how to acquire a 12-lead ECG. (pp 967-968, Skill Drill 2)

4. Demonstrate how to perform manual defibrillation. (pp 993-994, Skill Drill 3)

5. Demonstrate how to perform defibrillation with an AED. (pp 995-996, Skill Drill 4)

6. Demonstrate how to perform cardioversion. (pp 997-998, Skill Drill 5)

7. Demonstrate how to perform transcutaneous cardiac pacing. (pp 999-1000, Skill Drill 6)

8. Demonstrate how to manage symptomatic bradycardia. (pp 999-1001)

9. Demonstrate how to perform ACLS care. (pp 1004-1006)

10. Demonstrate how to perform postresuscitative care. (p 1010)

Introduction

Heart disease has been the number one killer in the United States almost every year since 1900. It was for the purpose of providing early, definitive treatment for patients with acute myocardial infarction (AMI) that the job of paramedic first came into being more than 30 years ago. Even with paramedic availability, more than 600,000 Americans die of heart disease every year; approximately half die in an emergency department (ED) or before reaching a hospital, during the first minutes and hours after the onset of symptoms. It is easy to see why the recognition and management of cardiovascular emergencies continue to receive strong emphasis in paramedic education.

This chapter will prepare you to integrate pathophysiologic principles and assessment findings to formulate a field impression and implement a treatment plan for patients with cardiovascular disease (CVD). You will first learn about the epidemiology of CVD in terms of its prevalence, mortality and morbidity, risk factors, and prevention strategies. After reviewing the anatomy and function of the cardiovascular system, the chapter covers some of the clinical manifestations of CVD. Considerable emphasis is given to the interpretation of cardiac <u>dysrhythmias</u> and their management within the context of the patient's overall clinical condition. Finally, you will learn about pharmacologic and other treatment modalities surrounding advanced cardiac life support (ACLS).

Epidemiology

According to the American Heart Association (AHA), about 34% of all US deaths in 2007 were attributable to heart disease. Risk factors for heart disease fall into two categories: those that are modifiable, at least to some extent, and those that are not `Table 1`. It was previously thought that heart disease primarily affected men, but statistics now show that more women die of heart disease than men.

Education and early recognition are also important prevention strategies. Educating people about the risk factors of heart disease may decrease mortality. This is an area of interest for EMS providers who are involved in community health promotion. `Table 2` lists methods for decreasing the risks for CVD.

Table 1 Risk Factors for Heart Disease

Modifiable	Nonmodifiable
Hypertension	Advanced age
Elevated cholesterol level	Family history
Smoking	Carbohydrate intolerance
Poor diet	Type A personality traits
Obesity	
Sedentary lifestyle	
Use of oral contraceptives	
Use of hormone replacement therapy	
High stress	

Table 2 Decreasing the Risk for Cardiovascular Disease

- Awareness
- Behavior modification
- Smoking cessation
- Blood pressure control
- Cholesterol management
- Lipid management
- Weight management
- Aerobic exercise

Anatomy and Physiology

Structure and Function

The cardiovascular system is composed of the heart and blood vessels. Its primary function is to deliver oxygenated blood and nutrients to every cell in the body. It is also responsible for delivering

---

YOU *are the Medic*   PART 1

You have just poured your first cup of coffee for the morning when your unit receives a call for "unknown medical." While you are en route, the dispatcher updates you as follows: "The patient is a 55-year-old woman who was awakened at approximately 0500 this morning with jaw pain. The patient has a history of diabetes." You look at your watch—it is now 0830. When you arrive on scene you find the patient lying in bed. She looks pale and diaphoretic. The patient tells you that she has an awful pain in her jaw that she cannot explain. "I was going to call my dentist when his office opens, but I really do not feel well," she says. You ask the patient if she is having pain anywhere else, to which she replies, "No."

1. What is your initial impression of this patient's condition?

2. What initial history do you need for your assessment of this patient?

chemical messages (hormones) within the body and for transporting the waste products of metabolism from the cells to sites of recycling or waste disposal.

The Heart

The driving force behind the cardiovascular system is the heart **Figure 1**. This remarkable pump sits in the chest, above the diaphragm, behind and slightly to the left of the lower sternum (**retrosternal**). The heart is not much larger than the owner's fist and weighs between 250 g and 300 g (about 9 oz). Despite its relatively small size, it is strong enough to circulate 7,000 L to 9,000 L of blood around the body every day!

On visualization of the chest, you may be able to see the apical thrust or **point of maximal impulse (PMI)**. The PMI is normally located on the left anterior part of chest, in the midclavicular line, at the fifth intercostal space. This thrust occurs when the heart's apex rotates forward with systole, gently beating against the chest wall and producing a pulsation.

The wall of the heart consists of three layers **Figure 2**:

- The **epicardium** consists of a thin membrane that forms the outmost layer of the heart.
- The **myocardium** is the muscular middle layer of the heart wall found between the epicardium and endocardium. The myocardium is composed of specialized cardiac fibers that can spontaneously contract.
- The **endocardium** consists of a thin membrane that lines the inside of the heart's cavities and forms the valves. The endocardium plays a vital role in reducing turbulence inside the heart as blood travels through the chambers.

Surrounding the heart is a tough, fibrous sac called the **pericardium**. It is designed to protect the heart and provide lubrication between the heart and surrounding structures. The superficial layer of the pericardium is called the parietal pericardium and it anchors the heart within the mediastinum and surrounding vessels. The deep layer is called the visceral pericardium; it is fused to the epicardium. Between the two layers exists a potential space. Certain infectious processes, cancer, and trauma can lead to an abnormal accumulation of fluid within the pericardial sac. A small accumulation of fluid is referred to as pericardial effusion. A large accumulation of fluid that causes a decrease in cardiac output, and eventually cardiovascular collapse, is called pericardial tamponade.

Like all cells in the body, myocardial cells require an uninterrupted supply of oxygen and nutrients. However, the cardiac demand for oxygen is particularly unremitting because the heart never stops to rest (not without catastrophic consequences), so it is essential that the heart have an absolutely reliable blood supply. Oxygenated blood reaches the heart through the **coronary arteries Figure 3**, which branch off the aorta at the coronary ostia, located just above the leaflets of the aortic valve. There are two main coronary arteries—left and right. The left main coronary artery (LMCA) subdivides into the left anterior descending artery (LAD) and **circumflex coronary artery** (LCx), both of

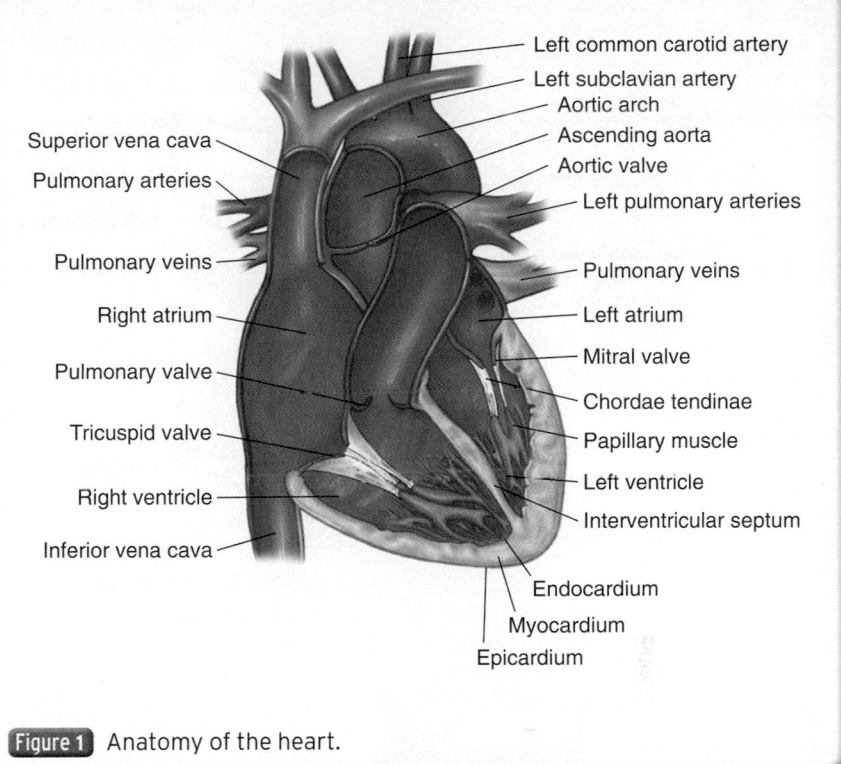

Figure 1 Anatomy of the heart.

which branch widely to supply the more muscular left ventricle of the heart along with the interventricular septum and part of the right ventricle. The right coronary artery (RCA) travels between the right atrium and right ventricle by way of the atrioventricular groove. These marginal arteries supply the right atrium and ventricle and part of the left ventricle with oxygen-rich blood. The numerous connections (anastomoses) between the arterioles of the various coronary arteries allow for the development of alternative routes of blood flow. In the early stages of coronary heart disease, the inside diameter of the coronary arteries begins to narrow as plaque deposits on the vessel walls. In response to the decreased ability to perfuse the myocardium, **collateral circulation** develops to overcome the imbalance. Collateral circulation is the formation of additional blood vessels connecting arterioles originating from other blood vessels. The result is an increase in oxygenated blood delivery to the myocardium.

The arteries and the main coronary vein cross the heart in a groove, called the **coronary sulcus**, that separates the atria from the ventricles. Venous blood empties into the **coronary sinus**, a large vessel in the posterior part of the coronary sulcus, which in turn ends in the right atrium of the heart.

Structurally, the heart consists of four chambers (see Figure 3). The upper chambers of the heart, or atria, are separated from their respective lower chambers, or ventricles, by **atrioventricular (AV) valves**, which prevent backflow during ventricular contraction. The **tricuspid valve** separates the right atrium from the right ventricle; the **mitral valve**, also called the bicuspid valve, separates the left atrium from the left ventricle. Anatomic guide wires, called **chordae tendineae**, attached to **papillary muscles** within the heart anchor the valve leaflets and keep them from inverting (prolapsing) during ventricular contraction. Injury

Two other valves in the heart Figure 4 , which are collectively known as **semilunar valves** because of their half-moon shape, are found at the junction of the ventricles and the pulmonary and systemic circulation. The **pulmonary semilunar valve** (pulmonic valve) separates the right ventricle from the pulmonary artery, preventing backflow from the artery into the right ventricle. The **aortic semilunar valve** (aortic valve) serves the same function for the left ventricle, preventing blood that has already entered the aorta from flowing back into the left ventricle.

The Cardiac Cycle

The **cardiac cycle** represents a complete depolarization and repolarization of the atria and ventricles. **Diastole** is a term used to describe the period of time when the atria or ventricles are resting. Atrial diastole refers to atrial rest, ventricular diastole, and ventricular rest. **Systole** is a term used to describe the period of time when the atria or ventricles are contracting. Atrial systole refers to atrial contraction, ventricular systole, and ventricular contraction.

During the relatively longer relaxation phase (normally 0.52 second [s]), the left atrium fills passively with blood, under the influence of venous pressure. Approximately 80% of ventricular filling also occurs during this time as blood flows through the open tricuspid and mitral valves.

With atrial contraction (normally both atria contract at the same time), the content of each atrium is squeezed into the respective ventricle to complete ventricular filling. The contribution to ventricular filling made by contraction

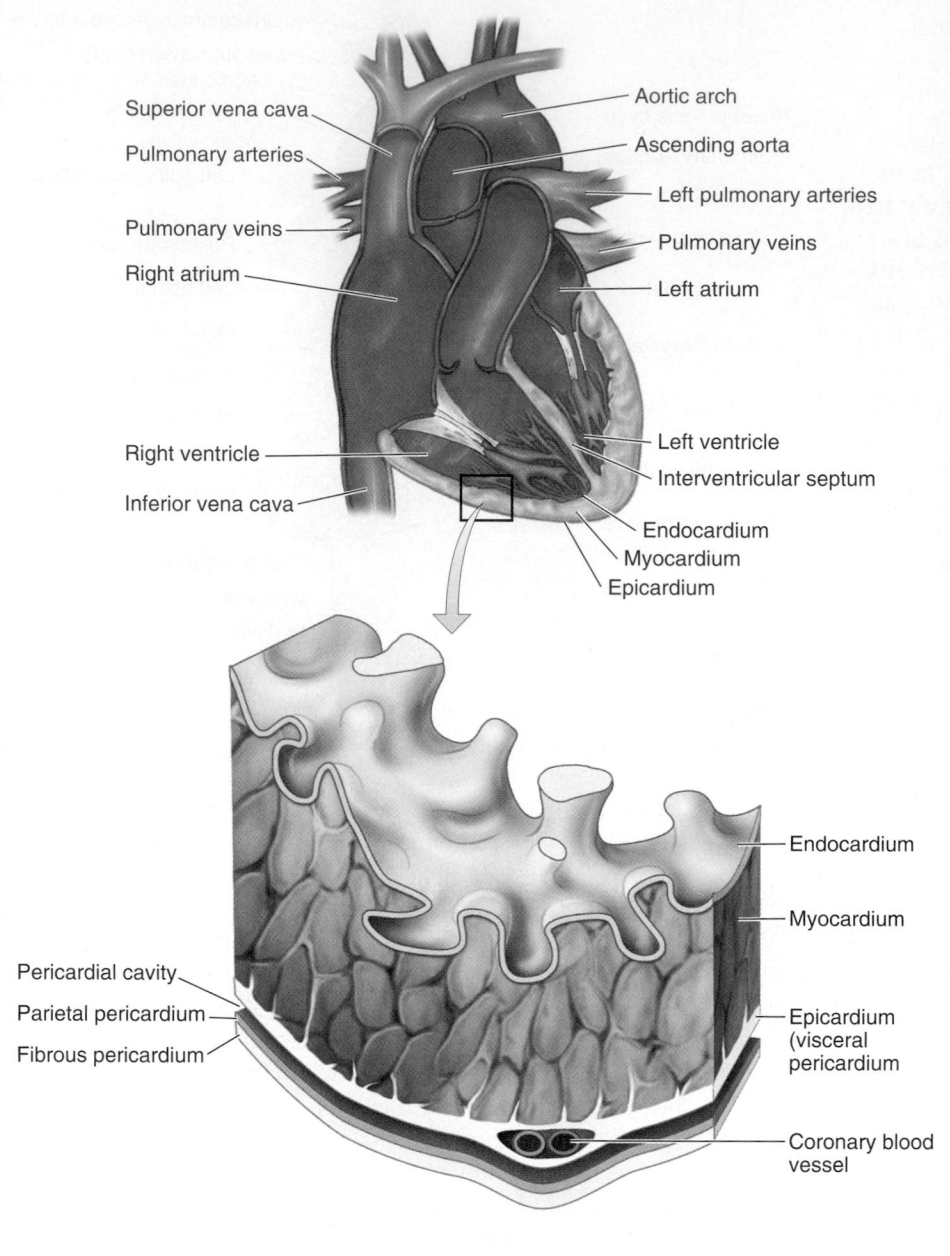

Superior vena cava
Pulmonary arteries
Pulmonary veins
Right atrium

Aortic arch
Ascending aorta
Left pulmonary arteries
Pulmonary veins
Left atrium

Right ventricle
Inferior vena cava

Left ventricle
Interventricular septum
Endocardium
Myocardium
Epicardium

Endocardium

Myocardium

Pericardial cavity
Parietal pericardium
Fibrous pericardium

Epicardium (visceral pericardium)

Coronary blood vessel

Figure 2 The three layers of the heart include the epicardium, the myocardium, and the endocardium.

or disease, however, may disrupt the chordae tendineae and permit a valve leaflet to prolapse, allowing blood to regurgitate from the ventricle into the atrium.

Words of Wisdom

The mitral valve is on the left side of the heart. The left side has higher pressure than the right. Because the mitral valve is involved in the higher pressure side, you can remember it as the "mighty" valve.

Words of Wisdom

The volume of blood that fills each ventricle depends on preload pressure. Preload pressure is affected by a number of factors including venous tone, circulating volume, venous blood pressure, and atrial kick. Atrial kick is defined as the increase in preload pressure as a result of atrial contraction and accounts for 10% to 40% of ventricular filling. Certain conditions such as atrial fibrillation prevent the atria from contracting, resulting in a significant decrease in cardiac output.

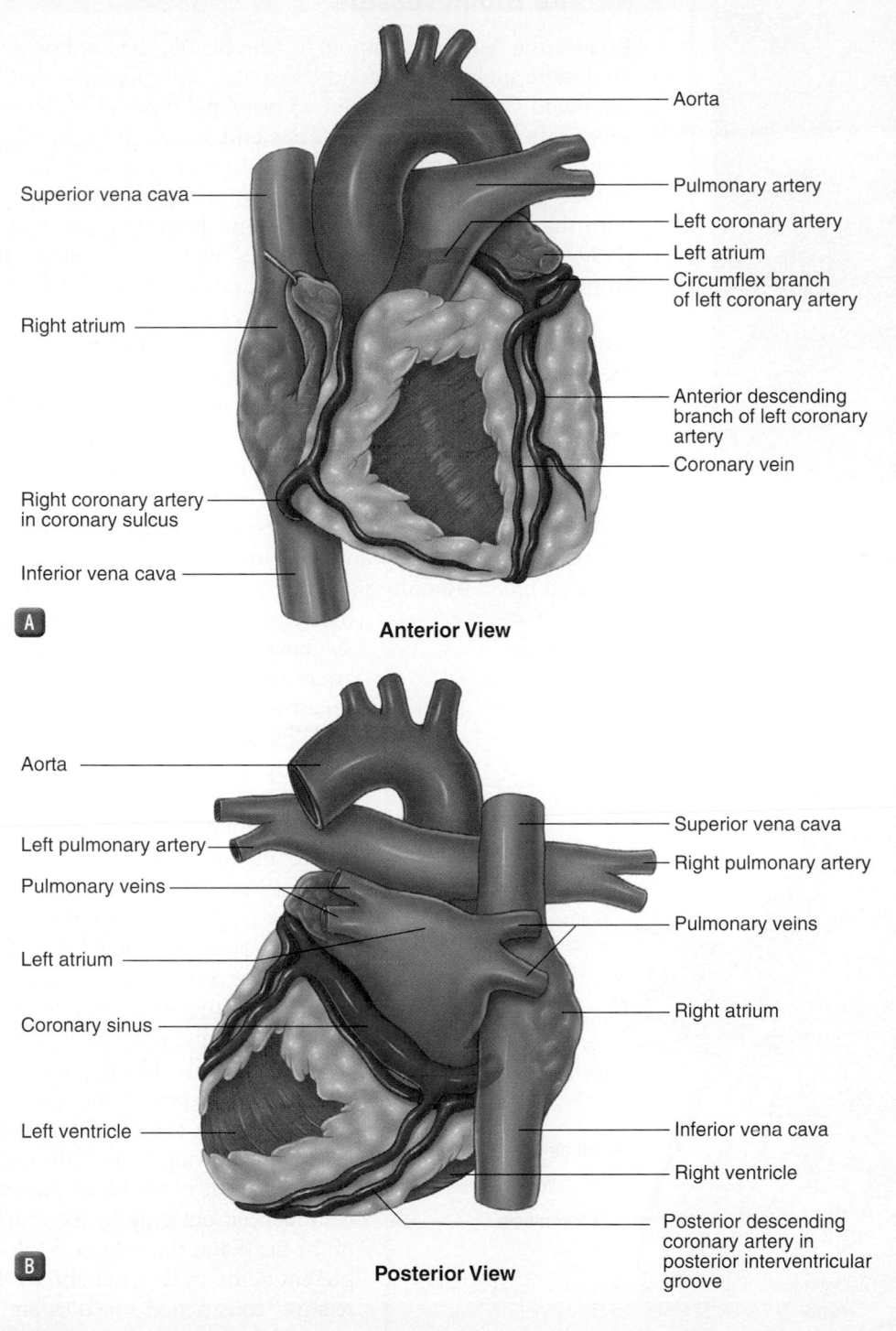

Anterior View

Aorta

Superior vena cava

Pulmonary artery

Left coronary artery

Left atrium

Circumflex branch of left coronary artery

Right atrium

Anterior descending branch of left coronary artery

Coronary vein

Right coronary artery in coronary sulcus

Inferior vena cava

A

Posterior View

Aorta

Left pulmonary artery

Pulmonary veins

Left atrium

Coronary sinus

Left ventricle

Superior vena cava

Right pulmonary artery

Pulmonary veins

Right atrium

Inferior vena cava

Right ventricle

Posterior descending coronary artery in posterior interventricular groove

B

Figure 3 Coronary arteries. **A.** Anterior view, showing takeoff point of left and right main coronary arteries from the aorta. **B.** View from below and behind, showing the coronary sinus.

through the pulmonic valve, and into the pulmonary arteries. Blood from the left ventricle is pushed through the aortic valve and out into the aorta. Systole is usually complete in a little more than half the time it takes to fill the ventricles, about 0.28 s.

Blood Flow Through the Heart

Although the heart has been referred to as a pump, that description is not entirely accurate. Functionally, the heart is actually *two* pumps—a right pump and a left pump, separated by a thin wall (the **interventricular septum**)—that just happen, for purposes of efficiency, to be housed in one organ and to work in parallel **Figure 5**.

The right side of the heart, which is composed of the right atrium and right ventricle, is a *low-pressure* pump: It pumps against the relatively low resistance of the pulmonary circulation. The superior **vena cava** collects deoxygenated blood from the upper half of the body, while the inferior vena cava collects deoxygenated blood from the lower portion of the body. Deoxygenated blood enters the **right atrium** and is pumped into the **right ventricle**. The right ventricle pumps the blood into the **pulmonary artery** for distribution to the lungs, where it is oxygenated.

The **pulmonary veins** collect the oxygen-rich blood and return it to the **left atrium**, which pumps it into the powerful **left ventricle**. The left side of the heart is a *high-pressure* pump; the initial stretching of the cardiac myocytes prior to contraction of this side of the heart is known as **preload**. It drives blood out of the heart against the relatively high resistance of the systemic arteries, which is known as **afterload**.

Because there are two pumps, there must be two sets of tubing into which the pumps empty. Thus, the human body, in effect, has two circulations. The **systemic circulation** **Figure 6A** consists of all blood vessels between the left ventricle and right atrium. The **pulmonary circulation** **Figure 6B** consists of all the blood vessels between the right ventricle and left atrium.

of the atrium is referred to as **atrial kick**—it is the amount of blood "kicked in" by the atrium. At the beginning of ventricular contraction, the AV valves snap shut, the two ventricles contract (ventricular systole), and the semilunar valves (also known as the aortic valve and the pulmonic valve) are forced open. Blood squeezed out of the right ventricle moves forward,

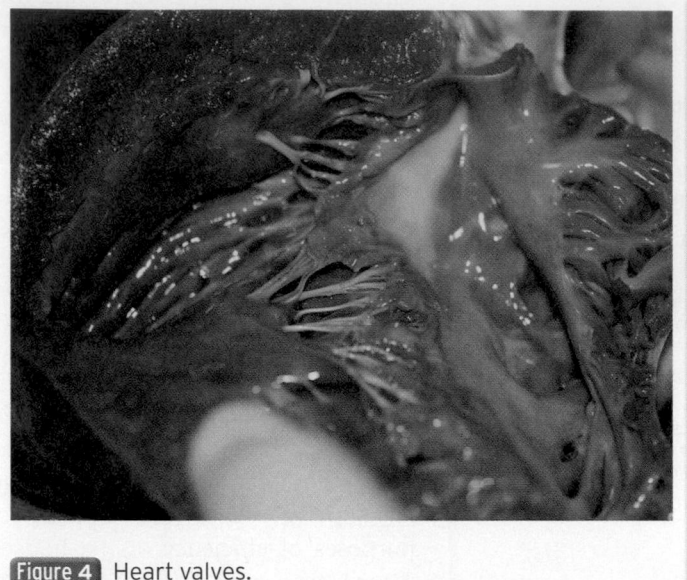

Figure 4 Heart valves.

The Blood Vessels

Besides the "cardio" component (the heart), the cardiovascular system includes a second, "vascular" component—that is, the blood vessels. There are two principal types of blood vessels in the human body—arteries and veins—both of which share a common structure **Figure 7** . A protective outer layer of fibrous tissue, the <u>tunica adventitia</u>, provides blood vessels with the strength needed to withstand high pressure against their walls. A middle layer of elastic fibers and muscle, the <u>tunica media</u>, gives strength and contractility to blood vessels. This medial layer is much thicker and more powerful in arteries than in veins. The innermost layer of the blood vessel, the <u>tunica intima</u>, is a smooth inner lining that is only one cell thick. The opening within the blood vessel is referred to as the <u>lumen</u>.

<u>Arteries</u> are thick-walled, muscular vessels—befitting pipes operating in a high-pressure system—that carry blood away from the heart. Usually, arteries carry *oxygenated* blood; the only exceptions are the pulmonary arteries, which carry oxygen-depleted blood from the right ventricle to the lungs (they carry blood away from the heart). Arteries range in size from the largest artery in the body, the <u>aorta</u>, to the tiniest arterial branch, or <u>arteriole</u>. **Figure 8** depicts the major arteries in the body.

Arterial walls are highly sensitive to stimulation from the autonomic nervous system. Indeed, in response to that stimulation, their diameter may change significantly as the arteries contract and relax. In that manner, the arteries help to regulate <u>blood pressure</u>—that is, the pressure exerted by the blood against the arterial walls. Blood pressure is generated by repeated forceful contractions of the left ventricle, which keep blood flowing through the body. The magnitude of the blood pressure is influenced not only by the output of the heart and the volume of blood present in the system, but also by the relative constriction or dilation of arteries.

<u>Veins</u>, which operate on the low-pressure side of the system, have thinner walls than arteries and, consequently, less capacity to decrease their diameter. The thinner walls also make the veins much more likely to distend when exposed to small increases in "backpressure." Veins carry blood to the heart—as a rule, deoxygenated blood. The only exceptions are the pulmonary veins, which carry oxygenated blood to the

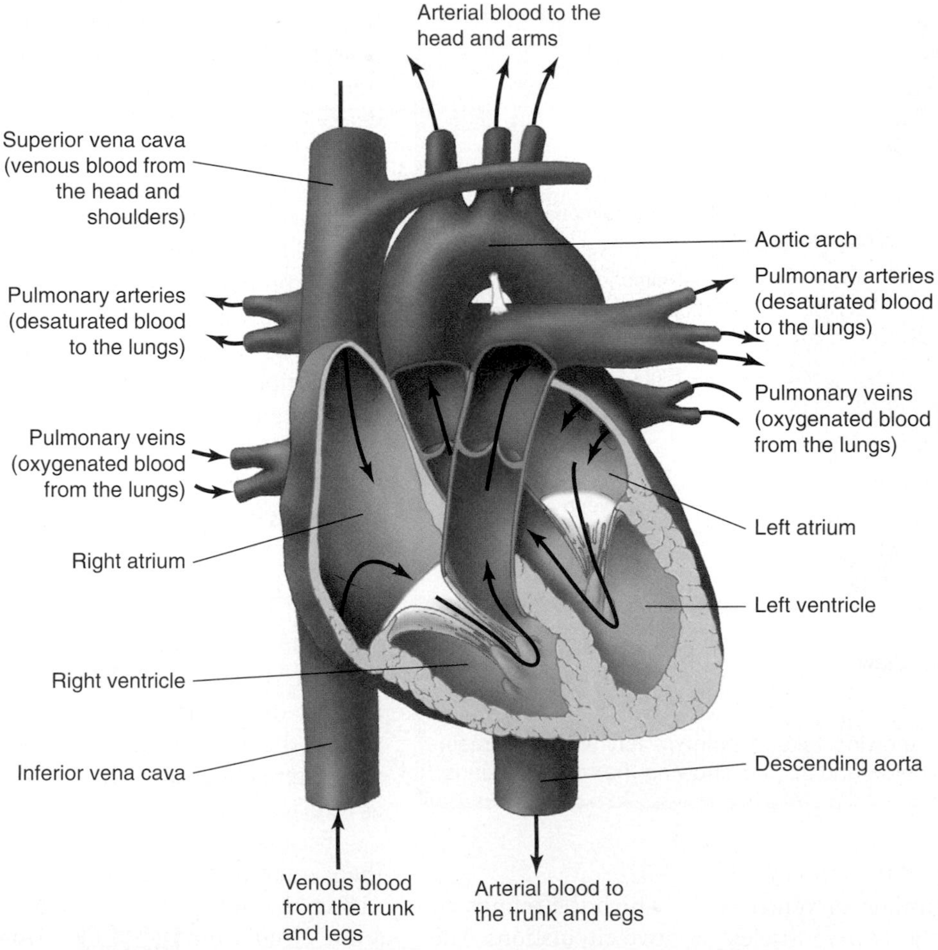

Arterial blood to the
head and arms

Superior vena cava
(venous blood from
the head and shoulders)

Aortic arch

Pulmonary arteries
(desaturated blood
to the lungs)

Pulmonary arteries
(desaturated blood
to the lungs)

Pulmonary veins
(oxygenated blood
from the lungs)

Pulmonary veins
(oxygenated blood
from the lungs)

Left atrium

Right atrium

Left ventricle

Right ventricle

Inferior vena cava

Descending aorta

Venous blood
from the trunk
and legs

Arterial blood to
the trunk and legs

Figure 5 Blood flow through the heart. Deoxygenated blood enters the right atrium from the venae cavae, proceeds to the right ventricle, and travels to the lungs via the pulmonary arteries. Oxygenated blood enters the left atrium from the pulmonary veins, proceeds to the left ventricle, and is pumped to the body via the aorta.

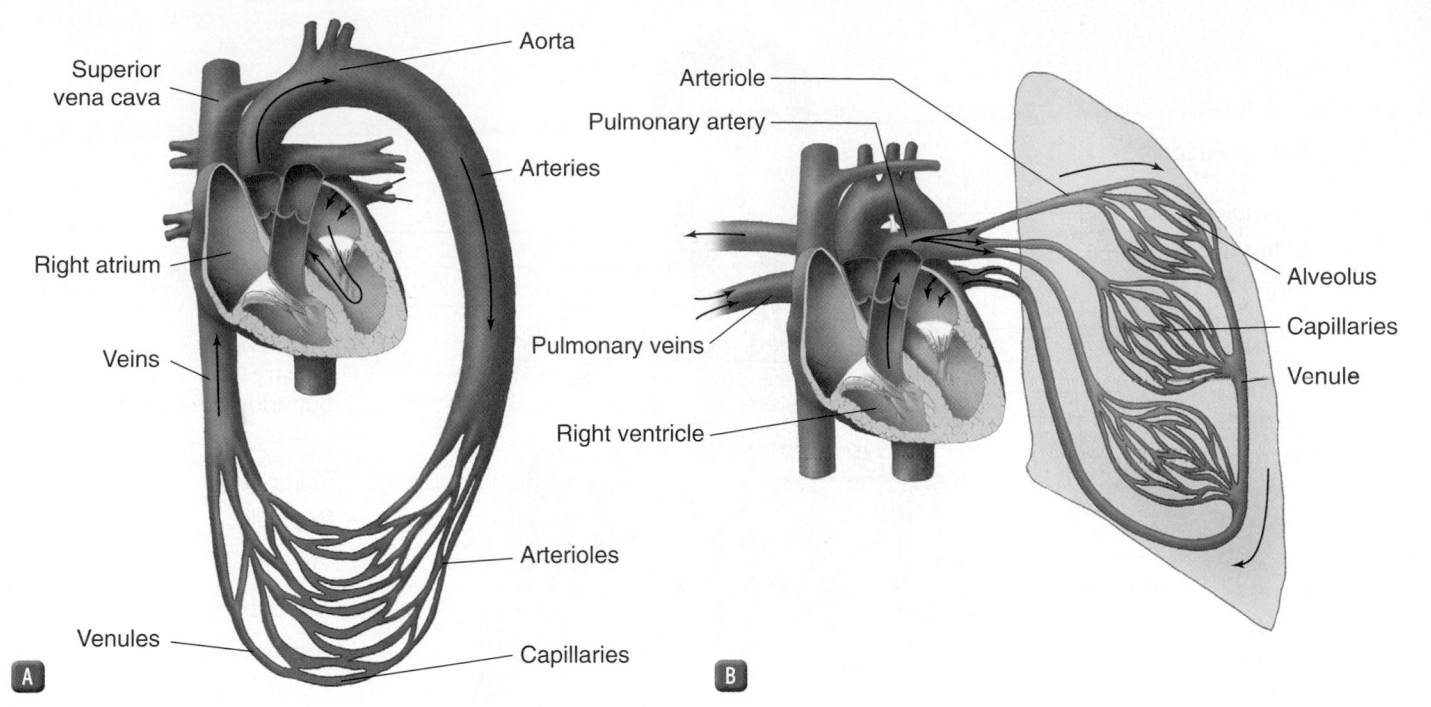

Figure 6 Dual human circulation. **A.** The systemic circulation consists of all blood vessels distal to the left ventricle. **B.** The pulmonary circulation consists of all blood vessels between the right ventricle and the left atrium.

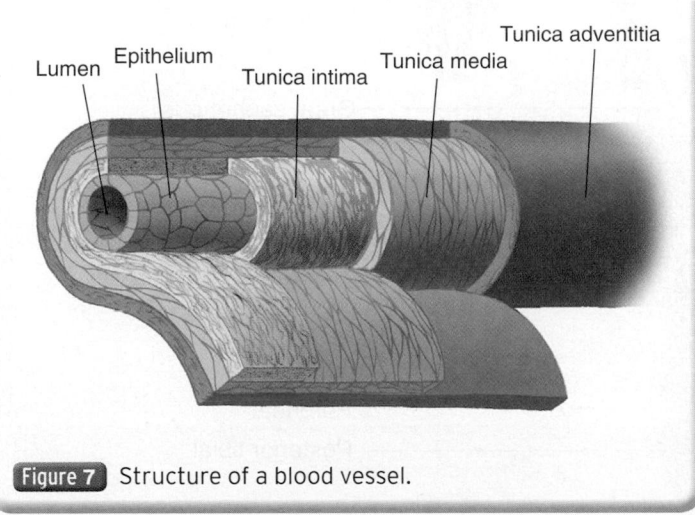

Figure 7 Structure of a blood vessel.

left side of the heart. The smallest veins, or **venules**, gradually empty into larger and larger veins, terminating in the two largest veins of the body, the inferior and superior venae cavae. Veins also contain valves (which are unnecessary in arteries); these valves keep the blood flowing in the forward direction only.

Between the tiny arterioles and venules is a network of microscopic blood vessels called **capillaries**. The walls of capillaries are extremely thin—only one cell thick—enabling the exchange of gases and nutrients across them; the capillary diameter is so small that red blood cells must pass through them single file.

■ The Pump at Work

The skeletal muscle and thoracoabdominal pumps are part of a system that aids in returning venous blood to the heart. Muscle contraction around the limb veins during normal movement propels blood toward the heart. Valves inside the veins prevent backward flow of blood.

To understand how the heart functions as a pump, it is necessary to learn some technical terms:

- **Cardiac output (CO).** The amount of blood that is pumped out by either ventricle. The left and right ventricles are approximately equal in interior size, so the two ventricles have relatively equivalent outputs. Normal CO for an average adult is 5 to 6 L/min.
- **Stroke volume (SV).** The amount of blood pumped out by either ventricle in a single contraction (heartbeat). Normally, the SV is 60 to 100 mL, but the healthy heart has considerable spare capacity and can easily increase SV by at least 50%.
- **Heart rate (HR).** The number of cardiac contractions (heartbeats) per minute—in other words, the pulse rate. The normal HR for adults is 60 to 100 beats/min.
- **Ejection fraction (EF).** The percentage of blood that leaves the heart each time it contracts. This measurement is usually taken from only the left ventricle because it is the primary pump for the heart. The left ventricular ejection fraction has a normal range of 55% to 70%, but may be lower if the heart sustains some type of damage (ie, myocardial infarction, heart valve disease, cardiomyopathy, or chronic hypertension).

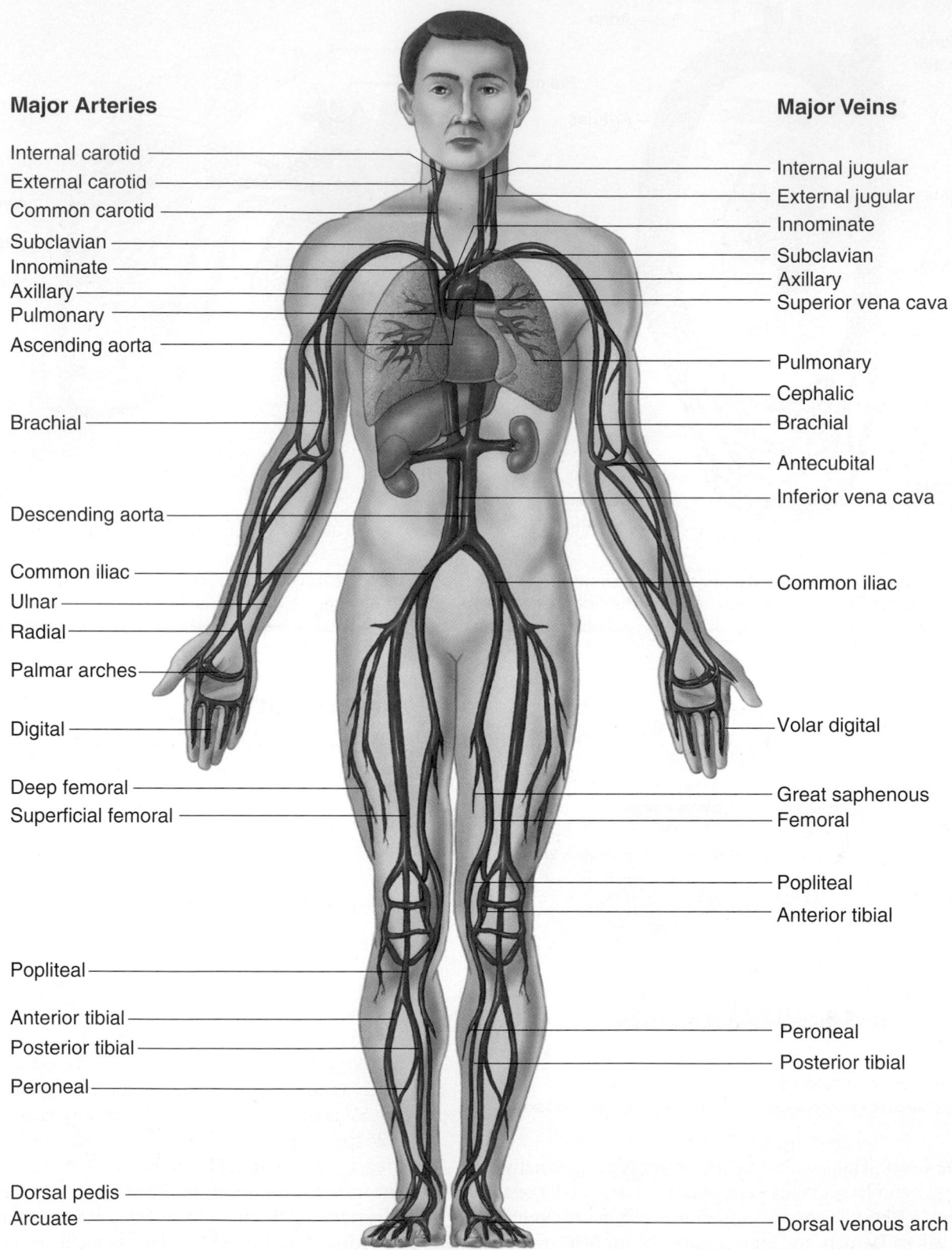

Major Arteries

Internal carotid
External carotid
Common carotid
Subclavian
Innominate
Axillary
Pulmonary
Ascending aorta

Brachial

Descending aorta

Common iliac
Ulnar
Radial
Palmar arches

Digital

Deep femoral
Superficial femoral

Popliteal

Anterior tibial
Posterior tibial
Peroneal

Dorsal pedis
Arcuate

Major Veins

Internal jugular
External jugular
Innominate
Subclavian
Axillary
Superior vena cava

Pulmonary
Cephalic
Brachial
Antecubital
Inferior vena cava

Common iliac

Volar digital

Great saphenous
Femoral

Popliteal
Anterior tibial

Peroneal
Posterior tibial

Dorsal venous arch

Figure 8 The major arteries and veins.

The volume of blood that either ventricle pumps out per minute equals the volume of blood it pumps out in a single contraction times the number of contractions per minute:

$$CO = SV \times HR$$

To meet changing demands, the heart must be able to increase its output several times over in response to the body's increased demand for oxygen—for example, during exercise. The CO equation tells us that the heart can increase its output by increasing its SV, increasing its rate, or both.

In a mechanical piston pump, the SV is a fixed quantity related to the distance traveled by the piston and the size of the cylinder. The heart, by contrast, has several ways of increasing SV. One characteristic of cardiac muscle is that, when it is stretched, it contracts with greater force to a limit—a property called the **Frank-Starling mechanism**. If an increased volume of blood is returned from the systemic veins to the right side of the heart or from the pulmonary veins to the left side of the heart, the muscle surrounding the cardiac chambers must stretch to accommodate the larger volume. The more the cardiac muscle stretches, the greater the force of its contraction, the more completely it empties, and, therefore, the greater the SV. From the CO equation, it is clear that any increase in SV, with the HR held constant, will cause an increase in the overall CO. Think of a latex balloon. If you blow the balloon up a bit and then let the air escape, it does so slowly and with little force. This is because the elastic walls of the balloon were not stretched very much. However, if you blow the balloon up as much as possible without popping it, and then let the air out, it does so very quickly and with much more force. The heart works the same way. If the walls are stretched a bit, a small amount of blood is released.

If the walls are stretched a great deal, a large amount of blood is released.

As mentioned earlier, the pressure under which a ventricle fills (the preload) is influenced by the volume of blood returned by the veins to the heart. In situations of increased oxygen demand, the body returns more blood to the heart (preload increases), and CO consequently increases through the Frank-Starling mechanism. In a diseased heart, the same mechanism is used to achieve a normal resting CO (which explains why some diseased hearts become enlarged).

Words of Wisdom

The Frank-Starling mechanism is named after the two men who first described it. In the late 19th century, Otto Frank discovered that in the frog heart, the strength of ventricular contraction was increased when the ventricle was stretched before contraction. In the 20th century, Ernest Starling expounded on this information with studies finding that increasing venous return, and, therefore, the filling pressure of the ventricle, led to increased SV in dogs.

The heart can also vary the degree of contraction of its muscle *without* changing the stretch on the muscle—a property called **contractility**. Changes in contractility may be induced by medications that have a positive or negative **inotropic effect** (inotropic refers to affecting the contractility of muscle tissue). The ventricles are never completely emptied of blood with any single beat. However, if the heart squeezes into a tighter ball when it contracts, a larger percentage of the

YOU *are the Medic*   PART 2

You and your partner begin your assessment. Your partner obtains vital signs while you assess the patient's blood glucose level. The meter reads "152". You ask for OPQRST and SAMPLE history, which indicate nothing unusual except for the pain in the patient's jaw. The patient says the pain feels like a dull ache that she rates "about a 5 out of 10" on a scale with 10 being the worst pain possible. Your partner reports that the patient's pulse feels irregular at a rate of 64 beats/min. You start an IV of normal saline and administer 2 mg of morphine via slow IV push.

Recording Time: 5 Minutes	
Appearance	Awake, pale, moist skin
Level of consciousness	Alert (oriented to person, place, and day)
Airway	Open
Breathing	Adequate
Circulation	Adequate

3. Having ruled out a diabetes-related problem, what is your next step?

4. What are the differences between the presentations of cardiac problems in men and women?

ventricular blood will be ejected, thereby increasing SV and overall CO. Nervous controls regulate the contractility of the heart from beat to beat. When the body requires increased CO, nervous signals increase myocardial contractility, thereby augmenting SV.

The heart can also increase its CO, given a constant SV, by increasing the number of contractions per minute—that is, by increasing the heart rate (positive **chronotropic effect**—increasing the heart's rate of contraction). As an example, consider a heart that has a resting SV of 70 mL/beat and a resting rate of 70 beats/min:

$$CO = 70\,mL \times 70\,beats/min = 4{,}900\,mL/min$$

Suppose that the owner of that heart begins to exercise. Oxygen demand increases, and nervous mechanisms stimulate the heart to increase its rate. If, for example, the heart rate increases to 110 beats/min without any change in the SV, the CO would increase as follows:

$$CO = 70\,mL/beat \times 110\,beats/min = 7{,}700\,mL/min$$

The Frank-Starling mechanism is an intrinsic property of heart muscle—that is, it is not under nervous system control. By contrast, contractility and changes in the heart rate are regulated by the nervous system.

The Electrical Conduction System of the Heart

Cardiac cells that help to make up heart muscle demonstrate four important properties that help the heart to function as an efficient machine: excitability, conductivity, automaticity, and contractility. **Excitability** allows these cells to respond to an electrical impulse. **Conductivity** enables cardiac cells to pass an electrical impulse from one cell to another. Heart muscle is unique among body tissues because it can generate its own electrical impulses without stimulation from nerves, a property known as **automaticity**. As mentioned previously, contractility refers to heart cells' ability to contract. In addition, the heart is endowed with specialized conduction tissue that can rapidly propagate electrical impulses to the muscular tissue of the heart. The area of conduction tissue in which the electrical activity arises at any given time is called the **pacemaker**, because it sets the pace (that is, rate) for cardiac contraction. This system as a whole is termed the **electrical conduction system**.

The Dominant Pacemaker: The Sinoatrial Node

Theoretically, any cell within the heart's electrical conduction system can act as a pacemaker. In the normal heart, however, the dominant pacemaker is the **sinoatrial (SA) node**, which is

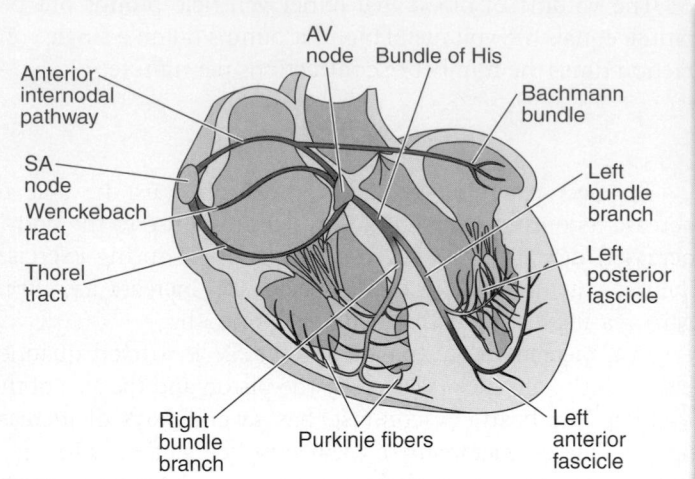

Figure 9 The electrical conduction system of the heart. Impulses that originate in the SA node spread through the atria and along the internodal pathways to the AV node. From the AV node, they travel down the bundle of His and right and left bundle branches and into the Purkinje network of the ventricles. Note that the Bachmann bundle is an interatrial pathway that initiates depolarization of the left atrium.

located in the right atrium, near the inlet of the superior vena cava **Figure 9**. The SA node receives blood from the RCA. If the RCA is occluded, as in a myocardial infarction (MI), the SA node will become ischemic. As a result, the SA node may fire slower than normal, or cease to fire completely.

The SA node is the fastest pacemaker in the heart. Electrical impulses generated in this node spread across the two atria through **internodal pathways** (including the Bachmann bundle) in the atrial wall in about 0.08 s, causing the atrial tissue to depolarize as they pass. The Bachmann bundle is the interatrial pathway that connects the right and left atria. A branch off the Bachmann bundle forms a pathway between the SA and AV nodes, and is called the anterior internodal pathway. The Wenckebach tract forms the middle internodal tract. The Thorel tract is the last of the internodal pathways and is represented by the posterior internodal pathway.

From the SA node, electrical impulses move to the **atrioventricular (AV) node** in the region of the **AV junction** (which includes the AV node and its surrounding tissue along with the **bundle of His**). The AV node serves as a "gatekeeper" to the ventricles. In 85% to 90% of people, its blood supply comes from a branch of the RCA; in 10% to 15% of people, it comes from a branch of the left circumflex artery. The conduction of the impulse is delayed in the AV node for about 0.12 s so that the atria can empty into the ventricles. Approximately 60% to 90% of the blood in the atria fills the ventricles by gravity; the remaining 10% to 40% comes from atrial contraction (atrial kick).

Some additional conduction pathways exist that allow the current to bypass the AV node. James fibers exist in the atrial internodal pathways and extend into the ventricles while bypassing the AV node. Mahaim fibers are contained within the AV node, the bundle of His, and the bundle branches. These fibers extend into the ventricles and provide a common pathway for re-entrant dysrhythmias. The bundle of Kent is an accessory pathway typically located between the left atrium and the left ventricle, although it may also sometimes be found between the right atrium and the right ventricle. The bundle of Kent enables the depolarization wave to bypass the AV node and trigger early depolarization of a section of ventricular tissue. Simultaneously, depolarization travels through the AV node and bundle of His to the bundle branches. These simultaneous depolarization events create a unique change on the ECG tracing called a delta wave. In certain instances, accessory pathways can trigger tachydysrhythmias that often require medical intervention to terminate.

When the atrial rate becomes very rapid, not all atrial impulses can get through the AV junction. Normally, however, impulses pass through it into the bundle of His and then move rapidly into the right and left bundle branches located on either side of the interventricular septum. Next, they spread into the <u>Purkinje fibers</u>, thousands of fibrils distributed through the ventricular muscle. It takes about 0.08 s for an electric impulse to spread across the ventricles, during which time the ventricles contract simultaneously. The effect on the velocity of conduction is referred to as the <u>dromotropic effect</u>.

Depolarization and Repolarization

<u>Depolarization</u> is the process by which muscle fibers are stimulated to contract. It occurs through changes in the concentration of electrolytes across cell membranes Figure 10A . Myocardial cells, like all cells in the body, are bathed in an electrolyte solution. Chemical pumps inside the cell maintain the concentrations of ions within the cell, in the process creating an electric gradient across the cell wall. As a consequence, a resting (polarized) cell normally has a net internal charge of −90 millivolts (mV) with respect to the outside of the cell (Figure 10, part A1). When the myocardial cell receives a stimulus from the conduction system (Figure 10, part A2), the permeability of the cell wall changes through opening of specialized channels in such a way that sodium ions (Na+) rush into the cell, causing the inside of the cell to become more positive. Calcium ions (Ca++) also enter the cell—albeit more slowly and through a different set of specialized channels—helping maintain the depolarized state of the cell membrane and supplying calcium ions for use in contraction of the cardiac muscle tissue. This reversal of electric charge—depolarization—starts at one spot in the cell and spreads in a wave along the cell until the cell is completely depolarized (Figure 10, part A3). As the cell depolarizes and calcium ions enter, mechanical contraction occurs.

If the cell were to remain depolarized, it could never contract again! However, the cell is able to recover from depolarization through a process called repolarization Figure 10B . Repolarization starts with the closing of the sodium and calcium channels, which stops the rapid inflow of these ions. Next, special potassium channels open, allowing a rapid escape of potassium ions (K+) from the cell. This helps restore the inside of the cell to its negative charge; the proper electrolyte distribution is then reestablished by pumping sodium ions out of the cell and potassium ions back in. After the potassium channels close, this sodium-potassium pump helps move sodium and potassium ions back to their respective locations. For every

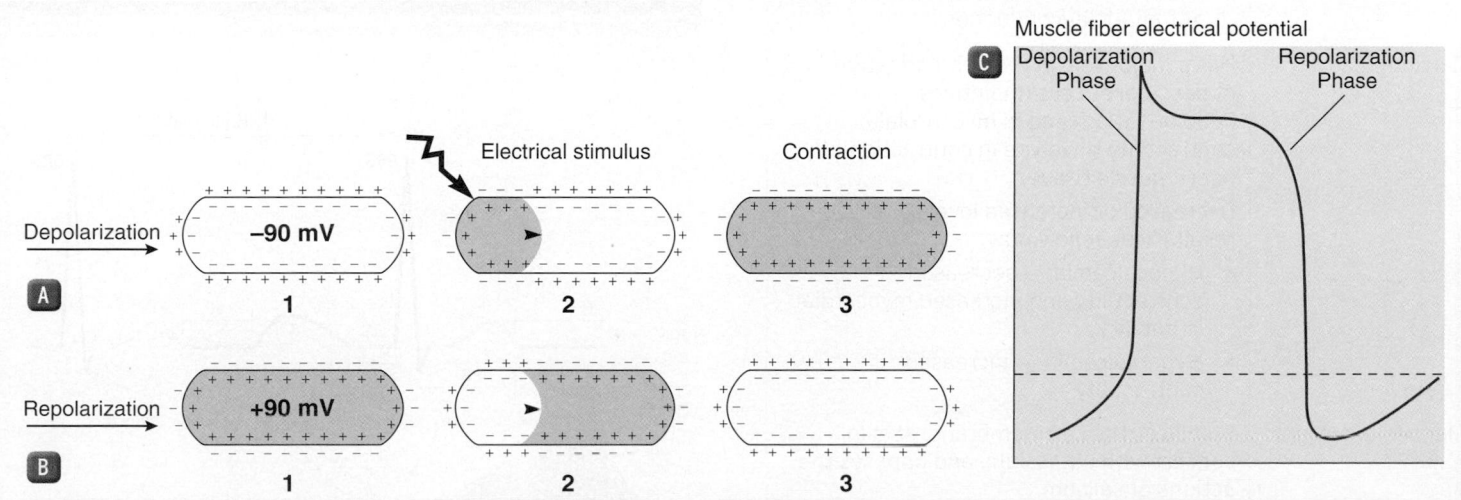

Figure 10 Movement of ions to produce a net current flow. **A.** Depolarization. (1) At rest, the cellular interior has a net charge of −90 mV. (2) The wave of depolarization begins as sodium ions pour into the cell. (3) Depolarized cell. **B.** Repolarization. (1) Depolarized cell. (2) The wave of repolarization begins as potassium ions leave the cell. (3) Repolarized cell. **C.** Changes in muscle fiber electrical potential associated with contraction.

three sodium ions this pump moves out of the cell, it moves two potassium ions into the cell, thereby maintaining the polarity of the cell membrane. To accomplish this task, the sodium-potassium pump moves ions against the natural gradient by a process called active transport, which requires the expenditure of energy.

Table 3 summarizes the roles of the various electrolytes in cardiac function.

A myocardial cell cannot respond to an electrical stimulus from the conduction system normally unless it is fully polarized. The period when the cell is depolarized or in the process of repolarizing—the so-called **refractory period**—consists of two phases. In the **absolute refractory period**, the heart muscle is completely depolarized and unable to respond to any stimulus. In the **relative refractory period**, the heart is partially repolarized and may respond to an electrical stimulus and depolarize. Only those cells that were repolarized will respond to the stimulus. The other cells will simply continue to repolarize and remain unaffected.

Secondary Pacemakers

The SA node normally has the most rapid intrinsic rate of firing (60 to 100 times/min), so it will literally outpace any slower conduction tissue. If it becomes damaged or is suppressed, any component of the conduction system may act as a secondary pacemaker. The farther removed the conduction tissue is from the SA node, the slower its intrinsic rate of firing. Thus, the AV junction, which is located near the border that separates the atria and ventricles, will spontaneously fire 40 to 60 times/min. The Purkinje system, which is located in the ventricles and is farther removed from the SA node, will spontaneously fire at rate of approximately 20 to 40 times/min.

Suppose that the SA node is damaged by ischemia (tissue injury caused by hypoxemia) and does not fire. When the AV node fails to receive impulses from the SA node, the AV junction might then begin firing at its own rate; thus, a "junctional rhythm" would occur at a rate of 40 to 60 beats/min. If both the SA and AV nodes fail to initiate an impulse, the Purkinje fibers will initiate an impulse, resulting in a "ventricular rhythm" at a rate of 20 to 40 beats/min **Table 4**.

Measuring the Heart's Electrical Conduction Activity

The electrical conduction events in the heart can be recorded on an ECG as a series of waves and complexes **Figure 11**. The depolarization of the atria produces the **P wave**. It is followed

Table 3 Role of Electrolytes in Cardiac Function

Electrolyte	Role in Cardiac Function
Sodium (Na⁺)	Flows into the cell to initiate depolarization
Potassium (K⁺)	Flows out of the cell to initiate repolarization Decreased or increased levels of potassium result in the following: ■ *Hypo*kalemia → increased myocardial irritability ■ *Hyper*kalemia → decreased automaticity/conduction
Calcium (Ca⁺⁺)	Has a major role in the depolarization of pacemaker cells (maintains depolarization) and in myocardial contractility (involved in contraction of heart muscle tissue) Decreased or increased levels of calcium result in the following: ■ *Hypo*calcemia → decreased contractility and increased myocardial irritability ■ *Hyper*calcemia → increased contractility
Magnesium (Mg⁺⁺)	Stabilizes the cell membrane; acts in concert with potassium, and opposes the actions of calcium Decreased or increased levels of magnesium result in the following: ■ *Hypo*magnesemia → decreased conduction ■ *Hyper*magnesemia → increased myocardial irritability

Table 4 Pacemaker Intrinsic Rates

Pacemaker	Rate (beats/min)
SA node	60 to 100
AV junction	40 to 60
Purkinje	20 to 40

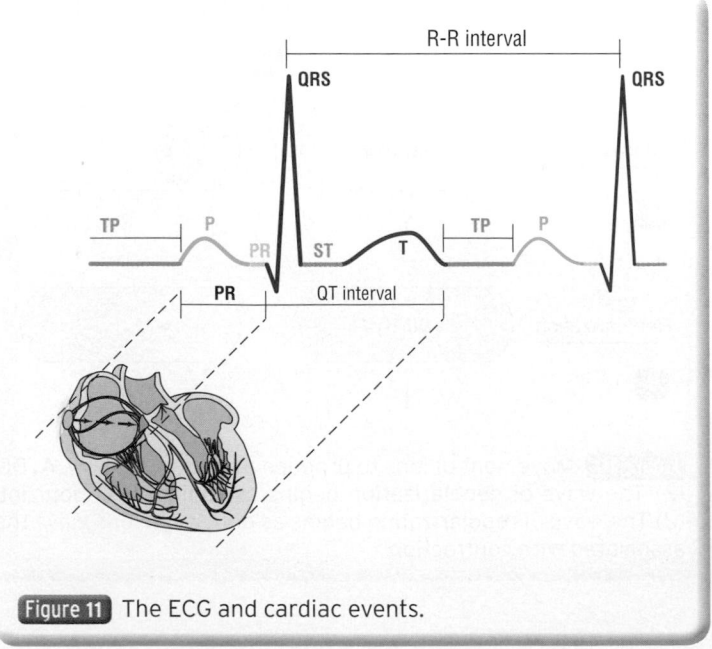

Figure 11 The ECG and cardiac events.

by a brief pause as conduction is momentarily slowed through the AV junction. Next, the **QRS complex** occurs, representing depolarization of the ventricles. Repolarization of the atria produces a wave that is too small to be seen on the ECG but occurs during the PR segment. The ventricles produce **T waves** that follow the QRS complex Table 5.

The intervals between waves and complexes also have names. The **PR interval** is the distance from the beginning of the P wave to the beginning of the QRS complex. It represents the time required for an impulse to traverse the atria and AV junction and is normally 0.12 to 0.20 s. The PR segment represents the amount of time the AV node delays transmission of atrial activity to the ventricles. When the AV node is diseased or hypoxic, the PR segment can elongate beyond normal limits. A prolonged PR interval is almost always due to a prolonged PR segment because the P wave rarely exceeds 110 ms duration. Prolonged PR intervals will be discussed later in the chapter when heart blocks are introduced. The **ST segment** is the line from the end of the QRS complex to the beginning of the T wave. The beginning of the ST segment is called the J point, or junction point, which indicates the end of ventricular depolarization and the beginning of ventricular repolarization. The ST segment should normally be at the same level as the baseline (**isoelectric line**). An elevated ST segment or a depressed ST segment may indicate myocardial ischemia or injury. The **R-R interval** is the time between two successive QRS complexes. It represents the interval between two ventricular depolarizations and can be used to calculate the heart rate. The QT interval represents one complete ventricular cycle and is measured from the beginning of the Q wave (or R wave if no Q wave exists) to the end of the T wave. A long QT interval can lead to ventricular dysrhythmias and sudden cardiac arrest.

■ The Autonomic Nervous System and the Heart

The **autonomic nervous system** is the part of the human nervous system that controls automatic (that is, involuntary) actions. Its importance can be gauged by considering the alternative: Suppose all body functions were solely under voluntary control. Sixty times a minute, 24 hours a day, you would have to remind your heart to beat. Twelve times a minute, 24 hours a day, you would be required to order your lungs to inflate and relax. You would have to warn your stomach that food was on the way, tell your pancreas and gallbladder to step up their activities, and urge your gut to speed up or slow down as necessary. Whenever you changed your level of activity—for example, during exercise—you would be forced to issue a complex series of orders to your cardiovascular system to ensure that CO increased sufficiently to meet increased metabolic demands.

Fortunately, these body functions are automatically accomplished without any conscious effort on the part of the person. As is often the case, the nervous system works better in pairs. Like a musical show comprised of actors and an orchestra, the voluntary nervous system and the involuntary (autonomic) nervous system work together and complement each other perfectly. The voluntary nervous system (aka the actors) allows a person's mind to consciously control the movement of muscles while the autonomic nervous system (aka the orchestra) allows body functions to proceed smoothly in the background, without thought.

As skilled as the orchestra is, it does not always function well without a conductor. The autonomic nervous system is unique in that it has two conductors: the sympathetic nervous system and parasympathetic nervous system. The sympathetic nervous system takes care of such tasks as speeding up the heart, constricting blood vessels, and dilating the bronchi and pupils. The parasympathetic nervous system regulates the body's vegetative functions: it slows the heart rate and encourages digestion. Together, these two systems work together to direct the orchestra to play at the perfect pace.

Figure 12 shows the organization of the human nervous system. Table 6 provides a review of the properties of the autonomic nervous system. Figure 13 shows where parasympathetic and sympathetic nerves originate (the craniosacral and the thoracolumbar section of the spine, respectively), and the end organs that they affect.

The Parasympathetic Nervous System

As mentioned previously, the **parasympathetic nervous system** is concerned primarily with vegetative functions and sends its messages mainly through the **vagus nerve**. Think of it as the "rest and digest" nervous system. The vagus nerve can be stimulated in a number of ways, including pressure on the carotid sinus, straining against a closed glottis (**Valsalva maneuver**), and distention of a hollow organ (such as the bladder or stomach).

At times, the brain may sense that the heart should slow its pace, perhaps because pressure is being applied over the carotid sinus or a person is straining during a bowel movement. A message in the form of an electrical impulse will now travel down the vagus nerve to the place where the nerve abuts on the SA node of the heart Figure 14. There, the electrical impulse causes the release of a naturally occurring chemical, **acetylcholine (ACh)**. (The parasympathetic nervous system derives its other name, the *cholinergic* nervous system, from this chemical.)

Table 5	Components of the ECG
ECG Representation	**Cardiac Event**
P wave	Depolarization of the atria
PR interval	Depolarization of the atria and delay at the AV junction
QRS complex	Depolarization of the ventricles
ST segment	Period between ventricular depolarization and beginning of repolarization
T wave	Repolarization of the ventricles
R-R interval	Time between two ventricular depolarizations

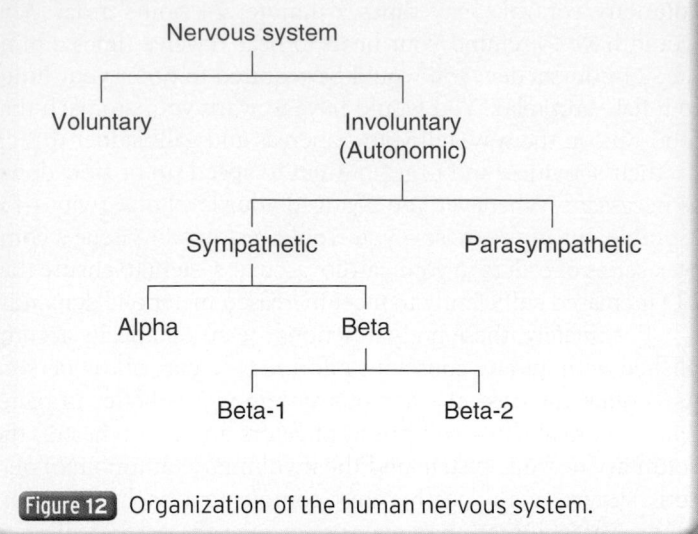

Figure 12 Organization of the human nervous system.

The ACh then crosses over to the SA node of the heart and signals the SA node, indicating that the brain is calling for a slowing of the heart via a transmission through the vagus nerve. To ensure that the message is received and acted on, another ACh molecule travels to the AV node of the heart. This action is, in effect, a "reminder" to the SA node to slow down, making sure no extra impulses get through to the ventricles. Following these actions, ACh is escorted away by acetylcholinesterase (AChE). Acetylcholinesterase is an enzyme that breaks down ACh so it can be recycled.

A commonly used drug that blocks the actions of the parasympathetic nervous system is **atropine**. In EMS, atropine is used to block the vagus nerve and thereby cause an increase in the heart rate.

Suppose the heart is slowing, beating at a rate of 50 beats/min, and you administer 0.5 mg of atropine intravenously. The atropine will travel through the bloodstream until it reaches the SA node, where it causes the SA node to speed up.

The Sympathetic Nervous System

The **sympathetic nervous system** prepares the body to respond to various stresses; it is the fight-or-flight system mentioned earlier. The parasympathetic nervous system works well for routine activities such as keeping the heart beating during rest or coordinating digestion, but it provides no mechanism for the body to adapt to changing demands. By contrast, the sympathetic nervous system increases the heart rate, strengthens the force of cardiac muscle contractions, and provides other adaptive responses to ensure that the tissues' increased oxygen demands are satisfied with increased CO.

Suppose you start running to catch a bus. After a few seconds, your muscles will have used up all the oxygen and nutrients immediately on hand. The muscles, now lacking these nutrients, send a message to the brain, requesting an increase in the delivery of oxygen.

Table 6 Autonomic Nervous System		
Features	**Parasympathetic**	**Sympathetic**
Other name	Cholinergic; "rest and digest," "feed and breed"	Adrenergic; "fight or flight"
Natural chemical mediator	Acetylcholine	Norepinephrine, epinephrine
Primary nerve(s) regulating cardiac function	Vagus	Nerves from the thoracic and lumbar ganglia of the spinal cord
Effect of stimulation	Decreases contractility (negative inotropic effect)	Increases contractility (positive inotropic effect)
	Slows conduction velocity (negative dromotropic effect)	Speeds conduction velocity (positive dromotropic effect)
	Slows the heart* (negative chronotropic effect)	Speeds the heart (positive chronotropic effect)
	Constricts pupils	Dilates pupils
	Increases salivation	Constricts blood vessels
	Increases gut motility	Slows the gut
		Dilates the bronchi
Agonists	Neostigmine, reserpine	Alpha: phenylephrine
		Beta: isoproterenol
		Beta-2: albuterol
		Alpha + beta: norepinephrine, epinephrine, dopamine
Antagonists	Atropine	Alpha: chlorpromazine, phentolamine
		Beta: propranolol, metoprolol, labetalol, atenolol

*Slowing occurs mostly at the SA node.

In response to this need, the brain sends a message through the sympathetic nerves, passing through the thoracic and lumbar ganglia, ultimately arriving at the heart. Whereas the vagus nerve releases ACh, sympathetic nerves convey their commands through release of **norepinephrine**. Norepinephrine travels to the SA node, AV node, and ventricles, spreading the command from the sympathetic nerves. To prevent a buildup of lactic acid, the heart speeds up, increasing CO and, therefore, delivering more oxygen and nutrients throughout the body.

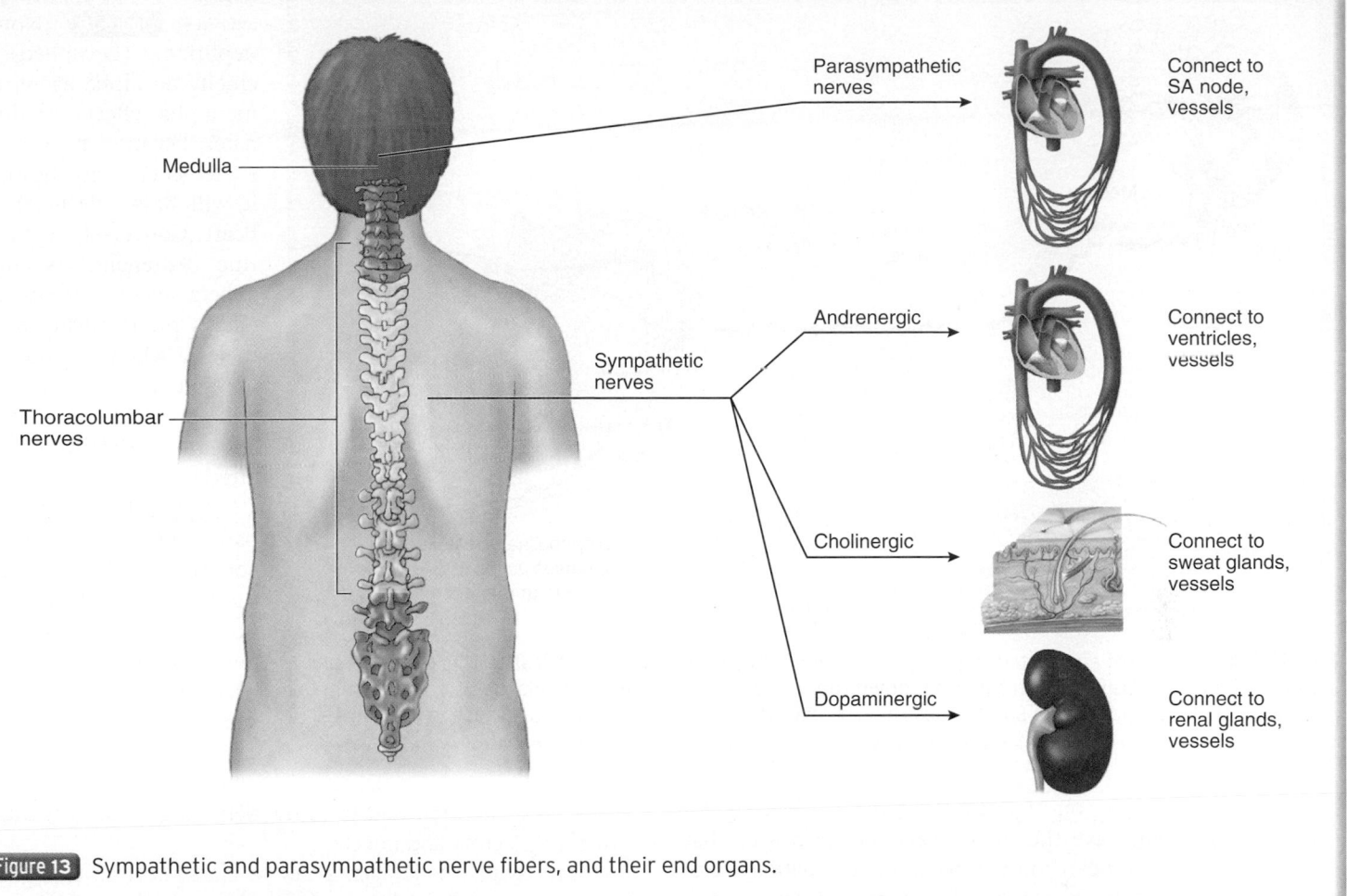

Figure 13 Sympathetic and parasympathetic nerve fibers, and their end organs.

Words of Wisdom

The below analogy, a legacy that originated with Dr. Nancy Caroline, demonstrates the effect of atropine on the parasympathetic nervous system.

"You're firing a little slowly today, aren't you?" says atropine.

"Just following orders," says the SA node. "The vagus told me to take it easy."

"Vagus, vagus–why are you always trying to slow everything down?"

"I'm just following orders from the brain. You know a job can't be done well if it's done too fast," says the vagus nerve.

"We don't have time for that. Speed up, SA," says atropine.

"But what about the vagus?" says the SA node.

"If you keep paying attention to the vagus, before you know it, you'll slow down so much that the brain won't get enough blood and oxygen and will shut down! Take my advice, bud, and open the gates wide. Let all the impulses through."

"Are you sure that's a good idea? The vagus said . . ."

"Forget about the vagus. He's just an old obstructionist."

"Okay," says the SA node, always eager to please when atropine is around. So the SA node speeds up.

Atropine then blocks the vagus nerve so he cannot interfere.

"I guess I've been overruled," says the vagus.

When intense stimulation of the sympathetic nervous system occurs, a special hormone—epinephrine—may be mobilized to spread the alarm and command the heart to speed up. Epinephrine is produced in the adrenal gland and is also called **adrenaline**, leading to the other name of the sympathetic system—the *adrenergic* system.

Drugs That Act on the Sympathetic Nervous System

Drugs that influence the sympathetic nervous system are classified according to the receptors with which they interact. A drug receptor can be visualized as analogous to the ignition switch in a car. When the proper key is inserted into the car's ignition and turned, a predictable sequence of events follows: The battery sends a current to the starter and the spark plugs, which fire; combustion of gasoline and air occurs; and the engine starts. Although many keys may fit into a specific car's ignition, not every key that fits will turn and start the car—but all that do turn cause the same reaction. Likewise, the organs of the body have a number of "ignition switches." In the sympathetic nervous system, those switches, or **receptors**, are labeled alpha and beta. Whenever one of those switches is activated by a "key" (a drug or hormone), a predictable sequence of responses will occur **Table 7** .

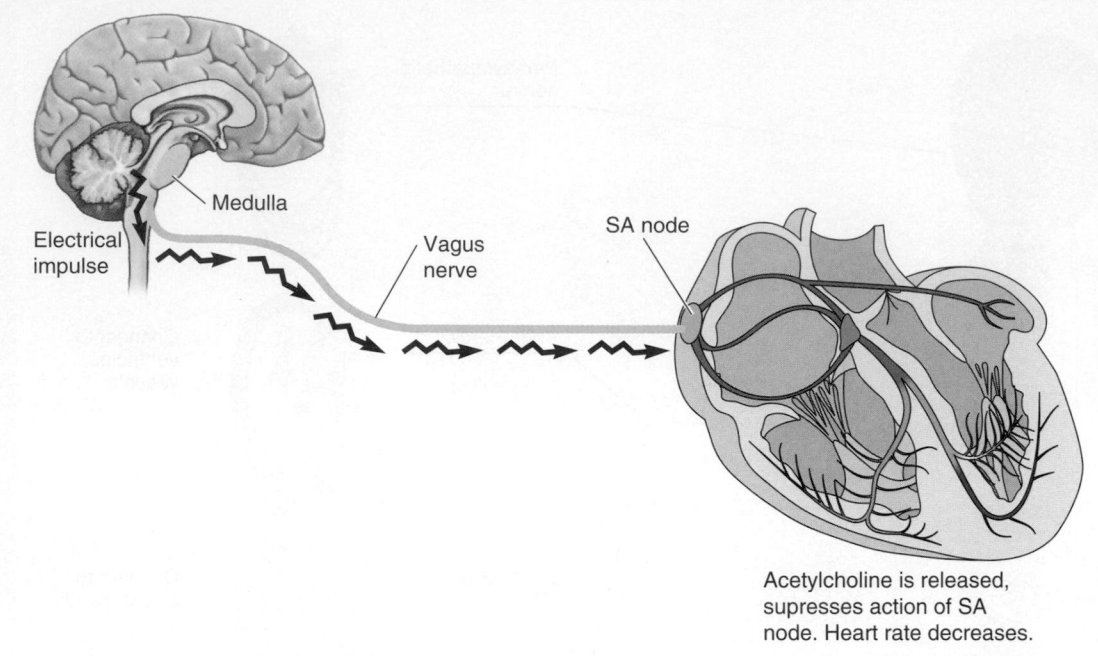

Acetylcholine is released, supresses action of SA node. Heart rate decreases.

Figure 14 Example of an electrical impulse that stimulates release of a chemical. In this example, an electrical impulse travels from the brain down the vagus nerve, causing the release of acetylcholine (ACh) near the SA node. ACh suppresses the action of the SA node, causing a decrease in heart rate.

degrees of alpha and beta activity **Figure 18**. Norepinephrine (Levophed) is chiefly an alpha agent, and its alpha effects predominate; because it also has some beta activity, however, it will have effects on the heart. Conversely, epinephrine (Adrenalin) is chiefly a beta agent, and its beta effects predominate; nevertheless, when administered in high doses, epinephrine will produce some alpha effects, especially on the arteries.

Table 8 lists several sympathomimetic agents that are commonly encountered in the field. Two of the drugs, norepinephrine and epinephrine, are also naturally occurring chemicals of the sympathetic nervous system. Their actions are the same whether they are produced in the body and released from the nervous system or manufactured in a factory and injected.

Beta sympathetic agents can be classified into two groups based on the subtle differences between the beta receptors in

The heart has only one ignition switch for a beta agent. Any beta agent will have the same effect on the heart—that is, it will increase the heart's rate, force, and automaticity. The arteries, by contrast, have receptors for alpha and beta agents. An alpha drug will turn on the switch that causes __vasoconstriction__; a beta agent will activate the switch that causes __vasodilation__. Similarly, the lungs have alpha and beta receptors. Alpha agents do not have much effect on the lungs; at most, they cause minor __bronchoconstriction__. By contrast, beta adrenergic agonists (such as drugs used to treat asthma) trigger significant __bronchodilation__. **Figure 15** represents these concepts schematically.

Drugs that have alpha or beta sympathetic properties are called sympathomimetic drugs because they imitate (mimic) the actions of naturally occurring sympathetic chemicals. If you know whether a sympathomimetic drug is an alpha or beta agent, you can predict the response by the heart, lungs, and arteries.

Consider isoproterenol (Isuprel). It is a pure beta agent. Armed with this knowledge, you can immediately recognize that isoproterenol acts in the manner shown in **Figure 16**—it stimulates the heart, dilates the bronchi, and dilates the arteries.

Phenylephrine (Neo-Synephrine), by contrast, is a pure alpha agent. It has no direct effect on the heart but causes slight bronchoconstriction and marked vasoconstriction **Figure 17**.

In reality, things are not always so simple. Although isoproterenol and phenylephrine are pure beta and alpha agents, respectively, most other sympathomimetic drugs have varying

Words of Wisdom

To remember the difference between beta-1 and beta-2, ask yourself, "How many hearts do I have?" One heart–beta-1. "How many lungs do I have?" Two lungs–beta-2.

Table 7 Responses to Sympathetic Stimulation

Organ	Sympathetic Stimulation
Heart	Increased heart rate (positive chronotropic effect) (beta-1) (Hint: one heart, beta 1)
	Increased force of contraction (positive inotropic effect) (beta-1)
	Increased conduction velocity (positive dromotropic effect) (beta-1)
Arteries	Constriction (alpha)
Lungs	Bronchial muscle relaxation (beta-2) (Hint: two lungs, beta 2)

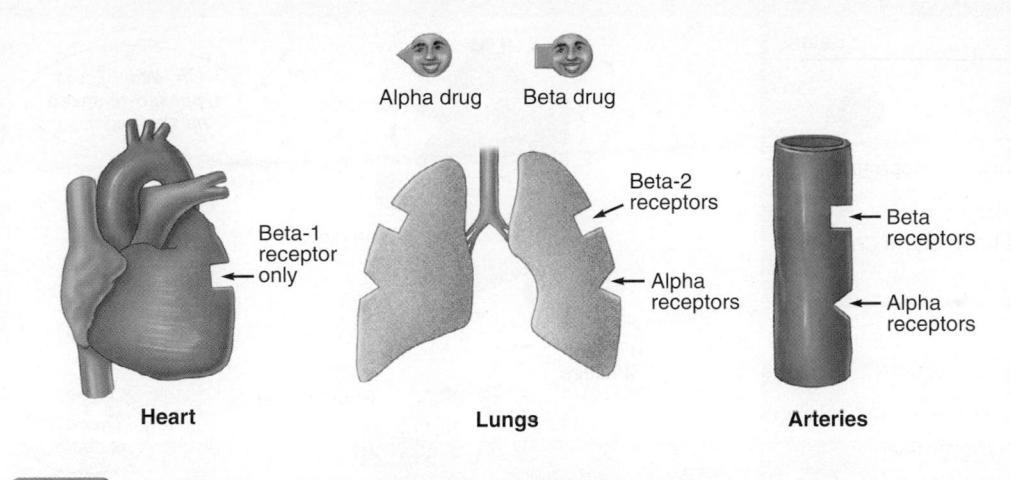

Figure 15 Receptor sites of the sympathetic nervous system in the heart, lungs, and arteries.

agonists. Commonly prescribed bronchodilators (beta 2 adrenergic agonists) include albuterol, formoterol, salbuterol, levalbuterol, and salmetorol.

Another class of drugs that acts on the sympathetic nervous system comprises the sympatholytic or sympathetic blockers. As their name implies, they block the action of sympathetic agents by beating them to the receptor sites and preventing these agents from turning on the ignition. The receptor sites cannot distinguish a blocker from a stimulator until it is too late. With the blocker occupying the receptor site, the stimulating agent cannot get in to turn on the switch **Figure 19** .

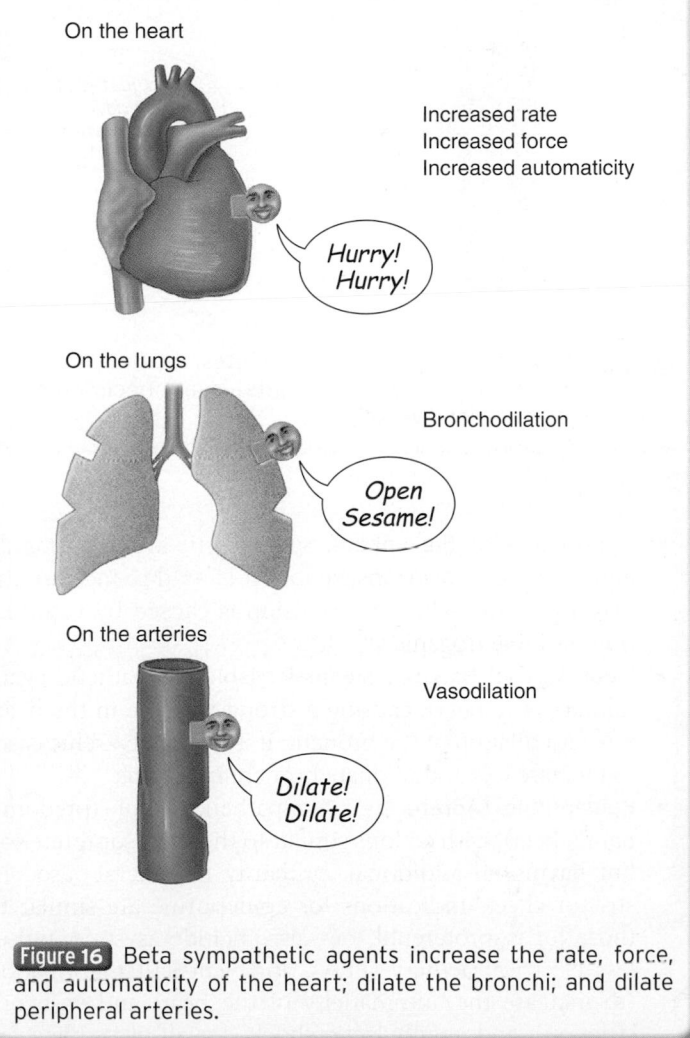

Figure 16 Beta sympathetic agents increase the rate, force, and automaticity of the heart; dilate the bronchi; and dilate peripheral arteries.

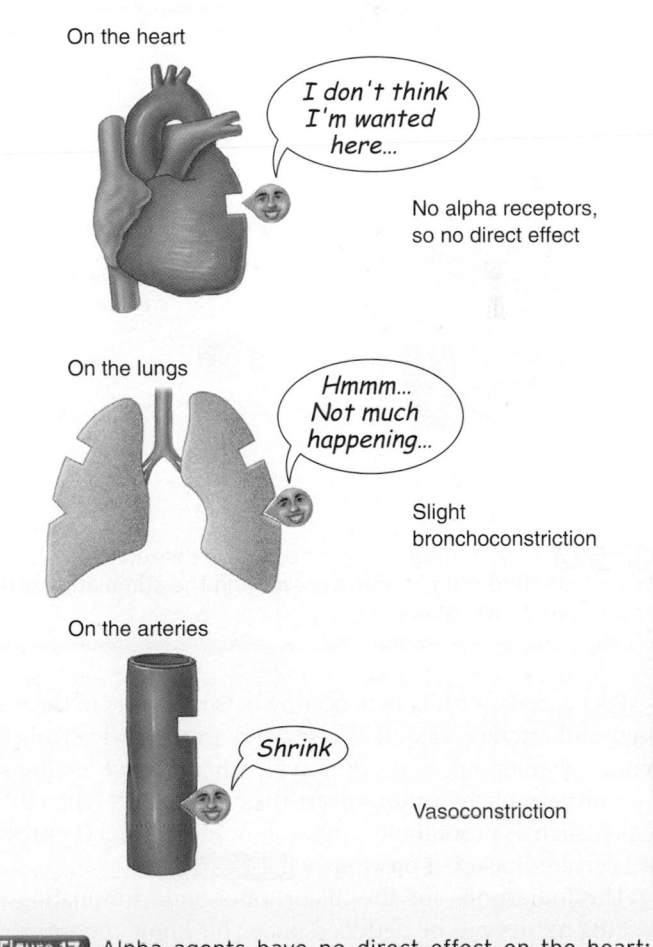

Figure 17 Alpha agents have no direct effect on the heart; they cause slight bronchoconstriction and marked vasoconstriction.

the heart and the lungs. Drugs that act primarily on cardiac beta receptors are called beta 1 adrenergic agonists; those that act chiefly on pulmonary beta receptors are called beta 2 adrenergic

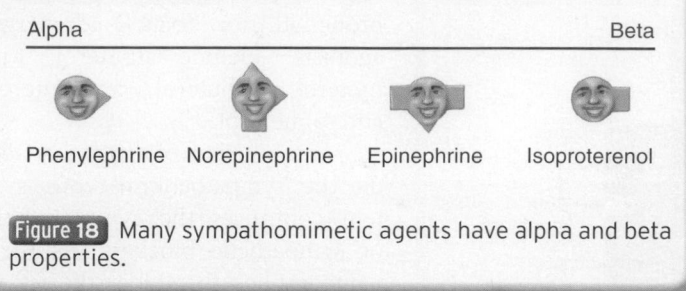

Figure 18 Many sympathomimetic agents have alpha and beta properties.

Table 8 Common Sympathomimetic Agents	
Alpha	Phenylephrine (Neo-Synephrine)
	Norepinephrine bitartrate (Levophed)
Alpha or beta, depending on dose	Dopamine
Beta	Epinephrine
	Albuterol (Proventil; beta-2-specific) Isoproterenol (Isuprel; pure beta-specific)

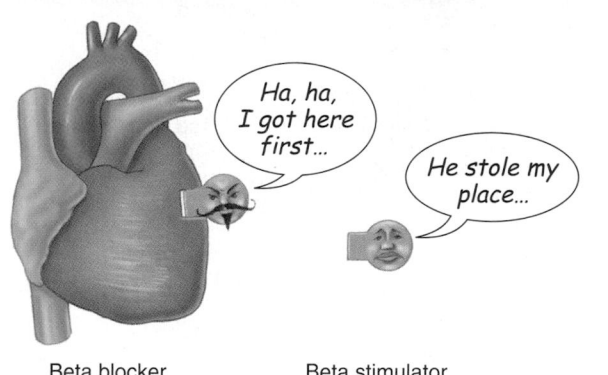

Figure 19 A sympathetic blocker occupies the receptor site for the stimulating drug, thereby preventing the stimulating drug from exerting its usual effect.

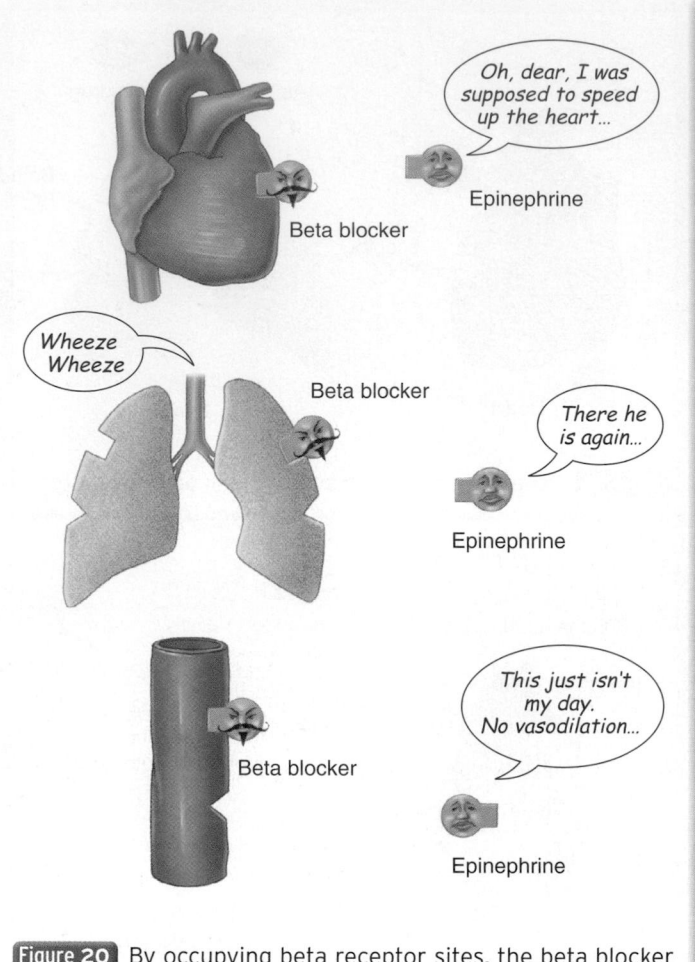

Figure 20 By occupying beta receptor sites, the beta blocker prevents epinephrine from exerting its usual effects on the heart, lungs, and blood vessels.

Beta adrenergic blockers occupy beta receptors in the heart, lungs, and arteries, as well as elsewhere in the body. Thus beta agents, whether released from sympathetic nerve endings or given intravenously, cannot exert their full effects when a beta blocker such as propranolol (Inderol) or metoprolol (Lopressor) has been administered previously **Figure 20**.

The indications for the major autonomic stimulating and blocking agents can be deduced once you know the properties of the drugs and the manner in which they interact with the autonomic nervous system:

- **Atropine.** Parasympathetic blocker, opposing the vagus nerve. It is used to speed the heart when excessive vagal firing has caused bradycardia.

- **Norepinephrine (Levophed).** Sympathetic agent (primarily alpha), causing vasoconstriction. It is used to increase the blood pressure when hypotension is caused by vasodilation (as in neurogenic shock).

- **Isoproterenol (Isuprel, Medihaler-Iso).** Sympathetic agent (almost pure beta), causing a strong increase in the heart rate and dilation of the bronchi. It is used in extreme cases to increase CO and to dilate bronchi in asthma.

- **Epinephrine (Adrenaline).** Sympathetic agent (predominantly beta), with actions similar to those of isoproterenol, but having an additional, primarily peripheral vasoconstrictor effect. Indications for epinephrine are similar to those for isoproterenol, but also include asystole, pulseless electrical activity (PEA), and ventricular fibrillation (to increase the automaticity of the heart and vasoconstriction); and anaphylactic shock (for all of its effects—bronchodilation, vasoconstriction, increased CO).

- **Dopamine (Intropin).** Sympathetic agent, used to increase renal perfusion, increase rate and force of myocardial contraction, and constrict peripheral blood vessels. Dopamine is a unique medication because it causes different physiologic effects at different dosages, as listed in **Table 9**.

Table 9 Physiologic Effects of Dopamine Categorized by Dose

Dose (µg/kg/min)	Receptor	Effect
1-2	Dopaminergic	Increased renal perfusion
2-10	Beta 1	Increased rate/force
10-20	Alpha	Vasoconstriction

- **Albuterol (Proventil, Ventolin), isoetharine (Bronchosol, Bronkometer), terbutaline (Brethine, Bricanyl, Brethaire, Terbulin).** Sympathetic beta-2 agents that act on the lungs. These agents are used to induce bronchodilation in asthma, chronic obstructive pulmonary disease, and other bronchospastic conditions.
- **Propranolol (Inderal).** Sympathetic beta blocker, opposing the actions of beta-stimulating agents. It is used clinically to slow the heart rate in certain tachydysrhythmias, to decrease the pain of chronic angina (by decreasing the work of the heart), and to depress irritability in the heart (by decreasing the tendency of the heart to fire automatically). Its use is contraindicated in asthma.

■ The Sympathetic Nervous System and Blood Pressure Regulation

The body attempts to maintain a fairly constant blood pressure to ensure perfusion of vital organs. At any given moment, the blood pressure is influenced by the CO and the resistance (degree of constriction) of the arterioles:

$$\text{Blood Pressure} = \text{CO} \times \text{Peripheral Vascular Resistance (PVR)}$$

Thus, the blood pressure can be increased by increasing the CO, the peripheral resistance, or both.

Under normal circumstances, the body balances flow and resistance to maintain a stable blood pressure. That is, alterations in one variable bring about compensatory changes in the other variable to restore blood pressure toward normal. Consider, for example, a situation in which CO decreases suddenly, as in hemorrhage. The fall in CO will inevitably lead to a fall in blood pressure unless the peripheral resistance is altered. The falling CO activates the sympathetic nervous system, however, which in turn causes the arterioles to constrict. Vasoconstriction increases the peripheral resistance, thereby tending to restore the blood pressure back toward normal.

To look at the blood pressure equation in a slightly different way, the following example divides both sides by the peripheral resistance, thus coming up with a new equation:

$$\text{CO} = \frac{\text{Blood Pressure}}{\text{Peripheral Vascular Resistance}}$$

This equation explains that, for any given blood pressure, the CO will vary inversely with the peripheral vascular resistance. In other words, the higher the peripheral resistance (that is, the more constricted the arterioles), the lower the CO. That makes intuitive sense, for clearly it is harder to push fluid through narrower pipes. The resistance against which the ventricle contracts is termed the afterload. The greater the afterload, the harder the ventricle must work to pump the blood. In conditions of chronically high afterload, such as

YOU are the Medic   PART 3

You ask your partner to place electrodes on the patient's chest to assess her ECG while you provide the patient high-flow oxygen. Lead II of the ECG shows a sinus rhythm with multifocal PVCs tracing at 8 to 10 per minute. Your partner sets up a 12-lead ECG, whose results are unremarkable for elevation or depression.

Recording Time: 10 Minutes	
Respirations	14 breaths/min
Pulse	64 beats/min, irregular
Skin	Warm, pale, moist
Blood pressure	100/60 mm Hg
Oxygen saturation (Spo$_2$)	89% on room air, 99% on O$_2$
Pupils	Equal and reactive

5. What are PVCs and what does "multifocal" mean?

6. What is your first-line treatment for PVCs?

arteriosclerosis-induced high blood pressure, the left ventricle may eventually grow exhausted from the extra work and cease pumping efficiently or even fail.

Patient Assessment

Patients experience a variety of symptoms when they have a cardiovascular problem. The most common complaints are chest pain, dyspnea, fainting, palpitations, and fatigue. If the patient is pulseless or breathless, basic life support (BLS) measures may be used. In some cases, ACLS procedures may be necessary. This section reviews the organized approach to assessing patients by focusing on their cardiac and pulmonary systems.

Note that the order of steps for performing primary assessment differs depending on the type of cardiac patient. Whereas the order of steps in the primary assessment is normally ABC (assess airway, breathing, and then circulation), if the patient is found unresponsive and is suspected of being in cardiac arrest, the order changes to CAB (first assess circulation, then airway and breathing). In this section, we will assume the patient is conscious and breathing and has a pulse.

Scene Size-up

The primary assessment begins with sizing up the scene and ensuring scene safety. In addition, you should try to anticipate the need for other resources such as extra personnel. As you enter the scene you should also be looking for any clues that may help identify what may have brought on the potential problem, such as medications, drug paraphernalia, alcohol, cigarettes, or living conditions.

Primary Assessment

Form a General Impression

Observe the patient's general appearance as you approach him or her, and assess for apparent life threats. The primary assessment is fairly consistent for all patients, but this discussion has a cardiac focus. Sometimes the primary assessment can be accomplished easily by merely greeting the patient and introducing yourself, assuming that the patient can answer you, is conscious, has an open airway, is breathing, and has a pulse. Determine the patient's level of consciousness (LOC) based on his or her response to your greeting, and use the AVPU scale by adding, "Do you know where you are and the day of the week?" to your interview.

Airway and Breathing

Determine the patency of the patient's airway. If the patient is talking to you, the airway is patent. The patient may be able to maintain an open airway or, depending on the LOC, may need help with clearing obstructions (debris, blood, or teeth) by you properly positioning the head and/or placing an airway adjunct. Note the rate, quality, and effort of the breathing. Is the respiratory rate abnormally rapid (tachypnea)? Is the patient laboring to breathe? If the breathing is in question, listen with your stethoscope for the presence and quality of breath sounds. Consider initiating oxygen therapy at this time. Respiratory distress in a cardiac patient suggests the possibility of congestive heart failure (CHF), with fluid in the lungs.

Circulation

Assessment of circulation is done primarily by checking the patient's pulse. For a conscious patient, you will typically check the radial pulse; if the patient is unconscious, check the carotid pulse. While you are checking the pulse, note the rate, regularity, and overall quality. Is it weak, bounding, or irregular? You may also choose to compare central and peripheral pulses at the same time to make sure that they are equal to rule out the possibility of internal bleeding.

While holding the patient's hand in yours, assess the skin color and condition. The skin is the largest organ of the body, so a good indication that the rest of the body is getting adequate circulation is that the skin and mucous membranes are pink and the skin is warm and dry. Is there edema, poor turgor, or skin "tenting"?

Transport Decision

The primary assessment ends with making a transport decision for your patient. Based on your findings to this point, you should be able to determine whether the patient requires immediate transport. If you are unsure, continue with the history taking and secondary assessment, and the correct decision may become more apparent as you work your way through the patient assessment process.

History Taking

History taking consists of an inquiry into the patient's medical history based on the patient's chief complaint; it is also referred to as the history of present illness. The SAMPLE history is included in this assessment. In patients with acute coronary syndromes (ACS), the most common chief complaints are chest pain, dyspnea, fainting, palpitations, and fatigue.

Symptoms

Chest pain is often the presenting symptom of an AMI. The patient's description of the pain is important for assessing its significance. The OPQRST format can be used to elaborate on the patient's chief complaint:

O What is the *Onset* or origin of the pain—that is, how did it begin (suddenly or gradually)? Has anything like this ever happened before?

P What *Provoked* the pain—that is, what, if anything, brought it on? Is it exertional or nonexertional? What was the patient doing at the time? Sitting in a chair? Changing a tire? Shoveling snow? Having an argument? Does anything make it worse? What palliates the pain—that is, does anything make it better? Patients with chronic CAD may take nitroglycerin for episodes of chest pain. Ask whether the patient did so and, if so, whether it helped.

P also stands for *palliation*—Is there anything that makes the pain go away or get better?

Q What is the *Quality* of the pain—that is, what does it feel like? Get the patient's narrative description. Dull? Sharp? Crushing? Heavy? Squeezing? Note the exact words the patient uses to describe the pain, and observe the patient's body language as he or she does so. Try not to lead the patient's description unless he or she is unable to describe the pain. In such cases, try to give alternatives, such as "Is it sharp, dull, or crampy?"

R Does the pain *Radiate*? From where to where? To the jaw? Down the left arm? Into the back?

S What is the *Severity* of the pain—that is, how bad is it? Use the pain scale of 1 to 10, with 10 being the worst. If the patient has chronic angina, ask him or her to compare the pain with the usual angina pain.

T What was the *Timing* of the attack—that is, when did it start? How long did it last? What time did it get worse or better? Was it continuous or intermittent?

Another chief complaint among patients with an ACS is dyspnea. In the context of ACSs, dyspnea may be the first clue to failure of the left side of the heart. To explore this possibility, ask the following questions:

- When did the dyspnea start? Did it awaken the patient from sleep? **Paroxysmal nocturnal dyspnea (PND)** is an acute episode of shortness of breath in which the patient suddenly awakens from sleep with a feeling of suffocation. Often the patient will report going to a window to get "more air" or will move from the bed to a recliner. PND is one of the classic signs of left-sided heart failure, although it may also occur in chronic lung diseases.
- Did the dyspnea come on gradually or suddenly?
- Is it continuous or intermittent?
- Does it happen during activity or while at rest?
- Does any position make the dyspnea better or worse? The dyspnea of pulmonary edema usually worsens when the patient is lying down (**orthopnea**), because blood pools in the lungs when the body is horizontal. Patients with significant orthopnea will often sleep with several pillows, or even sitting in a recliner, to maintain a semiupright position.
- Has the patient ever had dyspnea like this before? If so, under what circumstances?
- Does the patient have a cough? Is it dry or productive?
- Were there any associated symptoms?

Fainting (**syncope**) occurs when CO suddenly declines, leading to a reduction in cerebral perfusion. Cardiac causes of syncope include dysrhythmias, increased vagal tone, and heart lesions. There are also numerous noncardiac causes of syncope (discussed in the chapter, *Neurologic Emergencies*). As part of taking a history from someone who has fainted, try to sort out whether the patient fainted from cardiac or noncardiac causes:

- Under what circumstances did the syncopal episode occur? What was the patient doing at the time? A 20-year-old person who faints at the sight of blood is unlikely to have significant underlying cardiac disease; a 60-year-old person who faints after feeling some "fluttering" in the chest may have a dangerous cardiac dysrhythmia.

- Were there any warning feelings before the episode, or did the fainting spell occur suddenly and unexpectedly?
- What position was the patient in when he or she fainted? Standing? Sitting? Lying down? Losing consciousness while sitting or lying down has more ominous implications than fainting while standing up.
- Has the patient fainted before? If so, under what circumstances?
- Were there any associated symptoms, such as nausea, vomiting, urinary incontinence, or seizures?

Finally, patients with cardiac problems may present with a chief complaint of palpitations. **Palpitations** refer to the sensation of an abnormally fast or irregular heartbeat—except after extreme exertion, a person normally remains blissfully unaware of his or her heartbeat. The cause of palpitations is often a cardiac dysrhythmia. The patient may not use the word "palpitations" but may report feeling the heart "skip a beat" or use words to that effect. In such a case, inquire about the onset, frequency, and duration of this symptom and previous episodes of palpitations. Also ask about the presence of associated symptoms (such as chest pain, dizziness, and dyspnea).

Patients may report a variety of other related symptoms as you explore their history of present illness. They may have a "feeling of impending doom" or a sense that they will soon experience a life-changing event. Some patients report feeling nauseous or having vomited. Listen carefully for indications that trauma may be involved or that their activity has been limited as a result of their condition. Observe their faces as you listen to them tell their stories. Do you see a look of fear or anguish? Are they holding their chest? Most of the other associated complaints your patients may have are related to hypoxia or poor perfusion resulting from inadequate CO—for example, decreased LOC, diaphoresis, restlessness and anxiety, fatigue, headache, behavioral changes, and syncope.

After exploring the patient's chief complaint, inquire briefly about pertinent aspects of the patient's other medical history:

- Is the patient under treatment for any serious illnesses or conditions? Ask specifically whether he or she has ever been diagnosed with any of the following:
  - Coronary artery disease
  - Atherosclerotic heart disease: angina, previous MI, hypertension, congestive heart failure
  - Valvular disease
  - Aneurysm
  - Pulmonary disease
  - Diabetes
  - Renal disease
  - Vascular disease
  - Inflammatory cardiac disease
  - Previous cardiac surgery (such as coronary artery bypass graft or valve replacement)
  - Congenital anomalies
- Is the patient taking any medications regularly? History taking is a great opportunity to ask about which drugs have been prescribed and whether the patient is taking

them as instructed. Be sure to ask when the patient took the medications last. Is he or she taking medications that were prescribed for someone else (borrowed)? Also ask about any over-the-counter medications or any herbal supplements the patient uses. It may be appropriate to ask about recreational drug use. Take particular note of the groups of medications prescribed for the treatment of cardiac problems. Specific medications and categories of medications prescribed for heart disease are discussed later in this chapter. If you are unfamiliar with any medication, ask the patient what it was prescribed for. It is also a good idea to ask if the patient takes any medication for each medical condition he or she reports as part of the history and to verify that these medical conditions match the medications the patient is actually taking.

- Does the patient have known allergies to foods or medications? If so, ask what kind of reaction the patient has with each one.
- Ask the patient when he or she last had anything to eat or drink, and note the time that occurred. This information will prove helpful later in many situations.
- If you have not asked already, find out the history of the current event. Get any extra information about what was happening when the problem started and what was done before your arrival.

Medications Commonly Prescribed to Patients with Cardiovascular Diseases

Patients with diseases affecting the cardiovascular system may be taking a wide variety of medications for a number of reasons, and it is not always possible to identify the patient's specific problem on the basis of a medication that he or she is taking. Beta blockers, for example, are prescribed for relief of angina, to lower blood pressure in hypertension, and to prevent recurrence of AMI. Similarly, diuretic medications may be given simply to help rid the body of excess fluid in CHF or because of their effects in lowering blood pressure. Thus, you need to look at any given medication the patient is taking in the context of the patient's clinical history and the other medications he or she is taking Figure 21.

Digitalis Preparations

Digitalis preparations are prescribed for the treatment of chronic CHF or for certain rapid atrial dysrhythmias (such as rapid atrial flutter, atrial fibrillation, supraventricular dysrhythmias). Digitalis acts by increasing the strength of cardiac contractions, thereby improving CO, and slowing conduction through the AV junction (such as in atrial fibrillation or flutter, allowing fewer impulses to be conducted through to the ventricles so the overall heart rate slows). In at least 30% of patients taking digitalis, some symptoms of toxic effects of the drug develop—for example, loss of appetite, nausea, vomiting, headache, blurred vision, yellow vision, or various cardiac dysrhythmias. *Virtually any cardiac dysrhythmia may be caused by the toxic effects of digitalis*, so it is important to ask all patients with disturbances in cardiac rhythm to determine whether they are taking digitalis.

Patients taking digitalis are sensitive to calcium preparations. They are also highly sensitive to a decline in the serum potassium level, so caution must be exercised in giving agents that might reduce the body's potassium stores (such as diuretics or large quantities of sodium bicarbonate). Commonly used digitalis preparations include digoxin (Lanoxin) and digitoxin (Crystodigin).

Antianginal Agents

Three major classes of drugs are used to relieve the pain of angina: nitrates, beta blockers, and calcium channel blockers. All of them work exclusively or primarily on the demand side of the oxygen supply-demand equation; that is, all of them diminish, in one way or another, myocardial oxygen demand.

Nitrates

Nitrates were the first drugs to be used for the relief of angina. The prototype of this group is nitroglycerin, which comes as rapid-acting sublingual tablets, sustained-release oral tablets, topically applied ointment, and skin patches Table 10. If a patient reports that he or she takes a medicine that is put under the tongue, that medicine is mostly likely nitroglycerin.

Nitroglycerin is thought to exert its therapeutic effect by decreasing the work of the heart. The heart's need for oxygen is, therefore, decreased, as is the anginal pain that results from insufficient oxygenation. Nitroglycerin usually takes effect within 3 to 5 minutes of administration.

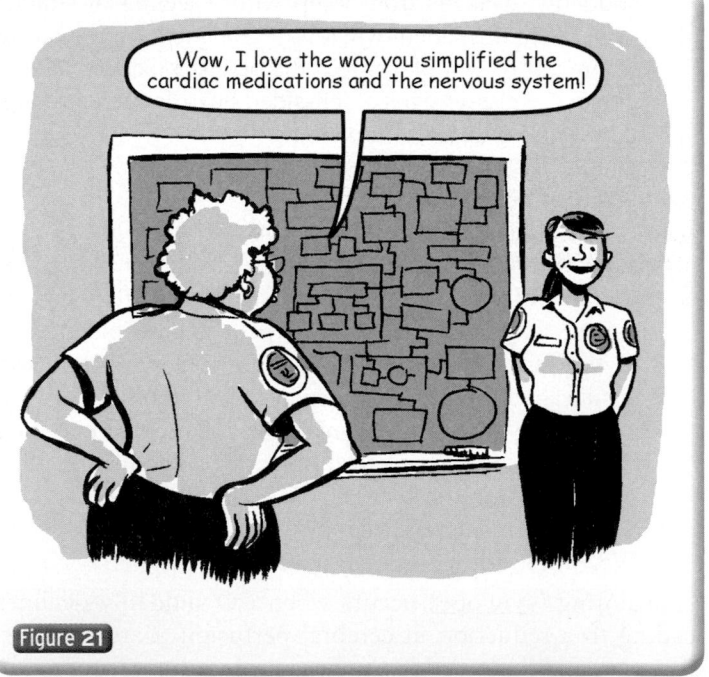

Figure 21

Table 10 Commonly Prescribed Nitrates	
Generic Name	**Trade Name**
Nitroglycerin	Nitrostat, Nitrolingual, Nitrogard, Nitroglycerin, Nitrong, Nitro-Bid, Nitro-Dur, Nitrol, Nitroglyn
Isosorbide dinitrate	Isordil, Sorbitrate

Nitroglycerin also causes significant vasodilation. For that reason, it is sometimes used in the field as an adjunctive therapy in the treatment of pulmonary edema secondary to left-sided heart failure. Used in that circumstance, nitroglycerin produces an "internal phlebotomy"—that is, a pooling of blood within the venous vessels that reduces the blood volume in the pulmonary vasculature just as if blood had been physically withdrawn from the body.

When a patient reports taking nitroglycerin for chest pain, you need to find out the answers to two questions: (1) How many nitroglycerin tablets/doses/sprays did the patient take? (2) Did the nitroglycerin relieve the pain? Failure of nitroglycerin to relieve anginal pain can occur for one of two reasons—the pain is of extraordinary severity, such as that associated with an AMI, or the nitroglycerin has been open too long and is no longer effective. Fresh, potent nitroglycerin has certain distinct side effects, including a transient, throbbing headache; a burning sensation under the tongue; and a bitter taste. If the patient did not find the pill bitter or did not experience a headache when he or she took the nitroglycerin, chances are the drug was outdated or ineffective, and you may consider administering nitroglycerin from your drug box per your local protocols. The patient's response to nitroglycerin does not predict a cardiac event, and must not be used to exclude any event. If the patient has a decrease in chest pain after administration of nitroglycerin, this does not mean that the pain must be cardiac. Often, patients with noncardiac chest pain experience a decrease in pain after nitroglycerin administration!

Beta Blockers

Drugs that block beta sympathetic receptors are also prescribed for the relief of angina Table 11. They work by decreasing the rate and strength of cardiac contractions, thereby decreasing the heart's demand for oxygen. Taking beta-blocking drugs on a regular basis usually leads to resistance to the action of beta-stimulating agents, such as epinephrine. When such patients

have a cardiac arrest, therefore, the administration of epinephrine during resuscitation attempts may not have the desired effect because the action of epinephrine may be blocked.

Calcium Channel Blockers

Calcium channel blockers, as their name implies, block the influx of calcium ions into cardiac muscle. These agents relieve angina in two ways: (1) by preventing spasm of the coronary arteries and (2) by weakening cardiac contraction, thereby decreasing myocardial oxygen demand. Hypotension may be a significant side effect. Table 12 lists calcium channel blockers.

Antidysrhythmic Agents

Antidysrhythmic drugs are used to control chronic disturbances in cardiac rhythm. Thus, when you encounter a patient taking one of these agents, you know the patient has had significant dysrhythmias in the past, which justifies particular surveillance for recurrent rhythm disturbances. Patients taking antidysrhythmic drugs should be monitored while under your care.

Some of the drugs mentioned under other categories are also used for their antidysrhythmic activity. Digitalis preparations, for example, are used to suppress atrial dysrhythmias. Beta blockers are sometimes prescribed for their suppressive effect on myocardial excitability, as are some of the calcium channel blockers. Finally, the seizure medication, phenytoin sodium (Dilantin), is occasionally used for cardiac dysrhythmias, particularly for dysrhythmias due to the toxic effects of digitalis. Table 13 lists antidysrhythmic drugs that are commonly used in emergencies.

Diuretics

Diuretics ("water pills") are prescribed to patients with chronic fluid overload, principally patients with chronic CHF, but are also used as primary or adjunctive therapy in the treatment of hypertension. Diuretics trick the kidneys into excreting more sodium

Table 11 Beta Blockers

Category	Generic Name*	Trade Name
Beta 1	Atenolol	Tenormin
	Bisoprolol	Zebeta
	Metoprolol	Lopressor, Toprol-XL
	Nevibolol	Bystolic
Nonselective (beta 1, beta 2, and alpha)	Carvedilol	Coreg
	Labetalol	Normodyne, Trandate
	Propranolol	Inderal, Inderal-LA
	Sotalol (also has Class 3 antidysrhythmic properties)	Betapace
	Nadolol	Corgard, Corzide

*The generic drug names in this class of medications end in "-olol" or "-alol".

Table 12 Calcium Channel Blockers

Category	Generic Name	Trade Name
Dihydropyridines (these medication names end in "-ipine")	Amlodipine	Norvasc
	Felodipine	Plendil
	Nicardipine	Cardene, Cardene SR
	Nifedipine	Adalat, Adalat CC, Procardia, Procardia XL
Nondihydropyridines	Diltiazem	Cardizem, Cardizem CD, Cardizem SR, Dilacor XR, Diltiazem XT, Tiazac
	Verapamil	Calan, Calan SR, Covera-HS, Isoptin, Isoptin SR, Verelan, Verelan PM

and water than usual (the desired effect). The kidneys also tend to dump out potassium along with the sodium (an undesired effect). Thus, patients taking diuretics often become depleted of potassium if they are not given potassium supplements. Patients in whom potassium deficits (hypokalemia) develop are prone to cardiac dysrhythmias—especially if they are also taking digitalis. Table 14 lists commonly prescribed diuretics.

Antihypertensive Agents

As the name implies, antihypertensive agents are used to treat hypertension (high blood pressure). Many of the diuretic agents already mentioned are also used as antihypertensives or in combination with antihypertensives for a synergistic effect. Similarly, beta blockers are used in the treatment of hypertension.

It is often difficult to regulate the dosage of antihypertensives so that the patient's blood pressure is lowered enough but not too much. As a consequence, some patients taking these agents may have symptoms of hypotension, including weakness and dizziness. Many will experience a feeling of giddiness with a change in position (such as when moving from a recumbent to a sitting or standing position); this phenomenon is termed orthostatic hypotension. Every patient taking antihypertensive

drugs, therefore, should have his or her blood pressure checked in the recumbent and sitting positions to detect orthostatic hypotension. Table 15 lists commonly prescribed antihypertensive agents.

Anticoagulant and Antiplatelet Agents

Anticoagulant drugs ("blood thinners") diminish the ability of the blood to clot. They are prescribed to patients who have had recurrent problems with blood clots (such as patients who have had pulmonary emboli) and to patients who might be prone to develop clots (such as some patients who have had a MI in the past; patients with artificial heart valves or valvular heart disease; patients whose normal heart rhythm is atrial fibrillation). Patients who take anticoagulants are apt to bleed excessively from minor trauma or even venipuncture, so you should be alert to that possibility. A commonly used oral anticoagulant drug is warfarin (Coumadin, Panwarfin). Warfarin requires that the patient's clotting ability be tested weekly. A newer agent, dabigatran (Pradaxa), is another anticoagulant medication that is gaining popularity because it does not require this testing. Patients undergoing home dialysis may be taking the IV anticoagulant, heparin, during their dialysis cycle.

Clopidogrel (Plavix) has become a drug that has gained popularity in its use in managing myocardial infarctions. Plavix is an antiplatelet drug, which means it keeps the platelets found in blood from sticking together. Table 16 lists anticoagulant and antiplatelet agents.

Other Medications

In addition to those discussed thus far, Table 17 lists additional medications that may be prescribed for patients with cardiac conditions.

Table 13 Commonly Used Antidysrhythmic Drugs

Generic Name	Trade Name
Amiodarone	Cordarone
Digoxin	Lanoxin
Lidocaine	Xylocaine
Procainamide	Procan, Pronestyl

Table 14 Commonly Prescribed Diuretics

Category	Generic Name	Trade Name
Loop diuretics	Furosemide Bumetanide Torsemide	Lasix Bumex Demadex
Potassium-sparing diuretics	Spironolactone Triamterene	Aldactone Dyrenium
Thiazide diuretics	Chlorothiazide Hydrochlorothiazide Metolazone	Diuril Esidrix, HydroDIURIL Diulo, Zaroxolyn
Vasodilator/Nitrate	Hydralazine	Apresoline
Combination drugs	Hydrochlorothiazide and spironolactone Triamterene and hydrochlorothiazide Triamterene and hydrochlorothiazide	Aldactazide Dyazide Maxzide

Table 15 Commonly Prescribed Antihypertensive Agents

Category	Generic Name	Trade Name
Nonselective beta blockers (have both beta 1 and beta 2 effects)	Labetalol Propranolol	Normodyne, Trandate Inderal
Angiotensin-converting enzyme inhibitors (ACEI) (The generic drug names in this class of medications end in "-pril")	Benazepril Captopril Enalapril Fosinopril Lisinopril Quinapril Ramipril	Lotensin Capoten Vasotec Monopril Prinivil, Zestril Accupril Altace
Alpha agonist	Clonidine Methyldopa	Catapres Aldomet
Alpha blocker	Prazosin	Minipress
Other antihypertensive	Reserpine	Sandril, Ser-Ap-Es, Serpasil

Table 16 Commonly Prescribed Anticoagulant and Antiplatelet Agents

Category	Drug
Antiplatelet agents	Clopidogrel (Plavix); ticlopidine (Ticlid); aspirin
Coumarin anticoagulant	Warfarin (Coumadin)
Direct thrombin inhibitor	Dabigatran (Pradaxa)

Table 17 Other Medicines Prescribed to Treat or Prevent Heart Disease

Category	Drug
Angiotensin II receptor blockers (ARB) (The generic drug names in this class of medications end in "-sartan")	Losartan (Cozaar); valsartan (Diovan); irbesartan (Avapro); candesartan (Atacand)
Cholesterol-lowering drugs	Statins: lovastatin (Altacor, Mevacor); fluvastatin (Lescol); pravastatin (Pravachol); atorvastatin (Lipitor); simvastatin (Zocor) Niacins: nicotinic acid (Niacor); extended-release niacin (Niaspan) Bile acid resins: colestipol (Colestid); cholestyramine (Questran); colesevelam (Welchol) Fibrates: clofibrate (Atromid); gemfibrozil (Lopid); fenofibrate (Tricor)
Cardiac glycoside	Digoxin (Lanoxin, Lanoxi-caps)
Vasodilators	Isosorbide dinitrate* (Dilatrate-SR, Iso-Bid, Isonate, Isorbid, Isordil, Isotrate, Sorbitrate); isosorbide mononitrate (Imdur); hydralazine* (Apresoline)

*Isosorbide dinitrate and hydralazine are given together.

■ Secondary Assessment

The physical exam during secondary assessment is similar for many medical patients. Nevertheless, certain aspects warrant greater emphasis in the patient whose chief complaint suggests a cardiac problem.

When you are observing the patient's general appearance, pay particular attention to the LOC, which is an excellent indicator of the adequacy of cerebral perfusion. If a patient is alert and oriented, the brain is getting enough oxygen, which in turn means the heart is doing its job as a pump. Conversely, stupor or confusion may indicate poor CO, which may be the result of myocardial damage or dysfunction. Skin color and temperature are also valuable indicators of the state of the patient's circulation: The cold, sweaty skin of many patients with MI reflects massive peripheral vasoconstriction.

Physical Exam

Begin the physical exam with inspection, auscultation, and palpation of the patient's respirations.

Inspect the neck and tracheal position. Is the trachea midline and mobile to gentle manipulation? Press down with your finger in the patient's suprasternal notch to verify that the trachea is midline.

Also inspect adjacent structures such as the neck veins. The external jugular veins reflect the pressure within the patient's systemic circulation. Normally, they are collapsed when a person is sitting or standing. If the function of the right side of the heart is compromised, however, blood will back up into the systemic veins behind the right side of the heart and distend those veins. To estimate the patient's jugular venous pressure, place the patient in a semi-Fowler position (45° angle) with the head slightly rotated away from the jugular vein you are examining; observe the height of the distended fluid column within the vein, and note how far up the distension extends above the sternal angle.

Continue the assessment by inspecting and palpating the chest. Look for surgical scars that might indicate previous cardiac surgery. Is there a nitroglycerin patch on the patient's skin? Is there a bulge under the patient's skin indicating a pacemaker or an automated implanted cardioverter defibrillator (AICD)? These devices are implanted just below the right or left clavicle and are about the size of a half-dollar **Figure 22**. Is the anterior-posterior diameter of the chest enlarged, as in a barrel-chested patient with chronic obstructive pulmonary disease? On palpation, do you observe any sign of crepitus?

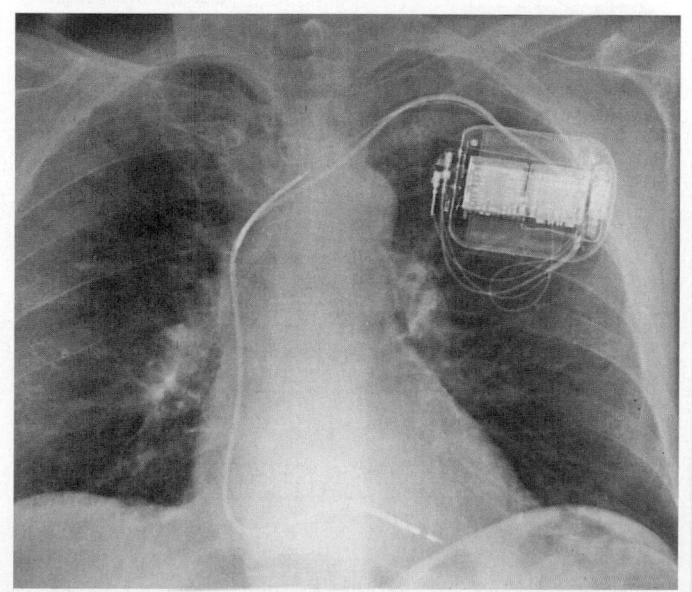

Figure 22 An AICD is attached directly to the heart and continuously monitors heart rhythm, delivering shocks as needed. The electricity from the AICD is so low that it has no effect on rescuers.

Listen carefully to the chest with your stethoscope. Crackles or wheezes may be suggestive of left-sided heart failure with pulmonary edema. Examine the extremities for pedal edema and examine the back for sacral edema; these are signs of failure of the right side of the heart.

Heart Sounds

During the physical exam, listen to the patient's heart sounds. The purpose of listening to heart sounds is to identify the "lub-dub" that indicates the cardiac valves are operating properly. The major heart sounds are the two normal sounds, S_1 and S_2 **Figure 23**, and the two abnormal sounds, S_3 and S_4 **Figure 24**.

S_1 occurs near the beginning of ventricular contraction (systole), when the tricuspid and mitral valves close. The closing of these two valves should occur simultaneously as the pressure within the ventricles increases. The S_1 sound should correspond to the pulse located at the carotid artery. The closing of the tricuspid valve can be louder in those patients who are experiencing pulmonary hypertension due to the increased pressure that exists past the valve. In patients who have anemia, a fever, or hyperthyroidism, louder S_1 sounds may be noted due to the valves being open when the ventricles contract. Patients who have stenosis of their mitral valve will also have a louder S_1. Patients who have a mitral valve that is subject to fibrosis or is calcified can have decreased S_1 heart sounds. Other conditions such as obesity, emphysema, and cardiac tamponade (fluid around the heart) can diminish S_1 heart sounds as well. Any delay in the closing of these two valves, heard as a split sound, is considered abnormal.

S_2 occurs near the end of ventricular contraction (systole), when the pulmonary and aortic valves close. As the ventricles relax, these valves close because of backward flow in the pulmonary artery and aorta. The two valves can close simultaneously or with a slight delay between them under normal physiologic circumstances. Patients with chronic high blood pressure or pulmonary hypertension may experience a higher closing pressure for these valves, resulting in the aortic valve that makes a louder sound when closing. Patients with hypotension will produce a decreased S_2 sound. The S_2 sound may be split if the patient has a right bundle branch, which results in the delay of the pulmonic valve closing. Left bundle branch blocks may cause a situation where the aortic valve is closing more slowly than the pulmonic valve.

S_3 is an extra, abnormal heart sound in adults. It is caused by vibrations of the ventricular walls, resulting from the rapid filling period of the ventricle during the beginning of diastole. An S_3 sound should occur 120 to 170 milliseconds (ms) after S_2, if it is heard at all. S_3 is generally heard in children and young adults. When it is heard in older adults, it often signifies heart failure.

S_4 is a rare heart sound heard just before S1. It is caused by turbulent filling of a stiff ventricle as seen in the case of hypertrophy and possibly myocardial infarction.

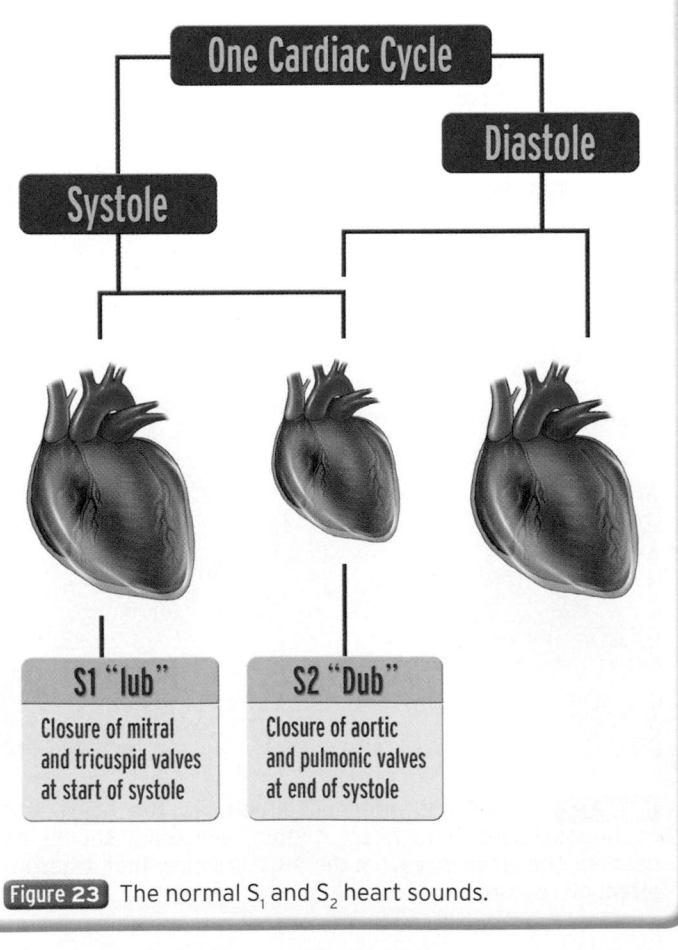

Figure 23 The normal S_1 and S_2 heart sounds.

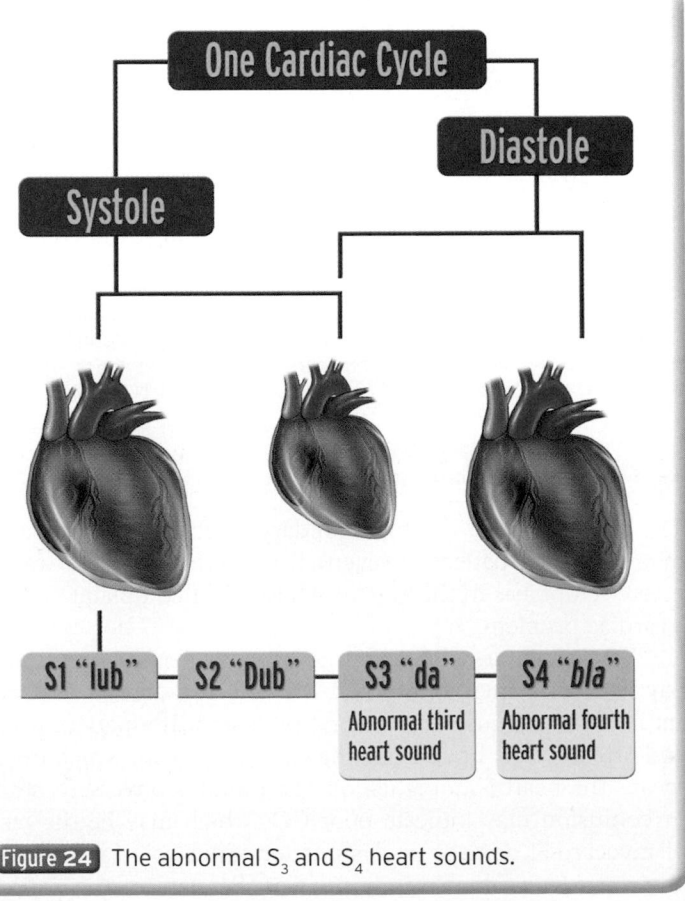

Figure 24 The abnormal S_3 and S_4 heart sounds.

Other abnormal heart sounds that are found in patients include an opening snap, ejection click, pericardial friction rub, murmur, thrill, and pericardial knock. An **opening snap** is indicative of a noncompliant valve, such as the mitral valve found in a patient who has a history of rheumatic fever. In an **ejection click**, a high-pitched sound occurs just after the S_1 sound; it may indicate a dilated pulmonary artery or septal defect. A **pericardial friction rub** creates a to-and-fro sound that can be heard in systole and diastole. The sound is heard in patients who have inflammation of the pericardial sac (pericarditis). In pericarditis, the pericardial sac is inflamed, causing the visceral and parietal surfaces of the pericardium to rub together. A **murmur** is an ambiguous sound that is associated with turbulent blood flow through the heart valves. This turbulent blood flow can be generated from increased blood flow across a normal valve, flow across an irregular or constricted valve, blood flow into an enlarged chamber of the heart, or blood flow going backwards through a compromised valve. A **thrill** is a vibration that occurs frequently and remains constant. A **pericardial knock** is a high-pitched sound during the diastole phase that indicates a thickened pericardium that is limiting how far the ventricle can expand during the diastole phase.

Vital Signs
Pulse

When you obtain the vital signs, make a careful assessment of the patient's pulse. Is it regular or irregular? Abnormally fast or slow? Strong or weak? An irregular pulse signals a disturbance in cardiac rhythm. A very rapid pulse (tachycardia) may simply indicate anxiety, but it can also occur secondary to severe pain, CHF, or a cardiac dysrhythmia. A weak, thready pulse suggests a reduction in CO.

You should be familiar with the potentially abnormal pulse findings. For example, the patient may have a **pulse deficit**. A deficit occurs when the palpated radial pulse rate is less than the apical pulse rate; it is reported numerically as the difference between the two. To assess for a deficit, check the peripheral radial pulse while listening to an apical pulse.

Another abnormal pulse finding is **pulsus paradoxus**. Pulsus paradoxus is an excessive drop (> 10 mm Hg) in the systolic blood pressure with each inspired breath. Pulsus paradoxus can sometimes be palpated as a decrease in the amplitude of the pulse waveform, which makes the affected pulse beats feel weaker than the others. This observation can best be made when the rhythm is regular. If the variation is slight, it can be detected only by use of a blood pressure cuff and stethoscope.

Finally, you might recognize **pulsus alternans**. This pulse alternates between strong and weak beats and typically is representative of left ventricular systolic damage.

Blood Pressure

In patients older than 50 years, a systolic blood pressure of more than 140 mm Hg is a much more important risk factor for CVD than the diastolic pressure. Patients with a systolic blood pressure of 120 to 139 mm Hg or a diastolic blood pressure of 80 to 89 mm Hg are considered "prehypertensive" and need to adopt a healthier lifestyle to prevent CVD.

In emergency situations, an elevated blood pressure may reflect the patient's anxiety or pain. A systolic blood pressure of less than 90 mm Hg might suggest serious hypotension and shock, depending on the patient's overall condition and chief complaint. The pulse pressure (the difference between the systolic and diastolic pressures) gives a rough indication of the elasticity of the arterial walls and the SV. In patients with arteriosclerosis, the arterial walls are stiffened, and the pulse pressure is increased. In cardiogenic shock or cardiac tamponade, the SV is reduced because the heart cannot pump effectively, so the pulse pressure is narrowed accordingly.

It may be beneficial to obtain the blood pressure in both arms and compare the readings. Some conditions such as stroke or aortic aneurysm may cause blood pressures to vary from the right to the left side.

Monitoring Devices

One of the most important and widely used tools in the prehospital setting is the ECG monitor-defibrillator. The ECG machine enables paramedics to monitor and record 3-lead ECG tracings, and record 12-lead ECGs in the field and transmit them to the receiving facility. Studies have shown that EMS has a tremendous positive impact on cardiac care, especially in patients with acute myocardial infarction (AMI). The ECG monitor enables prehospital providers to quickly identify suspected AMI, transmit the findings electronically, and make sound transport decisions based on the ECG findings. The ECG monitor-defibrillator also provides rescuers with the ability to defibrillate, cardiovert, and perform transcutaneous pacing in the prehospital setting.

As part of obtaining the vital signs, attach the cardiac monitor, waveform capnography, or pulse oximeter if you have not done so already. Use the ECG and oxygen saturation measurement just as you do other vital signs—that is, as tools to help you in your assessment and not as the only guide to treatment (treat the patient, not the monitor). When you are caring for a patient in relatively stable condition who does not require rapid assessment, the physical exam may be done while monitoring devices are in use on the patient. The steps for performing cardiac monitoring are discussed later in this chapter.

Reassessment

Once the history and vital signs have been obtained and the physical exam has been completed, treatment of the patient should be continued and transportation initiated. The reassessment is accomplished en route to the hospital. It begins with a repeat of the primary assessment (LOC and ABCs). The vital signs should be obtained every 5 minutes for critical patients or every 15 minutes for those patients who are determined to be in stable condition. A repeated physical exam should be accomplished to see if any changes have occurred or if any conditions were missed in the initial physical exam.

Assess the effectiveness of all interventions implemented. For example, is the IV fluid still flowing or has the pain diminished after nitroglycerin administration?

Finally, be sure to create proper documentation of the call, including notifying the receiving facility of any history findings, physical exam findings, and cardiac monitoring or ECG findings.

Finally, part of the care of the patient with STEMI should involve transmitting the 12-lead ECG to the catheterization lab to shorten the interval from the arrival time to treatment time. Be sure to transmit your findings.

Electrophysiology

Once the patient has been identified as having a cardiovascular problem, it becomes imperative to assess the nature of the specific problem. Cardiac rhythm disturbances or dysrhythmias Table 18 may arise from a variety of causes; they are not solely caused by AMI. A cardiac dysrhythmia is simply a disturbance in the normal cardiac rhythm, which may or may not be clinically significant. Sometimes dysrhythmias are caused by ischemia, electrolyte imbalances, disturbances or damage in the electrical conduction system resulting in escape beats, circus reentry, or enhanced automaticity. Thus, it is always necessary to evaluate the dysrhythmia in the context of the patient's overall clinical condition. It is the patient's clinical condition—not the lines and tracings on a piece of paper—that should ultimately determine whether treatment is necessary. Treat the patient, not the monitor!

One of the most important tasks in the prehospital care of a patient with an AMI is to anticipate, recognize, and treat life-threatening dysrhythmias. Dysrhythmias develop after an AMI for two principal reasons. First, irritability of the ischemic heart muscle surrounding the infarct may cause the damaged muscle to generate abnormal currents of electricity that cause abnormal cardiac contractions. When the dysrhythmia arises from irritable spots in the myocardium (ectopic foci), it is usually a rapid dysrhythmia (tachydysrhythmia), such as ventricular tachycardia, premature atrial contractions (PACs), or PVCs. Second, dysrhythmias may occur after an AMI because the infarct damages the conduction

Table 18 Causes of Cardiac Dysrhythmias

Myocardial ischemia or infarction
Other forms of heart disease
Rheumatic heart disease
Cor pulmonale
Generalized hypoxemia from any cause
Autonomic nervous system imbalance
Increased vagal tone
Increased sympathetic output
Distention of cardiac chambers (as in heart failure)
Electrolyte disturbances, especially those involving potassium, calcium, or magnesium
Drug toxicity
Certain poisons (such as organophosphate insecticides)
Central nervous system damage
Hypothermia
Metabolic imbalance
Normal variations
Trauma (such as cardiac contusions)

YOU are the Medic   PART 4

You lift the patient to the stretcher and move her to the unit for transport. While en route to the hospital, you notice that the PVCs have dropped from 8 to 10 per minute to 2 per minute, and they appear to be unifocal. The patient states that she is feeling a little bit better but she still reports pain in her jaw. She says it is "still a 5 on a 1 to 10 scale."

Recording Time: 15 Minutes	
Respirations	14 breaths/min
Pulse	70 beats/min, irregular
Skin	Warm, pale, moist
Blood pressure	110/66 mm Hg
Oxygen saturation (Sp_{O_2})	99% on oxygen
Pupils	Equal and reactive

7. What does the acronym MONA stand for?

8. Of the steps in MONA, which should you perform next?

tissues. In such a case, the abnormal rhythm is usually a block or a bradydysrhythmia.

ECG analysis is indicated in any patient who might have a cardiac-related condition. Any patient with chest pain should undergo ECG analysis, but this monitoring should also be instituted for any patient with a history of heart problems. Given that age is a contributing factor to heart disease, ECG analysis is appropriate for elderly patients in many situations. You should think of the ECG as another vital sign, similar to the blood pressure or pulse oximetry.

Cardiac Monitoring and ECG Use

The ECG monitor **Figure 25** serves several functions in the prehospital setting. The device can be used to continuously monitor the patient's cardiac rhythm during transport, print out a rhythm strip to perform dysrhythmia interpretation, and print out a 12-lead ECG for specific disease diagnosis.

Typically, continuous monitoring is performed using the three standard __limb leads__: leads I, II, and III. Continuous ECG monitoring may be used during transport to identify any changes in the patient's heart rhythm. When analyzing cardiac monitoring ECGs, the tracing from lead II is usually most useful.

The ECG device also enables paramedics to acquire and document a 12-lead ECG. The 12-lead ECG provides detailed information about the heart's conduction system and records the activity from 12 separate angles. In virtually all cases, when a paramedic records a 3-lead ECG, it is because he or she suspects the patient is experiencing a cardiac event; therefore, a 12-lead ECG should also be captured. Although the 3-lead ECG provides a great deal of information, it is very limited compared with the information obtained from a 12-lead tracing.

Cardiac monitors contain leads (wires) that are connected to electrodes that are placed on the patient. Each lead offers an electrical snapshot of a certain part of the heart. The cardiac monitor records an ECG tracing for each lead used; these tracings can then be reviewed by persons trained in interpreting the findings.

Devices capable of recording 12-lead ECGs also contain interpretation software. Such software is a good tool, but has many limitations. It is always best to rely on your own interpretation and not the automated interpretation when reading the ECG; think of automatic interpretation software as a nudge or hint as to what may be happening in the patient's heart. Some devices are also capable of transmitting ECGs to the hospital. This technology enables physicians in the emergency department to review the ECG prior to your arrival and prepare specialized resources for the patient.

Electrode Placement

In order for an ECG to be reliable and useful, the electrodes must be placed in consistent positions on each patient **Figure 26**. To maintain consistency in monitoring and obtaining a useful ECG, there are predetermined locations to place electrodes and leads.

Electrodes used in the prehospital setting are generally adhesive and have a gel center to aid in skin contact. Some manufacturers offer a "diaphoretic" electrode that sticks to a sweating patient more effectively. Whichever type is used, certain basic principles should be followed to achieve the best skin contact and minimize __artifact__ in the signal (artifact refers to an ECG tracing that is the result of interference, such as patient movement, rather than the heart's electrical activity). These principles are as follows:

- To maintain the correct lead placement, it may be necessary to shave body hair from the electrode site. Do not be fooled by a hairy chest. It may appear that you have good skin contact initially, but the electrode will rise off the skin and stick to the hair. Shaving should also be done when you are using hands-free adhesive defibrillation pads.
- To remove oils and dead tissues from the surface of the skin, rub the electrode site briskly with an alcohol swab before application. Wait for the alcohol to dry before electrode application or dry it with a quick wipe of a 4″ × 4″ gauze pad.

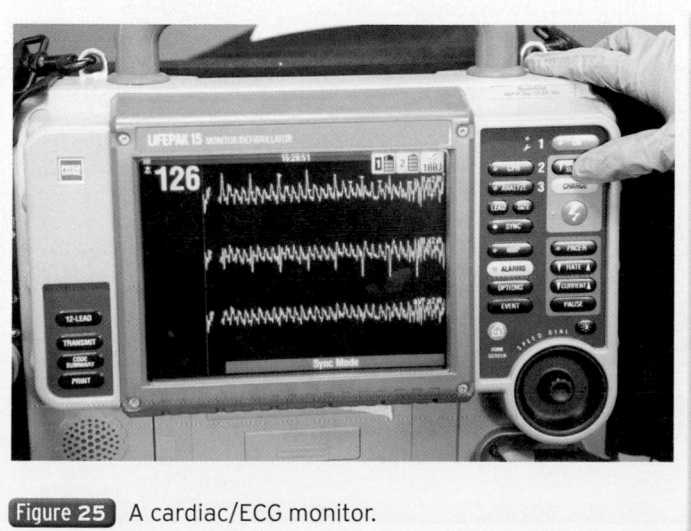

Figure 25 A cardiac/ECG monitor.

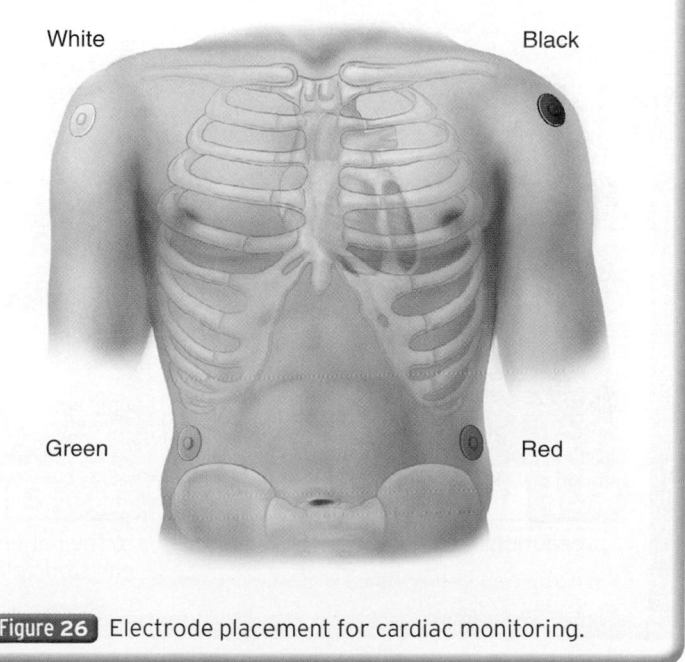

White   Black

Green   Red

Figure 26 Electrode placement for cardiac monitoring.

- Attach the electrodes to the ECG cables before placement. Confirm that the appropriate electrode now attached to the cable is placed at the correct location on the patient's chest or limbs (each cable is marked and color coded as to the correct location for placement).

- Once all electrodes are in place, switch on the monitor, and print a sample rhythm strip. If the strip shows any "interference" (artifact), verify that the electrodes are firmly applied to the skin and the monitor cable is plugged in correctly.

Artifact on the monitor can be tricky. A straight-line ECG in an alert, communicative patient indicates a loose or disconnected lead, not asystole (flat line). Similarly, a wavy baseline resembling ventricular fibrillation may be caused by patient movement or muscle tremor. Before you reach for the defibrillator paddles, look at the patient! If he or she is alert and in no obvious distress, recheck the leads and equipment. Remember to treat the patient, not the monitor.

Skill Drill 1 shows the steps for performing cardiac monitoring, which are listed here:

Skill Drill 1

1. Take standard precautions Step 1.
2. Explain the procedure to the patient. Prepare the skin for electrode placement Step 2.
3. Attach the electrodes to the leads before placing them on the patient Step 3.
4. Position the electrodes on the patient, on the torso if performing continuous monitoring, on the limbs if you will be acquiring a 12-lead Step 4.

5. If you plan to obtain a 12-lead tracing as well, place the limb leads Step 5.
6. Turn on the monitor Step 6.
7. Record tracings Step 7.
8. Label each strip Step 8.

The Leads

There are two main groups of **leads**: the limb leads and the **precordial leads**. The limb leads are leads I, II, III, and aVR, aVL, aVF. The limb leads are created by placing four electrodes on the body. If you are performing continuous cardiac monitoring, the four electrodes should be placed on the patient's torso in the following manner:

1. White – right upper chest near the shoulder
2. Black – left upper chest near the shoulder
3. Red – left lower abdomen
4. Green – right lower abdomen

If you are acquiring a 12-lead ECG, the four electrodes should be placed on the patient's limbs in the following manner:

1. White – right wrist
2. Black – left wrist
3. Red – left ankle
4. Green – right ankle

Placing these four electrodes on the patient enables the ECG device to record all six of the limb leads using Einthoven's theory. Einthoven was a physicist who discovered that every time the heart contracts, it emits a tiny amount of electrical energy that travels across the surface of the skin. Using electrodes and an ECG monitor, these waves of energy can be recorded and plotted on a piece of grid paper. Einthoven recorded three leads initially—leads I, II, and III, where lead I was formed between

Skill Drill 1

Performing Cardiac Monitoring

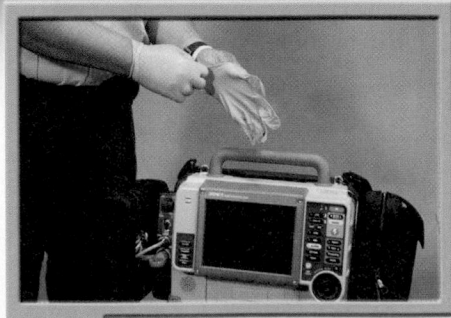

Step 1 Take standard precautions.

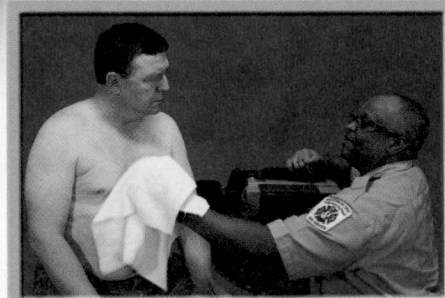

Step 2 Explain the procedure to the patient. Prepare the skin for electrode placement.

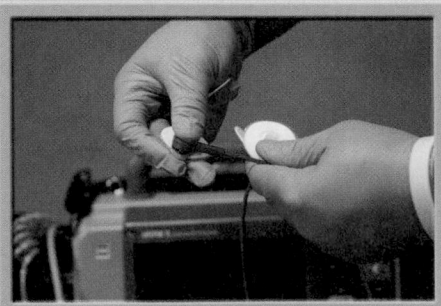

Step 3 Attach the electrodes to the leads before placing them on the patient.

Continues

Skill Drill 1

Performing Cardiac Monitoring, continued

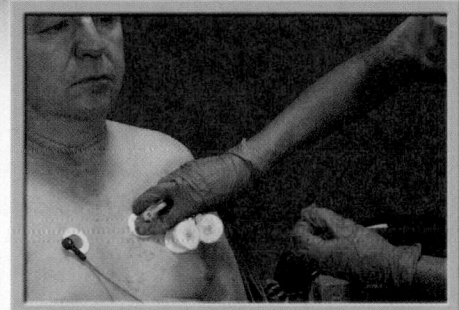

Step 4 Position the electrodes on the patient.

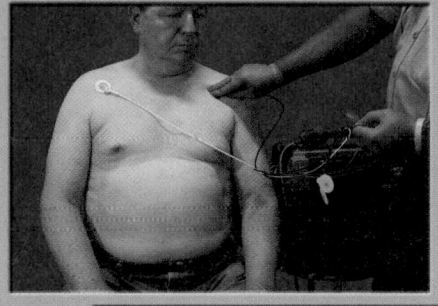

Step 5 If you plan to obtain a 12-lead tracing as well, place the limb leads.

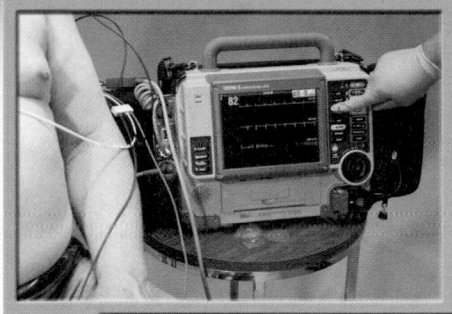

Step 6 Turn on the monitor and set lead II.

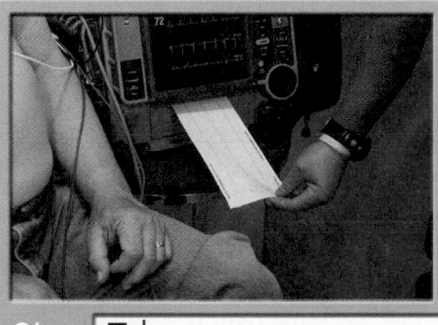

Step 7 Record tracings.

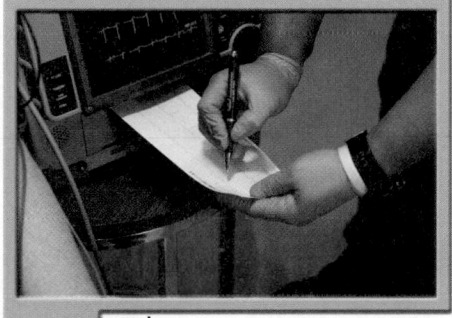

Step 8 Label each strip.

the right and left arms, lead II between the right arm and left leg, and lead III between the left arm and left leg **Figure 27**.

The augmented voltage or aV leads are also created using the four limb electrodes. Leads aVR, aVL, and aVF are created by combining two of the limb leads, thereby forming a new lead, and using the remaining lead as the other pole. For example, lead aVR is created between the right arm and the combination of the left arm and leg electrodes **Figure 28**. The green lead serves as a ground in all cases and is not used to create any lead.

The precordial leads consist of six additional electrodes placed on the anterior chest of the patient. It is critical to place the electrodes in the correct location to ensure an accurate ECG tracing. The electrodes for the precordial leads should be placed in the following manner **Figure 29**:

1. V_1 – Right of sternum, 4th intercostal space (ICS)
2. V_2 – Left of sternum, 4th ICS
3. V_4 – Midclavicular, 5th ICS
4. V_3 – Precisely between V_2 and V_4
5. V_6 – Midaxillary, 5th ICS
6. V_5 – Precisely between V_4 and V_6

Right-Sided ECGs Certain conditions require paramedics to record a right-sided ECG to evaluate the electrical activity of the right ventricle. In that case, the precordial leads are placed on the right anterior thorax. The electrodes for the right-sided ECG should be placed in the following manner **Figure 30**:

1. V_1R – Left of sternum, 4th intercostal space (ICS)
2. V_2R – Right of sternum, 4th ICS
3. V_4R – Right midclavicular, 5th ICS
4. V_3R – Precisely between V_2 and V_4
5. V_6R – Right midaxillary, 5th ICS
6. V_5R – Precisely between V_4 and V_6

Note: lead V_4R is the most sensitive and specific for right ventricular acute myocardial infarction and is often the only lead recorded on the right-sided ECG.

Posterior ECGs The posterior ECG is used to evaluate the electrical activity of the posterior wall of the left ventricle. In that case, three of the precordial leads are placed on the left posterior thorax. The electrodes for the posterior ECG should be placed in the following manner **Figure 31**:

1. V_7 – Between V_6 and V_8, 5th intercostal space
2. V_8 – Midscapular, 5th intercostal space
3. V_9 – Just to the left of the spine, 5th intercostal space

Note: The posterior ECG is rarely used in practice for two main reasons. First, isolated posterior wall myocardial infarction is very rare, only accounting for 2% to 4% of all ST segment elevation MI. It is almost always associated with inferior wall MI. Next, the electrical activity of posterior wall of the left ventricle can be seen through the "eyes" of leads V_1 through V_3. This will be discussed in great detail in the ischemia section later in this chapter.

15- and 18-Lead ECG Certain texts refer to the 15- and 18-lead ECGs. The 15-lead ECG is a phrase used to describe acquisition of the standard 12-lead ECG, plus leads V_4R, V_7, and V_8. The additional leads enable the paramedic to view the right ventricle and posterior wall of the left ventricle and determine if ischemia or injury is present. The 15-lead ECG involves recording a second tracing containing the additional leads. The new recording contains nine of the standard leads plus the three additional ones.

The 18-lead ECG is a phrase used to describe acquisition of the standard tracing, plus leads V_4R through V_6R and V_7 through V_9. This is not commonly acquired by EMS or in-hospital setting and is only mentioned to familiarize you with the terms in case you come across them in literature.

Unipolar Versus Bipolar Leads Leads I, II, and III are **bipolar leads**. Bipolar leads are leads that contain a positive and negative pole. Leads aVR, aVL, and aVF are **augmented unipolar leads**. Augmented unipolar leads contain one true pole, while the other end of the lead is referenced against a combination of other leads. For example, lead aVR is the white electrode at the right arm, referenced against the combination of the left arm and left leg. The precordial leads V_1 to V_6 are also unipolar leads. The precordial leads are referenced against a calculated point known as Wilson's central terminal **Figure 32**. Wilson's central terminal is created by bisecting the limb leads in Einthoven's triangle.

Lead Polarity The bipolar leads have a positive and negative end. Lead I is formed between the right and left arm electrodes. The left arm electrode is the positive terminal. Lead II is formed between the right arm and left leg. The left leg electrode is the positive terminal. Lead III is formed between the left arm and left leg. The left leg is the positive terminal **Figure 33**.

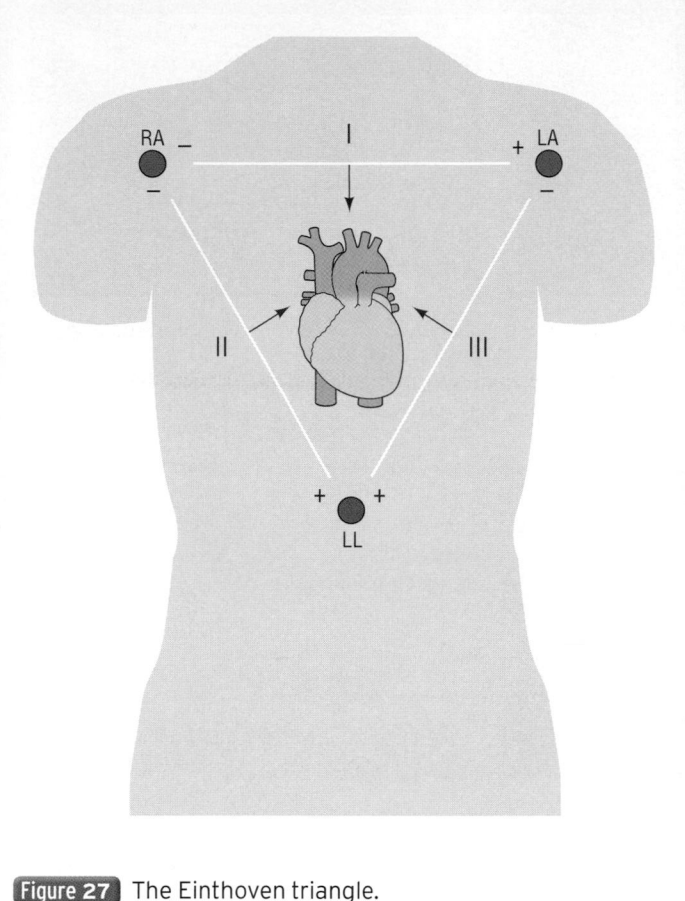

Figure 27 The Einthoven triangle.

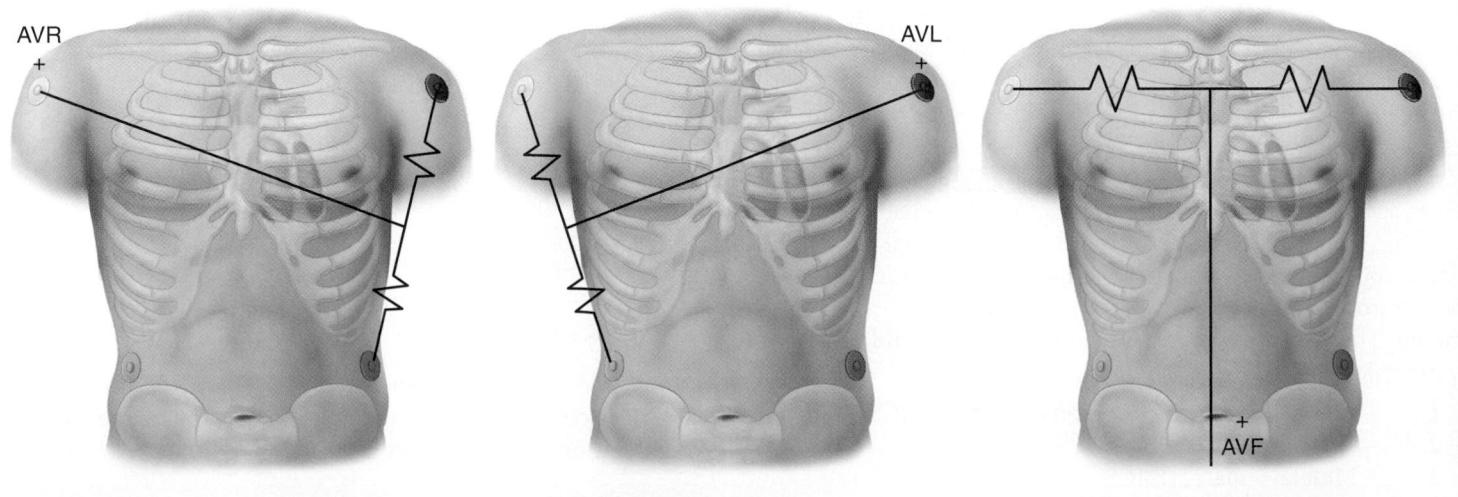

Figure 28 Augmented voltage leads are created from the limb leads, by using information from one lead, and a combination of information from the other two leads.

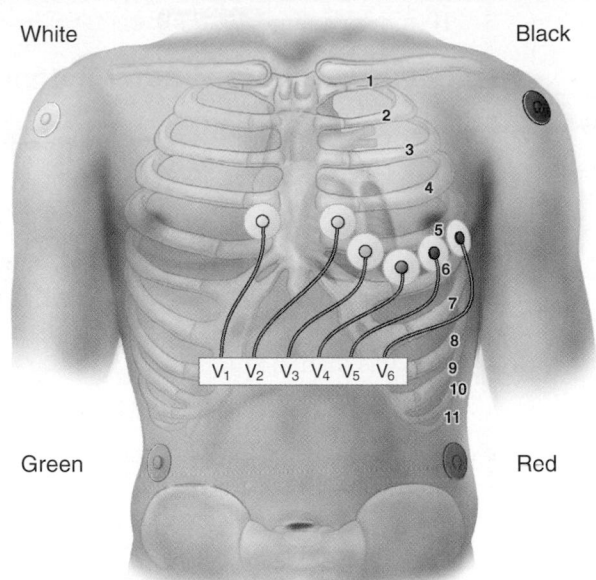

Lead	Location	View
V_1	4th intercostal space, right sternal border	Ventricular septum
V_2	4th intercostal space, left sternal border	Ventricular septum
V_3	Between V_2 and V_4	Anterior wall of left ventricle
V_4	5th intercostal space, midclavicular line	Anterior wall of left ventricle
V_5	Lateral to V_4 at the anterior axillary line	Lateral wall of left ventricle
V_6	Lateral to V_5 at the midaxillary line	Lateral wall of left ventricle

Figure 29 12-lead electrode placement.

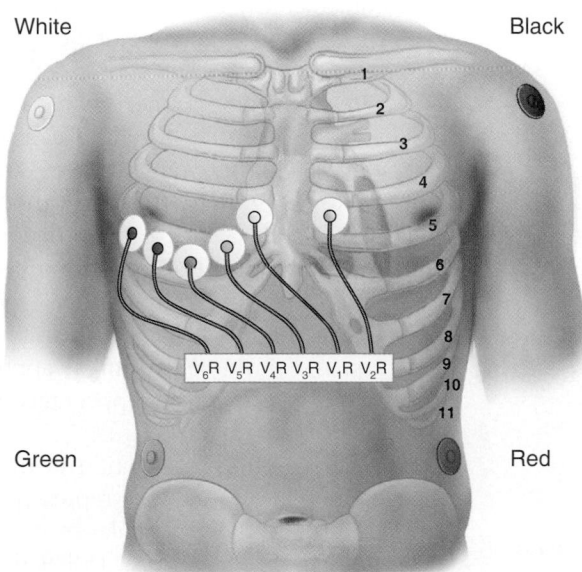

Lead	Location	View
V_1R	Left of sternum, 4th intercostal space (ICS)	Ventricular septum
V_2R	Right of sternum, 4th ICS	Ventricular septum
V_3R	Precisely between V_2 and V_1	Right ventricle
V_4R	Right midclavicular, 5th ICS	Right ventricle
V_5R	Precisely between V_4 and V_6	Right ventricle
V_6R	Right midaxillary, 5th ICS	Right ventricle

Figure 30 Placement of right-sided leads.

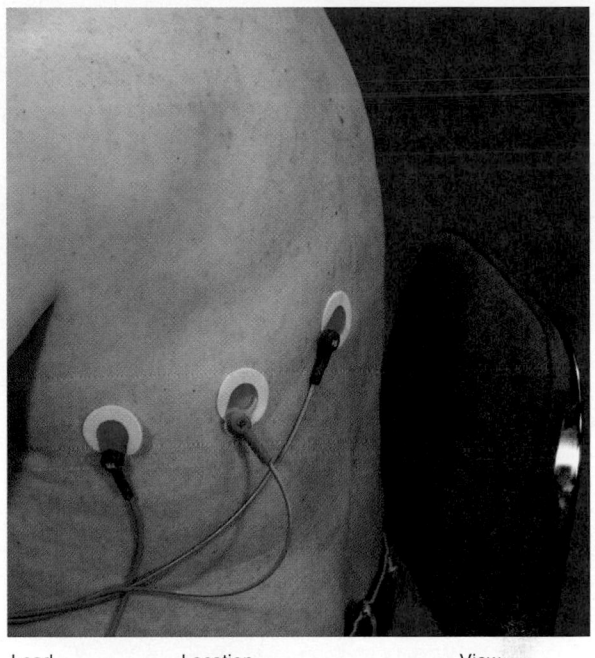

Lead	Location	View
V_7	Between V_6 and V_8, 5th intercostal space	Posterior wall of left ventricle
V_8	Midscapular, 5th intercostal space	Posterior wall of left ventricle
V_9	Just to the left of the spine, 5th intercostal space	Posterior wall of left ventricle

Figure 31 Placement of posterior leads.

The electrodes for the unipolar leads are the positive terminals for that lead. Recall that there is only one true pole in unipolar lead systems; the other end of the lead does not have polarity. For example, lead V_1 is positive at the V_1 electrode placement; the other end of the lead is Wilson's central terminal.

ECG Concepts

As mentioned, the ECG uses electrodes placed on the body to detect minute electrical waves traveling across surface of the skin. If an electrical wave moves in the direction of a positive electrode, this results in a deflection above baseline. Conversely, if an electrical wave moves in the direction of a negative electrode, this results in a deflection below baseline **Figures 34, 35, and 36**. The ECG baseline represents an electrically silent period during the cardiac cycle. The baseline is also referred to the **isoelectric** line, TP segment, and isomeric line.

A wave that travels perpendicularly to a lead results in one of two possibilities. The first is a perfectly flat line. The second is a wave that has a positive and a negative component. Waves containing both a positive and negative component are called biphasic waves.

The ECG Paper

ECGs are recorded on graph paper, which moves past a stylus at a standardized speed (25 mm/s). Thus, the horizontal distance on the graph paper represents a given time. Specifically, one small (1 mm) box is equivalent to 0.04 second (1/25th of a second), or 40 milliseconds, and one large box (which consists of five small boxes) is equivalent to 0.20 second, or 200 milliseconds

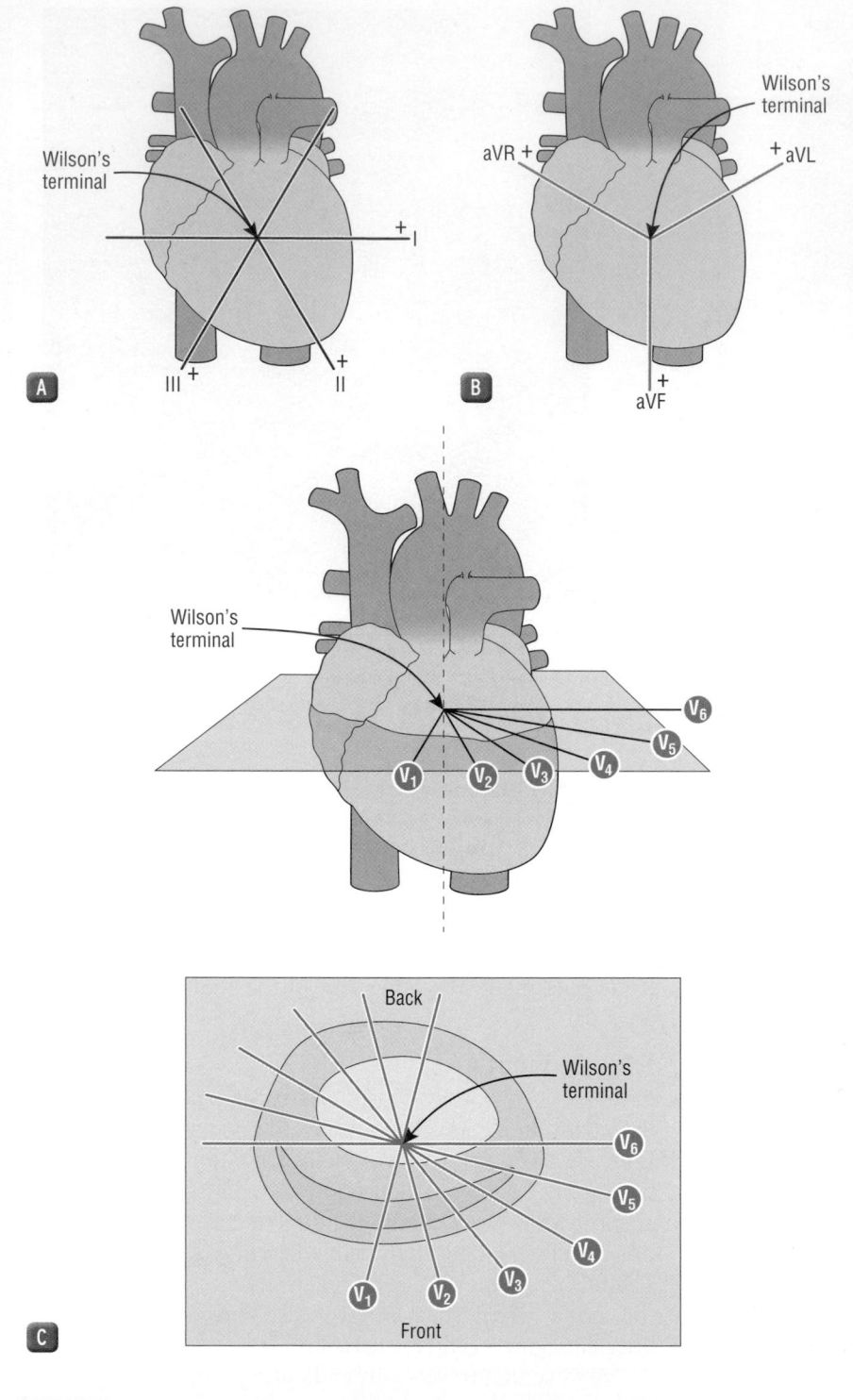

(0.04 × 5 = 0.20) **Figure 37** . The vertical axis on the graph paper represents the amplitude or "gain" of deflection in millivolts. The standard calibration for amplitude is 10 millimeters per millivolt. A calibration box is printed at the beginning of all ECGs. The calibration box informs the paramedic about the paper speed and amplitude and measures 5-mm wide by 10-mm tall, representing

the standard 25-mm/s paper speed and 10-mm/mV gain **Figure 38** .

Components of the ECG Rhythm

The components of an ECG rhythm correspond to electrical events occurring in the heart, as shown in **Figure 39** .

P Wave The P wave represents atrial depolarization and is characterized by a smooth, round, upright shape. The normal P wave duration is less than 110 ms and the amplitude less than 2.5 mm tall.

PR Interval The PR interval (PRI) includes atrial depolarization and the conduction of the impulse through the AV junction. It includes the slight delay that normally occurs when the impulse is held in the AV node, allowing time for ventricular filling **Figure 40** .

The PRI represents the amount of time it takes for the atria to depolarize and for the impulse to travel through the AV node. The PRI is measured from the start of the P wave to the point at which the QRS complex begins and has a normal duration of 0.12 to 0.20 s, or 120 to 200 ms (three to five small boxes on the ECG strip) **Figure 41** .

QRS Complex The QRS complex, which consists of three waveforms, represents depolarization of two simultaneously contracting ventricles. It is measured from the beginning of the Q wave to the end of the S wave and should follow each P wave in a consistent manner.

In healthy people, the QRS complex is narrow, with sharply pointed waves, and has a duration of less than 120 ms (three small boxes on the ECG strip). Such a complex indicates that conduction of the impulse has proceeded normally from the AV junction, through the bundle of His, left and right bundles, and the Purkinje system. If abnormal, the complex has a bizarre appearance and a duration of longer than 120 ms.

The first negative deflection in the QRS is called a Q wave; this wave represents conduction through the ventricular septum. The electricity spreads from right to left through the septum. The Q wave should last no more than 40 ms and should be less than one third the overall height of the QRS complex. The first upward deflection of the QRS is referred to as the R wave. Most of both ventricles are depolarized during the R wave. The S wave is any downward deflection after the R wave. If there is a second upward deflection, it is called an R-prime (R') wave.

J Point The J point is the point in the ECG where the QRS complex ends and the ST segment begins **Figure 42** . Thus, it

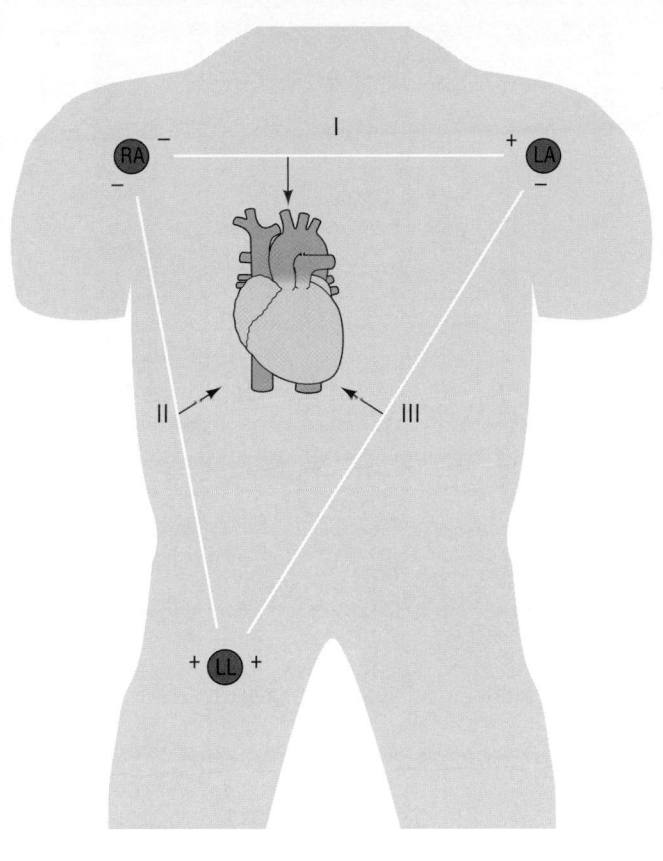

Figure 33 The bipolar leads each have a positive and negative end.

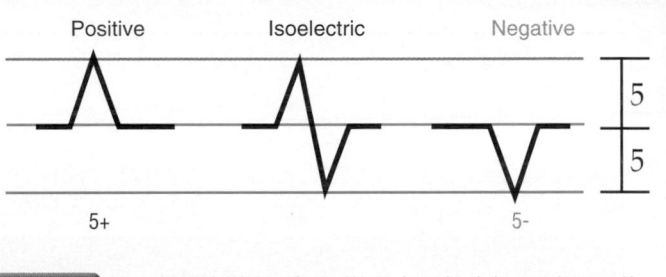

Figure 35 Representation of positive, isoelectric, and negative QRS deflections.

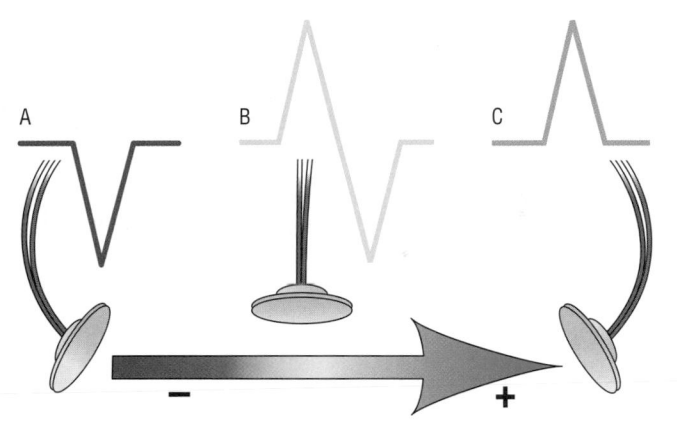

Figure 36 The size of a deflection on the ECG relates to the direction in which an electrical vector is moving, relative to the location of the electrode.

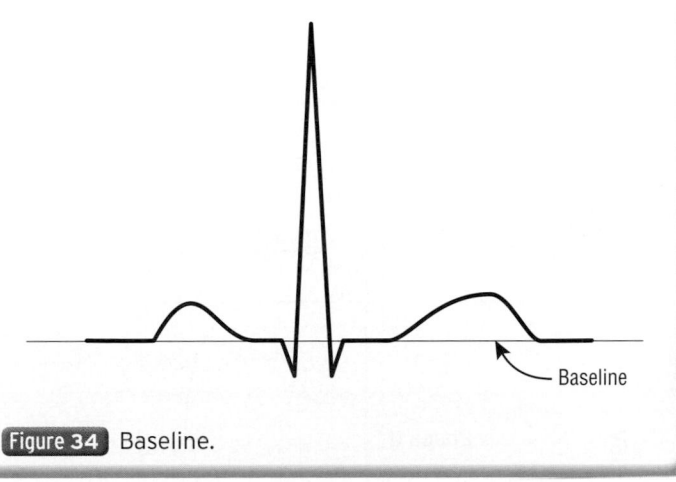

Figure 34 Baseline.

represents the end of depolarization and the apparent beginning of repolarization. The J point is significant because it often depresses or elevates when the myocardium is ischemic. J-point changes will be discussed later in this chapter.

ST Segment The ST segment begins at the J point and ends at the T wave. The ST represents early ventricular repolarization.

T Wave A T wave represents ventricular repolarization. The T wave should be asymmetric, be less than half the overall height of the QRS complex, and be oriented in the same direction as the overall QRS complex **Figure 43**. For example, if the QRS complex is predominantly upright, the T wave should be predominantly upright.

The T wave consists of two halves. The first half (closest to the QRS complex) represents a period of time called the absolute refractory period (ARP). During the ARP, the ventricles have not sufficiently repolarized to enable another depolarization. A helpful analogy is a flushing toilet. If you flush a toilet and then immediately try to flush it again, does the toilet flush? No! Why? Because the tank has not yet filled back up with water! The second half of the T wave represents the relative refractory period (RRP). The RRP indicates that some cells have repolarized sufficiently to depolarize again. Now think about flushing the toilet and waiting 15 seconds before flushing again. What happens this time? You get a partial flush because perhaps half the tank was able to fill with water before you flushed it again. So, during the ARP, nothing can stimulate the ventricles to contract again at that moment in time. During the RRP, however, a large stimulus can initiate depolarization of those cells that are repolarized.

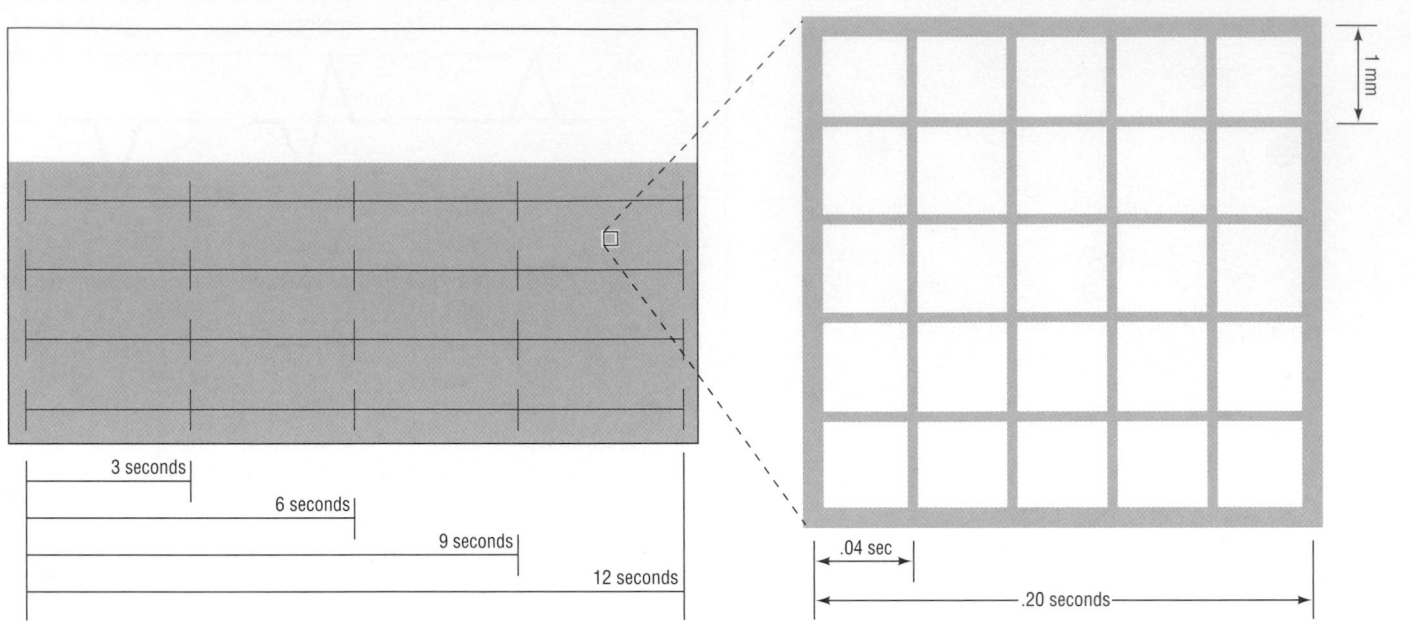

Figure 37 ECG paper. Height (amplitude) is measured in millimeters (mm) and width in milliseconds (ms) (.04 seconds equals 40 milliseconds; .20 seconds equals 200 milliseconds).

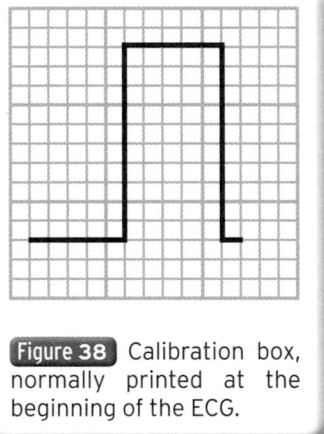

Figure 38 Calibration box, normally printed at the beginning of the ECG.

QT Interval The QT interval represents all the electrical activity of one complete ventricular cycle (that is, ventricular depolarization and repolarization). It begins with the onset of the Q wave and ends with the T wave as it comes back to the isoelectric line. If there is no Q wave, measurements begin with the R wave.

The QT interval normally lasts 360 to 440 ms.

■ Approach to Dysrhythmia Interpretation

Part of your role as a paramedic will be to interpret ECG strips from cardiac monitoring and be alert for dysrhythmia. Here, a five-step method is presented:

1. Identify the waves (P-QRS-T).
2. Measure the PRI.
3. Measure the QRS duration.
4. Determine rhythm regularity.
5. Measure the heart rate.

It is critical to follow this method each and every time so as not to overlook any important findings on the ECG tracing. You will usually exclusively use lead II to perform dysrhythmia interpretation.

We have already discussed where P, QRS, and T waves appear, and have discussed the PRI and QRS duration. When identifying whether there are P waves, note whether

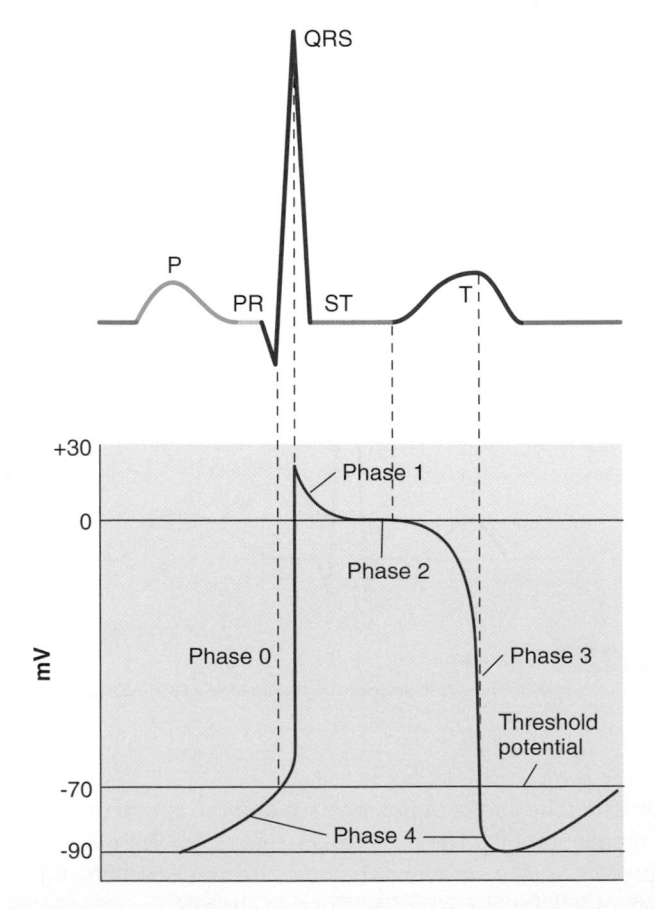

Figure 39 The components of an ECG rhythm correspond to the phases of myocyte stimulation.

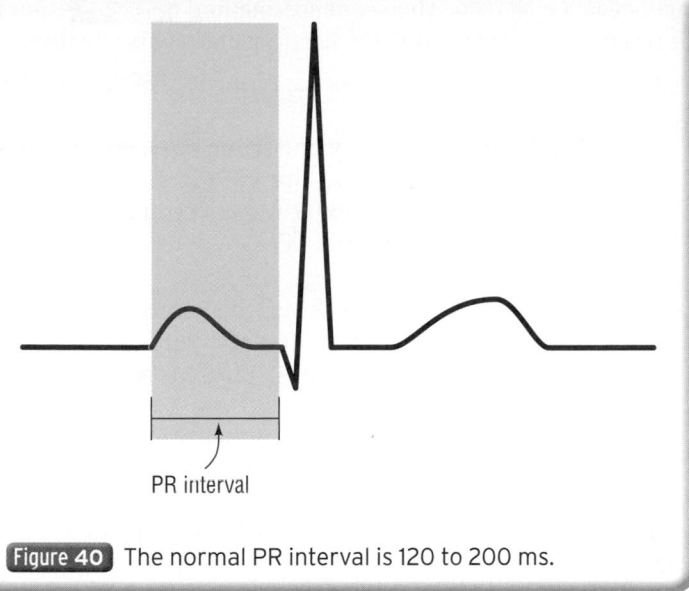

PR interval

Figure 40 The normal PR interval is 120 to 200 ms.

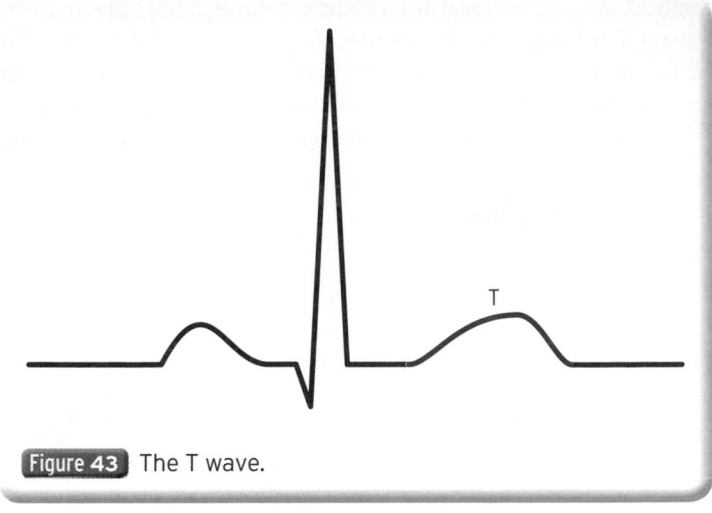

T

Figure 43 The T wave.

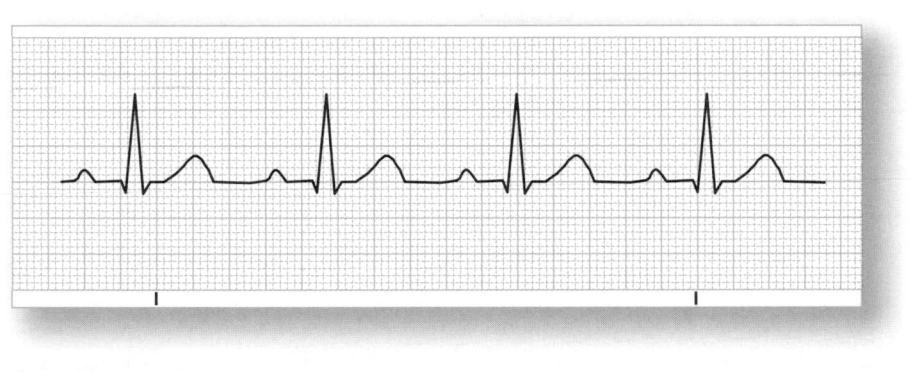

Figure 41 A PR interval greater than 200 ms is considered prolonged.

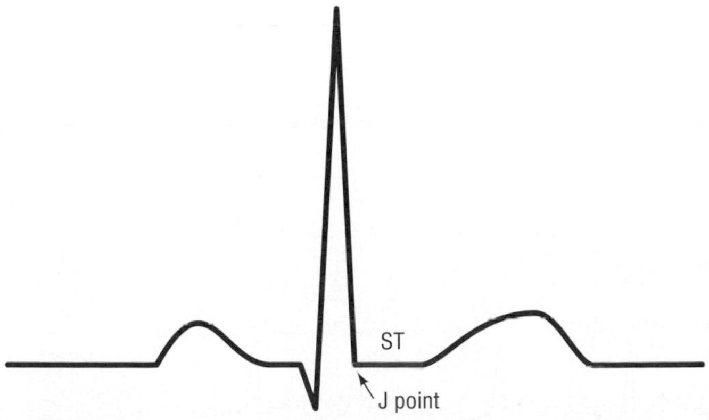

ST

J point

Figure 42 The J point.

Rhythm Regularity

A rhythm can be regular, regularly irregular, or irregularly irregular. Determining rhythm regularity is simple. Measuring the distance between R waves is one method used to evaluate rhythm regularity. If the distance is exactly the same between R waves, the rhythm is regular **Figure 44**. If no two R waves are equidistant, the rhythm is irregularly irregular **Figure 45**. If the R waves are irregular, but appear to follow a pattern, the rhythm is regularly irregular **Figure 46**. For example, you obtain the following data when measuring the distance between R waves: 25 mm, 27 mm, 30 mm, 25 mm, 27 mm, 30 mm. This represents a regularly irregular rhythm. ECG calipers can also be used to measure the distance between R waves, or the edge of a piece of paper may be used to create a "ruler."

Determining Heart Rate

This section describes some of the more common methods of determining the rate of a cardiac rhythm strip.

The 6-Second Method The 6-second method is the fastest method for measuring heart rate from the ECG. The 6-second

Words of Wisdom

Concordant precordial pattern refers to the direction of the QRS complexes in the precordial leads. For example, if all the QRS complexes are upright in leads V_1 to V_6, the QRS complexes exhibit concordance across the precordium. QRS concordance in the precordial leads can indicate several problems, including improper lead placement, anterior wall myocardial infarction, and ventricular tachycardia.

they are upright and within normal parameters. Is there only one P wave for every QRS complex? Next we will discuss how to determine rhythm regularity, and how to measure the heart rate.

method should be used for rhythms whose rates appear to be between 50 and 150 beats/min, and can be used on regular or irregular rhythms. In fact, the 6-second method is the best method for calculating heart rate involving irregular rhythms.

- Count the number of QRS complexes in a 6-second strip, and multiply that number by 10 to obtain the rate per minute Figure 47 .

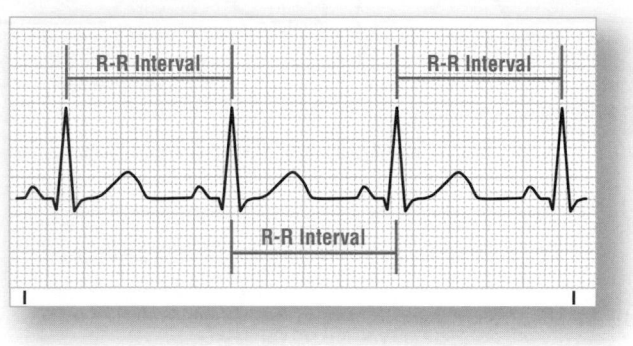

Figure 44   When the rhythm is regular, the R-R intervals are the same.

The Sequence Method The sequence method Figure 48 should be reserved for determining the heart rate of regular rhythms:

- First, memorize the following sequence: 300, 150, 100, 75, 60, 50.
- Find an R wave on a heavy line (large box), and count off "300, 150, 100, 75, 60, 50" for each large box you land on until you reach the next R wave. (Estimate the rate if the second R wave does not fall exactly on a heavy black line.)
- If the R-R interval spans fewer than three large boxes, the rate is greater than 100 (tachycardia). If it covers more than five large boxes, the rate is less than 60 (bradycardia).

The 1500 Method The 1500 method is the most accurate method for calculating heart rate from the ECG. It is typically used for heart rates in excess of 150 beats/min and can only be used on regular rhythms:

- Calculate the rate by counting the number of small boxes between any two QRS complexes (the R-R interval), and then divide that number into 1500.
- In Figure 49 , for example, there are approximately 23 small boxes between two successive QRS complexes; 1500/23 = 65, so this calculation shows that the rate is about 65 beats/min.

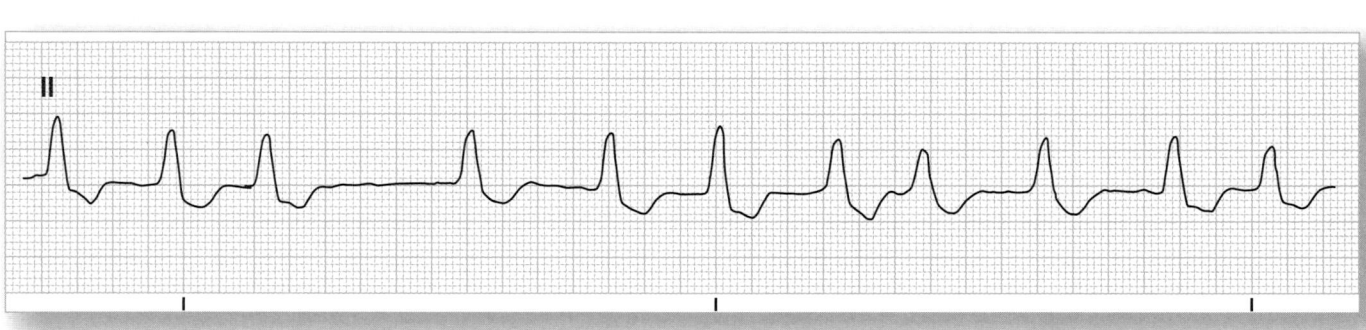

Figure 45   In an irregularly irregular rhythm, no two R-R intervals are the same.

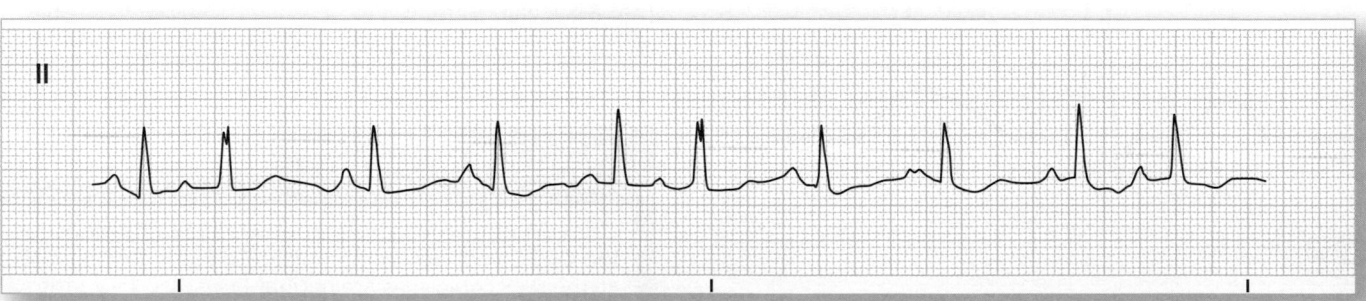

Figure 46   In a regularly irregular rhythm, there is a pattern in the R-R intervals.

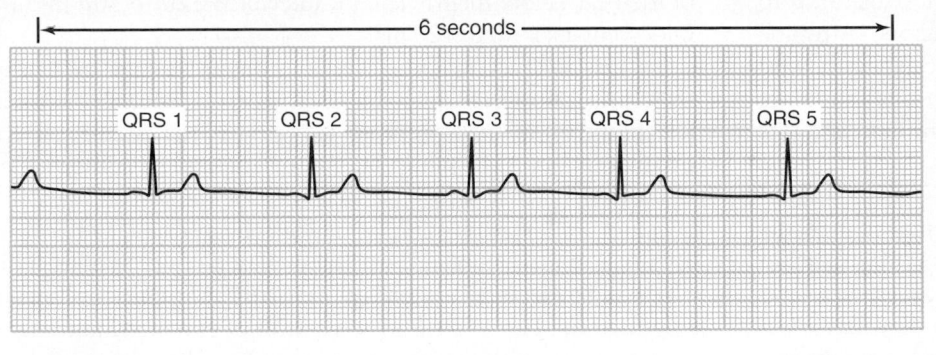

Figure 47 Calculation of rate. To calculate the rate, multiply the number of QRS complexes in a 6-second strip by 10.

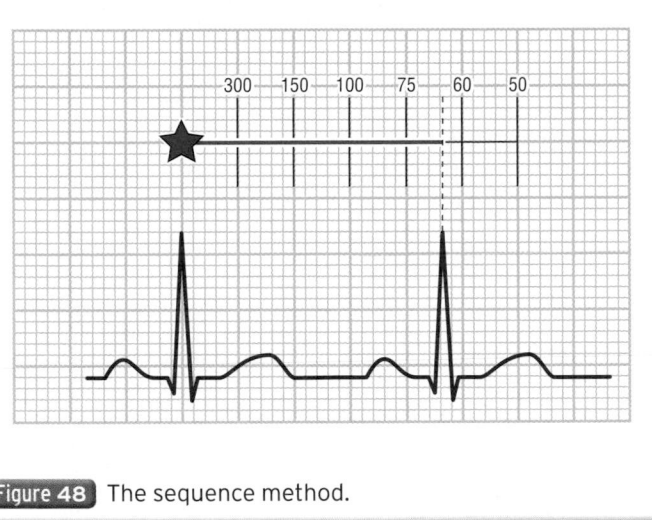

Figure 48 The sequence method.

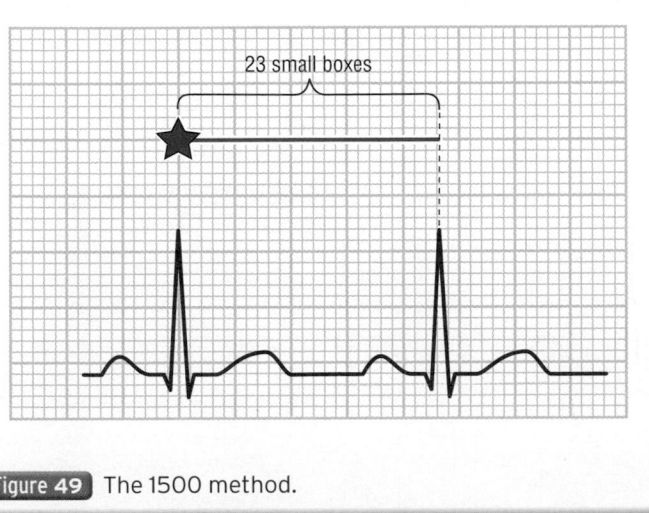

Figure 49 The 1500 method.

■ Specific Cardiac Dysrhythmias

Cardiac dysrhythmias can be induced by a variety of events. The flow of electricity through damaged or oxygen-deprived tissue is different than the flow through normal well-oxygenated tissue;

this sometimes appears as irregularities on the ECG. Many can be traced to ischemia in the heart, especially in areas related to the cardiac conduction system. Often ischemia will cause a particular area of the heart to spontaneously depolarize, resulting in a premature complex. These premature complexes interfere with the normal conduction of impulses and produce dysrhythmias. In other situations, the ischemia occurs within the conduction system itself, causing it to malfunction directly.

It is difficult to estimate the number of people affected by cardiac dysrhythmias because many dysrhythmias are well tolerated and cause no serious effects. It is well documented, however, that cardiac dysrhythmias are the most common cause of cardiac arrest.

There are nearly as many systems for classifying cardiac dysrhythmias as there are books written on the subject. Dysrhythmias may, for example, be categorized according to whether they are disturbances of automaticity or disturbances of conduction, whether they are tachydysrhythmias or bradydysrhythmias, or whether they are life threatening or non–life threatening. In this section, the cardiac dysrhythmias are addressed based on the site from which they arise (and as they appear in lead II). After looking at a normal sinus rhythm for comparison, the following section will cover the dysrhythmias that arise in the SA node, atrial tissue, AV node and junction, and ventricles. Lastly, paced rhythms will be explored.

Rhythms Originating in the SA Node
Normal Sinus Rhythm The SA node is the primary pacemaker for the heart. A **normal sinus rhythm** **Figure 50** has an intrinsic rate of 60 to 100 beats/min. The rhythm is regular, with minimal variation between R-R intervals. The P wave is present, is upright, and precedes each QRS complex. The PR interval will measure 120 to 200 ms. The QRS complex will measure 40 to 120 ms.

Sinus Bradycardia In **sinus bradycardia**, the pacemaker is still the SA node, but with a rate of less than 60 beats/min **Figure 51**. The rhythm is regular, and P waves are present and upright, preceding every QRS complex. The PR interval is 120 to 200 ms. The QRS complex is 40 to 120 ms.

Very slow heart rates (less than 40 to 50 beats/min) lead to inadequate CO and often precede electrical instability of the heart. Furthermore, when the sinus rate becomes very slow, ectopic pacemakers in the AV node or ventricles may fire and produce escape beats to assist in maintaining CO.

Sinus bradycardia can be an asymptomatic phenomenon in healthy adults and conditioned athletes and may be exhibited during sleep. More serious causes include hypothermia; SA node disease; AMI, which may stimulate vagal tone (parasympathetic stimulation); increased intracranial pressure; and use of beta blockers, calcium channel blockers, morphine, quinidine (including interactions between quinidine and some calcium channel blockers), or digitalis.

In general, treatment focuses on the patient's tolerance to the bradycardia and looking for causative factors. Atropine may be necessary if the patient is symptomatic. Patients who are symptomatic and do not respond to atropine may require a transcutaneous pacemaker to assist the heart in increasing its ventricular rate.

Sinus Tachycardia The SA node is still the pacemaker in <u>sinus tachycardia</u> but demonstrates a rate of more than 100 beats/min **Figure 52**. The rhythm is regular, and P waves are present and upright, preceding every QRS complex (although they may occasionally be difficult to see if they are partially buried in the T wave

of the beat before them). The PR interval is 120 to 200 ms. The QRS complex is 40 to 120 ms.

Sinus tachycardia may result from a variety of causes, including pain, fever, hypoxia, hypovolemia, exercise, stimulation of the sympathetic nervous system (such as by stress, fright, or anxiety), an AMI, pump failure, or anemia. In addition, certain drugs (such as atropine, epinephrine, amphetamines, and cocaine), caffeine, nicotine, and alcohol can cause tachycardia. Hypoxia, metabolic alkalosis, hypokalemia, and hypocalcemia can lead to electrical instability; cells that normally do not fire impulses can begin to do so. This kind of enhanced automaticity may occur with the use of drugs such as digitalis or atropine

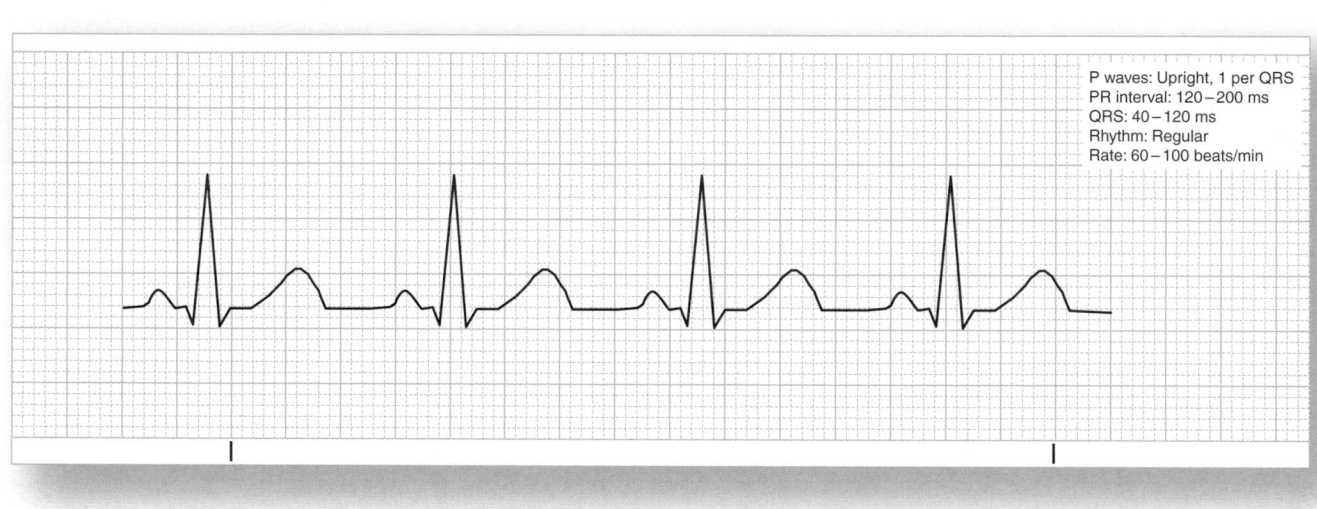

P waves: Upright, 1 per QRS
PR interval: 120–200 ms
QRS: 40–120 ms
Rhythm: Regular
Rate: 60–100 beats/min

Figure 50   Normal sinus rhythm.

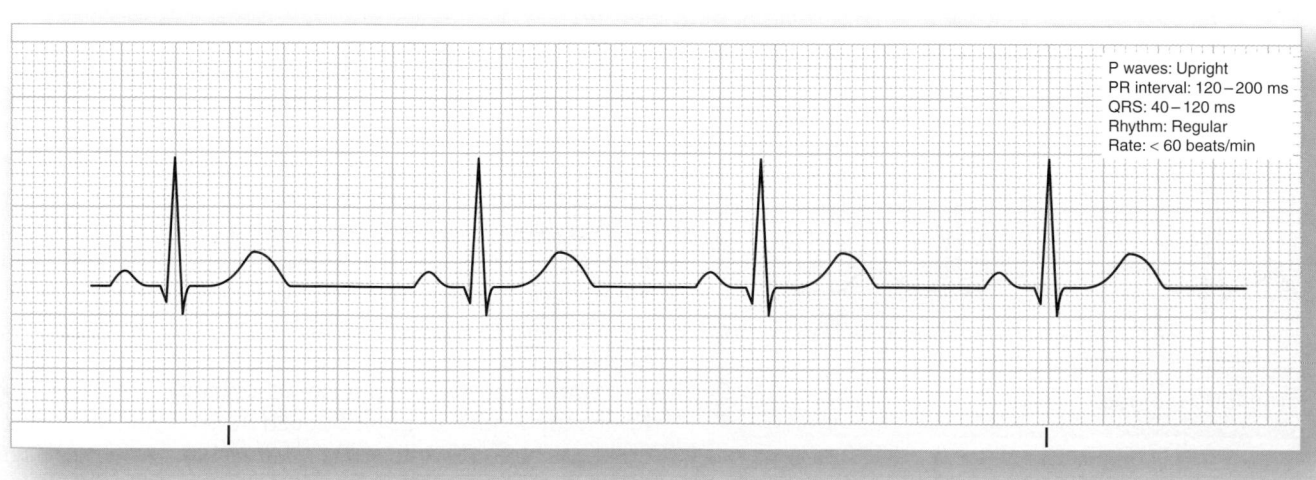

P waves: Upright
PR interval: 120–200 ms
QRS: 40–120 ms
Rhythm: Regular
Rate: < 60 beats/min

Figure 51   Sinus bradycardia.

and is manifested by ectopic beats anywhere in the heart. The result is the potential for tachycardias, flutters, and fibrillations in the atria or ventricles, heralding serious rhythms such as ventricular tachycardia and ventricular fibrillation. Circus reentry can also be a serious problem **Figure 53**. The AV node may be bombarded by more than one impulse—potentially blocking the pathway for one impulse and allowing the other to stimulate cardiac cells that have already depolarized. The danger here comes when these impulses get "stuck" in a pattern of repetition, causing multiple ectopic beats or ventricular fibrillation.

Prolonged tachycardia increases the work of the heart, leading to further ischemia and infarction during an AMI. In addition, CO may be significantly reduced when the heart rate exceeds 120 to 140 beats/min because the ventricles do not have enough time between contractions to fill completely with blood.

The treatment of sinus tachycardia is related to the underlying cause.

Sinus Dysrhythmia <u>Sinus dysrhythmia</u> is defined as a slight variation in cycling of a sinus rhythm, usually one that exceeds 120 ms between the longest and shortest cycles **Figure 54**. The SA node is still the pacemaker; P waves are present and upright, preceding every QRS complex; and a PR interval of 120 to 200 ms still exists. The QRS complex is 40 to 120 ms.

Sinus dysrhythmia is often somewhat more prominent with fluctuation in the respiratory cycle because the heart rate

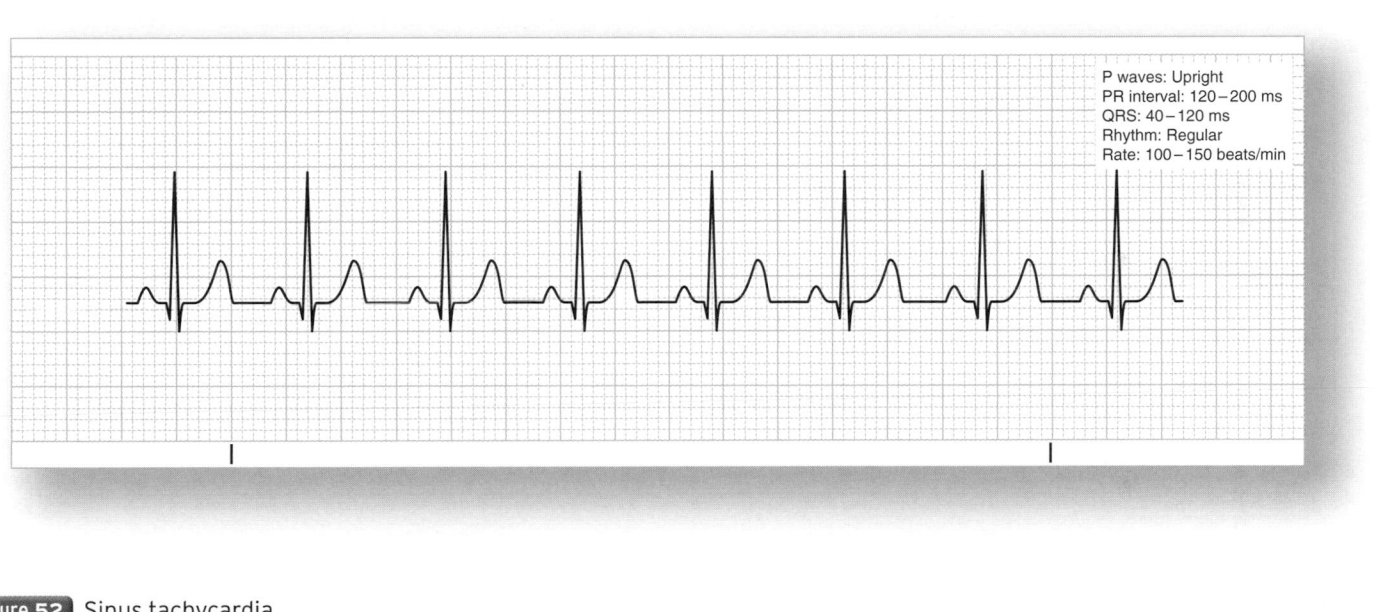

> P waves: Upright
> PR interval: 120–200 ms
> QRS: 40–120 ms
> Rhythm: Regular
> Rate: 100–150 beats/min

Figure 52 Sinus tachycardia.

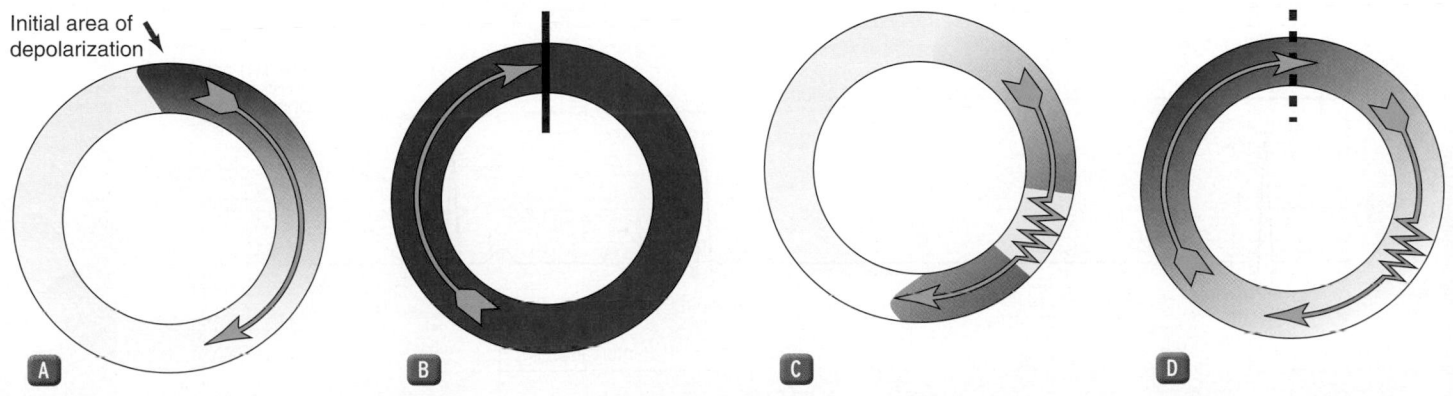

Figure 53 **A.** The original impulse site fires and triggers a depolarization wave that spreads throughout the rest of the cells in the direction shown. **B.** By the time the depolarization wave reaches the original site (represented by the black line) the original site is still refractory and cannot accept the new impulse. The depolarization wave essentially dies at this point. **C.** The area in yellow represents an area of slow conduction. The depolarization wave slows down as it traverses this area. **D.** By the time the depolarization wave reaches the original site (represented by the dotted black line), the original site is now ready to receive a new impulse. The result is a circus movement that is self-perpetuating.

accelerates with inspiration and slows with expiration. Increased filling pressures of the heart during inspiration stimulate the Bainbridge reflex, which increases the heart rate and is partially responsible for respiratory sinus dysrhythmia. The increased filling pressure on the heart increases SV (remember the Frank-Starling mechanism) and blood pressure. The increase in blood pressure stimulates the baroreceptor reflex (baroreflex), which attempts to block the rate increase caused by the Bainbridge reflex. In this way, the baroreflex inhibits the respiratory sinus dysrhythmia.

Sinus dysrhythmia is often a normal finding in children and young adults and tends to diminish or disappear with age.

Sinus Arrest Sinus arrest occurs when the SA node fails to initiate an impulse, eliminating the P wave, QRS complex, or/and T wave for one cardiac cycle **Figure 55**. After this missed set of complexes, the SA node resumes normal functioning just as if nothing ever happened. In sinus arrest, the atrial and ventricular rates are usually within normal limits and the rhythm is regular except for the absent complexes. P waves are present and upright, preceding every QRS complex, and the PR interval,

when present, is 120 to 200 ms. The QRS complex, when present, is 40 to 120 ms.

Common causes of sinus arrest include ischemia of the SA node, increased vagal tone, carotid sinus massage (discussed later in this chapter), and use of drugs such as digitalis and quinidine. Occasional episodes of sinus arrest are not significant; however, if the heart rate drops below 30 to 50 beats/min, the CO may fall and an ectopic focus from the ventricles may take over. In such a case, treatment is based on the overall heart rate and tolerance by the patient and may include a temporary pacemaker (a transvenous pacer in the field) or a permanent pacemaker once the patient is admitted to the hospital.

Sick Sinus Syndrome Sick sinus syndrome (SSS) encompasses a variety of rhythms that involve a poorly functioning SA node and is common in elderly patients. On an ECG, SSS announces itself in many ways, including sinus bradycardia, sinus arrest, SA block, and alternating patterns of extreme bradycardia and tachycardia (bradycardia-tachycardia syndrome). As a result of SSS, some patients may experience a syncopal or near-syncopal

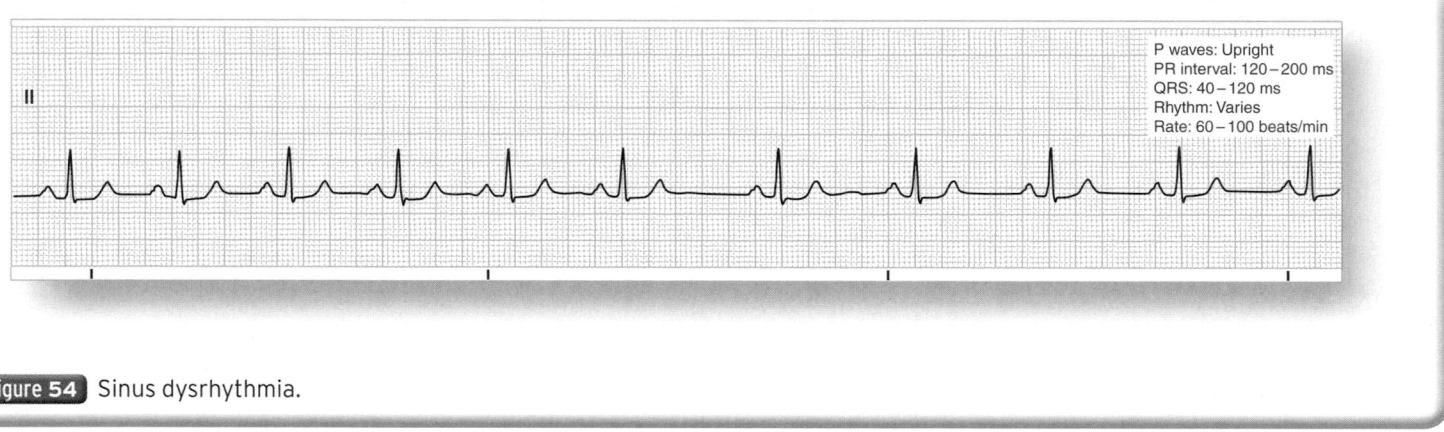

P waves: Upright
PR interval: 120–200 ms
QRS: 40–120 ms
Rhythm: Varies
Rate: 60–100 beats/min

Figure 54 Sinus dysrhythmia.

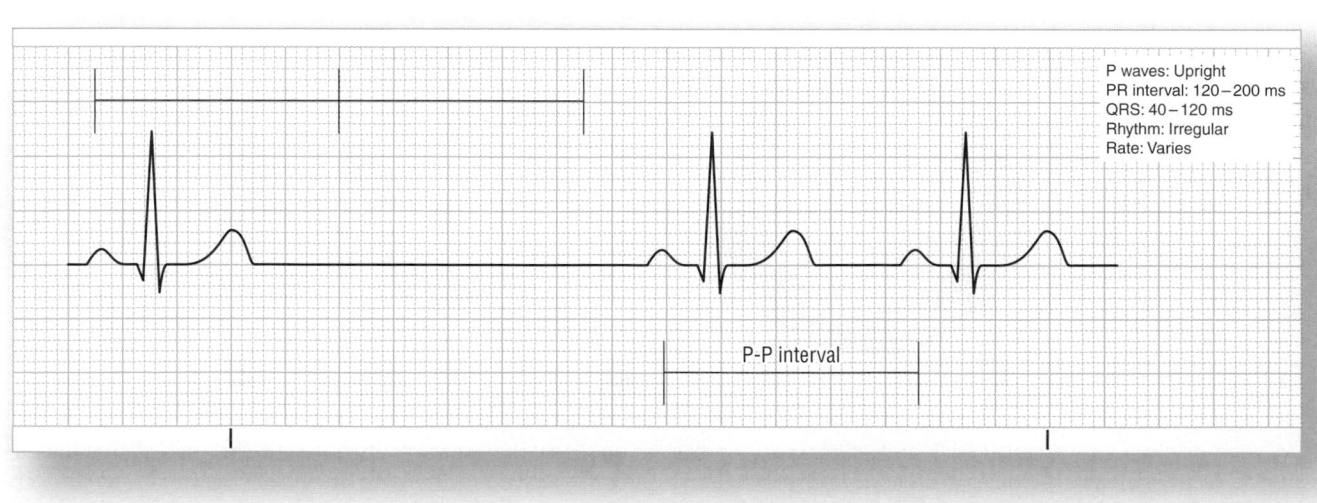

P waves: Upright
PR interval: 120–200 ms
QRS: 40–120 ms
Rhythm: Irregular
Rate: Varies

P-P interval

Figure 55 Sinus arrest.

episode, dizziness, and palpitations. Other patients remain asymptomatic.

Rhythms Originating in the Atria

Although the SA node is normally the pacemaker for the heart, any area in the atria may originate an impulse, thereby usurping the pacemaking authority of the SA node within the body's electrical conduction system. Rhythms originating from the atria will have upright P waves that precede each QRS complex but that are not as well rounded as those coming from the SA node. Atrial rhythms generally result in heart rates of 60 to 100 beats/min.

Atrial rhythms can be grouped into those that are common and those that are rare. This section is organized in that order, beginning with those that are common.

Atrial Flutter Atrial flutter is a rhythm in which the atria contract at a rate much too rapid for the ventricles to match **Figure 56**. The atrial complexes in atrial flutter are known as flutter or F waves rather than P waves. F waves have a distinctive shape, resembling a sawtooth or picket fence.

In atrial flutter, one or more of the F waves is blocked by the AV node, resulting in several flutter waves before each QRS complex. The rhythm may be regular (most common), with a constant (usually 2:1) conduction, or irregular if the conduction of impulses to the ventricles varies. The QRS complex will measure 40 to 120 ms.

Atrial flutter is usually a sign of a serious heart problem. In many cases, it is a transient rhythm that degenerates into atrial fibrillation. Treatment generally consists of medication or electrical cardioversion, although neither of these measures is usually attempted in the field unless the patient's condition is critical and transport time is long.

Atrial Fibrillation Atrial fibrillation is a rhythm in which the atria no longer contract but rather fibrillate or quiver without any organized contraction **Figure 57**. It occurs when many different cells in the atria depolarize independently rather than in response to an impulse from the SA node. The result of this random depolarization, which occurs throughout the atria, is a fibrillating or chaotic baseline.

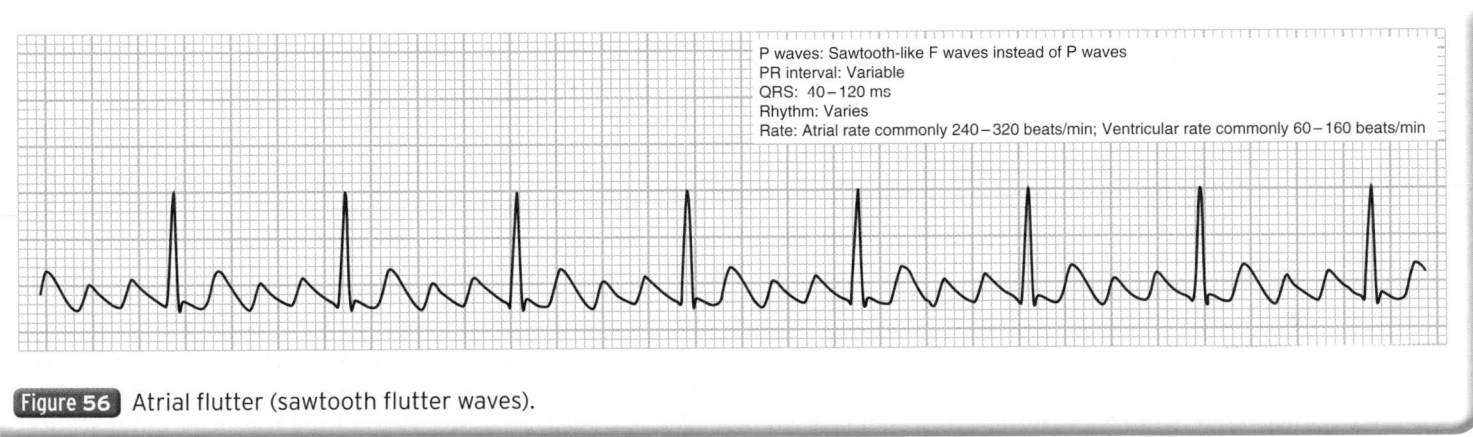

P waves: Sawtooth-like F waves instead of P waves
PR interval: Variable
QRS: 40–120 ms
Rhythm: Varies
Rate: Atrial rate commonly 240–320 beats/min; Ventricular rate commonly 60–160 beats/min

Figure 56 Atrial flutter (sawtooth flutter waves).

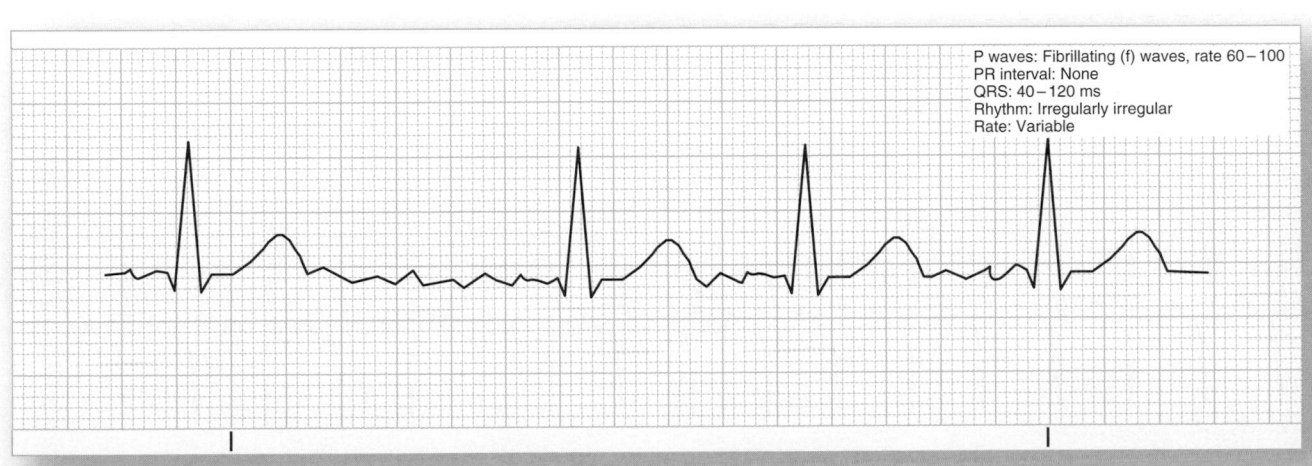

P waves: Fibrillating (f) waves, rate 60–100
PR interval: None
QRS: 40–120 ms
Rhythm: Irregularly irregular
Rate: Variable

Figure 57 Atrial fibrillation.

In atrial fibrillation, there are usually no visible P waves on the ECG strip and, hence, no PR interval to measure. Instead, one of the keys to identifying this condition is its "irregularly irregular" appearance. Because the AV node is bombarded with impulses from the fibrillating atria, it allows impulses to pass on to the ventricles in a random manner, which results in the highly irregular ventricular rhythm. The QRS complex will measure 40 to 120 ms.

Atrial fibrillation is usually a sign of a serious heart problem and is a fairly common rhythm among elderly patients. One of the main hazards associated with this dysrhythmia is that the blood moving through the fibrillating atria has a tendency to form small clots, which may then become emboli and block circulation elsewhere in the body. There is an increased risk of stroke in a patient with atrial fibrillation. Because of this risk, many elderly patients whose normal rhythm is atrial fibrillation take an anticoagulant medication such as warfarin (Coumadin), as well as other medications, such as digitalis, to regulate the rate of ventricular response. A newer class of drugs, direct thrombin inhibitors, is used to prevent blood clots in patients who are at risk, such as those with atrial fibrillation. Prehospital treatment of atrial fibrillation is rare because of the risks involved. If required, it consists of electrical cardioversion when the patient's condition is critical and transport time is long.

Supraventricular Tachycardia Supraventricular tachycardia (SVT) is defined as a tachycardic rhythm originating from a pacemaker above the ventricles Figure 58. Once called atrial tachycardia, it occurs when the true origin of a tachycardia is unknown (which is why the name was changed).

When tachycardias reach 150 to 180 beats/min, the P waves (if present) tend to be completely obscured by the T wave of the preceding beat. At lower heart rates, P waves can be identified; thus, to be considered SVT, a rhythm should have a rate exceeding 150 beats/min. The rhythm is regular, with essentially no variation between R-R intervals. SVT is known to originate from a point above the ventricles because the QRS complexes are of normal width. The PR interval is not measurable because the P wave is obscured. The QRS complex will measure 40 to 120 ms.

Patients who present with SVT can have a physical finding known as cannon "A" waves. Cannon "A" waves are created when there becomes dissociation between the atria and ventricles. This sign can also present itself when there is a right atrial contraction against a closed tricuspid valve. Larger "A" waves can present indicating that there is a decrease in the functionality of the right ventricle or an increase in the right ventricular end diastolic pressure. The physical sign can be found where the jugular veins are located; during the cannon "A" wave, a depression of the jugular veins occurs that forms an "A."

SVT is often referred to as paroxysmal SVT (PSVT), reflecting its tendency to begin and end abruptly (*paroxysmal* means "occurring in spasms"). Technically, to call this dysrhythmia a PSVT, you would need to witness the rhythm speed up on the ECG. The most up-to-date terminology used today is reentry SVT.

When the ventricular rate exceeds 150 beats/min, the ventricular filling time is greatly diminished, which will in turn greatly reduce the CO. For this reason, SVT should be treated promptly. The treatment, which is discussed later in this chapter, includes using medication or electrical therapy to slow the heart rate.

Premature Atrial Complex A premature atrial complex (PAC) is not, strictly speaking, a dysrhythmia, but rather the existence of a particular complex within another rhythm Figure 59. Premature atrial complexes are also known as ectopic complexes, meaning that they occur out of the normal location. A PAC occurs earlier in time than the next expected sinus complex, leading to an abnormally short R-R interval between it and the previous complex. Because the heart rate depends on the underlying rhythm, the presence of a PAC will make the rhythm irregular. The P wave is present and upright and precedes each QRS complex; however, its shape differs from the shapes of the P waves originating from the SA node, as an indication of its different site of origin. The PR interval will measure 120 to 200 ms but may

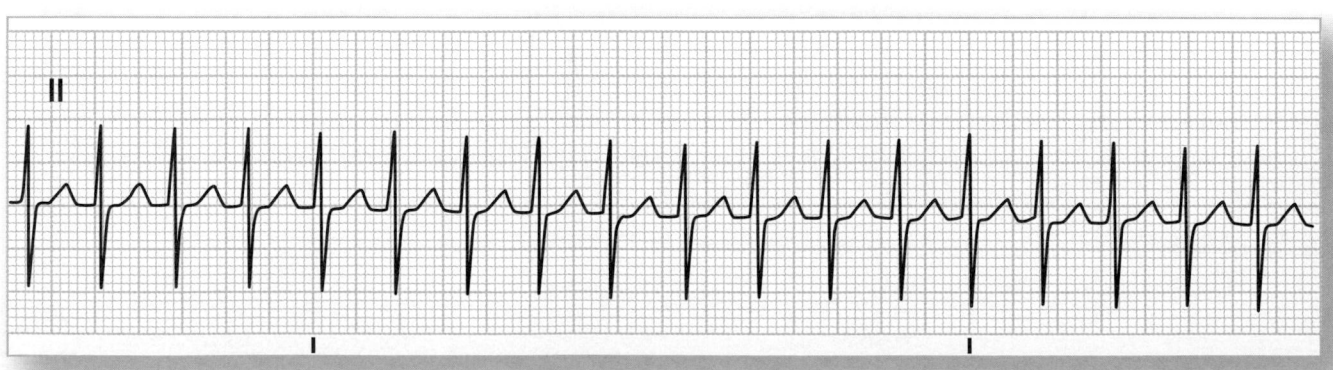

Figure 58 Supraventricular tachycardia.

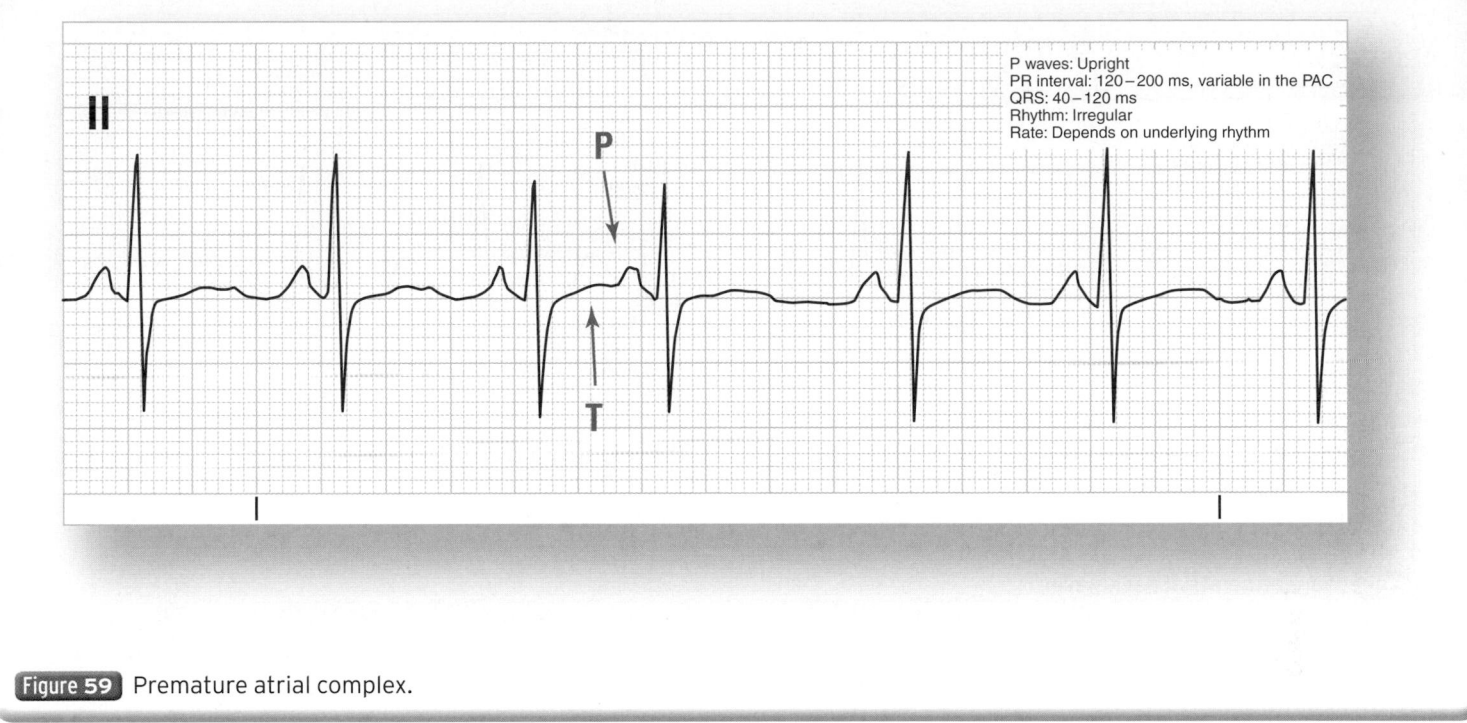

P waves: Upright
PR interval: 120–200 ms, variable in the PAC
QRS: 40–120 ms
Rhythm: Irregular
Rate: Depends on underlying rhythm

Figure 59 Premature atrial complex.

vary slightly based on the origin of the premature complex. The QRS complex will measure 40 to 120 ms.

Premature atrial complexes are not always conducted to the ventricles. The presence of a P wave that occurs early on the ECG and which is not followed by a QRS complex is referred to as a non-conducted PAC. These should not be confused with AV nodal heart blocks. The two are easily differentiated because non-conducted PACs generally occur infrequently and in no particular pattern (unlike heart block), and the P wave associated with the non-conducted PAC occurs early on the ECG. That is, if you measure the P-P interval, the P wave associated with non-conducted PAC will be shorter than the other P-P intervals (unlike heart block where the P-P interval is constant).

A PAC can be caused by use of a variety of drugs (including caffeine), or it may result from organic heart disease. It is not usually treated in the prehospital setting but may be a predictor of future cardiac dysrhythmias.

Wandering Atrial Pacemaker

In wandering atrial pacemaker, as the name suggests, the pacemaker of the heart **Figure 60** moves from the SA node to various areas within the atria. Wandering atrial pacemaker usually has a rate of 60 to 100 beats/min. The rhythm is slightly irregular, with variations between R-R intervals based on the site of the pacemaker for that particular complex. The P wave is present and upright and precedes each QRS complex; however, the shapes of the P waves vary as an indication of their different sites of origin. The definition of wandering atrial pacemaker depends on having at least three different shapes of P waves within one ECG strip. The PR interval will measure 120 to 200 ms, but will also vary slightly based on the origin of the particular complex. The QRS complex will measure 40 to 120 ms.

Wandering atrial pacemaker is most commonly seen in patients with significant lung disease. Treatment is usually not indicated in the prehospital setting, although the rhythm is an indication of likely future cardiac complications.

Multifocal Atrial Tachycardia

In multifocal atrial tachycardia (MAT), the pacemaker of the heart moves within various areas of the atria **Figure 61**. Multifocal atrial tachycardia is characterized by a rate of more than 100 beats/min and is, in effect, a tachycardic wandering atrial pacemaker. The rhythm is irregular, with variation between R-R intervals based on the site of the pacemaker for that particular complex. The P wave is present and upright and precedes each QRS complex; however, the shapes of the P waves vary as an indication of their different sites of origin. The PR interval will measure 120 to 200 ms, but also varies slightly based on the origin of the particular complex. If the MAT increases to a rate exceeding 150 beats/min, the P waves may no longer be visible; thus, the only indication of the rhythm may be the irregularity associated with the varying sites of origin within the atria. The QRS complex will measure 40 to 120 ms.

Like a wandering atrial pacemaker, MAT is most commonly seen in patients with significant lung disease. Treatment is usually not attempted in the prehospital setting, and therapies aimed at correcting SVT are usually ineffective with MAT.

Rhythms Originating in the AV Node or AV Junction

If the SA node—the body's dominant pacemaker—fails to initiate an impulse, the AV node will take over as pacemaker of the heart. Rhythms originating from the AV node are commonly referred to as "junctional" rhythms owing to the proximity of the AV node to the junction of the atria and ventricles. Junctional rhythms feature inverted or missing P waves but normal QRS complexes.

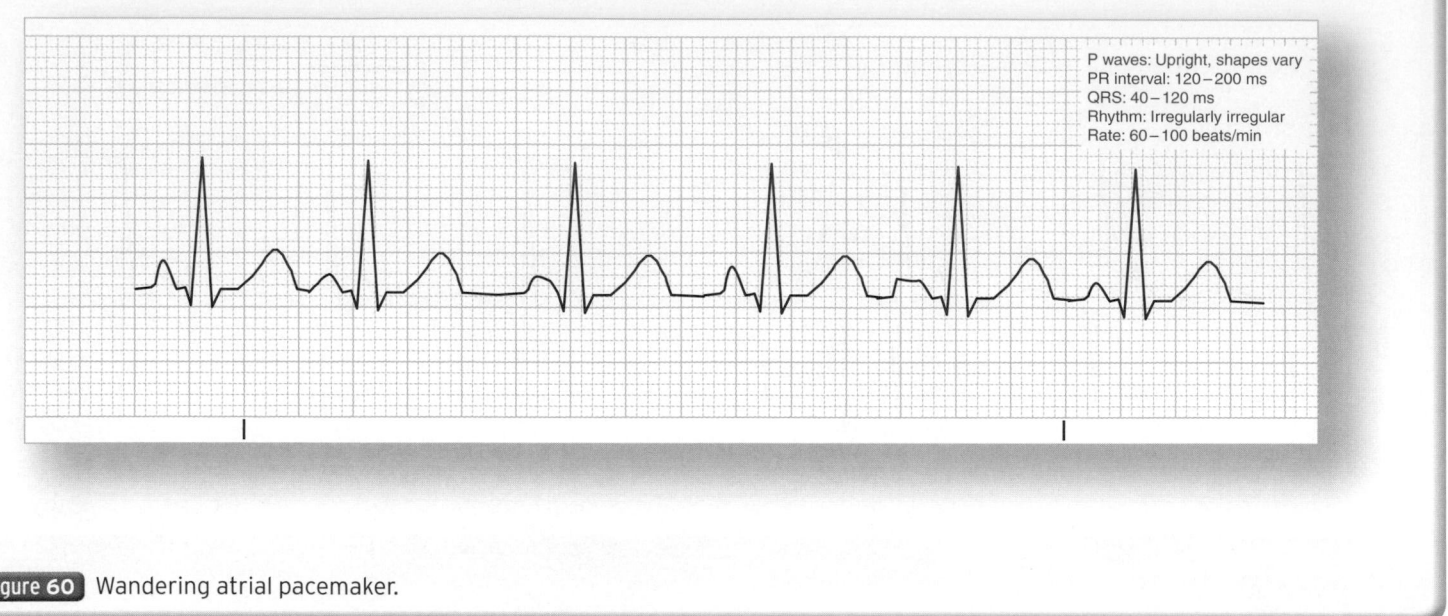

P waves: Upright, shapes vary
PR interval: 120–200 ms
QRS: 40–120 ms
Rhythm: Irregularly irregular
Rate: 60–100 beats/min

Figure 60 Wandering atrial pacemaker.

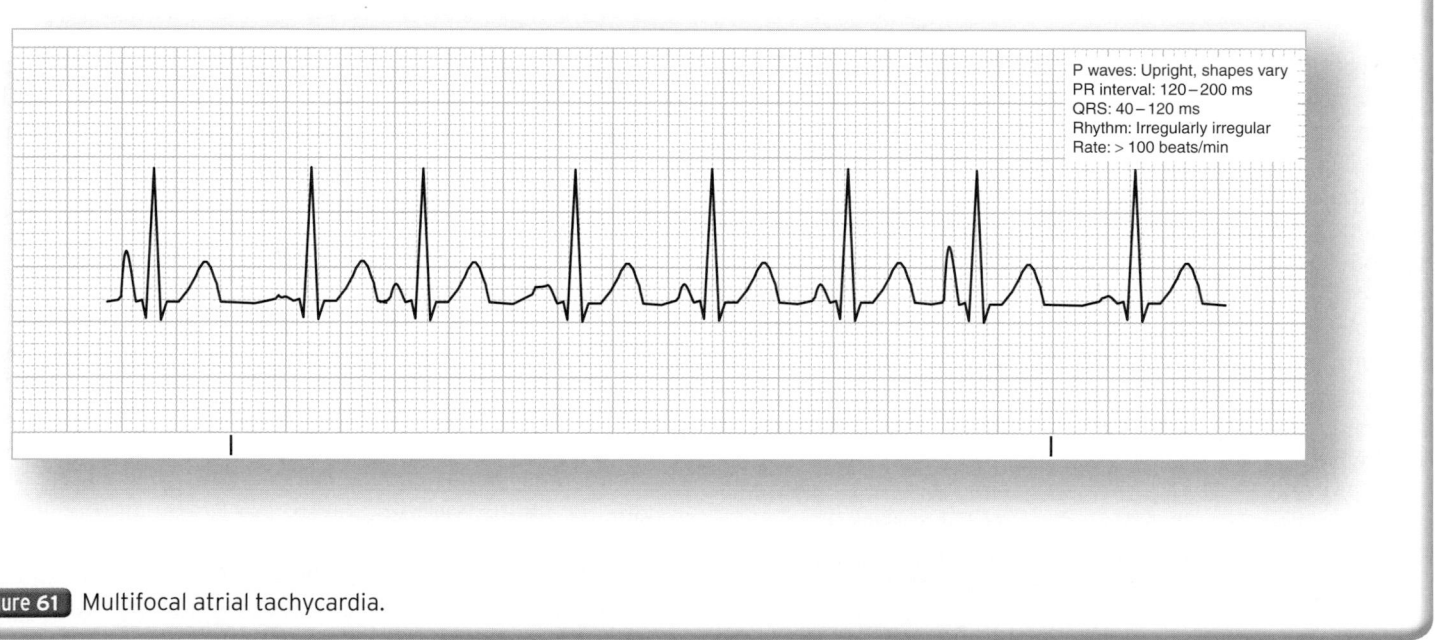

P waves: Upright, shapes vary
PR interval: 120–200 ms
QRS: 40–120 ms
Rhythm: Irregularly irregular
Rate: > 100 beats/min

Figure 61 Multifocal atrial tachycardia.

When an impulse is generated in the AV node, it travels down through the conduction system into the ventricles as if it had come from the SA node, resulting in normal QRS complexes. At the same time, the impulse travels upward through the atria and the internodal pathways toward the SA node. There are then three possible cases, none of which includes an upright P wave, but in which the QRS complex appears normal:

- If the impulse begins moving upward through the atria before the other part of it enters the ventricles, an upside-down P wave will be visible (upside down because the impulse is traveling in the opposite direction from that which causes normal upright P waves). This P wave is usually followed immediately by the QRS complex, without any pause between the two.

- If the impulse moving through the atria occurs at the exact same time as the impulse is traveling through the ventricles, the smaller inverted P wave will be buried within the larger QRS complex. This will give the appearance of a missing P wave—that is, the baseline remains flat until the beginning of a normal QRS complex.

- The impulse may start late through the atria and result in an inverted P wave appearing after the QRS complex.

Because the intrinsic rate of the AV node is 40 to 60, junctional rhythms normally present with rates of 40 to 60 beats/min.

Junctional (Escape) Rhythm A <u>junctional rhythm</u> occurs when the SA node ceases functioning and the AV node takes over as the pacemaker of the heart **Figure 62**. Because this allows the heart to "escape" from stopping completely, junctional rhythms are sometimes referred to as junctional escape rhythms. A normal junctional escape rhythm has a rate of 40 to 60 beats/min owing to the intrinsic rate of the AV node as a pacemaker. A junctional escape rhythm is usually regular, with little variation between R-R intervals. The P wave, if present, is inverted or upside down but may appear to be absent. The PR interval, if an inverted P wave is present, will measure less than 120 ms. The QRS complex will measure 40 to 120 ms.

Junctional rhythms are most commonly seen in patients with significant problems with the SA node. Treatment usually consists of a surgically implanted pacemaker. Thus, little can be done in the field other than to institute <u>transcutaneous pacing</u> if the patient's condition is severely compromised.

Accelerated Junctional Rhythm Occasionally, a junctional rhythm will present with a rate that exceeds its normal upper rate of 60 beats/min but remains less than 100 beats/min. Because the rhythm is greater than 60 beats/min, it cannot be considered a "normal" junctional rhythm; because it is less than 100 beats/min, it cannot be called tachycardia either. In this case, the name given the rhythm is accelerated junctional rhythm.

An accelerated junctional rhythm is also regular, with little variation between R-R intervals **Figure 63**. The P wave, if present, is inverted or upside down but may appear to be absent. The PR interval, if an inverted P wave is present, will measure less than 120 ms. The QRS complex will measure 40 to 120 ms.

Accelerated junctional rhythms are serious, but they seldom require treatment in the prehospital setting because the rate is usually fast enough to maintain a reasonable CO.

Junctional Tachycardia Occasionally, a junctional rhythm will present with a rate that exceeds 100 beats/min. Any rhythm that results in a ventricular rate of greater than 100 beats/min is referred to as tachycardia. In this case, the rhythm is termed junctional tachycardia.

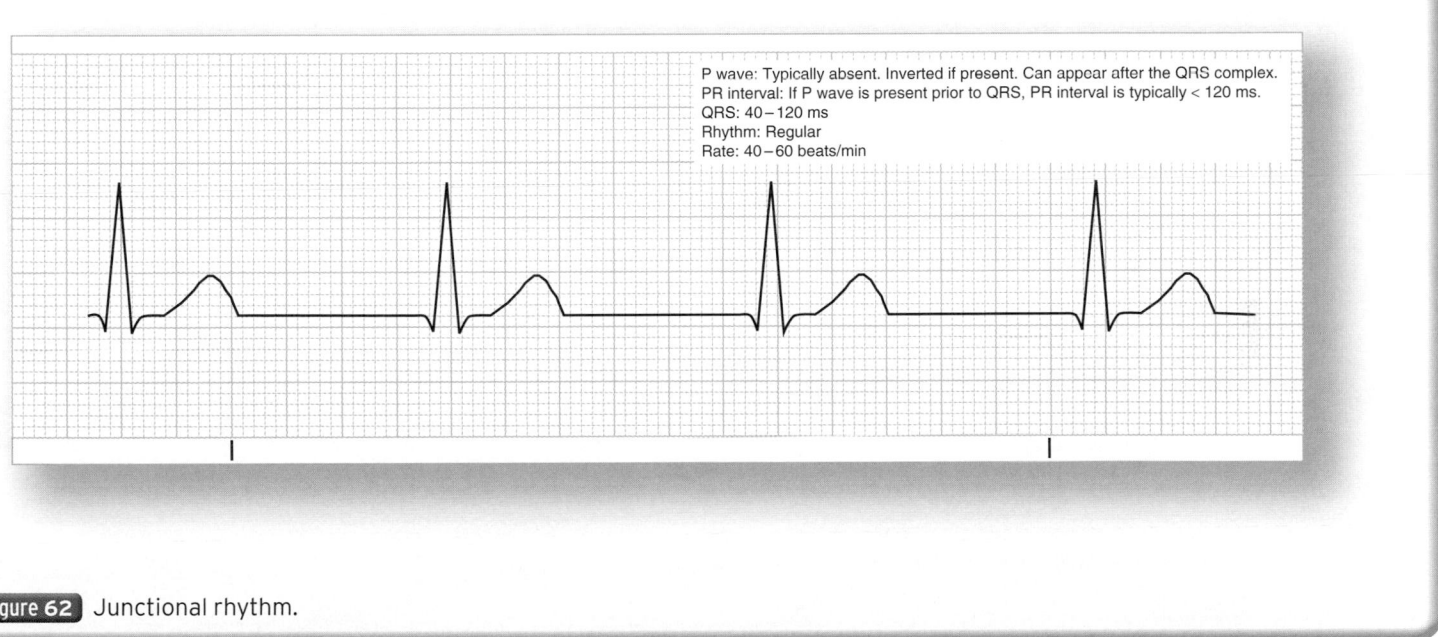

P wave: Typically absent. Inverted if present. Can appear after the QRS complex.
PR interval: If P wave is present prior to QRS, PR interval is typically < 120 ms.
QRS: 40–120 ms
Rhythm: Regular
Rate: 40–60 beats/min

Figure 62 Junctional rhythm.

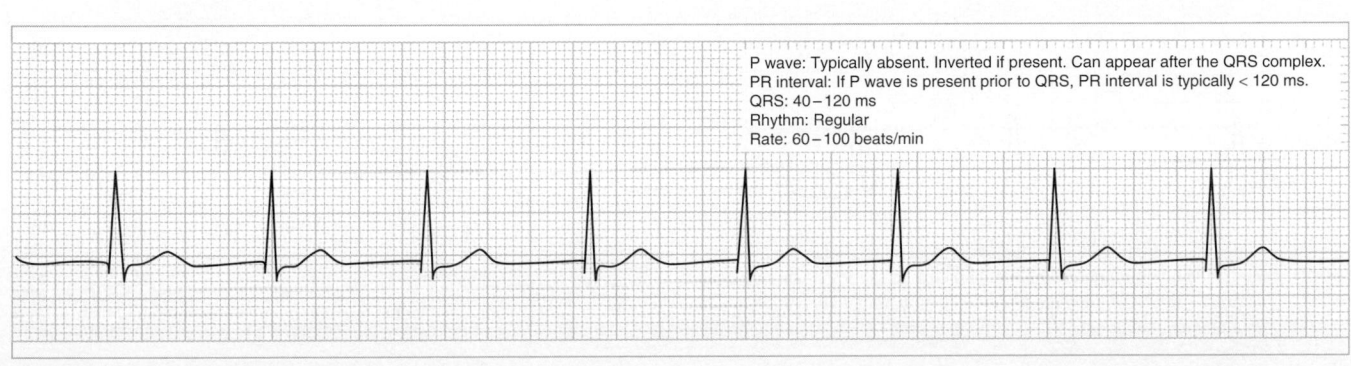

P wave: Typically absent. Inverted if present. Can appear after the QRS complex.
PR interval: If P wave is present prior to QRS, PR interval is typically < 120 ms.
QRS: 40–120 ms
Rhythm: Regular
Rate: 60–100 beats/min

Figure 63 Accelerated junctional rhythm.

Junctional tachycardia is also regular, with little variation between R-R intervals Figure 64 . The P wave, if present, is inverted or upside down but may appear to be absent. The PR interval, if an inverted P wave is present, will measure less than 120 ms. The QRS complex will measure 40 to 120 ms.

Junctional tachycardia is serious, but it seldom requires treatment in the prehospital setting because the rate is usually fast enough to maintain a reasonable CO. If the rate exceeds 150 beats/min, however, the CO could suffer. In such a case, the rhythm is rarely junctional and is referred to as SVT.

Premature Junctional Complex Premature junctional complex (PJC) is not, strictly speaking, a dysrhythmia (just as PAC is not), but rather the existence of a particular complex within another rhythm Figure 65 . Premature junctional complexes are also known as ectopic complexes, meaning that they occur out of the normal location. A PJC also occurs earlier in time than the next expected sinus complex, causing the R-R interval to be less between it and the previous complex.

The rate depends on the underlying rhythm, and the PJC will make the rhythm irregular. The P wave, if present, will be inverted or upside down, and it may precede or follow the QRS complex. The PR interval, if present, will measure less than 120 ms. The QRS complex will measure 40 to 120 ms.

Premature junctional complexes can be caused by many of the same problems that cause premature atrial contractions. They are rarely treated in the prehospital setting but may be a predictor of future cardiac dysrhythmias.

Heart Blocks

After the SA node initiates impulses, the impulses proceed through the atria and ventricles and result in contraction of the heart. When they reach the AV node, the impulses are delayed to allow the atria to contract and fill the ventricle. This delay is a normal function of the AV node and usually causes no problems. Occasionally, however, the impulses traveling through the AV node are delayed more than usual, resulting in heart blocks.

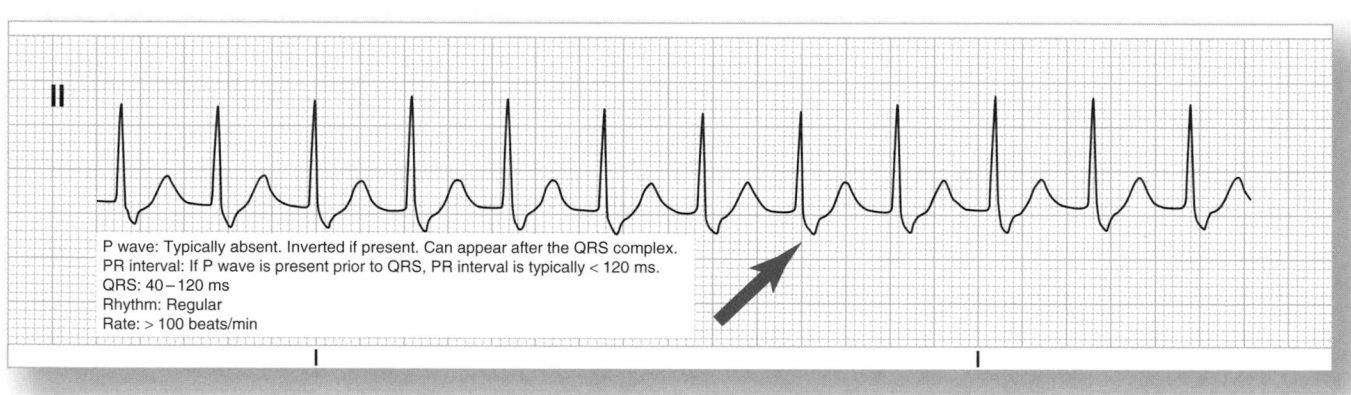

P wave: Typically absent. Inverted if present. Can appear after the QRS complex.
PR interval: If P wave is present prior to QRS, PR interval is typically < 120 ms.
QRS: 40–120 ms
Rhythm: Regular
Rate: > 100 beats/min

Figure 64 Junctional tachycardia. The blue arrow points to an inverted P wave after the QRS wave.

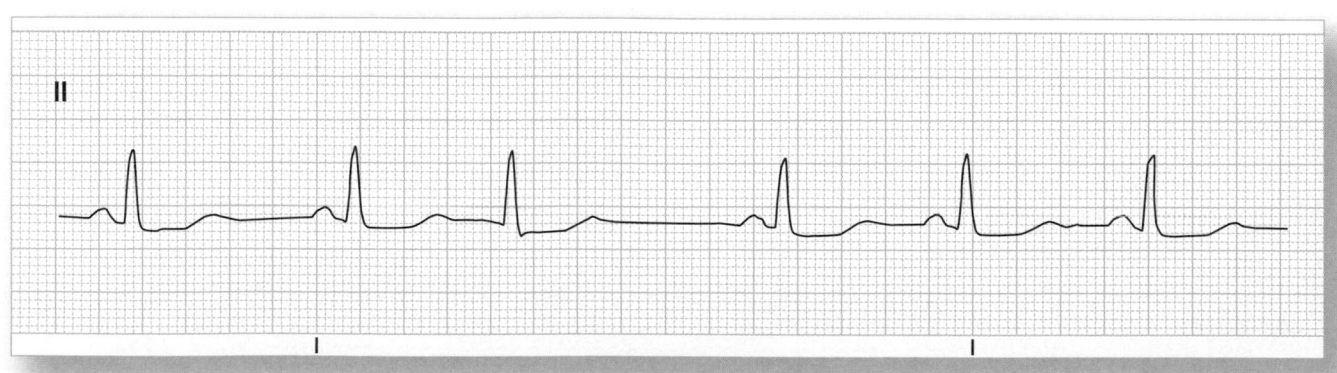

Figure 65 Premature junctional complexes.

Heart blocks are classified into different degrees based on the seriousness of the block and the amount of myocardial damage. The least serious heart block is a first-degree heart block; the most serious is a third-degree block. In between are two types of second-degree block.

First-Degree Heart Block A **first-degree heart block** occurs when each impulse reaching the AV node is delayed slightly longer than is expected and results in a PR interval of greater than 200 ms. Because each impulse eventually passes through the AV node and causes a QRS complex, this block is considered the least serious. Nevertheless, it is often the first indication of damage that has occurred to the AV node.

Because it originates from the normal pacemaker of the heart, first-degree heart block usually has an intrinsic rate of 60 to 100 beats/min, although it typically occurs at the low end of this range **Figure 66**. The rhythm is regular, with minimal variation between R-R intervals. The P wave is present and

upright, and it precedes each QRS complex. The PR interval will measure greater than 200 ms. The QRS complex will measure 40 to 120 ms. The only difference between first-degree heart block and normal sinus rhythm is the prolonged PR interval.

First-degree heart block is rarely treated in the prehospital setting unless it is associated with bradycardia that results in significantly reduced CO.

Second-Degree Heart Block: Mobitz Type I (Wenckebach) A second-degree heart block occurs when an impulse reaching the AV node is occasionally prevented from proceeding to the ventricles and causing a QRS complex. Second-degree heart block, Mobitz type I (Wenckebach), occurs when each successive impulse is delayed a little longer, until finally one impulse is not allowed to continue.

Because it begins from the normal pacemaker of the heart, second-degree heart block, type I, usually has an intrinsic rate of 60 to 100 beats/min, although it typically occurs at the low end of this range **Figure 67**. The rhythm is irregular, with a prolonged

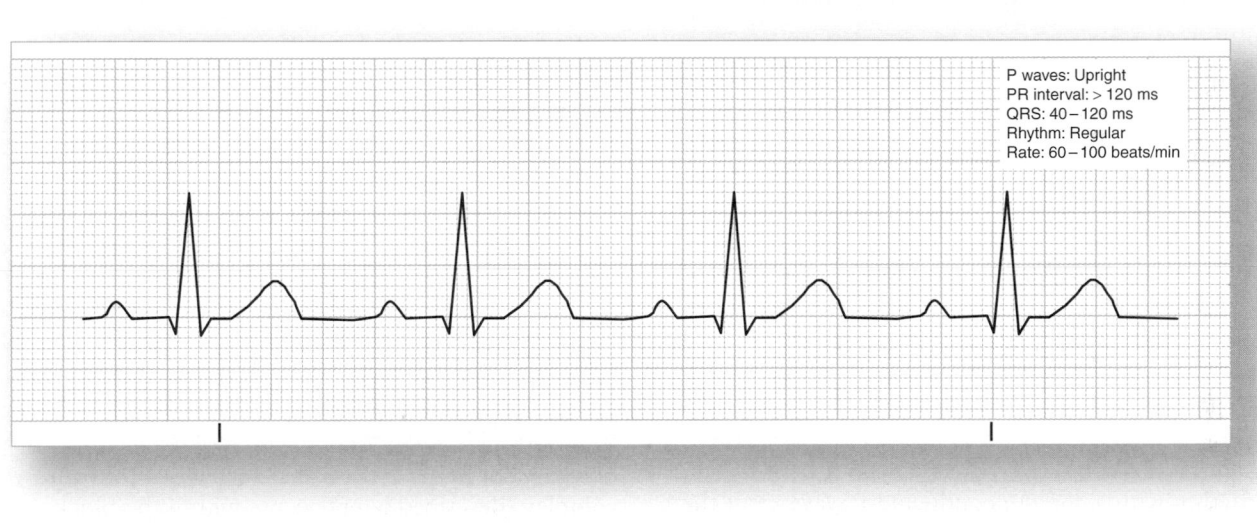

P waves: Upright
PR interval: > 120 ms
QRS: 40–120 ms
Rhythm: Regular
Rate: 60–100 beats/min

Figure 66 First-degree heart block.

P waves: Upright
PR interval: Elongates until QRS is dropped
QRS: 40–120 ms
Rhythm: Regularly irregular
Rate: 60–100 beats/min

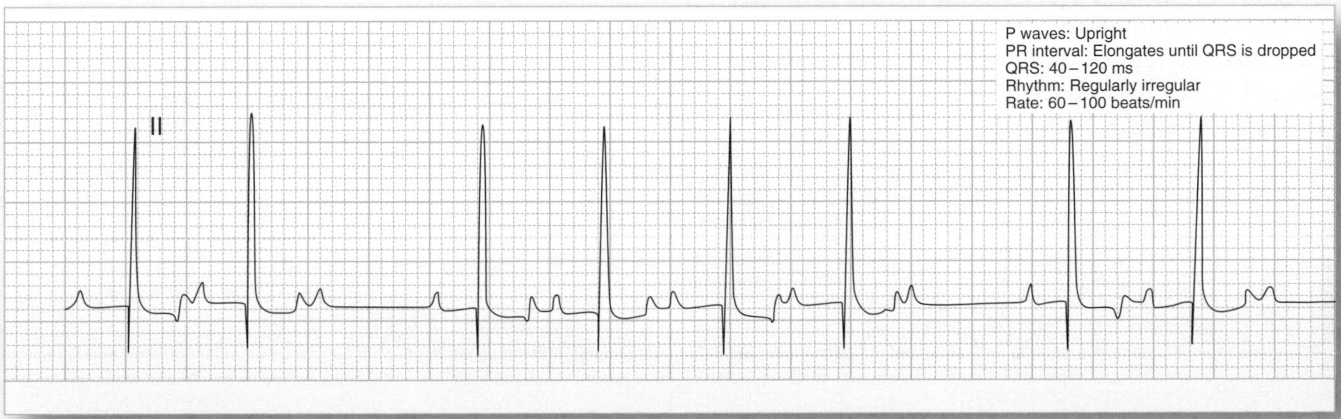

Figure 67 Second-degree heart block, Mobitz type I.

R-R interval occurring between the last QRS complex before the blocked P wave and the QRS complex after the first unblocked P wave. The P wave is present and upright, and it precedes most QRS complexes. The PR interval starts out within the normal limits of 120 to 200 ms but, with each successive P wave, grows longer. It finally results in a P wave that is followed not by a QRS complex, but by another P wave; this P wave is then followed by a QRS complex with a normal PR interval. This pattern repeats over and over in the rhythm. The QRS complex will measure 40 to 120 ms.

The key to identification of second-degree type I heart block is the recognition of the increasing PR interval followed by the P wave without a QRS complex. This rhythm is always irregular, and you can often easily see the wide R-R interval with the "extra" P wave located there.

Second-degree type I heart blocks are treated in the pre-hospital setting only if they are associated with bradycardia that results in significantly reduced CO.

Second-Degree Heart Block: Mobitz Type II (Classical)
Second-degree heart block, Mobitz type II, occurs when several impulses are not allowed to continue. It is sometimes called classical because it was well known before the Wenckebach heart block was discovered.

Because it originates from the normal pacemaker of the heart, second-degree heart block, type II, usually has an intrinsic rate of 60 to 100 beats/min, although it typically occurs at the low end of this range **Figure 68** . The rhythm may be regular, with every other P wave blocked, or irregular, with a prolonged R-R interval between the last QRS complex before the blocked P wave and the QRS complex after the first unblocked P wave. The P wave is present and upright, and it precedes some QRS complexes. The PR interval is always constant. In fact, this is the easiest way to identify a second-degree type II heart block. If you see a rhythm with some nonconducted P waves, but the PR interval is constant among all conducted P waves and their corresponding QRS complexes, you have identified a second-degree type II heart block.

It is important to remember that this block can be regular or irregular. Sometimes several normal beats will occur without a nonconducted P wave; sometimes two or more nonconducted P waves may appear before one P wave is conducted. In other situations, a pattern develops that consists of one conducted P wave followed by one nonconducted P wave.

Second-degree type II heart blocks are treated in the pre-hospital setting only if they are associated with bradycardia that results in significantly reduced CO.

Third-Degree Heart Block (Complete Heart Block)
A third-degree heart block occurs when all impulses reaching the AV node are prevented from proceeding to the ventricles and causing a QRS complex. Unlike in first- and second-degree heart blocks, in a third-degree heart block *all* impulses from the atria are prevented from traveling to the ventricles. As a consequence, this block is also known as a complete heart block. Because all impulses from the atria are blocked, the ventricles will develop their own pacemaker to continue circulation of blood, albeit at a greatly reduced rate.

Because it originates from the normal pacemaker of the heart, third-degree heart block usually has an intrinsic atrial rate of 60 to 100 beats/min, but the ventricular rate—which depends on the activity of a ventricular pacemaker—is less than 60 beats/min **Figure 69** . The rhythm is usually regular, with the P-P and R-R intervals being consistent. The P wave is present and upright. The PR interval in this type of heart block is non-existent.

The classic way of identifying a third-degree heart block is to identify the presence of nonconducted P waves and then to be unable to identify a relationship between the P waves and the QRS complexes. Because the ventricular rate depends on the presence of a ventricular pacemaker, it is common to see the QRS complexes in a third-degree heart block that are wider than 120 ms. When you see a rhythm with wide QRS complexes (and no narrow QRS complexes) along with P waves, you should suspect a third-degree heart block. If the rhythm is regular and the PR interval is not constant, it is almost certainly a third-degree heart block. The major issue with looking for third-degree heart blocks to be regular is the fact that if a premature ventricular complex (described later) occurs within the block, it will make the block appear irregular.

Third-degree heart blocks are treated in the prehospital setting only if they are associated with bradycardia that results in significantly reduced CO. In such a case, the patient will require TCP.

Rhythms Originating in the Ventricles
If the SA node fails to initiate an impulse, the AV node will usually take over as pacemaker. If the AV node cannot perform

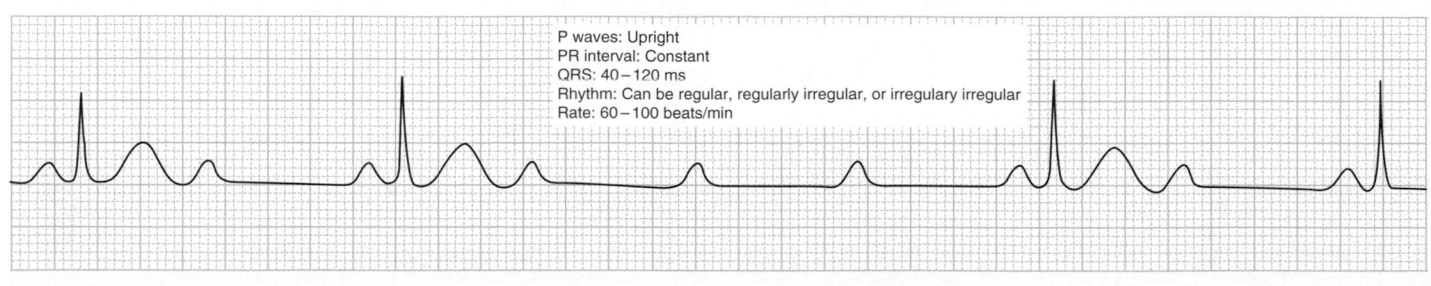

P waves: Upright
PR interval: Constant
QRS: 40–120 ms
Rhythm: Can be regular, regularly irregular, or irregulary irregular
Rate: 60–100 beats/min

Figure 68 Second-degree heart block, Mobitz type II.

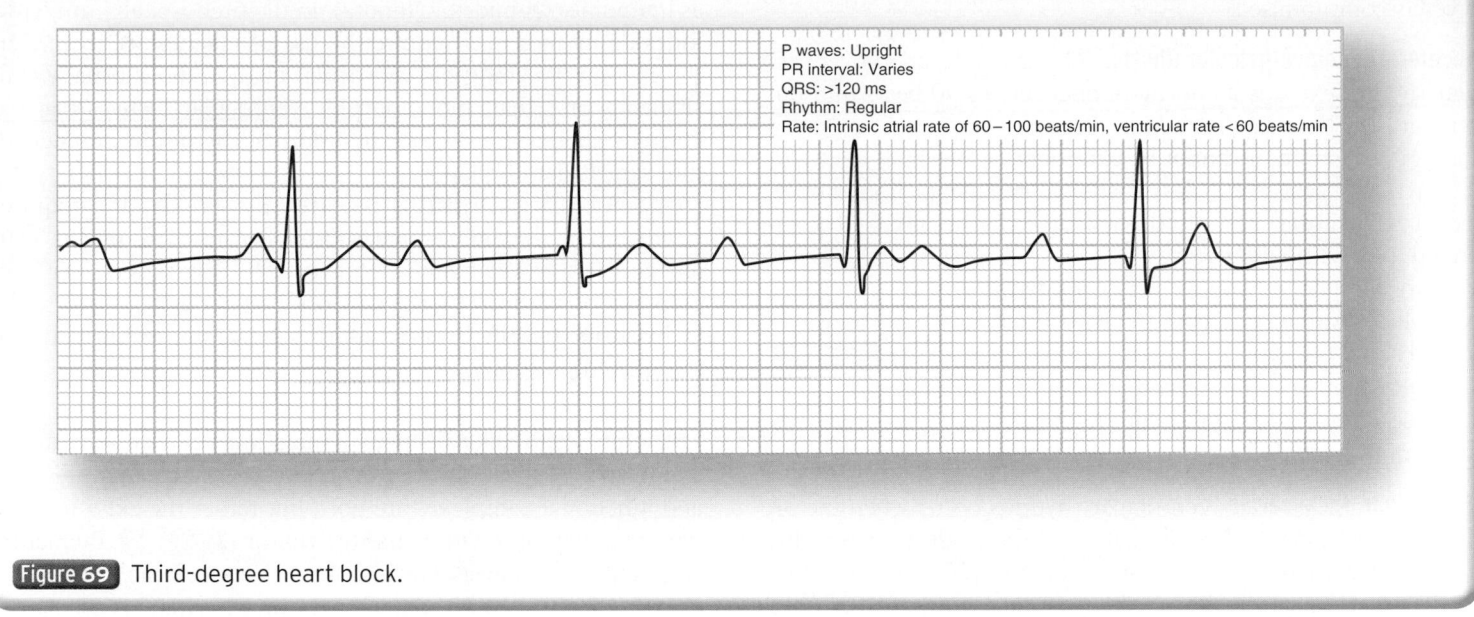

P waves: Upright
PR interval: Varies
QRS: >120 ms
Rhythm: Regular
Rate: Intrinsic atrial rate of 60–100 beats/min, ventricular rate <60 beats/min

Figure 69 Third-degree heart block.

this duty, however, the ventricles may begin to originate their own impulses and become the pacemaker of the heart. Such ventricular rhythms will have missing P waves and wide QRS complexes.

If an impulse is generated in the ventricles, it must travel through the ventricles in a cell-to-cell manner because the cell originating the impulse is unlikely to be located on the conduction system. Because impulses travel more slowly via cell-to-cell transmission than when they travel on the conduction system, ventricular-initiated impulses result in very wide QRS complexes—more than 120 ms in duration. Because the intrinsic rate of the ventricles is 20 to 40, ventricular rhythms normally demonstrate rates of 20 to 40 beats/min.

Idioventricular Rhythm An <u>idioventricular</u> (meaning only the ventricles or produced by the ventricles) rhythm occurs when the SA and AV nodes fail and the ventricles must take over pacing the heart **Figure 70**. It has a rate of 20 to 40 beats/min owing to the intrinsic rate of the ventricles as pacemakers. An idioventricular rhythm is usually regular, with little variation between R-R intervals. P waves are absent owing to the failure of the SA and AV nodes. Because there is no P wave, there is no PR interval. The QRS complex will measure greater than 120 ms because it originates in the ventricles.

Idioventricular rhythms are serious and may or may not result in a palpable pulse. Treatment is geared toward improving the CO by increasing the rate and, if possible, treating the

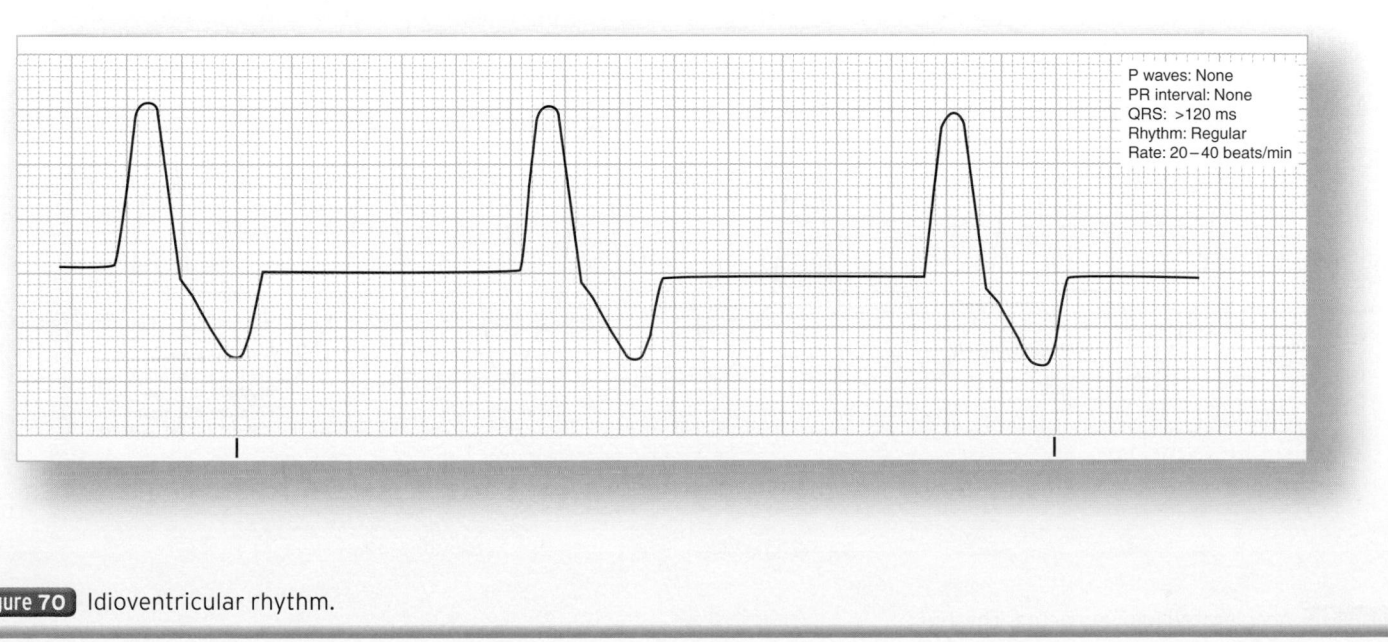

P waves: None
PR interval: None
QRS: >120 ms
Rhythm: Regular
Rate: 20–40 beats/min

Figure 70 Idioventricular rhythm.

underlying cause. In such a case, the patient's condition is usually severely compromised.

Accelerated Idioventricular Rhythm Occasionally, an idioventricular rhythm exceeds its normal upper rate of 40 beats/min but remains less than 100 beats/min. Because the rhythm is greater than 40 beats/min, it cannot be considered a "normal" ventricular rhythm; because it is less than 100 beats/min, it cannot be called tachycardia either. In this case, the rhythm is called accelerated idioventricular rhythm.

An accelerated idioventricular rhythm is also regular, with little variation between R-R intervals. The P waves are absent, so the PR interval does not exist **Figure 71**. The QRS complex will measure greater than 120 ms.

Accelerated idioventricular rhythms are serious, but they are seldom treated in the prehospital setting.

Ventricular Tachycardia Ventricular rhythms occur when the SA and AV nodes fail as the pacemakers of the heart. Occasionally, a ventricular rhythm has a rate that exceeds 100 beats/min. Any rhythm that results in a ventricular rate of greater than 100 beats/min is considered tachycardia. In this case, the rhythm is termed ventricular tachycardia.

Ventricular tachycardia is regular, with no variation between R-R intervals. The P waves are absent, so the PR interval also does not exist. The QRS complex will measure greater than 120 ms.

Ventricular tachycardia usually presents with QRS complexes that have uniform tops and bottoms; this type of ventricular tachycardia is referred to as **monomorphic** (having one common shape of QRS complex) **Figure 72**. Occasionally, ventricular tachycardia will present with QRS complexes that vary in height in an alternating pattern; this type of ventricular tachycardia is called polymorphic ventricular tachycardia. The most common polymorphic ventricular tachycardia is torsades de pointes, which is usually seen in patients who have a condition of a prolonged QT interval **Figure 73**. Torsades de pointes may be normal for

the patient or it may be induced by medications or drugs such as quinidine (Quinidex, Quinora). In the prehospital setting, torsades de pointes may require the use of magnesium to convert the rhythm. Polymorphic ventricular tachycardia is usually considered worse than monomorphic ventricular tachycardia and converts spontaneously back to a normal rhythm or degenerates into ventricular fibrillation.

Ventricular tachycardia is extremely serious, and requires treatment in the prehospital setting because the rate is usually too fast to maintain adequate CO. This reduced CO, in conjunction with the increased workload of the heart due to the tachycardia, usually leads to ventricular failure or fibrillation if not treated promptly.

Premature Ventricular Complex Premature ventricular complex is not, strictly speaking, a dysrhythmia (just as premature atrial and junctional complexes are not), but rather the existence of a particular complex within another rhythm **Figure 74**. Premature ventricular complexes are also known as ectopic complexes, meaning that they occur out of the normal location. A premature ventricular complex also occurs earlier than the next expected sinus complex, causing the R-R interval to be less between it and the previous complex.

Because the rate depends on the underlying rhythm, the premature ventricular complex will make the rhythm irregular. There is no P wave associated with the premature ventricular complex, so there is no PR interval. The QRS complex will measure greater than 120 ms.

Premature ventricular complexes may also be further distinguished as unifocal or multifocal. **Unifocal** premature ventricular complexes originate from the same spot or "focus" within the ventricle and will appear the same on the ECG **Figure 75**. Two premature ventricular complexes with different appearances are **multifocal**, meaning there is more than one focus initiating ventricular impulses **Figure 76**.

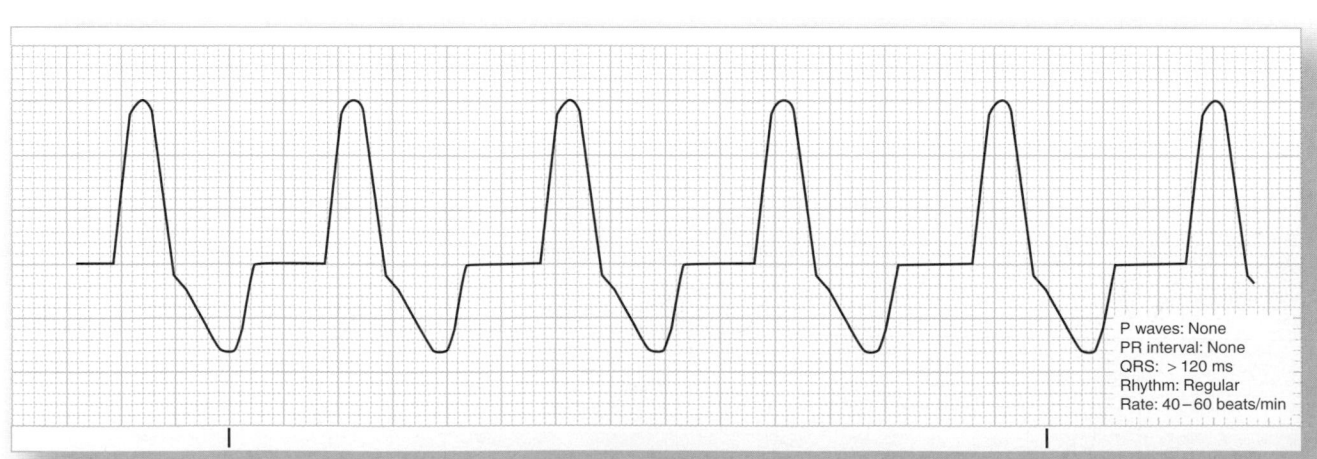

P waves: None
PR interval: None
QRS: > 120 ms
Rhythm: Regular
Rate: 40 – 60 beats/min

Figure 71 Accelerated idioventricular rhythm.

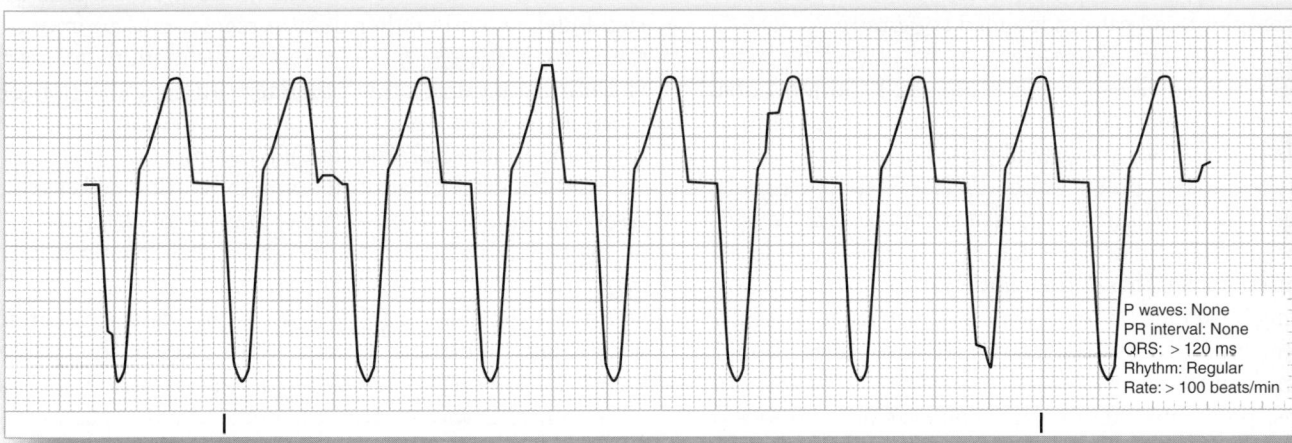

P waves: None
PR interval: None
QRS: > 120 ms
Rhythm: Regular
Rate: > 100 beats/min

Figure 72 Ventricular tachycardia. This example shows monomorphic ventricular tachycardia.

Sometimes two premature ventricular complexes may occur together without any pause between them. This pair of complexes is referred to as a **couplet** **Figure 77**. If three or more premature ventricular complexes occur in a row, they constitute a "run" of ventricular tachycardia; these are also referred to as salvos. Occasionally, these complexes will become so frequent that they alternate with normal complexes, causing a normal–premature ventricular complex–normal–premature ventricular complex pattern. This pattern is called **bigeminy** of pre-

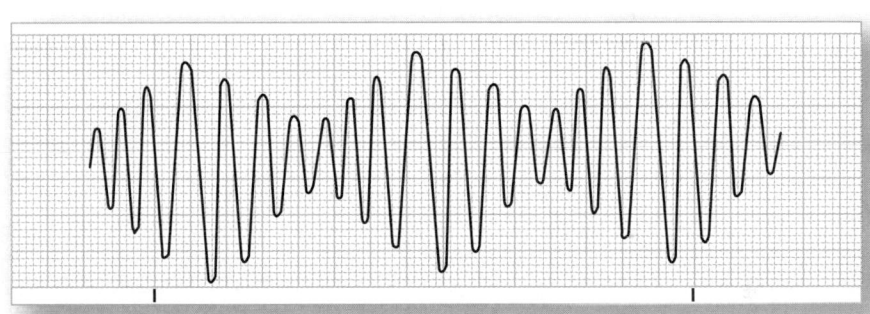

Figure 73 Torsades de pointes.

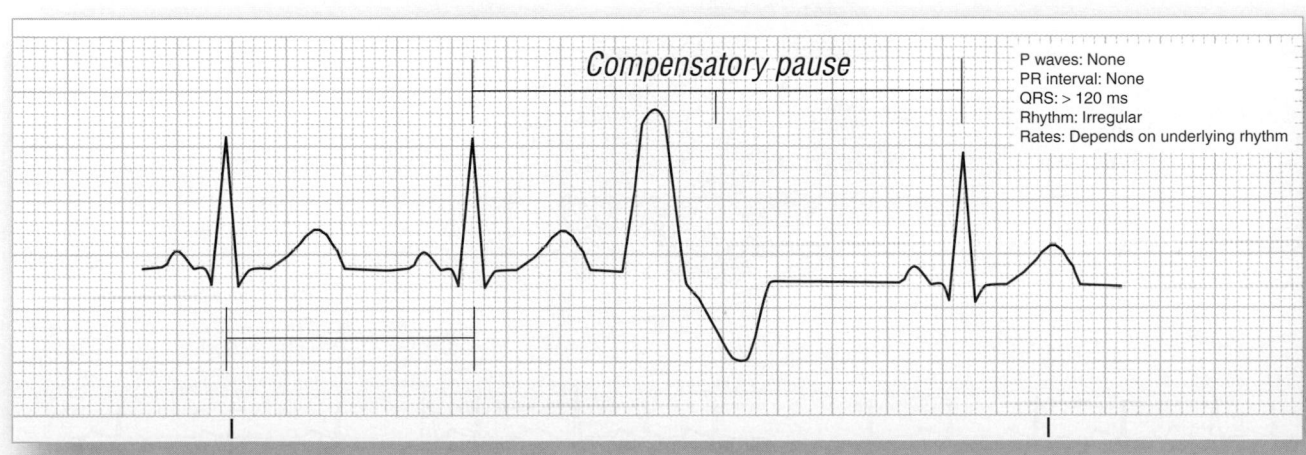

Compensatory pause

P waves: None
PR interval: None
QRS: > 120 ms
Rhythm: Irregular
Rates: Depends on underlying rhythm

Figure 74 Premature ventricular complex.

mature ventricular complexes Figure 78 . If every third beat is a premature ventricular complex (normal–normal–premature ventricular complex), the pattern is called **trigeminy**.

Premature ventricular complexes can be caused by many of the same problems that cause premature atrial and junctional contractions, but they most commonly originate from ischemia in the ventricular tissue. They are generally considered more serious than premature atrial or junctional complexes. Multifocal, couplet, and bigeminy premature ventricular complexes are considered more serious than unifocal premature ventricular complexes. One of the principal hazards of premature ventricular complexes is that they might occur at a time when the ventricles are not fully repolarized (as indicated by the T wave). This so-called R-on-T phenomenon often results in ventricular fibrillation. For this and other reasons, premature ventricular complexes are considered serious and an indication of serious underlying heart conditions. Nevertheless, this condition is not usually treated in the prehospital setting, unless it is significantly affecting CO, and even then it must be treated with caution.

Ventricular Fibrillation Ventricular fibrillation is a rhythm in which the entire heart is no longer contracting but rather fibrillating or quivering without any organized contraction. It occurs when many different cells in the heart become depolarized independently rather than in response to an impulse from the SA node Figure 79 . The result of this random depolarization is a fibrillating or chaotic baseline without indication of organized activity. As opposed to atrial fibrillation, there are no P waves, no PR interval, and no QRS complexes.

Early in ventricular fibrillation, the cardiac cells have energy reserves that allow a considerable amount of electrical energy to be expended and cause the height of the chaotic waves to be large. These large waves are sometimes referred to as "coarse" ventricular fibrillation Figure 80 . As the ventricles continue to go without circulation, the energy reserves of the cardiac cells are gradually used up, leading to a great reduction of the height of the chaotic waves. This phenomenon is sometimes called "fine" ventricular fibrillation Figure 81 .

Ventricular fibrillation is the rhythm most commonly seen in adults who go into cardiac arrest. Fortunately, it responds well to defibrillation performed with an automated or manual defibrillator within the first 3 to 4 minutes of an arrest. After 4 minutes or so, it is necessary to provide CPR compressions to help make the heart more susceptible to defibrillation and to increase the oxygen to the myocardial cells. Prehospital treatment of ventricular fibrillation is common and will be discussed in detail later in this chapter.

Asystole **Asystole** ("flat line"), the only true **arrhythmia**, is a rhythm in which the entire heart is no longer contracting but rather is sitting still within the thorax without any organized activity Figure 82 . It occurs when many cells of the heart have been hypoxic for so long that they no longer have any energy for any kind of contraction. Asystole

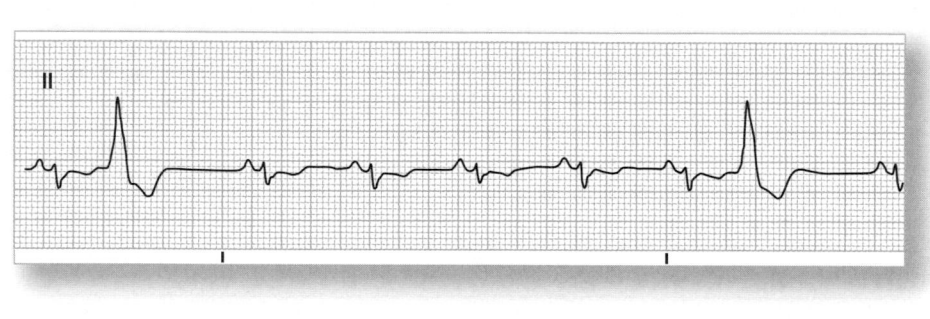

Figure 75 Unifocal premature ventricular complexes.

Multifocal
PVCs

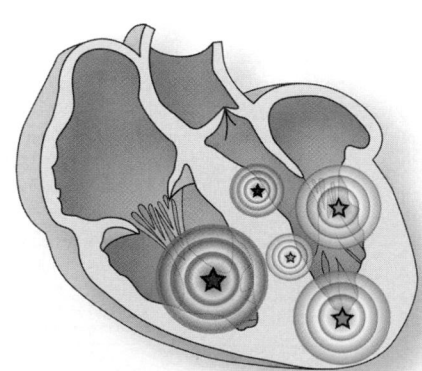

Figure 76 Multifocal premature ventricular complexes.

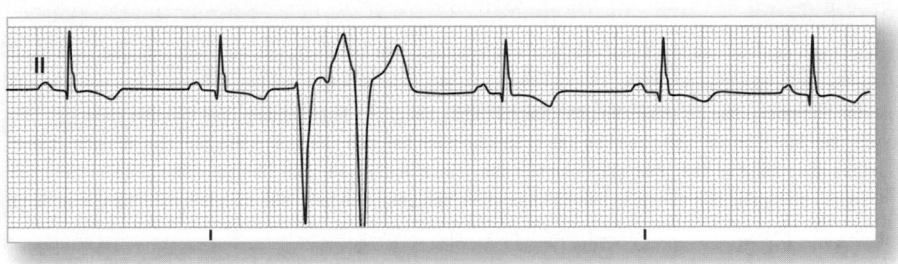

Figure 77 Couplet or grouped premature ventricular complexes.

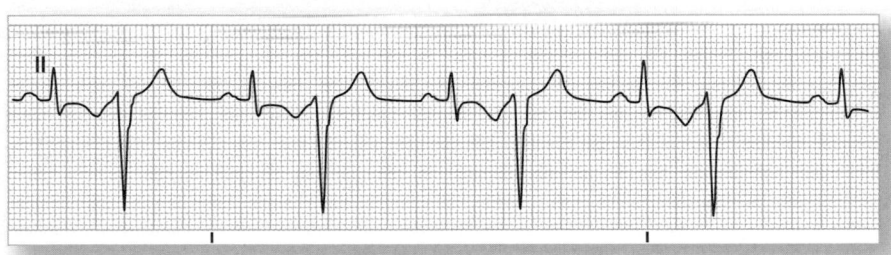

Figure 78 Premature ventricular complexes in a pattern of bigeminy or ventricular bigeminy.

presents with a complete absence of electrical activity: no P waves, no PR intervals, no QRS complexes, and no T waves.

In one variation of asystole, the flat baseline associated with asystole is interrupted by a small sinusoidal complex. This condition, which is termed **agonal rhythm**, is probably a result of residual electrical discharge from a dead heart (**agonal** means "pertaining to the period of dying"). Agonal rhythm should not be confused with an idioventricular rhythm **Figure 83**. An idioventricular rhythm may result in a palpable pulse, but an agonal rhythm will not.

Asystole is generally considered a confirmation of death, although in certain circumstances, it may be treated (as discussed later in this chapter).

Artificial Pacemaker Rhythms

Many of your patients will have experienced problems with their cardiac conduction systems and had artificial pacemakers implanted in their chest. When these patients are connected to the heart monitor, the presence of the artificial

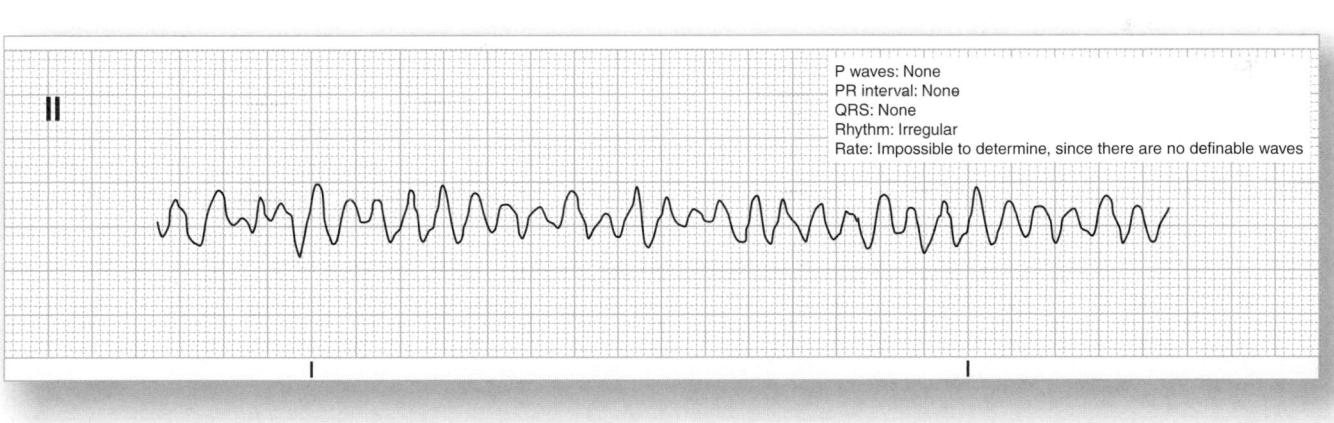

P waves: None
PR interval: None
QRS: None
Rhythm: Irregular
Rate: Impossible to determine, since there are no definable waves

Figure 79 Ventricular fibrillation.

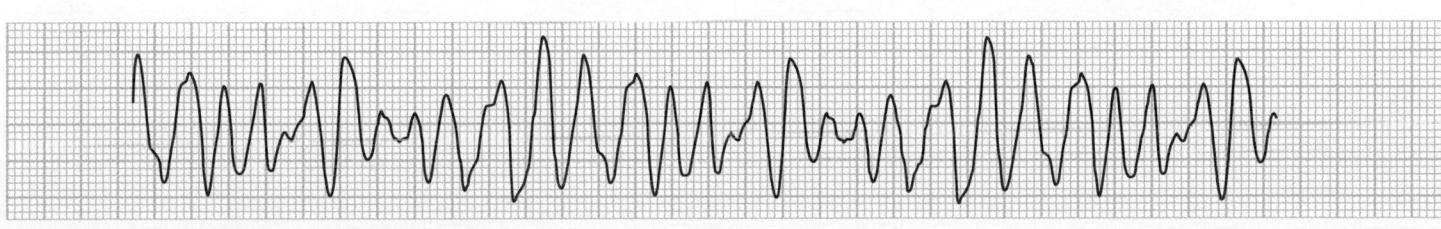

Figure 80 Coarse ventricular fibrillation.

pacemaker is obvious. The firing of an artificial pacemaker causes a unique vertical spike on the ECG tracing **Figure 84**. When you attach the cardiac monitor to a patient and see these sharp vertical spikes on the ECG, you can assume the patient has an artificial pacemaker **Figure 85**.

Many types of artificial pacemakers exist, and more are being developed. The most common type in the past has been the ventricular pacemaker, which is attached to the ventricles only; it causes a sharp pacemaker spike followed by a wide QRS complex resulting from the impulse traveling through the ventricles. Another type of pacemaker is attached to the atria and the ventricle; it produces a pacemaker spike that is followed by a P wave and another pacemaker spike followed by a wide QRS complex. Many of the newer pacemakers are equipped with sensors that can identify the rate of spontaneous depolarization of the heart. These "demand" pacemakers begin to generate pacing impulses only when they sense that the natural pace of cardiac impulses has slowed below a specific number (usually 60 per minute) **Figure 86**.

Occasionally, a patient may experience a problem with his or her pacemaker. If the patient's pacemaker is failing (eg, due to battery failure), the pacemaker spikes may still be visible, but they will not be followed by a QRS complex. This loss of

capture indicates the pacemaker is not operating properly. A loss of capture may also occur if the wire connecting the pacemaker to the patient's heart becomes dislodged. In either of these cases, the patient's heartbeat now depends on the natural pacemaker (usually the ventricles), resulting in greatly reduced CO. In such cases, patients need TCP instituted as quickly as possible (discussed later in this chapter).

Another type of pacemaker failure involves a "runaway" pacemaker. A runaway pacemaker presents as a very tachycardic pacemaker rhythm that must be slowed to preserve the patient's cardiac function. Usually a strong magnet placed over the pacemaker will "reset" a runaway pacemaker. This would be done in the ED by a cardiologist.

■ 12-Lead ECGs

Up to now, we have considered ECG rhythm strips obtained from monitoring a single lead. For purposes of rhythm interpretation and identification of lethal rhythms, a single lead (typically lead II) is usually sufficient. To localize the site of injury to heart muscle and to identify other cardiac abnormalities, however, you must be able to look at the heart from several angles. That is precisely the purpose of a 12-lead ECG.

Suppose you wanted to check out the condition of a used car you were thinking of buying. If you needed to know only whether the motor was running, you could stand anywhere near the car and listen (just as you can use any one lead to monitor the cardiac rhythm). But if you wanted to know what kind of shape the car body is in, you would have to walk around the car and look at it from all sides. The driver's side might be in mint condition, but on the passenger's side, the entire door frame might be caved in from a road crash.

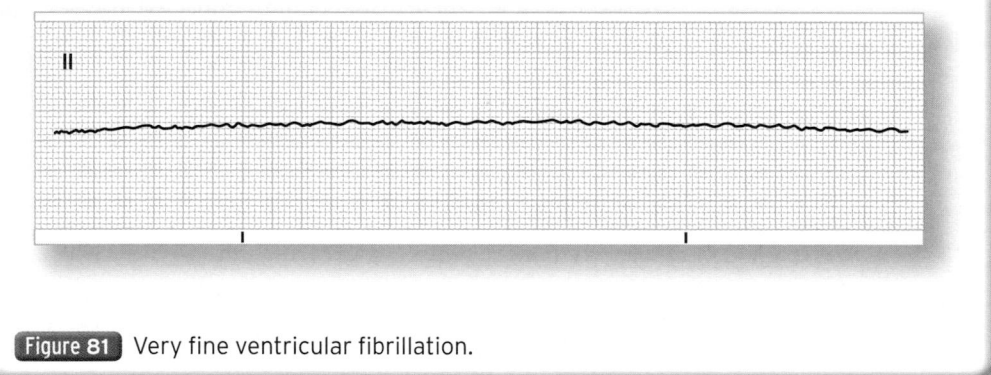

Figure 81   Very fine ventricular fibrillation.

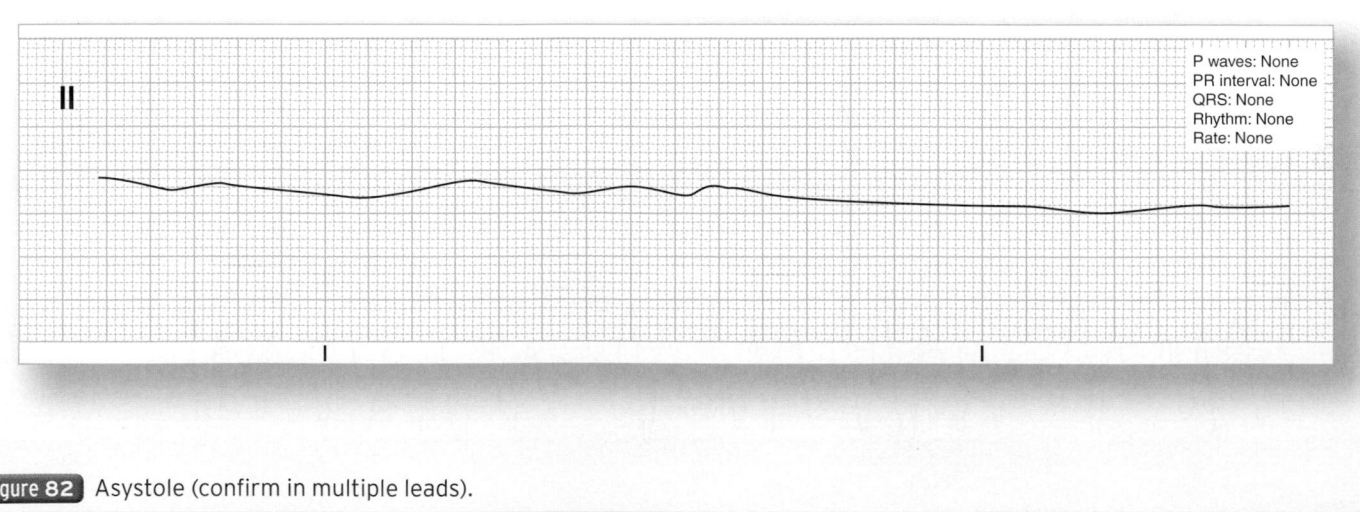

P waves: None
PR interval: None
QRS: None
Rhythm: None
Rate: None

Figure 82   Asystole (confirm in multiple leads).

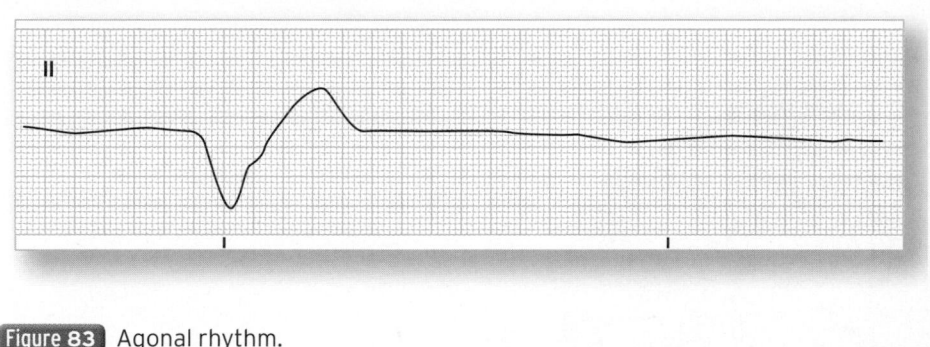

Figure 83 Agonal rhythm.

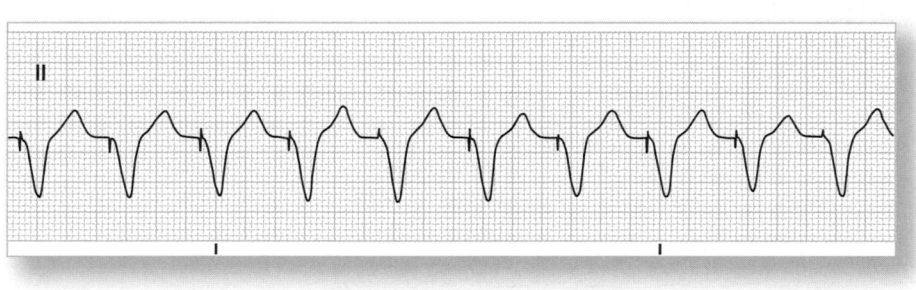

Figure 84 Artificial ventricular pacemaker rhythm.

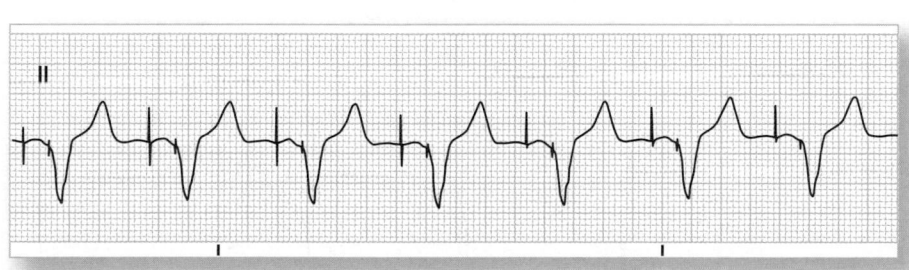

Figure 85 Artificial (AV sequential) pacemaker rhythm.

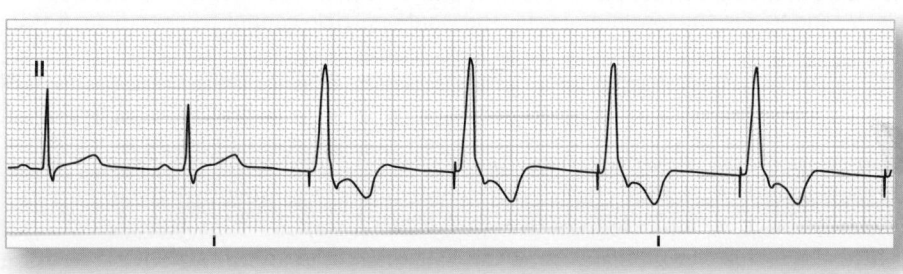

Figure 86 Artificial (demand pacemaker) pacemaker rhythm.

Similarly, each ECG lead looks at the heart from a different angle. Although one lead may detect a normal myocardium, another may be showing major damage.

In the standard 12-lead ECG, you record 12 leads—that is, 12 different pictures of the electrical activity of the heart. What does a lead "see" when it looks at the heart? A **lead** provides an electrical picture of the heart taken from a specified vantage point. Lead I, for example, "looks" at the heart from the left, so it "sees" the left side of the heart. Another lead, lead aVF, looks up at the heart from the feet (F stands for "foot"), so it sees the bottom of the heart. The word *lead*, as it is used in electrocardiography, can be somewhat confusing. Sometimes the word is used to refer to one of the cables and monitoring electrodes that connect the ECG machine to the patient (such as the "right arm lead").

Precordial Leads

Recall from the section on cardiac monitoring that there are three types of leads: bipolar limb leads, unipolar augmented limb leads, and precordial leads. A 12-lead ECG adds six **precordial leads** to the six limb leads discussed thus far. These six precordial leads (V_1 to V_6) are also called unipolar chest leads, anterior leads, or V leads. The six precordial leads are placed on the anterior and lateral chest walls, usually with adhesive electrodes, in the positions shown in **Figure 87**. These leads look at the heart in the horizontal plane (as shown in the inset to the figure), so they provide a picture of the heart taken from the front (anterior wall of the heart) and from the left side (anterolateral). More specifically, leads V_1 and V_2 look at the septum; V_3 and V_4 look at the anterior wall of the left ventricle; and V_5 and V_6 look at the lateral wall of the left ventricle.

Placement of 12-Lead ECG Electrodes

Recall that correct electrode placement is important in order to ensure that the lead is viewing the heart from the correct angle each time an ECG is recorded. ECGs are compared with previous ECGs. For the

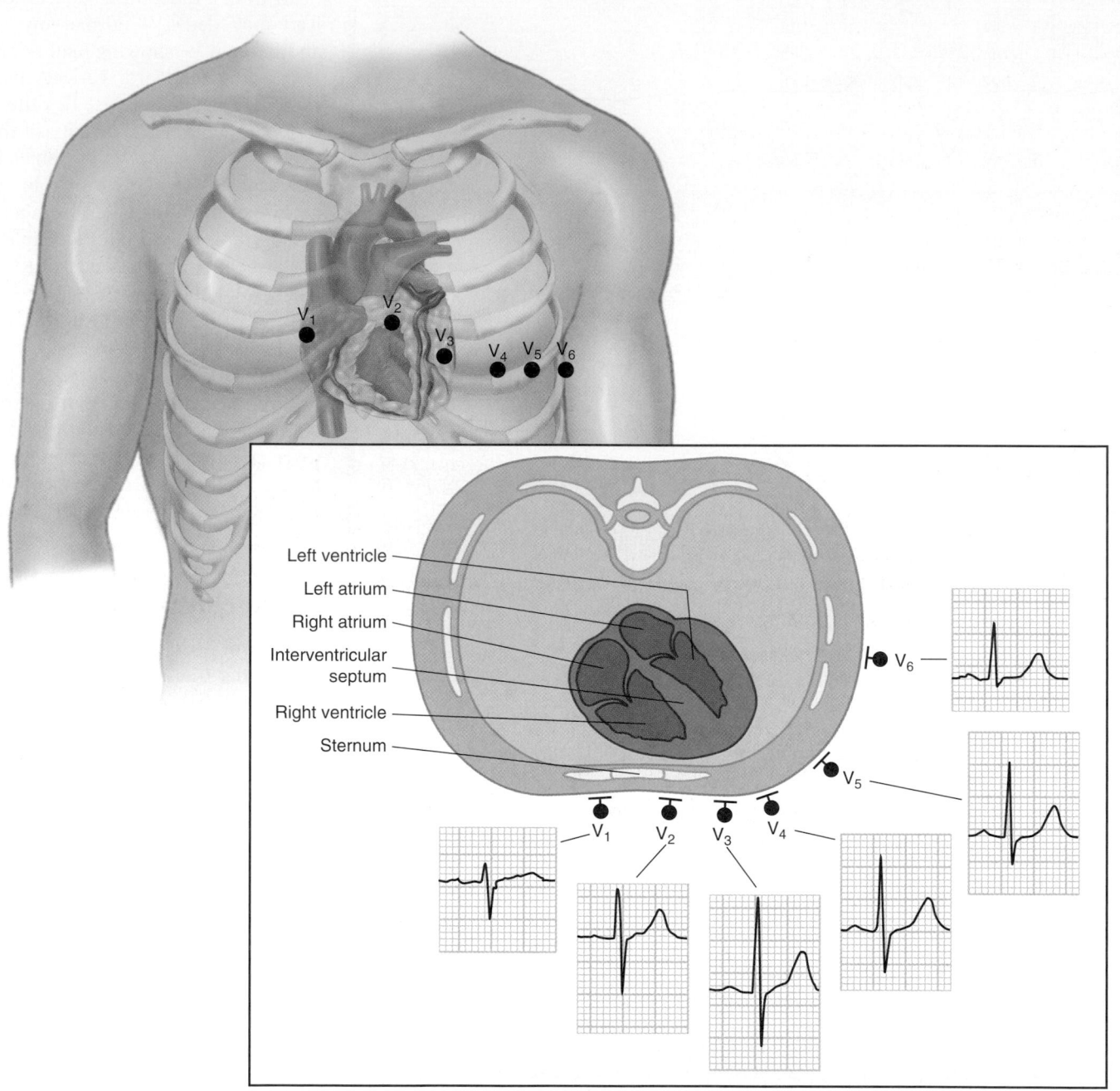

Figure 87 Precordial leads (chest leads) look at the heart in the horizontal plane. Inset: V_1 and V_2 look at the interventricular septum. V_3 and V_4 "see" the anterior wall of the left ventricle. V_5 and V_6 see the low lateral wall. The right ventricle cannot be seen from a standard tracing.

comparison to be reliable for identifying existing problems or highlighting the appearance of new problems (such as ST-segment elevation), the electrodes must be placed consistently.

Acquisition Modes

The ECG device can record tracings using different electromagnetic frequency ranges. For the purposes of rhythm interpretation, the ECG is recorded in monitor mode. Monitor mode employs electronic filters to remove artifact and unwanted information from the ECG tracing. Unfortunately, monitor mode also skews the shape and location of the ST segment and T wave. Monitor mode captures electrical information within the range of 1 to 30, 40, 100, or 150 hertz (Hz).

Diagnostic mode is the second acquisition mode that filters out very little electrical information, making it prone to having more artifact on the tracing. Diagnostic mode is always used to record a 12-lead ECG by default and cannot be changed. Many devices enable users to record 3-lead ECGs in diagnostic mode as well. The problem with doing this is that the 3-lead ECG is usually acquired in the early minutes of patient contact when there is a lot of movement. This results in high levels of artifact on the tracing and the inability to interpret the rhythm. Diagnostic mode captures electrical information within the range of 0.05 to 40 Hz. The pediatric right ventricle and artificial pacemakers emit an electrical signal with a higher frequency. Most devices capture pediatric ECG tracings within the range of 0.05 to 150 Hz. The frequency range is always printed near the bottom of the ECG tracing **Figure 88**.

Lead Placement

The best way to learn how to record a 12-lead ECG is to practice with the equipment itself.

Make sure the patient does not become chilled because shivering will produce artifact in the ECG tracing. Note that

x1.0 .05-150Hz 25mm/sec
P/N 805319

Figure 88 The electromagnetic frequency range is printed near the bottom of the ECG. Diagnostic mode is always used in 12-lead ECG tracings.

12-lead ECGs are more sensitive to artifact than 3-lead monitoring ECGs.

Skill Drill 2 lists the steps involved in acquiring a 12-lead ECG:

Skill Drill 2

1. Take standard precautions **Step 1**. Place the patient in a supine position.
2. Explain the procedure to the patient. Prepare the skin for electrode placement as you would for placing monitoring electrodes **Step 2**.
3. Attach the electrodes to the leads before placing them on the patient **Step 3**.
4. Position the electrodes on the patient **Step 4**. This involves connecting the four limb electrodes. Double-check that the correct electrode is on each limb (the "LA" electrode on the left arm, the "RA" electrode on the right arm, and so on). Confirm that the limb electrodes are on the arms and legs and *not* on the trunk of the body, as sometimes is the case for monitoring the ECG.

   Once the limb electrodes are connected, connect and apply the electrodes for the precordial leads:

   - V_1 – fourth intercostal space to the right of the sternum
   - V_2 – fourth intercostal space to the left of the sternum
   - V_3 – directly between leads V_2 and V_4
   - V_4 – fifth intercostal space at left midclavicular line
   - V_5 – level with lead V_4 at left anterior axillary line
   - V_6 – level with lead V_5 at left midaxillary line

Skill Drill 2

Acquiring a 12-Lead ECG

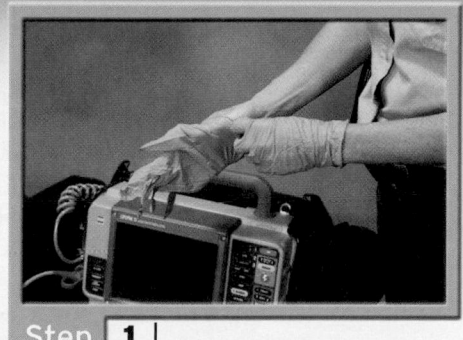

Step 1 Take standard precautions.

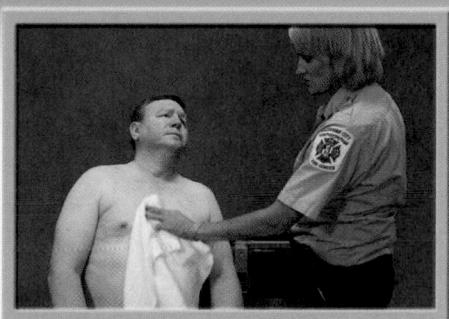

Step 2 Explain the procedure to the patient. Prepare the skin for electrode placement.

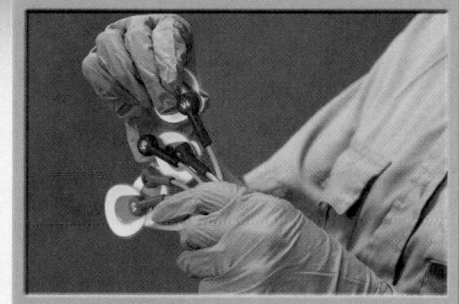

Step 3 Attach the electrodes to the leads before placing them on the patient.

Continues

Skill Drill 2

Acquiring a 12-Lead ECG, continued

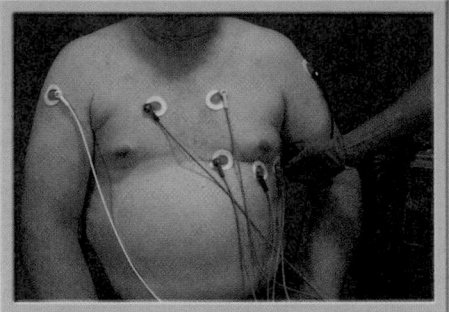

Step 4 Position the electrodes on the patient.

- V_1 - fourth intercostal space to the right of the sternum
- V_2 - fourth intercostal space to the left of the sternum
- V_3 - directly between leads V_2 and V_4
- V_4 - fifth intercostal space at left midclavicular line
- V_5 - level with lead V_4 at left anterior axillary line
- V_6 - level with lead V_5 at left midaxillary line

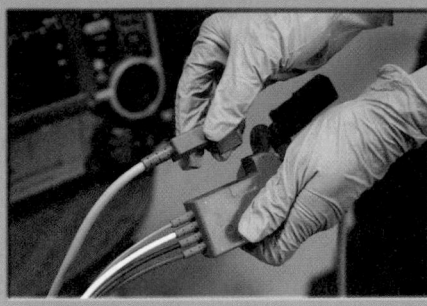

Step 5 Connect the cables to the monitor.

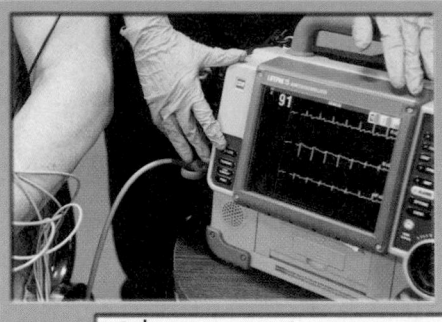

Step 6 Press the *12-lead Analyze* button.

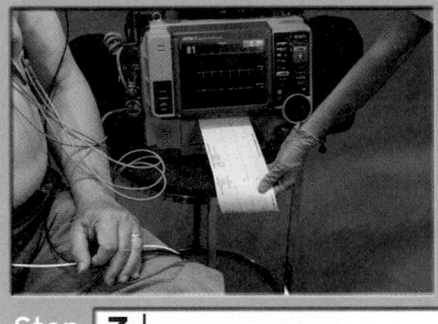

Step 7 Record tracings.

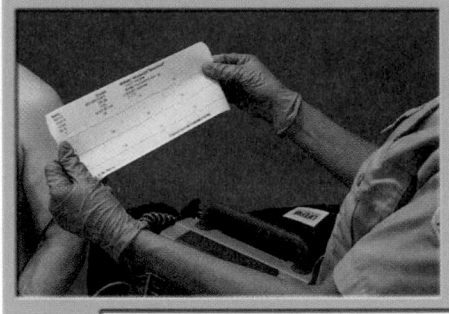

Step 8 Review the tracing. Determine whether additional views of the right and posterior walls (15- or 18-lead tracings) are needed. Label the tracing.

5. Connect the cables to the monitor Step 5.

6. Press the *12-lead Analyze* button Step 6.

7. Record tracings Step 7.

8. Review the tracing. Determine whether additional views of the right and posterior walls (15- or 18-lead tracings) are needed. Label the tracing Step 8.

12-Lead ECG Concepts

As discussed earlier, when a current is moving toward a lead, it creates a positive (upright) deflection on the ECG tracing of that lead. Thus, in Figure 89, the current depolarizing the ventricles is moving toward lead II, so what you see in lead II is an upright QRS complex (recall that the QRS complex is produced by depolarization of the ventricles). If the depolarizing current is moving toward lead II, then it must be moving away from lead aVR, so you would expect to see a negative deflection in aVR. And, indeed, the QRS complex in aVR is a downward deflection. That makes intuitive sense. For example, if you and a friend are standing facing each other at opposite ends of a football field, a ball thrown toward your friend will look bigger and bigger to the friend as it approaches; the same ball will meanwhile look smaller and smaller to you as it travels the same course. Similarly, leads II and aVR, being nearly opposite each other, will present nearly opposite pictures of the same wave of electrical depolarization. If a depolarizing wave is coming toward lead II, it will be going away from aVR.

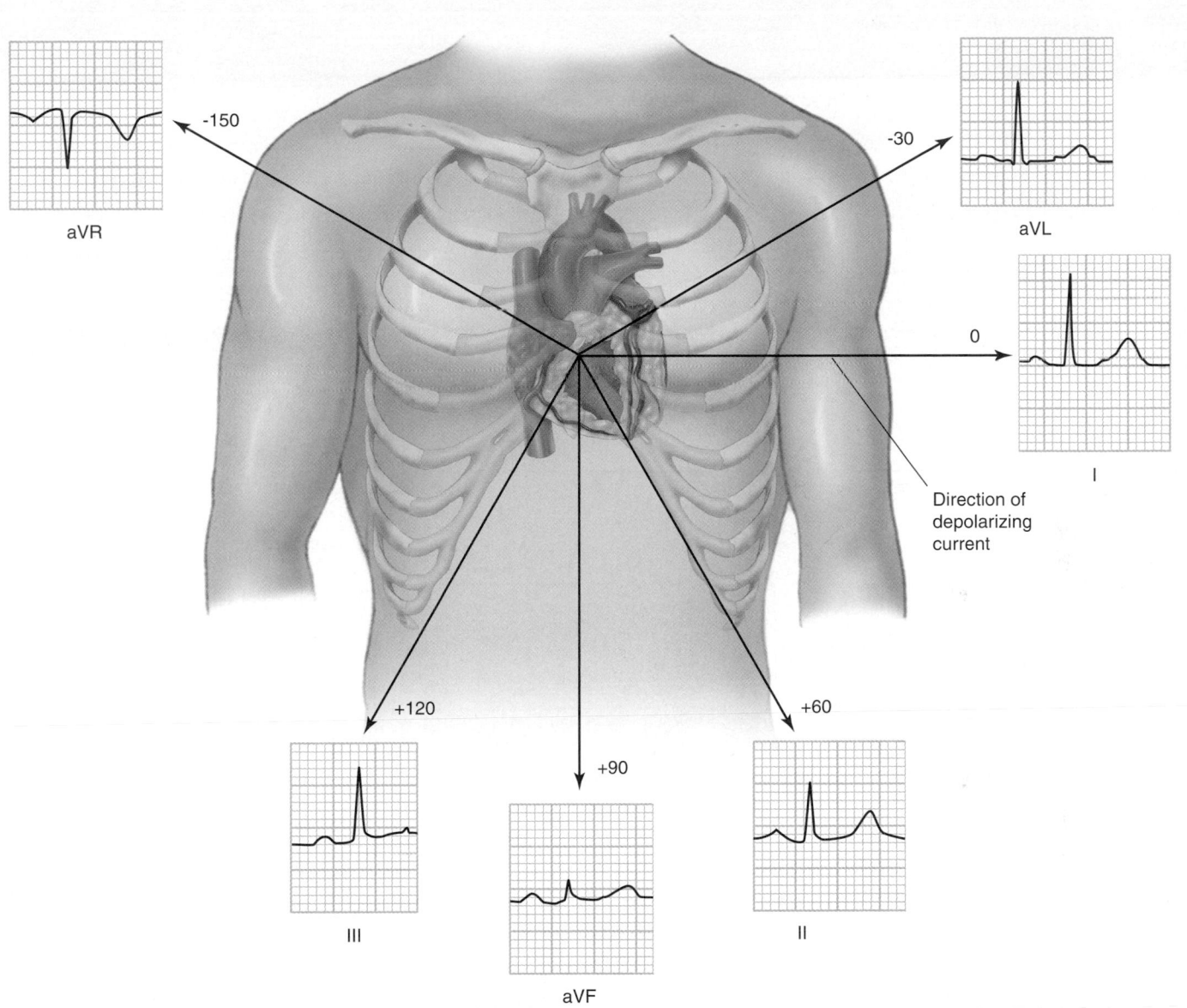

Figure 89 The morphology of QRS complexes varies based on the lead position and the direction of the electrical impulse movement within the heart. If the electrical impulses are moving primarily toward lead II, it will be upright as shown, while lead aVR will be inverted because the impulse is moving away from it.

Table 19 outlines where the different leads look and possible complications that can be seen with each lead.

Figure 90A shows colors associated with certain leads of the 12-lead ECG. Each of the colors has a purpose; that is, each color represents an area of the heart. From this figure, you can see which leads look at the same area of the heart. For example, leads II, III, and aVF all look at the inferior wall. Lead aVR is not used for this purpose, so no color is assigned to it. Figure 90B shows a normal ECG with standard 12-lead format.

Approach to Interpretation of the 12-Lead ECG

Similar to dysrhythmia interpretation, 12-lead ECG interpretation requires a systemic approach to ensure nothing is missed. A 7-step method to 12-lead ECG interpretation follows.

1. Snapshot
2. Dysrhythmia interpretation
3. Axis

Table 19 Focus of ECG Leads

Leads	Area Viewed	Coronary Artery Involved	Possible Complications
II, III, and aVF	Inferior wall LV	RCA: posterior descending	Hypotension, LV dysfunction
V_1 and V_2	Septum	LCA: LAD, septal	Infranodal blocks and BBBs
V_3 and V_4	Anterior wall LV	LCA: LAD, diagonal	LV dysfunction, CHF, BBBs, complete heart block, PVCs
V_5, V_6, I, and aVL	Lateral wall LV	LCA: circumflex	LV dysfunction, AV nodal block in some
V_4R	RV	RCA: proximal	Hypotension, infranodal and AV nodal blocks, atrial fibrillation, PACs

LV indicates left ventricle; LAD, left anterior descending; BBB, bundle branch block; RV, right ventricle; RCA, right coronary artery; LCA, left coronary artery; PAC, premature atrial contraction; PVC, premature ventricular contraction; CHF, congestive heart failure.

I	aVR	V_1	V_4
High lateral wall LV LCx		Interventricular septum LAD	Anterior wall LV LAD
II	**aVL**	**V_2**	**V_5**
Inferior wall LV RCA	High lateral wall LV LCx	Interventricular septum LAD	Low lateral wall LV LCx
III	**aVF**	**V_3**	**V_6**
Inferior wall LV RCA	Inferior wall LV RCA	Anterior wall LV LADt	Low lateral wall LV LCx

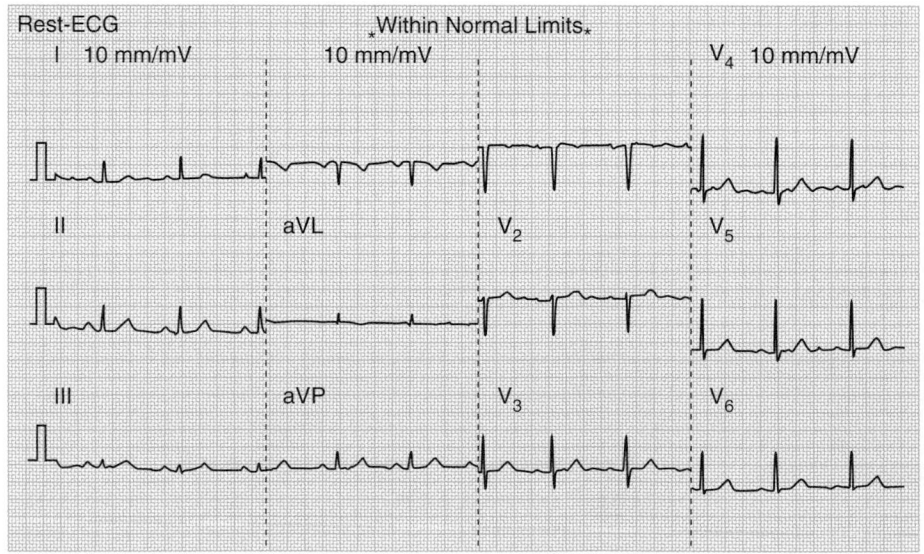

B

Figure 90 **A.** The areas on a 12-lead ECG correlate to different leads and therefore different areas of the heart. The coronary artery that supplies the wall for each lead is listed as well. **B.** A normal ECG with standard 12-lead format.

4. Conduction system
5. Chamber size
6. Ischemia, injury, infarction
7. Noncardiac

The Snapshot

First, take a look at the tracing and see if anything stands out. For example, is the rate extremely slow or fast? This step is a quick overall look at the 12-lead ECG to see if all the leads printed, if artifact is present, and if the rate is at one of the extremes.

Dysrhythmia Interpretation

This is the same 5-step process presented earlier in the chapter. Identify the underlying rhythm using these rules.

1. P waves (morphology, shape, direction, number)
2. QRS complexes (shape, duration)
3. PR intervals (duration)
4. Regularity
5. Rate (atrial, ventricular, calculation methods, parameters)

Axis

Every myocyte emits a small electrical charge when it depolarizes. If you added up all the electrical charges from all the myocytes at a specific moment in time, taking into account the direction and force of the charge, you would have a single value called a vector. A vector is a term used to describe a quantity, such as force, and has a magnitude and direction. The vector created by the ventricles during depolarization is referred to as the axis of depolarization Figure 91.

Figure 92 shows that, viewed from lead I, the QRS wave will be a positive deflection if it is heading toward the left arm and a negative deflection if it is heading toward the right arm.

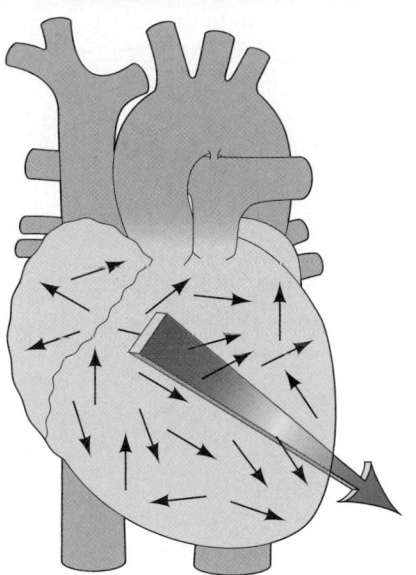

Figure 91 The sum of all ventricular vectors equals the electrical axis.

Figure 93 shows that, viewed from lead aVF, the QRS wave will be a positive deflection if it is heading toward the patient's feet and a negative deflection if it is heading toward the patient's head.

There are a number of methods that can be employed to determine the QRS axis. The easiest and fastest method involves using the QRS complexes in leads I and aVF. These two leads are used because they are the only perfectly horizontal and vertical leads, respectively. Using these leads, you can create a simple quadrant system.

Lead I is represented by the red line in **Figure 94** and lead aVF by the green line. Imagine placing these lines on top of one another and you have created a large + sign. Now, you have four quadrants where the center point or intersection of the two lines represents the origin of the impulse, and the four quadrants where the impulse can travel through. Using the direction of the QRS complexes in leads I and aVF, you can determine the QRS axis **Table 20**.

First, look at the QRS complexes in leads I and aVF and decide if the complex is positive or negative. If the QRS complexes are positive in lead I and aVF, the axis falls in quadrant 4 and lies between 0 and 90 degrees. This is the normal QRS axis. If the QRS complex is positive in lead I and negative in lead aVF, the axis falls in quadrant 2 and lies between 0 and −90 degrees. This is called left **axis deviation**. Right axis deviation is diagnosed by a negative QRS in lead I and positive QRS in lead aVF. Finally, extreme right axis deviation exists when QRS complexes are negative in leads I and aVF.

The QRS axis will always move in the direction of hypertrophy, and always move away from infarction. Recall that the P wave corresponds to electrical activity occurring in the SA node, whereas the QRS complex represents ventricular depolarization. Therefore, the direction of the QRS axis, or the axis deviation, relates to electrical activity in the ventricles. If one of the ventricles is enlarged (hypertrophy), it contributes more electrical energy, causing the overall electrical vector to point in the direction of the hypertrophy. Conversely, an infarcted area is dead tissue that has no electrical energy. Therefore, if an area of the ventricle is infarcted, the vector will point away from it.

Although axis deviation provides an important clue about electrical activity in the heart, it is not sensitive or specific for any particular diagnosis. Rather, it is used with other information to help clinicians understand what is happening in the heart.

Conduction System Disturbances

Next, look for conduction system disturbances on the 12-lead ECG. These include the bundle branch blocks, the fascicle or hemiblocks, and preexcitation.

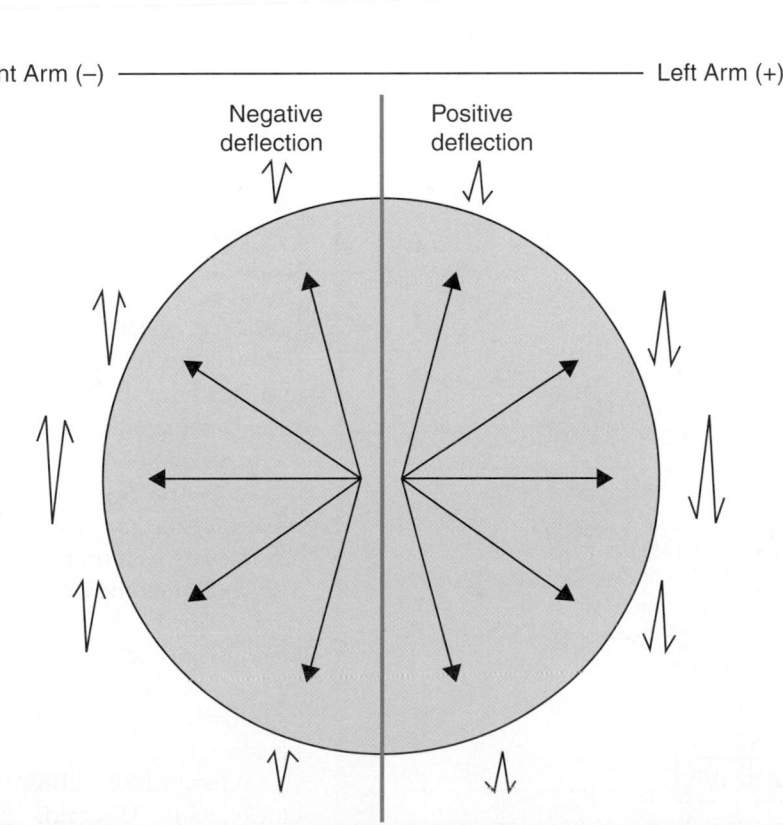

Lead I   Right Arm (−) ———————————————— Left Arm (+)

Negative deflection   Positive deflection

Figure 92 When lead I is viewed, a positive QRS deflection means the electrical vector is heading toward the left arm, whereas a negative QRS deflection means the electrical vector is heading toward the right arm.

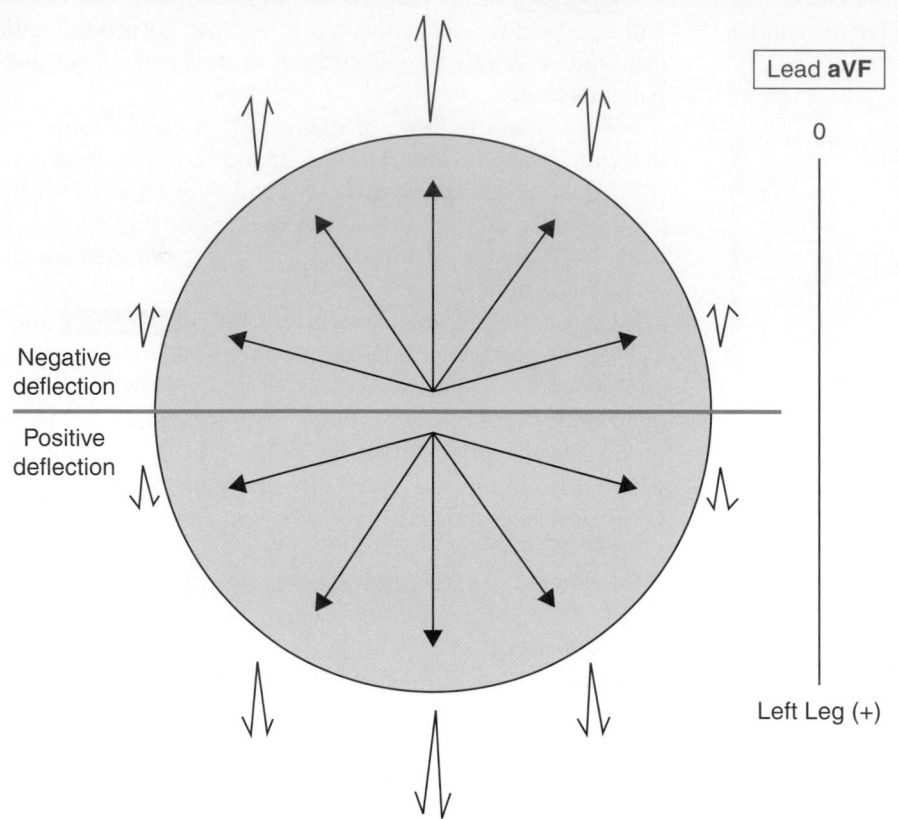

Figure 93 When lead aVF is viewed, a positive QRS deflection means the electrical vector is heading toward the feet, whereas a negative QRS deflection means the electrical vector is heading toward the head.

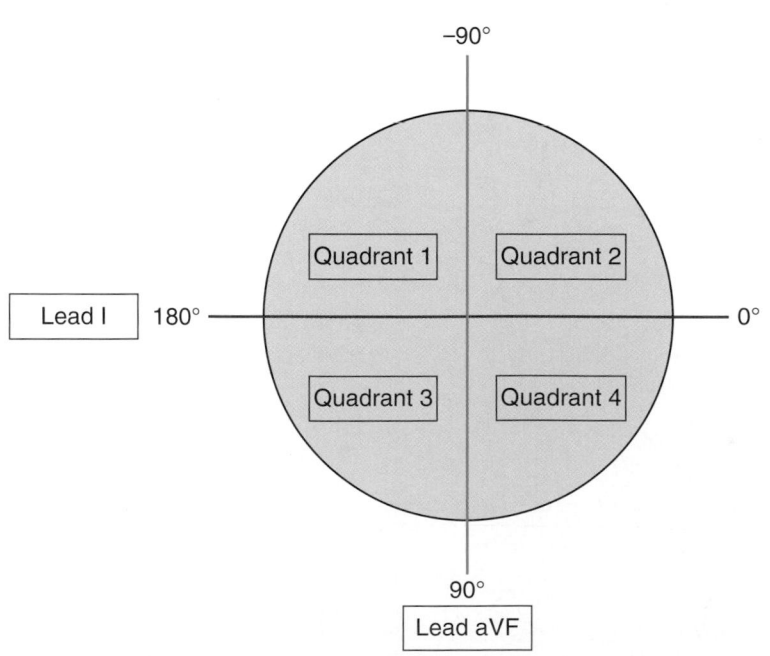

Figure 94 Four-quadrant system that can be used to determine the overall direction of an electrical vector in the ventricular region of the heart. This is an imaginary reference system to help find the axis deviation.

Bundle Branch Blocks A QRS complex with a bizarre appearance and a duration of longer than 120 ms signifies some abnormality in conduction through the ventricle as in a **bundle branch block**.

Right bundle branch blocks (RBBBs) and left bundle branch blocks (LBBBs) are some of the most commonly encountered findings on the 12-lead ECG. The names of these electrical conduction abnormalities identify where the electrical system is being delayed. Right bundle branch block is characterized by the presence of a wide QRS complex (duration greater than 120 ms), and a terminal R wave in lead V_1 (the second half of the QRS complex terminates in an R wave) **Figure 95**. Typically, the QRS complex in lead V_1 appears as an rSR' complex. (The ' symbol represents an R-prime wave. R-prime waves are never normal; they indicate trouble in the conduction system of the ventricle.) Terminal S waves are also seen in leads I, aVL, and V_6.

An LBBB is characterized by the presence of a wide QRS complex (duration greater than 120 ms) and a terminal S wave in lead V_1 (the second half of the QRS complex terminates in an S wave) **Figure 96**. Terminal R waves are also seen in leads I, aVL, and V_6.

The term RBBB or LBBB **aberration** is used to describe the shape of the QRS complex in aberrantly conducted beats. For example, if a particular complex has an rSR' shape, it is said to have RBBB morphology.

Fascicular Blocks (Hemiblocks) The left bundle branch bifurcates into the anterior and posterior fascicles. When these tissues become diseased or ischemic, they are unable to conduct electrical impulses, resulting in a **fascicular block**, or hemiblock. An anterior fascicular block is characterized by rS complexes in leads II, III, aVF, and qR complexes in leads I and aVL. A posterior fascicular block is rare and a diagnosis of exclusion. A posterior fascicular block is characterized by qR complexes in leads II, III, and aVF, and by rS complexes in lead I.

When RBBB, LBBB, anterior hemiblocks, and posterior hemiblocks are described, you will often hear the term bifascicular block. In a **bifascicular block**, a combination of two of the fascicles or conduction pathways is blocked. This

Table 20 Determining the QRS Axis Using Leads I and aVF

	Lead I		Lead aVF		
If...		and		then	**Normal** axis
If...		and		then	**Left** axis deviation
If...		and		then	**Right** axis deviation
If...		and		then	**Extreme right** axis deviation

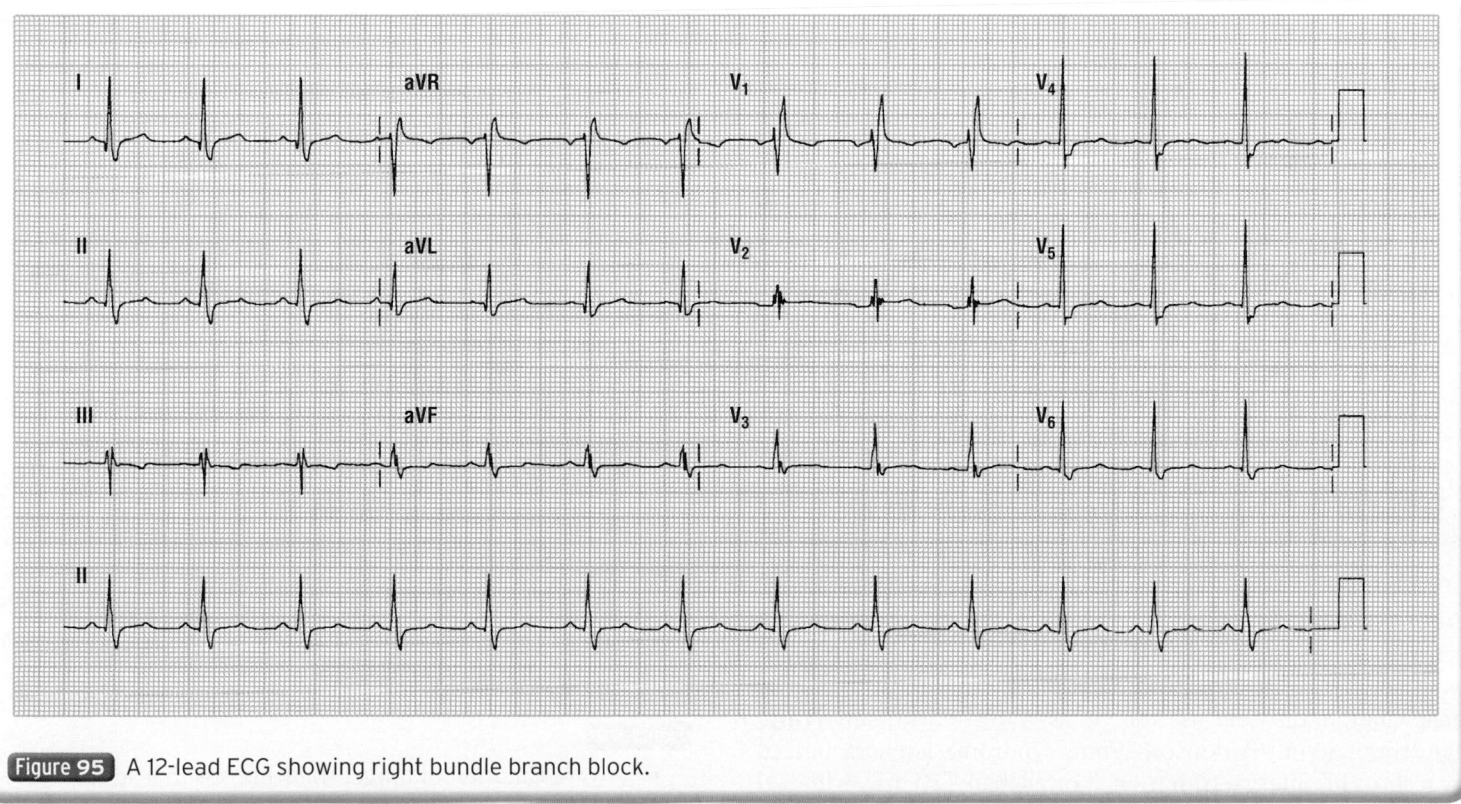

Figure 95 A 12-lead ECG showing right bundle branch block.

combination can vary and produces different effects in different patients. These combinations can be an RBBB and anterior hemiblock, an RBBB and posterior hemiblock, or an anterior hemiblock and posterior hemiblock, which is also known as an LBBB. A **trifascicular block** indicates that all three components that make up the ventricular conduction system are blocked or impaired but one still occasionally works to provide AV conduction.

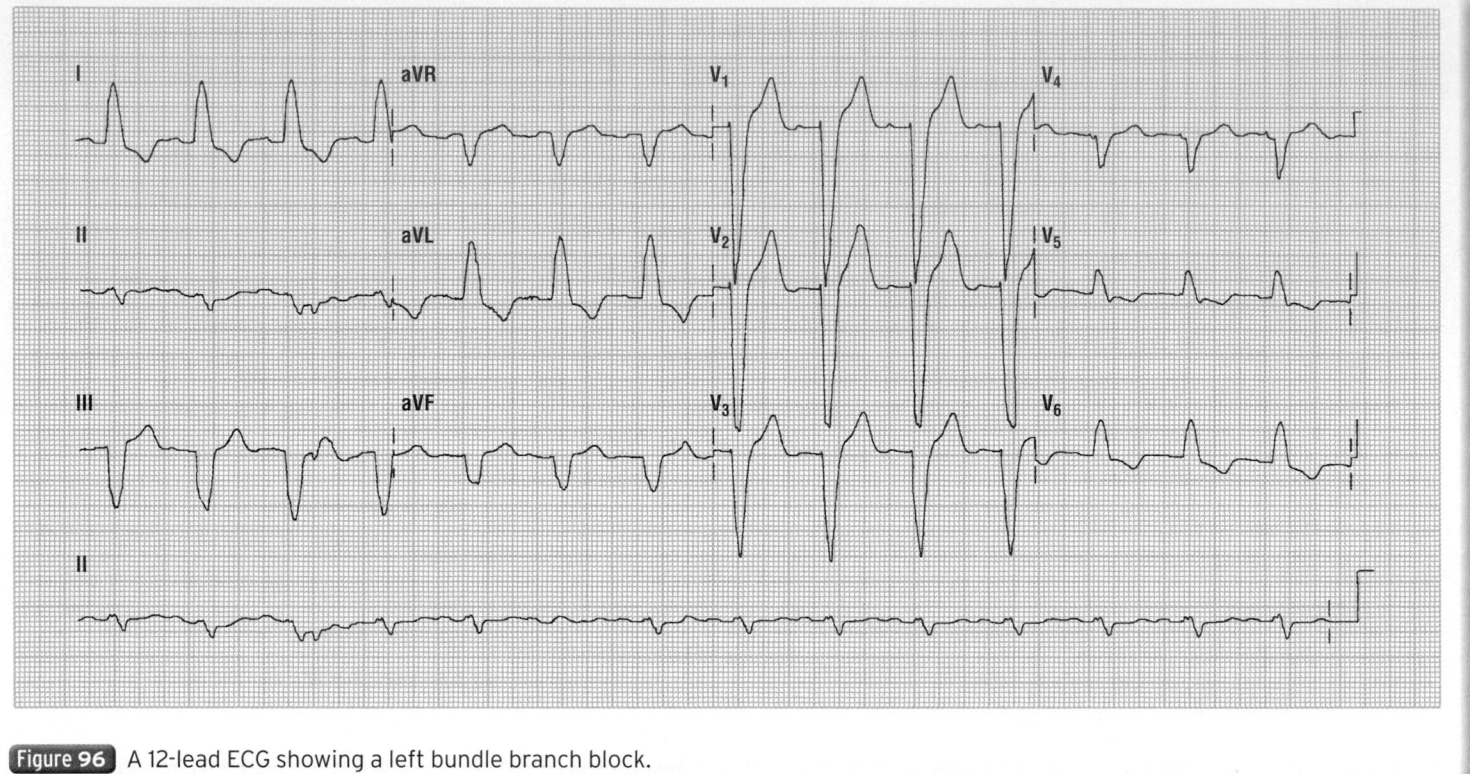

Figure 96 A 12-lead ECG showing a left bundle branch block.

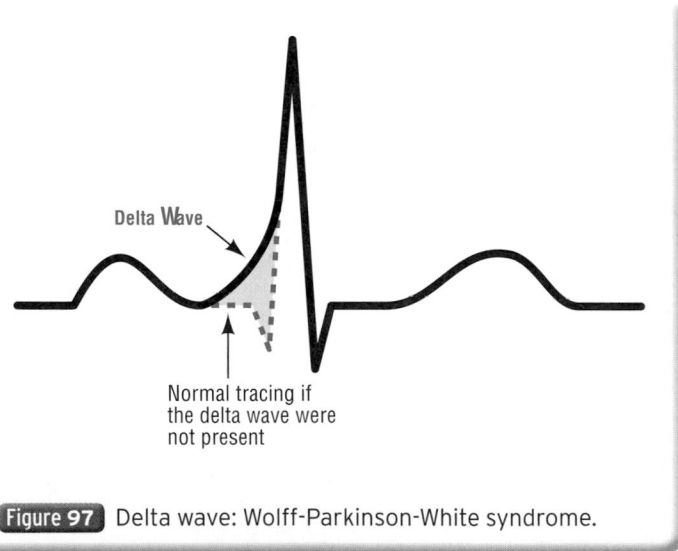

Figure 97 Delta wave: Wolff-Parkinson-White syndrome.

Preexcitation <u>Preexcitation</u> refers to early depolarization of ventricular tissue due to the presence of an accessory pathway between the atria and ventricles. The most common preexcitation disorder is known as <u>**Wolff-Parkinson-White syndrome**</u>. Wolff-Parkinson-White syndrome is characterized by a short PR interval (duration shorter than 120 ms), widened QRS complex, and the presence of a <u>**delta wave**</u>. The delta wave indicates an early departure from the PR segment as a result of conduction through the accessory pathway (Bundle of Kent) and subsequent early depolarization of ventricular tissue **Figure 97** . Patients with this syndrome are susceptible to tachydysrhythmias.

<u>**Lown-Ganong-Levine syndrome**</u> is another disorder that causes preexcitation of ventricular tissue. The syndrome is characterized by a short PR interval and a normal QRS duration on the ECG. Patients with Wolff-Parkinson-White syndrome and those with Lown-Ganong-Levine syndrome are predisposed to tachydysrhythmias.

Chamber Size

The 12-lead ECG can also provide information about the size of the heart's chambers. The R wave may be wide if the ventricle is enlarged and may be abnormally high if ventricular hypertrophy is present. If the S wave is abnormally deep, it may indicate hypertrophy of the ventricles.

The right atrium is a small, thin structure that is designed to function efficiently in a low-pressure environment. If returning venous pressure is elevated, or pulmonary pressures are high, the right atrium will dilate. Generally, <u>**right atrial enlargement**</u> (or right atrial dilation) results from chronic pulmonary disorders.

Right atrial enlargement is characterized by a P wave that has an amplitude higher than 2.5 mm in lead II and/or higher than 1.5 mm in lead V_1 **Figure 98** .

<u>**Left atrial enlargement**</u> is characterized by the following **Figure 99** :

- P wave duration of longer than 110 ms in lead II
- P wave with notched appearance
- Peak-to-peak duration of P wave longer than 40 ms
- P wave in lead V_1 predominantly negative

Left atrial enlargement has two primary causes: systemic hypertension, and mitral or aortic valve stenosis. It can also occur in an athletic heart.

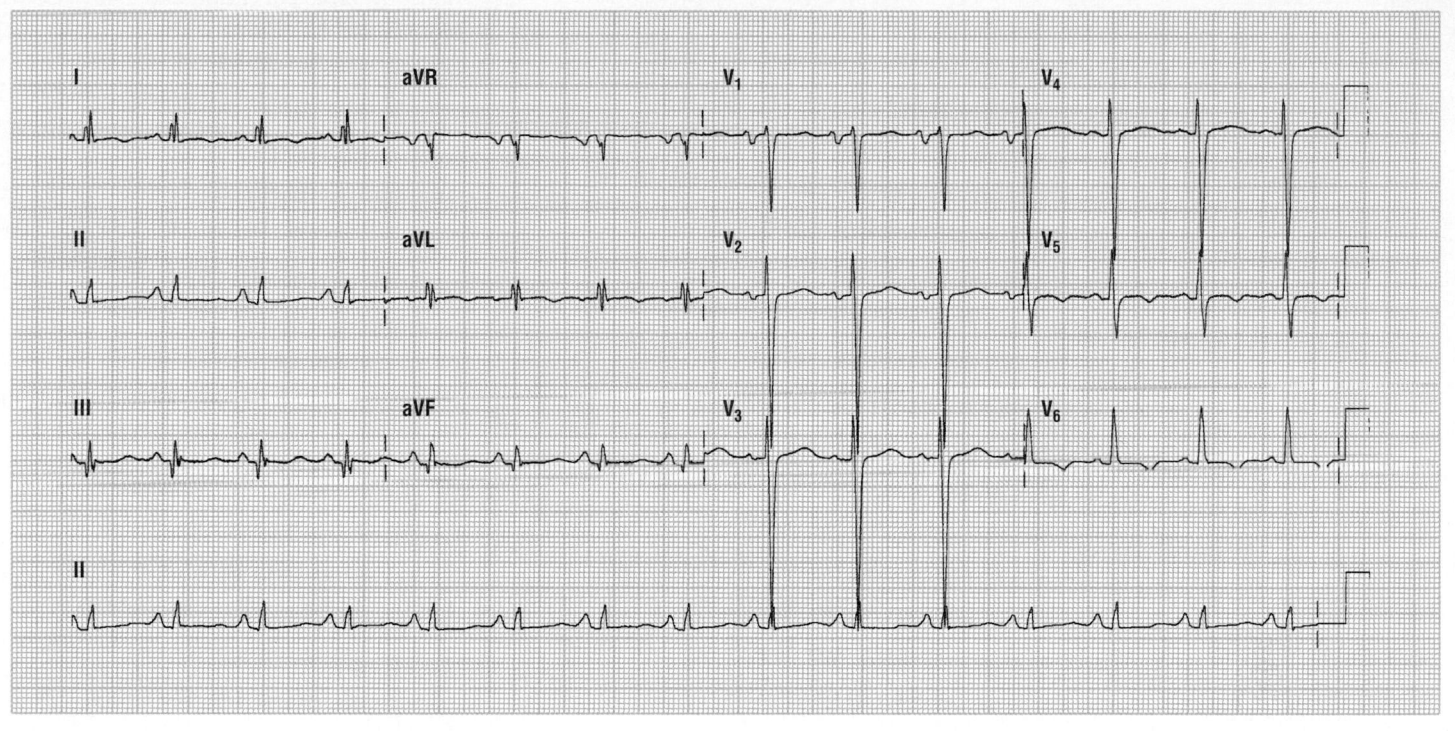

Figure 98 A 12-lead ECG showing right atrial enlargement.

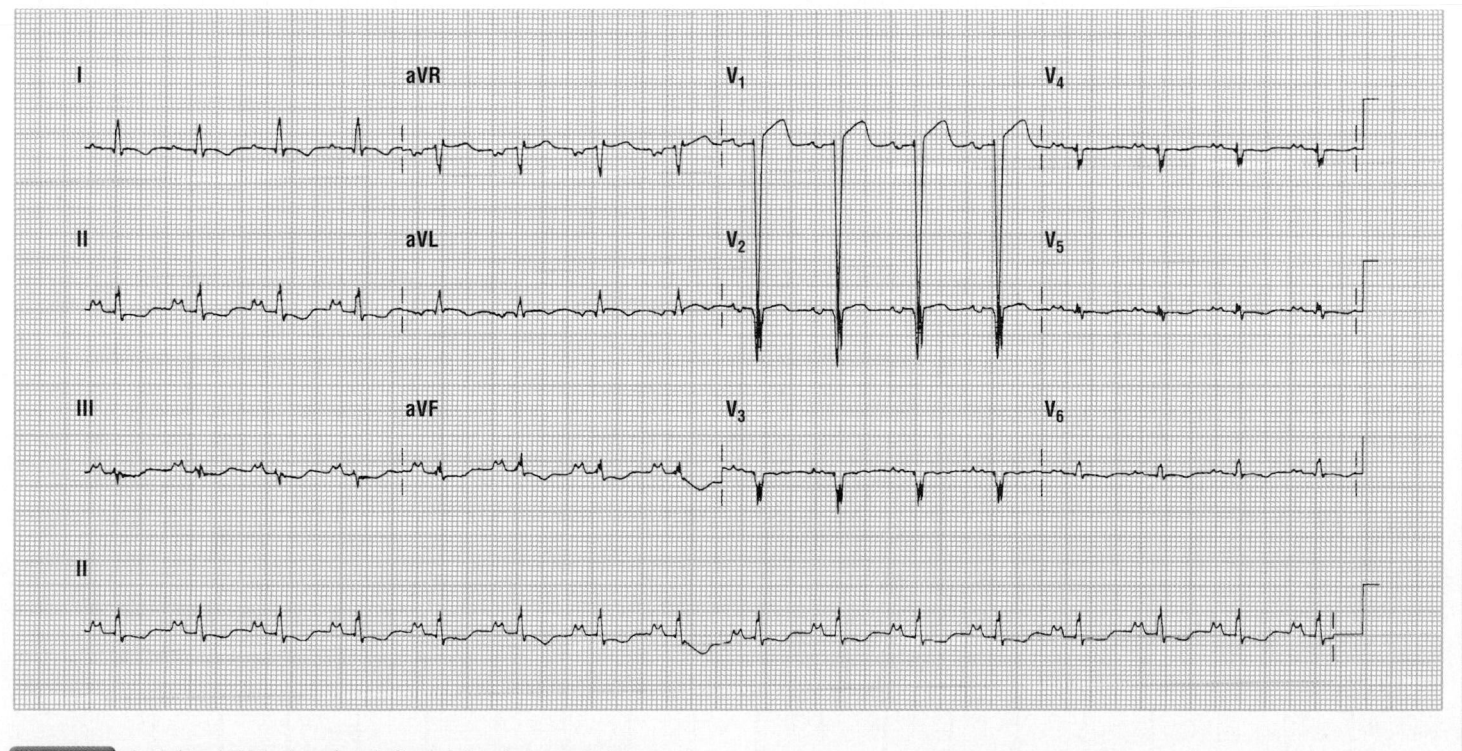

Figure 99 A 12-lead ECG showing left atrial enlargement.

In **right ventricular hypertrophy (RVH)**, the right ventricle becomes enlarged. This condition is usually caused by pulmonary hypertension. Right ventricular hypertrophy (think of it as dilation) is diagnosed using the following criteria **Figure 100**:

- Large R wave in lead V_1, and/or
- R wave in lead aVR with an amplitude taller than 5 mm
- QRS/T discordance in V_1

In **left ventricular hypertrophy (LVH)**, the left ventricle becomes enlarged, most commonly due to hypertension,

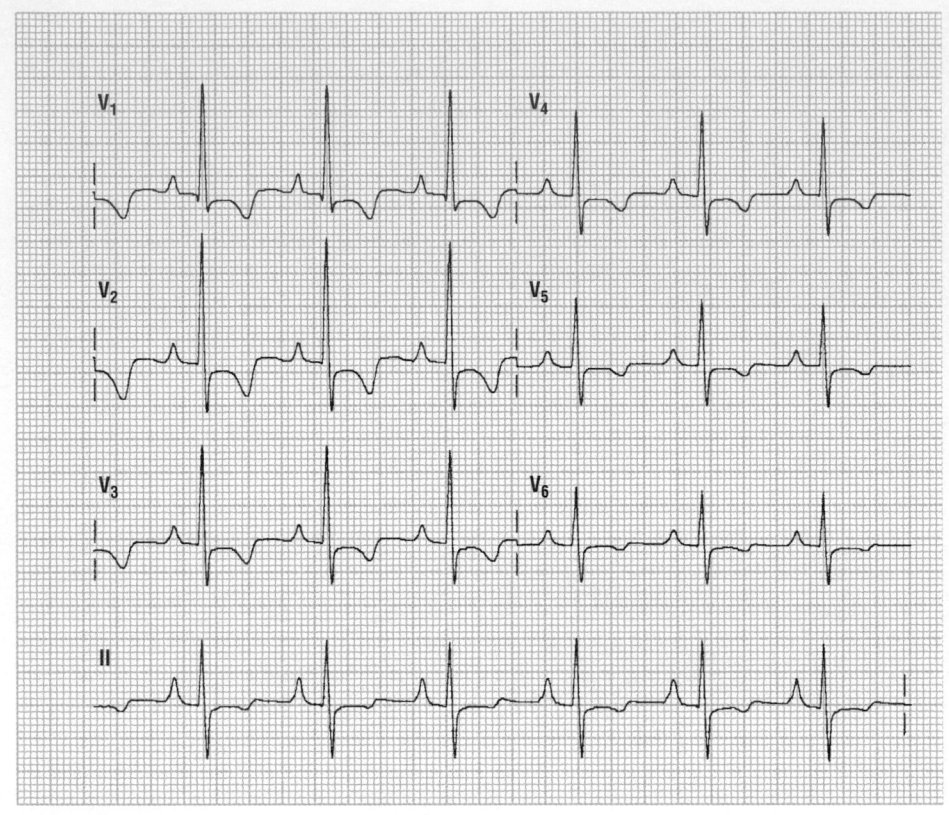

Figure 100 A 12-lead ECG showing right ventricular hypertrophy.

although this condition can also arise with some cardiac abnormalities. The left ventricle becomes enlarged because the left ventricular wall has increased due to the increase in the workload. The left ventricle will then lose elasticity and may fail to pump blood effectively, leading to CHF. Left ventricular hypertrophy is diagnosed using the following criteria **Figure 101** :

- Deepest S wave in lead V_1/V_2, plus
- Tallest R wave in V_5/V_6 taller than 35 mm, and/or
- R wave in lead aVL taller than 11 mm
- QRS/T discordance

Note: there are numerous methods of determining LVH from the ECG tracing. We have only presented two of them here. Diagnosis of LVH is made by echocardiogram, not ECG. It is not correct to say patients have LVH if they meet the criteria listed above. Rather, it is more appropriate to say the ECG meets the voltage criteria for LVH.

Ischemia, Injury, Infarction

In discussing ischemia, injury, and infarction, it is important to understand that it is critical to minimize EMS-to-balloon time,

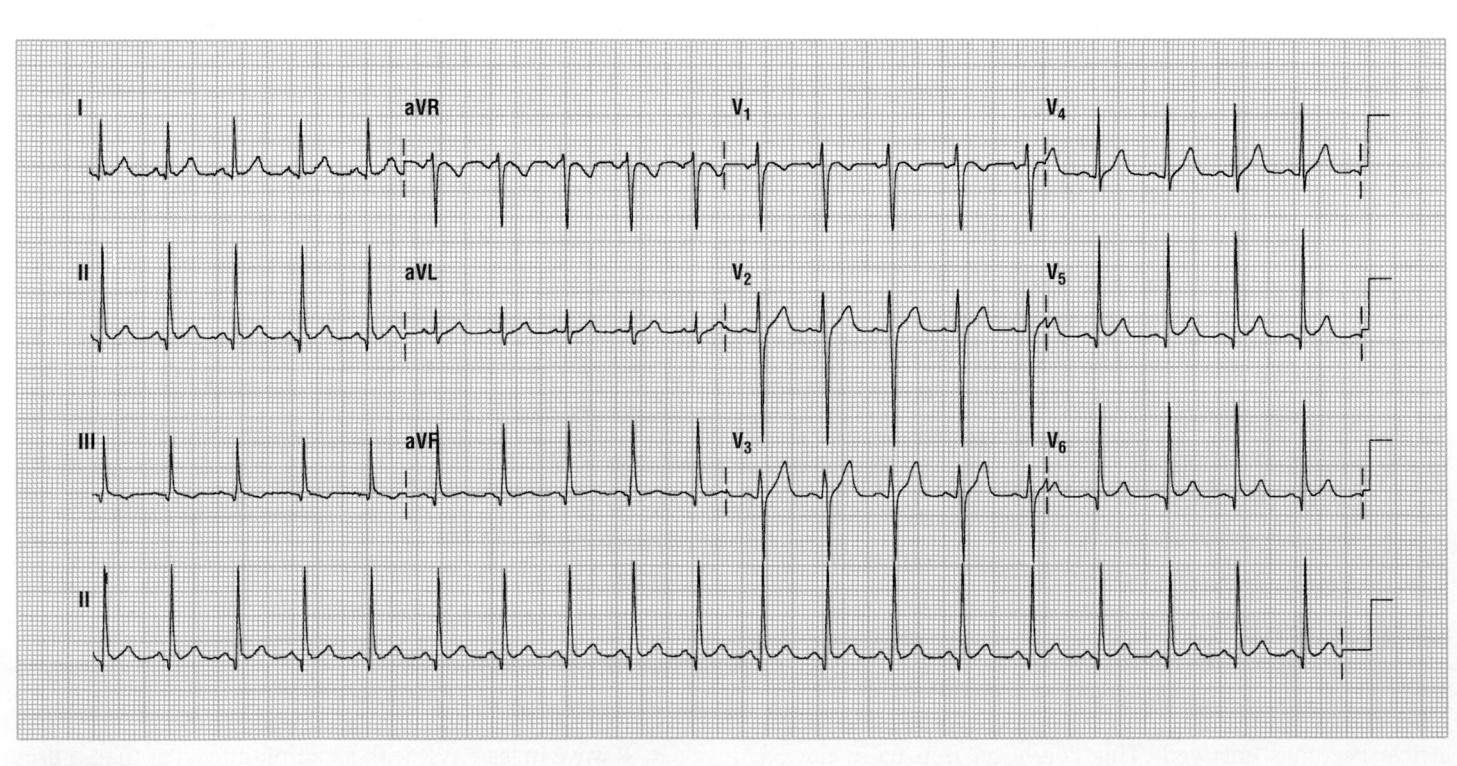

Figure 101 A 12-lead ECG showing left ventricular hypertrophy.

door-to-balloon time, and door-to-needle time. These concepts refer to the time frame that passes until the patient receives definitive therapy for the emergency condition. EMS-to-balloon time is the time frame that starts at the first moment of patient contact by EMS providers, and ends when definitive therapy occurs (when a catheter passes through the lesion in the affected coronary vessel). Door-to-balloon time is the time from patient presentation to the hospital and has the same endpoint as EMS-to-balloon time. Door-to-needle time starts when the patient presents at the ED and ends when a fibrinolytic medication is administered. Currently, the American Heart Association recommends a door-to-balloon time of less than 90 minutes and a door-to-needle time of less than 30 minutes.

Some of the most critical findings on the 12-lead ECG are myocardial ischemia, injury, and infarction. Rapid identification of a myocardial infarction is the single most important factor in decreasing the EMS-to-balloon time and mortality. There are several areas of the ECG that change dynamically during periods of ischemia; the Q wave, the J point, the ST segment, and the T wave. **Figure 102** shows the pattern of changes that indicate progression of a heart from normal state, to ischemia, to injury, to infarction.

Q waves are abnormal or pathologic if they are one small square (40 ms) wide on the ECG strip. Likewise, if they are deeper than one third of the total height (amplitude) of the

QRS complex (in lead II), they are abnormal. Such a finding is significant because it may indicate an AMI.

The J point is the junction point between QRS complex and the ST segment. It signifies the end of ventricular depolarization and the beginning of ventricular repolarization. For the purposes of this section, think of acute myocardial injury and infarction as a problem of repolarization. This will prompt you to look for anomalies on the right side of the QRS complex.

The ST segment begins at the J point and terminates at the T wave. The ST segment represents early repolarization of the ventricles. The ST segment can sink below, rise above, or stay in line with the isoelectric line during myocardial events. If the ST segment depresses below the isoelectric line, this is referred to as a pattern of ischemia. If the ST segment elevates above the isoelectric line, this is referred to as a pattern of injury. The lack of ST segment changes in the presence of acute coronary syndrome presentation is referred to as a nondiagnostic ECG. A nondiagnostic ECG does not rule out acute myocardial ischemia, injury or infarction; it simply means the tracing is nondiagnostic for those events. Serial blood work and additional testing is required.

The ST segment, which is the line between the QRS complex and the beginning of the T wave, is normally isoelectric. An ST segment whose amplitude is significantly (taller than 1 mm or one small box) above or below the isoelectric line is highly suggestive of myocardial ischemia or injury in three contiguous leads, although a full 12-lead ECG is required to determine the precise significance of ST segment elevation or depression.

Figure 103 depicts an injury (ST-segment elevation) in the leads that look at the anterior wall of the heart, leads V_3 and V_4, or V_1 through V_4. **Figure 104** shows the signs of ischemia (T-wave inversion) in the leads that look at the anterolateral wall of the heart, leads V_3 through V_6 and/or leads I and aVl.

Finally, the T wave is the most dynamic wave on the ECG. During ischemia, injury, and infarction, the T wave becomes

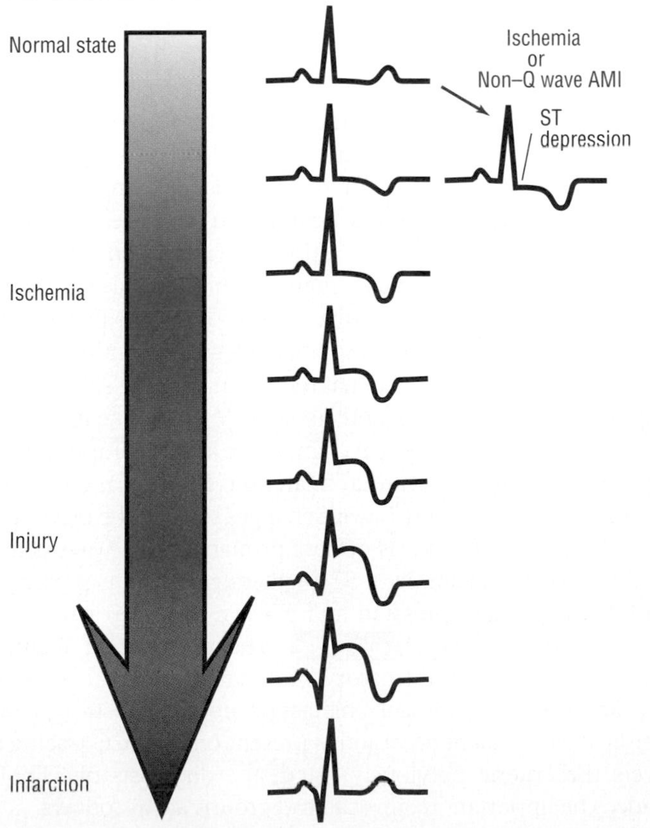

Figure 102 Evolutionary pattern or indicative changes of myocardial infarction.

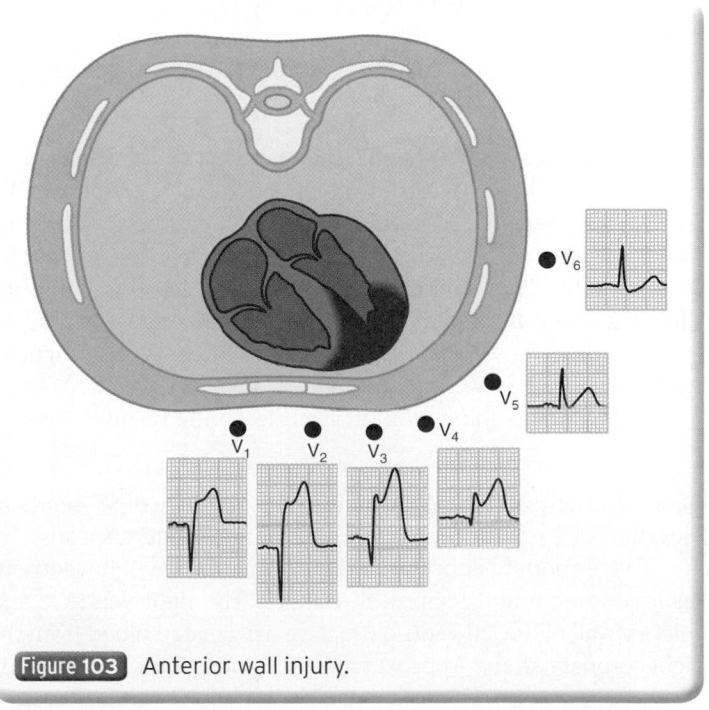

Figure 103 Anterior wall injury.

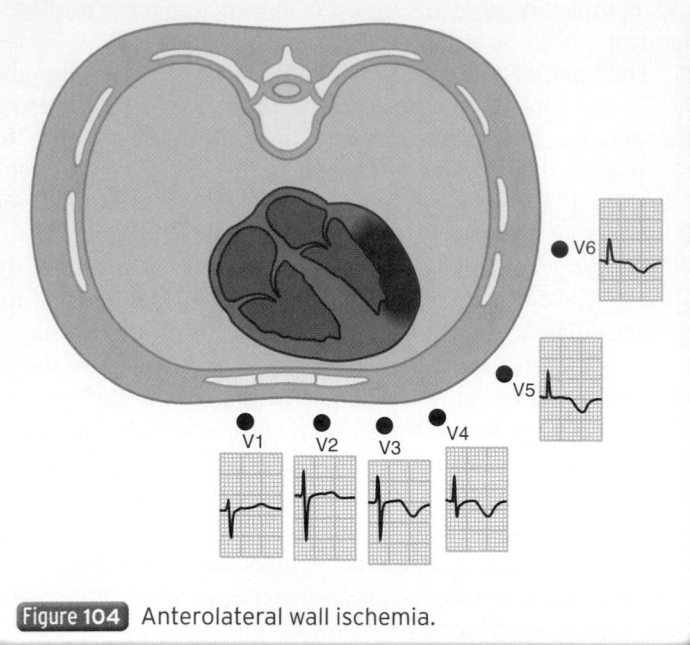

Figure 104 Anterolateral wall ischemia.

Table 21	Evolution of an Acute Myocardial Infarction on the ECG	
Stage	**ECG Changes**	**Timing**
Ischemia	T-wave inversion ST-segment depression	With the onset of ischemia
Injury	ST-segment elevation	Minutes to hours
Infarction	Q waves may appear or the tracing may normalize completely	Within several hours to several days

Note: Reciprocal changes will be seen in opposite leads.

Words of Wisdom

Recall that the 12-lead ECG shows STEMI in about 50% of those with evolving injury. The remaining 50% have nondiagnostic changes on the ECG. The ECG alone does not rule out myocardial ischemia, injury, or infarction!

very large (hyperacute), peaked or tented in shape, symmetric, and broad based. It is important to look for these changes on the ECG so you do not miss an ischemic event!

The terms TP segment, isoelectric line, isomeric line, and ECG baseline are synonyms. These terms refer to a period of "electrical silence" in the myocardium. Remember that although the baseline is neither positive nor negative, there is still electrical activity (movement of ions) in the myocardium. Perhaps a better phrase to describe the baseline would be a period of equal negative and positive electrical activity. The baseline is generally a flat, straight, horizontal line that begins at the end of the T wave and ends at the start of the P wave. The baseline is the reference point to which we compare the J point. A J point elevated by one or more millimeters with respect to the baseline is considered diagnostic for acute myocardial injury in the respective leads. Ischemia manifests itself as the J point depressed below baseline and/or T-wave inversion.

Ischemia Myocardial ischemia manifests itself as ST-segment depression and/or T-wave inversion on the diagnostic quality tracing. Furthermore, the area of ischemia can be localized by looking for changes in contiguous leads. **Contiguous leads** refer to leads that view geographically similar areas of the myocardium. Leads II, III, and aVF are contiguous. Leads V_1 and V_2, V_2 and V_3, V_3 and V_4, V_4 and V_5, and V_5 and V_6 are sets of contiguous leads. Leads I and aVL, and aVL and V_5 are also contiguous sets. **Table 21** lists the evolution from ischemia to infarction on an ECG.

Injury A diagnosis of AMI is made in the presence of ST-segment elevation of 1 mm or more in two or more contiguous leads.

Two important concepts in identifying MIs are right ventricular involvement and reciprocal changes. The right ventricle and inferior wall of the left ventricle receive oxygenated blood from the right coronary artery. Approximately 40% of patients experiencing

an **inferior wall MI** will also have right ventricular involvement. Right ventricular involvement is an important finding in the prehospital setting because of the impact on treatment. The indication for performing a right-sided ECG is the presence of inferior wall STEMI. Recall that the ECG changes of inferior wall STEMI include an ST elevation of 1 mm or more in leads II, III, and aVF.

A right-sided ECG is acquired by placing an electrode in the fifth intercostal space at the midclavicular line on the right side of the chest (V_4R). Unsnap the lead V_4 on the left side of the chest and snap it onto a new electrode on the right side, leaving all the other electrodes in place. Now press "acquire" on the 12-lead ECG monitor. If you see ST-segment elevation of greater than 1 mm in the V_4R lead on this second ECG, there is a high likelihood that you have identified a right ventricular MI. Of course, the ECG monitor does not know that this V_4 is right-sided, so on printing this ECG tracing, you should indicate that the tracing is right sided by writing an "R" next to the "V_4," and circle the V_4R to make it stand out.

As mentioned, reciprocal changes are another important concept in identifying myocardial infarction. Reciprocal changes are J-point, ST-segment, and T-wave changes seen on the ECG during STEMI. Reciprocal changes oppose primary J/ST/T-wave changes on the ECG. For example, if ST-segment elevation is present in a lead, ST-segment depression and T-wave inversion will be seen in the reciprocal leads **Figure 105**. The presence of reciprocal changes is highly confirmatory of acute myocardial infarction. The absence of reciprocal changes is not diagnostic. In other words, if ST-segment elevation is present on the ECG tracing and meets the criteria previously listed, the diagnosis of STEMI is made. The important reciprocal lead groups are as follows:

- Leads II, III, aVF, and Leads I, aVL
- Leads II, III, aVF, and Leads V_1 to V_3
- Leads V_7 to V_9 and Leads V_1 to V_3

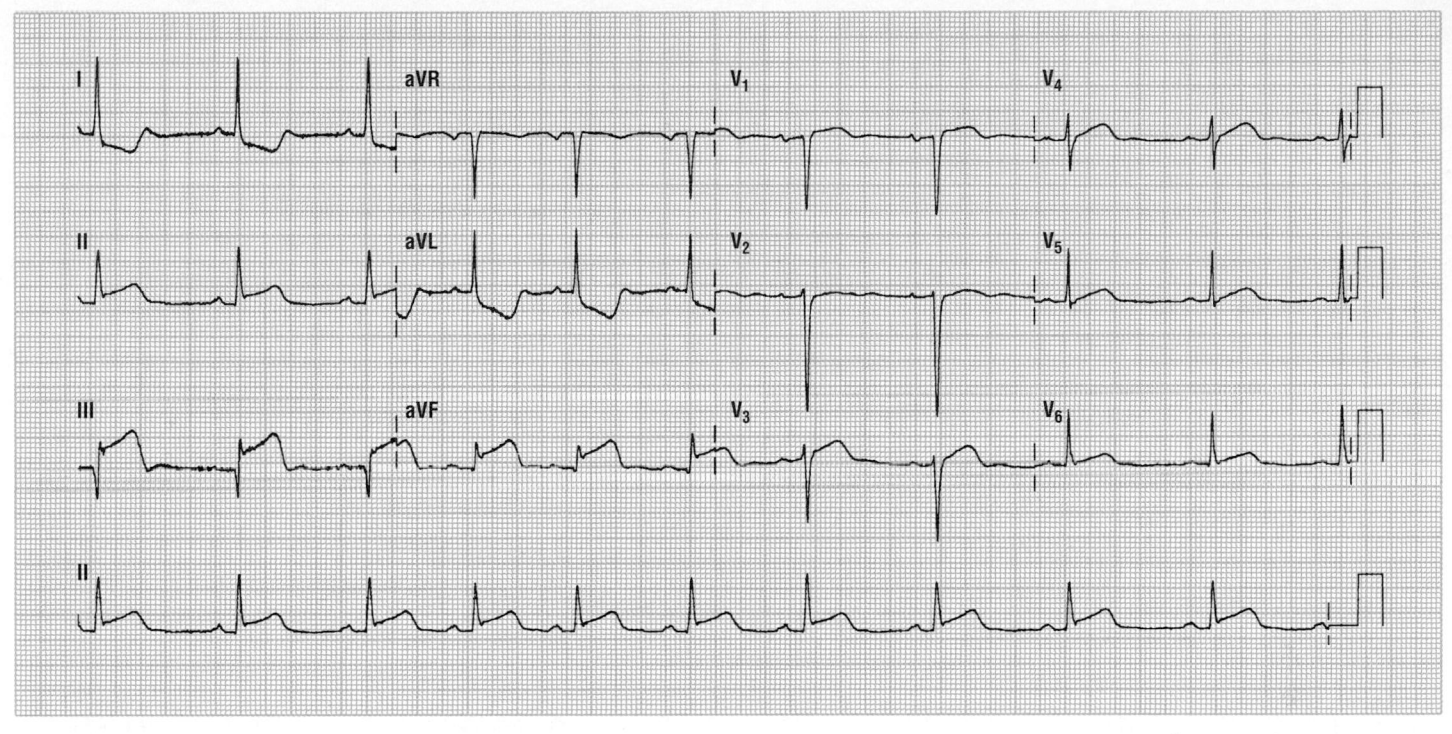

Figure 105 ST-segment elevation with ST-segment depression and T-wave inversion in reciprocal leads.

Typically, the following changes will be observed during myocardial injury:

1. ST-segment elevation in leads II, III, and aVF and reciprocal changes in leads I and aVL (ST-segment depression and T-wave inversion).

2. ST-segment elevation in leads V_1 to V_3 (and sometimes V_4) and reciprocal changes in leads II, III, aVF (ST-segment depression and T-wave inversion).

3. The final lead group involves the posterior wall of the left ventricle. Although you can record a posterior ECG by placing leads V_7 to V_9 on the posterior aspect of the left thorax, the same data can be derived from the reciprocal anterior leads. Diagnosis of posterior wall STEMI is made using the following criteria:

- QRS duration of shorter than 120 ms
- Large R waves in leads V_1 to V_3 (R wave larger than S wave)
- ST-segment depression and T-wave inversion in leads V_1 to V_3

Finally, the specific area of ischemia, injury, or infarct can be localized by noting which areas of the ECG show changes. Lead groups enable the paramedic to localize ischemic changes using the ECG. **Table 22** summarizes the leads corresponding to different locations of myocardial injury. **Figure 106** shows ECGs with these areas of damage localized.

Treatment The 12-lead ECG plays a crucial role in the diagnosis of STEMI in that it drives medical therapy based on the presence or absence of certain findings. Prehospital treatment of AMI follows the same treatment algorithm as the treatment of chest

Table 22 Localization of an Acute Myocardial Infarction

Site of Ischemia, Injury, Infarction	Seen in Leads
Inferior wall	II, III, and aVF
Septal	V_1 to V_2
Anterior	V_3 to V_4
Low lateral High lateral Right ventricle	V_5 to V_6 I and aVL V_4R
Posterior wall	V_7-V_9 and/or V_1-V_3

pain. Aspirin and nitroglycerin should be administered early in the absence of any contraindications. There is controversy over the safety and efficacy of oxygen and morphine administration in AMI. Follow your local protocols to ensure appropriate administration of morphine and oxygen for AMI.

STEMI treatment involves the rapid reperfusion of the affected lesion or lesions by way of mechanical methods (percutaneous coronary intervention [PCI]). The 12-lead ECG also allows for early and rapid detection of right ventricular injury in the face of inferior wall injury. This finding dictates the need for volume replacement prior to administration of nitrates to prevent large drops in systemic blood pressure (remember

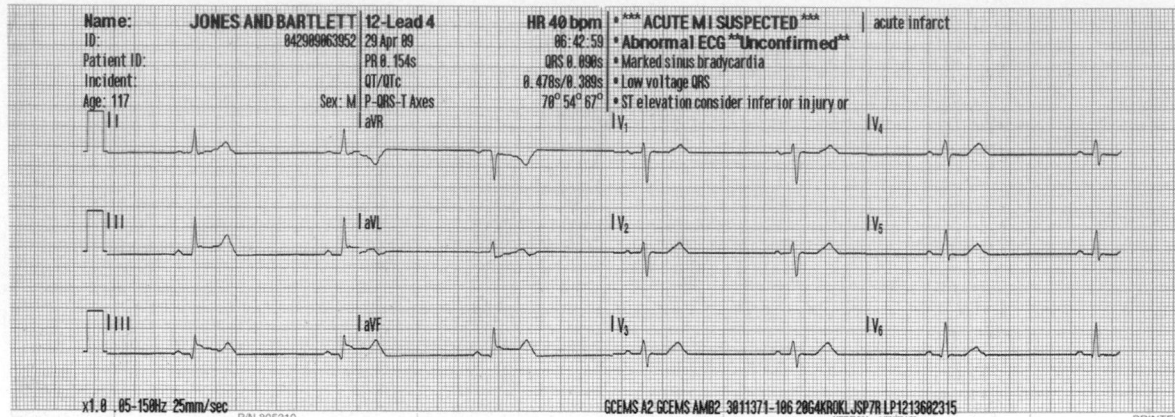

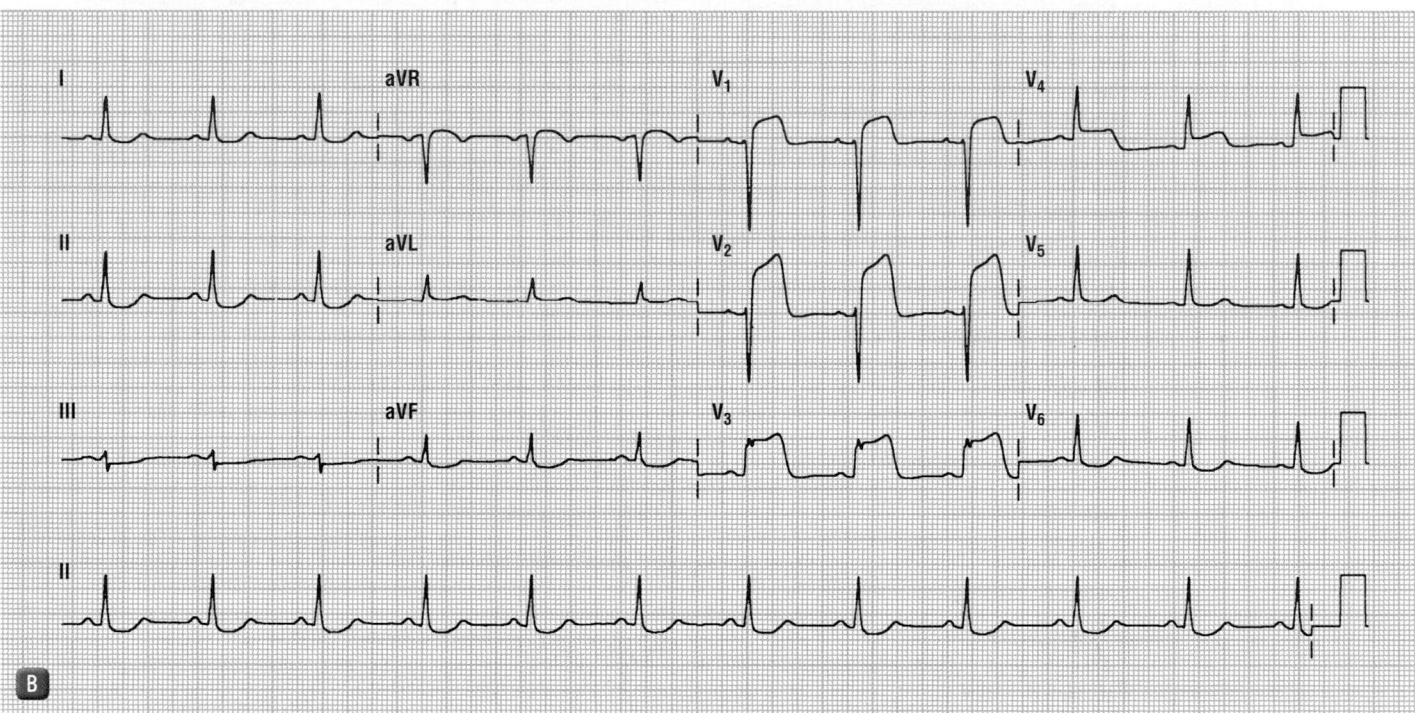

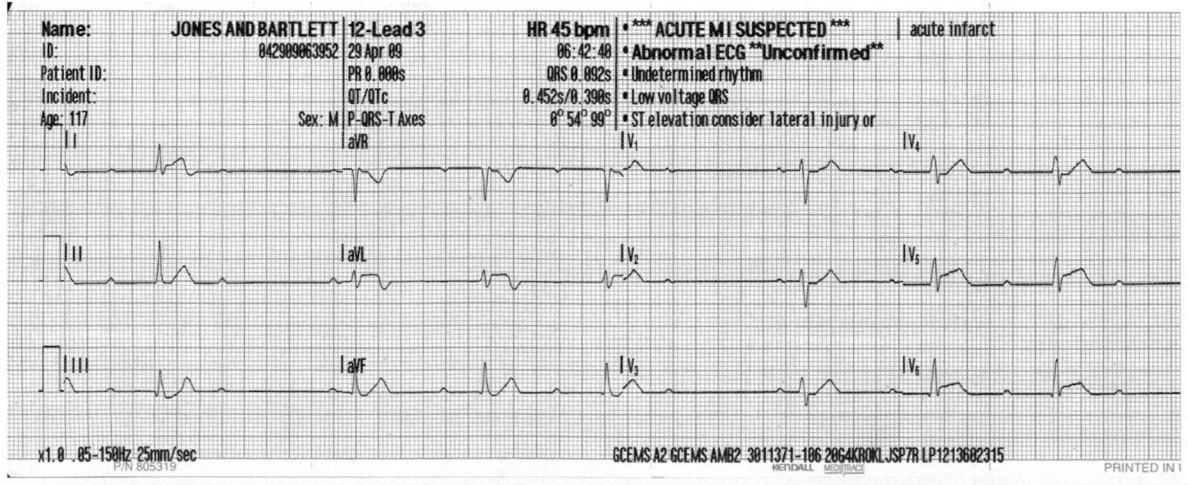

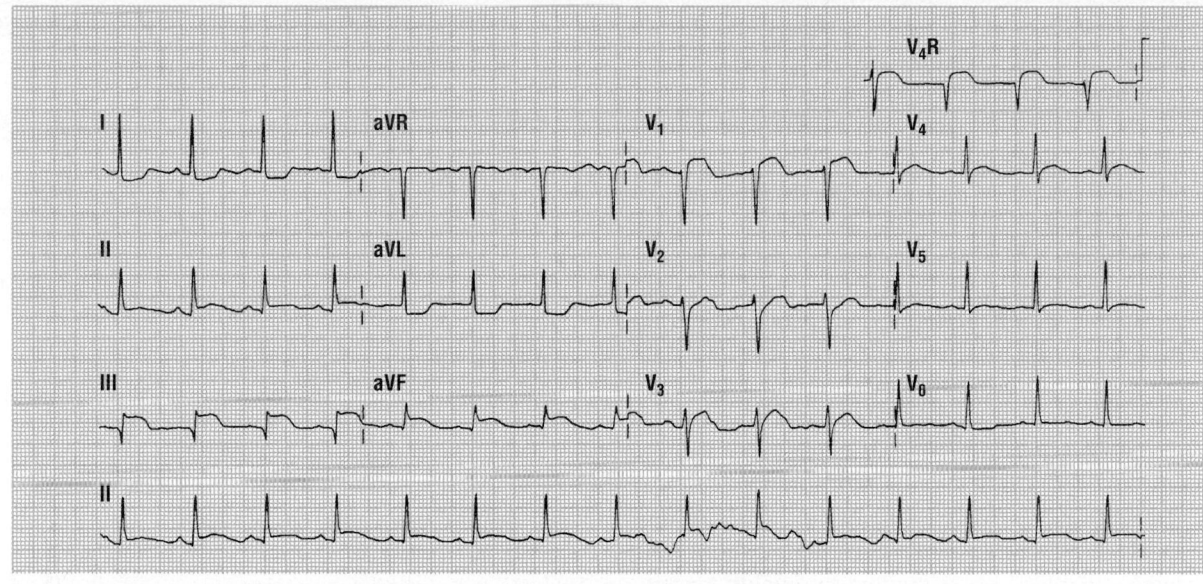

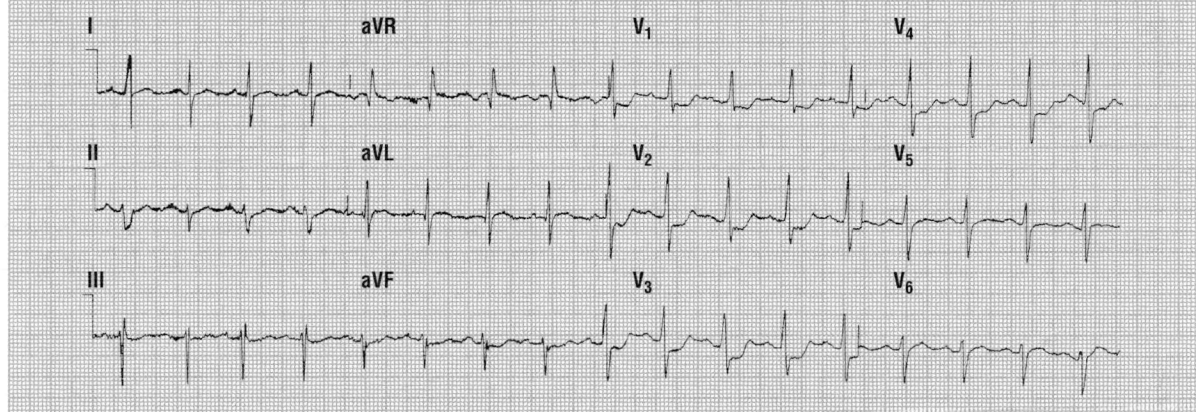

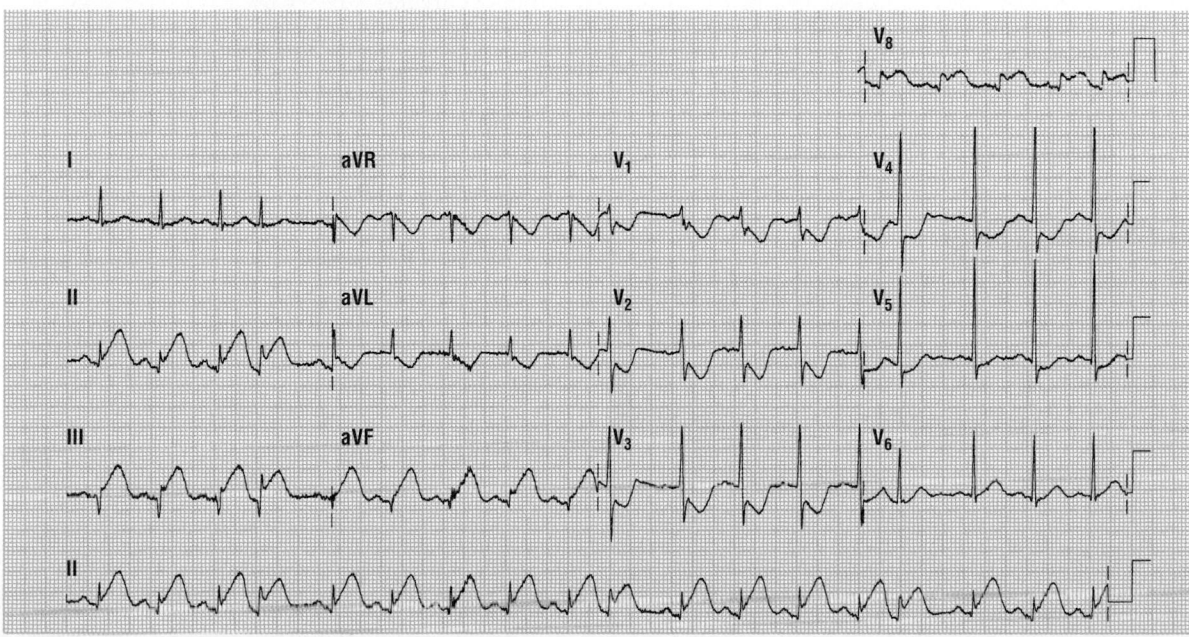

Figure 106 ECGs with these areas of damage localized. **A.** Inferior wall. **B.** Anteroseptal. **C.** Lateral. **D.** Right ventricle. **E.** Posterior wall. **F.** Inferior-right ventricular-posterior. Isolated posterior STEMI occurs rarely (2% to 4%); posterior wall infarction almost always occurs with inferior wall STEMI.

this group is preload dependent!). In patients presenting with classic, atypical, or angina-type pain, the 12-lead ECG allows for rapid stratification into one of three categories: STEMI (ST elevation in two or more contiguous leads, or new or suspected LBBB), NSTEMI (new ECG changes, non-ST elevation), and normal (nondiagnostic). Remember, a normal ECG does not rule out ischemia, injury, or infarction. Patients presenting with ST elevation are candidates for emergent primary percutaneous coronary intervention (pPCI) and should be transported to a facility capable of performing the procedure. As of the date of this printing, patients experiencing NSTEMI (nondiagnostic ECG, ACS presentation with positive cardiac biomarkers) are not candidates for urgent cardiac catheterization.

Cardiac catheterization is a minimally invasive procedure performed under fluoroscopy and is used to diagnose and treat blocked coronary arteries. Cardiac catheterization, pPCI, and percutaneous transluminal coronary angioplasty (PTCA) are used interchangeably to refer to cardiac catheterization. The 12-lead ECG tracing enables EMS providers to quickly identify STEMI in the prehospital setting, transmit the ECG to the receiving facility (or relay the findings over the phone or radio), decrease the door-to-balloon time, and decrease mortality. Some jurisdictions do not have a local hospital capable of performing cardiac catheterization. Most emergency departments can effectively treat patients with STEMI by administering fibrinolytic medications to dissolve blood clots. The process of dissolving blood clots is called __fibrinolysis__.

Prehospital 12-lead ECGs and advance notification to the receiving hospital can lead to faster diagnosis, decrease the time until fibrinolysis is administered, and potentially decrease mortality rates. The time savings in door-to-perfusion therapy ranges from 10 to 60 minutes. Therefore it is the standard of care for paramedics to efficiently acquire and transmit ECGs or communicate the findings to the emergency department with only a minimal increase (0.2 to 5.6 minutes) in on-scene time. The decision of where to transport patients with acute coronary syndrome (ACS) should be based on current guidelines and recommendations from national groups such as the AHA and the American College of Cardiology.

Words of Wisdom

A patient who reports heavy, crushing, squeezing, or choking chest pain may be experiencing an acute myocardial infarction even if the ECG is perfectly normal.

The Many Faces of Ischemia: Summary Figures 107 through 112 represent common ECG findings suggestive of myocardial ischemia. Throughout the text, we use the terms ischemia and injury interchangeably. Although the focus of 12-lead ECG interpretation in EMS is to quickly and accurately recognize STEMI so the patient can be transported to a facility capable of pPCI, it is equally important to recognize a tracing that indicates only ischemia. It is thought that this subset of patients does not necessarily benefit from emergent PCI, but does benefit from receiving treatment aimed at reducing myocardial ischemia and that may

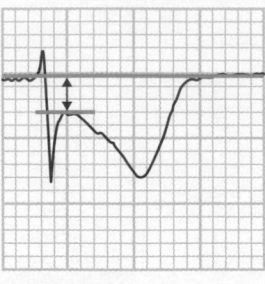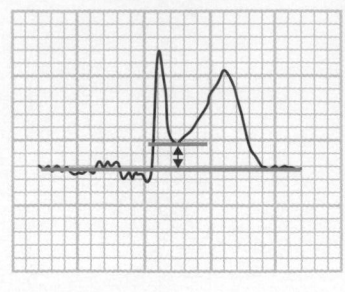

Figure 107 The "J" point.

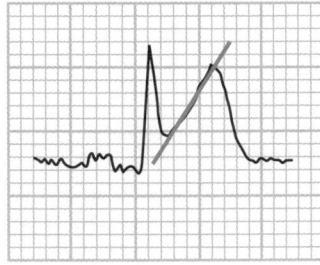

Figure 108 A convex ST segment indicates possible ischemia. Test for this by drawing a line from the J point to the peak of the T wave. If the line superimposes or if the T wave is above the line, the segment is convex.

prevent a myocardial infarction from occurring.

Other Cardiovascular Conditions
The 12-lead ECG can also provide information about noncardiovascular problems, including pulmonary embolism, acute intracranial hemorrhage, and electrolyte abnormalities.

__Benign early repolarization__, or early repolarization is thought to be a normal variant that affects approximately 1% of the population. The diagnosis of benign early repolarization is made by ECG and is almost always a coincidental finding. Frequently, the diagnosis is made while recording an ECG during a routine physical examination or during testing for an unre-

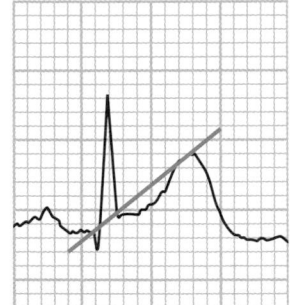

Figure 109 A concave ST segment indicates possible benign conditions, such as pericarditis and benign early repolarization; however, ischemia can *also* manifest with this pattern, as seen in STEMI.

lated condition. Benign early repolarization is characterized by ST-segment elevation (or J-point elevation), a J or fishhook appearance at the J point, and concave ST-segment morphology Figure 113. The changes are often seen exclusively in the left precordial leads

Up Sloping   Horizontal   Down Sloping

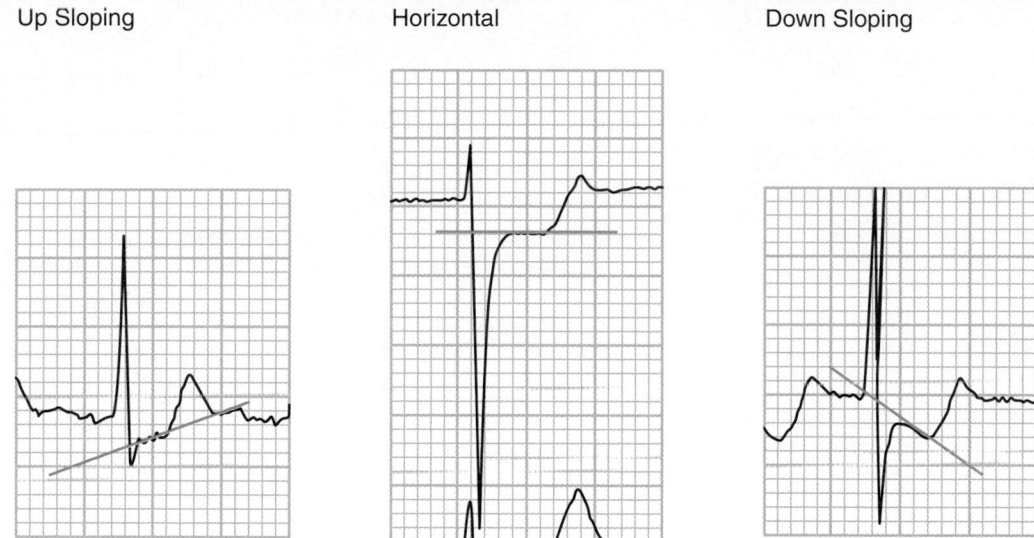

Figure 110 Direction of slope. All of these examples illustrate myocardial ischemia. Horizontal and down-sloping ST segments are always pathologic findings. A slow up-slope is most often a pathologic finding. A rapidly up-sloping ST segment is generally a normal electrocardiographic change, as demonstrated during exercise stress testing.

Peaked / tented – the apex of the T wave elevates and forms a "peaked" appearance

Hyperacute – the height of the T wave exceeds ½ the overall height of the QRS

Symmetry – the T wave becomes symmetrical with respect to the Y axis

Broad base – the base of the T wave elongates during ischemia

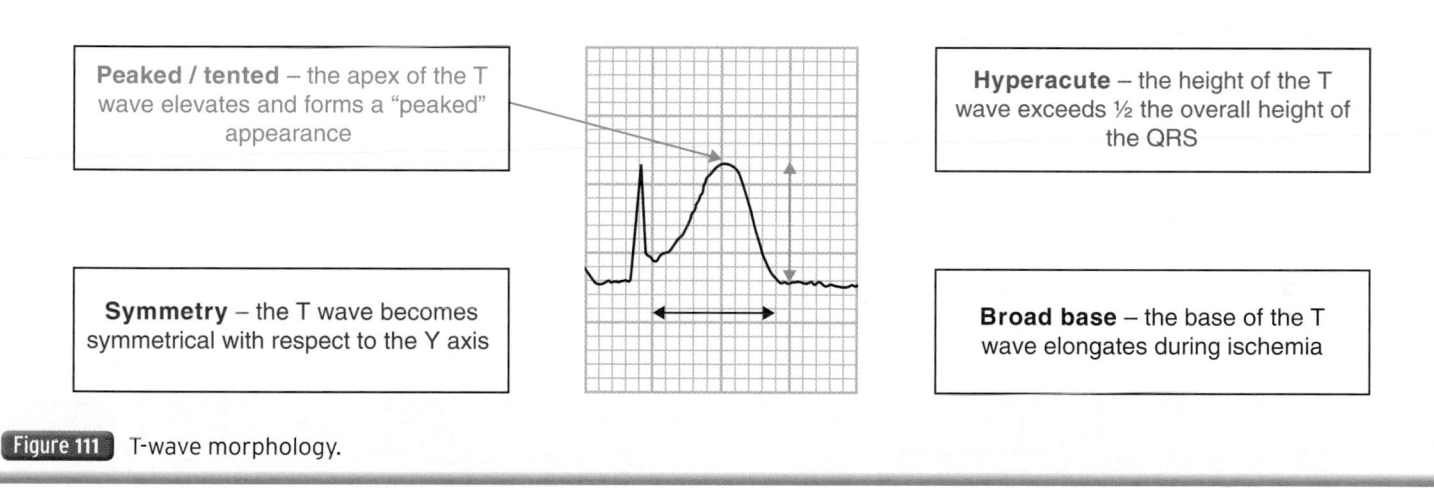

Figure 111 T-wave morphology.

Without ST-segment depression

With ST-segment depression

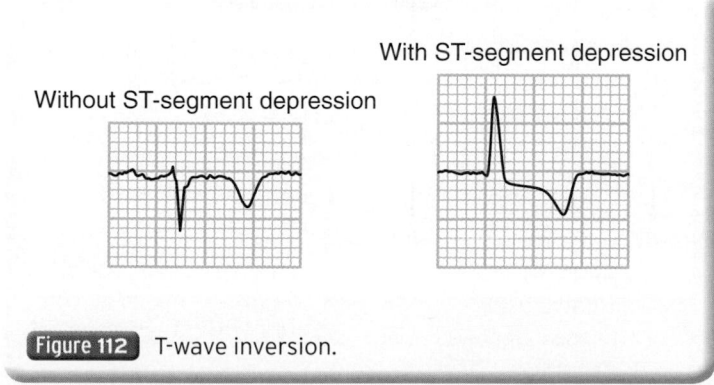

Figure 112 T-wave inversion.

(V_4 to V_6) and/or the inferior leads. Reciprocal changes are never seen in benign early repolarization.

<u>Pericarditis</u> is the inflammation of the pericardial sac as a result of an infection (bacterial, viral, or fungal) or trauma. Patients can present with positional chest pain (often alleviated by sitting forward), shortness of breath, and history of recent infection or fever. The condition is characterized by diffuse ST-segment elevation (not exceeding 5 mm) and a depressed or down-sloping PR segment **Figure 114**. The PR segment is elevated or up-sloping in lead aVR. The ST segment is concave in pericarditis, and reciprocal ST-segment depression is never seen.

Noncardiac Causes of ECG Abnormalities

The remaining ECG abnormalities to be discussed are noncardiac causes, including genetic disorders that affect the size or function of the heart.

Pulmonary Embolism A <u>pulmonary embolism</u> may also be identified on a 12-lead ECG. The criteria for suspecting this include the presence of an S1Q3T3 pattern, new RBBB, and ST-segment depression in leads V_1 to V_3 **Figure 115**. The pattern refers to a deep S wave in lead I, a deep, narrow Q wave in lead III, and T-wave inversion in lead III. This is also sometimes written as

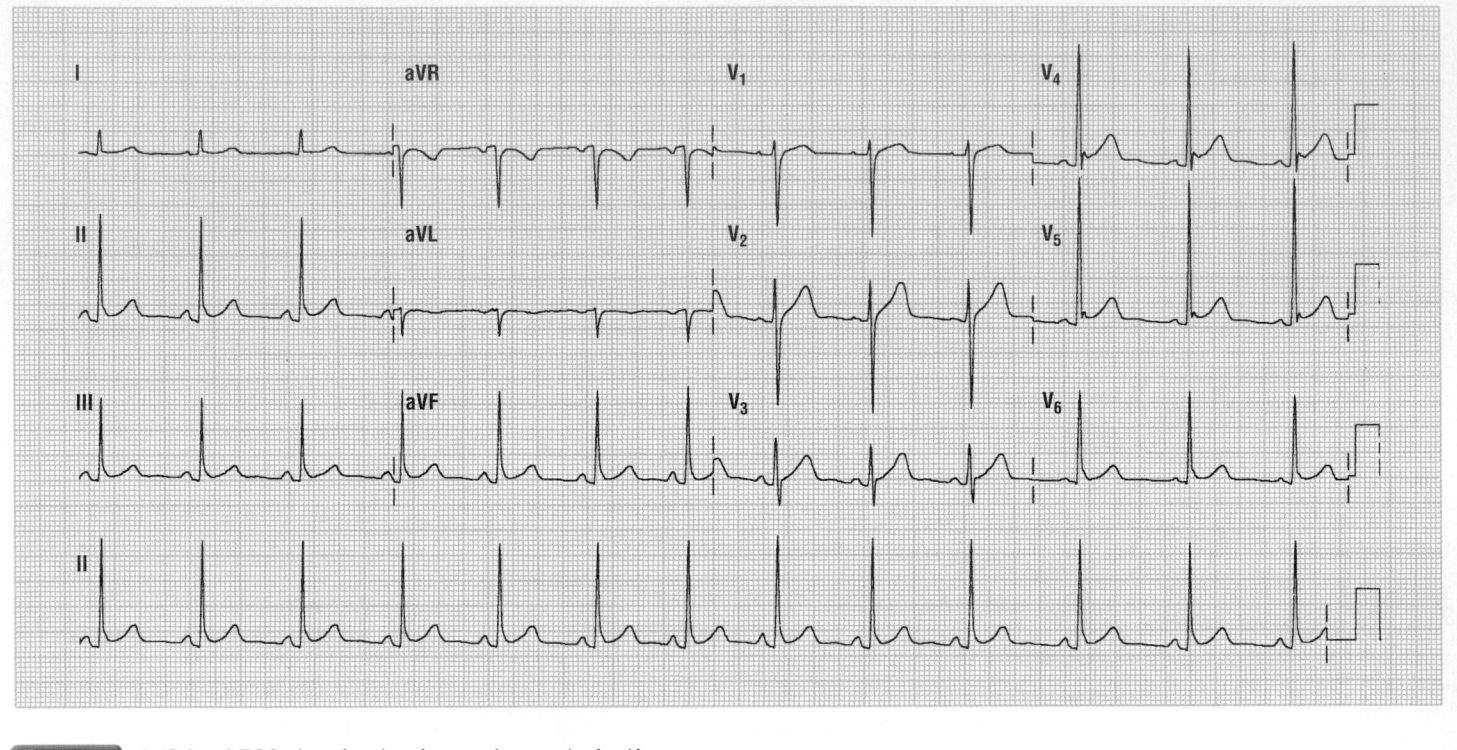

Figure 113 A 12-lead ECG showing benign early repolarization.

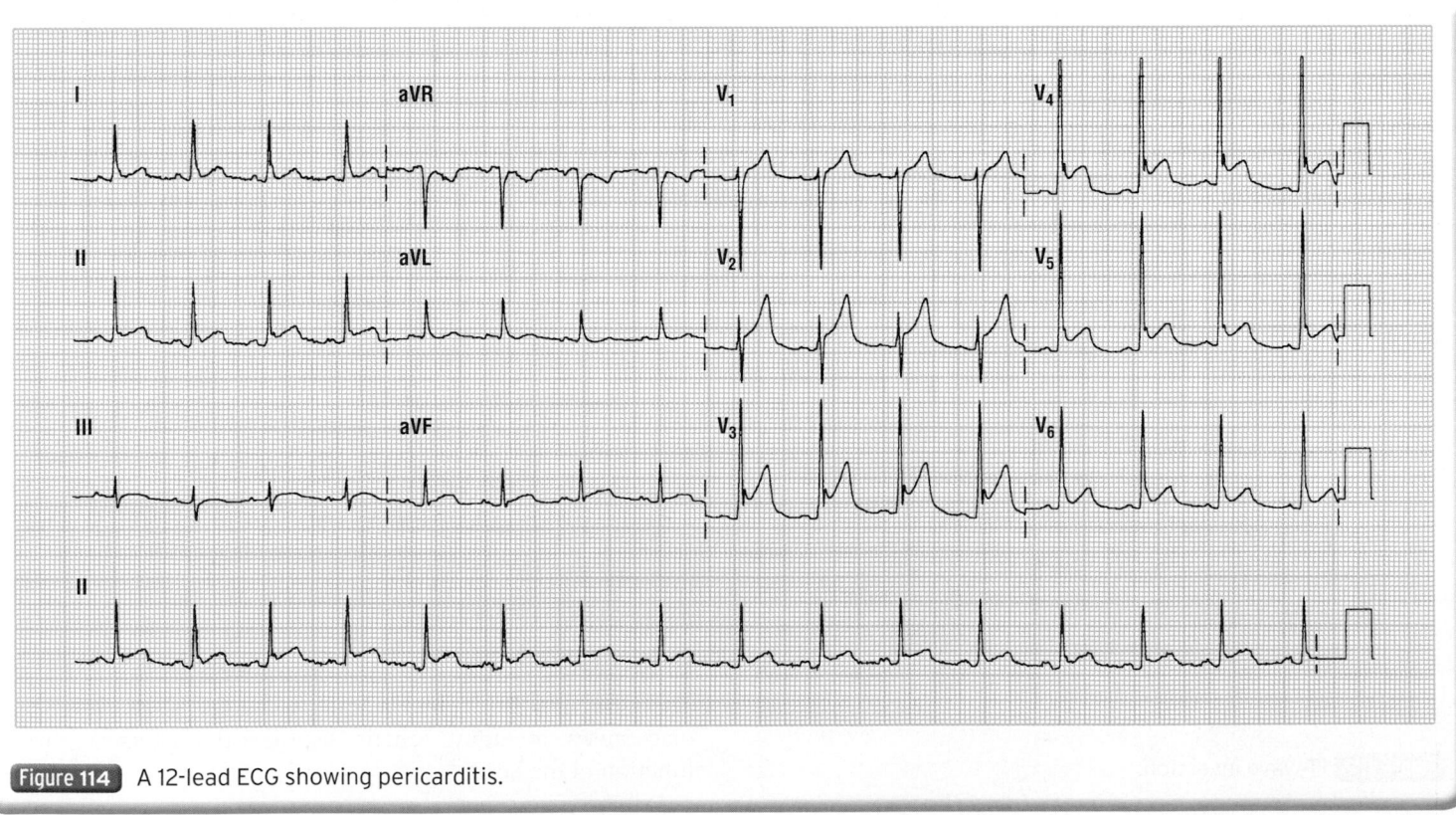

Figure 114 A 12-lead ECG showing pericarditis.

S1Q3T3, with the T upside-down, to indicate T-wave inversion. It is important to note that only approximately 12% of pulmonary embolisms have these ECG changes. Unfortunately, these changes are almost exclusively seen in cases of large pulmonary embolism. The absence of S1Q3L3 and RBBB on the surface ECG does not rule out a pulmonary embolism. Pulmonary embolism remains one of the most frequently missed conditions. It is critical to collect pertinent information about the patient's medical history, including any surgeries or medications, and current health status, including a family history, and to perform a thorough physical exam.

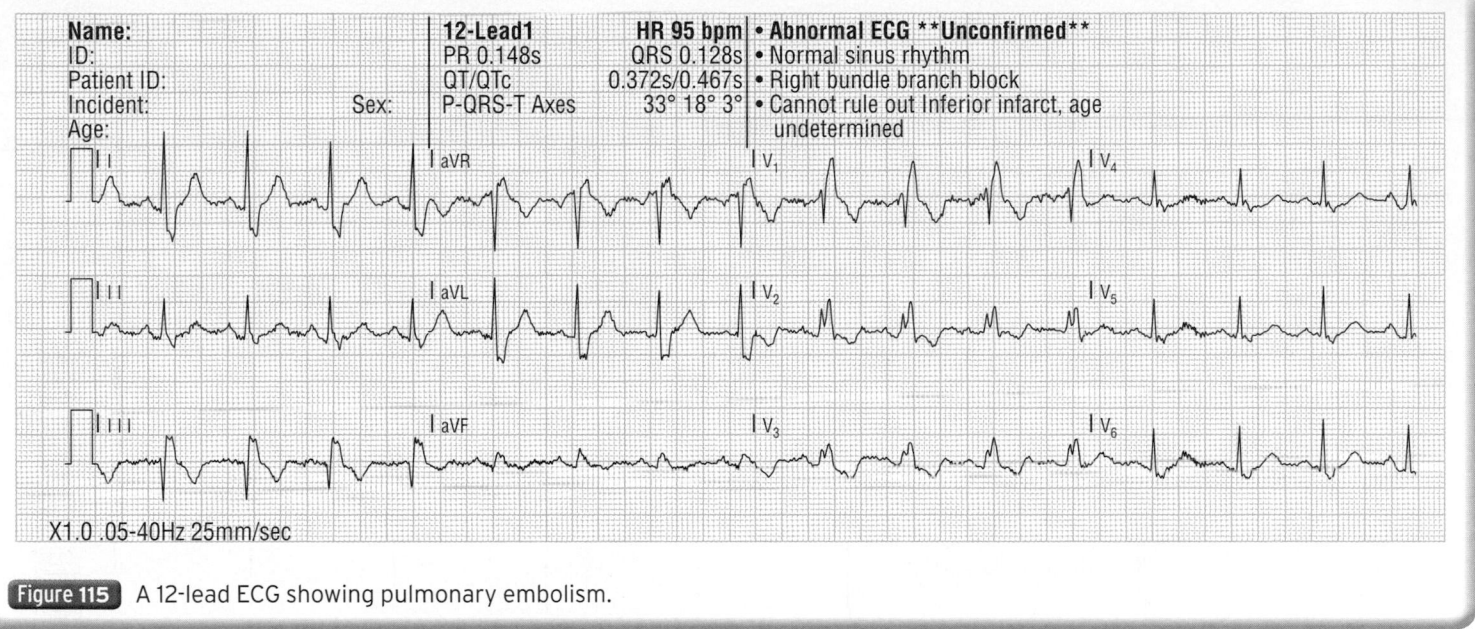

Name:		12-Lead1	HR 95 bpm	• Abnormal ECG **Unconfirmed**
ID:		PR 0.148s	QRS 0.128s	• Normal sinus rhythm
Patient ID:		QT/QTc	0.372s/0.467s	• Right bundle branch block
Incident:	Sex:	P-QRS-T Axes	33° 18° 3°	• Cannot rule out Inferior infarct, age
Age:				undetermined

X1.0 .05-40Hz 25mm/sec

Figure 115 A 12-lead ECG showing pulmonary embolism.

Patients experiencing severe hypothermia may develop J waves (Osborne) on the ECG. The J wave is often a large, upright wave that occurs on the terminal wave of the QRS complex. The ECG also typically appears as a bradycardic rhythm and baseline containing artifact from shivering and poor electrode adhesion to wet or cold skin **Figure 116**. The J wave may also be accompanied by ST-segment depression and T-wave inversion. Generally, the more serious the hypothermia, the larger the J wave. Evidence of a J wave should be considered only an indication of hypothermia; it is not enough to make a definitive diagnosis.

Electrolyte imbalances can also cause changes on the ECG. The two most common electrolyte imbalances involve potassium and calcium. **Hyperkalemia** causes specific ECG changes. First, tall, peaked, asymmetric T waves develop and the P waves can become flattened and eventually disappear from the tracing. In hyperkalemia, the T wave may be tall and sharply peaked. In more severe cases, wide QRS complexes appear on the tracing **Figure 117**. By contrast, **hypokalemia** usually presents with flat or apparently absent T waves along with the development of a **U wave**. The U wave is a small wave (smaller even than a P wave) that occurs after a T wave but before the next P wave. U waves are uncommon and may often be mistaken for extra P waves or another unknown abnormality **Figure 118**.

Hypercalcemia may cause a shortened QT interval, for example, whereas **hypocalcemia** may slightly lengthen the QT interval. It is important to note that the overall shortening or lengthening of the QT interval in hypercalcemia or hypocalcemia, respectively, is specifically due to the change in length of the

ST segment. The T wave itself is unaffected by changes in calcium concentrations. The isolated ST-segment change is attributed to the fact that the ST segment represents phase 2 of the myocardial action potential.

Hypertrophic cardiomyopathy is a condition in which the myocardial walls become very thick. Patients often experience shortness of breath, chest pain, or syncope, which is often associated with physical exercise. Patients are often diagnosed in their 30s or 40s. Hypertrophic cardiomyopathy is characterized by deep, narrow Q waves in the inferior leads and high lateral leads, and very tall R waves in the left precordial leads, similar to the changes seen in LVH **Figure 119**.

Brugada syndrome is a genetic disorder involving sodium channels in the heart.

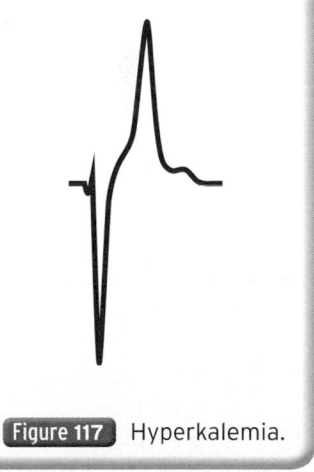

Figure 117 Hyperkalemia.

Osborn or J wave

Figure 116 Osborne (J) wave.

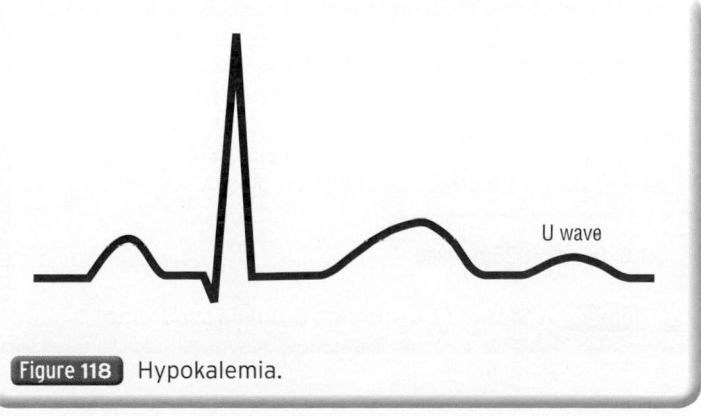

U wave

Figure 118 Hypokalemia.

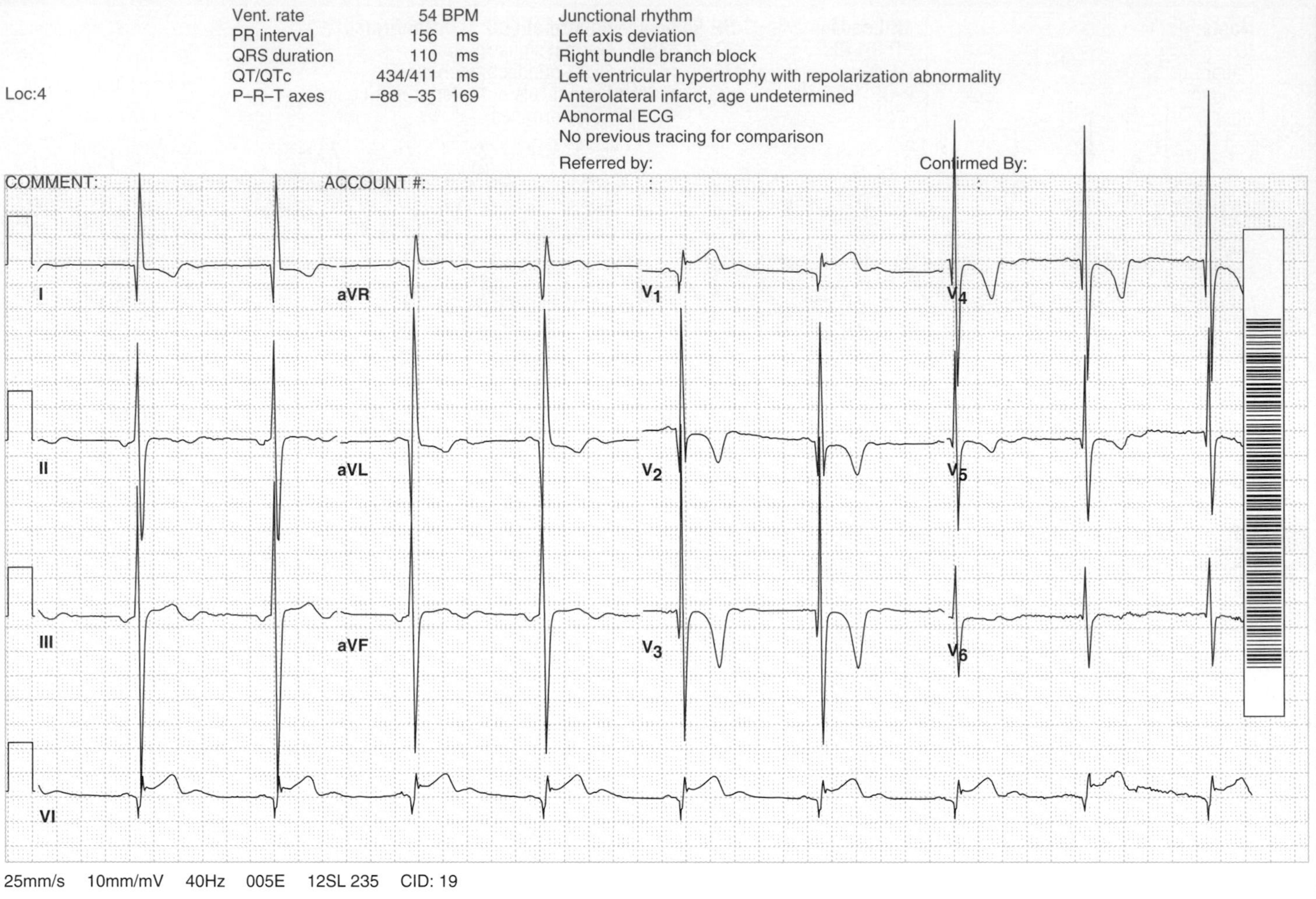

Loc:4

Vent. rate	54 BPM	Junctional rhythm
PR interval	156 ms	Left axis deviation
QRS duration	110 ms	Right bundle branch block
QT/QTc	434/411 ms	Left ventricular hypertrophy with repolarization abnormality
P–R–T axes	–88 –35 169	Anterolateral infarct, age undetermined
		Abnormal ECG
		No previous tracing for comparison

Referred by: Confirmed By:

COMMENT: ACCOUNT #:

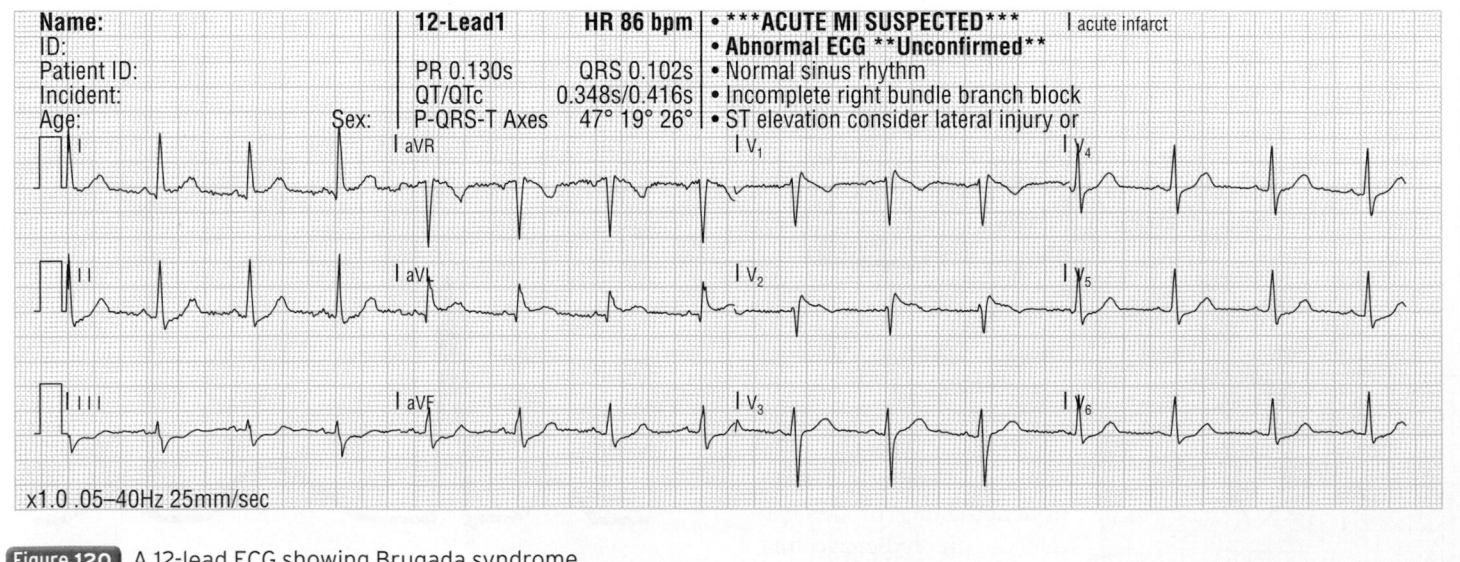

25mm/s   10mm/mV   40Hz   005E   12SL 235   CID: 19

Figure 119 A 12-lead ECG showing hypertrophic cardiomyopathy.

Name: **12-Lead1**   **HR 86 bpm**   • ***ACUTE MI SUSPECTED***   I acute infarct
ID: • **Abnormal ECG **Unconfirmed****
Patient ID: PR 0.130s   QRS 0.102s   • Normal sinus rhythm
Incident: QT/QTc   0.348s/0.416s   • Incomplete right bundle branch block
Age: Sex: P-QRS-T Axes 47° 19° 26°   • ST elevation consider lateral injury or

x1.0 .05–40Hz 25mm/sec

Figure 120 A 12-lead ECG showing Brugada syndrome.

Brugada syndrome is believed to be responsible for approximately 4% of all sudden cardiac arrest. It is most common in men of Southeast Asian origin. The disease is often diagnosed in a person's 40s or 50s, and often, patients are unaware of the condition until a sudden onset, in the form of syncope or cardiac arrest, prompts them to seek medical care. Brugada syndrome is characterized by incomplete RBBB (rSR pattern in lead V_1, QRS duration of shorter than 140 ms), and ST-segment elevation that aggressively returns to baseline **Figure 120**. These changes are seen exclusively in leads V_1 to V_2 (and possibly in V_3).

Long QT syndrome is a condition characterized by a QT interval exceeding approximately 450 ms **Figure 121**. A prolonged QT interval (long QT syndrome) indicates that the heart is experiencing an extended refractory period, making the ventricle more vulnerable to dysrhythmias. LQTS is a result of genetic mutation of several genes. LQTS syndrome may also occur with administration of certain drugs (such as amiodarone), and can result from certain conditions such as hypocalcemia, AMI, and pericarditis. Conversely, the QT interval may be shortened in hypercalcemia and in patients taking digitalis.

The QT interval is age-specific and gender-specific, so there is no single value for all patients. Long QT syndrome predisposes the patient to ventricular dysrhythmias, which can result in syncope and sudden cardiac arrest and can be a result of medication administration, myocardial ischemia, intracranial hemorrhage, or congenital disorders. Patients with LQTS are at increased risk for ventricular dysrhythmias, including torsade de pointes and ventricular fibrillation. EMS is often called to treat patient who experienced syncope, palpitations, or sudden death. It is critical to record an ECG on all patients experiencing syncope including younger patients.

Intracranial hemorrhage can also cause ECG changes. The mechanism by which the changes appear is not fully understood. Intracranial hemorrhage may cause deeply inverted, symmetric T waves in the precordial leads, along with a prolonged QT interval **Figure 122**. As a general rule, patients with these ECG changes resulting from intracranial hemorrhage almost always have neurologic symptoms including unresponsiveness.

The 12-lead ECG is an amazing tool that can provide insight about the function of the cardiac conduction system

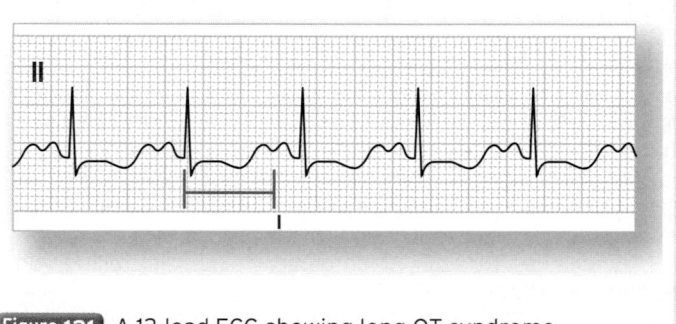

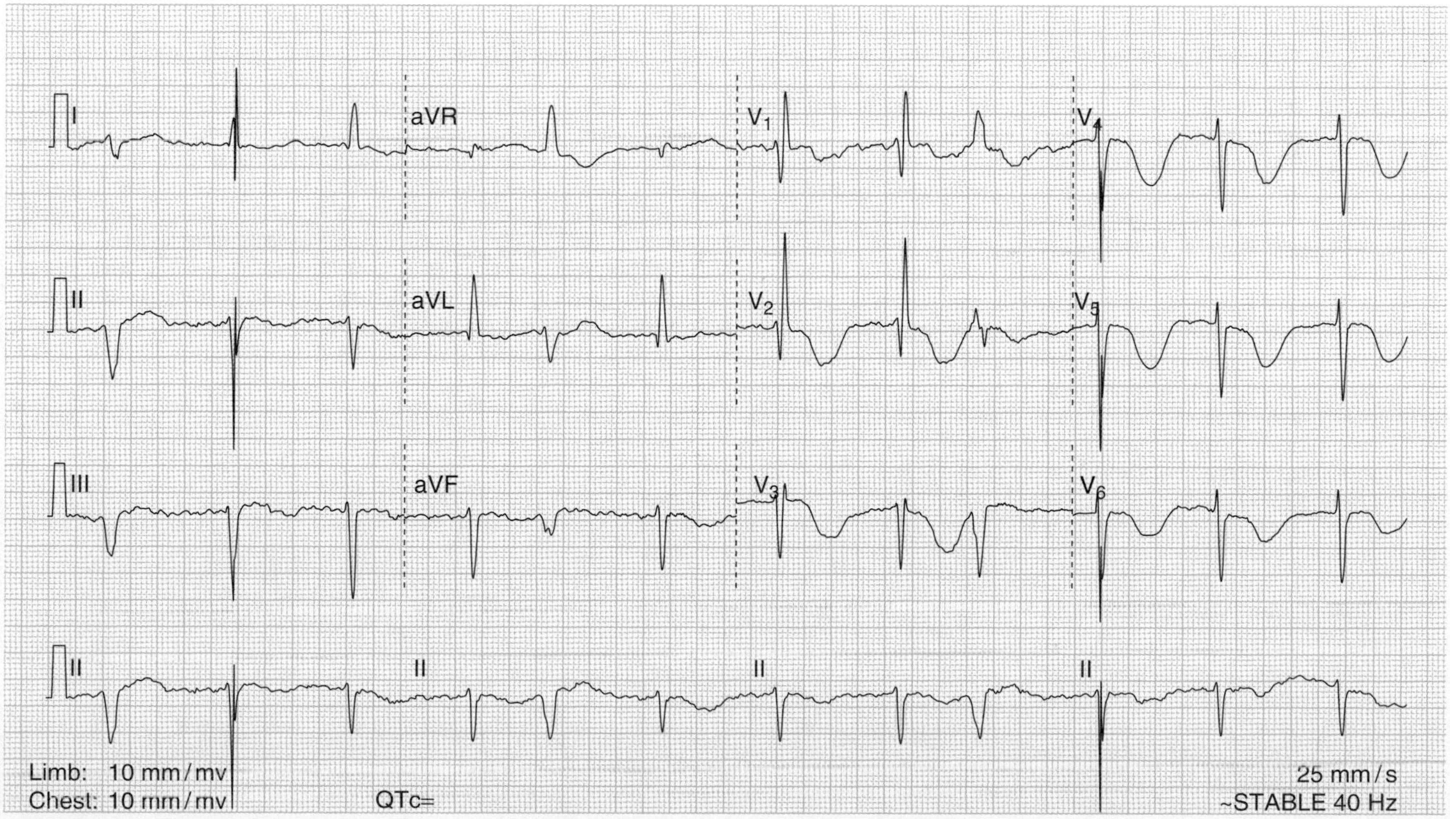

Figure 121 A 12-lead ECG showing long QT syndrome.

Figure 122 A 12-lead ECG showing intracranial hemorrhage.

Words of Wisdom

The following analogy by the late Dr. Nancy Caroline helps to illustrate the function of the electrical conduction system in the context of the three types of heart blocks.

Cast

Sidney Sinus. Sidney, the SA node, is boss of the heart. He ordinarily dispatches messengers 70 to 80 times per minute; the messengers are supposed to dash down the atria, slip through the AV junction, and depolarize the ventricles. Sidney is not terribly bright but is usually conscientious and reliable.

Albert and Alice Atria. Albert and Alice are the right and left atria. These somewhat temperamental little pouches normally contract in response to the messages sent by Sidney and squeeze their blood into the ventricles, providing the ventricles with an atrial kick. Their contraction is represented on the ECG by the P wave.

AV Abe. Abe, the AV node, is a lower-level pacemaker who secretly yearns to be boss of the heart. Unfortunately, because of his lower intrinsic rate, he rarely gets the opportunity to run the show. Abe stands at the threshold of the ventricles and checks out every messenger sent by Sidney Sinus. Normally, Abe lets the messengers pass into the ventricles after a brief security check (PR interval). However, as the node in charge of traffic control into the ventricles, Abe does regulate the flow of messengers and occasionally closes a few southbound lanes, especially when the traffic gets heavy or when he's not feeling well.

Vance and Virginia Ventricle. Vance and Virginia are big, tough, muscular types, also not very bright, who are charged with the enormous responsibility of pumping blood to the whole body. Normally, they take their orders from the messengers sent by Sidney Sinus, but sometimes the Ventricles grow irritable and contract without orders, especially when they run a little short on oxygen. They also tend to be impatient when they don't hear from Sidney on time; under that circumstance, they sometimes contract on their own.

Montgomery, Mimi, Mortimer, Millicent, et al. These messengers consist of tiny electric impulses. Earnest and dedicated, their job is to carry the orders for depolarization from Sidney's headquarters all the way to the ventricles.

First-Degree AV Block, or "The Little Messenger That Could"

One fine day, Sidney Sinus dispatched Mortimer Messenger with the usual order: "Depolarize the ventricles." Mortimer scampered down the atria without difficulty but arrived at the AV node to find a pile of debris blocking the entrance to the ventricles. "Sorry," said AV Abe, "we're closed for repairs."

"But I *have* to get through," said Mortimer.

"Impossible," said Abe.

But Mortimer was brave and determined. "I think I can. I think I can. I know I can," he said, gathering his few milliamps of strength. Finally, after a long struggle (prolonged PR interval), Mortimer crashed through the AV junction into the ventricles and breathlessly issued the order to contract **Figure 123**. The ventricles were depolarized, and everyone lived happily ever after, until . . .

Second-Degree AV Block, Type I

When Montgomery Messenger left for work that day, there was no sign there would be trouble. He took his first set of orders from Sidney Sinus, whistled down the atria, zipped through the AV node, and smartly ordered the ventricles to depolarize.

On the next trip down, however, Montgomery felt just a bit tired and slowed slightly as he crossed the AV junction. "Why break my neck?" he thought. "So, the PR interval will be a tiny bit prolonged. Who'll notice, anyway?"

On his third trip, Montgomery encountered several roadblocks in the region of the AV junction and had to pick his way around them. Glancing at his watch as he reached the ventricles, he scowled. "Nuts," he said, "240 ms. Boy, is Sidney going to be mad."

Making his fourth trip from the SA node, Montgomery found the gates to the ventricles closed and locked. Frantically, he banged on the gates. "Come on, Abe, I know you're around somewhere. Let me through." To no avail. The gates remained tightly shut. Defeated, Montgomery returned to the SA node, leaving a lonely P wave to chronicle his struggle **Figure 124**.

"What do you mean, you couldn't get through?" Sidney Sinus demanded.

"I couldn't get through," Montgomery said. "I'm telling you the gates were locked tight."

"Okay," said Sid, "off to the showers. You've had it for the day." So Sidney called Mimi Messenger. "Now look," he told her, "I want you to go straight down to the ventricles and give them this message, and no fooling around at the AV junction, understand?"

"Oh, yes sir," said Mimi, always eager to please. So off Mimi went, sailing down the atria, through the AV junction, and into the ventricles. "Hmm, 140 ms," she noted to herself. "Sid can't complain about that." On her second run, however, Mimi tripped over a shoelace and barely made it in under 200 ms. On the third trip, some highway construction held her up for 240 ms. But the fourth trip south was the worst, for she arrived at the AV junction to find that once again Abe had locked the gates. Mimi banged and banged on the gates. "Come on, Abe, open up. I'm going to lose my job." No response. Crestfallen, Mimi returned to the SA node.

"And what happened to you?" Sid demanded.

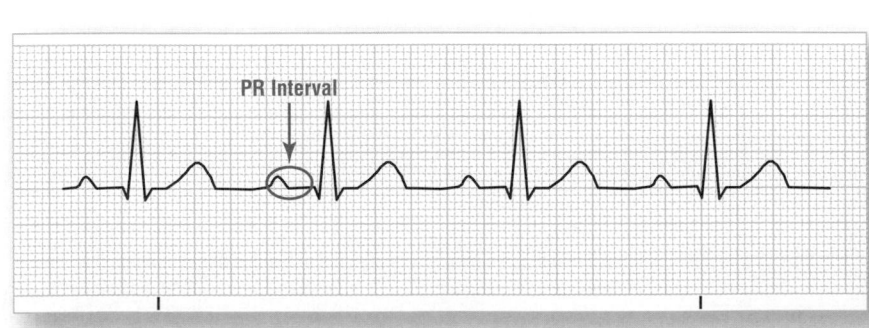

Figure 123 First-degree AV block. When there is trouble at the AV junction, it may take the messengers from the SA node longer to get through.

Words of Wisdom, continued

"I couldn't get through to the ventricles this time."

"Couldn't get through? Did you get lost, maybe?"

"But at least I made a nice P wave," Mimi ventured.

"A nice P wave! A nice *P wave*, she says. What good's a P wave without a QRS complex? Do you think the atria are going to supply blood to the whole body? They're strictly small-time. The big guns are in the ventricles. That's why I sent you to depolarize them. Now you get to the showers."

And so it went. Messenger after messenger faltered at the AV junction, but the worst was yet to come.

Second-Degree AV Block, Type II

It just wasn't Montgomery's week. Reporting for work the next day, he received the usual order from Sidney to depolarize the ventricles. Montgomery set out full of confidence and vigor, traversing the atria without difficulty. But when he arrived at the threshold of the ventricles, he found his path blocked by AV Abe.

"Let me through," Montgomery said. "I have an important message for the ventricles."

"Get lost," said Abe, who was feeling rather dyspeptic that day.

"But I have to get through. I've already used up 190 ms."

"Beat it, sonny. I'm the boss around here."

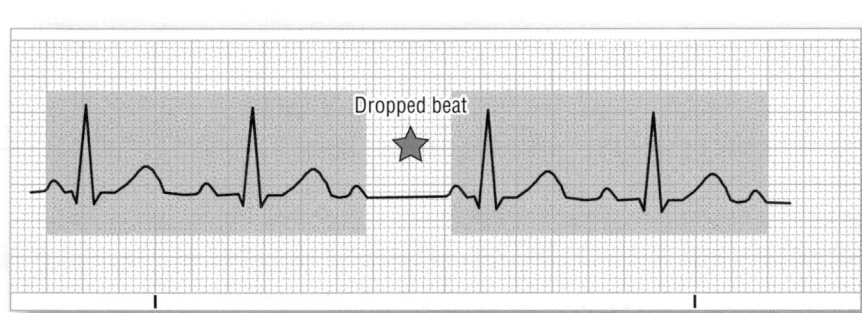

Figure 124 Second-degree AV block, type I (Wenckebach). Each transit through the AV junction is a bit slower, until finally the messenger cannot get through, and a beat is dropped.

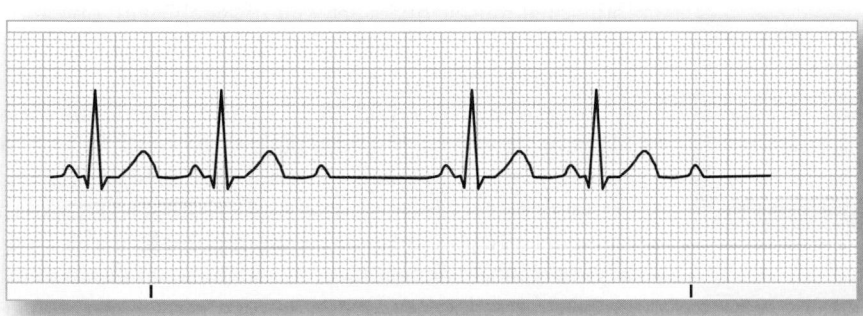

Figure 125 Second-degree AV block, type II. Every second impulse from the SA node is blocked at the AV junction.

Montgomery returned to Sidney Sinus disgraced. "What happened to you?" Sidney wanted to know. "You were supposed to order the ventricles to contract."

"I couldn't get past Abe," Montgomery replied.

"What do you mean, you couldn't get past Abe? I just sent your friend, Mimi Messenger down there, and she got through without any problem."

"But he wouldn't let me pass," whimpered Montgomery.

"I don't want to hear any excuses. You just go right back down there and deliver your message to the ventricles. I can't tolerate weaklings on my staff."

So Montgomery squared his shoulders, sailed down the atria again, and arrived once more at the gate of the ventricles.

"Are you here again?" said Abe. "I thought I told you to beat it."

"Please," said Montgomery, "I have to get through. You don't know what Sid is like when he gets upset."

"Sorry, sonny, I'm closed for lunch."

Montgomery returned to Sidney Sinus. "I couldn't make it," he said.

"Look, Montgomery," said Sidney, "Millicent Messenger just breezed by Abe right after you left. Now you march back down there and do your job."

"Yes, sir," said Montgomery.

Arriving again at the threshold of the ventricles, Montgomery once more found Abe blocking his path.

"Listen, Abe, I'm not kidding this time. If you don't let me through, I'm going to use some atropine and blast the gate open."

"Those are big words, sonny," said Abe, "but I'm not scared of a little atropine."

"The last time they used atropine, you were zonked for hours," Montgomery reminded him.

"I'll take my chances."

And so it went. Each time Montgomery reached the gate to the ventricle, AV Abe barred his path. Yet the messenger coming right after Montgomery kept getting through (2:1 block) **Figure 125**.

"Montgomery," cautioned Sidney, "if this keeps up, they're going to put in a pacemaker, and we'll all be out of a job. Shape up."

But the worst was yet to come.

Complete Heart Block (Third-Degree AV Block)

The next day was even worse for Sidney's operation. It was bad enough, Montgomery not getting through. "Every second P wave not followed by a QRS complex," wailed Sidney. "My reputation is being ruined!" But then, suddenly, the situation became even worse. Sidney had just sent Mildred Messenger down to the ventricles, and she

Words of Wisdom, continued

arrived at the AV junction to find the gate shut and bolted. A sign tacked to the gate read: "Closed until further notice."

"That's impossible," said Sidney when he heard the story. "Abe can't do that to me." So he sent another messenger, Marvin, to depolarize the ventricles. Marvin charged down the atria and ran smack into the closed gate. He banged and shouted, but there was no response.

"Impossible," said Sidney. "Abe must be sleeping." So he dispatched Melvin Messenger. Again the door was bolted tight.

"Oh, what I'd give for a bolus of atropine," sighed Sidney.

Meanwhile, the ventricles were starting to get nervous, and Vance, the right ventricle, said to Virginia, the left ventricle,

"Have you heard anything from the atria lately?"

"Not a thing."

"Funny. Those messengers are usually pretty prompt."

"Must have run into some problems with Abe."

"Yeah. Every time that guy has a little too much digitalis, he gets delusions of grandeur and starts hassling the messengers."

"How long do you suppose we ought to wait?"

"I don't know. It's already been more than a second, and the brain is starting to complain about not getting enough oxygen."

"The brain is always complaining about something."

"Yeah, but the kidneys don't sound happy either."

"Okay, okay. Let's go ahead and contract. I hate to do it without authorization from above. The last time we decided to go ahead and fire on our own, some of that disgusting lidocaine came barreling down the pipes. I was sick for a week."

So Vance and Virginia set off on their own, contracting slowly (about 30 times per minute) so as not to attract much attention, little appreciating that back in the atria Sidney was frantically sending messenger after messenger, all in vain, to assault the closed gate **Figure 126**.

"What's happened to Sidney?" Virginia said to Vance, as they plodded along slowly.

"I wish I knew," said Vance.

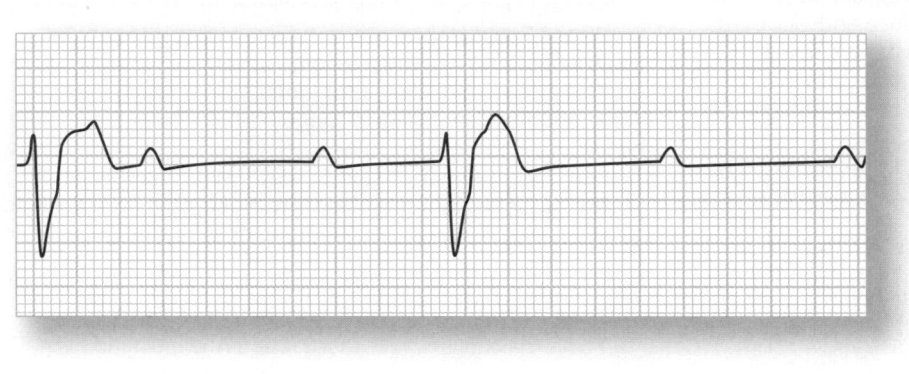

Figure 126 Third-degree AV block. The atria and ventricles are marching to the beat of different drummers.

---

and dysrhythmias. The QRS axis can also be measured from the ECG. Chamber size and ischemic changes can also be seen on the surface tracing. The ECG can also provide information about many noncardiac causes such as disorders of the lungs, kidneys, or brain.

Words of Wisdom

Impulse blockage within the SA node is referred to as sinoatrial block. Electrocardiographic changes associated with sinoatrial block are often very subtle or invisible on the surface ECG and require electrophysiologic study to diagnose.

Emergency Medical Care

This section profiles some of the devices and methods used in the treatment of patients with cardiac emergencies. Not all of the techniques or devices described are used in every EMS system, and not all are required for certification as a paramedic. Direct your attention to the material that is relevant to your local practice.

The 2010 AHA guidelines suggest that a checklist be used to assist in the triage of patients with ACS **Figure 127**.

■ Treating Dysrhythmias

Defibrillation

Defibrillation is the process by which a surge of electric energy is delivered to the heart. Recall that when the heart fibrillates, its individual muscle fibers get "out of synch" with one another and begin contracting individually. As a result, the heart as a whole ceases any useful movement. Indeed, if you were to look at a fibrillating heart, you would see movement resembling that of a bag of energetic worms. The idea behind defibrillation is to deliver a current to the heart that is powerful enough to depolarize all of its component muscle cells; ideally, when those cells repolarize after the shock, they will respond to an impulse from the SA node and begin organized depolarization, leading to cardiac contraction.

Defibrillation needs to be carried out as soon as possible in two rhythms—ventricular fibrillation and pulseless ventricular tachycardia—because the likelihood of its success declines rapidly with time (in seconds, not minutes!). If the arrest is not witnessed and CPR is not in progress, immediately start CPR and continue for 2 minutes before delivering the first shock. If the patient's rhythm converts to ventricular fibrillation or pulseless ventricular tachycardia and the defibrillator is already attached,

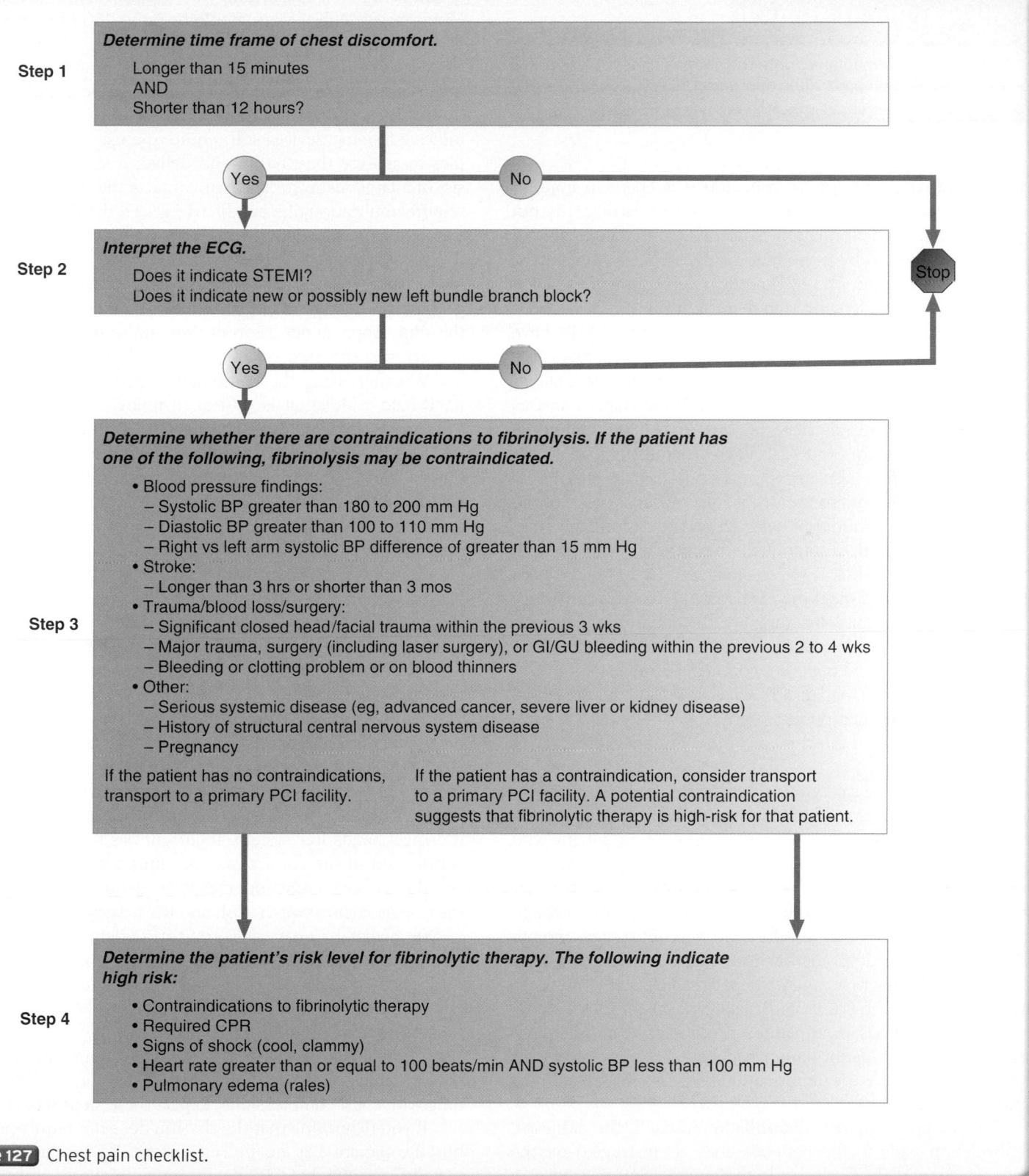

Step 1

Determine time frame of chest discomfort.

Longer than 15 minutes
AND
Shorter than 12 hours?

Yes — No

Step 2

Interpret the ECG.

Does it indicate STEMI?
Does it indicate new or possibly new left bundle branch block?

Yes — No

Stop

Step 3

Determine whether there are contraindications to fibrinolysis. If the patient has one of the following, fibrinolysis may be contraindicated.

- Blood pressure findings:
  - Systolic BP greater than 180 to 200 mm Hg
  - Diastolic BP greater than 100 to 110 mm Hg
  - Right vs left arm systolic BP difference of greater than 15 mm Hg
- Stroke:
  - Longer than 3 hrs or shorter than 3 mos
- Trauma/blood loss/surgery:
  - Significant closed head/facial trauma within the previous 3 wks
  - Major trauma, surgery (including laser surgery), or GI/GU bleeding within the previous 2 to 4 wks
  - Bleeding or clotting problem or on blood thinners
- Other:
  - Serious systemic disease (eg, advanced cancer, severe liver or kidney disease)
  - History of structural central nervous system disease
  - Pregnancy

If the patient has no contraindications, transport to a primary PCI facility.

If the patient has a contraindication, consider transport to a primary PCI facility. A potential contraindication suggests that fibrinolytic therapy is high-risk for that patient.

Step 4

Determine the patient's risk level for fibrinolytic therapy. The following indicate high risk:

- Contraindications to fibrinolytic therapy
- Required CPR
- Signs of shock (cool, clammy)
- Heart rate greater than or equal to 100 beats/min AND systolic BP less than 100 mm Hg
- Pulmonary edema (rales)

Figure 127 Chest pain checklist.

perform CPR only long enough to charge the defibrillator and then defibrillate. Defibrillation is *not* useful in asystole because there is no evidence that the myocardial cells are spontaneously depolarizing. Defibrillation of asystole is unlikely to be beneficial and is harmful (due to the unnecessary interruption of compressions). Thus, if you are unsure about asystole after checking more

than one lead, resume CPR and follow the asystole pathway in the pulseless arrest algorithm until the next pulse and rhythm check.

Manual Defibrillation Some defibrillators are combination units that can perform either manual or automated defibrillation. An **automated external defibrillator (AED)** interprets the cardiac

Special Populations

Remember to immediately note the patient's age. Use pediatric defibrillation pads when appropriate.

rhythm and determines if defibrillation is needed. In **manual defibrillation**, the paramedic interprets the cardiac rhythm and determines if defibrillation is needed. Automated external defibrillation is used by personnel who are not trained in ECG rhythm interpretation. The AED mode will recommend a shock and walk the responders through the procedure.

Paramedics may arrive to a scene at which EMTs have brought an AED that is set in AED mode. In such cases, the paramedics use the AED, but switch it to manual mode, allowing all electrical therapy functions to work (ie, transcutaneous pacing and synchronized cardioversion), as well as the multiple lead cardiac monitoring and 12-lead ECG acquisition.

Paramedics may also arrive at a scene where an AED is not in use, but the patient then goes into cardiac arrest. In that case, manual mode should be selected on the defibrillator unit. The paramedic can then look at the monitor and determine if the rhythm is shockable. If so, he or she can then proceed with charging the unit and shocking the patient. This saves time since CPR can continue until the moment the monitor is ready to shock; the paramedic does not need to wait for the AED mode to analyze the rhythm and make a recommendation.

Remember, with patients in cardiac arrest, it is essential to minimize any interruptions in chest compressions! A well-trained paramedic can interpret a cardiac rhythm more quickly than an AED can.

Follow the same safety measures when performing manual defibrillation as you would when using an AED. Ensure that no one is touching the patient. Do not defibrillate a patient who is in pooled water. There will be some danger to you if you are in the water, and also, the electricity will diffuse into the water instead of traveling between the defibrillation pads and through the patient's heart. Therefore, the heart will not receive enough electricity to cause defibrillation. You can defibrillate a soaking wet patient, but try first to dry the patient's chest. Do not defibrillate someone who is touching metal that others are touching.

If the patient has an implanted pacemaker or internal defibrillator, place the defibrillation pad below the pacemaker or defibrillator, or place the defibrillation pads in anterior and posterior positions.

To perform manual defibrillation, attach the adhesive defibrillation pads to the patient's chest as instructed on the package. As with ECG electrode placement, you may have to dry the skin before placing the defibrillation pads. Depending on the device, you may place the defibrillation pads before turning on the main power switch, or may turn the switch on once the pads are in place. After the pads are placed and the main power switch is turned on, set the energy level to 200 J (for biphasic devices), or follow the defibrillator manufacturer's

recommendations regarding the appropriate energy level. Monophasic defibrillators should be set to 360 J for the first and all successive shocks. Charge the defibrillator.

Today, most EMS agencies use combination pacing/defibrillation pads, which allow the paramedic to quickly assess the patient's cardiac rhythm and deliver an electrical shock, if indicated. Some devices still require the use of hand-held paddles to analyze the rhythm and deliver a shock. Paddles consist of a large metal surface that contacts the patient's skin, and require application of a conductive gel on the paddle surface to ensure maximum contact with the skin. Failure to use conductive gel on the paddles often results in burns to the skin and ineffective energy delivery to the heart. Use electrode paste or saline gel pads to make good electric contact between the paddles and the skin. Apply about 25 lb of pressure to hold the paddles in contact with the chest.

Whether using the combination pads or the older style, hand-held paddles, it is critical to follow manufacturer's recommended placement on the chest to avoid electrical arcing between the two contact points. Paramedics must also ensure that the devices are not placed over metal objects such as jewelry and internal pacemakers or medication patches as burns to the patient may result. From here on, we will use the term *defibrillation pads* to refer to pads, paddles, and combination pads.

Position the defibrillation pads so that the negative (sternum) pad is just to the right of the upper part of the sternum below the right clavicle and the positive (apex) pad is just below and to the left of the left nipple **Figure 128**. If using paddles, exert firm pressure (20 to 25 lb) on each paddle to make good skin contact.

When the defibrillator is charged, clear the area so that no one—including the operator—is in contact with the patient or stretcher. The operator should then announce, "All clear!" At this point, discharge the defibrillator by pressing the button on each handle simultaneously or pressing the button on the machine if using a hands-free system. If current has reached the patient, contraction of the chest and other muscles will be evident. If you do not see contraction, check the defibrillator to be certain the synchronizing switch is off and the battery is charged.

Immediately after delivering the defibrillating current, resume CPR. Continue CPR for 2 minutes or five cycles, and then pause to check for a pulse and reevaluate the rhythm. If at any point you see an organized rhythm on the monitor, check for a pulse (maximum of 10 seconds).

If you determine that the rhythm requires an additional shock, deliver one shock followed immediately by CPR, beginning with chest compressions. Repeat these steps if needed.

If you determine that the rhythm does not require a shock, but the patient has no pulse, perform five cycles (approximately 2 minutes) of CPR beginning with chest compressions. After five cycles (2 minutes) of CPR, reanalyze the patient's cardiac rhythm. If the rhythm is still not shockable, continue CPR. Transport the patient, and contact medical control as needed.

If you determine that the rhythm does not require a shock, and the patient has a pulse, check the patient's breathing.

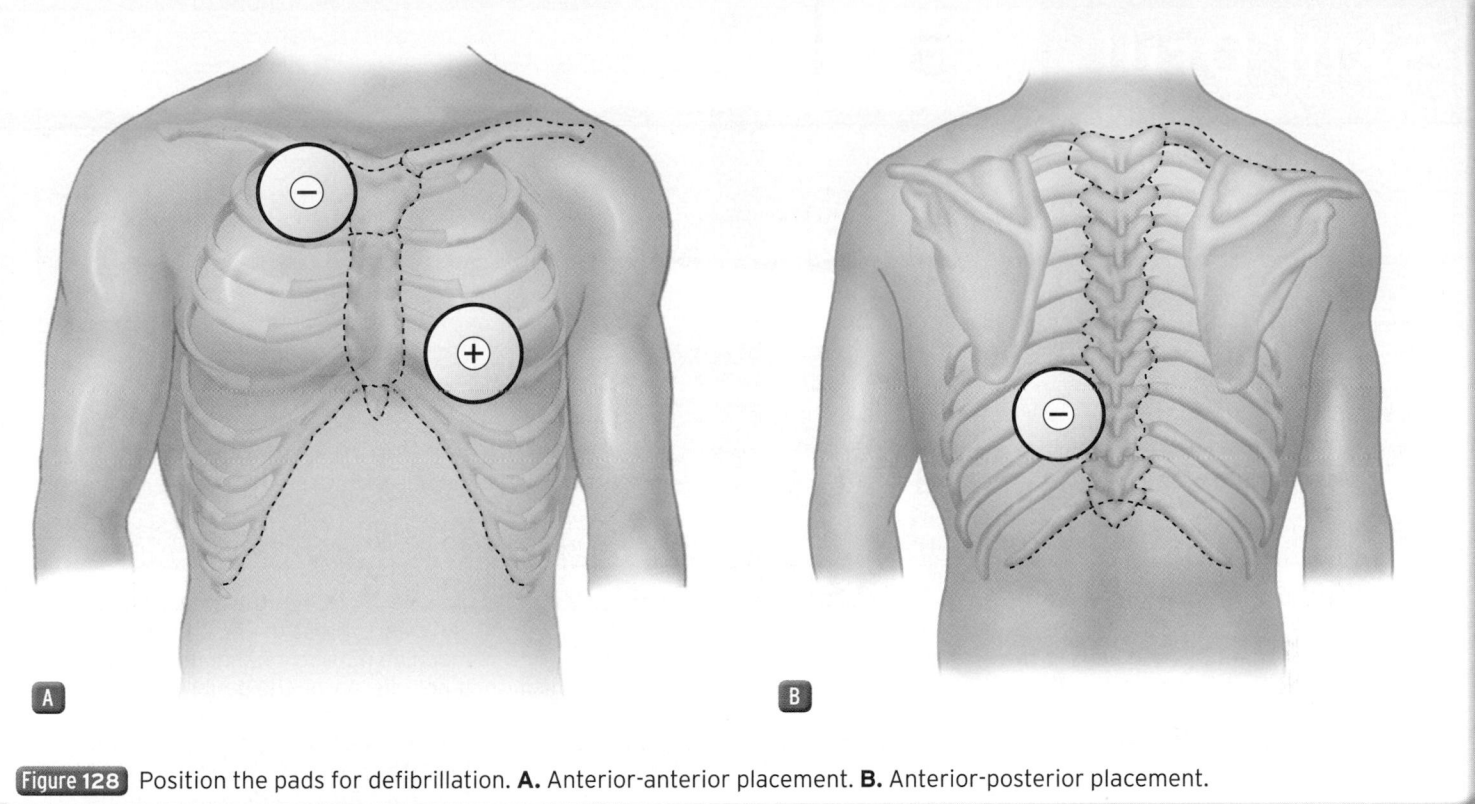

Figure 128 Position the pads for defibrillation. **A.** Anterior-anterior placement. **B.** Anterior-posterior placement.

Words of Wisdom

Manual defibrillation can be performed more quickly than defibrillation with an AED; when using an AED, you must wait while the machine analyzes rhythm. Therefore, manual defibrillation is the defibrillation method of choice for paramedics.

If the patient is breathing, but his or her Spo$_2$ is less than 94%, administer oxygen and transport.

An implanted artificial pacemaker—which you may detect from the pacemaker-produced spikes on the ECG or the bulge where its battery pack has been implanted under the patient's skin—is *not* a contraindication to defibrillation. Just make certain that you do not place the defibrillation pads directly over the pacemaker battery.

The defibrillator should be inspected at the beginning of each shift, using a checklist to cover all aspects of the apparatus and its gear. Inspection should include the defibrillation pads, cables and connectors, power supply, monitor, ECG recorder, and any ancillary supplies (such as electrode gel, pads, spare battery). The US Food and Drug Administration has developed an Operator's Shift Checklist for inspecting defibrillators. Conscientious use of the checklist should significantly reduce the incidence of defibrillator failures.

Skill Drill 3 summarizes the procedures for manual defibrillation:

Skill Drill 3

1. Take standard precautions.
2. Prepare the skin for placement of the defibrillation pads if needed. Attach the adhesive defibrillation pads to the patient's chest as instructed on the package Step 1. If using paddles, lubricate them with a conductive gel.
3. Turn on the main power switch.
4. Set the energy level to 200 J (for biphasic devices), or follow the defibrillator manufacturer's recommendations regarding the appropriate energy level Step 2. Monophasic defibrillators should be set to 360 J for the first and all successive shocks.
5. Charge the defibrillator.
6. If using paddles, exert firm pressure (20 to 25 lb) on each paddle to make good skin contact.
7. Ensure that no one is touching the patient. Remember not to defibrillate a patient who is in pooled water. Ensure that the patient is not touching metal.
8. Clear the area. Announce, "All clear!"
9. Press the button on the machine if using a hands-free system; if not, discharge the defibrillator by pressing the button on each handle simultaneously Step 3.

Skill Drill 3

Performing Manual Defibrillation

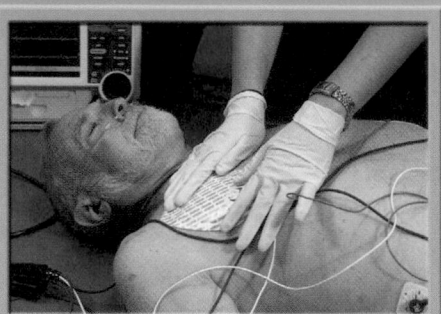

Step 1 Take standard precautions. Prepare the skin. Attach the adhesive defibrillation pads to the patient's chest as instructed on the package. If using paddles, lubricate them with a conductive gel.

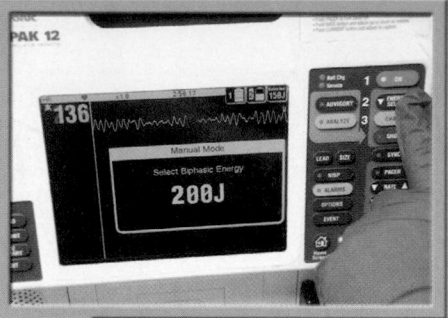

Step 2 Turn on the main power switch. Set the defibrillator to the proper energy setting. Charge the defibrillator. If using paddles, exert firm pressure to make good skin contact. Ensure that no one is touching the patient.

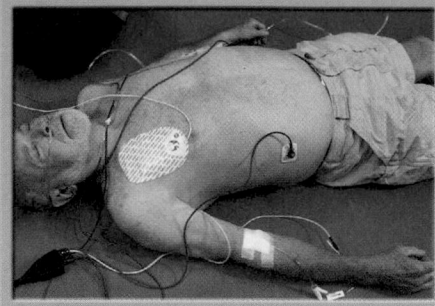

Step 3 Clear the area. Announce, "All clear!" Press the button on the machine if using a hands-free system; if not, discharge the defibrillator by pressing the button on each handle simultaneously. Observe for contraction of the patient's chest muscles. Resume CPR immediately. Continue CPR for 2 minutes or five cycles, and then pause to check for a pulse and reevaluate the rhythm. If at any point you see an organized rhythm on the monitor, check for a pulse (maximum of 10 seconds).

10. Observe for contraction of the patient's chest muscles. If you do not see contraction, check the defibrillator to be certain the synchronizing switch is off and the battery is charged.

11. Resume CPR immediately. Continue CPR for 2 minutes or five cycles, and then pause to check for a pulse and reevaluate the rhythm. If at any point you see an organized rhythm on the monitor, check for a pulse (maximum of 10 seconds).

Patients who do not regain a pulse on the scene of the cardiac arrest usually do not survive. What you do with these patients depends on your EMS system. Whether you should transport the patient should be dictated by the local protocols established by medical control.

Administration of CPR while patients are being moved or transported is usually not effective. The best chance for patient survival occurs when the patient is resuscitated where found, unless the location is unsafe.

If your local protocols agree, you should begin transport when one of the following occurs:

- The patient regains a pulse.
- Six to nine shocks have been delivered (or as directed by local protocol).

- The machine gives three consecutive messages (separated by 2 minutes of CPR) that no shock is advised (or as directed by local protocol).

If you transport a patient while performing CPR, you need a plan for managing the patient in the ambulance. Ideally, you will have two EMS providers in the patient compartment while a third drives. You may deliver additional shocks at the scene or en route with the approval of medical control. It is not as safe to defibrillate in a moving ambulance. Therefore, you should come to a complete stop if an additional shock is needed. Be sure you know and follow the protocol of your EMS service. The algorithm for cardiac arrest is shown later in this chapter, in the section, Treatment for Ventricular Fibrillation or Pulseless Ventricular Tachycardia.

Automated External Defibrillator As mentioned, paramedics usually perform manual defibrillation, but as a paramedic you may encounter AEDs when responding to a scene where law enforcement or other EMS providers have already attached an AED to the patient; therefore, you must know how to use AEDs.

The AED can analyze the patient's ECG rhythm and determine whether a defibrillating shock is needed. They assess the patient's rhythm and—if ventricular fibrillation or ventricular tachycardia is present—charge the pads and deliver countershocks, without any intervention by the rescuer. Some AEDs may be fully automated, though these are now rare. A semiautomated AED, on the other hand, detects ventricular fibrillation and rapid ventricular tachycardia, a voice prompt may say, "Shock advised. Press to shock." The rescuer must then depress the shock button to defibrillate the patient.

Remember to observe safety measures. Distance yourself from the patient. Do not defibrillate a patient who is in pooled water. Do not defibrillate a patient who is touching metal. Remove a nitroglycerin patch from a patient's chest and wipe the area with a dry towel before defibrillation to prevent ignition of the patch.

If you witness a patient's cardiac arrest, begin CPR starting with chest compressions and attach the AED as soon as it is available. However, if the patient's cardiac arrest was not witnessed, especially if the call-to-arrival time is longer than 4 minutes, you should perform five cycles (about 2 minutes) of CPR before applying the AED. The rationale for this is that the heart is more likely to respond to defibrillation within the first few minutes of the onset of ventricular fibrillation. If the arrest interval is prolonged, however, metabolic waste products accumulate within the heart, energy stores are rapidly depleted, and the chance of successful defibrillation is reduced. Therefore, a 2-minute period of CPR before applying the AED to patients with prolonged cardiac arrest (greater than 4 to 5 minutes) can "prime the pump," thus restoring oxygen to the heart, removing metabolic waste products, and increasing the chance of successful defibrillation.

The steps for using the AED are listed here and shown in Skill Drill 4:

Skill Drill   4

1. If CPR is in progress, assess the effectiveness of chest compressions by palpating for a carotid or femoral pulse. It is important to limit the amount of time compressions are interrupted. If the patient is responsive, do not apply the AED.

2. If the patient is unresponsive and CPR has not been started yet, begin providing chest compressions and rescue breaths at a ratio of 30 compressions to 2 breaths (beginning with compressions), continuing until an AED arrives and is ready for use (Step 1). It is important to start chest compressions and use the AED as soon as possible. Compressions provide vital blood flow to the heart and brain, improving the patient's chance of survival.

3. Turn on the AED now, or after pad placement, depending on manufacturer recommendations for the device you are using. Remove clothing from the patient's chest area. Apply the pads to the chest: one just to the right of the breastbone (sternum) just below the collarbone (clavicle), the other on the left lower chest area with the top of the pad 2″ to 3″ below the armpit (Step 2). Do not place the pads on top of breast tissue. If necessary, lift the breast out

of the way and place the pad underneath. Ensure that the pads are attached to the patient cables (and that they are attached to the AED in some models). Plug in the pads connector to the AED.

4. Stop CPR.

5. State aloud, "Clear the patient," and ensure that no one is touching the patient.

6. Push the *Analyze* button, if there is one, and wait for the AED to determine whether a shockable rhythm is present.

7. If a shock is not advised, perform five cycles (about 2 minutes) of CPR beginning with chest compressions and then reanalyze the cardiac rhythm. If a shock is advised, reconfirm that no one is touching the patient and push the *Shock* button.

8. After the shock is delivered, immediately resume CPR, beginning with chest compressions (Step 3).

9. After five cycles (about 2 minutes) of CPR, reanalyze the patient's cardiac rhythm (Step 4). Do not interrupt chest compressions for more than 10 seconds.

10. If the AED advises a shock, clear the patient, push the *Shock* button, and after the shock is delivered immediately resume CPR compressions. If no shock is advised, immediately resume CPR, beginning with chest compressions.

11. Gather additional information about the arrest event.

12. After five cycles (2 minutes) of CPR, reassess the patient.

13. Repeat the cycle of 2 minutes of CPR, one shock (if indicated), and 2 minutes of CPR.

14. Begin to transport (if ALS has not yet arrived), and contact medical control as needed.

The care of the patient after the AED delivers a shock depends on your location and EMS system; therefore, you should follow your local protocols. After the AED protocol is completed, one of the following is likely:

- Pulse is regained.
- No pulse is regained, and the AED indicates that no shock is advised.
- No pulse is regained, and the AED indicates that a shock is advised.

For each of these scenarios, the sequence of compressions and defibrillation is the same as described in the earlier section on manual defibrillation, with the only difference being that the AED determines whether the cardiac rhythm is shockable.

Cardiac Arrest During Transport If you are traveling to the hospital with an unresponsive patient, closely monitor the patient and watch for an ECG rhythm change as well as a pulse change. If a pulse is not present, take the following steps:

1. Stop the vehicle.
2. If the defibrillator is not immediately ready, perform CPR, beginning with chest compressions, until it is available.
3. Analyze the rhythm.
4. Deliver one shock, if indicated, and immediately resume CPR.
5. Continue resuscitation according to your local protocol.

Skill Drill | 4

Performing Defibrillation With an AED

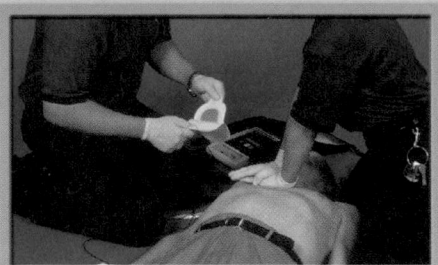

Step 1 Assess compression effectiveness if CPR is already in progress. If the patient is unresponsive and CPR has not been started yet, begin providing chest compressions and rescue breaths at a ratio of 30 compressions to 2 breaths, continuing until an AED arrives and is ready for use.

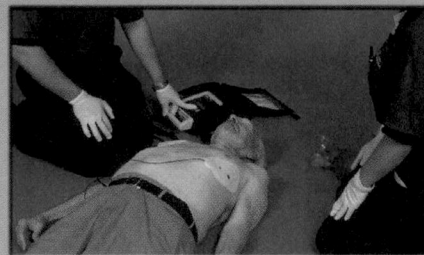

Step 2 Turn on the AED. Apply the AED pads to the chest and attach the pads to the AED. Stop CPR.

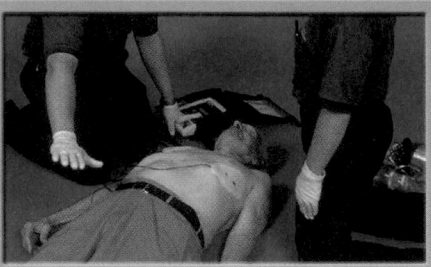

Step 3 Verbally and visually clear the patient. Push the *Analyze* button, if there is one. Wait for the AED to analyze the cardiac rhythm. If no shock is advised, perform five cycles (2 minutes) of CPR and then reanalyze the cardiac rhythm. If a shock is advised, recheck that all are clear, and push the *Shock* button. After the shock is delivered, immediately resume CPR beginning with chest compressions.

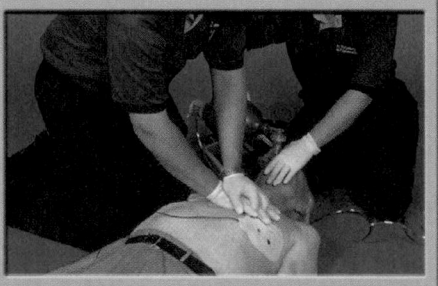

Step 4 After five cycles (2 minutes) of CPR, reanalyze the cardiac rhythm. Do not interrupt chest compressions for more than 10 seconds. If shock is advised, clear the patient, push the *Shock* button, and immediately resume CPR compressions. If no shock is advised, immediately resume CPR compressions. After five cycles (2 minutes) of CPR, reanalyze the cardiac rhythm. Repeat the cycle of five cycles (2 minutes) of CPR, one shock (if indicated), and 2 minutes of CPR. Begin transport (if ALS has not yet arrived), and contact medical control as needed.

If you are en route with a conscious adult patient who is having chest pain and becomes unconscious, take the following steps:

1. Check for a pulse.
2. Stop the vehicle.
3. If the defibrillator is not immediately ready, perform CPR, beginning with chest compressions, until it is ready.
4. Analyze the rhythm.
5. Deliver one shock, if indicated, and immediately resume CPR.
6. Begin compressions, and continue resuscitation according to your local protocol, including transporting the patient.

Cardioversion

Synchronized cardioversion is the use of the defibrillator to terminate hemodynamically unstable tachydysrhythmias. Unlike defibrillation where energy is delivered at any time during the cardiac cycle, synchronized cardioversion involves a "timed" energy delivery. The device identifies R waves on the ECG and will only deliver energy at the peak of the R wave. Recall from the electrophysiology section that the R wave indicates ventricular depolarization. The peak of the R wave is significant because the majority of myocardial tissue is already depolarized and refractory to outside stimulus. Delivering energy during this time period increases the probability of depolarizing any myocytes that are polarized, allowing the SA to resume the primary pacemaker function. Synchronized cardioversion is performed just as defibrillation except that the synchronize setting on the defibrillator is selected first.

Emergency cardioversion is indicated for rapid ventricular and supraventricular rhythms that are associated with severely compromised CO—such as rapid ventricular tachycardia or SVT.

In the field, cardioversion is carried out *only* for patients whose CO is severely impaired. These patients are usually unconscious, so premedication is not necessary. When cardioversion is performed electively on a conscious patient, the patient *must* be sedated first; cardioversion is a painful and terrifying experience for a patient who is awake. Medications commonly used for sedation in these circumstances include benzodiazepines such as diazepam (Valium) or midazolam (Versed) (follow your protocol).

The procedure for cardioversion is listed here and shown in Skill Drill 5 . Make sure the patient is placed supine; be prepared for the possibility that the patient could go into cardiac arrest.

Skill Drill | 5

1. Take standard precautions Step 1 .
2. Prepare the equipment Step 2 .
3. Place ECG electrodes and lead wires in the same position as you would if you were performing cardiac monitoring or acquiring a 12-lead ECG (either way is fine). The best lead to use is lead II, since the R wave is tallest in this lead.

   - White electrode: Right arm/shoulder
   - Black electrode: Left arm/shoulder
   - Red electrode: Left leg/lower chest
   - Green electrode: Right leg/lower chest

4. Place the multipurpose quick-connect pads in the proper positions. Turn the main power on, and assess the patient's rhythm Step 3 .
5. Turn the synchronize switch on the machine to the on position (unlike for defibrillation) Step 4 . Note that the limb leads and defibrillation pads must be in place in order to perform synchronized cardioversion as the device is unable to sense electrical activity *and* delivery electricity through the same cable.

6. Assess the pulse Step 5 . If pulse is absent, reevaluate the ECG rhythm and the need for other interventions. If a pulse is present, cardiovert.
7. Connect the pads to the monitor Step 6 .
8. Check the patient's blood pressure. Consider basic care, such as oxygen, if time permits. Sedate the patient Step 7 .
9. Confirm the rhythm by looking at the monitor Step 8 . It is best that this confirmation be made verbally so other caregivers are aware of the patient's situation.
10. Prepare and apply the pads or paddles as described for defibrillation.
11. Set the energy level as ordered by the physician. Note that the energy level could be set by the physician or by protocol. Energy levels required for cardioversion vary depending on the type of dysrhythmia and the type of defibrillator. Supraventricular tachycardia, for example, can often be converted with energy levels as low as 50 J; by contrast, ventricular tachycardia will usually require at least 100 J. In emergencies, if an initial attempt to convert a rapid rhythm with a low energy level fails, immediately turn the setting up (stepwise to 100, 200, 300, and then 360 J) and repeat the shock as needed.
12. Charge the pads.
13. Clear the area by announcing, "All clear!" Step 9
14. Reconfirm the rhythm by looking at the monitor.
15. Depress the shock buttons, and keep them depressed until the defibrillator discharges Step 10 . That may take a few seconds because the charge is synchronized to fire about 10 ms after the peak of the R wave.
16. Reassess the patient's condition (ECG rhythm and pulse) Step 11 . Repeat the cardioversion if necessary.
17. If a cardioversion shock produces ventricular fibrillation, immediately take the following steps:
    - Recharge the defibrillator to the setting for defibrillation.
    - Turn the synchronizer circuit to the off position if it has not defaulted to that position.
    - Deliver the defibrillation and then immediately begin chest compressions.

Transcutaneous Cardiac Pacing

Artificial pacemakers deliver repetitive electric currents to the heart. Like the tiny electric currents generated by natural pacemakers, the current from an artificial pacemaker can cause the myocardial tissue to depolarize. In this way, the artificial pacemaker can substitute for a natural pacemaker that has become blocked or nonfunctional.

The artificial pacemakers first developed for emergency use consisted of a small battery pack and a wire that had to be threaded through a vein into the right ventricle of the heart. Insertion of one of those transvenous pacemakers was a tricky and often time-consuming job, usually best undertaken in a coronary care unit. Recently, however, effective transcutaneous pacemakers—that is, pacemakers that deliver their current through the skin of the chest—have been developed and have come into widespread use. Indeed, most prehospital monitor-defibrillators now come equipped with TCP capability.

Skill Drill | 5

Performing Cardioversion

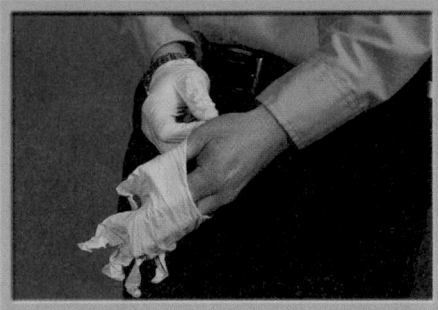

Step 1 Take standard precautions.

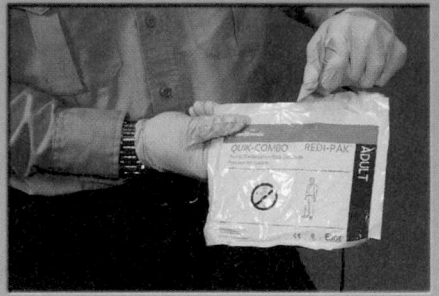

Step 2 Prepare the equipment. Place the electrodes in the same position as you would when performing cardiac monitoring or acquiring a 12-lead ECG.

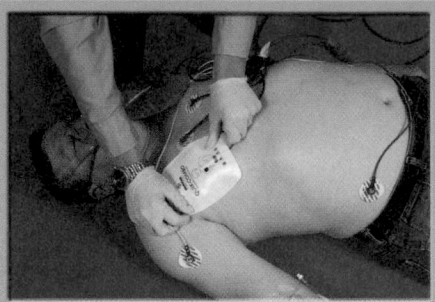

Step 3 Place the multipurpose quick-connect pads in the proper positions. Turn the main power on, and assess the patient's rhythm.

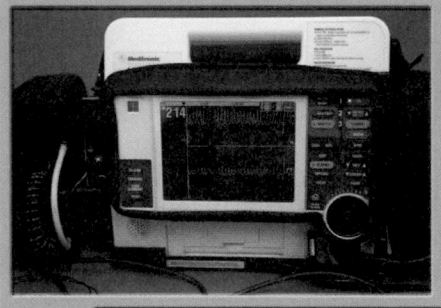

Step 4 Turn the synchronize switch on the machine to the on position (unlike for defibrillation).

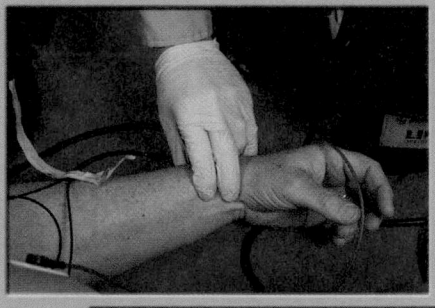

Step 5 Assess the pulse. If a pulse is present, prepare to cardiovert.

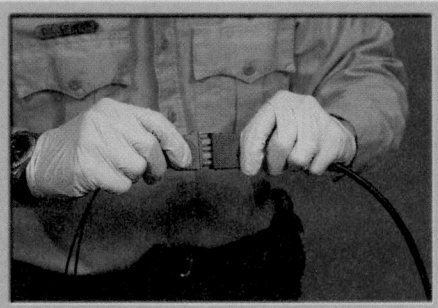

Step 6 Connect the pads to the monitor.

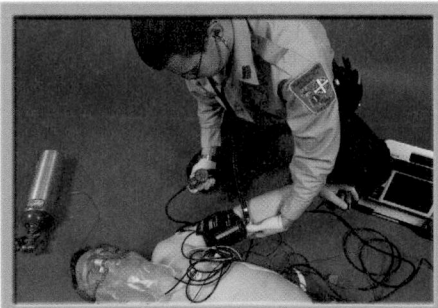

Step 7 Check the patient's blood pressure. Sedate the patient.

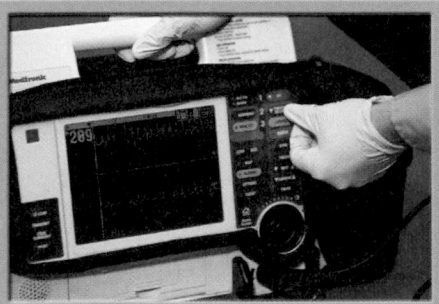

Step 8 Confirm the rhythm. Prepare and apply the pads or paddles as described for defibrillation. Set the energy level as ordered by the physician. Charge the pads. Note that the energy level could be set by the physician or by protocol.

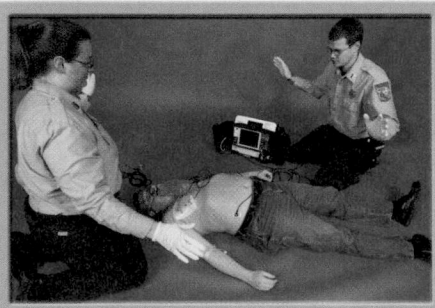

Step 9 Clear the area by announcing, "All clear!"

Continues

Skill Drill 5

Performing Cardioversion, continued

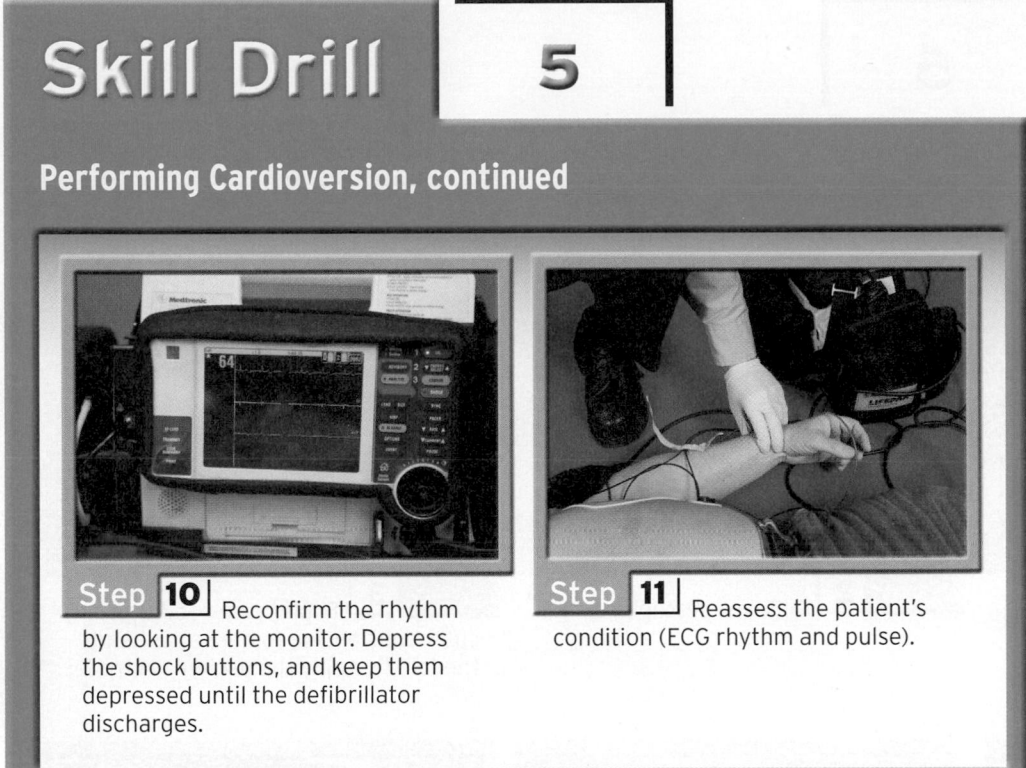

Step 10 Reconfirm the rhythm by looking at the monitor. Depress the shock buttons, and keep them depressed until the defibrillator discharges.

Step 11 Reassess the patient's condition (ECG rhythm and pulse).

In TCP, a small electrical charge is passed through the patient's skin across the heart between one externally placed pacing pad and another. The pacer is set for a specific rate, and the energy is increased until the heart just begins to respond to the stimulus. This phenomenon, which is termed "capture," is usually associated with depolarization of the ventricles, which appears as a wide QRS complex on the ECG and results in a corresponding pulse.

TCP may have several useful applications in prehospital care:

- Interhospital transfer of patients needing pacemaker implantation (for example, a patient with complete heart block admitted to a small community hospital that does not have the facilities to implant a permanent pacemaker)
- Symptomatic patients with artificial pacemaker failure
- Patients with bradydysrhythmias or blocks associated with severely reduced CO and that are unresponsive to atropine, before cardiac arrest

In any of those circumstances, TCP may buy time for the patient and enable him or her to reach the hospital in a state of optimal perfusion rather than in or near cardiac arrest.

Many brands of transcutaneous external cardiac pacemakers are available, and you must become familiar with the particular pacemaker used in your local EMS system. In general, the steps in initiating TCP are listed here and shown in Skill Drill 6:

Skill Drill 6

1. Take standard precautions Step 1.
2. Recognize the need for pacing. After connecting the patient to the ECG monitor and assessing the initial vital signs, determine the need for transcutaneous pacing based on the indications previously listed.
3. Obtain a precapture strip of the ECG tracing for documentation Step 2.
4. Explain the need for transcutaneous pacing to the patient and the family.
5. If you need to sedate the patient or pretreat the patient with IV medication, obtain IV access. Do not delay initiation of TCP to place an intravenous catheter!
6. Apply pacing electrodes Step 3. Often the defibrillation position is used when the same pads can be used for defibrillation and pacing. The alternative is to place one pad anteriorly left of the lower sternum and the other pad posteriorly just below the left scapula.
7. Attach the cables to the electrodes if not done previously.
8. Switch the pacer power on Step 4.
9. Set the pacing rate (70 to 80 beats/min is commonly chosen) Step 5.
10. Start increasing the current Step 6. Raise the current by 10 to 20 milliamps every few seconds.
11. Check for capture Step 7; that is, look for every pacemaker spike being followed by a (usually wide) QRS complex Figure 129. If the QRS is not present, the pacemaker current is not depolarizing the ventricles. Increase the current gradually until there is consistent capture.
12. Once capture is achieved, briefly lower the current until capture is lost, and then increase it by the smallest amount possible to restore capture Step 8. The purpose of this action is to find the lowest energy setting that achieves consistent capture.
13. Obtain rhythm strips for documentation.
14. Immediately transport the patient.

Transcutaneous pacemakers depolarize not only cardiac muscle, but also muscles in the chest wall beneath the pacing electrode. As a result, patients who are conscious when TCP is initiated (or who regain consciousness during pacing) usually experience chest discomfort and sometimes severe pain from the procedure. Some form of analgesia and sedation (such as diazepam [Valium] or morphine [Astramorph PF]) should be given to conscious patients when transcutaneous pacemakers are used.

Management of Symptomatic Bradycardia

A patient who presents with or develops symptomatic bradycardia needs to be treated in a manner that will increase the

Skill Drill   6

Performing Transcutaneous Pacing

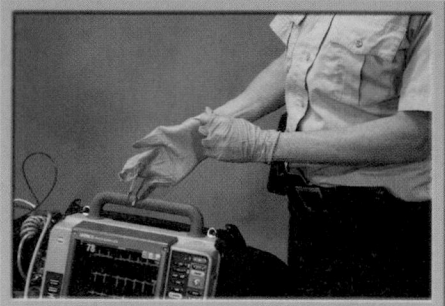

Step 1 Take standard precautions.

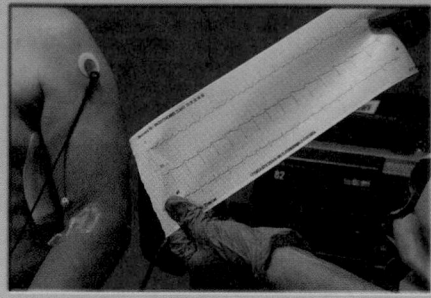

Step 2 Obtain a precapture strip.

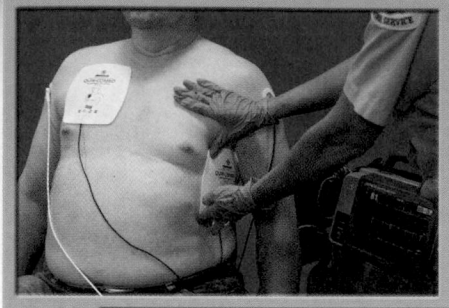

Step 3 Explain the need for transcutaneous pacing to the patient and the family. Apply the pacing electrodes.

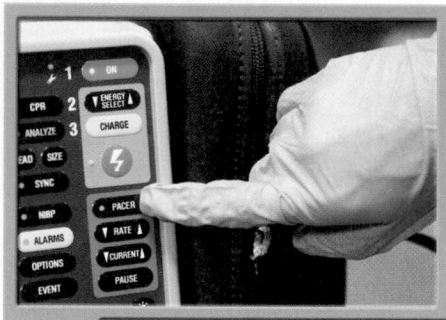

Step 4 Switch the pacer power on.

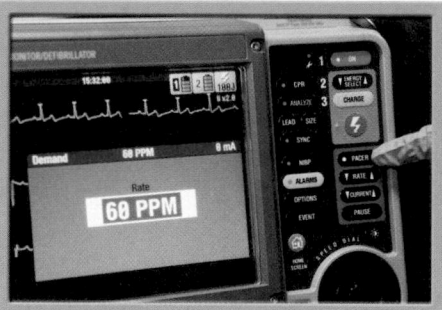

Step 5 Set the pacing rate.

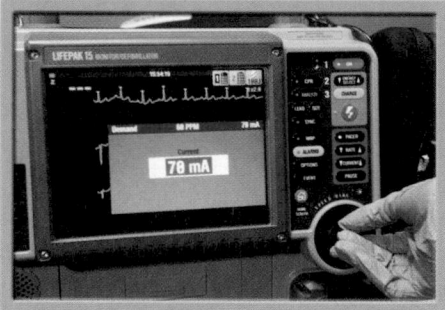

Step 6 Start increasing the current.

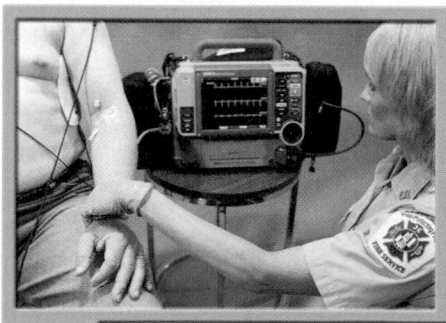

Step 7 Check for mechanical capture.

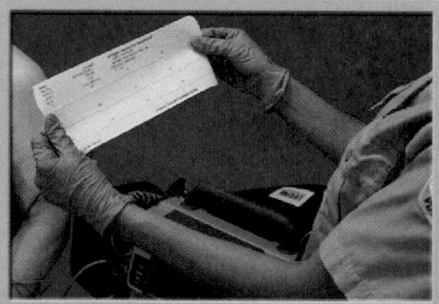

Step 8 Once capture is achieved, briefly lower the current until capture is lost, and then increase it by the smallest amount possible to restore capture. Obtain rhythm strips for documentation.

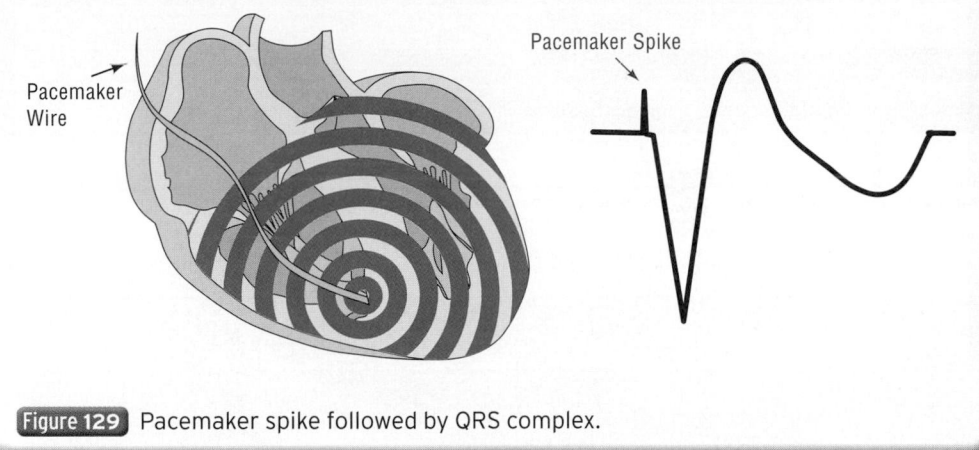

Figure 129 Pacemaker spike followed by QRS complex.

heart rate and improve CO. Symptoms such as altered mental status and hypotension are common indications for treatment of bradycardic patients. Assuming that airway and breathing have been supported:

1. Establish an IV line of normal saline.
2. Administer atropine, 0.5-mg IV bolus. You may repeat this dose every 3 to 5 minutes until the heart reaches the desired rate (usually 60 beats/min or faster) or until the maximum total dose of 0.04 mg/kg has been reached.
3. If the patient is in severely compromised condition or does not respond to the administration of atropine, establish TCP as quickly as possible. If the patient is in a second-degree type II or third-degree heart block, TCP is the first-line treatment.
4. If atropine and TCP are unsuccessful (or if TCP is unavailable), consider the administration of a sympathomimetic drug—most commonly, dopamine (Intropin) or epinephrine, albeit only as a drip in this situation. Dopamine, which is the milder of the two, is administered at a dose of 2 to 10 µg/kg/min. The epinephrine drip rate is 2 to 10 µg/min. To mix an epinephrine drip, put 1 mg of epinephrine into a 250-mL bag of normal saline, start the drip at 30 drops/min with a microdrip administration set, and titrate it to the desired heart rate.
5. Transport the patient to a hospital capable of transvenous pacing and surgical implantation of pacemakers.

Patients who are symptomatic and require TCP in the field often require the surgical implantation of a pacemaker in the hospital **Figure 130**. Early identification and hospital notification can often speed this process.

■ Management of Tachycardia

A patient who presents with or develops tachycardia presents a more complicated situation than one in bradycardia. Tachycardia can have a supraventricular pacemaker site or may be ventricular in origin. In addition, the patient may be mildly or severely symptomatic owing to the tachycardia or another condition. Because of the many possible variations in tachycardic patients,

several judgments must be made before treatment is begun.

The first decision relates to the seriousness of the signs or symptoms the patient is exhibiting. Patients who present with serious signs and symptoms such as chest pain, dyspnea, hypotension, or altered mental status should be considered in unstable condition and may need immediate treatment. First, however, you must determine whether these signs and symptoms are the result of the tachycardia or whether the tachycardia and signs and symptoms are the response to another condition.

Tachycardias with rates of less than 150 beats/min are rarely fast enough to cause serious signs and symptoms. For example, a patient who is experiencing an MI is likely to be mildly tachycardic, but obviously the MI—not the tachycardia—is causing the signs and symptoms. Conversely, a patient who was previously asymptomatic but becomes symptomatic only after the onset of the tachycardia is more likely presenting with symptoms resulting from the tachycardia. This brings to mind the adage: "Treat the patient, not the monitor." It is critical to make this distinction before beginning treatment, because slowing the heart rate of a patient whose heart is compensating for a medical condition may be a fatal mistake.

A patient in unstable condition whose signs and symptoms are determined to be the result of tachycardia needs cardioversion. Electrical cardioversion is similar to defibrillation and, as such, is a serious intervention. For this reason, it is limited to patients whose condition is so serious as to make them likely to arrest if the treatment is not administered quickly. Most of these patients will be unconscious. In the unlikely case of a conscious patient who needs cardioversion, sedation (usually with diazepam [Valium] or midazolam [Versed]) is a necessity. Wait an appropriate amount of time for the drugs to take effect before cardioversion. Should the patient become unconscious, sedation is no longer a concern.

When a patient in tachycardia has limited or mild signs and symptoms, a slower but safer treatment regimen is recommended. In these cases, it becomes necessary to determine the origin of the tachycardia or the pacemaker site of the rhythm. Generally speaking, wide QRS complexes are presumed to be ventricular in origin, whereas narrow QRS complexes (< 0.12 s) are presumed to be supraventricular in origin. SVTs may originate in the SA node, elsewhere in the atria, or in the AV node (junctional rhythms). The differentiation among these three pacemaker sites requires examining the P wave. In tachycardias with rates exceeding 150 beats/min, however, the P waves (if present) are usually "buried" within the T wave of the preceding beat. The inability to see P waves limits you to labeling these tachycardias as supraventricular rather than giving a specific site of origin.

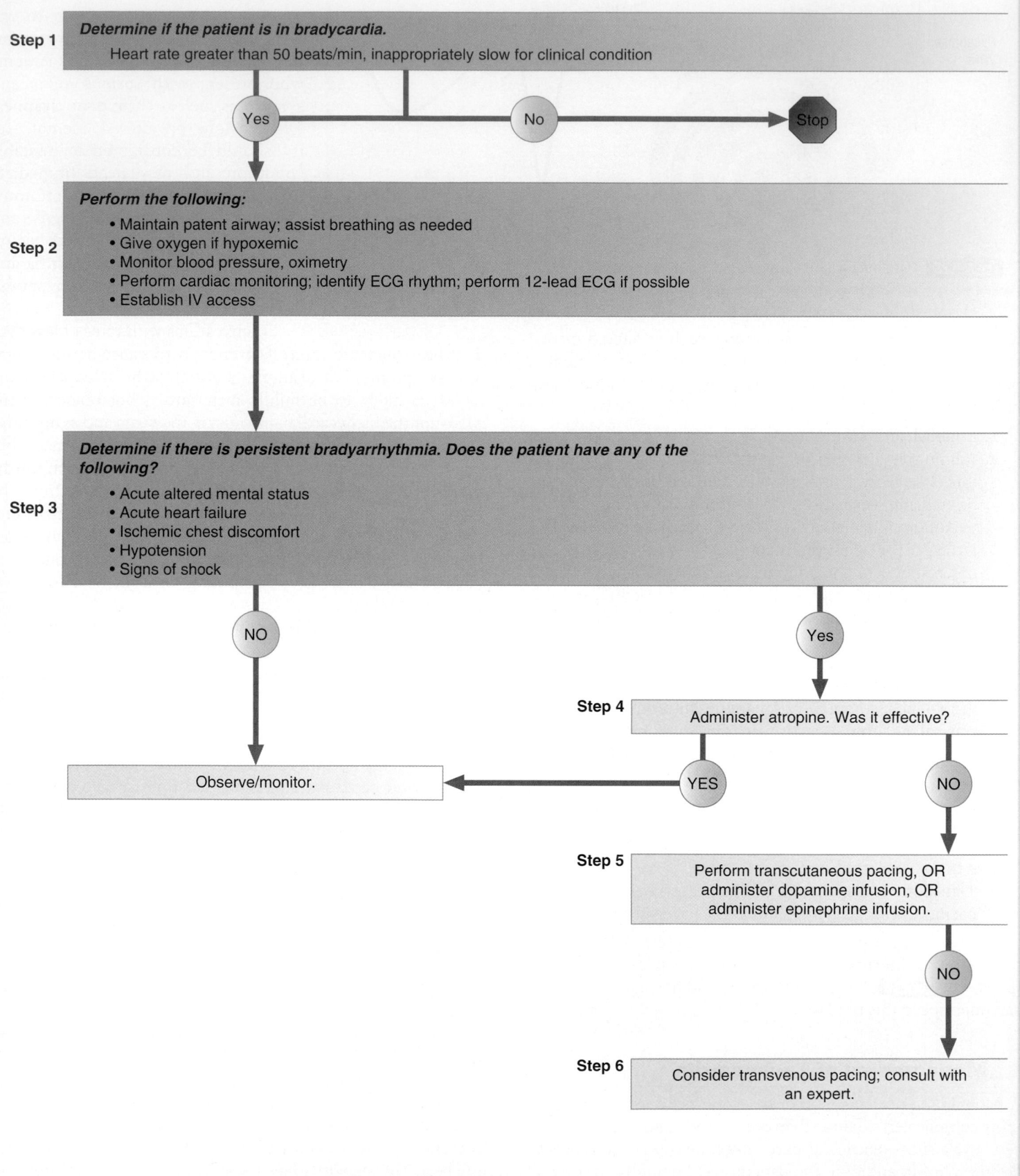

Step 1

Determine if the patient is in bradycardia.

Heart rate greater than 50 beats/min, inappropriately slow for clinical condition

Yes — No — Stop

Step 2

Perform the following:

- Maintain patent airway; assist breathing as needed
- Give oxygen if hypoxemic
- Monitor blood pressure, oximetry
- Perform cardiac monitoring; identify ECG rhythm; perform 12-lead ECG if possible
- Establish IV access

Step 3

Determine if there is persistent bradyarrhythmia. Does the patient have any of the following?

- Acute altered mental status
- Acute heart failure
- Ischemic chest discomfort
- Hypotension
- Signs of shock

NO

Yes

Observe/monitor.

Step 4 Administer atropine. Was it effective?

YES

NO

Step 5 Perform transcutaneous pacing, OR administer dopamine infusion, OR administer epinephrine infusion.

NO

Step 6 Consider transvenous pacing; consult with an expert.

Figure 130 Algorithm for bradycardia.

Occasionally, aberrant conduction of a supraventricularly originated beat will make it difficult to identify a tachycardia as truly ventricular or supraventricular. In most cases of uncertainty, the rhythm is ventricular rather than supraventricular and should be treated as such. In either case, you should administer oxygen and establish an IV line for normal saline.

In SVTs, you should attempt to stimulate the patient's vagus nerve. Many vagal stimulation techniques exist, including carotid sinus massage, which is shown in Figure 131, but the most common technique is having the patient bear down against a closed glottis. The patient is instructed to perform this technique as if attempting to have a bowel movement. The stimulation of the vagal nerve in turn stimulates the parasympathetic nervous system to slow the heart. *Never* massage both carotid arteries simultaneously as significant bradycardia or asystole may result Figure 132. One factor to consider when deciding whether to perform carotid massage is the patient's history. If the patient's condition involves risks that would override the potential rewards, do not perform the technique. For example,

a patient with advanced age, coronary artery disease, and high cholesterol would not be a good candidate for carotid massage because of the high risk of thromboembolism. If carotid massage is successful, the patient should still be transported for hospital evaluation because the condition is likely to recur. If it reappears, instruct the patient to repeat the vagal maneuver. If at any time the vagal stimulation proves unsuccessful, pharmacologic treatment should be attempted.

Next, administer adenosine (Adenocard), 6 mg, by rapid IV push. Adenosine is in the class of drugs called purine nucleosides. In EMS, adenosine is used to transiently induce AV nodal blockade in order to interrupt tachydysrhythmias involving the AV node. Before you begin this treatment, you should always recheck the history for allergies and advise the patient of the possible adverse effects of adenosine administration. To administer the medication, choose the closest IV site to the patient and insert the syringe of adenosine. In the same site, insert another syringe containing at least 20 mL of normal saline solution. After clamping off the IV line above the site, push the adenosine as rapidly as possible and then push the saline as soon as the adenosine plunger hits bottom. Be prepared to see a short run of asystole with the administration of adenosine (although this response does not always occur). If the first dose of adenosine is unsuccessful, you may administer it again in 1 to 2 minutes up to two times at 12 mg each. If the adenosine is unsuccessful in converting the patient's rhythm, transport expeditiously to the hospital without further treatment as long at the patient remains in stable condition.

If at any time the condition of a patient with SVT becomes unstable, you should move to the "unstable" or cardioversion algorithm. Remember that when cardioversion of SVT is required, you should start at a lower energy setting than with a ventricular rhythm.

If the patient is in stable condition but the rhythm is ventricular in origin, the patient should be transported to the hospital while you watch carefully for the development of serious signs and symptoms. If they appear, the patient should undergo cardioversion according to the unstable tachycardia algorithm. If your transport time to the hospital is long, medical control may order the administration of a ventricular antidysrhythmic medication such as amiodarone (Cordarone, Pacerone) or lidocaine (Xylocaine).

Any patient with a tachycardic rhythm should be monitored carefully Figure 133. A heart that is stressed by the requirements of excessive tachycardia is likely to become ischemic and is at high risk for arrest.

Management of Cardiac Arrest

Nothing gets the adrenaline pumping more furiously—in paramedics, even if not in the patient—than a "code," or **cardiopulmonary arrest**. Most cardiac arrest victims have evidence of atherosclerosis or other underlying cardiac disease. However, cardiac arrest can also occur after electrocution, drowning, and other types of trauma. Indeed, many cardiac arrest victims have

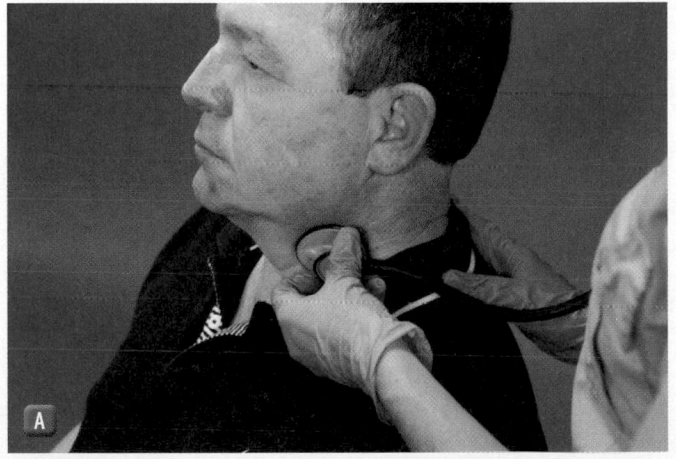

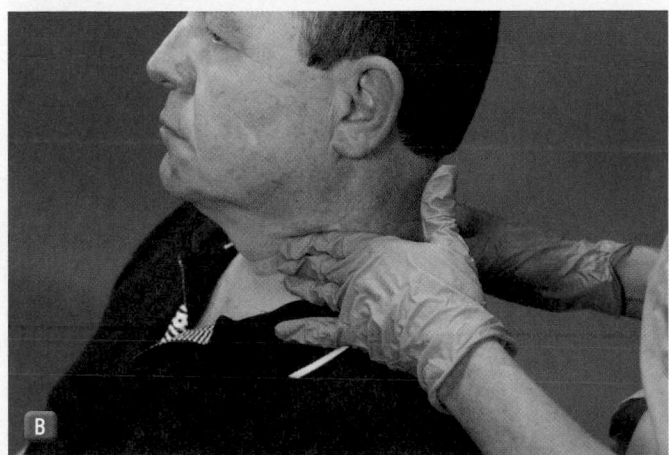

Figure 131 Carotid sinus massage. **A.** Listen for bruits. **B.** Massage the carotid artery.

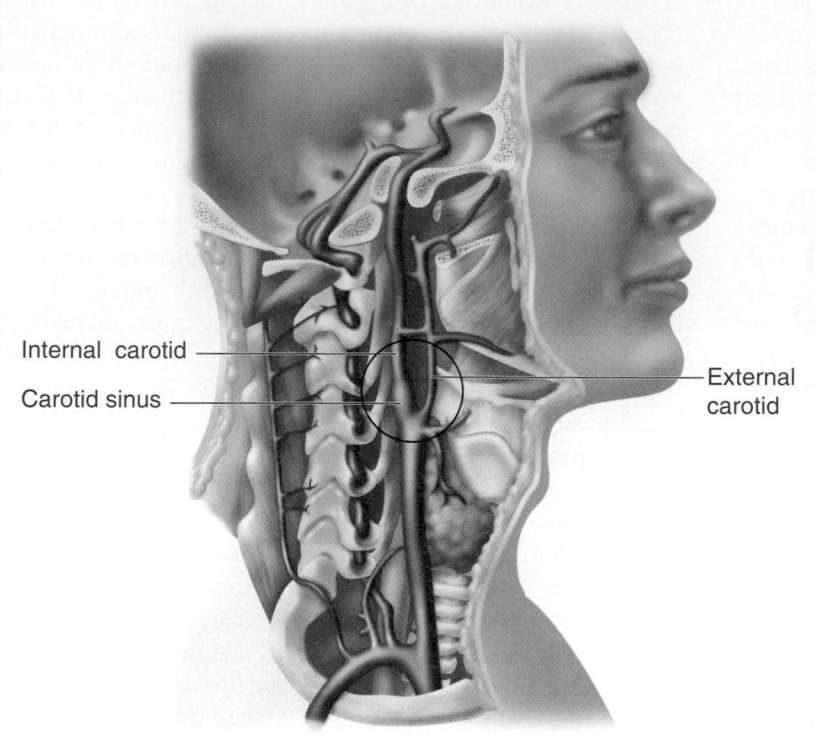

Internal carotid

Carotid sinus

External carotid

Figure 132 Never massage both the internal and external carotid arteries at the same time.

Words of Wisdom

The calcium channel blocker verapamil is often used by paramedics to achieve rate control of tachdysrhythmias. Verapamil's mechanism of action includes blocking conduction of electrical impulses through the AV node. AV nodal blockade is a safe and effective way to protect the ventricles from atrial tachydysrhythmias and to slow the overall heart rate. Wide QRS complexes on the ECG may be signs of bundle branch block, ventricular dysrhythmia, or preexcitation. Administration of verapamil to a patient with preexcitation can lead to VF or VT and sudden death. Therefore, administration of verapamil must be reserved for patients exhibiting narrow QRS complex tachydysrhythmias and should never be administered in wide complex tachycardias.

no warning before the event occurs. No matter what the cause, cardiac arrest is a stressful event for all involved. The best way to reduce the stress in providers and increase the potential for return of spontaneous circulation is to practice, practice, and practice so your team works like a pit crew. This concept is discussed further in the chapter, *Responding to the Field Code.*

Management of cardiac arrest requires you to deploy a great many of the advanced life support (ALS) skills that you have learned and to do so under urgent circumstances in which minutes may mean the difference between life and death. It is difficult to think clearly in such stressful circumstances,

especially when there are likely to be other stressed and panicky people at the scene (the patient's family, for example). For these reasons, it is absolutely essential for you to follow an orderly, systematic approach to cardiac arrest emergencies. That approach needs to be rehearsed repeatedly, in a team setting, until it is nearly automatic, and must include the steps of BLS and ALS.

BLS: A Review

The techniques and sequences of BLS should be familiar to all paramedic students. Remember, good ALS builds on good BLS, and good BLS builds on prompt bystander action. This section reviews the guidelines for ensuring maximally effective (and minimally damaging) CPR to adults in cardiac arrest. In the 2010 AHA Guidelines, there was a change from the "ABC" routine to "CAB." That is, CPR should now be initiated prior to the assessment of the airway and breathing in the unresponsive patient.

- Concentrate on high-quality compressions (deep enough–more than 2″, fast enough–100 times a minute, and with full chest recoil) with a minimum of interruptions.
- Avoid excessive volume and inflation pressure in artificial ventilation. Inflate just enough to observe visible chest rise.
- Keep your compressions smooth, regular, and uninterrupted.
    1. Maintain each compression for at least half the compression-release cycle.
  2. Avoid bouncing or jerky compressions,
  3. Keep your shoulders directly over the patient's sternum, and keep your elbows straight.
  4. Maintain proper hand position: fingers off the chest, and hands coming up off the sternum slightly between compressions to allow for complete chest recoil.
  5. Rotate fresh compressors every 2 minutes when help is available.
- As a single rescuer for adults, give 30 compressions to 2 ventilations at a rate of 100 compressions per minute. Once an advanced airway is placed, compressions continue at a rate of 100/min uninterrupted with 8 to 10 ventilations given with 100% supplemental oxygen.
- Do not interrupt CPR compressions except for advanced airway placement, defibrillation, or moving the patient. In all cases, minimize the duration of the interruption to 10 seconds or less. Any stop in compressions also stops perfusion—and perfusion is what it is all about!

Now you will learn how to integrate these well-rehearsed steps of BLS into the sequences of ACLS.

Advanced Cardiac Life Support

BLS is defined as maintenance of circulation and the airway and breathing without adjunctive equipment. Early quality compressions and defibrillation, both of which are BLS, are the measures that have been scientifically proven to have the greatest success for patients in ventricular fibrillation. In addition to

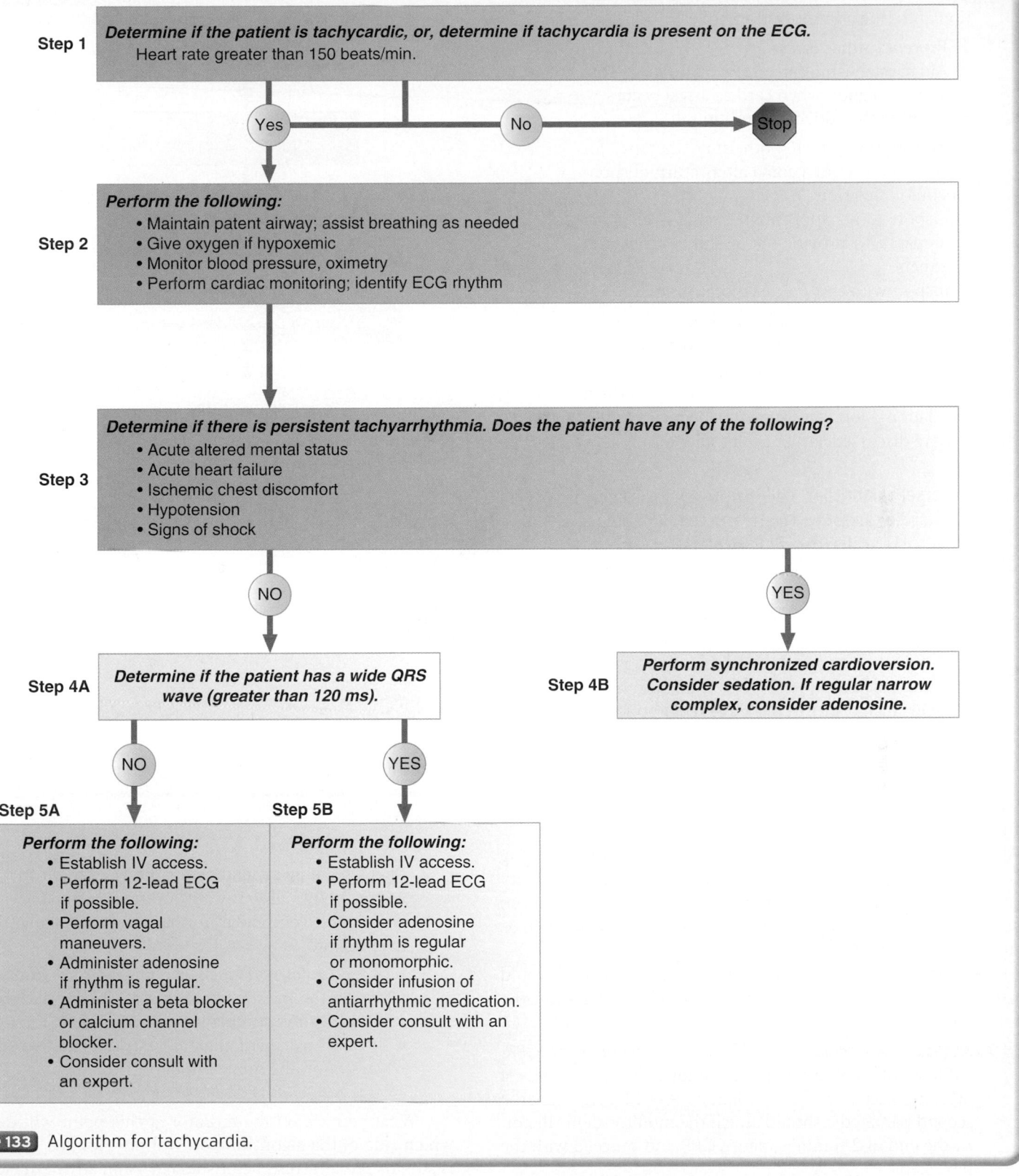

Step 1 — *Determine if the patient is tachycardic, or, determine if tachycardia is present on the ECG.*
Heart rate greater than 150 beats/min.

Yes → / No → Stop

Step 2 — *Perform the following:*
- Maintain patent airway; assist breathing as needed
- Give oxygen if hypoxemic
- Monitor blood pressure, oximetry
- Perform cardiac monitoring; identify ECG rhythm

Step 3 — *Determine if there is persistent tachyarrhythmia. Does the patient have any of the following?*
- Acute altered mental status
- Acute heart failure
- Ischemic chest discomfort
- Hypotension
- Signs of shock

NO / YES

Step 4A — *Determine if the patient has a wide QRS wave (greater than 120 ms).*

Step 4B — *Perform synchronized cardioversion. Consider sedation. If regular narrow complex, consider adenosine.*

NO / YES

Step 5A — *Perform the following:*
- Establish IV access.
- Perform 12-lead ECG if possible.
- Perform vagal maneuvers.
- Administer adenosine if rhythm is regular.
- Administer a beta blocker or calcium channel blocker.
- Consider consult with an expert.

Step 5B — *Perform the following:*
- Establish IV access.
- Perform 12-lead ECG if possible.
- Consider adenosine if rhythm is regular or monomorphic.
- Consider infusion of antiarrhythmic medication.
- Consider consult with an expert.

Figure 133   Algorithm for tachycardia.

high-quality BLS, you will be called on to deliver more definitive therapy as well, so the skills of ACLS must also become second nature, to be deployed swiftly and systematically in the event of cardiac arrest.

The AHA has defined ACLS for a patient in cardiac arrest (or a patient at immediate risk of cardiac arrest) as consisting of the following elements:

- Effective and minimally interrupted chest compression (for cardiac arrest)
- Use of adjunctive equipment for ventilation and circulation
- Cardiac monitoring for dysrhythmia recognition and control
- Establishment and maintenance of an IV infusion line

- Use of definitive therapy, including defibrillation and drug administration, to:
  1. Prevent cardiac arrest
  2. Aid in establishing an effective cardiac rhythm and circulation when cardiac arrest occurs
  3. Stabilize the patient's condition
- Administration of hypothermia therapy for patients who are in a coma after return of spontaneous circulation
- Transport to an appropriate facility—one that is prepared to provide successful resuscitation treatment
- Transport with continuous monitoring.

The use of airway adjuncts and equipment for artificial ventilation has already been discussed. In this section, the focus is on the sequence of actions in ACLS. Some of the specific techniques—such as defibrillation—for restoring an effective cardiac rhythm were discussed earlier in this chapter.

The Universal Algorithm The approach to every patient in cardiac arrest will start with the same steps, which the AHA calls the *BLS Healthcare Provider Algorithm* **Figure 134**. These basic steps are always deployed as soon as a person is found unresponsive and possibly in cardiac arrest. The BLS health care provider algorithm includes measures that bystanders should take before your arrival (such as "phone 9-1-1 or emergency number"), so you need to modify the universal algorithm a bit to make it applicable to emergency medical services personnel.

As always, you should bring your defibrillator with you when you initially approach the scene, as well as a portable oxygen cylinder and a "jump kit" that contains equipment for managing the airway. Also take the intubation kit, the IV equipment, and the drug box. If you are shorthanded, do not spend time carrying every piece of equipment from the ambulance to the patient; you can send someone to the ambulance for other equipment, such as the backboard and stretcher, later.

As soon as you reach the patient, one paramedic should ready the monitor-defibrillator while the other carries out the following steps:

1. **Assess the circulation.** *If there is no pulse, start CPR.* CPR should continue for 2 minutes or five cycles of 30 compressions and 2 ventilations. As CPR continues, the second paramedic should attach the monitor-defibrillator. At the end of 2 minutes, pause CPR and proceed with the next steps.
2. **Assess responsiveness.** If the patient is *not* responsive:
   - *Open the airway and assess for breathing.* If the patient is *not* breathing:
   - *Give two slow breaths.* Use the bag-mask device or a barrier device.

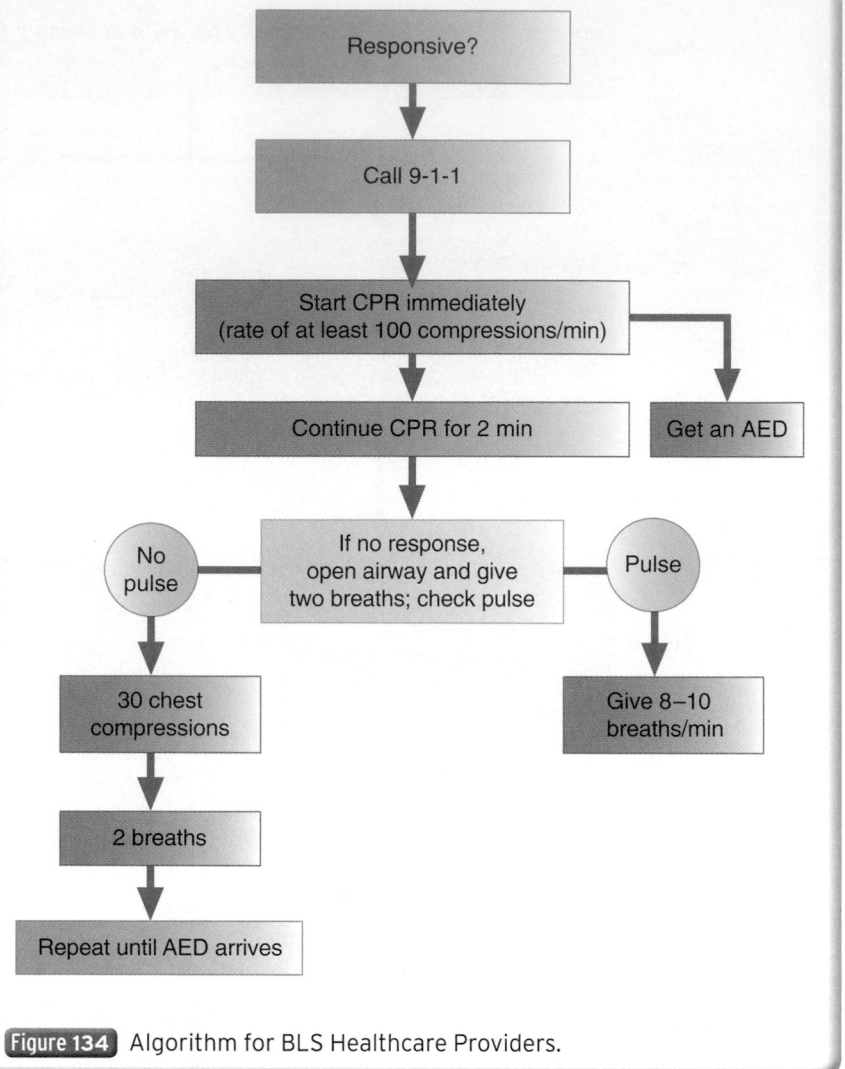

Figure 134 Algorithm for BLS Healthcare Providers.

3. **Check for a pulse, and check the rhythm on the monitor.** At this point, all you want to know is the answer to one question: Is ventricular fibrillation or ventricular tachycardia present?
   - *If ventricular fibrillation or ventricular tachycardia is present* on the monitor-defibrillator, follow the ventricular fibrillation/ventricular tachycardia arm of the algorithm.
   - *If ventricular fibrillation or ventricular tachycardia is not present* on the monitor-defibrillator, *resume CPR immediately.*

What you see on the monitor at this point will determine which side of the algorithm you will now follow. If the patient is still in cardiac arrest, he or she may be in any of the following situations:

- Ventricular fibrillation or pulseless ventricular tachycardia
- PEA (that is, you can see an organized rhythm on the monitor, but there is no detectable pulse)
- Asystole

Each of these situations requires a different, specific approach (a different pathway down the pulseless arrest algorithm).

Treatment for Ventricular Fibrillation or Pulseless Ventricular Tachycardia

Managing ventricular fibrillation or pulseless ventricular tachycardia is probably the most important algorithm for you to know because patients found in ventricular fibrillation or ventricular tachycardia are the most likely to be successfully resuscitated—*if* they receive timely and appropriate treatment. The steps of the ventricular fibrillation/ventricular tachycardia pathway down the pulseless arrest algorithm are presented schematically in Figure 135. Additionally, Table 23 lists possible causes and treatment of cardiac arrest rhythms.

The steps in managing ventricular fibrillation and pulseless ventricular tachycardia are as follows:

1. Address CAB issues.
2. Begin CPR immediately and attach the defibrillator simultaneously, if sufficient personnel are available. Continue CPR for 2 minutes if you did not witness the cardiac arrest.
3. Confirm ventricular fibrillation or ventricular tachycardia on the monitor-defibrillator.
4. Confirm absence of a pulse (in a maximum of 10 seconds). Other things besides ventricular fibrillation and ventricular tachycardia can make squiggly lines on a monitor, such as loose ECG leads or muscle tremor. Remember: Treat the patient, not the monitor.
5. Resume CPR while charging the defibrillator.
6. Clear the patient and then defibrillate the ventricular fibrillation or ventricular tachycardia:
   - If using a biphasic defibrillator, set it to 120 to 200 joules (J). This energy level depends on the manufacturer's recommendation. If the recommendation is unknown and the defibrillator is biphasic, use 200 J as the default energy dose.
   - If using a monophasic defibrillator, set it to 360 J.

As soon as the defibrillator discharges, resume CPR. It is important not to delay resuming CPR at this time to determine the rhythm. Continue CPR for 2 minutes or five cycles. Recent research indicates that even if an organized rhythm appears in the post-resuscitation period, the presence of an immediate pulse is unlikely. It has also been shown that 2 minutes of post-resuscitation CPR is unlikely to cause a return of ventricular fibrillation. After 2 minutes or five cycles, stop CPR, and assess the patient's circulation and check the rhythm on the monitor.

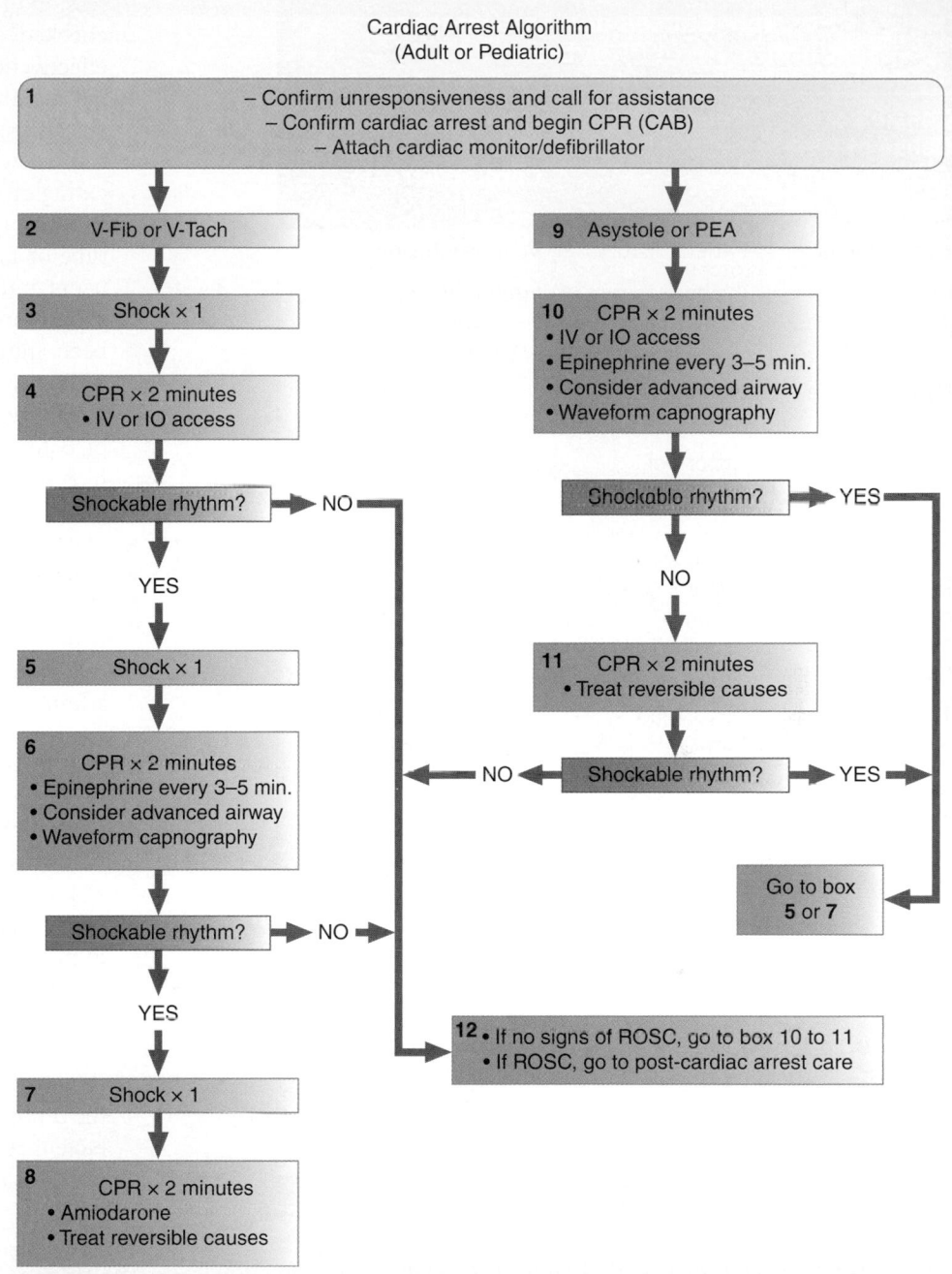

Figure 135 ACLS algorithm for cardiac arrest. Reversible causes in adults that can be treated include Hs and Ts: hypovolemia, hypoxia, hydrogen ion (acidosis), hypokalemia, hyperkalemia, hypothermia, tension pneumothorax, toxins, cardiac tamponade, and pulmonary and coronary thrombosis.

Table 23   Possible Causes and Treatment of Cardiac Arrest Rhythms

Possible Cause of PEA to Consider During Arrest	Clues to Cause	Treatment (Beyond Managing the Cardiac Arrest)
Hypovolemia	Patient history	Volume infusion
Hypoxemia	Cyanosis, airway problem	Intubation and ventilation with 100% oxygen
Hypoglycemia	Blood glucose level < 60 mg/dL	Dextrose 50% in water, 25 g
Hypothermia	History of exposure to cold	See hypothermia algorithm in the chapter, *Environmental Emergencies*
Hyperkalemia, hypokalemia, hydrogen ions (acidosis)	History, ECG changes	Immediate transport Consider sodium bicarbonate if certain of acidosis
Tension pneumothorax	History, no pulse with CPR, unequal breath sounds with hyperresonance to percussion on affected side	Needle decompression of the affected side of the chest
Cardiac tamponade	History, no pulse with CPR, jugular venous distention	Pericardiocentesis (immediate transport)
Others: Drug overdose, trauma, massive MI, pulmonary embolism	History	Consider need for immediate transport. Naloxone (Narcan) for opioid or narcotic overdose.

7. If a rhythm other than ventricular fibrillation or ventricular tachycardia appears on the monitor screen:

 - *Identify the new rhythm.*
 - If there is no pulse, move to the asystole-PEA pathway down the algorithm and resume CPR immediately.
 - If there is a pulse, move to the appropriate algorithm for the new rhythm.

8. If the rhythm continues to be ventricular fibrillation or ventricular tachycardia, *resume CPR while charging the defibrillator.*

9. *Clear the patient and then defibrillate* the ventricular fibrillation or ventricular tachycardia:

 - Use the same energy setting as for the initial shock.
 - *Resume CPR immediately*, and continue for 2 minutes after the shock. The CPR compressor and ventilator should change positions at the end of each 2-minute

session of CPR (while the rhythm and pulse are being checked) to avoid fatigue, which can reduce the effectiveness of chest compressions.

 - During these 2 minutes of CPR, you should *insert an advanced airway only if the BLS airway is not adequate*. Advanced airways include intraglottic and extraglottic devices including the endotracheal tube, King LT airway, laryngeal mask airway, and Combitube or EasyTube. After intubation, verify placement using multiple methods include waveform capnography, and secure the tube. Once the patient has been intubated, it is no longer necessary to pause CPR compressions for ventilation to be administered. Ventilations should be administered at a rate of 8 to 10 breaths per minute (one breath every 6 to 8 seconds or one breath after each 10 to 12 compressions). The rate of compressions is 100/min.
 - *Start an IV line* with normal saline.
 - *If unable to establish IV access, establish intraosseous (IO) access* via an adult IO access system. If IV access is not obtained but IO access is, all drugs and fluids that would normally be administered via IV should be administered via IO until IV access is established.
 - As soon as IV or IO access has been established, *administer a vasopressor drug*. The two recommended vasopressor drugs are epinephrine and vasopressin (Pitressin synthetic). *Epinephrine (1:10,000) is given as 1 mg IV push;* this dose should be repeated every 3 to 5 minutes as long as a pulse is absent. *Vasopressin is given as 40 units IV push, one time only*. Vasopressin can be given in place of the first or second dose of epinephrine (but not both). Whenever you give a medication through a peripheral IV line during CPR, follow it immediately with a 20- to 30-mL bolus of IV fluid and then elevate the extremity to facilitate delivery of the medication to the central circulation (which may take 1 to 2 minutes). Note that IO administration has the same effect of central circulation.

10. *At the end of 2 minutes of CPR, pause compressions to check for circulation and check the rhythm on the monitor.*

11. If ventricular fibrillation or ventricular tachycardia is still present, *resume CPR while charging the defibrillator.*

12. *Clear the patient and then defibrillate* the ventricular fibrillation or ventricular tachycardia:

 - Use the same energy setting as before.
 - Resume CPR immediately, and continue for 2 minutes after the shock. Remember to change CPR compressors after each rhythm check.
 - During these 2 minutes of CPR, you should *consider the administration of an antidysrhythmic medication*. The preferred antidysrhythmic medication is *amiodarone (Cordarone, Pacerone)*, which is given as a 300-mg bolus during CPR. Amiodarone may be repeated once at 150 mg in 3 to 5 minutes after the initial dose. If amiodarone is unavailable, you may administer *lidocaine*, 1 to 1.5 mg/kg IV push. Lidocaine (Xylocaine) can be repeated at 0.5

to 0.75 mg/kg every 5 to 10 minutes until the maximum dose of 3 mg/kg has been reached. It is important not to combine these two antidysrhythmic medications because this practice can actually cause dysrhythmias.

13. *At the end of 2 minutes of CPR, pause compressions to check for circulation and check the rhythm on the monitor.*
14. If *ventricular* fibrillation or ventricular tachycardia is still present, *resume CPR while charging the defibrillator.*
15. *Clear the patient and then defibrillate* the ventricular fibrillation or ventricular tachycardia:
    - Use the same energy setting as before.
    - Resume CPR immediately, and continue for 2 minutes after the shock. Remember to change CPR compressors after each rhythm check.
    - If ventricular fibrillation or ventricular tachycardia is still present, consider making a transport decision with the advice of medical control. Continue the cycle of defibrillation followed by immediate CPR for 2 minutes while administering repeated doses of medications.
16. If at any point during this sequence there is a return of spontaneous circulation:
    - Assess the patient's vital signs.
    - Support the airway and breathing, as required.
    - Provide medications as indicated for regulating the heart rate, controlling cardiac dysrhythmias, and maintaining the blood pressure.
17. Consider implementation of hypothermia protocol and transport to appropriate cardiac care center.

Treatment for Pulseless Electrical Activity The term <u>pulseless electrical activity (PEA)</u> refers to an organized cardiac rhythm (other than ventricular tachycardia) on the monitor that is not accompanied by any detectable pulse. This category includes what was once called electromechanical dissociation and conditions in which the heart beats so weakly that it cannot produce a palpable pulse, which may occur, for example, in cardiogenic or hypovolemic shock, cardiac tamponade, massive pulmonary embolism, disturbances of electrolyte imbalance, including hyperkalemia in renal failure, or drug overdose. Providing the appropriate treatment depends on identifying the cause of PEA in a specific case.

When the monitor is applied to a pulseless patient and a rhythm (other than ventricular fibrillation, ventricular tachycardia, or asystole) is seen:

1. *Immediately resume CPR.*
2. *Insert an advanced airway if the BLS airway is not adequate.*
3. *Start an IV line* with normal saline.
4. *If you are unable to establish IV access, consider establishing IO access.*
5. As soon as IV or IO access has been established, *administer a vasopressor drug.* The two recommended vasopressor drugs are epinephrine and vasopressin. *Epinephrine (1:10,000) is given as 1 mg IV push;* this dose should be repeated every 3 to 5 minutes for as long as a pulse is

absent. *Vasopressin (Pitressin synthetic) is given as 40 units IV push, one time only.* Vasopressin can be given in place of the first or second dose of epinephrine (but not both). Whenever you give a medication through a peripheral IV line during CPR, follow it immediately with a 20- to 30-mL bolus of IV fluid and then elevate the extremity to facilitate delivery of the medication to the central circulation (which may take 1 to 2 minutes).

6. *At the end of 2 minutes of CPR, pause the compressions to check for circulation and check the rhythm on the monitor.*
7. If PEA is still present:
   - *Continue CPR immediately.*
   - Search for and treat the possible causes ("Hs and Ts," discussed in Table 23).

Words of Wisdom

Sodium bicarbonate is in the class of drugs called alkalinizing agents. These drugs are used to increase the pH of blood and urine (alkalinize), for example in cases of acidosis.

Asystole Treatment A flat line on an ECG monitor may or may not be asystole. Thus, one of the first things to do when you see a flat-line ECG is to rule out causes other than asystole. Possible causes of a flat-line ECG include leads that are not connected to the patient, loose leads, leads that are not connected to the monitor-defibrillator, an incorrect monitor setting, very-low-voltage ventricular fibrillation, and true asystole.

When the monitor is applied to a pulseless patient and asystole is seen:

1. *Immediately resume CPR,* assuming you are not presented with a valid advance directive indicating *not* to perform CPR ("do not resuscitate" orders).
2. *Confirm asystole by checking for other causes of the flat line.* Make sure that all monitoring electrodes are firmly fastened to the patient and that the cables are hooked into the monitor. Switch to another lead to detect low-voltage ventricular fibrillation. If the rhythm is asystole, you need to be aware that the prognosis is grim and the chances for successful resuscitation are poor.
3. *Insert an advanced airway if the BLS airway is not adequate.*
4. *Start an IV line* with normal saline.
5. *If unable to establish IV access, consider establishing IO access.*
6. As soon as IV or IO access has been established, *administer a vasopressor drug.* The two recommended vasopressor drugs are epinephrine and vasopressin. *Epinephrine (1:10,000) is given as 1 mg IV push;* this dose should be repeated every 3 to 5 minutes for as long as a pulse is absent. *Vasopressin (Pitressin synthetic) is given as 40 units IV push, one time only.* Vasopressin can be given in place of the first or second dose of epinephrine (but not both). Whenever you give a medication through a peripheral IV line during CPR, follow it immediately with a 20- to 30-mL bolus of IV fluid and then elevate the extremity to facilitate

delivery of the medication to the central circulation (which may take 1 to 2 minutes).

7. *At the end of every 2 minutes of CPR, pause the compressions to check for circulation and to check the rhythm on the monitor.*

8. If asystole is still present:
   - *Immediately resume CPR.*
   - Search for and treat possible causes. Possible causes are the same as for PEA and are listed in Table 23.
   - *Seriously consider termination of the resuscitation with advisement from medical control and then focus on the survivors.*

Postresuscitative Care

If an effective cardiac rhythm is restored in the field, your next task is to make sure that the rhythm *stays* restored and that optimal conditions are provided to promote recovery of the patient's brain from the hypoxic insult of cardiac arrest.

First, the heart rate should be stabilized. If the rhythm is bradycardic or tachycardic in the postresuscitation period, the bradycardia or tachycardia algorithms should be followed.

Next, cardiac rhythm should be stabilized to the degree possible. If the arrest rhythm was ventricular fibrillation or ventricular tachycardia, consider administering a bolus of an anti-dysrhythmic drug, followed by an infusion of the same drug. Historically, lidocaine (Xylocaine) has been given in this situation, but if amiodarone (Cordarone, Pacerone) was given to the patient in arrest, then an infusion of amiodarone should be started and lidocaine should not be used. If severe bradycardia is present in the postarrest period, atropine or TCP may be required, and the hospital should be alerted to prepare a transcutaneous pacemaker.

Once the cardiac rhythm is stable, attention turns to the patient's brain and to ameliorating the effects of cardiac arrest on it. Marked hypotension needs to be corrected rapidly because the brain will not be adequately perfused if the blood pressure is very low. If the patient has marked hypotension and the transport time to the hospital will be prolonged, the physician may order an infusion of dopamine (Intropin). In an intubated patient, avoid tracheal suctioning unless absolutely necessary; suctioning tends to increase intracranial pressure. Finally, consider elevating the patient's head to about 30° to increase cerebral venous drainage.

Words of Wisdom

BiPAP increases intrathoracic pressure, which in turn stimulates baroreceptors in the aorta and causes a decrease in venous return and blood pressure. BiPAP must be used with extreme caution or withheld in patients who are borderline normotensive or hypotensive, respectively. Conversely, deep inspiration causes an increase in venous return because of the negative pressure in the thoracic cavity.

Postresuscitative care is an important component of caring for cardiac arrest patients. If an effective cardiac rhythm is restored in the field, transport immediately; the patient needs careful monitoring and titrated therapy that can most effectively be given in an intensive care unit. However, if the patient

is comatose after return of spontaneous circulation, begin hypothermia treatment immediately.

The following is a summary of postresuscitative care:

1. Stabilize the cardiac rhythm (give an antidysrhythmic drug for post–ventricular fibrillation or post–ventricular tachycardia; give atropine or use a transcutaneous pacemaker for symptomatic bradycardia).

2. Normalize the blood pressure (give a dopamine [Intropin] or norepinephrine infusion to raise the systolic pressure to at least 100 mm Hg).

3. Elevate the patient's head to 30° if the blood pressure allows.

When to Stop CPR

Since the dawn of paramedic-staffed ambulances in the early 1970s, many communities have *not* permitted the termination of CPR in the field. That policy was established because, in most jurisdictions, only a physician is authorized to pronounce a person dead (stopping CPR is considered equivalent to pronouncing a person dead). Cardiac arrest patients who were not successfully resuscitated at the scene were invariably transported urgently to the hospital, with some semblance of CPR occurring en route.

With the accumulation of vast experience from EMS systems throughout the United States, it soon became clear that transport to the ED of adults who did not respond to an adequate trial of prehospital ACLS was an exercise in futility: Fewer than 1% of patients ultimately survived. This policy was also given as the example of an unethical practice in the AHA's 2010 guidelines because it instills false hope in the family. Furthermore, rapid transport of patients in cardiac arrest, with CPR en route, involves considerable hazards to EMS personnel: The risks of vehicular crashes or of injuries while working in a moving ambulance are greatly increased during urgent transport.

AHA criteria for terminating CPR in the prehospital setting are listed in **Table 24**.

In some jurisdictions, state legislation will be required to permit pronouncement of death at the scene by a paramedic. Once such legislation is enacted, each EMS system will have to formulate its own criteria for the termination of CPR in the prehospital setting.

Gaining permission to stop CPR in the field will not necessarily make your life easier. Delicate issues are involved, such as the expectations of the patient's family or the disposition of the body. You may face enormous pressure from bystanders

Table 24 AHA Criteria for Terminating CPR in the Field
1. The arrest was not witnessed by anyone.
2. No bystander CPR was provided.
3. Spontaneous circulation did not return after complete ALS care in the field.
4. No shocks were administered.

to continue resuscitative efforts long after there is any medical justification for doing so. Stopping CPR may also be difficult for you; you may not be accustomed to having to tell a family that the person is dead and nothing more can be done. It is much easier to provide transport to the hospital with red lights flashing and sirens blaring and leave the emergency department staff with the "expectation of providing a miracle" and the unpleasant task of breaking bad news, as well as a very expensive ED bill.

If and when it becomes legal in your EMS system to terminate CPR in the field, it will be a good idea to meet with your medical director and "walk through" some of the scenes you may have to face. Role-play exercises can be particularly useful in helping you to pinpoint situations in which you feel uncomfortable and develop strategies in advance for dealing with those situations. Many jurisdictions have adopted protocols to assist providers in deciding when resuscitation attempts are futile and should be terminated.

Pathophysiology, Assessment, and Management of Specific Cardiovascular Problems

Coronary Artery Disease and Angina

Coronary artery disease (CAD) is the most common form of heart disease and the leading cause of death in US adults. The coronary arteries supply oxygen and nutrients to the myocardium. If one of these blood vessels becomes blocked, the muscle it supplies will be deprived of oxygen (ischemia). If this oxygen supply is not quickly restored, the ischemic area of heart muscle will eventually die (undergo infarction).

Atherosclerosis is of particular concern because it affects the inner lining of the aorta and cerebral and coronary blood vessels, leading to the narrowing of those vessels and reduction of blood flow through them. The atherosclerotic process begins, probably in childhood, when small amounts of fatty material are deposited along the inner wall (intima) of arteries, usually at points of turbulent blood flow (such as where the arteries bifurcate or where the arterial wall has been damaged). As the streak of fat enlarges, it becomes a mass of fatty tissue, an atheroma, which gradually calcifies and hardens into a plaque. The atheromatous plaque infiltrates the arterial wall and decreases its elasticity. At the same time, it narrows the arterial lumen and interferes with blood flow through the lumen. The narrowed, roughened area of the arterial intima provides a locus for the formation of a fixed blood clot, or thrombus, which may then obstruct the artery altogether (when in a coronary artery is known as a coronary thrombosis). In addition, calcium may precipitate from the bloodstream into the arterial walls, causing arteriosclerosis, which greatly reduces the elasticity of the arteries.

Risk Factors for Atherosclerosis

Although atherosclerosis is widespread in industrialized countries, certain factors increase the risk of developing atherosclerosis and CAD: hypertension (high blood pressure), cigarette smoking, diabetes, high serum cholesterol levels (which may be related to a high dietary intake of saturated fats and calories), lack of exercise, obesity, family history of heart disease or stroke, and male gender. Clearly, these risk factors include some things a person cannot do anything about. You cannot, for example, select your parents and grandparents or choose to be born female. Nevertheless, something can be done for about nearly half the risk factors for CAD, which are, therefore, called modifiable risk factors:

- Cigarette smoking is the most significant cause of preventable death in the United States, and a smoker's chances of sudden death are several times greater than those of a nonsmoker. The good news is that smokers who quit return rapidly to the same risk level as nonsmokers.
- Hypertension cannot be prevented or cured, but it can be controlled with changes in diet and with medications. A person with uncontrolled hypertension has two to three times the risk of CAD as a person with normal blood pressure.
- The levels of serum cholesterol are at least in part a consequence of dietary intake of saturated fats. In populations with low fat intake, the incidence of CAD is also low. Furthermore, lowering the serum cholesterol levels has been shown to reduce the incidence of heart attacks and other dangerous cardiac events. Cholesterol may also be controlled with medications, if necessary.
- One behavior that may have a role in elevating serum cholesterol is lack of exercise, which also has a variety of other untoward effects on the body. Exercise improves overall fitness, cardiac reserve, and collateral coronary circulation.
- Obesity may go hand in hand with several other risk factors (such as diabetes and hypertension). But obesity by itself also may contribute to an increased risk of CAD. Weight reduction, through consumption of a sensible diet and increased physical exercise, can reap several lifelong and life-extending benefits. Normalizing body weight will lower elevated blood pressure, elevated serum cholesterol levels, elevated blood glucose levels, and the risk of CAD.

Data suggest that risk factor modification can make a difference in the impact of CAD. According to the AHA, from 1993 to 2003, mortality from CAD declined 22% in the United States Figure 136 . From 2006 to 2007, mortality from diseases of the heart decreased by 4.6%. According to the CDC, in 2007, approximately 25% of deaths resulted from diseases of the heart. Although experts cannot say precisely what caused that decline (it would be rewarding to think that paramedic-staffed ambulances had a significant role!), reduction in smoking, better control of hypertension, changes in dietary habits, and an upsurge of interest in fitness undoubtedly made substantial contributions to this trend. Unfortunately, the incidence of obesity and type 2 diabetes is increasing, which will likely overshadow steps that have been taken to help decrease CAD.

Peripheral Vascular Disorders

Although atherosclerosis is rarely the primary cause of medical emergencies, it is a major contributor to other conditions that

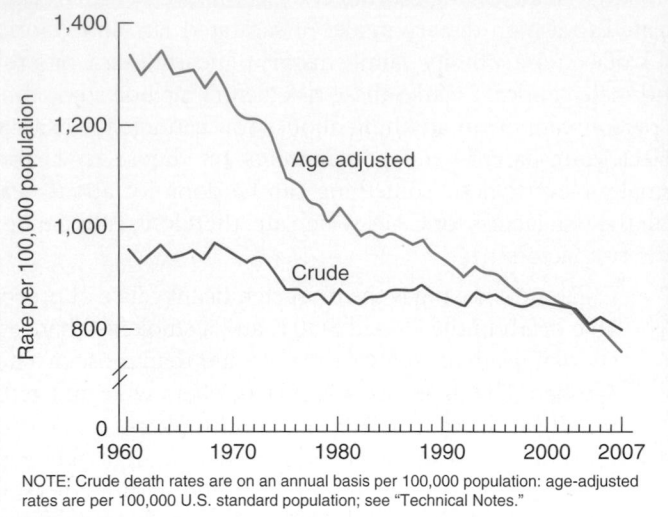

NOTE: Crude death rates are on an annual basis per 100,000 population: age-adjusted rates are per 100,000 U.S. standard population; see "Technical Notes."

Figure 136 Crude and age-adjusted death rates, United States, 1960-2007.

may become medical emergencies. For example, arterial <u>bruits</u> or "swishing" sounds (heard with a stethoscope placed over the carotid arteries) signal the presence of atherosclerosis and contraindicate the use of carotid sinus massage. Atherosclerosis can also contribute to <u>claudication</u>, a severe pain in the calf muscle caused by narrowing of the arteries in this muscle and leading to a painful limp. Finally, atherosclerosis may be associated with <u>phlebitis</u>—swelling and pain along the veins that can lead to the formation of blood clots called deep vein thrombosis (DVT). If dislodged, these thrombi become emboli that could travel to the heart and through its right side, lodging in the pulmonary arterial tree and causing a pulmonary embolism.

An estimated 5 to 20 million Americans are affected by significant peripheral vascular disorders annually. The most dangerous complication of these disorders is pulmonary embolism, which causes approximately 200,000 deaths each year. Risk factors for peripheral vascular disorders include age, oral contraceptive use, smoking, recent surgery, recreational IV drug use, trauma, and extended immobilization. Identification of these risk factors has a significant role in diagnosing peripheral vascular occlusions. Signs of peripheral vascular occlusion may include pain, redness, swelling, warmth, and tenderness in the extremity; these signs are present in only about half of all cases, however. The presence of claudication indicates a significant narrowing of the peripheral arteries associated with peripheral vascular disorders. Arterial bruits are another sign of vascular narrowing that can contribute to ischemia or stroke.

Because peripheral vascular disorders can have serious consequences, such as pulmonary embolism or loss of a limb through arterial occlusions, you must be familiar with the signs, symptoms, and risk factors for these conditions. Unfortunately, prehospital treatment of peripheral vascular conditions is limited. Beyond providing supplementary oxygen, obtaining IV access, and, possibly, aspirin administration, little can be done in the field if you suspect a peripheral vascular disorder.

Thromboembolism The development of a clot, or thrombus, either in the arteries or in the veins can lead to decreased blood flow to certain areas within the body. Furthermore, if the clot were to become dislodged, at which point it is termed a <u>thromboembolism</u>, it could produce a complete blockage of the vessel, resulting in a stoppage of the flow of oxygen-rich blood if the blockage occurs on the arterial side and a decreased venous return if it occurs in a vein. Prehospital treatment of thromboembolism includes supportive care. For example, if a pulmonary embolism is suspected, therapy is centered on oxygenation and ventilation to maintain appropriate oxygen saturation levels.

Angina Pectoris

The principal symptom of CAD is <u>angina pectoris</u> (literally "choking in the chest"). Angina occurs when the supply of oxygen to the myocardium is insufficient to meet the demand. As a result, the cardiac muscle becomes ischemic, and a switch to anaerobic metabolism leads to the accumulation of lactic acid and carbon dioxide. The concept of "supply and demand" is critical here. When at rest, a person with heart disease may have an adequate supply of oxygen to the heart to meet these sedentary needs, despite some narrowing of the coronary arteries. When the same person exercises or experiences some other stress, however, the blood flow to the myocardium may not be able to satisfy the heart's increased demand for oxygen; in that case, angina will result. Clearly, the patient who experiences angina at rest, when oxygen needs are minimal, has more severe CAD than a person who experiences angina only with vigorous exercise.

<u>Prinzmetal angina</u> results in chest pain at rest and is caused by coronary artery vasospasm. Although men and women can experience Prinzmetal angina, it is more common in women in their 50s. People with Prinzmetal angina have an increased risk of experiencing ventricular dysrhythmias, myocardial infarction, heart block, or sudden death. This condition can present itself with little adjustment in vital signs. Although most patients with this type of angina have significant CAD, some patients may have none.

When you are obtaining the history from a patient with chest pain, it is important to distinguish between stable angina and unstable angina. <u>Stable angina</u> follows a recurrent pattern: A person with stable angina experiences pain after a certain, predictable amount of exertion, such as climbing one flight of stairs or walking for three blocks. The pain also has a predictable location, intensity, and duration. The patient may report, for example, "Every time I walk up the hill to the bus stop, I get a squeezing pain under my breast bone, and I have to sit down for 2 or 3 minutes until it goes away."

Words of Wisdom

Other names for unstable angina include preinfarction angina, crescendo angina, and ACS.

Patients with chronic, stable angina often take nitroglycerin or some other form of "nitrate" for relief of anginal pain. In its usual formulation, nitroglycerin is supplied as a white tablet, which is placed under the tongue (sublingual) and allowed to dissolve there, or in a spray form that is sprayed under the tongue. It may also be given as sustained-release capsules taken two or three times a day, as a cream rubbed into the skin (topical), or as a patch worn on the skin. Regardless of which form is used, nitroglycerin will have a predictable effect in stable angina, producing relief of symptoms within a few minutes.

<u>Unstable angina</u> is much more serious than stable angina and indicates a greater degree of obstruction of the coronary arteries. It is characterized by noticeable changes in the frequency, severity, and duration of pain and often occurs without predictable stress. The patient may report that the anginal attacks have grown more frequent and severe during the past several days or weeks or that they awaken him or her from sleep or occur when otherwise at rest. It may or may not be relieved by rest or medications. Such attacks are often warning signs of an impending MI.

Acute Coronary Syndrome

<u>Acute coronary syndrome (ACS)</u> is the term used to describe any group of clinical symptoms consistent with acute myocardial ischemia. Acute myocardial ischemia typically presents as chest pain due to insufficient blood supply to the heart muscle, which itself is a result of CAD. The life-threatening ACS disorders are responsible for much of the emergency medical care and hospitalization in the United States.

Patients experiencing symptomatic, acute myocardial ischemia should receive a 12-lead ECG to determine whether they have an ST-segment elevation. Most patients whose ECG displays ST-segment elevation will ultimately develop a "Q-wave AMI" (heart attack), also known as STEMI (ST-elevation myocardial infarction). Patients who have ischemic discomfort (chest pain) without an ST-segment elevation are having unstable angina or a non–ST-segment elevation MI that usually leads to a non–Q-wave MI; these conditions are collectively known as UA/NSTEMI (unstable angina/non–ST-elevation myocardial infarction). Patients who experience angina may also present with ST-segment depression. Finally, some patients experiencing angina or MI may have *no* changes indicated by the ECG.

Management

Of course, not all chest pain is caused by cardiac ischemia or injury. Many other conditions—such as pulmonary embolism, pneumothorax, pneumonia, pericarditis, aortic dissection, indigestion, and peptic ulcer—may cause chest pain that can be mistaken for angina or an MI. It is important for you to perform a thorough physical exam, including history taking, to determine whether the cause of the complaint is likely cardiac in origin.

As a general rule, it is safe to assume that any patient who has called for an ambulance because of chest pain has, at the least, unstable angina and perhaps an evolving AMI. Patients with chronic, stable angina rarely call for help unless something has changed—often dramatically—for the worse. Because it is difficult and sometimes impossible to differentiate between angina and an MI in the field, the treatment of angina should be the same as for an MI. It is far better for you to overtreat angina as an MI than to undertreat an MI by assuming it is angina.

■ Acute Myocardial Infarction

Pathophysiology

An <u>acute myocardial infarction (AMI)</u>, or heart attack, occurs when a portion of the cardiac muscle is deprived of coronary blood flow long enough that portions of the muscle die (undergo <u>necrosis</u>, or infarct). Several things can diminish flow through coronary vessels, especially if the vessels are already narrowed by atherosclerotic disease: occlusion of a coronary artery by a blood clot (thrombus), spasm of a coronary artery, or reduction of overall blood flow from any cause (such as shock, dysrhythmias, or pulmonary embolism).

The location and size of a myocardial infarct depend on which coronary artery is blocked and where along its course the blockage occurred. Most infarcts involve the left ventricle. When the anterior, lateral, or septal walls of the left ventricle are infarcted, the source is usually occlusion of the left coronary artery or one of its branches. Inferior wall infarcts are usually the result of RCA occlusion. When the ischemic process affects only the inner layer of muscle, the infarct is referred to as a <u>subendocardial myocardial infarction</u>. When the infarct extends through the entire wall of the ventricle, it is a <u>transmural myocardial infarction</u>. The infarcted tissue is invariably surrounded by a ring of ischemic tissue—an area that is relatively deprived of oxygen but still viable. That ischemic tissue tends to be electrically unstable and is often the source of cardiac dysrhythmias.

Words of Wisdom

For purposes of treatment outside the hospital, the patient with chest pain must be assumed to be having an acute myocardial infarction until proven otherwise and should therefore be treated as any other patient with a suspected AMI.

Cardiovascular disease accounted for more than 191,000 deaths in 2005. Of deaths related to cardiovascular disease, AMI is the leading cause of death in the United States; 60% to 70% of AMIs occur outside the hospital, during the first 2 to 3 hours after the onset of symptoms. Of all deaths from AMI, 90% are due to dysrhythmias, usually ventricular fibrillation, which typically occur during the early hours of the infarct. Dysrhythmias can be prevented or treated, so *most deaths from AMI are preventable.*

Words of Wisdom

When a patient with chest pain calls for an ambulance, it means that the patient never had chest pain before or that his or her chronic chest pain has changed. Take all chest pain complaints seriously.

Assessment

Symptoms of AMI Although there is no "typical AMI patient," when most Americans think about the symptoms of an AMI, they envision the classic pain presentation usually associated with men. In fact, AMIs can occur in younger and older people and in men and women. The patient may be slightly overweight and may have recently overindulged at the dinner table or perhaps on the tennis court. Nevertheless, many heart attacks occur at rest or just after arising in the morning.

The most common symptom of AMI is chest pain. This pain is similar to that of angina but can be much more severe and last more than 15 minutes. A patient with chronic angina will be aware that something different from previous anginal attacks is happening. The pain of AMI is typically felt just beneath the sternum and is variously described as heavy, squeezing, crushing, or tight. Often the patient unconsciously clenches a fist when describing the pain (Levine sign) to convey in body language the squeezing nature of the pain. In 25% of patients, the pain radiates to the arms (most often the left arm) and into the fingers; it may also radiate to the neck, jaw, upper back, or epigastrium. Occasionally, a patient will mistake the pain of AMI for indigestion and may take antacids in an attempt to relieve the discomfort. The pain of AMI is not influenced by coughing, deep breathing, or other body movements, and may or may not be relieved by nitrates or rest.

Not every AMI patient has chest pain, however. In fact, 10% to 20% of patients with AMI *do not experience any chest pain.* Women, diabetics, the elderly, and heart transplant patients, for example, generally do not present with chest pain, a condition referred to as "silent MI." Instead, these patients may present with symptoms related to a drop in CO. It is not unusual for them to develop sudden dyspnea, progressing rapidly to **pulmonary edema**, a sudden loss of consciousness, an unexplained drop in blood pressure, an apparent stroke, or simply confusion.

Women with an AMI may present differently from men with the same condition. Women may experience nausea, lightheadedness, epigastric burning, or sudden onset of weakness or unexplained tiredness. Women may also have pain radiating down the right arm instead of the classic left arm pain. Because they are not experiencing the typical chest pain expected with an AMI, many women ignore their symptoms. Unfortunately, cardiovascular disease is the number one cause of death for US women.

Words of Wisdom

More men have heart disease, but more women die of heart disease, in part because their symptoms are less clear-cut.

When you are obtaining the history from a patient whose chief complaint is chest pain, ask the usual OPQRST questions to elaborate on the chief complaint, but also ask whether the patient has taken anything for the pain and, if so, whether it helped. If the patient reports having taken nitroglycerin without relief, it is important to establish *why* the patient did not obtain relief.

Two reasons might explain this failure. One possibility is that the patient is, indeed, having an AMI, for which

nitroglycerin would not provide complete pain relief. The other possibility is that the nitroglycerin has simply gone stale. To retain its potency, nitroglycerin must be stored in a dark, airtight container; if it is left out in the open for any period (for example, if the patient stores the medicine on the window sill above the kitchen sink), it loses its therapeutic effectiveness. To distinguish between the two explanations, ask the patient whether he or she noticed the usual effects of the nitroglycerin. Nitroglycerin tablets that are therapeutically active cause a slight burning under the tongue, may make the patient feel flushed, or may give the patient a transient throbbing headache. If the patient confirms that he or she felt one of those effects but the chest pain still would not go away, then you know there was nothing wrong with the nitroglycerin but there may be something very wrong with the patient.

Words of Wisdom

Start treatment immediately for any patient with chest pain.

As soon as you have elicited a chief complaint of a cardiac nature, you will need to start treatment of the patient; the more in-depth history taking and the secondary assessment can wait. For purposes of discussion, though, this section will continue to proceed through the history and secondary assessment. Besides pain (or, sometimes, instead of pain), a number of other symptoms are associated with AMI:

- Diaphoresis (sweating), often profuse, is principally the result of massive discharge by the autonomic nervous system. The patient may soak through his or her clothing and report a cold sweat.
- Dyspnea may be a warning of impending left-sided heart failure.
- Anorexia (loss of appetite), nausea, vomiting, or belching frequently accompanies MI. Hiccups may occasionally occur as well, due to irritation of the diaphragm by an inferior wall MI.
- Weakness may be profound, and the patient may describe this feeling with phrases such as "a limp rag."
- If CO is significantly diminished, dizziness may reflect the reduced circulation to the brain.
- Palpitations are sometimes experienced by patients with cardiac dysrhythmias as a sensation that the heart has skipped a beat.
- A feeling of impending doom is common among patients having an MI. The patient is frightened, looks frightened, and expresses his or her fear to other people—all of which adds to a general atmosphere of panic and dread.

Signs of AMI Although patients with an AMI often have abnormalities in the physical exam, many have relatively normal physical exam findings, and the diagnosis in the field (and in the emergency department) depends chiefly on the history. Nevertheless, it is important for you to take note of a few specific things during the physical exam to detect the development of complications to AMI, such as heart failure or cardiogenic shock.

- Pay attention to the patient's general appearance. Does the patient appear anxious? Frightened? In obvious pain?
- What is the patient's state of consciousness? Is he or she fully alert? Confused? Remember: Poor perfusion creates confusion. If the patient does not seem "all there," it may be because the heart is giving out and not enough oxygenated blood is reaching the brain.
- Is the skin pale, cold, and clammy?
- Assess the patient's vital signs. Is the pulse strong or weak? Regular or irregular? Is the respiratory rate abnormally rapid? Is the blood pressure abnormally high or low?
- Are there signs of left-sided heart failure (wheezes or crackles)? Signs of right-sided heart failure (distended neck veins, pedal or presacral edema)?

A typical patient with an AMI is apprehensive, with ashen-gray pallor and cold, wet skin. He or she *looks* scared. The pulse rate may be rapid unless heart block has occurred. The blood pressure may be decreased, reflecting decreased CO from the damaged heart, or it may be elevated from pain and anxiety.

Management of AMI and Suspected AMI in the Field

On your arrival at the scene, start treatment at once for any middle-aged or older patient with chest pain, even before you complete the history and secondary assessment. One of the most important components in the rapid identification and treatment of a cardiac event is the rapid acquisition of the 12-lead ECG. A 12-lead ECG should always be performed *before* the administration of any medication (except possibly aspirin and oxygen; in some regions, these are administered prior to taking a 12-lead ECG); data suggest that rapid acquisition of a 12-lead ECG in the prehospital environment decreases the door-to-balloon time by an average of 18 minutes. Therefore, a 12-lead ECG should be acquired immediately, then treatment can begin. If a medication is administered prior to the acquisition of the 12-lead ECG, certain conditions may be resolved by this treatment, so there may be no documentation of the initial condition that can assist in further treatment of the patient. For example, suppose a patient is experiencing chest pain and ST depression is apparent on the 12-lead ECG. If nitroglycerin was administered to that same patient prior to the 12-lead ECG, the ST elevation may not be present at the time of the monitoring.

The longest delay in treatment seems to be the phase from onset of symptoms to patient recognition, so your care must begin immediately. The goals of treatment are to limit the size of the infarct, to decrease the patient's fear and pain, and to prevent the development of serious cardiac dysrhythmias.

Place the Patient at Physical and Emotional Rest

The stress response causes the adrenal glands to squeeze out a surge of catecholamines (epinephrine and norepinephrine), which in turn can send the damaged heart racing. At the same time, the massive discharge throughout the fight-or-flight system puts the peripheral circulation in a state of severe vasoconstriction; thus, not only is the heart being pushed to go faster and faster, but it also has to work harder and harder against the increased

afterload. The heart's need for oxygen, therefore, soars precisely when it is already in a state of marked oxygen deprivation. This cycle can lead quickly to dysrhythmias and death. Prehospital deaths are related to dysrhythmias (often ventricular fibrillation), and most occur during the first 4 hours after onset of symptoms. Nevertheless, this deadly cycle can be interrupted by community education programs designed to assist citizens in early recognition of symptoms, early activation of EMS, and, if needed, CPR and early access to an AED.

To begin your treatment, put the patient physically at ease. Recall that one goal of treatment is to try to limit the size of the infarct; one way to do so is to decrease the amount of work that the heart must do, which will begin to decrease the patient's myocardial oxygen requirements immediately. The position in which cardiac work is minimal is the semi-Fowler position—that is, reclining on the stretcher with the back of the stretcher raised about 30°. Of course, the patient has to get to the stretcher and must not be permitted to do so alone. From the time you arrive, the patient must not do anything, including walking to the ambulance.

Administer Oxygen and Aspirin

The mnemonic MONA is used to help you remember the supportive treatments of Morphine, Oxygen, Nitroglycerin, and Aspirin for a patient with an ACS—but these treatments are not to be given in that order. MONA is administered in the following order, provided these measures are not contraindicated by hypotension: (1) oxygen, (2) aspirin, (3) nitroglycerin, and (4) morphine.

Oxygen may limit ischemic myocardial injury and reduce the amount of ST-segment elevation. Its effects on morbidity and mortality in acute infarction are unknown. Treatment with oxygen should be individualized and titrated to maintain the Sp_{O_2} level above 94%.

In most EMS systems, as long as the patient has no aspirin allergy or gastrointestinal bleeding, dispatchers may advise patients to chew baby aspirin (160 mg to 325 mg). If this has not been done before your arrival or the patient has not already taken aspirin on his or her own, then give the patient 160 mg to 325 mg of non–enteric-coated aspirin to chew.

Provide Pain Relief

Some form of pain relief must be provided because the pain of AMI is severe and places enormous stress on the patient's autonomic nervous system—stress that may contribute to complications. Nitroglycerin is a good place to start, but make sure the patient's blood pressure is adequate before its administration. In particular, before giving this medication, it is imperative that you ascertain whether the patient is taking phosphodiesterase-5 (PDE-5) inhibitors for erectile dysfunction **Table 25**. These drugs may worsen certain medical conditions and interact with a number of drugs, especially nitrate medications (such as nitroglycerin) prescribed to prevent or treat acute angina. Both types of medication dilate blood vessels, and their combined effects can cause dizziness, low blood pressure, and loss of consciousness.

Place a 0.4-mg tablet (or spray) of nitroglycerin under the patient's tongue. If the patient is experiencing an AMI and not simply angina, this medication is unlikely to relieve his or her

Table 25   PDE-5 Inhibitors

Brand Name	Generic Name	Duration of Effect
Viagra	Sildenafil citrate	Up to 4 h
Levitra	Vardenafil	Up to 4 h
Cialis	Tadalafil	24 to 36 h

pain, but it may help to reduce the size of the infarction. Do *not* give nitroglycerin if there is hypotension or bradycardia, and do *not* give it to patients having epigastric symptoms ("indigestion") or hiccups. Nitroglycerin may be repeated every 3 to 5 minutes, up to a total of three doses as long as the patient's condition remains stable.

If nitroglycerin provides no relief of pain and if authorized by medical command, morphine sulfate may be titrated in IV doses according to local protocols. Give this medication in 2- to 4-mg IV doses as needed for pain, being sure to reassess the patient's blood pressure, pulse, and respiratory rate after each dose, until the patient experiences relief of pain or experiences a drop in pulse or blood pressure. If bradycardia occurs, notify the physician immediately. Remember that morphine should *not* be given to patients with low blood pressure (less than about 100 mm Hg systolic or according to local protocol), dehydrated patients, or patients suspected of having an AMI involving the inferior wall of the heart. At least half of all patients with inferior wall MI will also experience a right ventricular infarction; as a consequence, they may already be hypotensive or the administration of nitroglycerin and morphine may cause hypotension.

In some EMS medical protocols, fentanyl (Sublimaze) is favored over morphine for pain not relieved with nitroglycerin because of its rapid onset and relatively short duration. Fentanyl also has fewer side effects than morphine.

Perform Cardiac Monitoring
Apply the ECG monitor, and run a strip to document the initial rhythm. As long as you are applying electrodes to the chest, also place your anterior chest leads in anticipation of obtaining a 12-lead ECG. Ideally, your monitor should have an audible tone that beeps with each QRS complex (also called systole beep), so that you can keep track of the patient's cardiac rhythm even when you have to take your gaze from the monitor to do other things. The ear, in any case, is far more sensitive than the eye to slight irregularities in rhythm, so the chances are that you will hear the beginning of a cardiac dysrhythmia much sooner than you will see it on the monitor. Keep the other cardiac drugs that you carry close at hand so you can reach them quickly if a cardiac dysrhythmia develops.

Words of Wisdom

Patients may not be forthcoming about taking medications. They may omit something from their list of home medications if they do not take the medicine daily. Be sure to ask.

Record the Vital Signs
Obtain vital signs, including pulse, respirations, blood pressure, and oxygen saturation. Measure the blood pressure, and repeat that measurement at least every 5 minutes. Measure the pulse rate. The ECG monitor provides information only about the electrical activity of the heart; it gives no information about the strength of the heartbeat (muscular activity) or even about whether the heart is beating at all! The ECG does not record mechanical function of the heart. It is, therefore, necessary to monitor the patient's pulse to assess peripheral blood flow, especially during transport, when blood pressure measurements are difficult to obtain and unreliable.

Take a History and Perform the Secondary Assessment
After you have completed the preceding steps (as appropriate), you should obtain a more detailed history and perform the secondary assessment. Find out if the patient has a history of cardiac disease; takes any heart medications, such as beta blockers, angiotensin-converting enzyme inhibitors, diuretics, or nitroglycerin (nitrates); or has had a previous heart attack or any heart surgery (such as coronary artery bypass graft). Also obtain a more complete description of the present symptoms, especially regarding their onset. It is also important to make sure to find out all past medical history that may be relevant to the existing problem—that is, differential diagnoses. Some examples can include but are not limited to cholecystitis, acute viral pericarditis, aneurysm, hiatal hernia, esophageal disease, gastric reflux, pulmonary embolism, peptic ulcer disease, pancreatitis, chest wall syndrome, costochondritis, acromioclavicular disease, pleural irritation, respiratory infection, aortic dissection, pneumothorax, dyspepsia, herpes zoster, chest wall tumors, and chest wall trauma.

Gathering that information should not delay transport to the hospital. Once you have taken the necessary precautions to stabilize the patient's condition (aspirin, oxygen, IV saline lock, monitor/12-lead ECG, analgesia), there is no reason to remain any longer at the scene unless a cardiac arrest or dysrhythmia requires immediate treatment. Obtain the rest of the history en route to the hospital. Remember that "time is muscle." Heart cells are being destroyed during the infarction before reperfusion is started in the hospital.

Transport the Patient
Once the patient is in stable condition, transport him or her to an appropriate hospital in a semi-Fowler position (unless the patient is in shock, in which case he or she should be supine). Do all you can to ensure that the patient is as relaxed and as comfortable as possible. En route, some additional treatment measures may be worthwhile, especially when transport time will be lengthy.

Safe and appropriate transport is what you need to strive for. *Do not rush* and *do not use sirens* when you are transporting the patient to the hospital. High speed and sirens send two clear messages to the patient: (1) Something is terribly wrong. (2) The personnel on the ambulance do not feel capable of dealing with the situation. Those are *not* the messages you want to convey to a frightened patient with a damaged heart! The patient needs to feel confident that those caring for him or her are in control of the situation.

If a serious dysrhythmia occurs during transport, consider stopping the vehicle, institute treatment immediately, and notify medical control. Except under unusual circumstances, treatment of life-threatening situations should not be attempted in a moving ambulance. Whenever possible, the driver should pull over to the side of the road and go to the back of the vehicle to help the other provider.

Reperfusion Techniques for AMI and Suspected AMI

Most AMIs occur as a result of thrombus (fixed blood clot) formation at the site of a preexisting atherosclerotic plaque. The thrombus occludes the coronary artery, preventing further blood flow through it. Thus, it seems reasonable to try to restore circulation through the occluded coronary artery, thereby restoring perfusion to the ischemic myocardium. Simply put, that is reperfusion.

The most immediate forms of reperfusion are fibrinolytic therapy and percutaneous intervention (PCI). All paramedics should be alert for patients who are good candidates for reperfusion, should know which hospitals in their area carry out fibrinolytic therapy and/or PCI, and should provide early notification (along with 12-lead ECG results) to the emergency department that a candidate for such therapy is en route.

Fibrinolysis One way in which to reperfuse the blocked coronary artery is to try to dissolve the occluding blood clot, thereby restoring circulation to the ischemic heart. That idea is the essence of **fibrinolytic therapy**.

In fact, this concept is not altogether new. Attempts to use fibrinolytic agents in the treatment of AMI were reported over 50 years ago, albeit without success. In retrospect, one reason the early attempts failed was that fibrinolytic therapy was started too late, after irreversible damage to the myocardium had already occurred. With that realization came the concept that "time is myocardium": The longer a segment of myocardium remains unperfused, the smaller the chances of salvaging that tissue and restoring its normal function. The obvious corollary is that the sooner fibrinolytic therapy can begin with respect to the onset of the blockage, the better the chances for saving the affected distal myocardium. Indeed, fibrinolytic treatment given within 30 to 60 minutes of the onset of symptoms can sometimes abort the MI altogether.

In the 1980s, providers began to start fibrinolytic treatment as soon as possible after the patient with an AMI reached the emergency department, rather than waiting until he or she was admitted to the coronary care unit. Inevitably, applying the doctrine that time is myocardium led to the idea of starting fibrinolytic treatment even earlier, in the prehospital phase of care.

Recent clinical trials have shown the benefit of starting fibrinolysis as soon as possible after the onset of ischemic-type chest pain in patients with STEMI or new or presumably new

left bundle branch block. Several prospective studies have also documented reduced time to administration of fibrinolytics and decreased mortality rates when prehospital fibrinolytics were given to patients with STEMI and no contraindications to fibrinolytics. Some EMS systems may opt to start fibrinolytic treatment in the field, and in rural areas with long transport times, prehospital initiation of fibrinolytic therapy may make a lot of sense. Even in EMS systems in which paramedics do not give fibrinolytic therapy, their ability to identify candidates for such therapy has a decisive role in helping emergency department personnel administer fibrinolytic therapy early enough to make a difference. For these reasons, all paramedics should thoroughly understand the principles of fibrinolytic therapy for AMI.

Fibrinolytic therapy seeks to administer, during the early hours of AMI, an agent that will activate the body's own internal system for dissolving clots, the fibrinolytic system. Once activated, that system can begin to dissolve the clot that has formed within the coronary artery, thereby reopening the artery (**recanalization**) and allowing the resumption of blood flow through it (**reperfusion**). Unfortunately, if an agent capable of promoting clot dissolution is given intravenously, its effects cannot be limited to the clot in the coronary artery; it can also act anywhere else in the body where clots are being formed and, therefore, may lead to bleeding. Thus, the benefit of fibrinolytic therapy—the possible salvage of myocardium—must always be weighed against its risks—principally, the risk of bleeding.

To determine the appropriate candidates for fibrinolytic agents, you need to be as certain as possible that your patient is experiencing an AMI. A patient having chest pain from another source would receive no potential benefit from fibrinolytic therapy—so he or she would be subjected to this therapy's risks for no reason. Although it is difficult in the early hours of an AMI to be certain of the diagnosis, inclusion criteria have been established to help select patients most likely to be having an AMI. At the same time, exclusion criteria are used to identify patients for whom the risk of fibrinolytic therapy is unacceptably high—for example, patients most likely to experience hemorrhagic complications. **Table 26** summarizes the inclusion and exclusion criteria for fibrinolytic therapy.

Most treatment regimens for fibrinolysis include one of three agents: alteplase (Activase; a tissue plasminogen activator), streptokinase (Streptase), or reteplase (Retavase; recombinant tissue). All of them work by converting, in one way or another, the body's own clot-dissolving enzyme from its inactive form, plasminogen, to its active form, **plasmin**.

According to the AHA's 2010 guidelines, the focus continues to be on the early recognition and notification of those patients who may benefit from fibrinolysis therapy early on in the process. A prehospital fibrinolytic program is recommended only in systems with well-established protocols, checklists, experience in ACLS, ability to communicate with the receiving institution, and a medical director with training and experience in the management of STEMI.

Percutaneous Intervention As an alternative to fibrinolysis, many institutions perform a **percutaneous coronary intervention (PCI)**. Patients with complex, multivessel disease or ACSs may

Words of Wisdom

Time is muscle (myocardium)!

Table 26   ST-Segment Elevation or New or Presumably New LBBB: Evaluation for Reperfusion

Step 1: Assess time and risk

- Time since onset of symptoms
- Risk of STEMI
- Risk of fibrinolysis
- Time required to transport to skilled PCI catheterization suite

Step 2: Select reperfusion (fibrinolysis or invasive) strategy

Note: If presentation < 3 hours and no delay for PCI, then PCI is preferred.

Fibrinolysis is generally preferred if:	An invasive strategy is generally preferred if:
<ul><li>≤ 3 hours from symptom onset</li><li>Invasive strategy is not an option (eg, lack of access to skilled PCI facility or difficult vascular access) or would be delayed<ul><li>Medical contact-to-balloon or door-to-balloon > 90 min</li><li>(Door-to-balloon) minus (door-to-needle) is > 1 hour</li></ul></li><li>No contraindications to fibrinolysis</li></ul>	<ul><li>Late presentation (symptom onset > 3 hours ago)</li><li>Skilled PCI facility available with surgical backup</li><li>Medical contact-to-balloon or door-to-balloon < 90 min</li><li>(Door-to-balloon) minus (door-to-needle) is < 1 hour</li><li>Contraindications to fibrinolysis, including increased risk of bleeding and intracranial hemorrhage</li><li>High risk from STEMI (CHF with acute pulmonary edema)</li><li>Diagnosis of STEMI is in doubt</li></ul>

Source: Modified from the 2010 American Heart Association *Guidelines for Cardiopulmonary Resuscitation and Emergency Cardiovascular Care.*

benefit from PCI. In this therapy, balloons, stents, or other devices are passed through a 2-mm-diameter catheter via a peripheral artery to recanalize and keep the blocked coronary artery open. The success rate is high, and the risks are low. PCI is often used for patients who are not candidates for fibrinolytic therapy.

Congestive Heart Failure

<u>Congestive heart failure (CHF)</u> (also known as chronic heart failure) occurs when the heart is unable, for any reason, to pump powerfully enough or fast enough to empty its chambers; as a result, blood backs up into the systemic circuit, the pulmonary circuit, or both. Although CHF may develop in situations other than AMI—for example, in a patient with chronic high blood pressure—the basic principles of diagnosis and treatment are similar, whatever the precipitating factors.

More than 2 million people in the United States have CHF, and an additional 500,000 cases are diagnosed each year. Nearly half of the patients with CHF classified as severe die within 1 year of diagnosis.

Left-Sided Heart Failure

Pathophysiology The left ventricle is most commonly damaged during an AMI. Likewise, in chronic hypertension, the left ventricle tends to suffer the long-term effects of having to pump against an increased afterload (constricted peripheral arteries). In both cases, the right side of the heart continues to pump relatively normally and to deliver normal volumes of blood to the pulmonary circulation. By comparison, the left side of the heart may no longer be able to pump the blood being delivered from the pulmonary vessels. As a result, blood backs up behind the left ventricle, and the pressure in the left atrium and pulmonary

veins increases. As the pulmonary veins become engorged with blood, serum is forced out of the pulmonary capillaries and into the alveoli. The serum mixes with air in the alveoli to produce foam (pulmonary edema). This is <u>left-sided heart failure</u>.

When fluid occupies the alveoli, oxygenation is impaired. The patient experiences that impairment as shortness of breath (dyspnea), particularly in the recumbent position (orthopnea). If left ventricular failure is the result of chronic overload (as opposed to AMI), the patient is likely to give a history of a week or two of paroxymal nocturnal dyspnea (PND). To compensate for the impairment in oxygenation, the patient's respiratory rate increases (tachypnea); even so, if the patient's condition is advanced enough, cyanosis may become evident. In some patients with pulmonary edema, especially elderly patients, Cheyne-Stokes respirations may be present.

Fluid from the pulmonary vessels also leaks into the interstitial spaces in the lungs, and increasing interstitial pressure causes narrowing of the bronchioles. Air passing through the narrowed bronchioles creates wheezing noises, whereas air bubbling through the fluid-filled alveoli produces crackles. Furthermore, the patient may cough up the edema fluid in the form of foamy, blood-tinged sputum. As the airways narrow and the lungs grow heavier from the accumulation of fluid, the work of breathing increases, which puts an even greater strain on the already floundering heart. Dyspnea and hypoxemia produce a state of panic, which induces the release of epinephrine from the adrenal glands. The heart is pushed even harder, and its oxygen demand is increased precisely when fluid in the alveoli is reducing the amount of oxygen available.

To make matters worse, the sympathetic nervous system response produces peripheral vasoconstriction: Peripheral resistance (afterload) increases, and the weakened, hypoxic heart now has to push blood out into smaller and smaller vessels. Clinically, peripheral vasoconstriction is apparent as pallor and elevated blood pressure. The massive sympathetic discharge also produces sweating of the pale, cold skin.

It is not unusual for a patient with left-sided heart failure to become frantic from air hunger. He or she may pace or thrash about or may even be combative and struggle with the rescue team. Furthermore, hypoxemia results in inadequate oxygen supply to the brain, often manifested as confusion or disorientation. If hypoxemia is severe, cardiac arrest may follow quickly.

Assessment The signs and symptoms of left-sided heart failure include extreme restlessness and agitation, confusion, severe dyspnea and tachypnea, tachycardia, elevated blood pressure, crackles and possibly wheezes, and frothy, pink sputum. Sometimes, it may be difficult to distinguish the wheezing of asthma from that of left-sided heart failure. Table 27 presents some of the features that can help you differentiate the two conditions.

The ECG may show cannon atrial waves. Also called cannon A waves, these are pulsations seen in the jugular veins. When the atria and ventricles contract simultaneously, there is a large surge in pressure back through the venous system resulting in jugular vein pulsations. Cannon A waves are often seen in patients with fluid overload and heart failure.

Management Prehospital treatment of left-sided heart failure is aimed at improving oxygenation and decreasing the workload of the heart, chiefly by reducing the volume of venous blood returned to the heart (the preload), so that the left ventricle is less overburdened.

Administer 100% supplemental oxygen, preferably by demand valve or bag-mask device with positive end-expiratory pressure, because positive pressure is helpful in driving fluid out of the alveoli. Continuous positive airway pressure (CPAP) has been showed to be an effective tool in the management of pulmonary edema as it pertains to CHF. CPAP provides a continuous increase of pressure in the lower airway passages. This in turn helps to improve gas exchange in the alveoli by reinflating the collapsed alveoli. CPAP will also increase the surface area of the alveoli, thereby providing a larger area over which gas exchange can take place. If the patient will not tolerate those modalities, use the nonrebreathing mask. The patient's respiratory

Table 27 Differentiation and Treatment of Asthma and Left-Sided Heart Failure

	Asthma	Left-Sided Heart Failure
History	Often a younger patient May have allergic history or family history of allergy Previous attacks of acute, episodic dyspnea May have had recent respiratory infection Unproductive cough Medications may include: ■ Inhalers: Isoproterenol (Medihaler-Iso, Isuprel), albuterol (Vaponefrin), epinephrine (Micronefrin), isoetharine (Bronkosol), ■ Pills: calcium carb/glycine chew (Tedral), pseudoephedrine (Sudafed), theophylline and guaifenesin (Quibron), triprolidine and pseudoephedrine (Actifed)	Often an older patient May have history of heart problems, hypertension Dyspnea worse when lying down (orthopnea) Recent rapid weight gain Cough with watery or foamy sputum Medications may include: ■ Digitalis glycosides: digoxin (Lanoxin), digitoxin ■ Diuretics: chlorothiazide (Diuril), furosemide (Lasix), hydrochlorothiazide (Esidrix), ethacrynic acid (Edecrin), trichlormethiazide (Metahydrin, Naquasone)
Possible physical findings	Wheezing Chest hyperinflated and hyperresonant Use of accessory muscles to breathe If bronchospasm severe, chest may be silent	Wheezing Crackles S_3 gallop Distended neck veins Pedal or presacral edema
Treatment	Oxygen (humidified) Intermittent positive-pressure breathing Monitor IV: normal saline Selective beta-2 adrenergic medications Sometimes bicarbonate (morphine and diuretics contraindicated)	Oxygen Intermittent positive-pressure breathing Monitor IV: normal saline to keep open or saline lock (adrenergics and bicarbonate usually contraindicated) Morphine Diuretics (furosemide) Nitroglycerin

status should be monitored via waveform capnography; if it is unavailable, the use of pulse oximetry will suffice.

Sit the patient up, with the feet dangling. That position encourages venous pooling in the legs, thereby reducing venous return to the heart. The sitting position also makes breathing easier for a patient in respiratory distress.

Start a saline lock or an IV line with normal saline at a keep-vein-open rate. Also, attach monitoring electrodes because patients in CHF are prone to dysrhythmias.

Pharmacologic therapy of left-sided heart failure may vary slightly from place to place, but the mainstays of drug therapy include the drugs mentioned below (in order of the author's preference). Refer to your usual protocols, and have the appropriate medications drawn up and ready, pending the physician's order to administer them. Remember to constantly monitor the blood pressure because many of these medications lower it.

Nitroglycerin, 0.4 mg sublingually, may be ordered as a vasodilator to create venous pooling, thereby reducing the volume of blood returned from the periphery to the heart. Before ordering this medication, the physician will want to know how much, if any, nitroglycerin the patient has already taken. The initial dose of 0.4 mg may be repeated at 5-minute intervals up to a total of 1.2 mg (three doses).

Furosemide (Lasix) is a diuretic that has two positive effects in left-sided heart failure. Initially (within the first 5 to 10 minutes), it has a venodilating effect, increasing peripheral pooling of blood. Subsequently, it removes excess fluid from the body by promoting its excretion by the kidneys. If ordered, furosemide is given in a dose of 20 to 40 mg or 0.5 to 1 mg/kg by IV bolus. If the patient already takes furosemide, the higher dose should be used. The use of furosemide in the prehospital setting remains a controversial topic. Several studies have found poor clinical outcomes in patients receiving prehospital diuretics.

Morphine sulfate has long been part of the standard treatment of cardiogenic pulmonary edema. Like nitroglycerin, morphine works as a vasodilator, increasing the pooling of blood in the periphery, but it also has a substantial calming effect on a frantic patient. If morphine is ordered, first check the patient's blood pressure (do not give morphine if the patient is hypotensive). Then administer approximately 3 mg slowly by IV bolus, and recheck the blood pressure. If the blood pressure remains stable, another 3 mg may be given. Proceed in that manner until the total dose ordered by the physician has been administered.

The presence of wheezing indicates that bronchoconstriction has developed from the excessive fluid. In such a case, bronchodilator drugs such as albuterol (Proventil, Ventolin, Volmax), metaproterenol sulfate (Alupent), or ipratropium (Atrovent) may be ordered.

Under special circumstances, when transport will be prolonged and the patient's blood pressure is low, the physician may order a pressor such as dopamine (Intropin), which will increase blood pressure and/or CO. The dose is based on protocol, and ranges from 2 to 20 µg/kg/min by IV drip titrated to the desired blood pressure.

Transport the patient to the hospital in a sitting position, with the legs dangling down.

Some patients who present with left-sided heart failure may receive a pacemaker in an effort to address an electrical conduction problem within the heart as well as the synchronization of the heart muscle. Heart synchronization therapy uses a special pacemaker that helps to stimulate or pace both of the heart's ventricles. This treatment improves the pumping function of the left ventricle so that it can pump more volume, which may help in alleviating some of the symptoms of left-sided heart failure, such as dysrhythmias or pulmonary edema.

A left ventricular assist device (LVAD) may be used in those patients who have sustained significant damage to their left ventricle such that it cannot meet the demands of the body. These patients require a heart transplant to meet these demands, but may have to wait for some time to find a compatible heart. This is where the LVAD comes into use: It can support the body while the patient is waiting for a donor heart to become available. With the LVAD, a tube is placed in the left ventricle that draws blood from the left ventricle into the device's pump. The pump then sends this oxygen-rich blood through another tube to the aorta.

The LVAD is typically inserted into the abdominal cavity of the patient. A tube from the pump goes through the abdominal wall to the outside, where it connects to the battery pack for the unit. EMS providers should be aware that if there is power to the battery pack, the issue is probably not the LVAD itself, but rather another underlying problem, such as infection.

Right-Sided Heart Failure

Right-sided heart failure most commonly occurs as a result of left-sided heart failure. As blood backs up from the left side of the heart into the lungs, the right side has to work increasingly harder to pump blood into the engorged pulmonary vessels. Eventually, the right side of the heart is unable to keep up with the increased workload, and it, too, fails. Right-sided heart failure may also occur as a result of pulmonary embolism or long-standing chronic obstructive pulmonary disease (COPD), especially chronic bronchitis.

When right-sided heart failure occurs, blood backs up behind the right ventricle and increases the pressure in the systemic veins, causing them to become engorged. Distention can be seen in the veins visible on the surface of the body, such as the external jugular veins, which should be assessed in the semi-Fowler position. Over time, as the pressure within the systemic veins increases, serum is forced out of the veins and into the surrounding tissues, producing edema. Edema is most likely to be visible in dependent parts of the body, such as the feet in a person who is sitting or standing or the lower back in a bedridden patient. Edema is also present in parts of the body that are *not* visible; a painful liver easily palpable in the right upper quadrant, for example, signals engorgement and swelling within that organ (hepatomegaly). Right-sided heart failure also causes fluid to leak into the peritoneal cavity causing abdominal distention. Ascites is the medical term used to describe the accumulation of fluid in the abdominal cavity.

The development of right-sided heart failure can actually improve left-sided heart failure because the failing right side of the heart can no longer pump as much blood into the lungs. The decrease in output from the right side, in essence, amounts to a decrease in preload for the left side of the heart and may lessen pulmonary congestion.

Right-sided heart failure, by itself, is seldom a life-threatening emergency. Usually it develops gradually over days to weeks; likewise, it requires days to weeks to reverse the process by slowly ridding the body of excess salt and water. Therefore, treatment in the field of a patient with right-sided heart failure is simply to make the patient comfortable, preferably in the semi-Fowler position. Monitoring is always indicated in any patient with significant cardiac disease. If signs of associated left-sided heart failure are present, treat them as outlined in the previous section.

■ Cardiac Tamponade

Pathophysiology

The pericardium is a tough, fibrous membrane with the ability to stretch only up to a point. Normally, a small amount of pericardial fluid separates the pericardium and the outer surface of the heart. Cardiac tamponade occurs when excessive fluid accumulates within the pericardium, limiting the heart's ability to expand fully after each contraction and resulting in reduced CO. If unrecognized and untreated, this condition will reduce cardiac filling to the point that the heart is unable to circulate the blood.

Assessment

Cardiac tamponade can occur as a result of tumors, pericarditis, or trauma to the chest. Rarely, cardiac tamponade can also occur after myocardial infarction as a result of cardiac rupture. Pericarditis, for example, can cause excessive amounts of fluid to accumulate in the pericardial space. Blunt or penetrating trauma can cause bleeding from blood vessels on the surface of the heart, allowing accumulation of blood in the pericardial space.

Signs and symptoms of cardiac tamponade vary depending on its cause. If the onset is gradual (as with pericarditis), the patient may initially report dyspnea and weakness. If the cause is traumatic, the chief complaint might be chest pain. As the volume of fluid increases in the pericardium, the SV decreases, causing an initial drop in the systolic blood pressure. Eventually, the diastolic pressure will slowly rise, resulting in the classic symptom of narrowing pulse pressure. The initial drop in blood pressure is usually followed by an increase in the heart rate, which leads to tachycardia. The heart sounds may be muffled or quieter than usual owing to the buildup of fluid, although this sign may be difficult to identify in the field. The patient may experience jugular vein distention as well, owing to the backup of blood from the right side of the heart. The combination of narrowing pulse pressure (hypotension) along with jugular vein distention and muffled heart sounds is commonly known as Beck's triad.

The ECG is of limited value to you in identifying cardiac tamponade. Aside from tachycardia, you might see electrical alternans (alternating small- and large-amplitude QRS complexes). In addition, you might identify pulsus alternans (alternating strong and weak pulses). Pulsus paradoxus—a drop in systolic blood pressure of more than 10 mm Hg with the patient's inhalation that may be associated with a weakening pulse during inhalation—may also be present.

Identification of cardiac tamponade requires a thorough assessment. Changes in blood pressure can be recognized only after at least three values have been obtained, usually 5 to 10 minutes apart. Muffled heart sounds, pulsus alternans, electrical alternans, and pulsus paradoxus are not common signs and so may be easily overlooked. Occasionally, you may have difficulty distinguishing between cardiac tamponade and tension pneumothorax. One way to differentiate between the two is to remember that in cardiac tamponade, the breath sounds will be equal and the trachea will be midline because the lungs are not affected.

Management

The ultimate treatment for cardiac tamponade is pericardiocentesis, which involves inserting a needle attached to a syringe into the chest far enough to penetrate the pericardium and then withdrawing fluid. Often, withdrawal of as little as 50 mL of fluid will result in significant improvement in the patient's condition. This technique is risky, however, and medical direction rarely allows it to be performed by paramedics. If pericardiocentesis is not allowed, you should provide rapid transport to a facility that can perform this procedure.

Supporting the patient's airway, breathing, and oxygenation during transport is essential. An IV fluid bolus of 500 mL of saline might be ordered by medical direction. When you are reporting to medical control, make sure that you identify all signs and symptoms that led you to believe the patient has cardiac tamponade so that the receiving hospital will be prepared to perform the pericardiocentesis.

■ Cardiogenic Shock

Pathophysiology

Cardiogenic shock occurs when the heart is so severely damaged that it can no longer pump a volume of blood sufficient to maintain tissue perfusion. An AMI nearly always produces some impairment of left ventricular function. When 25% of the left ventricular myocardium is involved in the AMI, left-sided heart failure usually develops. When 40% or more of the left ventricle has been infarcted, cardiogenic shock occurs. Thus, cardiogenic shock indicates extensive injury to the myocardium; accordingly, it is a high priority in the field. Transient cardiogenic shock can occur after resuscitation. Patients recovering from defibrillation for ventricular fibrillation, for example, often have signs of cardiogenic shock. Symptoms of cardiogenic shock include difficulty breathing, extreme fatigue, and general malaise.

Assessment

The signs and symptoms of cardiogenic shock are similar to those of most other kinds of shock. Because of the reduced cerebral perfusion, the patient is often confused or even comatose; if awake, he or she is likely to be restless and anxious. Massive peripheral vasoconstriction results in pale, cold skin, and poor renal perfusion is reflected in minimal or absent urine output. Respirations are rapid and shallow, with a possibility of adventitious breath sounds, and the pulse is racing and thready. The patient's ECG may be normal or reveal fast or slow dysrhythmias. The diagnosis of cardiogenic shock is made clinically, not by ECG changes.

As these compensatory mechanisms begin to fail, the blood pressure will fall, sometimes to less than 90 mm Hg systolic. However, this vital sign may be deceptive. In patients with preexisting hypertension, systolic pressures higher than 90 mm Hg may still be associated with cardiogenic shock. The goal in treatment of cardiogenic shock is to identify and support the patient before the blood pressure drops to the point where the shock becomes irreversible.

Management

Treatment of cardiogenic shock focuses on improving oxygenation and peripheral perfusion without adding to the work of the heart. Secure the patient's airway, and administer 100% supplemental oxygen by mask or bag-mask device. An advanced airway (endotracheal tube, laryngeal mask airway, King LT, or Combitube) will be necessary if the patient is unresponsive. Place the patient in a supine position unless pulmonary edema is present; in that case, the patient should be placed in the semi-Fowler position.

Start an IV line with normal saline at a keep-vein-open rate. The physician may order a trial of fluids to determine whether the shock includes a hypovolemic component. If so, rapidly infuse 100 to 200 mL of saline, and closely monitor the patient's pulse, blood pressure, and level of consciousness (LOC). Report those observations to the physician.

Apply monitoring electrodes and obtain a 12-lead ECG. Dysrhythmias may bring about hypotension by causing severe disturbances in CO; thus, until major dysrhythmias are corrected, you cannot be certain that the patient's hypotension is due to cardiogenic shock.

Depending on the distance to the hospital and local protocols, you may be asked to administer a vasopressor drug, such as one of those listed in Table 28. Dopamine might be preferred because, at beta doses, it maintains renal perfusion better than the other agents listed. To prepare a dopamine infusion, add 400 mg of dopamine to a 250-mL bag of normal saline, to yield a concentration of 1,600 µg/mL. The infusion rate will depend on the patient's weight and response, but it is usually initiated at 5 µg/kg/min. The administration of dopamine (Intropin) or any other vasopressor drug requires careful titration and frequent monitoring of the blood pressure. Measure the blood pressure at least every 5 minutes. Slow the infusion if the systolic pressure rises to more than 90 or 100 mm Hg; speed up the infusion if the systolic pressure falls below 70 mm Hg.

Except for the correction of life-threatening dysrhythmias, there are no measures that you can perform to stabilize the condition of a patient in cardiogenic shock in the field. Therefore, transport the patient expeditiously to the hospital.

■ Aortic Aneurysm

The word aneurysm comes from a Greek word meaning a widening; it refers to the dilation or outpouching of a blood vessel. The aneurysms of greatest concern to you are those that involve the aorta, particularly acute dissecting aneurysms of the thoracic aorta and expanding or ruptured aneurysms of the abdominal aorta.

Acute Dissecting Aneurysm of the Aorta

Pathophysiology The proximal aorta is subject to enormous hemodynamic forces. Anywhere from 60 to 100 times a minute, 60 minutes an hour, 24 hours a day—that is, around 40 million times a year—pulsatile waves of blood come pounding out of the left ventricle against the aortic walls. Over the years, that pounding takes its toll, producing degenerative changes in the media (the middle layer) of the aorta, especially the ascending aorta (the part of the aorta that rises from the heart toward the aortic arch). The degenerative changes are more pronounced with advancing age and in people with chronic high blood pressure, and their effect is to "unglue" the layers of the aortic wall from one another.

Eventually, the degenerative changes in the aortic media may lead to a disruption of the underlying intima (innermost layer of the artery). Tearing of the intima is most likely to occur in the portions of the thoracic aorta that are under the greatest stress—specifically, the ascending aorta just distal to the aortic valve (approximately 65% of cases) and the descending aorta just beyond the takeoff point of the left subclavian artery.

Once the intima is torn, the process of dissection, or separation of the arterial wall, often begins. With each ventricular systole, a jet of blood is forced into the torn arterial wall, creating a false channel between the intimal and medial layers of the wall. This channel is propagated distally and sometimes proximally along the length of the wall. If the dissection progresses back into the aortic valve, it may prevent the valve from closing, so that blood regurgitates back from the aorta into the

Table 28	**Vasopressor Agents**		
Drug	**Preparation**	**Concentration (µg/mL)**	**Rate**
Dopamine (Intropin)	400 mg in 250 mL normal saline	1,600	2 to 20 µg/kg/min
Norepinephrine (Levophed)	4 mg in 250 mL D$_5$W	16	0.1 to 0.5 µg/kg/min
Epinephrine (Adrenalin)	1 mL (1 mg) in 250 mL normal saline	4	0.1 to 0.5 µg/kg/min

left ventricle during systole. Recall that the coronary arteries branch off from the aorta just above the leaflets of the aortic valve; thus, if the valve is affected, coronary blood flow will likely be affected as well. If the dissection involves the takeoff point of the innominate, left common carotid, or left subclavian artery, blood flow through the affected artery or arteries will be compromised.

Two classification systems are used for determining the significance of an aneurysm. The Stanford classification distinguishes two types of aortic dissection: Type A, which involves the ascending aorta, and Type B, which does not. Type A will require surgical intervention while Type B can be managed medically. The DeBakey classification places aortic dissections into three categories: Type I involves the ascending aorta, aortic arch, and descending aorta; Type II is localized to the ascending aorta; and Type III focuses on dissections involving the descending aorta that is distal to the left subclavian artery. Type III is further broken down into Type IIIa and Type IIIb. Type IIIa dissections start at the left subclavian artery but extend both proximal and distally mostly above the diaphragm. Type IIIb dissections start distally to the left subclavian artery but extend only distally and may be below the diaphragm.

Assessment The typical patient with a dissecting aneurysm is a middle-aged or older man with chronic hypertension, although dissection may occur during pregnancy and in younger patients with Marfan syndrome. In Marfan syndrome, the walls of the major arteries—including the aorta—are weakened. When blood flow leaks through the tears of the weakened aortic wall, it results in an aortic dissection. By far, the most common chief complaint is chest pain, which is usually described as "the worst pain I have ever experienced," or as "ripping," "tearing," "sharp," or "like a knife." This pain comes on suddenly and is located in the anterior part of the chest or in the back between the shoulder blades.

On the basis of the patient's description, it may be difficult to differentiate the chest pain of a dissecting aneurysm from that of an AMI, but a number of distinctive features may help. The pain of an AMI is often preceded by other symptoms—nausea, "indigestion," weakness, and sweating—and tends to come on gradually, getting more severe with time and often being described as "pressure" rather than "stabbing." By contrast, the pain of a dissecting aneurysm usually comes on full force from one minute to the next, without prodromal symptoms. Table 29 summarizes the differences in the clinical presentations of AMI and dissecting aortic aneurysm.

Other signs and symptoms of dissecting aneurysm will depend on the site of the intimal tear and the extent of the dissection. In dissections of the ascending aorta, which tend to occur in younger patients previously in good health, one or more of the vessels of the aortic arch are usually compromised. Disruption of flow through the innominate artery, for example, is likely to produce a difference in blood pressure between the two arms. (If you do not routinely check the blood pressure in both arms of a patient, you will never pick up that sign!) You may also find that one femoral or carotid pulse is missing or weak. Disruption of blood flow into the left common carotid artery may produce signs and symptoms of a stroke. When the dissection extends proximally to the ostia of the coronary arteries, coronary blood flow is likely to be compromised, and ECG changes of myocardial ischemia are likely. Death from dissection of the ascending aorta is nearly always a result of aortic rupture into the pericardium and resultant cardiac tamponade. In such a case, you will see the characteristic signs of cardiac tamponade: distended neck veins, hypotension, narrow pulse pressure, and muffled heart sounds.

Dissection of the descending aorta occurs more commonly in older patients, especially those with a history of hypertension. The pain is likely to be somewhat less severe when the descending aorta is involved; indeed, the patient may wait a few days before seeking help. The dissection usually proceeds distally, so the aortic arch is spared, which means that blood pressure discrepancies between the two arms are not part of the picture. The pulses in the lower extremities, however, may be affected.

Management The goal of prehospital management in a suspected dissecting aneurysm is primarily to provide adequate pain relief. In the hospital setting, medications will be given to lower the patient's blood pressure and reduce myocardial contractility to take some of the hemodynamic load off the aorta. Only in unusual circumstances would such therapy be started in the field because it requires careful monitoring of intra-arterial pressure.

The steps of prehospital management in suspected dissecting aneurysm are as follows:

- Calm and reassure the patient.
- Administer 100% supplemental oxygen by nonrebreathing mask.
- Insert an IV line, and give a crystalloid solution.

Table 29 AMI Versus Dissecting Aortic Aneurysm

	AMI	Dissecting Aneurysm
Onset of pain	Gradual, with prodromal symptoms	Abrupt, without prodromal symptoms
Severity of pain	Increases with time	Maximal from the outset
Timing of pain	May wax and wane	Does not abate once it has started
Location of pain	Substernal; back is rarely involved	Back is often involved, between the shoulder blades
Clinical signs	Peripheral pulses equal	Blood pressure discrepancy between arms or decrease in a femoral or carotid pulse

- Apply monitoring electrodes and obtain an ECG rhythm strip.
- If the patient is not hypotensive, administer IV morphine sulfate, 2 mg at a time, up to a total dose of 10 mg during 10 to 15 minutes.
- Transport without delay. Nothing can be done to stabilize the patient's condition in the field. The patient will need aggressive therapy in the intensive care unit and possibly surgery.

Expanding and Ruptured Abdominal Aortic Aneurysms

Pathophysiology Abdominal aortic aneurysms (AAAs) affect approximately 2% of the US population older than 50 years and account for 15,000 deaths each year. Most commonly, the aneurysm is located just distal to the renal arteries. An expanding aneurysm is, as the name implies, an aneurysm that is getting larger and producing symptoms by compressing on adjacent structures, although the aortic wall remains intact. When an aneurysm starts expanding and producing symptoms, it can be assumed that rupture is imminent.

Assessment The typical patient with an AAA is a man in his late 50s or 60s. As long as the aneurysm remains stable, the patient usually will be asymptomatic. When the aneurysm starts to expand, however, the patient becomes symptomatic, with the sudden onset of abdominal or back pain. When the pain is principally in the abdomen, it tends to center on the umbilicus. Often, the pain may be located solely in the lower back, leading the patient to think he or she has "pulled a muscle" or otherwise injured the back. The pain is constant and moderate to severe; it cannot be relieved by changes in position. It tends to radiate into the thigh and groin. If the aneurysm is leaking blood into the retroperitoneal space, the patient may report an urge to defecate. In some patients, an episode of syncope heralds the onset of symptoms.

The most characteristic physical finding in a patient with an AAA is a pulsatile mass palpable in the abdomen. The patient is likely to be normotensive when first seen, but signs of shock, with or without hypotension, may develop rapidly if the aneurysm has ruptured.

Management Prehospital management of an expanding or ruptured aortic aneurysm is aimed at getting the patient to the hospital as expeditiously as possible because the definitive treatment requires urgent surgery. The key is to maintain a high index of suspicion whenever a middle-aged or older man presents with sudden back pain and a pulsatile abdominal mass. The more likely problem in the field in a conscious patient is a leaking aneurysm that has yet to rupture.

The steps of prehospital management of patients with an expanding or ruptured aortic aneurysm are as follows:

- Administer supplemental oxygen.
- Consider applying (but do not inflate) the pneumatic antishock garment (PASG)/military antishock trousers (MAST) if available.
- Transport without delay.

- Insert an IV line en route, and give normal saline or lactated Ringer's. Use a large-gauge catheter, but maintain the flow to keep the vein open unless signs of shock appear. If there are signs of shock, treat as for any other case of shock, with IV fluids.

■ Hypertensive Emergencies

Pathophysiology

Hypertension (high blood pressure) affects nearly 60 million Americans and is directly responsible for more than 30,000 deaths per year. In addition, it is a major contributing cause in many cases of MI, CHF, and stroke. Most hypertension is the result of advanced atherosclerosis or arteriosclerosis, which decreases the lumen of the arteries and reduces their elasticity. The resulting high afterload on the heart leads to an increase in filling volume and stimulates the Frank-Starling reflex, which raises the pressure behind the blood leaving the heart.

Hypertension is present when the blood pressure at rest is consistently greater than about 140/90 mm Hg. Many conditions, such as anxiety or pain, can transiently elevate a person's blood pressure (especially the systolic blood pressure), so a single blood pressure measurement taken during an emergency scarcely constitutes adequate grounds for telling a patient that he or she is hypertensive. Instead, you may say something like this: "Sir, your blood pressure is a little high right now. That may be because of the stress you are under and may not have any real significance. To be safe, you should have your blood pressure rechecked a couple of times in the next few months under less stressful circumstances."

Persistent elevation of the diastolic pressure, by contrast, is indicative of hypertensive disease. If left untreated, hypertension significantly shortens a person's life span and predisposes the person to a variety of other medical problems. The most common complications of hypertension include renal damage, stroke, and heart failure—the last a result of the left ventricle having to pump for years against a markedly increased afterload.

Assessment

In the majority of cases, hypertension is entirely asymptomatic and is detected by chance during a routine examination. By the time symptoms start to occur, hypertension is already in a more advanced stage and has probably produced at least some damage to organs such as the heart, kidneys, and brain.

The symptoms that occur in advanced hypertensive disease may be related to the elevated blood pressure or to secondary complications. Headache is the most common symptom directly related to blood pressure elevation; hypertensive headache is usually localized to the occipital region of the head and occurs when the patient first awakens in the morning, then subsides gradually over the next few hours. Other symptoms of moderately severe hypertension include dizziness, weakness, epistaxis, tinnitus, and blurring of vision. Rarely, seizures can result from severe hypertension. Often a patient with these hypertension-related signs and symptoms has already been prescribed medication for hypertension but is not taking it as prescribed.

Management

Hypertensive emergencies occur in about 1% of all hypertensive patients. A hypertensive emergency is defined as an acute elevation of blood pressure with evidence of end-organ damage. That last phrase is important, because it is the evidence of end-organ dysfunction that determines the urgency of the situation, not the reading on the sphygmomanometer. Two end-organ emergencies that may result from uncontrolled hypertension were discussed earlier in this chapter: left-sided heart failure and dissecting aortic aneurysm. A rare but much more devastating complication of hypertension is hypertensive encephalopathy.

Hypertensive encephalopathy (also known as acute hypertensive crisis) may complicate any form of hypertension. Hypertensive crisis is usually signaled by a sudden, marked rise in blood pressure to levels of greater than 200/130 mm Hg. The determining factor for hypertensive encephalopathy is usually the mean arterial pressure (MAP). The MAP is calculated by adding one third of the difference between the systolic blood pressure (SBP) and diastolic blood pressure (DBP) to the diastolic blood pressure.

$$MAP = DBP + 1/3 (SBP - DBP)$$

When the MAP exceeds 150 mm Hg, the pressure breaches the blood-brain barrier and fluid leaks out, increasing intracranial pressure. Usually the first symptoms noticed are severe headache, nausea, and vomiting. They are followed by seizures and alternations in mental status (that is, confusion to unresponsiveness). Sometimes patients may show focal neurologic signs, such as sudden blindness, aphasia (disturbances in speech production or comprehension), or hemiparesis. Widespread neuromuscular irritability may be signaled by muscle twitching.

The goal of treatment in hypertensive encephalopathy is to lower the blood pressure in a gradual, controlled manner during a 30- to 60-minute period so that cerebral blood flow is restored to normal. This is best accomplished under controlled conditions in a hospital. Thus, if you are within 20 to 30 minutes of the nearest hospital, provide supportive treatment only:

- Secure the airway, and administer supplemental oxygen by nasal cannula or nonrebreathing mask.
- Establish an IV line with normal saline at a keep-vein-open rate.
- Apply monitoring electrodes, and run an ECG rhythm strip (consider running a 12-lead ECG en route to the emergency department).
- Transport without delay.

Paramedics working in rural areas or other circumstances where long transport times to the hospital are unavoidable may have to initiate drug therapy for hypertensive encephalopathy in the field. One widely accepted drug for this purpose is labetalol (Normodyne, Trandate), which has alpha- and beta-blocking properties. As an alpha blocker, it prevents vasoconstriction, thereby decreasing the overall peripheral vascular resistance. Meanwhile, its beta-blocking actions prevent the reflex tachycardia that would otherwise occur in response to a drop in blood pressure. As a beta blocker, however, labetalol is relatively contraindicated in patients with asthma and COPD.

Labetalol can be given initially by slow IV push at 20 mg, repeated in 10 minutes as necessary, or an IV drip can be started. To administer a labetalol drip, add 250 mg to 250 mL of normal saline, yielding a concentration of 1 mg/mL. Start the infusion at a rate of 2 mg/min (2 mL/min), and watch the infusion carefully! A runaway IV could prove disastrous. Monitor the patient's blood pressure every 2 to 3 minutes. When the blood pressure has fallen to the target level specified by the physician, stop the infusion.

The other drug that may be ordered to lower a dangerously high blood pressure is nitroglycerin, 0.4 mg sublingual. This drug is not the first choice for this indication, but its use is acceptable if labetalol is not available.

Whenever you give a drug to lower a patient's blood pressure, keep the patient supine, and measure his or her blood pressure at least every 3 to 5 minutes. Record each measurement on a flowchart.

■ Infectious Diseases of the Heart

Endocarditis is an infection of the inner lining of the heart, characterized by inflammation of the endocardium (the inside lining of the heart chambers, including the heart valves). It is almost exclusively caused by staphylococcal or streptococcal infection. Patients with prosthetic heart valves and intravenous drug abusers top the list of those at highest risk for developing endocarditis. Typically this infection comes from another location of the body such as the mouth; it is spread through the bloodstream, ultimately reaching the heart. If left untreated, large growths on the valve leaflets can develop as a result of the infection, and can damage or even destroy the heart valves, which in turn can lead to life-threatening complications such as regurgitation and hemodynamic instability. Treatment for endocarditis typically consists of administration of antibiotics, but severe cases can require surgery.

Pericarditis is an acute inflammation of the pericardium that can last anywhere from several weeks to several months. The pericardial sac becomes red and swollen, and occasionally a buildup of fluid in the pericardial sac is noted. Patients report chest pain that is sharp and stabbing that can increase with coughing, swallowing, deep breathing, or lying flat. Patients may also indicate that the pain decreases if they are in the sitting position while leaning forward. Treatment for these patients consists of administration of nonsteroidal anti-inflammatory drugs (NSAIDs) or antibiotics.

Myocarditis is defined as inflammation of the myocardium. It can be caused by viral, bacterial, and fungal infections, and also from traumatic injury. Myocarditis can cause chest pain, dysrhythmias, heart failure, and sudden cardiac arrest.

Rheumatic fever is an inflammatory disease that is caused by streptococcal bacteria strains. This disease can cause a stenosis of the mitral valve or aortic valve, leading to heart complications.

Scarlet fever is a disease caused by the bacterium *Streptococcus pyogenes*. This is the same bacterium responsible for causing strep throat. The disease is characterized by a sore throat, fever, rash, and "strawberry tongue" (a white-colored tongue

with red speckles). Patients younger than 1 year are at greatest risk for developing the infection. Scarlet fever is treated with antibiotics and prehospital care is entirely supportive.

In conclusion, there are a few other cardiac conditions that may lead to emergencies. These include congenital heart disease and cardiomyopathy. Congenital heart disease is covered in the chapter, *Neonatal Care*. Cardiomyopathy is discussed in the chapter, *Pediatric Emergencies*.

YOU are the Medic | SUMMARY

1. What is your initial impression of this patient's condition?

Right now, the patient's condition is uncertain. There could be a number of causes for the pain in the patient's jaw. These range from a dental problem to recent trauma to referred pain from another condition. The patient looks sick with pale, moist skin, which is concerning. This could be related to the patient's diabetes, or may be unrelated to that. As always, you will need to do a thorough assessment to determine what is happening with this patient.

2. What initial history do you need for your assessment of this patient?

You should obtain baseline vital signs and OPQRST findings to assess the pain as soon as possible. Not every patient with an AMI has chest pain, however. People with diabetes, older people, and heart transplant patients, for example, generally do not present with chest pain. Because this patient has diabetes, her perception of pain will be altered.

3. Having ruled out a diabetes-related problem, what is your next step?

The blood glucose reading of 152 mg/dL is slightly elevated. Unexplained jaw pain in any patient should raise your index of suspicion for a possible cardiac event. Acquire a 12-lead ECG early and perform a focused cardiac examination.

4. What are the differences between the presentations of cardiac problems in men and women?

Women may experience different symptoms during AMI than men. Women may experience nausea, light-headedness, epigastric burning, or sudden onset of weakness or unexplained fatigue. Women may also have pain radiating down the right arm instead of the classic left arm pain. Because they may not experience the typical chest pain expected with an AMI, many women ignore their symptoms. Unfortunately, cardiovascular disease is the number one cause of death in US women.

5. What are PVCs and what does "multifocal" mean?

Premature ventricular complexes (PVCs) are ventricular beats that occur early in the cardiac cycle. Premature ventricular complexes are also known as ectopic complexes, meaning that

they occur outside of the normal conduction pathway. Premature ventricular complexes can be categorized into two groups: unifocal and multifocal. Unifocal PVCs originate from the same spot or "focus" within the ventricle and will have the same shape and direction on the ECG. Multifocal premature ventricular complexes originate from two or more irritated foci in the ventricles and will have differing morphologic features on the ECG.

6. What is your first-line treatment for PVCs?

If the Spo_2 is below 94%, the PVCs may be due to hypoxia. Administer oxygen and titrate to an Spo_2 of 98% to 100%. If the Spo_2 is above 94%, consider other causes of PVCs including myocardial infarction, cocaine and other drug use, alcohol, mitral valve prolapse, and caffeine.

7. What does the acronym MONA stand for?

The mnemonic MONA is used to help us remember treatments for acute coronary syndromes. MONA stands for Morphine, Oxygen, Nitroglycerin, and Aspirin. The mnemonic MONA is easy to remember, but it is important to note that the order of administration does not follow the order of letters in the acronym. The order of treatment can be controversial. Generally, the order should be: Oxygen (if the Spo_2 is 94% or lower), Aspirin, Nitroglycerin, and Morphine; however, always follow your local protocol.

8. Of the steps in MONA, which should you perform next?

You have already seen results from the oxygen administration: PVCs dropped from 8 to 10 per minute, to 2 per minute, and they appear to be unifocal. Therefore, the next step in treatment should be administration of aspirin. In most EMS systems, as long as the patient has no aspirin allergy or gastrointestinal bleeding, dispatchers may advise patients to chew baby aspirin (160 to 325 mg). If this has not been done before your arrival or the patient has not already taken aspirin on his or her own, then give the patient 160 to 325 mg of non-enteric-coated aspirin to chew. Aspirin prevents platelets from sticking to one another, minimizing the growth of clots. Morphine at 2 mg slow IV push is also appropriate in this patient.

YOU *are the Medic*   SUMMARY, *continued*

EMS Patient Care Report (PCR)

Date: 09-09-11	Incident No.: 889	Nature of Call: Cardiac		Location: 220 Halifax Ave	
Dispatched: 0828	En Route: 0828	At Scene: 0835	Transport: 0855	At Hospital: 0902	In Service: 0914

Patient Information

Age: 55 Sex: F Weight (in kg [lb]): 64 kg (140 lb)	Allergies: Patient denies Medications: Glyburide Past Medical History: Diabetic Chief Complaint: Jaw pain

Vital Signs

Time: 0845	BP: 100/60	Pulse: 64 irreg	Respirations: 14	Spo$_2$: 89% on room air, 99% on O$_2$
Time: 0850	BP: 110/66	Pulse: 70 irreg	Respirations: 14	Spo$_2$: 99% on O$_2$
Time:	BP:	Pulse:	Respirations:	Spo$_2$:

EMS Treatment
(circle all that apply)

Oxygen @ __15__ L/min via (circle one): NC (NRM) Bag-mask device	Assisted Ventilation	Airway Adjunct	CPR
Defibrillation	Bleeding Control	Bandaging	Splinting	Other

Narrative

Arrived to find a 55-year-old female pt lying supine in her bed. Pt states she was awakened from sleep by pain in her jaw. Pt called 9-1-1 after 2 hours duration. Pt describes the pain as a dull ache, 5/10 scale. Pt is conscious, alert, and oriented. Pt states her medical hx as diabetic and denies any other. Pt blood glucose level = 152. Skin warm, pale, and moist. Started IV of NS. ECG shows SR with multifocal PVCs at 8 to 10 per minute. O$_2$ 15 L/min via NRM applied. 2 mg MS IVP administered with pain relief noted. 12-lead unremarkable for elevation or depression. Pt lifted from bed to stretcher and moved to unit for transport to regional medical center. En route, pt PVCs decreased to 1 to 2 per minute and changed to unifocal. ASA 325 mg administered to pt during transport. Report to RMC upon arrival to Susan RN. **End of report**

Prep Kit

- Cardiovascular disease has been the number one killer in the United States almost every year since 1900.

- The cardiovascular system is composed of the heart and blood vessels. Its primary function is to deliver oxygenated blood and nutrients to every cell.

- The body attempts to maintain a fairly constant blood pressure to ensure perfusion of vital organs.

- Patients experience a variety of symptoms when they have a cardiovascular problem, the most common of which are chest pain, dyspnea, fainting, palpitations, and fatigue.

- Patients with cardiovascular disease are often prescribed several medications. Patients with advanced age typically experience more side effects from medications than do younger patients. Adverse drug events account for approximately 10% of all ED visits in the elderly.

- Cardiac rhythm disturbances (dysrhythmias) may arise from a variety of causes, including AMI.

- One of the most important tasks in the prehospital care of a patient with an AMI is to anticipate, recognize, and treat life-threatening dysrhythmias. In fact, ECG analysis is indicated in any patient who might have a cardiac-related condition.

- Most deaths from AMI are due to dysrhythmias, which typically occur during the early hours of the infarct.

- Cardiac monitors consist of leads that are connected to electrodes, which are placed on the patient. Each lead offers an electrical snapshot of a certain part of the heart. The cardiac monitor records the electrical activity acquired by each lead used, resulting in a 12-lead ECG tracing.

- Cardiac monitoring and ECG analysis are indicated in any patient who might have a cardiac-related condition. Any patient with chest pain or a history of heart problems should undergo ECG analysis.

- Cardiac monitoring usually involves using four limb leads to create an ECG printout showing lead I, II, and III to monitor the electrical activity in the patient's heart.

- Components of a rhythm strip produced by an ECG include the P wave, PR interval, QRS complex, J point, ST segment, T wave, and QT interval.

- Each component of the rhythm strip represents a phase of electrical activity within the heart. One whole complex on a rhythm strip represents one complete cycle of electrical conduction.

- Items to assess when you are analyzing a rhythm strip or ECG include the following: P waves, the PR interval, QRS duration, rhythm, and rate.

- The 12-lead ECG enables localization of cardiac ischemia to specific areas of the heart. The 12 leads include three limb leads (I, II, and III), three augmented limb leads (aVR, aVL, and aVF), and six precordial leads (V_1 to V_6).

- Leads that look at the same general area of the heart are called contiguous leads.

- Transmission of 12-lead ECG findings to the receiving facility is an important step that can lead to a faster diagnosis, decrease the time from emergency onset to definitive therapy (door-to-balloon time and door-to-needle time), and decrease mortality.

- Management of cardiac arrest involves BLS and ALS skills, including CPR, defibrillation, cardiac monitoring, IV fluid or medication infusion, post-resuscitative care, and cooling.

- Defibrillation is an intervention used to interrupt rapid chaotic rhythms such as ventricular tachycardia and ventricular fibrillation. Defibrillation simultaneously depolarizes all cardiac tissue in hopes of allowing the SA node to resume the function of primary pacemaker. Paramedics most often perform manual defibrillation rather than automated external defibrillation, because they are trained in interpreting cardiac rhythms.

- Synchronized cardioversion is an intervention used to interrupt rapid, organized, and hemodynamically unstable rhythms such as supraventricular tachycardia and atrial fibrillation. Unlike defibrillation, synchronized cardioversion is timed or "synchronized" to the patient's cardiac rhythm. Energy is delivered precisely at the peak of the R wave to capitalize on the already depolarized state of the ventricles. The energy delivered during synchronized cardioversion is aimed at depolarizing any tissue that remains polarized in hopes that the SA node resumes the primary pacemaking function.

- Transcutaneous pacing is an intervention used to depolarize heart muscle using an external stimulus. Pads placed on the patient's chest deliver electrical energy to the heart, causing muscle contraction. The external pacemaker serves as a bridge to permanent internal pacemaker implantation. Transcutaneous pacing is used to treat patients with hemodynamically unstable bradycardias.

- Treatment of hemodynamically unstable dysrhythmias should be centered on rate control of the dysrhythmia using electrical therapies.

- Most cardiac arrest victims have evidence of atherosclerosis or other underlying cardiac disease. However, cardiac arrest can also occur secondary to electrocution, submersion, and other types of trauma. Indeed, many cardiac arrest victims have no warning before the event occurs.

- Coronary artery disease is the most common form of heart disease and the leading cause of death in adults in the United States.

- Cardiac tamponade occurs when excessive fluid accumulates within the pericardium, limiting the heart's ability to fully expand. This can reduce cardiac filling to the point that the heart is unable to circulate blood. Emergent pericardiocentesis is lifesaving in patients with cardiac tamponade and hemodynamic instability. Transport the patient to the closest emergency facility.

- Cardiogenic shock results from extensive injury to the myocardium and carries a high mortality rate. Transport the patient expeditiously to the hospital. Except for the correction of life-threatening dysrhythmias, there are no measures that can stabilize the condition of a patient in cardiogenic shock in the field.

- Aortic aneurysms—particularly acute dissecting aneurysms of the thoracic aorta and expanding or ruptured aneurysms of the abdominal aorta—are of greatest concern to the EMS responder. The most common chief complaint is sudden severe ripping or tearing pain in the chest or abdomen.

- Treatment of hypertensive emergencies includes slow, controlled lowering of the patient's blood pressure. Management of elevated blood pressure should be reserved for the emergency department physician. Remember that systemic hypertension can be a result of increased intracranial pressure and is essential to maintain cerebral perfusion pressure.

■ Vital Vocabulary

abdominal aortic aneurysm (AAA) A sac or bulge in the wall of the abdominal portion of the aorta, resulting in weakening of that wall; it is considered life threatening if it ruptures.

aberration A term used to describe the shape of the QRS complex in aberrantly conducted beats.

absolute refractory period The early phase of cardiac repolarization, wherein the heart muscle cannot be stimulated to depolarize.

acetylcholine (ACh) A chemical mediator used in both the sympathetic and parasympathetic nervous systems.

acute coronary syndrome (ACS) Term used to describe any group of clinical symptoms consistent with acute myocardial ischemia.

acute myocardial infarction (AMI) A condition present when a period of cardiac ischemia caused by sudden narrowing or complete occlusion of a coronary artery leads to death (necrosis) of myocardial tissue.

adrenaline The hormone produced by the adrenal gland with alpha and beta sympathomimetic properties.

afterload The resistance against which the ventricle contracts.

agonal Pertaining to the period of dying.

agonal rhythm A cardiac dysrhythmia seen just before the heart stops altogether; essentially asystole with occasional QRS complexes that are not associated with cardiac output.

aneurysm A sac or bulge resulting from the weakening of the wall of a blood vessel or ventricle.

angina pectoris The sudden pain from myocardial ischemia, caused by diminished circulation to the cardiac muscle. The pain is usually substernal and often radiates to the arms, jaw, or abdomen and usually lasts 3 to 5 minutes and disappears with rest.

aorta The largest artery in the body, originating from the left ventricle.

aortic semilunar valve The valve between the left ventricle and the aorta; also called the aortic valve.

arrhythmia The lack of a cardiac rhythm; asystole.

arteries The muscular, thick-walled blood vessels that carry blood away from the heart.

arteriole A small blood vessel that carries oxygenated blood, branching into yet smaller vessels called capillaries.

arteriosclerosis A pathologic condition in which the arterial walls become thickened and inelastic.

artifact An artificial product; in cardiology, is used to refer to noise or interference in an ECG tracing.

asystole The absence of ventricular contractions; a "straight-line ECG."

atheroma A mass of fatty tissue.

atherosclerosis An accumulation of fat inside blood vessels resulting in narrowing of the lumen diameter.

atrial kick The volume (percentage) of blood pumped into the ventricles by the atria.

atrioventricular (AV) node A specialized structure located in the AV junction that slows conduction through the AV junction.

atrioventricular (AV) valves The mitral and tricuspid valves.

atropine A parasympathetic blocker; opposes the action of acetylcholine on the heart and elsewhere, causing an increase in heart rate.

augmented unipolar leads On an ECG, leads that only contain one true pole; the other is a combination of information from other leads; includes leads aVR, aVL, and aVF.

automated external defibrillator (AED) A "smart" defibrillator that can analyze the patient's ECG rhythm and determine whether a defibrillating shock is needed.

automaticity Spontaneous initiation of depolarizing electric impulses by pacemaker sites within the electric conduction system of the heart.

autonomic nervous system A subdivision of the nervous system that controls primarily involuntary body functions; comprised of the sympathetic and parasympathetic nervous systems.

AV junction The atrioventricular junction; the portion of the electric conduction system of the heart located in the upper part of the interventricular septum that conducts the excitation impulse from the atria to the bundle of His.

axis deviation A component of an ECG that looks at the direction of travel for the electricity going through the heart as it depolarizes.

Beck's triad The combination of narrowed pulse pressure, muffled heart tones, and jugular vein distention associated with cardiac tamponade.

benign early repolarization Early repolarization that is thought to be a normal variant; characterized by ST-segment elevation (or J-point elevation), a J or fishhook appearance at the J point, and concave ST-segment morphology.

bifascicular block Blockage of any combination of two of the fascicles or conduction pathways: a right bundle branch block (RBBB) and anterior hemiblock, a RBBB and posterior hemiblock, or an anterior hemiblock and posterior hemiblock.

bigeminy A dysrhythmia in which every other heartbeat is a premature contraction; can be atrial or ventricular.

bipolar leads On an ECG, leads that contain a positive and a negative pole; includes leads I, II, and III.

blood pressure The pressure exerted by the pulsatile flow of blood against the arterial walls.

bronchoconstriction Narrowing of the bronchial tubes.

bronchodilation Widening of the bronchial tubes.

Brugada syndrome A genetic disorder involving sodium channels in the heart; characterized by incomplete RBBB and ST-segment elevation that aggressively returns to baseline.

bruits Abnormal whooshing sounds indicating turbulent blood flow within a blood vessel.

bundle branch block A disturbance in electric conduction through the right or left bundle branch from the bundle of His.

bundle of His The portion of the electric conduction system in the interventricular septum that conducts the depolarizing impulse from the atrioventricular junction to the right and left bundle branches.

capillaries Extremely narrow blood vessels composed of a single layer of cells through which oxygen and nutrients pass to the tissues; these form a network between arterioles and venules.

cardiac cycle The period from one cardiac contraction to the next. Each cardiac cycle consists of ventricular contraction (systole) and relaxation (diastole).

cardiac output (CO) Amount of blood pumped by the heart per minute, calculated by multiplying the stroke volume by the heart rate per minute.

cardiac tamponade Restriction of cardiac contraction, failing cardiac output, and shock, caused by the accumulation of fluid or blood in the pericardium.

cardiopulmonary arrest The sudden and often unexpected cessation of adequate cardiac output.

chordae tendineae Fibrous strands shaped like umbrella stays that attach the free edges of the leaflets, or cusps, of the atrioventricular valves to the papillary muscles.

chronotropic effect The effect on the rate of contraction of the heart.

circumflex coronary artery One of the two branches of the left main coronary artery.

claudication A severe pain in the calf muscle that is caused by narrowing of the arteries in this muscle and that leads to a painful limp.

collateral circulation The mesh of arteries and capillaries that supplies blood to a segment of tissue whose original arterial supply has been obstructed.

concordant precordial pattern A pattern in which the QRS complexes are all in the same direction in the precordial leads.

conductivity The property that enables cardiac cells to pass an electrical impulse from one cell to another.

congestive heart failure (CHF) A condition that occurs when the heart is unable to pump powerfully enough or fast enough to empty its chambers; as a result, blood backs up into the systemic circuit, the pulmonary circuit, or both.

contiguous leads Leads that view geographically similar areas of the myocardium; useful for localizing areas of ischemia.

contractility The ability to shrink, shorten, or contract.

coronary arteries The blood vessels of the heart that supply blood to its walls.

coronary artery disease (CAD) A pathologic process caused by atherosclerosis that leads to progressive narrowing and eventual obstruction of the coronary arteries.

coronary sinus A large vessel in the posterior part of the coronary sulcus into which the coronary veins empty.

coronary sulcus The groove along the exterior surface of the heart that separates the atria from the ventricles.

couplet Two premature ventricular contractions occurring sequentially.

DeBakey classification A classification system for aortic dissections that includes three categories.

defibrillation The use of an unsynchronized direct current (DC) electric shock to terminate ventricular fibrillation.

delta wave The slurring of the upstroke of the first part of the QRS complex that occurs in Wolff-Parkinson-White syndrome.

depolarization The process of discharging resting cardiac muscle fibers by an electric impulse that causes them to contract.

diastole The period of ventricular relaxation during which the ventricles passively fill with blood.

digitalis preparations The drugs used in the treatment of congestive heart failure and certain atrial dysrhythmias.

dissection In reference to blood vessels, an aneurysm, or bulge, formed by the separation of the layers of an arterial wall.

dromotropic effect The effect on the velocity of conduction.

dysrhythmias Disturbances in the cardiac rhythm.

ejection click A high-pitched heart sound that occurs just after the S_1 sound.

ejection fraction (EF) The percentage of blood that leaves the heart each time it contracts.

electrical conduction system In the heart, the specialized cardiac tissue that initiates and conducts electric impulses; includes the SA node, internodal conduction pathways, atrioventricular junction, atrioventricular node, bundle of His, and the Purkinje network.

endocarditis Inflammation of the endocardium.

endocardium The thin membrane lining the inside of the heart.

epicardium The thin membrane lining the outside of the heart.

excitability The property that allows cells to respond to an electrical impulse.

fascicular block Disease or ischemia of either of the anterior and posterior fascicles of the electrical conduction system of the heart; also called hemiblock.

fibrinolysis The process of dissolving blood clots.

fibrinolytic therapy The therapy that uses medications that act to dissolve blood clots.

first-degree heart block A partial disruption of the conduction of the depolarizing impulse from the atria to the ventricles, causing prolongation of the PR interval.

Frank-Starling mechanism A characteristic of cardiac muscle that enables it, when stretched, to contract with greater force; the more cardiac muscle stretches, the greater the force of its contraction, the more completely it empties, and the greater the stroke volume.

heart rate (HR) The number of heart contractions per minute.

hyperkalemia An excessive amount of potassium in the blood.

hypertension High blood pressure, usually a diastolic pressure of greater than 90 mm Hg.

hypertensive emergency An acute elevation of blood pressure with evidence of end-organ damage.

hypertensive encephalopathy A condition that may complicate any form of hypertension, and which is usually signaled by a sudden, marked rise in blood pressure to levels greater than 200/130 mm Hg; also known as acute hypertensive crisis.

hypertrophic cardiomyopathy A condition in which the heart muscle is unusually thick, which means that the heart has to pump harder to get blood to leave.

hypocalcemia A low level of calcium in the blood.

hypokalemia A low concentration of potassium in the blood.

idioventricular Related to only the ventricles; produced by the ventricles.

infarction Death (necrosis) of a localized area of tissue caused by the cutting off of its blood supply.

inferior wall MI Death of myocardial tissue involving the lower (inferior) portion of the heart.

inotropic effect The effect on the contractility of muscle tissue, especially cardiac muscle.

internodal pathways The three pathways of the electrical conduction system found in the atria that transmit the impulse from the SA node to the AV node.

interventricular septum A thick wall that separates the right and left ventricles.

ischemia Tissue anoxia from diminished blood flow to tissue, usually caused by narrowing or occlusion of an artery.

isoelectric When referring to a wave, the wave is neither positive nor negative.

isoelectric line The baseline of the ECG.

junctional rhythm A dysrhythmia arising from ectopic foci in the area of the atrioventricular junction; often shows an absence of the P wave, P-wave inversion, a short PR interval, or a P wave appearing after the QRS complex.

leads The electrical cable attaching the electrode to the ECG monitor; the voltage difference between two points. For example, lead I is the voltage difference between the right and left arm electrodes.

left atrial enlargement Dilation of the left atrium that results either from systemic hypertension, mitral or aortic valve stenosis, or an athletic heart.

left atrium The upper left chamber of the heart; receives blood from the pulmonary veins.

left-sided heart failure A condition in which the left ventricle cannot effectively pump; this leads to a backup of blood behind the left ventricle, and eventually serum is forced out of the pulmonary capillaries and into the alveoli.

left ventricle The thick-walled, muscular, lower left chamber of the heart; receives blood from the left atrium and pumps it out through the aorta into the systemic arteries.

left ventricular hypertrophy (LVH) A cardiac condition in which the left ventricle becomes enlarged, most commonly due to hypertension.

limb leads The ECG leads attached to the limbs and that form the hexaxial system, along the frontal plane.

long QT syndrome A condition characterized by a QT interval exceeding approximately 450 ms.

Lown-Ganong-Levine syndrome A disorder that causes preexcitation of ventricular tissue and which is characterized on the ECG by a short PR interval and a normal QRS duration.

lumen The inside of an artery or other hollow structure.

manual defibrillation A mode available on automated external defibrillators, allowing the paramedic to interpret the cardiac rhythm and determine if defibrillation is needed (rather than the monitor making the determination).

mitral valve The valve located between the left atrium and the left ventricle of the heart.

monomorphic Having one common shape.

multifocal Arising from or pertaining to many foci or locations.

murmur An ambiguous heart sound that is associated with turbulent blood flow through the heart valves.

myocarditis Inflammation of the myocardium.

myocardium The cardiac muscle.

necrosis The death of tissue, usually caused by a cessation of its blood supply.

norepinephrine A neurotransmitter and drug sometimes used in the treatment of shock; produces vasoconstriction through its alpha stimulator properties.

normal sinus rhythm The normal rhythm of the heart, wherein the excitation impulse arises in the SA node, travels through the internodal pathways to the atrioventricular junction, down the bundle of His, through the bundle branches, and into the Purkinje network without interference.

opening snap A heart sound indicative of a noncompliant valve.

orthopnea Severe dyspnea experienced when lying down and relieved by sitting up.

orthostatic hypotension A fall in blood pressure when changing to an erect position.

P wave The first wave of the ECG complex, representing depolarization of the ventricles.

pacemaker The specialized tissue within the heart that initiates excitation impulses; an electronic device used to stimulate cardiac contraction when the electric conduction system of the heart is malfunctioning, especially in complete heart block; consists of a battery-powered pulse generator and a wire that transmits the electric impulse to the ventricles.

palpitations A sensation felt under the left breast of the heart "skipping a beat," usually caused by a premature ventricular contraction.

papillary muscles Protrusions of the myocardium into the ventricular cavities to which the chordae tendineae are attached.

parasympathetic nervous system A subdivision of the autonomic nervous system that is involved in control of involuntary, vegetative functions, mediated largely by the vagus nerve through the chemical acetylcholine.

paroxysmal nocturnal dyspnea (PND) Severe shortness of breath occurring at night after several hours of recumbency, during which fluid pools in the lungs; the person is forced to sit up to breathe; caused by left heart failure or decompensation of chronic obstructive pulmonary disease.

pericardial friction rub A to-and-fro sound that is an abnormal heart sound and which can be heard in systole and diastole; heard in patients who have pericarditis.

pericardial knock A high-pitched heart sound heard during diastole.

pericarditis Inflammation of the pericardium.

pericardium The double-layered sac containing the heart and the origins of the superior vena cava, inferior vena cava, pulmonary artery, and aorta.

percutaneous coronary intervention (PCI) A therapy in which balloons, stents, or other devices are passed through a catheter via a peripheral artery to recanalize and keep a blocked coronary artery open.

phlebitis Inflammation of the wall of a vein, sometimes caused by an IV line, manifested by tenderness, redness, and slight edema along part of the length of the vein.

plaque In cardiology, the white to yellow lesion found in atherosclerosis that is made up of lipids, cell debris, and smooth muscles cells; in older people, may also include calcium.

plasmin A naturally occurring clot-dissolving enzyme, usually present in the body in its inactive form, plasminogen.

point of maximal impulse (PMI) The palpable beat of the apex of the heart against the chest wall during ventricular contraction; normally palpated in the fifth left intercostal space in the midclavicular line.

PR interval The period between the beginning of the P wave (atrial depolarization) and the onset of the QRS complex (ventricular depolarization), signifying the time required for atrial depolarization and passage of the excitation impulse through the atrioventricular junction.

precordial leads Another term used to describe the chest leads in an ECG.

preexcitation Early depolarization of ventricular tissue due to the presence of an accessory pathway between the atria and ventricles.

preload The pressure under which the ventricle fills.

Prinzmetal angina A type of chest pain that occurs when a person is at rest, when oxygen needs are minimal.

pulmonary artery One of two arteries that carry deoxygenated blood from the right ventricle to the lungs.

pulmonary circulation The flow of blood from the right ventricle through the pulmonary arteries and all of their branches and capillaries in the lungs and back to the left atrium through the venules and pulmonary veins; also called the lesser circulation.

pulmonary edema Congestion of the pulmonary air spaces with exudate and foam, often secondary to left heart failure.

pulmonary embolism Obstruction of a pulmonary artery or arteries by solid, liquid, or gaseous material swept through the right side of the heart into the lungs.

pulmonary semilunar valve The valve between the right ventricle and the pulmonary artery; also called the pulmonic valve.

pulmonary veins The vessels that carry oxygenated blood from the lungs to the left atrium.

pulse deficit A situation in which the palpated radial pulse rate is less than the apical pulse rate; reported numerically as the difference between the two.

pulseless electrical activity (PEA) An organized cardiac rhythm (other than ventricular tachycardia) on an ECG monitor that is not accompanied by any detectable pulse.

pulsus alternans A pulse that alternates between strong and weak beats, characteristic of left ventricular systolic damage.

pulsus paradoxus A weakening or loss of a palpable pulse during inhalation, characteristic of cardiac tamponade and severe asthma.

Purkinje fibers A system of fibers in the ventricles that conducts the excitation impulse from the bundle branches to the myocardium.

QRS complex Deflections of the ECG produced by ventricular depolarization.

recanalization The opening up of new channels through a blocked artery.

receptors Specialized cells that respond to stimuli such as pressure, light, or chemicals.

refractory period A short period immediately after depolarization in which the myocytes are not yet repolarized and are unable to fire or conduct an impulse.

relative refractory period That period in the cell-firing cycle at which it is possible but difficult to restimulate the cell to contract.

reperfusion The resumption of blood flow through an artery.

retrosternal Situated or occurring behind the sternum.

rheumatic fever An inflammatory disease caused by streptococcal bacteria strains that can cause a stenosis of the mitral valve or aortic valve.

right atrial enlargement Dilation of the right atrium that results when returning venous pressure is elevated or pulmonary pressures are high.

right atrium The upper right chamber of the heart; receives blood from the venae cavae and supplies blood to the right ventricle.

right-sided heart failure A condition in which the right side has to work increasingly harder to pump blood into engorged pulmonary vessels, which eventually leads to an inability to keep up with the increased workload.

right ventricle The lower right chamber of the heart; receives blood from the right atrium and pumps blood out through the pulmonic valve into the pulmonary artery.

right ventricular hypertrophy (RVH) A cardiac condition in which the right ventricle becomes enlarged, most commonly due to pulmonary hypertension.

R-R interval The period between the onset of one QRS complex and the onset of the next QRS complex.

scarlet fever A disease caused by the bacterium *Streptococcus pyogenes*, and characterized by a sore throat, fever, rash, and "strawberry tongue."

semilunar valves The two valves, the aortic and pulmonic, that divide the heart from the aorta and pulmonary arteries.

sinoatrial (SA) node The dominant pacemaker of the heart, located at the junction of the superior vena cava and the right atrium.

sinus bradycardia A sinus rhythm with a heart rate of less than 60 beats/min.

sinus dysrhythmia A slight irregularity of the heart rate caused by changes in parasympathetic tone during breathing.

sinus tachycardia A sinus rhythm with a heart rate of greater than 100 beats/min.

ST segment The interval between the end of the QRS complex and the beginning of the T wave; often elevated or depressed with respect to the isoelectric line when there is significant myocardial ischemia.

stable angina Angina pectoris characterized by periodic pain with a predictable pattern.

Stanford classification A classification system for aortic dissections that includes two categories.

stroke volume (SV) The volume of blood pumped forward with each ventricular contraction.

subendocardial myocardial infarction A type of acute myocardial infarction in which the ischemic process affects only the inner layer of muscle.

sympathetic nervous system A subdivision of the autonomic nervous system that governs the body's fight-or-flight reactions, stimulating cardiac activity.

synchronized cardioversion The use of a synchronized direct current (DC) electric shock to convert tachydysrhythmias (such as atrial fibrillation) to normal sinus rhythm.

syncope Fainting; brief loss of consciousness caused by transiently inadequate blood flow to the brain.

systemic circulation The flow of blood from the left ventricle through the aorta, to all of its branches and capillaries in the tissues, and back to the right atrium through the venules, veins, and venae cavae; also called the greater circulation.

systole The period of time when the atria or ventricles are contracting; also called atrial systole.

T waves The upright, flat, or inverted wave following the QRS complex of the ECG, representing ventricular repolarization.

thrill A vibration heart sound that occurs frequently and remains constant.

thromboembolism A blood clot that has formed within a blood vessel and is floating within the bloodstream.

thrombus A fixed blood clot.

transcutaneous pacing The act of depolarizing myocardial tissue with a small electrical charge delivered by a device that sends a small electrical charge through the skin of the chest between one externally placed pacing pad and another.

transmural myocardial infarction A type of acute myocardial infarction in which the infarct extends through the entire wall of the ventricle.

tricuspid valve The valve between the right atrium and right ventricle of the heart.

trifascicular block A blockage or impairment of all three components of the ventricular conduction system, with one working occasionally to provide AV conduction.

trigeminy A premature complex in every third heartbeat.

tunica adventitia The outer layer of tissue of a blood vessel wall, composed of elastic and fibrous connective tissue.

tunica intima The smooth, thin, inner lining of a blood vessel.

tunica media The middle and thickest layer of tissue of a blood vessel wall, composed of elastic tissue and smooth muscle cells that allow the vessel to expand or contract in response to changes in blood pressure and tissue demand.

U wave A small flat wave sometimes seen after the T wave and before the next P wave.

unifocal Arising from a single site.

unstable angina Angina pectoris characterized by a changing, unpredictable pattern of pain, which may signal an impending acute myocardial infarction.

vagus nerve One of 12 nerves that comprise the parasympathetic nervous system and is responsible for decreasing heart rate.

Valsalva maneuver Forced exhalation against a closed glottis, the effect of which is to stimulate the vagus nerve and, thereby, slow the heart rate.

vasoconstriction Narrowing of the diameter of a blood vessel.

vasodilation Widening of the diameter of a blood vessel.

veins The blood vessels that carry blood to the heart.

vena cava The largest vein of the body; there are two, of which each return blood to the right atrium.

venules Very small veins.

Wolff-Parkinson-White syndrome A syndrome characterized by short PR intervals, delta waves, nonspecific ST-T wave changes, indicating the presence of an accessory pathway.

Assessment in Action

Your unit is dispatched to a single-family residence for a person with chest pain. The dispatcher tells you the patient is a 66-year-old man who has an extensive cardiac history. On arrival inside the residence, you see the patient is lying on the sofa in his living room. He tells you he has a history of two prior heart attacks and has had bypass surgery. He states he has pain that feels like previous heart attacks.

1. Cardiac output is defined as:
   A. the number of cardiac contractions (heartbeats) per minute.
   B. the amount of blood pumped out by either ventricle in a single contraction.
   C. the stroke volume times the heart rate.
   D. the percentage of blood that is leaving the heart each time it contracts.

2. What is a normal ejection fraction?
   A. 30% to 55%
   B. 55% to 70%
   C. 75% to 100%
   D. 80% to 90%

3. The pressure under which a ventricle fills is called:
   A. vascular resistance.
   B. preload.
   C. afterload.
   D. contractility.

4. You have obtained vital signs on this patient, which are: BP, 96/58 mm Hg; pulse, 82 beats/min; respirations, 16 breaths/min; and SpO_2, 96%. The patient's skin is pale, cool, and diaphoretic. What is the next step in the assessment of this patient?
   A. Obtain a list of current medications.
   B. Obtain an ECG strip of lead aVL.
   C. Obtain a 12-lead ECG.
   D. Obtain a blood draw for blood chemistry.

5. The 12-lead ECG assessment of this patient shows ST changes in leads II, III, and aVF. Changes in these leads reflect a problem with which anatomic region of the heart?
   A. Anterior
   B. Lateral
   C. Septal
   D. Inferior

6. The patient describes his pain as an 8 on a 1:10 scale. You have followed your protocol and administered nitroglycerin for pain relief. When you reassess after administration, the patient's pain level did not decrease. What is your next choice of medication for pain relief?
   A. Ativan
   B. Morphine
   C. Haldol
   D. Demerol

7. The patient now becomes unresponsive, stops breathing, and has no pulse. Your partner has already applied defibrillation pads on the patient's chest. What is your first course of action to treat this patient?
   A. Insert an endotracheal tube and ventilate the patient with 100% oxygen.
   B. Start an IV line of normal saline.
   C. Start CPR.
   D. Leave the patient and retrieve the AED.

8. The primary pacemaker of the heart is the:
   A. sinoatrial node.
   B. atrioventricular node.
   C. atrioventricular junction.
   D. bundle of Kent.

9. The process by which muscle fibers are stimulated to contract is called:
   A. inotrope.
   B. depolarization.
   C. repolarization.
   D. chronotrope.

10. What electrolytes are primarily responsible for depolarization?
    A. Sodium and potassium
    B. Sodium and calcium
    C. Potassium and calcium
    D. Potassium and magnesium

Additional Questions

11. Which drug is considered a vagolytic? What part of the nervous system does this drug act on?

12. What part of the nervous system does norepinephrine affect?

Neurologic Emergencies

National EMS Education Standard Competencies

Medicine

Integrates assessment findings with principles of epidemiology and pathophysiology to formulate a field impression and implement a comprehensive treatment/disposition plan for a patient with a medical complaint.

Neurology

Anatomy, presentations, and management of

- Decreased level of responsiveness (pp 1048-1050)

Anatomy, physiology, pathophysiology, assessment, and management of

- Stroke/transient ischemic attack (pp 1058-1065)
- Seizure (pp 1067-1069)
- Status epilepticus (p 1069)
- Headache (pp 1070-1071)

Anatomy, physiology, epidemiology, pathophysiology, psychosocial impact, presentations, prognosis, and management of

- Stroke/intracranial hemorrhage/transient ischemic attack (pp 1058-1065)
- Seizure (pp 1067-1069)
- Status epilepticus (p 1069)
- Headache (pp 1070-1071)
- Dementia (pp 1071-1072)
- Neoplasms (pp 1071-1073)
- Demyelinating disorders (pp 1073-1075)
- Parkinson disease (p 1075)
- Cranial nerve disorders (pp 1075-1076)
- Movement disorders (p 1077)
- Neurologic inflammation/infection (pp 1077-1079)
- Spinal cord compression (p 1079)
- Hydrocephalus (p 1080)
- Wernicke encephalopathy (p 1071)

Knowledge Objectives

1. Describe the incidence, morbidity, and mortality of neurologic emergencies. (p 1038)
2. Discuss the anatomy and physiology of the organs and structures that make up the nervous system. (pp 1038-1043)
3. Explain how neurons and related structures transmit impulses. (pp 1042-1043)
4. Differentiate between the central and peripheral nervous systems, and describe the functions of each. (p 1038)
5. State what a neoplasm is, and identify several types of neoplasms that affect the nervous system. (pp 1071-1073)

6. Specify the characteristics of a degenerative neurologic disease. (pp 1073-1075)
7. Define *developmental anomaly*, and explain how such conditions arise within the nervous system of the developing human embryo. (pp 1080-1081)
8. Identify the types of pathogenic organisms that can infect the nervous system, and list the signs and symptoms of a nervous system infection. (pp 1077-1079)
9. Specify the vascular causes of neurologic conditions. (pp 1058-1065)
10. Compare the causes, signs, and symptoms of vascular neurologic conditions that occur suddenly with those that develop gradually. (p 1066)
11. Identify the layers that make up the arterial wall. (p 1059)
12. Define *multifactorial condition* and describe several factors that influence the development of neurologic conditions. (p 1058)
13. Specify the contents that occupy the cranial vault and explain how their interaction determines intracranial pressure. (pp 1059-1060)
14. Discuss the two major problems that stem from increased intracranial pressure. (p 1060)
15. Consider the importance of observing standard precautions and securing the physical environment in ensuring your safety when caring for a neurologic patient. (pp 1043-1044)
16. Identify the abnormal respiratory patterns associated with central nervous system illness. (p 1045)
17. Compare how to investigate a chief complaint in an unresponsive patient with how you would do so in a conscious patient. (p 1046)
18. List and explain the components of the physical examination of a patient with a neurologic illness. (pp 1047-1056)
19. Describe how to determine level of consciousness when assessing a patient with a neurologic complaint. (pp 1048-1050)
20. Compare the characteristics of decorticate and decerebrate posturing, and consider the likely implications of each for the patient's outcome. (p 1050)
21. Specify several speech difficulties that can reveal a diminished level of consciousness. (pp 1053-1054)
22. Specify several movement difficulties that can reveal a diminished level of consciousness. (pp 1054-1056)
23. List and describe the most important interventions used to treat patients with neurologic conditions. (pp 1056-1058)
24. Outline standard guidelines for treating patients with neurologic complaints. (pp 1058-1081)
25. Define *stroke* and discuss its pathophysiology, assessment, and management. (pp 1058-1064)
26. Compare the pathophysiology of ischemic (occlusive) stroke with that of hemorrhagic stroke. (pp 1059-1060)
27. Discuss several instruments used to screen for stroke. (pp 1063-1064)
28. Define *transient ischemic attack* and explain its relationship to stroke. (pp 1064-1065)
29. Define *seizure* and discuss its pathophysiology, assessment, and management. (pp 1067-1069)

30. Explain how to differentiate stroke from seizure. (p 1046)

31. Compare generalized seizures with partial seizures, and analyze how seizures are further classified. (pp 1067-1069)

32. Define *status epilepticus* and discuss its pathophysiology, assessment, and management. (p 1069)

33. Define *syncope* and discuss its pathophysiology, assessment, and management. (pp 1069-1070)

34. List the most common types of headaches, and outline their pathophysiology, assessment, and management. (pp 1070-1071)

35. Define *dementia* and discuss its pathophysiology, assessment, and management. (p 1071)

36. Compare the causes, signs and symptoms, and typical course of several common types of dementia. (p 1071)

37. Define *demyelination* and analyze the common features of demyelinating conditions. (pp 1073-1074)

38. Define *multiple sclerosis* and discuss its pathophysiology, assessment, and management. (pp 1073-1074)

39. Define *Guillain-Barré syndrome* and discuss its pathophysiology, assessment, and management. (p 1074)

40. Define *amyotrophic lateral sclerosis* and discuss its pathophysiology, assessment, and management. (pp 1074-1075)

41. Define *Parkinson disease* and discuss its pathophysiology, assessment, and management. (p 1075)

42. List several cranial nerve disorders and evaluate their shared characteristics. (pp 1075-1076)

43. Define *dystonia* and discuss its pathophysiology, assessment, and management. (p 1077)

44. Compare encephalitis with meningitis in terms of pathophysiology, assessment, and management. (pp 1077-1079)

45. Define an *abscess* and discuss its pathophysiology, assessment, and management. (p 1079)

46. Define *poliomyelitis* and discuss its pathophysiology, assessment, and management. (p 1079)

47. Define *peripheral neuropathy* and discuss its pathophysiology, assessment, and management. (p 1079)

48. Define *hydrocephalus* and discuss its pathophysiology, assessment, and management. (p 1080)

49. Define *spina bifida* and discuss its pathophysiology, assessment, and management. (pp 1080-1081)

50. Define *cerebral palsy* and discuss its pathophysiology, assessment, and management. (p 1081)

Skills Objectives

1. Assess a patient's level of consciousness. (pp 1048-1050)

2. Perform a complete neurologic examination. (pp 1047-1056)

3. Use several commonly used screening tools to screen a patient suspected of having had a stroke. (pp 1063-1064)

Introduction

The National Center for Health Statistics lists 3 of the top 15 causes of death in 2007 as neurologic in nature. Stroke is the third leading cause of death in the United States. **Table 1** shows the occurrence of neurologic disorders throughout the United States. Prevalence refers to the total number of people in a given population, such as adults older than 65 years in the United States, with a particular disease. Incidence refers to the number of people newly diagnosed with a particular disorder in a given 1-year period.

Patients with neurologic problems are vulnerable and can be in danger. Many of the reflexes that protect an awake person can be temporarily inactive when the nervous system is depressed by any cause. The eyelids do not blink away dust and irritants. The larynx does not cause gagging and coughing in reaction to secretions oozing down the airway. The body does not seek a more comfortable position in response to compression of a limb in an awkward position. The tongue goes slack. The airway is at risk.

To help you better determine each patient's problem, a review of the anatomy and physiology of the nervous system is presented in this chapter. This information will create the proper foundation on which to later begin a discussion on assessment and treatment.

Anatomy and Physiology

Structure of the Nervous System

The nervous system is perhaps the most complex organ system within the human body. It comprises two major structures, the brain and spinal cord, and thousands of nerves that allow every part of the body to communicate. This system is responsible for fundamental functions such as controlling breathing, pulse rate, and blood pressure. But the true complexity of the nervous system is seen in its ability to allow higher level activity such as reading a book, enjoying music, having a discussion with a friend, and even watching television. All of these activities require the brain to engage memory, understanding, and thought.

The basic structure of the nervous system is portrayed in **Figure 1**. The major structures are divided into two main categories: the **central nervous system (CNS)**, which is responsible for thought, perception, feeling, and autonomic body functions, and the **peripheral nervous system (PNS)**, which is responsible for transmitting commands from the brain to the body and receiving feedback from the body.

As a review of the nervous system, consider the example of a child riding a bicycle. This common and seemingly simple activity is abounding with conscious and unconscious functions. The child has many things to do so that he or she does not fall or ride into a tree.

The Brain

Lobes On a summer morning the rider, Justin, goes to the garage to get his bike. Already the brain is hard at work. As Justin enters the garage, the brain must determine which object is a bike. As Justin scans the garage, the images produced by his eyes are transmitted via the optic nerve to the occipital lobe of the brain **Figure 2**. There, the image, which is transmitted upside down, needs to be reoriented. The occipital lobe now scans through tens of thousands of images that are stored to determine whether this image has been seen before.

Once the image is recognized, an exiting pathway is accessed to the temporal lobe. Here, language and speech are stored. As Justin walks through the garage, he is able to put names to what he sees—a car, a workbench, a bike. When Justin was learning to speak, he often became confused about the correct names of objects. As he practiced, he received reinforcement for the correct names and redirection for the names that were incorrect. In his brain, more and more pathways were laid down between the image of an object with two wheels, a seat, and pedals and stored in the occipital lobe as the word "bike."

As Justin gets his helmet, commands from the frontal lobe of the brain are sent to his arms so that he can pick up the helmet and place it on his head. The frontal lobe, which controls

YOU are the Medic   PART 1

Your unit is dispatched for the report of a person falling at a local apartment building. The police have already arrived on the scene and confirm that it is safe. You arrive to find a responsive 81-year-old man lying on the floor of his apartment. His two sons are present at his side. The elder son states that they visited their father last night and left him around 1900 hours as he was watching television. This morning, they returned and discovered him lying on the floor next to the chair he was sitting in last evening. The time is now 0900 hours. The sons state that their father "is not acting right."

1. How are you going to further define "not acting right"?

2. At this point, is your concern higher for a traumatic cause or a medical cause for the fall?

Table 1   Approximate Occurrence of Neurologic Disorders in the United States

Disorder	Estimated Occurrence	Incidence or Prevalence
Alzheimer disease	5,300,000 cases (> 14% of people older than 65 years and > 40% of people older than 80 years)	Prevalence
Amyotrophic lateral sclerosis	6 per 100,000 population	Prevalence
Bell palsy	25 per 100,000 population	Incidence
Acoustic neuroma	1 case per 100,000 population	Prevalence
Creutzfeldt-Jakob disease	1 case per million (approximately 300 cases in the United States)	Prevalence
Dystonia	About 300,000 people affected within North America	Incidence
Encephalitis	Various types and difficult to determine true numbers within the US; estimates are several thousand cases of viral encephalitis per year	Incidence
Glossopharyngeal neuralgia	1 per 100,000 population	Incidence
Guillain-Barré syndrome	1 per 100,000 population	Incidence
Headache	45 million experience chronic, recurring headaches	Prevalence
Hemifacial spasm	About 10 per 100,000 population	Incidence
Huntington disease	About 4 per 100,000 population	Prevalence
Hydrocephalus, congenital	1 in 1,000 live births	Prevalence
Ménière disease	15 per 100,000 population	Prevalence
Meningitis	1.5 cases per 100,000 population	Incidence
Multiple sclerosis	0.5-1.0 per 1,000 population	Incidence
Myasthenia gravis	0.5-14 per 100,000 population	Prevalence
Neoplasm, spinal	10,000 new cases per year	Incidence
Neoplasm, brain	7-19 per 100,000 population	Incidence
Parkinson disease	120 per 100,000 population	Prevalence
Peripheral neuropathy	9,000,000 people with diabetes who have neuropathy	Prevalence
Pick disease	Rare (As part of the group of frontotemporal dementias, it is the fourth leading cause of dementia)	Prevalence
Postpolio syndrome	100,000 cases	Prevalence
Seizures	3,000,000 cases	Prevalence
Spinal cord compression	There are many causes of spinal cord compression: trauma, tumor, improper alignment of the spine, etc. 90% of Americans will have lower back pain at some point in their lives, much of which is caused by spinal cord compression.	Prevalence
Stroke	700,000 new cases per year, third leading cause of death in the United States	Incidence
Syncope	3% of emergency department visits nationwide	Incidence
Trigeminal neuralgia	155 cases per 1 million population	Prevalence
Wernicke encephalopathy	About 1% of population	Incidence

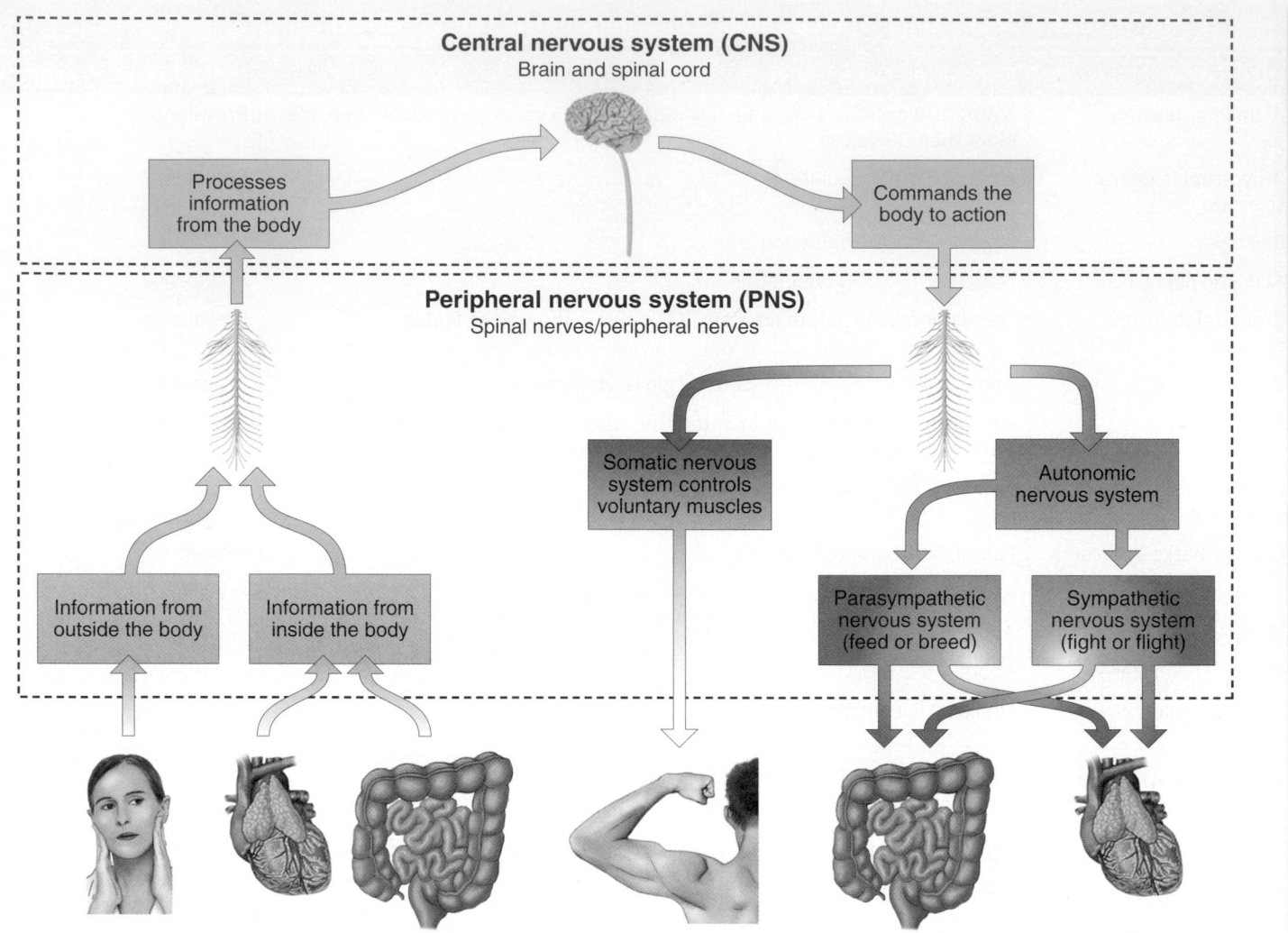

Figure 1 Organization of the nervous system. The central nervous system consists of the brain and spinal cord, which work together to process information. This information takes the form of signals generated in response to stimuli from both inside and outside the body. The peripheral nervous system commands the body to act. It consists of the somatic nervous system, which controls voluntary muscles, and the autonomic nervous system, which oversees sympathetic (fight or flight) and parasympathetic responses.

voluntary motion, sends signals out of the CNS along efferent nerves to the arms, shoulders, chest, and hands to perform the task of picking up the helmet. The **efferent nerves** leave the brain through the peripheral nervous system and convey commands to other parts of the body.

Which way should the helmet be applied? This motor memory is stored within the frontal lobe. The brain is storing memories in the areas that were initially stimulated. As the helmet is being applied, Justin needs to make fine adjustments to its position. His brain is receiving impulses from nerves within the skull and muscle of the head.

If the helmet is uncomfortable, Justin will sense pressure and possibly pain from the improperly placed helmet. These **afferent nerves** (nerves that send information to the brain) send signals of discomfort to the parietal lobe where the body's sense of touch and pain perception are found. Signals are sent from the parietal lobe to the frontal lobe to signal the body to adjust the helmet until the pressure signals have stopped.

Diencephalon and Brainstem How does the brain manage a massive amount of information without confusion and misdirection? One of the major roles of the **diencephalon** is to filter out unneeded information before it reaches the cerebral cortex. For example, the diencephalon keeps you from having to think about shifting your weight on a chair when it becomes uncomfortable. Instead, signals of pressure or pain sent through the peripheral nerves initially stop in the diencephalon, which dispatches the command to switch positions slightly without your being conscious of doing so.

How does a person know it is time to get up in the morning? The **midbrain** portion of the **brainstem** is responsible for helping to regulate the level of consciousness (LOC), including patterns of sleep and wakefulness. The reason that you get tired often at the same time of the day is due in part to the functions of the reticular activating system (RAS) in the midbrain **Figure 3**.

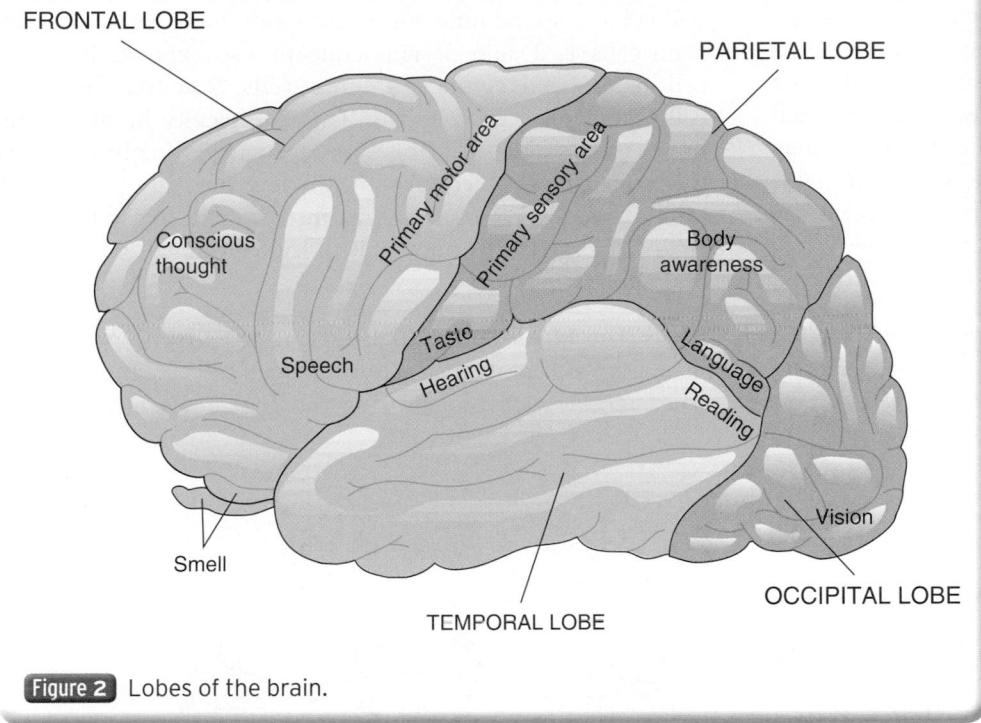

Figure 2 Lobes of the brain.

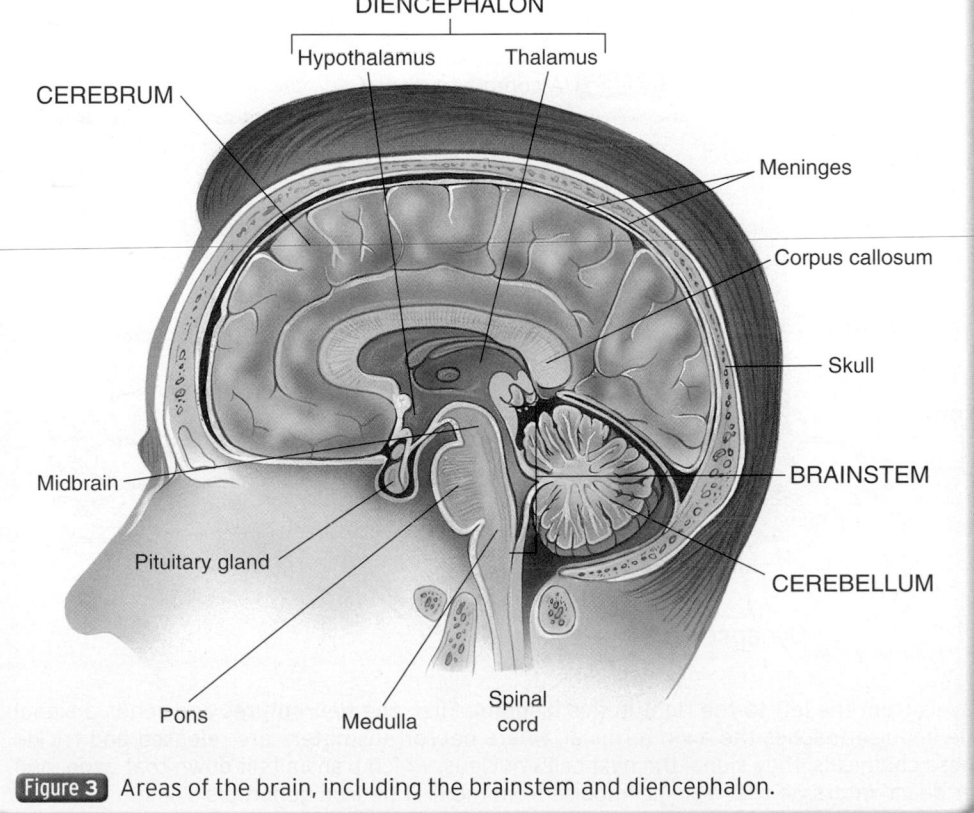

Figure 3 Areas of the brain, including the brainstem and diencephalon.

The brainstem is also responsible for controlling blood pressure, pulse rate, and respiratory rate and pattern. The **pons**, located just inferior to the midbrain, controls respiratory pace and depth. Blood pressure and pulse rate are controlled by the **medulla oblongata**. These functions obviously need to occur constantly, but Justin could not ride his bike if he needed to spend time and energy consciously controlling his pulse rate. The brainstem frees the cerebral cortex for higher activities.

Hypothalamus and Pituitary Gland Justin now mounts his bike and begins to ride. The smile on his face indicates that he is having a good time. Emotions come from two main areas within the brain: the **limbic system**, where rage and anger are generated, and the **hypothalamus**, a part of the diencephalon, where pleasure, thirst, and hunger are found. All emotions are then mediated by the prefrontal cortex so people can choose how they are going to act in response to how they feel.

Our rider begins to pick up speed. As he approaches a corner, he must turn or risk crashing into a tree. The excitement is increasing his pulse rate and blood pressure. The hypothalamus communicates to the **pituitary gland**, a member of the endocrine system. The pituitary gland then sends chemical commands to the **adrenal glands** to release epinephrine and norepinephrine. These chemicals, found in the sympathetic nervous system, give Justin the increased strength and cardiovascular reserves that he needs to handle the bike in a tight turn. As quickly as these chemicals act, they are shut off. This prevents the body from depleting its reserves. Additionally, too much epinephrine and norepinephrine can be damaging in the long term.

Cerebellum Justin is able to shift his weight and make the turn successfully due in large part to his **cerebellum**. This lobe of the brain, located in the posterior, inferior area of the skull, manages complex motor activity unconsciously. When Justin first learned to ride a bike, he had to think about what to do, where to shift his weight, and how to hold his upper body. Over time, and with practice, the frontal lobe of the brain tires of sending the same commands again and again, so this task is transferred to the cerebellum.

Neurons and Impulse Transmission

A neuron is the fundamental element of the nervous system. This cell comprises a cell body, axon, axon terminal, and dendrites. The cell body contains the nucleus. The axon is a projection from the nucleus that extends toward another cell carrying signals away from the nucleus. The axon may or may not contain myelin, a chemical insulator. The axon terminal is the portion of the axon where the neurotransmitters are manufactured. Dendrites project off the nucleus, but they carry signals from other cells toward the nucleus.

Synapses All of this complex activity is made possible by the **synapse**. Nerve cells do not actually come in direct contact with each other. There is a slight gap between each cell. This allows for a far greater level of fine control than if each cell were in direct contact with the next. The synapse, which is present wherever a nerve cell terminates, "connects" to the next cell by chemicals called *neurotransmitters*.

Neurotransmitters A host of **neurotransmitters** are present within the brain and throughout the body. Dopamine, acetylcholine, epinephrine, and serotonin are good examples. These chemicals take the electrically conducted signal from one nerve cell (a neuron) and relay it to the next cell. How do the chemical neurotransmitters achieve a greater degree of control as opposed to simply wiring the cells together? The answer is in the connections Figure 4.

It is important to remember that nerve cells respond in an all-or-nothing fashion. They either fire or they do not; a neuron cannot fire weakly. The complexity in the system is found in how the cells are connected. As you can see in Figure 4,

each cell is connected to the next in a straight line. This is a reliable method of getting a signal from point A to point B. To gain more control, however, a system must have more complexity. In Figure 5, you can see how three cells might convene at a single synapse with one other cell. This fourth cell will fail to respond unless it receives simultaneous stimulation from cells 1, 2, and 3. This concept also explains how one cell sends signals to many different cells. Note that the fourth cell stimulates cells 5 and 6. This complexity helps explain how Justin is able to see his bike, recognize the object, know the name of the object, instantly know how to use it, know how to make the muscles of his mouth work to say the word "bike," and appreciate how it will feel to ride the bike—all at the same time.

Axons The axons of many neurons are coated with **myelin**, an insulating substance that allows the cell to transmit its signal consistently, without "shorting out" or losing electricity to

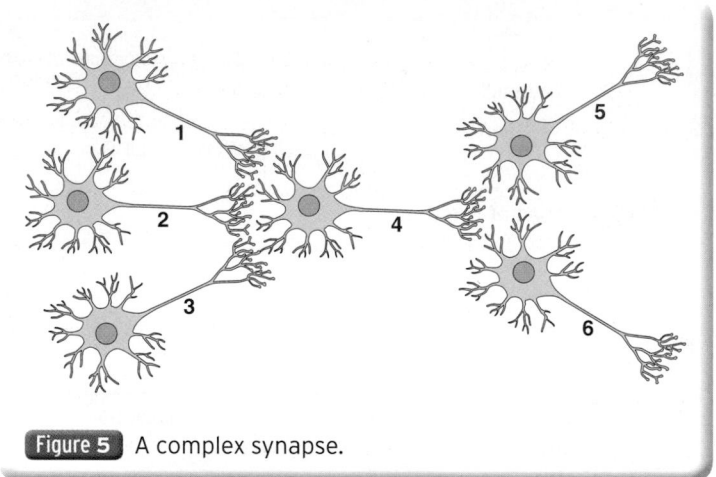

Figure 5   A complex synapse.

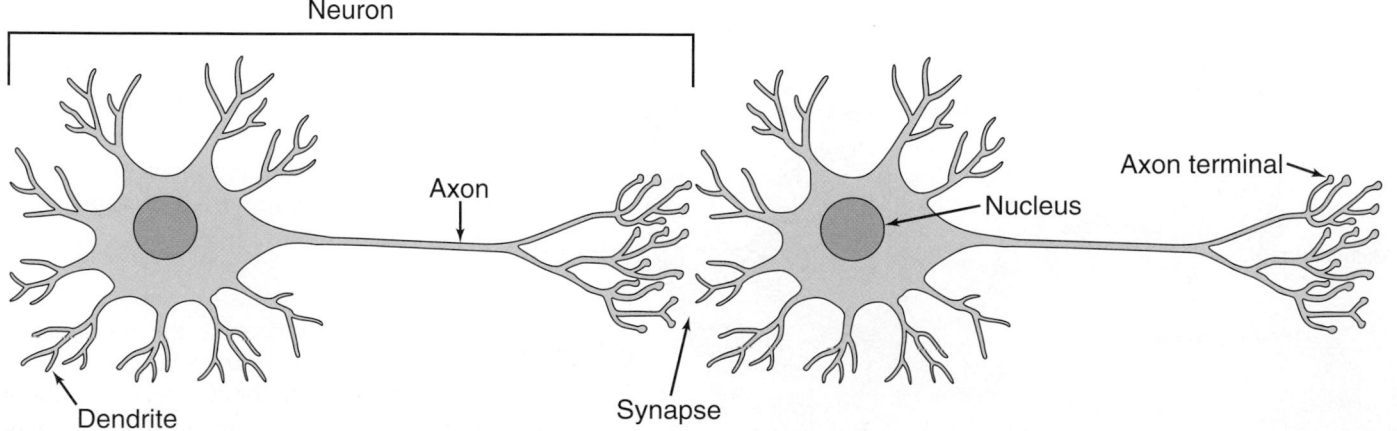

Figure 4   Neuron and synapse. The signal travels from the left to the right in this diagram: First, the neuron fires and sends a signal along its **axon** to the axon terminal. Next, the impulse reaches the axon terminal, where neurotransmitters are released and trickle across the synapse. When dendrites detect these chemicals, they signal the next cell's nucleus, which transmits it down that axon, and so on. Dendrites also release neurotransmitter deactivators, so that a single impulse from the first neuron generates a single response from the second.

surrounding fluids and tissues. Myelin also increases the speed of conduction. Where speed is important, neurons have myelin. Where speed is of less value, neurons do not have myelin. Most of the neurons within the body have myelin.

This review has touched on highlights of the various portions of the nervous system. A good basic reference is included in Table 2 .

■ Patient Assessment

The brain is the most sensitive organ within the body to variable temperatures and fluctuating levels of oxygen and glucose. Even small alterations can impair its function. Conversely, the brain is also surprisingly resilient to internal environmental changes. It does not simply shut down when the oxygen level falls. Assessment of a patient would most likely be easier if the patient were either completely awake or completely asleep. When you are trying to determine whether your patient has a neurologic problem, you need to look for both gross, or obvious, changes and also subtle, sometimes hidden changes that can indicate disease. The next section reviews the assessment process for the neurologic patient.

■ Scene Size-up

The purpose of standard precautions is to protect you from exposure to potentially harmful organisms or environments. For example, patients who have periodic tonic/clonic seizures may be incontinent. Gloves are a necessary standard approach for all patients. You should also ensure that additional equipment necessary for observing standard precautions is available, such as gowns and protective eyewear. The standard precautions you use should be based on the procedure you are conducting and the likelihood of being contaminated. Your patients may not know that they have a disease, may not be able to tell you, or worse, may hide this fact from you entirely. Be cautious, be consistent, and be safe!

The location of a neurologic patient can place you in scenes that may not be the safest environment for you. Some patients are unconscious because of a drug overdose. When people use illegal drugs, weapons and crime are likely to be close at hand. This fact may place you close to armed criminals, in the midst of a volatile situation.

Your assessment of the physical environment should begin at dispatch. What is the nature of the call? Do you need police assistance? Should you enter the scene without backup? Do not hesitate to call for additional resources to ensure your safety.

Table 2   Structures of the Nervous System and Their General Functions

System	Major Structure	Subdivision	General Functions
Central nervous system	Brain	Occipital	Vision and storage of visual memories
		Parietal	Sense of touch and texture and storage of tactile memories
		Temporal	Hearing and smell Language Storage of sound and odor memories
		Frontal	Voluntary muscle control and storage of spatial memories
		Prefrontal	Judgment and prediction of consequences of a person's actions Abstract intellectual functions
		Limbic system	Basic emotions Basic reflexes, such as chewing and swallowing
		Diencephalon (thalamus)	Relay center that prioritizes signals to hone in on important messages
		Diencephalon (hypothalamus)	Emotions Temperature control Interface with the endocrine system
	Brainstem	Midbrain	Level of consciousness Reticular activating system Muscle tone and posture
		Pons	Respiratory pattern and depth
		Medulla oblongata	Pulse rate, blood pressure, and respiratory rate
	Spinal cord		Reflexes Relay of information to and from the body
Peripheral nervous system	Cranial nerves		Special peripheral nerves that connect directly from the brain to body parts to relay information from the brain
	Peripheral nerves		Brain to spinal cord to body part Receive stimulus from body, send commands to body

Examine the scene from a wide perspective. As you approach the patient, know what is going on around you. Where are the bystanders? What obstacles are present? Do you have a quick retreat route?

Ensure that no matter what type of event is taking place, you have a way to remove yourself from the scene relatively easily. This certainly can be easier said than done, but the way to make this happen is to *think* about scene safety during the entire call. As you leave the ambulance, examine the environment for possible threats. Look for animals, obstacles, suspicious or threatening people, and trip hazards. Review the chapter, *Patient Assessment* for additional discussion of this important concept.

Initially, you must gather only basic information related to the event. Did the event occur suddenly or gradually? What is the primary complaint at this time? You should use this information to help determine what additional resources you may need and what types of equipment should be brought into the scene. Many departments have their equipment divided into various bags or boxes. The information provided at this stage tells you which bag or box you need.

Examine the scene to determine the number of patients. Clues can be obtained with the dispatch information. Consider the mechanism of injury (MOI)/nature of illness (NOI). Motor vehicle crashes typically involve more than one vehicle; therefore, you may have more than one patient. If there are many patients with similar signs and symptoms, you should be cautious. One patient with a headache does not stand out. However, if an entire family in the same house is reporting a headache, carbon monoxide exposure must be considered a possibility. The house may now become an unsafe scene. Ensure that you have the correct PPE.

Primary Assessment

Form a General Impression

The general impression gives you an overview of the patient and his or her current state. Determine the following information:

- Where is the patient?
- Does the patient appear to be in distress or pain?
- Is the patient standing, sitting, or lying down?
- Is the patient outside or inside?
- Does the patient have obvious injuries?
- What does the environment look like?
- Is there evidence of drug paraphernalia?
- What are the living conditions: clean, cluttered, dirty?
- Can the patient walk through the house without tripping?
- Is the patient conscious or unconscious?
- Is the patient in stable or unstable condition?

The answers to these questions can give you clues to the overall functioning of the patient's nervous system. Patients sitting in a home who state "It hurts right here" provide evidence of a functioning nervous system. Patients who are found unresponsive should be evaluated as being in unstable condition with obvious nervous system impairment. Examining the living conditions can provide insight into the general functioning of the brain. People who are emotionally depressed may not be able to manage cleaning the house. Cluttered or disorganized living conditions may be an indicator of a nervous system condition.

This information can be valuable because paramedics are an integral part of the total health care system. Your general impression of the patient not only provides you with assessment information needed to determine whether this is a critical patient, it also provides insight into the lives of your patients. This information can be used to help find the correct social service needs, help direct injury prevention education, assess what types of needs are present when the patient is discharged, and determine the effects of past interventions.

Airway and Breathing

Is the airway patent? Listen to the sound of air moving through the patient's mouth. Does it move freely? Is there any whistling sound? If the patient is awake, speak to him or her. One of the reasons that paramedics ask open-ended questions is to hear the patient speak. Listen to the sound of the patient's voice. Is the patient hoarse? Is his or her voice harsh or rough? Is this voice normal for the patient? If the patient is awake and speaking comfortably, it is obvious that he or she has a stable airway.

The trigeminal, glossopharyngeal, vagus, and hypoglossal nerves are responsible for airway control. These nerves allow for swallowing, controlling the tongue, and ensuring the muscles in the hypopharynx are slightly contracted. Alteration in the signals from these nerves can produce too much relaxation or too much constriction of the airway.

If the patient is not responding to stimuli, carefully assess the airway. Stridor is a classic sound that is created if a partial obstruction of the upper airway is present. This high-pitched sound, usually heard during inspiration, should cause you to investigate further. The patient may have tried to swallow food and aspirated instead. Another relatively common presentation is tightly clenched teeth. This state, called **trismus**, can make it difficult to manage the airway. Trismus can occur in conscious or unconscious patients. In the unconscious patient, this can indicate a seizure in progress, severe head injury, and/or cerebral hypoxia.

If you suspect an airway obstruction, evaluate the airway more closely. If the patient is not responding or is **posturing**, take a tongue blade or laryngoscope blade and closely examine the hypopharynx for obstructions. Have your Magill forceps ready to remove any objects. Be prepared to perform endotracheal intubation if after you clear the obstruction the patient is still having difficulty maintaining an airway. Ensure an oxygen saturation level of 94% or better. In the case of trismus, the patient may need to be sedated/paralyzed to relax the facial muscles causing the clenched teeth, allowing you to better control the airway. Finally, remember that routine hyperventilation of neurologic patients can be harmful. Provide hyperventilation only to those patients with documented unconsciousness *and* signs of increased intracranial pressure (ICP).

For additional information on rapid sequence intubation or airway obstruction clearance, refer to the chapter, *Airway Management and Ventilation*.

Table 3 Respiratory Patterns

Waveform	Pattern	Description	Causes
	Eupnea	Regular rate and pattern; inspiration and expiration are equal	Normal
	Tachypnea	Increased respiratory rate Regular pattern	Stimulants Exercise Excitement
	Bradypnea	Decreased respiratory rate Regular pattern	Narcotics
	Apnea	Absence of breathing	Severe hypoxia
	Hyperpnea	Rapid, regular, deep respirations	Stimulants Overdose Exercise
	Cheyne-Stokes	Gradual increases and decreases in respirations with periods of apnea	Pre-death pattern Brainstem injury
	Biot/Ataxic	Irregular respirations with periods of apnea; unpredictable	Brainstem injury
	Kussmaul	Extreme tachypnea and hyperpnea	Acidosis Diabetic ketoacidosis
	Apneustic	Prolonged inspiratory phase with shortened expiratory phase and bradypnea	Brainstem injury

As mentioned previously, the functions of breathing are controlled by the pons and the medulla oblongata. Check the rate and rhythm of the breathing. Breathing patterns are summarized in Table 3. Notice how the rhythms can have subtle changes or can be dramatically different from normal. The greater the deviation from normal, the more severely affected the nervous system is likely to be.

Circulation

Evaluate the peripheral and central pulse pressures. Are they the same? The absence of a peripheral pulse with a central pulse present should cause you to suspect shock. Shock is rarely caused *solely* by a neurologic problem. What is the characteristic of the skin? Is there evidence of gross bleeding? Is the pulse bounding?

If a patient has increased pressure within the cranium, there may be evidence from the vital signs. The blood pressure rises and the pulse rate and respiratory rate fall in the setting of increased ICP Table 4. This is called Cushing reflex, and is indicated by the following signs:

- Decreased pulse rate
- Decreased respiratory rate
- Widened pulse pressure (systolic hypertension)

This reflex is the opposite of what typically occurs in shock, when blood pressure falls and the pulse rate and respiratory rate climb. It is one of the hallmarks of increased ICP listed as follows:

- Cushing reflex
  - Bradycardia
  - Bradypnea
  - Widened pulse pressure (systolic hypertension)
- Decorticate posturing
- Decerebrate posturing
- Biot respirations
- Apneustic respirations
- Cheyne-Stokes respirations
- Anisocoria

Establish vascular access and administer normal saline or lactated Ringer's solution. Do not use solutions containing dextrose. Consider drawing blood samples for later analysis at the hospital. Check the patient's blood pressure and pulse rate.

Table 4 Vital Signs for Shock and Increased ICP

	Pulse Rate	Respiratory Rate	Blood Pressure	Pulse Pressure
Shock	↑	↑	↓	Narrowed
Increased ICP	↓	↓	↑	Widened

If the patient is hypotensive, support blood pressure to ensure adequate cerebral perfusion pressure (CPP). The target is a systolic blood pressure of 110 to 120 mm Hg. Perform continuous heart monitoring by means of a 12-lead ECG.

As the ICP rises, blood flow to the brain diminishes. To compensate, the medulla oblongata sends signals to the heart to increase the force of contraction. This causes systolic pressure to rise. If the ICP continues to increase, downward forces on the brainstem begin to damage the medulla's ability to send signals to the body. Diastole falls as the blood vessels relax or dilate. This results in a widened pulse pressure. Finally, this pressure also damages the ability to control the respiratory and pulse rates; consequently they both decrease.

Transport Decision

When you have completed the primary assessment, you now need to decide how to proceed. Is the patient in stable or unstable condition? Do you suspect a major underlying problem? Consider how to transport this patient. At this point, you have the following two choices:

1. Complete a rapid secondary assessment, which would involve a full head-to-toe approach, OR
2. Complete a secondary assessment and evaluate only the area(s) of the patient's complaint(s).

A rapid medical or trauma exam should be performed on any patient with an abdominal assessment, any patient with a significant MOI/NOI, or any patient whom you suspect may have a major problem. Examples would be a patient who is unconscious, is experiencing a seizure, or has a sudden loss of movement of the body.

If the patient is in stable condition, conducting a secondary assessment based on the complaint(s) is appropriate. These patients, such as those with headaches or non-traumatic back pain, have a completely normal primary assessment, have a minor MOI/NOI, and/or you suspect a local problem.

Be cautious, though. Just because a patient has a headache does not mean it is the result of a simple cause, such as stress. Stroke patients can also have headaches. If you suspect a more complicated problem, perform a rapid secondary assessment that covers the entire body. This expanded assessment will ensure that you are giving the patient the best possible care.

■ History Taking

Obtain a history from patients who are in stable condition and have only minor complaints. These include patients with a completely normal primary assessment and a minor MOI/NOI and for whom you suspect a localized problem.

If the patient is unresponsive, you will need to gather any history of the present illness from family or bystanders. If no one is around, quickly look for explanations for the altered mental status, including signs of trauma, medical alert tags, track marks, and environmental clues such as open alcohol or medication containers.

To determine the chief complaint in a responsive patient, begin by asking what happened. Look for signs and symptoms that may indicate the cause of the altered mental status, such as a stroke, and determine whether there is any evidence of the patient having had a seizure, such as incontinence or a bitten tongue. Evaluate the patient's speech. Is it slurred? Does the patient make sense?

If you know that the patient has had a seizure and is now in a postictal state, you will not be able to obtain a history. Look for any obvious explanation for why the patient had a seizure, such as trauma. If the patient has a headache, try to determine the patient's level of stress, the likelihood of infection, and the patient's history of headaches. If you believe a more complicated problem may be present, perform a more detailed evaluation.

YOU are the Medic   PART 2

The patient is awake and responding to his sons, although he is not acting normal. He recognizes his sons, but confuses their names. He knows where he is, but does not know the day of the week, the month, or even the year. His sons indicate this is unusual for him. He is speaking clearly in a loud voice.

Recording Time: 0 Minutes	
Appearance	Awake
Level of consciousness	Confused
Airway	Patent
Breathing	Adequate
Circulation	Adequate

3. **What assessment steps can you take to determine why the patient is confused?**
4. **What assumption should you make about the patient's communication with you and his sons?**

Determining the history from a child can be problematic. Age will determine how much interaction the pediatric patient is able to have. If the child is able to speak and understands the concept of time, talk to him or her to gather information. Also, talk to the parents. Parents can provide a lot of valuable information.

If the patient is responsive and breathing, obtain a SAMPLE history. Also try to speak with family or friends who can explain the events leading up to the altered mental status, remembering that time can be critical in a neurologic emergency. You may be the only person with the opportunity to obtain crucial information about the time of onset.

If family or friends report that the patient last seemed normal when he or she went to bed the night before, report that the time last seen normal was at bedtime, not when the patient awoke with symptoms. If the patient lives alone, talk to care providers, neighbors, or anyone else who might have had recent contact with the patient. Record family members' and friends' impressions of the patient's general state of health before the episode. List all medications the patient has taken, and gather the actual medication bottles if possible. Find out about the patient's medication allergies and when he or she last ate or drank anything, even water.

Documentation and Communication

Although a patient who has had a stroke might appear to be unresponsive and is unable to speak, he or she may still be able to hear and understand what is taking place. As with any patient, you should avoid making any remarks that might cause the patient distress. Look for indications that the patient understands you, such as a comprehending glance or gaze, a nod or other purposeful motion, pressure of the hand, or an effort to speak. Give the patient paper and a pen or pencil if he or she is able to write.

Reassure the patient that you understand that verbal communication may be difficult at this time but that you will keep him or her continually informed about what you and your team members are doing. Such compassionate communication can help you calm the patient and ease his or her fears, which are undoubtedly intensified by the inability to communicate.

Your SAMPLE history should reveal whether the patient has a history of seizures. If so, it is important to find out what tends to trigger them and whether this episode differs from previous ones. You should also find out what medications the patient takes. Phenytoin (Dilantin) and phenobarbital (for example, Solfoton) point strongly toward a seizure disorder. Your history may reveal that the patient has run out of medication or has stopped taking it. You may uncover coexisting conditions, such as diabetes. A patient who has diabetes and has a seizure may use up all the glucose in his or her body to fuel the seizure.

If a patient with no history of seizures is now experiencing a seizure for the first time, you should suspect a grave condition, such as a brain tumor, intracranial bleeding, or a serious infection. Determine whether the patient takes medications that lower the blood glucose level, such as insulin or oral hypoglycemic agents. Finally, inquire about drug use and exposure to toxins if appropriate.

Secondary Assessment

When you are performing the secondary assessment, it is important that you to conduct the physical examination in a consistent and organized fashion. This gives you a template for a quality assessment. Once you have memorized a standard assessment format, you can focus more on the abnormal findings than on what part of the body should be assessed next. Practice doing every assessment the same way. Repetition is the foundation of good assessment. This process keeps you from forgetting any assessment steps, such as assessing the pupils or listening to lung sounds. More importantly, it gives you more interaction with the patient, provides you with more "normal" findings so that you can more easily discover abnormal findings, and allows you to gain confidence in your skill in assessing routine patients. This hard work will pay off when you are confronted with a complex, critically ill patient who needs rapid, accurate assessment and treatment. Assess the patient in the following order:

1. **Head.** The head is the area in which you will spend the most time in a neurologic examination. Here is where you can gather critical information on the functioning of the nervous system. In addition, you will assess the head for trauma, including deformities, contusions, abrasions, penetrations, burns, tenderness, lacerations, and swelling (DCAP-BTLS). Even though this chapter focuses on the medical patient, a hands-on assessment for such anomalies provides you with valuable information.

2. **Neck.** Examine the neck for DCAP-BTLS. Look for symmetry. Are there masses? Examine the trachea. Is it midline? Look for jugular vein distention (JVD). Remember that JVD is best found along the lateral side of the neck near the ears. Palpate the posterior neck. Are the cervical vertebrae aligned?

3. **Chest.** Evaluate the chest for DCAP-BTLS. Look for symmetry in the chest's shape. Does the chest rise and fall equally? Many cardiac dysrhythmias can cause neurologic disorders by decreasing the amount of blood supplied to the brain. Apply the cardiac monitor and evaluate the ECG. If needed, obtain a 12-lead ECG. Examples of patients who will need a 12-lead include anyone with a sudden loss of consciousness. How much effort is the patient exhibiting to breathe? Is there any degree of respiratory distress? Listen to lung sounds. Evaluate for the presence of adventitious sounds and equality of sounds. If not already done, determine the pulse oximeter reading. Normal readings are 95% to 100%. Remember this number is affected by the amount of hemoglobin within the body and the presence of carbon monoxide.

4. **Abdomen.** Examine the abdomen for DCAP-BTLS. Are there any masses noted? Are any pulsations noted within the abdomen? Does the patient have any complaints within the abdomen? Signs of nausea and vomiting are common with some types of headaches.

5. **Pelvis.** Examine the pelvis for DCAP-BTLS. Is the pelvis stable to stress? If the patient is able to walk without assistance, the pelvis should be stable. Determine whether there is any incontinence. Urinary and/or fecal incontinence are common findings with seizures and fainting. Incontinence also acts as a relatively objective marker in determining the severity of illness in the unconscious patient. Obviously, patients are able to control their bowel and bladder functions when they are asleep. If incontinence is present, then the LOC has decreased below that of sleep.

6. **Extremities.** Examine for DCAP-BTLS and distal pulses, motor function, and sensation (PMS). Are there any signs of edema? Look for signs of recent venipuncture marks. Also note if these marks are at various stages of healing. Venipuncture marks may indicate recent illegal drug use.

7. **Back.** Examine the back for DCAP-BTLS. Examine the spine for appropriate curvature. The cervical vertebrae are curved posterior, the thoracic vertebrae are curved anterior, and the lumbar vertebrae are curved posterior. Feel along the spine to ensure the curves are in the correct places. Palpate each of the vertebrae, looking for pain, deformity, or instability.

As you perform the DCAP-BTLS assessment, notice the symmetry of the face. Is there any obvious facial droop? Look at the eyes. Are the eyelids even bilaterally? **Ptosis** is the medical term for the drooping, sagging, or prolapse of a part of the body. Eyelid ptosis can indicate Bell palsy or a stroke. **Figure 6** demonstrates facial droop and eyelid ptosis.

Level of Consciousness

There can be many variations in a patient's level of consciousness (LOC) and there are many ways to evaluate it. Your patient can be interacting appropriately with the environment or not at all. To better understand all the variations in LOC, refer to **Figure 7**. This figure shows a continuum from what most people would consider normal to a patient who has no responses whatsoever. The point on the extreme right side of the continuum (completely unresponsive to the environment) would be called coma. **Coma** is a state in which a person does not respond to verbal or painful stimuli. The points in between are guide markings. Patients do not stop at every point, of course, as the LOC increases or decreases. Nevertheless, these points provide you with an idea of the relationships among various levels of consciousness. Whereas the extremes of the scale are easy to understand, the points in the middle can be more difficult to interpret. The following section better explains these questionable areas.

AVPU Mnemonic

The **AVPU** mnemonic helps you make a broad assessment of the patient's LOC.

  A – Awake and alert (oriented to person, place, and day)
  V = Responds to verbal stimuli
  P = Responds to painful stimuli
  U = Unresponsive

This is a blunt assessment instrument designed to help you gather only the most basic information. For example, you are assessing a 43-year-old man who is sitting on a chair and he is reporting

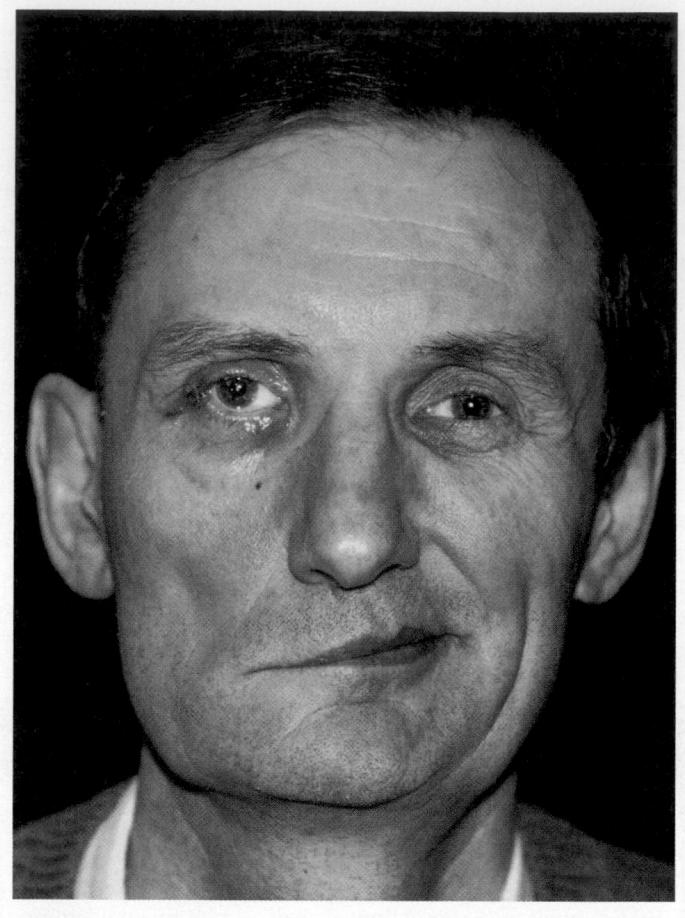

Figure 6 Facial droop and ptosis.

a headache. You introduce yourself and the patient immediately responds. He says that he has a headache and is in need of medical care. This patient would be evaluated as **A**wake. Now, assume the patient responds differently. He says that he is a famous rock star and asks you if you want his autograph. This patient would also be correctly evaluated as **A**wake and alert but clearly he is confused. **A**wake and alert means the patient is oriented to person, place, and day, and refers to the ability of the patient to respond to the environment with little external stimulation. Someone who is awake typically speaks to you and looks at you.

V is used for patients who are not spontaneously awake. When you arrive, you discover that the patient is not responding. The patient's eyes are closed. But when you approach the patient and announce yourself, the patient responds. Now the patient opens his eyes and makes eye contact—he may even speak to you. This patient would be appropriately evaluated as **V**erbal. Having an assessment of **V**erbal may indicate a seizure in progress, injury to the RAS, or merely that the patient was asleep.

Responding only to **P**ain is usually a more ominous finding. There are several ways for you to evaluate a patient's response to pain. For example, you have walked up to the patient and announced yourself, and the patient has not responded. Now, the goal is to elicit pain but not cause harm to the patient. For the patient to respond to pain, he or she needs a functioning brain,

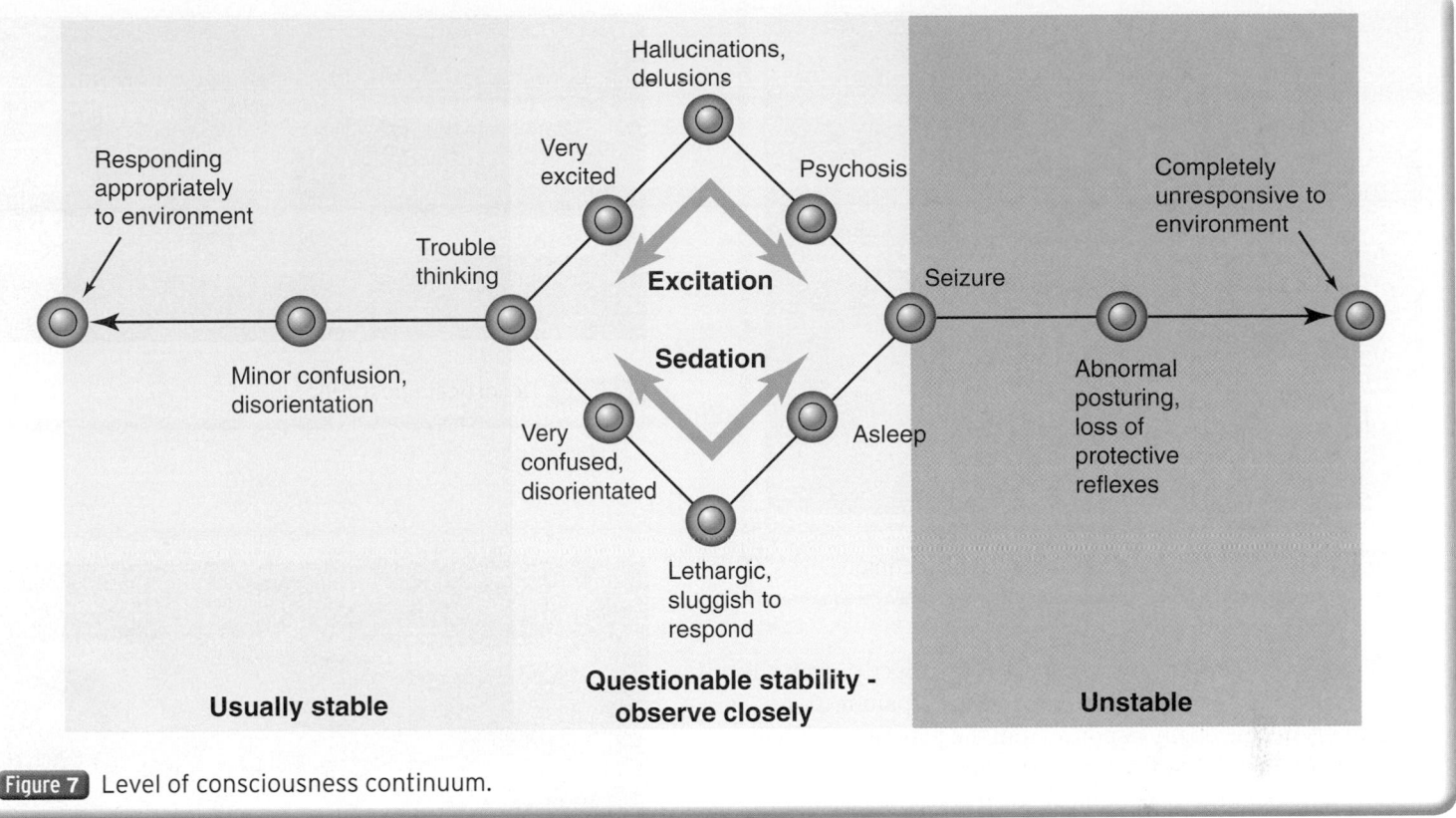

Figure 7 Level of consciousness continuum.

an intact spinal cord, and an intact peripheral nervous system. Here are some recommended methods for you to use to elicit noxious stimuli.

The first method is to apply fingernail pressure. Take a pen, penlight, or handle of a pair of trauma scissors. Hold one of the patient's fingers in your hand and place the finger between your index finger and your thumb. Now place the object between your thumb and the patient's finger. The object should be parallel to the nail bed. You want the object at the most proximal portion of the nail. Now squeeze the object against the nail. The more pressure applied, the more pain; however, the procedure should not cause trauma. The downside of this pain stimulation technique is that the patient must have an intact spinal cord to "feel" the pain Figure 8 .

Another assessment technique is to apply pressure to the **supraorbital foramen**. The supraorbital foramen is part of the frontal bone and feels like a notch near the bridge of the nose. Place your thumb in the upper, inner orbit and feel for a notch about 1 to 2 cm lateral to the bridge of the nose. With the tip of your thumb, apply pressure in an inward, upward manner over the top of this notch. This action will generate a significant amount of pain. This is another area of the body in which more pressure increases the degree of pain quickly. When done correctly, no trauma should occur to the patient. This response does not require that the patient have an intact spinal cord, so it is ideal pain stimulation for patients with back trauma or spina bifida within the thoracic spine Figure 9 .

There are some precautions you must take with this procedure. First you will be applying pressure to the head, so ensure that the patient does not have a facial fracture. Second, the

pressure should be applied along the upper, inner orbital ridge. Do not apply pressure directly onto the eye. Finally, this procedure is technique sensitive. If your thumb is too far to the left or right of the supraorbital foramen, the patient will not experience

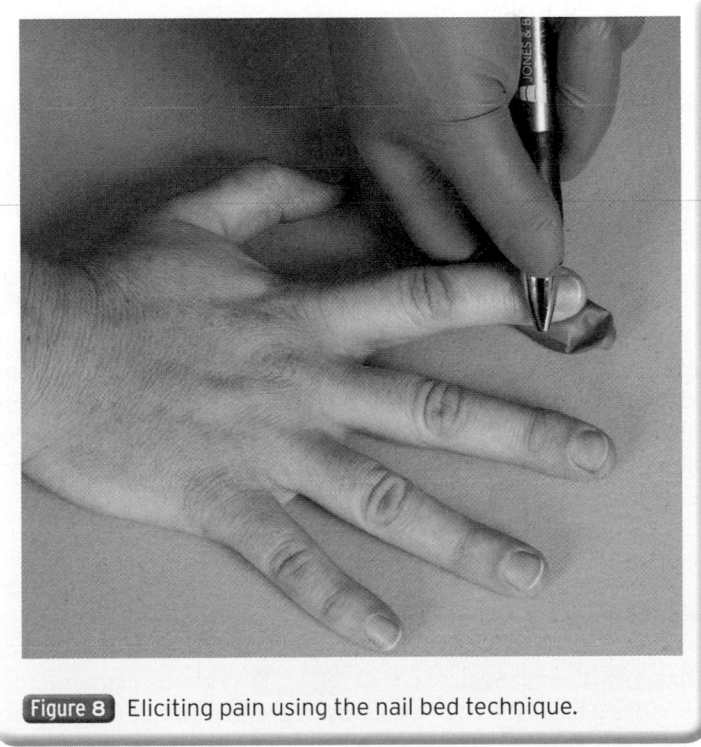

Figure 8 Eliciting pain using the nail bed technique.

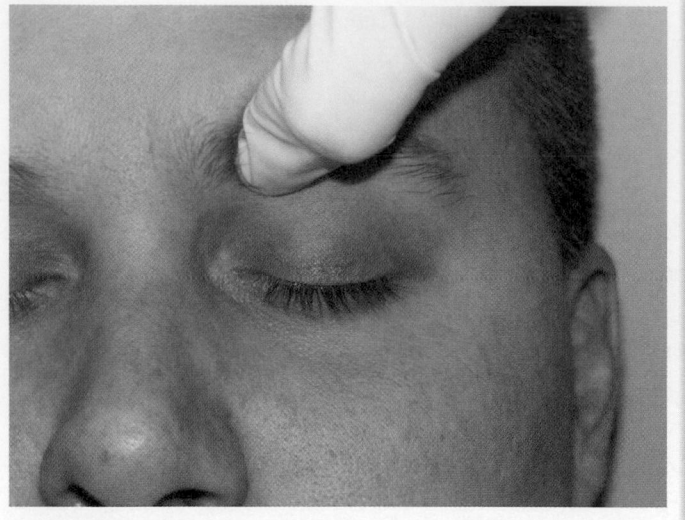

Figure 9 Eliciting pain using the supraorbital technique.

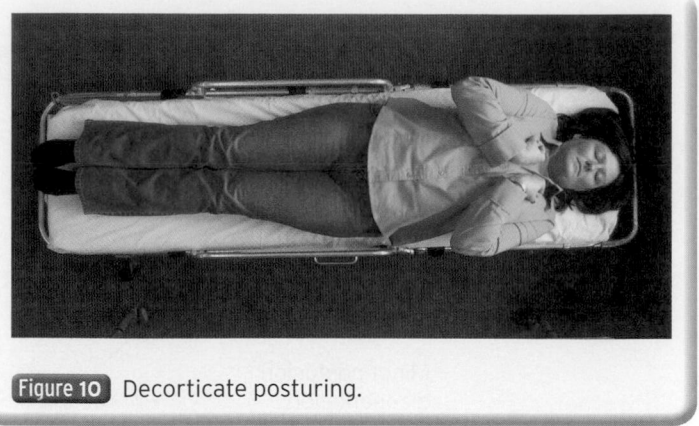

Figure 10 Decorticate posturing.

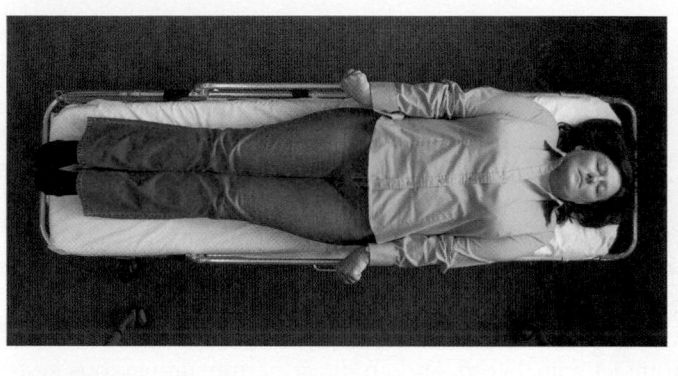

Figure 11 Decerebrate posturing.

great discomfort. Your thumb needs to be directly over the foramen (the notch) for this technique to elicit a pain response.

As you generate a pain response from the patient, what happens? Does the patient wake up? Does the patient move away from the pain? Does the patient move in an abnormal fashion? Is there abnormal posturing that occurs with any painful stimulation? There are two main abnormal postures that a patient can exhibit when exposed to painful stimulation. It is important to understand that this posturing occurs in patients who are otherwise unresponsive. You may notice these postures during IV insertion. The patient may involuntarily move once the painful stimulus occurs. These postures are not conscious and if you see either of these postures, you should immediately consider your patient to be critical.

The first posture is decorticate (remember bending the arms toward the "core" of the patient). In **decorticate posturing**, patients contract their arms and curl them toward their chest. At the same time, they point their toes. Finally the wrists are flexed. This is also called abnormal flexion. This posture may indicate damage to the area directly below the cerebral hemispheres **Figure 10**.

The other abnormal posture is called **decerebrate posturing** or abnormal extension. In this posture, patients again point their toes, but now extend their arms outward and rotate the lower arms in a palms-down manner (called **pronation**). The wrists are again flexed. This type of posturing is a more severe finding than decorticate posturing. In decerebrate, the level of damage is within or near the brainstem (diencephalon/pons/midbrain) **Figure 11**.

The final level of the AVPU system is **U**. The **U**nresponsive patient does not respond in any way to your stimulus.

Glasgow Coma Scale

One tool to assist with the consistent evaluation of LOC is the **Glasgow Coma Scale (GCS)** **Table 5**. This assessment tool provides a basis for you to determine the severity of the patient's

illness or injury. The GCS uses parameters that test a patient's eye opening, best verbal response, and best motor response. The three numeric scores are added together to form a total score that defines the patient's brain function.

This tool is useful in helping you determine how to proceed with patient care, what care should be given, and where the patient should be transported. **Table 6** provides general guidelines for using GCS scores. Mildly ill patients need care that conforms to standard care guidelines. Usually you can honor the patient's request to be transported to a particular hospital. Patients with moderate conditions require you to make more challenging decisions. They are not critically ill but are considered to be in unstable condition; therefore, your most appropriate action should be to perform close assessment and provide transport to the closest appropriate facility. Critically ill patients need airway management and rapid transportation to the closest appropriate hospital.

Orientation

As already discussed, you can use the AVPU system or the Glasgow Coma Scale to evaluate LOC. Another LOC system to consider is orientation. Orientation tests mental status by checking a patient's memory and thinking ability. The most common test evaluates a patient's ability in four areas:

Table 5 Glasgow Coma Scale

	Adult	Pediatric (<5 y)
Eye opening	4. Spontaneous	4. Spontaneous
	3. Voice	3. To shout/voice
	2. Pain stimulation	2. Pain stimulation
	1. None	1. None
Verbal	5. Oriented	5. Cry, smile, coo, words correct for age
	4. Disoriented	4. Cries, inappropriate words for age
	3. Inappropriate words	3. Inappropriate scream or cry
	2. Incomprehensible	2. Grunts
	1. None	1. None
Motor	6. Obeys	6. Spontaneous
	5. Localizes pain	5. Localizes pain
	4. Withdraws from pain	4. Withdraws from pain
	3. Decorticate	3. Decorticate
	2. Decerebrate	2. Decerebrate
	1. None	1. None

Table 6 Interpretations of Glasgow Coma Scale Scores

Score	Interpretation	Treatment	Facility
13-15	Mild	Ensure adequate oxygen, glucose, and temperature to promote proper nervous system functioning	Patient's or family's choice
9-12	Moderate	Close airway assessment Watch for decreasing consciousness	Closest appropriate facility
8 or less	Critical	May need airway/ ventilation control Decrease scene time	Closest appropriate facility

- **Person** The patient is able to give his or her name.
- **Place** The patient is able to identify his or her current location.

- **Time** The patient is able to tell you the current year, month, and approximate date.
- **Event** The patient is able to describe what happened (the MOI or NOI).

If the patient knows these facts, the patient is said to be alert. If you determine the patient does not know these facts, he or she is considered less than fully oriented.

Patients may be confused. Confusion may indicate a low blood glucose level, decreased oxygen level, overdose, or even decreased blood pressure. Ensure that you are asking questions to which you know the answers if you are trying to determine the level of confusion. Some degree of confusion may be appropriate for the situation. After waking someone from a deep sleep, some confusion is to be expected.

As you are determining a patient's level of orientation, examine the speed and intensity at which the patient responds. Generally, patients either undergo excitation or sedation. As you are talking, does the patient appear to be sleepy? Is the patient sluggish? Is the patient talking quickly and unable to sit still? How many words are in the sentences the patient uses? Do you have to speak loudly at the patient in order to get a response?

Common Reality

Hallucinations are sensory stimulation the patient experiences that are not based in a **common reality**. People use their senses to determine what is real. If you see flames, smell smoke, and feel heat, there must be a fire. But what if all of these sensations are purely in your mind? One way to determine that the sensations you are experiencing are real is to ask others what they are experiencing. If there are others who also see flames, smell smoke, and feel heat, then the fire is real. This is called a common reality: sensory stimulation that can be confirmed by others.

In **hallucinations**, patients can hear voices, see snakes, feel insects, smell burning paper, or taste metal. All of these experiences are completely within their mind. There are no outside observers who can also hear, see, feel, smell, or taste the same things. The patient believes the snakes on the ground are *real.* If the patient is afraid of snakes, he or she will be frightened. Tell the patient that you do not see the snake but you understand that he or she does see it. Your task here is to not reinforce the hallucination. Try to bring the patient back to a common reality, but do not argue if the patient is insistent. Reassure the patient that he or she is safe.

Delusions are similar to hallucinations. Delusions are thoughts or perceived abilities that are also not based in a common reality. Examples of delusions include persons who believe they can fly or that everyone is out to get them. As with hallucinations, you should try to redirect patients, but do not argue with them.

As delusions and hallucinations increase, the patient may move farther and farther away from a common reality. Eventually, the amount of shared reality between you and your patient becomes so minimal that the patient can no longer determine what is real and what is inside his or her mind. This state is called **psychosis**. Psychotic patients can be unpredictable. They are responding to a barrage of stimulation that no one else can experience. They are struggling to interact with a "world" in which the rules are constantly changing. Fear, anger, and helplessness are common emotions when a patient is in this state.

When caring for patients who are experiencing psychosis, ensure your safety. Because of the unpredictable nature of psychotic patients, ensure you are not alone with the patient and have a clear avenue of retreat. Your job is to decrease stimulation as much as possible. Limit the number of voices talking to the patient to one. Give clear, simple commands and be ready to patiently repeat those commands. Do not place the patient in a dimly lit room or ambulance. The shadows can be interpreted as harmful. Medication may be needed to help manage hallucinations, delusions, and psychosis. For more recommendations on the management of patients with hallucinations, delusions, and/or psychosis, see the chapter, *Psychiatric Emergencies.*

Other Changes

Changes in the patient's mood or the tempo of the nervous system should alert you to changes in the patient's neurologic status. The oxygen level or blood pressure could be falling. Body temperature could be climbing. A psychiatric condition can be escalating. The level of blood glucose could be critically low or high. Regardless of the underlying cause, this observation of a change requires you to further evaluate the patient to ensure the appropriate level of care. Mood or affect is another attribute that provides insight into the patient. Ask the patient how he or she feels. Frustration, anger, or aggression can be caused by a low glucose or oxygen level.

As you speak to the patient, ask how easy it is for him or her to think. A patient who has a decreased blood glucose level or is taking narcotics can have trouble concentrating. Low blood glucose levels and narcotics tend to sedate the nervous system. Patients who are taking cocaine can also have difficulty concentrating, but not because of slower functioning. Cocaine is a sympathomimetic so it increases nervous system activity. These patients experience mania. Their thoughts can tumble in quickly, so they find it hard to concentrate. If the speed of nervous system activity continues to increase, the patient may hallucinate, become delusional, or become psychotic.

Corneal Reflex

A quick, simple way for you to determine indirectly whether the patient's cough and gag reflexes are intact is to assess the **corneal reflex**, which protects the eyes from trauma. This reflex closes the eyelids, pulls the head posteriorly, and constricts the pupils when an object either touches the eyes or eyelids or moves quickly toward the eyes.

To see whether this reflex is present, tap between the patient's eyes. Patients who are asleep or pretending to be unconscious will blink reflexively with each tap. Even if the eyes are closed tightly, you should see the eyelids twitch.

If you tap lightly between the eyes and the patient does not blink or twitch, you should assume that the patient does not have an intact cough or gag reflex and will not be able to protect the airway. Insert an oral airway. If the patient does not cough or gag, you have confirmed that the airway is unprotected and should take measures to protect it. The presence of the corneal reflex does not guarantee that the cough and gag reflexes are intact. If you remain doubtful about the patient's ability to protect the airway, attempt to insert an oral airway.

Pupillary Response

When you are assessing the patient's eyes, you need to ensure that you are eliciting a reaction to light, and not movement. To limit the corneal reflex, take your light pen and approach the eyes from a 45° angle. This should ensure that the pupils are reacting to the light itself, rather than to the approach of the light pen.

Examine the pupils for shape, size, and reactivity. The pupils should be round, respond quickly to a light by constricting, and be equal in size, shape, and response. Pupillary shape can be changed by trauma, glaucoma, or increased ICP. Pupil size is measured in millimeters. A quick way to determine size is to imagine how many dimes can be stacked across the pupil. The width (thickness) of a dime is close to a millimeter. You can certainly use the gauge on the side of the light pen (if present) for a more accurate measurement.

Generally speaking, stimulants cause pupillary dilation. Remember the flight-or-fight sympathetic response caused by epinephrine. If someone is trying to attack you, you will need to see as much of the world as possible in order to defend yourself effectively or retreat. Your eyes, then, need as much light as

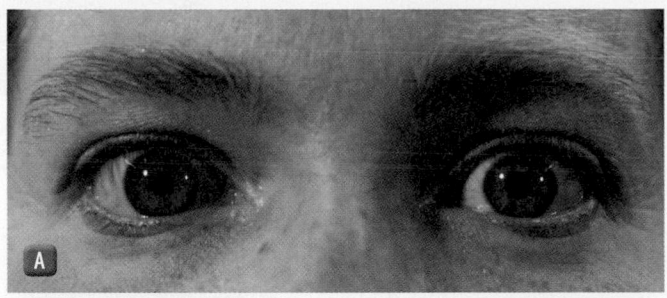

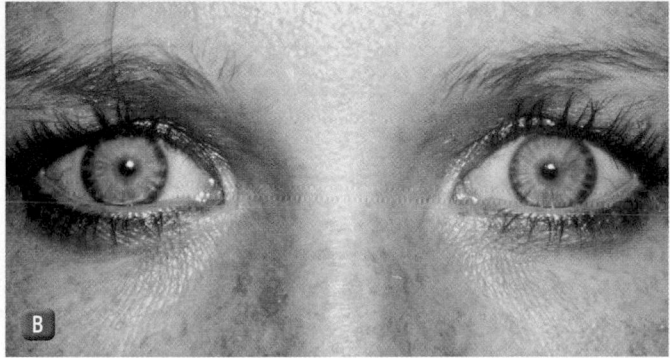

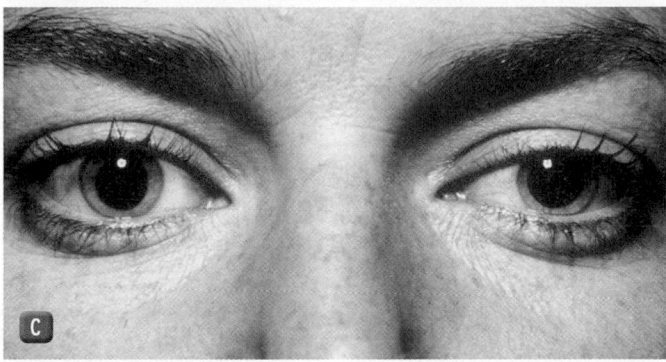

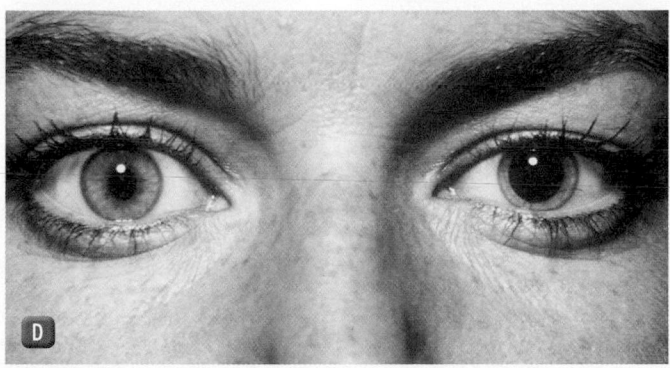

Figure 12 Pupil responses. **A.** Normal. **B.** Constricted. **C.** Dilated. **D.** Unequal (anisocoria).

possible. Cocaine, methamphetamines, and hallucinogens also tend to cause pupil dilation. Conversely, depressants tend to constrict the pupils.

Equality of pupils is an important observation. Unequal pupils are called <u>anisocoria</u>. Many people have a slight inequality in pupillary size. Anything greater than a 1-mm

difference is worth noting. As pressure increases within the skull, the brainstem can be squeezed. This squeezing can interrupt signals to one pupil, resulting in pupils that are dramatically different in size. Unequal pupils are a sign of increased ICP **Figure 12** .

Cranial Nerve Functioning

Assessment of the head includes gathering information on the functioning of the cranial nerves. These peripheral nerves control various portions of the body. Refer to **Table 7** for more information on the functions of the cranial nerves and how they are assessed. When performing this assessment, you are looking for the patient's ability to respond, strength of response, and symmetry. Patients with stroke, trigeminal neuralgia, <u>myasthenia gravis</u>, or other conditions may demonstrate abnormal cranial nerve functioning.

Speech

Listen to the quality of the patient's speech. Is it slurred? Slurring is a classic finding with stroke. It the speech appropriate? You need to focus on not only the quality of the words that are spoken but the appropriateness of those words. There are several situations in which speech may be clear but word choice is incorrect. Assess the patient's object recognition abilities.

When a patient has <u>agnosia</u>, he or she is unable to tell you the names of common objects. In agnosia (a = without, gnosis = knowledge), damage has occurred to the connections between visual interpretation of objects and the words that are associated with the objects. <u>Apraxia</u> (a = without, praxis = movement or action) refers to the inability to know how to use a common object. It is possible for patients to be speaking clearly and yet have these subtle knowledge deficits.

To test for these signs, show the patient your pen, or scissors, or a set of keys. Ask the patient, "What is the name of this object?" If the patient responds correctly, hand him or her the object and ask him or her to show you how he or she would use the object. Patients may have one of these signs without the other. One is not a more severe finding than the other. Both signs simply indicate that there is some degree of misfiring of neurons between the occipital lobe and temporal lobe (agnosia) or between the temporal lobe and the frontal lobe (apraxia). It is possible for patients to have both slurred speech and object recognition difficulties.

Language can be affected by injury or disease. In aphasia, a person's speech is affected. The three main forms of aphasia are as follows:

1. **Receptive aphasia.** A person with <u>receptive aphasia</u> is unable to understand (receive) speech, but is able to speak clearly. This dysfunction indicates damage to the temporal lobe. To determine whether the patient has receptive aphasia, ask questions to which you and the patient know the answer, such as "Who is the president?" and "What month is it?" You should not ask yes/no questions. If the patient speaks clearly but gives you incorrect answers, he or she may have receptive aphasia.

Table 7   Assessment of Cranial Nerve Function

Nerve	Function	Assessment Technique
I. Olfactory	Smell	Not usually assessed. Can use an ammonia inhalant or other known scent.
II. Optic	Vision	Place finger in front of patient's face. Can he or she see the finger?
III. Oculomotor	Movement of the eye, pupil, and eyelid	Have the patient follow your finger as you move it in an "H" shape. Have the patient blink.
IV. Trochlear	Movement of the eye	Have the patient follow your finger as you move it in an "H" shape. Have the patient blink.
V. Trigeminal	Chewing Pain Temperature Touch of the mouth and face	Have the patient smile.
VI. Abducens	Movement of the eye	Have the patient follow your finger as you move it in an "H" shape. Have the patient blink.
VII. Facial	Movement of the face Tears Salivation and taste	Have the patient smile.
VIII. Auditory	Hearing and balance	Have the patient follow your spoken commands.
IX. Glossopharyngeal	Swallowing, taste, and sensations in the mouth and pharynx	Have the patient smile and then swallow.
X. Vagus	Sensation and movement of the pharynx, larynx, thorax, and GI system	Have the patient swallow.
XI. Accessory	Movement of the head and shoulders	Have the patient shrug his or her shoulders (hold on to both shoulders at the same time to assess their symmetry).
XII. Hypoglossal	Movement of the tongue	Have the patient stick out his or her tongue.

2. **Expressive aphasia.** A person with <u>expressive aphasia</u> is unable to speak (express him- or herself) clearly, but is able to understand speech. This dysfunction is caused by damage to the frontal lobe, which controls the motor function of speech. Simply ask the patient to raise his arm. If he does, he can understand you. Then ask him his name. Lack of response or a slurred response indicates expressive aphasia.

3. **Global aphasia.** <u>Global aphasia</u> is characterized by features of both expressive and receptive aphasia. The patient cannot follow commands or answer questions. It is important to remember that such patients often can think clearly. They have needs, anxieties, and discomforts, but no way to express them. This dysfunction can be frightening to patients who cannot understand what you are saying and cannot respond to your questions despite being able to formulate the answers in their minds. Be sensitive to this

condition and reassure the patient by moving slowly and purposefully, using therapeutic touch, and maintaining good eye contact.

Body Movement
Hemiparesis and Hemiplegia
Observe how the patient moves. Does the body move equally on both sides? Patients with strokes can have weakness or paralysis of one side of the body. Weakness of one side of the body is called <u>hemiparesis</u>. Paralysis of one side of the body is called <u>hemiplegia</u>. At times, you will assess patients who have weakness on one side of the body but facial droop on the other side. This can occur because of the process of <u>decussation</u>, the crossing of nerves as they leave the cerebral cortex, move through the brainstem, and arrive at the spinal cord. Nerves that decussate originate on one side of the brain and cross over to control the opposite side of the body. In a patient who has had a left cerebral

stroke, for example, the patient would have right-sided arm and leg weakness, as well as right-sided facial droop because the left side of the brain controls the right side of the body.

Examining the functioning of the cerebellum can also give you information about possible damage to the brain. Have the patient close his or her eyes and hold out the arms in front of the body at the same level. With the eyes closed, the patient's only way to tell where his or her arms are located is from the sensations being processed by the cerebellum. If the patient has had a stroke, one of the arms may drift away from the other Figure 13.

Gait and Posture

Some patients have alterations in their gait (walking patterns). Ataxia is the term used to describe alteration of a person's ability to perform coordinated motions such as walking. A person's gait can become slow, shuffling, or scissors-like, for example.

Unless there is some medical reason to avoid it, have the patient walk for several steps. Assessing gait is another test of activity of the cerebellum. In reality, walking is actually a controlled fall because as you move your center of gravity

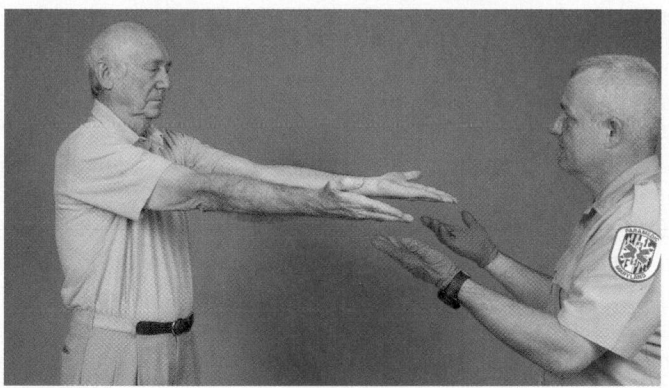

A

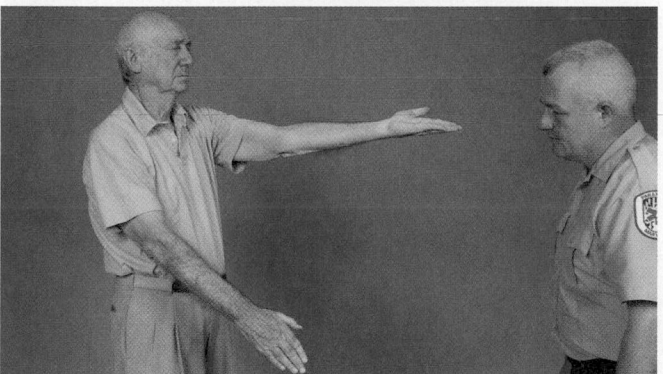

B

Figure 13   **A.** A person who has not had a stroke will be able to hold both arms in front of the body even with his or her eyes closed. **B.** A person who has had a stroke might not be able to maintain this position. One arm will drift down and turn toward the body.

forward, you must move a leg forward to catch yourself. Once you learn how to walk, your cerebellum controls the mechanics of this activity and allows you to focus on where you want to walk, not how to walk. If there is damage to the cerebellum, you may observe your patient walking erratically, stumbling, or even losing the ability to walk.

In addition to alterations in gait, a patient's posture may become rigid. Have your patient stand straight. Place one hand on the patient's chest and your other hand behind the patient's back. Now push on the chest. Normally, as you push backward, the patient compensates quickly by taking a step to keep from falling. In patients with certain disorders, such as **Parkinson disease**, the patient's rigidity does not allow him or her to compensate quickly enough, and you will push the patient over. It is important to have a hand behind the patient to keep the patient from falling.

Bizarre Movement

Patients can exhibit bizarre movement that indicates disruption within the nervous system. **Myoclonus** is a type of rapid, jerky muscle contraction that occurs involuntarily. Most people have experienced myoclonic jerks. A classic example of this phenomenon is the student who is about to fall asleep in class. As the student gets sleepier, the head begins to sag, until the head involuntarily jerks upward and the student wakes up. This startled response is called a *myoclonic jerk*.

Another form of bizarre movement is called **dystonia**. In this movement, a part of the body contracts and remains contracted. Dystonia is discussed later in this chapter.

Alterations in Smooth Motion

As you are assessing your patient, does he or she move smoothly? This type of action requires proper functioning of the frontal lobe, cerebellum, brainstem, spinal cord, and peripheral nerves. When these structures are functioning correctly, muscle groups alternately contract and relax, allowing the body to move. When this fine balance is upset, patients may have **rigidity** (stiffness of motion).

Tremors are another example of an alteration in smooth motion. This fine, oscillating (back and forth) movement usually occurs in the hands and head. Several types of tremor exist, named for the kind of activity that elicits them:

- **Rest tremor**—occurs with the patient at rest and not moving.
- **Intention tremor**—occurs when the patient is asked to reach out and grab an object. It is common for this tremor to increase as the patient gets closer to the object to be grabbed.
- **Postural tremor**—occurs when a body part is placed in a particular position and required to maintain that position for a long period of time. Most people have experienced this type of tremor when working hard for a long time. As fatigue sets in, the body parts being used the most begin to shake. A postural tremor can also occur when a person is standing. The body's muscles are constantly making tiny corrections to maintain posture. The head can oscillate back and forth as the person tries to keep it still.

A type of movement that may appear similar to a tremor is a seizure. Whereas a tremor is a fine movement, a seizure is a larger, less focused type of movement. Seizures are associated with either tonic or clonic activity, described as follows:

- Tonic activity is a rigid, contracted body posture. The arms, legs, neck, and back can contract so tightly that the body part shakes from the intensity of the contraction.
- Clonic activity is characterized by rhythmic contraction and relaxation of muscle groups. Clonic activity can be described as the bizarre, non-purposeful movement of any body part. Arms and legs may flail, teeth may clench, the head may bob, and the torso may convulse wildly.

Sensation

The last area for you to assess is sensation within the body. Many nervous system conditions can alter the ability to feel pain, temperature, pressure, or light touch. A sensation of numbness or tingling is called paresthesia. If the patient can feel nothing within a body part, this is called anesthesia.

Blood Glucose Level

Glucose is the fuel that runs the brain. The brain uses glucose faster than any other part of the body and it has no means to store glucose. All patients with a change in LOC should have their blood glucose level checked. A normal blood glucose reading is 60 to 120 mg/dL. As the glucose level falls, so does the LOC. The patient's LOC can be affected by a high blood glucose level; however, the level must increase significantly before the LOC is diminished. A glucose level of below 10 mg/dL is incompatible with brain functioning and is usually fatal. Generally, if the level of blood glucose falls below 30 mg/dL or rises above 300 mg/dL, the patient will become confused or unconscious. Blood glucose monitoring is now the standard of care for the patient with an altered LOC.

Vital Signs

In the patient who is having a stroke or seizure, check and document the pulse rate, rhythm, and quality; respiratory rate, rhythm, and quality; blood pressure; skin temperature, color, and condition; and pupil size and reactivity.

Given how critical normal cerebral perfusion is, you must closely monitor blood pressure in any patient with the potential for increased ICP. Frequent assessment becomes even more essential when the blood pressure has dropped. Ensure that the patient maintains a systolic blood pressure of at least 110 to 120 mm Hg. Ensure adequate respiratory rate and pattern, and effective pulse rate and rhythm.

Changes in pupil size or reactivity indicate significant bleeding and pressure on the brain. If the patient has an altered mental status, regardless of the cause, check the blood glucose level if you have a glucometer available. During most active seizures, it is impossible to evaluate vital signs, and doing so is not a priority. Unless the situation is unusual, vital signs obtained during the postictal state will be close to normal.

The patient's temperature can be difficult to determine in the prehospital setting. If hypothermia or hyperthermia is suspected, the standard of care is to use a thermometer to establish the patient's temperature. An oral, otic, transdermal, or rectal temperature can be used. You should avoid using the axillary method.

Not all EMS systems have the ability to check a patient's temperature with a thermometer. You can nevertheless gather information about the NOI that will allow you to identify a temperature alteration. For example, was the patient in the water or in wet clothing for a long period of time? Has the patient been in snow? Did the patient fall and lie on the floor of his or her home for several days? In such cases, you should consider hypothermia. It would be reasonable to cover the patient with blankets and turn up the heat in the patient compartment. Alternatively, are you treating a patient who has been in the hot sun for several hours? Is the patient's skin hot and dry? Does the patient have a history of fever? In such situations, it would be prudent to remove the patient's clothing, cover the patient with a sheet, and turn off the heat in the patient compartment.

Do not actively rewarm or cool such patients. Refer to the chapter, *Environmental Emergencies* for guidance in active rewarming and cooling for environmentally induced temperature alterations.

Reassessment

Interventions

Administration of Dextrose 50% (D_{50})

Follow your local protocol regarding what blood glucose reading is considered low. One guideline to consider is if the blood glucose level is below 60 mg/dL, glucose is needed. Two medications are available prehospital for the treatment of hyperglycemia: dextrose 50% in water (D_{50}) and glucagon. When you are administering D_{50}, an IV line must be established. This access site should be in a large vessel. An 18-gauge needle is preferred because D_{50} is thick and difficult to administer. Ensure that the IV is patent *before* administering the D_{50}. Extravasation of D_{50} into the interstitial space can cause severe damage or death to muscles, nerves, and skin. The usual dose of D_{50} is 25 g or one full syringe. The effects of D_{50} typically begin in 30 seconds to 2 minutes. If the D_{50} has no effect or if the patient's blood glucose level remains low, ensure adequate IV access and administer a second dose.

There have been cases of dextrose shortages throughout the country. One solution to this problem is to give D_{25} (12.5 g per syringe) but give two syringes. This would give the patient twice as much volume but the exact same amount of dextrose as is found within a D_{50}.

Thiamine may be needed before the administration of D_{50}. Patients who are severely malnourished, such as chronic alcoholics, may have insufficient supplies of vitamin B_1 (thiamine) to adequately metabolize dextrose. Thiamine is needed to convert dextrose to glucose. If extreme malnourishment is suspected, thiamine should be administered before D_{50}. In cases where you are unsure, thiamine can be administered. The typical dose in an emergent situation is 50 mg by slow IV bolus or IM. Thiamine can cause hypotension if administered too quickly. If IV access cannot be obtained, then administer 0.5 to 1 mg of glucagon subcutaneously or intramuscularly. This naturally occurring body chemical is responsible for converting the body's stores of glycogen into glucose. Thiamine is not needed for glucagon to be effective. You should see an increase in the LOC and blood glucose level within 20 minutes of administration. If the blood glucose level remains low, repeat the glucagon to a maximum of three doses.

If the blood glucose level is high, there is currently no safe way to decrease blood glucose in the prehospital setting. Administration of insulin can be problematic because it is easy to over-correct the imbalance, resulting in a hypoglycemic state. Ensure adequate support of blood pressure. Hyperglycemic patients are often dehydrated and may need volume support.

Finally, be cautious in patients whose blood glucose level cannot be checked. If the patient is unresponsive or has decreased LOC and no blood glucose monitor is available, administer 12.5 g (½ syringe) of D_{50} and then reassess the patient for response. Proceed with additional dextrose cautiously, based on responses to previous doses. Hyperglycemia can increase the morbidity of stroke patients.

Airway Management

Several conditions exist in which patients are unable to protect the airway adequately and cannot adequately ventilate themselves. The use of bag-mask devices, laryngeal mask airways (LMAs), King LT airway devices, Combitubes, or endotracheal intubation should be initiated to provide sufficient oxygen, ventilation, and airway protection. Endotracheal intubation is the most effective means by which to isolate and protect the trachea from aspiration, although you must be proficient in this skill for it to succeed. Ensure that the patient's pulse oximeter reading is 95% or better. Provide oxygen via nasal cannula or mask as needed. Provide ventilatory assistance as needed.

As mentioned previously, neurologic patients can have changes to their muscle tone within their face and mouth. If trismus is noted, initially determine how effectively the patient can be ventilated with a bag-mask device. If ventilation is poor or unsuccessful, a nasotracheal airway can be attempted, as long as the patient is still breathing on his or her own. If this is unsuccessful, consider a paralytic agent to relax the mouth and allow for airway management. If paralytics are not available or contraindicated and the patient cannot be ventilated, then transtracheal airway management is the only remaining option to prevent hypoxia and death. For further information on how to manage the complicated airway, refer to the chapter, *Airway Management and Ventilation*.

Administration of Naloxone

Naloxone (Narcan) is used for the treatment of unresponsive/ unknown patients or those with suspected narcotic overdose. The initial dose is 0.4 to 2 mg IVP. You may repeat this dose until you reach 10 mg. This narcotic antagonist competes with any circulating narcotic, displacing it from its receptors, and allowing the LOC to increase. Naloxone can result in quite dramatic effects when used. Patients who had a GCS score of 3 can move to 15 within 30 seconds. This rapid change in LOC can cause patients to become fearful and potentially angry or aggressive.

Ensure that you have either adequate support to restrain the patient or the ability to leave the scene quickly before you administer naloxone (Narcan). Administer the naloxone slowly until respiratory effort improves. Some EMS systems are waiting to administer enough naloxone to wake up the patient completely until they arrive at the emergency department. This ensures that adequate personnel are present if the patient becomes violent.

Airway management in relation to narcotic overdose can also be complicated. Airway and ventilation are the focus of a large percentage of the care that you provide. When you encounter a severely bradypneic, cyanotic patient, it is reflexive to want to establish an airway and intubate the patient quickly. When considering administering naloxone (Narcan), a slightly different approach is warranted.

Ensure airway control and adequate BLS ventilation but do not immediately intubate the patient. As you are oxygenating, establish an IV line and administer the naloxone (or consider IM dose if there are limited IV access sites). With such a short onset of action time for this drug and such a dramatic potential response, the patient may quickly wake up after the naloxone, grab the ET tube, and pull it out. This provides a mechanism for vocal cord or tracheal trauma during the violent extubation. If after you administer the medication there is no response, then intubation may be needed.

Rectal Administration of Diazepam

In patients who are experiencing a seizure and IV access cannot be established, diazepam (Valium) can be administered via the rectal route. The dose is 0.2 mg/kg. The procedure is as follows:

- Take standard precautions.
- Draw up the appropriate dose, then remove and dispose of the needle.
- Attach a 2″, 14-gauge angiocatheter to the end of the syringe only, then remove and dispose of the angio needle.
- Insert the plastic catheter into the rectum until the entire catheter is within the rectum. The entire syringe remains outside body.
- Inject the medication and remove catheter.
- Hold patient's buttocks together for at least 5 minutes.

Communication and Documentation

Notify the receiving facility of your patient's chief complaint and your assessment findings. Most designated stroke centers will want you to call a stroke alert for patients you have assessed and found to be having a stroke (check your local protocol). This will alert the stroke team members at the hospital and give them time to assemble their resources to treat the patient without delay. Be sure to communicate the time that the patient was last seen to be healthy, the findings of your neurologic examination, and the time you anticipate arriving at the hospital.

A key piece of information to document is the time of onset of the patient's signs and symptoms. If the diagnosis is an ischemic stroke, the time of onset of the signs and symptoms is critical in determining whether the patient is a candidate for treatment with clot-dissolving (fibrinolytic) drugs. It is also important to document your findings from your stroke scale and the score of the GCS, along with any changes you found during your reassessment. Document airway management and interventions performed, including the position in which the patient was placed. Also document any change in the patient during transport and the reason for the choice of hospital.

For patients who have had a seizure, give a description of the seizure activity, if known. Include bystanders' comments if they witnessed the seizure. Document the onset and duration of the seizure. Did the patient notice or express noticing an aura? Record any evidence of trauma and interventions performed. Document whether this is the patient's first seizure or whether the patient has a history of seizures. If the latter, how often does he or she have them, and is there any history of status epilepticus? When you document your interventions, record the time each intervention was performed, how the patient responded to the intervention, and what the findings of continued reassessments showed.

You may be the only provider to witness some patient activity, so accurate documentation is critical to the continuity of care. Avoid using words that can have multiple meanings, such as "lethargic," "sleepy," "obtunded," and "out of it." Describe the patient using active language, as in the following examples:

You performed an assessment and discovered this finding:

Confusing: Arrive to find male patient who is out-of-it.

Better: Arrive to find a male patient disoriented to place and time.

Confusing: Caring for a 43-year-old obtunded male.

Better: Caring for a 43-year-old male who is slow to respond to verbal or painful stimulation.

Special Populations

When you are applying assessment and history of present illness information to the older adult population, take into account the patient's past medical history. Patients with a history of dementia are complicated to manage. The primary question you need to answer is how much change has occurred in the patient's LOC. Do not evaluate the patient from the point of a normal LOC. Speak to family, friends, or other caregivers to determine the patient's baseline LOC. Document that level clearly using active language.

Medications can also create alterations in the LOC. Explore all medications that the patient is taking. Include prescription, nonprescription, herbal, supplements, homeopathic, and illegal medications. Older adult patients are at a higher risk for having many physicians, many conditions, and many medications. Combinations of medications can result in unexpected neurologic effects.

In the pediatric population, the child's developmental stage must be considered. A 1-year-old child should cry when you are conducting an assessment. This would be considered a normal reaction to strangers. A 5-year-old child who normally talks freely may be quiet with a stranger. Evaluate the child at his or her appropriate developmental level.

Special Populations

When you are assessing ICP in infants, consider the quality of the baby's cry. As ICP increases, the pitch of the cry rises as well, until it resembles a shriek similar to that of a cat. At the same time, the shape of the pupils can change from round to more oval. These two findings are the basis of the mnemonic related to infants and ICP: "Cat's eyes and cat's cries."

■ Pathophysiology, Assessment, and Management of Common Neurologic Emergencies

Most diseases or conditions, including neurologic disorders, are caused by more than one factor, so they are said to be *multifactorial*. If diseases had only one cause, then every person exposed to a particular pathogen would become infected. Every person with a high-fat diet would develop blocked arteries. But disease susceptibility is often related to a number of causes, such as the following:

- How the body system was created during development of the embryo/fetus
- How effective the body's defense and repair functions are
- How severe or prolonged the body's exposure is to the pathogen, toxin, or other damaging factor

During the following discussion on some common neurologic conditions, keep in mind that the reason for their development usually cannot be attributed to a single cause.

■ Stroke

A stroke is a serious medical condition in which blood supply to areas of the brain is interrupted, causing ischemia. People older than 65 years represent almost 75% of all patients who have strokes. For every decade after age 55 years, the risk of having a stroke more than doubles. Today, nearly half of all patients who have brain attacks, or strokes, deny their symptoms. Many fail to activate EMS and consequently delay care. The goal of treatment is early recognition and rapid, appropriate intervention. The longer the stroke continues, the less likely the patient will have a promising outcome. "Time is brain."

Pathophysiology

Neurologic conditions can also have a vascular origin. Vascular emergencies can occur suddenly or gradually. Sudden occurrences are typically the result of emboli or aneurysms **Figure 14** . If a blood vessel is suddenly blocked, as in an embolism, the cells beyond the blockage can become **ischemic**. As oxygen and glucose levels drop, brain cells turn to anaerobic metabolism to stay alive. This mechanism, however, is only a stopgap measure. Anaerobic metabolism creates only minuscule amounts of energy for the cell and produces acidic byproducts. If circulation is not returned quickly, the cell will not have enough fuel to survive.

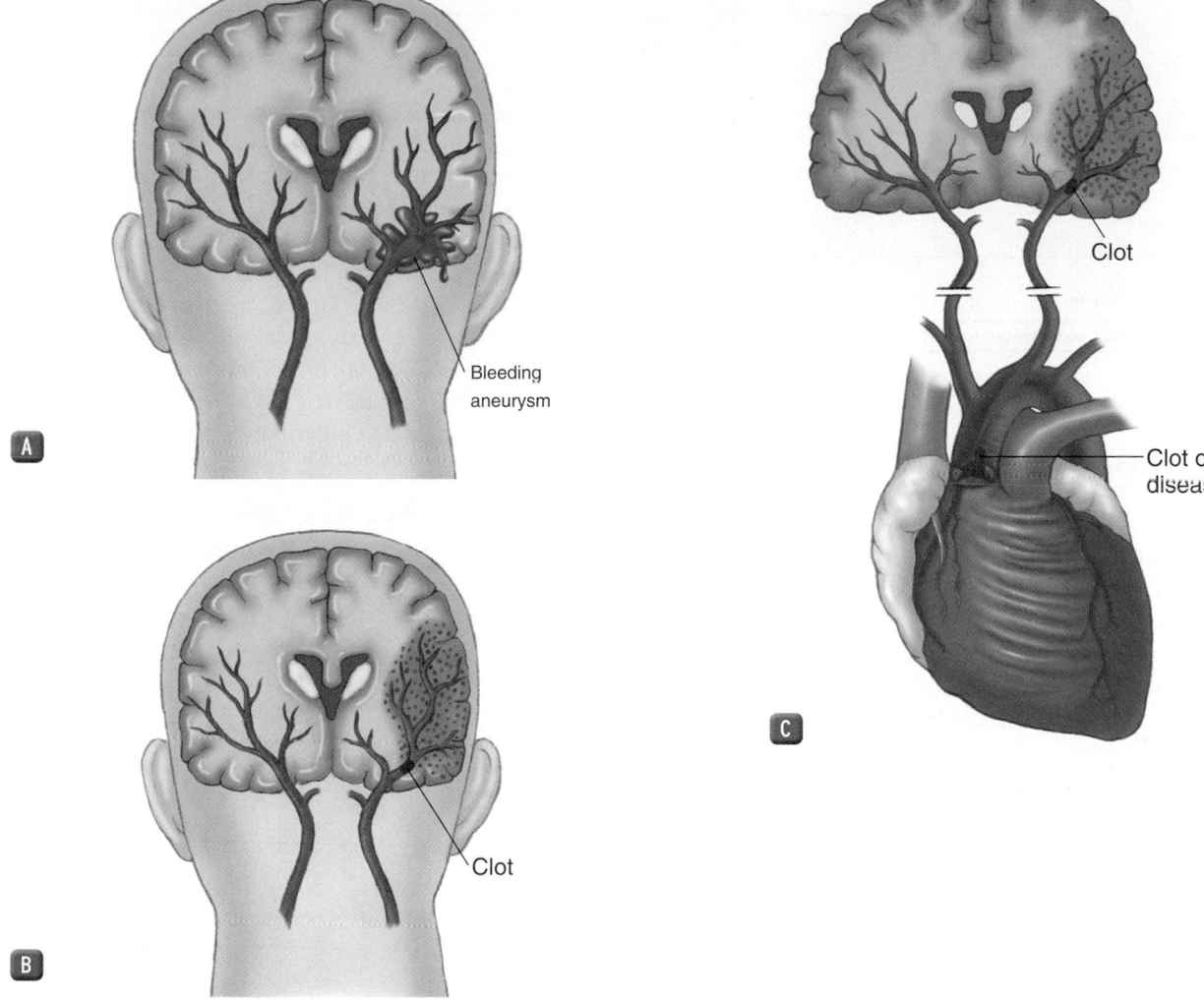

Figure 14 Vascular causes of neurologic conditions. **A.** An aneurysm is an area of weakness in the wall of an artery that can bulge out and eventually leak or rupture. **B.** Atherosclerosis can damage the wall of a cerebral artery, narrowing the artery or producing a clot. When the vessel is completely blocked, brain cells begin to die. **C.** An embolus is a blood clot formed elsewhere in the body, often on a diseased heart valve. It can travel through the vascular system and lodge in a cerebral artery, causing a stroke.

Artery walls consist of three layers of tissue that lie on top of each other. An aneurysm is a weakness in one or more of those layers. The process of aneurysm development is as follows:

1. Small tears or defects occur within the arterial wall.
2. Blood enters between the layers of the artery.
3. Pressure builds up, and the initial small tear increases in size.

If this process continues, the wall will become so damaged that it can no longer withstand the normal pressure of blood flowing through the artery. The weakened wall will begin to bulge. If the damage is severe, the bulging artery can leak or the wall can catastrophically fail, causing an intracranial hemorrhage.

Pathophysiology of Ischemic Stroke There are two basic types of strokes: ischemic (75%) and **hemorrhagic** (25%). Ischemic strokes are also called *occlusive strokes* because they are caused

by an occlusion, or blockage. This blockage can be caused by either a thrombus or embolus. These two causes of strokes have presentation patterns that differ. The graph seen in **Figure 15** provides some insight into the evolution of a stroke. In an ischemic stroke, a blood vessel is blocked so the tissue distal to the blockage becomes ischemic. Eventually that tissue will die if blood flow is not returned. But this pathology is self-limiting. Only the tissue beyond the blockage is affected, so the area(s) of the brain involved is limited.

Notice how the line representing signs and symptoms stops climbing and begins to stabilize. This stabilization does not imply that a patient cannot die from an ischemic stroke. The exact extent of the stroke and its severity are dictated by the artery involved and the portion of the brain being denied oxygen. For example, an ischemic stroke in which blood flow to the brainstem is blocked is certainly life threatening. The plateau indicates that signs and symptoms have reached a peak and leveled off because the area of the brain affected is no longer working.

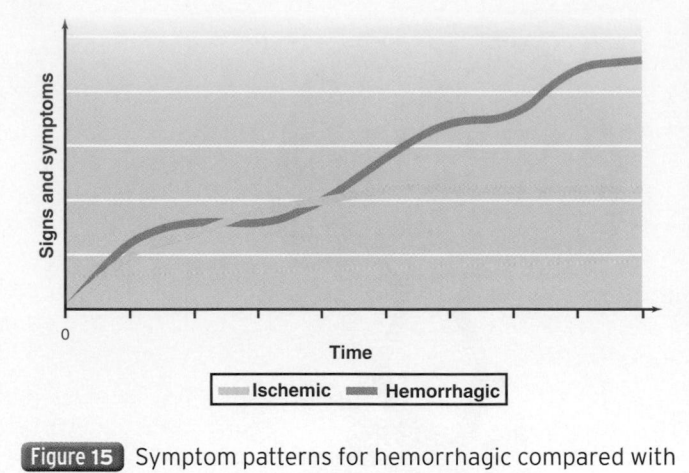

Figure 15 Symptom patterns for hemorrhagic compared with ischemic stroke.

Pathophysiology of Hemorrhagic Stroke Hemorrhagic strokes have a different pattern. They tend to get worse over time because of bleeding within the cranium. This bleeding can cause increased ICP and brainstem herniation. One of the hallmarks of a hemorrhagic stroke is the "worst headache of my life" complaint. If the patient reports a severe headache and later cannot speak, becomes difficult to arouse, and finally begins showing signs of increased ICP, you should strongly consider a hemorrhagic stroke.

It is important to understand the dynamics of ICP. The skull (cranial vault) is filled with three substances: brain, blood, and cerebrospinal fluid. These three substances exert pressure against the skull and the skull exerts a reflected pressure **Figure 16** . This exchange is balanced, allowing the brain to fit

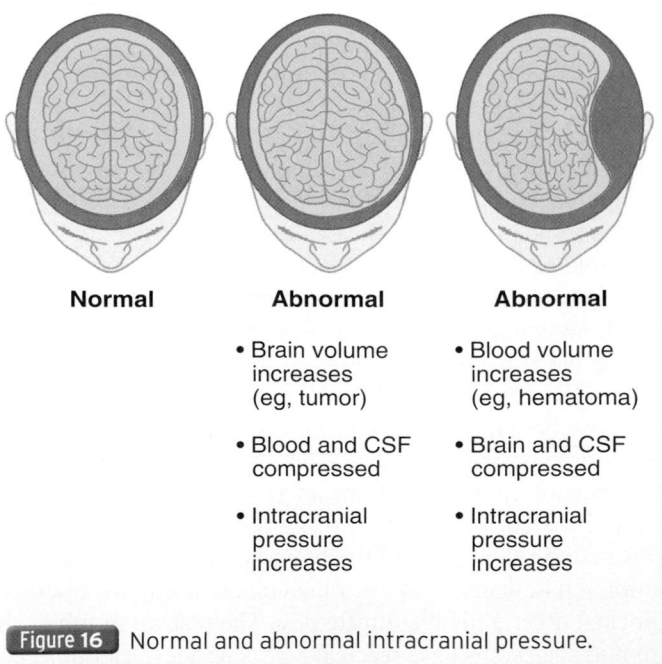

Figure 16 Normal and abnormal intracranial pressure.

Normal	Abnormal	Abnormal
	• Brain volume increases (eg, tumor)	• Blood volume increases (eg, hematoma)
	• Blood and CSF compressed	• Brain and CSF compressed
	• Intracranial pressure increases	• Intracranial pressure increases

snugly within with skull. If there were spaces or voids within the skull, the brain would slam into the skull with only minimal head movement. The pressure of these substances within the skull constitutes ICP. Normally, ICP measures between 1 to 10 mm Hg.

Two difficulties arise when the pressure within the cranial vault begins to climb and remains high. First, the brain may become ischemic because of a lack of blood supply and/or the brain may herniate. Herniation is the movement of a structure from its normal location into another space. Portions of the brain can be pushed into different locations, causing tissue damage and potential death. As ICP rises, the amount of blood available to the brain decreases. Cerebral perfusion pressure (CPP), the pressure of blood within the cranial vault, begins to fall. Normal CPP is 70 to 90 mm Hg. Below 50 mm Hg, the brain begins to become ischemic. CPP can be calculated by the following equation:

$$CPP = MAP - ICP$$

The MAP, or mean arterial pressure, is the average (mean) pressure within the blood vessels at any given time. Typically, MAP is about 80 to 90 mm Hg. Many newer cardiac monitors that have automatic blood pressure readings will display the MAP on the screen.

As with most readings within the body, ICP changes constantly. Coughing, vomiting, or bearing down, for instance, tends to increase ICP. These momentary spikes in ICP are not harmful. If there is blood, swelling, pus, or a tumor within the cranial vault, ICP will increase and remain high. The volume of the cranial vault is limited and inflexible, so the pressure increases as more and more substances are squeezed into this space. Patients can have life-threating issues when ICP rises sharply and/or blood pressure becomes critically low.

The second possible outcome of increased ICP is herniation, a shift of the intracranial contents within the cranial vault or displacement of the contents toward the foramen magnum, the large opening at the inferior portion of the skull through which the spinal cord exits. This will eventually compress the brainstem, at which point the patient will lose control of his or her vegetative functions.

Assessment

Stroke causes sudden-onset changes in neurologic status. Patients can exhibit any combination of the following signs and symptoms:

- **Language effects:** Slurred speech, aphasia, agnosia, and apraxia
- **Movement effects:** Hemiparesis, hemiplegia, arm drifting, facial droop, tongue deviation, swallowing difficulties, ptosis, and ataxia
- **Sensory effects:** Headache (hemorrhagic), sudden blindness, and sudden unilateral paresthesia

- **Cognitive effects:** Decreased LOC, difficulty thinking, seizures, and coma
- **Cardiac effects:** Hypertension

Documentation and Communication

Patients with strokes can present with a wide range of communication difficulties.
- Patients who are multilingual may lose understanding of one language but not another.
- Patients may be able to understand the written word but not the spoken word.
- Patients may not be able to understand any form of communication.
- Be open to trying various ways to communicate. Remember, communication problems do not indicate that the patient is not thinking. The problem is that the patient cannot get you to understand what he or she is thinking.

Management

In patients who are unconscious *and* demonstrate other signs of increased ICP, administer fluids as needed. Unless you are concerned about possible cervical spine injury, elevate the patient's head 30°. This change will cause a slight decrease in ICP. Ensure that the airway is clear, but do not vigorously suction because stimulating the cough and gag reflexes will increase ICP. Watch for seizures and be prepared with diazepam or lorazepam. The patient may be bradycardic. However, atropine and pacing are not indicated because of the systolic hypertension that accompanies the bradycardia. The ICP is causing the bradycardia, not the other way around. Notify the hospital and provide rapid transport.

It is important for you to monitor blood pressure closely in any patient with a potential problem with ICP. Frequent assessment becomes even more critical when a decrease in blood pressure is also present. For any patient at risk for ICP, ensure that the blood pressure remains at least 110 to 120 systolic.

Carbon dioxide and oxygen levels are important in patients with increased ICP. A high oxygen level causes constriction of the cerebral arteries. This vasoconstriction further impairs perfusion to the brain. Alternatively, a diminished level of carbon dioxide lowers ICP. This effect provides a more suitable environment for brain perfusion. Ventilation, then, decreases CO_2 (good) and increases O_2 (bad). This incompatibility can make decision making difficult because prehospital treatment is simply not effective at decreasing ICP. You should provide ventilatory support at a rate of 16 to 20 breaths per minute. Do not increase the rate any higher than 30 per minute. If you are using end tidal CO_2 readings, ventilate to maintain a PET CO_2 in the high 20s to low 30s mm Hg. Do not ventilate the patient to CO_2 readings of lower than the high 20s.

Consider the American Heart Association (AHA) algorithm showing goals for the management of patients with suspected stroke **Figure 17**. Treatment at the hospital takes different

---

YOU *are the Medic* | **PART 3**

The patient's speech is clear, and he has no facial droop. He is positive for arm drift and negative for ptosis. He is confused to time of day, but follows commands. His affect is calm and cooperative. Apraxia noted (shown pen; when asked what it does, patient tried to shave his face with the pen). He is negative for agnosias and negative for headache. Gait is not assessed because of a possible cervical spine injury. His blood glucose level is 92 mg/dL. The family says the patient's pants were soiled. Pulse oximetry reading is 92% on room air. The ECG shows atrial fibrillation at approximately 90 beats/min. A 12-lead ECG shows no acute ST changes and no Q waves.

Recording Time: 5 Minutes	
Respirations	24 breaths/min
Pulse	90 beats/min, irregular
Skin	Pale, warm, dry
Blood pressure	142/86 mm Hg
Oxygen saturation (Spo$_2$)	92% room air
Pupils	Equal and reactive

5. What are the two types of stroke?

6. Of the two types of stroke, which one's symptoms will progressively worsen over time?

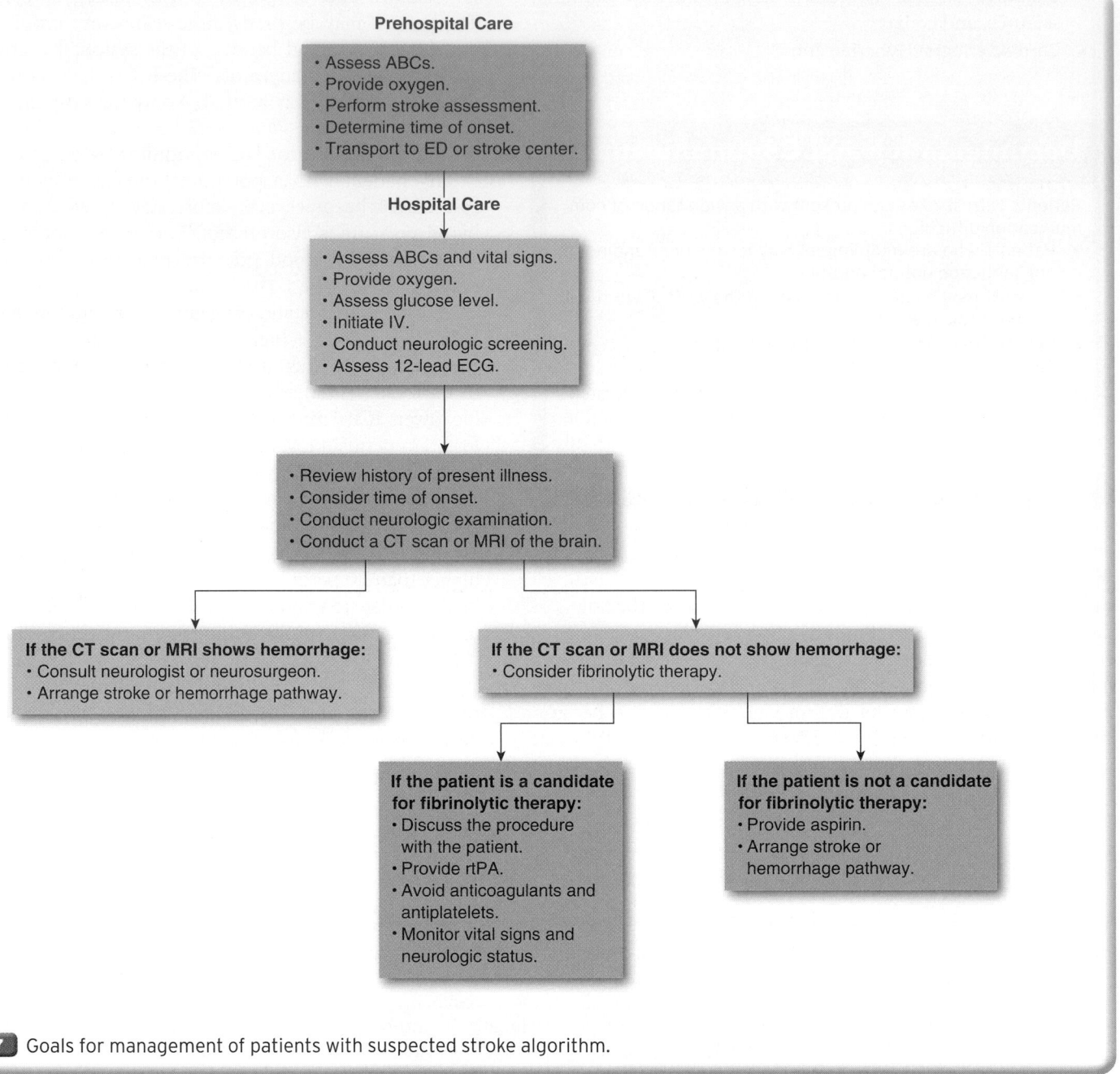

Prehospital Care

- Assess ABCs.
- Provide oxygen.
- Perform stroke assessment.
- Determine time of onset.
- Transport to ED or stroke center.

Hospital Care

- Assess ABCs and vital signs.
- Provide oxygen.
- Assess glucose level.
- Initiate IV.
- Conduct neurologic screening.
- Assess 12-lead ECG.

- Review history of present illness.
- Consider time of onset.
- Conduct neurologic examination.
- Conduct a CT scan or MRI of the brain.

If the CT scan or MRI shows hemorrhage:
- Consult neurologist or neurosurgeon.
- Arrange stroke or hemorrhage pathway.

If the CT scan or MRI does not show hemorrhage:
- Consider fibrinolytic therapy.

If the patient is a candidate for fibrinolytic therapy:
- Discuss the procedure with the patient.
- Provide rtPA.
- Avoid anticoagulants and antiplatelets.
- Monitor vital signs and neurologic status.

If the patient is not a candidate for fibrinolytic therapy:
- Provide aspirin.
- Arrange stroke or hemorrhage pathway.

Figure 17 Goals for management of patients with suspected stroke algorithm.

paths of care for each type of stroke. One feature, however, is common to both: Time is essential. For ischemic strokes, fibrinolytics need to be administered within 3 hours of onset. In hemorrhagic strokes, the more the patient bleeds into the cranium, the greater the potential for increased ICP and brainstem damage.

The AHA recommends a comprehensive approach to the care of the patient experiencing a stroke. The general public needs to be educated as to the signs and symptoms of stroke. The public then needs to call 9-1-1 so trained dispatchers can summon the appropriate prehospital resources. EMS personnel

need to have adequate training in the delivery of care to patients with strokes, including which patients would benefit from a stroke center. Once in the emergency department, a coordinated and comprehensive approach to care is essential. Some patients will benefit from fibrinolytics, some need intra-arterial clot removal, while others may need neurosurgery. Once care has been delivered and the stroke mitigated, appropriate rehabilitation needs to be considered to ensure the patient returns to the highest quality of life possible.

EMS providers need to be involved in educating the community about stroke signs and symptoms, the effects

Documentation and Communication

Neurologic emergencies can produce feelings of confusion, fear, anger, and helplessness. Therefore, you need to provide emotional support for the patient and family. A therapeutic gentle touch on the shoulder can communicate your compassion to the patient. Use a calm, reassuring voice to reorient the patient and tell him or her that you are there to help.

emergency department physician will need before fibrinolytics can be considered. During the assessment phase, EMS providers should use a standard stroke assessment tool to increase the accuracy of their field impressions. Use the Cincinnati Prehospital Stroke Scale Table 9 or the Los Angeles Prehospital Stroke Screen Table 10.

Standard stroke care includes titrating oxygen therapy to the patient's need. Evaluate the patient's pulse oximetry to maintain an Spo_2 of 95% or greater. Research is providing evidence that patients in hyperoxic states (high oxygen levels) can have greater cellular damage because of the increased oxygen level. Ensure that your Spo_2 reading is accurate. Use other assessment techniques to ensure your patient does not need large amounts of O_2. From a respiratory point of view, if the patient is in stable condition, the nasal cannula is probably sufficient.

There is currently no AHA guideline for the prehospital control of hypertension. Do not administer aspirin. Aspirin is helpful in patients with ischemic stroke but is harmful in patients with hemorrhagic stroke. Therefore, it should be administered after only a CT/MR scan has been obtained. Because patients may not be able to feel or move their arms or legs, make sure to protect them from injury.

of strokes, and how to activate EMS. Too many patients deny their complaints or drive themselves to emergency departments. Patients need to understand that immediately on discovering stroke symptoms, they must call EMS for assistance.

In addition, all levels of EMS providers should be trained to recognize stroke signs and symptoms. Rapid identification is imperative. Time is brain, and fibrinolytic agents must be administered within 3 hours of stroke onset. The checklist presented in Table 8 will help you focus on gathering information the

Table 8 Sample Prehospital Fibrinolytic Checklist for Stroke

Use this checklist in all patients suspected of stroke.

YES	NO	
❑	❑	Age 18 years or older?
❑	❑	Facial droop?
❑	❑	Slurred speech?
❑	❑	Arm drift? (Test performed with the patient's eye's closed)
❑	❑	When the signs and symptoms began, did the patient have a seizure?
❑	❑	Systolic BP > 185 mm Hg?
❑	❑	Diastolic BP > 110 mm Hg?
❑	❑	Right vs. left arm systolic BP differences > 15 mm Hg?
❑	❑	History of structural central nervous system disease (eg, stroke, aneurysm, arteriovenous malformation, brain tumor)?
❑	❑	Significant closed head/facial trauma or myocardial infarction within the past 3 months?
❑	❑	Recent (within 6 weeks) major trauma, surgery (including laser eye surgery), or GI/GU bleeding?
❑	❑	Bleeding or clotting problems or on blood thinners?
❑	❑	History of bleeding into the brain?
Date: _____ AM/PM: _____		Time signs and symptoms began (Record time) If unknown, answer next question.
Date: _____ AM/PM: _____		Time patient last known to be normal (Record time)
_____ mg/dL		Blood glucose reading (Record number)

Table 9 Cincinnati Prehospital Stroke Scale

Assessment	Normal	Abnormal
Facial Droop		
Ask the patient to smile and show his or her teeth.	Both sides of the face move equally.	One side of the face does not move as well as the other side.
Arm Drift		
Ask the patient to close eyes and hold arms out for 10 seconds.	Both arms move the same or neither arm moves.	One arm does not move or one arm drifts down compared with the other.
Abnormal Speech		
Ask patient to repeat the phrase "You can't teach an old dog new tricks."	Uses correct words, no slurring.	Slurs words, uses inappropriate words, or is unable to speak.

Interpretation: If any one is abnormal, probability of a stroke is 72%.

Table 10 Los Angeles Prehospital Stroke Screen

Criteria	Yes	Unknown	No
1. Age > 45	❑	❑	❑
2. History of seizures or epilepsy absent	❑	❑	❑
3. Symptoms < 24 hours	❑	❑	❑
4. At baseline, patient is not wheelchair bound or bedridden	❑	❑	❑
5. Blood glucose between 60 and 400	❑	❑	❑
6. Obvious asymmetry (right vs. left) in any of the following 3 exam categories (must be unilateral):	❑	❑	❑

	Equal	Right Weak	Left Weak
Facial smile/ grimace	❑	❑ Droop	❑ Droop
Grip	❑	❑ Weak Grip ❑ No Grip	❑ Weak Grip ❑ No Grip
Arm strength	❑	❑ Drifts Down ❑ Falls Rapidly	❑ Drifts Down ❑ Fall Rapidly

Interpretation: If criteria 1–6 are marked yes, specificity of a stroke is 97%.

Words of Wisdom

Keep in mind the following pearls regarding oxygen administration:

- Patients starving for O_2 (as evidenced by cyanosis, low Spo_2, and decreased LOC) should be administered large amounts of O_2.
- In patients with no evidence of hypoxia on assessment, large amounts of O_2 can have a choking effect on the patient.
- Whether the patient starves of oxygen or chokes on it, he or she may die either way.

Complete a fibrinolytic checklist, focusing on when the signs and symptoms began or when the patient was last seen normal. At times it can be difficult to pin down the exact time the stroke began. If no set time is available, use this "when they were last seen normal" as a beginning. If possible, transport a family member or significant other who can speak to medical personnel in the ED.

Transport Decisions Determine an appropriate facility for transport. Patients should be transported to stroke centers: facilities with stroke teams who are trained in the administration of fibrinolytics and in the diagnosis and management of various types of strokes. Contact the facility to ensure their CT/MRI capabilities are operational. Some facilities will need to contact scan technicians on call during night hours or weekends.

Early hospital notification to the ED can decrease the time that elapses before the patient receives a scan. If the patient is rapidly decompensating or you are considering a hemorrhagic stroke, consider transporting the patient to a facility that can perform neurosurgery. Call ahead to alert the hospital of the need for rapid evaluation.

■ Transient Ischemic Attacks

Pathophysiology

Transient ischemic attacks (TIAs) are episodes of cerebral ischemia without any permanent damage. Any of the typical presentations associated with a stroke can occur with TIAs. What makes these different from a stroke is the resolution of signs and symptoms within 24 hours. There is no residual damage

Health care in the United States is big business. The mission of hospitals is to provide high-quality patient care. But how can they provide quality care without having patients? Patients, through various means, provide the funding needed for hospitals to continue to operate. In some systems, the competing concepts of quality of care and number of patients served can become entangled. The stroke patient provides an excellent example of this dilemma.

Suppose a 62-year-old woman is having a stroke. Your assessment reveals left-sided weakness, slurred speech, and an arm drift (she has a positive result on the Cincinnati Prehospital Stroke Scale). These changes began around 08:15. You are caring for her, and it is now 08:45. She says she has the worst headache of her life. She is getting sleepy and becoming more and more difficult to arouse. You get the patient into the ambulance to transport her to the local hospital, and she begins to display decorticate posturing. What should you do? What type of care will she need when she arrives at the hospital?

Given the patient's history, your physical findings, and rapid deterioration of LOC, you should conclude tentatively that this patient is having a hemorrhagic stroke. If your field impression is correct, she will ultimately need a facility capable of neurosurgery. The closest hospital is 15 minutes away and cannot offer that service. The closest facility that offers the care she needs is 30 minutes away. Which is better for the patient: immediate transfer to a facility that you believe cannot completely manage the patient, or a lengthened transport time to a fully equipped facility?

Many EMS systems have progressive medical direction that recognizes the need to transport certain patients to facilities with specialized capabilities. In such systems, your local protocols will dictate where to take this type of patient. If your protocols do not specify where to take such patients, it is appropriate to discuss the destination with your medical director. Before your discussion, do your homework:

- Gather information about the presentation of different types of stroke.
- Research hemorrhagic stroke and its care.
- Become familiar with the capabilities of your local hospitals.
- Then create a template guideline to be discussed with the medical director.

During this conversation, control your emotions. Persuade the medical director with facts, and keep the aim of providing good patient care always in mind. Whatever guideline template you create, ensure that it is flexible. Do not go into the meeting without some ability to bend. If you present yourself well, you will pave the way for greater responsibility as a paramedic, increased respect for the profession, and improved patient care.

to brain tissue and subsequently no signs and symptoms after the episode ends. These mini-strokes are often signs of a serious vascular problem that requires medical evaluation. More than one third of patients with TIAs will have a stroke soon afterward. Think of the TIA/stroke relationship as the equivalent of the relationship between angina and myocardial infarction.

Assessment

Any of the signs and symptoms of strokes can occur with a TIA. Your assessment of the patient will therefore be the same whether the patient is experiencing a stroke or a TIA.

Management

In managing TIAs, follow the stroke management guidelines discussed earlier. Close neurologic assessment is needed. Patients may experience a multitude of TIAs, coming and going. Strongly encourage the patient to be transported. If the patient refuses transportation, appeal to the patient's family for assistance. If the patient still refuses, encourage him or her to seek medical care soon. It is important to reinforce with the patient that this TIA was a warning sign of a serious and potentially deadly problem with the blood vessels within the brain. Hypertension is the number one preventable cause of strokes and TIAs. Encourage the patient to talk with his or her doctor about blood pressure control and to take antihypertensive medications as prescribed.

■ Coma

Pathophysiology

The call for the unresponsive person is common. There are many causes of a decreased LOC. One way to remember the most common of these is to use the mnemonic AEIOUTIPS Table 11 . This memory aid will help you focus on general groups of causes.

Note from the table that each grouping has a different onset of signs and symptoms. As with most medical complaints, the history of present illness is vital to determining the underlying cause of the patient's complaints. An easy approach is to determine when the patient was last seen functioning normally.

Evaluate the speed of onset of the patient's altered LOC. Again, the onset will help to distinguish one cause from another. It would be exceedingly unusual for a person to be absolutely healthy one minute and unresponsive because of an infection the next. A seizure, though, is an excellent example of a condition that can cause unresponsiveness almost instantly.

Assessment

The common signs and symptoms of diminished LOC and imminent coma are as follows:

- **Cognitive effects:** Decreasing LOC, confusion, hallucinations, delusions, psychosis, difficulty thinking, and sleepiness
- **Speech effects:** Slurred speech, agnosia, apraxia, and aphasia
- **Movement effects:** Ataxia, seizures, and posturing
- **General CNS effects:** Total unresponsiveness (coma)

Management

The focus of care for comatose patients occurs in two stages. First, support vital functions. Following standard care guidelines

Table 11 AEIOU-TIPS: Altered Mental Status

Letter	Name	Onset	Treatment Focus
A	Alcohol	Acute (hours) Chronic (days)	Ensure oxygen, glucose, and temperature for proper brain functioning. Consider thiamine with D_{50}
	Acidosis	Acute (hours)	Ventilation Sodium bicarbonate
E	Epilepsy (seizure)	Sudden (seconds)	If prolonged, diazepam (Valium) or lorazepam (Ativan)
I	Insulin	Acute (hours)	D_{50} or glucagon
O	Overdose	Acute to gradual (hours to days, depending on agent)	Administration of selected drugs; consider naloxone (Narcan)
U	Uremia (kidney failure)	Gradual (days to weeks)	Ensure oxygen, glucose, and temperature for proper brain functioning.
T	Trauma	Sudden (seconds)	Take cervical spine precautions Ensure adequate blood pressure
I	Infection	Gradual (hours to days)	Ensure adequate blood pressure
P	Psychosis	Sudden (seconds) History of mental illness or substance abuse is typical	Ensure oxygen, glucose, and temperature for proper brain functioning.
S	Stroke	Sudden (seconds to hours)	Ensure oxygen, glucose, and temperature for proper brain functioning.

should allow you to secure and maintain airway, breathing, and circulation effectively. The second goal is to gather information about the possible cause of the altered LOC or coma. Gather past medical history, evaluate medications, look for signs of trauma, and determine the history of the present illness. This information will help you direct your care to the most likely cause.

It is not uncommon to have too little information to determine a cause. This fact should not deter you from looking for one. Are there medical identification tags? How was the patient acting before you were called? Was there drug paraphernalia near the patient? If there is any concern that the patient may have taken a narcotic, administer naloxone (Narcan),

YOU are the Medic   PART 4

While you are providing transport to the hospital, there is no change in the patient's condition. You continue your assessment and ensure that no new nervous system deficits develop. His vital signs show no evidence of increased ICP. Report to the receiving facility is given on your arrival.

Recording Time: 15 Minutes	
Respirations	22 breaths/min
Pulse	86 beats/min, irregular
Skin	Warm, dry, pink
Blood pressure	142/86 mm Hg
Oxygen saturation (Spo$_2$)	98% on 4 L/min O$_2$ NC
Pupils	Equal and reactive

7. Would aspirin be indicated for a possible stroke patient?

8. How does a TIA differ from a stroke?

0.4 to 2 mg IVP. This information can be critical to providing the continued, quality care this patient will need in order to return to health.

In-hospital care will focus on supporting airway, breathing and circulation, and attempting to discover or confirm a diagnosis. Patients will routinely need urine and blood analysis, conventional radiography, computed tomography, and magnetic resonance imaging.

◼ Seizures

Pathophysiology

A seizure is the sudden, erratic firing of neurons. Patients can experience a wide array of signs and symptoms when having seizures, such as muscle spasms, increased secretions, diaphoresis, and cyanosis. A seizure can be limited to the shaking of one hand or the taste of pennies in the mouth, or it can involve the movement of every limb or the complete loss of consciousness. Patients can be aware of the seizure or wake up afterwards not knowing what happened. Each of these experiences is defined as a seizure if it is brought on by the random firing of neurons.

If a seizure continues for a long period of time, profound changes occur within the brain and body. Cerebral glucose and oxygen supplies can be depleted. Systemic hypoxia, hypercarbia, blood pressure changes, and hyperthermia can occur. A single, short duration seizure is typically not a major life-threatening concern. However, if seizures group together and/or last for long periods of time, these complications can cause serious long-term effects to the patient, including death.

As with most medical patients, you should try to determine the cause of the problem—in this case, the seizure. Ask about medication compliance. Phenytoin (Dilantin), lorazepam (Ativan), carbamazepine (Tegretol), and valproic acid (Depakene) are common anticonvulsant medications. For various reasons, however, patients may have taken an insufficient amount of medication to prevent seizures. Patients may stop taking their medication because they have not had a seizure in several months and believe they are cured. Children can outgrow the dosage of their anticonvulsant medication. Older adult patients may be unable to afford the medication entirely.

Another common cause of seizure is fever in infants (febrile seizure). Febrile seizures will be covered in the chapter, *Pediatric Emergencies*. Seizure may occur in people with diabetes who have a low blood glucose level. Knowing the cause of the seizure will help you direct management. Some common causes of seizure are listed in Table 12.

Assessment of Generalized Seizures

Seizures can be classified as generalized, affecting large portions of the brain or partial, affecting a limited area of the brain. Within generalized seizures are tonic/clonic and absence types.

Tonic/Clonic Seizures Tonic/clonic seizures, also called *grand mal seizures,* present you with the greatest assessment challenges. This type of seizure has a peculiar pattern. Most tonic/clonic

Table 12 Common Causes of Seizures
◾ **Abscess**
◾ Alcohol
◾ Birth anomaly
◾ Brain infections (meningitis, encephalitis)
◾ Brain trauma
◾ Diabetes mellitus
◾ Febrile
◾ **Idiopathic** (no known cause)
◾ Inappropriate medication dosage
◾ Organic brain syndromes
◾ Recreational drug use
◾ Stroke or TIA
◾ Systemic infection
◾ Tumor
◾ Uremia (kidney failure)

seizures travel through each of these steps in sequence; there are cases, however, in which one or more steps are skipped:

1. Aura—This is a sensation the patient experiences before the seizure occurs. It might be a muscle twitch, a funny taste, or the perception of seeing lights or hearing a high-pitched noise.
2. Loss of consciousness.
3. Tonic phase—Systemic (body-wide) rigidity.
4. Hypertonic phase—Arched back, and rigid.
5. Clonic phase—Rhythmic contraction of major muscle groups. Arms, legs, head movement, lip smacking, biting, clenching teeth.
6. Postseizure—Major muscles relax, nystagmus may still be occurring. Eyes may be looking posterior (at back of head).
7. Postictal—Reset period of the brain. This can take several minutes to hours before the patient gradually returns to pre-seizure LOC. During this time patients often display the following signs:
   - Initially aphasic (unable to speak)
   - Confused/unable to follow commands
   - Emotional
   - Tired or sleeping
   - Headache
   - Gradually the brain begins to function normally

Tonic/clonic seizures are disconcerting for both family and health care providers to watch. During the seizure process, respiration may become erratic, loud, and obviously abnormal. Alternatively, the patient may stop breathing and become cyanotic. These periods of apnea are usually short lived and do not require intervention. If the patient is apneic for more than 30 seconds, immediately begin ventilatory assistance. Another disconcerting aspect of seizures, particularly for the patient, is incontinence.

Absence Seizures In contrast to tonic/clonic seizures, absence seizures (or *petit mal seizures*) present with little or no movement. The typical patient with absence seizures is a child. Classically, the child will simply stop—stop walking, stop speaking mid-sentence, or stop playing and freeze with a toy in the hand. The child rarely falls. These seizures usually last no more than several seconds. There is no postictal period and no confusion. The seizure may be brought on by flashing lights or hyperventilation.

Pseudoseizures Pseudoseizures are a generalized neurologic event. Symptomatically, you may not notice any difference from a tonic/clonic seizure. Tonic/clonic motion, loss of consciousness, and a postictal phase are all present in these events. The difference is that in pseudoseizures, the cause is of psychiatric origin. It is important to understand that in most cases of pseudoseizure, the patient is not intentionally causing the "seizure." The root cause may be psychiatric, but the patient is not willfully causing this behavior.

Pseudoseizures present with loss of consciousness. This is usually triggered by some emotional event, stress, lights, or pain. These seizures conspicuously occur with witnesses. This fact may lead health care providers to believe they are contrived. Motion that occurs during the seizure is relatively organized—side to side movement of the head, pedaling movements of the legs (like riding a bicycle), weeping, or stuttering. These patients often have a psychiatric history and/or other medical history, such as fibromyalgia, chronic pain, or chronic fatigue.

Assessment of Partial Seizures

Partial seizures affect a limited portion of the brain and can be further divided into simple partial or complex partial. The defining characteristic of a partial seizure is that only a limited portion of the brain is involved. These seizures can be localized to just one spot within the brain or they can begin in one spot and move wave-like to other locations. Like dropping a pebble in a still pond, this wave can spread and is called a <u>Jacksonian march</u>.

Simple partial seizures involve either movement of one part of the body (frontal lobe) or sensations in one part of the body (parietal lobe). An example of a Jacksonian march in a simple partial seizure is shaking of the left hand, which moves to the left arm, then shoulder, then head, then right arm, then right hand, and finally moves out of the body. Complex partial seizures involve subtle changes in LOC. Here the patient can become confused, lose alertness, have hallucinations, or become unable to speak. There may be some small movements of the head or eyes. Patients typically do not become unresponsive **Table 13** .

Whether they are generalized or partial, most seizures are self-limiting and all you need to do is monitor and protect patients from injuring themselves.

Management

In managing seizures, you should quickly determine whether trauma is a concern. Where was the patient before the seizure? What was the patient doing before the seizure? How did the

Table 13 **Classification of Seizures**

Grouping	Type	Presentation
Generalized	Tonic/clonic (grand mal)	Full-body, violent jerking movements
	Absence (petit mal)	Freezing or staring
	Pseudoseizures	Tonic/clonic but caused by a psychiatric mechanism—the patient is not faking the seizure
Partial	Simple partial	Shaking of one area of the body
		Sensation in one area of the body
	Complex partial	Subtle alterations in LOC

patient get to his or her current position? If trauma is unclear or confirmed, take C-spine precautions.

If you arrive during the seizure, do not restrain or try to stop the seizing movement. Remain calm and prevent the patient from striking objects and becoming injured. Do not place anything in the patient's mouth while the patient is seizing. If bystanders have placed objects in the patient's mouth (for example, a spoon or a butter knife inserted sideways), remove them. If you believe this to be a pseudoseizure, treat it like any other seizure. Do not dismiss this as a patient acting out. Correct hypoglycemia by giving intravenous glucose as needed; otherwise, most seizures are self-limiting. Ventilatory assistance may be necessary if the seizure or apnea is prolonged, but ventilation of a patient who is actively having a seizure is difficult. Performing oral or nasotracheal intubation is next to impossible during a seizure (see the discussion of status epilepticus).

After the seizure, it is important that you provide emotional support. Provide privacy for the patient and speak calmly and slowly. Be prepared to repeat yourself. Reorient the patient to place and time. If the seizure was febrile, encourage the patient or parents to administer medications for fever reduction (acetaminophen or ibuprofen).

Unless a clear and easily reversible cause for the seizure is found, all patients should be transported. Seizures can be a warning sign of more serious nervous system problem such as stroke, brain tumor, or severe metabolic imbalance. If the patient has a known history of seizures, he or she may not wish to go to the hospital. Advise the patient to follow up with his or her family doctor within 24 hours. The patient with diabetes who is awakened after administration of glucose may not wish to be transported. Advise the patient to eat a good meal and follow up with his or her family doctor.

If you are concerned that a patient may have a seizure during transport, establish vascular access so you are prepared to administer diazepam (Valium) or lorazepam (Ativan), the drugs of choice to stop seizures. Place blankets over the rails of the ambulance cot and over any hard surfaces near the patient. Ensure the patient's cot straps are not too tight.

In-hospital management involves determining the cause of the seizure. Hematologic studies, including drug level and blood glucose level, will be ordered. CT and/or MRI scans may be done.

■ Status Epilepticus

Pathophysiology

Status epilepticus can be defined as a seizure that lasts longer than 4 to 5 minutes or consecutive seizures without a return to consciousness between seizures. This time frame is arbitrary. Some authors suggest status epilepticus does not occur until 30 minutes of uninterrupted seizure activity. Refer to your local protocols for guidelines related to how long a seizure can continue before you should intervene. This circumstance should not be taken lightly. Nearly 20% of patients in status epilepticus will die.

During a seizure, neurons are in a hyper metabolic state (using large amounts of glucose and producing lactic acid). For a short period, this state does not produce long-term damage. If the seizure continues, the body becomes unable to remove the waste products effectively or to ensure adequate glucose supplies. The state can result in neurons being damaged or killed. The goal of prehospital care is to stop the seizure and to ensure adequate ABCs.

Assessment

Assessment of the patient with status epilepticus is the same as that of the patient expenencing a seizure. The only difference is the length of time that the seizure lasts.

Management

Follow standard care guidelines for seizures. Administer a benzodiazepine, either diazepam (Valium) 5 mg IV/IM or lorazepam (Ativan) 0.05 mg/kg, with a maximum dosage of 4 mg. If necessary, you may repeat a dose of diazepam every 10 to 15 minutes to a total dose of 30 mg. If you are unable to obtain IV access, diazepam can be given per rectum. If you are administering lorazepam, you may repeat the dose in 10 to 15 minutes, with a maximum dosage of 8 mg in 12 hours.

You should be prepared to control airway and ventilation completely because benzodiazepines can cause respiratory depression and arrest. Continue to use airway positioning and bag-mask ventilations until the medication has stopped the seizure. If the seizure cannot be quickly controlled by benzodiazepines and the patient cannot be ventilated, paralytics may be needed to allow for adequate airway management.

■ Syncope

Pathophysiology

Syncope is the sudden and temporary loss of consciousness with accompanying loss of postural tone. Syncope, or fainting, accounts for nearly 3% of all emergency department visits. The brain uses glucose at an astounding rate and has no ability to store glucose, so even a 3- to 5-second interruption in blood flow causes loss of consciousness. This is the underlying reason for syncope. The question is what caused the sudden decrease in cerebral perfusion? Table 14 provides the common causes of syncope.

Assessment

Classically, the patient with syncope is in a standing position when the event occurs. In younger adults, the pattern is usually one of vasovagal syncope. The adult experiences fear, emotional stress, or pain. The person then suddenly experiences a spinning sensation and passes out. This is why you should seat the patient before drawing blood or starting an IV line. In older adults, the more typical cause of syncope is a cardiac dysrhythmia. The patient has a sudden run of ventricular tachycardia, the blood pressure drops, and the patient falls to the floor. The rhythm terminates, blood pressure rises, and the patient feels fine. In either case, the whole process takes less than 60 seconds.

Patients with syncope usually experience a prodrome. These are the signs or symptoms that precede a disease or condition. For syncope, the prodromal signs and symptoms include feelings of dizziness, weakness, shortness of breath, chest pain, a headache, or the patient stating his or her vision went black. Incontinence is possible with syncope. Seizures and syncope can be difficult to differentiate if not actually witnessed. Table 15 offers some guidance.

Management

The first step in managing syncope is determining possible trauma during the patient's fall and whether cervical spine precautions are needed. Next, focus on blood pressure and cardiac causes. Evaluate the blood glucose level and oxygen saturation and obtain orthostatic vital signs. Provide emotional support; syncope can be embarrassing. Because you will not

Table 14	Causes of Syncope
Cardiac rhythm disturbances	Bradycardia of any type Sick sinus syndrome Supraventricular tachycardia Torsades de pointes Transient asystole Transient ventricular fibrillation Ventricular tachycardia
Other cardiac causes	Cardiomyopathy Myocardial infarction
Noncardiac causes	Dehydration Hypoglycemia Vasovagal response

Table 15 Differentiating Syncope From Seizure

Characteristic	Syncope	Seizure
Position of patient before event	Standing	Any position
Prodromal signs and symptoms	Dizziness, visual changes, shortness of breath, weakness	Odd taste in the mouth Seeing lights Hearing sounds Twitching
Activity during event	Relaxed	Generalized body movement
Response after event	Quick return of orientation	Slow return of orientation

know the exact cause of the syncope, it is important to transport any syncope patient to the hospital. Syncope can be a sign of life-threatening cardiac dysrhythmia, stroke, or other serious medical condition.

Headache

Everyone has had a headache at one time or another. What exactly is hurting? The brain and skull do not have pain receptors. Headaches originate from the nerves within the scalp, face, blood vessels, and muscles of the neck and head. The most common types of headaches are discussed in the next section. Other types of headaches are rare, but they may be caused by tumor, inflammation of the temporal artery, stroke, CNS infection, or hypertension. Presentation varies, depending on the underlying cause.

Pathophysiology and Assessment of Muscle Tension Headaches

Muscle tension headaches are caused by stress (tension), which causes residual muscle contractions (tension) within the face and head. Ninety percent of headaches are this type. The pain tends to be perceived on both sides of head, traveling from back to front, and can be characterized as a dull ache or a squeezing pain. The jaw, neck, or shoulders may also be stiff or sore.

Pathophysiology and Assessment of Migraine Headaches

Migraine headaches are caused by changes in the size of blood vessels at the base of the brain. The patient may report seeing an aura, or a perception of bright lights. The pain tends to be unilateral and focused, becoming more diffuse as the headache progresses. The patient often describes throbbing, pounding, pulsating pain and may have nausea and vomiting. He or she may prefer to remain in a dark, quiet environment. A migraine headache can last several days.

Pathophysiology and Assessment of Cluster Headaches

Cluster headaches are a rare vascular headache that begins in the face as a minor pain around one eye. The pain quickly intensifies and spreads to one side of the face. The headaches occur in groups, or clusters, and last only 30 to 45 minutes each. However, a person may have several per day. The headaches can recur for days and then stop entirely. They may return at the same time the following month or the same time the next day. It is unclear what is triggering these headaches, but serotonin and histamine are suspected of playing a role. The headaches are often accompanied by anxiety.

Pathophysiology and Assessment of Sinus Headaches

Sinus headaches are caused by inflammation or infection within the sinus cavities of the face. The pain is located in the superior portions of the face and increases when the patient bends over. Sinus headache pain is often worst on waking. This kind of headache may be accompanied by postnasal drip, a sore throat, and nasal discharge.

Management of the Headache Patient

When you are caring for a patient with a headache, be cautious because headaches can indicate a more serious problem **Figure 18**. If other signs indicate that a stroke may be in progress, treat the patient for stroke. Remember, a patient who reports the worst headache of his or her life may be having a stroke.

Ask what medications the patient has taken, such as ibuprofen, acetaminophen, and aspirin. Determine how much the patient took and when the last dose(s) was taken.

Medications for pain management might include ketorolac tromethamine (Toradol IM) (30 mg IVP), meperidine (Demerol) (25 mg slow IVP), and morphine (2 to 4 mg slow IVP). Most patients, however, do not require narcotics. Also consider

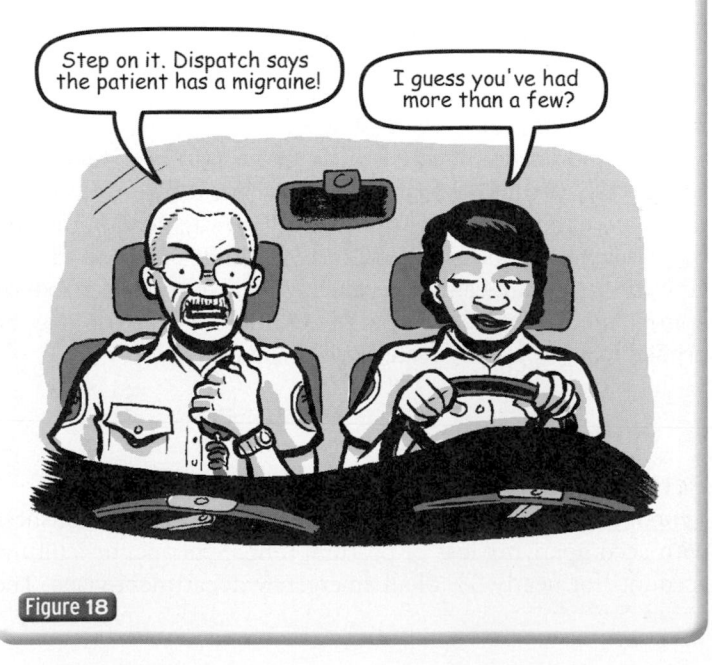

Figure 18

promethazine (Phenergan) (12.5 to 25 mg IVP) or ondansetron (Zofran) (4 mg IVP) for nausea and vomiting. In-hospital management includes administering analgesics and ruling out serious medical problems.

■ Dementia

Pathophysiology

Dementia is the chronic deterioration of memory, personality, language skills, perception, reasoning, or judgment, with no loss of consciousness. These changes can occur over weeks to years and can be subtle. The reasons for these neurologic changes are dramatically different. Wernicke encephalopathy presents with dementia and is caused by a vitamin B_1 deficiency. This condition occurs in patients who are chronically malnourished. The classic patient is a chronic alcoholic who ingests a diet mostly consisting of simple sugars. Without vitamin B_1, brain neurochemistry will not work correctly.

Compare this to Alzheimer disease, the most common form of dementia. Alzheimer disease is a progressive organic condition in which neurons die. When the affected brain tissue is examined under a microscope, it appears to be riddled with tangles and clumps of damaged tissue.

Dementia should not be confused with delirium. Delirium is a sudden state of confusion or disorientation. By definition, delirium is reversible, whereas many dementias are irreversible. If you have ever been to a bar and seen someone drunk, you have witnesed delirium: sudden onset confusion that is reversible.

Assessment

The initial demonstration of the disease can be dismissed as forgetfulness or "old age." It is important to note that Alzheimer disease is not a natural part of aging. As the disease progresses, it becomes obvious that this is not simple memory loss when patients cannot remember names, addresses, directions, or how to perform tasks. Patients can become aggressive and violent because the disease damages their judgment centers. Confusion is the hallmark sign. Eventually, the damage involves the ability to swallow. See **Table 16** for a comparison of types of dementia.

Management

Prehospital management follows standard care guidelines. Ensure that no reversible cause is present. Check the blood glucose level, oxygen level, and blood chemistry. Changes in any of these levels can cause confusion. You need to be compassionate and ready to repeat yourself. These conditions can be frustrating for the patient. In the early stages, patients realize that they are not able to think as efficiently as in the past. Depression and withdrawal are common.

Wernicke encephalopathy bears special mention. In this condition, the confusion and dementia are partially reversible. Remember that the brain needs vitamin B_1 to metabolize sugars, so in patients suspected of being malnourished, you should administer thiamine, 100 to 200 mg IVP, before any glucose is given. In patients with a vitamin B_1 deficit, giving glucose can actually cause confusion or worsen the patient's presentation if thiamine is not present.

These patients may have other malnutrition concerns, including hypomagnesemia, hypokalemia, and hyponatremia. It would be prudent to perform ECG monitoring and obtain blood chemistries.

In-hospital care of patients begins with diagnosis. Imaging scans, neurologic functioning tests, EEGs, and blood work are done to determine the cause. In many dementias, there is no definitive treatment for the destroyed neurons.

■ Neoplasms

Pathophysiology

Neoplasm is the medical term for growths within the body that serve no useful purpose and are caused by errors that occur during cellular reproduction. The human body is composed of trillions of cells. Each of these cells has a life expectancy. People are able to live for 70, 80, or 100 years because the body's cells can reproduce. This cellular reproduction, called *mitosis,* is the process by which one parent cell divides into two identical duplicates called daughter cells. This process of cell division occurs constantly as cells age and must be replaced. **Figure 19** illustrates the process of normal cell division.

When mitosis occurs, the daughter cells that are created are usually perfect copies of the parent cell. This duplication ensures continued functioning of bones, ventricles, lungs, and other vital structures. Occasionally, though, errors in duplication occur. These errors tend to happen during the untwining and reproduction of the cellular DNA. If the error is severe, the cell will have too much damaged DNA to survive. It will die, and the DNA error will die with it.

If the error is more subtle, however, the cell may survive. This daughter cell is said to contain a mutation and thus is not identical to the parent cell. This altered cell can reproduce and copy the error to its own daughter cells. Simply put, cancer is an error in one's own cell reproduction. The magnitude of the cancer depends on how effectively this new, altered cell is able to reproduce and obtain nutrients for growth.

Neoplasms can be categorized as either benign or malignant. Essentially, benign tumors are not cancerous and are not very aggressive. They tend to remain within a fibrous capsule, which limits their growth. They are also usually easy to remove. Malignant neoplasms, on the other hand, will take over blood supplies, grow unchecked, and move to other sites within the body. Neoplasms have finger-like projections that extend into surrounding tissue, spreading and invading new areas. This growth without regard to other cells is the main reason that many malignancies are fatal.

Within the context of the neurologic system, a neoplasm is a cancer of the brain or spinal cord.

Tumors can be classified according to whether they represent primary or metastatic disease. Primary neoplasms of the neurologic system are cancers that arise within the nervous system. Because mature neurons no longer divide, however, they rarely become cancerous. Primary CNS tumors, then, are usually caused by errors in mitosis within the support structures of the CNS, such as a meningioma.

Table 16 Comparison of Selected Types of Dementia

Disease	Cause	Presentation	Typical Course of Disease
Alzheimer disease	Multifactorial: Gradual buildup of plaques within the brain, which cause neuronal death. Eventual decrease in brain mass. Process begins 10 to 20 years before signs and symptoms appear.	Chronic, insidious memory loss is the earliest finding. In moderate disease, a decrease in attention, judgment, and language functions (people get lost, cannot balance a check book, repeat questions). In severe disease, cannot recognize people; eventually cannot communicate and become bedridden.	8 to 10 years
Pick disease	Unknown. Does have a genetic aspect. Disease has its roots in damage to neurons in the frontal and temporal lobes.	Occurs in people between ages 55 and 65 years, with insidious presentation of socially inappropriate behavior, such as stealing and obsessive behaviors. Patient may be apathetic, depressed, or inappropriately elated. Additionally, rest tremors, difficulty naming common objects (anomia), and incontinence may be present.	6 years
Huntington disease (Huntington chorea)	An adult-onset genetic disorder marked by severe loss of neurons.	Initially fidgetiness, abnormal eye movements, tics, myoclonus, irritability, and loss of interest. As the disease progresses, bradykinesia, difficulty standing, ataxia, slowing of thinking, and memory loss occur.	19 years
Creutzfeldt-Jakob disease	Prion infection, usually contracted by eating contaminated beef. Can rarely occur as a spontaneous change within the brain.	Myoclonic jerking, major cognitive deterioration, visual impairment, unstable gait (ataxia). Disease is always fatal.	8 months
Wernicke encephalopathy	Thiamine (vitamin B_1) deficiency. Occurs in patients with longstanding malnutrition, such as chronic alcoholics.	Ataxia, confusion, agitation, memory loss, nystagmus, generalized weakness, foot drop, and peripheral neuropathy.	Variable, depending on cause and extent of malnutrition

The process by which cancerous cells move to sites distant from their site of origin is called <u>metastasis</u>. Metastatic neoplasms of the neurologic system are tumors that arise elsewhere in the body, travel through the bloodstream or lymphatic system, and take up residence within nervous system tissues. Lung and breast cancers are the two most common types of cancer to metastasize to the CNS.

Assessment

Headache, nausea and vomiting, seizures, change in mental status, and stroke-like signs and symptoms are common in patients with brain tumors. The rate and intensity of these signs and symptoms depends on how quickly the cancer is growing and its location. Patients may have months of headaches or suddenly have a seizure without any prior complaints.

Patients with spinal tumors have signs and symptoms related to compression of the cord. Back pain is the most common symptom. Patients may also experience weakness, ataxia, loss of sensation in a limb, incontinence, and a deformity along the spine. Other symptoms related to compression of the spinal cord are discussed in the trauma chapters.

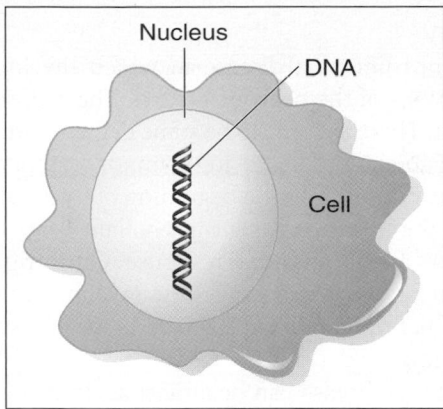

The parent cell prepares to reproduce.

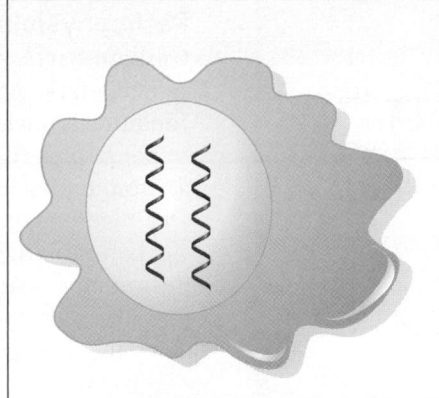

Intertwined strands of DNA separate.

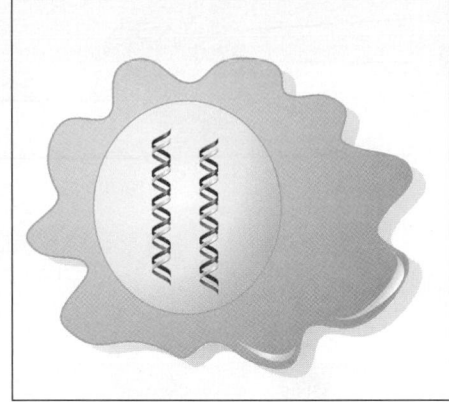

DNA copies itself, creating two identical DNA strands.

Figure 19 Normal mitosis.

Management

Prehospital management is supportive. Watch for status epilepticus. If needed, administer diazepam. These patients can have elevated ICP. All patients with new onset seizures or chronic headaches that cannot be managed need to be medically evaluated. If the patient has a spinal tumor, be prepared to protect limbs from injury. In-hospital management is complex depending on the type of cancer and location.

■ Pathophysiology, Assessment, and Management of Demyelinating and Motor Neuron Disorders

■ Multiple Sclerosis

Pathophysiology

Multiple sclerosis (MS) is an autoimmune condition in which the body attacks the myelin of the brain and spinal cord **Figure 20**. This results in demyelination, or destruction of the myelin. The resulting areas of scarring led to the name *multiple sclerosis* (from the Greek word *skleros,* meaning "hard"). As discussed in the chapter, *Pathophysiology,* the body has the ability to determine which proteins are "self" and which are "non-self." In an autoimmune disorder, the body begins to attack its own cells. The immune system is no longer able to distinguish friend from foe.

Consider the normal neuron. Myelin coats the axons of most nerve cells and allows for smooth transmission of signals to their target cell. In multiple sclerosis, the body believes that the proteins making up this insulation are foreign. It subsequently attacks that myelin, creating gaps in the insulation. These gaps cause characteristic signs and symptoms. It is believed that some as yet unknown environmental trigger, such as a virus, begins to focus the attention of the immune system on the myelin.

Assessment

The presentation of MS follows a pattern of attacks and remissions. In the initial attack, double vision and blurred vision are common complaints. The patient may have **nystagmus**, an involuntary, rhythmic eye movement.

The attacks can vary in intensity and remissions can vary in length. Patients experience muscle weakness; impairment of pain, temperature, and touch senses; pain (moderate to severe); ataxia; intention tremors; speech and vision disturbances; vertigo; bladder and bowel dysfunction; sexual dysfunction; depression; euphoria; cognitive abnormalities; and fatigue during attacks **Figure 21**. Patients may also experience a strange electrical sensation. When the head is flexed forward, patients experience an electrical sensation down their spine or extremities (Lhermitte sign).

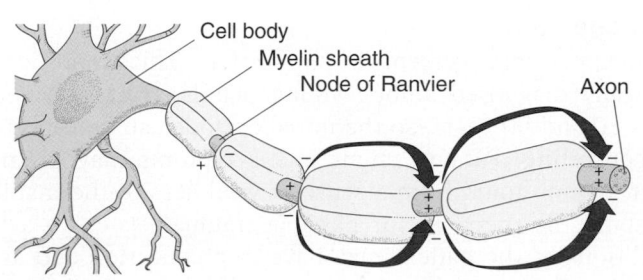

Figure 20 The myelin sheath insulates the axon, allowing impulses to jump from node to node, which accelerates the rate of signal transmission. In multiple sclerosis and other demyelinating conditions, this protective sheath is destroyed by inflammation and signals can no longer be transmitted smoothly.

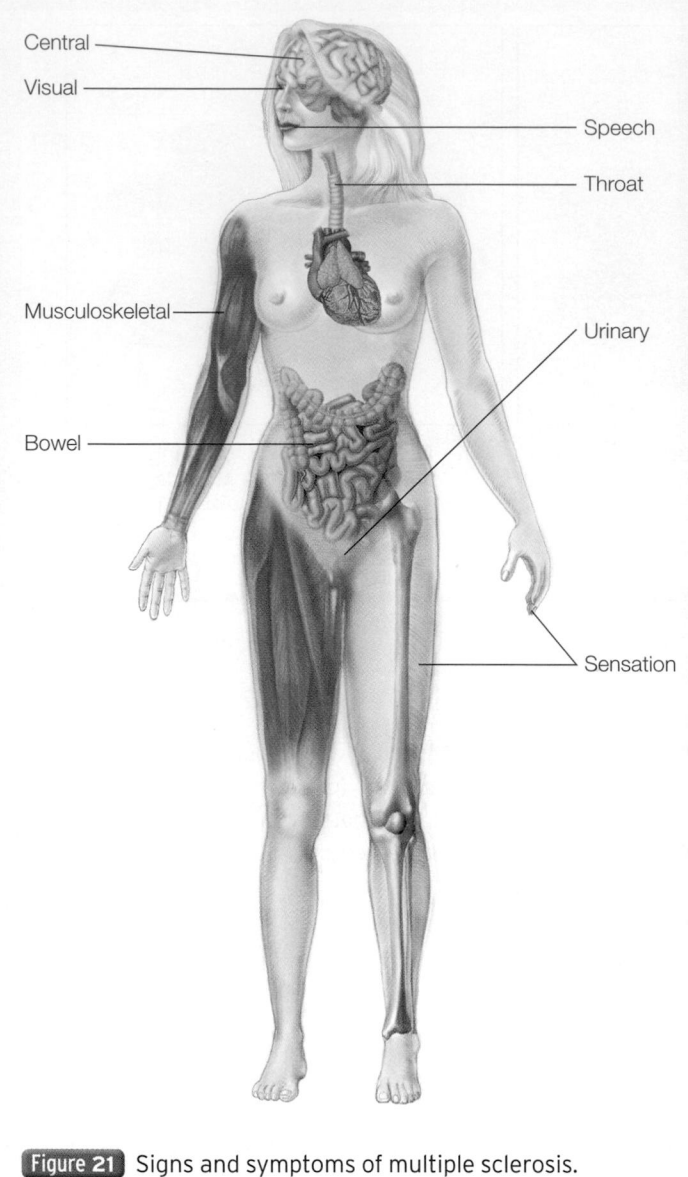

Central
Visual
Speech
Throat
Musculoskeletal
Urinary
Bowel
Sensation

Figure 21 Signs and symptoms of multiple sclerosis.

Management

Prehospital management is supportive. This condition is typically diagnosed among young people, usually between ages 20 and 50 years, so the initial episode can be especially disconcerting. Patients' signs and symptoms may progress over several hours from a sense of weakness to the inability to stand. Be prepared for possible trauma related to a fall. Additionally, the patient may have true confusion and anxiety—not because of some brain malfunction, but because this previously healthy person is trying to understand what is happening.

In-hospital treatment is directed at controlling the symptoms. Administration of anti-inflammatory medications may be used to decrease the length of the attack. There is currently no cure.

■ Guillain-Barré Syndrome

Pathophysiology

Guillain-Barré syndrome is a disease in which the immune system attacks portions of the nervous system. The cause of the condition is unclear. There appears to be some degree of immune response present. Patients report having a minor respiratory or gastrointestinal infection prior to the beginning of the weakness. One theory is that the infectious agent in Guillain-Barré (ghee-yan bah-ray) triggers an autoimmune response. Once triggered, the immune system attacks and damages the myelin, and therefore it is a demyelinating condition. Signals being transmitted along the axon are impaired.

The reversal of this disease can be almost as dramatic as its onset. Some patients recover completely without residual weakness in as little as several weeks. About one third of patients have some degree of weakness after 3 years. Some patients require ventilatory assistance for the rest of their lives.

Assessment

This rare condition is frightening for most patients. It begins as weakness and tingling sensations in the legs. This weakness moves up the legs and begins to affect the thorax and arms. The weakness can become severe and may lead to paralysis. This transition from being able to walk and speak to needing a ventilator to breathe can take as little as several hours. Most patients experience maximum muscle weakness or paralysis within 2 weeks of the onset of the disease. In addition to the peripheral motor neuron involvement, the autoregulatory systems can be involved. Patients are prone to severe swings in pulse rate and blood pressure.

Management

Prehospital management should include close assessment of the ability of the patient to effectively protect the airway and ventilate. Monitor the patient closely with ECG and repeat vital signs. Continuous end tidal CO_2 readings can provide evidence of impending respiratory failure. Be prepared to administer IV fluids to maintain blood pressure and treat hemodynamically significant bradycardia following AHA guidelines. It needs to be emphasized that patients can be experiencing terror as the condition progresses; therefore, use a comforting voice and a therapeutic touch as you care for the patient.

In-hospital management includes plasmapheresis (exchanging the plasma within the blood) and immunoglobulin injections. These therapies decrease the patient's recovery time.

■ Amyotrophic Lateral Sclerosis (ALS)

Pathophysiology

Amyotrophic lateral sclerosis (ALS) (Lou Gehrig disease) is a disease that strikes the voluntary motor neurons. It is unclear exactly what causes the death of the motor neurons. One theory is that the body's immune system selectively attacks and kills them. There is some evidence that genetics may play a role. The condition is more common in middle-aged men of any race.

Assessment

Initially this condition is rather subtle and progresses without being noticed. Fatigue, general weakness of muscle groups, and difficulty doing routine activities like eating, writing, and dressing will develop. Patients may also experience difficulty speaking. As the condition progresses, the ability to walk, move the arms, eat, and speak is lost. The speed of progression is different for every patient. Because this condition is motor neuron only, the patient is completely aware of his or her surroundings and the inability to move.

The average person diagnosed with this condition dies within 3 to 5 years. As the destruction of motor neurons continues, eventually patients are unable to breathe effectively without ventilatory assistance. Patients die from respiratory infections or other complications related to immobility.

Management

Prehospital treatment for these patients follows standard care guidelines. Assess the patient's ability to swallow and monitor the airway closely. Patients may rely on a variety of home medical technologies, including feeding pumps, IV pumps, long-term IV access ports, and ventilators. Transportation of such patients can become complicated. Ask for guidance from the family or home health care provider to operate any unfamiliar devices. If needed, disconnect the patient from the technology after consulting medical control and transport.

In-hospital care for ALS is geared toward supporting vital functions. Patients undergo physical therapy to help strengthen remaining neurons and muscles. Medications can be given to mitigate some of the symptoms; however, this condition has no cure.

■ Parkinson Disease

Pathophysiology

Parkinson disease is a neurologic condition in which past injuries to the brain can have an influence. A portion of the brain is responsible for production of dopamine. If this section is damaged or overused, Parkinson disease can result. The substantia nigra, the portion of the brain that produces dopamine, has been found to be damaged in patients with Parkinson disease. In some patients, the damage can be linked to past injuries, whereas in other patients, the damage is unexplainable at this time. Dopamine is a neurotransmitter that, among other things, is needed for muscles to contract smoothly. Patients with Parkinson disease used to have a mortality rate three times that of the general population. With appropriate treatment, however, that mortality rate has been cut in half.

Assessment

A gradual onset of symptoms over months to years is typical. The initial signs are often unilateral tremors. Over time, as the dopamine level falls, more areas of the body are involved. Genetics play an important role. Parkinson-like activity can be observed in head injuries and some overdose patients.

The classic presentation of Parkinson disease involves the following four characteristics:

1. **Tremor.** Rest tremors and postural tremors are common among patients with Parkinson disease.
2. **Postural instability.** Patients have a stiff posture in which they are stooped over, and the disease alters their gait. This combination makes these patients more unsteady when walking, and they are therefore at an increased risk of falling.
3. **Rigidity.** Rigidity, a condition in which muscles do not contract and relax smoothly, causes the patient to move in fits and starts.
4. **Bradykinesia.** Parkinson patients have a classic type of gait. They tend to shuffle in a straight line, with their feet close together. When asked to turn, they take small steps until the turn is complete. This is called bradykinesia, the slowing down of routine motions.

Other symptoms of Parkinson disease include depression, difficulty swallowing, speech impairments, and fatigue. Prognosis is poor as the condition advances. Patients in later stages are at a much greater risk of death from aspiration, pneumonia, falls, or complications due to immobility.

Management

Prehospital management is supportive. Remember that these patients may be depressed or even have some degree of dementia. Reorient the patient if needed. A compassionate gesture can be very helpful. If the patient has trauma, those injuries will need to be managed as well. In-hospital management includes levodopa, which helps to temporarily restore dopamine levels. Other medications, surgery, and modification of diet and exercise are other options.

■ Cranial Nerve Disorders

Pathophysiology

In this portion of the chapter, relatively rare disorders will be discussed. You must understand that some disorders can mimic other conditions.

Someone with severe facial pain or sudden-onset facial paralysis is not necessarily having a stroke. Not everyone with left ventricular hypertrophy is having a myocardial infarction. Cranial nerve disorders are no different: They may not be as clear-cut as they first appear.

All of these conditions involve one or more of the cranial nerves, typically of the facial region. Table 17 provides an overview of these disorders.

Assessment

You can also test for vertigo. However, this test can only be done in patients who are at no risk of cervical spine trauma or other neck disease. Have the patient lie supine. Place your hands on either side of the head and move the head rapidly from side to side once. Then return the head to the neutral position. This maneuver causes the liquid within the inner ear to move. Next, look at the patient's eyes. If the patient has vertigo, you should

Table 17   Cranial Nerve Disorders

Disorder	Cause/Cranial Nerve Involved	Presentation
Trigeminal neuralgia Also called *tic douloureux* (tik' doo-loo-roo')	The usual cause is irritation by an artery lying too close to the nerve. Over time, as the artery changes diameter to meet blood supply needs, this motion can grate the myelin sheath off of the nerve. With the insulation partially gone, the nerve can "short out," causing pain without trauma to the area. Cranial nerve involved is the trigeminal nerve (cranial nerve V).	Severe, shock-like, or stabbing pain, usually on one side of the face. Attacks can last for several minutes to several months. Triggered by touching the face, speaking, brushing teeth, eating, putting on clothing, the wind—essentially any activity in which the face is stimulated. No loss of taste, hearing, or facial sensation or motor control of the face.
Hemifacial spasm	Dilated blood vessels irritate the facial nerve, cranial nerve VII.	Involuntary unilateral facial movements. Tics, myoclonic contractions, jaw distortion, and facial tremors. There is no pain associated with this condition.
Acoustic neuroma	Neoplasm (tumor) at the base of the brain. As the tumor grows, it can apply pressure to nerves, prevent movement of cerebrospinal fluid, or compress blood vessels, causing ischemia. This process takes years because this tumor grows slowly. Affects cranial nerve VIII or VII (vestibulocochlear and facial nerves).	Unilateral hearing loss, headache, tinnitus, facial numbness, and balance disorders.
Glossopharyngeal neuralgia	Irritation of the glossopharyngeal nerve (cranial nerve IX). Cause of irritation is unknown.	Attacks of severe, sharp unilateral pain in the tongue, at the back of the throat, in the middle ear, and in the tonsil area. Pain can last from seconds to several minutes, with multiple attacks possible in one day. Attacks can be triggered by swallowing, eating cold food or drinks, sneezing, or coughing.
Ménière disease	Cause is unclear but the disease is believed to be related to an increase in fluid pressure within the inner ear. This pressure stimulates the VIII cranial nerve (vestibulocochlear nerve).	Unilateral tinnitus, dizziness, hearing loss, and a sensation of fullness in the ear. Episodes tend to last 2 to 4 hours. Repeated attacks can cause permanent deafness.
Bell palsy	Minor infection of the facial nerve, cranial nerve VII.	The attack is sudden and can easily be confused with a stroke. Signs and symptoms are eyelid ptosis, facial droop or weakness, excessive salivation, loss of the ability to taste. Episodes can last up to 2 weeks.

Documentation and Communication

When discussing cranial nerve disorders, it is important to make a clear distinction between vertigo and dizziness. Vertigo, which involves the cranial nerves, is the sensation that you are moving when you are not, like the feeling you had as a child rolling down a hill. It is typically caused by inner ear disease. Vertigo is not the same as dizziness. Dizziness is a sensation of lightheadedness typically related to low blood pressure in the brain. So how can you differentiate the two? Talk with the patient. Ask him or her to describe the sensation without using the word "dizzy." Listen carefully to the words the patient chooses. Words and phrases like "spinning," "whirling," and "off balance" point toward vertigo, whereas descriptors such as "fuzzy" and "blackout" suggest dizziness. Good communication with your patient can help you draw accurate conclusions.

see nystagmus. Also, the motion of the head will typically increase the patient's sensation of vertigo.

Management

Treatment for cranial nerve disorders is mainly supportive. Patients may need promethazine (Phenergan) (12.5 to 25 mg IVP) or ondansetron (Zofran) (4 mg IVP) for the nausea and vomiting that may be present with some cranial nerve disorders. Benzodiazepines such as diazepam (Valium) may provide some relief from the vertigo.

In-hospital management of these conditions is related to the specific condition and its cause. Care is focused on ensuring that a serious condition, such as a brain tumor, is not present. Therapy is then directed at making the patient comfortable and treating the underlying cause. Carbamazepine (Tegretol) and gabapentin (Neurontin) are often used to treat these conditions. Antivirals and cortisteroid medications may also be used.

■ Dystonia

Pathophysiology

Dystonias are severe, abnormal muscle spasms that cause bizarre contortions, repetitive motions, or postures. Primary dystonias occur for an unknown reason. A defect in the body's ability to process neurotransmitters is thought to be the core of the problem. These patients have normal intelligence and no psychiatric medical history. Spasmodic torticollis Figure 22, in which the neck muscles contract, twisting the head to one side and usually pulling it forward or backward, is a common example of a primary dystonia. The head then remains painfully frozen in that position. Facial dystonia can take several forms.

Assessment

These spasms are involuntary and are often painful. Dystonia can be both a sign and a symptom. Some patients who take antipsychotic medications may have a sudden onset of bizarre contortions of the face or body. This would be a secondary dystonia and would more appropriately be considered a sign than a symptom.

Words of Wisdom

Regardless of the underlying cause, dystonias are socially upsetting because patients suddenly twist and writhe uncontrollably. It is critical that you provide compassionate care.

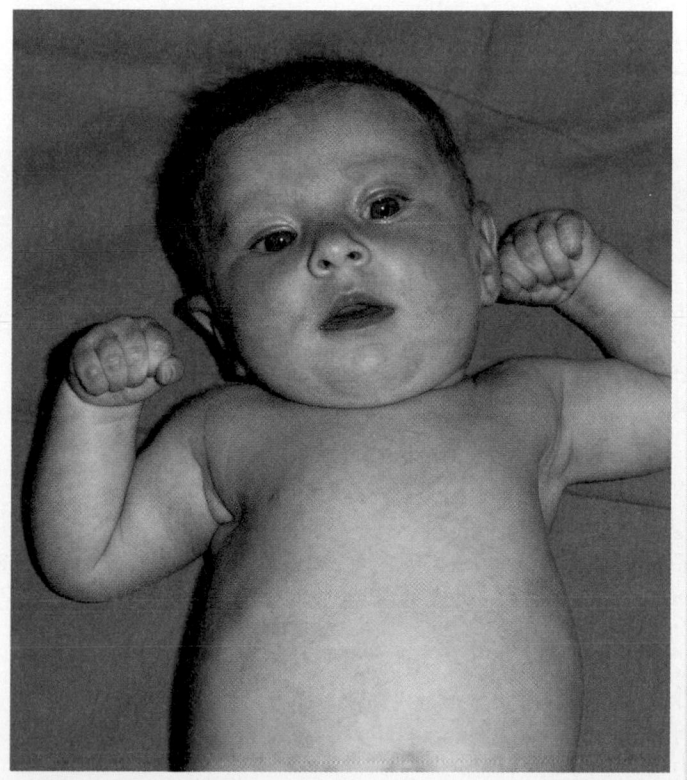

Figure 22 Example of torticollis or "wry neck" dystonia.

Management

Prehospital management should be focused on ruling out other problems like seizures, strokes, or psychiatric medication reaction. If you suspect a dystonic reaction to antipsychotic medications, diphenhydramine (Benadryl) (25 mg IVP) is the drug of choice to stop the contraction. Unfortunately, this medication is ineffective in primary dystonias. Regardless of their cause, dsytonias can be very unnerving and even painful. Pain management may be considered appropriate. Talk with your patient and let him or her know you are trying to help. Be calm and reassuring. In-hospital management involves a variety of medication options to control the condition.

■ Central Nervous System Infections/Inflammation

Pathophysiology

To begin the discussion on central nervous system infections and inflammation, it is important for you to understand some fundamental definitions. Encephalitis is inflammation of the brain. Meningitis is the inflammation of the meninges, the outer covering of the central nervous system. Clinically, these infections are difficult, if not impossible, to distinguish in the prehospital arena. Both infections can result from a variety of causes, including infectious, chemical, and/or metabolic. Infectious pathology is the most common form of both conditions when it presents in the acute phase.

Infectious causes for conditions are the result of bacteria, viruses, fungi, or prions gaining access to the body, reproducing and causing damage. These organisms have a basic goal—to continue to live. To do so, all organisms need food and must reproduce. As the organism begins to attack the body, it is looking for fuel with which to create the next generation of bacteria, viruses, or other pathogens. The damage that these organisms create occurs due to several mechanisms. Either the damage is caused by the body's reaction to the infection or by the activities of the attacking organisms.

The most common sign of infectious disease is the presence of a fever. Many pathogenic organisms prefer to grow within a narrow temperature range, so even a 2° to 3° climb in body temperature can slow the reproduction of some viruses or bacteria. This allows the immune system to gain control, providing valuable time for neutrophils (the body's defenses) to find and kill the invading organisms. It also signals the rest of the body that an attack is underway. More white blood cells are produced and chemical mediators are released to improve the body's effectiveness at finding and eliminating the organisms. Fevers are good.

If the temperature of the body becomes too high, the brain can be affected. Remember the last time you felt ill and had a fever. The increased temperature made your thinking dull, it was difficult to concentrate, and you may have had a headache. These effects are common with fevers. Neurons are sensitive to temperature changes. As the temperature rises, the effects on the neurons can become more profound. Eventually, a person may hallucinate, become delusional, or lose consciousness. Another possibility is the random firing of neurons, which in this case would be referred to as a febrile seizure.

Another mechanism by which infectious agents can cause damage to the body is through destruction of cells. Organisms can produce **endotoxins** or **exotoxins** that can damage living cells. Endotoxins are proteins that are released by gram-negative bacteria when they die. Exotoxins are proteins that are secreted by some bacteria or fungi to aid in the death and digestion of other cells. In poliomyelitis, the virus responsible for the disease attacks the axons directly and destroys them. The virus is also rather specific. It does not attack just any axon. It has a preference for motor axons—neurons that are responsible for making muscles contract. Without these axons in place, the patient can experience weakness, paralysis, and respiratory arrest.

Assessment

Table 18 shows that the presentation of encephalitis and meningitis is similar. Both illnesses begin with flu-like symptoms. As the organism reproduces and causes more damage, a stiff neck, photophobia, lethargy, an altered LOC, and seizures are possible. Kernig sign Figure 23A or Brudzinski sign Figure 23B may be elicited in meningitis.

Management

Treatment for these conditions is mainly supportive. Patients with suspected meningitis should have a mask placed over their mouths to limit the spread of organisms. You should also wear a mask if the patient is coughing. Be prepared for seizures and treat accordingly. One of the risks, particularly for bacterial meningitis, is increased ICP. Another risk of these conditions is septicemia. This indicates the infection is now present within the bloodstream. Septicemia can cause ruptures of capillaries and loss of vasomotor control of blood vessels. See the chapter, *Infectious Diseases* for more information on septicemia.

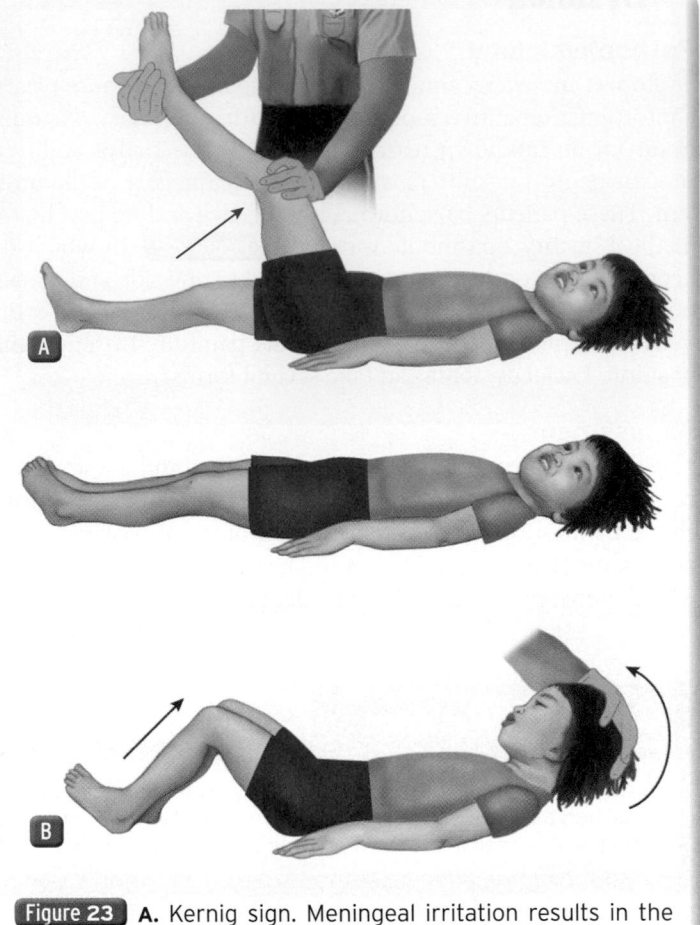

Figure 23 **A.** Kernig sign. Meningeal irritation results in the inability to straighten the leg with the hips flexed. **B.** Brudzinski sign. Meningeal irritation results in an involuntary flexion of the knees when the head is flexed toward the chest.

Table 18	Comparison of Encephalitis and Meningitis		
Condition	**Organisms Usually Responsible**	**Presentation**	**Timeline**
Encephalitis	Herpes simplex virus: Most common sporadic form. Arboviruses: Most common episodic form. These viruses are transmitted by vectors and cause outbreaks of illnesses. Examples include West Nile virus, rabies, and Japanese virus encephalitis.	First signs and symptoms are fever, headache, nausea/vomiting, and general malaise. As the condition progresses, changes in LOC occur, including behavioral and personality changes, nuchal rigidity (stiff neck), photophobia, lethargy, confusion, and seizure.	Several days, depending on the specific virus involved.
Meningitis	Neonates: *Streptococci* and *Escherichia coli.* Infants/children: *Haemophilus influenzae* (more common in children), *Streptococcus pneumoniae*, and *Neisseria meningitidis.* Adults: *S. pneumoniae, N. meningitides* (more common in adults), and *H. influenzae.*	First signs and symptoms are upper respiratory infection (runny nose, cough, malaise). As the condition progresses, the patient may have headache, nuchal rigidity, fever and chills, photophobia, vomiting, seizures, confusion, Kernig sign, and Brudzinski sign. Infants are irritable when held, and have a high-pitched cry (cat's cry) and bulging fontanelles.	Bacterial pathogen: presentation within 24 hours Viral pathogen: presentation in 1 to 7 days.

Encephalitis is not particularly contagious from person to person but meningitis can be. Follow-up care for the paramedic may involve preventive antibiotic treatment for possible bacterial meningitis. It is important for you (or your supervisor) to stay in contact with the infection control officer from the hospital to which the patient was transported. Hospital treatment is directed at decreasing swelling in the brain and spinal cord, fighting the infection, and supporting the patient's vital signs.

Abscesses

Pathophysiology

Abscesses are the caused by an infectious agent within the brain or spinal cord. When an infectious agent attacks brain or spinal cord cells and destroys tissue, the immune system responds by attempting to kill the pathogen. If it cannot, the body's second line of defense is to erect a wall to prevent the pathogen from spreading. This capsule envelops the infectious agent, as well as dead or dying brain or spinal cord cells, dead white blood cells, and white blood cells that are still fighting the infection. Over time, with continued tissue destruction and immune system response, swelling can occur. The result is an abscess.

The underlying reason for an infection within the brain or spinal cord is varied. Such an infection is often preceded by an infection of the sinuses, throat, gums, or ear. The pathogenic organism can also be introduced to the brain when head or spinal cord trauma occurs.

Assessment

The two main consequences of the infection are damage to an area of the brain or spinal cord and the presence of an abscess within the cranial vault or spinal cord. These two factors dictate the presentation of a patient with a CNS abscess. Look for a low- or high-grade fever, persistent headache (often localized), drowsiness, confusion, generalized or focal seizures, nausea and vomiting, focal motor or sensory impairments, and hemiparesis.

Management

Follow standard care guidelines. Pay close attention for evidence of increased ICP. Take seizure precautions. Evaluate temperature. If it is low, cover the patient, turn on the heat, and prevent heat loss. If it is high, remove the patient's clothing, cover the patient with a sheet, and turn off the heat in the patient compartment.

In-hospital management involves antibiotics, seizure precautions, and sometimes surgical removal of the abscess.

Poliomyelitis and Postpolio Syndrome

Pathophysiology

Poliomyelitis is a viral infection transmitted by the fecal-oral route. Its incidence peaked in the United States in the 1950s. Since then, an effective vaccine has been developed. There have been no cases of wild polio within the United States since 1979. It is believed that polio will be eradicated worldwide within 10 years. Most patients who contract the virus do not become ill.

Assessment

Signs and symptoms for those people who become infected begin in as little as 1 week after exposure. In the most severe cases, they include sore throat, nausea, vomiting, diarrhea, stiff neck, and muscle weakness/paralysis.

Management

In-hospital care for patients with the acute illness is directed at hydration, ventilation, and calorie support until the infection has been managed by the immune system. The way the virus damages the nervous system places patients at risk for problems decades after the initial infection. The virus attacks motor neurons within the brain and brainstem. This causes the classic signs of weakness and paralysis. The remaining neurons now begin to send out new axons to try to compensate for this loss. This allows the patient to regain function.

Over time, these neurons are doing more work than they are accustomed and they can begin to break down and die. This creates postpolio syndrome. Patients who had polio in the early- to mid-20th century may now have difficulty swallowing, weakness, fatigue, or breathing problems. Typically, the location in which the patient had symptoms when they were infected now presents with milder fatigue and weakness than the original infection caused.

Prehospital treatment emphasizes managing possible airway obstruction due to swallowing difficulties. In-hospital treatment for postpolio syndrome includes physical therapy and some experimental medications.

Peripheral Neuropathy

Pathophysiology

Peripheral neuropathy is a group of conditions in which the nerves leaving the spinal cord are damaged. The signals moving to or from the brain become distorted. There are many causes for this group of conditions including trauma, toxins, tumors, autoimmune attacks, and metabolic disorders. Trigeminal neuralgia and Guillain-Barré syndrome are examples. The remainder of this discussion will be limited to the most common form, which is diabetic neuropathy.

Assessment

As the blood glucose level rises, damage can occur to the peripheral nerves. The result is misfiring and shorting of signals. Patients may have sensory or motor impairment. Loss of sensation, numbness, burning, pain, paresthesia, and muscle weakness are common. Patients may eventually lose the ability to feel their feet or other areas. The condition is progressive and is accelerated by high blood glucose levels.

Management

Management in the prehospital setting is supportive. In-hospital management includes pain medication. The use of antidepressants and anticonvulsants seems to have a positive effect on calming the peripheral nerves.

■ Hydrocephalus

Pathophysiology

Hydro- means water and *cephalus* refers to the head. This "water on the head" condition is primarily, though not exclusively, a pediatric condition. It is the result of an error in the manufacture, movement, or absorption of cerebrospinal fluid (CSF). As you recall, the brain is bathed in CSF. Only about 120 mL of CSF is present within the central nervous system. That is only 4 ounces of liquid. Our bodies produce about 0.3 mL/min. This production rate, however, is matched by the absorption rate, so that the net volume of fluid within the brain remains constant.

There are two main types of hydrocephalus. Normal-pressure hydrocephalus is a rare condition that occurs in older adults and its mechanism is unclear. The other type of hydrocephalus results in increased pressure within the cranial vault. The most common cause of increased ICP hydrocephalus is the slowed movement of CSF. Congenital malformations in the aqueducts for CSF, tumors, trauma, intracranial hemorrhage, and meningitis are the most common reasons why the flow of fluid slows. Even though movement of CSF decreases, production does not; therefore, total CSF volume increases.

Assessment

The signs and symptoms of increased ICP hydrocephalus can develop gradually, over months, or suddenly, over days. These signs and symptoms will also vary, however, depending on the cause and the age of the patient. An infant has a relatively soft skull and so the increased pressure results in increased head circumference. Infants also experience lethargy, irritability, vomiting, sun-setting eyes (a downward deviation of the eyes, as shown in **Figure 24**), tense or bulging fontanelles, and seizures.

Older children and adults do not have the flexibility of the skull that infants have and so their symptoms are slightly different. Headache, nausea, projectile vomiting, blurry or double vision, ataxia, poor coordination, and memory and personality impairments are seen in this population.

Management

A shunt is placed in most patients with hydrocephalus. This tube is placed in the ventricle within the brain, where CSF is stored. The tube drains CSF out of the skull and typically into the abdomen (called a ventriculoperitoneal [VP] shunt). This drainage allows the increased CSF to be safely removed and normal ICP to be maintained.

Complications of these shunts are inappropriate drainage of CSF. Too much drainage and the brain can collapse because of its own weight. This causes tearing and intracranial hemorrhage.

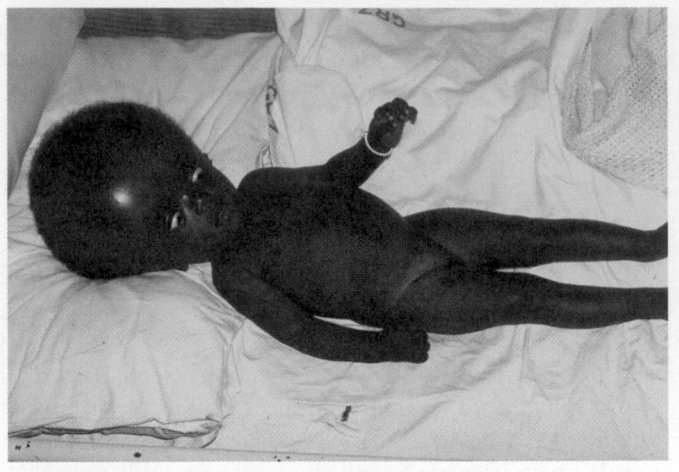

Figure 24 The "sunsetting sign" is so called because pressure on cranial nerves forces the eyes downward, leaving only a crescent visible beneath the sclera. This is a late sign of increased ICP hydrocephalus.

Too little drainage causes increased ICP. Obviously, placing a catheter within the brain breaks the skin and therefore increases the chance for infection. Finally, these shunts are often placed in children. As the children grow, the length of the tube becomes shorter than needed.

Care for these patients involves standard care. Be prepared for seizures and increased ICP. Because the patient is typically a child with multiple medical problems, the family can be a great resource. Use of invasive medical technology, including feeding tubes and ventilators, is not uncommon. Use the experience of the family in helping to care for these medically complicated children. Do not manipulate the VP shunt. The emergency department physician will access the shunt if needed.

■ Spina Bifida

Pathophysiology

Soon after conception, the blastocyst is no more than a ball of cells, each cell identical to the other. The changes that occur are rapid. Within just 8 days, the once uniform ball of cells is now ready to give rise to an embryo. One of the critical changes that must occur is the formation of the neural tube. In patients with **spina bifida**, the neural tube fails to close fully, and part of the nervous system remains outside the body.

The early embryo consists of a flat plate of cells. Around day 15 to 20, a layer of cells folds in to form a hollow tube. This neural tube will become the entire nervous system. In spina bifida, several cells do not fold correctly. These cells are outside the neural tube. This creates an outcropping of nervous system cells. As the embryo grows into a fetus and eventually a baby, these errant cells can become nervous tissue outside of its normal location **Figure 25**.

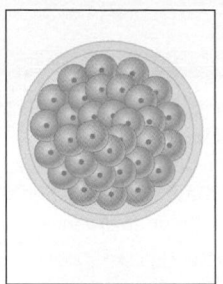

Morula

Soon after fertilization, the products of conception become a uniform ball of cells called a *morula*. This ball is 4 days old.

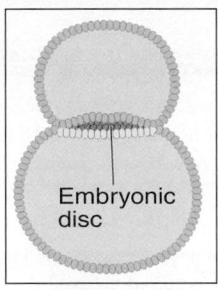

Blastocyst

On about day 5, the ball of cells separates into regions. It is now called a *blastocyst*. A plate of cells that will become the embryo is formed.

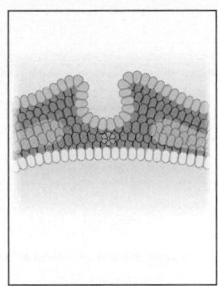

Begin to fold

The embryonic disc has three cell layers. This plate begins to fold on about day 15.

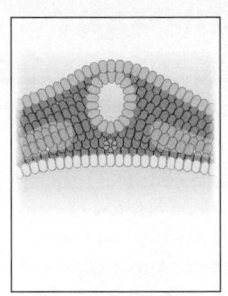

Neural tube

The folds now come together, forming a tube. This neural tube is the basis of the nervous system.

Figure 25 Embryonic development of the human nervous system.

technology, including feeding tubes, long-term IV access, ventilatory support, ambulatory assistive devices, and intraventricular shunts to drain excess CSF from the brain's ventricles. To avoid complications, consult with family and other home health care personnel when attempting to transport the patient. In-hospital management is supportive. It is possible to reimplant the spinal cord, even while the fetus remains within the uterus, but the damage to the previously exposed nerve tissue is permanent.

This condition has been linked to a low intake of folic acid during early pregnancy. This is one of the reasons why multivitamins are standard during pregnancy.

Even if the fetus forms correctly, problems may still occur. If an infection or chemical agent gains access to the growing fetus, areas of the brain can be damaged. A temporary decrease in oxygen can also damage the brain.

Spina bifida is a developmental condition resulting from a neural tube defect. It is unclear why the neural tube does not close, but due to this fact a portion of the spinal cord remains outside of its normal location. The severity of the condition is based on where the defect lies on the cord and how displaced it is from normal. Interestingly, many patients with spina bifida have allergies to latex. This creates patient care difficulties if your equipment is not latex free.

Assessment

This condition can present with no complications to complete loss of motor and sensory functions below the level of the defect. In the most severe forms, the defect also interferes with normal movement of CSF. CSF is made within the brain, circulates through the meninges, and is then reabsorbed. Hydrocephalus (water on the brain) is common in children with severe spina bifida because the CSF continues to be produced but cannot effectively be circulated. Pressure builds within the brain and these children have increased ICP problems and seizures.

Management

Prehospital management is supportive. In the most severe cases, these children are in need of multiple types of medical

Cerebral Palsy

Pathophysiology

Cerebral palsy (CP) is a developmental condition in which damage is done to the brain (often the frontal lobe). Scientists once believed that perinatal (around the time of birth) hypoxia was the primary cause of the disease. Recent research has shown, however, that perinatal hypoxia accounts for less than 10% of cases. Though its causes are currently unclear, infections, jaundice, or Rh incompatibility may be involved. The condition is self-limiting and therefore will not get worse over time. Infants who have a low birth weight, are premature, or are delivered breech, and those who are part of a multiple birth (twins or triplets, for example) are at higher risk of CP.

Assessment

The presentation of CP begins as an infant. Developmental milestones, such as walking or crawling may be delayed. The type and extent of damage soon becomes apparent. Patients with the spastic form of cerebral palsy often walk with a stiff, scissors-like gait, with the toes pointed inward and the knees nearly touching. This form of CP, in which muscles are in a nearly constant state of contraction, accounts for 70% to 80% of the cases. Other types of CP involve slow, uncontrolled writhing movements, tremor, and coordination difficulties.

Management

Prehospital management is supportive. In-hospital management is symptom based. There is no cure or correction for the damage. Care is directed at maximizing the child's abilities through surgery on the affected limbs and physical and occupational therapy.

YOU *are the Medic*   SUMMARY

1. How are you going to further define "not acting right"?

The three major elements that the brain needs to function are oxygen, glucose, and normal temperature. Use these principles to guide your assessment and pinpoint which of these elements may be causing the patient's altered mental status. Use the AVPU system or the Glasgow Coma Scale to evaluate the patient's LOC. Also, the patient may be confused. Confusion may indicate a low blood glucose level, decreased oxygen, an overdose, or even decreased blood pressure.

2. At this point, is your concern higher for a traumatic cause or a medical cause for the fall?

At this point in your assessment, you cannot make a decision either way. To aid in the process of discovery, obtain a general impression for this patient. Your general impression includes answers to the following questions:

- Where is the patient?
- Does the patient appear to be in distress or pain?
- Is the patient standing, sitting, or lying down?
- Is the patient outside or inside?
- Does the patient have obvious injuries?
- What does the environment look like?
- Is there evidence of drug paraphernalia?
- Is the house cluttered?
- Can the patient walk through the house without tripping?
- Is the patient responsive or unresponsive?
- Is the patient in stable or unstable condition?

3. What assessment steps can you take to determine why the patient is confused?

During the assessment phase, you should use a standard stroke assessment tool to increase the accuracy of your field impression. Use the Cincinnati Prehospital Stroke Scale or the Los Angeles Prehospital Stroke Screen as recommended by the American Heart Association.

4. What assumption should you make about the patient's communication with you and his sons?

Listen to the quality of the patient's speech. Is it slurred? Slurring is a classic finding with stroke. Is the speech appropriate? You need to focus on not only the quality of the words that are spoken, but the appropriateness of those words. There are several situations in which speech may be clear but word choice is incorrect. Assess the patient's object recognition abilities. In agnosia, patients will be unable to tell you the name of common objects. Agnosia relates to damage to the connections between visual interpretation of objects and the words that are associated with the object. Apraxia refers to the inability to know how to use a common object. It is possible for patients to be speaking clearly yet have these subtle knowledge deficits that may indicate a neurologic condition or emergency.

5. What are the two types of stroke?

There are two basic types of strokes: Ischemic (75%) and hemorrhagic (25%). Ischemic strokes can be caused by either a thrombus or embolus. The presentation patterns of these types of stroke differ. In ischemic stroke, a blood vessel is blocked, causing tissue distal to the blockage to become ischemic. Only the tissue beyond the blockage is affected, so the area(s) of the brain involved are limited. In the hemorrhagic stroke, a blood vessel ruptures, causing blood to be pumped into an enclosed space, increasing the ICP.

6. Of the two types of stroke, which one's symptoms will progressively worsen over time?

Hemorrhagic stroke tends to worsen over time because of bleeding within the cranium. This will cause increased ICP and herniation of the brainstem. One of the hallmarks of a hemorrhagic stroke is a report of the "worst headache of my life." If the patient reports a severe headache, and then later cannot speak, becomes difficult to arouse, and finally shows signs of increased ICP, you should strongly consider the possibility of a hemorrhagic stroke and provide rapid transport.

7. Would aspirin be indicated for a possible stroke patient?

Do not administer aspirin when you suspect a patient is having a stroke. The aspirin will help the patient with an ischemic stroke and cause harm in the patient with a hemorrhagic stroke. Aspirin should be administered only after a CT scan or MRI is performed to determine the location and type of brain injury.

8. How does a TIA differ from a stroke?

TIAs are episodes of cerebral ischemia without any permanent damage. Any of the typical presentations associated with a stroke can occur with TIAs. What distinguishes a TIA from a stroke is the resolution of signs and symptoms within 24 hours. With a TIA, there is no residual damage to brain tissue and, subsequently, no signs and symptoms after the episode ends. These mini-strokes are often signs of a serious vascular problem that requires medical evaluation. Over one third of patients with TIAs will experience a stroke soon afterwards. Think of the TIA/stroke relationship as being similar to the angina/myocardial infarction relationship.

YOU *are the Medic*   SUMMARY, *continued*

EMS Patient Care Report (PCR)

Date: 11-06-11	Incident No.: 3986		Nature of Call: Fall		Location: 1070 First St #2	
Dispatched: 0853	En Route: 0854	At Scene: 0858	Transport: 0916	At Hospital: 0923		In Service: 0940

Patient Information

Age: 81	Allergies: Opiates
Sex: M	Medications: Diltiazem, warfarin (Coumadin)
Weight (in kg [lb]): 63 kg (140 lb)	Past Medical History: A-fib
	Chief Complaint: Disoriented

Vital Signs

Time: 0902	BP: 142/86	Pulse: 90	Respirations: 24	Spo$_2$: 92% RA
Time: 0915	BP: 142/86	Pulse: 86	Respirations: 22	Spo$_2$: 98% on 4 L/min
Time:	BP:	Pulse:	Respirations:	Spo$_2$:

EMS Treatment
(circle all that apply)

Oxygen @ __4__ L/min via (circle one): (NC) NRM Bag-mask device	Assisted Ventilation	Airway Adjunct	CPR
Defibrillation	Bleeding Control	Bandaging	Splinting	Other

Narrative

Arrived to find this 81-year-old male pt lying supine on the floor. Two of the pt's sons are on the scene. The sons advised they were visiting with their father last evening and left his presence at approx 1900 hours. Per the sons, pt showed nothing unusual last night. When they arrived just prior to calling 9-1-1, pt was found down on the floor. Pt is awake, alert, and confused concerning the identity of his sons, day, time, week, and year. Both sons state this is not normal for pt. Speech is clear, no facial droop. Positive arm drift, neg. ptosis, confused to time of day, follows commands, affect is calm and cooperative, apraxia noted, agnosia noted, neg. headache, blood glucose 92 mg/dL. Family states pt's pants were soiled. ECG shows atrial fibrillation at approx. 90 beats/min. 12-lead shows no acute ST changes, no Q waves. O$_2$ applied at 4 L/min NC. Pt moved for transport to Community Hospital. Pt showed no signs of change during transport. Report upon arrival to Tammy RN. **End of report**

Prep Kit

- Neurologic problems can be dangerous because depressed reflexes leave the airway and other body systems vulnerable.

- The central nervous system has two major structures: the brain and the spinal cord. They communicate with a neural network to regulate breathing, pulse rate, blood pressure, and complex cognitive functions such as memory and understanding.

- The peripheral nervous system consists of the somatic nervous system, which controls voluntary muscles, and the autonomic nervous system, which oversees sympathetic (fight-or-flight) and parasympathetic responses.

- Each portion of the brain is responsible for specific functions. The occipital lobe receives and stores images. The temporal lobe makes language and speech possible. The frontal lobe controls voluntary motion. The parietal lobe allows perception of the sensations of touch and pain. The diencephalon filters out unneeded information from the cerebral cortex. The midbrain helps to regulate the level of consciousness. The brainstem regulates the blood pressure, pulse rate, and respiratory rate and pattern. The hypothalamus and pituitary control the release of epinephrine and norepinephrine from the endocrine system. The cerebellum allows unconscious management of complex motor activity.

- Nerve cells, or neurons, transmit signals along their axons and across synapses by means of chemical neurotransmitters.

- A variety of disease processes can cause neurologic dysfunction, including cancer, degenerative conditions, developmental anomalies, infectious diseases, and vascular conditions. Most neurologic diseases are thought to be multifactorial— that is, a number of factors combine to induce vulnerability to a particular disease process.

- Intracranial pressure is determined by the volume of the intracranial contents: the brain, blood, and cerebrospinal fluid.

- The primary dangers of increased intracranial pressure are ischemia and brain herniation.

- The neurologic assessment identifies small alterations that can impair nervous system function.

- Investigating the neurologic patient's chief complaint requires taking a history to determine the mechanism of injury or the nature of the illness. This task is more difficult when the patient is unresponsive, but environmental clues and the reports of family, friends, and bystanders can be helpful.

- It is critical to determine when the patient was last seen normal because the amount of time elapsed since the onset of symptoms will dictate the treatments available.

- Level of conscious can be evaluated using the Glasgow Coma Scale, the AVPU mnemonic, a test of corneal reflex or pupillary response, evaluation of cranial nerve functioning, assessment of the patient's orientation and alertness, assessment of the patient's speech and ability to recognize and name objects, evaluation of the patient's movement, testing of the patient's sensory perceptual abilities, testing of the blood glucose level, and measurement of the vital signs.

- Following a set of standard care guidelines can help you address common neurologic problems in a systematic way.

- Stroke is a condition in which the blood supply to the brain is interrupted. In ischemic stroke, the blood supply may be blocked by a clot (thrombus or embolus). In hemorrhagic stroke, a damaged artery bleeds into the brain instead of carrying the blood to the brain,

- Stroke causes sudden-onset changes in neurologic status, including effects on language, movement, sensation, level of consciousness, and blood pressure.

- Time is brain. Fibrinolytic (clot-busting) agents need to be administered within 3 hours of the onset of a stroke in order for the agents to be effective. To achieve this target, a stroke must be recognized and EMS dispatched quickly, and the patient must be transported rapidly to an appropriate facility, such as a stroke center.

- Transient ischemic attacks are episodes of cerebral ischemia that resolve within 24 hours, leaving no permanent damage. They may, however, signal an underlying vascular problem that can lead to a stroke. Prompt medical evaluation is essential.

- A diminished level of consciousness is marked by increasing deficits in cognition and speech and changes in movement and posture. The patient may become comatose without timely medical intervention.

- Seizures are cause by the sudden, erratic firing of neurons. Lengthy seizures can have devastating effects on the brain and body and can even be life threatening.

- Seizures have a wide range of causes, from drug use to tumors.

- Seizures are classified as either generalized, affecting large portions of the brain, or partial, affecting only a limited area of the brain.

- Generalized seizures are divided into tonic/clonic (grand mal) seizures, which follow a particular sequence; absence (petit mal) seizures, which are characterized not by movement but by the absence of it; and pseudoseizures, which have a psychiatric origin.

- Simple partial seizures involve either movement of one part of the body (frontal lobe) or sensations in one part of the body (parietal lobe). Complex partial seizures subtly diminish the level of consciousness, causing confusion, a lack of alertness, or an inability to speak.

- Status epilepticus can be defined as a seizure that lasts longer than 4 to 5 minutes or consecutive seizures without consciousness returning between seizures.

- Syncope, or fainting, is caused by a brief interruption in cerebral blood flow that can be traced to cardiac rhythm disturbances, other cardiac causes, or noncardiac causes.

- Headaches can be classified as muscle tension, migraine, cluster, or sinus headaches. Each has a different cause and a different presentation. Other types of headache may occur as well.

- Dementia is not a single illness, but a chronic process that can take many forms. It is characterized by deterioration of memory, personality, language skills, perception, reasoning, or judgment, with no loss of consciousness. Management is similar for the various dementias and is primarily supportive.

- Tumors of the neurologic system affect the brain and spinal cord and are classified as either primary or metastatic disease.

- Demyelinating conditions attack the insulating sheath that surrounds and protects the axon, so that nerve impulses can no longer travel smoothly.

- Multiple sclerosis is an autoimmune condition in which episodic attacks are followed by periods of remission. Patients with multiple sclerosis can have a range of neurologic deficits, from incontinence to significant sensory impairments.

- Amyotrophic lateral sclerosis (Lou Gehrig disease) is a disease that strikes the voluntary motor neurons, causing progressive paralysis and death.

- Parkinson disease damages the substantia nigra, the portion of the brain that produces dopamine, which is needed for muscle contraction.

- Cranial nerve disorders have a range of signs and symptoms and are often mistaken for other disorders.

- Dystonias are severe, abnormal muscle spasms that cause bizarre contortions, repetitive motions, or postures. They can affect the neck, face, jaw, or other muscles, and they are often painful.

- Encephalitis and meningitis are central nervous system infections that cause inflammation of the brain and meninges, respectively.

- Abscesses indicate the presence of an infectious agent within the brain or spinal cord.
- Polio is a viral infection that can cause long-term damage to the brain and brainstem, leading to muscle weakness and paralysis.
- Peripheral neuropathy is a group of conditions in which the nerves leaving the spinal cord are damaged by trauma, toxins, tumors, autoimmune attack, and metabolic disorders, or other processes.
- Normal-pressure hydrocephalus is a rare condition that occurs in older adults for unknown reasons. Increased intracranial pressure hydrocephalus occurs primarily among infants with congenital malformations. It causes increased pressure within the cranial vault.
- Cerebral palsy is a developmental condition characterized by damage to the frontal lobe of the brain. Its cause is unclear.

■ Vital Vocabulary

abscess An area in the brain or spinal cord in which cells have been attacked, typically by an infectious agent. The immune system erects a wall to prevent spread of the infection, creating a pus-filled pocket within the nervous system tissue.

adrenal glands Endocrine glands located on top of the kidneys that release adrenalin when stimulated by the sympathetic nervous system.

afferent nerves Nerves that send information to the brain.

agnosia Inability to connect an object with its correct name.

Alzheimer disease A progressive organic condition in which neurons in the brain die, causing dementia.

amyotrophic lateral sclerosis (ALS) ALS, also known as Lou Gehrig disease, strikes the voluntary motor neurons, causing their death. The disease is characterized by fatigue and general weakness of muscle groups; eventually the patient becomes unable to walk, eat, or speak.

anesthesia Lack of feeling within a body part.

anisocoria Unequal pupils with a greater than 1-mm difference.

apraxia Inability to connect an object with its proper use.

ataxia Alteration in the ability to perform coordinated motions like walking.

aura Sensations experienced before an attack occurs. Common in seizures and migraine headaches.

AVPU Evaluation tool used to determine a patient's level of consciousness.

axon The long, slender filament projecting from a nerve cell that conducts impulses to adjacent cells.

Bell palsy A temporary paralysis of the facial nerve (cranial nerve VII), which controls the muscles on each side of the face.

bradykinesia The slowing down of voluntary body movements. Found in Parkinson disease.

brainstem The area of the brain between the spinal cord and the cerebrum, surrounded by the cerebellum. It controls functions that are necessary to sustain life, such as respiration.

central nervous system (CNS) The brain and spinal cord.

cerebellum The region of the brain essential in coordinating muscle movement.

cerebral palsy (CP) A developmental condition in which damage is done to the brain. It presents during infancy as a delay in walking or crawling, and can take on a spastic form in which muscles are in a nearly constant state of contraction.

clonic activity Type of seizure movement involving the contraction and relaxation of muscle groups.

coma A state in which a person does not respond to verbal or painful stimuli.

common reality Sensory stimulation that can be verified by others.

corneal reflex A protective movement that results in blinking, moving the head posteriorly, and pupillary constriction.

daughter cells The two identical cells produced when a parent cell divides by mitosis.

decerebrate posturing Abnormal extension of the arms with rotation of the wrists along with toe pointing. This indicates brainstem damage.

decorticate posturing Abnormal flexion of the arms toward the chest with the toes pointed. It indicates lower cerebral damage.

decussation Movement of nerves from one side of the brain to the opposite side of the body.

delusions Thoughts, ideas, or perceived abilities that have no basis in common reality.

dementia The slow, progressive onset of disorientation, shortened attention span, and loss of cognitive function.

diencephalon The part of the brain that lies between the brainstem and the cerebrum and includes the thalamus and hypothalamus.

dystonia Contractions of body into bizarre positions.

efferent nerves Nerves that leave the brain through the peripheral nervous system and convey commands to other parts of the body.

endotoxin A toxin released by some bacteria when they die.

exotoxin A toxin secreted by living cells to aid in the death and digestion of other cells.

expressive aphasia Damage or loss in the ability to speak.

gait Walking or ambulating.

Glasgow Coma Scale (GCS) Evaluation tool used to determine level of consciousness. Effective in determining patient outcomes.

global aphasia Damage or loss of both the ability to speak and the ability to understand speech.

Guillain-Barré syndrome A rare condition that begins as a sensation of weakness and tingling in the legs, moving to the arms and thorax; the disorder can lead to paralysis within 2 weeks.

hallucinations Sensory stimulation that cannot be verified by others.

hemiparesis Weakness to one side of the body.

hemiplegia Paralysis to one side of the body.

hemorrhagic One of the two main types of stroke; occurs as a result of bleeding inside the brain.

hypothalamus Comprising the most inferior portion of the diencephalon, the hypothalamus controls many essential functions, including pulse rate, digestion, sexual development, temperature regulation, hunger, thirst, and the sleep-wake cycle.

idiopathic Of no known cause.

incidence The number of people in a given population, such as the United States, who are newly diagnosed with a particular disease or disorder in a specified 1-year period.

intention tremor A tremor that occurs when trying to accomplish a task.

ischemic One of the two main types of stroke, sometimes called an *occlusive stroke*; occurs when blood flow to a particular part of the brain is cut off by a blockage—that is, an occlusion, such as a blood clot—within an artery.

Jacksonian march The wave-like movement of a seizure from a point of focus to other areas of the brain.

limbic system Structures within the cerebrum and diencephalon that influence emotions, motivation, mood, and sensations of pain and pleasure.

medulla oblongata The inferior portion of the midbrain, which serves as a conduction pathway for ascending and descending nerve tracts.

metastasis The process by which cells from a malignant neoplasm break away from their site of origin, such as the lung, and move through the bloodstream or lymphatic system to other body sites, such as the brain.

midbrain The part of the brain responsible for helping to regulate level of consciousness.

multiple sclerosis (MS) An autoimmune condition in which the body attacks the myelin that insulates the brain and spinal cord, causing scarring.

mutation A change in the sequence of a cell's DNA that damages the cell's structure or impedes its ability to function.

myasthenia gravis A condition in which the body generates antibodies against its own acetylcholine receptors, causing muscle weakness, often in the face.

myelin An insulating sheath that envelops certain types of neurons, allowing the cells to transmit electricity along their axons without dissipation of the signal as it moves through surrounding fluids and tissues.

myoclonus Jerking motions of the body.

neoplasm A tumor.

neurotransmitter A chemical produced by the body that stimulates electrical reactions in adjacent neurons.

nystagmus The rhythmic shaking of the eyes.

paresthesia Sensation of tingling, numbness, or "pins and needles" in a body part.

Parkinson disease A neurologic condition in which the portion of the brain responsible for production of dopamine has been damaged or overused, resulting in tremors.

peripheral nervous system (PNS) The part of the nervous system that consists of 31 pairs of spinal nerves and 12 pairs of cranial nerves. These nerves may be sensory, motor, or connecting nerves.

peripheral neuropathy A group of conditions in which the nerves that exit the spinal cord are damaged, distorting signals to or from the brain. One type of peripheral neuropathy is caused by diabetes; peripheral nerves are damaged as the blood glucose level rises, resulting in lack of sensation, numbness, burning, pain, paresthesia, and muscle weakness.

pituitary gland The gland that secretes hormones that regulate the function of many other glands in the body; also called the *hypophysis*.

poliomyelitis A viral infection that attacks and destroys nerve axons, especially motor axons. The disease can cause weakness, paralysis, and respiratory arrest. Because an effective vaccine has been developed, the incidence of the disease is now rare.

pons The portion of the brainstem that lies below the midbrain and contains nerve fibers that affect sleep and respiration.

postictal The period of time after a seizure in which the brain is reorganizing activity.

postpolio syndrome The death of nerve fibers as a late consequence of polio; the syndrome is characterized by swallowing difficulties, weakness, fatigue, and breathing problems.

postural tremor A tremor that occurs as the person holds a body part still.

posturing Abnormal body positioning that indicates damage to the brain.

prevalence The total number of people in a given population who have a particular disease.

prodromal/prodrome The early signs and symptoms that occur before a disease or condition fully appears, eg, dizziness before fainting.

pronation Turning of the lower arms in a palm downward manner.

psychosis Breaking with common reality and existing mainly within an internal world.

ptosis Prolapse of a body part; often refers to drooping of the eyelid.

receptive aphasia Damage to or loss of the ability to understand speech.

rest tremor A tremor that occurs when the body part is not in motion.

rigidity Stiffness or hardness (in motion). Found in patients with Parkinson disease.

spina bifida A developmental anomaly in which a portion of the spinal cord or meninges protrudes outside the spinal column or even outside the body, usually in the area of the lumbar spine (the lower third of the spine).

status epilepticus A condition in which seizures recur every few minutes, or in which seizure activity lasts more than 30 minutes.

supraorbital foramen A small notch located on the frontal bone near the inner, upper area of each orbit.

synapses Gaps between nerve cells, across which nervous stimuli are transmitted.

syncope A fainting spell or transient loss of consciousness.

tonic activity A type of seizure movement involving the constant contraction and trembling of muscle groups.

transient ischemic attack (TIA) A disorder in which brain cells temporarily stop working because of insufficient oxygen, causing stroke-like symptoms that resolve completely within 24 hours of onset.

tremors Fine involuntary, rhythmic movements, usually involving the hands or head.

trismus The involuntary contraction of the mouth resulting in clenched teeth. Occurs during seizures and head injuries.

uremia Severe renal failure resulting in the buildup of waste products within the blood. Eventually brain functions will be impaired.

Assessment in Action

Your unit is dispatched to a motor vehicle crash. After ensuring scene safety, you don your personal protective equipment and approach the vehicle. You find a man sitting in the driver's seat. The patient does not respond to you and is snoring loudly. You see bleeding from the patient's ears, and his arms are drawn in toward his chest.

1. Clenching of the teeth is called:
   A. posturing.
   B. trismus.
   C. torticollis.
   D. bruxism.

2. The respiratory pattern with gradual increases and decreases with periods of apnea is called:
   A. tachypnea.
   B. ataxic.
   C. Cheyne-Stokes.
   D. apneustic.

3. A decreased pulse rate, decreased respiratory rate, and widened pulse pressure (systolic hypertension) indicate which of the following condition?
   A. Posturing
   B. Trismus
   C. Einthoven triangle
   D. Cushing reflex

4. This patient is exhibiting flexion posturing. What is the term for this?
   A. Decerebrate posturing
   B. Decorticate posturing
   C. Focal posturing
   D. Sympathetic posturing

5. Extension posturing is called:
   A. decerebrate posturing.
   B. decorticate posturing.
   C. focal posturing.
   D. sympathetic posturing.

6. What could a lack of a corneal reflex indicate?
   A. Damage is within or near the brainstem.
   B. Damage is to the area directly below the cerebral hemispheres.
   C. Patient is faking unconsciousness.
   D. Patient does not have an intact cough or gag reflex.

Diseases of the Eyes, Ears, Nose, and Throat

National EMS Education Standard Competencies

Medicine

Integrates assessment findings with principles of epidemiology and pathophysiology to formulate a field impression and implement a comprehensive treatment/disposition plan for a patient with a medical complaint.

Diseases of the Eyes, Ears, Nose, and Throat

Knowledge of the anatomy, physiology, epidemiology, pathophysiology, psychosocial impact, presentations, prognosis, and management of

- Common or major diseases of the eyes, ears, nose, and throat, including nose bleed (pp 1094-1102, 1103-1106, 1107-1108, 1110-1115)

Knowledge Objectives

1. Explain facial anatomy and relate physiology to facial injuries. (pp 1091-1092, 1102, 1106, 1108-1110)
2. Differentiate between the following types of facial injuries, highlighting the defining characteristics of each:
   a. Eye (pp 1094-1102)
   b. Ear (pp 1103-1106)
   c. Nose (pp 1107-1108)
   d. Throat (pp 1110-1115)
   e. Mouth (pp 1110-1115)
3. Explain the pathophysiology of eye injuries. (pp 1094-1102)
4. Relate assessment findings associated with eye injuries and disorders to pathophysiology. (pp 1094-1102)
5. Integrate pathophysiologic principles to the assessment of a patient with an eye injury or eye disorder. (pp 1092-1102)
6. Formulate a field impression for a patient with an eye injury based on the assessment findings. (pp 1092-1094)
7. Develop a patient management plan for a patient with an eye injury based on the field impression. (pp 1092-1094)

8. Explain the pathophysiology of ear injuries and disorders. (pp 1103-1106)
9. Relate assessment findings associated with ear injuries and disorders to pathophysiology. (pp 1102-1106)
10. Integrate pathophysiologic principles to the assessment of a patient with an ear injury. (pp 1102-1106)
11. Formulate a field impression for a patient with an ear injury based on the assessment findings. (pp 1102-1106)
12. Develop a patient management plan for a patient with an ear injury based on the field impression. (pp 1102-1106)
13. Explain the pathophysiology of nose injuries and disorders. (pp 1107-1108)
14. Relate assessment findings associated with nose injuries and disorders to pathophysiology. (pp 1106-1108)
15. Integrate pathophysiologic principles to the assessment of a patient with a nose injury. (pp 1106-1108)
16. Formulate a field impression for a patient with a nose injury based on the assessment findings. (pp 1106-1108)
17. Develop a patient management plan for a patient with a nose injury based on the field impression. (pp 1106-1108)
18. Explain the pathophysiology of throat and mouth injuries and disorders. (pp 1110-1115)
19. Relate assessment findings associated with throat and mouth injuries and disorders to pathophysiology. (pp 1108-1115)
20. Integrate pathophysiologic principles to the assessment of a patient with a throat or mouth injury. (pp 1108-1115)
21. Formulate a field impression for a patient with a throat or mouth injury based on the assessment findings. (pp 1108-1115)
22. Develop a patient management plan for a patient with a throat or mouth injury based on the field impression. (pp 1108-1115)

Skills Objectives

There are no skills objectives for this chapter.

Introduction

Disorders of the eye, ear, nose, and throat (EENT) are becoming more of an issue for emergency personnel. Paramedics may respond to calls that involve these important structures.

A significant number of calls for EMS involving EENT structures are a result of trauma; such injuries will be discussed in the chapter, *Face and Neck Trauma*. This chapter covers medical conditions that could result in a call to 9-1-1, or which you could notice when you are assessing a patient who called 9-1-1 for an unrelated reason. On such calls, familiarity with these conditions will help you during assessment of the patient. Knowledge of these conditions also allows you the opportunity to educate the patient on prevention or potential care for a condition that the patient may have.

Oftentimes, when you encounter a patient with an EENT disorder, it makes sense to transport the patient possibly to an emergency department with access to an eye specialist or an ear, nose, and throat specialist for further evaluation. For example, any time an object is lodged in the eye, ear, nose, or throat, the patient must receive transport.

This chapter begins by discussing general considerations when you are assessing a patient with a complaint related to conditions of the eyes, ears, nose, and throat. You will also learn about specific conditions and their field treatment, if any.

The Eye

Every year, more than 2.5 million Americans sustain eye injuries that require medical attention. Some of the emergencies associated with eye disease include glaucoma, macular degeneration, and diabetic retinopathy. Usually patients having these diseases have a long-standing history of an underlying condition that predisposes them to the disorder (comorbidity). From a standpoint of mortality, incidence is low.

Anatomy and Physiology of the Eye

The <u>globe</u>, or eyeball, is a spherical structure measuring about 1 inch in diameter that is housed within the eye socket, or orbit.

Special Populations

According to the CDC, vision disability is one of the top 10 disabilities among children.

In the geriatric population, you are likely to encounter patients who have undergone laser-assisted eye surgery (lasik surgery). Lasik surgery uses a special laser to slice a flap in the cornea and adjust the shape of the middle section of the cornea (stroma). This surgery can reduce the need for corrective lenses. The latest techniques can be done without the "flap" in the cornea. Immediately following the surgery and for the next few weeks, patients are instructed to not let air blow directly into their eyes and wear goggles while they sleep so they do not scratch their cornea. Geriatric patients are also more likely to undergo cataract surgery and eye surgery for glaucoma.

Older people may also experience eye injuries from falls. Eye conditions and problems are part of the list of comorbid factors simultaneously occurring in the geriatric population. Diabetic retinopathy affects one third of those older than 40 years who have diabetes mellitus.

The eyes are held in place by loose connective tissue and several muscles. These muscles also control eye movements. The <u>oculomotor nerve</u> (third cranial nerve) innervates the muscles that cause motion of the eyeballs and upper eyelids. It also carries parasympathetic nerve fibers that cause constriction of the pupil and accommodation of the lens. The <u>optic nerve</u> (second cranial nerve) provides the sense of vision Figure 1.

The structures of the eye include the following:

- The <u>sclera</u> ("white of the eye") is a tough, fibrous coat that helps maintain the shape of the eye and protect the contents of the eye. In some illnesses, such as hepatitis, the sclera becomes yellow (icteric) from staining by bile pigments.
- The <u>cornea</u> is the transparent anterior portion of the eye that overlies the iris and pupil. Clouding of the cornea during aging results in a condition known as <u>cataract</u>.
- The <u>conjunctiva</u> is a delicate mucous membrane that covers the sclera and internal surfaces of the eyelids but not the iris. Cyanosis can be detected in the conjunctiva

YOU are the Medic   PART 1

You are dispatched to a local school for a child with a sore throat. It is very cold outside and you are wondering what prompted this call to 9-1-1. When you arrive on scene, you are directed to the administrative office. You and your partner enter the office to see a small child, approximately 5 years old. The child is sitting upright and leaning slightly forward. He is breathing through his mouth and looks very sick. The administrator says they are trying to contact the child's parents and that the school nurse took the child's temperature, which was 102° F.

1. What is your primary concern after scene safety is established?

2. Do you have concerns that the patient's parents have not been contacted?

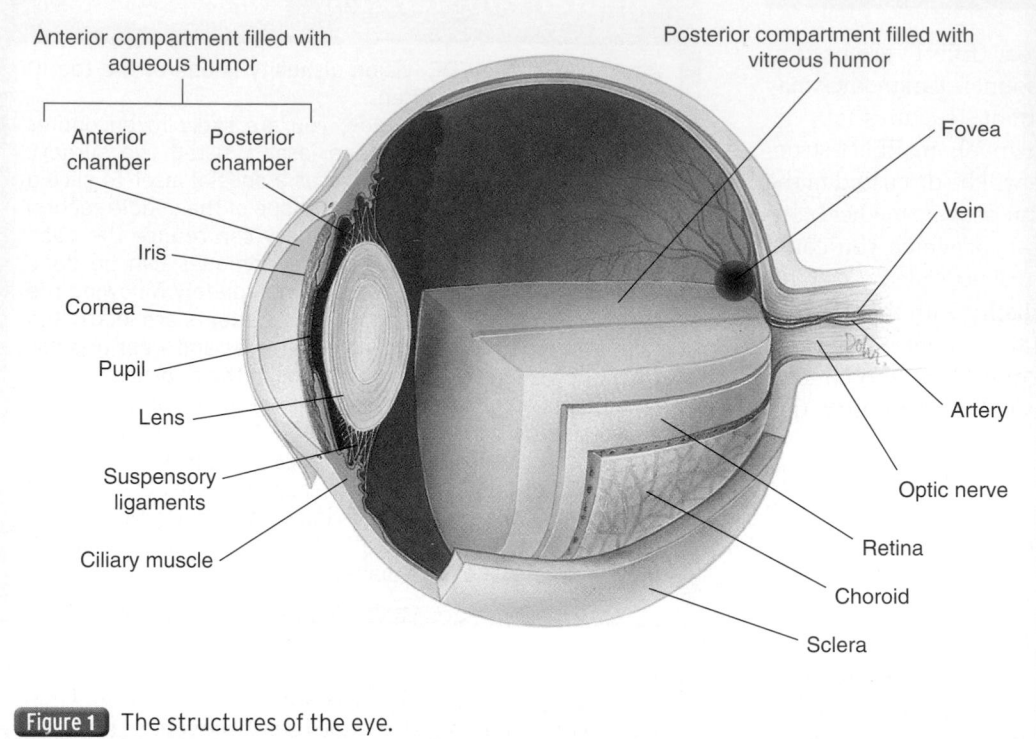

Figure 1 The structures of the eye.

There are two types of vision: central and peripheral. **Central vision** facilitates visualization of objects directly in front of you and is processed by the macula, the central portion of the retina. The remainder of the retina processes **peripheral vision**, which enables visualization of lateral objects while a person is looking forward.

The **lacrimal apparatus** secretes and drains tears from the eye. Tears produced in the lacrimal gland drain into lacrimal ducts, then into lacrimal sacs that pass into the nasal cavity via the **nasolacrimal duct**. Tears moisten the conjunctivae **Figure 2**.

Patient Assessment

Making sure you and other responders are safe from the many hazards on trauma scenes, and the often hidden dangers on medical scenes, should stand first in your order of priorities. Fear and panic from loss of vision can cause dangerous and bizarre behavior in your patient. Keep your patient calm. The scene size-up is an opportunity to discover clues to the cause of the complaint, while avoiding potential hazards.

As you form a general impression of the patient, note environmental clues at the scene, the approximate age and sex of the patient, and his or her degree of distress. Do not let the high degree of distress or concern over the potential visual

when it is not easily assessed on the skin of dark-skinned patients.

- The **iris** is the pigmented part of the eye that surrounds the pupil. It consists of muscles and blood vessels that contract and expand to regulate the size of the pupil.
- The **pupil** is the circular adjustable opening within the iris through which light passes to the lens. A normal pupil dilates in dim light to permit more light to enter the eye and constricts in bright light to decrease the light entering the eye.
- Behind the pupil and iris is the **lens**, a transparent structure that can alter its thickness to focus light on the retina at the back of the eye.
- The **retina**, which lies in the posterior aspect of the interior globe, is a delicate, 10-layered structure of nervous tissue that extends from the optic nerve. It receives light impulses and converts them to nerve signals that are conducted to the brain by the optic nerve and interpreted as vision.

The **anterior chamber** is the portion of the globe between the lens and the cornea. It is filled with **aqueous humor**, a clear watery fluid. If aqueous humor is lost through a penetrating injury to the eye, it will gradually be replenished.

The **posterior chamber** is the portion of the globe between the iris and the lens that is filled with **vitreous humor**, a jelly-like substance that maintains the shape of the globe. If vitreous humor is lost, it cannot be replenished, and blindness may result.

Light rays enter the eyes through the pupil and are focused by the lens. The image formed by the lens is cast on the retina, where sensitive nerve fibers form the optic nerve. The optic nerve transmits the image to the brain, where it is converted into conscious images in the **visual cortex**.

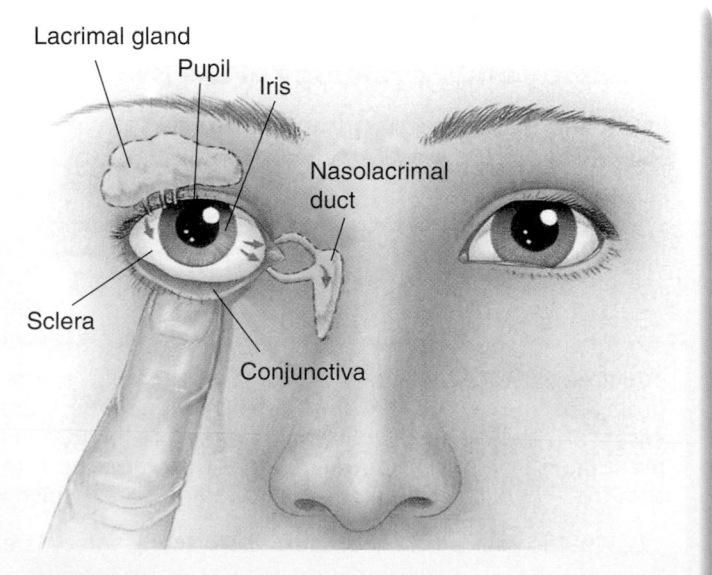

Figure 2 The lacrimal system consists of tear glands and ducts. Tears act as lubricants and keep the anterior part of the eye from drying.

impairment sidetrack your observations of the scene and those dangers that may have caused an injury or condition.

Primary assessment of airway and breathing should take precedence, as should ruling out any life threats. Do not be distracted by a swollen, irritated, or deformed eye to the extent that you bypass the highest priorities. You must ensure that the patient has an open and adequate airway, that the patient is breathing, that there are no threats to ventilation, and that the patient has an adequate pulse. Ensure that there are no life threats to circulation that need your immediate attention.

Depending on the severity of the eye condition, an early transport decision to the right facility can improve outcomes. Level 1 trauma centers have the skilled services necessary to treat a serious eye problem. Covering both eyes can limit damage to the affected eye. Consider pain management and, if necessary, mild sedation during transport.

Cardiac monitoring is recommended. Ocular pressure can stimulate the vagus nerve, and a vagal response in your patient. Eye drops and eye medication can cause side effects such as low or high blood pressure.

Your demeanor should be supportive and calm. Remember, a patient facing potential long-term vision loss will need emotional care as well; this can be a life-changing event for your patient.

Obtain the chief complaint from the patient and begin to elaborate on it using OPQRST. When you are obtaining the history, determine how and when the symptoms began, and what symptoms the patient is experiencing. Are both eyes affected? Does the patient have any underlying diseases or conditions of the eye (such as glaucoma)? Does the patient take medications for his or her eyes? Diabetes is the leading cause of new cases of blindness in adults according to the Centers for Disease Control and Prevention (CDC). One in three of diabetic adults older than 40 years has a disease called **diabetic retinopathy**. Forty-two million adults have diabetic retinopathy, and 655,000 have vision alteration due to this condition. Diabetic retinopathy affects the small blood vessels in the retina. Vision disturbances can include blurred vision, floaters, blind spots, or blindness.

A variety of symptoms may indicate a serious ocular condition:

- *Visual loss* that does not improve when the patient blinks is an important symptom. It may indicate damage to the globe or to the optic nerve.
- *Double vision* usually points to trauma involving the extraocular muscles, such as a fracture of the orbit.
- *Severe eye pain* is a symptom of a significant eye injury.
- A *foreign body sensation* usually indicates superficial injury to the cornea or the presence of a foreign object trapped behind the eyelids.

Assessment of specific eye conditions begins with a thorough examination to determine the extent and nature of the situation. Always perform your examination using standard precautions, taking great care to avoid aggravating the affected area. Be sure to assess for pain or tenderness, swelling, abnormal or loss of movement, sensation changes, circulatory changes, deformity, visual changes, and airway compromise.

Physical examination of the eyes includes assessment of the visible ocular structures, as well as ocular function. This evaluation is shown in the chapter, *Patient Assessment*. Assess the ocular structures for the following:

- **Orbital rim:** for ecchymosis, swelling, lacerations, and tenderness
- **Eyelids:** for ecchymosis, swelling, lacerations, or any abnormalities
- **Corneas:** for foreign bodies
- **Conjunctivae:** for redness, pus, inflammation, and foreign bodies
- **Globes:** for redness, abnormal pigmentation, and lacerations. Inspect the eye surface for growths, discoloration, and differences between the eyes.
- **Pupils:** for size, shape, equality, and reaction to light. Note whether they are symmetric.

When you are assessing ocular function, perform the following:

- **Visual acuity.** Assess the patient's ability to see large and small letters, for example by reading the writing on a prescription bottle, or by using a hand-held visual acuity chart such as the Snellen chart (shown in the chapter, *Patient Assessment*). Test each eye separately and document the results.
- **Peripheral vision.** Evaluate the peripheral vision by testing the ability to recognize an object entering the extremes of the visual field (confrontation).
- **Ocular motility.** Check the ability to move the eyes in all directions. Check for paralysis of gaze or discoordination between the movements of the two eyes (**dysconjugate gaze**).

In addition to the physical examination, during the secondary assessment you should obtain a full set of baseline vital signs.

During reassessment, vital signs should be monitored every 5 to 15 minutes depending on the severity of the patient's condition. Continuing assessment allows you to track any trends that may be occurring.

Note that a patient may experience more side effects if he or she uses multiple eye medications. Also, if a patient uses too much of one or several medications, he or she may experience side effects because the medication can enter the bloodstream via the nasolacrimal system, which serves the function of draining tears. Side effects can be systemic if enough medication enters the bloodstream.

Ask patients how they administered their eye medications. Sometimes part of the problem is that the patient did not follow the instructions for the specific medication, ie, it is usually recommended to wait approximately 5 minutes between administering the first and second drop. Of course, this 5-minute rule does not apply to emergency measures such as administering tetracaine prior to inserting a Morgan lens.

There are many medications to address a variety of eye problems. Eye drops can be used for conjunctivitis, dry eyes, red eyes, eye pain, glaucoma, eye surgery, herpes simplex, itchy eyes, and corneal abrasions. Eye lubricants are available for protecting eyes that do not produce tears (as a result of

Words of Wisdom

<u>Anisocoria</u>, a condition in which the pupils are not of equal size, is a significant finding in patients with ocular injuries or closed head trauma. However, simple or physiologic anisocoria occurs in approximately 20% of the population. Therefore, about one person out of five has some degree of difference in the sizes of their pupils. Usually, the patient's pupils differ in size by less than 1 mm; however, approximately 4% of people have pupils that vary in size by more than 1 mm. This is not a clinically significant finding.

Unilateral cataract surgery may also cause inequality of pupil size. The pupil of the eye affected by the cataract will be nonreactive to light.

seventh nerve damage). Eye drops and lubricants are most often applied by gently squeezing the lower eyelid to make a pouch and applying the medicine into the lower lid. The patient then should close his or her eyes and roll the eyes downward with eyes closed. Gentle pressure should be applied to the corner of the eyes to prevent drainage of the medicine from the eye. Irrigation of the eyes may be necessary for chemical burns or thermal burns. Treatment consists of irrigating the eye with sterile water or isotonic saline solution, flushing the liquid from the inside corner to the outside of the eye, except when a Morgan lens is being used (described below). Eye injuries should be seen in the emergency department. Children may need to be treated under anesthesia. Many eye injuries will need a topical anesthetic and antibiotic, which is not generally performed by a paramedic.

Eye injuries may be irreversible, and patients may or may not be aware of the seriousness of the event. Patients may exhibit denial, anger, fear, hysteria, and depression. Communication is key to keeping your patient calm and informed. Remember that early decisions to transport to the appropriate facility can improve outcomes in some patients, and early communication with a medical control physician can help direct your care and help with transport decisions.

Words of Wisdom

When patients ask you what you think is wrong, remember you are serving them. Remind them that you do not have definitive answers and that you are not a physician, but tell them what you think is going on. Be honest and sincere about what you are telling them, with the goal of keeping your patient both informed and calm.

Pathophysiology, Assessment, and Management of Specific Conditions

Burns of the Eye and Adnexa

Burns to the eye account for somewhere between 7% and 15% of eye injuries. Chemicals, heat, and light rays can all burn the delicate tissues of the eye and <u>adnexa</u> (the surrounding structures and accessories), often causing permanent damage. Your role is to stop the burning process and prevent further damage.

Thermal burns occur when a patient is burned in the face during a fire, although the eyes usually close rapidly because of the heat. This reaction is a natural reflex to protect the eyes from further injury. However, the eyelids remain exposed and are frequently burned **Figure 3**.

Infrared rays, eclipse light (if the patient has looked directly at the sun), and laser burns can cause significant damage to the sensory cells of the eye when rays of light become focused on the retina. Retinal injuries that are caused by exposure to extremely bright light are generally not painful but may result in permanent damage to vision.

Superficial burns of the eye can result from ultraviolet rays from an arc welding unit, prolonged exposure to a sunlamp, or reflected light from a bright snow-covered area (snow blindness). This kind of burn may not be painful initially but may become so 3 to 5 hours later, as the damaged cornea responds to the injury. Severe conjunctivitis usually develops, along with redness, swelling, and excessive tear production.

Assessment and Management Eye injuries are a substantial distracting injury. If the mechanism of injury suggests a high index of suspicion for a spinal injury, all spinal precautions must be followed. Spine and head stabilization may be necessary, as

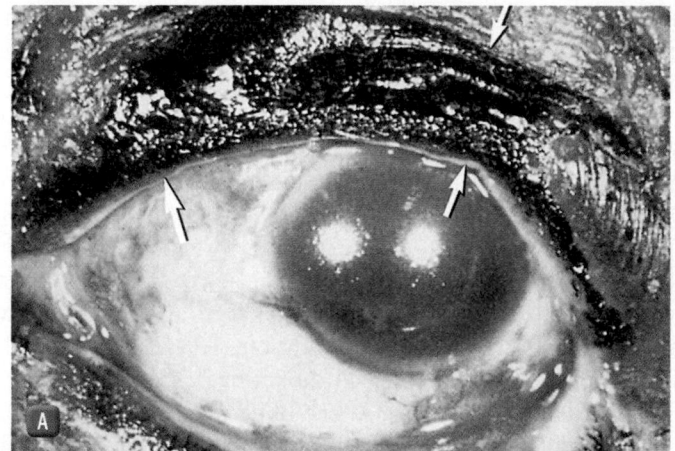

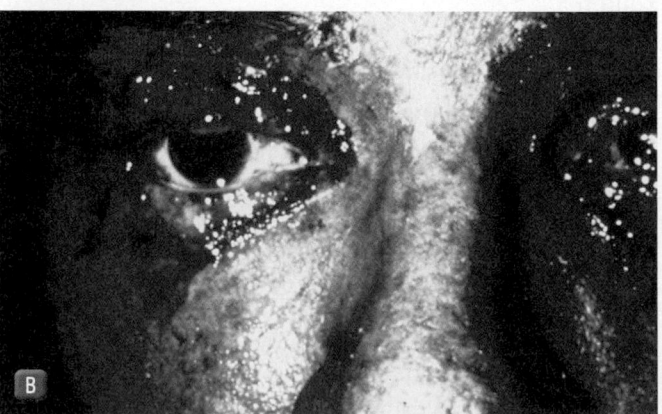

Figure 3 Thermal burns occasionally cause significant damage to the eyelids. **A.** Arrows show some full-thickness burns. **B.** Burns of the eyelids require immediate hospital care.

well as correcting any life threats. Assessment may be difficult because the patient may be forcibly keeping his or her eyes closed. You will need to gain the patient's trust and open the lid to irrigate the eye with sterile water or saline solution. You may not be able to adequately assess the patient's eye until the pain has been managed. When full examination is possible, assessment should include checking whether the eye can move to the following six cardinal positions of gaze: right, right up, right down, left, left up, and left down (following in a Z or H pattern). Assessment should also include checking pupil dilation to light, and checking the patient's vision when he or she looks to the left and to the right. Peripheral vision can be checked by having patients look straight ahead while you provide motion at the extreme left and right of their view. You can move your hand into the field of vision, from beyond the field of vision, asking the patient to acknowledge when he or she sees your hand. The chapter, *Patient Assessment* shows how to perform an eye examination with an ophthalmoscope. Finally, document all changes.

Burns to the eye that are caused by ultraviolet light are most effectively treated by covering the eye with a sterile, moist pad and an eye shield. The application of cool compresses *lightly* over the eye may provide some pain relief if the patient is in extreme distress. Place the patient in a supine position during transport, and protect the patient from further exposure to bright light.

Chemical burns, which are usually caused by acid or alkali solutions, require immediate emergency care because they can rapidly lead to blindness Figure 4 . The most important prehospital treatment in such cases is to *begin immediate irrigation* with sterile water or saline solution. *Never use any chemical antidotes (such as vinegar, baking soda) when you are irrigating the patient's eye; use sterile water or saline only.*

The goal when you are irrigating the eye is to direct the greatest amount of solution or water into the eye as gently as possible. Because opening the eye spontaneously may cause the patient pain, you may have to force the lids open to irrigate the eye adequately. Ideally, you should use a bulb or irrigation syringe, a nasal cannula, or some other device that will allow you to control the flow Figure 5 . In some circumstances, you may have to pour water into the eye by holding the patient's head under a gently running faucet. You can have the patient immerse his or her face in a large pan or basin of water and rapidly blink the affected eyelid. If only one eye is affected, take care to avoid contaminated water getting into the unaffected eye.

Irrigate the eye for at least 5 minutes. If the burn was caused by an alkali or a strong acid, irrigate the eye continuously for 20 minutes because these substances can penetrate deeply. One common possibility occurs where anhydrous ammonia is used during the process of cooking methamphetamine. If the eyes are not irrigated promptly and efficiently, permanent damage is likely. Whenever you have to irrigate the eye(s), continue to irrigate the eye en route to the hospital if possible.

You may have access to an eye irrigation device called the Morgan lens. The Morgan lens is appropriate for use with eye burns from acids, alkalis, or solvents, and can also be used to help remove a foreign body as long as it is not embedded or impaled in the eye. Follow these steps when you are using a Morgan lens:

1. Administer with a topical anesthetic such as tetracaine (Pontocaine, Dicaine).
2. Connect the Morgan lens to the bag of IV fluid of choice: 0.9% saline, lactated Ringer's, or sterile water and let it begin to drip.
3. Pull tension on the upper eyelid and slide the Morgan lens under the upper eyelid.
4. Cup the lower eyelid and slide the Morgan lens under the lower eyelid.

YOU *are the Medic*   PART 2

Your patient feels very hot to the touch. While your partner is obtaining vital signs, you ask the administrator if she could provide any information as to what happened to the patient. She states that the patient's teacher said that he was leaning forward and drooling like he was going to vomit. She also says the patient has been coughing and it "sounds funny." She says the child's name is Jimmy.

Recording Time: 0 Minutes	
Appearance	Awake
Level of consciousness	Alert (oriented to person, place, and day) but is drowsy
Airway	Open
Breathing	Sounds obstructed
Circulation	Adequate

3. What do you need to know about the patient's cough?

4. What steps will you take in your further assessment of this patient?

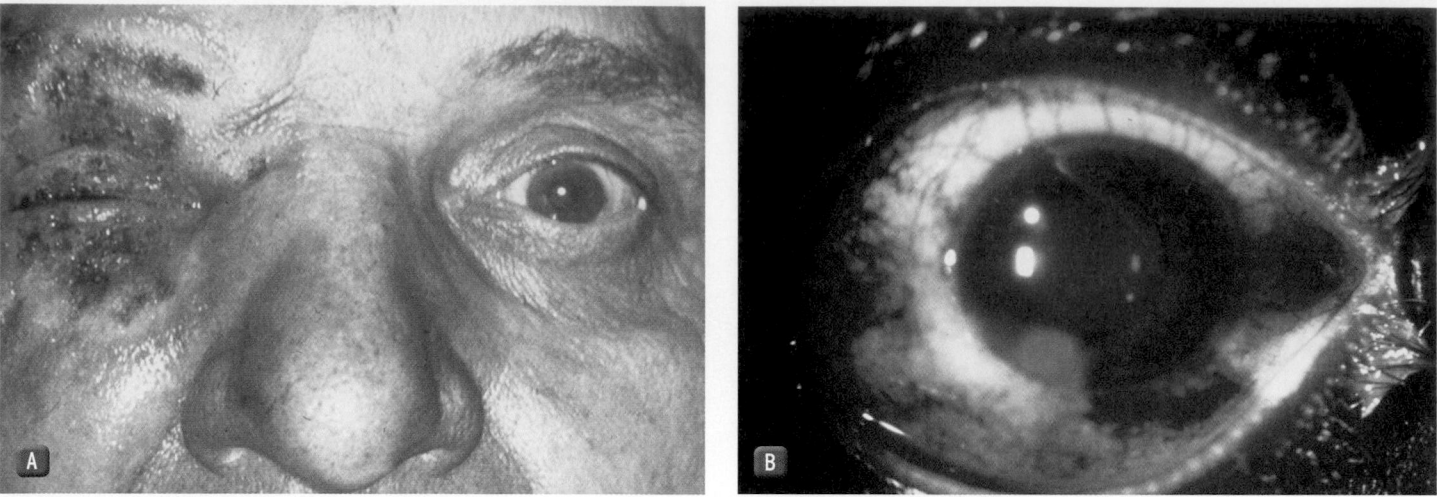

Figure 4   **A.** Chemical burns typically occur when an acid or alkali is splashed into the eye. **B.** A chemical burn from lye, an alkaline solution.

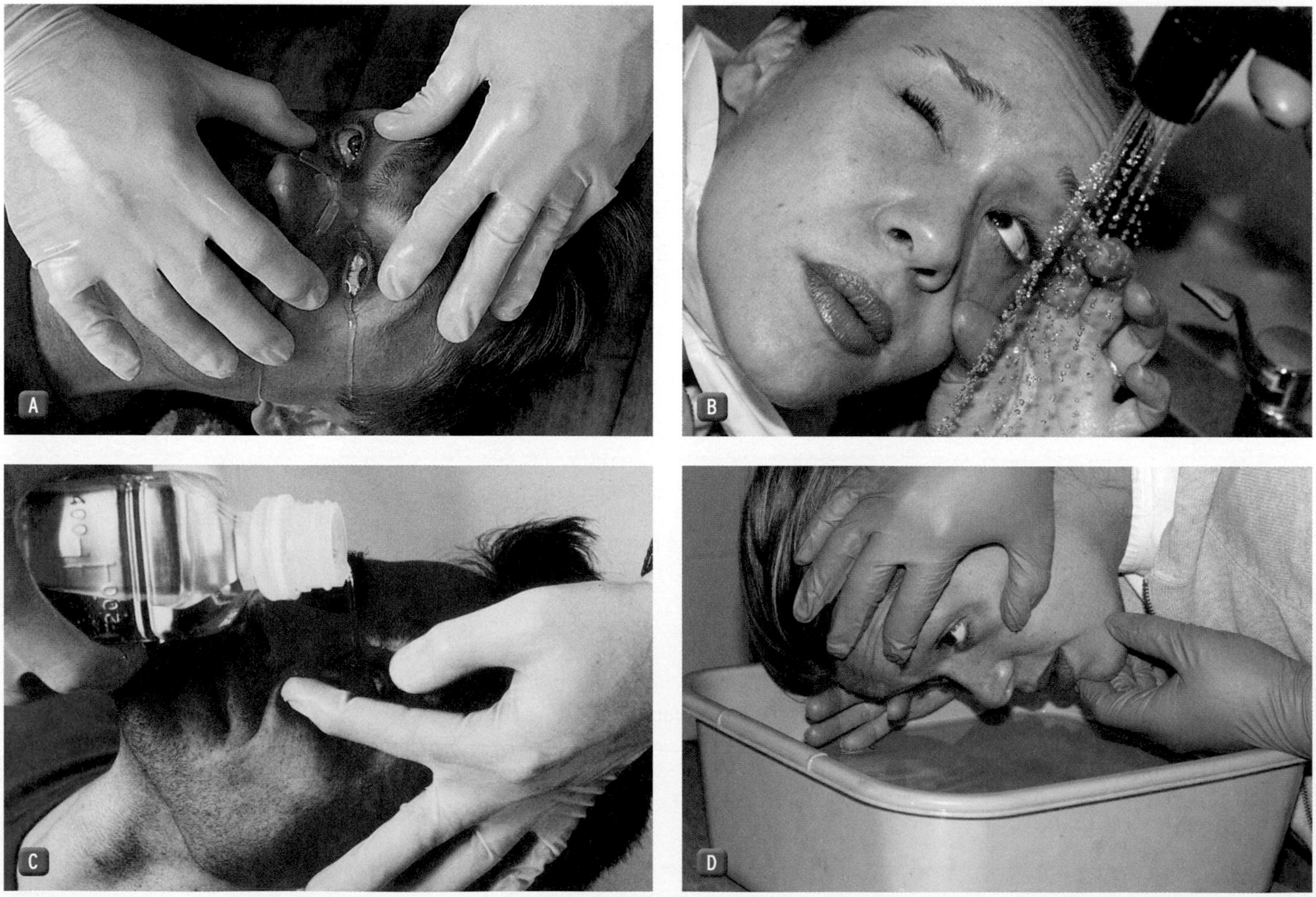

Figure 5   Four ways to effectively irrigate the eye. **A.** Nasal cannula. **B.** Shower. **C.** Bottle. **D.** Basin. Always protect the uninjured eye from the irrigating solution to prevent exposure to the substance.

5. Run the fluid at the desired rate.

6. *Continue to run the fluid* while the Morgan lens is in place. Do not stop the fluid.

The Morgan lens should generally not be removed in the field. It is best to use the lens with continuous fluid until arrival at the emergency department where a physician can consider use of an eye lubricant and removal of the lens.

Transport considerations for eye burn patients include preventing one eye from draining into the unaffected eye, which would contaminate it. If irrigation is in progress, the unaffected eye should be in a protected position. Specialized treatment and care for burns to the eyes can be found at level 1 trauma centers.

You may encounter patients who wear contact lenses. In general, if the eye is injured, you should not attempt to remove contact lenses because you may further aggravate the injury. The only indication for removing contact lenses in the prehospital setting is a chemical burn of the eye. In this situation, the lens can trap the offending chemical and make irrigation difficult, thus worsening the injury.

There are three types of contact lenses: hard, rigid gas-permeable, and soft (hydrophilic). Small, hard contact lenses usually are tinted, making them relatively easy to see. Large, soft contact lenses are clear and can be difficult to see, even more so if they "float" up or down under an eyelid.

To remove a hard contact lens, use a small suction cup, moistening the end with saline **Figure 6A**. To remove soft lenses, place one to two drops of saline in the eye **Figure 6B**, gently pinch the lens between your gloved thumb and index finger, and lift it off the surface of the eye **Figure 6C**. Place the contact lens in a container with sterile saline solution. Always advise emergency department staff if a patient is wearing contact lenses.

Occasionally, you may care for a patient who is wearing an eye prosthesis (artificial eye). You should suspect an eye of being artificial when it does not respond to light, move in concert with the opposite eye, or appear quite the same as the opposite eye. If you are unsure as to whether the patient has an eye prosthesis, ask the patient. No harm will be done if you care for an artificial eye as you would a normal one; however, you should make every attempt to accurately determine the patient's eye function.

Conjunctivitis

<u>Conjunctivitis</u> or "pink eye" is a condition where the conjunctiva becomes inflamed and red **Figure 7**. Conjunctivitis most often starts in one eye and spreads to the other eye. The conjunctiva is a thin layer that lines the inside of the eyelids and the white part of the eye. Inflammation causes the white part of the eye to take on a red or pink tint. Most often this is caused by bacteria, viruses, allergies, or foreign bodies present in the eye. Viral and bacterial causes are highly contagious and can become an epidemic. Conjunctivitis accounts for the most absences in daycare or school settings according to the CDC. Allergic conjunctivitis is caused by a trigger or irritating allergen. Viral conjunctivitis is often associated with an upper respiratory virus or cold. Bacterial conjunctivitis is caused by various bacterial infections. Newborns are susceptible to conjunctivitis from sexually transmitted diseases passed on by the mother, irritation to antibiotic eye drops at birth, or an infection from a clogged tear

duct. If conjunctivitis is due to a foreign body, the eye will begin to produce tears in an attempt to flush out the object.

Assessment and Management Assessment of the patient's condition should occur after ruling out any life threats to the patient or dangers to the crew. A general assessment of the patient's vision should be performed, including assessment of visual acuity, assessment of the external eye, assessment of the pupils, assessment of peripheral vision, and assessment of eye movement, as described earlier.

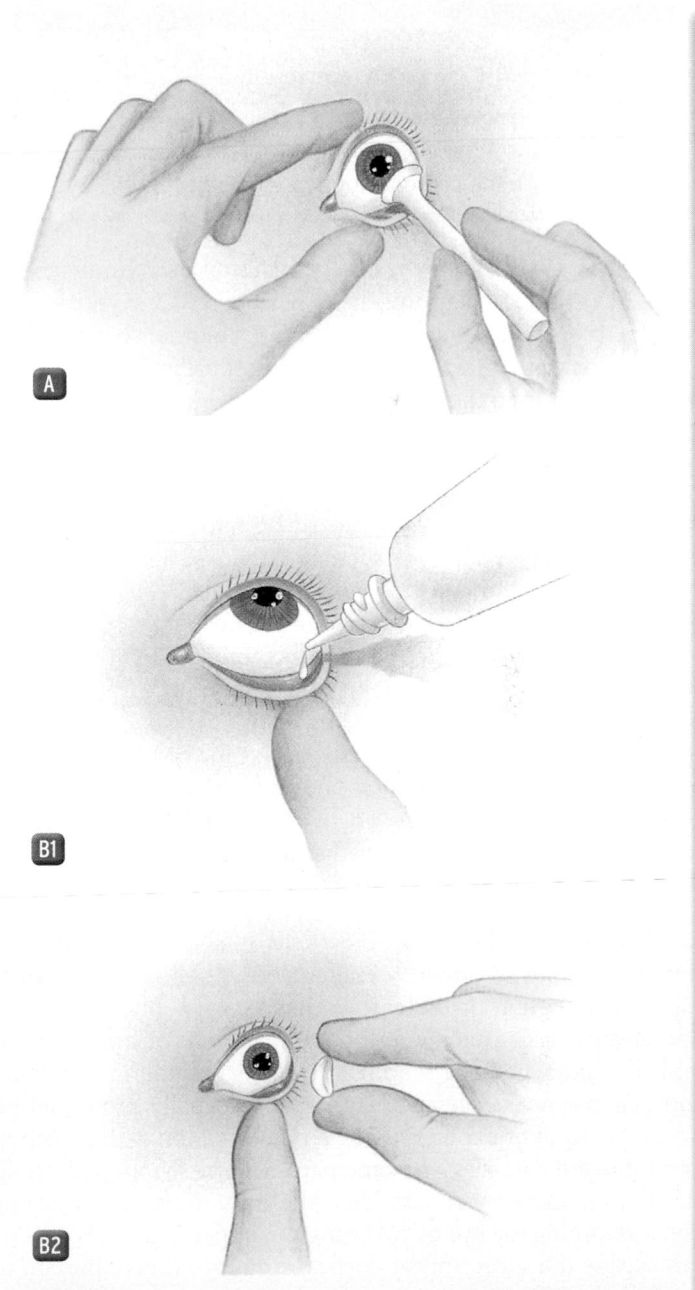

Figure 6 Removing contact lenses should be limited to patients with chemical burns to the eye. **A.** To remove hard contact lenses, use a specialized suction cup moistened with sterile saline solution. **B.** Step 1: To remove soft contact lenses, instill 1 or 2 drops of saline or irrigating solution. Step 2: Pinch off the lens with your gloved thumb and index fingers.

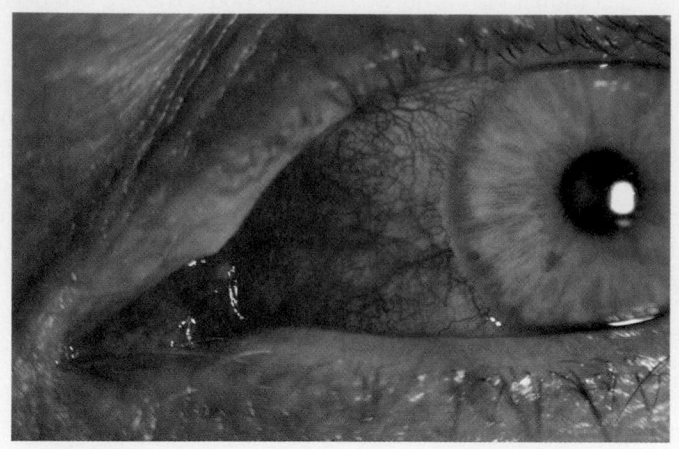

Figure 7 Conjunctivitis is inflammation of the eye. It may be associated with the presence of a foreign object in the eye.

Viral conjunctivitis normally resolves on its own. It can last up to 2 weeks but usually reaches a peak in 3 to 5 days. Bacterial conjunctivitis requires a topical antibiotic in order to heal. Allergic conjunctivitis may need a topical antihistamine prescribed by the physician in the emergency department.

Corneal Abrasion

Abrasions or scrapes to the outer surface of the eye can be quite painful. They are commonly caused by fingernails, paper, and airborne objects from construction activities. Metal filings are particularly inflammatory because they cause a "rust ring" after 24 hours, which must be removed in the hospital.

Corneal abrasions are the most common eye injury seen in emergency departments. They are due to superficial trauma to the cornea, often from a foreign body, but may also be due to excessive rubbing, chemical burns, or being poked in the eye by a finger or makeup brush. If the redness and discomfort does not resolve after an object has been removed, or after the eye has been flushed with water or saline, the patient should be seen in the emergency department and referred to an ophthalmologist if necessary.

Assessment and Management Patients will likely experience significant pain, sensitivity to light (photophobia), and tearing. Close examination of the cornea may reveal a line or scratch. The cornea heals quickly and abrasion sensation may vary. It may feel like a grain of sand in the eye or a stabbing sensation and can promote excessive tearing. It is usually more painful when the injury is exposed to the air. Lubrication with irrigation or a lubricant can alleviate some pain. Taping the injured eyelid closed with paper tape can keep the injured eye from drying out. Examining the eye by inverting the upper and lower eyelids can expose the source of the corneal abrasion. It is important to carefully look for a foreign body in the eye.

A topical anesthetic like tetracaine can relieve some symptoms. Supportive care in the prehospital setting may include irrigation, which may also help remove the object. If the cause of the abrasion is still present, it may need to be removed at an appropriate facility. If movement of the eye causes severe discomfort, it may be necessary to cover both eyes. A lubricant can

resolve some of the pain along with closing and covering the injured eye. Taping the eyelid closed with paper tape can allow the patient to relax without forcibly holding the injured eye shut. These injuries, especially those involving metal fragments, may need to be examined under a special microscope. In-hospital treatment consists of removing the fragment (if still present), treating the eye with topical antibiotics, and patching the eye.

Foreign Body

Dust, dirt, splinters, and other particles are commonly involved in eye injuries. Although most are not threatening to sight, they can cause significant pain. Most foreign objects in the eye occur as a result of occupational injury; however, you may also treat patients whose injury is hobby-related.

The use of grinders, sanders, nailers, weed whackers, and other machines commonly cause these injuries. As the machinery is working, it can dislodge and eject particles a long distance, and if safety glasses are not worn, foreign objects can enter the eyes. Foreign objects in the eye can also be due to auto crashes, firearm use, and recreational activities.

Assessment and Management Using a light, evaluate the entire eye. Note any blood or discoloration of the sclera. Gentle irrigation usually will not wash out foreign bodies that are stuck to the cornea or lying under the upper eyelid. To examine the undersurface of the upper eyelid, pull the lid upward and forward. If you spot a foreign object on the surface of the eyelid, you may be able to remove it with a moist, sterile, cotton-tipped applicator. *Never attempt to remove a foreign body that is stuck or imbedded in the cornea.*

Foreign bodies ranging in size from a pencil to a sliver of metal may be impaled in the eye **Figure 8** . Clearly, these objects must be removed by a physician.

To ease pain and assist with dislodging the foreign body, begin by irrigating the eye with a sterile saline solution. This will frequently flush away loose, small foreign objects lying on the surface of the eye. Always flush from the nose side of the eye toward the outside to avoid flushing material into the other eye. After its removal, a foreign body will often leave a small abrasion on the surface of the conjunctiva, which leads to continued irritation; for this reason, you should transport the patient to the hospital for further assessment and treatment.

When a foreign body is impaled in the globe, *do not remove it!* Stabilize it in place. Cover the eye with a moist, sterile dressing; place a cup or other protective barrier over the object, and secure it in place with bulky dressing **Figure 9** . Cover the unaffected eye to prevent further damage caused by **sympathetic eye movement**, and promptly transport the patient to the hospital.

Inflammation of the Eyelid (Chalazion and Hordeolum)

The eyelid has oil glands and oil ducts that provide a protective film across the eye. Occasionally these ducts and/or glands become blocked, causing a small swollen bump or pustule on the external eyelid (**chalazion**) **Figure 10** . A red tender lump in the eyelid or at the lid margin may be due to a blocked oil duct (**hordeolum**), commonly known as a stye **Figure 11** .

Words of Wisdom

Large and small foreign bodies, particularly small metal fragments, can become completely embedded in the globe. The patient may not even be aware of the cause of the problem. Suspect such an injury when the history includes metal work (such as hammering, exposure to splinters, grinders, vigorous filing) and when you observe signs of ocular injury (such as redness, irritation, inflammation).

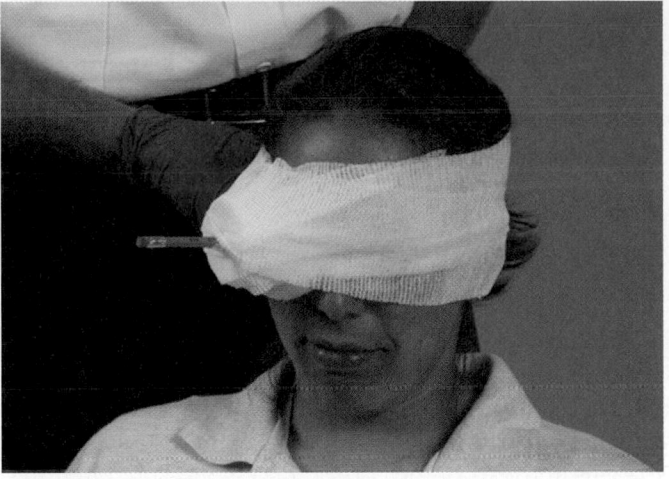

Figure 9 Secure an impaled object in the eye with a protective barrier and bulky dressing.

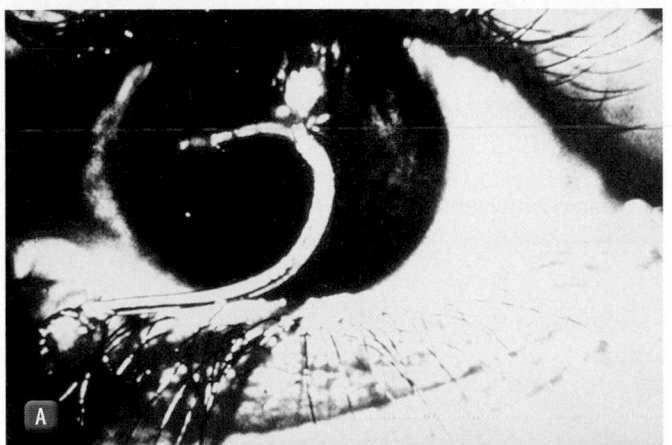

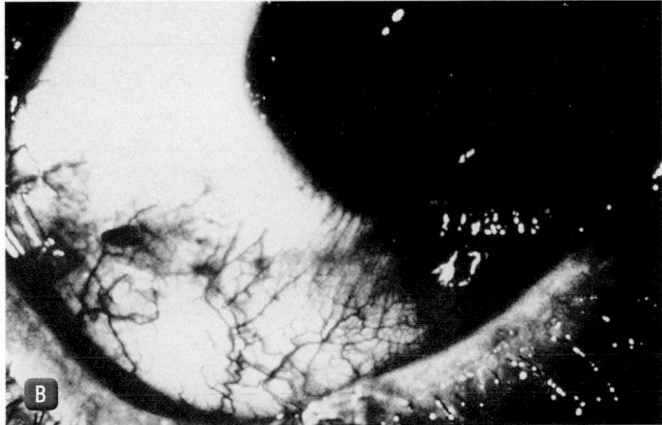

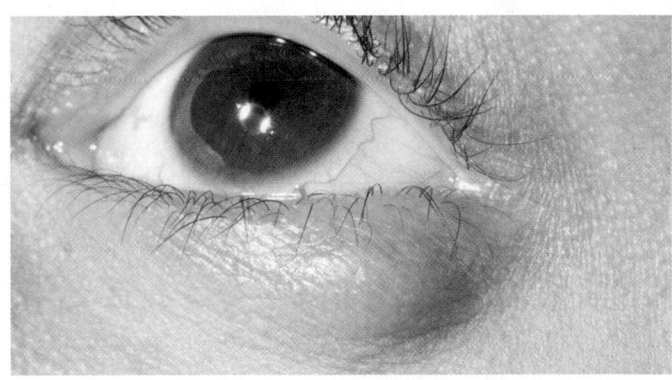

Figure 10 A chalazion is a small, swollen bump or pustule on the external eyelid.

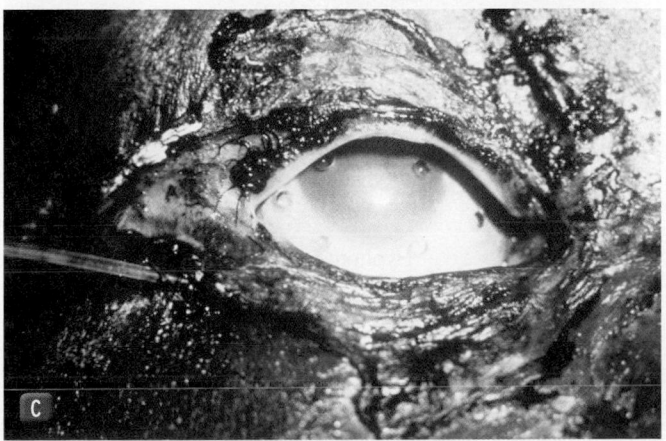

Figure 8 Any number of objects can be impaled in the eye. **A.** Fishhook. **B.** Sharp, metal sliver. **C.** Knife blade.

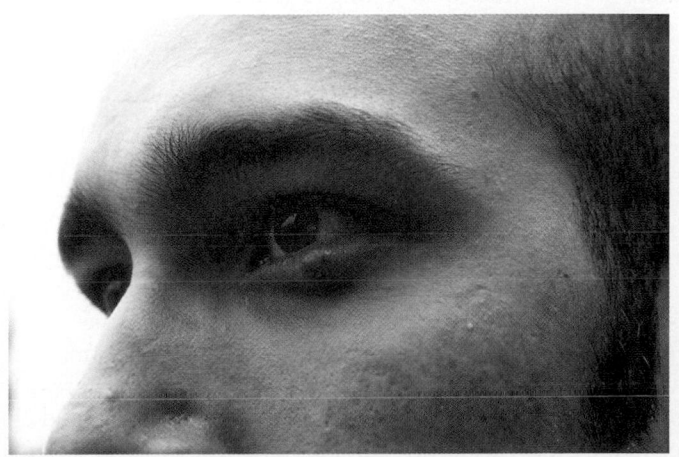

Figure 11 A hordeolum, or stye, is a red, tender lump in the eyelid or at the lid margin.

Assessment and Management The infection that occurs as a result of the clogged ducts is often painful. Infection can progress to become systemic. A thorough assessment of vital signs and history is warranted especially when the patient may now have systemic symptoms.

Paramedics can treat eyelid inflammation with a warm moist washcloth over the affected area, simulating warm soaks that the patient can do at home. The patient should be transported to the emergency department for topical antibiotics and pain management if necessary.

Glaucoma

Glaucoma is a group of conditions that lead to increased intraocular pressure. It is one of the leading causes of blindness. The white fluid in the eye (vitreous humor) circulates nutrients to the lens and part of the cornea. Excess pressure buildup can cause damage to the optic nerve. Glaucoma is usually treated with eye drops to reduce ocular pressures.

Assessment and Management Prehospital complaints may involve the patient reporting a loss of field of vision or a blind spot toward the center of vision. Assessment should rule out any trauma or physical injury to the eye. You will perform a general eye assessment as described earlier, evaluating vision, motility, and any abnormalities of the external eye or anterior surface. Document any pertinent negatives and all abnormal findings. An ophthalmologist will perform a much more comprehensive exam, assessing inner eye pressure, the shape and color of the optic nerve viewed through a dilated pupil, the angle in the eye where the iris meets the cornea, and the thickness of the cornea, and will perform a test to assess the complete field of vision. Because paramedics are not normally trained to do this comprehensive eye exam, all patients with eye injuries or conditions should be taken to the emergency department for follow-up.

Depending on the cause of the pressure buildup, eye drops are usually prescribed to reduce the pressure. Glaucoma increases in incidence with the elderly, but can occur any time from birth forward. Always ask patients which medications they have taken prior to your arrival on the scene. Administration of eye medications in the prehospital setting is usually limited to tetracaine (Pontocaine, Dicaine) for pain relief, or emergency irrigation for removal of a damaging or irritating substance from the eyes. As the population of geriatric patients increases, the scope of practice for the paramedic may change to include limited eye care.

Hyphema

Blunt trauma can cause serious eye injuries, ranging from swelling and ecchymosis **Figure 12** to rupture of the globe. Hyphema is bleeding into the anterior chamber of the eye that obscures vision, partially or completely **Figure 13**. It may be the result of blunt trauma to the eye or a medical cause. It may be a marker of damage to other structures of the eye and, therefore, requires a full ophthalmologic examination. One of the concerns is blood clotting in the canal connecting the anterior chamber to the posterior chamber, causing an acute rise in intraocular pressure. Approximately 25% of hyphemas are associated with globe injuries.

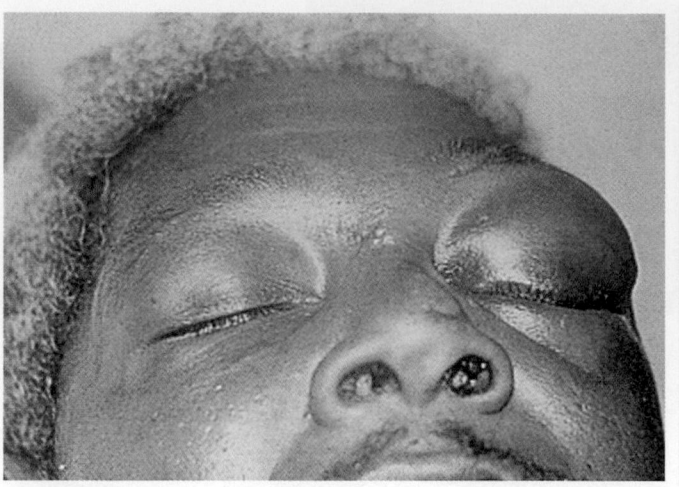

Figure 12 Swelling and ecchymosis are hallmark findings associated with blunt trauma to the eye.

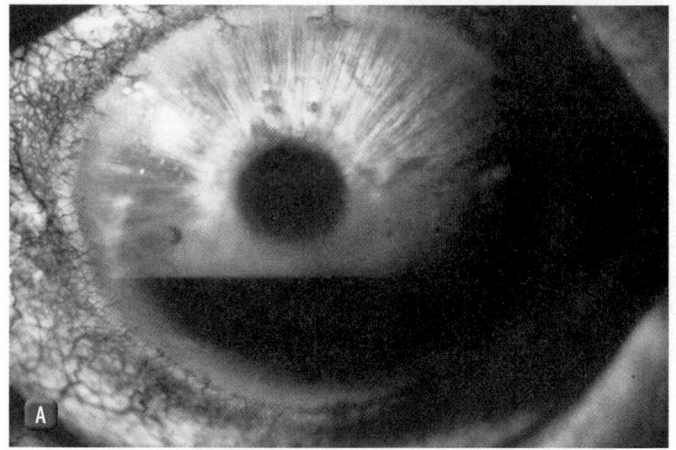

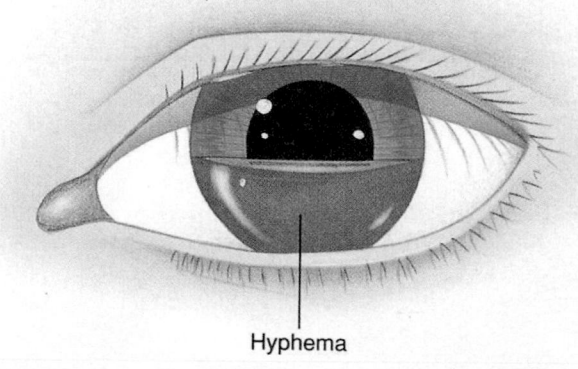

Hyphema

Figure 13 A hyphema, characterized by bleeding into the anterior chamber of the eye, can occur following blunt trauma to the eye. This condition should be considered a sight-threatening emergency. **A.** Actual hyphema. **B.** Illustration.

Assessment and Management A patient with hyphema is likely to experience pain and possibly blurred vision. The patient will report reduced vision directly proportional to the size of the hyphema. Often the blood is directly visible, but shining a penlight obliquely at the globe may help you to visualize the blood, which will pool with gravity.

If hyphema or rupture of the globe is suspected, take spinal motion restriction precautions. Such injuries indicate that a significant amount of force was applied to the face and, thus, may include a spinal injury. Elevate the head of the backboard approximately 40° to decrease intraocular pressure (IOP) and discourage the patient from performing activities that may increase IOP (eg, coughing).

If there are no other contraindications, transport should be performed with the patient sitting as upright as possible and both eyes should be patched. Pain should be managed with acetaminophen with or without codeine and aspirin; other medications with antiplatelet effects should be avoided. An anxiolytic may facilitate transport.

Iritis

Iritis is inflammation of the iris 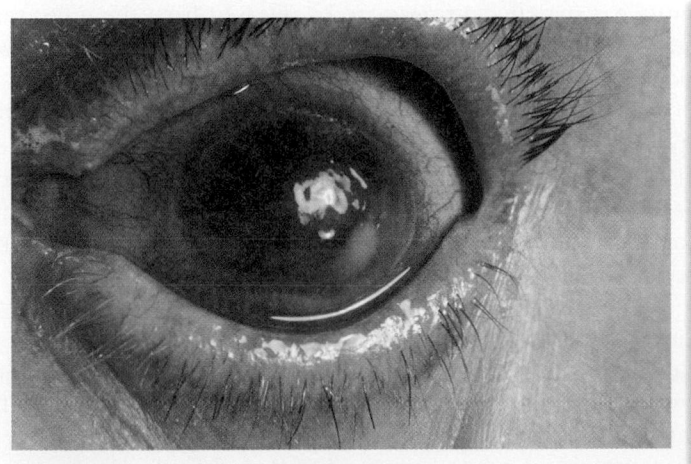 **Figure 14** . This is also termed anterior uveitis. Uveitis is the third leading preventable cause of blindness.

Iritis can be acute or chronic. When acute, it can be caused by trauma or irritants, and usually affects only one eye. Autoimmune diseases, different types of arthritis, irritable bowel disease, and Crohn disease can predispose patients to developing iritis. Infectious causes include Lyme disease, tuberculosis, and sexually transmitted diseases.

Assessment and Management Iritis presents as a red area surrounding the iris, cloudy vision, or an unusually shaped pupil. The assessment should focus on history. Many ophthalmologists are not trained to recognize iritis. Patients should be directed to a uveitis specialist or an ocular immunologist.

Acute iritis usually responds well to topical corticosteroids as long as the cause is not fungal, viral, or bacterial. There are

Figure 14 Iritis is inflammation of the iris.

over 90 different pathogens or autoimmune processes that have a relationship to chronic or recurrent iritis. These patients should be referred to a specialist. Failure to treat iritis can result in permanent disability.

Papilledema

Papilledema results from swelling or inflammation of the optic nerve at the rear part of the eye. The optic nerve communicates between the eyes and the brain. Patients experience headaches, nausea with possible vomiting, temporary vision loss, or narrowing vision fields. They may also experience a "graying" in their field of vision.

The increased pressure in the brain, which causes optic nerve swelling and inflammation, may have several different causes. Space-occupying lesions like abscesses and tumors can create intracranial pressure increases. An inner ear infection, lung infection, or dental infection can cause pus accumulation in the brain, causing an abscess that presses on the optic nerve. Meningitis, fever, brain tumors, hypertensive crisis, chronic high blood pressure, and other diseases such as Guillain Barré syndrome may all result in an increase in cerebrospinal fluid (CSF) pressures, leading to papilledema.

Assessment and Management The diagnosis of papilledema is made by an ophthalmologist, or emergency department physician, who has been trained to examine the patient's retina with an ophthalmoscope. If swelling is present, red spots will also indicate bleeding.

Prehospital management consists of treating the symptoms and transporting the patient. As always, assess the ABCs to ensure that there are no life threats. Depending on the severity of anxiousness or pain, the patient may benefit from analgesics or a mild sedative. Vision loss can become permanent if treatment does not begin within a few days of onset; therefore, immediate treatment should be encouraged. Treatment is aimed at the underlying cause of the intracranial pressure increase. Paramedics who have an expanded scope of practice that includes use of an ophthalmoscope should receive further training in the use of this device from their medical director.

Retinal Detachment and Defect

Another potential result of blunt eye trauma is retinal detachment, or separation of the inner layers of the retina from the underlying choroid (the vascular membrane that nourishes the retina). Retinal detachment is often seen in sports injuries, especially boxing.

Assessment and Management This painless condition produces flashing lights, specks, or "floaters" in the field of vision, and a cloud or shade over the patient's vision. Because it can cause devastating damage to vision, retinal detachment is an ocular emergency and requires *immediate* medical attention. Transport the patient to the most appropriate emergency department.

Cellulitis of the Orbit: Periorbital and Orbital Cellulitis

Periorbital and orbital cellulitis are both most commonly caused by staphylococcus and streptococcus bacterial infections. The location of these infections determines which type is present.

Periorbital cellulitis is more prevalent in children than adults. Also known as preseptal cellulitis or eyelid cellulitis, it presents as a painful, red, swollen eyelid. Fever may also be a symptom along with redness of the white part of the eyes (conjunctivitis). Insect bites, upper respiratory disorders, and trauma increase the potential to develop periorbital cellulitis.

Orbital cellulitis is an infection within the eye socket and is considered a medical emergency because it can lead to permanent vision problems and blindness. The goal of treatment is to avoid the formation of an abscess. Predisposed risk factors include sinusitis, tooth infections, facial or middle ear infections, trauma, and sinus infections.

Assessment and Management   Treatment in children is usually IV antibiotics for both forms of cellulitis. Adults are treated with oral antibiotics; however, if symptoms are severe, IV antibiotics are used for adults as well.

Prehospital management is directed at ruling out life threats with a thorough history and transporting the patient to the appropriate care.

■ The Ear

The ear is the primary structure for hearing and balance, but is also integral to self-protection. When you think of ear problems, you most likely think of hearing loss. But hearing is not all the ear affects; the ear also plays in important part in balance and orientation. Disorders and injury to the ear can leave a person unable to communicate, react, and maintain equilibrium. For example, scuba divers are susceptible to vertigo from cold water moving into the ear canal during pressure equalization. A tumor that grows on the eighth cranial nerve (acoustic neuroma) can affect the inner ear and balance. The tumor is usually slow growing, but if it grows larger, other cranial nerves can be affected, including the fifth, sixth, and seventh. This can affect facial sensation, eye movement, facial movement, taste, and hearing.

Loss of hearing is a large health problem for adults, most likely associated with occupational noise injury. Hearing loss can affect a child's ability to develop communication, language, and social skills. The earlier children with hearing loss start receiving services, the more likely they are to reach their full potential.

■ Anatomy and Physiology of the Ear

The ear is divided into three anatomic parts: external, middle, and inner Figure 15 . The external ear consists of the pinna, external auditory canal, and the exterior portion of the tympanic membrane or what is commonly known as the eardrum. The middle ear consists of the inner portion of the tympanic membrane and the ossicles while the inner ear consists of the cochlea and semicircular canals.

Sound waves enter the ear through the auricle, or pinna, the large cartilaginous external portion of the ear. They then travel through the external auditory canal to the tympanic membrane. Vibration of sound waves against the tympanic membrane sets up vibration in the ossicles, the three small bones on the inner side of the tympanic membrane. These vibrations are transmitted to the cochlear duct at the oval window, the opening between the middle ear and the vestibule. Movement of the oval window causes fluid within the cochlea, a shell-shaped structure in the inner ear, to vibrate. Within the cochlea at the organ of Corti, vibration stimulates hair movements that form nerve impulses that travel to the brain via the auditory nerve. The brain then converts these impulses into sound.

Special Populations

Hearing loss is more common in the older population than vision loss. With age, changes in the structures of hearing result in loss of high-frequency hearing, or even deafness. If an older patient uses a hearing aid for everyday activity, it is best to keep it in place to provide for better communication during transport to the hospital.

Consider learning American Sign Language so that you can better communicate with patients who are deaf.

■ Patient Assessment

Initial observation of the scene must rule out hazards to EMS personnel and crew. Blast injuries warrant special consideration as to approach, staging, and scene safety; these are discussed in the chapter, *Trauma Systems and Mechanism of Injury*.

Foreign objects forced into the auditory canal can damage the eardrum. Ear infections may cause the eardrum to blister and bleed. Inner ear infections can cause excessive pressures behind the eardrum. Blast pressure waves can burst the eardrum. When altitudes are rapidly changing, equalizing pressures can be difficult if the eustachian tubes are clogged from a cold, allergy, or inflammation. When a person moves to a higher altitude, expanding air needs to be released from the inner ear. Swallowing and plugging the nose and blowing against a closed glottis can relieve the pressure.

As you approach the patient, aside from determining the approximate age, sex, environmental conditions, and degree of distress, note whether the patient has a hearing aid. Sometimes patients do not sleep with their hearing aid in and they may seem confused until you are told by someone else that the patient cannot hear you!

Assessment and management of the patient with an ear condition begins by ensuring airway patency, breathing adequacy, circulation, and managing any threats to life. Although patients with ear conditions may be in pain or have a hearing deficit, they generally are not considered the highest priority nor have a life threat that needs to be immediately dealt with.

Typically, medical conditions involving the ears are not life threats unless they are a symptom of a much more serious problem (eg, ear damage from a blast injury or head trauma).

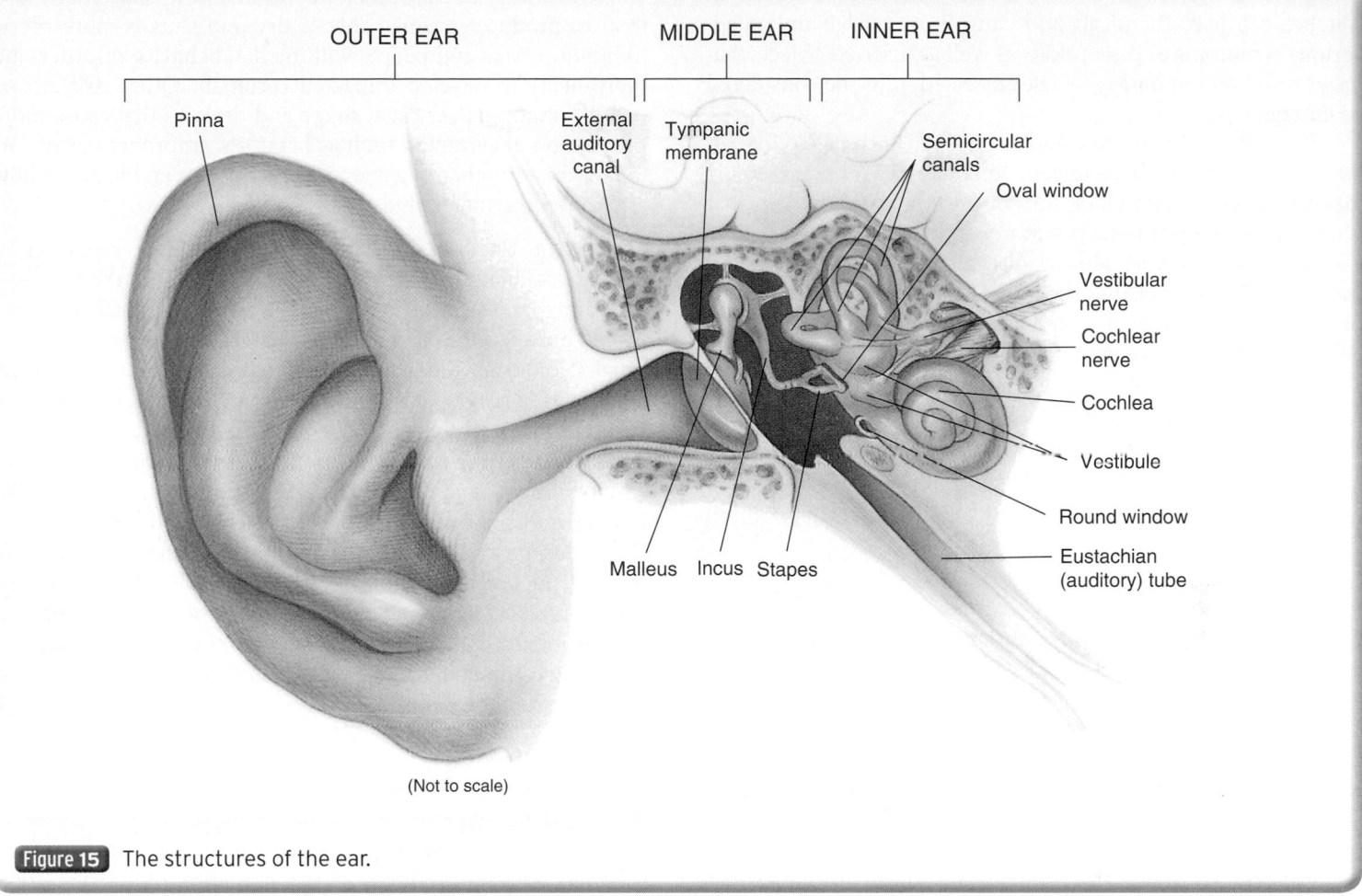

Figure 15 The structures of the ear.

These patients may be very uncomfortable and their condition cannot be resolved in the field. Therefore, transport these patients to the emergency department where they can receive the appropriate physical examination, diagnosis, and treatment.

Take a complete history and find out if the patient has had this condition before. Observe the ears for drainage, excess cerumen, and inflammation or swelling. If the patient has pain, it should be quantified on a pain scale and identified by region and cause. When asking OPQRST assessment questions, P, provocation, should include pertinent negatives, such as "Does it hurt when you swallow, sneeze, cough, or when you bend over?" History of the events leading up to the complaint can help provide clues to the onset of symptoms. The patient may describe unusual pressure changes with "ear popping," itching in the ears, a recent respiratory infection or cold, or a scuba diving trip. Paramedics generally will treat only the discomfort caused by the symptoms and will pass on the history to the treating facility.

Assess for new aberrations in hearing perception. If hearing is affected, changes should be noted and reassessed during transport. Ask the patient if he or she has experienced tinnitus (ringing in the ears) or dizziness. Inspect and palpate for wounds, swelling, or drainage (pus, blood, cerebrospinal fluid). Often the mastoid process of the skull, which is palpated immediately posterior to the auricle, is assessed for discoloration and tenderness (**Battle sign**). Abnormalities of the external canal and tympanic membrane are visualized by use of an otoscope. This skill is shown in the chapter, *Patient Assessment*. Trauma to the ears is discussed in the chapter, *Face and Neck Trauma*.

An adequate assessment of the external ear canal and middle ear cannot be performed in the field. Transport the patient, and as always, be sure to document your findings and communicate as appropriate with the receiving facility.

■ Pathophysiology, Assessment, and Management of Ear Injuries

Foreign Body

Foreign bodies in the ear are most likely to be seen in the pediatric population. The majority of the objects are solid, such as beads, stones, or even erasers. However, it is possible for an insect to crawl into the ear canal or for a child to put vegetative matter in the ear.

Assessment and Management Assessment of the foreign body should determine the nature of the object and the urgency of treatment. The assessment of a foreign body in the ear in the prehospital environment is limited to visual clues if the object can be seen. Look for bleeding, redness or inflammation, and symptoms associated with infection. Some objects such as organic matter and food will swell from moisture and may become more entrapped as they swell. Small batteries such as those found in watches can leak chemicals and cause burns if left untreated. Serious symptoms or discomfort, as well as inserted objects that may cause harm or damage if left untreated, must be considered an emergency.

The ear canal is narrow and angulated. Probing for foreign bodies in the ear is discouraged. In some areas the paramedic may use an otoscope to look further into the ear; however, that is outside the scope of practice in most regions.

As is the case with almost all foreign bodies, observe and document, but do not pull the impaled object out. Rather, simply stabilize it in place. The pediatric ear canal is small and any effort to retrieve the foreign object may do more harm.

Due to the potential for infection and damage to the ear drum, these patients should be seen by a physician in the ED. Management of both adults and children is to transport to the appropriate facility in the position of comfort. Severe pain or anxiousness can be treated with pain management medication and/or mild sedation.

Impacted Cerumen

Cerumen is the yellowish oily substance found in the outer ear canal. It helps prevent dirt and water from entering the middle ear canal and may protect the ear from bacteria or fungus. Cerumen may present as "wet," which is a sticky brown color, or "dry" as a greyish flaky substance. Commonly known as "earwax," cerumen can become impacted and cause pressure against the eardrum. Impaction occurs when too much cerumen builds up and gets stuck in the outer ear canal.

Normally cerumen flows outwardly toward the outer ear and gets washed away. It helps remove dead skin cells from the ear canal. Cerumen impaction is more common in the elderly,

where hearing aids may block the normal flow. The elderly also tend to produce cerumen that is dry and thus is more prone to buildup. Men and people with mental behavior disorders are more likely to develop impacted cerumen. Other risk factors include abnormal ear canal shape and diseases that cause more production of cerumen, such as keratosis. Improper use of cotton swabs and other hygiene tools or objects can block the flow and cause a cerumen plug.

Assessment and Management Symptoms include sensation of pressure or fullness in the ear, dizziness, ringing in the ears, loss of hearing, and pain or itching in the ear. Prehospital treatment should include a thorough history and visual inspection of the ear canal. Because an elderly person may have many different medical conditions, it may be difficult to rule out other serious problems. It may be likely that elderly patients with impacted cerumen may not have seen a physician lately for various socioeconomic reasons.

Treatment is aimed at removing the excess cerumen. An otoscope will be used by a physician to identify the problem. Once found, irrigation or tools designed to remove the wax will be used. Suction and eardrops such as wax softeners may also be used. Untreated, cerumen can cause infection and irritation that can potentially damage the eardrum and hearing. The process of removing cerumen may also cause injury, so follow-up is necessary after the procedure.

Labyrinthitis

Labyrinthitis is most recognized as the feeling of vertigo or loss of balance after an ear infection or upper respiratory infection. Irritation and swelling in the inner ear affects the nerves of the inner ear and produces a loss of balance. Other symptoms include ringing in the ears (tinnitus), dizziness, loss of hearing, nausea, and vomiting. Permanent hearing loss can occur.

YOU are the Medic | PART 3

You ask, "Jimmy, are you having a hard time swallowing?" Instead of answering, Jimmy slowly nods his head. You ask him if he can talk to you. When Jimmy tries, he ends up coughing. It sounds high pitched and painful. Jimmy looks like he is working hard to breathe. The administrator says she was able to contact Jimmy's mom and that she will meet you at Parkside Hospital.

Recording Time: 3 Minutes	
Respirations	20 breaths/min
Pulse	120 beats/min
Skin	Hot, pale, moist
Blood pressure	106/82 mm Hg
Oxygen saturation (Spo$_2$)	97% room air
Pupils	Equal and reactive

5. What do you suspect is wrong with the patient?

6. Do you have any additional concerns because this child appears drowsy but is working hard to breathe?

Assessment and Management Severe symptoms usually resolve within a week. Prehospital treatment is directed at reducing the severity of the nausea and vomiting and transporting the patient in a position of comfort. The differential diagnoses for vertigo with associated nausea include neurologic disorders such as Meniere disease and acoustic neuroma. These serious disorders will need to be ruled out by a CT scan and an MRI. You should be able to recognize the serious implications of the symptoms and suggest the patient be seen at the emergency department.

Hospital treatment of labyrinthitis includes an antiemetic for nausea and vomiting, an antihistamine to reduce swelling, anti-vertigo medicine, and diazepam (Valium) as a sedative/muscle relaxant. Prompt treatment of respiratory and ear infections reduces the risk of labyrinthitis.

Meniere Disease

Meniere disease is an inner ear disorder, usually affecting adults (mostly those older than 50 years), in which endolymphatic rupture creates increased pressure in the cochlear duct, which then leads to damage to the organ of Corti and the semicircular canal. Meniere disease may have an abrupt onset. Dilation of the endolymphatic spaces occurs after rupture and healing. Hypersecretion or underabsorption occurs, which results in excess fluid in the endolymphatic space. Patients will likely experience severe vertigo (dizziness), tinnitus (perception of sound in the inner ear with no external environmental cause), and sensorineuronal hearing loss.

Assessment and Management Assessment of a patient with Meniere disease is not likely to be performed in the field. The symptoms of hearing loss, ear pressure, vertigo, dizziness, nausea, and vomiting have a number of causes, including viral, bacterial, and neurologic causes, among others. In the prehospital setting, care is focused on treating the nausea and vomiting with an antiemetic. In the clinical setting, after diagnosis, the physician may treat the fluid buildup with diuretics and the nausea with an antiemetic (Compazine). There are surgical procedures that have had limited success. In most patients, Meniere disease resolves very gradually over 2 to 8 years.

Otitis Externa and Media

Otitis is an infection that results from bacterial growth in the ear canal. It can be categorized into otitis externa and otitis media. These are infections of the outer and middle ear cavity, respectively. This is more common in children than in adults partially because as humans grow, the angle of the tube becomes more vertical, allowing the tubes to drain more easily. The angle of the eustachian tube in some children is almost horizontal, preventing the tube from properly draining and allowing infective material to collect. In children younger than 5 years, otitis media is the most common affliction requiring medical intervention.

Otitis externa and otitis media are most commonly bacterial infections, but otitis externa can also be an allergic or fungal reaction and otitis media can be virally induced, developing when sinusitis or rhinitis spreads along the eustachian tubes. Also, auditory canal blockage from excessive cerumen or lack of enough cerumen can lead to bacterial growth that can cause infection.

Assessment and Management

Both otitis externa and media are painful conditions. Allergic or fungal otitis externa may be accompanied by itching, and examination of the external ear canal will show edema and erythema. Patients with otitis media may experience diminished hearing acuity, and examination with an otoscope will reveal an inflamed, bulging tympanic membrane (eardrum). The otoscope is a device designed to look in a patient's ears Figure 16. Use of this device is covered in the chapter, *Patient Assessment*. Typically paramedics do not use these devices unless they work in an expanded scope of practice in which they have received additional training from their medical director. Both disorders are common in children and prior to language development, children will often indicate ear pain by pulling at or rubbing the infected ear. In severe cases the tympanic membrane may tear or rupture, revealing blood in the external ear canal. Untreated infections can cause permanent hearing loss.

Prehospital treatment should be directed at relieving unbearable symptoms. The physician will treat the patient with topical antibiotics and possibly corticosteroids to reduce inflammation. The paramedic should monitor the patient's condition and administer pain medication when necessary. In the hospital setting, if the symptoms are tolerated, the patient's condition is monitored. If no improvement occurs, antibiotics are administered. When the physician can see a bulging tympanic membrane from excess fluid buildup in the middle ear, additional antibiotics may be administered. When several trials

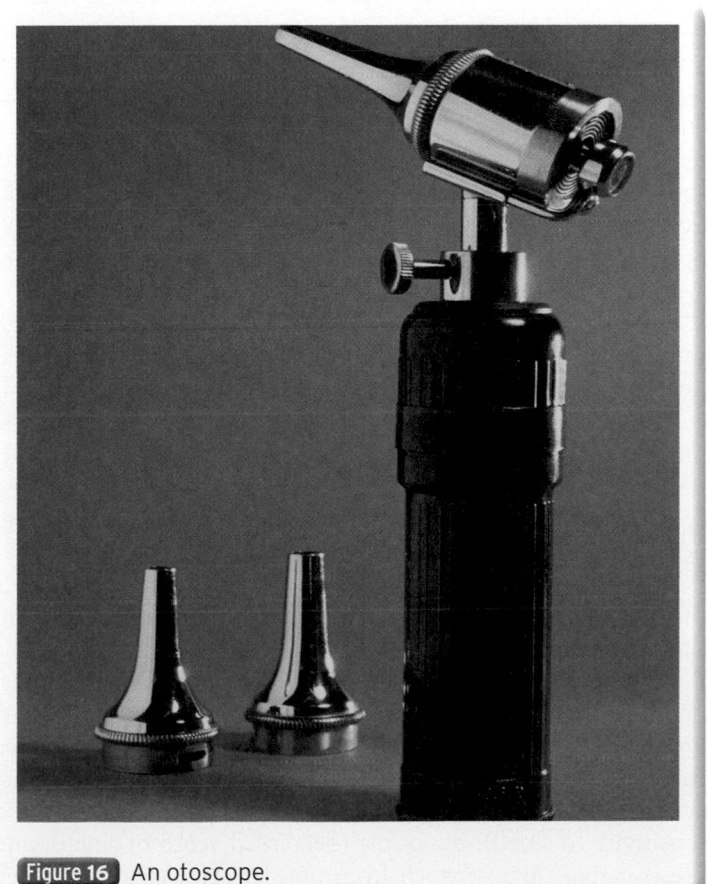

Figure 16 An otoscope.

of antibiotics have been unsuccessful, such as in children who have immune deficiencies, tympanocentesis (needle aspiration) is performed by a physician. The middle ear fluid that has been aspirated is cultured. This aids in specific treatment for the bacteria present. The results of the culture will indicate the type of bacteria present and aid in determining the treatment necessary.

Perforated Tympanic Membrane

Perforation of the tympanic membrane (ruptured eardrum) can result from foreign bodies in the ear or from pressure-related injuries, such as blast injuries resulting from an explosion, or diving-related injuries that result in barotrauma to the ear. Blast injuries are covered in more detail in the chapter, *Terrorism*. Diving injuries are covered in the chapter, *Environmental Emergencies*.

Assessment and Management Signs and symptoms of a perforated tympanic membrane include loss of hearing and blood drainage from the ear. Although the injury is extremely painful for the patient, the tympanic membrane typically heals spontaneously and without complication. Nevertheless, a careful assessment should be performed to detect and treat other injuries, some of which may be life threatening. Transport the patient for further evaluation. Pain management should be considered in severe cases.

■ The Nose

The nose is subject to increased rates of injury because of its prominent location on the human face. Your nose is a filter, humidifier, and heater for the air that enters the body. Allergens, particles, and chemicals can cause inflammation, infection, and injury. Because the sinus cavities are in the forehead and face, and drain to the back of the throat, complications from nasal disorders are common. Sinus headaches from pressure, scratchy throat from drainage, and respiratory infection from the aspiration of draining, infected material all lead to other manifestations and systemic infections. You may encounter a myriad of symptoms that may have begun as a nasal infection.

The inside of the nose is extremely vascular. Although this can cause it to bleed, this also makes intranasal medication administration an excellent route for some medicines. It is also a common route for drug abuse such as cocaine. The nasal mucosa is also a short route to the brain. The blood-brain barrier can be bypassed through the nasal mucosa by entering the spinal fluid. This makes the intranasal route faster than intravenous administration with some medicines.

As any person knows, another main function of the nose is the ability to smell. Loss of smelling sensation has many different causes, including aging, smoking, allergies, rhinitis, polyps, the flu, medications, and traumatic brain injury (damage to cranial nerve 1 [the olfactory nerve]). Different types of smelling disorders include anosmia (total loss of sense of smell), dysosmia (distorted sense of smell in which the person perceives unpleasant odors when the odors do not exist), hyperosmia (increased sensitivity to smell), hyposmia (decreased sense of smell), and presbyosmia (loss of smell from normal aging). Loss of smell also affects a person's sense of taste.

■ Anatomy and Physiology of the Nose

The nose is one of the two primary entry points for oxygen-rich air to enter the body. The **nasal septum**—the separation between the nostrils—is located in the midline Figure 17. Often, it bulges slightly to one side or the other. The external portion of the nose is formed mostly of cartilage.

Within each nasal chamber are layers of bone called the **turbinates**, which are covered with a moist lining. Both chambers have a superior turbinate, a middle turbinate, and an inferior turbinate. As a person breathes, air moves through the nasal chambers and is humidified as it passes over the turbinates. Directly above the nose are the frontal sinuses and, on either side, the orbit of the eye.

Several bones associated with the nose contain cavities known as the **paranasal sinuses** Figure 18. These hollowed sections of bone, which are lined with mucous membranes, decrease the weight of the skull and provide resonance for the voice. The contents of the sinuses drain into the nasal cavity.

■ Patient Assessment

An ambulance summoned for a complaint of the nose could have several etiologies. The condition of the residence as you approach can give clues to exposure. A factory spewing toxins, the scent of cleaning agents in the hallway, or other unpleasant odors can alert the paramedic to possible dangers to the crew. Until the seriousness of the problem is known, standard precautions are key to limiting the spread of respiratory infections.

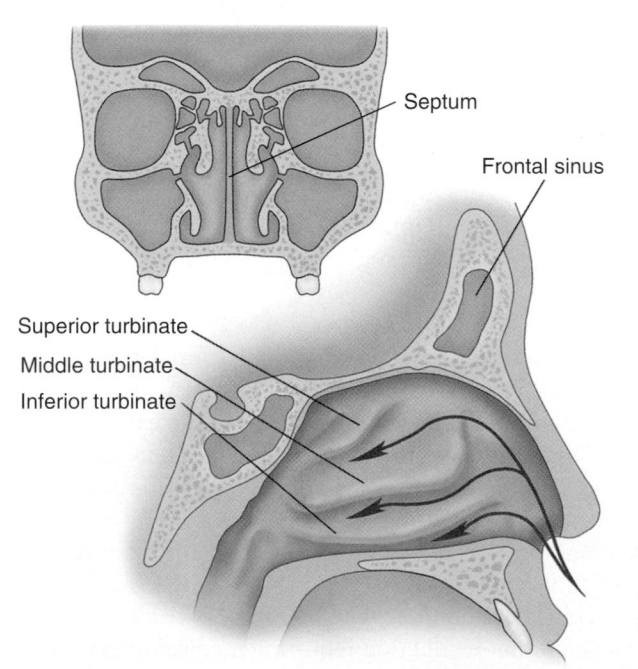

Septum

Frontal sinus

Superior turbinate

Middle turbinate

Inferior turbinate

Figure 17 The nose has two chambers, divided by the septum. Each chamber is composed of layers of bone called turbinates. Above the nose are the frontal sinuses and, on either side, the orbit of the eye.

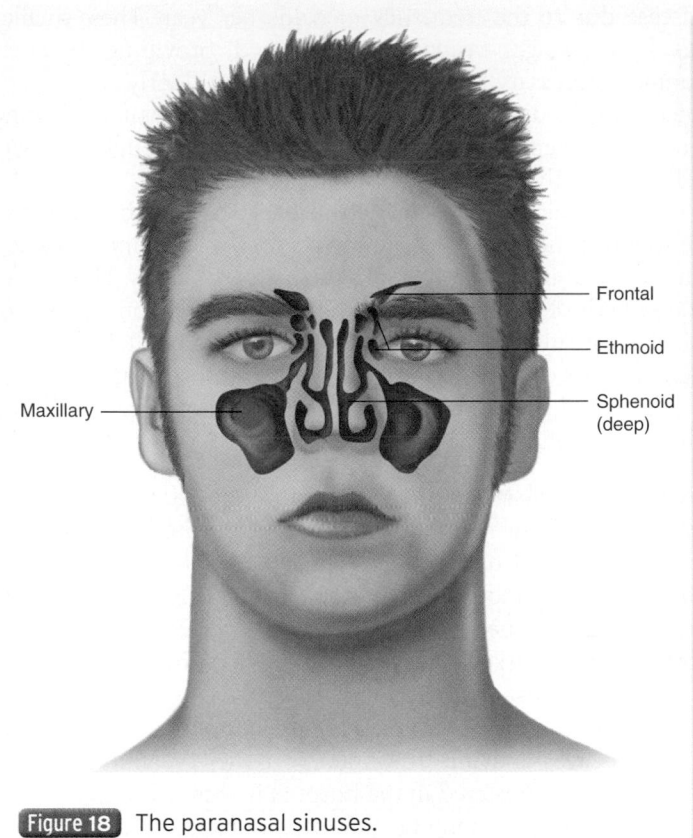

Figure 18 The paranasal sinuses.

Frontal

Ethmoid

Sphenoid (deep)

Maxillary

When the scene is determined to be safe for the crew to respond, the first impression of the patient can tell you if airway and breathing are sufficient, and you can note the amount of distress your patient is experiencing. Environmental clues, as well as your own nose, can identify possible irritants. Remember, a sneezing, sniffling, coughing patient easily spreads airborne germs in water droplets.

The vascular nature of the nasal cavities make them susceptible to bleeding. A severe nosebleed or condition that blocks the airway with swelling or blood is a life-threatening condition. You must be able to determine whether the patient has a general medical condition or if the condition is or could become life threatening.

Insert an airway adjunct as needed to maintain airway patency. However, *do not insert a nasopharyngeal airway or attempt nasotracheal intubation in any patient with suspected nasal fractures or in patients with CSF or blood leakage from the nose.* After establishing and maintaining a patent airway, assess the patient's breathing and intervene appropriately.

Inquire about a previous history of nose conditions or bleeding that needed to be packed and quartered in the emergency department. Always consider hypertensive crisis when an elderly person has a nosebleed.

■ Pathophysiology, Assessment, and Management of Specific Conditions

Epistaxis

Epistaxis, or nosebleed, is a common problem that can occur spontaneously or from trauma. One of the most common causes

Words of Wisdom

Blood or CSF drainage from the nose (cerebrospinal rhinorrhea) suggests a skull fracture. *Do not make any attempt to control this bleeding*; doing so may increase intracranial pressure (ICP) if the patient has a concomitant brain injury. Furthermore, the insertion of nasal airway adjuncts and nasotracheal intubation should be avoided in patients with suspected nasal fractures, especially if rhinorrhea is present. A nasally inserted airway device could enter the cranial vault through an occult fracture (such as a cribriform plate fracture) and penetrate the brain, further worsening the situation.

of nosebleeds is digital trauma (picking the nose with a finger); other causes include dryness and hypertension. Nosebleeds are further classified into anterior and posterior epistaxis. Anterior nosebleeds usually originate from the area of the septum and bleed fairly slowly. These are usually self-limiting and resolve quickly. Posterior nosebleeds are usually more severe and often cause blood to drain into the patient's throat, causing nausea and vomiting.

Assessment and Management For a nontrauma patient who is bleeding from the nose, you should place the patient in a sitting position, leaning forward, and pinch his or her nostrils together **Figure 19** . Direct the patient not to sniffle or blow his or her nose. For a detailed discussion of the care for epistaxis in the context of trauma, see the chapter, *Bleeding.*

Foreign Body

Foreign bodies in the nose are most likely to be seen in the pediatric population and are commonly solid objects, such as beads, stones, marbles, or small pieces of food. Children age 2 to 5 years have the greatest incidence of exploring their nasal cavities with foreign objects. At age 9 months, a child's grip is sufficient to grasp an object and direct it up one or both nares. Food, toys,

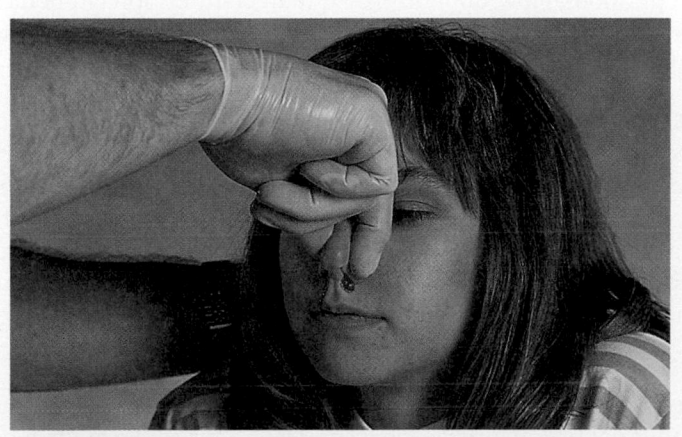

Figure 19 Control bleeding from the nose by pinching the nostrils together.

rocks, and beads may become lodged or travel to the mouth through the nasal pharyngeal cavity. Those objects that make it to the mouth become a risk for inhalation or may become lodged in the esophagus if swallowed. Objects lodged in place can cause other complications. Pressure in the delicate nasal passage can cause tissue necrosis, inflammation, and swelling. The inflammatory process can cause tissue ulceration and epistaxis. Nasal blockage can lead to sinusitis. Rhinotillexomania (nose picking) in adults is a cause of nasal infections and the introduction of irritants to the nasal mucosa. (There is even limited evidence that spontaneous epistaxis from nose picking has led to motor vehicular crashes!)

Assessment and Management In all patients, the paramedic must determine if the foreign body presents a life-threatening condition. Nasal foreign bodies are usually visible in the anterior nares, but some may be far enough into the nares as to not be seen on visual examination. If you do see the object, you may only see one end of the object; the other end may be lodged in place. Any persistent, foul-smelling, purulent discharge from the nares should lead to suspicion of a foreign body. If you note a discharge from the nose, let it drain, treat it as potentially infective material, and transport the patient. Remember to always use standard precautions.

Any lodged object should be removed in the hospital after radiography. Transport the patient in the position of comfort with an emphasis on limiting the ability of gravity to introduce the object further into the cavity. Preventing aspiration is a priority. Where the object is an extreme irritant, pain management may be necessary. Sedation may be necessary in rare cases. Consultation with medical control is advised.

Rhinitis

Rhinitis is a nasal disorder that is most common during childhood and adolescence. There are many causes of this common complaint. It is generally caused by allergens (pollen, dust, house mites, animal dander). Once inhaled, the body's store of immunoglobulin E (IgE) binds to the allergens, which then produce chemicals that can cause inflammation. Rhinitis can also be caused by viruses, certain medications (high blood pressure medications), low humidity, cold temperatures, foreign bodies, irritants in the air (smoke, chemicals), the "common cold" (nasal infection), and hormonal changes in pregnancy.

Assessment and Management Signs and symptoms of rhinitis include nasal congestion, sneezing, itchy runny nose, itchy eyes, postnasal drip (which may feel like a tickle in the throat), and possibly cough. Because there is little you can perform in the way of treatment, keep the patient in a Fowler position and provide transport. Physician-directed treatment is aimed at treating the cause of the rhinitis.

Sinusitis

People with sinusitis experience thick nasal discharge, sinus and facial pressure, headache, and fever. This is one of the most common conditions in the United States, affecting 31 million people per year. Young children are more susceptible to the disease due to the frequency of colds per year. Their smaller nasal air passages easily become clogged, providing the environment necessary for bacterial growth. The elderly also experience sinusitis due to their dry nasal passages. Their weakening immune system, coupled with a diminished cough and gag reflex, make them prone to respiratory infections.

The nasal passages are rich in bacteria, but the paranasal sinuses have no bacteria. Infection occurs to cause sinusitis when an obstruction or growth blocks the paranasal sinus. This allows the growth of bacteria and, ultimately, an infection. Causes of blockage include nasal congestion from a cold or allergy, abnormal passages or growths, and changes in atmospheric pressures. Swelling and inflammation from an infection further block the sinus passages.

Assessment and Management The duration of the symptoms determines if the condition is chronic, acute, or recurrent. Treatment is aimed at reducing inflammation and draining the sinuses. Mild to moderate symptoms lasting 7 to 10 days can be treated with a saline rinse and a decongestant. Decongestants can dry the nasal passage and delay healing if overused. Antibiotics are prescribed usually only after 7 to 10 days.

Complications occur when the infection moves beyond the nasal passages and into the brain or bone. IV antibiotics will need to be administered in the hospital in this case.

Sinusitis is the complication of a blockage. Patient history is important. Prehospital management should include treatment of any respiratory compromise and transport to an appropriate facility.

■ The Throat

Disorders of the pharynx and larynx may represent acute inflammation and infections, chronic inflammation, or abnormal growths. Specific disorders include vocal cord polyps and nodules, contact ulcers, vocal cord paralysis, laryngoceles, laryngeal papillomas, and cancer.

Throat infections (pharyngitis) are particularly common among children, although adults may be affected as well. Causes, symptoms, and treatment are similar in both except that in adults and sexually abused children, gonorrhea, a sexually transmitted disease, may affect the throat.

Throat problems can be exacerbated by swallowing problems (dysphagia). Cranial nerves VI, VII, IX, and XII all play a role in swallowing. Neurologic problems associated with stroke or trauma can cause swallowing difficulty. Facial nerve paralysis (nerve VII) can cause unilateral facial and gag reflex paralysis. Aspiration pneumonia is a life-threatening condition. Patients who survive the episode have a high risk of death from aspiration pneumonia. The geriatric population has a high incidence of pneumonia-related death. As high as 71% of these deaths are associated with aspiration. Sixty-one percent of aspirations are classified as silent and unwitnessed. Prehospital treatment of aspiration involves maintaining a patent airway. Intubation may be necessary.

Esophageal disorders can affect the throat. The valve at the end of the esophagus (lower esophageal sphincter) keeps the acidic stomach contents from coming back up the throat after swallowing. In the case of esophageal reflux, the valve only partially closes, or opens too often. The symptoms include a burning sensation in the chest and indigestion. If the stomach acids come up the throat to the vocal cords, voice tone may change from inflammation and swelling. This can cause a precancerous condition from tissue scarring in the esophagus.

Anatomy and Physiology of the Throat

The normal adult mouth contains 32 permanent teeth. The primary or deciduous teeth are lost during childhood. Adult teeth are distributed about the maxillary and mandibular arches. The teeth on each side of the arch are mirror images of each other and form four quadrants: right upper, left upper, right lower, and left lower. Each quadrant contains one central incisor, one lateral incisor, one canine, two premolars, and three molars Figure 20A. The third molars, or what are called wisdom teeth, do not appear until late adolescence.

The top portion of the tooth, external to the gum, is the **crown**, containing one or more **cusps**. Below the crown lie the neck and the root. The pulp cavity fills the center of the tooth and contains blood vessels, nerves, and specialized connective tissue, called **pulp**. Dentin and enamel surround the pulp cavity and protect the tooth from damage. **Dentin**, which forms the principal mass of the tooth, is much denser and stronger than bone. The bony sockets for the teeth that reside in the mandible and maxilla are called **alveoli**. The ridges between the teeth, the **alveolar ridges**, are covered by the gingiva, or gums, which are thickened connective tissue and epithelium. Teeth are attached to the alveolar bone by a periodontal membrane Figure 20B.

The Mouth

Digestion begins in the mouth with **mastication**, or the chewing of food by the teeth. During mastication, food is mixed with secretions from the salivary glands.

The tongue, a muscular process in the floor of the mouth, is the primary organ of taste; it is also important in the formation of speech and in chewing and swallowing of food. The tongue is attached at the mandible and hyoid bone, is covered by a mucous membrane, and extends from the back of the mouth upward and forward to the lips Figure 21.

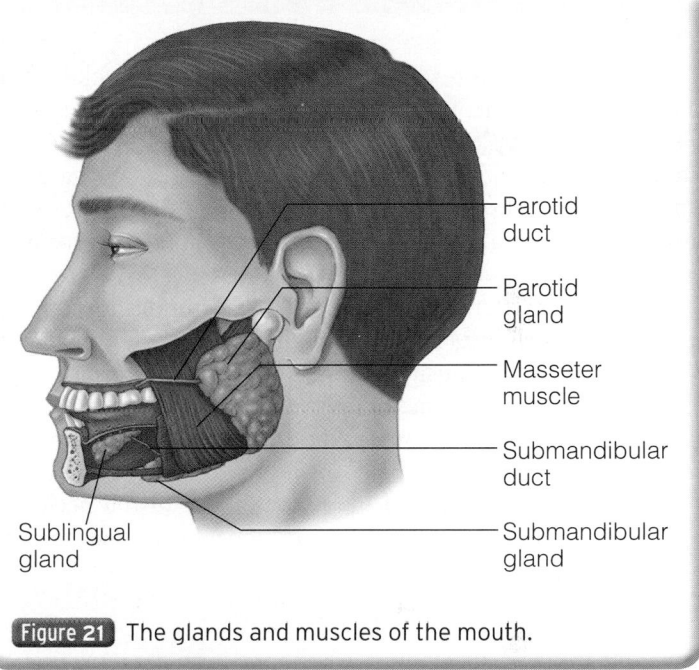

Figure 21   The glands and muscles of the mouth.

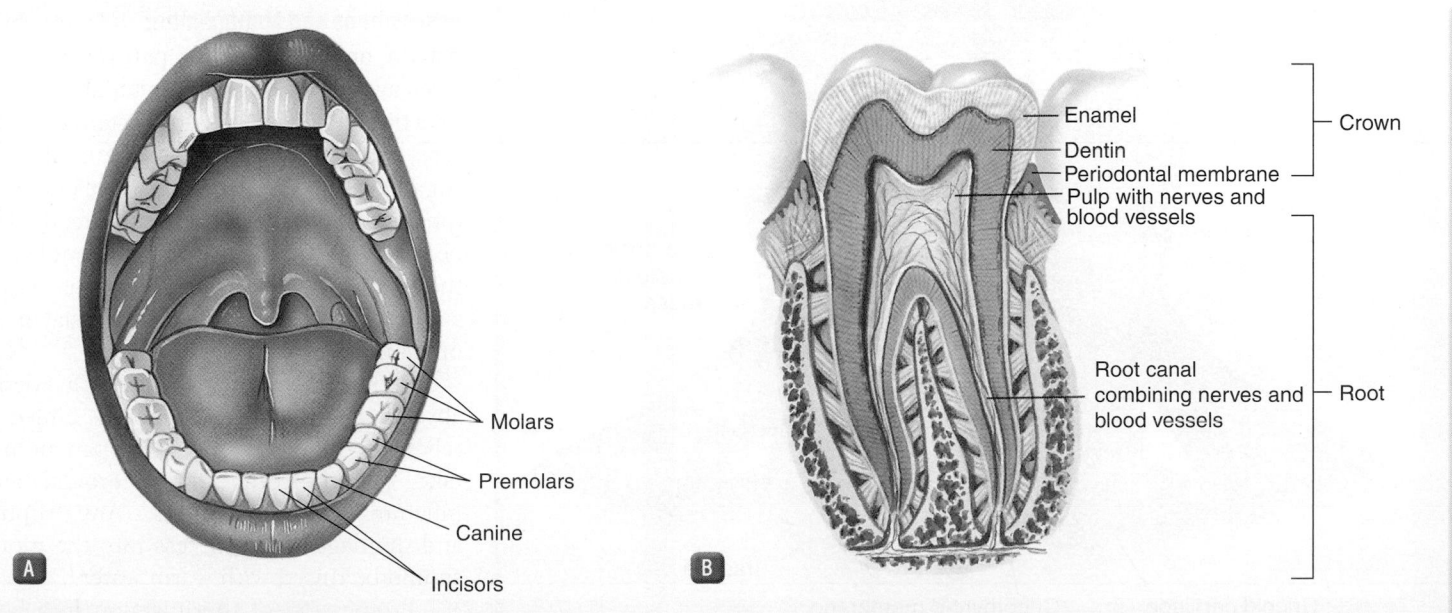

Figure 20   The teeth of the adult mouth. **A.** The incisors are used for biting. Canines are used for tearing food. The premolars and molars are used for grinding and crushing. **B.** Each tooth contains nerves and blood vessels.

The hypoglossal, glossopharyngeal, trigeminal, and facial nerves supply the mouth and its structures. The **hypoglossal nerve** (cranial nerve XII) provides motor function to the muscles of the tongue. The **glossopharyngeal nerve** (cranial nerve IX) provides taste sensation to the posterior portions of the tongue and carries parasympathetic fibers to the salivary glands on each side of the face. The mandibular branch of the **trigeminal nerve** (cranial nerve V) provides motor innervation to the muscles of mastication. The facial nerve (cranial nerve VII), in addition to supplying motor activity to all muscles of facial expression, provides the sense of taste to the anterior two thirds of the tongue and cutaneous sensations to the tongue and palate.

The Neck

The principal structures of the anterior part of the neck include the thyroid and cricoid cartilage, trachea, and numerous muscles and nerves `Figure 22`. The major blood vessels in this area are the internal and external carotid arteries `Figure 23` and the internal and external jugular veins `Figure 24`. The vertebral arteries run laterally to the cervical vertebrae in the posterior part of the neck.

The major arteries of the neck—the carotid and vertebral arteries—supply oxygenated blood directly to the brain. Therefore, in addition to causing massive bleeding and hemorrhagic shock, injury to any of these major vessels can produce cerebral hypoxia, infarct, air embolism, and/or permanent neurologic impairment.

Other key structures of the anterior part of the neck that may sustain injury from blunt or penetrating mechanisms include the vagus nerves, thoracic duct, esophagus, thyroid and parathyroid glands, lower cranial nerves, brachial plexus (which is responsible for function of the lower arm and hand), soft tissue and fascia, and various muscles.

■ Patient Assessment

Patients with swallowing abnormalities or copious mucous production should be placed in a position to allow drainage. A lateral recumbent position or recovery position will allow mouth drainage and help protect the airway. Stroke patients may not be able to swallow as a result of neurologic deficit. Assessing these patients must include early recognition of threats to their airway and prompt action to alleviate the risks. Abscesses can develop rapidly and block the airway. Medical problems of the mouth, neck, and throat can have serious consequences to breathing. Assessments should consider epiglottitis if there are symptoms of sore throat, drooling, and a head that is hung forward.

■ Pathophysiology, Assessment, and Management of Specific Conditions

Dentalgia and Dental Abscess

Dentalgia or "toothache" can be the starting point for the development of a dental abscess. A cavity in a tooth harbors bacteria, resulting in rapid decay of the tooth. Eventually the integrity of the tooth is compromised, giving access to the tooth root and nerve. This can cause inflammation, swelling, and intense pain.

A **dental abscess** occurs when the bacteria growth spreads directly from the cavity into the gums, facial tissue, bones, and/or neck `Figure 25`. Pain is relieved somewhat when the abscess ruptures and drains pus, thus reducing the swelling. An abscess may have to be drained surgically.

Assessment and Management If fever, chills, nausea, and vomiting are part of the symptoms accompanying the dental abscess, the infection may have become systemic. In this case, a physician will prescribe antibiotics. An abscess in the throat, neck, or under the tongue can affect the ability to breath. This becomes a true emergency. Depending on the location of the abscess, it may have to be surgically drained under anesthesia in the operating room.

Prehospital treatment of a dental abscess or dentalgia it mostly aimed at relieving the symptoms. The patient may take over-the-counter nonsteroidal anti-inflammatory medications. Any rupture and drainage of an abscess into the mouth should be rinsed with warm water.

Progression of the infection into bone and surrounding tissue can have serious complications. You should encourage transport to an appropriate facility.

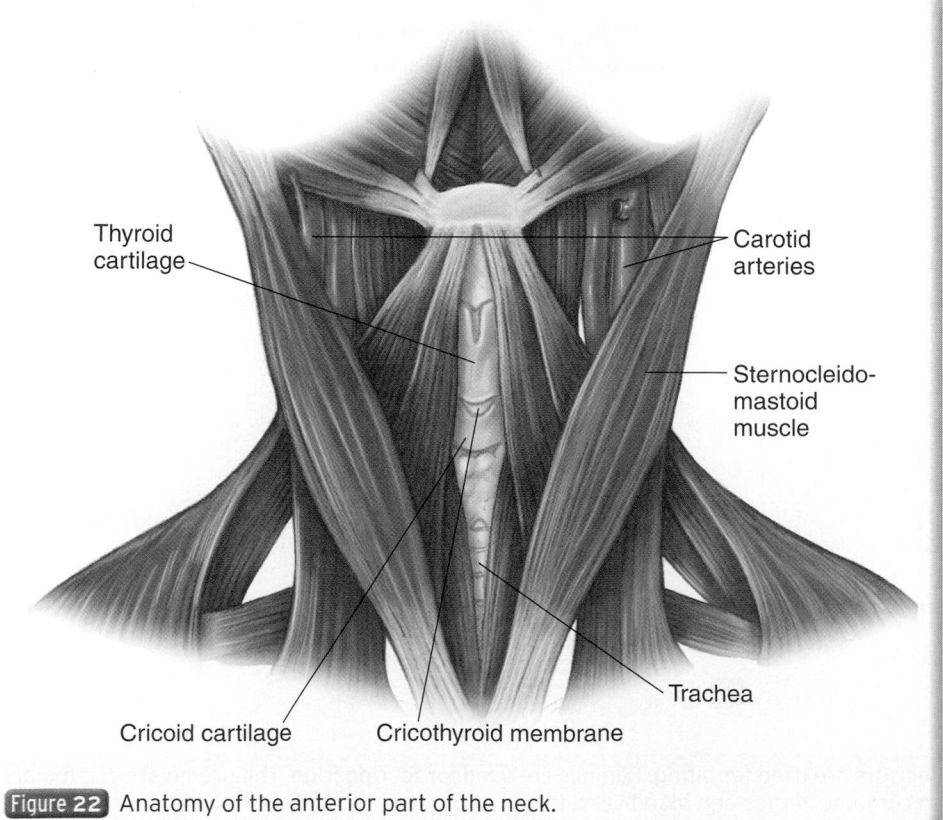

Figure 22 Anatomy of the anterior part of the neck.

- Thyroid cartilage
- Carotid arteries
- Sternocleidomastoid muscle
- Trachea
- Cricoid cartilage
- Cricothyroid membrane

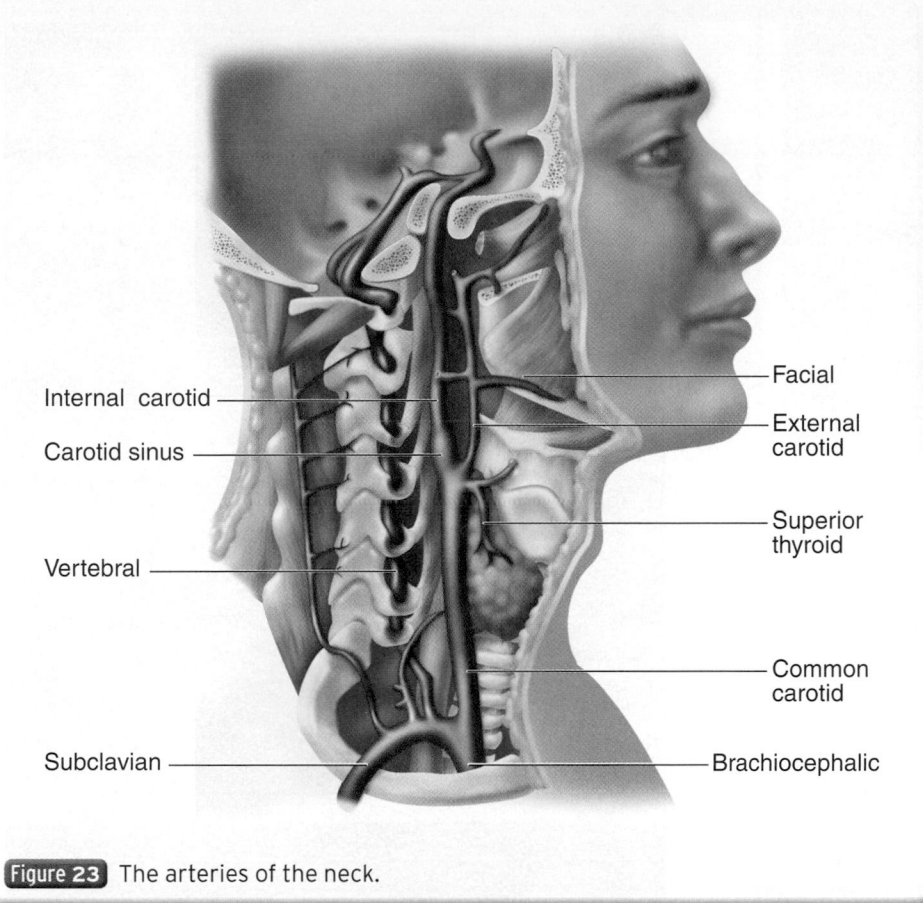

Internal carotid
Carotid sinus
Vertebral
Subclavian

Facial
External carotid
Superior thyroid
Common carotid
Brachiocephalic

Figure 23 The arteries of the neck.

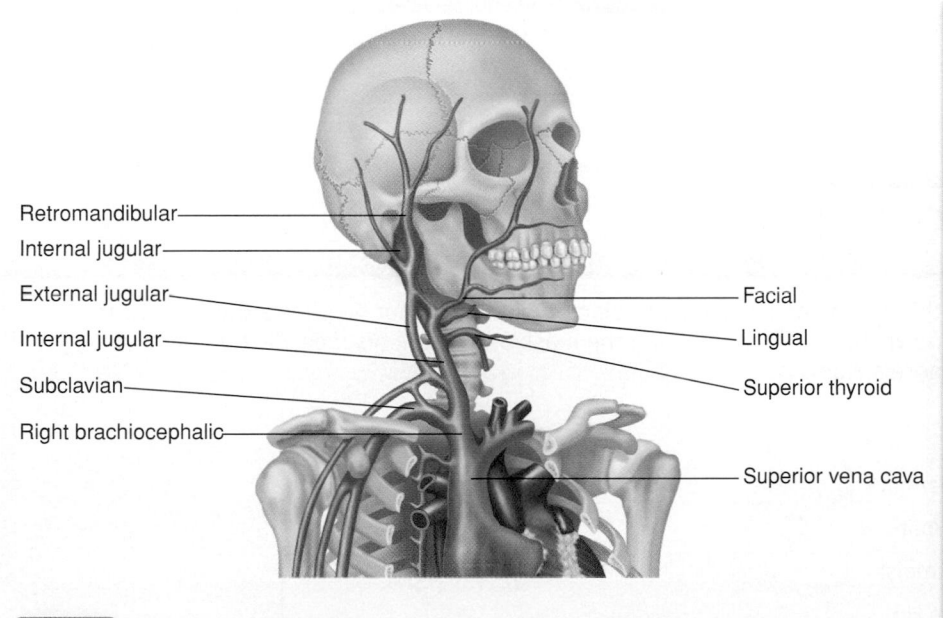

Retromandibular
Internal jugular
External jugular
Internal jugular
Subclavian
Right brachiocephalic

Facial
Lingual
Superior thyroid
Superior vena cava

Figure 24 The veins of the neck.

Diseases of Oral Soft Tissue

Diseases of the soft tissue of the mouth can be the root cause to other health problems. Gum disease has been linked to heart disease, stroke, diabetes, osteoporosis, and low birth weight babies. Infective endocarditis, which affects the lining of the heart and heart valves, can be linked directly to tooth infection and gum disease. Ninety percent of the diseases affecting the human body may have oral manifestations. A good dental examination may find these potential diseases in the early stages. Diabetes, leukemia, cancer, heart disease, and kidney disease may manifest with mouth ulcers, swollen gums, and dry mouth. The condition of the mouth reflects the condition of the human body. Poor oral health also affects the digestive system and may be a cause of irritable bowel syndrome.

Some common mouth disorders include the following:

- Cold sores: painful sores on the lips and around the mouth caused by a type of herpes virus
- Canker sores: Painful sores in the mouth or on the gums caused by bacteria or virus
- Thrush: A yeast infection that causes white patches in the mouth or on the tongue (this is discussed further in the chapter, *Infectious Diseases*)
- Leukoplakia: A smoker's disease that causes excess cell growth in the mouth, cheek, or gums and presents as white patches
- Gingivitis: Red swollen gums that bleed easily during brushing
- Bad breath: Usually linked to impacted plaque and poor oral hygiene. Bacteria release sulfur compounds that account for the foul smell. Fruity breath odor can be linked to diabetes and high blood glucose levels. Breath that smells like feces can be caused by a bowel obstruction. Breath odor that smells of urine or that smells "fishy" may be caused by chronic renal failure.

Assessment and Management Sores and diseases of the mouth can be embarrassing to the patient. The patient may not want to tell you about them. Be sure to rule out urticaria and allergic reactions when you are assessing lumps and sores of the mouth.

Oral Candidiasis

More commonly called "thrush," <u>oral candidiasis</u> is a condition in which the fungus *Candida albicans* accumulates on the lining of the mouth. When a patient has oral thrush, he or she will have creamy white lesions on the tongue and inner cheeks **Figure 26** . These lesions may be painful and bleed as they are scraped, causing their spread to the roof of the mouth, gums, posterior pharynx, and the tonsils.

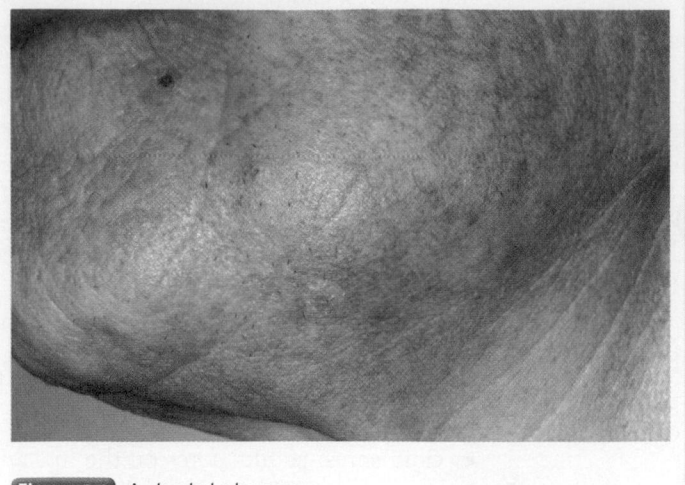

Figure 25 A dental abscess.

Assessment and Management Thrush is most likely to be found in babies, patients with compromised immune systems, patients who wear dentures, and patients who use inhaled corticosteroids (eg, prednisone). In addition to the white lesions and slight bleeding, signs and symptoms of thrush include pain, cracking and redness at the corners of the mouth, and a loss of taste. Patients often describe a "cottony" feeling in the mouth. In severe cases, the lesions can spread down the esophagus, causing the sensation that food is getting stuck in the throat when swallowing. Patients with a medical history of HIV/AIDS, cancer, diabetes, and vaginal yeast infections are more prone to develop thrush.

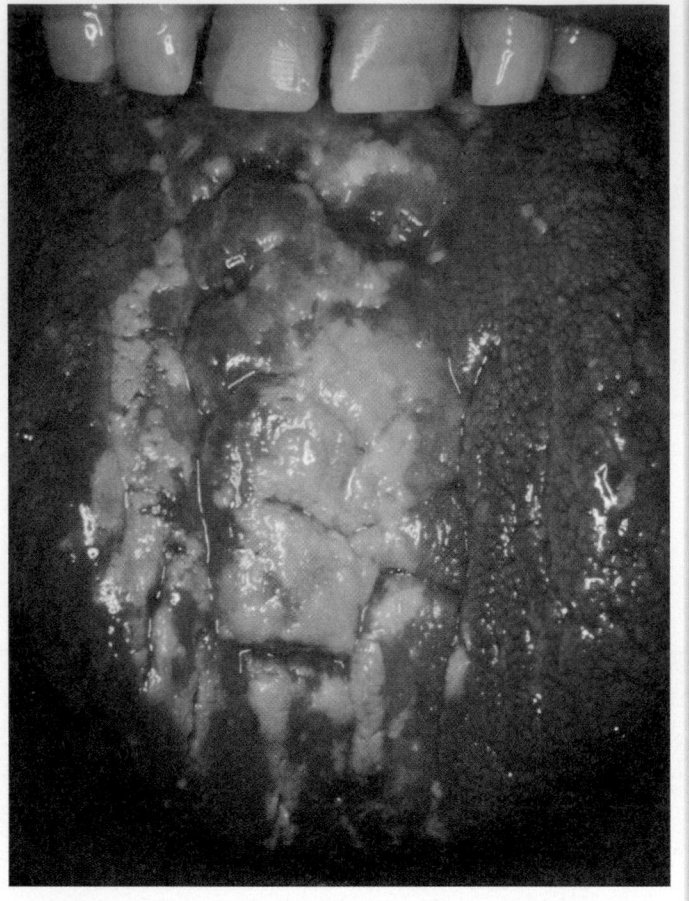

Figure 26 Oral candidiasis.

YOU *are the Medic* | PART 4

Your partner prepares a pediatric nonrebreathing mask and attempts to place it on Jimmy, but he pulls away and starts coughing violently. You attempt to calm him down, but he keeps shoving the mask away from his face. Each time he struggles, his ability to breathe worsens and you hear more stridor.

Recording Time: 8 Minutes	
Respirations	22 breaths/min
Pulse	120 beats/min
Skin	Hot, pale, moist
Blood pressure	110/86 mm Hg
Oxygen saturation (Spo$_2$)	97% room air
Pupils	Equal and reactive

7. It is obvious that Jimmy needs additional oxygen. How are you going to get him to tolerate it?

8. Should you inspect the airway and attempt intubation?

This is not a condition that requires paramedic care aside from treating higher priorities, making the patient comfortable, and encouraging him or her to follow up with a physician. You are likely to come across patients with thrush when treating or transporting immune deficient patients under physician care for the conditions already mentioned. Always use standard precautions when managing a patient with thrush.

Ludwig Angina

Ludwig angina is a type of cellulitis caused by bacteria from an infected tooth root (tooth abscess) or mouth injury. It occurs on the floor of the mouth under the tongue. Because of swelling, which may be rapid, there can be an airway obstruction. A physical exam may show redness and swelling of the neck or under the chin. The tongue may also be swollen. In severe cases, this is a potential life threat. You may have to provide an airway through the nasal passages to avoid the affected and swollen tissue. A tracheostomy may have to be surgically performed to adequately ventilate these patients. The abscess may also have to be surgically drained.

Assessment and Management Symptoms may include difficulty breathing, difficulty swallowing, neck pain, neck swelling, fever, drooling, and altered speech sounds. Prehospital treatment requires aggressive management of the patient's airway in severe cases. Early treatment with steroids may slow the inflammatory process and reduce swelling. Early contact with a medical control physician is important to determine your management options. Treatment may include dental surgery to repair the source of the infection at the tooth root.

Ludwig angina is painful and frightening for the patient because symptoms may develop rapidly. You should remain calm and organized as you attend to the basic ABCs while formulating a plan for aggressive airway management. Pay careful attention to the condition and smells originating in the mouth to alert you to other disease processes that may be in progress.

Foreign Body in the Throat

Assessment and Management Foreign bodies lodged in the mouth should alert the paramedic to the potential for airway obstruction and aspiration. It is paramount to keep the patient calm and in a position where if the object becomes dislodged, gravity will allow it to fall out.

Patients often panic from objects lodged in the throat, thinking they cannot breathe. As the patient speaks to you, comfort him or her by explaining; "By the sound of your voice, I can tell your airway is open. The object lodged in your throat may be very uncomfortable, but you seem to be breathing fine." Transport the patient in a position of comfort.

Epiglottitis

Epiglottitis is an inflammation of the epiglottis (the flap at the base of the tongue that covers the trachea). As the epiglottis swells, it blocks the trachea and obstructs the airway. Epiglottitis used to most commonly occur in pediatric patients (ages 1 to 5 years), but is now occurring more often in adults who did not receive inoculation for this disease. Often a result of the

H influenzae type b virus, incidence has decreased over time due to the Hib vaccine.

Assessment and Management Patients with epiglottitis experience fever, sore throat, painful swallowing (dysphagia), stridor, and respiratory distress. A patient with epiglottitis looks sick and will be anxious, will sit upright in the classic "tripod" position or in the sniffing position with the chin thrust forward to allow for maximal air entry, and is often drooling because of an inability to swallow secretions. Work of breathing is increased, and pallor or cyanosis may be evident.

Transport a patient with suspected epiglottitis to an appropriate hospital while maintaining the patient's airway. Because rapidly progressive disease carries a risk for acute airway obstruction and respiratory arrest, you should minimize your scene time and not attempt procedures that might agitate the patient. Remember not to attempt to look in the mouth because this can precipitate complete airway obstruction. Alert personnel at the receiving facility to the suspected diagnosis and patient's condition because they will need to mobilize a team for the management of this difficult airway.

Laryngitis

Swelling and inflammation of the larynx is associated with hoarseness or loss of voice. It can be the result of overuse, where the vocal cords and larynx are inflamed, causing hoarseness. The most common form of laryngitis is caused by a virus, similar to the cold or flu. It can also be caused by pneumonia, irritants and chemicals, GERD, bronchitis, allergies, and bacterial infection. Typically laryngitis is not serious unless it leads to croup or epiglottitis, which can be serious and are covered in the chapter, Respiratory Emergencies.

Assessment and Management The symptoms the patient will present with are fever, hoarseness, and swollen lymph nodes or glands in the neck. Obtain a good history to rule out evolving upper airway obstruction or an allergic reaction. If the patient speaks in a quiet tone and has a raspy voice, he or she may have sustained a hyoid bone fracture from a blow to the anterior neck. Otherwise, typically laryngitis is a symptom of an ongoing upper respiratory infection and the patient should follow up with a physician.

Tracheitis

Tracheitis is a bacterial infection of the trachea. It is caused by the bacterium Staphylococcus aureus. Tracheitis frequently occurs in young children following a recent viral upper respiratory infection. In small children the trachea is easily blocked by swelling, so this can be a life-threatening condition.

Assessment and Management The symptoms of tracheitis include a deep "croup-like" cough, difficulty breathing, high fever, and high-pitched stridor with breathing. As the illness progresses, the child may exhibit tripod positioning and intercostal retractions, and can proceed from respiratory distress to failure if not managed quickly.

Prehospital care is supportive, minimizing stress to the child and administering 100% oxygen. Use pulse oximetry and monitor vital signs en route. Be prepared for a difficult intubation and have the correct size ET tube as well as the next smaller size available based on your length-based tape measurement of the child (Broselow). Transport the child as soon as possible to a facility capable of handling critically ill children.

In the critical care setting, many of these children will be managed with ET tube placement and administration of IV antibiotics.

Tonsillitis

Tonsillitis is swelling and inflammation of the tonsils, which are the two oval-shaped pads of tissue at the back of the throat Figure 27 . Most cases of tonsillitis are caused by viral infections, although tonsillitis has been known to be caused by bacteria. As the tonsils become inflamed, they swell and cause difficulty swallowing.

Assessment and Management The symptoms of tonsillitis include swollen tonsils, a sore throat, and difficulty swallowing. The patient will have red, swollen tonsils, white or yellow coating or patches on the tonsils, a fever, and a sore throat. Patients may also present with pain when swallowing, enlarged and tender lymph nodes in the neck, bad breath, headache, and a stiff neck. In severe cases, drooling indicates difficulty swallowing. Surgery used to be common but today is usually only done with patients who have frequent bouts of tonsillitis that do not respond to drugs. Serious cases causing partial airway obstruction are also an indication for surgery. You should transport all patients with suspected tonsillitis to the emergency department for further evaluation.

Pharyngitis

Pharyngitis is an inflammation of the pharynx, which is the back of the throat between the tonsils and the larynx Figure 28 . Pharyngitis is often due to a rapid onset of sore throat with discomfort or pain on swallowing.

Assessment and Management Symptoms of pharyngitis also include a fever, pharyngeal erythema, headache, purulent patchy yellow, gray, or white exudate, nasal congestion, hoarseness, cough, and ulcers on the soft palate.

The treatment involves follow-up in the emergency department so the patient can be examined, with cultures obtained to assess for strep, and a decision will be made as to the usefulness of antibiotics. Your major prehospital concern is assessment for partial airway obstruction in severe cases with difficulty swallowing.

Peritonsillar Abscess

Peritonsillar abscess is a collection of infected material around the tonsils Figure 29 . It is a complication of tonsillitis most often cause by bacterial infection. Usually a condition found in older children through young adults, it has become rare due to antibiotics being used to treat tonsillitis.

Assessment and Management With peritonsillar abscess, one or both tonsils are infected. The roof of the mouth and neck or chest may also be infected. The patient may have chills, difficulty opening the mouth, and pain with opening the mouth. He or she may have facial swelling, fever, drooling or inability

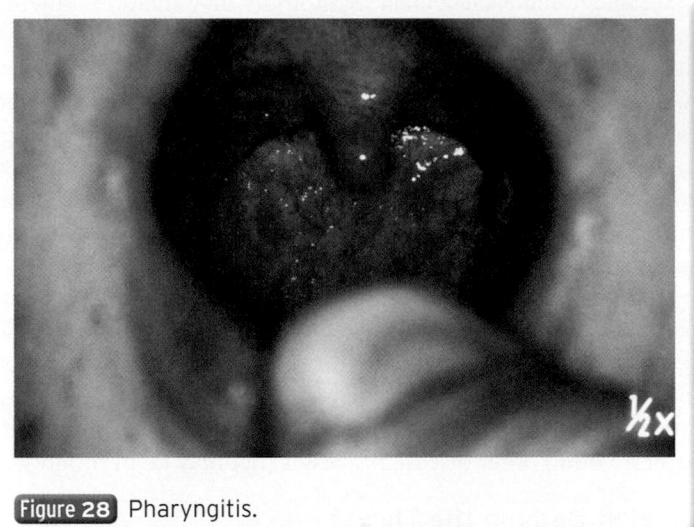

Figure 28 Pharyngitis.

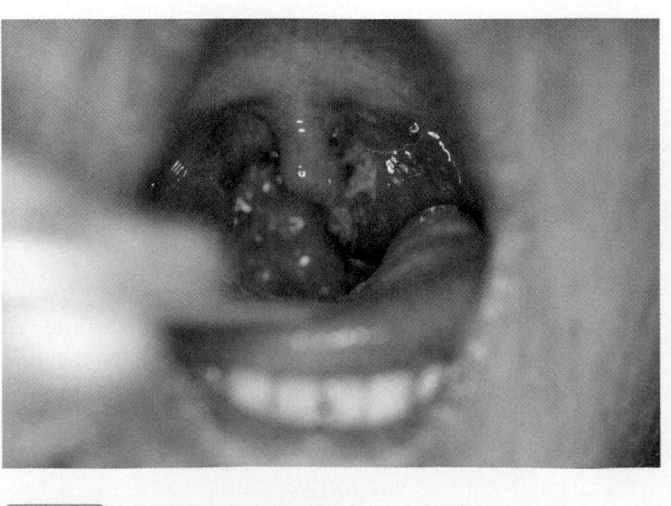

Figure 27 Tonsillitis.

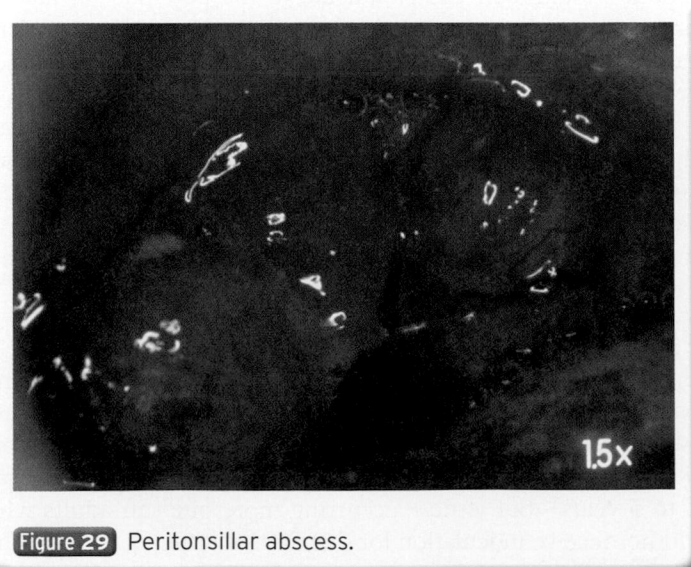

Figure 29 Peritonsillar abscess.

to swallow saliva, headache, muffled voice, sore throat (usually on one side), and tender glands of the jaw and throat. Treatment involves antibiotics and draining the abscess, and may include a tonsillectomy, so it is important to take these patients to the hospital. In some cases the condition could be life threatening if the swollen tissues block the airway.

Temporomandibular Joint Disorders
The mandible is the large bone forming the lower jaw and containing the lower teeth. Numerous muscles of chewing attach to the mandible and its rami. The posterior condyle of the mandible articulates with the temporal bone at the temporomandibular joint (TMJ), allowing movement of the mandible **Figure 30**. The TMJ allows a person to talk, chew, and yawn. When patients report jaw pain, clicking when they "jut" their jaw, or headaches, they often have been diagnosed, or may soon be, with a <u>temporomandibular joint disorder</u>.

Causes of TMJ include arthritis damage to the joint's cartilage, jaw injury, and jaw muscle fatigue from grinding or clenching of the teeth, especially during sleep. The disk can erode or move out of its proper alignment, leading to TMJ disorder.

Assessment and Management The symptoms of TMJ include headache, jaw pain, aching around the ear, an uneven bite and/or painful bite, difficulty chewing, and locking of the joint causing difficulty either opening or closing the mouth. The symptoms are usually managed by over-the-counter pain medications.

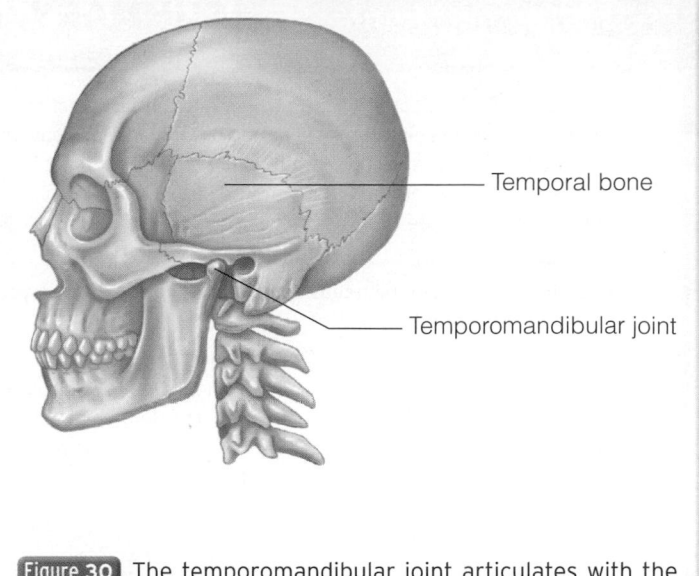

— Temporal bone

— Temporomandibular joint

Figure 30 The temporomandibular joint articulates with the temporal bone.

In severe cases, TMJ disorders may require dental or surgical intervention. As a paramedic you should be aware of TMJ, the symptoms it causes, and the fact that it is usually managed by the patient's physician or dentist.

YOU are the Medic   SUMMARY

1. What is your primary concern after scene safety is established?

The child appears to be very ill. His positioning and mouth breathing indicate you should have concern for the patency of the child's airway.

2. Do you have concerns that the patient's parents have not been contacted?

You should have concern about caring for this patient above all else. Most schools have signed agreements with parents that state that treatment can be rendered in case of emergency. The administrator would have access to these documents. In the event the school does not provide this documentation and the patient's condition warrants, provide treatment and transport as state law allows. Contact medical control if in doubt.

3. What do you need to know about the patient's cough?

Because you are getting the information about the patient's cough third-hand, you should continue a thorough assessment of the patient. Visual clues should tell you something significant is happening with the airway. The patient is sitting upright, leaning forward, and drooling.

4. What steps will you take in your further assessment of this patient?

In this patient, lung sounds and listening to the patient's upper airways will provide you with information on the status of the patient's respiratory system. You may hear significant stridor, wheezing, or a combination of sounds that will direct your further treatment.

5. What do you suspect is wrong with the patient?

The child has classic signs of epiglottitis. He is sitting upright, leaning forward (tripod position), drooling, has a high fever, and has been ill. He looks very sick. Epiglottitis is an inflammation of the epiglottis (the flap at the base of the tongue that covers the trachea). As the epiglottis swells, it blocks the trachea and obstructs the airway. Epiglottitis can occur in pediatric patients (ages 1 to 5 years) who have not been vaccinated.

6. Do you have any additional concerns because this child appears drowsy but is working hard to breathe?

Any patient who appears drowsy in combination with signs and symptoms of a significant respiratory problem should be a

YOU are the Medic   SUMMARY, continued

great concern. This patient has been working hard to breathe through a swollen epiglottis for a period of time and his body is starting to tire. This could be an indication of hypoxia, muscle fatigue, or a combination. Either way, the patient is losing his ability to compensate.

7. It is obvious that Jimmy needs additional oxygen. How are you going to get him to tolerate it?

It is essential that patients with suspected epiglottitis are handled in a calm, caring manner. Upsetting the child and causing him to work harder to breathe will further irritate the epiglottis. This could cause additional swelling, which could completely occlude the child's airway. Many manufacturers make airway adjuncts that look like toys or items that are more readily

accepted by children. In the event that you do not have anything like this on board, use connection tubing to deliver oxygen in a "blow-by" fashion. If all else fails, cut the mask off of the tubing and use the remaining tube.

8. Should you inspect the airway and attempt intubation?

Under no circumstances should you look in the patient's mouth or throat if you suspect that he or she has epiglottitis. Additionally, do not try to place an oral airway or visualize the airway using a laryngoscope. This could cause the airway to swell or spasm to the point that it is completely closed. If this should happen, obtaining an airway will be extremely difficult if not impossible without surgical intervention.

EMS Patient Care Report (PCR)

Date: 12-10-11	Incident No.: 93542	Nature of Call: Respiratory		Location: 100 School Street	
Dispatched: 1115	En Route: 1116	At Scene: 1121	Transport: 1128	At Hospital: 1135	In Service: 1153

Patient Information

Age: 5 Sex: M Weight (in kg [lb]): 20 kg (45 lb)	Allergies: Unknown Medications: Unknown Past Medical History: Unknown Chief Complaint: Difficulty breathing

Vital Signs

Time: 1124	BP: 106/82	Pulse: 120	Respirations: 20	Spo$_2$: 97% RA
Time: 1129	BP: 110/86	Pulse: 120	Respirations: 22	Spo$_2$: 97% RA
Time:	BP:	Pulse:	Respirations:	Spo$_2$:

EMS Treatment
(circle all that apply)

Oxygen @ __15__ L/min via (circle one): NC (NRM) Bag-mask device	Assisted Ventilation	Airway Adjunct	CPR
Defibrillation	Bleeding Control	Bandaging	Splinting	Other: Oxygen (blow-by)

Narrative

Arrived to find 5-yo-M in the administrative office of Parker School with administrator Ann Smith present. Pt was in classroom and teacher reported the pt was having difficulty breathing. Pt is sitting upright in a chair in tripod position. Pt has a very high-pitched cough and is actively drooling from his mouth. Pt seems unwilling to speak but nods his head when asked if he has trouble swallowing. School nurse reported pt temp as 102°F, skin is hot, pale, and moist. Pt has stridor noted in upper airways, and is using accessory muscles to breathe. Pt appears drowsy but will respond and is oriented to person, place, and day. Pt would not tolerate NRBM so switched to blow-by for O$_2$ administration to keep the patient calm. Mother contacted by Ms. Smith and she advised she would meet our crew at Parkside Hospital. No attempt made to visualize the pt's airway due to potential for epiglottitis. Report called to Parkside Hospital. Pt had no change during transport. Report given to charge nurse on arrival. **End of report**

Prep Kit

■ Ready for Review

- A patient may call EMS with an emergency related to a disorder of the eye, ear, nose, or throat (EENT), or paramedics may encounter patients with these disorders while assessing an unrelated emergency. Paramedics should be familiar with these important structures and diseases that affect them.

- Be sure to assess the eye for pain or tenderness, swelling, abnormal or loss of movement, sensation changes, circulatory changes, deformity, and visual changes. Obtain a thorough history including when the problem began, whether both eyes are affected, and a description of the symptoms.

- Early transport decision to the right facility can improve outcomes. Consider transport to a facility that has skilled services necessary to treat a serious eye problem. Consider pain management and mild sedation during transport.

- Remember to provide emotional care to patients with eye conditions. Fear and panic from loss of vision can cause dangerous and bizarre behavior, which may be alleviated if you practice good, calming communication skills.

- Flush burns to the eye with copious amounts of sterile saline or sterile water. Never use chemical antidotes when treating burn injuries to the eye.

- Specific conditions of the eye include conjunctivitis, corneal abrasion, foreign body, inflammation, glaucoma, hyphema, iritis, papilledema, retinal detachment and defect, and cellulitis of the orbit. Become familiar with these conditions so that you can recognize them in the field and transport the patient as needed.

- The ear is the primary structure for hearing and balance. Disorders of the ear can leave a person unable to communicate, react, and maintain equilibrium.

- Adequate assessment of the external ear canal and middle ear cannot be performed in the field. Treatment is to transport the patient so that he or she can be evaluated at the receiving facility.

- Specific conditions of the ear include foreign body, impacted cerumen, labyrinthitis, Meniere disease, otitis, and perforated tympanic membrane.

- The nose is a vascular structure and contains nasal mucosa that is a short route to the brain.

- Never insert a nasopharyngeal airway or attempt nasotracheal intubation in any patient with suspected nasal fractures or in patients with cerebrospinal fluid or blood leakage from the nose. It could penetrate the brain and cause further damage.

- Specific problems related to the nose include epistaxis, foreign body, rhinitis, and sinusitis.

- Disorders of the throat (pharynx and larynx) may represent acute inflammation and infections, chronic inflammation, or abnormal growths. Throat infections are particularly common among children.

- When you are assessing a patient with a throat complaint, note whether the patient is able to swallow. If not, position the patient to allow drainage. Be sure to assess for threats to the airway and breathing.

- Specific disorders include dentalgia, dental abscess, Ludwig angina, foreign body, epiglottitis, laryngitis, tracheitis, oral candidiasis, peritonsillar abscess, pharyngitis/tonsillitis, and temporomandibular joint disorders.

■ Vital Vocabulary

adnexa The surrounding structures and accessories of an organ; for the eye: the eyelids, lashes, lacrimal structures.

alveolar ridges The ridges between the teeth, which are covered with thickened connective tissue and epithelium.

alveoli In the context of facial anatomy, small pits or cavities, such as the sockets for the teeth.

anisocoria A condition in which the pupils are not of equal size.

anterior chamber The anterior area of the globe between the lens and the cornea that is filled with aqueous humor.

aqueous humor The clear, watery fluid in the anterior chamber of the globe.

auricle The large outside portion of the ear through which sound waves enter the ear; also called the pinna.

Battle sign Bruising over the mastoid bone behind the ear commonly seen following a basilar skull fracture; also called retroauricular ecchymosis.

cataract A clouding of the lens of the eye that is normally a result of aging.

central vision The visualization of objects directly in front of you.

cerebrospinal rhinorrhea Cerebrospinal fluid drainage from the nose.

cerumen Ear wax.

chalazion A small, swollen bump or pustule on the external eyelid, resulting when the eyelid's oil glands or ducts become blocked.

cochlea The shell-shaped structure within the inner ear that contains the organ of Corti.

cochlear duct A canal within the cochlea that receives vibrations from the ossicles.

conjunctiva A thin, transparent membrane that covers the sclera and internal surfaces of the eyelids.

conjunctivitis An inflammation of the conjunctivae that usually is caused by bacteria, viruses, allergies, or foreign bodies; should be considered highly contagious; also called pink eye.

cornea The transparent anterior portion of the eye that overlies the iris and pupil.

crown The part of the tooth that is external to the gum.

cusps Points at the top of a tooth.

dental abscess A collection of pus that forms in the gums, facial tissue, bones, and/or neck.

dentalgia Toothache.

dentin The principal mass of the tooth, which is made up of a material that is much more dense and stronger than bone.

diabetic retinopathy A condition associated with diabetes, in which the small blood vessels of the retina are affected; can eventually lead to blindness.

dysconjugate gaze Paralysis of gaze or lack of coordination between the movements of the two eyes.

dysphagia Pain when swallowing.

epiglottis The small flap of skin at the base of the tongue that covers the trachea and keeps food from entering the windpipe.

epistaxis Nosebleed.

external auditory canal The area in which sound waves are received from the auricle (pinna) before they travel to the eardrum; also called the ear canal.

external ear One of three anatomic parts of the ear; it contains the pinna, the ear canal, and the external portion of the tympanic membrane.

glaucoma A group of conditions that lead to increased intraocular pressure, causing damage to the optic nerve; a leading cause of blindness.

globe The eyeball.

glossopharyngeal nerve Ninth cranial nerve; supplies motor fibers to the pharyngeal muscle, providing taste sensation to the posterior portion of the tongue, and carrying parasympathetic fibers to the parotid gland.

hordeolum A red tender lump in the eyelid or at the lid margin; commonly known as a stye.

hyphema Bleeding into the anterior chamber of the eye; results from direct ocular trauma.

hypoglossal nerve Twelfth cranial nerve; provides motor function to the muscles of the tongue and throat.

inner ear One of three anatomic parts of the ear; it consists of the cochlea and semicircular canals.

iris The colored portion of the eye.

iritis Inflammation of the iris; also called anterior uveitis.

labyrinthitis Irritation and swelling in the inner ear that produces a loss of balance and possibly tinnitus, dizziness, loss of hearing, nausea, and vomiting.

lacrimal apparatus The structures in which tears are secreted and drained from the eye.

laryngitis Swelling and inflammation of the larynx that is associated with hoarseness or loss of voice.

lens A transparent body within the globe that focuses light rays.

Ludwig angina A type of cellulitis that occurs on the floor of the mouth under the tongue; caused by bacteria from an infected tooth root (tooth abscess) or mouth injury.

mastication The process of chewing with the teeth.

Meniere disease An inner ear disorder in which endolymphatic rupture creates increased pressure in the cochlear duct, which then leads to damage to the organ of Corti and the semicircular canal; symptoms include severe vertigo, tinnitus, and sensorineuronal hearing loss.

middle ear One of three anatomic parts of the ear; it consists of the inner portion of the tympanic membrane and the ossicles.

nasal septum The separation between the right and left nostrils.

nasolacrimal duct The passage through which tears drain from the lacrimal sacs into the nasal cavity.

oculomotor nerve Third cranial nerve; innervates the muscles that cause motion of the eyeballs and upper eyelid.

optic nerve Either of the second cranial nerves that enter the eyeball posteriorly, through the optic foramen.

oral candidiasis A condition that presents as white lesions on the tongue and inner cheeks, caused by the fungus *Candida albicans*; also called thrush.

orbital cellulitis An infection within the eye socket.

organ of Corti A structure located in the cochlea that contains hairs that are stimulated by vibrations to form nerve impulses that travel to the brain and are perceived as sound.

ossicles The three small bones in the inner ear that transmit vibrations to the cochlear duct at the oval window.

otitis An infection of either the outer or middle ear cavity.

oval window An oval opening between the middle ear and the vestibule.

papilledema An eye condition that results from increased pressure on the optic nerve at the rear part of the eye, and whose symptoms include headaches, nausea with possible vomiting, temporary vision loss, or narrowing vision fields.

paranasal sinuses The sinuses, or hollowed sections of bone in the front of the head, that are lined with mucous membrane and drain into the nasal cavity.

periorbital cellulitis An infection of the eyelid; also known as preseptal cellulitis or eyelid cellulitis.

peripheral vision Visualization of lateral objects while looking forward.

peritonsillar abscess A collection of infected material around the tonsils.

pharyngitis Inflammation of the pharynx.

pinna The large outside portion of the ear through which sound waves enter the ear; also called the auricle.

posterior chamber The posterior area of the globe between the lens and the iris.

pulp Specialized connective tissue within the pulp cavity of a tooth.

pupil The circular opening in the center of the eye through which light passes to the lens.

retina A delicate 10-layered structure of nervous tissue located in the rear of the interior of the globe that receives light and generates nerve signals that are transmitted to the brain through the optic nerve.

retinal detachment Separation of the inner layers of the retina from the underlying choroid, the vascular membrane that nourishes the retina.

rhinitis A nasal disorder generally caused by allergens, which, once inhaled, result in production of chemicals that can cause inflammation.

sclera The white part of the eye.

sinusitis An infection of the sinuses, characterized by thick nasal discharge, sinus and facial pressure, headache, and fever.

sympathetic eye movement The movement of both eyes in unison.

temporomandibular joint disorders A collection of disorders that present with jaw pain, and which occur when the connection between the temporal bone and the temporomandibular joint erodes or moves out of proper alignment.

tinnitus The perception of sound in the inner ear with no external environmental cause; often reported as "ringing" in the ears, but may be roaring, buzzing, or clicking.

tonsillitis Inflammation of the tonsils.

tracheitis Bacterial infection of the trachea.

trigeminal nerve The fifth cranial nerve; its mandibular branch provides motor innervation to the muscles of mastication.

turbinates Three bony shelves that protrude from the lateral walls of the nasal cavity and extend into the nasal passageway, parallel to the nasal floor; serve to increase the surface area of the nasal mucosa, thereby improving the processes of warming, filtering, and humidification of inhaled air.

tympanic membrane A thin membrane that separates the middle ear from the inner ear and sets up vibrations in the ossicles; also called the eardrum.

vertigo A type of dizziness in which a person experiences the sensation of movement when standing still or of the environment moving around himself or herself; often due to an inner ear disorder.

visual cortex The area in the brain where signals from the optic nerve are converted into visual images.

vitreous humor A jellylike substance found in the posterior compartment of the eye between the lens and the retina.

Assessment in Action

Y ou are responding to an elderly patient with a nosebleed. On arrival you find a 70-year-old man who is holding a towel to his face. The patient states that he has been bleeding from the nose for about 10 minutes and he cannot get it to stop. The patient tells you that his doctor has put him on a new medication called warfarin for his atrial fibrillation.

1. What is the first step you should take in the care of this patient?
   A. Assess the nose and apply a bandage.
   B. Make sure the patient can maintain his airway.
   C. Have the patient lay supine.
   D. Pack the nose with gauze.

2. Warfarin is classified as which of the following?
   A. Anticoagulant
   B. Antiemetic
   C. Calcium channel blocker
   D. Anticonvulsant

3. What is the preferred method for stopping a nosebleed?
   A. Pack the nose with gauze.
   B. Pinch the nares closed and hold for a minimum of 15 minutes.
   C. Have the patient lean forward and allow the bleeding to stop on its own.
   D. Insert a nasopharyngeal airway.

4. What is another name for a nosebleed?
   A. Hemophilia
   B. Hematemesis
   C. Anisocoria
   D. Epistaxis

5. What may happen if this patient swallows a large amount of blood?
   A. The blood will be digested without problem.
   B. The patient may vomit.
   C. The patient may develop dysrhythmias.
   D. Nothing will happen.

Additional Questions

6. What is conjunctivitis?

Abdominal and Gastrointestinal Emergencies

National EMS Education Standard Competencies

Medicine

Integrates assessment findings with principles of epidemiology and pathophysiology to formulate a field impression and implement a comprehensive treatment/disposition plan for a patient with a medical complaint.

Abdominal and Gastrointestinal Disorders

Anatomy, presentations, and management of shock associated with abdominal emergencies

- Gastrointestinal bleeding (pp 1139-1142)

Anatomy, physiology, epidemiology, pathophysiology, psychosocial impact, presentations, prognosis, and management of

- Acute and chronic gastrointestinal hemorrhage (pp 1138-1142)
- Liver disorders (pp 1148-1149)
- Peritonitis (p 1142)
- Ulcerative diseases (pp 1140-1141, 1145)
- Irritable bowel syndrome (p 1146)
- Inflammatory disorders (pp 1145-1146)
- Pancreatitis (pp 1144-1145)
- Bowel obstruction (pp 1149-1150)
- Hernias (p 1150)
- Infectious diseases (pp 1147-1149)
- Gall bladder and biliary tract disorders (pp 1142-1143)
- Rectal abscesses (p 1148)
- Rectal foreign body obstruction (p 1151)
- Mesenteric ischemia (p 1151)

Knowledge Objectives

1. Describe the incidence, morbidity, and mortality of gastrointestinal emergencies. (p 1125)
2. Identify the primary risk factors for gastrointestinal disease. (p 1125)
3. Describe lifestyle changes that reduce the likelihood of developing gastrointestinal disease. (p 1124)
4. Discuss the anatomy and physiology of the organs and structures of the gastrointestinal system. (pp 1124-1128)
5. Explain how to size up scene safety when responding to a patient with a gastrointestinal emergency. (pp 1128-1130)
6. Analyze the nature of the illness for a broad range of gastrointestinal disorders. (p 1130)
7. List the personal protective equipment that is likely to be necessary during a call in response to a patient with a gastrointestinal emergency. (pp 1128-1129)

8. Explain how to integrate pathophysiologic principles and assessment findings to formulate a field impression and implement a treatment plan for the patient with a gastrointestinal emergency. (pp 1130-1136)
9. Evaluate the mechanisms by which airway patency and circulation might be compromised in the patient with a gastrointestinal emergency. (p 1130)
10. Indicate the considerations that go into making a transport decision for the patient with a gastrointestinal emergency. (pp 1130-1131)
11. Explore ways of investigating the chief complaint of a patient with a gastrointestinal disorder, including how to take the patient's history using the SAMPLE mnemonic. (p 1131)
12. Describe the technique for performing a comprehensive physical examination on a patient with abdominal pain, including percussion and auscultation of bowel sounds and palpation to evaluate for pain and masses. (pp 1132-1135)
13. Define somatic, visceral, and referred pain as they relate to gastroenterology. (p 1134)
14. Discuss how orthostatic vital signs can help assess the extent of abdominal bleeding. (p 1135)
15. List monitoring devices used to evaluate patients with gastrointestinal disorders. (p 1135)
16. Consider the proper extent of pain management for the gastrointestinal patient. (pp 1135-1136)
17. Examine ways in which you can communicate effectively with the patient with an abdominal emergency. (p 1131)
18. Specify how to manage airway, breathing, and circulation in patients with gastrointestinal or abdominal emergencies. (pp 1136-1137)
19. Discuss the pathophysiologic mechanisms that can cause hypovolemia. (p 1138)
20. Compare the pathophysiology, assessment, and management of upper gastrointestinal bleeding with that of lower gastrointestinal bleeding. (pp 1139-1142)
21. Define esophagogastric varices and discuss their pathophysiology, assessment, and management. (pp 1139-1140)
22. Define Mallory-Weiss syndrome and discuss its pathophysiology, assessment, and management. (p 1140)
23. Define peptic ulcer disease and discuss its pathophysiology, assessment, and management. (pp 1140-1141)
24. Define hemorrhoids and discuss their pathophysiology, assessment, and management. (p 1141)
25. Define anal fissures and discuss their pathophysiology, assessment, and management. (pp 1141-1142)
26. Explain how the immune system responds to acute and chronic inflammation within the gastrointestinal tract. (p 1142)
27. Define cholecystitis and discuss its pathophysiology, assessment, and management. (pp 1142-1143)
28. Define appendicitis and discuss its pathophysiology, assessment, and management. (p 1143)
29. Define diverticulitis and discuss its pathophysiology, assessment, and management. (pp 1143-1144)

30. Define pancreatitis and discuss its pathophysiology, assessment, and management. (pp 1144-1145)

31. Define ulcerative colitis and discuss its pathophysiology, assessment, and management. (pp 1145-1146)

32. Define irritable bowel syndrome and discuss its pathophysiology, assessment, and management. (p 1146)

33. Define Crohn disease and discuss its pathophysiology, assessment, and management. (pp 1146-1147)

34. Explain why the gastrointestinal system is vulnerable to infection and how the immune system reacts to infection within the gastrointestinal tract. (p 1147)

35. Explain the pathophysiologic mechanisms involved in nausea, vomiting, and diarrhea. (p 1138)

36. Define acute gastroenteritis and discuss its pathophysiology, assessment, and management. (pp 1147-1148)

37. Define rectal abscess and discuss its pathophysiology, assessment, and management. (p 1148)

38. Define cirrhosis and discuss its pathophysiology, assessment, and management. (pp 1148-1149)

39. Define hepatic encephalopathy and discuss its pathophysiology, assessment, and management. (p 1149)

40. Define small- and large-bowel obstruction and discuss their pathophysiology, assessment, and management. (pp 1149-1150)

41. Define hernia and discuss its pathophysiology, assessment, and management. (p 1150)

42. Compare the four types of abdominal hernias: reducible, incarcerated, strangulated, and incisional. (p 1150)

43. Describe rectal foreign body obstruction and discuss its pathophysiology, assessment, and management. (p 1151)

44. Compare rectal foreign body obstructions caused by swallowed objects with obstructions caused by inserted objects. (p 1151)

45. Identify the special challenges children face when an abdominal or gastrointestinal emergency arises. (pp 1151-1153)

46. Describe the gastrointestinal anomalies gastroschisis and intestinal malrotation, and explain how they are managed. (p 1152)

47. Discuss the incidence of congenital gastrointestinal anomalies in the United States. (p 1152)

48. Define pyloric stenosis and discuss its pathophysiology, assessment, and management. (p 1152)

49. Identify the special challenges older adults face when an abdominal or gastrointestinal emergency arises. (p 1153)

Skills Objectives

1. Demonstrate how to palpate the abdomen to assess for pain, rebound tenderness, and masses. (pp 1133-1134)

2. Demonstrate how to palpate the right upper quadrant to assess for Murphy sign, indicating cholecystitis. (pp 1134-1135)

3. Demonstrate how to auscultate the abdomen to assess for diminished, absent, or abnormal bowel sounds. (pp 1132-1133)

■ Introduction

Gastrointestinal (GI) problems, in and of themselves, are rarely life threatening. Nevertheless, systemic problems can originate from untreated or undertreated disorders of the GI system. For example, the appendix, a small, inconsequential portion of the intestine, has no known function. Yet when this small, fleshy pouch becomes infected, the consequences can be deadly.

This chapter will review the structures that perform **digestion** and their functions and locations Figure 1 . After a brief review of the general assessment process for a patient with an **acute abdomen** (sudden onset of abdominal pain) or other abdominal emergency, the pathophysiology, assessment, and management of several common GI conditions will be discussed. To begin, you need to gain an appreciation for the scope of GI emergencies.

At one time or another, everyone has had abdominal pain or a case of the flu. **Diarrhea**, nausea, and vomiting are the undesirable signs and symptoms of such an illness. They might cause intense discomfort, and indicate an underlying condition. In other words, they cannot themselves be considered conditions or illnesses.

The number of disorders responsible for causing abdominal pain, diarrhea, and nausea is impressive. Table 1 presents some statistics on the incidence (the number of new cases of a disease diagnosed in a given year) and prevalence (the number of people who are currently living with a particular disease) of GI disorders in the United States. Fortunately, most GI disorders are not deadly. With the exception of septicemia (a generalized infection of the bloodstream that could be caused by a GI disorder), GI disorders are not among the top 10 diseases that cause death within the United States.

The current population of the United States is over 300 million. Using this number as a basis for comparison, an astounding 60 million people have gastroesophageal reflux disease (GERD). This certainly accounts for the number of advertisements for heartburn relief medications on television, in magazines, and on health-related websites. All GI disorders combined represent 1 in 4 people in the United States. It is clear that paramedics will be called on frequently to treat patients with GI disorders.

As you explore these conditions, knowing which behaviors and characteristics may predispose patients to GI disorders can assist you with the care or prevention of future GI problems. Two known behavioral risk factors are smoking and excessive alcohol consumption. Both nicotine and alcohol increase the release of gastric acid in the stomach. This is why a *small* amount of wine or a beer taken before a meal is known as an *apéritif*, from a French word meaning "to open": it primes the stomach for the forthcoming meal. Smoking or chronic alcohol consumption, however, increases the acidity of the stomach beyond the ability of the mucosal lining to protect it. The result is an increased risk for ulcers of the upper GI tract.

Other activities that place patients at increased risk are listed in Table 2 . You can use this information to help educate patients about ways in which they can decrease or even eliminate their GI discomfort. To effectively counsel your patients, a review of normal anatomy and physiology is in order.

■ Anatomy and Physiology

To help illustrate the structures and functions of the GI system, the process of eating a meal will be examined. For example, you are enjoying a garden salad of lettuce, tomatoes, cucumbers, raisins, peanuts, croutons, carrots, and shrimp with ranch dressing—a nutritious meal. Examining the salad's journey through the digestive system will help to illustrate normal anatomy and physiology.

YOU *are the Medic*   PART 1

Your unit is dispatched for an unresponsive person at a local residence. The dispatcher tells you the patient is a 64-year-old woman who lost consciousness in her bathroom. You arrive at the residence and are met at the door by the patient's husband. The husband leads you to the upstairs bathroom where you find the patient lying next to the toilet. There is a foul odor in the room and you notice about 250 mL of melenotic stool covering the patient's clothing and around the floor near her buttocks. The patient is responsive when you approach. The husband explains that his wife had been sleeping, woke up, and asked him to help her to the bathroom because she had to have a bowel movement. He said when they reached the bathroom she passed out so he helped her to the floor next to the toilet. The patient said the last thing she remembers is walking to the bathroom with her husband. The patient has been feeling ill with stomach cramps for the past several days.

1. What is melena?
2. What part of the GI system do you believe might be affected?

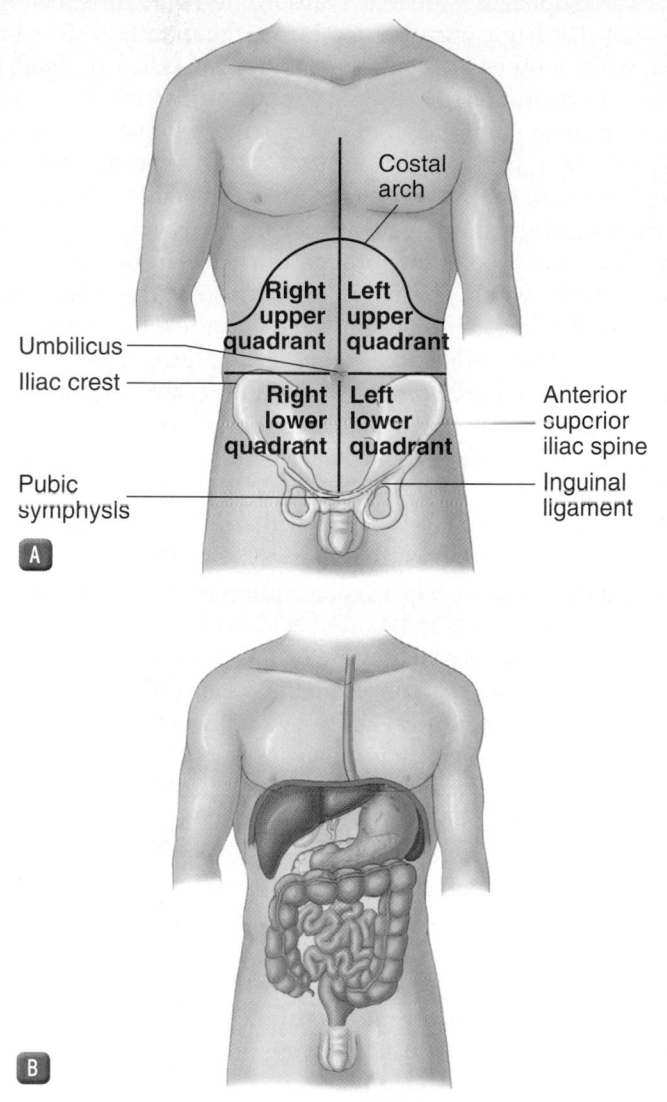

Figure 1 The anatomy of the abdomen. **A.** The four quadrants of the abdomen. **B.** Abdominal organs can lie in more than one quadrant. Note that though the kidneys are in the abdomen, they are not part of the gastrointestinal system, and are covered in the chapter, *Genitourinary and Renal Emergencies*.

As you take a bite of the lettuce, carrots, and cucumbers, you feel a pleasant cool and crisp sensation in your mouth that encourages you to chew. Your front teeth are mainly used to tear or cut the food. While chewing, the food is worked toward the back of the mouth, where the flat surfaces of the molars crush and grind the food into a more easily swallowed consistency. This mechanical activity eases food down the esophagus during swallowing and helps to prevent aspiration of food into the lungs. This chewing process is referred to as *mastication* **Figure 2**.

While chewing, saliva mixes with the salad. Saliva is secreted in the mouth to help lubricate food. Shrimp, which are already somewhat slippery, would have little trouble slipping down the esophagus. Conversely, croutons are dry and hard.

Table 1 Incidence and Prevalence of GI Disorders

Disorder	Incidence/Prevalence*
All GI disorders	60-70 million (236,000 deaths per year, 14 million hospitalizations per year)
Constipation	63 million
Crohn disease	359,000
Diverticular disease (diverticulosis, diverticulitis)	2.2 million
Gallstones	20 million
Gastritis	3.7 million
GI infections	Non-foodborne: 135 million Foodborne: 76 million
GERD	20% of the US population
Hemorrhoids	8.5 million
Hepatitis A	2,979 new cases
Hepatitis B	4,519 new cases
Hepatitis C	849 new cases
Hernia, abdominal wall	4.7 million
Irritable bowel syndrome	15.3 million
Liver disease	2.6 million
Pancreatitis	1.1 million
Peptic ulcer disease	14.5 million
Ulcerative colitis	619,000

*Data represent the number of new cases of a disease diagnosed in a given year in the US.

Data source: Centers for Disease Control and Prevention.

Table 2 Behaviors and Corresponding Risk Factors for GI Disease

Behavior	Risk Factor
Smoking	Stomach/esophageal disease
Ingestion of caustic agents	Stomach/esophageal disease
Low-fiber diet	Colon disease/constipation
Alcohol	Stomach/esophageal/liver disease
Ingestion of certain medications: acetylsalicylic acid, nonsteroidal anti-inflammatory drugs (NSAIDs), anticoagulants	Stomach/esophageal disease
Stress	Disease throughout the GI tract

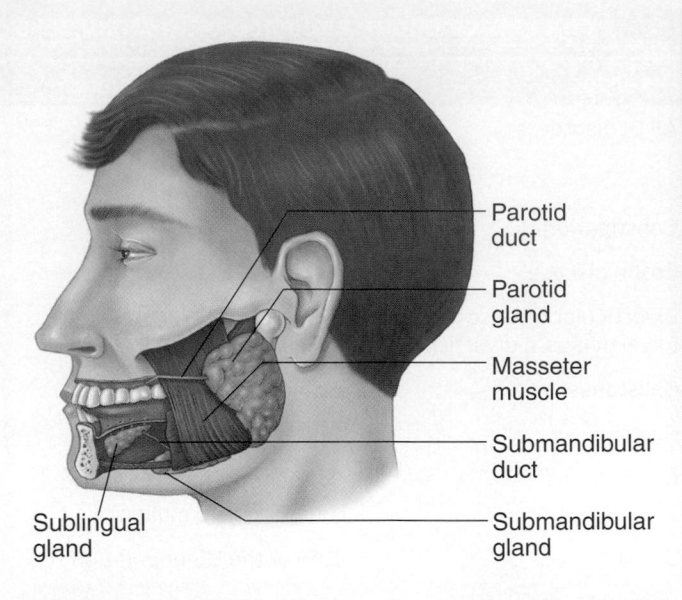

Parotid duct

Parotid gland

Masseter muscle

Submandibular duct

Sublingual gland

Submandibular gland

Figure 2 Mastication, or the process of chewing, is the first step in the process of digestion.

Without saliva to lubricate them and mastication to pulverize them into a smooth bolus, these bread cubes would become lodged in the esophagus.

In addition to its role in helping food travel through the esophagus, saliva contains enzymes that begin the chemical breakdown of starches, or complex carbohydrates. These carbohydrates can be broken down into simple sugars, which the body can more easily absorb. As you eat the raisins in your salad, simple sugars are released and rapidly absorbed by capillaries in the tongue and mouth. This is why you get a quick "sugar rush" when you eat a chocolate bar. Some initial breakdown of triglycerides occurs in the mouth as well.

Once the food has been ground down, you prepare to swallow. The esophagus is located in the posterior portion of the hypopharynx. It is a muscular tube that typically lies collapsed in on itself, like a dry fire hose. This deflated position allows air to flow easily into the lungs, and not into the stomach. The esophagus dilates, however, when food or liquid travels through it.

The collapsed position of the esophagus explains how gastric distention can occur during ventilation. If a patient requires positive-pressure ventilation, a bag-mask device can be used to push air into the lungs. If, however, the pressure of the ventilation is too great, the esophagus will dilate. Air follows the path of least resistance. Given the choice of moving through a broad tube into a large open space—the stomach—or wending its way down through a series of progressively smaller tubes, from the trachea into the bronchi, the air will flow into the stomach. This causes gastric distention that can impede lung expansion.

The esophagus is unable to absorb nutrients. It is merely a conduit that helps transport food from the mouth to the stomach, using a series of rhythmic contractions called **peristalsis**. Intertwined around the esophagus are veins that drain into another, more complex series of veins that ultimately converge to form the **portal vein**. The purpose of the portal vein is to transport venous blood from the GI tract directly to the liver for processing of the nutrients that have been absorbed. For a variety of reasons, blood flow through the liver can be slow. There are no valves within this series of veins, so as the blood backs up, it is able to communicate throughout the entire GI system. The veins surrounding the stomach and esophagus become dilated. Even a small amount of pressure can cause leaking or rupture of these vessels. This bleeding can be minor or severe. This problem will be discussed later in the pathology section for each condition.

The food now travels through the diaphragm and comes to a sphincter that serves as a doorway connecting the esophagus and the stomach. The **cardiac sphincter**, so called because people who have regurgitation of acid from the stomach to the esophagus often feel as if they are having a heart attack, controls the amount of food that moves up the esophagus.

The meal is about to begin its second major transformation. When empty, the stomach is rather small, but it has the capacity to stretch to many times its normal size to accommodate meals **Figure 3**. As the food enters this muscular organ, the stomach begins to secrete hydrochloric acid. This powerful chemical helps to break down the food. The stomach contracts to help mix the acid with the food more evenly, churning the acid and food mixture together until a relatively smooth consistency is achieved. The material that exits the pyloric sphincter, the doorway between the inferior portion of the stomach and the entry to the small intestine, is called **chyme**.

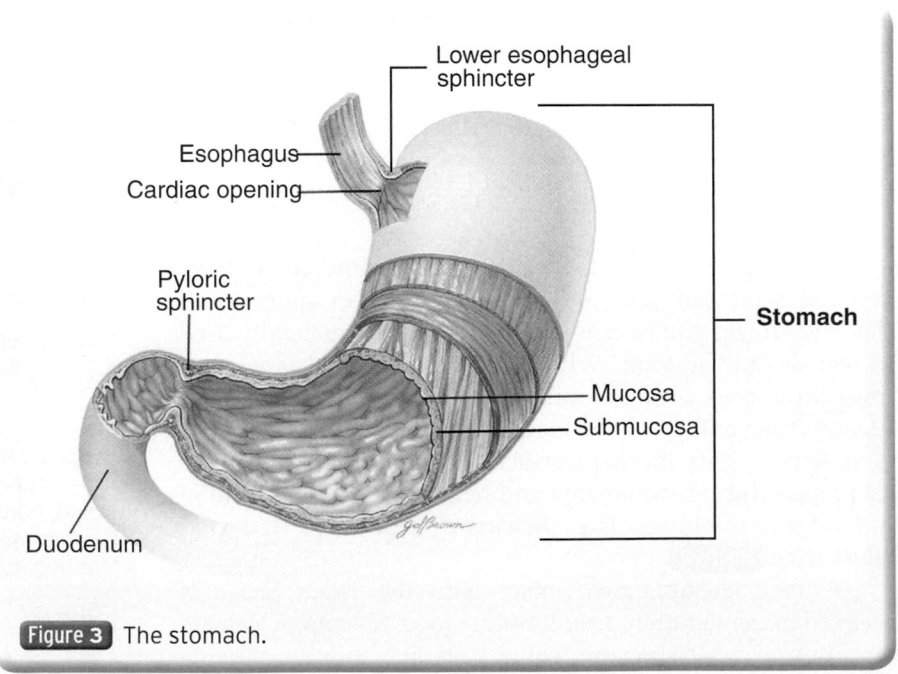

Lower esophageal sphincter

Esophagus

Cardiac opening

Pyloric sphincter

Stomach

Mucosa

Submucosa

Duodenum

Figure 3 The stomach.

As you eat, you are enjoying your salad, and you eat a large serving of it—far too much food to be accommodated by the duodenum, the portion of the small intestine in which absorption begins. To help manage this volume of food, the stomach is designed to release only small amounts of the food into the duodenum, allowing the small intestine to better manage the job of digestion.

Some absorption occurs in the stomach. Water- and fat-soluble substances, such as alcohol, are absorbed there. If wine is consumed with the salad, alcohol absorption begins in the stomach but the rate is rather slow. Alcohol is absorbed more rapidly in the duodenum. The longer the alcohol remains in the stomach, the slower the rate of absorption into the bloodstream. To delay absorption of alcohol, eating a fatty meal will delay gastric emptying because fat is more difficult to break down than other nutrients, such as sugars, and the stomach has to work to digest the fat. Your meal of salad is relatively low in fat, so you will feel the effects of the alcohol relatively quickly as the food leaves your stomach through the pyloric sphincter and heads to the duodenum.

But why are you eating in the first place? As the levels of nutrients available to your cells start to drop, you begin to feel hungry. You eat in order to replenish your energy resources, keeping your cells supplied with proteins, sugars, fats, electrolytes, and vitamins. The main function of the GI system is to absorb these products of digestion to fuel the cells within the body.

The duodenum is the first part of the small intestine. It connects the pancreas, liver, and gallbladder to the digestive system. The exocrine portion of the pancreas secretes several enzymes into the duodenum. These enzymes assist with digestion of fats, proteins, and carbohydrates. Additionally, pancreatic juice, as it is called, helps to neutralize gastric acid.

The liver has one direct effect and several indirect effects on the GI system. Bile is produced by the liver and stored inside the gallbladder. Bile is an enzyme used by the body to help break down fats. The shrimp, ranch dressing, peanuts, and croutons in your salad contain fat that must be broken down before it can be absorbed into the bloodstream. Bile is released into the duodenum, where it helps to emulsify, or dissolve, the fats.

An indirect effect of the liver on the GI system is to promote carbohydrate metabolism. If the blood glucose level falls, the liver can convert glycogen into glucose. Dramatic decreases in glucose stores will prompt the liver to convert fats and proteins into glucose. Remember, your brain cells can burn only one fuel source—glucose. As blood flows through the liver, fat and protein metabolism continues. Without a functioning liver, you would be dead in a few days because your body would not be able to use any of the proteins absorbed through the GI system. Finally, the liver detoxifies drugs, completes the breakdown of dead red and white blood cells, and stores vitamins and minerals.

The real workhorse of the digestive system is the small intestine, where 90% of all absorption occurs. It would be difficult to stay properly nourished if a section of your small intestine had to be removed because of Crohn disease, cancer, or some other disease process.

The small intestine is about 20′ long and divided into three sections: the duodenum, which is the last section of what is called the upper GI system; the jejunum, the first part of the lower GI system; and the ileum. In the small intestine, water-soluble and fat-soluble vitamins are absorbed by diffusion into the bloodstream for use by cells. The small intestine also produces enzymes that work with the pancreatic enzymes to turn chyme into substances that can be directly absorbed into the bloodstream through the capillaries on its surface **Figure 4**.

Blood enriched with these energy molecules now exits the intestinal circulation and flows to the liver, where fat and protein metabolism takes place. The blood then leaves the liver and enters the subclavian vessels.

The large intestine, or colon, is about 5′ long **Figure 5**. By now, all nutrients have been broken down and absorbed by the body. The remaining waste products are now called *feces*.

The ileocecal valve joins the ileum to the first portion of the large intestine, called the *cecum*. Lying directly posterior to the ileocecal valve is the appendix. The appendix is a small, saclike outcropping that has no known function, but may become infected with retained fecal material. Appendicitis is discussed in detail later in this chapter.

Rising up from the cecum is the ascending colon. It attaches to the transverse colon, which runs from right to left. A 90° turn occurs, and the descending colon begins. The end of the colon, then, lies near the left lower quadrant. The sigmoid colon then takes an "S" turn. The most inferior portion of the sigmoid colon lies in the center of the abdomen. Finally, the sigmoid colon is

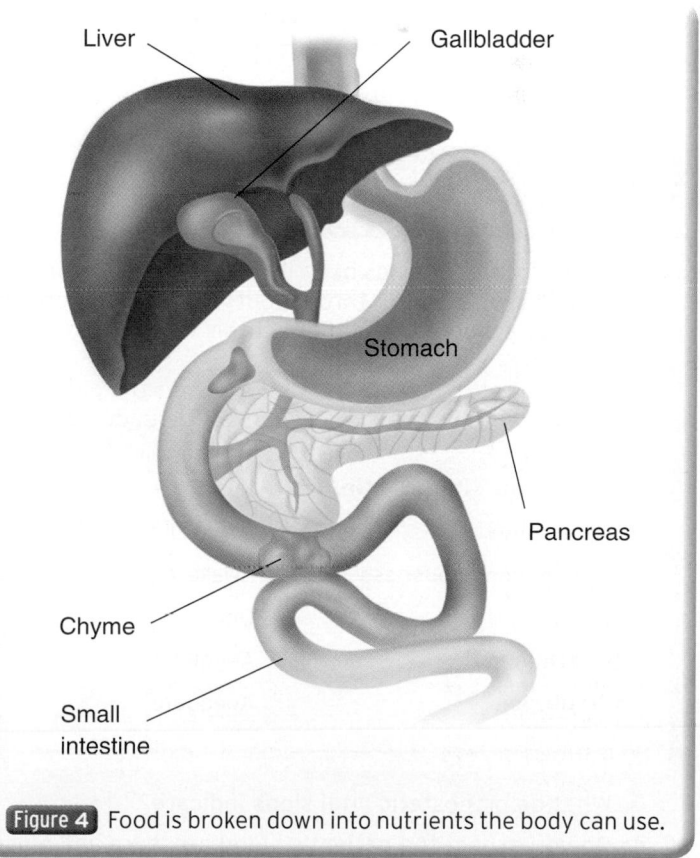

Figure 4 Food is broken down into nutrients the body can use.

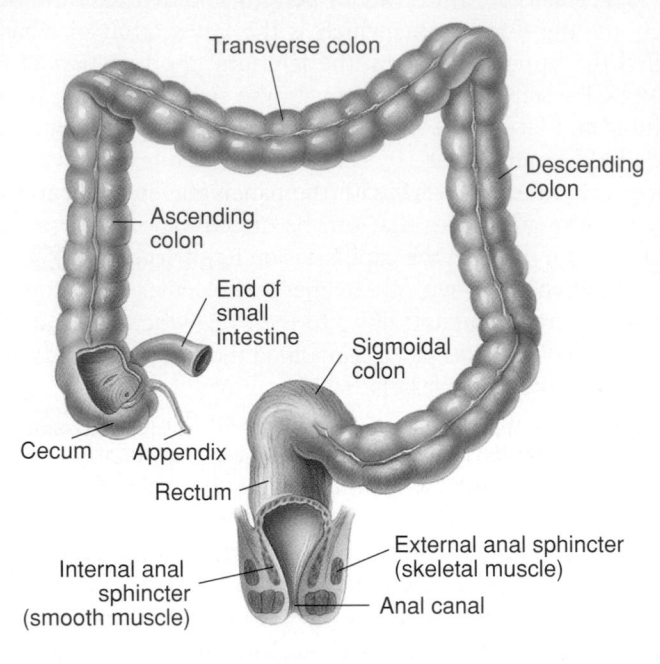

Figure 5 The colon is the next destination for the remaining products of digestion.

adjacent to the rectum, the last portion of the colon. The colon terminates at a sphincter called the *anus*, through which feces is expelled from the body.

The main role of the large intestine is to complete the reabsorption of water. Most water is reabsorbed in the small intestine. This osmotic function of the colon helps to solidify the stool. Failure of this bowel function results in **soft stool** or diarrhea.

The colon is also the site of bacterial digestion. Bacteria normally found in the colon help to complete the breakdown of chyme. This process produces gas as a by-product. Flatulence may be considered impolite, but it is certainly normal.

The entire journey from mouth to anus, summarized in Table 3, takes 8 to 72 hours. At this pace, a normal number of bowel movements is between three per day and one every 3 days. Of course, this number varies according to the types of food you eat, the amount of water consumed, the amount of exercise you get, and how much stress your body is under.

Patient Assessment

Scene Size-up

Assessment of the GI system begins with the scene size-up. Caution must be exercised to ensure that all EMS providers remain safe.

As you observe the scene, look for indicators of the mechanism of injury or nature of illness to help you determine your field impression. Multiple patients are not a common occurrence with GI patients; however, vigilance is essential to ensure scene safety.

In today's society, hazards vary and may include chemical and biologic agents, and when coupled with the threat of terrorism, you must critically evaluate the dispatch information. A call for assistance to an office building where several patients are reporting abdominal pain should lead you to consider a scene where an agent has been released.

Standard precautions are particularly important when treating a patient with GI problems because of the high likelihood of contact with infectious agents. Don PPE, including

YOU are the Medic   PART 2

The patient states she has been ill for several days with dark, smelly stools twice every day for the past 3 days. She denies any vomiting but reports pain throughout her entire abdomen. She states the pain can be bad enough to wake her. She did not go to the hospital because she thought this was just a case of the flu.

You obtain a set of orthostatic vital signs. As the patient sits up with your assistance, she reports being dizzy. Assessment of the abdomen reveals normal bowel sounds. The abdomen is soft, but tender in all four quadrants.

Recording Time: 0 Minutes	
Appearance	Awake, lying on bathroom floor
Level of consciousness	Awake, oriented
Airway	Open
Breathing	Adequate
Circulation	Adequate

3. What do orthostatic vital signs indicate?

4. Do you expect the patient's blood pressure and pulse rate to increase or decrease when the patient is moved?

Table 3   **Location and Functions of the GI System-Related Organs**

Organ/Structure	Location	Function
Mouth	Head	Mechanically breaks down food; begins chemical breakdown of food with saliva.
Esophagus	Substernal, **epigastric**	Tube that moves food from the mouth to the stomach. Muscular and vascular structure.
Stomach	Left upper quadrant, epigastric	Performs mechanical and chemical breakdown of food. Food in, chyme out.
Rectum	Superpubic, hypogastric	
Anus	Most inferior portion of the large intestine	Sphincter to control release of feces.
Liver	Upper abdomen. Mainly right with central upper abdomen.	Produces bile; assists with carbohydrate, protein, and fat metabolism; vitamin storage and manufacture; blood detoxification; waste elimination.
Pancreas Exocrine	Posterior to the stomach	Produces enzymes for protein, carbohydrate, and fat breakdown within the duodenum.
Endocrine		Produces insulin, somatostatin, and glucagon.
Gallbladder	Inferior surface of the liver	Storage of bile.
Spleen	Left upper abdomen	Filtering of blood, recycling of dead red blood cells.
Aorta	Central upper abdomen	Main artery supplying blood to the lower body.
Bladder	Suprapubic area	Storage of urine.
Uterus	Suprapubic area	Reproduction.
Iliac arteries	Central abdomen and lower right/left quadrants	Supply blood to the legs and pelvis.
Small intestine		
Duodenum	Central, upper **umbilical**	Major site for chemical breakdown of food; major site of water, fat, protein, carbohydrate, and vitamin absorption.
Jejunum	Central, umbilical	
Ileum	Central, hypogastric to lower right abdomen	
Large intestine		
Ascending colon	Right lower quadrant, hypogastric into epigastric	Water reabsorption, formation of feces, bacterial digestion of food.
Transverse colon	Right to left upper quadrant, epigastric	
Descending colon	Left upper and lower quadrant, epigastric to umbilical	
Sigmoid colon	Left lower quadrant, hypogastric	

goggles or a face shield, ahead of time when you anticipate coming into contact with sprays or splashes of blood or body fluids. Gloves are always needed. However, with the possibility of coming into contact with vomitus, diarrhea, blood, and soiled patient clothing, additional PPE may be necessary. Gowns can be very helpful when dealing with patients who have become incontinent. Masks can help with noxious odors. Cleaning the patient helps provide some degree of dignity to a person humiliated by the circumstances of his or her disease. In addition to gloves, gowns, and masks, the following equipment

is essential to providing good patient hygiene while maintaining personal safety:

- Eye protection
- Towels and wash rags
- Extra linens
- Absorbent pads (Chux)
- Emesis basin
- Disposable basin
- Biohazard bags
- Sterile water for irrigation

Proper cleaning and maintenance of equipment and uniforms soiled during a call is essential to ensuring the health of the EMS crew and the health of the next patient. Remember, hepatitis B can remain infectious even in dried blood for over a week.

Primary Assessment

Form a General Impression

As you begin to form your initial general impression of the patient, closely examine where he or she is found. The patient's body posture or position can give you hints as to what happened. Was the patient walking to the bathroom when he or she passed out? Has the patient been in bed sick for several days? Was the patient at work when a sudden bout of pain caused him or her to double over? Look to the environment for clues as to the length and degree of illness the patient is experiencing.

One aspect of the general impression of the patient with GI problems is odor. What is the smell of the room or location of the patient? Few conditions create such a noxious odor as upper GI bleeding. The foul-smelling stool often present during these calls can make even experienced EMS providers nauseated.

A tip when dealing with these strong odors is to hold your ground. The sense of smell is the most acute for about 1 minute. After that time, more than 50% of the intensity of an odor is lost due to the olfactory nerve becoming tired of sending the same signal. If you are faced with a strong odor on a call, stay in the environment. After about 2 to 5 minutes, your nose will tire of sending the same odor signal, and the smell may be hardly noticeable.

Examine the location where you find the patient. Is it dirty, disorganized, or unsanitary? How is the patient dressed? Does the patient have adequate hygiene? This information can help you determine if the problem is chronic or acute. It can also provide you a valuable foundation for whether the patient's emergency is isolated to the GI system. Unsanitary living conditions could indicate dementia, failure of the patient's support systems, and/or multiple medical issues. In these settings a social service intervention is certainly warranted.

As you approach the patient, focus on the level of consciousness. Many GI complaints are associated with pain or hemorrhage, which can diminish the patient's level of consciousness (LOC). Is the patient awake and alert? Does he or she obey commands? Someone who is talking automatically provides you with some foundational physiologic information. Talking means an open airway. To talk, the patient must also be breathing, have adequate blood pressure to maintain brain activity, and have a sufficient blood glucose level. To stand and walk requires even more physiologic stability. This is not to say that all patients who walk are stable. You must apply your understanding of normal physiology so the correct interpretation of physical examination results can be made.

Airway and Breathing

Airway patency becomes more pertinent in a patient with GI problems. A patient who is vomiting has a greater chance of aspiration. Open the airway using the appropriate maneuvers—jaw thrust for trauma, head tilt–chin lift for medical patients. Closely inspect the airway for foreign bodies. Remove or suction obstructions. While evaluating the airway, take note of any unusual odors from the mouth. Patients who have extremely advanced bowel obstructions can have **feculent** breath, smelling of stool.

Breathing is rarely directly affected by GI problems. If a breathing problem is encountered, it typically stems from a severe complication. Again, ensure that the airway is clear. If the patient has aspirated, the ability to oxygenate and ventilate can be impaired.

Circulation

Assessment of the circulatory system is essential in understanding the impact of GI disease on the body. As with all patients, assess skin color, temperature, and moisture. Note findings that would be consistent with shock. Determine the pulse rate. Evaluate the peripheral pulses and how they compare with central pulses.

Many GI diseases involve pain or hemorrhage. As blood volume begins to drop, the body compensates by releasing catecholamines (ie, epinephrine and norepinephrine) to vasoconstrict the periphery, increase the pulse rate, and increase the force of left ventricular contraction. Pain stimulates similar body responses. Either problem can leave the patient with tachycardia, diminished peripheral pulses, diaphoresis, and pale, cool, clammy skin.

You should ensure that the reading you obtain for the patient's blood pressure is accurate. Be cautious with the use of automatic blood pressure monitors. These labor-saving devices are outstanding at performing a task over and over; however, they can be inaccurate. To ensure the most accurate initial measurement of the patient's blood pressure, obtain a manual pressure before the use of automated blood pressure machines. You must obtain orthostatic vital signs in order to determine the extent of any bleeding; this is discussed later.

When you are examining patients for gross bleeding, it is not unusual to find large amounts of blood. Take note of the amount of blood. Many people grossly exaggerate the volume of blood lost; practice volume estimation skills during your training, for example by spilling various amounts of water and observing the size of the resulting puddle.

Transport Decision

When making your transportation decision, integrate the information gathered from the primary assessment. If the patient has positive orthostatic vital signs (vital signs vary with a change in position), give close consideration to how the patient will be moved. Can the patient sit up in a stair chair or will this cause the patient to pass out? Be cautious when transporting any patient in severe pain because syncope, simply from increased pain, is a real possibility.

Transportation of the patient with GI disease rarely requires lights and sirens. Choose the mode of ambulance transportation consciously. Using lights and sirens increases the risk of injury to both you and the patient. Using lights and sirens saves only a few minutes during the average transport. Is your patient so unstable that every second is needed?

History Taking

Gathering information about the patient's medications, allergies, and past medical history can provide information about the cause of the patient's signs and symptoms. Many people with GI complaints have longstanding medical problems, so the information provided can help you to determine an appropriate field impression. Many GI disorders can quickly increase in intensity after months of minimal problems. Ask if this emergency has ever occurred before. Gather information, asking the patient to compare a past episode to the one that is occurring today. A patient with a history of gastric ulcers who reports abdominal pain, for instance, must be asked if the pain is his or her "typical" pain from the gastric ulcer. Additionally, if a patient states that he or she takes esomeprazole (Nexium) or lansoprazole (Prevacid), you can conclude that the patient has a past history of GI problems.

The mnemonic SAMPLE helps you gather information about the history of present illness and past medical history Figure 6 . When asking the patient about his or her complaints, you might need to discuss subjects that do not often come up in everyday conversation. It is important that you and your patient have a common frame of reference. For example, one person's diarrhea is another person's soft stool. Table 4 presents standardized language you can use so that the health care providers taking over care from you will have the same understanding of the patient's condition as you do.

Be sure to ask whether the patient has had a recent change in bowel habits or in the color or quality of his or her stool. Find out if the patient has had a recent onset of diarrhea, constipation, or nausea and vomiting. Ask about any recent weight loss. Finally, ask about the patient's last meal. Some types of meals are associated

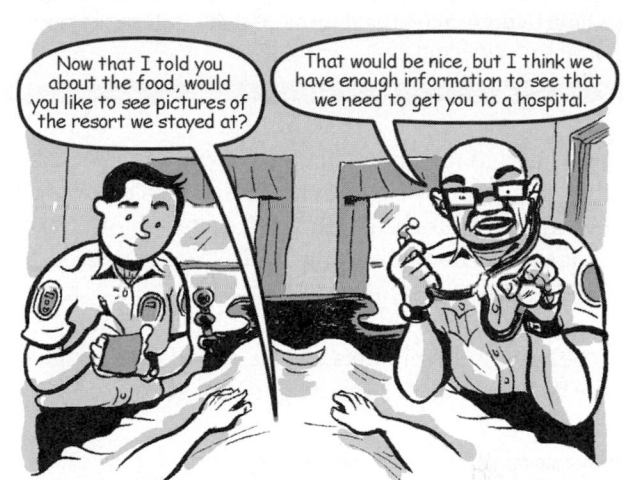

Gather information about even subtle changes in bowel habits, eating habits, new foods, travel, new medications, or low-grade fevers.

Figure 6

Table 4 Body Substances Originating in the Gastrointestinal Tract		
Substance	**Description**	**Possible Cause**
Vomitus	Food and partially digested food. Strong acidic odor mixed with the odor of food.	Influenza, food intolerance.
Hematemesis or "coffee grounds" emesis	Black or very dark red granular material. This slurry may contain food, but the food and blood are indistinguishable.	Blood from the mouth, esophagus, or stomach that has been digested by stomach acids and then vomited.
Vomitus with gross blood	Vomitus in which red blood is obvious. Food and blood are distinguishable.	Bleeding from the mouth or esophagus that has not been exposed to stomach acids.
Diarrhea	Frequent liquid stool with the consistency of water. It can range in color from clear to dark brown.	Intestinal infections, bowel obstructions. Usually associated with small intestinal problems. Is always considered abnormal.
Acholic stools	Tan-colored, formed stools. May be softer than typical.	Liver problem. Bile is released by the liver into the small intestine. Bile gives stool its normally dark color.
Steatorrhea	Foamy, foul-smelling, mushy, yellow to grey stools. These oily stools usually float within water.	Liver or pancreas disease causing excessive excretion of fat within the stool.
Soft stools	Bowel movement that is the consistency of soft-serve ice cream. Can range in color from tan to dark brown.	Normal variant for some people. Caused by new foods or a rapid change in diet.
Hematochezia	Stool and blood that are incorporated together into the same substance, yet are easily distinguished from each other.	Bleeding from the lower GI tract.
Melena	Black, tarry, sticky, and very odorous stool and blood blended together into one substance. Blood cannot be distinguished from stool.	Bleeding from the upper GI tract.

Documentation and Communication

When you are recording information about the patient's body substances, be as accurate as possible. Describe the substances in detail. Saying a patient had feces covering his legs is adequate if melena is not present. If you see the diarrhea, use terms to describe how liquid it is. This information can help to determine the degree of dehydration the patient may be experiencing.

with particular conditions. When a patient has cholecystitis, a flare-up of this condition is often associated with a fatty meal that was eaten several hours before the pain occurred. Ask the patient how he or she has been tolerating meals. Does nausea occur after eating? Any abnormal symptoms? Ask the patient if these signs and symptoms have been occurring at greater frequencies than usual. The signs and symptoms may be related to food intolerance or can be an indication of a more significant condition.

■ Secondary Assessment

For patients whose conditions are unstable, the head-to-toe examination gives you ample opportunity to discover clues to the problem or problems.

Beginning at the patient's head, you will perform the standard primary examination. There are no major changes within the examination of the head, neck, or chest. The major effects from GI disease on the nervous, cardiovascular, or respiratory systems result from pain, hypovolemia, and/or infection.

Examining the abdomen requires more detail. This examination sometimes can be embarrassing for both you and the patient. Be professional and talk calmly. As you prepare to conduct this part of the examination, place a pillow under the patient's knees if the patient's condition is stable, Have the patient relax the arms at his or her side. Straight legs with arms over the head flexes the abdominal muscles, which can distort your examination. Make sure your hands are warm before you touch the abdomen. If the patient is uncomfortable with this examination, try carrying on a casual conversation as a distraction. If the patient's condition is unstable, proceed with the examination in a quick and compassionate manner.

Look at the skin for irregularities. Are there scars indicating trauma or past surgery? If so, ask the patient about the scarring. Do you notice stretch marks also called **striae** Figure 7 ? These indicate a change in the size of the abdomen over a short period of time. Recent increases or decreases in weight, pregnancy, or severe abdominal edema can all cause striae.

Is the abdomen symmetric? Looking down at a supine patient, the abdomen should lie flat and gently slope from the ribs with a gentle upward slope as you approach the pelvis. Tumors, hernia, enlarged or distended organs, pregnancy, and other masses can cause asymmetry.

What is the shape of the abdomen? Is it flat, round, **protuberant**, or **scaphoid**? Has the patient recently had any changes in weight? As people gain weight, some of it is localized to the

abdomen. This increase will cause a round abdomen. If weight gain becomes excessive, the abdomen may protrude or become protuberant. Other causes of protuberance are fluid buildup within the abdomen called **ascites** Figure 8 , pregnancy, or organ

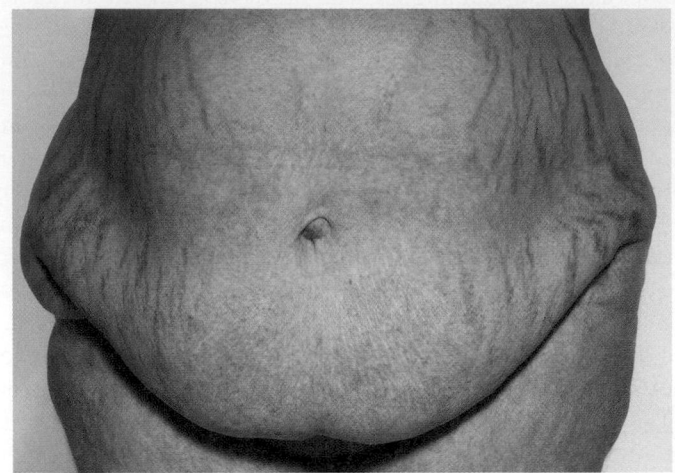

Figure 7 Striae. These vertical lines usually indicate a relatively rapid change in weight or a large amount of fluid accumulation in the abdomen.

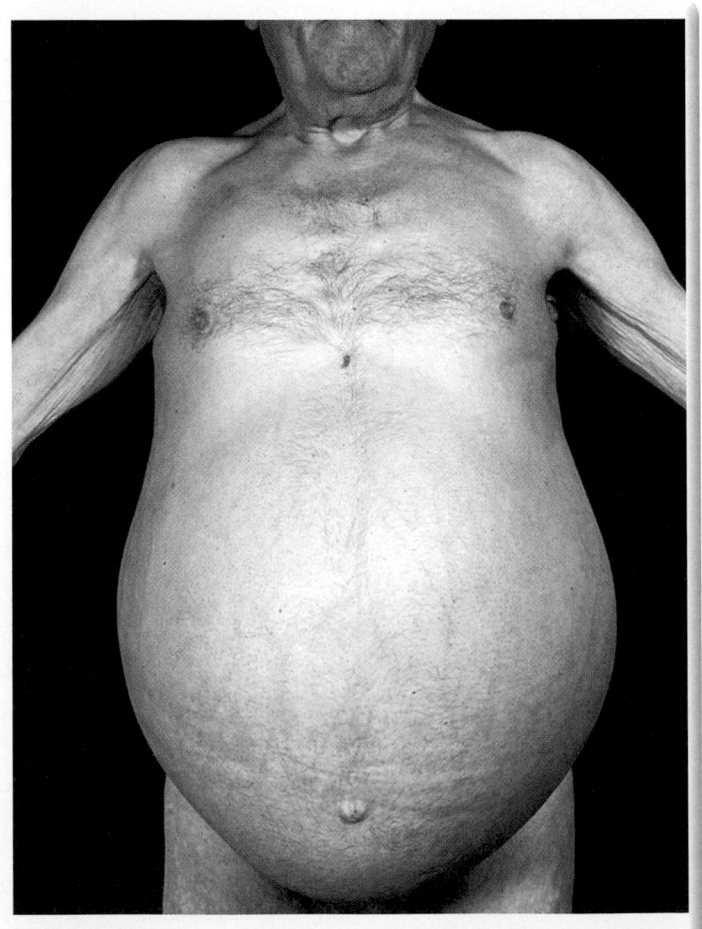

Figure 8 Protuberant abdomen caused by fluid buildup: ascites.

enlargement. The term *scaphoid* is used to describe an abdomen that is concave. This is the result of decreased abdominal volume, such as that associated with abdominal evisceration or diaphragmatic hernia.

Auscultate the abdomen. This must be done before you touch the abdomen. Palpation of the abdomen can alter the bowel sound patterns. Bowel sounds are transmitted easily through the abdominal cavity. Auscultating one location, such as the right lower quadrant is usually all that is needed. Place your stethoscope lightly on the abdominal wall and listen.

Normal bowel sounds sound like gurgles and clicks. These sounds occur between 5 and 30 times per minute. You are merely listening for the presence or absence of these sounds. Sometimes you will hear loud, prolonged sounds. This "stomach growling" is called **borborygmi**. It indicates strong contractions of the intestines. This can be normal or be present with diarrhea. Interestingly, **hyperperistalsis** can also be present in patients with early bowel obstruction. In this case, the bowel is contracting forcefully to try to overcome the obstruction.

Decreased bowel sounds, auscultating over the right lower quadrant and hearing nothing after 15 to 20 seconds, can indicate decreased peristalsis of the intestines. This lack of movement can lead to bowel obstruction. Absent bowel sounds may be difficult to note in the prehospital setting. These are characterized by no sounds heard for 2 minutes. The absence of bowel sounds indicates the intestines are not contracting; therefore, any material within them is not in motion. Bowel sounds are summarized in **Table 5**.

Percussion of the abdomen can reveal information about its contents. Typically the abdomen should be **tympanic** (empty sounding) to percussion, due to the gas in the abdominal cavity. A duller sound is generated around the upper left and upper right quadrants, due to the location of the spleen and liver, respectively. Percussion of the epigastrium may reveal tympany (empty stomach) or dullness (full stomach). Similarly, when percussing the suprapubic area, the bladder will generate these results. If the liver or spleen is enlarged, the areas of dullness can also increase.

Unfortunately, the intestines are able to mask or augment any of these findings based on their contents. Large amounts of gas in the intestines can mask the presence of splenomegaly during percussion. In patients with constipation, hepatomegaly may be falsely diagnosed on percussion because of the feces found within the intestines. These hidden or exaggerated effects are not localized to one side of the abdomen. Intestinal contents can dramatically modify the sounds heard on percussion. Use the results of your percussion as just one more piece of information: no more or less important than any other.

Remember, rarely does one assessment finding have any true meaning. As a good paramedic, you should continue to gather information and compare assessment findings looking for trends and associations. This is how to determine the correct field impression.

Palpation of the abdomen can reveal important information. Place your hand flat on the wall of the abdomen with your

Table 5 Bowel Sounds

Name	Description	Possible Causes
Normal	Soft gurgles or clicks occurring at 5–30/min	Normal movement of material through the intestines.
Borborygmi	Loud gurgles, often heard without a stethoscope often occurring at greater than 30/min	Hyperperistalsis. Can be normal. If prolonged, can indicate increased intestinal contractions, as with diarrhea of any cause.
Decreased	Quiet sounds occurring at less than 1 sound per 15 to 20 sec	**Hypoperistalsis**. Can indicate impending intestinal obstruction.
Absent	No sounds after 2 min of continuous listening	Bowel obstruction/intestinal paralysis.

fingers together. Begin your assessment in the quadrant farthest away from the patient's complaint, and end in the quadrant in which the complaint is located. Doing so will decrease the anxiety of the patient as you gain trust with each palpation. A more cautious approach to an abdominal assessment will reveal more accurate information and allow the patient to focus his or her attention on other portions of the abdomen that may not have been considered because of the discomfort the patient is experiencing. As you palpate the abdomen, it should be soft and nontender.

With your hand sitting on the wall of the abdomen, raise your wrist so you indent the abdominal wall with your fingers about 2″ to 4″. As you are palpating, you are assessing for the presence of rigidity, discomfort, or masses. Sometimes patients may feel ticklish or otherwise guard their abdomen with flexed muscles. This can make it difficult to determine whether the abdomen is rigid or just muscularly guarded. A rigid abdomen can indicate hemorrhage or infection.

Have the patient breathe with an open mouth. It becomes more difficult to hold your stomach contracted during mouth breathing. This can help relax the abdomen and allow for a more accurate assessment. You can also hold your fingers slightly depressed into the abdomen during the respiratory cycle to accomplish the same result.

When the patient exhales, the abdomen often relaxes. You can also try to coach the patient to relax the abdomen, but this is not always successful. However, if you are going to report a rigid abdomen, it is important that you have taken reasonable steps to ensure your assessment finding is accurate.

Pain is often an important finding in patients with abdominal complaints. It can indicate trauma, hemorrhage, infection, obstruction, or other serious problems. As with the standard assessment process, you should determine the OPQRST of the complaint. All of these pieces of the medical puzzle are important in determining the nature of the patient's condition.

There are several types of pain: <u>visceral pain</u>, <u>parietal pain</u> (rebound), <u>somatic pain</u>, and <u>referred pain</u>. Table 6 presents an overview of those types of pain.

<u>Rebound tenderness</u> (parietal pain) can sometimes accompany abdominal pain. Rebound tenderness occurs when the peritoneum is irritated because of either hemorrhage or infection. Evaluating for rebound tenderness involves a particular technique. Once you discover an area of the abdomen that is tender to the patient, depress the skin with your fingertips about 2″ to 4″. Now, very quickly pull your fingers off of the abdominal wall. Speed is essential. If you pull the fingers off too slowly, you will not be able to get the desired movement of the peritoneum. If possible, check for rebound tenderness in the quadrant opposite of where the patient is reporting pain.

The peritoneum is a thin layer within the abdominal cavity that envelops most of the abdominal organs. A small amount of fluid is normally found within this protective membrane. What you are trying to do is to vibrate the peritoneum. If the peritoneum is irritated, the vibration will cause a sudden increase in pain. There can also be a sudden relocation of pain to another region of the abdomen. Note this response in your assessment. Remember, rebound tenderness suggests serious and possibly life-threatening pathology.

An alternative method for assessing rebound tenderness is the Markle heel drop test. In the prehospital environment, this can be performed with the patient lying supine, while the paramedic percusses the heel of the patient's foot. If the peritoneum is irritated, this small movement will cause pain that is disproportionate with the touch.

Some consider checking for rebound tenderness to be akin to torture; this topic is somewhat controversial. Check local protocols before evaluating for rebound tenderness, and contact medical control if in doubt.

The abdomen should be rather smooth on light palpation Figure 9 . Whereas deep palpation can help you identify some of the organs and structures within the cavity, this requires a level of technique rarely used in the prehospital setting. As you palpate the abdomen, note the presence of any masses. These will feel like areas of increased density compared with the soft surrounding tissue. A mass may indicate an engorged liver, bowel distention, aortic aneurysm, or a cancerous tumor.

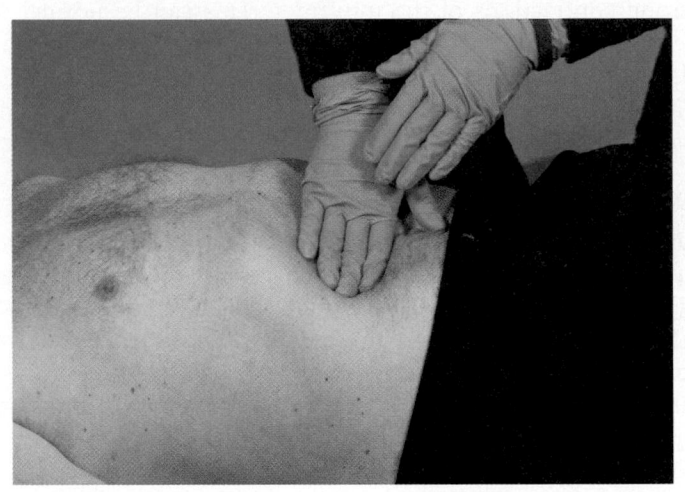

Figure 9 Palpating the four quadrants of the abdomen.

Table 6	Types of Abdominal Pain			
Types of Abdominal Pain	**Origin**	**Description**	**Cause**
Visceral pain	Hollow organs	Difficult to localize. Described as burning, cramping, gnawing, or aching. Usually felt superficially.	Organ contracts too forcefully or is distended (stretched)
Parietal pain/rebound pain	Peritoneum	Steady, achy pain. Easier to localize than visceral pain. Pain increases with movement.	Inflammation of the peritoneum (caused by bleeding or infection)
Somatic pain	Peripheral nerve tracts	Localized pain, usually felt deeply.	Irritation of or injury to tissue, causing activation of peripheral nerve tracts
Referred pain	Peripheral nerve tracts	Pain originating in the abdomen and causing the perception of pain in distant locations. Attributable to similar paths for the peripheral nerves of the abdomen and those in the distant location.	Usually occurs after an initial visceral, parietal, or somatic pain

Murphy sign is an assessment procedure to help with the field impression of cholecystitis (discussed later in this chapter). If the patient has right upper quadrant pain, this assessment technique may be used. Ask the patient to breathe out. Then take the tips of your fingers and palpate deeply along the intercostal margin of the right upper quadrant. You are now applying pressure to the liver and subsequently to the gallbladder.

Next, ask the patient to inhale deeply. As inspiration continues, the diaphragm will drop and eventually come into contact with the gallbladder. If the patient has cholecystitis, he or she may suddenly stop inspiring because of a sharp increase in pain, or a positive Murphy sign. Although not conclusive for only cholecystitis, Murphy sign, along with additional assessment information, can help to provide a solid foundation for the field impression of this condition.

It is critical to obtain the patient's **orthostatic vital signs** to gauge the extent of any bleeding. First, have the patient assume a position of comfort. Usually this is either seated or lying down. Obtain an accurate blood pressure and pulse rate. Then have the patient change positions by having the patient stand or sit up. Use caution when you change the patient's position. It is possible for the patient to lose consciousness with a positional change. Now that the patient is in another position, quickly repeat the blood pressure and pulse rate. Normally, there should be little variation in the blood pressure or pulse rate with this change in position. When a patient has a significant loss of fluid within the vascular space, however, you will note a 10-beat increase in the pulse rate or a 10-mm Hg drop in blood pressure. Either finding indicates a significant volume loss.

Many GI diseases have the potential to affect electrolyte levels. With point-of-service lab testing a reality, EMS providers are now able to determine laboratory findings at the scene in as little as 3 to 5 minutes. If the function of the GI system is impaired, its ability to eliminate waste will be impaired as well. Sodium and potassium levels in particular can change rapidly so be sure to monitor these patients, as these conditions could lead to cardiac irritability. Handheld blood analyzers such as the i-STAT allow paramedics to test these levels in the back of the ambulance. Hyperkalemia or hypokalemia can cause deadly dysrhythmias or cardiac arrest. Finding these chemical imbalances early provides the paramedic with the information needed to institute preventive therapy.

Ultrasonography and intra-abdominal pressure testing are two additional tools that may be available to the EMS provider; however, published research does not support their use in the prehospital setting at this time. These are more typically seen in the critical care transport setting. The information gathered from these devices can be used to effectively triage patients to the correct medical facility, avoiding interfacility transfers. Patients are also able to receive the definitive care they need more quickly.

▶ Reassessment

The purpose of the reassessment is to monitor your patient for changes. Routine monitoring should include pulse rate,

electrocardiogram, blood pressure, respiratory rate, and pulse oximetry. If the patient has GI bleeding, it is important to continue to assess for signs of shock. It is equally important to know the effects of your treatment on the patient. Before giving additional fluid boluses, for example, it is certainly a good habit to auscultate lung sounds. In the prehospital setting, this is valuable information in determining if the patient is deteriorating into congestive heart failure.

Many patients with abdominal pain are given pain medication. How effective was your treatment? Does the patient need more medication? How is his or her blood pressure and respiratory rate? These findings will help you evaluate the effectiveness of your treatment and form the foundation of future treatments.

Controversies

Should paramedics provide pain relief for patients with abdominal pain? This question may provoke some debate. In the past, surgeons relied on the location, quality, and intensity of abdominal pain to guide them during exploratory surgery. In medicine today, techologies such as CT scans and ultrasound allow abdominal tissues to be viewed more clearly. The images provided by these technologies show incredibly detailed information about disease.

One reason often given for withholding pain medication from a patient is the risk of addiction. The specter of drug addiction can be a powerful force that must be weighed when considering alleviation of pain. Now, however, pain management can be provided without the risk of addiction because of the availability of non-narcotic medications.

With all of these advances, it is most humane to make a patient in pain more comfortable. Administer analgesia and antiemetics per local medical control.

When you are providing pain management for GI problems, the goal should be to make the patient more comfortable, not to abolish the pain. Enough medication to completely remove the pain may result in severe hemodynamic compromise. The following five medications provide you with tools to manage abdominal pain.

- Meperidine hydrochloride (Demerol) 50 to 150 mg IV/IO/IM. This is a synthetic narcotic and therefore can cause hypotension and respiratory depression. This drug is often given with hydroxyzine to decrease its nausea side effects.
- Morphine 5 to 10 mg IV/IO/IM. This narcotic can cause hypotension and respiratory depression.
- Ketorolac (Toradol) 15 to 60 mg IV/IO/IM (IV dose not in excess of 30 mg). This medication is a non-narcotic and therefore does not tend to cause hypotension and respiratory depression.
- Nalbuphine (Nubain) 10 mg IV/IO/IM. This is a synthetic narcotic and therefore can cause hypotension and respiratory depression.

- Fentanyl (Sublimaze) 1 mcg/kg. This is a commonly used opioid agonist. It is very potent, rapid acting, and has a short half-life.

The following medications may be administered to address nausea:

- Ondansetron (Zofran) 0.4 mg IV/IO/IM. This medication should be administered slowly over at least 2 minutes.
- Diphenhydramine (Benadryl) 10 to 50 mg IV/IO/IM. This medication is typically used for allergic reactions, but also has antiemetic properties. Be cautious when using this medication because it can cause drowsiness and a drop in blood pressure.
- Hydroxyzine (Vistaril) 25 to 100 mg IM. Be cautious when administering this medication to patients who have taken any medication that has central nervous system (CNS) depressive effects. Hydroxyzine increases the CNS depressive effects of other medications.
- Promethazine (Phenergan) 12.5 to 25 mg IV/IO/IM. Be cautious when administering this medication to patients who have taken any medication that has CNS depressive effects. Like hydroxyzine, promethazine increases the CNS depressive effects of other medications. Also, this medication tends to cause a marked burning sensation during injection. Administer slowly.

Talk with the patient during your initial care and transport. Patient care is more than just administering medications and watching IV rates. Patients with GI complaints are often upset and embarrassed. Be kind and treat the patient with respect. When creating your documentation, try to be objective about your visual findings. Avoid terms like "covered in blood" when describing your visual findings of the patient and/or scene. It is best for you to use more descriptive sentences like, "Blood noted on the floor, toilet, and patient's clothing." "Patient's clothing saturated with blood" also helps the reader to understand the quantity that was seen.

Emergency Medical Care

If there is a sudden dramatic change in the patient's condition, repeat the assessments as if you were assessing a new patient. Starting from the beginning will give you the best chance of modifying your care to adequately manage any worrisome new developments.

Often there is little you can do about the GI disease itself, but you are able to care for the effects of the disease. Patients may have severe pain; they may be experiencing severe **dehydration**, hypotension, or extreme nausea. The patient may be thirsty, but you must inform the patient that he or she cannot have anything to eat or drink at this time. GI complaints can result in the need for surgery, and ingestion of food or drink could delay needed medical treatment. Your main goals are observation of standard precautions, maintenance of ABCs, and management of pain/nausea.

Airway Management

For the patient with GI problems, airway concerns include possible aspiration or obstruction of the airway because of the presence of vomit or blood. Although rare, these situations do pose real concerns for the paramedic.

- Place the patient so as to ensure adequate drainage of material out of the mouth. If trauma is considered, be prepared to tilt the long board. This means the patient must be packaged and padded well so spinal movement is minimized during the board movement.

YOU are the Medic   PART 3

Your patient has a past medical history for diabetes, hypertension, and atrial fibrillation. She is currently taking propranolol, diltiazem, warfarin, and glyburide. She has no allergies to medications. She has also been taking an over-the-counter bismuth solution hoping to relieve the pain.

Recording Time: 5 Minutes	
Respirations	20 breaths/min
Pulse	120 beats/min, lying down; 136 beats/min sitting
Skin	Cool, pale, moist
Blood pressure	106/82 mm Hg, lying down; 92/78 mm Hg, sitting
Oxygen saturation (Spo$_2$)	98% with oxygen at 15 L/min via nonrebreathing mask
Pupils	Equal and reactive

5. On the basis of the patient's orthostatic vital signs, what is your suggested treatment?

6. Which of the patient's medications are you most concerned with?

- Portable suction should be part of every department's "first in" equipment.
- Management of GI bleeding may require the use of a nasogastric tube. This tube, placed in the stomach, allows stomach contents to be removed via suctioning. Its use can be beneficial in patients with severe upper GI bleeding or to decompress the stomach.

Breathing

Breathing concerns are not common with GI problems. If breathing problems are present, they are often associated with a decreased hemoglobin level caused by bleeding.

- **Administer high-concentration oxygen.** Do not rely on oxygen saturation readings as evidence that oxygen is not needed. A patient who has been bleeding internally may have a severely decreased level of hemoglobin. The oxygen saturation may read 96%, but if the hemoglobin level is low, oxygen is still needed.
- **Prevent aspiration.** Oxygen masks can cause some patients to experience a sense of confinement. This is problematic with patients who are experiencing nausea. Monitor patients using a mask to ensure they are able to remove it quickly if they need to vomit.
- **Auscultate lung sounds.** Obtain baseline information and continue to monitor lung sounds to ensure the safe administration of fluids.

Circulation

The two main circulation concerns are dehydration and hemorrhage. In patients who are dehydrated, the overall goal of treatment is to refill the cellular space. The degree of hemodynamic stability will dictate whether to use a hypotonic or isotonic solution. A patient in stable condition should receive a hypotonic solution. A one-half normal saline solution will effectively move fluids from the vascular space into the interstitial and finally into the intracellular space, refilling the cells. In these patients, an infusion rate of 125 mL/h is usually sufficient to slowly rehydrate cells without causing dramatic swings in either fluid volume or electrolyte balance.

If the patient is more profoundly dehydrated, isotonic fluid would be needed to re-expand the vascular space first. Though the cells in this setting are dehydrated, the resultant decrease in blood volume can be life threatening, so refilling the vascular space takes priority over rehydrating the cells. This step is essential to ensuring adequate perfusion to the vital organs of the body. The guidelines for emergent filling of the vascular space and refilling the vascular space due to hemorrhage are the same.

As with the severely dehydrated patient, care for the patient with hemorrhaging is directed at maintaining perfusion of vital organs. This can be a rather controversial subject. Internal hemorrhaging falls into the category of hemorrhaging that cannot be controlled. Volume replacement is critical to ensuring adequate circulation to the vital organs. However, very aggressive volume replacement can result in dramatic

hemodilution (dilution of the blood). Without an adequate supply of blood, its oxygen supply, and clotting capabilities, the patient will die. As blood pressure falls, the amount of bleeding decreases; therefore, the body actually retains more blood. Low pressure equals decreased perfusion, *but* retention of clotting factors and hemoglobin. Titrate fluids to a blood pressure of 90 to 100 mm Hg; do not normalize the blood pressure.

If the blood pressure cannot be maintained at adequate levels to maintain peripheral perfusion, then you may need to consider the use of vasoactive medications. Dopamine and epinephrine are the two more common medications used in the prehospital setting for blood pressure support through vasoconstriction. These medications should only be used in circumstances where it has been determined that the patient has sufficient fluid volume to squeeze against. Fluid resuscitation should be accomplished before these medications are considered.

Once the patient arrives at the hospital, blood administration will be critical to stabilization. If you are assisting with an interfacility transfer, be prepared to manage blood products. Patients with GI bleeding often require blood replacement.

Words of Wisdom

When you are treating a patient who has had significant bleeding, remember that pulse oximetry reads the percentage of circulating hemoglobin that is saturated (typically with oxygen). If the patient's hemoglobin is 7 g/100 mL, the oxygen saturation may read 100%. This indicates that 100% of the available hemoglobin is saturated; however, if the patient has lost half of his or her blood supply, he or she would have half the normal amount of hemoglobin. This reading, then, is dangerously misleading.

Pathophysiology, Assessment, and Management of Specific Abdominal and Gastrointestinal Emergencies

The paramedic must have an understanding of many conditions to care effectively for the abdominal patient. Some of these conditions are difficult, if not impossible, to differentiate from one another in the prehospital setting. In addition, many of the conditions cannot be treated in the field. However, you must expend the effort to learn about each of them because EMS is changing, as are the demands being placed on paramedics.

In the near future, paramedics will be asked to help online medical directors decide if the patient should be transported to a hospital, to a family physician, or to a clinic or pharmacy, for example. The sophistication with which you assess patients must increase if you are to meet the demands of this new role. Another reason to change is economics. It is less expensive to have a paramedic safely triage a patient to a family physician or a clinic than to transport every patient to the emergency department.

The other main reason that you need to know about these conditions is patient education. How the body is maintained and how it functions are often key factors that affect whether a disease is well controlled or life threatening. GI conditions are no different. Patients make choices that can increase or diminish the severity of their diseases.

Consider the patient with cholecystitis. Medical experts would agree that such patients need to closely monitor the types of food they eat. If these patients eat very fatty meals, they are more likely to have an attack of pain and discomfort. Patients may need to try small amounts of fatty food to see which ones they should avoid. This education is essential to improving the well-being of patients with cholecystitis. By learning about GI diseases, you may be able to help patients make better choices so they can stay healthy.

Table 7 outlines the major diseases of the GI system, which will be discussed in the following pages. It provides information about each specific disease, its main cause, and its primary effects on the body.

Remember to consider hypovolemia when managing a GI emergency. Hypovolemia is caused by either dehydration or hemorrhage. Dehydration occurs from vomiting and/or diarrhea. As the patient loses fluid, the body continues to shift water from inside the cells to interstitial space and finally into the vascular space to maintain adequate fluid volume in the blood vessels, until the patient has reached the limits of effectively moving fluid.

During this process, electrolytes levels are also affected. Although persistent vomiting decreases the amount of food ingested, diarrhea causes more dramatic swings in the levels of electrolytes. The main electrolytes affected by diarrhea are sodium and potassium. Diarrhea can either increase or decrease electrolytes, depending on the water content of the diarrhea. Table 8 outlines the effects of electrolyte imbalances on the body.

The second cause of hypovolemia in GI patients is hemorrhage. Bleeding in the GI system typically occurs from either the rupture or the destruction of a structure. The GI system is well supplied with blood. This fact is essential to the underlying function of getting nutrients out of what is eaten and then transporting the nutrients to the cells that need replenishing. Without blood, the entire process of digestion would accomplish very little. This close proximity to the blood supply, however, makes damage to the GI system more likely to cause severe hemorrhage.

Trauma is an obvious mechanism for bleeding in the GI system. Other mechanisms include erosion of the protective mucosal layers, chemical destruction of tissue, and dilation of blood vessels. It is possible to experience a fatal hemorrhage from GI bleeding. The bleeding can occur slowly, over several

Table 7 Gastrointestinal Diseases by Type of Condition and Presenting Problem

Disease	Type of Condition	Common Presenting Problem
Acute gastroenteritis	Infectious	Diarrhea, dehydration, pain
Acute hepatitis	Infectious	Pain, liver failure
Appendicitis	Acute inflammation	Pain, sepsis
Bowel obstruction	Decreased motility	Pain, sepsis
Cholecystitis	Acute inflammation	Pain
Colitis	Chronic inflammation	Pain, diarrhea, dehydration
Crohn disease	Chronic inflammation	Pain, diarrhea, dehydration
Diverticulitis	Acute inflammation	Pain, sepsis
Esophagogastric varices	Hemorrhagic	Pain, hemorrhage
Gastroenteritis	Erosive	Diarrhea, dehydration, pain
Hemorrhoids	Hemorrhagic	Pain, hemorrhage
Pancreatitis	Acute inflammation	Pain, hemorrhage
Peptic ulcer disease	Erosive/ infectious	Pain, hemorrhage

Table 8 Electrolyte Imbalances Due to Diarrhea

Condition	Effects	Signs and Symptoms
Hyponatremia: Low sodium	Swelling of cells	Muscle weakness, cramps, coma, convulsions
Hypernatremia: High sodium	Shrinking of cells caused by excessive water loss	Coma, convulsions
Hypokalemia: Low potassium	More stimulation needed to fire nerve/muscle cells	Muscle cramps, weakness, paralysis, heart failure, dysrhythmia, prolonged Q-T interval, flattened T waves
Hyperkalemia: High potassium	Less stimulation needed to fire nerve/muscle cells	Muscle weakness and cramps, bradycardia, asystole, shortened Q-T interval, tented T waves

days or weeks, or it can be sudden, with a large volume of blood loss. In either case, assessment is the key to correctly identifying and treating these patients.

In patients with diarrhea or hemorrhage, an absolute loss of volume occurs. Consequently, classic signs and symptoms of shock are typically present. The brain is the first organ to show the effects of shock, and the patient becomes anxious and restless. Pale, cool, clammy skin and tachycardia are common. The pulse pressure is usually narrowed because the epinephrine causes vasoconstriction. The respiratory rate increases. All of these changes occur with a near-normal blood pressure. A drop in the patient's blood pressure indicates that a significant volume of blood has been lost, and the body's efforts to compensate have failed. Such a patient is critically ill. See the management section of each condition for advice on how to manage these problems.

Pathophysiology, Assessment, and Management of Gastrointestinal Bleeding

Bleeding in the GI tract is a symptom of another disease, not a disease itself. Causes of GI bleeding are shown in **Table 9**. The presentation differences between upper and lower GI bleeding are predominately related to the consistency and characteristics of the vomit and stool that may be present. Upper GI bleeding is far more common than lower GI bleeding.

Presentation of GI bleeding is variable. Each of the many conditions that can cause GI bleeding has its own pattern of disease progression. For example, diverticular disease has a rather gradual onset and tends to affect people in their 50s, 60s, or older. Mallory-Weiss syndrome has a sudden onset and affects people of any age. Gathering the information about how the patient moved from being healthy to needing an ambulance is critical in determining the correct field impression.

The patient's past medical history and other possible events of abdominal pain or bleeding from the GI tract are also important. Find out the medications the patient is taking. As previously mentioned, several medications can cause irritation to the GI tract, precipitating bleeding. Question the patient about the length of time he or she has been having complaints.

Treatment for the patient with GI bleeding consists of several general management guidelines. Fluid resuscitation is common. In most patients, even those with stable vital signs, it is prudent to establish an IV line, providing 1,000 mL of normal saline solution or lactated Ringer's using a macro drip tubing. This type of IV will allow you to quickly resuscitate the patient with fluids should conditions change. Specific conditions that cause GI bleeding will be discussed next.

Upper Gastrointestinal Bleeding: Esophagogastric Varices

Pathophysiology

Esophagogastric varices are caused by pressure increases in the blood vessels that surround the esophagus and stomach. These esophageal blood vessels drain into the portal system.

Table 9 Gastrointestinal Bleeding by Organ and Cause

Organ	Causes	Location	Substances
Esophagus	Inflammation (esophagitis) Varices Tear (Mallory-Weiss syndrome) Cancer Dilated veins (cirrhosis, liver disease) Gastroesophageal reflux disease (GERD)	Upper GI	Melena, hematemesis, Vomitus with gross blood
Stomach	Ulcers Cancer Inflammation (**gastritis**)	Upper GI	Melena, hematemesis, vomitus with gross blood
Small Intestine	Ulcer (duodenal)	Upper GI	Melena, hematemesis, vomitus with gross blood
	Cancer Inflammation (irritable bowel disease)	Upper or Lower GI	Melena, hematemesis, vomitus with gross blood
Large Intestine	Infections	Lower GI bleed	Hematochezia
	Inflammation (ulcerative colitis) Colorectal polyps Colorectal cancer Diverticular disease		
Rectum	Hemorrhoids	Lower GI bleeding	Hematochezia, gross bleeding

However, if the liver is damaged and blood cannot flow through it easily, the blood will begin to back up into the portal vessels, which can ultimately lead to rupture of the vessels. In the Westernized world, alcohol used to be the main cause of **portal hypertension**. Today, hepatitis C is the primary cause.

Assessment

Presentation of esophagogastric varices has a two-fold appearance. Initially, the patient exhibits signs of liver disease. Examples include fatigue, weight loss, jaundice, anorexia, an edematous abdomen, **pruritus**, abdominal pain, nausea, and vomiting. The disease process is gradual, taking months to years to reach a state of extreme discomfort.

Rupture of the varices is far more sudden. The patient will report an abrupt onset of discomfort in the throat. He or she may have severe dysphagia, vomiting of bright red blood, hypotension, and signs of shock. If the bleeding is less dramatic, <u>hematemesis</u> and <u>melena</u> are likely. Regardless of the speed of bleeding, damage to these vessels can be life threatening. The patient's hemoglobin level and hematocrit value will drop. These laboratory results can help determine the severity of the hemorrhaging. As with any patient who has liver disease, elevated levels of liver enzymes (alanine aminotransferase [ALT] and aspartate aminotransferase [AST]) should be expected.

Management

Treatment for these patients in the prehospital setting includes use of the general management guideline. As with any GI bleeding disorder, accurate assessment of the degree of blood loss is critical. Be prepared for a hemodynamically unstable patient needing volume resuscitation and aggressive suctioning of the airway. If the patient's level of consciousness begins to decrease, consider securing the airway to prevent aspiration.

In-hospital treatment involves stopping the bleeding and aggressive fluid resuscitation. It may be necessary to perform an <u>endoscopy</u>. In this procedure, an endoscope is advanced into the esophagus and a flexible fiberoptic tube is advanced into the stomach. Internal structures can then be seen, and specimens can be taken. The physician will then attempt to control the bleeding directly at the site of hemorrhage by either using chemicals to cauterize the bleeding veins or a type of rubber band to constrict them. Once bleeding has been controlled, surgical management may be an option. If the primary problem is liver failure, the only real cure for this condition may be liver transplantation.

◼ Upper Gastrointestinal Bleeding: Mallory-Weiss Syndrome

Pathophysiology

<u>Mallory-Weiss syndrome</u> is a special type of esophageal condition in which severe hemorrhage can occur. In this condition, the junction between the esophagus and the stomach tears, causing severe bleeding and potentially death. The reason for the tearing is that during the act of vomiting, pressure in the stomach can increase so greatly as to cause a failure of the structure of the esophagus. Mallory-Weiss syndrome affects both men and women equally. It tends to occur in older adults and older children.

Assessment

The presentation is linked to vomiting. In women, it may be associated with hyperemesis gravidarum, a condition of severe vomiting related to pregnancy. The extent of the bleeding can be small, resulting in little blood loss to severe bleeding and extreme hypovolemia. In extreme cases, patients will have signs and symptoms of shock, epigastric abdominal pain, hematemesis, and melena.

Management

Management is the same as with esophagogastric varices and is directed at determining the extent of blood loss. In this case, the patient may be dehydrated from the repeated vomiting so blood loss can be exaggerated in its effects. In-hospital management may include volume resuscitation as needed, endoscopy to visualize the extent of the damage, and possibly an attempt to repair the tear. However, in most patients with Mallory-Weiss syndrome, the tears will resolve spontaneously.

◼ Upper Gastrointestinal Bleeding: Peptic Ulcer Disease

Pathophysiology

The stomach and duodenum are subjected to high levels of acidity. To help prevent damage, protective layers of mucous line both organs. In <u>peptic ulcer disease (PUD)</u>, the protective layer has been eroded, allowing the acid to eat into the organ itself. This erosion typically occurs over weeks, months, or even years.

PUD was once thought to be related to a person's diet. However, there are many cultures worldwide that have a diet far spicier than the typical American diet. If spiciness by itself were the cause of stomach ulcers, a higher prevalence of ulcers would be expected in those countries rather than in England, Norway, or the United States. In fact, the reverse is true—PUD is more common in developing countries.

PUD, which affects men and women equally, is now known to come from a variety of causes. The most common cause is an infection of the stomach with the bacterium *Helicobacter pylori*. Another major cause is erosive gastritis. The chronic use of NSAIDs is the most frequent cause of this condition, in which the mucosal lining of the stomach slowly erodes and ulcerates. Patients who have sustained severe burns or other types of trauma are susceptible to this disease. These extreme stress states increase gastric acid production. Alcohol and smoking can also affect the severity of PUD by increasing gastric acidity.

> ### Special Populations
>
> Older adults are more vulnerable to the primary and secondary causes of peptic ulcer disease (PUD). As a result, PUD tends to affect an older population. As people age, the immune system's ability to fight infection decreases, making infection with *Helicobacter pylori* more likely. In addition, older adults frequently use NSAID medications for arthritis and other musculoskeletal conditions. Thus, older adults are more likely to develop erosive gastritis.

Assessment

Patients will experience a classic sequence of pain in the stomach that subsides or diminishes immediately after eating and then reemerges 2 to 3 hours later. The pain is described as burning or gnawing. Nausea, vomiting, belching, and heartburn are common. If the erosion is severe, gastric bleeding can occur with the result of hematemesis and melena.

Management

The major focus for prehospital management is for you to accurately assess the degree of blood loss and prepare to manage any hypotension that is present. Orthostatic vital signs are critical in determining fluid needs and transportation/packaging issues.

In-hospital management will include acid neutralization and reduction therapies. Antibiotic therapy is often effective at stopping any new erosion. Management for erosion of the GI tract will be tailored to the degree of damage to the GI tract. Patients will often undergo endoscopy of the esophagus. The stomach wall can then be directly assessed for damage. Surgical repair of the damaged stomach lining in concert with medication therapy are often effective.

■ Upper Gastrointestinal Bleeding: Gastroesophageal Reflux Disease (GERD)

Pathophysiology

Gastroesophageal reflux disease (GERD) is a condition in which the sphincter between the esophagus and the stomach opens, allowing stomach acid to move superiorly. This condition, also referred to as acid reflux disease, can cause a burning sensation within the chest (heartburn). Various factors can make some people more prone to this condition. Smoking, obesity, and pregnancy all increase the chances of GERD. Eating fatty fried foods, drinking alcohol, and eating citrus fruits are also factors that are associated with GERD. If the reflux continues over a long period of time, damage can occur to the esophageal wall. This damage could result in weakened portions that are more prone to bleeding.

Assessment

Heartburn is the predominant clinical finding for this condition. This pain may be increased with positional changes—sitting upright is preferred whereas lying flat makes the condition worse. Some patients may not have pain, but experience coughing or have difficulty swallowing. Bleeding can occur if the damage is long term, resulting in hematemesis and melena.

Management

Prehospital treatment is supportive in nature. Medical treatment is focused on decreasing the acidity of the material within the esophagus by neutralizing it or preventing the acid from being produced. Antacids, proton pump inhibitors, and H$_2$ blockers are the common classifications of medications used for this condition. If these medications fail to control the discomfort, then surgical repair may be needed.

One confounding circumstance that can occur is when the patient with a history of GERD begins to have a myocardial infarction. Such a patient may confuse the pain in his or her chest with GERD. Patients may begin to self-medicate, taking large amounts of antacid to try to control the pain. If you have a patient who reports chest pain and has a white "milk moustache," the coating around his or her mouth may be an antacid. Ask how much antacid the patient has taken. Large amounts of antacid can cause metabolic alkalosis.

■ Lower Gastrointestinal Bleeding: Hemorrhoids

Pathophysiology

A number of conditions can cause lower GI bleeding. Hemorrhoids are a type of GI bleeding that results from the swelling and inflammation of the blood vessels surrounding the rectum. These are a common problem. By the age of 50 years, nearly one half of all people have experienced or continue to experience problems from hemorrhoids. These can be caused by either conditions that increase pressure on the rectum or cause irritation of the rectum. Pregnancy, straining at stool, and chronic constipation cause increased pressure. Anal intercourse and diarrhea cause irritation and lower GI bleeding.

Assessment

Hemorrhoids present with bright red blood during defecation. This hematochezia, or gross bleeding, tends to be minimal and is easily controlled. Additionally, patients may experience itching and a small mass on the rectum. Typically this mass is a clot formed in response to the mild bleeding.

Management

Prehospital management is supportive. In isolation, hemorrhoids are more of an inconvenience than they are a life-threatening condition. Some patients may be at greater risk for serious consequences. Cautiously assess the patient who has any bleeding disorder or is taking anticoagulants. In this setting, even a minor bleeding problem can become life threatening. To ensure the patient is hemodynamically stable, obtain orthostatic vital signs.

Most hemorrhoids will resolve within 2 to 3 days, even without treatment. In-hospital management may include creams to help shrink the inflamed tissues. If the condition becomes chronic, surgical removal is a possibility. The best management for hemorrhoids is prevention, which includes eating a high-fiber diet.

■ Lower Gastrointestinal Bleeding: Anal Fissures

Pathophysiology

Another cause of lower GI bleeding is anal fissures. These are linear tears to the mucosal lining in and near the anus Figure 10. The exact reason why a fissure is created near the anus is unclear. It is thought to be precipitated by the passage of large, hard stools. Patients who have diets that are low in raw fruits and vegetables are at highest risk.

Assessment

Patients present with painful defecation. There may be a small amount of bright red blood noted on the toilet paper, but rarely do these fissures cause significant blood loss. The pain persists

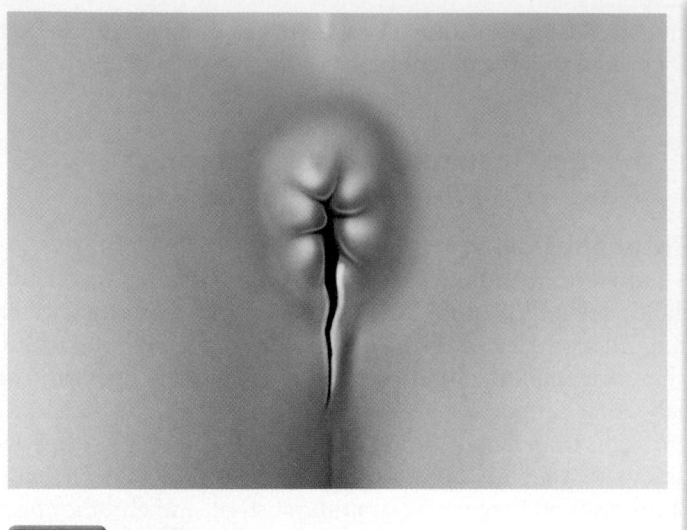

Figure 10 Anal fissures.

for several minutes to several hours after the bowel movement. Any time this area is stretched, the fissure stretches, causing pain and more tearing. Pain is common with every bowel movement.

This pain creates a vicious cycle. Because it hurts to have a bowel movement, patients delay as long as possible. This delay causes the feces to become larger and harder, thus making them more difficult to pass. Eventually, when the movement is inevitable, the large stool causes more stretching, more tearing, and consequently more pain. This painful bowel movement precipitates an even greater reluctance to have a bowel movement.

Management

Treatment of anal fissures is the same as for hemorrhoids: supportive care. To facilitate patient comfort, a 5 × 9 dressing can be placed over the patient's anus to help pad the area. Do not under any circumstances pack dressings into the fissure or the anus. Remember, bleeding for this condition, as with hemorrhoids, is typically minimal and non-life threatening.

The next section will discuss acute inflammatory conditions and chronic inflammatory conditions.

■ Pathophysiology, Assessment, and Management of Acute Inflammatory Conditions

Inflammation is a natural response to injury. If the body is attacked by one of the infectious agents discussed in the previous section, then vasodilation, mobilization of white blood cells, and changes in cellular metabolic processes will result. All of these effects allow the cell to move from a normal operating mode into one of being under siege. The purpose of inflammation is to assist the white blood cells in either destroying the invading agent or, at the least, seal it off so it cannot spread.

The redness, swelling, and tenderness that occur during an infection are the result of inflammation. The change in vascular permeability and vasodilation will cause redness and swelling.

Swelling can cause pressure, which causes pain. Vasodilation and increased capillary permeability enable white blood cells to more effectively get to the area of damage.

Inflammation in the GI system can occur at many levels. Localized inflammation will cause localized signs and symptoms. For example, patients with <u>hepatitis</u>, an inflammation of the liver, can experience pain in the right upper quadrant of the abdomen. This pain can be due to mild swelling of the liver. In <u>peritonitis</u>, inflammation and irritation occurs to the peritoneum throughout the abdomen, so the patient may experience generalized pain that is rebound in nature. If the inflammation is caused by an infectious agent, the peritonitis can be a sign of movement of bacteria into the abdomen and eventually into the bloodstream. This infection is called sepsis.

The body will respond to sepsis with a more generalized inflammatory response. One of the severe consequences of sepsis is the depletion of resources to manage the infection. In sepsis, infection is almost literally everywhere in the body. The body is trying to fight many battles but does not have adequate white blood cells, histamine, blood, and energy. Soon the battles being fought are inadequate, resulting in possible detriment to the patient. If a balance between resource demand and supply cannot soon be restored, death will occur.

Many of the diseases of the GI system are caused by inflammation. The difference is there is no defined reason for the inflammation. The body is attacking and killing its own cells. This is referred to as an autoimmune condition.

There are a variety of reasons postulated for this misdirected attack, but no conclusive cause and effect relationship has been found. One theory is that the patient ingests some type of food with a little-known antigen present. This protein substance is identified as foreign and antibodies are created. Another speculation is the patient comes in contact with a virus that triggers an immune response. White blood cells begin to destroy a portion of the GI system, causing damage. The body works to rebuild the damaged areas, but scarred portions of the GI tract may result.

■ Cholecystitis and Biliary Tract Disorders

Pathophysiology

<u>Biliary tract disorders</u> involve inflammation of the gallbladder. Biliary tract disorders are a group of conditions including <u>cholangitis</u>, an inflammation of the bile duct; <u>cholelithiasis</u>, the presence of stones within the gallbladder; <u>cholecystitis</u>, inflammation of the gallbladder; and <u>acalculus cholecystitis</u>, inflammation of the gallbladder without the presence of gallstones. Cholangitis can cause acalculus cholecystitis.

It is unclear why gallstones are formed; it is believed to be either due to increased production of bile or decreased emptying of the gallbladder. Other causes of gallbladder inflammation arise from decreased flow of biliary materials. These include major trauma, sepsis, sickle cell disease, and prolonged fasting.

Women have cholecystitis two to three times more often than men. Caucasians have a higher prevalence than do African

Americans. Other persons at risk are older people and people who are overweight or obese or have had a recent extreme weight loss.

The gallbladder's function is to store bile, an enzyme used to break down fat, and then contract, releasing that bile. When fatty foods are present in the duodenum, the gallbladder contracts, but if a blockage is present, extreme pain in the right upper quadrant, radiating to the right shoulder, will occur. This pain can be quite severe. In addition to the pain, the patient may demonstrate a positive Murphy sign. Nausea, vomiting, fever, jaundice, and tachycardia are also present with this disease.

Assessment

The presentation of this condition also takes on a pattern. The classic pattern is for the patient to have no pain until a fatty meal is eaten. Two to three hours later the patient begins to develop severe upper right quadrant abdominal pain. This pattern is not absolute. The variability in presentation is based on the consistency of the food that is eaten. A fatty steak will remain in the stomach longer than a cheesy casserole. The faster the food is emptied from the stomach, the sooner the pain begins after the meal.

Management

Prehospital treatment for this condition is directed at making the patient comfortable. Rarely is this condition life threatening, though the pain from cholecystitis can make the patient experience vasovagal stimulation.

Medications to control pain include meperidine and morphine. There is some contention about which medication is best to use for this condition. Morphine is believed to cause a contraction of the sphincter of Oddi, the valve controlling bile movement out of the gallbladder. This contraction can increase pain in this condition. To be cautious, meperidine is an acceptable alternative. Nausea should be controlled using the medications listed earlier. IV fluids are also indicated because the patient is often vomiting.

In-hospital treatment will include antibiotics, pain medication, ultrasound, and potential removal of the gallbladder through surgery.

◼ Appendicitis

Pathophysiology

Appendicitis is a condition most people are familiar with and it is a frequent cause of acute abdomen. The condition occurs when fecal matter or other material accumulates in the appendix. When the organ can no longer flush out this material normally, pressure builds. This pressure decreases the flow of blood and lymph fluid, hindering the body's ability to fight infection. The combination of bacteria in the feces and diminished ability to combat local infection creates an ideal environment for the uncontrolled reproduction of bacteria. If left unchecked, over-pressurization of the appendix will eventually cause it to rupture, resulting in peritonitis, sepsis, and death.

Appendicitis occurs in every age group. The peak time for the occurrence of this condition is during adolescence. Though the elderly experience appendicitis less often, they have a higher mortality rate. Men are slightly more prone to appendicitis than women.

Assessment

The presentation of appendicitis can be divided into three stages: early, ripe, and rupture.

- **Early.** Periumbilical pain. Nausea, vomiting, low-grade fever, loss of appetite.
- **Ripe.** Pain in lower right quadrant (McBurney's point)
- **Rupture.** Decrease in pain (decreased pressure); generalized pain, rebound tenderness

In early stages, patients classically present with poorly defined periumbilical pain. Nausea, vomiting, anorexia, and a low-grade fever are typically present. The vomiting tends to occur after the pain starts and not before. Over several hours, the appendix will swell and eventually pressure will increase. This takes approximately 48 to 72 hours. The patient is now in the ripe stage. During this time, the pain will migrate to localized right lower quadrant pain and become more severe. If the appendix ruptures, the rupture stage is entered.

In this stage, at first there may be a sudden decrease of pain with a sense of relief because of the sudden decreased pressure. Now the infectious material has access to the entire abdominal cavity. During this stage the pain becomes generalized throughout the abdomen. Rebound tenderness is a sign of perforation of the appendix with resultant peritonitis. Dunphy sign, severe abdominal pain in the right lower quadrant with coughing, is another way for you to evaluate the patient for peritonitis.

Additional diagnostic information can be obtained through blood work and imaging studies. Patients with appendicitis will have an elevated white blood cell count (WBC) and C-reactive protein levels. C-reactive protein is a chemical created by the liver in response to infection or inflammation. Ultrasonography and CT scans provide the physician with images of the abdomen and are valuable in diagnosing appendicitis.

Management

Prehospital management of appendicitis should include a cautious assessment for septicemia. If this blood infection is present, septic shock can occur. Volume resuscitation may not be adequate to restore blood pressure. Be prepared to use dopamine if crystalloids are not effective. Administration of pain and antinausea medications are clearly indicated with these patients.

In-hospital treatment includes antibiotics and typically surgical removal of the appendix.

◼ Diverticulitis

Pathophysiology

To understand diverticulitis, you must first know what a diverticulum is—a weak area in the colon that begins to have small outcroppings that turn into pouches. These pockets are called diverticula (the plural of *diverticulum*). The condition of having diverticula is referred to as diverticulosis. When these diverticula become inflamed, it is called diverticulitis.

What causes these pouches is unclear, but research has shown that people in the Westernized world tend to get diverticulitis, whereas people from Africa and Asia do not. The disease was first recognized around 1900, when the type of foods people were eating began to dramatically change. The amount of fiber in the US diet plummeted as the amount of processed foods eaten increased.

What is believed is that as the amount of fiber in a person's diet decreases, the consistency of the normal stool becomes more solid. This hard stool takes more contractions to move and subsequently increases colon pressure. In this environment, small defects in the colonic wall that would otherwise never pose a problem now fail, resulting in bulges in the wall.

The next step is similar to appendicitis. As feces travel through the colon, some may be trapped in the pouch. Bacteria can grow and cause localized inflammation and infection. As the body attempts to manage this infection, scarring, adhesions, and even fistulas can develop. A __fistula__ is an abnormal connection between two cavities. The common location for fistulas in diverticulitis is between the colon and the bladder. Significant infections can develop from having feces in the bladder.

The typical patient is older than 60 years. More important than sex or race is the amount of fiber in the patient's diet. Decreased amounts of fiber increase the patient's risk for this disease.

Assessment

Presentation of diverticulitis is abdominal pain that tends to be localized to the left side of the lower abdomen. Classic signs of infection include: fever, malaise, body aches, chills, nausea, and vomiting. Bleeding is rare with this condition. Patients can have either diarrhea or constipation. Because of the local infections of these pouches, adhesions can develop, thus narrowing the diameter of the colon. This can result in constipation, and potentially bowel obstruction. Though this condition typically results in left-sided pain, the problem can occur anywhere within the colon. Thus, diverticulitis can look like many other abdominal pain conditions.

Management

Management of this condition is directed at making the patient comfortable. Examine the patient closely to ensure severe infection is not present. Sepsis can occur easily in patients with fistulas to the urinary bladder. These patients may need large amounts of fluids and/or dopamine to maintain blood pressure. The general management guidelines will assist in helping the patient's comfort. In-hospital treatment will include antibiotics, allowing the GI tract to rest by giving the patient a liquid diet, and possibly surgery to remove the pouches and repair any fistulas.

■ Pancreatitis

Pathophysiology

The enzymes the pancreas creates are designed to break down the food into substances that can be absorbed by the intestines. If the tube carrying these enzymes becomes blocked, the enzymes will perform their chemical process on the protein and fat of the pancreas itself. This is referred to as *autodigestion of the pancreas.*

Autodigestion leads to inflammation of the pancreas, or __pancreatitis__. This process can occur suddenly or over many months. Patients can have single attacks or episodic attacks and remissions for a long time. Men tend to have this condition more commonly than women. It also occurs more often in African Americans aged 35 to 64 years. The main causes of this condition are increased alcohol consumption and gallstones. Other causes include medication reactions, trauma, cancer, and high triglyceride levels.

Assessment

The pain of this condition tends to be localized to the epigastric area or right upper abdomen. It can be sharp and may be quite severe. Radiation of the pain to the back is not uncommon. In addition to the pain, the patient may experience nausea,

YOU *are the Medic* | PART 4 |

You establish an IV line and administer a 250-mL fluid challenge after listening to lung sounds in all fields. The patient continues to report abdominal pain, which she describes as an 8 on a 1:10 scale. The patient is still unable to sit up and appears restless.

Recording Time: 10 Minutes	
Respirations	18 breaths/min
Pulse	110 mm Hg, lying down
Skin	Cool, pale, moist
Blood pressure	110/86 mm Hg, lying down
Oxygen saturation (Spo$_2$)	98% with oxygen at 15 L/min via nonrebreathing mask
Pupils	Equal and reactive

7. Knowing that your patient has postural vital signs, how are you going to move the patient downstairs?

8. Should you administer a pain medication to make your patient more comfortable?

vomiting, fever, tachycardia, hypotension, and muscle spasms in the extremities. This condition tends to cause hypocalcemia, low blood calcium, which can lead to muscle spasms.

The most alarming concern of this condition is internal hemorrhage. If autodigestion is advanced, blood vessels in and near the pancreas can be compromised. Severe and uncontrolled hemorrhage can ensue. In these patients, hemodynamic instability can be present. In addition, Cullen sign (bruising around the umbilicus) **Figure 11** or Grey Turner sign (bruising in the flanks) **Figure 12** may be present, indicating severe internal bleeding.

Laboratory findings of importance with this condition include lipase and amylase levels. These levels are indicative of pancreatic damage: the higher the levels the more severe the damage. Also important would be hemoglobin and hematocrit to determine the extent of any potential hemorrhage.

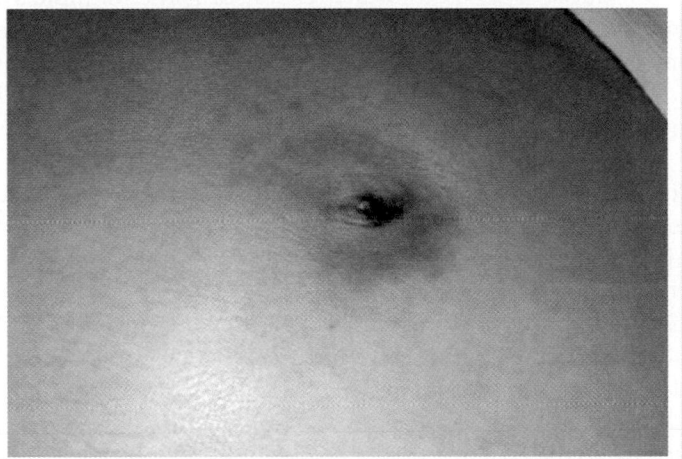

Figure 11 Periumbilical ecchymosis, or Cullen sign, indicating intraperitoneal hemorrhage.

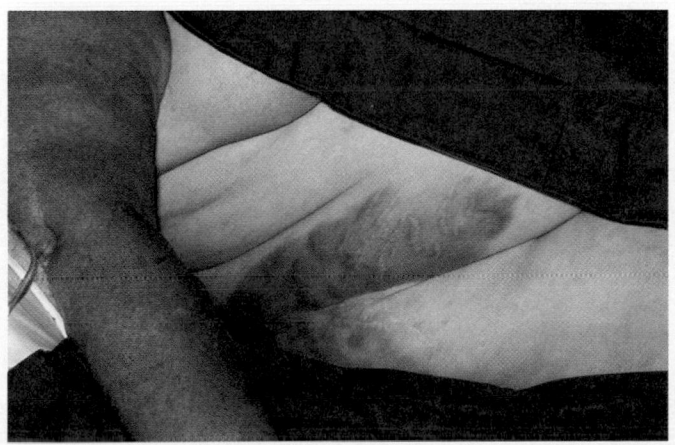

Figure 12 Flank ecchymosis, or Grey Turner sign, indicating retroperitoneal hemorrhage.

Management

Treatment for the prehospital patient with pancreatitis should be directed by general management guidelines. Pay special attention to assessing the patient for signs of severe hemorrhage. If present, begin fluid resuscitation. Because some of these patients will also have gallstones, the most conservative choice for the management of abdominal pain is meperidine. Morphine may cause spasms of the gallbladder, thus increasing the patient's pain.

In-hospital management includes GI rest and fluid resuscitation. In some patients, antibiotics and surgery can be helpful. Though the pancreas cannot be removed unless it is immediately replaced (ie, during a transplant), surgery can be done to control bleeding or manage the gallstones and subsequent blockage of bile from the liver.

■ Pathophysiology, Assessment, and Management of Chronic Inflammatory Conditions

■ Ulcerative Colitis

Pathophysiology

Ulcerative colitis is caused by inflammation of the colon. The inflammation is generalized and does not occur in patches, as in Crohn disease. It is unclear what causes the chronic inflammation, though genetics, stress, and autoimmunity have been speculated. In this condition, the inflammation causes a thinning of the wall of the intestine, resulting in a weakened, dilated rectum. This damaged lining of the colon is now prone to infections by bacteria and bleeding. These two states establish the foundation on which the signs and symptoms develop.

In the typical patient with ulcerative colitis, the disease peaks between ages 15 and 25 years and then again between 55 and 65 years. It occurs more often in women than men. There is a strong family history component for this disease with 20% of patients reporting a family member with this disease. This fact reinforces that genetics plays some role in this disease. The disease is more prevalent in Caucasians and people of Jewish descent.

Assessment

The presentation of this condition is gradual onset of bloody diarrhea, hematochezia, and mild to severe abdominal pain. Other signs and symptoms can be joint pain and skin lesions. These effects lend credence to the idea of an autoimmune component to the disease. Finally, the patient can experience fever, fatigue, and loss of appetite from the infection.

Management

Management consists of determining the degree of hemodynamic instability. Look for signs of shock. If the diarrhea and bleeding have caused sufficient volume loss to make the patient's condition unstable, administer fluids to return the patient to a near-normal volume balance. Otherwise, care is supportive. Follow the general management guideline.

In-hospital care for these patients will include anti-inflammatory medications, antibiotics, antidiarrheals, and potentially surgical removal of the diseased sections of the colon. This is a long-term disease where many people have periods of diarrhea and abdominal pain for years. A large number of these patients will have part of their colon removed.

Irritable Bowel Syndrome

Pathophysiology

Irritable bowel syndrome (IBS) is a condition in which patients have abdominal pain and changes in their bowel habits. One diagnostic criterion is that patients have pain at least 3 days a month for at least 3 months. The pathology of the disease is unclear. The following three main factors are prevalent in patients with IBS.

- Hypersensitivity of bowel pain receptors. Normal stretching of the bowel can cause pain in these patients.
- Hyperresponsiveness of the smooth muscles in the bowel. This produces the cramping sensations and diarrhea.
- Psychiatric disorder connection and irritable bowel syndrome. It is unclear if the bowel disorder causes the psychiatric disorder or vice versa.

Hyperresponsiveness of the bowel in irritable bowel syndrome can cause areas of spasm. These spasms can stop fecal movement, creating constipation and bloating. Conversely, if the spasms are more wavelike than localized, the patient can experience diarrhea as the feces are moved quickly through the bowel.

Patients typically begin to have problems with bowel habits during childhood. In Western countries, women are more prone to this disease. Interestingly, in the Indian subcontinent, the typical patient is a man. This condition strikes most cultures evenly.

This condition can be triggered by various stimuli. Stress, large meals, and certain foods, such as wheat, rye, chocolate, alcohol, milk products, and caffeinated drinks, can trigger an attack.

Assessment

IBS is a chronic condition. Prehospital presentations will typically involve a flare-up of the condition. Patients may present with abdominal pain or discomfort. This pain is relieved by a bowel movement. When the pain starts, there is usually a change in the frequency and consistency of bowel movements. Patients may experience diarrhea, steatorrhea, or constipation. They may also feel bloated.

Management

Management of these patients is supportive. The paramedic must understand that a coexisting psychiatric condition may be present. Be kind and compassionate. Do not minimize the patient's pain or discomfort. Your assessment must include the patient's mood and thought content. Consider whether the patient is severely depressed. If depression and/or suicide are noted, treat those accordingly. Analgesia may be needed in patients with irritable bowel syndrome.

Crohn Disease

Pathophysiology

Crohn disease is similar to ulcerative colitis; however, the entire GI tract can be involved. The main part of the GI tract that tends to be involved is the ileum. This is the last portion of the small intestine before it joins the large intestine. There are several theories as to the cause, though no definitive cause has been identified.

The typical patients are between 20 and 30 years. Men are diagnosed as often as women. African Americans tend not to have this condition whereas people of Jewish descent have an increased incidence.

Of interest with Crohn disease and colitis is the presence of signs and symptoms outside the GI system. This evidence helps to support the theory that an autoimmune component is operating within this disease. It is unclear what is causing this immune reaction. Does the presence of antigens in the GI tract trigger an immune response? Is the immune system itself is not working correctly? Another theory is that the immune system creates antibodies for an antigen that does not exist, thus creating a cascade of reactions to a nonexistent invader.

Family history and genetics play a role with this disease. Medical researchers are discovering that how the body is made and how it is able to function are important characteristics in whether a person gets a disease and how that disease progresses. The fact that many of the people with Crohn disease have family members who have some type of bowel disease suggests a familial/genetic component. Crohn disease helps prove most conditions are both nature and nurture.

Regardless of the underlying reason, the result is a series of attacks by the immune system on the GI tract. This activity of white blood cells damages all layers of the portion of GI tract involved. The result is most often a scarred, narrowed, stiff, and weakened portion of the small intestine. This patch of damage is found among areas of intestine that are normal. This narrowing can cause bowel obstruction.

Assessment

Patients with this condition present with a chronic complaint of abdominal pain, often in the lower right area. This pain corresponds to the location of the ileum. Rectal bleeding, weight loss, diarrhea, arthritis, skin problems, and fever may also be present with this condition. Bleeding tends to be small amounts over a long period of time. Acute severe hemorrhage is rare, but chronic bleeding resulting in anemia and hypotension does occur. Patients can have episodes of mild to severe signs and symptoms.

Management

Management in the prehospital setting is focused on the general management guideline. Volume resuscitation may be needed if diarrhea and chronic hemorrhage are occurring. Control of nausea and pain are commonly required by patients with Crohn disease. In-hospital care will focus on stopping the inflammation, correcting any fluid imbalances that are present, managing infections, and creating an environment where the GI tract can heal itself. The damage to the intestines can at times be so severe that surgical removal of portions is needed.

■ Pathophysiology, Assessment, and Management of Acute Infectious Conditions

Many foods are teeming with bacteria, viruses, and fungi. These microorganisms are present throughout the food chain. Infections in the GI system typically occur either when contaminated food is ingested or when the GI tract ruptures. For a person to become ill, either the immune system is overwhelmed by the number or complexity of the organism, or the immune system is weakened and cannot effectively defend the body.

Most people who become ill have stomach aches, vomiting, or diarrhea. According to the Centers for Disease Control and Prevention, in the United States, it is estimated that 48 million people will contract a foodborne illness every year. Of this group, 3,000 will die; in other words, only 0.006% of those who become ill, die. So what makes that small group different from the vast majority? People who are immunocompromised, very old, and very young generally have a more difficult time combating an infection of any type. Types of patients who are immunocompromised would include people with AIDS or certain types of cancers, people undergoing chemotherapy, and transplant patients.

In the United States, the food chain is very clean. Compared with other countries, the number of people who fall ill or die of foodborne disease is low. Traveling to other countries can place patients at greater risk for food intolerances or foodborne infections. Traveler's diarrhea can occur in as many as 33% of all people who travel to countries where food cleanliness is less than adequate. Travel within North America and Europe is generally safer than travel throughout South America, Asia, and Africa in terms of the risk of foodborne illness.

Damage to the GI system is another way infection can occur. A breach in the container allows GI contents filled with organisms to move into the surrounding tissues. In appendicitis, feces moving through the intestines become trapped in the appendix. The normal flushing of this structure is now prevented and fecal bacteria multiply. Pus and gas—by-products of bacterial activity—can cause pressure on the appendix. If the pressure is too high, the structure will fail, spilling material laden with pus and feces into the peritoneum. This can cause peritonitis, or inflammation of the protective lining of the abdominal cavity. The major symptom of peritonitis is severe pain, and the chief clinical signs are abdominal tenderness and distention.

Regardless of the cause, the body will begin to defend itself. Fever will develop in an attempt to slow down reproduction of the invading organism. White blood cells will be directed to the site of infection to attack the invaders. The patient will begin to feel malaise, weakness, chills, and a decreased ability to concentrate. Abdominal pain is another symptom. If the pain is caused by an infection in the peritoneum, rebound tenderness may be present. As the infection continues to multiply, it can leave the confines of the peritoneum or GI system and can enter the bloodstream. Once in the bloodstream, the invading organism is able to infect distant portions of the body. This is referred to as *sepsis*. Sepsis and its hemodynamic complications will be discussed in the chapter, *Infectious Diseases*.

■ Acute Gastroenteritis

Pathophysiology
Acute gastroenteritis is a family of conditions all revolving around a central theme of infection with fever, abdominal pain, diarrhea, nausea, and vomiting. These illnesses can be caused by a wide variety of organisms, as shown in Table 10. These agents typically enter the body via the fecal-oral route through contaminated food or water.

Cholera, relatively unknown in the United States, is common in other parts of the world. The norovirus virus is responsible for most cases of acute viral gastroenteritis in adults, whereas rotavirus causes the same condition in children. Various parasites may be contracted by swimming in water contaminated with them.

Assessment
Depending on the organism involved, patients may begin to experience GI upset and diarrhea in as little as several hours or days after contact with the contaminated food or water. The disease can run its course in 2 to 3 days or continue for several weeks.

The presentation involves diarrhea of various types. Patients can experience large dumping type diarrhea or frequent small liquid stools. The diarrhea can contain blood and/or pus, and it may have a foul odor or be odorless. Abdominal cramping is frequent as hyperperistalsis continues. Nausea and vomiting, fever, and anorexia are also present.

If the diarrhea continues, dehydration and hemodynamic instability will result. As the volume of fluid loss increases, the likelihood of potassium and sodium imbalance also increases. You should be watching for changes in level of consciousness and other profound signs of shock, which clearly indicate a critical volume loss.

Table 10 Gastroenteritis: Causative Organisms

Type of Organism	Organism
Viruses	*Norovirus*: Norwalk virus *Rotavirus*
Parasites	*Giardia lamblia* (protozoan) *Cryptosporidium parvum* *Cyclospora cayetanensis*
Bacteria	*Escherichia coli* *Klebsiella pneumonia* *Enterobacter* *Campylobacter jejuni* *Vibrio cholera* *Shigella* *Salmonella*

Management

Prehospital management is directed by the general management guideline. Special attention should be paid to determining the degree of fluid deficit the patient is experiencing. If the patient's condition is stable, one-half normal saline solution may be indicated to begin rehydration. Additionally, patients often feel markedly better after rehydration. Fluid resuscitation may be needed; therefore, obtain orthostatic vital signs to best determine the need for isotonic fluids. Analgesic and antiemetic medications are also indicated for these patients. One of the most critical issues in managing this condition is patient education. You need to instruct patients about safe food and water use to prevent future infections.

In-hospital care is directed at rehydration, control of vomiting and diarrhea, identification of the organism involved, antibiotic therapy, and stabilization of electrolyte imbalances.

■ Rectal Abscess

Pathophysiology

The rectum creates mucus to lubricate feces during defecation. If the ducts through which this mucus travels are blocked, a <u>rectal abscess</u> can result. This area has large amounts of bacteria present. The blockage can allow bacteria to grow and spread around the anus. Men are twice as likely to have this problem as women. The most common age groups are people in their 30s and 40s.

Assessment

Patients present with rectal pain that increases with defecation and then diminishes. The pain will continue between defecations. Fever and rectal drainage are also common findings. Bleeding is typically not a problem. Patients may become constipated and unwilling to defecate because of increased pain.

Management

Management in the prehospital setting involves keeping the patient comfortable. Transport the patient in a position of comfort. The lateral position may be preferable to supine or Fowler's position. In the hospital, patients will typically need surgery to explore the exact extent of this abscess. Drainage, repair, and antibiotics typically follow.

■ Liver Disease: Cirrhosis

Pathophysiology

The liver is a very resilient and important organ. Beyond its role in the metabolism of fats, proteins, and glucose, the liver is responsible for detoxifying the blood, creating coagulation factors, recycling dead red blood cells, storing vitamins, and creating hormones needed in growth. Damage to this organ can result in severe imbalances in the body. Few portions of the body are able to operate normally without a functioning liver.

When the liver is damaged by infection, it is referred to as *hepatitis*. This disease will be discussed in the chapter, *Infectious Diseases*. Other ways to damage the liver are from direct trauma, toxic ingestion, and autoimmune disorders. Regardless of the cause, if the damage to the liver is severe, the patient will experience the beginning stages of liver failure. Early failure is referred to as <u>cirrhosis</u>.

As the liver is damaged, it works to rebuild itself. The liver is so resilient, it is possible for adults to donate a portion of the liver to someone else. The donated portion will grow to normal size and the remaining portion will return to normal size and function. During the regeneration process, fibrotic tissue can result. This dense material will prevent proper filtering and flow of blood. Consequently, the hallmarks of cirrhosis are portal hypertension (discussed earlier in this chapter), deficiencies with coagulation, and diminished detoxification, which can result in hepatic encephalopathy.

Assessment

Clinically, the disease has two phases. In the first phase, patients experience joint aches, weakness, fatigue, nausea, vomiting, anorexia, <u>urticaria</u>, and pruritus (itching). During this phase, the patient may be misdiagnosed as having influenza or gastroenteritis.

The second clinical phase involves sufficient damage to the liver. The damage must reach a point where liver failure results. It is characterized by <u>acholic stools</u>, darkening of the urine, jaundice, <u>icteric</u> conjunctiva (yellow eyes) **Figure 13**, and ascites (see Figure 7). Abdominal pain found in the right upper quadrant, along with an enlarged liver, are also present at this time.

Laboratory findings may reveal abnormal liver functions. Aminotransferases (alanine aminotransferase, or ALT, and aspartate aminotransferase, or AST), alkaline phosphatase, albumin, and bilirubin are common blood tests used to gauge liver function. Additionally, coagulation studies are needed to determine the effect of the liver failure on coagulation.

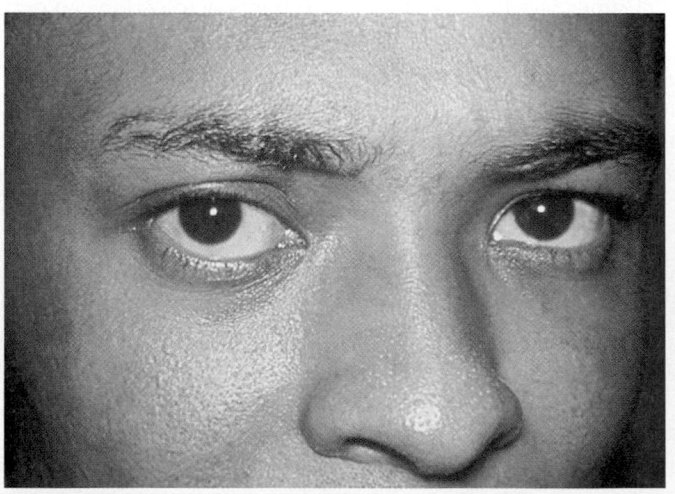

Figure 13 Jaundiced skin and icteric sclera caused by the buildup of bilirubin in the skin and conjunctiva.

Management

The prehospital management for cirrhosis is supportive. Follow the general management guideline for the patient with GI problems. Some important areas of focus involve bleeding control and medication administration. With the damaged liver, the ability for blood clotting may be impaired. Be cautious with all venipunctures.

Because of the liver's detoxification functions, any drug that is given will remain active in the body far longer than anticipated when the liver is compromised. When administering medications to patients with signs of liver failure, use the lower ends of the normal dose range. Give medications at longer intervals and watch for signs of cumulative effects.

In-hospital management is directed at supporting liver function. There is no artificial liver available and without a functioning liver, death is days away. In extreme cases, a liver transplant is the only viable treatment.

Liver Disease: Hepatic Encephalopathy

Pathophysiology

As the functions of the liver continue to diminish, eventually brain function will be impaired. This is called hepatic encephalopathy. There are several theories as to the underlying cause of the brain dysfunction. Ammonia levels tend to rise as liver functions fail. Ammonia can affect neurons by changing the flow of materials across the semipermeable membrane. Diminished functions of the nervous system may be due to simply diminished cellular energy supplies. The liver has a pivotal role in providing cellular substrates necessary for metabolism. Diminished liver function equals diminished metabolism. The decrease in function may also be caused by a change in the blood-brain barrier permeability. If this barrier were able to be easily breached, neurotoxins could cause cellular damage resulting in an altered LOC. Regardless of the underlying cause, the brain is affected.

Assessment

The mental status of a patient with hepatic encephalopathy can range from mild loss of memory to coma.

The patient's clinical findings are more important than laboratory results. Most patients will have ammonia levels checked, but these results are not always a good indicator of the severity of brain impairment. The results of CT and MRI scans are inconclusive for this disease. Patients may have the encephalopathy precipitated by an infection, renal failure, GI bleeding, or constipation. Opiates, benzodiazepines, and psychotropic medications can worsen the presentation.

Management

Treatment is primarily supportive. One of the most important issues is for you to ensure that some other reversible cause for an altered LOC is not present. Check the patient's blood glucose level and vital signs. Assess for trauma and overdose. These patients will typically have a significant past medical history for cirrhosis. Gather detailed information about the history of present illness. What is normal for this patient? How long has the patient been sick? Focus on infections, renal function, bleeding, and constipation because these issues can precipitate hepatic encephalopathy.

■ Pathophysiology, Assessment, and Management of Obstructive Conditions

The cardinal sign of bowel obstruction is decreased intestinal motility, a condition in which the intestines become unable to move material through the digestive tract. Two main reasons for this problem are paralysis of the intestines or a change in the diameter of their lumen. Paralysis can be caused by infection, kidney disease, impaired blood flow to the intestines, or medications. Narcotics and anesthetics are specific types of medications that can paralyze the intestinal muscles. This is why patients who have major surgery often will not be released from the hospital until they have had at least one bowel movement.

Intestinal lumen diameter compromise can be caused by neoplasms, tumors of the intestines, objects that the patient has swallowed, or strictures (narrowing of the lumen due to damage in the intestinal wall). Other causes include hernia (intestine trapped and compressed), intussusception (telescoping of the intestines into themselves), or volvulus (twisting of the intestines). The end result is that the diameter of the intestines is narrowed or blocked.

■ Small-Bowel Obstruction

Pathophysiology

In the small intestine, postoperative adhesions are the most common cause of obstruction. When a patient undergoes a surgical procedure that requires opening the abdomen, the resulting inflammation results in scarring as the body heals. These weblike bands of tissue, called *adhesions*, can constrict the diameter of the intestine or decrease the ability of the intestine to dilate. Other causes of small-bowel obstruction include cancer, Crohn disease, hernias, and foreign bodies (objects that have been swallowed).

Assessment

The presentation of a small-bowel obstruction begins with abdominal pain. The pain tends to be crampy and intermittent. Patients will initially experience diarrhea, nausea, and vomiting because of the increased pressure on the intestine. As the patient continues to eat, some food is able to advance beyond the blockage. This causes increased intestinal pressure. The result is the increased peristalsis to try to move the blockage. Constipation will eventually occur because limited food will be unable to get beyond the blockage. The material that is vomited may be feculent, having the smell of feces. Fever and tachycardia are also associated with small-bowel obstruction, and a history of abdominal surgery can be related. Patients can experience a small-bowel obstruction decades after undergoing abdominal surgery.

A blockage of the small intestines can cause several localized changes. The area involved becomes irritated; therefore, swelling occurs. This further complicates the blockage. If the bowel becomes twisted or for any other reason blood supply is compromised, ischemia can occur. This is referred to as a *strangulated obstruction*. Mortality in the untreated strangulated obstruction is near 100%. If treated early, the mortality rate is markedly lower.

Management

Treatment is supportive. As with most problems involving the GI tract, there is a concern related to sepsis. Monitor blood pressure and be prepared for volume resuscitation and administration of dopamine as needed. A nasogastric tube may be used to decompress the stomach of any material. Antiemetics are clearly indicated with this problem.

In-hospital management will include antibiotic therapy. Imaging studies will be done to help determine the cause of the obstruction. If needed, surgery will be performed to help ensure adequate blood supply and a restoration of bowel movement.

Large-Bowel Obstruction

Pathophysiology

As with small-bowel obstructions, large-bowel obstructions are caused by either mechanical obstruction or dilation of the colon resulting in decreased internal diameter. In the case of mechanical obstruction, the most common causes are colon cancer and diverticulitis. Both of these conditions are more closely associated with older patients; therefore, large-bowel obstructions are more common in that age group. Another cause is a volvulus, or twisting of the bowel until a kink occurs, blocking flow. In pediatric populations, intussusception is a more common diagnosis than in adults.

Imaging studies are used to determine the location and extent of the obstruction. Finding the exact cause will direct eventual hospital treatment. Once located, many obstructions can be easily treated. Untreated, the mortality can be high if cancer is the cause of the obstruction. In addition, the blockage can lead to increased permeability of the intestinal wall, which allows intestinal bacteria to gain access to the bloodstream and septicemia can occur.

Assessment

Assessment reveals a patient with abdominal pain. Nausea and vomiting are also common. The abdomen is distended and typically bowel sounds are absent. Percussion of the abdomen should reveal hyperresonance. If the obstruction has ruptured into the peritoneum, the classic signs of peritonitis (fever, tachycardia, and pain) will be present. Gather information about the patient's recent bowel habits and weight. If the obstruction is related to cancer, recent unexplained weight loss and gradually increasing difficulty in having bowel movements tend to occur.

Management

The treatment for large-bowel obstruction is the same as that for small-bowel obstruction.

Hernia

Pathophysiology

A <u>hernia</u> is a protrusion of an organ or structure into an adjacent cavity. During a physical examination, a physician will often place his or her fingers on the wall of the lower abdomen as the patient is instructed to cough. Coughing increases intra-abdominal pressure. If there is a weakness in the wall of the abdomen, it can be felt as bulging during the cough. This procedure is done to check for an inguinal hernia. Inguinal simply refers to the location of the protrusion. In this case, the protruding organ is typically the intestines. About 1 million hernia repairs are done each year in the United States, with the inguinal hernia being the most common form.

Any condition or state that increases intra-abdominal pressure can facilitate the creation of a hernia. Obesity, standing for long periods, heavy lifting, straining during a bowel movement, or chronic obstructive pulmonary disease can precipitate this condition. Chronic obstructive pulmonary disease is associated with hernias because of the increased work of breathing and subsequent use of the abdominal muscles.

Assessment

In the abdomen there are four types of hernias and several common locations Figure 14 .

- **Reducible.** A hernia that will return to its normal location either spontaneously or by manual manipulation. The patient typically experiences little discomfort unless he or she has increasing intra-abdominal pressure. The patient may perceive a fullness or swelling, or report achiness at the hernia site.
- <u>Incarcerated</u>. Consider the nonmedical meaning of the word *incarcerate*: to place in jail. In this type of hernia, the organ is trapped in the new location. The most common problem in this case is bowel obstruction. Incarcerated hernias are more painful as a result of the obstruction.
- <u>Strangulated</u>. A strangulated hernia is one in which the intestine is trapped and squeezed to the point that blood supply to the area is diminished. Consequently, this kind of hernia is considered an emergency. Patients experience severe pain and sepsis and require urgent transport.
- <u>Incisional</u>. In another type of hernia, called an incisional hernia, patients who are recovering from abdominal surgery will have intestinal contents herniate through the incision. This is similar to the trauma condition known as evisceration.

Management

Prehospital treatment for hernias is supportive with care directed at pain management. Place the patient in a comfortable position. Lying supine will probably not be comfortable because this stretches the abdominal wall. Closely assess the patient for sepsis. In the hospital, reduction of the hernia may be attempted in the emergency department. If unsuccessful or not appropriate, surgical repair will be explored.

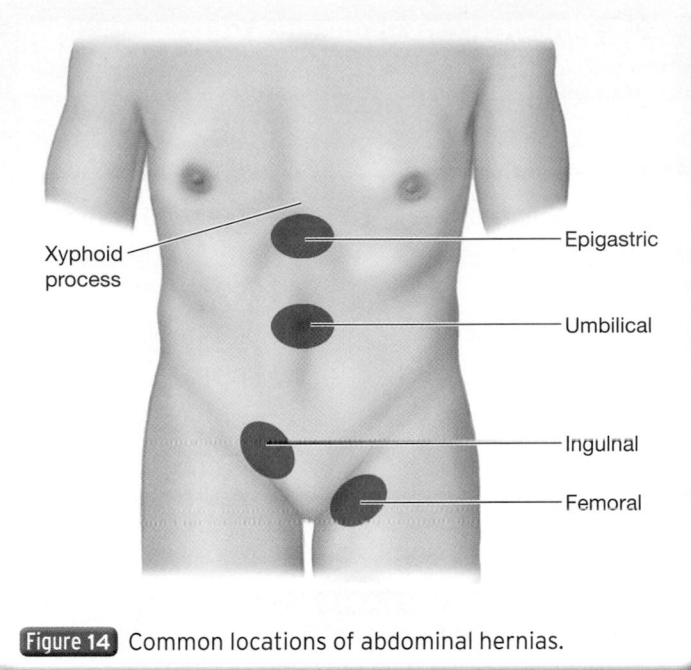

Xyphoid process

Epigastric

Umbilical

Inguinal

Femoral

Figure 14 Common locations of abdominal hernias.

Rectal Foreign Body Obstruction

Pathophysiology

A foreign body in the rectum interferes with defecation. Objects can be introduced from the upper GI tract or by anal insertion. Indigestible swallowed objects may have difficulty passing. Chicken bones, toothpicks, and various other materials may pass through the entire GI tract without difficulty and become lodged in the rectum during defecation. Prisoners, for example, may swallow objects during an inspection or search. Fecaliths can also cause obstructions. A fecalith is a very hard piece of feces (fecal = feces, lith = stone). Finally, other objects that pass through the GI tract, such as gallstones, can cause obstructions.

Most rectal obstructions occur when an object is inserted into the rectum. Men are 28 times more likely to engage in this activity than women. The average age of these patients is in their 20s. The primary reason for the activity is erotic stimulation. Older men may insert objects into their rectum to help relieve urinary difficulties caused by an enlarged prostate.

Assessment

These two types of causes create two very different patient presentations. If the obstruction originated from the upper GI tract, the patient will present with a sudden onset of rectal pain with defecation. Rarely is bleeding or abdominal pain noted in the acute phase. If the object has perforated the rectum, peritonitis is possible. Peritonitis would in turn lead to fever, diffuse abdominal pain, and possible sepsis.

Most patients who have rectal obstructions seek medical care for removal of an intentionally placed object. Knowing what type of object was inserted and whether the patient has attempted to remove the object can be important. This information can help you determine whether the patient's rectum is perforated. During your history taking, ensure that the patient was

not assaulted. Rectal insertion during an assault can cause severe and possibly life-threatening internal damage.

In either case, physical findings may be limited to the patient's report of rectal pain. If perforation has occurred, peritonitis and consequent sepsis may be present. Depending on the size and shape of the object, it may be apparent on physical examination.

Management

Even when the inserted object is visible on physical examination, you should not attempt to remove it. Treatment in the prehospital setting should be limited to ensuring that the patient is comfortable. Allow the patient to sit laterally, if possible, in order to reduce the pressure on the rectum. If the patient is in pain, analgesia is indicated. As with other abdominal complaints in which peritonitis is a possibility, close monitoring of vital signs is important.

Mesenteric Ischemia

Pathophysiology

Mesenteric ischemia is not related to bowel motility. In patients with this condition, the blood supply to the mesentery is interrupted. In one third of cases, an arterial embolism is the cause. These emboli tend to come from a cardiac thrombus. Another third of cases are caused by a thrombosis. These patients have underlying thrombotic disease. Finally, a third of cases result from profound vasospasm, which can occur with the use of cocaine, with ergot poisoning, or in severe shock. Mesenteric ischemia occurs in both sexes and is more prevalent among older patients. It is a rare but serious condition, with a mortality rate of between 60% and 100%.

Assessment

Depending on the exact cause of the abdominal pain, it may have a gradual or sudden onset. The location of the pain within the abdomen tends to be ill-defined and is severe. Nausea, vomiting, and diarrhea are also common. Blood may be present in the stool. The disease is difficult to diagnose. Its cardinal presentation includes severe abdominal pain with normal abdominal examination results. A thorough history is needed. If the patient has ingested something, this information will dramatically change the in-hospital therapy. Discovering the cause of the ischemia is essential to offering correct lifesaving therapy in the hospital.

Management

Treatment for these patients requires rapid transportation. Monitor these patients closely, checking vital signs for evidence of sepsis. If shock is present, fluid resuscitation should be initiated. Analgesics may be indicated. In-hospital treatment will include imaging studies and antibiotics. Depending on the cause, surgery or vasodilators will be used.

Gastrointestinal Conditions in Pediatric Patients

GI complaints are common in children. Most parents are comfortable managing nausea, vomiting, and complaints of stomach aches. Gastroenteritis, as discussed earlier, occurs frequently in children, with rotavirus being a common cause. As with most conditions that cause fluid loss, it is essential not to underestimate the effects of vomiting, diarrhea, or bleeding on children. Children are at risk for severe changes in their sodium and potassium levels because of fluid loss. Additionally, children have limited fuel stores and, when faced with persistent vomiting or diarrhea, hypoglycemia or shock becomes a grave possibility.

A major difference in the management of the pediatric patient with GI complaints is the increased possibility of a patient with severe birth defects. As the embryo develops, one of the layers called the endoderm will become the GI tract. The development of this body system takes many weeks. The embryo will fold on itself around 16 weeks. If this folding does not occur correctly, portions of the GI tract can be misplaced. An example of a misplaced problem is called **gastroschisis**. Here, portions of the abdominal cavity are located outside of the abdominal wall Figure 15 . During later stages of development, the intestines, which are located in the correct position, may not rotate correctly. This creates intestinal **malrotation**, which can result in intestinal obstruction. These two conditions are associated with each other. Children with malrotation have similar presentations to those of a bowel obstruction: vomiting, abdominal pain, and abdominal distention.

Table 11 lists several congenital GI anomalies and their occurrence rates within the United States. These conditions are all caused by some degree of incorrect formation of the embryo and/or fetus during development.

Pyloric stenosis is the most common cause of infantile intestinal obstruction. It involves a hypertrophy of the pyloric

Table 11 Incidence of Congenital Gastrointestinal Anomalies	
Condition	**Incidence**
Anorectal malformation	1 in 5,000 live births
Congenital diaphragmatic hernia	1 in 2,000–3,000 live births
Gastroschisis	1 in 2,000 live births
Hirschsprung disease	1 in 5,000 live births
Intussusception	1 in 2,000 live births
Malrotation	1 in 500 live births
Pyloris stenosis	2–4 per 1,000 live births

sphincter of the stomach Figure 16 . As this tissue grows, it can begin to impact the movement of material out of the stomach. This particular condition occurs more often in Caucasian males. Pyloric stenosis presents with projectile vomiting and dehydration, often accompanied by malnutrition. As the infant eats, food cannot advance. The stomach contracts to attempt to force the food through, thus causing the projectile vomiting. The inability to get nutrients beyond the obstruction leads to dehydration.

Children can also experience GI bleeding. The signs and symptoms are very similar to those found in adults: hematemesis, melena, and/or hematochezia depending on the location of the bleeding.

Close attention to assessment is critical. Check skin turgor, pulse rate, and peripheral pulse status. Is the child crying? If so, are tears being created? If the child has fontanelles, check to see if they are sunken. Is the child having wet diapers? Neurologic

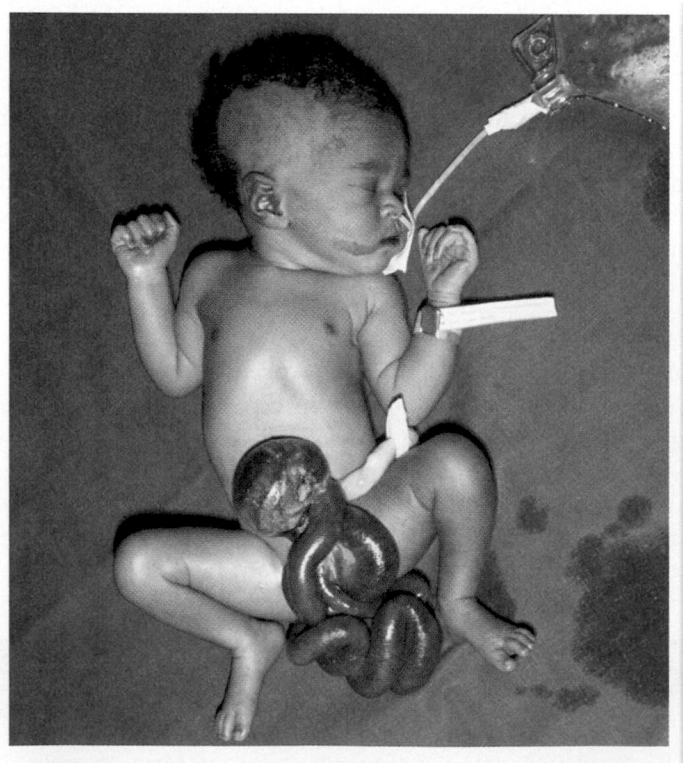

Figure 15 Gastroschisis.

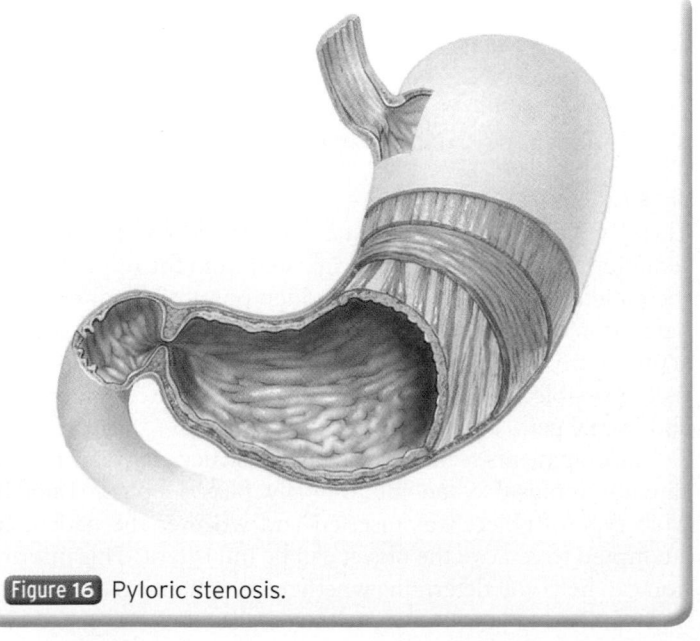

Figure 16 Pyloric stenosis.

status provides prime evidence related to how well the child is coping with the fluid loss. If the patient has a diminished LOC, you should assume that a severe issue is occurring. Standard fluid resuscitation is 20 mL/kg of an isotonic fluid. If possible, check the child's glucose, sodium, and potassium levels, and osmolality. The osmolality will provide information about how dehydrated the child is. It is also important in interpreting the glucose, sodium, and potassium readings.

Management of the pediatric patient with GI complaints relies on you gathering a detailed assessment. Talk with the parents. The parents will be an excellent resource related to past medical history, medications, and treatments. If the patient has pyloric stenosis, fluid resuscitation is required at 20 mL/kg. Monitor blood glucose and electrolytes to ensure adequate levels. Sodium and potassium levels can be greatly affected by any condition that changes the speed of materials moving through the GI tract. As with adults, both elevated and depressed levels are possible.

Patients with complicated medical histories may have a tube placed for long-term feeding. These gastrostomy tubes can become dislodged or clogged. If the tube is dislodged, simply place a sterile dressing over the site and continue your care. Do not try to reinsert the tube into the abdomen. If the feeding tube is clogged, talk with the parents about ways to clear the tube. Be careful not to pull on the tube as to dislodge it from the patient's abdominal wall. If there is no easy way to manage the blockage, turn off the patient's feeding and clamp the tube. Transport the patient to the emergency department for further evaluation and repair of the gastrostomy tube.

Gastrointestinal Conditions in Older Adults

Many of the conditions discussed in this chapter are more prevalent in the elderly. The elderly can have diminished abilities to detect pain, and as a result they may not display rigidity or guarding. This can hamper diagnosis but more importantly, it can delay access to health care. If an elderly patient does not feel pain, he or she may not know why a fever has occurred. The patient may try to treat it at home and by the time EMS is activated, the patient is already septic and seriously ill.

Abdominal pain can also be a symptom of a cardiac condition. Imagine how difficult it would be to initially distinguish the source of abdominal pain in a 75-year-old man with a history of gastric ulcers, diverticulitis, and heart disease. Additionally, vascular pathology such as an abdominal aortic aneurysm can cause abdominal pain.

Words of Wisdom

A good rule of thumb when caring for any patient with comorbid factors (patient having many diseases at once) is to be conservative. Listen to the patient and assume the worst. Understand that one disease can either hide or augment the signs and symptoms of another.

Comorbidity creates great difficulties for health care providers, but success can be achieved by obtaining a thorough history and performing a thorough physical examination. Consider obtaining a 12-lead ECG and establishing IV access on most patients with abdominal pain who have comorbid factors. Finally, monitor vital signs and be ready for any changes in the patient's status.

Prevention Strategies

As EMS evolves, it becomes more important for paramedics to consider the prevention of diseases. EMS is moving from a service that is strictly related to the delivery of 9-1-1 services, to a system that augments nonemergency aspects of health care. There are many patient behaviors that can limit the intensity or entirely prevent the onset of many GI diseases. Table 12 lists some of the behaviors and the diseases that can be affected.

Following a healthy diet is one of the best ways to prevent GI disorders. A diet that is high in fiber and low in fat will facilitate movement of materials through the GI tract. Good sources of dietary fiber are listed in Table 13. Not only does such a diet help improve bowel health, but it also has a strong connection to

Table 12 Prevention of Selected Gastrointestinal Conditions

Condition	Prevention Strategy
Constipation	Increase fiber and fluid content in diet / Exercise / Chew food fully
Diverticulitis	Increase fiber and fluid content in diet / Exercise / Chew food fully
Gallstones	Most gallstones cannot be prevented, but a lower-fat diet may provide some protection
Heartburn	Avoid smoking / Avoid eating close to bedtime / Avoid chocolate, peppermint, caffeine
Hemorrhoids	Increase fiber and fluid content in diet
Liver disease	Limit alcohol / Avoid high doses of vitamins unless prescribed / Follow directions on cleaning supplies (ventilation/gloves/masks)
Peptic ulcers	Manage stress well / Limit caffeine / Limit alcohol

heart health. Another heart-healthy behavior that has a positive effect on the GI system is to eliminate smoking and to control the amount of alcohol consumed. Finally, the connection between stress and disease is clear. Meditating, exercising, and practicing relaxation techniques can have a profound effect on a person's quality and quantity of life.

Table 13   Selected Sources of Dietary Fiber

Fruits	Vegetables	Other Good Fiber Choices
Artichokes	Beans (baked, black, lima, pinto)	Barley
Apples, pears (with skin)	Broccoli	Bread, muffins (whole wheat, bran)
Berries (blackberries, blueberries, raspberries)	Chickpeas	Cereals (bran flakes, bran, oatmeal, shredded wheat)
Dates	Lentils	Coconut
Figs	Parsnips	Crackers (rye, whole wheat)
Prunes	Peas	Nuts (almonds, Brazil, peanuts, pecans, walnuts)
	Pumpkin	Rice (brown)
	Rutabaga	Seeds (pumpkin, sunflower)
	Squash (winter)	

YOU are the Medic   SUMMARY

1. What is melena?

Melena is black, tarry, sticky, and very odorous stool and blood blended together into one substance. You are unable to distinguish blood from stool.

2. What part of the GI system do you believe might be affected?

Melena is common when there is bleeding from the esophagus, stomach, or proximal small intestine.

3. What do orthostatic vital signs indicate?

Orthostatic vital signs will help you to determine the extent of bleeding that has occurred. First, have the patient assume a position of comfort. Usually this is either seated or lying down. You will need to obtain an accurate blood pressure and pulse rate. Then have the patient change positions; have the patient stand or sit up. Use caution when you change the patient's position. It is possible for the patient to lose consciousness with a positional change. Now that the patient is in another position, quickly repeat the blood pressure and pulse rate check. Normally, there should be little change in the blood pressure or pulse rate with this change.

4. Do you expect the blood pressure and pulse rate to increase or decrease when the patient is moved?

When a patient has a significant loss of fluid within the vascular space, there will be a 10-beat increase in the pulse rate and/or a 10-mm Hg drop in blood pressure. Either finding indicates a significant volume loss.

5. On the basis of the patient's orthostatic vital signs, what is your suggested treatment?

The patient's vital signs indicate that she is hypovolemic. The patient should be given IV fluids as long as no findings are present that would contraindicate it. You should also attempt to keep the patient lying as flat as possible to keep the postural effects minimized.

6. Which of the patient's medications are you most concerned with?

You should be concerned with the warfarin because it is an anticoagulant. Volume replacement is still your treatment of choice, but warfarin should increase your suspicion of substantial bleeding somewhere in the GI tract. Bismuth solutions (Pepto Bismol) will also color stools black without any bleeding.

7. Knowing that your patient has postural vital signs, how are you going to move the patient downstairs?

The best method to help the patient's comfort level would be to maintain a lying position if at all possible. A stair chair would not be a good choice for this patient. A Reeves device or a scoop stretcher may be your best choice.

8. Should you administer a pain medication to make your patient more comfortable?

Because this patient is already hemodynamically compromised, fentanyl or tramadol may be a better choice than morphine or meperidine (which cause vascular pooling), if your local protocols allow. Consult medical control regarding the best choice.

YOU *are the Medic* | SUMMARY, *continued* |

EMS Patient Care Report (PCR)

Date: 08-10-11	Incident No.: 73542	Nature of Call: Unresponsive		Location: 215 Brooks Street	
Dispatched: 0115	En Route: 0116	At Scene: 0121	Transport: 0146	At Hospital: 0153	In Service: 0211

Patient Information

Age: 64	Allergies: No known drug allergies
Sex: F	Medications: Propranolol, diltiazem, warfarin, glyburide, bismuth OTC
Weight (in kg [lb]): 91 kg (200 lb)	Past Medical History: Diabetic, HTN, A-fib
	Chief Complaint: GI bleeding

Vital Signs

Time: 0126	BP: 106/82 lying, 92/78 sitting	Pulse: 120 lying, 136 sitting	Respirations: 20	Spo$_2$: 98% 15 l/min
Time: 0134	BP: 110/86 lying	Pulse: 110 lying	Respirations: 18	Spo$_2$: 98% 15 L/min
Time:	BP:	Pulse:	Respirations:	Spo$_2$:

EMS Treatment
(circle all that apply)

Oxygen @ __15__ L/min via (circle one): NC (NRM) Bag-mask device	Assisted Ventilation	Airway Adjunct:	CPR
Defibrillation	Bleeding Control	Bandaging	Splinting	Other

Narrative

Arrived to find 64-year-old woman in an upstairs bathroom at her residence. Husband states the pt has been feeling ill for a few days. Pt awoke and he assisted her to the bathroom when she became syncopal. The husband helped her down to the floor and she did not fall. Pt has approx 250 mL of melena on the floor near her position. Pt reports abdominal pain an 8 on 1:10 scale. Pt denies any vomiting. Abd assessment equals soft, tender in all quads. Pt orthostatic vital signs show postural changes. IV established and 250-mL challenge administered. Pt lifted off floor with a scoop stretcher and carried down stairs to ambulance. Pt had no change during transport to Charity Hospital. Report given to charge nurse on arrival. **End of report**

Prep Kit

- Gastrointestinal problems, in and of themselves, are rarely life threatening. This fact does not minimize the systemic problems that can erupt from untreated or undertreated disease of the GI system.

- The structures and functions of the GI system perform digestion, which begins in the mouth, and continues through a multitude of organs and structures: the esophagus, portal vein, stomach, duodenum, pancreas, liver, gallbladder, small intestine, large intestine, appendix, and the anus.

- During calls for patients with suspected abdominal or GI emergencies, it is likely you will come into contact with blood, vomitus, urine, or feces. A complete size-up of scene safety requires a survey of the personal protective equipment required for protection against infectious agents.

- Your general impression of the patient with a suspected abdominal or GI emergency is formed by observing the patient's posture, his or her environment, any foul odors present, and the patient's level of consciousness.

- Airway patency and adequate circulation must be maintained, and the extent of any bleeding must be assessed by obtaining the patient's orthostatic vital signs.

- Transport decisions are made by weighing the patient's stability against the risk of injury to the patient and the paramedic by electing to use rapid transport with lights and sirens.

- Your field impression of the patient and the information you gather about the patient's medications, allergies, past medical history, and precipitating events can provide information about the cause of the patient's chief complaint.

- Secondary assessment is accomplished with a comprehensive physical examination in which you pay special attention to the appearance of the shape, size, color, and other characteristics of the abdomen, auscultate bowel sounds, and perform percussion and palpation to assess for dullness, rigidity, guarding, pain or discomfort, rebound tenderness, fluid accumulation, and masses.

- When taking a patient's orthostatic vital signs, a 10-beat increase in the pulse rate or a 10-mm Hg drop in blood pressure indicates a significant volume loss caused by uncontrolled bleeding.

- Reassessment includes monitoring for changes in pulse rate, ECG readings, blood pressure, respiratory rate, oxygen saturation, or signs of shock.

- Advances in technology allow pain relief to be offered to most patients with abdominal or GI emergencies. It is also important to manage nausea and, by extension, vomiting.

- Talking with patients and their families to keep them calm and informed is the foundation of compassionate, high-quality care. Documenting your observations and the results of all assessments, examinations, and tests is also essential to delivering excellent patient care.

- Sudden, worrisome changes in a patient's condition warrant performing comprehensive and detailed new assessments and examinations.

- Airway management includes delivery of high-concentration oxygen, prevention of aspiration, and auscultation of lung sounds, as dictated by the patient's condition.

- Circulation may be compromised in a patient with a GI emergency by dehydration or hemorrhage. Fluid resuscitation to replace volume and maintain perfusion may be a lifesaving intervention.

- Paramedics must learn about individual GI diseases in order to keep pace with the rising stature of the EMS field and the increasing level of responsibility paramedics must be prepared to assume. Such knowledge is also necessary in order to educate patients about their own or a loved one's disease.

- Four major conditions are responsible for abdominal and GI emergencies:
  - Hypovolemia caused by dehydration or hemorrhage
  - Acute or chronic inflammation
  - Infection
  - Obstruction

- Bleeding within the GI tract is a symptom of another disease, not a disease itself. Presentation of GI bleeding is variable because it can reflect the presence of a number of diseases. Each of these conditions has its own pattern of disease progression.

- Pediatric patients face special challenges during abdominal and GI emergencies because of their size and physiology, particularly when a congenital anomaly is present.

- Comorbidities, multiple medications, and other factors can complicate the care of older adults with abdominal or GI emergencies.

Vital Vocabulary

acalculus cholecystitis Inflammation of the gallbladder without the presence of gallstones.

acholic stools Light, clay-colored stools indicative of liver failure.

acute abdomen A condition of sudden onset of pain within the abdomen, usually indicating peritonitis; demands immediate medical or surgical treatment.

acute gastroenteritis A family of conditions that revolve around a central theme of infection with fever, abdominal pain, diarrhea, nausea, and vomiting.

anal fissures Linear tears to the mucosal lining in and near the anus, possibly caused by the passage of large, hard stools; a cause of lower GI bleeding.

appendicitis Inflammation of the appendix.

ascites Abdominal edema typically signaling liver failure.

biliary tract disorders A group of disorders that involve inflammation of the gallbladder; these include cholangitis, cholelithiasis, cholecystitis, and acalculus cholecystitis.

borborygmi A bowel sound characterized by increased activity within the bowel; also called *hyperperistalsis*.

cardiac sphincter Sphincter that serves as a door way connecting the esophagus and the stomach; controls the amount of food that moves up the esophagus.

cholangitis Inflammation of the bile duct.

cholelithiasis The presence of stones within the gallbladder.

cholecystitis Inflammation of the gallbladder.

cirrhosis Early failure of the liver; characterized by portal hypertension, coagulation deficiencies, and diminished detoxification.

chyme The term given to the slurry of food that has been partially digested, then exits the stomach and enters the duodenum.

Crohn disease Inflammation of the ileum and possibly other portions of the GI tract, in which the immune system attacks portions of the intestinal walls, causing them to become scarred, narrowed, stiff, and weakened.

dehydration A state in which the body lacks adequate fluids because of inadequate water intake or excessive fluid loss.

diarrhea Liquid stool.

digestion The mechanical and chemical breakdown of the large molecules in food into small molecules that can be absorbed in the GI tract and converted to energy for cellular function.

diverticulitis Inflammation of pouches in the colon; these pouches form as a result of difficulty moving feces through the colon.

Once the pouches are formed, bacteria can become trapped in the pouch, leading to inflammation and infection.

diverticulum A weak area in the colon that begins to have small outcroppings that turn into pouches; plural is diverticula.

Dunphy sign Severe abdominal pain in the right lower quadrant with coughing; a method for evaluating a patient for peritonitis.

endoscopy Insertion of a flexible fiberoptic tube into the esophagus to visualize, remove, or repair damaged or diseased tissue.

epigastric The region of the abdomen directly inferior to the xyphoid process and superior to the umbilicus.

esophagogastric varices Dilated blood vessels of the esophagus, commonly caused by difficulty in blood flow through the liver; the presence of these can lead to vessel rupture.

feculent Smelling of feces.

fistula An abnormal connection between two cavities.

gastritis Inflammation of the stomach.

gastroesophageal reflux disease (GERD) A condition in which the sphincter between the esophagus and the stomach opens, allowing stomach acid to move superiorly; can cause a burning sensation within the chest (heartburn); also called acid reflux disease.

gastroschisis A congenital malformation in which an embryo develops improperly and a portion of the GI tract develops outside of the abdominal wall instead of inside.

hematemesis Vomit with blood; can either look like coffee grounds, indicating the presence of partially digested blood, or contain bright-red blood, indicating active bleeding.

hematochezia The passage of stool in which bright red blood can be distinguished; caused by lower GI bleeding.

hepatic encephalopathy Impairment of brain function resulting from failure of the liver.

hepatitis Inflammation of the liver, usually caused by a virus, that causes fever, loss of appetite, jaundice, fatigue, and altered liver function.

hernia The protrusion of a loop of an organ or tissue through an abnormal body opening.

hyperperistalsis A bowel sound characterized by increased activity within the bowel; also called borborygmi.

hypoperistalsis Decreased bowel sounds.

icteric Yellowish coloration of the conjunctiva (the whites of the eyes) caused by the buildup of bilirubin in the blood during liver failure.

incarcerated A type of hernia in which an organ is trapped in the new location; most commonly obstructs the bowel.

incisional A type of hernia in which intestinal contents herniate through an incision, for example after abdominal surgery.

intussusception Telescoping of the intestines into themselves.

irritable bowel syndrome (IBS) A condition in which patients have abdominal pain and changes in their bowel habits; generally the pain must be present for at least 3 days a month for at least 3 months to be considered this disease.

Mallory-Weiss syndrome A condition in which the junction between the esophagus and the stomach tears, causing severe bleeding and, potentially, death.

malrotation Incorrect rotation of the intestines, for example as a result of a congenital anomaly such as gastroschisis; can result in intestinal obstruction.

melena Dark, tarry, malodorous stools caused by upper GI bleeding.

mesenteric ischemia An interruption of the blood supply to the mesentery.

Murphy sign Pressure applied to the right upper quadrant of the abdomen to help detect gallbladder problems.

orthostatic vital signs Assessment of vital signs in two different patient positions to determine the degree of hypovolemia.

pancreatitis Inflammation of the pancreas.

parietal pain Pain caused by inflammation of the parietal peritoneum that is generally described as steady, aching, and aggravated by movement.

peptic ulcer disease (PUD) A disease in which the mucous lining of the stomach and duodenum have been eroded, allowing the acid to eat into these organs.

peristalsis Rhythmic contraction of the intestines and esophagus that allows material to move through them.

peritonitis Inflammation of the peritoneum, the protective membrane that lines the abdominal and pelvic cavities.

portal hypertension Increased pressure in the portal veins; caused by the inability of blood to normally flow through the liver; can lead to rupture of these vessels.

portal vein A large vessel created by the intersection of blood vessels from the GI system. The portal vein drains into the liver.

protuberant Term used to describe an abdomen with a convex, or distended, shape; can be caused by edema.

pruritus Itching.

pyloric stenosis Hypertrophy (enlargement) of the pyloric sphincter of the stomach; ultimately leads to intestinal obstruction, often in infants.

rebound tenderness Pain that the patient feels when pressure is released as opposed to when pressure is applied; characteristic of appendicitis.

rectal abscess An infection involving a collection of pus in the rectal walls that results from blockage of the rectal mucus ducts.

referred pain The pain felt in an area of the body other than the area where the cause of pain is located.

scaphoid A concave shape of the abdomen; can be caused by evisceration.

soft stool A bowel movement that is the consistency of soft-serve ice cream; can range in color from tan to dark brown.

somatic pain Localized pain, usually felt deeply, which represents irritation or injury to tissue, causing activation of peripheral nerve tracts.

steatorrhea Foamy, fatty stools associated with liver failure or gallbladder problems.

strangulated Complete obstruction of blood circulation in a given organ as a result of compression or entrapment; an emergency situation causing death of tissue.

striae Vertical stretch marks that occur when a person loses or gains weight rapidly.

tympanic A loud, high-pitched sound, similar to the sound of a drum, heard on percussion of a hollow space (eg, the empty stomach or a puffed out cheek).

ulcerative colitis Generalized inflammation of the colon that results in a weakened, dilated rectum, making it prone to infection and bleeding.

umbilical The region of the abdomen surrounding the umbilicus.

urticaria An itching rash.

visceral pain Crampy, aching pain deep within the body, the source of which is usually difficult to pinpoint; common with urologic problems.

volvulus Twisting of the bowel until a kink occurs; results in blocked flow.

Assessment in Action

Your unit is dispatched to a local park for a man down. Law enforcement has cleared the scene so it is safe to enter. You find a man lying unconscious on a park bench. There is copious blood coming from his mouth. You recognize him as a frequent patient who has alcoholism and who stays at the local mission.

You have transported the man before for problems related to cirrhosis of the liver that are the result of his chronic alcoholism. The physician who treated him last time told the patient he had the beginning stages of varices. As you approach the patient, you find he is incontinent of urine and feces. There is a dark, tarry look to the fecal matter.

1. What does the portal vein do?
   A. Transports blood to the lungs
   B. Transports blood to the liver
   C. Transports blood to the legs
   D. Transports blood to the brain

2. An increase in hepatic pressure through the portal vein can cause leaking of blood in the esophagus. This is called:
   A. esophageal erosion.
   B. esophagogastric varices.
   C. cholecystitis.
   D. gastroenteritis.

3. Because you suspect this patient has upper GI bleeding, which sign would you not expect to see?
   A. Hematemesis
   B. Melena
   C. Hematochezia
   D. Bright red stools

4. Because this patient may be bleeding from ruptured esophagogastric varices, what is the most important step in management of his airway?
   A. Suction
   B. Oxygen via a nonrebreathing mask
   C. Insertion of a dual-lumen airway device
   D. Endotrachael intubation

5. A sharp pain on inspiration when pressure is applied to the right upper quadrant is called:
   A. Biot sign.
   B. hematemesis.
   C. Beck sign.
   D. Murphy sign.

6. Autodigestion of the pancreas results in:
   A. Mallory-Weiss syndrome.
   B. pancreatitis.
   C. autoimmune disorder.
   D. diabetes.

Additional Question

7. You are dispatched to a private residence for a person with abdominal pain. When you arrive on scene, the patient is doubled over in pain and reports point tenderness to the upper right quadrant. The patient's vital signs are: pulse rate, 108 beats/min with sinus tachycardia; blood pressure, 110/70 mm Hg; respiratory rate, 24 breaths/min; and pulse oximetry, 100% on room air. What management is required for this patient?

Genitourinary and Renal Emergencies

National EMS Education Standard Competencies

Medicine

Integrates assessment findings with principles of epidemiology and pathophysiology to formulate a field impression and implement a comprehensive treatment/disposition plan for a patient with a medical complaint.

Genitourinary/Renal

- Blood pressure assessment in hemodialysis patients (pp 1174-1175)

Anatomy, physiology, pathophysiology, assessment, and management of

- Complications related to
  - Renal dialysis (pp 1174-1176)
  - Urinary catheter management (not insertion) (pp 1167, 1169)
- Kidney stones (pp 1169-1170)

Anatomy, physiology, epidemiology, pathophysiology, psychosocial impact, presentations, prognosis, and management of

- Complications of
  - Acute renal failure (pp 1170-1172)
  - Chronic renal failure (pp 1172-1173)
  - Dialysis (pp 1174-1176)
- Renal calculi (pp 1169-1170)
- Acid-base disturbances (p 1171)
- Fluid and electrolytes (pp 1163, 1174)
- Infection (p 1169)
- Male genital tract conditions (pp 1176-1177)

Knowledge Objectives

1. Describe the anatomy and physiology of the male and female urinary systems: kidneys, ureters, urinary bladder, and urethra. (pp 1161-1164)
2. Describe the primary and secondary assessment processes for patients with renal and genitourinary emergencies. (pp 1165-1166)
3. Specify factors that influence transport decisions for such patients. (pp 1166, 1167)
4. Discuss the questions that must be asked in order to obtain thorough historical information from a patient. (p 1166)
5. Indicate the components of the physical examination for a patient with a renal or genitourinary complaint. (p 1166)
6. Name the components of an effective treatment plan. (pp 1166-1167)
7. Specify best practices for documenting renal and genitourinary emergencies and communicating with the receiving facility. (pp 1166-1167)
8. Compare visceral pain with referred pain, and explain how each contributes to the field diagnosis. (p 1168)
9. Outline the pathophysiology, assessment, and management of common diseases and conditions of the renal and genitourinary systems, including urinary tract infections, kidney stones, acute renal failure, chronic renal failure, and end-stage renal disease. (pp 1169-1174)
10. Discuss the purpose and types of renal dialysis. (p 1174)
11. Identify the possible complications of dialysis and the prehospital interventions associated with each. (pp 1174-1176)
12. Discuss the pathophysiology, assessment, and management of conditions related to the male genital tract, including epididymitis, Fournier gangrene, phimosis, priapism, benign prostate hypertrophy, testicular masses, and testicular torsion. (pp 1176-1177)

Skills Objectives

There are no skills objectives for this chapter.

Introduction

The urinary system performs two main functions for the body. First, it acts as the body's accounting firm, balancing the levels of electrolytes, water, acids, and bases in the blood. Second, it performs the essential job of serving as the blood's sewage treatment plant, removing metabolic wastes, drug metabolites, and excess fluids. The kidneys perform these tasks continuously, filtering 200 L of blood every day. In addition, the kidneys also produce hormones that generate new red blood cells and help the liver convert glycogen to glucose.

The most common renal disorder is kidney disease, which affects more than 20 million Americans. Approximately 50,000 Americans die of kidney disease each year, and more than 30,000 require dialysis. The most common acute renal disease is renal calculi (kidney stones), with 2 million cases diagnosed each year. Other common types of renal disease include urinary tract infections, which occur in more than 50% of all women, and noncancerous enlargement of the prostate, which 60% of men will develop by age 50. Many of these conditions can be prevented by practicing proper hygiene, following a healthy diet, and staying adequately hydrated.

Anatomy and Physiology

The urinary system consists of the **kidneys**, which filter the blood and produce **urine**; the **ureters**, which transport urine from the kidneys to the bladder; the **urinary bladder**, which stores the urine until it is released from the body; and

the **urethra**, the route by which urine leaves the bladder and exits the body.

Kidneys

The bean-shaped kidneys are tucked into the retroperitoneal space (behind the peritoneum), which extends from the twelfth thoracic vertebra to the third lumbar vertebra. The right kidney is positioned slightly lower than the left because of the position of the liver. The medial side of the kidney is concave, forming a cleft called the **hilus**, where the ureters, renal blood vessels, lymphatic vessels, and nerves enter and leave the kidney **Figure 1A**.

A fibrous capsule envelops the kidney and protects it against infection. Surrounding this capsule is a fatty mass of adipose tissue, which cushions the kidney and holds it in place in the abdomen. A layer of dense fibrous connective tissue called the **renal fascia** anchors the kidney to the abdominal wall **Figure 1B**.

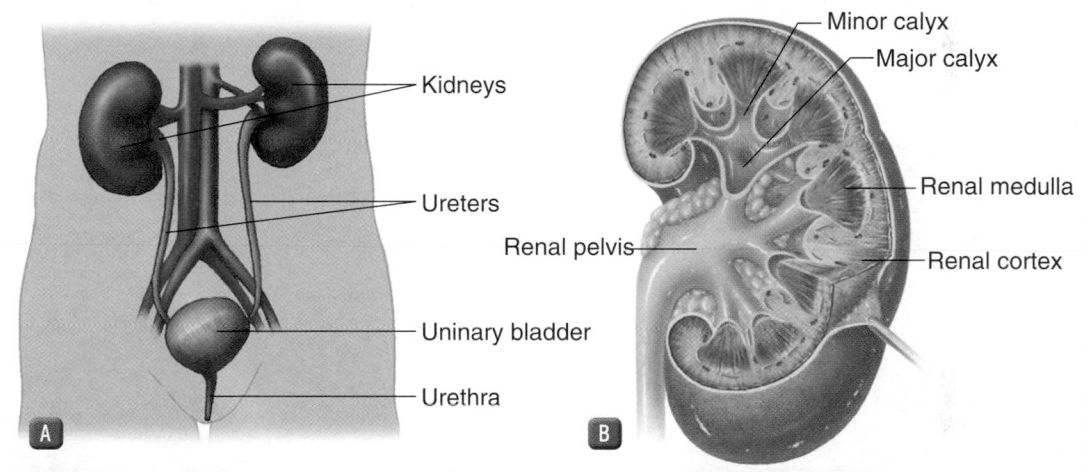

Figure 1 The urinary system. **A.** Anterior view showing the relationship of the kidneys, ureters, urinary bladder, and urethra. **B.** Cross-section of the human kidney showing the renal cortex, renal medulla, and renal pelvis.

YOU are the Medic   PART 1

At about 0600 hours you are dispatched to 327 West Main Street for a woman reporting back pain. You arrive to find a slender, gray-haired man waiting for you at the front door of the turn-of-the-century residence. He motions for you and says, "It's my daughter. She's very sick. I would have taken her to the hospital myself, but I can't carry her. She's in the upstairs bedroom." The stairway is dark and narrow. As you walk up the steps, you hear a young woman say, "Dad, I'm going to be sick again."

1. What concerns may you have about the scene?

2. Although you have not seen your patient yet, what information do you already know that is part of the primary assessment?

The internal anatomy of the kidney can be divided into three distinct regions: the cortex, the medulla, and the pelvis. The **cortex** is the lighter-colored outer region closest to the capsule. The **medulla** (middle layer) includes the cone-shaped **renal pyramids** (parallel bundles of urine-collecting tubules), and inward extensions of cortical tissue that surround the pyramids, called the **renal columns**. The **renal pelvis** is a flat, funnel-shaped tube that fills the sinus at the level of the hilus. The major and minor **calyces** branch off the pelvis and connect with the renal pyramids to receive the urine that drains from the collecting tubules. This arrangement has been said to resemble several strands of uncooked spaghetti (the collecting tubules) sitting in a thimble (the papilla, or tip, of the renal pelvis). The collected urine flows through the renal pelvis and into the ureter on its way to the bladder.

Approximately one fourth of the body's systemic cardiac output flows through the kidney each minute. Blood ejected from the heart flows from the abdominal aorta into the kidney by way of the renal artery. Once it enters the kidney at the hilus, the artery branches several times to become the **afferent arteriole**. The afferent arteriole quickly branches into a tuft of capillaries called a **glomerulus**, the kidney's main filter. From the glomerulus, the blood enters the **efferent arteriole**, which branches into the **peritubular capillaries**, where tubular reabsorption occurs. This secondary set of capillaries is unique to the kidney; no other organ in the body has two distinct capillary beds. The capillaries then merge, forming venules and veins, until the renal vein leaves the hilus, carrying the cleansed blood to the inferior vena cava.

Nephrons, found in the cortex, are the structural and functional units of the kidney that form urine. Each nephron is composed of the glomerulus; the **glomerular (Bowman's) capsule**, which surrounds the glomerulus; the **proximal convoluted tubule (PCT)**; the **loop of Henle**; and the **distal convoluted tubule (DCT)**, which connects with the kidney's collecting tubules. Each kidney contains approximately 1.25 million nephrons Figure 2 .

The glomerular capsule is a double-layered cup in which the inner layer infiltrates and surrounds the capillaries of the glomerulus. Special cells in the inner membrane called **podocytes** wrap around the capillaries in the glomerulus, forming filtration slits. The filtrate passes through these slits, across the

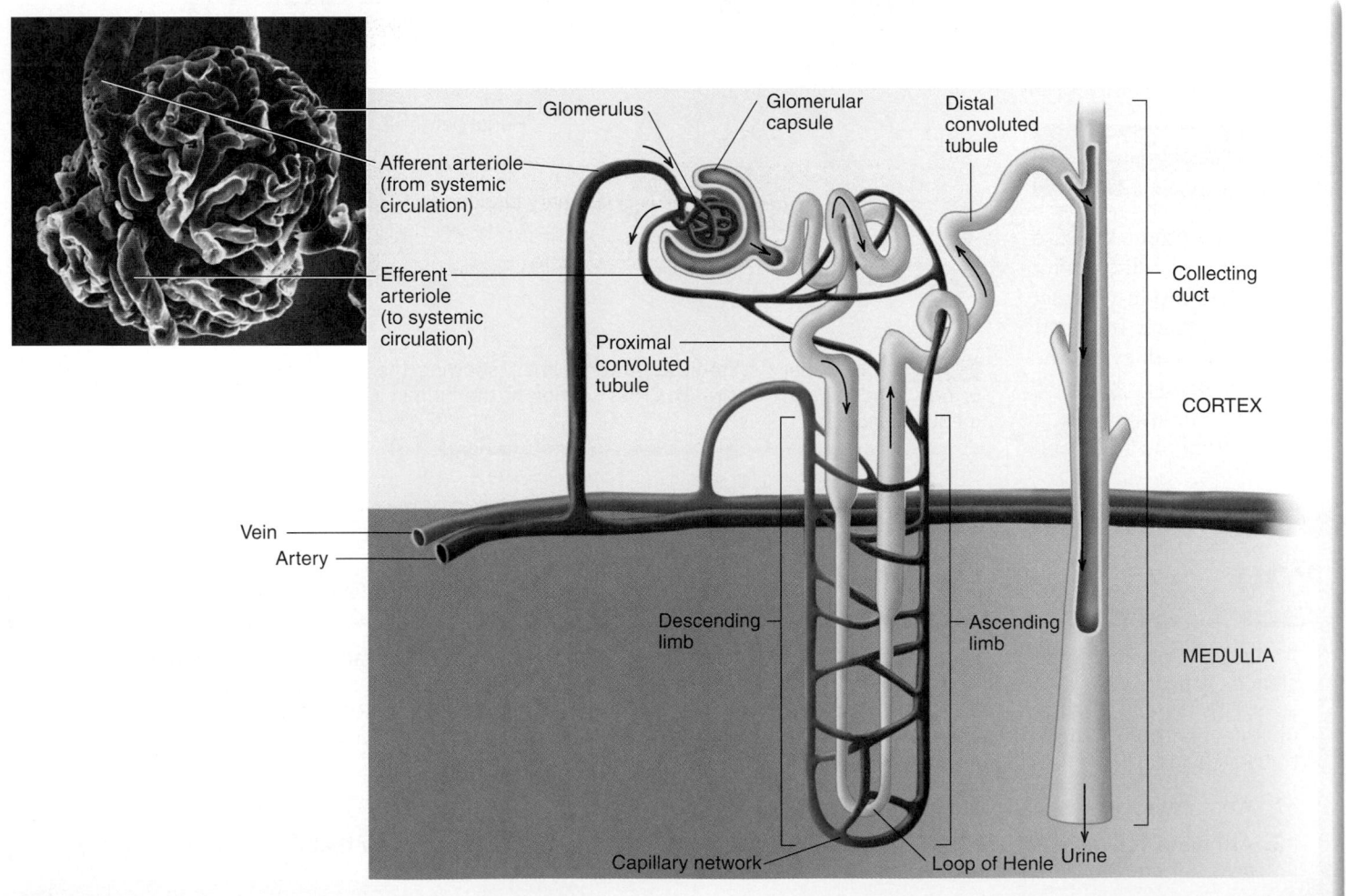

Figure 2 The nephrons of the kidney. Part of the nephron is located in the cortex, and part is located in the medulla. The inset at left is an electron micrograph of a glomerulus from a human nephron.

filtration membrane, and into the capsule. In this manner, the filtration membrane prevents large molecules, such as proteins, from entering the capsule.

Imagine watering your garden with an open-ended hose. If you place your finger over half of the hose's opening, the same amount of water must now pass through half the space. As a consequence, the pressure increases and you can spray the water farther. The same thing happens at the glomerulus. As blood moves from the relatively large afferent arteriole into the smaller capillaries of the glomerulus, the pressure increases. This effect, along with the smaller diameter of the efferent arteriole, causes the pressure in the glomerulus to rise enough to force the filtrate from the blood into the glomerular capsule **Figure 3**.

The amount of filtrate produced, called the **glomerular filtration rate (GFR)**, is maintained at a relatively constant rate of 125 mL/min in healthy adults. Changes in the GFR cause many of the renal emergencies encountered in the prehospital setting.

Initially, the filtrate contains everything that can pass through the filtration membrane: salts, minerals, glucose, water, and metabolic wastes. As the filtrate passes through the rest of the nephron, tubular reabsorption and tubular secretion convert the filtrate into urine. As the fluid passes through the PCT, the cells lining the PCT remove all organic nutrients and plasma proteins, as well as some ions, from the filtrate. These compounds are deposited in the interstitial fluid surrounding the PCT. As these solutes accumulate, the concentration of

the surrounding fluid becomes higher than that of the filtrate. Water will then move from the filtrate by osmosis. The fluid and nutrients in the interstitial fluid, in turn, move into the peritubular capillaries around the PCT. This process reestablishes the homeostatic balance in the blood and reduces the volume of the tubular filtrate.

Additional reabsorption of water and electrolytes occurs in the loop of Henle. The loop of Henle has two sections—the descending limb, extending toward the medulla, and the ascending limb, moving toward the cortex. The cells in the descending limb are permeable to water, but impermeable to sodium and chloride ions; the cells in the ascending limb are permeable to sodium and chloride ions, but impermeable to water. As a consequence, when the sodium and chloride ions move out of the ascending limb, they increase the solute concentration of the fluid surrounding the descending limb. Water moves by osmosis from the descending limb into the surrounding tissue and eventually into the **vasa recta**, a series of peritubular capillaries that surround the loop of Henle. This **countercurrent multiplier** process allows the body to produce either concentrated or diluted urine, depending on the body's needs.

After leaving the loop of Henle, the fluid enters the DCT. At this point, about 80% of the water and 85% of the solutes originally forced out of the glomerulus have been reabsorbed. As the urine passes through the DCT and the collecting ducts to which it is attached (both of which are impermeable to solutes), its composition undergoes its final adjustments. Ions are actively secreted or reabsorbed, and the body alters the permeability of the DCT and collecting ducts to water as necessary, depending on the body's homeostatic needs. These adjustments to the final composition of the urine facilitate the removal of metabolic wastes while maintaining the body's fluid-electrolyte balance.

At the site where the efferent arteriole comes in contact with the DCT, a structure called the **juxtaglomerular apparatus** is formed. The pressure-sensitive cells in the efferent arteriole (called juxtaglomerular cells) monitor the blood pressure. The cells in the DCT (called macula densa cells) are sensitive to chemical changes and monitor the concentration of the filtrate in the DCT. When triggered by changes in the blood pressure of the filtrate content, the juxtaglomerular cells release **renin**. This enzyme initiates a cascade of reactions in the body by converting the plasma protein angiotensinogen into angiotensin I. Other enzymes present in the blood then convert angiotensin I into angiotensin II. A potent blood vessel constrictor, angiotensin II promotes smooth muscle contraction in the arterioles throughout the body. This constriction raises the blood pressure by increasing peripheral resistance. Angiotensin II also increases the reabsorption of sodium from the PCT. Given that water tends to follow sodium, by increasing sodium reabsorption, the kidney increases water reabsorption and, in turn, blood pressure.

The final adjustments to the composition of the urine at the DCT and collecting duct are controlled primarily by two hormones: **antidiuretic hormone (ADH)** and **aldosterone**. ADH is produced by the hypothalamus and stored in the posterior lobe of the pituitary; aldosterone is produced in the **adrenal glands**.

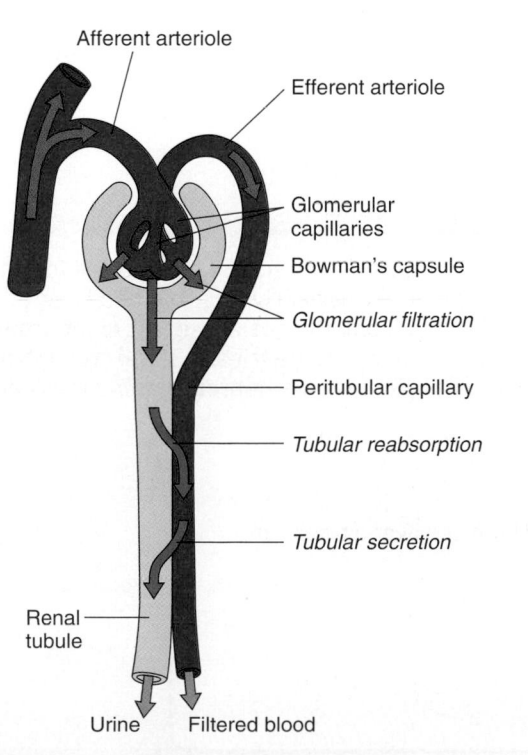

Figure 3 The glomerulus of the kidneys. The nephron carries out three blood-filtering processes: glomerular filtration, tubular reabsorption, and tubular secretion.

Neurons in the hypothalamus monitor the solute concentration of the blood. When the solute concentration of the blood increases (eg, due to sweating or decreased fluid intake), ADH is released into the bloodstream. This hormone travels to the DCT and collecting ducts, increasing these structures' permeability to water. Water therefore leaves the DCT and collecting ducts, and reenters the bloodstream. As the solute concentration returns to normal, secretion of ADH will stop.

Aldosterone increases the rate of active reabsorption of sodium and chloride ions into the blood; a corresponding increase occurs in water reabsorption. This hormone also decreases the reabsorption of potassium ions, resulting in excess potassium being secreted in the urine.

Diuretics, chemicals that increase urinary output, work in a variety of ways. A substance that is not reabsorbed from the filtrate, for example, will increase the amount of water retained in the urine. An example of such an osmotic diuretic is glucose in a patient with diabetes mellitus. Alcohol encourages diuresis, or increased urine output, by inhibiting the production of ADH. Other diuretics, including caffeine and the diuretics commonly prescribed for hypertension and congestive heart failure (Lasix, Diuril), inhibit the sodium importers in the DCT and collecting ducts.

◼ Ureters

Once the urine enters the collecting ducts (the renal pyramids of the medulla), it passes through the minor calyx, into the major calyx, and then into the renal pelvis. From there, the urine moves through the ureter and is stored in the urinary bladder. Like the kidneys, the ureters are paired structures, with one descending from each kidney. The two kidneys and two ureters compose the upper urinary tract.

◼ Urinary Bladder

Most of the bladder rests in the anterior abdominal cavity, but the dome of the bladder sits in the posterior abdominal cavity, or retroperitoneum, where the ureters and kidneys reside. When empty, the bladder collapses, and the muscular walls fold over onto themselves. In contrast, as urine accumulates, the bladder expands and becomes pear-shaped. The stretching of the bladder walls ultimately stimulates nerve impulses to produce the **micturition reflex**. This spinal reflex causes contraction of the bladder's smooth muscle, which in turn produces the urge to void as pressure is exerted on the internal urinary sphincter. Normally, the brain controls this urge, keeping the external urinary sphincter contracted until conditions are favorable for urination. At this point, inhibition of the external urinary sphincter is reduced and the urine passes from the urinary bladder into the urethra.

◼ Urethra

The urinary bladder and the urethra make up the lower urinary tract. The beginning of the urethra, through which urine is expelled, sits at the inferior aspect of the bladder. In females, the urethra exits at the site of the external genitalia. The female urethra is shorter than the male urethra (4 cm versus 20 cm) Figure 4 .

The male urethra can be divided into three regions:

- The *prostatic urethra* begins at the bladder and extends through the prostate gland.
- The *membranous urethra* extends from the prostate gland through the abdominal wall and into the penis.
- The *spongy, or penile, urethra* passes through the penis to the external urethral opening.

YOU *are the Medic*   PART 2

As you reach the bedroom door, you hear the sound of vomiting. You turn to your partner to request that he call for additional personnel and the stair chair. The father opens the door, and you see a woman in her early 20s, in a bed covered with several blankets. The father tells you that she has been feeling ill for a few days, but she got worse last night around midnight. He said that she's been vomiting throughout the night and feels very dizzy when she tries to stand. You introduce yourself and ask if you can take her vital signs. She nods yes. You apply oxygen at 15 L/min via nonrebreathing mask and continue your assessment.

Recording Time: 0 Minutes	
Appearance	Lying on her right side, head hanging off the bed over a trash can
Level of consciousness	Alert
Airway	Patent with active vomiting
Breathing	Rapid
Circulation	Flushed, sweaty skin

3. What concerns do you have about her history, signs, and symptoms?

4. What should be done with the emesis?

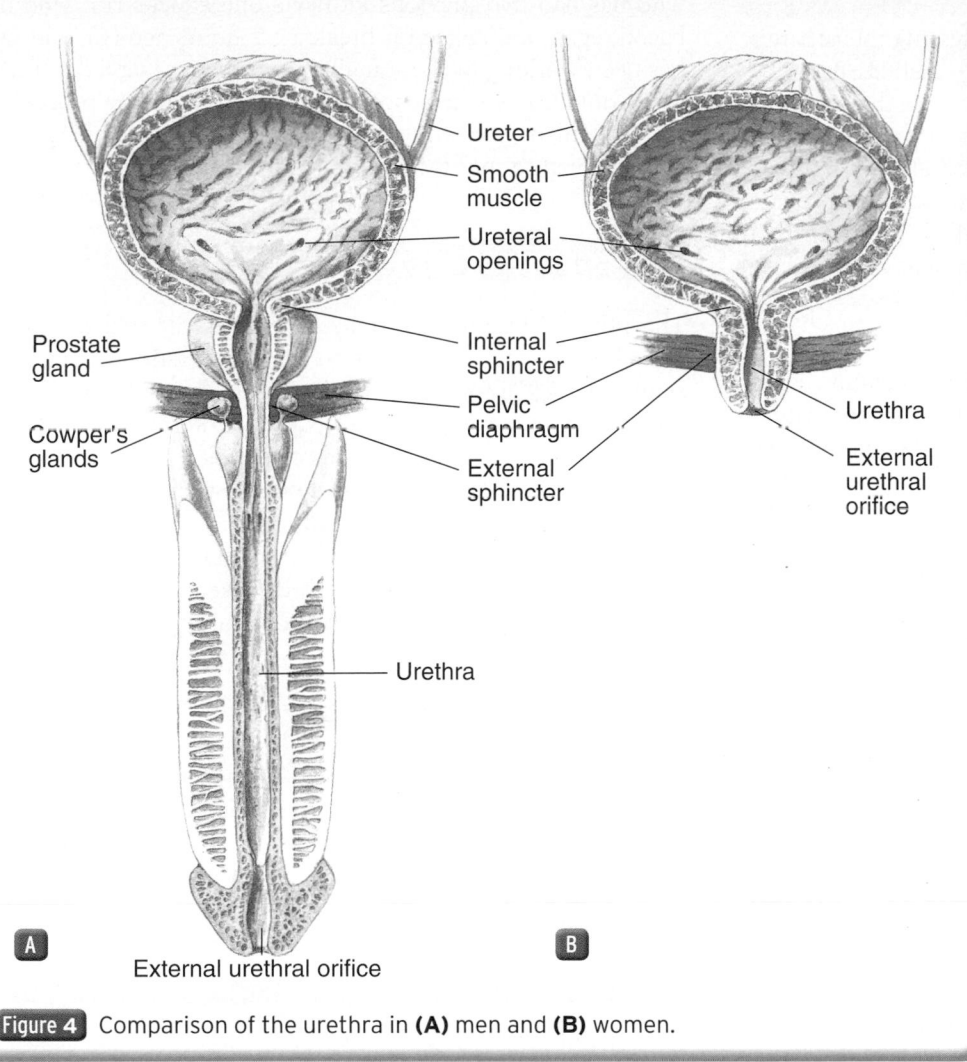

Figure 4 Comparison of the urethra in **(A)** men and **(B)** women.

- Ureter
- Smooth muscle
- Ureteral openings
- Prostate gland
- Internal sphincter
- Cowper's glands
- Pelvic diaphragm
- External sphincter
- Urethra
- External urethral orifice
- Urethra
- External urethral orifice
- **A**
- **B**

Patient Assessment

Assessment of a patient with a renal and genitourinary emergency is the same as for any other medical patient. Begin with the scene size-up, perform a primary assessment, obtain a history, perform a secondary assessment including physical examination, form a field impression, make a treatment decision, and reassess the patient continuously en route to the hospital.

Scene Size-up

In the scene size-up, you should not only ensure that the scene is safe for you and your fellow providers, but also consider the mechanism of injury, assess for hazards and the need for additional help, and determine the number of patients. Remember that urine is a body fluid and that, as always, you must take standard precautions to avoid contact.

Patients who are experiencing renal problems may exhibit many of the same symptoms as a patient with other abdominal problems—nausea and vomiting, constipation or diarrhea, weight loss, loss of appetite, chest pain, and abdominal pain.

Because pain is a common symptom in both abdominal and urologic ailments, it is often difficult to determine the source of the pain. Urologic pain can have many origins—eg, bacterial infection, extension of the ureter by a kidney stone, or distention of the bladder because of prostate enlargement. However, assessment of urologic emergencies, as with all abdominal emergencies, is designed to detect and prevent life threats and provide supportive care for the patient. Do not waste valuable time trying to determine the exact cause of the pain in the prehospital setting.

Primary Assessment

Form a General Impression

In the primary assessment, you form a general impression of the patient and check for life-threatening conditions. A patient with genitourinary or renal problems may exhibit extremes of activity. Is the patient constantly changing positions in an attempt to find a comfortable position ("the kidney stone dance")? Or is the patient sitting very still with the knees drawn up to the chest? Is the patient in obvious pain? Does he or she appear pale or jaundiced? What is the patient's level of consciousness? Your observation of the patient's body movements, posture, skin color, breathing pattern, mental acuity, and other factors will give you a good overall sense of the severity of the patient's condition.

Documentation and Communication

Establish and document your baseline impression early in the assessment process. Document any changes in mental status or level of consciousness as you reevaluate the patient, and note how he or she responds to administration of supplemental oxygen, fluids, pain medication, and other interventions. Stay in close contact with medical control, and notify the receiving facility as soon as possible if life threats are apparent. Record the findings of your serial assessments in your report to the receiving facility, concluding with your overall impression of the patient's condition at the time of transfer.

Airway and Breathing

You should now check for life threats by assessing the patient's mental status and airway, breathing, and circulation. Begin by observing the patient's breathing and ensure that the airway is patent. Do you see signs of respiratory distress or failure, such as shallow breathing, a rapid respiratory rate, sweating, nasal flaring, chest retractions, or wheezing? Clear the airway and provide suctioning, bag-mask ventilation, or high-flow supplemental oxygen if necessary, as indicated by the patient's respiratory status.

Circulation

Next, assess skin color, heart rate, and blood pressure. Does the patient show signs of profuse bleeding or circulatory compromise? Is the abdomen distended or rigid? Look for signs of shock, such as a rapid heart rate and low blood pressure. If you discover any life-threatening conditions, take immediate steps to correct them and provide urgent transport to an appropriately equipped receiving facility. Advise the facility en route to begin mobilizing resources and staff so that they will be on standby at the time of transfer.

Transport Decision

When making your transport decision, integrate the information you obtained in the primary assessment. Determine as quickly as possible whether urgent transport is warranted for life threats such as air embolism, hyperkalemia, or subdural hematoma. Consider how you will move the patient, especially if doing so is likely to cause a drop in blood pressure with the change of position. Take into account any special equipment needed to handle the patient, such as a bariatric stretcher. Also keep in mind which receiving facility has the diagnostic or treatment equipment that will be necessary after transfer, such as a lithotripsy unit.

Ensure that the ride during transport is as gentle as possible for the patient. Drive smoothly and steadily. Rapid driving can result in increased vehicle movement, potentially aggravating and possibly worsening the patient's abdominal pain.

History Taking

In genitourinary patients, the history and physical examination will provide the information you need to successfully manage the patient. Because 80% of all medical diagnoses are based on the patient's history, it is imperative that you ask the right questions during this examination. Determining that the patient's pain actually started in the flank, for example, and not in its present location in the lower right quadrant, could mean the difference between a correct field diagnosis of a kidney stone and an incorrect field diagnosis of appendicitis. Similarly, determining that the patient has a history of diabetes and hypertension along with signs of uremia can help confirm your impression of chronic kidney failure.

The SAMPLE mnemonic (signs and symptoms, allergies, medications, pertinent past medical history, last oral intake, events leading to the injury or illness) can guide you in obtaining pertinent historical information from the patient. For example, a patient who reports flank pain and is agitated (S); who has had two previous kidney stone attacks (P); who had bacon, eggs, and coffee for breakfast 7 hours ago (L); and who has been working in the sun all day (E) has presented a history that would lead you to suspect kidney stones. Before proceeding with treatment, you would obviously want to assess allergies (A) and any medications (M) the patient has taken.

Secondary Assessment

The physical examination may be focused or you may move from head to toe, depending on the presentation of signs and symptoms. **Figure 5** shows the division of the abdominal region into either four quadrants overlying the internal organs (**A**) or nine anatomic segments (**B**). A more detailed physical examination may be performed en route if not done at the scene.

Monitoring the patient's vital signs is part of the physical examination. You should obtain serial vital signs at least every 5 minutes if renal failure is suspected. Take prompt action if you note any deterioration in the patient's vital signs or level of consciousness.

Special Populations

Abnormal vital signs in an older adult patient may be particularly worrisome. An elderly patient with a fever, for instance, should receive especially close scrutiny for other signs of infection. In your interpretation of abnormal readings, however, be sure to account for age-related variations.

Finally, consider the link between abnormal vital signs and the patient's history. For example, a diuretic or other medication might be responsible for a patient's low blood pressure. Diabetes, chronic obstructive pulmonary disease (COPD), or another chronic condition noted in the patient's history might explain other abnormal findings and provide clues to the patient's current genitourinary or renal diagnosis.

ECG monitoring is extremely important in any patient with a suspected urologic emergency because of the possibility of electrolyte imbalances that may affect the heart. In a patient with hyperkalemia, for example, the ECG monitor will show a series of tall, peaked T waves.

Reassessment

Patients with urologic emergencies, especially those with signs and symptoms of renal failure, require reassessment. The electrolyte imbalances caused by the buildup of toxins can cause rapid deterioration in the functioning of the body's organs. The heart is particularly susceptible to electrolyte changes, so cardiac monitoring should be established for every renal patient.

The information obtained from the history and physical examination is used to formulate a more nuanced field impression and to select a treatment plan. The interventions might be

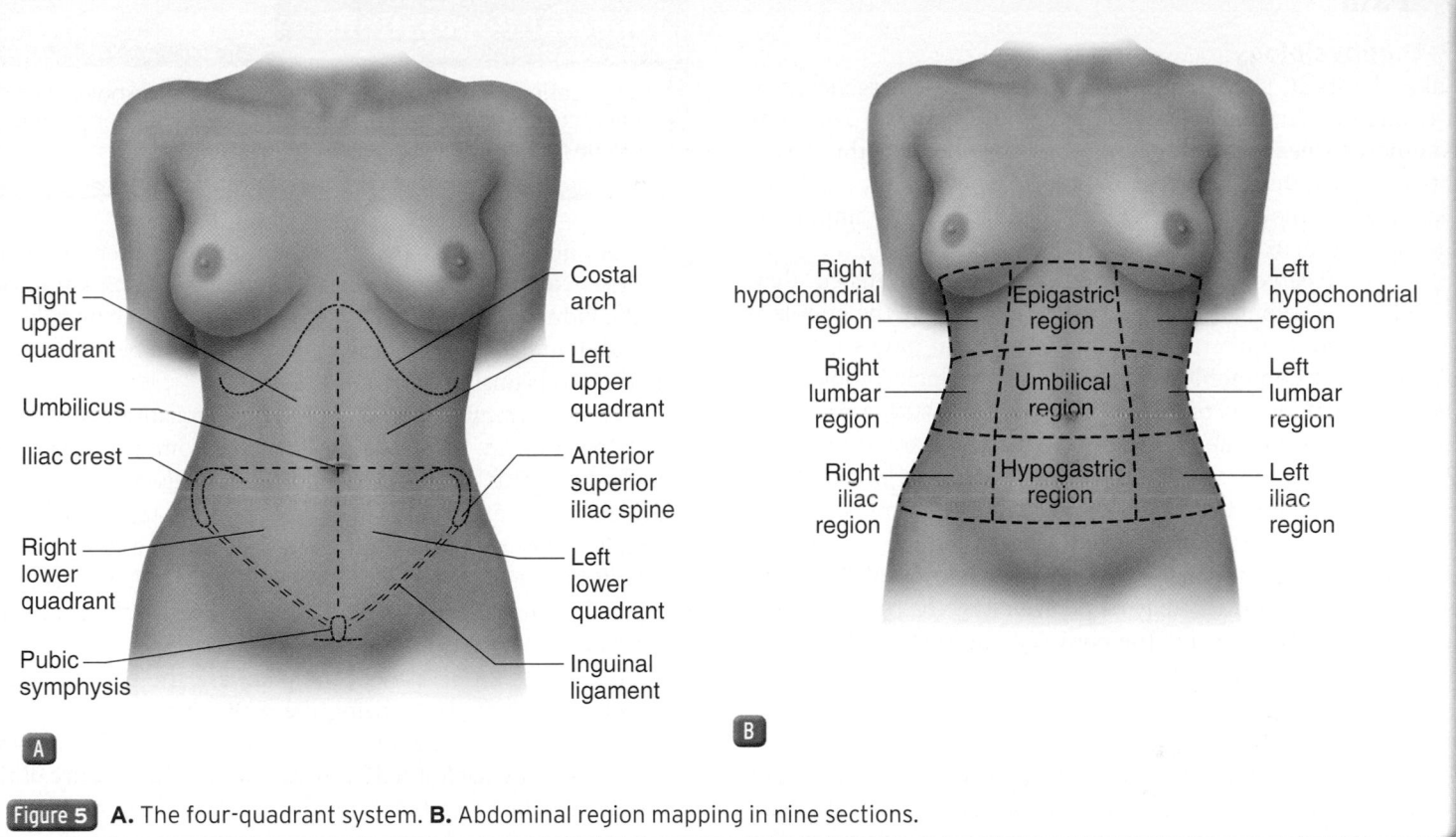

Right upper quadrant

Umbilicus

Iliac crest

Right lower quadrant

Pubic symphysis

Costal arch

Left upper quadrant

Anterior superior iliac spine

Left lower quadrant

Inguinal ligament

A

Right hypochondrial region

Right lumbar region

Right iliac region

Epigastric region

Umbilical region

Hypogastric region

Left hypochondrial region

Left lumbar region

Left iliac region

B

Figure 5 **A.** The four-quadrant system. **B.** Abdominal region mapping in nine sections.

as simple as monitoring the ABCs and providing circulatory support to a patient with a urinary tract infection (UTI), or as complex as adjusting medications and providing support (with medical consultation and direction) for a patient with renal failure, identified on the basis of ECG changes. The treatment plan includes the transport decision, which may be made at any time during the assessment process. If the disease process requires immediate medical procedures (ie, removal of a urinary catheter, adjustment of a fistula or shunt, etc) that go beyond the scope of the prehospital setting, perform the primary assessment and transport, reassessing the patient en route to the hospital.

Serial vital signs should be obtained and documented on the prehospital care report, at least every 5 minutes in patients with possible renal failure. Note any trends in the vital signs and level of consciousness because they can be indicators of disease progression. Patients with possible urologic disease should not be given anything by mouth because this may induce vomiting or complicate surgical procedures. Document all vital signs and report any apparent trends to the receiving facility.

Words of Wisdom

Patients with renal failure who miss their dialysis treatments are prone to hyperkalemia, among other conditions. You should suspect hyperkalemia if the patient has severe muscle weakness and tall, peaked T waves appear on the ECG.

Pathophysiology, Assessment, and Management of Specific Emergencies

Diseases and problems of the renal and urologic systems range from mild (urinary tract infections) to true emergencies (acute renal failure). Although the prehospital care for many urologic diseases is supportive, your ability to recognize the signs and symptoms of these conditions, especially when they are genuine emergencies, is critical to providing your patients with the best chance of a positive outcome. Many conditions discussed in this section can cause **urinary retention**— incomplete emptying of the bladder, or even a complete lack of ability to empty the bladder. These conditions are listed in Table 1.

Table 1 Conditions That May Cause Urinary Retention

Renal calculi
Acute renal failure
Benign prostate hypertrophy
Urethral obstructions
Urinary tract infections
Nerve damage

Pain

Pathophysiology

Taken by itself, pain cannot be considered an emergency, but it is often the cardinal sign of one. Because pain is a symptom common to nearly all the conditions presented in this chapter, understanding its pathophysiology is helpful in the field. Determining the origin of referred pain can be an important diagnostic tool in some urologic and renal diseases.

When receptors at the affected organs are stimulated, they send impulses along the nerves to the brain, where the impulses are evaluated and interpreted as pain. <u>Visceral pain</u>—the type of pain most commonly associated with urologic problems—usually occurs when receptors in the hollow structures, such as the ureters, urinary bladder, and urethra, are stimulated. Pinpointing the source of such pain is challenging because only a few nerve fibers may be involved in the pain transmission. Because many different nerve fibers travel to the brain through the spinal cord, pain that originates in one area of the body (eg, the urinary bladder) may be perceived by the brain as coming from a different area of the body (eg, the neck or shoulder). This is called <u>referred pain</u>.

Assessment Findings

The OPQRST (onset, provocation, quality, region/radiation/referral, severity, timing) mnemonic is used to evaluate the type and severity of pain. *Onset* involves questions about when the pain started and what the patient was doing at the time. The patient may describe visceral pain, such as that caused by a kidney stone, as a crampy or aching sensation deep within the

body. It often begins as a vague discomfort and then gradually increases. Next, determine what, if anything, *provokes* the pain (eg, the kidney stone dance or statue stillness). To help rule out other abdominal causes of pain, take note of any relationship between food consumption and the pain.

After determining the onset and provocation, assess the *quality* of the pain. As stated earlier, pain from a kidney stone usually begins as vague discomfort that becomes extremely sharp pain within an hour. The *R* stands for *region (location), radiation,* or *referral*; for example, the pain from a kidney stone moves from the flank anteriorly, toward the groin. The fact that the pain has moved also suggests that a kidney stone is passing through the system.

To evaluate the *severity* of the pain, ask the patient, "On a scale of 1 to 10, with 10 being the worst pain you have ever experienced, how would you rate the pain?" Although this number is helpful, by itself it tells you very little. The severity of the pain may not be consistent with the severity of the problem. It is important to repeat the pain severity assessment to look for trends or to verify the efficacy of treatment.

The final pain evaluation is to inquire about the *timing* of the pain. Did the pain come on suddenly, or more gradually? Has it

YOU *are the Medic*   PART 3

Your partner returns with the stair chair and tells you additional personnel are en route and should be arriving in a few minutes. You ask your partner to obtain the patient's temperature while you finish obtaining the SAMPLE history and assemble your supplies to start an IV line. The patient tells you that she has had burning with urination for a few days and that she has had urinary tract infections in the past. At one point, her physician put her on prophylactic Cipro. She decided that was not a good idea, and now just takes herbal supplements containing cranberry when she feels an infection is starting.

Recording Time: 5 Minutes	
Respirations	24 breaths/min
Pulse	110 beats/min
Skin	Flushed, sweaty
Blood pressure	108/60 mm Hg; lying down
Oxygen saturation (Spo$_2$)	95%
Pupils	PEARRL

5. What additional assessment techniques might you use?

6. Why is assessing her temperature important?

been constant, or does it come and go? In the case of a kidney stone, you would expect fairly constant pain that varies in severity and moves as the stone travels through the system.

Management

Once you have checked and established adequate airway, breathing, and circulation (the ABCs), allow the patient to assume a position of comfort. Patients in severe pain may have nausea and vomiting, so be prepared to suction and be ready for the possibility of aspiration. Analgesia may be provided if necessary, but remember that the masking of abdominal pain is not a desired result of prehospital care. Consult medical control before administering pain medication. Establish an IV line. If kidney function is present, administer a bolus of fluid to the patient with a UTI as well as to the patient with a kidney stone. The fluid will rehydrate the UTI patient, and increased urine will help flush the infection from the system. For the patient who has a renal calculus, the increased urine formation will help move the stone through the system.

■ Urinary Tract Infections

Urinary tract infection (UTI) results in over six million physician visits per year. It is most common in females after infancy. After the age of 50, there is an increase in UTIs in men because of obstruction of the urethra by the prostrate. Definitive treatment requires antibiotics. Mild cases respond well to oral antibiotics, whereas severe cases may require IV administration.

Pathophysiology

Urinary tract infections (UTIs) usually develop in the lower urinary tract (urethra and bladder) when normal flora (bacteria that naturally populate the skin) enter the urethra and grow. These infections are more common in women because of the relatively short urethra and its close proximity to the vagina and rectum. UTIs in the upper urinary tract occur most often when lower UTIs go untreated. Upper UTIs can lead to pyelonephritis (inflammation of the kidney linings) and abscesses, which eventually reduce kidney function. In severe cases, untreated UTIs can lead to sepsis.

Assessment Findings

Patients with UTIs display a classic triad of symptoms: painful urination, frequent urges to urinate, and difficulty in urination. The pain usually begins as a visceral discomfort, but soon becomes an extreme, burning pain, especially during urination. The pain, which remains localized in the pelvis, is often perceived as bladder pain in women and as prostate pain in men. Sometimes the pain is referred to the shoulder or neck. In addition, the urine will have a foul odor and may appear cloudy.

Patients with UTIs appear to be restless and uncomfortable. The skin ranges from pale, cool, and moist in a patient with a lower UTI to warm and dry in a patient with an upper UTI, such as pyelonephritis. Vital signs vary with the degree of illness, but palpation of the abdomen usually reveals tenderness over the pubis or pain in the flank, depending on the area of the infection.

Management

Management of patients with UTIs consists mainly of supportive care of the ABCs. Allow the patient to ride in a position of comfort, but be prepared for nausea and vomiting. Analgesics will probably be needed only in severe cases of pyelonephritis. For most patients, nonpharmacologic pain management with breathing and relaxation techniques is usually sufficient. Establish an IV line and administer a fluid bolus, which will promote blood flow through the kidney and dilute the urine. Transport the patient to the nearest appropriate facility for evaluation.

■ Urinary Catheters

Many patients who are hospitalized for a urinary problem or other medical disease receive catheterization. Bladder catheterization involves introducing a latex or plastic tube through the urethra and into the bladder. The tube is connected to a drainage bag, which is attached to the bed frame or wheelchair at a level below the bladder. The catheter allows a continuous outflow of urine and provides a means of measuring urine output in hemodynamically unstable patients.

When you are transporting a catheterized patient, urine backflow is a concern. If the drainage bag is raised above the level of the patient's bladder, urine can backflow into the bladder, increasing the chance of infection. Care should be taken not to lift the drainage bag while loading, positioning, or otherwise handling the patient.

■ Urinary Incontinence

Urinary incontinence is loss of bladder control—the inability to control the release of urine from the bladder. Whereas urinary incontinence can occur in anyone (for example from sneezing or a forceful cough), it may be a sign of a medical problem if it falls into one of the following two categories:

- **Urge incontinence.** This is a sudden, intense urge to urinate and then within seconds to minutes, involuntary urine loss occurs. Urination is frequent—for example, throughout the night. Urge incontinence has many potential medical causes, including urinary tract infection, bladder irritants, bowel problems, Parkinson disease, Alzheimer disease, stroke, injury, or nervous system damage associated with multiple sclerosis.
- **Overflow incontinence.** This is a constant, continual slow flow of urine. Overflow incontinence can have medical causes, such as a damaged bladder, blocked urethra, or nerve damage from diabetes and in men with prostate gland problems.

■ Renal Calculi (Kidney Stones)

Pathophysiology

Kidney stones are extremely common and originate in the renal pelvis. They form when an excess of insoluble salts or uric acid crystallizes in the urine Figure 6 . According to the National Institutes of Health, more than 600,000 patients visited emergency departments for kidney stones in the year 2000.

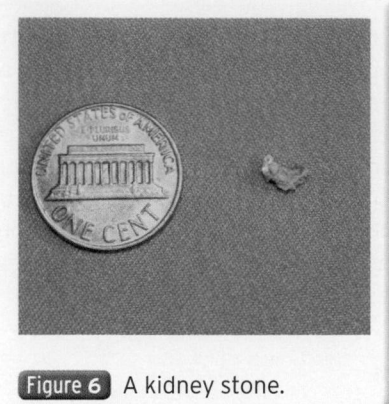

Figure 6 A kidney stone.

The excess of salts can typically be attributed to water intake that is insufficient to dissolve the salts. The stones consist of different types of chemicals, depending on the precise imbalance in the urine.

The most common stones—calcium stones—occur more frequently in men than in women. Their formation may have a hereditary component. These stones also form in patients with hormonal or metabolic disorders, such as gout. Struvite stones are more common in women and may be associated with chronic UTI or frequent catheterization. Uric acid and cystine stones are the least common. Uric acid stones tend to run in families, especially those with a history of gout. Cystine stones are associated with a condition that causes large amounts of amino acids and proteins to be excreted in the urine.

Assessment Findings

Patients who have kidney stones are almost always in pain. It usually starts in the flank but may migrate forward, toward the groin, as the stone passes through the system. The patient may feel vague discomfort that progresses to become intense pain within 30 to 60 minutes. In fact, many patients rate kidney stone pain as an 11 on a scale of 1 to 10.

Some patients appear agitated and restless, pacing and moving about in an attempt to relieve the pain. Other patients try to remain motionless to guard the abdomen. Either behavior makes palpation of the abdomen difficult. Vital signs vary according to the severity of pain. The greater the pain, the higher the patient's blood pressure and pulse will be.

Most kidney stones can be treated without surgery. To help the kidney stones pass through the urinary system, the usual protocol consists of the patient consuming plenty of water (2 to 3 quarts a day) to help move the stone along. If a kidney stone becomes lodged in the lower ureter, the patient may have signs and symptoms of a UTI (frequency and urgency of urination, painful urination, and/or **hematuria**) but will not have a fever. Extracorporeal lithotripsy uses shock waves to pulverize the stone into passable fragments. Direct endoscopy may also be used to remove some stones. If a kidney stone is suspected, be sure to obtain a patient history and a family history; both can supply important information.

Management

The prehospital management of kidney stones centers on pain relief. After ensuring the ABCs, allow the patient to assume a position of comfort. Administer analgesia; if your local protocols do not allow for this, contact medical control regarding pain relief options. Pain relief is crucial for the patient with a kidney stone, but there are some instances in which narcotics should not be given, such as if there is a possibility of a gastrointestinal condition. Nitrous oxide is an alternative treatment to narcotics. Pain management may also be accomplished by using breathing techniques like those used for women during labor. Establish an IV line and administer fluids to accelerate movement of the stone through the system. Transport the patient to an appropriate facility with a lithotripsy unit if possible, providing supportive care as necessary.

■ Acute Renal Failure

Acute renal failure (ARF) is a sudden decrease in the rate of filtration through the glomeruli, causing toxins to accumulate in the blood. This loss of function may occur over a period of several days. In 2008, the National Kidney and Urological Disease Information Clearinghouse reported that ARF accounts for between 2% and 7% of all hospitalizations in the United States. Critically ill patients with ARF have an overall mortality rate of 50% to 80% but the disease is reversible if diagnosed and treated early.

Urine output of less than 500 mL/day is called **oliguria**. Complete cessation of urine production is called **anuria**. Whenever ARF occurs, the patient may experience generalized edema, acid buildup, and high levels of nitrogenous and metabolic wastes in the blood. If left untreated, ARF can lead to heart failure, hypertension, and metabolic acidosis.

ARF is classified into three types, based on the area in which the failure occurs: prerenal, intrarenal, and postrenal. The signs and symptoms of each type are summarized in **Table 2**.

Pathophysiology

The toxic buildup of nitrogenous wastes and salts in the blood associated with ARF causes impaired mentation, hypotension, fluid retention, tachycardia, acid/base imbalances, and increased PR and QT intervals associated with hyperkalemia.

Prerenal ARF is caused by hypoperfusion of the kidneys. In other words, not enough blood passes into the glomeruli for them to produce filtrate. The most common causes of prerenal ARF are hypovolemia (low blood volume caused by hemorrhage or dehydration), trauma, shock, sepsis, and heart failure (congestive heart failure, myocardial infarction). Prerenal ARF is often reversible if the underlying condition can be treated and perfusion restored to the kidney.

Words of Wisdom

Patients with kidney stones usually have severe, nearly unbearable pain, and should be given narcotic analgesics (ie, morphine, fentanyl) in the prehospital setting. Because higher-than-usual doses are often required, naloxone (Narcan) must be readily available in the event that central nervous system depression occurs. Follow local protocols or contact medical control as needed regarding pain relief for these patients.

Table 2 Signs and Symptoms of Acute Renal Failure

Type of Acute Renal Failure	Signs and Symptoms
Prerenal	Hypotension Tachycardia Dizziness Thirst
Intrarenal	Flank pain Joint pain Oliguria Hypertension Headache Confusion Seizure
Postrenal	Pain in lower flank, abdomen, groin, and genitalia Oliguria Distended bladder Hematuria Peripheral edema

Intrarenal acute renal failure (IARF) involves damage to one of three areas in the kidney: the glomeruli capillaries and small blood vessels, the cells of the kidney tubules, or the renal parenchyma (the interstitial cells around the nephrons). Damage to the small vessels and glomeruli hinders blood flow through these vital parts of the nephrons. This damage is often caused by immune-mediated diseases (eg, type 1 diabetes mellitus). Tubule damage can be caused by prerenal ARF or toxins (eg, heavy metals). Chronic inflammation of the interstitial cells surrounding the nephrons (interstitial nephritis) can also produce IARF. This type of renal failure may be caused by medications such as antibiotics, anticancer drugs, alcohol, and drugs of abuse (eg, cocaine).

Postrenal ARF is caused by obstruction of urine flow from the kidneys. The source of this obstruction is often a blockage of the urethra by an enlarged prostate, renal calculi, or strictures. This blockage raises pressure in the nephrons, which eventually shuts them down. At this point, the kidneys can no longer carry out their cleansing functions, resulting in the development of hyperkalemia (an increase in the blood potassium level) and/or metabolic acidosis (an increase in the hydrogen ion content of the blood). Both conditions are life-threatening emergencies that can lead to fatal cardiac dysrhythmias.

Assessment Findings

The skin will be pale, cool, and moist, and edema of the extremities and face will be apparent. The patient may report tinnitus, excessive urinary output at night, and a metallic taste in the mouth. Other possible findings include decreased urinary output, neuropathies of the hands and feet, anorexia, hypertension, an altered mental status, prolonged bleeding, and flank pain.

When you are inspecting the abdomen, look for any scars, ecchymosis, or distention. If the abdomen is distended, note whether the swelling is symmetric. Palpate the abdomen for any pulsing masses, which could indicate an aortic aneurysm. A hematocrit and urinalysis (if available) may be helpful in

YOU are the Medic — PART 4

Additional crew members have arrived to assist you with moving, lifting, and patient care. You explain to your patient that her condition requires that blood be drawn, and that it is necessary to establish an IV line to perform the blood draw and to administer fluids. Your team members have assembled the stair chair, listened to lung sounds, and placed her on the cardiac monitor. After you initiate the IV line and draw blood samples, you tell her, "We are going to put you in this chair with wheels to take you down the stairs." Her father tells you that is probably not a good idea because she "doesn't do well sitting up."

Recording Time: 10 Minutes	
Respirations	24 breaths/min
Pulse	112 beats/min
Skin	Flushed, sweaty
Blood pressure	108/60 mm Hg; lying down
Oxygen saturation (Spo$_2$)	98%
Pupils	PEARRL
Blood glucose	56 mg/dL

7. What should you consider with regard to moving the patient to the ambulance based on the father's comment?

8. What other questions may you have for the patient?

identifying such causes as acute anemia, chronic hemorrhage, or pyelonephritis.

Management

Because the metabolic changes caused by ARF can be life-threatening, it is imperative that the treatment plan support the ABCs. Administer high-flow supplemental oxygen and, if necessary, provide ventilatory support with bag-mask ventilation. Place the patient in the position dictated for shock by your local protocol. Consider administering an IV bolus if the patient exhibits signs of shock, but use caution to prevent pulmonary edema. If possible, and with medical direction and appropriate training, you may perform a fluid lavage for patients who undergo peritoneal dialysis.

The increase of metabolites in patients with ARF may be toxic to the kidneys. Many medications can be nephrotoxic (toxic to the kidneys), including many analgesics and antibiotics. Consult medical control if you suspect ARF and are transporting a patient with antibiotic or analgesic drips. If medical control is unavailable, discontinue the medication and transport the patient to the nearest appropriate facility.

Many patients with ARF have other comorbid diseases that may complicate treatment and lead to depression. As with any medical patient, patients with ARF need psychological support. Talk with your patient and inform him or her of what you are doing and what is occurring. Be confident and calm in your responses to questions, and reassure the patient that he or she is receiving the best care possible.

▮ Chronic Renal Failure

In the United States, over 300,000 people are on long-term dialysis. According to the National Health and Nutrition Examination Survey performed between 1999 and 2004, approximately 23 million adults (11.5%) age 20 years and up have signs and symptoms of chronic kidney disease.

Pathophysiology

Chronic renal failure (CRF) is progressive and irreversible inadequate kidney function that is the result of permanent loss of nephrons. This disease develops over months or years. More than half of all cases are a consequence of systemic disease, such as diabetes or hypertension. CRF can also be caused by congenital disorders or prolonged pyelonephritis.

As the damaged nephrons cease to function, scarring occurs in the kidneys. The tissue begins to shrink and waste away as the scarring progresses, leading to a loss of nephrons and renal mass. As kidney function diminishes, waste products and fluid build up in the blood. Uremia (an increased concentration of urea and other waste products in the blood) and azotemia (an increased level of nitrogenous wastes in the blood) develop, leading to systemic complications such as hypertension, congestive heart failure, anemia, and electrolyte imbalances.

Assessment Findings

Patients with CRF have an altered level of consciousness caused by electrolyte imbalances and their effects on transmission of nerve impulses in the brain. Patients may also present with

lethargy, nausea, headaches, cramps, signs of anemia, weakness, vomiting, anorexia, increased thirst, pruritus, and hypertension. Their urine may appear rusty-brown. In the late stages, seizures and coma are possible.

In a patient with CRF, the skin is pale, cool, and moist, and the patient may appear jaundiced because of the buildup of nitrogenous wastes. A powdery accumulation of uric acid called uremic frost may also be present, especially on the face. The skin may appear to be bruised, and muscle twitching may be present.

Patients with CRF exhibit edema in the extremities and face because of fluid imbalances; they are also hypotensive and tachycardic. As hyperkalemia develops, the heart's electrical conduction will decrease. The ECG monitor will show lengthening PR and QT intervals. As the hyperkalemia progresses, these dysrhythmias may evolve into an idioventricular rhythm. Pericarditis and pulmonary edema are also common in patients with CRF and should be evaluated during auscultation of the chest.

Management

Management of a patient with CRF is initially similar to management of a patient with ARF. Support the ABCs. Administer high-flow supplemental oxygen and, if necessary, provide ventilatory support with bag-mask ventilation. Place the patient in the position dictated for shock by your local protocol. If there are no signs of pulmonary edema, consider administering an IV bolus if the patient shows signs of shock. Because CRF patients are prone to third-space shock (because of fluid shifts) and major electrolyte changes, treatment strategies should center on the regulation of fluid imbalances and cardiovascular function. For example, if hypotension occurs, a vasopressor may be administered, or medical control may order the administration of sodium bicarbonate to correct acidosis. Ultimately, patients with CRF will require renal dialysis. After life threats have been addressed, transport the patient to the appropriate facility for treatment. Because patients with CRF already have electrolyte imbalances in their blood, be conservative with your treatment plans for these patients.

Transport should be undertaken in a calm manner; talk quietly and confidently with the patient. If the patient has an altered mental status, be sure to assess his or her orientation frequently and record any changes.

■ End-Stage Renal Disease

Pathophysiology

If left untreated, acute or chronic renal failure will progress to end-stage renal disease (ESRD). In a patient with ESRD, the kidneys have lost all ability to function, and toxic waste materials build up in the patient's blood. ESRD is fatal unless treated by dialysis or renal transplant. In 2007, over 527,000 people in the United States were undergoing treatment for ESRD and over $35 billion was spent on dialysis.

Assessment Findings

Confusion, shortness of breath, peripheral edema, bruising, chest pain, and bone pain are initial signs of ESRD. As toxins continue to accumulate, pruritus, nausea and vomiting, muscle twitching and tremors, and hallucinations may occur. Patients may also present with lethargy, headaches, cramps, and signs of anemia. The skin is pale, cool, and moist, and may appear jaundiced or bruised. Uremic frost may be present around the face. Edema of the extremities and face is apparent, and patients are hypotensive and tachycardic. The ECG monitor shows lengthening PR and QT intervals. As hyperkalemia increases, these dysrhythmias may become an idioventricular rhythm. Pericarditis and pulmonary edema are also common and should be evaluated during auscultation of the chest. In the late stages, seizures and coma are possible and the patient may ultimately die.

Management

Treatment for patients with ESRD is limited to renal dialysis or kidney transplant. Provide supportive care. Administer high-flow supplemental oxygen and be ready to provide ventilatory support with bag-mask ventilation if the patient shows signs of respiratory distress. Place the patient in the shock position dictated by your local protocol. Under the direction of medical control, regulate fluid imbalances, electrolyte abnormalities, and cardiovascular function.

Words of Wisdom

Patients with ESRD often have an altered level of consciousness; therefore, maintain a calm demeanor during transport. Speak quietly and confidently to the patient, and assess his or her orientation frequently. Be sure to document your findings and let the receiving facility know that the patient has an impaired mental status.

YOU are the Medic   PART 5

Because family members serve as invaluable sources of information, you thank the patient's father. You then explain that it is necessary to move her in order to treat her properly, but that you will handle her very gently and you will prepare for changes in her condition. As you help the patient slowly sit up, she reports some dizziness, but seems to tolerate the position. You buckle her into the stair chair and explain how she will be moved down the stairs. You reach the front door, transfer her to the gurney, and cover her with blankets. You reassess her in the ambulance, and she tells you she feels better lying down. You note that her orthostatic vital signs are positive for change. After contacting medical control, you are advised to administer another 500-mL bolus of normal saline. You are further advised to administer odansetron (Zofran), 4 mg, if she continues to vomit and 25 g of dextrose 50% if she has a decrease in her level of consciousness.

Recording Time: 15 Minutes	
Respirations	24 breaths/min
Pulse	120 beats/min
Skin	Flushed, sweaty
Blood pressure	100/50 mm Hg; lying down
Oxygen saturation (Spo$_2$)	98%
Pupils	PEARRL
IV fluids	500-mL NS; repeated

9. What may you consider requesting from medical control in addition to dextrose and antiemetics?

10. How will her condition affect transport?

Renal Dialysis

Although not truly a urologic disorder, <u>renal dialysis</u> and problems associated with it may require prehospital interventions. Renal dialysis is a technique for filtering toxic wastes from the blood, removing excess fluid, and restoring the normal balance of electrolytes **Figure 7**.

There are two types of dialysis—peritoneal dialysis and hemodialysis. In peritoneal dialysis, large amounts of specially formulated dialysis fluid are infused into (and then drained from) the abdominal cavity. This fluid remains in the cavity for 1 to 2 hours, allowing equilibrium to occur as waste diffuses across the peritoneal membrane and into the fluid. Peritoneal dialysis is very effective but carries a high risk of peritonitis; consequently, aseptic technique is essential. With proper training, however, peritoneal dialysis can be performed in the home.

In hemodialysis, the patient's blood circulates through a dialysis machine that functions in much the same way (albeit not as elegantly) as the normal kidneys. Most patients undergoing chronic hemodialysis have some sort of shunt, ie, a surgically created connection between a vein and an artery. The patient is connected to the dialysis machine through this shunt, which allows blood to flow from the body into the dialysis machine and back to the body. A Scribner shunt, for example, consists of two plastic tubes: one fastened in the radial artery, the other in the cephalic vein. These two tubes are joined near the wrist by a Teflon connector. A Thomas shunt is similar, but this device is usually placed in the groin. Other patients have a small, button-shaped device called a HemaSite, which has a rubber septum that can be punctured with dialysis needles during treatment. HemaSites are usually placed in the upper arm or proximal anterior thigh. Finally, some patients have an <u>internal shunt</u> (an arteriovenous [AV] fistula), which is an artificial connection between a vein and an artery that is usually located in the forearm or upper arm **Figure 8**.

In patients with a life-threatening emergency, the internal shunt may be used for IV access. In all other instances, an alternative IV site should be selected. AV shunts should not be used for routine blood draws.

The only time you will most likely see a dialysis machine is if your service transports patients to and from dialysis centers. If there is a dialysis machine in a private residence, treatments will most likely be performed by a trained dialysis technician or possibly by the patient or family members.

Patients requiring chronic dialysis usually undergo the process every 2 or 3 days for 3 to 5 hours. Many receive dialysis in the hospital or in community dialysis facilities, but a significant number have home dialysis units. Patients undergoing dialysis at home usually have extensive training in the procedures, and often someone else in the home has also been trained. If a problem with the machine occurs, the patient may know a lot more about it than you do, so always ask what the patient has done prior to your arrival.

Whereas patients undergoing chronic dialysis can experience the same spectrum of illnesses and injuries as other patients, they are particularly vulnerable to certain problems, either because of the dialysis itself or because of the underlying renal failure. Problems associated with dialysis may result from accidental disconnection from the machine, malfunction of the machine, or rapid shifts in fluids and electrolytes that produce hypotension, potassium imbalances, and disequilibrium syndrome. The management of medical emergencies resulting from dialysis is summarized in **Table 3**.

Persons who miss dialysis treatments will often present with signs of electrolyte imbalance, including weakness of muscles, cramping, pulmonary edema, and uremic frost. Other general complications of dialysis include muscle cramps, nausea and vomiting, and infections at the IV site.

Hypotension and Shock

A sudden drop in blood pressure is not uncommon during or immediately after a patient undergoes dialysis, but it can lead to cardiac arrest if not promptly detected and treated.

> ### Words of Wisdom
>
> When you measure the blood pressure in a dialysis patient, use the arm that does not have the shunt!

The patient may feel light-headed or become confused, and often he or she yawns more than usual. Because dialysis alters the blood's chemistry, the patient may experience an electrolyte imbalance. For this reason, you should always monitor dialysis patients for cardiac dysrhythmias. Shock secondary to bleeding is also possible from any number of causes. Patients with CRF, for example, are very prone to duodenal ulcers; bleeding from these ulcers is not unusual. Bleeding may also occur at the site of the dialysis cannula.

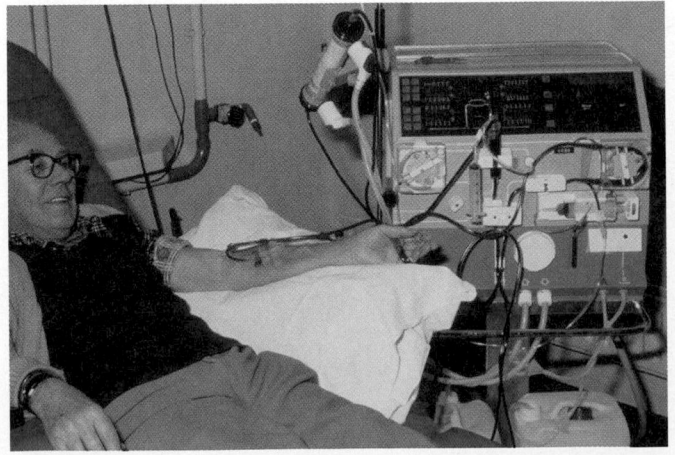

Figure 7 A patient undergoing dialysis.

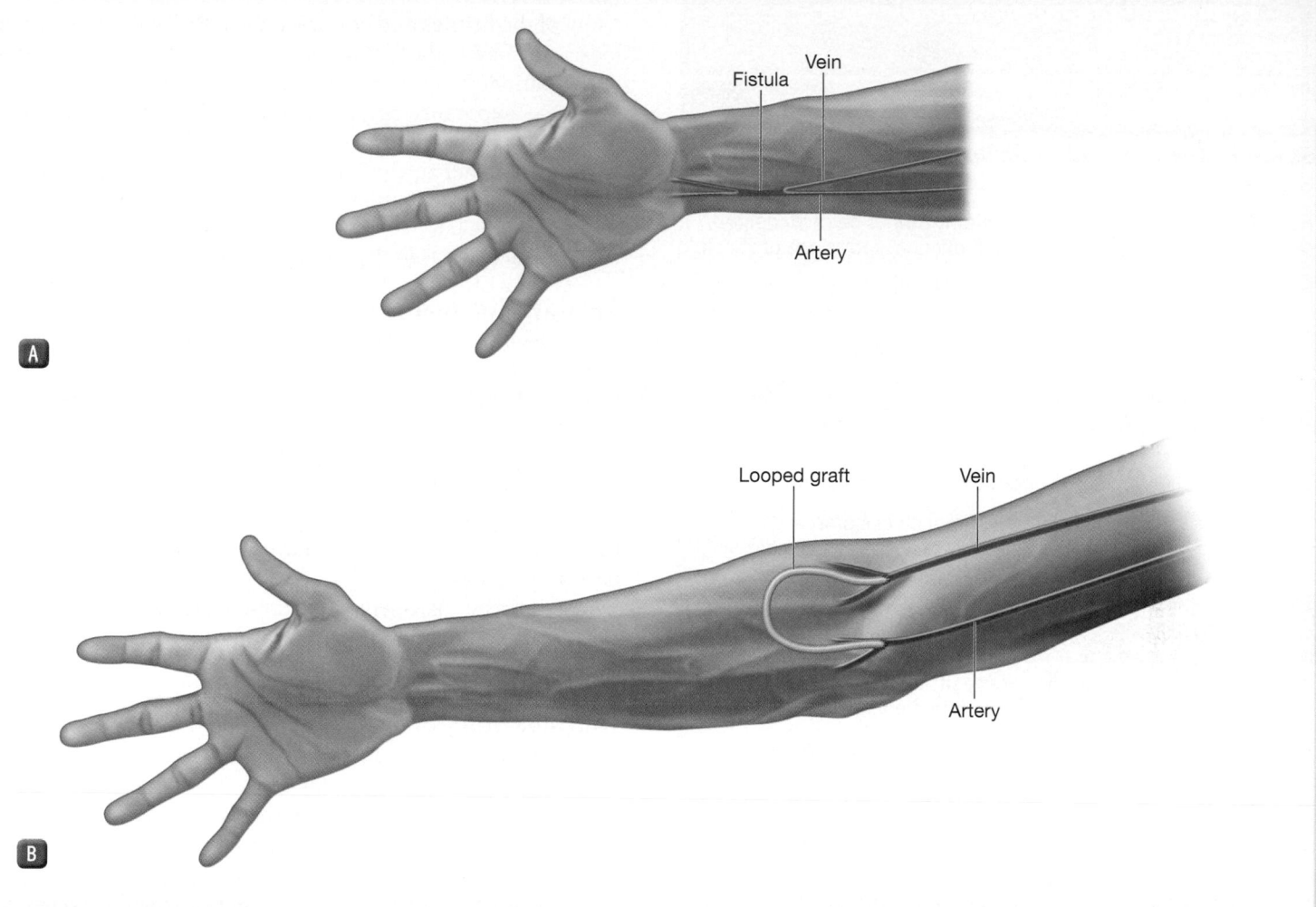

Figure 8 **A.** With an arteriovenous (AV) fistula, a bulge is created beneath the skin by arterial pressure at the site where the artery and vein have been directly connected. **B.** An AV graft creates a raised area beneath the skin that looks like a large vessel.

When you find a shunt leaking during the dialysis cycle, attempt to tighten up the connection. If it has become disconnected at the vein, clamp the cannula and disconnect the patient from the machine. In a suicide attempt, the patient may open up the cannula and allow himself or herself to exsanguinate. Keep in mind that these patients have often endured numerous medical interventions to simply survive. If you encounter this situation, immediately *clamp off the cannula* and apply direct pressure.

Potassium Imbalance

One consequence of renal impairment is the inability to excrete ingested potassium. As a consequence, CRF patients are prone to the development of hyperkalemia, especially in circumstances of increased potassium intake or catabolic stress. Such a patient may present with profound muscular weakness. On the ECG, the classic signs of hyperkalemia are peaked T waves **Figure 9**, a prolonged QRS complex, and sometimes disappearance of the P waves. Complete heart block and asystole may occur. If you see these signs, treatment is urgently required and must be undertaken in the field if you are any distance from the hospital.

Hypokalemia may also occur as a consequence of overaggressive dialysis. The potassium level is most likely to fall during or immediately after a dialysis cycle. The patient may be hypotensive, and cardiac dysrhythmia (usually bradycardia) is almost always present. Treat the dysrhythmia if it is hemodynamically significant (see the chapter, *Cardiovascular Emergencies*).

Disequilibrium Syndrome

Dialysis rapidly lowers the concentration of urea in the blood, whereas the concentration of solutes in the cerebrospinal fluid (CSF) remains high. Water, of course, moves by osmosis from a solution of lower concentration into a solution of higher concentration. Thus, as a consequence of dialysis, water initially shifts from the bloodstream into the CSF, thereby mildly increasing intracranial pressure. In such a circumstance, the patient may experience <u>disequilibration syndrome</u>, a condition characterized by nausea, vomiting, headache, and confusion. After a few hours, the fluid will re-equilibrate between the blood and CSF, and the patient's symptoms will improve on their own.

Table 3 Medical Emergencies in Dialysis Patients

Problem	Prehospital Management
Problems related to dialysis itself:	
Hypotension	Administer 50 mL of normal saline IV
Hemorrhage from the shunt	If the shunt cannot be reconnected, clamp it off; check for signs of shock
Potassium imbalance	For hypokalemia: treat bradycardia with atropine
	For hyperkalemia: calcium and bicarbonate may be considered
Disequilibrium syndrome	Supportive treatment only
Air embolism	Left lateral recumbent position in about 10° of head-down tilt
Machine dysfunction	Turn off machine; clamp ends of shunt; disconnect patient from machine; transport
Problems to which dialysis patients are more vulnerable:	
Congestive heart failure	Oxygen; sitting position; rapid transport to dialysis facility
Myocardial infarction and cardiac dysrhythmias	Treat as any other patient, but use caution in administering any medications
Hypertension	Transport only; the treatment is dialysis
Pericardial tamponade	Emergency transport as soon as detected
Uremic pericarditis	Oxygen; position of comfort; transport

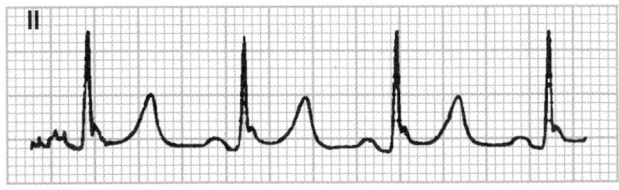

Figure 9 Peaked T waves, as shown in this rhythm strip, are a classic sign of hyperkalemia.

Words of Wisdom

In the field, it may be impossible to distinguish between disequilibrium syndrome and subdural hematoma, to which dialysis patients are particularly vulnerable. In such a case, transport the patient to the hospital immediately for a full neurologic evaluation.

Air Embolism

If any of the fittings and connections in the dialysis system are loose, air may enter the system, producing an <u>air embolism</u> in the patient. Symptoms of an air embolism include sudden dyspnea, hypotension, and cyanosis. If you suspect an air embolism, disconnect the patient from the dialysis machine, place him or her in the left lateral recumbent position with about 10° of head-down tilt, and transport immediately.

■ Male Genital Tract Conditions

Epididymitis and Orchitis

One possible complication of male UTI is <u>epididymitis</u>, an infection that causes inflammation of the epididymis along the posterior border of the testis. When one or both testes become infected, this is called <u>orchitis</u>. With orchitis, the infection causes one or both testes to become enlarged and tender, causing pain and swelling in the scrotum. Swelling may occur in the groin on the affected side. The pain may increase during bowel movements. The patient will have a fever, and the urine will have a foul odor.

Prehospital management of these conditions is supportive. Because the patient is likely in pain, consider administering analgesics.

Fournier Gangrene

If bacteria enter the scrotum or perineum because of a laceration, <u>Fournier gangrene</u> may occur. This infection causes necrosis of the subcutaneal tissue and muscle in the scrotum. The scrotum will be spongy to the touch, the scrotal tissues will become gray-black, drainage will occur from the wound site, and fever and scrotal pain will be present. This is a true emergency and prompt transport to the hospital is indicated. If left untreated, the infection can enter the bloodstream, causing sepsis. Patients with Fournier gangrene should receive prompt transport and be assessed and treated for shock.

Priapism

<u>Priapism</u>, a painful, tender, persistent erection, can result from diseases such as leukemia and tumors, from blunt perineal trauma, spinal cord injury, abuse of cocaine, or erectile dysfunction drugs. This condition is discussed in more detail in the chapter, *Abdominal and Genitourinary Trauma*. Be sure to maintain the patient's privacy and do not make assumptions

Words of Wisdom

A patient who sustained blunt renal trauma often presents with flank pain and hematuria (blood in the urine) that usually goes undetected until evaluation in the emergency department. Obvious hematomas or ecchymoses over the upper abdomen, middle back, or lower rib cage may also suggest renal injuries. Keep this in mind when assessing a patient with a urologic emergency (discussed in detail in the chapter, *Abdominal and Genitourinary Trauma*).

about the cause of the condition. Whatever the cause, treat all patients with respect, and administer analgesics for pain. If a spinal cord injury is suspected, ensure proper immobilization techniques.

Phimosis and Paraphimosis

Phimosis is the inability to retract the distal foreskin over the glans penis. This condition is usually associated with poor hygiene and scarring of the foreskin by bacterial infection. Prehospital treatment includes cold compresses and transport.

Paraphimosis results when the foreskin is retracted over the glans penis and becomes entrapped. Because of the tightness of the foreskin, the glans swells even further, making it even harder to slide the foreskin back into the normal position. Paraphimosis usually occurs in elderly men, but can occur after piercings of the glans penis. Paraphimosis is a true emergency. Failure to relieve the paraphimosis can result in necrosis of the glans.

Benign Prostate Hypertrophy

Benign prostate hypertrophy (BPH) is an age-related nonmalignant (noncancerous) enlargement of the prostate gland. It occurs in about 50% of men older than age 60. It may be asymptomatic, or it may lead to difficulty starting urine flow, a slow weak urine flow once started, incomplete emptying of the bladder, increased urination at night, and urinary retention.

Testicular Masses

Testicular masses rarely require prehospital treatment. They may be painful or painless, and if painful, the pain may radiate up the spermatic cord or be localized to a specific scrotal point. Most are benign cystic masses or a varicocele—a painless mass of dilated veins posterior to the testicle. Testicular cancer usually presents as a painless solid lump on the testicle. Incidence of testicular cancer is on the rise and reported cases have doubled since 1975. In 2005, the American Cancer Society reported 8,000 new cases in the United States.

Testicular Torsion

Testicular torsion is a twisting of the testicle on the spermatic cord, from which it is suspended. This condition is associated with the sudden onset of scrotal pain and swelling. It is a medical emergency if the twisting of the vessels reduces blood flow to the testis. The torsion is usually unilateral, occurring in only one testis at a time. Torsions may occur with or without blunt trauma, a testicular lump, or blood in the semen. Patients should be carefully and promptly transported and allowed to assume the position of greatest comfort. Analgesics may be given for pain control.

YOU are the Medic   SUMMARY

1. What concerns may you have about the scene?

Performing a scene assessment is essential to ensure the safety of you and your crew. Knowing this is an older home with a narrow stairwell and the patient is on the second floor should prompt you to consider requesting additional personnel and a stair chair, Reeves stretcher, or other items required for safe moving and lifting.

2. Although you have not seen your patient yet, what information do you already know that is part of the primary assessment?

Because you heard your patient call out for her father telling him she was about to "be sick again," you know that she is alert, has a patent airway, and is breathing. This information may change rapidly, but you have gathered a lot of information before seeing her.

3. What concerns do you have about her history, signs, and symptoms?

More information is needed to narrow your differential diagnosis. Causes for concern include her skin signs, pointing to fever/infection as well as dizziness while standing. She is likely to have positive orthostatic vital signs and is significantly dehydrated because of the vomiting.

4. What should be done with the emesis?

Do not forget to look at the emesis for any signs of blood. Follow local protocols regarding transport of specimens to the hospital.

5. What additional assessment techniques might you use?

One technique used to assess for kidney infection or pyelonephritis is to locate the costovertebral angle. Then, place your fist over this site and gently tap with the other hand. If the kidney is infected, this will elicit a painful response; therefore, you should use this technique with caution.

6. Why is assessing her temperature important?

Temperature assessment is important and should not be forgotten in the prehospital setting. Having appropriate thermometers can provide a wealth of information in hypothermic and hyperthermic patients. Assessing this patient's temperature, along with other assessment findings, can assist you in treating and documenting infection.

7. What should you consider with regard to moving the patient to the ambulance based on the father's comment?

You should be prepared for neurologic symptoms including syncope. You may have to adjust your method of moving her to the ambulance. Prehospital providers have a wide range of moving and lifting options to accommodate patient needs, and access/egress challenges. In this scenario, moving the patient via a Reeves sleeve may be another option if she becomes too symptomatic while sitting up in a stair chair.

8. What other questions may you have for the patient?

Because she is a woman of childbearing age, questions about her last menstrual cycle should be asked. Also ask about

YOU are the Medic   SUMMARY, continued

urination, color, frequency, odor, the presence of blood, or other symptoms.

9. What may you consider requesting from medical control in addition to dextrose and antiemetics?

Pain management in the kidney patient is an important part of patient care. Many protocols will specifically address pain associated with kidney stones, but may not in this case. Follow local protocols.

10. How will her condition affect transport?

This patient is not demonstrating signs and symptoms of a life-threatening renal emergency. Therefore, she should be transported in a position of comfort with minimal jostling and slow, careful driving to avoid excessive bumps, sudden acceleration, deceleration, or turns.

EMS Patient Care Report (PCR)

Date: 04-11-12	**Incident No.:** 20227	**Nature of Call:** Medical		**Location:** 327 West Main Street	
Dispatched: 0600	**En Route:** 0603	**At Scene:** 0608	**Transport:** 0632	**At Hospital:** 0645	**In Service:** 0650

Patient Information

Age: 23 Sex: F Weight (in kg [lb]): 70 kg (154 lb)	Allergies: No known drug allergies Medications: Cipro, OTC cranberry supplement Past Medical History: UTIs Chief Complaint: Lower back pain

Vital Signs

Time: 0613	**BP:** 108/60	**Pulse:** 110	**Respirations:** 24	**Spo$_2$:** 95%
Time: 0618	**BP:** 108/60	**Pulse:** 112	**Respirations:** 24	**Spo$_2$:** 98%
Time: 0623	**BP:** 100/50	**Pulse:** 120	**Respirations:** 24	**Spo$_2$:** 98%

EMS Treatment
(circle all that apply)

Oxygen @ _____ L/min via (circle one): NC (NRM) Bag-mask device	Assisted Ventilation	Airway Adjunct	CPR
Defibrillation	**Bleeding Control**	**Bandaging**	**Splinting**	**Other**

Narrative

Dispatched to female reporting lower back pain at 327 West Main Street. Pt 23 yo female lying on her right side in bed, vomiting into trash can. Alert, skin diaphoretic, very warm, flushed. Pt reporting lower back pain, stated she's been "feeling ill" for the past 2–3 days including burning with urination and n/v since last night around midnight. Urinating makes the pain worse. Pt describes lower back pain as "achy" radiating from flank to pubic bone. Pt rates severity as 4 on scale of 1 to 10 with 10 being the worst. Pt last ate yesterday 2100 hours.

Vital signs lying down as noted above. Temp 38.3°C, blood glucose level 58 mg/dL, PEARRL, HEENT atraumatic, breath sounds clear and equal bilaterally. Abd has overactive bowel tones, soft, diffuse tenderness in all 4 quadrants with increased tenderness of both lower, right flank pain, p/m/s/X4. Suspect possible pyelonephritis.

Administered O$_2$ at 15 L/min NRM. Established IV 18g NS 500-mL bolus. ECG ST w/o further ectopy. Moved pt with stair chair. Transported to WWMC. Contacted MCC for instructions to administer additional 500-mL bolus NS. Continued to monitor en route w/o changes. Arrived at ED transfer of care to J. Smith, RN. **End of report**

Prep Kit

■ Ready for Review

- Chronic kidney disease is the most common renal disorder. Kidney stones and urinary tract infections also affect many people.

- The genitourinary system includes the kidneys, urinary bladder, ureters, urethra, male and female reproductive organs, and specific structures within the kidneys.

- Blood flows through the kidney into the afferent arteriole and then through the glomerulus, the main filter. It then enters the efferent arteriole, followed by the peritubular capillaries, where it is reabsorbed.

- Urine forms in the nephrons. The nephrons are composed of the glomerulus, the glomerular capsule, the proximal convoluted tubule, the loop of Henle, and the distal convoluted tubule.

- In the glomerular capsule, filtrate from the blood—which contains salts, minerals, glucose, water, and metabolic wastes—passes through a membrane. Next, it passes through the rest of the nephron, after which it is converted into urine. This urine passes through the proximal convoluted tubule and the loop of Henle to be further concentrated.

- In the distal convoluted tubule, the composition of urine is further refined based on the body's needs. Two hormones, antidiuretic hormone and aldosterone, are involved in adjusting the urine composition.

- The juxtaglomerular apparatus in the kidneys releases renin, an enzyme that causes reactions in the body such as an increase in blood pressure.

- Diuretics are chemicals that increase urinary output.

- As urine collects in the bladder, the micturition reflex causes the bladder to contract, stimulating the urge to void.

- The anatomy of the urethra is different in males and females. The female urethra is shorter and therefore more prone to urinary tract infections.

- In the physical examination, use the four-quadrant system and abdominal region mapping. Perform cardiac monitoring, and do not give urologic patients anything by mouth.

- Visceral pain is the type most often associated with genitourinary problems. Referred pain originates in one organ or tissue but is perceived by the patient to be located in a different area of the body.

- The OPQRST (onset, provocation, quality, region/radiation/referral, severity, timing) mnemonic is used during the primary and secondary assessments to evaluate and reevaluate the type and severity of pain.

- Pain is managed with patient positioning, analgesics and fluids as indicated, and supportive care.

- Symptoms of urinary tract infection include painful urination, frequent urges to urinate, difficulty urinating, and possibly referred pain in the shoulder or neck. The urine may have a foul odor and be cloudy. Management of patients with UTIs consists mainly of supportive care of the ABCs, allowing the patient to remain in a position of comfort, administering IV fluid, and possibly administering analgesics.

- Catheterization of the bladder allows a continuous outflow of urine and provides a means of measuring urine output in hemodynamically unstable patients. To avoid backflow of urine, the drainage bag should not be lifted above the level of the patient's bladder.

- Kidney stones result when an excess of insoluble salts or uric acid crystallizes in the urine. Symptoms include severe flank pain that may migrate to the groin. The pain may produce a spike in blood pressure and pulse rate.

- Acute renal failure is a sudden decrease in filtration through the glomeruli, resulting in a release of toxins into the blood. The three types of acute renal failure are prerenal, intrarenal, and postrenal. Signs and symptoms range from hypotension, tachycardia, dizziness, and thirst, to pain, oliguria, distended bladder, hematuria, and peripheral edema.

- Chronic renal failure is progressive and irreversible inadequate kidney function. Nephrons become damaged, losing their functionality and causing a buildup of wastes and fluid in the blood. Symptoms can include an altered level of consciousness, lethargy, nausea, headaches, cramps, anemia, bruised skin, edema in the extremities and face, hypotension, tachycardia, and possibly seizures or coma.

- Patients with acute or chronic renal failure require support of airway, breathing, and circulation; administration of medications to regulate acidosis, electrolyte imbalances, and fluid volume; and calm transport with psychological support.

- If left untreated, acute or chronic renal failure will progress to end-stage renal disease, meaning that the kidneys have lost all ability to function. Toxic waste materials build up in the patient's blood, leading to a multitude of potential signs and symptoms and possibly dysrhythmias. Prehospital care is supportive, including treating for shock and, under medical direction, regulating fluid imbalances, electrolyte abnormalities, and cardiovascular function.

- Renal dialysis is a procedure for removing toxic wastes and excess fluid from the blood. Dialysis patients usually have a shunt through which they are connected to the dialysis machine. Such patients are vulnerable to problems such as hypotension, potassium imbalance, disequilibrium syndrome, and air embolism.

- Always monitor dialysis patients for cardiac dysrhythmias. Shock secondary to bleeding is also possible from any number of causes. Watch for peaked T waves on the ECG. These are a classic sign of hyperkalemia.

- When you find a shunt leaking during the dialysis cycle, attempt to tighten the connection. If it has become disconnected at the vein, clamp the cannula and disconnect the patient from the machine.

- Specific conditions that may occur in the male genital tract include epididymitis, Fournier gangrene, priapism, phimosis, benign prostate hypertrophy, testicular masses, and testicular torsion. Prehospital management for most of these conditions is supportive. Because the patient is likely in pain, consider administering analgesics, and transport gently.

■ Vital Vocabulary

acute renal failure (ARF) A sudden decrease in filtration through the glomeruli.

adrenal glands Triangular paired structures located on top of the kidneys that produce essential hormones to help regulate body processes.

afferent arteriole The structure in the kidney that supplies blood to the glomerulus.

air embolism The presence of air in the venous circulation, which forms a gas bubble that can block the outflow of blood from the right ventricle to the lung; can lead to cardiac arrest, shock, or other life-threatening complications.

aldosterone One of the two main hormones responsible for adjustments to the final composition of urine, aldosterone increases the rate of active reabsorption of sodium and chloride ions into the blood and decreases reabsorption of potassium.

antidiuretic hormone (ADH) One of the two main hormones responsible for adjustments to the final composition of urine, ADH causes ducts in the kidney to become more permeable to water.

anuria A complete cessation of urine production.

azotemia Increased nitrogenous wastes in the blood.

benign prostate hypertrophy (BPH) Age-related nonmalignant (noncancerous) enlargement of the prostate gland.

calyces (singular: calyx) Large urinary tubes that branch off the renal pelvis and connect with the renal pyramids to collect the urine draining from the collecting tubules.

chronic renal failure (CRF) Progressive and irreversible inadequate kidney function caused by the permanent loss of nephrons.

cortex Part of the internal anatomy of the kidney; the lighter-colored outer region closest to the capsule.

countercurrent multiplier The process by which the body produces either concentrated or diluted urine, depending on the body's needs.

disequilibration syndrome A condition characterized by nausea, vomiting, headache, and confusion, which results when, as a consequence of dialysis, water initially shifts from the bloodstream into the cerebrospinal fluid, mildly increasing intracranial pressure.

distal convoluted tubule (DCT) Connects with the kidney's collecting tubules.

diuretics Chemicals that increase urinary output.

efferent arteriole The structure in the kidney where blood drains from the glomerulus.

end-stage renal disease (ESRD) A condition in which the kidneys have lost all ability to function, and toxic waste materials build up in the patient's blood; occurs after acute or chronic renal failure.

epididymitis An infection that causes inflammation of the epididymis along the posterior border of the testis; a possible complication of male urinary tract infection.

Fournier gangrene A condition that results from bacteria entering a laceration to the scrotum or perineum, causing infection and subsequent necrosis of the subcutaneal tissue and muscle in the scrotum.

glomerular (Bowman's) capsule A double-layered cup with the inner layer infiltrating and surrounding the capillaries of the glomerulus.

glomerular filtration rate (GFR) The rate at which blood is filtered through the glomeruli.

glomerulus A tuft of capillaries located in the kidney that serves as the main filter of the blood in the kidney.

hematuria The presence of blood in the urine.

hilus A cleft where the ureters, renal blood vessels, lymphatic vessels, and nerves enter and leave the kidney.

internal shunt Also called an arteriovenous (AV) fistula, this device is an artificial connection between a vein and an artery, usually in the forearm or upper arm.

interstitial nephritis A chronic inflammation of the interstitial cells surrounding the nephrons.

intrarenal acute renal failure (IARF) A type of acute renal failure characterized by damage in the kidney itself, often caused by immune-mediated diseases, prerenal ARF, toxins, heavy metals, some medications, or some organic compounds.

juxtaglomerular apparatus A structure formed at the site where the efferent arteriole and distal convoluted tubule meet.

kidneys Solid, bean-shaped organs housed in the retroperitoneal space that filter blood and excrete body wastes in the form of urine.

kidney stones Solid crystalline masses formed in the kidney, resulting from an excess of insoluble salts or uric acid crystallizing in the urine; may become trapped anywhere along the urinary tract.

loop of Henle The U-shaped portion of the renal tubule that extends from the proximal to the distal convoluted tubule; concentrates the filtrate and converts it to urine.

medulla Part of the internal anatomy of the kidney; the middle layer.

micturition reflex A spinal reflex that causes contraction of the bladder's smooth muscle, producing the urge to void as pressure is exerted on the internal urinary sphincter.

nephrons The structural and functional units of the kidney that form urine; composed of the glomerulus, the glomerular (Bowman's) capsule, the proximal convoluted tubule, the loop of Henle, and the distal convoluted tubule.

oliguria Urine output of less than 500 mL/day.

orchitis A complication of a male urinary tract infection in which one or both testes become infected, enlarged, and tender, causing pain and swelling in the scrotum.

paraphimosis A condition that results when the foreskin is retracted over the glans penis and becomes entrapped; constriction of the glans causes it to swell even further.

peritubular capillaries A set of capillaries unique to the kidney that branch off from the efferent arteriole; the site of tubular reabsorption.

phimosis Inability to retract the distal foreskin over the glans penis.

podocytes Special cells in the inner membrane of the glomerulus that wrap around the capillaries in the glomerulus, forming filtration slits.

postrenal ARF A type of acute renal failure caused by obstruction of urine flow from the kidneys, commonly caused by a blockage of the urethra by an enlarged prostate gland, renal calculi, or strictures.

prerenal ARF A type of acute renal failure that is caused by hypoperfusion of the kidneys, resulting from hypovolemia (hemorrhage, dehydration), trauma, shock, sepsis, and heart failure (congestive heart failure, myocardial infarction); often reversible if the underlying condition can be found and perfusion restored to the kidney.

priapism A painful, tender, persistent erection of the penis; can result from spinal cord injury, erectile dysfunction drugs, or sickle cell disease.

proximal convoluted tubule (PCT) One of two complex sections of the nephron, the PCT includes an enlargement at the end called the glomerular capsule.

pyelonephritis Inflammation of the kidney linings.

referred pain Pain that originates in one area of the body but is perceived as coming from a different area of the body.

renal columns Inward extensions of cortical tissue that surround the renal pyramids.

renal dialysis A technique for filtering the blood of its toxic wastes, removing excess fluids, and restoring the normal balance of electrolytes.

renal fascia Dense, fibrous connective tissue that anchors the kidney to the abdominal wall.

renal pelvis Part of the internal anatomy of the kidney; a flat, funnel-shaped tube filling the sinus at the level of the hilus.

renal pyramids Parallel cone-shaped bundles of urine-collecting tubules that are located in the medulla of the kidneys.

renin A hormone produced by cells in the juxtaglomerular apparatus when the blood pressure is low.

testicular torsion Twisting of the testicle on the spermatic cord, from which it is suspended; associated with scrotal pain and swelling, and is a medical emergency.

uremia The presence of excessive amounts of urea and other waste products in the blood.

uremic frost A powdery buildup of uric acid, especially on the skin of the face.

ureters A pair of thick-walled, hollow tubes that transport urine from the kidneys to the bladder.

urethra A hollow tubular structure that drains urine from the bladder, expelling it from the body.

urinary bladder A hollow muscular sac in the midline of the lower abdominal area that stores urine until it is released from the body.

urinary incontinence The inability to control the release of urine from the bladder; loss of bladder control.

urinary retention Incomplete emptying of the bladder, or a complete lack of ability to empty the bladder.

urinary tract infections (UTIs) Infections, usually of the lower urinary tract (urethra and bladder), that occur when normal flora (bacteria that naturally populate the skin) enter the urethra and multiply.

urine Liquid waste products filtered out of the body by the urinary system.

vasa recta A series of peritubular capillaries that surround the loop of Henle, into which water moves after passing through the descending and ascending limbs of the loop of Henle.

visceral pain Crampy, aching pain deep within the body, the source of which is usually hard to pinpoint; common with genitourinary problems.

Assessment in Action

I t is a beautiful sunny, summer day. You are at a friend's house for a barbecue and are enjoying your day off. As you sit and sip your iced tea, you watch some of your friends playing football in a park across the busy street. You notice that the game seems to be getting fairly competitive.

During one of the plays, one of the men, Jon, jumps up to catch a pass, spins around, catches the ball, and lands quite hard on the ground. You see several of the other men surrounding Jon as he continues to lie on the ground. The crowd looks over at you and motions for you to come over.

As you arrive, Jon states that he has severe pain in the abdomen and groin. You direct a bystander to call 9-1-1. As you begin assessing Jon, he whispers to you that the pain is in the testicular area. You politely ask the gathered bystanders to move away so you can talk with the patient in privacy.

1. What is your chief concern?
   A. Duty to act
   B. Expectations of friends
   C. Calling 9-1-1
   D. Scene safety

2. According to your differential diagnosis, you would expect this patient to experience:
   A. sudden, severe pain.
   B. intermittent pain.
   C. no pain.
   D. referred pain.

3. As you approach the crowd, you see that Jon is lying on the ground in the fetal position. Of the following injuries, which would be considered a true emergency?
   A. Spiral tibia fracture
   B. Testicular torsion
   C. Torn anterior cruciate ligament
   D. Peroneal tendon tear

4. From your choice in the preceding question, what treatment will be required?
   A. Cast and pain medication
   B. Surgical intervention
   C. Rest, ice, compression, elevation
   D. Steroids

5. What time of year is this injury most likely to occur?
   A. Spring
   B. Summer
   C. Fall
   D. Winter

Additional Questions

6. What immediate safety concerns do you have?

7. Is there a duty to act?

8. What other issues or questions may arise from this diagnosis?

Gynecologic Emergencies

National EMS Education Standard Competencies

Medicine

Integrates assessment findings with principles of epidemiology and pathophysiology to formulate a field impression and implement a comprehensive treatment/disposition plan for a patient with a medical complaint.

Gynecology

Recognition and management of shock associated with
- Vaginal bleeding (pp 1192-1193)

Anatomy, physiology, assessment findings, and management of
- Vaginal bleeding (pp 1192-1193)
- Sexual assault (to include appropriate emotional support) (pp 1200-1201)
- Infections (pp 1195-1196)

Anatomy, physiology, epidemiology, pathophysiology, psychosocial impact, presentations, prognosis, and management of common or major gynecologic diseases and/or emergencies
- Vaginal bleeding (pp 1192-1193)
- Sexual assault (pp 1200-1201)
- Infections (pp 1195-1196)
- Pelvic inflammatory disease (pp 1195-1196)
- Ovarian cysts (p 1197)
- Dysfunctional uterine bleeding (pp 1192-1193)
- Vaginal foreign body (pp 1201, 1203)

Knowledge Objectives

1. Describe the anatomy and physiology of the female reproductive system. (pp 1185-1186)
2. Discuss the pathophysiology of gynecologic emergencies, including pelvic inflammatory disease, sexually transmitted diseases, ruptured ovarian cyst, ectopic pregnancy, vaginal bleeding, traumatic abdominal pain, and sexual assault. (pp 1192-1201)
3. Describe the assessment process for patients with gynecologic emergencies. (pp 1188-1191)
4. Discuss the importance of history taking when assessing a patient with a gynecologic emergency. (pp 1190-1191)
5. Discuss the general management of a patient with a gynecologic emergency. (p 1192)
6. Discuss assessment and management of specific gynecologic emergencies, including pelvic inflammatory disease, sexually transmitted diseases, ruptured ovarian cyst, ectopic pregnancy, vaginal bleeding, and traumatic abdominal pain. (pp 1192-1201)
7. Discuss special concerns, assessment, and management, including pharmacologic treatment, when working with a patient who encountered sexual assault. (pp 1200-1201)

Skills Objectives

There are no skills objectives for this chapter.

Introduction

The *Merriam-Webster Dictionary* defines gynecology as "a branch of medicine that deals with the diseases and routine physical care of the reproductive system of women" and obstetrics as "a branch of medical science that deals with birth and with its antecedents and sequels." Although the medical specialties of obstetrics and gynecology are separate fields of study, the two are so inextricably entwined—as these definitions make clear—that it is virtually impossible to write about one without referencing the other.

This chapter first discusses the female anatomy and physiology, and then outlines issues that are unique to female patients, including problems that may be encountered in the emergency setting. The chapter also covers the gynecologic causes of abdominal pain in women and looks in detail at life-threatening conditions. Also briefly discussed is the topic of vaginal bleeding, both traumatic and organic, and how it should be managed in the field. Finally, the principles of managing a woman or girl who has been the victim of sexual assault are discussed.

Female Reproductive System

Anatomy

The female external genitalia, collectively called the **pudendum** or vulva, are the structures seen from the outside of the body **Figure 1**. The **mons pubis** is an anatomic landmark that is a rounded pad of fatty (adipose) tissue that overlies the symphysis pubis, located anterior to the urethral and vaginal openings. Coarse, dark hair normally appears here in early puberty, becoming sparser later in life with the advent of menopause. The **labia majora** and **labia minora**, described as "lips," surround and protect the vaginal opening together with the more anterior opening of the urethra. The labia majora are covered with pubic hair, but the labia minora are not. The area between the vaginal opening and the anus is called the **perineum**. The **clitoris** is located at the anterior junction of the labia minora, just below a layer of skin called the **prepuce**. The clitoris is a small,

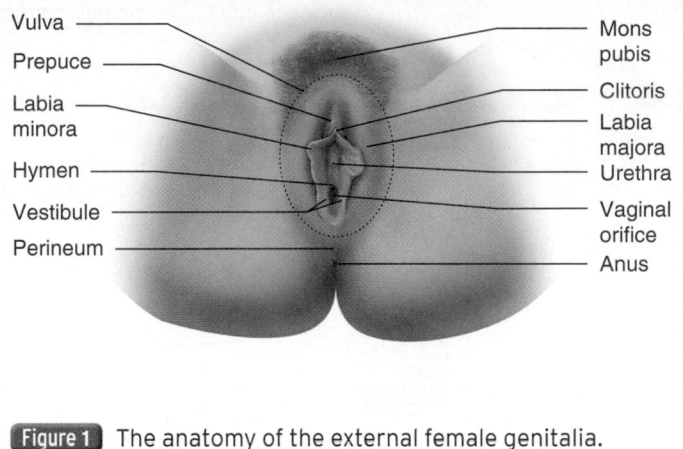

Figure 1   The anatomy of the external female genitalia.

cylindrical mass of erectile tissue and nerves that is similar to the glans penis of the male. Like the male penis, the clitoris becomes enlarged with blood flow on tactile stimulation, and it has an important role in the sexual excitement of the female.

Between the labia minora is a cleft referred to as the **vestibule**. Located within the vestibule is the urethral opening (orifice), the vaginal opening, and the hymen. The urethra, which leads to the bladder, allows for passage of urine. The length of the urethra in females averages approximately 4 cm. This short length is one reason why women are more prone than men to urinary tract infections and bladder infections.

The anatomy of the female reproductive system is shown in **Figure 2**. The **vagina**, or lower portion of the birth canal, serves as a passage for menstrual flow and as the receptacle of the penis during sexual intercourse. Just inside the lower vagina are two tiny openings that lead to the **Bartholin glands**. These glands secrete mucus that acts as a lubricant during intercourse.

Before first intercourse, the vaginal orifice is protected by the **hymen**. This membrane forms a border around the vaginal orifice, partially enclosing it. The hymen may be ruptured

YOU *Are the Medic*   PART 1

Your unit is dispatched for a patient with abdominal pain. While en route, the dispatcher tells you the patient is a 24-year-old woman who is complaining of lower abdominal pain and vaginal bleeding. When you arrive at the residence, you are met by the patient's husband. He tells you that his wife has had "problems with her period for months." He called 9-1-1 because she is in a lot of pain today.

1. What are you looking for in your scene size-up?
2. What are you looking for in your primary assessment?

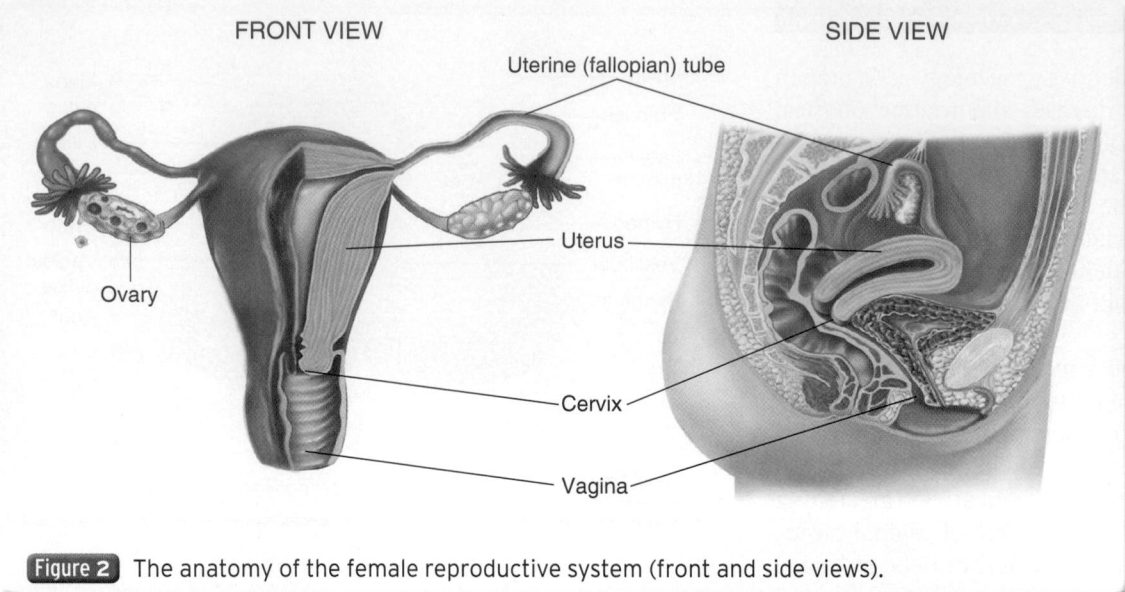

FRONT VIEW   SIDE VIEW

Uterine (fallopian) tube

Uterus

Ovary

Cervix

Vagina

Figure 2 The anatomy of the female reproductive system (front and side views).

The birth canal consists of the lower portion of the uterus called the **cervix** and the vagina. The vagina is the outermost cavity of the female reproductive system and forms the lower part of the birth canal. It is about 8 to 12 cm in length, begins at the cervix, and ends as an external opening of the body.

Menstruation

Also called the menses, period, or menstrual cycle, **menstruation** is the cyclic and periodic vaginal discharge of 25 to 65 mL of blood, epithelial cells, mucus, and tissue. The duration of the cycle differs from woman to woman, ranging from an average of 24 days to 35 days.

before first intercourse by trauma or by events such as horseback riding, gymnastics, or other sports. Pain and vaginal bleeding will generally be present in such an event; because this usually occurs in young women, it may be of concern to the patient and her parents. In some cases, the hymen may completely cover the vaginal orifice, a condition called **imperforate hymen**. If it remains undetected until puberty, this condition will block the flow of first menses, resulting in relatively acute pain, with severe constipation and low back pain. Such a condition may lead to endometriosis or cause other secondary painful effects as well. Imperforate hymen can also be caused by childhood sexual abuse, in which the imperforation results from scarring from digital or penile penetration.

The female reproductive system also includes the ovaries, the fallopian tubes, uterus, cervix, and vagina. The ovaries are two glands, one on each side of the uterus, that are similar in function to the male testes. Each **ovary** contains thousands of follicles and each follicle contains an **oocyte**. During each menstrual cycle, there will only be one follicle that is successful at maturing and is able to release an oocyte. The remaining follicles will die off and are reabsorbed by the body. The processes that the follicle goes through and the actual release of the oocyte (ovulation) are both stimulated by the release of specific hormones in the female body.

Normally, there is one **fallopian tube** associated with each ovary. When the oocyte is released, it travels through the fallopian tube to the uterus. The actual fertilization of the oocyte by a sperm usually occurs when the oocyte is inside the fallopian tube. The fertilized oocyte then continues to the uterus where it continues to develop into an embryo (early stages of the fetus) and implants into the wall of the uterus.

The **uterus**, or womb, is the muscular organ where the embryo grows. It is responsible for contractions during labor and ultimately helps to push the infant through the birth canal.

The **menstrual cycle** is composed of two phases, the ovarian cycle (ovarian changes) and the uterine cycle (changes in the uterus).

The first phase of the ovarian cycle is called the follicular phase (days 1 to 13) and is the time from the first day of menstruation until ovulation. The second phase of the ovarian cycle is called the luteal phase and occurs during days 14 to 28. This is the time from when the oocyte is released from the ovary (ovulation) until the first day of menstruation.

The uterus is also undergoing changes during this time. The uterine cycle is divided into the **proliferative phase** (days 5 to 14) and the **secretory phase** (days 14 to 28). The proliferative phase is the time after menstruation and before the next ovulation occurs. It is during this phase that the uterine lining (endometrium) increases significantly in thickness in preparation to receive a fertilized oocyte. The time after ovulation until menstruation is the secretory phase and occurs when the oocyte is not fertilized. When fertilization does not occur, estrogen and progesterone levels decrease and the thick lining of the uterus is shed from the woman's body. Based on a 28-day cycle, the menstrual phase (discharge) lasts about 5 days **Figure 3** .

During the menstrual cycle, a woman experiences several systemic changes as her hormonal levels ebb and flow. She may experience a weight gain of several pounds because of extracellular edema (fluid retention) that tends to localize in the abdomen, fingers, and ankles; muscle sensitivity because of the extracellular edema (hypertonicity); vascular alterations that increase her susceptibility to bruising; breast pain and tenderness resulting from swelling; mild to severe headache, including "menstrual migraine" (a vascular headache resulting from the hormonal "dump"); severe cramping; and emotional changes, such as agitation, irritability, depression, anger, and moodiness.

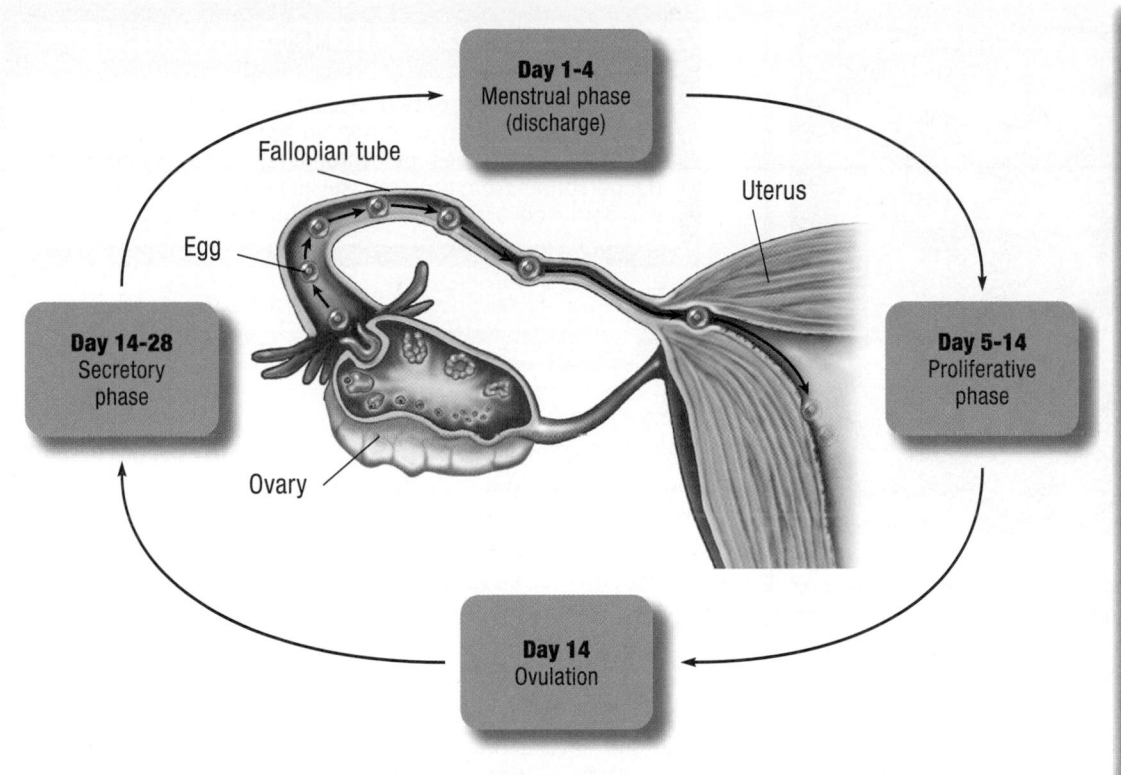

Figure 3 The menstrual cycle, based on an average 28-day cycle. The length of the cycle and number of days in each phase vary from woman to woman, but generally fall within a range of 24 to 35 days.

of the bladder and urethral mucosa can result in urinary frequency, nocturia, and incontinence.

Menstruation is predominantly related to the discussion of obstetrics, but is also a necessary component of the gynecologic examination. Disorders of the menstrual cycle may be seen in the prehospital setting **Figure 4**.

Premenstrual syndrome (PMS) is a cluster of all or some of the troubling symptoms mentioned in the discussion of the menstrual cycle. It normally occurs 7 to 14 days before the onset of the menstrual flow, and then generally subsides once the flow begins. Premenstrual syndrome affects about one third of all premenopausal women, particularly in the 30- to 40-year-old group, and may be significantly debilitating. Stress, diet, alcohol consumption, and prescription or nonprescription drug use may exacerbate symptoms. In addition, some women may experience reactive hypoglycemia, resulting in increased fatigue. This may be a strong clue as to what is troubling the patient, especially if the history elicits a recent intense craving for sweets or decreased alcohol tolerance. Prehospital treatment is predominantly supportive. Supportive field treatment may include administration of oral or IV glucose, if blood glucose levels support the need, or administration of a small dose of analgesics or anxiolytics to reduce patient anxiety.

The onset of the first menses, when a female reaches childbearing age, is called menarche. Depending on genetics, socioeconomic factors, and individual health, this event may take place anywhere between the ages of 11 and 14 years. You should consider this a possibility when your patient is this age and has a chief complaint of vaginal bleeding. The last menses, when a woman has reached the end of childbearing age, is called menopause. The advent of menopause typically begins between the ages of 40 and 50, with menstrual cycles becoming less frequent.

Owing to gradually decreasing production of estrogen and other hormones during this time, a woman may experience a range of symptoms because of hormonal imbalance. These symptoms may be as benign as copious diaphoresis, hair loss, and hot flashes (sometimes accompanied by tachycardia) or as ominous as the symptoms seen often in the emergency setting such as severe muscle aches and pains, headache, dyspnea, vertigo, digestive problems, and emotional instability. It is important to remember that this age group can still become pregnant, so your history taking and assessment should include this possibility.

Postmenopausal women no longer have to deal with the discomfort and irritation of monthly menses, but the decreased hormone production makes them more susceptible to atherosclerosis, osteoporosis, and coronary heart disease. Diminished estrogen may also result in atrophy of genitourinary organs, resulting in vaginal dryness and discomfort. Atrophy

Some women may experience abdominal pain and cramping in the 2 weeks before the beginning of menses. This pain and its accompanying symptoms result from the ovulatory process and are collectively called mittelschmerz (pronounced "MITT-ul-shmurz"; German for "middle pain"). Mittelschmerz, which may start at any time during ovulation (midcycle), affects approximately 20% of women. In most cases, the pain is not severe; it may last only a few minutes or as long as 48 hours (average, 6 to 8 hours). Signs and symptoms include sharp, cramping pain in the lower abdomen, localized to one side, beginning midcycle, with a history of similar pain episodes during previous periods. The pain may also be reported as "switching sides" from month to month. Some women also report feeling nauseated or experiencing minor blood spotting. The condition itself is not serious, and the pain can often be relieved by over-the-counter analgesics. Any persistent pain or any abnormal symptoms are cause for concern and should be evaluated by a physician.

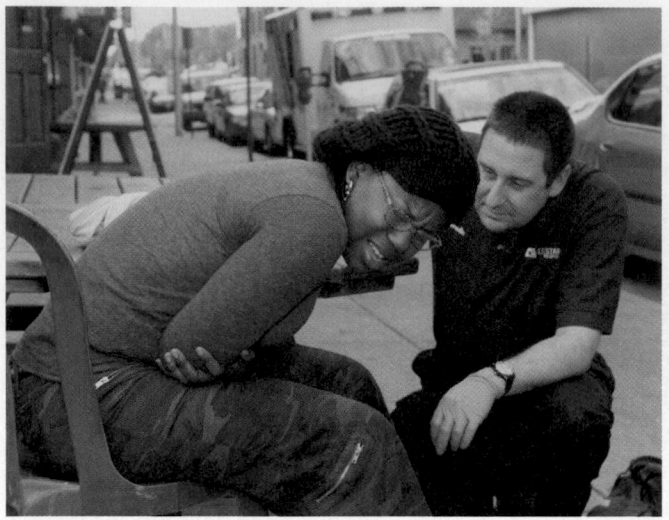

Figure 4 A patient may call EMS because she perceives her condition to be an emergency. Make sure you take each call seriously.

<u>Amenorrhea</u> is the absence or cessation of menses. This condition may be caused by a number of factors, but *the most common cause is pregnancy*. Exercise-induced amenorrhea is common in female athletes, particularly those who participate in physically intense sports. Amenorrhea may occur when a woman's body fat drops below a certain percentage. Amenorrhea can also be caused by emotional problems or extreme stress. In an adolescent or young adult, the condition may have its origination in anorexia nervosa; in this case, it is a symptom of the patient's malnutrition and emotional state.

Words of Wisdom

The most common cause of amenorrhea is pregnancy.

Patient Assessment

Obtaining an accurate and detailed patient assessment is of utmost importance when dealing with gynecologic issues. You may not be able to make a specific diagnosis in the field, but a thorough detailed examination and patient history will help determine whether the patient is experiencing a life-threatening emergency.

Women have many of the same conditions that cause abdominal pain in men—for example, renal colic, ulcers, gastroenteritis, cholecystitis, diverticulitis, pancreatitis, appendicitis, mesenteric ischemia, and dissecting aneurysm. In addition, there are numerous gynecologic causes of abdominal pain. An old medical axiom states, "Anyone who neglects to consider a gynecologic cause in a woman of childbearing age who complains of abdominal pain will miss the diagnosis at least 50% of the time." Missing the diagnosis may be fatal for the patient.

Documentation and Communication

Your attempts to obtain accurate, truthful information from the patient may be hindered by the presence of family members, loved ones, or bystanders. Removing nonessential personnel from the area will increase the likelihood that you obtain accurate information from the patient.

Scene Size-up

Every emergency call—including calls involving gynecologic emergencies—begins with a thorough scene size-up. Is the scene safe? Will you need assistance? Is it a medical call, a trauma call, or both? How many patients do you have? Have you taken proper standard precautions? Gynecologic emergencies can involve large amounts of blood and body fluids that can be contaminated with communicable diseases.

What is the mechanism of injury or nature of illness? Where is the patient found? If she is at home, what is the condition of the residence? Is it clean, filthy, or wrecked? Do you see evidence of a fight? Are alcohol, tobacco products, or drug paraphernalia present? Does the patient live alone or with other people? All information you obtain will contribute to your assessment of the patient's overall health and the safety of the scene. In case of a crime scene, you may also be required to testify in court regarding the conditions at the scene.

Primary Assessment

What is the overall presentation of the patient? Does your rapid scan reveal any obvious life threats? Is she conscious? Does she have obvious breathing difficulty or evidence of injury? Does she appear pale, cyanotic, red, or gray? Is she alert and oriented or confused? Is she calm or distraught? What is her emotional state? What is her physical appearance—well kempt or dirty? Do you find the patient sitting up, lying down, prone, supine, in the fetal position, in the tripod position, in the bathtub, or on all fours?

Once you have answered these basic questions and treated any immediate threats to airway, breathing, or circulation, you can proceed with a secondary assessment and obtain more history of the present illness.

Try to protect the patient's modesty at all times while obtaining your history and conducting your assessment. Gynecologic emergencies can be highly embarrassing for the patient, and many women may be extremely uncomfortable about discussing their sexual history in front of strangers or even close family members **Figure 5**. A teenage or adolescent girl may want to keep her sexual history from her parents, and few women are comfortable with having their genitals exposed to a crowd of family, neighbors, paramedics, police officers, or fire fighters. Limit the crowd to personnel required to perform the necessary tasks, and show the patient you respect her by being the advocate for her modesty. You also serve as a role model for other EMS providers when you act this way.

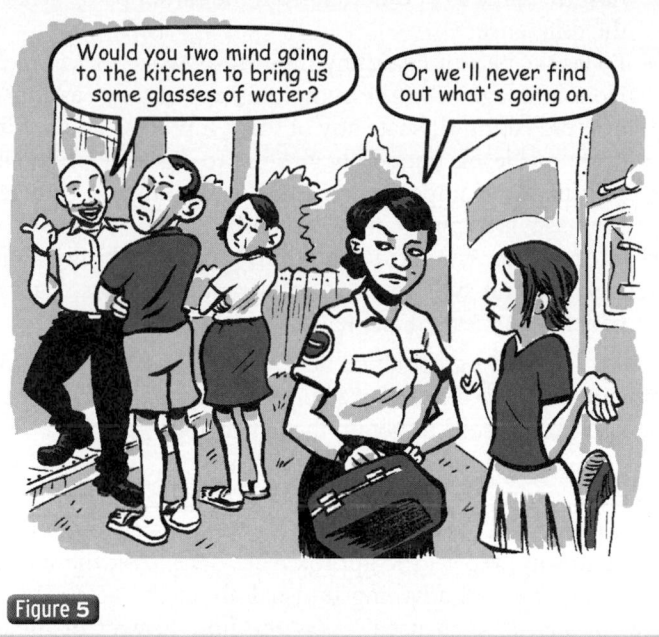

Figure 5

Form a General Impression

As always, you should begin with an assessment of the patient's level of consciousness. Note whether the patient is generally in stable or unstable condition. You will use this information to help you as you proceed with your further assessment.

Airway and Breathing

You should always evaluate the airway and breathing immediately to ensure that they are adequate, and treat any airway or breathing problem that is identified according to established guidelines and local protocol. Identifying and treating life threats takes precedence over all other assessment and treatment.

Circulation

It is important to carefully assess the circulation in all patients. What is the color of the skin and mucous membranes? Is there any cyanosis, pallor, or flushing? Cyanosis is a sign of respiratory insufficiency. Pallor can indicate shock, and flushing may be seen with fever from infection. Palpating a pulse and evaluating skin color, temperature, and moisture can help identify the patient who might have blood loss. If the patient has experienced a significant blood loss because of vaginal bleeding, she may not be demonstrating obvious signs of shock but may still be hypovolemic. If the patient has a weak or rapid pulse or has pale, cool, or diaphoretic skin, place the patient in the position dictated by local protocol for shock patients. Cover the patient to keep her warm, and then provide transport to the emergency department for treatment.

Transport Decision

Most cases of gynecologic emergencies are not life threatening. However, if signs of shock exist because of bleeding, then rapid transport is warranted. In such cases, the remainder of the assessment can be performed en route to the hospital.

Words of Wisdom

In the woman with abdominal pain, the most important things to look for are signs of shock.

Documentation and Communication

By properly documenting your general impression, level of consciousness, chief complaint, life threats, and ABCs (the primary assessment), you provide vital information that is necessary for good, ongoing patient care.

YOU are the Medic   PART 2

Your patient is lying on the sofa and is conscious, alert, and cooperative. The patient tells you she has been having lower back and pelvic pain for at least 3 months. She has had a very heavy menstrual flow with spotting between periods. She adamantly denies any possibility she could be pregnant.

Recording Time: 0 Minutes	
Appearance	Awake
Level of consciousness	Alert, oriented
Airway	Open
Breathing	Adequate
Circulation	Adequate

3. What three life-threatening gynecologic conditions present with pain?

4. What steps will you take in your further assessment of this patient?

History Taking

What is the patient's chief complaint? If it is excessive bleeding, you can move on to obtaining the gynecologic history. If the chief complaint is abdominal pain, you need to find out more about the pain itself. Although the OPQRST (Onset; Provoking factors; Quality of pain; Region of pain and whether it radiates or refers; Severity; and Time [duration]) method discussed in previous chapters works well, a more specific approach is the LORDS TRACHEA mnemonic.

- **L** What is the *Location* of the pain? Can the patient point to where the pain originates? Are multiple areas producing pain? Pain located in the midline may indicate spontaneous abortion (miscarriage). An achy pain that is diffused throughout the lower abdomen may be pelvic inflammatory disease. Pain localized to one side of the abdomen may be an ectopic pregnancy.

- **O** What was the *Onset* of the pain? When did the pain start? What activity was the patient performing when the pain started? A patient who reports the pain began during exercise may have a ruptured ovarian cyst.

- **R** Does the pain *Radiate*? That is, does the pain stay centralized or does it travel? Pain that radiates to the shoulder may indicate large amounts of blood in the abdomen.

- **D** What is the *Duration* of the pain? Is it constant or intermittent? If intermittent, how long does the pain last?

- **S** What is the *Severity* of the pain, on a scale of 0 to 10? Is the pain excruciating or tolerable? Excruciating pain usually points to a non-gynecologic cause, such as renal colic or aortic dissection.

- **T** What is the *Timing* of the pain? Did it start after the patient took an oral contraceptive? Is there a relationship between the onset of the pain and the last menstrual period? Pain that originates with pelvic inflammatory disease generally starts after the last menstrual flow. Which symptoms presented first? In cases of spontaneous abortion, pain generally *follows* bleeding. With ectopic pregnancy, the pain usually develops *before* bleeding.

- **R** Does anything *Relieve* the pain? Does holding still, posturing a particular way, or lying down diminish the pain? Has the patient taken any medication for the pain? If so, what? Did the medication help?

- **A** What *Aggravates* the pain? Does physical activity such as walking, sitting, or turning make the pain worse? Is the pain aggravated by physiologic activities, such as urinating, defecating, breathing, or swallowing? A patient with pelvic inflammatory disease may (or may not) volunteer that the pain is made worse by sexual intercourse.

- **C** What is the *Character* of the pain? Is it crampy? Aching? Sharp? Dull? Squeezing? Shooting? Stabbing? A patient experiencing a spontaneous abortion generally presents with "cramping" pain. The pain of pelvic inflammatory disease will most likely be dull and steady.

- **H** Is there a *Historic* precedent? Has the patient ever had this pain before? If yes, what was the cause? Is the pain now the same as or different from the earlier pain? What is the difference?

- **E** Has the patient *Eaten* anything? If so, what? How much? How long ago? Did the symptoms appear after eating? If not, did eating alleviate any of the symptoms? Fluctuating hormonal levels frequently give rise to digestive problems, so it is just as important to rule out the obvious (indigestion) as it is to pinpoint the obscure.

- **A** Are there *Associated* symptoms? Ask specifically about bleeding and symptoms of significant blood loss. Has the patient experienced any nausea, vomiting, or vertigo?

Once you have ascertained all that you can about the chief complaint and have developed an understanding for the patient's pain, you can proceed to obtain the gynecologic history. Probably the single most important question to ask is, "When did you have your last menstrual period (LMP)?" If the patient knows for certain, record the beginning and ending dates of the LMP. If she is unsure, record the approximate dates. Ask the patient whether she noticed anything unusual about the LMP. Was it longer or shorter than usual? Was the flow heavier or lighter than usual? Was there more or less cramping involved? Was the period late or on time? Did she have any spotting or bleeding between periods? Was any unusual pain involved?

Does the patient suspect that she might be pregnant, or is there any possibility of pregnancy? Many patients may find this question highly personal and may be uncomfortable answering it. They do not want you making a character judgment of their sexual history. Be patient, reassuring, professional, and nonjudgmental in your questioning. If the answer is a strong "No way," find out why. Younger, sexually active women may incorrectly presume that birth control methods are 100% effective against pregnancy; in truth, most current methods are only 98% effective at best, and only if used correctly. If not using any contraceptive, 25% of women will become pregnant within 1 month and 85% within 1 year. If the patient insists she cannot be pregnant, ask about other symptoms such as breast enlargement and tenderness, morning sickness (nausea and vomiting on waking), weight gain, and urinary frequency.

Words of Wisdom

Use the mnemonic ACHES-S to help isolate the "symptom cluster" associated with oral contraceptives: Abdominal pain, Chest pain, Headache (severe), Eyes (blurred vision), Spotting, and Sharp leg pain.

Does the patient use contraception and, if so, what kind? Does the patient use birth control pills and, if so, what kind? Are they uniquely prescribed for her or does she borrow them from a friend? Did the patient just start using birth control pills? (Vaginal spotting is sometimes a side effect of a new prescription.) Does she use spermicides, condoms, or a diaphragm? Does she use an implanted device (such as, Norplant) or an

Words of Wisdom

Vaginal bleeding is a sign of internal bleeding and should not be taken lightly. Apply a pad over the vaginal area, and transport all used pads with the patient to the hospital for analysis.

intrauterine device (IUD)? Women who use an IUD (also called the "loop" or "coil") are more prone to pelvic inflammatory disease and ectopic pregnancy. The IUD may also perforate the uterus, causing pain and bleeding.

Determine whether the patient has experienced vaginal bleeding. If yes, try to quantify the amount of blood. Try to obtain an accurate description of the bleeding. Is the blood bright red, dark, or a combination? Are there clots? When did the bleeding start? Is it intermittent or continuous? Is the bleeding excessive? Are signs of shock present? If so, initiate standard fluid therapy with a large-bore IV catheter and infuse at a rate following local protocol. An initial fluid bolus of 100 to 200 mL should be considered to improve the patient's perfusion status.

Has the patient experienced any vaginal discharge? If so, what was its nature? Did the discharge have an odor? What color was it? Was it clear fluid or mucus? Was it frothy, lumpy, or stringy? Was any blood observed with the fluid? Has the patient or her partner ever had a sexually transmitted disease (STD)? If yes, which one? Has she ever been treated for an STD?

What is the woman's obstetric history? A woman's obstetric history may be documented with G (gravida), P (para), and A (abortive history). <u>Gravida</u> describes the number of times a woman has been pregnant, <u>para</u> denotes the number of times a pregnant woman has delivered a viable newborn, and abortive history is the number of elective abortions the woman has had. For example, if a woman has been pregnant twice, but had a miscarriage during her first pregnancy and one healthy child, she would be G2P1A0.

Additional questions should include the following: Has she ever been pregnant? How many times? Has she ever had a live birth? How many? Have any of the deliveries been complicated? How? Were any of the pregnancies complicated? How? What kind of deliveries did she experience—vaginal or cesarean? How much time passed between pregnancies? Has she had any miscarriages and, if so, how many? Has she had any abortions? Were they spontaneous or elective? If elective, what form of abortion was used—medical or surgical? Elective abortion statistically increases the risks of future miscarriage, ectopic pregnancy, and development of certain cancers. A recent elective abortion may also be the underlying cause of the current emergency.

Does the patient have a history of gynecologic problems? Are there any known issues such as bleeding or infections? Is there any history of an ectopic pregnancy?

Does the patient have any known medical conditions? Is the patient being treated for a known medical condition? Does she take antihypertensives, anticoagulants, or diuretics? Make sure all of the components of the SAMPLE history are completed at this point.

Gynecologic emergencies often have the same signs and symptoms as emergencies involving other abdominal organs. Assess the patient carefully to determine the nature and extent of the problem. Be sure to follow the SAMPLE mnemonic. What, if any, associated signs and symptoms are noted: fever, diaphoresis, syncope, diarrhea, constipation, dysuria? Other medical problems may present as an abdominal problem. For example, cardiac pain may be misinterpreted as epigastric pain.

Secondary Assessment

When you are conducting an assessment of a woman with abdominal pain, your chief concern is to identify any signs of shock. Therefore, determining the following information should be your main focus:

- What is the patient's general presentation? Does she appear anxious? Is she restless or apprehensive? Is she fatigued? Is she thirsty?
- What is the condition of the skin and mucous membranes? Is the skin warm and dry? Feverish? Diaphoretic? Cold and clammy? Is there pallor or cyanosis? Does the patient appear dehydrated? Are the mucous membranes pale?

Next, examine the patient's abdomen. Inspect the abdomen for signs of abuse, such as bruising. Also note bruising in other areas, which could indicate possible abuse (an estimated 30% to 50% of pregnant woman are abused; the likelihood of a woman being abused increases when she is pregnant). The abdomen is a favorite target of abusers, especially if a woman is pregnant. Do you see any surgical scarring from abdominal surgery or previous cesarean section or stretch marks from previous pregnancies? Is evidence of needle tracks from illicit drug use apparent? The abdomen is a favorite injection spot for chronic drug abusers because clothing hides the evidence. Also look for a positive Cullen sign (ecchymosis at the umbilicus) or Grey Turner sign (ecchymosis at the flanks); either is indicative of internal bleeding. Is the abdomen swollen and distended (possibly indicative of pregnancy, internal bleeding, bowel obstruction, or liver problems)? Is it flat and flaccid? Is there any guarding of the abdomen? Are any rashes or lesions present? Is the abdomen symmetrical? Is the liver or spleen enlarged and protruding from under the rib cage?

Palpate the abdomen. Examine all quadrants, starting at the quadrant farthest from the pain and working toward the quadrant where the pain is located. Examine this quadrant last. Is the abdomen rigid (possibly indicative of internal bleeding)? Is there point tenderness? Does the palpation elicit more pain? Is rebound tenderness present (indicative of infection, such as may be associated with appendicitis)? Are there masses present? If yes, are they pulsating (abdominal aortic aneurysm)?

What are the patient's vital signs? Are there any variations in the pulse? Is it fast, slow, or irregular? Strong or weak and thready? Is the blood pressure normal, low, or elevated? What is normal for the patient? Check the pressure in sitting and standing positions. Are there significant orthostatic changes? If yes, the patient must be presumed to be in shock.

General management of abdominal pain is mostly psychologically supportive. Local protocols may allow for narcotic administration pain management. Prophylactically gain IV access in any woman of child bearing age with abdominal pain. Pain-free or reduced pain transport will greatly reduce your patient's anxiety.

Reassessment

En route to the hospital, recheck your interventions and note any improvement (or decline) in the patient's condition. Remember to obtain serial vital signs. Pay specific attention to the needs of your patient, and accommodate her desire for conversation or silence.

Communication and documentation are important, but in gynecologic cases, do not focus on your paperwork during the call. Your main focus must be on the patient, including providing emotional care. You are caring for a human being—the paperwork can wait until the patient has been delivered to the receiving facility.

Emergency Medical Care

Primary management of a gynecologic patient is directed at mitigating life threats, being supportive and compassionate, and protecting the patient's modesty. In most gynecologic emergencies, your role will be primarily investigatory. The more accurate and detailed the history and examination are, the better you will be at differentiating gynecologic and nongynecologic pathology. For all patients, assess and supply the appropriate oxygen needs. Obtain vital signs, and continue to monitor vital signs throughout your patient care. Initiate fluid therapy, providing for pharmacologic interventions (pain management) or volume replacement as necessary. Provide transport. Protect the patient's modesty, and provide psychological care with a supportive attitude.

Management of Gynecologic Trauma

The female genital area is highly vascular and very susceptible to trauma. Trauma sustained from motor vehicle crashes, sporting events, assault, and even consensual sex are common mechanisms of injury. Bleeding from genital trauma may be profuse (and very painful), and, if the patient is currently having her period, trying to differentiate between menstrual blood and trauma-related blood can be difficult.

Applying simple external pressure over the area of the laceration is usually sufficient to control bleeding. Bleeding from the *internal* genitalia, by contrast, can be massive and very difficult to control. Blindly packing the vagina is dangerous and is *not* recommended or even useful. A woman with exsanguinating vaginal hemorrhage must be treated as any other injured patient with exsanguinating hemorrhage—that is, she must be treated for shock and rapidly transported to the hospital, preferably one with obstetric and gynecologic services.

Assessment of a patient with gynecologic trauma will focus on the following questions: What are her symptoms? Is there a mechanism of injury? Is the patient pale, cool, and diaphoretic? Does she appear fatigued? Anxious? Irritable? Is the patient using sanitary pads or tampons? Can she tell you how many pads have been soaked? An average pad holds about 30 mL of blood and a tampon about 20 mL. Is the blood a normal color? Is it brighter or darker than normal? Do any clots appear in the flow? Is the abdomen tender or distended (for example, from internal bleeding)? Affirmative answers may indicate that the patient is in the early stages of shock. Ensure an adequate airway, administer oxygen, provide IV fluid resuscitation, and monitor the ECG **Figure 6**. Assess vital signs frequently. Consider transport in the Trendelenburg position. Do *not* perform an interior vaginal examination. Examination of the external genitalia is warranted in the presence of genital trauma only.

Pathophysiology, Assessment, and Management of Specific Emergencies

Of the several diverse gynecologic conditions that you may be called on to treat, only three are truly life-threatening emergencies: ectopic pregnancy, ruptured ovarian cyst, and tubo-ovarian abscess. Each of these manifests with similar symptoms, so they are virtually impossible to definitively diagnose in the field. You may also be called on to treat conditions related to pelvic inflammatory disease.

Vaginal Bleeding

Pathophysiology

Dysmenorrhea is painful menses. It is classified into two categories: primary and secondary. Primary dysmenorrhea

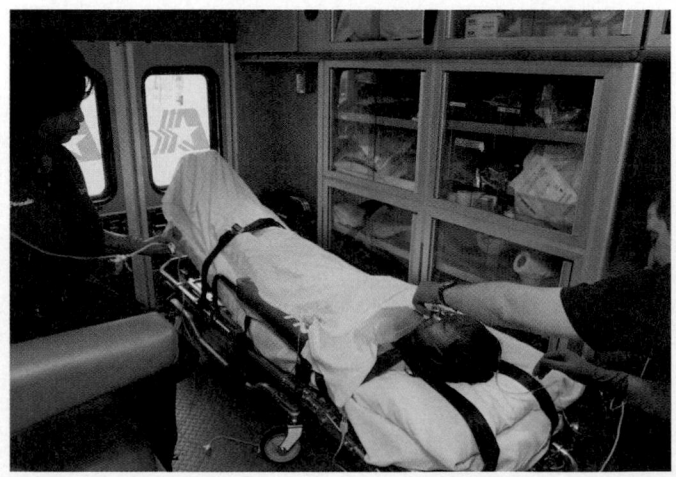

Figure 6 A patient with gynecologic trauma should be kept lying down. Manage the airway, administer supplemental oxygen and IV fluids, and monitor the ECG.

occurs with the advent of the menstrual flow and normally lasts for the first 1 to 2 days with gradual relief. Severe cramping may precede the period, with pain originating in the area of the symphysis pubis and radiating downward to the vulva and outward to the thighs. Nausea, vomiting, and diarrhea may accompany the pain. Primary dysmenorrhea accounts for about 80% of patients presenting with painful menses and accompanies a "regular" period. Secondary dysmenorrhea is pain that is present before, during, and after the menstrual flow. It is generally organic in nature (not hormonal) and may signal an underlying illness or dysfunction.

Vaginal bleeding or dysfunctional uterine bleeding is one of the most frequent reasons that women consult a gynecologist and can occur at any age. Vaginal bleeding, when not in the course of regular menstruation, is always an abnormal finding. Dysfunctional uterine bleeding is irregular vaginal bleeding that is not caused by pregnancy, infection, or tumors. The cause may be as benign as emotional stress or as serious as pelvic, cervical, or uterine cancer. Likewise, a disturbance in the normal menstrual cycle is cause for concern.

If the flow of blood lasts several days longer than normal or is excessive, the condition is called hypermenorrhea. If the blood flow occurs more often than a 24-day interval, it is termed polymenorrhea (usually caused by physical or emotional stress). Blood flow or intermittent spotting of blood occurring irregularly but frequently is termed metrorrhagia. Metrorrhagia is of greatest concern to paramedics because its causes range from hormonal imbalance to malignancies to spontaneous abortion (miscarriage).

Assessment

The assessment of a patient with vaginal bleeding depends largely on whether there is a mechanism of injury. Assess for hypovolemic shock. Although it may be awkward for you and for the patient, your assessment should include questions about any incidents or events that led up to the patient requesting EMS. With the patient's assistance, determine the amount of blood loss. If significant, assess for signs and symptoms of hypovolemic shock. Determine if the patient has any pain or discharge associated with the bleeding.

Management

Management of a patient with vaginal bleeding will depend on whether there is a mechanism of injury. Prehospital treatment of vaginal bleeding is largely supportive. Manage any signs and symptoms of shock with high-flow oxygen, keep the patient warm, and provide IV fluid therapy. If the bleeding is severe, apply dressings to the vaginal area. Maintain your professionalism and empathy with the patient because some women may be embarrassed with having a male EMS provider assist in this type of situation; even female EMS providers must take the patient's emotional state into consideration.

Ectopic Pregnancy

Pathophysiology

The word *ectopic* means "located away from a normal position." In ectopic pregnancy, a fertilized oocyte is implanted somewhere other than the uterus Figure 7. In 97% of cases, the oocyte is fertilized inside one of the fallopian tubes and has been blocked from passing into the uterus, generally by an obstruction, such as PID-related tubal scarring or as a result of tubal surgery (ligation or reverse ligation). The other 3% of ectopic pregnancies occur in the abdomen, within the cervix, or on an ovary. Ectopic pregnancy is the leading cause of maternal death in the first trimester, accounting for approximately 10% of pregnancy-related deaths. Ectopic pregnancies occur in 1% to 2% of all pregnancies with more than 100,000 cases in the United States each year. Although PID is the most common cause of ectopic pregnancy, other causes include pelvic surgery, smoking, IUD use (IUDs do not cause ectopic pregnancy but, by blocking uterine pregnancy, may cause fertilization to occur higher up), fibroids, tumors, or cysts in the tubes, fallopian endometriosis, and hormonal imbalance.

With a tubal pregnancy, the fertilized oocyte implants in the fallopian tube, then begins to grow and produce hormones in the same way a normally implanted oocyte does, taking nourishment from the maternal blood supply. Owing to the production of hormones, the woman begins to experience the early physiologic changes of pregnancy. Her period stops, her breasts become enlarged and tender, and the uterine environment changes just as it would with a normal pregnancy. The fallopian tube, lacking the expansive muscle capacity of the uterus, has little stretching ability, so the developing embryo will soon run out of growing room. When this occurs, the tube is likely to rupture, causing massive intra-abdominal hemorrhage and shock.

Assessment

Nearly all women with ectopic pregnancy will present with a chief complaint of abdominal pain. This pain will generally be

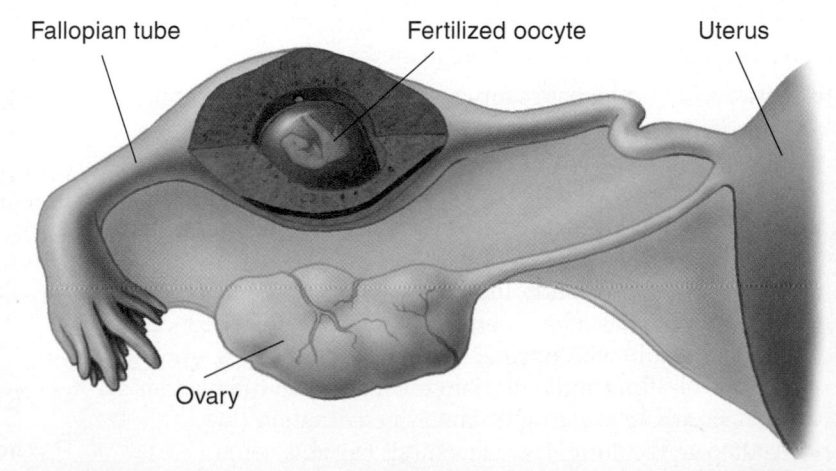

Fallopian tube   Fertilized oocyte   Uterus

Ovary

Figure 7 In an ectopic pregnancy, a fertilized oocyte implants somewhere other than the uterus. Here it is implanted in one of the fallopian tubes.

localized to one side of the abdomen and, in the early stages, will be described as crampy and intermittent. As the pregnancy progresses, the embryo will abort or the tube will rupture. Either event will produce severe abdominal pain, localized to one side. By the time EMS is involved, the patient is likely to be in constant pain, which will be diffused throughout the abdomen. Diffuse pain is especially likely if there is significant <u>hemoperitoneum</u> (blood in the abdominal cavity). Referred pain to the shoulder is ominous because it indicates massive hemoperitoneum. Vaginal bleeding is another sign of ectopic pregnancy, occurring in approximately 65% of women. This bleeding will usually occur *after* onset of pain in ectopic pregnancy, in contrast with spontaneous abortion, in which bleeding usually *precedes* pain.

Part of the blood volume in ectopic pregnancy originates in the shedding of the uterine lining as the embryo is displaced from its site of implantation and the production of hormones ceases. Vaginal bleeding may itself be light, so it is not a good indicator of internal blood loss. Look for a positive Cullen sign or Grey Turner sign and for signs of shock and abdominal distention and tenderness to help gauge the extent of internal bleeding.

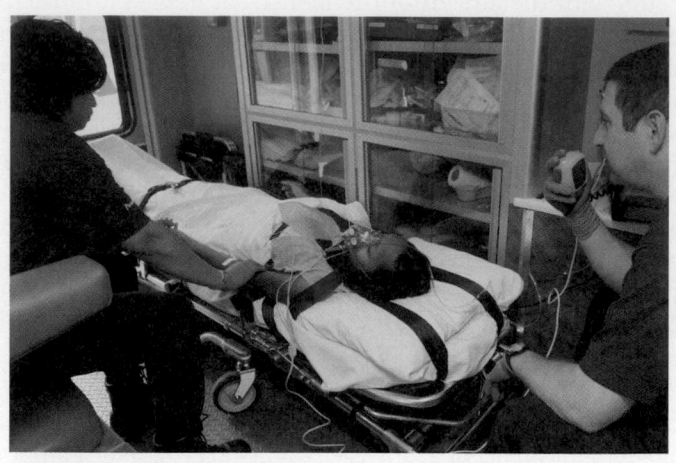

Figure 8 Always treat for shock in any woman with abdominal pain and vaginal bleeding.

Words of Wisdom

In ectopic pregnancy, bleeding usually occurs after the onset of pain.

The classic triad for diagnosing ectopic pregnancy is amenorrhea (75% of patients), vaginal bleeding, and abdominal pain. A history of ectopic pregnancy, IUD use, and a history of PID also significantly raise the index of suspicion.

Management

Always treat for shock in any woman presenting with abdominal pain and vaginal bleeding, regardless of whether shock symptoms are actually present **Figure 8**. Follow these steps in the management of a patient with a suspected ectopic pregnancy:

- Ensure an adequate airway, and administer high-concentration supplemental oxygen.
- Keep the patient left laterally recumbent, even if unconscious and intubated.
- Initiate IV fluid therapy with a large-bore IV line following local protocol.
- Give nothing by mouth, including water.
- If local protocols allow, consider urethral catheterization, filling the bulb with normal saline. This can help tamponade the bleeding and will drain the bladder. A full bladder can exacerbate bleeding from uterine relaxation.
- Anticipate vomiting. Have an emesis bag and suction close at hand.
- Keep the patient warm.
- Monitor the patient's ECG.
- Transport.

- Notify the receiving hospital of the patient's suspected diagnosis, her condition, and your estimated time of arrival.
- Recheck vital signs frequently during transport.

Endometritis

Pathophysiology

<u>Endometritis</u> is an inflammation or irritation of the <u>endometrium</u> (uterine lining). Women are more likely to have endometritis after having a baby or after a miscarriage. This condition is most commonly caused by infection, frequently by an STD (gonorrhea and chlamydia, predominantly).

Assessment

Symptoms of endometritis may include malaise, fever (high- or low-grade), constipation or uncomfortable bowel movements, vaginal bleeding or discharge (or both), abdominal distention, and lower abdominal or pelvic pain. Abdominal auscultation may reveal decreased bowel sounds, and pain may be elicited by palpation of the abdomen.

Management

Endometritis is treated with antibiotics. Provide reassurance to your patient and transport in a position of comfort. If necessary, start an IV and titrate to the patient's vital signs. Left untreated, endometritis may lead to septic shock or cause spontaneous abortion in a pregnant patient. Most patients fully recover after antibiotic treatment.

Endometriosis

Pathophysiology

Over 5 million women in the United States are diagnosed with <u>endometriosis</u> every year. This condition can be extremely painful, or there may be no symptoms. It results when endometrial tissue grows outside the uterus, generally on the surface of abdominal and pelvic organs. Organs of the pelvic cavity are the most common locations for the ectopic growths, but endometrial tissue can occasionally be found in the lungs or other parts of the body. This condition is one of the leading causes of infertility in women, with 30% to 40% of affected women unable to conceive. Many women do not even realize they have endometriosis until they encounter difficulties trying to get pregnant.

Assessment

In women who experience symptoms, the most common complaint is pain (sometimes chronic pain), generally localized in the lower back, pelvic, and abdominal regions. Other symptoms include painful intercourse (during and after), gastrointestinal pain, dysuria and painful bowel movements during the menstrual cycle, fatigue (perhaps leading to misdiagnosis as chronic fatigue syndrome), extremely painful and escalating menstrual cramping, and very heavy menstrual periods. Patients may also experience bleeding between periods or report premenstrual spotting.

Management

Prehospital care for endometriosis is based on the patient's signs and symptoms. If the patient reports severe pain, you should provide pain relief with analgesics if allowed in your protocol. Let the patient position herself so she is as comfortable as possible. Use dressings or towels as needed to absorb any significant vaginal bleeding.

■ Pelvic Inflammatory Disease

Pathophysiology

Approximately one of every seven women in the United States, or more than 1 million women per year, will contract pelvic inflammatory disease (PID) at some point. It is estimated that

70% of women diagnosed with PID are 25 years old or younger. PID is one of the most common causes of women calling 9-1-1 with a chief complaint of abdominal pain. One of every four women who contract PID will have severe abdominal pain or experience sterility or childbirth complications. Many women may have PID for years but do not realize it until they learn they are infertile.

PID is an infection of the female upper organs of reproduction—specifically, the uterus, ovaries, and fallopian tubes—that occurs almost exclusively in sexually active women. Disease-causing organisms enter the vagina, generally by the process of sexual activity, and migrate through the opening of the cervix and into the uterine cavity, where they invade the mucosa. The infection may then expand to the fallopian tubes (producing scarring that can lead to life-threatening ectopic pregnancy or infertility), eventually involving the ovaries (leading to the development of a life-threatening tubo-ovarian abscess) and the peritoneal cavity. Although PID itself is seldom a threat to life, its ultimate consequences can be lethal.

Risk factors for PID include the use of an IUD as a <u>contraceptive device</u> Figure 9 , frequent sexual activity with multiple partners, and a history of previous PID. The disease is most prevalent in the collegiate age group (20 to 24 years)

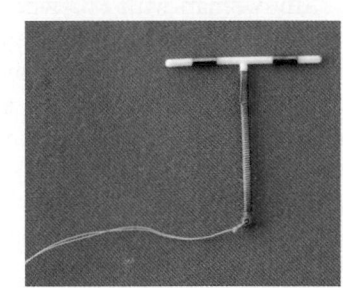

Figure 9 The IUD contraceptive device can increase a woman's risk of developing PID and ectopic pregnancy and may cause pain and bleeding.

YOU *are the Medic* | PART 3

Your partner administers oxygen to the patient via a nonrebreathing mask and begins assessing her vital signs. The patient states she is not under a doctor's care for this problem because it seemed normal at first. She tells you that she has been taking ibuprofen in an attempt to alleviate the pain but it has not been working. She describes the pain as a dull ache in her pelvis and lower back that does not go away.

Recording Time: 5 Minutes	
Respirations	18 breaths/min
Pulse	80 beats/min
Skin	Pink, warm, and dry
Blood pressure	128/60 mm Hg
Oxygen saturation (Spo$_2$)	98% on 4 L/min via a nonrebreathing mask
Pupils	Equal and reactive

5. What is the LORDS TRACHEA mnemonic?

6. What is the next question you should ask this patient?

and statistically decreases after age 30 years (the typical monog-amy and marriage years).

Assessment

A patient with PID will present with abdominal pain in virtually every scenario encountered by paramedics. The pain generally starts during or after normal menstruation, so eliciting the LMP is an important component of the history. The pain is typically diffuse and is spread over both quadrants of the lower abdomen. It may be described as "achy," and the patient may volunteer that the pain is made worse by walking or by sexual intercourse. The latter revela-tion usually indicates cervical involvement in the infective process. Pain localized to the right upper quadrant is indicative of infection that has spread to the abdominal cavity. Associated symptoms may include vaginal discharge, fever and chills, and pain or burning on urination (dysuria).

Any woman with PID who feels sick enough to call for an ambulance probably has a severe infection and is likely to pres-ent as febrile and look sick. Physical examination findings may be sparse or may include the entire textbook profile. Be alert for signs of peritoneal irritation (that is, the patient winces on palpation of the abdomen or every time the ambulance hits a bump). Be very gentle should you decide to palpate this patient's abdomen as part of the examination.

Management

PID cannot be treated in the field because it generally requires administration of an appropriate antibiotic for 10 to 14 days. The best you can do is obtain a thorough history, make the patient as comfortable as possible, and transport with as gentle a ride as can be managed.

Words of Wisdom

The ambulance does not carry the appropriate supplies and equipment for a definitive diagnosis of a gynecologic problem in the field. Look for life threats, treat for shock, and transport in a position of comfort.

■ Vaginitis

Pathophysiology

Vaginitis, by definition, is an inflammation of the vagina that is caused by an infection and is a common condition seen in women. There are several different types of vaginitis, including vaginal yeast infections.

Vaginal yeast infections are typically caused by the *Can-dida albicans* fungus. Yeasts are tiny organisms that normally live in small numbers inside the vagina and on the skin. The normal acidic environment of the vagina helps keep yeast from growing. If the vagina becomes less acidic, however, the yeast population may increase dramatically and result in infection. Conditions that may alter the acidic balance of the vagina include the use of oral contraceptives, menstruation, pregnancy, diabetes, and

some antibiotics. Moisture and irritation of the vagina also seem to encourage yeast growth. Stress from lack of sleep, illness, or poor diet are other contributing factors. Women with immuno-suppressive diseases such as HIV infection or diabetes are also at increased risk. Approximately 75% of all women will likely experience at least one infection during their lifetime.

Vulvovaginitis is an inflammation of the external vulva. Patients with this condition should be evaluated by a physician.

Assessment

Although some patients may be asymptomatic, common symp-toms of vaginitis include itching, irritation, discharge, odor, painful intercourse, and lower abdominal pain.

Regarding vaginal yeast infections, symptoms may include itching, burning, soreness in the vagina and around the vulva, and vulvar swelling. Some women may report a thick, white vaginal discharge ("cottage cheese" appearance), pain during sexual intercourse, and burning on urination.

Symptoms of vulvovaginitis include redness, pain, swelling, discharge, burning, and itching.

Management

If not treated, vaginitis can lead to infertility, preterm birth, endometritis, PID, and an increased risk for STDs. Antibiotics are required for definitive treatment. Prehospital management is generally limited to a supportive role. Treatment of vulvovagini-tis includes antibiotics and topical creams.

■ Bartholin Abscess

Pathophysiology

Approximately 2% of women in the United States are diagnosed and treated for a Bartholin abscess every year. Just inside the lower vagina are two small ducts, one on each side, that lead to the Bartholin glands. These glands secrete mucus that acts as a lubricant during intercourse. Bacterial infection, particularly gonorrhea, may cause these openings to become abscessed and cystic.

Assessment

The Bartholin abscess is usually unilateral and the patient reports a painful lump, irritation (swelling and redness), painful intercourse, and possibly fever.

Management

If the abscess becomes a pus-filled cyst, the cyst will have to be removed by a physician. Physicians will typically drain any abscesses and prescribe antibiotics.

■ Gardnerella Vaginitis

Pathophysiology

The *Gardnerella* bacterium normally resides in the genital area in women. It can cause an infection called Gardnerella vagi-nitis if the bacteria become too numerous. Young, sexually active women are the most likely to be affected (one in three women can be affected), but it can develop in any female—adult or child. This infection can also occur in the urethra of males. It can be associated with PID, and recent use of antibiotics can increase the risk of contracting the infection. Gardnerella vaginitis can cause complications in pregnant women.

Assessment

Gardnerella vaginitis is often confused with a yeast infection. Signs and symptoms include a "fishy" vaginal odor, itching, irritation, and a smooth, thin, sticky, white or gray discharge. Patients often describe their symptoms as being worse after intercourse or menstruation.

Management

Although patients are not in acute distress, they should be seen by a physician, who will most likely treat the condition with antibiotics.

■ Ruptured Ovarian Cyst, Ovarian Torsion, and Tubo-ovarian Abscess

Pathophysiology

An ovarian cyst is essentially a fluid-filled sac that forms on or within an ovary. Most sources state that almost every female has ovarian cysts, but most are considered functional and noncancerous. Of the many types of cysts, the most common is the *functional cyst*, which generally develops during the menstrual cycle. During the cycle, the ovaries form tiny sacs (cysts) to hold the oocytes. Once an oocyte matures, the sac breaks open and releases the oocyte, which then begins its journey through the fallopian tube for fertilization; the sac itself dissolves. If the sac fails to break open, however, the oocyte may continue to mature and form a *follicular cyst.* Under normal circumstances, this type of cyst spontaneously disappears within a 1- to 3-month period. A *corpus luteum cyst* develops if the sac seals itself after release of the oocyte. Fluid then accumulates inside the cyst, and the cyst continues to grow. Fertility drugs can increase the chances of corpus luteum cysts developing.

If the cycle of forming sacs is repeated excessively and the oocytes do not release, *polycystic ovaries* may develop. This hormonal reproductive disorder is characterized by lack of progesterone and high levels of androgens (male hormone). It can have a negative impact on normal insulin production, leading to diabetes (especially gestational). It can also initiate heart and blood vessel problems, such as hypertension, and produce pelvic pain and irregular menstrual cycles.

Ovarian torsion occurs when a cyst does not self-resolve and grows to a significant size. Ovarian cysts can grow as large as 4″. Ovarian torsion is the fifth most common gynecologic emergency that requires surgery. Large ovarian cysts can actually twist the ovary and cause bleeding and pain. Signs and symptoms include a sudden onset of severe unilateral lower abdominal pain that may radiate to the back or thigh. Nausea and vomiting are very common with this condition.

Tubo-ovarian abscess is encountered secondary to a primary infectious agent—typically, the ones that cause PID. The most common underlying cause is gonorrhea. Diverticulitis and appendicitis have also been found to be causative agents. In this condition, the fallopian tubes or ovaries become blocked by an infectious mass, which grows and forms an abscess.

Assessment

A patient with an ovarian cyst may report dull, achy pain in the lower back and thighs, abdominal pain or pressure, nausea and vomiting, breast tenderness, abnormal bleeding and painful menstruation, and painful intercourse. A ruptured ovarian cyst usually presents with a sudden onset of abdominal pain and can be related to the menstrual cycle. A ruptured cyst can lead to shock from internal bleeding and infection. Signs and symptoms include lower abdominal pain (usually described as sharp), abdominal distention, and tenderness. Some patients may report dizziness, or weakness, or experience a syncopal episode.

A patient with a tubo-ovarian abscess may present with severe abdominal pain, guarding and rebound tenderness, nausea and vomiting, abdominal distention, and fever. If the abscess ruptures, infectious matter can spread throughout the entire body. With any of these conditions, the patient may have internal hemorrhage.

Management

The prehospital management of ruptured ovarian cyst and tubo-ovarian abscess is the same as for ectopic pregnancy. Assess and treat for shock. If local protocol allows, administer pain management medications to the patient. For patients with ovarian torsion, you should start an IV line for pain medications and dehydration from vomiting, and also administer antiemetics.

■ Prolapsed Uterus

Pathophysiology

A condition known as prolapsed uterus occurs when the uterus drops from its normal position. Within the pelvic cavity, there are muscles, ligaments, and connective tissues that support the organs inside the cavity (bladder, uterus, and intestines). These structures can become weakened by age, childbirth, obesity, and decreased estrogen levels. Almost half of all women who have been through childbirth experience this condition, with greatest risk in women who have delivered seven or more viable infants. There is an expected increase for this condition as our population ages. This condition may also be chronic and asymptomatic in elderly woman. Uterine prolapse is not common in women who have not been through childbirth. When it does occur, the organs inside the pelvic cavity move or drop from their original location. With a prolapsed uterus, the uterus drops into the vaginal opening. There are varying degrees of prolapse, from the uterus dropping into the vagina, to a portion of the uterus protruding from the vagina, to the complete uterus being outside of the body.

Assessment

Patients with prolapsed uterus often report vaginal and pelvic pain, low back pain, dysuria, incontinence, discharge, infections, and varying degrees of a feeling like something is falling out of or bulging from their vagina. Your assessment should include a thorough history and inspection of the vagina if the patient reports that tissue is protruding from her vagina. Assess for any signs of shock.

Management

Prehospital treatment of prolapsed uterus is limited to pain management (if local protocol allows), treatment for shock if present, and care for any tissue or the uterus itself if it is exposed. Do not replace any tissue. Cover any protruding tissue with warm, moist dressings. If at all possible, do not let the patient walk; assist her to the stretcher. A professional and reassuring manner will greatly reduce the anxiety and possible embarrassment the patient may be experiencing. Definitive treatment for this condition includes devices to hold the organs in place or surgery.

■ Toxic Shock Syndrome

Pathophysiology

Toxic shock syndrome (TSS) is a form of septic shock. The disease has been identified as having *Streptococcus pyogenes* (group A strep) or *Staphylococcus aureus* as the causative agent. TSS affects men and women, and it can involve several of the body's systems, including the hepatic, cardiovascular, central nervous, and renal systems. It can result when minor infections of the lungs, sinuses, skin lesions, or the vagina progress to actual TSS, which can be lethal. Menstruating women appear particularly prone to developing TSS—hence, the original association between the syndrome and tampon use. The incidence of TSS has decreased dramatically since the 1980s as a result of tampon manufacturers improving their products. Currently, the incidence of toxic shock syndrome is approximately two cases per 100,000 people.

Assessment

Initial symptoms of TSS include syncope, myalgia, diarrhea, vomiting, headache, fever, and sore throat. Other symptoms may include diverse petechiae, light rash, and scleral injection (bloodshot eyes). As the disease progresses, signs of systemic shock will begin to appear. Disseminated intravascular coagulation, severe hypotension, adult respiratory distress syndrome, and dysrhythmias may develop, and the patient may show signs of kidney and liver failure.

Management

Rapid transport is indicated in cases of TSS. Provide high-flow supplemental oxygen, IV therapy, pressors if necessary, and cardiac monitoring. Little more can be done for a patient with TSS in the field because aggressive antibiotic therapy and possible surgical intervention are required.

■ Sexually Transmitted Diseases

As mentioned earlier, PID results from infective organisms crossing the cervix. It is typically a secondary infection, with the primary infection being a sexually transmitted disease (STD)—often chlamydia or gonorrhea. STDs are reviewed briefly here, with the exception of the human immunodeficiency virus (HIV), which is discussed in the chapter on *Infectious Diseases*.

In general, there is no specific prehospital treatment for STDs. Protect your patient's privacy and modesty. Your assessment will reveal the signs and symptoms that require treatment.

The most common complaints that would require treatment include pain, nausea and vomiting, bleeding, and fever. If indicated, apply oxygen, control bleeding, start an IV line (titrate to vital signs), and administer analgesics and antiemetics.

Bacterial Vaginosis

Bacterial vaginosis is one of the most common conditions to afflict women. In this infection, normal bacteria in the vagina are replaced by an overgrowth of other bacterial forms. Symptoms of bacterial vaginosis may include itching, burning, or pain and may be accompanied by a "fishy," foul-smelling discharge. Left untreated, bacterial vaginosis can lead to premature birth or low birthweight in cases of pregnancy, make the patient more susceptible to more serious infections, and result in PID. It is treated with metronidazole, an antibiotic. If the patient consumes alcohol while taking this therapy, severe nausea and vomiting may develop.

Chancroid

Chancroid is caused by infection with the bacterium *Haemophilus ducreyi*. This is a highly contagious yet curable disease. Chancroid is known to facilitate the transmission of HIV. This disease causes painful sores (ulcers), usually of the genitals. Swollen, painful lymph glands or inguinal buboes in the groin area may be present as well. Women may be asymptomatic and, thus, unaware they have the disease. Prehospital treatment is supportive only.

Chlamydia

Chlamydia is caused by the bacterium *Chlamydia trachomatis*. It is a very common STD that is considered the most widespread STD in the United States, with a reported annual diagnosis of over 1.2 million. Although symptoms of chlamydia are usually mild or absent, some women may have symptoms including lower abdominal pain, low back pain, nausea, fever, pain during intercourse, or bleeding between menstrual periods. Chlamydial infection of the cervix can spread to the rectum, leading to rectal pain, discharge, or bleeding. If not treated, chlamydia can progress to PID. In rare cases, chlamydia causes arthritis that may be accompanied by skin lesions and inflammation of the eye and urethra (Reiter syndrome).

Cytomegalovirus

Cytomegalovirus (CMV) is a member of the herpesvirus family. This very common viral infection has no known cure, and the virus can remain dormant in the body for years. An estimated 80% of the US population has been exposed to CMV. In its active stages, CMV may produce symptoms including prolonged high fever, chills, headache, malaise, extreme fatigue, and an enlarged spleen. People with an increased risk for developing active infection and more serious complications (such as fever, pneumonia, liver infection, and anemia) include those with immune disorders, people receiving chemotherapy, and pregnant women. Newborns who acquire CMV are susceptible to lung problems, blood problems, liver problems, swollen glands, rash, and poor weight gain.

Genital Herpes

Genital herpes is an infection of the genitals, buttocks, or anal area caused by herpes simplex virus, type I or type II. Type I, which is the most common form, infects the mouth and lips, causing cold sores or "fever" blisters; it may also produce sores on the genitals. Type II, the more serious infection, can affect the mouth as well, but is more commonly known as the primary cause of genital herpes. Genital herpes infection is more prevalent in women than in men. While over one in five Americans have genital herpes, one in four women in the United States are infected with type II herpes.

In an active herpes infection (called an outbreak), symptoms generally appear within 2 weeks of primary infection and can last for several weeks. Symptoms may include tingling or sores near the area where the virus has entered the body, such as on the genital or rectal area, on the buttocks or thighs, or on other parts of the body where the virus has entered through broken skin. In women, the sores may occur inside the vagina, on the cervix, or in the urinary passage. Small red bumps appear first, develop into small blisters, and finally become itchy, painful sores that might develop a crust and heal without leaving a scar. Other symptoms that may accompany the first outbreak, and possibly subsequent outbreaks, include fever, muscle aches and pains, headache, dysuria, vaginal discharge, and swollen glands in the groin area.

Gonorrhea

Gonorrhea is caused by *Neisseria gonorrhoeae*, a bacterium that can grow and multiply rapidly in the warm, moist areas of the reproductive tract, including the cervix, uterus, and fallopian tubes in women and in the urethra in women and men. The bacterium can also grow in the mouth, throat, eyes, and anus.

Symptoms of gonorrhea, which are generally more severe in men than in women, appear approximately 2 to 10 days after exposure. Women may be infected with gonorrhea for months but experience virtually no symptoms until the infection has spread to other parts of the reproductive system. When symptoms do appear in women, they generally manifest as dysuria (painful urination), with associated burning or itching, a yellowish or bloody vaginal discharge, usually with a foul odor, and occult blood associated with vaginal intercourse. More severe infections may present with cramping and abdominal pain, nausea and vomiting, and bleeding between periods; these symptoms indicate that the infection has progressed to PID. Rectal infections generally present with anal discharge and itching, plus occasional painful bowel movements with fecal blood spotting. Infection of the throat (for which oral sex is the introducing factor) is called gonococcal pharyngitis. Its symptoms are usually mild, consisting of painful or difficulty swallowing, sore throat, swollen lymph glands, and fever. Headache and nasal congestion may also be present. If a gonorrhea infection is not treated, the bacterium may enter the bloodstream and spread to other parts of the body, including the brain—a condition known as disseminated gonococcemia.

Genital Warts

Genital warts (also called condylomata acuminata and venereal warts) are caused by the human papillomavirus (HPV). Of the more than 100 types of HPV that have been identified (most are harmless), about 30 types are spread through sexual contact. HPV is the most common STD, with millions of new cases being reported every year. Sources estimate that 75% to 80% of all people in the United States will be infected with HPV at some time in their life. HPV has been identified as a causative agent in cervical, vulvar, and anal cancers. In pregnant women, warts may develop

YOU are the Medic   PART 4

The patient tells you her last menstrual period was 7 days ago. The flow was very heavy and she was in a great deal of pain. She is still having the pain, but now she is also spotting. You determine the hospital of choice for the patient and she agrees to transport. Prior to placing the patient on your stretcher, you have your partner assess her vital signs, which show no change. En route, the patient rests comfortably with no change in signs or symptoms.

Recording Time: 10 Minutes	
Respirations	18 breaths/min
Pulse	80 beats/min, lying; 82 beats/min, sitting
Skin	Pink, warm, dry
Blood pressure	128/60 mm Hg, lying; 128/60 mm Hg, sitting
Oxygen saturation (Spo$_2$)	98% on 4 L/min via nonrebreathing mask
Pupils	Equal and reactive

7. What is the general patient care for this patient?

8. Can you accurately diagnose a difference between a gynecologic and abdominal problem in the field?

that become large enough to impede urination or obstruct the birth canal. If the virus is passed to the fetus, the child may develop *laryngeal papillomatosis* (throat warts that block the airway), a potentially life-threatening condition. Some people infected with genital warts have no symptoms. In others, multiple growths develop in the genital areas—that is, the vagina, vulva, cervix, or rectum, or the penis and scrotum in men.

Syphilis

Syphilis is caused by the bacterium *Treponema pallidum*. Because many of its signs and symptoms mimic other diseases, syphilis is sometimes called the "great imitator" by clinicians. The disease manifests in three stages: primary, secondary, and late. Approximately 40,000 cases of syphilis are reported each year in the United States, mostly in the 20- to 40-year-old group. Transmission occurs through direct contact with open sores, which may arise anywhere on the body, but tend to appear on the genitals, anus, rectum, lips, or mouth. A person with syphilis may remain asymptomatic for years, not realizing that his or her sores are manifestations of a disease.

The primary stage of syphilis is usually marked by the appearance of a single sore (a chancre), although in some people, multiple sores develop. The chancre is usually painless and is small, firm, and round. It usually goes away after 3 to 6 weeks, at which point the disease has progressed to the second stage.

The secondary stage of syphilis is characterized by the development of mucous membrane lesions and a skin rash. The characteristic rash may manifest on the palms of the hands and the bottoms of the feet as rough, red or reddish brown spots. Alternatively, it may be barely discernible or resemble rashes from other diseases. The rash generally does not itch. Symptoms of secondary syphilis may include fever, swollen lymph glands, sore throat, patchy hair loss, headaches, weight loss, muscle aches, and fatigue. Like the chancre of the primary stage, these symptoms will resolve without treatment. Left untreated, the secondary stage invariably leads to late-stage syphilis.

In the late stage, syphilis has no signs or symptoms, but internal damage is accumulating. Syphilis attacks the brain, nerves, eyes, heart, blood vessels, liver, bones, and joints, although the damage may not become evident for years. Paralysis, numbness, dementia, gradual blindness, and difficulty coordinating muscle movements are possible physical manifestations and may be serious enough to cause death. Pregnant women with syphilis may have stillborn babies, babies who are born blind, developmentally delayed babies, or babies who die shortly after birth.

Trichomoniasis

Trichomoniasis is caused by a single-celled protozoan parasite, *Trichomonas vaginalis*. This parasite is transmitted through sexual contact, with the vagina being the most common site of infection. Left untreated, the infection can lead to low birthweight or premature birth in pregnant women and to increased susceptibility to HIV infection. Approximately 7 million cases of trichomoniasis are reported in the United States each year. The person infected with trichomoniasis may be asymptomatic or may experience signs and symptoms including a frothy, yellow-green vaginal discharge with a strong odor. The infection may also cause irritation and itching of the female genital area, discomfort during intercourse, dysuria, and lower abdominal pain. When present, symptoms usually appear in women within 5 to 28 days of exposure to *T. vaginalis*.

■ Sexual Assault

Pathophysiology

Sexual assault can take many forms, but the most common is rape. In the United States, one of every three women will be raped in her lifetime (though only one in five file a crime report), and one of every four will be sexually molested, often before the age of 12 years.

Because rape is a *crime*, you can generally expect police involvement early in the situation. In many cases, EMS may be called by the police. Police officers generally have rudimentary medical training, with many states requiring at least basic training at the first responder level. Nevertheless, primary training for police officers focuses on *investigation*, not patient care.

A rape victim has just experienced a purposeful "major vehicle crash" of her mind and body. The act was most likely perpetrated by someone she knew and trusted. The last thing she wants to do is give a concise, detailed report of what she has just experienced, and attempting to elicit information in this manner most likely will cause the victim to "shut down." Whenever possible, a female rape victim should be given the option of being treated by a female paramedic because the patient may be experiencing ambivalent feelings toward men in general; these feelings will hinder assessment and the patient's well-being.

It is the job of law enforcement officers to solve the crime, arrest the perpetrator, and see justice served. The job of paramedics is to manage the medical aspects of the case and to act as the patient advocate. In this capacity, it is important for you to focus on several key issues.

Assessment

Paramedics called on to treat a victim of sexual assault, molestation, or actual or alleged rape face many complex issues, ranging from obvious medical ones to serious psychological and legal issues. In particular, you may be the first person the victim has contact with after the encounter, and how the situation is managed from first contact throughout treatment and transport may have lasting effects for the patient and you. Professionalism, tact, kindness, and sensitivity are of paramount importance. First, ask the patient if he or she would be more comfortable with a female or male paramedic, and make every effort to fulfill this request.

Limit any physical examination to a brief survey for life-threatening injuries. Expose and examine the vaginal area only if there is evidence of bleeding that needs to be treated. Do everything possible to protect the patient's privacy and give some sense of control back to the patient. Examine and interview the patient with a minimum of people present, moving her to the ambulance if necessary.

The first issue is the medical treatment of the patient. Is she physically injured? Are any life-threatening injuries present? Does the patient complain of any pain?

The second issue is your psychological care of the patient. Do not cross-examine her or attempt to elicit information for the benefit of the police. These issues will be handled later in the emergency department. Do not pass judgment on the patient, and protect her from the judgment of others on the scene. It does not matter how the patient is dressed, what her local reputation is, where she was, or what she was doing when the assault occurred. The concept of a woman "deserving" to be raped is just as ludicrous as you "deserving" to be assaulted for wearing the colors of a rival sports team. A crime has been committed, and you need to remain cognizant of that fact. Many women report feeling "re-raped" when subjected to interrogation, criticism, or incredulity.

Management

Remember that you are at a crime scene. Although your job is to treat the *medical* aspects of the incident and not collect evidence, you still have a responsibility to *preserve* evidence. Do not cut through any clothing or throw away anything from the scene. Place bloodstained articles in separate paper (not plastic) bags. Obtain evidentiary bags from the police if necessary. Paper bags allow wet items to dry naturally, whereas plastic allows mold to grow and may destroy biologic evidence.

It may also be necessary to gently persuade the patient to *not* clean herself up. This will be a natural desire on the part of the patient, stemming from the desire to "wash away" the humiliation and embarrassment of the assault. Valuable evidence can be destroyed in this process. The patient also needs to be discouraged from using hand sanitizer, urinating, changing clothes, moving her bowels, or rinsing out her mouth. She will need to be photographed by law enforcement personnel as well, and the photographic record needs to be as accurate as possible. If the patient cannot be dissuaded from taking these actions, respect her feelings.

Some patients may refuse transport altogether. For adults who are mentally competent, this is the patient's right. In such cases, you should follow your system's refusal of treatment policy or procedure for sexual assault victims without judging or being condescending to the patient. In no instance should you simply accept the patient's refusal and leave. Offer to call the local rape crisis center for the patient. Many communities have rape crisis centers, with victim advocates on-call. Getting a professional advocate to the scene may help the patient deal with the trauma, and the advocate can better explain the necessities of evidence preservation in more compassionate detail. Many victim advocates are rape-trauma survivors themselves.

Follow your protocol concerning this type of call. Some EMS systems may consider administering a sedative to a patient in this situation.

The patient care report is a legal document and, should the case result in an arrest and subsequent trial, may be subpoenaed. Keep the report concise, and record only what the patient stated in her own words. Use quotation marks to indicate that you are reporting the patient's version of events. Do

not insert your own opinion as to whether the patient was raped or offer any conclusions that would validate or invalidate the patient's account of the event. Focus on the facts. Record your observations during the physical examination—the patient's emotional state, the condition of her clothing, and any obvious injuries. Bear in mind that rape is a *legal* diagnosis, not a medical diagnosis. The medical team can establish only whether sexual intercourse occurred; a court must decide whether intercourse was inflicted forcibly on the victim, against her will.

Drugs Used to Facilitate Rape

It is not uncommon for drugs to be involved when a rape or other sexual assault has taken place. In fact, alcohol is the most common element to rape scenes. But other drugs of choice for commission of the crime of rape are "club drugs" such as gamma-hydroxybutyric acid (GHB), ketamine, ecstasy, and Rohypnol. These drugs are summarized in Table 1.

Sexual Practices and Vaginal Foreign Bodies

Pathophysiology

There is a variety of ways that men and women engage in sexual acts. Your exposure to these practices will most likely occur when these private sexual practices go bad, resulting in an embarrassing call to 9-1-1.

The most common sexual gynecologic emergency you may encounter is simply a foreign object (a soda pop or beer bottle or a sex toy) that has become stuck in the vagina or anus. For example, a bottle may develop a vacuum inside of the body and stick to an interior structure. Attempts at removal by the patient may result in intense pain or even vaginal bleeding as internal structures tear. Bleeding and pain cause the patient to panic. With this type of call, keep the patient calm, protect his or her dignity as much as possible, and transport. Do not attempt to remove any foreign objects from the vagina or anus. If at all possible, do not let the patient walk. Overpenetration of any item may lead to internal injury, and should be managed as such.

Table 1 Drugs Used to Facilitate Rape

Drug	Street Names	General Information	Symptoms	Emergency Care
Gamma-hydroxybutyric acid (GHB)	■ Georgia home boy ■ Grievous bodily harm ■ Easy lay ■ G ■ Scoop ■ Liquid X ■ Soap ■ Salty water	■ Depressant, has amnestic properties ■ Common in the "rave" and "club" crowds ■ Colorless liquid ■ Generally has a salty taste that is disguised when mixed in a drink	■ Range from sleepiness, loss of muscle tone, and forgetfulness to seizurelike activity ■ Respirations and pulse rate are depressed, progressing to a comalike state that generally lasts about 2 hours	■ Supportive ■ Make sure that adequate ventilatory support is initiated for patients in respiratory depression. ■ There is no current antidote for GHB ingestion. ■ Naloxone (Narcan) and flumazenil (Romazicon, a benzodiazepine agonist) are of no benefit.
Ketamine hydrochloride (Ketalar, Ketaset)	■ Special K ■ Vitamin K ■ Cat Valium ■ Fort Dodge	■ Predominantly marketed in the United States as a veterinary anesthetic ■ Blocks pain pathways ■ May produce frightening hallucinations ■ Available in liquid and powder form ■ Can be inhaled, injected, or mixed into a drink	■ Loss of coordination ■ Muscle rigidity ■ Slurred speech ■ Catatonic or blank stare ■ General sense of numbness ■ Can lead to aggressive and violent behavior and an exaggerated sense of strength ■ Symptoms of overdose include nausea and vomiting, hypertension, and respiratory impairment leading to oxygen deprivation of the brain	■ There is no field antidote for ketamine; transport
Ecstasy (methylenedioxy methamphetamine [MDMA])	■ XTC ■ Adam ■ X ■ Lover's speed ■ Clarity	■ Methamphetamine derivative with hallucinogenic properties; a stimulant ■ Generally sold in capsule or tablet form ■ Can also be found as a powder ■ Can be injected, inhaled, ingested, or smoked ■ Regular users may use paraphernalia such as rubber or candy pacifiers to ease the effects ■ A surgical mask smeared with Vicks VapoRub is also a clue of ecstasy use because the vapors reportedly increase the effect of the "rush" ■ Logos that may appear on tablets: Superman, Batman, Nike, Mercedes, Rolls Royce	■ Similar to those of cocaine and speed ■ Rapid pulse rate ■ Rapid increase of body temperature, often to deadly levels ■ Anxiety ■ Hypertension ■ Blurred vision ■ Mental confusion ■ Nausea ■ Excessive sweating, leading to dangerous levels of dehydration ■ Rapid eye movement ■ Tremors ■ Bruxism (teeth clenching)	■ Transport

Continues

Table 1 Drugs Used to Facilitate Rape, continued

Drug	Street Names	General Information	Symptoms	Emergency Care
Rohypnol	■ Roofies ■ Roof ■ Roachies ■ Rocha ■ Mexican Valium	■ Has sedative-hypnotic, amnestic, and anesthetic properties ■ Legally marketed outside the United States by Roche Pharmaceuticals as a sedative and preoperative anesthetic ■ White, scored tablet, with the word "Roche" appearing on one side ■ Tablet can be dissolved in a drink, where it is undetectable ■ Roche Pharmaceuticals has recently added a color base of royal blue to the tablet; if the drug is mixed with a drink, the color will appear	■ Impaired judgment and motor skills ■ Loss of social inhibitions ■ Decreased blood pressure ■ Drowsiness ■ Dizziness ■ Confusion ■ Memory loss (victim will have no memory of approximately the last 15 to 20 minutes before blacking out)	■ Supportive, with possible administration of flumazenil ■ Naloxone (Narcan) has no effect on Rohypnol, but its administration may be considered because Rohypnol is sometimes used in conjunction with other drugs

Some cases of bottle insertion may be associated with rape, so bear in mind that the patient may be an assault victim. Some gangs have been known to insert beer bottles in a woman's vagina after rape, then take turns punching the woman in the lower abdomen until the bottle breaks. If this is the case, use extreme care and do not move the patient more than necessary to prevent even more internal damage.

Among some of the more bizarre practices you may encounter includes a technique known as "fisting," which involves placing the closed fist and wrist into a body orifice (vagina or rectum) for sexual stimulation. Whether the patient is male or female, organ rupture (rectum, vagina) is likely. Life-threatening peritonitis may result. Another sexual practice is the insertion of live animals into the vagina, including fish, eels, snakes, worms, and hamsters. The patient becomes alarmed when the animal goes in but does not come out.

Assessment

Assessment in this situation is sensitive. Maintain your patient's privacy. Depending on the circumstances, you may need to inspect the genital area for bleeding, wounds, or objects that may need to be stabilized. Avoid focusing on only one part of your patient; you still need to conduct a thorough patient assessment including vital signs and history.

Management

Treat such a case as you would with any other foreign object, remain nonjudgmental, and transport. Do not attempt to retrieve the object, even if it is an animal, from inside the vagina. Transport the patient in a knees-flexed, legs-together position.

Documentation and Communication

As with other sexually related injuries, patients involved in fisting or the insertion of live animals are often reluctant to divulge correct historic information.

YOU *are the Medic* | **SUMMARY**

1. What are you looking for in your scene size-up?

Every emergency call—including calls involving gynecologic emergencies—begins with a thorough scene size-up. Is the scene safe? Will you need assistance? Is it a medical call, a trauma call, or both? How many patients do you have? Have you taken proper standard precautions? Gynecologic emergencies can be messy, sometimes involving large amounts of blood and body fluids contaminated with communicable diseases. In the case of a crime scene, you may also be required to testify in court regarding the conditions at the scene.

2. What are you looking for in your primary assessment?

What is the overall presentation of the patient? Does your rapid scan reveal any obvious life threats? Is she conscious? Does she have obvious breathing difficulty or evidence of injury? Does she appear pale, cyanotic, red, or gray? Is she alert and oriented or confused? Is she calm or distraught? What is her emotional state? What is her physical appearance—well kempt or dirty? Do you find the patient sitting up, lying down, prone, supine, in the fetal position, in the tripod position, in the bathtub, or on all fours?

Once you have answered these basic questions and treated any immediate threats to airway, breathing, or circulation, you can proceed with a secondary assessment and obtain more history of the present illness.

3. What three life-threatening gynecologic conditions present with pain?

Only three life-threatening gynecologic conditions present with pain (ectopic pregnancy, ruptured ovarian cyst, and tubo-ovarian abscess), all of which typically present with similar findings. Other gynecologic causes of pain are not immediately (if at all) life-threatening, but any manifestation of pain will naturally be worrisome to the patient.

4. What steps will you take in your further assessment of this patient?

What is the patient's chief complaint? If it is excessive bleeding, you can move on to obtaining the gynecologic history. If the chief complaint is abdominal pain, you need to find out more about the pain itself, using the OPQRST method (Onset; Provoking factors; Quality of pain; Region of pain and whether it radiates or refers; Severity; and Time [duration]).

5. What is the LORDS TRACHEA mnemonic?

The LORDS TRACHEA mnemonic covers the following assessment points:

L What is the Location of the pain?
O What was the Onset of the pain?
R Does the pain Radiate?
D What is the Duration of the pain?
S What is the Severity of the pain, on a scale of 0 to 10?
T What is the Timing of the pain?
R Does anything Relieve the pain?
A Aggravates the pain?
C What is the Character of the pain?
H Is there a Historic precedent?
E Has the patient Eaten anything?
A Are there Associated symptoms?

6. What is the next question you should ask this patient?

Once you have ascertained all that you can about the chief complaint and have developed an understanding of the patient's pain, you can proceed to obtain a gynecologic history. Probably the single most important question to ask is, "When did you have your last menstrual period (LMP)?" If the patient knows for certain, record the beginning and ending dates of the LMP. If she is unsure, record the approximate dates. Ask the patient whether she noticed anything unusual about the LMP.

7. What is the general patient care for this patient?

The management of a gynecologic patient is generally simple because there are few interventions you can initiate in the field. Primary management will be directed at mitigating life threats, being supportive and compassionate, and protecting the patient's modesty. For all patients, assess and supply the appropriate oxygen needs. Obtain the patient's vital signs, and continue to monitor her vital signs throughout her care.

8. Can you accurately diagnose a difference between a gynecologic and abdominal problem in the field?

Gynecologic emergencies often have the same signs and symptoms as emergencies involving other abdominal organs. Assess the patient carefully to determine the nature and extent of the problem. Be sure to follow the SAMPLE mnemonic. What, if any, associated signs and symptoms are noted: fever, diaphoresis, syncope, diarrhea, constipation, dysuria? Other medical problems may present as an abdominal problem. For example, cardiac pain may be misinterpreted as epigastric pain.

YOU are the Medic   SUMMARY, continued

EMS Patient Care Report (PCR)

Date: 05-31-11	**Incident No.:** 78865	**Nature of Call:** Abdominal pain		**Location:** 1065 Meadow Lane	
Dispatched: 1005	**En Route:** 1005	**At Scene:** 1010	**Transport:** 1040	**At Hospital:** 1047	**In Service:** 1058

Patient Information

Age: 24 **Sex:** F **Weight (in kg [lb]):** 91 kg (200 lb)	**Allergies:** No known drug allergies **Medications:** OTC ibuprofen **Past Medical History:** Denies **Chief Complaint:** Abdominal/pelvic pain

Vital Signs

Time: 1012	**BP:** 128/60	**Pulse:** 80	**Respirations:** 18	**Spo₂:** 98% 4 L/min
Time: 1017	**BP:** 128/60 lying/sitting	**Pulse:** 80 lying, 82 sitting	**Respirations:** 18	**Spo$_2$:** 98% 4 L/min
Time:	**BP:**	**Pulse:**	**Respirations:**	**Spo$_2$:**

EMS Treatment
(circle all that apply)

Oxygen @ __4__ L/min via (circle one): NC (NRM) Bag-mask device	**Assisted Ventilation**	**Airway Adjunct**	**CPR**
Defibrillation	**Bleeding Control**	**Bandaging**	**Splinting**	**Other**

Narrative

Arrived to find 24-year-old woman complaining of abdominal and pelvic pain. Pt states the pain is a dull ache located in her pelvis and lower back that has been present for 3 months. Pt also complains of increased menstrual flow with spotting between periods. Pt states LMP was 7 days ago. Pt states pain is constant and does not change with movement or OTC medication. Pt is not under a doctor's care for same. Pt states she is not pregnant. Pt vital signs assessed including postural, which shows no change. Pt agreed to transport to Community Hospital. Pt rested comfortably during transport with no change in condition noted. Report to Dr. Sullivan on arrival in ED bed 4. **End of report**

Prep Kit

- Gynecology is the study of and care for diseases of the female reproductive system.

- The external anatomy of the female genitalia, sometimes referred to as the pudendum, includes the mons pubis, labia majora, labia minora, perineum, clitoris, prepuce, and vestibule.

- The internal anatomy of the female genitalia includes the vagina, Bartholin glands, cervix, uterus, fallopian tubes, and ovaries.

- Menstruation (menses or period) is the vaginal discharge of primarily blood that generally occurs every 24 to 35 days in premenopausal women.

- A woman can experience physical changes during the menstrual cycle that result in fluid retention, breast pain and tenderness, headache, cramping, and more intense emotional states. This premenstrual syndrome can be debilitating.

- The last menses is called menopause; it generally occurs between the ages of 40 and 50 years. Women may experience physical symptoms of menopause, including diaphoresis, hair loss, hot flashes, muscle aches and pains, headache, dyspnea, vertigo, digestive problems, and emotional instability.

- When assessing a patient with a gynecologic emergency, begin by focusing on the ABCs.

- Protect the patient's modesty at all times. Gynecologic emergencies can be very embarrassing for the patient.

- If the chief complaint is abdominal pain, investigate the pain by following the mnemonic LORDS TRACHEA: Location, Onset, Radiation, Duration, Severity, Timing, Relief, Aggravation, Character, History, Eating, and Associated symptoms.

- Determine when the patient had her last menstrual period, if it is unusual in any way, whether she could be pregnant, and whether she uses contraception.

- Vaginal bleeding that does not occur during the course of regular menstruation is cause for concern. Consider whether there is a mechanism of injury. Try to obtain an accurate description of the bleeding.

- During the patient history, obtain the patient's obstetric history, including any previous pregnancies, miscarriages, or abortions. If the patient has a vaginal discharge, obtain a description of it.

- General management for gynecologic emergencies is simple, including addressing life threats, being supportive, and protecting the patient's modesty.

- The three life-threatening gynecologic emergencies are ectopic pregnancy, ruptured ovarian cyst, and tubo-ovarian abscess. Patients will present with abdominal pain and possibly vaginal bleeding, nausea, vomiting, or fever. Identify when each symptom began. Management includes airway maintenance, supplemental oxygen, positioning the patient on the left side, IV fluids, keeping the patient warm, monitoring the ECG, and transporting.

- Mittelschmerz is abdominal pain and cramping that occur about 2 weeks before menstruation. Dysmenorrhea is painful menstruation. Prehospital treatment is supportive.

- Amenorrhea is the absence or cessation of menses. The most common cause is pregnancy. Amenorrhea can also occur in athletes and in people with anorexia nervosa or emotional problems.

- Endometritis is inflammation or irritation of the endometrium. Symptoms include malaise, fever, bowel problems, vaginal bleeding, abdominal distention, and lower abdominal or pelvic pain.

- Endometriosis is the growth of endometrial tissue outside of the uterus. It can cause infertility. Symptoms include low back, pelvic, or abdominal pain; painful coitus; elimination problems during menstruation; menstrual cramping; and heavy menstruation.

- Pelvic inflammatory disease (PID) is an infection of the female upper reproductive organs. One of the most common causes of abdominal pain in women, it can cause infertility.

- Patients with pelvic inflammatory disease will present with abdominal pain starting during or after menstruation. Obtain a thorough history and transport gently.

- Vaginitis and vulvovaginitis are inflammations of the vaginal tissues and external vulva caused by an infection. Symptoms include itching, irritation, discharge, odor, painful intercourse, and lower abdominal pain. Both of these common conditions are treated with antibiotics.

- A patient with a Bartholin gland abscess will report a painful lump, irritation (swelling and redness), painful intercourse, and possibly fever. The abscess is usually on one side of the vaginal opening and may need to be drained by a physician.

- In ectopic pregnancy, a fertilized oocyte implants somewhere other than the uterus, usually in a fallopian tube, which can lead to rupture of the fallopian tube.

- Ruptured ovarian cyst, tubo-ovarian abscess, and ovarian torsion are other gynecologic conditions that can become an emergency.

- A prolapsed uterus is when the uterus drops into the vagina. There are varying degrees of prolapse from a small protrusion of visible tissue to the entire uterus being outside of the vagina. Treat with warm, moist dressings and emotional support.

- Toxic shock syndrome is a form of septic shock that can result from an infection in the body. Symptoms include syncope, myalgia, diarrhea, vomiting, headache, fever, sore throat, petechiae, rash, and bloodshot eyes. Transport patients rapidly.

- Sexually transmitted diseases (STDs) can cause pelvic inflammatory disease. STDs include bacterial vaginosis, chancroid, chlamydia, cytomegalovirus, genital herpes, gonorrhea, syphilis, and trichomoniasis.

- Symptoms of sexually transmitted diseases can include itching, burning, pain, fishy smelling discharge, sores around the genitals, swollen or painful lymph glands, lower abdominal or back pain, nausea, fever, painful intercourse, bleeding between menstrual periods, fatigue, headache, and painful urination.

- Sexual assault is a category of crime that includes molestation and rape. Your compassion and professionalism in these situations are of the utmost importance.

- It may be difficult to obtain a history from a victim of rape. Have a same-sex paramedic treat the patient when possible.

- Remember that your job is to medically treat the patient. Ask only medical questions, and do not judge the patient. Limit the physical examination to addressing life-threatening injuries.

- Preserve evidence when possible. Try to persuade the rape victim not to clean herself.

- Document cases of sexual assault properly and professionally. On your patient care report, report the patient's words in quotation marks. Record facts obtained from the physical examination.

- Drugs used to facilitate rape include gamma-hydroxybutyric acid, ketamine hydrochloride, Ecstasy, and Rohypnol. These drugs can cause sleepiness, forgetfulness, numbness, loss of inhibitions, or rapid pulse rate and increase in body temperature, depending on the drug.

- Sexual emergencies may involve foreign objects stuck in the vagina or anus, which may potentially lead to internal injury. Do not remove the object. Remain professional, and transport the patient.

■ Vital Vocabulary

amenorrhea Absence of menstruation.

bacterial vaginosis An overgrowth of bacteria in the vagina, characterized by itching, burning, or pain, and possibly a "fishy" smelling discharge.

Bartholin glands The glands that secrete mucus for sexual lubrication.

cervix The narrowest portion (lower third of neck) of the uterus that opens into the vagina.

chancroid A highly contagious sexually transmitted disease caused by the bacteria *Haemophilus ducreyi*, which causes painful sores (ulcers), usually of the genitals.

chlamydia A sexually transmitted disease caused by the bacterium *Chlamydia trachomatis*.

clitoris A small, cylindrical mass of erectile tissue and nerves located at the anterior junction of the labia minora, similar to the glans penis of the male.

contraceptive device A device used to prevent pregnancy.

cytomegalovirus (CMV) A herpesvirus that can produce the symptoms of prolonged high fever, chills, headache, malaise, extreme fatigue, and an enlarged spleen.

dysfunctional uterine bleeding Abnormal vaginal bleeding that is irregular and is not caused by pregnancy, infection, or tumor.

dysmenorrhea Painful menstruation.

ecstasy A drug officially named methylenedioxymethamphetamine (MDMA) that is sometimes used to facilitate date rape; a methamphetamine derivative with hallucinogenic properties; street names include XTC, Adam, X, lover's speed, and clarity.

ectopic pregnancy A pregnancy in which the ovum implants somewhere other than the uterine endometrium.

endometriosis A condition in which endometrial tissue grows outside the uterus.

endometritis An inflammation of the endometrium that often is associated with a bacterial infection.

endometrium The inner mucous membrane of the uterus.

fallopian tube The anatomic structure that connects each ovary with the uterus and provides a passageway for the ova.

gamma-hydroxybutyric acid (GHB) A drug used to facilitate date rape; is colorless with a salty taste disguised when mixed with a drink; street names include Georgia home boy, grievous bodily harm, easy lay, G, scoop, liquid X, soap, and salty water.

Gardnerella vaginitis An infection caused by a bacterium that normally resides in the genital area in women but that can cause infection if the bacteria become too numerous; signs and symptoms include a vaginal odor that may be fishy, itching, irritation, and, possibly, a smooth, thin, sticky, white or gray discharge.

genital herpes An infection of the genitals, buttocks, or anal area caused by herpes simplex virus (HSV), which may cause sores of the genitals, mouth, or lips.

genital warts Warts caused by the human papillomavirus (HPV), a sexually transmitted disease; also called condylomata acuminata or venereal warts.

gonorrhea A sexually transmitted disease caused by *Neisseria gonorrhoeae*.

gravida A term used to describe the number of times a woman has been pregnant.

hemoperitoneum Blood in the peritoneal cavity.

hymen A membrane that protects the vaginal orifice before first intercourse.

hypermenorrhea Menstrual blood flow that lasts several days longer than it should or flow that is abnormally excessive.

imperforate hymen A situation in which the hymen completely covers the vaginal orifice.

ketamine hydrochloride A drug used to facilitate date rape but that is predominantly marketed in the United States as a veterinary anesthetic and is a phencyclidine hydrochloride derivative; street names include special K, vitamin K, cat Valium, and Fort Dodge.

labia majora Outer fleshy "lips" covered with pubic hair that protect the vagina.

labia minora Inner fleshy "lips" devoid of pubic hair that protect the vagina.

menarche The beginning phase of a woman's life cycle of menstruation.

menopause The ending phase of a woman's life cycle of menstruation.

menstrual cycle The entire monthly cycle of menstruation from start to finish.

menstruation Monthly flow of blood.

metrorrhagia Irregular but frequent vaginal bleeding.

mons pubis A rounded pad of fatty tissue that overlies the symphysis pubis and is anterior to the urethral and vaginal openings.

oocyte The precursor to a mature egg.

ovarian cyst A fluid-filled sac that forms on or within an ovary.

ovarian torsion A painful condition in which the ovary becomes twisted.

ovary A female reproductive organ that produces an oocyte (ovum) that if fertilized will develop into a fetus.

para A term used to describe the number of times a woman has delivered a viable (live) newborn.

pelvic inflammatory disease (PID) An infection of the female upper organs of reproduction, specifically the uterus, ovaries, and fallopian tubes.

perineum The area between the vaginal opening and the anus.

polymenorrhea Menstrual blood flow that occurs more often than a 24-day interval.

premenstrual syndrome (PMS) A cluster of all or some of the troubling symptoms that occur during a woman's menstrual phase that can include fluid retention, breast pain and tenderness, headache, severe cramping, and emotional changes, including agitation, irritability, depression, and anger.

prepuce In the anatomy of the female genitalia, a layer of skin directly above the clitoris.

prolapsed uterus A condition in which the uterus moves or drops into the vagina due to weakened pelvic muscles and connective tissues.

proliferative phase The first phase of the uterine cycle and marks the time after menstruation and before the next ovulation occurs. The uterine lining increases in thickness in preparation to receive a fertilized oocyte.

pudendum The female external genitalia.

rape Sexual intercourse inflicted forcibly on another person, against that person's will.

Rohypnol A benzodiazepine used to facilitate date rape and that can create memory loss; street names include roofies, roof, roachies, rocha, and Mexican Valium.

ruptured ovarian cyst A fluid-filled sac within the ovary that bursts from internal pressure.

secretory phase The second phase of the uterine cycle and is the time after ovulation until menstruation (occurs when oocyte is not fertilized).

sexual assault An attack against a person that is sexual in nature, the most of common of which is rape.

syphilis A sexually transmitted disease caused by the bacterium *Treponema pallidum*, which manifests in three stages—primary, secondary, and late—and is transmitted through direct contact with open sores.

toxic shock syndrome (TSS) A form of septic shock caused by *Streptococcus pyogenes* (group A strep) or *Staphylococcus aureus*; initial symptoms include syncope, myalgia, diarrhea, vomiting, headache, fever, and sore throat.

trichomoniasis A parasitic infection.

tubo-ovarian abscess An infectious mass growing within the ovaries and fallopian tubes.

uterus The muscular organ where the fetus grows, also called the womb. It is found between the urinary bladder and the rectum.

vagina The lower portion of the birth canal, which also serves as a passage for menstrual flow and as the receptacle of the penis during sexual intercourse.

vaginal bleeding Bleeding from the vagina.

vaginal yeast infection An infection caused by the fungus, *Candida albicans*, in which fungi overpopulate the vagina.

vaginitis An inflammation of the vagina that is caused by an infection.

vestibule A cleft between the labia minora, where the urethral opening (orifice), the vaginal opening (orifice), and the hymen are located.

vulvovaginitis An inflammation of the external vulva.

Assessment in Action

Your unit is dispatched for a patient with abdominal pain. While en route, the dispatcher tells you the patient is a 24-year-old woman who is complaining of severe abdominal pain and vaginal bleeding. When you arrive on scene, you find that the patient looks very ill. She is pale, lying in a fetal position on the floor, and in severe pain. Her pants are wet with blood in the vaginal area. The patient tells you that she has been trying to get pregnant, but she knows something is terribly wrong.

1. Cullen sign is:
   A. discoloration over the pelvic bone.
   B. discoloration of the periumbilical skin.
   C. a change in blood pressure.
   D. a change in the pulse rate.

2. Bleeding followed by pelvic pain in a patient who is less than 20 weeks' pregnant may be caused by:
   A. a spontaneous abortion.
   B. an ectopic pregnancy.
   C. Braxton-Hicks contractions.
   D. pelvic inflammatory disease.

3. The primary predisposing factor in the development of an ectopic pregnancy is:
   A. a prolapsed uterus.
   B. pelvic inflammatory disease.
   C. mittelschmerz.
   D. dysmenorrhea.

4. When you are assessing this patient, look for the classic ectopic pregnancy triad. That triad includes which of the following?
   A. Amenorrhea, vaginal bleeding, and cystitis
   B. Amenorrhea, vaginal bleeding, and no abdominal pain
   C. Amenorrhea, no vaginal bleeding, and abdominal pain
   D. Amenorrhea, vaginal bleeding, and abdominal pain

5. The primary focus in the care of this patient is:
   A. treatment for pain.
   B. treatment for shock.
   C. treatment for abdominal pain.
   D. treatment depending on the severity of the signs and symptoms.

Additional Questions

6. What is toxic shock syndrome and does it only affect women?

7. The primary concern for the treatment of a victim of sexual assault is medical treatment based on any injuries. What is the secondary concern in this situation?

Endocrine Emergencies

National EMS Education Standard Competencies

Medicine

Integrates assessment findings with principles of epidemiology and pathophysiology to formulate a field impression and implement a comprehensive treatment/disposition plan for a patient with a medical complaint.

Endocrine Disorders

Awareness that

- Diabetic emergencies cause altered mental status (pp 1218, 1221, 1224)

Anatomy, physiology, pathophysiology, assessment, and management of

- Acute diabetic emergencies (pp 1221-1230)

Anatomy, physiology, epidemiology, pathophysiology, psychosocial impact, presentations, prognosis, and management of

- Acute diabetic emergencies (pp 1221-1230)
- Diabetes (pp 1221-1225)
- Adrenal disease (pp 1231-1233)
- Pituitary and thyroid disorders (pp 1233-1236)

Knowledge Objectives

1. Describe the incidence, morbidity, and mortality of endocrine emergencies. (pp 1221-1222)
2. Discuss the anatomy and physiology of the organs and structures of the endocrine system. (pp 1212-1217)
3. Explain how to size up scene safety when responding to a patient with an endocrine system emergency. (p 1218)
4. Analyze the nature of the illness for a broad range of endocrine disorders. (p 1218)
5. Indicate the considerations that go into making a transport decision for the patient with an endocrine emergency. (p 1219)
6. Specify how to investigate the chief complaint of a patient with an endocrine disorder, including how to take the patient's history using the SAMPLE mnemonic. (pp 1219-1220)

7. Describe the technique for performing a comprehensive physical examination on a patient with an endocrine emergency. (p 1220)
8. Examine ways in which you can communicate effectively with patients who have endocrine disorders. (pp 1219-1221)
9. Specify how to manage airway, breathing, and circulation in patients with endocrine system emergencies. (pp 1218-1219)
10. Define and explain the terms *diabetes, low blood glucose,* and *high blood glucose.* (pp 1221, 1226-1230)
11. Compare the pathophysiology, assessment, and management of type 1 diabetes with that of type 2 diabetes. (pp 1223-1225)
12. Discuss the role of glucose as a major source of energy for the body, and explain the relationship of glucose to insulin. (pp 1221-1223)
13. Compare hyperglycemic and hypoglycemic diabetic emergencies, including their pathophysiology, assessment, and management. (pp 1226-1230)
14. Outline some age-related considerations to keep in mind when managing a pediatric patient who is experiencing a hypoglycemic crisis. (p 1228)
15. Discuss the steps in conducting a primary and secondary assessment of a patient with a diminished level of consciousness who is suspected of having diabetes. (pp 1218-1220)
16. Describe the interventions for providing emergency medical care during a hypoglycemic crisis to conscious and unconscious patients who have a history of diabetes. (pp 1226-1227)
17. Provide the generic and trade names, form, dose, administration, indications, and contraindications for administering 50% dextrose to a patient with hypoglycemia. (p 1227)
18. Explain some age-related considerations to keep in mind when managing an older adult patient who is thought to have undiagnosed diabetes. (p 1223)
19. Define *hyperosmolar nonketotic coma/hyperosmolar hyperglycemic nonketotic coma (HONK/HHNC),* and name the signs characteristic of the condition. (p 1230)
20. Define *hyperglycemia* and discuss its pathophysiology, assessment, and management. (pp 1227-1230)
21. Describe the interventions for providing emergency medical care during a hyperglycemic crisis to conscious and unconscious patients who have a history of diabetes. (pp 1229-1230)
22. List the signs and symptoms of diabetic ketoacidosis (DKA) and describe its relationship to hyperglycemia. (pp 1227-1230)

23. Identify the special challenges children face during an episode of DKA. (p 1228)

24. Compare primary and secondary adrenal insufficiency, including their incidence, morbidity and mortality, pathophysiology, assessment, and management. (pp 1231–1232)

25. Define *addisonian crisis*, discuss what triggers this emergency, and identify its chief clinical manifestation and other signs and symptoms. (p 1232)

26. Define *Cushing syndrome*, list the physical manifestations characteristic of the disorder, and discuss its pathophysiology, assessment, and management. (p 1233)

27. Discuss the clinical presentation of a patient with an adrenal gland tumor. (p 1233)

28. Define *congenital adrenal hyperplasia*. (p 1233)

29. Compare the effects of hypothyroidism and hyperthyroidism on the cardiovascular, metabolic, neurologic, musculoskeletal, and gastrointestinal systems, and discuss the general somatic and emotional effects of each condition. (pp 1233–1236)

30. Explain the relationship of Graves disease to hyperthyroidism, and discuss the characteristic physical signs of the disease. (p 1234)

31. Explain the relationship of Hashimoto disease to hyperthyroidism, and compare Hashimoto disease with Graves disease. (p 1234)

32. Outline the characteristic signs of myxedema coma, and describe its relationship to hypothyroidism. (pp 1234–1235)

33. Discuss the incidence, morbidity, and mortality associated with myxedema coma, explain why it is considered to be an emergency, and outline appropriate treatment. (pp 1234–1235)

34. Describe thyrotoxicosis and thyroid storm, and specify their relationship to hyperthyroidism. (p 1235)

35. Define *inborn errors of metabolism*, explain how they are categorized, and give examples from each category. (p 1236)

Skills Objectives

1. Demonstrate the assessment and care of a patient with hypoglycemia and a decreased level of consciousness. (pp 1226–1227)

2. Demonstrate how to administer glucose to a patient with an altered mental status. (pp 1226–1227)

3. Demonstrate how to administer 50% dextrose to a patient with hypoglycemia. (pp 1226–1227)

4. Demonstrate how to administer glucagon to a patient with hypoglycemia. (p 1227)

Introduction

Few other systems in the body share the level of responsibility assigned to the endocrine system. This system directly or indirectly influences almost every cell, organ, and function of the body. Consequently, patients with an endocrine disorder often have a broad range of signs and symptoms, necessitating a thorough assessment and immediate treatment to avert life-threatening emergencies.

Anatomy and Physiology

The endocrine system comprises a network of glands that produce and secrete chemical messengers called hormones. The main function of the endocrine system and its hormone messengers is to maintain homeostasis and to promote permanent structural changes. Maintaining homeostasis requires a response to any change in the body, such as low glucose or calcium levels in the blood.

Exocrine glands (*exo-*means "outside") secrete chemicals for elimination. These glands have ducts that carry their secretions to the surface of the skin or into a body cavity. Sweat glands, salivary glands, and the liver are examples of exocrine glands.

Endocrine glands (*endo* means "inside") secrete or release chemicals that are used inside the body. These glands lack ducts, so they release hormones directly into the surrounding tissue and blood. Hormones act on the body's cells by increasing or decreasing the rate of cellular metabolism. They transfer information from one set of cells to another to coordinate body functions, such as the regulation of mood, growth and development, metabolism, tissue function, and sexual development and function.

Whereas the nervous system—the body's major controlling system—uses nerve impulses to activate and monitor the faster processes of the body, hormones of the endocrine system—considered the body's second great controlling system—are released directly into the bloodstream and act more slowly to achieve their effects. The hormones travel through the bloodstream to target tissues **Figure 1** . Each target cell has specific receptor sites on the cell membrane, or inside the cell, to which the specific hormone can attach or bind. These receptors have two main functions: to recognize and bind to their particular hormones and to initiate an appropriate signal. Once the hormone has attached to the receptor site of the cell, the "message" to alter the cellular function is delivered.

Many cells contain multiple receptors and act as targets for several hormones—or for molecules introduced into the body as therapy. Agonists are molecules that bind to a cell's receptor and trigger a response by that cell; they produce some kind of action or biologic effect. Antagonists are molecules that bind to a cell's receptor and block the action of agonists. Hormone antagonists are widely used as drugs.

Mechanisms of Hormonal Regulation

Hormones operate within feedback systems (either positive or negative) to maintain an optimal internal operating environment in the body. Release of hormones is regulated by chemical factors, other hormonal factors, and neural control. Endocrine regulation, through negative feedback, is the most important method by which hormonal secretion is maintained within a physiologic range.

One example of this negative feedback mechanism is the release of epinephrine from the adrenal medulla in response to stress. When stress stimulates the body's neural regulation by means of the sympathetic nervous system, it releases epinephrine into the bloodstream from the adrenal medulla to help the body respond. When the stressor is removed, nervous system stimulation decreases and less epinephrine is released **Figure 2** .

Disease occurs when normal cell signaling is interrupted and positive feedback is given. As a consequence, the system stops providing the critical negative feedback required to regulate function. Cell signaling is covered in more detail in the chapter, *Pathophysiology.*

YOU *are the Medic*   **PART 1**

You are dispatched to a local grocery store for a man "sitting in the butter." When you arrive, you are greeted by an elderly woman who tells you there is a large man sitting in one of the refrigerated sections of the store. The woman points down the dairy aisle and says, "There he is. We found him like that. He was shaking all over. I tried to help him, but now I have to go."

From a distance, you see an obese man casually sitting on top of a refrigerated dairy case. As you approach, you notice numerous large white tablets scattered on the aisle floor and what appears to be a food wrapper next to his feet. When you call out to him, he does not respond.

1. What key information is provided from the dispatch and scene size-up?

2. What types of medical conditions can cause an altered mental status?

levels of ADH stimulate the renal tubules to reabsorb sodium and water. At the same time, ADH acts as a vasopressor.

Components of the Endocrine System

The major components of the endocrine system include the hypothalamus; the pineal, pituitary, thyroid, thymus, parathyroid, and adrenal glands; the pancreas; and the gonads including the ovaries and testes. The pancreas has a role in hormone production as well as in digestion.

Hypothalamus

The hypothalamus is not a gland, but a small region of the brain that contains several control centers for body functions and emotions. It is the primary link between the endocrine system and the nervous system.

Pineal Gland

The pineal gland is located in the posterior end of the third ventricle of the brain. It synthesizes and secretes melatonin, which is a hormone that has an effect on sleep/wake patterns and seasonal functions (behavior patterns that occur in mammals, such as the mating season).

Pituitary Gland

The pituitary gland is often referred to as the "master gland" because its secretions orchestrate the activity of other endocrine glands. It is located at the base of the brain and is about the size of a grape. A thin tissue connects the pituitary gland to the hypothalamus. The pituitary is divided into the following two regions, or lobes:

1. The anterior pituitary, which produces and secretes seven hormones (growth hormone, thyroid-stimulating hormone, adrenocorticotropin hormone, melatonin-stimulating hormone, and three gonadotropic hormones).

2. The posterior pituitary, which secretes two hormones (ADH and oxytocin) but does not produce them Figure 3 ADH and oxytocin are synthesized in hypothalamic neurons but are stored in the posterior pituitary gland until the hypothalamus sends nerve signals to the pituitary to release them.

Table 1 lists the eight hormones secreted by the pituitary gland. Six of these hormones stimulate other endocrine glands

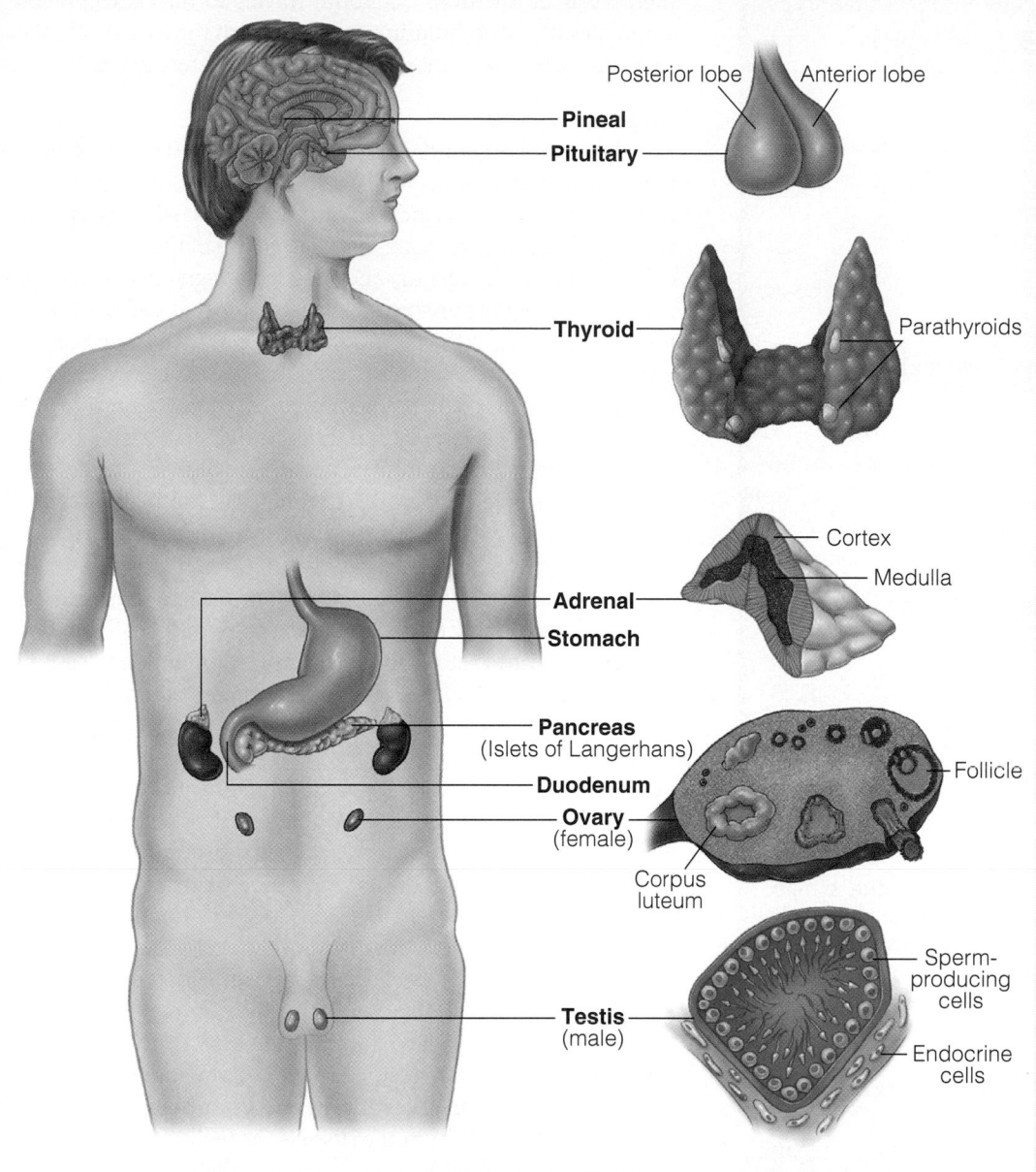

Figure 1 The endocrine system uses the various glands within the system to deliver chemical messages to organ systems throughout the body.

The hypothalamus and pituitary gland are intimately related through the vascular system. The hypothalamic–pituitary system controls the function of multiple peripheral endocrine organs (eg, thyroid, adrenal cortex, gonads, and breasts). Although technically a part of the nervous system, the hypothalamus is often considered a part of the endocrine system. It represents the junction between the nervous system and the endocrine system. The hypothalamus also produces its own regulatory (releasing and inhibitory) hormones. The regulatory hormones control the release of hormones by the pituitary gland.

Some of these hormones have physiologic effects that depend on their concentration. For example, a decrease in the body's water content triggers the release of antidiuretic hormone (ADH). The hypothalamus senses the concentration of salt in body fluids and signals the posterior pituitary to increase ADH secretion. Increased

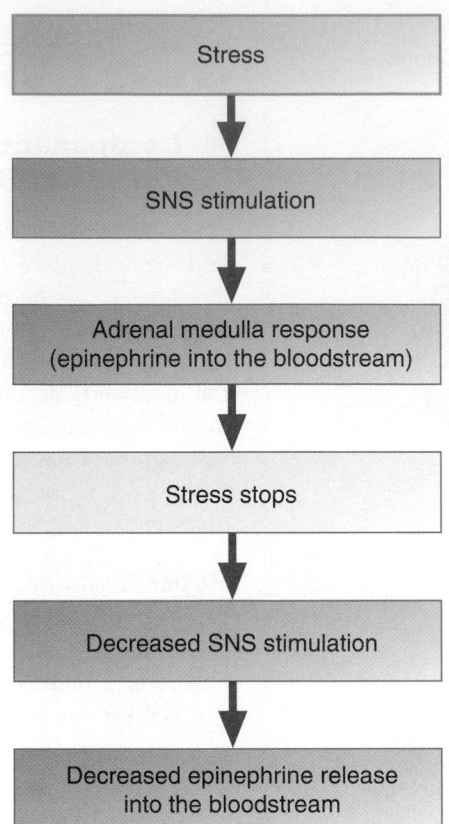

Figure 2 Stress stimulates neural regulators in the sympathetic nervous system (SNS) to signal the adrenal medulla to release epinephrine into the bloodstream to assist the body's "flight or fight" response. When the stimulus is eliminated, the neural regulating mechanism decreases its signals to the adrenal medulla and less epinephrine is released (negative feedback loop).

and are referred to as "tropic" (from the Greek *tropos*, meaning "to turn" or "change") hormones. The other two hormones control other body functions. The production and secretion of pituitary hormones can be influenced by factors such as emotions and seasonal changes.

Thyroid Gland

The thyroid gland secretes thyroxine when the body's metabolic rate decreases. Thyroxine, the body's major metabolic hormone, stimulates energy production in cells, which increases the rate at which cells consume oxygen and use carbohydrates, fats, and proteins. When the body gets cold, for example, the increased cellular metabolism creates heat. Iodine is an important component of thyroxine. Without the proper level of dietary iodine intake, thyroxine cannot be produced, and the person's physical and mental growth are diminished. Thyroxine production is regulated by a negative feedback mechanism that inhibits the hypothalamus from stimulating the thyroid when levels become high.

The thyroid gland also secretes calcitonin, which helps maintain normal calcium levels in the blood. This hormone is secreted directly into the bloodstream when the thyroid detects high levels of calcium. Calcitonin travels to the bones, where it stimulates the bone-building cells to absorb the excess calcium. It also stimulates the kidneys to absorb and excrete excess calcium.

Thymus Gland

The thymus gland, or *thymus*, is a component of the immune system that is located anteriorly and superiorly in the chest, posterior to the sternum. The gland can shrink rapidly when subjected to chronic illness or severe stress. The function of the gland is to help the immune system identify and destroy foreign intruders. In studies involving organ transplants in baby mice that had their thymus removed, the organ that was transplanted was not rejected; however, the mice became highly susceptible to disease-causing pathogens and to various pathogenic processes, such as cancer.

Lymphocytes are white blood cells that assist the lymphatic system with immunity. T lymphocytes, or T cells, evolve from stem cells located in the thymus that are produced in the bone marrow. These cells provide cell-mediated immunity and respond to defend against viruses, fungi, parasites, tumor cells, and some bacteria. The term *cell mediated* refers to the ability of the T cells to directly target and destroy an antigen. This process is different from that of humoral immunity, which uses B lymphocytes and antibodies to respond to most bacterial invasions.

There are three different types of T-cells, killer T cells, helper T cells, and suppressor T cells. The killer T cell, or cytotoxic T cell, attacks the antigen directly and triggers phagocytosis, thus preventing its reproduction. If you recall your medical terminology, *cyto*-means "cell" and *toxic* means capable of causing injury or death. The helper T cell, on the other hand, is not an instrument of destruction, but of information. It releases lymphokines, chemical mediators that deliver messages about antigens to the B cells. Because the immune system has the ability to cause injury, the suppressor T cells contain the immune response. If uncontrolled, the immune system causes excessive inflammation that may result in severe tissue damage. It is possible that a failure in the suppressor system contributes to the development of autoimmune diseases as well.

Controversies

Although it has long been thought that as we age the immune system does not function as well and infections are more likely, current research does not appear to support this theory. Increased morbidity and mortality secondary to infection, however, do exist. Anatomic and functional deterioration of systems is thought to be the reason. For example, urinary retention leads to an increase in urinary tract infections.

Parathyroid Glands

The parathyroid glands also assist in the regulation of calcium. However, the parathyroid hormone (PTH), when secreted by the parathyroid, acts as an antagonist to calcitonin. PTH is secreted when calcium blood levels are low. It stimulates the bone-dissolving cells to break down bone and release calcium into the bloodstream. In the kidneys, PTH decreases the amount of calcium released in the urine.

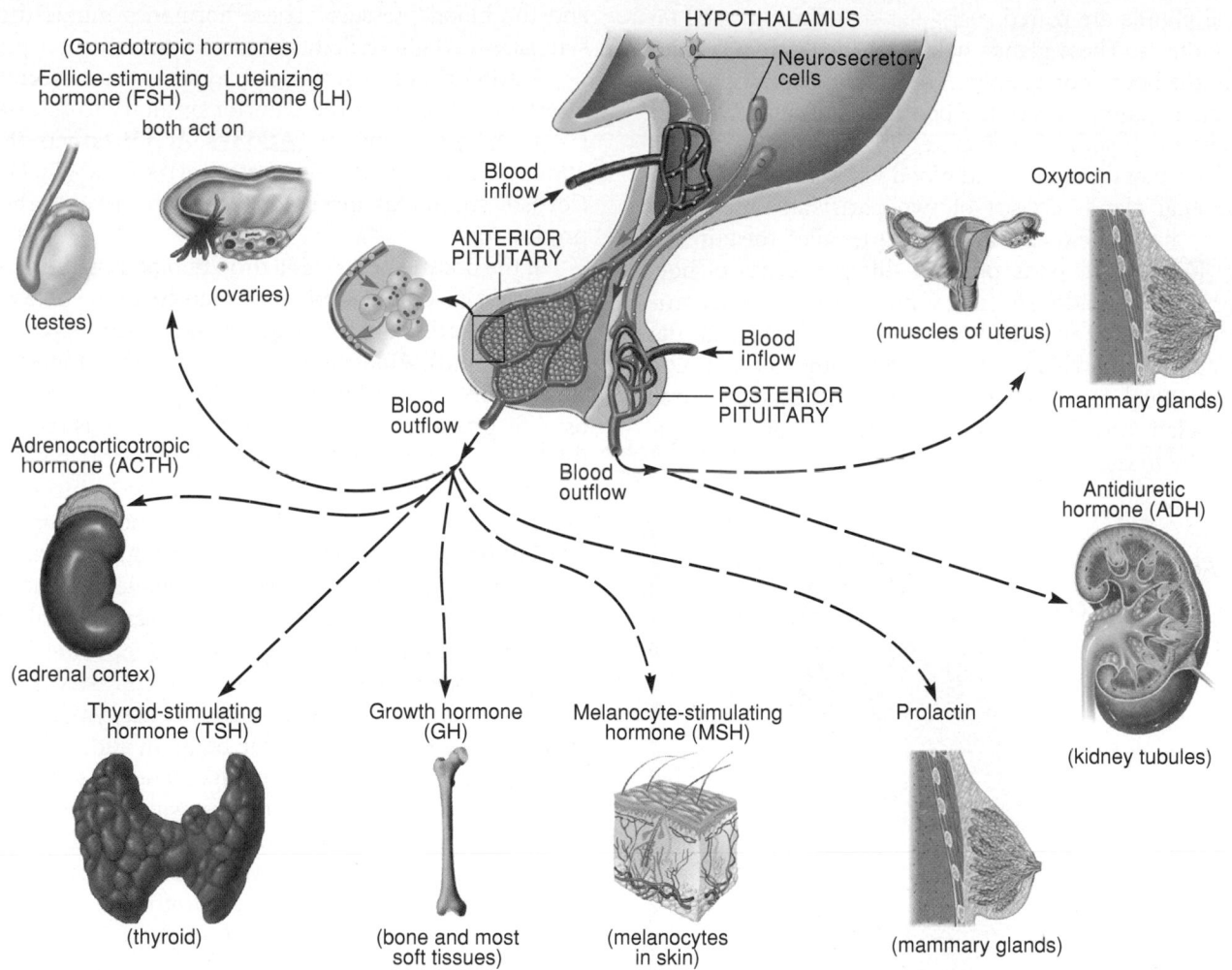

Figure 3 The pituitary gland secretes hormones from its two regions: the anterior pituitary lobe and the posterior pituitary lobe.

Table 1 Hormones Secreted by the Pituitary Gland

Hormone	Functions
Growth hormone (GH)	Regulates metabolic processes related to growth and adaptation to physical and emotional stressors
Thyroid-stimulating hormone (TSH)	Increases production and secretion of thyroid hormones
Adrenocorticotropic hormone (ACTH)	Stimulates the adrenal gland to secrete cortisol and adrenal proteins that contribute to the maintenance of the adrenal gland
Luteinizing hormone (LH)	In women: ovulation, progesterone production In men: regulates spermatogenesis, testosterone production
Follicle-stimulating hormone (FSH)	In women: follicle maturation, estrogen production In men: spermatogenesis
Prolactin	Milk production
Antidiuretic hormone (ADH)	Controls plasma osmolality; increases the permeability of the distal renal tubules and collecting ducts, which leads to an increase in water reabsorption
Oxytocin	Contracts the uterus during childbirth and stimulates milk production

Adrenal Glands

The <u>adrenal glands</u> are paired triangular structures located on top of the kidneys. These glands help coordinate several functions within the body. For example, they secrete hormones that suppress inflammation, govern the body's use of nutrients, and regulate how much sodium is excreted in the urine, which in turn modulates blood pressure and blood volume.

The adrenal glands consist of two parts: an outer part, called the <u>adrenal cortex</u>, and an inner part, called the <u>adrenal medulla</u> Figure 4 . Both parts produce different types of hormones Table 2 . The adrenal cortex produces mineralocorticoids, glucocorticoids, and sex hormones, which regulate the body's metabolism, its balance of salt and water, the immune system, and sexual function. The adrenal medulla produces hormones called <u>catecholamines</u> (epinephrine and norepinephrine), which assist the body in coping with physical and emotional stress by increasing the pulse and respiratory rates and the blood pressure. These hormones mimic those of the sympathetic (fight or flight) nervous system.

During times of stress, the hypothalamus secretes a hormone that stimulates the anterior pituitary to release <u>adrenocorticotropic hormone (ACTH)</u>. ACTH targets the adrenal cortex and causes it to secrete <u>cortisol</u> (a glucocorticoid). Cortisol stimulates most body cells to increase their energy production.

If the body experiences a drop in blood pressure or volume, a decrease in sodium level, or an increase in the potassium level, the adrenal cortex is stimulated to secrete <u>aldosterone</u> (a mineralocorticoid). Aldosterone stimulates the kidneys to reabsorb sodium from the urine and excrete potassium by altering the osmotic gradient in the blood. When sodium is reabsorbed into the blood, water follows; this action increases both blood volume and blood pressure. Aldosterone also reduces the amount of salt and water lost through the sweat and salivary glands.

The body's reaction to physical or emotional stress is referred to as the "fight or flight" response. Following stimulation from the hypothalamus, the adrenal medulla secretes small amounts of <u>norepinephrine</u> and large amounts of <u>epinephrine</u>. Norepinephrine raises blood pressure by causing blood vessels and skeletal muscles to constrict. Epinephrine stimulates sympathetic nervous system receptors throughout the body. In addition, it stimulates the liver to convert glycogen to glucose for use as energy in the cells. The action of both hormones results in increased levels of oxygen and glucose in the blood and faster circulation of blood to the brain, heart, and muscles, which in turn enables the body to respond to the short-term emergency situation.

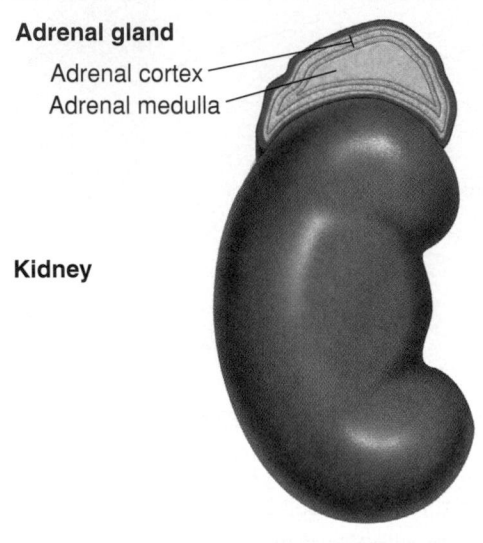

Adrenal gland
Adrenal cortex
Adrenal medulla

Kidney

Figure 4 The adrenal glands, which sit on top of the kidney, consist of two parts—the adrenal cortex and the adrenal medulla.

Table 2 Hormones of the Adrenal Glands

Hormone	Class	Functions
Cortisol	Glucocorticoid	Increases metabolic rate, using fat and protein for energy
Aldosterone	Mineralocorticoid	Reabsorbs sodium and water from the urine, and excretes excess potassium
Epinephrine/ norepinephrine	Catecholamines	Stimulates sympathetic nervous system receptors

Pancreas

The <u>pancreas</u> is a digestive gland that is considered both an endocrine gland and an exocrine gland. It secretes digestive enzymes into the duodenum through the pancreatic duct. The exocrine component is responsible for the secretion of the digestive enzymes. The endocrine component comprises the <u>islets of Langerhans</u>. These cell groups within the pancreas act like "an organ within an organ." The main hormones they secrete are <u>glucagon</u>, secreted by the alpha cells, and <u>insulin</u>, secreted by the beta cells. Glucagon and insulin are responsible for the regulation of blood glucose levels. <u>Somatostatin</u>, secreted by delta cells, is responsible for the inhibition of insulin and glucagon secretion Figure 5 .

When the body's blood glucose level falls, such as between meals, glucagon (a starch form of the sugar glucose made up of thousands of glucose units) is secreted to raise the glucose level and bring the body's energy back to normal. When it enters the bloodstream, glucagon stimulates the liver to change glycogen into sugar and secrete it into the bloodstream, where cells can use it for energy.

Insulin is responsible for the transport of glucose from the blood for storage as glycogen, fats, and protein. When blood glucose levels are elevated, the islets of Langerhans, in the pancreas, secrete insulin, which is carried by the bloodstream to the cells Table 3 . Cell membrane permeability is increased by insulin allowing the movement of glucose into the cells. The cells

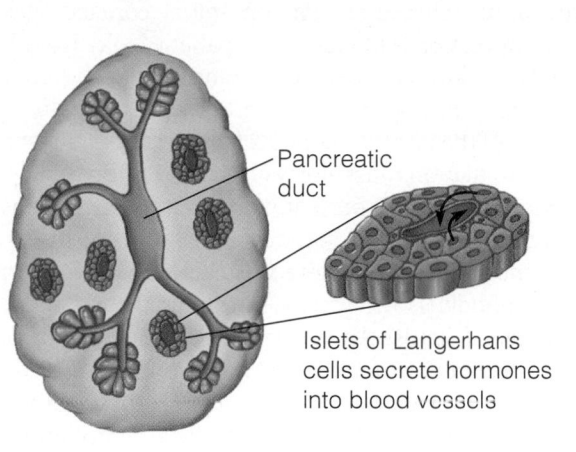

Figure 5 The islets of Langerhans secrete hormones into blood vessels.

Pancreatic duct

Islets of Langerhans cells secrete hormones into blood vessels

Table 4 Hormones of the Gonads

Hormone	Functions
Male	
Testosterone	Main sex hormone in males Responsible for secondary sex characteristics: voice deepening, growth of facial hair, muscle development, pubic hair, growth spurts
Female	
Estrogen	Responsible for secondary sex characteristics: breast growth, fat accumulation at hips and thighs, pubic hair, growth spurts Involved in pregnancy Regulation of menstrual cycle
Progesterone	Involved in pregnancy Regulation of menstrual cycle Prevents maturation of additional egg during ovulation

Table 3 Hormones of the Pancreas

Hormone	Functions
Insulin	Excreted when blood glucose is high (hyperglycemia) Increases conversion of glucose to glycogen Assists glucose across cell membrane
Glucagon	Excreted when blood glucose level is low (hypoglycemia) Increases conversion of glycogen to glucose (glycogenolysis)
Somatostatin	Excreted with increased levels of insulin and glucagon Decreases insulin and glycogen secretion Slows the absorption of nutrients

then take in more glucose and use it to produce energy. Insulin also stimulates the liver to take in more glucose and store it as glycogen for later use by the body. Insulin is the *only* hormone that decreases the blood glucose levels. Insulin is essential for glucose to enter and nourish the cells. Once the blood glucose levels have returned to normal, the islets of Langerhans discontinue the secretion of insulin.

Gonads

The <u>gonads</u> are the main source of sex hormones **Table 4**. In men, the gonads, or <u>testes</u>, are located in the scrotum and produce hormones called <u>androgens</u>. The most important androgen in men is <u>testosterone</u>. Androgens regulate body changes associated with sexual development (puberty), including growth spurts, deepening of the voice, growth of facial and pubic hair, and muscle growth and strength.

In women, the gonads are the <u>ovaries</u>, which release the eggs and secrete the hormones <u>estrogen</u> and <u>progesterone</u>. Estrogen signals the anterior pituitary gland to secrete <u>luteinizing hormone (LH)</u> when an egg is developing in an ovarian follicle. Estrogen and progesterone also assist in the regulation of the menstrual cycle. At puberty, estrogen also supports development of the secondary sex characteristics: enlargement of the breasts, uterine enlargement, fat deposits in the hips and thighs, and development of hair under the arms and in the pubic area.

Patient Assessment

The difficult part of assessing patients with endocrine emergencies is that their problems tend to affect many organ systems and the seriousness of their presentations varies greatly. Many of the patients will have had their conditions for some time and may already be receiving treatment. These patients or their family members will likely share with you that there is a history of an endocrine problem; this information, in addition to the common signs and symptoms associated with each endocrine emergency, should help you determine the cause of the current problem. In any event, do not take these calls lightly because poor outcomes can result quickly.

Words of Wisdom

Although specific pathophysiology varies for each disease, endocrine emergencies are usually caused by the following:

- Failure of normal hormone production
- Excessive hormone production
- Failure of feedback inhibition systems involving the hypothalamus, pituitary gland, endocrine gland, and the target organ

Scene Size-up

Scene safety should always be a primary concern as you arrive on scene. Make sure that all hazards are addressed and that you follow standard precautions.

Your observations of the scene can also give valuable information regarding what might have happened. Check bureau tops, bedside tables, and medicine cabinets for medications that might give a clue as to the patient's underlying illness. Check the refrigerator for insulin **Figure 6**. Bring any medication bottles along with the patient to the hospital. They can help pinpoint the patient's underlying medical problems and identify his or her physician, who should be able to provide more information.

Primary Assessment

The primary assessment begins with the basics: airway, breathing, and circulation. Patients experiencing an endocrine emergency may be in serious distress, so it is essential that you identify and manage any life threats immediately. In patients with an altered mental status, check for a medical identification bracelet or necklace that may list allergies or known conditions.

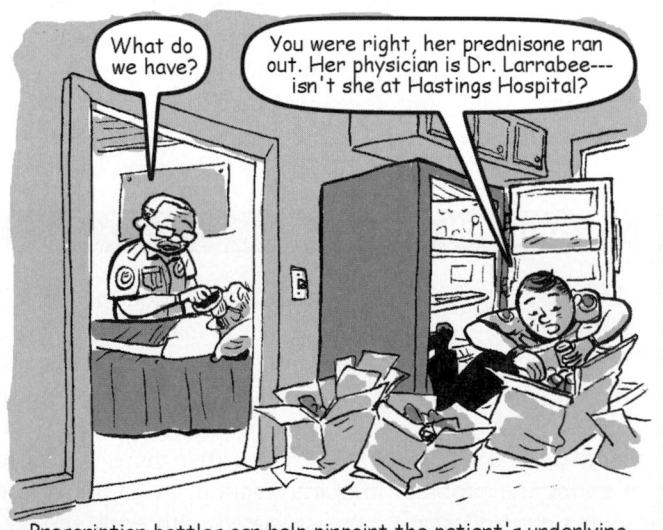

Prescription bottles can help pinpoint the patient's underlying medical problems and identify his or her physician.

Figure 6

Form a General Impression

As you approach the patient on initial contact, you form a general impression. How does the patient look? Does he or she have normal skin color and appearance, make eye contact, and answer questions appropriately without any difficulty speaking? Regardless of the patient's condition or the cause, airway, breathing, and circulation must always be assessed first.

Endocrine diseases present with signs and symptoms that are dependent on the hormone production or secretion that is affected. The patient's position may give you clues as to the severity of his or her condition. Is the patient alert or is there a change in the normal mental status? An unresponsive patient is obviously in a critical state and may be experiencing an endocrine crisis, such as hypoglycemia, hyperglycemia, or a myxedema coma with severe thyroid deficiency. Diaphoresis is usually a sign of severe distress and is present in thyrotoxicosis, along with pulmonary edema.

Your general impression can assist you in initiating the process of forming a field impression. A "buffalo hump," "moon face," and acne are telltale signs of Cushing disease. Mottled skin may be associated with pancreatitis. Enlarged or abnormal body parts may occur with conditions such as edema with syndrome of inappropriate antidiuretic hormone (SIADH) or anasarca with myxedema coma. Underweight or overweight patients may indicate an endocrine dysfunction such as hypothyroidism, hyperthyroidism, or diabetes. Exophthalmos is present in Graves disease, which causes hyperthyroidism. Children with panhypopituitarism may have abnormal development.

Your general impression combined with a thorough physical assessment and patient history is essential in helping you to identify the causes of your patient's distress.

Airway and Breathing

Check the patient's airway to ensure that it is patent. Any abnormal sounds associated with breathing should be investigated for obstructions. When patients present with an altered level of consciousness, they may be unable to protect their airway. Many will be very ill and have chronic episodes of vomiting. Maintain the airway as needed through patient positioning, suctioning, or basic airways.

Patients with endocrine emergencies may present with a variety of breathing levels. You should immediately assess the patient's effort of breathing. Breathing should be effortless. A rate of greater than 24 breaths/min or less than 8 breaths/min indicates that oxygen administration is necessary, such as with a nasal cannula or nonrebreathing mask. Supplemental oxygen is recommended in all cases of suspected respiratory involvement. Although pulse oximetry is commonly used, do not let a normal reading persuade you to withhold oxygen.

Circulation

Assess the patient's skin color, moisture, and temperature, and obtain the patient's blood pressure. Skin condition can assist you in determining the patient's medical status. A patient with pale, cool, moist skin may be in shock or have hypoglycemia, whereas a patient with hot, dry skin may have a fever or hyperglycemia. A patient in hypoglycemic crisis will have a rapid, weak pulse. Because endocrine emergencies may affect the body's compensating systems, IV administration or blood component replenishment may be necessary. Follow your local protocols.

Transport Decision

Many patients with endocrine disorders are being treated by specialists, and they should be transported to a facility that specializes in these conditions. If the patient's condition is unstable or shows signs of becoming unstable, such as a diminished level of consciousness, transport the patient rapidly to the closest facility for stabilization first.

Documentation and Communication

Communication with hospital staff is important for continuity of care. Hospital personnel need to be informed about the patient's history, the present situation, assessment findings, and your interventions and the results. Your run report is the only legal document you have to say that appropriate care was provided. Document clearly your assessment findings as the basis for your treatment. Patients who refuse transport because you "cured" them with oral glucose may require even more thorough documentation. Follow your local protocols for patients who refuse treatment or transport.

History Taking

In diabetic emergencies in particular, the family history can provide important information. Because diabetes is a genetic disease (passed down through family members), learning that a parent or grandparent has a history of diabetes is a major clue and may prove to be invaluable in your treatment decision. This is especially true if the patient is a child and has a new onset of altered mental status.

Investigate the chief complaint or the history of the present illness. While you are assessing the chief complaint, you should consider the patient's signs and symptoms and any pertinent negatives.

If a patient is unresponsive, obtain a blood glucose level and manage any abnormalities appropriately. Do not assume that because a patient does not have a history of diabetes he or she does not have a new onset of the disease.

Follow the SAMPLE mnemonic. Gather as much information as possible from the scene and any family members or bystanders present.

Observe the patient for any signs that may assist you in confirming the patient's reported symptoms. Signs and symptoms of endocrine disorders include those mentioned in the general impression section, as well as many symptoms such as polyphagia, polyuria, and polydipsia in patients with undiagnosed or poorly managed diabetes. Tachycardias, PVCS, PACs, and atrial dysrhythmias may all occur with hyperthyroidism and thyrotoxicosis.

It is essential to ascertain any allergies the patient may have prior to medication administration. Document all medications the patient is currently taking on a regular basis and whether the patient has been compliant with the regimen. Medications are often a clue to already diagnosed conditions. Is the patient taking medications associated with diabetes (such as insulin)? Or, is the patient undergoing thyroid hormone replacement therapy for hypothyroidism or using glucocorticoids to manage Cushing disease?

Pertinent past medical history is very significant when diagnosing and managing the patient with an endocrine condition. Many conditions have been diagnosed prior to your arrival and the patient may have a significant amount of information regarding his or her condition. Family members are also often well versed in these conditions.

In addition to inquiring about last oral intake, ask females of childbearing age about their last menstrual period (LMP). This

---

YOU are the Medic   PART 2

As you introduce yourself and ask him what is wrong, you see he has chocolate all over his mouth and an ice cream sandwich melting in his hand. He does not respond to you until you pinch the back of his hand. He then pushes your hand away.

Recording Time: 0 Minutes	
Appearance	Sitting upright with a blank stare
Level of consciousness	P (responsive to painful stimulus)
Airway	Open
Breathing	Adequate chest rise and volume
Circulation	Weak, rapid radial pulse

3. Although the patient is cooperative, what do you need to consider when you treat any patient with an altered mental status?

4. What could be the cause of his reported shaking?

information may be significant, for example, for patients with hypothyroidism who may have a history of light or absent periods.

The patient, family members, or bystanders may be able to give additional information regarding anything that may have happened prior to the current situation. For example, a diabetic patient may not have eaten that day or may have been under a high level of emotional stress or physical activity.

Secondary Assessment

Begin the physical examination by observing the patient's general appearance and the position in which he or she is found. Patients found in awkward positions often have brainstem damage; conversely, a natural posture tends to be a good sign. Decorticate or decerebrate posturing should also be noted, if present; both are signs of serious illness.

Your physical examination should be geared toward identifying as many atypical findings as possible. Unless the patient had an endocrine emergency that caused some form of trauma, a focused assessment is usually not necessary. In this situation, a comprehensive full-body scan is more appropriate, although life threats should always be managed first.

The physical exam will reveal the finer abnormalities that will help determine your treatment. For example, the condition of the patient's skin provides important information. Cold, clammy skin is a classic sign of shock but may also signal severe hypoglycemia, as from an insulin reaction and the body's response to catecholamine release. Cold, dry skin may indicate an overdose of sedative drugs or alcohol intoxication. Hot, dry skin suggests hyperglycemia, fever, or possibly heat stroke.

The goals of the physical examination in the comatose patient are twofold. First, you want to determine the patient's level of consciousness with precision so that later assessments can readily determine whether the patient's condition is improving or deteriorating. Second, you should look for signs that might provide clues to the source of coma.

When you check the patient's vital signs, look for the combination of hypertension and bradycardia, which suggests increased intracranial pressure. Be alert for abnormal respiratory patterns. Cheyne-Stokes breathing usually points to a nonneurologic source of the coma. Kussmaul respirations are often present in patients experiencing a diabetic ketoacidosis (DKA) event. It is one of the body's compensatory mechanisms to "blow off" excess acid that is produced in this condition.

More worrisome are other abnormal breathing patterns, such as central neurogenic ventilation or huffing and puffing that do not seem to move much air. Look for pararespiratory motions, such as sneezing and yawning. An intact brainstem is required to produce a sneeze or a yawn, so both of those actions have positive prognostic significance. Hiccupping and coughing, by contrast, may indicate brainstem damage.

Reassessment

Once you have initiated your treatment plan, continually reassess the patient to check for obvious and subtle changes. For every action you take, there should be a response. No response *is* a response. Critical patients should be reassessed at least every 5 minutes, whereas noncritical patients may be reassessed every 15 minutes. Document your findings along the way.

YOU *are the Medic*   PART 3

Your protocol requires obtaining a blood glucose reading for any patient with a decreased level of consciousness. You find this patient's blood glucose level is 30 mg/dL. Your partner attempts to apply a nonrebreathing mask but the patient fights it, so your partner applies 6 L/min of oxygen via nasal cannula instead. You obtain IV access and prepare to administer dextrose 50%. A bystander comes up to you and says, "Is he going to be okay? When another shopper and I found him there, I called 9-1-1. An older lady said he was probably diabetic, so she tried to shove ice cream in his mouth, but it didn't seem to help."

Recording Time: 5 Minutes	
Respirations	24 breaths/min
Pulse	100 beats/min, weak, and regular
Skin	Cool, pale, and diaphoretic
Blood pressure	160/94 mm Hg
Oxygen saturation (Spo$_2$)	97% on room air
Pupils	PEARRL

5. **What concerns you about the bystander's statement?**

6. **If your partner was unable to obtain IV access, what additional treatment options exist for correcting the patient's blood glucose level?**

Management of the ABCs should have been carried out during the primary assessment. Remember that a patient whose gag reflex is absent cannot protect his or her own airway from aspiration. You should be prepared to suction the airway. If the patient does not regain consciousness with treatment (eg, a hypoglycemic patient receives glucose and remains unresponsive), intubation should be considered. If breathing is abnormally slow or shallow, assist breathing with bag-mask ventilation. Give supplemental oxygen whether the patient is breathing spontaneously or being ventilated. Be sure to obtain blood specimens early in patients with diabetes, because any administration of prehospital dextrose or other medications will significantly change the chemical makeup of subsequent blood samples.

If the patient has an altered mental status, establish an IV with 0.9% NS or a saline lock. Make an immediate determination of the blood glucose level and initiate treatment if the reading is less than 60 mg/dL. Give 12.5 g to 25 g of D_{50} (50 g of dextrose in every 100 mL); this dose will reverse most cases of hypoglycemia.

If the patient's condition does not improve after a dose of D_{50} and if you have a reason to suspect a narcotics overdose (pinpoint pupils, needle tracks on the arms, depressed respirations), consider administering naloxone (Narcan).

An important aspect of patient care is to address the patient's emotional needs. Diabetes can be a stressful condition to manage, and diabetics have an increased risk of depression. Be empathetic and responsive to the patient's needs and provide emotional support as needed.

Monitor the cardiac rhythm of every comatose patient. During neurologic assessment, the most important consideration is not a single measurement at a single point in time but rather the *trend* shown by several measurements. Recheck the patient's vital signs, pupils, and level of consciousness (every 5 minutes in unstable patients and every 15 minutes in stable patients) and *record your findings* immediately. Every patient you transport should have at least two sets of vital signs documented regardless of the length of the transport.

Documentation is an important part of your job. The record you write is a legal document and becomes a permanent part of the patient's medical record. It is important that you document accurately and thoroughly to ensure the appropriate continuity of care and to protect yourself in the event of a future court case.

Emergency Medical Care

Transport the comatose patient *supine* with a cervical collar in place if the patient is intubated to decrease the risk of unintentional extubation during transport; otherwise, you may transport the patient in the stable side position (unless injuries preclude that position). If there are indications of increasing intracranial pressure such as Cushing triad, posturing, or unequal pupils, transport with the head elevated to 30° to 45° and the head midline to assist in venous return and minimize intracranial pressure. Always keep the mouth and pharynx suctioned free of secretions, vomitus, and blood.

Pathophysiology, Assessment, and Management of Glucose Metabolic Derangements

Endocrine disorders are caused by either hypersecretion or insufficient secretion of a gland. Hypersecretion presents as overactivity of the target organ regulated by the gland. Insufficient secretion results in underactivity of the organ controlled by the gland. Glucose metabolic derangements, or disorders, are caused by dysfunction of the pancreas, which impairs the body's ability to metabolize glucose.

The effects of a disturbance of endocrine gland function are determined by the degree of dysfunction of the gland and by the age and sex of the patient. Pancreatic dysfunction may range from barely detectable to extreme. Most glucose derangements and other clinically significant endocrine emergencies result in compromise of the ABCs, improper fluid balance, deteriorating mental status, and abnormal vital signs and blood glucose levels.

Diabetes Mellitus

Medically, the term *diabetes* refers to a metabolic disorder in which the body's ability to metabolize simple carbohydrates (glucose) is impaired. It is characterized by the following:

- Polyphagia, an increased appetite caused by the inability of glucose to be transported across the cell membrane.
- Polydipsia, a significant thirst caused by dehydration brought about by an increase in diuresis
- Polyuria, the passage of large quantities of urine containing glucose. Excess glucose is excreted and attracts water, resulting in excessive diuresis.

Glucose (also known as *dextrose*) is one of the basic sugars in the body and, along with oxygen, is the primary fuel for cellular metabolism.

Insulin, a hormone produced by the islets of Langerhans in the pancreas, assists in the metabolism of carbohydrates and the transport of glucose into the cells. Diabetes is a pathologic condition in which there is a flaw in the production or function of insulin, or both.

Diabetes mellitus is characterized by the body's inability to sufficiently metabolize glucose. *Mellitus*, from the Greek word for honeybee, means "sweet"—a reference to the presence of glucose in the urine. In people with this disease, the pancreas does not produce enough insulin or the body's cells do not respond to the effects of the insulin that is produced. In either case, the result is the same: an elevated level of glucose in the blood and glucose in the urine. Glucose builds up in the blood, overflows into the urine, and flows out of the body. Thus cells can starve even when the blood contains large amounts of glucose **Figure 7**.

The National Institute of Diabetes and Digestive and Kidney Diseases (NIDDK) estimates that the total prevalence of diabetes in the United States in 2010 was 25.8 million people (8.3% of the population). Of those, 18.8 million people have

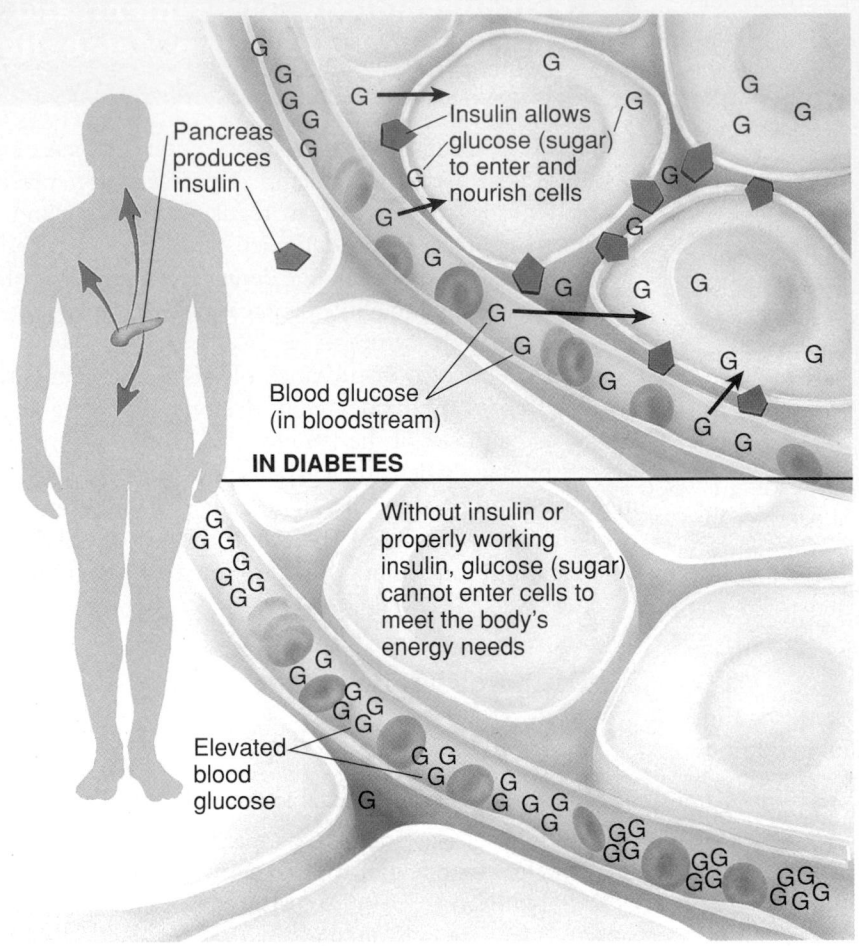

Pancreas produces insulin

Insulin allows glucose (sugar) to enter and nourish cells

Blood glucose (in bloodstream)

IN DIABETES

Without insulin or properly working insulin, glucose (sugar) cannot enter cells to meet the body's energy needs

Elevated blood glucose

Figure 7 Diabetes is defined as a lack of or ineffective action of insulin. Without insulin, cells begin to "starve" because insulin is needed to allow glucose to enter and nourish the cells.

been diagnosed with the disease, and the other 7 million have diabetes but do not yet know it **Figure 8**.

As these statistics reveal, diabetes is thought to be under-diagnosed, according to the NIDDK. In 2007, diabetes was the seventh leading cause of death in the United States. The disease is responsible for a myriad of life-altering complications, a few of which are listed below:

- **Kidneys.** Diabetes is the principal cause of kidney failure, accounting for 44% of new cases in 2008. The glomeruli of the kidney become sclerotic, causing **necrosis** of the papillary tissue and leading to nephropathy (end-stage renal disease) and renal failure. High levels of glucose in the blood cause the kidneys to work harder than normal and may result in decreased kidney function over a period of time.
- **Heart.** Adults with diabetes are two to four times more likely to die of heart disease or to have a stroke than those who do not have diabetes. When diabetes is poorly controlled, the process of **lipolysis** (from *lipo-*, meaning "fat," and *-lysis*, meaning "breakdown") raises the level of fat in the blood. As a result of this **dyslipidemia**, the risk of atherosclerosis and coronary artery disease

increases. The fat circulating through the bloodstream adheres to the vessel walls, eventually causing them to be stiff and brittle. In addition, glucose crystals are sharp and frequent elevation in blood glucose levels also damages vessels. The microscopic deterioration of the vessel walls, called **microangiopathy**, is a condition in which swelling of basement membrane cells restricts the flow of blood to organs and tissues. Inadequate blood flow, called **ischemia**, causes necrosis, or tissue death. Chronic heart failure develops over a period of several years and is twice as prevalent among people with diabetes than among those without the disease. Finally, central nerve damage can cause cardiac dysrhythmias.

- **Cerebrovascular disease, stroke, and hypertension.** Vessels damaged by microangiopathy characterize cerebrovascular disease and are associated with an increased incidence of stroke. Peripheral artery disease is also common in persons with diabetes and impairs circulation to the lower extremities. Hypertension is present in two out of three persons with diabetes. Hypertension is associated with an increased risk of heart disease, stroke, kidney disease, and blindness.
- **Eyes.** In adults ages 20 to 74 years, diabetes is the chief cause of new cases of blindness as a result of retinopathy. High glucose levels in the blood damage the vessels of the eye, causing swelling, wall weakness, and obstruction. Scar tissue may form that pulls the retina from the eye or retinal detachment. Cataracts are a cloudy film that forms when fructose and sorbitol are deposited in the lens of the eye.
- **Neuropathy.** Neuropathy is nerve damage that results in a loss of sensation and function in the area innervated by the affected nerves. The damage can cause sexual impotence, neurogenic bladder, constipation, or diarrhea. Neuropathy associated with diabetes often affects peripheral nerves, causing diminished sensation and function in the extremities. Persons with peripheral neuropathy often have paresthesia, a pinprick sensation in the hands, feet, arms, or legs. Paresthesia and dysesthesia—the absence of sensation—can blunt pain perception, making it possible for foot ulcers to go unnoticed until they become seriously infected. Because many of these persons also have poor circulation in the extremities, gangrene may develop in adjacent tissues and infection may spread to the bone. In fact, more than 60% of nontraumatic lower limb amputations can be attributed to diabetes.

Because of the impact diabetes has on all systems of the body, any preexisting condition will be more complex to

Estimated number of new cases of diagnosed
diabetes among people ages 20 years or older,
by age group, United States, 2010

About 1.9 million people ages 20 years or older
were newly diagnosed with diabetes in 2010.

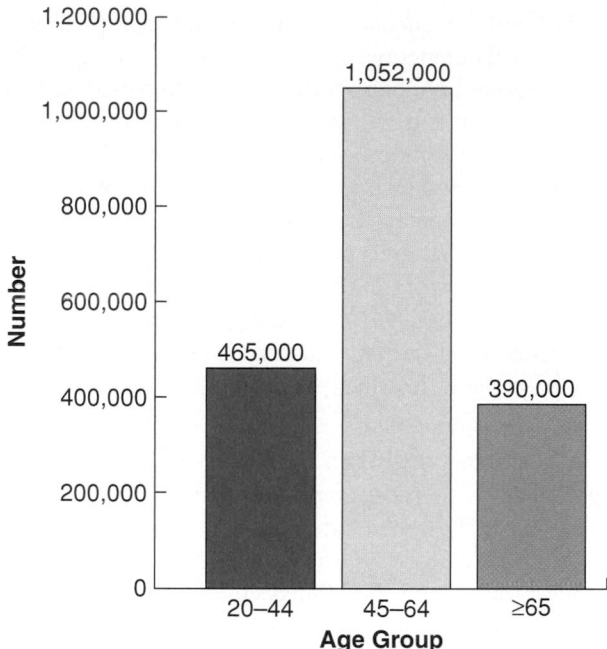

Figure 8 Incidence of diabetes in the United States, 2010.
Numbers shown are the number of new diagnoses of diabetes
in the United States among people ages 20 and older (approximately 1.9 million were newly diagnosed in 2010).

Source: 2007-2009 National Health Interview Survey estimates projected to
the year 2010.

Special Populations

You might encounter an older patient who has undiagnosed
diabetes. These patients report that they have not been feeling well for a while but have not seen a physician. A patient
with undiagnosed diabetes or one who is in denial or ignores
the advice of his or her physician may call 9-1-1 when the
signs and symptoms get worse. Nonhealing wounds, blindness, renal failure, and other complications are associated
with poorly controlled or uncontrolled diabetes. It is important that you recognize the signs and symptoms of diabetes
because you might be the first health care provider to suggest medical treatment to an older adult patient who might
otherwise ignore the condition.

Elderly patients and those with diabetes commonly present atypically with an acute myocardial infarction. They
often do not present with chest pain or pressure because of
the neuropathy associated with increasing age and diabetes. Elderly patients also generally have a higher tolerance
for pain compared with younger patients. Other causes of
an altered perception of pain may include impaired cognition or slowed nerve conduction. You should maintain a
high index of suspicion when these populations experience
a syncopal episode, fatigue, shortness of breath, or nausea
and diaphoresis.

Elderly patients are also more susceptible to dehydration
and infections. As we age, our bodies tend to lose approximately 10% of the total body fluid. Elderly patients may not
become thirsty or react to thirst until they are very dehydrated. Medications may also cause an increase in diuresis,
compounding the problem.

---

manage. The more compliant patients are with the management
of their diabetes, the better the outcome of other conditions.
Conditions that develop subsequent to the onset of diabetes
will respond more effectively with appropriate diabetes management as well. Many conditions associated with the presence of
diabetes can be delayed or prevented with appropriate lifestyle
changes and continued management of diabetes.

Any kind of distress can also have an impact on the patient
and result in a 9-1-1 call because blood glucose levels are more
difficult to control when there is an increase in physical activity
or emotional stress.

In addition to this human toll, the direct and indirect economic costs of diabetes continue to escalate. It is estimated
that in 2007, diabetes cost the nation about $174 billion. This
figure reflects the indirect costs associated with disability, lost
productivity, and premature mortality, as well as the direct
costs of managing the complex health problems associated
with diabetes.

Chronic as well as acute complications are associated
with diabetes mellitus. Although these complications are present in both forms of the disease, they have a tendency to be
more severe in people with diabetes who require insulin. Left

untreated, diabetes leads to organ system dysfunction, wasting
of body tissues, and death. Even with excellent medical care,
some patients with particularly aggressive forms of diabetes
will die relatively young from complications of the disease. The
severity of diabetic complications correlates with the average
blood glucose level and with the age of onset. Although most
patients with well-controlled diabetes have a normal life span,
they must be willing to adjust their lives to the demands of the
disease, especially their eating habits and physical activity. There
is no cure for the disease, so treatment focuses on maintaining
the level of blood glucose within the normal range.

Two forms of diabetes mellitus exist: type 1 and type 2. The
terms "juvenile-onset" and "adult-onset" diabetes have been
replaced by type 1 and type 2 diabetes. The age of onset of the
patient's symptoms is less important than whether the patient
requires insulin to survive. Both types are serious conditions
that affect many tissues and functions other than the glucose-
regulating mechanism, and both require life-long medical management.

Type 1 Diabetes Mellitus

Pathophysiology Type 1 diabetes has historically been referred
to as insulin-dependent diabetes mellitus, IDDM, or juvenile
diabetes because it generally affects children. Although type 1
diabetes has a hereditary predisposition, it is now believed that
environmental factors may be part of the cause—for example, an
infection that triggers an autoimmune disorder (ie, antibodies

destroy the islets of Langerhans). In type 1 diabetes the beta cells in the islets of Langerhans have been destroyed and no longer produce insulin. Because these cells are the only source of insulin, the insulin must then be administered by injection or pump.

In type 1 diabetes, the endocrine system of most patients does not produce any insulin. These patients require daily injections of supplementary, synthetic insulin throughout their lives to control their levels of blood glucose. In addition to daily insulin injections, strict dietary control must be observed; this can be difficult with young children. Increased activity and alcohol consumption can lead to low blood glucose levels (alcohol depletes glycogen stores in the liver). In adults with type 1 diabetes, therefore, alcohol consumption must also be controlled.

Assessment Assessment of a patient with a history of diabetes will be much the same as your assessment of any other medical patient; however, there are some considerations you will want to keep in mind. Determine whether the patient is compliant with the management of the disease.

If the patient has an altered mental status, suspect a low blood glucose level **Figure 9**. Hypoglycemia is a potentially life-threatening event. Patients with diabetes also may potentially have additional chronic conditions such as renal failure, congestive heart failure, CAD, hypertension, and vision and hearing impairment. Because patients may have an altered perception of pain, particularly in their extremities, it is important to assess for any signs of sores or infections. It is also important to ask about tingling, numbness, or swelling of the extremities. Patients with long-standing diabetes may have an amputated limb that may become infected or septic.

Ask the patient about any vision changes, headaches, dizziness, bleeding, or sores in the mouth. Also ask whether there has been a recent change in the patient's bowel or eating habits.

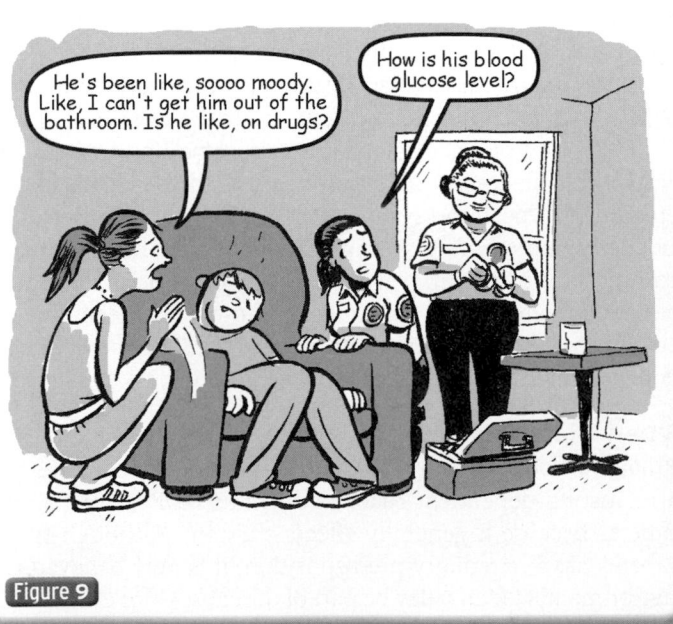

Figure 9

Management You will likely encounter patients with diabetes who use insulin pumps to treat their disease. These small devices consist of an infusion set, a reservoir for insulin, and the pump itself. A promising alternative to multiple daily injections of insulin, insulin pumps provide improved control of blood glucose levels for many patients.

Type 1 diabetes always requires the use of insulin that is administered by injection or an insulin pump, also called continuous subcutaneous insulin infusion therapy. Insulin cannot be ingested orally because the digestive process will render it inactive. An insulin pump replaces the need for multiple daily injections. It is more accurate in regulating blood glucose levels and is reported to improve quality of life. Except in persons with type 1 diabetes, the body produces insulin. Currently, there are several different types of insulin available in the United States: rapid-acting insulin, regular or short-acting insulin, intermediate-acting insulin, and long-acting insulin. Insulin differs in its onset of action, duration, and peak time. All of these types of insulin are synthetic; however, animal insulin can be imported.

Type 2 Diabetes Mellitus

Pathophysiology The most common form of diabetes is <u>type 2 diabetes</u> (formerly called adult-onset diabetes), a condition in which blood glucose levels are elevated. About 90% of all people with diabetes in the United States have type 2 diabetes, which typically develops later in life, usually when the patient is middle-aged, although the disease is becoming more common in younger people. Type 2 diabetes may be related to *metabolic syndrome*, a cluster of characteristics including excessive fat in the abdominal area, elevated blood pressure, and high levels of blood lipids. Risk factors for developing metabolic syndrome include excess weight, lack of physical activity, and genetic factors.

In many people with type 2 diabetes, the pancreas actually produces enough insulin; however, for reasons not fully understood, the body cannot effectively use it. This condition is known as <u>insulin resistance</u>. One possible explanation is that the insulin receptor cells located on the target cells have changed in some way and are no longer able to receive the insulin when it arrives at the target cell. Type 2 diabetes can also be caused by a deficiency in insulin production.

Assessment Symptoms of type 2 diabetes may include the following:

- Fatigue
- Nausea
- Frequent urination
- Thirst
- Unexplained weight loss
- Blurred vision
- Frequent infections and slow healing of wounds
- Being cranky, confused, or shaky
- Unresponsiveness
- Seizure

These symptoms tend to develop gradually and usually become noticeable in middle age. In fact, the onset of type 2 diabetes may be so insidious that patients may not realize they have the disease. In some instances, the symptoms can develop over several years in overweight adults older than 40 years. A small percentage of persons do not display any symptoms.

Words of Wisdom

New-onset weakness in a patient known to have diabetes must be considered a myocardial infarction until proven otherwise. Many patients with type 1 and type 2 diabetes have an acquired dysfunction in the peripheral nervous system (neuropathy). Also, increased insulin levels result in increased blood lipid levels. This combination often leads to an earlier onset of coronary artery disease. People with diabetes do not always have typical clinical symptoms of acute coronary syndrome because of an alteration in sensation. They are more likely to present with general body weakness.

Management Weight loss is an important factor in helping to control type 2 diabetes. Exercise and a well-balanced, nutritious diet are key components in combating the complications of diabetes. To maintain glucose levels within the normal range, food intake must be spread throughout the day in coordination with daily medications/insulin injections. You can help patients by reinforcing this message to the patient and by helping the family understand how to reduce the patient's risk of diabetic complications.

Oral medications used to manage type 2 diabetes may be used alone or in combination because they exhibit different mechanisms of action. As with all medications, there is always the risk of interaction with other medications. A physician or pharmacist should be consulted prior to the addition of any medication, whether over the counter or prescription. These oral medications can be divided into six classes, as shown in Table 5 .

Gestational Diabetes

Pathophysiology

Gestational diabetes is a form of glucose intolerance that occurs during pregnancy. This condition has been identified more often in African American, Hispanic/Latino, and Native American populations, as well as in women who are obese or with a family history of diabetes. Women who experience gestational diabetes during pregnancy have an increased risk of 40% to 60% of type 2 diabetes within a decade. For most women, gestational diabetes will resolve before delivery. In a few women, however, diabetes will not resolve or type 2 diabetes will develop.

Gestational diabetes is usually diagnosed at 28 weeks of gestation or later in the third trimester of pregnancy. It is thought that hormones produced by the placenta during pregnancy impede the function of insulin. Because this condition does not occur until later in pregnancy, it does not produce birth defects

Table 5 Oral Agents Used to Treat Type 2 Diabetes Mellitus

Medication Class	Function	Examples
Sulfonylureas	Stimulate beta cells to produce more insulin	Chlorpropamide (Diabinese) Glipizide (Glucotrol and Glucotrol XL) Glyburide (Micronase, Glynase, and DiaBeta) Glimepiride (Amaryl)
Meglitinides	Stimulate beta cells to produce more insulin	Repaglinide (Prandin) Nateglinide (Starlix)
Biguanides	Decrease the amount of glucose produced by the liver	Metformin (Glucophage)
Thiazolidinediones	Increase insulin effectiveness in the muscle and decrease liver glucose production	Rosiglitazone (Avandia) Pioglitazone (ACTOS)
Alpha-glucosidase inhibitors	Prevent the breakdown of starches	Acarbose (Precose) Miglitol (Glyset)
DPP-4 inhibitors	Inhibit the breakdown of GLP-1, a naturally occurring compound in the body that reduces blood glucose levels	Sitagliptin (Januvia) Saxagliptin (Onglyza)

but it often results in macrosomia, or a large baby. These infants are at higher risk for obesity and diabetes in their lifetime.

Assessment

Blood glucose crosses the placental barrier. When a pregnant woman is hyperglycemic, high levels of glucose enter the fetus, causing an increased production of insulin by the fetus to normalize blood glucose levels. The extra glucose is converted into fat, and women experiencing gestational diabetes often deliver large babies and may encounter difficult deliveries. Often cesarean sections are required.

Management

Management should be initiated as soon as possible to stabilize blood glucose levels and minimize potential complications to both mother and baby. Management includes diet modification, exercise, and blood glucose testing. Insulin injections may be required.

Hypoglycemia

Pathophysiology

Hypoglycemia in persons with insulin-dependent diabetes often is the result of having taken too much insulin, too little food, or both. The tissues of the central nervous system (including the brain), unlike other tissues that can usually metabolize fat or protein in addition to sugar, depend entirely on glucose as their source of energy. If the level of glucose in the blood drops dramatically, the brain is literally starved.

Assessment

The patient will tremble, have a rapid pulse rate, sweat, and feel hungry. These symptoms reflect the disordered function of hungry brain cells and the alarm reaction (sympathetic nervous system discharge) set off by the brain's distress signals. If hypoglycemia persists, cerebral dysfunction progresses quickly to permanent brain damage. Additional signs and symptoms associated with hypoglycemia include headache, mental confusion, memory loss, incoordination, slurred speech, irritability, dilated pupils, and seizures and coma in severe cases.

Normal blood glucose levels range from approximately 70 to 120 mg/dL; hypoglycemia occurs when blood glucose levels drop to 45 mg/dL or less. Hypoglycemia develops *very rapidly*, from minutes to a few hours and should be suspected in any patient with diabetes who presents with bizarre behavior, neurologic signs, or coma. Often the hypoglycemic patient appears intoxicated because of slurred speech and lack of coordination and may be paranoid, hostile, and aggressive.

Of course, people with diabetes are not the only persons who are prone to episodes of hypoglycemia. Patients with alcoholism, patients who have ingested certain poisons or overdosed with certain drugs (notably aspirin), and patients with certain cancers, liver disease, kidney disease, and some other conditions may also experience hypoglycemic episodes. Do not discount the possibility of hypoglycemia in a comatose patient just because the patient is not known to have diabetes. Conversely, do not let a known diagnosis of diabetes prevent you from considering other causes of coma. Persons with diabetes may also experience head injury, stroke, seizures, meningitis, and other traumatic injuries or conditions. Keep an open mind and assess the patient thoroughly.

Management

Whenever you suspect hypoglycemia, treat it *immediately*: Permanent cerebral damage may ensue if blood glucose levels are not rapidly restored. Measure the patient's blood glucose level, especially if you are treating an older adult or a patient whose clinical history suggests that the problem may be stroke—administration

Words of Wisdom

The longer a patient remains unconscious from hypoglycemia, the more likely there will be permanent brain damage! If more than 20 to 30 minutes go by, toxic compounds (free radicals) in the brain are produced that can cause permanent neuronal damage.

YOU are the Medic   PART 4

As you administer dextrose, you notice the patient begin to look around. After a few minutes he says, "Oh! That one snuck up on me!" He tells you that he is an insulin-dependent diabetic, and he felt his blood glucose level dropping. He tried to open his package of glucose tablets, and that was the last thing he remembers. You assist him up out of the refrigerator case and reassess his vital signs, including his blood glucose level. His blood glucose level is now 120 mg/dL.

The patient's 21-year-old son arrives. The patient tells you, "Thanks very much. I'll be fine now." After discussing the case with medical control and receiving their agreement to leave the patient with his son, you inform dispatch the patient refused further treatment and transport and your medic unit is available for calls. You assist your patient to the food court where he orders a hamburger and fries.

Recording Time: 10 Minutes	
Respirations	20 breaths/min; regular
Pulse	90 beats/min, regular
Skin	Slightly cool, pale, diaphoretic
Blood pressure	156/92 mm Hg
Oxygen saturation (Spo₂)	98% on room air
Pupils	PEARRL

7. What challenges often occur on calls such as this one?

8. How would you document this patient contact?

of concentrated glucose solutions in a suspected stroke situation may exacerbate cerebral damage **Figure 10**. When the comatose patient is older than 55 years or the family gives a history of recent transient ischemic attacks, perform a field glucose test to rule out hypoglycemia. A field glucose test involves obtaining a small amount of blood and using a blood glucose monitor to determine the patient's blood glucose level.

1. Clean the site to be punctured with alcohol.
2. Allow the patient's arm to hang briefly to allow blood to flow to the fingertips.
3. Grasp the finger near the area to be pricked (the side of the finger is less painful to prick than the top) and squeeze for 3 seconds.
4. Use the lancet device quickly and apply adequate pressure to puncture the skin.
5. Keep the hand down, prick the side of the fingertip, and squeeze gently until you obtain a drop of blood. Be careful not to squeeze too hard.
6. Apply the blood to the test strips according to the manufacturer's instructions.

Words of Wisdom

If you are uncertain of a patient's blood glucose level, always err on the "low side" and assume that hypoglycemia is present. A period of hypoglycemia is more dangerous to the patient than an equivalent period of hyperglycemia.

If the patient is alert, able to swallow, and has an intact gag reflex, administer sugar by mouth. Provide a candy bar, a glass of warm water to which a few teaspoons of sugar have been added, a nondiet cola drink—any of those should improve the patient's condition. Do *not* give anything by mouth to a patient whose level of consciousness is depressed!

If the patient is in a coma, treat him or her as you would any other comatose patient, with attention to the airway and supplemental oxygen. Do not use an advanced airway (ie, endotracheal tube, King LT, Combitube, laryngeal mask airway) until you have given the patient D_{50} (50% dextrose); if the patient awakens in response to the D_{50}, the endotracheal tube will be pulled out immediately by the patient!

Start an IV with a *small-bore catheter* in a *big vein*, and begin a 0.9% normal saline (NS) infusion. Check the IV carefully to confirm that it is patent and flowing freely. Inject a test bolus of 10 to 20 mL of NS infusion fluid, making sure the IV is not prone to infiltration. Recheck its status by lowering the IV bag and looking for backflow of blood into the infusion set. D_{50} is both hypertonic and acidic and can cause serious damage if it infiltrates out of the vein and enters the surrounding tissue.

If you are certain the IV is reliable, administer 12.5 to 25 g of D_{50} *slowly*, over at least 3 minutes. To ensure the patency of the line, draw back on the D_{50} syringe to observe a blood return. If the cause of coma is hypoglycemia, the patient will often awaken rapidly—although in cases of severe hypoglycemia, another 25 g of D_{50} may be required to restore a normal level of consciousness.

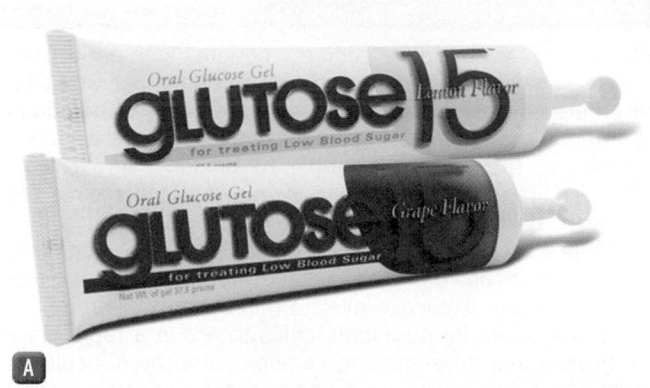

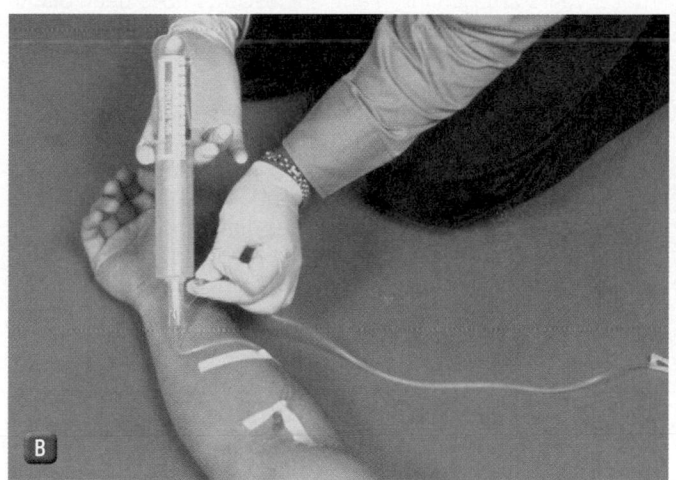

Figure 10 Administering glucose is appropriate in diabetic emergencies unless you have a reliable blood glucose measurement indicating normal or high blood glucose levels. Available forms include oral glucose paste **(A)** and 50% glucose solution for IV administration **(B)**.

If the patient is unresponsive and hypoglycemic and you are unable to obtain appropriate IV access, you should administer glucagon IM. Hypoglycemia is a life-threatening event and glucose administration should not be delayed if an IV line cannot be established. An unresponsive patient should never be given oral glucose or anything by mouth due to the risk of choking and aspiration.

Glucagon increases blood glucose levels and also relaxes smooth muscle located in the gastrointestinal tract if administered parenterally. Patients with type 1 diabetes may not have as great an increase in blood glucose levels as those with stable type 2 diabetes. Therefore, patients with type 1 diabetes require immediate access to oral carbohydrates or additional glucose administration. See the chapter, *Emergency Medication* for more information on glucagon.

Hyperglycemia and Diabetic Ketoacidosis

Pathophysiology

Hyperglycemia (a high blood glucose level) is one of the classic symptoms of diabetes mellitus. Common early signs

Special Populations

When you are caring for pediatric patients with endocrine-related emergencies, it is important to remember that children are not just "small adults." Children and young adults are much more commonly diagnosed with type 1 diabetes; therefore, they are susceptible to diabetic ketoacidosis (DKA), a life-threatening event. Events of hypoglycemia can be particularly damaging to the developing brain.

Children are at varying stages of cognitive development, depending on age and maturity; therefore, consistent maintenance of blood glucose levels within the normal range can be challenging. By definition, children are in a rapid state of growth and development, compounding the difficulty in controlling blood glucose levels. Researchers have found that 2 years after children and adolescents have been diagnosed with diabetes, they have a twofold increased incidence of depression and adjustment issues when compared with their peers.

A low socioeconomic status is associated with an increased incidence of DKA, poor blood glucose control, and lengthier hospital admissions. Children and adolescents have unique needs, and it is essential that the family be involved and supportive to increase compliance.

Additional complications of diabetes in children include cerebral edema associated with DKA, increasing mortality by 20% to 90%. Patients who survive have a 20% to 40% risk of neurologic impairment. Signs and symptoms include an altered mental status, headache, nausea, vomiting, bradycardia, and hypertension. Seizures, changes in pupils, incontinence, and respiratory arrest signal rapid deterioration. These conditions usually present clinically 4 to 12 hours after treatment has been initiated; however, they may occur even prior to treatment. Successful management includes the IV administration of 5 to 10 mL/kg of 3% NaCl over 30 minutes or 0.25 to 1 g/kg of mannitol over 20 minutes. Intubation and ventilation may be necessary, however; hyperventilation should be used with caution or avoided. Neurologic improvement is rapid. Dehydration associated with DKA in the pediatric patient should be managed slowly over 48 hours to diminish the potential for cerebral edema.

In DKA, the deficiency of insulin prevents cells from taking up the extra glucose. The cells are starving, and a distress signal goes out over the sympathetic nervous system, causing the release of various stress hormones. Because the body cannot use glucose, it turns instead to other sources of energy—principally, fat. The metabolism of fat generates *acids* and *ketones* as waste products. (The ketones give the characteristic fruity odor to the breath of a patent in DKA, but not all providers are able to smell this.) Because glucose must be excreted in the urine in solution, the body loses excessive amounts of water and electrolytes (sodium and potassium). This may lead to disturbances in water balance and acid-base balance. Disturbances in acid-base balance and the compensatory role of the kidneys are covered in more detail in the chapter, *Pathophysiology*.

can be caused by excessive food intake, insufficient insulin dosages, infection or illness, injury, surgery, and emotional stress. Reassess the patient frequently for the presence of these underlying causes so that definitive treatment can be given. Onset may be rapid (within minutes) or gradual (hours to days), depending on the cause. For example, excessive food intake may cause blood glucose to rise quickly, whereas an infection or illness will result in hyperglycemia over the course of several days.

If left untreated, hyperglycemia will progress to diabetic ketoacidosis (DKA), which is associated predominately in people with type 1 diabetes. A life-threatening condition, DKA occurs when certain acids accumulate in the body because insulin is not available Figure 11. Common causes of DKA include infection, injury, alcohol use, emotional discord, and illness, such as stroke or myocardial infarction. Patients who have this condition tend to be young—teenagers and young adults.

Meanwhile, glucose continues to accumulate in the blood. As the blood glucose rises, the patient undergoes massive osmotic diuresis (passing large amounts of urine because of the high solute concentration of the blood); this, together with vomiting, causes dehydration and even shock.

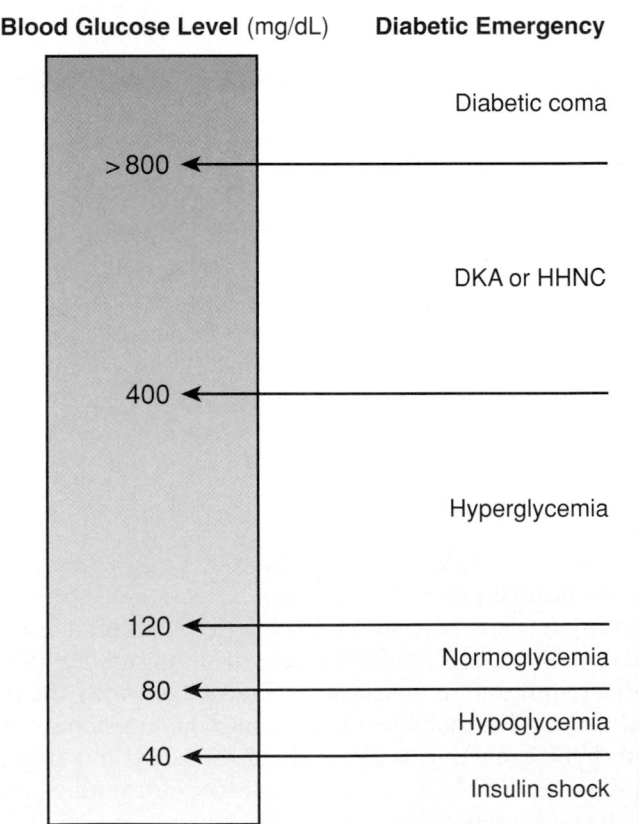

Figure 11 The two most common diabetic emergencies, diabetic ketoacidosis and insulin shock, develop when the patient has too much or too little glucose in the blood, respectively.

include frequent and excessive thirst accompanied by frequent and excessive urination. Hyperglycemia occurs when levels of glucose in the blood exceed the normal range (80 to 120 mg/dL). In patients with diabetes, physicians try to maintain glucose levels at less than 160 mg/dL. Hyperglycemia

Assessment

A hyperglycemic condition without other classic symptoms is not dispositive of a diagnosis of diabetes mellitus, but hyperglycemia is also an independent medical condition with other causes. The signs and symptoms of hypoglycemia and hyperglycemia can be similar (Table 6).

Hyperglycemia usually progresses slowly, over a period of 12 to 48 hours, with the patient's level of consciousness deteriorating only gradually. Patients in DKA are seldom deeply comatose, so if the patient is totally unresponsive, look for another source of the coma, such as head injury, stroke, or drug overdose.

There is no predictable correlation between the increase in a patient's blood glucose level and the degree of ketoacidosis in the blood. Rely on the patient's clinical presentation rather than on test results.

The signs and symptoms of DKA are generally predictable from the underlying pathophysiology:

- Polyuria (excessive urine output), because of osmotic diuresis
- Polydipsia (excessive thirst), because of dehydration
- Polyphagia (excessive eating), probably related to inefficient utilization of nutrients

- Nausea and vomiting, the latter worsening the patient's dehydration
- Tachycardia as a consequence of dehydration
- Deep, rapid respirations (Kussmaul respirations)—the body's attempt to compensate for acidosis by blowing off carbon dioxide
- Warm, dry skin and dry mucous membranes, also reflecting dehydration
- Fruity odor of ketones on the breath
- Abdominal pain, hypotension, and sometimes fever

Management

The treatment of DKA in the field depends on making the correct diagnosis. If the patient's history and physical examination are consistent with DKA and your field measurement of the patient's glucose level reveals that it is markedly elevated (more than 300 mg/dL), the physician will probably order treatment for DKA. The goals of prehospital treatment are to begin rehydration and to correct the patient's electrolyte and acid–base abnormalities. In most instances, specific treatment with insulin should await the patient's arrival at the hospital, where therapy can be closely monitored with laboratory determinations of blood glucose and ketones.

Table 6   Comparison of Hyperglycemia and Hypoglycemia

	Hyperglycemia	Hypoglycemia
History		
Food intake	Excessive	Insufficient
Insulin dosage	Insufficient	Excessive
Onset	Gradual (hours to days)	Rapid, within minutes
Skin	Warm and dry	Pale and moist
Infection	Common	Uncommon
Gastrointestinal tract		
Thirst	Intense	Absent
Hunger	Absent	Intense
Vomiting	Common	Uncommon
Respiratory system		
Breathing	Rapid, deep (Kussmaul respirations)	Normal or rapid
Odor of breath	Sweet, fruity (nailpolish remover/acetone smell)	Normal
Cardiovascular system		
Blood pressure	Normal to low	Low
Pulse	Normal or rapid and full	Rapid, weak
Nervous system		
Consciousness	Restless merging to coma	Irritability, confusion, seizure, or coma
Urine		
Sugar	Present	Absent
Acetone	Present	Absent
Treatment		
Response	Gradual, within 6 to 12 hours following medical treatment	Immediately after administration of glucose

Follow the procedure for any comatose patient with regard to airway maintenance and oxygen. Be particularly alert for *vomiting*, and have suction ready. Start an IV and infuse up to 1 L of NS during the first half hour or at the rate suggested by protocol or online medical control. Remember, a patient in DKA is severely dehydrated, often to the point of shock, and needs volume, usually at a rate of about 1 L/h for at least the first few hours.

Monitor cardiac rhythm. Changes in serum potassium caused by DKA can lead to marked myocardial instability. Note the contour of the T waves on the rhythm strip; if they are sharply peaked, the patient's potassium level may be dangerously high, and you may need to administer sodium bicarbonate. As potassium levels rise, the QRS complex will widen and may blend with the T wave, developing into a <u>sine wave</u> and becoming bradycardic. At this point, management with calcium chloride or gluconate may be indicated to antagonize potassium at the receptor site. If ordered to do so, proceed with caution—even a little too much can cause serious problems or death.

Complications of DKA are frequently associated with its management. The infusion of insulin may lead to hypoglycemia, so blood glucose levels should be monitored continuously. Hypokalemia may result when insulin shifts potassium back into cells, lowering blood serum levels; therefore, management of hyperkalemia should be considered cautiously. Cerebral edema may occur if blood glucose levels shift too rapidly; however, this complication is more prevalent in pediatric patients, particularly newborns and premature infants.

Hyperosmolar Nonketotic Coma

Pathophysiology

<u>Hyperosmolar nonketotic coma (HONK)</u>, also called <u>hyperosmolar hyperglycemic nonketotic coma (HHNC)</u>, is a metabolic derangement that occurs principally in patients with type 2 diabetes. This condition is characterized by hyperglycemia, hyperosmolarity, and an absence of significant ketosis.

Oddly enough, fewer than 10% of patients present in a comatose state. Instead, most patients have severe dehydration and focal or global neurologic deficits. In addition, acute myocardial infarction is frequently associated with HONK/HHNC. The clinical features of HONK/HHNC and DKA tend to overlap and are often observed simultaneously.

HONK/HHNC often develops in patients with diabetes who have some secondary illness that leads to reduced fluid intake.

> **Words of Wisdom**
>
> Certain medications, including diuretics, beta blockers, histamine-2 (H_2) blockers, dialysis, total parenteral nutrition, and dextrose-containing fluids, may contribute to the development of HONK/HHNC by raising serum glucose, inhibiting insulin, or causing dehydration. Hyperglycemia and hyperosmolarity lead to osmotic diuresis and an osmotic shift of fluid to the intravascular space, resulting in further intracellular dehydration.

Although infection (in particular, pneumonia and urinary tract infection) is the most common cause, many other conditions can cause altered mentation or dehydration. In most cases, the secondary illness is not identified.

Assessment

Unlike patients with DKA, patients with HONK/HHNC do not experience ketoacidosis. Although most patients diagnosed with HONK/HHNC have a known history of diabetes (usually type 2), approximately 30% do not have a prior diagnosis of diabetes. The stress response to any acute illness tends to increase hormones that favor elevated glucose levels; cortisol, catecholamines (epinephrine and norepinephrine), glucagon, and many other hormones have effects that tend to counter those of insulin. Various neurologic changes may be found, including drowsiness and lethargy, delirium and coma, focal or generalized seizures, visual disturbances, hemiparesis, and sensory deficits.

Not all patients with increased blood glucose levels have DKA or HONK/HHNC. Many people have glucose intolerance and hyperglycemia with no symptoms. Look at the patient, not at the number.

Management

The treatment of HONK/HHNC in the prehospital setting follows the pathway for dehydration and altered mental status. Airway management is the top priority. The comatose patient is often unable to maintain and protect his or her airway. For this reason, endotracheal intubation may be indicated and should be completed as early as possible. Cervical spine immobilization should be used for all unresponsive patients found lying down, unless witnesses can validate that no fall occurred. Large-bore IV access should be gained as soon as possible, but do not delay transfer while initiating the IV. If necessary, obtain IV access during transport to the emergency department. Also, obtain a blood glucose level as soon as possible.

> **Words of Wisdom**
>
> Although oral corticosteroid therapy is the most common cause of exogenous adrenal suppression, inhaled corticosteroids (used for asthma or chronic obstructive pulmonary disease) may also have a similar effect.

Once you have initiated the IV, a bolus of 500 mL 0.9% NS is appropriate for nearly all adults who are clinically dehydrated. In patients with a history of congestive heart failure and/or renal insufficiency, a 250-mL bolus may be a more appropriate starting point. Fluid deficits in patients with HONK/HHNC may amount to 10 L or more. These patients may receive 1 to 2 L within the first hour. If the glucose level is less than 60 to 80 mg/dL, then (depending on your local protocols), administer 12.5 to 25 g of D_{50} as soon as possible.

Pathophysiology, Assessment, and Management of Other Disorders of the Pancreas

Pancreatitis

Pathophysiology

Pancreatitis is an inflammation of the pancreas, can occur as either an acute or a chronic condition, and is more common in men. Acute pancreatitis is a medical emergency and can lead to dehydration and hypotension. The most common causes of pancreatitis are gallstones, which cause bile duct obstruction, and chronic alcohol abuse. As in acute pancreatitis, years of alcohol abuse is the most common cause of chronic pancreatitis. These two etiologies account for 60% to 80% of acute pancreatitis cases, with alcohol abuse being more common in younger patients and obstruction more common in older adults. Other potential causes of pancreatitis include the use of certain medications, trauma, pancreatic cancer, and genetic predisposition.

Chronic pancreatitis refers to a progressive disease that destroys the pancreas, eventually leading to the loss of all endocrine and exocrine functions. It often causes chronic pain. Computed tomography (CT) is used to diagnosis the presence of this condition.

Assessment

Patients with acute pancreatitis present with what is described as a constant dull, boring flank and/or epigastric pain that worsens if the patient is placed in a supine position. Tachycardia, fever, and jaundice may also be present. Typically an attack is a result of a large, heavy meal or excessive drinking. Nausea and vomiting are present in 75% to 80% of patients, whereas 50% to 90% of patients have abdominal distention or muscle spasms. Necrosis and organ failure may develop in 20% to 30% of patients who experience acute pancreatitis. Laboratory tests used to diagnose acute pancreatitis include determinations of serum amylase, lipase, and trypsin if available.

Management

Once diagnosed, most patients are managed with supportive care. Patients should not eat until nausea and vomiting have subsided. Patients should be transported and pain management can be considered, although it is not always effective with pancreatitis. Endoscopic retrograde cholangiopancreatography (ERCP) is used for patients who have cholelithiases. No other treatments are shown to decrease pain or hospital stay length.

For patients with chronic pancreatitis, lifestyle changes, including changes in diet and the termination of alcohol and tobacco use, are critical to management. Analgesics are used to control pain, pancreatic enzymes assist with steatorrhea and malabsorption, and finally surgical intervention may be considered. Patients should be monitored for pancreatic cancer because there is a higher incidence of this disease noted in patients suffering from chronic pancreatitis.

Pathophysiology, Assessment, and Management of Adrenal Insufficiency

Adrenal insufficiency is characterized by decreased function of the adrenal cortex and consequent underproduction of cortisol and aldosterone. A decrease in either of these adrenal hormones will result in weakness, dehydration, and an inability of the body to maintain adequate blood pressure or to properly respond to stress.

Cortisol affects almost every organ and tissue in the body. Although its primary role is to assist with the body's response to stress, this adrenal hormone also helps maintain blood pressure and cardiovascular function; regulates the metabolism of carbohydrates, proteins, and fats; modulates glucose levels in the blood by balancing the effects of insulin; and functions as an anti-inflammatory agent by slowing the inflammatory response.

Secretion of aldosterone is regulated chiefly by the renin–angiotensin system, but is also stimulated by increased serum potassium concentrations. Abnormal adrenal cortical function produces abnormalities in the metabolism of carbohydrates and protein as well as disturbances in salt and water metabolism.

Adrenal insufficiency is usually well tolerated unless the clinical picture is complicated by coexisting factors such as infection or stress. It affects about 4 persons per 100,000 in the United States, strikes an equal number of men and women, and is found in patients of all races and ages. Adrenal insufficiency is classified as either primary or secondary.

Primary Adrenal Insufficiency

Pathophysiology

Primary adrenal insufficiency (also known as Addison disease) is caused by atrophy or destruction of both adrenal glands, leading to deficiency of all the steroid hormones these glands produce. A rare disease (occurring in approximately

1/100,000 persons in the United States), it is usually the result of idiopathic atrophy, an autoimmune process in which the immune system creates antibodies that attack the adrenal cortex, leading to its gradual destruction. This phenomenon accounts for approximately 70% of cases of Addison disease in the United States. Adrenal insufficiency occurs when at least 90% of the adrenal cortex has been destroyed. Less commonly (approximately 30% of cases), the adrenal destruction is caused by tuberculosis; a bacterial, viral, or fungal infection; adrenal hemorrhage; or cancer of the adrenal glands. Patients with Addison disease who receive treatment have a normal life expectancy.

Assessment

Signs of chronic adrenal insufficiency include unexplained weight loss, fatigue, vomiting, diarrhea, anorexia, salt craving, muscle and joint pain, abdominal pain, postural dizziness, and increased pigmentation in the extensor surfaces, palmar creases, and oral mucosa Figure 12 . In patients with Addison disease, the body improperly regulates the content of sodium, potassium, and water in body fluids. Blood volume and pressure fall, as does the sodium concentration of the blood; blood potassium rises. The blood volume may become so reduced that the circulation can no longer be maintained efficiently.

Management

Treatment of patients experiencing an adrenal crisis includes the assessment and management of airway, breathing and circulation. If needed, use the coma protocol of glucose, thiamine, and naloxone (Narcan) as indicated. Aggressive fluid replacement using 5% dextrose in normal saline should be initiated. Hydrocortisone, 100 mg IV, is indicated in the acute management of a crisis. Electrolyte imbalances are common and may not be obvious in the prehospital environment.

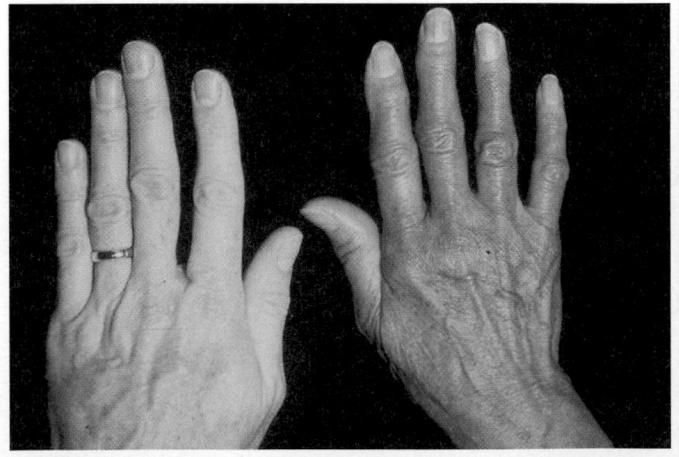

Figure 12 The hand of a patient with Addison disease (right) compared with the hand of a normal subject (left).

■ Secondary Adrenal Insufficiency

Pathophysiology

Secondary adrenal insufficiency is a relatively common condition characterized by a lack of adrenocorticotropic hormone (ACTH) secretion from the pituitary gland. ACTH, a pituitary messenger, stimulates the adrenal cortex to manufacture and secrete cortisol. If ACTH secretion is insufficient, cortisol production is not stimulated. Patients who abruptly stop taking corticosteroids (eg, prednisone) may also experience secondary adrenal insufficiency. Corticosteroid treatments suppress natural cortical production; however, aldosterone production is usually not affected in this form of adrenal insufficiency.

Assessment

Signs and symptoms of acute adrenal insufficiency may appear suddenly, which is called an addisonian crisis. An addisonian crisis may be triggered by an acute exacerbation of chronic insufficiency, usually brought on by stress, trauma, surgery, or severe infection. Corticosteroid withdrawal is the most common cause.

Although most patients with acute adrenal insufficiency have symptoms severe enough to prompt them to seek medical treatment before a crisis occurs, about 25% of patients first experience symptoms during an addisonian crisis. The chief clinical manifestation of adrenal crisis is shock. Patients may also manifest nonspecific symptoms, including weakness; lethargy; confusion or loss of consciousness; low blood pressure (vascular collapse); elevated temperature; severe pain in the lower back, legs, or abdomen; and severe vomiting and diarrhea that leads to dehydration.

Management

An unrecognized, untreated episode of acute adrenal insufficiency may be fatal. Death is usually attributable to hypotension or cardiac dysrhythmias caused by hyperkalemia. Treatment is based on clinical presentation and findings and is geared toward maintaining the airway, breathing, and circulation until arrival at the emergency department. With regard to airway maintenance and supplemental oxygen, follow the procedure for a patient who has altered mental status or is comatose. Be alert for vomiting, and have suction ready.

Other goals of prehospital treatment are to begin rehydrating the patient and to correct the electrolyte and acid–base abnormalities. Start an IV and infuse up to 1 L of 0.9% NS. If the patient is hypotensive, administer an NS bolus at 20 mL/kg. Remember, a patient in adrenal insufficiency may be severely dehydrated, often to the point of shock, and needs volume.

Check the patient's glucose level. Administer 25 to 50 g of D_{50} to correct the hypoglycemia. D_5NS is the preferred IV fluid, but administering D_5W through a second IV can help maintain the patient's blood glucose level. Monitor cardiac rhythm because changes in serum electrolytes can lead to marked myocardial instability.

Pathophysiology, Assessment, and Management of Other Adrenal Emergencies

Cushing Syndrome

Pathophysiology

Cushing syndrome is caused by an excess of cortisol production by the adrenal glands or by excessive use of cortisol or other similar corticosteroid (glucocorticoid) hormones. Tumors of the pituitary gland or adrenal cortex can stimulate the production of excess hormone, for example, and lead to Cushing syndrome. Administration of large amounts of cortisol or other glucocorticoid hormones (eg, hydrocortisone, prednisone, methylprednisolone, or dexamethasone) for the treatment of life-threatening illnesses, such as asthma, rheumatoid arthritis, systemic lupus, inflammatory bowel disease, and some allergies, can also cause this syndrome.

Regardless of the cause, excess cortisol causes characteristic changes in many body systems. Metabolism of carbohydrate, protein, and fat is disturbed, such that the blood glucose level rises. Protein synthesis is impaired so that body proteins are broken down, which leads to loss of muscle fibers and muscle weakness. Bones become weaker and more susceptible to fracture.

Assessment

Other common signs and symptoms related to excess cortisol include the following:

- Weakness and fatigue
- Depression and mood swings
- Increased thirst and urination
- Low blood glucose level
- Weight gain, especially on the abdomen, face ("moon face"), neck, and upper back ("buffalo hump")
- Thinning of the skin, with easy bruising and pink or purple stretch marks (striae) on the abdomen, thighs, breasts, and shoulders
- Increased acne, facial hair growth, and scalp hair loss in women, and cessation of menstrual periods
- Darkening of skin (acanthosis) on the neck
- Obesity and poor growth in height in children

Management

Management is designed to decrease the level of cortisol in the body, which is difficult in the prehospital environment. Assess and manage the patient's airway, breathing, and circulation and manage any life-threatening conditions immediately. Prehospital treatment is generally supportive. Obtain a blood glucose level and administer D_{50} if indicated.

Adrenal Gland Tumor

Pheochromocytoma is a tumor of the adrenal gland, usually in the medulla, that causes excessive release of the hormones epinephrine and norepinephrine. Less than 10% of such tumors are malignant (cancerous).

The tumors may occur at any age, but they are most common in young adult to mid-adult life. A common clinical presentation is a combination of symptoms (ie, hypertension, anxiety, chest pain, abdominal pain, fatigue, weight loss, vision problems, and sometimes seizures) that may be frequent but sporadic, and may increase in frequency, duration, and severity.

Congenital Adrenal Hyperplasia

Congenital adrenal hyperplasia (CAH) is a condition of the adrenal gland in which there is inadequate production of cortisol and aldosterone. Some states require testing of infants for this condition at birth. People born with severe CAH have masculine features whereas those with a mild form may never be diagnosed. Persons with CAH are susceptible to infection and stress because they are unable to produce an adequate amount of hormones. The lack of cortisol may result in an acute adrenal crisis.

Children may present with undefined signs and symptoms, so diagnosis may be difficult. Multiple signs listed as follows may be associated with CAH.

- Female infants may have enlarged parts of the vagina or it may resemble a penis.
- Male infants may be asymptomatic; however, they may exhibit signs of puberty as a toddler, including increased musculature, penis growth, pubic hair, and a lowering of the voice.
- The child may exhibit excessive facial and/or body hair and initial rapid growth.
- Numerous respiratory infections and illnesses and high blood pressure may be present.
- Salt wasting caused by insufficient aldosterone levels may lead to dehydration, low blood pressure, low sodium levels, and high potassium levels in the blood.
- The child may also exhibit short stature and severe acne.

Children will usually require lifetime treatment with cortisol and/or aldosterone replacement therapy. Times of increased stress will require higher doses of cortisol. Surgery can correct genital deformities early in life. Dexamethasone may be prescribed to a pregnant woman prior to the infant's delivery if the condition is diagnosed early in the first trimester of pregnancy.

Pathophysiology, Assessment, and Management of Thyroid, Parathyroid, and Pituitary Gland Disorders

Hypothyroidism and Hyperthyroidism

Thyroid hormone is secreted in response to the stimulation of the thyroid gland by the anterior pituitary gland. The anterior pituitary gland secretes thyroid-stimulating hormone (TSH) in response to the hypothalamus's secretion of thyrotropin-releasing hormone (TRH). **Table 7** summarizes the major effects of hypothyroidism and hyperthyroidism. Approximately 20 million Americans have some kind thyroid disorder, and many of them will be unaware of their condition.

Table 7	**Comparison of Major Effects of Hypothyroidism and Hyperthyroidism**	
	Hypothyroidism	**Hyperthyroidism**
Cardiovascular effects	Slow pulse, reduced cardiac output	Rapid pulse, increased cardiac output
Metabolic effects	Decreased metabolism, cold skin, weight gain	Increased metabolism, skin hot and flushed, weight loss
Neuromuscular effects	Weakness, sluggish reflexes	Tremor, hyperactive reflexes
Mental, emotional effects	Mental processes sluggish, personality placid	Restlessness, irritability, emotional lability
Gastrointestinal effects	Constipated	Diarrhea
General somatic effects	Cold, dry skin	Warm, moist skin

Patients with hyperthyroidism and hypothyroidism are likely to require supplemental oxygen. Hyperthyroid metabolic activity increases oxygen demand. Hypothyroid conditions may lead to diminished respiratory effort that may require positive-pressure ventilation.

Graves Disease

The most severe and common cause of hyperthyroidism is Graves disease. This disorder is more common in women than in men, with an overall incidence of 1.4 cases per 1,000 persons. Graves disease tends to follow a chronic course of remission and relapse. If left untreated, it may be fatal.

Graves disease is an autoimmune disorder in which the thyroid gland hypertrophies, or enlarges, as its activity increases. The hypertrophied thyroid gland produces a visible mass called a goiter in the anterior part of the neck. The overactive gland secretes an excessive amount of thyroxine, causing the hyperthyroidism that characterizes Graves disease. In addition to having a goiter, signs and symptoms of the condition include a substantially increased appetite with marked weight loss that may progress to cachexia. Patients also have polydipsia as a result of dehydration caused by diarrhea and excessive sweating. They may also present with exophthalmos, or protruding eyeballs. This condition is caused by edema of the tissue behind the eyes. Another sign of Graves disease is pretibial myxedema, an "orange peel" appearance and nonpitting edema of the skin on the anterior part of the leg below the knee. Finally, the hypermetabolism that accompanies Graves disease increases stress on the heart and may lead to heart failure.

Hashimoto Disease

Hashimoto disease is another cause of hyperthyroidism that is also more common in women. The thyroid gland is enlarged as a result of the infiltration of T lymphocytes and plasma cells. Like Graves disease, Hashimoto disease is an autoimmune disorder that affects the TSH (thyroid-stimulating hormone) receptors; however, it is milder than Graves disease. The hyperthyroidism is transient, with a subsequent hypothyroidism after antibodies destroy the follicles.

Myxedema Coma

Thyroid hormones are critical for cell metabolism and organ function. If their supply becomes inadequate, organ tissues do not grow or mature (due to the decreased metabolic rate), energy production declines (a cause of the decreased metabolic rate), and the actions of other hormones are affected.

Adult hypothyroidism is sometimes called *myxedema*. Frequently, patients have localized accumulations of mucinous material in the skin, which gives the disease its name (the prefix *myx-* refers to "mucin," and *edema* means "swelling") **Figure 13** . The condition is manifested by a general slowing of the body's metabolic processes due to the reduction or absence of thyroid hormone. All organ systems may exhibit symptoms of the disorder, and the severity of the symptoms will be consistent with the degree of the hormone deficiency.

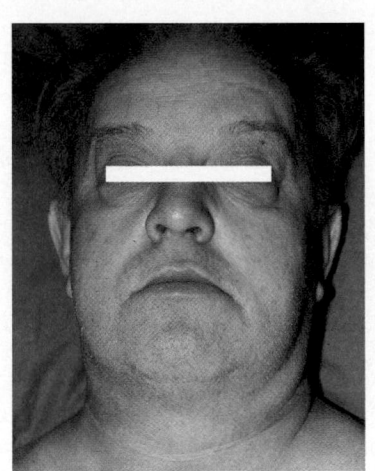

Figure 13 Localized accumulations of mucinous material in the neck of a hypothyroid patient.

Symptoms of hypothyroidism include fatigue, feeling cold, weight gain, dry skin, and sleepiness. Because these symptoms are often subtle and can be mistaken for other conditions, the disease may go undiagnosed. Continued decrease of the hormone levels may lead to myxedema coma, an extreme manifestation of untreated hypothyroidism that is accompanied by physiologic decompensation. When hypothyroidism is long standing, physiologic adaptations occur, such as reduced metabolic rate and decreased oxygen consumption, which in turn lead to peripheral vasoconstriction. Triggers such as infection (especially pulmonary and urinary tract infections), exposure to cold, trauma, surgery, and certain medications are often precipitating factors in the progression to myxedema coma.

The hallmark of myxedema coma is deterioration of the patient's mental status. Although family members may not be overly concerned about more subtle changes, such as apathy or decreased intellectual function, more obvious changes, such as confusion, psychosis, and coma, will most certainly elicit a call for emergency assistance.

Most cases of myxedema coma occur during the winter in women older than 60 years. The condition is four to eight times more common in women than in men. Just as the incidence of hypothyroidism increases with age, myxedema coma occurs primarily in elderly patients. One consistent finding is hypothermia, and you may need to use a thermometer that records temperatures of less than 90°F in cases of myxedema coma. Thus, absence of fever in the presence of infection is a common finding.

Hypothyroidism decreases intestinal motility, and the decreased metabolic rate associated with this condition can lead to drug toxicity, especially in the elderly. A slower metabolic rate causes the levels of medications, especially those that affect the central nervous system, to rise to toxic levels in the blood. This accidental overdose in the hypothyroid patient can actually precipitate myxedema coma.

Myxedema coma is a metabolic and cardiovascular emergency. If not diagnosed and treated immediately, the mortality rates are approximately 50%. Thus the patient's condition must be stabilized as soon as possible.

Administer supplemental oxygen therapy to correct hypoxia. Intubation and ventilation are indicated for patients with diminished respiratory drive or those who are unable to protect their airway; these measures will help prevent respiratory failure.

Monitor the patient's cardiac status. Hypotension may respond to crystalloid therapy, and vasopressive agents may be necessary (dopamine [Intropin]). Administer 25 to 50 g of D_{50} if glucose levels are less than 60 mg/dL.

Treat hypothermia with passive rewarming methods because aggressive rewarming may lead to vasodilation and hypotension. Hemodynamically unstable patients with profound hypothermia, however, will require active rewarming. Avoid sedatives, narcotics, and anesthetics because of the delayed metabolism.

Thyrotoxicosis

Thyrotoxicosis is a toxic condition caused by excessive levels of circulating thyroid hormone. Although hyperthyroidism can cause thyrotoxicosis in some patients, the two conditions are not identical. Thyrotoxicosis may also be caused by goiters, autoimmune disorders such as Graves disease, or thyroid cancer.

Words of Wisdom

Both hyperthyroidism and hypothyroidism can adversely affect the electrical status of the myocardium. Application of the cardiac monitor may reveal tachydysrhythmias in hyperthyroidism or bradydysrhythmias in hypothyroidism. Treat all dysrhythmias according to local protocol, while keeping in mind that these dysrhythmias may be difficult to correct without first fixing the underlying disorder.

A thyroid storm is a rare, life-threatening condition that may occur in patients with thyrotoxicosis. The condition is usually triggered by a stressful event or increased volume of thyroid hormones in the circulation. In addition to the normal signs and symptoms of hyperthyroidism, patients may present with fever, severe tachycardia, nausea, vomiting, altered mental status, and possibly heart failure.

Hyperparathyroidism

The increased parathyroid hormone level that occurs in hyperparathyroidism will result in increased levels of blood calcium, hypercalcemia, and decreased phosphate blood levels. Causes of hyperparathyroidism can be divided between primary and secondary causes. Primary causes are those that result from the gland itself while secondary causes occur elsewhere in the body and affect gland secretion. The most common cause is a benign neoplasia on the gland called an adenoma.

Signs and symptoms can be vague, as in many of the endocrine conditions. Fatigue, weakness, nausea, vomiting, and confusion may be present. Occasionally, pathologic fractures may occur secondary to thinning bones or kidney stones due to an increase in calcium and phosphorous in the urine. Surgery to remove the enlarged gland is definitive management and successful 95% of the time. Patients with mild forms of the disease require monitoring of calcium blood levels. Prehospital management involves the management of ABCs and supportive care as indicated.

Panhypopituitarism

Panhypopituitarism is the inadequate production or absence of the pituitary hormones, including adrenocorticotropic hormone (ACTH), cortisol, thyroxine (T4), luteinizing hormone (LH), follicle-stimulating hormone (FSH), growth hormone, and antidiuretic hormone (ADH). The anterior pituitary gland is responsible for the production of several different hormones; therefore, clinical presentation varies depending on the hormone(s) that are lacking. Figure 14 summarizes these hormones and the symptoms associated with each deficiency.

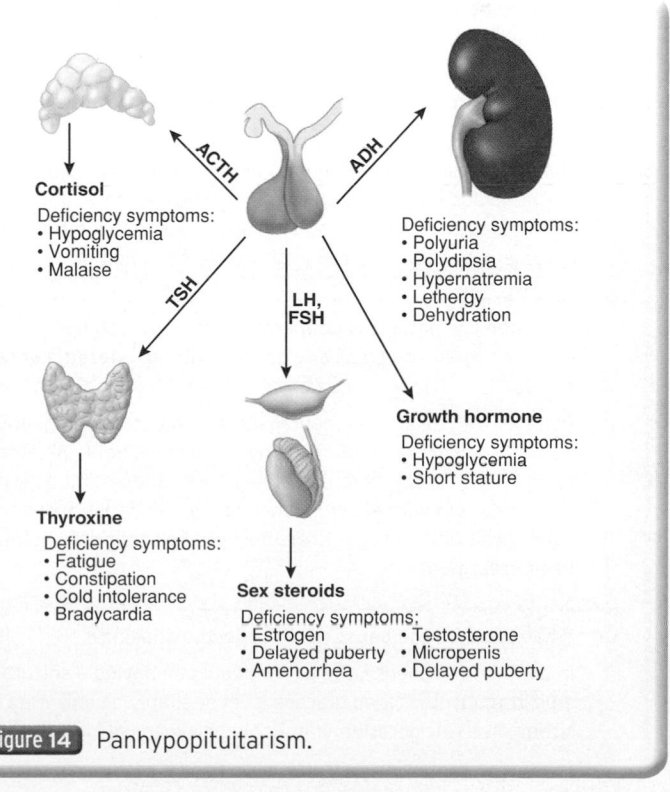

Figure 14 Panhypopituitarism.

It is important for a pediatric endocrinologist to manage children diagnosed with panhypopituitarism. Often these conditions are a result of the hypothalamus, rather than the pituitary gland, functioning abnormally. These hormones control growth and sexual maturation, and once hormone therapy is initiated, children can generally live a normal life. Hormone replacement therapy will need to be continually monitored throughout the patient's life.

Diabetes Insipidus

Diabetes insipidus (DI) includes some of the same characteristics as diabetes, such as polyuria and polydipsia. It is a relatively uncommon disorder, unlike diabetes mellitus (DM). The body is unable to regulate fluid caused by the lack of ADH (central diabetes insipidus) or the kidneys are unable to respond appropriately (nephrogenic diabetes insipidus). One difference in DI and DM is the amount of glucose present in the urine. In DI the urine is very diluted, whereas in DM there is an excess of glucose present in the urine. It seems obvious that dehydration and electrolyte imbalances may occur; however, there is also the risk of water intoxication as well and hyponatremia. Management may include synthetic ADH.

Inborn Errors of Metabolism

Inborn errors of metabolism are hereditary diseases that result in the body being unable to transform food to energy. Identification of these conditions may be difficult because patients present with vague signs such as failure to thrive and poor feeding in infants. These signs vary, depending on the specific condition. A neonate with sepsis or who is critically ill should be assessed for an __inborn error of metabolism (IEM)__. Usually identified in infancy, these conditions are grouped into two categories:

- Disorders that result in toxic accumulations
    - Maple syrup urine disease—a genetic disorder that causes a buildup of the amino acids leucine, isoleucine, and valine
    - Phenylketonuria—the body's inability to break down the amino acid phenylalanine
- Disorders of energy production or utilization
    - Hereditary fructose intolerance—a lack of aldolase B, the enzyme responsible for breaking down fructose
    - Galactosemia—the inability to break down the simple sugar galactose

YOU are the Medic   SUMMARY

1. What key information is provided from the dispatch and scene size-up?

The dispatch information indicated unusual circumstances or bizarre behavior. Your scene size-up has confirmed a patient with an altered mental status. The presence of medication and an ice cream wrapper lead you to suspect the patient could have hypoglycemia.

2. What types of medical conditions can cause an altered mental status?

Numerous medical emergencies can cause an altered mental status, including a seizure, stroke, or drug overdose. It is essential to perform a thorough patient assessment. Make no assumptions about the cause of a patient's condition.

3. Although the patient is cooperative, what do you need to consider when you treat any patient with an altered mental status?

Patients with an altered mental status can become combative, particularly those experiencing hypoglycemia. Some patients stare off into space, whereas others curse and exhibit bizarre or sometimes violent behavior. When you are in doubt about scene safety, wait until police officers declare the scene safe before you begin treatment.

4. What could be the cause of his reported shaking?

In addition to epilepsy, the patient could be having a seizure from an extremely low blood glucose level or simply be shivering from sitting on a refrigeration unit. Look for a medical identification

bracelet for additional information and perform a thorough assessment, noting the presence or absence of incontinence. Seizures due to hypoglycemia are an ominous sign.

5. What concerns you about the bystander's statement?

Often, laypersons are well-intentioned but do not know what to do. Patients with an altered mental status frequently have airway problems and sometimes require airway management beyond the application of oxygen. It is possible that in addition to hypoglycemia, he has aspirated food into his lungs.

6. If your partner was unable to obtain IV access, what additional treatment options exist for correcting the patient's blood glucose level?

Patients with diabetes often have fragile veins. Also, your patient is obese, and obtaining IV access could be difficult. Another treatment option is to administer glucagon intramuscularly. Glucagon is an endogenous hormone secreted by the alpha cells in the islets of Langerhans. This hormone stimulates glycolysis, or the breakdown of glycogen into glucose. The typical dosage is 1 unit, or 1 mg, and requires adequate glycogen stores in the liver to be effective.

7. What challenges often occur on calls such as this one?

Often, patients with diabetes do not wish to be transported. It is vitally important that the patient eat a meal as soon as possible. Administration of IV dextrose is only a temporary measure. If the patient does not eat a meal containing complex carbohydrates, his or her blood glucose level will likely drop again, and another 9-1-1 call will be necessary.

YOU are the Medic   SUMMARY, continued

8. How would you document this patient contact?

Many seasoned paramedics believe that a refusal of treatment and/or transport is the most difficult call to document. A patient cannot refuse care unless he or she is an adult of sound mind. It is imperative to thoroughly document not only the patient assessment findings and interventions provided, but also the consequences of refusal of treatment and/or transport to document that the patient refusal was an informed decision. Document the contact and discussion with medical control in which you obtained authorization to refuse transport (or treatment). Also document

that you left the patient in the care of his son, with instructions to call back if needed.

Diabetic emergencies, specifically hypoglycemia, are frequent calls in EMS. It is important to avoid complacency, particularly with scene safety and documentation of refusals. Patients with diabetes can experience significant trauma injuries that can prevent you from discovering the medical emergency precipitating the traumatic event. It is vital to remain diligent in your assessments and care.

EMS Patient Care Report (PCR)

Date: 05-30-11	**Incident No.:** 53011	**Nature of Call:** Altered mental status		**Location:** Walt's Grocery	
Dispatched: 0900	**En Route:** 0901	**At Scene:** 0903	**Transport:** N/A	**At Hospital:** N/A	**In Service:** 0930

Patient Information

Age: 40 **Sex:** M **Weight (in kg [lb]):** 160 kg (353 lb)	**Allergies:** Penicillin **Medications:** Insulin (Humulin N) **Past Medical History:** IDDM **Chief Complaint:** Hunger

Vital Signs

Time: 0905	**BP:** 160/94	**Pulse:** 100	**Respirations:** 24	**Spo$_2$:** 97% on room air
Time: 0910	**BP:** 156/92	**Pulse:** 90	**Respirations:** 20	**Spo$_2$:** 98% on room air
Time:	**BP:**	**Pulse:**	**Respirations:**	**Spo$_2$:**

EMS Treatment
(circle all that apply)

Oxygen @ 6 **L/min via (circle one):** (NC) NRM Bag-mask device	**Assisted Ventilation:** N/A	**Airway Adjunct:** none	**CPR:** N/A
Defibrillation	**Bleeding Control**	**Bandaging**	**Splinting**	**Other**

Narrative

Dispatched to "man sitting in the butter" at a grocery store. Pt, a 40-year-old man, was found sitting in the refrigerated section by a woman bystander. Woman reported the pt was "shaking all over." On arrival, pt was found sitting upright in the dairy section with chocolate all over his face and an ice cream sandwich melting in his hand. Medication tablets were on the floor. Airway was open and breathing adequate. Weak, rapid radial pulse present. Pt was responsive to pain (a pinch to the back of his hand); skin was cool, pale, and diaphoretic; no trauma noted to head, eyes, ears, nose, or throat; PEARRL; chest rise and volume adequate, no apparent trauma and bilateral breath sounds present/no adventitious lung sounds; no trauma noted to abdomen. Pt had an altered mental status secondary to hypoglycemia. Blood glucose level was 30 mg/dL; 6 L/min of oxygen administered via nasal cannula after pt resisted NRM, IV line started with 18-gauge R AC, normal saline to keep the vein open. Pt administered 25 g of dextrose 50. Pt's blood glucose level increased to 120 mg/dL. Pt's 21-year-old son arrived. Pt refused transport; IV and oxygen discontinued. Pt advised IV dextrose will not prevent glucose level from dropping again and he could have aspirated food into his lungs. Pt assisted to food court where he ordered a hamburger and fries. Signature obtained for refusal of care; advised pt he could call back if he changed his mind. Pt released to self and left in care of 21-year-old son; notified medical control and dispatch. **End of report**

Prep Kit

- The endocrine system directly or indirectly influences almost every cell, organ, and function of the body.

- Patients with an endocrine disorder often have a broad range of signs and symptoms, necessitating a thorough assessment and immediate treatment to avert life-threatening emergencies.

- The endocrine system comprises a network of glands that produce and secrete hormones. The main function of the endocrine system and its hormonal messengers is to maintain homeostasis and promote permanent structural changes.

- Hormones travel through the bloodstream to target tissues.

- The major components of the endocrine system are the hypothalamus, pineal gland, pituitary, thyroid, thymus, parathyroid, adrenals, pancreas, and reproductive organs (gonads). The pancreas has a role in hormone production as well as in digestion.

- The hypothalamus is the primary link between the endocrine system and the nervous system.

- The pineal gland synthesizes and secretes melatonin, a hormone that helps regulate sleep/wake patterns.

- The pituitary gland is often referred to as the "master gland" because its secretions control, or regulate, the activity of other endocrine glands.

- The thyroid secretes thyroxine, the body's major metabolic hormone, in order to stimulate energy production in cells, increasing the rate at which cells consume oxygen and use carbohydrates, fats, and proteins. The thyroid gland also secretes calcitonin, which helps maintain normal calcium levels in the blood.

- The thymus gland helps the immune system identify and destroy pathogens, disease-causing pathogens, and various pathogenic processes, such as cancer.

- Three types of T cells evolve from stem cells in the thymus: killer T cells, helper T cells, and suppressor T cells. These specialized white blood cells boost immunity by helping the lymphatic system defend the body against pathogenic organisms.

- The parathyroid gland helps regulate blood calcium levels by secreting parathyroid hormone, a hormone that directs specialized cells to dissolve bone, thereby releasing calcium.

- The adrenal glands, paired triangular structures located atop the kidneys, consist of an outer covering, or cortex, and an inner portion, the medulla. These glands produce hormones that help regulate the body's metabolism, its balance of salt and water, the immune system, and sexual function. Adrenal hormones also help the body cope with physical and emotional stress by increasing the pulse, respiratory rate, and blood pressure.

- The pancreas secretes digestive enzymes as well as the hormones glucagon and insulin, which are responsible for the regulation of blood glucose levels.

- The gonads—the testes in men and the ovaries in women—are the main source of sex hormones.

- The testes are located in the scrotum and produce hormones called *androgens*. The most important androgen in men is testosterone, which regulates sexual development during puberty, including growth spurts, deepening of the voice, growth of facial and pubic hair, and muscle growth and strength.

- The ovaries release ova (eggs) and secrete the hormones estrogen and progesterone. These hormones regulate sexual development in women and also assist in regulating the menstrual cycle and pregnancy.

- Diabetes is a metabolic disorder in which the body's ability to metabolize glucose is impaired. It is characterized by the passage of large quantities of urine containing glucose, significant thirst, and deterioration of body function.

- Endocrine emergencies can be difficult to assess because they affect many organ systems. Do not take these calls lightly because poor outcomes can result quickly.

- In type 1 diabetes, most patients do not produce insulin. They require daily injections of supplemental synthetic insulin throughout their lives to control blood glucose levels.

- When checking vital signs, be alert for signs of increased intracranial pressure, unusual breathing patterns, and pararespiratory motions.

- Management of an endocrine emergency may require intubation, administration of supplemental oxygen, infusion of dextrose, or other measures. All findings must be thoroughly documented.

- In type 1 diabetes, the beta cells in the islets of Langerhans have been destroyed and no longer produce insulin. Type 1 diabetes mellitus requires close monitoring of blood glucose and at least daily administration of insulin by injection or pump.

Prep Kit, continued

- The most common form of diabetes is type 2 diabetes (formerly called "adult-onset diabetes"), in which the blood glucose level is elevated.

- Hypoglycemia in a person with insulin-dependent diabetes is often the result of having taken too much insulin, eaten too little food, or both. As a result of the actions of epinephrine, the patient will tremble, have a rapid pulse rate, sweat, and feel hungry.

- Hyperglycemia (high blood glucose level) is one of the classic symptoms of diabetes mellitus. Common early signs include frequent and excessive thirst accompanied by frequent and excessive urination.

- If left untreated, hyperglycemia progresses to the life-threatening condition known as *diabetic ketoacidosis (DKA)*. DKA occurs when certain acids accumulate in the body because insulin is not available.

- Hyperosmolar nonketotic coma/hyperosmolar hyperglycemic nonketotic coma (HONK/HHNC) is a metabolic derangement that occurs principally in patients with type 2 diabetes. This condition is characterized by hyperglycemia, hyperosmolarity, and an absence of significant ketosis.

- Gestational diabetes is a form of glucose intolerance that usually manifests itself late in pregnancy.

- Adrenal insufficiency is characterized by underproduction of cortisol and aldosterone, which leads to weakness, dehydration, and the body's inability to maintain adequate blood pressure or to properly respond to stress. Primary adrenal insufficiency (also known as *Addison disease*) is caused by atrophy or destruction of both adrenal glands, leading to deficiency of all the steroid hormones produced by these glands.

- Secondary adrenal insufficiency is defined as a lack of adrenocorticotropic hormone (ACTH) secretion from the pituitary gland.

- Acute adrenal insufficiency is referred to as an *addisonian crisis*, which may result from an acute exacerbation of chronic insufficiency, usually brought on by a period of stress, trauma, surgery, or severe infection.

- Cushing syndrome is caused by an excess of cortisol production by the adrenal glands or by excessive use of cortisol or other similar corticosteroid (glucocorticoid) hormones.

- Pheochromocytoma is generally a nonmalignant tumor of the adrenal gland, usually in the medulla, that causes excessive release of the hormones epinephrine and norepinephrine.

- Congenital adrenal hyperplasia (CAH) is a condition of the adrenal gland in which there is not enough production of cortisol and aldosterone.

- Thyroid hormones are critical for cell metabolism and organ function. If their supply becomes inadequate, organ tissues do not grow or mature (due to the decreased metabolic rate), energy production declines (a cause of the decreased metabolic rate), and the actions of other hormones are affected.

- Graves disease is the most severe and common cause of hyperthyroidism. The disease can produce goiter, exophthalmos, and pretibial myxedema.

- Hashimoto disease, another cause of hyperthyroidism, is an autoimmune disease in which the thyroid gland is enlarged as a result of the infiltration of T lymphocytes and plasma cells.

- Symptoms of hypothyroidism include feeling fatigued, feeling cold, gaining weight, having dry skin, and being sleepy. Continued decrease of thyroid hormone levels may lead to myxedema coma.

- Myxedema coma is a condition in which a general slowing of the body's metabolic processes occurs in the setting of reduced or absent thyroid hormone.

- Thyrotoxicosis is a toxic condition caused by excessive levels of circulating thyroid hormone. A thyroid storm is a rare, life-threatening condition that may occur in patients with thyrotoxicosis.

- In hyperparathyroidism, blood calcium levels increase, resulting in hypercalcemia and decreased phosphate blood levels.

Prep Kit, continued

<u>addisonian crisis</u> Acute adrenal insufficiency.

<u>adrenal cortex</u> The outer part of the adrenal glands that produces corticosteroids.

<u>adrenal glands</u> Paired glands located above the kidneys; each adrenal gland consists of an inner adrenal medulla and an adrenal cortex.

<u>adrenal medulla</u> The inner part of the adrenal glands that produces catecholamines (epinephrine and norepinephrine).

<u>adrenocorticotropic hormone (ACTH)</u> Hormone that targets the adrenal cortex to secrete cortisol (a glucocorticoid).

<u>agonists</u> Molecules that bind to a cell's receptor and trigger a response by that cell. Agonists produce some kind of action or biologic effect.

<u>aldosterone</u> Hormone that stimulates the kidneys to reabsorb sodium from the urine and excrete potassium by altering the osmotic gradient in the blood.

<u>androgens</u> Male sex hormones that regulate body changes associated with sexual development (puberty), including growth spurts, deepening of the voice, growth of facial and pubic hair, and muscle growth and strength.

<u>antagonists</u> Molecules that bind to a cell's receptor and block the action of agonists. Hormone antagonists are widely used as drugs.

<u>antidiuretic hormone (ADH)</u> A hormone secreted by the posterior pituitary lobe of the pituitary gland, ADH constricts blood vessels and raises the blood pressure; also called *vasopressin*.

<u>calcitonin</u> The hormone secreted by the thyroid gland that helps maintain normal calcium levels in the blood.

<u>catecholamines</u> Hormones produced by the adrenal medulla (epinephrine and norepinephrine) that assist the body in coping with physical and emotional stress by increasing the pulse and respiratory rates and the blood pressure.

<u>congenital adrenal hyperplasia (CAH)</u> Inadequate production of cortisol and aldosterone by the adrenal gland.

<u>corticosteroids</u> Hormones that regulate the body's metabolism, the balance of salt and water in the body, the immune system, and sexual function.

<u>cortisol</u> Hormone that stimulates most body cells to increase their energy production.

<u>Cushing syndrome</u> A condition caused by an excess of cortisol production by the adrenal glands or by excessive use of cortisol or other similar corticosteroid (glucocorticoid) hormones.

<u>diabetes mellitus</u> Disease characterized by the body's inability to sufficiently metabolize glucose. The condition occurs either because the pancreas does not produce enough insulin or the cells do not respond to the effects of the insulin that is produced.

<u>diabetic ketoacidosis (DKA)</u> A form of acidosis in uncontrolled diabetes in which certain acids accumulate when insulin is not available.

<u>dyslipidemia</u> An excessive level of lipids (fats) circulating in the blood, increasing the risk of atherosclerosis and coronary artery disease.

<u>endocrine glands</u> Glands that secrete or release chemicals that are used inside the body. Endocrine glands lack ducts and release hormones directly into the surrounding tissue and blood.

<u>epinephrine</u> Hormone produced by the adrenal medulla that plays a vital role in the function of the sympathetic nervous system.

<u>estrogen</u> One of the three major female hormones. At puberty, estrogen brings about the secondary sex characteristics.

<u>exocrine glands</u> Glands that excrete chemicals for elimination.

<u>exophthalmos</u> Protrusion of the eyes from the normal position within the socket.

<u>gestational diabetes</u> Diabetes that develops during pregnancy in women who did not have diabetes before pregnancy.

<u>glands</u> Cells or organs that selectively remove, concentrate, or alter materials in the blood and then secrete them back into the body.

<u>glucagon</u> Hormone produced by the pancreas that is vital to the control of the body's metabolism and blood glucose level. Glucagon stimulates the breakdown of glycogen to glucose.

<u>goiter</u> A visible mass in the anterior part of the neck caused by enlargement of the thyroid gland.

<u>gonads</u> The reproductive glands; the main source of sex hormones.

<u>Graves disease</u> An autoimmune disorder that causes thyroid gland hypertrophy and severe hyperthyroidism.

<u>Hashimoto disease</u> A type of hyperthyroidism in which the thyroid gland becomes enlarged as it is infiltrated by T lymphocytes and plasma cells.

helper T cells A type of T lymphocyte that is involved in both cell-mediated and antibody-mediated immune responses. The cells secrete cytokines that stimulate the B cells and other T cells.

homeostasis A tendency to constancy or stability in the body's internal environment.

hormones Chemicals secreted by the body that regulate many body functions, such as growth, reproduction, temperature, metabolism, and blood pressure.

hyperglycemia Abnormally high blood glucose level.

hyperosmolar hyperglycemic nonketotic coma (HHNC) Also known as hyperosmolar nonketotic coma (HONK), HHNC is a metabolic derangement that occurs principally in patients with type 2 diabetes. The condition is characterized by hyperglycemia, hyperosmolarity, and an absence of significant ketosis.

hyperosmolar nonketotic coma (HONK) See *hyperosmolar hyperglycemic nonketotic coma (HHNC)*.

hypoglycemia Abnormally low blood glucose level.

hypothalamus A small region of the brain that contains several control centers for the body functions and emotions. It is the primary link between the endocrine system and the nervous system.

inborn errors of metabolism (IEM) A group of congenital conditions that cause either accumulation of toxins or disorders of energy metabolism in the neonate. These conditions are characterized by an infant's failure to thrive and by vague signs such as poor feeding.

insulin Hormone produced by the pancreas that is vital to the control of the body's metabolism and blood glucose level. Insulin causes sugar, fatty acids, and amino acids to be taken up and metabolized by cells.

insulin resistance Condition in which the pancreas produces enough insulin but the body cannot effectively use it.

iodine An essential element in the diet and an important component of thyroxine. Without the proper level of iodine intake, thyroxine cannot be produced, and physical and mental growth are diminished.

ischemia Tissue anoxia from diminished blood flow to tissue, usually caused by narrowing or occlusion of the artery.

islets of Langerhans A specialized group of cells in the pancreas where insulin and glucagon are produced.

killer T cells Cytotoxic T cells that attack and phagocytize antigens in order to halt their reproduction.

lipolysis The metabolism (breakdown or destruction) of stored fat that has been released into the circulation.

luteinizing hormone (LH) Hormone that regulates the production of both eggs and sperm, as well as production of reproductive hormones.

lymphocytes White blood cells that assist the lymphatic system with immunity.

lymphokines Cytokines released by lymphocytes, including many of the interleukins, gamma interferon, tumor necrosis factor beta, and chemokines.

microangiopathy Microscopic deterioration of vessel walls caused primarily by adherence of blood lipids to vessel walls.

myxedema coma A rare condition that can occur in patients who have severe, untreated hypothyroidism.

necrosis Tissue death, usually caused by a cessation of blood supply.

norepinephrine Hormone produced by the adrenal glands that is vital in the function of the sympathetic nervous system.

ovaries Female gonads; ovaries release eggs and secrete the female hormones.

pancreas The digestive gland that secretes digestive enzymes into the duodenum through the pancreatic duct. The pancreas is considered both an endocrine gland and an exocrine gland.

panhypopituitarism The inadequate production or absence of the pituitary hormones, including adrenocorticotropic hormone (ACTH), cortisol, thyroxine, luteinizing hormone (LH), follicle-stimulating hormone (FSH), estrogen, testosterone, growth hormone, and antidiuretic hormone (ADH).

parathyroid hormone (PTH) A hormone secreted by the parathyroids that acts as an antagonist to calcitonin. PTH is secreted when calcium blood levels are low.

pheochromocytoma A tumor of the adrenal gland, usually in the medulla, that causes excessive release of the hormones epinephrine and norepinephrine.

pineal gland A gland in the brain that synthesizes and secretes melatonin, a hormone that affects patterns of sleep and wakefulness.

pituitary gland Gland whose secretions control, or regulate, the secretions of other endocrine glands. Often called the "master gland."

pretibial myxedema An "orange peel" appearance and nonpitting edema of the skin on the anterior part of the leg below the knee.

primary adrenal insufficiency Also known as Addison disease. A rare condition in which the adrenal glands produce an insufficient amount of adrenal hormones.

progesterone One of the three major female hormones.

secondary adrenal insufficiency A common condition characterized by a lack of adrenocorticotropic hormone (ACTH, also called corticotrophin) secretion from the pituitary gland.

sine wave An unusual waveform that has a repetitive, uniform see-saw pattern, representing an alternating current; also known as a *sinusoidal waveform.*

somatostatin A hormone that inhibits insulin and glucagon secretion by the pancreas.

suppressor T cells Lymphocytes that modulate the immune response to avoid injury to body systems.

target tissues Tissues on which hormones are directed to act.

testes Male gonads located in the scrotum that produce hormones called androgens.

testosterone The most important androgen in men.

thymus gland A gland that helps the immune system identify and destroy components foreign to the body.

thyroid Large gland located at the base of the neck that produces and excretes hormones that influence growth, development, and metabolism.

thyroid-stimulating hormone (TSH) Hormone that controls the release of thyroid hormone from the thyroid gland.

thyroid storm A rare, life-threatening condition that may occur in patients with thyrotoxicosis. The condition is usually triggered by a stressful event or increased volume of thyroid hormones in the circulation.

thyrotoxicosis A toxic condition caused by excessive levels of circulating thyroid hormone.

thyroxine The body's major metabolic hormone. Thyroxine stimulates energy production in cells, which increases the rate at which the cells consume oxygen and use carbohydrates, fats, and proteins.

type 1 diabetes The type of diabetic disease that usually starts in childhood and requires daily injections of supplemental synthetic insulin to control blood glucose; sometimes called *juvenile diabetes* or *juvenile-onset diabetes.*

type 2 diabetes The type of diabetic disease that usually starts in later life and often can be controlled through diet and oral medications; sometimes called adult-onset diabetes.

Assessment in Action

Your response area includes a large number of poverty-stricken families. Many persons in the area do not receive medical care. Although your agency does not have a high call volume, when you are dispatched, it is often for extremely ill or significantly injured patients.

One morning, you hear frantic knocking on the station door. You open it to find a frightened teenager who tells you, "My mom needs help! She's not acting right, and can't stop throwing up. We were evicted from our apartment a few days ago. Please help us." As you have your partner pull the ambulance out and notify dispatch, you approach the vehicle to find an approximately 30-year-old woman in the passenger seat. She is confused and febrile to the touch. Her radial pulse is very rapid, weak, and irregular. When you assess her pupils, you notice her eyes are bulging.

1. What is your primary concern regarding this patient's condition?
   A. Decreased level of consciousness
   B. Fast, irregular pulse rate
   C. Fever
   D. Bulging eyes

2. Which interventions may be required?
   A. Epinephrine
   B. Atropine
   C. Beta blockers
   D. Nitrous oxide

3. This condition is often precipitated by what type of event?
   A. Sudden, transient loss of consciousness
   B. Stressful event
   C. Severe abdominal pain
   D. Sudden blindness

4. Given her condition, what are the possible differential diagnoses?
   A. Narcotic overdose
   B. Thyroid storm
   C. Malignant hypothermia
   D. All of the above

5. Which additional signs and symptoms could have been experienced by the patient prior to this event?
   A. Palpitations
   B. Slow pulse rate
   C. Weight gain
   D. Hair growth

6. Which medical conditions may this patient have?
   A. Thyroid cancer
   B. Goiter
   C. Graves disease
   D. All of the above

7. Which procedure is required to diagnose this condition?
   A. Chest radiograph
   B. Skin biopsy
   C. Thyroidectomy
   D. Blood testing

Additional Questions

8. When you are forming a general impression, why is it important to make note of a patient's vital statistics, dress/grooming and hygiene, and breath or body odors?

9. Why is it important to perform a rapid full-body scan?

Hematologic Emergencies

National EMS Education Standard Competencies

Medicine

Integrates assessment findings with principles of epidemiology and pathophysiology to formulate a field impression and implement a comprehensive treatment/disposition plan for a patient with a medical complaint.

Hematology

Anatomy, physiology, pathophysiology, assessment, and management of

- Sickle cell crisis (pp 1252–1253)
- Clotting disorders (pp 1256–1257)

Anatomy, physiology, epidemiology, pathophysiology, psychosocial impact, presentations, prognosis, and management of common or major hematological diseases and/or emergencies

- Sickle cell crisis (p 1252)
- Blood transfusion complications (pp 1257–1258)
- Hemostatic disorders (p 1257)
- Lymphomas (p 1255)
- Red blood cell disorders (pp 1253, 1256)
- White blood cell disorders (pp 1254–1255)
- Coagulopathies (pp 1256–1257)

Knowledge Objectives

1. Discuss the composition and functions of blood's essential components: red blood cells, white blood cells, and platelets. (pp 1245–1248)
2. Summarize the role of white blood cells in the normal inflammatory process. (pp 1245, 1246–1247)
3. Distinguish between cell-mediated immunity and humoral immunity. (p 1247)
4. Define hemostasis, and discuss the mechanisms essential to its maintenance in the body. (pp 1248–1249)
5. Outline the steps in the primary assessment and management of a patient with a hematologic disorder. (p 1249–1250)
6. Describe the pathophysiology, assessment, and management of sickle cell disease. (pp 1252–1253)
7. Define three types of sickle cell crisis. (p 1252)
8. Outline the pathophysiology, assessment, and management of other common diseases and conditions of the blood, including anemia, leukopenia, thrombocytopenia, leukemia, lymphomas, polycythemia, disseminated intravascular coagulation (DIC), hemophilia, and multiple myeloma. (pp 1253–1257)
9. Discuss the causes, symptoms, assessment, and management of blood transfusion complications. (pp 1257–1258)

Skills Objectives

There are no skills objectives for this chapter.

Introduction

Most EMS systems rarely respond to hematologic emergencies. The term <u>hematologic disorder</u> refers to any disorder of the blood. Within this categorization, <u>hemolytic disorders</u> refer to disease processes that cause the breakdown of red blood cells, and <u>hemostatic disorders</u> refer to bleeding and clotting abnormalities. These disorders can be complex, difficult to assess, and challenging to treat in the prehospital setting. Although you may be able to provide only limited interventions, your actions may not only offer support, but also save the patient's life. As a paramedic you should have a basic understanding of the <u>hematopoietic system</u> (the blood components and the organs involved in their development and production) and hematologic disorders and know how to respond to these kinds of emergencies appropriately. The hematopoietic system consists of organs and tissues, primarily bone marrow, spleen, and lymph nodes, involved in the production of blood components.

Anatomy and Physiology

Blood and Plasma

Blood is "the fluid of life": Without it, we would not be able to live. Blood performs the following functions:

- **Respiratory function.** Transports oxygen from the lungs to the tissues and carbon dioxide from the tissues to the lungs
- **Nutritional function.** Carries nutrients (glucose, proteins, and fats) from the digestive tract to cells throughout the body
- **Excretory function.** Ferries the waste products of metabolism from the cells where they are produced to the excretory organs
- **Regulatory function.** Transports hormones to their target organs and transmits excess internal heat to the surface of the body to be dissipated
- **Defensive function.** Carries defensive cells and <u>antibodies</u>, which protect the body against foreign organisms

Blood is made up of two main components: plasma and formed elements (cells). <u>Plasma</u> is essentially 92% water and 6% to 7% proteins; the remainder consists of a variety of other elements (including electrolytes, clotting factors, and glucose). Plasma accounts for 55% of the total blood volume. The formed elements account for 45% of the total blood volume. These elements include red blood cells (RBCs), or <u>erythrocytes</u>; white blood cells (WBCs), or <u>leukocytes</u>; and platelets, or <u>thrombocytes</u>. Most of these elements (99%) are RBCs.

The production of RBCs occurs within stem cells; this production is stimulated by a protein (called erythropoietin) secreted by the kidneys in response to circulatory need. The RBCs may take as long as 5 days to mature and have an average life of about 4 months. Within the RBCs, iron-rich hemoglobin is responsible for carrying oxygen to the tissues. Oxygen attached to hemoglobin gives blood its characteristic red color, although many other factors can change the color of blood (such as carbon monoxide poisoning, when blood changes to bright red).

Three laboratory tests are commonly performed on blood: RBC count, hemoglobin level, and hematocrit measurement. The RBC count measures the number of RBCs in a sample of blood. The <u>hemoglobin</u> level identifies the amount of hemoglobin found within the RBCs. The measurement of <u>hematocrit</u> gives the overall proportion of RBCs in the blood. The patient's blood is considered balanced (even if the numbers are too high or low) if the hemoglobin level is one third of the hematocrit value and the RBC count is one third of the hemoglobin level. **Table 1** describes these tests in more detail.

The WBCs, which are larger than RBCs, provide the body with immunity against "foreign invaders." They are derived from the <u>stem cells</u>, or cells that develop into other types of cells in the body. Several types of WBCs exist, each of which performs a specific task in relation to maintaining the immune system.

Platelets are the smallest of the formed elements and are responsible for the clotting of the blood. Platelets form the initial plug following vascular injury. The clotting proteins then toughen and complete the blood clot. <u>Hemostasis</u> is a highly complex process that allows the body to stop bleeding

---

YOU *are the* **Medic**   **PART 1**

Your unit is dispatched to a private residence for a "general medical" complaint. The dispatcher informs you that the patient is a 73-year-old man with a history of leukemia who is feeling "poorly." When you arrive on scene, you find a man who appears frail. Family members confirm the patient was diagnosed with leukemia years ago. A family member states the patient has a fever (temperature of 102°F) and is feeling pain all over. You notice bruising on the patient's arms.

1. Where in the body does leukemia develop?
2. What do you need to know about the patient's status?

Table 1   Red Blood Cell and Platelet Counts

Name	Normal Values	Examples of Conditions Associated With Low Readings	Examples of Conditions Associated With High Readings
RBC count (×10⁶/μL)	4.5-6.0 in adults; 3.3-5.5 in children	Anemia, hemorrhage, certain leukemias, overhydration, chronic infections	Polycythemia, cardiovascular disease, hemoconcentration, dehydration
Hemoglobin (g/dL)	12.0-16.0 in females; 14.0-18.0 in males; 10.7-17.1 in children	Anemia, hyperthyroidism, liver disease, hemorrhage, hemolytic reactions	COPD, CHF, polycythemia, high-altitude sickness
Hematocrit (%)	35-45 in females; 40-50 in males; 32-55 in children	As for RBCs and hemoglobin, including leukemia, lupus, endocarditis, rheumatic fever, nutritional disorders	Polycythemia and usually anything that produces severe dehydration
Thrombocytes (platelets)	150,000-400,000 cells/μL	Thrombocytopenia, certain cancers, certain leukemias, sickle cell disease, systemic lupus erythematosus	Pulmonary embolism, polycythemia, acute hemorrhage, metastatic cancer, surgical stress

COPD indicates chronic obstructive pulmonary disease; CHF, congestive heart failure. The normal ranges provided are not intended to be definitive. Each laboratory determines its own values and normal ranges are method dependent.

through vascular spasm, coagulation, and platelet plugging. The opposite of hemostasis is hemorrhage. Approximately two thirds of the platelets circulate throughout the blood; the rest are stored in the spleen. Platelets are also derived from stem cells. They have an average life span of about 5 to 11 days.

Blood-Forming Organs and RBC Production

Although many parts and organs of the human body can alter or affect the hematologic system, the major players are the bone marrow, liver, and spleen **Figure 1**.

The bone marrow is the primary site for cell production within the human body. Bone marrow is found in most of the long bones plus the pelvis, skull, and vertebrae.

The liver produces the <u>clotting factors</u> found in the blood. It filters the blood, removing toxins, and is essential to normal metabolism and homeostasis. As old RBCs enter the liver, they are broken down into bile. The liver is a highly vascular organ that also stores some blood.

The spleen is also quite vascular. It is involved with the filtering and breakdown of erythrocytes, assists with the production of lymphocytes (one type of WBC), and has an important role in providing homeostasis and infection control. If the spleen, which stores about one third of the platelets, is removed, the platelets formed after that time remain in the blood throughout their life span.

The Inflammatory Process

At birth, all of the body's cells and blood contain <u>antigens</u>—substances within the body that can activate the immune system. Typically, the body keeps these antigens in memory and, when exposed to something for which it already has antibodies, will not initiate a reaction (see the chapter on *Pathophysiology*).

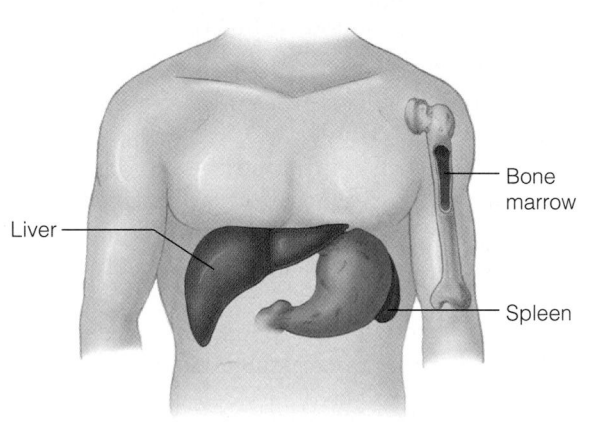

Figure 1   The bone marrow, liver, and spleen are major organs responsible for producing and regulating the blood and its components.

However, when the body is exposed to something it cannot identify in its base antigens, it produces antibodies to counteract the foreign or unidentified antigen. This reaction can also occur in patients with an <u>autoimmune disease</u>, such as lupus

Words of Wisdom

To check for a possible low RBC count, ask the patient to outstretch his or her palm and look at the creases. *White creases could mean a low hematocrit value or RBC count.* This test works only on normal-temperature skin.

Words of Wisdom

"Clot busters" (fibrinolytic therapy given in cases of acute myocardial infarction and stroke) activate the body's fibrinolytic system, resulting in clot decomposition (also known as lysis). Such therapy must be monitored closely in patients with hematologic disorders because clot busters may cause excess bleeding.

or multiple sclerosis. In patients with such diseases, the body identifies its own antigen as a foreign body.

The Immune System

The immune system is a highly complex biologic system whose processes protect the body from pathogens and other unwanted material. It must be able to distinguish the body's own tissue from outside organisms.

The immune system consists of two types of immunity: native immunity (also called innate immunity) and acquired immunity (also called adaptive immunity). Native immunity provides a nonspecific, maximal response to any disturbance. It operates as the first line of defense against pathogens. Most native immunity is associated with the initial inflammatory response.

Acquired immunity is specific to vertebrates, and provides a pathogen-specific response. This response arises when the body is exposed to a foreign substance or disease and produces antibodies to that invader.

Immune system responses can be categorized into **humoral immunity** and **cell-mediated immunity**. Humoral immunity refers to the secretion of antibodies called immunoglobulins, which recognize a specific antigen. In cell-mediated immunity, macrophages and T cells attack and destroy pathogens or foreign substances.

A primary component of the immune system is the WBCs. Like other blood cells, WBCs are produced in the bone marrow. A small number of WBCs are always circulating in the bloodstream, but a larger reserve is ready to spring into action whenever pathogens are detected in the blood. Specific laboratory values relating to WBCs and measurement of essential subcomponents—namely, neutrophils, lymphocytes, basophils, and eosinophils—can provide valuable information about the status of the immune system **Table 2**. Higher levels generally indicate the possible presence of infection, although in severe infections, such as overwhelming sepsis, the WBC count may actually drop, as destruction of WBCs exceeds the rate of WBC production.

The baseline WBC count is measured when the body is in a normal state (during times of no known infection or

Table 2 WBC Count and Differential

Name	Normal Values	Examples of Conditions Associated With Low Readings	Examples of Conditions Associated With High Readings
WBC count	5,000-10,000 cells/μL in adults; 4,500-15,500 cells/μL in children; 9,400-34,000 cells/μL in infants	Viral infections, bone marrow diseases or disorders, leukemia, radiation, late-stage AIDS	Viral and bacterial infections, hemorrhage, traumatic tissue injuries, leukemia, cigarette smoking
Neutrophils (segmented and unsegmented)	50%-60%*; 2,500-8,000 cells/μL	Leukemia, infections, rheumatoid arthritis, vitamin B$_{12}$ deficiency, enlarged spleen	Bacterial infections, tissue breakdown, hemolytic reactions, tumors, MI, surgical stress, cancer
Basophils (also known as mast cells)	0.5%-1%*; 25-100 cells/μL	Allergic reactions, hyperthyroidism, MI, bleeding ulcers, stress	Certain leukemias, inflammations, allergy, polycythemia, hemolytic anemia
Eosinophils	1%-4%*; 50-500 cells/μL	Mononucleosis, CHF, Cushing disease	Addison disease, tumors, skin infections, allergies
Lymphocytes	20%-40%*; 1,000-4,000 cells/μL	Hodgkin disease, burns, trauma, lupus, Cushing disease, immunodeficiency states	Numerous bacterial and viral infections, hepatitis, leukemia, toxoplasmosis, Graves disease
Monocytes	2%-6%*; 100-700 cells/μL	Corticosteroid use, infections, rheumatoid arthritis, HIV	Numerous bacterial and parasitic infections, recovery of acute infections, TB, hematologic disorders

MI indicates myocardial infarction; CHF, congestive heart failure; TB, tuberculosis. The normal ranges provided are not intended to be definitive. Each laboratory determines its own values and normal ranges are method dependent.

*Percentage of the total WBC count.

Example: If the WBC is 5,000, neutrophils should account for 2,500 to 3,000 of this count.

inflammation). The normal range is 5,000 to 10,000 cells/µL. Women tend to have higher baseline WBC counts, especially during childbearing years, owing to changes that occur during menstrual periods.

Blood Classifications

To ensure compatibility and prevent medical problems during blood component replacement, blood-type classifications have been developed. In the ABO system, the RBC classification types are "O," "A," "B," and "AB", which indicate the antigens found in the plasma membrane Table 3 . Type O blood, because it has no ABO antigens, can be given to anyone; a person with type O blood is known as a "universal donor." A person with type AB blood can receive blood from any donor without having an ABO reaction because type AB blood has no ABO antibodies; therefore, the person is known as a "universal recipient."

Blood contains a secondary antigen, known as the Rh antigen (the name signifies that the antigen was first found in the rhesus monkey). In the United States, 85% to 90% of all Caucasians and African Americans have this antigen. Thus, if a person has the blood type A-positive (A+), the blood contains the Rh antigen. Not having the Rh antigen is important in pregnancy because a woman without the antigen (Rh−) who is carrying a fetus with the antigen (Rh+) might become sensitized to the antigen and develop antibodies against the RBCs of the fetus, resulting in hemolytic disease.

Hemostasis

As mentioned, hemostasis is the highly complex process of stopping bleeding through vasoconstriction, platelet plugging, and coagulation. Alterations in the hemostasis process are known as hemostatic disorders, and are discussed later in this chapter.

The immediate physiologic response to hemorrhage is vasoconstriction—narrowing of the blood vessel—to clamp down and cut off blood flow at the affected site. Locally, vasoconstrictors such as thromboxane are released. Should the hemorrhage prove a significant threat to homeostasis, the adrenal glands release epinephrine, a potent vasoconstrictor, leading to systemic vasoconstriction.

The secondary response to hemorrhage is platelet plugging. Platelets are small cellular fragments that stick to collagen and

Table 3 Blood Types

Blood Type	ABO Antigens	ABO Antibodies	Acceptable Blood Donor Types
A	A	Anti-B	A, O
B	B	Anti-A	B, O
AB	A, B	None	A, B, AB, O
O	None	Anti-A Anti-B	O

YOU are the Medic PART 2

You begin your assessment of the patient while your partner obtains more information from the family. The patient is alert and cooperative with your questioning. You ask the patient what he is experiencing right now. The patient states, "My bones hurt, and I do not feel well." The patient also tells you that he takes chemotherapy and his most recent treatment was 4 days ago. You notice numerous used facial tissues that appear to have blood on them.

Recording Time: 0 Minutes	
Appearance	Awake, frail
Level of consciousness	Alert and oriented
Airway	Open
Breathing	Adequate
Circulation	Adequate

3. What is thrombocytopenia?

4. How will a patient with leukemia typically present?

become activated. Collagen exists within the deep membranes of blood vessels, and a cut or rupture exposes it to the platelets within circulation. The first platelets to be activated release chemicals that cause the aggregation of additional platelets to the site of injury. This growing number of platelets causes a plug to form, helping to stop bleeding.

This process of coagulation involves about a dozen clotting factors that are activated when the body is injured. These factors each require the presence and activation of the preceding factor to work. Clots themselves are made up of fibrin. When injury is detected, thrombin converts fibrinogen to fibrin, and the clotting process begins. Calcium acts as a binding agent, holding fibrin fibers close together to form the meshwork of the clot.

The <u>clotting cascade</u>—the term that refers to the process by which clotting factors work together to ultimately form fibrin—can be initiated through either an intrinsic or an extrinsic pathway. The intrinsic pathway is triggered by elements within the blood itself. This could be as a result of damage to the lumen of a blood vessel. The extrinsic pathway is activated by tissue damage outside of the blood vessels themselves. Any process that interferes with the activation or continuation of the clotting cascade or hemostasis is known as a <u>coagulopathy</u>. Coagulopathies are bleeding disorders that can lead to heavy or prolonged bleeding.

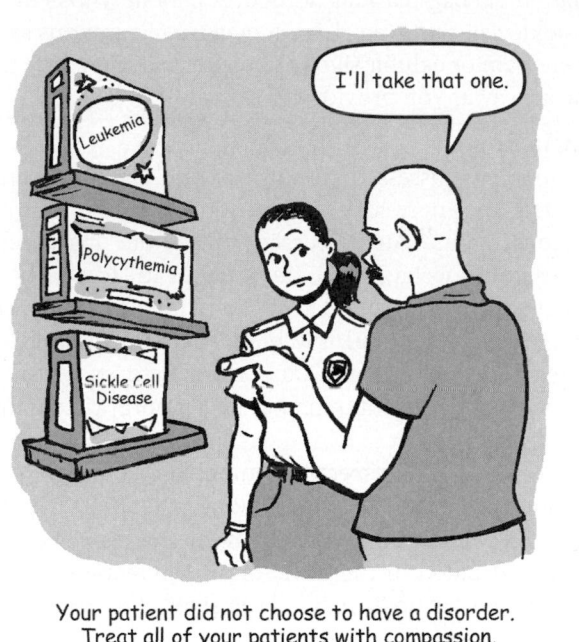

Your patient did not choose to have a disorder. Treat all of your patients with compassion.

Figure 2

Special Populations

As in all medical care, particular attention must be paid during the assessment and care of at-risk populations such as pediatric patients and the elderly. Many hematologic disorders manifest themselves in childhood; these require more refined assessment and treatment skills. The elderly have a greater incidence of decompensation due to a disease process or treatment regimens, and likewise require finesse and careful observation.

Patient Assessment

Assessment of a patient suspected of having a hematologic disorder should be no different from assessment of any other patient, albeit with a few additional items to consider and questions to ask. During the primary assessment, note any signs and symptoms that may be immediately life threatening. A major purpose of taking a history and performing the secondary assessment is to clearly and thoroughly understanding the chief complaint, which requires asking in-depth and relevant questions about the patient's history and SAMPLE history and following up on the responses to questions. Because some patients with a blood disorder may be unwilling to disclose the condition for fear of being treated differently from people without the disorder, a nonjudgmental approach is essential Figure 2 .

Scene Size-up

As always, ensure that the scene is safe for entry, consider the mechanism of injury, determine the number of patients, and assess for hazards and the need for additional help. Standard precautions should consist of gloves and eye protection at a minimum. Remember to evaluate each situation quickly and make sure the necessary personal protective equipment is readily available.

Note that although your report from dispatch may be for a patient with an unknown medical problem, most patients presenting with a sickle cell crisis have had a crisis before and will relay that information to the dispatcher.

Primary Assessment

An African American patient or any patient of Mediterranean descent who reports severe pain may have undiagnosed sickle cell disease.

Perform cervical spine stabilization, if necessary. Remember that even though a person has a history of sickle cell disease, sickle cell disease may not be causing the current problem; trauma or another type of medical emergency may be the cause. For this reason, you must always perform a thorough, careful primary assessment, paying attention to the ABCs and immediately correcting any life-threatening issues.

Form a General Impression
Perform a rapid scan of the patient to form an initial general impression. How does the patient look? Does the patient appear anxious, restless, or listless? Is the patient apathetic or irritable? Determine the patient's level of consciousness.

Airway and Breathing
As you are forming your general impression, assess the patient's airway and breathing. Patients showing signs of inadequate breathing or altered mental status should receive high-flow

oxygen at 12 to 15 L/min via a nonrebreathing mask or ventilation via bag-mask as needed. A patient who is experiencing a sickle cell crisis may have increased respirations as a result of severe pain or exhibit signs of pneumonia. Continue to monitor the airway as you provide care.

Circulation

Once you have assessed the airway and breathing and have performed the necessary interventions, check the patient's circulatory status. An increased pulse rate may indicate a compensatory mechanism, in an attempt to "force" the sickled cells through smaller vasculature. Look for signs of shock, such as a rapid pulse rate and low blood pressure. If you find any life-threatening conditions, take immediate steps to manage them and provide urgent transport to an appropriately equipped receiving facility.

In patients with suspected hemophilia, be alert for signs of acute blood loss such as pallor, a weak pulse, and hypotension. Note any bleeding of unknown origin, such as nosebleeds, bloody sputum, and blood in the urine or stool. Owing to blood loss, patients with hemophilia may exhibit signs of hypoxia or shock.

Transport Decision

Whether you decide to rapidly transport the patient will depend on the severity of the patient's condition and the patient's wishes. Transport to the closest, most appropriate facility should always be recommended to any patient who is experiencing a sickle cell crisis or uncontrolled bleeding.

Remember that patients with a history of sickle cell disease, but who have not had a crisis in some time, may require emotional support.

■ History Taking

It is extremely important to understand the chief complaint; to do so, you may need to be overly inquisitive about the patient's history and SAMPLE history. When you are obtaining the patient's history, you may discover previous or current sickle cell disease or hemophilia conditions.

Do not take a call for a person having a sickle cell crisis lightly. Patients are often in life-threatening situations, characterized by shortness of breath and signs of pneumonia. Their skin will show signs of inadequate perfusion, accompanied by hypotension. Physical signs, such as swelling of the fingers and toes, priapism, and jaundice may also guide you in determining whether the patient is experiencing a sickle cell crisis.

During history taking, look for changes in level of consciousness and symptoms such as vertigo, feelings of fatigue, and syncopal episodes. Has the patient had dyspnea, chest pain, changes in pulse rate and rhythm, or coughing up of blood? Has the patient experienced visual disturbances, muscle pain, or stiffness?

Ascertain whether the pain is isolated to a single location or if pain is felt throughout the entire body. Has the patient experienced skin changes such as color changes, burning, or itching? Bleeding from the nose, gums, and ulcers, or blood in the urine or stool? Be alert for signs of acute blood loss (pallor, weak pulse, and hypotension). History of liver problems or pain for

unknown reasons? Problems with the genitourinary system? Is the patient experiencing any gastrointestinal problems, such as nausea, vomiting, or abdominal cramping? In a patient with known sickle cell disease, ask the following questions in addition to obtaining a SAMPLE history:

- Have you had a crisis before?
- When was the last time you had a crisis?
- How did your last crisis resolve?
- Have you had any illness, unusual amount of activity, or stress lately?

■ Secondary Assessment

The secondary assessment may be performed on scene, en route to the emergency department, or not at all. This will depend on transport time and the patient's condition.

When treating a patient with a known or suspected blood disorder, you will need to perform a physical exam. In such cases, it is extremely important to have a basic understanding of some of the common findings in blood disorders Table 4.

Systematically examine the patient, focusing on major joints at which cells congregate, and obtain your patient's baseline vital signs including a measurement of the patient's oxygen saturation level. However, keep in mind that the oxygen saturation reading you obtain may be inaccurate as a result of the patient's anemic state. Evaluate and document mental status using the AVPU scale.

In patients experiencing a sickle cell crisis, respirations are normal to rapid, the pulse is weak and rapid, and the skin is typically pale and clammy with a low blood pressure.

Table 4 Common Findings With Blood Disorders	
System	**Examples of Common Findings**
Level of consciousness	Alterations in level of consciousness, ranging from excitability, agitation, and combativeness, to complete unresponsiveness
Skin	Uncontrolled bleeding, unexplained or chronic bruising, itching, pallor, or jaundice (yellow appearance usually indicates liver problems)
Visual disturbances	Visual disturbances, including blurred vision, decreased vision, tunnel vision, and seeing black or grey spots
Gastrointestinal	Epistaxis (bloody nose), bleeding or infected gums, ulcers, melena (blood in the stool), and liver failure (causes jaundice)
Skeletal	Chronic joint or bone pain or rigidity
Cardiovascular	Dyspnea, tachycardia, chest pain, hemoptysis (coughing up blood)
Genitourinary	Hematuria, menorrhagia, chronic or recurring infections

Documentation and Communication

Many anti-inflammatory drugs (such as aspirin and ibuprofen) and some herbals (such as ginkgo, garlic, ginger, ginseng, and feverfew) decrease platelet aggregation. Although this effect may be beneficial (such as in the prevention of myocardial infarction and stroke), these drugs may also increase the tendency to bleed. Always ask patients about medications, including over-the-counter and herbal medications.

Reassessment

It is important to reassess the patient frequently to determine if there have been changes in his or her condition. For example, are there changes in the patient's mental status? Are the ABCs still intact? How is the patient responding to the interventions performed? Should you adjust or change the interventions? In many patients, you will note marked improvement with appropriate treatment.

Supplemental oxygen should be administered via nonrebreathing mask at 12 to 15 L/min in an attempt to hypersaturate the remaining hemoglobin and increase the level of perfusion that has been decreased by the sickled cells or hemophilia. Ventilation should be provided when respirations are insufficient.

Place the patient in a position of comfort and cover to maintain body temperature. Administer IV fluid for hydration and nitrous oxide for pain as allowed by local protocol. Once the patient has arrived at the hospital, care for sickle cell disease can include analgesics for pain, penicillin to prevent infection, and, depending on the severity of the crisis, a blood transfusion.

Distinguishing a true sickle cell crisis from other nonspecific causes of pain can be difficult. In these situations, perform a thorough assessment and contact the hospital to help sort out the signs and symptoms. Medical control should be a resource for you to help problem-solve situations and provide guidance on how to manage your patient.

Prehospital care for a patient with hemophilia may include IV therapy to treat hypotension. Provide appropriate supplemental oxygen and cover the patient to maintain body temperature. At the hospital, the patient may receive a transfusion or plasma.

Communication with hospital staff is important for continuity of care. Hospital personnel need to be informed about the patient's history, the present situation, your assessment findings, and your interventions and their results.

Your run report is the only legal document that shows appropriate care was provided. Be sure to thoroughly document each assessment, your findings, treatment, the time of the interventions, and any changes in the patient's condition. Follow your local protocols for patients who refuse treatment or transport.

Emergency Medical Care

Emergency medical care for any patient with problems related to a blood disorder should include the following:

- **Oxygen.** The amount needed and how it is given (that is, bag-mask ventilation or nonrebreathing mask) depend on the severity of the patient's condition and respiratory status.
- **Fluids.** Initiate intravenous (IV) fluid replacement as indicated for the specific disorder or chief complaint.
- **Electrocardiogram (ECG).** Monitor and treat symptomatic cardiac rhythm disturbances as needed.

YOU are the Medic   PART 3

Your partner returns and tells you the family was unsure of what to do. A home health care agency that has been assisting with his supportive care was contacted, and general comforting methods were described for the patient. The patient has a DNR (do not resuscitate), and documents show supportive measures should be undertaken as required. The family is concerned that the patient is not responding well to "supportive measures" and wants the patient transported to the Downtown Hospital oncology unit.

Recording Time: 5 Minutes	
Respirations	20 breaths/min
Pulse	100 beats/min
Skin	Cool, pale, and moist
Blood pressure	100/60 mm Hg
Oxygen saturation (Spo₂)	97% while breathing room air
Pupils	Equal and reactive

5. Are you concerned with the patient's vital signs at this point?

6. What are "supportive measures" for this patient?

- **Transport.** Transport to the closest, most appropriate facility.
- **Comfort.** Place the patient in a position of comfort, and cover to maintain body temperature.
- **Pharmacology.** Pain management is often necessary, especially in a sickle cell crisis.
- **Psychological support.** Be supportive of and communicate therapeutically with the patient.

Pathophysiology, Assessment, and Management of Specific Emergencies

The aforementioned general steps in emergency medical care apply to all patients with an emergency related to a blood disorder. Depending on the specific blood disorder, you will need to refine your assessment and management as discussed in the next sections. While not the most common complaint encountered by the prehospital care provider, hematologic disorders are serious and often life threatening. Over 245,000 people in the United States alone are afflicted with hematologic disorders and experience increased morbidity and mortality as a result.

Sickle Cell Crisis

Pathophysiology

Sickle cell disease is—by far—the leading inherited blood disorder. Although it primarily affects African American, Puerto Rican, and European populations, it can occur in anyone. In the United States, approximately 70,000 to 100,000 Americans have sickle cell disease. The numbers are much greater in Africa, where the World Health Organization estimates that 200,000 infants are born with the disease each year. Mortality at younger ages is common, with an average life expectancy of 45 years. In general, women tend to live slightly longer than men with this disease.

Sickle cell disease starts with a gene defect of the adult-type hemoglobin (HbA). This mutation can be inherited from both parents (HbSS) or one parent (HbS). When the gene is inherited from both parents, there is a high probability that their offspring will be prone to sickle cells (that is, the person actually has the disease) or the sickle cell trait (the person is a carrier of the mutation).

The defective RBCs have an oblong shape instead of a smooth, round shape **Figure 3**. This shape makes the RBC a poor oxygen carrier, which means a patient with this disease is highly susceptible to hypoxia. Because sickle cells also have a much shorter life span than normal RBCs, the patient is also more prone to having anemia.

Sickle cell disease may lead to an aplastic crisis, or hemolytic crisis. In an aplastic crisis, the body temporarily stops RBC production, causing the patient to become easily tired, anemic, pale, and short of breath. A hemolytic crisis arises when there is acute red blood cell destruction leading to jaundice. In both cases, the patient may have rapidly evolving anemia, leukocytosis, and fever. The odd shape may also cause RBCs to lodge in small blood vessels, leading to thrombosis. A sickle cell crisis may manifest in several ways:

- Vasoocclusive crisis results from blood flow to an organ becoming restricted, causing pain, ischemia, and often organ damage. Most vasoocclusive crises last between 5 and 7 days. Frequently, circulation to the spleen becomes obstructed as a result of its narrow vessels and function

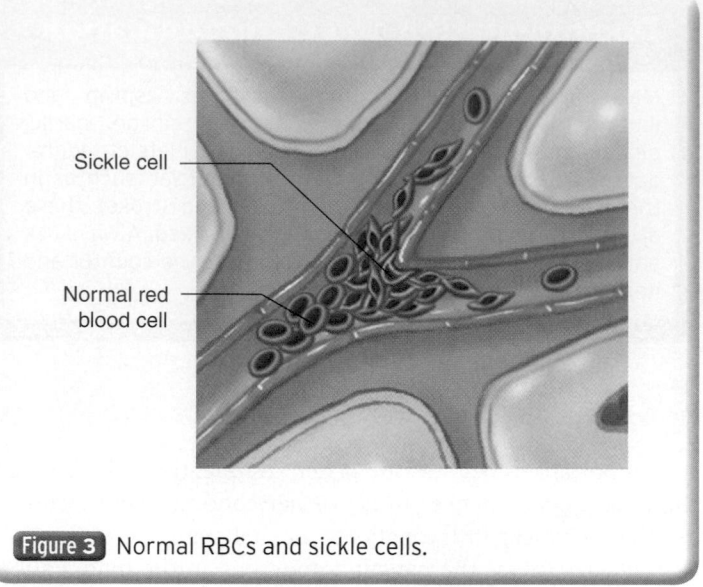

Figure 3 Normal RBCs and sickle cells.

of removing damaged RBCs. The organ may swell to the point of rupture, which can lead to death.

- Acute chest syndrome is a vasoocclusive crisis that can be associated with pneumonia. Common signs and symptoms include chest pain, fever, and cough. Vasoocclusion in the brain may result in a cerebrovascular accident, or stroke.
- Splenic sequestration crisis is caused by sickle cells within the spleen blocking blood from leaving the spleen, which results in painful, acute enlargement of the spleen and a hard and bloated abdomen. In acute splenic sequestration syndrome, RBCs become trapped in the spleen, causing a dramatic fall in hemoglobin available in the circulation. Patients will present not only with a painful, acute abdomen, but with sudden weakness, pallor, tachypnea, and tachycardia. It usually occurs in infants or toddlers. Within the US, the occurrence of acute splenic sequestration syndrome is approximately 7.5%, with mortality rates up to 12% for those experiencing a first attack. Recurrent crises arise in approximately 50% of cases, with an increased mortality rate.

Assessment

Do not take a call for a person having a sickle cell crisis lightly. Patients are often in life-threatening situations, characterized by shortness of breath and signs of pneumonia. Their skin will show signs of inadequate perfusion, accompanied by hypotension. There may be signs of jaundice and yellowing in the eye (icteric sclera). Signs of mild dehydration and many other complaints are often present.

In acute crises, patients may have significant pain resulting from congested vessels that do not allow the passage of oxygen and nutrients into tissues and joints. Patients may report multiple system involvement, including chest, abdominal, and arthritic-type pain, although some may report only fatigue or achiness along with fever. Pediatric patients will typically present with initial pain in the hands and feet, whereas adult patients will report back and proximal extremity pain.

Management

Administer high levels of oxygen to prevent further destruction of the RBCs due to hypoxia, and rapidly transport to an appropriate facility. You may also need to give IV fluid therapy to counter the patient's dehydration and aid in flushing of damaged RBCs from organs and peripheral tissues. It is important that the patient's body temperature be maintained; cold can contribute to sickling of the cells, and warm compresses may reduce further sickling. Patients may have lived with the disease for a long time and, thus, may have a very high pain threshold. As a consequence, they often require a higher level of analgesia due to a developed tolerance. Recommend that the patient rest as much as possible during transport.

Anemia

Pathophysiology

Anemia is defined as a hemoglobin or an erythrocyte level that is lower than normal Figure 4. Usually it is associated with some type of underlying disease process. Anemia may also result from acute or chronic blood loss or a decrease in production or increase in destruction of erythrocytes. Anemia may be an outcome of a preexisting hemolytic disorder (a disorder related to the breakdown of RBCs).

Iron deficiency anemia is the most common type of anemia, affecting 50 of 1,000 men, 140 of 1,000 women, and 470 of 1,000 children between 1 and 2 years of age. Typical causes include gastrointestinal blood loss, menstrual bleeding (the most common cause in US women, affecting primarily African American women), and blood loss due to frequent donations or diagnostic tests for patients hospitalized for long periods. In children, it is most often related to premature birth or low birth weight.

Anemia may be caused by an inherited hemolytic disorder, including sickle cell disease and thalassemia. In these disorders, when the RBCs are first developing their membranes, they may become rigid and deformed. The RBCs may then become lodged in small blood vessels, leading to a thrombosis (blood clot). Anemia may also be caused by hematologic disorders resulting from a deficiency of an enzyme known as glucose-6-phosphate dehydrogenase. This enzyme helps protect RBCs during infections. When levels of this enzyme are low, cells can become damaged. Although glucose-6-phosphate dehydrogenase deficiency is most commonly seen in African Americans, it can arise in people of any race.

The most common type of acquired anemia develops when the flow of RBCs is disrupted owing to problems with blood vessel linings (such as aneurysms and weaknesses) or blood clots. In autoimmune disorders, RBCs are destroyed by the body's own antibodies, which erroneously think that the normal blood cells are foreign. The RBCs can also be destroyed by microorganisms in the blood.

Anemia can also have serious consequences for people who travel to high-altitude areas. The combination of the lower number of RBCs and reduced partial pressure of oxygen in the atmosphere

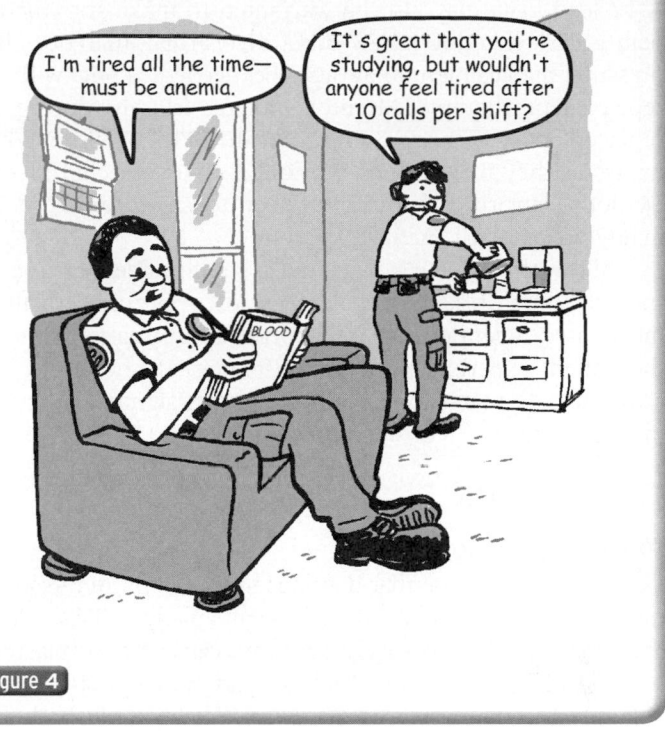

Figure 4

can lead to serious conditions that a healthy person would not experience, such as hypoxia, difficulty breathing, and chest pain.

Assessment

Your basic assessment should be the same for all patients, although you may want to ask some specific questions when anemia is suspected. Most commonly, patients with anemia will complain of feeling worn down, having no energy, or feeling as if they have overexerted themselves. Patients may also report that they "can't catch their breath." Owing to the reduction of hemoglobin, some may have anginal-type chest pain related to the reduction in oxygen availability to the heart muscle. Also common in patients with anemia are leukopenia (reduction in WBCs) and thrombocytopenia (reduction in platelets); both conditions can induce more frequent infections, fevers, cutaneous bleeding, and nosebleeds.

Management

In cases of anemia, check and monitor the airway and the patient's breathing closely, administering high-flow oxygen when necessary. Check vital signs frequently. In cases of chest pain, apply a cardiac monitor and closely watch the rhythm. A 12-lead ECG may also be warranted to make sure the chest pain is not related to a new-onset myocardial infarction. Blood pressure management may also be needed, along with fluid replacement therapy. Monitor patients closely during fluid replacement—IV fluids do not contain RBCs or blood components, so they may induce unwanted or unexpected bleeding. Do not be surprised if you have to control significant nosebleeds in any patient with anemia.

Allow the patient to rest in a comfortable position, and transport him or her to the closest, most appropriate facility. In most cases, a gentle, easy transport is appropriate. However, if the patient experiences an abrupt change in the level of consciousness, hypotension develops, or other significant perfusion inadequacies arise, consider rapid transport.

Leukemia

Pathophysiology

Leukemia is a disease that develops in the lymphoid system. In this type of cancer, blood cells—particularly WBCs—develop abnormally and/or excessively. Leukemia can cause anemia, thrombocytopenia (decrease in platelets), and leukocytosis (increased WBCs). Chemotherapy used to treat leukemia typically leads to leukopenia (decreased WBCs). Patients with leukemia experience frequent bleeding, bruising, infections, and fever Figure 5 .

Leukemia can be classified as acute or chronic. In most situations, but especially in chronic cases, the disease tends to develop more frequently in older populations (65 years or older). In acute leukemia, bone marrow is replaced with abnormal lymphoblasts. In chronic leukemia, abnormal mature lymphoid cells accumulate in the bone marrow, lymph nodes, spleen, and peripheral blood. This form of leukemia is typically found by chance during routine blood tests; suspicions are raised when the tests reveal a high lymphocyte count.

Survival of a person with leukemia depends on factors such as the stage at which the disease is detected, the patient's underlying medical condition, and the response to treatment. Acute and chronic leukemia are treated with chemotherapy and radiation therapy. In most cases, treatment results in remission, especially when the condition was identified early. Indeed, approximately 80% of children will be cured when their leukemia is diagnosed and treated early. Owing to the higher occurrence of genetic abnormalities and leukemic lymphoblasts as a result of the aging process, the adult cure rate is approximately 55%.

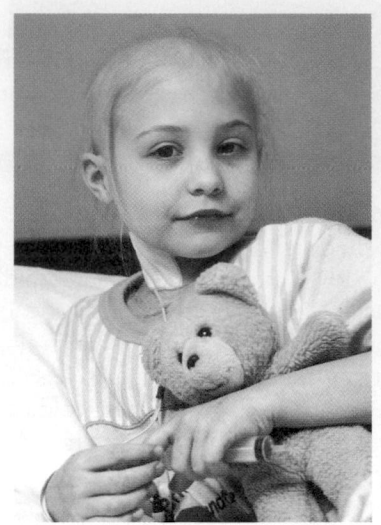

Figure 5 People with leukemia may have frequent bleeding, bruising, infections, and fever.

Assessment

How patients with leukemia present depends on the stage of the leukemia and the patient's current treatment. Patients typically complain of fatigue, headaches, or dyspnea and may have signs of neurologic defects. During the detailed physical exam, fever, bone pain, and diaphoresis may be found. Patients may complain of feeling full, soreness in the mid part of the chest, and unexplained

---

YOU *are the Medic* PART 4

Your partner administers oxygen to the patient at 12 L/min via nonrebreathing mask and looks for a location to insert an IV line. The patient is agreeable to being transported to the hospital for evaluation. The patient is still feeling considerable pain throughout his body. You lift the patient to the stretcher and move the patient to the ambulance for transport.

Recording Time: 10 Minutes	
Respirations	20 breaths/min
Pulse	100 beats/min
Skin	Cool, pale, and moist
Blood pressure	98/60 mm Hg
Oxygen saturation (Spo$_2$)	99% with oxygen at 12 L/min by nonrebreathing mask
Pupils	Equal and reactive

7. What should you do for the patient's pain level?

8. Do you think the patient's family has called you unnecessarily?

bleeding. You should monitor all basic vital signs (blood pressure, pulse, respirations, and temperature) and the cardiac rhythm. Hypotension and tachycardia are often present; therefore, vital signs may be consistent with signs of shock.

Management

Management of leukemia includes providing airway support and oxygen therapy as appropriate. IV fluid therapy and analgesics for comfort may be needed as well. Patients typically need constant positive support because many have a negative outlook toward their condition. The patient's loved ones may be quite concerned, especially during advanced stages of the disease; be supportive to them as well. In some cases, you may be called because the patient's condition has deteriorated and the family is uncertain about what to do. In such a scenario, your assessment may indicate normal findings for the patient. The patient or family may change their minds about transport or may have never wanted transport but rather professional insight and support. Discuss this situation with medical control, document all findings before leaving, and have a refusal and/or release form signed if the patient or family member decides against transport.

Few calls for patients with leukemia require extreme measures or rapid transport; however, be alert to rapid changes in the patient's condition. If you transport, be aware that the patient could go into arrest. Make sure you find out the patient's and family's wishes about what to do in this situation.

Lymphomas

Pathophysiology

Lymphomas are a group of malignant diseases that arise within the lymphoid system. They are classified in two categories: non-Hodgkin lymphoma (accounting for the majority of cases) and Hodgkin lymphoma.

Non-Hodgkin lymphoma can occur at any age in any person and can be hereditary. Furthermore, these types of cancer may be characterized based on the progression of the disease: indolent, aggressive, or highly aggressive. With very slow (indolent) progression, the disease may never leave the lymphoid system. In the highly aggressive form, the disease may affect multiple organs in a relatively short period, usually within several months. How well the disease responds to treatment depends on the specific type of non-Hodgkin lymphoma and how early it is recognized and classified.

Hodgkin lymphoma is a painless, progressive enlargement of the lymphoid glands, most commonly affecting the spleen and the lymph nodes. A highly rare form of lymphoma, it is suspected to have some hereditary components. The incidence of Hodgkin lymphoma has two peaks: one between 15 and 35 years of age and a second peak after age 55 to 60 years. The disease is twice as common in men as in women. Patients may not show any symptoms for many years, with the disease being found only after patients complain of night sweats, chills, persistent cough, and swelling of various lymph nodes (usually in the neck first). They may also note loss of appetite for an unknown reason, significant weight loss, generalized itching, fatigue, and/or bone pain. With aggressive treatment, symptoms may disappear for long periods; 60% to 90% of patients may actually be cured.

Assessment

Generally speaking, lymphomas require specialized levels of treatment involving some form of chemotherapy or radiation therapy. How well the disease responds to these treatments depends on the stage of the disease and its classification. As a rule, lymphomas respond well to chemotherapy; in fact, aggressive lymphomas respond better than indolent ones. Even if an indolent lymphoma is not cured with chemotherapy, many patients may survive as long as 10 years.

When you are assessing patients with lymphoma, ask specific questions such as "What type of lymphoma (cancer) do you have?" and "What type of treatment are you receiving?" As you perform your assessment, you will usually note pallor. The airway will usually be patent and breathing adequate, although sometimes you may note some congestion in the lower lung fields. The patient may describe being first hot and then cold or even both in different areas of the body. Signs of inadequate perfusion are common, including low blood pressure accompanied by an elevated pulse rate. Abnormal ECG rhythms may also be evident.

Management

Patients with lymphoma may be in constant, extreme pain; therefore, if pain management is needed and available, it may have to be aggressive because the patient will likely already be receiving a high-dose analgesic regimen. Treat inadequate perfusion with fluid therapy, and provide supplemental oxygen **Figure 6** . If necessary, treat abnormal heart rhythms. If the

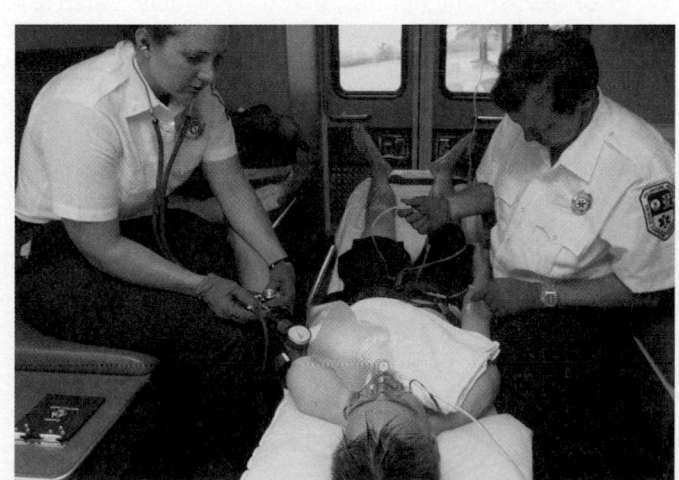

Figure 6 Patients with lymphoma who are in extreme pain should receive fluid therapy, oxygen, and analgesics.

patient's condition does not improve or even deteriorates following these measures, initiate rapid transport to the closest facility. As with leukemia, you may be called to offer support but no transport. Be supportive, discuss your findings with medical control, explain the options to the patient and family, and allow them to make a decision.

Polycythemia

Pathophysiology

Polycythemia is characterized by an overabundance or over-production of RBCs. The increased RBC production can be caused by a rare disorder originating in a single stem cell or an existing disease such as congestive heart failure or hypertension. It can also arise in persons who live in high-altitude areas for long periods. The disease essentially causes hyperviscosity of the circulatory system.

The overabundance of the blood components associated with polycythemia may lead to many other conditions, such as strokes, transient ischemic attacks, headaches, and abdominal pain (usually associated with an enlarged spleen). Many times this disease is found incidentally when blood cell counts are performed after a patient reports frequent episodes of signs and symptoms associated with hematologic diseases. Cases of polycythemia are more frequently found in adults 60 to 80 years of age.

Clinical treatment usually includes phlebotomy to try to maintain hematocrit levels at less than 45% in men and less than 42% in women. Other treatments have included cancer-type therapy intended to slow the production of new RBCs within the bone marrow. Survival is less than 18 months when the disease goes untreated but can be as long as 15 years for treated patients.

Assessment

Owing to the nature of polycythemia and its plethora of symptoms, your assessment findings may vary widely. Altered levels of consciousness may be evident due to stroke or transient ischemic attack–like events or hypoxia due to poor circulation because of lesions within the circulatory system. Respiratory distress is common, as are changes in peripheral pulses, pulse rate, and skin color. Tachycardia is the most common change in heart rhythm. Patients also tend to have purplish skin with red hands and feet.

As you assess the patient, note the extent and duration of dyspnea. Has the patient experienced uncontrolled itching (**pruritus**) or noted changes in skin temperature? Make sure to obtain a thorough medical history in cases of known or suspected polycythemia.

Management

Prehospital care largely consists of supportive care and transporting the patient to an appropriate facility. Administer oxygen as needed. Establish IV access for possible pharmacologic interventions for pain or pulse rate control as appropriate. Be supportive to the patient and family.

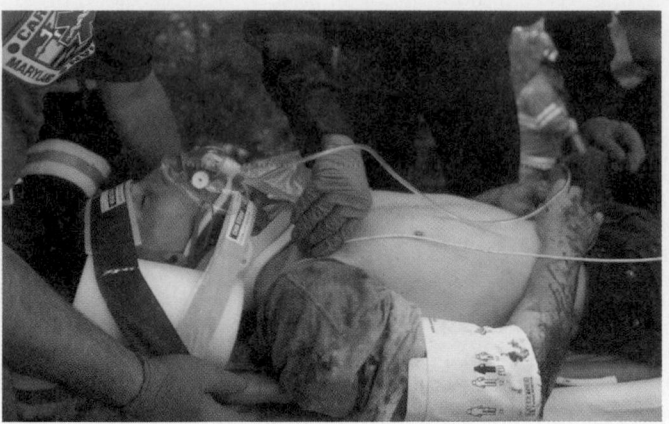

Figure 7   Severe trauma and extended hypotension can result in DIC.

Disseminated Intravascular Coagulation

Pathophysiology

Disseminated intravascular coagulation (DIC) may result from any number of life-threatening conditions such as massive injury and hypotension due to trauma **Figure 7**. Sepsis and obstetric complications also may cause DIC.

The condition progresses in two stages. First, free thrombin and fibrin deposits in the blood increase, and platelets begin to aggregate. In this stage of the condition, owing to excessive bleeding, massive blood loss, or tissue injury, defibrination, or a breakdown of the fibrin clots, occurs. In the second stage of the condition, uncontrolled hemorrhage results from the severe reduction in clotting factors.

The mortality rate of patients with DIC is quite high, especially in acute cases; some studies have shown it to be up to 75%. The primary causes of death relate to uncontrolled bleeding, hypotension, and shock.

Assessment

As you assess and care for critically injured or ill patients, keep in mind the issues that may lead to DIC. Your goal is to identify signs and symptoms commonly associated with DIC or progression toward it. In cases involving severe trauma, patients may have episodes of respiratory difficulty, signs of shock, and skin changes ranging from cold and clammy to pallor to small black-and-blue marks (purpura) on the chest and abdomen.

Management

It is important to identify the cause underlying the patient's presenting condition and establish treatment early, while not delaying transport to an appropriate facility. Maintain an airway, administer supplemental oxygen, and treat the patient for shock (keep the patient warm, control bleeding, administer IV fluids for hypotension) per local protocol. Pharmacologic interventions may entail pain management and treatment for abnormal heart rhythms, although treatment for altered heart rhythms should come last. Patients who have DIC due to severe trauma have a poor survival rate; they and family members need strong support. Be optimistic but honest with patients and family, and do not give false hope regarding survival.

Words of Wisdom

Patients with DIC have a failure of multiple organs (such as kidneys, lungs, and heart) at once, accompanied by bleeding from IV sites, bleeding into joints, and, possibly, intracranial hemorrhage.

Hemophilia

Pathophysiology

Hemophilia is a bleeding disorder in which clotting does not occur or occurs insufficiently (as in von Willebrand disease). It is usually associated with an X-linked recessive inheritance pattern, albeit one that is poorly understood. The disease is classified into two primary types: type A, which is due to low levels of factor VIII (antihemophilic globulin and antihemophilic factor), and type B, which is associated with a deficiency of factor IX (plasma thromboplastin component, also known as the Christmas factor). This disease is primarily found in the male population. The levels of factors VIII and IX determine the severity of the disease.

Type A and type B have the same signs and symptoms. Acute and chronic bleeding can occur at any time and may or may not be life threatening. Any injury or illness that can cause bleeding should not be taken lightly in a person with hemophilia. Spontaneous intracranial bleeding is common in hemophilia and is a major cause of death. Patients with significant acute bleeding episodes require hospitalization for transfusion and often require infusion of factors VIII and IX. If a patient has just had or needs surgery, the levels of these factors should be 100% at the beginning of the procedure and should be maintained to levels up to 50% for several weeks thereafter.

Assessment

When you are obtaining the patient's history, you may learn that the patient has a history of conditions associated with hemophilia. In addition to taking care of the ABCs, be alert for signs of acute blood loss (pallor, weak pulse, and hypotension). Note any bleeding of unknown origin, such as nosebleeds, bloody sputum, and blood in the urine or stool (melena). Owing to blood loss, patients may exhibit signs of hypoxia due to the reduction in oxygen-carrying capacity.

Management

Any patient who complains of respiratory problems should receive high-flow oxygen. Note ECG findings, and treat symptomatic dysrhythmias as appropriate. In cases of unstable hypotension, IV therapy may be necessary, but understand that the patient actually needs a transfusion of blood or plasma. Some patients will have significant pain, so analgesics may be appropriate. Although you may be called to treat someone with bleeding of unknown cause only to find that the bleeding stopped before you arrived on scene, you should suggest that the patient get immediate hospital or physician follow-up.

Multiple Myeloma

Pathophysiology

In multiple myeloma, the number of plasma cells (B cells that form antibodies) in the bone marrow increases abnormally, forming tumors in the bone. The tumors impair the ability of the bone marrow to function normally, so RBC, WBC, and platelet formation is decreased. Anemia and susceptibility to infection result. Neoplastic cells may also accelerate protein development in the bloodstream, leading to organ failure (primarily the kidneys) and eventually death. This disease rarely occurs early in life—most patients are older than 40 years. Men have this disease more frequently than do women.

As the disease progresses further and tumors grow or become more numerous, patients may have weakness in the bones, resulting in spontaneous fractures. Pain in the bones and back is also common. In advanced cases of myeloma, chemotherapy and other anticancer-type treatment may be given but may not cure the disease. Morbidity and mortality primarily depend on the extent of the disease and any underlying medical conditions.

Assessment

Findings during your assessment and management of multiple myeloma depend on the stage of the disease. Early stage complaints may be as simple as fatigue or mild pain. Later-stage disease may be evidenced by unexplained hemorrhage and significant weight loss, frequent bone fractures, and pain in any number of locations.

Management

Management is similar to that for other blood disorders: IV fluid therapy, pain management, and supportive care. Do not assume that the patient is ready to or is going to die; he or she may be having a complication of the myeloma. Definitive care at an appropriate facility may improve the patient's condition.

Transfusion Reactions

Pathophysiology

Emergency care may be required in response to a patient's reaction to a blood transfusion. Transfusion reactions occur in approximately 1 in 250,000 RBC transfusions. Transfusion reactions are similar to an anaphylactic reaction—they occur rapidly and can cause severe circulatory collapse and even death. When a patient receives a blood transfusion, it is important to monitor the patient very closely for the first 30 to

60 minutes because transfusion reactions typically begin within this time frame.

It is important to determine a patient's blood type and the type of blood received. When a patient receives blood or plasma that matches his or her blood type (for example, A+ given to an A+ patient) or the universal donor blood type (O), problems rarely arise. However, if a patient receives a blood type that is different from his or her own—for example, a patient with type A receives type B blood—a transfusion reaction will occur. Also, if a patient with A− blood receives an A+ transfusion, a transfusion reaction could occur, but this is rare.

Assessment

Signs and symptoms are generally easy to spot in a responsive patient, but they may be more subtle in an unresponsive or intubated patient. In the acute reaction, the patient experiences a rapid onset of chills, fever, back pain, vomiting, tachycardia, and hypotension. Transfusion reactions may be delayed up to 7 days after the transfusion; however, these events tend to be less severe than the typical acute reaction.

Complications generally fall into the following categories:

- **Hemolytic.** An acute hemolytic reaction is the greatest threat to the patient during blood transfusion. The primary cause is incompatibility between the recipient and the donor blood. Careful screening of the patient and the blood product can typically prevent this reaction from occurring.
- **Febrile.** A simple febrile reaction is the most common transfusion complication. It is usually benign, and is treated with an antipyretic and observation.
- **Allergic.** In addition to the transfusion reaction, the patient may also experience an anaphylactic reaction to preservatives or other agents in the product being transfused. Onset is typically within the first few minutes of transfusion and follows classic signs and symptoms of an anaphylactic state.
- <u>**Transfusion-related lung injury**</u>. Transfusion-related lung injury is a noncardiogenic pulmonary edema caused by increased capillary permeability post transfusion. Treatment is focused on supporting the ABCs. Because this is not a cardiac failure or fluid overload issue, diuretics are generally not effective.
- **Circulatory overload.** The rapid infusion of blood products can lead to circulatory overload, mimicking congestive heart failure. This typically occurs in patient populations with preexisting cardiomyopathy or ventricular dysfunction. Treatment consists of relieving the system of its excess fluids through diuresis, and with the use of oxygen, nitrates, and morphine.
- **Bacterial infection.** Bacterial infection is typically a result of poor blood product handling, or contamination during the infusion process. This occurs most commonly in platelet transfusions because platelets are kept at room temperature. This infection can lead to full systemic sepsis, requiring antibiotic administration and supportive care.

Management

In general, the severity of the reaction is directly correlated to the amount of blood volume transfused. Whereas there is no specific antidote or remedy for a transfusion reaction, care is centered on immediately stopping the transfusion, providing hemodynamic supportive care to counteract shock, and maximizing kidney perfusion.

In a patient in hemodynamically unstable condition, early invasive monitoring, vasopressors, and the promotion of diuresis with isotonic fluids and a loop diuretic (furosemide) are indicated. Dopamine in a renal dose regimen (2 to 4 μg/kg/min) may be helpful. Other treatments such as steroids, mannitol, or heparin are controversial due to the indecisive results of studies on their use.

High-flow oxygen should be administered, and administration of epinephrine and diphenhydramine should be considered to counteract the reactive process. Epinephrine and diphenhydramine are essential components of any anaphylactic treatment regimen, and should be administered according to local protocol.

YOU *are the Medic*   SUMMARY

1. Where in the body does leukemia develop?

Leukemia is a disease that develops in the lymphoid system. In this type of cancer, blood cells–particularly WBCs–develop abnormally and/or excessively.

2. What do you need to know about the patient's status?

The family and patient should be prepared to provide you with written documentation concerning the patient's status. The documentation should include the patient's information such as "code" status and what care should be provided to the patient. Many states have standard forms that are designed for use by medical care providers. Make sure you know the legal requirements for documentation of patients on home care for your area.

3. What is thrombocytopenia?

Thrombocytopenia is a decrease in the number of platelets. Leukemia can cause anemia, thrombocytopenia, and leukocytosis (increased WBCs). Chemotherapy used to treat leukemia typically leads to leukopenia (decreased WBCs).

YOU *are the Medic* | SUMMARY, *continued*

4. How will a patient with leukemia typically present?

Patients with leukemia experience frequent bleeding, bruising, infections, and fever.

5. Are you concerned with the patient's vital signs at this point?

Although the vital signs would commonly indicate shock or impending shock, they may be "normal" for this patient. Anemia can lead to an increased pulse rate and respirations as the body tries to compensate for the inadequate number of RBCs, which carry the hemoglobin, the oxygen-carrying component of blood. It is essential to carefully observe the patient's vital signs throughout your care and to contact medical control for advice about analgesic doses, but unless there is a substantial or sudden change, symptomatic treatment, such as oxygen, IV fluids, and analgesics, is sufficient.

6. What are "supportive measures" for this patient?

Management of this patient's care includes providing airway support and oxygen therapy as appropriate. Intravenous fluid therapy and analgesics for comfort may be needed as well. Patients need positive support because they may be discouraged about their condition, but be honest and do not give false hope.

7. What should you do for the patient's pain level?

You should consult your local protocol concerning the administration of analgesics to any patient under your care. With this particular patient, there should be consideration for the patient's vital signs. Consult with medical control for any direction you may need.

8. Do you think the patient's family has called you unnecessarily?

You should not think the call for service was unwarranted. The patient's loved ones are concerned, especially because the patient is in the advanced stages of the disease; be supportive to the family members as well as the patient. In some cases, you may be called because the patient's condition has deteriorated and the family is uncertain about what to do.

EMS Patient Care Report (PCR)

Date: 11-06-11	Incident No.: 9875	Nature of Call: General medical		Location: 11384 Castle Rock Road	
Dispatched: 1840	En Route: 1841	At Scene: 1845	Transport: 1908	At Hospital: 1918	In Service: 1940

Patient Information

Age: 73 Sex: M Weight (in kg [lb]): 59 kg (130 lb)	Allergies: No known drug allergies Medications: Numerous, see list Past Medical History: Leukemia Chief Complaint: Fever/body pain

Vital Signs

Time: 1850	BP: 100/60	Pulse: 100	Respirations: 20	Spo$_2$: 97%, room air
Time: 1855	BP: 98/60	Pulse: 100	Respirations: 20	Spo$_2$: 99%, with O$_2$
Time:	BP:	Pulse:	Respirations:	Spo$_2$:

EMS Treatment
(circle all that apply)

Oxygen @ __12__ L/min via (circle one): NC **(NRM)** Bag-mask device	Assisted Ventilation	Airway Adjunct	CPR
Defibrillation	Bleeding Control	Bandaging	Splinting	Other

Narrative

This unit dispatched to this address for a 73-year-old man with a history of leukemia. Pt is experiencing general body pain and a temperature of 102°F. Pt is receiving chemotherapy and had last treatment on 11-02-11. Pt is under home health agency care and has advance directive for supportive care only. Family presented appropriate written documentation verifying same. Family contacted home health agency and received instructions to reduce fever and manage the pt's pain. Family stated they became concerned when these measures were not effective and called 9-1-1 for response. Pt is conscious, alert, oriented, and cooperative. O$_2$ 12 L/min via NRM and IV established TKO. Pt agreed to transport to Downtown Hospital. Medical control contacted concerning administration of analgesic for pain, B/P is low. Medical control advised to administer 1 mg of morphine sulfate IV titrated to effect. Pain decreased, and pt rested comfortably during transport. Report to charge nurse on arrival. **End of report**

Prep Kit

- Most EMS systems rarely respond to hematologic emergencies.
- Blood performs respiratory, nutritional, excretory, regulatory, and defensive functions.
- Blood is made up of plasma and formed elements, or cells, including red blood cells, white blood cells, and platelets.
- Laboratory tests commonly performed on blood are red blood cell count, hemoglobin level, and hematocrit measurement.
- Blood tests that measure subtypes of white blood cells can provide valuable information about the status of the immune system.
- The ABO system is commonly used to classify blood types.
- During the primary assessment of a patient with a hematologic disorder, note any signs and symptoms that may be immediately life threatening.
- While taking a history and during the secondary assessment, look for changes in the level of consciousness such as vertigo, feelings of fatigue, or syncopal episodes.
- General management for any patient with problems related to a blood disorder should include the following elements: oxygen, fluids, ECG, transport, medications, and psychological support.
- Hematologic disorders include sickle cell crisis, anemia, leukopenia, thrombocytopenia, leukemia, lymphomas, polycythemia, DIC, hemophilia, multiple myeloma, and complications of blood transfusions.
- A patient experiencing a sickle cell crisis will experience significant pain due to congested vessels and may have a serious infection that can lead to sepsis and death.

- A patient with anemia has a hemoglobin or red blood cell level that is lower than normal. Anemia may be caused by an underlying hematologic or hemolytic disorder.
- Leukopenia is a reduction in the number of white blood cells and thrombocytopenia, a reduction in the number of platelets; both are conditions often seen in patients with anemia or leukemia.
- Leukemia is a type of cancer that affects the production of white blood cells. Patients often experience bleeding, bruising, infections, and fever.
- Lymphomas are a group of malignant disorders that arise within the lymphoid system. The two types are non-Hodgkin (making up the majority of cases) and Hodgkin lymphoma.
- Polycythemia is characterized by an overabundance or overproduction of red blood cells, causing hyperviscosity of the circulatory system.
- Disseminated intravascular coagulation (DIC) may result from a massive injury, sepsis, or obstetric complications. In the first stage, too much blood clotting results from an over-activated coagulation system. In the second stage, the body's natural reaction to breaking up these clots causes uncontrolled hemorrhage.
- Hemophilia is a bleeding disorder found primarily in the male population in which clotting does not occur or occurs insufficiently. Type A is due to a low level of factor VIII, and type B is due to a deficiency in factor IX.
- Multiple myeloma is a cancer of the bone marrow caused by malignant plasma cells.
- Complications of blood transfusions are similar to anaphylactic reactions and are caused by a mismatch of the patient's blood type to that received or an allergic reaction to preservatives or agents in the transfused product.

■ Vital Vocabulary

ABO system The commonly used blood classification system, based on the antigens present or absent in the blood.

acute chest syndrome A vasoocclusive crisis that can be associated with pneumonia; common signs and symptoms include chest pain, fever, and cough; associated with sickle cell disease.

acute splenic sequestration syndrome A condition in which red blood cells become trapped in the spleen, causing a dramatic fall in hemoglobin available in the circulation; usually occurs in infants or toddlers.

anemia A lower than normal hemoglobin or erythrocyte level.

antibodies Molecules in the body that react against foreign antigens in the body.

antigens Substances (usually protein) identified as foreign to the body.

aplastic crisis A temporary stop in the production of red blood cells; may occur as a result of sickle cell disease.

autoimmune disease A type of disease in which the body identifies its own antigen as a foreign body and activates the inflammatory system, sending out antibodies to destroy the antigen.

cell-mediated immunity The immune process in which macrophages and T cells attack and destroy pathogens or foreign substances.

clotting cascade The term that refers to the process by which clotting factors work together to ultimately form fibrin.

clotting factors Substances in the blood that are necessary for clotting; also called coagulation factors.

coagulation Clotting of the blood.

coagulopathy Any type of bleeding disorder that interferes with the activation or continuation of the clotting cascade or hemostasis.

disseminated intravascular coagulation (DIC) A life-threatening condition commonly found in severe trauma.

erythrocytes Red blood cells.

hematocrit The proportion of RBCs in total blood volume.

hematologic disorder Any disorder of the blood.

hematopoietic system The system that includes all blood components and the organs involved in their development and production.

hemoglobin The iron-rich protein in the blood that carries oxygen.

hemolytic crisis A condition in which red blood cells break down quickly; may occur as a result of sickle cell disease.

hemolytic disorder A disorder relating to the breakdown of RBCs.

hemophilia A bleeding disorder that is primarily hereditary, in which clotting does not occur or occurs insufficiently.

hemostasis The body's natural blood-clotting mechanism.

hemostatic disorder A bleeding and clotting abnormality.

humoral immunity The immune process in which antibodies recognize foreign antigens and stimulate an attack on the foreign body.

iron deficiency anemia The most common type of anemia in which iron stores are low or lacking and the serum iron concentration is low.

leukemia Cancer or malignancy of the blood-forming organs, particularly affecting the WBCs that develop abnormally and/or excessively at the expense of normal blood cells.

leukocytes White blood cells.

leukopenia A reduction in the number of WBCs.

lymphoblasts Lymphocytes transformed because of stimulation by an antigen.

lymphoid system The system primarily made up of the bone marrow, lymph nodes, and spleen that participates in formation of lymphocytes and immune responses.

lymphomas Malignant diseases that arise within the lymphoid system; includes non-Hodgkin and Hodgkin lymphomas.

melena Blood in the stool.

multiple myeloma A disease in which the number of plasma cells in the bone marrow increases abnormally, causing tumors to form in the bones.

neoplastic cells Another term for cancerous cells.

petechiae Tiny purple or red spots that appear on the skin due to bleeding within the skin or under mucous membranes.

plasma A component of blood, made of 92% water, 6% to 7% proteins, and electrolytes, clotting factors, and glucose; plasma makes up 55% of the total blood volume.

polycythemia An overabundance or production of RBCs, WBCs, and platelets.

pruritus Unspecified itching.

reticuloendothelial system The system in the body that is primarily used to defend against infection.

sickle cell crisis A condition in which a patient with sickle cell disease experiences significant pain due to insufficient passage of oxygen and nutrients into tissues and joints because of vessel congestion.

sickle cell disease A disease that causes the RBCs to be misshapen, resulting in poor oxygen-carrying capability and potentially resulting in lodging of the RBCs in blood vessels or the spleen.

splenic sequestration crisis An acute, painful enlargement of the spleen caused by sickle cell disease.

stem cells Cells that can develop into other types of cells in the body.

thalassemia A type of anemia in which not enough hemoglobin is produced, or the hemoglobin is defective.

thrombocytes Platelets.

thrombocytopenia A reduction in the number of platelets.

transfusion reactions A physiologic response that is similar to an anaphylactic reaction, in which the body reacts to the infusion of blood; occurs rapidly and can cause severe circulatory collapse and death.

transfusion-related lung injury A transfusion reaction characterized by increased pulmonary capillary permeability, resulting in noncardiogenic pulmonary edema.

vasoconstriction Narrowing of a blood vessel, such as with hypoperfusion or cold extremities.

vasoocclusive crisis Ischemia and pain caused by sickle-shaped red blood cells that obstruct blood flow to a portion of the body.

Assessment in Action

Your unit is transporting a patient on an interfacility transfer. Onboard you have an unresponsive patient who had a reaction to a blood transfusion. The patient was given the transfusion 6 hours ago during elective surgery.

1. Substances within the body that can activate the immune system are called:
   A. eosinophils.
   B. antigens.
   C. lymphocytes.
   D. antibodies.

2. Red blood cells are classified using the _____ system.
   A. ABO
   B. ABC
   C. RBC
   D. WBC

3. What is the secondary antigen carried in the blood?
   A. Inflammatory antigen
   B. RBC antigen
   C. ABO antigen
   D. Rh antigen

4. When you are assessing a patient whom you suspect is having a reaction to a blood transfusion, what condition will the signs and symptoms be similar to?
   A. Asthma
   B. Anaphylaxis
   C. Acute myocardial infarction
   D. Overdose

5. What are the three goals of treatment for a transfusion reaction?
   A. Stop transfusion, counteract shock, cardioversion
   B. Stop transfusion, counteract shock, kidney perfusion
   C. Stop transfusion, counteract shock, liver perfusion
   D. Stop transfusion, counteract shock, peripheral perfusion

6. What is the renal dose of dopamine?
   A. 2 to 4 µg/kg/min
   B. 4 to 10 µg/kg/min
   C. 10 to 20 µg/kg/min
   D. Greater than 20 µg/kg/min

Additional Questions

7. Is it true that sickle cell disease affects only the African American population?

8. How should you address analgesia with patients who have lymphoma?

Immunologic Emergencies

National EMS Education Standard Competencies

Medicine

Integrate assessment findings with principles of epidemiology and pathophysiology to formulate a field impression and implement a comprehensive treatment/disposition plan for a patient with a medical complaint.

Immunology

Recognition and management of shock and difficulty breathing related to

- Anaphylactic reactions (p 1275)

Anatomy, physiology, pathophysiology, assessment, and management of hypersensitivity disorders and/or emergencies

- Allergic and anaphylactic reactions (pp 1275-1277)

Anatomy, physiology, epidemiology, pathophysiology, psychosocial impact, presentations, prognosis, and management of common or major immunologic system disorders and/or emergencies

- Hypersensitivity (p 1265)
- Allergic and anaphylactic reactions (pp 1275-1277)
- Anaphylactoid reactions (p 1267)
- Collagen vascular diseases (pp 1267-1268, 1277-1279)
- Transplant-related problems (pp 1279-1280)

· ·

Knowledge Objectives

1. Describe the purpose of the immune system. (p 1268)
2. Discuss the process that begins when a foreign substance is detected in the body (primary response). (p 1269)
3. Explain the role of basophils and mast cells in the immune response process. (p 1269)
4. Explain the roles of chemical mediators including histamines and leukotrienes, in the immune response process. (pp 1269, 1273-1274)
5. Describe the process that occurs when the body undergoes a secondary response. (p 1270)

6. Discuss acquired immunity and natural immunity. (p 1270)
7. Understand and define the terms allergic reaction, anaphylaxis, and anaphylactoid reaction. (pp 1265-1267)
8. List and compare the signs and symptoms of an allergic reaction with those of anaphylaxis. (pp 1265-1267, 1275)
9. Describe the assessment process for a patient with an allergic reaction. (pp 1270-1271)
10. Explain the importance of managing the care of a patient who is having an allergic reaction. (pp 1275-1277)
11. Review the process for providing emergency medical care to a patient who is experiencing an allergic reaction. (pp 1275-1277)
12. Explain the factors involved when making a transport decision for a patient having an allergic reaction. (pp 1271, 1273, 1277)
13. Explain the difference between a local and a systemic response to allergens. (p 1265)
14. Explain the rationale, including communication and documentation considerations, when determining whether to administer epinephrine to a patient who is having an allergic reaction. (pp 1272, 1273, 1276, 1277)
15. Explain the various treatment options and pharmacologic interventions used to manage anaphylaxis. (pp 1275-1277)
16. Discuss autoimmune disorders and collagen vascular diseases, including systemic lupus erythematosus and scleroderma. (pp 1267-1268, 1277-1279)
17. Describe the principles of organ transplantation and disorders related to organ transplants. (pp 1279-1280)
18. Understand the importance of patient education in the management of anaphylaxis and allergic reactions. (p 1280)

Skills Objectives

1. Demonstrate how to remove a stinger from a bee sting and proper patient management following its removal. (p 1275)
2. Demonstrate how to use an EpiPen to deliver medication. (p 1277)
3. Demonstrate how to administer epinephrine using an auto-injector. (p 1277)

Introduction

Every year, at least 1,500 Americans die of acute allergic reactions. As much as 15% of the US population is at risk for experiencing an anaphylactic reaction, which can be fatal for approximately 1% of the people exposed. In dealing with allergy-related emergencies, you must be aware of the possibility of acute airway obstruction and cardiovascular collapse and be prepared to treat these life-threatening complications. You must also be able to distinguish between the body's usual response to a sting or bite and an allergic reaction, which may require epinephrine. Your ability to recognize and manage the many signs and symptoms of allergic reactions may be the only thing standing between life and imminent death for a patient.

This chapter begins by describing the physiology of the body's immune response and the pathophysiology of an allergic reaction—how an immune response can become a potentially life-threatening event. These problems include anaphylaxis, anaphylactoid reactions, allergic reactions, hypersensitivity, collagen vascular diseases, hypersensitivity, and transplant-related disorders.

The first task is to clarify the many terms associated with allergic and anaphylactic reactions. An **allergen** is a substance that produces allergic symptoms in a patient. Most allergens are usually harmless substances that do not pose a threat to other people—for example, milk, eggs, chocolate, and strawberries. An **antibody** is a protein the body produces in response to an **antigen**. This protein (globulin) is found in the plasma—hence, its other name *immunoglobulin* (Ig). **Table 1** lists the common antibodies, their actions, and locations.

An **allergic reaction** is an abnormal immune response the body develops when the person has been previously exposed or sensitized to a substance or allergen. In most people, exposure to this substance would not be a problem; in a person who is sensitive to this allergen, however, a local or systemic reaction may occur. In a **local reaction**, the body limits its response to a specific area after being exposed to a foreign substance; the swelling around an insect bite is an example. A **systemic reaction** occurs throughout the body, possibly affecting multiple body systems.

Table 1	Antibodies or Immunoglobulins	
Antibody	**Action**	**Location**
IgA	Provides localized protection to mucous membranes. Stress can lower the IgA level, making the body more susceptible to infection.	Tears, saliva, mucus, breast milk, gastrointestinal secretions, blood, and lymph
IgD	Thought to stimulate antibody-producing cells to make antibodies.	Blood, lymph, and the surface of B cells
IgE*	Responds in allergic reactions.	Located on mast and basophil cells
IgG	Provides protection against bacteria and viruses; enhances phagocytosis; neutralizes toxins; triggers the complement system.	Blood, lymph, and intestines
IgM	One of the first to appear; causes agglutination and lysis of microbes. ABO agglutinins are IgM antibodies.	Blood, lymph, and surface of B cells

*The IgE antibody is the primary antibody you need to be concerned with during allergic and anaphylactic reactions.

This reaction is seen when a person who is allergic to strawberries, for example, has swelling and hives all over his body after eating strawberry shortcake. **Hypersensitivity** occurs when a person reacts with exaggerated or inappropriate allergic symptoms after coming into contact with a substance perceived by the body to be harmful. **Anaphylaxis** is an extreme systemic form of an allergic reaction involving two or more body systems. This term was first used in 1902, when Portier and Richet were

YOU are the Medic   PART 1

Your unit is dispatched to a local restaurant for a man down. The dispatcher tells you that there is no further information because the call was made from the manager's office. When you enter the restaurant, you see the tables have been moved and a small male child is lying supine on the floor. The child appears to be about 2 years old and the parents are present. When you look at the child, his skin appears red and rashy, and his mouth looks swollen. The child is responsive but is not following you with his eyes as you enter the room.

1. What is your first impression of this patient?
2. What is your preliminary determination of the chief complaint?

Words of Wisdom

The term anaphylaxis is not really accurate; the fundamental problem in an anaphylactic reaction is not a lack of protection but rather overprotection. That is, anaphylaxis is a form of allergy—a very extreme and devastating form—and allergy represents the body's protective immune system gone overboard.

vaccinating dogs with sea anemone toxin. After the second dose of the toxin, one of the dogs died. Because this response was against protection, it was referred to as anaphylaxis (meaning "without protection").

Although it is estimated that millions of Americans are at risk for anaphylaxis, no exact cause for this life-threatening event can be determined in up to two thirds of patients. To anticipate anaphylaxis, of course, it would be useful to be able to identify people at greatest risk. Neither race nor gender seems to affect the incidence of anaphylaxis. The incidence of anaphylaxis from insect stings tends to be higher in men. Women have a greater incidence of anaphylactic reactions to latex, aspirin, and IV muscle relaxants. Anaphylactic reactions have been documented in children as young as 6 months and adults as old as 89 years. Children are more likely to have severe food allergies, whereas adults tend to have anaphylactic reactions to insect stings, anesthetics, and radiocontrast media. Table 2 lists the common substances associated with anaphylaxis.

Table 2 Common Causes of Anaphylactic Reactions

General Type of Antigen	Specific Antigen	Examples/Comments
Drugs	Penicillin (antibiotic)	Causes most IgE-mediated drug interactions in the United States.
	Beta-lactam antibiotics (cephalosporins)	Possibly a cross-reaction in patients allergic to penicillin.
	Other antibiotics	Ampicillin
	Sulfa drugs (antibiotic)	Sulfonamide, sulfisoxazole
	Muscle relaxants, hypnotics, opioids	Cyclobenzaprine, diazepam, acetaminophen with codeine, morphine, meperidine
	Salicylates	Aspirin
	Colloids	Albumin, hetastarch, dextran
	Local anesthetics	Procaine
	Enzymes	Chymotrypsin, penicillinase
	Mismatched blood transfusion	For example, providing A⁺ blood to a B⁻ recipient
	Iodinated radiocontrast dyes used in taking radiographs	IV pyelogram
	Biologic extracts and hormones	Insulin, heparin
	Vaccines	
Insect stings	Bees, yellow jackets, hornets, wasps, and fire ants	0.5%–3% of the population will have a systemic reaction after being stung.
Foods (problem worldwide—most common cause of anaphylaxis)	Peanuts	As little as 100 µg of peanut protein can cause a reaction.
	Tree nuts, fish, and shellfish	Most common to all age groups.
	Some fruits	Mango, strawberries
	Egg, soy, and milk	Most common in children.
Latex (may be seen in myelodysplasia, spina bifida, genitourinary anomalies, patients with frequent exposure to latex, and sensitized health care workers)	Gloves and other materials made from latex	The incidence rate is decreasing due to awareness and better manufacturing practices. People with allergies to bananas, kiwi, and strawberries may have a cross-reaction to latex.
Immunotherapy	Allergen immunotherapy, skin testing (Note: Patients with atopic diseases (diseases related to hypersensitivity and, therefore, allergies) are at greater risk for anaphylaxis.)	Rare, associated with asthma, errors in administration, overdose, and beta blocker use during immunotherapy.
Animals	Dander	Long-haired animals
	Animal serum products	Horse serum, gamma globulins

Adapted from Dreskin et al, Anaphylaxis, eMedicine, *www.emedicine.com/med/topic128.htm*. Accessed 5/26/06.

Words of Wisdom

EMS providers are required to be prepared for latex allergies in the field and to consider a latex-free or latex-safe environment. The National Institute for Occupational Safety and Health (NIOSH) offers publications on preventing allergic reactions to latex in the workplace.

Words of Wisdom

Anaphylaxis and anaphylactoid responses are clinically indistinguishable and should be treated in the same manner because both can be life threatening.

Diseases related to allergies, such as allergic rhinitis, asthma, and atopic dermatitis, increase the potential for anaphylactic reactions. One third to one half of patients with anaphylaxis have a history of these which are called atopic diseases.

The other major factors associated with anaphylaxis are the route of exposure to the allergen and time between exposures. It is important to note the route, though a severe reaction can occur by any route. Also, the longer the time between exposures to a substance, the less likely a severe anaphylactic reaction will occur. This is thought to be due to the decreased production of the specific immunoglobulin (Ig) or antibody cells in the body over time.

Anaphylaxis is classified as a response mediated by IgE antibodies, while an __anaphylactoid reaction__ is a response that does not involve IgE antibody mediation. The exact mechanism is unknown, but an anaphylactoid event may occur without the patient being previously exposed to the offending agent. Examples of causes of anaphylactic reactions are nuts, fish, and latex. Anaphylactoid causes include some contrasts given before radiography, morphine-derivative medications, and aspirin. Even though the process that causes the reaction is different, the patient presentation is the same.

In anaphylaxis and allergic reactions, the body responds to a foreign invader as the enemy, but not so with collagen vascular diseases. __Collagen vascular diseases__ are considered autoimmune, which means that the body perceives its own tissues or cells—in this case collagen tissue—as a dangerous invader and sets out to attack that tissue. The attack can be chronic, causing long-term inflammation, or severe enough to result in death. This chapter addresses two collagen vascular diseases: systemic lupus erythematosus and scleroderma.

__Systemic lupus erythematosus__ (SLE or lupus) is a multisystem autoimmune disease that occurs more commonly in women than men. In the United States, 5.1 cases per 100,000 are diagnosed yearly. African American women are four times more likely to have lupus than Caucasian women, and Asian women have a higher incidence of lupus than Caucasian women as well. Lupus is most often diagnosed in young women, particularly young African American women of childbearing age, and can be a debilitating and life-threatening problem. In lupus, multiple systems are under attack—dermatologic, renal, neurologic, cardiac, pulmonary, gastrointestinal, and hematologic—and the disease may also result in rheumatologic problems. The survival rate has improved over the years to 15 years and is expected for 80% of patients. Patients with lupus tend to die of infections and complications of the disease if they are diagnosed in their 20s; death is often the result of a myocardial infarction or stroke if they are diagnosed after age 35. Paramedics, therefore, should assess for these life threats when caring for patients with lupus.

__Scleroderma__ (*sclero* meaning hard and *derma* meaning skin) is an autoimmune connective tissue disease that causes fibrotic (scar tissue–like) changes to the skin, blood vessels, muscles, and

YOU are the Medic   PART 2

While your partner sets up the oxygen equipment to start treating the child, you ask the parents what happened. The mother states that her son was eating french fries when he started choking. She opened his mouth and did not see anything. She noticed the child's mouth appeared to be swelling and he was getting a rash. You ask if this had ever happened before, and she said "yes," but only with seafood. She assures you that he did not eat any seafood today.

Recording Time: 0 Minutes	
Appearance	Awake
Level of consciousness	Not alert
Airway	Open
Breathing	Audible wheezing without stethoscope
Circulation	Adequate

3. What is your determination of the patient's condition now?

4. Can this be an allergic reaction if the child did not consume seafood?

internal organs. There are two types of scleroderma—localized and systemic. Of the estimated 300,000 cases of scleroderma in the United States, one third are the systemic form of the disease. Children are more likely to have localized scleroderma, whereas adults tend to have the systemic form. Women have a higher incidence of scleroderma than men. Patients with scleroderma are at greatest risk of dying from organ damage during the first 3 years after skin symptoms begin. The life-threatening complications of scleroderma involve the lungs, heart, and kidneys, so assessment should focus on these systems.

With lupus and scleroderma, the patient's condition stems from the body attacking itself because of an overactive immune system. Treatment may include the administration of medications to *suppress* the immune system and decrease the attack.

Patients who have had organ transplants also receive immune system suppression medications, but for a very different reason—they have received an organ from an outside source; the body recognizes the transplanted organ as foreign and tries to destroy or reject it. Suppression of the immune system is key to the survival of these patients. The overall 1-year survival rate for solid organ transplant recipients is 80%. Solid organ transplants include the heart, liver, kidney, pancreas, and lungs. In the United States, the most common organ transplant is the kidney. No matter what type of transplant the patient has received, the EMS provider must understand the anatomic considerations and must be prepared to identify signs of rejection, infection, and medication toxicity.

When the body receives a new organ, the organ comes without its previous connections and message-relaying ability. This means that the organ may not behave "normally" when it is having problems. Pain is one of the symptoms; the organ cannot relay information to its new host, so pain, such as angina, is not a reliable indicator of problems as it may have been previously. In addition, the new organs will be tethered to the structures in the body such as blood vessels, other organs, and tissues. Knowing where and how an organ is placed and attached may also be useful in identifying problems.

With any organ transplant, infection is the greatest threat to survival, so you must be constantly aware of the potential for infection. Rejection of the organ immediately after the surgery is less common than in the past because of improved donor-recipient matching. It is essential that patients take their immunosuppressant medications. The failure to take even one dose may result in rejection of the organ. Drug toxicity is also a problem for transplant patients. The three common medications administered are outlined in Table 3. You should be aware of the medications and possible effects with each.

■ Anatomy and Physiology

■ The Normal Immune Response

The immune system protects the human body from substances and organisms that are considered foreign. Without your immune system for protection, life as you know it would not exist. You would be under constant attack from any bacterium,

Table 3	Drug Toxicity With Immunosuppressant Medications
Cyclosporine	Multiple drug interactions ■ Erythromycin and ketoconazole increase the effect and the potential for toxicity ■ Rifampin increases metabolism, which can cause episodes of organ rejection Toxic effects ■ Renal toxicity ■ Liver toxicity ■ Hyperkalemia ■ Hirsutism (hair growth where hair does not typically grow) ■ Tremor ■ Gingival hyperplasia
Azathioprine	Toxic effects ■ It is a bone marrow toxin that can cause a decrease in white blood cell count ■ Liver dysfunction ■ Gastrointestinal disturbances
Corticosteroids	Toxic effects ■ Osteoporosis ■ Cataracts ■ Gastrointestinal bleeding ■ Glucose intolerance ■ Bone disease ■ Adrenal suppression

virus, or other type of invader that wanted to make your body their home. Luckily, for the majority of the population, the body is equipped with an amazing immune system that is on patrol 24 hours a day, 7 days a week, to detect unauthorized visits or invading attacks by foreign substances.

The body protects itself via two types of systems: cellular immunity and humoral (that is, related to the body's fluids) immunity. In **cellular immunity**, also called *cell-mediated immunity*, the body produces special white blood cells called T cells that attack and destroy invaders. In **humoral immunity**, B cell lymphocytes produce antibodies that dissolve in the plasma and lymph to wage war on invading organisms. The cells producing immunity are located throughout the body in the lymph nodes, spleen, and gastrointestinal tract. Their goal is to intercept foreign forces as they enter the body, thereby limiting the spread and damage of invaders.

■ Routes of Entry for Allergens

Substances can invade the body through the skin, the respiratory tract, or the gastrointestinal tract. Invasion through the skin may come in the form of injection or absorption. In **injection**, the invading substance pierces the skin and deposits foreign material into the skin. Bees and hornets are often the cause of this type of invasion. <u>Absorption</u> occurs when foreign material is deposited on the skin and slowly absorbed through the skin. Invasion by allergens does not stop at the skin; they may also enter the respiratory tract as the patient quietly breathes. This is referred to as an <u>inhalation</u> exposure. The foreign substance advances through the respiratory system and launches its attack from the lungs. Cat hair and dander, peanuts, and many plants are involved in this type of exposure. The final way allergens attack the body is through the gastrointestinal tract via <u>ingestion</u>. Foods such as strawberry shortcake, a mushroom and cheese omelet, or a peanut butter pie, can cause an allergic reaction.

Physiology

Once a foreign substance invades the body, the body goes on alert and initiates a series of responses. The first encounter with the foreign substance begins the <u>primary response</u>. Cells (macrophages) immediately confront and engulf the invaders to determine if they are allowed in the body. If the body is unable to identify the substance, it uses immune cells to record the salient features of the outside substance. These cells record one or two of the proteins on the surface of the invading substance and then design specific proteins to match each substance. These proteins—called antibodies—are intended to match up with the invader—the antigen—and inactivate it.

Through the primary response, the body develops <u>sensitivity</u>—that is, the ability to recognize the foreigner the next time it is encountered. To determine whether the substance is "one of us," the body records enough details to assist in future identification of the substance and production of antibodies to perfectly fit the invading antigen. The body then sends out these details to the rest of the body. These details are distributed by placing the specific antibodies on two types of cells: <u>basophils</u> and <u>mast cells</u>. Basophils are stationed in specific sites within the tissues. Mast cells are on patrol through the connective tissues, bronchi, gastrointestinal mucosa, and other vulnerable border areas that act as barriers to foreign invaders.

The basophils and mast cells produce the body's "chemical weapons"—that is, <u>chemical mediators</u> Table 4. These cells contain granules filled with a host of powerful substances that are ready to be released to fight invading forces of antigens. As long as the body is not invaded by one of the previously identified foreign substances, the granules are kept encapsulated in their protective walls and remain inactive. If an antigen invades the body and combines with one of the antibodies, however, the granules are ejected from the mast cells and detonated. The chemical mediators are then released into the surrounding tissue and the bloodstream Figure 1.

The chemical mediators launch and maintain the immune response. They summon more white blood cells to the area to battle the invading force. They also increase blood flow to the area under attack by dilating the blood vessels and increasing the capillary permeability. These actions are useful when a small invasion occurs to a limited area but can be extremely

Table 4 **Chemical Mediators**

Mediator	Physiologic Effects
Histamine	■ Systemic vasodilation ■ Increased permeability of blood vessels ■ Decreased cardiac contractility ■ Decreased coronary blood flow ■ Dysrhythmias ■ Bronchoconstriction ■ Pulmonary vasoconstriction
Eosinophil chemotactic factor	■ Attracts eosinophils and neutrophils
Arachidonic acid (precursor of the following):	These factors act to produce other inflammatory mediators:
Prostaglandin	■ Smooth muscle contraction

Leukotrienes (slow-reacting substance of anaphylaxis [SRS-A])	■ Vascular permeability
	■ Bronchoconstriction
	■ Decreased force of cardiac contraction
	■ Decreased coronary blood flow
	■ Dysrhythmias
	  - More potent than histamine (thousands of times)
	  - React more slowly than histamine

Platelet-activating factor	■ Platelet aggregation ■ Causes histamine release
Serotonin	■ Pulmonary vasoconstriction ■ Bronchoconstriction
Proteoglycans:	
Heparin Chondroitin sulfate	■ Control the release of histamine. These mediators as a whole work to activate the kinin system and are thought to contribute to prolonged and biphasic reactions.
Chemokines Cytokines	■ These mediators trigger inflammatory pathways and increase the recruitment of inflammatory cells.
Kinins	■ Bradykinin is one of the stronger kinins and is responsible for increased vascular permeability.

dangerous when they spread throughout the body. When they have systemic effects, the chemical mediators cause the signs and symptoms of the allergic and anaphylactic reactions seen in the body.

As health care providers, you exploit the body's ability to protect itself. For example, you administer vaccines to produce <u>immunity</u> against a disease. The body develops antibodies in

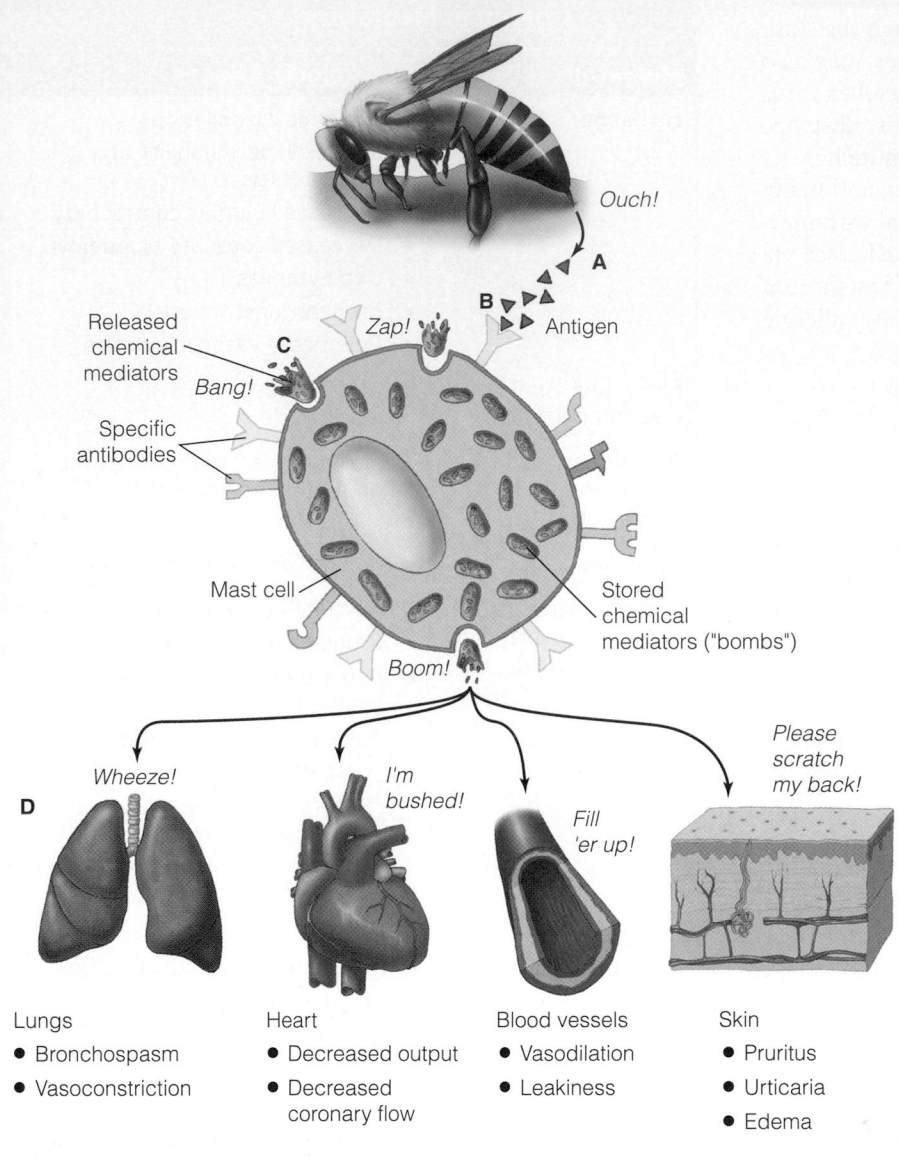

Ouch!

Released chemical mediators

Zap!

A

B Antigen

C

Specific antibodies

Bang!

Mast cell

Stored chemical mediators ("bombs")

Boom!

D

Wheeze!

I'm bushed!

Fill 'er up!

Please scratch my back!

Lungs
- Bronchospasm
- Vasoconstriction

Heart
- Decreased output
- Decreased coronary flow

Blood vessels
- Vasodilation
- Leakiness

Skin
- Pruritus
- Urticaria
- Edema

Figure 1 The sequence of events in anaphylaxis. **A.** The antigen is introduced into the body. **B.** The antigen-antibody reaction at the surface of a mast cell. **C.** Release of mast cell chemical mediators. **D.** Chemical mediators exert their effects on end organs.

traces of the invasion. This intense response to the invading virus is called the **secondary response**. Meanwhile, the "contaminated," immunized person remains unaware of the battle raging inside his or her body.

This battle is termed **acquired immunity**. In this type of immunity, the administration of a vaccine allows the body to produce antibodies without having to experience the disease. Vaccinations against measles, mumps, and polio are examples of acquired immunity. In **natural immunity**, by contrast, the body encounters the antigen and experiences a full immune response with all the pathology of the disease. Having the measles, for example, causes the body to produce antibodies to this pathogen, but the drawback is that the person has the itching, rash, and high fever associated with the disease.

Use of the polio vaccine has resulted in herd immunity, which occurs when a group of persons are immunized against a substance. This immunization protects the entire group by decreasing the number of people able to contract the disease, thus protecting all members of the group. Other vaccines that have led to herd immunity include measles, mumps and rubella, as well as pertussis. Herd immunity can be lost when there is a decrease in pediatric immunizations.

Patient Assessment

Scene Size-up

Assess the scene for safety issues—an angry swarm of bees may put you and the patient at risk. Once you have ensured that the scene is safe, you should determine the nature of the illness by observing for any potential exposure problems. For example, if the patient was gardening, a bee sting might be a cause of the problem. Dinner at a seafood restaurant might make you suspicious of the shellfish menu items or food fried in peanut oil. Because anaphylaxis is a life-threatening event, taking the time to survey the scene for potential hazards for anaphylaxis is important.

Primary Assessment

A patient may have bite or sting marks that may accompany other signs and symptoms of an allergic reaction. Allergic symptoms are almost as varied as the allergens themselves. Your assessment of a patient experiencing an allergic reaction should include evaluations of the level of consciousness, the

response to the vaccine so it can produce an immune response to neutralize the invading disease before it can establish itself and damage the body. Thus, the body develops antibodies in a controlled way. When the hepatitis B vaccine is administered, for example, a small amount of the hepatitis B virus (HBV) enters the body. The body identifies this virus and produces antibodies to it; these antibodies are then distributed throughout the body. Should an immunized person later be exposed to HBV, the virus will invade the body. Once in the body, the virus begins to set up residency and reproduce. At this point, the wandering immune cell identifies the HBV as something that does not belong in the area. The alarm is sounded, and the body begins aggressive production of the "antihepatitis" antibodies, sending them in to kill the HBV and clean up residual

respiratory system, the circulatory system, mental status, and the skin. As mentioned earlier, allergic reactions can range from local to systemic. They can be categorized as mild, moderate, or severe. Mild reactions affect a local area of the body and do not spread to other areas. Itchy, watery eyes or a rash are examples of a mild reaction. Slight congestion would also be considered a mild reaction. Moderate reactions begin as mild reactions, but the symptoms do spread to other parts of the body. For example, your patient initially reports itchy, watery eyes and then develops tightness in the chest with trouble breathing. Severe reactions are considered anaphylactic reactions, and they result in potentially life-threatening emergencies. Severe reactions are systemic; for example, the patient may report congestion that progresses to respiratory distress, and hypotension. Onset may be sudden and affect the entire body.

Form a General Impression

Observe the patient. The patient's presentation will give you an indication of the severity of the problem. Does the patient's condition appear stable or unstable? If the patient is unable to speak, assess the airway for patency before assuming a neurologic problem. Level of consciousness is an indicator of the patient's severity and a reflection of the patient's oxygenation and circulatory status. Restlessness, confusion, anxiety, and combativeness are common signs of hypoxia. As the carbon dioxide levels rise and oxygen levels diminish, the patient will become less responsive. Any change in mental status in an anaphylactic patient should direct you to immediate airway evaluation and management.

Breathing and Airway

A noisy upper airway is a concern in any patient, but even more so in an anaphylactic patient because it may be an early sign of impending airway occlusion due to swelling.

You should listen for stridor and hoarseness. In addition, the patient may report a tight feeling or a "lump in the throat." Observe the patient for tachypnea, labored breathing, accessory muscle use, abnormal retractions, and prolonged expiration. The severity of these findings predicts the stability of the patient's condition. Lung sounds are also a predictor of severity. Initially, you will hear wheezing. As the patient's condition deteriorates and the lungs become tighter and less ventilated (hypoventilation), the diminished lung sounds will be present and the chest may become silent. A silent chest is an ominous finding.

Circulation

Evaluate the skin for erythema, rashes, edema, moisture, pruritis, and urticaria. These symptoms are more commonly associated with an anaphylactic reaction due to histamine release. Pallor and cyanosis may be present as well.

Transport Decision

As you are completing the primary assessment, you should be making the decision whether to remain on the scene, load the patient and initiate treatment in the vehicle, begin immediate transport, or even call for air transport. In addition, you should be determining which facility the patient should be transported to based on the patient's need for services.

■ History Taking

The patient history should include investigation of the chief complaint, SAMPLE, and OPQRST. The history should be specifically directed at this incident. Some steps may be skipped or collected later if a life threat exists. Does the patient have any allergies? Has the patient ever had an allergic or anaphylactic

---

YOU *are the Medic* | **PART 3** |

Your partner administers oxygen to the patient, who appears very drowsy. The audible wheezing you were hearing is becoming quiet and the patient's face is swelling more. The father hands you an adult EpiPen and tells you that, although this auto-injector belongs to him, it was the only one he had with him at the time because he also has allergies, so he used it on his child.

Recording Time: 5 Minutes	
Respirations	36 breaths/min, very shallow
Pulse	150 beats/min
Skin	Red, warm, dry
Blood pressure	90/58 mm Hg
Oxygen saturation (Spo$_2$)	92% on room air
Pupils	Equal and reactive

5. What is the difference between an adult EpiPen and an EpiPen Jr?

6. What effect can you expect the adult EpiPen to have on this patient?

reaction? If so, how severe was the incident and how rapidly did it progress? Comparing it to this incident by asking how severe this incident is and how rapidly it is progressing is a useful tool as well. You may want to interview the patient to determine whether he or she had a previous exposure to the antigen; for example, if the patient just ate peanuts, asking about previous ingestions may be useful. A severe reaction may occur at the second exposure to an antigen, so the patient might not know about the allergy. Asking about medications, in particular new medications, may help identify the antigen.

In anaphylactoid reactions, a previous exposure may not be present. In some cases, you may not be able to identify the offending antigen. When in doubt, in the presence of a severe reaction, intervention takes precedence over identifying the antigen. To help determine where the patient is in the reaction process, ask when the symptoms began. Because the airway is a major concern, ask about feelings of dyspnea.

You should also determine whether the patient or first responders have administered any treatment before your arrival. This may include using an EpiPen, taking diphenhydramine (Benadryl), or using an inhaler with a beta-agonist (such as albuterol or metaproterenol) or aerosolized epinephrine (such as Primatene Mist or racemic epinephrine) **Figure 2** . If the patient has an EpiPen or used one, be aware that some EpiPens come with two doses. Do not discard the second dose.

◼ Secondary Assessment

Physical Examinations

Next, perform a physical examination. The classic presentation of anaphylaxis includes respiratory symptoms and hypotension. Gastrointestinal symptoms such as abnormal cramping, nausea, vomiting, and diarrhea may be present. If the patient is identified as having life-threatening problems, a physical examination should be performed; however, it should be done en route to the hospital.

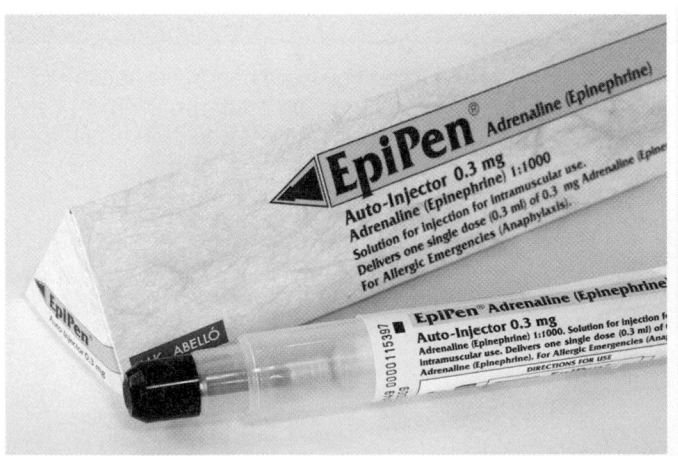

Figure 2 Patients who experience severe allergic reactions often carry their own epinephrine, which comes predosed in an auto-injector or a standard syringe. An EpiPen® auto-injector is shown here.

The secondary assessment may help direct treatment. As in all emergencies, your assessment of a patient experiencing an allergic reaction should include a systematic head-to-toe or focused assessment to determine hidden trauma or other unrelated medical problems.

Perform evaluations of the respiratory system. Thoroughly assess breathing, including increased work of breathing, use of accessory muscles, head bobbing, tripod positioning, nostril flaring, and grunting. Carefully auscultate the trachea and the chest.

Wheezing may be present during an allergic reaction. It occurs because excessive fluid and mucus are secreted into the bronchial passages, and muscles around these passages tighten in response to the release of histamines and leukotrienes induced by the allergen. Exhalation, normally the passive, relaxed phase of breathing, becomes increasingly difficult as the patient tries to cough up the secretions or move air past the constricted airways. The combination of fluid in the air passages and the constricted bronchi produce the wheezing sound. Breathing rapidly becomes more difficult, and the patient may even stop breathing. Prolonged respiratory difficulty can cause a rapid heartbeat (tachycardia), shock, respiratory failure, and death. Stridor, a harsh, high-pitched inspiratory sound, occurs when swelling in the upper airway (near the vocal cords and throat) closes off the airway and can eventually lead to total obstruction.

Assess the circulatory system. Remember, the presence of hypoperfusion (shock) or respiratory distress indicates that the patient is having a severe enough allergic reaction that death can result.

Carefully assess the skin for swelling, rash, hives, and signs of the source of the reaction: bite, sting, or contact marks. A rapidly spreading rash can be concerning because it may indicate a systemic reaction. Red, hot skin may also indicate a systemic reaction as the blood vessels lose their ability to constrict and blood moves to the extremities. If this reaction continues, the body will have difficulty supplying blood and oxygen to the vital organs, and one of the first signs will be altered mental status as the organs are deprived of oxygen and glucose.

Vital Signs

Vital signs help determine whether the body is compensating for stress. Assess baseline vital signs, including pulse, respirations, blood pressure, skin, pupils, and oxygen saturation. Rapid, labored breathing indicates airway obstruction. Rapid respiratory and pulse rates may indicate respiratory distress or systemic shock. Fast pulse rates and hypotension are ominous signs, indicating systemic vascular collapse and shock. Skin signs may be an unreliable indicator of hypoperfusion because of rashes and swelling.

Monitoring Devices

You should use tools such as a cardiac monitor in your assessment because dysrhythmias may be associated with anaphylaxis. A 12-lead ECG should be considered during the assessment to monitor for cardiac ischemia. End-tidal carbon dioxide levels should be monitored because they may be elevated in anaphylaxis. Watch for a "shark fin" waveform on the $ETCO_2$

monitor, which is due to bronchoconstriction. Monitoring by pulse oximetry may alert you to low oxygen saturation, which will assist in identifying the degree of respiratory distress. However, it is important to remember that pulse oximetry is just another tool in your tool box. Factors such as decreased circulation and exposure to carbon monoxide can alter pulse oximetry readings. The decision to administer oxygen to a patient experiencing an allergic reaction should be based on a careful assessment of the patient's airway and breathing, not solely on the pulse oximetry readings.

Reassessment

Reassessment is conducted typically en route to the emergency department. A patient experiencing a suspected allergic reaction should be monitored with vigilance because deterioration of the patient's condition can be rapid and fatal. Special attention should be given to any signs of airway compromise, including increasing work of breathing, stridor, and wheezing. The patient's anxiety level should be monitored because increased anxiety is a good indication that the reaction may be progressing. Also, watch the skin for signs of shock, including pallor and diaphoresis, as well as for flushing because of vascular collapse. Serial vital signs are important indicators when evaluating your patient's status. Any increase in the respiratory or pulse rate or decrease in blood pressure should be noted. Finally, reassess the chief complaint.

Interventions

To treat allergic reactions, you must first identify how much distress the patient is experiencing. Some allergic reactions will produce severe signs and symptoms in a matter of minutes and threaten the patient's life. Other allergic reactions have a slower onset and cause less severe distress. Epinephrine and ventilatory support are required for severe reactions. Milder reactions, without respiratory or cardiovascular distress, may require only supportive care, such as oxygen. In either situation, the patient should be transported to a medical facility for further evaluation.

Recheck your interventions. If you administered epinephrine, what was the effect? Is the patient's condition improving? Do you need to consider a second dose? You may need to give more than one injection of epinephrine if you note that the patient has decreasing mental status, increased breathing difficulty, or a decreasing blood pressure. Be sure to consult medical control first. Identify and treat changes in the patient's condition.

In case of anaphylaxis, check interventions (such as the need for another dose of epinephrine, oxygen therapy, Trendelenburg position for patients in anaphylaxis with hypotension, and reassessment of the patient's lung sounds). When the patient has a mild anaphylactic reaction, the patient may be placed in the semi-Fowler position.

During transport, you will call in the report on the patient to the receiving facility. With a severe condition, the more time you can give the staff at the facility to prepare for the patient, the better. You will want to communicate the patient's status, interventions completed, the patient's response to interventions, and an estimated time of arrival. Once your transport is complete, documentation of the call should not only include the signs and symptoms found during your assessment, but also clearly show why you chose to provide the care you did. A written handoff report is important to ensure accurate information on the status of the patient and the care you provided.

Pathophysiology, Assessment, and Management of Specific Emergencies

Anaphylactic Reactions

Pathophysiology

An ever-watchful and responsive immune system is essential to life and health. Unfortunately, sometimes the immune system becomes overzealous in defending the body. The resulting problems may range in severity from hay fever to anaphylaxis and exist along the spectrum from a simple annoyance to a life-threatening crisis. During these abnormal reactions, the immune system becomes hypersensitive to one or more substances. The body often has these reactions to substances that should not be identified as harmful by the immune system—substances such as ragweed, strawberries, and penicillin **Figure 3** . The immune cells of the allergic person are more sensitive than the immune cells of a person without allergies. Although these cells are able to recognize and react to dangerous invaders such as bacteria and viruses, they also identify harmless substances as posing a threat.

When the invading substance enters the body, the mast cells recognize it as potentially harmful and begin releasing chemical mediators. **Histamine**, one of the primary chemical weapons, causes the blood vessels in the local area to dilate and the capillaries to leak. Leukotrienes, which are even more powerful, are released and cause additional dilation and leaking. White blood

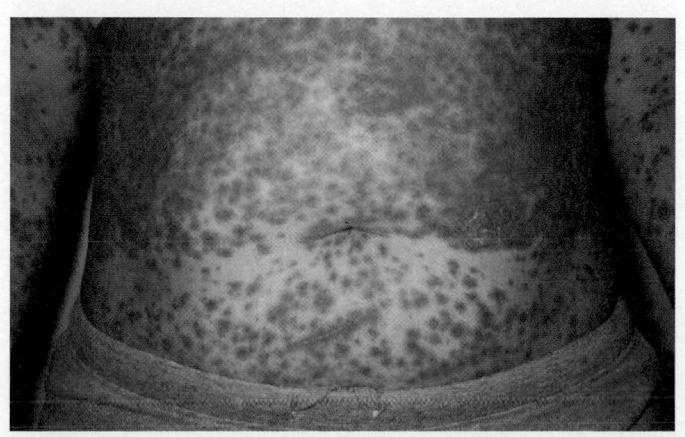

Figure 3 A severe allergic reaction to medication. This patient was allergic to penicillin and most other antibiotics.

cells are called to the area to help engulf and destroy the enemy, and platelets begin to collect and clump together. In most cases, this overreaction to harmless invaders is usually restricted to the local area being invaded. The runny, itchy nose and swollen eyes associated with hay fever are examples of a local allergic reaction.

In the case of anaphylaxis, the person is not so lucky. Chemical mediators are released, and the effect involves more than one system throughout the body. An initial effect may be seen from the histamine release, with secondary effects following a few hours later when the remainder of the chemicals are released.

Histamine release causes immediate vasodilation, which often presents as erythematous skin and hypotension. It also increases vascular permeability, which results in edema, fluid secretion, and fluid loss. The edema can present as urticaria **Figure 4** , airway constriction, and increased fluids in the airway. Histamine likewise causes smooth muscle contraction, especially in the respiratory system and gastrointestinal system. This results in laryngospasm or bronchospasm and abdominal cramping. Finally, histamine decreases the inotropic effects of the heart. When this effect is coupled with vasodilation, the person may experience profound hypotension. Dysrhythmias due to hypoperfusion and hypoxia are also common.

Later responses from the much more powerful leukotrienes compound the effects of histamine. The person's respiratory status will become even more dire as these highly potent bronchoconstrictors are released. In addition, leukotriene release causes coronary vasoconstriction, which contributes to a worsening cardiac condition and myocardial irritability. Leukotrienes are also associated with increased vascular permeability, contributing to a further state of hypoperfusion.

The remaining chemical mediators continue to worsen the situation as they undertake what they see as steps to protect the body from this foreign invader. As a result of these activities, when the body undergoes an anaphylactic reaction, it may not survive without immediate intervention.

Clinical Symptoms of Anaphylaxis

The skin is the body's first line of defense against would-be invaders, so skin symptoms are often the first indications of anaphylaxis. Initially, the person may be aware of feeling warm and flushed. <u>Pruritus</u> (itching) is another early sign that is due to vasodilation and capillary leaking. The area around the eyes is often susceptible to this effect, which causes swollen, red eyes. Swelling of the face and tongue (angioedema) may contribute to airway compromise. Edema of the hands and feet may also be noted. Histamine is responsible for the <u>urticaria</u> (hives) experienced by the patient with anaphylaxis.

The most common complaints are usually respiratory symptoms, which often present as shortness of breath or dyspnea and tightness in the throat and chest. Stridor and/or hoarseness may also be noted. These signs and symptoms are often due to upper airway swelling in the laryngeal and epiglottic areas. Affected patients may report a lump in the throat. The lower airway is often involved as well. Bronchoconstriction and increased secretions may result in wheezes and crackles. It is not uncommon for the patient to cough or sneeze as the body tries to clear the airway. These symptoms may progress slowly or alarmingly fast. You may have only 1 to 3 minutes to halt this rapid, life-threatening process.

Cardiovascular symptoms are serious complications of anaphylaxis. As noted earlier, histamine and leukotrienes work directly on the heart to decrease its contractility. The resulting decrease in cardiac output is complicated by vasodilation and increased capillary permeability, which further decrease the amount of fluid returned to the heart. As cardiac output declines, perfusion decreases, leading to ischemia and bringing the potential for cardiac dysrhythmias. As the fluid leaks out of the capillaries, the intravascular system is left short on fluid. (As much as 50% of the vascular volume can be shifted to the extravascular space within 10 minutes of exposure to an antigen.) Instead of responding normally to the fluid loss and constricting, the blood vessels do just the opposite: they dilate. The already low vascular volume becomes totally inadequate, and hypotension reigns. In response to the low blood pressure, the heart rate increases, putting stress on an already compromised heart. In this situation, tachycardia, flushed skin, and hypotension are synonymous with anaphylactic shock.

Gastrointestinal symptoms may also be part of an anaphylactic response, particularly if the offending antigen has been ingested. Abdominal cramping is a common presentation, but nausea, bloating, vomiting, abdominal distention, and profuse, watery diarrhea may also be present.

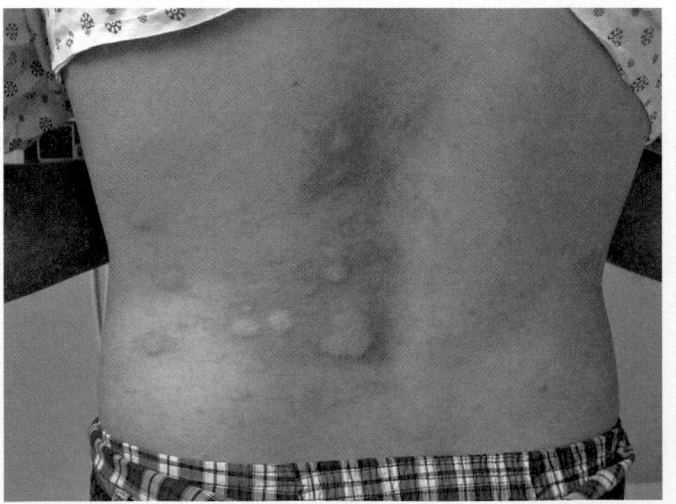

Figure 4 Urticaria, or hives, may appear following a sting and are characterized by multiple, small, raised areas on the skin.

Words of Wisdom

Flushing (from vasodilation) and tachycardia are so characteristic of anaphylactic shock that it is very questionable to make the diagnosis without these two signs being present.

Patients may present with central nervous system symptoms in response to decreased cerebral perfusion and hypoxia. These symptoms include headache, dizziness, confusion, and anxiety. A sense of "impending doom" aptly represents the patient's sense of being near death. A patient who expresses a sense of impending doom requires rapid assessment and treatment.

Table 5 summarizes the signs and symptoms of anaphylaxis. Anaphylaxis may present as affecting any two or more of these body systems, so the picture can be confusing at times. Think of a patient with anaphylaxis as experiencing three types of shock: (1) cardiogenic shock due to decreased cardiac output, (2) hypovolemic shock due to fluids leaking into the tissues, and (3) neurogenic shock due to inability of the blood vessels to constrict. You will need to use your assessment skills to identify the potential for anaphylaxis and take aggressive action to manage the patient and stop the anaphylactic process as rapidly as possible.

Assessment

Assessment of a patient with an anaphylactic reaction can be highly challenging. You may have to simultaneously assess the patient, identify the problem, and intervene within seconds of arriving on the scene to save the patient's life. Index of suspicion for anaphylaxis must be high on your list if any of the symptoms discussed previously are present. You may not have a second opportunity because the patient's condition may deteriorate before your eyes.

Management

People having allergic reactions are separated into two groups for management purposes. The first group includes patients who have signs of an allergic reaction—for example, hives—but no respiratory distress or dyspnea. The drug of choice is diphenhydramine (Benedryl). Continue to monitor for changes in the patient's condition, but most patients in this group will recover with no further problems.

The second group includes patients with signs of an allergic reaction and dyspnea. These patients require oxygen, epinephrine, and antihistamines (usually diphenhydramine [Benedryl]). Whenever dyspnea is present with signs of an allergic reaction, you should administer epinephrine and monitor the patient for the development of anaphylaxis.

Remove the offending agent. When possible, remove the patient from the situation involving the antigen or the antigen from the patient. For example, if the patient is allergic to peanuts and is being exposed to peanuts through inspiration, you may need to remove the patient from the room because you may not be able to eliminate the peanut allergen from the air. If the patient has a stinger from a bee sting still in place, you will need to remove the stinger. Remember to scrape the stinger off because you can inject more venom into the patient if you pinch or squeeze the stinger Figure 5.

Table 5 Signs and Symptoms of Anaphylaxis*	
System	**Signs and Symptoms**
Skin	■ Warm ■ Flushed ■ Itching (pruritus) ■ Swollen, red eyes ■ Swelling of the face and tongue ■ Swelling of the hands and feet ■ Hives (urticaria)
Respiratory	■ **Dyspnea** ■ Tightness in the throat and chest ■ Stridor ■ Hoarseness ■ Lump in throat ■ Wheezes ■ Crackles ■ Coughing ■ Sneezing
Cardiovascular	■ Dysrhythmias ■ **Hypotension** ■ **Tachycardia**
Gastrointestinal	■ Abdominal cramping ■ Nausea ■ Bloating ■ Vomiting ■ Abdominal distention ■ Profuse, watery diarrhea
Central nervous	■ Headache ■ Dizziness ■ Confusion ■ Anxiety and restlessness ■ Sense of impending doom ■ Altered mental status
*Key indicators are represented by bold type.	

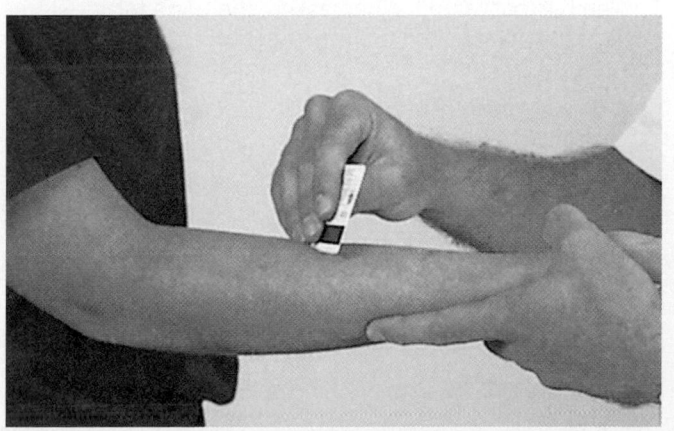

Figure 5 To remove the stinger of a honeybee, gently scrape the skin with the edge of a sharp, stiff object such as a credit card.

Maintain the airway. The airway is always a priority in every situation. You will need to be prepared to intubate. If the airway is already swollen shut, you may need to perform a cricothyrotomy to ventilate the patient. Assessing for the presence of stridor and hoarseness should indicate the severity of the airway compromise. If the patient is still awake, allow him or her to assume a position that does not compromise breathing. Use an appropriate oxygen device for supplemental oxygen administration, and consider early transport. Be prepared to assist breathing as needed. *Early administration of epinephrine should be a priority.*

Words of Wisdom

In the absence of an IV/IO site, intramuscular (IM) administration of epinephrine is preferred because it provides more rapid absorption. Administration in the thigh is preferred over the deltoid site for more rapid absorption. Subcutaneous (SQ) administration of epinephrine is unpredictable and may have delayed effects in the presence of shock.

Administer epinephrine. Use the IV, IO, IM, or SQ route to administer epinephrine as soon as possible if airway or respiratory compromise and/or hypotension are present. Epinephrine is the drug of choice for anaphylactic reactions because it stops the process of mast cell degranulation. The action of epinephrine is immediate; it can rapidly reverse the effects of anaphylaxis. In addition, epinephrine reverses the effects of the chemical mediators released via this degranulation. The alpha-adrenergic properties cause the blood vessels to constrict, which reverses vasodilation and hypotension. This, in turn, elevates the diastolic pressure and improves coronary blood flow. The beta-1 adrenergic effects increase cardiac contractility, reversing the depressing effects on the heart and improving the strength of cardiac contractions. The beta-2 adrenergic effects cause bronchodilation, relieving bronchospasm in the lungs. Many patients and EMTs carry epinephrine in the form of an EpiPen and may have administered it before your arrival. The patient may have taken other medications as well, so it is important to obtain a medication history.

Maintain circulation. Insert at least one large-bore IV catheter to administer an isotonic solution (lactated Ringer's or normal saline) at a wide-open rate. Ideally, you should place two IV lines en route to the emergency department. This step is crucial, especially if the patient is hypotensive and does not respond to the epinephrine. Initially, 1 to 2 L should be administered. If there is no response, you may need to administer up to 4 L. If the patient does not respond after 4 L of fluid, consider administering a vasopressor in conjunction with fluid administration.

Special Populations

Because epinephrine can stress the heart, it is important to use this drug only as needed in older patients and patients with a cardiovascular disease history. Monitor patients closely for cardiac problems or hypertension.

Initiate pharmacologic therapy. Administer high-flow oxygen, epinephrine, antihistamines, anti-inflammatory and immunosuppressant agents, and a vasopressor. Be prepared to assist ventilation. Patients who receive epinephrine must be monitored closely for adverse effects. Use a cardiac monitor to watch for dysrhythmias, and reassess the patient's vital signs at least every 5 minutes.

YOU *are the Medic*   PART 4

Your partner sets up for endotracheal intubation while you reassess vital signs. It appears that any effect from the adult EpiPen has not lasted. When asked, the boy's father states that the dose was administered prior to calling 9-1-1. Your partner successfully places the endotracheal tube (ETT) and administers epinephrine 1:1,000 intramuscularly to the patient. You move the patient to your vehicle for immediate transport.

Recording Time: 10 Minutes	
Respirations	Assisted to 20
Pulse	140 beats/min
Skin	Red, warm, dry
Blood pressure	90/56 mm Hg
Oxygen saturation (Spo$_2$)	98% assisted
Pupils	Equal and reactive

7. What is your next medication choice considering there is airway involvement?

8. What is the pediatric dose for that medication?

Allergic reactions that are *not* accompanied by signs of cardiovascular collapse (that is, hypotension) or airway compromise can be adequately treated with epinephrine 1:1,000 via the SQ route. For adults, give 0.3 to 0.5 mg of epinephrine; for children, give 0.01 mg/kg.

The adult EpiPen **Figure 6** delivers 0.3 mg of a 1:1,000 solution of epinephrine intramuscularly. The EpiPen Jr, which contains 0.15 mg of a 1:2,000 solution, is used for children who weigh less than 33 lb (15 kg).

Epinephrine should be administered intravenously as soon as possible if hypotension or a reaction involving the airway or respiratory system is suspected or occurring. For adults with mild allergic reactions and asthma, administer 0.3–0.5 mg (0.3–0.5 mL 1:1,000) SQ. For anaphylaxis, administer 1 mg (10 mL of 1:10,000) IV, IO over 5 minutes.

Antihistamine administration should be considered only after epinephrine has been administered. Antihistamines block the histamine 1 (H_1) and 2 (H_2) receptor sites. Diphenhydramine (Benadryl) is commonly used in the prehospital setting following the administration of epinephrine. This medication does not prevent histamine release, but rather blocks histamine effects at the H_1 receptor sites. The typical dose of diphenhydramine (Benadryl) is 25 to 50 mg administered slowly via the IM or IV route. H_2 blockers such as cimetidine (Tagamet) and ranitidine (Zantac) are also indicated but are more commonly used in the hospital setting. It is recommended that H_1 and H_2 blockers be administered until the anaphylactic symptoms resolve.

Corticosteroids do not have an immediate effect but are useful in preventing late-phase anaphylactic reactions and should be administered early in the treatment process. Common corticosteroids include methylprednisolone (Solu-Medrol), hydrocortisone (Solu-Cortef), and dexamethasone (Decadron).

Glucagon may also be indicated for an anaphylactic patient, especially if the patient does not respond to epinephrine or is taking a beta blocker. The usual dose is 1 to 2 mg IM or IV every 5 minutes. Glucagon increases cardiac contractility, and

is primarily used for patients with hypoglycemia in whom IV access cannot be obtained.

Vasopressors such as dopamine (Intropin) should be considered if the patient does not respond to fluid administration to treat the hypotension.

Inhaled beta-adrenergic agents such as albuterol (Ventolin) may also be included as part of the care regimen if bronchospasm is present.

Special Populations

Patients taking beta blockers have been reported to have more severe and frequent anaphylactic reactions and can develop a paradoxical reaction to epinephrine. Glucagon and ipratropium (Atrovent) should be considered for these patients.

Psychological support is a crucial component of management. Anaphylaxis can progress rapidly and has the potential to be a life-threatening event. Patients and their families will need reassurance as you perform the necessary interventions. Many of the patients have experienced similar events and may recognize how serious their condition has become. For others, this may be a first-time event. You need to be professional and reassuring and focus on early intervention and transport.

Words of Wisdom

Steroids include both corticosteroids, such as prednisone or its derivative, and anabolic steroids, which are substances used to promote muscle growth and development and have little legitimate medical use.

Consider early transport if the patient needs resources beyond your capabilities. Even if you are able to stop the reaction and the patient begins to recover, it is recommended that patients be observed in a medical facility. As many as 20% of patients will have a recurrence of the symptoms within the next 8 hours, even if they have been free of symptoms for a time. Once the patient has been symptom free for 4 hours, he or she can be released from the facility but should be instructed to return or call an ambulance if the symptoms recur.

■ Collagen Vascular Diseases

Pathophysiology

Systemic Lupus Erythematosus Systemic lupus erythematosus (SLE or lupus) should be suspected in women of childbearing age who present with fever, rash, and joint pain. It is not your job to diagnose lupus, but awareness of the signs, symptoms, and life threats associated with lupus are important. Lupus is a multisystem autoimmune disease, and the effects on the various body systems are outlined in **Table 6**.

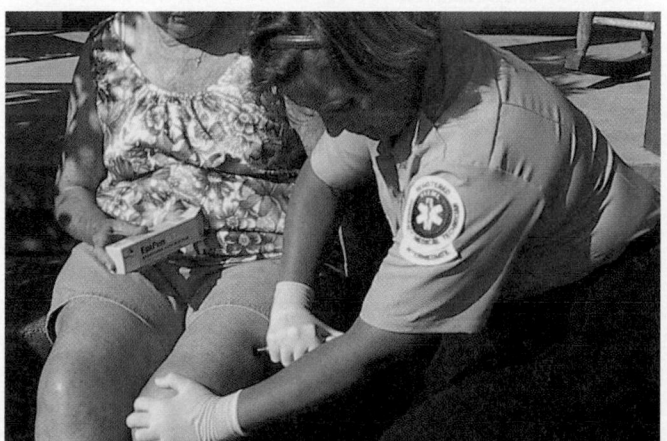

Figure 6 Administration of epinephrine with an auto-injector involves stabilizing the leg, pushing the auto-injector firmly against the thigh, and holding it in place until all of the medication is injected.

Table 6 Signs, Symptoms, and Prehospital Implications of Lupus

System	Signs and Symptoms	Prehospital Implications
Cutaneous	<ul><li>Rash that is aggravated by sunlight</li><li>Butterfly-like rash across the cheeks and nose</li><li>Sores or lesions in the mouth</li><li>Hair loss</li><li>Bruising</li></ul>	<ul><li>Patients are sensitive to the sun; protect them from prolonged exposure to the sun.</li></ul>
Musculoskeletal	<ul><li>Joint pain and swelling</li><li>Muscle aches and pain</li><li>Inflammation of the hands causing symmetric hand pain</li><li>Lesions on the extremities that result in gangrene</li></ul>	<ul><li>Do not let the complaints of joint and muscle pain distract you from assessing for a life threat.</li><li>Assess potential for infection.</li></ul>
Pleural	<ul><li>Pleurisy, pleural effusions, or pleural rub</li><li>Pulmonary hemorrhage with hemoptysis</li><li>Pneumonia</li><li>Pulmonary emboli</li><li>Pulmonary hypertension</li></ul>	<ul><li>Assess for any of these conditions if a patient reports fever, tachypnea, cough, or worsening of chest pain.</li></ul>
Pericardial	<ul><li>Pericarditis (most common)</li><li>Myocardial infarction</li><li>Pericardial effusion</li><li>Hypertension</li><li>Endocarditis</li><li>Myocarditis</li><li>Vasculitis</li><li>Valvular heart disease</li></ul>	<ul><li>Obtain a 12-lead ECG and assess for signs of pericarditis or ischemia.</li></ul>
Neurologic	<ul><li>Stroke</li><li>Seizures</li><li>Behavioral changes</li><li>Psychosis</li><li>Migraines</li><li>Peripheral neuropathies</li><li>Meningitis</li></ul>	<ul><li>Monitor for stroke and initiate seizure precautions when neurologic symptoms are present.</li></ul>
Renal	<ul><li>Nephritis</li><li>Proteinuria</li><li>Renal failure that may require dialysis</li><li>Urinary tract infection</li><li>Fluid and electrolyte imbalance</li><li>Edema</li></ul>	<ul><li>Assess for history of renal failure and electrolyte imbalance.</li><li>Assess for urinary tract infections.</li></ul>
Hematologic	<ul><li>Anemia</li><li>Decreased white blood cell count</li><li>Thrombocytopenia</li></ul>	<ul><li>Recognize potential for hypoxia due to anemia and risk for infection.</li></ul>
Gastrointestinal	<ul><li>Oral ulcers</li><li>Abdominal cramping</li><li>Pseudo-obstruction</li><li>Pancreatitis</li><li>Vasculitis that may result in perforation</li><li>Gangrene and peritonitis</li></ul>	<ul><li>Collect a history to include bloody stools. Maintain a high index of suspicion.</li></ul>

Lupus affects the entire body. The priority of care should be directed at monitoring for life threats should the patient present with any change in his or her normal presentation. Because these patients may be on medications to suppress their immune system, slight changes such as fever, cough, or an increase in pain should alert you to be prepared to treat these patients aggressively as their conditions warrant.

Scleroderma Patients with scleroderma present with tightening, thickening, and scarring of the skin. Patients will often have symptoms of Raynaud phenomenon (pain, blanching, cyanosis or redness of the fingers and toes when stress occurs or when exposed to the cold). Pulmonary presentations are due to the stiffness of the lungs and blood vessels resulting in pulmonary fibrosis and pulmonary hypertension. Renal damage from scleroderma may result in hypertension and renal crisis. One of the major complications of scleroderma is damage to the heart muscle. Assessment for dysrhythmias, palpitations, and congestive heart failure is a priority when caring for these patients. When cardiac involvement occurs, patients with scleroderma have a lower survival rate.

Assessment

Assessment of patients with lupus or scleroderma should focus on ruling out life threats. These patients may have extensive multisystem problems, so avoid attributing their complaints to their chronic conditions until life threats can be ruled out.

Management

Management should be directed at treating any life threats. Monitor patients for signs of infection. Because each patient may present with different system involvement, you will need to determine the patient's care according to the affected system.

■ Organ Transplant Disorders

Pathophysiology

When a patient's organs are severely damaged, a transplant may be performed. The problem with a transplant is that the body sees the replacement organ as an invader, and even though the body could not survive without the new organ, the immune system will work to eliminate the organ or "reject it." In order to prevent the rejection, patients are placed on anti-rejection medications that prevent the immune system from attacking the new organs. It sounds like a perfect fix—give the patient a new organ and a medication to tell the body to leave the new organ alone, and all is well. The difficulty with these medications, however, is that the person is now at greater risk for infection. The medications cause the self-defense mechanism to either not recognize other threats or to shut down portions of its function, putting the body at risk for infection and/or sepsis.

As a paramedic, you will encounter patients who have undergone organ transplants. The organs most likely transplanted include the heart, liver, kidney, pancreas, and lungs. As you care for these patients, it is important to address the priorities in caring for the specific organ that has been transplanted.

Heart Transplant Approximately 2,000 heart transplants are performed in the United States each year. During the procedure, the recipient's heart is usually removed and replaced by the donor heart, but in some cases the native heart may be left in place. On the ECG, you may notice tachycardia at the rate of 100 to 110 beats/min due to denervation of the vagus nerve. In addition, two P waves are common, one from the patient's native heart and one from the transplanted heart. The second P wave is conducted in most patients. Chest pain is uncommon because the denervated heart cannot generate angina-like pain. Therefore, a patient with ischemia tends to present with signs of congestive heart failure or dysrhythmias rather than angina. Atropine is not indicated for bradycardia or heart blocks (a delay or disruption of the normal electrical signals that cause the heart to beat). Because the implanted heart does not have vagus nerve innervation, the heart would not respond to the vagolytic action of atropine. Sympathomimetic drugs tend to work well for heart transplant patients. If hypertension occurs, antihypertensive medications tend to work even in crisis situations. Norepinephrine and isoproterenol (Isuprel) may have a slightly increased response in heart transplant patients.

Up to 85% of acute rejections occur in the first 3 months. The signs and symptoms may be subtle and require a biopsy for confirmation. Common problems include sepsis and pneumonia. Paramedics should assess for fever, shortness of breath, hypoxia, hypotension pressure, poorly controlled hypertension, or the development of a new dysrhythmia, as these are indicators of infection.

Liver Transplant Liver transplants are the second most common solid organ procedure. If rejection occurs, the loss of function results in rapid deterioration of the patient and possibly death. Infection, in particular opportunistic infection, is a problem for liver transplant patients.

Kidney Transplant Kidney transplants are the most common type of transplant in the United States and are extremely successful. Infection is one of the major concerns for these patients as with all transplants. These patients also have a tendency to develop hepatitis C and later liver disease. Rejection of the graft presents as fever, with tenderness and swelling over the implanted kidney, which is located in the anterior area of the retroperitoneal pelvis.

Lung Transplant Lung transplants are performed alone or in conjunction with a heart transplant. In most cases, lung transplants are performed unilaterally, so unequal breath sounds are a common finding. Adhesions may be present that may complicate the placement of the chest tube on the side of the lung transplant. Signs of rejection include cough, dyspnea, fever, rales, rhonchi, and a decrease in oxygenation. Infection presents similar to the signs of rejection and requires immediate intervention.

Pancreas Transplant Pancreas transplants have a high rate of complications and a lower survival rate than the other single-organ transplants at 1 year. Most pancreas transplants are for diabetic patients and are often performed along with kidney transplants. The pancreas has an exocrine function, so a route to drain the exocrine component must be placed. Generally the secretions are drained into the bladder, which results in urinary tract signs and symptoms such as infections and hematuria. In addition, these patients have a chronic non-anion gap acidosis because the bicarbonate the pancreas produces is drained directly into the bladder for excretion. This information is important for clinicians to remember when evaluating the patient's arterial blood gases, so as not to be confused with lactic acidosis. Infection and rejection are common problems for patients with pancreas transplants.

Assessment

Assessment of the patient who has had an organ transplant requires an awareness of subtle signs and symptoms. Keep a high index of suspicion for infection and rejection. Signs and symptoms of organ rejection vary depending on the organ; for example, rejection of a transplanted kidney may cause the patient to excrete less urine. Patients who are experiencing organ transplant rejection will usually have general discomfort and feel ill. Remember that if a transplant patient calls for EMS, the condition is usually serious. Consider contacting the patient's transplant center if you have any questions regarding the assessment or findings in these patients.

Management

The priorities of care for transplant patients are focused on the organ transplanted, the medications, recognition of infection or rejection, and transport to the most appropriate facility. Care for patients with transplants varies depending on the organ that is transplanted. It is therefore essential that you familiarize yourself with the priorities of patient care with each type of transplant. Before you administer medication, make sure you know how the medication will interact with the medications the patient is taking and how the medication will be metabolized to ensure that toxicity will not develop. Because patients who have undergone transplants may be immunosuppressed, you should monitor for signs and symptoms of infection or organ rejection. Remember, missing even one dose of their immunosuppressive medications is an emergency. Finally, consider transporting the patient to a transplant facility when possible, or consulting the facility about care when transport to the facility is not possible.

■ Patient Education

■ Anaphylaxis

The best management of anaphylaxis and allergic reactions is to educate patients about prevention and self-preservation. At a minimum, discuss the following topics:

- **Avoid the antigen.** Review information on the offending item. For example, if the patient is allergic to penicillin, he or she should be provided with a list of drugs that include penicillin and the alternative names for penicillin. Drugs that may produce a cross-reaction should also be discussed. Food allergies can be even more difficult to avoid. Peanuts are an example of a food that may be a problem. Peanut oil may be used to prepare foods that do not actually contain peanuts, and peanut butter may be an ingredient in various foods. Some patients are so allergic to peanuts that just using the same devices to process non-peanut-containing foods can cause a reaction. Patients must be educated to avoid the allergen, read labels, and ask about how food is prepared to avoid exposure. Latex allergies are also a concern, so advising patients to notify care providers of latex allergies is essential. Many services are latex free, but not all of them, so patients must inform providers of their allergies so exposures can be avoided.
- **Notify all health personnel of the allergy.** Review the need to alert health personnel to the allergy. This is important because people often think only a physician would need this information, not an EMS provider.
- **Wear identification tags or bracelets.** These items notify providers of allergies in case the patient is unable to do so.
- **Carry an anaphylaxis kit.** A reaction may happen rapidly or worsen before help can arrive. Make sure the patient and his or her family know how to use the kit.
- **Report symptoms early.** Ideally, intervention should begin before the situation becomes life threatening. The patient should recognize that reactions can occur more rapidly and with greater severity with repeated exposures.

■ Collagen Vascular Diseases and Organ Transplants

Education for patients with collagen vascular diseases or organ transplants should include the following topics:

- **Encourage self-monitoring.** Patients should be encouraged to monitor themselves for signs of infection or rejection and take these signs seriously.
- **Consult a physician before taking a new medication.** Emphasize the fact that patients should not take any new medications without consulting their physician.
- **Comply with the immunosuppressive regimen.** Encourage patients to always take their oral dose of immunosuppressive medications. Missing even one dose is an emergency; their physician or contact should be notified if this occurs.
- **Know who to contact.** Patients should know to call the transplanting facility to seek prehospital care, as directed by their physician or transplant contact.

YOU are the Medic   SUMMARY

1. What is your first impression of this patient?

Looking at the patient can give you an indication of the severity of the problem. Does the patient's condition appear stable or unstable? The status of the brain (level of consciousness) is reflected in the patient's oxygenation and circulatory status. A restless, confused, anxious, or combative patient most likely has hypoxia. As the patient's condition deteriorates and the oxygen level decreases or the carbon dioxide level increases, you are likely to find a patient who has a decreased level of consciousness or is completely unresponsive. In this situation, the patient is supine, his skin appears red, and although he is conscious, he is not following you with his eyes. This suggests that his level of consciousness is beginning to decrease.

2. What is your preliminary determination of the chief complaint?

Initially, you should suspect that this is an allergic reaction of some sort. When you review the patient's history and signs and symptoms, most point to allergic reaction. Red skin, urticaria, and swelling of the patient's mouth are strong indications of an allergic reaction.

3. What is your determination of the patient's condition now?

At this point, you should have made a determination of anaphylaxis. You should also take into consideration that, according to the mother, the patient was choking. When you are placing a definitive airway, visualize as much as possible to ensure that food is not blocking the airway.

4. Can this be an allergic reaction if the child did not consume seafood?

It is entirely possible the patient is having an anaphylactic event because of seafood. If the child is severely allergic to seafood, it is possible he could be having a reaction because the food he ate was prepared in the same environment where seafood was also being prepared. It may also be possible the child is allergic to peanut oil which is sometimes used to fry foods like french fries.

5. What is the difference between an adult EpiPen and an EpiPen Jr?

The adult EpiPen delivers 0.3 mg of a 1:1,000 solution of epinephrine intramuscularly. The EpiPen Jr, which contains 0.15 mg of a 1:2,000 solution, is used for children who weigh less than 33 lb (15 kg). This child is a toddler and would need the junior dose if the pen is used by a family member or EMT. Paramedics will simply follow their treatment protocols.

6. What effect can you expect the adult EpiPen to have on this patient?

You can expect the following:

- Alpha effect: vasoconstriction
- Beta-1 effect: positive inotropic and chronotropic and dromotropic
- Beta-2 effect: bronchial smooth muscle relaxation and dilation of skeletal vasculature
- Blocking of histamine receptors

Also, because the dose administered is double the amount at a higher concentration, you should expect a pronounced effect on the patient's vital signs.

7. What is your next medication choice considering there is airway involvement?

Epinephrine should be administered intravenously as soon as possible if hypotension or a reaction involving the airway or respiratory system is suspected or occurring. The advantage of an IV infusion is that the dose can be more easily controlled if the patient reacts negatively to the epinephrine (eg, nausea, vomiting, headache). This approach may eliminate the need for repeated doses. In this case, the toddler is not hypotensive so the IM route should be used while attempting to obtain IV access, which could be more difficult in a child this age.

8. What is the pediatric dose for that medication?

Allergic reactions that are *not* accompanied by signs of cardiovascular collapse (that is, hypotension) or airway compromise can be adequately treated with epinephrine 1:1,000 via the IM route. For children, administer 0.01 mg/kg.

YOU *are the Medic*   SUMMARY, *continued*

EMS Patient Care Report (PCR)

Date: 06-30-11	**Incident No.:** 4563	**Nature of Call:** Anaphylaxis	**Location:** 100 N. Main Street
Dispatched: 1810	**En Route:** 1810	**At Scene:** 1816 **Transport:** 1832	**At Hospital:** 1841 **In Service:** 1856

Patient Information

Age: 2 **Sex:** M **Weight (in kg [lb]):** 11 kg (25 lb)	**Allergies:** Seafood **Medications:** Family denies **Past Medical History:** Allergic reaction **Chief Complaint:** Anaphylaxis

Vital Signs

Time: 1821	**BP:** 90/58	**Pulse:** 150	**Respirations:** 36	**Spo$_2$:** 92% on room air
Time: 1826	**BP:** 90/56	**Pulse:** 140	**Respirations:** Assisted to 20	**Spo$_2$:** 98% O$_2$
Time:	**BP:**	**Pulse:**	**Respirations:**	**Spo$_2$:**

EMS Treatment
(circle all that apply)

Oxygen @ __15__ L/min via (circle one): NC NRM (Bag-mask device)	**Assisted Ventilation**	**Airway Adjunct**	**CPR**
Defibrillation	**Bleeding Control**	**Bandaging**	**Splinting**	**Other**

Narrative

Arrived at the Main Street Grill for a reported man down. Upon arrival, we found a 2-year-old boy lying on the floor of the restaurant. Mother and father are present with the child. Family states the pt was eating french fries when he started choking. The mother laid the child on the floor where she discovered the pt's skin was red, warm, dry and the child's mouth appeared to be swelling. Father states he administered an adult EpiPen to the pt prior to calling 9-1-1. Pt is awake and not alert, obvious swelling noted to pt's face and mouth. Audible wheezing present and pt moving little air. ETT placed with good lung sounds all fields, confirmed by waveform capnography, and no gastric sounds noted before and after securing the ETT in place. Administered 0.11 mg Epi 1:1,000 IM and obtained IV access prior to moving pt for emergency transport to Town Hospital. En route, slight improvement noted with IM Epi. Continued improvement noted until arrival at ED. Report to Dr. Morrison on arrival. **End of report**

Prep Kit

■ Ready for Review

- An antigen is a substance the body recognizes as foreign. This recognition causes the body to produce antibodies to destroy the foreign substance.

- The immune system is responsible for the antigen–antibody response.

- An allergic response occurs when the body produces the antigen–antibody response when exposed to a substance that is usually harmless. An allergic response is usually limited to one body system or a local area.

- Anaphylaxis is an extreme form of systemic allergic response involving two or more body systems.

- A person must be sensitized to an antigen before an allergic or anaphylactic reaction can occur.

- An anaphylactoid reaction may occur without the patient being previously exposed to the offending agent.

- The routes of exposure to an antigen include injection, absorption, inhalation, and ingestion.

- Mast cells release chemical mediators to stimulate the allergic reaction.

- Chemical mediators produce signs and symptoms through their effects on the skin, cardiovascular, respiratory, neurologic, and gastrointestinal systems.

- Skin effects include erythema, urticaria, and pruritis. Cyanosis and pallor may also be present.

- Cardiovascular effects include vasodilation, hypotension, decreased cardiac output, cardiac ischemia, and dysrhythmias.

- Respiratory effects include upper airway edema and stridor, hoarseness, bronchoconstriction, increased bronchial secretions, wheezes, and hypoxia.

- Neurologic symptoms include altered level of consciousness, anxiety, restlessness, combativeness, and unconsciousness.

- Gastrointestinal symptoms include nausea, vomiting, diarrhea, and cramping.

- As part of your assessment, you should evaluate the scene, patient history, level of consciousness, upper airway, lower airway, skin, and vital signs.

- Treatment of anaphylaxis includes removing the offending agent; maintaining the airway; administering medications such as epinephrine, antihistamines (diphenhydramine, cimetidine, ranitidine), corticosteroids, inhaled beta-adrenergic agents, and vasopressors; resuscitating with IV fluids; and initiating rapid transport.

- Epinephrine is first-line drug therapy for anaphylaxis.

- Patient education to prevent reexposure, to understand symptoms, and to understand the need to use an anaphylaxis kit is essential.

- Collagen vascular diseases and other autoimmune diseases may require treatment that involves administering medications to suppress the immune system and decrease the attack.

- Organ transplant disorders can present a multitude of problems in patients. It is important to know the treatment priorities when you care for patients who have undergone organ transplants.

■ Vital Vocabulary

<u>absorption</u> In allergic reactions, when foreign material is deposited on and moves into the skin.

<u>acquired immunity</u> The immunity the body develops as part of exposure to an antigen.

allergen A substance that produces allergic symptoms in a patient.

allergic reaction An abnormal immune response the body develops when reexposed to a substance or allergen.

anaphylactoid reaction An extreme allergic response that does not involve IgE antibody mediation. The exact mechanism is unknown, but an anaphylactoid event may occur without the patient being previously exposed to the offending agent.

anaphylaxis An extreme systemic form of an allergic reaction involving two or more body systems.

antibody A protein the body produces in response to an antigen; an immunoglobulin.

antigen An agent that, when taken into the body, stimulates the formation of specific protective proteins called antibodies.

basophils White blood cells that work to produce chemical mediators during an immune response.

cellular immunity The immunity provided by special white blood cells called T cells that attack and destroy invaders.

chemical mediators Chemicals that work to cause the immune or allergic response; for example, histamine.

collagen vascular diseases A group of autoimmune disorders that affect the collagen in tendons, bones, and connective tissues.

histamine A chemical found in mast cells that, when released, causes vasodilation, capillary leaking, and bronchiole constriction.

humoral immunity The use of antibodies dissolved in the plasma and lymph to destroy foreign substances.

hypersensitivity Occurs when a patient reacts with exaggerated or inappropriate allergic symptoms after coming into contact with a substance the body perceives as harmful.

immune system The system that protects the body from foreign substances.

immunity The body's ability to protect itself from acquiring a disease.

ingestion Eating or drinking materials for absorption through the gastrointestinal tract.

inhalation In allergic reactions, foreign substances are breathed in through the respiratory system.

injection In allergic reactions, when the skin is pierced, and foreign material is deposited into the skin.

local reaction When the body limits a response to a specific area after being exposed to a foreign substance.

mast cells Basophils that are located in the tissues.

natural immunity The immunity the body develops as part of being exposed to an antigen and developing antibodies—for example, exposure to measles, having the measles, and developing immunity to the measles.

primary response The first encounter with the foreign substance to begin the immune response.

pruritus Itching.

scleroderma An autoimmune connective tissue disease that causes fibrotic (scar tissue–like) changes to the skin, blood vessels, muscles, and internal organs.

secondary response The body's reaction when it is exposed to an antigen for which it already has antibodies, in which it responds by killing the invading substance.

sensitivity The ability to recognize a foreign substance the next time it is encountered.

systemic lupus erythematosus A multisystem autoimmune disease.

systemic reaction A reaction that occurs throughout the body, possibly affecting multiple body systems.

urticaria Hives or reddened elevated patches on the skin.

Assessment in Action

Your unit is dispatched to an apartment building for a woman with lupus. Dispatch tells you the patient is 36 years old and is having severe pain. When you arrive on scene, the patient looks very uncomfortable. You see a bright rash on the patient's face.

1. What type of disease is systemic lupus erythematosus (SLE)?
   A. Cardiac
   B. Endocrine
   C. Autoimmune
   D. Cutaneous

2. What occurs in Raynaud phenomenon?
   A. Patient cannot move fingers.
   B. Patient's fingertips change color when cold.
   C. Patient experiences tetany when exposed to cold.
   D. Patient has blood in urine.

3. As you assess the patient, you note that she has numerous oral ulcers. This indicates that which body system has been affected by her disease?
   A. Renal
   B. Cutaneous
   C. Neurologic
   D. Gastrointestinal

4. An abnormal decrease in the number of total platelets in a patient's blood count is a common hematologic finding of lupus and is called:
   A. thrombocytopenia.
   B. thromboembolism.
   C. thrombocytosis.
   D. thrombophlebitis.

5. The patient reports severe pain in her hands, arms, hips, and legs. What should be your treatment priority for this patient?
   A. Administer analgesia.
   B. Assess and treat immediate life threats.
   C. Keep the patient out of the sunlight.
   D. Administer diphenhydramine.

6. When the immune system attacks its own collagen tissue, this is known as:
   A. collagen degeneration disease.
   B. collagen vascular disease.
   C. cutaneous degeneration disease.
   D. cutaneous vascular disease.

Additional Questions

7. Why are immunosuppressant medications prescribed to patients who already have a malfunctioning immune system?

8. Why are immunosuppressant medications prescribed as an anti-rejection medication for transplant patients?

Infectious Diseases

National EMS Education Standard Competencies

Medicine

Integrates assessment findings with principles of epidemiology and pathophysiology to formulate a field impression and implement a comprehensive treatment/disposition plan for a patient with a medical complaint.

Infectious Diseases

Awareness, assessment, and management of

- A patient who may have an infectious disease (pp 1288-1289, 1295-1296)
- How to decontaminate equipment after treating a patient (p 1289)

Assessment and management of

- How to decontaminate the ambulance and equipment after treating a patient (p 1289)
- A patient who may be infected with a bloodborne pathogen (pp 1290, 1292)
  - Human immunodeficiency virus (HIV) (pp 1305-1306)
  - Hepatitis B (pp 1304-1305)
- Antibiotic-resistant infections (pp 1311-1313)
- Current infectious diseases prevalent in the community (pp 1288-1290, 1296)

Anatomy, physiology, epidemiology, pathophysiology, psychosocial impact, presentations, prognosis, and management of

- HIV-related disease (pp 1305-1307)
- Hepatitis (pp 1303-1305, 1308)
- Pneumonia (pp 1298-1299)
- Meningococcal meningitis (p 1297)
- Tuberculosis (pp 1297-1298)
- Tetanus (p 1311)
- Viral diseases (pp 1307-1309)
- Sexually transmitted diseases (pp 1301-1303)
- Gastroenteritis (p 1307)
- Fungal infections (p 1296)
- Rabies (p 1310)
- Scabies and lice (p 1303)
- Lyme disease (p 1309)
- Rocky Mountain spotted fever (pp 1309-1310)
- Antibiotic-resistant infections (pp 1311-1313)

Knowledge Objectives

1. Define communicable disease. (p 1288)
2. Name the agencies responsible for protecting the public health in the United States, and outline their functions at the national, state, and local levels. (pp 1288-1289)
3. Describe the paramedic's obligation to protect the public from infection and what steps the paramedic can take in order to meet it. (p 1289)
4. Describe how communicable diseases are transmitted by direct and indirect contact, droplet transmission, and airborne transmission. (pp 1289-1290)
5. List the personal protective equipment a paramedic may need in specific circumstances to prevent exposure to communicable and other infectious diseases. (pp 1290-1292)
6. Describe the steps to take for personal protection from airborne and bloodborne pathogens. (pp 1290-1292)
7. Explain proper follow-up after exposure to a patient's blood or body fluids, including documentation of the event and communication with an infection control officer and public health authorities. (pp 1292-1293)
8. Understand the standard precautions the paramedic must follow in order to prevent infection during patient care activities. (p 1294)
9. List the general assessment and management principles for a patient with an infectious disease. (pp 1295-1296)
10. Describe the cycle of infection, and list factors that affect susceptibility to infectious disease. (pp 1295-1296)
11. Discuss the pathophysiology, assessment, and management of a patient with meningitis. (p 1297)
12. Discuss the pathophysiology, assessment, and management of a patient with tuberculosis. (pp 1297-1298)
13. Discuss precautions paramedics should take to protect themselves from exposure to tuberculosis. (pp 1297-1298)
14. Compare the types of pneumonia caused by viruses, bacteria, and fungi in terms of their pathophysiology, risk factors, and complications. (pp 1298-1299)
15. Discuss general principles of assessment and management for a patient with pneumonia. (pp 1298-1299)
16. Discuss the pathophysiology, assessment, and management of a patient with respiratory syncytial virus. (p 1299)
17. Discuss the pathophysiology, assessment, and management of patients with bronchitis, laryngitis, and epiglottitis. (pp 1299-1300)
18. Discuss the pathophysiology, assessment, and management of a patient with mononucleosis. (p 1300)
19. Discuss the pathophysiology, assessment, and management of a patient with influenza. (pp 1300-1301)
20. Discuss general principles of assessment and management for a patient with a sexually transmitted disease. (pp 1301-1303)
21. Discuss the pathophysiology, assessment, and management of patients with gonorrhea, syphilis, genital herpes, and chlamydia. (pp 1301-1303)
22. Describe the risk factors, incidence, pathophysiology, assessment, and management of scabies and lice infestation. (p 1303)
23. Compare the types of viral hepatitis, and outline general assessment findings and management principles for the patient with hepatitis. (pp 1303-1305)
24. Discuss precautions paramedics should take to protect themselves from exposure to hepatitis, and describe postexposure follow-up. (pp 1303-1305)

25. Discuss the pathophysiology, assessment, and management of a patient with human immunodeficiency virus/acquired immunodeficiency syndrome (HIV/AIDS). (pp 1305-1307)

26. Discuss precautions paramedics should take to protect themselves from exposure to HIV, and describe postexposure follow-up. (pp 1305-1307)

27. Discuss the pathophysiology, assessment, and management of a patient with gastroenteritis. (p 1307)

28. Discuss general principles of assessment and management for a patient with a fungal infection. (p 1296)

29. Discuss the pathophysiology, assessment, and management of patients with West Nile virus, Lyme disease, Rocky Mountain spotted fever, hantavirus, rabies, and tetanus. (pp 1308-1311)

30. Compare the most common antibiotic-resistant organisms and explain what steps paramedics and patients can take to curb their spread. (pp 1311-1313)

31. Discuss the pathophysiology, assessment, and management of bronchiolitis, croup, measles, rubella, mumps, and chickenpox. (pp 1313-1316)

32. Discuss general principles of assessment and management for patients with severe acute respiratory syndrome (SARS) and avian flu. (p 1317)

33. Describe age-related variations that affect patients with communicable and other infectious diseases. (pp 1297, 1300, 1306, 1311, 1315-1317)

Skills Objectives

1. Clean and disinfect the ambulance interior and equipment. (p 1289)

Introduction

In 1913, Randolph Borne said, "We can become as much slaves to precaution as we can to fear." This statement is particularly relevant to EMS care today because many care providers are fearful when caring for patients who have or are suspected of having a <u>communicable disease</u>—that is, an <u>infectious disease</u> that can be passed from one person to another. A paramedic who does not understand how communicable diseases are transmitted and how to take sensible precautions will be hesitant in caring for some patients, no matter what the cause of their illness. This chapter explores the ways in which such diseases are transmitted and outlines some measures a paramedic can take to protect against them. The communicable diseases that paramedics are most likely to encounter in the course of their work are examined, as are the illnesses that create the greatest anxiety among EMS personnel and the public at large.

Protecting Public Health

Responsibilities of Public Health Agencies

A number of government agencies are responsible for protecting the health of the general public. Agencies at the national level include the Occupational Health and Safety Administration (OSHA), which has promulgated rules and regulations designed to protect the employees of public and private organizations. This chapter refers to several OSHA regulations, for example, CFR 1910.1030, commonly known as the Bloodborne Pathogen Standard. Data on the numbers of patients infected and research and guidance for health care providers and the general public are available from the Centers for Disease Control and Prevention (CDC). Another federal law, the Ryan White Comprehensive AIDS Resources Emergency (CARE) Act, Part G, requires that medical facilities notify emergency response personnel of airborne- and droplet-transmitted disease involving patients they transported. This notification must happen as soon as possible, and no longer than 48 hours from the time they have a "suspect" case. The diseases listed in the original act include human immunodeficiency virus, hepatitis B, tuberculosis, meningococcal disease, diphtheria, pneumonic plague, viral hemorrhagic fevers, and rabies. In August 2011, the CDC published an expanded list of diseases covered under this mandate. The diseases added include hepatitis C, measles, rubella, SARS-CoV, pertussis, cutaneous anthrax, chickenpox, mumps, vaccinia, novel influenza A viruses, and potentially life-threatening diseases caused by biologic agents.

The CDC also added hepatitis C to the list of bloodborne diseases covered in the law. Now, there is much broader coverage for emergency responders to be notified and followed for exposures.

On the state and local levels, state and county public health departments bear the responsibility for protection of the public from disease, prevention of epidemics, and management of outbreaks. Although paramedics may not believe that supervision of water quality, cleanliness of restaurants, and routine immunization and vaccination programs relate directly to emergency care, it is beneficial for EMS agencies to know their local public health officials and to work with them. When potential threats to a community's health exist—such as the aftermath from Hurricane Katrina, the anthrax and smallpox scares past September 11, and Avian flu—a close working relationship between EMS providers and public health agencies is essential. If you do not know the public health professionals and officials in your county or parish, reach out to them and learn who they are.

YOU *are the Medic* | PART 1

Your unit is dispatched to an assisted care facility for a patient who is vomiting and has had diarrhea for a few days. While you are en route, the dispatcher states that the nurse on scene says a few of their patients have flulike symptoms, and the patient you are responding to has been severely ill for about 48 hours. When you arrive on scene, staff members meet you at the door. As they are guiding you to the room, one of the nurses tells you that the staff physician thinks a few of their patients have Norwalk, or norovirus.

1. What is your first concern at this scene?

2. What is norovirus?

State and local public health departments are responsible for many activities related to infectious diseases, including collecting data on the incidence of diseases, performing contact follow-up, and running TB and immunization clinics. The public health department monitors reportable disease weekly, monthly, and annually. This surveillance helps public health officials identify any upswing in the incidence of a particular disease. If the incidence of cases of a specific disease in a particular geographic area remains steady over time, that figure is said to be the endemic number of cases for that area. A rising case load may signal the beginning of an underlined epidemic. When a disease infects large numbers of people and spreads all over the world, it is considered a underlined pandemic. Public health departments have a major role in investigating epidemics and pandemics.

The public health department collects all disease statistics for each locality and shares the information with the state health department, which then sends the state totals to the CDC.

Responsibilities of Paramedics

Paramedics have an obligation to protect patients from health care–associated (nosocomial) infections (infections acquired from a health care setting—in this case, an ambulance). One way to protect patients is by complying with work restriction guidelines: Reporting for work when you have a sore throat or the flu is *not* in the best interest of your patients or your coworkers.

Another way to protect patients from health care–associated infections is to keep the ambulance interior and its equipment clean and disinfected. When cleaning and disinfecting equipment, select cleaning solutions to fit the equipment category:

- **Critical equipment.** Items that come in contact with mucous membranes: laryngoscope blades, endotracheal tubes, and Combitubes. High-level disinfection (that is, use of Environmental Protection Agency [EPA]-registered chemical "sterilants") is the minimum level for this equipment.
- **Semicritical equipment.** Items that come in direct contact with intact skin: stethoscopes, blood pressure cuffs, splints, uniforms, personal protection equipment (PPE), and pneumatic antishock garments. Clean with solutions that have a label claiming to kill hepatitis B virus (HBV). Bleach and water at a 1:100 dilution fits this requirement.
- **Noncritical equipment.** Cleaning surfaces, floors, ambulance seats, and work surfaces: For this equipment, a mixture of EPA-registered hospital-grade cleaner or bleach and water is effective.

General cleaning routines need to be listed in the department's exposure control plan. A basic rule of thumb is to follow the steps below after *every* call:

1. Strip used linens from the stretcher immediately after use, and place them in a plastic bag or the designated receptacle in the emergency department.
2. In an appropriate receptacle, discard all disposable equipment used for care of a patient that meets your state's definition of medical waste. Most items will be considered general trash. Refer to your state law on medical waste disposal.
3. Wash contaminated areas with soap and water. For disinfection to be effective, cleaning must be done first.
4. Disinfect all nondisposable equipment used in the care of a patient. For example, disassemble the bag-mask device, and place the components in a liquid sterilization solution as recommended by the manufacturer.
5. Clean the stretcher with an EPA-registered germicidal-virucidal solution or bleach and water at a 1:100 dilution.
6. If any spillage or other contamination occurred in the ambulance, clean it up with the same germicidal-virucidal or bleach-water solution.
7. Create a schedule for routine full cleaning for the vehicle, as required by the exposure control plan. Name the brands of solution to be used.
8. Have a written policy and procedure for cleaning each piece of equipment. Refer to the manufacturer's recommendations as a guide.

Protecting Health Care Providers

Although the risk of contracting a communicable disease is real, it should not be exaggerated and certainly should not be a source of fear and stress. Fear comes from lack of proper education and training, and there is no reason a paramedic should not be properly educated about disease transmission.

Communicable Disease Transmission

By the very nature of their work, health care providers come in contact with sick people; a certain proportion of the sick people have contagious diseases. Communicable diseases are diseases that can be transmitted from one person to another under certain conditions. These conditions are listed in the formula for infection and are dependent on dose, virulence, mode of entry, and the health status of the host. Infectious diseases cause illness in the patient but do not always pose a risk to the health care provider.

To understand the principles of prevention, you must first understand how diseases are spread. Infectious diseases are caused by pathogenic microorganisms—usually bacteria or viruses, but sometimes fungi and parasites. They spread from person to person by several specific mechanisms:

- Contact transmission. Direct contact with an infected person may be brief, such as touching a patient. Most cases of the common cold are thought to be transmitted through casual direct contact. Venereal diseases, such as syphilis and gonorrhea, are transmitted principally by direct sexual contact and are, therefore, referred to as sexually transmitted diseases (STDs).

  Direct contact also includes puncture by a contaminated needle or other sharp instrument. Punctures may occur if a health care provider is not using needle-safe or needleless devices.

  Direct contact may also occur by transfusion of contaminated blood products from one patient to another.

Screening tests for bloodborne disease have vastly reduced the risks of contracting illnesses from contaminated blood. However, donated blood is not 100% safe from **bloodborne pathogens**.

Indirect contact occurs by touching or handling an infected object or by coming into contact with a person who is contaminated with pathogens from an infected person or his or her secretions. For example, a paramedic can become infected by touching a bloody stretcher railing with an open cut or sore on his or her hand or by shaking hands with a father who has just wiped his infected child's nose. Objects that harbor microorganisms and can transmit them to others, such as the stretcher railing in the preceding example, are called **fomites**. Towels used by a patient are a good illustration of fomites that could transmit infection.

- **Droplet transmission**. Droplet transmission occurs with inhalation of infected droplets, such as those released into the surroundings when a person with pulmonary TB coughs or sneezes. With these diseases, there is generally a 3- to 6-foot rule. Droplets fall after traveling a distance.
- **Airborne transmission**. Pathogens transmitted by the airborne route are carried in microscopic particles that become aerosolized when an infected person coughs, sneezes, or exhales. This vapor of infectious particles can remain suspended in the air for long periods and can drift to new locations far from their source.

Disease transmission can also occur by means other than person-to-person transmission. A **vector** is an organism that harbors pathogens that are harmless to the organism but cause disease when transmitted to a human host. For example, a mosquito infected with West Nile virus that bites a susceptible person may transmit the disease.

Personal Protective Equipment and Practices

PPE serves as a secondary protective barrier beyond what your body provides. The selection and use of PPE depends on the task and procedure at hand. Your department's exposure control plan and respiratory protection plan should contain a listing of its risk procedures and the recommended use of PPE. The CDC has also developed guidelines for PPE **Table 1**.

Hand hygiene, including handwashing, is your major protective measure **Figure 1**. The current standard for handwashing is the use of antimicrobial, alcohol-based foams or gels. Use of antibacterial products is not recommended. The friction used to get alcohol-based foams and gels to evaporate removes surface organisms and kills viruses but leaves the normal flora intact.

Table 1 **Recommended Personal Protective Equipment for Preventing Transmission of Human Immunodeficiency Virus and Hepatitis B Virus in the Prehospital Setting**

Task or Activity	Disposable Gloves	Gown	Mask	Protective Eyewear
Bleeding control with spurting blood	Yes	Yes	Yes	Yes
Bleeding control with minimal bleeding	Yes	No	No	No
Emergency childbirth	Yes	Yes	Yes, if splashing is likely	Yes, if splashing is likely
Drawing blood samples	Not required by CDC, but recommended for EMS	No	No	No
Inserting an IV line	Yes	No	No	No
Endotracheal intubation, laryngeal mask airway, Combitube use	Yes	No	No, unless splashing is likely*	No, unless splashing is likely*
Oral/nasal suctioning, manually cleaning airway	Yes	No	No, unless splashing is likely*	No, unless splashing is likely*
Handling and cleaning instruments with microbial contamination	Yes	No, unless soiling is likely	No	No
Measuring blood pressure	No	No	No	No
Measuring temperature	No	No	No	No
Giving an injection	Not required by CDC, but recommended for EMS	No	No	No

*Splashing is often likely, so use personal protective equipment accordingly.

Adapted from: Centers for Disease Control and Prevention (CDC): *Morbidity and Mortality Weekly Report (MMWR)*. Vol. 38, No. S-6. Table 4. Available at: http://wonder.cdc.gov/wonder/prevguid/p0000114/p0000114.asp. Published June 23, 1989. Accessed November 10, 2011.

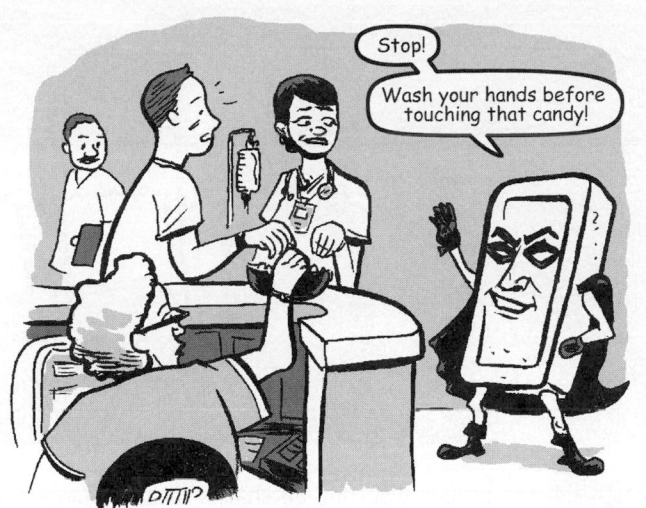

The cycle of infection can often be easily broken by handwashing.

Figure 1

Words of Wisdom

Wash your hands before and after every call.

According to the CDC, OSHA, and NFPA (National Fire Protection Association) 1581, *Standard on Fire Department Infection Control Program*, health care providers who have open cuts or sores on their hands should cover the area with a dressing. If the area is too large to cover, the provider should not perform high-risk tasks and procedures. Health care providers caring for high-risk patients are not permitted to wear artificial nails or nail extensions. Studies reported in the CDC Hand Hygiene Guidelines (2002) document the transmission of bacterial and fungal infections from health care workers wearing these nails.

The PPE used should include, but not be limited to, disposable gloves, protective eyewear, cover gowns, surgical masks, N95 respirators (P100 respirators required in California under certain circumstances), waterless handwashing alcohol-based foam or gel, needle-safe or needleless devices, biohazard bags, and resuscitative equipment.

A particulate respirator filters particles that come in through the mask. Never place a respirator on a patient. A full respiratory protection program that complies with the OSHA respiratory protection program 1910.134 must be in place if N95 or P100 respirators are on EMS vehicles. A respirator may be more valuable than a simple surgical mask in protecting against airborne particles in aerosols generated during emergency procedures.

Gloves are not needed for intramuscular or subcutaneous injections or contact with sweat. However, they are recommended for starting IVs, suctioning, intubation, contact with blood or **other potentially infectious materials (OPIM)**, and

Controversies

Surgical masks protect against splatter into the mouth or nose. Patients thought to have airborne or droplet-transmitted diseases may be asked to wear them because they filter what goes out through the mask. According to the CDC, N95 or P100 respirators are indicated for emergency intubation and open suctioning. Some health officials suggest that such procedures generate aerosols that could transmit airborne/droplet particles. No evidence-based studies support the assertion that using an N95 or P100 respirator offers more protection than wearing a surgical mask in most cases. In fact, three well-controlled studies indicate that surgical masks are as effective as respirators in protecting against infection. For more information, review the CDC guidelines "Prevention Strategies for Seasonal influenza in Healthcare Settings" (September 2010).

contact with patient mucous membranes or nonintact skin. For cleaning activities, OSHA requires the use of utility-style gloves (dishwashing gloves). These are washable and reusable as long as they are free of tears and holes **Figure 2** . Hands should be washed after glove removal because gloves are not a primary protection. Many gloves contain holes and absorb viruses and bacteria.

Words of Wisdom

Blood is not the only fluid that poses a threat of infection. Other potentially infectious materials (OPIM) include cerebrospinal fluid, pericardial fluid, amniotic fluid, synovial fluid, peritoneal fluid, and any fluid containing visible blood. Use gloves if it is possible you will come into contact with any of them.

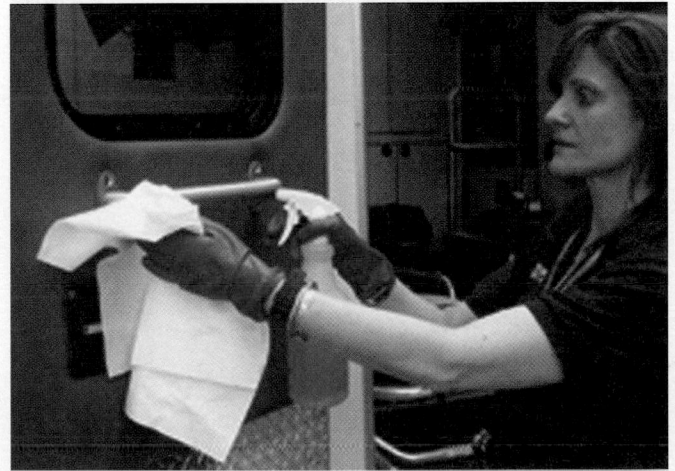

Figure 2 Utility-style gloves are washable and reusable as long as they are free of tears and holes.

Protective eyewear blocks splatter into the eye. Prescription glasses may be worn with disposable or reusable side shields. Goggles should not be worn over prescription glasses because vision may be distorted **Figure 3**.

Cover garments are recommended for large-splash situations. These garments could be washable or disposable jackets or gowns. Uniforms may also serve as PPE if the employer purchases, maintains, and launders them. Booties and hair covers are not needed in the prehospital setting. Pocket masks and/or respiratory assistive devices (for example, bag-mask devices) must be readily available.

More than 80% of exposures of health care providers to infectious agents come through sharps injuries. In 2000, Congress passed the Needlestick Safety and Prevention Act, which required that all sharps be needle-safe or **needleless systems**. The systems that have adopted needle-safe and needleless devices have reported no sharps injuries. All sharps must be placed into sharps containers that are puncture-resistant, closable, leakproof, and contain the biohazard symbol **Figure 4**.

Postexposure Medical Follow-up

Postexposure medical follow-up is your third line of defense against the effects of communicable diseases. If an exposure occurs, the **designated infection control officer (DICO)** will

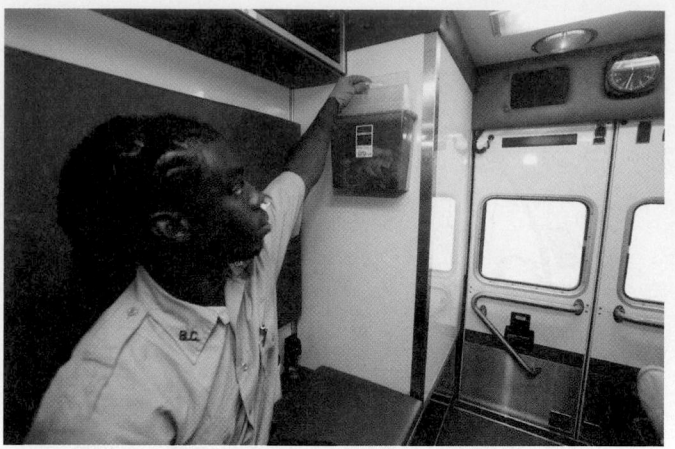

Figure 4 For proper disposal, all sharps must be placed in containers that are puncture-resistant, closable, leakproof, and that bear the biohazard symbol.

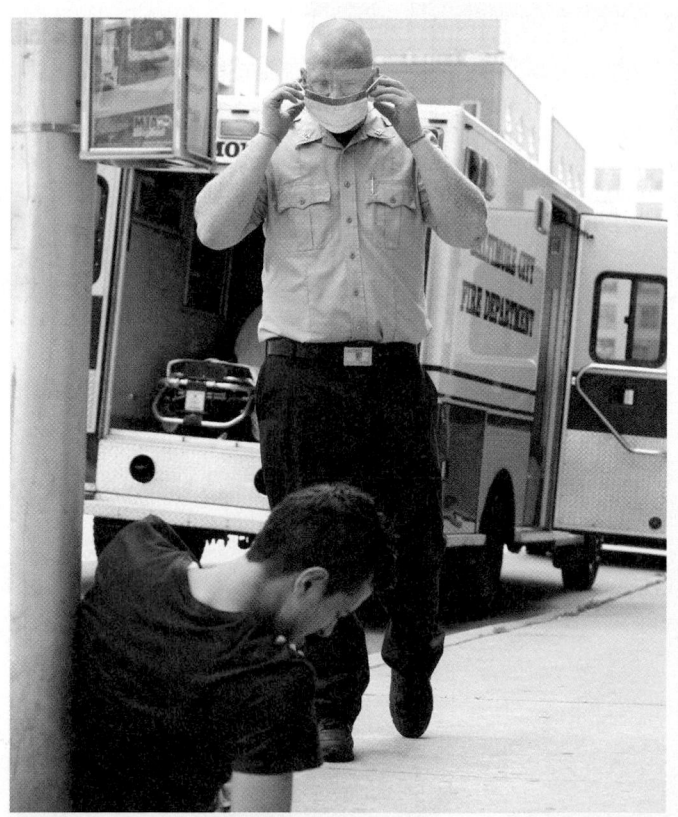

Figure 3 Wear eye protection and a mask to prevent blood and oral secretions from splattering into your eyes, nose, and mouth.

ensure that you receive proper postexposure medical treatment, including counseling, to reduce your chances of developing the disease to which you were exposed. Postexposure medical prophylaxis (prevention) is available for many communicable diseases, except hepatitis C virus (HCV) infection.

Exposure to bloodborne pathogens can occur in a number of different ways:

- A contaminated needlestick injury
- Blood or OPIM splattered into the eye, nose, or mouth
- Blood or OPIM in contact with an open area of the skin (a fresh cut, an abrasion, an area of dermatitis)
- Cuts with a sharp object covered with blood or OPIM
- Human bites involving blood exposure (The source is the person who is bleeding, not the biter.)

If any of these events occurs, you should immediately contact your DICO.

For airborne- and/or droplet-transmissible diseases, the DICO will review the following criteria: the organism involved, the amount of time spent with the patient, the provider's distance from the patient, the procedure or task being performed, and the ventilation present.

Words of Wisdom

Contaminated laundry has been soiled with blood or OPIM or may contain sharps. A contaminated sharp is any contaminated object that can penetrate the skin.

According to a 1999 OSHA statement, postexposure medical management begins with the **source individual**, not the exposed employee. Employers must pay for all costs related to exposure events, including testing the source individual.

Blood work for the source patient should include rapid testing for the human immunodeficiency virus (HIV), HBV antigen, rapid HCV antibody, and, if the HIV or HCV test is positive, syphilis testing. The HIV and HCV results should be available in less than 1 hour, and HBV results usually are available by the following day. Because most care providers have been vaccinated against some diseases already, however, the time frame is not a major concern. Testing for HIV requires patient consent in roughly half the states in the United States, but state law often makes exceptions for occupational exposure of health care providers. In the other states, there is "deemed consent"—that is, the state assumes consent to be tested.

Under the Ryan White Comprehensive AIDS Resources Emergency (CARE) Act (otherwise known as the Ryan White notification law), the medical facility must release the source patient's test results to the DICO; this release is not considered a violation of privacy under the Health Information Portability and Accountability Act. The Ryan White CARE Act, Part G, also requires medical facilities to notify the DICO if a patient is transported who is suspected of having or known to have TB or meningitis.

This information is shared with the exposed employee, and proper care and counseling begin. The blood work done as a baseline for an exposed paramedic does not yield information on the exposure that just occurred; rather, it documents whether the paramedic already has one of these diseases. Postexposure medical counseling and treatment should begin within 24 to 48 hours, unless testing of the source patient yields information that necessitates more rapid follow-up.

Designated Infection Control Officer

The federal Ryan White CARE Act, Part G, requires that every emergency response agency have a DICO. This person is charged with ensuring that proper postexposure medical treatment and counseling are provided to the exposed employee or volunteer.

Postexposure medical treatment is offered to reduce the chances that an exposed health care provider will contract the disease to which he or she was exposed. Treatment should be offered within 24 to 48 hours following an exposure, with the actual time frame based on the diagnosis. Exposure to bacterial meningitis, for example, would require treatment within 24 hours.

The DICO tracks and monitors compliance with the correct time frames, serves as a liaison between the exposed employee and the medical facility, ensures that confidentiality is maintained, and ensures that documentation adheres to guidelines. This role of the DICO is important for workers' compensation issues and, in some states, presumption issues.

The communication network for exposure reporting involves three people: the exposed paramedic, the DICO, and the treating physician. A paramedic who believes an exposure has occurred should call the DICO directly. It is the DICO's job to determine whether an actual exposure occurred. Each department must have a reporting system that complies with the Ryan White notification law and the OSHA-required exposure control plan.

The public health department acts as a backup for exposure notification and determination of the need for medical follow-up treatment. Under the Ryan White notification law, the local public health department must know the identity of the DICO for each EMS department. The public health department director serves as a liaison for problems that may arise regarding exposure notification by the medical facility and the sharing of source-patient testing results.

YOU *are the Medic*   **PART 2**

You and your partner arrive at the patient's room, which is shared with another resident. Your patient is an 86-year-old woman who appears very ill. She is pale and appears very weak but is alert and able to answer questions. The staff member tells you the patient has been vomiting and having watery, nonbloody diarrhea for 2 days. The patient leans forward to vomit into a basin, and nothing comes up. The staff member not wearing gloves takes a tissue from a container and wipes the patient's mouth and then discards it in the trash can.

Recording Time: 1 Minute	
Appearance	Awake
Level of consciousness	Alert (oriented to person, place, and day)
Airway	Open
Breathing	Adequate
Circulation	Adequate

3. What can you determine about the patient's condition now?

4. Because a diagnosis of norovirus infection has not actually been made for this patient, are you concerned about exposure?

Standard Precautions

The term **standard precautions** describes infection control practices that reduce the opportunity for an exposure to occur in the daily care of patients. It replaces the older terms "universal precautions" and "body substance isolation (BSI)." The BSI precautions have been taught to EMS providers for the past decade; this approach assumes that all blood and body fluids are infectious. Standard precautions add another element: protection from moist body substances that may transmit other bacterial or viral infections. For example, a paramedic with a cut on a finger who suctions a patient with oral herpes lesions and does not wear a glove could become infected with herpes. Standard precautions apply to all body substances except sweat.

CDC-Recommended Immunizations and Vaccinations

Vaccines are suspensions of whole (live or inactivated) or fractionated bacteria or viruses that have been rendered nonpathogenic; they bring about immunity by causing the immune system to produce antibodies. Keeping current with recommended **vaccinations** boosts host resistance and the immune response. In 1997, the CDC published an **immunization** schedule for health care providers. A Tdap booster is required because of the increasing incidence of pertussis (whooping cough) in the United States. **Table 2** lists the CDC recommendations for health care providers. In 1999, OSHA began enforcing the CDC guidelines.

Each employer must offer the CDC-recommended vaccinations to staff and pay for them. Individual paramedics have the right to decline them but will be required to sign a declination form.

It is important for each new employee and volunteer to obtain his or her vaccination records. These records can be obtained from a personal physician, high school, college, training program, or previous employer. Current staff also need to obtain these records. To comply with privacy regulations, records must be requested by the employee or volunteer from one of the aforementioned sources.

Department Responsibilities

Under the OSHA mandate and the Ryan White CARE Act, Part G, to protect staff from exposure to bloodborne pathogens, meningitis, and TB, each EMS department is required to have a comprehensive exposure control plan. This document lays out the specifics of how the department plans to reduce the risk of exposure to infectious agents and provide postexposure medical follow-up, if needed. Key elements of the exposure control plan include proper education and training related to bloodborne pathogens and TB and establishment of postexposure medical follow-up procedures **Table 3**.

Another key component of the plan is compliance monitoring. Management must make spot checks to ensure that staff members are following the exposure control plan and that the plan is working effectively. Although management is responsible for developing and implementing the plan, OSHA has made it clear that the employees are required to follow the plan.

A part of the exposure control plan that benefits department personnel and patients is the work restriction guidelines. These guidelines, which were published by the CDC and are enforced by OSHA, indicate when employees with various illnesses may or may not be at work and when they may not care for high-risk patients. Work restriction guidelines require employees to use sick time unless the illness is the result of an occupational exposure, in which case it is covered under workers' compensation. Following work restriction guidelines is of particular importance during the flu (respiratory influenza) season.

It is important to distinguish between contamination and infection. An object that has microorganisms on or in it is **contaminated**. This term applies to water, food, dressing materials, linens, sharps, equipment, and even the ambulance. A person is not infected, however, unless the microorganisms actually produce an illness. With some diseases, such as HBV or HCV infection, a person may have the disease and not be aware of it; there are no signs or symptoms, and the person is not ill. However, such **carriers** can pass the disease to others through their blood and through sexual contact.

Table 2 Recommended Vaccinations for Health Care Providers
Hepatitis B
Measles, mumps, rubella (MMR)
Varicella (chickenpox)
Tuberculosis (TB) testing
Tetanus, diphtheria, and pertussis (Tdap): one-time dose followed by a booster every 10 years thereafter
Influenza (annually)
Adapted from: Centers for Disease Control and Prevention: Healthcare Personnel Vaccination Recommendations, March 2011.

Table 3 Exposure Control Plan Components
Exposure determination
Education and training
Hepatitis B vaccine program
Tuberculosis testing program
Personal protective equipment
Engineering controls and work practices
Postexposure management
Medical waste management
Compliance monitoring
Record keeping

Patient Assessment

The assessment of a patient suspected of having an infectious disease should be approached much like that of any other medical patient. First, the scene must be sized up and standard precautions taken. Once you have ensured that the scene is safe, proceed with the primary assessment by following the ABC plan—assess the patient's airway, breathing, circulation, and mental status, and prioritize treatment of the patient. With most patients who have a potentially infectious disease and are being seen in the prehospital setting, the next step is to take the patient's history, using OPQRST (Onset, Provocation/palliation, Quality, Radiation, Severity, Time of onset) to elaborate on the chief complaint. Typical chief complaints include fever, nausea, rash, pleuritic chest pain, and difficulty breathing. Be sure to obtain a SAMPLE history and a set of baseline vital signs, paying particular attention to medications the patient is currently taking, the events leading up to today's problem, and whether the patient has recently traveled. Always show respect for the feelings of patients, family, and others at the scene. Then proceed to the secondary assessment, including the physical exam.

Pathophysiology, Assessment, and Management of Common Infectious Diseases

Chain of Infection

Infection involves a chain of events through which the communicable disease spreads. In some cases, solving the puzzle of why a specific disease developed in a particular person or group of people may be as simple as retracing steps to find the source of exposure. In other cases, the puzzle is more difficult to solve, with infectious disease experts taking years to find a pattern in the spread of a disease and then plan a strategy to break the chain of the infection. The study of infectious diseases takes into consideration population demographics that can affect the spread of a disease, such as age distributions; genetic factors; income levels; ethnic groups; workplaces and schools; geographic boundaries; and the expansion, decline, or movement of the disease.

Here is a scenario that illustrates how easily disease may spread. In a local hospital pediatric unit, a visitor brought a box of candy for a child. Because of the "no food" rule, an attentive nurse placed the candy at the nurses' station. Another nurse had emptied a bedpan of stool from a child admitted for a hepatitis A infection but was in such a rush that she forgot to wash her hands. She then noticed the box of candy, poked at a few selections with her fingernails, and finally found one she wanted to eat. The candy was consumed throughout the morning. Subsequently, another nurse came down with hepatitis A, a disease that is typically spread by the oral-fecal route. The chain of infection in this scenario could have been broken by handwashing.

Exposure and the Risk of Infection

Several factors determine a person's risk of contracting an infection following an exposure. An organism's mere presence presents a risk. However, other factors influence the level of risk, including the dose of the organism, the virulence of the organism, its mode of entry, and the host resistance of the exposed person.

Type of Organism

Pathogenic organisms include bacteria, viruses, fungi, and parasites. They differ in the ways in which they infect the host, grow and reproduce within host tissues, and cause illness. **Table 4** compares these organisms.

Dose of the Organism

A certain number of organisms must be present for infection to occur. For example, the laboratory report on a urine specimen sent for culture may note "greater than 100,000 colonies of bacteria per milliliter" of urine indicating infection. A value of equal to or less than 100,000 is considered as not indicating infection.

Virulence of the Organism

<u>Virulence</u> is the ability of an organism to invade and create disease in a host. It also encompasses the organism's ability to survive outside the living host. For example, HIV does not pose a risk outside the human body because it dies when it is exposed to light and air.

Mode of Entry

If the organism does not enter the body by the "correct" route, infection cannot occur. For example, a respiratory virus that enters the body through a cut will not cause a respiratory viral infection and likely will not cause any infection. On the other hand, an inhaled respiratory virus could cause respiratory illness. Thus, if you apply a mask to a patient who might have a communicable respiratory disease, you will not inhale the droplets.

Host Resistance

The healthier you are, the less susceptible you are to infection. Your ability to fight off infection is called <u>host resistance</u>. Your immune system will help protect you from acquiring disease even though all of the other risk factors may be present. Wellness programs and immunization programs serve to boost host resistance.

Once a susceptible person has been exposed to an organism, it takes time for the organism to multiply within the body and produce symptoms. That period between exposure to the organism and the first symptoms of illness is called the <u>incubation period</u>. For example, it usually takes 12 to 26 days from a susceptible person's exposure to the mumps virus until the person begins to feel feverish and ill. The incubation period for the influenza virus is much shorter—usually 24 to 72 hours.

Most communicable diseases are contagious only during a portion of the illness. A person may be sick with chickenpox for 2 to 3 weeks but is capable of transmitting the virus to another person for only about 1 week—from 1 day before the <u>vesicles</u> appear on the skin to about 6 days after. The period during which a person can transmit the illness to someone else is called the <u>communicable period</u>.

Table 4   Comparison of Selected Pathogenic Organisms

Organism	Life Cycle	Effect on Host	Example
Bacteria	Grow and reproduce outside the human cell in an environment characterized by the appropriate temperature and nutrients	Cause disease when they invade and multiply within the host's tissues	*Salmonella* bacteria can multiply in potato salad that has been unrefrigerated, leading to human illness when the food is eaten
Viruses	Much smaller than bacteria and can multiply only inside a host; die when exposed to the environment	Cause disease when they invade and multiply within the host's tissues	Human immunodeficiency virus (HIV) does not multiply or maintain its infectiousness outside a living host
Fungi	Similar to bacteria in that they can grow rapidly in the presence of nutrients and organic material	Most infections acquired from contact with decaying organic matter or airborne spores in the environment; often cause opportunistic infections in people with compromised immune systems	Range from relatively harmless infections of the skin, such as athlete's foot (*Tinea pedis*), to life-threatening systemic infections, such as pneumonia (*Pneumocystis jirovecii*, formerly known as *Pneumocystis carinii*) in people with acquired immunodeficiency syndrome (AIDS)
Parasites	Live in or on another living creature	Take advantage of their host by feeding off the host cells and tissues	Scabies and lice **Protozoa**: single-celled, usually microscopic, eukaryotic organisms such as amoebas, ciliates, flagellates, and sporozoans. *Entamoeba histolytica*, for example, causes dysentery Helminths (commonly called worms): invertebrates with long, flexible, rounded or flattened bodies; *Ascaris lumbricoides*, for example, causes hookworm

In the context of communicable disease, a **reservoir** is a place where organisms may live and multiply. In institutional settings, for example, air-conditioning systems and showerheads have been identified as reservoirs for the bacterium that causes Legionnaires disease. In ambulances, the oxygen humidifier is commonly implicated as a reservoir for infection. Health care personnel are responsible not only for protecting themselves from contracting communicable diseases, but also ensuring, to the extent possible, that they and their equipment do not transmit illness to others.

Host Defense Mechanisms

The human body provides built-in protection from pathogenic organisms with several defenses that protect against **infection**. Skin, which covers the entire exterior of the body, offers a primary protective barrier blocking pathogens' ability to enter through the intact surface. The normal secretions of the skin also provide an antibacterial property that protects against pathogen entry. Antibacterial handwashing solutions should not be used because they kill all bacteria on the skin, including normal flora.

Mucous membranes offer another protective barrier. For example, the eyes produce tears that dilute and remove foreign substances. The mucous membranes that line the urinary, respiratory, and gastrointestinal (GI) tracts also trap and remove organisms. Cells that line the respiratory tract secrete lysozymes that destroy bacteria, while macrophages trap and destroy bacteria; thus, these mucous membranes serve as a first line of defense against airborne and droplet-transmitted diseases. Goblet cells lining the GI tract produce highly acidic and alkaline secretions, which form barriers that prevent penetration by bacteria and some viruses.

The immune system contains proteins that kill viruses. Immune response ignites the production of antibodies that are directed against specific invading organisms. B cells and T cells work together to fight infection.

■ General Management Principles

The general management of a patient with a suspected communicable disease first focuses on any life-threatening conditions that were identified in the primary assessment (airway maintenance, oxygen and ventilatory assistance, bleeding control, and circulatory support). Remember to be empathetic. Because most patients with a communicable disease will have a fever of an unexplained origin or mild breathing problems, place the patient in a position of comfort on the stretcher and keep him or her warm. If the patient has early signs of dehydration, a preliminary IV and a fluid infusion of normal saline or lactated Ringer's solution may be appropriate. Remember to use standard precautions for your own safety and to properly dispose of sharps, even needle-safe devices. Always follow your agency's exposure control plan for cleaning the suction unit and any reusable equipment, and properly discard any disposable supplies and linens.

Meningitis

Meningitis is an inflammation of the membranes that cover the brain and spinal cord, called the *meninges*. Two types of meningitis are distinguished: bacterial and viral. The bacterial form is communicable, and the viral form is not. Meningitis is not transmitted through the air, but rather is a droplet-transmitted disease. The most common bacterial organisms implicated in meningitis are *Neisseria meningitidis, Streptococcus pneumoniae, Haemophilus influenzae*, group B *Streptococcus*, and *Listeria monocytogenes*.

The type of meningitis most often involved in epidemic outbreaks is **meningococcal meningitis**, which is caused by *N meningitidis*. Sporadic cases of meningococcal meningitis occur most frequently during winter and spring, but epidemic outbreaks can occur at any time, especially when people live together in crowded conditions, such as in college dorms, homeless shelters, or military barracks.

Pathophysiology

Transmission occurs following direct contact with the nasopharyngeal secretions of an infected person (mouth-to-mouth, suctioning, or intubation with spraying of secretions) or prolonged contact time of 8 or more hours. The incubation period for meningococcal meningitis is between 2 and 10 days. The communicable period is variable; it lasts as long as meningococcal bacteria are present in the patient's nasal and oral secretions. The microorganisms generally disappear from the patient's upper respiratory tract within 24 hours after antibiotic treatment begins.

Words of Wisdom

Meningitis is not transmitted by airborne means. Viral meningitis is infectious but not communicable.

Assessment

The classic signs and symptoms of meningitis are the same for the viral and bacterial forms: sudden-onset fever, severe headache, stiff neck, Kernig sign (the patient cannot extend his or her leg at the knee when the thigh is flexed because of stiffness in the hamstrings), Brudzinski sign (passive flexion of the leg on one side causes a similar movement in the opposite leg), photosensitivity, and a pink rash that becomes purple. The patient almost always experiences changes in mental status, ranging from apathy to delirium. Projectile vomiting is common. Diagnosis is made by Gram stain, a simple test in which CSF is placed on a slide, crystal violet stain is added to the CSF, and there is an initial identification of whether a bacterium or virus is present.

Management

When you are treating a patient with meningitis, ask the patient to wear a surgical mask or a nonrebreathing mask. If this is not possible, you should wear a surgical mask. Routine standard precautions, including gloves and good handwashing

Special Populations

Meningitis in infants and children has decreased in incidence and mortality with the development and administration of vaccines. Vaccines protect against *Haemophilus influenzae* type b, *Streptococcus* pneumonia, and *Neisseria meningitidis*. Vaccine administration is started at age 2 months. However, in a child who has not been vaccinated, meningitis remains a major emergency that requires antibiotic treatment.

The health care provider must assess the patient for signs and symptoms suggestive of meningitis, which include fever, vomiting, irritability, and lethargy. In infants, a bulging fontanelle may also be noted. The paramedic should assess the patient for respiratory distress, which may indicate the need for intubation en route, oxygen administration, and rapid transport.

technique, are also important. Diagnosis is not made until a lumbar puncture is performed, so precautions must be maintained throughout your interactions with the patient.

Additional treatment will be added based on symptoms. Patient needs may include oxygen, airway management, and ventilation support. Medical control may order IV fluids based on patient signs and symptoms, and medications may be ordered en route if seizures occur or the patient shows signs of shock. Only patients with severe signs and symptoms would require rapid transport to a medical facility.

Transmission from patient to health care provider is rare. Postexposure treatment typically includes ciprofloxacin (one dose given orally) or rifampin for 2 days. This treatment is not appropriate if the person is taking birth control pills, and it should not be offered to pregnant patients. The meningitis vaccine is not recommended for any health care provider group; it is recommended for college students entering dormitory living for the first time, military recruits, and middle school and high school students. Ciprofloxacin-resistant bacterial meningitis has been documented in the United States. It is important to offer postexposure treatment only when an actual exposure has occurred.

Tuberculosis

Tuberculosis (TB) is an important cause of disability and death in much of the developing world. This disease was once widespread in the United States, but no longer. In 2009, the lowest incidence of TB in US history was documented. About 52% of all cases reported in the United States occurred in California, New York, Florida, Illinois, and Texas.

Pathophysiology

TB is *not* a highly communicable disease. Three types of TB exist: typical, which is communicable, and atypical and extrapulmonary (TB of the bone, kidney, lymph glands, and so on), which are not communicable. Persons at risk for contracting TB include the malnourished, such as the homeless, and incarcerated persons, due to overcrowded conditions and poor health care. The immunocompromised are also at risk due to suppressed immune response.

TB infection (latent TB) means that a person has tested positive for exposure to TB but does not have, and may never develop, active disease. People with TB infection do not pose a risk to others. *TB disease* means that the person has active TB disease verified by laboratory testing and a positive chest radiograph.

The first case of multidrug-resistant TB (MDR-TB) was identified in Boston, Massachusetts, in 1985. Although it was initially an untreatable disease, therapies for it are now available. MDR-TB means that the bacterium is resistant to two or more of the first-line drugs (of several available) used to treat TB. MDR-TB occurs in immunocompromised people who have not completed the full course of treatment, but its incidence is quite low. In 2008, 107 cases were reported in the United States (of a total population of more than 300 million people). In 2007, extensively drug-resistant TB (XDR-TB) was identified in the United States. There were two cases reported in 2007; however, there were no reported cases in 2008 or 2009. XDR-TB means that the bacterium is resistant to two of the first-line oral medications and two of the first-line injectable medications, but there are other medications available. MDR-TB and XDR-TB are treatable diseases.

Transmission occurs by large, airborne particles from a person with active untreated disease. In general, that type of spread occurs among people who have continued, intimate exposure to the infected person (primarily people living in the same household). For paramedics, such intense exposure is likely to occur only when mouth-to-mouth ventilation is given to a patient with active untreated TB.

The incubation period for TB is 4 to 12 weeks. The disease is communicable only when an active lesion develops in the lungs and bacteria are expelled into the air by coughing. Of patients who are treated, 10% are no longer communicable after 2 days of treatment. After 14 days of treatment, virtually all patients are no longer communicable.

Early infection with TB can be detected by a **tuberculin skin test** or by the QuantiFERON-TB Gold blood test. All health care providers, including paramedics, should have a tuberculin test at the beginning of employment and periodically based on the TB risk assessment for the department. The TB risk assessment is based on the number of patients with active-untreated TB the department transported in the previous 12 months, not on the number of patients in the community served. If a known positive history is present when a person is hired, a questionnaire must be completed by the employee. This is then reviewed by the designated physician. It is important to note that TB develops in only 10% of persons with a positive TB test. Disease activation would depend on the overall health status of the person later in life. A chest radiograph is indicated only for a first positive test.

Assessment

Signs and symptoms of TB include a persistent cough for more than 3 weeks plus one of more of the following: night sweats, headache, fever, fatigue, weight loss, hemoptysis, hoarseness, or chest pain.

Management

As a preventive measure, place a surgical mask on a patient suspected of having TB. If the patient cannot be masked, place a surgical mask on yourself to block transmission of TB. N95 or HEPA respirators are not needed or required for EMS transport of a suspected TB patient (CDC, 2005 TB Guidelines). The patient may require high-concentration oxygen administration and/or airway or ventilation support based on assessment. If preventive measures were not taken, report the incident to your DICO. Given that the incubation period for TB is 4 to 12 weeks, a paramedic who suspects he or she has been exposed to TB should assess the need for baseline testing and then be retested in 8 to 10 weeks. If the test has become positive at that time, the paramedic needs to have a chest radiograph to rule out infection and usually will be offered a 6- to 9-month course of antibiotic therapy. Because these drugs are toxic to the liver, the paramedic should not consume alcohol while taking the drugs, and liver function tests should be conducted monthly.

No special measures are required after transporting a patient suspected of having active TB. The vehicle should be cleaned as usual. No airing is required.

■ Pneumonia

Pathophysiology

Each year more than 60,000 people in the United States die of **pneumonia**, which is an inflammation of the lungs. The cause of pneumonia may be bacteria, viruses, fungi, or other organisms. More than 50 types of pneumonia have been identified, ranging from mild to life threatening. Most cases of pneumonia are not communicable. Cases caused by *Staphylococcus* or *Streptococcus* may be communicable and would be transmitted via respiratory secretions.

Assessment

People who are most susceptible to pneumonia are older adults, people who smoke heavily, people with alcoholism, people with chronic illnesses, and immunocompromised people. Worldwide, pneumonia is a leading cause of death in pediatric patients, particularly infants.

Patients may present with high fever, chest pain, cough (productive), and respiratory distress. If this is noted, check for diminished breath sounds. In this case, proper airway management and ventilation support may be indicated. Oxygen administration and IV treatment should be administered.

Management

Although antibiotics have been very successful in treating the most common forms of bacterial pneumonia, some antibiotic-resistant strains pose a serious therapeutic challenge.

A mask on the patient or a surgical mask on the paramedic would reduce any exposure.

■ Respiratory Syncytial Virus

Pathophysiology

Respiratory syncytial virus (RSV) is the leading cause of lower respiratory tract infections in infants, older people, and immunocompromised people. This virus spreads in the hospital environment and in the community. In the community setting, outbreaks generally occur in late fall, winter, and early spring.

Transmission may occur in two ways: (1) by direct contact with large droplets that do not extend more than 3', or (2) by indirect contact with contaminated hands or contaminated items. Research has shown that RSV on hands will die within 1 hour; however, the virus has been shown to survive on other surfaces for as long as 30 hours. The incubation period ranges from 2 to 8 days.

Assessment

Signs and symptoms include those of upper respiratory infection—sneezing, runny nose, nasal congestion, cough, and fever. The disease progresses to the lower respiratory tract, leading to pneumonia, bronchiolitis, and tracheobronchitis. Hypoxemia and apnea are often seen in infants and are usually the leading cause for a child's hospitalization.

Management

Prevention of RSV transmission relies on proper use of PPE. Gloves should be worn when caring for an RSV-infected patient, and their removal must be followed by good handwashing. The use of alcohol-based foams or gels is acceptable. Post-transport cleaning of the vehicle is important, but special cleaning solutions are not required.

Postexposure treatment consists of supportive care. If you have been exposed, your DICO will monitor your health status. Health care providers in whom RSV infection develops should be placed on work restrictions—in particular, they should not care for immunocompromised patients.

■ Other Respiratory Conditions

A number of other respiratory conditions may (or may not) be associated with a fever and may (or may not) be infectious.

YOU are the Medic | PART 3

You begin your assessment of the patient. When asked, she says that she has been vomiting and having diarrhea for a few days. She also says she is too weak to stand and has not been able to keep water down. When your partner feels for the patient's pulse, there is obvious tenting when the skin on her forearm is pinched.

Recording Time: 5 Minutes	
Respirations	18 breaths/min
Pulse	106 beats/min
Skin	Pale, cool, dry; tenting noted
Blood pressure	98/58 mm Hg
Oxygen saturation (Spo$_2$)	97% on room air
Pupils	Equal and reactive

5. After oxygen, what is your first choice of treatment for this patient?
6. Are there any notifications you should make concerning the scene?

These conditions run the gamut from mildly annoying symptoms to potentially life-threatening conditions.

Bronchitis arises when the inner walls of the bronchioles become inflamed, usually due to infection. Symptoms include soreness in the chest and throat, congestion, wheezing, dyspnea, and a slight fever. This condition may be caused by the same virus that causes the common cold and gastric reflux disease (GERD) and/or by common pollutants and smoking or second-hand smoke. Patients are considered to have chronic bronchitis if they cough most days for spans of 3 months or more a year, for 2 or more consecutive years. Chronic bronchitis is discussed further in the chapter, *Respiratory Emergencies*.

Laryngitis is an inflammation of the voice box due to overuse, irritation, or infection. Its cause is usually viral but can be bacterial. Symptoms include hoarseness, weak voice, sore throat, dry throat, and cough.

Epiglottitis is a life-threatening condition that causes the epiglottis and supraglottic tissues to swell. The pus-filled flap of tissue then partially or completely occludes the glottic opening. Although this disease can affect any age group, it is most prevalent in 2- to 7-year-olds. Its incidence has fallen sharply since 1985, when administration of the *Haemophilus influenzae* type b (Hib) vaccine to 2-month-old infants became routine. Symptoms include difficulty breathing and swallowing with stridor and drooling. Patients are very anxious, are cyanotic, and have a muffled voice and fever. Epiglottitis is caused by the Hib bacteria and is contagious by the droplet route via coughing and sneezing.

The common cold is an infection of the upper respiratory system characterized by a runny nose, sore throat, cough, congestion, and watery eyes. Any one of 200 viruses can cause the cold, so symptoms may vary. Patients do not have a fever. Colds are especially common in preschoolers but can occur in people of all ages. Colds usually last about a week and are spread by droplets, coughing, hand-to-hand contact, and shared utensils.

■ Mononucleosis

Pathophysiology

Mononucleosis is caused by the Epstein-Barr virus (EBV), a herpes virus. This virus is also suspected of causing a related disease, chronic fatigue syndrome. The virus grows in the epithelium of the oropharynx and sheds into saliva—hence the name "kissing disease." In most of the cases of mononucleosis there are no symptoms, which means the EBV infection is subclinical. Studies show that EBV infects about 50% of children by the age of 5; they also show that about 90% of such cases are subclinical. This illness is not reportable in all states.

Transmission occurs via direct contact with the saliva of an infected person. Some cases have also been linked to contaminated blood transfusions. The incubation period is 4 to 6 weeks following exposure, with a prolonged communicable period.

Assessment

Signs and symptoms of mononucleosis include sore throat, fever, secretions from the pharynx, swollen lymph glands (especially the posterior cervical glands), malaise, anorexia, headache,

muscle pain, and an enlarged liver and spleen. Pharyngeal secretions may persist for 1 year or more after infection. In severe cases, complications may include anemia, dehydration, spleen rupture, seizures, or pneumonia.

Management

Prevention of mononucleosis involves the use of gloves and good handwashing techniques when in direct contact with a patient's oral secretions. No special cleaning solutions are required following transport of a patient.

> ### Words of Wisdom
>
> A paramedic with a cold or flu can be extremely hazardous to a patient who is immunocompromised.

■ Seasonal Influenza

Influenza (flu) viruses cause acute respiratory illnesses generally presenting as winter epidemics. In the United States, the flu causes approximately 36,000 deaths each year.

> ### Special Populations
>
> Infection rates are high in children, but the most deaths occur among adults older than 65 years, especially people with medical conditions such as chronic pulmonary or heart disease.

nH1N1 (novel H1N1) influenza began in California and was first believed to be poised to cause a major pandemic. Fortunately, however, it proved to be a new seasonal flu virus that did not result in a significant number of deaths worldwide. The comparison to the number of deaths in the United States each year from normal seasonal flu makes this very clear. Each year in the United States, at least 36,000 people die of seasonal flu. For nH1N1 worldwide, the World Health Organization (WHO) reported fewer than 19,000 deaths.

Pathophysiology

For this droplet-transmitted disease, transmission was thought to be airborne. However, further research has shown transmission to be hand-to-nose-to-mouth-to-eye. The incubation period is about 1 to 4 days following exposure. The communicable period in adults lasts from the day before symptoms begin until about 5 days after the onset of the illness.

Assessment

Signs and symptoms of influenza include systemic fever, shaking chills, headache, muscle pain, malaise, and loss of appetite. Respiratory symptoms include dry, often protracted coughing; hoarseness; and nasal discharge. The duration of illness is about 3 to 4 days, and complications may include viral or bacterial pneumonia.

Management

Prevention of influenza involves placing a surgical mask or non-rebreathing mask on the patient. This has been a mild disease over the past 2 years. Very few patients have required IV fluids for dehydration or ventilation assistance during transport. The key preventive measure, however, is an annual "flu shot." Each year, a new vaccine is developed based on the anticipated strains for that year. The injectable form of the vaccine does not contain live virus, so you cannot get the disease from the flu shot. An alternative to the injectable form is the nasal spray, which contains live attenuated virus. There is no work restriction needed for a paramedic who takes the nasal spray. The nasal spray is an option for people younger than 49 years. If you do not take a flu shot, you must sign a declination form. This provision is set forth by OSHA, NFPA 1581, and the CDC. An effort is under way to make seasonal flu vaccination mandatory for all health care providers as a patient safety issue.

If you have not been vaccinated and have an exposure, antiviral drugs may be offered within 48 hours to reduce the severity of the flu should you contract it.

Pathophysiology, Assessment, and Management of Sexually Transmitted Diseases

As the name implies, sexually transmitted diseases (STDs) are usually acquired by sexual contact. Although the term *STD* ordinarily conjures up diagnoses such as gonorrhea or syphilis, the range of diseases transmitted sexually is wide and includes such conditions as herpes, hepatitis, and HIV infection. Hepatitis, HIV infection, and acquired immunodeficiency syndrome (AIDS) are considered separately in this chapter. This section reviews the features of gonorrhea, syphilis, scabies, and genital herpes infections. In most cases, you will not know that a patient has an STD; therefore, standard precautions and good handwashing are appropriate.

Gonorrhea

Pathophysiology

Gonorrhea is an infection caused by the gonococcal bacteria, *Neisseria gonorrhoeae*. In 2009, more than 300,000 cases of gonorrhea were reported to the CDC. Transmission occurs sexually, by contact with the pus-containing fluid from mucous membranes of infected persons. Therefore, anyone who engages in unprotected sexual contact is at risk. The incubation period is usually 2 to 7 days but may be longer. This infection is communicable for months if not treated. If treated, the disease is noncommunicable within hours.

Assessment

Signs and symptoms of gonorrhea differ between males and females. Males usually experience a pus-containing discharge from the urethra and often report pain on urination (dysuria) starting a few days after exposure. In women, the initial inflammation of the urethra or cervix may be so mild that it passes unnoticed, and the illness may progress to pelvic inflammatory disease, with signs and symptoms of an acute abdomen. Depending on the patient's sexual practices, gonorrheal infection may also involve the anus and throat.

Management

The risk of acquiring any STD through a route other than sexual contact is remote. Prevention includes glove use if touching drainage from the genital area and thorough handwashing.

Syphilis

Pathophysiology

Syphilis is caused by the spiral shaped bacterium *Treponema pallidum*. Because the disease progresses in three stages, it is considered to be an acute and a chronic disease. Its incidence has been increasing in the United States for the past several years. The groups with the highest incidence rates are people aged 20 to 35 years. High numbers of cases are also reported in urban areas. This disease has been increasing in major areas: California, Texas, Florida, and New York City. Generally, men who have sex with men have a high incidence rate, but in Florida the highest rate is in a large retirement community. The CDC initially published a plan to eliminate this disease in the United States by 2010. However, due to new STD guidelines, this has now been set for 2015.

Transmission occurs by direct contact with the infectious fluids of the primary lesion(s). The bacteria can be transmitted across the placenta from an infected mother to her fetus, by sexual contact, or through blood transfusion. The incubation period is 10 days to 3 months; the communicable period is variable. If treated with penicillin, the person is considered noncontagious within 48 hours.

Assessment

The primary infection with syphilis produces an ulcerative lesion, called a chancre, of the skin or mucous membrane at the site of infection Figure 5 . Chancres are most commonly located in the genital region. *Secondary infection* is the term used to describe the presence of skin rash, patchy hair loss, and swollen lymph glands. Complications of syphilis in the tertiary (third) stage can include cardiac, ophthalmic, auditory, and central nervous system complications and lesions of the tissues and bone.

Management

Prevention measures include use of gloves and good handwashing techniques. No special cleaning precautions are required.

Genital Herpes

Pathophysiology

Genital herpes is a chronic, recurrent illness produced by infection with the herpes simplex virus. The herpes simplex virus is further classified into two types: type 1 is generally transmitted via contact with oral secretions, and type 2 is spread through sexual contact. All sexually active persons are at risk for this infection. Cases of genital herpes do not have to be reported to the CDC, so data on incidence are not available. Herpes simplex

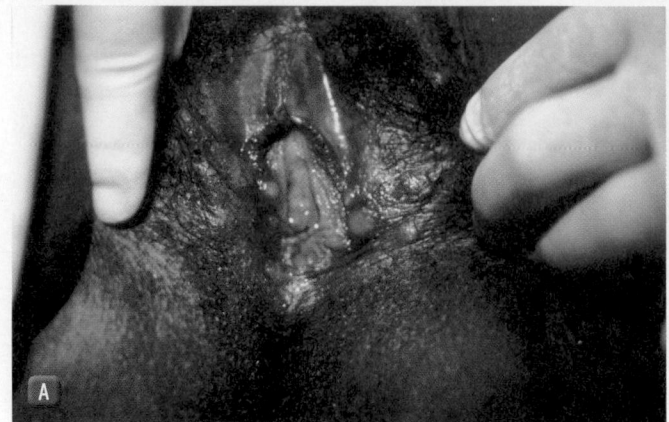

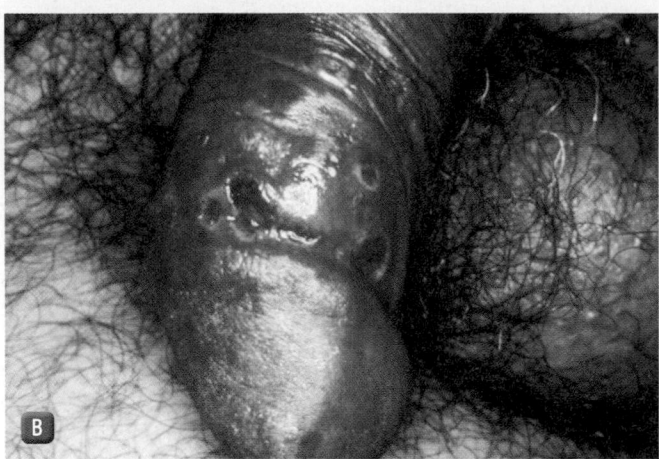

Figure 5 A chancre is a painless ulceration that arises at the site of syphilis infection, such as the rectum or genitals. It often appears on the vulva or vagina in women **(A)** or on the penis in men **(B)**. This small round lesion heralds the primary stage of the disease.

type 1 infection is usually activated from a dormant status by stress and febrile illness. It causes a blister-like sore, usually on the lips or inside the mouth.

Paramedics need to use gloves and use good handwashing practices if they come in contact with the lesions. If a paramedic has an open cut on the hand or finger and is in contact with the drainage, the paramedic may develop herpetic whitlow (herpes infection of the finger), which is considered an occupational risk. To avoid such risks, use of gloves is important when suctioning or intubating a patient with oral lesions. There is no postexposure treatment for this infection.

Assessment

Genital herpes is characterized by vesicular lesions **Figure 6** . In women, the vesicles occur initially on the cervix; during recurrent infections, vesicles may also appear around the vulva, legs, and buttocks. In men, lesions commonly occur on the penis, as

well as around the anus, depending on sexual practices. Lesions may also be present on the mouth as the result of oral sex.

Transmission usually occurs through sexual contact, but infants may become infected if delivered through the birth canal of a woman with active disease. The incubation period is 2 to 12 days. Secretion of the virus in saliva has been noted to persist for up to 7 weeks following the appearance of a lesion. Genital lesions are infectious for 4 to 7 days.

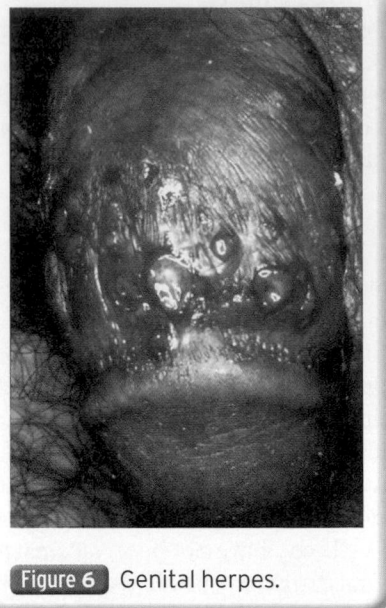

Figure 6 Genital herpes.

This disease is elusive; it can suddenly become reactivated, often repeatedly, over many years. Outbreaks are often stress-related.

Management

There is no cure for genital herpes. However, it can be treated with acyclovir, valacyclovir, or famciclovir for 7 to 10 days to reduce outbreaks. Preventive measures include the use of gloves when touching drainage from lesions and good handwashing techniques. No special cleaning precautions are necessary.

Chlamydia

Pathophysiology

Chlamydia infections have the highest incidence of all STDs. In 2009, more than 1 million cases were reported to the CDC; the growth in this number is believed to be the result of the availability of more sensitive screening tests and the trend toward routine screening.

Transmission occurs through sexual contact. Perinatal infections may result in premature rupture of membranes, premature birth, or stillbirth. The incubation period is believed to be 7 to 14 days or longer. The communicable period is unknown.

Assessment

In most women with chlamydia, the infection initially remains asymptomatic. However, in many women infected with *Chlamydia trachomatis*, pelvic inflammatory disease eventually develops. In men, infection may lead to epididymitis, prostatitis, proctitis, and proctocolitis.

Signs and symptoms include inflammation of the urethra, epididymis, cervix, and fallopian tubes when the infection is acquired through sexual transmission. Urethral discharge may be gray or white. The amount of discharge is variable.

Management

Chlamydia infection is treated with antibiotics. Preventive measures include wearing gloves when in contact with discharge from the genital area and using good handwashing techniques. There are no special cleaning requirements for the EMS vehicle or linens.

◼ Scabies

Pathophysiology

Scabies is caused by infection with *Sarcoptes scabiei*, a parasite. The incidence of this disease has been increasing during the past few years in the United States and Europe. This infection commonly affects families, children, sexual partners, chronically ill patients, and people in group homes. People of every race and social class are vulnerable to scabies infection.

Transmission occurs via direct skin-to-skin contact, such as through wrestling, sexual contact, and by sharing undergarments, towels, and linens. The incubation period is 4 to 6 weeks for persons with no prior exposure to the pathogen. A second or subsequent infestation may appear in as little as a few days. The communicable period lasts until the mites and eggs are destroyed by treatment. The female mite can live on a human host for several weeks. Without a host, the parasite dies in 2 to 4 days.

Assessment

Signs and symptoms of scabies include a rash of small, raised red bumps where the mite has burrowed into the skin, causing intense itching, especially at night. The rash appears on the hands, flexor aspects of the wrists, axillary folds, ankles, toes, genital area, buttocks, and abdomen **Figure 7**. The patient may develop sores from scratching the rash.

Management

Prevention consists of wearing gloves and practicing good handwashing techniques. Vehicle linens require only routine

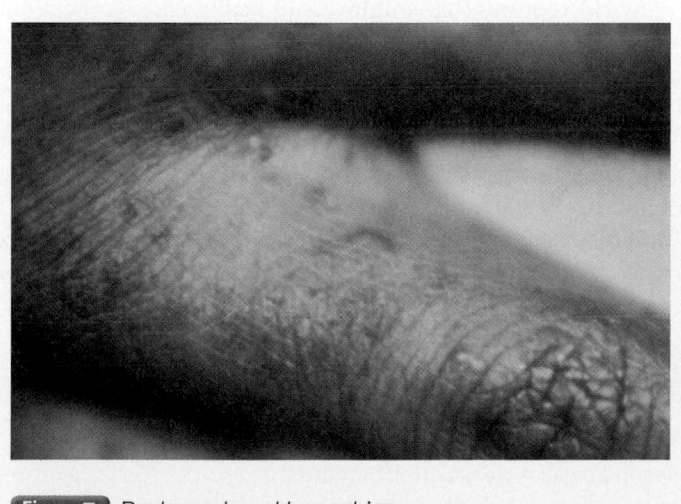

Figure 7 Rash produced by scabies.

washing in hot water, with routine cleaning of the vehicle after patient transport. Lindane is a topical treatment for scabies, but no treatment cream or lotion should be applied on a routine basis because of reports of lindane toxicity. In case of documented exposure, treatment will be undertaken and work restrictions from patient care may be ordered.

◼ Lice

Pathophysiology

Lice are small insects that crawl through the hair and feed on blood through the skin. They cannot hop or fly. There are three types of lice: the head louse (*Pediculus humanus capitis*), body louse (*Pediculus humanus corporis*), and pubic louse (*Phthirus pubis*).

All types of lice are acquired through direct contact with an infested person. Head and body lice can also be acquired from objects such as hats, combs, or clothes infested with lice. Lice eggs look like small white or tan dots on the skin. The eggs hatch after about 1 week, and the new lice mature in 1 to 2 weeks. Thereafter, an adult will begin to reproduce and will lay eggs over the next 28 days. Head lice can be found in the hair and on in other hairy areas of the head, such as eyebrows, eyelashes, mustaches, and beards. Body lice are usually found in the seams of clothing and can transfer certain diseases.

When discussing **lice** as an STD, the focus is on pubic or crab lice. *Phthirus pubis* is a parasite that is usually grayish. Lice are common in people with poor hygiene, people living in group homes, and people with multiple sexual partners.

Transmission of pubic lice occurs through intimate physical or sexual contact. The incubation period lasts approximately 8 to 10 days after the eggs hatch. The communicable period ends when all lice and eggs are destroyed by treatment.

Assessment

Signs and symptoms of pubic lice include slight to severe itching and irritation and, possibly, sores. Nits (eggs) can be seen clinging to the pubic, perianal, or perineal hair. Pubic lice can also infest eyelashes, eyebrows, axillae, scalp, and other body hairs.

Management

Preventive measures include wearing gloves and practicing good handwashing techniques. Routine cleaning of the vehicle after transport is sufficient. In case of documented exposure, treatment with permethrin cream may be prescribed, and restrictions from patient care may be indicated until the paramedic is free of lice.

◼ Pathophysiology, Assessment, and Management of Common Bloodborne Diseases

◼ Types of Viral Hepatitis

Viral hepatitis is an inflammation of the liver produced by a virus. Five distinct forms of viral hepatitis (A, B, C, D, and E) exist.

They are produced by different viruses and vary somewhat in their means of transmission. However, all types present with the same signs and symptoms, so the type causing illness is ultimately determined by blood testing. Hepatitis A and hepatitis E are discussed as enteric (intestinal) diseases in this chapter, because they are not bloodborne infections.

Hepatitis B Virus Infection

Hepatitis type B virus (HBV), also known as <u>serum hepatitis</u>, is transmitted through sexual contact, blood transfusion, or puncture of the skin with contaminated needles. Until immunization programs began in the United States in 1982, health care providers, especially those involved in surgery, dentistry, and emergency medicine, were deemed to have a particularly high risk of contracting hepatitis through accidental needlestick injuries. Since then, the incidence of occupationally acquired HBV infection has fallen by 95%. In 2009, the CDC announced that infection with HBV is now infrequent among health care workers. Immunization programs targeting children and young adults have reduced the incidence of HBV in the general population.

Pathophysiology

Needles, including those used for tattooing and acupuncture, and occasionally other objects, such as shared razors, have been implicated in transmission of HBV. Type B hepatitis is particularly common among intravenous (IV) drug users who share needles.

Limited data suggest that the HBV can survive outside the body in the medium of dried blood for as long as 7 days. The incubation period for HBV varies widely—from 45 to 200 days. The communicable period starts weeks before the first symptoms appear and may persist for years in chronic carriers. An estimated 2% to 10% of all HBV-infected people will become chronic carriers. In about 3% to 5% of people infected with HBV, cirrhosis of the liver or liver cancer will eventually develop.

Assessment

Signs and symptoms of HBV infection include loss of appetite, nausea, vomiting, general fatigue and malaise, low-grade fever, vague abdominal discomfort, and, sometimes, aching in the joints. The very smell of food may provoke nausea, and smokers often notice a sudden distaste for cigarettes. At this point, signs and symptoms subside for 50% to 60% of infected persons, which explains why many infected people never know that they have acquired the disease. For people whose disease progresses into the second phase, their urine begins to turn dark. A day or two later, <u>jaundice</u>, a yellowing of the skin, and scleral <u>icterus</u>, a yellowing of the sclera (the whites of the eyes), develop in the patient Figure 8 . Type B hepatitis usually lasts several weeks, although complete recovery may take 3 to 4 months.

Management

Prevention of HBV transmission focuses on using gloves when handling blood, OPIM, or materials containing visible blood. Good handwashing technique is also essential. Paramedics should be immunized against HBV when hired.

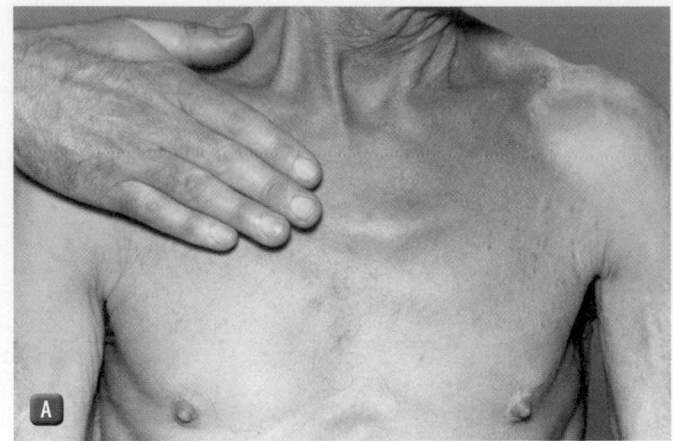

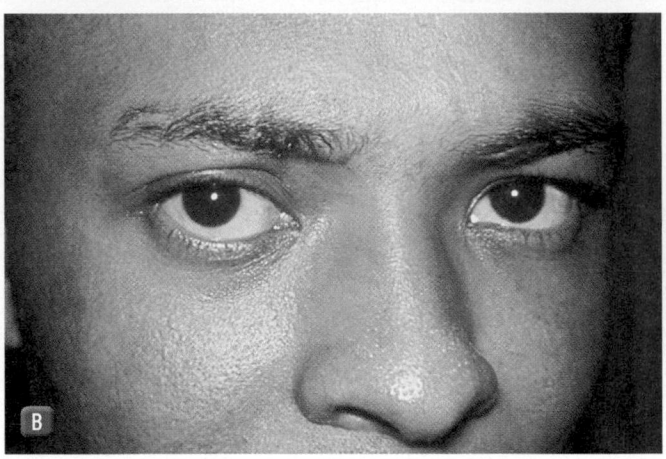

Figure 8 Signs of HBV infection. **A.** Jaundice. **B.** Scleral icterus.

Vaccination, which is safe and effective, protects against HBV for life; it also protects indirectly against hepatitis D virus (HDV) infection, because a person must be infected with type B to acquire type D.

OSHA requires that employers of health care workers offer the HBV immunization at no cost to at-risk staff members. If you are allergic to yeast or mercury (thimerosal), notify the vaccine administrator, and arrangements will be made to obtain the proper vaccine to meet your needs. The vaccine is administered in a three-dose series Table 5 . When the series has been completed, you should have a blood test (titer) performed 1 to 2 months later to ensure that your immune system responded. Periodic titer testing is neither required nor recommended.

Table 5 Hepatitis B Vaccination Series
Initial dose
Second dose: 4 weeks after first dose
Third dose: 6 months after first dose
Titer: 1 to 2 months after completion of the three-dose series

Practice routine standard precautions. If you are exposed, notify your DICO. The DICO will verify the source patient's test results. If you have a positive titer on file, no follow-up treatment is needed. If you do not have a titer report on file and the patient is positive for HBV infection, a titer test will be ordered for you. Treatment will depend on the results of the titer testing. If you have not been vaccinated and the patient is positive for HBV, you will be offered hepatitis B immune globulin and the vaccine series. The risk of infection is 6% to 30% only if you were not vaccinated and did not report the exposure event.

Hepatitis C Virus Infection

Hepatitis type C virus is the most common chronic bloodborne infection and the leading cause of liver transplantation in the United States. An estimated 1% to 4% of health care providers are antibody-positive for HCV. However, this disease is not efficiently transmitted through occupational exposure, and no health care provider group is at increased risk for occupationally acquired HCV infection. Instead, occupational risk is related to a contaminated deep needlestick with visible blood on the sharp, a sharp that has been in the patient's vein or artery, a hollow-bore needle, and a source patient with a high viral load. The risk for contracting HCV infection from a high-risk needlestick injury is 1.5%.

Pathophysiology
Transmission may occur by blood-to-blood contact with an open area of the skin, sexual contact, blood transfusion, organ donation, unsafe medical practices, and from an infected mother to her infant. Transmission through mucous membrane or nonintact skin exposure is rare. The virus cannot survive in the environment long enough to pose a risk for any means of transmission except via bloodborne contact.

In approximately 75% to 80% of HCV-infected people, the disease progresses to long-term chronic infection. The incubation period ranges from 2 to 24 weeks (average, 6-7 weeks).

Assessment
Signs and symptoms are the same as those for HBV infection: lack of appetite, nausea and vomiting, low-grade fever, abdominal distress, joint discomfort, and a general feeling of illness and listlessness. The diagnosis is established by testing for HCV antibody. Some 75% of infected persons remain unaware that they acquired the infection because phase 2 signs and symptoms, such as dark urine, jaundice, and scleral icterus, do not develop.

A new group at risk are "baby boomers," those born during the period following World War II from the mid 1940s to the late 1960s; people in this age group may have increased their risk by experimenting with drugs during the 1960s and 1970s. The Institute of Medicine (IOM) has recommended testing for this group for HCV.

Management
To prevent HCV transmission, use gloves when in direct contact with blood or OPIM, and use needle-safe or needleless devices. No special cleaning requirements apply—perform routine cleaning of the vehicle and equipment.

If you have sustained an exposure, testing will begin with the source patient; permission to test for hepatitis C is not required. Rapid HCV testing should be performed on the source with results in 1 hour. If the source is HCV positive, you will have a baseline HCV antibody test and liver function test. You should have an HCV-RNA test 2 weeks following the exposure event. If it is negative, you did not acquire HCV from the exposure. If it is positive, you will be offered treatment. Newly diagnosed persons are offered 24 weeks of treatment with a three-drug "cocktail." This new treatment has resulted in a 75% cure rate for HCV infection.

There is currently no medication to offer after exposure to prevent infection; however, treatment is available that is highly successful in curing this infection. A vaccine for prevention of HCV infection is currently in human clinical trials in Sweden. In some cases, it is being offered to people with newly diagnosed HCV infection as part of the trials. This is currently a "therapeutic" vaccine because it is only given to newly diagnosed persons.

Hepatitis D Virus Infection

Hepatitis type D, also called delta hepatitis, requires that the host be infected with hepatitis B for hepatitis D virus (HDV) infection to occur. For this reason, HDV is considered a parasite for HBV. Approximately 5,000 to 7,000 cases of HDV infection occur each year in the United States, with the highest incidence noted in IV drug users.

Pathophysiology
Transmission is generally by percutaneous exposure, because HDV is not effectively transmitted through sexual contact. Perinatal transmission is rare. The incubation period for HDV infection ranges from 30 to 180 days. Blood is considered to be infectious during all phases of the illness.

Assessment
Signs and symptoms are the same as those associated with HBV infection.

Management
To protect against HDV transmission, use gloves when in contact with blood or OPIM, use needle-safe or needleless devices, and perform routine cleaning of the vehicle following patient transport. Do not go through the pockets of known IV drug users who are found unconscious because they may contain contaminated sharps. If a documented exposure occurs, testing begins with the source patient in accordance with state testing laws. If the source is positive for HDV and you are protected against HBV, no further treatment is indicated.

Human Immunodeficiency Virus Infection

Human immunodeficiency virus (HIV), type 1, was first identified in the late 1970s. Today, millions of people worldwide are infected with this virus. In the United States, reporting of HIV infection to public health authorities is not legally mandated in all states. Because of testing and treatment, persons with HIV and AIDS are living many years after diagnosis as productive members of society.

Pathophysiology

In addition to other means of transmission by contact with blood and body fluids, including sexual transmission, HIV can be transmitted through blood transfusions. Such transmission has occurred at a very low rate, however, since the initiation of testing for the presence of P24 (a protein present from the beginning of the HIV life cycle) in donated blood. With P24 testing, the virus can now be detected 1 to 6 days after infection.

HIV is not transmitted through casual or even household contact. Even among people who routinely share eating utensils, toothbrushes, and razors with HIV-infected patients, there is no evidence of an increased rate of HIV infection. This disease is not transmitted by airborne or droplet means.

The HIV pathogen envelops infected cells and attacks the immune system and other body organs. As a result, the immune system is unable to assist in protecting an infected person from other diseases. It takes about 7 days for the virus to envelop a cell, and this process may occur 4 to 6 weeks after the exposure event. The communicable period is unknown but is believed to span from the onset of infection possibly throughout life.

Assessment

Signs and symptoms may include acute febrile illness, malaise, swollen lymph glands, headache, and, possibly, rash. Following initial infection with HIV, most people present with enlargement of the lymph nodes but appear otherwise healthy. However, if the infection is left untreated, the number of T-helper lymphocytes (CD4 cells) gradually declines. T-helper cells are essential components of the immune system that mediate cellular and humoral immunity. Seroconversion, meaning that antibodies can be detected in the blood, occurs, usually within the first 3 months following exposure. Persons who are **seropositive** for HIV are prescribed antiretroviral drug treatment.

Management

Prevention focuses on the use of gloves when in direct contact with patient blood or OPIM, the use of needle-safe or needleless devices, good handwashing technique, and routine cleaning of the vehicle after transport. Postexposure medical follow-up is covered in the AIDS section that follows.

The risk for acquiring HIV infection for health care providers is related to handling and disposal of sharps. As of December 2008, documented occupationally acquired HIV infection had developed in 57 health care providers; none were fire or EMS

personnel. Of these occupational infections, 49 were the result of a high-risk exposure. A high-risk exposure to HIV includes *all* of the following: a deep stick with a large-gauge hollow-bore needle, visible blood on the device, an HIV-positive patient with a high viral load, and a device that had been in the patient's vein or artery. Following this type of exposure, the risk of transmission is 0.3% for exposure to the mucous membrane of the eye and 0.09% for nonintact skin (only one case has been reported and documented).

Acquired Immunodeficiency Syndrome

Acquired immunodeficiency syndrome (AIDS) is the end-stage disease process caused by HIV. A patient with AIDS is extremely vulnerable to numerous **opportunistic infections** that would not affect a person with an intact immune system. In 2010, the CDC reported that there were 35,741 newly diagnosed cases of HIV infection in the United States; the number of cases of AIDS has not been released. Patients who respond to the cocktail drug treatment render the virus unable to multiply, and thus 96% cannot transmit the disease.

Pathophysiology

The incubation period of AIDS spans the time between documented infection (that is, becoming HIV-positive) and development of the end-stage disease; it is determined by the CD4 cell count and the presence of opportunistic infections. The communicable period is presumed to last as long as the patient is seropositive, *even before development of one of the clinically apparent AIDS-defining conditions*. Surveys of patients presenting to emergency departments have shown that around 6% of seriously ill or injured patients are HIV-positive.

Assessment

The development of specific opportunistic bacterial, viral, and fungal infections defines the transition from HIV infection to AIDS. The conditions are known accordingly as *AIDS-defining* or *AIDS-related conditions*. They include PCP pneumonia in infants or people with compromised immune systems; cytomegalovirus, which can cause blindness; reddish or purple skin cancers known as Kaposi sarcoma; atypical TB; and cryptococcal meningitis.

Management

Prevention involves following standard precautions. Use gloves when in contact with blood or OPIM, use needle-safe or needleless devices, and perform routine cleaning of the vehicle and equipment. There is no need to restrict pregnant care providers from contact with patients with known HIV infection or AIDS.

If an exposure occurs, the source patient will be tested in accordance with state law, ideally using the rapid HIV testing method. Its results are accurate and available in less than 1 hour. If the test is negative, no further testing is indicated. If the source is positive, a blood sample is sent for assessment of viral load and the paramedic may be offered antiretroviral drugs for a period of 4 weeks. The criteria for use of these drugs are published by the CDC; they are not given automatically.

The CDC guidelines for postexposure prophylaxis are enforced by OSHA under the bloodborne pathogens regulation (CFR 1910.1030).

Words of Wisdom

> Unless they contain visible blood, the following body fluids do not transmit bloodborne disease: tears, sweat, urine, stool, vomitus, nasal secretions, and sputum.

Antiretroviral drugs are toxic, so careful and complete counseling should be provided to exposed health care providers. The CDC recommends that a physician knowledgeable in the use of these drugs be consulted. If one is not available, then the physician should contact the 24-hour Post-Exposure Prophylaxis (PEP) Hotline at 1-888-448-4911 before prescribing these drugs. Before initiating antiretroviral therapy, baseline laboratory testing should be done—CBC and liver and kidney function tests. For a female of childbearing age, pregnancy testing is appropriate. These tests should be repeated every 2 weeks during drug therapy.

Words of Wisdom

> Diseases acquired through contact with bloodborne pathogens are considered "protected handicaps" under the Americans with Disabilities Act.

Pathophysiology, Assessment, and Management of Enteric (Intestinal) Diseases

Norovirus Infection

Pathophysiology
Previously termed Norwalk agent, norovirus causes about 90% of epidemic nonbacterial outbreaks of gastroenteritis in the world. Norovirus may be responsible for up to 50% of all food-borne outbreaks in the United States. This virus affects persons of all ages.

When norovirus enters the body, it begins to multiply in the small intestines. Transmission can be person-to-person, by ingestion of food or water that has been contaminated by infected feces (the fecal-oral route), or by aerosols created when a person vomits or has diarrhea. Symptoms may appear within 1 to 2 days. Acute symptoms usually begin in 24 to 28 hours and may last 24 to 60 hours. The virus can be shed for weeks after infection.

Assessment
Patients will present with nausea, forceful vomiting, watery diarrhea, abdominal pain, weakness, and low-grade fever; they are rarely admitted to the hospital.

Management
Wear gloves and practice good handwashing technique using soap and water. Alcohol sanitizers are not considered effective against norovirus. Cleaning after transport will require the use of a chlorine-based product such as bleach diluted with water.

YOU are the Medic | PART 4

You move the patient to your unit for transport after starting an IV and administering fluid. The transport is uneventful, and you report to receiving facility staff on arrival. The patient's blood pressure improves slightly in response to the fluid administration. After you transfer your patient to the hospital bed, you notice the sheets on your stretcher are wet.

Recording Time: 10 Minutes	
Respirations	18 breaths/min
Pulse	96 beats/min
Skin	Cool, pale, and dry
Blood pressure	102/60 mm Hg
Oxygen saturation (Spo$_2$)	98% on oxygen
Pupils	Equal and reactive

7. What decontamination measures should you use for your stretcher?
8. What decontamination measures should you use for yourself?

Hepatitis A Virus Infection

Pathophysiology

Hepatitis type A (HAV), or <u>infectious hepatitis</u>, is the most common type of hepatitis in the United States. In the past, outbreaks of this disease have been reported in several states. Transmission is by the fecal-oral route. Epidemic outbreaks are most often traced to contaminated drinking water, milk, sliced meats, and undercooked shellfish. The incidence has been declining, however, and no cases related to flood water have been reported since the early 1980s.

Infection with HAV is often described as a "benign" disease because acquiring it provides lifelong immunity to it. Since 2000, children in the United States have been immunized to protect them from contracting this disease. The vaccine is usually administered at age 12 months (between 12 and 23 months of age). Children who have not been vaccinated by 2 years of age should be vaccinated as soon as possible.

The incubation period is usually about 2 to 4 weeks, although it can range from 15 to 50 days after ingestion of the virus. The communicable period probably starts toward the end of the incubation period and continues for a few days after the patient becomes jaundiced.

Assessment

Signs and symptoms in phase 1 include fatigue, loss of appetite, fever, nausea, and abdominal pain; smokers will lose their interest in smoking. In phase 2, patients have jaundice, dark-colored urine, and whitish stools.

Depending on the type of hepatitis contracted, chronic liver disease or liver cancer may develop. This is true for HBV and HCV. Hepatitis A, however, is not associated with long-term disease and is considered a "mild" disease because it resolves after several weeks.

Management

Prevention includes the use of good handwashing technique, and, if in contact with patient stool, gloves. No special cleaning of the vehicle is needed. Hepatitis A vaccine is recommended for Federal Emergency Management Agency (FEMA) response team members who may work outside the United States, but not for any other health care provider groups.

Hepatitis D Virus Infection

Pathophysiology

Hepatitis D virus (HDV), also known as "delta hepatitis," is an incomplete virus. This means that in order for HDV to replicate, HBV must be present; therefore, HDV only occurs among people who are infected with HBV. HDV is transmitted through percutaneous or mucosal contact with infected blood and can be acquired either as a coinfection with HBV or as a superinfection (an infection that results subsequent to an earlier infection) in persons with HBV. This disease is not common in the United States.

Management

There is no vaccine for HDV infection, but it can be prevented by administration of a hepatitis B vaccination in persons who are not already infected.

Hepatitis E Virus Infection

Pathophysiology

Hepatitis E virus (HEV) is also referred to as enterically transmitted non-A, non-B hepatitis (ET-NANB). HEV accounts for an estimated 50% of hepatitis cases in developing countries, where it is strongly associated with floods and poor sanitation and hygiene.

Transmission typically occurs via the fecal-oral route by ingestion of contaminated water. In developing countries, rare cases of transmission via blood transfusion have been documented, and sexual transmission has also been documented.

This disease is not chronic and has an incubation period of approximately 15 to 64 days. The communicable period is believed to be the same as for HAV infection.

Assessment

Signs and symptoms of HEV infection are the same as for other forms of hepatitis.

Management

Prevention includes the use of gloves when in contact with stool, good handwashing technique, and cleaning contaminated equipment.

Pathophysiology, Assessment, and Management of Vector-borne and Zoonotic (Animal-borne) Diseases

Introduction

Diseases that are transmitted through a vector (vector-borne diseases) are usually transmitted by ticks or mosquitoes and include diseases such as Rocky Mountain spotted fever, Lyme disease, and West Nile virus. These diseases may also be referred to as <u>zoonotic</u> diseases.

West Nile Virus

<u>West Nile virus (WNV)</u> is a relatively new disease in the United States. The virus was first discovered in Uganda in the 1930s; its first identified appearance in the Western hemisphere was in New York City in 1999. The number of cases in the United States has been dropping for the past several years. In 2010, 363 cases were reported nationwide. It seems that the incidence of this disease may be declining as people and birds develop immunity.

Pathophysiology

Transmission occurs via a bite from a mosquito carrying the virus (only about 1% of mosquitoes carry WNV). This infection is not transmitted from person to person, so there is no period of communicability. WNV has been transmitted via donated blood and organs and during hemodialysis; two cases have involved needlestick injuries in laboratory workers working with WNV. The incubation period is from 3 to 14 days after transmission.

Assessment

In the majority of cases, this disease is mild and uneventful; 80% of persons who acquire WNV infection remain unaware that they have it. The 20% of persons who are symptomatic exhibit fever, headache, body rash, and swollen lymph glands. Mild symptoms appear in older people and immunocompromised people. In healthy people, the immune system fights off the disease. Severe reactions, such as neurologic complications and death, occur in about 1 in 150 symptomatic people.

Management

Use needle-safe devices to avoid a contaminated sharps injury when WNV infection is suspected. If you sustain a contaminated sharps injury involving a patient with WNV, notify your DICO. There is no recommended medical follow-up treatment. No special cleaning of the vehicle is needed or recommended.

Lyme Disease

Lyme disease is named for Lyme, Connecticut, the town where the disease was first identified. It is the most common tick-borne disease in the United States. The deer tick can be a vector for the bacterium *Borrelia burgdorferi*. The tick's bite injects the pathogen into the bloodstream of a human host. In 1982, a national reporting system was established for this infection. The highest prevalence of Lyme disease is found along the Atlantic coast, in the upper Midwest, and along the Pacific coast. The peak season is between June and August; incidence rates decrease in the early fall. In 2010 there were 22,561 confirmed cases of Lyme disease in the United States.

Pathophysiology

Lyme disease occurs more often in children younger than 10 years and in middle-aged adults. It is not transmitted from person to person. The incubation period ranges from 3 to 32 days.

Assessment

Lyme disease primarily affects the skin, heart, joints, and nervous system. Some patients remain asymptomatic. For patients in whom signs and symptoms develop, the disease is usually divided into three stages: early localized, early disseminated, and late manifestations:

1. **Early localized stage.** The early stage is characterized by a round, red skin lesion. This bull's-eye rash (so called because it extends outward with a ring in the center) is most common in the area of the groin, thigh, or axilla **Figure 9**. If present, it is warm to the touch and may blister or scab.
2. **Early disseminated stage.** In the early disseminated stage, secondary lesions may develop within days, and the patient may report flu-like symptoms—fever, chills, headache, malaise, and muscle pain. Nonproductive cough, testicular swelling, sore throat, enlarged spleen, and enlarged

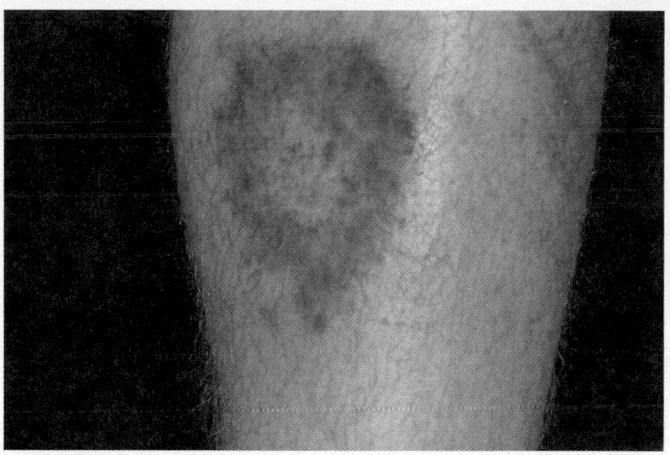

Figure 9 The bull's-eye rash of Lyme disease is most common in the area of the groin, thigh, or axilla.

lymph nodes may be present. Neurologic involvement, including meningoencephalitis and cranial and peripheral neuropathy, occurs in 15% to 20% of untreated patients within 2 to 8 weeks. Cardiac involvement, including pericarditis, myocarditis, and atrioventricular conduction difficulties, occurs in 10% of untreated patients.

3. **Late manifestations.** In the third stage of the illness, arthritis occurs in about 60% of untreated patients, beginning days to years after the initial infection. Intermittent joint pain affects about 50% of patients and lasts from days to months. Chronic neurologic symptoms are uncommon. In the United States, memory impairment, depressed mood, and severe fatigue are the most common symptoms of Lyme disease.

Management

Prevention includes wearing long sleeves and pants when in tick-infested areas, plus use of insecticides that contain carabaril, diazinon, chlorpyrifos, or cyfluthrin. If you sustain a tick bite, use proper technique for removing ticks. Postexposure treatment with antibiotics is not warranted or recommended.

Rocky Mountain Spotted Fever

Rocky Mountain spotted fever (RMSF) is a tick-borne disease caused by the bacterium *Rickettsia rickettsii*. This organism is a cause of potentially fatal human illness in North and South America. Transmission to humans occurs by the bite of infected tick species. In the United States, these include the American dog tick (*Dermacentor variabilis*), Rocky Mountain wood tick (*Dermacentor andersoni*), and brown dog tick (*Rhipicephalus sanguineus*). There were approximately 1,985 cases in 2010 but only 156 were confirmed, with the highest incidence in Missouri and Tennessee.

Pathophysiology

RMSF can be a severe or even fatal illness if not treated in the first few days of symptoms. Patients who had a particularly severe infection requiring prolonged hospitalization may have long-term health problems caused by this disease.

Assessment

Typical symptoms include fever, headache, abdominal pain, vomiting, and muscle pain. A rash may also develop, but is often absent in the first few days, and in some patients a rash never develops.

The initial diagnosis is made based on clinical signs and symptoms and medical history and can later be confirmed by using specialized laboratory tests. RMSF and other tick-borne diseases can be prevented.

Management

Doxycycline is the first-line treatment for adults and children of all ages, and it is most effective if started before the fifth day of symptoms.

RMSF is not a communicable disease. It is not transmitted from patient to health care provider. To be exposed, a person needs to be bitten by the tick.

■ Hantavirus Infection

Hantavirus infection, also known as *hemorrhagic fever with pulmonary syndrome*, is associated with the deer mouse, white-footed mouse, and cotton rat. Hantavirus pulmonary syndrome may also occur and is characterized by flulike symptoms that can progress rapidly to potentially life-threatening breathing problems. It has also been found in rats in urban areas. This disease was first identified in Korea in the early 1950s and in the southwestern United States in 1993. By 2000, about 330 cases had been reported in the United States. In 2009, 242 cases of hantavirus infection were diagnosed in the United States.

Pathophysiology

Hantavirus is found in the urine, feces, and saliva of chronically infected rodents. Transmission occurs via direct contact with rodent waste matter, often through aerosol inhalation, which can occur when cleaning up infested areas such as households, barns, and sheds. The incubation period usually lasts 12 to 16 days following exposure but has been noted to range from 5 to 42 days. This disease is not transmitted from person to person, so there is no period of communicability.

Assessment

Signs and symptoms of hantavirus infection begin with the sudden onset of fever, which lasts 3 to 8 days. It is accompanied by headache, abdominal pain, loss of appetite, and vomiting. For pulmonary syndrome, signs and symptoms present in two stages. In stage 1, complaints may include fever, chills, headaches, muscle aches, vomiting, diarrhea, and abdominal pain. In stage 2, the patient may present with a cough that produces secretions, shortness of breath, and fluid accumulation within the lungs. Low blood pressure and cardiac insufficiency may also be noted.

Management

Prevention focuses on standard precautions. Routine cleaning of the vehicle is all that is indicated. Depending on the stage of illness and presenting symptoms, other supportive measures may be needed. Assisted respiration, through intubation or mechanical ventilation, may be indicated. Oxygen therapy may also be needed. Rapid transport is paramount, as a diagnosis will be made at the medical facility following antibody testing for hantavirus.

■ Rabies

Rabies (hydrophobia) is found worldwide and accounts for about 300,000 deaths each year in developing countries. In the United States, cases have been declining since rabies control programs began in the 1940s. In 2009, four human cases of rabies were reported in the United States. The vaccination of domestic animals and the development of a vaccine and rabies immunoglobulin have greatly reduced the number of deaths in humans who contract rabies.

Pathophysiology

Transmission of rabies is primarily related to the direct bite of an infected animal. The virus is shed in the saliva of the infected animal from the time it becomes infected. Animals most commonly identified to have rabies include raccoons, skunks, foxes, coyotes, and insectivorous bats. Another route of transmission is contamination of mucous membranes (eyes and mouth); one case suspected of having been contracted during a cornea organ transplant has been reported. In general, however, non-bite exposures to rabies—scratches, abrasions, open wounds, or mucous membranes contaminated with saliva or other potentially infectious material from a rabid animal—are rare. There are no documented cases of human-to-human transmission of rabies. The incubation period is usually 2 to 8 weeks but varies depending on the severity of the bite and the location of the wound.

Assessment

Signs and symptoms in human infection are generally nonspecific: fever, chills, sore throat, malaise, headache, and weakness. Paresthesia (skin sensation with no apparent cause) may develop at or near the site of exposure. Following these initial signs, the neurologic phase of the disease begins—hyperactivity, seizures, bizarre behavior, and hydrophobia. Patients may also have fear of the sight of water or while drinking it as a result of severe spasms of the throat and masseter (chewing) muscles. As the disease progresses, paralysis may develop and mental status may deteriorate, leading to coma. Although rabies is generally viewed as a fatal disease, several cases of survival have been reported recently even after symptoms had appeared. Generally, there are fewer than five cases reported in the United States each year.

Management

For prevention, follow standard precautions for patient care and cleaning of the vehicle. If you are bitten or scratched by a suspect animal, you will be offered human rabies vaccine if deemed appropriate. The CDC does not recommend rabies vaccination for fire and EMS personnel on a routine basis. Follow-up would include wound care. Remember, first aid always comes before reporting.

Tetanus

In 2010, 26 cases of tetanus (lockjaw) were reported. Tetanus is more common in agricultural areas and in underdeveloped areas, where contact with animal waste is common and immunization is inadequate.

Pathophysiology

The tetanus bacillus is found in the intestines of horses and other animals, but some cases have been linked to use of IV drugs.

Transmission occurs when tetanus spores enter the body by either of two means: (1) a puncture wound contaminated with animal feces, street dust, or soil; or (2) contaminated street drugs. Tetanus is not transmitted from person to person. Occasionally, cases have occurred postoperatively or following seemingly minor injuries.

The incubation period is usually about 14 days from the exposure but has been documented to be as short as 3 days. The cases that have short incubation periods tend to have a higher level of contamination.

Assessment

Signs and symptoms begin at the site of the wound, followed by painful muscle contractions or rigidity (tetany) in the neck, face, jaw, and trunk muscles. The key sign that suggests tetanus, particularly in children, is abdominal rigidity, although this rigidity may be confined to the location of the injury. Dysphagia, hydrophobia, drooling, and respiratory distress may also occur.

Management

Prevention involves the use of gloves when treating any patient wounds and managing drainage. A patient with tetanus may require airway and ventilation support en route. Oxygen may be ordered along with IV fluids. Tetanus immune globulin (TIG) is recommended for treatment of tetanus. A single intramuscular dose of 3,000 to 5,000 units is generally recommended for children and adults, with part of the dose infiltrated around the wound if it can be identified. Paramedics should be offered tetanus booster doses every 10 years for protection. No special cleaning routines are necessary after transport of a patient with tetanus.

Pathophysiology, Assessment, and Management of Infection With Antibiotic-Resistant Organisms

The overuse and misuse of antibiotics have led some pathogens to develop resistance to the antibiotic drugs commonly prescribed to eradicate them. There is concern in the medical community that there may soon be infections that are not treatable. Currently, there are only two new antibiotics under development. As a consequence, medical facility pharmacies and the CDC now restrict the use of many antibiotics. There has also been an attempt to educate the population regarding the risks associated with the overuse of antibiotics.

Patients infected with some types of antibiotic-resistant organisms, particularly vancomycin-resistant *enterococci* (VRE) and methicillin-resistant *Staphylococcus aureus* (MRSA), may be protected by the Americans With Disabilities Act (infection with these organisms is discussed in the sections that follow), depending on the definition of "disability" in state law. It is important not to use more PPE than is reasonably required when treating patients with such infections because doing so may be considered discrimination.

Methicillin-Resistant *Staphylococcus aureus*

Staphylococcus aureus became resistant to penicillin in the late 1950s. The drug methicillin became available in the early 1960s to treat infections with *S aureus*. By the mid 1970s, MRSA was present in US hospitals; it has since moved into the community. Today, almost 90% of cases are community-acquired MRSA. The number of health care–associated cases of MRSA is starting to decline with the increased focus on infection control. In 2010, encouraging results from a CDC study published in the *Journal of the American Medical Association* showed that life-threatening MRSA infections in health care settings are declining. Invasive MRSA infections that began in hospitals declined 28% from 2005 through 2008. Decreases in infection rates were even greater for patients with bloodstream infections. In addition, the study showed a 17% drop in invasive MRSA infections that were diagnosed before hospital admissions (community onset) in people with recent exposures to health care settings.

Strains of MRSA are also resistant to some other antibiotics, including cephalosporins, erythromycins, clindamycin (Cleocin), tetracyclines, and aminoglycosides. Although vancomycin (Vancocin) has been shown to treat MRSA effectively, some mild strains are showing resistance to this drug as well. Other drugs used to treat MRSA include a quinupristin-dalfopristin combination (Synercid), linezolid (Zyvox), and daptomycin (Cubicin).

> ### Special Populations
>
> Community-acquired (CA)-methicillin-resistant *Staphylococcus aureus* (MRSA) infection with clone USA300 is a major cause of infectious disease in children. It presents primarily as a superficial soft-tissue infection and can be easily treated by incision and drainage without the use of antibiotics.

Pathophysiology

In health care settings, MRSA is believed to be transmitted from patient to patient via unwashed hands of health care providers. Studies have shown that 50% to 90% of health care providers carry MRSA in their nares; the pathogen can subsequently be transferred to skin and other areas of the body through a break in the skin, causing infection **Figure 10**. Surfaces contaminated with MRSA do not seem to be important in transmission. The presence of MRSA in ambulances and fire stations has been documented, which suggests that cleaning routines and good

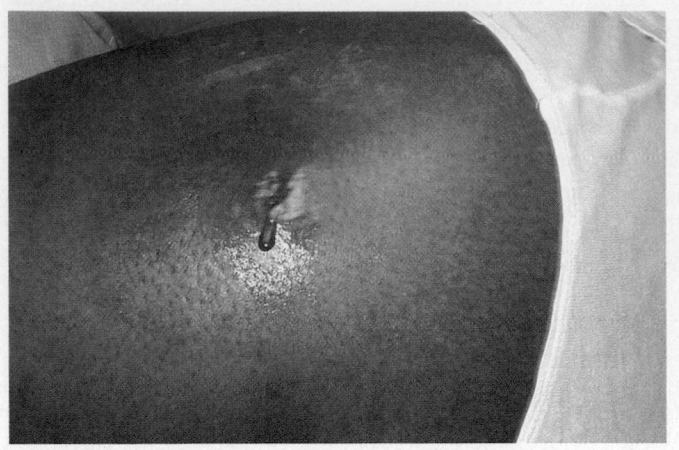

Figure 10 A draining, purulent skin abscess on the thigh caused by MRSA.

handwashing techniques are not being followed. Factors that increase the risk for developing MRSA include antibiotic therapy, prolonged hospital stays, a stay in an intensive care or a burn unit, and exposure to an infected patient. Many patients who contract MRSA live in long-term care facilities.

Assessment

Patients with MRSA may be <u>colonized</u> with this organism or infected. The incubation period seems to be between 5 and 45 days. The communicable period varies; patients who have active infection may carry MRSA for months. In community-acquired cases, MRSA results in soft-tissue infections. Manifestations of MRSA may include localized skin abscesses and cellulites, empyemas, and endocarditis. Sepsis is found in older patients with *S aureus* infections. After bloodstream infection with MRSA, secondary infections such as osteomyelitis and septic arthritis may develop at sites other than the initial site of MRSA infection.

Management

Patients will undergo incision and drainage for soft-tissue infections. No antibiotics need to be prescribed. This treatment is in accordance with the guidelines published by the Infectious Disease Society of America. It is estimated that more than 90% of MRSA soft-tissue infections will clear following incision and drainage alone. To prevent MRSA transmission, use standard precautions (gloves and good handwashing technique) when in contact with wounds and nonintact skin. If you are in direct contact with wound drainage but your skin is intact, no exposure will occur. If you have a true exposure, no postexposure treatment is recommended. The incident must still be documented, however.

■ **Vancomycin-Resistant *Staphylococcus aureus***

Vancomycin is one of the leading drugs for treating *Staphylococcus* infections. However, once the organism has become resistant to this drug, it is no longer effective in treating the infections.

Like MRSA, vancomycin-resistant *Staphylococcus aureus* (VRSA) infections present as pimples, boils, and other skin conditions. VRSA infections can become severe, resulting in sepsis; however, the incidence of infection is rare in the United States. To date, only two cases have been reported: one in Pennsylvania in 2002 and one in Michigan in the same year.

Pathophysiology

Persons at risk for the development of VRSA infections include those with several underlying health conditions (such as diabetes and kidney disease), previous infections with MRSA, indwelling catheters (such as Foley catheters), recent hospitalizations, and recent exposure to vancomycin or other antimicrobial agents.

Assessment

Signs and symptoms may include localized skin abscesses and cellulites, pneumonia, bloodstream infections, meningitis, or osteomyelitis. Fever, chills, or body weakness and pain, cough, chest pain, and trouble breathing are commonly present, but other signs and symptoms will depend on the location of the infection.

Management

This form of infection is currently treatable with antibiotics. Standard precautions and routine cleaning of the vehicle and patient care equipment after each call are important, as is routine handwashing. Make sure all open cuts on your skin are covered. No postexposure treatment is recommended, but if you are exposed, notify your DICO.

■ **Vancomycin-Resistant Enterococci**

<u>*Enterococcus*</u> is a common, normal organism of the gastrointestinal (GI) tract, urinary tract, and genitourinary tract. More than 450 species of enterococci exist, many of which are resistant to antimicrobial agents. These organisms grow under reduced oxygen and oxygenated conditions. When they become resistant to the main drug used for treating enterococcal infection, vancomycin, the patient is said to have vancomycin-resistant enterococci (VRE).

According to recent National Nosocomial Infections Surveillance surveys, enterococci remain in the top three most common pathogens that cause nosocomial infections in the United States. These infections have occurred in the general hospitalized population, and from the late 1980s to mid 1990s, the rate of VRE isolates increased 34-fold among intensive care unit hospitalizations. Currently, one fourth of all enterococcal isolates are vancomycin resistant.

Pathophysiology

Infection with VRE is primarily a <u>nosocomial infection</u> (that is, a health care–associated infection). Patients identified with VRE infections outside the hospital setting typically reside in nursing homes or visit hemodialysis centers. In fact, people are not susceptible to VRE infection unless they are already ill or immunocompromised. Patients in the ICU and transplant recipients are especially vulnerable, for example.

VRE may be found in urinary tract infections (UTIs) and bloodstream infections; it has also been identified in livestock stool, uncooked chicken, and persons who work at farms or processing plants. The infectious organisms can live on surfaces for long periods, so transmission may occur by direct contact with contaminated surfaces or equipment.

A person can be colonized or infected with VRE, but only infected patients can transmit the organism. Thus transmission may occur when you have direct contact with wound drainage and an open cut or sore allows entry of the organism. Infection with VRE can be treated with a new synthetic antibiotic, linezolid.

Assessment

VRE can cause UTIs, particularly in patients who have urinary catheters. Other kinds of catheters, such as central lines, can serve as a port of entry for VRE, causing bacteremia that sometimes evolves into a dangerous systemic bloodstream infection called *sepsis*. Surgical wounds, especially in patients who have had abdominal or chest surgery, may also become infected with VRE.

Management

Prevention relies on the use of standard precautions, gloves, and good handwashing technique when in contact with wound drainage. A cover gown is necessary only if your uniform may come in contact with wound drainage. Post-transport cleaning of all areas that came in contact with the patient is important, but no special cleaning solution is required. If you sustain direct contact with an open wound and body fluids from a patient with a VRE infection, notify your DICO and complete an exposure report. No postexposure medical treatment is indicated.

▪ *Clostridium difficile*

Clostridium difficile (commonly referred to as *C diff*) is not a multidrug-resistant organism but is being treated like one. It can occur after antibiotic treatment because some antibiotics can destroy the normal bacteria in the intestine, and the *C difficile* organisms take over. Infections with *C difficile* are generally related to a stay in a health care facility.

Pathophysiology

The spore-forming bacterium *C difficile* produces two endotoxins that cause watery diarrhea, the chief symptom of infection. Transmission occurs by contact with surfaces contaminated with feces. The bacterium can be transmitted to patients by contact with the unwashed hands of health care providers. Diagnosis is usually made by stool culture. Illness resolves 2 to 3 days after discontinuing antibiotics.

Assessment

Infection with *C difficile* causes frequent watery, green, foul-smelling diarrhea; nausea and vomiting; fever; loss of appetite; and abdominal discomfort. Diseases associated with *C difficile* infection include pseudomembranous colitis, sepsis, and colonic perforation. For patients presenting with these signs

and symptoms, a paramedic should ask about the patient's medications, especially any antibiotics he or she is taking.

Management

Glove use, good handwashing technique, and cleaning of contaminated surfaces with an appropriate cleaning agent are important in managing *C difficile*. Because *C difficile* is a spore-forming agent, a chlorine-based cleaning solution is required. Report contamination of open skin areas to your DICO. No medical follow-up is recommended.

▪ Pathophysiology, Assessment, and Management of Common Communicable Diseases of Childhood

The most striking aspect of "common" communicable diseases of childhood is that they have returned—there are increased numbers of cases of these preventable diseases across the United States. Some are related to religious waivers from vaccination, and others are related to fears that vaccines might lead to autism in children (which has been disproven in multiple scientific studies). Mumps, chickenpox, and pertussis were the cause of several outbreaks across the United States in 2008 and 2009. In California in 2010, 10 children died of pertussis—a disease that is preventable by vaccination. The United States has a goal to vaccinate all children against diseases preventable by vaccine. The CDC website lists a recommended vaccination schedule, as well as other useful information to help the paramedic educate parents.

Common childhood communicable diseases are also discussed in more detail in the chapter, *Pediatric Emergencies*.

Words of Wisdom

Place a surgical mask on any patient who presents with fever and a rash. Most droplet and airborne disease exposure can be prevented by following this simple rule.

▪ Bronchiolitis

Bronchiolitis is an infection of the lungs and airways that usually occurs in children ages 3 to 6 months.

Pathophysiology

The cause of bronchiolitis is usually viral (for example, respiratory syncytial virus, parainfluenza virus, or influenza virus). Transmission of bronchiolitis generally occurs by inhaling droplets of infected mucus or respiratory secretions.

Assessment

Remember to take standard precautions. Initial symptoms are a runny nose and slight fever. After 2 to 3 days, wheezing and coughing, tachypnea, and tachycardia are present. Because the signs and symptoms of bronchiolitis can be difficult to distinguish from asthma, obtain a thorough history and assess the respiratory rate.

Management

Management of bronchiolitis is supportive. Oxygen may be administered with IV fluids if dehydration is present. Be prepared to assist ventilation with bag-mask ventilation or endotracheal intubation if needed.

▇ Croup

Croup is the inflammation of the larynx and airway just below it. It primarily affects children 5 years and younger.

Pathophysiology

Croup is caused by a virus similar to the virus that causes the common cold and by other viruses (for example, parainfluenza virus, respiratory syncytial virus, "measles virus," and adenovirus). It is spread by respiratory secretions or droplets from coughing, sneezing, and breathing. Droplets are small particles that only travel a short distance.

Assessment

Croup comes on strongest in the nighttime and may last 3 to 7 days. Symptoms include a loud, harsh, barking cough; fever; noisy inhalations; hoarse voice; and mild to moderate dyspnea.

Management

Prehospital management of croup is the same as for most respiratory emergencies. Depending on the severity of symptoms, nebulized epinephrine administration may be effective. In severe cases, nebulized epinephrine alone may not be adequate and assisted ventilation may be necessary. Assisted ventilation with bag-mask ventilation will often succeed in overcoming the upper airway obstruction.

There is no definitive treatment for the viruses that cause croup. Drug treatment is directed toward decreasing airway edema, and supportive care is directed toward the provision of respiratory support and the maintenance of hydration. Most cases are mild and cared for in the home.

▇ Measles

Pathophysiology

Measles—also known as rubeola, hard measles, or red measles—is a highly communicable viral disease transmitted by airborne aerosolized droplets or by direct contact with the nasal or pharyngeal secretions of an infected person. Less commonly, measles can be spread by indirect contact if an uninfected person handles articles recently soiled by the patient's nasal or throat sections (tissues, for example).

Measles was thought to have been eliminated in the United States in 2000. However, in 2010, 63 cases were reported. Most of these cases were imported by people traveling from foreign countries (whether they were visiting the United States or returning from travel abroad) or were the result of unvaccinated contacts.

The incubation period is about 10 days. The onset of fever is generally between days 7 and 18 (after exposure), and the rash appears about day 14 after exposure. The communicable period begins when the first symptoms appear (about 4 days before the rash) and then diminishes rapidly, ending about 2 days after the rash appears.

About 30% of cases of measles develop one or more complications, including pneumonia, which is the complication most often associated with the cause of death in young children. Ear infections occur in about 1 in 10 cases, which can result in permanent loss of hearing. Diarrhea is reported in about 8% of cases. These complications are more common among children younger than 5 years and adults older than 20 years.

Assessment

Measles in the early (prodromal) phase is characterized by fever, conjunctivitis, and coryza (acute rhinitis). This is followed by onset of coughing, a blotchy red rash (which often starts on the head), and whitish gray spots on the buccal (mouth) mucosa (known as Koplik spots) **Figure 11**.

Management

Care of a patient with measles is supportive. Although placing a mask on the patient may prevent droplet transmission, the only certain protection against measles is immunity. Exposure is defined as transport of a patient or being in the same room as the patient, so the patient should remain isolated, though this may not be realistic when transporting a patient in an ambulance.

Anyone who has had measles or who received two doses of live virus measles vaccine after 1968 should be able to document immunity to measles. If you did not receive live virus vaccine, you should be revaccinated. It is important to assess the immunity status of all new hires. Postexposure treatment includes vaccination if you are not immune.

No special disinfection measures are required for the ambulance after transporting a patient known to have measles. Simply washing patient contact areas and laundering any soiled linens are sufficient.

▇ Rubella

Pathophysiology

Rubella, also known as German measles or 3-day measles, is caused by a virus and occurs most commonly during the winter and spring. It is highly communicable to susceptible people.

Figure 11 A blotchy red rash is characteristic of measles.

Transmission occurs by direct contact with the nasopharyngeal secretions of an infected person—by droplet spread or by touching the patient or articles freshly contaminated with the patient's secretions. This disease was considered to have been eliminated from the United States in 2000. However, five cases were reported in 2010. The incubation period for rubella is 14 to 23 days. The communicable period starts about a week before the rash appears and continues until 4 days after the rash becomes evident.

Special Populations

Because of their relatively immature immune systems, infants and small children are especially susceptible to infectious diseases. Pediatric immunizations prevent disease in children who receive them and protect those who come into contact with unvaccinated people. Although the incidence of vaccine-preventable diseases has decreased in the United States, the viruses and bacteria that cause them still exist. According to the CDC, all children should be immunized against the following diseases:

- Measles, mumps, and rubella
- Diphtheria, pertussis, and tetanus
- HAV infection
- HBV infection
- Polio
- *Haemophilus influenzae* type b
- Seasonal influenza

Vaccinations are recommended for other diseases in children in addition to those listed above. Refer to the CDC website—www.cdc.gov—for the most current pediatric immunization schedule.

Assessment

Rubella is characterized by a low-grade fever, headache, runny nose, swollen lymph glands, and usually a diffuse maculopapular rash that may look a bit like the rash of measles. When it occurs in children, rubella is ordinarily a mild, uncomplicated illness. When it occurs in women during the first 3 to 4 months of pregnancy, however, rubella may cause severe abnormalities in the developing fetus, including deafness, cataracts, mental retardation, and heart defects.

Management

There is no treatment for rubella. Offer supportive care. As with measles, the only certain protection against rubella is immunity. In accordance with the *CDC Guidelines for Immunization and Vaccination of Healthcare Workers*, all paramedics except women who are pregnant or planning to become pregnant within 3 months should be vaccinated against rubella before starting employment unless immunity has been established.

No special measures are needed to disinfect the ambulance after transporting a patient known to have rubella. Prevention measures include placing a surgical mask on the patient. Postexposure treatment includes vaccination if you are not immune. Practice standard precautions and routine cleaning after transport of a rubella patient.

Mumps

Mumps is a viral disease that occurs most commonly in winter and spring. Anyone who has not been vaccinated is at risk for this disease. In 2010, there were more than 2,600 cases of mumps reported in the United States, including two outbreaks at summer camps in New York State. One of the outbreaks resulted in more than 2,000 cases in several states.

Pathophysiology

Transmission of mumps occurs by droplet spread or direct contact with the saliva of an infected person. Mumps is not an airborne-transmitted disease. The incubation period is 12 to 26 days. The communicable period lasts 9 days after the salivary glands swell.

Assessment

Signs and symptoms in children include fever plus swelling and tenderness of one of the salivary glands, usually the parotid. Mumps in males past the age of puberty may have a very painful complication: inflammation of the testicles occurs in up to 25% of cases, although it does not result in sterility. Thus, while rubella is a matter of particular concern for female paramedics of childbearing age, as explained in the previous section, mumps should worry any male paramedic who did not have the illness or was not vaccinated against it against it as a child. All paramedics should be vaccinated against mumps before starting employment if they are not already immune. However, female paramedics of childbearing age will need to be counseled not to become pregnant for 4 weeks following each dose of vaccine. The mumps vaccine is a live virus vaccine and will not be administered to women who are already pregnant.

Management

As a precaution, place a surgical mask on a patient with the mumps. Wear gloves when in contact with drainage, and carry out routine cleaning following patient transport. Only supportive care is needed for transport. Once diagnosed, the patient will be cared for in his or her home. A hospital stay is not generally needed. Postexposure vaccination is not recommended because it has not been found to be effective. An employee, if not immune, will need to remain on work restriction from days 12 to 26 after the exposure. If exposure occurred on the job, the time off work will be covered by workers' compensation.

Chickenpox

Pathophysiology

Chickenpox, also known as varicella zoster, is a viral illness that produces a distinctive rash of itchy, fluid-filled vesicles. The virus is transmitted by direct contact or droplet spread of respiratory secretions from patients with chickenpox. Contact with the vesicular fluid of patients with chickenpox or herpes zoster and, probably, contact with articles recently contaminated by the fluid can also transmit the virus. Therefore, this illness has two modes of transmission—airborne and direct contact transmission. Anyone who is not vaccinated is at risk for infection. In 2010, there were more than 15,000 cases of chickenpox reported in the United States. The incubation period for chickenpox is 10 to 21 days. The communicable period starts 1 to 2 days before the appearance of the rash and lasts about 5 days after the first vesicles become apparent. Having chickenpox as a child usually provides lifelong immunity against infection.

Assessment

Chickenpox is a highly contagious viral disease that produces listlessness, a slight fever, photosensitivity, and a vesicular rash that gradually crusts over, leaving a series of scabs `Figure 12`. The raised, fluid-filled vesicles arise in crops, moving from the clothing-covered areas of the body to uncovered areas.

Management

When you are transporting a patient suspected to have chickenpox, place a surgical mask on the patient. Treatment is supportive. Following diagnosis at the medical facility, patients with chickenpox will be cared for in their own home. Wear gloves

Special Populations

The varicella zoster virus can lead to herpes zoster ("shingles") in older adults. The chickenpox virus takes up residence in nerve root ganglia and becomes dormant, often for decades. Herpes zoster arises when the dormant varicella virus becomes active again, often during times of physical or emotional stress. Lesions appear in a discernible pattern along the affected nerve pathway and can be extremely painful. If identified within 48 hours of onset, shingles can be treated with a medication; thereafter, it cannot.

Adults older than 60 years have an increased risk of herpes zoster, especially if they had chickenpox during the first year of life. Susceptibility to shingles is also greater among older adults whose immune systems have been compromised by illness or weakened by certain medications. A herpes zoster vaccine is available to persons older than 50 years.

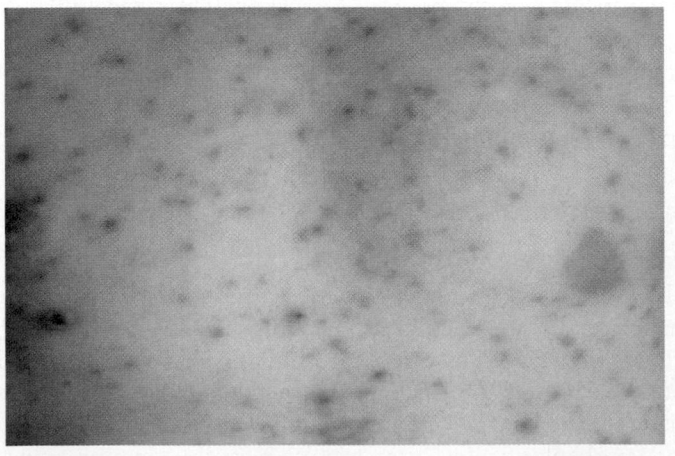

Figure 12 The distinctive rash produced by chickenpox is composed of small, blisterlike vesicles that arise in clusters.

when in contact with discharges or drainage from lesions. The vehicle does not require airing out or any special cleaning solution or technique.

Postexposure treatment includes vaccination if not immune. In the past, varicella zoster immune globulin (VZIG) was offered if an exposed person was pregnant or immunocompromised. However, the supply is almost depleted and VariZIG is now being offered in its place. All paramedics not immune to chickenpox should be offered the vaccination when hired. Pregnant female paramedics are an exception to this rule because they cannot receive a live virus vaccine. Vaccination will be offered following delivery.

Pertussis

Pertussis (whooping cough) is an infection caused by the bacterium *Bordetella pertussis*. This disease was also thought to have been eliminated from the United States through vaccination; however, as with certain other diseases, it was not. Anyone who has not been vaccinated is at risk. More than 27,000 cases were reported in 2010 in the United States. Many health care workers have not had a booster since age 11 and need to receive additional boosters if there is no serologic proof of immunity.

Assessment

Pertussis has an insidious onset and is characterized by an irritating cough that becomes paroxysmal in about 1 to 2 weeks; this cough may last for 1 to 2 months. A high-pitched "whoop" sound occurs on inspiration. The patient's eyes may have broken blood vessels, or there may be bruising around the eyes, as a result of the coughing attacks. Some cases have occurred in previously vaccinated persons who have diminished immunity.

Special Populations

In recent years, the incidence of pertussis has been increasing in adolescents and young adults. For many persons immunity has decreased over the years and a booster dose is needed. This disease has been involved in outbreaks across the United States. In 2009 and 2010, several children died during a major outbreak in California.

Pathophysiology

Transmission takes place through direct contact with discharge from mucous membranes and/or airborne droplets. The incubation period is 7 to 14 days. This disease is highly communicable in its early stages, before the cough becomes paroxysmal, and then its effects become negligible in about 3 weeks.

Complications from pertussis include apnea in up to 50% of cases and pneumonia in 20% of cases. For children younger than 1 year who contract pertussis, pulmonary hypertension is a common, severe complication that contributes to death; encephalopathy occurs in approximately 20% of cases.

Management

Prevention of pertussis includes placing a surgical mask on the patient. If coughing makes this placement difficult, try a nonrebreathing mask. Provide supportive care. Postexposure care may include antibiotic treatment. Good handwashing and routine cleaning of the vehicle are the only special measures required after transporting a patient with pertussis.

All paramedics should be assessed for immunity to diphtheria, pertussis, and tetanus (DPT). The CDC recommends a one-time booster dose of TDaP (tetanus, diphtheria, acellular pertussis) vaccine for all health care workers, especially those who work with children.

Pathophysiology, Assessment, and Management of New and Emerging Diseases

In the past, a disease would "jump" from animals to humans every 20 to 30 years. Today, this transmission occurs much more frequently. Recent examples include HIV infection, monkeypox, severe acute respiratory syndrome (SARS), and avian flu. The latter two are discussed here.

Severe Acute Respiratory Syndrome

Severe acute respiratory syndrome (SARS) is a new disease that arose from the merger of two viruses, one from mammals and one from birds. The source of this virus has been identified as bats found in Hong Kong. SARS was first reported in Asia in February 2003. Within a few months, the disease had spread from Asia to Canada, South America, and Europe. By spring 2003, the World Health Organization (WHO) reported a total of 8,098 cases worldwide and 774 deaths. In the United States, there were eight confirmed cases (all mild) and no deaths; all of the US cases involved people who had traveled to areas where SARS cases had been reported. The last cases of SARS were reported in April 2004 in China and resulted from a laboratory accident. In the United States, no health care providers have contracted SARS.

Pathophysiology

Transmission of SARS is by close personal contact—that is, living with and caring for a person with the disease or having direct contact with respiratory secretions or body fluids of an infected person (for example, kissing or hugging, sharing eating utensils, or standing within 3′ of an infected person who is talking). The incubation period is about 10 days from the date of exposure; the communicable period has not been well defined.

Assessment

Signs and symptoms include a fever of greater than 100.4°F, headache, overall feeling of discomfort, and body aches. Initially, SARS resembles any general flu-like illness; however, after 2 to 7 days, a dry cough appears, and severe cases may progress to pneumonia; patients may need respiratory support.

Management

Caring for a person suspected of having SARS consists of using adequate PPE, including an N95 or P100 respirator that has been properly fit-tested, notifying the DICO, completing an exposure form, and perhaps being placed on a 10-day quarantine.

Avian Flu

The first cases of avian (bird) flu in humans were reported in Hong Kong in 1997; 18 people became infected and 6 died in this outbreak. In the cases that have occurred since then, the death rate has been approximately 25%.

Pathophysiology

Avian flu is caused by a virus that occurs naturally in the bird population. This virus is carried in the intestinal tract of wild birds and does not usually cause illness. However, in domestic bird populations (for example, chickens, ducks, and turkeys), it is very contagious. Birds acquire the illness from contact with contaminated excretions or surfaces that are contaminated with excretions. If an infected bird is used for food and is cooked, it does not pose a risk to the people who eat it.

No rapidly spread human-to-human cases of this disease have been reported. Instead, the cases occurring in humans have involved close contact with infected birds. The transmission risk for humans is quite low.

Some concern exists that someone infected with a regular type A flu virus may become coinfected with avian flu, allowing the two to merge and form a new virus. In August 2011, the United Nations stated that it appeared that the avian flu was once again on the rise in Asia.

Assessment

Signs and symptoms of avian flu include fever, sore throat, cough, and muscle aches; some eye infections have also been noted. Illness may eventually progress to pneumonia and severe respiratory distress.

Management

Preventive measures include placing a surgical mask on the patient to contain secretions. If the patient's condition does not permit this action, you can wear a surgical mask for protection. Follow current CDC guidelines regarding protection for health care providers. Under the current information-sharing system, the medical facility is required to notify the DICO if a patient transported is later given a diagnosis of avian flu. If an exposure is documented, an antiviral drug may be offered within 48 hours of exposure. Antiviral drugs do not prevent the flu, but rather reduce the severity of the illness. It is also important to get an annual flu shot to ensure protection from type A viruses.

Words of Wisdom

The lead agency for responding to potential pandemic diseases in the United States is the Department of Health and Human Services. The CDC is part of this agency.

YOU *are the Medic* | SUMMARY

1. What is your first concern at this scene?

Based on information that a few patients may be ill with the same signs and symptoms, you should be thinking about some sort of viral-based disorder. This possibility will be unconfirmed unless you actually assess all of the patients, but your suspicion should be heightened.

2. What is norovirus?

Norwalk is the name given to certain viruses. The name Norwalk was first used because the virus was identified after a disease outbreak in Norwalk, Ohio. The Norwalk virus and Norwalk-like viruses cause viral gastroenteritis, also called the stomach flu. These viruses are extremely contagious but do not multiply outside of the body. The Norwalk virus, now termed norovirus, is found in contaminated food or drinking water and may be transmitted to others by not thoroughly washing hands after coming in contact with feces or after a bowel movement. Norovirus infection has been in the news because it sometimes appears on cruise ships, in convention centers, and at similar locations.

3. What can you determine about the patient's condition now?

Staff members have advised that the patient has been ill for a few days and has been vomiting and having diarrhea. You witnessed the patient attempt to vomit, and nothing was produced. This information, along with the tenting of the skin on the forearm, should lead you to believe that substantial dehydration exists.

4. Because a diagnosis of norovirus infection has not actually been made for this patient, are you concerned about exposure?

Gastroenteritis, also known as the stomach flu, comprises many types of infections and irritations of the gastrointestinal tract, including those caused by norovirus. Patients experience symptoms such as nausea and vomiting, fever, abdominal cramps, and diarrhea. In healthy people, gastroenteritis is usually not serious. In children, elderly persons, and patients with chronic illness, severe complications such as dehydration may develop. Some of the viral strains are extremely contagious.

5. After oxygen, what is your first choice of treatment for this patient?

You should be working on fluid replacement because of the evidence of dehydration. You should consider a fluid challenge after assessing lung sounds. Consider starting at 250 mL and repeating until the desired effect is reached or whatever is appropriate in your protocol.

6. Are there any notifications you should make concerning the scene?

The federal Ryan White Law, Part G (2009), requires that every emergency response agency have a designated infection control officer (DICO). This person is charged with ensuring that proper postexposure medical treatment and counseling are provided to exposed employees and volunteers. Postexposure medical treatment is offered to prevent an exposed health care provider from contracting the disease to which he or she was exposed. Treatment should be offered within 24 to 48 hours following an exposure, with the actual time frame based on the diagnosis. Exposure to bacterial meningitis, for example, would require treatment within 24 hours.

7. What decontamination measures should you use for your stretcher?

Strip used linens from the stretcher immediately after use, and place them in a plastic bag or in the designated receptacle in the emergency department. Clean the stretcher with an EPA-registered germicidal/virucidal solution or bleach and water at 1:100 dilution. If any spillage or other contamination occurred in the ambulance, clean it up with the same germicidal/virucidal or bleach/water solution.

8. What decontamination measures should you use for yourself?

You should have already been using standard precautions. These precautions apply to all body substances except sweat. You should also wash your hands well and use a hand sanitizer as available. If your uniform was contaminated, you should change into a clean uniform and wash exposed skin. If you have a significant exposure, notify your DICO or follow your company policy.

YOU *are the Medic*   **SUMMARY,** *continued*

EMS Patient Care Report (PCR)

Date: 07-30-11	Incident No.: 9678	Nature of Call: Vomiting		Location: 550 Healthcare Blvd	
Dispatched: 0950	En Route: 0950	At Scene: 0955	Transport: 1015	At Hospital: 1020	In Service: 1040

Patient Information

Age: 86 **Sex:** F **Weight (in kg [lb]):** 54 kg (120 lb)	**Allergies:** Denies **Medications:** Diltiazem (Cardizem) **Past Medical History:** Heart disease, diabetes **Chief Complaint:** Nausea and vomiting for 48 h

Vital Signs

Time: 1008	BP: 98/58	Pulse: 106	Respirations: 18	Spo₂: 97% on room air
Time: 1013	BP: 102/60	Pulse: 96	Respirations: 18	Spo₂: 98% on oxygen
Time:	BP:	Pulse:	Respirations:	Spo₂:

EMS Treatment
(circle all that apply)

Oxygen @ __15__ L/min via (circle one): NC (NRM) Bag-mask device	Assisted Ventilation		Airway Adjunct	CPR
Defibrillation	Bleeding Control	Bandaging	Splinting	Other

Narrative

Arrived at The Springs assisted living facility for an 86-year-old woman complaining of nausea and vomiting for 48 h. Staff advise that the facility has a number of pts with the same signs and symptoms. Staff member reports a staff physician believes it may be related to norovirus but this is unsubstantiated by evaluation. Pt appears weak and reports she is unable to stand because of weakness. Pt attempted to vomit, but nothing was produced. Assessment reveals tenting of skin on the pt's forearm. Oxygen at 15 L/min by NRM started and IV established with a 250-mL challenge per protocol. Lung sounds are clear in all fields before and after challenge. Pt has slight improvement in vital signs during transport to receiving hospital. Report given to company DICO concerning potential for multiple pts. **End of report**

Prep Kit

- Government agencies such as the Occupational Safety and Health Administration (OSHA), the Centers for Disease Control and Prevention (CDC), and state and county public health departments bear the responsibility for protection of the public health, prevention of epidemics, and management of outbreaks.
- Clean and disinfect the ambulance and your equipment to protect patients from infection.
- A patient suspected of having an infectious disease is assessed like any other medical patient.
- Infection involves a typical chain of events through which a communicable disease spreads.
- Communicable diseases can be transmitted from one person to another under certain conditions.
- The risk of infection depends on the type and dose of the organism, its virulence, its mode of entry, and the host's resistance.
- The human body offers several defenses to protect against infection, such as skin, the mucous membranes, and the immune system.
- Protection against and reduction of the occurrence of communicable diseases involve the designated infection control officer (DICO), the public health department, standard precautions, immunizations and vaccinations, personal protective equipment (PPE), postexposure medical follow-up, and an exposure control plan.
- Sexually transmitted diseases (STDs) are usually acquired by sexual contact and are caused by a wide range of organisms.
- Enteric diseases are infectious diseases that affect the gastrointestinal tract. The organisms that cause enteric infections include rotaviruses, parasites, and bacteria.
- Bloodborne diseases include viral hepatitis, HIV, and AIDS.
- A vector is a living organism, such as an insect or rodent, that carries a disease-causing human pathogen. This pathogen does not harm the organism itself, but it can be transmitted to humans by means of a bite, inhalation of contaminated animal feces, or other means.
- The overuse and misuse of antibiotics has made some pathogens resistant to the antibiotic drugs commonly prescribed to eradicate them.
- Serious communicable childhood diseases that had become uncommon in recent decades are making a resurgence because some parents refuse to have their children vaccinated. Research showing a link between vaccines and the development of autism in children has been discredited.
- New and emerging diseases of concern include severe acute respiratory syndrome (SARS) and the avian flu.

acquired immunodeficiency syndrome (AIDS) The end-stage disease process caused by the human immunodeficiency virus (HIV); results in extreme vulnerability to numerous opportunistic bacterial, viral, and fungal infections that would not affect a person with an intact immune system.

airborne transmission The transmission of an infectious agent by inhalation of small particles that become aerosolized when the infected person coughs, sneezes, talks, or exhales; particles remain suspended in this vapor and can be carried a short distance, usually 3' to 6'.

avian (bird) flu A disease caused by a virus that occurs naturally in the bird population; signs and symptoms include fever, sore throat, cough, and muscle aches.

bacteria Small organisms that can grow and reproduce outside the human cell in the presence of the needed temperature and nutrients and cause disease by invading and multiplying in the tissues of the host.

bloodborne pathogens Pathogenic microorganisms that are present in human blood and can cause disease in humans. These pathogens include, but are not limited to, hepatitis B virus (HBV), human immunodeficiency virus (HIV), and hepatitis C (HCV).

carriers People who harbor an infectious agent and, although not personally ill, can transmit the infection to other people.

chancre The primary hard lesion or ulcer of syphilis that occurs at the entry site of the infection.

chickenpox A very contagious disease caused by the varicella zoster virus, which is part of the herpes virus family, occurring most often in the winter and early spring.

chlamydia A sexually transmitted disease (STD) with the highest incidence in sexually transmitted diseases; signs and symptoms include inflammation of the urethra, epididymis, cervix, and fallopian tubes, and discharge from the urethra.

colonized A pathogen is present but has produced no illness in the host; often progresses to active infection; a colonized host is often called a *carrier* because he or she can transmit the pathogen to others.

communicable disease An infectious disease that can be transmitted from one person to another by direct contact or by indirect contact through a vector or fomite; also called contagious disease.

communicable period The period during which an infected person can transmit a communicable disease to someone else.

contact transmission The transmission of an infectious agent by means of direct or indirect contact with the infected persons, such as skin-to-skin contact or contact with the patient's environment.

contaminated The presence or the reasonably anticipated presence of blood or other potentially infectious materials on an item or surface.

designated infection control officer (DICO) A person trained to ensure that proper postexposure medical treatment and counseling are provided to an exposed employee or volunteer.

droplet transmission The transmission of an infectious agent by inhalation of relatively large particles generated when an infected person coughs or sneezes; these particles travel a short distance through the air before falling to the ground.

endemic Consistently present or prevalent in a population or geographic area.

epidemic An outbreak of disease that substantially exceeds what is expected based on recent experience.

Enterococcus A common, normal organism of the gastrointestinal (GI) tract, urinary tract, and genitourinary tract that can be pathogenic and become resistant to vancomycin.

fomites Inanimate objects contaminated with microorganisms that serve as a means of transmitting an illness.

fungi Small organisms that can grow rapidly in the presence of the needed nutrients and organic material and can cause infection related to contact with decaying organic matter or from airborne spores in the environment such as molds; singular term, fungus.

gastroenteritis A term that comprises many types of infections and irritations of the gastrointestinal tract; symptoms include nausea and vomiting, fever, abdominal cramps, and diarrhea; also called stomach flu.

gonorrhea A sexually transmitted disease (STD) that results in infection caused by the gonococcal bacteria, *Neisseria gonorrhea*; signs and symptoms include pus-containing discharge from the urethra and painful urination in males and signs and symptoms of an acute abdomen in females.

hantavirus A type of virus found in wild rodents, which can also cause disease in humans, characterized by fever, headache, abdominal pain, loss of appetite, and vomiting; diseases caused are hemorrhagic fever with renal syndrome and hantavirus pulmonary syndrome.

host resistance One's ability to fight off infection.

human immunodeficiency virus (HIV) The virus that may lead to acquired immunodeficiency syndrome (AIDS); cells in the immune system are killed or damaged so that the body is unable to fight infections and certain cancers.

icterus Jaundice; the yellow appearance of the skin and other tissues caused by an accumulation of bile pigments.

immunization The process of producing widespread immunity to a specific infectious disease among a targeted group by inoculating individual members of the population; can also refer to a set of vaccinations given together or on a recommended schedule.

incubation period The period between exposure to an organism and the first symptoms of illness, during which the organism multiplies within the body and starts to produce symptoms. This period is when the disease can be transmitted to another person.

infection The invasion of a host or host tissue by pathogenic organisms such as bacteria, viruses, or parasites that produces illness that may or may not have clinical manifestations.

infectious disease A disease caused by pathogenic organisms.

infectious hepatitis Another name for hepatitis A; an inflammation from a virus that causes mild fatigue, loss of appetite, fever, nausea, abdominal pain, and, eventually, jaundice, dark-colored urine, and whitish stools.

influenza The flu, a respiratory infection caused by a variety of viruses; differs from the common cold in that the flu involves a fever, headache, and extreme exhaustion.

jaundice The presence of excessive bile pigments in the bloodstream that give the skin, mucous membranes, and eyes a distinct yellow color; often associated with liver disease.

lice Tiny, wingless, parasitic insects that feed on blood; an infestation is easily spread through close personal contact; types include head, body, and pubic lice.

Lyme disease A tick-borne disease that primarily affects the skin, heart, joints, and nervous system and is characterized by a round, red lesion or bull's-eye rash.

measles An infectious viral disease that occurs most often in late winter and spring; begins with a fever followed by a cough, running nose, and pink eye; a rash spreads from the face and neck down the back and trunk.

meningitis An inflammation of the meningeal coverings of the brain and spinal cord; usually caused by a virus or bacterium; the viral type is less severe than the bacterial; the bacterial type can result in brain damage, hearing loss, learning disability, or death.

meningococcal meningitis A type of meningitis caused by the meningococcal bacterium, *Neisseria meningitidis*.

mononucleosis Infectious mononucleosis or mono (glandular fever); caused by the Epstein-Barr virus, is often called the kissing disease; also spread by coughing or sneezing.

mumps A viral infection that primarily affects the parotid glands, which are one of the three pairs of salivary glands, causing swelling in front of the ears.

needleless systems Devices that do not use needles for the collection of body fluids or withdrawal of body fluids after initial venous or arterial access is established, the administration of medication or fluids, or any other procedure involving the potential for occupational exposure to bloodborne pathogens by percutaneous injuries from contaminated sharps.

nosocomial infection An infection acquired from a health care setting.

opportunistic infections The infections in which an organism thrives when the immune system has been compromised by illness, chemotherapeutic medications, or antirejection drugs in an organ transplant recipient. These fungi, bacteria, viruses, and parasites are normally held in check by a healthy immune system.

other potentially infectious materials (OPIM) Cerebrospinal fluid (CSF), pericardial fluid, amniotic fluid, synovial fluid, peritoneal fluid, and any fluid containing visible blood.

pandemic An outbreak of disease that occurs on a global scale.

parasites Any living organisms in or on any other living creature; take advantage of the host by feeding off cells and tissues.

pertussis An acute infectious disease characterized by a catarrhal stage, followed by a paroxysmal cough that ends in a whooping inspiration; also called whooping cough.

pneumonia An inflammation of the lungs caused by bacterial, viral, or fungal infections or infections with other microorganisms.

protozoa Single-celled, usually microscopic, eukaryotic organisms such as amoebas, ciliates, flagellates, and sporozoans; a type of parasite.

rabies A fatal infection of the central nervous system caused by a bite from an animal that has been infected with the rabies virus.

reservoir In the context of communicable disease, a place where organisms may live and multiply.

respiratory syncytial virus (RSV) A labile paramyxovirus that infects the upper and lower respiratory tracts, but disease, namely pneumonia and bronchiolitis, is more prevalent in the lower respiratory tract.

rubella A viral disease similar to measles, best known by the distinctive red rash on the skin; not nearly as infectious or severe as measles.

scabies An infestation of the skin with the mite *Sarcoptes scabiei*; spreads rapidly with skin-to-skin contact.

seropositive Having a positive blood test for an infectious agent, such as human immunodeficiency virus (HIV) or hepatitis B or C virus.

serum hepatitis Infection with the hepatitis B virus (HBV), which is transmitted through sexual contact, blood transfusion, or puncture of the skin with contaminated needles; signs and symptoms include loss of appetite, nausea, vomiting, general fatigue and malaise, low-grade fever, vague abdominal discomfort, and sometimes aching in the joints; eventually, jaundice occurs.

severe acute respiratory syndrome (SARS) A potentially life-threatening viral infection that usually starts with flu-like symptoms.

sexually transmitted diseases (STDs) A group of diseases usually acquired by sexual contact and that include gonorrhea, syphilis, chlamydia, scabies, pubic lice, herpes, hepatitis, and HIV infection.

source individual Any person, living or dead, whose blood or other potentially infectious materials may be a source of occupational exposure to another person; examples include but are not limited to, hospital and clinic patients; clients in institutions for the developmentally disabled; trauma victims; clients of drug and alcohol treatment facilities; residents of hospices and nursing homes; human remains; and people who donate or sell blood or blood components.

standard precautions The term currently used to describe the infection control practices that will reduce the opportunity for exposure of providers in the daily care of patients; consider all body fluids, except sweat, to present a possible risk.

Staphylococcus aureus A strain of bacteria that became resistant to the drug methicillin, creating a new strain called methicillin-resistant *S aureus*; symptoms include infection and possibly localized skin abscesses and cellulites, empyemas, and endocarditis.

syphilis A sexually transmitted disease (STD) caused by the spiral-shaped bacteria *Treponema pallidum* with signs and symptoms that include an ulcerative lesion or chancre of the skin or mucous membrane at the site of infection, commonly in the genital region.

tetanus A disease caused by spores that enter the body through a puncture wound contaminated with animal feces, street dust, or soil or that can enter through contaminated street drugs; signs and symptoms include pain at the wound site and painful muscle contractions in the neck and trunk muscles.

tuberculin skin test (TST) A test to determine if a person has ever been infected with tuberculosis.

tuberculosis (TB) An infection that can progress to a disease characterized by a persistent cough for > 3 weeks plus night sweats, headache, weight loss, hemoptysis, and/or chest pain.

vaccinations Inoculations with a vaccine, usually by injection or inhalation, to bring about immunity to a specific disease in a person.

vaccines The products formulated to bring about immunity by introducing into the body a killed or weakened virus to which the immune system produces antibodies.

vector An animal or insect that carries a disease-causing organism and transmits it to a human host, without itself becoming ill.

vesicles Tiny fluid-filled sacs; small blisters.

viral hepatitis An inflammation of the liver produced by one of five distinct forms a virus—A, B, C, D, and E. The types differ in transmission but present with the same signs and symptoms.

virulence The ability of an organism to invade and create disease in a host; also refers to the ability of an organism to survive outside the living host.

viruses Small organisms that can multiply only inside a host, such as a human, and cause disease.

West Nile virus (WNV) A type of virus that is transmitted by mosquitos, and usually causes only mild disease in humans but can cause encephalitis, meningitis, and death; symptoms, if any, include fever, headache, body rash, and swollen lymph glands.

zoonotic Refers to infectious diseases of animals that can be transmitted to humans and cause disease.

Assessment in Action

You are called to a local rehab center for a person vomiting. When you arrive, the staff nurse tells you the patient has a history of hepatitis. The patient has been vomiting most of the day, has a fever, and is very weak. When you enter the patient's room, you notice the patient's skin appears yellow.

1. Before you physically assess this patient, what type of precautions should be taken?
   A. Standard precautions
   B. Special precautions
   C. Barrier precautions
   D. Cutaneous precautions

2. The yellow coloring to the patient's skin is caused by:
   A. a decrease in the red blood cell count.
   B. an increase in the bilirubin level in the blood.
   C. a decrease in the bilirubin level in the blood.
   D. an increase in the red blood cell count.

3. The most common chronic bloodborne infection and the leading reason for liver transplantation in the United States is:
   A. hepatitis A.
   B. hepatitis B.
   C. hepatitis C.
   D. hepatitis D.

4. If you had a positive exposure to confirmed HBV while treating this patient and you have a positive titer test on file, what follow-up treatment is recommended?
   A. A follow-up titer test to make sure of immunity
   B. None because you show immunity to HBV
   C. Precautionary antibiotics as soon as possible
   D. Repeating the three-vaccination series

5. Which of the following types of hepatitis is enteric?
   A. A
   B. B
   C. C
   D. D

6. The ability of an organism to invade and create disease in a host is called:
   A. indirect transmission.
   B. direct transmission.
   C. vector transmission.
   D. virulence.

Additional Questions

7. What are the requirements for the designated infection control officer (DICO)?

8. What is the role of the public health department in infectious disease outbreaks?

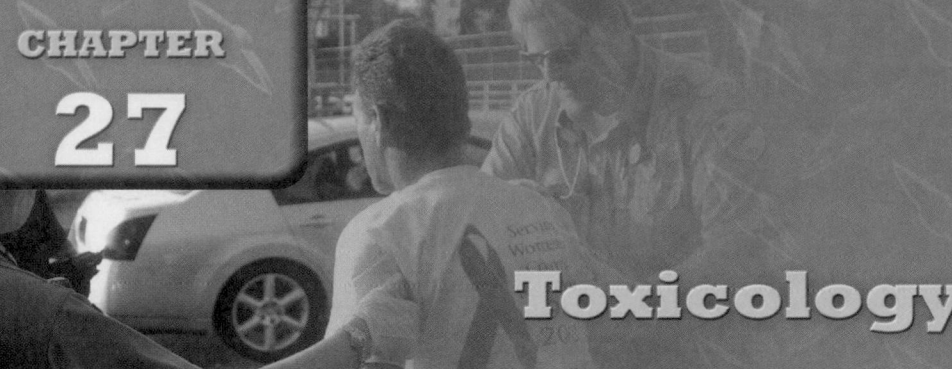

Toxicology

National EMS Education Standard Competencies

Medicine

Integrates assessment findings with principles of epidemiology and pathophysiology to formulate a field impression and implement a comprehensive treatment/disposition plan for a patient with a medical complaint.

Toxicology

Recognition and management of

- Carbon monoxide poisoning (pp 1344-1345)
- Nerve agent poisoning (p 1344)

How and when to contact a poison control center (p 1326)

Anatomy, physiology, pathophysiology, assessment, and management of

- Inhaled poisons (pp 1327-1328, 1337-1338, 1344-1347)
- Ingested poisons (pp 1327, 1333-1347)
- Injected poisons (pp 1328, 1336-1337)
- Absorbed poisons (pp 1328, 1344-1348)
- Alcohol intoxication and withdrawal (pp 1333-1336)
- Opiate toxidrome (pp 1341-1342)

Anatomy, physiology, epidemiology, pathophysiology, psychosocial impact, presentations, prognosis, and management of the following toxidromes and poisonings:

- Cholinergics (pp 1329, 1344)
- Anticholinergics (pp 1329, 1353)
- Sympathomimetics (pp 1329, 1336-1340)
- Sedative/hypnotics (pp 1329, 1340-1341)
- Opiates (pp 1329, 1341-1342)
- Alcohol intoxication and withdrawal (pp 1333-1336)
- Over-the-counter and prescription medications (pp 1355-1356)
- Carbon monoxide (pp 1344-1345)
- Illegal drugs (pp 1336-1339)
- Herbal preparations (p 1361)

Knowledge Objectives

1. Define toxicology, poison, and overdose. (pp 1325-1326)
2. Describe routes of entry of toxic substances into the body, including ingestion, inhalation, injection, and absorption. (pp 1327-1328)

3. Discuss major toxidromes and their use in assessment and management of toxicologic emergencies. (pp 1328-1329)
4. Identify the common signs and symptoms of poisoning. (pp 1329- 1330)
5. Describe the assessment and management of the patient with suspected poisoning. (pp 1344-1348, 1349-1353, 1357-1361)
6. Describe the assessment and management of the patient with suspected overdose. (pp 1331-1344, 1348-1349, 1353-1357)
7. Understand the role of airway management in the patient with suspected poisoning or overdose. (p 1331)
8. Discuss substance abuse and concepts associated with it. (pp 1329-1331)
9. Discuss emergencies related to severe intoxication, including alcoholism. (pp 1333-1361)
10. Explain the use of activated charcoal, including indications, contraindications, and the need to obtain approval from medical control before its administration. (pp 1341, 1348, 1350, 1353, 1354)
11. Identify the main types of specific poisons and their effects, including alcohol, stimulants, marijuana, hallucinogens, sedative-hypnotic drugs, narcotics (opiates and opioids), cardiac medications, organophosphates, carbon monoxide, chlorine gas, cyanide, caustics, drugs abused for sexual purposes, poisonous alcohols, hydrocarbons, psychiatric medications, nonprescription pain medications, theophylline, and metals and metalloids. (pp 1333-1358)
12. Describe the assessment and management of the patient with suspected plant or mushroom poisoning. (pp 1339-1340, 1358-1361)
13. Describe the assessment and management of the patient with suspected food poisoning. (p 1361)

Skills Objectives

1. Demonstrate the steps in the assessment and management of the patient with suspected poisoning. (pp 1331-1333)
2. Demonstrate the steps in the assessment and management of the patient with suspected overdose. (pp 1331-1333)

Introduction

Rarely will an entire shift pass without a paramedic treating one or more patients who are abusing <u>licit</u> (legal) or <u>illicit</u> (illegal) drugs. In the United States, alcohol—which can be bought on an over-the-counter (OTC) basis—is the most common substance of abuse **Figure 1**. Another licit substance that is often abused is oxycodone, which is available by prescription only. On the illegal side of drug use and abuse, it is impossible to accurately identify how many "users" of such substances as heroin or ecstasy exist. Although research indicates that the use of street drugs seems to have stabilized in smaller communities in recent years, larger cities have seen increases in heroin and cocaine use. Methamphetamine abuse seems to increase and decrease depending on the availability of the chemicals required to produce methamphetamine. When pseudoephedrine and anhydrous ammonia are easily obtained, it is virtually guaranteed that persons making methamphetamines will be in full production mode.

To begin, it is important to define some key terms. A <u>poison</u> is a substance that is toxic by nature, no matter how it gets into the body or how much is taken. At a minimum, a poison will make people ill; in the worst-case scenario, it will kill them. By contrast, a <u>drug</u> is a substance that has some therapeutic effect (such as reducing inflammation, fighting bacteria, or producing euphoria) when given in the appropriate circumstances and in the appropriate dose. When a drug (either licit or illicit) is taken in excess, the person is said to have "overdosed." This can be a true toxicologic emergency because the person has been potentially "poisoned." To put it concisely, a poison is *always a poison*, whereas a licit or illicit substance *may poison a person* if it is taken to excess.

The term "bioavailability" is used to describe the extent to which any given drug is present in sufficient amounts to produce the desired result. "Half-life" describes the point when the bioavailability of a given drug has decreased to 50%; it is usually given in minutes, but may sometimes last for hours or even days. Lastly, the term "excretion" is used to describe how a drug is removed from the body.

Types of Toxicologic Emergencies

<u>Toxicologic emergencies</u> usually fall under one of two general headings: intentional and unintentional. Poisoning in adults is

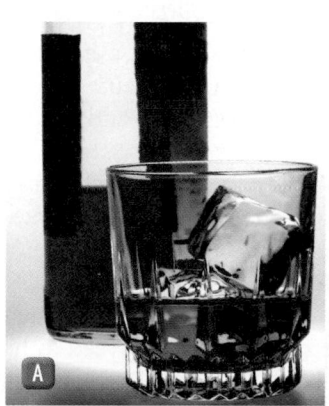
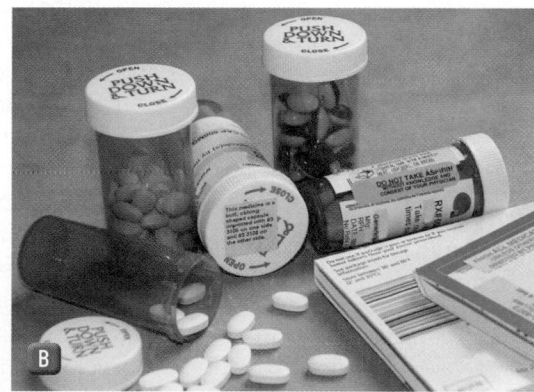
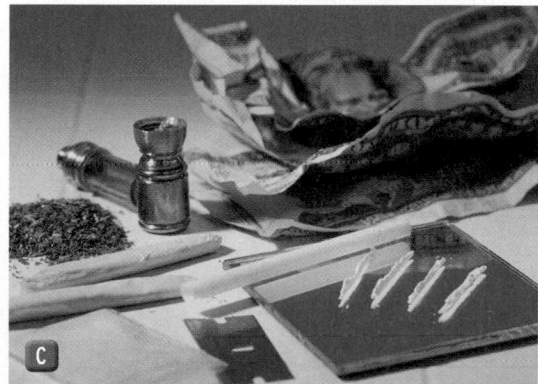

Figure 1 **A.** Alcohol is a legal substance that is a drug. **B.** Medications are legal substances that can be abused. **C.** Illegal drugs can also be abused.

YOU *are the Medic* — PART 1

Your unit is dispatched to an apartment for a possible overdose. The dispatcher tells you that law enforcement personnel are already on scene and that a woman was found unconscious on the sidewalk in front of the apartments. The officer reports that the patient is breathing but is unresponsive. When you arrive, you find a young woman lying supine on the sidewalk. Your primary assessment reveals that the patient is barely breathing but has a strong pulse. You see linear scar tissue on both arms. According to the law enforcement officer, witnesses say this patient was dropped off by a car that sped away.

1. What is your first impression of this patient?
2. What is your priority for patient care?

commonly intentional. In particular, suicide is often accomplished with the use of drugs.

An unintentional toxicologic emergency can occur in many ways. For example, medication dosing errors are common problems in clinical practice. If you inadvertently move a decimal point just one place to the right, 2.0 mg of morphine becomes 20.0 mg of morphine—10 times the intended dose! In some cases a drug event may be idiosyncratic: 2 mg of midazolam (Versed) may simply relax one patient but cause respiratory arrest in another.

Childhood poisonings are quite common, especially in younger children who will put anything into their mouths **Figure 2** . For example, the colorful berries on a house or garden plant may draw a toddler's attention. Likewise, a parent's prescription medication may be mistaken for candy.

Even nature is fraught with toxicologic perils—just ask any hiker who has inadvertently wandered through a patch of poison ivy. Wild mushrooms, once in the body, can produce a wide spectrum of results—from being a tasty treat, to being nauseating, or, in some cases, to being deadly.

The workplace also harbors its share of toxic hazards. Unfortunately, many industrial hazards are not identified until after the exposure has occurred and persons who are ill start seeking medical attention. For example, countless workers in the electric energy field worked with polychlorinated biphenyls (PCBs) on a daily basis and developed cancer later in life. Similarly, asbestosis (mesothelioma) developed in thousands of people after their continued exposure to asbestos in the workplace.

Unintentional toxicologic emergencies can also occur from simple neglect or oversight. Consider a geriatric person with diabetes, possibly combined with early-onset dementia or Alzheimer disease, who takes his or her insulin in the morning, but later cannot remember whether the dose was taken, and so takes another dose. The result: a call to 9-1-1 for an "unconscious, unresponsive" person in need of assistance.

Intentional poisoning or overdose commonly occurs during what might be termed "intimate crimes." Chloral hydrate ("knockout drops") has been used to commit assault for decades, and other pharmacologic agents have been used in homicide as well. In recent years, "date rape" drugs such as flunitrazepam (Rohypnol) have been used to facilitate sexual assault. Flunitrazepam is a powerful benzodiazepine that has both antegrade and retrograde amnesiac properties; in other words, it erases the person's memory for the next 4 or 5 hours as well as 3 or 4 of the immediate past hours, leaving the victim and the police with little information to go on in pressing a case against the assailant.

■ Poison Centers

Given the variety of illicit drugs coupled with the continued growth of licit drugs, even the most well-read veteran paramedic may find it difficult to keep current with the myriad drugs sold in the streets today. For this reason, Poison Centers (1-800-222-1222) may be an indispensable aid, along with smart phone applications such as Epocrates.

Suppose you are called to a home in which a frantic mother is hovering over a toddler who sits beside the remains of a potted philodendron, with two large leaves that are well chewed on and mostly gone. Is the plant poisonous? How poisonous? Should you make the child vomit? Is an antidote available? In such a scenario, you can call the Poison Center and get a fast rundown on the ingestion, its toxic potential, and steps to negate its effects, thereby providing proper patient care.

Poison Centers are a virtual goldmine of information that you should add to your paramedic toolbox. Never hesitate to tap these resources when you are confronted with *any toxin* for which you have limited or no familiarity. *When in doubt, call!*

At the same time, your call helps the center collect data on poisonings in your region. These data may be analyzed to help detect trends, spot developing public health problems, and evaluate current treatment protocols for different poisonings.

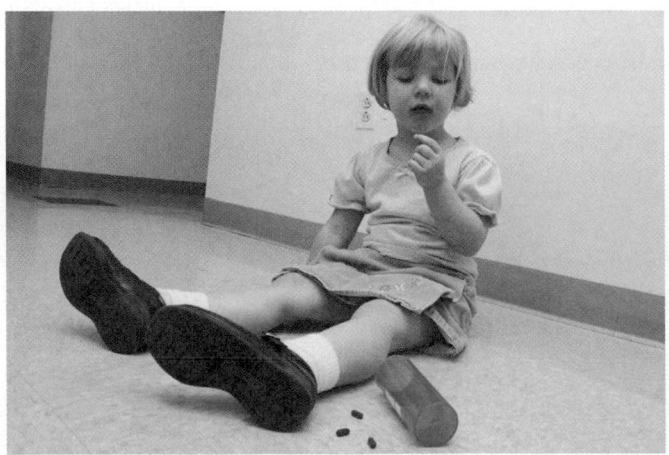

Figure 2 Toddlers will put anything into their mouths, including dangerous medications.

Words of Wisdom

The National Capital Poison Center was founded in 1980 to help prevent poisonings, limit injuries from poisonings, and save lives. As EMS providers should know, the Center offers 24-hour guidance for poisoning by certified specialists in poison information. Board-certified physician toxicologists back up the team of specialists and help manage each case. The Poison Center assists with the management of roughly 70% of all poisonings.

In addition to knowing how to reach the Poison Center, paramedics should familiarize themselves with information on poisoning available at the Centers for Disease Control and Prevention (CDC) website. The *Poisoning in the United States: Fact Sheet* addresses the scope of problem, costs associated with poisonings, the groups at greatest risk, additional sources of information, and related publications.

Words of Wisdom

Record all your findings about a poisoned patient, even if you do not know their significance. Someone at the Poison Center will know.

■ Anatomy and Physiology

■ Routes of Absorption

Toxins cannot exert their effects until they enter the human body. The four primary methods of entry are *ingestion, inhalation, injection,* and *absorption.* Just as each of these methods of entry is unique, so is the rate at which a given toxin is absorbed into the body. Once a toxin is in the body, the combination of the amount of toxin and the relative speed at which it is metabolized affect both the bioavailability of the toxin and the excretion rate.

Poisoning by Ingestion

Ingested poisons may produce immediate damage to tissues, or their toxic effects may be delayed for several hours. With ingestions of a caustic substance (that is, a strong acid or alkali) damage occurs immediately. By contrast, some poisons must be absorbed into the bloodstream before they can produce their toxic effects. *Medications* around the home and *household chemicals* (such as cleaning agents) are two of the most common sources of poisoning by ingestion.

Poisoning by ingestion is marked by a wide range of possibilities in regard to *what* is actually ingested and *why* it was ingested. Consider, for example, the curious child who eats the bright red berries off a holly plant or the trumpet-like flowers of a purple foxglove **Figure 3**. Now consider a person who is taking acetaminophen for pain relief, and then takes another medication also containing acetaminophen. This person may inadvertently increase his or her intake to a toxic level, possibly to the point of destroying the liver and leading to death.

Although both this scenario and the preceding one would be considered accidental, intentional poisoning by ingestion is also common. For example, a person may take a lethal quantity or combination of drugs in a suicide attempt.

Assessment clues pointing toward ingestion can be as obvious as a plant with partially chewed leaves or a section of plant with

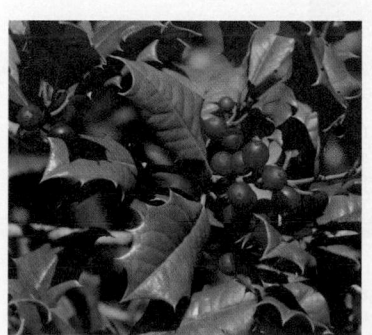

Figure 3 Certain berries and flowers are poisonous, such as those of the holly plant and the purple foxglove.

berries missing. Look for stained fingers, lips, or tongues. Any patient reporting the sudden onset of stomach cramps with or without nausea, vomiting, or diarrhea may have an ingestion-related problem. Empty pill bottles are another obvious clue, as is the date on which the prescription was filled. The bottle for a prescription filled 6 months ago probably was not anywhere close to full today; an empty bottle for a prescription filled yesterday is a far more ominous clue.

A toxin that enters the body by the oral route generally provides a more forgiving time frame for identification and treatment of the offending agent. Little absorption occurs in the stomach; the ingested substance may stay there for a variable period, with most absorption actually taking place in the small intestine. As a consequence, much of the management of poisoning by ingestion aims to remove or neutralize the poison before it gains access to the intestines.

Poisoning by Inhalation

A person can be poisoned by inhalation when the toxic agent is present in the surrounding atmosphere. That fact, obvious as it seems, has important implications. First, so long as the patient remains in the toxic environment, he or she will keep inhaling the poison—and so will any paramedic who enters that environment without the appropriate protective breathing apparatus. Second, when poisoning occurs because of a toxic environment, you are likely to encounter more than one patient at the emergency scene. Home medications and household chemical products (such as bleach and cleaning agents) are responsible for the most common types of inhalation emergencies.

Poisoning by inhalation may be either accidental or intentional. Consider carbon monoxide (CO) poisoning. Leaving the garage door shut while seated in an automobile with the engine running provides a quick, painless method of suicide. By contrast, an automatic damper on a furnace that fails to open or a bird's nest that blocks a chimney can allow a house to quickly fill with colorless, odorless, deadly CO, quietly, quickly, and efficiently poisoning those inside.

Emergency responders should be aware of an emerging method of suicide in the United States that is placing EMS, fire, and law enforcement officers at risk. Suicidal persons have killed themselves by mixing certain household chemicals inside an automobile with all of the doors and windows closed. As the chemicals mix, toxic gases are created, which harm or kill the occupants of the vehicle.

The resulting chemicals are often colorless and may or may not have a recognizable odor. Emergency responders are at risk of serious injury when attempting to access the vehicle or patient after observing an unresponsive person inside. In some instances, the suicidal person has left a note, warning bystanders and emergency responders of the presence of toxic chemicals. In other instances, bystanders attempting to render aid and emergency responders have been exposed to extremely hazardous chemicals while trying to access and assess a victim who is already dead.

From the anatomic and physiologic perspective, inhaled toxins reach the alveoli quickly, providing almost instant access to the circulation. CO, for example, binds to hemoglobin on the red blood cells about 250 times more readily than do oxygen molecules. As a result, rapid systemic distribution of carbon monoxide can occur with an equally rapid onset of signs and symptoms. For this reason, the window of opportunity for problem identification and subsequent treatment is limited.

When you are dealing with an inhalation emergency, the first general management consideration is that of scene safety. After donning the appropriate breathing apparatus, remove the patient(s) to a safe environment before beginning any assessment or treatment.

Words of Wisdom

Scene safety is your primary concern when you are called to an inhalation incident. Whenever you encounter more than one sick patient, where the patients exhibit similar symptoms, but you find no evidence of any mechanism of injury (MOI), be suspicious of some form of poisoning. Toxic fumes may be odorless and colorless, and they do not discriminate between rescuers and victims. Be suspicious of a potentially toxic environment when you are responding to a report of one or more patients with changes in level of consciousness (LOC), especially at an industrial site or enclosed space.

Inhaled toxins produce a wide range of signs and symptoms, many of which are unique to the toxin involved. A patient with CO poisoning does not exhibit the same signs and symptoms as a person who has sniffed glue, who in turn looks nothing like a patient poisoned by a furniture stripper containing methylene chloride. Frequently, the emergency scene often contains much information to help you identify the toxin that made your patient(s) ill, such as MSDS paperwork, a shipping manifest, a bill of lading, or transportation placards. That information, coupled with the assistance of the Poison Center and direction from the medical control physician, will drive your treatment plan. Correction of hypoxia is a must; deliver oxygen to the patient to maintain a saturation level in the 95% range. Establish vascular access, apply an electrocardiographic (ECG) monitor, and perform pulse oximetry and capnography.

Words of Wisdom

Always treat the patient and not the diagnostic tool. Pulse oximeters may give false readings when patients have been exposed to carbon monoxide.

Poisoning by Injection

Injected poisons usually gain access to the body as the result of stings or bites from a variety of insects and animals. Abuse of intravenously administered drugs such as heroin, cocaine,

Words of Wisdom

All tools used to inject substances should be considered biohazards. These needles or devices may have been shared with other drug users and may carry the human immunodeficiency virus (HIV) or other pathogens.

amphetamines, and "speedballs" (heroin and cocaine together) is also a common event in the prehospital setting.

Depending on the geographic location, possibilities for poisoning by injection frequently exist in the environment. Whereas snake bites and scorpion stings are more prevalent in the southwestern United States, paramedics in coastal areas are more likely to encounter patients stung by jellyfish, Portuguese man-of-war, sea urchins, or anemones. Wasps, yellow jackets, and hornets have a wider geographic distribution, and stings from these insects are common occurrences throughout most of the United States.

Some of these injected poisons are neurotoxic, whereas others produce localized or systemic reactions. When a bite or sting hits a vein or artery and results in a toxin immediately entering the bloodstream, the outcome is much more dangerous than when the same toxin enters a muscle mass such as the calf, from which the toxin has a much slower rate of absorption and distribution.

When you are assessing bites and stings, physical findings will usually provide the most numerous clues, especially local reactions such as pain at the wound site. Depending on the specific toxin, signs and symptoms can vary greatly. Frequently, the patient may be able to identify the culprit, greatly simplifying the assessment process.

Poisoning by Absorption

Some poisons gain access to the body by being absorbed through the skin. Of the poisonings that occur by absorption, those caused by pesticides such as organophosphates and similar substances are often the most serious.

Words of Wisdom

Absorption of toxic substances through the skin is a common problem in agriculture and manufacturing. Most solvents and "cides"—insecticides, herbicides, and pesticides—are toxic and can be readily absorbed through the skin.

■ Understanding and Using Toxidromes

Although the sheer number of potential substances of abuse is daunting, the good news is that many drugs, on entering the body, result in similar signs and symptoms. Consider narcotics. Irrespective of whether it is a natural product derived from opium (an opiate) or a synthetic, non–opium-derived narcotic (an opioid), all drugs in this group work in a similar manner, so they produce similar signs and symptoms. The syndrome-like symptoms of a class or group of similar poisonous agents are termed a toxic syndrome or **toxidrome**. Toxidromes are useful for remembering the assessment and management of different substances that fall under the same clinical umbrella. Six major toxidromes exist: stimulants, narcotics, cholinergics, anticholinergics, sympathomimetics, and sedative/hypnotics Table 1 .

Table 2 lists common signs and symptoms of poisoning. If you look at your history and physical examination findings in conjunction with the vital signs, more often than not you can develop a working diagnosis that will allow you to provide appropriate care until you can deliver the patient to the receiving facility.

Overview of Substance Abuse

Human beings have a long history of abusing drugs and alcohol. With the passing of time, the physiologic and societal effects

Table 1 Major Toxidromes

Toxidrome	Drug Examples	Signs and Symptoms
Stimulant	Amphetamine, methamphetamine, cocaine, diet aids, nasal decongestants, bath salts	Restlessness, agitation, incessant talking; insomnia, anorexia; dilated pupils, tachycardia; tachypnea, hypertension or hypotension; paranoia, seizures, cardiac arrest
Narcotic (opiate and opioid)	Heroin, opium, morphine, hydromorphone (Dilaudid), fentanyl, oxycodone-aspirin combination (Percodan), zolpidem tartrate (Ambien), secobarbital	Constricted (pinpoint) pupils, marked respiratory depression; needle tracks (IV abusers); drowsiness, stupor, coma
Sympathomimetic	Pseudoephedrine, phenylephrine, phenylpropanolamine, amphetamine, and methamphetamine	Hypertension, tachycardia, dilated pupils (mydriasis), agitation and seizures, hyperthermia
Sedative/Hypnotics	Phenobarbital, diazepam (Valium), thiopental, midazolam (Versed), lorazepam	Drowsiness, disinhibition, ataxia, slurred speech, mental confusion, respiratory depression, progressive central nervous system depression, hypotension
Cholinergic	Acephate (Orthene), diazinon (Basudin, Knox Out, Spectracide), and malathion (Celthion, Cythion), parathion, sarin, tabun, VX	Increased salivation, lacrimation, gastrointestinal distress, diarrhea, respiratory depression, apnea, seizures, coma
Anticholinergic	Atropine, scopolamine, antihistamines, antipsychotics	Dry, flushed skin, hyperthermia, dilated pupils, blurred vision, tachycardia; mild hallucinations, dramatic delirium

Table 2 Common Signs and Symptoms of Poisoning

Sign or Symptom	Type	Possible Causative Agents
Odor	Bitter almonds	Cyanide
	Garlic	Arsenic, organophosphates, phosphorus
	Acetone	Methyl alcohol, isopropyl alcohol, aspirin, acetone, diabetes
	Wintergreen	Methyl salicylate
	Pears	Chloral hydrate
	Violets	Turpentine
	Camphor	Camphor
	Alcohol	Alcohol
Pupils	Constricted	Narcotics, organophosphates, Jimson weed, nutmeg, propoxyphene (Darvon)
	Dilated	Barbiturates, atropine, amphetamine, glutethimide (Doriden), lysergic acid diethylamide (LSD), cyanide, CO
Mouth	Salivation	Organophosphates, arsenic, strychnine, mercury, salicylates
	Dry mouth	Atropine (belladonna), amphetamines, diphenhydramine (Benadryl), narcotics
	Burns in mouth	Formaldehyde, iodine, lye, toxic plants, phenols, phosphorous, pine oil, silver nitrate, acids

Continues

Table 2 Common Signs and Symptoms of Poisoning, continued

Sign or Symptom	Type	Possible Causative Agents
Skin	Pruritus	Jimson weed, belladonna, boric acid
	Dry, hot skin	Atropine (in belladonna), botulism, nutmeg
	Sweating	Organophosphates, arsenic, aspirin, amphetamines, barbiturates, mushrooms, naphthalene
Respiratory	Depressed respirations	Narcotics, alcohol, propoxyphene, CO, barbiturates
	Increased respirations	Aspirin, amphetamines, boric acid, cyanide, kerosene, methyl alcohol, nicotine
	Pulmonary edema	Organophosphates, petroleum products, narcotics, CO
Cardiovascular	Tachycardia	Alcohol, amphetamines, arsenic, atropine, aspirin, cocaine, some antiasthma drugs
	Bradycardia	Digitalis, gasoline, nicotine, mushrooms, narcotics, cyanide, mistletoe, rhododendron
	Hypertension	Amphetamines, lead, nicotine, antiasthma drugs
	Hypotension	Barbiturates, narcotics, tranquilizers, house plants, mistletoe, nitroglycerin, antifreeze
Central nervous system	Seizures	Amphetamines, camphor, cocaine, strychnine, arsenic, CO, petroleum products, scorpion sting
	Coma	All depressant drugs (such as narcotics, barbiturates, tranquilizers, alcohol), CO, cyanide
	Hallucinations	Atropine, LSD, mushrooms, organic solvents, phencyclidine (PCP), nutmeg
	Headache	CO, alcohol, disulfiram (Antabuse)
	Tremors	Organophosphates, CO, amphetamine, tranquilizers, poisonous marine animals
	Weakness or paralysis	Organophosphates, botulism, eel, hemlock, puffer fish, pine oil, rhododendron
Gastrointestinal	Cramps, nausea, vomiting, and/or diarrhea	Many, if not most, ingested poisons

of alcohol abuse have become well known and thoroughly documented. Unfortunately, the area of medicine dealing with drugs of abuse is highly challenging because of uncertainty about the prevalence of the problem and the continual evolution of the substances themselves. In the 1980s, creative chemists took existing pharmacologic agents and structurally manipulated them to create new or different drugs ("designer drugs") that were often far more potent than the original drugs. For example, cocaine was made into crack, a far more addictive form of the drug.

Part of the definition of substance abuse is cultural; indeed, there is great variation in what is considered "abuse." In our society, for example, it is acceptable to administer narcotics under medical supervision for the relief of pain; conversely, self-administration of the same drugs for the purpose of inducing euphoria is regarded as drug abuse.

Any given society's definition of abuse may have little relation to the potential harm from the abused substance. For example, other than defining a legal age to purchase tobacco, our culture places no restrictions on the long-term and compulsive use of this substance, even though it is a major contributor to cardiovascular and respiratory disease **Figure 4**. By comparison, use of marijuana, which has less damaging effects, is often punishable by fines or imprisonment.

The following list formally defines some basic terms and concepts related to substance abuse:

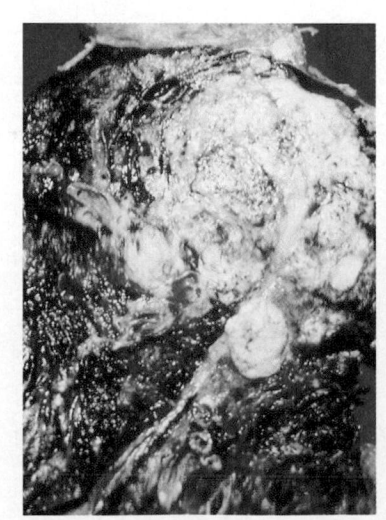

Figure 4 A diseased lung as a result of tobacco use.

- **Drug abuse**. Any use of drugs that causes physical, psychological, economic, legal, or social harm to the user or to others affected by the drug user's behavior.
- **Habituation**. Psychological dependence on a drug or drugs.

Words of Wisdom

Substance abuse is broadly defined as the self-administration of either licit or illicit substances in a manner not in accord with approved medical or social practice.

- **Physical dependence**. A physiologic state of adaptation to a drug, usually characterized by tolerance to the drug's effects and a withdrawal syndrome if the drug is stopped, especially if it is stopped abruptly.
- **Psychological dependence**. The emotional state of craving a drug to maintain a feeling of well-being.
- **Tolerance**. Physiologic adaptation to the effects of a drug such that increasingly larger doses of the drug are required to achieve the same effect.
- **Withdrawal syndrome**. A predictable set of signs and symptoms, usually involving altered central nervous system (CNS) activity, that occurs after the abrupt cessation of a drug or after rapidly decreasing the usual dosage of a drug.
- **Drug addiction**. A chronic disorder characterized by the compulsive use of a substance resulting in physical, psychological, or social harm to the user, who continues to use the substance despite the harm.
- **Antagonist**. Something that counteracts the action of something else. In relation to drugs, a drug that is an antagonist has an affinity for a cell receptor; by binding to that receptor, the antagonist prevents the cell from responding.
- **Potentiation**. Enhancement of the effect of one drug by taking it with another drug.
- **Synergism**. The action of two substances, such as drugs, in which the total effects are greater than the sum of the independent effects of the two substances (that is, 2 + 2 = 5).

Drug abuse is not limited to members of the younger generation or to any particular stratum of society. It occurs in all age groups and at all social levels.

Patient Assessment

Generally, patients with toxicologic emergencies are considered medical patients, although toxicologic emergencies may lead to trauma, too. The general assessment approach is the same for all patients: scene size-up, primary assessment, history taking, secondary assessment, and reassessment. If the mental status is altered, monitor the patient's airway and breathing diligently to ensure that he or she does not aspirate and is adequately filling the chest with air. If the patient is responsive, use the OPQRST mnemonic to elaborate on the chief complaint, obtain the patient's vital signs, obtain a SAMPLE history, and perform a rapid scan and then a more thorough physical examination. If the patient is not responsive, obtain vital signs and complete a rapid medical assessment; obtain the OPQRST and SAMPLE history from bystanders and family members, if possible.

Scene Size-up

Patients who have taken an overdose may be extremely dangerous, so make sure you perform a scene size-up in every case. If necessary, call for law enforcement backup or a crisis unit to minimize potential for injury to you and your team.

Primary Assessment

The primary assessment of a patient who has overdosed on drugs or has been poisoned begins with you forming a general impression. It can be as simple as "a young adult man on his back, snoring in a public bathroom stall." The primary assessment seeks to rapidly identify concerns with mental status, airway, breathing, and circulation. Threats to life need to be quickly managed by measures such as sealing defects of the chest wall, performing the head tilt–chin lift maneuver, suctioning, or assisting ventilations with a bag-mask device. The primary assessment should identify the mechanism of injury (MOI) or nature of illness (NOI) as well as the need for additional units, along with setting the priority and "tone" of the call.

History Taking

Most poisoning and overdose cases involve patients with medical conditions, so you will need to elaborate on their chief complaint using the OPQRST questions as part of history taking. As noted earlier, if the patient is capable of answering questions, you should obtain a SAMPLE history directly from the patient. If he or she is not conscious, obtain the OPQRST and SAMPLE history from bystanders and family members, if possible.

To choose the appropriate course of action in a toxicologic emergency, obtain at least the following specific information:

- *What is the agent?* If the patient has overdosed on a prescription drug, take the pill bottle and the remaining pills in with the patient **Figure 5**. If the substance was a commercial product, take the container and its remaining contents to the emergency department (ED). If the patient ingested a plant, find out what part (roots, leaves, stem, flower, or fruit) and take a sample of the plant to the ED for identification. If the patient vomits, save a sample of the vomitus in a clean, closed container, and take it with you to the ED.
- *When was the poison ingested, injected, absorbed, or inhaled?* The decision to induce vomiting (infrequently done—check local protocols) or to flush out (lavage) the stomach is strongly influenced by the amount of time that has elapsed since the exposure. The likelihood of retrieving significant quantities of the poison from the stomach decreases rapidly after the first 30 to 60 minutes. Also, acute-onset events often indicate a more serious patient scenario—for example, if the patient smoked crack cocaine 15 minutes ago and immediately began to have crushing chest pain.

Documentation and Communication

Have someone count the medications left in the prescription bottle to figure out the maximum number the patient might have taken.

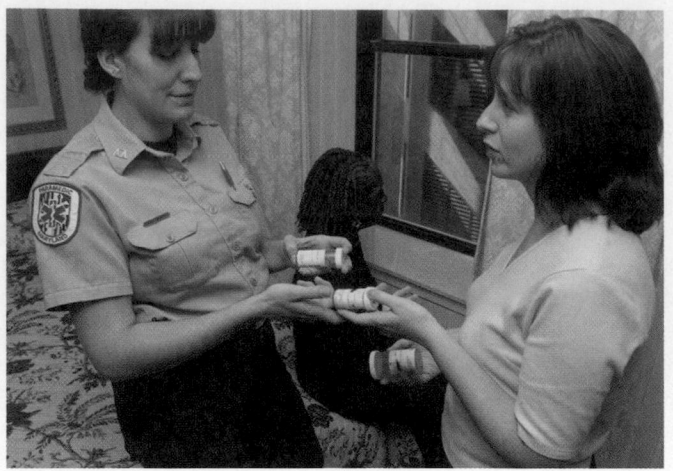

Figure 5 Take any bottles, containers, and their remaining contents to the emergency department.

- *Has the patient vomited or aspirated?* If so, how soon after the ingestion or exposure? How much?
- *Why was the substance taken?* Although you may not get a reliable answer from someone abusing illicit drugs, this is still a question worth asking. Do not assume that every patient is trying to get high. Drug use could be a coping mechanism for a person who is being abused, or it could be a suicide attempt. Put the reason in "quotation marks" on your patient care report.

Documentation and Communication

While at the scene, make thorough (and legible) notes about the nature of the poisoning. You can then quickly state the type and amount of substance and the time and route of exposure in your radio, verbal, and written reports. Clear notes that can be handed over on arrival will be appreciated by the hospital staff.

- *How much was taken, injected, absorbed, or inhaled?* Street drugs are commonly sold in single-dose "hits" or "tabs" (tablets). If the patient says he has taken "three hits of acid," you know he has taken three times the "normal dose" of LSD. If the patient says that she took four tabs of ecstasy, that is four times a single dose. There is almost always a distinct correlation between dose and toxic effects.
- *What else was taken?* A majority of intentional self-poisonings (suicide attempts) or illicit drug overdoses involve polydrug ingestions, often with alcohol as one of the drugs. The patient may also have tried to take something as an antidote (that is, something to counteract the effect of the poison). This information can be invaluable to ED staff when deciding which tests to order.

■ Secondary Assessment

After completing the primary assessment, begin the secondary assessment. With a trauma case, you will need to classify the patient as having a significant or nonsignificant MOI.

For a patient who has trauma with a significant MOI (as may occur in an overdosed or a poisoned patient who fell, was assaulted, or decided he or she could "fly" and jumped off the third-story fire escape), you must quickly perform a rapid trauma assessment of the major body regions—head, neck, chest, abdomen, pelvis, back, buttocks, and four extremities. Obtain a set of baseline vital signs as well. Such a patient should also receive a more detailed physical exam en route to the hospital.

YOU *are the Medic*   PART 2

While your partner sets up equipment to start assisting the patient's respirations, which were assessed at 6 breaths/min, you assess the patient's pulse. You find a strong radial pulse—100 beats/min.

Recording Time: 2 Minutes	
Appearance	Unconscious
Level of consciousness	Unresponsive in AVPU
Airway	Open
Breathing	Very slow
Circulation	Adequate

3. If this patient has overdosed, which drug classification would be your focus?

4. Give some examples of drugs that would meet this classification.

Special Populations

In an accidental overdose or poisoning, a geriatric patient may have become confused about his or her drug regimen. The person may have forgotten that the medication had been taken and repeat the dose one or more times. The patient could also have forgotten the doctor's instructions to discard leftover medication and might have taken both the current medication and the older drug, resulting in increased effects or unwanted drug interactions. A geriatric patient may also intentionally overdose in a suicide attempt.

If the patient does not have a significant MOI, perform a more thorough physical exam of the injured body part at the scene. During this exam, evaluate the patient's distal pulse, motor, and sensory functions, and range of motion.

At the completion of your physical exam, prioritize the injuries, manage them appropriately, and document your findings on the patient care report.

Controversies

If a pediatric patient is in stable condition and has a history of a single small ingestion of a low-risk agent, some EMS systems allow the transport to be canceled after agreement from medical control. Although this approach may be medically sound, it eliminates an opportunity for assessment of psychosocial and risk factors in the emergency department.

Reassessment

Reassessment focuses on monitoring the patient's condition, reprioritizing the patient's status if necessary, and checking the effectiveness of interventions provided. It is typically done in the ambulance while en route to the ED. Continually monitor all patients who have ingested, injected, absorbed, or inhaled a poisonous substance, and be aware that they may vomit at any point.

Emergency Medical Care

From a management perspective, ALS care for toxicologic emergencies builds on the basics:

- Ensure that the scene is safe for access and egress.
- Maintain the airway.
- Ensure that breathing is adequate.
- Ensure that circulation is not compromised (that is, by hypoperfusion or dysrhythmia).
- Administer high-concentration supplemental oxygen to achieve saturation levels of 95%.

- Establish vascular access.
- Be prepared to manage shock, coma, seizures, and dysrhythmias.
- Transport the patient as soon as possible. Place the patient in the left lateral recumbent position if there is any risk of vomiting to reduce the risk of aspiration.

Table 3 provides a list of normal laboratory values for selected medications; levels above these may be considered toxic.

Pathophysiology, Assessment, and Management of Abuse of and Overdose With Specific Substances

Alcohol

Alcohol is the most widely abused drug in the United States. More than 100 million Americans regularly consume alcohol, of whom slightly more than 10% have **alcoholism**.

Alcoholism occurs in all social strata of almost every culture, but only a small minority of people with alcoholism fit the classic "skid row" stereotype. Red flags pointing to alcoholism include the following:

- Drinking early in the day
- Drinking alone or in "secret"
- Periodic binges
- Loss of memory or "blackouts"

Table 3   Normal Serum Values for Selected Medications

Medication	Normal Serum Level
Acetaminophen (Tylenol)	Consult nomogram; greater than 150 mg/L 4 hours after ingestion is considered toxic; consult specialist for questions of chronic toxicity or unusual circumstances
Amiodarone (Cordarone)	0.5-2.5 mg/L
Aspirin	15-30 mg/L
Carbamazepine (Tegretol)	4-12 µg/mL
Digoxin	0.8-2 ng/mL
Lithium	0.6-1.2 mEq/L
Phenytoin (Dilantin)	10-20 µg/mL
Valproic acid (Depakote)	50-125 µg/mL

Source: Courtesy of Andrew Bartkus.

- Tremulousness and anxiety
- Cigarette burns on clothing from falling asleep with a lit cigarette
- "Green tongue syndrome," caused by the use of chlorophyll-containing compounds to disguise the smell of alcohol on the breath
- Chronically flushed face and palms

Pathophysiology

Alcoholism usually evolves through two distinct phases. The first phase is problem drinking, during which alcohol is used increasingly more often to relieve tensions or other emotional difficulties. Because of the disinhibition, relaxation, and sense of well-being mediated by alcohol, some degree of psychological dependence often develops with its use. Unfortunately, many people become so dependent on the psychological influences of alcohol that they become compulsive drinkers. As a person becomes more dependent on drinking, his or her performance at work and relationships with friends, family, and coworkers may deteriorate. Increased absence from work, emotional disturbances, and automobile crashes become more frequent.

Physical dependence also results from the regular consumption of large quantities of alcohol. At this level of dependence, should a person abruptly stop consuming alcohol, withdrawal symptoms will result. The severity of the withdrawal can vary according to the severity of the alcoholic habit. Minor withdrawal is characterized by restlessness, anxiousness, sleeping problems, agitation, and tremors. For seriously addicted drinkers, sudden abstinence can cause major withdrawal symptoms—for example, increased blood pressure, vomiting, and hallucinations.

Delirium tremens (DTs), or alcohol withdrawal delirium, results in fever, disorientation, confusion, and seizures, and can be fatal.

Words of Wisdom

If you find a patient who is stuporous and has the smell of alcohol on his or her breath, do not assume that he or she is intoxicated.

Because of the toxic effects of alcohol, a person with alcoholism is considerably more prone than sober counterparts to a number of serious illnesses and injuries Table 4 . Alcoholism remains one of the top five causes of death in the United States. Furthermore, because of its harmful effects on organs, including the liver, stomach, heart, pancreas, brain, and CNS, alcoholism decreases a person's life span by 10 to 20 years. In addition, people with alcoholism tend to have chronic malnutrition, and they fall frequently, increasing the likelihood of traumatic brain injury or other trauma.

Chronic damage to the CNS, for example, leads to deterioration in higher mental functions, such as memory and logical thinking. Damage to the cerebellum results in problems with balance, which in turn contributes to the frequent falls experienced by alcoholics. Damage to peripheral nerves leads to decreased sensation in the extremities, making the person prone to burns and similar injuries that an intact pain sense would ordinarily prevent.

YOU are the Medic   PART 3

Your partner is assisting ventilations with a bag-mask device while you perform a rapid assessment. The patient has no response to painful stimuli and is cyanotic around the lips. The Spo₂ prior to administering oxygen was 90%. You do not see much improvement in the patient, despite assisting her ventilations. When you look at the patient's pupils, you note that they are pinpoint.

Recording Time: 5 Minutes	
Respirations	6 breaths/min
Pulse	100 beats/min
Skin	Cyanosis around lips, dry, cool
Blood pressure	100/58 mm Hg
Oxygen saturation (Spo₂)	90% room air
Pupils	Pinpoint, nonreactive

5. Should you intubate this patient?

6. What is your next step in treating this patient after the airway is controlled?

Table 4 Medical Problems to Which People With Alcoholism are Particularly Susceptible

Condition	Contributing Factors
Subdural hematoma	Frequent falls; impaired clotting mechanisms
GI bleeding	Irritant effect of alcohol on the stomach lining (leading to gastritis); impaired clotting mechanisms; cirrhosis of the liver, leading to engorgement of esophageal veins (esophageal varices)
Pancreatitis	Indirect effect of alcohol on the pancreas
Hypoglycemia	Damage to the liver, which normally mobilizes glucose into the blood
Pneumonia	Aspiration of vomitus occurring during intoxication and coma; suppression of immune system by alcohol
Burns	Relative insensitivity to pain occurring during intoxication; falling asleep with a lit cigarette while intoxicated
Hypothermia	Insensitivity to extremes of temperatures while intoxicated; falling asleep outside in the cold
Seizures	Effect of withdrawal from alcohol
Dysrhythmias	Toxic effects of alcohol on the heart
Cancer	Mechanism not known (perhaps related to suppression of the immune system), but people with alcoholism are 10 times more likely than the general population to have cancer
Esophageal varices (abnormally enlarged veins in the lower part of the esophagus)	Develop when normal blood flow to the liver is blocked and blood backs up into smaller, more fragile blood vessels in the esophagus; do not produce symptoms unless they rupture and bleed (a life-threatening condition that requires immediate medical care; can be fatal when not controlled)

As alcohol travels through the digestive system, it irritates tissue and can damage the lining of the stomach by causing acid imbalances, inflammation, and acute gastric distress. Often, the result is gastritis (an inflamed stomach), gastric esophageal reflux disease (GERD), or heartburn. The more frequently someone drinks, the more likely that the GI system will be irritated, as evidenced by the fact that one of every three heavy drinkers has chronic gastritis. Heavy drinkers also have double the risk of cancer of the mouth and esophagus. Prolonged heavy use of alcohol may cause ulcers, hiatal hernias, and cancers throughout the digestive tract.

The toxic effects of alcohol on the liver produce a variety of complications, such as coagulopathies (easy bleeding and poor clotting ability), hypoglycemia, and GI bleeding. In addition,

alcoholics are at high risk of acute pancreatitis, pneumonia, and cardiomyopathy.

Any of the conditions previously mentioned may contribute to an emergency. In addition, acute abstinence from alcohol by a person with alcoholism may produce serious problems, including withdrawal seizures.

Acute Alcohol Intoxication

Severe alcohol intoxication is a form of poisoning and carries the same lethal potential as poisoning with any other CNS depressant. Death from alcohol intoxication has been reported with blood alcohol levels of 400 mg/dL, which can be attained by the relatively rapid consumption of as little as a half-pint of whiskey. The most immediate danger to an acutely intoxicated person is death from respiratory depression and/or aspiration of vomitus or stomach contents secondary to a suppressed gag reflex.

If an intoxicated patient is unconscious, treat him or her as you would any unconscious patient. As always, first establish and maintain the airway. With an intact gag reflex, place the patient in left lateral recumbent position with suction ready. If there is no gag reflex, intubate the patient. In addition, give high-concentration supplemental oxygen, and assist ventilation as needed. Establish vascular access. Monitor the ECG rhythm. Assess the patient's blood glucose level, treating hypoglycemia if it is found. If directed to do so by medical control, administer thiamine 100 mg via slow intravenous (IV) push. Finally, transport the patient to an appropriate facility.

Words of Wisdom

The patient with alcohol on his or her breath may be ill or injured from other causes. Do not let the smell of alcohol impair your judgment as well as the patient's.

Withdrawal Seizures

A person who has been drinking heavily for an extended period and suddenly stops drinking may experience a variety of withdrawal phenomena. Seizures usually occur within about 12 to 48 hours of the last drink. Use the same care plan described for alcohol intoxication, and consult with medical control about administering benzodiazepines for seizure control.

Delirium Tremens

One of the most serious and lethal complications of alcohol withdrawal is delirium tremens (DTs). Symptoms usually start 48 to 72 hours after the last alcohol intake, although a week to 10 days may pass before the onset of symptoms in some cases. Delirium tremens is a serious and potentially fatal syndrome with mortality reported as high as 15%. Signs and symptoms include confusion, tremors, restlessness, fever, diaphoresis, hallucinations (extremely frightening—such as snakes, spiders, and rats), and hypotension, often secondary to dehydration.

The treatment for a patient in DTs is aimed at protecting the patient from injury and supporting the cardiovascular system. The often-terrifying hallucinations associated with DTs typically make for an agitated, often combative patient. Try to keep the patient calm. In addition, you should administer supplemental oxygen by nasal cannula and establish vascular access. Manage hypotension with an infusion of normal saline, and, during the reassessment, check breath sounds. Maintain an ongoing dialogue with the patient throughout transport to help orient and reassure the patient.

Stimulants

Few drugs compare with stimulants in potential for abuse—particularly cocaine, amphetamines, and methamphetamine. A first-time user may become addicted to one of these substances within just a few days. If the person decides to quit using stimulants, the success rate of overcoming the addiction is extremely low. Unfortunately, for some drug addicts, the only way out of methamphetamine or cocaine addiction is often an early death.

Depending on the formulation, stimulant drugs may be taken orally, smoked, or injected intravenously. The clinical presentation of the stimulant abuser includes excitement, delirium, tachycardia, hypertension with a fast pulse rate or hypotension with a fast pulse rate, and dilated pupils. As toxic levels are reached, the patient may experience outright psychosis, hyperpyrexia, tremors, seizures, and cardiac arrest.

The chronic "speed freak" or "tweaker" is easily recognized by a wild-eyed but thin-as-a-rail appearance, nervous or jittery movements, and often picked-raw skin. For a serious stimulant abuser, week-long runs without sleeping are not unusual, and the person often goes days without eating during such a period. As the days pass, increasing paranoia makes encounters risky. Patients are usually "amped up" when you encounter them, and it often takes little to set off a violent tirade. When stimulant abuse is suspected, stay alert for signs of violence or a destabilizing scene.

Cocaine

Cocaine is a naturally occurring alkaloid that is extracted from the *Erythroxylon coca* plant leaves found in South America. Once processed into cocaine hydrochloride, the active ingredient in the leaves increases from 2% to 100% pure, drastically increasing its toxic potential and lethality.

Use of cocaine has had devastating effects on the US population. Since 1988, ED visits by cocaine abusers have tripled, and more than 50 tons of cocaine makes its way into the United States every year. Cocaine is sold under many street names (blow, flake, lady, nose candy, snow, toot). When the National Survey on Drug Use and Health was conducted in 2009, approximately 1.6 million Americans admitted to being current cocaine users. Once addicted to the drug, people will spend large sums of money trying to replicate the intensity and unique euphoria from their first cocaine experience. Cocaine addicts will often sell everything they own, turn to stealing to support their addiction, and inevitably lose their jobs, their homes, and their family and friends.

Pathophysiology Cocaine is a local anesthetic and a CNS stimulant. It also has the ability to create a euphoria that features enhanced alertness and a tremendous sense of well-being.

Collectively, this constellation of effects makes cocaine one of—if not the most—psychologically addictive drugs available.

Today, cocaine has limited use in clinical medicine, mostly in ear, nose, throat, and eye surgery. This water-soluble hydrochloride salt is quickly absorbed across all mucosal membranes, allowing it to be applied topically, insufflated (snorted), swallowed, or injected intravenously. Another form of cocaine, crack cocaine, is simply cocaine mixed with two inexpensive ingredients, baking soda and water. Once mixed together into a pastelike slurry and cooked or baked, the end result is smokable cocaine (crack).

When cocaine is snorted nasally, effects are felt within 1 to 2 minutes, and peak effects occur in 20 to 30 minutes. After the intense, initial high, only 15 to 30 minutes passes before the user wants to redose. When cocaine is smoked and the alveoli are literally bathed in cocaine-laden smoke, the onset of effects is much more rapid (in the 8- to 10-second range) and the high is even more intense than when cocaine is snorted.

When the effects of cocaine wear off, a predictable cycle of events occurs. The user experiences a "crash," which is characterized by depression, irritability, sleeplessness, and exhaustion. To avoid this crash, the user will often seek more cocaine. Adding to the problem, a cocaine addict who is trying to escape the unpleasant effects of a crash often takes a sedative (such as diazepam [Valium], alcohol, or heroin). Thus, a chronic cocaine user almost certainly practices polypharmacy and may be dependent on more substances than cocaine, increasing the likelihood that he or she will need EMS care because of a possible overdose on uppers, downers, and alcohol—or all three.

Speedballing refers to the combined use of heroin and cocaine simultaneously. Heroin addicts may use cocaine to withdraw or detoxify themselves from heroin by gradually decreasing the amounts of heroin taken while increasing the amounts of cocaine used. Addicts claim that cocaine provides relief from the unpleasant withdrawal effects that accompany heroin abstinence.

Assessment A person who has overdosed on cocaine may exhibit any of the signs and symptoms for stimulants in general (discussed earlier). Furthermore, cocaine has been reported to cause a variety of serious—sometimes fatal—complications: lethal ECG dysrhythmias, acute myocardial infarction, seizures, stroke, apnea, and hyperthermia. In addition, a crack smoker risks pneumothorax and pneumomediastinum.

You should give particular attention to the ECG rhythm in a patient in whom you suspect cocaine overdose. Cocaine has quinidinelike effects on cardiac conduction, causing widening of the QRS and QT prolongation. With increased dosing levels, cocaine exerts potentially deadly, toxic effects on the myocardium, which may present as wide-complex dysrhythmias, negative inotropic effects with decreased cardiac output, hypotension, or tachycardia initially, followed by bradycardia.

Amphetamine, Methamphetamine, and Amphetamine-like Drugs

Amphetamines are structurally similar to the derivatives of phenylethylamine and include methamphetamine (crank or ice), methylenedioxyamphetamine (MDA, Adam), and methylenedioxymethamphetamine (MDMA, Eve, ecstasy). Amphetamine and amphetamine-like drugs have a number of legitimate clinical applications. Most nasal decongestants and diet pills are members of this family, as are the drugs used to treat narcolepsy, attention-deficit disorder (ADD), and attention-deficit/hyperactivity disorder (ADHD) **Figure 6** .

Methamphetamine is problematic because it is a low-cost, long-acting (up to 12 hours) stimulant that is extremely addictive. This drug has become a problem in the United States because the ingredients to cook methamphetamine are available locally and the drug is easily and quickly made. Therefore, those who manufacture the drug avoid the hassle, risk, and high cost associated with importing cocaine. "Meth labs" are dangerous and should be treated as a hazardous materials incident (see the chapter, *Hazardous Materials*).

The clinical presentation of the patient abusing amphetamine or methamphetamine is almost identical to that of a person abusing cocaine, with the primary exception that the effects of the former drugs last many hours longer than those of cocaine. Patient management remains the same as well. In most patients, prehospital management is primarily supportive. Never forget about the potential emotional and psychological instability seen in drug abusers, particularly in patients who have been on a "run." With each passing day of no sleep and little or no food, they become increasingly paranoid and even psychotic. Their behavior can quickly become violent, so consider the situation a potential hazard. At the first hint of trouble, contact law enforcement personnel for support. (See the chapter, *Psychiatric Emergencies* for details on the issue of restraint.)

Bath Salts

Newcomers to the world of substance abuse include some products marketed as "bath salts," under unique names such as "Blaze," that contain an active ingredient that is a pseudoephedrine (Sudafed) reduction drug called methcathinone or a similar methamphetamine knock-off. Users typically snort, smoke, or ingest this drug, which couples the intensity and long-acting

effects of methamphetamine with the euphoric effects of crack cocaine. The more serious side effects of this designer drug include agitation, hallucinations, and paranoia. Although this drug actually has nothing in common with bath salts, selling it under this umbrella label has (so far) allowed its manufacturers and users to escape the legal restrictions imposed on illicit drugs. Many states are moving quickly to get legislation on the books to make it illegal to manufacture or possess this drug.

Management of Stimulant Abuse

The treatment for patients abusing cocaine, amphetamine, or methamphetamine is fundamentally the same: Maintain maximum oxygen saturation levels, prevent seizures with adequate sedation, and monitor serial vital signs.

- Establish and maintain the airway. Consider an advanced airway as needed.
- Give high-concentration, supplemental oxygen to achieve and maintain saturations levels of 95%.
- Establish vascular access.
- Apply the ECG monitor, pulse oximeter, and capnometer.
- To control anxiety and seizures, administer benzodiazepines per local protocol.
- Manage hypotension with serial fluid infusions of normal saline.
- For uncontrolled hypertension, contact medical control regarding administration of nitroprusside.
- For violent behavior, contact medical control for consideration of intramuscular (IM) haloperidol (Haldol; chemical restraint).
- Transport to the appropriate facility.

For patients with excessive pulse rates, preload time can drop drastically, resulting in a drop in blood pressure. In the past, use of beta blockers was contraindicated for fear of the patient having a corresponding alpha crisis, in which the blood pressure could potentially rise to lethal levels. As such, a combined alpha-beta blockade drug such as labetalol was considered the drug of choice. Several recent studies have since shown that a beta blocker alone can safely be used to control overly fast pulse rates in patients with stimulant overdose. Follow your local protocols.

In severe cases of stimulant overdose, the patient may present with hyperthermia, as a part of what is termed "agitated or excited delirium," which can be lethal. Application of ice packs or misting the patient's skin may reduce his or her temperature.

Throughout the resuscitation process, it is essential to maintain urine output with aggressive fluid therapy. Regular assessment of breath sounds to avoid inadvertent overhydration is a must.

If the patient has a seizure, benzodiazepines constitute first-line therapy. Haloperidol (Haldol) is another choice because it can be given IM without having to gain vascular access. Should the situation worsen into status epilepticus, phenobarbital (Luminal) or IV or rectal diazepam (Valium) may be administered. In addition, neuromuscular blockade may be needed to control motor activity to avoid hyperthermia, acidosis, and, potentially, rhabdomyolysis.

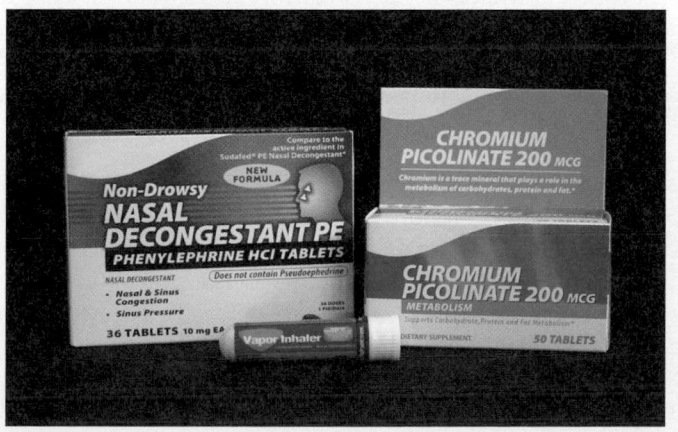

Figure 6 Drugs such as nasal decongestants and diet pills generally fall into the category of amphetamines.

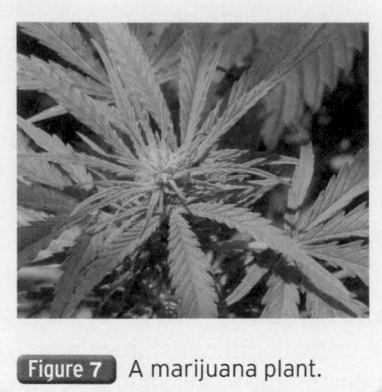

Figure 7 A marijuana plant.

Marijuana and Cannabis Compounds

When the leaves and flower buds of the *Cannabis sativa* plant are harvested and dried, the end product is referred to as **marijuana** (also known as weed, pot, dope, and smoke; **Figure 7**). The resin produced by the maturing flower tops can also be harvested and used to produce hashish (also known as hash). Clinical uses of marijuana are limited but include the treatment of glaucoma and relief of nausea and appetite loss for patients undergoing chemotherapy.

Pathophysiology

The primary psychoactive ingredient in marijuana and hashish is delta 9-tetrahydrocannabinol. Marijuana is usually smoked but can be ingested (such as when baked in cookies or brownies). The onset of effects from smoking marijuana is a matter of minutes; oral ingestion slows the onset time to several hours. When smoked, the effects generally last 2 to 4 hours. When ingested, the effects can last twice as long, or sometimes even longer.

Although classified as a hallucinogen, marijuana does not produce true hallucinations (unlike PCP, LSD, and mescaline), but users may have a distorted sense of time and space and, occasionally, a feeling of unreality. Smoking marijuana results in bronchodilation and slight tachycardia. Other signs and symptoms of marijuana use include euphoria, drowsiness, decreased short-term memory, diminished motor coordination, increased appetite, and bloodshot eyes.

Assessment and Management

Assessment and management focuses on supportive care because the likelihood of serious medical complication is small. A novice user may exhibit some behavioral symptoms such as paranoia and (rarely) psychosis. Psychological first aid and reassurance generally suffice to address either issue. If the patient remains anxious, low-dose benzodiazepines may be administered. Transport for continued evaluation is rarely warranted, but providing information for support and counseling services can be helpful.

Spice

Another recent entry into the illicit drug world is a drug called **Spice**, which is sold as incense in efforts to skirt existing drug laws. This drug is a blend of synthetic cannibinoids (knock-offs of the natural occurring psychoactive elements in marijuana). Unlike marijuana, which typically has relaxing, laidback effects, Spice can make people delirious and produce both short-term and long-term psychotic effects. In some cases, these effects have been noted to last as long as 3 months.

Hallucinogens

A **hallucinogen** is a substance that causes some distortion of sense perception—seeing, hearing, or feeling things that are not actually present. These outcomes are termed psychedelic effects. Experiences involving hallucinogens can vary markedly, with people taking the same dose of the same drug from the same batch experiencing totally different effects. The overall drug experience is affected by the user's previous drug experience, the dose taken, the user's expectations, and the social setting.

A wide variety of substances have been used over the centuries for their hallucinogenic properties, and these substances can be classified into two categories: synthetic and naturally occurring. The synthetic class includes LSD, PCP, and ketamine. Naturally occurring hallucinogens include mescaline, psilocybin mushroom, and the seeds of the Jimson weed plant.

LSD

In 1947, Dr Albert Hoffman discovered what would be the prototype for synthetic hallucinogens, lysergic acid diethylamine (LSD). Use of this drug peaked in the 1960s, subsequently faded, and then rebounded in the 1990s. LSD is considered a non–habit-forming drug, although tolerance can occur if it is taken for several days in a row.

Pathophysiology LSD primarily affects the senses rather than changing physiologic functions. Synthesthesias (crossing of the senses) often prompt a user to respond to the question, "What were you doing?" with a reply such as, "I was watching the music play" or "I was listening to that painting." Users often experiment with LSD for self-exploration, for religious reasons, or to experience its often stunning visual and auditory effects.

Because of LSD's high potency, as little as 25 µg can produce significant CNS effects. A single dose or "hit" is 25 to 100 µg, although many users take three or more hits. As dosing increases to about 1,000 µg, there is a proportional increase in the drug's effects, which may last for 12 hours or more, although 3 to 4 hours is more typical.

From a physiologic perspective, the effects of LSD are mostly sympathomimetic, often consisting of mild tachycardia, mild hypertension, and dilated pupils. In a "bad trip," the user has a frightening experience, resulting in an acute anxiety attack and the physical effects secondary to increased anxiety.

Assessment and Management The treatment for a patient using LSD is primarily supportive, focusing on the psychological aspects of the drug experience. For the person having a bad trip, it is like being in a bad dream that is as real as reality; unlike a regular dream that ends the moment you awaken, however, this dream does not end until the drug wears off.

During transport of a patient who has taken LSD, try to limit sensory stimulation as much as possible—for example, by avoiding the use of emergency lights and sirens. Routine transport to the appropriate facility and providing psychological support are usually all that is required for these patients.

Phencyclidine

Phencyclidine (PCP), also called angel dust or dust, was developed in the late 1950s. In clinical trials, problems with the drug—namely, delirium and psychotic symptoms—led to PCP being relegated to use as an animal tranquilizer. PCP abuse was first noted in the 1970s. The majority of PCP available on the streets today is manufactured in clandestine laboratories, so variations in potency and purity are common. PCP is also a contaminant in many other street drugs.

Pathophysiology Although PCP is grouped with the hallucinogens here, it is actually classified as a dissociative anesthetic. It is typically smoked or snorted, although it can be injected. Small doses (25–50 mg) can produce signs and symptoms of intoxication in an adult, with the high from a single dose typically lasting 4 to 6 hours. Slurred speech, staggering gait, tachycardia, hypertension, staring blankly for extended periods, and horizontal nystagmus (involuntary, rhythmic movement of the eyes) are common with PCP use. Muscle rigidity and especially grinding of the teeth prompt many users to resort to pacifiers in an effort to avoid pronounced jaw aches.

More problematic are the mind-body separation, related hallucinations, and violent outbreaks that are hallmarks of PCP use. Users may make bizarre comments such as "I can fly" and then jump off a balcony to prove it. Users have an almost unfathomable ability to take pain with no reaction and exhibit almost superhuman strength. In one case, it took four large fire fighters to subdue and contain a young woman weighing approximately 100 pounds who was intoxicated on PCP. Police who use Tasers often tell stories of PCP victims not even being bothered by these devices' effects.

Assessment and Management PCP can cause some of the most violent and difficult behavior you will encounter in the field because a patient can go from being mildly nervous and jumpy to being aggressively violent in just seconds. For that reason, a continuous concern when responding to calls involving PCP users is the safety of the EMS team. Care focuses on trying to calm the patient and addressing any wounds. Given that no PCP antagonist exists, there is little reason to insert an IV line—especially given that even the slightest event can send a PCP abuser into a violent tirade. If you can safely establish vascular access, you will have a route to administer benzodiazepines if the patient's behavior becomes overly aggressive or violent. Haloperidol (Haldol) can be given by the IM route in an emergency situation. Administer high-flow oxygen, monitor vital signs, and provide safe transport to an appropriate facility.

Ketamine

Ketamine (special K, vitamin K; also discussed in the chapter, *Psychiatric Emergencies*) is an analog of PCP. Most ketamine available on the street is stolen from veterinary clinics, although this drug is actually used in clinical medicine, primarily in pediatric patients. Ketamine, which is colorless and odorless, is commonly found in powdered form. It is often mixed in a drink, although it can be snorted. It is physically and psychologically addicting.

Pathophysiology Ketamine is a dissociative anesthetic. Typical oral dosing is 75 to 300 mg. When snorted, the dose is reduced slightly, to 15 to 200 mg. At low doses, a user presents with mild inebriation, dreamy or erotic thoughts, and increased sociability. At higher doses, a patient may have pronounced nausea, difficulty moving, and a complaint of "entering another reality." In extreme cases, users will enter the "K hole," which involves out-of-body experiences that may never resolve.

Assessment and Management Although violent outbreaks in patients are much less likely with ketamine than with PCP, the principles of management are the same for patients who have used either drug. Secure the patient well, assess and manage the ABCs, provide oxygen therapy, establish vascular access if the patient is receptive, and provide safe transport to the appropriate facility. Keep a close eye on the patient, because violent behavior can suddenly occur.

Peyote and Mescaline

Native tribes in the southwestern United States and Mexico have been using hallucinogens for thousands of years, primarily for religious purposes, with their primary drug of choice being mescaline.

Pathophysiology Ingesting between 3 and 12 of the dried flower "buttons" of the peyote cactus delivers a dose of roughly 200 to 500 mg of mescaline **Figure 8** . The buttons have a bitter taste and are a potent gastric irritant, with profound vomiting occurring shortly after their ingestion. The psychedelic experience then typically begins with feelings of increased sensitivity to sensory stimulation. Flashes of color, commonly in geometric patterns, are noted, although images of animals and people may also arise. Users experience a distortion of time and space, and out-of-body experiences are commonly reported.

The chemical structure of mescaline does not resemble that of LSD, although the two drugs produce similar psychedelic effects. Structurally, mescaline looks more like amphetamine, which accounts for its physical effects: dilated pupils, increased pulse rate, mild hypertension, and increased body temperature.

Assessment and Management Care in the field setting is primarily supportive. Pay attention to the ABCs, administer supplemental oxygen therapy, monitor vital signs, provide positive psychological support, and arrange safe transport to the receiving facility.

Psilocybin Mushrooms

After LSD, psilocybin mushrooms **Figure 9** are probably the most frequently used hallucinogens in the United States. Hallucinogenic mushrooms come from several different genera,

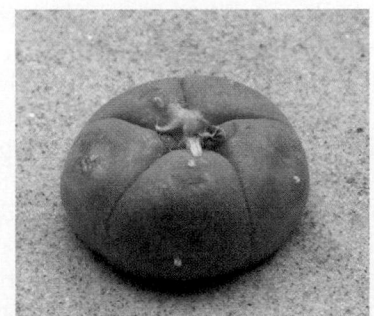

Figure 8 Dried flower buttons of the peyote cactus contain mescaline and produce a hallucinogenic effect if ingested.

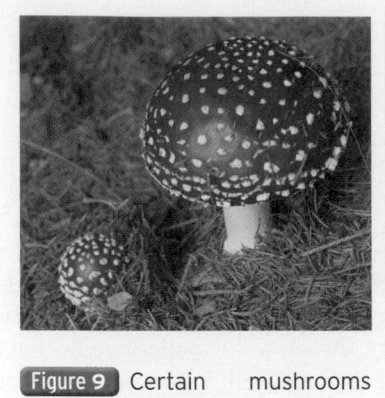

Figure 9 Certain mushrooms are hallucinogenic if ingested.

including *Psilocybe*. In the United States, the most commonly abused are the *Psilocybe mexicana* and *Psilocybe cyaescens* varieties. The typical dose is estimated to be 4 to 10 mg (approximately 2 to 4 mushrooms). Consumption of 100 mushrooms or more as a single dose has been reported.

Pathophysiology The onset of symptoms and hallucinogenic effects (similar to LSD but less intense) is within 30 minutes of ingestion, and effects usually last 4 to 6 hours. Signs and symptoms include nausea and vomiting, mydriasis, mild tachycardia, and mild hypertension. The likelihood of any serious medical side effects is low, although the literature describes seizures and hyperthermia in some patients.

Assessment and Management Treat the patient with supportive care. Attention to the ABCs and monitoring vital signs are usually all that is required, along with safe transport to the appropriate facility. If time and circumstances allow, establish vascular access to facilitate seizure control with benzodiazepines, if necessary.

Sedatives and Hypnotics

The drugs in the <u>sedative-hypnotic</u> category have a wide range of applications. Drugs with sedative qualities are used to reduce anxiety and to calm agitated patients. Drugs with hypnotic qualities are used as sleep aids, helping produce drowsiness and sleep. In either case, sedative-hypnotic drugs function primarily as CNS depressants.

Barbiturates

The <u>barbiturates</u> have a long history of use as sleep aids, anti-anxiety drugs, and seizure control medications. Barbiturate use and abuse reached their peak in the late 1970s, when these drugs were often tagged with street names that coincided with the color of the pill or capsule: reds (secobarbital), yellows or yellow jackets (pentobarbital), blues or blue heavens (amobarbital), and rainbows (amobarbital plus secobarbital).

The frequent combination of alcohol and barbiturates as a suicide mechanism, coupled with the high incidence of accidental overdoses, pushed researchers to develop sedative-hypnotic drugs that had fewer depressive effects on the respiratory system and were less lethal. Today, the likelihood of death after the ingestion of a single-entity sedative-hypnotic such as diazepam (Valium) is small.

Pathophysiology Barbiturates come in four basic configurations: long-acting, intermediate-acting, short-acting, and ultra–short-acting. The long-acting barbiturates tend to be less lipid soluble,

which results in a delayed onset and long duration of action. By comparison, the short- and ultra–short-acting barbiturates are highly lipid soluble, so they can quickly move across the blood-brain barrier and exert their effects in a matter of minutes. Phenobarbital (Luminal), for example, is a long-acting barbiturate, which makes it ideal for use in seizure control. If the patient delays taking this medication for a few hours, there is no real impact. Conversely, delaying a dose of an ultra–short-acting barbiturate might lead to a seizure. The liver metabolizes most barbiturates into inactive waste products, although barbiturates that bind less tightly to proteins tend to be excreted unchanged in the urine.

Assessment Your assessment findings will reflect the dosing and the configuration of the barbiturate. With mild to moderate barbiturate intoxication, patients present much like alcohol intoxication; their symptoms include drowsiness, decreased inhibitions, ataxia, mental confusion, and staggering gait. As the dose increases, the patient moves farther down the scale of CNS depression, becoming increasingly lethargic and demonstrating an increasingly lower level of responsiveness until he or she is comatose (that is, no neurologic response and a Glasgow Coma Scale score of 3).

Management Care for a patient who has overdosed on barbiturates follows a logical and predictable path. Because of the CNS depressant effects of these drugs, airway control is the first management priority, often requiring intubation to secure the airway and prevent aspiration should the patient vomit. Next, you should administer high-concentration supplemental oxygen, monitor the ECG rhythm, and establish venous access. Use pulse oximetry and capnography to monitor hemoglobin saturation and the effectiveness of respiration and ventilations.

If shock develops, rapid infusion of 1 to 2 L of crystalloids may be needed—specifically, as sequential boluses of 200 to 400 mL of normal saline. Assess breath sounds *before and after each bolus,* rather than simply infusing an entire liter and then assessing breath sounds. The bolus approach is particularly indicated for older patients and for patients with renal disease or decreased cardiac function. If the patient has received adequate fluid replacement but hypotension persists, administer a vasopressor such as dopamine (Intropin).

For the long-acting barbiturates such as phenobarbital (Luminal), administering a dose of 1 to 2 mEq of sodium bicarbonate helps alkalinize the urine and traps the drug in its ionized form, promoting effective excretion in the urine. This therapy is not effective for shorter-acting barbiturates, however. Use of fluid loading coupled with forced diuresis can further supplement urine alkalinization efforts, but again is limited to the long-acting barbiturates. Administration of IV furosemide (Lasix) will accomplish the task but is contraindicated for patients who are already hypotensive or showing signs or symptoms of shock.

Gastric emptying is not recommended unless you have reason to believe that the patient ingested a life-threatening dose of barbiturates *and* the procedure can be implemented within 60 minutes of ingestion. In such a case, perform intubation to protect the airway before instituting gastric lavage. For patients outside the 1-hour window, use of activated charcoal is a more practical option. Studies have shown that activated charcoal is at least as effective as gastric lavage and may be a better option because it almost immediately reduces serum barbiturate levels.

Words of Wisdom

While one provider explains the use of activated charcoal to the patient, the other can prepare a large plastic garbage bag to hang on the patient as a bib. This will help contain the charcoal solution if the patient vomits.

Barbiturate abusers quickly develop tolerance and require ever-larger doses to produce the desired effects. Long-term use results in physical addiction. Abrupt cessation in a long-term barbiturate abuser will produce typical signs and symptoms of withdrawal syndrome in approximately 24 hours, with potentially life-threatening signs and symptoms arising during a period of several days to a week. In the case of minor withdrawal, the patient may present with symptoms similar to those observed in a patient with alcohol withdrawal: restlessness and anxiety, depression, insomnia, diaphoresis, abdominal cramping, and nausea and vomiting. With severe cases of withdrawal, expect delirium, hallucinations, psychosis, seizures, hyperthermia, and cardiovascular collapse.

If you encounter barbiturate abstinence syndrome in the prehospital setting, focus your treatment efforts on preventing seizures (IV benzodiazepines are a common choice) and cardiovascular collapse (use serial fluid boluses). Rapid transport to an ED, with subsequent intensive care, will be required to best manage the patient over the long-term.

Words of Wisdom

Consider the possibility of a drug-related problem in any patient presenting with unexplained behavioral changes, stupor, coma, or seizures.

Benzodiazepines

Benzodiazepines are also members of the sedative-hypnotic family. They are most commonly used to treat anxiety, seizures, and alcohol withdrawal. In recent years, the use of fast-acting benzodiazepines such as zolpidem tartrate (Ambien) for treatment of insomnia has grown rapidly. Drugs such as Ambien can be easily obtained from Internet sources, increasing the likelihood of their abuse.

Pathophysiology Benzodiazepines exert their effects by stimulating the gamma-aminobutyric acid pathways, resulting in sedation, reduced anxiety, and relaxation of striated muscle. When taken orally, these medications are readily absorbed from the GI tract. IV administration allows for more rapid onset of action and more controlled dosing. Because IM injections of

benzodiazepines other than lorazepam (Ativan) and midazolam (Versed) often result in variable rates of absorption, the IV route is more desirable when you are administering benzodiazepines in the prehospital setting. These drugs are metabolized primarily by the liver.

Assessment Assessment of a patient who is abusing benzodiazepines can be complicated because the person is also likely to use other drugs as well as alcohol. In a single-entity overdose, benzodiazepines have a relatively low rate of morbidity and mortality. The most common clinical effects of benzodiazepine overdose include altered mentation, drowsiness, confusion, slurred speech, ataxia, and general incoordination. For a suspected overdose in which the patient presents with severe respiratory depression, hypotension, or coma, you need to think beyond a simple benzodiazepine event to other CNS depressants and alcohol. On occasion, extrapyramidal reactions may occur in tandem with hepatotoxic or hematologic reactions.

Management Treatment of benzodiazepine overdose is relatively straightforward:

- Assess and manage the airway, inserting an advanced airway as needed.
- Administer high-concentration supplemental oxygen.
- Establish vascular access.
- Apply the ECG monitor, pulse oximeter, and capnometer.
- Consider administering flumazenil (a benzodiazepine antagonist) via slow IV push (0.2 mg IV/min) up to a total of 3 mg. Flumazenil (Romazicon) is contraindicated for patients with head injuries and elevated intracranial pressure.
- Transport to the appropriate facility.

■ Narcotics, Opiates, and Opioids

A narcotic is a drug that produces sleep or altered mental status. Historically, narcotics have been classified into two major divisions: opiates and opioids. The term opiate is used to describe natural drugs derived from opium (that is, from poppy juice); the term opioid refers to non–opium-derived synthetics. In this text, the term opioids is used to describe licit therapeutic agents and illicit substances in this group.

Narcotics have a long history of use and abuse that continues to the present, with abuse of narcotics remaining one of the most common causes of overdose deaths reported to Poison Centers.

Narcotic agents include morphine, codeine, heroin, fentanyl (Sublimaze), hydrocodone, oxycodone (OxyContin), meperidine (Demerol), propoxyphene (Darvon), and dextromethorphan (Robitussin DM, Benylin, Delsym). Although these drugs share certain commonalities, they exhibit highly diverse effects and vary widely in their potency. Opioids are used primarily in clinical medicine for analgesia, whereas the illicit drug heroin is abused for the unique euphoria it produces. In terms of potency, 80 to 100 mg of meperidine (Demerol) produces analgesia for 2 to 4 hours; 10 mg of morphine or 2 mg of hydromorphone (Dilaudid) induces analgesia for a similar time frame.

Pathophysiology

Opioids produce their major effects on the CNS by binding with receptor sites in the brain and other tissues. The highest concentrations of receptor sites are found in the limbic system, frontal and temporal cortices, thalamus, hypothalamus, midbrain, and spinal cord.

Opioids are readily absorbed from the GI tract but can also be absorbed from the nasal mucosa (when snorted) or from the lungs (opium smoking). When taken orally, the effects of these drugs are lessened owing to their significant first-pass metabolism through the liver compared with their effects when given parenterally. When heroin makes its first pass through the liver, it is metabolized into acetyl-morphine, which continues to exert narcotic effects that may outlast the effects of naloxone (Narcan). It is important to remember that a dose of naloxone (Narcan) may not permanently reverse the effects of the heroin, and the patient may lapse into unconsciousness again 15 or 20 minutes later.

Morphine is a commonly used analgesic in the prehospital setting and is a potent vasodilator. When given to young adults, its half-life is roughly 2 to 3 hours, but it typically takes longer to metabolize in older adults.

Assessment

The classic presentation of opioid use features euphoria, hypotension, respiratory depression, and pinpoint pupils. Depending on the particular agent, nausea, vomiting, and constipation may occur as well. Allergic phenomena may also occur with opioid use, albeit rarely. With increased doses, coma, seizures (usually secondary to hypoxia), and cardiac arrest (usually secondary to respiratory arrest) are common.

Morphine and heroin produce an impressive dreamlike state. Shortly after injecting heroin, a user will appear to pass out (in street terms, "going on the nod"). However, the user is typically quite lucid and remains acutely aware of what is being done or said even though he or she appears to have dozed off.

Management

Because of the CNS depressant effects, patient management initially focuses on establishing and maintaining a patent airway and providing adequate ventilation. A patient who has overdosed on opioids is almost always hypoventilating, sometimes breathing as few as 3 or 4 breaths/min. In addition, respirations are shallow, resulting in inadequate removal of CO_2 and a hypercarbic state. Rather than moving immediately to intubation, you should place an oropharyngeal airway and provide bag-mask ventilation with 15 L/min of supplemental oxygen.

Next, establish vascular access and administer 0.4 to 2 mg of naloxone (Narcan). For street heroin, which can range in purity from 5% to 30%, as little as 0.4 mg of naloxone may bring a patient back to consciousness before you can remove the needle from the injection port. This abrupt reversal can have clinical and safety implications—the patient may be angry that you reversed the drug's effects. The best approach is to draw up 2 mg of naloxone in a 10-mL syringe and fill the rest of the syringe with normal saline. Administer the naloxone just to the point that the patient's respirations improve, rather than waking the patient up completely.

Sometimes the patient may not respond to naloxone. If the patient has taken a potent synthetic drug such as fentanyl (Sublimaze), a much higher dose of naloxone may be required to reverse its effects. In one case, a patient presented with the classic signs and symptoms of opioid overdose. When he showed no response to 2.0 mg of naloxone, medical control ordered 10 mg of naloxone, which aroused the patient for only approximately 30 seconds, after which he became unconscious again. Ultimately, it took 40 mg of naloxone at the hospital to bring the patient back to consciousness. It was determined that the patient had taken a dose of a fentanyl analog that was several thousand times more potent than a typical dose of heroin.

A second possibility if the patient does not respond to naloxone is that the person has a "mixed-bag overdose"—that is, the patient may have taken multiple drugs, some of which were not opioids and will not respond to naloxone. Alternatively, the coma may be from another source altogether, such as a head injury. In such a scenario, you should insert an advanced airway and provide other care as needed, and transport the patient to an appropriate facility.

■ Cardiac Medications

Pathophysiology

Paramedics administer a variety of medications that alter the function or electrical rhythm of the heart. Patients also receive these medications for long-term management of cardiovascular disorders. The major classes of drugs used as part of these treatment regimens include antidysrhythmics, beta blockers, calcium channel blockers, cardiac glycosides, and angiotensin-converting enzyme inhibitors. Many patients take a combination of drugs, sometimes three or more, in attempts to control hypertension, ECG rhythm disturbances, or other problems. Many of these medications have serious and potentially life-threatening adverse effects, even at prescribed therapeutic doses. Overdoses with these drugs are usually accidental—a result of the multidrug approach to cardiac care—because these types of drugs do not produce effects desirable to recreational drug abusers. Accidental or intentional overdose of more than twice the prescribed daily dose should automatically be considered potentially life-threatening. A single adult pill or tablet of many of these medications can cause serious effects or death in small children and infants.

Type 1 Antidysrhythmic Medications This group includes procainamide (Pronestyl) and lidocaine. These medications inhibit fast sodium channels within the heart, affecting depolarization and impulse conduction. Overdose of these medications will produce a variety of symptoms including myocardial depression, impaired conduction, and decreased contractility.

The treatment of overdose or toxicity is usually supportive. In certain instances, intravenous sodium bicarbonate may be used to treat QT prolongation, bradycardia, and hypotension by reversing the inhibition of fast sodium channels within cardiac cells.

Type II Antidysrhythmic (Beta-Adrenergic Antagonist/Beta Blocker) Medications Beta-adrenergic blocker medications are primarily used to control pulse rate and blood pressure by preventing catecholamines from activating beta$_1$-adrenergic receptors in the heart and blood vessels. Patients with beta-adrenergic blocker toxicity typically present with hypotension, bradycardia, and many related symptoms such as dizziness, syncope, or altered mental status. Hypoglycemia and hyperkalemia also occur following an overdose of beta-adrenergic blocking medications. Bronchospasm is possible following beta-adrenergic blocker overdose in patients with reactive airway disease.

Intravenous glucagon is considered the antidote to beta-adrenergic blocker toxicity. High doses of glucagon (5 to 10 mg) are administered by IV bolus, followed by an IV infusion at 1 to 5 mg/h. This usually requires more glucagon than is generally available on most ALS ambulances. Additionally, there is a risk of toxicity from the phenol that is used to reconstitute the dry glucagon powder when large doses of glucagon are administered. In these instances, paramedics should reconstitute glucagon with sterile water. Atropine, epinephrine infusions, and cardiac pacing may be required in severe overdose situations.

Type III Antidysrhythmic Medications Type III antidysrhythmic medications block cardiac cell potassium channels causing a prolongation of the cardiac action potential and increasing the effective refractory period. Amiodarone (Cordorone) is a type III antidysrhythmic medication used in the prehospital setting and for long-term management of various atrial and ventricular dysrhythmias.

Acute toxicity from amiodarone may present as hypotension, bradycardia, or certain ventricular dysrhythmias. Patients receiving long-term therapy with amiodarone may experience damage to a wide variety of internal organs including a potentially fatal pulmonary fibrosis. The treatment for acute amiodarone toxicity is primarily supportive although intravenous magnesium sulfate may be used to treat torsades de pointes.

Type IV Antidysrhythmic (Calcium Channel Blocker) Medications Calcium channel blocker medications are used widely in health care for control of pulse rate and blood pressure as well as a wide variety of seemingly unrelated medical conditions. Paramedics may administer verapamil (Calan) or diltiazem (Cardizem) in the prehospital setting.

These medications slow calcium influx into cells present in the heart, blood vessels, and other types of smooth muscle. Therapeutic use and toxicity causes a decrease in pulse rate, decreased myocardial contractility, and vasodilation. Calcium channel blockers may also cause hyperglycemia, nausea, vomiting, altered mental status, and metabolic acidosis.

Intravenous calcium chloride or calcium gluconate is the initial treatment for calcium channel blocker toxicity. Intravenous glucagon can improve both the pulse rate and myocardial contractility following calcium channel blocker overdose. Refractory hypotension and bradycardia can be treated with an intravenous epinephrine infusion.

Assessment and Management

Signs and symptoms of overdose with cardiac drugs vary but may include hypotension, weakness or confusion, nausea and vomiting, rhythm disturbances (most commonly bradycardia or heart block), headache, and difficulty breathing. As with all emergencies, ensure a patent airway, provide adequate ventilation, and administer high-flow supplemental oxygen.

YOU *are the Medic* **PART 4**

Your partner uses an oral airway and a bag-mask device to maintain the airway. You start an IV line on the patient and check her blood glucose level, which is 120 mg/dL. You look for any obvious signs of trauma; this check is negative. The patient's skin color continues to deteriorate and her pupils remain pinpoint. You take a closer look at the patient's arms, which have obvious track marks.

Recording Time: 10 Minutes	
Respirations	Assisted
Pulse	100 beats/min
Skin	Cyanotic
Blood pressure	98/56 mm Hg
Oxygen saturation (Spo$_2$)	96% assisted
Pupils	Pinpoint and nonreactive

7. What is your medication choice and dosage to treat this patient?

8. What should you do if this medication does not correct the overdose?

Establish vascular access in case of overdose with these agents because several therapeutic interventions and antidotes are available if the specific agent is identified. For a beta blocker overdose, glucagon is the drug of choice but often requires dosing in excess of what is typically carried in an ambulance. For a calcium channel blocker overdose, calcium gluconate and calcium chloride are options. Among the most problematic cardiac medications in regard to toxicity levels are the cardiac glycosides (such as digoxin), which typically have small therapeutic windows. For an overdose with these agents, digoxin immune Fab (Digibind) is the antidote of choice. In a patient with hypotension, sequential fluid boluses of normal saline will often bring the blood pressure into an acceptable range.

Because of the sophistication of cardiac drugs and the likelihood that the patient may be taking multiple cardiac and other medications, making contact with medical control to consult with a physician is prudent.

Organophosphates

Organophosphates are a major component in many insecticides used in agriculture and in the home; they include acephate (Orthene), diazinon (Basudin, Knox Out, Spectracide), and malathion (Celthion, Cythion), carbamates, warfarins, and pyrethrums (Raid). Similar-performing compounds are used in chemical warfare. Introduced as replacements for organophosphates, carbamates cause thousands of cases of poisoning each year, with about 10% of victims requiring hospitalization. The death rate is around 10% for adults and nearly 50% for children.

Suicide attempts account for a considerable share of organophosphate poisonings. When suicide is the goal, the poison is usually taken by mouth. Accidental agricultural exposure is another common source, and persons involved in the manufacture of organophosphates and similar compounds are also at risk. In one case, a farmer decided to burn the empty chemical bags after applying the pesticide and then did some work downwind of the fire. The smoke contained enough organophosphate residue to result in a 9-1-1 call and a trip to the ED.

US soldiers serving in the Persian Gulf, along with civilian populations within range of Iraqi missiles, were put at risk of mass organophosphate poisoning during the Gulf War. The nerve gases used in chemical weapons are members of the same family as agricultural pesticides, with nerve gases used in the military setting differing chiefly by having increased potency.

Pathophysiology

Organophosphates exert their toxic effects at junctions (synapses) of the nerve cells of the autonomic nervous system. The conduction of an impulse from one nerve to another occurs through the release of acetylcholine at the synapse. Acetylcholine works as a chemical messenger, crossing the synapse to depolarize the nerve on the other side of the junction. Once it has delivered its message, the acetylcholine molecule must be inactivated or it will continue to stimulate the target nerve cell indefinitely, leaving the nerve cell unable to receive another message from the brain.

The symptoms of organophosphate poisoning are fundamentally the same regardless of entry by ingestion, inhalation, or absorption: anxiety and restlessness; headache, dizziness, and confusion; tremors or seizures; dyspnea, diffuse wheezing, and respiratory depression; and loss of consciousness. A patient poisoned with organophosphates will usually present with signs and symptoms within the first 8 hours. In addition, the CNS signs and symptoms associated with cholinergic excess are often expressed; the SLUDGE mnemonic, Salivation, Lacrimation, Urination, Defecation, Gastric upset, and Emesis, is helpful in the assessment and diagnosis.

Assessment and Management

Assessment and management of a patient with organophosphate poisoning start with decontamination and removal of all contaminated clothing *before* initiating care or loading the patient into the ambulance. Contaminated clothing should be placed in plastic bags and disposed of as hazardous materials. Ideally, the patient should be scrubbed with soap and water. After that, patient care includes the following measures:

- Establish and maintain the airway. Consider an advanced airway as needed.
- Suction as needed.
- Deliver high-flow oxygen to achieve and maintain saturation levels of 95%.
- Establish vascular access.
- Administer 1.0 mg atropine IV push, and repeat the dose every 3 to 5 minutes until symptom reversal (that is, atropinization) occurs.
- Administer 1 to 2 g of pralidoxime (2-PAM) infused with normal saline during 5 to 10 minutes.
- Apply the ECG monitor, pulse oximeter, and capnometer.
- Immediately transport to the appropriate facility.

Carbon Monoxide

CO causes more poisoning deaths than any other toxic substance. CO is produced during the incomplete combustion of organic fuels, such as in an automobile engine or a home-heating device. CO poisoning is often a winter phenomenon, occurring when a flue or ventilating system becomes blocked. However, approximately half of successful adult suicides are caused by CO: An automobile running in a closed garage can generate a lethal concentration of CO in as little as 30 minutes. CO is also a major contributor to death in house fires.

Pathophysiology

CO is a colorless, odorless, tasteless gas, so people exposed to this toxin have no idea that they are inhaling a toxic substance until it is too late. The toxicity rises quickly primarily from CO's affinity for hemoglobin in RBCs; CO displaces oxygen, thereby preventing the RBCs from carrying oxygen to the tissues and leading to suffocation at the cellular level. Hemoglobin's affinity for CO is more than 250 times its affinity for oxygen, so the atmospheric level of CO does not need to be very high for poisoning to occur. Even relatively small concentrations of CO in the atmosphere can convert a significant proportion of hemoglobin into carboxyhemoglobin (hemoglobin combined with carbon dioxide), making it ineffective as an oxygen carrier.

Because the overall ability of the blood to transport oxygen is so drastically reduced when CO reaches toxic levels, anything that increases the body's oxygen requirements, such as physical exertion or a fever, will increase the severity of the poisoning. Children, whose metabolic rate is intrinsically higher than that of adults, tend to have more severe symptoms at any given level of exposure.

Assessment

CO poisoning can be difficult to diagnose in the field unless it is the direct result of an easily identifiable cause such as a fire or intentional exposure to exhaust fumes from an automobile. Its signs and symptoms are highly variable and quite vague, often resembling early onset of the flu—for example, headache, nausea, and vomiting. With acute CO poisoning, the patient may be confused and unable to think clearly. Complaints of a sensation of pressure in the head or roaring in the ears are common. Physical examination often reveals bounding pulses, dilated pupils, and pallor or cyanosis. The cherry red color of the skin that is mentioned in many textbooks is a late sign of CO poisoning. Consider the possibility of CO poisoning whenever you are confronted with several (possibly many) people who have shared the same accommodations for any period, especially if they have been quartered together in a closed area, such as one house in the winter.

> ### Words of Wisdom
>
> CO is a hazard for rescuers as well as for patients. An encounter with multiple patients with similar complaints—at the same time and inside the same building or area—equals poisoning until proven otherwise! Move the patients to your ambulance for assessment and treatment.

Recent developments in technology have given paramedics the ability to perform noninvasive identification of CO poisoning (% Spco) in the field, which helps address the problem of delayed diagnosis. Note that pulse oximetry *will not* provide a true assessment of arterial oxygenation under these circumstances because the device cannot determine whether it is CO or oxygen that is bound to the hemoglobin. A reading of 99% on the pulse oximeter would be excellent in a normal environmental setting but would be a grave error in the presence of carboxyhemoglobin because the hemoglobin is saturated with the wrong chemical! Application of the ECG monitor to assess for cardiac ischemia can further support diagnostic and treatment efforts when CO is the suspected culprit.

Management

Treatment of CO poisoning in the field is aimed at providing the highest concentration of oxygen possible to attempt to displace CO molecules from the hemoglobin. For patients with only mild symptoms, such as headache, nausea, and flulike symptoms, the

elimination half-time of carboxyhemoglobin is roughly 4 hours. By comparison, if the patient is breathing 100% oxygen, the half-time can be reduced to about 1.5 hours. Hyperbaric oxygen therapy at 2.5 atmospheres of pressure can further reduce the elimination time to 15 to 20 minutes.

If you suspect CO poisoning, take the following actions:

- Remove the patient from the exposure environment.
- Establish and maintain the airway, inserting an advanced airway as needed.
- Give high-flow supplemental oxygen by a tight-fitting nonrebreathing mask to achieve and maintain a saturation level of 95%.
- Establish vascular access.
- Keep the patient quiet and at rest to minimize oxygen demand.
- Monitor the ECG rhythm and LOC.
- Transport to the appropriate facility. If the patient is unresponsive or has signs of serious CO poisoning, direct transport to a facility capable of providing hyperbaric medicine is preferred.
- For patients with injuries or illness from a structural or vehicular fire, consider the possibility of combined CO/cyanide poisoning, especially if the patient has signs of shock. Contact medical control for an order to administer amyl nitrate or sodium thiosulfate, if available.

CO poisoning can be reversed if it is diagnosed and treated in time. Even if the patient recovers, however, acute CO poisoning may result in permanent damage to vital organs and lead to mild to severe neurologic deficits.

■ Chlorine Gas

Incidents involving chlorine gas are relatively common because of the widespread use of chlorine compounds in the home and occupational settings. Household exposures usually occur when someone mixes a cleaning agent containing sodium hypochlorite (such as bleach) with a strong acid in an overzealous attempt to "really clean" a toilet bowl Figure 10 . The resulting chemical reaction releases chlorine gas, often in concentrations high enough to be toxic. Most cases of chlorine gas exposure occur outside the home, however. The chlorination of large swimming pools, which tends to rely on gaseous rather than liquid or solid forms of chlorine, has led to mass exposures at hotels and community recreation centers. Leakage of chlorine gas from an industrial storage tank, truck, or rail car can also result in a multiple-casualty incident.

Pathophysiology

The signs and symptoms of chlorine gas exposure depend on the concentration of the inhaled gas and the duration of exposure. Chlorine gas is extremely irritating to all mucous membranes. When it comes in contact with the moisture on those surfaces, it can form hydrochloric and other acids that are damaging to human tissue. With a minor exposure, the patient will experience burning sensations in the eyes, nose, and throat along with a slight cough. More intense exposure to chlorine gas causes

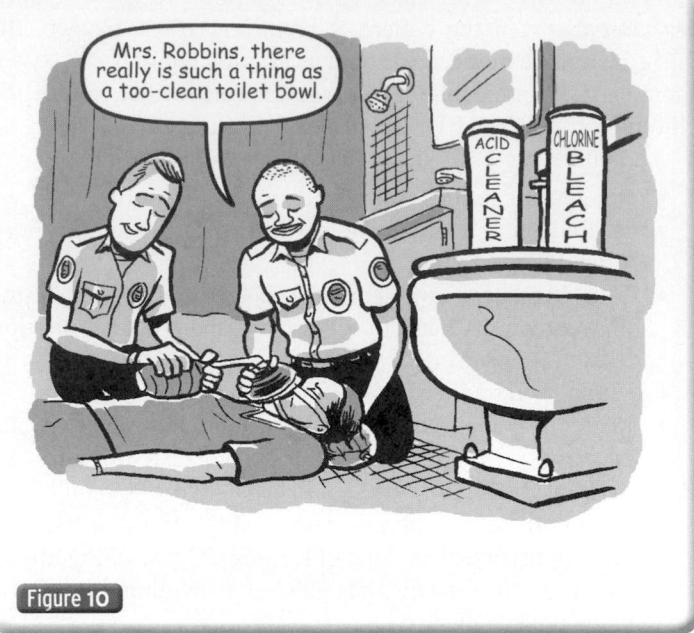

Figure 10

chest tightness, choking, paroxysmal cough, headache, nausea and vomiting, and diffuse wheezing. Patients with more severe exposures may also develop cyanosis, crackles in the chest, shock, seizures, and loss of consciousness.

Assessment and Management

When you are treating patients who have been exposed to chlorine gas, your first priority is to remove them from the area of exposure. If the incident involves a serious gas spill, an upwind location for parking the ambulance is a must. Also make sure that all rescuers wear protective breathing apparatus.

Once in a safe environment, quickly triage the patients. People with dyspnea, wheezing, severe cough, or other signs of respiratory distress are priority patients and should ideally receive high-concentration, humidified oxygen by mask. Intubation and rapid-sequence intubation (RSI) are considerations as well for patients who are fatigued and can no longer compensate. Irrigate burning or itching eyes with water, as well as any areas of the skin that have come in contact with the chlorine.

▉ Cyanide

Cyanide is used in industry for electroplating, ore extraction, and fumigation of structures. In addition to industrial exposures, poisoning can occur after ingestion of cyanide contained in commercial products such as silver polish or from the seeds of cherries, apples, pears, and apricots. More commonly, cyanide poisoning occurs when a household fire results in the combustion of nitrogen-containing materials (such as plastic items or furnishings, wool carpeting, polyurethane silk).

Pathophysiology

Cyanide is one of the most rapid-acting and deadly poisons. This toxin does its damage by combining with a crucial cellular enzyme, cytochrome oxidase, which in turn blocks the utilization of oxygen at the cellular level. The results are cellular suffocation and death of the patient within seconds if the cyanide was inhaled or within minutes to possibly an hour or two if it was ingested.

Assessment

Physical examination of a patient who has been poisoned with cyanide may reveal an altered mental state. If awake enough to answer questions, the patient may report a headache, palpitations, or dyspnea. The classic odor of bitter almonds on the patient's breath is highly suggestive of cyanide poisoning but is not diagnostic. Respirations are usually rapid and labored early on; as the poisoning progresses, they become slow and gasping. The pulse is usually rapid and thready. Vomiting, seizures, and coma are common. The patient's venous blood and sometimes the patient's body may be bright red—even though oxygen is available in the bloodstream, it is not being taken up by the tissues.

Management

Cyanide poisoning is a dire emergency, and treatment must be instituted as fast as possible. The aim of treatment is to displace the cyanide from the cytochrome oxidase by introducing another chemical that will "attract" the cyanide. In the prehospital setting, that is usually amyl nitrite because of the ease of administration. If given in time, the treatment is usually effective.

If the cyanide poisoning occurred as the result of a toxic inhalation, remove the patient from the source of the cyanide (the toxic environment). Establish an airway, and administer 100% supplemental oxygen, assisting ventilations as necessary.

If you have the commercially available cyanide antidote kit (manufactured by Eli Lilly), follow the instructions supplied with the kit, which includes IV administration of 50 mL of sodium thiosulfate solution. If you do not stock the kits, break a vial of amyl nitrite into a gauze pad and hold it over the patient's nose for about 20 seconds, and then remove it to allow the patient to breathe a high concentration of oxygen for about 40 seconds. Thus, in each minute, the patient should inhale the amyl nitrite one third of the time and breathe oxygen two thirds of the time. Keep switching between the amyl nitrite and the oxygen while maintaining this ratio. While you are administering the amyl nitrite, your partner should establish vascular access.

Words of Wisdom

The most important aspect of treatment in toxic inhalations is to remove the patient from the toxic environment, but do not enter a known toxic environment without protective breathing apparatus.

Anticipate hypotension as a consequence of amyl nitrite therapy, and keep the patient supine with the legs elevated. If the systolic blood pressure falls below 80 mm Hg, consult medical control about whether to administer an IV vasopressor.

Monitor the ECG rhythm carefully. Notify the receiving hospital of the probable diagnosis so staff can begin preparation of sodium thiosulfate. Transport the patient without delay to an appropriate facility.

Hydroxocobalamin Hydroxocobalamin is a safe alternative or adjunct to the traditional treatment of cyanide poisoning. The commercially available "Cyanokit" contains hydroxocobalamin, an IV preparation of vitamin B$_{12}$, along with an IV infusion set. In the event of cyanide exposure, patients are given 5 g (or 70 mg/kg) of hydroxocobalamin IV over 30 minutes. The hydroxocobalamin binds with cyanide molecules to form the compound cyanocobalamin that is relatively nontoxic.

Hydroxocobalamin is considered a relatively safe antidote, with allergy/anaphylaxis as the primary concern. Patients may also experience some temporary skin changes such as itching or redness after hydroxocobalamin administration. Other adverse effects have not been widely reported.

Methylene Blue Methylene blue is an antidote used to treat methemoglobinemia, that may occur during the treatment of cyanide poisoning with sodium nitrite. In severe cases of cyanide poisoning, methemoglobinemia, an alteration of the structure of hemoglobin, is induced by the administration of amyl nitrite and sodium nitrite in order to bind with cyanide molecules in the body. In mild cases of cyanide poisoning, methemoglobinemia may cause its own severe or fatal toxicity and should be avoided. Methylene blue is typically administered in acute health care settings under the guidance of expert consultation. Paramedics may transport patients who have received methylene blue as treatment for methemoglobinemia from treatment of cyanide poisoning or from another unrelated cause.

▪ Caustics

Caustics include strong acids (pH < 2.0) and strong alkalis (pH > 12.0). Both types of chemicals are commonly used in industry, agriculture (anhydrous ammonia), and the home **Table 5** and **Figure 11** . According to the American Association of Poison Control Centers (AAPCC), approximately 100,000 caustic exposures occur each year in the United States. Most cases involve accidental dermal or ocular exposure, although occasionally you may encounter oral ingestions. If the patient is an adult, oral ingestion of caustics is usually an intentional suicide attempt. Although many serious burns occur from caustics, including results such as cataracts and blindness, only about 20 people die each year of caustic exposure.

Pathophysiology

Caustic substances cause direct chemical injury to the tissues they contact. Signs and symptoms of a caustic exposure include severe pain, burns, difficulty talking or swallowing (with oral ingestions), and hypoperfusion or shock (rarely, usually secondary to internal bleeding).

The widespread practice of storing such substances in beverage containers (such as soft drink or milk bottles), usually because the original container has started to leak, increases the

Table 5	Common Caustic Substances	
Substance	**Example**	**Source**
Acids	Hydrochloric acid	Toilet bowl cleaners, swimming pool cleaners
	Sulfuric acid	Battery acid, toilet bowl cleaners (as bisulfate)
	Others	Bleach disinfectants, slate cleaners
Alkalis	Lye (sodium or potassium hydroxide)	Paint removers, washing powders, drain cleaners (such as Drano, Liquid-Plumr, Plunge), button-shaped batteries, Clinitest tablets
	Sodium hypochlorite	Bleach (Clorox)
	Sodium carbonate	Bleach (Purex), nonphosphate detergents
	Ammonia	Hair dyes, jewelry cleaners, metal cleaners or polishes, antirust agents
	Potassium permanganate	Electric dishwasher detergents

likelihood that a child will regard the substance as something to drink. As the liquid enters the mouth and begins to burn, the child may simultaneously remove the bottle and turn the head, resulting in burns to the mouth, tongue, and face and neck.

Assessment and Management

Most patients who have swallowed caustic substances present with severe pain in the mouth, throat, or chest. Usually the airway is not a problem; nor is the patient in shock. Respiratory distress, if present, is most probably due to soft-tissue swelling in the larynx, epiglottis, or vocal cords, which means that the patient is in immediate danger of complete airway obstruction. For a caustic ingestion in an alert patient, giving milk—at least 6 to 8 ounces for a child and 8 to 12 ounces for an adult—may help if the Poison Center or medical control agrees. Establish vascular access, usually en route, because immediate transport to the ED is indicated.

Words of Wisdom

If a patient who swallowed a caustic agent is in respiratory distress, provide immediate transport to the hospital. Have your cricothyrotomy kit ready.

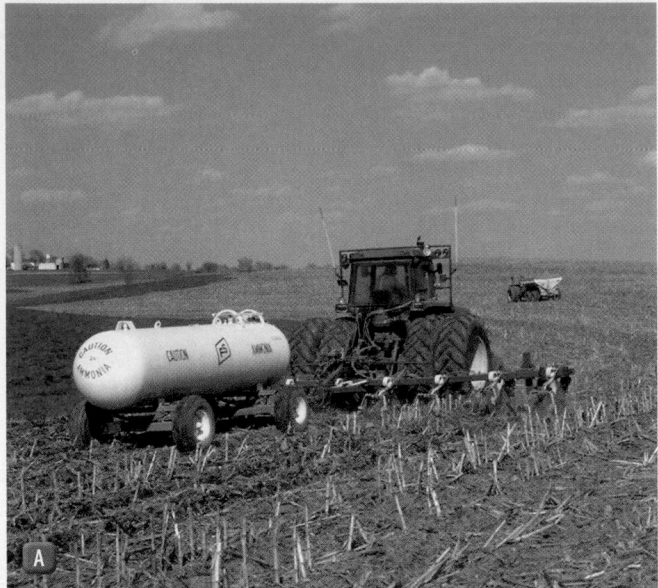

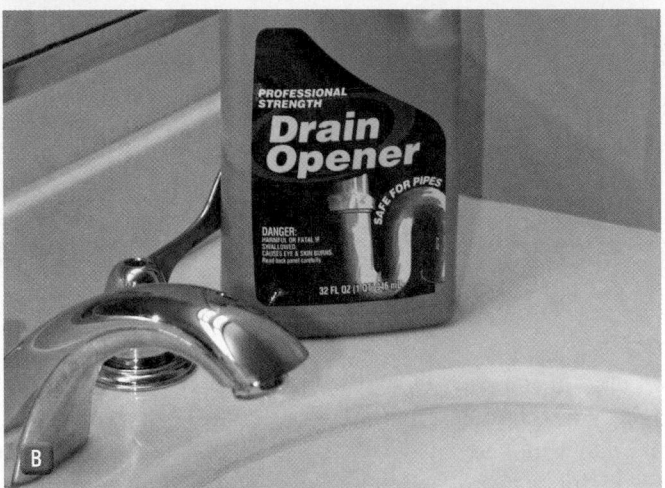

Figure 11 Caustic chemicals are commonly used in industry. **A.** Anhydrous ammonia tank used in agriculture. **B.** Plumbing agents used in the home.

With dermal exposure to a strong acid, the result is immediate and excruciating pain. For a strong alkali, the onset of pain is somewhat delayed, allowing more time before the patient reacts and increasing the severity of the burn. In such an injury, diluting and flushing away the caustic substance is the main goal of field treatment. Acids tend to be more water-soluble than alkalis, so they can often be diluted relatively quickly.

Words of Wisdom

Some chemicals react vigorously with water, so be sure to check the relevant warnings or placard for information you really need.

With alkalis, it is more important to keep water continually flowing because it usually takes much longer to rinse an alkali away (compared with an acid).

For an eye exposure, cut off the prong section of a nasal cannula, place it on the bridge of the patient's nose, and plug in a macro IV administration set and run it wide open to provide continuous irrigation. This also frees you up to perform other tasks. A Morgan lens may also be used after the initial gross flushing has been accomplished. Use of a Morgan lens is covered in the chapter, *Diseases of the Eyes, Ears, Nose, and Throat.*

One of the most common caustic exposures in the agricultural setting involves anhydrous ammonia. The exposure usually occurs during the hook-up or disconnection of a nurse tank. Farmers often keep a small water bottle in the shirt pocket, allowing them to immediately rinse their eyes should an exposure occur. Without treatment, eye exposure to anhydrous ammonia can cause devastating damage in less than a minute, resulting in cataracts or blindness.

The following are significant "do not's" for caustic ingestions:

- *Do not* give any "neutralizing substances." Some product laboratories incorrectly advise neutralizing the caustic agent—for example, by giving lemon juice or dilute vinegar (both weak acids) to a patient who has swallowed an alkali. Mixing an acid and an alkali produces *heat,* adding a thermal injury to the chemical injury.
- *Do not* induce vomiting—what burned on the way down will burn again on the way up.
- *Do not* perform gastric lavage.
- *Do not* give activated charcoal. It is not effective in acid or alkali ingestion, and it may interfere with the patient's subsequent care by blackening the field of vision when an endoscope is used to inspect the esophagus and stomach for damage.

Common Household Items

From a toxicologic perspective, the average home is full of dangerous substances. Many houseplants have poisonous leaves or berries. All pesticides and herbicides used in lawn and garden care are potentially poisonous. All hydrocarbon products (such as paint thinners, solvents, gas) can cause permanent neurologic damage or death if inhaled or huffed in toxic amounts. The same is true of glue fumes. Many household cleaning agents are also toxic if ingested.

It is not possible within the scope of this chapter to discuss all of the possibilities when it comes to household poisonings. Some of the more likely culprits are covered in several of the other sections to assist in preparing you to handle the myriad possibilities. As always, keep in mind that the Poison Center is an invaluable resource.

Drugs Abused for Sexual Purposes

Drugs that are abused for sexual purposes include those that increase sexual gratification and those that are used to facilitate sexual assault.

Drugs That Increase Sexual Gratification

Drugs that increase sexual gratification constitute a long and varied list. Clearly, the most dangerous include erectile dysfunction medications such as sildenafil (Viagra), which are contraindicated for patients who take nitrites for cardiac problems. Their use by people taking nitrites may result in severe hypotension or total cardiovascular collapse, potentially leading to death. For hypotension, repeated boluses of normal saline can bring the blood pressure up to an acceptable level. If cardiac arrest occurs, follow your protocols.

For some people, the relaxed dreamy high of marijuana is desirable for sexual gratification. There is no overdose potential for marijuana. Supportive care is all that is required.

Cocaine and other stimulant drugs (such as amphetamines and methamphetamine) are popular choices for people seeking a more intense sexual experience. Should the patient develop tachycardia in such a case, hypotension can occur as a result of inadequate preload. Be alert for this possibility when the pulse rate is in the range of 170 to 180 beats/min or higher, although a rate in the 150s could cause problems for a patient with an extensive cardiac history. Serial boluses of normal saline will usually stabilize the blood pressure. If fluid boluses are not effective in stabilizing hypotension, a vasopressor (such as dopamine [Intropin] or dobutamine [Dobutrex]) may be required.

Another drug that increases sexual gratification is amyl nitrite (also known as poppers, rush, happy snaps). This organic nitrate drug can be crushed and inhaled, again producing an intense sexual experience. As with any nitrate, hypotension may result from blood pooling in the periphery owing to the drug's vasodilatory effects.

One of the most unique drugs in this group is ecstasy (the love drug, hug drug). Although this so-called club drug is an analog of methamphetamine, its effects hardly resemble the actions of methamphetamine. Ecstasy would be more correctly termed an "empathogenic"—it creates an incredible sense of well-being.

Dextromethorphan (DXM), which is found in almost 150 over-the-counter (OTC) cough suppressants, can produce a euphoric floating sensation or out-of-body experience. At a plateau level of approximately six tablets (180-mg dose), DXM produces a mild stimulant effect that may enhance a sexual experience. DXM or "Robo" (Robitussin) abusers are often called "Roboheads"; this kind of abuse is common among teenagers because this drug is readily available in pharmacies and online. Consuming large quantities of DXM can lead to hallucinations, psychedelic visions, loss of motor control, confusion, blurred vision, dreamlike euphoria, and out-of-body sensations.

Drugs Used to Facilitate Sexual Assault

Drugs used to facilitate sexual assault are often administered to an unsuspecting woman, frequently in an alcoholic drink. These substances are used by sexual predators, which explains why they are called "date rape" drugs. They are discussed further in the chapter, *Psychiatric Emergencies*.

GHB Gamma-hydroxybutyrate (GHB) is an endogenous metabolite of gamma-aminobutyric acid, a neuromodulator involved with sleep cycles, memory retention, and emotional control. GHB was used as anesthetic in Europe for approximately 40 years before it appeared in the United States, where it was originally sold in health food stores as GLB (which metabolizes into GHB) for body-building purposes (it supposedly "burned fat" while the person was sleeping). By the late 1980s, GHB had gained popularity with young people as a club drug, earning the name "liquid ecstasy" from its euphoric effects at raves (all-night dance parties). In the mid 1990s, GHB became increasingly associated with sexual assaults. In 1990, the US Food and Drug Administration banned this drug from OTC sales. In 1996, the federal government enacted the Drug-Induced Rape Prevention and Punishment Law. This law allows prison terms of up to 20 years for anyone who commits a violent crime, including sexual assault, with the assistance of any controlled substance.

Although GHB is available as an odorless and colorless liquid, it has a salty taste. Reportedly, it cannot be tasted when placed in a drink such as a margarita in a salt-rimmed glass. Once ingested, GHB quickly crosses the blood-brain barrier, exerting its effects within 30 to 60 minutes. As little as 0.5 mg of this drug can produce a pronounced hypnotic effect along with disinhibition, severe passivity (that is, a lack of the will to resist), and antegrade amnesia. When taken with alcohol, GHB increases the risk of potentially lethal CNS depression (culminating in coma or death). When taken with methamphetamine and similar drugs, GHB increases the risk of seizures.

Treatment for GHB intoxication focuses on the CNS depression and the risks of the patient being unable to protect the airway. First, establish and maintain the airway, inserting an advanced airway as needed. Carefully monitor the patient's LOC. Assist breathing as necessary, and administer high-flow supplemental oxygen. Establish vascular access. Apply the ECG monitor, pulse oximeter, and capnometer. Finally, provide rapid transport to the ED.

Rohypnol Rohypnol (also known as roofies) is a potent benzodiazepine that is also used to facilitate sexual assault. This drug is illegal to make or distribute, so most of the supply found in the United States enters the country from Mexico.

Poisonous Alcohols

The form of alcohol consumed by humans in alcoholic beverages is ethyl alcohol (or ethanol). It is not conventionally recognized as a poison, even though it has many properties of a poison when ingested in sufficient quantities. Instead, "poisonous alcohols" are generally considered to encompass alcohols manufactured for industrial or nongastronomic purposes, such as methyl alcohol and ethylene glycol.

Methyl Alcohol

Methyl alcohol (also known as wood alcohol or methanol) is present in paints, paint remover, windshield washer fluids, varnishes, antifreeze, and canned fuels such as Sterno **Figure 12**. Methanol poisoning can occur after inadvertently drinking contaminated whiskey or moonshine, or from intentional ingestion in a suicide attempt. Methanol is a popular substitute for ethanol among

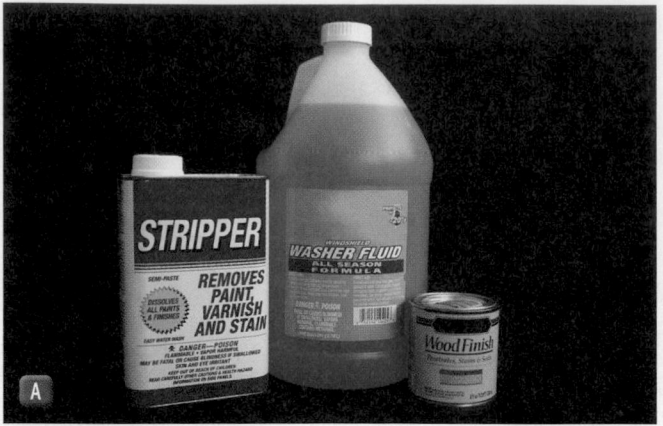

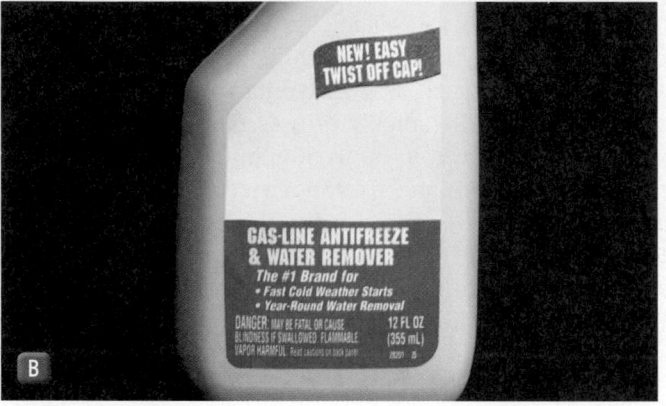

Figure 12 Methyl alcohol is present in paints, paint remover, windshield washer fluids, and varnishes **(A)** and in antifreeze and canned fuels **(B)**.

desperate people with alcoholism when they do not have the means to obtain ethanol. This colorless liquid has a unique odor.

Pathophysiology Methanol itself is not harmful. Rather, its metabolic breakdown products, formaldehyde and formic acid, are responsible for the characteristic signs and symptoms of methanol poisoning. A dose of as little as 30 mL (2 tablespoons) can produce toxicity and even death. Once ingested, methanol is quickly absorbed from the GI tract, with peak blood levels attained within 30 to 90 minutes. In mild toxicity, the half-life of methanol is 14 to 20 hours. As toxicity increases, the half-life increases to 24 to 30 hours. The liver eliminates 90% to 95% of the methanol.

Assessment The symptoms of methanol poisoning do not usually appear immediately but begin from 12 to 18 hours, occasionally up to 72 hours, after ingestion. As a consequence, the patient may or may not connect the symptoms to what he or she drank yesterday or several days ago. Patient complaints include nausea and vomiting (in almost 50% of cases), headache or vertigo, abdominal pain (often from pancreatitis), and blurred vision ("looks like a snowstorm") or possibly blindness. Findings on the physical exam may include an odor of alcohol on the breath, altered mental status ranging from drunken

behavior to seizures or coma, dilated pupils with sluggish or no reaction, hyperpnea and tachypnea from metabolic acidosis, and bradycardia and hypotension (very late signs).

Management Field care for methanol poisoning is primarily supportive. Establish and manage the airway, considering advanced airway placement as needed. Establish vascular access. Assess the blood glucose level, and administer glucose if the patient has hypoglycemia. In addition, administer thiamine per local protocol. Consult medical control for consideration of sodium bicarbonate. Provide immediate transport to an appropriate facility.

If the patient is alert, the ingestion took place within the last 30 minutes, and if local protocol allows it, insert a nasogastric tube and attempt to aspirate the gastric contents. You should also assess the patient for other drug involvement. Administration of activated charcoal is contraindicated unless other drugs have been ingested that are adsorbable, in which case you should follow your local protocol.

Ethylene Glycol

Ethylene glycol is a colorless, odorless liquid found in a variety of commercial products, including antifreeze, coolant, deicers, polishes, and paints. Its relatively pleasant taste has made it a favorite substitute among people with alcoholism when the beverage of choice is unavailable. The lethal dose of ethylene glycol is estimated to be 2 mL/kg, or as little as 150 mL in the average-size adult.

Pathophysiology Ethylene glycol is water-soluble. With oral intake, it is absorbed rapidly, with peak blood levels attained within 1 to 4 hours after ingestion. The liver and kidneys metabolize ethylene glycol into a number of toxic metabolites, including aldehydes, lactate, oxalate, and glycolate. In turn, these metabolites produce metabolic acidosis.

Assessment Toxicity from ethylene glycol occurs in three stages, so the signs and symptoms vary depending on when you encounter the patient relative to the time of ingestion:

- **Stage 1:** 20 minutes to 12 hours after ingestion. The patient presents with CNS depression and may appear intoxicated, as evidenced by slurred speech and ataxia, although the odor of ethanol on the breath is notably absent. The patient may also experience nausea, vomiting, seizures, or coma.
- **Stage 2:** 12 to 24 hours after ingestion. Pulmonary edema can result in tachypnea, tachycardia, mild hypertension, and rales (or crackles). In severe cases, acute respiratory distress syndrome, congestive heart failure, and cardiovascular collapse may occur.
- **Stage 3:** 24 to 72 hours after ingestion. The renal damage produced by the ethylene glycol becomes evident with patients reporting flank pain and anuria (absence of urine formation).

Management The care plan for a patient with suspected ethylene glycol poisoning is the same as for methanol poisoning, with the exception of possibly getting an order from medical control to administer 10 mL of 10% calcium gluconate via slow IV push to treat the hypocalcemia that accompanies ethylene glycol toxicity. This medication is usually ordered only after good urine flow is established and after the IV line is flushed clear of sodium bicarbonate. Once at the hospital, care focuses on correction of acidosis, administration of fomepizole (Antizol) or ethanol (to reduce the conversion of the methanol to its toxic metabolites), and, potentially, renal dialysis.

Hydrocarbons

Hydrocarbons are compounds made up principally of hydrogen and carbon atoms, with most, but not all, obtained from the distillation of petroleum. Hydrocarbons are found in a variety of products around the home, including cleaning and polishing agents, glues, spot removers, lighter fluids, paints, paint thinners and paint removers, other fuels, and pesticides.

Hydrocarbon Inhalation

The vast majority of intentional hydrocarbon inhalations are "recreational." Frequently, people who "bag" or huff are young—middle-school age and, occasionally, younger children. The profile adds up with deadly simplicity: Young children who see their siblings and parents abuse alcohol or drugs may seek to emulate that behavior but not having the cash to purchase these items, they turn to everyday products such as paint thinner, solvents, paint strippers, gasoline, nonstick cooking spray (such as Pam), and glues. The rich alveolar capillary network makes the lungs a highly efficient mechanism for providing a quick and inexpensive drug high. Unfortunately, long-term inhalant abuse can lead to permanent loss of mental function as evidenced by a variety of neuropathies, such as loss of hearing, loss of fine motor function, balance and equilibrium disorders, and occasionally death.

The modern epidemic of inhalation began in the early 1960s with glue sniffing. Within a short time, the number of agents being inhaled to get high had increased exponentially, as had the techniques for inhalation. Simple sniffing over the opening of a glue bottle did not provide an intense enough exposure for serious abusers. Pouring the volatile material onto a rag, placing it in a trash bag, and holding the bag over one's face to breathe in the fumes produced a more intense high more quickly. Breathing fumes directly off a soaked rag or towel is termed huffing, whereas the use of a trash bag is termed bagging. Table 6 lists commonly abused inhaled compounds.

The primary goals when you are caring for a patient who has inhaled hydrocarbons focus on removal from the noxious environment, administering high-concentration supplemental oxygen, and prompt transport to the appropriate facility.

Table 6 Compounds Commonly Abused by Sniffing and Bagging

Example	Sources	Signs and Symptoms of Toxicity
Halogenated hydrocarbons		
1,1,1-Trichloroethane (methylchloroform)	Cleaning solvents, typewriter correction fluid, aerosol propellant	Eye irritation, lightheadedness, incoordination, CNS depression, respiratory failure, cardiac dysrhythmias, sudden death
Trichloroethylene	Degreasing solvent, aerosol propellant, rubber cement, plastic cement	Euphoria, anesthesia, weakness, vomiting, abdominal cramps, loss of coordination, neuropathy, blindness, cardiac dysrhythmias, "degreaser's flush" (flushed face, neck, and shoulders when taken along with alcohol)
Tetrachloroethylene (perchloroethylene)	Solvent, dry cleaning agent	Drunken behavior, dizziness, lightheadedness, difficulty walking, numbness, sleepiness, visual disturbances, memory impairment, eye irritation, cutaneous flushing, sudden death
Methylene chloride (dichloromethane)	Refrigerant, paint remover, aerosol propellant	Fatigue, weakness, chills, sleepiness, nausea, dizziness, incoordination, pulmonary edema
Carbon tetrachloride	Cleaning fluid	Narcosis, sudden death
Petroleum hydrocarbons		
Benzene	Cable cleaner, industrial solvents, rubber cement	Delirium, agitation, seizures, sudden death
Toluene	Spray paint, model and plastic cements, lacquer thinner	Narcosis, hallucinations, mania; loss of fine motor skills; impulsive, destructive, accident-prone behavior; sudden death
Gasoline	Gas tank/portable gas can	Sudden death

Hydrocarbon Ingestion

Pathophysiology Because of the ready accessibility of hydrocarbons and the high likelihood that they might be mistaken for potable beverages, hydrocarbon poisonings are common among children younger than 5 years. The potential hazards of swallowing a given hydrocarbon are directly related to the viscosity of the agent: The lower the viscosity, the higher the risk of aspiration and other complications. Most hydrocarbon ingestions do *not* produce lasting damage. Patients who develop symptoms within a few minutes of ingestion are likely to have aspirated and need immediate attention.

Low-viscosity hydrocarbons (such as kerosene, naphtha, and toluene) can easily enter the lungs during swallowing. If the patient reports coughing, choking, or vomiting immediately after swallowing the substance, assume that aspiration occurred. Similarly, any signs of respiratory distress—air hunger, intercostal retractions, tachypnea, cyanosis—must be considered danger signals.

Low viscosity also facilitates the uptake of a hydrocarbon by tissues of the CNS and, therefore, its anesthetic effects. At first, the patient may experience excitement and euphoria, followed by weakness, incoordination, drowsiness, confusion, and coma. Some petroleum products—notably gasoline—can produce hypoglycemia and cardiac dysrhythmias, so you should continuously monitor the patient's ECG rhythm.

Many hydrocarbon products cause gastric irritation, which results in severe abdominal pain, diarrhea, and belching, sometimes lasting for hours after the incident. Conversely, just a single hydrocarbon substance exposure may cause life-threatening toxicity and, on occasion, sudden death.

Assessment and Management If a patient who has swallowed a hydrocarbon product is asymptomatic when you arrive and remains so while you are on scene, he or she is unlikely to experience significant complications. In such a scenario, and after discussion with medical control, some patients may not warrant transport because they can be safely observed at home. In one study involving 211 patients suspected of hydrocarbon ingestion, fewer than 1% required physician intervention.

By contrast, all symptomatic patients suspected of ingesting a hydrocarbon product—especially patients with respiratory symptoms—should be transported immediately to the ED for further evaluation and care. Management should include the following measures:

- Remove contaminated clothing and decontaminate the patient, ideally before placing the patient in the ambulance.
- Establish and maintain the airway, and ensure adequate ventilation.
- Administer high-flow supplemental oxygen to achieve and maintain blood saturation levels of 95%.
- Establish vascular access.
- Continuously monitor the ECG rhythm; consider running a 12-lead.
- Administer sequential bolus infusions of normal saline to treat hypotension.
- Transport the patient to the most appropriate facility.

▪ Hydrofluoric Acid/Hydrogen Fluoride

Pathophysiology

Hydrofluoric acid is hydrogen fluoride (HF) that has been placed into an aqueous solution. This potent caustic substance can cause devastating local and systemic toxicity from exposure to an extremely small amount of concentrated liquid. The fluoride in HF leaches calcium and magnesium from body tissues, resulting in profound, often lethal hypocalcemia and hypomagnesemia. These electrolyte alterations also prompt a massive release of sequestered potassium into the systemic circulation.

HF may cause throat discomfort, bronchospasm, stridor, and local airway injury following inhalation. Lung auscultation reveals wheezes, rhonchi, or rales. Serious inhalation exposures can cause delayed chemical pneumonitis or pulmonary edema.

Ingestion of HF may cause vomiting, abdominal pain, and gastritis, in addition to profound systemic toxicity. Ingestions of large amounts or concentrated solutions of HF are often lethal. Systemic effects from HF poisoning are primarily related to hypocalcemia and electrolyte imbalance. Dysrhythmias, tetany, muscle spasm, vasospasm, and acidemia are common.

Assessment and Management

Patients exposed to HF may deteriorate rapidly, so careful monitoring is critical. As always, manage the ABCs. For ingestion exposure, provide immediate stomach evacuation with a nasogastric or orogastric tube. Administer a calcium- or magnesium-containing substance such as milk, antacids, magnesium citrate, or magnesium hydroxide.

▪ Hydrogen Sulfide

Pathophysiology

A highly toxic, colorless gas, hydrogen sulfide (HS) is usually identified by its distinctive rotten-egg odor. Poisoning by HS usually occurs by inhalation. Hydrogen sulfide affects all organs, but has the most impact on the lungs and central nervous system.

Workers in industrial settings may be exposed to low levels over a long period of time. Chronic exposure to this gas may cause patients to lose their ability to smell the gas. Low-level exposures cause eye, nose, and throat irritation, as well as headaches and bronchitis. When patients are exposed to high concentrations of the gas, they present with nausea and vomiting, confusion, dyspnea, and loss of consciousness. Seizures, shock, coma, and cardiopulmonary arrest may result from exposure to very high concentrations.

Assessment and Management

There is no proven antidote for HS poisoning. Therefore, you should quickly remove the patient from the contaminated area. Once the patient has been moved to a safe area, management is largely supportive, monitoring and assisting the patient's respiratory and cardiovascular functions.

▪ Oxides of Nitrogen

The group of gases known as nitrogen oxides includes nitric oxide and nitrogen dioxide. Nitric oxide is colorless or brownish at room temperature and has a sweet smell. Nitrogen dioxide is also normally colorless or brownish and is generally described as having a harsh odor. These gases are common pollutants. Patients may be exposed to very high concentrations from kerosene heaters in their homes or in an occupational setting in facilities that produce nitric acid.

Pathophysiology

Exposure to oxides of nitrogen can result in irritation of the throat and upper respiratory tract, buildup of fluid in the lungs, and difficulty breathing.

Assessment and Management

Take precautions, including a self-contained breathing apparatus, before entering the scene. Prehospital treatment includes immediately removing the patient from the environment. Provide supportive care, gain IV access, and be prepared to perform endotracheal intubation.

Psychiatric Medications

Psychiatric medications are designed to alter dysfunctions of mood and affect (most commonly depression) and of thought, orientation, or perception; thus, they are sophisticated pharmacologic agents. When patients taking psychiatric medications have toxicologic emergencies, you should expect to be challenged with matters of patient care and scene management.

Tricyclic Antidepressants

Pathophysiology Tricyclic antidepressants (TCAs) were once the drugs of choice to treat depression. Unfortunately, TCAs require close attention to compliance with dosing regimens—and patients who need them have difficulty following the regimen. Patients are depressed, and many also have problems with alcohol (a CNS depressant). Consequently, they are at high risk of both intentional and unintentional overdose.

Making matters worse, TCAs have a small therapeutic window—that is, the difference between "minimum dosing" (the least amount of drug needed for the desired effect) and "maximum dosing" (the amount at which the drug becomes toxic). With some drugs, the therapeutic window may span several thousand milligrams. With TCAs, even minimal dosing errors may produce toxic effects.

According to one report from the American Association of Poison Control Centers (AAPCC), TCAs were involved in more deaths than any other class of medication. Of the eight TCAs currently available in the United States, the five most likely to be involved in drug-related events are amitriptyline (40%), imipramine (Tofranil; 17%), doxepin (Sinequan, Zonalon; 14%), nortriptyline (Aventyl, Pamelor; 12%), and desipramine (Norpramin, Pertofrane; 6%). Although they are no longer first-line therapy for depression, TCAs still have other applications, such as pain management.

Assessment The signs and symptoms of TCA overdose may vary dramatically among patients. One patient may present with only a mild antimuscarinic symptom such as a dry mouth, whereas another may have cardiotoxic effects, such as life-threatening or fatal dysrhythmias. The most common signs and symptoms of a TCA overdose are altered mental status (drowsy, confused, slurred speech), dysrhythmias (usually sinus tachycardia or supraventricular tachycardia), dry mouth, blurred vision or dilated pupils, urinary retention, constipation, and pulmonary edema. With a more serious toxic exposure, you should be alert for ventricular tachycardia, hypotension, respiratory depression, QT prolongation on the ECG Figure 13, and seizures.

When TCAs exert their toxic effects, the most common cause of death is cardiac dysrhythmia. A significant number of the drug overdoses involving TCAs also involve other drugs and frequently alcohol, which contributes to increased morbidity and mortality. A patient who presents with serious signs and symptoms within 6 hours of the ingestion should be considered in critical condition.

Management Management of patients with a TCA overdose includes the following measures:

- Maintain the airway. If the patient's mental status suddenly deteriorates, as is often the case, insert an advanced airway.
- Administer high-flow supplemental oxygen to achieve and maintain blood saturation levels of 95%.
- Establish vascular access.
- Provide continuous ECG monitoring (watch for widening of the QRS).
- Administer activated charcoal per medical control orders.
- Consult with medical control to consider sodium bicarbonate administration (if the QRS interval begins to widen).
- Manage hypotension with sequential boluses of normal saline. Be alert to the possibility of pulmonary edema; it occurs frequently in patients with TCA overdose.
- Assess blood glucose levels. Give D_{50} if the patient is hypoglycemic.
- Rule out head trauma as a possible cause of decreased mental status.
- Be alert for agitation or violence. Manage this problem with reassurance and benzodiazepines.

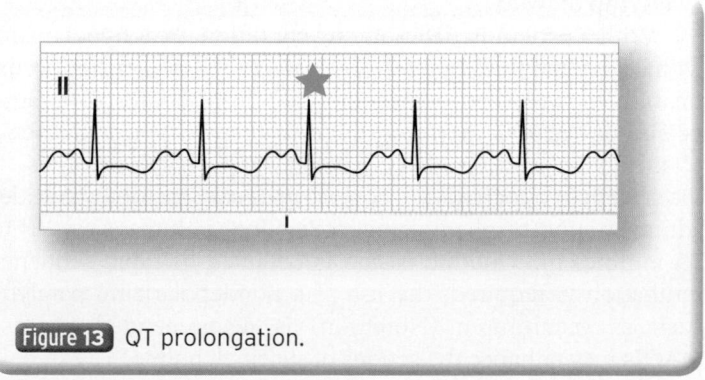

Figure 13 QT prolongation.

- *Do not give* flumazenil (Romazicon; may cause seizures) or physostigmine (Eserine, Antilirium).
- For seizures, consider administration of benzodiazepines, and consider rapid-sequence intubation (RSI) or endotracheal intubation.
- Provide rapid transport to the appropriate facility.

Monoamine Oxidase Inhibitors

Pathophysiology Monoamine oxidase inhibitors (MAOIs) are used primarily to treat atypical depression. They work by increasing norepinephrine and serotonin levels within the CNS. Unfortunately, the potential for drug interactions is a major issue for patients receiving MAOI therapy. A tight therapeutic window also contributes to the limited popularity of MAOIs—as little as 2 mg/kg may produce a life-threatening event. In addition, MAOIs can precipitate a hypertensive crisis if taken in conjunction with tyramine-containing foods (such as beer, wine, aged cheese, chopped liver, pickled herring, sour cream, yogurt, fava beans). When taken in toxic levels, MAOIs can be lethal because they can produce hyperkalemia, metabolic acidosis, and rhabdomyolysis.

Assessment Symptoms of MAOI toxicity are often delayed, occurring 6 to 12 hours after ingestion and, in some cases, as long as 24 hours later. Once signs and symptoms begin to appear, you should prepare to manage a life-threatening event. When death occurs from an MAOI overdose, it is usually secondary to multiple-system organ failure.

Early signs and symptoms of MAOI overdose include hyperactivity, dysrhythmias (usually sinus tachycardia or SVTs), hyperventilation, and nystagmus. With increased levels of toxicity, be alert for chest pain, palpitations, hypertension, diaphoresis, agitated or combative behavior, marked hyperthermia, and hallucinations. With a severe MAOI overdose, expect bradycardia, hypotension, seizures, worsening hyperthermia, pulmonary edema, coma, or cardiac arrest.

Management Unfortunately, there is no antidote available for an MAOI overdose. With any suspected MAOI overdose, you should establish and maintain the airway, inserting an advanced airway as needed. In addition, administer high-flow supplemental oxygen. Establish large-bore vascular access. Monitor the ECG rhythm, staying alert for changes indicative of hyperkalemia. After consultation with medical control, you may administer a single dose of activated charcoal. However, you should *not* give syrup of ipecac.

With a patient in deteriorating condition, treat hypotension with sequential fluid boluses of normal saline. If seizures occur, treat them with benzodiazepines per local protocol because persistent seizures may contribute to the combined problems of metabolic acidosis, hyperkalemia, and rhabdomyolysis. If the patient is hypertensive, contact medical control to consider administration of phentolamine (Regitine) boluses every 10 to 15 minutes until normotension is obtained. If rapid sequence intubation is required, the use of a nondepolarizing paralytic such as vecuronium (Norcuron) is recommended because MAOIs may enhance the actions of succinylcholine.

Selective Serotonin Reuptake Inhibitors

Pathophysiology A larger therapeutic window, which increases their safety margin, has helped make selective serotonin reuptake inhibitors (SSRIs) a top choice for managing depression. In addition, SSRIs have far fewer anticholinergic and cardiac effects than the TCAs. Popular SSRIs include fluoxetine (Prozac), paroxetine (Paxil), and sertraline (Zoloft).

Assessment As many as 50% of adult patients may be asymptomatic with an SSRI overdose. However, when symptoms are present, the most commonly seen include nausea, vomiting, dysrhythmias (usually sinus tachycardia), sedation, and tremors. Other symptoms that occur much less often include dilated pupils, agitation, blood pressure changes (hypotension or hypertension), seizures, and hallucinations, When SSRIs are taken in conjunction with alcohol, look for tachycardia, mild hypotension, and generally lethargy as the most common signs and symptoms.

Management A pure SSRI overdose with no other drugs or alcohol involved usually produces limited toxic effects, with the exception of seizures or serotonin syndrome (discussed later in this section). As such, management of an SSRI overdose follows the general approach for poisoned patients:

- Establish and maintain the airway.
- Administer high-flow supplemental oxygen to achieve and maintain blood saturation levels of 95%.
- Establish vascular access.
- Provide continuous ECG monitoring.
- Consider a single dose of activated charcoal per medical control orders.
- Treat seizure activity with benzodiazepines per local protocol.
- Should widening of the QRS occur, consult with medical control for consideration of sodium bicarbonate administration.
- Transport to the appropriate facility.

Serotonin Syndrome Serotonin syndrome is an idiosyncratic complication that occasionally occurs with antidepressant therapy. This condition is not limited to patients taking SSRIs, but also can occur when patients take any combination of drugs that increase central serotonin neurotransmission. Because no laboratory test can pinpoint serotonin syndrome and the symptomatology is vague, it is a difficult diagnosis based on clinical suspicion after other psychiatric or medical causes have been ruled out. Lower extremity muscle rigidity is one of the few classic signs, with approximately half of patients presenting with confusion or disorientation and one third with agitation.

Although serotonin syndrome is rare, it is potentially lethal: 1 of every 10 patients dies. The primary treatment is to discontinue drug therapy, which is clearly not a field intervention. In the field, management is primarily supportive. Pay close attention to the patient's ability to protect the airway because 25% of patients with serotonin syndrome eventually require intubation.

Lithium

Despite the major advances made in many areas of psychiatric medicine, lithium remains the cornerstone drug for the treatment of bipolar disorder. In 1949, lithium salts made their debut for the treatment of mania. Eventually, they were found to be much more efficacious for the treatment of bipolar disorder, and they retain their position as the main treatment for this condition.

Pathophysiology Lithium is almost completely absorbed in the GI tract roughly 8 hours after ingestion. Bioelimination occurs relatively slowly, with approximately 95% of the lithium eliminated in the urine; although two thirds of the lithium dose is excreted within 12 hours after ingestion, the remainder is excreted during the next 2 weeks. Given its small therapeutic window and slow excretion process, the threat of toxic levels and overdosing is ever present.

Assessment Early signs and symptoms of lithium overdose include nausea, vomiting, hand tremors, excessive thirst, and slurred speech. With increased toxicity come increased neurologic symptoms: ataxia, muscle weakness and incoordination, blurred vision, and hyperreflexia (twitching). Eventually, the patient may have seizures and become comatose.

Management Management of a patient suspected of a lithium overdose is mostly supportive. Establish and maintain the airway, inserting an advanced airway as needed. Provide high-concentration supplemental oxygen, and establish vascular access. If the patient experiences hypotension, administer serial boluses of normal saline. Maintain continuous ECG monitoring, being alert for AV blocks and ventricular dysrhythmias. Finally, transport the patient to an appropriate facility.

◼ Nonprescription Pain Medications

Medications used for pain management make up a large part of the OTC drug market. In the OTC and prescription drug markets, nonsteroidal anti-inflammatory drugs (NSAIDs) are some of the most popular options for pain relief, fever control, and anti-inflammatory action. Their convenient dosing schemes and large therapeutic windows, coupled with their safe track records relative to acute ingestion and overdose, enhance their popularity.

Pathophysiology

NSAIDs are rapidly absorbed from the GI tract before being eliminated from the body in urine and feces. The half-lives of these agents vary widely, ranging from 2 to 4 hours for ibuprofen, to approximately 15 hours for selective cyclooxygenase-2 inhibitors, to 50 hours for some long-acting agents. Patients who take lithium and NSAIDs have slowed renal clearance of the lithium, increasing the likelihood that they will inadvertently reach a toxic lithium level.

Most of the problems associated with NSAID use involve long-term use; patients may experience GI bleeding and kidney dysfunction. Acute ingestion and overdoses are rare, with ibuprofen being the NSAID most commonly encountered in the acute setting.

Assessment

At toxic levels, the signs and symptoms of NSAID overdose may include headache, altered mentation (cognitive difficulties, behavioral changes), seizures, bradydysrhythmia, hypotension, abdominal pain, nausea, and vomiting. However, many patients who experience NSAID overdose remain asymptomatic.

Management

For symptomatic patients, care in the prehospital setting is usually supportive. Establish and maintain the airway, inserting an advanced airway as needed. Administer high-concentration supplemental oxygen, and establish vascular access. If hypotension develops, administer fluid boluses of normal saline. If hypotension persists after sequential fluid boluses, consider giving a vasopressor. Treat seizures with benzodiazepines per local protocol. Finally, transport the patient to an appropriate facility.

A unique side effect of NSAID use is aseptic meningitis, in which a patient presents with complaints of a stiff neck, headache, and fever within several hours after taking an NSAID. Discontinuing the NSAID therapy generally resolves the problem, but patients must be evaluated at the hospital to rule out other causes.

Salicylates

Although aspirin (acetylsalicylic acid, or ASA) can be involved in a toxic event, more typically OTC products containing salicylates cause toxicity. For example, a single 30-mL dose of Pepto-Bismol (bismuth subsalicylate) contains 261 mg of salicylate (two thirds the total dose of one aspirin). Similarly, many of the liniments used with hot-air vaporizers contain high levels of methyl salicylate. With continued use of these products for a period of days, infants or young toddlers may ingest toxic levels of the salicylate.

Pathophysiology The clinical presentation of salicylate overdose can change based on three primary variables: the patient's age, the dose ingested, and the duration of the exposure. Ingestion of 150 mg/kg or less will usually make a person "mildly toxic." At this level, chief complaints are usually nausea, vomiting, and abdominal pain. With a dosing range of 150 to 300 mg/kg, moderate toxicity results, with signs and symptoms including vomiting, diaphoresis, hyperpnea, ringing in the ears, pulmonary edema, and acid-base disturbances. At levels of 300 mg/kg, severe toxicity may produce metabolic acidosis or combined respiratory alkalosis–metabolic acidosis.

When pediatric patients have an acute salicylate episode, the ingestion is usually accidental, the symptoms are mild, and they recover swiftly. A chronic event (possibly from several days of vaporizer use) is usually much more serious in pediatric patients.

By comparison, an acute salicylate event with an adult usually involves an intentional overdose, with the most common patient profile being young women with a history of drug abuse or psychiatric problems. A fatal event is possible if an adult with suspected salicylate overdose is unresponsive during the primary assessment and presents with a high fever, seizures, or cardiac dysrhythmias.

Assessment and Management No salicylate antidote or antagonist is available, so field management is primarily supportive. Establish and maintain the airway, inserting an advanced airway as needed. Provide high-concentration supplemental oxygen, and establish vascular access. Because of the fast, deep tachypnea often associated with aspirin overdose, stay alert for signs of respiratory fatigue. If hypotension develops (from volume depletion), administer serial boluses of normal saline. Monitor carbon dioxide levels with capnometry. Following consultation with medical control, administer one dose of activated charcoal. In addition, consult with medical control regarding urine alkalinization with sodium bicarbonate. Finally, transport the patient to an appropriate facility.

Acetaminophen

Acetaminophen is a well-tolerated drug with few side effects that is available on an OTC basis. These characteristics have made this drug one of the best-selling analgesics in the United States—and a common culprit in toxic exposures. In one publication, the Toxic Drug Exposure System revealed that acetaminophen was involved in 5% of all toxic exposures and produced 23% of all deaths from this cause. Its lethality is believed to stem from two sources: a widely held belief that acetaminophen is not a dangerous drug and a general lack of awareness that acetaminophen is an ingredient in many other preparations.

Pathophysiology Once ingested, acetaminophen is rapidly absorbed from the GI tract, producing peak serum levels in 30 to 120 minutes. Absorption slows when the drug is combined with diphenhydramine (Tylenol PM) or with propoxyphene (Darvocet). One unique aspect of acetaminophen toxicity is that the signs and symptoms appear in four distinct stages **Table 7**.

Assessment and Management It is important for you to try to accurately estimate the time of ingestion because this information drives the decision-making process for patient care in the field and the hospital. Although an antidote for acetaminophen toxicity exists—namely, acetylcysteine (Acetadote)—ideally this drug should be given less than 8 hours after the ingestion.

Table 7 Signs and Symptoms of Acetaminophen Toxicity

Stage	Time Frame	Signs and Symptoms
I	< 24 h	Nausea, vomiting, loss of appetite, pallor, malaise
II	24–72 h	Right upper quadrant abdominal pain; abdomen tender to palpation
III	72–96 h	Metabolic acidosis, renal failure, coagulopathies, recurring GI symptoms
IV	4–14 d (or longer)	Recovery slowly begins, or liver failure progresses and the patient dies

Typically, however, it is administered based on the patient's laboratory results; as such, it is not a field intervention.

Management of the patient in the field first focuses on establishing and maintaining the airway, with an advanced airway being inserted as needed. Administer high-concentration supplemental oxygen, and establish vascular access. For recent ingestions, administer activated charcoal after consulting with medical control. Finally, transport the patient to an appropriate facility.

▪ Theophylline

Theophylline, caffeine, and theobromine are naturally occurring alkaloids found in a variety of plants around the world; they belong to the family of drugs called methylated xanthines. It is estimated that half the world's population drinks tea, which contains caffeine and theophylline. Cocoa and chocolate contain caffeine and theobromine as well.

Pathophysiology

For many years, theophylline was used to treat patients with chronic obstructive pulmonary disease and asthma, primarily because of its bronchodilatory effects. In addition, theophylline is a potent CNS stimulant. Even when taken in normal therapeutic doses, it can cause a variety of ECG rhythm disturbances, including sinus or atrial tachycardia, frequent premature atrial contractions, atrial fibrillation, and atrial flutter. Even more problematic is the occurrence of premature ventricular contractions and ventricular dysrhythmias, including ventricular tachycardia. Theophylline has a small therapeutic window. This narrow safety range, coupled with the prevalence of CNS and cardiovascular side effects and the continued development of beta-2 agonists for chronic obstructive pulmonary disease and asthma treatment, has led to decreased use of theophylline.

Peak levels of theophylline are reached within 90 to 120 minutes after ingestion, except in the case of sustained-release preparations, which may take as long as 8 hours to produce peak serum levels. Absorption rates increase if the drug is taken on an empty stomach or with large amounts of fluids, but also can decrease when theophylline is taken with certain foods. Approximately 85% to 90% of the drug is metabolized by the liver, with the remainder excreted in the urine.

Assessment and Management

Most toxic exposures of theophylline in adults involve unintentional overdoses, usually resulting from the drug's variable absorption rate and small therapeutic window. The toxic effects may range from mild GI distress (nausea and vomiting) to life-threatening or fatal cardiac dysrhythmias. A patient taking theophylline can quickly go from being asymptomatic to a life-threatening state with little to no warning. Complaints of restlessness, insomnia, tremors, agitation, and other signs and symptoms of CNS overstimulation are common, as are cardiac dysrhythmias.

Because of the rapidity with which a patient's condition may deteriorate, prompt intervention is essential, especially in regard to the use of activated charcoal, which can greatly reduce the half-life of theophylline. First, establish and maintain the airway, inserting an advanced airway as needed. Administer high-flow supplemental oxygen, and establish vascular access. Continuously monitor the ECG rhythm. After consulting with medical control, administer activated charcoal, repeating the dosing as necessary. If hypotension develops, administer fluid boluses; if they fail to relieve the problem, administer a vasopressor. You may also consider low-dose beta blockers, per your local protocol. For symptomatic reentry supraventricular tachycardia, you may give adenosine, but stay alert for bronchospasm (a potential side effect of adenosine). Finally, treat dysrhythmias per ACLS (see the chapter, *Cardiovascular Emergencies*).

Metals and Metalloids

Although acute metal and metalloid toxic exposures are relatively rare, when they occur, they can produce devastating results, usually because of delayed diagnosis or misdiagnosis. The difficulty reaching the correct diagnosis may contribute to increased mortality or morbidity because of delayed or inadequate treatment. Toxic exposures involving metals or metalloids usually manifest by affecting four body systems: neurologic, hematologic, renal, and GI.

Lead

Despite the bans on lead in gasoline, paint, canning processes, and plumbing, lead poisoning remains the leading cause of chronic metal poisoning. It has long been known that elevated lead levels may significantly hamper intellectual development in children.

Pathophysiology With inorganic lead, absorption usually occurs via the respiratory or GI tract. Once in the body, approximately 90% of the lead is stored in bone. From this site, it eventually makes its way into the bloodstream. Inorganic lead can also cross the placental barrier and negatively affect fetal development. Its excretion from the body is incredibly slow, with the half-life of lead in bone estimated at 30 years.

Most organic lead (tetraethyl lead) exposures occur in the occupational setting, although they can also occur from gas sniffing where leaded gasoline is available. Once in the body, tetraethyl lead is metabolized to inorganic lead and triethyl lead, with triethyl lead the primary cause of CNS toxicity.

Assessment and Management Lead poisoning is associated with a long list of signs and symptoms (Table 8). In particular, encephalopathy is a major cause of mortality and morbidity from lead poisoning.

In the field, you have few treatment options for lead poisoning. Your most helpful move may be identification of the source of the lead, which can assist the appropriate government agency to prevent more occurrences by removing the toxin. When you are managing the patient, first establish and maintain the airway, inserting an advanced airway as needed. Administer high-flow supplemental oxygen. Establish vascular access with a saline or heparin lock. Unless hypotension is present, do not provide fluid therapy—it may worsen cerebral edema. Transport the patient to an appropriate facility.

Table 8 Systems Affected by Lead Poisoning

System	Signs and Symptoms
CNS	Altered mentation, including irritability, mood changes, memory deficit, sleep disturbances; headache; seizures; ataxia
GI	Abdominal pain (usually occurs with acute poisoning); constipation; diarrhea
Renal	Renal insufficiency; hypertension; gout
Hematologic	Anemia

Iron

A recent AAPCC annual report identified 30,000 calls specific to iron supplement ingestion. Although only a small amount of iron is required as part of a healthy diet, many adult and pediatric multivitamins contain iron. Children younger than 6 years have frequent iron exposures, usually secondary to ingesting chewable vitamins. By comparison, most toxic exposures in adults are intentional.

Pathophysiology In the average 70-kg adult, the body's entire iron supply consists of only about 4 g. Of that total, roughly 65% is found in hemoglobin, with the remainder sequestered elsewhere. Because of its toxic potential, iron is stored in the body by several mechanisms, which permit access to the supply as needed. The body of a healthy person does not contain "free" (unbound) iron.

From a practical perspective, the toxic effects of an iron exposure reflect the amount of elemental iron ingested. With ingestion of 20 to 60 mg/kg, mild to moderate toxicity should be expected. With dosing of more than 60 mg/kg, severe and potentially lethal toxicity is a possibility.

Assessment and Management Two broad categories of iron poisoning can be distinguished: GI and systemic. With GI toxicity, the symptoms consist of abdominal pain, vomiting (the most common sign), and diarrhea. With systemic toxicity, patients may be hypotensive or in frank shock from coagulopathy and vomiting blood. They are commonly in metabolic acidosis and become tachypneic as the body attempts to adjust pH by increasing the elimination of carbon dioxide.

Children typically remain asymptomatic when they have a low-level iron exposure. However, children who ingest a large dose of iron are at risk of dying unless aggressive and timely interventions take place. Unfortunately, there is little you can do in the field for iron poisoning, other than provide basic attention to the ABCs and transport the patient to the hospital for further evaluation and laboratory studies.

Mercury

Mercury exists in a variety of organic and inorganic forms. In the human body, all forms produce toxic effects. Although accidental exposures to mercury often occur in the occupational setting, mercury can be found in the home in thermometers and in some switches used in heating and air conditioning.

Pathophysiology Organic mercury is lipid-soluble and quickly accumulates in the liver, CNS, and kidneys. It can also cross the placental membrane into the fetus.

Assessment Mercury poisoning can present differently depending on the type of mercury and its route of entry into the body. Most signs and symptoms involve the CNS and GI and renal systems. CNS alterations may include anxiety, depression, irritability, sleep disturbances, and memory loss. In addition, tremors, ataxia, paresthesias, muscle weakness or rigidity, and excessive drooling may develop.

Management In the occupational setting, safe removal of the patient from the exposure source is the primary intervention. In all cases of suspected mercury poisoning, your management is supportive and includes basic attention to the ABCs and transport to the hospital. In the hospital setting, the patient may undergo aggressive GI decontamination and receive dimercaprol (BAL), succimer (DMSA), or other agents.

Arsenic

The most common cause of acute metal poisoning and the second leading cause of chronic metal poisoning is arsenic. This metal is used in a variety of industries and appears in a variety of compounds, so it is often the source of unintentional exposures. Intentional exposures include the use of arsenic in homicide and suicide.

Pathophysiology Arsenic can enter the body by ingestion, inhalation, and absorption and dermally through a wound. It is eliminated from the body through the kidneys.

Assessment The clinical presentation of arsenic poisoning depends on the type, amount, and concentration of arsenic that enters the body and the rate of absorption and elimination. In general, symptoms appear within 30 minutes to several hours of arsenic ingestion. Arsenic poisoning should be suspected with patients who present with hypotension of unknown cause following a bout of severe gastroenteritis.

Signs and symptoms of arsenic poisoning include severe abdominal pain, nausea, explosive diarrhea, "metal taste" in the mouth, skin rash, general malaise, weakness, hypotension secondary to fluid loss, pulmonary edema, rhabdomyolysis, and renal failure. ECG changes and dysrhythmias (usually sinus tachycardia or SVTs) may be apparent, but nonspecific ST-segment and T-wave changes are also possible, as is QT prolongation. Ventricular tachycardia and torsades de pointes can occur as well.

Management A patient with acute arsenic toxicity is in critical condition and requires aggressive interventions. Establish and maintain the airway, inserting an advanced airway as needed. Administer high-flow supplemental oxygen, and establish vascular access. For hypotension, administer sequential boluses of normal saline. If the hypotension proves refractory to fluid therapy, administer a vasopressor (dopamine [Inotropin] or dobutamine [Dobutrex]). Continuously monitor the ECG,

and follow ACLS algorithms for dysrhythmias—uncorrected hypotension dysrhythmias may lead to death. For torsades de pointes, consider administration of 2 to 4 grams of magnesium sulfate after consulting with medical control. Finally, provide rapid transport to an appropriate facility.

British anti-Lewisite (also known as BAL and dimercaprol) and Unitol (DMPS) can be used as chelating agents to bind many heavy metals and promote excretion by the body. Treatment with these agents occurs in a health care setting and requires expert consultation. BAL is administered by deep IM injection and Unitol is typically administered by IV infusion, although alternative routes may be used in unusual situations.

■ Poisonous Plants

Of the thousands of plant varieties, only a few are poisonous Figure 14. Oddly enough, poisonous plants represent some of the most common ornamental garden shrubs and houseplants. Perhaps for that reason, 70% to 80% of plant-related exposures involve children younger than 6 years. In the AAPCC's 2001 report, plant ingestions ranked fourth on the list of most common reasons to contact a Poison Center. Thankfully, deaths from plant ingestions are rare (< 0.001% of all cases). Table 9 lists plants that can cause toxic results and, in some cases, death.

Pathophysiology

The ubiquitous <u>dieffenbachia</u> is a lovely green plant with broad, variegated leaves. It is nicknamed "dumb cane," because eating dieffenbachia can result in a person being unable to speak. All parts of the dieffenbachia plant—leaves, stems, roots—contain sharp caladium oxalate crystals. When ingested, the crystals cause burns of the mouth and tongue and, sometimes, paralysis of the vocal cords. In severe cases, edema of the tongue and larynx may lead to airway compromise.

<u>Caladium</u>, with its stunning multicolored leaves, is another hazardous plant. Like dieffenbachia, it contains caladium oxalate crystals and produces the same results when ingested. Nausea, vomiting, and diarrhea commonly occur after ingestion of either plant.

<u>Lantana</u> (also known as red sage or wild sage) is a perennial flowering shrub with clusters of little red berries. These berries—particularly when ripe—can lead to serious poisoning. Even when still green, the berries contain lantadene A, a poison that causes stomach upsets, muscle weakness, shock, and sometimes death.

Another dangerous plant is the <u>castor bean</u>. The seeds of this attractive shrub are highly poisonous—chewing on just a few seeds (and, in some cases, just one) can kill a child. Ricin, the poison in castor beans, causes a variety of toxic effects: burning of the mouth and throat; nausea, vomiting, diarrhea, and severe stomach pains; prostration; failing vision; and kidney failure (the usual cause of death).

<u>Foxglove</u>, which has beautiful trumpetlike flowers, contains cardiac glycosides and is used in making the drug digitalis.

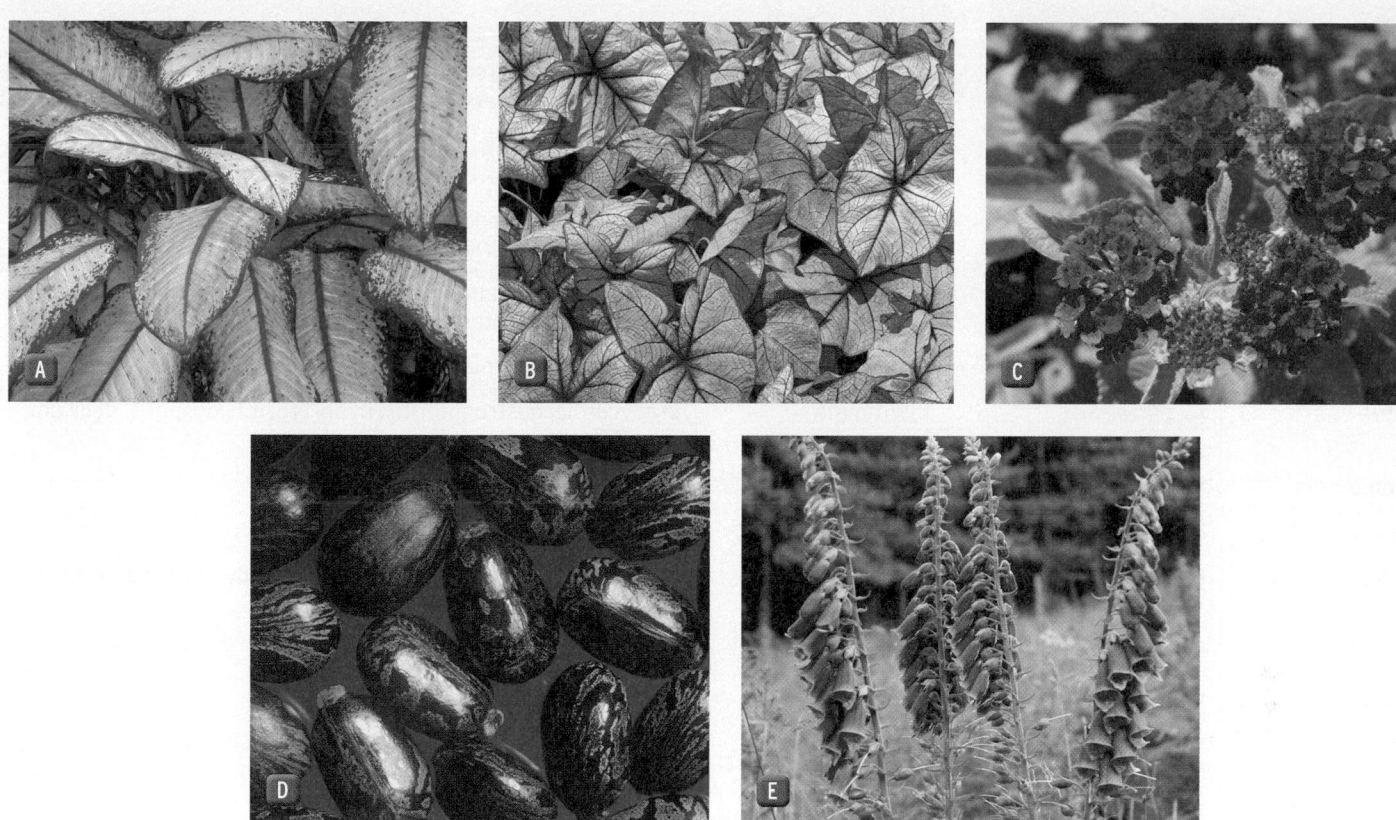

Figure 14 Poisonous plants. **A.** Dieffenbachia. **B.** Caladium. **C.** Lantana. **D.** Castor beans. **E.** Foxglove.

Table 9 Poisons in Some Common Plants

Plant	Poisonous Part	Poison	Signs and Symptoms of Poisoning
Apricot	Seeds	Cyanide	Headache, dizziness, weakness, nausea, vomiting, coma, seizures
Autumn crocus	Entire plant	Colchicine	Cramps, nausea, hematuria, diarrhea, coma, shock
Bird of paradise	Pod	Multiple	Vomiting, diarrhea
Bloodroot	Root	Sanguinarine	Cramps, diarrhea, dizziness, paralysis, coma
Buttercup	Entire plant	Protoanemonin	Gastroenteritis, seizures
Caladium	Leaves and roots	Calcium oxalate	Burning of mucous membranes, swelling of the tongue and throat, salivation, gastroenteritis
Cherry	Bark, leaves, seed	Amygdalin	Stupor, vocal cord paralysis, seizures, coma
Chinaberry	Berry; leaves and bark to a lesser extent	Tetranortriterpene neurotoxins	Vomiting, diarrhea, sometimes excitement or depression
Daffodil	Bulb	Multiple	Gastroenteritis
Deadly nightshade	Berry, leaf, root	Atropine	Fever; tachycardia; dilated pupils; hot, red, dry skin
Dieffenbachia	Leaves and roots	Calcium oxalate	Same as for caladium
Elderberry	Leaf, shoot, bark	Sambunigrin	Gastroenteritis
Holly	Berries	Ilicin	Gastroenteritis, coma

Continues

Table 9 Poisons in Some Common Plants, continued

Plant	Poisonous Part	Poison	Signs and Symptoms of Poisoning
Hyacinth	Bulb	Multiple	Severe gastroenteritis
Jack-in-the-pulpit	All parts	Calcium oxalate	Severe gastroenteritis
Jimson weed	All parts	Atropine	Dry mouth; hot, red skin; headache; hallucinations; tachycardia; hypertension; delirium; seizures
Laurel	All parts	Andromedotoxin	Salivation, lacrimation, rhinorrhea, vomiting, seizures, bradycardia, hypotension, paralysis
Lily of the valley	Leaf, flowers	Glycosides	Cardiac dysrhythmias, nausea
Mistletoe	All parts	Tyramine	Bradycardia, gastroenteritis, hypertension, dyspnea, delirium, sweating, shock
Morning glory	Seeds	LSD	Hallucinations
Narcissus	Bulb	Multiple	Gastroenteritis
Oleander	Entire plant	Oleanin	Cramps, bradycardia, dilated pupils, bloody diarrhea, coma, apnea (one leaf is lethal)
Philodendron	Entire plant	Calcium oxalate	Edema of tongue, throat
Poinsettia	Leaves, stem, sap	Multiple	Contact dermatitis, gastroenteritis
Potato	Green tubers, new sprouts	Solanine	Severe gastroenteritis, headache, apnea, shock
Rhododendron	Entire plant	Andromedotoxin	Salivation
Rhubarb	Leaves only	Oxalic acid	Cramps, nausea, vomiting, anuria
Wisteria	Pods	Glycoside	Severe gastroenteritis, shock

Along with nausea, vomiting, diarrhea, and abdominal cramps, ingestion of foxglove can produce hyperkalemia and cardiac dysrhythmias, usually bradydysrhythmias.

Assessment

When you encounter a case of plant poisoning, get all the information you can from the parent, and then consult your regional Poison Center for advice:

- *When was the plant ingested?* If it was more than 12 hours ago and the patient is still asymptomatic, it is likely that the patient will not experience any medical problems. Most plant poisonings produce signs and symptoms of toxicity, if they are going to do so, within 4 hours of ingestion. One notable exception is the castor bean, for which symptoms may not appear until 1 to 3 days after ingestion.
- *What, exactly, did the child eat?* Try to find out not just which type of plant, but also which parts of the plant (leaves, root, stem, flower, or fruit) were eaten. If possible, estimate how much was ingested (such as a bite or two from a leaf, three or four leaves). If you transport the child to the hospital, take the offending plant—or whatever is left of it—with you.
- *What signs or symptoms, if any, does the child have?*

Management

Most plant-related exposures require no treatment—a decision that can be made after consulting with the Poison Center and medical control per local protocol. If there is a responsible adult who can keep a close eye on the child for at least 4 to 6 hours after the ingestion, there is no need to transport the child to the hospital. Conversely, a child with any signs or symptoms should be evaluated in the ED.

■ Poisonous Mushrooms

Four groups of people are most likely to be the victims of poisoning related to mushroom ingestion: wild mushroom pickers, people looking for hallucinogenic mushrooms to get high, people attempting suicide or homicide, and young children who eat them by accident. Even among educated people who like to gather their own mushrooms in the wild, mistakes can happen. In 2001, Poison Centers received 8,400 calls related to mushroom ingestions, with 70% occurring in children younger than 6 years. Thankfully, most of these events result in limited or no toxic effects.

Pathophysiology

A variety of factors determine whether a mushroom ingestion will produce toxic results: the age of the mushroom, the season

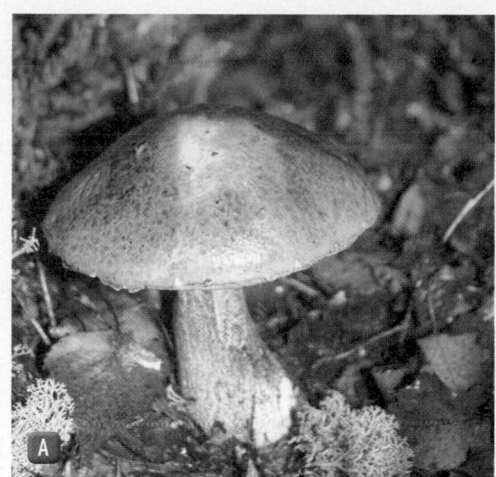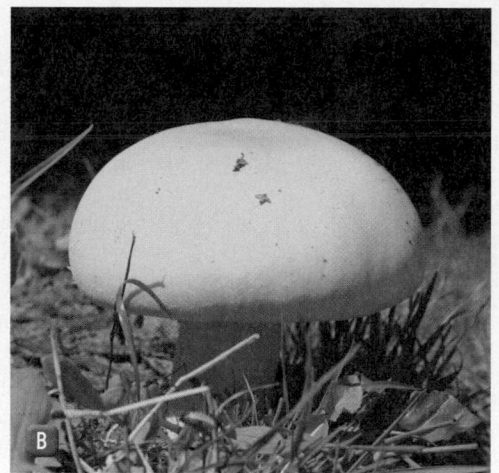

Figure 15 **A.** The deadly *Amanita* mushroom. **B.** A nonpoisonous, edible mushroom.

take place in restaurants, cafeterias, and delicatessens.

Pathophysiology

Three toxins—*Salmonella, Listeria,* and *Toxoplasma*—produce roughly 35% of all food-related deaths. Poisoning with *Clostridium botulinum,* an extremely deadly toxin, is usually the result of improper food storage or canning. In addition, the toxins produced by dinoflagellates in "red tides" may contaminate bivalve shellfish such as oysters, clams, and mussels and produce life-threatening or fatal paralytic shellfish poisoning. Cooking does not kill these toxins.

in which it was gathered, the amount ingested, and the preparation method. Toxic effects vary from mild GI signs and symptoms to severe cytotoxic—even lethal—effects. In the United States, many deaths due to mushroom ingestion involve the *Amanita* species (*Amanita phalloides, Amanita virosa,* and *Amanita verna*) **Figure 15** .

Assessment

Time of symptom onset can serve as a predictor of potential severity. If the patient presents with symptoms within approximately 2 hours of ingestion, the event is most likely to be non–life-threatening. By comparison, if symptom onset occurs 6 hours or later, there is a much greater likelihood the event will be serious and potentially fatal. The most common patient complaints involve GI signs or symptoms, including abdominal cramping and watery or bloody diarrhea. Patients may also experience chills or headaches.

Management

Management for a symptomatic patient with a toxic mushroom ingestion includes supportive measures. Establish and maintain the airway, and establish vascular access. For hypotension secondary to vomiting and diarrhea, administer fluid boluses of normal saline. Contact the Poison Center and medical control per local protocol, and administer activated charcoal if directed to do so. Finally, transport the patient to an appropriate facility.

Food Poisoning

Whenever you encounter two or more people sick at the same time and at the same scene with similar symptoms, think food poisoning or CO poisoning—your hunch will likely be correct. In the United States, an estimated 76 million food-related illnesses occur each year, requiring 325,000 hospitalizations and producing 5,000 deaths. Almost half of these food poisonings

Assessment

Depending on the toxin, onset of signs and symptoms can range from several hours after ingestion to days or weeks. The longer the time until symptom onset, the more difficult it will be to link the patient's problem to the event at which the toxin was ingested. Gastrointestinal complaints are the most common and include abdominal pain and cramping, nausea, vomiting, and diarrhea. With prolonged episodes of vomiting or diarrhea, hypotension secondary to fluid loss and electrolyte imbalance becomes likely. Respiratory distress or arrest can occur with toxins such as *C botulinum* or those found in paralytic shellfish poisoning.

Management

Management for patients with food poisoning is usually supportive because most cases you encounter will not be life threatening, and the signs and symptoms of acute gastroenteritis are typically self-limiting. Establish and maintain the airway, inserting an advanced airway as needed. Administer high-flow supplemental oxygen, and establish vascular access. For hypotension secondary to fluid loss, administer fluid boluses of normal saline. Consider administration of antiemetics, per local protocol. For patients with facial flushing (most likely secondary to histamine release), consider administration of diphenhydramine per local protocol. Finally, transport the patient to an appropriate facility.

Words of Wisdom

Herbal preparations can cause potentially serious interactions with traditional medications. There have been cases of overdose which involved herbal preparations. Be sure to determine all medications the patient may have taken, including herbal medications or supplements.

YOU are the Medic   SUMMARY

1. What is your first impression of this patient?

This patient is a critical, load-and-go patient. You may or may not assume an overdose at this point, but from what you do know it is possible. Some of the signs that may lead you to an assumption of an overdose are the scar tissue on the arms, the suspicious way the patient was left at the scene, and the lack of respiratory sufficiency with a strong pulse.

2. What is your priority for patient care?

Maintaining a patent airway and providing adequate ventilation for this patient are imperative measures that should be done prior to anything else. Whatever is causing the patient to hypoventilate will cause her to arrest from hypoxia in a short amount of time.

3. If this patient has overdosed, which drug classification would be your focus?

The classic presentation of opioid use consists of euphoria, hypotension, respiratory depression, and pinpoint pupils. Depending on the particular agent, nausea, vomiting, and constipation may occur as well. With increased doses, coma, seizures (usually secondary to hypoxia), and cardiac arrest (usually secondary to respiratory arrest) are common.

4. Give some examples of drugs that would meet this classification.

Narcotic agents include morphine, codeine, heroin, fentanyl (Sublimaze), oxycodone (OxyContin), meperidine (Demerol), propoxyphene (Darvon), and dextromethorphan. Although these drugs share certain commonalities, they exhibit highly diverse effects and vary widely in their potency. Opioids are used primarily in clinical medicine for analgesia, whereas the illicit drug heroin is abused for the unique euphoria it produces.

5. Should you intubate this patient?

A patient who has overdosed on opioids is almost always hypoventilating, sometimes breathing as few as 4 or 5 breaths/

min, and is consequently hypoxic and hypercarbic. Rather than moving immediately to intubation, you should place an oropharyngeal airway and provide bag-mask ventilation with 15 L/min of supplemental oxygen. If this is an opioid overdose, you may be able to correct it and reverse the hypoventilation in a matter of minutes.

6. What is your next step in treating this patient after the airway is controlled?

You should establish IV access and assess for other causes for the patient's condition. Is the patient wearing a medic alert tag or any other medical identification? Is drug paraphernalia present at the scene? If you are preparing to give a medication, make sure it is appropriate by obtaining as much information as possible.

7. What is your medication choice and dosage to treat this patient?

Administer 0.4 to 2 mg of naloxone (Narcan). For street heroin, which can range in purity from 5% to 30%, as little as 0.4 mg of naloxone may bring a patient back to consciousness before you can remove the hub from the injection port. This abrupt reversal can have clinical and safety implications, so titrate the dose. The best approach is to draw up 2 mg of naloxone in a 10-mL syringe and fill the rest of the syringe with normal saline. Administer the naloxone just to the point that the patient's respirations improve.

8. What should you do if this medication does not correct the overdose?

Sometimes the patient may not respond to naloxone. Perhaps the patient has taken a potent synthetic drug such as fentanyl, which may require a much higher dose of naloxone to reverse its effects. This may also be a mixed overdose in which more than one drug was taken. If allowed by protocol, repeat the naloxone dose or call for orders to increase the dose.

EMS Patient Care Report (PCR)

Date: 08-10-11	**Incident No.:** 4563	**Nature of Call:** OD		**Location:** 6th and Main	
Dispatched: 0310	**En Route:** 0311	**At Scene:** 0317	**Transport:** 0337	**At Hospital:** 0345	**In Service:** 0400

Patient Information

Age: Approx 20 **Sex:** F **Weight (in kg [lb]):** 50 kg (110 lb)	**Allergies:** Unknown **Medications:** Unknown **Past Medical History:** Unknown **Chief Complaint:** Possible overdose

Vital Signs

Time: 0322	**BP:** 100/58	**Pulse:** 100	**Respirations:** 6	**Spo₂:** 90% on room air
Time: 0327	**BP:** 98/56	**Pulse:** 100	**Respirations:** Assisted	**Spo₂:** 96% O₂
Time: 0337	**BP:** 100/60	**Pulse:** 98	**Respirations:** 10	**Spo₂:** 97% O₂

YOU are the Medic   SUMMARY, continued

EMS Treatment (circle all that apply)				
Oxygen @ __15__ L/min via (circle one): NC **(NRM)** Bag-mask device		Assisted Ventilation	Airway Adjunct OPA	CPR
Defibrillation	Bleeding Control	Bandaging	Splinting	Other

Narrative
Arrived on scene with PD present at the corner of 6th Street and Main Street for a possible overdose. This pt appears to be an approximately 20-year-old woman that was found down on the sidewalk. PD reports the pt was dropped off from a vehicle that left the scene. Pt is unconscious with a resp of 6 per min. The pt has a strong radial pulse and visible track marks on her forearms. Airway maintained with OPA and BVM at 15 L/min assisted to a rate of 14 breaths per min. IV established, BGL is 120 off of the hub. Naloxone (Narcan) administered at 0.4 mg IVP without change. Dose repeated × 1 per protocol with an increase in respiratory effort noted. Pt responds to painful stimuli post Narcan and oral airway removed due to increased gag reflex. Pt transported emergency to regional hospital. Report to Dr. Smith on arrival. **End of report**

Prep Kit

Ready for Review

- Toxicologic emergencies usually fall under one of two general headings: intentional and unintentional.

- Given the variety of illicit drugs coupled with the continued growth of licit drugs, even the most well-read veteran paramedic may find it difficult to stay current with the myriad drugs sold in the streets today. For this reason, Poison Centers may be an indispensable aid.

- The four primary methods whereby a toxin commonly enters the body are ingestion, inhalation, injection, and absorption.

- Although the sheer number of substances of abuse may seem daunting, the good news is that many drugs of similar design, on entering the body, produce similar signs and symptoms as the original parent drug.

- Human beings have a long history of abusing drugs and alcohol. With the passing of time, the physiologic and societal effects of alcohol abuse have become well known and thoroughly documented. Unfortunately, the area of medicine dealing with drugs of abuse is challenging because of uncertainty about the prevalence of the problem and the continual evolution of the substances themselves.

- Alcohol is the most widely abused drug in the United States.

- Generally, patients with toxicologic emergencies are considered medical patients, although toxicologic emergencies may lead to trauma, too.

- From a management perspective, ALS care for toxicologic emergencies builds on the basics:
  - Ensure the scene is safe for access and egress.
  - Maintain the airway; secure it as needed.
  - Ensure that breathing is adequate.
  - Ensure that circulation is not compromised (by hypoperfusion or dysrhythmia).
  - Maintain adequate blood/oxygen saturations (95%).
  - Establish vascular access.
  - Be prepared to manage shock, coma, seizures, and dysrhythmias.
  - Transport the patient as soon as possible. Place the patient in the left lateral recumbent position if there is any risk of vomiting to reduce the risk of aspiration.

Vital Vocabulary

alcoholism A state of physical and psychological addiction to ethanol.

amphetamines A class of drugs that increase alertness and excitation (stimulants); includes methamphetamine (crank or ice), methylenedioxyamphetamine (MDA, Adam), and methylenedioxymethamphetamine (MDMA, Eve, ecstasy).

antagonist Something that counteracts the action of something else; in relation to drugs, a drug that is an antagonist has an affinity for a cell receptor and, by binding to it, the cell is prevented from responding.

barbiturates Potent sedative-hypnotics historically used as sleep aids, antianxiety drugs, and as part of the regimen for seizure control.

benzodiazepines The family of sedative-hypnotics most commonly used to treat anxiety, seizures, and alcohol withdrawal.

caladium A common houseplant that contains caladium oxalate crystals; ingestion leads to nausea, vomiting, and diarrhea.

castor bean A seed that contains the poison ricin; causes a variety of toxic effects: burning of the mouth and throat; nausea, vomiting, diarrhea, and severe stomach pains; prostration; failing vision; and kidney failure, which is the usual cause of death.

caustics Chemicals that are acids or alkalis; cause direct chemical injury to the tissues they contact.

cocaine A stimulant; a naturally occurring alkaloid that is extracted from the *Erythroxylon coca* plant leaves found in South America.

delirium tremens (DTs) A severe withdrawal syndrome seen in people with alcoholism who are deprived of ethyl alcohol; characterized by restlessness, fever, sweating, disorientation, agitation, and seizures; can be fatal if untreated.

dieffenbachia A common houseplant that resembles "elephant ears"; ingestion leads to burns of the mouth and tongue and, possibly, paralysis of the vocal cords and nausea and vomiting; in severe cases, may be edema of the tongue and larynx, leading to airway compromise.

drug Substance that has some therapeutic effect (such as reducing inflammation, fighting bacteria, or producing euphoria) when given in the appropriate circumstances and in the appropriate dose.

drug abuse Any use of drugs that causes physical, psychological, economic, legal, or social harm to the user or others affected by the user's behavior.

drug addiction A chronic disorder characterized by the compulsive use of a substance that results in physical, psychological, or social harm to the user who continues to use the substance despite the harm.

foxglove A plant that contains cardiac glycosides used in making digitalis; ingestion of leaves causes nausea, vomiting, diarrhea, abdominal cramps, hyperkalemia, and a variety of dysrhythmias.

habituation The situation in which there is a physical tolerance and psychological dependence on a drug or drugs.

hallucinogen An agent that produces false perceptions in any one of the five senses.

hydrocarbons Compounds made up principally of hydrogen and carbon atoms mostly obtained from the distillation of petroleum.

illicit In relation to drugs, illegal drugs such as marijuana, cocaine, and LSD.

lantana A perennial flowering shrub with clusters of red berries that can lead to serious and even fatal poisoning. Also known as red sage or wild sage; ingestion causes stomach upsets, muscle weakness, shock, and, sometimes, death.

licit In relation to drugs, legalized drugs such as coffee, alcohol, and tobacco.

lithium The cornerstone drug for the treatment of bipolar disorder.

marijuana The dried leaves and flower buds of the *Cannabis sativa* plant that are smoked to achieve a high.

methamphetamine A highly addictive drug in the amphetamine family.

monoamine oxidase inhibitors (MAOIs) Psychiatric medication used primarily to treat atypical depression by increasing norepinephrine and serotonin levels in the central nervous system.

narcotic The generic term for opiates and opioids, drugs that act as a CNS depressant and produce insensibility or stupor.

opiate Various alkaloids derived from the opium or poppy plant.

opioid A synthetic narcotic not derived from opium.

organophosphates A class of chemical found in many insecticides used in agriculture and in the home.

physical dependence A physiologic state of adaptation to a drug, usually characterized by tolerance to the drug's effects and a withdrawal syndrome if use of the drug is stopped, especially abruptly.

poison A substance whose chemical action could damage structures or impair function when introduced into the body.

potentiation Enhancement of the effect of one drug by another drug.

psychological dependence The emotional state of craving a drug to maintain a feeling of well-being.

rhabdomyolysis The destruction of muscle tissue leading to a release of potassium and myoglobin.

salicylates Aspirin-like drugs.

sedative-hypnotic A drug used to reduce anxiety, calm agitated patients, and help produce drowsiness and sleep (CNS depressants).

selective serotonin reuptake inhibitors (SSRIs) A class of antidepressants that inhibit the reuptake of serotonin.

serotonin syndrome An idiosyncratic complication that occurs with antidepressant therapy in which patients have lower extremity muscle rigidity, confusion or disorientation, and/or agitation.

Spice An illicit drug consisting of a blend of synthetic cannibinoids; it can produce delirium and short- and long-term psychotic effects.

synergism The action of two substances such as drugs, in which the *total effects are greater than the sum of the independent effects* of the two substances.

theophylline A naturally occurring alkaloid found in a variety of plants (such as tea leaves).

tolerance Physiologic adaptation to the effects of a drug such that increasingly larger doses of the drug are required to achieve the same effect.

toxicologic emergencies Medical emergencies caused by toxic agents such as poison.

toxidrome The syndrome-like symptoms of any given class or group of poisonous agents.

tricyclic antidepressants (TCAs) A group of drugs used to treat severe depression and manage pain; minimal dosing errors can cause toxic results.

withdrawal syndrome A predictable set of signs and symptoms, usually involving altered central nervous system activity, that occurs after the abrupt cessation of a drug or after rapidly decreasing the usual dosage of a drug.

Assessment in Action

Your unit has responded to a structure fire. The engine company crew has rescued a resident from the structure and moved him outside of the hot zone, so the scene is safe. The patient is a man who is having difficulty breathing. The patient has soot around his nose and mouth, and is coughing forcefully.

1. Prior to placing oxygen on the patient, you assess his Spo_2 level; the pulse oximeter shows this level to be 100%. How do you account for this reading?
   - **A.** The patient is breathing adequately.
   - **B.** The patient is a smoker and can tolerate the exposure.
   - **C.** The pulse oximeter is accurately measuring the saturation of hemoglobin.
   - **D.** The pulse oximeter is not accurately measuring the saturation of hemoglobin.

2. A substance that is toxic by nature, no matter how it gets into the body or in what quantity, is called a:
   - **A.** drug.
   - **B.** poison.
   - **C.** toxin.
   - **D.** substance.

3. Ingestion, inhalation, injection, and absorption are examples of:
   - **A.** routes of administration.
   - **B.** hazardous materials.
   - **C.** methods of identification.
   - **D.** methods of entry.

4. What is the primary treatment for the patient in this scenario?
   - **A.** Correct the patient's hypoxia with oxygen administration.
   - **B.** Administer hydroxocobalamin.
   - **C.** Establish vascular access.
   - **D.** Consider rapid sequence intubation.

5. The syndrome-like symptoms of a poisonous agent are termed:
   - **A.** delirium tremens.
   - **B.** a drug.
   - **C.** a dermatome.
   - **D.** a toxidrome.

6. The action of two substances, such as drugs, in which the total effects are greater than the sum of the independent effects of the two substances, is termed:
   - **A.** dependence.
   - **B.** synergy.
   - **C.** agonism.
   - **D.** antagonism.

Additional Questions

7. What does the mnemonic SLUDGE stand for and which type of chemical exposure causes it?

8. Why do patients who experience a tricyclic antidepressant overdose develop a widened QRS complex?

Psychiatric Emergencies

National EMS Education Standard Competencies

Medicine

Integrates assessment findings with principles of epidemiology and pathophysiology to formulate a field impression and implement a comprehensive treatment/disposition plan for a patient with a medical complaint.

Psychiatric

Recognition of

- Behaviors that pose a risk to the EMS provider, patient, or others (pp 1369-1370)

Assessment and management of

- Basic principles of the mental health system (pp 1369-1370)
- Suicidal/risk (p 1384)

Anatomy, physiology, epidemiology, pathophysiology, psychosocial impact, presentations, assessment, prognosis, and management of

- Acute psychosis (pp 1382-1383)
- Agitated delirium (pp 1383-1384)
- Cognitive disorders (pp 1383-1384)
- Thought disorders (pp 1382, 1383, 1387-1388)
- Mood disorders (p 1386)
- Neurotic disorders (pp 1388-1389)
- Substance-related disorders/addictive behavior (pp 1389-1390)
- Somatoform disorders (p 1390)
- Factitious disorders (p 1390)
- Personality disorders (p 1391)
- Patterns of violence/abuse/neglect (pp 1385-1386)
- Organic psychoses (p 1371)

Knowledge Objectives

1. Discuss the potential causes of behavioral emergencies, including organic and environmental causes. (p 1371)
2. Define normal, abnormal, overt, and covert behavior. (p 1369)

3. Discuss medicolegal considerations and their relevance in psychiatric emergencies. (p 1370)
4. Describe the assessment process for patients with psychiatric emergencies, including safety guidelines and specific questions to ask. (pp 1372-1376)
5. Discuss the importance of history taking when assessing a patient with a psychiatric emergency. (p 1375)
6. Discuss general management of a patient with a psychiatric emergency. (pp 1376-1377)
7. Describe situations where restraint may be justified. (pp 1379-1382)
8. Describe methods used to restrain patients. (pp 1379-1382)
9. Compare physical restraint with chemical restraint and provide examples of when each may be the preferred option, should restraint be necessary. (pp 1379-1382)
10. Describe the care for a psychotic patient. (pp 1382-1383)
11. Define agitated delirium and describe the care for a patient with agitated delirium. (pp 1383-1384)
12. Explain how to recognize the behavior of a patient at risk of suicide, and discuss the management of such a patient. (pp 1384-1385)
13. Discuss risk factors that help indicate whether a patient may become violent. (pp 1385-1386)
14. Explain the safe management of a potentially violent patient. (pp 1385-1386)
15. List specific psychiatric disorders that can play a role when a patient experiences acute psychosis or agitated delirium. (pp 1386-1391)
16. Discuss assessment and management of specific psychiatric emergencies. (pp 1386-1391)
17. Discuss medications used in the treatment of psychiatric disorders. (pp 1391-1393)

Skills Objectives

1. Demonstrate the techniques used to mechanically restrain a patient. (pp 1380-1381)

Introduction

The mind and the body are not separate entities; they are inseparable parts of a whole human being. When a person becomes ill with any disease, that illness will inevitably affect the person's behavior—often making him or her anxious or depressed. Similarly, changes in mental state influence the body's physical health. A depressed person, for example, may lose appetite or become more susceptible to bodily disease. Thus, whenever you examine a patient, it is important to view the patient as a whole person and try to understand both the physical and the mental factors that contribute to the patient's distress.

As a paramedic, you can expect to be called on to care for patients undergoing a psychological or behavioral crisis. This chapter covers various kinds of behavioral emergencies, including those involving overdoses, violent behavior, and mental illness. It will also cover legal concerns when caring for disturbed patients.

Definition of Behavioral Emergency

The concept of <u>behavior</u> has been debated over the years, with most experts defining it as the way people act or perform—for example, how they respond to a situation. Behavior includes all the things people do and the reasons why they do those things. Who defines when the behavior becomes abnormal is also a source of debate, as is who defines what is normal behavior—society in general, a particular community or social group, a parent, a boss, a friend, or even a stranger. Both normal and abnormal behavior may be overt; <u>overt behavior</u> is open and generally understood by those around the person. <u>Covert behaviors</u> are those that have hidden meanings or intentions that only the person understands. Abnormal behavior in and of itself may not be a medical problem and is hardly cause for alarm. The real questions are "When does abnormal behavior require medical intervention?" and "When does it require EMS?" Almost all disordered behavior represents the person's effort to adapt to some stress, whether internal or external. In most cases the disruptive behavior is a temporary action, abating when the person has managed to mobilize his or her psychological defense mechanisms.

<u>Behavioral emergencies</u> are situations in which the patient's presenting problem is some disorder of mood, thought, or behavior that interferes with his or her <u>activities of daily living (ADLs)</u>; ADLs are normal, everyday activities such as getting dressed and taking out the garbage. When a person becomes so depressed that he or she cannot get up in the morning, shower, and make breakfast, or when someone has delusions or hallucinations that prohibit holding a job, a behavioral emergency exists.

A <u>psychiatric emergency</u> exists when the abnormal behavior threatens a person's health and safety or the health and safety of another person. The most extreme examples are situations in which a person becomes suicidal, homicidal, or psychotic. In a psychotic episode, a person often experiences <u>delusions</u> (false beliefs) or <u>hallucinations</u> and illusions (errors in perception) that result in loss of contact with reality. For example, a patient who has taken illicit drugs may experience an alteration of reality—a "bad trip." Psychotic episodes can have dangerous consequences for the patient, bystanders, and the paramedic because of <u>violent behavior</u>, usually from exaggerated fear or paranoia.

No matter how a textbook may define a psychiatric emergency, the *operative* definition of a behavioral or psychiatric emergency is provided by the person who dials 9-1-1. Often what makes a psychiatric emergency an "emergency" is panic on the part of the patient, the family, bystanders, or all of these parties. That panic, in turn, may translate into a demand for action on your part, and you may therefore face intense pressure to do something (such as transport the patient to an emergency department with a crisis unit). Paradoxically, it is precisely in this situation—when the patient is behaving strangely and

YOU are the Medic — PART 1

You are dispatched to the third floor of an apartment building for a 44-year-old man who says he is fearing for his life. You are advised that police have been on scene with this patient for 20 minutes and the patient will not leave his apartment. The apartment building is known to house residents with psychiatric disorders. On arrival at the building, an officer directs you to the elevator and informs you that the patient is not armed, but officers are remaining on scene in case he becomes violent.

You go to the third floor where you are met by another officer. He informs you that they were called to the scene by the patient who had stated that someone was trying to kill him. He told officers that he overheard information he should not have heard, and now someone is going to kill him. The door to the apartment is open and the patient is visible. He does not appear to have a weapon but is refusing to leave the apartment or let anyone in.

1. What are the initial components of the assessment for this patient?

2. What are your safety concerns in dealing with this patient?

bystanders are clamoring for action—that you may feel least able to do something.

It can be difficult to perform to the utmost of your ability when you are trying to understand a person's confused and frayed feelings that are often present during a psychiatric emergency. Dealing with more straightforward problems such as fractures of the legs, cardiac dysrhythmias, or narcotic overdoses may be more comfortable for some paramedics. Paramedics tend to be action-oriented people who like to see tangible results—a hypoglycemic patient improving after a bolus of glucose, or a clinically dead patient restored to life by CPR and defibrillation. What tangible rewards can there be in escorting a confused, hallucinating patient to the hospital, or caring for a belligerent and violent patient who is screaming obscenities?

In fact, prehospital behavioral intervention is possible and often critical in these emergencies. You can make a difference in the life of a disturbed patient, and the skills for doing so can be learned just like any other skill. Indeed, the skills for dealing with abnormal behavior may ultimately be much more important to your work than skills such as endotracheal intubation because, in reality, how many of your calls require that you place an advanced airway? Many more calls require you to care for people who are angry, depressed, agitated, panicky, or out of control. Clearly, it is of benefit to you to learn how to take an organized and systematic approach to emergencies that involve abnormal behavior.

Prevalence

According to the Centers for Disease Control and Prevention (CDC), the average number of mentally unhealthy days (those including stress, depression, and problems with emotions) for Americans has increased. In 1993, Americans reported an average of 2.9 mentally unhealthy days per month, whereas in 2004, this number increased to 3.5 days, where it remains today.

According to the 2009 National Survey on Drug Use and Health: Mental Health Findings published by the U.S. Department of Health and Human Services, Substance Abuse and Mental Health Services Administration (SAMHSA), Office of Applied Studies, there were an estimated 45.1 million adults aged 18 or older in the United States with any mental illness in the past year. This represents 19.9% of all adults in this country. Eleven million adults aged 18 years and older, representing 4.8% of the American population, are estimated to have had a serious mental illness within the last year. The prevalence among specific age groups and ethnicities is shown in Table 1. Results from the 2009 National Survey on Drug Use indicated 21.8 million Americans, aged 12 years and older, an estimated 8.7% of the population, are considered current illicit drug users, a compounding factor in many mental illnesses.

Medicolegal Considerations

Every call has the potential for legal complications, especially calls for behavioral emergencies. When a patient's behavior,

Table 1   Prevalence of Serious Mental Illness in Subgroups of the US Population

Population	Prevalence of Serious Mental Illness (% of population)
Sex	
Women, 18 years or older	6.4
Men, 18 years or older	3.2
Employment	
Unemployed adults	7.1
Employed adults, part-time	5.6
Employed adults, full-time	3.6
Race	
Caucasian	5.3
Native American or Alaska Native	5.3
Hispanic	4.0
African American	3.7
Asian	2.0

speech, and thoughts are erratic and disorganized, it can be difficult for you to communicate clearly and understand the situation. Be prepared to spend time with the disturbed patient. Do not be in a hurry; rather, convey the message that you have the time and concern to learn what is bothering the patient. Obtain consent as with any other patient when possible. If the patient refuses, continue to talk with him or her about the situation, explaining your responsibilities now that you have been called and have responded.

If the patient refuses transportation, follow your local guidelines and standing orders for providing transport against the patient's will. You will often need assistance from law enforcement personnel. In most jurisdictions, paramedics (or anyone else) are not allowed to restrain or transport persons against their will except possibly at the express order of a county mental health physician.

Be clear in your explanations about administering treatments and medications. Do not assume the patient is unable to understand what you are trying to do, regardless of the patient's state of mind. You should still include the patient in his or her own care as much as possible. Taking extra time to assess and manage a patient with mental health concerns requires that you also take extra time to make a thorough and complete record of the call. Be objective and factual, and include comments made by the patient. Good communication, following standards and protocols, and having patience will be your best protection against legal action.

Pathophysiology

Causes of Abnormal Behavior

Abnormal behavior typically results from a complex interaction of biologic or organic causes, developmental factors, psychological stressors, emotional stimuli, and sociocultural influences. Those causes can be classified into four broad categories: (1) causes that are biologic or organic in nature, (2) causes resulting from the person's environment, (3) causes resulting from acute injury or illness, and (4) causes that are substance-related.

Biologic or Organic Causes

Many patients who present with psychiatric symptoms are actually being affected by biologic or organic influences that interfere with normal cerebral function. Such patients are generally classified as having **organic brain syndrome**. Examples of biologic or organic causes of abnormal behavior are many and include such conditions as chronic hypoxia, seizure, traumatic brain injury, chronic alcohol and drug abuse, and brain tumors **Table 2**. These conditions alter the normal functioning of the brain and may cause derangements in behavior. Probably the most common offenders are alcohol and drugs; however, dementia or delirium should be considered.

Environmental Causes

A person's environment exerts a tremendous influence on behavior. Typically, that environment includes both psychosocial and sociocultural influences on behavior.

When people are consistently exposed to stressful psychosocial events (eg, childhood trauma) or developmental influences (eg, parents who deprived them of love, caring, support, and encouragement), they may develop abnormal reactions. When a person's basic needs are threatened, that person faces a crisis. A person in crisis has two alternatives for dealing with this threat: (1) cope with it, finding ways to alter the situation or his or her perception of it so that it is no longer so stressful, or (2) attempt to alleviate the discomfort by escaping from the stress. Escape may take many forms, including alcohol, drugs, psychiatric symptoms, and even suicide.

Humans are social, preferring to live in groups. Not surprisingly, then, sociocultural factors directly affect biology, behavior, and responses to the stress of emergencies. For example, the effects of assault, rape, and racial attacks or the death of a loved one may produce significant changes in a person's behavior.

Injury and Illness as Causes

Acute illness can overwhelm a person, causing changes in his or her behavior. Medical problems such as severe infections, electrolyte abnormalities, and many types of metabolic disorders result in stress on coping mechanisms and can cause abnormal behaviors.

The number of traumatic events occurring in the general population has increased in both frequency and intensity in recent years. An acute traumatic situation creates a great deal

Table 2	Selected Disease States That May Produce Psychotic Symptoms
Disease State	**Psychotic Symptoms**
Toxic and deficiency states	Drug-induced psychoses, especially from: ■ Digitalis ■ Steroids ■ Disulfiram ■ Amphetamines ■ LSD, PCP, and other psychedelics Nutrition disorders: ■ Alcohol abuse ■ Vitamin deficiencies Poisoning with bromide or other heavy metals Kidney failure Liver failure
Infections	Syphilis Parasites Viral encephalitis (eg, after measles) Brain abscess
Neurologic disease	Seizure disorders (especially temporal lobe seizures) Primary and metastatic tumors of the brain Dementia Stroke Closed head injury
Cardiovascular disorders	Low cardiac output (eg, in heart failure)
Endocrine disorders	Thyroid hyperfunction (thyrotoxicosis) Adrenal hyperfunction (Cushing syndrome)
Metabolic disorders	Electrolyte imbalances (eg, after severe diarrhea) Hypoglycemia Diabetic ketoacidosis

of stress for the person experiencing the trauma as well as those around them. You are not immune to this stress. **Posttraumatic stress disorder (PTSD)** is a severe form of anxiety that stems from a traumatic experience; it is characterized by the individual reliving the stress of the original situation. Causes of PTSD can range from combat military service and terrorist attacks to a car crash or sexual assault **Figure 1**.

Substance-Related Causes

Substance-related disorders include the use of alcohol, cigarettes, illicit drugs, and other substances that change the way a person feels, behaves, or thinks. These disorders cost thousands of lives and billions of dollars annually. It was not until 1980 that substance-related disorders were recognized as a complex biologic and psychological problem rather than a sign of moral weakness.

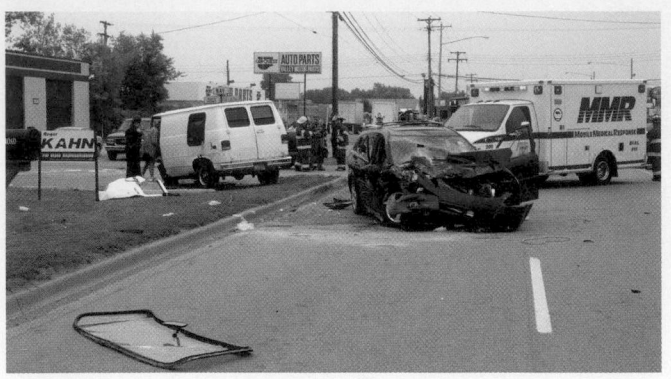

Figure 1 Posttraumatic stress disorder can be caused by a traumatic event such as a car crash with a fatality.

mental health is challenged, similar psychological mechanisms or behaviors mobilize to help return the person's mental state to homeostasis. These defensive mechanisms present as various types of psychiatric signs and symptoms or behaviors that you may also observe.

Like the symptoms and signs of physical illness, psychiatric symptoms and signs can be grouped according to the "systems" they affect. Here, however, the focus is on systems of psychological (rather than physiologic) functioning. The psychological functions involved are consciousness, motor activity, speech, thought, affect, memory, orientation, and perception. Psychiatric signs and symptoms can affect the following areas: consciousness, motor activity, speech, thinking, mood and affect, memory, orientation, perception, and intelligence. The signs and symptoms of these disorders are listed in Table 3 .

Psychiatric Signs and Symptoms

When a person's physical health is challenged, the human body mobilizes various defenses to correct the abnormality. The patient experiences the effects of those abnormalities and corrective measures as symptoms, and you observe them as signs. Physical symptoms and signs reflect the body's attempts to maintain its balance in the face of physical stress. When a person's

Patient Assessment

Assessment of the patient with a behavioral emergency differs in at least two ways from the methods of patient assessment studied so far. In assessing the patient with trauma or acute illness, you use a variety of diagnostic instruments to measure vital functions and detect abnormalities, such as a stethoscope to evaluate breath sounds and a sphygmomanometer to measure

---

YOU *are the Medic* | **PART 2**

As you approach the apartment, you note the patient is pacing back and forth just inside the doorway. He is clenching and unclenching his fists. You hear him repeating, "They're coming for me" in a low voice. Speaking calmly, you ask the patient his name and tell him you are with emergency services and are here to help him. He stops pacing, turns to you, and tells you his name. He tells you that you cannot help him because they are going to kill him.

You repeat that you want to help him and ask if he will tell you why he feels this way. He looks around nervously and says he has to whisper because they can hear him. He continues to refuse to come into the hall because he says he will be an easier target there. You ask if you can come in and sit with him. He allows you in and you sit in a chair near the door so that your access to the exit is not blocked. The apartment appears neat. There is no evidence of alcohol present in the kitchen or living area that you can see. The patient is fully dressed in wrinkled clothes that appear clean. You do not note any unusual odors. You are limited to a visual assessment of the patient at this time.

Recording Time: 0 Minutes	
Appearance	Agitated, anxious
Level of consciousness	Alert and oriented to person and place, distracted by delusions
Airway	Patent
Breathing	Appears adequate, occasionally rapid
Circulation	Skin color appears normal

3. What is your initial impression of this patient? What factors, signs, or symptoms would lead you to this conclusion?

4. Does this patient need to be evaluated at a hospital?

Table 3 Classification of Psychiatric Signs and Symptoms

Disorder	Psychiatric Signs and Symptoms
Disorders of consciousness	Distractibility and inattention Confusion Delirium Stupor and coma
Disorders of motor activity	Restlessness Stereotyped movements (repetition of movements that do not seem to serve any useful purpose) Compulsions (repetitive actions that are carried out to relieve the anxiety of obsessive thoughts) Slow movements
Disorders of speech	Slow speech Acceleration or pressure of speech (the pouring out of words like water escaping under pressure) Neologisms (words the patient invents) Echolalia (the patient echoes words he or she hears) Mutism (the patient does not speak at all)
Disorders of thinking	Disordered thought progression: ■ Flight of ideas (accelerated thinking in which the mind skips very rapidly from one thought to the next) ■ Slowness of thought ■ Perseveration (repetition of the same idea over and over again) ■ Circumstantial thinking Disordered thought content: ■ Delusions ■ Obsessions ■ Phobias (obsessive, irrational fears of specific things or situations, such as fear of heights, fear of open places, fear of confined spaces, or fear of certain animals)
Disorders of mood and affect	Anxiety Euphoria Depression Inappropriate affect (emotion that is out of synch with the situation; for example, wearing a waxy smile while discussing a parent's death) Flat affect (the absence of emotion; appearing to feel no emotion at all)
Disorders of memory	Amnesia Confabulation (inventing experiences to fill gaps in memory)
Disorders of orientation	Disoriented to person, place, and time
Disorders of perception	Illusions Hallucinations
Disorders of intelligence	Difficulty learning

the blood pressure. In assessing the disturbed patient, *you* are the diagnostic instrument. You must use your thinking processes to evaluate someone else's thinking processes, your perceptions to test the validity of someone else's perceptions, your feelings to measure someone else's feelings. This takes practice, because most EMS providers are not accustomed to using their feelings in this way. For example, if someone makes you feel angry, your natural instinct may be to talk back to him or her. In working an emergency call, however, a more useful paradigm is "That patient infuriates me, so it is quite likely he is paranoid, because paranoid patients often elicit anger in others."

A second way in which the assessment of a patient with a behavioral emergency differs from that of a patient with an acute illness or trauma is that the assessment is part of the treatment. As soon as you speak to the patient, your voice and manner will influence his or her condition, for better or worse. The process of listening to the patient describe the issue at hand can also mitigate the problem.

Assess the patient wherever the emergency occurs. Do not rush off immediately to the hospital because the hospital is likely to be a strange, intimidating place for the patient. Your haste to get there may reinforce the patient's belief that something is terribly wrong. Let the patient attempt to recover his or her bearings in familiar surroundings when medically possible.

Scene Size-up

The safety concerns surrounding a behavioral emergency may not appear to be as threatening as a hazardous chemical spill in an industrial setting or an accident on a busy highway where vehicles are twisted and damaged in a crash, but a situation involving a distraught person with severe depression or a drug addict experiencing an acute psychotic break poses its own unique threats. Although every situation you encounter has the potential for surprises and unexpected events, the situations you respond to that have a strong behavioral component will most likely have the most sudden and unexpected turn of events of any type of call. At first look, these calls may appear to be simple "injury with bleeding" or "breathing difficulty" calls, but the problem may be the result of the patient's own drastic behavior.

Observe the situation to determine whether it is unduly dangerous to you and your partner. If so, immediately summon law enforcement personnel. Observe the scene carefully for weapons, remembering that almost anything—a chair, a lamp, or a book—can be used as a weapon. If you have any questions about your ability to manage the situation safely, call for assistance. Follow the general guidelines listed in Table 4 to ensure your safety at the scene of a behavioral emergency.

Assessment of the environment can help give clues to the patient's condition or the cause of the emergency. Is the home too hot or too cold? Is the home well kept and secure? Are there hazardous conditions? Look for potential clues from the patient's social history; general living conditions; availability of social and family support; activity level; medications; overall appearance with respect to nutrition, general health, cleanliness, and personal hygiene; and attitude and mental well-being.

Finally, consider the mechanism of injury and/or nature of illness. For example, a patient with diabetes may have an altered mental status because of a low blood glucose level.

Primary Assessment

Identify yourself clearly. Tell the patient who you are and what you are trying to do. If the patient is confused or delusional, you may have to explain who you are at frequent intervals. Do so in a nonargumentative, emotionally neutral tone of voice. ("No, Mr. Jones, I'm not from the CIA. I'm a paramedic with the city ambulance service, and I'm here to help you.")

Form a General Impression
The patient's overall condition and the nature of his or her psychiatric problem will determine how much of the assessment you are able to perform. A disturbed patient may prefer not to be touched, and you must respect that wish unless there is a compelling medical reason for doing otherwise (eg, profuse bleeding from slashed wrists or a decreased level of consciousness from

Table 4	**Safety Guidelines for Behavioral Emergencies**

Assess the scene. If the patient is armed or has potentially harmful objects in his or her possession, have these removed by law enforcement personnel before you provide care.

Be prepared to spend extra time. It may take longer to assess, listen to, and prepare the patient for transport.

Have a definitive plan of action. Decide who will do what. If restraint is needed, how will it be accomplished?

Identify yourself calmly. Try to gain the patient's confidence. If you begin shouting, the patient is likely to shout louder or become more excited. A low, calm voice is often a quieting influence.

Be direct. State your intentions and what you expect of the patient.

Stay with the patient. *Do not let the patient leave the area, and do not leave the area yourself unless law enforcement personnel can and will stay with the patient.* Otherwise, the patient may go to another room and obtain weapons, lock himself or herself in the bathroom, or take pills.

Encourage purposeful movement. Help the patient get dressed and gather appropriate belongings to take to the hospital.

Express interest in the patient's story. Let the patient tell you what happened or what is going on now in his or her own words. However, do not play along with auditory or visual disturbances.

Keep a safe distance from the patient. Everyone needs personal space. Furthermore, you want to be sure you can move quickly if the patient becomes violent or tries to run away. Do not physically talk down to or directly confront the patient. A squatting, 45° angle approach is usually not confrontational; however, it may hinder your movements. Do not allow the patient to get between you and the exit.

Avoid fighting with the patient. You do not want to get into a power struggle. Remember, the patient is not responding to you in a normal manner; he or she may be wrestling with internal forces over which neither of you has control. You and others may be stimulating these inner forces without knowing it. If you can respond with understanding to the feeling that the patient is expressing, whether this is anger, fear, or desperation, you may be able to gain his or her cooperation. If it is necessary to use force, ensure that you have adequate help and move toward the patient quietly and with assured firmness.

Be honest and reassuring. If the patient asks whether he or she has to go to the hospital, the answer should be, "Yes, that is where you can receive medical help."

Do not judge. You may see behavior that you dislike. Set those feelings aside, and concentrate on providing emergency medical care.

an overdose). At the very least, you should be able to assess the patient's general appearance—for example, the patient's dress, cleanliness, and grooming, all of which provide clues to the way the patient perceives himself or herself. Pay attention to the patient's posture. Does the patient appear frustrated, angry, sobbing, or <u>catatonic</u> (lacking expression or movement, or appearing rigid)?

You should also assess the pupils carefully because they may indicate other causes of altered mental status. For example, constricted pupils may indicate opiate ingestion, or unequal pupils may indicate cerebral trauma.

When performing your assessment, it is important to limit the number of people around the patient. Remember to stay alert to potential danger. A patient in unstable condition may become violent at any time. Watch for signs of agitation or aggression. It is important to separate the patient from bystanders or family members who seem to be exacerbating the patient's condition. You may ask them to step into another room and speak to your partner, or you may take your patient to the ambulance before beginning your primary assessment, if appropriate.

Airway and Breathing

Attend first to priority problems—airway, breathing, or circulatory concerns. Assess the airway to make sure it is patent and adequate. Next, evaluate the patient's breathing. Provide any appropriate interventions on the basis of your assessment findings. In most patients with behavioral emergencies, the problem will be more psychiatric than physiologic in presentation. However, your assessment must look for signs and symptoms of abnormal functioning, abnormal behavior, or threatening gestures.

Circulation

Next, you will need to assess the pulse rate, quality, and rhythm. Obtain the systolic and diastolic blood pressures when possible. Assessing a patient's circulation includes an evaluation for the presence of shock and bleeding. Assess the patient's perfusion level by evaluating skin color, temperature, and condition.

Transport Decision

Patients who are seriously disturbed should be seen by a physician and evaluated for possible hospitalization. Many of these patients will agree to their transport to the hospital. Others may not want your help and will try to prevent you from taking them to a hospital. Because transporting a patient against his or her will deprives the patient of his or her civil liberties, it must never be undertaken lightly. Even an experienced psychiatrist may find it difficult to define what kind of behavior justifies removing a person from society or what constitutes "dangerous behavior." Furthermore, laws vary from one region to another, so it is important to be familiar with the legal requirements in your community.

As a general rule, a conscious adult must consent to be taken to the hospital. If the patient withholds this consent, he or she may be taken against his or her will only at the express request of the police or the county mental health physician (in many jurisdictions). The same policy applies to the use of forcible restraint. Where such measures are deemed necessary, law enforcement officers should be summoned. In addition, every ambulance service should have clearly defined protocols, drawn up with legal advice, for dealing with patients who require involuntary commitment. Follow those protocols to the letter and consult medical command as necessary.

■ History Taking

The <u>mental status examination (MSE)</u> is a key part of your assessment of a patient who is experiencing an acute psychiatric problem. To conduct the MSE, you must check each of the "systems" of mental function in an orderly way. A useful mnemonic for the elements of the MSE is COASTMAP Figure 2 :

- **Consciousness.** Determine the patient's level of consciousness (alert, confused, responds to pain, unresponsive). Note the patient's ability to *pay attention* to a discussion and *concentrate*. Is the patient easily distracted, or can he or she focus on the events at hand?
- **Orientation.** Ask what the year or month is. Ask the patient to state where he or she is at the moment—the country, state, town, or specific location. If the patient is not sure, have the patient make a best guess.
- **Activity.** Examine the patient's behavior. Is the patient restless and agitated, pacing up and down? Experiencing tremors? Sitting still, scarcely moving at all? Making any strange or repetitive movements (scanning of the environment, odd or repetitive gestures)?
- **Speech.** Identify the form, rather than the content of the patient's speech. Note the rate, volume, flow, articulation, and intonation of speech. Is it too fast or too slow? Too loud or too soft? Is the speech garbled or slurred (dysarthria)? Is the patient stuttering or mumbling? Using any strange words?
- **Thought.** Listen to the patient's story. What is on his or her mind? Is the patient making sense? Is there anything unusual about his or her reasoning? Is the patient expressing apparently false ideas (delusions), such as a belief that the CIA is after him/her? Is the patient experiencing any false sensory impressions (hallucinations), such as hearing voices? Is he/she experiencing a flight of ideas?

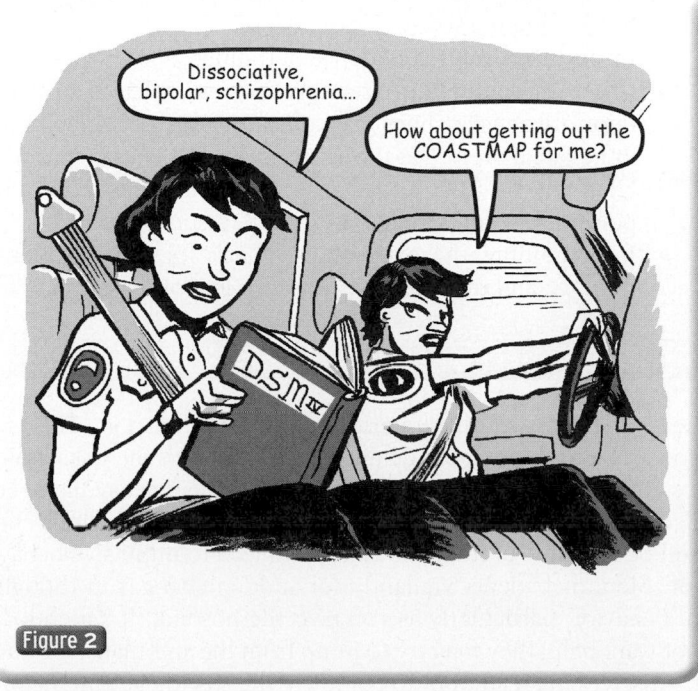

Figure 2

- **Memory.** Form an impression of the patient's memory—recent, remote, and immediate. If memory loss is present, determine whether it is constant or variable. Some patients may create memories to take the place of things they cannot recall (confabulation).
- **Affect and mood.** The patient's mood may be objectively noted via body language. Is the mood euphoric or sad? Is it <u>labile</u>? Does the affect—the expression of inner feelings—seem appropriate to the situation or is it animated, angry, flat, or withdrawn?
- **Perception.** Detecting disorders of perception may be difficult, because patients often hesitate to answer direct questions about hallucinations or illusions. Sometimes it is helpful to ask the patient, "Do you ever hear things that other people cannot hear?"

You can conduct nearly all of the MSE just by watching and listening (and knowing what to watch and listen *for*). Only the assessment of memory, orientation, and perhaps perception requires you to ask some direct questions. Practice being an observer. As you sit in a restaurant, eavesdrop on the waitress talking to other customers and systematically go through the COAST-MAP sequence to evaluate her mental status. Get into the habit of noticing how other people talk, move, and express their feelings, and practice describing those things to your partner.

Secondary Assessment

Whereas much of your assessment involves interviewing the patient about psychiatric history and performing the MSE, you must also look for signs of an organic cause of the patient's behavior:

- Obtain the vital signs to look for fever or indications of increased intracranial pressure.
- Examine the skin temperature and moisture, and note any prominent tattoos. Scars may indicate self-mutilation in **borderline personality disorders**.
- Inspect the head for evidence of trauma.
- Check the pupils for size, equality, and reaction to light. Pupillary abnormalities may indicate a toxic ingestion or an intracranial process as the source of the patient's behavior.
- Note any unusual odors on the patient's breath such as poisons, alcohol, or ketones from diabetic ketoacidosis.
- In examining the extremities, check for needle tracks, tremors, and unilateral weakness or loss of sensation.

Reassessment

Reassessment is routinely performed during transport. This is a good time to assess more details of your patient's mental status.

Many times patients with abnormal behavior may have settled down physically by the time you arrive, but their minds may still be in a state of flux, and this could lead to impulsive behavior. Monitor patients vigilantly for sudden changes in thought or behavior, particularly as you near the hospital. If patients do not want help, they may try to jump from the ambulance or hurt themselves in an attempt to complete the suicide gesture before

arriving at the hospital. They may even turn that aggressive and impulsive behavior toward you.

Your radio report to the hospital should include your usual report of medical and mental health history, medications prescribed, and your assessment findings as based on local protocols and guidelines. Be sure to include pertinent information from the mental status examination to provide a clear picture of the patient you are caring for. Discuss with the hospital the need for restraints or medications necessary to control behavior prior to instituting these interventions when possible; otherwise inform the hospital staff of measures used to protect the patient and providers or other standing orders you have instituted. If your patient is aggressive or potentially violent, you should provide advance notice to the emergency department staff so they can mobilize security or additional help prior to your arrival.

Emergency Medical Care

Management of the patient with a psychiatric problem follows the approach stressed throughout this text. Ensure scene safety and focus on life-threatening conditions. If the erratic behavior might possibly be caused by a medical disorder (eg, hypoglycemia, overdose, or hypoxia), treat the patient for the medical disorder before presuming that the patient's behavior is due to an emotional or psychiatric cause. These measures may include oxygen therapy, testing of the blood glucose level, and administration of D_{50} (50 grams of dextrose in every 100 mL), as well as general interventions for hypothermia or shock management.

Communication Techniques

As mentioned earlier, good communication is part of the treatment of a patient with a psychiatric emergency.

When evaluating a trauma patient, you can generally obtain enough information to provide appropriate initial treatment just based on the physical examination findings, even if the patient is unresponsive and cannot provide a history. Conversely, when evaluating a patient with a behavioral emergency, virtually all of the diagnostic information (and much of the therapeutic benefit) must come from you talking with the patient. Skill in interviewing a patient with a behavioral crisis, therefore, is central to dealing with psychiatric emergencies. Set some ground rules for your interview. Let the patient know what you expect, and what he or she may expect of you. ("It's okay to cry or even scream, but we aren't going to let you hurt yourself or anyone else.") Allow the patient to tell the story in his or her own way. Do not attempt to direct the conversation, but allow the patient to vent his or her feelings. The following are some guidelines:

- **Begin with an open-ended question.** An open-ended question does not provide possible answers for the patient, but rather allows the patient to give the answer. For example, say "It's clear you've been feeling bad. Tell me something about the kind of troubles you've been having." (You may begin with more direct questioning when it is essential to obtain specific information in a hurry, such as "What kind of pills did you take? How many?")

- **Let the patient talk** and tell the story in his or her own way, even if it takes a little more time. Letting patients talk allows them to gain some control over themselves and their situation. At the same time, it enables you to assess the patient's speech, affect, and thought processes.
- **Listen, and show that you are listening.** Your facial expression, posture, eye contact, an occasional nod—all of these things can convey to the patient that you are paying close attention to what he or she is saying **Figure 3**.
- **Do not be afraid of silences,** even though they may seem intolerably long. Maintain an attentive and relaxed attitude until the patient takes up the story again. It is especially important to be silent when the patient stops speaking because of overwhelming emotion. Avoid the temptation to jump into the silence with a hasty "There, there," to forestall the patient's expressions of emotion, such as crying. The expression of feelings is often therapeutic in itself, and the patient will likely be better able to express himself or herself after intense emotion has been released. Furthermore, your silence gives patients a chance to get control of themselves in their own way.
- **Acknowledge and label the patient's feelings.** The disturbed patient may feel overwhelmed by intense and chaotic feelings. Identifying those feelings and giving them a name (eg, "You seem angry") can help the patient gain control over them.

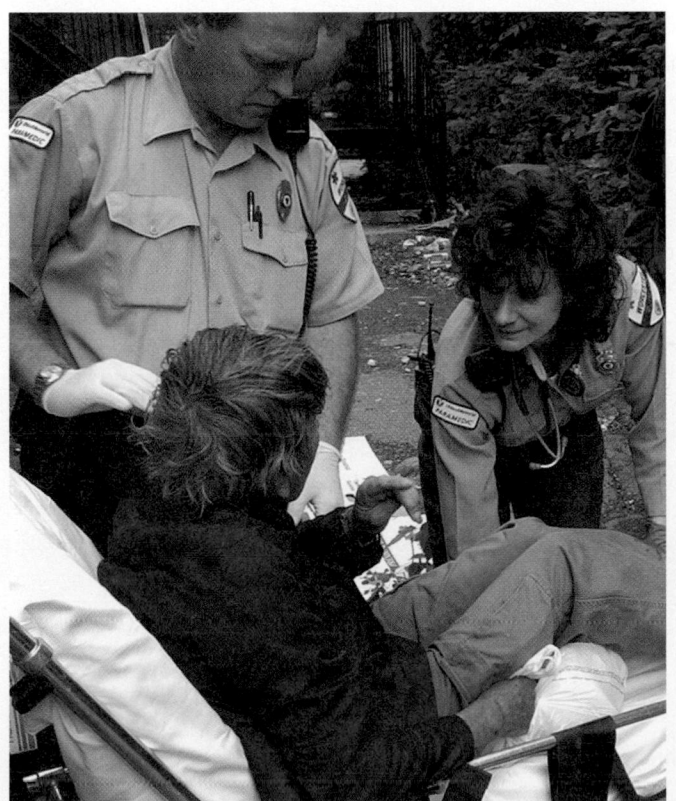

Figure 3 Making eye contact with a patient can provide useful clues about his or her emotional state—but do not stare at the patient.

- **Do not argue.** If the patient misperceives reality, make note of the misperceptions, but do not try to talk the patient out of them. When a misperception is frightening or distressing to the patient, you might try just once to provide a simple and factual statement, in a neutral tone of voice ("Yes, that does look a lot like a snake, but actually it's just a shadow."). But do not get into a dispute on the nature of reality.
- **Facilitate communication.** Facilitation is a technique of encouraging the patient to communicate by using gestures or noncommittal words, such as a nod of the head or a phrase like "Go on," "I see," or "What happened after that?" You can also use facilitation to return the patient to a topic on which you would like some elaboration. For example, a patient may have made a passing reference to suicidal thoughts and then moved on to another subject. When the patient finishes, you might comment, "You say you've had thoughts of suicide?" This remark tells the patient that you have been paying attention to the story and would like to learn more.
- **Direct the patient's attention.** Confrontation refers to pointing out something of interest in the patient's conversation or behavior, thereby directing the patient's attention to something he or she may have been unaware of. Confrontations describe how the patient appears to the interviewer based on observations, *not* judgments. For example, you might remark, "You seem worried" or "You look sad." Such comments often elicit a freer expression of feelings from the patient. Confrontations must be carefully phrased, so they do not sound nagging or condescending.
- **Ask questions.** When the patient finishes giving the initial account of the problem, you will have to ask questions. Keep the questions as nondirective as possible. Avoid asking questions that can be answered with a yes or no ("Are you angry?") or asking leading questions ("Do you think that your husband is a part of the problem?"). *How* and *what* questions are preferred ("How did you feel when that happened?").
- **Adjust your approach as needed.** Some patients find it difficult to deal with the unstructured situation of nondirective questioning and may become anxious during silences. That response is particularly likely among adolescents, severely depressed patients, and confused or disorganized patients. When your open-ended questions meet with uncomprehending silence, try another approach and perform a more structured interview.

Crisis Intervention Skills

The following guidelines apply to the care of *any* patient with a psychiatric problem:

- **Be as calm and direct as possible.** Disturbed patients are often frightened of losing self-control. Your behavior should indicate that you have confidence in the patient's ability to maintain control. One of the main purposes of the interview is to help the patient reestablish some self-mastery. If you show anxiety or panic, you merely affirm the patient's conviction that the situation is overwhelming.

- **Exclude disruptive people.** In most cases, you should interview the patient alone, while relatives and bystanders wait in another room (your partner can interview them). Some patients, however, will become anxious if separated from an important person—a parent, or perhaps a friend. If another person has a calming effect on the patient, ask that person to remain present.
- **Sit down.** Sit down to interview the patient, preferably at a 45° angle from the patient so you do not encroach on the patient's "personal space" Figure 4 .
- **Maintain a nonjudgmental attitude.** Accept the patient's right to have his or her own feelings about things, and do not blame, judge, or criticize the patient for those feelings.
- **Provide honest reassurance.** Give supportive, truthful information—for example, "Many people experience periods of hopelessness like you're having, but today there are effective treatments for those feelings." Avoid excessive reassurance, however, such as "Everything's going to be all right." Such statements will merely convince the patient that you do not understand how bad things are.
- **Develop a plan of action.** After the patient has finished telling his or her story and you have concluded your assessment, develop a definite plan of action. This step gives the patient the feeling that something is being done to help, which in turn relieves anxiety. Furthermore, people in crisis need direction. Do not present the patient with an array

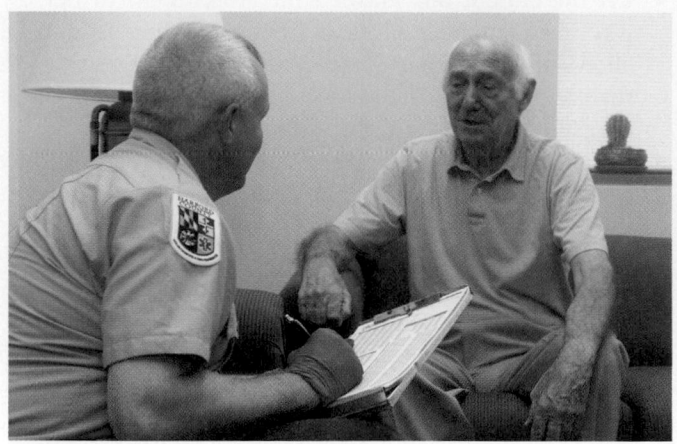

Figure 4 When interviewing the patient, sit at a 45° angle to avoid encroaching on personal space.

of decisions (eg, "Do you want to go to the hospital, or would you rather stay at home and call your doctor tomorrow?"); rather, state what you think is the best course of action ("I think it's important for you to go to the hospital. There are doctors there who can help you."). Once the plan is determined and you have begun to carry it out, allow the patient to make choices and thereby exercise some control over the situation. You might ask the patient, for example,

YOU are the Medic   PART 3

The patient agrees to sit in a chair opposite you. You ask the patient if he knows what day it is. He correctly informs you of the day of week. You continue your mental status assessment of this patient using the COASTMAP method. The patient is restless in his seat. He is gripping the edge of the chair and rocking back and forth. You ask the patient if he has any medical problems. He tells you that he sees his doctor regularly because he has schizophrenia. He is supposed to take medication every day but he has not taken any for the past week because he overheard them at the drug store when he was refilling his prescriptions. Once he realized that they knew he overheard them, he stopped taking his medications because they were poisoned. He explains to you that he wanted to take them but he is afraid. He says he cannot go out to get more.

You ask the patient if your partner can check his vital signs while you look at the medications he takes. He consents and directs you to a basket on the table with medicine bottles. You locate two new bottles. The patient should take thioridazine (Mellaril), 200 mg twice daily, and mesoridazine (Serentil), 50 mg twice daily. The bottles indicate they are for treatment of schizophrenia.

Recording Time: 8 Minutes	
Respirations	20 breaths/min
Pulse	110 beats/min
Skin	Warm, pink, dry
Blood pressure	130/84 mm Hg
Oxygen saturation (Spo$_2$)	99% on room air
Pupils	Equal, round, and reactive to light

5. What conclusions might you make about medication compliance and the patient's medical history?

6. As a paramedic, what options should you consider if the patient refuses to be transported?

whether he or she prefers to be carried on a stretcher or to walk to the ambulance on his or her own. These small decisions may seem minor, but they allow the patient to attain a measure of autonomy and self-respect.

- **Encourage some motor activity.** Moving about often helps ease anxiety. If you are taking the patient to the hospital, accompany the patient while he or she gathers the things he or she wants to bring along. Let the patients do as much for themselves as possible, to reinforce the feeling that you expect them to improve.
- **Stay with the patient at all times.** Once you have responded to the emergency, the patient's safety becomes your responsibility. Do not allow the patient to leave you or to go to the bathroom alone. This could allow the patient to swallow the contents of a bottle of pills, for example.
- **Bring all of the patient's medications to the hospital.** If the patient is receiving treatment for psychiatric problems, knowing which medications have been prescribed can help physicians identify the condition for which the patient has been treated.
- **Never assume that it is impossible to talk with any patient until you have tried to do so.** Even if the patient sits silently and appears unaware of your presence, assume that he or she can hear and understand everything you say.

◼ Use of Force and Types of Restraint

When verbal interventions fail to reduce severe agitation in a patient, consider the use of chemical or physical restraint.

Physical Restraint

Some devices used for physical restraint may be improvised from materials on the ambulance; others are commercially made from leather or nylon that is padded for comfort and safety. Most commercial restraints are applied to the wrists and ankles to prevent movement of the arms and legs. Some are placed around the waist to restrict movement of the torso. Vest-type restraints are applied from the front of the patient and may include sleeves to restrain the arms from moving. Make sure you are familiar with the restraints used by your agency before you enter a situation requiring their application.

Make sure you have sufficient personnel before you attempt to overpower and restrain the patient. You must have overwhelming force to apply a physical restraint, which means a *minimum* of four trained, able-bodied people—one for each limb (assign a specific limb in advance to each responder) and one for the head. Appoint one leader, who will direct the team and maintain verbal contact with the patient. Before you begin, discuss the plan of action. Law enforcement personnel should be included when physically restraining violent patients. They are well trained in techniques, both verbal and physical, used to subdue violent people. They also provide an objective perspective of the situation.

When subduing a disturbed patient, use the minimum force necessary. You should avoid acts of physical force that may cause injury to the patient. Do not move toward the patient immediately; give him or her a chance to choose a nonviolent alternative behavior.

If the show of force does not calm the patient down, responders must move quickly to restrain the patient. First, remove any equipment or jewelry from your own person that could be used as a weapon (eg, name badge, scissors worn on the belt, key chain, earrings). Make sure you have adequate restraining devices—preferably padded leather or nylon restraints—immediately available. Then, at a signal from the leader, move in *fast* from the patient's sides. Grasp the patient at the elbows, knees, and head, and apply restraints to all four extremities.

The best position in which to secure the patient to the stretcher is supine, with both legs and both arms secured to one side of the stretcher, with the patient's head turned to the side. This positioning will prevent aspiration in case of vomiting. Never tie the patient's ankles and wrists together as one; this type of restraint has been known to result in death. Never "hobble tie" a patient (tying just the feet together). Placing a patient face down in a Reeves stretcher can also be dangerous and lead to positional asphyxia or aspiration.

Throughout the process, someone, preferably you or your partner, should talk with the patient. Remember to treat the patient with dignity and respect at all times. This will decrease the amount of stimuli experienced by the patient. Avoid being bitten by the patient during the restraining procedure. Once the restraints are in place, do not remove them. Do not negotiate or make deals. If the patient is spitting, you can place a surgical mask over the face.

Once the patient is restrained, continuously monitor the patient for airway and breathing, vomiting, airway obstruction, and cardiovascular stability. Drug or alcohol intoxication initially may cause violent behavior but then can also lead to physical problems such as vomiting and aspiration or respiratory depression. Never place your patient face down because it is impossible to adequately monitor the patient and this positioning may inhibit the breathing of an impaired or exhausted patient. Be careful not to place restraints in such a way that the patient's respirations are compromised.

Check the patient's peripheral circulation every few minutes to make sure the restraints are not too tight **Figure 5**. Check the radial pulses in the arms and the dorsalis pedis pulses in the feet.

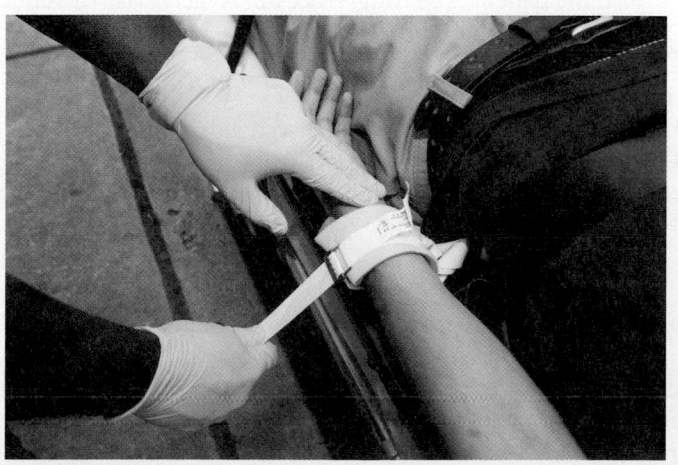

Figure 5 Assess circulation frequently while a patient is restrained.

Be careful if a combative patient suddenly becomes calm and cooperative. This is not the time to relax; you should continue to remain vigilant. The patient may suddenly become combative again and injure someone.

Document everything in the patient's chart—the reasons for using restraints (be specific, giving examples of the patient's behavior and the indications of the violence potential); the number of people used to subdue the patient; the restraining devices used; and the status of the peripheral circulation after restraints were applied. Keep in mind that you may use reasonable force to defend yourself against an attack by an emotionally disturbed patient. It is extremely helpful to have (and document) witnesses in attendance, even during transport, to protect against false accusations.

Proper physical restraint is summarized in the following steps, shown in **Skill Drill 1** :

Skill Drill 1

1. Approach the patient cautiously **Step 1** . If possible, corner the patient in a safe area with the least obstruction and no glass.

2. Assemble four or five rescuers and have the stretcher or carrying device and soft restraints (wide cloth or commercial leather restraints) nearby **Step 2** .

3. Designate a leader who will communicate with both the team and the patient.

4. Assign positions to each team member: four extremities and the head.

5. On the direction of the team leader, who will be talking to the patient calmly, move together toward the patient.

6. Each team member should grasp the assigned body part and carefully, with the least amount of force, bring the patient to the ground.

7. Carefully place the patient on the stretcher or carrying device in a face-up position **Step 3** .

8. Consider tying the patient with soft restraints at each wrist and ankle as well as over the chest and pelvis with sheets **Step 4** .

9. If the patient is spitting, place an oxygen mask or surgical mask on his or her face. **Step 5**

Chemical Restraint

Physical restraint for aggressive and psychotic behavior can be complicated and hazardous. One alternative to physical restraint is to use chemical restraint—the use of medication to subdue a patient. This option should be used only with approval from medical control and following clearly established local protocols and guidelines.

The most common drugs used for chemical restraint include short-acting benzodiazepines, haloperidol (Haldol), or droperidol (Inapsine). The Food and Drug Administration has issued a black box warning for droperidol (Inapsine) due to its association with prolonged QT syndromes; a black box warning indicates that the drug may have serious adverse effects. Benzodiazepines and haloperidol carry their own risks. Haloperidol (Haldol) is a traditional antipsychotic and may cause extrapyramidal symptoms or seizures. It is administered either IM (5 to 10 mg) or IV (2 to 5 mg) with

Controversies

Many law enforcement agencies use TASER® devices to immobilize people who are behaving in a violent or aggressive manner **Figure 6** . TASER® devices were designed as an alternative to more violent immobilization methods. There is some controversy in the use of these weapons in the in-custody death phenomenon. There are data supporting the assertion that these weapons are temporally, but not causally, related to these deaths in custody. More studies are being done. EMS personnel need to be aware that many of the patients subjected to a TASER® exposure are at high risk for medical problems due to the underlying condition affecting their behavior. It is important for EMS personnel to identify these underlying conditions and to ensure appropriate medical care. Conditions to be vigilant for include: drug overdose syndromes, excited delirium, acute psychiatric decompensation, hypoglycemia, heatstroke, hepatic encephalopathy, seizure disorders, dementia, and encephalitis. Police officers are not routinely trained to recognize these conditions and will rely on EMS personnel to make appropriate disposition decisions at the scene.

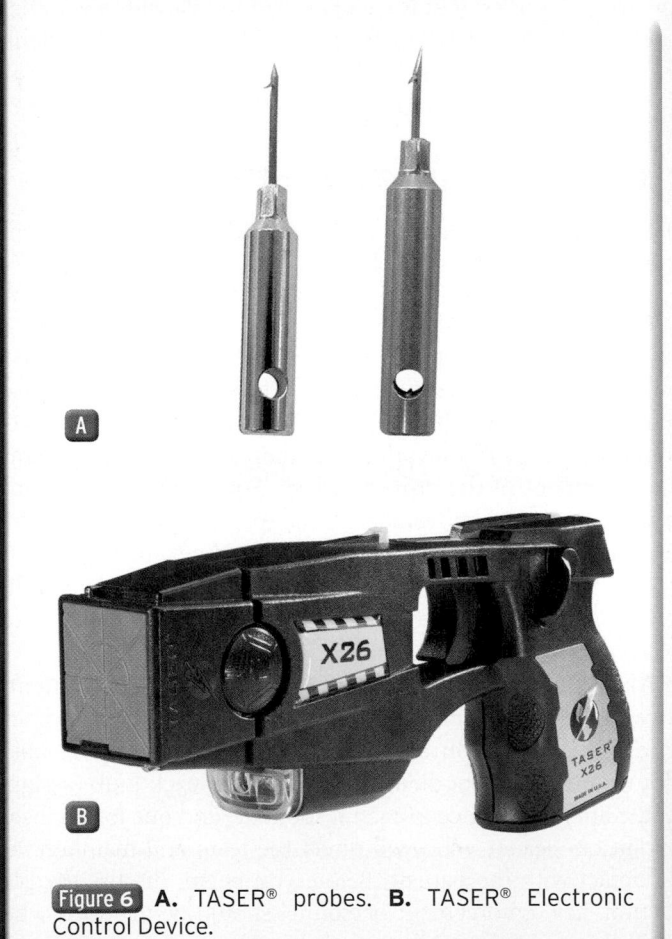

Figure 6 **A.** TASER® probes. **B.** TASER® Electronic Control Device.

an onset of action of 5 to 20 minutes depending on the route of administration. Haloperidol should not be administered to patients younger than 14 years, those with a suspected head injury, or those who may be pregnant. As with administering medications to most

Skill Drill 1

Restraining a Patient

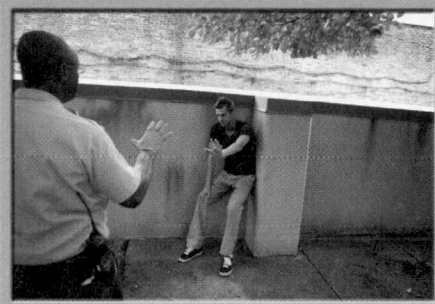

Step 1 Approach the patient cautiously. If possible, corner the patient in a safe area.

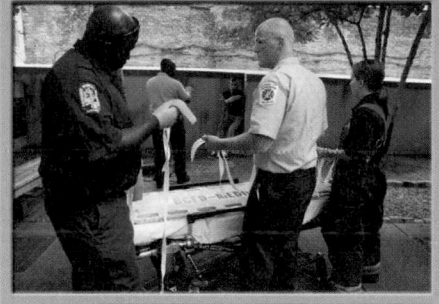

Step 2 Assemble four or five rescuers and have the stretcher or carrying device and soft restraints nearby. Designate a leader. Assign positions to each team member: four extremities and the head.

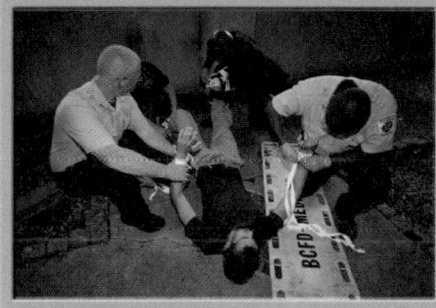

Step 3 On the direction of the team leader, move together toward the patient. Each team member should grasp the assigned body part and carefully, with the least amount of force, bring the patient to the ground. Carefully place the patient on the stretcher or carrying device in a face-up position.

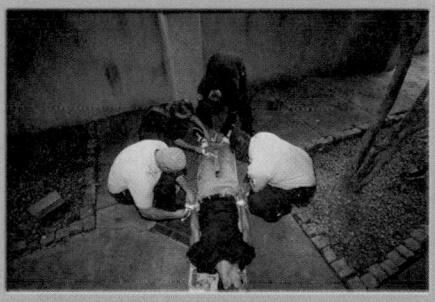

Step 4 Consider tying the patient with soft restraints at each wrist and ankle as well as the chest and pelvis with sheets.

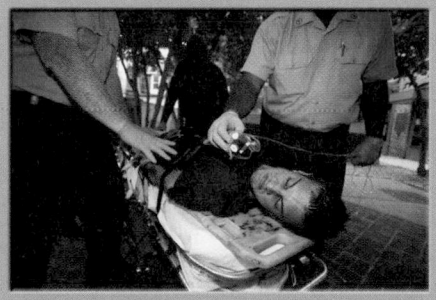

Step 5 If the patient is spitting, place an oxygen mask or surgical mask on his or her face.

elderly patients, it is recommended to begin with lower doses and repeat based on the advice of medical control.

Because aggressive and dangerous behaviors are often caused by illicit drug use (cocaine, methamphetamines, PCP), benzodiazepines are usually a safer and more effective form of chemical restraint when compared with other medications. Shorter acting benzodiazepines, such as midazolam (Versed), may be given intranasally, for example by using a mucosal atomizer device. This method provides easy preparation and quick administration with less risk to providers than intramuscular or IV injections. The usual dose and administration of intranasal midazolam is 0.2 mg/kg, up to 10 mg of a 5-mg/mL solution, delivered by an atomizer device with half the total dose administered in each nostril.

The only benzodiazepines that have reliable intramuscular absorption are midazolam and lorazepam (Ativan). As stated, the typical dose of midazolam is 0.2 mg/kg up to 10 mg IM; via the IV route, the typical dose of midazolam is 0.1 mg/kg IV up to 5 mg. The usual dose of lorazepam for uncooperative patients is 1 to 2 mg IM or IV. The side effects of benzodiazepines are usually mild and easily treated. Drowsiness, decreased mental alertness, sedation, and ataxia are the most common side effects. Although infrequent, paradoxical responses to benzodiazepines, such as insomnia and agitation, are more common in the elderly.

Follow the direction of medical control and standing orders when patient treatment includes using drugs to control behavior. The patient's pulse rate, blood pressure, and respiratory rate should be monitored closely, particularly if both chemical and physical restraint are used. Be prepared to support ventilation as needed any time you administer a sedating medication.

Pathophysiology, Assessment, and Management of Specific Emergencies

Many factors contribute to disturbances of behavior. Some of these influences are easily identified and treated, whereas others may never be clearly understood. The causes, signs, symptoms, and management of abnormal behavior can be grouped into several common areas, shown in Table 5. The most relevant areas in paramedicine are acute psychosis, agitated delirium, suicide,

Table 5 Psychiatric Disorders Categorized by Type

Category	Specific Disorder
Cognitive disorders	Agitated delirium
Thought disorders	Schizophrenia Acute psychosis
Mood disorders	Bipolar mood disorder Manic behavior Depression
Neurotic disorders	Generalized anxiety disorder Phobias Panic disorder
Substance-related disorders and addictive behavior	Substance use Substance intoxication Substance abuse Substance dependence Eating disorders (bulimia nervosa, anorexia nervosa)
Somatoform disorders	Hypochondriasis Conversion disorder (physical problem that has no identifiable pathophysiology; results from faking a physical disorder)
Factitious disorders	Intentionally making oneself sick Münchausen syndrome (when a parent intentionally makes his or her child sick; also called factitious disorder by proxy)
Impulse control disorders	Intermittent explosive disorder Kleptomania Pyromania Pathologic gambling
Personality disorders	Odd or eccentric disorders Dramatic, erratic, or emotional disorders Anxious or fearful disorders

and patterns of violence, abuse, and neglect. Finally, specific psychiatric disorders will be discussed.

Acute Psychosis

Pathophysiology

Psychosis is a state of delusion in which the person is out of touch with reality. Affected people are tuned into their own internal reality of ideas and feelings, which they mistake for the reality of the external world. To the person experiencing an acute psychotic episode, the line differentiating reality from fantasy is blurred—not distinct, as it is in those people without psychoses. That internal reality may make patients belligerent and angry toward others. Alternatively, they may become mute and withdrawn as they give all their attention to the voices and feelings within.

Psychoses or psychotic episodes occur for many reasons, some biologic or organic and others due to mental illness or drug abuse. The use of mind-altering substances is one of the most common causes, and that experience may be limited to the time that the substance is being metabolized within the body. Other causes more related to the patient's environment or mental illness include intense stress, delusional disorders, and, more commonly, schizophrenia. Some psychotic episodes last for brief periods; others last a lifetime.

Disorganization and disorientation are *not* diagnoses, but rather ways in which various conditions such as schizophrenia or organic brain syndromes may present themselves. These presentations account for a large number of ambulance calls, particularly those involving older people. Although you do not need to make a specific diagnosis in such cases, you do need to know how to manage these patients in the field.

Assessment

The most characteristic feature of psychosis is a profound thought disorder, often accompanied by disturbances in mood and perception. Patients are usually incoherent or rambling in their speech, although they may be oriented to person and place. Often these patients are found wandering aimlessly down the street, dressed oddly, uttering meaningless words and sentences. A thorough examination of the patient is rarely possible, and your principal objective is to transport the patient to the hospital in an atraumatic fashion.

The following list, using the COASTMAP acronym, outlines common signs and symptoms of the psychotic patient.

- **Consciousness.** The psychotic patient is awake and alert, but may be easily distracted, especially if paying attention to hallucinations. If the level of consciousness is fluctuating, suspect an organic brain syndrome.
- **Orientation.** Disturbances in orientation are more common in organic disorders than in psychoses, but the severely psychotic patient may be disoriented as to time and place.
- **Activity.** Activity is most commonly accelerated, with agitation and hyperactivity, but it may also be diminished. Bizarre, stereotyped movements are common.
- **Speech.** Speech may be pressured or sound strange because of unusual words that the patient has invented (neologisms).

- **Thought.** Thought is disturbed in progression and content and may show any of the following disorders:
  - Flight of ideas, with the patient's mind plunging from one thought to another.
  - Loosening of associations, in which the logical connection between one idea and the next becomes obscure, at least to the listener. In extreme cases, the patient's speech may be entirely incomprehensible.
  - Delusions, especially of persecution.
  - **Thought broadcasting** (the belief that thoughts are broadcast aloud and can be heard by others).
  - **Thought insertion** (the belief that thoughts are being thrust into his or her mind by another person) and **thought withdrawal** (the belief that thoughts are being removed).
- **Memory.** Memory can be relatively or entirely intact in psychosis. It may be difficult to obtain the cooperation of the patient for formal memory testing.
- **Affect and mood.** Mood is likely to be disturbed in psychosis. The disturbance may take the form of euphoria, sadness, or wide swings in mood; affect may reflect those inner states or be flat.
- **Perception.** Auditory hallucinations are common in psychosis. Patients hear voices commenting on their behavior or telling them what to do. Suspect that patients are hearing such voices when they seem to be attending a conversation other than yours or talking to themselves.

Management

Dealing with an acutely psychotic patient is difficult. The usual methods of reasoning with a patient are unlikely to be effective because the psychotic person has his or her own rules of logic that may be quite different from those that govern nonpsychotic thinking. Furthermore, you are likely to feel uncomfortable in the presence of a psychotic person. Those uncomfortable feelings are one of your built-in diagnostic instruments. They are elicited by the fear, suspicion, and hostility that the patient is broadcasting through body language. Use your uncomfortable feelings to help make a tentative diagnosis of a psychotic problem.

The disorganized patient needs structure. You should explain in plain language what is being done and what the patient's role will be. Directions should be simple, consistent, and firm. It may be impossible to try to obtain a detailed history; a name and address may be all information that you can obtain. Explain to these patients that they need to be seen by a doctor, and that you will take them to the hospital to get help.

In managing the disoriented patient, the key is to *keep orienting the patient* to time, place, and the people in the environment. Tell the patient who you are, and explain what you are doing. You may have to repeat that information several times en route. Reassure the patient, and point out landmarks to help orient the patient.

The nonpharmacologic techniques discussed earlier in the chapter, such as maintaining an emotional distance, explaining each step of the assessment, and involving people the patient trusts, should be the methods you try first.

Words of Wisdom

Be forewarned! The patient who hears voices that command him or her to hurt himself or herself or others must be considered dangerous.

When a patient's behavior becomes so excited it threatens his or her own well-being or the safety of others, more aggressive means should be sought to prevent injury, including either physical or chemical restraint and, at times, both. When you are considering the need for restraint, also consider involving law enforcement personnel if you have not already contacted them.

Special Populations

Some communities have crisis intervention teams (CIT) staffed by law enforcement officers with specialized training in recognizing and managing people experiencing a mental health crisis. The primary role of the CIT is to keep patients from revolving through the criminal justice system and the hospital. The program has been successful in establishing long-term care and solutions for people with chronic and persistent mental health issues that may not otherwise have the resources or support to get that help.

For the person experiencing a psychotic episode, compliance with treatments, especially medication administration, may be difficult. Such a patient often will not hold still long enough to have an IV line started and a sedating agent administered. The person might have the delusion that you are injecting him or her with something that will cause more harm. Nonpharmacologic interventions should be employed first, as discussed earlier. Developing trust is an important therapy but may be difficult to achieve with a patient who is in an acutely psychotic and agitated state.

When these methods fail, safely restraining the patient and administering a medication to help with the behavior may be appropriate. If it can safely be administered, an antianxiety drug such as a benzodiazepine (eg, midazolam) given intranasally, or an antipsychotic drug such as haloperidol (Haldol) given intramuscularly, should help calm the patient. Follow your medical control direction and standing orders when using drugs to control behavior.

■ Agitated Delirium

Pathophysiology

Delirium is a state of global cognitive impairment that is acute in onset and associated with fluctuations in mental status and behavior, inattention, disorganized thinking, and an altered level of consciousness. It is usually caused by toxic and metabolic problems or infections. Dementia is a more chronic process that produces severe deficits in memory, abstract thinking, and judgment.

People who experience delirium may become agitated and violent when stressors overwhelm them or they are unable to maintain homeostasis because of the disease process. The result is similar to that in a patient who is experiencing an acute psychotic state. Common risk factors that may preclude delirium include medical histories of hypertension, COPD, alcohol abuse, and smoking.

Assessment

Depending on the level of impairment, you should first try to reorient patients to their surroundings and circumstances. Perform a thorough assessment, including past medical history and medications, to help differentiate between delirium and dementia or identify other causes.

Management

Identifying the stressor or metabolic problem may help identify possible treatments (for example, reducing fevers, administering glucose for hypoglycemia, treating dysrhythmias to improve hypoperfusion). Be cautious when administering morphine or antipsychotics to patients with a known history of dementia because complications may be common.

▇ Suicidal Ideation

Pathophysiology

<u>Suicide</u> is any willful act designed to end one's own life. It is the third leading cause of death among 15- to 24-year-olds and the second leading cause of death in 25- to 34-year-olds. For persons between 45 and 54 years of age, suicide is the fifth leading cause of death. Suicide is more common among men, especially those who are Caucasian and single, widowed, or divorced. The risk of suicide is also high among depressed patients, one sixth of whom will succeed in taking their own lives. Alcoholism is another important risk factor. Notably, more than half of all successful suicides have made a previous attempt, and three fourths have given a clear warning of their intent to kill themselves. Table 6 summarizes the risk factors for suicide.

Suicide attempts typically occur when a person feels that close emotional attachments are endangered or when the person has lost someone or something important in his or her life. The suicidal person may also have feelings characteristic of depression—feelings of worthlessness, lack of self-esteem, and a sense of being unable to manage his or her life.

Table 6 Risk Factors for Suicide

▪ Depression, or sudden improvement in depression	▪ Expresses suicidal thoughts and concrete plans for carrying them out
▪ Male gender, age < 55	▪ Caucasian
▪ Single, widowed, or divorced	▪ Social isolation
▪ Alcohol or other drug abuse	▪ Previous suicide attempt(s)
▪ Recent loss of spouse or significant relationship	▪ Financial setback or job loss
▪ Chronic, debilitating illness	▪ Family history of suicide
▪ Schizophrenia	

Assessment

The assessment of *every* depressed patient must include an evaluation of the suicide risk. Many paramedics are reluctant to ask a patient directly about suicidal thoughts because they fear that they might "put ideas into the patient's head" Figure 7. You should realize, however, that suicide is not such an original idea that a depressed patient will not have thought of it. Most depressed patients, in fact, are relieved when the topic is brought up because this discussion gives them "permission" to talk about their suicidal ideas. Often it is easier for both you and the patient to broach the subject in a stepwise fashion. You might start by asking, "Have you ever thought that life wasn't worth living?" From there, you may proceed by degrees: "Did you ever feel that you would be better off dead? Have you ever thought of harming yourself? Do you feel that way now? Do you have a plan of how you would go about it? Do you have the things you need to carry out the plan? Has anyone in your family ever committed suicide? Have you ever tried to kill yourself before?" Patients who have made previous attempts; who have fashioned detailed, concrete plans for suicide; or who have a history of suicide among close relatives are at higher risk and must be evaluated at the hospital.

Many patients make last-minute efforts to communicate their suicidal intentions. When a person phones to threaten suicide, someone should stay on the line until the rescue squad has reached the scene. On arrival, quickly survey the area for any implements that the patient might use for self-injury and discreetly remove those items. Make certain that you account for your own safety. Talk with the patient, and encourage him or her to discuss feelings. Ask the same questions mentioned earlier regarding the patient's suicidal ideas and plans.

Management

Whenever you find a patient to be severely depressed or you have another reason to suspect that a patient is at risk of suicide, follow these guidelines:

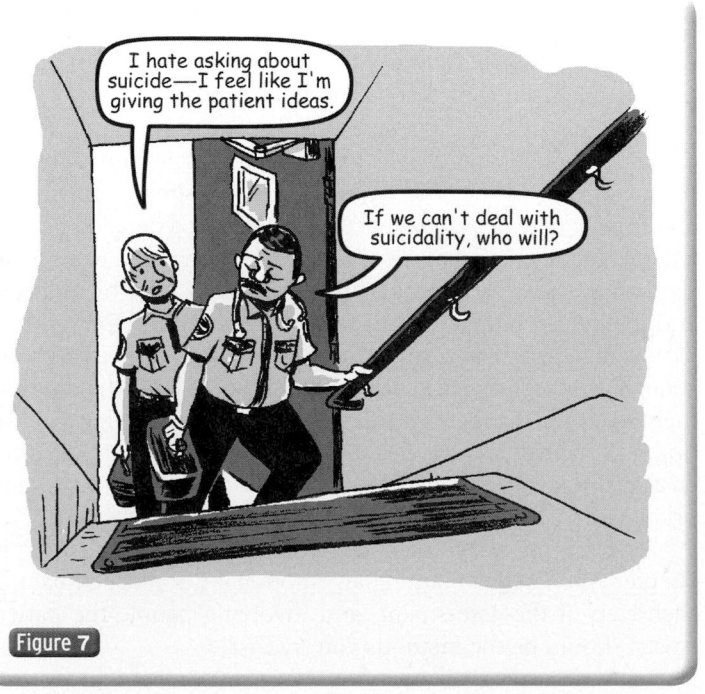

Figure 7

- **Do not leave the patient alone.** The patient's well-being is your responsibility until he or she is transferred to the care of another medical professional.
- **Collect implements.** Bring any implements of potential self-destruction you may have found at the scene (pill bottles, weapons) to the hospital.
- **Acknowledge the patient's feelings.** Do not argue with the wish to die, but provide honest reassurance. ("It's not unusual for a person to feel like you do after losing someone close to them. Sometimes it helps to talk about it.")
- **Encourage transport.** If the patient refuses transport, try to get the people who are close to him or her to help the patient cooperate. If the patient continues to resist, it may be necessary to obtain law enforcement assistance.

When a person has *attempted* suicide, medical treatment has priority. The patient who has taken an overdose of sedative or depressant drugs must be managed for possible respiratory depression or circulatory collapse; the patient who has slashed his or her wrists must be treated to control bleeding and restore circulating volume. Nonetheless, if the patient is conscious, try to establish communication and ask the patient to talk about the situation.

A person who attempts suicide is in enormous distress. Among the most important skills that any health care provider can acquire is the ability to see beyond another person's behavior to the underlying distress. When you are called to treat a person who has attempted suicide, it is worthwhile to say to the person, and to remind yourself, "You must have been unhappy to do something like this. It's time to get some help."

■ Patterns of Violence, Abuse, and Neglect

Few situations are as difficult for the paramedic as dealing with a hostile, angry patient, or a victim of abuse or neglect. It takes a great deal of maturity and a lot of experience to understand your own personal feelings in these situations and remain professional, positive, and still provide the best care you can to all parties involved.

Abuse and Neglect

Victims and perpetrators of violence and abuse may themselves have a mental illness that contributes to the situation. An astute paramedic will not only assess the patient, but will also assess the environment and other persons involved in order to look for indicators that suggest abuse, neglect, or patterns of violence. Document your findings so they may be appropriately used to support a case of neglect or abuse. Report your concerns for abuse and neglect according to your local protocols. Safety and management of acute medical and trauma concerns are your priorities in these situations.

Violence

Anger may be a response to illness and aggressive behavior may be the patient's way of dealing with feelings of helplessness. Sometimes the patient seems to be implying, "There's something wrong with me, and you're not doing everything possible to help." The temptation is to respond with anger, but doing so rarely serves any useful purpose. Most angry patients can be calmed by a trained person who conveys an impression of confidence that the patient will behave well. It may be helpful to ask the patient directly

about his or her anger: "Can you explain why you're so angry with me?" Giving the patient a chance to talk about these feelings often enables the patient to gain mastery over those feelings.

A patient who is violent or threatening violence poses one of the most difficult management problems for EMS personnel. EMS personnel should prepare themselves beforehand—both psychologically and tactically—to deal with hostile or violent behavior. Furthermore, the encounter with a violent patient carries the constant risk that someone may get hurt—the patient, a bystander, the paramedics, or all of them. The best way to ensure that no one is harmed is to take preventive action—that is, to assess the potential for violence in *every* call and to take steps to prevent violence from happening.

Assessing the potential for violence is not merely an academic exercise. The majority of paramedics are exposed to some form of violence during their career; this could include verbal intimidation, verbal abuse, physical abuse, sexual harassment, or sexual assault. It is crucial that paramedics stay alert for possible violent encounters and take measures to prevent them before they occur.

Identifying Situations With the Potential for Violence

Preventive action starts with being psychologically prepared for a possible violent encounter and keeping that possibility somewhere in the back of your mind in your response to *every* call. Do not rely too heavily on the information you get from your dispatcher. Being psychologically prepared for violence does *not* mean becoming paranoid or treating every patient with distrust. It *does* mean developing a "nose for danger," also known as "survival awareness."

Risk Factors for Violence

Scenarios in which violence is more likely to occur include any situation where alcohol or illicit drugs are being consumed (eg, tavern, party), crowd incidents, and incidents in which violence has already occurred (eg, shooting, stabbing, domestic disturbances). People who are more likely to be violent include those who are intoxicated with alcohol or drugs (especially PCP, LSD, amphetamines, and cocaine), experiencing withdrawal from alcohol or drugs, psychotic (especially manic and paranoid types), or delirious from any cause (eg, hypoglycemia, sepsis).

The most important clues to the patient's potential for violence are found in the person's behavior and body language. Look for the following warning signals:

- **Posture**—the patient who sits tensely at the edge of the chair or grips at the armrest.
- **Speech**—loud, critical, threatening, full of profanity.
- **Motor activity**—unable to sit still; pacing back and forth or in circles; easily startled.
- **Other body language**—clenched fists, avoidance of eye contact, turning away when spoken to.
- **Your own feelings**—your own "gut" response to the patient. If your instinct tells you that you are in danger, pay attention!

Management of the Violent Patient

Once you have concluded, for *any* reason, that there is a potential for violence in a situation, take the following steps:

Assess the whole situation. Are factors in the surroundings contributing to the escalation of violence (eg, friends who are egging the patient on)? Can those factors be removed? Does evidence suggest drug use, alcohol use, head injury, or diabetes? Can anyone present give you some background information? (Did the patient's behavior come on gradually or suddenly? Does he or she have a history of violent behavior? Are there any known medical problems, such as diabetes?)

Observe your surroundings. Make sure you have an escape route. Place yourself between the patient and the door, but do not move behind an agitated patient. Do not turn your back on the patient, even for a moment. Note any furniture or other potential barriers. Scan the area for anything that could be used as a weapon (eg, heavy or sharp objects) if the level of violence escalates. If a violent patient is armed with a weapon, do not try to deal with the situation yourself; back off and notify law enforcement authorities. Make sure that others at the scene are not endangered while you await the arrival of the police.

Maintain a safe distance. Moving too close to a potentially violent patient is likely to increase his or her anxiety level. Maintain a safety zone of two arm lengths; if the patient is backing away from you, it is a sign that you are too close. Let the patient find a comfortable distance. Do not position yourself directly face-to-face with the patient but rather slightly to the side at a 45° angle, with your escape route unobstructed.

Try verbal interventions first. Anger and aggressive behavior are often responses to illness or to feelings of helplessness. Just talking to the angry person in a calm, sympathetic way may defuse some of the anger.

- Take a moment to concentrate your own thoughts so that you can convey an impression of calmness and self-control to the patient.
- Identify yourselves as medical personnel who are there to try to help. Keep your voice low—that forces the patient to stop what he or she is doing to focus on what you are saying.
- Acknowledge the patient's behavior, and restate your willingness to help. ("You look upset. How can we help you?").
- Encourage the patient to talk about what is bothering him or her. Listen to what is said, and show that you are listening by paraphrasing the words back to the patient. ("I think I understand. Are you saying that . . .?")
- Ask the patient specifically if he or she might lose control or is carrying any sort of weapon.
- Define your expectations of the patient's behavior. Acknowledge his or her potential to do harm ("You could really hurt someone with that crowbar . . ."), but assure the patient that losing control will not be permitted.
- If "verbal de-escalation" is not working, back off and get help. ("Sir, I think we need to take a break to see if you can get hold of yourself, but I'm not leaving. We'll try talking again in a few minutes. If that doesn't work, I'm going to have some people with me to keep you from hurting anyone.")

Specific Psychiatric Disorders

The following disorders will be not diagnosed by a paramedic, but it is helpful to be familiar with these as potential causes for acute psychosis or agitated delirium. Assessment and treatment of patients with these conditions follows the general principles discussed earlier in this chapter.

Mood Disorders

Mood disorders, formally known as affective disorders, are among the most prevalent psychiatric disorders. As much as 10% of the US population will experience a mood disorder, such as a manic-depressive illness or a major depression, at some point in their lives. Although feelings such as depression and joy are universal, mood disorders differ from normal bouts of sadness or happiness. In mood disorders, the changes in affect are accompanied by other symptoms, and the net effect is to cause a major disturbance in the person's ability to function. Patients who experience either depression or mania have a unipolar mood disorder; that is, their mood remains at only one pole of the depression-mania continuum. Patients who alternate between mania and depression (both poles of the continuum) have bipolar mood disorder. Most patients with a unipolar mood disorder are depressed. Unipolar mania is relatively rare.

YOU are the Medic   PART 4

The patient appears to have tolerated having his vital signs taken but continues to glance nervously at the officers outside of his apartment. You explain to the patient that you can help him by transporting him to the hospital. He can obtain safe medication and treatment. You explain that he needs to continue taking his medication to treat his illness. You offer to drive him in the ambulance where he will be safe. He appears to consider this but continues to be apprehensive.

The patient becomes more agitated and refuses transport to the hospital. He tells you that it is not safe for him to leave his apartment. The officers express concern about allowing him to refuse transport because of the potential of harm to himself or others should his condition worsen. You consider your options and contact medical control for the recommendations. The physician orders administration of haloperidol (Haldol) 5 mg IM. You are concerned about how the patient may react to this decision, but explain to the patient that the physician at the hospital feels he should be evaluated and treated for his condition and has ordered administration of medication that will help him relax.

7. What are your considerations and concerns for administration of this medication to an uncooperative patient?

8. What are some legal implications of taking this patient to the hospital without his consent?

Manic Behavior <u>Mania</u> is one of the most striking psychiatric conditions. Typically a bystander or family member calls for an ambulance because the patient is unlikely to believe that anything is wrong. To the contrary, the manic patient is more apt to report being "on top of the world—never felt better in my life." Persons experiencing mania typically have abnormally exaggerated happiness, joy, or euphoria with hyperactivity and insomnia.

Manic patients are typically awake and alert but are easily distracted. They are also often markedly hyperactive and may report being unable to concentrate. Almost all manic patients report a significantly decreased need for sleep, and they may go for days without sleeping. In conversation, persons experiencing mania are talkative, with pressured and rapid speech. Flight of ideas and delusions of grandeur make it difficult for them to focus on one thing. Patients may report that their thoughts are racing; their monologues may skip rapidly from one topic to another (<u>tangential thinking</u>). Their ideas are often grandiose, such as unrealistic plans to embark on a large business venture or to run for high public office. Patients may also believe that they have special powers or they are famous and wealthy. Their memory is usually intact but may be distorted by underlying delusions. Their affect is elated (the hallmark of mania). The patient seems to be on a "high," and is unusually and infectiously cheerful. The good cheer may be quite brittle, however, and the person may quickly become irritable, sarcastic, and hostile with little provocation. A person having an acute manic episode may show psychotic symptoms such as hallucinations.

Persons experiencing acute manic episodes have a high probability of getting themselves into trouble of one sort or another—for example, going on wild spending sprees, making foolish business investments, driving recklessly, committing sexual indiscretions, or picking fights. Generally it is when the person has gotten into some sort of trouble, or when his or her behavior has become intolerably disruptive, that an ambulance is summoned.

Because manic patients are unlikely to consider themselves ill, they may not agree that they need treatment. In dealing with the manic patient, be calm, firm, and patient; do not argue or get into a power struggle. Minimize external stimulation. Talk to the patient in a quiet place, away from other people. (Meanwhile, have your partner obtain the history separately from relatives or bystanders.) When it is time to transport the patient, do not use sirens.

If the patient refuses transport, consult medical control. Obtain law enforcement assistance for transport if your medical director indicates that hospital evaluation is necessary.

Depression Depression is the leading cause of disability in people between ages 15 and 44 years. It affects women more frequently than men and may occur at any age (the mean age of onset is 32 years). The depressed patient is often readily identified by a sad expression, bouts of crying, and listless or apathetic behavior. He or she expresses feelings of worthlessness, guilt, and pessimism. These patients may want to be left alone, asserting that no one understands or cares and that their problems are hopeless.

Depression may occur in episodes with a sudden onset and limited duration; this is common in major depressive disorder, in which the patient feels substantial suffering and pain that interfere with social or occupational functioning. In other cases, the onset of depression may be insidious and chronic in nature. When a person experiences signs and symptoms of depression for more days than not for a period of at least 2 years, he or she may be experiencing a chronic form of depression known as dysthymic disorder. The signs and symptoms of dysthymic disorder cause social and occupational distress but rarely require hospitalization unless the person becomes suicidal.

The diagnostic features of depression are most easily remembered by the mnemonic GAS PIPES:

- **Guilt** and self-reproach are characteristic features of depression. One way to try to get at the patient's guilt feelings is to ask a question such as "Are you down on yourself?" or "Do you ever feel as if you're worthless?"
- **Appetite** is abnormal in depression. Usually it is decreased, but a minority of depressed patients may report increased appetite.
- **Sleep** disturbance usually takes the form of insomnia. The typical depressed patient will report that he or she awakens at 3:00 or 4:00 AM and cannot get back to sleep.
- **Paying attention.** The depressed patient has an impaired ability to concentrate; the impairment is sometimes severe. Ask the patient, "When you're reading a book or a newspaper, can you get all the way through what you're reading, or does your mind start to wander after a couple of minutes?"
- **Interest.** The depressed patient loses interest in things that were once important. He or she can no longer summon enthusiasm for work or hobbies. You might ask the patient, "Are you a [local team name] fan?" If the answer is yes, ask, "How are they doing this season?" The depressed patient will tell you, "Well, I haven't really been following them lately."
- **Psychomotor abnormalities.** In the depressed patient, psychomotor abnormalities can be increased (from agitation) or slowed. Although many depressed patients seem to do everything in slow motion, a significant percentage show agitated behavior, such as pacing, wringing their hands, or picking at themselves.
- **Energy.** Depressed people have no energy. They are tired all the time and do not feel like doing anything.
- **Suicidal thoughts.** Most worrisome, depressed people tend to have pervasive and recurrent thoughts of suicide.

Schizophrenia

<u>Schizophrenia</u> is a complex disorder that is neither easily defined nor readily treated, yet has a dramatic effect on society. One in 100 people will be affected by schizophrenia in their lifetimes. An estimated 0.2% to 1.5% of the world's population has schizophrenia. The typical onset occurs during early adulthood, with dysfunctional symptoms becoming more prominent over time. Some persons diagnosed with schizophrenia display signs during early childhood; their disease may be associated with brain damage sustained early in life. Other influences thought to contribute to this disorder include genetics, neurobiologic influences, and psychological and social influences.

Persons with schizophrenia may experience delusions, hallucinations, apathy, mutism, a flat affect, a lack of interest in pleasure, erratic speech, emotional responses, and motor behavior (either a lack of motor behavior, or excessive motor behavior).

Neurotic Disorders

Neurotic disorders are a collection of psychiatric disorders without psychotic symptoms and lacking the intense psychopathology of other mood disorders. These disorders cause many problems for persons, their families, and society in general. Treating neurotic disorders comes at a subantial price; however, the cost to society of not treating these disorders (in terms of lost production and lost efficiency) is probably more.

This category of conditions includes **anxiety disorders**, mental disorders in which the dominant moods are fear and apprehension. Everyone experiences anxiety occasionally, and a certain amount of anxiety helps people adapt constructively to stress. Patients with anxiety disorders, by contrast, experience persistent, incapacitating anxiety in the absence of external threat. Almost one fifth of adults will experience some form of anxiety disorder in any given year. Several types of anxiety disorders, including generalized anxiety disorder, phobias, and panic disorder, are likely to elicit a call for an ambulance or affect the delivery of prehospital care.

Generalized Anxiety Disorder Although some anxiety in everyday activity is normal, when a person worries about everything for no particular reason, or if that worrying is unproductive and the person cannot decide what to do about an upcoming situation, the person may be experiencing **generalized anxiety disorder (GAD)**. To make a diagnosis of GAD, symptoms (anxiety and worry) must be present more days than not for a period of at least 6 months and the worry must be difficult to turn off or control. GAD is one of the most common anxiety disorders. Patients experiencing GAD are often treated with both pharmacologic agents and counseling. The acute symptoms of anxiety and worry can become overwhelming in GAD, however, prompting a family member or coworker to call for an ambulance.

When you are dealing with a patient with GAD, identify yourself in a calm, confident manner. Listen attentively to the patient and talk with the person generally about his or her feelings.

Phobias **Phobic disorders** involve an unreasonable fear, apprehension, or dread of a specific situation or thing. The patient with a **simple phobia** focuses all his or her anxieties onto one class of objects (eg, mice, spiders, dogs) or situations (eg, high places, darkness, flying). Almost one tenth of adults have social phobias, or fear of everyday social situations such as fear of going to parties, meeting new people, speaking, or eating in public. When confronted with the feared object or situation, the phobic person experiences intolerable anxiety and all of the autonomic symptoms that anxiety brings. The patient usually recognizes that the fear is unreasonable but is unable to do anything about it.

In managing a phobic patient, explain each step of treatment in detail before you carry it out **Figure 8** : "First we'll give you oxygen to help you breathe. Then we're going to move you onto the stretcher, so that we can carry you downstairs."

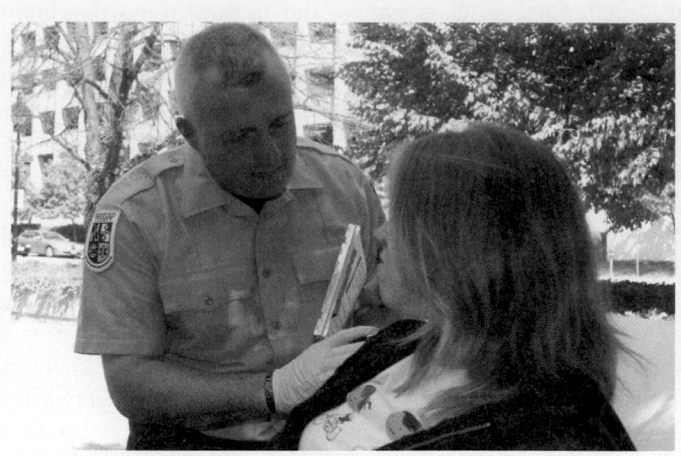

Figure 8 With a phobic patient, explain each step of treatment in detail before carrying it out.

Table 7 Signs and Symptoms of a Panic Attack	
- Shortness of breath or a sensation of being smothered	- Dizziness or feeling faint
- Palpitations or tachycardia	- Trembling
- Sweating	- Feeling of choking
- Nausea or abdominal distress	- Paresthesias
- Flushes or chills	- Chest pain or discomfort
- Fear of dying	- Fear of going crazy
- Feelings of unreality or of being detached from oneself	

Source: Adapted from American Psychiatric Association, *Diagnostic and Statistical Manual of Mental Disorders, Fourth Edition, Text Revision.* Washington, DC: APA, 2000.

Panic Disorder **Panic disorder** is characterized by sudden, usually unexpected, and overwhelming feelings of fear and dread, accompanied by a variety of other symptoms produced by a massive activation of the autonomic nervous system. Women are two thirds more likely to be affected by this condition than are men, and the disorder tends to run in families. The attacks usually begin when the patient is in his or her 20s. Most affected persons can identify a stressful event that preceded their first attack, such as an illness or loss of a loved one. Thereafter, the attacks may come "out of the blue," without any apparent precipitating stress. If allowed to continue, panic attacks may cause severe restrictions in the patient's lifestyle. The person becomes afraid to go to work, to go shopping, or to leave the house at all, out of fear that an attack will occur away from home. The fear of going into public places is called **agoraphobia** (literally, "fear of the marketplace").

The classic signs and symptoms of panic disorder are summarized in **Table 7** . A large percentage of the signs and symptoms—such as palpitations and sweating—are a consequence of autonomic nervous system discharge, whereas others (chest discomfort, paresthesias) may reflect hyperventilation. The symptoms usually peak in intensity within about 10 minutes and last around an hour altogether.

By the time you arrive at the scene, the patient having a panic attack may be surrounded by many anxious and excited people, who will themselves contribute to the problem. Accordingly, you will need to take the following steps to control the situation quickly:

- **Separate the patient from panicky bystanders.** If you can find a calm friend or member of the patient's family, however, having this person present may be helpful.
- **Provide a calm environment.** The environment should be as calm as possible as you transport the patient to the hospital.
- **Be tolerant of the patient's disability.** The patient having an anxiety attack may not be able to cooperate or answer questions at first because of intense fear and distress. Your manner must convey that everything is under control.
- **Reassure the patient that he or she is safe.** The word "safe" can be a magic pill that will often de-escalate symptoms to a more manageable level: "We're going to take you down these stairs on the stretcher. It's going to be okay; we'll go slowly and be careful to keep you safe while we move you."
- **Give the patient's symptoms a name.** Once you have checked the vital signs and the electrocardiogram (ECG) monitor, you should be in a position to reassure the patient that he or she is not in immediate danger of dying: "I know that your feeling of panic is distressing, but it is not life-threatening."
- **Help the patient regain control.** Encourage the patient to do things for himself or herself to the extent that he or she is able, to help regain a sense of being in control.

Panic attacks may mimic a range of physical disorders in their presentation. Conversely, symptoms of anxiety may be the presenting complaint in medical conditions such as cardiac dysrhythmias, withdrawal states, anaphylaxis, hyperthyroidism, and certain tumors. For that reason, any patient experiencing a panic attack—especially a first panic attack—should be fully evaluated in the hospital. Hyperventilating patients should not be treated with "paper bag therapy." Patients whose anxiety results from an unsuspected pulmonary embolism or cardiac problem may experience serious complications and even die of hypoxemia if a paper bag is used. Hyperventilation is best managed by coaching patients to slow their breathing until they regain control.

Substance-Related Disorders and Addictive Behavior

Disorders of substance use, addiction, and personal control generally evolve over a relatively long period of time. Because of the chronic nature of these problems, EMS will typically be called when an acute exacerbation of the underlying problem occurs—for example, when a bulimic patient experiences electrolyte imbalances that produce a sudden onset of weakness, dizziness, cardiac or respiratory problems, or seizures, or when an alcoholic experiences respiratory depression from binge drinking. Emergency management of these patients typically focuses on treating symptomatic complaints and the presenting signs and symptoms.

Substance-Related Disorders Substance-related disorders include psychological disorders associated with the use of alcohol, cigarettes, illicit drugs, and other substances that change the way a person feels, behaves, or thinks. These disorders cost thousands of lives and billions of dollars annually. It was not until 1980 that substance-related disorders were recognized as a complex biologic and psychological problem rather than a sign of moral weakness. An estimated 8.7% of the US population used illegal drugs in 2009.

Substance-related disorders are regarded on four levels. In **substance use**, a person may use moderate amounts of a substance without seriously affecting ADLs (eg, a social drinker). **Substance intoxication** describes use that results in impaired thinking and motor function (eg, a drunk driver). **Substance abuse** occurs when the use of a substance disrupts ADLs (eg, a person has difficulty with work, school, or relationships). **Substance dependence** describes an addiction to a substance. The person is physiologically dependent and requires increasingly larger amounts to produce the same effect. An addict may display "drug-seeking behaviors" such as the repeated use of the substance or taking desperate measures to ingest more of the substance (stealing money, standing out in the cold to smoke a cigarette).

Determining the most effective treatment for substance-related disorders requires an integrative approach of examining the social, biologic, cultural, cognitive, and psychological dimensions of the problem. As a paramedic, it will be difficult for you to explore these areas during a short transport to the hospital, particularly given that much of your time will be devoted to ensuring the safety of your crew and the patient's ABCs. Understanding the complex nature of substance-related disorders is the first step in providing professional, competent, and compassionate care to the homeless drug addict as well as the substance-dependent businessperson.

Eating Disorders Eating disorders have been around for many decades, although their incidence began to increase rapidly in the 1950s and 1960s. Today, eating disorders are widespread in the developed world and are emerging as a problem in developing countries: Some countries are experiencing a fourfold increase in eating disorders. Persons most likely to be affected by these disorders are young females of upper middle class or upper class socioeconomic status who live in socially competitive surroundings.

There are two major types of eating disorders: **bulimia nervosa** and **anorexia nervosa**. In both forms, persons may experience severe electrolyte imbalances leading to cardiac problems, seizures, and renal failure as well as erosion of dental enamel and salivary gland enlargement. Anxiety, depression, and substance abuse disorders are noted in as many as two thirds of those persons diagnosed with eating disorders.

Bulimia nervosa is characterized by consumption of large amounts of food, typically more junk food than fruits and vegetables; many persons with this disorder describe their eating as "out of control." Most patients compensate for the binge eating by using purging techniques such as vomiting, laxatives, diuretics, or excessive exercise. Persons with bulimia are humiliated by both their problem and their lack of control.

People with anorexia differ from those with bulimia in one important characteristic—they are successful at losing weight.

Unfortunately, they are so effective at losing weight that they jeopardize their health and even their lives. They may even binge, albeit on smaller quantities of food. These persons diet by exerting extraordinary control over their eating. The typical anorexic has decreased body weight based on age and height, demonstrates an intense fear of obesity even though the person is underweight, and experiences amenorrhea (the absence of menstruation).

Somatoform Disorders

People who are overly concerned with their physical health and appearance may have a <u>somatoform disorder</u> if their preoccupation dominates their life. A hypochondriac provides the classic example of a somatoform disorder. In hypochondriasis, patients have a great deal of anxiety or fear that they may have a serious disease. They are so convinced that they are ill that even a physician cannot convince them otherwise. Although the problem in hypochondriasis is anxiety, the person is preoccupied with other supposed symptoms. With somatization disorder, patients also have multiple complaints, but are more concerned with the symptoms than with their meaning. In conversion disorders, a physical problem (eg, paralysis, blindness, or seizures) has no identifiable pathophysiology, but results from malingering or faking a physical disorder.

Factitious Disorders

A <u>factitious disorder</u>, also called Münchausen syndrome, is one in which a person intentionally produces or feigns physical or psychological signs or symptoms. In such cases, the patient wishes to be sick. There could be various motives for such behavior, for example to avoid legal responsibility, or to gain attention. The symptoms the patient is experiencing are under voluntary control and there is no obvious physiologic reason for the symptoms.

The symptoms the patient experiences may be physical, psychological, or both; are usually quite dramatic; and indicate an immediate need for care. Patients will typically present at night or on weekends in hopes of finding less skilled health care providers or of having difficulty obtaining insurance or medical records.

One type of factitious disorder is factitious disorder by proxy, also called Münchausen syndrome by proxy. This refers to a situation in which a parent intentionally makes a child sick to garner attention and pity. This is an atypical form of child abuse.

Impulse Control Disorders

Persons who have <u>impulse control disorders</u> lack the ability to resist a temptation or cannot avoid acting on a drive. Examples of impulse control disorders include intermittent explosive disorder (acting on aggressive impulses involving

YOU *are the Medic*   PART 5

The patient attempts to rise and move past you as you prepare the medication. Your partner has already explained what has been ordered to the officers and they quickly move to restrain the patient to the chair. They continue to secure him while you administer the medication to a site on the rectus femoris muscle through his slacks. You expect to see changes in the patient within 10 minutes, so the officers continue to restrain the patient to the chair while your partner prepares the stretcher and you obtain another set of vital signs including a blood glucose level. You continue to tell the patient what is happening, and collect his medications and identification. The patient is secured to the stretcher and has become much less agitated.

You and your partner move him to the ambulance with the assistance of two officers. During transport, an officer agrees to ride with you. You reassess the patient's vital signs every 5 minutes, watching for potential side effects from the medication. On arrival, you give your report to the receiving nurse and place the patient in the psychiatric treatment area of the emergency department. You complete your patient care report with the awareness of the importance of good documentation for the patient with a behavioral emergency.

Recording Time: 20 Minutes	
Respirations	14 breaths/min
Pulse	88 beats/min
Skin	Warm, pink, and dry
Blood pressure	118/78 mm Hg
Oxygen saturation (Spo$_2$)	98% on room air
Pupils	Equal, round, and reactive to light
Blood glucose level	96 mg/dL

9. Why is it important to check for blood glucose levels in a patient with a behavioral emergency?

10. What is the most common side effect that can occur with administration of haloperidol and how do you treat it?

11. What are some important aspects related to documentation of a patient having a behavioral emergency that you should consider?

the destruction of property), kleptomania (acting on the urge to steal things), pyromania (acting on the urge to set fires), and pathologic gambling.

Of course, not every arsonist is a pyromaniac, nor is everyone who steals a kleptomaniac. Impulse control disorders are typically associated with other disorders, such as depression, antisocial or borderline personality disorders, and Alzheimer disease. This group of disorders is rare; only 4% of arsonists are diagnosed with pyromania, for example.

In-hospital treatment relies on cognitive and behavioral interventions to identify underlying triggers and influences.

Personality Disorders

According to the American Psychiatric Association, <u>personality disorders</u> are "enduring patterns of perceiving, relating to, and thinking about the environment and one's self that are exhibited in a wide range of social and personal contexts" and are "inflexible and maladaptive, and cause significant functional impairment or subjective distress." Common definitions of "personality" include the ways a person behaves or thinks. How people think or behave in the world and with others may be suspicious, outgoing, fearful, or overly dramatic. When these ways of relating to others become dysfunctional or cause distress to other people, that person is considered to have a personality disorder. Many times the person with the personality disorder does not feel any subjective distress, whereas others feel such distress acutely.

True personality disorders are rare in the general population. When a person does have a personality disorder, another psychiatric illness is likely to be present at the same time. Such patients tend to do poorly during treatment. For example, patients who are depressed in addition to having a personality disorder usually have more difficulty managing the depression when compared with patients who have no personality disorder.

EMS providers have difficulty influencing personality disorders over the long term because of their limited interaction with patients. Nevertheless, it is important for you to understand these abnormal behaviors so that you are aware of how to react appropriately in the current situation. For example, a patient with an antisocial personality will not hesitate to hurt you if agitated, whereas one with a histrionic personality may be demanding and dictate the level of care. Be calm and professional in your interactions with patients exhibiting these traits.

Medications for Psychiatric Disorders and Behavioral Emergencies

Patients with psychiatric problems may be taking any of several types of <u>psychotropic drugs</u>—that is, drugs that affect mood, thought, or behavior. During your assessment, determine which medications have been prescribed for your patient and whether he or she is actually taking them. Psychotropic drugs are among the most widely prescribed medications in the United

States. Most of these medications target the autonomic nervous system by either inhibiting or enhancing the sympathetic or parasympathetic nervous systems. It is important that you have a thorough understanding of these two systems as well as knowledge of how the drugs in your paramedic's kit may potentially interact with these types of medications.

Psychiatric Medication Types

Antidepressants

Antidepressants are prescribed to combat the symptoms of depressive illness (Table 8). The main types of antidepressants are serotonin reuptake inhibitors, tricyclic antidepressants, and monoamine oxidase (MAO) inhibitors.

The mechanism of action for most antidepressants lies within their ability to alter levels of neurotransmitters in the autonomic nervous system such as serotonin, norepinephrine, or dopamine. The most commonly prescribed antidepressant in the United States is fluoxetine, a selective serotonin reuptake inhibitor (SSRI). Other SSRIs currently available include sertraline and paroxetine. SSRIs are primarily used to treat major depressive episodes but are also useful in anxiety disorders, including generalized anxiety disorder, panic disorder, and obsessive-compulsive disorder. Side effects are minimal, and because they lack the anticholinergic and cardiac effects typical of other antidepressants, overdose of SSRIs does relatively

Table 8 Medications for Depression

Class	Generic Name	Trade Name
Heterocyclic (tricyclic and tetracyclic) antidepressants and related drugs	Amitriptyline	Amitril, Endep, Elavil
	Amoxapine	Asendin
	Desipramine	Norpramin, Pertofrane
	Doxepin	Adapin, Sinequan
	Imipramine	Imavate, Janimine, Pramine, Presamine, Tofranil
	Maprotiline	Ludiomil
	Nortriptyline	Aventyl, Pamelor
	Protriptyline	Vivactil
	Trimipramine	Surmontil
MAO inhibitors	Isocarboxazid	Marplan
	Phenelzine	Nardil
	Tranylcypromine	Parnate
Selective serotonin reuptake inhibitors	Fluoxetine	Prozac
	Paroxetine	Paxil
	Sertraline	Zoloft
Others	Trazodone	Desyrel
	Bupropion	Wellbutrin

little harm. Side effects include symptomatic bradycardia with fluoxetine, whereas other more common side effects are headaches, dizziness, sexual dysfunction, nausea, diarrhea, insomnia, and agitation.

Heterocyclic (tricyclic and tetracyclic) antidepressants are a group of medications, some in use since the 1950s, that have been primarily used for major depression, but may also be effective for panic disorder, agoraphobia, obsessive-compulsive disorder, enuresis, and school phobia. Examples include amitriptyline, desipramine, imipramine, and nortriptyline. Side effects are common and often occur even though serum levels may be within the designated therapeutic range. Most side effects are either anticholinergic (dry mouth, metallic taste, blurred vision, constipation, sedation, mydriasis, agitation, and delirium) or cardiotoxic (eg, nonspecific T-wave changes, prolonged QT interval, varying degrees of atrioventricular block, and atrial and ventricular dysrhythmias). Orthostatic hypotension is common in the elderly. Heterocyclic antidepressants are not frequently prescribed today because of these serious side effects.

A third class of antidepressant, monoamine oxidase inhibitors, are recommended for atypical major depressive episodes. They are also occasionally useful in selected cases of heterocyclic-refractory major depression and panic disorder. One potential side effect is orthostatic hypotension, which, although occasionally severe, usually responds to supportive therapy. Other side effects include CNS irritability, including agitation, motor restlessness, and insomnia.

Benzodiazepines

Several classes of medications are effective in the treatment of anxiety disorders, including many antidepressants **Table 9**.

A physician may prescribe benzodiazepines in the treatment of a person experiencing severe emotional distress, even if the patient is not psychotic or an imminent threat to himself or herself or others. Even so, benzodiazepines are not a substitute for more formal therapy, and short-term medication therapy may be helpful in the anxious patient experiencing crisis or acute panic reactions. Other uses include muscle relaxation; controlling seizures; and treating alcohol, sedative, or hypnotic withdrawal. Benzodiazepines are contraindicated in patients with known hypersensitivity to benzodiazepines and in patients with acute, narrow-angle glaucoma. Pregnancy, particularly in the first trimester, is a relative contraindication. Some benzodiazepines have long half-lives and gradually accumulate in the body and therefore have a greater potential for causing sedation and confusion, particularly in the elderly.

Antipsychotics

Antipsychotic drugs were first introduced in the 1950s to treat mental health illnesses such as schizophrenia and other psychoses. They revolutionized the management of these types of disorders with their effect on the patient's neurologic function, which led to the term neuroleptics. These older medications, while still in use today, are known to have varying degrees of adverse effects. Newer antipsychotic medications have less risk of adverse effects and are more effective at treating the cognitive

Table 9 Medications for Anxiety

Class	Generic Name	Trade Name
Antidepressants		
Selective serotonin reuptake inhibitors	Citalopram	Celexa
	Escitalopram	Lexapro
	Fluoxetine	Prozac
	Fluvoxamine	Luvox
	Paroxetine	Paxil
	Sertraline	Zoloft
Monoamine oxidase inhibitors	Phenelzine	Nardil
Serotonin-norepinephrine reuptake inhibitors	Venlafaxine	Effexor
Anxiolytics		
Benzodiazepines	Alprazolam	Xanax
	Chlordiazepoxide	Librium
	Clonazepam	Klonopin
	Clorazepate	Tranxene
	Diazepam	Valium
	Lorazepam	Ativan
Nonbenzodiazepines	Buspirone	Buspar
Other Classes		
Antihistamines	Hydroxyzine	Atarax, Vistaril
Beta blockers	Propanolol	Inderol
Anticonvulsants	Carbamazepine	Tegretol
	Gabapentin	Neurontin
	Valproic acid	Depakote

dysfunction associated with psychoses. This new class of antipsychotics is known as atypical antipsychotic (AAP) drugs, whereas the original, older medications are referred to as typical antipsychotic drugs. The pharmacokinetics of all antipsychotic medications are similar. **Table 10** lists antipsychotic medications.

The AAP agents are often used as first-line therapy because they not only relieve symptoms such as delusions and hallucinations but also enhance the quality of life by improving the affective symptoms of anxiety and depression and decreasing suicidal tendencies. However, the AAP medications may cause metabolic side effects such as glucose deregulation, hypercholesterolemia, and hypertension.

The cardiovascular effects of both typical and atypical antipsychotics depend on the specific medication. They directly affect the heart and blood vessels and indirectly act through CNS and autonomic reflexes to produce other cardiovascular changes. The results are as varied as simple orthostatic hypotension and as complex as ECG changes. A subcategory of traditional

Table 10	Antipsychotic Medications	
Type	**Generic Name**	**Trade Name**
Atypical antipsychotic (AAP) agents	Aripiprazole	Abilify
	Clozapine	Clozaril
	Olanzapine	Zyprexa
	Quetiapine	Seroquel
	Risperidone	Risperidal
	Ziprasidone	Geodon
Traditional antipsychotics	Chlorpromazine	Thorazine
	Chlorprothixene	Taractan
	Fluphenazine	Prolixin, Permitil
	Haloperidol	Haldol
	Loxapine	Loxitane, Daxolin
	Mesoridazine	Serentil
	Molindone	Moban
	Perphenazine	Trilafon
	Thioridazine	Mellaril
	Thiothixene	Navane
	Trifluoperazine	Stelazine

antipsychotics, known as phenothiazines, may reduce contractility of the heart. Haloperidol (Haldol), commonly used in paramedicine for treatment of acute psychosis, is found in this class. ECG changes include prolongation of the QT and PR intervals, blunting of T waves, and depression of the ST segment.

Patients taking antipsychotic agents may occasionally experience an **acute dystonic reaction**, in which the patient develops muscle spasms of the neck, face, and back within a few days of starting treatment with the drug. An acute dystonic reaction can be rapidly corrected by giving diphenhydramine (Benadryl), 25 to 50 mg IV, but the muscle spasms are likely to recur after the diphenhydramine wears off.

Typical antipsychotic medications also have **atropine-like effects** (anticholinergic effects), so patients taking antipsychotic medications may experience the side effects associated with atropine use, such as dry mouth, blurred vision, urinary retention, and cardiac dysrhythmias.

Amphetamines

Amphetamines are powerful central nervous system (CNS) and parasympathetic nervous system (PNS) stimulants similar to other sympathomimetic drugs (eg, epinephrine). Amphetamines (eg, Adderall) are prescribed to help with attention deficit disorder with hyperactivity in both adults and children. It is also used to treat narcolepsy in adults. When taken, they raise both systolic and diastolic blood pressure while the pulse rate often is slowed; with large doses, cardiac dysrhythmias may occur. The psychological effects depend on the dose, mental state, and personality of the patient. The results are alertness, reduced sense of fatigue, elevated mood, increased concentration, euphoria, and increased motor and speech activities.

Problems Associated With Medication Noncompliance

Most psychotropic medications are designed to alter a patient's mental state, most often to sedate or calm the patient. Dulling of the senses and slowed thinking are common reasons patients choose to be noncompliant (not stay on their medications). Another factor may also be the cost of the medications. For example, patients who have been prescribed amphetamines but who cannot afford them or do not have health insurance may consume energy drinks with high doses of caffeine or herbal supplements containing ephedra (ma huang) to compensate. This **medication noncompliance** often results in frequent confrontation with others when abnormal behaviors develop.

Changes in behavior are not always a result of the abuse of drugs. Behavior changes may also occur when medications have been prescribed and even dispensed to treat mental health symptoms but the person chooses to not take them. Noncompliance with medications, together with substance abuse, increases the likelihood that a person with a severe mental illness will commit a violent act. When you are obtaining the patient's medication history, previously prescribed medications and missed doses should always be included.

Emergency Use of Medications

To a greater or lesser degree, every call you respond to will have a behavioral component mixed in with the patient's trauma or medical problem. For example, the businessman having a heart attack may appear calm and collected, but he is still anxious. In this situation, treatment for an acute coronary syndrome includes oxygen, aspirin, nitroglycerin, and morphine as indicated. The morphine not only helps reduce the patient's anxiety, it also reduces discomfort and improves cardiac output. A woman who experiences intense anxiety after confronting her cheating husband may benefit from a small dose of a benzodiazepine if permitted by medical control.

The situations that require emergency use of medications are often those in which the behavioral component gives rise to violence in the situation—for example, the patient who is experiencing an acute psychotic episode or an agitated state of delirium. In these situations the potential danger to the patient, bystanders, and health care professionals is too great not to intervene, and the emergency use of medications may be indicated. The intensity of the situation and the patient's response to you will determine whether verbal, physical, or chemical intervention is necessary. Depending on your protocols and the situation, you may opt to administer medications for chemical restraint, as discussed earlier in this chapter. Before using medications to control behavior, you should complete your assessment with a thorough understanding of the patient's chief complaint and attention to allergies as well as medical and medication history. Antipsychotics or benzodiazepines are beneficial in situations involving aggression, but their use also comes with risks.

Special Populations

Pediatric Behavioral Problems

Fifty percent of childhood mental illnesses will present by age 14 years with 75% presenting by age 24. Many of these problems begin as simple complaints and are not easily recognized by health care providers. When not treated properly, such a problem will most likely persist into adulthood. Given that suicide is the third leading cause of death in adolescents and the fourth leading cause of death in children between ages 10 and 14 years, increased attention has been given to mood disorders, anxiety, and other behavioral problems in this population. Children are also more likely to have coexisting problems (eg, attention deficit hyperactivity disorder, conduct disorder, and oppositional defiant disorder) along with the more traditional mental health disorders.

Mental health problems in children are difficult to diagnose because the lines between normal and abnormal behavior are less clear in this population. Diagnosis and treatment may be difficult when trying to distinguish between organic, genetic, and environmental causes. Cultural and ethnic factors also blur the line between normal and abnormal coping mechanisms. The mental status assessment of the child is similar to that of an adult, but takes the child's developmental level into consideration. Abnormal findings in the developmental and MSE are often related to adjustment disorders and stress rather than the more serious disorders. Your assessment must include an assessment of suicide risk in any child Figure 9 .

Geriatric Behavioral Problems

As people age, they are exposed to new experiences and alterations to routines that may have become well established over the course of many years. Some of these experiences may result in physical and psychological changes in the older adult.

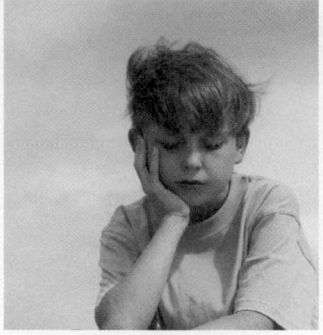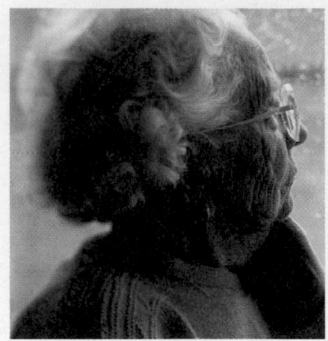

Figure 9 Children as well as older adults are affected by behavioral problems.

For example, dementia may result from Alzheimer disease, chronic alcohol abuse, aftereffects of multiple strokes, or nutritional deficiencies. The loss of loved ones or family moving away may cause loneliness. Financial worries, dissatisfaction with living arrangements, or doubts about the significance of one's life accomplishments may become a significant concern as well. These issues often produce psychological distress and physical pain, which may manifest as abnormal behavior.

An elderly person is less likely to be diagnosed accurately with a mental illness than is a similarly affected younger person. All too often, anxiety and depression are incorrectly considered a normal part of aging. Ageism is discrimination against older people because of their age. To avoid engaging in ageism and to provide proper care for the geriatric population, particularly those with mental health issues, you must first take stock of your own attitudes toward older people and the mentally ill. With this awareness, you will be able to perform a complete physical and psychosocial assessment without bias, and will understand the complex issues surrounding the care of older people.

YOU are the Medic   SUMMARY

1. What are the initial components of the assessment for this patient?

Provider safety is essential. The scene should be carefully assessed for potential hazards or weapons. Forming your general impression of the scene is important to help you identify possible clues to the patient's condition/behavior. You should form a general impression of the patient including behavior, personal hygiene, and posture. A visual assessment of life threats such as signs of alteration in breathing, inadequate circulation, or obvious hemorrhage should be done.

2. What are your safety concerns in dealing with this patient?

This patient is exhibiting behaviors suggestive of an acute psychotic episode. He is experiencing delusions and has an altered perception of reality. He is exhibiting signs that indicate there are risk factors for violence, such as refusing to allow the police officers in his apartment, refusal to come out of his apartment, delusions of violence against himself, and low socioeconomic status/potential for history of psychiatric illness based on his residence.

3. What is your initial impression of this patient? What factors, signs, or symptoms would lead you to this conclusion?

The patient appears to be having an acute psychotic episode, possibly schizophrenic. He appears agitated which is demonstrated by his pacing. He is exhibiting repetitive behavior by clenching and unclenching his fists. He is having delusions that are paranoid of people wanting to kill him. His mood appears anxious, and he is wary of strangers.

YOU are the Medic   SUMMARY, continued

4. Does this patient need to be evaluated at a hospital?

This patient needs to be evaluated at the hospital because he is having an acute episode. Because of his delusions, he may be a threat to himself or others. He may not be competent to refuse treatment and transport in his current condition.

5. What conclusions might you make about medication compliance and the patient's medical history?

Based on the fact that the patient is aware of his illness, states that he sees a physician regularly, and filled his prescription recently, it is likely the patient is normally compliant with his medications. Similar to results seen in medication noncompliance, the patient is likely experiencing this episode of psychotic behavior as a result of not taking medications for approximately 1 week. Therapeutic levels may have fallen to the degree that this patient's condition has exacerbated or behavior has become abnormal.

6. As a paramedic, what options should you consider if the patient refuses to be transported?

As a paramedic, you may have local protocols that address this situation with regard to use of restraint or law enforcement intervention. Local statutes may require that law enforcement personnel intervene as a result of concerns for the patient and the safety of others based on his condition. There are legal implications that should be considered, including the competence of the patient to make decisions. Medical control is an excellent resource. Orders to apply physical restraints or administer medications for the purposes of chemical restraint may be granted.

7. What are your considerations and concerns for administration of this medication to an uncooperative patient?

Benzodiazepines are typically considered to be the safest class of drug because of the ability to administer intranasally. Administration of medication such as haloperidol (Haldol) IM means that you will have a large exposed needle. If the patient is unrestrained or restrained ineffectively, you could be harmed during the administration attempt. The patient may view any medication administered as dangerous or a threat to his person. All medications have risks of side effects. As a potential benefit, haloperidol may be administered through clothing in this type of situation.

8. What are some legal implications of taking this patient to the hospital without his consent?

The patient may be determined to be competent later and your actions may constitute violating his rights. Adverse outcomes may generate other potential for litigation as well as harm to the patient.

9. Why is it important to check for blood glucose levels in a patient with a behavioral emergency?

Blood glucose levels can be obtained easily and allow you to rule out a medical disorder such as hypoglycemia as a cause for the abnormal behavior. Patients experiencing psychiatric disturbances may not be maintaining adequate nutrition; hypoglycemia may be present and may potentially contribute to the patient's condition.

10. What is the most common side effect that can occur with administration of haloperidol and how do you treat it?

The most common side effect is extrapyramidal symptoms, which include a wide array of symptoms such as involuntary movements, tremors, rigidity, muscle contractions, restlessness, and changes in breathing and pulse rate. If such symptoms occur, diphenhydramine hydrochloride (Benadryl) may be administered in a dose of 25 to 50 mg depending on local protocols. Because of the risk of this side effect, and assuming this is allowed per protocols, you should have diphenhydramine hydrochloride readily available after administration of haloperidol (Haldol).

11. What are some important aspects related to documentation of a patient having a behavioral emergency that you should consider?

Extra care and time should be spent completing a thorough patient care report. Document all assessment findings. Be objective in your findings and factual in your statements. Use direct quotes to incorporate any comments made by the patient. Identify all personnel who provided care for the patient, including the name of the physician providing any orders. Document all efforts to convince the patient to consent to treatment and/or transport.

EMS Patient Care Report (PCR)

Date: 08-14-11	**Incident No.:** 201035684	**Nature of Call:** Psychiatric emergency	**Location:** 906 Abbott Street, Apt 312		
Dispatched: 1528	**En Route:** 1529	**At Scene:** 1535	**Transport:** 1604	**At Hospital:** 1610	**In Service:** 1630

Patient Information

Age: 44 **Sex:** M **Weight (in kg [lb]):** 76.4 kg (168 lb)	**Allergies:** No known drug allergies **Medications:** Mellaril 200 mg twice daily, Serentil 50 mg twice daily **Past Medical History:** Schizophrenia **Chief Complaint:** Paranoid delusions

YOU *are the Medic*   SUMMARY, *continued*

Vital Signs				
Time: 1543	**BP:** 130/84	**Pulse:** 110	**Respirations:** 20	**Spo₂:** 99%
Time: 1555	**BP:** 118/78	**Pulse:** 88	**Respirations:** 14	**Spo₂:** 98%
Time:	**BP:**	**Pulse:**	**Respirations:**	**Spo₂:**

EMS Treatment (circle all that apply)				
Oxygen @ _____ L/min via (circle one): NC NRM Bag-mask device		**Assisted Ventilation**	**Airway Adjunct:**	**CPR**
Defibrillation	**Bleeding Control**	**Bandaging**	**Splinting**	**(Other:)** 5 mg haloperidol

Narrative
EMS requested to above location for a man fearing for his life. On arrival, pt found inside apartment, anxious and agitated, pacing in the living area. Multiple officers on scene in the hallway. Pt refused to leave apartment. Pt stating repeatedly, "They're coming for me." EMS allowed into apartment by pt. Pt sat in chair continuing to clench hands and appear restless. Pt advised he has a history of schizophrenia, but has not taken his medications for approximately 1 week because he "knows it's poisoned." EMS advised pt of need for transport to hospital for evaluation and treatment. Pt refused transport. Medical direction contacted. Dr. Jones ordered administration of 5 mg haloperidol IM for agitation and transport to City Memorial Medical Center for further evaluation and treatment. Pt placed on stretcher and loaded into ambulance for non-emergent transport. Officer accompanied EMS during transport. Blood glucose level 96 mg/dL. Pt became more relaxed and was calm during transport. Pt reassessed en route without changes. Report called to emergency department prior to arrival, which included pt's current condition and ETA. On arrival, pt was placed on the ED stretcher, rails up both sides, and report given to RN. Physician signature obtained for medication order. **End of report**

Prep Kit

Ready for Review

- Behavioral emergencies such as overdoses, violent behavior, and mental illness can present unique challenges in patient management. Panic on the part of the patient, the family, bystanders, or all of these parties may translate into a demand for action on your part. Focus on reducing the patient's stress without exposing yourself to unnecessary risks.

- A behavioral or psychiatric emergency is any reaction to events that interferes with activities of daily living. A person who is no longer able to respond appropriately to the environment and whose abnormal behavior threatens the health and safety of either himself or herself or another may be having a true psychiatric emergency.

- Not all behavioral emergencies involve a mental health problem. Some emergencies are a temporary response to a traumatic event.

- Calls for behavioral emergencies have special medical and legal considerations, including the need to obtain consent, to follow local guidelines and standing orders for transporting against the patient's will, and to obtain law enforcement assistance when appropriate to do so.

- You have limited legal authority to require a patient to undergo emergency medical care in the absence of a life-threatening emergency. Most states have provisions allowing law enforcement personnel to place mentally impaired persons in custody so that such care can be provided. Always involve law enforcement personnel any time you are called to assist a patient with a severe behavioral or psychiatric crisis.

- If a patient poses an immediate threat, leave the area until law enforcement personnel secure the scene. Always consult medical control and contact law enforcement for help.

- Underlying causes of behavioral emergencies fall into four broad categories: biologic (organic) causes, causes resulting from the person's environment, causes resulting from acute injury or illness, and causes that are substance related.

- Psychiatric signs and symptoms occur when a person's mental health is challenged and psychological mechanisms or behaviors mobilize to help return the person's mental state to homeostasis. Psychiatric signs and symptoms can be grouped according to the systems of psychological (rather than physiologic) functioning they affect: consciousness, motor activity, speech, thought, affect, memory, orientation, and perception.

- Assessing a patient with a behavioral emergency differs from other methods of patient assessment, in that with the disturbed patient, you are the diagnostic instrument, using your thinking processes, perceptions, and feelings to evaluate and measure the patient. With a behavioral emergency, assessment is also part of the treatment because your voice and manner affect the patient's response.

- In providing emergency medical care for a patient having a behavioral emergency, be direct, honest, and calm; have a definitive plan of action; stay with the patient at all times, but do not get too close; and express interest in the patient's story, but do not judge his or her behavior. Always treat patients with respect.

- When you are sizing up the scene, pay special attention to potential dangers and threats (objects that may be used as potential weapons, hazardous chemicals, and the like). Potentially harmful objects should be removed. Situations with a strong behavioral component have great potential for sudden and unexpected turns of events, so it is essential to follow established safety guidelines when responding.

- Primary assessment of a behavioral emergency includes identifying yourself clearly, forming a general impression of the patient's overall condition and the nature of the psychiatric problem, assessing the ABCs, making a decision about transport, and taking a history via the mental status examination (MSE). A useful mnemonic for the MSE is COASTMAP: consciousness, orientation, activity, speech, thought, memory, affect/mood, and perception.

- Secondary assessment involves looking for signs of an organic cause of the patient's behavioral emergency. This includes inspecting the patient for head trauma, checking pupil size, noting any unusual odors on the patient's breath, and examining the extremities for needle tracks, tremors, or unilateral weakness/loss of sensation.

- Management of the patient with a behavioral emergency is focused on ensuring scene safety and maintaining awareness of life-threatening conditions, while treating the patient for any medical disorders before assuming an emotional or psychiatric cause for the problem.

- Effective communication techniques for a behavioral emergency include beginning with an open-ended question, allowing the patient to talk, showing that you are listening, allowing silence when appropriate, acknowledging and labeling the patient's feelings, avoiding argument, facilitating communication, directing the patient's attention, asking questions, and adjusting your approach as needed.

- Crisis intervention skills include staying calm and being as direct as possible, excluding any disruptive people from the scene, sitting down to interview the patient, maintaining a nonjudgmental attitude, providing honest reassurance, developing a plan of action, encouraging some motor activity, staying with the patient at all times, bringing all of the patient's medications to the hospital, and assuming that the patient can hear and understand everything you say.

- Use of chemical or physical restraints is reserved for times when verbal intervention fails to reduce severe agitation. It is important to be familiar with the type of restraints and medications used by your agency before you encounter a situation in which they are needed. If restraints are required, use the minimum force necessary. Assess the airway, breathing, and circulation frequently while the patient is restrained, and maintain a constant dialogue with the patient throughout the restraining process. Maintain constant vigilance for safety and document everything that is done.

- Pathophysiologic factors that contribute to behavioral disturbances include cognitive impairment (agitated delirium), thought disorders (including schizophrenia and psychosis), mood disorders (bipolar mood disorder, manic behavior, and depression), neurotic disorders (generalized anxiety disorder, phobias, and panic disorder), substance-related disorders and addictive behavior, somatoform disorders (hypochondriasis and conversion disorder), factitious disorders, impulse control disorders, and personality disorders. Each condition has its own unique pathophysiology as well as standards for assessment and management, so it is important to be familiar with each.

- You may encounter patients with psychosis, a thought disorder characterized by a state of delusion in which the person is out of touch with reality. Patients may be belligerent and angry, or silent and withdrawn. The usual methods of reasoning with a patient are unlikely to be effective with psychotic patients, so be sure to learn the guidelines in caring for a psychotic patient, including being calm, direct, straightforward, and nonconfrontational.

- You may also encounter patients with agitated delirium. This is impairment of cognitive function that can present with disorientation, hallucinations, or delusions, and is characterized by restless and irregular physical activity. One of the most important factors to consider when caring for these patients is your personal safety. Use careful interviewing techniques and refrain from upsetting the patient further.

- The threat of suicide requires immediate intervention. Depression is the most significant risk factor for suicide. Other risk factors include personal or family history of suicide attempts, chronic debilitating illness, financial setback, and severe mental illness. Guidelines for managing the suicidal patient include never leaving the patient alone, collecting any implements of self-destruction, acknowledging the patient's feelings, and providing transport.

- Situations involving violence, abuse, and neglect can be a particular challenge for you because of their potential for escalation and the possibility of evoking emotional responses in you. Violent patients make up only a small percentage of those undergoing a behavioral or psychiatric crisis, but it is important for you to assess for risk factors for such a patient: history, posture, the scene, speech patterns and other vocal activity, agitation, depression, and physical activity can show clues as to the likelihood of the patient becoming violent. Management of the violent patient includes assessing the whole situation, observing your surroundings, maintaining a safe distance, and trying verbal interventions first, and of course requesting law enforcement personnel if they are not already present.

- Patients with psychiatric emergencies may be taking any of several types of psychotropic drugs. During assessment, it is important to determine which medications have been prescribed for the patient and whether he or she is actually taking them. Types of psychiatric medications include antidepressants, benzodiazepines, antipsychotics, and amphetamines. The patient's medication noncompliance often results in abnormal behaviors and confrontational behavior toward others.

■ Vital Vocabulary

activities of daily living (ADLs) The basic activities a person usually accomplishes during a normal day, such as eating, dressing, and washing.

acute dystonic reaction A syndrome that may occur in patients taking typical antipsychotic agents. The patient develops muscle spasms of the neck, face, and back within a few days of starting treatment with the drug.

affect The outward expression of a person's inner feelings (happy, sad, angry, fearful, withdrawn).

agoraphobia Literally, "fear of the marketplace"; fear of entering a public place from which escape may be impeded.

anorexia nervosa An eating disorder in which a person diets by exerting extraordinary control over his or her eating, and loses weight to the point of jeopardizing his or her health and life.

anxiety disorder A mental disorder in which the dominant mood is fear and apprehension.

atropine-like effects Results of some antipsychotic medications that include side effects similar to atropine, resulting in dry mouth, blurred vision, urinary retention, and cardiac dysrhythmias.

behavior How a person functions or acts in response to his or her environment.

behavioral emergency The point at which a person's reactions to events interfere with activities of daily living; becomes a psychiatric emergency when it causes a major life interruption, such as attempted suicide.

bipolar mood disorder A disorder in which a person alternates between mania and depression.

borderline personality disorder A disorder characterized by disordered images of self, impulsive and unpredictable behavior, marked shifts in mood, and instability in relationships with others.

bulimia nervosa An eating disorder characterized by consumption of large amounts of food, and for which the patient then sometimes compensates by using purging techniques.

catatonic Lacking expression or movement, or appearing rigid.

circumstantial thinking Situation in which the patient includes many irrelevant details in his or her account of things.

compulsions Repetitive actions carried out to relieve the anxiety of obsessive thoughts.

confabulation The invention of experiences to cover gaps in memory, seen in patients with certain organic brain syndromes.

confrontation Pointing out something of interest in the patient's conversation or behavior, thereby directing the patient's attention to something he or she may have been unaware of.

covert behavior Behavior that has a hidden meaning or intention that only the person understands.

delirium An acute confessional state characterized by global impairment of thinking, perception, judgment, and memory.

delusion A fixed belief that is not shared by others of a person's culture or background and that cannot be changed by reasonable argument; a false belief.

dementia The slow onset of progressive disorientation, shortened attention span, and loss of cognitive function.

depression A mental health disorder characterized by a persistent mood of sadness, despair, and discouragement; it may be a symptom of many different mental and physical disorders, or it may be a disorder on its own.

disorganization A condition in which a person is characterized by uncontrolled and disconnected thought, is usually incoherent or rambling in speech, and may or may not be oriented to person and place.

disorientation A condition in which a person may be confused about his or her identity, the location, and the time of day; one of the ways in which various conditions such as schizophrenia or organic brain syndrome may present.

echolalia Meaningless echoing of the interviewer's words by the patient.

factitious disorder A disorder in which a person wishes to be sick and intentionally produces or feigns physical or psychological signs or symptoms. Symptoms are under voluntary control, with no obvious physiologic reason.

flat affect The absence of emotion; appearing to feel no emotion at all.

flight of ideas Accelerated thinking in which the mind skips very rapidly from one thought to the next.

generalized anxiety disorder (GAD) A disorder in which a person worries about everything for no particular reason, or the worrying is unproductive and the person cannot decide what to do about an upcoming situation.

hallucination A sense perception not founded on objective reality; a false perception.

impulse control disorder A condition in which a person lacks the ability to resist a temptation or cannot stop acting on a drive.

inappropriate affect Emotion that is out of synch with the situation (for example, wearing a waxy smile while discussing a parent's death).

labile Rapidly shifting among different emotional states.

loosening of associations A situation in which the logical connection between one idea and the next becomes obscure, at least to the listener.

mania A mental disorder characterized by abnormally exaggerated happiness, joy, or euphoria with hyperactivity, insomnia, and grandiose ideas.

manic-depressive illness A bipolar disorder in which mood fluctuates between depression and mania. The alterations in mood are usually episodic and recurrent.

medication noncompliance A situation in which a patient chooses not to stay on his or her prescribed medications, for reasons that may include undesirable side effects or prohibitive cost.

mental status examination (MSE) A way of measuring the "mental vital signs" in a disturbed patient. The mnemonic COASTMAP can be used to conduct this exam, assessing consciousness, orientation, activity, speech, thought, memory, affect and mood, and perception.

mood disorder A group of disorders in which the disturbance of mood is accompanied by full or partial manic or depressive syndrome.

mutism The absence of speech.

neologism An invented word that has meaning only to its inventor.

neurotic disorders A collection of psychiatric disorders without psychotic symptoms and lacking the intense psychopathology of other mood disorders; includes anxiety disorders, phobias, and panic disorder.

organic brain syndrome Temporary or permanent dysfunction of the brain, caused by a disturbance in the physical or physiologic functioning of brain tissue.

overt behavior Behavior that is open and generally understood by those around the person.

panic disorder A disorder characterized by sudden, usually unexpected, and overwhelming feelings of fear and dread, accompanied by a variety of other symptoms produced by a massive activation of the autonomic nervous system.

perseveration Repeating the same idea over and over again.

personality disorder The condition a person has when he or she behaves or thinks in a way that is dysfunctional or causes distress to other people.

phobia An abnormal and persistent dread of a specific object or situation.

phobic disorders Disorders involving an unreasonable fear, apprehension, or dread of a specific situation or thing.

posttraumatic stress disorder (PTSD) A severe form of anxiety that stems from a traumatic experience; characterized by the reliving of the stress and nightmares of the original situation.

pressure of speech Speech in which words seem to tumble out under immense emotional pressure.

psychiatric emergency An emergency in which abnormal behavior threatens a person's health and safety or the health and safety of another person, for example when a person becomes suicidal, homicidal, or has a psychotic episode.

psychosis A mental disorder characterized by the loss of contact with reality.

psychotropic drugs Drugs that affect mood, thought, or behavior.

schizophrenia A complex, difficult-to-identify mental disorder whose typical onset is during early adulthood. Dysfunctional symptoms typically become more prominent over time and include delusions, hallucinations, apathy, mutism, flat affect, a lack of interest in pleasure, erratic speech, emotional responses, and motor behavior.

simple phobia A fear that is focused on one class of objects (eg, mice, spiders, dogs) or situations (eg, high places, darkness, flying).

somatoform disorder A condition in which a person is overly concerned with physical health and appearance to the point that it dominates his or her life; an example is hypochondria.

stereotyped movements Repetitive movements that do not appear to serve any purpose.

substance abuse Use of a substance that disrupts activities of daily living.

substance dependence Use of a substance that results in addiction and physiologic dependence on the substance.

substance intoxication Use of a substance that results in impaired thinking and motor function.

substance use Use of moderate amounts of a substance without seriously affecting activities of daily living.

suicide Any willful act designed to bring an end to one's own life.

tangential thinking Leaving the current topic midconversation to talk about something else, inhibiting interpersonal communication.

thought broadcasting The belief that thoughts are broadcast aloud and can be heard by others.

thought insertion The belief that thoughts are being thrust into one's mind by another person.

thought withdrawal The belief that thoughts are being removed from one's mind.

violent behavior Behavior that presents a threat of injury or destruction; usually a result of exaggerated fear or paranoia.

Assessment in Action

Y ou are the paramedic on a unit dispatched at 11:00 AM to an assisted-living facility. Dispatch information indicates you are responding to a 72-year-old woman whom staff describes as having aggressive behavior and mood swings. On arrival at the reception area of the facility, you are greeted by a social worker who informs you that the patient refused to leave her room, has threatened staff, and refused all meals and medications since breakfast. She leads you through the facility to a room down the hall.

On arrival at the patient's room, you note that the door is open and she is seated on a chair in a living area just inside the small apartment. She is rubbing a pillow in her lap and watching the doorway as you enter. She appears anxious. You introduce yourself and ask her name. She correctly provides her name, but then asks if you know where her husband is. You look to the social worker who indicates he is recently deceased. You ask the patient if you may sit with her and talk. She allows this but again asks if you know where her husband is. You calmly explain that he has died recently and ask if she remembers this. She becomes angry and informs you that he is being kept from her and is not dead. You notice that she becomes rigid in her seat and squeezes the pillow tightly.

1. Which of the four categories of causes of behavioral emergencies does this patient fall under?
   A. Biologic or organic
   B. Environment
   C. Acute injury or illness
   D. Substance-related

2. Your first step in the assessment and treatment of the patient having a behavioral emergency is to:
   A. determine the patient's mental status.
   B. obtain vital signs, including a blood glucose level to rule out a medical cause.
   C. assess the scene carefully.
   D. contact medical control for orders to apply chemical or physical restraints in case the patient becomes violent.

3. _____ is a state of delusion in which the person is out of touch with reality.
   A. Depression
   B. Panic disorder
   C. Organic brain syndrome
   D. Psychosis

4. What is the safest type of medication to use for chemical restraints?
   A. Antipsychotics
   B. Benzodiazepines
   C. Opiates
   D. Antidepressants

5. Which of the following is not typically a cause of agitated delirium?
   A. Alzheimer disease
   B. Drug toxicity
   C. Sepsis
   D. Metabolic disorders

6. Which of the following is the most appropriate way to respond to this patient's impaired perception of reality?
   A. Agree with the patient's belief that she is being kept apart from her husband and make up a reason for why this is happening.
   B. Ignore her questions and avoid addressing the issue because it clearly upsets her.
   C. Continue to attempt to reorient her to reality, and remind her that her husband is deceased while providing reassurance.
   D. Tell her that the people at the hospital are waiting to take her to her husband so she will agree to be transported.

7. Which of the following would not be an appropriate interview technique with a patient experiencing a behavioral emergency?
   A. Ask open-ended questions.
   B. Do not argue with the patient.
   C. Allow silence.
   D. Ask closed-ended questions.

8. Which of the following is a false assumption about the legal considerations concerning the patient with a behavioral emergency?
   A. You should include the patient in the assessment and treatment as much as possible.
   B. You should spend time with the patient and avoid rushing into treatment and/or transport.
   C. You should remove the patient from the environment as soon as possible to prevent the patient from becoming violent.
   D. You should document all aspects of the assessment of the scene and patient well, including quoting the patient's specific comments.

Additional Questions

9. Why is it important to provide a thorough physical assessment of the patient having a behavioral emergency?

10. What are some considerations related to the age of this patient?

11. If physical restraints are necessary to transport this patient, what factors should be considered?

Glossary

3-3-2 rule   A method used to predict difficult intubation. A mouth opening of less than three fingers wide, a mandible length of less than three fingers wide, and a distance from hyoid bone to thyroid notch of less than two fingers wide indicate a possibly difficult airway.

abandonment   Termination of care for the patient without giving the patient sufficient opportunity to find another suitable health care professional to take over his or her medical treatment.

abdomen   The body cavity that contains the major organs of digestion and excretion. It is located below the diaphragm and above the pelvis.

abdominal aortic aneurysm (AAA)   A sac or bulge in the wall of the abdominal portion of the aorta, resulting in weakening of that wall; it is considered life threatening if it ruptures.

abdominal thrust maneuver   Abdominal thrusts performed to relieve a foreign body airway obstruction.

abduction   Motion of a limb away from the midline.

aberration   A term used to describe the shape of the QRS complex in aberrantly conducted beats.

ABO system   The commonly used blood classification system, based on the antigens present or absent in the blood.

abscess   A collection of pus in a sac, formed by necrotic tissues and an accumulation of white blood cells; the immune system creates the sac to prevent spread of the infection.

absolute refractory period   The early phase of cardiac repolarization, wherein the heart muscle cannot be stimulated to depolarize; also known as the effective refractory period.

absorption   The process by which the molecules of a substance are moved from the site of entry or administration into systemic circulation; also refers to the process of foreign materials being deposited onto and moving into the skin.

acalculus cholecystitis   Inflammation of the gallbladder without the presence of gallstones.

access port   A sealed hub on an administration set designed for sterile access to the IV fluid.

accessory muscles   The muscles not normally used during normal breathing; include the sternocleidomastoid muscles of the neck, the chest pectoralis major muscles, and the abdominal muscles.

acetabulum   The depression on the lateral pelvis where its three component bones join, in which the femoral head fits snugly.

acetylcholine (ACh)   A chemical neurotransmitter which servers as a mediator in both the sympathetic and parasympathetic nervous systems.

acetylcholinesterase   The enzyme that causes muscle relaxation by helping to break down acetylcholine.

acholic stools   Light, clay-colored stools indicative of liver failure.

acid   Any molecule that can give up a hydrogen ion (H^+), and therefore increases the concentration of hydrogen ions in a water solution.

acidosis   A pathologic condition resulting from the accumulation of acids in the body (blood pH less than 7.35).

acquired immunity   The immunity that occurs when the body is exposed to a foreign substance or disease and produces antibodies to the invading antigen.

acquired immunodeficiency syndrome (AIDS)   The end-stage disease process caused by the human immunodeficiency virus (HIV); results in extreme vulnerability to numerous opportunistic bacterial, viral, and fungal infections that would not affect a person with an intact immune system.

acromioclavicular separation (AC separation)   An injury caused by distraction of the clavicle away from the acromion process of the scapula.

acromion process   The tip of the shoulder and the site of attachment for both the clavicle and various shoulder muscles.

action potentials   An electrochemical event where stimulation of a nearby cell could cause excitation of another cell.

activation   Mediators of inflammation trigger the appearance of molecules known as selectins and integrins on the surfaces of endothelial cells and polymorphonuclear neutrophils, respectively.

active hyperemia   The dilation of arterioles after transient arteriolar constriction, which allows influx of blood under increased pressure.

active metabolite   A medication that has undergone biotransformation and is able to alter a cellular process or body function.

active transport   A method used to move compounds across a cell membrane to create or maintain an imbalance of charges, usually against a concentration gradient and requiring the expenditure of energy.

activities of daily living (ADLs)   The basic activities a person usually accomplishes during a normal day, such as eating, dressing, and washing.

acute abdomen   A condition of sudden onset of pain within the abdomen, usually indicating peritonitis; demands immediate medical or surgical treatment.

acute chest syndrome   A vasoocclusive crisis that can be associated with pneumonia; common signs and symptoms include chest pain, fever, and cough; associated with sickle cell disease.

acute coronary syndrome (ACS)   Term used to describe any group of clinical symptoms consistent with acute myocardial ischemia.

acute dystonic reaction   A syndrome that may occur in patients taking typical antipsychotic agents. The patient develops muscle spasms of the neck, face, and back within a few days of starting treatment with the drug.

acute gastroenteritis   A family of conditions that revolve around a central theme of infection with fever, abdominal pain, diarrhea, nausea, and vomiting.

acute myocardial infarction (AMI)   A condition present when a period of cardiac ischemia caused by sudden narrowing or complete occlusion of a coronary artery leads to death (necrosis) of myocardial tissue.

acute renal failure (ARF)   A sudden decrease in filtration through the glomeruli.

acute splenic sequestration syndrome   A condition in which red blood cells become trapped in the spleen, causing a dramatic fall in hemoglobin available in the circulation; usually occurs in infants or toddlers.

acute stress reaction   Reaction to stress that occurs during a stressful situation.

Adam's apple   The firm prominence in the upper part of the larynx formed by the thyroid cartilage. It is more prominent in men than in women.

adaptation   The temporary or permanent reduction of sensitivity to a particular stimulus.

adaptive (specific) defense   Immunity; it targets specific pathogens and acts more slowly than innate defenses.

addisonian crisis   Acute adrenal insufficiency.

adduction   Motion of a limb toward the midline.

adenoid   The pharyngeal tonsil; located on the posterior nasopharyngeal wall.

adenosine triphosphate (ATP)   The nucleotide involved in energy metabolism; used to store energy.

adhesion   The attachment of polymorphonuclear neutrophils to endothelial cells, mediated by selectins and integrins.

adipose tissue   Fat tissue that lies beneath the skin, between muscles, around the kidneys, behind the eyes, in certain abdominal membranes, on the heart's surface, and around certain joints.

administration set Tubing that connects to the IV bag access port and the catheter to deliver IV fluid.

adnexa The surrounding structures and accessories of an organ; for the eye: the eyelids, lashes, lacrimal structures.

adolescents Persons who are 13 to 17 years of age.

adrenal cortex The outer layer of the adrenal gland; it produces hormones that are important in regulating the water and salt balance of the body.

adrenal glands Paired endocrine glands located on top of the kidneys that release adrenalin when stimulated by the sympathetic nervous system; each adrenal gland consists of an inner adrenal medulla and an adrenal cortex.

adrenal medulla The inner part of the adrenal glands that produces catecholamines (epinephrine and norepinephrine).

adrenaline Hormone with alpha and beta sympathomimetic properties, produced by the adrenal glands that mediates the "fight-or-flight" response of the sympathetic nervous system; also called epinephrine.

adrenergic receptor A type of receptor that is associated with the sympathetic nerves and that is stimulated by epinephrine and norepinephrine; activation causes a sympathetic response.

adrenocorticotropic hormone (ACTH) Hormone that targets the adrenal cortex to secrete cortisol (a glucocorticoid).

advance directive A written document or oral statement that expresses the wants, needs, and desires of a patient in reference to future medical care; examples include living wills, do not resuscitate (DNR) orders, and organ donation choices.

adventitious A type of breath sound that occurs in addition to the normal breath sounds; examples are crackles and wheezes.

adventitious breath sounds Abnormal breath sounds such as wheezes, rhonchi, rales, stridor, and pleural friction rubs.

adverse reaction/side effect Abnormal or harmful effect to an organism caused by exposure to a chemical. It is indicated by some result such as death, a change in food or water consumption, altered body and organ weights, altered enzyme levels, or visible illness.

aerobic metabolism Metabolism that can proceed only in the presence of oxygen.

affect The outward expression of a person's inner feelings (happy, sad, angry, fearful, withdrawn).

afferent arteriole The structure in the kidney that supplies blood to the glomerulus.

afferent nerves Nerves that send information to the brain.

affinity The ability of a medication to bind with a particular receptor site.

after-image The perception of a stimuli is still present after the stimuli is removed.

afterload The pressure in the aorta against which the left ventricle must pump blood; increasing this can decrease cardiac output.

agnosia Inability to connect an object with its correct name.

agonal Pertaining to the period of dying.

agonal gasps Slow, gasping respirations, indicating life-threatening cerebral injury or ischemia.

agonal rhythm A cardiac dysrhythmia seen just before the heart stops altogether; essentially asystole with occasional QRS complexes that are not associated with cardiac output.

agonist A substance that mimics the actions of a specific neurotransmitter or hormone by binding to the specific receptor of the naturally occurring substance; triggers a response, producing some kind of action or biologic effect.

agonist medications The group of medications that initiates or alters a cellular activity by attaching to receptor sites, prompting a cellular response.

agoraphobia Literally, "fear of the marketplace"; fear of entering a public place from which escape may be impeded.

agranulocytes Leukocytes that lack granules.

air embolism The presence of air in the venous circulation, which forms a gas bubble that can block the outflow of blood from the right ventricle to the lung; can lead to cardiac arrest, shock, or other life-threatening complications.

airborne transmission The transmission of an organism or infectious agent by inhalation of small particles that become aerosolized when the infected person coughs, sneezes, talks, or exhales; particles remain suspended in this vapor and can be carried a short distance, usually 3' to 6'.

albumins The smallest of plasma proteins; they make up around 60% of these proteins by weight.

alcoholic ketoacidosis The metabolic acidotic state that manifests because of the inadequate nutritional habits associated with chronic alcohol abuse. The liver and body experience inadequate fuel reserves of glycogen and, thus, have to switch to fatty acid metabolism.

alcoholism A state of physical and psychological addiction to ethanol.

aldosterone One of the two main hormones responsible for adjustments to the final composition of urine; increases the rate of active reabsorption of sodium and chloride ions into the blood and decreases reabsorption of potassium.

alert and oriented (A × O) A determination made when assessing mental status by looking at whether the patient is oriented to four elements: person, place, time, and the event itself. Each element provides information about different aspects of the patient's memory.

alkalosis A pathologic condition resulting from the accumulation of bases in the body (blood pH greater than 7.45).

alleles Variant forms of a gene, which can be identical or slightly different in DNA sequence.

allergen A substance that causes a hypersensitivity reaction or an allergic reaction; also referred to as an antigen.

allergic reaction An abnormal immune response the body develops when reexposed to a substance or allergen.

allergy A hypersensitivity reaction to the presence of an agent (allergen) that is intrinsically harmless.

alpha cells Cells located in the islets of Langerhans that secrete glucagon.

alpha effects Stimulation of alpha receptors that results in vasoconstriction.

alternative time sampling Time parameters that are set during a research project.

alveolar ducts Ducts formed from division of the respiratory bronchioles in the lower airway; each duct ends in clusters known as alveoli.

alveolar minute volume (VA) The amount of air that actually reaches the alveoli per minute and participates in gas exchange.

alveolar ridges The ridges between the teeth, which are covered with thickened connective tissue and epithelium.

alveolar volume Volume of inhaled air that reaches the alveoli and participates in gas exchange; equal to tidal volume minus dead space volume and is approximately 350 mL in an average adult; also called alveolar ventilation.

alveoli The air sacs of the lungs in which the exchange of oxygen and carbon dioxide takes place (singular, alveolus). In the context of facial anatomy, small pits or cavities, such as the sockets for the teeth.

alveolocapillary membrane The very thin membrane, consisting of only one cell layer, that lies between the alveolus and capillary, through which respiratory exchange between the alveolus and the blood vessels occurs.

Alzheimer disease A progressive organic condition in which neurons in the brain die, causing dementia.

amblyopia Lazy eye; the eyes may be oriented correctly but one fails to send adequate signals to the vision centers, also causing a loss of depth perception and poor-quality images.

amenorrhea Absence of menstruation.

amphetamines A class of drugs that increase alertness and excitation (stimulants); includes methamphetamine (crank or ice), methylenedioxyamphetamine (MDA, Adam), and methylenedioxymethamphetamine (MDMA, Eve, ecstasy).

ampules Small glass containers that are sealed and the contents sterilized.

amyotrophic lateral sclerosis (ALS) ALS, also known as Lou Gehrig disease, strikes the voluntary motor neurons, causing their death. The disease is characterized by fatigue and general weakness of muscle groups; eventually the patient becomes unable to walk, eat, or speak.

anabolism The synthesis of larger molecules from smaller ones.

anaerobic metabolism The metabolism that takes place in the absence of oxygen; the principal byproduct is lactic acid.

anal fissures Linear tears to the mucosal lining in and near the anus, possibly caused by the passage of large, hard stools; a cause of lower GI bleeding.

anaphylactic shock A severe hypersensitivity reaction that involves bronchoconstriction and cardiovascular collapse.

anaphylactoid reaction An extreme allergic response that does not involve IgE antibody mediation. The exact mechanism is unknown, but an anaphylactoid event may occur without the patient being previously exposed to the offending agent.

anaphylaxis An extreme systemic form of an allergic reaction involving two or more body systems.

anatomic position The position of reference in which the patient stands facing you, arms at the side, with the palms of the hands forward.

anatomy The study of the structure of an organism and its parts.

androgens Male sex hormones mostly produced by the testicular interstitial cells, and which regulate body changes associated with sexual development (puberty), including growth spurts, deepening of the voice, growth of facial and pubic hair, and muscle growth and strength.

anemia A lower than normal hemoglobin or erythrocyte level.

anesthesia Lack of feeling within a body part.

aneurysm A swelling or enlargement of part of a blood vessel, resulting from weakening of the vessel wall.

angina pectoris The sudden pain from myocardial ischemia, caused by diminished circulation to the cardiac muscle. The pain is usually substernal and often radiates to the arms, jaw, or abdomen and usually lasts 3 to 5 minutes and disappears with rest.

angioedema A vascular reaction that may have an allergic cause and may result in profound swelling of the tongue and lips.

angiogenesis The growth of new blood vessels.

anion An ion that contains an overall negative charge.

anisocoria Unequal pupils with a greater than 1-mm difference.

anorexia nervosa An eating disorder in which a person diets by exerting extraordinary control over his or her eating, and loses weight to the point of jeopardizing his or her health and life.

anoxia An absence of oxygen.

antagonist A molecule that blocks the ability of a given chemical to bind to its receptor, preventing a biologic response.

antagonist medications The group of medications that prevent endogenous or exogenous agonist chemicals from reaching cell receptor sites and initiating or altering a particular cellular activity.

antecubital The anterior aspect of the elbow.

anterior The front surface of the body; the side facing forward in the anatomic position.

anterior cavity Aqueous chamber; portion of the eyeball filled with aqueous humor, a fluid whose quantity determines the intraocular pressure, which is critical to sight.

anterior chamber The anterior area of the globe between the lens and the cornea that is filled with aqueous humor.

anterograde amnesia An inability to remember events after the onset of amnesia.

antibiotics The medications used to fight infection by killing the microorganisms or preventing their multiplication to allow the body's immune system to overcome them.

antibody (immunoglobulin) A protein secreted by certain immune cells that reacts against foreign antigens in the body by binding to the antigens, making them more visible to the immune system.

anticoagulant A substance that prevents blood from clotting.

antidiuretic hormone (ADH) Secreted by the posterior pituitary lobe of the pituitary gland, this hormone constricts blood vessels and raises the blood pressure, and also is responsible for adjustments to the final composition of urine by causing ducts in the kidney to become more permeable to water; also called *vasopressin*.

antifungals The medications used to treat fungal infections.

antigen A substance or molecule that, when taken into the body, stimulates immune system response and causes formation of specific protective proteins called antibodies.

antimicrobials The medications used to kill or suppress the growth of microorganisms.

antiseptics Chemicals used to cleanse an area before performing an invasive procedure, such as starting an IV line; not toxic to living tissues; examples include isopropyl alcohol and iodine.

anuria A complete cessation of urine production.

anxiety disorder A mental disorder in which the dominant mood is fear and apprehension.

anxiolysis The relief of anxiety.

anxious avoidant attachment A bond between an infant and his or her parent or caregiver in which the infant is repeatedly rejected and develops an isolated lifestyle that does not depend on the support and care of others.

aorta The principal artery leaving the left side of the heart and carrying freshly oxygenated blood to the body; this is the largest artery in the body.

aortic arch One of the three described portions of the aorta; the section of the aorta between the ascending and descending portions that gives rise to the right brachiocephalic (innominate), left common carotid, and left subclavian arteries.

aortic semilunar valve The valve between the left ventricle and the aorta; also called the aortic valve.

aortic valve The semilunar valve that regulates blood flow from the left ventricle to the aorta.

apex (plural: apices) The pointed extremity of a conical structure.

aphasia The impairment of language that affects the production or understanding of speech and the ability to read or write.

aphonia The inability to speak.

aplastic crisis A temporary stop in the production of red blood cells; may occur as a result of sickle cell disease.

apneustic center A portion of the pons that assists in creating longer, slower respirations.

apneustic respirations Prolonged gasping inspirations followed by extremely short, ineffective expirations; associated with brainstem insult.

apoptosis Normal, genetically programmed cell death.

appendicitis Inflammation of the appendix.

appendicular skeleton The portion of the skeletal system that comprises the arms, legs, pelvis, and shoulder girdle.

appendix A small tubular structure that is attached to the lower border of the cecum in the lower right quadrant of the abdomen.

apraxia Inability to connect an object with its proper use.

aqueous humor Watery fluid filling the anterior eye cavity; the quantity determines the intraocular pressure, which is critical to sight.

arachnoid The middle membrane of the three meninges that enclose the brain and spinal cord.

areolar tissue The type of tissue that binds skin to underlying organs and fills in spaces between muscles.

arrhythmia The lack of a cardiac rhythm; asystole.

arteries The muscular, thick-walled blood vessels that carry blood away from the heart.

arteriole A small blood vessel that carries oxygenated blood, branching into yet smaller vessels called capillaries.

arteriosclerosis A pathologic condition in which the arterial walls become thickened and inelastic.

Arthus reaction A localized reaction involving vascular inflammation in response to an IgG-mediated allergic response.

artifact An artificial product; in cardiology, is used to refer to noise or interference in an ECG tracing.

arytenoid cartilages Pyramid-like cartilaginous structures that form the posterior attachment of the vocal cords.

ascending aorta The first of three portions of the aorta; originates from the left ventricle and gives rise to two arteries, the right and left main coronary arteries.

ascites Abnormal accumulation of fluid in the peritoneal cavity; typically signals liver failure.

aseptic technique A method of cleansing used to prevent contamination of a site when you are performing an invasive procedure, such as starting an IV line.

aspiration The entry of fluids or solids into the trachea, bronchi, and lungs; the act of drawing material in or out by suction.

assault To create in another person a fear of immediate bodily harm or invasion of bodily security.

asthma A chronic inflammatory lower airway condition resulting in intermittent wheezing and excess mucus production.

astigmatism Condition where parts of the image are out of focus and others are in focus; caused by irregularities in the shape of the eye lens.

astrocytes Neuroglia found usually between neurons and blood vessels.

asymmetric chest wall movement Unequal movement of the two sides of the chest; indicates decreased airflow into one lung.

asystole The absence of ventricular contractions; a "straight-line ECG."

ataxia Alteration in the ability to perform coordinated motions like walking; staggered walk or gait.

atelectasis The collapse of the alveolar air spaces of the lungs.

atheroma A mass of fatty tissue.

atherosclerosis A disorder in which cholesterol and calcium build up inside the walls of the blood vessels, forming plaque, which eventually leads to partial or complete blockage of blood flow.

atlanto-occipital joint The joint formed at the articulation of the atlas of the vertebral column and the occipital bone of the skull.

atlas The first cervical vertebra (C1), which provides support for the head.

atomic number A whole number representing the number of positively charged protons in the nucleus of an atom.

atomic weight The total number of protons and neutrons in the nucleus of an atom.

atoms The smallest complete units of an element that have the element's properties; they vary in size, weight, and interaction with other atoms.

atopic The medical term for having an allergic tendency.

atrial kick The volume (percentage) of blood pumped into the ventricles by the atria.

atrioventricular (AV) node A specialized structure located in the AV junction that slows conduction through the AV junction.

atrioventricular (AV) valves The mitral and tricuspid valves through which blood flows from the atria to the ventricles.

atrium One of the two upper chambers of the heart.

atrophy A decrease in cell size due to a loss of subcellular components.

atropine A parasympathetic blocker; opposes the action of acetylcholine on the heart and elsewhere, causing an increase in heart rate.

atropine-like effects Results of some antipsychotic medications that include side effects similar to atropine, resulting in dry mouth, blurred vision, urinary retention, and cardiac dysrhythmias.

auditory ossicles The bones that function in hearing and are located deep within cavities of the temporal bone.

augmented unipolar leads On an ECG, leads that only contain one true pole; the other is a combination of information from other leads; includes leads aVR, aVL, and aVF.

aura Sensations experienced before an attack occurs. Common in seizures and migraine headaches.

aural Pertaining to the ear.

auricle The large outside portion of the ear through which sound waves enter the ear; also called the pinna.

auscultation The method of listening to sounds within the body with a stethoscope.

authoritarian A parenting style that demands absolute obedience.

authoritative A parenting style that balances parental authority with the child's freedom by setting and enforcing rules, but also allowing the child to have some freedom.

autoantibodies Antibodies directed against the person's own proteins.

autocrine hormone A hormone that acts on the cell from which it has been secreted.

autoimmune disease A type of disease in which the body identifies its own antigen as a foreign body and activates the inflammatory system, sending out antibodies to destroy the antigen.

autoimmunity The production of antibodies or T cells that work against the tissues of a person's own body, producing autoimmune disease or a hypersensitivity reaction.

automated external defibrillator (AED) A "smart" defibrillator that can analyze the patient's ECG rhythm and determine whether a defibrillating shock is needed.

automatic transport ventilator (ATV) A portable mechanical ventilator attached to a control box that allows the variables of ventilation (such as rate and tidal volume) to be set.

automaticity A state in which cardiac cells are at rest, waiting for the generation of a spontaneous impulse from within.

autonomic nervous system (ANS) A subdivision of the nervous system that controls primarily involuntary body functions; comprised of the sympathetic and parasympathetic nervous systems.

autosomal dominant A pattern of inheritance that involves genes that are located on autosomes or the nonsex chromosomes. Inheritance of only one copy of a particular form of a gene is needed to show the trait.

autosomal recessive A pattern of inheritance that involves genes located on autosomes or the nonsex chromosomes. Inheritance of two copies of a particular form of a gene is needed to show the trait.

autosomes The chromosomes that do not carry genes that determine sex.

AV junction The atrioventricular junction; the portion of the electric conduction system of the heart located in the upper part of the interventricular septum that conducts the excitation impulse from the atria to the bundle of His.

avascular Lacking blood vessels.

avian (bird) flu A disease caused by a virus that occurs naturally in the bird population; signs and symptoms include fever, sore throat, cough, and muscle aches.

AVPU A method of assessing mental status by determining whether a patient is Awake and alert, responsive to Verbal stimuli or Pain, or Unresponsive; used principally in the primary assessment.

axial skeleton The part of the skeleton comprising the skull, spinal column, and rib cage.

axillary vein The vein that is formed from the combination of the basilic and cephalic veins; it drains into the subclavian vein.

axis The second cervical vertebra; the point that allows the head to turn.

axis deviation A component of an ECG that looks at the direction of travel for the electricity going through the heart as it depolarizes.

axon The long, slender filament projecting from a nerve cell that conducts impulses to adjacent cells.

azotemia Increased nitrogenous wastes in the blood.

B lymphocytes (B cells) Lymphocytes that exist in the blood, and are abundant in the lymph nodes, bone marrow, intestinal lining, and spleen.

bacteria Small organisms that can grow and reproduce outside the human cell in the presence of the needed temperature and nutrients and cause disease by invading and multiplying in the tissues of the host.

bacterial vaginosis An overgrowth of bacteria in the vagina, characterized by itching, burning, or pain, and possibly a "fishy" smelling discharge.

bag-mask device A manual ventilation device that consists of a bag, mask, reservoir, and oxygen inlet; capable of delivering up to 100% oxygen.

barbiturates Potent sedative-hypnotics historically used as sleep aids, anti-anxiety drugs, and as part of the regimen for seizure control; include drugs such as thiopental (Pentothal, Trapanal) and methohexital (Brevital).

baroreceptors Receptors in the blood vessels, kidneys, brain, and heart that respond to changes in pressure in the heart or main arteries to help maintain homeostasis.

barotrauma Trauma resulting from increased pressure, for example from too much pressure in the lungs.

Bartholin glands The glands that secrete mucus for sexual lubrication.

basal metabolic rate The rate at which nutrients are consumed in the body.

base Any molecule that can accept a hydrogen ion (OH⁻), and therefore decreases the concentration of hydrogen ions in a water solution.

base station Assembly of radio equipment consisting of at least a transmitter, receiver, and antenna connection at a fixed location.

basement membrane Anchors epithelial tissue to connective tissue.

basilic vein One of the two major veins of the arm; it combines with the cephalic vein to form the axillary vein.

basophils White blood cells that work to produce chemical mediators during an immune response; make up approximately 1% of leukocytes.

battery Any act of touching another person without that person's consent.

Battle sign Bruising over the mastoid process, which may be indicative of a basilar skull fracture; also known as retroauricular ecchymosis and raccoon eyes.

Beck triad The combination of a narrowed pulse pressure, muffled heart tones, and jugular venous distention associated with cardiac tamponade; usually resulting from penetrating chest trauma.

behavior How a person functions or acts in response to his or her environment.

behavioral emergency The point at which a person's reactions to events interfere with activities of daily living; becomes a psychiatric emergency when it causes a major life interruption, such as attempted suicide.

Bell palsy A temporary paralysis of the facial nerve (cranial nerve VII), which controls the muscles on each side of the face.

benign early repolarization Early repolarization that is thought to be a normal variant; characterized by ST-segment elevation (or J-point elevation), a J or fishhook appearance at the J point, and concave ST-segment morphology.

benign prostate hypertrophy (BPH) Age-related nonmalignant (noncancerous) enlargement of the prostate gland.

benzodiazepines The family of sedative-hypnotics that provide muscle relaxation and mild sedation; most commonly used to treat anxiety, seizures, and alcohol withdrawal; include drugs such as diazepam (Valium) and midazolam (Versed).

beta cells Cells located in the islets of Langerhans that secrete insulin.

beta effects Stimulation of beta receptors that results in inotropic, dromotropic, and chronotropic states.

beta-2 agonist A pharmacologic agent that stimulates the beta-2 receptor sites found in smooth muscle; includes common bronchodilators such as albuterol and levalbuterol.

bifascicular block Blockage of any combination of two of the fascicles or conduction pathways: a right bundle branch block (RBBB) and anterior hemiblock, a RBBB and posterior hemiblock, or an anterior hemiblock and posterior hemiblock.

bigeminy A dysrhythmia in which every other heartbeat is a premature contraction; can be atrial or ventricular.

bilateral In anatomy, a body part that appears on both sides of the midline.

bile ducts The ducts that convey bile between the liver and the intestine.

biliary tract disorders A group of disorders that involve inflammation of the gallbladder; these include choleangitis, cholelithiasis, cholecystitis, and acalculus cholecystitis.

bilirubin A waste product of red blood cell destruction that undergoes further metabolism in the liver.

binocular vision The merging of two images into one.

bioavailability The percentage of the unchanged medication that reaches systemic circulation.

Biot (ataxic) respirations Irregular pattern, rate, and depth of respirations with intermittent periods of apnea; result from increased intracranial pressure.

biotelemetry Transmission of physiologic data, such as an ECG, from the patient to a distant point of reception (commonly referred to in EMS as "telemetry").

biotransformation A process with four possible effects on a medication absorbed into the body: (1) An inactive substance can become active, capable of producing desired or unwanted clinical effects. (2) An active medication can be changed into another active medication. (3) An active medication may be completely or partially inactivated. (4) A medication is transformed into a substance (active or inactive) that is easier for the body to eliminate.

bipolar leads On an ECG, leads that contain a positive and a negative pole; includes leads I, II, and III.

bipolar mood disorder A disorder in which a person alternates between mania and depression.

bivalent An ion that contains two charges.

blind panic A fear reaction in which a person's judgment seems to disappear entirely; it is particularly dangerous because it may precipitate mass panic among others.

blinding The method of not giving the specifics of a project to the people participating in a research or study.

blood The fluid tissue that is pumped by the heart through the arteries, veins, and capillaries and consists of plasma and formed elements or cells, such as red blood cells, white blood cells, and platelets.

blood pressure (BP) The measurement of the force exerted against the walls of the blood vessels as the heart contracts and relaxes; it is calculated as the product of cardiac output and peripheral vascular resistance.

blood tubing A special type of macrodrip administration set designed to facilitate rapid fluid replacement by manual infusion of multiple IV bags or IV-blood replacement combinations.

bloodborne pathogens Pathogenic microorganisms that are present in human blood and can cause disease in humans; include, but are not limited to, hepatitis B virus (HBV), hepatitis C virus (HCV), and human immunodeficiency virus.

bolus A term used to describe "in one mass"; in medication administration, a single dose given by the IV or IO route; may be a small or large quantity of the drug.

bonding The formation of a close, personal relationship.

bone The most rigid type of connective tissue, with high mineral content that makes it harder than the other types.

Bone Injection Gun (BIG) A spring-loaded device that is used for inserting an IO needle into the proximal tibia in adult and pediatric patients.

bone marrow Specialized tissue found within bone that manufactures most erythrocytes.

bony labyrinth The collection of hollows in the bone of the inner ear that provide protection to the structures of the inner ear from damage and from extraneous stimulation.

borborygmi A bowel sound characterized by increased activity within the bowel; also called hyperperistalsis.

borderline personality disorder A disorder characterized by disordered images of self, impulsive and unpredictable behavior, marked shifts in mood, and instability in relationships with others.

botulism Poisoning from eating food containing botulinum toxin.

Bourdon-gauge flowmeter An oxygen flowmeter that is commonly used because it is not affected by gravity and can be placed in any position.

Boyle's law States that the pressure of a gas is inversely proportional to its volume.

brachial artery The major vessel in the upper extremity that supplies blood to the arm.

bradykinesia The slowing down of voluntary body movements. Found in Parkinson disease.

bradypnea A slow respiratory rate.

brain The controlling organ of the body and center of consciousness; functions include perception, control of reactions to the environment, emotional responses, and judgment.

brainstem The area of the brain between the spinal cord and cerebrum, surrounded by the cerebellum; controls functions that are necessary for life, such as respiration.

bronchi The main branches of the trachea; subdivide into smaller bronchi and bronchioles that conduct air into and out of the lungs.

bronchioles Fine subdivisions of the bronchi that give rise to the alveolar ducts; made of smooth muscle and dilate or constrict in response to various stimuli.

bronchoconstriction Narrowing of the bronchial tubes.

bronchodilation Widening of the bronchial tubes.

bronchophony A test of decreased breath sounds performed by placing the diaphragm of the stethoscope over the area in question while the patient says "ninety-nine"; a loud, clear sound indicates lung consolidation.

bronchospasm Severe constriction of the bronchial tree.

bronchovesicular sounds A combination of the tracheal and vesicular breath sounds; heard where airways and alveoli are found, the upper part of the sternum and between the scapulas.

Brugada syndrome A genetic disorder involving sodium channels in the heart; characterized by incomplete RBBB and ST-segment elevation that aggressively returns to baseline.

bruits Abnormal whooshing sounds indicating turbulent blood flow within a narrowed blood vessel, usually heard in the carotid arteries.

buccal Between the cheek and gums.

buffer system Fast-acting defenses for acid-base changes, providing almost immediate protection against changes in the hydrogen ion concentration of extracellular fluid.

buffers Molecules that modulate changes in pH to keep it in the physiologic range; they do this by reversibly binding with H^+.

bulbourethral glands Cowper's glands; glands that lie inferior to the prostate gland and secrete a lubricating fluid that prepares the penis for sexual intercourse.

bulimia nervosa An eating disorder characterized by consumption of large amounts of food, and for which the patient then sometimes compensates by using purging techniques.

bundle branch block A disturbance in electric conduction through the right or left bundle branch from the bundle of His.

bundle of His The portion of the electric conduction system in the interventricular septum that conducts the depolarizing impulse from the atrioventricular junction to the right and left bundle branches.

burnout The exhaustion of physical or emotional strength.

BURP maneuver The backward, upward, rightward pressure used during intubation to improve the laryngoscopic view of the glottic opening and vocal cords; also called external laryngeal manipulation.

bursa A small fluid-filled sac located between a tendon and a bone that cushions and protects the joint.

butterfly catheter A rigid, hollow, venous cannulation device identified by its plastic "wings" that act as anchoring points for securing the catheter.

butyrophenones Potent, effective sedatives; include drugs such as haloperidol (Haldol) and droperidol (Inapsine).

caladium A common houseplant that contains caladium oxalate crystals; ingestion leads to nausea, vomiting, and diarrhea.

calcaneous The heel bone.

calcitonin The hormone secreted by the thyroid gland that helps maintain normal calcium levels in the blood.

calorie The amount of heat needed to raise the temperature of a gram of water by 1°C.

calyces (singular: calyx) Large urinary tubes that branch off the renal pelvis and connect with the renal pyramids to collect the urine draining from the collecting tubules.

cancellous bone A type of bone that consists of a lacy network of bony rods called trabeculae.

cannulation The insertion of a catheter, such as into a vein to allow for fluid flow.

cape cyanosis Deep cyanosis of the face and neck and across the chest and back; associated with little or no blood flow; a particularly ominous sign.

capillaries The tiny blood vessels between the arterioles and venules, composed of a single layer of cells, that permit transfer of oxygen, carbon dioxide, nutrients, and waste between body tissues and the blood.

capillary refill time A test done on the fingernails or toenails by briefly squeezing the toenail or fingernail and evaluating the time it takes for the color to return.

capnographer A device that attaches between the endotracheal tube and bag-mask device; provides graphic information about the presence of exhaled co_2.

capnography A noninvasive diagnostic tool that can quickly and efficiently provide information on a patient's ventilatory and circulatory status.

capnometer A device that performs the same function and attaches in the same way as a capnographer but provides a digital reading of the exhaled co_2.

capnometry The use of a capnometer, a device that measures the amount of expired carbon dioxide.

carbohydrates Substances (including sugars and starches) that provide much of the energy required by the body's cells, as well as helping to build cell structures.

carboxyhemoglobin (COHb) Hemoglobin loaded with carbon monoxide (CO).

cardiac cycle The period from one cardiac contraction to the next. Each cardiac cycle consists of ventricular contraction (systole) and relaxation (diastole).

cardiac muscle tissue A special striated muscle of the myocardium, containing dark intercalated disks at the junctions of abutting fibers.

cardiac output (CO) Amount of blood pumped by the heart per minute, calculated by multiplying the stroke volume by the heart rate per minute.

cardiac sphincter Sphincter that serves as a doorway connecting the esophagus and the stomach; controls the amount of food that moves up the esophagus.

cardiac tamponade Restriction of cardiac contraction, failing cardiac output, and shock, caused by the accumulation of fluid or blood in the pericardium.

cardiogenic shock A condition caused by loss of 40% or more of the functioning myocardium; the heart is no longer able to circulate sufficient blood to maintain adequate oxygen delivery.

cardiopulmonary arrest The sudden and often unexpected cessation of adequate cardiac output.

carina A ridgelike projection of tracheal cartilage located where the trachea bifurcates into the right and left mainstem bronchi.

carotid artery The major artery that supplies blood to the head and brain.

carotid bifurcation The point of division at which the common carotid artery branches at the angle of the mandible into the internal and external carotid arteries.

carpometacarpal joint The joint between the wrist and the metacarpal bones; the thumb joint.

carpopedal spasm Contorted position of the hand or foot in which the fingers or toes flex in a clawlike manner; may result from hyperventilation or hypocalcemia.

carriers People who harbor an infectious agent and, although not personally ill, can transmit the infection to other people.

cartilage The support structure of the skeletal system that provides cushioning between bones; also forms the nasal septum and portions of the outer ear.

cartilaginous joints Those connected by hyaline cartilage, or fibrocartilage, such as the joints that separate the vertebrae.

case study A type of research in which a single case is investigated and documented over a period of time.

castor bean A seed that contains the poison ricin; causes a variety of toxic effects: burning of the mouth and throat; nausea, vomiting, diarrhea, and severe stomach pains; prostration; failing vision; and kidney failure, which is the usual cause of death.

catabolism The breakdown of larger molecules into smaller ones.

cataract A clouding of the lens of the eye or its surrounding transparent membrane; normally a result of aging.

catatonic Lacking expression or movement, or appearing rigid.

catecholamines Hormones produced by the adrenal medulla (epinephrine and norepinephrine) that assist the body in coping with physical and emotional stress by increasing the heart and respiratory rates and the blood pressure.

catheter shear Occurs when a needle is reinserted into the catheter, and it slices through the catheter, creating a free-floating segment.

cation An ion that contains an overall positive charge.

caustics Chemicals that are acids or alkalis; cause direct chemical injury to the tissues they contact.

cecum The first part of the large intestine, into which the ileum opens.

cell membrane The cell wall; a selectively permeable layer of cells that surround intracellular contents and control movement of substances into and out of the cell.

cell signaling The process by which cells communicate with one another.

cell-mediated immunity The immune process by which T-cell lymphocytes and macrophages attack and destroy pathogens or foreign substances; the process involves recognizing antigens, then secreting cytokines (specifically lymphokines) that attract other cells or stimulate the production of cytotoxic cells that kill the infected cells.

cellular immune response Cell-mediated immunity; it occurs when T cells attach to foreign, antigen-bearing cells such as bacterial cells, and interact with direct cell-to-cell contact.

cellular immunity The immunity provided by special white blood cells called T cells that attack and destroy invaders.

cellular metabolism Process within a cell where nutrients can be broken down from complex to simpler forms or complex forms can be built from those building blocks.

cellular respiration A biochemical process resulting in the production of energy in the form of adenosine triphosphate; also called metabolism.

cellular telephones Low-power portable radios that communicate through an interconnected series of repeater stations called "cells."

Celsius scale A scale for measuring temperature where water freezes at 0° and boils at 100°.

central nervous system (CNS) The brain and spinal cord.

central shock A type of shock caused by central pump failure, including cardiogenic shock and obstructive shock.

central vision The visualization of objects directly in front of you.

cephalic vein One of the two major veins of the arm that combine to form the axillary vein.

cerebellum One of the three major subdivisions of the brain, sometimes called the "little brain"; coordinates the various activities of the brain, particularly fine body movements.

cerebral palsy (CP) A developmental condition in which damage is done to the brain. It presents during infancy as a delay in walking or crawling, and can take on a spastic form in which muscles are in a nearly constant state of contraction.

cerebrospinal fluid (CSF) Fluid produced in the ventricles of the brain that flows in the subarachnoid space and bathes the meninges.

cerebrospinal otorrhea Cerebrospinal fluid drainage from the ears.

cerebrospinal rhinorrhea Cerebrospinal fluid drainage from the nose.

cerebrum The largest part of the three subdivisions of the brain, sometimes called the "gray matter"; made up of several lobes that control movement, hearing, balance, speech, visual perception, emotions, and personality.

certification A process in which a person, an institution, or a program is evaluated and recognized as meeting certain predetermined standards to provide safe and ethical care.

cerumen Ear wax.

cervical spine The portion of the spinal column consisting of the first seven vertebrae that lie in the neck.

cervix The narrowest portion (lower third of neck) of the uterus that opens into the vagina.

chalazion A small, swollen bump or pustule on the external eyelid, resulting when the eyelid's oil glands or ducts become blocked.

chancre The primary hard lesion or ulcer of syphilis that occurs at the entry site of the infection.

chancroid A highly contagious sexually transmitted disease caused by the bacteria *Haemophilus ducreyi*, which causes painful sores (ulcers), usually of the genitals.

CHARTE method A narrative writing method that allows the narrative to be broken down into logical sections similar to the steps of the EMS assessment; components include chief complaint, history, assessment, treatment, transport, and exceptions.

chelating agents Medications that bind with heavy metals in the body and create a compound that can be eliminated; used in cases of ingestion or poisoning.

chemical mediators Chemicals that work to cause the immune or allergic response; for example, histamine.

chemoreceptors Sense organs that monitor the levels of oxygen and carbon dioxide and the pH of the CSF and blood and provide feedback to the respiratory centers to modify the rate and depth of breathing based on the body's needs at any given time.

chemotaxins Components of the activated complement system that attract leukocytes from the circulation to help fight infections.

chemotaxis The movement of additional white blood cells to an area of inflammation in response to the release of chemical mediators, such as neutrophils, injured tissue, and monocytes.

Cheyne-Stokes respirations A gradually increasing rate and depth of respirations followed by a gradual decrease with intermittent periods of apnea; associated with brainstem insult.

chickenpox   A very contagious disease caused by the varicella zoster virus, which is part of the herpes virus family, occurring most often in the winter and early spring.

chief complaint   The problem for which the patient is seeking help.

chlamydia   A sexually transmitted disease (STD) caused by the bacterium *Chlamydia trachomatis*; has the highest incidence in sexually transmitted diseases; signs and symptoms include inflammation of the urethra, epididymis, cervix, and fallopian tubes, and discharge from the urethra.

choleangitis   Inflammation of the bile duct.

cholecystitis   Inflammation of the gallbladder.

cholelithiasis   The presence of stones within the gallbladder.

cholinergic   A term used to describe the fibers in the parasympathetic nervous system that release a chemical called acetylcholine.

chordae tendineae   Thin bands of fibrous tissue that attach to the valves in the heart and prevent them from inverting.

choroid   The vascular, pigmented middle layer of the eye wall.

choroid plexus   Specialized capillaries within hollow areas in the ventricles of the brain that produce cerebrospinal fluid.

chromosomes   Structures formed from condensed DNA fibers and protein; they are thread-like, and are contained within the nucleus of the cells.

chronic bronchitis   A chronic inflammatory condition affecting the bronchi that is characterized by excessive mucus production as a result of overgrowth of the mucous glands in the airways.

chronic obstructive pulmonary disease (COPD)   A progressive and irreversible disease of the airway marked by decreased inspiratory and expiratory capacity of the lungs.

chronic renal failure (CRF)   Progressive and irreversible inadequate kidney function caused by the permanent loss of nephrons.

chronotropic effect   The effect on the rate of contraction of the heart.

chyme   The name given to the substance that leaves the stomach once food is digested; it is a combination of all of the eaten foods with added stomach acids.

cilia   The hairlike microtubule projections on the surface of a cell that can move materials over the cell surface.

ciliary body   The structure associated with the choroid layer of the eye that secretes aqueous humor and contains the ciliary muscle.

circulatory system   The complex arrangement of connected tubes, including the arteries, arterioles, capillaries, venules, and veins, that moves blood, oxygen, nutrients, carbon dioxide, and cellular waste throughout the body.

circumflex coronary artery   One of the two branches of the left main coronary artery.

circumstantial thinking   Situation in which the patient includes many irrelevant details in his or her account of things.

cirrhosis   Early failure of the liver; characterized by portal hypertension, coagulation deficiencies, and diminished detoxification.

civil suit   An action instituted by a private person or corporation against another private person or corporation.

class   How a medication is categorized as compared to other medications. This is usually done by grouping those medications with similar characteristics, traits, or primary components.

claudication   A severe pain in the calf muscle that is caused by narrowing of the arteries in this muscle and that leads to a painful limp.

clavicle   The collarbone; it is lateral to the sternum and anterior to the scapula.

clitoris   In females, a small, cylindrical mass of erectile tissue and nerves located at the anterior junction of the labia minora, similar to the glans penis of the male.

clonic activity   Type of seizure movement involving the contraction and relaxation of muscle groups.

closed-ended question   A question that is specific and focused, demanding either a yes or no answer or an answer chosen from specific options.

clotting cascade   The term that refers to the process by which clotting factors work together to ultimately form fibrin.

clotting factors   Substances in the blood that are necessary for clotting; also called coagulation factors.

coagulation   Clotting of the blood.

coagulation system   The system that forms blood clots in the body and facilitates repairs to the vascular tree.

coagulopathy   Any type of bleeding disorder that interferes with the activation or continuation of the clotting cascade or hemostasis.

Cobra perilaryngeal airway (CobraPLA)   A supraglottic airway device with a shape that allows the device to slide easily along the hard palate and to hold the soft tissue away from the laryngeal inlet.

cocaine   A stimulant; a naturally occurring alkaloid that is extracted from the *Erythroxylon coca* plant leaves found in South America.

coccyx   The last three or four vertebrae of the spine; the tailbone.

cochlea   The shell-shaped structure within the inner ear that contains the organ of Corti.

cochlear duct   A canal within the cochlea that receives vibrations from the ossicles.

cohort research   A type of research that examines patterns of change, a sequence of events, or trends over time within a certain population of study subjects.

collagen vascular diseases   A group of autoimmune disorders that affect the collagen in tendons, bones, and connective tissues.

collateral circulation   The mesh of arteries and capillaries that supplies blood to a segment of tissue whose original arterial supply has been obstructed.

colloid solutions   Solutions that contain molecules (usually proteins) that are too large to pass out of the capillary membranes and, therefore, remain in the vascular compartment.

colonized   A pathogen is present but has produced no illness in the host; often progresses to active infection; a colonized host is often called a *carrier* because he or she can transmit the pathogen to others.

colorimetric capnographer   A device that attaches between the endotracheal tube and bag-mask device; uses special paper that should turn from purple to yellow during exhalation, indicating the presence of exhaled CO_2.

coma   A state in which a person does not respond to verbal or painful stimuli.

Combitube   A multilumen airway device that consists of a single tube with two lumens, two balloons, and two ventilation ports; an alternative device if endotracheal intubation is not possible or has failed.

common reality   Sensory stimulation that can be verified by others.

communicable disease   An infectious disease that can be transmitted from one person to another by direct contact or by indirect contact through a vector or fomite; also called contagious disease.

communicable period   The period during which an infected person can transmit a communicable disease to someone else.

compact bone   A type of bone that is mostly solid.

competitive antagonists   The medications that temporarily bind with cellular receptor sites, displacing agonist chemicals.

competitive depolarizing   A term used to describe paralytic agents that act at the neuromuscular junction by binding with nicotinic receptors on muscles, causing fasciculations and preventing additional activation by acetylcholine.

complement   A group of proteins in plasma and other body fluids that interact to cause inflammation and phagocytic activities.

complement system   A group of plasma proteins whose function is to do one of three things: attract leukocytes to sites of inflammation, activate leukocytes, and directly destroy cells.

compounds   Molecules made up of different bonded atoms.

compulsions   Repetitive actions carried out to relieve the anxiety of obsessive thoughts.

concentration The amount of a medication that is present in the ampule or vial; usually expressed in milligrams, grams, or grains.

concentration gradient The natural tendency for substances to flow from an area of higher concentration to an area of lower concentration, within or outside the cell.

concept formation Pattern of understanding based on initially obtained information.

concordant precordial pattern A pattern in which the QRS complexes are all in the same direction in the precordial leads.

conductivity The property that enables cardiac cells to pass an electrical impulse from one cell to another.

cones One of two photoreceptors of the retina that can distinguish colors, but requires a greater amount of light to activate and create an image.

confabulation The invention of experiences to cover gaps in memory, seen in patients with certain organic brain syndromes.

confrontation Pointing out something of interest in the patient's conversation or behavior, thereby directing the patient's attention to something he or she may have been unaware of.

congenital adrenal hyperplasia (CAH) Inadequate production of cortisol and aldosterone by the adrenal gland.

congestive heart failure (CHF) A condition that occurs when the heart is unable to pump powerfully enough or fast enough to empty its chambers; as a result, blood backs up into the systemic circuit, the pulmonary circuit, or both.

conjunctiva A thin, transparent membrane that covers the sclera and internal surfaces of the eyelids.

conjunctivitis An inflammation of the conjunctivae that usually is caused by bacteria, viruses, allergies, or foreign bodies; should be considered highly contagious; also called pink eye.

connective tissues Tissues that bind, support, protect, frame, and fill body structures; they also store fat, produce blood cells, repair tissues, and protect against infection.

consent Agreement by the patient to accept a medical intervention.

contact transmission The transmission of an infectious agent by means of direct or indirect contact with the infected persons, such as skin-to-skin contact or contact with the patient's environment.

contaminated The presence or the reasonably anticipated presence of blood or other potentially infectious materials on an item or surface.

contaminated stick The puncturing of an emergency care provider's skin with a needle or catheter that was used on a patient.

contiguous leads Leads that view geographically similar areas of the myocardium; useful for localizing areas of ischemia.

continuous positive airway pressure (CPAP) A method of ventilation used primarily in the treatment of critically ill patients with respiratory distress; can prevent the need for endotracheal intubation.

continuous quality improvement (CQI) A system of internal and external reviews and audits of all aspects of an EMS system.

contraceptive device A device used to prevent pregnancy.

contractility The strength of heart muscle contraction.

contraindication Any condition, especially any condition of disease, that renders some particular line of treatment improper or undesirable.

contributory negligence Act(s) committed by plaintiff that contributes to adverse outcomes.

convenience sampling A type of research in which subjects are manually assigned to a specific person or crew, rather than being randomly assigned; the least-preferred component of research.

conventional reasoning A type of reasoning in which a child looks for approval from peers and society.

conversion hysteria A reaction in which a person subconsciously transforms his or her anxiety into a bodily dysfunction; the person may be unable to see or hear or may become partially paralyzed.

cookbook medicine Blindly following a protocol or algorithm without thinking about what you are doing and whether or not it is working.

CO-oximeter A device that measures absorption at several wavelengths to distinguish oxyhemoglobin from carboxyhemoglobin.

cor pulmonale Heart disease that develops because of chronic lung disease, affecting primarily the right side of the heart.

cornea The transparent anterior portion of the eye that overlies the iris and pupil.

corneal reflex A protective movement that results in blinking, moving the head posteriorly, and pupillary constriction.

coronal plane An imaginary plane where the body is cut into front and back parts.

coronary arteries Arteries that arise from the aorta shortly after it leaves the left ventricle and supply the heart with oxygen and nutrients.

coronary artery disease (CAD) A pathologic process caused by atherosclerosis that leads to progressive narrowing and eventual obstruction of the coronary arteries.

coronary sinus Veins that collect blood that is returning from the walls of the heart.

coronary sulcus The groove along the exterior surface of the heart that separates the atria from the ventricles.

corpus callosum A deep bridge of nerve fibers connecting the brain hemispheres.

corpus luteum Yellow body; a temporary glandular structure created from enlarged follicular cells because of the release of luteinizing hormone.

cortex Part of the internal anatomy of the kidney; the lighter-colored outer region closest to the capsule.

corticosteroids Hormones secreted by the adrenal gland, and which regulate the body's metabolism, the balance of salt and water in the body, the immune system, and sexual function.

cortisol A hormone of the middle adrenal cortex that influences protein and fat metabolism and stimulates glucose to be synthesized from noncarbohydrates; stimulates most body cells to increase their energy production.

countercurrent multiplier The process by which the body produces either concentrated or diluted urine, depending on the body's needs.

couplet Two premature ventricular contractions occurring sequentially.

covalent bond A chemical bond where atoms complete their outer electron shells by sharing electrons.

covert behavior Behavior that has a hidden meaning or intention that only the person understands.

crackles The breath sounds produced as fluid-filled alveoli pop open under increasing inspiratory pressure; can be fine or coarse; formerly called rales.

cranial nerves The 12 pairs of nerves that arise from the base of the brain.

cranial vault The bones that encase and protect the brain, including the parietal, temporal, frontal, occipital, sphenoid, and ethmoid bones.

cranium The area of the head above the ears and eyes; the skull. The cranium contains the brain.

creatine phosphate An organic compound in muscle tissue that can store and provide energy for muscle contraction.

crenation Shrinkage of a cell that results when too much water leaves the cell through osmosis.

crepitus Crackling, grating, or grinding that is often felt or heard when two ends of bone rub together.

cretinism A disease caused by lack of thyroid hormone during pregnancy; it results in severely stunted physical and mental development.

cribriform plate A horizontal bone perforated with numerous foramina for the passage of the olfactory nerve filaments from the nasal cavity.

cricoid cartilage A firm ridge of cartilage that forms the lower part of the larynx; the first ring of the trachea and the only upper airway structure that forms a complete ring; also called the cricoid ring.

cricothyroid membrane A thin, superficial membrane located between the thyroid and cricoid cartilage that is relatively avascular and contains few nerves; the site for emergency surgical and nonsurgical access to the airway.

criminal prosecution An action instituted by the government against a private person for violation of criminal law.

crista galli A prominent bony ridge in the center of the anterior fossa to which the meninges are attached.

critical incident An event that overwhelms the ability to cope with the experience, either at the scene or later.

critical incident stress management (CISM) A process that confronts responses to critical incidents and defuses them.

Crohn disease Inflammation of the ileum and possibly other portions of the GI tract, in which the immune system attacks portions of the intestinal walls, causing them to become scarred, narrowed, stiff, and weakened.

cross section The product of slicing an object across or perpendicular to its long axis.

cross-sectional design A data collection method in which all data at one point in time are collected, essentially serving as a "snapshot" of events and information.

cross-tolerance A process in which repeated exposure to a medication within a particular class causes a tolerance that may be "transferred" to other medications in the same class.

croup A common disease of childhood due to upper airway obstruction and characterized by stridor, hoarseness, and a barking cough.

crown The part of the tooth that is external to the gum.

crystalloid solutions Solutions of dissolved crystals (for example, salts or sugars) in water; contain compounds that quickly dissociate in solution.

cumulative action Several smaller doses of a particular medication capable of producing the same clinical effects as a single larger dose of that same medication.

cumulative stress reaction Prolonged or excessive stress.

current health status A composite picture of a number of factors in a patient's life, such as dietary habits, current medications, allergies, exercise, alcohol or tobacco use, recreational drug use, sleep patterns and disorders, and immunizations.

curved laryngoscope blade A blade designed to fit into the vallecula, indirectly lifting the epiglottis and exposing the vocal cords; also called the Macintosh blade.

Cushing reflex The combination of a slowing pulse, rising blood pressure, and erratic respiratory patterns; a grave sign for patients with head trauma or cerebrovascular accident.

Cushing syndrome A condition caused by an excess of cortisol production by the adrenal glands or by excessive use of cortisol or other similar corticosteroid (glucocorticoid) hormones.

cusps In the context of the heart, the flaps that comprise the heart valves; in the context of the oral cavity, the points at the top of a tooth.

cutaneous membrane The skin; it covers the entire surface of the body.

cyanosis A bluish-gray skin color that is caused by inadequate levels of oxygen in the blood.

cytochrome P-450 system A hemoprotein involved in the detoxification of many drugs.

cytokines The products of cells that affect the function of other cells.

cytokinesis The division of the cytoplasm of a cell.

cytomegalovirus (CMV) A herpesvirus that can produce the symptoms of prolonged high fever, chills, headache, malaise, extreme fatigue, and an enlarged spleen.

cytoplasm The gel-like material that fills out a cell; it makes up most of the cell's volume, and suspends the cell's organelles.

cytosol The clear liquid portion of the cytoplasm.

D_2W An intravenous solution made up of 5% dextrose in water.

damages Compensation for injury awarded by a court.

data interpretation The process of reaching conclusions based on comparing the patient's presentation with information from your training, education, and past experiences.

daughter cells The two identical cells produced when a parent cell divides by mitosis.

DCAP-BTLS A mnemonic for assessment in which each area of the body is evaluated for Deformities, Contusions, Abrasions, Punctures/penetrations, Burns, Tenderness, Lacerations, and Swelling.

dead space Any portion of the airway that contains air and cannot participate in gas exchange, such as the trachea and bronchi.

dead space volume (V_D) Any portion of the airway that does not contain air and cannot participate in gas exchange.

DeBakey classification A classification system for aortic dissections that includes three categories.

decerebrate posturing Abnormal extension of the arms with rotation of the wrists along with toe pointing. This indicates brainstem damage.

decision-making capacity The patient's ability to understand and process the information you give him or her about your proposed plan of care.

decomposition A reaction that occurs when bonds within a reactant molecule break, forming simpler atoms, molecules, or ions.

decorticate posturing Abnormal flexion of the arms toward the chest with the toes pointed. It indicates lower cerebral damage.

decussation Movement of nerves from one side of the brain to the opposite side of the body.

deep Further inside the body and away from the skin.

defamation Intentionally making a false statement, through written or verbal communication, which injures a person's good name or reputation.

defendant In a civil suit, the person against whom a legal action is brought.

defense mechanisms Psychological ways to relieve stress; they are usually automatic or subconscious. Defense mechanisms include denial, regression, projection, and displacement.

defibrillation The use of an unsynchronized direct current (DC) electric shock to terminate ventricular fibrillation.

dehydration Depletion of the body's systemic fluid volume.

delayed stress reaction Reaction to stress that occurs after a stressful situation.

delirium An acute confusional state characterized by global impairment of thinking, perception, judgment, and memory.

delirium tremens (DTs) A severe withdrawal syndrome seen in people with alcoholism who are deprived of ethyl alcohol; characterized by restlessness, fever, sweating, disorientation, agitation, and seizures; can be fatal if untreated.

delta cells Cells within the pancreas that produce somatostatin, which helps to regulate the endocrine system.

delta wave The slurring of the upstroke of the first part of the QRS complex that occurs in Wolff-Parkinson-White syndrome.

delusions Thoughts, ideas, or perceived abilities that have no basis in common reality.

dementia The slow, progressive onset of disorientation, shortened attention span, and loss of cognitive function.

dendrites The parts of neurons that receive impulses from the axon and contain vesicles for release of neurotransmitters.

denial An early response to a serious medical emergency, in which the severity of the emergency is diminished or minimized. Denial is the first coping mechanism for people who believe they are going to die.

dense connective tissue White fibrous tissue that makes up tendons and ligaments, and exists in the eyeballs and deep skin layers.

dental abscess A collection of pus that forms in the gums, facial tissue, bones, and/or neck.

dentalgia   Toothache.

dentin   The principal mass of the tooth, which is made up of a material that is much more dense and stronger than bone.

dependence   The physical, behavioral, or emotional need for a medication or chemical in order to maintain "normal" physiologic function.

depolarization   The rapid movement of electrolytes across a cell membrane that changes the cell's overall charge. This rapid shifting of electrolytes and cellular charges is the main catalyst for muscle contractions and neural transmissions.

depolarizing neuromuscular blocker   A drug that competitively binds with the acetylcholine receptor sites but is not affected as quickly by acetylcholinesterase; succinylcholine is the only one.

depressant   A chemical or medication that decreases the performance of the central nervous system or sympathetic nervous system.

depression   A mental health disorder characterized by a persistent mood of sadness, despair, and discouragement; it may be a symptom of many different mental and physical disorders, or it may be a disorder on its own.

dermatomes   Distinct areas of skin that correspond to specific spinal or cranial nerve levels where sensory nerves enter the central nervous system.

dermis   The inner layer of the skin, containing hair follicles, sweat glands, nerve endings, and blood vessels.

descending aorta   One of the three portions of the aorta, it is the longest portion and extends through the thorax and abdomen into the pelvis.

descriptive   A research format in which an observation of an event is made, but without attempts to alter or change it.

designated infection control officer (DICO)   A person trained to ensure that proper postexposure medical treatment and counseling are provided to an exposed employee or volunteer.

desired dose   The quantity of a medication that is to be administered to a patient; the drug order; usually expressed in milligrams, grams, or grains.

despair phase   The second phase of an infant's response to a situational crisis; characterized by monotonous wailing.

diabetes mellitus   A metabolic disorder in which the ability to metabolize carbohydrates (sugar) is impaired due to lack of insulin or failure of the cells to use insulin properly.

diabetic ketoacidosis (DKA)   A form of acidosis in uncontrolled diabetes in which certain acids accumulate when insulin is not available.

diabetic retinopathy   A condition associated with diabetes, in which the small blood vessels of the retina are affected; can eventually lead to blindness.

diapedesis   A process whereby leukocytes leave blood vessels to move toward tissue where they are needed most.

diaphoresis   Excessive sweating; it is often associated with shock.

diaphragm   A muscular dome that forms the undersurface of the thorax, separating the chest from the abdominal cavity. Contraction of the diaphragm (and the chest wall muscles) brings air into the lungs. Relaxation allows air to be expelled from the lungs.

diaphysis   The shaft of a long bone.

diarrhea   Liquid stool.

diastole   The period of ventricular relaxation during which the ventricles passively fill with blood.

diastolic pressure   The result of residual pressure in the circulatory system while the left ventricle is relaxing (ie, in diastole).

dieffenbachia   A common houseplant that resembles "elephant ears"; ingestion leads to burns of the mouth and tongue and, possibly, paralysis of the vocal cords and nausea and vomiting; in severe cases, may be edema of the tongue and larynx, leading to airway compromise.

diencephalon   The part of the brain that lies between the brainstem and the cerebrum and includes the thalamus and hypothalamus.

differential diagnosis   The process of weighing the probability of one disease versus other diseases by comparing clinical findings that could account for a patient's illness.

differentiation   The process of specialization of a cell.

diffusion   A process where molecules move from an area of higher concentration to an area of lower concentration.

digestion   The mechanical and chemical breakdown of the large molecules in food into small molecules that can be absorbed in the GI tract and converted to energy for cellular function.

digital intubation   A method of intubation that involves directly palpating the glottic structures and elevating the epiglottis with the middle finger while guiding the endotracheal tube into the trachea by using the sense of touch.

digital radio   The microwave transmission of digital signals through space or the atmosphere instead of transmission by radio waves.

digitalis preparations   The drugs used in the treatment of congestive heart failure and certain atrial dysrhythmias.

diluent   A solution (usually water or normal saline) used for diluting a medication.

diploid   Cells that carry two of each of the 23 chromosomes—one from the father and one from the mother.

diplopia   Double vision.

direct contact   Exposure to or transmission of a communicable disease from one person to another by physical contact.

direct laryngoscopy   Visualization of the airway with a laryngoscope.

disaccharides   A simple sugar comprised of two monosaccharides.

disequilibration syndrome   A condition characterized by nausea, vomiting, headache, and confusion, which results when, as a consequence of dialysis, water initially shifts from the bloodstream into the cerebrospinal fluid, mildly increasing intracranial pressure.

disinfectants   Chemicals used on nonliving objects to kill organisms; toxic to living tissues.

disorganization   A condition in which a person is characterized by uncontrolled and disconnected thought, is usually incoherent or rambling in speech, and may or may not be oriented to person and place.

disorientation   A condition in which a person may be confused about his or her identity, the location, and the time of day; one of the ways in which various conditions such as schizophrenia or organic brain syndrome may present.

dispatch   To send to a specific destination or to send on a task.

displacement   Redirection of an emotion from yourself to another person.

dissection   In reference to blood vessels, an aneurysm, or bulge, formed by the separation of the layers of an arterial wall.

disseminated intravascular coagulation (DIC)   A life-threatening condition commonly found in severe trauma.

dissociates   Process of losing a hydrogen atom in the presence of water. Acids are classified as strong or weak, depending on how completely they dissociate.

distal   Farther from the trunk or nearer to the free end of the extremity.

distal convoluted tubule (DCT)   Connects with the kidney's collecting tubules.

distribution   The movement and transportation of a medication throughout the bloodstream to tissues and cells and, ultimately, to its target receptor.

distributive shock   The type of shock that occurs when there is widespread dilation of the resistance vessels (small arterioles), the capacitance vessels (small venules), or both.

diuresis   The production of large amounts of urine by the kidney.

diuretic   A chemical that increases urinary output.

diverticulitis   Inflammation of pouches in the colon; these pouches form as a result of difficulty moving feces through the colon. Once the pouches are formed, bacteria can become trapped in the pouch, leading to inflammation and infection.

diverticulum   A weak area in the colon that begins to have small outcroppings that turn into pouches; plural is diverticula.

do not resuscitate (DNR) order A type of advance directive that describes which life-sustaining procedures should be performed in the event of a sudden deterioration in a patient's medical condition.

dorsal The posterior surface of the body, including the back of the hand.

dorsal respiratory group (DRG) A portion of the medulla oblongata where the primary respiratory pacemaker is found.

dorsalis pedis artery The artery on the anterior surface of the foot between the first and second metatarsals.

dose-response curve A graphic illustration of the response of a drug according to the dose administered.

dosing The specified amount of a medication to be given at specific intervals.

down-regulation The process in which a mechanism reducing available cell receptors for a particular medication results in tolerance.

drip chamber The area of the administration set where fluid accumulates so that the tubing remains filled with fluid.

dromotropic effect Related to the effect of the heart's conduction rate.

droplet transmission The transmission of an infectious agent by inhalation of relatively large particles generated when an infected person coughs or sneezes; these particles travel a short distance through the air before falling to the ground.

drug Substance that has some therapeutic effect (such as reducing inflammation, fighting bacteria, or producing euphoria) when given in the appropriate circumstances and in the appropriate dose.

drug abuse Any use of drugs that causes physical, psychological, economic, legal, or social harm to the user or others affected by the user's behavior.

drug addiction A chronic disorder characterized by the compulsive use of a substance that results in physical, psychological, or social harm to the user who continues to use the substance despite the harm.

drug interactions Any potential effects that a medication may have when administered in conjunction or in the presence of another medication already in the patient's system, a medication delivery device, or fluid.

drug reconstitution Injecting sterile water or saline from one vial into another vial containing a powdered form of the drug.

due process A right to a fair procedure for a legal action against a person or agency; has two components: Notice and Opportunity to be Heard.

Dunphy sign Severe abdominal pain in the right lower quadrant with coughing; a method for evaluating a patient for peritonitis.

duplex Radio system using more than one frequency to permit simultaneous transmission and reception.

dura mater The outermost of the three meninges that enclose the brain and spinal cord; it is the toughest membrane.

duration of action Three values are given: (1) onset: the estimated amount of time it will take for the medication to enter the body/system and begin to take effect, (2) peak effect: the estimated amount of time it will take for the medication to have its greatest effect on the patient/system, and (3) duration: the estimated amount of time that the medication will have any effect on the patient/system.

duration of effect The time a medication concentration can be expected to remain above the minimum level needed to provide the intended action.

duty Legal obligation of public and certain other ambulance services to respond to a call for help in their jurisdiction.

dysconjugate gaze Paralysis of gaze or lack of coordination between the movements of the two eyes.

dysfunctional uterine bleeding Abnormal vaginal bleeding that is irregular and is not caused by pregnancy, infection, or tumor.

dyslipidemia An excessive level of lipids (fats) circulating in the blood, increasing the risk of atherosclerosis and coronary artery disease.

dysmenorrhea Painful menstruation.

dysphagia Pain when swallowing.

dysphonia Difficulty speaking.

dysplasia An alteration in the size, shape, and organization of cells.

dyspnea Difficult or labored breathing.

dysrhythmias Disturbances in the cardiac rhythm.

dystonia Contractions of body into bizarre positions.

dystonic Pertaining to voluntary muscle movements that are distorted or impaired because of abnormal muscle tone.

ear canal The cavity leading from the exterior atmosphere to the tympanum.

early adults Persons who are 18 to 40 years of age.

ecchymosis Localized bruising or blood collection within or under the skin.

echolalia Meaningless echoing of the interviewer's words by the patient.

ecstasy A drug officially named methylenedioxymethamphetamine (MDMA) that is sometimes used to facilitate date rape; a methamphetamine derivative with hallucinogenic properties; street names include XTC, Adam, X, lover's speed, and clarity.

ectopic foci Sites of generation of electrical impulses other than normal pacemaker cells.

ectopic pregnancy A pregnancy in which the ovum implants somewhere other than the uterine endometrium.

efferent arteriole The structure in the kidney where blood drains from the glomerulus.

efferent nerves Nerves that leave the brain through the peripheral nervous system and convey commands to other parts of the body.

efficacy In a pharmacologic context, the ability of a medication to produce the desired effect.

egophony A test of decreased breath sounds performed by placing the diaphragm of the stethoscope over the area in question while the patient says "ee"; an "ay" sound indicates lung consolidation.

ejaculation The forcing of semen through the urethra to outside of the body.

ejaculatory duct A structure formed by the vasa deferentia uniting with the duct of a seminal vesicle; this type of duct passes through the prostate gland to empty into the urethra.

ejection click A high-pitched heart sound that occurs just after the S_1 sound.

ejection fraction (EF) The percentage of blood that leaves the heart each time it contracts.

elastic cartilage A flexible type of cartilage that provides framework for the ears and larynx.

electrical conduction system In the heart, the specialized cardiac tissue that initiates and conducts electric impulses; includes the SA node, internodal conduction pathways, atrioventricular junction, atrioventricular node, bundle of His, and the Purkinje network.

electrolytes Salt or acid substances that become ionic conductors when dissolved in a solvent (ie, water); chemicals dissolved in the blood; used in the body to perform certain critical metabolic functions.

electrons Single, negatively charged particles that revolve around the nucleus of an atom.

elements Fundamental substances, such as carbon, hydrogen, and oxygen, that compose matter.

elimination In a pharmacologic context, the removal of a medication or its by-products from the body.

emancipated minor A person who is under the legal age in a given state, but is legally considered an adult because of other circumstances.

emergency medical dispatch First aid instructions given by specially trained dispatchers to callers over the telephone while an ambulance is en route to the call.

emergency medical dispatcher (EMD) A person who receives information and relays that information in an organized manner during the emergency.

emergency medical services (EMS) A health care system designed to bring immediate on-scene care to those in need along with transport to a definitive medical care facility.

emission   The movement of sperm cells from the testes, and secretions of the prostate gland and seminal vesicles, into the urethra.

emphysema   The infiltration of any tissue by air or gas; a chronic obstructive pulmonary disease characterized by distention of the alveoli and destructive changes in the lung parenchyma.

EMTALA   The Emergency Medical Treatment and Active Labor Act enacted in 1986 to combat the practice of patient dumping (hospitals refusing to admit seriously ill patients or women in labor who could not pay, forcing EMS providers to dump the patients at another hospital). EMTALA regulates hospitals that receive Medicare funding and severely fines hospitals or doctors who violate its provisions.

encapsulated nerve endings   Nerve endings in the skin surrounded by connective tissue that measure mechanical inputs.

encoded   A message is put into a code before it is transmitted.

endemic   Consistently present or prevalent in a population or geographic area.

endocarditis   Inflammation of the endocardium.

endocardium   The thin membrane lining the inside of the heart.

endochondrial ossification   The process of bone formation.

endocrine glands   Glands that secrete or release chemicals that are used inside the body; these lack ducts and release hormones directly into the surrounding tissue and blood.

endocrine hormones   The hormones that are carried to their target or cell group in the bloodstream.

endocrine system   The complex message and control system that integrates many body functions, including the release of hormones.

endogenous   Originating from within the organism (body).

endolymph   The fluid containing nerve receptors that resides inside the membranous labyrinth. Sound waves converted into pressure waves are transmitted through this fluid to the auditory nerves.

endometriosis   A condition in which endometrial tissue grows outside the uterus.

endometritis   An inflammation of the endometrium that often is associated with a bacterial infection.

endometrium   The inner layer of the uterine wall.

endoscopy   Insertion of a flexible fiberoptic tube into the esophagus to visualize, remove, or repair damaged or diseased tissue.

endosteum   A layer that lines the inner surfaces of bone.

endothelial cells   Specific types of epithelial cells that line the blood vessels.

endotoxin   A toxin released by some bacteria when they die.

endotracheal (ET) tube   A tube that is inserted into the trachea for definitive airway maintenance; equipped with a distal cuff, proximal inflation port, a 15/22-mm adapter, and centimeter markings on the side.

endotracheal intubation   Inserting an endotracheal tube through the glottic opening and sealing the tube with a cuff inflated against the tracheal wall.

end-stage renal disease (ESRD)   A condition in which the kidneys have lost all ability to function, and toxic waste materials build up in the patient's blood; occurs after acute or chronic renal failure.

end-tidal carbon dioxide   The carbon dioxide contained in the last few milliliters of exhaled air; the unit of measure is a percentage.

end-tidal CO_2 ($ETCO_2$) monitors   Devices that detect the presence of carbon dioxide in exhaled air.

enhanced 9-1-1 system   An emergency call-in system in which additional information such as the phone number and location of the caller is recorded automatically through sophisticated telephone technology and the dispatcher need only confirm the information on the screen.

enteral medications   Medication administration that involves the medication passing through a portion of the gastrointestinal tract.

Enterococcus   A common, normal organism of the gastrointestinal (GI) tract, urinary tract, and genitourinary tract that can be pathogenic and become resistant to vancomycin.

enzymes   Substances designed to speed up the rate of specific biochemical reactions.

eosinophils   White blood cells with a major role in allergic reactions and bronchoconstriction during an asthma attack; make up approximately 1% to 3% of leukocytes.

ependymal cells   Neuroglia that cover specialized brain parts and form inner linings enclosing spaces inside the brain and spinal cord; they secrete cerebrospinal fluid.

epicardium   The thin membrane lining the outside of the heart; also referred to as the visceral pericardium.

epidemic   An outbreak of disease that substantially exceeds what is expected based on recent experience.

epidermis   The outermost layer of the skin that acts as the body's first line of defense.

epididymides   Tightly coiled tubes connected to ducts within a testis; they become the vas deferens.

epididymitis   An infection that causes inflammation of the epididymis along the posterior border of the testis; a possible complication of male urinary tract infection.

epigastric   The region of the abdomen directly inferior to the xyphoid process and superior to the umbilicus.

epiglottis   A leaf-shaped cartilaginous structure that closes over the trachea during swallowing.

epinephrine   A hormone produced by the adrenal medulla that has a vital role in the function of the sympathetic nervous system.

epiphyseal plate   The growth plate of a bone; a major site of bone development during childhood.

epiphyses   The growth plate of a long bone; also called the epiphyseal plate.

epistaxis   Nosebleed.

epithelial membranes   Membranes that cover body surfaces and line body cavities.

epithelial tissues   Body tissues that cover organs, form the inner lining of cavities, and line hollow organs.

epithelium   A type of tissue that covers all external surfaces of the body.

erection   The swelling and elongation of the penis in preparation for sexual intercourse.

erythrocytes   Red blood cells.

erythropoiesis   The process by which red blood cells are made.

esophageal detector device   A bulb or syringe that is attached to the proximal end of the endotracheal (ET) tube; a device used to confirm proper ET tube placement.

esophagogastric varices   Dilated blood vessels of the esophagus, commonly caused by difficulty in blood flow through the liver; the presence of these can lead to vessel rupture.

esophagus   A collapsible tube that extends from the pharynx to the stomach; contractions of the muscle in the wall of the esophagus propel food and liquids through it to the stomach.

estrogen   A hormone released from the ovaries that stimulates the uterine lining during the menstrual cycle.

ethical   A behavior expected by a person or group following a set of rules.

ethics   A set of values in society that differentiates right from wrong.

etomidate   A nonnarcotic, nonbarbiturate hypnotic-sedative drug; also called Amidate.

eustachian tube   A branch of the internal auditory canal that connects the middle ear to the oropharynx.

evaluation   Collection of the methods, skills, and activities necessary to determine whether a service or program is needed, likely to be used, conducted as planned, and actually helps people.

evidence-based practice   The use of practices that have been proven to be effective in improving patient outcomes.

exchange reaction   A chemical reaction where parts of the reacting molecules are shuffled around to produce new products.

excitability   The property that allows cells to respond to an electrical impulse.

exhalation   Passive movement of air out of the lungs; also called expiration.

exocrine glands   Glands that excrete chemicals for elimination.

exocrine hormones   The hormones that are secreted through ducts into an organ or onto epithelial surfaces.

exogenous   Originating outside the organism (body).

exophthalmos   Protrusion of the eyes from the normal position within the socket.

exotoxin   A toxin secreted by living cells to aid in the death and digestion of other cells.

expiratory reserve volume   The amount of air that can be exhaled following a normal exhalation; average volume is about 1,200 mL.

expressed consent   A type of informed consent that occurs when the patient does something, either through words or by taking some sort of action, that demonstrates permission to provide care.

expressive aphasia   Damage or loss in the ability to speak.

extension   The straightening of a joint.

external auditory canal   The area in which sound waves are received from the auricle (pinna) before they travel to the eardrum; also called the ear canal.

external ear   One of three anatomic parts of the ear; it contains the pinna, the ear canal, and the external portion of the tympanic membrane.

external jugular (EJ) vein   Large neck vein that is lateral to the carotid artery.

external respiration   The exchange of gases between the lungs and the blood cells in the pulmonary capillaries; also called pulmonary respiration.

external rotation   Rotating an extremity at its joint away from the midline.

extracellular fluid (ECF)   Fluid outside of the cell, in which most of the body's supply of sodium is contained; accounts for 15% of body weight.

extravasation   Seepage of blood and medication into the tissue surrounding the blood vessel.

extrinsic muscles   Referring to the eye; six muscles that attach to the exterior of the globe and are controlled by the cranial nerves.

extubation   The process of removing the tube from an intubated patient.

eyelash reflex   Contraction of a patient's lower eyelid when the upper eyelashes are gently stroked; a fairly reliable indicator of the presence or absence of an intact gag reflex.

EZ-IO   A hand-held, battery-powered driver to which a special IO needle is attached; used for insertion of the IO needle into the proximal tibia of children and adults.

face-to-face intubation   Performing intubation at the same level as the patient's face; used when the standard position is not possible. In this position, the laryngoscope is held in the provider's right hand and the endotracheal tube in the left.

facilitated diffusion   Process whereby a carrier molecule moves substances in or out of cells from areas of higher to lower concentration.

factitious disorder   A disorder in which a person wishes to be sick and intentionally produces or feigns physical or psychological signs or symptoms. Symptoms are under voluntary control, with no obvious physiologic reason.

Fahrenheit scale   A scale for measuring temperature where water freezes at 32° and boils at 212°.

fallopian tube   The anatomic structure that connects each ovary with the uterus and provides a passageway for the ova.

false imprisonment   The intentional and unjustified detention of a person against his or her will.

fascia   A sheet or band of tough fibrous connective tissue that covers, supports, and separates muscles, and which also covers arteries, veins, tendons, and ligaments.

fascicular block   Disease or ischemia of either of the anterior and posterior fascicles of the electrical conduction system of the heart; also called hemiblock.

fasciculation   Brief, uncoordinated, visible twitching of small muscle groups; may be caused by the administration of a depolarizing neuromuscular blocking agent (namely, succinylcholine).

FAST1   A sternal IO device used in adults; stands for First Access for Shock and Trauma.

feculent   Smelling of feces.

Federal Communications Commission (FCC)   The federal agency that has jurisdiction over interstate and international telephone and telegraph services and satellite communications, all of which may involve EMS activity.

feedback inhibition   Negative feedback resulting in the decrease of an action in the body.

femoral artery   The principal artery of the thigh, a continuation of the external iliac artery. It supplies blood to the lower abdominal wall, external genitalia, and legs. It can be palpated in the groin area.

femoral head   The proximal end of the femur, articulating with the acetabulum to form the hip joint.

femoral vein   A continuation of the saphenous vein that drains into the external iliac vein.

femur   The thighbone; the longest and one of the strongest bones in the body.

fibrin   A whitish, filamentous protein formed by the action of thrombin on fibrinogen; the protein that polymerizes (bonds) to form the fibrous component of a blood clot.

fibrinogen   A plasma protein that is important for blood coagulation.

fibrinolysis   The process of dissolving blood clots.

fibrinolysis cascade   The breakdown of fibrin in blood clots and the prevention of the polymerization of fibrin into new clots.

fibrinolytic therapy   The therapy that uses medications that act to dissolve blood clots.

fibroblast   A star-shaped fixed cell that produces fibers via protein secretion into the extracellular matrix.

fibrocartilage   A tough type of cartilage that absorbs shock in the spinal column, knees, and pelvic girdle.

fibrous joints   Those that lie between bones that closely contact each other, joined by thin, dense connective tissue.

fibula   The long bone on the lateral aspect of the lower leg.

field impression   A determination of what you think is the patient's current problem, usually based on the patient history and the chief complaint.

fight-or-flight syndrome   A physiologic response to a profound stressor that helps a person deal with the situation at hand; features increased sympathetic tone and results in dilation of the pupils, increased heart rate, dilation of the bronchi, mobilization of glucose, shunting of blood away from the gastrointestinal tract and cerebrum, and increased blood flow to the skeletal muscles.

filtration   Use of hydrostatic pressure to force water or dissolved particles through a semipermeable membrane.

first-degree heart block   A partial disruption of the conduction of the depolarizing impulse from the atria to the ventricles, causing prolongation of the PR interval.

first-order elimination   The process in which the rate of elimination is directly influenced by plasma levels of a substance.

fistula   An abnormal connection between two cavities.

flash chamber   The area of an IV catheter that fills with blood to help indicate when a vein is cannulated.

flat affect   The absence of emotion; appearing to feel no emotion at all.

flexion   The bending of a joint.

flight of ideas   Accelerated thinking in which the mind skips very rapidly from one thought to the next.

fluid balance The process of maintaining homeostasis through equal intake and output of fluids.

focused assessment A type of physical assessment that is typically performed on patients who have sustained an isolated injury or on responsive medical patients. This type of examination is based on the chief complaint and focuses on one body system or part.

fomites Inanimate objects contaminated with microorganisms that serve as a means of transmitting an illness.

fontanelles Areas where the infant's skull has not fused together; usually disappear at approximately 18 months of age.

foramen magnum A large opening at the base of the skull through which the brain connects to the spinal cord.

foramen ovale An opening between the two atria that is present in the fetus but normally closes shortly after birth.

foramina Small openings, perforations, or orifices in the bones of the cranial vault.

fossa ovalis A depression between the right and left atria that indicates where the foramen ovale had been located in the fetus.

Fournier gangrene A condition that results from bacteria entering a laceration to the scrotum or perineum, causing infection and subsequent necrosis of the subcutaneal tissue and muscle in the scrotum.

fovea centralis The region of the retina of the eye that has densely packed cones and provides the greatest visual activity.

Fowler's position A sitting position with the head elevated to 90° (sitting straight upright).

foxglove A plant that contains cardiac glycosides used in making digitalis; ingestion of leaves causes nausea, vomiting, diarrhea, abdominal cramps, hyperkalemia, and a variety of dysrhythmias.

fraction of inspired oxygen (Fio$_2$) The percentage of oxygen in inhaled air.

Frank-Starling mechanism A characteristic of cardiac muscle that enables it, when stretched, to contract with greater force; the more cardiac muscle stretches, the greater the force of its contraction, the more completely it empties, and the greater the stroke volume.

free nerve endings Fine receptors responsible for sensing light touch and smaller vibrations.

free radicals Molecules that are missing one electron in their outer shell.

frequency In radio communications, the number of cycles per second of a signal; inversely related to the wavelength.

full-body exam A systematic head-to-toe examination that is performed during the secondary assessment of a patient who has sustained a significant mechanism of injury, is unresponsive, or is in critical condition.

functional reserve capacity The amount of air that can be forced from the lungs in a single exhalation.

fungi Small organisms that can grow rapidly in the presence of the needed nutrients and organic material and can cause infection related to contact with decaying organic matter or from airborne spores in the environment such as molds; singular term, fungus.

gag reflex An automatic reaction when something touches an area deep in the oral cavity that helps protect the lower airway from aspiration.

gait Walking or ambulating.

gallbladder A sac on the undersurface of the liver that collects bile from the liver and discharges it into the duodenum through the common bile duct.

gametes Sex cells; in humans, sperm and ovaries.

gamma-hydroxybutyric acid (GHB) A drug used to facilitate date rape; is colorless with a salty taste disguised when mixed with a drink; street names include Georgia home boy, grievous bodily harm, easy lay, G, scoop, liquid X, soap, and salty water.

ganglion neurons Responsible for transmitting information from the rods and cones of the eye through the optic nerve.

Gardnerella vaginitis An infection caused by a bacterium that normally resides in the genital area in women but that can cause infection if the bacteria become too numerous; signs and symptoms include a vaginal odor that may be fishy, itching, irritation, and, possibly, a smooth, thin, sticky, white or gray discharge.

gas exchange The process by which oxygen-depleted blood from the pulmonary circulation releases carbon dioxide and is enriched with oxygen; occurs by diffusion at the interface of the alveoli and the pulmonary capillary bed; newly oxygen-enriched blood enters the cardiac circulation for distribution to the body's tissues.

gastric distention The enlargement or expansion of the stomach, often with air; can be a complication of ventilating the esophagus instead of the trachea.

gastric tube A tube that is inserted into the stomach to remove its contents or decompress it.

gastritis Inflammation of the stomach.

gastroenteritis A term that comprises many types of infections and irritations of the gastrointestinal tract; symptoms include nausea and vomiting, fever, abdominal cramps, and diarrhea; also called stomach flu.

gastroesophageal reflux disease (GERD) A condition in which the sphincter between the esophagus and the stomach opens, allowing stomach acid to move superiorly; can cause a burning sensation within the chest (heartburn); also called acid reflux disease.

gastroschisis A congenital malformation in which an embryo develops improperly and a portion of the GI tract develops outside of the abdominal wall instead of inside.

gauge The internal diameter of an IV catheter or needle.

general adaptation syndrome A three-stage description of the body's short-term and long-term reactions to stress.

general impression The overall initial impression that determines the priority for patient care; based on the patient's surroundings, the mechanism of injury, signs and symptoms, and the chief complaint.

general senses Sensations monitored throughout the body by receptors scattered throughout many different tissues.

generalized anxiety disorder (GAD) A disorder in which a person worries about everything for no particular reason, or the worrying is unproductive and the person cannot decide what to do about an upcoming situation.

genital herpes An infection of the genitals, buttocks, or anal area caused by herpes simplex virus (HSV), which may cause sores of the genitals, mouth, or lips.

genital system The reproductive system in males and females.

genital warts Warts caused by the human papillomavirus (HPV), a sexually transmitted disease; also called condylomata acuminata or venereal warts.

genotype The arrangement of person's genes and thier characteristics is based on the combination of alleles, for one gene or many.

germinal layer The deepest layer of the epidermis where new skin cells are formed.

gestational diabetes Diabetes that develops during pregnancy in women who did not have diabetes before pregnancy.

glands Cells or organs that selectively remove, concentrate, or alter materials in the blood and then secrete them back into the body.

glandular epithelium Specialized tissue that produces and secretes substances into ducts or body fluids.

glans penis The cone-shaped end of the penis that covers the ends of the corpora cavernosa and opens as the external urethral orifice.

Glasgow Coma Scale (GCS) An evaluation tool used to determine level of consciousness, which evaluates and assigns point values (scores) for eye opening, verbal response, and motor response, which are then totaled; effective in helping predict patient outcomes.

glaucoma A disease of the eye caused by an increase in intraocular pressure; when severe enough, this may damage the optic nerve and potentially cause permanent loss of vision.

glenoid fossa   The part of the scapula that forms the socket in the ball-and-socket joint of the shoulder.

global aphasia   Damage or loss of both the ability to speak and the ability to understand speech.

globe   The eyeball.

globulins   Antibodies made by the liver or lymphatic tissues that make up around 36% of the plasma proteins.

glomerular (Bowman's) capsule   A sac-like structure that surrounds the glomerulus, from which it receives filtered fluid.

glomerular filtrate   Mostly water, it has the same components as blood plasma except for large protein molecules; it is received by the glomerular capsule.

glomerular filtration   The process that initiates urine formation.

glomerular filtration rate (GFR)   The rate at which blood is filtered through the glomeruli.

glomerulus   A tuft of capillaries located in the kidney that serves as the main filter of the blood in the kidney.

glossoepiglottic ligament   The ligament between the tongue and the epiglottis.

glossopharyngeal nerve   Ninth cranial nerve; supplies motor fibers to the pharyngeal muscle, providing taste sensation to the posterior portion of the tongue, and carrying parasympathetic fibers to the parotid gland.

glottis   The vocal cords and the opening between them.

glucagon   Hormone produced by the pancreas that is vital to the control of the body's metabolism and blood glucose level. Glucagon stimulates the breakdown of glycogen to glucose.

gluconeogenesis   A process that stimulates both the liver and the kidneys to produce glucose from noncarbohydrate molecules.

glycogen   A long polymer from which glucose is converted in the liver (animal starch).

glycogenolysis   The breakdown of glycogen to glucose.

glycolysis   A process that involves a series of enzymatically catalyzed reactions in which glucose is broken down to yield lactic acid or pyruvic acid.

goblet cells   The mucus-producing cells found mainly in the respiratory and intestinal tracts.

goiter   A visible mass in the anterior part of the neck caused by enlargement of the thyroid gland.

gonadotropins   Hormones secreted by the anterior pituitary gland, which include luteinizing hormone and follicle-stimulating hormone.

gonads   The reproductive glands; the main source of sex hormones.

gonorrhea   A sexually transmitted disease (STD) that results in infection caused by the gonococcal bacteria, *Neisseria gonorrhea*; signs and symptoms include pus-containing discharge from the urethra and painful urination in males and signs and symptoms of an acute abdomen in females.

Good Samaritan law   A statute providing limited immunity from liability to persons responding voluntarily and in good faith to the aid of an injured person outside the hospital.

gram-negative   A reaction of bacteria to a Gram stain in which the bacteria do not retain the dark purple stain; this type of bacteria has cell walls that consist largely of lipids, and have pathogenic qualities that make them especially problematic for humans.

gram-positive   A reaction of bacteria to a Gram stain in which the bacteria retain the dark purple stain; this type of bacteria has thick cell walls composed of many layers.

granulocytes   A type of leukocyte that has large cytoplasmic granules that are easily seen with a simple light microscope.

Graves disease   An autoimmune disorder that causes thyroid gland hypertrophy and severe hyperthyroidism.

gravida   A term used to describe the number of times a woman has been pregnant.

greater trochanter   A bony prominence on the proximal lateral side of the thigh, just below the hip joint.

Greenfield filter   A mesh filter placed in the inferior vena cava to catch blood clots in patients who are at high risk of pulmonary embolus.

gross negligence   Negligence that is willful, wanton, intentional, or reckless; a serious departure from the accepted standards.

growth plates   Structures located on either end of an infant's bone that aid in lengthening bones as the child grows.

gtt   A unit of measure that indicates drops.

guarding   Contraction of the abdominal muscles in patients.

Guillain-Barré syndrome   A disease of unknown cause that involves progressive paralysis that moves from the feet to the head (ascending paralysis); if paralysis reaches the diaphragm, the patient may require respiratory support; can lead to paralysis within 2 weeks.

gum elastic bougie   A flexible device that is inserted between the glottis under direct laryngoscopy; the endotracheal tube is threaded over the device, facilitating its entry into the trachea.

gut-associated lymphoid tissue   The lymphoid tissue that lies under the inner lining of the esophagus and intestines.

habituation   The situation in which there is a physical tolerance and psychological dependence on a drug or drugs.

Haddon matrix   A framework developed by William Haddon, Jr, MD, as a method to generate ideas about injury prevention that address the host, agent, and environment and their impact in the pre-event, event, and post-event phases of the injury process.

hair follicles   The small organs that produce hair.

half-life   The time needed in an average person for metabolism or elimination of 50% of a substance in the plasma.

hallucination   A sense perception not founded on objective reality; a false perception.

hallucinogen   An agent that produces false perceptions in any one of the five senses.

hantavirus   A type of virus found in wild rodents, which can also cause disease in humans, characterized by fever, headache, abdominal pain, loss of appetite, and vomiting; diseases caused are hemorrhagic fever with renal syndrome and hantavirus pulmonary syndrome.

haploid cells   Cells that carry genetic instructions via 23 individual chromosomes.

hapten   A substance that normally does not stimulate an immune response but can be combined with an antigen and at a later point initiate an antibody response; found in certain drugs, dust particles, animal dander, and various chemicals.

Hashimoto disease   A type of hyperthyroidism in which the thyroid gland becomes enlarged as it is infiltrated by T lymphocytes and plasma cells.

head tilt–chin lift maneuver   Manual airway maneuver that involves tilting the head back while lifting up on the chin; used to open the airway of an unresponsive nontrauma patient.

health care power of attorney   A legal document that allows another person to make health care decisions for the patient, including withdrawal or withholding of care, when the patient is incapacitated.

health care professional   A person who follows specific professional attributes that are outlined in this profession.

Health Insurance Portability and Accountability Act (HIPAA)   The law enacted in 1996 that provides for criminal sanctions as well as civil penalties for releasing a patient's protected health information (PHI) in a way not authorized by the patient.

heart   A hollow muscular organ that pumps blood throughout the body.

heart rate (HR)   The number of heart contractions per minute.

heave   A sensation felt upon palpation of the chest wall, in which the heart beats extremely strongly; suggests hypertrophy; also called a lift.

helper T cells   A type of T lymphocyte that is involved in both cell-mediated and antibody-mediated immune responses; these secrete cytokines that stimulate the B cells and other T cells.

hematemesis Vomit with blood; can either look like coffee grounds, indicating the presence of partially digested blood, or contain bright-red blood, indicating active bleeding.

hematochezia The passage of stool in which bright red blood can be distinguished; caused by lower GI bleeding.

hematocrit The percentage of red blood cells in a blood sample.

hematologic disorder Any disorder of the blood.

hematoma An accumulation of blood in the tissues beneath the skin; a potential complication of IV therapy.

hematopoeisis The creation of all formed elements.

hematopoietic system The system that includes all blood components and the organs involved in their development and production.

hematuria The presence of blood in the urine.

hemiparesis Weakness to one side of the body.

hemiplegia Paralysis to one side of the body.

hemochromatosis An inherited disease in which the body absorbs more iron than it needs and stores it in the liver, kidneys, and pancreas.

hemoglobin (Hb) An iron-containing protein within red blood cells that has the ability to combine with oxygen.

hemolysis The destruction of red blood cells by disruption of the cell membrane.

hemolytic anemia A disease characterized by increased destruction of the red blood cells. It can occur from an Rh factor reaction (primarily in Rh-positive neonates born to sensitized Rh-negative mothers), exposure to chemicals, or a disorder of the immune system.

hemolytic crisis A condition in which red blood cells break down quickly; may occur as a result of sickle cell disease.

hemolytic disorder A disorder relating to the breakdown of RBCs.

hemoperitoneum Blood in the peritoneal cavity.

hemophilia A bleeding disorder that is primarily hereditary, in which clotting does not occur or occurs insufficiently.

hemoptysis Coughing up blood.

hemorrhagic One of the two main types of stroke; occurs as a result of bleeding inside the brain.

hemostasis Control of bleeding by formation of a blood clot; the body's natural blood-clotting mechanism.

hemostatic disorder A bleeding and clotting abnormality.

Henry's law A law of gas that states that the amount of a gas in a solution varies directly with the partial pressure of a gas over the solution.

heparin A substance found in large amounts in basophils that inhibits blood clotting.

hepatic encephalopathy Impairment of brain function resulting from failure of the liver.

hepatic portal system A specialized part of the venous system that drains blood from the stomach, intestines, and spleen.

hepatic veins The veins to which blood empties after liver cells in the sinusoids of the liver extract nutrients, filter the blood, and metabolize various drugs.

hepatitis Inflammation of the liver, usually caused by a virus, that causes fever, loss of appetite, jaundice, fatigue, and altered liver function.

Hering-Breuer reflex A protective mechanism that terminates inhalation, thus preventing overexpansion of the lungs.

hernia Protrusion of any organ through an opening into a body cavity where it does not belong.

hertz (Hz) Unit of frequency equal to 1 cycle per second.

hilum The point of entry for the bronchi, vessels, and nerves into each lung.

hilus A cleft where the ureters, renal blood vessels, lymphatic vessels, and nerves enter and leave the kidney.

HIPAA The Health Insurance Portability and Accountability Act that was enacted in 1996, providing for criminal sanctions as well as for civil penalties for releasing a patient's protected health information (PHI) in a way not authorized by the patient.

histamine A chemical found in mast cells that, when released, causes vasodilation, capillary leaking, and bronchiole constriction.

history of the present illness Information about the chief complaint, obtained using the OPQRST mnemonic.

homeostasis A tendency to constancy or stability in the body's internal environment.

homologous chromosome A chromosome of the same numbered pair from the opposite parent.

hordeolum A red tender lump in the eyelid or at the lid margin; commonly known as a stye.

hormones Substances formed in specialized organs or glands and carried to another organ or group of cells in the same organism; regulate many body functions, including metabolism, growth, and body temperature.

host resistance One's ability to fight off infection.

hostile environment Situation in which an employer or an employer's agent either creates or allows to continue an offensive practice related to sex that makes it uncomfortable or impossible for an employee to continue working.

human chorionic gonadotropin (hCG) One of three major female hormones; it is produced by a developing embryo after conception.

human immunodeficiency virus (HIV) The virus that may lead to acquired immunodeficiency syndrome (AIDS); cells in the immune system are killed or damaged so that the body is unable to fight infections and certain cancers.

humerus The supporting bone of the upper arm.

humoral immune response When antibodies react to destroy antigens or antigen-containing particles.

humoral immunity The immune process in which antibodies recognize foreign antigens and stimulate an attack on the foreign body; uses antibodies made by B-cell lymphocytes.

hyaline cartilage The type of cartilage on the ends of bones in many joints, the soft portion of the nose, and in the respiratory passages' supporting rings; it is the most common type of cartilage.

hydrocarbons Compounds made up principally of hydrogen and carbon atoms mostly obtained from the distillation of petroleum.

hydrogen bond The attraction of the positive hydrogen end of a polar molecule to the negative nitrogen or oxygen end of another polar molecule.

hydrophilic Attracted to water molecules.

hydrostatic pressure The pressure of water against the walls of its container.

hymen A fold of mucous membrane that partially covers the entrance to the vagina.

hyoepiglottic ligament The ligament between the hyoid bone and the epiglottis.

hyoid bone A small, horseshoe-shaped bone to which the jaw, tongue, epiglottis, and thyroid cartilage attach.

hypercalcemia An elevated blood calcium level.

hypercarbia Increased carbon dioxide levels in the bloodstream.

hypercholesterolemia An elevated blood cholesterol level.

hyperextension When a body part is extended to the maximum level or beyond the normal range of motion.

hyperflexion When a body part is flexed to the maximum level or beyond the normal range of motion.

hyperglycemia Abnormally high blood glucose level.

hyperkalemia An excessive amount of potassium in the blood.

hypermagnesemia An increased serum magnesium level.

hypermenorrhea Menstrual blood flow that lasts several days longer than it should or flow that is abnormally excessive.

hypernatremia A serum sodium level greater than 145 mEq/L.

hyperopia Farsighted; the ability to see distant objects with difficulty focusing on objects close.

hyperosmolar hyperglycemic nonketotic coma (HHNC) Also known as hyperosmolar nonketotic coma (HONK), HHNC is a metabolic derangement that occurs principally in patients with type 2 diabetes. The condition is characterized by hyperglycemia, hyperosmolarity, and an absence of significant ketosis.

hyperosmolar nonketotic coma (HONK) See *hyperosmolar hyperglycemic nonketotic coma (HHNC)*.

hyperperistalsis A bowel sound characterized by increased activity within the bowel; also called borborygmi.

hyperphosphatemia An elevated serum phosphate level.

hyperplasia An increase in the actual number of cells in an organ or tissue, usually resulting in an increase in the size of the organ or tissue.

hypersensitivity Occurs when a patient reacts with exaggerated or inappropriate allergic symptoms after coming into contact with a substance the body perceives as harmful.

hypertension High blood pressure, usually a diastolic pressure of greater than 90 mm Hg.

hypertensive emergency An acute elevation of blood pressure with evidence of end-organ damage.

hypertensive encephalopathy A condition that may complicate any form of hypertension, and which is usually signaled by a sudden, marked rise in blood pressure to levels greater than 200/130 mm Hg; also known as acute hypertensive crisis.

hypertonic Concentration of solute is higher within the cell as compared to outside the cell.

hypertonic solution A solution that has a greater concentration of sodium than does the cell; the increased osmotic pressure can draw water out of the cell and cause it to collapse.

hypertrophic cardiomyopathy A condition in which the heart muscle is unusually thick, which means that the heart has to pump harder to get blood to leave.

hypertrophy An increase in the size of the cells due to synthesis of more subcellular components, leading to an increase in tissue and organ size.

hyperventilation A condition in which an increased amount of air enters the alveoli; carbon dioxide elimination exceeds carbon dioxide production.

hyphema Bleeding into the anterior chamber of the eye; results from direct ocular trauma.

hypocalcemia A low level of calcium in the blood.

hypocarbia Decreased carbon dioxide content in arterial blood.

hypoglossal nerve Twelfth cranial nerve; provides motor function to the muscles of the tongue and throat.

hypoglycemia Abnormally low blood glucose level.

hypokalemia A low concentration of potassium in the blood.

hypomagnesemia A decreased serum magnesium level.

hyponatremia A serum sodium level that is less than 135 mEq/L.

hypoperfusion A condition that occurs when the level of tissue perfusion decreases below that needed to maintain normal cellular functions.

hypoperistalsis Decreased bowel sounds.

hypophosphatemia A decreased serum phosphate level.

hypothalamic-pituitary-adrenal axis A major part of the neuroendocrine system that controls reactions to stress. It is the mechanism for a set of interactions among glands, hormones, and parts of the midbrain that mediate the general adaptation syndrome.

hypothalamus A small region of the brain that is the primary link between the endocrine system and the nervous system; contains several control centers for emotions and body functions, including pulse rate, digestion, sexual development, temperature regulation, hunger, thirst, and the sleep-wake cycle.

hypothyroidism Myxedema; lowered levels of thyroid hormones.

hypotonic Concentration of solute is lower within the cell as compared to outside the cell.

hypotonic solution A solution that has a lower concentration of sodium than does the cell; the increased osmotic pressure lets water flow into the cell, causing it to swell and possibly burst.

hypoventilate To move inadequate volumes of air into the lungs.

hypoventilation A condition in which a decreased amount of air enters the alveoli; carbon dioxide production exceeds the body's ability to eliminate it by ventilation.

hypovolemic shock A condition that occurs when the circulating blood volume is inadequate to deliver adequate oxygen and nutrients to the body.

hypoxemia A decrease in arterial oxygen level.

hypoxia A dangerous condition in which the supply of oxygen to the tissues is reduced.

hypoxic drive A situation in which a person's stimulus to breathe comes from a decrease in Pao_2 rather than the normal stimulus, an increase in $Paco_2$.

I/E ratio Inspiratory/expiratory ratio; an expression for comparing the length of inspiration with that of expiration, normally 1:2, meaning that expiration is twice as long as inspiration (not measured in seconds).

iatrogenic Related to a side effect or complication of treatment.

icteric Yellowish coloration of the conjunctiva (the whites of the eyes) caused by the buildup of bilirubin in the blood during liver failure.

icterus Jaundice; the yellow appearance of the skin and other tissues caused by an accumulation of bile pigments.

idiopathic Of no known cause.

idiosyncratic In a pharmacologic context, abnormal susceptibility to a medication, possibly due to genetic traits or dysfunction of a metabolic enzyme, that is peculiar to an individual patient (and usually unexplained).

idioventricular Related to only the ventricles; produced by the ventricles.

ilium One of three bones that fuse to form the pelvic ring.

illicit In relation to drugs, illegal drugs such as marijuana, cocaine, and LSD.

immune response The body's defense reaction to any substance that is recognized as foreign.

immune system The body system that includes all of the structures and processes designed to mount a defense against foreign substances and disease-causing agents.

immunity Physiologically, refers to the body's ability to protect itself from acquiring disease. Legally, refers to legal protection from penalties that could normally be incurred under the law.

immunization The process of producing widespread immunity to a specific infectious disease among a targeted group by inoculating individual members of the population; can also refer to a set of vaccinations given together or on a recommended schedule.

immunodeficiency An abnormal condition in which some part of the body's immune system is inadequate, and, consequently, resistance to infectious disease is decreased.

immunogen An antigen that is capable of generating an immune response.

immunoglobulins Antibodies secreted by the B cells.

imperforate hymen A situation in which the hymen completely covers the vaginal orifice.

implanted vascular access devices (VAD) Devices that are implanted in surgery, sutured under the skin, for the purpose of long-term medication administration, total parenteral nutrition, chemotherapy, blood product administration, and venous blood sampling; an arteriovenous fistula is an example.

implementation plan   A strategy for carrying out an intervention; includes goals, objectives, activities, evaluation measures, resource assessment, and time line.

implied consent   Assumption on behalf of a person unable to give consent that he or she would have done so.

impulse control disorder   A condition in which a person lacks the ability to resist a temptation or cannot stop acting on a drive.

in loco parentis   Phrase used to describe situations in which a designated authority figure makes medical treatment and transport decisions for a minor child when a parent is not available.

inactive metabolite   A medication that has undergone biotransformation and now is no longer able to alter a cell process or body function; not pharmacologically active.

inappropriate affect   Emotion that is out of synch with the situation (for example, wearing a waxy smile while discussing a parent's death).

inborn errors of metabolism (IEM)   A group of congenital conditions that cause either accumulation of toxins or disorders of energy metabolism in the neonate. These conditions are characterized by an infant's failure to thrive and by vague signs such as poor feeding.

incarcerated   A type of hernia in which an organ is trapped in the new location; most commonly obstructs the bowel.

incidence   The number of new cases of a disease in a population in a specified 1-year period.

incisional   A type of hernia in which intestinal contents herniate through an incision, for example after abdominal surgery.

incubation period   The period between exposure to an organism and the first symptoms of illness, during which the organism multiplies within the body and starts to produce symptoms. This period is when the disease can be transmitted to another person.

indication   A circumstance that points to or shows the cause, pathology, treatment, or issue of an attack of disease; that which points out; that which serves as a guide or warning.

indirect contact   Exposure or transmission of disease from one person to another by contact with a contaminated object.

infants   Persons who are from 1 month to 1 year of age.

infarction   Death (necrosis) of a localized area of tissue caused by the cutting off of its blood supply.

infection   The invasion of a host or host tissue by pathogenic organisms such as bacteria, viruses, or parasites that produces illness that may or may not have clinical manifestations.

infection control   Procedures to reduce transmission of infection among patients and health care personnel.

infectious disease   A disease that is caused by infection or one that is capable of being transmitted with or without direct contact.

infectious hepatitis   Another name for hepatitis A; an inflammation from a virus that causes mild fatigue, loss of appetite, fever, nausea, abdominal pain, and, eventually, jaundice, dark-colored urine, and whitish stools.

inferential   A research format that uses a hypothesis to prove one finding from another.

inferior   Below a body part or nearer to the feet.

inferior vena cava   One of the two largest veins in the body; carries blood from the lower extremities and the pelvic and the abdominal organs to the heart.

inferior wall MI   Death of myocardial tissue involving the lower (inferior) portion of the heart.

infiltration   The escape of fluid into the surrounding tissue; the result of vein perforation during IV cannulation.

inflammatory response   A reaction by tissues of the body to irritation or injury, characterized by pain, swelling, redness, and heat.

influenza   The flu, a respiratory infection caused by a variety of viruses; differs from the common cold in that the flu involves a fever, headache, and extreme exhaustion.

informed consent   A patient's voluntary agreement to be treated after being told about the nature of the disease, the risks and benefits of the proposed treatment, alternative treatments, or the choice of no treatment at all.

ingestion   Eating or drinking materials for absorption through the gastrointestinal tract.

inhalation   The active process of moving air into the lungs; also called inspiration. This is also a medication delivery route.

inhibin   Hormone that helps to regulate the menstrual cycle in females and may play a role in regulating sperm production in the male.

injection   In allergic reactions, when the skin is pierced, and foreign material is deposited into the skin.

innate (nonspecific) defense   One that protects the body from pathogens involving mechanical barriers, chemical barriers, natural killer cells, inflammation, phagocytosis, fever, or species resistance.

inner ear   One of three anatomic parts of the ear; it consists of the cochlea and semicircular canals.

inorganic   Not having both carbon and hydrogen atoms.

inotropic effect   The effect on the contractility of muscle tissue, especially cardiac muscle.

insertion   A moveable part of the body to which a skeletal muscle is fastened at a moveable joint; its action opposes that of an origin.

inspection   Looking at the patient, either in general or at a specific area (ie, a patient's overall appearance from the doorway, versus looking specifically at the chest wall for abnormalities/deformities).

inspiratory reserve volume   The amount of air that can be inhaled after a normal inhalation; the amount of air that can be inhaled in addition to the normal tidal volume.

institutional review board (IRB)   A group or institution that follows a set of requirements for review that were devised by the US Public Health Service.

insulin   Hormone produced by the pancreas that is vital to the control of the body's metabolism and blood glucose level. Insulin causes sugar, fatty acids, and amino acids to be taken up and metabolized by cells.

insulin resistance   Condition in which the pancreas produces enough insulin but the body cannot effectively use it.

intention tremor   A tremor that occurs when trying to accomplish a task.

intentional injuries   Injuries that are purposefully inflicted by a person on himself or herself or on another person; examples include suicide or attempted suicide, homicide, rape, assault, domestic abuse, elder abuse, and child abuse.

interatrial septum   A membrane that separates the right and left atria.

interference   One medication or chemical taken by a patient that undermines the effectiveness of another medication taken by or administered to a patient.

interferon   A protein produced by cells in response to viral invasion that is released into the bloodstream or intercellular fluid to induce healthy cells to manufacture an enzyme that counters the infection.

interleukins   Chemical substances that attract white blood cells to the sites of injury and bacterial invasion.

internal respiration   The exchange of gases between the blood cells and the tissues.

internal rotation   Rotating the anterior surface of an extremity toward the midline.

internal shunt   Also called an arteriovenous (AV) fistula, this device is an artificial connection between a vein and an artery, usually in the forearm or upper arm.

internodal pathways   The three pathways of the electrical conduction system found in the atria that transmit the impulse from the SA node to the AV node.

interpersonal communications   The exchange of information between two or more persons.

interstitial cells   The cells of Leydig; they lie in spaces between the seminiferous tubules, producing and secreting male sex hormones.

interstitial fluid The fluid located outside of the blood vessels in the spaces between the body's cells; accounts for about 10.5% of body weight and includes special fluid collections such as cerebrospinal fluid and intraocular fluid.

interstitial nephritis A chronic inflammation of the interstitial cells surrounding the nephrons.

interstitial space The space in between the cells.

interventions In the context of prevention, specific measures or activities designed to meet a program objective; categories include education/behavior change, enforcement/legislation, engineering/technology, and economic incentives.

interventricular septum A thick wall that separates the right and left ventricles.

intracellular fluid (ICF) Fluid within cells in which most of the body's supply of potassium is contained; accounts for 45% of body weight.

intradermal The layer of the dermis, just beneath the epidermis; a medication delivery route.

intramembranous ossification Process where bones develop from connective tissue membranes, are replaced by spongy bone, and then compact bone, to form flat bones.

intramuscular (IM) Into a muscle; a medication delivery route.

intranasal Within the nose.

intraosseous Within the bone.

intraosseous (IO) infusion A technique of administering fluids, blood and blood products, and medications into the intraosseous space of a long bone, usually the proximal tibia.

intraosseous (IO) space The spongy cancellous bone of the epiphyses and the medullary cavity of the diaphysis, collectively.

intrapulmonary shunting Bypassing of oxygen-poor blood past nonfunctional alveoli.

intrarenal acute renal failure (IARF) A type of acute renal failure characterized by damage in the kidney itself, often caused by immune-mediated diseases, prerenal ARF, toxins, heavy metals, some medications, or some organic compounds.

intravascular fluid (plasma) The noncellular portion of blood found within the blood vessels; accounts for about 4.5% of body weight; also called plasma.

intravenous Within a vein.

intravenous (IV) therapy Cannulation of a vein with an IV catheter to access the patient's vascular system.

intussusception Telescoping of the intestines into themselves.

involuntary consent An oxymoron, as consent is never involuntary; often used to describe a figure of authority dictating medical care be given to someone in custody, incapacitated, or a minor.

involuntary muscle The muscle over which a person has no conscious control. It is found in many automatic regulating systems of the body.

iodine An essential element in the diet and an important component of thyroxine. Without the proper level of iodine intake, thyroxine cannot be produced, and physical and mental growth are diminished.

ionic bond A chemical bond where oppositely charged ions attract each other.

ionic concentration The amount of charged particles found in a particular area.

ions Atoms that have become positively or negatively charged by giving up or acquiring an electron.

iris The muscle and surrounding tissue behind the cornea that dilate and constrict the pupil, regulating the amount of light that enters the eye; pigment in this tissue gives the eye its color.

iritis Inflammation of the iris; also called anterior uveitis.

iron deficiency anemia The most common type of anemia in which iron stores are low or lacking and the serum iron concentration is low.

irritable bowel syndrome (IBS) A condition in which patients have abdominal pain and changes in their bowel habits; generally the pain must be present for at least 3 days a month for at least 3 months to be considered this disease.

ischemia Tissue anoxia from diminished blood flow to tissue, usually caused by narrowing or occlusion of the artery.

ischemic One of the two main types of stroke, sometimes called an *occlusive stroke*; occurs when blood flow to a particular part of the brain is cut off by a blockage—that is, an occlusion, such as a blood clot—within an artery.

ischium One of three bones that fuse to form the pelvic ring.

islets of Langerhans A specialized group of cells in the pancreas where insulin and glucagon are produced.

isoelectric When referring to a wave, the wave is neither positive nor negative.

isoelectric line The baseline of the ECG.

isoimmunity The formation of antibodies or T cells that are directed against antigens or another person's cells.

isotonic Concentrations on either side of the membrane are equal.

isotonic crystalloids Intravenous solutions that do not cause a fluid shift into or out of the cell; examples include normal saline and lactated Ringer's solutions.

isotonic solution A solution that has the same concentration of sodium as does the cell. In this case, water does not shift, and no change in cell shape occurs.

isotope One of two (or more) forms of an element having the same number of protons and electrons, but different numbers of neutrons; they may or may not be radioactive.

Jacksonian march The wave-like movement of a seizure from a point of focus to other areas of the brain.

jaundice The presence of excessive bile pigments in the bloodstream that give the skin, mucous membranes, and eyes a distinct yellow color; often associated with liver disease.

jaw-thrust maneuver A technique to open the airway by placing the fingers behind the angle of the jaw and bringing the jaw forward; used when a patient may have a cervical spine injury.

joint (articulation) The place where two bones come into contact.

joint capsule The fibrous sac that encloses a joint.

jugular vein The two main veins that drain the head and neck.

jugular venous distention (JVD) The visible bulging of the jugular veins when a patient is in semi-Fowler's or full Fowler's position; indicates inadequate blood movement through the heart and/or lungs.

junctional rhythm A dysrhythmia arising from ectopic foci in the area of the atrioventricular junction; often shows an absence of the P wave, P-wave inversion, a short PR interval, or a P wave appearing after the QRS complex.

juxtaglomerular apparatus A structure formed at the site where the efferent arteriole and distal convoluted tubule meet; also called a juxtaglomerular complex.

ketamine hydrochloride A drug used to facilitate date rape but that is predominantly marketed in the United States as a veterinary anesthetic and is a phencyclidine hydrochloride derivative; street names include special K, vitamin K, cat Valium, and Fort Dodge.

ketoacidosis An acidotic state created by the production of ketones via fat metabolism.

ketones Acidic by-products of fat metabolism.

kidney stones Solid crystalline masses formed in the kidney, resulting from an excess of insoluble salts or uric acid crystallizing in the urine; may become trapped anywhere along the urinary tract.

kidneys Two retroperitoneal organs that excrete the end products of metabolism as urine and regulate the body's salt and water content.

killer T cells Cytotoxic T cells that attack and phagocytize antigens in order to halt their reproduction.

kilocalories Commonly known as calories, the amount of energy that can be obtained from the nutrients you eat.

King LT airway A single-lumen airway that is blindly inserted into the esophagus; when properly placed in the esophagus, one cuff seals the esophagus, and the other seals the oropharynx.

kinin system A general term for a group of polypeptides that mediate inflammatory responses by stimulating visceral smooth muscle and relaxing vascular smooth muscle to produce vasodilation.

Korotkoff sounds Sounds related to blood pressure measurement that are heard by stethoscope.

Kussmaul respirations A respiratory pattern characteristic of diabetic ketoacidosis, with marked hyperpnea and tachypnea.

kyphosis Outward curve of the thoracic spine.

labia majora Two prominent, rounded folds of skin lateral to the labia minora of the female external genitalia.

labia minora A pair of skin folds in the female external genitalia that border the vestibule.

labile Rapidly shifting among different emotional states.

labored breathing The use of muscles of the chest, back, and abdomen to assist in expanding the chest; occurs when air movement is impaired.

labyrinthitis Irritation and swelling in the inner ear that produces a loss of balance and possibly tinnitus, dizziness, loss of hearing, nausea, and vomiting.

lacrimal apparatus The structures in which tears are secreted and drained from the eye.

lacrimal glands The glands that produce fluids to keep the eye moist; also called tear glands.

lacrimal sac Depository for debris, bacteria, or other material that is swept from the surface of the eye.

lactated Ringer's (LR) solution A sterile isotonic crystalloid IV solution of specified amounts of calcium chloride, potassium chloride, sodium chloride, and sodium lactate in water.

lactic acid A metabolic end product of the breakdown of glucose that accumulates when metabolism proceeds in the absence of oxygen.

lactic acidosis Anaerobic cellular respiration due to hypoperfusion of tissues and organs.

landline Communications system linked by wires, usually in reference to a conventional telephone system.

lantana A perennial flowering shrub with clusters of red berries that can lead to serious and even fatal poisoning. Also known as red sage or wild sage; ingestion causes stomach upsets, muscle weakness, shock, and, sometimes, death.

large intestine The portion of the digestive tube that encircles the abdomen around the small bowel, consisting of the cecum, the colon, and the rectum; it helps regulate water balance and eliminate solid waste.

laryngeal mask airway (LMA) A device that surrounds the opening of the larynx with an inflatable silicone cuff positioned in the hypopharynx; an alternative device to bag-mask ventilation.

laryngectomy A surgical procedure in which the larynx is removed.

laryngitis Swelling and inflammation of the larynx that is associated with hoarseness or loss of voice.

laryngoscope A device that is used in conjunction with a laryngoscope blade to perform direct laryngoscopy.

laryngospasm Spasmodic closure of the vocal cords.

laryngotracheobronchitis Inflammation of the larynx, trachea, and bronchi.

larynx A complete structure formed by the epiglottis, thyroid cartilage, cricoid cartilage, arytenoid cartilage, corniculate cartilage, and cuneiform cartilage; the voice box.

late adults Persons who are 61 years old or older.

lateral In anatomy, parts of the body that lie farther from the midline; also called outer structures.

lateral malleolus An enlargement of the distal end of the fibula, which forms the lateral wall of the ankle joint.

leads The electrical cable attaching the electrode to the ECG monitor; the voltage difference between two points. For example, lead I is the voltage difference between the right and left arm electrodes.

left anterior descending (LAD) artery One of the two branches of the left main coronary artery that is the largest and shortest of the myocardial blood vessels; this vessel and the circumflex coronary arteries supply blood to the left ventricle and other areas.

left atrial enlargement Dilation of the left atrium that results either from systemic hypertension, mitral or aortic valve stenosis, or an athletic heart.

left atrium The upper left chamber of the heart; receives blood from the pulmonary veins.

left ventricle The thick-walled, muscular, lower left chamber of the heart; receives blood from the left atrium and pumps it out through the aorta into the systemic arteries.

left ventricular hypertrophy (LVH) A cardiac condition in which the left ventricle becomes enlarged, most commonly due to hypertension.

left-sided heart failure A condition in which the left ventricle cannot effectively pump; this leads to a backup of blood behind the left ventricle, and eventually serum is forced out of the pulmonary capillaries and into the alveoli.

lens The transparent part of the eye through which images are focused on the retina.

lesser trochanter The projection on the medial/superior portion of the femur.

leukemia Cancer or malignancy of the blood-forming organs, particularly affecting the WBCs that develop abnormally and/or excessively at the expense of normal blood cells.

leukocytes White blood cells.

leukocytosis Elevation of the white blood cell count, often due to inflammation.

leukopenia A reduction in the number of WBCs.

leukotrienes Arachidonic acid metabolites that function as chemical mediators of inflammation; also known as slow-reacting substances of anaphylaxis.

liability A finding in civil cases that the preponderance of the evidence shows the defendant was responsible for the plaintiff's injuries.

libel Making a false statement in written form that injures a person's good name.

lice Tiny, wingless, parasitic insects that feed on blood; an infestation is easily spread through close personal contact; types include head, body, and pubic lice.

licensure The process whereby a state allows qualified people to perform a regulated act.

licit In relation to drugs, legalized drugs such as coffee, alcohol, and tobacco.

life expectancy The average amount of years a person can be expected to live.

lift A sensation felt upon palpation of the chest wall, in which the heart beats extremely strongly; suggests hypertrophy; also called a heave.

ligament A band of fibrous tissue that connects bones to bones. It supports and strengthens a joint.

ligands Any molecules that bind to a receptor to form a more complex structure.

limb leads The ECG leads attached to the limbs and that form the hexaxial system, along the frontal plane.

limbic system Structures within the cerebrum and diencephalon that influence emotions, motivation, mood, and sensations of pain and pleasure.

limited data set   Information necessary for public health and research such as some geographic information, birth dates, and dates of treatment.

lipids   Fats, fat-like substances (cholesterol and phospholipids), and oils that supply energy for body processes and building of certain structures.

lipolysis   The metabolism (breakdown or destruction) of stored fat that has been released into the circulation.

lipophilic   Attracted to fats and lipids.

literature review   A form of research in which the existing literature is reviewed, and the researcher analyzes the collection of research to draw a conclusion.

lithium   The cornerstone drug for the treatment of bipolar disorder.

liver   A large solid organ that lies in the right upper quadrant immediately below the diaphragm; it produces bile, stores glucose for immediate use by the body, and produces many substances that help regulate immune responses.

living will   A type of advance directive, generally requiring a precondition for withholding resuscitation when the patient is incapacitated.

local reactions   Reactions that occur in a localized area; a potential complication of IV therapy.

long QT syndrome   A condition characterized by a QT interval exceeding approximately 450 ms.

longitudinal design   A data collection method in which information is collected at various set time intervals, and not just at one time.

longitudinal section   The view of an object cut along its long axis.

loop of Henle   The U-shaped portion of the renal tubule that extends from the proximal to the distal convoluted tubule; concentrates the filtrate and converts it to urine.

loose connective tissue   Adipose, areolar, and reticular connective tissue.

loosening of associations   A situation in which the logical connection between one idea and the next becomes obscure, at least to the listener.

lordosis   Inward curve of the lumbar spine just above the buttocks. An exaggerated form of lordosis results in the condition known as swayback.

Lown-Ganong-Levine syndrome   A disorder that causes preexcitation of ventricular tissue and which is characterized on the ECG by a short PR interval and a normal QRS duration.

Ludwig angina   A type of cellulitis that occurs on the floor of the mouth under the tongue; caused by bacteria from an infected tooth root (tooth abscess) or mouth injury.

lumbar spine   The lower part of the back, formed by the lowest five non-fused vertebrae; also called the dorsal spine.

lumen   The inside of an artery or other hollow structure.

lung compliance   The ability of the alveoli to expand when air is drawn into the lungs during negative-pressure ventilation or positive-pressure ventilation.

lungs   The two primary organs of breathing.

luteinizing hormone (LH)   Hormone that regulates the production of both eggs and sperm, as well as production of reproductive hormones.

Lyme disease   A tick-borne disease that primarily affects the skin, heart, joints, and nervous system and is characterized by a round, red lesion or bull's-eye rash.

lymph   A thin, plasma-like liquid formed from interstitial or extracellular fluid that bathes the tissues of the body.

lymph nodes   Round or bean-shaped structures interspersed along the course of the lymph vessels, which filter the lymph and serve as a source of lymphocytes.

lymph vessels   Thin-walled vessels through which lymph circulates through the body; they travel close to the major veins.

lymphatic system   A network of capillaries, vessels, ducts, nodes, and organs that helps to maintain the fluid environment of the body by producing lymph and transporting it through the body.

lymphoblasts   Lymphocytes transformed because of stimulation by an antigen.

lymphocytes   The white blood cells responsible for a large part of the body's immune protection.

lymphoid system   The system primarily made up of the bone marrow, lymph nodes, and spleen that participates in formation of lymphocytes and immune responses.

lymphokines   Cytokines released by lymphocytes, including many of the interleukins, gamma interferon, tumor necrosis factor beta, and chemokines.

lymphomas   Malignant diseases that arise within the lymphoid system; includes non-Hodgkin and Hodgkin lymphomas.

lysis   The process of disintegration or breakdown of cells that occurs when excess water enters the cell through osmosis.

macrodrip sets   Administration sets named for the large orifice between the piercing spike and the drip chamber; allow for rapid fluid flow into the vascular system; allow 10 or 15 gtt/mL, depending on the manufacturer.

macrophages   Cells that develop from the monocytes that provide the body's first line of defense in the inflammatory process.

macula   Also known as the macula lutea; a yellowish depression in the retina where acute vision arises.

Magill forceps   A special type of forceps that is curved, thus allowing paramedics to maneuver it in the airway.

mainstem bronchi   The part of the lower airway below the larynx through which air enters the lungs.

malfeasance   Unauthorized act committed outside the scope of medical practice defined by law.

Mallampati classification   A system for predicting the relative difficulty of intubation based on the amount of oropharyngeal structures visible in an upright, seated patient who is fully able to open his or her mouth.

Mallory-Weiss syndrome   A condition in which the junction between the esophagus and the stomach tears, causing severe bleeding and, potentially, death.

malrotation   Incorrect rotation of the intestines, for example as a result of a congenital anomaly such as gastroschisis; can result in intestinal obstruction.

mandible   The bone of the lower jaw.

mania   A mental disorder characterized by abnormally exaggerated happiness, joy, or euphoria with hyperactivity, insomnia, and grandiose ideas.

manic-depressive illness   A bipolar disorder in which mood fluctuates between depression and mania. The alterations in mood are usually episodic and recurrent.

manual defibrillation   A mode available on automated external defibrillators, allowing the paramedic to interpret the cardiac rhythm and determine if defibrillation is needed (rather than the monitor making the determination).

manubrium   The upper quarter of the sternum.

margination   The loss of fluid from the blood vessels into the tissue, causing the blood left in the vessels to have increased viscosity, which in turn slows the flow of blood and produces stasis.

marijuana   The dried leaves and flower buds of the *Cannabis sativa* plant that are smoked to achieve a high.

mast cells   The cells that resemble basophils but do not circulate in the blood; have a role in allergic reactions, immunity, and wound healing.

mastication   The process of chewing with the teeth.

mastoid process   A prominent bony mass at the base of the skull behind the ear.

matrix   A combination of connective tissue, blood vessels, and minerals that compose bone.

matter   Liquids, gases, and solids both inside and outside of the human body; it takes up space and has weight.

maxillae   The upper jawbones that assist in the formation of the orbit, the nasal cavity, and the palate and hold the upper teeth.

measles   An infectious viral disease that occurs most often in late winter and spring; begins with a fever followed by a cough, running nose, and pink eye; a rash spreads from the face and neck down the back and trunk.

mechanism of action   The way in which a medication produces the intended response.

mechanism of injury (MOI)   The series of events that result in traumatic injuries; the forces that act on the body to cause damage.

medial   Parts of the body that lie closer to the midline; also called inner structures.

medial malleolus   The distal end of the tibia, which forms the medial side of the ankle joint.

median effective dose (ED$_{50}$)   The weight-based dose of a medication that was effective in 50% of the humans and animals tested.

median lethal dose (LD$_{50}$)   The weight-based dose of a medication that caused death in 50% of the animals tested.

median toxic dose (TD$_{50}$)   The weight-based dose of a medication that demonstrated toxicity in 50% of the animals tested.

mediastinum   The space between the lungs, in the center of the chest, that contains the heart, trachea, mainstem bronchi, part of the esophagus, and large blood vessels.

medical ambiguity   Vague or unclear aspects of medicine.

medical asepsis   A term applied to the practice of preventing contamination of the patient by using aseptic technique.

medical direction   Direction given to an EMS service or provider by a physician.

medical necessity   A standard used by Medicare to determine whether a patient's condition requires ambulance transport in a particular situation.

Medical Practice Act   An act that usually defines the minimum qualifications of those who may perform various health services, defines the skills that each type of practitioner is legally permitted to use, and establishes a means of licensure or certification for different categories of health care professionals.

medication monograph   A document that gives detailed information about drugs, such as the indications and uses, dosing information, precautions, contraindications, and adverse effects.

medication noncompliance   A situation in which a patient chooses not to stay on his or her prescribed medications, for reasons that may include undesirable side effects or prohibitive cost.

medication sensitivity   A mild to severe reaction after the first exposure to a medication or other substance, often with many of the same signs and symptoms as an immune-mediated reaction.

medulla   Part of the internal anatomy of the kidney; the middle layer.

medulla oblongata   Nerve tissue that is continuous inferiorly with the spinal cord; serves as a conduction pathway for ascending and descending nerve tracts; coordinates heart rate, blood vessel diameter, breathing, swallowing, vomiting, coughing, and sneezing.

medullary cavity   An internal cavity that contains bone marrow.

meiosis   A type of cell division that includes first and second divisions.

melena   Dark, tarry, malodorous stools caused by upper GI bleeding.

membrane attack complex   Molecules that insert themselves into the bacterial membrane, leading to weakened areas in the membrane.

membranous labyrinth   A collection of passageways and reservoirs within the bony labyrinth of the inner ear.

menarche   The beginning phase of a woman's life cycle of menstruation.

Meniere disease   An inner ear disorder in which endolymphatic rupture creates increased pressure in the cochlear duct, which then leads to damage to the organ of Corti and the semicircular canal; symptoms include severe vertigo, tinnitus, and sensorineuronal hearing loss.

meninges   A set of three tough membranes, the dura mater, arachnoid, and pia mater, that enclose the entire brain and spinal cord.

meningitis   An inflammation of the meningeal coverings of the brain and spinal cord; usually caused by a virus or bacterium; the viral type is less severe than the bacterial; the bacterial type can result in brain damage, hearing loss, learning disability, or death.

meningococcal meningitis   A type of meningitis caused by the meningococcal bacterium, *Neisseria meningitidis*.

menopause   The ending phase of a woman's life cycle of menstruation.

menstrual cycle   The entire monthly cycle of menstruation from start to finish.

menstruation   Monthly flow of blood.

mental status examination (MSE)   A way of measuring the "mental vital signs" in a disturbed patient. The mnemonic COASTMAP can be used to conduct this exam, assessing consciousness, orientation, activity, speech, thought, memory, affect and mood, and perception.

mesenteric ischemia   An interruption of the blood supply to the mesentery.

metabolic   Pertaining to the breakdown of ingested foodstuffs into smaller and smaller molecules and atoms that are used as energy sources for cellular function.

metabolic acidosis   A pathologic condition characterized by a blood pH of less than 7.35, and caused by accumulation of acids in the body from a metabolic cause.

metabolic alkalosis   A pathologic condition characterized by a blood pH of greater than 7.45 and caused by an accumulation of bases in the body from a metabolic cause.

metabolism   The chemical processes that provide the cells with energy from nutrients.

metacarpals   The bones of the palms of the hand.

metaplasia   A reversible, cellular adaptation in which one adult cell type is replaced by another adult cell type.

metastasis   The process by which cells from a malignant neoplasm break away from their site of origin, such as the lung, and move through the bloodstream or lymphatic system to other body sites, such as the brain.

metatarsals   The bones of the soles of the feet; they form the foot arches.

metered-dose inhaler (MDI)   A pressurized canister that delivers a specific dose of a medication; commonly used for beta-agonist bronchodilators.

methamphetamine   A highly addictive drug in the amphetamine family.

methemoglobin (metHb)   A compound formed by oxidation of the iron on hemoglobin.

metric system   A decimal system based on tens for the measurement of length, weight, and volume.

metrorrhagia   Irregular but frequent vaginal bleeding.

microangiopathy   Microscopic deterioration of vessel walls caused primarily by adherence of blood lipids to vessel walls.

microdrip sets   Administration sets named for the small needlelike orifice between the piercing spike and the drip chamber; allow for carefully controlled fluid flow and are ideally suited for medication administration; allow for 60 gtt/mL.

microglial cells   Neuroglia found throughout the central nervous system.

micturition reflex   A spinal reflex that causes contraction of the bladder's smooth muscle, producing the urge to void as pressure is exerted on the internal urinary sphincter.

midbrain   The part of the brain that is responsible for helping to regulate the level of consciousness.

middle adults   Persons who are 41 to 60 years of age.

middle ear   One of three anatomic parts of the ear; it consists of the inner portion of the tympanic membrane and the ossicles.

midsagittal plane (midline)   An imaginary vertical line drawn from the middle of the forehead through the nose and the umbilicus (navel) to the floor.

milliequivalent (mEq)   Unit of measure for electrolytes.

minerals   Inorganic elements essential for human metabolism.

minimum data set   The mandatory clinical assessment standard information that must be documented on every emergency call as set by Medicare and Medicaid, and per the National Highway Traffic Safety Administration (NHTSA) for the purpose of the national data system.

minute volume (VM)   The amount of air that moves in and out of the lungs per minute minus the dead space; also called minute ventilation.

misfeasance   Appropriate act performed in an improper manner, such as a medication administered at the wrong dose.

mitochondria   The metabolic center or powerhouse of the cell; small and rod-shaped organelles.

mitosis   The division of chromosomes in a cell nucleus.

mitral valve   The valve in the heart that separates the left atrium from the left ventricle.

mixed acidosis   A pathologic condition in which there is a low pH, an elevated P_{CO_2} level, and low bicarbonate level, and which occurs when there is both a respiratory and metabolic cause present at the same time.

mixed alkalosis   A pathologic condition in which there is an elevated pH, a low P_{CO_2} level, and an elevated bicarbonate level, which occurs when there is both a respiratory and metabolic cause present at the same time.

Mix-o-Vial   A single vial divided into two compartments by a rubber stopper; methylprednisolone sodium succinate (Solu-Medrol) is stored this way.

mobile intensive care units (MICUs)   An early title given to an ambulance-style unit.

molecule   Particles made up of two or more joined atoms.

monoamine oxidase inhibitors (MAOIs)   Psychiatric medication used primarily to treat atypical depression by increasing norepinephrine and serotonin levels in the central nervous system.

monocytes   Mononuclear phagocytic white blood cells derived from myeloid stem cells that circulate in the bloodstream for about 24 hours and then move into tissues to mature into macrophages.

monomorphic   Having one common shape.

mononuclear phagocytic system   Phagocytic cells that remove foreign particles from the lymph and blood.

mononucleosis   Infectious mononucleosis or mono (glandular fever); caused by the Epstein-Barr virus, is often called the kissing disease; also spread by coughing or sneezing.

monophonic   The sound of one note during wheezing, caused by the vibration of a single bronchus.

monosaccharides   The most simple carbohydrate molecule.

monovalent   An ion that contains one charge.

mons pubis   A rounded pad of fatty tissue that overlies the symphysis pubis and is anterior to the urethral and vaginal openings.

mood disorder   A group of disorders in which the disturbance of mood is accompanied by full or partial manic or depressive syndrome.

morality   Pertaining to conscience, conduct, and character.

morbid obesity   An excessively unhealthy accumulation of body fat, defined as a body mass index of greater than or equal to 40 kg/m².

morbidity   Number of nonfatally injured or disabled people; usually expressed as a rate, meaning the number of nonfatal injuries in a certain population in a given time period divided by the size of the population.

moro reflex   An infant reflex in which, when an infant is caught off guard, the infant opens his or her arms wide, spreads the fingers, and seems to grab at things.

mortality   Deaths caused by injury and disease; usually expressed as a rate, meaning the number of deaths in a certain population in a given time period divided by the size of the population.

motor end plate   The flattened end of a motor neuron that transmits neural impulses to a muscle.

motor nerves   Nerves that carry information from the CNS to the muscles of the body.

motor neurons   Nerve cells that transmit instructions from the CNS to the end organs; also known as efferent neurons.

motor pathways   In the peripheral nervous system, common routes by which motor nerve impulses are transmitted.

motor unit   A motor neuron and the muscle fibers that it controls.

mottling   A blotchy pattern on the skin; a typical finding in states of severe protracted hypoperfusion and shock.

mucosa-associated lymphoid tissue   The lymphoid tissue associated with the skin and the respiratory, urinary, and reproductive traits as well as the tonsils.

mucosal atomizer device (MAD)   A device that attaches to the end of a syringe that is used to spray (atomize) certain medications via the intra-nasal route.

mucous membranes   The lining of body cavities and passages that communicate directly or indirectly with the environment outside the body.

mucus   The opaque, sticky secretion of the mucous membranes that lubricates the body openings.

multifocal   Arising from or pertaining to many foci or locations.

multilumen airways   Airway devices with a single long tube that can be used for esophageal obturation or endotracheal tube ventilation, depending on where the device comes to rest following blind positioning.

multiple myeloma   A disease in which the number of plasma cells in the bone marrow increases abnormally, causing tumors to form in the bones.

multiple organ dysfunction syndrome (MODS)   A grave but sometimes reversible condition in an acutely ill patient characterized by the progressive dysfunction of two or more organs or organ systems not affected by the patient's initial illness or injury.

multiple sclerosis (MS)   An autoimmune condition in which the body attacks the myelin that insulates the brain and spinal cord, causing scarring.

multiplex   Method by which simultaneous transmission of voice and ECG signals can be achieved over a single radio frequency.

mumps   A viral infection that primarily affects the parotid glands, which are one of the three pairs of salivary glands, causing swelling in front of the ears.

murmur   An abnormal "whoosh"-like sound heard over the heart that indicates turbulent blood flow around a cardiac valve.

Murphy sign   Pressure applied to the right upper quadrant of the abdomen to help detect gallbladder problems.

Murphy's eye   An opening on the side of an endotracheal tube at its distal tip that permits ventilation to occur even if the tip becomes occluded by blood, mucus, or the tracheal wall.

muscle impulse   One that passes in many directions over a muscle fiber membrane after stimulation by acetylcholine.

muscle tissues   Contractile tissue consisting of filaments of actin and myosin, which slide past each other, shortening cells.

musculoskeletal system   The bones and voluntary muscles of the body.

mutation   A change in the sequence of a cell's DNA that damages the cell's structure or impedes its ability to function.

mutism   The absence of speech.

myasthenia gravis   A condition in which the body generates antibodies against its own acetylcholine receptors, causing muscle weakness, often in the face.

myelin   An insulating sheath that envelops certain types of neurons, allowing the cells to transmit electricity along their axons without dissipation of the signal as it moves through surrounding fluids and tissues.

myocardial infarction   Blockage of the arteries that supply oxygen to the heart, resulting in death to a portion of the myocardium.

myocarditis Inflammation of the myocardium.

myocardium The cardiac muscle.

myoclonus Jerking motions of the body.

myoglobin A pigment synthesized in the muscles to give skeletal muscles their reddish-brown color.

myometrium The thick muscular middle layer of the uterine wall.

myopia Nearsighted; the ability to see objects close with difficulty seeing objects far away.

myxedema Hypothyroidism; lowered levels of thyroid hormones.

myxedema coma A rare condition that can occur in patients who have severe, untreated hypothyroidism.

narcotic The generic term for opiates and opioids, drugs that act as a CNS depressant and produce insensibility or stupor.

nasal cannula A device that delivers oxygen via two small prongs that fit into the patient's nostrils; with an oxygen flow rate of 1 to 6 L/min, an oxygen concentration of 24% to 44% can be delivered.

nasal cavity The chamber inside the nose that lies between the floor of the cranium and the roof of the mouth.

nasal septum The rigid partition composed of bone and cartilage that separates the right and left nostrils.

nasogastric (NG) tube A gastric tube is inserted into the stomach through the nose.

nasolacrimal duct The passage through which tears drain from the lacrimal sacs into the nasal cavity.

nasopharyngeal (nasal) airway A soft rubber tube about 6″ long that is inserted through the nose into the posterior pharynx behind the tongue, thereby allowing passage of air from the nose to the lower airway.

nasopharynx The nasal cavity (portion of the pharynx that lies above the level of the roof of the mouth); formed by the union of the facial bones.

nasotracheal intubation Insertion of an endotracheal tube into the trachea through the nose.

natural immunity The immunity the body develops as part of being exposed to an antigen and developing antibodies—for example, exposure to measles, having the measles, and developing immunity to the measles.

nature of illness (NOI) The general type of illness a patient is experiencing.

nebulizer A device for producing a fine spray or mist that is used to deliver inhaled medications.

necrosis The death of tissue, usually caused by a cessation of the blood supply.

needle cricothyrotomy Insertion of a 14- to 16-gauge over-the-needle IV catheter (such as an Angiocath) through the cricothyroid membrane and into the trachea.

needleless systems Devices that do not use needles for the collection of body fluids or withdrawal of body fluids after initial venous or arterial access is established, the administration of medication or fluids, or any other procedure involving the potential for occupational exposure to bloodborne pathogens by percutaneous injuries from contaminated sharps.

negative feedback The concept that once the desired effect of a process has been achieved, further action is inhibited until it is needed again; also called feedback inhibition.

negative-pressure ventilation Drawing of air into the lungs; airflow from a region of higher pressure (outside the body) to a region of lower pressure (the lungs); occurs during normal (unassisted breathing).

negligence Professional action or inaction on the part of the health care worker that does not meet the standard of ordinary care expected of similarly trained and prudent health care practitioners and that results in injury to the patient.

negligence per se Inexcusable violation of a statute, such as practicing without a valid license or certification.

neologism An invented word that has meaning only to its inventor.

neoplasm A tumor.

neoplastic cells Another term for cancerous cells.

nephrons The structural and functional units of the kidney that form urine; composed of the glomerulus, the glomerular (Bowman's) capsule, the proximal convoluted tubule, the loop of Henle, and the distal convoluted tubule.

nerve fibers Groups of nerve cells bundled together to form nerves.

nerve impulse Electrochemical changes transmitted by neurons to other neurons and to cells outside the nervous system.

nerve plexus Nerves that exit the spinal cord and follow similar tracts through the body.

nervous system The system that controls virtually all activities of the body, both voluntary and involuntary.

nervous tissues Neurons and neuroglia.

net filtration pressure Usually a positive pressure, it forces substances out of the glomerulus.

neurogenic shock A type of shock that usually results from spinal cord injury; loss of normal sympathetic nervous system tone and vasodilation occur.

neuroglia Supporting cells that provide a supporting skeleton for neural tissue, isolate and protect the cell membranes of neurons, regulate the composition of interstitial fluid, defend neural tissue from pathogens, and aid in the repair of injury.

neuroglial cells The supporting tissue cells of the nervous system that provide insulation, physical support, and nutrients to neurons.

neuromuscular junction The connection between a motor neuron and a muscle fiber.

neurons The basic nerve cells of the nervous system, containing a nucleus within a cell body and extending one or more processes; they exist in masses to form nervous tissue.

neuropathy Damage to nerve endings causing a wide range of symptoms including weakness, tremors, mild pain or "pins and needles," to such hypersensitivity that some parts of the body cannot be touched; also referred to as peripheral neuropathy.

neurotic disorders A collection of psychiatric disorders without psychotic symptoms and lacking the intense psychopathology of other mood disorders; includes anxiety disorders, phobias, and panic disorder.

neurotransmitter A chemical produced by the body that stimulates electrical reactions in adjacent neurons.

neutrons Uncharged or "neutral" particles in the nucleus of an atom.

neutrophils One of the three types of granulocytes; they have multi-lobed nuclei that resemble a string of baseballs held together by a thin strand of thread; they destroy bacteria, antigen-antibody complexes, and foreign matter.

nodes of Ranvier Narrow gaps between Schwann cells.

noise In radio communications, interference in a radio signal.

noncompetitive antagonists Medications that permanently bind with receptor sites and prevent activation by agonist chemicals.

nondepolarizing A term used to describe drugs that produce muscle relaxation by interfering with impulses between the nerve ending and muscle receptor.

nondepolarizing neuromuscular blockers Drugs that bind to acetylcholine receptor sites; they do not cause depolarization of the muscle fiber; examples are vecuronium (Norcuron) and pancuronium (Pavulon).

nonelectrolytes Solutes that have no electrical charge; include glucose and urea; measured in milligrams (mg).

nonfeasance Failing to perform a required or expected act.

nonionic Uncharged.

nonrebreathing mask A combination mask and reservoir bag system in which oxygen fills a reservoir bag attached to the mask by a one-way valve permitting a patient to inhale from the reservoir bag but not to exhale into it; at a flow rate of 15 L/min, it can deliver 90% to 100% inspired oxygen.

non-tunneling devices   Devices that have been inserted by direct venipuncture through the skin directly into a selected vein, for the purpose of long-term medication administration, total parenteral nutrition, chemotherapy, and venous blood sampling; peripheral inserted central catheters and central venous catheters are examples.

norepinephrine   A neurotransmitter and drug sometimes used in the treatment of shock; produces vasoconstriction through its alpha-stimulator properties.

normal saline   A solution of 0.9% sodium chloride; an isotonic crystalloid.

normal sinus rhythm   The normal rhythm of the heart, wherein the excitation impulse arises in the SA node, travels through the internodal pathways to the atrioventricular junction, down the bundle of His, through the bundle branches, and into the Purkinje network without interference.

nosocomial infection   An infection acquired from a health care setting.

nucleic acids   Large organic molecules, or macromolecules, that carry genetic information or form structures within cells, and include DNA and RNA.

nucleus   In the context of the cell, a cellular organelle that contains the genetic information; controls the function and structure of a cell. In the context of an atom, the central portion of an atom that contains protons and neutrons.

nutrients   Carbohydrates, lipids, proteins, vitamins, minerals, and water.

nystagmus   The rhythmic shaking of the eyes.

obesity   An unhealthy accumulation of body fat, defined as a body mass index of greater than or equal to 30 kg/m².

objective information   Information that you observe and that is measurable, such as a patient's blood pressure.

obstructive shock   The type of shock that occurs when blood flow to the heart or great vessels is obstructed.

occlusion   Blockage, usually of a tubular structure such as a blood vessel or IV catheter.

ocular   Pertaining to the eye.

oculomotor nerve   The third cranial nerve; innervates the muscles that cause motion of the eyeballs and upper eyelid.

off-line medical control   Medical direction given through a set of protocols, policies, and/or standards.

olfactory bulb   The cranial nerve for smell.

olfactory cells   Cells in the superior nasopharynx that respond to smell.

oligodendrocytes   Neuroglia found aligned along nerve fibers.

oligosaccharide   A simple sugar composed of 2 to 10 monosaccharides.

oliguria   Urine output of less than 500 mL/day.

oncotic pressure   The pressure of water to move, typically into the capillary, as the result of the presence of plasma proteins.

online (direct) medical control   Medical direction given in real time to an EMS service or provider.

onset   The time needed for the concentration of the medication at the target tissue to reach the minimum effective level.

oocyte   The precursor to a mature egg, formed in the ovaries.

oogenesis   The process of egg cell formation, which begins at puberty.

open cricothyrotomy   An emergency incision of the cricothyroid membrane with a scalpel and insertion of an endotracheal or a tracheostomy tube directly into the subglottic area of the trachea; also called surgical cricothyrotomy.

open-ended question   A question that does not have a yes or no answer, and that does not give the patient specific options from which to choose.

opening snap   A heart sound indicative of a noncompliant valve.

ophthalmoscope   An instrument used to look into a patient's eyes and view the retina and aqueous fluid; consists of a concave mirror and a battery-powered light that is usually contained in the handle.

opiate   Various alkaloids derived from the opium or poppy plant.

opioid   A synthetic narcotic not derived from opium, with sedative properties; examples are fentanyl (Sublimaze) and alfentanil (Alfenta); also called narcotics.

opportunistic infections   The infections in which an organism thrives when the immune system has been compromised by illness, chemotherapeutic medications, or antirejection drugs in an organ transplant recipient. These fungi, bacteria, viruses, and parasites are normally held in check by a healthy immune system.

opsonization   The process by which an antibody coats an antigen to facilitate its recognition by immune cells.

optic chiasm   Location where approximately half of the nerve fibers from each eye cross over to the opposite side of the brain.

optic disk   Area of the retina where nerve fibers (axons) exit to become part of the optic nerve.

optic nerve   Either of the second cranial nerves that enter the eyeball posteriorly, through the optic foramen.

oral candidiasis   A condition that presents as white lesions on the tongue and inner cheeks, caused by the fungus *Candida albicans*; also called thrush.

orbit   The eye socket, made up of the maxilla and zygoma.

orbital cellulitis   An infection within the eye socket.

orchitis   A complication of a male urinary tract infection in which one or both testes become infected, enlarged, and tender, causing pain and swelling in the scrotum.

ordinary negligence   Negligence that is a failure to act, or a simple mistake that causes harm to a patient.

organ of Corti   The organ that is the primary receptor for sound, and is made up of thousands of individual cilia, each with their own associated nerve.

organelles   The internal cellular structures that carry out specific functions for the cell.

organic   Having both carbon and hydrogen atoms.

organic brain syndrome   Temporary or permanent dysfunction of the brain, caused by a disturbance in the physical or physiologic functioning of brain tissue.

organophosphates   A class of chemical found in many insecticides used in agriculture and in the home.

orgasm   Physiologic and psychological release that is the culmination of sexual stimulation; accompanied by emission and ejaculation—in females there is a lesser expulsion of fluid.

origin   A relatively immovable part of the body where a skeletal muscle is fastened at a moveable joint; its action opposes that of an insertion.

orogastric (OG) tube   A gastric tube inserted into the stomach through the mouth.

oropharyngeal (oral) airway   A hard plastic device that is curved so that it fits over the back of the tongue with the tip in the posterior pharynx.

oropharynx   A tubular structure that forms the posterior portion of the oral cavity, extending vertically from the back of the mouth to the esophagus and trachea.

orotracheal intubation   Insertion of an endotracheal tube into the trachea through the mouth.

orthopnea   Severe dyspnea experienced when recumbent and relieved by sitting or standing up.

orthostatic hypotension   A fall in blood pressure when changing to an erect position.

orthostatic vital signs   Assessing vital signs in two different patient positions (for example, from a lying to a sitting position) to determine the degree of hypovolemia; also called a tilt test.

osmolarity   The concentration of osmotically active particles in solution expressed as osmoles of solute per liter of solution.

osmosis The movement of a solvent, such as water, from an area of low solute concentration to one of high concentration through a selectively permeable membrane to equalize concentrations of a solute on both sides of the membrane.

osmotic Characterized by the movement of a solvent, such as water, across a semipermeable membrane (for example, the cell wall) from an area of lower to higher concentration of solute molecules.

osmotic pressure The tendency of water to move by osmosis across a membrane.

ossicles The three small bones in the inner ear that transmit vibrations to the cochlear duct at the oval window.

ossification The formation of bone by osteoblasts.

osteoblasts Cells involved in the formation of bony tissue.

osteocytes Mature bone cells.

osteogenesis imperfecta A congenital bone disease that results in fragile bones.

osteomyelitis Inflammation of the bone and muscle caused by infection.

other potentially infectious materials (OPIM) Cerebrospinal fluid (CSF), pericardial fluid, amniotic fluid, synovial fluid, peritoneal fluid, and any fluid containing visible blood.

otitis An infection of either the outer or middle ear cavity.

otoliths A pair of fluid-filled sacs within the inner ear that are used by the CNS to collect information about movement and orientation in space.

otoscope A tool used to examine the ears of a patient; consists of a head and a handle. The head contains an electric light source and a low-power magnifying lens.

outcome (impact) objectives State the intended effect of the program on participants or on the community in such terms as the participants' increased knowledge, changed behaviors or attitudes, or decreased injury rates.

oval window An oval opening between the middle ear and the vestibule.

ovarian cyst A fluid-filled sac that forms on or within an ovary.

ovarian torsion A painful condition in which the ovary becomes twisted.

ovary A female gland that produces sex hormones and ova (eggs).

overhydration An increase in the body's systemic fluid volume.

overt behavior Behavior that is open and generally understood by those around the person.

over-the-needle catheter A Teflon (plastic) catheter inserted over a hollow needle.

overweight An unhealthy accumulation of body fat, defined as a body mass index of 25 to 29.9 kg/m^2.

ovulation The development of a secondary oocyte and first polar body via oogenesis of the primary oocyte.

oxidation The process by which oxygen combines with another chemical, is involved in the removal of hydrogen, or loses electrons.

oxygen debt The amount of oxygen that liver cells need to convert lactic acid into glucose, as well as the amount needed by muscle cells to restore ATP and creatine phosphate levels.

oxygen humidifier A small bottle of water through which the oxygen leaving the cylinder is moisturized before it reaches the patient.

oxygenation The process of adding oxygen, such as for delivery to the cells.

oxyhemoglobin (Hbo$_2$) Hemoglobin that is occupied by oxygen.

P wave The first wave of the ECG complex, representing depolarization of the ventricles.

pacemaker The specialized tissue within the heart that initiates excitation impulses; an electronic device used to stimulate cardiac contraction when the electric conduction system of the heart is malfunctioning, especially in complete heart block; consists of a battery-powered pulse generator and a wire that transmits the electric impulse to the ventricles.

palate The structure that forms the roof of the mouth and separates the oropharynx and nasopharynx.

palatine tonsils One of three sets of lymphatic organs that constitute the tonsils; located in the back of the throat, on each side of the posterior opening of the oral cavity; help protect the body from bacteria introduced into the mouth and nose.

palatoglossal arch The posterior border of the oral cavity.

palatopharyngeal arch The entrance from the oral cavity into the throat.

palliative care A type of care intended to provide comfort and relief from pain.

pallor Paleness.

palmar The forward facing part of the hand in the anatomic position.

palmar grasp An infant reflex that occurs when something is placed in the infant's palm; the infant grasps the object.

palpation Physical touching for the purpose of obtaining information.

palpitations A sensation felt under the left breast of the heart "skipping a beat," usually caused by a premature ventricular contraction.

pancreas A flat, solid organ that lies below the liver and the stomach, and which is a digestive gland that secretes digestive enzymes into the duodenum through the pancreatic duct; considered both an endocrine gland and an exocrine gland.

pancreatitis Inflammation of the pancreas.

pancuronium A nondepolarizing neuromuscular blocking agent; used to maintain paralysis following succinylcholine-facilitated intubation; also called Pavulon.

pandemic An outbreak of disease that occurs on a global scale.

panhypopituitarism The inadequate production or absence of the pituitary hormones, including adrenocorticotropic hormone (ACTH), cortisol, thyroxine, luteinizing hormone (LH), follicle-stimulating hormone (FSH), estrogen, testosterone, growth hormone, and antidiuretic hormone (ADH).

panic disorder A disorder characterized by sudden, usually unexpected, and overwhelming feelings of fear and dread, accompanied by a variety of other symptoms produced by a massive activation of the autonomic nervous system.

papillary muscles Specialized muscles that attach the ventricles to the cusps of the valves by muscular strands called chordae tendineae.

papilledema An eye condition that results from increased pressure on the optic nerve at the rear part of the eye, and whose symptoms include headaches, nausea with possible vomiting, temporary vision loss, or narrowing vision fields.

para A term used to describe the number of times a woman has delivered a viable (live) newborn.

paracrine hormones The hormones that diffuse through intracellular spaces to their target.

paradoxical Opposite from expected.

paradoxical motion The inward movement of the chest during inhalation and outward movement during exhalation; the opposite of normal chest wall movement during breathing.

paralytics Drugs that paralyze skeletal muscles; used in emergency situations to facilitate intubation; also called neuromuscular blocking agents.

parameters Outlined measures that may be difficult to obtain in a research project.

paranasal sinuses The sinuses, or hollowed sections of bone in the front of the head, that are lined with mucous membrane and drain into the nasal cavity; the frontal and maxillary sinuses.

paraphimosis A condition that results when the foreskin is retracted over the glans penis and becomes entrapped; constriction of the glans causes it to swell even further.

parasites Any living organisms in or on any other living creature; take advantage of the host by feeding off cells and tissues.

parasthesias Tingling feeling or sensory change.

parasympathetic nervous system A subdivision of the autonomic nervous system, involved in control of involuntary, vegetative functions, mediated largely by the vagus nerve through the chemical acetylcholine.

parathyroid glands Four glands that are embedded in the posterior portion of each lobe of the thyroid; they produce and secrete parathyroid hormone.

parathyroid hormone (PTH) Hormone produced and secreted by the parathyroid glands; it maintains normal levels of calcium in the blood and normal neuromuscular function.

parenchyma The functional portions of a gland or solid organ.

parenteral route A route of medication administration that involves any route other than the gastrointestinal tract.

paresthesia Sensation of tingling, numbness, or "pins and needles" in a body part.

parietal pain Pain caused by inflammation of the parietal peritoneum that is generally described as steady, aching, and aggravated by movement.

parietal pleura The membrane that lines the pleural cavity.

Parkinson disease A neurologic condition in which the portion of the brain responsible for production of dopamine has been damaged or overused, resulting in tremors.

paroxysmal nocturnal dyspnea (PND) Severe shortness of breath occurring at night after several hours of recumbency, during which fluid pools in the lungs; the person is forced to sit up to breathe; caused by left heart failure or decompensation of chronic obstructive pulmonary disease.

partial agonist A chemical that binds to the receptor site but does not initiate as much cellular activity or change as other agonists do; lowers the efficacy of other agonist chemicals present at the cells.

partial laryngectomy Surgical removal of a portion of the larynx.

partial pressure The amount of gas in air or dissolved in fluid, such as the blood; measured in millimeters of mercury (mm Hg) or torr.

partial pressure of carbon dioxide (Paco$_2$) A measurement of the amount of carbon dioxide in the blood.

partial pressure of oxygen (Pao$_2$) A measurement of the amount of oxygen in the blood.

partial rebreathing mask A mask similar to the nonrebreathing mask but without a one-way valve between the mask and the reservoir; room air is not drawn in with inspiration; residual expired air is mixed in the mask and rebreathed.

passive interventions Something that offers automatic protection from injury or illness, often without requiring any conscious change of behavior by the person; child-resistant bottles and air bags are some examples.

past medical history Information obtained during the history-taking process, such as the patient's general state of health, childhood and adult diseases, surgeries and hospitalizations, psychiatric and mental illnesses, or traumatic injuries, which may relate to the patient's current problem.

patella The kneecap; a specialized bone that lies within the tendon of the quadriceps muscle.

patent Open.

pathologic fracture A fracture that occurs when normal forces are applied to abnormal bone structures.

pathophysiology The study of how normal physiologic processes are affected by disease.

patient autonomy The right to direct one's own care, and to decide how you want your end-of-life medical care provided.

patient care report (PCR) A written record of the incident that describes the nature of the patient's injuries or illness at the scene and the treatment provided; also known as the prehospital care report.

patient history Information about the patient's chief complaint, present symptoms, and previous illnesses.

peak In a pharmacologic context, the point of maximum effect of a drug.

peak expiratory flow An approximation of the extent of bronchoconstriction; used to determine whether therapy (such as with inhaled bronchodilators) is effective.

peer review The process used by medical magazines, journals, and other publications to ensure quality and validity of an article before publishing it, and which involves sending the article to subject matter experts for review of the content and research methods.

pelvic inflammatory disease (PID) An infection of the female upper organs of reproduction, specifically the uterus, ovaries, and fallopian tubes.

pelvis The attachment of the lower extremities to the body, consisting of the sacrum and two pelvic bones.

penis The cylindrical male sex organ; it conveys urine and semen through the urethra.

Penrose drain A type of surgical drain often used as a constricting band.

peptic ulcer disease (PUD) A disease in which the mucous lining of the stomach and duodenum have been eroded, allowing the acid to eat into these organs.

peptides Protein molecules consisting of amino acids held together by peptide bonds.

perception Brought to conscious thought.

percussion Gently striking the surface of the body, typically overlying various body cavities, to detect changes in the densities of the underlying structures.

percutaneous Through the skin or mucous membrane.

percutaneous coronary intervention (PCI) A therapy in which balloons, stents, or other devices are passed through a catheter via a peripheral artery to recanalize and keep a blocked coronary artery open.

perfusion The circulation of oxygen and nutrients at the cellular level and removal of waste products of metabolism for elimination.

pericardial friction rub A to-and-fro sound that is an abnormal heart sound and that can be heard in systole and diastole; heard in patients who have pericarditis.

pericardial knock A high-pitched heart sound heard during diastole.

pericardial tamponade The impairment of diastolic filling of the right ventricle due to significant amounts of fluid in the pericardial sac surrounding the heart, leading to a decrease in the cardiac output.

pericarditis Inflammation of the pericardium.

pericardium The double-layered sac containing the heart and the origins of the superior vena cava, inferior vena cava, pulmonary artery, and aorta.

perilymph Fluid within the bony labyrinth that surrounds and protects the membranous labyrinth while allowing transmission of pressure waves caused by sound.

perimetrium The outer serosal layer of the uterine wall.

perineum The area between the vaginal opening and the anus.

periorbital cellulitis An infection of the eyelid; also known as preseptal cellulitis or eyelid cellulitis.

periosteum A double layer of connective tissue that lines the outer surface of the bone.

peripheral nerves All of the nerves of the body extending from the brain and spinal cord.

peripheral nervous system (PNS) The part of the nervous system that consists of 31 pairs of spinal nerves and 12 pairs of cranial nerves. These nerves may be sensory, motor, or connecting nerves.

peripheral neuropathy A group of conditions in which the nerves that exit the spinal cord are damaged, distorting signals to or from the brain. One type is caused by diabetes; peripheral nerves are damaged as the blood glucose level rises, resulting in lack of sensation, numbness, burning, pain, paresthesia, and muscle weakness.

peripheral shock A term that describes shock caused by peripheral circulatory abnormalities; includes hypovolemic shock and distributive shock.

peripheral vein cannulation Cannulating veins of the periphery, that is, those that can be seen and/or palpated. Examples of peripheral veins include those of the hand, arm, and lower extremity and the external jugular vein.

peripheral vision Visualization of lateral objects while looking forward.

peristalsis The wavelike contraction of smooth muscle in tubular organs or structures, such as the esophagus, intestines, and ureters, by which they a propel their contents.

peritonitis Inflammation of the peritoneum, the protective membrane that lines the abdominal and pelvic cavities.

peritonsillar abscess A collection of infected material around the tonsils.

peritubular capillaries A set of capillaries unique to the kidney that branch off from the efferent arteriole; the site of tubular reabsorption.

permissive A parenting style in which the parent does not impose many rules, if any, on the child; two subcategories include indifferent and indulgent.

perseveration Repeating the same idea over and over again.

personality disorder The condition a person has when he or she behaves or thinks in a way that is dysfunctional or causes distress to other people.

pertinent negatives A lack of certain signs and symptoms one would normally expect to see specific to illnesses or conditions; these findings warrant no medical care or intervention, but demonstrate the thoroughness of the patient examination and history.

pertussis An acute infectious disease characterized by a catarrhal stage, followed by a paroxysmal cough that ends in a whooping inspiration; also called whooping cough.

pervasive developmental disorders (PDDs) A group of disorders that cause delays in many areas of childhood development, such as the development of skills to communicate and interact socially, and may include repetitive body movements and difficulty with changes in routine; includes autism and Asperger syndrome, among others.

petechiae Tiny purple or red spots that appear on the skin due to bleeding within the skin or under mucous membranes.

pH The measure of acidity or alkalinity of a solution.

phagocytes The cells that engulf and consume foreign material such as microorganisms and debris.

phagocytosis The process in which one cell "eats" or engulfs a foreign substance to destroy it.

phalanges The small bones of the digits of the fingers and toes.

phantom pain A sensation of pain in a part of the body that is no longer present.

pharmacodynamics The biochemical and physiologic effects and mechanism of action of a medication in the body.

pharmacokinetics The fate of medications in the body, such as distribution and elimination.

pharmacology The scientific study of how various substances interact with or alter the function of living organisms.

pharyngitis Inflammation of the pharynx.

pharynx The cavity lying posterior to the mouth connecting to the esophagus; the throat.

phenotype The appearance, health condition, or other characteristics associated with a particular genotype.

pheochromocytoma A tumor of the adrenal gland, usually in the medulla, that causes excessive release of the hormones epinephrine and norepinephrine.

phimosis Inability to retract the distal foreskin over the glans penis.

phlebitis Inflammation of the wall of a vein, sometimes caused by an IV line, manifested by tenderness, redness, and slight edema along part of the length of the vein.

phobia An abnormal and persistent dread of a specific object or situation.

phobic disorders Disorders involving an unreasonable fear, apprehension, or dread of a specific situation or thing.

phospholipid A type of lipid molecule that comprises the cell membrane.

phospholipid bilayer The cell membrane's double layer, consisting of a hydrophilic outer layer composed of phosphate groups, and a hydrophobic inner layer made up of lipids, or fatty acids. It is this structure and composition that allows the cell membrane to have selective permeability.

physical dependence A physiologic state of adaptation to a drug, usually characterized by tolerance to the drug's effects and a withdrawal syndrome if use of the drug is stopped, especially abruptly.

physiologic dead space Additional dead space created by intrapulmonary obstructions or atelectasis.

physiologic fracture A fracture that occurs when abnormal forces are applied to normal bone structures.

physiology The study of the body functions of the living organism.

pia mater The innermost of the three meninges that enclose the brain and spinal cord; it rests directly on the brain and spinal cord.

piercing spike The hard, sharpened plastic spike on the end of the administration set designed to pierce the sterile membrane of the IV bag.

pineal gland A gland in the brain that synthesizes and secretes melatonin, a hormone that affects patterns of sleep and wakefulness.

pinna The large outside portion of the ear through which sound waves enter the ear; also called the auricle.

pinocytosis A process by which cells ingest the extracellular fluid and its contents.

piriform fossae Two pockets of tissue on the lateral borders of the larynx.

pituitary gland An endocrine gland whose secretions control, or regulate, the secretions of other endocrine glands; often called the "master gland"; also called the hypophysis.

placebo effect In a pharmacologic context, the positive and negative effects of an inactive medication on a person that are related to the person's expectations and other factors.

plaintiff In a civil suit, the person who brings a legal action against another person.

plantar The bottom surface of the foot.

plaque In cardiology, the white to yellow lesion found in atherosclerosis that is made up of lipids, cell debris, and smooth muscles cells; in older people, may also include calcium.

plasma A sticky, yellow fluid that carries the blood cells and nutrients and transports cellular waste material to the organs of excretion; makes up 55% of the total blood volume.

plasma cells Cells that produce antibodies (immunoglobulins) to destroy antigens or antigen-containing particles; formed from divided and differentiated B cells.

plasma protein binding A process in which medication molecules temporarily attach to proteins in the blood plasma, significantly altering medication distribution in the body.

plasmin A naturally occurring clot-dissolving enzyme, usually present in the body in its inactive form, plasminogen.

platelets Tiny, disk-shaped elements that are much smaller than the cells; they are essential in the initial formation of a blood clot, the mechanism that stops bleeding.

pleura The serous membranes covering the lungs and lining the thoracic cavity, completely enclosing a potential space known as the pleural space.

pleural effusion Excessive accumulation of fluid in the pleural space.

pleural friction rubs Squeaking or grating sounds that occur when the pleural linings rub together, which may be heard on inspiration, expiration, or both, commonly caused by inflammation of the pleura.

pleural space The potential space between the parietal pleura and the visceral pleura. It is described as "potential" because under normal conditions, the space does not exist.

pneumonia An inflammation of the lungs caused by bacterial, viral, or fungal infections or infections with other microorganisms.

pneumonitis Inflammation of the lung; implies lung inflammation from an irritant such as a chemical, dust, or radiation, or from aspiration.

pneumotaxic (pontine) center A portion of the pons that assists in creating shorter, faster respirations.

podocytes Special cells in the inner membrane of the glomerulus that wrap around the capillaries in the glomerulus, forming filtration slits.

point of maximal impulse (PMI) The palpable beat of the apex of the heart against the chest wall during ventricular contraction; normally palpated in the fifth left intercostal space in the midclavicular line.

poison A substance whose chemical action could damage structures or impair function when introduced into the body.

polarized When a cell is at rest, ions are actively transported into and out of the cell to create an electrochemical gradient across the cell membrane.

poliomyelitis A viral infection that attacks and destroys nerve axons, especially motor axons. The disease can cause weakness, paralysis, and respiratory arrest. Because an effective vaccine has been developed, the incidence of the disease is now rare.

polycythemia The production of more red blood cells over time, making the blood "thick"; a characteristic of people who have chronic lung disease and chronic hypoxia.

polymenorrhea Menstrual blood flow that occurs more often than a 24-day interval.

polymorphonuclear neutrophils (PMNs) The type of white blood cells formed by bone marrow tissue that have a nucleus consisting of several parts or lobes connected by fine strands.

polypeptide Formed from many amino acids bound into a chain. When a polypeptide has more than 100 molecules, it is considered to be a protein. Certain protein molecules have more than one polypeptide.

polyphonic The sound of multiple notes during wheezing; caused by the vibrations of many bronchi.

polysaccharides Complex carbohydrates that contain many simple joined sugar units, such as plant starch. Some polysaccharides such as cellulose cannot be broken down for nutrition in humans but play important roles in digestion.

polyuria Frequent and plentiful urination.

pons An organ that lies below the midbrain and above the medulla and contains numerous important nerve fibers, including those for sleep, respiration, and the medullary respiratory center.

popliteal artery A continuation of the femoral artery at the knee.

popliteal vein The vein that forms when the anterior and posterior tibial veins unite at the knee.

portal hypertension Increased pressure in the portal veins; caused by the inability of blood to normally flow through the liver; can lead to rupture of these vessels.

portal vein A large vessel created by the intersection of blood vessels from the GI system. The portal vein drains into the liver.

positive end-expiratory pressure (PEEP) Mechanical maintenance of pressure in the airway at the end of expiration to increase the volume of gas remaining in the lungs.

positive-pressure ventilation Forcing of air into the lungs.

postconventional reasoning A type of reasoning in which a child bases decisions on his or her conscience.

posterior In anatomy, the back surface of the body; the side away from you in the standard anatomic position.

posterior cavity Vitreous chamber; portion of the eyeball filled with vitreous humor, a jellylike fluid that helps the globe maintain its shape without distorting light.

posterior chamber The posterior area of the globe between the lens and the iris.

posterior column pathway Sensory pathway responsible for sending information about localized fine touch, pressure, vibration, and proprioception to the brain.

posterior tibial artery The artery just behind the medial malleolus; supplies blood to the foot.

postictal The period of time after a seizure in which the brain is reorganizing activity.

postpolio syndrome The death of nerve fibers as a late consequence of polio; the syndrome is characterized by swallowing difficulties, weakness, fatigue, and breathing problems.

postrenal ARF A type of acute renal failure caused by obstruction of urine flow from the kidneys, commonly caused by a blockage of the urethra by an enlarged prostate gland, renal calculi, or strictures.

postsynaptic terminal Portion of the postsynaptic cell that contains receptor sites and receives the neurotransmitter.

posttraumatic stress disorder (PTSD) A delayed stress reaction to a previous incident, often the result of one or more unresolved issues concerning the incident.

postural hypotension Symptomatic drop in blood pressure related to the patient's body position; detected by measuring pulse and blood pressure while the patient is lying supine, sitting up, and standing. An increase in pulse rate and a decrease in blood pressure in any one of these positions is considered a positive sign for this condition.

postural tremor A tremor that occurs as the person holds a body part still.

posturing Abnormal body positioning that indicates damage to the brain.

potency The relationship between the desired response of a medication and the dose required to achieve the response.

potentiation Enhancement of the effect of one drug by another drug.

PR interval The period between the beginning of the P wave (atrial depolarization) and the onset of the QRS complex (ventricular depolarization), signifying the time required for atrial depolarization and passage of the excitation impulse through the atrioventricular junction.

preconventional reasoning A type of reasoning in which a child acts almost purely to avoid punishment to get what he or she wants.

precordial leads Another term used to describe the chest leads in an ECG.

preexcitation Early depolarization of ventricular tissue due to the presence of an accessory pathway between the atria and ventricles.

prefilled syringes Medication syringes that are prepackaged and prepared with a specific concentration.

preload The volume of blood returned to the heart; also referred to as the pressure of blood that is returned to the heart (venous return).

premenstrual syndrome (PMS) A cluster of all or some of the troubling symptoms that occur during a woman's menstrual phase that can include fluid retention, breast pain and tenderness, headache, severe cramping, and emotional changes, including agitation, irritability, depression, and anger.

prepuce In the anatomy of the female genitalia, a layer of skin directly above the clitoris.

prerenal ARF A type of acute renal failure that is caused by hypoperfusion of the kidneys, resulting from hypovolemia (hemorrhage, dehydration), trauma, shock, sepsis, and heart failure (congestive heart failure, myocardial infarction); often reversible if the underlying condition can be found and perfusion restored to the kidney.

presbyopia The increased difficulty in focusing on objects that occurs with aging.

preschoolers Persons who are 3 to 5 years of age.

pressure infuser device A sleeve that is placed around the IV bag and inflated to force fluid to flow from the IV bag and into the tubing.

pressure of speech Speech in which words seem to tumble out under immense emotional pressure.

pressure-compensated flowmeter An oxygen flowmeter that incorporates a float ball in a tapered calibrated tube; the float rises or falls according to the gas flow in the tube; is affected by gravity and must remain in an upright position for an accurate reading.

presynaptic terminal Portion of the presynaptic cell that contains and releases the neurotransmitter.

pretibial myxedema An "orange peel" appearance and nonpitting edema of the skin on the anterior part of the leg below the knee.

prevalence The number of cases of a disease in a specific population within a given period.

priapism A painful, tender, persistent erection of the penis; can result from spinal cord injury, erectile dysfunction drugs, or sickle cell disease.

primary adrenal insufficiency Also known as Addison disease. A rare condition in which the adrenal glands produce an insufficient amount of adrenal hormones.

primary assessment The part of the assessment process that focuses on identifying immediately or potentially life-threatening conditions so that you can initiate lifesaving care.

primary follicles Matured primordial follicles; the site of gene transcription in the growth of the oocyte.

primary prevention Keeping an injury or illness from occurring.

primary respiratory drive The normal stimulus to breathe; based on fluctuations in Paco$_2$ and pH of the cerebrospinal fluid.

primary response The first encounter with the foreign substance to begin the immune response.

primary taste sensations Sweet, salty, sour, and bitter.

primitive reflexes Reflex reactions such as Babinski, grasping, and sucking signs normally found in young patients.

primordial follicles Structures in developing female fetuses that contain a primary oocyte surrounded by follicular cells.

Prinzmetal angina A type of chest pain that occurs when a person is at rest, when oxygen needs are minimal.

process objectives State how a program will be implemented, describing the service to be provided, the nature of the service, and to whom it will be directed.

prodromal/prodrome The early signs and symptoms that occur before a disease or condition fully appears, eg, dizziness before fainting.

profession A specialized set of knowledge, skills, and/or expertise.

progesterone A hormone released from the ovaries that stimulates the uterine lining during the menstrual cycle.

projection Blaming unacceptable feelings, motives, or desires on others.

prolapsed uterus A condition in which the uterus moves or drops into the vagina due to weakened pelvic muscles and connective tissues.

proliferative phase The first phase of the uterine cycle and marks the time after menstruation and before the next ovulation occurs. The uterine lining increases in thickness in preparation to receive a fertilized oocyte.

pronation Turning the palms downward (toward the ground).

prone Lying flat, and face down.

proprioception The ability to perceive the position and movement of one's body or limbs.

prospective research A type of research that gathers information as events occur in real time.

prostaglandins Lipids made from arachidonic acid that usually act more locally than hormones, are very potent, stimulate hormone secretions, and help to regulate blood pressure.

prostate gland A small gland that surrounds the male urethra where it emerges from the urinary bladder; it secretes a fluid that is part of the ejaculatory fluid.

protected health information (PHI) Data that contain the patient's name, address, and other specific identifiers.

proteins Created from amino acids, they include enzymes, plasma proteins, muscle components (actin and myosin), hormones, and antibodies.

protest phase An infant's initial response to a situational crisis; characterized by loud crying.

prothrombin An alpha globulin made in the liver that is converted into thrombin.

protocol A treatment plan developed for a specific illness or injury.

protons Single, positively charged particles inside the nucleus of an atom.

protozoa Single-celled, usually microscopic, eukaryotic organisms such as amoebas, ciliates, flagellates, and sporozoans; a type of parasite.

protuberant Term used to describe an abdomen with a convex, or distended, shape; can be caused by edema.

proximal Closer to the trunk.

proximal convoluted tubule (PCT) One of two complex sections of the nephron, the PCT includes an enlargement at the end called the glomerular capsule.

proximate cause The specific reason that an injury occurred; one of the items that must be proven in order for a paramedic to be held liable for negligence.

pruritus Itching.

pseudomembrane A false membrane formed by a dead tissue layer; seen in the posterior pharynx of patients with diphtheria.

pseudostratified columnar epithelium Tissue that lines respiratory system passages and is layered in appearance and involved in secretion.

psychiatric emergency An emergency in which abnormal behavior threatens a person's health and safety or the health and safety of another person, for example when a person becomes suicidal, homicidal, or has a psychotic episode.

psychological dependence The emotional state of craving a drug to maintain a feeling of well-being.

psychosis A mental disorder characterized by the loss of contact with reality.

psychotropic drugs Drugs that affect mood, thought, or behavior.

ptosis Prolapse of a body part; often refers to drooping of the eyelid.

puberty The time during development when the body becomes reproductively functional.

pubic symphysis A hard bony and cartilaginous prominence found at the midline in the lowermost portion of the abdomen where the two halves of the pelvic ring are joined by cartilage at a joint with minimal motion.

pubis One of three bones that fuse to form the pelvic ring.

public health An industry whose mission is to prevent disease and promote good health within groups of people.

pudendum The female external genitalia.

pulmonary artery One of two arteries that carry deoxygenated blood from the right ventricle to the lungs.

pulmonary circulation The flow of blood from the right ventricle through the pulmonary arteries and all of their branches and capillaries in the lungs and back to the left atrium through the venules and pulmonary veins; also called the lesser circulation.

pulmonary edema Congestion of the pulmonary air spaces with exudate and foam, often secondary to left heart failure.

pulmonary embolism A blood clot or foreign matter trapped within the pulmonary circulation.

pulmonary semilunar valve The valve between the right ventricle and the pulmonary artery; also called the pulmonic valve.

pulmonary veins The four veins that return oxygenated blood from the lungs to the left atrium of the heart.

pulmonic valve The semilunar valve that regulates blood flow between the right ventricle and the pulmonary artery.

pulp Specialized connective tissue within the pulp cavity of a tooth.

pulse The wave of pressure created as the heart contracts and forces blood out the left ventricle and into the major arteries; palpated at a point where an artery passes close to a bone.

pulse deficit A situation in which the palpated radial pulse rate is less than the apical pulse rate; reported numerically as the difference between the two.

pulse oximeter A device that measures oxygen saturation (Spo_2).

pulse oximetry An assessment tool that measures oxygen saturation of hemoglobin in the capillary beds.

pulse pressure The difference between the systolic and diastolic pressures.

pulseless electrical activity (PEA) An organized cardiac rhythm (other than ventricular tachycardia) on an ECG monitor that is not accompanied by any detectable pulse.

pulsus alternans A pulse that alternates between strong and weak beats, characteristic of left ventricular systolic damage.

pulsus paradoxus A weakening or loss of a palpable pulse during inhalation, equivalent to a drop in the systolic blood pressure of 10 mm Hg or more; commonly seen in patients with pericardial tamponade or severe asthma.

punitive damages Compensation, usually monetary, awarded to a plaintiff for intentional or reckless acts committed by the defendant.

pupil The circular opening in the center of the eye through which light passes to the lens.

Purkinje fibers A system of fibers in the ventricles that conducts the excitation impulse from the bundle branches to the myocardium.

purulent Full of pus; having the character of pus.

pyelonephritis Inflammation of the kidney linings.

pyloric stenosis Hypertrophy (enlargement) of the pyloric sphincter of the stomach; ultimately leads to intestinal obstruction, often in infants.

pyrogenic reaction A reaction characterized by an abrupt temperature elevation (as high as 106°F [41°C]) with severe chills, backache, headache, weakness, nausea, and vomiting; a potential complication of IV or IO therapy.

pyrogens Chemicals or proteins that travel to the brain and affect the hypothalamus and stimulate a rise in the body's core temperature.

QRS complex Deflections of the ECG produced by ventricular depolarization.

quadrants The way to describe the sections of the abdominal cavity. Imagine two lines intersecting at the umbilicus dividing the abdomen into four equal areas.

qualified immunity Protection in which the paramedic is only held liable when the plaintiff can show that the paramedic violated clearly established law of which he or she should have known.

qualitative A type of descriptive statistic in research that does not use numeric information.

quality control The responsibility of the medical director to ensure that the appropriate medical care standards are met by EMS personnel on each call.

quantitative A type of measurement in research that uses a mean, median, and mode.

quid pro quo Circumstance in which a person in authority attempts to exchange some work-related benefit, such as a raise or promotion, for sexual favors.

rabies A fatal infection of the central nervous system caused by a bite from an animal that has been infected with the rabies virus.

radioisotopes Also known as radioactive isotopes or radionuclides, they are atoms with unstable nuclei.

radiopaque Feature of an IV catheter (or any other object) that allows it to appear on a radiograph.

radius The bone on the thumb side of the forearm.

rales Rattling, bubbling, or crackling lung sounds indicative of fluid in the small airways; also known as crackles.

range of motion The arc of movement of an extremity at a joint in a particular direction.

rape Sexual intercourse inflicted forcibly on another person, against that person's will.

rapid exam A 60- to 90-second nonsystematic review and palpation of the patient's body to identify injuries that must be managed or protected immediately; conducted during the primary assessment and includes the mnemonic DCAP-BTLS.

rapid-sequence intubation (RSI) A specific set of procedures, combined in rapid succession, to induce sedation and paralysis and intubate a patient quickly.

reactive airway disease A term used to describe any condition that causes hyperreactive bronchioles and bronchospasm.

reassessment The part of the assessment process in which problems are reevaluated and responses to treatment are assessed.

rebound tenderness Pain that the patient feels when pressure is released as opposed to when pressure is applied; characteristic of appendicitis.

recanalization The opening up of new channels through a blocked artery.

receptive aphasia Damage to or loss of the ability to understand speech.

receptor A specialized area in tissue that initiates certain actions after specific stimulation.

reciprocity The process of granting licensure or certification to a provider from another state or agency.

recovery position Left-lateral recumbent position; used in all unresponsive nontrauma patients who are able to maintain their own airway spontaneously and are breathing adequately.

rectal abscess An infection involving a collection of pus in the rectal walls that results from blockage of the rectal mucus ducts.

rectum The lowermost end of the colon.

red blood cells Cells that carry oxygen to the body's tissues; also called erythrocytes.

reduced hemoglobin The hemoglobin after the oxygen has been released to the cells.

referred pain Pain that feels as if it is originating from a body part other than the site being stimulated.

reflex arc The simplest type of nerve pathway, consisting of only a few neurons.

reflexes Involuntary motor responses to specific sensory stimuli, such as a tap on the knee or stroking the eyelash.

refracting system A series of transparent structures within the eye that redirect light as it passes through mediums of different densities.

refractory period A short period immediately after depolarization in which the myocytes are not yet repolarized and are unable to fire or conduct an impulse.

registration Providing information to an entity that stores it in some form of record book. In the context of EMS, records of your education, state or local licensure, and recertification are held by a recognized board.

regression A return to more childish behavior while under stress.

relative refractory period That period in the cell-firing cycle at which it is possible but difficult to restimulate the cell to contract.

remote console A terminal that receives transmissions of telemetry and voice from the field and transmits messages back, usually through the base station.

renal arteries The vessels that supply the kidneys with blood for filtration; they arise from the abdominal aorta.

renal columns Inward extensions of cortical tissue that surround the renal pyramids.

renal corpuscle The initial blood-filtering component of the nephron.

renal cortex The outer portion of each kidney; it forms renal columns and has tiny tubules associated with the nephrons.

renal dialysis A technique for filtering the blood of its toxic wastes, removing excess fluids, and restoring the normal balance of electrolytes.

renal fascia Dense, fibrous connective tissue that anchors the kidney to the abdominal wall.

renal medulla The inner portion of each kidney; it is made of conical renal pyramids, and has striations.

renal pelvis A cone-shaped collecting area that connects the ureter and the kidney.

renal pyramids Parallel cone-shaped bundles of urine-collecting tubules that are located in the medulla of the kidneys.

renal tubule The portion of the nephron containing the tubular fluid filtered through the glomerulus.

renal vein The vessel from the kidneys that joins the inferior vena cava.

renin A hormone produced by cells in the juxtaglomerular apparatus when the blood pressure is low.

renin-angiotensin system System that helps to regulate fluid balance and blood pressure through actions in the kidney.

renin-angiotensin-aldosterone system (RAAS) A complex feedback mechanism responsible for the regulation of sodium in the body by the kidneys.

repeater Miniature transmitter that picks up a radio signal and rebroadcasts it, extending the range of a radio communications system.

reperfusion The resumption of blood flow through an artery.

repolarization The process by which ions are moved across the cell wall to return to a polarized state.

res ipsa loquitur Theory of negligence that assumes an injury can only occur when a negligent act occurs.

research agenda The specific question(s) that a study aims to answer, and the precise methods in which the data will be gathered.

research consortium A group of agencies working together to study a particular topic.

research domain The area (clinical, systems, or education) that will be impacted by a study.

reservoir In the context of communicable disease, a place where organisms may live and multiply.

residual volume The air that remains in the lungs after maximal expiration.

respiration The inhaling and exhaling of air; the physiologic process that exchanges carbon dioxide from fresh air.

respiratory acidosis A pathologic condition characterized by a blood pH of less than 7.35, and caused by accumulation of acids in the body from a respiratory cause.

respiratory alkalosis A pathologic condition characterized by a blood pH of greater than 7.45, and resulting from the accumulation of bases in the body from a respiratory cause.

respiratory rate The number of times a person breathes in 1 minute.

respiratory syncytial virus (RSV) A labile paramyxovirus that infects the upper and lower respiratory tracts, but disease, namely pneumonia and bronchiolitis, is more prevalent in the lower respiratory tract.

respiratory system All the structures of the body that contribute to the process of breathing, consisting of the upper and lower airways and their component parts.

rest tremor A tremor that occurs when the body part is not in motion.

restrictive lung diseases Diseases that limit the ability of the lungs to expand appropriately. Skeletal abnormalities (kyphosis and scoliosis) are a common example of restrictive lung disease.

reticular activating system Located in the upper brainstem; responsible for maintenance of consciousness, specifically one's level of arousal.

reticular connective tissue The type of tissue that helps to create a framework inside internal organs such as the spleen and liver.

reticuloendothelial system The system in the body that is primarily used to defend against infection.

retina A delicate 10-layered structure of nervous tissue located in the rear of the interior of the globe that receives light and generates nerve signals that are transmitted to the brain through the optic nerve.

retinal detachment Separation of the inner layers of the retina from the underlying choroid, the vascular membrane that nourishes the retina.

retractions Skin pulling between and around the ribs and clavicles during inhalation; a sign of respiratory distress.

retrograde intubation A technique in which a wire is placed through the trachea and into the mouth with a needle via the cricoid membrane; the endotracheal tube is then placed over the wire and guided into the trachea.

retroperitoneal Behind the abdominal cavity.

retroperitoneum The space behind the peritoneum.

retrospective research Research performed from current available information.

retrosternal Situated or occurring behind the sternum.

reversible reaction A chemical reaction where the products of the reaction can change back into the reactants they originally were.

Rh factor An antigen present in the erythrocytes (red blood cells) of about 85% of people.

rhabdomyolysis The destruction of muscle tissue leading to a release of potassium and myoglobin.

rheumatic fever An inflammatory disease caused by streptococcal bacteria strains that can cause a stenosis of the mitral valve or aortic valve.

rhinitis A nasal disorder generally caused by allergens, which, once inhaled, result in production of chemicals that can cause inflammation.

rhonchi Coarse, low-pitched breath sounds heard in patients who chronically have mucus in the airways (singular, rhonchus).

ribonucleic acid (RNA) A nucleic acid associated with controlling cellular activities.

right atrial enlargement Dilation of the right atrium that results when returning venous pressure is elevated or pulmonary pressures are high.

right atrium The upper right chamber of the heart; receives blood from the venae cavae and supplies blood to the right ventricle.

right ventricle The lower right chamber of the heart; receives blood from the right atrium and pumps blood out through the pulmonic valve into the pulmonary artery.

right ventricular hypertrophy (RVH) A cardiac condition in which the right ventricle becomes enlarged, most commonly due to pulmonary hypertension.

right-sided heart failure A condition in which the right side has to work increasingly harder to pump blood into engorged pulmonary vessels, which eventually leads to an inability to keep up with the increased workload.

rigidity Stiffness or hardness (in motion). Found in patients with Parkinson disease.

risk A potentially hazardous situation that puts people in a position in which they could be harmed.

risk factors Characteristics of people, behaviors, or environments that increase the chances of disease or injury; some examples are alcohol use, poverty, smoking, or gender.

rocuronium A nondepolarizing neuromuscular blocking agent; used to maintain paralysis following succinylcholine-facilitated intubation; also called Zemuron.

rods One of two photoreceptors of the retina sensitive to light, but does not discriminate colors, producing a picture that is somewhat less focused and essentially black and white.

Rohypnol A benzodiazepine used to facilitate date rape and that can create memory loss; street names include roofies, roof, roachies, rocha, and Mexican Valium.

rooting reflex An infant reflex that occurs when something touches an infant's cheek, and the infant instinctively turns his or her head toward the touch.

R-R interval The period between the onset of one QRS complex and the onset of the next QRS complex.

rubella A viral disease similar to measles, best known by the distinctive red rash on the skin; not nearly as infectious or severe as measles.

rubor Redness; one of the classic signs of inflammation.

ruptured ovarian cyst A fluid-filled sac within the ovary that bursts from internal pressure.

saccule An enlarged region of the membranous labyrinth of the inner ear.

sacroiliac joint The connection point between the pelvis and the vertebral column.

sacrum One of three bones (sacrum and two pelvic bones) that make up the pelvic ring; consists of five fused sacral vertebrae.

saddle joint Two saddle-shaped articulating surfaces oriented at right angles to each other so that complementary surfaces articulate with each other, such as is the case with the thumb.

safe residual pressure The pressure at which an oxygen cylinder should be replaced with a full one; often is 200 psi.

sagittal (lateral) plane An imaginary line where the body is cut into left and right parts.

salicylates Aspirin-like drugs.

saline locks Special types of IV devices that eliminate the need to hang a bag of IV fluid; also called a buff cap or INT (intermittent); commonly used for patients who do not require fluid boluses but may require medication therapy.

salivary glands The glands that produce saliva to keep the mouth and pharynx moist.

sampling errors Expected errors that occur in the sampling phase of research.

saphenous vein The longest vein in the body, it drains the leg, thigh, and dorsum of the foot.

scabies An infestation of the skin with the mite *Sarcoptes scabiei*; spreads rapidly with skin-to-skin contact.

scaffolding An instructional technique that builds on what has already been learned.

scalp The thick skin covering the cranium, which usually bears hair.

scaphoid A concave shape of the abdomen; can be caused by evisceration.

scapula The shoulder blade.

scarlet fever A disease caused by the bacterium *Streptococcus pyogenes*, and characterized by a sore throat, fever, rash, and "strawberry tongue."

scene size-up A quick assessment of the scene and its surroundings made to provide information about scene safety and the mechanism of injury or nature of illness, before you enter and begin patient care.

schizophrenia A complex, difficult-to-identify mental disorder whose typical onset is during early adulthood. Dysfunctional symptoms typically become more prominent over time and include delusions, hallucinations, apathy, mutism, flat affect, a lack of interest in pleasure, erratic speech, emotional responses, and motor behavior.

Schlemm's canal Responsible for maintaining the proper pressure of aqueous humor, draining excess into the bloodstream.

school age A person who is 6 to 12 years of age.

Schwann cells Neuroglial cells in the peripheral nervous system that form a myelin sheath around axons.

sclera The white, fibrous outer layer of the eyeball.

scleroderma An autoimmune connective tissue disease that causes fibrotic (scar tissue–like) changes to the skin, blood vessels, muscles, and internal organs.

scoliosis Sideways curvature of the spine.

scope of practice What a state permits a paramedic practicing under a license or certification to do.

scrotum A pouch of skin and subcutaneous tissue hanging from the lower abdominal region, posterior to the penis.

sebaceous glands Glands that produce an oily substance called sebum, which discharges along the shafts of the hairs.

secondary adrenal insufficiency A common condition characterized by a lack of adrenocorticotropic hormone (ACTH, also called corticotrophin) secretion from the pituitary gland.

secondary assessment The process by which more detailed, quantifiable, objective information is obtained from a patient about his or her overall state of health.

secondary bronchi Airway passages in the lungs that are formed from the division of the right and left mainstem bronchi.

secondary prevention Reducing the effects of an injury or illness that has already happened.

secondary response The body's reaction when it is exposed to an antigen for which it already has antibodies, in which it responds by killing the invading substance.

secretory phase The second phase of the uterine cycle and is the time after ovulation until menstruation (occurs when oocyte is not fertilized).

secure attachment A bond between an infant and his or her parent or caregiver, in which the infant understands that parents or caregivers will be responsive to his or her needs and provide care when help is needed.

sedation The reduction of a patient's anxiety, induction of amnesia, and suppression of the gag reflex, usually by pharmacologic means.

sedative-hypnotic A drug used to reduce anxiety, calm agitated patients, and help produce drowsiness and sleep (CNS depressants).

Seldinger technique A technique that involves inserting a needle with a syringe, then inserting a guide wire into the needle, removing the needle, making an incision, and inserting a catheter over the guide wire; the guide wire is then removed.

selective permeability The ability of the cell membrane to selectively allow compounds into the cell based on the cell's current needs.

selective serotonin reuptake inhibitors (SSRIs) A class of antidepressants that inhibit the reuptake of serotonin.

self-concept A person's perception of himself or herself.

self-esteem How a person feels about himself or herself, and how a person feels about how he or she fits in with peers.

self-sealing blood tubes Glass tubes with self-sealing rubber caps; used to obtain blood samples for laboratory analysis.

semen Seminal fluid ejaculated from the penis and containing sperm.

semilunar valves The two valves, the aortic and pulmonic, that divide the heart from the aorta and pulmonary arteries.

seminal vesicles Storage sacs for sperm and seminal fluid, which empty into the urethra at the prostate.

seminiferous tubules Highly coiled structures inside each lobule of a testis; they form a network of channels, then ducts, which join the epididymis.

semipermeable Property of the cell membrane that describes the ability to allow certain elements to pass through while not allowing others to do so.

sensitivity The ability to recognize a foreign substance the next time it is encountered.

sensory nerves The nerves that carry sensations of touch, taste, heat, cold, pain, and other modalities from the body to the central nervous system.

sensory receptors Structures located in the dermis that initiate nerve impulses that can reach our conscious awareness.

septic shock The type of shock that occurs as a result of widespread infection, usually bacterial; untreated, the result is multiple organ dysfunction syndrome and often death.

seropositive   Having a positive blood test for an infectious agent, such as human immunodeficiency virus (HIV) or hepatitis B or C virus.

serotonin   A vasoactive amine that increases vascular permeability to cause vasodilation.

serotonin syndrome   An idiosyncratic complication that occurs with antidepressant therapy in which patients have lower extremity muscle rigidity, confusion or disorientation, and/or agitation.

serous membrane   Membranes that line body cavities that lack openings to the outside.

serum hepatitis   Infection with the hepatitis B virus (HBV), which is transmitted through sexual contact, blood transfusion, or puncture of the skin with contaminated needles; signs and symptoms include loss of appetite, nausea, vomiting, general fatigue and malaise, low-grade fever, vague abdominal discomfort, and sometimes aching in the joints; eventually, jaundice occurs.

serum sickness   A condition in which antigen-antibody complexes formed in the bloodstream deposit in sites around the body, most notably the kidneys, with resultant inflammatory reactions.

severe acute respiratory syndrome (SARS)   A potentially life-threatening viral infection that usually starts with flu-like symptoms.

sex cells   Germ (reproductive) cells; in males they are known as sperm and in females are known as oocytes (eggs).

sex chromosomes   The X and Y chromosomes, which determine sex.

sexual assault   An attack against a person that is sexual in nature, the most of common which is rape.

sexually transmitted diseases (STDs)   A group of diseases usually acquired by sexual contact and that include gonorrhea, syphilis, chlamydia, scabies, pubic lice, herpes, hepatitis, and HIV infection.

sharps   Any contaminated item that can cause injury; includes IV needles and catheters, broken ampules or vials, or anything else that can penetrate or lacerate the skin.

Shiley   A type of tracheostomy tube.

shock   An abnormal state associated with inadequate oxygen and nutrient delivery to the metabolic apparatus of the cell

shock position   The position that has the head and torso (trunk) supine and the lower extremities elevated 6″ to 12″. This helps to increase blood flow to the brain; also referred to as the modified Trendelenburg position.

shoulder girdle   The proximal portion of the upper extremity, made up of the clavicle, the scapula, and the humerus.

shunt   A situation in which a portion of the output of the right side of the heart reaches the left side of the heart without being oxygenated in the lungs; may be caused by atelectasis, pulmonary edema, or a variety of other conditions. In hemodialysis, an anastomosis between a peripheral artery and vein.

sickle cell crisis   A condition in which a patient with sickle cell disease experiences significant pain due to insufficient passage of oxygen and nutrients into tissues and joints because of vessel congestion.

sickle cell disease   A disease that causes the RBCs to be misshapen, resulting in poor oxygen-carrying capability and potentially resulting in lodging of the RBCs in blood vessels or the spleen.

signs   Indications of illness or injury that the examiner can see, hear, feel, smell, and so on.

simple columnar epithelium   Single-layer tissue found in female reproductive tubes, the uterus, and most digestive tract organs; involved in secretion and absorption.

simple cuboidal epithelium   Single-layer tissue covering the ovaries and lining kidney tubules and glandular ducts; involved in secretion and absorption.

simple phobia   A fear that is focused on one class of objects (eg, mice, spiders, dogs) or situations (eg, high places, darkness, flying).

simple squamous epithelium   Single-layer tissue lining the alveoli, capillary walls, blood and lymph vessels, and body cavities.

simplex   Method of radio communication using a single frequency that enables transmission reception of voice or an ECG signal but is incapable of simultaneous transmission and reception.

sine wave   An unusual waveform that has a repetitive, uniform seesaw pattern, representing an alternating current; also known as a *sinusoidal waveform*.

sinoatrial (SA) node   The dominant pacemaker of the heart, located at the junction of the superior vena cava and the right atrium.

sinus bradycardia   A sinus rhythm with a heart rate of less than 60 beats/min.

sinus dysrhythmia   A slight irregularity of the heart rate caused by changes in parasympathetic tone during breathing.

sinus tachycardia   A sinus rhythm with a heart rate of greater than 100 beats/min.

sinuses   Cavities formed by the cranial bones that trap contaminants from entering the respiratory tract and act as tributaries for fluid to and from the eustachian tubes and tear ducts.

sinusitis   An infection of the sinuses, characterized by thick nasal discharge, sinus and facial pressure, headache, and fever.

situational crisis   A crisis caused by a specific set of circumstances.

skeletal muscle tissue   Voluntary muscle tissue attached to bones and composed of long thread-like cells that have light and dark striations.

skeleton   The framework that gives the body its recognizable form; also designed to allow motion of the body and protection of vital organs.

skull   The structure at the top of the axial skeleton that houses the brain and consists of the 28 bones that comprise the auditory ossicles, the cranium, and the face.

slander   Verbally making a false statement that injures a person's good name.

sliding filament model   A method of action of muscle contraction involving how sarcomeres shorten, with thick and thin filaments sliding past each other toward the center of the sarcomere from both ends.

slow-reacting substances of anaphylaxis   Biologically active compounds derived from arachidonic acid called leukotrienes.

small intestine   The portion of the digestive tube between the stomach and the cecum, consisting of the duodenum, jejunum, and ileum.

smooth muscle   The nonstriated involuntary muscle found in vessel walls, glands, and the gastrointestinal tract.

smooth muscle tissue   Unstriated, involuntary muscle tissue with a "spindle"-shaped appearance; it composes hollow internal organ walls.

snoring   A noise made during inhalation when the upper airway is partially obstructed by the tongue.

SOAP method   A narrative writing method in which information is organized into four categories, including subjective information, objective information, assessment, and treatment plan.

sodium-potassium (Na$^{\pm}$-K$^{\pm}$) pump   The mechanism by which the cell brings in two potassium (K$^+$) ions and releases three sodium (Na$^+$) ions.

soft stool   A bowel movement that is the consistency of soft-serve ice cream; can range in color from tan to dark brown.

solute   The dissolved particles contained in the solvent.

solution   Combination of dissolved elements (solutes) and water (solvent).

solvent   The fluid that does the dissolving, or the solution that contains the dissolved components.

somatic cells   All of the other cells in the human body besides the sex cells.

somatic nervous system   The part of the nervous system that regulates activities over which there is voluntary control.

somatic pain   Localized pain, usually felt deeply, which represents irritation or injury to tissue, causing activation of peripheral nerve tracts.

somatoform disorder A condition in which a person is overly concerned with physical health and appearance to the point that it dominates his or her life; an example is hypochondria.

somatostatin A hormone that helps to regulate the endocrine system and has a wide range of effects throughout the body, including inhibiting insulin and glucagon secretion by the pancreas.

source individual Any person, living or dead, whose blood or other potentially infectious materials may be a source of occupational exposure to another person; examples include but are not limited to, hospital and clinic patients; clients in institutions for the developmentally disabled; trauma victims; clients of drug and alcohol treatment facilities; residents of hospices and nursing homes; human remains; and people who donate or sell blood or blood components.

spacers The devices that collect medication as it is released from the canister of a metered-dose inhaler, allowing more medication to be delivered to the lungs and less to be lost to the environment.

sperm Male sex cells; they are formed in the testes.

spermatogenesis The process by which sperm cells are formed.

spermatogenic cells Those that form sperm cells and line the seminiferous tubules.

spermatogonia Undifferentiated spermatogenic cells in a male embryo.

sphincters Muscles arranged in circles that are able to decrease the diameter of tubes. Examples are found within the rectum, bladder, and blood vessels.

sphygmomanometer A blood pressure cuff.

Spice An illicit drug consisting of a blend of synthetic cannibinoids; it can produce delirium and short- and long-term psychotic effects.

spina bifida A developmental anomaly in which a portion of the spinal cord or meninges protrudes outside the spinal column or even outside the body, usually in the area of the lumbar spine (the lower third of the spine).

spinal cord An extension of the brain, composed of virtually all the nerves carrying messages between the brain and the rest of the body. It lies inside of and is protected by the spinal canal.

spinal nerves 31 pairs of nerves each responsible for sending and receiving sensory and motor messages to and from the CNS from a portion of the body.

spleen The largest lymphatic organ; filters the blood via the actions of lymphocytes and macrophages.

splenic sequestration crisis An acute, painful enlargement of the spleen caused by sickle cell disease.

splitting In the context of heart sounds, the situation in which events on the right side of heart occur slightly later than those on the left side, and create two discernible sounds rather than one heart sound.

ST segment The interval between the end of the QRS complex and the beginning of the T wave; often elevated or depressed with respect to the isoelectric line when there is significant myocardial ischemia.

stable angina Angina pectoris characterized by periodic pain with a predictable pattern.

standard of care What a reasonable paramedic with training would do in the same or a similar situation.

standard precautions The term currently used to describe the infection control practices that will reduce the opportunity for exposure of providers in the daily care of patients; consider all body fluids, except sweat, to present a possible risk.

standing order A type of protocol that is a written document signed by the EMS system's medical director that outlines specific directions, permissions, and sometimes prohibitions regarding patient care that is rendered prior to contacting medical control.

Stanford classification A classification system for aortic dissections that includes two categories.

Staphylococcus aureus A strain of bacteria that became resistant to the drug methicillin, creating a new strain called methicillin-resistant *S aureus*; symptoms include infection and possibly localized skin abscesses and cellulites, empyemas, and endocarditis.

status asthmaticus A severe, prolonged asthma attack that cannot be stopped with conventional treatment, such as the administration of epinephrine.

status epilepticus A condition in which seizures recur every few minutes, or in which seizure activity lasts more than 30 minutes.

statutes of limitations Laws that limit the time within which a lawsuit may be filed.

steatorrhea Foamy, fatty stools associated with liver failure or gallbladder problems.

stem cells Cells that can develop into other types of cells in the body, allowing for continual growth and renewal.

stenosis A narrowing, such as of a blood vessel or stoma.

stereotyped movements Repetitive movements that do not appear to serve any purpose.

sterile The destruction of all living organisms; achieved by using heat, gas, or chemicals.

sternocleidomastoid muscles The muscles on either side of the neck that allow movement of the head.

sternum The breastbone.

steroid Molecules with four connected rings of carbon atoms, including cholesterol, estrogen, progesterone, testosterone, cortisol, and estradiol.

Stevens-Johnson syndrome A severe, possibly fatal reaction that mimics a burn; may be due to a medication.

stimulant A medication or chemical that temporarily enhances central nervous system and sympathetic nervous system functioning.

stoma In the context of the airway, the resultant orifice of a tracheostomy that connects the trachea to the outside air; located in the midline of the anterior part of the neck.

strabismus Loss of perception of depth and overlapping or doubled images.

straight laryngoscope blade A blade designed to lift the epiglottis and expose the vocal cords; also called the Miller blade.

strangulated Complete obstruction of blood circulation in a given organ as a result of compression or entrapment; an emergency situation causing death of tissue.

stratified columnar epithelium Thick tissue found in the male urethra, vas deferens, and areas of the pharynx.

stratified cuboidal epithelium Thick tissue that lines the mammary gland ducts, sweat glands, salivary glands, pancreas, ovaries, and seminiferous tubules.

stratified squamous epithelium Thick tissue that forms the epidermis and lines the mouth, esophagus, vagina, and anus.

stratum corneal layer The outermost or dead layer of the skin.

stress A nonspecific response of the body to any demand made on it.

stressor Any agent or situation that causes stress.

striae Vertical stretch marks that occur when a person loses or gains weight rapidly.

stridor A harsh, high-pitched inspiratory sound representing air moving past an obstruction within or immediately above the glottic opening; associated with severe upper airway obstruction.

stroke volume (SV) The volume of blood pumped forward with each ventricular contraction.

stylet In the context of intubation, a semirigid wire inserted into an endotracheal tube to mold and maintain the shape of the tube.

subarachnoid hemorrhage A hemorrhage between the arachnoid membrane and the pia mater.

subarachnoid space The space located between the pia mater and the arachnoid membrane.

subclavian artery The proximal part of the main artery of the arm, which supplies the brain, neck, anterior chest wall, and shoulder.

subclavian vein The proximal part of the main vein of the arm, which unites with the internal jugular vein.

subcutaneous (SC) Into the tissue between the skin and muscle; a medication delivery route.

subcutaneous tissue Tissue, largely fat, that lies directly under the dermis and serves as an insulator of the body.

subendocardial myocardial infarction A type of acute myocardial infarction in which the ischemic process affects only the inner layer of muscle.

subjective information Information that is told to you, but which cannot be seen, such as the symptoms a patient describes.

sublingual Under the tongue; a medication delivery route.

substance abuse Use of a substance that disrupts activities of daily living.

substance dependence Use of a substance that results in addiction and physiologic dependence on the substance.

substance intoxication Use of a substance that results in impaired thinking and motor function.

substance use Use of moderate amounts of a substance without seriously affecting activities of daily living.

substrate The target of enzyme action.

succinylcholine chloride A depolarizing neuromuscular blocker frequently used as the initial paralytic during rapid-sequence intubation; causes muscle fasciculations; also called Anectine.

sucking reflex An infant reflex in which the infant starts sucking when his or her lips are stroked.

suicide Any willful act designed to bring an end to one's own life.

superficial Closer to or on the skin.

superior Above a body part or nearer to the head.

superior vena cava One of the two largest veins in the body; carries blood from the upper extremities, head, neck, and chest into the heart.

supination Turning the palms upward (toward the sky).

supine The position in which the body is lying face up.

suppressor T cells Lymphocytes that modulate the immune response to avoid injury to body systems.

supraorbital foramen A small notch located on the frontal bone near the inner, upper area of each orbit.

surfactant A liquid protein substance that coats the alveoli in the lungs, decreases alveolar surface tension, and keeps the alveoli expanded; a low level in a premature baby contributes to respiratory distress syndrome.

surrogate decision maker A person designated by a patient to make health care decisions as the patient would want when the patient becomes incapable of making decisions.

surveillance The ongoing systematic collection, analysis, and interpretation of injury data essential to the planning, implementation, and evaluation of public health practice.

suspensory ligaments Ligaments that anchor the lens to the cornea allowing the various muscles of the eye to pull the lens into varying degrees of refraction.

sutures Attachment points in the skull where the cranial bones join together.

sweat glands The glands that secrete sweat, located in the dermal layer of the skin.

sympathetic eye movement The movement of both eyes in unison.

sympathetic nervous system A subdivision of the autonomic nervous system that governs the body's fight-or-flight reactions by inducing smooth muscle contraction or relaxation of the blood vessels and bronchioles.

sympathomimetics Medications administered to stimulate the sympathetic nervous system.

symphysis A type of joint that has grown together forming a very stable connection.

symptoms The pain, discomfort, or other abnormality that the patient feels.

synapses Gaps between nerve cells, across which nervous stimuli are transmitted.

synaptic cleft The space between neurons.

synaptic vesicles Vesicles that contain neurotransmitters.

synchronized cardioversion The use of a synchronized direct current (DC) electric shock to convert tachydysrhythmias (such as atrial fibrillation) to normal sinus rhythm.

syncopal episodes Fainting; brief losses of consciousness caused by transiently inadequate blood flow to the brain.

syncope A fainting spell or loss of consciousness caused by transiently inadequate blood flow to the brain.

synergism The action of two substances such as drugs, in which the *total effects are greater than the sum of the independent effects* of the two substances.

synovial fluid The small amount of liquid within a joint used as lubrication.

synovial joints Complex joints that allow free movement and are lubricated with synovial fluid.

synovial membrane The lining of a joint that secretes synovial fluid into the joint space.

synthesis reaction A reaction that occurs when two or more reactants (atoms) bond to form a more complex product or structure.

syphilis A sexually transmitted disease caused by the bacterium *Treponema pallidum*, which manifests in three stages—primary, secondary, and late—and is transmitted through direct contact with open sores; characterized by an ulcerative lesion or chancre of the skin or mucous membrane at the site of infection, commonly in the genital region.

systematic sampling A computer-generated list of subjects or groups for research.

systemic circulation The portion of the circulatory system outside of the heart and lungs.

systemic complications Reactions that affect systems of the body.

systemic lupus erythematosus A multisystem autoimmune disease.

systemic reaction A reaction that occurs throughout the body, possibly affecting multiple body systems.

systemic vascular resistance (SVR) The resistance that blood must overcome to be able to move within the blood vessels. SVR is related to the amount of dilation or constriction in the blood vessel.

systole The period of time when the atria or ventricles are contracting; also called atrial systole.

systolic pressure Blood pressure created by the left ventricle while it is contracting (ie, in systole).

T killer cells The cells released during a type IV allergic reaction that kill antigen-bearing target cells.

T lymphocytes (T cells) Specialized lymphocyte precursors that make up the majority of circulated blood lymphocytes.

T waves The upright, flat, or inverted wave following the QRS complex of the ECG, representing ventricular repolarization.

tachyphylaxis A condition in which repeated doses of medication within a short period rapidly cause tolerance, making the medication virtually ineffective.

tactile fremitus Vibrations in the chest that can be felt with a hand on the chest as the patient breathes.

talus The bone that articulates with the tibia and fibula to form the ankle.

tangential thinking Leaving the current topic midconversation to talk about something else, inhibiting interpersonal communication.

target tissues Tissues on which hormones are directed to act.

tarsals The bones of the ankles.

taste receptors   Receptors on the taste buds that respond to sweet, salty, sour, and bitter; help us to identify foods that are satiating and substances that are potential poisons.

temporomandibular joint (TMJ)   The joint where the mandible meets with the temporal bone of the cranium just in front of each ear.

temporomandibular joint disorders   A collection of disorders that present with jaw pain, and which occur when the connection between the temporal bone and the temporomandibular joint erodes or moves out of proper alignment.

ten-code   A radio code system using the number 10 plus another number.

tendons   The fibrous connective tissue that attaches muscle to bone.

tenting   A condition in which the skin slowly retracts after being pinched and pulled away slightly from the body; a sign of dehydration.

terminal drop hypothesis   The theory that a person's mental function declines in the last 5 years of life.

tertiary bronchi   Airway passages in the lungs that are formed from branching of the secondary bronchi.

testes   The male reproductive organs that produce sperm and secrete male hormones; also called testicles.

testicular torsion   Twisting of the testicle on the spermatic cord, from which it is suspended; associated with scrotal pain and swelling, and is a medical emergency.

testosterone   The most important male sex hormone (androgen).

tetanus   A disease caused by spores that enter the body through a puncture wound contaminated with animal feces, street dust, or soil or that can enter through contaminated street drugs; signs and symptoms include pain at the wound site and painful muscle contractions in the neck and trunk muscles.

thalassemia   A type of anemia in which not enough hemoglobin is produced, or the hemoglobin is defective.

theophylline   A naturally occurring alkaloid found in a variety of plants (such as tea leaves).

therapeutic communication   Communicating with the patient.

therapeutic index   The relationship between the median effective dose and the median lethal dose or median toxic dose; also known as the therapeutic ratio.

therapy regulator   A device that attaches to the stem of the oxygen cylinder and reduces the high pressure of gas to a safe range (about 50 psi).

thermoregulation   The process of maintaining homeostasis of temperature.

third spacing   The shifting of fluid into the tissues, creating edema.

thoracic cage   The chest or rib cage.

thoracic duct   One of two great lymph vessels; it empties into the superior vena cava.

thoracic spine   The 12 vertebrae that lie between the cervical vertebrae and the lumbar vertebrae. One pair of ribs is attached to each of the thoracic vertebrae.

thorax   The chest cavity that contains the heart, lungs, esophagus, and great vessels.

thought broadcasting   The belief that thoughts are broadcast aloud and can be heard by others.

thought insertion   The belief that thoughts are being thrust into one's mind by another person.

thought withdrawal   The belief that thoughts are being removed from one's mind.

threshold level   In a pharmacologic context, the concentration of medication at which initiation or alteration of cellular activity begins.

thrill   A humming vibration that can be palpated through the chest wall; suggests an underlying bruit or murmur.

thrombin   An enzyme that causes the conversion of fibrinogen to fibrin, which binds to the platelet plug, forming the final mature clot.

thrombocytes   Platelets.

thrombocytopenia   A reduction in the number of platelets.

thromboembolism   A blood clot that has formed within a blood vessel and is floating within the bloodstream.

thrombophlebitis   Inflammation of a vein.

thromboplastin   A chemical that stimulates clotting of blood.

thrombus   A fixed blood clot.

through-the-needle catheters   Plastic catheters inserted through a hollow needle; referred to as Intracaths.

thymus   A gland that is larger in children but shrinks with age; it secretes thymosins, which are important in early immunity by affecting production and differentiation of lymphocytes.

thymus gland   A gland that helps the immune system identify and destroy components foreign to the body.

thyroepiglottic ligament   The attachment of the thyroid cartilage to the epiglottis.

thyroid   Large gland located at the base of the neck that produces and excretes hormones that influence growth, development, and metabolism.

thyroid cartilage   A firm prominence of cartilage that forms the upper part of the larynx; the Adam's apple.

thyroid gland   A large endocrine gland that is located at the base of the neck and produces and excretes hormones that influence growth, development, and metabolism.

thyroid-stimulating hormone (TSH)   Hormone that controls the release of thyroid hormone from the thyroid gland.

thyroid storm   A rare, life-threatening condition that may occur in patients with thyrotoxicosis. The condition is usually triggered by a stressful event or increased volume of thyroid hormones in the circulation.

thyrotoxicosis   A toxic condition caused by excessive levels of circulating thyroid hormone.

thyroxine   The body's major metabolic hormone. Thyroxine stimulates energy production in cells, which increases the rate at which the cells consume oxygen and use carbohydrates, fats, and proteins.

tibia   The shin bone, the larger of the two bones of the lower leg.

tidal volume (VT)   A measure of the depth of breathing; the volume of air that is inhaled or exhaled during a single respiratory cycle.

tinnitus   The perception of sound in the inner ear with no external environmental cause; often reported as "ringing" in the ears, but may be roaring, buzzing, or clicking.

tissue plasminogen activator (t-PA)   A major component in the fibrinolytic system, in which clots that have already formed are lysed or disrupted, converting plasminogen to plasmin.

toddlers   Persons who are 1 to 3 years of age.

tolerance   Physiologic adaptation to the effects of a drug such that increasingly larger doses of the drug are required to achieve the same effect.

tongue-jaw lift maneuver   A manual maneuver that involves grasping the tongue and jaw and lifting; commonly used to suction the airway and to place certain airway devices.

tonic activity   A type of seizure movement involving the constant contraction and trembling of muscle groups.

tonicity   The tension exerted on a cell due to water movement across the cell membrane.

tonsillitis   Inflammation of the tonsils.

tonsil-tip catheter   A hard or rigid suction catheter; also called a Yankauer catheter.

topographic anatomy   The superficial landmarks of the body that serve as guides to the structures that lie beneath them.

torso   The trunk without the head and limbs.

tort   A wrongful act that gives rise to a civil suit.

total body water (TBW) Total amount of water in the human body; accounts for approximately 60% of the weight of an average man; divided into various compartments.

total laryngectomy Surgical removal of the entire larynx.

total lung capacity The total volume of air that the lungs can hold; approximately 6 L in an average man.

toxic shock syndrome (TSS) A form of septic shock caused by *Streptococcus pyogenes* (group A strep) or *Staphylococcus aureus*; initial symptoms include syncope, myalgia, diarrhea, vomiting, headache, fever, and sore throat.

toxicologic emergencies Medical emergencies caused by toxic agents such as poison.

toxidrome The syndrome-like symptoms of any given class or group of poisonous agents.

trabeculae Bony rods that form the lacy network in cancellous bones and are oriented to increase weight-bearing capacity of long bones.

trace elements Essential minerals found in very small amounts; include chromium, cobalt, copper, fluorine, iodine, iron, manganese, selenium, and zinc.

trachea The conduit for all entry into the lungs; a tubular structure that is approximately 10 to 12 cm long and composed of a series of C-shaped cartilaginous rings; also called the windpipe.

tracheal breath sounds Breath sounds heard by placing the stethoscope diaphragm over the trachea or sternum; also called bronchial breath sounds.

tracheitis Bacterial infection of the trachea.

tracheobronchial suctioning Inserting a suction catheter into the endotracheal tube to remove pulmonary secretions.

tracheostomy A surgical opening into the trachea.

tracheostomy tube A plastic tube placed within the tracheostomy site (stoma).

tracheotomy Surgically opening the trachea to create an airway.

track marks The visible scars from repeated cannulation of a vein; commonly associated with illicit drug use.

transceiver A radio transmitter and receiver housed in a single unit; a two-way radio.

transcutaneous pacing (TCP) The act of depolarizing myocardial tissue with a small electrical charge delivered by a device that sends a small electrical charge through the skin of the chest between one externally placed pacing pad and another.

transdermal Across the skin; a medication delivery route.

transfusion reactions A physiologic response that is similar to an anaphylactic reaction, in which the body reacts to the infusion of blood; occurs rapidly and can cause severe circulatory collapse and death.

transfusion-related lung injury A transfusion reaction characterized by increased pulmonary capillary permeability, resulting in noncardiogenic pulmonary edema.

transient ischemic attack (TIA) A disorder in which brain cells temporarily stop working because of insufficient oxygen, causing stroke-like symptoms that resolve completely within 24 hours of onset.

transillumination intubation A method of intubation that uses a lighted stylet to guide the endotracheal tube into the trachea.

transitional epithelium Tissue that changes in appearance due to tension; it lines the urinary bladder, ureters, and superior urethra.

translaryngeal catheter ventilation A method used in conjunction with needle cricothyrotomy to ventilate a patient; requires a high-pressure jet ventilator.

transmigration (diapedesis) The polymorphonuclear neutrophils permeate through the vessel wall, moving into the interstitial space.

transmission The way in which an infectious agent is spread: contact, airborne, by vehicles (for example, food or needles), or by vectors.

transmural myocardial infarction A type of acute myocardial infarction in which the infarct extends through the entire wall of the ventricle.

transverse (axial) plane An imaginary line where the body is cut into top and bottom parts.

trauma systems The collaboration of prehospital and in-hospital medicine that focuses on optimizing the use of resources and assets of each with a primary goal of reducing the mortality and morbidity of trauma patients.

tremors Fine involuntary, rhythmic movements, usually involving the hands or head.

Trendelenburg position The position in which the body is supine with the head lower than the feet.

triage Process of establishing treatment and transportation priorities according to severity of injury and medical need.

trichomoniasis A parasitic infection.

tricuspid valve The valve between the right atrium and right ventricle of the heart.

tricyclic antidepressants (TCAs) A group of drugs used to treat severe depression and manage pain; minimal dosing errors can cause toxic results.

trifascicular block A blockage or impairment of all three components of the ventricular conduction system, with one working occasionally to provide AV conduction.

trigeminal nerve The fifth cranial nerve; its mandibular branch provides motor innervation to the muscles of mastication.

trigeminy A premature complex in every third heartbeat.

triglycerides A subcategory of lipids that includes fat and oil.

trismus The involuntary contraction of the mouth resulting in clenched teeth. Occurs during seizures and head injuries.

tropomyosin An actin-binding protein that regulates muscle contraction and other actin-related mechanical functions of the body.

troponin A regulatory protein in the actin filaments of skeletal and cardiac muscle that attaches to tropomysin.

trunking Sharing of radio frequencies by multiple agencies or systems.

trust and mistrust A phrase that refers to a stage of development from birth to approximately 18 months of age, during which infants gain trust of their parents or caregivers if their world is planned, organized, and routine.

tuberculin skin test (TST) A test to determine if a person has ever been infected with tuberculosis.

tuberculosis (TB) A chronic bacterial disease caused by *Mycobacterium tuberculosis* that usually affects the lungs but can also affect other organs such as the brain and kidneys.

tubo-ovarian abscess An infectious mass growing within the ovaries and fallopian tubes.

tubular reabsorption The process that moves substances from the tubular fluid into the blood, within the peritubular capillary.

tubular secretion The process that moves substances from the blood in the peritubular capillary into the renal tubule.

tunica adventitia The outer layer of tissue of a blood vessel wall, composed of elastic and fibrous connective tissue.

tunica intima The smooth, thin, inner lining of a blood vessel.

tunica media The middle and thickest layer of tissue of a blood vessel wall, composed of elastic tissue and smooth muscle cells that allow the vessel to expand or contract in response to changes in blood pressure and tissue demand.

turbinates Three bony shelves that protrude from the lateral walls of the nasal cavity and extend into the nasal passageway, parallel to the nasal floor; they increase the surface area of the nasal mucosa, thereby improving warming, filtering, and humidification of inhaled air.

turgor Loss of elasticity in the skin.

tympanic　A loud, high-pitched sound, similar to the sound of a drum, heard on percussion of a hollow space (eg, the empty stomach or a puffed-out cheek).

tympanic membrane　A thin membrane that separates the middle ear from the inner ear and sets up vibrations in the ossicles; also called the eardrum.

type 1 diabetes　The type of diabetic disease that usually starts in childhood and requires daily injections of supplemental synthetic insulin to control blood glucose; sometimes called *juvenile diabetes* or *juvenile-onset diabetes*.

type 2 diabetes　The type of diabetic disease that usually starts in later life and often can be controlled through diet and oral medications; sometimes called adult-onset diabetes.

U wave　A small flat wave sometimes seen after the T wave and before the next P wave.

ulcerative colitis　Generalized inflammation of the colon that results in a weakened, dilated rectum, making it prone to infection and bleeding.

ulna　The inner bone of the forearm, on the side opposite the thumb.

ultrahigh frequency (UHF) band　The portion of the radio frequency spectrum between 300 and 3,000 mHz.

umbilical　The region of the abdomen surrounding the umbilicus.

unblinded study　A type of study in which the subjects are advised of all aspects of the study.

unifocal　Arising from a single site.

unilateral　Occurring on only one side of the body.

unintentional injuries　Injuries that occur without intent to harm (commonly called accidents); some examples are motor vehicle crashes, poisonings, drownings, falls, and most burns.

universal precautions　Protective measures that have traditionally been developed by the CDC for use in dealing with objects, blood, body fluids, or other potential exposure risks of communicable disease.

unstable angina　Angina pectoris characterized by a changing, unpredictable pattern of pain, which may signal an impending acute myocardial infarction.

untoward effect　A clinical change caused by a medication that causes harm or discomfort to a patient; also known as adverse effect.

upper airway　Consists of all anatomic airway structures above the level of the vocal cords.

urea　The result of amino acid catabolism; it filters into the renal tubule, with most of it reabsorbed and the balance excreted in the urine.

uremia　Severe renal failure resulting in the buildup of waste products within the blood. Eventually brain functions will be impaired.

uremic frost　A powdery buildup of uric acid, especially on the skin of the face.

ureters　A pair of thick-walled, hollow tubes that transport urine from the kidneys to the bladder.

urethra　A hollow tubular structure that drains urine from the bladder, expelling it from the body.

uric acid　The result of metabolism of certain organic bases in nucleic acids, mostly reabsorbed via active transport from the glomerular filtrate.

urinary bladder　A hollow muscular sac in the midline of the lower abdominal area that stores urine until it is released from the body.

urinary incontinence　The inability to control the release of urine from the bladder; loss of bladder control.

urinary retention　Incomplete emptying of the bladder, or a complete lack of ability to empty the bladder.

urinary system　The organs that control the discharge of certain waste materials filtered from the blood and excreted as urine.

urinary tract infections (UTIs)　Infections, usually of the lower urinary tract (urethra and bladder), that occur when normal flora (bacteria that naturally populate the skin) enter the urethra and multiply.

urine　The final product of tubular reabsorption and secretion; it is a clear, yellow-colored fluid that carries wastes out of the body.

urticaria　Multiple small, raised areas on the skin that may be one of the warning signs of impending anaphylaxis; also known as hives.

uterine tubes　Fallopian tubes, or oviducts; they open near the ovaries, penetrate the uterus, and open into the uterine cavity.

uterus　In females, the muscular organ where the fetus grows; found between the urinary bladder and the rectum; also called the womb.

utricle　An enlarged portion of the labyrinth of the inner ear.

uvula　A soft-tissue structure that resembles a punching bag; located in the posterior aspect of the oral cavity, at the base of the tongue.

V/Q mismatch　An imbalance in the amount of oxygen received in the alveoli and the amount of blood flowing through the alveolar capillaries.

vaccinations　Inoculations with a vaccine, usually by injection or inhalation, to bring about immunity to a specific disease in a person.

vaccines　The products formulated to bring about immunity by introducing into the body a killed or weakened virus to which the immune system produces antibodies.

Vacutainer　A cylindrical device that attaches to an 18- or 20-gauge sampling needle; accommodates self-sealing blood tubes when blood samples are being obtained.

vagina　The lower portion of the birth canal, which also serves as a passage for menstrual flow and as the receptacle of the penis during sexual intercourse.

vaginal bleeding　Bleeding from the vagina.

vaginal yeast infection　An infection caused by the fungus, *Candida albicans*, in which fungi overpopulate the vagina.

vaginitis　An inflammation of the vagina that is caused by an infection.

vagus nerve　The cranial nerve (X) that is responsible for decreasing heart rate, and which provides motor functions to the soft palate, pharynx, and larynx and carries taste bud fibers from the posterior tongue, sensory fibers from the inferior pharynx, larynx, thoracic, and abdominal organs, and parasympathetic fibers to thoracic and abdominal organs.

vallecula　An anatomic space, or "pocket," located between the base of the tongue and the epiglottis; an important anatomic landmark for endotracheal intubation.

Valsalva maneuver　Forced exhalation against a closed glottis, the effect of which is to stimulate the vagus nerve and, thereby, slow the heart rate.

varicose veins　Veins on the leg that are large, twisted, and ropelike and can cause pain, swelling, or itching.

vasa deferentia　The spermatic duct of the testicles; also called vas deferens.

vasa recta　A series of peritubular capillaries that surround the loop of Henle, into which water moves after passing through the descending and ascending limbs of the loop of Henle.

vasculitis　An inflammation of the blood vessels.

vasoactive amines　Substances such as histamine and serotonin that increase vascular permeability.

vasoconstriction　Narrowing of the diameter of a blood vessel.

vasodilation　Widening of the diameter of a blood vessel.

vasoocclusive crisis　Ischemia and pain caused by sickle-shaped red blood cells that obstruct blood flow to a portion of the body.

Vaughan-Williams　A classification scheme based on the mechanism of action rather than on specific medication groups.

vector　An animal or insect that carries a disease-causing organism and transmits it to a human host, without itself becoming ill.

vecuronium　A nondepolarizing neuromuscular blocking agent; used to maintain paralysis following succinylcholine-facilitated intubation; also called Norcuron.

veins　The blood vessels that carry blood to the heart.

vena cava　The largest vein of the body; there are two, which each return blood to the right atrium.

venous sinuses　Spaces between the membranes surrounding the brain that are the primary means of venous drainage from the brain.

venous thrombosis　The development of a stationary blood clot in the venous circulation.

ventilation   The process of exchanging air between the lungs and the environment; includes inhalation and exhalation.

ventral   The anterior surface of the body.

ventral respiratory group (VRG)   A portion of the medulla oblongata that is responsible for modulating breathing during speech.

ventricle   One of two lower chambers of the heart.

Venturi mask   A mask with a number of interchangeable adapters that draws room air into the mask along with the oxygen flow; allows for the administration of highly specific oxygen concentrations.

venules   Very small veins.

vertebrae   The 33 bones that make up the spinal column.

vertebral column   The spine or primary support structure of the body that houses the spinal cord and the peripheral nerves.

vertigo   A type of dizziness in which a person experiences the sensation of movement when standing still or of the environment moving around himself or herself; often due to an inner ear disorder.

very high frequency (VHF) band   The portion of the radio frequency spectrum between 30 and 150 mHz.

vesicles   Tiny fluid-filled sacs; small blisters.

vesicular breath sounds   Soft, muffled breath sounds in which the expiratory phase is barely audible.

vesicular sounds   Normal breath sounds made by air moving in and out of the alveoli; heard over a normal lung.

vestibular gland   One of two glands that lies on each side of the vaginal opening; it secretes mucus into the vestibule to moisten and lubricate the vagina for insertion of the penis.

vestibular system   A system within the inner ear composed of a pair of fluid-filled sacs (otoliths) and three fluid-filled, looping passageways (semicircular canals) used by the central nervous system to collect information about movement and orientation in space.

vestibule   In the context of female genitourinary anatomy, this is the structure into which the vagina opens posteriorly, and the female urethra opens into in the midline. In the context of the ear, this is the central part of the labyrinth, behind the cochlea and in front of the semicircular canals.

vials   Small glass or plastic bottles that contain medication; may contain single or multiple doses.

violent behavior   Behavior that presents a threat of injury or destruction; usually a result of exaggerated fear or paranoia.

viral hepatitis   An inflammation of the liver produced by one of five distinct forms a virus—A, B, C, D, and E. The types differ in transmission but present with the same signs and symptoms.

virulence   The ability of an organism to invade and create disease in a host; also refers to the ability of an organism to survive outside the living host.

viruses   Small organisms that can multiply only inside a host, such as a human, and cause disease.

visceral pain   Crampy, aching pain deep within the body, the source of which is usually difficult to pinpoint; common with genitourinary problems.

visceral pleura   The pleural membrane that covers the lungs.

visual acuity   The ability or inability to see, and how well one can see.

visual cortex   The area in the brain where signals from the optic nerve are converted into visual images.

vital capacity   The amount of air moved in and out of the lungs with maximum inspiration and exhalation.

vitamins   Organic compounds required for normal metabolism.

vitreous humor   A jellylike fluid filling the posterior eye cavity that helps the globe maintain its shape without distorting light.

vocal cords   White bands of tough tissue that are the lateral borders of the glottis.

volume   The amount of a fluid that is present in the ampule or vial in which the medication is dissolved. This is usually expressed in milligrams, grams, or grains.

volume of distribution   The extent to which a medication will spread within the body.

volume on hand   The amount of fluid you have on hand, such as the amount of fluid in an IV bag or the amount of fluid in a vial of medication.

voluntary muscle   Muscle that is under direct voluntary control of the brain and can be contracted or relaxed at will; skeletal, or striated, muscle.

Volutrol   A special type of microdrip set that features a 100- or 200-mL calibrated drip chamber; used for fluid regulation in patients prone to circulatory overload, such as pediatric and elderly patients; also called a Buretrol.

volvulus   Twisting of the bowel until a kink occurs; results in blocked flow.

vulva   The external accessory female organs, including the labia majora, labia minora, clitoris, and vestibular glands; they surround the openings of the urethra and vagina.

vulvovaginitis   An inflammation of the external vulva.

water-soluble   A property that indicates a material can be dissolved in water.

waveform capnography   A monitoring method that measures the exhaled carbon dioxide level and displays the value numerically and as a waveform tracing.

wavelength   The distance in a propagating wave from one point to the corresponding point on the next wave.

West Nile virus (WNV)   A type of virus that is transmitted by mosquitos, and usually causes only mild disease in humans but can cause encephalitis, meningitis, and death; symptoms, if any, include fever, headache, body rash, and swollen lymph glands.

wheezing   A high-pitched whistling sound that may be heard on inspiration, expiration, or both; indicates air movement through a constricted lower airway, as with asthma.

whispered pectoriloquy   A test of decreased breath sounds performed by placing the diaphragm of the stethoscope over the area in question while the patient whispers "ninety-nine"; a loud, clear sound indicates lung consolidation.

whistle-tip catheters   Soft plastic, nonrigid catheters; also called French catheters.

white blood cells   Blood cells that have a role in the body's immune defense mechanisms against infection; also called leukocytes.

white matter   Bundles of myelinated nerves.

withdrawal   In the context of infant behavior, the final phase of an infant's response to a situational crisis; characterized by apathy and boredom.

withdrawal syndrome   A predictable set of signs and symptoms, usually involving altered central nervous system activity, that occurs after the abrupt cessation of a drug or after rapidly decreasing the usual dosage of a drug.

Wolff-Parkinson-White syndrome   A syndrome characterized by short PR intervals, delta waves, nonspecific ST-T wave changes, indicating the presence of an accessory pathway.

xiphoid process   The narrow, cartilaginous lower tip of the sternum.

years of potential life lost   A way of measuring and comparing the overall impact of deaths resulting from different causes; calculated based on a fixed age minus the age at death.

yield   The amount of drug in 1 mL.

zero-order elimination   A process in which a fixed amount of a substance is removed during a certain period, regardless of the total amount in the body.

zoonotic   Refers to infectious diseases of animals that can be transmitted to humans and cause disease.

zygomas   The quadrangular bones of the cheek, articulating with the frontal bone, the maxillae, the zygomatic processes of the temporal bone, and the great wings of the sphenoid bone.

zygote   A large fertilized egg cell produced after contacting a male sperm cell; the first cell of a future offspring, it contains 23 chromosomes from the father and 23 chromosomes from the mother.

Index

Figures and tables are indicated with *f* and *t* following the page numbers.

A

AAAs (Abdominal aortic aneurysms), 1024
AAOS (American Academy of Orthopaedic Surgeons), 6
AAPCC. *See* American Association of Poison Control Centers
AAP (Atypical antipsychotic) drugs, 1392, 1393*t*
Abandonment, 103
Abciximab (ReoPro), 458
ABCs management. *See also* Airway management; Breathing; Circulation
    abdominal and gastrointestinal emergencies, 1135
    allergic reactions and, 494
    cardiovascular emergencies, 928
    patient assessment, 597, 677, 685
    psychiatric emergencies, 1388
    toxicology and, 1340, 1352, 1358
Abdomen and gastrointestinal system, 1122–1159. *See also* Acute inflammatory conditions
    acute infectious diseases, 1147–1149, 1147*t*, 1148*f*
    airway management and, 1136–1137
    anatomy and physiology, 250–251, 251*f*, 277–279, 279*f*, 657–658*f*, 657–661, 1124–1136, 1125–1128*f*, 1125*t*, 1129*t*, 1131–1132*f*, 1131*t*, 1133*t*, 1134*f*
    bleeding and airway management, 1140
    chronic inflammatory conditions, 1145–1147
    disorders, 364–365
    emergency medical care, 1136–1137
    examination of, 873
    gastrointestinal bleeding, 351, 1138–1139*t*, 1139–1142, 1142*f*
    history taking, 1131–1132, 1131*f*, 1131*t*
    lower gastrointestinal bleeding, 1141–1142, 1142*f*
    medications
        absorption, 437–438, 438*t*
        antiemetic medications, 437–438, 438*t*, 459–460
        histamine-2 receptor antagonists, 459
        octreotide (Sandostatin), 460
    motility and pregnancy, 431
    obstructive conditions, 1149–1151, 1151*f*
    older adults, 1153
    patient assessment, 1128–1136, 1131–1132*f*, 1131*t*, 1133*t*, 1134*f*
    pediatric patients, 1151–1153, 1152*f*, 1152*t*
    prevention strategies, 1153–1154, 1153–1154*t*
    primary assessment, 1130
    reassessment, 1135–1136
    scene size-up, 1128–1130
    secondary assessment, 1132–1135, 1132*f*, 1133–1134*t*, 1134*f*
    specific emergencies, 1137–1139, 1138*t*
    upper gastrointestinal bleeding, 1139–1141
Abdominal aorta, 247, 249*f*
Abdominal aortic aneurysms (AAAs), 1024
Abdominal edema, 1132, 1132*f*
Abdominal evisceration, 1133
Abdominal muscles, 235, 888
Abdominal thrust maneuver (Heimlich maneuver), 749
Abducens nerve, 269, 269*f*
Abduction, 186, 186*f*
Aberration, RBBB or LBBB, 972
ABG. *See* Arterial blood gas (ABG) analysis
Abnormal behavior, 1369, 1371–1372, 1371*t*, 1372*f*
Abnormal cell death, 356–357
Abortion, 1191
ABO system, 1248, 1248*t*
Abscesses, 886, 887*t*, 1067, 1067*t*, 1079
Absence seizures, 1068
Absolute refractory period, 450, 920

Absorption
    administration route bioavailability, 436
    as body process, 427
    exposure, 1269
    factors affecting, 431
    poisoning, 1328
Abuse and neglect, 72–73, 156–158, 617–618, 618*f*, 1385
Acalculus cholecystitis, 1142
Accelerated idioventricular rhythm, 960, 960*f*
Accelerated junctional rhythm, 955, 955*f*
Accessory muscles and respiration, 718, 729, 864, 864*f*, 865*t*
Access port, 479
"Accidental Death and Disability" (National Academy of Sciences/National Research Council), 6, 67
Accidents. *See* Unintentional injuries
ACE. *See* Angiotensin-converting enzyme
ACE inhibitors, 425, 452
Acetabulum, 223, 224*f*
Acetadote, 1356
Acetaminophen (Tylenol, APAP), 460, 1356, 1356*t*
Acetylcholine (ACh), 228, 448, 811, 812*t*, 921–922, 924*f*, 1344
Acetylcholinesterase, 229, 453
Acetylcholinesterase inhibitor toxicity, 453
Acetyl coenzyme A, 303–304
Acetylcysteine (Acetadote), 1356
Acetylsalicylic acid. *See* Aspirin
ACh. *See* Acetylcholine
ACHES-S mnemonic for oral contraceptives, 1190
Acholic stools, 1148
Acid-base disorders, 349–352, 350*f*, 352*f*
Acidosis, 191, 347–349, 474
Acids
    acid-base balance, 347–348*f*, 347–352, 350*f*, 352*f*, 728
    bases, pH scale and, 191, 191*f*
    defined, 191, 347, 347*t*
ACL (Anterior cruciate ligament), 224, 225*f*
Acne, 408
Acoustic stethoscopes, 630
Acquired immunity, 374, 1247, 1270
Acquired immunodeficiencies, 387, 387*f*
Acquired immunodeficiency syndrome (AIDS), 387, 1306–1307
Acquisition modes for 12-lead ECGs, 966–967, 967*f*
Acromioclavicular separation (AC separation), 222
Acromion process, 221, 221*f*
Acrosomal membranes, 294, 296
AC separation (Acromioclavicular separation), 222
ACTH (Adrenocorticotropin hormone), 283, 1216, 1240
Actidose. *See* Activated charcoal
Actin molecules, 228
Action potentials, 228
Activase, 458, 549–550
Activated charcoal (EZ-Char; Actidose; Liqui-Char), 443, 548, 1340–1341, 1348
Active hyperemia, 379
Active listening, 132–133
Active metabolites, 442
Active transport, 199–200, 290, 441, 475, 475*f*
Activities of daily living (ADLs), 1369, 1388
Acute abdomen, 1124
Acute alcohol intoxication, 1335
Acute chest syndrome, 1252
Acute coronary syndrome (ACS), 457, 982, 1013
Acute dissecting aneurysm of the aorta, 1022–1023, 1023*t*
Acute dystonic reaction, 1393
Acute gastroenteritis, 1147–1148, 1147*t*
Acute infectious diseases, 1147–1149, 1147*t*, 1148*f*
Acute inflammation, 379–383, 381*t*, 382*f*
Acute inflammatory conditions
    appendicitis, 1143
    cholecystitis and biliary tract disorders, 1142–1143

diverticulitis, 1143–1144
    pancreatitis, 1144–1145, 1145*f*
Acute leukemia, 1254
Acute myocardial infarction (AMI)
    assessment, 1014–1015
    ECG monitor-defibrillator and, 935
    evolution on the ECG, 977*f*, 978*t*
    fibrinolytics and, 458
    management in field, 1015–1017, 1016*t*
    pathophysiology, 1013
    reperfusion techniques, 1017–1018, 1018*t*
    signs, 1014–1015
    symptoms, 982, 1014
Acute phase proteins, 355
Acute psychosis, 1382–1383
Acute renal failure (ARF), 1170–1172, 1171*t*
Acute respiratory distress syndrome (ARDS), 895
Acute splenic sequestration syndrome, 1252
Acute stress reactions, 39
ADA. *See* Americans with Disabilities Act of 1990
Adalat, 567–568
Adam (Methylenedioxyamphetamine), 1337
Adam's apple, 218
Adaptation, nervous system, 271
Adaptive (specific) defense, 257
Adaptive (acquired) immunity, 260, 260*t*, 374, 1247
Addiction. *See* Drug abuse and addiction
Addictive behavior, 1389
Addison's disease and Addisonian crisis, 286, 1231–1232
Adduction, 186, 186*f*
Adenocarcinoma, 1231
Adenocard. *See* Adenosine
Adenoid, 715, 715*f*
Adenosine (Adenocard), 443, 450, 451–452, 548–549
Adenosine diphosphate (ADP), 228
Adenosine triphosphate (ATP), 201, 474, 724
Adhesion of neutrophils, 381, 1149
Adipocytes, 203, 205
Adipose tissue, 205–206, 337
ADLs (Activities of daily living), 1369, 1388
Administration set, 480
Administrative regulations, 92
Adnexa, 1094
Adolescents
    in history taking, 624
    pertussis and, 1316
    physical changes, 408, 408*f*
    privacy and modesty, 139
    psychosocial changes, 408–409, 408–409*f*
Adopted Names Council, US, 425
Adosine, 451–452
ADP (Adenosine diphosphate), 228
Adrenal cortex, 285, 285*f*, 1216, 1216*f*, 1216*t*
Adrenal glands, 285–286, 285*f*, 1041, 1163–1164, 1216
Adrenal gland tumor, 1233
Adrenalin. *See* Epinephrine
Adrenaline, 285
Adrenal insufficiency, 1231–1233, 1232*f*
Adrenal medulla, 1216, 1216*f*, 1216*t*
Adrenal suppression, 445
Adrenergic receptors, 337
Adrenocorticotropin hormone (ACTH), 283, 1216, 1240
Adult-onset diabetes. *See* Diabetes
Advanced airway management. *See also* Digital intubation; Intubation; Orotracheal intubation by direct laryngoscopy; Transillumination intubation techniques
    difficult airway, predicting, 69–70*f*, 775–776
    endotracheal intubation, 776–778, 777–778*f*
    face-to-face intubation, 801–802
    failed intubation, 802–803
    field extubation, 803–804
    nasotracheal intubation, 786–792, 789–790*f*

Photo Credits

Assessment in Action Courtesy of Jason Pack/ FEMA

Section Openers

2 © Victoria Alexandrova/ShutterStock, Inc.;
3 © Mark C. Ide; 4 © Mark C. Ide;
5 © Mark C. Ide.

Chapter 1

Opener © Mark C. Ide; 1-1 © Mark C. Ide; 1-2 © National Library of Medicine; 1-3 Courtesy of Eugene L. Nagel and the Miami Fire Department; 1-4 © Peter Casolino/Alamy Images; 1-5 © Matt Dunham/AP Photos; 1-6 © Amanda Herron, The Jackson Sun/AP Photos; 1-8 © Mark C. Ide; 1-10B © Dan Myers; 1-11 Courtesy of Captain David Jackson, Saginaw Township Fire Department.

Chapter 2

Opener © Mark C. Ide; 2-1 Reprinted with permission. www.heart.org. © 2011 American Heart Association, Inc.; 2-2 Courtesy of USDA; 2-3 © ShutterStock, Inc.; 2-8 Courtesy of Island Photography/U.S. Air Force; 2-10 © Hugh Van der Poorten/Alamy Images; 2-11 © David Buffington/ Photodisc/Getty Images; 2-13 © Photodisc; 2-16 © Glen E. Ellman; 2-18 © Mark C. Ide.

Chapter 3

Opener © National Museum of Health and Medicine, Armed Forces Institute of Pathology, (NCP1603); 3-1A © Ryan McVay/Photodisc/ Getty Images; 3-1B © Carolyn Brule/ShutterStock, Inc.; 3-3 © Steven Pepple/ShutterStock, Inc.; 3-5 © Capifrutta/ShutterStock, Inc.; 3-6 Courtesy of the American Public Heath Assocation. Photographed by David Fouse.; 3-7 © Dewitt/ ShutterStock, Inc.; 3-8 © Steven Townsend/ Code 3 Images; 3-9A Courtesy of Henry Pollak; 3-9B © Vladimir Korostyshevskiy/ShutterStock, Inc.; 3-9C Courtesy of Captain David Jackson, Saginaw Township Fire Department; 3-10A © Cristina Fumi/ShutterStock, Inc.; 3-10B © Photos.com; 3-10C © Andreas Nilsson/ShutterStock, Inc.; 3-12 © Mikael Karlsson/On Scene Photography; 3-13 © SuperStock/age fotostock; 3-14 © Steven Townsend/Code 3 Images; 3-15 © Mikael Karlsson/Alamy Images; 3-16 © Craig Jackson/IntheDarkPhotography.com.

Chapter 4

Opener © Mark C. Ide; 4-1 © Brand X Pictures/ Creatas; 4-7 Courtesy of Oregon State Police; 4-8 © Dan Myers; 4-9 © Photodisc; 4-12 © Gary Kazanjian/AP Photos; 4-13 © Brian Snyder/Reuters/ Landov; 4-17 © Jack Dagley Photography/ ShutterStock, Inc.; 4-19 © UPI/HO/Landov; 4-24 Courtesy of the MedicAlert Foundation®. © 2006, All Rights Reserved. MedicAlert® is a federally registered trademark and service mark.

Chapter 5

5-2 Courtesy of Anthony Caliguire, NREMT-P; 5-8 © Glen E. Ellman; 5-10 © Craig Jackson/InthDarkPhotography.com

Chapter 6

Opener © Mark C. Ide; 6-1 Courtesy of the Utah Department of Health; 6-2A Courtesy of Inspironix; 6-3 Courtesy of Rhonda Beck.

Chapter 7

Opener © Phil Date/Dreamstime.com; 7-4A–7-4C Courtesy of Rhonda Beck; 7-7 Adapted from Shier, D.N., Butler, J.L., and Lewis, R. Hole's Essentials of Human Anatomy and Physiology, Tenth Edition, McGraw-Hill Higher Education, 2009; 7-20A © Donna Beer Stolz, PhD, Center for Biologic Imaging, University of Pittsburgh Medical School; 7-20C © Donna Beer Stolz, PhD, Center for Biologic Imaging, University of Pittsburgh Medical School; 7-20E © Donna Beer Stolz, PhD, Center for Biologic Imaging, University of Pittsburgh Medical School; 7-21A © Donna Beer Stolz, PhD, Center for Biologic Imaging, University of Pittsburgh Medical School; 7-21C © Donna Beer Stolz, PhD, Center for Biologic Imaging, University of Pittsburgh Medical School; 7-21E © Donna Beer Stolz, PhD, Center for Biologic Imaging, University of Pittsburgh Medical School; 7-21H © Donna Beer Stolz, PhD, Center for Biologic Imaging, University of Pittsburgh Medical School; 7-23A © Donna Beer Stolz, PhD, Center for Biologic Imaging, University of Pittsburgh Medical School; 7-23C © Donna Beer Stolz, PhD, Center for Biologic Imaging, University of Pittsburgh Medical School; 7-23E © Donna Beer Stolz, PhD, Center for Biologic Imaging, University of Pittsburgh Medical School; 7-23G © Donna Beer Stolz, PhD, Center for Biologic Imaging, University of Pittsburgh Medical School; 7-23I © Donna Beer Stolz, PhD, Center for Biologic Imaging, University of Pittsburgh Medical School; 7-23K © Dr. John D. Cunningham/Visuals Unlimited; 7-24A © Donna Beer Stolz, PhD, Center for Biologic Imaging, University of Pittsburgh Medical School; 7-24C © Donna Beer Stolz, PhD, Center for Biologic Imaging, University of Pittsburgh Medical School; 7-24E © Donna Beer Stolz, PhD, Center for Biologic Imaging, University of Pittsburgh Medical School; 7-33 Adapted from Shier, D. N., Butler, J. L., and Lewis, R. Hole's Essentials of Human Anatomy & Physiology, Tenth edition. McGraw-Hill Higher Education, 2009; 7-34A © Ralph Hutchings/Visuals Unlimited.

Chapter 8

Opener © Jupiterimages/Brand X/Alamy Images; 8-14A–B From An Introduction to Human Disease, 7th edition. Photo courtesy of Leonard V. Crowley, MD, Century College; 8-16B Courtesy of Rocky Mountain Laboratory, NIAID, NIH; 8-20A–B Courtesy of Leonard Crowley; 8-23 Courtesy of Leonard Crowley; 8-24A–B Courtesy of Leonard Crowley; 8-26A–B Courtesy of Leonard Crowley.

Chapter 9

Opener © digitalskillet/ShutterStock, Inc.; 9-1 © Johanna Goodyear/ShutterStock, Inc.; 9-2 Courtesy of Marianne Gausche-Hill, MC, FACEP, FAAP; 9-4 Courtesy of Howard E. Huth, III, BA, EMT-P; 9-5 © Kevin Levit/ShutterStock, Inc.; 9-7 © Maxim Bolotnikov/ShutterStock, Inc.; 9-8 © EML/ ShutterStock, Inc.; 9-10 © Trout55/ShutterStock, Inc.; 9-11 © Jamie Wilson/ShutterStock, Inc.; 9-12 © SW Productions/Jupiterimages; 9-14 © Rubberball Productions; 9-15 © Photodisc; 9-16 © Photodisc; 9-20 © Photodisc.

Chapter 10

Opener Courtesy of Rhonda Beck

Chapter 11

Opener © Mark C. Ide; 11-9 © Medical-on-Line/ Alamy Images; 11-14–11-17 Courtesy of Rhonda Beck; 11-19 Courtesy of Rhonda Beck; 11-26 Courtesy of Rhonda Beck; 11-27 Courtesy of Rhonda Beck; 11-28 © Mark Boulton/Alamy Images; 11-29 Courtesy of Rhonda Beck; 11-30 Courtesy of Rhonda Beck; 11-35 Courtesy of VidaCare Corporation; 11-40 Used with permission of the American Academy of Pediatrics, Pediatric Education for Prehospital Professionals, (c) American Academy of Pediatrics, 2000; 11-50 Used with permission of the American Academy of Pediatrics, Pediatric Education for Prehospital Professionals, (c) American Academy of Pediatrics, 2000; 11-55 Courtesy of Baxter International Inc.; 11-56 Courtesy of Baxter International Inc.; 11-58 Courtesy of Wolfe Tory Medical, Inc.; Skill Drill 11-11 and Skill Drill 11-12 Courtesy of Rhonda Beck.

Chapter 13

Opener Courtesy of Rhonda Beck; 13-2 © Adam Alberti, NJFirePictures.com; 13-3 Courtesy of Anthony Caliguire, NREMT-P; 13-4 Courtesy of Tempe Fire Department; 13-5 © Paul Chiasson, CP/AP Photos; 13-6 Courtesy of James Tourtellotte/ U.S. Customs & Border Control; 13-11 © Glen E. Ellman; 13-13A © Mark C. Ide; 13-13B © Corbis; 13-13D © Dan Myers; 13-13E © Jack Dagley Photography/ShutterStock, Inc.; 13-13F © Larry St. Pierre/ShutterStock, Inc.; 13-13G © micheal ledray/ShutterStock, Inc.; 13-15 © Thinkstock/Getty Images; 13-19 © Jack Dagley Photography/ShutterStock, Inc.; 13-26 © Denis Pepin/ShutterStock, Inc.; 13-27 © WizData, Inc./ShutterStock, Inc.; 13-28 © Kenneth Chelette/ ShutterStock, Inc.; 13-31 © Biophoto Associates/ Photo Researchers, Inc.; 13-32 © E. M. Singletary, M.D. Used with permission; 13-34 © German Ariel Berra/ShutterStock, Inc.; 13-51 © Dr. P. Marazzi/ Photo Researchers, Inc.; 13-58 © Wellcome Trust Library/National Medical Slide Bank/Custom Medical Stock Photo; 13-59 © Dr. P. Marazzi/ Photo Researchers, Inc.; 13-60 © Southern Illinois University/Photo Researchers, Inc.; 13-63 From Arrhythmia Recognition: The Art of Interpretation, courtesy of Tomas B. Garcia, MD; 13-65A–C Courtesy of Physio-Control, Inc.

Chapter 14

14-1 © Mark C. Ide; 14-4 © Peter Willott, The St. Augustine Record/AP Photos; 14-5 © Craig Jackson/InTheDarkPhotography.com; 14-6 © Craig Jackson/InTheDarkPhotography.com; 14-9 © Mark C. Ide.